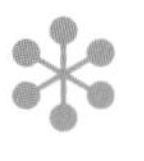

Brief Contents

Unit 1
Maternal and Child Health Nursing Practice 1

Chapter 1
A Framework for Maternal and Child Health Nursing 3

Chapter 2
Sociocultural Aspects of Maternal and Child Health Nursing 26

Chapter 3
The Childbearing & Childrearing Family 39

Chapter 4
The Childbearing & Childrearing Family in the Community 60

Unit 2
The Nursing Role in Preparing Families for Childbearing and Childrearing 81

Chapter 5
The Nursing Role in Reproductive and Sexual Health 83

Chapter 6
Assisting the Family with Reproductive Life Planning 117

Chapter 7
The Nursing Role in Genetic Assessment and Counseling 146

Chapter 8
Nursing Care of the Subfertile Couple 168

Unit 3
The Nursing Role in Caring for Families During Normal Pregnancy, Birth, the Postpartum, and Newborn Period 187

Chapter 9
The Growing Fetus 189

Chapter 10
Psychological and Physiologic Changes of Pregnancy 217

Chapter 11
Assessing Fetal and Maternal Health: Prenatal Care 244

Chapter 12
Promoting Fetal and Maternal Health 274

Chapter 13
Promoting Nutritional Health During Pregnancy 299

Chapter 14
Preparing a Family for Childbirth and Parenting 322

Chapter 15
Nursing Care of a Family During Labor and Birth 343

Chapter 16
Providing Comfort During Labor and Birth 395

Chapter 17
Nursing Care of a Postpartal Family 415

Chapter 18
Nursing Care of a Family with a Newborn 447

Chapter 19
Nutritional Needs of a Newborn 487

Unit 4
The Nursing Role in Caring for a Family During a Complicaton of Pregnancy, Birth, or the Postpartal Period 509

Chapter 20
Nursing Care of a Family Experiencing a Pregnancy Complication from a Pre-existing or Newly Acquired Illness 511

Chapter 21
Nursing Care of a Family Experiencing a Sudden Pregnancy Complication 549

Chapter 22
Nursing Care of a Pregnant Family with Special Needs 592

Chapter 23
Nursing Care of a Family Experiencing a Complication of Labor or Birth 623

Chapter 24
Nursing Care of a Family During Cesarean Birth 652

Chapter 25
Nursing Care of a Family Experiencing a Postpartal Complication 674

Chapter 26
Nursing Care of a Family with a High-Risk Newborn 698

Chapter 27
Nursing Care of the Child Born with a Physical or Developmental Challenge 743

Unit 5
The Nursing Role in Health Promotion for a Childrearing Family 781

Chapter 28
Principles of Growth and Development 783

Chapter 29
Nursing Care of a Family With an Infant 808

Chapter 30
Nursing Care of a Family With a Toddler 840

Chapter 31
Nursing Care of a Family With a Preschool Child 862

Chapter 32
Nursing Care of a Family With a School-Age Child 885

Chapter 33
Nursing Care of a Family With an Adolescent 914

Chapter 34
Child Health Assessment 947

Chapter 35
Communication and Teaching With Children and Families 1003

Unit 6
The Nursing Role in Supporting the Health of Ill Children and Their Families 1031

Chapter 36
Nursing Care of a Family With an Ill Child 1033

Chapter 37
Nursing Care of a Family When a Child Needs Diagnostic or Therapeutic Modalities 1066

Chapter 38
Nursing Care of a Family When a Child Needs Medication Administration or Intravenous Therapy 1097

Chapter 39
Pain Management in Children 1116

Unit 7
The Nursing Role in Restoring and Maintaining the Health of Children and Families With Physiologic Disorders 1135

Chapter 40
Nursing Care of a Family When a Child Has a Respiratory Disorder 1137

Chapter 41
Nursing Care of a Family When a Child Has a Cardiovascular Disorder 1188

Chapter 42
Nursing Care of a Family When a Child Has an Immune Disorder 1230

Chapter 43
Nursing Care of a Family When a Child Has an Infectious Disorder 1258

Chapter 44
Nursing Care of a Family When a Child Has a Hematologic Disorder 1289

Chapter 45
Nursing Care of a Family When a Child Has a Gastrointestinal Disorder 1318

Chapter 46
Nursing Care of a Family When a Child Has a Renal or Urinary Tract Disorder 1356

Chapter 47
Nursing Care of a Family When a Child Has a Reproductive Disorder 1387

Chapter 48
Nursing Care of a Family When a Child Has an Endocrine or Metabolic Disorder 1413

Chapter 49
Nursing Care of a Family When a Child Has a Neurologic Disorder 1445

Chapter 50
Nursing Care of a Family When a Child Has a Vision or Hearing Disorder 1484

Chapter 51
Nursing Care of a Family When a Child Has a Musculoskeletal Disorder 1510

Chapter 52
Nursing Care of a Family When a Child Has an Unintentional Injury 1543

Chapter 53
Nursing Care of a Family When a Child Has a Malignancy 1579

Unit 8
The Nursing Role in Restoring and Maintaining the Mental Health of Children and Families 1613

Chapter 54
Nursing Care of a Family When a Child Has a Cognitive or Mental Health Disorder 1615

Chapter 55
Nursing Care of a Family in Crisis: Abuse and Violence in the Family 1636

Chapter 56
Nursing Care of a Family When a Child Has a Long-Term or Terminal Illness 1659

Maternal & Child Health Nursing: Care of the Childbearing & Childrearing Family

Maternal & Child Health Nursing: Care of the Childbearing & Childrearing Family

Adele Pillitteri, PhD, RN, PNP
Associate Professor
University of Southern California
Los Angeles, California
Former Director, Neonatal Nurse Practitioner Program
State University of New York at Buffalo
Buffalo, New York

Edition 6

Wolters Kluwer Health | Lippincott Williams & Wilkins
Philadelphia • Baltimore • New York • London
Buenos Aires • Hong Kong • Sydney • Tokyo

Acquisitions Editor: Jean Rodenberger
Development Editor: Helene Caprari
Marketing Manager: Laura Meiskey
Art Director: Joan Wendt
Illustration Coordinator: Brett McNaughton
Manufacturing Coordinator: Karin Duffield
Production Services: Maryland Composition/ASI

6th edition

9 8 7 6 5 4

Printed in China

Library of Congress Cataloging-in-Publication Data

Pillitteri, Adele.
Maternal and child health nursing : care of the childbearing and childrearing family/Adele Pillitteri.—6th ed.
p. ; cm.
Rev. ed. of: Maternal & child health nursing. 5th ed. c2007.
Includes bibliographical references and index.
ISBN 978-1-58255-999-5
1. Maternity nursing. 2. Pediatric nursing. I. Pillitteri, Adele. Maternal & child health nursing. II. Title.
[DNLM: 1. Maternal-Child Nursing. 2. Family Health. WY 157.3 P641m 2009]
RG951.P637 2009
618.2′0231—dc22

2008052578

Care has been taken to confirm the accuracy of the information presented and to describe generally accepted practices. However, the author, editors, and publisher are not responsible for errors or omissions or for any consequences from application of the information in this book and make no warranty, expressed or implied, with respect to the currency, completeness, or accuracy of the contents of the publication. Application of this information in a particular situation remains the professional responsibility of the practitioner; the clinical treatments described and recommended may not be considered absolute and universal recommendations.

The author, editors, and publisher have exerted every effort to ensure that drug selection and dosage set forth in this text are in accordance with the current recommendations and practice at the time of publication. However, in view of ongoing research, changes in government regulations, and the constant flow of information relating to drug therapy and drug reactions, the reader is urged to check the package insert for each drug for any change in indications and dosage and for added warnings and precautions. This is particularly important when the recommended agent is a new or infrequently employed drug.

Some drugs and medical devices presented in this publication have Food and Drug Administration (FDA) clearance for limited use in restricted research settings. It is the responsibility of the health care provider to ascertain the FDA status of each drug or device planned for use in his or her clinical practice.

LWW.com

CCS1112

To my husband Joseph and my family: Rusty, Dawn, Bill, Heather, J. J., Lauren, Thomas, Lynn, Henry, and Lila

with love

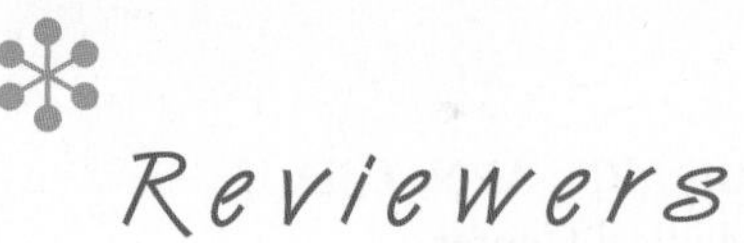

Reviewers

Kim Abel, MSN
Nursing Instructor
Illinois Valley Community College
Oglesby, IL

Susan Adrian, RN, MS, CPNP
Assistant Professor
Trocaire College
Buffalo, NY

Terri Ashcroft, RN, MN
Instructor II
University of Manitoba
Winnipeg, Manitoba

Jennifer Beck, MS, RN
Associate Professor and Chair of Undergraduate Studies
Our Lady of the Lake College
Baton Rouge, LA

Mary Ann Breen, RN, MEd, MS
Associate Professor
Director, AS & Professional Track Nursing Programs
Rivier College
Nashua, NH

Pam Bowden, RN, MS, PNP
Faculty
North Hennepin Community College
Brooklyn Park, MN

Theresa Broderick, MSN, ARNP
Assistant Professor
Bellarmine University
Louisville, KY

Mary Ann Cantrell, PhD, RN
Associate Professor
Villanova University
Villanova, PA

Katrina H. Carter, RNC, MS
Assistant Professor
McNeese State University
Lake Charles, LA

Linda Chipp, RN, BScN
Nursing Faculty
Vanier College
Saint Laurent, Quebec

Karen Luana Davis, MSN, RN, CNE, LNC
Assistant Clinical Professor
University of Arkansas for Medical Sciences
Little Rock, AR

Pamela P. DiNapoli, RN, PhD
Associate Professor
University of New Hampshire
Durham, NH

Kathleen Dolin, MSN, BSN, AAS
Northampton Community College
Bethlehem, PA

Marian Theresa Doyle, RN, MSN, MS
Associate Professor
Northampton Community College
Bethlehem, PA

Laura Dulski, RNC-HROB, MSN, CNE
Assistant Professor
West Suburban College of Nursing
Oak Park, IL

Cheryl Feenstra, RNC, PhD
Professor
Calvin College
Grand Rapids, MI

Ada Franklin, RN, MSN
Seattle Central Community College
Seattle, WA

Carole Fusco, BSN, MSN
Illinois Eastern Community College
Robinson, IL

Dawn Lee Garzon, PhD, APRN, BC, CPNP
Assistant Professor
University of Missouri – St. Louis
St. Louis, MO

Allison Green, MSN, BSN
Neumann College
Aston, PA

Yolanda Green, RN, MSN
Associate Professor of Nursing
Chattanooga State Community College
Chattanooga, TN

Marsha L. Heims, RN, EdD
Associate Professor Emeritus
Oregon Health & Science University
Portland, OR

Rachel Hofstetter, RN
Corning Community College
Corning, NY

Nancy Johnston, PhD, CRNP
Assistant Professor
Cedar Crest College
100 College Drive
Allentown, PA

Susan M. Koos, MS, RN, CNE
Professor of Nursing
Heartland College Community
Normal, IL

Dorothy Bishop Kurylo, MSN, RN
Pediatric Nursing Instructor
Citizens School of Nursing
West Penn Allegheny Health System
Pittsburgh, PA

Robyn Leo, RN, MS
Associate Professor
Worcester State College
Worcester, MA

Sharon McCleave, BSc (Hons), Dip (Med Tech)
Seneca College
King City, ON

Joanna McGrath, RN, MSN
Assistant Clinical Faculty
Villanova University
Villanova, PA

Lucille K. Morrison, MEd, MSN, CRNP (Current DNP student)
Assistant Professor
Mercyhurst College
Erie, PA

Margaret O'Connor, MS, RN
Assistant Clinical Professor
Lawrence Memorial/Regis College Nursing Program
Medford, MA

Michelle R. Offutt, MSN, ARNP
Assistant Professor
St. Petersburg College
St. Petersburg, FL

Katherine Perrozi, MSN, RN
Robert Morris University Coraopolis
Moon Township, PA

Karen Reach, MS, RN, LCCE, FACCE
Instructor and Curriculum Chairperson
Ellis Hospital School of Nursing
Schenectady, NY

Suzan Shane, RN, APN, EdD
St. Francis Medical Center
Peoria, IL

Koreen W. Smiley, RN, MSN, MSEd
Professor
St. Charles Community College
Cottleville, MO 63376

Cordia A. Starling, RN, BSN, MS, EdD
Professor and Dean
Dalton State College
Dalton, GA

Glenda F. Tali, RN, MSN, WHCNP-BC
Campus College Chair, Nursing & Health Administration
University of Phoenix, Hawaii Campus
Honolulu, HI

Mary Thibault, RN, MSN, MEd
Professor
Owens State Community College
Toledo, OH

Sharon Tighe, EdD, MN, BSN, AA, AS
Daytona Beach Community College
Daytona Beach, FL

Maureen Tippen, RN, C, MS
University of Michigan Flint
Clinical Assistant Professor
Flint, MI

Maureen Waller, MSN, RN
Professor
College of DuPage
Glen Ellyn, IL

Kate Walter, MSN, RNC-OB
Nursing Instructor
University of Pittsburgh Medical Center, Shadyside School of Nursing
Pittsburgh, PA

Wendy M. Wheeler, RN, BScN, MN
Instructor
Red Deer College
Red Deer, AB

Threasia L. Witt, EdD, MSN, BSN
Chairperson, Department of Nursing
Director, LPN-BSN Program
Director, RN-BSN Program
Director, International Nursing Program
Alderson-Broaddus College
Philippi, WV

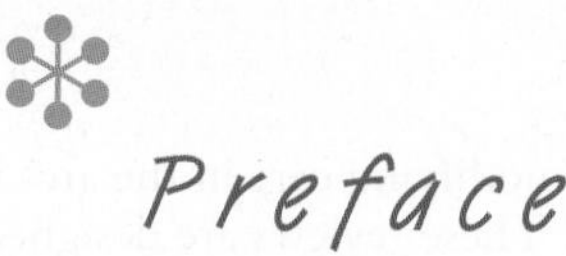

Preface

Maternal-newborn and child health nursing are expanding areas as a result of the broadening scope of practice within the nursing profession and the recognized need for better preventive and restorative care in these areas. The importance of this need is reflected in the fact that many of the health goals for the nation focus on these areas of nursing.

At the same time that the information in these areas of nursing is increasing, less time is available in nursing programs for teaching it. It's difficult for students to read all of the material contained in overlapping textbooks.

Maternal and Child Health Nursing: Care of the Childbearing and Childrearing Family, Sixth Edition, is written with this challenge in mind. It views maternal-newborn and child health care not as two separate disciplines but as a continuum of knowledge. It is designed to present the content of the two disciplines comprehensively but not redundantly. It is based on a philosophy of nursing care that respects clients as individuals, yet views them as part of families and society.

The book is designed for undergraduate student use in either a combined course in maternal-newborn and child health or for a curriculum in which these courses are taught separately. It provides a comprehensive, in-depth discussion of the many facets of maternal and child health nursing, while promoting a sensitive, holistic outlook on nursing practice. As such, the book will also be useful for practicing nurses or graduate students who are interested in reviewing or expanding their knowledge in these areas.

Basic themes that are integrated into this text include the experience of wellness and illness as family-centered events, the perception of pregnancy and childbirth as periods of wellness, and the importance of knowing normal child development in the planning of nursing care. Also included are themes reflective of changes in health care delivery and the importance of meeting the needs of a culturally diverse population.

THE CHANGING HEALTH CARE SCENE

Managed care has drastically changed the health care delivery system, increasing the role of the nurse from a minor to a major player. It has made understanding multidisciplinary approaches to care more important than ever before. An increasingly multicultural population is reflected among both nurses and the clients they care for, necessitating fine-tuning of culturally sensitive care. In order that nurses can be prepared for this new level of responsibility, educational changes have to keep pace with this health care reform by emphasizing expected outcomes, a greater focus on communication, therapeutic interventions, and critical thinking.

Nursing issues that grow out of the current climate of change include:

- **An emphasis on National Health Goals:** As a way to focus care and research, National Health Goals have gained wider attention at a time when there is a greater need than ever to be wise in the choice of how dollars are spent. Students can familiarize themselves with these goals by referring to the Focus on National Health Goals displays that appear at the beginning of each chapter.
- **The importance of health teaching with families as a cornerstone of nursing responsibility:** The teaching role of the nurse has greater significance in the new health care milieu as the emphasis on preventive care and short stays in the acute care setting create the need for families to be better educated in their own care. Focus on Family Teaching displays present detailed health information for the family, emphasizing the importance of a partnership between nurses and clients in the management of health and illness.
- **The importance of individualizing care according to sociocultural uniqueness:** This is a reflection of both greater cultural sensitivity and an increasingly diverse population of caregivers and care recipients. Greater emphasis is being placed on the implications of multiple sociocultural factors in terms of how they affect responses to health and illness. Focus on Communication boxes are included in each chapter to give examples of effective and less effective communication.
- **The importance of basing nursing care on nursing process and evidence based practice:** The variety of new care settings, as well as the diversity of roles in which nurses practice, is reflected both in the proliferation of community-based nursing facilities and also in the increase in the numbers of nurse-midwives and pediatric and neonatal nurse practitioners. This new edition places emphasis on the need for nurses to practice based on solid evidence in all settings. Focus on Evidence-Based Practice boxes in each chapter supply concrete examples of research and how it could be applicable to nursing practice. Focus on Nursing Care Planning boxes detail the use of nursing process in multidisciplinary oriented care.
- **Nursing process:** Nursing process serves as the foundation for nursing practice. Nursing Process Overview boxes included in each chapter provide a strong theoretical underpinning for nursing process and ways to use the nursing process in clinical practice.

ORGANIZATION OF THE TEXT

Maternal and Child Health Nursing follows the family from the pregnancy period, through labor, delivery, and the postpartal period; it then follows the child in the family from birth through adolescence. Coverage includes ambulatory and in-patient care and focuses on primary as well as secondary and tertiary care.

The book is organized in eight units:

Unit I provides an introduction to maternal and child health nursing. A framework for practice is presented, as well as current trends and the importance of considering childbearing and childrearing within a diverse socioeconomic and family/community context.

Unit II examines the nursing role in preparing families for childbearing and childrearing, and discusses reproductive and sexual health, the role of the nurse as a genetic counselor, reproductive life planning, and the concerns of the subfertile family.

Unit III presents the nursing role in caring for a pregnant family during pregnancy, birth and the postpartal period and serving as a fetal advocate. A separate chapter details the role of the nurse in providing comfort during labor and birth.

Unit IV addresses the nursing role when a woman develops a complication of pregnancy, labor or birth, or has a complication during the postpartal period. Separate chapters address the role of the nurse when a woman has a preexisting illness, develops a complication during pregnancy or the postpartal period, has a special need, or chooses or needs a cesarean birth. A final chapter details care of the high risk newborn or a child born with a physical or developmental challenge.

Unit V discusses the nursing role in health promotion during childhood. The chapters in this unit cover principles of growth and development and care of the child from infancy through adolescence, including child health assessment and communication and health teaching with children and families.

Unit VI presents.the nursing role in supporting the health of children and their families. The effects of illness on children and their families, diagnostic and therapeutic procedures, medication administration, and pain management are addressed, with respect to care of the child and family in hospital, home, and ambulatory settings.

Unit VII examines the nursing role in restoring and maintaining the health of children and families when illness occurs. Disorders are presented according to body systems so that students have a ready orientation for locating content.

Unit VIII discusses the nursing role in restoring and maintaining the mental health of children and families. Separate chapters discuss the role of the nurse when intimate partner or child abuse or mental, long-term, or fatal illness is present.

PEDAGOGIC FEATURES

Each chapter in the text is organized to provide a complete learning experience for the student. Numerous pedagogic features are included to help a student understand and increase retention. Important elements include:

- **Chapter Objectives:** Learning objectives are included at the beginning of each chapter to identify outcomes expected after the material in the chapter has been mastered.
- **Key Terms:** Terms that would be new to a student are listed at the beginning of each chapter in a ready reference list. When the terms first appear in the text, they are shown in boldface type and then defined. Definitions appear again in the Glossary.
- **Chapter-Opening Scenarios:** Short scenarios appear at the beginning of each chapter. These vignettes are designed to help students appreciate that nursing care is always individualized and provide a taste of what is to come in the chapter. At the end of the chapter, Critical Thinking questions related to the scenario bring the chapter full circle.
- **Nursing Process Overview:** Each chapter begins with a review of nursing process in which specific suggestions, such as examples of nursing diagnoses and outcome criteria helpful to modifying care in the area under discussion, are presented. These reviews are designed to improve students' preparation in clinical areas so they can focus their care planning and apply principles to practice.
- **Nursing Diagnoses and Related Interventions:** A consistent format highlights the nursing diagnoses and related interventions throughout the text. A special heading draws the students' attention to these sections where individual nursing diagnoses and outcome evaluation are detailed for the major conditions and disorders discussed.
- **Tables and Displays:** Numerous tables and displays summarize important information or provide extra detail on topics so that a student has ready references to this information.
- **Focus on National Health Goals:** To emphasize the nursing role in accomplishing the health care goals of our nation, these displays state specific ways in which maternal and child health nursing can provide better outcomes for both mother and child. They help the student to appreciate the importance of national health planning and the influence that nurses can have in creating a healthier nation.
- **Focus on Evidence-Based Practice:** These displays summarize research on topics related to maternal and child health nursing. They appear throughout the text to accentuate the use of evidence-based practice as the basis for nursing care.
- **Focus on Communication:** This feature presents case examples of less effective communication and more effective communication, illustrating for the student how an awareness of communication can improve the patient's understanding and positively impact outcomes.
- **Focus on Family Teaching:** These boxes present detailed health teaching information for the family, emphasizing the importance of a partnership between nurses and clients in the management of health and illness.
- **Focus on Pharmacology:** These boxes provide quick reference for medications that are commonly used for the health problems described in the text. They give the drug name (brand and generic, if applicable), dosage, pregnancy category, side effects, and nursing implications.
- **Focus on Nursing Procedures:** Techniques of procedures specific to maternal and child health care are boxed in an easy-to-follow two-column format, often enhanced with color figures.
- **Focus on Assessment:** These visual guides provide head-to-toe assessment information for overall health status or specific disorders or conditions.
- **Focus on Nursing Care Planning: Multidisciplinary Care Maps:** Because nurses rarely work in isolation, but rather as a member of a health care team or unit, Multidisciplinary Care Maps written for specific clients are included throughout the text to demonstrate the use of the nursing process, provide examples of critical thinking, and clarify nursing care for specific client needs. Multidisciplinary care maps not only demonstrate nursing process but also accentuate the increasingly important role of the nurse as a coordinator of client care.
- **Checkpoint Questions:** Throughout the text, multiple-choice Checkpoint Questions appear to help readers check progress and comprehension. They ask readers to use the knowledge just gained in the last few pages, helping them retain this information. Answers are supplied in the accompanying CD.

- **"What If" Questions:** "What If" (critical-thinking) questions also appear in each chapter in the text. These ask readers to apply the information just acquired in an "actual" situation. Readers must process the information and apply it to the new situation, thus maximizing learning and emphasizing critical thinking. Suggested solutions are supplied in the accompanying CD.
- **Key Points:** A review of important points is highlighted at the end of each chapter, to help students monitor their own comprehension.
- **Critical Thinking Exercises:** To involve a student in the decision-making realities of the clinical setting, several thought-provoking questions are posed at the end of each chapter. These could also serve as a basis for conference or class discussion. Suggested considerations are supplied in the accompanying CD.
- **Critical Thinking Scenarios:** An accompanying CD-ROM contains a patient care scenario detailing a full health history and examination findings pertinent to the chapter content as well as 20 related multiple-choice RN-CLEX types of questions to answer for further chapter review. These could also be used for classroom or clinical instruction.
- **References and Suggested Readings:** These provide a student with the information needed to do more in-depth reading of the sources noted in the text, as well as other relevant articles on the topics included in the chapter.
- **Appendices:** Appendices provide a quick reference to laboratory values, growth charts, vital sign parameters, nutrition pyramids, and drugs safe for use during lactation.

ANCILLARY PACKAGE

A complete learning and teaching package accompanying the text includes:

- **Free Interactive Self-Study CD-ROM:** Found on the inside front cover of each book, this free CD contains 300 **multiple-choice NCLEX-style questions** to challenge the student's comprehension and application of the material in the textbook. Feedback is provided for each answer.
- **Instructor's Resource DVD:** The perfect complement to classroom teaching strategies, this resource contains useful lecture points, discussion questions, and assignments for each chapter. Also included is a **computerized test bank,** containing more than 1000 multiple-choice NCLEX-style questions; an **image bank** containing art from the text; and **PowerPoint presentations** for every chapter.
- **Study Guide:** This companion to the text challenges the student's retention of key concepts and encourages critical thinking and application of information to actual nursing situations.
- **thePoint*:** Students and teachers can find additional resources to enhance learning at http://thePoint.lww.com/Pillitteri6e

Adele Pillitteri, PhD, RN, PNP

*thePoint is a trademark of Wolters Kluwer Health.

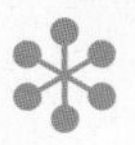

Acknowledgments

I would like to express my sincere appreciation to Helene Caprari, Development Editor; Jean Rodenberger, Senior Acquisitions Editor; Helen Ewan, Senior Production Manager; Tom Gibbons, Senior Production Editor; Joan Wendt, Art Director; and all the members of the Production Services Group involved with this text for their assistance and guidance throughout the project.

A.P.

Contents

Unit 1

Maternal and Child Health Nursing Practice 1

Chapter 1

A Framework for Maternal and Child Health Nursing 3

GOALS AND PHILOSOPHIES OF MATERNAL AND CHILD HEALTH NURSING 4
STANDARDS OF MATERNAL AND CHILD HEALTH NURSING PRACTICE 5
A FRAMEWORK FOR MATERNAL AND CHILD HEALTH NURSING CARE 5
A CHANGING DISCIPLINE 8
ADVANCED-PRACTICE ROLES FOR NURSES IN MATERNAL AND CHILD HEALTH 21
LEGAL CONSIDERATIONS OF MATERNAL-CHILD PRACTICE 22
ETHICAL CONSIDERATIONS OF PRACTICE 23

Chapter 2

Sociocultural Aspects of Maternal and Child Health Nursing 26

Nursing Process Overview for Respecting Sociocultural Aspects of Care 28

SOCIOCULTURAL DIFFERENCES AND IMPLICATIONS FOR DIVERSITY IN MATERNAL AND CHILD HEALTH NURSING 29

Chapter 3

The Childbearing & Childrearing Family 39

Nursing Process Overview for Promotion of Family Health 40

THE FAMILY 41
FAMILY FUNCTIONS AND ROLES 45
ASSESSMENT OF FAMILY STRUCTURE AND FUNCTION 51

Chapter 4

The Childbearing & Childrearing Family in the Community 60

Nursing Process Overview for the Pregnant Woman or Child on Home Care 61

THE FAMILY AS PART OF A COMMUNITY 66
HOME CARE 67
BEGINNING HOME CARE 68

Unit 2

The Nursing Role in Preparing Families for Childbearing and Childrearing 81

Chapter 5

The Nursing Role in Reproductive and Sexual Health 83

Nursing Process Overview for Promotion of Reproductive and Sexual Health 84

REPRODUCTIVE DEVELOPMENT 86
ANATOMY AND PHYSIOLOGY OF THE REPRODUCTIVE SYSTEM 87
MENSTRUATION 99
SEXUALITY AND SEXUAL IDENTITY 104
HUMAN SEXUAL RESPONSE 108
SEXUAL HARASSMENT 113
DISORDERS OF SEXUAL FUNCTIONING 113

Chapter 6

Assisting the Family with Reproductive Life Planning 117

Nursing Process Overview for Reproductive Health 118

METHODS OF CONTRACEPTION 119
THE COUPLE WITH A PHYSICAL OR COGNITIVE CHALLENGE 137
FUTURE TRENDS IN CONTRACEPTION 137
ELECTIVE TERMINATION OF PREGNANCY (INDUCED ABORTION) 139

Chapter 7

The Nursing Role in Genetic Assessment and Counseling 146

Nursing Process Overview for Genetic Assessment and Counseling 147

GENETIC DISORDERS 148
GENETIC COUNSELING 155
COMMON CHROMOSOMAL DISORDERS RESULTING IN PHYSICAL OR COGNITIVE DEVELOPMENTAL DISORDERS 163

Chapter 8

Nursing Care of the Subfertile Couple 168

Nursing Process Overview for the Couple With Subfertility 169

SUBFERTILITY 170
FERTILITY ASSESSMENT 174
SUBFERTILITY MANAGEMENT 178
ALTERNATIVES TO CHILDBIRTH 184

Unit 3

The Nursing Role in Caring for Families During Normal Pregnancy, Birth, the Postpartum, and Newborn Period 187

Chapter 9
The Growing Fetus 189

Nursing Process Overview to Help Ensure Fetal Health 190

STAGES OF FETAL DEVELOPMENT 191
EMBRYONIC AND FETAL STRUCTURES 192
ORIGIN AND DEVELOPMENT OF ORGAN SYSTEMS 197
ASSESSMENT OF FETAL GROWTH AND DEVELOPMENT 205

Chapter 10
Psychological and Physiologic Changes of Pregnancy 217

Nursing Process Overview for Healthy Adaptation to Pregnancy 218

PSYCHOLOGICAL CHANGES OF PREGNANCY 219
THE PSYCHOLOGICAL TASKS OF PREGNANCY 220
THE DIAGNOSIS OF PREGNANCY 227
PHYSIOLOGIC CHANGES OF PREGNANCY 230

Chapter 11
Assessing Fetal and Maternal Health: Prenatal Care 244

Nursing Process Overview for Prenatal Care 245

HEALTH PROMOTION DURING PREGNANCY 246
HEALTH ASSESSMENT DURING THE FIRST PRENATAL VISIT 247
SIGNS INDICATING COMPLICATIONS OF PREGNANCY 268

Chapter 12
Promoting Fetal and Maternal Health 274

Nursing Process Overview for Health Promotion of a Fetus and Mother 275

HEALTH PROMOTION DURING PREGNANCY 277
PREVENTING FETAL EXPOSURE TO TERATOGENS 288
PREPARATION FOR LABOR 296

Chapter 13
Promoting Nutritional Health During Pregnancy 299

Nursing Process Overview for Promoting Nutritional Health in a Pregnant Woman 300

RELATIONSHIP OF MATERNAL NUTRITION TO INFANT HEALTH 301
ASSESSMENT OF NUTRITIONAL HEALTH 307
PROMOTING NUTRITIONAL HEALTH DURING PREGNANCY 309

Chapter 14
Preparing a Family for Childbirth and Parenting 322

Nursing Process Overview for Childbirth and Parenting Education 323

CHILDBIRTH EDUCATION 324
THE CHILDBIRTH PLAN 326
PRECONCEPTION CLASSES 326
EXPECTANT PARENTING CLASSES 327
THE BIRTH SETTING 334
ALTERNATIVE METHODS OF BIRTH 340

Chapter 15
Nursing Care of a Family During Labor and Birth 343
Nursing Process Overview for a Woman in Labor 344
THEORIES OF LABOR ONSET 345
SIGNS OF LABOR 345
COMPONENTS OF LABOR 346
STAGES OF LABOR 359
MATERNAL AND FETAL RESPONSES TO LABOR 362
MATERNAL AND FETAL ASSESSMENT DURING LABOR 366
FETAL HEART RATE AND UTERINE CONTRACTION RECORDS 377
CARE OF A WOMAN DURING THE FIRST STAGE OF LABOR 381
CARE OF A WOMAN DURING THE SECOND STAGE OF LABOR 384
CARE OF A WOMAN DURING THE THIRD AND FOURTH STAGES OF LABOR 391
UNIQUE CONCERNS OF A WOMAN IN LABOR 392

Chapter 16
Providing Comfort During Labor and Birth 395
Nursing Process Overview for Pain Relief During Childbirth 396
EXPERIENCE OF PAIN DURING CHILDBIRTH 397
COMFORT AND PAIN RELIEF MEASURES 399
NURSING CARE TO PROMOTE THE COMFORT OF A WOMAN DURING LABOR 409

Chapter 17
Nursing Care of a Postpartal Family 415
Nursing Process Overview for a Postpartal Woman and Family 416
PSYCHOLOGICAL CHANGES OF THE POSTPARTAL PERIOD 417
PHYSIOLOGIC CHANGES OF THE POSTPARTAL PERIOD 421
NURSING CARE OF A WOMAN AND FAMILY DURING THE FIRST 24 HOURS AFTER BIRTH 426
NURSING CARE OF A WOMAN AND FAMILY IN PREPARATION FOR DISCHARGE 438
NURSING CARE OF A WOMAN AND FAMILY AFTER DISCHARGE 441
NURSING CARE OF A POSTPARTAL WOMAN AND FAMILY WITH UNIQUE NEEDS 442

Chapter 18
Nursing Care of a Family with a Newborn 447
Nursing Process Overview for Health Promotion of the Term Newborn 448
PROFILE OF A NEWBORN 449
APPEARANCE OF A NEWBORN 458
ASSESSMENT FOR WELL-BEING 467
CARE OF A NEWBORN AT BIRTH 472
NURSING CARE OF A NEWBORN AND FAMILY IN THE POSTPARTAL PERIOD 476
ASSESSMENT OF FAMILY'S READINESS TO CARE FOR A NEWBORN AT HOME 480

Chapter 19
Nutritional Needs of a Newborn 487
Nursing Process Overview for Promoting Nutritional Health in a Newborn 488
NUTRITIONAL ALLOWANCES FOR A NEWBORN 489
BREASTFEEDING 491
FORMULA FEEDING 504
DISCHARGE PLANNING 506

Unit 4

The Nursing Role in Caring for a Family During a Complicaton of Pregnancy, Birth, or the Postpartal Period 509

Chapter 20

Nursing Care of a Family Experiencing a Pregnancy Complication from a Pre-existing or Newly Acquired Illness 511

Nursing Process Overview for Care of a Woman With a Pre-existing or Newly Acquired Illness 512

IDENTIFYING A HIGH-RISK PREGNANCY 514
CARDIOVASCULAR DISORDERS AND PREGNANCY 514
HEMATOLOGIC DISORDERS AND PREGNANCY 521
RENAL AND URINARY DISORDERS AND PREGNANCY 525
RESPIRATORY DISORDERS AND PREGNANCY 527
RHEUMATIC DISORDERS AND PREGNANCY 530
GASTROINTESTINAL DISORDERS AND PREGNANCY 531
NEUROLOGIC DISORDERS AND PREGNANCY 534
MUSCULOSKELETAL DISORDERS AND PREGNANCY 535
ENDOCRINE DISORDERS AND PREGNANCY 535
CANCER AND PREGNANCY 545
MENTAL ILLNESS AND PREGNANCY 545

Chapter 21

Nursing Care of a Family Experiencing a Sudden Pregnancy Complication 549

Nursing Process Overview for a Woman Who Develops a Complication of Pregnancy 550

BLEEDING DURING PREGNANCY 551
PRETERM LABOR 568
PRETERM RUPTURE OF MEMBRANES 574
PREGNANCY-INDUCED HYPERTENSION 575
HELLP SYNDROME 582
MULTIPLE PREGNANCY 583
HYDRAMNIOS 585
OLIGOHYDRAMNIOS 585
POST TERM PREGNANCY 585
PSEUDOCYESIS 586
ISOIMMUNIZATION (RH INCOMPATIBILITY) 586
FETAL DEATH 587

Chapter 22

Nursing Care of a Pregnant Family with Special Needs 592

Nursing Process Overview for Care of a Pregnant Woman With Special Needs 593

THE PREGNANT ADOLESCENT 595
THE PREGNANT WOMAN OVER AGE 40 601
THE PREGNANT WOMAN WHO IS PHYSICALLY OR COGNITIVELY CHALLENGED 606
A WOMAN WHO IS SUBSTANCE DEPENDENT 610
TRAUMA AND PREGNANCY 613

Chapter 23
Nursing Care of a Family Experiencing a Complication of Labor or Birth 623
Nursing Process Overview for a Woman With a Labor or Birth Complication 624
COMPLICATIONS WITH THE POWER (THE FORCE OF LABOR) 625
PROBLEMS WITH THE PASSENGER 637
PROBLEMS WITH THE PASSAGE 645
ANOMALIES OF THE PLACENTA AND CORD 648

Chapter 24
Nursing Care of a Family During Cesarean Birth 652
Nursing Process Overview for a Woman Having a Cesarean Birth 653
CESAREAN BIRTH 654
NURSING CARE OF A WOMAN ANTICIPATING A CESAREAN BIRTH 656
NURSING CARE OF A WOMAN HAVING AN EMERGENT CESAREAN BIRTH 660
INTRAOPERATIVE CARE MEASURES 660
POSTPARTAL CARE MEASURES 662

Chapter 25
Nursing Care of a Family Experiencing a Postpartal Complication 674
Nursing Process Overview for a Woman Experiencing a Postpartal Complication 675
POSTPARTAL HEMORRHAGE 676
PUERPERAL INFECTION 683
THROMBOPHLEBITIS 686
MASTITIS 689
URINARY SYSTEM DISORDERS 689
CARDIOVASCULAR SYSTEM DISORDERS 693
REPRODUCTIVE SYSTEM DISORDERS 693
EMOTIONAL AND PSYCHOLOGICAL COMPLICATIONS OF THE PUERPERIUM 693

Chapter 26
Nursing Care of a Family with a High-Risk Newborn 698
Nursing Process Overview for the Family of a High-Risk Newborn 699
NEWBORN PRIORITIES IN FIRST DAYS OF LIFE 700
THE NEWBORN AT RISK BECAUSE OF ALTERED GESTATIONAL AGE OR BIRTH WEIGHT 707
ILLNESS IN THE NEWBORN 724
THE NEWBORN AT RISK BECAUSE OF MATERNAL INFECTION OR ILLNESS 736

Chapter 27
Nursing Care of the Child Born with a Physical or Developmental Challenge 743
Nursing Process Overview for Care of a Physically or Developmentally Challenged Child 744
IMMEDIATE CARE AT THE BIRTH OF AN INFANT BORN PHYSICALLY OR DEVELOPMENTALLY CHALLENGED 745
PHYSICAL AND DEVELOPMENTAL DISORDERS OF THE GASTROINTESTINAL SYSTEM 746
PHYSICAL AND DEVELOPMENTAL DISORDERS OF THE NERVOUS SYSTEM 759
PHYSICAL AND DEVELOPMENTAL DISORDERS OF THE SKELETAL SYSTEM 770

Unit 5

The Nursing Role in Health Promotion for a Childrearing Family 781

Chapter 28

Principles of Growth and Development 783

Nursing Process Overview for Promotion of Normal Growth and Development 784

GROWTH AND DEVELOPMENT AND THE ROLE OF THE NURSE 785
PRINCIPLES OF GROWTH AND DEVELOPMENT 786
FACTORS INFLUENCING GROWTH AND DEVELOPMENT 786
THEORIES OF DEVELOPMENT 795
USING GROWTH AND DEVELOPMENT IN PRACTICE 804

Chapter 29

Nursing Care of a Family With an Infant 808

Nursing Process Overview for Healthy Development of an Infant 809

GROWTH AND DEVELOPMENT OF AN INFANT 811
HEALTH PROMOTION OF AN INFANT AND FAMILY 821

Chapter 30

Nursing Care of a Family With a Toddler 840

Nursing Process Overview for Healthy Development of a Toddler 841

GROWTH AND DEVELOPMENT OF A TODDLER 842
HEALTH PROMOTION FOR A TODDLER AND FAMILY 847

Chapter 31

Nursing Care of a Family With a Preschool Child 862

Nursing Process Overview for Healthy Development of the Preschooler 863

GROWTH AND DEVELOPMENT OF A PRESCHOOLER 864
HEALTH PROMOTION FOR A PRESCHOOLER AND FAMILY 868

Chapter 32

Nursing Care of a Family With a School-Age Child 885

Nursing Process Overview for Healthy Development of a School-Age Child 886

GROWTH AND DEVELOPMENT OF A SCHOOL-AGE CHILD 887
HEALTH PROMOTION FOR A SCHOOL-AGE CHILD AND FAMILY 895

Chapter 33

Nursing Care of a Family With an Adolescent 914

Nursing Process Overview for Healthy Development of an Adolescent 915

GROWTH AND DEVELOPMENT OF AN ADOLESCENT 916
HEALTH PROMOTION FOR AN ADOLESCENT AND FAMILY 923

Chapter 34

Child Health Assessment 947

Nursing Process Overview for Health Assessment of the Child and Family 948

HEALTH HISTORY: ESTABLISHING A DATABASE 949
PHYSICAL ASSESSMENT 958
ASSESSING VISION, HEARING, AND SPEECH 979
ASSESSING DEVELOPMENTAL MILESTONES 989
IMMUNIZATION STATUS 992
CONCLUDING A HEALTH ASSESSMENT 999

Chapter 35

Communication and Teaching With Children and Families 1003

Nursing Process Overview for Health Teaching With Children 1004

COMMUNICATION 1005
HEALTH TEACHING IN A CHANGING HEALTH CARE ENVIRONMENT 1014
DEVELOPING AND IMPLEMENTING A TEACHING PLAN 1018
HEALTH TEACHING FOR A SURGICAL EXPERIENCE 1026

Unit 6

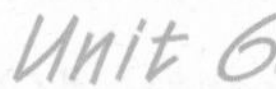

The Nursing Role in Supporting the Health of Ill Children and Their Families 1031

Chapter 36

Nursing Care of a Family With an Ill Child 1033

Nursing Process Overview for an Ill Child 1034

THE MEANING OF ILLNESS TO CHILDREN 1035
CARE OF THE ILL CHILD AND FAMILY IN THE HOSPITAL 1036
NURSING RESPONSIBILITIES FOR CARE OF AN ILL CHILD AND FAMILY 1048
PROMOTING NUTRITIONAL HEALTH OF AN ILL CHILD 1050
PROMOTING SAFETY FOR AN ILL CHILD 1052
PROMOTING ADEQUATE SLEEP FOR AN ILL CHILD 1053
PROMOTING ADEQUATE STIMULATION FOR AN ILL CHILD 1055
PROMOTING PLAY FOR AN ILL CHILD 1056

Chapter 37

Nursing Care of a Family When a Child Needs Diagnostic or Therapeutic Modalities 1066

Nursing Process Overview for a Child Who Needs Diagnostic or Therapeutic Procedures 1067

NURSING RESPONSIBILITIES WITH DIAGNOSTIC AND THERAPEUTIC TECHNIQUES 1068
MEASURING VITAL SIGNS 1074
REDUCING ELEVATED TEMPERATURE IN CHILDREN 1075
COMMON DIAGNOSTIC PROCEDURES 1076
COLLECTING SPECIMENS FOR ANALYSIS 1081
HOT AND COLD THERAPY 1086
NUTRITIONAL CARE 1086
ASSISTANCE WITH ELIMINATION 1092
WOUND CARE 1094

Chapter 38
Nursing Care of a Family When a Child Needs Medication Administration or Intravenous Therapy 1097
Nursing Process Overview for a Child Needing Medication/Intravenous Therapy 1098
MEDICATION ADMINISTRATION 1099
INTRAVENOUS THERAPY 1107

Chapter 39
Pain Management in Children 1116
Nursing Process Overview for a Child in Pain 1117
PHYSIOLOGY OF PAIN 1118
ASSESSING TYPE AND DEGREE OF PAIN 1119
PAIN ASSESSMENT 1121
PAIN MANAGEMENT 1124
NONPHARMACOLOGIC PAIN MANAGEMENT 1125
PHARMACOLOGIC PAIN RELIEF 1129
ONGOING PAIN RELIEF 1132

Unit 7

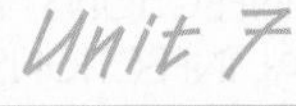

The Nursing Role in Restoring and Maintaining the Health of Children and Families With Physiologic Disorders 1135

Chapter 40
Nursing Care of a Family When a Child Has a Respiratory Disorder 1137
Nursing Process Overview for a Child With a Respiratory Disorder 1138
ANATOMY AND PHYSIOLOGY OF THE RESPIRATORY SYSTEM 1139
ASSESSING RESPIRATORY ILLNESS IN CHILDREN 1140
HEALTH PROMOTION AND RISK MANAGEMENT 1146
THERAPEUTIC TECHNIQUES USED IN THE TREATMENT OF RESPIRATORY ILLNESS IN CHILDREN 1147
DISORDERS OF THE UPPER RESPIRATORY TRACT 1158
DISORDERS OF THE LOWER RESPIRATORY TRACT 1170

Chapter 41
Nursing Care of a Family When a Child Has a Cardiovascular Disorder 1188
Nursing Process Overview for Care of a Child With a Cardiovascular Disorder 1189
THE CARDIOVASCULAR SYSTEM 1190
ASSESSMENT OF HEART DISORDERS IN CHILDREN 1190
HEALTH PROMOTION AND RISK MANAGEMENT 1195
NURSING CARE OF THE CHILD WITH A CARDIAC DISORDER 1195
CONGENITAL HEART DISORDERS 1206
ACQUIRED HEART D1ISEASE 1214
CARDIOPULMONARY ARREST 1225

Chapter 42

Nursing Care of a Family When a Child Has an Immune Disorder 1230

Nursing Process Overview for a Child With an Immune Disorder 1231

THE IMMUNE SYSTEM 1232
HEALTH PROMOTION AND RISK MANAGEMENT 1235
IMMUNODEFICIENCY DISORDERS 1237
ALLERGY 1241
COMMON IMMUNE REACTIONS 1245
ATOPIC DISORDERS 1248
DRUG AND FOOD ALLERGIES 1253
STINGING INSECT HYPERSENSITIVITY 1254
CONTACT DERMATITIS 1255

Chapter 43

Nursing Care of a Family When a Child Has an Infectious Disorder 1258

Nursing Process Overview for a Child With an Infectious Disorder 1259

THE INFECTIOUS PROCESS 1260
HEALTH PROMOTION AND RISK MANAGEMENT 1262
CARING FOR THE CHILD WITH AN INFECTIOUS DISEASE 1263
VIRAL INFECTIONS 1265
BACTERIAL INFECTIONS 1275
OTHER INFECTIOUS PATHOGENS 1283

Chapter 44

Nursing Care of a Family When a Child Has a Hematologic Disorder 1289

Nursing Process Overview for a Child With a Hematologic Disorder 1290

ANATOMY AND PHYSIOLOGY OF THE HEMATOPOIETIC SYSTEM 1291
ASSESSMENT OF AND THERAPEUTIC TECHNIQUES FOR HEMATOLOGIC DISORDERS 1294
HEALTH PROMOTION AND RISK MANAGEMENT 1298
DISORDERS OF THE RED BLOOD CELLS 1298
DISORDERS OF THE WHITE BLOOD CELLS 1311
DISORDERS OF BLOOD COAGULATION 1311

Chapter 45

Nursing Care of a Family When a Child Has a Gastrointestinal Disorder 1318

Nursing Process Overview for a Child With a Gastrointestinal Disorder 1319

ANATOMY AND PHYSIOLOGY OF THE GASTROINTESTINAL SYSTEM 1320
DIAGNOSTIC AND THERAPEUTIC TECHNIQUES 1321
HEALTH PROMOTION AND RISK MANAGEMENT 1321
FLUID, ELECTROLYTE, AND ACID–BASE IMBALANCES 1322
COMMON GASTROINTESTINAL SYMPTOMS OF ILLNESS IN CHILDREN 1324
COMMON DISORDERS OF THE STOMACH AND DUODENUM 1330
HEPATIC DISORDERS 1333
INTESTINAL DISORDERS 1339
DISORDERS OF THE LOWER BOWEL 1346
DISORDERS CAUSED BY FOOD, VITAMIN, AND MINERAL DEFICIENCIES 1351

Chapter 46

Nursing Care of a Family When a Child Has a Renal or Urinary Tract Disorder 1356

Nursing Process Overview for Care of a Child With a Renal or Urinary Tract Disorder 1357

ANATOMY AND PHYSIOLOGY OF THE KIDNEYS 1358
ASSESSMENT OF RENAL AND URINARY TRACT DYSFUNCTION 1360
THERAPEUTIC MEASURES FOR THE MANAGEMENT OF RENAL DISEASE 1363
HEALTH PROMOTION AND RISK MANAGEMENT 1366
STRUCTURAL ABNORMALITIES OF THE URINARY TRACT 1366
INFECTIONS OF THE URINARY SYSTEM AND RELATED DISORDERS 1368
DISORDERS AFFECTING NORMAL URINARY ELIMINATION 1371
KIDNEY TRANSPLANTATION 1382

Chapter 47

Nursing Care of a Family When a Child Has a Reproductive Disorder 1387

Nursing Process Overview for Care of a Child With a Reproductive Disorder 1388

ASSESSING REPRODUCTIVE DISORDERS IN CHILDREN 1389
HEALTH PROMOTION AND RISK MANAGEMENT 1391
DISORDERS CAUSED BY ALTERED REPRODUCTIVE DEVELOPMENT 1391
REPRODUCTIVE DISORDERS IN MALES 1393
REPRODUCTIVE DISORDERS IN FEMALES 1395
BREAST DISORDERS 1400
SEXUALLY TRANSMITTED INFECTIONS 1402

Chapter 48

Nursing Care of a Family When a Child Has an Endocrine or Metabolic Disorder 1413

Nursing Process Overview for Care of a Child With an Endocrine or Metabolic Disorder 1414

HEALTH PROMOTION AND RISK MANAGEMENT 1415
THE PITUITARY GLAND 1416
PITUITARY GLAND DISORDERS 1416
THE THYROID GLAND 1420
THYROID GLAND DISORDERS 1421
THE ADRENAL GLAND 1423
ADRENAL GLAND DISORDERS 1424
THE PANCREAS 1427
THE PARATHYROID GLANDS 1439
METABOLIC DISORDERS 1440

Chapter 49

Nursing Care of a Family When a Child Has a Neurologic Disorder 1445

Nursing Process Overview for Care of a Child With a Neurologic System Disorder 1446

ANATOMY AND PHYSIOLOGY OF THE NERVOUS SYSTEM 1447
ASSESSING THE CHILD WITH A NEUROLOGIC DISORDER 1449
HEALTH PROMOTION AND RISK MANAGEMENT 1454
INCREASED INTRACRANIAL PRESSURE 1454
NEURAL TUBE DISORDERS 1458
NEUROCUTANEOUS SYNDROMES 1458
CEREBRAL PALSY 1459
INFECTION 1462
INFLAMMATORY DISORDERS 1466
PAROXYSMAL DISORDERS 1467
ATAXIC DISORDERS 1476
SPINAL CORD INJURY 1476

Chapter 50
Nursing Care of a Family When a Child Has a Vision or Hearing Disorder 1484
Nursing Process Overview for Care of a Child With a Vision or Hearing Disorder 1485
HEALTH PROMOTION AND RISK MANAGEMENT 1486
VISION 1488
DISORDERS THAT INTERFERE WITH VISION 1489
STRUCTURAL PROBLEMS OF THE EYE 1491
INFECTION OR INFLAMMATION OF THE EYE 1493
TRAUMATIC INJURY TO THE EYE 1496
INNER EYE CONDITIONS 1498
THE CHILD UNDERGOING EYE SURGERY 1499
THE HOSPITALIZED CHILD WITH A VISION DISORDER 1500
STRUCTURE AND FUNCTION OF THE EARS 1500
DISORDERS OF THE EAR 1502
THE HOSPITALIZED CHILD WITH A HEARING IMPAIRMENT 1507

Chapter 51
Nursing Care of a Family When a Child Has a Musculoskeletal Disorder 1510
Nursing Process Overview for Care of a Child With a Musculoskeletal Disorder 1511
THE MUSCULOSKELETAL SYSTEM 1512
ASSESSMENT OF MUSCULOSKELETAL FUNCTION 1513
HEALTH PROMOTION AND RISK MANAGEMENT 1513
THERAPEUTIC MANAGEMENT OF MUSCULOSKELETAL DISORDERS IN CHILDREN 1514
DISORDERS OF BONE DEVELOPMENT 1520
INFECTIOUS AND INFLAMMATORY DISORDERS OF THE BONES AND JOINTS 1524
DISORDERS OF SKELETAL STRUCTURE 1527
DISORDERS OF THE JOINTS AND TENDONS: COLLAGEN-VASCULAR DISEASE 1531
DISORDERS OF THE SKELETAL MUSCLES 1534
INJURIES OF THE EXTREMITIES 1536

Chapter 52
Nursing Care of a Family When a Child Has an Unintentional Injury 1543
Nursing Process Overview for Care of a Child With an Unintentional Injury 1544
HEALTH PROMOTION AND RISK MANAGEMENT 1546
HEAD TRAUMA 1546
ABDOMINAL TRAUMA 1555
DENTAL TRAUMA 1556
NEAR DROWNING 1557
POISONING 1558
FOREIGN BODY OBSTRUCTION 1564
BITES 1565
THERMAL INJURIES 1566

Chapter 53

Nursing Care of a Family When a Child Has a Malignancy 1579

Nursing Process Overview for Care of a Child With a Malignancy 1580

HEALTH PROMOTION AND RISK MANAGEMENT 1581
NEOPLASIA 1581
ASSESSING CHILDREN WITH CANCER 1583
OVERVIEW OF CANCER TREATMENT MEASURES USED WITH CHILDREN 1584
THE LEUKEMIAS 1594
THE LYMPHOMAS 1597
NEOPLASMS OF THE BRAIN 1599
BONE TUMORS 1604
OTHER CHILDHOOD NEOPLASMS 1606

Unit 8

The Nursing Role in Restoring and Maintaining the Mental Health of Children and Families 1613

Chapter 54

Nursing Care of a Family When a Child Has a Cognitive or Mental Health Disorder 1615

Nursing Process Overview for Care of a Child With a Cognitive Challenge or Mental Illness 1616

HEALTH PROMOTION AND RISK MANAGEMENT 1617
CLASSIFICATION OF MENTAL HEALTH DISORDERS 1618
DEVELOPMENTAL DISORDERS 1618
ATTENTION-DEFICIT AND DISRUPTIVE BEHAVIOR DISORDERS 1623
ANXIETY DISORDERS OF CHILDHOOD OR ADOLESCENCE 1628
EATING DISORDERS 1629
TIC DISORDERS 1631
ELIMINATION DISORDERS 1632
OTHER PSYCHIATRIC DISORDERS AFFECTING CHILDREN 1632

Chapter 55

Nursing Care of a Family in Crisis: Abuse and Violence in the Family 1636

Nursing Process Overview for Care of a Family That Experiences Abuse 1637

HEALTH PROMOTION AND RISK MANAGEMENT 1638
CHILD ABUSE 1639
SEXUAL ABUSE 1648
RAPE 1650
INTIMATE PARTNER ABUSE 1653

Chapter 56

Nursing Care of a Family When a Child Has a Long-Term or Terminal Illness 1659

Nursing Process Overview for Care of a Family Coping With a Long-Term or Terminal Illness 1660

THE CHILD WITH A LONG-TERM ILLNESS 1661
THE CHILD WHO IS TERMINALLY ILL 1666

A The Rights of Children and Childbearing Women 1677
B Composition of Infant Formulas (per 100 mL) 1680
C Drug Effects in Lactation 1682
D Temperature and Weight Conversion Charts 1685
E Growth Charts 1687
F Standard Laboratory Values 1696
Pulse, Respiration, and Blood Pressure Values 1707
Denver II [illegible]
I Standard Infection Precautions 1710
J Recommended Childhood and Adolescent Immunization Schedule, United States, 2009 1712
K The Food Guide Pyramid 1717

Glossary 1719

Index 1739

- Care of infants during the perinatal period (6 weeks before conception to 6 weeks after birth)
- Care of children from birth through adolescence
- Care in settings as varied as the birthing room, the pediatric intensive care unit, and the home

In all settings and types of care, keeping the family at the center of care or considering the family as the primary unit of care is an essential goal. This is because the level of a family's functioning affects the health status of its members (Vonderheid, Norr, & Handler, 2007). If a family's level of functioning is low, the emotional, physical, and social health and potential of individuals in that family can be adversely affected. A healthy family, on the other hand, establishes an environment conducive to growth and health-promoting behaviors that sustain family members during crises. Similarly, the health of an individual and his or her ability to function strongly influence the health of family members and overall family functioning. For these reasons, a family-centered approach enables nurses to better understand individuals and their effect on others and, in turn, to provide holistic care. Box 1.2 provides a summary of key measures for the delivery of family-centered maternal and child health care.

BOX 1.2 ✻ Common Measures to Ensure Family-Centered Maternal and Child Health Care

Principles

- The family is the basic unit of society.
- Families come in many different forms and sizes and represent racial, ethnic, cultural, and socioeconomic diversity.
- Children grow both individually and as part of a family.

Nursing Interventions

- Consider the family as a whole as well as its individual members.
- Assess families for strengths as well as for specific needs or challenges.
- Respect diversity in families as a unique quality of that family.
- Share or initiate information on health planning with family members so that care is family oriented.
- Encourage family bonding through rooming-in in both maternal and child health hospital settings.
- Encourage families to give care to a newborn or ill child.
- Family members affect other members; individual members affect the total family group.
- Encourage family and sibling visits in the hospital to promote family contacts.
- Participate in early hospital discharge programs to reunite families as soon as possible.
- Include developmental stimulation in nursing care.
- Encourage families to reach out to their community so that family members are not isolated from their community or from each other.

STANDARDS OF MATERNAL AND CHILD HEALTH NURSING PRACTICE

The importance a society places on human life can best be measured by the concern it places on its most vulnerable members—its elderly, disadvantaged, and youngest citizens. To promote consistency and ensure quality nursing care and outcomes in these areas, specialty organizations have developed guidelines for care in their specific areas of nursing practice. In maternal-child health, standards have been developed by the Division of Maternal-Child Health Nursing Practice of the American Nurses Association in collaboration with the Society of Pediatric Nurses. These standards are shown in Box 1.3.

The Association of Women's Health, Obstetric, and Neonatal Nurses (AWHONN) has developed similar standards for the nursing care of women and newborns. These are summarized in Box 1.4. Notice how both these practice directives speak to family-centered care.

A FRAMEWORK FOR MATERNAL AND CHILD HEALTH NURSING CARE

Maternal and child health nursing can be visualized within a framework in which nurses, using nursing process, nursing theory, and evidence-based practice, care for families during childbearing and childrearing years through four phases of health care:

- Health promotion
- Health maintenance
- Health restoration
- Health rehabilitation

Examples of these phases of health care as they relate to maternal and child health are shown in Table 1.1.

The Nursing Process

Nursing care, at its best, is designed and implemented in a thorough manner, using an organized series of steps, to ensure quality and consistency of care (Carpenito, 2007). The nursing process, a form of problem solving based on the scientific method, serves as the basis for assessing, making a nursing diagnosis, planning, organizing, and evaluating care. That the nursing process is applicable to all health care settings, from the prenatal clinic to the pediatric intensive care unit, is proof that the method is broad enough to serve as the basis for nursing care.

Because nurses rarely work in isolation but rather as a member of a health care team or unit, multidisciplinary care maps are included throughout the text to demonstrate the use of the nursing process for selected clients, provide examples of critical thinking, and clarify nursing care for specific client needs. These also serve to accentuate the increasingly important role of the nurse as a coordinator of client care and member of a collaborative team.

Evidence-Based Practice

Evidence-based practice is the conscientious, explicit, and judicious use of current best evidence in making decisions about the care of patients (Foxcroft & Cole, 2009). Evidence can be a combination of research, clinical expertise, and

BOX 1.3 * American Nurses Association/Society of Pediatric Nurses Standards of Care and Professional Performance

Standards of Care

Comprehensive pediatric nursing care focuses on helping children and their families and communities achieve their optimum health potentials. This is best achieved within the framework of family-centered care and the nursing process, including primary, secondary, and tertiary care coordinated across health care and community settings.

Standard I: Assessment

The pediatric nurse collects patient health data.

Standard II: Diagnosis

The pediatric nurse analyzes the assessment data in determining diagnoses.

Standard III: Outcome Identification

The pediatric nurse identifies expected outcomes individualized to the child and the family.

Standard IV: Planning

The pediatric nurse develops a plan of care that prescribes interventions to obtain expected outcomes.

Standard V: Implementation

The pediatric nurse implements the interventions identified in the plan of care.

Standard VI: Evaluation

The pediatric nurse evaluates the child's and family's progress toward attainment of outcomes.

Standards of Professional Performance

Standard I: Quality of Care

The pediatric nurse systematically evaluates the quality and effectiveness of pediatric nursing practice.

Standard II: Performance Appraisal

The pediatric nurse evaluates his or her own nursing practice in relation to professional practice standards and relevant statutes and regulations.

Standard III: Education

The pediatric nurse acquires and maintains current knowledge and competency in pediatric nursing practice.

Standard IV: Collegiality

The pediatric nurse interacts with and contributes to the professional development of peers, colleagues, and other health care providers.

Standard V: Ethics

The pediatric nurse's assessment, actions, and recommendations on behalf of children and their families are determined in an ethical manner.

Standard VI: Collaboration

The pediatric nurse collaborates with the child, family, and other health care providers in providing client care.

Standard VII: Research

The pediatric nurse contributes to nursing and pediatric health care through the use of research methods and findings.

Standard VIII: Resource Utilization

The pediatric nurse considers factors related to safety, effectiveness, and cost in planning and delivering patient care.

American Nurses Association and Society of Pediatric Nurses. (2003). *Scope and standards of pediatric clinical practice.* Washington, DC: American Nurses Association Publishing House.

patient preferences when all three combine in decision making. The worth of evidence is ranked according to:

- **Level I:** Evidence obtained from at least one properly designed randomized controlled trial.
- **Level II:** Evidence obtained from well-designed controlled trials without randomization, well-designed cohort or case-control analytic studies, or multiple time series with or without an intervention. Evidence obtained from dramatic results in uncontrolled trials might also be regarded as this type of evidence.
- **Level III:** Opinions of respected authorities, based on clinical experience, descriptive studies, or reports of expert committees (U.S. Preventive Services Task Force, 2005).

Use of evidence-based practice helps to move all health care actions to a more solid, and therefore safer, scientific base. The Cochrane Database of Systematic Reviews is good source for discovering evidence-based practices as the organization consistently reviews, evaluates, and reports the strength of health-related research.

Nursing Research

Bodies of professional knowledge grow and expand to the extent that people in that profession plan and carry out research. **Nursing research,** the controlled investigation of problems that have implications for nursing practice, provides evidence for practice and justification for implementing activities for outcome achievement, ultimately resulting in improved and cost-effective patient care.

A classic example of how the results of nursing research can influence nursing practice is the application of the research carried out by Rubin (1963) on a mother's approach to her newborn. Before the publication of this study, nurses assumed that a woman who did not immediately hold and cuddle her infant at birth was a "cold" or unfeeling mother. After observing a multitude of new mothers, Rubin concluded that attachment is not a spontaneous procedure; rather, it more commonly begins with only fingertip touching. Armed with Rubin's findings and integrating these findings into practice, nurses became better able to differentiate

BOX 1.4 ✻ Association of Women's Health, Obstetric, and Neonatal Nurses Standards and Guidelines

Standards of Professional Performance

Standard I: Quality of Care
The nurse systematically evaluates the quality and effectiveness of nursing practice.

Standard II: Performance Appraisal
The nurse evaluates his/her own nursing practice in relation to professional practice standards and relevant statutes and regulations.

Standard III: Education
The nurse acquires and maintains current knowledge in nursing practice.

Standard IV: Collegiality
The nurse contributes to the professional development of peers, colleagues, and others.

Standard V: Ethics
The nurse's decisions and actions on behalf of patients are determined in an ethical manner.

Standard VI: Collaboration
The nurse collaborates with the patient, significant others, and health care providers in providing patient care.

Standard VII: Research
The nurse uses research findings in practice.

Standard VIII: Resource Utilization
The nurse considers factors related to safety, effectiveness, and cost in planning and delivering patient care.

Standard IX: Practice Environment
The nurse contributes to the environment of care delivery within the practice settings.

Standard X: Accountability
The nurse is professionally and legally accountable for his/her practice. The professional registered nurse may delegate to and supervise qualified personnel who provide patient care.

Association of Women's Health, Obstetric, and Neonatal Nurses. (1998). *Standards for the nursing care of women and newborns* (5th ed.). Washington, DC: Author.

healthy from unhealthy bonding behavior in postpartum women. Women who did not follow this step-by-step pattern of attachment were no longer categorized as unfeeling. By documenting these healthy and unhealthy parameters, nurses can identify women who do not follow a healthy pattern, and interventions can be planned and instituted to help these mothers gain a stronger attachment to their new infants. Additional nursing research in this area (discussed in Chapter 17) has provided further substantiation about the importance of this original investigation.

Evidence-based practice requires ongoing research to substantiate current actions as well as to provide guidelines for future actions. Some examples of current questions that warrant nursing investigation in the area of maternal and child health nursing include the following:

- What is the most effective stimulus to encourage women to come for prenatal care or parents to bring children for health maintenance care?
- How much self-care should young children be expected (or encouraged) to provide during an illness?
- What is the effect of market-driven health care on the quality of maternal-child nursing care?
- What active measures can nurses take to reduce the incidence of child or intimate partner abuse?

TABLE 1.1 ✻ Definitions and Examples of Phases of Health Care

Term	Definition	Examples
Health promotion	Educating clients to be aware of good health through teaching and role modeling	Teaching women the importance of rubella immunization before pregnancy; teaching children the importance of safer sex practices
Health maintenance	Intervening to maintain health when risk of illness is present	Encouraging women to come for prenatal care; teaching parents the importance of safeguarding their home by childproofing it against poisoning
Health restoration	Promptly diagnosing and treating illness using interventions that will return client to wellness most rapidly	Caring for a woman during a complication of pregnancy or a child during an acute illness
Health rehabilitation	Preventing further complications from an illness; bringing an ill client back to an optimal state of wellness or helping a client to accept inevitable death	Encouraging a woman with gestational trophoblastic disease to continue therapy or a child with a renal transplant to continue to take necessary medications

diseased cells with new growth cells; new fertility drugs and techniques allow more couples than ever before to conceive; and the ability to delay preterm birth and improve life for premature infants has grown dramatically. In addition, a growing trend toward health care consumerism, or self-care, has made childbearing and childrearing families active participants in their own health monitoring and care. Health care consumerism has also moved care from hospitals to community sites such as retail shopping malls and from long-term hospital stays to overnight surgical and emergent care settings.

Even in light of these changes, much more still needs to be done. National health care goals are established every 10 years for the following decade to continuously stress the importance of maternal and child health to overall community health (U.S. Department of Health and Human Services [DHHS]). Although health care may be more advanced, it is still not accessible to everyone. These and other social changes and trends have expanded the roles of nurses in maternal and child health and, at the same time, have made the delivery of quality maternal and child health nursing care a continuing challenge.

National Health Goals

In 1979, the U.S. Public Health Service first formulated health care objectives. These goals are ongoing and modified every 10 years (http://www.nih.gov). Many of these objectives directly involve maternal and child health care, because improving the health of this young age group will have such long-term effects. Two overarching national goals are to (a) increase quality and years of healthy life and (b) eliminate health disparities. The 10 leading health indicators or important secondary goals are shown in Box 1.6. Ongoing goals specific for each content area are highlighted in later chapters. National health goals are intended to help citizens more easily understand the importance of health promotion and disease prevention and to encourage wide participation in improving health in the next decade. It is important for maternal and child health nurses to be familiar with these goals because nurses play such a vital role in helping the nation achieve these objectives through both practice and research. The goals also serve as the basis for grant funding and financing of evidence-based practice.

Trends in the Maternal and Child Health Nursing Population

The maternal and child population is constantly changing because of changes in social structure, variations in family lifestyle, and changing patterns of illness. Table 1.2 summarizes some of the social changes that are altering health care priorities for maternal and child health nurses. Client advocacy, participating in cost-containment measures, focusing on health education, and creating new nursing roles are ways in which nurses have adapted to these changes. **Client advocacy** is safeguarding and advancing the interests of clients and their families. The role includes knowing the health care services available in a community, establishing a relationship with families, and helping them make informed choices about what course of action or service would be best for them. Some examples of English-Spanish communication that could be helpful are included at http://thePoint.lww.com.

Measuring Maternal and Child Health

Measuring maternal and child health is not as simple as defining a client as ill or well because individual clients and health care practitioners may have different perspectives on illness and wellness. For example, some children with chronic but controllable asthma think of themselves as well; others with the same degree of involvement consider themselves ill. Although pregnancy is generally considered a well state, some women think of themselves as ill during this period. A more objective view of health is provided by using national or regional health statistics.

A number of statistical terms are commonly used to express the outcomes of pregnancies and births and to describe maternal and child health (Box 1.7). Such statistics are useful for comparisons among states and for planning of future health care needs. Statistics require accurate recording, collection, and analysis, and nurses play a major role in the accurate collection and recording of these data that allow the nation's present and future health to be described.

Birth Rate

The birth rate in the United States has gradually decreased over the past 100 years from a high of 30.2 per 1000 population in 1909 to 13.9 per 1000 population at present (Eldridge & Sutton, 2009) (Fig. 1.2). Currently, the average family in the United States has 1.2 children. Boys are born more often than are girls, at a rate of 1050 boys to every 1000 girls (Eldridge & Sutton, 2009). Births to teenaged mothers are steadily declining (presently at 40.4 per 1000 from a high of 61.8 per 1000 in 1961). Births to women older than 40 years are steadily increasing (presently at 9.4 per 1000 from a low of almost no births in this age group).

Fertility Rate

The term **fertility rate** reflects what proportion of women who could have babies are having them. Fertility rates may be low in countries troubled by famine, war, or disease. The fertility rate in the United States is currently 66.7%, a rate that reflects a healthy postindustrial country (Eldridge & Sutton, 2009).

Fetal Death Rate

Fetal death is defined as the death in utero of a child (fetus) weighing 500 g or more, roughly the weight of a fetus of 20 weeks' or more pregnancy. Fetal deaths may occur because of maternal factors such as maternal disease, premature cervical dilation, or maternal malnutrition or fetal factors such as fetal disease, chromosome abnormality, or poor placental attachment. Many fetal deaths occur for reasons that are unknown. The fetal death rate is important in evaluating the health of a nation because it reflects the overall quality of maternal health and prenatal care. The emphasis on both preconceptual and prenatal care has helped to reduce this rate from a number as high as 18% in 1950 to 6.2% at present (Eldridge & Sutton, 2009).

Neonatal Death Rate

The first 28 days of life are known as the *neonatal period*, and an infant during this time is known as a **neonate.** The neonatal death rate reflects not only the quality of care available to women during pregnancy and childbirth but also the quality of care available to infants during the first month of life.

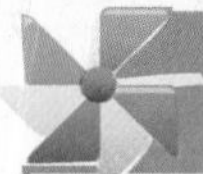

BOX 1.6 ✻ Focus on National Health Goals

Leading Health Indicators

Physical Activity

Regular physical activity throughout life is important for maintaining a healthy body, enhancing psychological well-being, and preventing premature death. The objectives selected to measure progress in this area are:

- Increase the proportion of adolescents who engage in vigorous physical activity that promotes cardiorespiratory fitness 3 or more days per week for 20 or more minutes per occasion.
- Increase the proportion of adults who engage regularly, preferably daily, in moderate physical activity for at least 30 minutes per day.

Overweight and Obesity

Overweight and obesity are major contributors to many preventable causes of death. The objectives selected to measure progress in this area are:

- Reduce the proportion of children and adolescents who are overweight or obese.
- Reduce the proportion of adults who are obese.

Tobacco Use

Cigarette smoking is the single most preventable cause of disease and death in the United States. Smoking results in more deaths each year in the United States than AIDS, alcohol, cocaine, heroin, homicide, suicide, motor vehicle crashes, and fires—combined. The objectives selected to measure progress in this area are:

- Reduce cigarette smoking by adolescents.
- Reduce cigarette smoking by adults.

Substance Abuse

Alcohol and illicit drug use are associated with many of this country's most serious problems, including violence, injury, and HIV infection. The objectives selected to measure progress in this area are:

- Increase the proportion of adolescents not using alcohol or any illicit drugs during the past 30 days.
- Reduce the proportion of adults using any illicit drug during the past 30 days.
- Reduce the proportion of adults or adolescents engaging in binge drinking of alcoholic beverages during the past month.

Responsible Sexual Behavior

Unintended pregnancies and sexually transmitted infections (STIs), including infection with the human immunodeficiency virus that causes AIDS, can result from unprotected sexual behavior. The objectives selected to measure progress in this area are:

- Increase the proportion of adolescents who abstain from sexual intercourse or use condoms if currently sexually active.
- Increase the proportion of sexually active adults who use condoms.

Mental Health

Approximately 20% of the U.S. population is affected by mental illness during a given year; no one is immune. Of all mental illnesses, depression is the most common disorder. More than 19 million adults in the United States suffer from depression. Major depression is the leading cause of disability and is the cause of more than two thirds of suicides each year. The objective selected to measure progress in this area is to:

- Increase the proportion of adults including postpartum depression who receive treatment.

Injury and Violence

More than 400 Americans die each day from injuries, due primarily to motor vehicle crashes, firearms, poisonings, suffocation, falls, fires, and drowning. The risk of injury is so great that most persons sustain a significant injury at some time during their lives. The objectives selected to measure progress in this area are:

- Reduce deaths caused by motor vehicle crashes.
- Reduce homicides.

Environmental Quality

An estimated 25% of preventable illnesses worldwide can be attributed to poor environmental quality. In the United States, air pollution alone is estimated to be associated with 50,000 premature deaths and an estimated $40 billion to $50 billion in health-related costs annually. The objectives selected to measure progress in this area are:

- Reduce the proportion of persons exposed to air that does not meet the U.S. Environmental Protection Agency's health-based standards for ozone.
- Reduce the proportion of nonsmokers exposed to environmental tobacco smoke.

Immunization

Vaccines are among the greatest public health achievements of the 20th century. Immunizations can prevent disability and death from infectious diseases for individuals and can help control the spread of infections within communities. The objectives selected to measure progress in this area are:

- Increase the proportion of young children who receive all vaccines that have been recommended for universal administration.
- Increase the proportion of noninstitutionalized adults who are vaccinated annually against influenza and ever vaccinated against pneumococcal disease.

Access to Health Care

Strong predictors of access to quality health care include having health insurance, a higher income level, and a regular primary care provider or other source of ongoing health care. Use of clinical preventive services, such as early prenatal care, can serve as indicators of access to quality health care services. The objectives selected to measure progress in this area are:

- Increase the proportion of persons with health insurance.
- Increase the proportion of persons who have a specific source of ongoing care.
- Increase the proportion of pregnant women who begin prenatal care in the first trimester of pregnancy.

From http://www.nih.gov.

TABLE 1.2 ❋ Trends in Maternal and Child Health Care and Implications for Nurses

Trend	Implications for Nursing
Families are not as extended so are smaller than previously.	Fewer family members are present as support people in a time of crisis. Nurses are called on to fulfill this role more than ever before.
Single parents have become the most common type of parent in the United States.	A single parent may have fewer financial resources than dual employed parents; this is more likely if the parent is a woman. Nurses can help by informing parents of care options and providing a backup opinion when needed.
Ninety percent of women work outside the home at least part-time.	Health care must be scheduled at times a working parent can come for care for herself or bring a child for care. Problems of latch-key (self-care) children and the selection of child care centers need to be addressed.
Families are more mobile than previously; there is an increase in the number of homeless women and children.	Good interviewing and health monitoring are necessary with mobile families so a health database can be established and there can be continuity of care.
Both child and intimate partner abuse is increasing in incidence.	Screening for child or intimate partner abuse should be included in all family contacts. Nurses must be aware of the legal responsibilities for reporting abuse.
Families are more health conscious than ever before.	Families are ripe for health education; providing this can be a major nursing role.
Health care must respect cost containment.	Comprehensive care is necessary in primary care settings because referral to specialists may no longer be an option. Health insurance is not available for all families.

The leading causes of infant mortality during the first 4 weeks of life are prematurity (early gestational age or low birth weight of less than 2500 g ([17%]) and congenital malformations (20%). Approximately 80% of infants who die within 48 hours after birth weigh less than 2500 g (5.5 lb). The proportion of infants born with low birth weight is about 12.5% of all births. This number rises slightly each year due to the increase in multiple births and better prenatal care that allows infants who would have died in utero (fetal death) to be born and survive (Hamilton et al., 2007).

Perinatal Death Rate

The perinatal period is the time period beginning when a fetus reaches 500 g (about week 20 of pregnancy) and ending about 4 to 6 weeks after birth. The perinatal death rate is the sum of the fetal and neonatal rates.

Infant Mortality Rate

The infant mortality rate of a country is an index of its general health because it measures the quality of pregnancy care, nutrition, and sanitation as well as infant health. This rate is the traditional standard used to compare the health care of a nation with that of previous years or of other countries.

Because of health care advances and improvements in child care, the infant mortality rate in the United States has been steadily declining in recent years to reach a record low of 6.6 per 1000 population (Eldridge & Sutton, 2009) (Fig. 1.3). Unfortunately, infant mortality is not equal for all people. The mortality rate for African American infants, for example, is almost 15%. This difference in infant deaths is thought to be related to the higher proportion of births to young African American mothers, unequal provision of health care, and the higher percentage of low-birth-weight babies born to African American women: 12%, compared with approximately 5% for white and Asian women (Eldridge & Sutton, 2009). Because teenage pregnancy leads to increased premature births, this can result in infants being born who are not as well prepared as others to face extrauterine life (Hamilton et al., 2007).

BOX 1.7 ❋ Statistical Terms Used to Report Maternal and Child Health

Birth rate: Number of births per 1000 population.

Fertility rate: Number of pregnancies per 1000 women of childbearing age.

Fetal death rate: Number of fetal deaths (weighing more 500 g) per 1000 live births.

Neonatal death rate: Number of deaths per 1000 live births occurring at birth or in the first 28 days of life.

Perinatal death rate: Number of deaths of fetuses weighing more than 500 g and within the first 28 days of life per 1000 live births.

Maternal mortality rate: Number of maternal deaths per 100,000 live births that occur as a direct result of the reproductive process.

Infant mortality rate: Number of deaths per 1000 live births occurring at birth or in the first 12 months of life.

Childhood mortality rate: Number of deaths per 1000 population in children, 1 to 14 years of age.

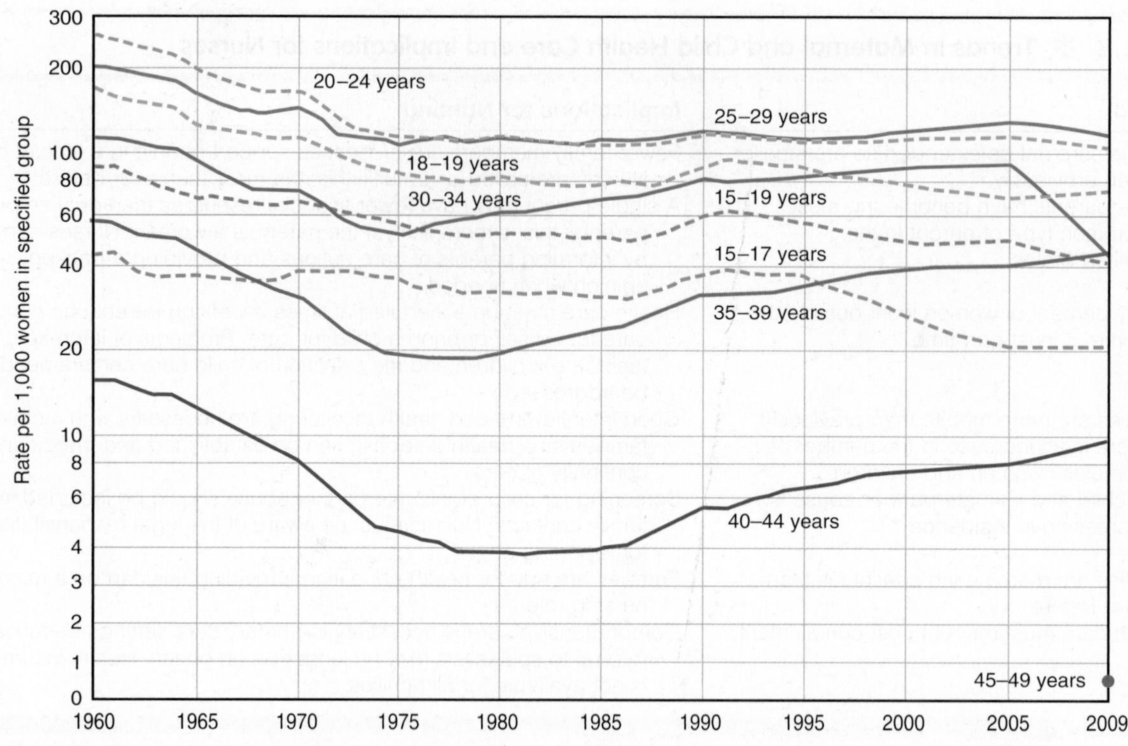

FIGURE 1.2 Birth rates by age of mother: United States, 1960–2009. (From National Center for Health Statistics. [2009]. Births, marriages, divorces and deaths. *National Vital Statistics Report, 57*[1], 6.)

The infant mortality rate also varies greatly from state to state within the United States (Table 1.3). For example, in the District of Columbia, the area with the highest infant mortality, the rate is almost three times higher than that of Massachusetts, the state with the lowest rate.

Table 1.4 shows the ranking of the United States compared with other countries. One would expect that a country such as the United States, which has one of the highest gross national products in the world and is known for its technological capabilities, would have the lowest infant mortality rate. The U.S. infant mortality rate is higher, however, than that of 32 other countries (United Nations Statistics Division, 2007).

Two factors that may contribute to national differences in infant mortality are the number of infants born to adolescent mothers (38% of U.S. infants are born to women under 20 years of age) and the type of health insurance and care available. In Sweden, for example, a comprehensive health care program provides free maternal and child health care to all residents. Women who attend prenatal clinics early in pregnancy receive a monetary award, a practice that almost guarantees that women come for prenatal care. This

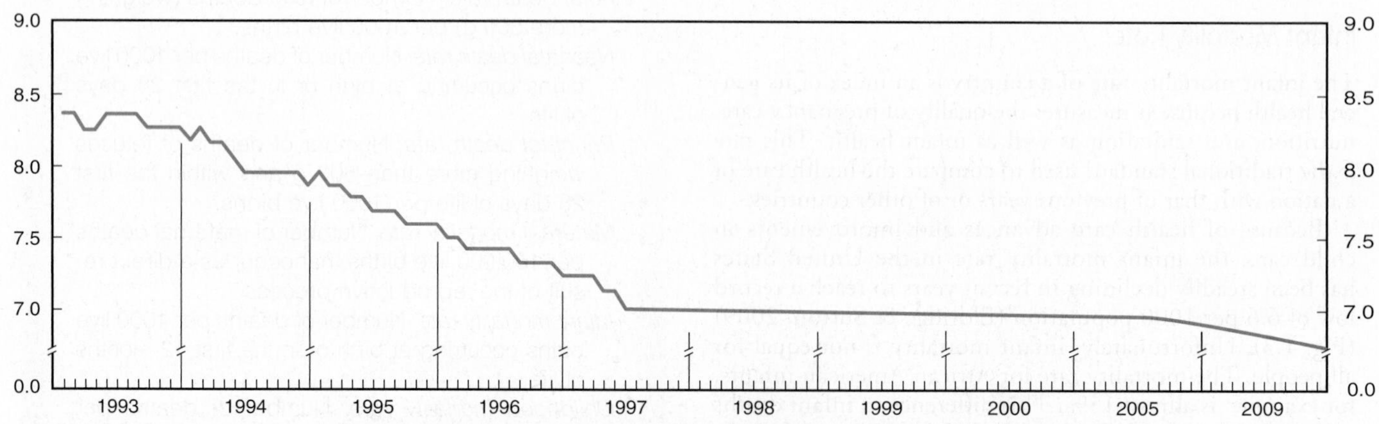

FIGURE 1.3 Infant mortality rates per 1000 live births for successive 12-month periods ending with month indicated: United States, 2009. (From National Center for Health Statistics. [2009]. Births, marriages, divorces and deaths. *National Vital Statistics Report, 57*[1], 2.)

TABLE 1.3 ✻ Infant Mortality Rates per 1000 by State

State	Rate	State	Rate
Massachusetts	4.8	Kansas	7.0
New Hampshire	4.9	Nebraska	7.0
Maine	5.1	Florida	7.2
Utah	5.3	Hawaii	7.2
California	5.4	Virginia	7.2
Minnesota	5.5	Pennsylvania	7.3
Oregon	5.5	Indiana	7.7
Vermont	5.5	Maryland	7.7
Washington	5.5	Missouri	7.7
Iowa	5.8	Ohio	7.7
Texas	5.9	Illinois	7.8
Colorado	6.0	North Dakota	7.8
Nevada	6.0	West Virginia	7.9
New Jersey	6.1	Oklahoma	8.0
New York	6.1	Michigan	8.1
Connecticut	6.4	Arkansas	8.3
New Mexico	6.4	North Carolina	8.4
South Dakota	6.4	Georgia	8.7
Wyoming	6.5	South Carolina	9.0
Idaho	6.6	Tennessee	9.0
Arizona	6.7	Alabama	9.3
Kentucky	6.7	Puerto Rico	9.4
Rhode Island	6.7	Delaware	9.6
Alaska	6.8	Louisiana	9.8
Montana	6.9	Mississippi	10.5
Wisconsin	6.9	District of Columbia	11.4

National Center for Health Statistics. (2007). *Births, marriages, divorces, and deaths.* Hyattsville, MD: Author.

TABLE 1.4 ✻ Infant Mortality Rate (Deaths per 1000 Live Births) for Selected Countries, 2000

Country	Rate	Country	Rate
1. Iceland	3	18. Ireland	5
2. Japan	3	19. Italy	5
3. Singapore	3	20. Israel	5
4. Sweden	3	21. Luxembourg	5
5. Andorra	4	22. Netherlands	5
6. Belgium	4	23. New Zealand	5
7. Finland	4	24. Slovenia	5
8. France	4	25. Spain	5
9. Germany	4	26. United Kingdom	5
10. Hong Kong SAR	4	27. Brunei Darussalam	6
11. Norway	4	28. Cuba	6
12. Republic of Korea	4	29. Cyprus	6
13. Switzerland	4	30. Czech Republic	6
14. Australia	5	31. Greece	6
15. Austria	5	32. Portugal	6
16. Canada	5	33. United States	6
17. Denmark	5		

United Nations Statistics Division. (2007). *Statistics & indicators on women & men.* New York: Author.

policy varies sharply with the availability of health care in an occupation-linked insurance system such as the U.S.

Fortunately, the proportion of pregnant women who receive prenatal care in the United States is increasing (about 83% now begin care in the first trimester). Early prenatal care is important, because it identifies potential risks and allows preventive strategies to help reduce complications of pregnancy.

The main causes of infant death in the United States are problems that occur at birth or shortly thereafter. Before antibiotics and formula sterilization practices became available, gastrointestinal disease was a leading cause of infant death. By advocating breastfeeding and teaching mothers strict adherence to good sanitary practices, health care practitioners help ensure that gastrointestinal infection does not again become a major factor in infant mortality.

Today, prematurity, low birth weight, congenital malformations, and sudden infant death syndrome (SIDS) are all major causes of mortality. SIDS is the sudden death of an infant less than 1 year of age that cannot be explained after a thorough investigation of the cause of death is conducted (Sahni, Fifer, & Myers, 2007). Although other factors that contribute to SIDS are yet to be determined, the recommendation to place infants on their back or side and to allow infants to sleep with a pacifier, made by the American Academy of Pediatrics, has led to an almost 50% decrease in its incidence (Centers for Disease Control and Prevention [CDC], 2007a). Nurses have been instrumental in reducing the number of these deaths as they are the health professionals who most often discuss newborn care with new parents (Esposito, Hegyi, & Ostfeld, 2007).

Maternal Mortality Rate

The maternal mortality rate is the number of maternal deaths that occur as a direct result of the reproductive process per 100,000 live births. Early in the 20th century, this rate in the United States reached levels as high as 600 per 100,000 live births. It is still high in developing countries such as Afghanistan (over 3500 per 100,000 births) (Eldridge & Sutton, 2009). In the United States at present, the maternal mortality rate has declined to a low of 6.5 per 100,000 live births (Fig. 1.4). This dramatic decrease can be attributed to improved preconceptual, prenatal, labor and birth, and postpartum care such as

- Increased participation of women in prenatal care
- Greater detection of disorders such as ectopic pregnancy or placenta previa and prevention of related complications through the use of ultrasound
- Increased control of complications associated with hypertension of pregnancy
- Decreased use of anesthesia with childbirth

For most of the 20th century, uterine hemorrhage and infection were the leading causes of death during pregnancy and childbirth. This has changed because of the increased ability to prevent or control hemorrhage and infection; now hypertensive disorders have become the leading causes of death in childbirth. Pregnancy-induced hypertension adds to preexisting hypertensive disorders, especially in older women. Nurses who are alert to the signs and symptoms of hypertension are invaluable guardians of the health of pregnant and postpartum women.

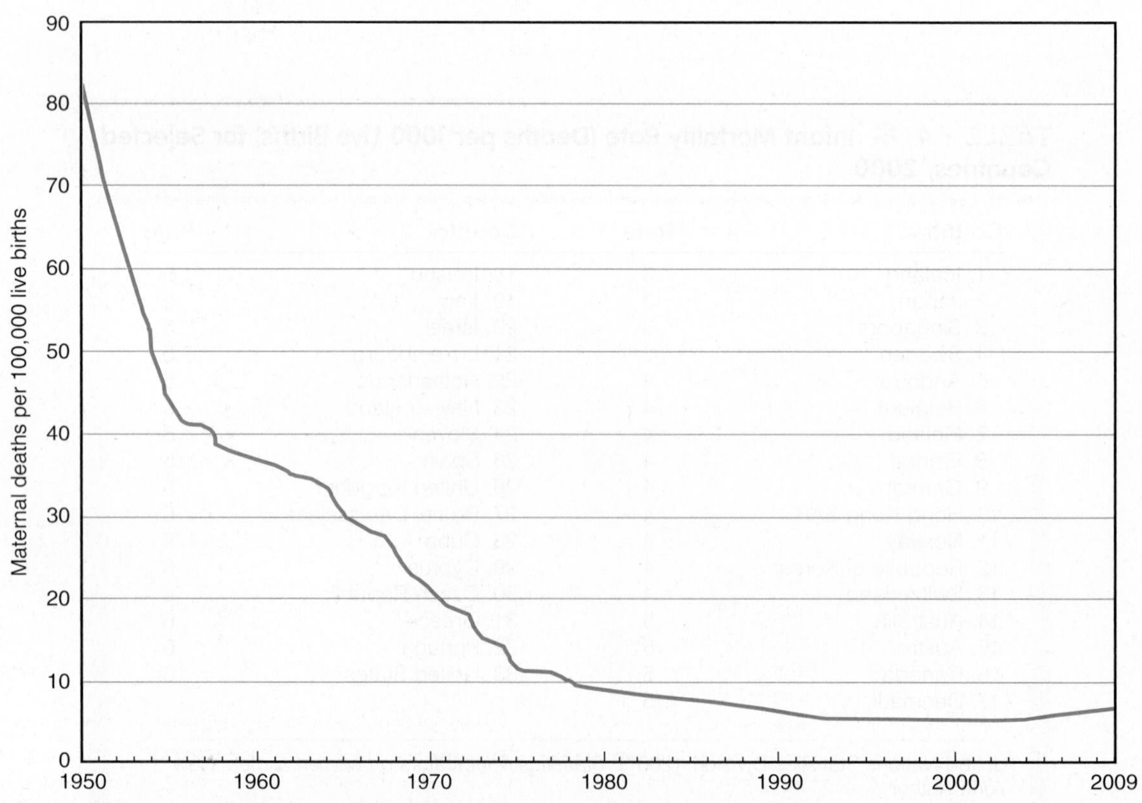

FIGURE 1.4 Maternal mortality rates. (From National Center for Health Statistics. [2009]. Births, marriages, divorces and deaths. *National Vital Statistics Report, 57*[1], 3.)

✓ Checkpoint Question 1.2

Nursing is changing because social change affects care. Which of the following is a trend that is occurring in nursing because of social change?

a. Children are treated in emergent care clinics, so nurses are hardly needed.
b. Immunizations are now available for all childhood infectious diseases.
c. The use of skilled technology has made nursing care more complex.
d. Pregnant women are so healthy today that they rarely need prenatal care.

Childhood Mortality Rate

Like the infant mortality rate, the childhood mortality rate in the United States is also declining. In 1980, for example, the mortality rate was about 6.4% for children aged 1 to 4 years and 3.1% for children aged 4 to 14 years; today, it is 2.9% and 1.4%, respectively (National Vital Statistics Service, 2009a). The risk of death in the first year of life is higher than that in any other year before age 55. Children in the prepubescent period (aged 5–14 years) have the lowest mortality rate of any child age group (Hamilton et al., 2007).

The most frequent causes of childhood death are shown in Box 1.8. Motor vehicle crashes remain the leading cause of death in children, although many of these accidents are largely preventable through education about the value of car seats and seat belt use, the dangers of drinking/drug abuse and driving, and the importance of pedestrian safety.

A particularly disturbing mortality statistic is the high incidence of homicide and suicide in the 10- to 19-year-old age group (more girls than boys attempt suicide, but boys are more often successful). Although school-aged children and adolescents may not voice feelings of depression or anger during a health care visit, such underlying feelings may actually be a primary concern (Hempstead, 2007). Nurses who are alert to cues of depression or anger can be instrumental in detecting these emotions and lowering the risk of suicide.

BOX 1.8 ✻ Major Causes of Death in Childhood

Under 1 Year

1. Congenital malformations and chromosomal abnormalities
2. Disorders related to short gestation age and low birth weight
3. Sudden infant death syndrome
4. Newborn affected by maternal complications of pregnancy
5. Unintentional injuries (accidents)

1–4 Years

1. Unintentional injuries (accidents)
2. Congenital malformations and chromosomal abnormalities
3. Malignant neoplasms
4. Assault or homicide
5. Diseases of the heart

5–14 Years

1. Unintentional injuries (accidents)
2. Malignant neoplasms
3. Assault or homicide
4. Intentional self-harm (suicide)
5. Congenital malformations and chromosomal abnormalities

15–24 Years

1. Unintentional injuries (accidents)
2. Assault or homicide
3. Intentional self-harm (suicide)
4. Malignant neoplasms
5. Diseases of the heart

National Center for Health Statistics. (2009a). *Trends in the health of Americans.* Hyattsville, MD: Author.

Childhood Morbidity Rate

Health problems commonly occurring in large proportions of children today include respiratory disorders (including asthma and tuberculosis), gastrointestinal disturbances, and consequences of injuries. Obesity has become such a health problem in some communities that more 20% of school-aged children are obese (National Vital Statistics Service, 2009b). Obesity in school-aged children can lead to cardiovascular disorders, self-esteem issues, and type 2 diabetes (Hussain et al., 2007). Nurses can be instrumental in teaching better nutrition and encouraging increased exercise to help decrease this incidence (Summerbell et al., 2009).

As more immunizations become available, fewer children in the United States are affected by common childhood communicable diseases. For instance, the incidence of poliomyelitis (once a major killer of children) is now zero because almost all children in the United States are immunized against it (National Vital Statistics Service, 2009a). Measles flared in incidence in the early 1990s but now is scheduled as a disease to be completely eradicated by 2010. It is important that this change happen, because measles encephalitis can be lethal. Continued education about the benefits of immunization against rubella (German measles) is also needed, because if a woman contracts this form of measles during pregnancy, her infant can be born with severe congenital malformations. The new vaccine against human papillomavirus (HPV) suggested for prepubertal girls should help prevent HPV infections that can have the same disastrous results (American Academy of Pediatrics, 2009).

Although the decline in the overall incidence of preventable childhood diseases is encouraging, as many as 25% of children younger than 4 years in some communities are still not fully immunized (CDC, 2009). There is a potential for the incidence of childhood infectious diseases to increase again if immunization is not maintained as a high national priority.

The advent of human immunodeficiency virus (HIV) infection has changed care considerations in all areas of nursing, but it has particular implications for maternal and child health nursing. Sexually active teenagers are at risk for becoming infected with HIV through sexual contact or exposure to blood and blood products (Purswani et al., 2007). Infected women may transmit the virus to a fetus during pregnancy through placental exchange (Paintsil & Andiman, 2007).

Nurses play a vital role in helping prevent the spread of HIV by educating adolescents and young adults about safer sexual practices (see Chapter 5). Follow standard infection precautions in maternal and child health nursing, as in other areas of nursing practice, to safeguard yourself, other health care providers, and clients from the spread of infection.

Other infectious diseases that are increasing in incidence include syphilis; genital herpes; hepatitis A, B, and C viruses; and tuberculosis. The rise of syphilis, hepatitis C virus, and genital herpes probably stems from an increase in nonmonogamous sexual relationships and lack of safer sex practices. The increase in hepatitis B virus infection is due largely to drug abuse and the use of infected injection equipment. One reason for the increase in hepatitis A virus is shared diaper-changing facilities in day care centers. Tuberculosis, once considered close to eradication, has experienced a resurgence, occurring today at approximately the same rate as measles in young adults. One form occurs as an opportunistic disease in HIV-positive persons and is particularly resistant to the usual therapy (Fraser et al., 2009).

Trends in Health Care Environment

The settings and philosophy of maternal and child health care are both changing to better meet the needs of increasingly well-informed and vocal consumers.

Initiating Cost Containment

Cost containment refers to systems of health care delivery that focus on reducing the cost of health care by closely monitoring the cost of personnel, use and brands of supplies, length of hospital stays, number of procedures carried out, and number of referrals requested while maintaining quality care (Callens, Volbragt, & Nys, 2007).

The advent of managed care has direct implications for maternal and child health nursing because lack of financial ability to pay is a major reason why women do not obtain prenatal care or children do not receive well-child care. A woman may fear that not working during pregnancy may lead to loss of insurance coverage, thereby reducing her ability to pay for services. As a result, she may continue to work long hours or in unfit conditions during pregnancy. Nurses are challenged to help reduce costs while maintaining quality care so that prenatal care remains available.

Before the philosophy of cost containment became prominent, health care insurance companies paid separately for each procedure or piece of equipment a client received. Under managed care, the agency receives a certain sum of money for a client's care, no matter how many supplies, procedures, or personnel are used in the client's care. In a managed care environment, helping to curtail cost yet provide quality care is an important nursing function. Suggestions such as using generic-brand supplies, never breaking into kits of supplies to remove a single item, and urging the use of disposable supplies so that less personnel time will be spent on cleaning and sterilizing items are welcome, cost-effective suggestions.

Cost containment has had dramatic effects on health care, most noticeably in limiting the number of hospital days, decreasing the number of uncompensated patients accepted by agencies, and changing the roles of personnel (McKay & Meng, 2007). Before managed care, for example, women stayed in a hospital for 3 or 4 days after childbirth; today, they rarely stay longer than 48 hours. Before managed care, nurses completed all care procedures for patients, no matter how small or unskilled the task. With managed care, ancillary personnel (e.g., unlicensed assistive personnel) perform many tasks under the supervision of the nurse. This system is designed to move the registered nurse (RN) to a higher level of function, because it makes the RN accountable for a fuller range of services to patients. It accentuates point-of-service care. It also increases the accountability and responsibility of RNs to delegate tasks appropriately. As a result of managed care, the new advanced-practice role of case manager was created.

It is important to know the legal aspects of delegation, as identified in individual state nursing practice acts, because some laws address specific tasks and activities that RNs may or may not delegate in that state. Accountability for completion and quality of the task remains with the nurse, so the nurse is responsible for knowing that the condition of the patient and the skill level of the assistive person are conducive to safe delegation. Four rules to follow when delegating are to

- Delegate the right task for the situation
- Delegate to the right person to complete the task
- Use right communication concerning what is to be done
- Ask for right feedback or evaluation that the task was completed

Examples of delegation responsibility that can occur in maternal and child health are highlighted in the multidisciplinary care maps located throughout this text.

Increasing Alternative Settings and Styles for Health Care

During the past 100 years, there have been several major shifts in settings for maternity care. At the turn of the 19th century, most births took place in the home, with only the very poor or ill giving birth in "lying-in" hospitals. By 1940, about 40% of live births occurred in hospitals; today, the figure has risen to 99%. At least 10% of these births are attended by certified nurse-midwives, not physicians (National Vital Statistics Service, 2009a). Today, a less dramatic but no less important trend that is occurring is an increase in the number of families once more choosing childbirth at home or in alternative birth settings rather than hospitals. These alternative settings provide families with increased control of the birth experience and options for birth surroundings that are unavailable in hospitals. One strength of this movement is its encouragement of family involvement in birth. It also increases nursing responsibility for assessment and professional judgment and provides expanded roles for *advanced practice nurses* such as the nurse-midwife and the nurse practitioner (nurses educated at the master's or doctoral level) (Declercq, 2007).

Hospitals have responded to consumers' demand for a more natural childbirth environment by refitting labor and delivery suites as birthing rooms, often called labor-delivery-recovery (LDR) or labor-delivery-recovery-postpartum (LDRP) rooms. Partners, family members, and other support people are invited to stay with the woman in labor so they feel a part of the

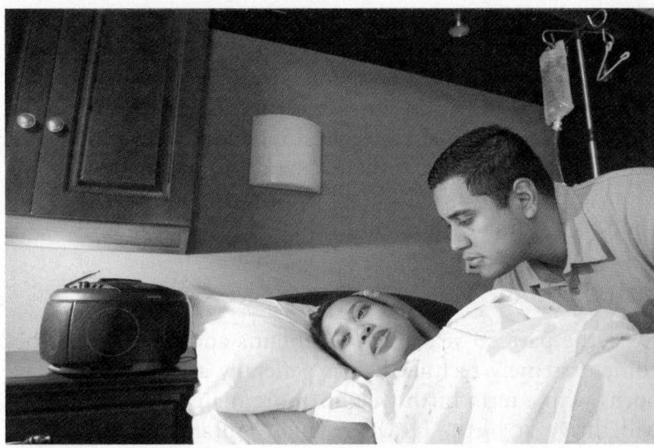

FIGURE 1.5 A couple, soon to be parents, share a close moment in a birthing room.

childbirth. The room is designed as a homelike environment (Fig. 1.5). Couplet care—care for both the mother and newborn by the primary nurse—is encouraged after the births. LDRP rooms promote a holistic, family-centered approach to maternal and child health care and are appealing to many families who might otherwise have opted against a hospital birth. Hospitals are continuing to search for the best labor, birth, and postpartum options. Whether childbirth takes place at home, in a birthing center, or in a hospital, the goal is to keep it as natural as possible while ensuring the protection that experienced health care providers can provide.

Health care settings for children are also changing. Clients' homes, community centers, school-based or retail setting emergent care clinics, and group homes are examples of settings in which comprehensive health care may be administered. In these settings, a nurse may provide immunizations, screenings, health and safety education, counseling, crisis intervention for teens, parenting classes, and care of ill children and families. This form of community-based care can provide cost-effective health promotion, disease prevention, and patient care to a large number of children and families in an environment that is familiar to them.

More and more children and women who are experiencing a pregnancy complication, who might otherwise have been admitted to a hospital, are now being cared for in ambulatory clinics or at home. Separating a child from his or her family during a long hospitalization has been shown to be potentially harmful to the child's development, so any effort to reduce the incidence of separation has a positive effect (see Chapter 36). Avoiding long hospital stays for women during pregnancy is also a preferable method of care, because it helps to maintain family contact.

Ambulatory or non–hospital-based care requires intensive health teaching by the nursing staff and follow-up by home care or community health nurses. Teaching parents of an ill child or a woman with a complication of pregnancy what danger signs to watch for that will warrant immediate attention includes not only imparting the facts of self-care but also providing support and reassurance that the client or parents are capable of this level of care. Retail clinics or emergent care clinics located in shopping malls are often staffed by nurse practitioners, so nurses play a vital role in seeing that such health care settings do not limit continuity of care (Berman, 2007).

What if... Melissa Chung has to remain in the hospital after the birth of her new baby while her baby is transported to a regional center for care? How could you help her keep in touch with her new baby?

Including the Family in Health Care

Health promotion with families during pregnancy or childrearing is a family-centered event, because teaching health awareness and good health habits is accomplished chiefly by role modeling. When children must be admitted to the hospital for extended stays, open visiting hours allow parents to visit as much as possible and sleep overnight in a bed next to their child. Encourage parents in such a setting to do as much for their child as they wish, such as feeding and bathing their child or administering oral medicine. Most of a parent's time, however, should be spent simply being close by to provide a comfortable, secure influence on their child. For the same reasons, the most important role of parents on a maternity unit is to room-in and give total care to their newborn (Box 1.9).

Family-centered nursing this way increases the number of clients a nurse cares for—that is, not four children, for ex-

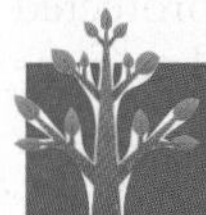

BOX 1.9 ✻ Focus on Family Teaching

Tips for Selecting a Health Care Setting

Q. Melissa Chung, the patient you met at the beginning of the chapter, asks you, "With so many health care settings available, how do we know which one to choose?"

A. When selecting a health care setting, asking the following questions can help you decide what is best for your family:

- Can it be reached easily? (Going for preventive care when well or for continuing care when ill should not be a chore.)
- Will the staff provide continuity of care so you will always see the same primary care provider if possible?
- Does the physical setup of the facility provide for a sense of privacy, yet a sense that health care providers share pertinent information so you do not have to repeat your history at each visit?
- Are the cost of care and the number of referrals to specialists explained clearly?
- Are preventive care and health education stressed (keeping well is as important as recovering from illness)?
- Is health education done at your learning level?
- Do health care providers respect your opinion and ask for your input on health care decisions?
- Do health care providers show a personal interest in you?
- Will the facility still be accessible if a family member becomes disabled?

ample, but four children plus four sets of parents; not just a single newborn, but his or her two parents as well. Caring for families rather than individuals, however, has an immeasurable effect on the health of children and parents and client satisfaction (Mullen et al., 2007).

Illness in a child is automatically a family-centered event. Parents may need to adjust work schedules to allow one of them to stay with the ill child; siblings may have to sacrifice an activity such as a birthday party or having a parent watch their school play; and family finances may have to be readjusted to pay for hospital and medical bills. When a mother is pregnant, family roles or activities may have to change to safeguard her health. A family may feel drawn together by the fright and concern of an acute illness. On the other hand, if an illness becomes chronic, it may pull a family apart or destroy it.

By adopting a view of pregnancy, childbirth, or illness as a family event, nurses can be instrumental in including family members in events from which family members were once totally excluded, such as an unplanned cesarean birth. They can help child health care to be family centered by consulting with family members about a plan of care and providing clear health teaching so that family members can monitor their own care (Fig. 1.6).

The U.S. government recognizes that the care of individual family members should be viewed as a family-centered event. The Family and Medical Leave Act of 1993 is a federal law that requires employers with 50 or more employees to provide a minimum of 12 weeks of unpaid, job-protected leave to employees under four circumstances crucial to family life:

- Birth of the employee's child
- Adoption or foster placement of a child with the employee
- Need for the employee to care for a parent, spouse, or child with a serious health condition
- Inability of the employee to perform his or her functions because of a serious health condition

A *serious health condition* is defined as "an illness, injury, impairment, or physical or mental condition involving such circumstances as inpatient care or incapacity requiring 3 workdays' absence" (U.S. Department of Labor, 1995).

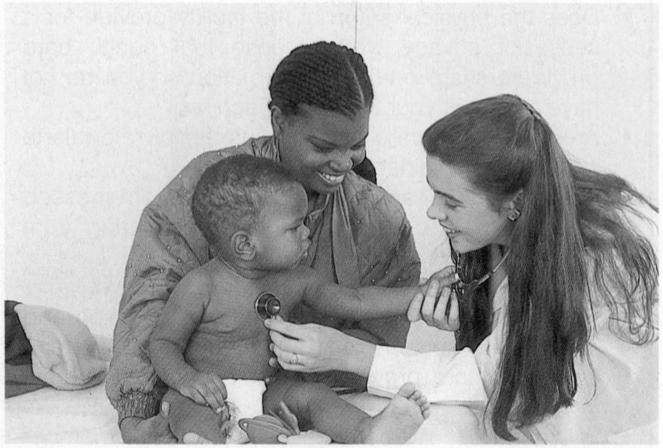

FIGURE 1.6 A nurse involves the mother in a physical exam to promote family-centered care. (© Barbara Proud.)

Specifically mentioned in the law is any period of incapacity due to pregnancy or for prenatal care with or without treatment. Illness must be documented by a health care provider. Nurse practitioners and nurse-midwives are specifically listed as those who can document a health condition. Although not as generous a program as that of many other developed countries, unpaid leave helps appreciably with the care of an ill child or a woman who is ill during pregnancy.

Increasing the Number of Intensive Care Units

Over the past 20 years, care of infants and children has become extremely technical. It is generally assumed that newborns with a term birth weight (more than 2500 g or 5.5 lb) will thrive at birth. However, many infants are born each year with birth weights lower than 2500 g or who are ill at birth and do not thrive. Such infants are regularly transferred to a neonatal intensive care unit (NICU) or intensive care nursery (ICN). Children who are undergoing cardiac surgery or recovering from near-drownings or multi-injury accidents are cared for in a pediatric intensive care unit (PICU). Intensive care at this early point in life is one of the most costly types of hospitalization. Expenses of $1000 to $2000 a day, or $20,000 to $100,000 for a total hospital stay, are not unusual for care during a high-risk pregnancy or care for a high-risk infant. As the number of these settings increases, the opportunities for advanced-practice nurses also increase (Riendeau, 2007).

Regionalizing Intensive Care

To avoid duplication of care sites, communities establish centralized maternal or pediatric health services. Such planning creates one site that is properly staffed and equipped for potential problems rather than a number of less well-equipped sites. When a newborn, older child, or parent is hospitalized in a regional center, the family members who have been left behind need a great deal of support. They may feel they have "lost" their infant, child, or parent unless health care personnel keep them abreast of the ill family member's progress by means of telephone calls or snapshots and encourage the family to visit as soon as possible.

When regionalization concepts of newborn care were first introduced, transporting the ill or premature newborn to the regional care facility was the method of choice (Fig. 1.7). Today, if it is known in advance that a child may be born with a life-threatening condition, it may be safer to transport the mother to the regional center during pregnancy, because the uterus has advantages as a transport incubator that far exceed those of any commercial incubator yet designed.

An important argument against regionalization for pediatric care is that children will feel homesick in strange settings, overwhelmed by the number of sick children they see, and frightened because they are miles from home. An important argument against regionalization of maternal care is that being away from her community and support network places a great deal of stress on the pregnant woman and her family and limits her own physician's participation in her care. These are important considerations. Because nurses more than any other health care group set the tone for hospitals, they are responsible for ensuring that clients and families feel as welcome in a regional center as they would have been in a small hospital. Staffing should be adequate to allow sufficient

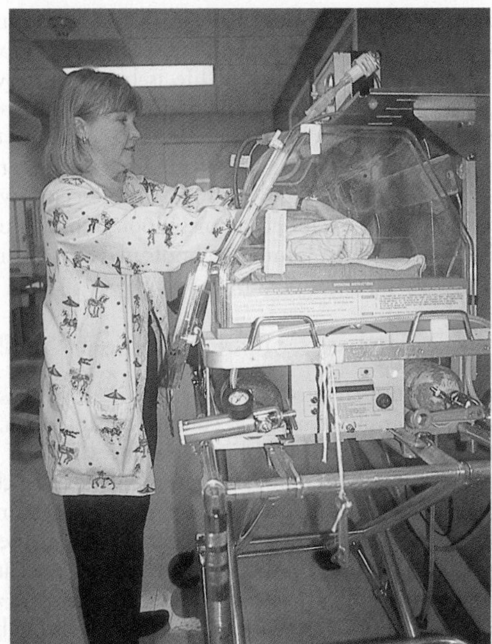

FIGURE 1.7 A nurse prepares an infant transport incubator to move a premature infant to a regional hospital. Helping with safe movement of pregnant women and ill newborns to regional centers is an important nursing responsibility. (© Caroline Brown, RNC, MS, DEd.)

time for nurses to comfort frightened children and prepare them for new experiences or to support the pregnant woman and her family. Documenting the importance of such actions allows them to be incorporated in critical pathways and preserves the importance of the nurse's role.

Increasing Comprehensive and Collaborative Care Settings

Comprehensive or collaborative health care is designed to meet all of a child's or woman's needs in one setting. In the past, a woman with a complication of pregnancy found herself visiting both an internist and an obstetrician for care. A child born with an illness such as myelomeningocele or cerebral palsy might have been followed by a corps of specialists such as a neurologist, a physical therapist, an occupational therapist, a psychologist for intelligence quotient testing, a speech therapist, an orthopedic surgeon, and, finally, a special education teacher. The parents might have needed to find a special dentist who accepts clients with multiple disabilities. Unfortunately, each specialist would look at only one area of the child's needs rather than the whole child's development. Without extra guidance, parents could find themselves lost in a maze of visits to different health care personnel. If they were not receiving financial support for their child's care, they may not have been able to afford all the necessary services at one time and had to make decisions as to which of their child's problems needed to be treated immediately and which could be left untreated without worsening and developing into a permanent disability. Although specialists are still important to care, a trusted primary care provider to help a family coordinate these specialized services is essential in today's managed care environment. In many settings, this primary care provider, who follows the woman or child through all phases of care, is an advanced-practice nurse such as a family nurse practitioner, pediatric nurse practitioner, or women's health nurse practitioner working in collaboration with a physician. Nurses can be helpful in seeing that both women and children become empowered to seek out a family-centered setting that will be best for their health.

Increasing Use of Alternative Treatment Modalities

There is a growing tendency for families to use alternative forms of therapy, such as acupuncture or therapeutic touch, in addition to, or instead of, traditional health care. Nurses have an increasing obligation to be aware of complementary or alternative therapies as these have the potential to either enhance or detract from the effectiveness of traditional therapy (Smith et al., 2007).

Health care providers who are unaware of the existence of some alternative forms of therapy may lose an important opportunity to capitalize on the positive features of that particular therapy. For instance, it would be important to know that an adolescent who is about to undergo a painful procedure is experienced at meditation, because asking the adolescent if she wants to meditate before the procedure could help her relax. Not only could this decrease the child's discomfort, but it could also offer her a feeling of control over a difficult situation. People are using an increasing number of herbal remedies, so asking about these at health assessment is important to prevent drug interactions. Ginger, for example, is frequently taken during pregnancy to relieve morning sickness (White, 2007).

Increasing Reliance on Home Care

Shortened hospital stays have resulted in the return home of many women and children before they are optimally ready to care for themselves. Ill children and women with complications of pregnancy may choose to remain at home for care rather than be hospitalized. This has created a "second system" of care requiring many additional care providers (Shepperd et al., 2009). Nurses are instrumental in assessing women and children on hospital discharge to help plan the best type of continuing care, devise and modify procedures for home care, and sustain clients' morale. Because home care is a unique and expanding area in maternal and child health nursing, it is discussed in Chapter 4.

Increasing Use of Technology

The use of technology is increasing in all health care settings. The field of assisted reproduction technology such as in vitro fertilization with the possibility of stem cell research is forging new pathways (Garrett & Yoder, 2007). Charting by computer, seeking information on the Internet, and monitoring fetal heart rates by Doppler ultrasound are other examples. In addition to learning these technologies, maternal and child health nurses must be able to explain their use and their advantages to clients. Otherwise, clients may find new technologies more frightening than helpful to them.

Freebirthing

Freebirthing refers to women giving birth without any health care provider supervision (Cooper & Clarke, 2008). Women may also refer to it as unassisted birth or couples birth. Using this technique, a woman may learn pregnancy care from sources including the Internet and then arrange to have her child at home in complete privacy or may invite family or friends to share the experience with her. Women choose an unassisted birth for a number of reasons:

- A belief that birth is a normal function of the female body and so does not require medical interventions and that some medical interventions have the potential to cause more harm than good.
- A belief that women are able to sense the natural flow of birth and so can recognize the optimal position or technique for birth if they are allowed to do this in an undisturbed birth setting.
- A belief that birth is a potentially orgasmic experience that will be experienced best with privacy.
- A belief that unassisted birth will increase the ability to bond with and take responsibility for her child.
- Lack of health insurance that makes home birth without health care supervision an economic advantage.
- Lack of information about patient rights in modern maternity units.

Freebirthing is potentially dangerous because if a complication of birth should occur, the woman may not recognize that the complication is occurring until damage to her child or herself results. Even after she recognizes that a problem is occurring, there is a space of time before emergency help can arrive to assist her. Freebirthing is particularly dangerous if a woman avoids prenatal care as well or depends solely on Internet information. Educating women that not all Internet information is reliable and that supervised birth does not mean that they have no choice in their care, such as whether they want pain relief or to use a special position for birth, are effective ways to help women make safer choices about birth.

Health Care Concerns and Attitudes

Health care made great strides in the past century. As we progress through the 21st century, there are likely to be even more changes as the United States actively works toward effective health goals and improved health care for all citizens. These steps can create new concerns.

Increasing Emphasis on Preventive Care

A generally accepted theory is that it is better to keep individuals well than to restore health after they have become ill. Counseling parents on ways to keep their homes safe for children is an important form of this type of prevention. Research supporting the facts that accidents are still a major cause of death in children and that women still do not receive preconceptual or prenatal care are testaments to the need for much more anticipatory guidance in maternal and child health.

Increasing Concern for the Quality of Life

In the past, health care of women and children was focused on maintaining physical health. Today, a growing awareness that quality of life is as important as physical health has expanded the scope of health care to include the assessment of psychosocial facets of life in such areas as self-esteem and independence. Good interviewing skills are necessary to elicit this information at health care visits. Nurses not only can help obtain such information but also can plan ways to improve quality of life in the areas the client considers most important.

One way in which quality of life is being improved for children with chronic illness is the national mandate to allow them to attend regular schools, guaranteeing entrance despite pregnancy, severe illness, or use of medical equipment such as a ventilator (Public Law 99-452). Adolescents who are pregnant cannot be excluded from school. School nurses or nurses asked to be consultants to schools play important roles in making these changes possible.

Increasing Awareness of the Individuality of Clients

Maternal and child clients today do not fit easily into any set mold. Varying family structures, cultural backgrounds, socioeconomic levels, and individual circumstances lead to unique and diverse clients (Jarvis, 2007). Some women having children are younger than ever before, and an increasing number of women are experiencing their first pregnancies after the age of 35 (Hamilton et al., 2007). About 38% of babies born are born to women outside of marriage. Gay and lesbian couples are also beginning to raise families, conceiving children through artificial insemination or adoption. As a result of advances in research and therapy, women who were once unable to have children, such as those with cystic fibrosis, are now able to manage a full-term pregnancy. Individuals with cognitive and physical challenges who once would have been isolated from childbearing are now able to establish families and rear children.

Many families who have emigrated from other countries enter the U.S. health care system for the first time during a pregnancy or with a sick child. This requires sensitivity to sociocultural aspects of care on the part of health care providers as people not used to non–government-sponsored health care can be easily lost in the U.S. system. They may have different cultural beliefs about health and illness than a health care provider. As the level of violence in the world increases, more and more families are exposed to living in violent communities. All of these concerns require increased nursing attention.

Empowerment of Health Care Consumers

In part because of the influence of market-driven care and a strengthened focus on health promotion and disease prevention, individuals and families have recently begun to take increased responsibility for their own health. This begins with learning preventive measures to stay well. For most families, this means following a more nutritious diet and planning regular exercise; for some families, this means adopting an entire new lifestyle. When a family member is ill, empowerment means learning more about the illness, participating in the treatment plan, and preventing the illness from returning. Parents want to stay with their ill child in the hospital. They are eager for information about their child's health and want to contribute to the decision-making process. They may question treatments or care plans that they believe are not in their child's best interest. If health care providers do not provide answers to a client's questions or are insensitive to needs, many health care consumers are willing to take their business to another health care setting or rely totally on alternative therapies.

Nurses can promote empowerment of parents and children by respecting their views and concerns, regarding parents as important participants in their own or their child's health, and keeping them informed and helping them to make decisions about care. Although a nurse may have seen 25 clients already in a particular day, he or she can make each client feel as important as the first by showing a warm manner and keen interest. Family Teaching displays are presented throughout this text to provide insight into ways in which nurses can help empower families.

What if... Melissa Chung demands that her 6-year-old, diagnosed with pneumonia, be hospitalized, even though it is your clinic's policy to have such children cared for at home by their parents? Would you advocate for hospitalization or not?

ADVANCED-PRACTICE ROLES FOR NURSES IN MATERNAL AND CHILD HEALTH

As trends in maternal and child health care change, so do the roles of maternal and child health nurses. In all settings, maternal and child health nurses function as caregivers, client advocates, researchers, case managers, and educators. Many nurses with a specified number of years of direct patient care, clinical expertise, and validated completion of pertinent continuing education programs are certified in a specialty. Those with advanced education function in advanced-practice roles.

Clinical Nurse Specialist

Clinical nurse specialists are nurses prepared at the master's or doctorate degree level who are capable of acting as consultants in their area of expertise, as well as serving as role models, researchers, and teachers of quality nursing care. Examples of areas of specialization are neonatal, maternal, child, and adolescent health care; genetics; childbirth education; and lactation consultation (McArthur & Flynn, 2008).

Consider the care necessary when a 4-year-old child with diabetes mellitus who has been admitted to the hospital becomes difficult to care for because he is both fearful of hospitalization and perplexed because his parents seem to be having such difficulty accepting his diagnosis. A clinical nurse specialist could be instrumental in helping a primary nurse organize care and in meeting with the parents to help them accept what is happening. Neonatal nurse specialists manage the care of infants at birth and in intensive care settings; they provide home follow-up care to ensure the newborn remains well. Childbirth educators teach families about normal birth and how to prepare for labor and birth. Lactation consultants educate women about breastfeeding and support them while they learn how to do this. **Genetic nurse counselors** consult with families about patterns of inheritance and offer support to families with a child who has inherited a genetic disorder.

Case Manager

A **case manager** is a graduate-level nurse who supervises a group of patients from the time they enter a health care setting until they are discharged from the setting or, in a seamless care system, into their homes as well, monitoring the effectiveness, cost, and satisfaction of their health care. They help prevent fragmentation of care and ensure that such important qualities as continuity of care and providing a feeling of "medical home" are included in care. Case management can be a vastly satisfying nursing role, because if the health care setting is "seamless," or one that follows people both during an illness and on their return to the community, it involves long-term contacts and lasting relationships and creates a high degree of satisfaction among clients (Hodnett, 2009).

Nurse Practitioner

Nurse practitioners are nurses educated at the master's or doctoral level. Recent advances in technology, research, and knowledge have amplified the need for longer and more in-depth education for nurse practitioners as they play pivotal roles in today's health care system. Doctor of nursing practice programs are designed to prepare nurse practitioners with the highest level of practice expertise integrated with the ability to translate scientific knowledge into complex clinical interventions. Preparing nurse practitioners at the doctor of nursing practice level has the potential to expand the scientific basis for practice as well as create leaders for organization and system management, quality improvement, health policy development, and interdisciplinary collaboration (Fain, Asselin, & McCurry, 2008).

Women's Health Nurse Practitioner

A women's health nurse practitioner has advanced study in the promotion of health and prevention of illness in women. Such a nurse plays a vital role in educating women about their bodies and sharing with them methods to prevent illness; in addition, they care for women with illnesses such as sexually transmitted infections, and offer information and counsel them about reproductive life planning. They play a large role in helping women remain well so that they can enter a pregnancy in good health and maintain their health throughout life.

Pediatric Nurse Practitioner

A pediatric nurse practitioner (PNP) is a nurse prepared with extensive skills in physical assessment, interviewing, and well-child counseling and care. In this role, a nurse interviews parents as part of an extensive health history and performs a physical assessment of the child (Fig. 1.8). If the

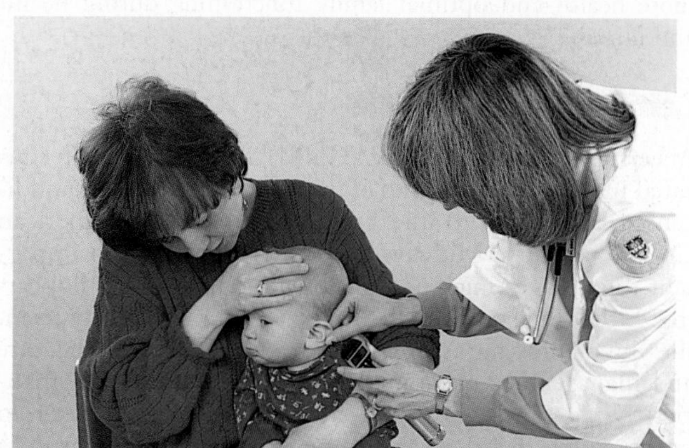

FIGURE 1.8 A pediatric nurse practitioner examines a 1-year-old child. (© Barbara Proud.)

nurse's diagnosis is that the child is well, he or she discusses with the parents any childrearing concerns mentioned in the interview, administers any immunizations needed, offers necessary anticipatory guidance (based on the plan of care), and arranges a return appointment for the next well-child checkup. The nurse has served as a primary health caregiver or as the sole health care person the parents and child see at that visit.

If the PNP determines that a child has a common illness (such as iron deficiency anemia), he or she orders the necessary laboratory tests and prescribes appropriate drugs for therapy. If the PNP determines that the child has a major illness (such as congenital subluxated hip, kidney disease, heart disease), he or she consults with an associated pediatrician; together, they decide what further care is necessary. Nurse practitioners may also work in inpatient or specialty settings such as genetics or cardiac care or emergency department settings providing continuity of care to children and adults (Percy & Sperhac, 2007). PNPs employed by schools provide care to all children in a given community or school setting.

Neonatal Nurse Practitioner

A neonatal nurse practitioner (NNP) is an advanced-practice role for nurses who are skilled in the care of newborns, both well and ill. NNPs may work in level 1, level 2, or level 3 newborn nurseries, neonatal follow-up clinics, or physician groups. The NNP's responsibilities include managing and caring for newborns in intensive care units, conducting normal newborn assessments and physical examinations, and providing high-risk follow-up discharge planning (Bowen, 2007). They also are responsible for transporting ill infants to these different care settings.

Family Nurse Practitioner

A family nurse practitioner (FNP) is an advanced-practice role that provides health care not only to women and children but also to the family as a whole. In conjunction with a physician, an FNP can provide prenatal care for a woman with an uncomplicated pregnancy. The FNP takes the health and pregnancy history, performs physical and obstetric examinations, orders appropriate diagnostic and laboratory tests, and plans continued care throughout the pregnancy and for the family afterward. FNPs then monitor the family indefinitely to promote health and optimal family functioning during health and illness.

Certified Nurse-Midwife

A **certified nurse-midwife** (CNM) is an individual educated in the two disciplines of nursing and midwifery and licensed according to the requirements of the American College of Nurse-Midwives (ACNM) who plays an important role in assisting women with pregnancy and childbearing. Either independently or in association with a physician, the nurse-midwife assumes full responsibility for the care and management of women with uncomplicated pregnancies. Nurse-midwives play a large role in making birth an unforgettable family event as well as helping to ensure a healthy outcome for both mother and child (Declercq, 2007) (Fig. 1.9).

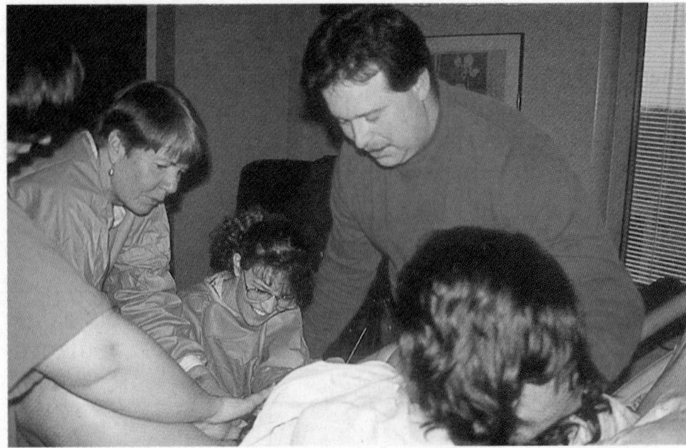

FIGURE 1.9 A certified nurse-midwife plays an important role in ensuring a safe and satisfying birth. (© Caroline Brown, RNC, MS, DEd.)

LEGAL CONSIDERATIONS OF MATERNAL-CHILD PRACTICE

Legal concerns arise in all areas of health care. Maternal and child health nursing carries some legal concerns that extend above and beyond other areas of nursing, because care is often given to an "unseen client"—the fetus—or to clients who are not of legal age for giving consent for medical procedures. In addition, labor and birth of a neonate are considered "normal" events, so the risks for a lawsuit are greater when problems arise (O'Grady et al., 2007). Nurses are legally responsible for protecting the rights of their clients, including confidentiality, and are accountable for the quality of their individual nursing care and that of other health care team members. New regulations on patient confidentiality guarantee that patients can see their medical record if they choose but health information must be kept confidential from others (DHHS, 2007). In a society in which child abuse is of national concern, all health care providers are becoming increasingly responsible for identifying and reporting incidents of suspected abuse in children (Newton & Vandeven, 2007).

Understanding the scope of practice and standards of care can help nurses practice within appropriate legal parameters.

Documentation is essential for protecting a nurse and justifying his or her actions. This concern is long-lasting, because children who feel they were wronged by health care personnel can bring a lawsuit at the time they reach legal age. This means that a nursing note written today may need to be defended as many as 21 years into the future. Nurses need to be conscientious about obtaining informed consent for invasive procedures and determining that pregnant women are aware of any risk to the fetus associated with a procedure or test. In divorced or blended families (those in which two adults with children from previous relationships now live together), it is important to establish who has the right to give consent for health care. Adolescents who support themselves or who are pregnant are termed "emancipated minors" or "mature minors" and have the right to sign for their own health care. Personal liability insurance is strongly recommended for all nurses, so that they do not incur great financial losses during a malpractice or professional negligence suit.

The specific legal ramifications of procedures or care are discussed in later chapters that describe procedures or treatment modalities. In some states, obstetric services are facing a crisis situation as more physicians and nurse-midwives find the cost of malpractice insurance to guard against "wrongful birth" is making their practice no longer profitable. A wrongful birth is the birth of a disabled child when the parents would have chosen to end the pregnancy if they had been informed about the disability during pregnancy. "Wrongful life" is a claim that negligent prenatal testing on the part of a health care provider resulted in the birth of an unperfect child. "Wrongful conception" denotes a contraceptive measure that failed, allowing an unwanted child to be conceived and born (O'Grady et al., 2007). Because many genetic disorders can be identified prenatally, the scopes of both "wrongful birth" and "wrongful life" grow yearly.

If a nurse knows that the care provided by another practitioner was inappropriate or insufficient, he or she is legally responsible for reporting the incident. Failure to do so can lead to a charge of negligence or breach of duty.

ETHICAL CONSIDERATIONS OF PRACTICE

Some of the most difficult ethical quandaries in health care today are those that involve children and their families. Examples are

- Conception issues, especially those related to in vitro fertilization, embryo transfer, ownership of frozen oocytes or sperm, cloning, stem cell research, and surrogate mothers
- Abortion, particularly partial-birth abortions
- Fetal rights versus rights of the mother
- Use of fetal tissue for research
- Resuscitation (for how long should it be continued?)
- Number of procedures or degree of pain that a child should be asked to endure to achieve a degree of better health
- Balance between modern technology and quality of life

Legal and ethical aspects of issues are often intertwined, which makes the decision-making process complex. Because maternal and child health nursing is so strongly family centered, it is common to encounter some situations in which the interests of one family member are in conflict with those of another. Maintaining privacy while aiding problem solving can be difficult (Recupero, 2008). It is not unusual for the values of a client not to match those of a health care provider. For example, if a pregnancy causes a woman to develop a serious illness, the family must make a decision either to terminate the pregnancy and lose the child or to keep the pregnancy and work to support the mother through the crisis. If the fetus is also at risk from the illness, the decision may be easier to make; however, the circumstances usually are not clear cut, and the decisions that need to be made are difficult. These and other issues are bound to emerge during the course of practice. Nurses can help clients who are facing such difficult decisions by providing factual information and supportive listening and helping the family clarify their values.

The Pregnant Woman's Bill of Rights and the United Nations Declaration of Rights of the Child (see Appendix A) provide guidelines for determining the rights of clients in regard to health care.

✔ Checkpoint Question 1.3

What is a legal implication pertinent to maternal and child health?

a. Informed consent is rarely needed as children are unable to understand this.
b. All adolescents over age 14 are able to sign consent for their own health care.
c. Children who feel they have been wronged can sue years into the future.
d. Pregnant women are not legally mandated to protect the health of their fetus.

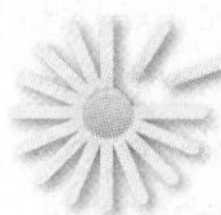

Key Points for Review

- Standards of maternal and child health nursing practice have been formulated by the American Nurses Association, the Society of Pediatric Nurses, and AWHONN to serve as guidelines for practice.
- Nursing research and use of evidence-based practice are methods by which maternal and child health nursing expands and improves.
- The most meaningful and important measure of maternal and child health is the infant mortality rate. It is the number of deaths among infants from birth to 1 year of age per 1000 live births. This rate is declining steadily, but in the United States it is still higher than in 32 other nations.
- Trends in maternal and child health nursing include changes in the settings of care, increased concern about health care costs, improved preventive care, and family-centered care.
- Advanced-practice roles in maternal and child health nursing include women's health, family, neonatal, and pediatric nurse practitioners; nurse-midwives; clinical nurse specialists; and case managers. All of these expanded roles contribute to make maternal and child health care an important area of nursing and health care.
- Maternal and child health care has both legal and ethical considerations and responsibilities over and above those in other areas of practice because of the role of the fetus and child.

CRITICAL THINKING EXERCISES

1. How might family-centered care help the Chung family, described in the beginning of the chapter? How can you explain recent changes in health care so that Melissa might understand why her hospital stay is so short? How can you empower the family so that they feel more in control of what is happening to them?
2. Mrs. Chung says she has trouble paying for health care. Some other countries in the world have a health care delivery system based not on profit but on provision of

care for all citizens through a tax-supported program. The infant mortality rate in many of these countries is lower than that in the United States. What are some reasons that might contribute to these lower rates?

3. The age at which women are having babies is increasing. For many women such as Melissa Chung, this age is now 35 years or older. How do you anticipate that this trend will change health care in the future? Are there special services that should be provided for such women? How will this trend influence childrearing in the future?
4. Examine the national health goals related to maternal, newborn, and child health. Most government-sponsored money for nursing research is allotted based on these goals. What would be a possible research topic to explore, pertinent to these goals, that would be applicable to the Chung family and could also advance evidence-based practice?

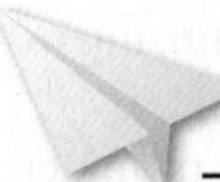

CRITICAL THINKING SCENARIO

Open the accompanying CD-ROM or visit http://thePoint.lww.com and read the Patient Scenario included for this chapter, then answer the questions to further sharpen your skills and grow more familiar with NCLEX types of questions related to trends in maternal and child health care. Confirm your answers are correct by reading the rationale for answers.

REFERENCES

American Academy of Pediatrics. (2009). *Recommendations for preventive pediatric health care.* Washington, DC: Author.

American Nurses Association and Society of Pediatric Nurses. (2003). *Scope and standards of pediatric clinical practice.* Washington, DC: Authors.

Association of Women's Health, Obstetric, and Neonatal Nurses. (1998). *Standards for the nursing care of women and newborns* (5th ed.). Washington, DC: Author.

Berman, S. (2007). Continuity, the medical home and retail-based clinics. *Pediatrics, 120*(5), 1123–1125.

Bowen, N. C. (2007). The role of the NNP in facilitating family-centered care. *Neonatal Network: The Journal of Neonatal Nursing, 26*(4), 271–272.

Callens, S., Volbragt, I., & Nys H. (2007). Legal thoughts on the implications of cost-reducing guidelines for the quality of health care. *Health Policy, 80*(3), 422–431.

Carpenito, L. J. (2007). *Handbook of nursing diagnosis* (12th ed.). Philadelphia: Lippincott Williams & Wilkins.

Centers for Disease Control and Prevention (CDC). (2007a). *Sudden infant death syndrome.* Atlanta, GA: Author.

Centers for Disease Control and Prevention (CDC). (2009). *Vaccine safety and adverse events.* Atlanta, Ga: Author.

Cooper, T., & Clarke, P. (2008). Freebirthing. Birthing alone: a concern for midwives? *Midwives, 11*(4), 34–35.

Declercq E. (2007). Trends in CNM-attended births. *Journal of Midwifery & Women's Health, 52*(1), 87–88.

Department of Health and Human Services, Office of Civil Rights. (2007). *Medical privacy—national standards to protect the privacy of personal health information: the Health Insurance Portability and Accountability Act.* Hyattsville, MD: Author.

Eldridge, R. I., & Sutton, P. D. (2009). Births, marriages, divorces, and deaths. *National Vital Statistics Reports, 59*(1), 1. Hyattsville, MD: National Center for Health Statistics.

Esposito, L., Hegyi, T., & Ostfeld, B. M. (2007). Educating parents about the risk factors of sudden infant death syndrome: the role of neonatal intensive care unit and well baby nursery nurses. *Journal of Perinatal and Neonatal Nursing, 21*(2), 158–164.

Fain, J. A., Asselin, M., & McCurry, M. (2008). The DNP ... why now? *Nursing Management, 39*(7), 34–37.

Foxcroft, R. R., & Cole, N. (2009). Organizational infrastructures to promote evidence based nursing practice. *Cochrane Database of Systematic Reviews, 2009*(1), (CD00212).

Fraser, A., et al. (2009). Drugs for preventing tuberculosis in people at risk of multiple-drug-resistant pulmonary tuberculosis. *Cochrane Database of Systematic Reviews, 2009*(1), (CD005435).

Garrett, D., & Yoder, L. H. (2007). Cancer: caring and conquering. An overview of stem cell transplant as a treatment for cancer. *MEDSURG Nursing, 16*(3), 183–190.

Hamilton, B. E., et al. (2007). Annual summary of vital statistics. *Pediatrics, 119*(2), 345–360.

Hempstead, K. (2007). The geography of self-injury: spatial patterns in attempted and completed suicide. *Social Science & Medicine, 62*(12), 3186–3196.

Hodnett, E. D. (2009). Continuity of caregivers for care during pregnancy and childbirth. *Cochrane Database of Systematic Reviews, 2009*(1), (CD000062).

Hussain, A., et al. (2007). Prevention of type 2 diabetes: a review. *Diabetes Research and Clinical Practice, 76*(3), 317–326.

Jarvis, J. (2007). The more things change: the pivotal role of nursing leadership in achieving cultural transformation. *Neonatal, Paediatric & Child Health Nursing, 10*(1), 3–4.

McArthur, L., & Flynn A. (2008). Evaluating the clinical nurse specialist role in child health. *Nursing Times, 104*(33), 28–29.

McKay, N. L., & Meng, X. (2007). The effect of managed care on hospitals' provision of uncompensated care. *Inquiry, 44*(1), 114–124.

Moher, M., Hey, K., & Lancaster, T. (2009). Workplace interventions for smoking cessation. *Cochrane Database of Systematic Reviews, 2009*(1), (CD003440).

Mullen, K., et al. (2007). Family-centered maternity care: one hospital's quest for excellence. *Nursing for Women's Health, 11*(3), 282–290.

National Vital Statistics Service. (2009a). *Trends in the health of Americans.* Hyattsville, MD: Author.

National Vital Statistics Service. (2009b). *Prevalence of overweight among children and adolescents: United States.* Hyattsville, MD: Author.

Nearns, J. (2009). Health insurance coverage and prescription contraceptive use among young women at risk for unintended pregnancy. *Contraception, 79*(2), 105–110.

Newton, A. W., & Vandeven, A. M. (2007). Update on child maltreatment. *Current Opinion in Pediatrics, 19*(2), 223–229.

O'Grady, J. P., et al. (2007). The borderland between law and medicine. In Fortner, K. B., et al. (Eds.). *The Johns Hopkins manual of gynecology and obstetrics.* Philadelphia: Lippincott Williams & Wilkins.

Paintsil, E., & Andiman, W. A. (2007). Care and management of the infant of the HIV-1-infected mother. *Seminars in Perinatology, 31*(2), 112–123.

Percy, M. S., & Sperhac, A. M. (2007). State regulations for the pediatric nurse practitioner in acute care. *Journal of Pediatric Health Care, 21*(1), 29–43.

Purswani, M. U., et al. (2007). A blinded survey of the seroprevalence of HIV-1 infection in an inner-city adolescent and young adult population attending a community hospital in the United States. *Journal of Adolescent Health, 40*(2), 182–184.

Recupero, P. R. (2008). Ethics of medical records and professional communications. *Child & Adolescent Psychiatric Clinics of North America, 17*(1), 37–51.

Riendeau, D. (2007). Advanced practice: where are you going and how do you get there? *Imprint, 54*(1), 50–57.

Rubin, R. (1963). Maternal touch. *Nursing Outlook, 11*(2), 828–829.

Sahni, R., Fifer, W. P., & Myers, M. M. (2007). Identifying infants at risk for sudden infant death syndrome. *Current Opinion in Pediatrics, 19*(2), 145–149.

Shepperd, S., et al. (2009). Discharge planning from hospital to home. *Cochrane Database of Systematic Reviews, 2009*(1), (CD000313).

Smith, C. A., et al. (2009). Complementary and alternative therapies for pain management in labour. *Cochrane Database of Systematic Reviews, 2009*(1), (CD003521).

Summerbell, C. D., et al. (2009). Interventions for treating obesity in children. *Cochrane Database of Systematic Reviews, 2009*(1), (CD001872).

United Nations Statistics Division. (2000). *The world's women 2000: trends and statistics.* New York: Author.

U.S. Department of Health and Human Services. Available online at http://www.nih.gov.

U.S. Department of Labor. (1995). Family and Medical Leave Act. *Federal Register, 60*(4), 2179.

U.S. Preventive Services Task Force. (2005). *Strength of recommendations and quality of evidence. Guide to clinical preventive services* (3rd ed.). Rockville, MD: Author.

Vonderheid, S. C., Norr, K. F., & Handler, A. S. (2007). Prenatal health promotion content and health behaviors. *Western Journal of Nursing Research, 29*(3), 258–276.

White, B. (2007). Ginger: an overview. *American Family Physician, 75*(11), 1689–1691.

SUGGESTED READINGS

Bell, A. F. (2007). Nurse-midwife and scientist: stuck in the middle? *JOGNN: Journal of Obstetric, Gynecologic, and Neonatal Nursing, 36*(1), 71–73.

Callister, L. C. (2007). How much does the world value children? *MCN, American Journal of Maternal Child Nursing, 32*(2), 124.

Cheng, C., Fowles, E. R., & Walker, L. O. (2007). Postpartum maternal health care in the United States: a critical review. *Journal of Perinatal Education, 15*(3), 34–42.

Currell, R., & Urquhart, C. (2009). Nursing record systems effects on nursing practice and health care outcomes. *Cochrane Database of Systematic Reviews, 2009*(1), (CD002099).

Haidar, E. (2007). Role of the advanced nurse practitioner in prescribing and general practice. *Nurse Prescribing, 5*(2), 74–78.

Mitchell, J. M., & Gaskin, D. J. (2007). Caregivers' ratings of access: do children with special health care needs fare better under fee-for-service or partially capitated managed care? *Medical Care, 45*(2), 146–153.

Partin, B. (2007). A new vision of advanced practice nursing. *Nurse Practitioner, 32*(7), 9.

Thompson, L. (2008). The role of nursing in governmentality, biopower and population health: family health nursing. *Health & Place, 14*(1), 76–84.

Tylee, A., et al. (2007). Youth-friendly primary-care services: how are we doing and what more needs to be done? *Lancet, 369*(9572), 1565–1573.

Wilkinson, S., & Walker, A. (2007). Healthy Start: improving maternal, infant and child health. *Nursing Standard, 21*(20), 48–56.

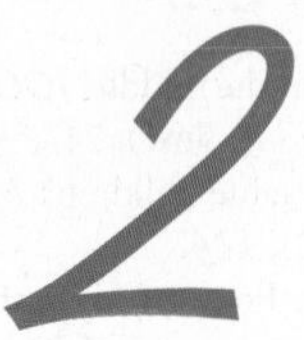

Chapter 2 Sociocultural Aspects of Maternal and Child Health Nursing

KEY TERMS

- acculturation
- assimilation
- cultural values
- culture
- discrimination
- diversity
- ethnicity
- ethnocentrism
- minority
- mores
- norms
- prejudice
- stereotyping
- taboos
- transcultural nursing

OBJECTIVES

After mastering the contents of this chapter, you should be able to:

1. Describe ways that sociocultural influences affect maternal and child health nursing.
2. Identify National Health Goals related to sociocultural considerations that nurses can help the nation achieve.
3. Use critical thinking to analyze how sociocultural aspects of care affect family functioning and health and develop ways to make nursing care more family centered.
4. Assess a family for sociocultural influences that might influence the way it responds to childbearing and childrearing.
5. Formulate nursing diagnoses related to culturally influenced aspects of nursing care.
6. Develop outcomes to assist families who have specific cultural needs to thrive in their community.
7. Plan nursing care that respects the sociocultural needs and wishes of families.
8. Implement nursing care to assist a family adapt to today's changing sociocultural environment.
9. Evaluate expected outcomes for achievement and effectiveness of care.
10. Identify areas of care related to sociocultural considerations that could benefit from additional nursing research or application of evidence-based practice.
11. Integrate sociocultural aspects of care with nursing process to achieve quality maternal and child health nursing care.

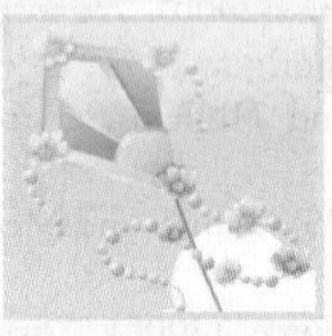

Maria Rodriques is a 12-year-old who is hospitalized for surgical repair of a broken tibia. She has a cast on her leg and will be on bed rest for 3 days, then allowed to learn crutch walking.

In planning care for Maria, you assume that because her culture is Hispanic, her family orientation will be male-dominant, her time focus will be on the present, and her nutrition preferences will be Mexican American. Based on this, you consult with Maria's father regarding the major aspects of her care. You concentrate on talking mainly about her current problem (bed rest) rather than her return to school. You caution her to avoid milk, because lactase deficiency is present in many Mexican Americans.

You are surprised on the second day of Maria's hospital stay to hear her say that she feels "second class." No one asks her for input in her care; she'd like some milk to drink and doesn't feel bed rest is a problem but is concerned that she won't be able to play soccer by next month.

The previous chapter described the standards and philosophy of maternal and child health nursing. This chapter adds information on caring for families from diverse cultures.

What went wrong with Maria's care? What would have been a better approach for determining this child's cultural preferences?

Culture is a view of the world and a set of traditions that a specific social group uses and transmits to the next generation. **Cultural values** are preferred ways of acting based on those traditions. **Ethnicity** refers to the cultural group into which a person was born, although the term is sometimes used in a narrower context to mean only race. *Race* refers to a category of people who share a socially recognized physical characteristic. The term is rarely used today as the research on the human genome shows no basic differences in structure among people.

Assessing sociocultural status, ethnicity, and cultural beliefs of families and clients can reveal why people take the type of preventive health measures that they do or seek a particular type of care for illness, because the way people react to health care is a cultural value (Crombleholme, 2009).

Cultural values differ from nation to nation because they often arise from environmental conditions (in a country where water is scarce, daily bathing is not valued; in a country where meat is scarce, ethnic recipes use little meat). The usual values of a group are termed **mores** or **norms.** Expecting women to come for prenatal care and parents to bring children for immunizations are examples of norms in the United States, but these are not beliefs worldwide (Niederhauser & Markowitz, 2007). Actions that are not acceptable to a culture are called **taboos.** Three taboos that are universal are murder, incest, and cannibalism. Issues such as abortion, robbery, and lying are controversial because these are taboos only to some people, not to everyone.

Cultural values are formed early in life and strongly influence the manner in which people plan for childbearing and childrearing, as well as the way they respond to health and illness (Whitley & Kirmayer, 2008). In a culture in which men are the authority figures, for example, it might be the father rather than the mother who expects to answer questions about an ill child at a health care visit. If you are from a culture in which women usually provide all child care, and were not aware of this family's norms, you might direct your questions to the wrong parent during a health interview. The way people respond to pain is heavily culturally influenced. If you believe that stoic behavior is the "proper" response to pain, and were unaware that there are cultural differences, you might be impatient with a woman who has been raised to believe that expressing discomfort during childbirth is "proper." When doing research, nurses need to be mindful to include all cultural groups in research samples, so that more can be learned about cultural preferences in relation to nursing interventions and care (Abuidhail & Fleming, 2007).

Cultural differences occur not only across different ethnic backgrounds but also different lifestyle behaviors such as drinking alcohol or smoking cigarettes (Angstman et al., 2007). Adolescents, urban youth, the hearing-challenged, and gay or lesbian couples have separate cultures from the mainstream, and respecting these cultures is just as important as respecting ethnic differences. A parent who has been deaf since birth, for example, expects her deaf culture to be respected by having health care professionals locate a sign language interpreter for her while she is in labor. A mother who is lesbian at a well-child visit would appreciate being asked, "Is your partner here?" rather than, "Is your husband here?"

Differing cultural values can be a major source of conflict between parents and children as children see opposing values in friends and school peers. Nurses can be instrumental in helping relieve this type of conflict by always including a cultural assessment at a health care visit (Gound et al., 2007).

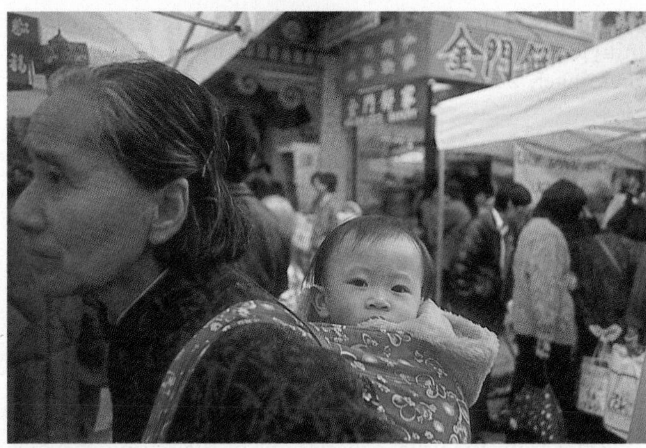

FIGURE 2.1 Various cultural preferences are evident in childrearing. In some cultures, extended family members such as grandparents are the primary caregivers. (© Kathy Sloane.)

Diversity means there is a mixture or variety of lifestyles and beliefs in a population (Fig. 2.1). The United States is a country of such varied cultural groups and socioeconomic conditions that you are likely to see a wide range of behaviors exhibited in any health care setting. National Health Goals in reference to cultural influences are shown in Box 2.1.

BOX 2.1 ✻ Focus on National Health Goals

Several National Health Goals are concerned with health practices that may be influenced by cultural factors:

- Increase the proportion of pregnant women who receive early and adequate prenatal care from a baseline of 74% to a target of 90%.
- Increase the proportion of mothers who breastfeed their babies in the early postpartum period from a baseline of 64% to a target of 75%, and increase the number to at least 60% (from a baseline of 43%) the proportion of mothers who breastfeed exclusively through 3 months.
- Increase the proportion of healthy full-term infants who are put down to sleep on their backs from a baseline of 35% to a target of 70%.
- Increase the proportion of young children who receive all vaccines that have been recommended for universal administration from a baseline of 73% to a target of 80% (http://www.nih.gov).

Nurses can help the nation achieve these goals by helping design prenatal and child care services that take into account cultural diversity and by promoting the nutritional and immunologic advantages of breastfeeding in a culturally sensitive manner. Additional nursing research is needed on ways to make prenatal care and child health services more appealing to culturally diverse populations and on the educational methods that best reach people who may not be proficient in English.

Nursing care that is guided by cultural aspects and respects individual differences is termed **transcultural nursing** (Leininger, 2007).

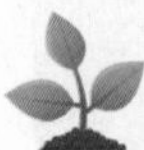

Nursing Process Overview

For Respecting Sociocultural Aspects of Care

Assessment

Assessment of sociocultural factors is important to be certain that care is planned based not on predetermined assumptions but on the actual preferences of a family. To do this, assess each client individually, not as one of a group. Note particularly any cultural characteristics that differ from the usual expectations of the setting in which care is being provided so that potential conflicts can be acknowledged and culturally competent care can be planned. Learn as much as you can about different cultures by reading about or talking to members of as many different ethnic groups as possible. Specific areas to assess, along with important findings in these areas, are shown in Table 2.1.

Assessing the culture of a community is as important as assessing individual families because families are intrinsically joined to their community. An important area to assess is whether the family matches the dominant culture in their community. This can be important because the type of foods stocked in supermarkets, the type of entertainment events that are available, and the values and history that are stressed in schools and work settings are all influenced by the dominant culture.

Communities age, the same as families. When homes are first built, many families tend to be young adults with children. Over the years, these families "settle in" to middle age and later the homes are filled with families at retirement. Older adults may find it difficult to relate if they move into a "young" community. A family who moves into a retirement-age community with young children may feel equally out of place. In all instances, a family that is of a culture other than the dominant one may have strong ties within the family but may have difficulty making strong, effective relationships in the community; this causes it to be more isolated than it would like to be. The importance of community assessment is further discussed in Chapter 4.

Nursing Diagnosis

Several nursing diagnoses speak to the consequences of ignoring cultural preferences in care:

- Powerlessness related to expectations of care not being respected
- Powerlessness related to sociocultural isolation
- Impaired verbal communication related to limited English proficiency
- Nutrition, less than body requirements, related to unmet cultural food preferences
- Anxiety related to a cultural preference for not bathing while ill
- Fear related to possible discrimination related to ethnicity

Outcome Identification and Planning

Planning needs to be very specific for individual families because sociocultural preferences tend to be very personal. Care may begin with in-service education for health care providers who are unfamiliar with a particular cultural practice and its importance to the specific family involved. The plan of care may include arranging for variations in policy, such as the length of family visiting hours, types of food served, or type of child care provided. Such planning is beneficial not only because it can make health care more acceptable to a child or family but also because it can motivate providers to examine policies, question the rationale

TABLE 2.1 ✻ Assessing for Cultural Values

Area of Assessment	Questions to Ask or Observations to Make
Ethnicity	What is the family's cultural preference?
Communication	What is the main language used in the home?
Touch	Do the family members typically touch each other? Do they use intimate or conversational space?
Time	Is being on time important? Is planning for the future important?
Occupation	Is work important to the family? Do they plan leisure time or leave it unstructured?
Pain	Does the family express pain or remain stoic when faced with it? What do they believe relieves pain best?
Family structure	Is the family nuclear? Extended? Single-parent? Are family roles clear? Can an individual name a family member he or she would call on for support in a crisis?
Male and female roles	Is the family male or female dominant?
Religion	What is the family's religion? Do they actively practice their religion?
Health beliefs	What does the family believe about health? What do they believe causes illness? Makes illness better? Do they use alternative therapies or traditional medical practices?
Nutrition	Does the family eat mainly ethnic foods? Are the foods they enjoy available in their community?
Community	Is the predominant culture in the community the same as the family's? Can they name a neighbor they could call on in a crisis?

behind them, and initiate more diverse care. Reputable websites to use for additional information on the importance of diversity are the National Association of Hispanic Nurses (http://www.the hispanicnurses.org), the National Black Nurses Association (http://www.nbna.org), and the Transcultural Nursing Society (http://www.tcns.org).

Implementation

Appreciate that cultural values are usually unchangeable. An example of implementing care might be to make arrangements for a new Native American mother to take home the placenta after birth of her child if that is important to her or planning home care for a Chinese American child whose family believes in herbal medicine. It might be to establish a network of health care agency personnel or personnel from a nearby university or importing firm to serve as interpreters. It might be to educate a child, family, or community about the reason for a hospital practice. There may be situations in which the health care provider or agency is unable to adapt to the particular cultural situation. This may call for both sides to adjust (cultural negotiation).

Outcome Evaluation

Assessing whether expected outcomes have been met should reveal that a family's sociocultural preferences were considered and respected during care. If this was not achieved, procedures may need to be modified until this can be realized. Examples of expected outcomes that might be established include:

- Parents list three ways they are attempting to preserve cultural traditions in their children.
- Child states she no longer feels socially isolated because of cultural differences.
- Family members state they have learned to substitute easily purchased foods for traditional foods unavailable in local stores to obtain adequate nutrition.
- Child with severe hearing impairment writes that he feels communication with ambulatory care staff has been adequate.

SOCIOCULTURAL DIFFERENCES AND IMPLICATIONS FOR DIVERSITY IN MATERNAL AND CHILD HEALTH NURSING

Given the cultural mix in the world today, almost any behavior can be considered appropriate for some individuals at some time and place. **Stereotyping** means expecting a person to act in a characteristic way without regard to his or her individual traits. It is generally derogatory in nature. Statements such as, "Men never diaper babies well" or "Japanese women are never assertive," are examples of stereotyping. Stereotyping occurs largely because of lack of exposure to enough people in a particular group and, consequently, a lack of understanding of the wide range of differences among people. In these examples, the first statement, having seen one man change diapers poorly, assumes that this represents the entire male population. The second example demonstrates lack of knowledge of a changing culture. Stereotyping can interfere with effective care because it can prevent you from planning care that is accurate, individualized, and valued (Box 2.2).

On the other hand, it is important not to ignore cultural characteristics in an attempt to not stereotype, because most people take pride in their cultural heritage. It is possible to acknowledge and celebrate a client's culture without stereotyping by admiring the way in which he or she expresses cultural characteristics, such as appreciating the ways a woman cooks an ethnic meal once a week to remind her family of their ethnic roots.

Women are often called the "keepers of the culture" or the people most influential in passing on cultural traditions from one generation to another. Respecting sociocultural values in this way is particularly important in maternal and child health care, because childbearing and childrearing are times in life that are surrounded by many cultural traditions (Andrews & Boyle, 2007).

In the past, the United States was viewed as a giant cultural "melting pot," where all new arrivals gave up their native country's traditions and values and became "Americans." **Acculturation** refers to the loss of ethnic traditions in this

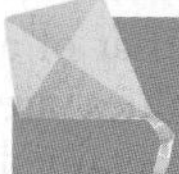

BOX 2.2 ✻ Focus on Evidence-Based Practice

Do children's stereotypes about obesity differ across cultures?

Stereotyping behavior can be evident in children as early as 3 years of age. Because children in mainland China see less obvious obesity than do children in the United States, it follows that U.S. children might show more bias or stereotyping of obese children than those living in China.

To investigate this question, researchers recruited 60 Caucasian children 7 years or 10 years of age from Virginia or Colorado and 61 children of the same ages from Guilin, China. Children were shown eight bottles of supposedly new drinks and asked to sample them for taste. Each bottle actually held identical fluid but the color of the fluid and the labels on the bottles were each different. The labels included a child's photograph and an explanation that the child pictured had created that flavor of drink. When asked afterward which drink tasted worst or was most apt to make them ill, both Chinese and American children most often chose the bottle of drink with an obese child pictured on the label. Chinese children reported consistent findings between age groups; the older group of Caucasian children were even more opposed to the drink created by the obese child than the younger group, or their bias against obese children increased with age.

Would the results of this study influence the way you plan care for obese children?

Source: Klaczynski, P. A. (2008). There's something about obesity: culture, contagion, rationality, and children's responses to drinks "created" by obese children. *Journal of Experimental Child Psychology, 99*(1), 58–74.

way. Cultural **assimilation** means that people have adopted the values of the dominant culture.

In the past, many Americans were intolerant of any behavior that was not like that of middle-class Americans, because they believed that the American way (which actually was the northern European way) was the "best" way. This belief that one's own culture is superior to all others is referred to as **ethnocentrism.**

Ethnocentrism can lead to **prejudice** (believing that some people are less than others based on their physical or cultural traits) because the feelings and ways of other cultures cannot be understood or appreciated without the philosophy that the world is large enough to accommodate a diversity of ideas and behaviors and that there is probably no "best" way to accomplish anything. **Discrimination** is the act of treating people differently based on their physical or cultural traits. Traditionally, people whose culture differs most drastically from the dominant culture suffer the greatest amount of rejection, because they are least able to assimilate. Over years of familiarity, mutual cultural assimilation does occur. As an example, when many Italians moved into American communities in the early 1900s, the average Italian family learned to speak English and the average American family learned to cook spaghetti with Italian sauce.

Today, many people question the idea that America ever was a melting pot; instead, the preferred concept is that of a "salad bowl," in which cultural traditions and values are tossed together but with all their crispness and flavor retained to make a perfect mix. Retaining ethnic traditions strengthens and enriches family life. It provides security to younger family members to realize that they are one of a continuing line of people who have a past and will have a future (Fig. 2.2, Box 2.3).

Cultural competence, or respecting cultural differences, allows you to plan culturally competent care and the integration of cultural elements into care, a goal worth achieving (Schim et al., 2007). Numerous levels of cultural intolerance or acceptance continue to persist, however, because many people continue to hold different beliefs along a cultural competence continuum (Fig. 2.3).

As a nurse, you will have the opportunity to meet many people who hold cultural values different from your own. When planning nursing care, try to not only respect people's cultural differences but also help people share their cultural beliefs with health care providers so that their beliefs can be considered and respected.

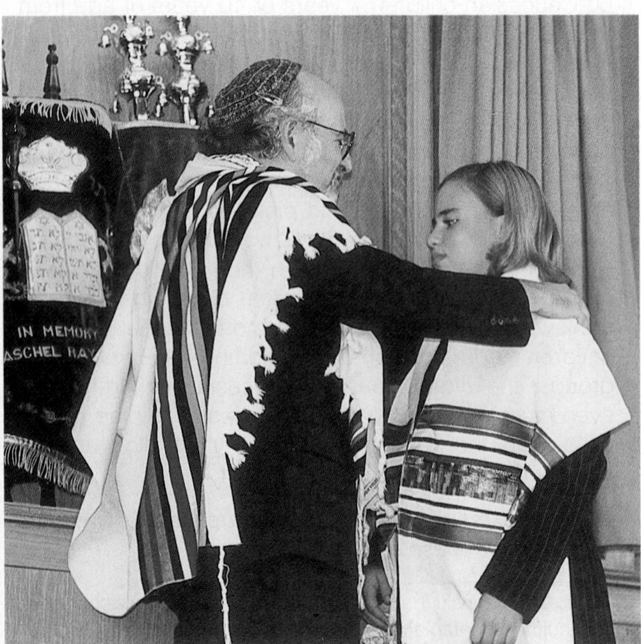

FIGURE 2.2 Cultural traditions offer a sense of security to children. (© Caroline Brown, RNC, MS, DEd.)

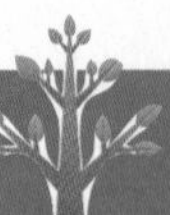

BOX 2.3 * Focus on Family Teaching

Preserving Cultural Heritage

Q. Mrs. Rodriques says, "I'm proud of my family's ethnic traditions. How can I help my family preserve these?"

A. Preserving your individual heritage when living in another culture calls for creative planning. Some common suggestions for doing this are as follows:

- Plan an "ethnic night" once a week when only ethnic food is served. Encourage children to invite friends for the meal and discuss the traditions behind the various foods.
- If a foreign language is part of your traditions, reserve one night a week when family members speak only the native language so they will value two languages.
- Choose books for children that are written by authors from your culture or that advantageously describe your culture. Read them together as a family.
- Monitor television for programs that focus positively on your culture. Watch them with your children.
- As bedtime stories or "talk time," talk to your children about your childhood and traditions and values so they can appreciate how long these values have been revered by your family.
- Celebrate holidays in your traditional manner. Including cultural influences in holiday celebrations adds a rich ingredient and feeling of security to these occasions.

✔ Checkpoint Question 2.1

While she is in the hospital, Maria Rodriques makes the following statements. Which is the best example of stereotyping?

a. My doctor is funny; he tells jokes and makes me laugh.
b. I'm glad I'm Mexican because all Mexicans are smart.
c. I'm sure my leg will heal quickly; I'm always healthy.
d. I like Mexican food, although not if it tastes too spicy.

Sociocultural Assessment

Almost all nations have a set of people who are its dominant or advantaged group. They hold the greater share of wealth in the nation and hold the majority of political offices. Almost all nations also have **minority** or disadvantaged groups—groups not necessarily fewer in number but who

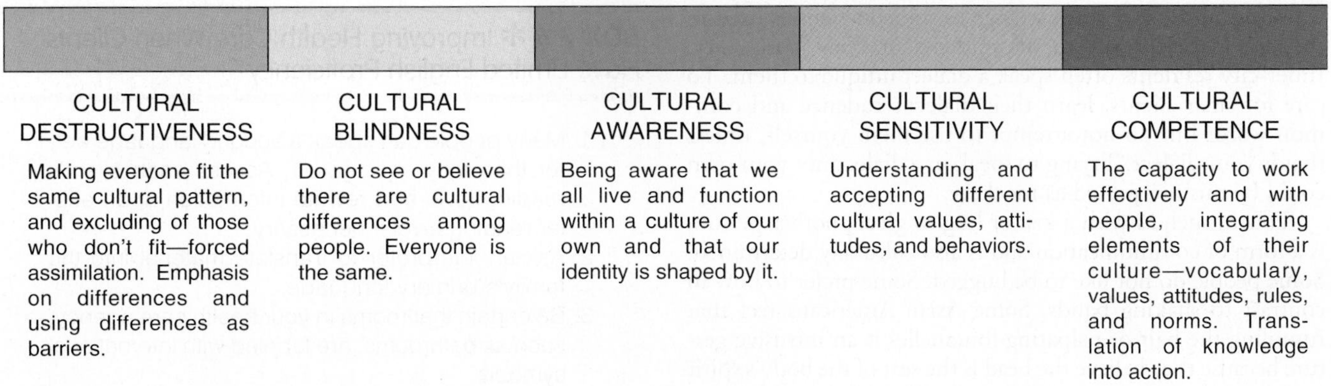

CULTURAL DESTRUCTIVENESS	CULTURAL BLINDNESS	CULTURAL AWARENESS	CULTURAL SENSITIVITY	CULTURAL COMPETENCE
Making everyone fit the same cultural pattern, and excluding of those who don't fit—forced assimilation. Emphasis on differences and using differences as barriers.	Do not see or believe there are cultural differences among people. Everyone is the same.	Being aware that we all live and function within a culture of our own and that our identity is shaped by it.	Understanding and accepting different cultural values, attitudes, and behaviors.	The capacity to work effectively and with people, integrating elements of their culture—vocabulary, values, attitudes, rules, and norms. Translation of knowledge into action.

FIGURE 2.3 Cultural competence continuum. (Courtesy of the National Council of La Raza.)

hold less power and wealth. When assessing families regarding whether there are socioeconomic or cultural influences that will make special considerations of care necessary, several categories of information related to the structure (composition) and function (roles and actions) of a family can be examined.

Communication Patterns

Communication patterns (not only what people say but also how they say it) are culturally determined. People whose primary language is not English can have great difficulty detailing a health history in English to a health care provider. Language barriers can be particularly significant for people who must give health histories when they or their child is ill, because their ability to cope and express themselves in any language when they are stressed may be at a low point (Darby, 2007). Even if people are able to converse well in English in social situations, they may not be able to give a health history as well as they would like because they cannot recall the English words for symptoms such as nausea or dizziness, words not commonly taught in English as a second language class. Unless you appear receptive, this person might omit mentioning a symptom rather than try to pantomime it or describe it in a different way. Listening to English instructions and translating them into another language can also cause confusion. The statement, "I need you to wait," for example, is easy to translate as "I need your weight." The word "hallmark" translates as "mark on the hall," or graffiti.

Children who are embarrassed or bashful about speaking another language may simply not talk, so their needs may go unmet. As a general rule, it is unfair to ask children to interpret for their parents. If a child is frequently asked to interpret for his or her parents, the child may be forced to miss days of school. Translating also can place a child in situations that require adult judgment and knowledge. In some cultures, it might be unacceptable for a younger person to serve as an interpreter for an older person, because this shifts authority.

The terms "Hispanic" and "Latina" or "Latino" refer to people who identify with a Spanish culture. There are about 18 million documented persons of Mexican, Puerto Rican, Cuban, or other Spanish-speaking origin in the United States. When added to the number of Spanish-speaking people who are undocumented or living illegally in the country, this group numbers close to 44 million, or about 14.8% of the total U.S. population (U.S. Census Bureau, 2009). Health care providers and Hispanic communities are encouraged to work together to bridge communication gaps by helping both community members who are not English proficient to learn more English and health care providers who are not Spanish proficient to learn to communicate better in Spanish. The type of health care provider that people choose is yet another trait that is not uniform across cultures. For some Hispanics, turning to a *yerbero* or *curandero* is preferable to professional health care because these people may not charge a fee but accept a donation or an exchange of goods or services. Also, relating health problems to them is not difficult because there is no language problem. Box 2.4 explains these terms.

Communication problems arise not only from foreign languages but also from dialects within a country. Something as simple as a New Englander adding an "r" sound to the end of words (saying "idear" instead of "idea") may make an explanation difficult to follow. The slow cadence of a person

BOX 2.4 ✻ English–Spanish Communication

Common Terms to Describe Hispanic Health Care Providers

brujo: Person who can not only revoke evil spells but also turn them around onto others

curandero: Person who heals by the use of herbs or diet

el que sabe ("the one who knows"): Trusted family member to whom family members turn to first for consultation and approval to seek therapy

espiritualisto: Person who can treat supernaturally caused illnesses

el enfermero or *la enfermera:* Nurse

médico or *médica:* Doctor

partera: Midwife who cares for women during pregnancy and birth

yerbero (herbalist): Person outside the family structure who grows herbs and instructs people in the use of herbs or cures

from the South may seem strange to someone who is used to the rapid speech pattern of residents of New York City. Inner-city residents often speak a dialect unique to them. To care for such clients, learn their dialect's cadence and common words but do not attempt to use them yourself, unless that is your dialect. Trying to speak in a dialect not your own could be misinterpreted as mockery.

Touch, such as with a kiss or hug to greet another person, is a form of communication and is also culturally determined. Some people do not like to be hugged. Some prefer to bow in contrast to shaking hands. Some Asian Americans feel that rumpling the hair or palpating fontanelles is an intrusive gesture because they believe the head is the seat of the body's spirit and should not be touched (Giger & Davidhizar, 2008).

Whether people look at one another when talking is also culturally determined. Chinese Americans, for example, may not make eye contact during a conversation. This social custom shows respect for the position of the health care professional and is a compliment, not an avoidance issue.

Cultural variations such as these should be respected in written as well as oral communications. In many instances, written communication is even more problematic than oral communication: many people can speak a second language but cannot write or read it. Using short, easy sentences and being certain not to use words with double meanings are important techniques (Boxes 2.5 and 2.6).

BOX 2.5 * Focus on Communication

Anna Rodriques brings her 4-year-old son, Pedro, to your pediatric clinic because she thinks he has an ear infection. She has brought a neighbor as an interpreter.

Less Effective Communication

Nurse: What's the reason you're here today?
Neighbor: She thinks her son has an ear infection.
Nurse: Is he pulling or tugging at it?
Neighbor: Not that I've seen.
Nurse: Does he have any pain?
Neighbor: She hasn't said anything about that.
Nurse: Well, I'll take his temperature, but I doubt it's an infection.

More Effective Communication

Nurse: What's the reason you're here today?
Neighbor: She thinks her son has an ear infection.
Nurse: Ask if he has been pulling or tugging at it.
Neighbor: I haven't seen him doing that.
Nurse: Would you ask if his mother has?

[The neighbor addresses Anna and then reports back.]

Neighbor: She says he's been pulling at it all morning.
Nurse: Ask Pedro if he has any pain.

[The neighbor addresses the child and then reports back.]

Neighbor: He says yes.
Nurse: Those are symptoms of an ear infection, all right.

Effectively using an interpreter adds additional responsibility to history taking. The nurse in the first scenario asked her first question of the mother but then directed all other questions to the interpreter. This means she secured a secondary history. When using an interpreter, be certain that the interpreter is "interpreting," not giving the history.

BOX 2.6 * Improving Health Care When Clients Have Limited English Proficiency

1. Many people can speak a second language better than they can read it. Assess each client's reading level and rewrite information at an easier reading level if necessary.
2. Ask an interpreter to translate material into the family's primary language.
3. Be certain that rooms in your health care agency, such as bathrooms, are labeled with international symbols.
4. Learn a few phrases, such as "Good morning" or "This won't hurt," from other languages, and use them in interactions with clients.
5. Use hand gestures or draw a figure, if need be, to communicate better. Imparting health information is what is important for safe care, not worrying how you look.
6. When using an interpreter, do not ignore the person seeking health care in preference to the interpreter. Observe their facial expressions for confirmation that they understand instructions. Use short sentences; avoid slang words that do not interpret cleanly.

Use of Conversational Space

People of different cultures use the space around them differently. In the Western world, physical examinations are conducted in a very tight (intimate) space, because palpation is a part of the examination. Conversation, on the other hand, is usually held at a distance of between 18 inches and 4 feet. Business is most often conducted at a 4-foot distance, as that allows room for a desk between parties. Any space beyond that, such as shouting across a parking lot, is public space. Use of the Internet or telephone can vary from private space ("I have a secret to tell you") to public space (conversation in a chat room). Everyone has had the uncomfortable experience of speaking to someone who moves closer to them than they expected or invades their intimate space while talking to them. Likewise, everyone has had someone shout something they wanted to be kept confidential (violation of public space). Being aware that use of space is culturally determined and can vary from person to person helps you to respect the use of space for clients.

Respect for modesty is a way to respect close space. Be aware that women from Middle Eastern cultures adhere to a level of modesty exceeding what you may be used to.

Time Orientation

The cultural pattern in the United States is geared toward punctuality regarding appointments. "Time is money" is an often-quoted axiom. Other cultures, however, may not have this concern for time. They may have, instead, a concept that time is to be enjoyed. For such a person, there is no such thing as wasted time. In some South Asian cultures, being late for appointments is a sign of respect (giving the person you are meeting time to organize and be prepared for your arrival). Women who do not have a strict time orientation may view the hospital's practice of feeding infants at designated times such as 10 AM or 2 PM as strange. People who are not accustomed to adhering to schedules in this way may have difficulty following a strict medical regimen. If they are told, for example, to give a child a medication at 8 AM, noon, and 6 PM daily and to return for another appointment at 2 PM in a week's time, you may have to stress that the medication should be taken three times a day, not necessarily at the specific times. Also stating that returning for a checkup at a set time is important because their physician is only in the health care facility at that time is also helpful.

Another way that time orientation differs is in whether a culture concentrates on the past, the present, or the future. The dominant U.S. culture is oriented to the present and future. People are expected not only to take care of themselves at the present moment but also to make plans and save money for the future. Other cultures are oriented toward the past: they carefully preserve traditions, allowing only the slightest changes or variations in practices. Still others are oriented toward the present; saving money for college (a future-oriented action) may not be a high priority in these cultures. If a family's orientation is for the present or the past, members may have difficulty accepting a long-term rehabilitation plan (e.g., by 6 months after an accident a boy will be walking with crutches, but it will be a full year before he will be fully ambulatory again). They may need to be motivated by present indications of progress (e.g., this afternoon the child will be allowed to sit up for the first time; this evening he can begin to have periods of time without oxygen).

The Amish are an example of a past-oriented culture: they adhere to time-honored traditions that do not include technologic advances such as immunizations. Some Native Americans also hold a past orientation. People from lower socioeconomic groups tend to be more present oriented than those in middle or higher socioeconomic groups because of the struggle just to get through each day. They may make different health care decisions because of this (Horodynski et al., 2007). People with strong religious convictions may be future oriented (looking forward to a future existence better than their present one). Knowledge of these different time orientations helps to plan effective care.

Work and School Orientation

The predominant culture in the United States stresses that everyone should be employed productively (called the Protestant work ethic) and that work should be a pleasure and valued in itself (as important as the product of the work). Other cultures do not value work in itself but see it as only a means to an end (you work to get money or food, not satisfaction). Suppose that a pregnant woman you care for has been told that she must be at home on bed rest for the remainder of her pregnancy. It is easy to think that she will be most concerned because this will not allow her to continue her job as a grade school teacher. A woman with a different work orientation might be more distressed to learn that she cannot continue her hobby (going to baseball games). This could be misconstrued as being unproductive when it is actually a cultural difference.

Because people in the United States are expected to work, they also are expected to finish school so they can learn an occupation and support themselves in their adult life. Work orientation has come to include using leisure time effectively, such as exercising or learning a new skill rather than just passively watching television. Because cultural influences dictate leisure time activity this way, and values differ, assessment will reveal differences in what people prefer to do during their leisure time and also the effect this can have on their overall health if sufficient exercise is not included (Brandes, 2007).

Family Orientation

Family structure and the roles of family members are other lifestyles that are culturally determined. In most cultures, the nuclear family (mother, father, and children) is most common. In other cultures, extended families (nuclear family plus grandparents, aunts, uncles, and cousins) and single-parent families (one parent and child) may be more common. Some cultures stress that information about a family should be carefully guarded (as a way of keeping the family intact and unique and perhaps also as a reflection of mistrust for health care providers). Other cultures willingly share the same information. When caring for children, be certain to identify a child's primary caregiver before giving health care instructions because who cares for children in a family can vary by culture. Identifying the family decision-maker can also be important, because this role can vary greatly among families.

Male and Female Roles

In most cultures, the man is the dominant figure. In such a culture, if approval for hospital admission or therapy is needed, the man is the one to give this approval. In a culture in which men are very dominant and women are extremely passive, a woman may be unable to offer an opinion of her own health or be embarrassed to submit to a physical examination, especially from a male physician or nurse practitioner, unless a female nurse is also present. The incidence of intimate partner violence may be higher in male-dominant cultures. In an extremely male-dominated family, a woman's pregnancy may have resulted not from a mutual decision but from sexual relations she felt she could not refuse.

In contrast, in some cultures, the woman may be the dominant person in the family. The oldest woman in the home would be the one to give consent for treatment or hospital admission.

It is important to evaluate male and female roles in this way, because knowing the identity of the dominant person in the household also helps you to understand the impact of the illness on a family. If a woman is the family's dominant person and can no longer make her usual decisions because she is ill during pregnancy, the entire family may be thrown into confusion. If the woman is a nondominant member, you may have to act as an advocate for her rights with a more dominant person.

In most health care settings today, a father is expected to play an active role during labor, as well as during a child's hospital stay. However, a man who sees his role as a passive one may be uncomfortable participating in labor or visiting a hospital to play with an ill child. Awareness that male and female roles differ from country to country in this way can help you find a middle ground for a parent's participation in pregnancy and child care.

What if... Mr. Rodriques says he does not wish to participate in labor when his wife has her new baby? Would you encourage him to time contractions (a typical role for fathers) or allow him to sit quietly in a corner of the room, as he prefers?

Religion

There are wide variations in religious practices, and many of these are culturally determined. Because religion guides a person's overall life philosophy, it influences how people feel about health and illness, what foods they eat, and their preferences about birth and death rituals (Miklancie, 2007). Knowing what religion a family practices helps you locate a religiously important support person when needed. It helps you in planning care because many nutritional practices, such as whether the family eats meat, can be dictated by religious beliefs. It also can have important implications for decision making during a difficult pregnancy or for childhood terminal care.

Health Beliefs

Health beliefs are not universal. For example, most people are familiar with the current controversy about whether male circumcision is necessary. More surprising to many people is a belief that female circumcision (amputation of the clitoris and perhaps a portion of the vulva) is thought to be necessary in some cultures (Braddy & Files, 2007).

It is generally assumed in developed countries that illness is caused by documented factors such as bacteria, viruses, or trauma. In other cultures, however, illness may be viewed primarily as a punishment from God or an evil spirit, or as the work of a person who wishes harm to the sick person. An example of this is a belief among some Hispanics that an "evil eye" (*mal ojo*) can cause illness. People who believe that their own sins caused an illness may not be highly motivated to take medication or other measures to get well again as they do not believe that a spoonful of penicillin will cure them. People with such beliefs may receive more comfort from a spiritualist or counselor than from their physician or nurse practitioner. They may believe it is necessary to suffer pain to be rid of the illness and so may be reluctant to ask for pain medication. Understanding different beliefs of this kind allows you to understand differing attitudes toward procedures and to work out mutual goals, even when the patient's views are not those you would choose for yourself or for a member of your family (see Focus on Nursing Care Planning Box 2.7).

As another example, women's concept of whether pregnancy is a time of wellness or illness and whether breastfeeding is advocated or not differs in various cultures (Oetzel et al., 2007). Most American women visit health care facilities early in pregnancy, follow prenatal directives, and, at birth, allow a health care provider to supervise the birth. In other cultures, pregnancy and childbearing are considered such natural processes that a health care provider is unnecessary. The woman knows the special rules and taboos she must follow to ensure a safe birth and a healthy child and depends on other women rather than on health care providers to guide her safely through labor and birth. She may plan to breastfeed until the next child is born, or for as long as 5 years. Unless differences such as these are respected, it is difficult to plan prenatal care that meets individual women's needs.

The type of therapy people choose to restore health is also dependent on culture. When one person wakes up with an upper respiratory infection, for example, he or she may immediately call a health care provider for a formal prescription. Another person with the same symptoms would not call at all but depend on an herbal or "natural" self-help method. Be aware when taking health histories that many people today from all cultures rely on complementary or alternative therapies. Ask if people use these to be certain that a prescribed medication will not counteract or be synergistic with these or if they want some advice on what would work better for them (Smith et al., 2009).

What if... The Rodriques family tells you that they believe the accident that caused Maria's broken leg was "God's will," not Maria's fault? Would it be appropriate to educate Maria about street safety, or would doing so interfere with the family's cultural beliefs?

Nutrition Practices

Foods and their methods of preparation are strongly culturally related. In many instances, people cannot find any food on a hospital menu that appeals to them because of cultural preferences. A Japanese diet, for example, includes many vegetables such as bean sprouts, broccoli, mushrooms, water chestnuts, and alfalfa. Children with this preference tire quickly of the macaroni and cheese common to a middle-class American childhood diet. Fortunately, in most instances, a child's family can provide food that is appealing culturally and is still within prescribed dietary limitations (Fig. 2.4).

When counseling a woman about nutrition during pregnancy, remember that respect for culturally preferred foods is

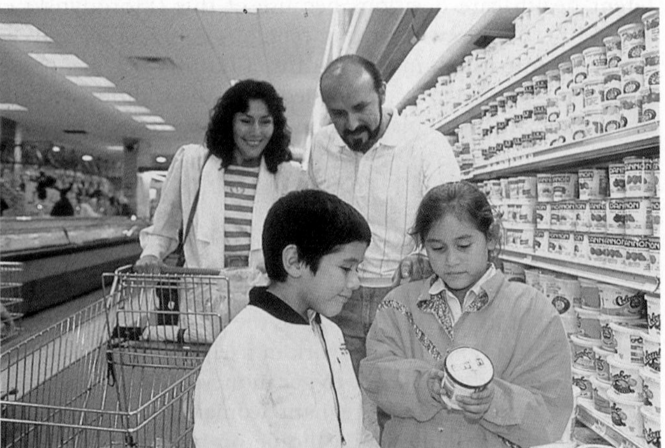

FIGURE 2.4 Families differ regarding what food selections they prefer because of sociocultural preferences. (© Photo Researchers/Jeffrey Greenberg.)

BOX 2.7 ✻ Focus on Nursing Care Planning

A Multidisciplinary Care Map for a Child Needing Sociocultural Care

Maria Rodriques is a 12-year-old child who is hospitalized following surgical repair of a broken tibia that was broken when she rode her bicycle into a busy street. She has a cast on her right leg and will be on bed rest for 3 days and then allowed to learn crutch walking.

Family Assessment ✻ Maria lives with her mother, Anna, her father, Carlos, and a 4-year-old brother, Pedro. She attends a local grade school and enjoys playing video games and reading Harry Potter books. Her mother is 4 months pregnant.

Client Assessment ✻ Temperature, 99.4° F; pulse, 86 beats/min; respirations, 24/min. Observed lying on side, gritting teeth as if in pain. Hands clenched and eyes tearing. When asked if she has pain, she quietly stated, "No. I'm okay." Father was overheard saying to her, "We're proud you're so brave." Cast on right leg dry and intact. Toes warm to touch. Intravenous fluid infusing without difficulty. Oral intake primarily tea and soup. Client's mother states, "She needs 'hot' foods to get better. Don't you have anything hotter?"

Nursing Diagnosis ✻ Pain related to tissue trauma of surgery, with cultural belief to not voice pain.

Outcome Criteria ✻ Client accepts pain medication when offered; nonverbal expressions of pain are minimal to absent. Client begins to eat and manage self-care.

Team Member Responsible	Assessment	Intervention	Rationale	Expected Outcome
		Self-Care Activities		
Nurse/physical therapist	Assess what self-care activities child feels ready to begin.	Plan a program of self-care that is possible within constraints of limited ambulation.	Ability to complete self-care can add to self-esteem and supply physiologic benefits.	Client feeds self, is out of bed in 3 days, and completes hygiene measures at 12-year-old level.
		Consultations		
Nurse	Assess pain level on a 1-to-10 scale. Determine what child feels would relieve pain best.	Consult with pain management team to establish a total pain relief plan for client.	Optimal health care is often a collaborative practice.	Child states that pain management plan is acceptable to her. Rates her pain level as below 2 on a 1-to-10 scale.
		Procedures/Medications		
Nurse	Assess for both verbal and nonverbal indicators of pain.	Offer pain medication as prescribed before pain becomes acute.	Offering medications relieves the client of the need to ask for relief when her belief is that she should not express pain. It also allows the child to have some choice and control in her care.	Child's chart documents that pain medication was offered every 4 hours during waking hours throughout hospital stay.
		Nutrition		
Nurse/nutritionist	Assess whether the child has food preferences that are not being met by hospital service.	Encourage the family to bring in foods from home that meet their cultural preferences.	Allowing the family to bring in foods demonstrates respect for their culture and increases the child's sense of security and being cared for.	Client increases nutrient intake by including foods brought from home.

(continued)

BOX 2.7 ✻ Focus on Nursing Care Planning (continued)

Team Member Responsible	Assessment	Intervention	Rationale	Expected Outcome
		Patient/Family Education		
Nurse	Assess the child's knowledge of broken bones and of why trauma leads to pain.	Explain the physiology of pain to family members as a way of explaining why the client is experiencing it.	Explanations help a child of this age understand what is happening so minimize fear.	Client describes what pain is and acknowledges that she will have some until healing is complete and that asking for something to relieve it is expected and acceptable.
		Spiritual/Psychosocial/Emotional Needs		
Nurse	Assess whether child has unmet needs other than pain relief.	Explain to child that you want to help but that she needs to verbally express her needs to enable you to do so.	Children may imagine that health care providers are all-knowing.	Child agrees to participate in expressing the presence of other factors, such as loneliness or fear.
		Discharge Planning		
Nurse	Assess with child what modifications she will need to make in her daily routine to adjust to cast.	Discuss with parents that their child may need modifications in daily routine to return to school.	Well-informed parents and children are able to make informed decisions.	Child attends school daily because of modifications in usual lifestyle.

important. People from some cultures, for example, tend to eat much less meat than do those from other cultures. Adequate protein can be ingested, however, by mixing sources of incomplete protein such as beans and rice. Some women may omit various foods during pregnancy because they believe a particular food will mark a baby (e.g., strawberries cause birthmarks, raisins cause brown spots), or they believe that it is necessary to eat "hot" or "cold" foods to ensure fetal growth. Pregnancy is usually considered a "hot" condition, so it may be difficult for a woman who is trying to eat only "cold" foods to agree to increase her intake of meat, usually considered a "hot" food. Asian women may believe in a similar pattern of required balances (yin and yang).

Before beginning nutrition counseling, become aware of what is the dominant type of food available in your health care agency's local food stores. Women who cannot buy the foods you recommend in their own neighborhood may not eat well because of the inconvenience involved in shopping elsewhere.

A trait present in many people that is ethnically determined is lactose intolerance. This is the absence of lactase, the enzyme that breaks down the sugar (lactose) in milk so milk can be used by the body. People with lactose intolerance (including many Asians and blacks) develop diarrhea and stomach cramps if they drink milk because of lactase deficiency (Bauchner, 2007). Be certain when counseling during pregnancy that you do not advise a woman who is lactose intolerant to drink milk. She can obtain adequate calcium through supplements or other foods high in calcium such as dark green vegetables. Adding a lactase additive to milk is yet another suggestion.

Pain Responses

A person's response to pain is a final category that is both individually and culturally determined (Jacob et al., 2008). Although all people may have the same threshold sensation (the amount of stimulus that results in pain), their pain threshold (the point at which the individual reports that a stimulus is painful) and pain tolerance (the point at which an individual withdraws from a stimulus) vary greatly.

Caring for a person having pain can be problematic when the caregiver's concept of "proper" responses to pain differs from the patient's concept. One woman in labor might report labor contractions as "agonizing" each time she feels one, whereas a woman in the room next to her, experiencing the same degree of pain, might report her pain as tolerable and barely change her facial expression with contractions because of her different cultural attitude toward expressing pain. Because there are so many possible responses to pain, it is important to assess each person individually.

Strategies to help recognize cultural influences on pain perception are to (a) appreciate that the meaning of pain varies among cultures, (b) appreciate that not all people communicate or express their level of pain in the same way, (c) recognize that communication of pain may not even be acceptable within a culture, (d) develop an awareness of your personal values and beliefs and that they may affect how you respond to people in pain, and (e) use an assessment tool, such as a 1-to-10 scale, to assist in measuring pain so you are certain that you are being as objective as possible (Giger & Davidhizar, 2008). Further assessment of pain and its meaning to people is discussed in Chapters 16 and 39.

✔ Checkpoint Question 2.2

Maria Rodriques is the 12-year-old student you met at the beginning of the chapter. Which statement by her is the best example of ethnocentrism?

a. My school, Stevens Park, is the best in the city.
b. Many schools in my city have good soccer teams.
c. Children from many cultures attend my school.
d. I want to go to a public, not a private, college.

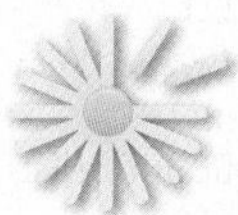

Key Points for Review

- Culture is an organized structure that guides behavior into acceptable ways for that group. Usual customs are termed "mores" or "norms." Actions that are not acceptable to a culture are "taboos."
- Stereotyping is expecting a person to act in a characteristic way without regard to his or her individual traits. Prejudice is thinking that people are different in some way, or is an *intellectual* act. Discrimination is treating people differently based on their physical or cultural traits, or is a *doing* act.
- Each culture differs to some degree from every other. Most people are proud of these differences or cultural traits.
- Cultural practices arise from environmental conditions and are transmitted by both formal and informal ways from generation to generation.
- Although cultural concepts adapt from time to time, they tend to remain constant.
- There is wide variation within a culture concerning values and actions, because individuals make up the group and individually express their cultural heritage.
- People bring cultural values and beliefs to nursing interactions, and these affect nursing and health care.
- Cultural aspects that are important to assess are communication patterns; use of conversational space; response to pain; time, work, and family orientation; and social organization including nutrition, family roles, and health beliefs.

CRITICAL THINKING EXERCISES

1. Maria Rodriques is the 12-year-old child you met at the beginning of the chapter. *What could the nurse have done differently in the plan of care for this child?* What would have been a better approach for determining this family's cultural preferences? Supposing Maria is present oriented: how would you approach discussions of a long-term rehabilitation program with her?
2. When you talk to Mrs. Rodriques, you realize that she is pregnant but has not gone for prenatal care. She states that before coming to the clinic she wants to visit a *yerbero,* who will both predict her child's sex and guarantee a safe birth. Would recommending that she have a sonogram (which also could predict the fetal sex) likely be as satisfying for her?
3. Although you know Maria is being raised as a vegetarian for religious reasons, suppose at lunch time you notice a hamburger on her meal tray. What would be your best action? Would you ask her to eat it because she needs protein for healing? Or ask for another food choice for her?
4. Examine the National Health Goals related to sociocultural aspects of health care. Most government-sponsored money for nursing research is allotted based on these goals. What would be a possible research topic to explore pertinent to these goals that would be applicable to the Rodriques family and also advance evidence-based practice?

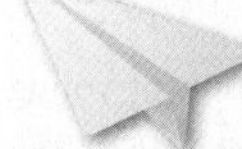

CRITICAL THINKING SCENARIO

Open the accompanying CD-ROM or visit http://thePoint.lww.com and read the Patient Scenario included for this chapter; then answer the questions to further sharpen your skills and grow more familiar with NCLEX types of questions related to cultural influences. Confirm your answers are correct by reading the rationales.

REFERENCES

Abuidhail, J., & Fleming, V. (2007). Beliefs and practices of postpartum infant care: review of different cultures. *British Journal of Midwifery, 15*(7), 418–421.

Andrews, M. M., & Boyle, J. S. (2007). *Transcultural concepts in nursing care.* Philadelphia: Lippincott Williams & Wilkins.

Angstman, S., et al. (2007). Tobacco and other substance use among Alaska Native youth in western Alaska. *American Journal of Health Behavior, 31*(3), 249–260.

Bauchner, H. (2007). Lactose intolerance: a common problem. *Archives of Disease in Childhood, 92*(5), 464–465.

Braddy, C. M., & Files, J. A. (2007). Female genital mutilation: cultural awareness and clinical considerations. *Journal of Midwifery & Women's Health, 52*(2), 158–163.

Brandes, A. H. (2007). Leisure time activities and obesity in school-based inner city African American and Hispanic children. *Pediatric Nursing, 33*(2), 97–102.

Crombleholme, W. R. (2009). Obstetrics. In S. J. McPhee & M. A. Papadakis (Eds.). *Current medical diagnosis & treatment.* Columbus, OH: McGraw-Hill.

Darby, S. B. (2007). Pre- and perinatal care of Hispanic families: implications for nurses. *Nursing for Women's Health, 11*(2), 160–169.

Giger, J. N., & Davidhizar, E. (2008). *Transcultural nursing: assessment and intervention.* New York: Elsevier Publishing.

Gound, M., et al. (2007). Attitude mismatching: discrepancies in the sexual attitudes of African American mothers and their pre-adolescent children. *AIDS and Behavior, 11*(1), 113–122.

Horodynski, M., et al (2007). Low-income mothers' decisions regarding when and why to introduce solid foods to their infants: influencing factors. *Journal of Community Health Nursing, 24*(2), 101–118.

Jacob, E., et al. (2008). Intensity, location, and quality of pain in Spanish-speaking children with cancer. *Pediatric Nursing, 34*(1), 45–52.

Klaczynski, P. A. (2008). There's something about obesity: culture, contagion, rationality, and children's responses to drinks "created" by obese children. *Journal of Experimental Child Psychology, 99*(1), 58–74.

Leininger, M. (2007). Theoretical questions and concerns: response from the theory of culture care diversity and universality perspective. *Nursing Science Quarterly, 20*(1), 9–13.

Miklancie, M. A. (2007). Caring for patients of diverse religious traditions: Islam, a way of life for Muslims. *Home Healthcare Nurse, 25*(6), 413–417.

Niederhauser, V. P., & Markowitz, M. (2007). Barriers to immunizations: multiethnic parents of under- and unimmunized children speak. *Journal of the American Academy of Nurse Practitioners, 19*(1), 15–23.

Oetzel, J., et al. (2007). Hispanic women's preferences for breast health information: subjective cultural influences on source, message, and channel. *Health Communication, 21*(3), 223–233.

Schim, S. M., et al. (2007). Culturally congruent care: putting the puzzle together. *Journal of Transcultural Nursing, 18*(2), 103–110.

Smith, C. A., et al. (2009). Complementary and alternative therapies for pain management in labour. *Cochrane Database of Systematic Reviews, 2009*(1), (CD003521).

U.S. Census Bureau. (2009). *Population projection program.* Washington, D.C.: Author, Population Division.

Whitley, R., & Kirmayer, L. J. (2008). Perceived stigmatisation of young mothers: an exploratory study of psychological and social experience. *Social Science & Medicine, 66*(2), 339–348.

SUGGESTED READINGS

Abdulwadud, O. A., & Snow, M. E. (2009). Interventions in the workplace to support breastfeeding for women in employment. *Cochrane Database of Systematic Reviews, 2009*(1), (CD006177)

Doumit, G., et al. (2009). Local opinion leaders: effects on professional practice and health care outcomes. *Cochrane Database of Systematic Reviews, 2009*(1), (CD000125).

Giger, J., et al. (2007). Developing cultural competence to eliminate health disparities in ethnic minorities and other vulnerable populations. *Journal of Transcultural Nursing, 18*(2), 95–102.

Greene, M. J. (2007). Strategies for incorporating cultural competence into childbirth education curriculum. *Journal of Perinatal Education, 16*(2), 33–37.

Hunt, R. J., & Swiggum, P. (2007). Being in another world: transcultural student experiences using service learning with families who are homeless. *Journal of Transcultural Nursing, 18*(2), 167–174.

Lee-Lin, F., et al. (2007). Breast cancer beliefs and mammography screening practices among Chinese American immigrants. *JOGNN: Journal of Obstetric, Gynecologic, and Neonatal Nursing, 36*(3), 212–221.

Lincroft, Y. (2007). Easing immigrant families' fears. *Children's Voice, 16*(4), 21.

Sadler, C., & Huff, M. (2007). African-American women: health beliefs, lifestyle, and osteoporosis. *Orthopaedic Nursing, 26*(2), 96–103.

Savage, C. L., et al. (2007). The culture of pregnancy and infant care in African American women: an ethnographic study. *Journal of Transcultural Nursing, 18*(3), 215–223.

Uman, L., et al. (2009). Psychological interventions for needle-related procedural pain and distress in children and adolescents. *Cochrane Database of Systematic Reviews, 2009*(1), (CD005179).

Chapter 3 The Childbearing and Childrearing Family

KEY TERMS

- ecomap
- family
- family nursing
- family of orientation
- family of procreation
- family theory
- genogram
- polygamy
- polygyny

OBJECTIVES

After mastering the contents of this chapter, you should be able to:

1. Describe family structure, function, and roles, and ways that these are changing.
2. Identify National Health Goals related to the family and specific ways that nurses can help the nation achieve these goals.
3. Use critical thinking to analyze additional ways that nursing care can be more family centered or that family members can be better integrated into maternal-child health care.
4. Assess a family for structure and healthy function.
5. Formulate nursing diagnoses related to family health.
6. Develop expected outcomes to help a family achieve optimal health.
7. Plan health teaching strategies, such as helping a family modify its lifestyle to adjust to a pregnancy, accommodate an ill child, or face a major life event such as loss of a job.
8. Implement nursing care, such as teaching a family more effective wellness behaviors.
9. Evaluate outcome criteria for achievement and effectiveness of nursing care to be certain that expected outcomes have been achieved.
10. Identify areas of care related to family nursing that could benefit from additional nursing research or the application of evidence-based practice.
11. Integrate knowledge of family nursing with nursing process to promote quality maternal and child health nursing care.

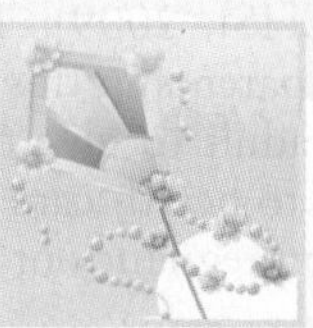

Marlo Hanovan is a 32-year-old who has a 10-year-old child, Carey, from a first marriage. Carey has been sick since birth with cystic fibrosis. He attends the local grade school although he needs daily respiratory therapy. Stone, Marlo's present husband, has a 2-year-old son, Brian, from his first marriage who is also part of the family. Stone is currently unemployed because of an accident at work a year ago. He has some income from selling woodworking products at craft shows. Mrs. Hanovan, a freelance writer, is pregnant now with a second child. She states that on many weeks she is forced to choose between health care and groceries.

The previous chapters discussed the philosophy of maternal and child health nursing and how cultural mores affect care. This chapter adds information about families and how nurses can help ensure healthy outcomes for families. Inadequate family support, which can occur in a dysfunctional family, can contribute to poor pregnancy outcome or poor childrearing practices.

Is the Hanovan family a well family?
Is their structure typical of other American families?

Humans have always lived in families, but the types of families formed and family goals established have changed as the rest of the world has changed. For example, when the largest number of families lived on farms, families were extended or had a wealth of relatives close by for both physical and psychological support. As more people moved into cities, families became typically nuclear with only two parents and children present. Less support was available to families. Today, the most frequent type of family seen in the United States is a single-parent family (National Center for Health Statistics [NCHS], 2009). This has important implications for nurses as parents in this type of family may not even have one other adult to give them support. This makes families look more to health care providers for guidance when a problem with pregnancy or childrearing occurs (Crombleholme, 2009).

Families are important to a country as no other social group has the potential to provide the same level of support and long-lasting emotional ties as a person's own family. What people learn in their family determines how they relate to people, what moral values they learn, and their perspective on both the present and the future (Clay et al., 2007).

Maintaining healthy family life is so important to the health and welfare of the nation that several National Health Goals speak directly to maintaining healthy family and community life (Box 3.1). Because the family has such an influence on the individual, nursing care that considers the family, not the individual **(family nursing)**—is a focus of modern nursing practice. **Family theory** details a set of perspectives from the family's point of view that can help nurses address the important health issues of childbearing and childrearing families.

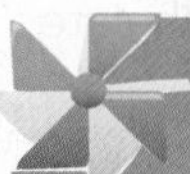

BOX 3.1 ✻ Focus on National Health Goals

Several National Health Goals focus on ways to improve the quality of family or community life. Representative of these are:

- Lower the current baseline of 25.2 per 1000 children younger than age 18 who are maltreated.
- Reduce physical abuse directed at women by male partners to no more than 27 per 1000 couples from a current baseline of 30 per 1000 couples.
- Eliminate the prevalence of blood lead levels exceeding 10 μg/dL in children aged 1 month to 6 years from a baseline of 4.4% (http://www.nih.gov).

Nurses can help to see that goals such as these for healthier family living are met by assessing families and their environment to identify families at risk, assisting with counseling, and maintaining contact with families to ensure that as a family grows its changing needs can be recognized and met. Intimate partner and child abuse are further discussed in Chapter 55; lead poisoning from excessive lead in the environment is discussed in Chapter 52.

For a family to adjust to a new family member, the family must have structure and roles that are flexible enough to adjust to the changes that pregnancy and a newborn will bring. An ill family member or one who is going through a difficult developmental period, such as adolescence, can put a tremendous strain on a family as well. The roles individuals assume in the family and their ability to adjust to new roles can influence a family's perception of the child's illness, as well as the family's ability to adjust to new situations and work through difficult times to a positive family outcome. Because families do not live in isolation, the family's ability to thrive in a community and gain strength from the community is equally important. For this reason, the modern concept of maternal and child health nursing is not limited to assessing individuals or individual circumstances but rather examines them first from a family and community standpoint (Shields, et al., 2009).

Family-centered maternal and child health nursing considers the strengths, vulnerabilities, and patterns of families to support families during childbirth and childrearing and to encourage healthy coping mechanisms in families facing a crisis. Health assessment and intervention planning is best when it includes considerations of the family's social, emotional, spiritual, and financial resources, as well as the physical and emotional condition of the home and the community.

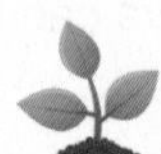

Nursing Process Overview

For Promotion of Family Health

Assessment

Assessment of the structure, function, strengths, and challenges of families provides information on the ability of a family to remain well during both calm and stressful times. It can reveal the meaning of a current health situation as well as the emotional support an individual family member can expect from other members or the community. This can be vital to understanding what a pregnancy or childhood illness will mean to different family members, especially if not all members appear to be in agreement.

Nursing Diagnosis

Nursing diagnoses formulated for families generally relate to a family's ability to handle stress and to provide a positive environment for growth and development of members. Examples are:

- Parental role conflict related to prolonged separation from child during long hospital stay
- Interrupted family processes related to emergency hospital admission of oldest child
- Impaired parenting related to unplanned pregnancy
- Ineffective family coping related to inability to adjust to mother's illness during pregnancy
- Readiness for enhanced family coping related to improved perceptions of child's capabilities
- Health-seeking behaviors related to birth of first child

"Impaired parenting" and "parental role conflict" are diagnoses that suggest parents need additional help with parenting. The first family coping diagnosis ("ineffective

- How can nurses best help families cope with the stress of long-term illness?
- How can nurses help prevent violence such as homicide in communities and modify the effects of violence on families?
- What do maternal-child health nurses need to know about alternative therapies such as herbal remedies to keep their practices current?

The answers to these and other questions provided by research help to bolster a foundation for specific actions and activities that have the potential to improve maternal and child health care. The Focus on Evidence-Based Practice boxes included in chapters throughout the text contain summaries of current maternal and child health research studies and are designed to assist you in developing a questioning attitude regarding current nursing practice and in thinking of ways to incorporate research findings into care (Box 1.5).

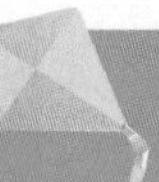

BOX 1.5 ✻ Focus on Evidence-Based Practice

Do nonsmoking programs actually reduce the level of smoking?

Cigarette smoking is strongly associated with heart and respiratory disease. If interventions to stop smoking could be employed in workplace settings, potentially thousands more individuals could be reached with such programs.

To see if workplace nonsmoking intervention programs are effective, researchers analyzed the outcome of a group of programs targeting individual smokers: 10 studies of group therapy, 7 studies of individual counseling, 9 studies of self-help materials, and 5 studies of nicotine replacement therapy. Workplace interventions aimed at the workforce as a whole included 14 studies of tobacco bans, 2 studies of social support, 4 studies of environmental support, 5 studies of incentives, and 8 studies of comprehensive (multicomponent) programs. Following the analysis, the authors concluded:

1. Interventions directed toward individual smokers such as advice from health care professionals or the use of pharmacological treatments increase the likelihood of individuals quitting smoking.
2. There is limited evidence that including competition or incentives organized by an employer can increase participation in programs.
3. There is consistent evidence that workplace tobacco policies and bans can decrease cigarette consumption during the working day by smokers and exposure of nonsmoking employees to environmental tobacco smoke at work. Such bans, however, may not decrease the overall prevalence of smoking or overall consumption of tobacco by smokers.

Suppose you are interested in reducing cigarette smoking in a family you care for? Could you use these findings to help plan a program for them?

Source: Moher, M., Hey, K. & Lancaster, T. (2009). Workplace interventions for smoking cessation. *Cochrane Database of Systematic Reviews, 2009*(1), (CD003440).

Nursing Theory

One of the requirements of a profession (together with other critical determinants, such as member-set standards, monitoring of practice quality, and participation in research) is that the concentration of a discipline's knowledge flows from a base of established theory.

Nursing theorists offer helpful ways to view clients so that nursing activities can best meet client needs—for example, by seeing a pregnant woman not simply as a physical form but as a dynamic force with important psychosocial needs, or by viewing children as extensions or active members of a family as well as independent beings. Only with this broad theoretical focus can nurses appreciate the significant effect on a family of a child's illness or of the introduction of a new member.

Another issue most nursing theorists address is how nurses should be viewed or what the goals of nursing care should be. Extensive changes in the scope of maternal and child health nursing have occurred as health promotion, or keeping parents and children well, has become a greater priority.

With health promotion as a major nursing goal, teaching, counseling, supporting, and advocacy are also common roles (Vonderheid et al., 2007). Nurses care for clients who are more critically ill than ever before. Because care of women during pregnancy and of children during their developing years helps protect not only current health but also the health of the next generation, maternal-child health nurses fill these expanded roles to a unique and special degree.

✔ Checkpoint Question 1.1

Suppose Melissa Chung asks you whether maternal-child health nursing is a profession. What qualifies an activity as a profession?

a. Members supervise other people.
b. Members use a distinct body of knowledge.
c. Members enjoy good working conditions.
d. Members receive relatively high pay.

A CHANGING DISCIPLINE

At the beginning of the 20th century, the infant **mortality rate** in the United States (i.e., the number of infants per 1000 births who die during the first year of life) was greater than 100 per 1000. In response to efforts to lower this rate, health care shifted from a treatment focus to a preventive one, dramatically changing the scope of maternal and child health nursing. Research on the benefits of early prenatal care led to a major national effort to provide prenatal care to all pregnant women through prenatal nursing services (home visits) and clinics. Today, thanks to these and other community health measures (such as efforts to encourage breastfeeding, increased immunization, and injury prevention), as well as many technological advances, the U.S. infant mortality rate has fallen to 6.6 per 1000 (Eldridge & Sutton, 2009).

Medical technology has contributed to a number of important advances in maternal and child health: childhood diseases such as measles and poliomyelitis are almost eradicated through immunization; specific genes responsible for many inherited diseases have been identified; stem cell therapy may make it possible in the next few years to replace

family coping") indicates that a family is not functioning at an optimal level; the second ("readiness for enhanced family coping") suggests a family that is ready for new growth because of a specific event, such as sudden illness in a child or discovery of an unplanned pregnancy. "Readiness for enhanced parenting" and "health-seeking behaviors" are diagnoses that apply to families who are investigating more effective ways to manage their present situation and improve family/community functioning.

Outcome Identification and Planning

Planning for nursing care is most effective if it includes a design that is family centered and so is both appropriate and desired by the majority of family members; otherwise, opposing family members may have difficulty following the plan. Be certain that plans also consider the community. For example, it is not helpful to suggest that a family take regular walks together to encourage shared decision making and improve family communication if walking in their neighborhood park is unsafe; participation in a family aerobics class at a local YMCA might be a more practical suggestion. To help women balance family and work, an interesting website to visit is The National Partnership for Women & Families (http://www.nationalpartnership.org).

Implementation

Implementations to improve family health should flow smoothly if family members have agreed on a plan of action out of support for one another. It may be necessary in some instances, however, to encourage family members to agree on a plan or to abide by a chosen plan. Otherwise, they can expend needless energy carrying out an activity that is counterproductive or in direct opposition to their major goal.

Outcome Evaluation

Evaluation should reveal not only that a goal was achieved but also that the family feels more cohesive after working together toward the goal. If evaluation does not reveal these two factors, reassess the goal as necessary to determine whether further interventions are required. Examples of expected outcomes that might be established are:

- Family members state they are adapting well to the presence of a newborn.
- Mother states she feels prepared to manage home care of her ill child.
- Father states he has arranged the family finances to accommodate new health care expenses for his family.
- Grandmother states she will omit trans-fatty acids from cooking to better safeguard the health of her family.

THE FAMILY

How well a family works together and how well it can organize itself against potential threats depend on its structure (who its members are) and its function (the activities or roles family members carry out). Recognizing different family structures can help you focus on family-centered care or provide a family-friendly environment for health care (Crea, Barth, & Chintapalli, 2007).

Defining the Concept of Family

A **family** is defined by the U.S. Census Bureau (2009) as "a group of people related by blood, marriage, or adoption living together." This definition is workable for gathering comparative statistics but is limited when assessing a family for its health concerns or the support people available, because some families are made up of unrelated couples, and at certain points in life not all family members may live together. Allender and Spradley (2008) define the family in a much broader context as "two or more people who live in the same household (usually), share a common emotional bond, and perform certain interrelated social tasks." This is a better working definition for health care providers because it addresses the broad range of types of families that could be encountered in any health care setting.

Family Types

Many types or structures of families exist, and family structures change over time as they are affected by birth, work, death, divorce, and the growth of family members. For the purposes of assessing families in maternal and child health nursing, two basic family types can be described:

- **Family of orientation** (the family one is born into; or oneself, mother, father, and siblings, if any)
- **Family of procreation** (a family one establishes; or oneself, spouse or significant other, and children)

Almost all families, regardless of type, share common activities (Cherlin, 2008). They influence the health and activities of their members (Chen, Shiao, & Gau, 2007). Specific descriptions of family types vary greatly depending on family roles, generational issues, means of family support, and sociocultural influences.

The Dyad Family

A dyad family consists of two people living together, usually a woman and a man, without children. Newly married couples, as an example, are dyad families. This category also refers to single young same sex adults who live together as a dyad in shared apartments, dormitories, or homes for companionship and financial security while completing school or beginning their careers. Dyad families are generally viewed as temporary arrangements, but if the couple chooses child-free living, this can also be a lifetime arrangement.

The Cohabitation Family

Cohabitation families are composed of heterosexual couples, and perhaps children, who live together but remain unmarried. Although such a relationship may be temporary, it may also be as long-lasting and as meaningful as a more traditional alliance. Many couples choose cohabitation as a way of getting to know a potential life partner better before marriage as it seems as if this might make their eventual marriage stronger. Statistically, however, couples who cohabit before marriage have a higher divorce rate than those who do not (Cherlin, 2008). This may occur because cohabitation couples enter the union without a real commitment. That is a contrast to married couples who enter a union with a "until death do I part" philosophy. The feeling that a union can be easily broken may influence a couple not to work at a marriage but merely walk away from that as well.

When in place, an effective cohabitation arrangement offers psychological comfort and financial security similar to marriage. Long-term cohabitation unions of this type are growing in number. The increasing numbers to adhere to a monogamous relationship through cohabitation could help contribute to decreasing sexually transmitted infections and decrease the financial burdens on the cohabiters. Because cohabitation unions simulate dyads, they offer the same companionship and security as dyad families.

The Nuclear Family

The traditional nuclear family structure is composed of a husband, wife, and children. In the past, it was the most common structure seen worldwide. Today, however, in the United States, the number of nuclear families has declined to about 49% of families. This is because of the increase in divorce, acceptance of single parenthood, and the greater acceptance of alternative lifestyles (NCHS, 2009). An advantage of a nuclear family is its ability to provide support to family members, because, with its small size, people know each other well and can feel genuine affection for each other. In a time of crisis, this same characteristic may become a challenge to a family as there are few family members to share the burden and offer support. Helping nuclear families locate and reach out to support people during a crisis can be an important nursing responsibility.

The Polygamous Family

Although **polygamy** (a marriage with multiple wives) has been illegal in the United States since 1978 and so is rarely seen today, such marriages are not that unusual an arrangement worldwide. New immigrants, particularly those from the Middle East, may have been raised in this type of family (Elbedour, Bart, & Hektner, 2007).

Polygyny (a marriage with one man and several wives) tends to occur in nations where women have low social status or are not valued for their individual talents. It can be attractive for men as it allows for sexual variety. It can serve as the mark of a wealthy man as wives cost money. With more than one wife having children, it also increases the chance that the marriage will produce a male heir. Advantages to women are that women in polygyny marriages are able to have fewer children than if they were a lone wife so it lowers their chance of dying in childbirth, a concern for women in nations where prenatal care is not a high national priority. If differences in wealth are great, women may prefer polygyny to being the wife of a poor man. Problems that can arise are jealousy and rivalry between wives because of perceived favoritism (Gibson & Mace, 2007).

The Extended (Multigenerational) Family

An extended family includes not only the nuclear family but also other family members such as grandmothers, grandfathers, aunts, uncles, cousins, and grandchildren. An advantage of such a family is that it contains more people to serve as resources during crises and provides more role models for behavior or values. A possible disadvantage of an extended family is that family resources, both financial and psychological, must be stretched to accommodate all members. In a typical extended family, although many members are present, there is usually only one main income provider and that can strain the family's resources. When assessing such families, remember that because many members are present, a parent's strongest support person may not be a spouse or intimate partner, and a child's primary caregiver may not be his or her own mother or father. The grandmother or an aunt or another sibling, for example, may provide the largest amount of support or child care, even though spouses and the child's parents are also present every day.

The Single-Parent Family

The incidence of single-headed families has increased from 10% of all families in 1960 to almost 51% today. Of these families, 17% have a man as the single parent (NCHS, 2009). A health problem in a single-parent family is almost always compounded. If the parent is ill, there is no back-up person for child care. If a child is ill, there is no close support person to give reassurance or a second opinion on whether the child's health is worsening or improving.

Low income is often an additional problem encountered by single-parent families, because the parent is most often a woman. Traditionally, women's incomes are lower than men's by about 33% (Cherlin, 2008). Single parents also may have difficulty with role modeling or clearly identifying their role in the family (i.e., they must provide duplicate roles, or financial support as well as child care). Trying to fulfill several central roles in this way is not only time-consuming but also mentally and physically exhausting and, in many instances, not rewarded. Such a parent may develop low self-esteem if things are not going well, especially if a spouse left them for another or if the other parent refuses to help with child support. Single-parent fathers may have difficulty with home management or child care if they had little experience with these roles before the separation. Such feelings have the potential to interfere with decision making and impede daily functioning.

Single-parent families have a special strength in that such a family can offer the child a special parent–child relationship and increased opportunities for self-reliance and independence. If there has been a divorce, one parent may have been given legal custody of the children or both parents may have joint custody. Either way, both parents often participate in decision making. At a time of illness, both may stay with the ill child in the hospital and be eager to receive reports of the child's progress. Identifying who is the custodial parent is especially important when consent forms for care are signed.

The Blended Family

In a blended family, or a remarriage or reconstituted family, a divorced or widowed person with children marries someone who also has children. Advantages of blended families include increased security and resources for the new family. Another benefit is that the children of blended families are exposed to different customs or culture and may become more adaptable to new situations.

Childrearing problems may arise in this type of family from rivalry among the children for the attention of a parent. In addition, each spouse may encounter difficulties in helping rear the other's children. Often stepparents believe they have been thrust into a limited or challenged role of authority. Children may not welcome a stepparent because they have not yet resolved their feelings about the separation of their biologic parents (through either divorce or death); the stepparent may differ from the biologic parent, particularly in terms of discipline and caregiving; or they may believe that the stepparent threatens their relationship with their biologic parent. They also may have heard so many stories about evil stepparents that they come to the new family prejudiced against their new parent. They may become extremely distressed at seeing their other biologic parent move into another home and become a stepparent to other children.

Although blended families usually lessen financial difficulties, finances can be severely limited, especially if one or both parents are obligated to pay child support for children from a previous marriage while supporting the children of the current marriage. If there is economic disparity between the biologic parents, conflicts and distorted expectations can occur. Nurses can be instrumental in offering emotional support to members of a remarriage family until the adjustments for mutual living can be made.

The Communal Family

Communes are formed by groups of people who choose to live together as an extended family. Their relationship to each other is motivated by social or religious values rather than kinship (Cherlin, 2008). The values of commune members may be more oriented toward freedom and free choice than those of a traditional family. Some communes are described as cults or composed of a group of people who follow a charismatic leader. Adolescents, because they are in the process of determining what values to adopt for their future life, may find this type of commune particularly appealing.

People living in a commune may have difficulty following traditional health care regimens, preferring instead to use complementary or alternative therapies (health care may be seen as an established system that they are rejecting). On the other hand, people who reject traditional values may be the most creative people in a community, the most interested in participating in their own care, and ripe for health teaching and learning.

The Gay or Lesbian Family

In homosexual unions, individuals of the same sex live together as partners for companionship, financial security, and sexual fulfillment. Such a relationship offers support in times of crisis comparable to that offered by a nuclear or cohabitation family. Some lesbian and gay families include children from previous heterosexual marriages or through the use of artificial insemination, adoption, or surrogate motherhood. Laws governing homosexual partners can affect health care if they limit health insurance coverage. Lack of understanding by health care providers of the strength and richness of these unions can further impede health care (Short, 2007).

✔ Checkpoint Question 3.1

The Hanovan family was a single-parent family before Mrs. Hanovan remarried. What is a common concern of single-parent families?

a. Reading disorders are common.
b. Finances are inadequate.
c. Children miss many days of school.
d. Children do not know any other family like theirs.

The Foster Family

Children whose parents can no longer care for them may be placed in a foster or substitute home by a child protection agency (Risley-Curtiss & Stites, 2007). Foster parents may or may not have children of their own. They receive remuneration for their care of the foster child. Foster home placement is theoretically temporary until children can be returned to their own parents. If return is impossible or is not imminent, children, unfortunately, may be raised to adulthood in foster care. Such children can experience almost constant insecurity, concerned that soon they will have to move again. In addition, they may have some emotional difficulties related to the reason they were removed from their original home (Rubin et al., 2007).

Most foster parents are as concerned with health care as the biologic parents. They can be entrusted to follow health care instructions as needed. When caring for children from foster homes, be certain to determine who has legal responsibility to sign for health care for the child (many times the child protection agency is the one with legal responsibility).

The Adoptive Family

Many types of families (nuclear, extended, cohabitation, single-parent, gay and lesbian) adopt children today. No matter what the family structure, adopting brings several challenges to the adopting parents and the child, as well as to any other children in the family (Fontenot, 2007).

Methods of Adoption

Agency Adoption. In traditional agency adoption, a couple usually contacts an agency by first attending an informational meeting. If the couple decides to apply to the agency, they are then put on a waiting list for processing that will include extensive interviewing and a home visit by an agency social worker to determine whether the couple can be relied on to provide a safe and nurturing environment for an adopted child. Once approved by the agency, the couple is placed on a second waiting list until a child is available. Depending on the area of the country and the couple's particular requests, this second waiting period may extend from a few months to 5 or 6 years. There are children in every state waiting for adoption and who can be placed immediately into adopting homes, but most of these children are older, have special care needs, or are of a different ethnic or cultural background from the prospective adoptive parents. They often have lived with many foster families or have gone back and forth between the homes of their birth parents and foster care many times to reach this point in life. Although adopting special needs children is not an option that is appealing for every couple, adoption of such children can be extremely rewarding for the right couple and can achieve an immediate family for them. Counsel parents to obtain a clear health history of any child they adopt so they can be aware of potential health problems and better prepared to help with health care decisions about their child.

Historically, there was little or no communication between a woman placing her baby for adoption and an adopting couple. This was seen as an advantage because the birth mother could then not interfere in the new couple's lives. Today, the disadvantage of this arrangement for the child is being realized: should a child want to learn his or her birth family's name or medical history or location, this information is not available. This has led to "open adoption" procedures, in which the identity of neither the birth mother nor the adoptive parents is kept secret, allowing as much interaction as desired between the two sets of parents (Wolfgram, 2008).

International Adoption. As many as 20,000 children are adopted to the United States from other countries yearly (Hellerstedt et al., 2008). International adoption can often provide a baby in less time than a traditional agency adoption but may create unanswered questions about prenatal health care or the birth parent's background. In addition, countries that are willing to permit abandoned or orphaned children to be adopted internationally are often economically disadvantaged or war torn, meaning the child's health or development may have suffered. War conditions may allow children to be released from the country one day but not the next. This means that couples who are waiting for an international adoption must be ready at a moment's notice to travel to the foreign country or to a neutral location to pick up their child or to give up the adoption because political reforms have stopped the release of children.

A home visit from a local agency and a significant amount of paperwork and communication with the international agency are usually required before a family can be approved for this type of adoption. Typically, the adoption is final before the child enters the country or shortly afterward. Encourage parents to examine their feelings ahead of time about having a child from a different culture. Help them explore ways to respect the child's natural heritage and deal with possible prejudice toward the child by neighbors and family who are not as culturally accepting as they are. Local support groups consisting of other families who have successfully adopted internationally can be helpful to couples considering this option. In addition, many of the international adoption agencies provide follow-up support. It may be difficult for internationally adopted children to learn about or locate their natural parents in years to come, because records of their birth may have been destroyed or changed in their native countries. In some countries, the birth certificate is deliberately changed to reflect the adoptive couple as the birth parents.

Private Adoption. For families who have exhausted other options or who cannot wait for the traditional agency adoption process, private adoption is another alternative. With private adoption, the adopting parents usually agree to pay a certain amount of money to a birth mother, part of which presumably goes toward the birth mother's prenatal and medical expenses. Sometimes, strict anonymity is maintained between the two parties; in other instances, the adopting couple and birth mother come to know each other well. Some pregnant women prefer to place their child for adoption directly with a couple this way rather than through an agency, so they can approve of the couple and maintain contact with the child afterward. The adopting parents might even attend the child's birth if the birth mother wishes.

The Internet has become a source where women wanting to place a baby for adoption can contact couples who want to adopt. Usually, a lawyer serves as the go-between to make certain all the legal ramifications of adoption have been considered by each party. It is important to caution adopting parents that Internet sites may not be reliable. They need to be certain to obtain a reliable health history on the child and discuss what will be their legal responsibility if the child is born with a health problem or dies at birth.

In some instances, close familiarity between the two parties creates difficulties later on: some couples may want to have the birth mother or father play a continued role in their lives, but others do not. If not, the birth mother may find it difficult to lose contact not only with the baby she has carried for 9 months but also with her new friends, who may have been extremely supportive of her during her pregnancy. These issues need to be worked out legally well in advance of the birth, because it is possible for a birth mother to change her mind about giving up her baby before the adoption is finalized. There is little that an adopting couple can do in this circumstance, because court decisions tend to favor the rights of the birth mother. Parents who adopt by this route may live in fear for years that the birth mother will change her mind. Although many states have laws that place a time limit on the period during which the birth mother can change her mind, many courts have ruled in favor of returning an adopted child to the birth mother no matter what period of time has elapsed.

Caring for Adoptive Families

Regardless of the type of adoption, new parents should visit a health care facility shortly after a child is placed in their home so that a baseline of health information on the child can be obtained, potential problems can be discussed, and solutions can be explored. If the birth mother of an adopted child ate inadequately or received little prenatal care, for example, the adopted child is at a higher risk for abnormal neurologic development than he or she would normally be. Children from countries that are war torn or poverty stricken have a greater risk of having illnesses such as hepatitis B, intestinal parasites, and growth restriction. They may lack immunizations (Bramlett, Radel, & Blumberg, 2007).

When assessing a family with a newly adopted child, determine the stage of parenting the parents have reached. The average parents have 9 months to prepare physically and emotionally for a coming baby. Although adoptive parents may have been planning on a baby for much longer than 9 months, the actual appearance of a child can occur suddenly. In a few days' time, the adoptive parents are asked to make the mental steps toward parenthood that biologic parents make over 9 months. There may be a great need at health care visits to explore their feelings about this change in their lives and their feelings about being parents so suddenly. If they have low self-esteem because they were unable to conceive or married a partner who was unable to conceive, they may need reassurance at health care visits that they are functioning well as parents. With the increase in foreign adoptions, parents often express a conflict between trying to preserve the child's native culture and socializing the child into the community and appreciate having this problem addressed.

Also be sure to assess siblings' responses to the adopted child. Biologic children (whether born before or after the adoption) may feel inferior to the adopted child because they were "just born," not "chosen." On the other hand, they may feel superior because they are the "real" children of the parents. These feelings can interfere with their relationship with the adopted child as well as their parents.

It is generally accepted that adopted children should be told as early as they can understand that they are adopted.

Knowing this from early childhood is not nearly as stressful as accidentally stumbling onto the information when they are school-aged or adolescents. By 3 years old, children are able to understand the story of their adoption. It is important for parents not to criticize the birth mother as part of the explanation to help build the child's self-esteem.

When children are first told they are adopted, they may exhibit "honeymoon behavior" or may try to behave perfectly for fear of being given away again. After this honeymoon period, children may deliberately test their parents to see whether, despite bad behavior such as disobeying or even shoplifting, the parents will still keep them. It helps parents to put this behavior in perspective if they are aware that it may happen and that nonadoptive children may use the same testing strategies on some occasions.

Counseling an adopted child or forming a relationship with one as a health care provider carries additional responsibility by making certain that the relationship is not ended abruptly or without closure. When ending a relationship, try to introduce the person who will continue health supervision for the child so the child does not feel abandoned. When hospitalized, all preschoolers worry about being abandoned and left in the hospital. Preschoolers who have just been told they are adopted, that they were chosen by their adoptive parents "from all the babies in the hospital nursery," may be terribly afraid that they are now being returned to the hospital to be given back. Parents of an adopted child may need additional help in preparing the child for the hospital experience and to be encouraged to stay with the child in the hospital as much as possible to reduce these types of postadoption fears.

As adopted children enter puberty and begin to think about having children of their own, they may begin to worry whether they will make good parents. Some children of this age have difficulty establishing a sense of identity because they do not know who their birth parents were. It is common for them to spend time tracing records and trying to locate their birth parents. Counsel adopting parents that this is not a rejection of them but a normal consequence of being adopted. Children seek their birth parents not because they do not love their adoptive parents but because they need that information to know where they fit into the eternal scheme of life.

FAMILY FUNCTIONS AND ROLES

A family is a small community group, and, as a group, it works best if it can designate certain people to complete certain tasks. Otherwise, it is easy for work to be duplicated or never completed. The family roles that people view as appropriate are usually the ones they saw their own parents fulfilling. As each new generation takes on the values of the previous generation, family traditions and culture pass to the next generation.

Because family roles are more flexible and often not as well defined as in the past, an important part of family assessment is to identify the roles of family members. Most families, for example, can identify an individual who serves as the wage earner or who supplies the bulk of the income for the family. In the past, this was the father, but today, it may just as easily be the mother. Also identified can be a financial manager (the person who pays the bills), a problem-solver, a decision-maker, a nurturer, a health manager, an environmentalist, a culture bearer, and a gatekeeper or the person who allows information into and out of the family. Knowing who fulfills these roles in a family helps you to work most effectively with the family.

If a hospitalized child will need continued care after he or she returns home, for example, it would be important to identify and contact the nurturing member of the family, because this person is probably the one who will supervise or give the needed care at home. Be careful not to make assumptions about role fulfillment based on gender or stereotyping, because every family operates differently. Although nurturing has typically been thought of as a female characteristic, many men fill this role today.

✔ Checkpoint Question 3.2

Mrs. Hanovan serves many roles in her family. If, when you talk to Carey, her 10-year-old son, she interrupts to say, "Don't tell our family secrets," she is fulfilling what family role?

a. Decision-maker
b. Gatekeeper
c. Problem-solver
d. Safety officer

Family Tasks

Duvall and Miller (1990) identified eight tasks that are essential for a family to perform to survive as a healthy unit. These tasks differ in degree from family to family and depend on the growth stage of the family, but they are usually present to some extent in all families. Wellness behaviors such as these may decrease during periods of heightened stress. Therefore, assessing families for these characteristics is helpful in establishing the extent of stress on a family and empowering the family to move toward healthier behaviors.

- *Physical maintenance:* A healthy family provides food, shelter, clothing, and health care for its members. Being certain that a family has enough resources to provide for a new or ill member is an important assessment.
- *Socialization of family members:* This task involves preparing children to live in the community and to interact with people outside the family. It means the family has an open communication system among family members and outward to the community. A family that lives in a community with a culture or values different from its own may find this a difficult task.
- *Allocation of resources:* Determining which family needs will be met and their order of priority is allocation of resources. In healthy families, there is justification, consistency, and fairness in the distribution. Resources include not only material goods but also affection and space. In some families, resources are limited, so, for example, no one has new shoes. A danger sign would be a family in which one child is barefoot while the others wear $100 sneakers.
- *Maintenance of order:* This task includes establishing family values, establishing rules about expected family responsibilities and roles, and enforcing common regulations for family members such as using "time out" for toddlers. Determining the place of a new infant and what rules will pertain to him or her may be an important task for a developing family. In healthy families, members know the family rules and respect and follow them.

- *Division of labor:* Healthy families evenly divide the work load among members and are flexible enough that they can change work loads as needed. Pregnancy or the illness of a child may change this arrangement and cause the family to have to rethink family tasks.
- *Reproduction, recruitment, and release of family members:* Often not a great deal of thought is given to this task; who lives in a family often happens more by changing circumstances than by true choice. Having to accept a new infant into an already crowded household may make a pregnancy a less-than-welcome event or cause reworking of this task.
- *Placement of members into the larger society:* Healthy families realize that they do not have to operate alone but can reach out to other families or their community for help when needed. Because they have the ability to be sensitive to the needs of individual family members they are able to select community activities, such as schools, religious affiliation, or a political group, that correlate with the family's beliefs and values. Selecting a birth setting, a special school setting, or choosing a hospital or hospice setting is part of this task.
- *Maintenance of motivation and morale:* Healthy families are able to maintain a sense of unity and pride in the family. When this is created, a sense of pride helps members defend the family against threats as well as serve as support people for each other during crises. It means that parents are growing with and through the experience of their children the same as children are growing through contact with the parents. Assessing whether this feeling is present tells you a lot about the overall health of a family.

Family Life Cycles

Families, like individuals, pass through predictable developmental stages (Duvall & Miller, 1990). To assess whether a family is using stage-appropriate health promotion activities, it is helpful to first determine a family's developmental stage. The age of the oldest child marks the stage. Because families are delaying the age at which they have a first child and parents are living longer, the lengths of stages 1, 7, and 8 are growing.

Stage 1: Marriage

Although Duvall referred to this stage as marriage, what occurs during it is also applicable to couples forming cohabitation, lesbian/gay, or single alliances. During this first stage of family development, members work to:

- Establish a mutually satisfying relationship
- Learn to relate well to their families of orientation
- If applicable, engage in reproductive life planning

Establishing a mutually satisfying relationship includes merging the values that the couple brings into the relationship from their families of orientation. This includes not only adjusting to each other in terms of routines (e.g., sleeping, eating, housecleaning) but also sexual and economic aspects. This first stage of family development is a tenuous one, as evidenced by the high rate of divorce or separation of partners at this stage. The illness of a family member or an unplanned pregnancy at this stage may be enough to destroy the still lightly formed bonds if the partners do not receive support from their former family members or health care providers do not recognize a problem exists.

Stage 2: The Early Childbearing Family

The birth or adoption of a first baby is usually both an exciting and a stressful event because it requires both economic and social role changes. An important nursing role during this period is health education about well-child care and how to integrate a new member into a family. It is a further developmental step for a family to change from being able to care for a well baby to being able to care for an ill one. One way of determining whether a parent has made this change is to ask what the new parent has tried to do to solve a childrearing or health problem. Even if what the person answers is not therapeutic or the best solution to the problem, as long as it is sensible (not "I don't do anything when the baby's sick; just take her right to my mother" but instead, "I've been trying to give her a little water and keep her temperature down"), it probably means the parent has mastered this developmental step. Parents who have difficulty with this step need a great deal of support and counseling from health care providers to be able to care for an ill child at home or to manage a difficult pregnancy.

Stage 3: The Family With a Preschool Child

A family with preschool children is a busy family because children at this age demand a great deal of time. Their imagination is at such a peak that safety considerations such as avoiding unintentional injuries (accidents) become a major health concern. If a child is hospitalized because of an accident, parents may have difficulty giving care because they feel they should have done more to prevent the child's injury. It may be difficult for parents to room in at the hospital because they have other young children at home who need care. If the child returns home for further care, a family in this stage may need continued support and help from a community health nurse to provide necessary health care for the ill child.

Stage 4: The Family With a School-Age Child

Parents of school-age children have the important responsibility of preparing their children to function in a complex world while at the same time maintaining their own satisfying marriage relationship. That makes this a trying time for many families. Family support systems seem strong but also can be deceptive: family members may be physically present but provide little or no emotional support if internal tension exists. Illness imposed at this stage adds to the burdens already present and may be enough to dissolve a family. Many families during this period need to turn to a tertiary level of support, such as friends, a religious affiliation, or counseling, for adequate support.

Important nursing concerns during this family stage are monitoring children's health in terms of immunization, dental care, and health care assessments; monitoring child safety related to home or automobile accidents; and encouraging a meaningful school experience that will make learning a lifetime concern, not one of merely 12 years.

Stage 5: The Family With an Adolescent

The primary goal for a family with a teenager differs considerably from the goal of the family in previous stages, which was to strengthen family ties and maintain family unity.

Now the family must loosen family ties to allow adolescents more freedom and prepare them for life on their own. As technology advances at a rapid rate, the gap between generations increases. Life when the parents were young was very different from what it is for their teenagers. This can make stage 5 a trying stage for both children and adults.

Violence—accidents, homicide, and suicide—is the major cause of death in adolescents (NCHS, 2009). As adolescents become sexually active, they risk contracting sexually transmitted infections such as human immunodeficiency virus (HIV) and gonorrhea. A nurse working with families at this stage needs to spend time counseling members on safety (driving defensively and not under the influence of alcohol; safer sex practices; proper care and respect for firearms) and the dangers of chemical abuse. If there is a "generation gap" between the parents and an adolescent, the adolescent may not be able to talk to the parents about these problems, particularly those of a controversial nature such as sexual responsibility. A nurse can be a neutral person to assist families at this stage when communication can be difficult while maintaining confidentiality between the family members.

Stage 6: The Launching Stage Family: The Family With a Young Adult

For many families, the stage at which children leave to establish their own households is the most difficult stage because it appears to represent the breaking up of the family. Parental roles change from those of mother or father to once-removed support people or guideposts. The stage may represent a loss of self-esteem for parents, who feel themselves being replaced by other people in their children's lives. They may feel old for the first time and less able to cope with responsibilities. Illness imposed on a family at this stage can be detrimental to the family structure, breaking up an already disorganized and noncohesive group.

Many young adults return home to live with their family after college until they can afford their own apartment or get married. They are termed a "boomerang" generation. As a general rule, this arrangement works best if there are no young children in the home and if the young adult has a job to supply some income. Males tend to remain home longer than females and females are generally asked to do more work around the house and are chaperoned more closely by parents.

A nurse can serve as an important counselor to such a family. He or she can help the parents see that what their children are doing is what they have spent a long time preparing them to do, or that leaving home is a positive, not a negative, step in family growth.

Stage 7: The Family of Middle Years

When a family returns to a two-partner unit, as it was before childbearing, the partners may view this stage either as the prime time of their lives (an opportunity to travel, economic independence, and time to spend on hobbies) or as a period of gradual decline (lacking the constant activity and stimulation of children in the home, finding life boring without them, or experiencing an "empty nest" syndrome). They may realize that they have grown in such different ways that they have very little in common any more. Women tend to experience less "empty nest" feelings than previously because few women in developed countries measure their worth by only their ability to care for children (Cherlin, 2008).

Because the family has returned to a two-partner union, support people may not be as plentiful as they were. Having children return home to live after college or a failed relationship can create a "sandwich family," or parents who are squeezed into taking care of both their aging parents and these returning young adults.

Stage 8: The Family in Retirement or Older Age

Families of retirement age account for approximately 15% to 20% of the population (NCHS, 2009). Although families at this stage are not having children, they remain important in maternal and child health because they can offer a great deal of support and advice to young adults who are just beginning their families. Many grandparents care for their grandchildren while the parents are at work. This can be a strain on older adults as they struggle to meet young children's needs in relation to both energy level and finances needed.

✔ Checkpoint Question 3.3

The Hanovan family consists of two parents plus Carey, age 10, and Brian, 2. Mrs. Hanovan is 5 months pregnant. Which of Duvall's family life stages is the family currently experiencing?

a. Pregnancy stage
b. Preschool stage
c. School-age stage
d. Launching stage

Changing Patterns of Family Life

Family life has changed significantly in the United States during the past 50 years because of many complex and interrelated factors, such as the increased mobility of families, an increase in the number of families in which both parents work outside the home (dual-earner families), an increase in the number of single-parent families, and an increase in shared childrearing responsibilities. Many couples delay marriage and childrearing until they are completely finished with school and established in their careers. This delay has implications for fertility and the need for assisted reproduction strategies. Some parents, believing they were finished with childrearing, are surprised to find their grown children returning home after college to live with them again. Others find themselves playing duel rules by caring for both children and aging parents. Understanding the impact these changes have on family structure and family life can help you create care plans that are realistic and meet the needs of today's families.

Increasing Mobility Patterns

Population movement has an important influence on the quality of family life. During the 20th century, vast numbers of rural families moved to urban communities, and many urban families moved to the suburbs. Today, families are moving back to inner cities to fill remodeled buildings that once held factories or served as warehouses (gentrification). This pattern of mobility is expected to continue into the future. This can mean that an area with many maternal and child health care facilities may find itself with few women and children to use them in the future; conversely, areas with many women and children may find few nearby facilities. This can cause a problem as parents will travel a great distance to obtain health care for an ill child or during a pregnancy with complications, but they are less likely to do so for health maintenance or health promotion; therefore, prenatal care or routine immunizations may be neglected. When assessing families, always ask if a family has ready accessibility to health care (Box 3.2).

Families of immigrants or migrant farm workers can have difficulty finding consistent health care because of their seasonal movement (Connor et al., 2007). Children from these families may also be at high risk for intestinal parasites, low socioeconomic status, and lack of immunizations. New immigrants have special problems in that they must adjust not only to a new country but also to a differently structured health care system than they have become accustomed to in their home country. If they entered the country illegally, their ability to even locate health care can be further compromised. Nurses can be instrumental in seeing that health care organizations consider these issues and institute innovative measures, such as providing transportation to facilities, changing locales or services so facilities and needs remain balanced, or setting up outreach and translator programs so families who are not proficient in English can receive adequate health care.

BOX 3.2 ✻ Focus on Communication

The Hanovan family consists of Mr. and Mrs. Hanovan and two children, Carey, age 10, and Brian, 2. You are concerned because Brian has missed so many health maintenance visits that he is underimmunized.

Less Effective Communication

Nurse: It's good to see you in clinic today, Ms. Hanovan. I know money is a problem, but you've got to start coming more often until your child gets caught up with immunizations.

Ms. Hanovan: It's hard with a 2-year-old—

Nurse: Babies, you know, have almost no natural immunity. That's why they need immunizations.

Ms. Hanovan: It's hard—

Nurse: It's hard to understand any reason important enough not to get him immunized.

Ms. Hanovan: I'll do better. I promise.

More Effective Communication

Nurse: It's good to see you in clinic today, Ms. Hanovan. I know money is a problem, but you've got to start coming more often until Brian gets caught up with his immunizations.

Ms. Hanovan: It's hard with a 2-year-old—

Nurse: Is there something I could do to make coming to the clinic easier?

Ms. Hanovan: I should never come. Brian's outgrown his car seat and it's illegal for me to drive him here.

Nurse: Let me give you the number of an agency to call to borrow a seat, not only so you can come to the clinic but so you can take him out safely at other times.

In our zeal to educate people about good health practices, it is easy to rush in and teach without first assessing a family's most important needs. Unless these needs are met, people may agree to comply with a better health regimen but then be unable to do so because their original need was not met.

Changing Cultural Patterns

Although families are more mobile today than formerly, cultural values and characteristics remain constant. Knowing some of the basic norms and taboos of different cultural groups is important as it allows you to understand and accept different practices of families. It helps you understand the family's value system and the degree of support family members are apt to have available.

Poverty tends to be a problem for nondominant (minority) ethnic groups. Characteristic responses that are sometimes described as cultural limitations are actually the consequences of poverty—for example, a mother seeking medical care for her child late in the course of an illness or late in pregnancy for herself is just as apt to be a financial influence as a cultural one. Solving this type of problem may be a question of locating financial resources rather than overcoming cultural influences.

Increasing Poverty

Although the United States is a large and wealthy country, extreme poverty also exists, and in some areas, the incidence is growing. As many as 20% of families with children have incomes that fall below the poverty line. This places children and families at risk for a variety of health problems (Kilanowski & Ryan-Wenger, 2007). A pregnant woman living in poverty, for example, is less likely to receive prenatal care or be able to afford important prenatal vitamins.

Each year the government determines the poverty level by computing the cost of food for a family of four. An average family spends about one-third of their income on food. A family that earns less than triple that defined price of food, therefore, earns significantly less than optimally or is said to be below the poverty line.

A family that must choose between buying groceries and paying for a child's immunizations will obviously buy groceries; the child's immunizations must wait until another time. If a family is forced to make this same choice week after week, the child could reach adulthood without protection against a number of potentially lethal diseases such as measles. Poverty allows acute illness to become chronic, forces families to live in dangerous neighborhoods, and, because of the high stress level always present, may increase the incidence of intimate partner abuse (Joly, 2007).

Reducing Government Aid Programs

Current legislation aimed at reducing the duration of government assistance to families and encouraging people receiving such assistance to begin or return to work was designed to stimulate parental productivity. Although some families who ordinarily would not qualify for Medicaid funding qualify for aid if the mother is pregnant, these laws reduce the number of people eligible for aid and so create child care problems and possibly increase poverty for individual families (Kaushal & Kaestner, 2007).

Health care providers can help families secure benefits such as food stamps or funding from the Women, Infants, and Children Special Supplemental Food Program (WIC) and free or scaled-payment health care programs to obtain health care despite their limited financial resources. Encouraging families to secure more education so they can better increase their earning capability and no longer need government assistance can also be helpful (Cricco-Lizza, 2008).

Increasing Numbers of Homeless Families

More than 3.5 million people in the United States today are homeless (NCHS, 2009). Although there is diversity in homeless families, as in all others, many homeless families are headed by a woman, and an increasing number are headed by pregnant and parenting adolescents (Tischler, Rademeyer, & Vostanis, 2007). The frequency of drug and alcohol abuse and severe psychiatric problems is greater among homeless families. Many mothers of homeless families were physically abused as children and have been battered by an intimate partner (Joly, 2007). Such families may not use health care providers or community agencies as effectively as other families because of their inexperience with bureaucracies or lack of transportation and money.

At least half of homeless children are younger than 5 years. Because of decreased environmental stimulation and lack of exposure to normal play activities, such children tend to not perform as well as others on standard developmental screening tests such as the Denver II. They tend to have more physical illnesses, such as anemia, pneumonia, dental problems, and restricted growth.

When caring for homeless families, remember that every day represents a struggle for such families. They often lack support people, so they may need a health care provider to serve in this capacity to help them achieve a healthier lifestyle or to give them active support during times of stress such as illness.

Increasing Divorce Rate

Divorce is rarely easy for anyone involved. Because parents are so emotionally entangled and their perceptions of their roles are changing so drastically, they may be unable to give their children the support they need during a divorce. This can leave marked long-term, negative effects on children or make the loss of a parent through divorce little different from the loss of a parent through death. Severing ties with grandparents or other relatives can also be difficult (Ahrons, 2007).

Children react in different ways to divorce depending on their developmental age and the explanations that parents give them. Divorce, as a rule, has three separate phases, and children's responses follow a course similar to grief. The first phase of divorce for parents is an antagonistic phase when parents realize they are no longer compatible; this is a time of quarreling, hurt feelings, and often whispered conversations. This can be an upsetting period for children because they do not understand what is happening. They may react with denial or anger and may believe that the impending divorce is their fault.

The second phase of divorce is the actual separation stage. Everyone in the family is asked to take on an unfamiliar role and perhaps a new home and a marked difference in financial arrangements. It is a time for grieving for the missing parent. Although it is comforting to be free from a house filled with tension and arguing, children may also wish they had their old life back (similar to the bargaining stage of grieving).

The third phase of divorce involves reshaping. Parents may remarry; financial arrangements stabilize. Children realize that their lives are permanently changed and they cannot go back to the time before the divorce (similar to the acceptance stage of grieving).

Boys may have emotional turmoil if the mother has custody and they lose their gender role model. All children may manifest their grief with physical symptoms such as nausea or fatigue. Their school performance may suffer. Most children report that when the noncustody parent remarries, it is one of the hardest moments for them because at that point they have to accept the divorce is final (Ahrons, 2007).

Although divorce is a stressful time for children, a redeeming feature may be that the period following a divorce may actually be less stressful to children than living in a home where there is a high level of conflict between parents. Children need an explanation of why the divorce has occurred and assurance that it was not their fault. If they do not receive this, they may have difficulty in the future thinking of themselves as good people; they may feel a loss of self-esteem if they believe one of their parents is a "bad person." The parent who will now be raising them may need help in avoiding saying any derogatory comments about the former partner. You can help by showing the parent that, although the former spouse was not a good marriage partner, he or she may have been a good parent and may be well loved and missed by the children.

Decreasing Family Size

The birth rate in the United States has declined steadily from 1900 to the present, putting the United States at a rate of almost zero population growth or with fewer births each year than deaths. The average number of children in families has decreased to 2.1 children (NCHS, 2009). Although small families mean fewer child care requirements for parents, this also limits the parents' experience in childrearing, so the amount of childrearing counseling time per parent may increase. As children have fewer older role models, they may need more counseling in behaviors such as how to manage stress or survive a failure at school.

Increasing Dual-Parent Employment

As many as 60% of women of childbearing age work at a full-time job outside the home today, and as many as 90% work at least part-time (Cherlin, 2008). The implication of this trend for health care providers is that health care facilities need to schedule appointments at times when parents are free to come (parents are willing to miss work if their child is sick, but not necessarily for a health maintenance or a routine prenatal visit). Instructions about how to take medications must take into account a child's schedule. For instance, help parents tailor administration of medicine to the times that they will be with the child to supervise the administration (e.g., before breakfast, following after-school child care, and at bedtime) rather than just "three times a day."

Dual-parent employment has increased the number of children attending day care centers or after-school programs (Trost, Rosenkranz, & Dzewaltowski, 2008). This may have an impact on health care, because children attending day care centers have an increased incidence of illnesses. Help parents choose a quality day care center or after-school program that takes the necessary precautions against infection (see Chapter 31). School-age children often return home from school before their parents return from work. Helping parents prevent loneliness in these "latchkey" or "self-care" children as well as helping children make good use of their time alone is another nursing responsibility (see Chapter 32).

What if... Mrs. Hanovan, who works outside her home from 9 AM to 5 PM, needs to supervise Carey taking a medication four times a day. At what times would you suggest he take the medication?

Increasing Family Responsibility for Health Monitoring

In the past, parents relied on health care providers to monitor their children's health, and they accepted advice about health care without asking many questions or expressing opinions. Today, most parents take (and should be encouraged to take) an active role in monitoring their children's and their own health and participating in planning and goal setting. Changes in health care such as short hospital stays and an increased focus on health promotion and maintenance add to the increased responsibility for families to be knowledgeable health care consumers.

Because of this new consumer awareness, be sure to include parents and children in health care decisions. Using the nursing process for planning helps to accomplish this because the goal-setting step encourages patient participation. Health teaching, such as reducing smoking in the home, increasing the fiber content in meals, and omitting trans-fatty acids from cooking, becomes more effective if the learners are interested in improving their health.

Increasing Technology

Family life today is loaded with technological innovations such as television, computers, cellular phones, and iPods. Such technology has opened up a world to children that they were never exposed to in years past—a world that brings encyclopedias of knowledge to their fingertips but also can bring the danger of predators (Wolak, Mitchell, & Finkelhor, 2007). On a typical day, as many as 75% of children watch television; 32% watch videos/DVDs for approximately 1 hour 20 minutes. Twenty-seven percent of 5- to 6-year-olds use a computer for about 50 minutes on a typical day. Many young children (one fifth of 0- to 2-year-olds and more than one third of 3- to 6-year-olds) have a television in their bedroom (Vandewater et al., 2007). So much time spent in sedentary activities such as television watching is one reason that obesity in children is at epidemic proportions (Gable, Chang, & Krull, 2007).

It is important for children to learn to live in a fast-paced world, but parents need to be certain they are monitoring how fast the world is being presented to their children. News of world events travels so fast today that information about an event is flashed across a television screen only minutes after the event has occurred. News is then reported over and over. That type of repetition can frighten children as it may seem as if 100 planes have gone down instead of one being reported over and over.

It can be difficult for parents to limit the amount of news their children are exposed to as news alerts often interrupt children's programs. Discussing the importance of blocking inappropriate television programs and limiting and monitoring viewing time are important to reduce the level of stress from television to which children are exposed to daily.

An additional danger of too much technology is that it can interfere with communication in a family. Everyone has seen a family strolling through a mall, but instead of talking to each other, everyone is listening to music or text messaging. At the end of the afternoon, although the family has spent the entire afternoon together, they have really communicated very little with each other. Technology has the potential to enrich children's lives, but it also may limit their ability to interact with others, a skill they need to thrive in a school or work setting. Discussing the role of technology in homes can help parents evaluate whether they need to limit technology times and encourage more time in activities, discussing the day's events or participating in an activity where all family members are brought together (Box 3.3).

BOX 3.3 * Focus on Family Teaching

Tips to Improve Family Communication

Q. Suppose Mrs. Hanovan tells you, "My family doesn't communicate well. How can I improve this?"

A. Traditionally, families gathered for an evening meal, and this practice allowed a set period each day for interaction, problem solving, and conflict resolution while problems were still small. If family meals are not possible because of busy work or school schedules, suggestions for better communication might include:

- Plan a time (even 15 minutes) daily when all family members "touch base" with each other.
- Use a telephone answering tape to leave daily messages.
- Set up a bulletin board or a chalk board that family members check each day for messages.
- Have all members check in daily by e-mail or a text message.
- Plan an earlier wake-up time two or three mornings a week so all family members can have breakfast together.
- Reserve one night a week as "family night," when the family plans a special activity to do together such as play a board game or watch a favorite movie.
- Agree that the night is off limits to cell phones, television, CDs, computers, iPods, etc., so family members are not distracted by outside sources.
- Plan special activities for holidays or weekends that involve the whole family.
- Participate in each other's activities (e.g., if one is playing in a ball game, all come and watch).

Increasing Obesity, Reduced Exercise, and Fast Foods

The level of exercise of families today is greatly reduced compared with what families enjoyed in the past. Children are often bused or given rides to school. They spend their time after school playing computer games instead of playing active games such as tag or sandlot baseball. After-school programs are structured around desk work rather than exercise (Box 3.4). Because families are busy and fast food is so available, families fix fast food lunches and dinners. Although this type of food solves problems of time management, it causes families to ingest more fat daily than may be good for them. The combined lack of exercise and consumption of fatty foods has led to a national epidemic of obesity in both adults and children (Biagioli et al., 2007). This has led to disorders such as morbid obesity and diabetes mellitus type 2 occurring in what otherwise would be problem-free pregnancies. Counseling families about their exercise program and nutrition should be on the agenda for all well-child and prenatal health care visits.

Increasing Abuse in Families

An alarming statistic in today's families is that the incidence and reports of domestic abuse (both child and intimate partner) are increasing yearly (Barlow et al., 2007). Detecting abuse begins with the awareness that it does occur. Both intimate partner and child abuse are discussed in Chapter 55.

> **BOX 3.4 ✻ Focus on Evidence-Based Practice**
>
> ***What environmental factors would best encourage urban teenagers to increase their level of physical exercise?***
>
> More children today are obese than ever before. An important component to reducing this obesity epidemic is encouraging adolescents to participate more in physical exercise. To discover what were deterrents to physical exercise among inner city youth, researchers presented 397 children between the 9th and 12th grade in two inner-city magnet high schools with 77 items that might interfere with physical activity and asked them to rate the items regarding their importance.
>
> When selecting items that encouraged physical activity, both boys and girls rated highest the following items: places for activities, friends with whom you can be physically active, physical activity or sports programs outside of school, open fields or free space in the neighborhood, and siblings encouraging you to be active. Items that were most apt to deter physical activity for boys were concrete items such as unsafe facilities and no lights on basketball courts. Girls, in contrast, rated more communitywide deterrents such as crime, violence, sexual offenders, drugs and drug dealers, gangs, and dark outside when you get home from school.
>
> ***Suppose you join a committee assigned to design a new inner-city recreation center. Would the results of this study be a help in planning?***
>
> Source: Ries, A. V., et al. (2008). Adolescents' perceptions of environmental influences on physical activity. *American Journal of Health Behavior, 32*(1), 26–39.

ASSESSMENT OF FAMILY STRUCTURE AND FUNCTION

Family characteristics can be assessed on a variety of levels and in varying degrees of detail. The type of family data collected and the method of collection should match the way in which the assessment data will be used.

General characteristics of family type and functioning can be assessed using observation and general history questions (Table 3.1). If more detailed information about family environment and roles is required, using an assessment tool specifically developed for that purpose is most effective.

The Well Family

Assessment of psychosocial family wellness requires measurement of how the family relates and interacts as a unit, including communication patterns, bonding, roles and role relationships, division of tasks and activities, governance, decision making, problem solving, and leadership within the family unit. Assessment also looks at how the family relates to the outside community.

The **genogram,** a diagram that details family structure, provides information about the family's history and the roles of various family members over time, usually through several generations. It can provide a basis for discussion and analysis of family interaction (Fig. 3.1).

The Family APGAR (Smilkstein, 1978) is a screening tool of the family environment (Fig. 3.2). A Family APGAR form is administered to each family member, and their scores are then compared. The tool is easy to use and can complement a family history.

Another aspect of family assessment is to document the "fit" of a family in their community. This is done by means of an **ecomap,** a diagram of family and community relationships (Fig. 3.3). To construct such a map, first draw a circle in the center to represent the family. Around the outside draw circles that represent the family's community contacts such as church, school, neighbors, or other organizations. Families that "fit" well into their community usually have many outside circles or community contacts. A mark of abusive families is that they have few community contacts as they deliberately keep outside people remote from them. Constructing such a map helps you assess the emotional support available to a family from the community. A family whom you assess as having few connecting lines between its members and the community may need increased nursing contact and support to remain a well family (see Focus on Nursing Care Planning Box 3.5).

Although family assessment is best done when a family is managing well, assessment of a family often first occurs when a family is in crisis. The way families react to a crisis depends largely on the particular crisis, their past experiences with problem solving, their perception of the event (whether they can clearly see what is the problem), and the resources available to them to help solve the problem. McCubbin and

(text continues on page 56)

TABLE 3.1 ✻ Family Assessment

Area of Assessment	Questions to Ask
Type of family	Who lives in the home? Is the family nuclear, extended, or other?
Family finances	Are finances adequate? Is money divided evenly among family members?
Safety	Is the home safe from fire or unintentional injuries (are smoke alarms present and police and fire telephone numbers posted?)
Health	Does the family eat a nutritious diet? Do they receive adequate sleep? Are immunizations current? Is there a balance between work and recreation? Can they cope with problems adequately?
Emotional support	
Within family	Do members eat together or spend an equal amount of time with each other daily? Do they band together to defend each other from outsiders?
Outside family	Is the family active in community organizations or activities? Do they visit (or are they visited by) friends and relatives? Can the family name one outside person they can always rely on for help in a time of crisis?
Family roles	
Nurturer	Who is the primary caregiver to children or any physically or cognitively challenged member?
Provider	Who brings in the bulk of the family's income?
Decision-maker	Who makes decisions, particularly in the area of lifestyle and leisure time?
Financial manager	Who supervises the family finances (pays the bills, provides for future savings)?
Problem-solver	On whom does the family depend to provide the solution to problems?
Health manager	Who ensures that family members keep health appointments, immunizations are kept current, and preventive care such as a mammogram for the mother is scheduled?
Culture bearer	Who maintains family and community customs to give children a sense of where they belong in history?
Environmentalist	Who is responsible for recycling, for not wasting electricity or water?
Gatekeeper	Who determines what information will be released from the family or what new information can be introduced?

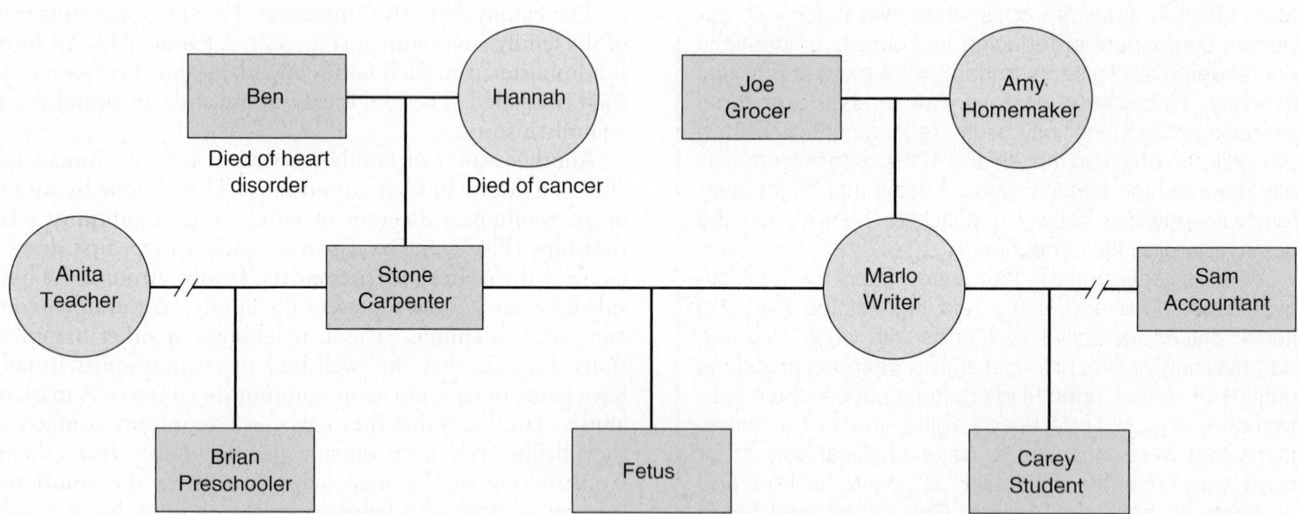

FIGURE 3.1 A Hanovan family genogram showing three generations. Males are shown by squares, and females by circles.

The Family APGAR Questionnaire

	Almost always	Some of the time	Hardly ever
I am satisfied with the help that I receive from my family* when something is troubling me.	______	______	______
I am satisfied with the way my family discusses items of common interest and shares problem solving with me.	______	______	______
I find that my family accepts my wishes to take on new activities or make changes in my lifestyle.	______	______	______
I am satisfied with the way my family expresses affection and responds to my feelings such as anger, sorrow and love.	______	______	______
I am satisfied with the way my family and I spend time together.	______	______	______

SCORING

Scoring: The patient checks one of three choices, which are scored as follows: 2 points for "Almost always," 1 point for "Some of the time" and 0 for "Hardly ever." The scores for each of the five questions are then totaled. A score of 7 to 10 suggests a highly functional family. A score of 4 to 6 suggests a moderately dysfunctional family. A score of 0 to 3 suggests a severely dysfunctional family.

WHAT IS MEASURED

Adaptation	How resources are shared, or the member's satisfaction with the assistance received when family resources are needed.
Partnership	How decisions are shared, or the member's satisfaction with mutuality in family communication and problem solving.
Growth	How nurturing is shared, or the member's satisfaction with the freedom available within the family to change roles and attain physical and emotional growth or maturation.
Affection	How emotional experiences are shared, or the member's satisfaction with the intimacy and emotional interaction within the family.
Resolve	How time* is shared, or the member's satisfaction with the time commitment that has been made to the family by its members.

*Besides sharing time, family members usually have a commitment to share space and money. Because of its primacy, time was the only item included in the Family APGAR; however, the nurse who is concerned with family function will enlarge understanding of the family's resolve by inquiring about family member's satisfaction with shared space and money.

FIGURE 3.2 The Family APGAR Questionnaire. (From Smilkstein, G. [1978]. The family APGAR: a proposal for a family function test and its use by physicians. *Journal of Family Practice, 6*(6), 1231–1239.)

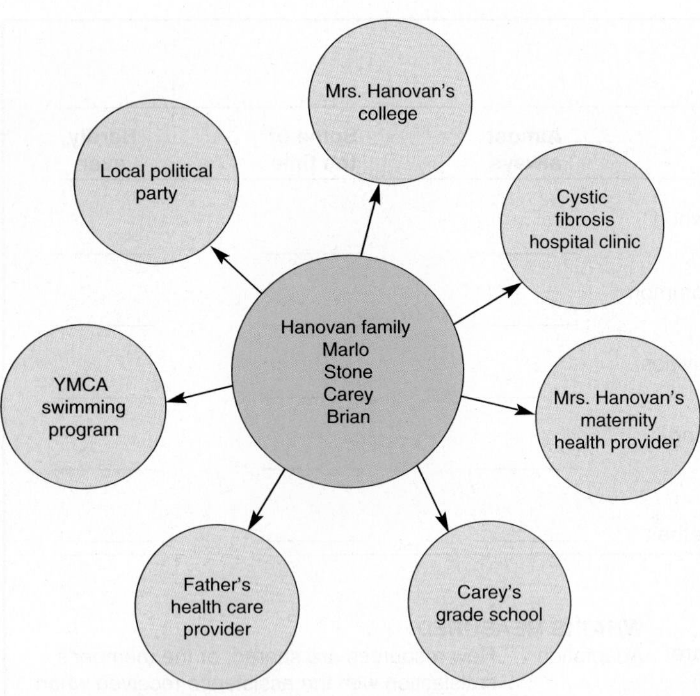

FIGURE 3.3 An ecomap of the Hanovan family's relationship to its community. The family members are shown in the center circle; the outer circles show community contacts.

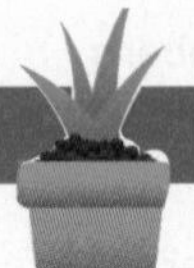

BOX 3.5 ✻ Focus on Nursing Care Planning

A Multidisciplinary Care Map for a Family With an Ill Child

Carey Hanovan is a 10-year-old child with cystic fibrosis. His mother tells you, "He's been acting out in school for the last month and doesn't always eat like he should, take his medicines, or do his treatments. He refuses to help around the house." Carey states, "Everybody's so busy, nobody has time for me. And I'm not like other kids. I'm always sick. Things will get even worse when the new baby comes."

Family Assessment ✻ Blended middle-class family that lives in an older three-bedroom home in the central city. Father is disabled from on-the-job accident; does not participate in community activities. Mother attends community college full-time with financial aid; is 5 months pregnant and active in local political party. Client is oldest child with one stepbrother, age 2 years. Mother swims weekly at the local YMCA; client refuses to go with her. Client is responsible for homework and cleaning kitchen after school while he is home alone. Client has few close friends. Two neighbors are available in case of emergency during his alone time.

Client Assessment ✻ Client's respiratory rate: 26 breaths per minute. Appears thin and pale. Productive cough with tenacious sputum. Medications last taken this morning. Lungs with fine bilateral rales.

Nursing Diagnosis ✻ Interrupted family processes related to effect of child's illness and situational stressors

Outcome Criteria ✻ Family demonstrates greater participation in family activities and positive methods of communication by 3 months' time. Client says he feels more family attachment and personal self-esteem by 3 months' time.

Team Member Responsible	Assessment	Intervention	Rationale	Expected Outcome
		Activities of Daily Living		
Nurse	Interview family regarding family structure and family roles.	Complete a family APGAR and genogram. Prioritize needs for each family member.	Family APGAR provides information about how families relate and interact. A genogram details family structure and roles. Priority setting promotes more focused, directed care for outcome achievement.	Family and health care providers complete a family APGAR and genogram with needs of family prioritized by next health-care visit.

Nurse	Help family explore and decide on a common activity enjoyed by all members.	Encourage participation in this activity, initially once a month, then twice a month, then weekly.	Participation in a group activity fosters bonding. Gradually increasing the frequency of the activity promotes integration into the family routine.	Client maintains a schedule documenting his participation at least once a week in a family activity.
		Consultations		
Nurse	Assess the number of contacts the family has in the community.	Draw and evaluate family's ecomap.	Ecomapping helps to assess the community support available to the family.	Ecomap reveals possible sources of community contacts that could serve as emotional support.
Social worker/ nurse	Assess what community agencies are available in the Hanovan family's community that could serve as additional sources of support.	Contact local community organizations with client and set up a visit. Possibly enlist the aid of the school nurse and guidance counselor in providing contacts.	Contacting the organization with the client offers support and helps reduce his possible anxiety with new situations. School personnel provide additional support and reassurance.	Client visits local or school agencies that provide community contacts.
		Procedures/Medications		
Nurse	Assess and list all of child's required exercises and medications.	Demonstrate exercise and medication procedures, if necessary, and have client return demonstration. Help client incorporate regimens into usual routine.	Review and redemonstration helps to reinforce measures and ensure client is doing them correctly. Incorporating them into client's routine helps to promote positive adjustment and decrease feelings of being different.	Client is able to redemonstrate procedures with 90% accuracy. Combines at least one exercise or medication with usual routine.
Nurse in conjunction with physical therapist	Help family assess which family member could serve as backup support for child's exercise and medication regimens.	Meet with family and plan a schedule that will allow a backup family member to supervise and participate in child's exercise and medication regimens.	Family involvement divides the responsibility and minimizes the risk of added stress on the family system.	Family members state that they cooperate with and encourage client to follow treatment regimen. Client says that he is adhering to treatment regimen 90% of time.
		Nutrition		
Nurse/ nutritionist	Assess nutrition needs based on medical prescriptions.	Review special diet needed by client with client and father (food preparer).	The food preparer needs to be as well informed about a special diet as the client.	Both client and father state that they understand that a special diet is necessary and describe a typical breakfast, lunch, and dinner for diet.
Nurse/ nutritionist	Assess family's eating habits.	Encourage family to eat together as a family unit at least two times a week.	Eating together should not only help client to comply with nutrition plan but provide a time for family sharing and communication.	Family reports they eat together at least twice a week or, if not possible, arrange for a substitute "sharing time."

(continued)

BOX 3.5 ✻ Focus on Nursing Care Planning (continued)

		Patient/Family Education		
Nurse	Assess client's present knowledge of his illness.	Review with client and parents an explanation of illness based on their present knowledge base.	Building on a client's knowledge base facilitates teaching and learning and minimizes repetition.	Client and family state that they understand the underlying cause of illness and rationale for treatments.
Nurse	Assess with client what a typical day consists of.	Brainstorm with client ways that he can "fit" into school routine better.	A feeling of "being different" can be detrimental to high self-esteem.	Client states that he has made at least one new friend by 2 months' time.
		Psychosocial/Spiritual/Emotional Needs		
Nurse	Help each family member identify the area of his or her greatest stress.	Help family members reduce stress by teaching better problem-solving techniques.	Identifying problems is the first step in effective problem solving.	Family members identify the greatest stressors in their family life and potential means to decrease stress.
Nurse	Assess stress-reducing measures currently being used.	Help family members develop strategies such as better time management to assist each other in meeting priority needs.	Use of therapeutic measures assists in clarifying family needs and expectations and also helps reduce stress.	Family members state that they are using strategies such as time management to better meet priorities.
		Discharge Planning		
Nurse	Meet with family to identify areas of needed support. Encourage family members to verbalize needs and feelings.	Help family identify a common activity enjoyed by all members that can be used to encourage family bonding. Encourage weekly participation in this activity.	Working together on a common task can foster group interaction, communication, trust, and bonding.	Family members state that they all participate in at least one enjoyable home activity by 2 months' time.
Nurse/case manager	Assess home rules and delegation of responsibilities.	Encourage joint cooperation in household tasks so client does not feel so isolated when home alone.	Joint ownership of household tasks encourages a sense of family.	Family members demonstrate they have a family schedule that evens out tasks and involves all members.
Nurse/case manager	Assess what resources are available in the Hanovans' community, such as the Cystic Fibrosis Foundation, that could be used as support resources.	Meet with family to see if members are interested in using any identified community organizations as resources.	Community resources provide additional support in areas of need.	Family members state that they have attended at least one Parents of Cystic Fibrosis Children meeting by 3 months' time.

colleagues (2000) suggest that assessing these factors is vital to predicting the probable extent of the crisis for the family. As a crisis can change a family's perceptions and the resources available to them, renewed assessment is necessary at the end of the crisis to see how the family has weathered the impact (a double ABCX model of assessment; Fig. 3.4).

To use this model, first assess what is the stressor (the event or transition that has the potential to influence the family's dynamics) and, then, how it is affecting the family. A house fire or illness of a family member is an example of a crisis situation. After identifying the stressor, assess the family's perception of the event. If the family states, for example,

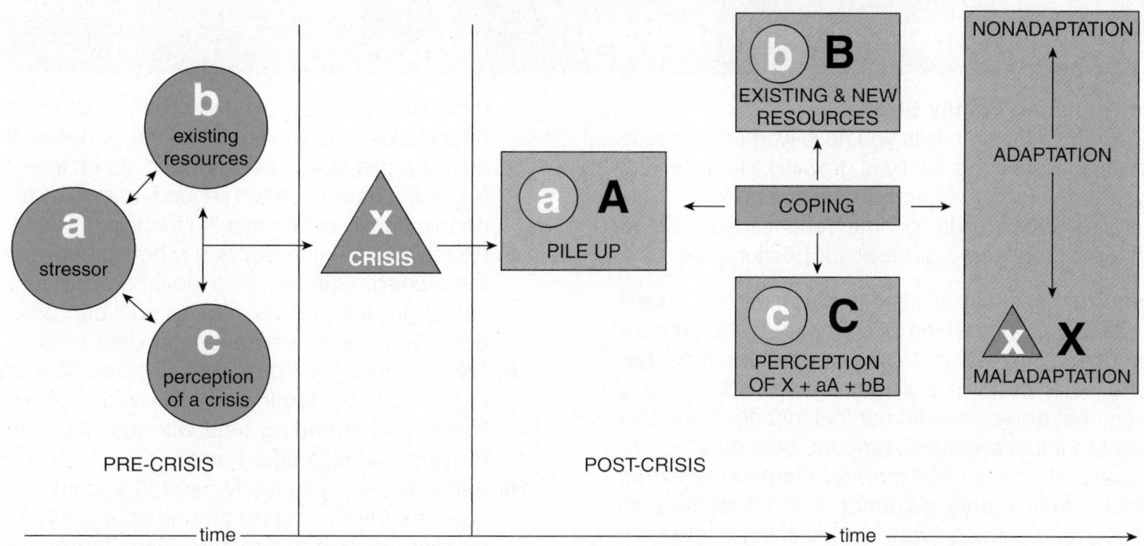

FIGURE 3.4 The ABCX System for Family Assessment. (From McCubbin, H. I., Thompson, E. A., Thompson, A. L., et al. [2000]. *The dynamics of resilient families.* Thousand Oaks, CA: Sage Publications.)

that they have adequate home or health insurance so the expense of replacing the house or a long hospitalization will be minimal, the stressor may have little effect. On the other hand, if they feel overwhelmed by the loss of their home and possessions or the strain of caring for someone so ill, the stressor is causing a major effect. The third step is to evaluate the resources available to the family, both internal and external. What are their challenges? What is the family type? What are their strengths? Do they have friends who can give them support? Do they belong to a church or temple that will help? Every family makes some kind of adjustment to a problem. What type of adjustment did they make? This adjustment and the resulting changed perception of the event reveal whether the family has weathered this event and may actually have become stronger or whether they need further assessment and guidance about steps to take.

This model is a useful one for family assessment, because it does not assume that just because a stressor happens, an automatic outcome will occur. It respects the individuality of families, an important factor to remember in family assessment.

Listing a family's strengths and coping abilities as well as its possible challenges actually strengthens a family as it brings out insights and better prepares family members to cope with their current level of stress and the difficult decisions that may be ahead. Box 3.6 provides practical suggestions to help families endure periods of stress.

What if... Your assessment of one child who is ready for hospital discharge shows that his family has multiple connections with the community, but the assessment of Carey and the Hanovan family shows only the hospital as a connection? Which family might need more discharge planning?

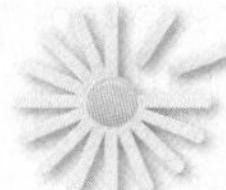

Key Points for Review

- A family is a group of people who share a common emotional bond and perform certain interrelated social tasks.
- Because families work as a unit, the unmet needs of any member can spread to become the unmet needs of all family members.
- Common types of families include nuclear, extended, single-parent, blended, cohabitation, single alliance, gay and lesbian, foster, and adopted families.
- Common family tasks are physical maintenance, socialization of family members, allocation of resources, maintenance of order, division of labor, reproduction, recruitment and release of members, placement of members into the larger society, and maintenance of motivation and morale.
- Common life stages of families are marriage; early childbearing; families with preschool, school-age, and adolescent children; launching stage; middle-years families; and the family in retirement.
- Changes in patterns of family life that are occurring are increased mobility, dual-parent employment, increased divorce, social problems such as abuse and poverty, reduced family size, and the addition of technology.
- Considering a family as a unit (a single client) helps in planning nursing care that meets the family's total needs.
- Families exist within communities; assessment of the community and the family's place in the community yields further information on family functioning and abilities.
- Families do not always function at their highest level during periods of crisis; reassessing them during a period of

BOX 3.6 ✻ Focus on Family Teaching

Tips for Reducing Family Stress

Q. Suppose Mr. Hanovan tells you he is worried because the tension level in his family is growing. He asks you, "How can my family better manage stress?"

A. Managing stress calls for interventions specific to each family, but some general suggestions are:

1. Recognize that stress levels differ from person to person. Because one person is not upset by some condition does not mean that another person will not be. On the other hand, if a situation does not annoy a person, that person should not feel that he or she has to react to it just because someone else does.
2. Anticipate life events and plan for them to the extent possible. Anticipatory guidance will not totally prepare you for a coming event but will at least serve notice that distress over the situation is normal.
3. Face a situation as honestly as possible. As a rule, knowing the exact nature of a threat is less stressful than a "something-is-out-there" feeling. On the other hand, do not feel compelled to face intense threats, such as a serious complication of pregnancy or a fatal illness in a child, until you have had time to mobilize your defenses, or you can feel overwhelmed.
4. Learn to change those things you cannot accept and accept those things you cannot change. Trial and error is often required to determine the difference.
5. Often a total change is unnecessary; a simple modification in one thing will be enough to make a difference.
6. Try to describe why you feel so stressed. Almost nothing limits the extent of a threat more than being able to describe it accurately. Detailing a problem is the beginning of problem solving.
7. Reach out for support. When you are under stress, it is easy to be so involved in the problem that you do not realize that people around you want to help. Sometimes people closest to you are under the same threat and so are no longer able to offer support. When this happens, you might have to call on second- or third-level support people (family or community) for help.
8. Reach out to give support when others are being threatened. Survival is a collaborative function of social groups; a favor offered now can be called in when you are in need at a later date.
9. Try to reduce the number of stressors that are coming at you by turning off television, dimming the lights, and spending time with just your inner self. Praying can also offer comfort.
10. Ask yourself if you really need to accomplish all the tasks that are piling up around you. Do you need to be room mother this month? Does the garage need to be cleaned this week?
11. Remember that unintentional injuries increase when people are under stress. A person worrying about a complication of pregnancy, for example, is more apt to have an automobile accident than a person who is stress free. Children are more apt to poison themselves when the family is under stress because parents are more apt to leave pills on counters during this time.
12. Action feels good during stress because doing something brings a sense of control over feelings of helplessness and disorganization. Action often is so satisfying that people do things such as write threatening letters or shout harmful remarks that they later regret. Channel your energy into therapeutic action (such as going for a long walk and quietly reflecting) instead.
13. Do not rush decisions or make final adaptive outcomes to a stressful situation. As a rule, major decisions should be delayed at least 6 weeks after an event; 6 months is even better.

stability may reveal a stronger family than appeared on first assessment.

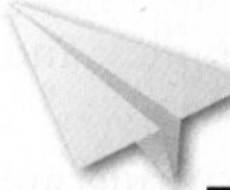

CRITICAL THINKING EXERCISES

1. You met the Hanovan family at the beginning of the chapter. Why is this a particularly unfortunate time for the Hanovans to have to choose between health care and groceries? Would their needs change if they were an extended family? A single-parent family? A cohabitation family?
2. The Hanovan family is a family under stress because of a poor financial base, a serious family illness, and limited family communication stemming from busy life roles. What other health care providers would it be helpful to include in a team approach for problem solving with this family?
3. As communities change, a family may find that it is the only family with children on a street or the only family who does not work at the local factory. What if you discovered the Hanovan family was "out of sync" with its community this way? How could you help such a family?
4. Examine the National Health Goals designed to improve the health of families. Most government-sponsored money for nursing research is allotted based on these goals. What would be a possible research topic to explore pertinent to these goals that would advance evidence-based practice in relation to the Hanovan family?

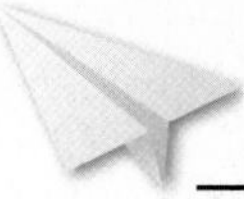

CRITICAL THINKING SCENARIO

Open the accompanying CD-ROM or visit http://thePoint.lww.com and read the Patient Scenario included for this chapter; then answer the questions to further sharpen your skills and grow more familiar with NCLEX types of questions related to family health. Confirm your answers are correct by reading the rationales.

REFERENCES

Ahrons, C. R. (2007). Family ties after divorce: long-term implications for children. *Family Process, 46*(1), 53–55.

Allender, J. A., & Spradley, B. W. (2008). *Community health nursing: Concepts and practice* (6th ed.). Philadelphia: Lippincott Williams & Wilkins.

Barlow, J., et al. (2007). Role of home visiting in improving parenting and health in families at risk of abuse and neglect: results of a multicentre randomised controlled trial and economic evaluation. *Archives of Disease in Childhood, 92*(3), 229–233.

Biagioli, F. E., et al. (2007). Managing overweight adolescents. *Contemporary Pediatrics, 24*(6), 37–43.

Bramlett, M. D., Radel, L. F., & Blumberg, S. J. (2007). The health and well-being of adopted children. *Pediatrics, 119*(Suppl 1), S54–S60.

Chen, M. Y., Shiao, Y. C., & Gau, Y. M. (2007). Comparison of adolescent health-related behavior in different family structures. *Journal of Nursing Research, 5*(1), 1–10.

Cherlin, A. J. (2008). *Public and private families.* New York: McGraw-Hill.

Clay, C. M., et al. Black women and white women: do perceptions of childhood family environment differ? *Family Process, 46*(2), 243–256.

Connor, A., et al. (2007). Increasing the delivery of health care services to migrant farm worker families through a community partnership model. *Public Health Nursing, 24*(4), 355–360.

Crea, T. M., Barth, R. P., & Chintapalli, L. K. (2007). Home study methods for evaluating prospective resource families. *Child Welfare, 86*(2), 141–160.

Cricco-Lizza, R. (2008). Voices from the battlefield: reports of the daily experiences of urban Black mothers. *Health Care for Women International, 29*(2), 115–134.

Crombleholme, W. R. (2009). Obstetrics. In S. J. McPhee & M. A. Papadakis (Eds.). *Current medical diagnosis & treatment.* Columbus, OH: McGraw-Hill.

Duvall, E. M., & Miller, B. (1990). *Marriage and family development.* Philadelphia: Lippincott Williams & Wilkins.

Elbedour, S., Bart, W., & Hektner, J. (2007). The relationship between monogamous/polygamous family structure and the mental health of bedouin Arab adolescents. *Journal of Adolescence, 30*(2), 213–230.

Fontenot, H. B. (2007). Transition and adaptation to adoptive motherhood. *JOGNN: Journal of Obstetric, Gynecologic, and Neonatal Nursing, 36*(2), 175–182.

Gable, S., Chang, Y., & Krull, J. L. (2007). Television watching and frequency of family meals are predictive of overweight onset and persistence in a national sample of school-aged children. *Journal of the American Dietetic Association, 107*(1), 53–61.

Gibson, M. A., & Mace, R. (2007). Polygyny, reproductive success and child health in rural Ethiopia. *Journal of Biosocial Science, 39*(2), 287–300.

Hellerstedt, W., et al. (2008). The International Adoption Project: population-based surveillance of Minnesota parents who adopted children internationally. *Maternal and Child Health Journal, 12*(2), 162–171.

Joly, L. (2007). Homeless women: trauma and abuse. *Primary Health Care, 17*(6), 34–35.

Kaushal, N., & Kaestner, R. (2007). Welfare reform and health of immigrant women and their children. *Journal of Immigrant & Minority Health, 9*(2), 61–74.

Kilanowski, J. F., & Ryan-Wenger, N. A. (2007). Health status in an invisible population: carnival and migrant worker children. *Western Journal of Nursing Research, 29*(1), 100–120.

McCubbin, H. I., et al. (2000). *The dynamics of resilient families.* Thousand Oaks, CA: Sage Publications.

National Center for Health Statistics (NCHS). (2009). *National Vital Statistics Reports, 58*(17), 9.

Ries, A. V., et al. (2008). Adolescent's perceptions of environmental influences on physical activity. *American Journal of Health Behavior, 32*(1), 26–39.

Risley-Curtiss, C., & Stites, B. (2007). Improving healthcare for children entering foster care. *Child Welfare, 86*(4),123–144.

Rubin, D. M., et al. (2007). The impact of placement stability on behavioral well-being for children in foster care. *Pediatrics, 119*(2), 336–344.

Shields, L., et al. (2009). Family-centered care for children in hospital. *Cochrane Database of Systematic Reviews, 2009*(1), (CD004811).

Short, L. (2007). Lesbian mothers living well in the context of heterosexism and discrimination: resources, strategies and legislative change. *Feminism & Psychology, 17*(1), 57–75.

Smilkstein, G. (1978). The family APGAR. *Journal of Family Practice, 6*(8), 1231.

Tischler, V., Rademeyer, A., & Vostanis, P. (2007). Mothers experiencing homelessness: mental health, support and social care needs. *Health and Social Care in the Community, 15*(3), 246–253.

Trost, S. G., Rosenkranz, R. R., & Dzewaltowski, D. (2008). Physical activity levels among children attending after-school programs. *Medicine and Science in Sports and Exercise, 40*(4), 622–629.

U.S. Census Bureau. (2009). *Statistical abstract of the United States.* Washington, DC: U.S. Department of Commerce.

Vandewater, E. A., et al. (2007). Digital childhood: electronic media and technology use among infants, toddlers, and preschoolers. *Pediatrics, 119*(5), e1006–e1015.

Wolak, J., Mitchell, K., & Finkelhor, D. (2007). Unwanted and wanted exposure to online pornography in a national sample of youth Internet users. *Pediatrics, 119*(2), 247–257.

Wolfgram, S. M. (2008). Openness in adoption: what we know so far—a critical review of the literature. *Social Work, 53*(2), 133–142.

SUGGESTED READINGS

Esperat, C., et al. (2007). Health behaviors of low-income pregnant minority women. *Western Journal of Nursing Research, 29*(3), 284–300.

Flaherty, E. G., et al. (2007). Effect of early childhood adversity on child health. *Archives of Pediatrics & Adolescent Medicine, 160*(12), 1232–1238.

Forsythe, P. L., et al. (2007). The long road home. SAFE discharge for infants with high-risk home environments. *Advances in Neonatal Care, 7*(2), 69–77.

Hall, W. A. (2007). Imposing order: a process to manage day-to-day activities in two-earner families with preschool children. *Journal of Family Nursing, 13*(1), 56–82.

Hoop, J. G., Smyth, A. C., & Roberts, L. W. (2008). Ethical issues in psychiatric research on children and adolescents. *Child & Adolescent Psychiatric Clinics of North America, 17*(1), 127–148.

Howard, K. R. (2007). Childhood overweight: parental perceptions and readiness for change. *Journal of School Nursing, 23*(2), 73–79.

Lee, P. (2007). Care and services for the unwell child in the community. *Primary Health Care, 17*(1), 41–46.

McClellan, C. B., & Cohen, L. L. (2007). Family functioning in children with chronic illness compared with healthy controls: a critical review. *Journal of Pediatrics, 150*(3), 221–223.

Piskosz, Z. (2007). One pediatric emergency department's successful approach to family-centered care. *Journal of Emergency Nursing, 33*(2), 169–171.

Thomas, R., et al. (2009). Family-based programmes for preventing smoking by children and adolescents. *Cochrane Database of Systematic Reviews, 2009*(1), (CD004493).

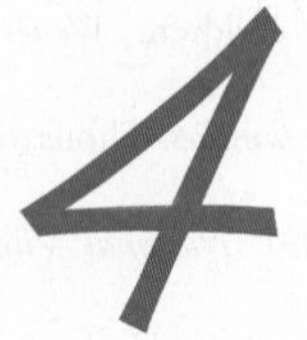

Chapter 4 The Childbearing and Childrearing Family in the Community

KEY TERMS

- community
- direct care
- home care
- hospice care
- indirect care
- perinatal home care
- skilled home nursing care

OBJECTIVES

After mastering the contents of this chapter, you should be able to:

1. Describe a healthy community and usual nursing and client concerns when home care is required during pregnancy or childhood.
2. Identify National Health Goals related to home care during pregnancy or childhood that nurses can help the nation achieve.
3. Use critical thinking to analyze how home care influences family functioning, and develop ways to make home nursing care more family centered.
4. Assess a pregnant woman or child and their community for likely success for home care.
5. Formulate nursing diagnoses related to care of a child or pregnant client at home.
6. Identify expected outcomes for a family requiring home care.
7. Plan nursing care appropriate to meet the needs of a home care client such as suggesting ways to keep in contact with significant others.
8. Implement nursing care to meet the needs of a pregnant woman or child on home care such as teaching techniques of intravenous therapy.
9. Evaluate expected outcomes for effectiveness and achievement of care.
10. Identify areas of home care nursing that could benefit from additional nursing research or application of evidence-based practice.
11. Integrate knowledge of home care with nursing process to achieve quality maternal and child health nursing care.

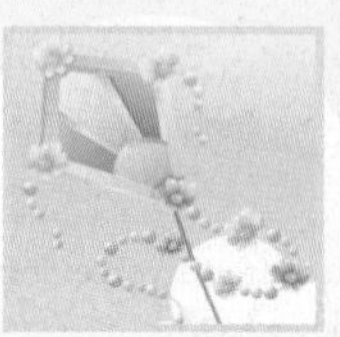

Lee Puente, a 16-year-old who is 20 weeks pregnant, lives with her parents. She was admitted to the hospital for 3 days at 14 weeks of her pregnancy and placed on a program of total parenteral nutrition because she has been vomiting at least four times daily since the beginning of pregnancy. She managed well on parenteral nutrition until last week, when her blood pressure rose to 160/90 mm Hg and she was diagnosed with hypertension of pregnancy. Bed rest with fetal and uterine surveillance at home was added to her care. She tells you it's impossible for her to rest at home: she's bored and wants to be back in school with her friends. She has missed three doses of her hypotensive agent because she forgot to take them. She wants to be hospitalized again for care.

Previous chapters discussed common types of families and how cultural traditions affect families. This chapter adds information about families and their community as they prepare to care for an ill family member at home.

Is Lee a good candidate for home care? What additional interventions does she need to help make home care more successful?

Home care is care of persons in their own home, provided by or supervised through a certified home health care or community health care agency. In recent years, as hospital stays have decreased in length, the need for home rehabilitation periods of this type has grown substantially.

Acute care or postsurgical clients often need follow-up home visits. Pregnant women with conditions that require monitoring and bed rest but not critical care can also be cared for at home. Children with chronic conditions such as bronchial pulmonary dysphasia, cystic fibrosis, and childhood cancer are cared for at home rather than in hospital settings when at all possible so they are not separated from their family. Many children in terminal stages of disease are also cared for at home (**hospice care**).

There is a strong economic incentive to provide care in the home (it is less costly for health care plans). Several factors have contributed to the success of the home as a health care setting. Technological advances have made it possible for potentially complicated procedures, such as the administration of total parenteral nutrition and ventilation therapy, to be performed safely at home. Perhaps the greatest benefit of home care for women and children is the opportunity it brings to include the entire family in health care planning and the ability to focus not only on a specific health problem but also on promoting healthy behaviors for the entire family (Pignone & Salazar, 2009).

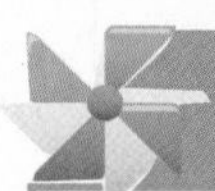

BOX 4.1 ✻ Focus on National Health Goals

National Health Goals are concerned with eliminating common infectious diseases of childhood and reducing complications of pregnancy both by encouraging better adherence to immunization programs for children and by better monitoring and preventing complications during pregnancy.

Both prevention of common childhood infectious illnesses and pregnancy complications would reduce the hours spent in home care. Examples of National Health Goals that speak to this area of concern are:

- Increase to at least 90% the proportion of all pregnant women who receive early and adequate prenatal care, from a baseline of 74%.
- Reduce the rate of preterm births, from a baseline of 11% to a target of 7.6%.
- Reduce or eliminate indigenous cases of vaccine-preventable diseases such as mumps, poliomyelitis, and diphtheria (http://www.nih.gov).

Nurses can help the nation achieve these goals by helping women better accept and adhere to home care if it is advised during pregnancy. They can remind parents that routine immunizations for children are important. Nursing research topics to address in this area are: What are the most effective ways to relieve a woman's anxiety about home care? What is the ideal frequency for home visits? When nursing care time is included in costs, is home care cost-effective? What is a good reminder system to help parents schedule immunization visits on time?

Whether home care is successful can be influenced by cultural expectations, especially male–female roles. In a family in which men and women share responsibility, for example, care tasks as well as time away from the stress of home care can be distributed equally. In contrast, in cultures in which the male is dominant and child care is strictly delegated to the woman, women can become exhausted from trying to keep house, prepare meals, care for other children, and also care for themselves or a medically fragile child.

Evaluating families individually is important to see what the family's usual childrearing practices are as well as how care is given during illness.

It is well documented that women who receive prenatal care have better pregnancy outcomes than those who do not (Bernstein & Weinstein, 2007). Because home care can be a means of increasing prenatal care, especially in the areas of additional health teaching and monitoring, National Health Goals that speak to prenatal and child care also apply to home care (Box 4.1).

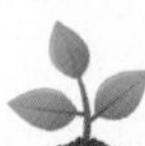

Nursing Process Overview

For the Pregnant Woman or Child on Home Care

Assessment

Being able to assess communities becomes more and more important as, because of personal preferences or short hospital stays, more children spend time at home recuperating from illnesses than ever before. Fewer pregnant women with a complication of pregnancy are hospitalized and are also using home care. Most women and children who will be scheduled for home care are first seen in an ambulatory health care setting or an acute care facility for initial diagnosis and then discharged from that facility with a referral to a home care program.

Home care is not a level of care adequate for everyone or every situation, so evaluating whether a family is a good candidate for home care is the first assessment needed. Figure 4.1 shows a typical assessment tool used to qualify women for home care. Using this tool, women or children can be divided into three levels of care based on the identification of factors, both physical and psychosocial, that may affect care and final outcome. Those categorized as low risk (level I) probably need only weekly visits; those at intermediate risk (level II), one to three visits per week; and those at high risk (level III), as many as four to seven visits per week. Both women and children need to be reevaluated about every 30 days to see if their risk level, and therefore the number of home visits needed, has changed.

Assessment for home care begins with an interview to identify ways a family thinks the illness and care at home will change their lives. This could include a wide range of situations such as increased expenses, the need for one parent to take a leave from work to care for an ill child or spouse at home, the need to schedule frequent ambulatory visits, consultation to handle body image changes, and the need to arrange for child care for other children. Because these needs change as the course of an illness changes, assessment must be ongoing.

A first home visit usually includes a thorough health history and physical examination to document a woman's

(text continues on page 65)

Client Data

Client's name ______

Nickname ______

Client's DOB ___/___/___ Client's Age ______

Client's ins. type & no. ______

Client's SS no. ______

Client's race ___ White ___ Black

___ Hispanic ___ Other

EDC ______ Weeks gestation ______

Primary language ______

___ Home ___ Shelter ___ Homeless

___ Staying with relatives

Current residence address:

______
Street

______
City Zip

Phone ______

Best time to contact ______

Diagnoses

1. ______

2. ______

3. ______

Emergency Contact Person/s

Name ______
Age

Relationship ______

Phone ______

Address ______
Street

______
City Zip

Doctor (must use PCP if applicable)

Name ______

Hospital ______

Phone ______

Address ______
Street

______
City Zip

Consulting Doctors on Care

Phone ______

1. ______

2. ______

3. ______

Other consultants:

1. SW ______

2. other ______

Exacerbating potentials:

______

1. Planned hospital for delivery ______

2. History of prenatal care this pregnancy ______

3. Planned delivery:

Vaginal C-section

______

I. Prior OB history: G ______ P ______

FIGURE 4.1 A perinatal home needs assessment tool.

PIH __________ GDM __________ IDDM __________ Eclampsia __________

No. of children living with her, and their ages: ____________________

____

Any children in foster care, or living elsewhere: ____________________

____

____

II. Current State of Health:

1. Physical
2. Mental
3. Emotional
4. Social
5. Hospitalizations/Surgeries
6. Diet/Nutrition/weight prior to pregnancy; weight gain so far
7. Activity
8. Physical limitations
9. Support systems
10. Limitations
11. Medications—Time, Frequency, Amount, Purpose, Side effects
12. Teaching Needed

___ Transportation ___ Self-treatment

___ Changes during pregnancy

___ Nutrition ___ Home Safety ___ Community Resources

___ utilities

___ phone

___ housing

___ cooking

___ water

___ respite

___ ref.

___ others

___ Growth/Dev.

___ Parenting Education

___ Budgeting of financial resources

___ Parenting skills ___ Parenting education

___ Gestational diabetes ___ Premature labor

___ Rupture of membranes ___ Signs/Symptoms of Labor

13. Referrals already made: ____________________

14. Referrals needed: ____________________

___ WIC ___ Wheels

____

FIGURE 4.1 *(continued)*

IV. Family Data/Support Network:
1. Other household members (name, age, medical issues)
2. Other significant others/extended family members
   Are they available to assist with care of child—when delivered?
3. Summary of household function—Do people work together?
   Do they get along? Who is in charge?
4. Evidence of drug/ETOH use
5. Smoker

Housing Information

1. Current residence __ Permanent __ Temporary
2. Type of residence __ House __ Apt. __ Shelter __ Other explain ____________
3. Length of time in current residence ____________
4. Are there Plans to Move? __ Yes __ No __ When? ____________
   New Address: ____________
5. Layout of House:
   no. of bedrooms ____ no. of bathrooms ____
   __ Kitchen __ Dining area __ Living area __ Furniture
   Condition of House: ____________
   Safety Issues at House:
   Outlets: __ 2 Prong __ 3 Prong __ Adeq. nos.
   __ Inadeq. nos.
   Smoke alarms: __ Yes __ No no. of alarms: ____________
   Stable railings: __ Yes __ No
   Adequate lighting: __ Yes __ No (specify)
   Emergency nos. Posted: __ Yes __ No
   Sanitation: no. of Bathrooms: __
   A. Is kitchen sanitary? __ Yes __ No (specify)
   B. Pest Control: Are the following present:
      __ Roaches __ Rats/Mice __ Flies
   C. Plumbing problems ____________
      Medication storage: Specify plan for storage, if refrigeration needed
      Infection control needs surrounding care:
      Summary of client home needs assessment
      ____
      Problem list—Preliminary
      ____
      Plan

FIGURE 4.1 *(continued)*

or child's current status and an environmental, community, and social assessment. Other assessments focus on likely adherence to medical, preventive, or medication regimens; whether the family will be able to continue to monitor the client's health at home; and what other services or resources the family needs such as the services of a home health care assistant or further nursing visits to ensure that home care is optimal. Future visits focus on continuing assessment and evaluation of patient progress and readiness to move to another level of health care.

The term "resources" refers not only to material objects (e.g., hospital bed, oxygen, fetal home monitor) but also to whether a family can deal with the chronic stress of home care. Women often have to quit work to become home care patients. One parent of an ill child usually has to do the same. This can reduce a family's income dramatically and cause financial problems. Environmental considerations also can add to the stress of the situation. Assess if the home's physical surroundings are adequate for home care. Is there enough floor space for a hospital bed? Is there space for a fetal heart monitor or oxygen equipment? Is there a telephone that can be reached by the pregnant woman or child? Is there adequate heat or air conditioning so an ill person can be comfortable?

Typically, women receiving care are taught how to self-assess various health parameters such as blood pressure, temperature, pulse, perhaps urine for protein or glucose, fundal height, fetal movement, fetal heart rate, and uterine contractions in preparation for home care. Parents or other family members of an ill child need to assess vital signs, comfort level, and side effects of medications. When teaching these assessments, spend enough time with the woman or family to assess the learning capabilities of the family so you know they thoroughly understand both the reason for the assessment and the priority procedures necessary for care. Assess at home care visits not only the results of the measurements but whether they are being done correctly and consistently.

Because the structure of families is culturally determined, home care is easier for some families than for others. If the family is extended, for example, a mother may be so involved in the care of other family members, such as an older adult, that she is unable to rest adequately at home or add enough time to care for an ill child to her other responsibilities. On the other hand, in such a family, there may be many people to offer care and support, so home care will be ideal.

In male-dominant cultures, the thought of the man giving care to his wife or an ill child contradicts a usual pattern. If a woman is the dominant member of the household, becoming a passive, cared-for partner may be extremely difficult for her.

Some cultures stress that women must be active during pregnancy to help ensure a small baby and therefore an easier birth. That makes bed rest difficult for a family to enforce. The culture of a particular community might oppose the use of technology, so a family living there might not like having a van come to supply needed oxygen or intravenous equipment. Assess each family individually to determine how home care may affect that particular family.

Nursing Diagnosis

Nursing diagnoses for home care may address the physiologic reason for supervised home care or the effect of the experience on the family, such as:

- Deficient knowledge related to complication of pregnancy and necessary procedures and treatments
- Interrupted family processes related to need for home care
- Ineffective role performance related to bed rest at home
- Social isolation related to need for home care
- Anxiety related to complication of pregnancy requiring home care

Home care of a child can place a heavy burden on a family. The stress of being responsible for an ill child's daily health status can have a negative impact on a parent's self-esteem or a couple's marriage, or it can prevent parents from spending time with their other children. Examples of possible nursing diagnoses that arise out of these factors are:

- Readiness for enhanced family coping related to increased time together because of home care
- Health-seeking behaviors related to skills needed to continue home care
- Risk for delayed growth and development related to lack of usual childhood activities
- Interrupted family processes related to dependence of ill child
- Disabled family coping related to changes in family routine brought about by home care needs of ill child

Outcome Identification and Planning

Outcome identification and planning for home care require close collaboration between a health care agency and health care providers supervising care at home. Typically, the initial referral from the health care agency provides the foundation from which the home care or community health nurse develops a plan of care. A major portion of this planning involves reviewing with a family exactly what their needs are, what will be expected of them, and what they can expect of the nurse and developing outcomes that address these needs and expectations such as extending the length of the pregnancy or increasing the comfort of a child on home care. If this is not carefully done, some families will assume that not going outside the home is all that is required by home care, when what is actually required is complete bed rest. "Walking through a day" helps a family determine at what points during the day they will need additional assistance so the pregnant woman or ill child can remain in bed at home. For example, a woman on bed rest may need assistance with meal preparation or hygiene while her partner is at work. In this situation, a referral for a home health assistant would probably be appropriate. She also may need help with transporting her children to school or activities. Discussing these issues with her helps her call on resources such as other family members, neighbors, or community volunteer groups.

Children need to continue with school if at all possible so they maintain contact with friends, do not fall behind a grade level, and have the stimulation of learning. This means parents must either make some sort of arrangement for this through their local school district (many schools are able to establish a telecommunication setup for children ill at home) or investigate their ability to home school the child.

Determining family roles (see Chapter 3), such as who is the wage earner, the decision maker, the nurturer, or the problem solver, is important for planning. Home care is most successful when these family roles are not disrupted but strengthened to support whatever new activities or concerns need to be addressed. Good Internet referral sites for families regarding come care are The International Association for Hospice & Palliative Care (http://www.hospicecare.com) and The National Association of Home Care and Hospice (http://www.nahc.org).

Implementation

Women and children receiving home care have the advantage over those hospitalized of being in their own environment with their families. Because home care provides only intermittent visits, however, there is the possible disadvantage of not being constantly supervised by health care personnel. Reassure women and children after assessment that their condition has not changed and it is safe for them to remain at home on the present program, assuming that is true. If changes have occurred, introduce new interventions and evaluate their effectiveness.

Interventions performed for a client at home are little different from those performed in an acute care facility. They range from teaching and counseling to hands-on care. To do this, home care nurses need to have the same background and level of expertise as acute care nurses. In addition, they may need to be more flexible and adaptable because each home visit may be very different from the one just before or after.

Nursing interventions for home care often involve teaching family members how to give care. This may include encouraging members to voice the frustration they feel at being constantly confined at home or what they perceive to be a lack of progress in their child's or partner's condition. If a child has a terminal illness, parents may need support to express their grief. They can grow discouraged because the work they are accomplishing is making the child comfortable but not preventing death.

Outcome Evaluation

Because a home setting is less structured than a health care facility, evaluation will show that some goals for care are more difficult to accomplish in the home. For the same reason, because there is more room for innovation at home, some goals will be more easily accomplished. Evaluation may reveal that circumstances have changed such as the client's condition requiring more monitoring than originally believed, the demands are greater than the family is willing to undertake, or family composition changes, making a responsible caregiver no longer available.

Outcome evaluation for the pregnant woman receiving home care includes determining whether a woman and fetus are remaining well at home and whether a woman feels comfortable and secure with the arrangement. For many women, successful home care can mean the difference between too early a birth and a successful term pregnancy.

Examples of outcome criteria for pregnant women could include:

- Client demonstrates adequate skill at performing home monitoring procedures.
- Client verbalizes changes in condition she will need to report to her health care provider.
- Client participates as a member of the family within limitations imposed by pregnancy complication.
- Family members state they have adjusted to home care of mother.
- Client states she is able to maintain contact with friends and family despite complete bed rest at home.

Examples of outcome criteria for an ill child might include:

- Parents state they have been able to make adjustments to accommodate care of ill child at home.
- Child states he or she enjoys respite care in hospice setting one weekend a month.
- Parents state they are actively trying to supply adequate growth experiences for siblings in light of home care of oldest child.

THE FAMILY AS PART OF A COMMUNITY

Families rarely live alone on islands, so they have to interact with a surrounding community to get food, use transportation, and receive wages for work (Monsen & Finley, 2007). A **community** can be defined in many ways, but it is generally accepted to refer to a limited geographic area in which the residents relate to and interact among themselves (Allender & Spradley, 2008). When asked what community they are from, people may mention an entire city, a school district, a geographic district ("the East Side"), a street name ("Pine Street area"), or a natural marking ("the Lower Creek area").

Because the health of individuals is influenced by the health of their community, it is important to become acquainted with the community in which you practice. Community assessment can reveal if there are aspects about a community that contributed to an illness (and therefore need to be corrected) and determine whether the person will be able to return to the community without extra help and counseling after recovering from an illness.

Knowing the individual aspects of families or a community can help you understand why some people reach the illness level they do before they come for health care (e.g., a woman has no transportation available to her until her husband comes home from work so this prevents her from coming for daytime prenatal care; a 5-year-old child develops measles because there are no free immunization services in the community).

Community assessment consists of examining the various systems that are present in almost all communities to see whether they are functioning adequately as well as features that are unique to a client's community (Conway, McClune, & Nosel, 2007). It is easier for you to prepare a woman or child for return to a community after childbirth or a hospital stay if, for example, you know the specific features of their community (Does the Pine Street area have well or city water? How many flights of stairs does someone from the

TABLE 4.1 ✻ Community Assessment

Area of Assessment	Questions to Ask
Age span	Is the family within the usual age span of the community and thereby assured of support people? Is the community a "young," a "settled-in," or a "retired" one? Is it at the same stage as the family?
Education	If the family has school-age children, are there schools nearby? Is there a public library for self-education? Is there easy access to such places if the person becomes physically challenged? If a special program such as diet counseling is needed, does it exist?
Environment	Are environmental risks present, such as air pollution? Busy highways? Train yards? Pools of water where drowning could occur? Could hypothermia be a problem?
Financial status	Is there a high rate of unemployment in the community? What is the average occupation? Will this family have adequate finances to manage comfortably in this neighborhood? Are supplemental aid programs available?
Health care	Is there a health care agency the family can use for comprehensive care? Is it convenient, in terms of finances and time?
Housing	Are houses primarily privately owned or apartments? Are homes close enough together to afford easy contact? Are they in good repair? Will new construction or deteriorated housing be a safety problem?
Political	Is the community active politically? Can adults reach a local polling place to vote, or do they know how to apply for absentee ballots?
Recreational	Are recreational activities of interest available? Are they economically feasible?
Religion	Is there a facility where the family can worship as they choose? Is there easy transportation to it?
Safety	Is there adequate protection so family members can feel safe to leave home or remain home alone? Do they know about available hotlines and local police and fire department numbers? Are there smoke alarms in the bedrooms and near the kitchen?
Sociocultural	What is the dominant culture in the community? Does the family fit into this environment? Are foods that are culturally significant available?
Transportation	Is there public transportation? Will family members have access to it if they become physically challenged?

Stevens Plaza area have to walk to reach an apartment? Is there public transportation so the mother can take her toddler for emergent care?). Table 4.1 summarizes areas to examine in community assessment. Drawing an ecomap or a diagram of a family's relationship to their community (see Chapter 3, Fig. 3.3) can help identify what community contacts are available for a family. Different communities may or may not have resources for families with special needs such as home physical therapists or occupational therapists to assist children whose growth or development is delayed.

HOME CARE

Home care providers work out of agencies that can be either freestanding or allied with a health care facility. Specialized services such as providing supplies for total parenteral nutrition, fetal monitoring, or laboratory analysis may be furnished by special service companies. Voluntary agencies often provide services such as transportation to and from health care agency assessments or respite care so parents can have time free from continual care (Yantzi, Rosenberg, & McKeever, 2007).

In some settings, telephone contacts and e-mail and chat room contacts are used to link health care providers with families during home care. In many instances, nurses need to be assertive enough to help a family secure adequate funding and resources for home care.

Perinatal home care is care of pregnant women in their homes. Many public health departments have maternal–newborn projects that provide home care this way during pregnancy, allowing women to maintain contact with their families rather than being hospitalized for long periods and provide psychological and social support as well as aspects of medical care (Roman et al., 2007).

Care at home may include **direct care,** in which a nurse remains in continual attendance or visits frequently and actually administers care, or **indirect care,** in which a nurse plans and supervises care given by others, such as home care assistants.

Nursing care is considered **skilled home nursing care** if it includes physician-prescribed procedures such as dressing changes, administration of medication, health teaching, or observation of a woman or child's progress or status through such activities as monitoring vital signs or fetal heart rate. Whether nursing care is categorized as skilled or not can determine whether it will be paid for by third-party reimbursement.

Home care is most successful if there are effective support people from the family or community to offer help. Otherwise, both women and children can experience such loneliness and low self-esteem that it interferes with their ability to remain on continuous bed rest or continue with a medical regimen.

It works best when a family is strongly committed to home care and well prepared to cooperate with health care providers. Pregnant women with complications such as preterm labor that has been halted, hyperemesis gravidarum (excessive nausea and vomiting of pregnancy), and hypertension of pregnancy are examples of pregnant women usually able to remain at home with supervision and periodic visits by a community or home care nurse. Frequent home visits are also helpful to monitor the health of newborns who were born with low birthweights or who arrived prematurely (Donovan et al., 2007). Although it is not well documented that bed rest prolongs such pregnancies, women with multiple pregnancies may be another example (Crowther, 2009).

Low birthweight occurs in newborns when preterm labor begins early and cannot be halted. In other women, labor can be halted but the woman needs careful monitoring for the rest of her pregnancy to be certain that the fetus is doing well in utero and labor is not beginning again. Nurses can be instrumental in seeing that women who are candidates for monitoring at home receive enough orientation and support that they are able to remain on home care and possibly prevent low birthweight. They can also be influential in seeing that time spent during home care is not wasted time but a time of preparation for birth and childrearing.

There may be an advantage of placing women with premature ruptured membranes on home care rather than hospital care because of the decreased exposure to infection in their own homes compared to hospitals. Children with chronic illnesses who need monitoring but not critical care are equally good candidates. It is possible that having a caring person such as a community health nurse visit frequently and take an interest in a family could have long-term effects, such as lowering the incidence of child abuse and child injury (Barlow et al., 2007).

Among the advantages of home care for a family are:

- It prevents extensive disruption of the family unit. For children who are acutely but not terminally ill, this extra emotional support may not be as immediately important as physical care. For those who are chronically ill or dying, being close to their family and friends may be the most important aspect of their care. For these children, home care is ideal (Tuffrey, Finlay, & Lewis, 2007).
- It can increase a woman's or child's self-confidence because it allows for more self-care and often more control of circumstances.
- Families can be better assessed in their own environment than in an agency, because family interactions, values, and priorities are more obvious than in a health care setting.
- Home visits provide a private, one-on-one opportunity for health teaching.
- Home care can reduce the cost of care when monitoring is the main type of care necessary.

In most instances, it is less costly to the health care delivery system to care for pregnant women or children at home rather than in a hospital setting because the number of health care personnel needed is so reduced. Cost containment, however, has to be weighed against the safety and quality of care. Not all home settings are safe for care and not all families have the commitment necessary, so it is not an alternative for all families. In addition, although home care is cost-effective for health care agencies, it may not be cost-effective for the family. Costs that health insurance would have paid for, such as dressings and medications, for example, had the client been hospitalized may no longer be covered once the person is transferred to home care.

Disadvantages of home care can be:

- It can actually increase the cost for an individual family if the family's insurance does not cover the cost of nursing visits or necessary supplies.
- It can cause increased anxiety and concern because pregnant women or family members are asked to assume a much greater responsibility for monitoring their own or a child's condition.
- The physical care required (e.g., tracheal suctioning or a complicated medication regimen) can be overwhelming for family caregivers.
- The financial strain of at least one parent or a spouse having to quit work and, therefore, not earning an income can cause a great financial strain on a family.
- Bed rest at home can cause social isolation and the disruption of normal family life.

Orienting families to home care, making home visits, supervising and coordinating home health personnel, providing health teaching in relation to pregnancy and childrearing, and evaluating whether home care remains appropriate are all important nursing responsibilities.

BEGINNING HOME CARE

Discharge planners in acute care settings can be instrumental in setting the stage for home care by discussing the need for continued health supervision with families and helping them begin establishing personal goals for home care. Several steps are then necessary for the actual home visit to be successful. These steps can be divided into previsit, visit, and postvisit phases.

Preparing for a Home Visit

Typically, a first home visit is made within 24 hours of discharge from an acute care facility or after notice from the ambulatory care facility. Be certain to obtain a copy of the client's referral form to familiarize yourself with the treatment course and plan of care. Obtain any supplies that may be needed for the visit. Keep in mind that you are going to be a guest in the client's home, so respect for the client's and family's privacy, beliefs, lifestyles, routines, culture, and requests is crucial.

As a part of individualizing care, make a telephone call to a client or family in advance to arrange a time for a visit so it will be convenient for the client and the fam-

BOX 4.2 ✻ Safety Tips for Home Health Care Travel and Visits

- Plan your trip in advance using a reliable map of the area so you do not become lost in a strange neighborhood.
- Let someone know where you are going and when you expect to return.
- Keep your automobile in good repair and filled with gasoline so you can avoid having to make stops at unfamiliar service stations.
- Park your car in a well-lighted, busy area. Lock the car door.
- Do not leave valuable objects such as an expensive CD player in your car, so it is not a target for car thieves.
- Lock any valuables in the trunk of your car *before* you leave the health care agency, not after you park in front of a home to visit, so no one sees you do this.
- Learn the location of public telephones in the area, or keep a cellular phone with you.
- If you suspect that someone is following you in your car, drive to the nearest police or fire station.
- If you suspect that someone is following you while you are walking, walk into a business establishment.
- Do not carry a purse or backpack that suggests you are carrying a large sum of money or drugs or valuables.
- Carry only minimal supplies so your hands are free to defend yourself.
- Drive or walk on main or busy streets; avoid shortcuts through alleys or unoccupied areas.
- Avoid approaching homes by a dark back alley; use the front door or a busy hallway.
- Use special caution in stairwells and elevators. Leave a stairwell or elevator if a potentially threatening person enters, with an excuse such as, "I've forgotten my red pen."
- Walk determinedly, as if you have a purpose and are in charge of your environment and situation.
- When you first enter a home, assess it for personal safety. Ask who is at home. If there are animals in the house, ask if they are friendly.
- If there are animals, take precautions to avoid getting flea bites (sit on a kitchen chair, not an upholstered chair).
- Be cautious about accepting food or drink if you are not certain about the hygiene of the dishes or food. Decline it gracefully with an excuse such as, "I'm trying to cut down on the amount of coffee I drink," or "It's against my agency's rules."
- Have your car keys in your hand when you leave the house so you can unlock and enter your car quickly.
- Look under your car when approaching it and in the back seat before entering it to be certain no one is there. Relock your car door immediately once inside.
- Leave a home immediately if you feel threatened or unsafe.
- If both you and the client are in personal danger, call the community emergency number, such as 911, for help.

ily. Obtain necessary instructions to reach the home. To avoid disrupting family routines, try not to visit at mealtime unless observing what a client is eating for a typical meal is necessary for assessment. Keep in mind that the ethical and legal aspects of nursing care, such as confidentiality, informed consent, decision making, and client rights, commonly associated with acute care nursing are also applicable to home care. Remember this especially when transporting a chart or notes or when discussing the visit with others.

Ensuring Personal Safety

Because home care visits are often made alone, take measures to ensure your personal safety on the way to a client's home, during a visit, and afterward. Safety tips for traveling in an unfamiliar community are shown in Box 4.2.

✔ Checkpoint Question 4.1

You need to schedule a first home visit for Lee Puente following a hospital stay. When is a first home-care visit typically made?

a. Within 1 hour after discharge
b. Within 24 hours after discharge
c. Within 4 days after discharge
d. Within 1 week of discharge

Making the Visit

Depending on the location of a client's home, the facilities and resources available may vary. The setting also varies from a house, apartment, mobile home, or shelter. On arrival at a client's home, knock or ring the bell and wait for someone to let you in. Greet the client and any other family members present. Greet family pets if they come to greet you (but do not pet strange dogs). Dogs typically serve a guard function, and you want them to view you as a friendly, not a threatening, visitor. Sometimes special advance arrangements, such as having a neighbor let you in, may be necessary if a woman lives alone and cannot walk down a stairway or a long hallway to answer the door.

As in any health care setting, wash your hands before touching a client for assessment, and follow standard infection precautions while giving care. Many home care nurses carry liquid soap and paper towels or disposable wipes with them for handwashing if the facilities in a home are inconvenient or unavailable.

What if... Lee Puente's family lives in a trailer park? Their nearest neighbor stops you every time you visit to ask you how Lee is doing. How would you answer her?

Assessing the Client

Typically, on a first home visit, a thorough health assessment is necessary, including a health history and physical examination, as well as evaluation of the social environment, medications, nutrition, safety, and adherence to treatment this far. In addition, a consent for treatment and release of information form may need to be signed (Fig. 4.2).

Provide privacy and confidentiality when obtaining the health history and performing a physical examination. At all times, despite the informality of the setting, good interviewing and physical assessment skills are important (Box 4.3). Some homes may be too cool early in the morning for physical assessment because the heat has been turned down during the night. Arranging for a visit later in the day alleviates this problem. If a home has few rooms, finding a private location can be difficult. Be certain to include assessment not only of physical aspects but of mental or psychosocial ones as well to detect depression, which can occur out of worry or loneliness (Secco et al., 2007). Families receiving home care are usually anxious to have a nurse confirm that they are well and that the self-assessments they have been making have been accurate. Throughout the assessment, evaluate the client's needs and provide instructions and reinforcement about any specific areas that are necessary.

If bed rest is required, ask how women or children occupy their time. A woman is not really resting if she is concerned about her family or finances, is caring for older children, or is bored. Children are not really resting if they are sitting up playing active video games.

Before leaving, be certain to evaluate the family's understanding of the illness and what danger signs to report immediately if they should occur. Be certain that the family has a means of obtaining refills on prescriptions and knows what measures to take if the woman's or child's condition should worsen, such as calling 911, the hospital, or a primary care provider. Many clients or families feel more comfortable calling the home care agency rather than the primary care provider's office if the agency has nurses on call around the clock. The nurse on call can then help the client determine what action would be best to take.

As a final check, be certain that families know what their responsibilities will be, when home care personnel will visit again, any modifications of their home that need to be made, the dates and times of return visits to a health care facility, and whether they have transportation for these visits.

Client Name: ____________________

Address: ____________________

City: __________ State: __________ Zip: __________ Phone: (   ) __________
Insurance Company: ____________________ Insurance I.D.#

I, the ____________________ (of the patient), intending to be legally bound, hereby:

1. Consent to such care and treatment by ____________________, and its employees and agents (collectively, the "Agency"), as prescribed by the client's physician or dictated by the client's condition.
2. Authorize the Agency to release any medical records in its possession concerning the client as may be required by law or to pay benefits on the client's behalf. I authorize the client's physicians, insurers, and hospitals to release such medical records to the Agency at the Agency's request.
3. Authorize my insurer to disclose to the Agency the terms and extent of my coverage, and the amount of payments made to me for services provided by the Agency.
4. Assign, transfer, and set over to the Agency all of my or the client's rights to insurance proceeds or other funds to which I am or the patient is or will become entitled as a result of the services rendered by the Agency.
5. Consent to and authorize payment, which would otherwise be payable to me or the client, to be made directly to the Agency. The Agency may issue a receipt for such payment which shall discharge the insurance company of its obligations under the policy to the extent of such payment.
6. Agree that I remain individually responsible to pay the Agency for all charges not paid for any reason by the insurer or other third-party payer. I understand that payment in full is due upon receipt of my bill. If payment for the Agency's service is made directly to me by my insurer, I agree to endorse the check to ____________________ and forward it to the Agency within three days of receipt.

A photocopy of this document, if executed, shall be considered as effective and valid as the original.

The effect of this form and the Client's Rights and Responsibilities on the back of this form have been explained to me by the Agency and I understand its content and significance.

Date: ____________________ Signature: ____________________

Name: ____________________

(Please Print)

FIGURE 4.2 A form for consent for treatment, release of information, assignment of benefits, and notice of client rights.

BOX 4.3 * Focus on Communication

Lee Puente is receiving home care because of hyperemesis of pregnancy and elevated blood pressure. She lost 15 pounds at the beginning of pregnancy but now, at 20 weeks, has gained back the lost pounds, plus 2 extra pounds, since beginning supplemental enteral feedings every day. A home health care assistant visits her three times a week to supervise her nutrition. She always seems pleased to be visited by a home care nurse once a week.

Less Effective Communication

Nurse: Hello, Lee. Is everything going all right?
Lee: Great.
Nurse: Are you eating everything you're supposed to?
Lee: Sure.
Nurse: Not throwing up any more, are you?
Lee: No.
Nurse: Good. I'm glad you're doing so well.

More Effective Communication

Nurse: Hello, Lee. How is everything?
Lee: Great.
Nurse: Are you eating everything you're supposed to?
Lee: Sure.
Nurse: What did you eat for breakfast this morning?
Lee: A slice of toast.
Nurse: What happened afterward?
Lee: I threw it up. I do that about once—maybe twice—a day.
Nurse: I need to do a more thorough assessment.

Because home settings are more informal than those of health care agencies, it is easy to forget that a home is a health care setting and to let a relationship become more relaxed than therapeutic. In the first scenario, the nurse lapsed into using leading questions rather than structured ones for a health interview. Lee responded to the leading questions by supplying answers she thought the nurse wanted to hear, not necessarily the true answers.

Assessing the Environment

During a visit, observe whether the house is safe for home care. This means there is adequate water, electricity, heat, and refrigeration. Are there smoke detectors in the home? Are they in working order? Are there drafts or broken windows? Are there rodents or insects or lead-based paint in the house that make the environment unsafe?

Evaluate how far the bathroom is from the client's bed. A bedside commode may be necessary to avoid a long walk. Check that there is a telephone nearby so the client has a means of calling someone, both to prevent loneliness and to secure emergency help. If a client needs assistance with personal hygiene, evaluate the floor plan of the bathroom or evaluate the need for a referral for a home health assistant.

Be sure that medical equipment brought into the home can be accommodated (Fig. 4.3). Hospital beds can be rented from medical supply companies. If a family cannot afford one, they can elevate a house bed on wooden or concrete blocks. Many home mattresses are not firm; a piece of plywood slid under the mattress improves firmness. A cardboard box or additional pillows can be placed under the mattress to elevate the head of a regular bed to a gatch position. Bed trays can be purchased at any department store or made from a heavy cardboard box.

If the client will use a wheelchair to ambulate, family members need to consider what adaptations of their home will be necessary. A local carpenter can build a ramp across the house steps to allow wheelchair access. Unless the person will be using a motorized wheelchair, the ramp should have a railing that can be grasped to pull the chair upward or to stop the wheelchair from moving downward too fast. Wheelchair lifts or elevators can be purchased and mounted alongside house steps, but they are usually more expensive.

Because it is difficult to move a wheelchair across a high-pile carpet, covering the carpet with plastic is helpful. Throw rugs usually have to be removed because they become tangled in wheelchair wheels. Placing furniture along the walls allows increased safe turning space for a wheelchair.

It is often impossible to reach high shelves from a wheelchair. A pair of tongs can be helpful to do this. Family members may have to move supplies that are used often, such as boxes of cereal, to a lower cabinet so the wheelchair challenged family member can reach them. If a kitchen counter is too high to prepare foods, placing a board across the wheelchair arms provides a workspace. If a stove has controls at the back, it is difficult for a person in a wheelchair to turn it on or off. Caution parents that if a child attempts to reach across a hot burner to reach the controls, he or she could be badly burned. A microwave oven placed on a low table can be a solution that allows a person to warm up meals and prepare snacks independently. Installing a safety rail by the toilet in the bathroom helps a person

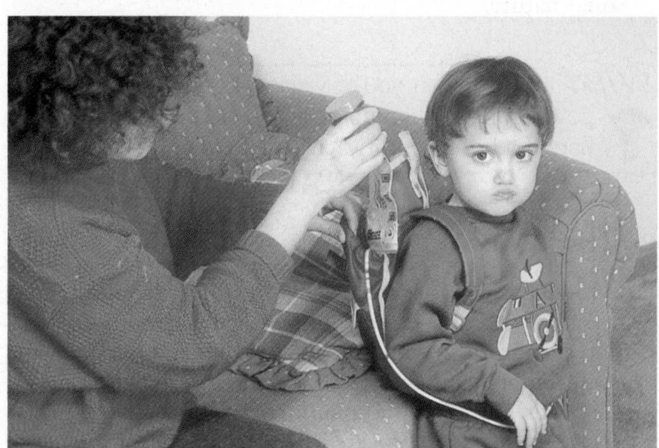

FIGURE 4.3 Procedures at home need to be modified to adjust to the setting. Here a young boy uses a backpack to carry an ambulatory bag for his gastrostomy tube feeding. (John Meyer/Custom Medical Stock Photograph.)

transfer from wheelchair to toilet. A chair placed in the bathtub alongside safety rails allows the person to transfer to the bathtub.

Federal law mandates that all public buildings provide easy access for people in wheelchairs or using walkers. In some towns, buildings may not be equipped this way because no one has ever asked for the service before. Urge the family to contact their city council if a problem exists. Serve as an advocate if the family's approach is met with less-than-prompt action so that everyone who uses a wheelchair will have access to facilities such as the public library, zoo, museums, and shopping malls.

Home Care Assistants

Effective home care requires a team of health care providers, including the supervising physician, home care nurses, health equipment suppliers, and home care assistants. Home health assistants are an invaluable help in providing home health care because they can supply the bulk of personal care services, such as assisting with or providing hygiene, assisting with ambulation, and providing adequate nutrition. Home care assistants have varied levels of education depending on the home health care or community health care agency policies and the level of care they are being asked to provide.

When working with unlicensed assistive personnel:

- Be sure you are familiar with their level of ability and education so you do not assign a task to them that is above their ability or one that prevents them from using their full potential.
- When making assignments, be certain they understand that making an assessment (e.g., recording a blood pressure) is not the same as evaluating the meaning of the assessment. That requires professional expertise.
- When they are in a client's house, remind them that they are a guest in the house and need to respect the values and patterns of that household.
- When a client no longer needs home care and the time comes to terminate the relationship, they may need your help with ending the relationship and saying good-bye because, often, their services have been of such a personal nature.

What if... When you're visiting Lee Puente, you discover large mouse holes in the bedroom that will be used by her new baby? What would you do?

Postvisit Planning

Postvisit planning consists of documenting all information gained from the visit in relation to a client's condition, completing agency forms so billing for supplies and nursing time can be accurate, and evaluating a client's current status and future needs. It may include communicating a change in status to the primary health care provider, asking for a renewal of orders, or updating and revising the plan of care. Although the forms may vary, the rules for accurate documentation in home care are the same as for any health care facility and just as essential.

Follow-up Visits

Subsequent home visits are planned depending on a client's circumstances and the amount of health education and supervision needed. A second visit could be scheduled as often as the next day or as infrequently as once a month. Frequent assessments accomplished at subsequent visits include vital signs, nutrition assessment, medication adherence, and nursing actions such as health education.

✔ Checkpoint Question 4.2

In the middle of a visit to Lee Puente's home, her former boyfriend arrives and threatens you and Lee. What would be your best action?

a. Tell him that threatening someone is not mature behavior and he should stop.
b. Suggest that Lee change all of her home locks so this man cannot visit again.
c. Leave the home and notify your agency that you were in unsafe circumstances.
d. Call 911 and report that you and a client are being threatened.

Nursing Diagnoses and Related Interventions

Nursing Diagnosis: Interrupted family process related to stress of caring for ill family member at home

Outcome Evaluation: Family members state they feel able to manage home care; family meets weekly to discuss problems and share accomplishments.

Nursing responsibilities for women and children receiving home care vary greatly because the reason for home care and the actions needed to be taken vary greatly. Typical interventions carried out in homes are concerned with promoting a healthy environment and healthy family function.

Ensure Bed Rest

Women and children on bed rest react in several ways, but many report feeling "tied down," "like a prisoner," and "as if I'm missing out." One solution to help them cope with the stress of the experience is for them to keep busy or use their time to learn a new skill. Most women can name activities they would like to do but have never had time to begin to do. For example, if a woman likes to read but does not always have the time, bed rest at home may provide an ideal time for her to catch up on her reading (Fig. 4.4). If she has other children, she can spend part of her time reading to them. She could also use the time to take a home-study course, learn a new hobby, write a short story, or study for a certifying examination related to her work. In any event, helping her plan meaningful activities such as these can help her view home care not as wasted time but as time invested in her family or career (Box 4.4).

Children need to involve themselves in school work or play, perhaps learning a new game or Sudoku or crossword puzzles. Otherwise, they may spend their time simply watching television or napping. Although play is a universal activity

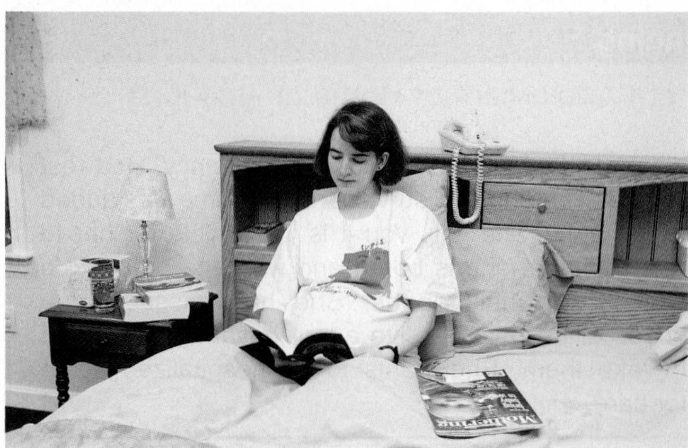

FIGURE 4.4 Bed rest can be stressful. Helping a woman who is on bed rest identify enjoyable and productive activities to pass the time can help ease stress.

of children, not all parents realize how important it is to children. Children's play activities vary greatly depending on cultural and socioeconomic circumstances. When a child is not proficient in English and that is the language of health care providers, games such as stacking blocks or building with Tinker Toys can be played despite communication difficulty. Playing CDs or tapes of well-loved children's songs can also be effective, because the child does not need to be able to understand the words to enjoy the music or clap with the rhythm.

Identify a Child's Primary Caregiver

Although traditionally the primary caregiver for an ill child is the mother, in today's families, if a father works more flexible hours, he may be the parent best able to give the bulk of care. In some homes, a grandparent or an older sibling will be the person primarily responsible for care. Arrange to include this person in planning and problem solving because this person knows best what strategy of care will be most effective with the child, as well as what strategy will be most appropriate in light of the physical layout of the home and the family's financial ability and lifestyle.

Determine Knowledge Level of Family

Before anyone can be cared for at home, teaching may be required so the family understands the illness and principles of care. Include in the Nursing Care Plan both the things to be learned immediately and additional care measures that will need to be taught as the client's condition changes (Box 4.5).

Identify Available Resources

The term "resources" refers not only to material objects (e.g., hospital bed, portable oxygen, or glucometer) but also to whether family members are able to deal with the chronic stress of fatiguing or around-the-clock nursing care. Assess physical surroundings: Is there adequate floor space for a hospital bed, oxygen equipment, and so forth? Is a fire company nearby, able to respond in case cardiopulmonary resuscitation (CPR) is needed? Is a backup resource available to power needed equipment if a blackout should occur? Does the family have a telephone? Could the patient be evacuated easily in case of a fire? Does the family have transportation to a health care facility for follow-up care? Table 4.2 lists additional important assessments to make, depending on the age of a child.

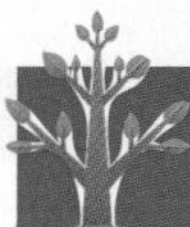

BOX 4.4 * Focus on Family Teaching

Suggestions for Best Use of Time While on Bed Rest

Q. Lee Puente tells you, "I feel like I'm wasting my time just being home this way. What can I do to keep busy?"

A. Try these suggestions:

- Concentrate on school work; make this a time to really delve into a subject.
- Ask your teacher if there is a special project you could work on from home while on bed rest.
- Renew an old hobby or begin a new one.
- Ask someone to bring you books on newborn care from the library so you can pass the time reading.
- Telephone your friends. Rest next to a telephone so friends know they will not be disturbing you when they return calls.
- Catch up on your correspondence. Friends and family will be surprised and delighted to hear from you.
- Investigate whether there is a local community project (e.g., making telephone calls for a political campaign, urging neighbors to write letters of support for a new playground) you could work on while on bed rest.
- If you have Internet access, spend time online looking for information about pregnancy, childbirth, or childrearing or just chatting with friends or others (if you have a dial-up connection, be conscious of the telephone bill that might result).
- Learn a second language; many books are available on this.
- Take a mail-order course on something you want to learn more about (e.g., creative writing; learning to be a paralegal).
- Ask your home care nurse about preparation-for-childbirth information. By conscientiously practicing breathing exercises while on bed rest, you can become well prepared for labor and birth.

Promote Healthy Family Functioning

A family that is supportive of all family members and provides an environment conducive to each member's continued growth and development is more likely to be able to manage home care than is a family with a history of ineffective or destructive coping strategies—that is, a family in which parents have unrealistic expectations of family members, one with a history of abusive relationships, or one that is coping ineffectively with other stressors in their lives. Even a family that appears to be functioning well, however, may be so adversely affected by the stress of home care that its members' ability to be successful with home care can be limited. For example, the loss of employment income, resentment over missed promotions, or cramped living space could put a family at risk for ineffective coping. Remember that every family operates differently and handles stress in different ways. Events that may seem overwhelming for a visiting health care provider may actually be easy for the family to handle. Conversely,

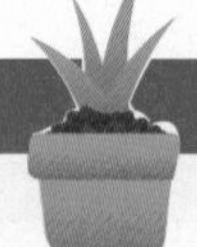

BOX 4.5 ✻ Focus on Nursing Care Planning

A Multidisciplinary Care Map for a Pregnant Adolescent at Home on Bed Rest

Lee Puente, a 16-year-old, who is 20 weeks pregnant, lives with her parents. She was admitted to the hospital for 3 days at 14 weeks of her pregnancy and placed on a program of total parenteral nutrition because she has been vomiting at least four times daily since the beginning of pregnancy. She managed well on parenteral nutrition until last week, when her blood pressure rose to 160/90 mm Hg and she was diagnosed with hypertension of pregnancy. Bed rest with fetal and uterine surveillance at home was added to her care. She tells you it is impossible for her to rest at home: she is bored and wants to be back in school with her friends. She has missed three doses of her hypotensive agent because she forgot to take them. She wants to be hospitalized again for care.

Family Assessment ✻ Child lives with parents in a two-story home. Child's bedroom is on second floor with bathroom located approximately 20 feet from child's bed. Child's mother is primary wage earner in the family; works full-time as a travel agent. Father is full-time doctoral student receiving only a student stipend. He stays home until noon daily.

Client Assessment ✻ Vital signs: Temperature 98.4° F; pulse 76; respirations 22; blood pressure 144/94; FHR 148. Mild facial edema; +1 protein in urine; 2-pound weight gain in 1 week.

Nursing Diagnosis ✻ Anxiety related to need for bed rest secondary to nausea and hypertension of pregnancy

Outcome Criteria ✻ Client identifies methods to continue in school while maintaining bed rest; expresses increased satisfaction with imposed bed rest; maintains bed rest until fetal maturity. Blood pressure remains 140/80 or less; FHR within acceptable parameters; urine for protein remains +1 or less; weight gain limited to 1 lb/week; edema limited and without increase for the duration of pregnancy.

Team Member Responsible	Assessment	Intervention	Rationale	Expected Outcome
		Activities of Daily Living		
Nurse	Assess vital signs, including heart rate, BP, and FHR at every visit.	Instruct client how to take own vital signs. Instruct how to do a "count-to-ten" assessment daily to document fetal activity.	Assessment of vital signs, especially BP and fetal activity, provides a baseline for future comparison and evidence of the client's and fetus's status.	Client demonstrates she is able to accurately obtain own pulse, BP, and fetal activity. Findings compare with nurse's weekly findings.
		Consultations		
Physician/nurse	Assess what services will be most appropriate for client.	Arrange for home care visiting by hospital home care team. Care assistant: daily; RN 1× week.	Home care functions best when it is part of a "seamless" service.	Client agrees to services of hospital home care team.
		Procedures/Medications		
Nurse	Assess random urine specimen for protein at each home visit. Assess what client interprets home bed rest to mean.	Instruct client to assess urine specimen and weigh herself every day. Review concept of complete bed rest. Arrange for a bedside commode if necessary.	Proteinuria +3 indicates severe edema. Increasing weight suggests tissue fluid retention. Varying degrees of bed rest may be necessary to reduce symptoms of hypertension of pregnancy.	Client voices an understanding of need for bed rest and adheres to restrictions. Demonstrates ability to carry out procedures accurately.

Nutrition				
Nutritionist/ nurse	Obtain a 24-hour recall pattern to determine nutritional intake.	Encourage a diet high in protein and adequate fluid intake.	Protein may affect the degree of hypertension of pregnancy.	Client lists a 24-hour intake that is adequate for pregnancy.
Patient/Family Education				
Social worker/ nurse	Assess what client feels are her chief needs to allow her to remain on bed rest at home.	Assist client with planning effective bed rest; discuss possible sources of help from friends and family in addition to daily health care assistant.	Planning concrete methods to make bed rest more tolerable alleviates stress.	Client demonstrates ways she has adapted to bed rest restrictions. Voices plan for creative uses of her time
		Urge parents to arrange for telephone jack or wireless connection so client can arrange computer connection to continue school activities.	Helping establish a means of communication provides stimulation and a better possibility of continuing in school.	Client demonstrates how she will use telephone, computer, and fax machine to continue to participate in school.
Psychosocial/Spiritual/Emotional Needs				
Nurse	Discuss with client areas of concern.	Encourage the client to plan frequent periods of quiet time for herself. Suggest activities such as reading and listening to music.	Discussion provides baseline information to identify client's needs, beliefs, and responsibilities.	Client describes any areas of concern that could interfere with bed rest. Client lists at least three restful activities that she can use to occupy her day.
Discharge Planning				
Nurse	Assess for readiness to participate in home monitoring.	Instruct client and family members in signs and symptoms of increased hypertension, such as increased edema, increased protein in urine, headache, dizziness, blurred vision, increased weight gain, or decreased urine output. Advise client to call the home care agency or primary health care provider if these occur.	Knowledge of danger signs and symptoms allows for early identification and prompt intervention to prevent threats to the mother and fetus.	Client lists signs and symptoms of elevated blood pressure and telephone number she will call if pressure is over 140/80.

problems that seem minor could be disruptive enough to affect the family's ability to provide adequate care at home.

Many women fulfill multiple roles in their family, such as financial manager, peacemaker, problem solver, nurturer, and decision maker. Even when a woman is on bed rest, help her to continue in these roles to ensure the family's usual functioning, because support people often have great difficulty assuming these roles in her place. In some families, older children fill these roles so need to be encouraged to continue in these roles if they are the ill family member being cared for at home.

As a rule, support people can only be supportive if they understand the need for the home care program and the importance of their role. Arranging for a homemaker service to help care for children or an aging parent or to help with light housework may be necessary to prevent support people from feeling stretched so thin they cannot function. Often support people are not present at the time of a home visit for a

TABLE 4.2 ✻ Assessment Criteria for Home Care by Age Group

Age	Points to Assess
All age groups	Are there adequate three-pronged plugs needed for the care equipment available? If oxygen will be used, is there a sign to omit smoking in the room? Is the oxygen away from a fireplace, gas space heater, or stove? Does the family know not to light candles near oxygen in a power failure or for a birthday? Is there adequate space for supplies? Is there a smoke detector in the patient's room? If a special diet is necessary, does the person who will cook have adequate knowledge of food preparation? Do caregivers know the emergency call system procedure in their community? How to reorder supplies? Has the power company been notified if an electrical appliance is necessary for life support? What would be the caregiver's actions in a power failure? What emergency steps should the caregiver take if the patient is suddenly worse?
Infant	Is there a suitable sleeping place? Do side rails of a crib lock securely? Can the infant be heard from the parents' room at night? Is there a functioning refrigerator if formula will be used? Is there protection from mosquitoes? Is the home free of rodents that might attack a small infant?
Toddler and preschooler	Is there a safe area for play free from stairs and poisoning possibilities? Are there screens or locks on windows to prevent a child from crawling onto a ledge? Is there provision for stimulation and learning activities?
School-age child and adolescent	What is the provision for schooling (possibly an intercom with a regular classroom or home tutor)? Is peer interaction possible? If adolescent is self-medicating, will reminder sheets or some other reminder system be necessary?

pregnant woman because they work during the day. Ask a woman at home visits how her support people are coping and if there are ways this experience could be made easier for them as well as for her. The ability to make decisions about her own care such as this can make a significant difference in whether a woman thinks her home care experience is satisfactory.

Provide Health Teaching

A home care visit can provide many more opportunities for one-on-one health teaching than a health care agency setting. An important aspect of teaching for a pregnant woman might be providing childbirth education, because a woman on bed rest will not be able to attend formal classes. For a child, it could be teaching the whole family about the child's illness and why the current therapy is needed.

Provide for Safe Medicine Administration

Most people receiving home care are prescribed some type of medicine, such as a tocolytic for pregnant women to halt preterm labor or an antibiotic for a child to cure an infection. Review the rules of safe medication administration with the family to minimize mistakes such as taking the medicine more frequently than prescribed or forgetting to take it (Box 4.6).

Manage Pain

Children who are on home care post surgery or those with a chronic or terminal illness may need efficient pain management while they are cared for at home. Be certain that parents understand the principles of pain management such as giving medication before pain becomes acute (Box 4.7). Other aspects of pain management are discussed in Chapter 39.

Provide for Adequate Nutrition and Hydration

A woman who is on home care often needs help maintaining adequate nutrition. If ordinarily she is the person who plans menus, shops for food, and cooks for the family, with her on bed rest, other family members must assume these roles. If other family members are inexperienced at cooking, the entire family, including the pregnant woman, may not be eating enough healthy foods.

BOX 4.6 ✻ Safety Tips for Safely Taking Medicine at Home

- Keep drugs in a safe place. In most homes, this is in a locked medicine cabinet or drawer above the height a child could reach.
- Remind parents that most childhood poisonings occur when a family is under stress; during these times, the family can forget usual procedures such as locking away a drug. Reinforce the need to take special precautions to lock away medications at these times.
- Never take medicine in front of children (children can imitate this action with the parent's medication).
- Do not pour or prepare medicine in the dark. Because almost all medicine bottles dispensed from local pharmacies look and feel the same, it is easy to pour the wrong liquid, extract the wrong pills, or read the bottle instructions incorrectly without adequate light.
- Make out a reminder sheet and hang it in a prominent place. Cross off each time the medication is taken.
- Purchase a medicine box with an individual compartment for each day of the week. Fill it at the beginning of the week. Such boxes help to eliminate confusion over whether medicine was taken or not.

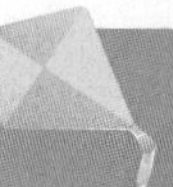

BOX 4.7 ✻ Focus on Evidence-Based Practice

Do parents adequately manage pain in children who are on home care after a tonsillectomy?

Tonsillectomy is one of the most common surgical procedures performed on children. It is done routinely on an ambulatory or day-surgery basis so most children spend only 3 to 4 hours in the ambulatory center. This puts the major responsibility for postoperative care including adequate pain management on the parents after the child returns home.

To investigate whether children usually receive adequate pain management while at home, nurse researchers asked 76 children ranging in age from 7 to 12, who were undergoing tonsillectomy to record their pain level, the type and timing of analgesics they received, and whether they received pain relief from the medicine while they were at home.

The children's diaries revealed that most children rated their pain level as "moderate." Ninety-six percent of the 25 children who were prescribed hydrocodone/acetaminophen (Vicodin), an opioid analgesic, were given by parents a dose below the recommended standard. Only 69% of the 22 children who were prescribed codeine and acetaminophen (Tylenol) received the recommended dose; 6.3% received less than the recommended dose, and 25% received more than the recommended dose. Drinking fluid can help relieve edema and therefore also reduce pain. Only 11% of children met the recommended amount of fluid intake in the first 24 hours after surgery.

The authors conclude that parents may need more information on hospital discharge regarding how to administer pain medication. A telephone call from the surgery setting in the first 24 hours might be helpful to assist parents with adequate pain management.

How would you use the above study findings if you were visiting a child in his home after surgery?

Source: Huth, M. M., & Broome, M. E. (2007). A snapshot of children's postoperative tonsillectomy outcomes at home. *Journal for Specialists in Pediatric Nursing, 12*(3), 186–195.

As ill children do not get as much activity as usual, they may not be hungry at mealtime. You may need to make suggestions for healthy snacks so a child's total daily intake is adequate even if not a lot of food is eaten at formal meals.

All women during pregnancy should drink six to eight full glasses of fluid a day to obtain adequate fluid for effective kidney function and placental exchange (Rojas, Wood, & Blakemore, 2007). Be certain women on bed rest have a supply of fluid close to their bed so they can do this easily.

Intravenous Administration

Many women and children on home care receive intravenous therapy as a route of medication administration (Balaguer & Gonzales de Dios, 2009). Women with hyperemesis gravidarum (uncontrolled vomiting during pregnancy) receive it as a means of hydration (Lamondy, 2007). Women and children with blood dyscrasias may receive blood transfusions in the home.

Intravenous medication and fluid administration can be accomplished by either a peripheral or central insertion site. Because peripheral intravenous lines frequently become dislodged, in the home setting, intravenous fluid is often administered by a central line or a peripherally inserted catheter threaded to a central blood vessel (a PICC line). Specially pressurized fluid containers allow for fast and easy administration of special solutions. To be certain that fluid infuses slowly and accurately, an intravenous infusion pump is strongly recommended. Many drugs, especially antibiotics, are given through bagged "piggyback" infusions that are kept frozen until the time of administration. Be certain a woman or a family member knows how to monitor intravenous insertion sites for inflammation and infiltration, how to protect the site from becoming infected (e.g., cover it with plastic rather than letting it get wet), and how to monitor the amount and kind of fluid or medication infused.

Home Enteral Nutrition

Chronically ill children and women who have hyperemesis gravidarum may receive nutrition by a nasogastric tube. The supplies necessary for enteral feedings, such as feeding tubes and enteral pumps, are available for rent or purchase through pharmacies or medical supply houses or the home care agency. Such tubes are usually changed every 2 to 4 weeks. The home care nurse will most likely be the person responsible for changing the tube, but this depends on the home care agency's policies. In addition to assessing the amount of formula infused by this route, be sure that a woman or family member is familiar with all aspects of care for the tube, equipment, and administration of the feeding. Caution the family to monitor the amount of formula for the feedings on hand so they do not run out, especially over weekends. Clients on enteral feedings probably will need to weigh themselves periodically and record the weight. Be certain they use the same scale, wear consistent clothing, and know when to call for advice if they are having difficulty or are unsure if their weight is remaining adequate.

Total Parenteral Nutrition

Total parenteral nutrition (TPN) is yet another way to supply complete nutrition and fluid to clients on home care. Usually the home care agency or a separate private vendor will furnish and deliver the formula, tubing, clean dressings, and an infusion pump. The formula, which consists of amino acids, hypertonic glucose, vitamins, and minerals in solution, needs to be stored in the client's refrigerator until 1 to 2 hours before use; it is then removed from the refrigerator and allowed to warm to room temperature. Women and children requiring this type of intravenous nutritional therapy usually have a central venous access device such as a central venous catheter or PICC line inserted. The home care nurse plays a key role in teaching family members about the therapy and also in assessing the woman or child's response to therapy.

Throughout therapy, be sure the client or a family member monitors the infusion of the solution and the patency of the tube, knows how to change dressings, observes the insertion site, and assesses body temperature for signs of possible infection. They also must be aware of any restrictions that should be adhered to (e.g., no baths if the water level will rise above the catheter insertion site) and the interval at which blood should be drawn for monitoring. Because TPN solutions are hypertonic, the woman or a family member needs to obtain fingerstick blood glucose levels as necessary, about every 6 hours, and keep a record of these. Be sure the family knows what findings should be reported immediately to a health care provider.

Promote Elimination

Promoting elimination in anyone receiving home care can call for advance planning. Assess if the place where the person is going to rest is close by a bathroom so the person can reach this easily. If strict bed rest is required, a bedside commode may be necessary.

Constipation occurs at a high rate during pregnancy and can occur in children on bed rest from lack of exercise. Encourage a diet high in fiber and fluid daily to minimize this problem.

Teach Monitoring of Vital Signs

Monitoring vital signs in the home does not differ from monitoring them in a health care agency except mercury thermometers may be used in place of electronic ones. If the family will be using a mercury/glass thermometer, caution them that mercury is a toxic contaminant if the thermometer breaks and that this type of thermometer takes a full 3 minutes to register rather than the more convenient few seconds needed by electronic thermometers. To avoid risk of mercury ingestion, they should not be used with children under 5 years of age.

Blood pressure is best measured if the person is in the same position (lying down or sitting up) and the pressure is taken on the same arm each time. Using an automated cuff simplifies taking blood pressure. These can be purchased at pharmacies or from home care agencies.

Teach Self-Monitoring of Uterine Height, Contractions, and Fetal Heart Rate

Uterine (fundal) height during pregnancy is measured by using a paper tape measure according to McDonald's rule (see Chapter 11). If a woman is asked to record serial fundal height measurements, demonstrate the correct technique and have her give a return demonstration, as this measurement varies greatly depending on where the tape measure is placed. Be sure a woman is measuring the height in the same location each time. It may be necessary to mark the points to measure with a permanent ink pen to ensure consistent and accurate measurements.

Many women conduct count-to-10 assessments daily (count the number of fetal movements they feel in a designated time period; see Chapter 21) to help assess fetal well-being (Chang & Blakemore, 2007). Fetal heart rate (FHR) is usually recorded by the home care nurse at each home visit. In addition, a client may be taught how to obtain this herself. FHR can be recorded by listening with a Doppler, a fetoscope, a regular stethoscope (although FHR may be very difficult to hear), or an electronic monitoring device supplied as part of her home care program.

The client can self-monitor uterine contractions using a uterine monitor, the same as in a health care facility, or by palpation (see Chapter 9). A rhythm strip or nonstress test can be conducted using a portable monitor approximately the size of an MP3 player or cell phone. A woman straps this device to her abdomen for 20 to 30 minutes at a set time every day, or at any time she feels contractions or is concerned about the lack of fetal movement (Fig. 4.5). The monitor records both uterine contractions and FHR. At the conclusion of the monitoring period, the monitor is held next to a telephone and the tracing is transmitted to a central facility for evaluation.

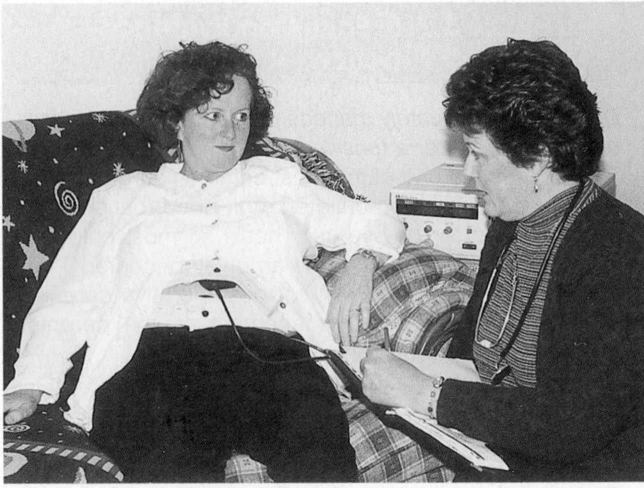

FIGURE 4.5 Fetal heart rate and uterine contractions can be recorded successfully by women at home. (Photograph by Melissa Olson, with permission of Healthy Home Coming, Inc., Bensalem, PA.)

Teach Self-Monitoring by Serum or Urine Testing

Women who develop diabetes mellitus during pregnancy are required to monitor their serum glucose levels using a test strip and glucometer at least once daily (Hampton, 2007). Children with diabetes need to do the same (Hill, 2007). Most people are reluctant to learn this procedure because they do not like the thought of having to pierce the skin of a finger to draw blood. Automated lancet devices are available to help with this.

Provide Long-term Home Care

Although many families are good candidates for home care, they continue to need advice to adapt constructively to the crisis of illness and home management, as the stress and problems that can occur from being responsible for an ill family member can lower people's self-esteem. The time involved can harm a marital relationship or prevent parents from spending time with other children. Physical care requirements can disrupt the normal family routines and shift the focus of attention onto the ill child and away from other children in the family (Fig. 4.6).

Help families maintain healthy functioning by promoting communication and encouraging family members to identify and share their feelings about the new situation at home. Encourage members to voice the frustration they feel at being constantly confined at home or what they perceive to be a lack of progress in the ill person's condition. If a child has a terminal illness, support parents to express their grief and not

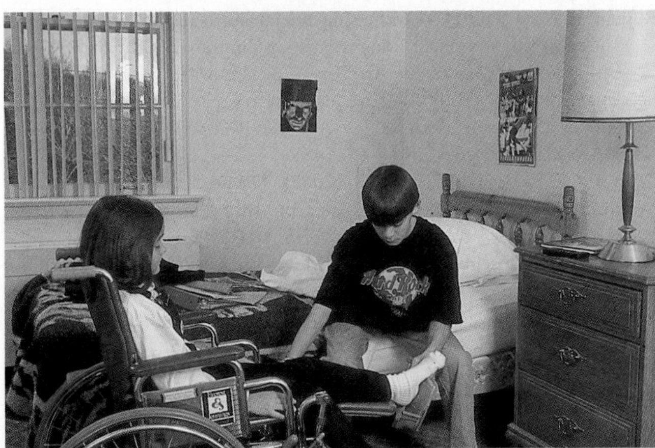

FIGURE 4.6 Home care of a child is family care. Here a brother helps his sister settle into her wheelchair.

grow discouraged, because the work they are accomplishing is making the child comfortable before death. Continued successful coping will require the family to acknowledge and take seriously the impact of home care on each family member and work together to solve identified problems. They may need to renegotiate roles and responsibilities within the family or seek outside help.

When a family is not functioning well at the beginning of home care or does not adjust to home care, nursing measures to support family functioning become even more important. A family whose coping strategies are maladaptive and ineffective may not be able to care for a sick family member at home for long.

✔Checkpoint Question 4.3

Lee Puente is developing constipation from being on bed rest. What measure would you suggest she take to help prevent this?

a. Drink more milk, as increased calcium prevents constipation.
b. Walk for at least half an hour daily to stimulate peristalsis.
c. Drink eight full glasses of a fluid such as water daily.
d. Eat more frequent small meals instead of three large ones daily.

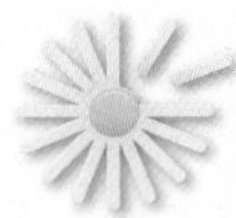

Key Points for Review

- Families exist within communities; assessment of the community and the family's place in the community yields further information on family functioning and abilities.
- Home care is increasing as a way of providing care to chronically ill children and women with complications of pregnancy. It has the advantages of being cost-effective and providing meaningful comfort and support.
- Disadvantages of home care are that families can become fatigued, the loss of a job for the primary caregiver can cause financial hardship, and social isolation and disruption of normal home life may occur.
- Home care requires careful planning and a combined effort between a home care agency and a health care provider to ensure collaboration and continuity.
- Not all homes are ideal for home care. Assess that a primary care provider is present; the family is knowledgeable about the care necessary; necessary resources are available; and safety features such as a smoke detector, a safe area for oxygen storage, and a safe refrigerator for food or medicine are present.
- Home care can be exhausting for families. Be certain a family devises a schedule of care that allows them enough rest. Advocate for medicine or treatment schedules that allow for administering medications during the day rather than a schedule that requires medication administration at night.
- Parents may need respite care to continue to be effective care providers for children the same as professionals need time off. Help parents to take turns giving care so that each has some free time during the week.

CRITICAL THINKING EXERCISES

1. Lee Puente is the adolescent you met at the beginning of the chapter. Was she a good candidate for home care? What additional interventions would she need to make home care more successful for her? Her mother is concerned that she will become exhausted because of the need for Lee's round-the-clock care. What suggestions could you offer to make care easier?
2. When you are visiting Lee in her home, do standard precautions to prevent the spread of infection apply? Explain your answer.
3. Lee Puente's father stays home from work until noon. A school friend visits every afternoon. Her mother stays with her in the evening. What would be the best time of the day to schedule a home visit?
4. Examine the National Health Goals related to home care. Most government-sponsored money for nursing research is allotted based on these goals. What would be a possible research topic to explore pertinent to these goals that would be applicable to the Puente family and also advance evidence-based practice?

CRITICAL THINKING SCENARIO

Open the accompanying CD-ROM or visit http://thePoint.lww.com and read the Patient Scenario included for this chapter; then answer the questions to further sharpen your skills and grow more familiar with NCLEX types of questions related to community assessment and home care. Confirm your answers are correct by reading the rationales.

REFERENCES

Allender, J. A., & Spradley, B. W. (2008). *Community health nursing: concepts and practice* (6th ed.). Philadelphia: Lippincott Williams & Wilkins.

Balaguer, A., & Gonzalez de Dios, J. (2009). Home intravenous antibiotics for cystic fibrosis. *Cochrane Database of Systematic Reviews, 2009*(1), (CD001917).

Barlow, J., et al. (2007). Role of home visiting in improving parenting and health in families at risk of abuse and neglect: results of a multicentre randomised controlled trial and economic evaluation. *Archives of Disease in Childhood, 92*(3), 229–233.

Bernstein, H. B., & Weinstein, M. (2007). Normal pregnancy and prenatal care. In A. H. Decherney & L. Nathan (Eds.). *Current diagnosis and treatment in obstetrics and gynecology* (10th ed.). Columbus, OH: McGraw-Hill.

Chang, D., & Blakemore, K. (2007). Fetal assessment. In K. B. Fortner, et al. (Eds.). *The Johns Hopkins manual of gynecology and obstetrics.* Philadelphia: Lippincott Williams & Wilkins.

Conway, A. E., McClune, A. J., & Nosel, P. (2007). Down on the farm: preventing farm accidents in children. *Pediatric Nursing, 33*(1), 45–48.

Crowther, C. A. (2009). Hospitalisation and bed rest for multiple pregnancy. *Cochrane Database of Systematic Reviews, 2009*(1), (CD000110).

Donovan, E. F., et al. (2007). Intensive home visiting is associated with decreased risk of infant death. *Pediatrics, 119*(6), 1145–1151.

Hampton, T. (2007). Study finds newborn outcomes affected by blood glucose levels during pregnancy. *JAMA: Journal of the American Medical Association, 298*(6), 613–614.

Hill, J. (2007). Treating type 1 diabetes in primary care. *Practice Nurse, 33*(11), 20–26.

Huth, M. M., & Broome, M. E. (2007). A snapshot of children's postoperative tonsillectomy outcomes at home. *Journal for Specialists in Pediatric Nursing, 12*(3), 186–195.

Lamondy, A. M. (2007). Managing hyperemesis gravidarum. *Nursing, 37*(2), 66–68.

Monsen, R. B., & Finley, S. (2007). The child in the community: nursing makes a difference. *Journal of Pediatric Nursing: Nursing Care of Children and Families, 22*(3), 231–232.

Pignone, M., & Salazar, R. (2009). Prevention and health maintenance. In S. J. McPhee & M. A. Papadakis (Eds.). *Current medical diagnosis and treatment.* Columbus, OH: McGraw-Hill.

Rojas, F., Wood, E., & Blakemore, K. (2007). Preconception counseling and prenatal care. In K. B. Fortner, et al. (Eds.). *The Johns Hopkins manual of gynecology and obstetrics.* Philadelphia: Lippincott Williams & Wilkins.

Roman, L. A., et al. (2007). Addressing mental health and stress in Medicaid-insured pregnant women using a nurse-community health worker home visiting team. *Public Health Nursing, 24*(3), 239–248.

Secco, M. L., et al. (2007). Factors affecting postpartum depressive symptoms of adolescent mothers. *JOGNN: Journal of Obstetric, Gynecologic, and Neonatal Nursing, 36*(1), 47–54.

Tuffrey, C., Finlay, F., & Lewis, M. (2007). The needs of children and their families at end of life: an analysis of community nursing practice. *International Journal of Palliative Nursing, 13*(2), 64–71.

Yantzi, N. M., Rosenberg, M. W., & McKeever, P. (2007). Getting out of the house: the challenges mothers face when their children have long-term care needs. *Health and Social Care in the Community, 15*(1), 45–55.

SUGGESTED READINGS

Davis, C. (2007). Caring for children at home. *Nursing Standard, 21*(36), 20–21.

Doggett, C., Burrett, S., & Osborn, D. A. (2009). Home visits during pregnancy and after birth for women with an alcohol or drug problem. *Cochrane Database of Systematic Reviews, 2009*(1), (CD004456).

Farasat, H., & Hewitt-Taylor, J. (2007). Learning to support children with complex and continuing health needs and their families. *Journal for Specialists in Pediatric Nursing, 12*(2), 72–83.

Jewell, D., & Young, G. (2009). Interventions for nausea and vomiting in early pregnancy. *Cochrane Database of Systematic Reviews, 2009*(1), (CD000145).

Lewis, M., & Noyes, J. (2007). Discharge management for children with complex needs. *Paediatric Nursing, 19*(4), 26–30.

Macdonald, G., et al. (2009). Home-based support for disadvantaged teenage mothers. *Cochrane Database of Systematic Reviews, 2009*(1), (CD006723).

Paulus, A. T., & van Raak, A. J. (2008). The impact of integrated care on direct nursing home care. *Health Policy, 85*(1), 45–59.

Peterson, C. A., et al. (2007). Enhancing parent-child interactions through home visiting: promising practice or unfulfilled promise? *Journal of Early Intervention, 29*(2), 119–140.

Polaschek, L., & Polaschek, N. (2007). Solution-focused conversations: a new therapeutic strategy in well child health nursing telephone consultations. *Journal of Advanced Nursing, 59*(2), 111–119.

Tandon, D., et al. (2007). Promotion of service integration among home visiting programs and community coalitions working with low-income, pregnant, and parenting women. *Health Promotion Practice, 8*(1), 79–87.

Unit 2

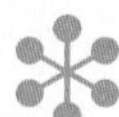

The Nursing Role in Preparing Families for Childbearing and Childrearing

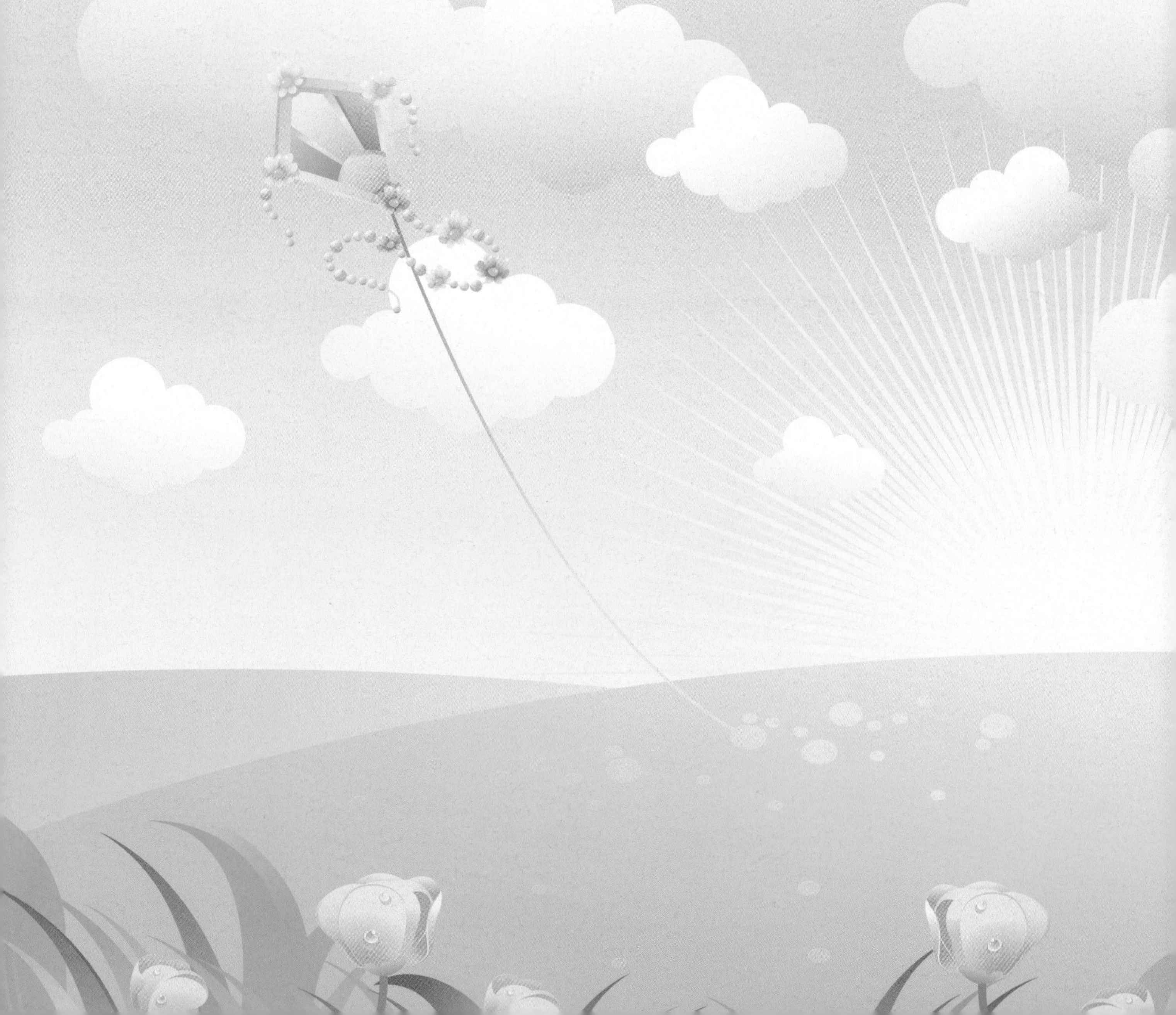

Chapter 5 The Nursing Role in Reproductive and Sexual Health

KEY TERMS

- adrenarche
- andrology
- anteflexion
- anteversion
- aspermia
- bicornuate uterus
- biologic gender
- culdoscopy
- cystocele
- dyspareunia
- erectile dysfunction
- gender identity
- gender role
- gonad
- gynecology
- gynecomastia
- laparoscopy
- menarche
- menopause
- menorrhagia
- metrorrhagia
- oocyte
- premature ejaculation
- rectocele
- retroflexion
- retroversion
- thelarche
- transsexual
- transvestite
- vaginismus
- voyeurism

OBJECTIVES

After mastering the contents of this chapter, you should be able to:

1. Describe anatomy and physiology pertinent to reproductive and sexual health.
2. Identify National Health Goals related to reproductive health and sexuality that nurses can help the nation achieve.
3. Use critical thinking to analyze ways in which clients' reproductive and sexual health can be improved for healthier childbearing and adult health within a family-centered framework.
4. Assess a couple for anatomic and physiologic health, biologic gender, gender role, gender identity, and readiness for childbearing.
5. Formulate nursing diagnoses related to reproductive and sexual health.
6. Identify appropriate outcomes for reproductive and sexual health education.
7. Plan nursing care related to anatomic and physiologic readiness for childbearing or sexual health, such as helping adolescents discuss concerns in these areas.
8. Implement nursing care related to reproductive and sexual health, such as educating middle school children about menstruation.
9. Evaluate expected outcomes for achievement and effectiveness of care.
10. Identify areas of care in relation to reproductive and sexual health that could benefit from additional nursing research or application of evidence-based practice.
11. Integrate knowledge of reproductive health and sexuality with nursing process to achieve quality maternal and child health nursing care.

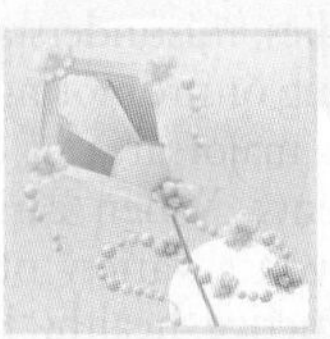

Suzanne and Kevin Matthews, a young adult couple, 12 weeks' pregnant, come to your antepartal clinic for a sixth-month visit. Suzanne, in tears, states, "My husband isn't interested in me anymore. We haven't had sex since I became pregnant." Kevin states, "I'm afraid I'll hurt the baby." Previous chapters presented the scope of maternal and child health and how the structure, function, and culture of families can have an impact on health. This chapter adds information about how to educate children, women, and their partners about anatomy, physiology, and sexuality to better prepare them for childbearing and childrearing.

How would you counsel Suzanne and Kevin Matthews?

Regardless of whether someone is planning on childbearing, everyone is wiser by being familiar with reproductive anatomy and physiology and his or her own body's reproductive and sexual health. Women and their partners who are planning on childbearing may be especially curious about reproductive physiology and the changes a pregnant woman will undergo during pregnancy, so this is an opportune time to educate both partners about reproductive and gynecologic health (Allen & Fountain, 2007).

Although the general public is becoming increasingly sophisticated about their bodies, misunderstandings about sexuality, conception (preventing or promoting), and childbearing still abound. Sexuality is a major area of concern for school-age children and adolescents. When caring for children of these ages, they may ask you a variety of detailed questions about sexuality or reproductive health. For instance, many young adults want to know what is considered a "normal" sexual response or the "normal" expected frequency for sexual relations. A general rule in answering this question is that normal sexual behavior includes any act mutually satisfying to both sexual partners. Actual frequency and type of sexual activity vary widely (MacKay, 2009).

One of the greatest contributions nurses can make is to encourage clients to ask questions about sexual and reproductive functioning. With this attitude, problems of sexuality and reproduction are brought out into the open and made as resolvable as other health concerns or problems. If this is an area that you were raised to not discuss freely, learning to be comfortable with the topic and your own sexuality can be the first step needed.

Nurses who can clearly explain the physical and emotional changes of puberty to the adolescent, the physiologic changes of pregnancy to a young adult couple, or the expected changes of menopause to a middle-aged woman provide much-needed health teaching information. Several National Health Goals that speak directly to improving reproductive or sexual health are shown in Box 5.1.

BOX 5.1 ✻ Focus on National Health Goals

Several National Health Goals speak directly to reproductive and sexual health:

- Reduce the proportion of adolescents who, by age 15, have engaged in sexual intercourse to no more than 15%, from a baseline rate of 27% of girls and 33% of boys.
- Increase to at least 50% the proportion of sexually active, unmarried people who used a condom at last sexual intercourse, from a baseline rate of 19%.
- Reduce deaths from cancer of the uterine cervix to no more than 1.3 per 100,000 women, from a baseline rate of 2.8 per 100,000.
- Reduce breast cancer deaths to no more than 20.6 per 100,000 women, from a baseline rate of 23 per 100,000 (http://www.nih.gov).

Nurses can help the nation achieve these goals by educating adolescents about abstinence and refusal skills, safer sex practices, and the advantage of obtaining a vaccine against the human papillomavirus (HPV), the virus associated with cervical cancer. Women need to participate in screening activities such as breast mammography and vulvar self-examination.

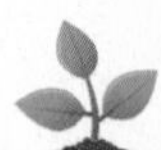

Nursing Process Overview

For Promotion of Reproductive and Sexual Health

Assessment

Problems of sexuality or reproductive health may not be evident on first meeting a client, because it may be difficult for a person to bring up the topic until he or she feels more secure. This makes good follow-through and planning important, because a person may find the courage to discuss a problem once but then be unable to do so again. If the problem is ignored or forgotten through a change in caregivers, it may never be addressed again.

Any change in physical appearance (such as occurs with puberty or with pregnancy) can intensify or create a sexual or reproductive concern. The person with a sexually transmitted infection (STI), excessive weight loss or gain, a disfiguring scar from surgery or an accident, hair loss such as occurs with chemotherapy, surgery or inflammation or infection of reproductive organs, chronic fatigue or pain, spinal cord injury, or the presence of a retention catheter needs to be assessed for problems regarding his or her sexual role as well as other important areas of reproductive functioning.

Assessing sexuality may not be appropriate as a routine part of every health assessment. However, it should be included when appropriate, such as when discussing adolescent development or before providing reproductive life planning information, during pregnancy, and after childbirth. At other times, it is wise to listen for verbal or nonverbal clues that suggest a person wants to discuss a sexual or reproductive concern. These clues are often subtle: "I guess marriage isn't for everyone"; "I'm not the woman I used to be"; "Are there ever funny effects from this medicine I'm taking?" Telling a seemingly inappropriate sexual joke may be yet another clue. Nonverbal clues may include extreme modesty or obvious embarrassment in response to a question about voiding or perineal pain or stitches.

Assessment in the area of reproductive health begins with interviewing to determine what a client knows about the reproductive process and STIs. Any concerns they might have about their own reproductive functioning or safer sex practices should be explored. This area of health interviewing takes practice and the conviction that exploring sexual health is as important as exploring less emotionally involved areas of health, such as dietary intake or activity level. The 14-year-old girl who is not yet menstruating, for instance, may be anxious about that fact but may be reluctant to say so unless asked directly. A statement such as the following invites discussion: "Although many of your friends at school may be menstruating, it's not at all uncommon for some girls not to begin their periods until age 15 or 16. How do you feel about not yet having your period?" This combination of providing information and questioning may encourage an adolescent to discuss not only her possible concern about delayed **menarche** (the beginning of menstruation) but also other areas that will show her knowledge or lack of knowledge about reproductive health. Specific questions to include in a sexual history are shown in Box 5.2.

It is important to include in a physical examination observation for normal distribution of body hair such as triangle-shaped pubic hair in women and diamond-shaped pubic hair in men, for normal genital and breast development, and for signs and symptoms of STIs. Many STIs are asymptomatic, so it is important to assess whether the client is at risk for contracting an STI (see Chapters 33 and 47 for documentation of stages of sexual development and signs of STIs).

Nursing Diagnosis

Common nursing diagnoses used in regard to reproductive health include:

- Health-seeking behaviors related to reproductive functioning
- Anxiety related to inability to conceive after 6 months without birth control
- Pain related to uterine cramping from menstruation
- Disturbance in body image related to early development of secondary sex characteristics

Diagnoses relevant to sexuality could include:

- Sexual dysfunction related to as-yet-unknown cause
- Altered sexuality patterns related to chronic illness
- Self-esteem disturbance related to recent reproductive tract surgery
- Altered sexuality patterns related to fear of harming the fetus
- Anxiety related to fear of contracting an STI
- Health-seeking behavior related to learning responsible sexual practices

Outcome Identification and Planning

A major part of nursing care in this area is to empower clients to feel control over their bodies. Plan health teaching to provide clients with knowledge about their reproductive system and specific information about ways to alleviate discomfort or prevent reproductive disease. It may also be important to plan interventions to strengthen the person's gender identity or role behavior. It is essential to design care that demonstrates acceptance of all gender-related lifestyles equally. A helpful referral organization for clients is the Children of Lesbians and Gays Everywhere group (http://www.colage.org) or http://www.sexualityandu.ca, a site with helpful tips on both sexuality and reproductive life planning.

Implementation

A primary nursing role concerning reproductive anatomy and physiology is education. This is a major role, because both female and male clients may feel more comfortable asking questions of nurses than of other health care providers. To help clients understand reproductive functioning and sexual health throughout their life, specific teaching might include:

- Encouraging women over 40 to have mammograms
- Explaining to a school-age boy that nocturnal emissions are normal
- Teaching an early adolescent what is normal and abnormal in relation to menstrual function
- Teaching a young adolescent safer sex practices
- Explaining reproductive physiology to a couple who wish to become pregnant

Teaching is often enhanced by the use of illustrations from books or journals, clips from videos or compact disks, or models of internal and external reproductive organs. Nursing interventions in this area, however, include much more than just distributing educational materials. For example, empathy for a woman's concern about increased tension before menstruation may help validate her concern that she has premenstrual dysphoric syndrome. Serving as a role model for gender roles can also be a valuable intervention, particularly for young clients. Discussing the subject of reproduction in a matter-of-fact way, or treating menstruation as a positive sign of growth in a woman rather than as a burden, may help clients assume a positive attitude about these subjects.

Interventions that strengthen an individual's sense of maleness or femaleness may improve a client's gender identity or gender role. A woman who believes that part of a female role is to be assertive needs opportunities in her care plan for making decisions and self-care; a hospitalized adolescent who views a man's role as being a person who watches Monday night football needs time structured for this activity at the same priority level as other activities. Unless such activities are structured, they can be easily omitted by busy health care providers.

BOX 5.2 ✻ Specific Questions to Include in a Sexual History

- Are you sexually active?
- Is your sexual partner of the same or different gender?
- How many sexual partners have you had in the past 6 months?
- Are you satisfied with your sex life? If not, why not?
- Do you have any concerns about your sex life? If so, what would you change?
- Do you practice "safer sex"?
- Have you ever contracted a sexually transmitted infection or are you worried that you have one now?
- Have you ever experienced a problem such as erectile dysfunction, failure to achieve orgasm, or pain during intercourse?
- Are you using a method to prevent pregnancy or sexually transmitted diseases?
- Are you satisfied with your current reproductive planning method, or do you have any questions about it?
- (For girls), Have you had a vaccine against human papillomavirus (HPV)?

Men who have sex with men (MWM) or women who have sex with women (WWW) or others with alternative lifestyles usually reveal their sexual orientation to health care providers because they want help dealing with friends or family who are having difficulty accepting their gender identity. In addition to support, provide health education that addresses potential concerns of clients with all lifestyles. For example, include a discussion about anal or oral-genital sex practices when presenting information on safer sex.

Outcome Evaluation

Evaluation in the area of reproductive health must be ongoing, because health education needs change with circumstances and increased maturity. For example, the needs of a woman at the beginning of a pregnancy may be totally different from her needs at the end.

How people feel about themselves sexually may have a great deal to do with how quickly they recover from an illness, how quickly they are ready to begin self-care after childbirth, or even how well motivated they are as adolescents to accomplish activities in other life phases that depend on being sure of sexuality or gender role.

Examples of expected outcomes are:

- Client states he is taking precautions to prevent contracting an STI.
- Client states she is better able to manage symptoms of premenstrual dysphoric syndrome.
- Couple states they have achieved a mutually satisfying sexual relationship.
- Client states he is ready to tell family about MWM gender identity.

REPRODUCTIVE DEVELOPMENT

Reproductive development and change begin at the moment of conception and continue throughout life.

Intrauterine Development

The sex of an individual is determined at the moment of conception by the chromosome information supplied by the particular ovum and sperm that joined to create the new life. A **gonad** is a body organ that produces the cells necessary for reproduction (the ovary in females, the testis in males). At approximately week 5 of intrauterine life, primitive gonadal tissue is already formed. In both sexes, two undifferentiated ducts, the mesonephric (wolffian) and paramesonephric (müllerian) ducts, are present. By week 7 or 8, in chromosomal males, this early gonadal tissue differentiates into primitive testes and begins formation of testosterone. Under the influence of testosterone, the mesonephric duct begins to develop into the male reproductive organs, and the paramesonephric duct regresses. If testosterone is not present by week 10, the gonadal tissue differentiates into ovaries, and the paramesonephric duct develops into female reproductive organs. All of the **oocytes** (cells that will develop into eggs throughout the woman's mature years) are already formed in ovaries at this stage (MacKay, 2009).

At about week 12, the external genitals develop. In males, under the influence of testosterone, penile tissue elongates and the urogenital fold on the ventral surface of the penis closes to form the urethra; in females, with no testosterone present, the urogenital fold remains open to form the labia minora; what would be formed as scrotal tissue in the male becomes the labia majora in the female. If, for some reason, testosterone secretion is halted in utero, a chromosomal male could be born with female-appearing genitalia. If a woman should be prescribed a form of testosterone during pregnancy or if the woman, because of a metabolic abnormality, produces a high level of testosterone, a chromosomal female could be born with male-appearing genitalia (Torresani & Biason-Lauber, 2007).

Pubertal Development

Puberty is the stage of life at which secondary sex changes begin. These changes are stimulated when the hypothalamus synthesizes and releases gonadotropin-releasing hormone (GnRH), which in turn triggers the anterior pituitary to begin the release of follicle-stimulating hormone (FSH) and luteinizing hormone (LH). FSH and LH initiate the production of androgen and estrogen, which in turn initiate secondary sex characteristics, the visible signs of maturity. Girls are beginning dramatic development and maturation of reproductive organs at earlier ages than ever before (9 to 12 years) (McDowell, Brody, & Hughes, 2007). Although the mechanism that initiates this dramatic change in appearance is not well understood, the hypothalamus, under the direction of the central nervous system, may serve as a gonadostat or regulation mechanism set to "turn on" gonad functioning at this age. Although it is not proved, the theory is that a girl must reach a critical weight of approximately 95 lb (43 kg) or develop a critical mass of body fat before the hypothalamus is triggered to send initial stimulation to the anterior pituitary gland to begin the formation of gonadotropic hormones. Studies of female athletes and girls with anorexia nervosa reveal that a lack of fat can delay or halt menstruation. The phenomenon of why puberty occurs is even less well understood in boys.

Role of Androgen

Androgenic hormones are the hormones responsible for muscular development, physical growth, and the increase in sebaceous gland secretions that causes typical acne in both boys and girls. In males, androgenic hormones are produced by the adrenal cortex and the testes; in females, by the adrenal cortex and the ovaries.

The level of the primary androgenic hormone, testosterone, is low in males until puberty (approximately age 12 to 14 years). At that time, testosterone levels rise to influence the further development of the testes, scrotum, penis, prostate, and seminal vesicles; the appearance of male pubic, axillary, and facial hair; laryngeal enlargement and its accompanying voice change; maturation of spermatozoa; and closure of growth in long bones.

In girls, testosterone influences enlargement of the labia majora and clitoris and formation of axillary and pubic hair. This development of pubic and axillary hair because of androgen stimulation is termed **adrenarche.**

Role of Estrogen

When triggered at puberty by FSH, ovarian follicles in females begin to excrete a high level of the hormone estrogen. This hormone is actually not one substance but three compounds (estrone [E1], estradiol [E2], and estriol [E3]).

It can be considered a single substance, however, in terms of action.

The increase in estrogen levels in the female at puberty influences the development of the uterus, fallopian tubes, and vagina; typical female fat distribution and hair patterns; breast development; and an end to growth because it closes the epiphyses of long bones. The beginning of breast development is termed **thelarche.**

Secondary Sex Characteristics

Adolescent sexual development is categorized into stages (Tanner, 1990). There is wide variation in the time required for adolescents to move through these developmental stages; however, the sequential order is fairly constant. In girls, pubertal changes typically are manifest as:

1. Growth spurt
2. Increase in the transverse diameter of the pelvis
3. Breast development
4. Growth of pubic hair
5. Onset of menstruation
6. Growth of axillary hair
7. Vaginal secretions

The average age at which menarche (the first menstrual period) occurs is 12.4 years (McDowell et al., 2007). It may occur as early as age 9 or as late as age 17, however, and still be within a normal age range. Irregular menstrual periods are the rule rather than the exception for the first year. Menstrual periods do not become regular until ovulation consistently occurs with them (menstruation is not dependent on ovulation), and this does not tend to happen until 1 to 2 years after menarche. This is one reason why estrogen-based oral contraceptives are not commonly recommended until a girl's menstrual periods have become stabilized or are ovulatory (to prevent administering a compound to halt ovulation before it is firmly established).

In boys, production of spermatozoa does not begin in intrauterine life as does the production of ova, nor are spermatozoa produced in a cyclic pattern as are ova; rather, they are produced in a continuous process. The production of ova stops at menopause (the end of the fertile period in females). In contrast, sperm production continues from puberty throughout the male's life.

Secondary sex characteristics of boys usually occur in the order of:

1. Increase in weight
2. Growth of testes
3. Growth of face, axillary, and pubic hair
4. Voice changes
5. Penile growth
6. Increase in height
7. Spermatogenesis (production of sperm)

✔ Checkpoint Question 5.1

Suzanne Matthews tells you she used to worry because her breasts developed at puberty later than those of most of her friends. Breast development is termed:

a. Adrenarche
b. Mamarche
c. Thelarche
d. Menarche

ANATOMY AND PHYSIOLOGY OF THE REPRODUCTIVE SYSTEM

Although the structures of the female and male reproductive systems differ greatly in both appearance and function, they are homologues—that is, they arise from the same or matched embryonic origin (Fig. 5.1). The study of the female reproductive organs is called **gynecology. Andrology** is the study of the male reproductive organs.

Male Reproductive System

The male reproductive system consists of both external and internal divisions (Fig. 5.2).

Male External Structures

External genital organs of the male include the testes (which are encased in the scrotal sac) and the penis.

Scrotum. The scrotum is a rugated, skin-covered, muscular pouch suspended from the perineum. Its functions are to support the testes and to help regulate the temperature of sperm. In very cold weather, the scrotal muscle contracts to bring the testes closer to the body; in very hot weather, or in the presence of fever, the muscle relaxes, allowing the testes to fall away from the body. In this way, the temperature of the testes can remain as even as possible to promote the production and viability of sperm.

Testes. The testes are two ovoid glands, 2 to 3 cm wide, that lie in the scrotum. Each testis is encased by a protective white fibrous capsule and is composed of several lobules, with each lobule containing interstitial cells (Leydig's cells) and a seminiferous tubule. Seminiferous tubules produce spermatozoa. Leydig's cells are responsible for the production of testosterone.

Testes in a fetus first form in the pelvic cavity. They descend, late in intrauterine life (about the 34th to 38th week), into the scrotal sac. Because this descent occurs so late in pregnancy, many male preterm infants are born with undescended testes. These infants need to be monitored closely to see that the testes do descend when the infant reaches what would have been the 34th to 38th week of gestational age, because testicular descent does not occur as readily in extrauterine life as it does in utero. Testes that remain in the pelvic cavity may not produce viable sperm and are associated with a 4 to 7 times higher incidence of testicular cancer (Ellsworth, 2009).

Although spermatozoa are produced in the testes, they reach maturity, surrounded by semen, in the external structures through a complex sequence of regulatory events. First, the hypothalamus releases GnRH, which in turn influences the anterior pituitary gland to release FSH and LH. FSH is then responsible for the release of androgen-binding protein (ABP). LH is responsible for the release of testosterone. ABP binding of testosterone promotes sperm formation. As the amount of testosterone increases, a feedback effect on the hypothalamus and anterior pituitary gland is created that slows the production of FSH and LH and ultimately decreases or regulates sperm production.

In most males, one testis is slightly larger than the other and is suspended slightly lower in the scrotum than the other (usually the left one). Because of this, testes tend to slide past

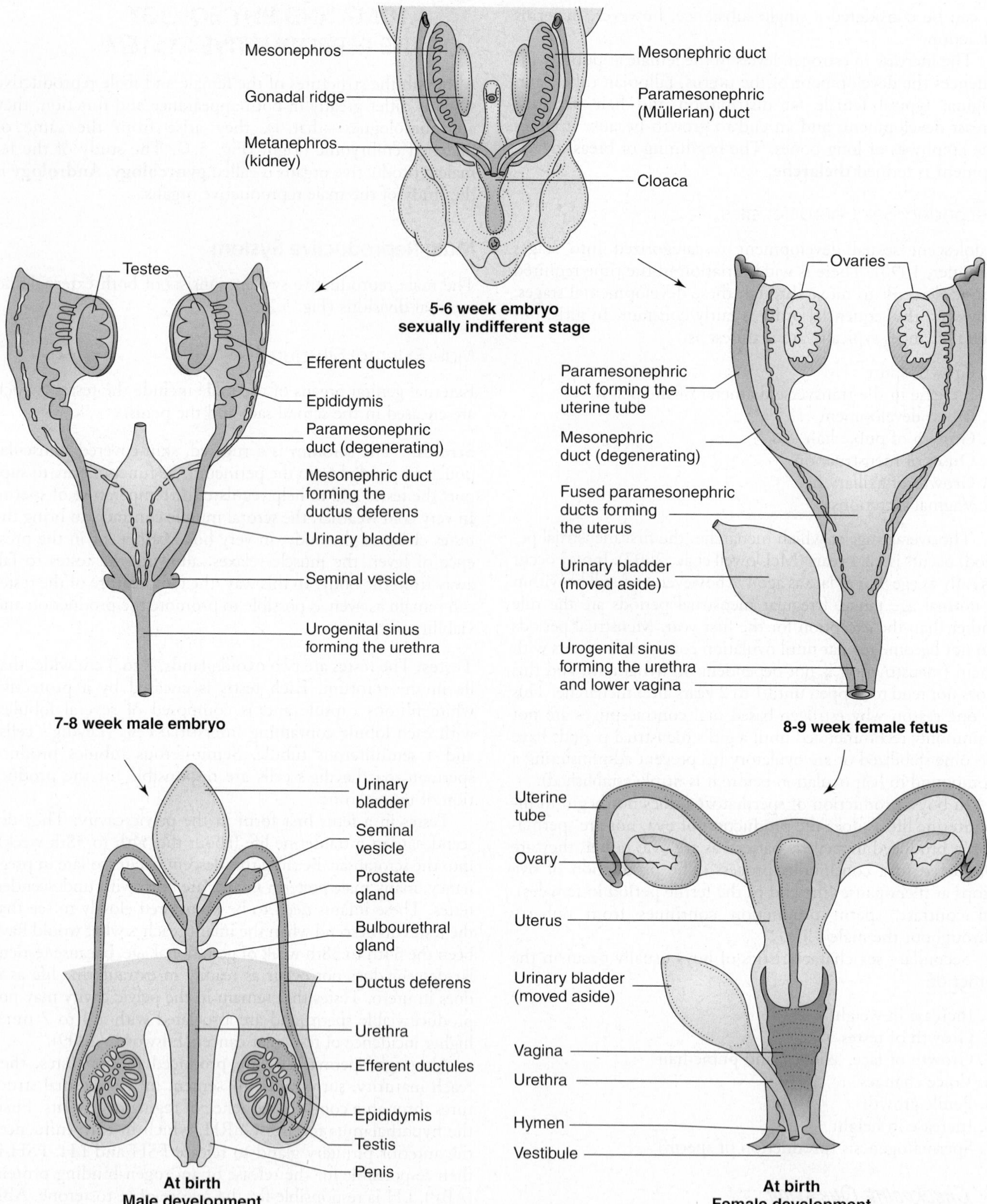

FIGURE 5.1 Development of the internal and external reproductive organs.

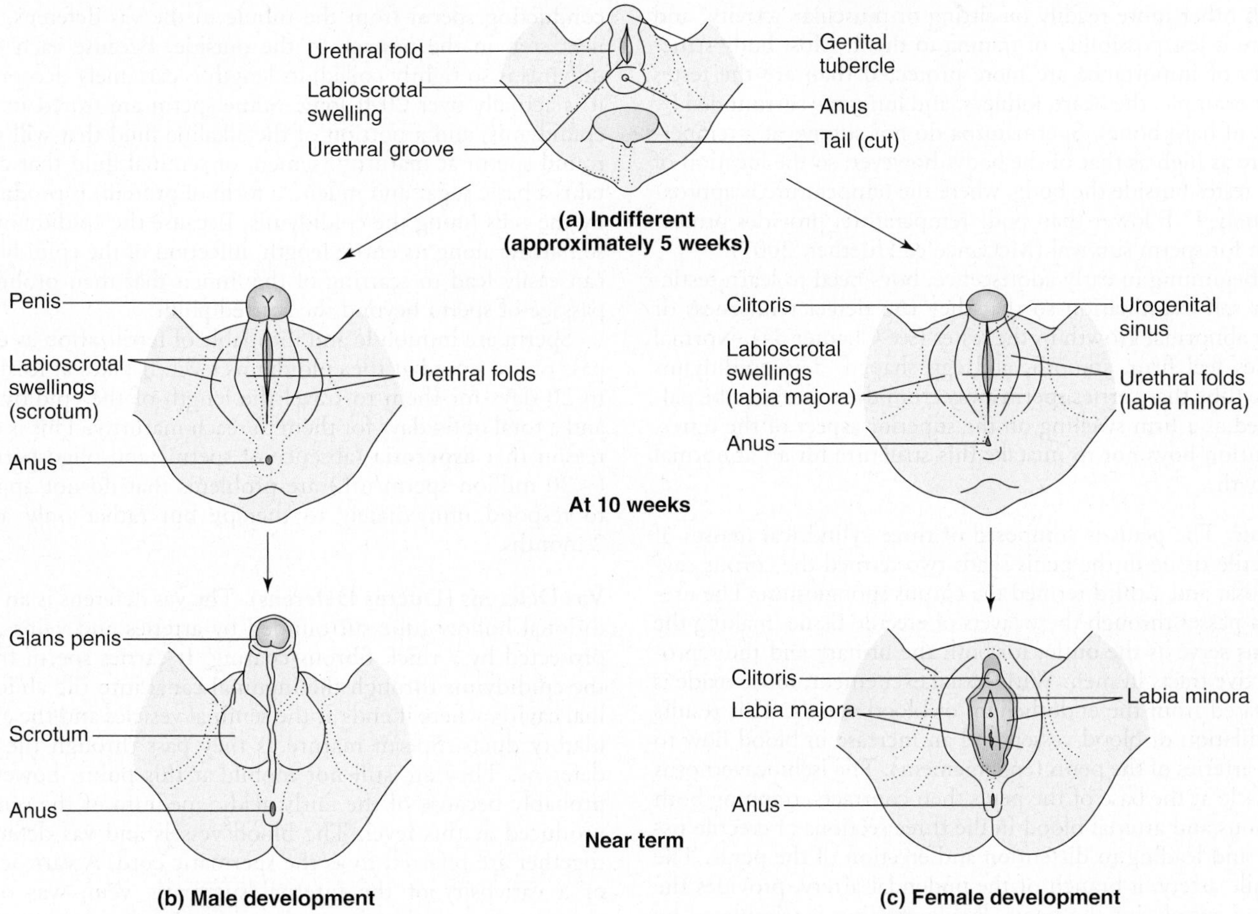

Urethral fold
Labioscrotal swelling
Urethral groove
Genital tubercle
Anus
Tail (cut)
(a) Indifferent
(approximately 5 weeks)
Penis
Labioscrotal swellings (scrotum)
Urethral folds
Anus
At 10 weeks
Clitoris
Labioscrotal swellings (labia majora)
Anus
Urogenital sinus
Urethral folds (labia minora)
Glans penis
Scrotum
Anus
Near term
Clitoris
Labia majora
Anus
Labia minora
(b) Male development
(c) Female development

FIGURE 5.1 *(continued)*

Rectum
Seminal vesicle
Ejaculatory duct
Prostate gland
Anus
Bulbourethral gland
Bulb of penis
Epididymis
Testis
Scrotum
Vas deferens
Urinary bladder
Symphysis pubis
Penis:
Corpus cavernosum
Corpus spongiosum
Urethra
Glans
Prepuce

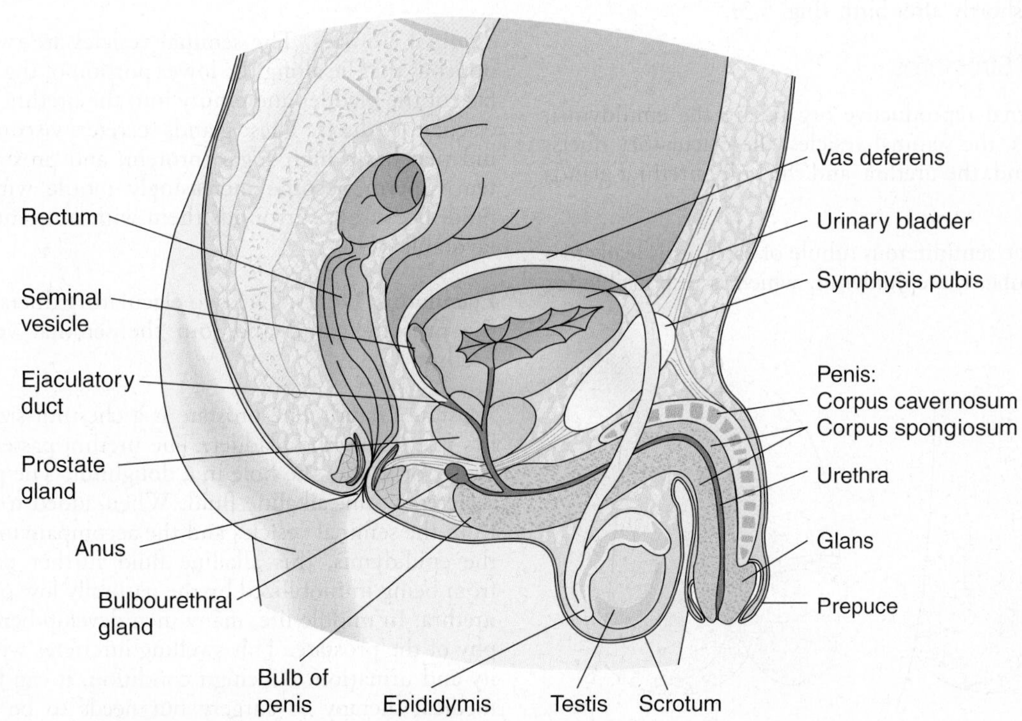

FIGURE 5.2 Male internal and external reproductive organs.

each other more readily on sitting or muscular activity, and there is less possibility of trauma to them. Most body structures of importance are more protected than are the testes (for example, the heart, kidneys, and lungs are surrounded by ribs of hard bone). Spermatozoa do not survive at a temperature as high as that of the body, however, so the location of the testes outside the body, where the temperature is approximately 1° F lower than body temperature, provides protection for sperm survival (McCance & Huether, 2007).

Beginning in early adolescence, boys need to learn testicular self-examination so that they can detect tenderness or any abnormal growth in the testes (see Chapter 34). Normal testes feel firm, smooth, and egg shaped. The epididymis (the tube that carries sperm away from the testes) can be palpated as a firm swelling on the superior aspect of the testes. Caution boys not to mistake this structure for an abnormal growth.

Penis. The penis is composed of three cylindrical masses of erectile tissue in the penis shaft: two termed the corpus cavernosa, and a third termed the corpus spongiosum. The urethra passes through these layers of erectile tissue, making the penis serve as the outlet for both the urinary and the reproductive tracts in men. With sexual excitement, nitric oxide is released from the endothelium of blood vessels. This results in dilation of blood vessels and an increase in blood flow to the arteries of the penis (engorgement). The ischiocavernosus muscle at the base of the penis then contracts, trapping both venous and arterial blood in the three sections of erectile tissue and leading to distention and erection of the penis. The penile artery, a branch of the pudendal artery, provides the blood supply for the penis. Penile erection is stimulated by parasympathetic nerve innervation.

At the distal end of the organ is a bulging, sensitive ridge of tissue, the glans. A retractable casing of skin, the prepuce, protects the nerve-sensitive glans at birth. Many infants in the United States have the prepuce tissue removed surgically (circumcision) shortly after birth (Fig. 5.3).

Male Internal Structures

The male internal reproductive organs are the epididymis, the vas deferens, the seminal vesicles, the ejaculatory ducts, the prostate gland, the urethra, and the bulbourethral glands (see Fig. 5.2).

Epididymis. The seminiferous tubule of each testis leads to a tightly coiled tube, the epididymis, which is responsible for conducting sperm from the tubule to the vas deferens, the next step in the passage to the outside. Because each epididymis is so tightly coiled, its length is extremely deceptive: it is actually over 20 ft long. Some sperm are stored in the epididymis, and a portion of the alkaline fluid that will surround sperm at maturity (semen, or seminal fluid that contains a basic sugar and mucin, a form of protein) is produced by the cells lining the epididymis. Because the epididymis is so narrow along its entire length, infection of the epididymis can easily lead to scarring of the lumen that then prohibits passage of sperm beyond the scarred point.

Sperm are immobile and incapable of fertilization as they pass or are stored at the epididymis level. It takes at least 12 to 20 days for them to travel the length of the epididymis and a total of 64 days for them to reach maturity. This is one reason that **aspermia** (absence of sperm) and oligospermia (<20 million sperm/mL) are problems that do not appear to respond immediately to therapy but rather only after 2 months.

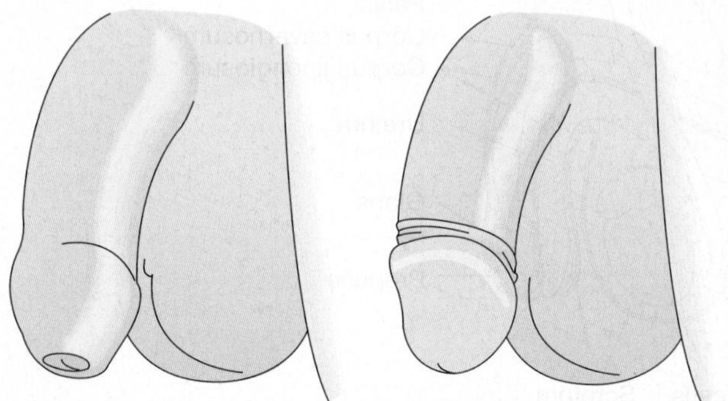

FIGURE 5.3 Uncircumcised and circumcised penis.

Vas Deferens (Ductus Deferens). The vas deferens is an additional hollow tube surrounded by arteries and veins and protected by a thick fibrous coating. It carries sperm from the epididymis through the inguinal canal into the abdominal cavity, where it ends at the seminal vesicles and the ejaculatory ducts. Sperm mature as they pass through the vas deferens. They are still not mobile at this point, however, probably because of the fairly acidic medium of the semen produced at this level. The blood vessels and vas deferens together are referred to as the spermatic cord. A varicocele, or a varicosity of the internal spermatic vein, was once thought to contribute to male subfertility by causing congestion with increased warmth in the testes but this appears to actually make little difference (Evers & Collins, 2009). Vasectomy (severing of the vas deferens to prevent passage of sperm) is a popular means of male birth control (Cook et al., 2009).

Seminal Vesicles. The seminal vesicles are two convoluted pouches that lie along the lower portion of the posterior surface of the bladder and empty into the urethra by way of the ejaculatory ducts. These glands secrete a viscous alkaline liquid that has a high sugar, protein, and prostaglandin content. Sperm become increasingly motile with this added fluid, because it surrounds them with nutrients and a more favorable pH.

Ejaculatory Ducts. The two ejaculatory ducts pass through the prostate gland and join the seminal vesicles to the urethra.

Prostate Gland. The prostate is a chestnut-sized gland that lies just below the bladder. The urethra passes through the center of it, like the hole in a doughnut. The prostate gland secretes a thin, alkaline fluid. When added to the secretion from the seminal vesicles and the accompanying sperm from the epididymis, this alkaline fluid further protects sperm from being immobilized by the naturally low pH level of the urethra. In middle life, many men develop benign hypertrophy of the prostate. This swelling interferes with both fertility and urination. A benign condition, it can be relieved by medical therapy or surgery but needs to be differentiated from prostate cancer (Parsons, 2007).

Bulbourethral Glands. Two bulbourethral or Cowper's glands lie beside the prostate gland and empty via short ducts into the urethra. Like the prostate gland and seminal vesicles, they secrete an alkaline fluid that helps counteract the acid secretion of the urethra and ensure the safe passage of spermatozoa. Semen, therefore, is derived from the prostate gland (60%), the seminal vesicles (30%), the epididymis (5%), and the bulbourethral glands (5%).

Urethra. The urethra is a hollow tube leading from the base of the bladder, which, after passing through the prostate gland, continues to the outside through the shaft and glans of the penis. It is approximately 8 in (18 to 20 cm) long. Like other urinary tract structures, it is lined with mucous membrane.

✔ Checkpoint Question 5.2

Suppose Kevin Matthews tells you that he is considering a vasectomy after the birth of his new child. Vasectomy is incision of which organ?

a. The testes
b. The vas deferens
c. The epididymis
d. The scrotum

Female Reproductive System

The female reproductive system, like the male system, has both external and internal components (Anderson & Genadry, 2007).

Female External Structures

The structures that form the female external genitalia are termed the vulva (from the Latin word for "covering") and are illustrated in Figure 5.4.

Mons Veneris. The mons veneris is a pad of adipose tissue located over the symphysis pubis, the pubic bone joint. It is covered by a triangle of coarse, curly hairs. The purpose of the mons veneris is to protect the junction of the pubic bone from trauma.

Labia Minora. Just posterior to the mons veneris spread two hairless folds of connective tissue, the labia minora. Before menarche, these folds are fairly small; by childbearing age, they are firm and full; after menopause, they atrophy and again become much smaller. Normally the folds of the labia minora are pink; the internal surface is covered with mucous membrane, and the external surface with skin. The area is abundant with sebaceous glands, so localized sebaceous cysts may occur here. Women who perform monthly vulvar examinations are able to detect infection or other abnormalities of the vulva such as sebaceous cysts.

Labia Majora. The labia majora are two folds of adipose tissue covered by loose connective tissue and epithelium that are positioned lateral to the labia minora. Covered by pubic hair, the labia majora serve as protection for the external genitalia and the distal urethra and vagina. They are fused anteriorly but separated posteriorly. Trauma to the area, such as occurs from childbirth or rape, can lead to extensive edema formation because of the looseness of the connective tissue base.

Other External Organs. The vestibule is the flattened, smooth surface inside the labia. The openings to the bladder (the urethra) and the uterus (the vagina) both arise from the vestibule. The clitoris is a small (approximately 1 to 2 cm), rounded organ of erectile tissue at the forward junction of the labia minora. It is covered by a fold of skin, the prepuce. The clitoris is sensitive to touch and temperature and is the center of sexual arousal and orgasm in a woman. Arterial blood supply for the clitoris is plentiful. When the ischio-

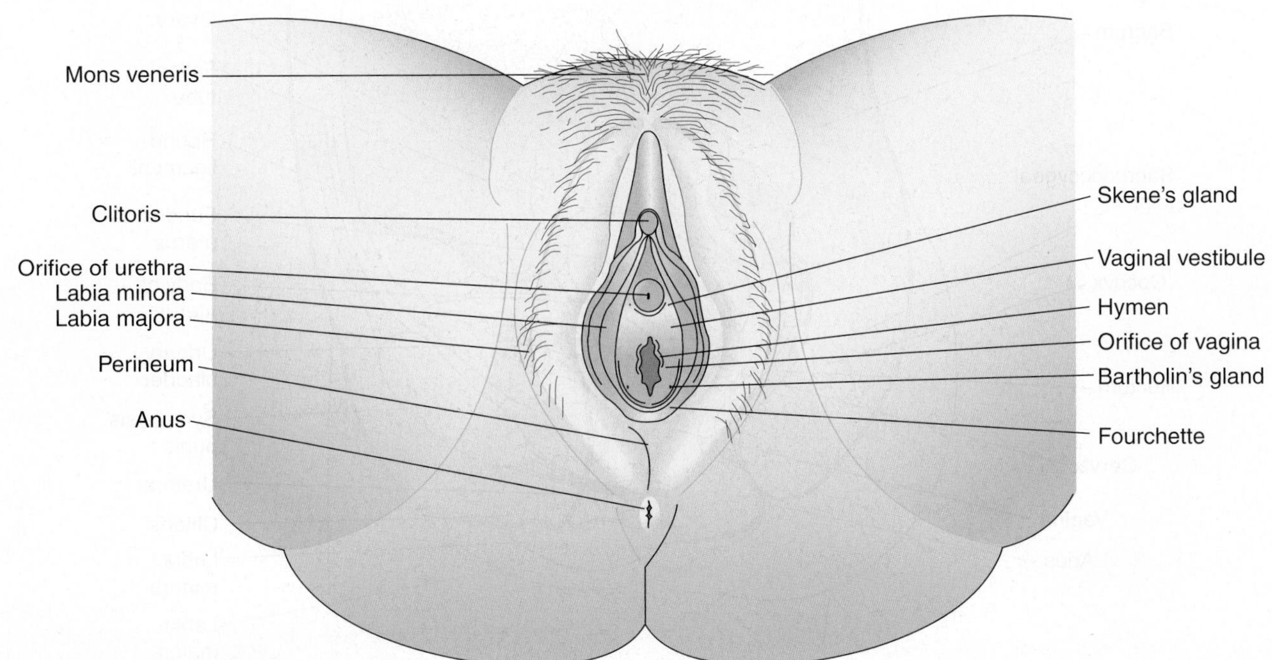

FIGURE 5.4 Female external genitalia.

cavernosus muscle surrounding it contracts with sexual arousal, the venous outflow for the clitoris is blocked, leading to clitoral erection.

Two Skene's glands (paraurethral glands) are located just lateral to the urinary meatus, one on each side. Their ducts open into the urethra. Bartholin's glands (vulvovaginal glands) are located just lateral to the vaginal opening on both sides. Their ducts open into the distal vagina. Secretions from both of these glands help to lubricate the external genitalia during coitus. The alkaline pH of their secretions helps to improve sperm survival in the vagina. Both Skene's glands and Bartholin's glands may become infected and produce a discharge and local pain.

The fourchette is the ridge of tissue formed by the posterior joining of the two labia minora and the labia majora. This is the structure that is sometimes cut (episiotomy) during childbirth to enlarge the vaginal opening.

Posterior to the fourchette is the perineal muscle or the perineal body. Because this is a muscular area, it is easily stretched during childbirth to allow for enlargement of the vagina and passage of the fetal head. Many exercises suggested for pregnancy (such as Kegel's, squatting, and tailor-sitting) are aimed at making the perineal muscle more flexible to allow easier expansion during birth without tearing of this tissue.

The hymen is a tough but elastic semicircle of tissue that covers the opening to the vagina in childhood. It is often torn during the time of first sexual intercourse. However, because of the use of tampons and active sports participation, many girls who have not had sexual relations do not have intact hymens at the time of their first pelvic examination. Occasionally, a girl has an imperforate hymen, or a hymen so complete that it does not allow for passage of menstrual blood from the vagina or for sexual relations until it is surgically incised (Dane et al., 2007).

Vulvar Blood Supply. The blood supply of the external genitalia is mainly from the pudendal artery and a portion of the inferior rectus artery. Venous return is through the pudendal vein. Pressure on this vein by the fetal head can cause extensive back-pressure and development of varicosities (distended veins) in the labia majora. Because of the rich blood supply, trauma to the area, such as occurs from pressure during childbirth, can cause large hematomas. This ready blood supply also contributes to the rapid healing of any tears in the area after childbirth (McCance & Huether, 2007).

Vulvar Nerve Supply. The anterior portion of the vulva derives its nerve supply from the ilioinguinal and genitofemoral nerves (L1 level). The posterior portions of the vulva and vagina are supplied by the pudendal nerve (S3 level). Such a rich nerve supply makes the area extremely sensitive to touch, pressure, pain, and temperature. Normal stretching of the perineum with childbirth causes temporary loss of sensation in the area. Anesthesia for childbirth may be administered locally to block the pudendal nerve, further eliminating pain sensation at the perineum during birth.

Female Internal Structures

Female internal reproductive organs (Fig. 5.5) are the ovaries, the fallopian tubes, the uterus, and the vagina.

Ovaries. The ovaries are approximately 4 cm long by 2 cm in diameter and approximately 1.5 cm thick, or the size and shape of almonds. They are grayish white and appear pitted, or with minute indentations on the surface. An unruptured, glistening, clear, fluid-filled graafian follicle (an ovum about to be discharged) or a miniature yellow corpus luteum (the structure left behind after the ovum has

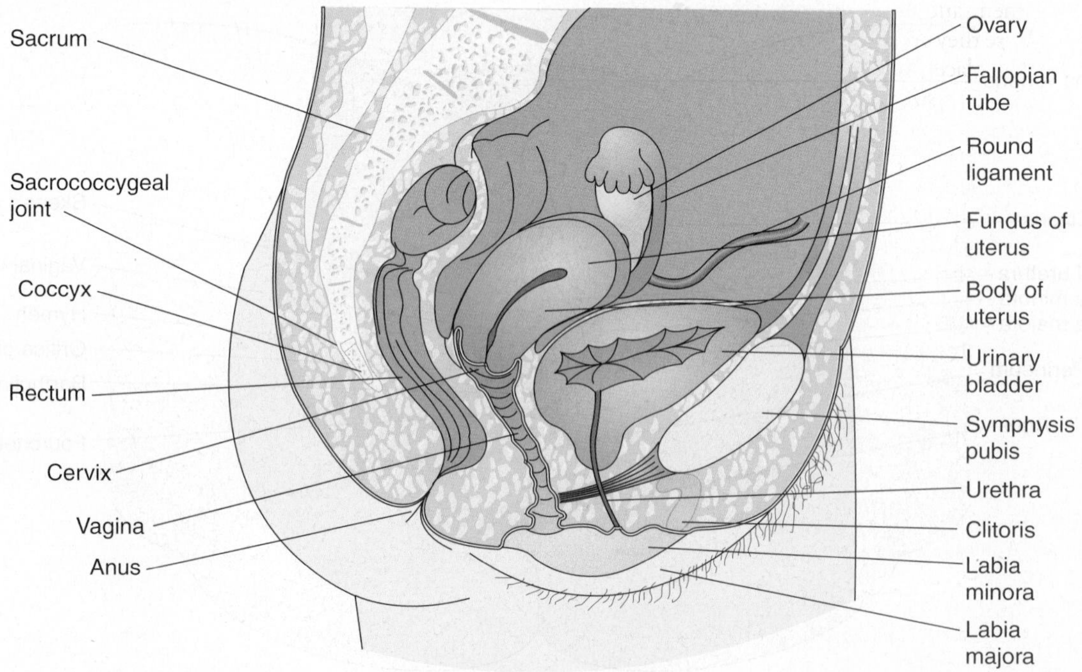

FIGURE 5.5 Female internal reproductive organs.

been discharged) often can be observed on the surface of an ovary.

Ovaries are located close to and on both sides of the uterus in the lower abdomen. It is difficult to locate them by abdominal palpation because they are situated so low in the abdomen. If an abnormality is present, such as an enlarging ovarian cyst, the resulting tenderness may be evident on lower-left or lower-right abdominal palpation.

The function of the two ovaries (the female gonads) is to produce, mature, and discharge ova (the egg cells). In the process, the ovaries produce estrogen and progesterone and initiate and regulate menstrual cycles. If the ovaries are removed before puberty (or are nonfunctional), the resulting absence of estrogen prevents breasts from maturing at puberty; in addition, pubic hair distribution assumes a more male pattern than normal. After menopause, or cessation of ovarian function, the uterus, breasts, and ovaries all undergo atrophy or a reduction in size because of a lack of estrogen. Ovarian function, therefore, is necessary for maturation and maintenance of secondary sex characteristics in females. The estrogen secreted by ovaries is also important to prevent osteoporosis, or weakness of bones, because of withdrawal of calcium from bones. This frequently occurs in women after menopause, making women prone to serious spinal, hip, and wrist fractures. Because cholesterol is incorporated into estrogen, the production of estrogen is thought to also keep cholesterol levels reduced, thus limiting the effects of atherosclerosis (artery disease) in women. Estrogen used to be prescribed for women at menopause to help prevent osteoporosis and cardiovascular disease. However, this type of long-term estrogen supplementation may contribute to breast cancer and cerebrovascular accidents, so it is no longer routinely recommended (Kulp & Zacur, 2007).

The ovaries are held suspended and in close contact with the ends of the fallopian tubes by three strong supporting ligaments attached to the uterus or the pelvic wall. They are unique among pelvic structures in that they are not covered by a layer of peritoneum. Because they are not encased in this way, ova can escape from them and enter the uterus by way of the fallopian tubes. Because they are suspended in position rather than being firmly fixed in place, an abnormal tumor or cyst growing on them can enlarge to a size easily twice that of the organ before pressure on surrounding organs or the ovarian blood supply leads to symptoms of compression. This is the reason that ovarian cancer continues to be one of the leading causes of death from cancer in women (i.e., the tumor grows without symptoms for an extended period) (Neves-E-Castro, 2007).

Ovaries have three principal divisions:

1. Protective layer of surface epithelium
2. Cortex, where the immature (primordial) oocytes mature into ova and large amounts of estrogen and progesterone are produced
3. Central medulla, which contains the nerves, blood vessels, lymphatic tissue, and some smooth muscle tissue

Division of Reproductive Cells (Gametes). At birth, each ovary contains approximately 2 million immature ova (oocytes), which were formed during the first 5 months of intrauterine life. Although these cells have the unique ability to produce a new individual, they basically contain the usual components of cells: a cell membrane, an area of clear cytoplasm, and a nucleus containing chromosomes.

The oocytes, like sperm, differ from all other body cells in the number of chromosomes they contain in the nucleus. The nucleus of all other human body cells contains 46 chromosomes, consisting of 22 pairs of autosomes (paired matching chromosomes) and 1 pair of sex chromosomes (two X sex chromosomes in the female, an X and a Y sex chromosome pair in the male). Reproductive cells (both ova and spermatozoa) have only half the usual number of chromosomes, so that, when they combine (fertilization), the new individual formed from them will have the normal number of 46 chromosomes. If both the ova and the spermatozoa carried the full complement of chromosomes, a new individual formed from them would have twice the normal number. There is a difference in the way reproductive cells divide that causes this change in chromosome number.

Cells in the body, such as skin cells, undergo cell division by mitosis, or daughter cell division. In this type of division, all the chromosomes are duplicated in each cell just before cell division, giving every new cell the same number of chromosomes as the original parent cell. Oocytes divide in intrauterine life by one mitotic division. Division activity then appears to halt until at least puberty, when a second type of cell division, meiosis (cell reduction division), occurs. In the male, this reduction division occurs just before the spermatozoa mature. In the female, it occurs just before ovulation. After this reduction division, an ovum has 22 autosomes and an X sex chromosome, whereas a spermatozoon has 22 autosomes and either an X or a Y sex chromosome. A new individual formed from the union of an ovum and an X-carrying spermatozoon will be female (an XX chromosome pattern); an individual formed from the union of an ovum and a Y-carrying spermatozoon will be male (an XY chromosome pattern).

Maturation of Oocytes. Each oocyte lies in the ovary surrounded by a protective sac, or thin layer of cells, called a primordial follicle. Between 5 and 7 million ova form in utero. The majority never develop beyond the primitive state and actually atrophy, so that by birth only 2 million are present. By age 7 years, only approximately 500,000 are present in each ovary; by 22 years, there are approximately 300,000; and by menopause, none are left (all have either matured or atrophied). "The point at which no functioning oocytes remain in the ovaries" is one definition of menopause.

Fallopian Tubes. The fallopian tubes arise from each upper corner of the uterine body and extend outward and backward until each opens at its distal end, next to an ovary. Fallopian tubes are approximately 10 cm long in a mature woman. Their function is to convey the ovum from the ovaries to the uterus and to provide a place for fertilization of the ovum by sperm.

Although a fallopian tube is a smooth, hollow tunnel, it is anatomically divided into four separate parts (Fig. 5.6). The most proximal division, the interstitial portion, is that part of the tube that lies within the uterine wall. This portion is only about 1 cm in length; the lumen of the tube is only 1 mm in diameter at this point. The isthmus is the next distal portion. It is approximately 2 cm in length and like the interstitial tube, is extremely narrow. This is the portion of the tube that is cut or sealed in a tubal ligation, or tubal sterilization

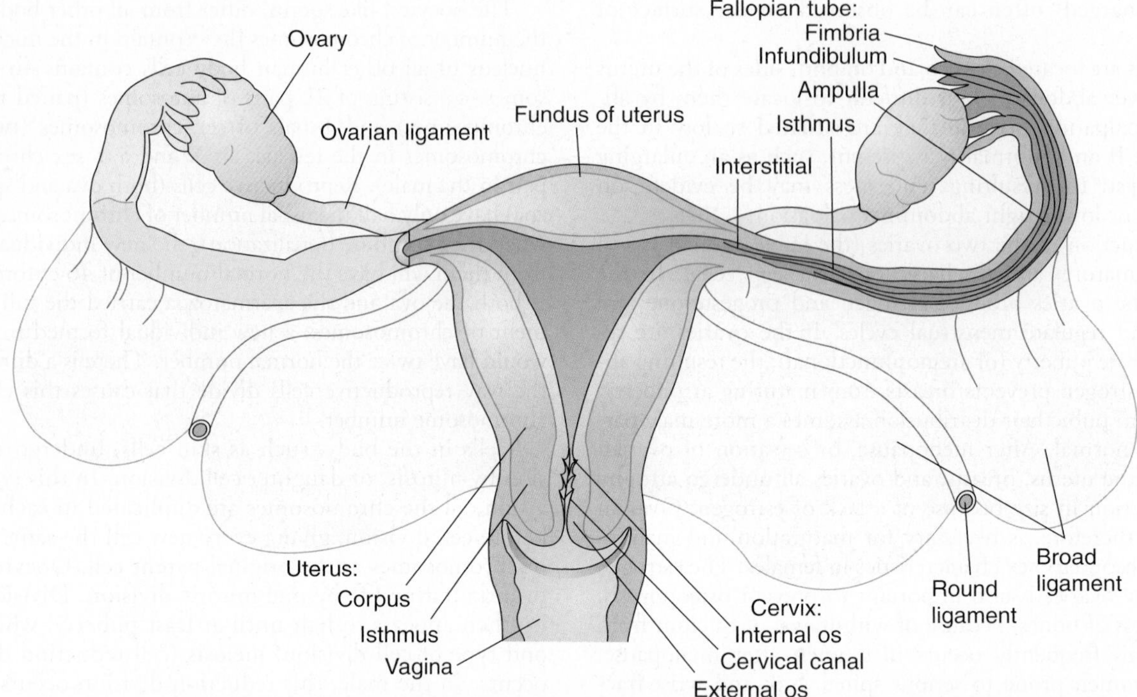

FIGURE 5.6 Anterior view of female reproductive organs showing relationship of fallopian tubes and body of the uterus.

procedure. The ampulla is the third and also the longest portion of the tube. It is approximately 5 cm in length. It is in this portion that fertilization of an ovum usually occurs. The infundibular portion is the most distal segment of the tube. It is approximately 2 cm long and is funnel shaped. The rim of the funnel is covered by fimbria (small hairs) that help to guide the ovum into the fallopian tube.

The lining of the entire fallopian tube is composed of mucous membrane, which contains both mucus-secreting and ciliated (hair-covered) cells. Beneath the mucous lining is connective tissue and a circular muscle layer. The muscle layer of the tube produces peristaltic motions that help conduct the ovum the length of the tube. Migration of the ovum is also aided by the action of the ciliated lining and the mucus, which acts as a lubricant. The mucus produced may also act as a source of nourishment for the fertilized egg, because it contains protein, water, and salts.

Because the fallopian tubes are open at their distal ends, a direct pathway exists from the external organs, through the vagina to the uterus and tubes, to the peritoneum. This pathway makes conception possible. It can also lead to infection of the peritoneum (peritonitis) if disease spreads from the perineum through the tubes to the pelvic cavity. For this reason, careful, clean technique must be used during pelvic examinations or treatment. Vaginal examinations during labor and birth are done with sterile technique to ensure that no organisms can enter.

Uterus. The uterus is a hollow, muscular, pear-shaped organ located in the lower pelvis, posterior to the bladder and anterior to the rectum. During childhood, it is approximately the size of an olive, and its proportions are reversed from what they are later (i.e., the cervix is the largest portion of the organ; the uterine body is the smallest). When a girl reaches approximately 8 years of age, an increase in the size of the uterus begins. An adolescent is closer to 17 years old before the uterus reaches its adult size. This may be a contributing factor to the low-birth-weight babies typically born to adolescents younger than this age.

With maturity, a uterus is approximately 5 to 7 cm long, 5 cm wide, and, in its widest upper part, 2.5 cm deep. In a nonpregnant state, it weighs approximately 60 g. The function of the uterus is to receive the ovum from the fallopian tube; provide a place for implantation and nourishment; furnish protection to a growing fetus; and, at maturity of the fetus, expel it from a woman's body.

After a pregnancy, the uterus never returns to its nonpregnant size but remains approximately 9 cm long, 6 cm wide, 3 cm thick, and 80 g in weight.

Anatomically, the uterus consists of three divisions: the body or corpus, the isthmus, and the cervix. The body of the uterus is the uppermost part and forms the bulk of the organ. The lining of the cavity is continuous with that of the fallopian tubes, which enter at its upper aspects (the cornua). During pregnancy, the body of the uterus is the portion of the structure that expands to contain the growing fetus. The portion of the uterus between the points of attachment of the fallopian tubes is termed the fundus. The fundus is also the portion that can be palpated abdominally to determine the amount of uterine growth occurring during pregnancy, to measure the force of uterine contractions during labor, and to assess that the uterus is returning to its nonpregnant state after childbirth.

The isthmus of the uterus is a short segment between the body and the cervix. In the nonpregnant uterus, it is only 1 to 2 mm in length. During pregnancy, this portion also enlarges greatly to aid in accommodating the growing fetus. It is the portion of the uterus that is most commonly cut when a fetus is born by a cesarean birth.

The cervix is the lowest portion of the uterus. It represents approximately one third of the total uterus size and is approximately 2 to 5 cm long. Approximately half of it lies above the vagina and half extends into the vagina. Its central cavity is termed the cervical canal. The opening of the canal at the junction of the cervix and isthmus is the internal cervical os; the distal opening to the vagina is the external cervical os. The level of the external os is at the level of the ischial spines (an important relationship in estimating the level of the fetus in the birth canal).

Uterine and Cervical Coats. The uterine wall consists of three separate coats or layers of tissue: an inner one of mucous membrane (the endometrium), a middle one of muscle fibers (the myometrium), and an outer one of connective tissue (the perimetrium).

The endometrium layer of the uterus is the one that is important for menstrual function. It is formed by two layers of cells. The layer closest to the uterine wall, the basal layer, remains stable, uninfluenced by hormones. In contrast, the inner glandular layer is greatly influenced by both estrogen and progesterone. It grows and becomes so thick and responsive each month under the influence of estrogen and progesterone that it is capable of supporting a pregnancy. If pregnancy does not occur, this is the layer that is shed as the menstrual flow.

The mucous membrane lining the cervix is termed the endocervix. The endocervix, continuous with the endometrium, is also affected by hormones, but changes are manifested in a more subtle way. The cells of the cervical lining secrete mucus to provide a lubricated surface so that spermatozoa can readily pass through the cervix; the efficiency of this lubrication increases or wanes depending on hormone stimulation. At the point in the menstrual cycle when estrogen production is at its peak, as much as 700 mL of mucus per day is produced; at the point that estrogen is very low, only a few milliliters are produced. Because mucus is alkaline, it helps to decrease the acidity of the upper vagina, aiding in sperm survival. During pregnancy, the endocervix becomes plugged with mucus, forming a seal to keep out ascending infections (the operculum).

The lower surface of the cervix and the lower third of the cervical canal are lined not with mucous membrane but with stratified squamous epithelium, similar to that lining the vagina. Locating the point at which this tissue changes from epithelium to mucous membrane is important when obtaining a Papanicolaou smear (a test for cervical cancer), because this tissue interface is most often the origin of cervical cancer.

The myometrium, or muscle layer of the uterus, is composed of three interwoven layers of smooth muscle, the fibers of which are arranged in longitudinal, transverse, and oblique directions. This network offers extreme strength to the organ. The myometrium serves the important function of constricting the tubal junctions and preventing regurgitation of menstrual blood into the tubes. It also holds the internal cervical os closed during pregnancy to prevent a preterm birth. When the uterus contracts at the end of pregnancy to expel the fetus, equal pressure is exerted at all points throughout the cavity because of its unique arrangement of muscle fibers. After childbirth, this interlacing network of fibers is able to constrict the blood vessels coursing through the layers, thereby limiting the loss of blood in the woman. Myomas, or benign fibroid (leiomyoma) tumors, arise from the myometrium (McCance & Heuther, 2007).

The perimetrium, or the outermost layer of the uterus, serves the purpose of adding strength and support to the structure.

Uterine Blood Supply. The large descending abdominal aorta divides to form two iliac arteries; main divisions of the iliac arteries are the hypogastric arteries (Fig. 5.7). These further divide to form the uterine arteries and supply the uterus. Because the uterine blood supply is not far removed from the aorta, it is copious and adequate to supply the growing needs of a fetus. As an additional safeguard, after supplying the ovary with blood, the ovarian artery (a direct subdivision of the aorta) joins the uterine artery as a fail-safe system to ensure that the uterus will have an adequate blood supply. The blood vessels that supply the cells and lining of the uterus are tortuous against the sides of the uterine body in nonpregnant women. As a uterus enlarges with pregnancy, the vessels "unwind" and so can stretch to maintain an adequate blood supply as the organ enlarges. The uterine veins follow the same twisting course as the arteries; they empty into the internal iliac veins.

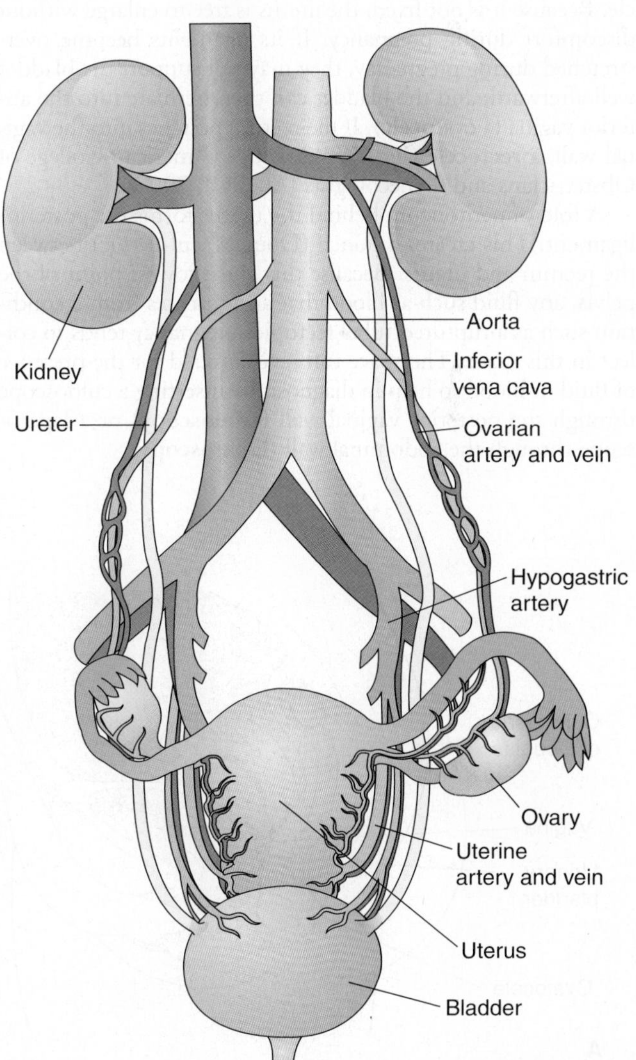

FIGURE 5.7 Blood supply to the uterus.

An important organ relationship to be aware of is the association of uterine vessels and the ureters. The ureters from the kidneys pass directly in back of the ovarian vessels, near the fallopian tubes. As shown in Figure 5.7, they cross just beneath the uterine vessels before they enter the bladder. This close anatomic relationship has implications in procedures such as tubal ligation, cesarean birth, and hysterectomy (removal of the uterus), because a ureter may be injured by a clamp if bleeding is controlled by clamping of the uterine or ovarian vessels.

Uterine Nerve Supply. The uterus is supplied by both efferent (motor) and afferent (sensory) nerves. The efferent nerves arise from the T5 through T10 spinal ganglia. The afferent nerves join the hypogastric plexus and enter the spinal column at T11 and T12. The fact that sensory innervation from the uterus registers lower in the spinal column than does motor control has implications in controlling pain in labor. An anesthetic solution can be injected near the spinal column to stop the pain of uterine contractions at the T11 and T12 levels without stopping motor control or contractions (registered higher, at the T5 to T10 level). This is the principle of epidural and spinal anesthesia (see Chapter 16).

Uterine Supports. The uterus is suspended in the pelvic cavity by several ligaments that also help support the bladder and is further supported by a combination of fascia and muscle. Because it is not fixed, the uterus is free to enlarge without discomfort during pregnancy. If its ligaments become overstretched during pregnancy, they may not support the bladder well afterward, and the bladder can then herniate into the anterior vagina (a **cystocele**). If the rectum pouches into the vaginal wall, a **rectocele** (Fig. 5.8) develops (American College of Obstetricians and Gynecologists [ACOG], 2007).

A fold of peritoneum behind the uterus forms the posterior ligament. This creates a pouch (Douglas' cul-de-sac) between the rectum and uterus. Because this is the lowest point of the pelvis, any fluid such as blood that accumulates from a condition such as a ruptured tubal (ectopic) pregnancy tends to collect in this space. The space can be examined for the presence of fluid or blood to help in diagnosis by inserting a culdoscope through the posterior vaginal wall (**culdoscopy**) or a laparoscope through the abdominal wall (**laparoscopy**).

The broad ligaments are two folds of peritoneum that cover the uterus front and back and extend to the pelvic sides to help steady the uterus. The round ligaments are two fibrous, muscular cords that pass from the body of the uterus near the attachments of the fallopian tubes, through the broad ligaments and into the inguinal canal, inserting into the fascia of the vulva. The round ligaments act as additional "stays" to further steady the uterus. If a pregnant woman moves quickly, she may pull one of these ligaments. This causes a quick, sharp pain of frightening intensity in one of her lower abdominal quadrants that can be mistaken for labor pain.

What if... Suzanne Matthews decides to have a tubal ligation (clamping of the fallopian tubes) after the birth of her baby? Why is observing women for urine output after uterine or fallopian tube surgery of this kind always a critical assessment?

Uterine Deviations. Several uterine deviations (shape and position) may interfere with fertility or pregnancy. In the fetus, the uterus first forms with a septum or a fibrous division, longitudinally separating it into two portions. As the fetus matures, this septum dissolves, so that typically at birth no remnant of the division remains. In some women, the septum never atrophies, and so the uterus remains as two separate compartments. In others, half of the septum is still present. Still other women have oddly shaped "horns" at the junction of the fallopian tubes, termed a **bicornuate uterus.** Any of these malformations may decrease the ability to conceive or to carry a pregnancy to term (Krantz, 2007). Some variations of uterine formation are shown in Figure 5.9. The specific effects of these deviations on fertility and pregnancy are discussed in later chapters.

Ordinarily, the body of the uterus is tipped slightly forward. Positional deviations of the uterus commonly seen are:

- **Anteversion,** a condition in which the entire uterus is tipped far forward
- **Retroversion,** a condition in which the entire uterus is tipped backward

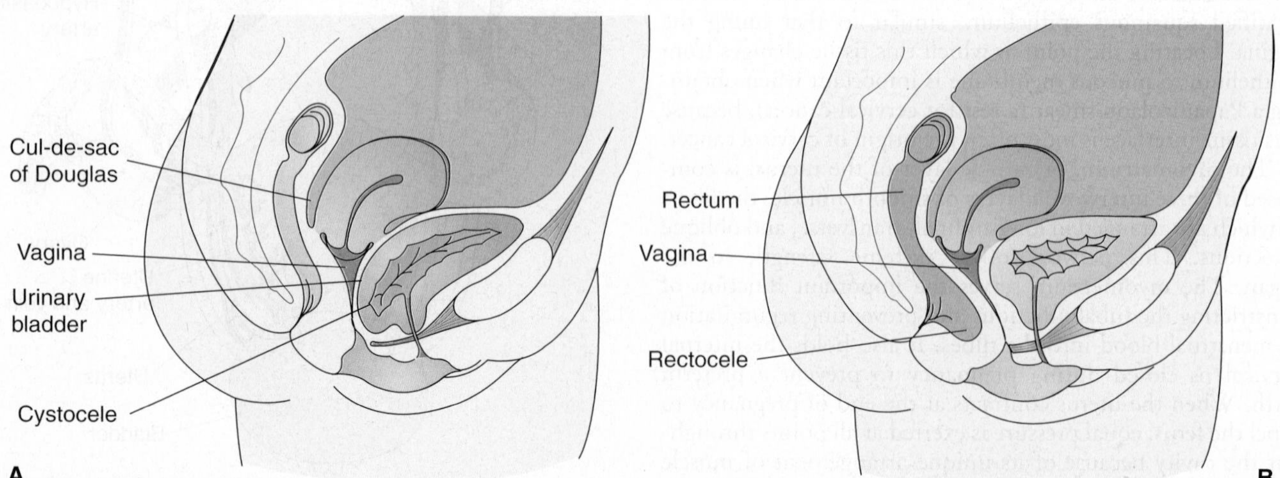

FIGURE 5.8 (**A**) Cystocele. The bladder has herniated into the anterior wall of the vagina. (**B**) Rectocele. The rectum has herniated into the posterior vaginal wall.

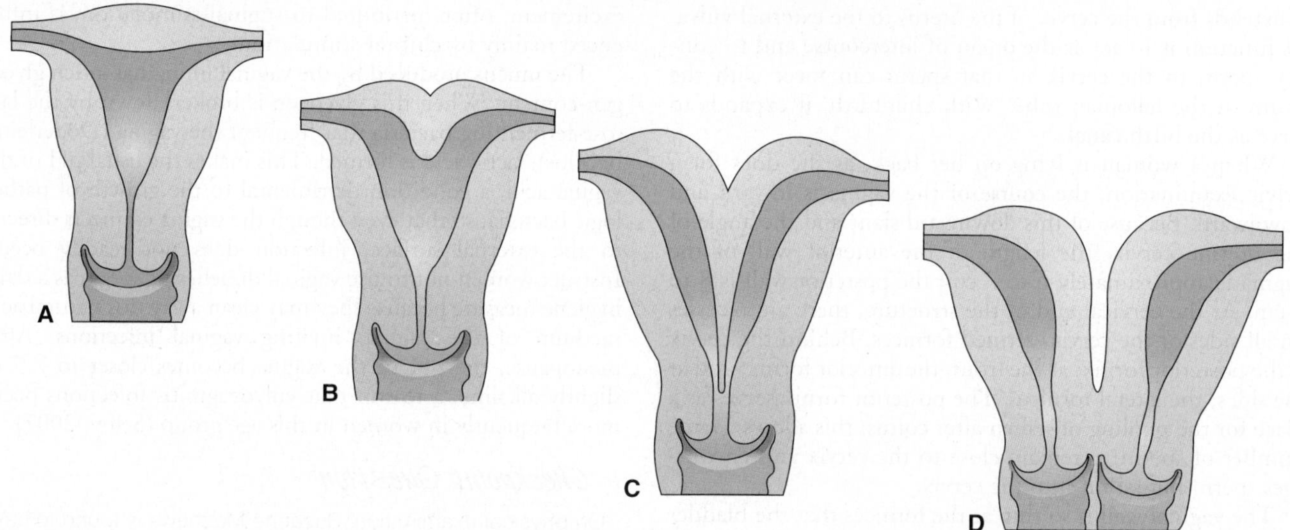

FIGURE 5.9 (**A**) Normal uterus. (**B**) Bicornuate uterus. (**C**) Septum dividing uterus. (**D**) Double uterus. Abnormal shapes of uterus allow less placenta implantation space.

- **Anteflexion,** a condition in which the body of the uterus is bent sharply forward at the junction with the cervix
- **Retroflexion,** a condition in which the body is bent sharply back just above the cervix

Minor variations of these positions do not cause reproductive problems. Extreme abnormal flexion or version positions may interfere with fertility, because they can block the deposition or migration of sperm. Examples of these abnormal uterine positions are shown in Figure 5.10.

Vagina. The vagina is a hollow, musculomembranous canal located posterior to the bladder and anterior to the rectum.

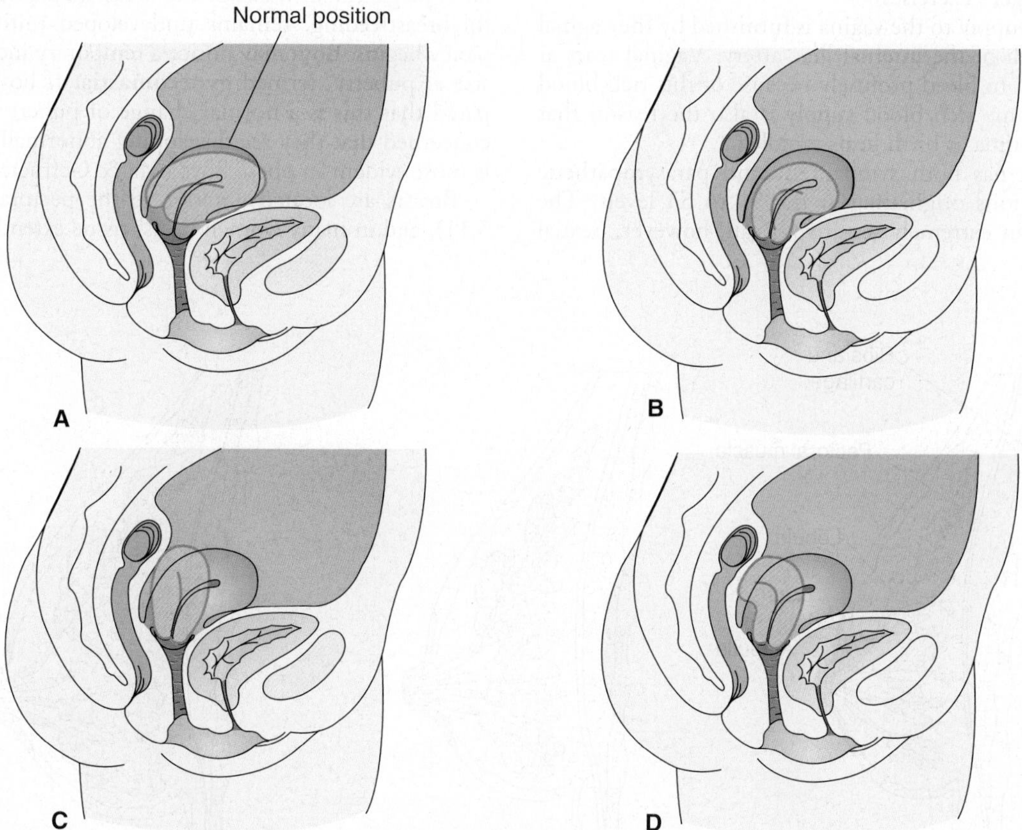

FIGURE 5.10 Uterine flexion and version. (**A**) Anteversion. (**B**) Anteflexion. (**C**) Retroversion. (**D**) Retroflexion.

It extends from the cervix of the uterus to the external vulva. Its function is to act as the organ of intercourse and to convey sperm to the cervix so that sperm can meet with the ovum in the fallopian tube. With childbirth, it expands to serve as the birth canal.

When a woman is lying on her back, as she does for a pelvic examination, the course of the vagina is inward and downward. Because of this downward slant and the angle of the uterine cervix, the length of the anterior wall of the vagina is approximately 6 to 7 cm; the posterior wall is 8 to 9 cm. At the cervical end of the structure, there are recesses on all sides of the cervix, termed fornices. Behind the cervix is the posterior fornix; at the front, the anterior fornix; and at the sides, the lateral fornices. The posterior fornix serves as a place for the pooling of semen after coitus; this allows a large number of sperm to remain close to the cervix and encourages sperm migration into the cervix.

The vaginal wall is so thin at the fornices that the bladder can be palpated through the anterior fornix, the ovaries through the lateral fornices, and the rectum through the posterior fornix. The vagina is lined with stratified squamous epithelium similar to that covering the cervix. It has a middle connective tissue layer and a strong muscular wall. Normally, the walls contain many folds or rugae that lie in close approximation to each other. These folds make the vagina very elastic and able to expand at the end of pregnancy to allow a full-term baby to pass through without tearing. A circular muscle, the bulbocavernosus, at the external opening of the vagina acts as a voluntary sphincter. Relaxing and tensing this external vaginal sphincter muscle a set number of times each day makes it more supple for birth and helps maintain tone after birth (Kegel's exercises).

The blood supply to the vagina is furnished by the vaginal artery, a branch of the internal iliac artery. Vaginal tears at childbirth tend to bleed profusely because of this rich blood supply. The same rich blood supply is also the reason that any vaginal trauma at birth heals rapidly.

The vagina has both sympathetic and parasympathetic nerve innervations originating at the S1 to S3 levels. The vagina is not an extremely sensitive organ, however. Sexual excitement, often attributed to vaginal stimulation, is influenced mainly by clitoral stimulation.

The mucus produced by the vaginal lining has a rich glycogen content. When this glycogen is broken down by the lactose-fermenting bacteria that frequent the vagina (Döderlein's bacillus), lactic acid is formed. This makes the usual pH of the vagina acid, a condition detrimental to the growth of pathologic bacteria, so that even though the vagina connects directly to the external surface, infection does not readily occur. Instruct women not to use vaginal douches or sprays as a daily hygiene measure because they may clean away this natural acid medium of the vagina, inviting vaginal infections. After menopause, the pH of the vagina becomes closer to 7.5 or slightly alkaline, a reason that vulvovaginitis infections occur more frequently in women in this age group (Selby, 2007).

✔ Checkpoint Question 5.3

On physical examination, Suzanne Matthews is found to have a cystocele. A cystocele is:

a. A sebaceous cyst arising from a vulvar fold.
b. Protrusion of the intestine into the vagina.
c. Prolapse of the uterus and cervix into the vagina.
d. Herniation of the bladder into the vaginal wall.

Breasts

The mammary glands, or breasts, form from ectodermic tissue early in utero. They then remain in a halted stage of development until a rise in estrogen at puberty produces a marked increase in their size. The size increase occurs mainly because of an increase of connective tissue plus deposition of fat. The glandular tissue of the breasts, necessary for successful breastfeeding, remains undeveloped until a first pregnancy begins. Boys may notice a temporary increase in breast size at puberty, termed **gynecomastia.** If boys are not prepared that this is a normal change of puberty, they may be concerned that they are developing abnormally. The change is most evident in obese boys (Ma & Geffner, 2008).

Breasts are located anterior to the pectoral muscle (Fig. 5.11), and in many women breast tissue extends well into the

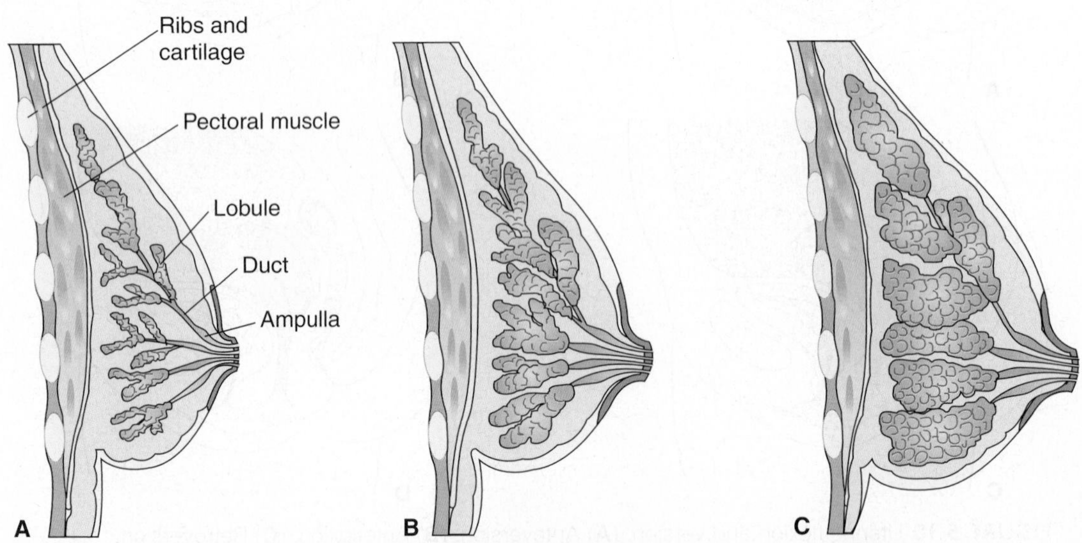

FIGURE 5.11 Anatomy of the breast. (**A**) Nonpregnant. (**B**) Pregnant. (**C**) During lactation.

TABLE 5.1 ✻ Characteristics of Normal Menstrual Cycles

Characteristic	Description
Beginning (menarche)	Average age at onset, 12.4 years; average range, 9–17 years
Interval between cycles	Average, 28 days; cycles of 23–35 days not unusual
Duration of menstrual flow	Average flow, 2–7 days; ranges of 1–9 days not abnormal
Amount of menstrual flow	Difficult to estimate; average 30–80 mL per menstrual period; saturating pad or tampon in less than an hour is heavy bleeding
Color of menstrual flow	Dark red; a combination of blood, mucus, and endometrial cells
Odor	Similar to that of marigolds

axilla. Breast self-examinations are not as effective in detecting early breast lesions as once believed and so are no longer routinely recommended (Kosters & Gotzsche, 2007). Women should have a yearly breast examination done by a health care professional, however, as this can detect breast disease. When palpating for breast health this way, always include the axillary region in the examination, or some breast tissue can be missed.

Milk glands of the breasts are divided by connective tissue partitions into approximately 20 lobes. All of the glands in each lobe produce milk by acinar cells and deliver it to the nipple via a lactiferous duct. The nipple has approximately 20 small openings through which milk is secreted. An ampulla portion of the duct, located just posterior to the nipple, serves as a reservoir for milk before breastfeeding.

A nipple is composed of smooth muscle that is capable of erection on manual or sucking stimulation. On stimulation, it transmits sensations to the posterior pituitary gland to release oxytocin. Oxytocin acts to constrict milk gland cells and push milk forward into the ducts that lead to the nipple. The skin surrounding the nipples is darkly pigmented out to approximately 4 cm and is termed the areola. The area appears rough on the surface because it contains many sebaceous glands, called Montgomery's tubercles.

The blood supply to the breasts is profuse because it is supplied by thoracic branches of the axillary, internal mammary, and intercostal arteries. This effective blood supply is important in bringing nutrients to the milk glands and makes possible a plentiful supply of milk for breastfeeding. However, it also aids in the metastasis of breast cancer if this is not discovered early with breast examination or mammography (McCance & Huether, 2007).

MENSTRUATION

A menstrual cycle (a female reproductive cycle) is episodic uterine bleeding in response to cyclic hormonal changes. The purpose of a menstrual cycle is to bring an ovum to maturity and renew a uterine tissue bed that will be responsible for the ova's growth should it be fertilized. It is the process that allows for conception and implantation of a new life. Because menarche may occur as early as 9 years of age, it is good to include health teaching information on menstruation to both school age children and their parents as early as fourth grade as part of routine care. It is a poor introduction to sexuality and womanhood for a girl to begin menstruation unwarned and unprepared for the important internal function it represents.

The length of menstrual cycles differs from woman to woman, but the average length is 28 days (from the beginning of one menstrual flow to the beginning of the next). It is not unusual for cycles to be as short as 23 days or as long as 35 days. The length of the average menstrual flow (termed menses) is 4 to 6 days, although women may have periods as short as 2 days or as long as 7 days (MacKay, 2009).

Because there is such variation in length, frequency, and amount of menstrual flow and such variation in the onset of menarche, many women have questions about what is considered normal. Contact with health care personnel during a yearly health examination or prenatal visit may be their first opportunity to ask questions they have had for some time. Table 5.1 summarizes the normal characteristics of menstruation for quick reference.

Physiology of Menstruation

Four body structures are involved in the physiology of the menstrual cycle: the hypothalamus, the pituitary gland, the ovaries, and the uterus. For a menstrual cycle to be complete, all four structures must contribute their part; inactivity of any part results in an incomplete or ineffective cycle (Fig. 5.12).

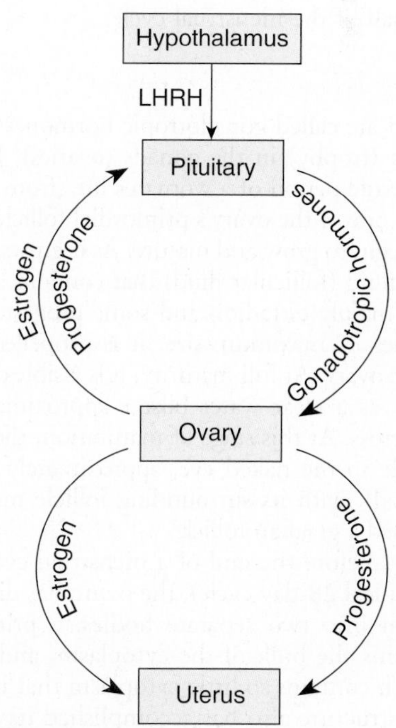

FIGURE 5.12 The interaction of pituitary-uterine-ovarian functions in a menstrual cycle.

Hypothalamus

The release of GnRH (also called luteinizing hormone–releasing hormone, or LHRH) by the hypothalamus initiates the menstrual cycle. When the level of estrogen (produced by the ovaries) rises, release of the hormone is repressed, and menstrual cycles do not occur (the principle that birth control pills use to eliminate menstrual flow). During childhood, the hypothalamus is apparently so sensitive to the small amount of estrogen produced by the adrenal glands that release of the hormone is suppressed. Beginning with puberty, the hypothalamus becomes less sensitive to estrogen feedback; this results in the initiation every month in females of the hormone GnRH. GnRH is transmitted from the hypothalamus to the anterior pituitary gland and signals the gland to begin producing the gonadotropic hormones FSH and LH. Because production of GnRH is cyclic, menstrual periods also cycle.

Diseases of the hypothalamus that cause deficiency of this releasing factor can result in delayed puberty. Likewise, a disease that causes early activation of GnRH can lead to abnormally early sexual development or precocious puberty (Kaplowitz, 2007) (see Chapter 47). In addition to the inhibitory feedback mechanism of estrogen and progesterone that halts production of the releasing factor for the remainder of each month, high levels of pituitary-based hormones such as prolactin, FSH, or LH can also inhibit the production of GnRH.

Pituitary Gland

Under the influence of GnRH, the anterior lobe of the pituitary gland (the adenohypophysis) produces two hormones that act on the ovaries to further influence the menstrual cycle: (a) FSH, a hormone that is active early in the cycle and is responsible for maturation of the ovum, and (b) LH, a hormone that becomes most active at the midpoint of the cycle and is responsible for ovulation, or release of the mature egg cell from the ovary, and growth of the uterine lining during the second half of the menstrual cycle.

Ovary

FSH and LH are called gonadotropic hormones because they cause growth (trophy) in the gonads (ovaries). Every month during the fertile period of a woman's life (from menarche to menopause), one of the ovary's primordial follicles is activated by FSH to begin to grow and mature. As it grows, its cells produce a clear fluid (follicular fluid) that contains a high degree of estrogen (mainly estradiol) and some progesterone. As the follicle reaches its maximum size, it is propelled toward the surface of the ovary. At full maturity, it is visible on the surface of the ovary as a clear water blister approximately 0.25 to 0.5 inches across. At this stage of maturation, the small ovum (barely visible to the naked eye, approximately the size of a printed period), with its surrounding follicle membrane and fluid, is termed a graafian follicle.

By day 14 before the end of a menstrual cycle (the midpoint of a typical 28-day cycle), the ovum has divided by mitotic division into two separate bodies: a primary oocyte, which contains the bulk of the cytoplasm, and a secondary oocyte, which contains so little cytoplasm that it is not functional. The structure also has accomplished its meiotic division, reducing its number of chromosomes to the haploid (having only one member of a pair) number of 23.

After an upsurge of LH from the pituitary, prostaglandins are released and the graafian follicle ruptures. The ovum is set free from the surface of the ovary, a process termed ovulation. It is swept into the open end of a fallopian tube. Teach women that ovulation occurs on approximately the 14th day before the onset of the next cycle, not necessarily at a cycle's midpoint. Because periods are typically 28 days, making the 14th day the middle of the cycle, many women believe incorrectly that the midpoint of their cycle is their day of ovulation. If their cycle is only 20 days long, however, their day of ovulation would be day 6 (14 days from the end of the cycle). If a cycle is 44 days long, ovulation would occur on day 30, not day 22.

After the ovum and the follicular fluid have been discharged from the ovary, the cells of the follicle remain in the form of a hollow, empty pit. The FSH has done its work at this point and now decreases in amount. The second pituitary hormone, LH, continues to rise in amount and acts on the follicle cells of the ovary. It influences the follicle cells to produce lutein, a bright-yellow fluid. Lutein is high in progesterone and contains some estrogen, whereas the follicular fluid was high in estrogen with some progesterone. This yellow fluid fills the empty follicle, which is then termed a corpus luteum (yellow body).

The basal body temperature of a woman drops slightly (by 0.5° to 1° F) just before the day of ovulation, because of the extremely low level of progesterone that is present at that time. It rises by 1° F on the day after ovulation, because of the concentration of progesterone (which is thermogenic) that is present at that time. The woman's temperature remains at this level until approximately day 24 of the menstrual cycle, when the progesterone level again decreases (McCance & Huether, 2007).

If conception (fertilization by a spermatozoon) occurs as the ovum proceeds down a fallopian tube and the fertilized ovum implants on the endometrium of the uterus, the corpus luteum remains throughout the major portion of the pregnancy (approximately 16 to 20 weeks). If conception does not occur, the unfertilized ovum atrophies after 4 or 5 days, and the corpus luteum (called a "false" corpus luteum) remains for only 8 to 10 days. As the corpus luteum regresses, it is gradually replaced by white fibrous tissue, and the resulting structure is termed a corpus albicans (white body). Figure 5.13 shows the times when ovarian hormones are secreted at peak levels during a typical 28-day menstrual cycle.

Uterus

Figure 5.13 also illustrates uterine changes that occur monthly as a result of stimulation from the hormones produced by the ovaries.

First Phase of Menstrual Cycle (Proliferative). Immediately after a menstrual flow (which occurs during the first 4 or 5 days of a cycle), the endometrium, or lining of the uterus, is very thin, approximately one cell layer in depth. As the ovary begins to produce estrogen (in the follicular fluid, under the direction of the pituitary FSH), the endometrium begins to proliferate. This growth is very rapid and increases the thickness of the endometrium approximately eightfold. This increase continues for the first half of the menstrual cycle (from approximately day 5 to day

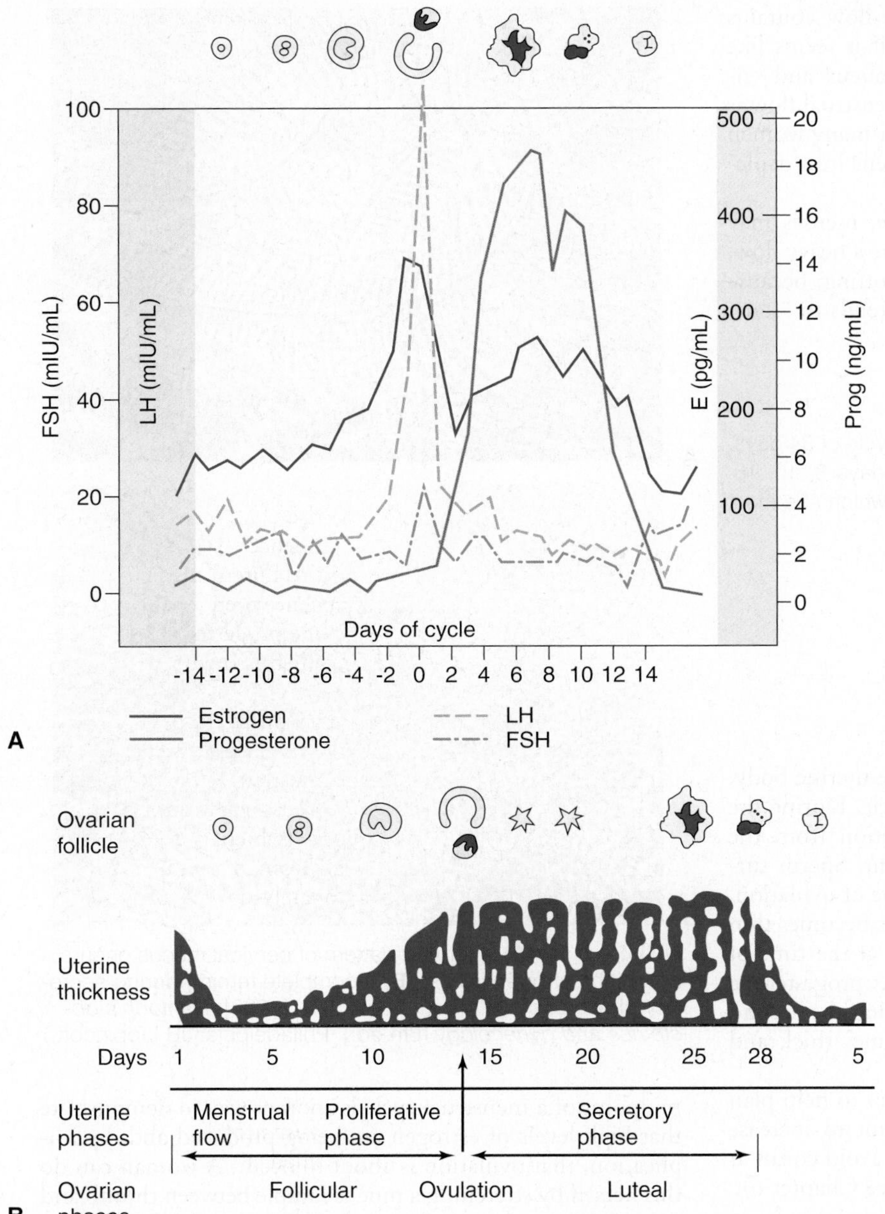

FIGURE 5.13 (**A**) Plasma hormone concentrations in the normal female reproductive cycle. (**B**) Ovarian events and uterine changes during the menstrual cycle.

14). This half of a menstrual cycle is termed interchangeably the proliferative, estrogenic, follicular, or postmenstrual phase.

Second Phase of Menstrual Cycle (Secretory). After ovulation, the formation of progesterone in the corpus luteum (under the direction of LH) causes the glands of the uterine endometrium to become corkscrew or twisted in appearance and dilated with quantities of glycogen (an elementary sugar) and mucin (a protein). The capillaries of the endometrium increase in amount until the lining takes on the appearance of rich, spongy velvet. This second phase of the menstrual cycle is termed the progestational, luteal, premenstrual, or secretory phase.

Third Phase of Menstrual Cycle (Ischemic). If fertilization does not occur, the corpus luteum in the ovary begins to regress after 8 to 10 days. As it regresses, the production of progesterone and estrogen decreases. With the withdrawal of progesterone stimulation, the endometrium of the uterus begins to degenerate (at approximately day 24 or day 25 of the cycle). The capillaries rupture, with minute hemorrhages, and the endometrium sloughs off.

Fourth Phase of a Menstrual Cycle (Menses). Menses, or the menstrual flow, is composed of:

- Blood from the ruptured capillaries
- Mucin from the glands
- Fragments of endometrial tissue
- The microscopic, atrophied, and unfertilized ovum

Menses is actually the end of an arbitrarily defined menstrual cycle. Because it is the only external marker of the cycle, however, the first day of menstrual flow is used to mark the beginning day of a new menstrual cycle.

Contrary to common belief, a menstrual flow contains only approximately 30 to 80 mL of blood; if it seems like more, it is because of the accompanying mucus and endometrial shreds. The iron loss in a typical menstrual flow is approximately 11 mg. This is enough loss that many women need to take a daily iron supplement to prevent iron depletion during their menstruating years.

In women who are beginning menopause, menses may typically consist of a few days of spotting before a heavy flow, or a heavy flow followed by a few days of spotting, because progesterone withdrawal is more sluggish or tends to "staircase" rather than withdraw smoothly.

✔ Checkpoint Question 5.4

Suzanne Matthews typically has a menstrual cycle of 34 days. She tells you she had sexual intercourse on days 8, 10, 15, and 20 of her last cycle. Which is the day on which she most likely conceived?

a. Day 8
b. Day 10
c. Day 15
d. Day 20

Cervix

The mucus of the uterine cervix, as well as the uterine body, changes each month during the menstrual cycle. During the first half of the cycle, when hormone secretion from the ovary is low, cervical mucus is thick and scant. Sperm survival in this type of mucus is poor. At the time of ovulation, when the estrogen level is high, cervical mucus becomes thin and copious. Sperm penetration and survival at the time of ovulation in this thin mucus are excellent. As progesterone becomes the major influencing hormone during the second half of the cycle, cervical mucus again becomes thick and sperm survival is again poor.

Women can analyze cervical mucus changes to help plan coitus to coincide with ovulation if they want to increase their chance of becoming pregnant or plan to avoid coitus at the time of ovulation to prevent pregnancy (see Chapter 6).

Fern Test. When high levels of estrogen are present in the body, as they are just before ovulation, the cervical mucus forms fernlike patterns caused by the crystallization of sodium chloride on mucus fibers when it is placed on a glass slide and allowed to dry. This pattern is known as arborization or ferning (Fig. 5.14). When progesterone is the dominant hormone, as it is just after ovulation, when the luteal phase of the menstrual cycle is beginning, a fern pattern is no longer discernible. Cervical mucus can be examined at midcycle to detect whether ferning, which suggests a high estrogen surge, is present. Women who do not ovulate continue to show the fern pattern throughout the menstrual cycle (i.e., progesterone levels never become dominant), or they never demonstrate it because their estrogen levels never rise.

Spinnbarkeit Test. At the height of estrogen secretion, cervical mucus not only becomes thin and watery but also can be stretched into long strands. This stretchability is in contrast to its thick, viscous state when progesterone is the dominant hormone. Performing this test, known as spinnbarkeit, at the midpoint of a menstrual cycle is another way to demonstrate that high levels of estrogen are being produced and, by implication, that ovulation is about to occur. A woman can do this herself by stretching a mucus sample between thumb and finger, or it can be tested in an examining room by smearing a cervical mucus specimen on a slide and stretching the mucus between the slide and coverslip (Fig. 5.15).

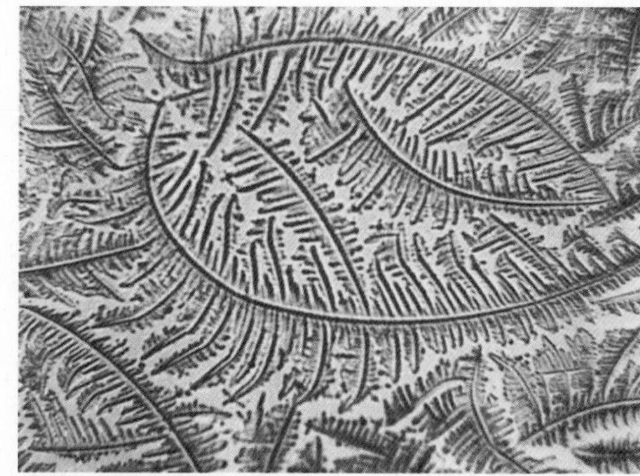
A

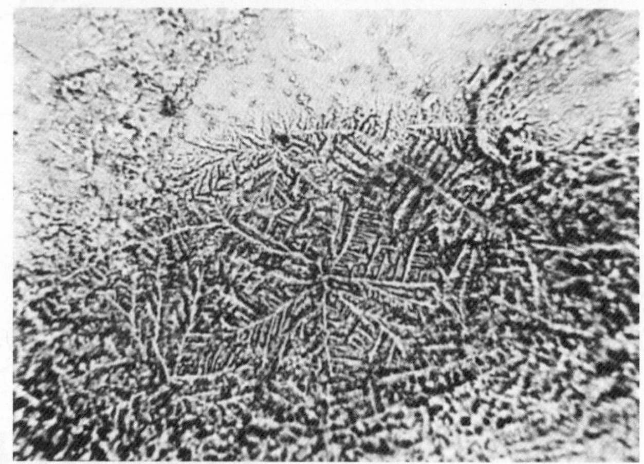
B

FIGURE 5.14 (**A**) A ferning pattern of cervical mucus occurs with high estrogen levels. (**B**) Incomplete ferning during secretory phase of cycle. (From Scott, J. R. [1990]. *Danforth's obstetrics and gynecology* [6th ed.]. Philadelphia: JB Lippincott.)

Education for Menstruation

Education about menstruation is an important component of comprehensive sexuality education. Many myths about menstruation still exist, such as that women should not get a hair permanent during menses, that they should not plant vegetables because the vegetables will die, or that they should not eat sour foods because this will cause cramping. Early preparation for menstruation to dispel these myths is important to a girl's concept of herself as a woman, because it teaches her to trust her body or to think of menstruation as a mark of pride or growing up rather than a burden. Education regarding menstruation is equally important for boys so they can appreciate the cyclic process that a woman's reproductive system activates and can be active participants in helping plan or prevent the conception of children.

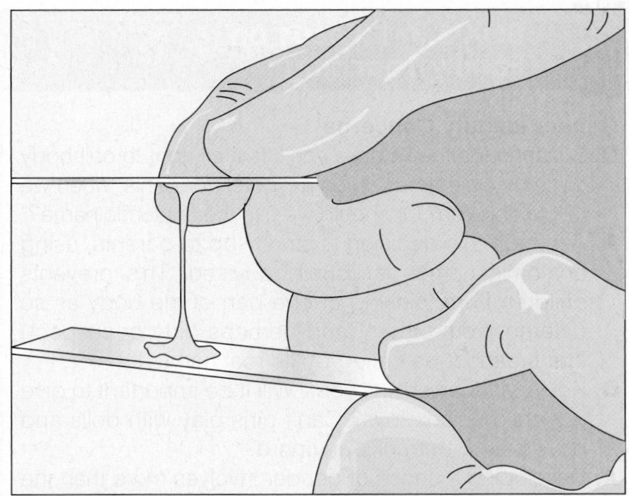

FIGURE 5.15 Spinnbarkeit is the property of cervical mucus to stretch a distance before breaking.

Girls who are well prepared for menstruation and view it as a positive happening are more likely to cope with any menstrual discomfort effectively, which results in fewer missed school days than those who view menstruation as an ill time. Important teaching points for girls at menarche regarding menstruation are summarized in Table 5.2. Menstrual disorders, including dysmenorrhea (painful menstruation), **menorrhagia** (abnormally heavy menstrual flows), **metrorrhagia** (bleeding between menstrual periods), menstrual migraines, and premenstrual dysphoric syndrome, are discussed in Chapter 47 with other reproductive system disorders.

Menopause

Menopause is the cessation of menstrual cycles. *Perimenopausal* is a term used to denote the period during which menopausal changes occur. *Postmenopausal* describes the time of life following the final menses. The age range at which menopause occurs is wide, between approximately 40 and 55 years of age with a mean age of 51.3.

The age at which menopause symptoms begin appears to be genetically influenced or at least is not associated with age of menarche. Women who smoke tend to have earlier menopause (Baram & Basson, 2007).

An older term to describe menopause was "change of life," because it marks the end of a woman's ability to bear children and the beginning of a new phase of life. Such a role change can produce psychological stress, although, through health teaching, nurses can help a woman appreciate that her role in life is greater than just bearing children; loss of uterine function may make almost no change in her life; and, for a woman with dysmenorrhea (painful menstruation) or with no desire for more children, menopause can be a welcome change. Menopause can cause physiologic stress as ovaries are a woman's chief source of estrogen. When ovaries begin to atrophy, reducing estrogen production, "hot flashes," vaginal dryness, or osteoporosis (lack of bone mineral density [BMD]) occurs. Urinary incontinence from lack of bladder support can also occur (Freeman et al., 2007).

Hot flashes can be accompanied by heart palpitations and can occur up to 20 to 30 episodes a day; episodes commonly last for 3 to 5 minutes at a time. An immediate aid in reducing this sudden overheated feeling is to sip at a cold drink or use a hand fan.

At one time, hormone replacement therapy (HR) was prescribed extensively to decrease menopause symptoms because it was believed that this therapy reduced cardiovascular complications such as atherosclerosis or heart attacks as well. HR is no longer prescribed routinely as such therapy does not appear to reduce cardiac risk or prevent osteoporosis and may be associated with endometrial cancer, cerebrovascular accidents (strokes), and perhaps breast cancer (Gabriel-Sanchez, et al., 2009).

HR may be prescribed on a short-term basis (1 to 2 years) if a woman has symptoms so severe that they interfere with her life plans but women should not receive estrogen replacement therapy indefinitely because of the possible adverse effects.

Women who notice excessive vaginal dryness can be advised to use a lubricating jelly such as KY Jelly prior to sexual

TABLE 5.2 ✻ Teaching About Menstrual Health

Area of Concern	Teaching Points
Exercise	Moderate exercise during menses promotes a general sense of well-being. Sustained excessive exercise, such as professional athletes maintain, can cause amenorrhea.
Sexual relations	Not contraindicated during menses although the male should wear a condom to prevent exposure to body fluid. Heightened or decreased sexual arousal may be noticed during this time. Orgasm may increase the amount of menstrual flow. It is improbable but not impossible for conception to occur from coitus during menses.
Activities of daily life	Nothing is contraindicated (many people believe incorrectly that activities such as washing the hair or bathing are harmful).
Pain relief	Prostaglandin inhibitors such as ibuprofen (Motrin) are most effective for menstrual pain. Applying local heat may also be helpful. If a migraine headache occurs, specific drugs for this are now available, such as sumatriptan (Imitrex). Adolescents under age 18 should not take aspirin because of the association between this and Reye's syndrome.
Rest	More rest may be helpful if dysmenorrhea interferes with sleep at night.
Nutrition	Many women need iron supplementation to replace iron lost in menses. Eating pickles or cold food does not cause dysmenorrhea.

relations. Other possibilities are application of estrogen cream or insertion of a vaginal ring that dispenses low-dose estrogen. Low-dose estrogen or testosterone can also be prescribed to increase sexual libido. Practicing Kegel's exercises (see Chapter 12) can help strengthen bladder supports and reduce urinary incontinence.

Osteoporosis occurs in as many as 13% to 18% of women over age 50. It is seen most frequently in women who are Asian, have a low body weight, have a positive family history, participate in few weight-bearing exercises, have a low intake of calcium, are cigarette smokers, have an early surgical menopause, or take certain anticonvulsant medications or corticosteroids. As calcium is withdrawn from bones, women notice a decrease in height and back pain from shortening of the vertebral column. If they fall, they are more prone to fractures than are younger women (Bessette et al., 2008).

BMD scans are helpful in diagnosis. To help prevent osteoporosis, women should be sure to ingest 1200 mg calcium daily along with 400 to 800 IU of vitamin D, in addition to beginning a program of weight-bearing exercises such as walking or low-impact aerobics. Calcitonin, a thyroid hormone that regulates body calcium, may be prescribed as a nasal spray. Other drugs commonly prescribed are selective estrogen receptor modulators (SERMS) such as Evista and bisphosphonates such as Fosamax that regulate calcium by aiding bone reabsorption.

If a woman lives to be 80, she will spend a third of her life postmenopausal. Women appreciate learning the normal parameters of menopause so they understand what will happen to them as changes occur and to be able to continue to monitor their health during this time.

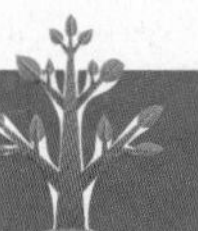

BOX 5.3 ✻ Focus on Family Teaching

Gender Identity Concerns

Q. Suzanne Matthews asks you, "Is it all right to call body parts by nicknames, such as 'peter' for penis, when we talk to children? Or should we use the anatomic name?"

A. Although this decision is strictly up to parents, using anatomic names is usually advised. This prevents children from thinking of one part of the body as so different from others (and perhaps dirty or suspect) that it cannot be called by its real name.

Q. Kevin Matthews asks you, "Will it be important to give our child unisex toys? Can't girls play with dolls and boys play with trucks anymore?"

A. Developing a sense of gender involves more than the toys that children use for play. If parents are concerned with instituting unisex roles in children, they need to begin by monitoring their own perspective on what they believe are female and male roles. Once they project a feeling that roles are interchangeable, such as both genders participating in sports and doing the same household chores, the general home milieu becomes more important than any one action in teaching this principle to children in their family.

SEXUALITY AND SEXUAL IDENTITY

Sexuality is a multidimensional phenomenon that includes feelings, attitudes, and actions. It has both biologic and cultural components. It encompasses and gives direction to a person's physical, emotional, social, and intellectual responses throughout life.

Biologic gender is the term used to denote a person's chromosomal sex: male (XY) or female (XX). **Gender identity** or sexual identity is the inner sense a person has of being male or female, which may be the same as or different from biologic gender. **Gender role** is the male or female behavior a person exhibits, which, again, may or may not be the same as biologic gender or gender identity (Box 5.3).

Development of Gender Identity

Several theories exist regarding whether gender identity arises from primarily a biologic or a psychosocial focus. The amount of testosterone secreted in utero (a process termed *sex typing*) may affect how gender develops. How appealing parents or other adult role models portray their gender roles may also influence how a child envisions himself or herself. For example, both sons and daughters may relate better to whichever parent is kinder and more caring. This could result in a son's assuming characteristics often regarded as feminine or a daughter's developing interests typically regarded as masculine.

Gender role is also culturally influenced. In Western society, women have in the past been viewed as having intrinsic nurturing qualities with sole responsibility for childrearing and homemaking. Men were viewed as financial providers. Gender roles today are more interchangeable: women pursue all types of jobs and careers without loss of femininity, and men participate in childrearing and household duties without loss of masculinity.

An individual's sense of gender identity develops throughout an entire life span, but the stage is set by expectations even before a child is born. Although parents usually respond to the question, "Do you want a boy or a girl?" with the answer, "It doesn't matter as long as it's healthy," many parents actually do have strong preferences for a male or female child. Although some parents may be disappointed if the child is not the gender they hoped for, most adapt quickly and will say later that they always wanted a child of that sex. Children who suspect that their parents wanted a child of the opposite sex are more likely to adopt roles of the opposite sex than if they are confident their parents are pleased with them as they are.

Infancy

From the day of birth, female and male babies are treated differently by their parents. People generally bring girls dainty rattles and dresses with ruffles; on the whole, they are treated more gently by parents and held and rocked more than male babies. People tend to buy boys bigger rattles and sports-related jogging suits. Admonitions given babies can be different. A girl might be told, "Don't cry. You don't look pretty when you cry." A boy might be told, "You've got to learn to be tougher than that if you're going to make it in this world." By the end of the first year, differences in play are usually strongly evident. Boys demonstrate more innate aggression, even at this early stage, than do girls. For more about the infant period, see Chapter 29.

Preschool Period

Children can distinguish between males and females as early as 2 years of age. By age 3 or 4 years, they can say what sex they are, and they have absorbed cultural expectations of that sex role. Often, boys will play rough-and-tumble games with other boys, and girls will play more quietly, although the two frequently mix at this age.

Sex role modeling is reinforced through behavior toward and expectations of the child, as well as from such things as the color and décor of the child's room and the child's clothing. Social contacts between the child and significant adults contribute to sexual identification and should be encouraged in this developmental period. A positive self-concept grows from parental love, effective relationships with others, success in play activities, and gaining skills and self-control.

Most American parents are not too rigid about what clothing or colors are appropriate for boys and girls. They strive to teach both sons and daughters about expressing feelings, performing household tasks, and engaging in the same play activities. However, some parents have fixed role identifications. Comments such as, "What kind of mommy are you going to be, treating a doll that way?" or "Is that the way a lady sits?" from parents and well-meaning friends help to govern girls' choice of actions. Common sayings such as "all boy" or "boys will be boys" represent the differences expected between the two sexes. The suggestions in Box 5.3 can help parents promote a positive and more unisex gender identity in their child.

Although the development of an Oedipus complex (the strong emotional attachment of a preschool boy for his mother or a preschool girl for her father) may have been overstated by Freud as a result of sexual bias, many children exhibit behavior that suggests such a phenomenon does occur during this time. The preschool boy shows signs of competing with his father for his mother's love and attention; the preschool girl competes with her mother for her father's attention and love. Parents may need reassurance that this phenomenon of competition and romance in preschoolers is normal and is only one step in the development of their child's gender role identity. Preschooler development is further discussed in Chapter 31.

School-Age Child

Early school-age children typically spend play time imitating adult roles as a way of learning gender roles (Fig. 5.16). They form strong impressions of what a female or male role should be. Where once schools promoted differences between males and females by separating activities into those only for girls and those only for boys and promoting beliefs such as expecting boys to be poorer readers, to write less neatly, and to act rougher in the school hallways, grade schools have become more attuned to unisex activities.

Girls may participate in activities that were once male dominated, such as Little League and auto repair courses; boys may take cooking or ballet lessons, formerly the province of girls. For more information about school-age development, see Chapter 32.

Adolescent

At puberty, as the adolescent begins the process of establishing a sense of identity, the problem of final gender role identification surfaces again. Most early adolescents maintain strong ties to their gender group, boys with boys and girls with girls. The advent of menstruation may provide a common bond for girls at this stage. Some adolescents choose a child of their own gender a few years older than themselves to use as their model of gender role behavior. This is a way that adolescents can be certain that they understand and feel comfortable with their own sex before they reach out and interact with members of the opposite sex.

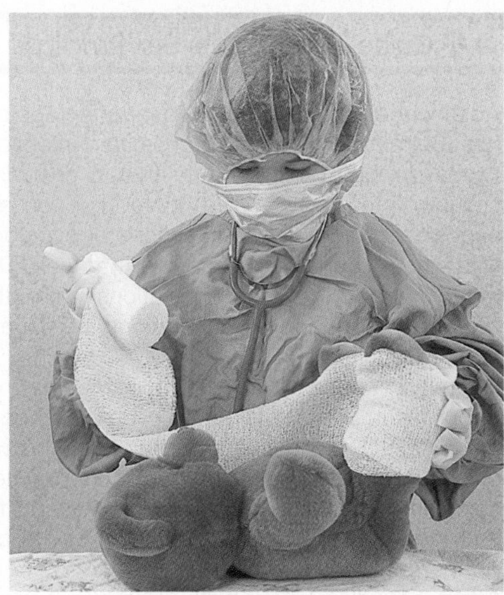

FIGURE 5.16 Early school-age children imitate adult roles to learn more about them. Here a girl "tries on" what being a nurse will feel like. (© Barbara Proud.)

When interviewing adolescents for a sexual history, appreciate that this is a new and sensitive area for them so they may feel embarrassed at being questioned about this area of their life. Although behavior varies in different communities, as many as 50% of adolescents past the age of 15 are already sexually active (Centers for Disease Control and Prevention [CDC], 2009). This means that children as young as the early teen years need guidelines for safer sex (Box 5.4). Including such instructions as part of sexual counseling should help to reduce the incidence of STIs as well as empower adolescents with better self-care skills. When discussing safer sex practices, be certain that adolescents understand not only when but how they can incorporate them into their lifestyle. One of the reasons that preventive measures for human immunodeficiency virus (HIV) and other STIs have not been as successful as first predicted may be that adolescents' total lifestyle and interpretation of sexuality were not at first considered (Box 5.5).

Adolescence can be a very stressful time for the boy who first realizes that he is gay or the girl who first realizes that she is a lesbian. Part of the reason for the high suicide rate in adolescence may be because homosexual teenagers feel so lost in a heterosexual-dominant culture (Kipke et al., 2007). Chapter 33 discusses adolescence in greater detail.

Young Adult

When young adults move away from home to attend college or establish their own home, the change in their eating patterns can increase or decrease their weight that lead to

BOX 5.4 ✻ Guidelines for Safer Sex Practices

1. Abstinence is the only 100% guarantee against not contracting a sexually transmitted infection.
2. If you do have sex, be selective in choosing sexual partners. When you have sex, you are exposing yourself to the infections of everyone with whom your partner has ever had sex. The more partners you have relations with, the greater your danger of contracting a sexually transmitted infection.
3. Do not be reluctant to ask a sexual partner about his or her sexual lifestyle before engaging in sexual relations. If a partner has a history of casual contacts or bisexual or unprotected sex, there is a greater hazard of infection for you than if your partner is also choosy about partners.
4. Avoid sexual relations with intravenous drug users or prostitutes (male or female) or sexual partners who have had sexual relations with such people, because such people have a greater than usual chance of carrying the human immunodeficiency virus (HIV) and hepatitis B or C infection.
5. Inspect your sexual partner for any lesions or abnormal drainage in the genital area. Do not engage in sexual relations with anyone who exhibits these signs.
6. The use of a condom is the best protection against infection. Condoms should be latex; the chance of the condom tearing is less if it is a prelubricated brand. Use water-based lubricants such as KY Jelly on condoms, because oil-based lubricants can weaken the rubber.
7. Condoms should be protected from excessive heat to avoid rubber deterioration and should be inspected to be certain they are intact before use. Do not inflate condoms before use to test for intactness, because this weakens the rubber.
8. Condoms should be fitted over the erect penis with a small space left at the end to accept semen. The condom should be held against the sides of the penis while the penis is withdrawn to prevent spillage of semen.
9. Void immediately after sexual relations to help wash away contaminants on the vulva or in the urinary tract.
10. Anal intercourse carries a high risk for HIV and hepatitis infection as well as infection from intestinal organisms. Always use a condom. Use lubricants for anal penetration to keep bleeding and condom resistance to a minimum.
11. Do not engage in oral-penile sex unless the male wears a condom, because even preejaculatory fluid may contain viruses and bacteria. For safer oral-vaginal sex, a condom split in two or a plastic dental dam (like that used for pediatric dentistry) covering the mouth should be used to protect against the exchange of body fluids.
12. Hand-to-genital contact may be hazardous if open cuts are present on hands. Use a latex glove or finger cot for protection.
13. To decrease the possibility of transferring germs, do not share sexual aids such as vibrators.
14. If you think you have contracted a sexually transmitted infection, do not engage in sexual relations until you have contacted a health care provider and are again infection free. Alert any recent sexual partners that you might have an infection so they also can receive treatment.

changes in their body image (Box 5.6). During this time, they choose the way they will express their sexuality along with other life patterns. Many young adults marry with a commitment to one sexual partner. Others establish relationships (cohabitation) that are less binding by legal definitions but perhaps equally binding in concern and support. Young adults may view cohabitation as a means of learning more about a possible marriage partner on a day-to-day basis, in the hope that a future marriage will then be stronger and more lasting. Homosexuality or bisexuality may be overtly expressed for the first time during this period.

Conflicts in parenting can occur if an individual's gender role does not meet the expectations of a family, or if an individual's partner has different expectations regarding gender role. It is time well spent for parents-to-be to take time to discuss with each other the views they have on parenting to see whether they agree on male and female roles and their relationship with their children. A single parent may be concerned about how both roles can be fulfilled and can benefit from talking with a health care provider about this area of concern. Conflicts in the roles parents have chosen often come to light for the first time during pregnancy, as they worry about what type of parents they are going to be or whether they are adequately prepared to be parents. Being able to talk to health care personnel about the gender roles they have adopted in life can be a major step in promoting feelings of adequacy and preparing themselves to raise a child.

Young adulthood is the time when many couples begin childbearing. Early in pregnancy, a woman may experience a decreased desire for coitus because of the increased estrogen in her body. As pregnancy advances and her abdomen increases in size, she and her sexual partner may need to use new positions for intercourse such as a side-by-side position or the woman in a superior position. Caution women with a nonmonogamous sexual partner that she or her partner need to use a condom to prevent transmission of an STI during pregnancy (Katsufrakis & Workowski, 2008).

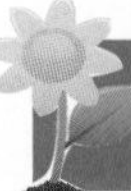

BOX 5.5 * Focus on Communication

Kevin brings his 16-year-old nephew, Mark, into your health care clinic because Mark has had painful urination for 2 days. A culture is taken to determine whether he has contracted a sexually transmitted infection (STI).

Less Effective Communication

Nurse: Mark, because you're sexually active you may have a sexually transmitted infection.
Mark: Uh-huh.
Nurse: Do you practice safer sex?
Mark: Uh, yeah.
Nurse: I assume that means you always use a condom.
Mark: Right.
Nurse: It would be hard to contract an STI if you always do.
Mark: Guess I'm just unlucky.

More Effective Communication

Nurse: Mark, because you're sexually active you may have a sexually transmitted infection.
Mark: Uh-huh.
Nurse: Do you practice safer sex?
Mark: Uh, yeah.
Nurse: What measures do you use?
Mark: My girlfriend's on the pill, so we don't really need to use anything else.
Nurse: The pill will help prevent pregnancy, but it won't protect you from contracting an STI.
Mark: No kidding.
Nurse: Let's talk about the different protection needed to prevent pregnancy and STIs.

Adolescents are often so concerned about protecting their privacy from adults that they may offer as little information as possible at a health care visit, especially in regard to sexual issues. Asking them specific, open-ended questions is important to ensure a positive exchange of information and effective health teaching. As they offer details, remain nonjudgmental to encourage them to continue to elaborate.

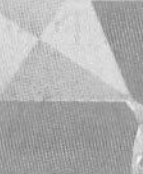

BOX 5.6 * Focus on Evidence-Based Practice

Does gender affect college weight gain?

It is often noted that college freshmen gain "freshman fifteen" or a significant weight gain during their first college year. To examine whether college weight gain is affected by gender, researchers asked 396 college freshman to complete a 40-item health survey and measured their height and weight at the study beginning and again at the end.

Results of the study showed that the amount of weight gained by the differing genders was not greatly different but the reason for the gains varied greatly. In this study, the average weight gain for men was 5.04 lb. It was 5.49 lb for women. Gains in weight for men were associated with increased alcohol consumption. An increased study workload was credited for the reason for weight gain in women.

Would the results of this study influence the way you would counsel college students who are interested in avoiding a freshmen weight gain?

Source: Economos, C. D., Hildebrandt, M. L., & Hyatt, R. R. (2008). College freshman stress and weight change: differences by gender. *American Journal of Health Behavior, 32*(1), 16–25.

Middle-Age Adult

For many women and men in midlife, sexuality has achieved a degree of stability. A sense of masculinity or femininity and comfortable patterns of behavior have been established. This increased security in identity can promote greater intimacy in sexual and social relationships. This may also be a time when adults allow themselves more freedom in exploring and satisfying sexual needs.

Although menopause alters reproductive functioning, it does not physically inhibit sexual functioning. Generally, a woman with a strong self-image, positive sexual and social relationships, and knowledge regarding her body and menopause is likely to progress through this natural biologic stage without problems and remain sexually active and satisfied. Nurses can be instrumental in teaching women what to expect at menopause so that it is not a surprise and in helping them maintain self-esteem through this natural process.

During midlife, men may begin to experience changes in sperm production, erectile power, achievement of orgasm, and sex drive, although these changes usually do not significantly alter reproductive or sexual functioning. Some men feel that these changes threaten their sexuality and "maleness" and may respond negatively. Other men feel that these changes make sex more pleasurable and intimate and often respond positively. Actual sexual dysfunctions, as a result of physical or psychosocial changes, may arise at this time. Teaching men about normal biophysical changes, providing them with methods to improve sexual functioning, and offering them support are important health education roles.

Midlife is often a time when both men and women reexamine life goals, careers, accomplishments, value systems, and familial and social relationships. As a result, some people adapt, whereas others experience stress or a crisis. This reexamination can positively or negatively affect an individual's gender identity and sexuality. For example, a woman may realize that she is not able to be both a homemaker and a career person. She may either modify her belief that it is important for a woman to assume both roles or try harder to achieve both goals, believing that she has personally failed. The increased incidence of sexual encounters that men have with younger women at this age may be a man's way of reassuring himself of his attractiveness and virility and denying that he is aging.

Certain medications, such as antihypertensives, antianxiety agents, and narcotics, may diminish sexual response in both men and women. Being aware of this fact is important not only for clients, so that they can understand that it is an expected response, but also for their partners.

The individual who comments about the need to maintain a reduced activity level at work or a reduced social schedule may also be seeking information and direction in other important areas of life, such as sexual relations.

Some women have surgery at midlife such as hysterectomy (removal of the uterus). If both ovaries are also removed (oophorectomy), an immediate surgical menopause occurs. For some women, the loss of a uterus and ovaries can be synonymous with the loss of femininity. Women who have such surgery need sensitive caregivers to listen to their concerns about the meaning of the experience for them.

Older Adult

Both male and female older adults continue to enjoy active sexual relationships. Some men experience less erectile firmness or ejaculatory force than when they were younger, but others discover that they are able to maintain an erection longer. Older women may have less vaginal secretions because they have less estrogen after menopause. Use of a water-soluble lubricant before coitus can enhance their comfort and enjoyment. Both sexes need to follow safer sex practices throughout life. Because males remain fertile throughout life, they must continue to be responsible sex partners in terms of reproductive planning.

The Individual Who Is Physically Challenged

Individuals who are physically challenged have sexual desires and needs the same as all others (Piotrowski & Snell, 2007). However, they may have difficulty with sexual identity or sexual fulfillment because of their condition. Males with upper spinal cord injury may have difficulty with erection and ejaculation, because these actions are governed at the spinal level. Manual stimulation of the penis or psychological stimulation achieves erection in most men with spinal cord lesions, allowing the man a satisfying sexual relationship with his partner. Most women with spinal cord injuries cannot experience orgasm but are able to conceive and have children.

Anyone who interprets a procedure such as a colostomy as disfiguring may be reluctant to participate in sexual activities, fearing that the sight of an apparatus will diminish their partner's satisfaction or enjoyment. People with chronic pain (e.g., arthritis) may be too uncomfortable to enjoy sexual relations. Individuals with urinary catheters may be concerned about their ability to enjoy coitus with the catheter in place. For women, a retention catheter should not interfere with sexual intercourse. Men can be taught how to replace their own catheter, so that they can remove it for sexual relations. In all instances in which one sexual partner is disabled in some way, the response of a loving partner does much to enhance body image and feelings of adequacy of a mate. Encouraging these clients to ask questions and work on specific difficulties is a nursing role.

Sexuality is a facet of rehabilitation that has not always received attention. If a person can accomplish activities of daily living such as eating, elimination, and mobility, then he or she is considered to be leading a normal or near-normal life. Establishment of a satisfying sexual relationship is an important part of living, however, so should be included in assessments of clients in rehabilitation programs.

HUMAN SEXUAL RESPONSE

Sexuality has always been a part of human life, but it is only in the past few decades that it has been studied scientifically. One common finding of researchers has been that feelings and attitudes about sex vary widely: the sexual experience is unique to each individual, but sexual physiology (i.e., how the body responds to sexual arousal) has common features (Baram & Basson, 2007).

Sexual Response Cycle

Two of the earliest researchers of sexual response were Masters and Johnson. In 1966, they published the results of a major study of sexual physiology based on more than 10,000 episodes of sexual activity among more than 600 men and women (Masters, 1998). In this study, they described the human sexual response as a cycle with four discrete stages: excitement, plateau, orgasm, and resolution. Stages may actually be more individualized than Masters proposed; they may blend together much more into one smooth process of desire, arousal, and orgasm.

Excitement

Excitement occurs with physical and psychological stimulation (i.e., sight, sound, emotion, or thought) that causes parasympathetic nerve stimulation. This leads to arterial dilation and venous constriction in the genital area. The resulting increased blood supply leads to vasocongestion and increasing muscular tension. In women, this vasocongestion causes the clitoris to increase in size and mucoid fluid to appear on vaginal walls as lubrication. The vagina widens in diameter and increases in length. The nipples become erect. In men, penile erection occurs, as well as scrotal thickening and elevation of the testes. In both sexes, there is an increase in heart and respiratory rates and blood pressure.

Plateau

The plateau stage is reached just before orgasm. In the woman, the clitoris is drawn forward and retracts under the clitoral prepuce; the lower part of the vagina becomes extremely congested (formation of the orgasmic platform), and there is increased nipple elevation.

In men, the vasocongestion leads to distention of the penis. Heart rate increases to 100 to 175 beats per minute and respiratory rate to approximately 40 respirations per minute.

Orgasm

Orgasm occurs when stimulation proceeds through the plateau stage to a point at which the body suddenly discharges accumulated sexual tension. A vigorous contraction of muscles in the pelvic area expels or dissipates blood and fluid from the area of congestion. The average number of contractions for a woman is 8 to 15 contractions at intervals of 1 every 0.8 seconds. In men, muscle contractions surrounding the seminal vessels and prostate project semen into the proximal urethra. These contractions are followed immediately by three to seven propulsive ejaculatory contractions, occurring at the same time interval as in the woman, which force semen from the penis.

As the shortest stage in the sexual response cycle, orgasm is usually experienced as intense pleasure affecting the whole body, not just the pelvic area. It is also a highly personal experience: descriptions of orgasms vary greatly from person to person.

Resolution

Resolution is a 30-minute period during which the external and internal genital organs return to an unaroused state. For the male, a refractory period occurs during which further orgasm is impossible. Women do not go through this refractory period, so it is possible for women who are interested and properly stimulated to have additional orgasms immediately after the first.

Controversies About Female Orgasm

The female orgasm has been a topic of much controversy over the years, beginning with Freud, who deducted that there were two types of female orgasms: clitoral and vaginal. He believed that clitoral orgasms (originating from masturbation or other noncoital acts) represented sexual immaturity and that only vaginal orgasms were the authentic, mature form of sexual behavior in women. Accordingly, he considered women to be neurotic if they could not achieve orgasm through intercourse.

Masters (1998) showed that there is no physiologic difference between an orgasm achieved through intercourse and one achieved by direct stimulation of the clitoris. Women have reported a difference in intensity and character between orgasms achieved through coitus and through other means, and some prefer one to the other, but there is no physiologic difference between them. For most women, adequate time for foreplay is essential for them to be orgasmic.

In recent years, a subject of controversy regarding female sexuality has arisen: the existence or not of "the G spot." First described in 1950 by the German physician Gräfenberg, the G spot, presumably located on the inner portion of the vaginal wall, halfway between the pubic bone and the cervix, has been promoted as an area of heightened erotic sensitivity (Baram & Basson, 2007). Several studies carried out in the past 10 years have not been able to verify the existence of this particular anatomic site, although some women do claim to possess such an erotic trigger.

Influence of the Menstrual Cycle on Sexual Response

During the second half of the menstrual cycle—the luteal phase—there is increased fluid retention and vasocongestion in a woman's lower pelvis. Because some vasocongestion is already present at the beginning of the excitement stage of the sexual response, women appear to reach the plateau stage more quickly and achieve orgasm more readily during this time. Women also may be more interested in initiating sexual relations at this time.

Influence of Pregnancy on Sexual Response

Pregnancy is another time in life when there is vasocongestion of the lower pelvis because of the blood supply needed by a rapidly growing fetus. This causes some women to experience a first orgasm during their first pregnancy. Following a pregnancy, many women experience increased sexual interest because the new growth of blood vessels during pregnancy lasts for some time and continues to facilitate pelvic vasocongestion. This is why discussing sexual relationships is an important part of health teaching during pregnancy. At a time when a woman may want sexual contact very much, she needs to be free of myths and misconceptions, such as the notion that orgasm will cause a spontaneous miscarriage (see Focus on Nursing Care Planning Box 5.7). Although the level of oxytocin does appear to rise in women after orgasm, this rise is not sufficient to lead to worry that sexual relations will lead to premature labor in the average woman.

For some women, the increased breast engorgement that accompanies pregnancy results in extreme breast sensitivity during coitus. Foreplay that includes sucking or massaging of the breasts may cause the release of oxytocin, but it is not contraindicated unless the woman has a history of premature labor (Purinton & Goldstein, 2007).

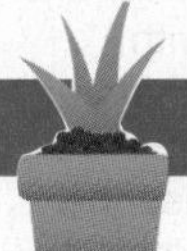

BOX 5.7 ✻ Focus on Nursing Care Planning

A Multidisciplinary Care Map for a Couple Needing Sexual Counseling

Suzanne and Kevin Matthews, a young adult couple, 6 months pregnant, come to your antepartal clinic for a routine visit. Suzanne, in tears, states, "My husband isn't interested in me anymore. We haven't had sex since I became pregnant." Couple engaged in coitus two to three times per week prior to this pregnancy. Kevin states, "I'm afraid I'll hurt the baby."

Family Assessment ✻ Couple has been married for 4 years; lives in two-bedroom apartment in refurbished downtown loft. Husband works as a high school teacher; wife works as a baker in a local coffeehouse.

Client Assessment ✻ A previous pregnancy, 2 years ago, ended at 8 weeks with a spontaneous miscarriage. Blood pressure today is 118/70 mm Hg; overall health is good.

Nursing Diagnosis ✻ Altered sexuality pattern related to pregnancy and fear of harming fetus.

Outcome Criteria ✻ Couple states that they recognize coitus is not harmful in normal pregnancy; reports engaging in sexual intercourse as well as pleasurable noncoital sexual activities by next visit.

(continued)

BOX 5.7 ✻ Focus on Nursing Care Planning (continued)

Team Member Responsible	Assessment	Intervention	Rationale	Expected Outcome
Activities of Daily Living				
Nurse	Assess lifestyle and sexual concerns.	Encourage couple to continue routine prenatal care. Discuss alternative sexual activities, such as cuddling or massage, at each visit.	As pregnancy progresses, discomfort, fatigue, and increasing abdominal size and pressure may interfere with a satisfying sexual relationship. Advanced planning prepares the couple for adaptations that may be necessary.	Couple continues prenatal care. Describes other ways of sexual expression.
Consultations				
Nurse	Assess signs and symptoms of pregnancy; note any indication of complications.	Consult with team primary care provider to be certain the client has no contraindications to remaining sexually active during pregnancy.	In a few women who have had previous miscarriages, or if vaginal bleeding is present, sexual relations may be contraindicated or the pregnancy will be threatened.	The couple's primary care provider supplies information on ability of couple to remain sexually active throughout pregnancy.
Procedures/Medications				
Nurse	Assess whether alternative types of sexual activity would fulfill couple's needs.	Review alternative sexual positions for optimal comfort and pleasure.	Alternative sexual positions may be necessary to provide comfort late in pregnancy as the woman's abdomen expands.	Couple describes alternative positions or ways they relate to each other.
Patient/Family Education				
Nurse in consultation with physician	Assess what couple understands about reproductive anatomy and usual sexual response.	Explain that sexual relations are allowed during pregnancy until labor begins. Use charts and illustrations to show how the fetus is protected in utero.	Barring complications, couples can engage in coitus to the extent that it is comfortable and desired. Visual aids enhance learning.	Couple states they understand sexual relations are allowed during a normal pregnancy and they understand that minimal contractions may occur with orgasm but that these are not harmful unless the woman has a history of premature labor.
Spiritual/Psychosocial/Emotional Needs				
Nurse	Assess whether couple knows that hormones can change sexual desire during pregnancy.	Encourage the couple to talk openly about their feelings, concerns, desires, and changes in interest to each other throughout the pregnancy.	Physical and psychological changes occur in both the pregnant woman and her partner throughout pregnancy. Open communication enhances the relationship.	Couple reports that they are able to voice their feelings and concerns during the pregnancy.

Nurse	Assess what communication pattern couple uses to share information with each other.	Teach importance for a couple of maintaining communication.	Beginning a sound communication pattern during pregnancy can lay a foundation for a sound future relationship.	Couple reports that they appreciate the importance of good communication for their ongoing relationship.
Discharge Planning				
Nurse	Assess whether couple's questions and concerns were answered satisfactorily.	Review concern about sexual relations at each visit.	Continued interest in a couple's problem allows them to continue to voice concerns.	Chart documents that questions were asked and answered at continuing visits.

Types of Sexual Orientation

Sexual gratification is experienced in several ways. What is considered normal varies greatly among cultures, although general components of accepted sexual activity are that it is an activity of adults and privacy, consent, and lack of force are included. Most individual value systems are closely aligned to these cultural norms.

Heterosexuality

A heterosexual is a person who finds sexual fulfillment with a member of the opposite gender. Because interest in the opposite sex and sexual relationships may begin as early as the beginning of puberty, it is important to provide information on safer sex practices and planning for their use to children as young as 10 to 12 years of age. Otherwise, this knowledge comes too late to be most helpful.

Homosexuality

A homosexual is a person who finds sexual fulfillment with a member of his or her own sex. Many homosexual men prefer to use the term "gay." "Lesbian" refers to a homosexual woman. More recent terms are "men who have sex with men" (abbreviated as "MWM") and "women who have sex with women" (WWW).

Why homosexual gender identity develops is unknown, although evidence that this orientation is genetically determined or develops because of the effect of an unusual level of estrogen or testosterone in utero is increasing. Even before puberty, most individuals who are homosexual know they are "different" in that they are not interested in opposite-sex classmates. It is during adolescence, in seeking a sense of identity, that they realize that the reason they feel "different" is because they are homosexual. This can be a stressful time, because a homosexual identity may not be easy to reveal to family or friends. Although attitudes are changing, some people refuse to associate with homosexuals to such an extent that a fear termed *homophobia* still exists (Newman, 2007).

Although men who have sex with men and women who have sex with women often have demonstrated behavior that is inconsistent with expected gender roles from early childhood, young adulthood is the time most persons begin to assume a homosexual lifestyle. Many young adults are worried about the stigma of being labeled homosexual and therefore keep their identity secret from heterosexual acquaintances. Others "commit" or "come out" or are able to reveal their sexual identity to friends and family (Avery et al., 2007).

Because the period of identity confusion during adolescence can be so traumatic to people with alternative lifestyles, it is important for health care providers to be extremely sensitive to needs in this area. Men who have sex with men may need additional counseling to help them avoid acquiring HIV and other STIs, because issues such as avoiding contact through anal intercourse may not be routinely covered in sex education classes (Sandfort, Melendez, & Diaz, 2007). If women who have sex with women cohort with bisexuals, they have the same risk of STIs as other people. If they avoid partners who are bisexual, they may be at less risk for STIs because of the low incidence of these diseases in a strictly female population.

Bisexuality

People are said to be bisexual if they achieve sexual satisfaction from both homosexual and heterosexual relationships. Like men who have sex with men, bisexual men may be at greater risk for HIV and STIs than are others. Female partners of bisexual men need to be aware that they are also at increased risk for HIV and other STIs.

Transsexuality

A **transsexual** or transgender person is an individual who, although of one biologic gender, feels as if he or she is of the opposite gender (Jain & Bradbeer, 2007). Such people may have sex change operations so that they appear cosmetically as the gender they feel that they are. Such operations do not change the person's chromosomal structure, however, so although capable of sexual relations in this new role (a synthetic vagina or penis is created), the person is incapable of reproduction. The incidence of sex change operations has decreased in recent years because of potential disappointment after the surgery:

despite a new outward appearance, people realize that they are still not totally the person they wished to become. Children of a transsexual parent may have a great deal of difficulty understanding why their parent changed from male to female or female to male (White & Ettner, 2007).

Types of Sexual Expression

Because people are individuals, types of sexual expression are individualized.

Sexual Abstinence

Sexual abstinence (celibacy) is separation from sexual activity (Ott, Labbett, & Gold, 2007). It is the avowed state of certain religious orders. It is also a way of life for many adults and one that is becoming fashionable among a growing number of young adults. It is the main point of many high school sex education classes (Kelly & Schwartz, 2007). The theoretical advantage of sexual abstinence is the ability to concentrate on means of giving and receiving love other than through sexual expression and, of course, is the most effective way to prevent pregnancy or an STI.

Masturbation

Masturbation is self-stimulation for erotic pleasure; it can also be a mutually enjoyable activity for sexual partners. It offers sexual release, which may be interpreted by the person as overall tension or anxiety relief. Masters (1998) reported that women may find masturbation to orgasm the most satisfying sexual expression and use it more commonly than men. Children between 2 and 6 years of age discover masturbation as an enjoyable activity as they explore their bodies. Children who are under a high level of tension may become accustomed to using masturbation as a means of falling asleep at night or at naptime. They do this without any attempt at concealment because they have not yet been affected by society's view that such activity should not be public.

School age children continue to use masturbation for enjoyment or to relieve tension, but they perform such activities in private. Counseling parents about masturbation is discussed in Chapters 31 through 33. In a hospital setting, a school age child may assume that he or she has more privacy than actually exists. Such an assumption means that a child may be discovered masturbating if someone walks unannounced into the room.

After reproductive tract surgery or childbirth, many adult men and women voice concern about how soon they will be able to have sexual relations again without feeling pain. They may masturbate to orgasm to test whether everything in their body is still functioning, much as the preschooler does.

Autoerotic asphyxia is the extreme practice of causing oxygen deficiency (usually by hanging) during masturbation with the goal of producing a feeling of extreme sexual excitement. Not aware that the act can be fatal, adolescents are killed by this practice each year (Musshoff et al., 2007).

Erotic Stimulation

Erotic stimulation is the use of visual materials such as magazines or photographs for sexual arousal. Although this is thought to be mostly a male phenomenon, there is increasing interest in centerfold photographs in magazines marketed primarily to women. Some parents of adolescents may need to be assured that an interest in this type of material is developmental and normal. Respect this type of reading material when straightening patients' rooms in a health care facility.

Fetishism

Fetishism is sexual arousal resulting from the use of certain objects or situations. Leather, rubber, shoes, and feet are frequently perceived to have erotic qualities. The object of stimulation does not just enhance the experience; rather, it becomes a focus of arousal and a person may come to require the object or situation for stimulation (Scorolli et al., 2007).

Transvestism

A **transvestite** is an individual who dresses in the clothes of the opposite sex. Transvestites can be heterosexual, homosexual, or bisexual. Many are married. Some transvestites, particularly married heterosexuals, may be under a great deal of strain to keep their lifestyle a secret from friends and neighbors.

Voyeurism

Voyeurism is obtaining sexual arousal by looking at another person's body. Almost all children and adolescents pass through a stage when voyeurism is appealing; this passes with more active sexual expressions. That some voyeurism exists in almost everyone is illustrated by the large number of R-rated movies shown on television and in movie theaters and by the erotic descriptions in modern novels. If voyeurism is practiced to the exclusion of other sexual experiences, such an extreme probably reflects insecurity or the inability to feel confident enough to relate to others on more personal levels. Stalking, a crime that includes elements of voyeurism, is discussed in Chapter 33.

Sadomasochism

Sadomasochism involves inflicting pain (sadism) or receiving pain (masochism) to achieve sexual satisfaction. It is a practice generally considered to be within the limits of normal sexual expression as long as the pain involved is minimal and the experience is satisfying to both sexual partners.

Other Types of Sexual Expression

A multitude of other types of sexual expression exist (e.g., exhibitionism, making obscene telephone calls, bestiality, and pedophilia). Exhibitionism is revealing one's genitals in public. Bestiality is sexual relations with animals. Pedophiles are individuals who are interested in sexual encounters with children. Known pedophiles are registered as sex offenders. When they move into a new community, families are notified of the move according to Megan's Law, a national law designed to alert citizens to the presence of a sex offender in a community. Ways to keep children safe from sex offenders are discussed in Chapter 31, along with other aspects of community safety for young children.

What if... When Kevin unpacks his suitcase at a hospital admission, you discover that he has brought a wardrobe of women's clothing? What would you do?

SEXUAL HARASSMENT

Sexual harassment is unwanted and repeated sexual advances, remarks, or behavior toward another that (a) is offensive to the recipient and (b) interferes with job or school performance. It can involve actions as obvious as a job superior demanding sexual favors or a job superior sending sexist jokes by e-mail to a person supervised. In school it can refer to bullying (Gruber & Fineran, 2007).

Two types exist. One is *quid pro quo* (an equal exchange), in which an employer asks for something in return for sexual favors, such as a hiring or promotion preference. The second is *hostile work environment,* in which an employer creates an environment in which an employee feels uncomfortable and exploited (e.g., being addressed as "honey," asked to wear revealing clothing, working where walls are decorated with sexist posters).

Sexual harassment rules apply to same-gender as well as opposite-gender harassment. In addition to causing occupational disruption, sexual harassment may be so distressing that it leads to short- and long-term psychosocial consequences for victims and their families such as emotional distress (anxiety, depression, posttraumatic stress disorder, substance abuse), interpersonal conflict, and impaired intimacy and sexual functioning (Street et al., 2007). Sexual harassment has been illegal in the United States since 1964. Clients who report being subjected to harassment should be advised to report the situation to their personnel supervisor. Nurses should be aware of the sexual harassment guidelines in their own work setting and likewise report such behavior to keep their workplace free of this type of strain.

DISORDERS OF SEXUAL FUNCTIONING

Disorders involving sexual functioning can be lifelong (primary) or acquired (secondary). They can have a psychogenic origin (produced by psychic rather than organic factors), a biogenic origin (produced by biologic processes), or both. They occur in both men and women.

Inhibited Sexual Desire

Lessened interest in sexual relations is normal in some circumstances, such as after the death of a family member, a divorce, or a stressful job change. The support of a caring sexual partner or relief of the tension causing the stress allows a return to sexual interest.

Decreased sexual desire can also be a side effect of many medicines. Chronic diseases, such as peptic ulcers or chronic pulmonary disorders, that cause frequent pain or discomfort may interfere with a man's or a woman's overall well-being and interest in sexual activity. Obese men and women may not feel as much satisfaction from sexual relations as others, because they have difficulty achieving deep penetration because of the bulk of their abdomens. An individual with an STI such as genital herpes may choose to forgo sexual relations rather than inform a partner of the disease. Some women experience a decrease in sexual desire during perimenopause. Administration of androgen (testosterone) to women may be helpful at that time, because it can improve interest in sexual activity (MacKay, 2009).

Failure to Achieve Orgasm

The failure of a woman to achieve orgasm can be a result of poor sexual technique, concentrating too hard on achievement, or negative attitudes toward sexual relationships. Treatment is aimed at relieving the underlying cause. It may include instruction and counseling for the couple about sexual feelings and needs.

Erectile Dysfunction

Erectile dysfunction (ED), formerly referred to as impotence, is the inability of a man to produce or maintain an erection long enough for vaginal penetration or partner satisfaction (Wessels et al., 2007). Most causes of ED are physical, such as aging, atherosclerosis, or diabetes, which limit blood supply. It may also occur as a side effect of certain drugs (Basson & Schultz, 2007). The problem is compounded by doubt about the ability to perform and reluctance to discuss the problem with health care providers. Examples of drugs prescribed today for ED are sildenafil (Viagra), tadalafil (Cialis), and vardenafil (Levitra), which are taken up to once a day to stimulate penile erection (Karch, 2009) (Box 5.8). If

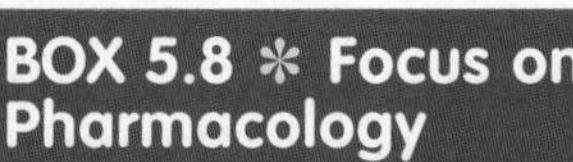

BOX 5.8 * Focus on Pharmacology

Sildenafil Citrate (Viagra)

Classification: A phosphodiesterase (PDE) inhibitor. Prescribed as therapy for erectile dysfunction; also pulmonary artery hypertension

Action: Causes smooth muscle relaxation and inflow of blood to the corpus cavernosum of the penis, achieving erection (Karch, 2009)

Dosage: 50 mg PO prn 1 hour before sexual activity, up to one dose per day

Possible Adverse Effects: The most common side effects are headache, facial flushing, and upset stomach. Less commonly, ventricular arrhythmia, bluish vision, blurred vision, impairment of blue/green discrimination, or sensitivity to light may briefly occur. Advise patients not to take this drug within 4 hours of taking an alpha-blocker agent.

Nursing Implications

- Assess patient for pre-existing cardiovascular risk.
- Caution patient that dose should be limited to one time per day; use is contradicted if the patient is taking nitrates or an alpha-blocker.
- Erection lasting more than 4 hours (priapism) can occur. Caution patient to alert health care provider if this occurs to avoid penile tissue damage.
- Caution patients that this drug does not protect against sexually transmitted infections or pregnancy, so the user must continue to use safer sex practices.
- In rare instances, men taking PDE5 inhibitors have reported a sudden decrease or loss of vision. Caution patient that if he experiences sudden decrease or loss of vision to stop taking the medication and call a doctor right away.

these are not successful (they are contradicted in men with a risk of cardiovascular illness and in those who are taking medications that contain nitrates), a surgical implant to aid erection by the use of vacuum pressure is a possible alternative (Hossein, 2007). Testosterone injections may be helpful in some men. In all instances, frank discussion about the cause of the problem and currently available therapies is helpful. Various herbal products such as fennel extracts are available for women that may improve sexual libido. Vibration or vacuum devices are also available to increase clitoral enlargement and sexual arousal in women. Sildenafil citrate (Viagra) can be used with women taking serotonin reuptake inhibitors who notice decreased sexual arousal (Nurberg, et al., 2008).

Premature Ejaculation

Premature ejaculation is ejaculation before penile–vaginal contact (Docherty, 2007). The term also is often used to mean ejaculation before the sexual partner's satisfaction has been achieved. Premature ejaculation can be unsatisfactory and frustrating for both partners.

The cause, like that of ED, can be psychological. Masturbating to orgasm (in which orgasm is achieved quickly because of lack of time) may play a role. Other reasons suggested are doubt about masculinity and fear of impregnating a partner, which prevent the man from sustaining an erection. Sexual counseling for both partners to reduce stress, as well as serotonergic antidepressants such as Mirtazapine, may be helpful in alleviating the problem.

Persistent Sexual Arousal Syndrome

Persistent sexual arousal syndrome (PSAS) is excessive and unrelenting sexual arousal in the absence of desire (Mahoney & Zarate, 2007). It may be triggered by medications or psychological factors. When assessing someone with the disorder, be certain to ask if the person is taking any herbal remedies such as *Ginkgo biloba* because some of these can have arousal effects.

Pain Disorders

Because the reproductive system has a sensitive nerve supply, when pain occurs in response to sexual activities, it can be acute and severe and impair a person's ability to enjoy this segment of their life.

Vaginismus

Vaginismus is involuntary contraction of the muscles at the outlet of the vagina when coitus is attempted that prohibits penile penetration (Engman, Wijma, & Wijma, 2007). Vaginismus may occur in women who have been raped. Other causes are unknown, but it could also be the result of early learning patterns in which sexual relations were viewed as bad or sinful. As with other sexual problems, sexual or psychological counseling to reduce this response may be necessary.

Dyspareunia and Vestibulitis

Dyspareunia is pain during coitus. This can occur because of endometriosis (abnormal placement of endometrial tissue), vestibulitis (inflammation of the vestibule), vaginal infection, or hormonal changes such as those that occur with menopause and cause vaginal drying. A psychological component may be present. Treatment is aimed at the underlying cause. Encouraging open communication between sexual partners can be instrumental in resolving the problem.

✓ Checkpoint Question 5.5

The Matthews' neighbor Cindy is a woman who has sex with women. When you see Cindy in your clinic, you would want to teach her:

a. Falling estrogen levels are apt to cause her an early menopause.
b. She does not need to practice safer sex as she does not have male partners.
c. Her risk for contracting an STI is less than if she were heterosexual.
d. As she will never be sexually active, she needs no advice in this area.

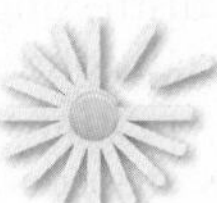

Key Points for Review

- The reproductive and sexual organs form early in intrauterine life; full functioning occurs at puberty.
- The female internal organs of reproduction include the ovaries, fallopian tubes, uterus, and vagina.
- The female external organs of reproduction include the mons veneris, labia minora and majora, vestibule, clitoris, fourchette, perineal body, hymen, and Skene's and Bartholin's glands.
- The male external reproductive structures are the penis, scrotum, and testes. Internal organs are the epididymis, vas deferens, seminal vesicles, ejaculatory ducts, prostate gland, urethra, and bulbourethral glands.
- A menstrual cycle is periodic uterine bleeding in response to cyclic hormones. Menarche is the first menstrual period. Menopause is the end of menstruation. Menstrual cycles are possible because of the interplay between the hypothalamus, pituitary, ovaries, and uterus.
- Biologic gender is determined by a person's chromosomes (XX or XY) and is set at conception. Gender identity is a person's concept of being male or female. This develops over a lifetime. Gender role is yet a third aspect and is the behavior a person demonstrates based on his or her gender identity as male or female.
- Masters and Johnson identified a sexual response cycle consisting of excitement, plateau, orgasm, and resolution stages. Disorders of sexual dysfunction include failure to achieve orgasm, vaginismus, dyspareunia, inhibited sexual desire, premature ejaculation, and erectile dysfunction.
- People assume varying sexual orientations, such as heterosexual, homosexual (women who have sex with women or men who have sex with men), or bisexual. Common sexual expressions are voyeurism, fetishism, and celibacy.
- Educating people about reproductive function is an important primary health strategy because it teaches people to better monitor their own health through vulvar or testicular self-examination.

- Teach adolescents that with sexual maturity comes sexual responsibility. They need to be aware of safer sex practices as protection against both an STI or an unintentional pregnancy.

CRITICAL THINKING EXERCISES

1. At the beginning of the chapter, you met Suzanne and Kevin Matthews, a young adult couple, 6 months pregnant, who came to your antepartal clinic for a routine visit. Suzanne, in tears, stated, "My husband isn't interested in me anymore. We haven't had sex since I became pregnant." Kevin states, "I'm afraid I'll hurt the baby." How would you counsel them?
2. Kevin's adolescent nephew Mark comes into the clinic because he has an STI. What would you advise Mark regarding safer sex practices?
3. Suzanne tells you that she hopes her new daughter won't be a "tomboy." She asks you the best way to convince a girl to be more of a "lady." What advice would you give her? Suppose she was concerned because a son was not "boyish" enough? Would your answer be any different?
4. Examine the National Health Goals related to reproductive tract or sexual functioning. Most government-sponsored money for nursing research is allotted based on these goals. What would be a possible research topic to explore pertinent to these goals that could advance evidence-based practice in relation to the Matthews family?

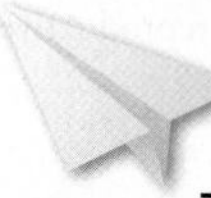

CRITICAL THINKING SCENARIO

Open the accompanying CD-ROM or visit http://thePoint.lww.com and read the Patient Scenario included for this chapter, then answer the questions to further sharpen your skills and grow more familiar with NCLEX types of questions related to reproductive and sexual health. Confirm your answers are correct by reading the rationales.

REFERENCES

Allen, L., & Fountain, L. (2007). Addressing sexuality and pregnancy in childbirth education classes. *Journal of Perinatal Education, 16*(1), 32–36.

American College of Obstetricians and Gynecologists [ACOG] Committee on Practice Bulletins. (2007). Pelvic organ prolapse. *Obstetrics and Gynecology, 109*(2 Pt 1), 461–473.

Anderson, J. R., & Genadry, R. (2007). Anatomy and embryology. In J. S. Berek (Ed.). *Berek & Novak's gynecology.* Philadelphia: Lippincott Williams & Wilkins.

Avery, A., et al. (2007). America's changing attitudes toward homosexuality, civil unions, and same-gender marriage. *Social Work, 52*(1), 71–79.

Baram, D. A., & Basson, R. (2007). Sexuality, sexual dysfunction and sexual assault. In J. S. Berek (Ed.). *Berek & Novak's gynecology.* Philadelphia: Lippincott Williams & Wilkins.

Basson, R., & Schultz, W. W. (2007). Sexual sequelae of general medical disorders. *Lancet, 369*(9559), 409–424.

Bessette, L., et al. (2008). The care gap in diagnosis and treatment of women with a fragility fracture. *Osteoporosis International, 19*(1), 79–86.

Centers for Disease Control and Prevention (CDC). (2009). *Adolescent pregnancy.* Washington, DC: Author.

Cook, L. A., et al. (2009). Vasectomy occlusion techniques for male sterilization. *Cochrane Database of Systematic Reviews, 2009*(1), (CD003991).

Dane, C., et al. (2007). Imperforate hymen—a rare cause of abdominal pain: two cases and review of the literature. *Journal of Pediatric & Adolescent Gynecology, 20*(4), 245–247.

Docherty, B. (2007). Reproductive system, part two—male physiology and function. *Nursing Times, 103*(14), 26–27.

Economos, C. D., Hildebrandt, M. L., & Hyatt, R. R. (2008). College freshman stress and weight change: differences by gender. *American Journal of Health Behavior, 32*(1), 16–25.

Ellsworth, P. I. (2009). Cryptorchidism. In F. J. Domino (Ed.). *The 5-minute clinical consult.* Philadelphia: Lippincott Williams & Wilkins.

Engman, M., Wijma, K., & Wijma, B. (2007). Itch and burning pain in women with partial vaginismus with or without vulvar vestibulitis. *Journal of Sex & Marital Therapy, 33*(2), 171–186.

Evers, J. L., et al. (2009). Surgery or embolisation for varicocele in subfertile men. *Cochrane Database of Systematic Reviews, 2009*(1), (CD000479).

Freeman, E. W., et al. (2008). Symptoms in the menopausal transition: hormone and behavioral correlates. *Obstetrics & Gynecology, 111*(1), 127–136.

Gabriel-Sanchez, R., et al. (2009). Hormone replacement therapy for preventing cardiovascular disease in post-menopausal women. *Cochrane Database of Systematic Reviews, 2009*(1), (CD002229).

Gruber, J. E., & Fineran, S. (2007). The impact of bullying and sexual harassment on middle and high school girls. *Violence Against Women, 13*(6), 627–643.

Hossein, S. N. (2007). Penile prosthesis surgery: a review of prosthetic devices and associated complications. *Journal of Sexual Medicine, 4*(2), 296–309.

Jain, A., & Bradbeer, C. (2007). Gender identity disorder: treatment and post-transition care in transsexual adults. *International Journal of STD & AIDS, 18*(3), 147–150.

Kaplowitz, P. B. (2007). Is it precocious puberty? *Contemporary OB/GYN, 52*(3), 42–44.

Karch, A. M. (2009). *Lippincott's nursing drug guide.* Philadelphia: Lippincott Williams & Wilkins.

Katsufrakis, P. J., & Workowski, K. A. (2008). Sexually transmitted diseases. In J. E. South-Paul, S. C. Matheny, & E. L. Lewis (Eds.) (2nd ed.). *Current diagnosis & treatment in family medicine.* Columbus, OH: McGraw-Hill.

Kelly, P. J., & Schwartz, L. R. (2007). Abstinence-only programs as a violation of adolescents' reproductive rights. *International Journal of Health Services, 37*(2), 321–331.

Kipke, M., et al. (2007). The health and health behaviors of young men who have sex with men. *Journal of Adolescent Health, 40*(4), 342–350.

Kosters, J. P., & Gotzsche, P. C. (2009). Regular self-examination or clinical examination for early detection of breast cancer. *Cochrane Database of Systematic Reviews, 2009*(1), (CD003373).

Krantz, K. E. (2007). Anatomy of the female reproductive system. In A. H. DeCherney & L. Nathan (Eds.). *Current diagnosis & treatment obstetrics & gynecology* (10th ed.). Columbus, OH: McGraw-Hill.

Kulp, J., & Zacur, H. (2007). Menopause & hormone replacement therapy. In K. B. Fortner, et al. (Eds.). *The Johns Hopkins manual of gynecology and obstetrics* (3rd ed.) Philadelphia: Lippincott Williams & Wilkins.

Ma, N. S., & Geffner, M. E. (2008). Gynecomastia in prepubertal and pubertal men. *Current Opinion in Pediatrics, 20*(4), 465–470.

MacKay, H. T. (2009). Gynecology. In S. J. McPhee, Papadakis, M. A. (Eds). *Current medical diagnosis & treatment.* Columbus, OH: McGraw-Hill.

Mahoney, S., & Zarate, C. (2007). Persistent sexual arousal syndrome: a case report and review of the literature. *Journal of Sex & Marital Therapy, 33*(1), 65–71.

Masters, W. H. (1998). *Heterosexuality.* New York: Smithmark Publishing.

McCance, K. L., & Huether, S. E. (2007). *Pathophysiology* (5th ed.). New York: Elsevier.

McDowell, M. A., Brody, D. J., & Hughes, J. P. (2007). Has age at menarche changed? Results from the National Health and Nutrition Examination Survey. *Journal of Adolescent Health, 40*(3), 227–231.

Musshoff, F., et al. (2007). Accidental autoerotic death by volatile substance abuse or nonsexually motivated accidents? *American Journal of Forensic Medicine & Pathology, 27*(2), 188–192.

Neves-E-Castro, M. (2007). An analysis of ovarian cancer in the Million Women Study. *Gynecological Endocrinology, 23*(7), 410–413.

Newman, B. S. (2007). College students' attitudes about lesbians: what difference does 16 years make? *Journal of Homosexuality, 52*(3–4), 249–265.

Nurnberg, H. G., et al. (2008). Sildenafil treatment of women with antidepressant-associated sexual dysfunction: a randomized controlled trial. *JAMA: Journal of the American Medical Society, 300*(4), 395–404.

Ott, M. A., Labbett, R. L., & Gold, M. A. (2007). Counseling adolescents about abstinence in the office setting. *Journal of Pediatric & Adolescent Gynecology, 20*(1), 39–44.

Parsons, J. K. (2007). Modifiable risk factors for benign prostatic hyperplasia and lower urinary tract symptoms: new approaches to old problems. *Journal of Urology, 178*(2), 395–401.

Piotrowski, K., & Snell, L. (2007). Health needs of women with disabilities across the lifespan. *JOGNN: Journal of Obstetric, Gynecologic, and Neonatal Nursing, 36*(1), 79–87.

Purinton, S. C., & Goldstein, A. (2007). Female sexual function & dysfunction. In Fortner, K. B., et al. (Eds.). *The Johns Hopkins manual of gynecology and obstetrics* (3rd ed.). Philadelphia: Lippincott Williams & Wilkins.

Sandfort, T. G., Melendez, R. M., & Diaz, R. M. (2007). Gender nonconformity, homophobia, and mental distress in Latino gay and bisexual men. *Journal of Sex Research, 44*(2), 181–189.

Scorolli, C., et al. (2007). Relative prevalence of different fetishes. *International Journal of Impotence Research, 19*(4), 432–437.

Selby, M. (2007). Menstrual problems: from menarche to menopause. *Practice Nurse, 33*(5), 33–34.

Street, A. E., et al. (2007). Gender differences in experiences of sexual harassment: data from a male-dominated environment. *Journal of Consulting & Clinical Psychology, 75*(3), 464–474.

Tanner, J. M. (1990). *Fetus into man: physical growth from conception to maturity* (2nd ed.). Cambridge, MA: Harvard University Press.

Torresani, T., & Biason-Lauber, A. (2007). Congenital adrenal hyperplasia: diagnostic advances. *Journal of Inherited Metabolic Disease, 30*(4), 563–575.

Wessells, H., et al. (2007). Erectile dysfunction. *Journal of Urology, 177*(5), 1675–1681.

White, T., & Ettner, R. (2007). Adaptation and adjustment in children of transsexual parents. *European Child & Adolescent Psychiatry 16*(4), 215–221.

SUGGESTED READINGS

Bersamin, M. M., et al. (2007). Defining virginity and abstinence: adolescents' interpretations of sexual behaviors. *Journal of Adolescent Health, 41*(2), 182–188.

Bralock, A. R., & Koniak-Griffin, D. (2007). Relationship, power, and other influences on self-protective sexual behaviors of African American female adolescents. *Health Care for Women International, 28*(3), 247–267.

Gettman, H. J., & Gelfand, M. J. (2007). When the customer shouldn't be king: antecedents and consequences of sexual harassment by clients and customers. *Journal of Applied Psychology, 92*(3), 757–770.

Janssen, D. F. (2007). First stirrings: cultural notes on orgasm, ejaculation, and wet dreams. *Journal of Sex Research, 44*(2), 122–134.

Lichtenstein, B., et al. (2008). HIV risk among long-haul truckers in the USA. *Culture, Health & Sexuality, 10*(1), 43–56.

Lisa, R., Taylor, M., & Hawton, K. (2009). Strategies for managing sexual dysfunction induced by antidepressant medication. *Cochrane Database of Systematic Reviews, 2009*(1), (CD003382).

McLaughlin, M., et al. (2007). Inequalities in the provision of sexual health information for young people. *Journal of Family Planning & Reproductive Health Care, 33*(2), 99–105.

Nelson, C. J., & Mulhall, J. P. (2007). Male orgasmic disorders: what do we know? *Contemporary Urology, 19*(2), 12–16.

Pastore, L., Owens, A., & Raymond, C. (2007). Postpartum sexuality concerns among first-time parents from one U.S. academic hospital. *Journal of Sexual Medicine, 4*(1), 115–123.

Williams, J. (2007). Midwifery basics: women's health needs: reproductive issues and choices. *Practising Midwife, 10*(2), 30–35.

Chapter 6 Assisting the Family With Reproductive Life Planning

KEY TERMS

- abstinence
- barrier methods
- basal body temperature
- cervical cap
- coitus
- coitus interruptus
- condom
- contraceptive
- diaphragm
- elective termination of pregnancy
- fertile days
- fertility awareness
- intrauterine device
- laparoscopy
- natural family planning
- reproductive life planning
- spermicide
- transdermal contraception
- tubal ligation
- vaginal ring
- vasectomy

OBJECTIVES

After mastering the contents of this chapter, you should be able to:

1. Describe common methods of reproductive life planning and the advantages, disadvantages, and risk factors associated with each.
2. Identify National Health Goals related to reproductive life planning that nurses can help the nation achieve.
3. Use critical thinking to analyze ways that family-centered reproductive life planning can be accomplished.
4. Assess clients for reproductive life planning needs.
5. Formulate nursing diagnoses related to reproductive life planning concerns.
6. Identify expected outcomes for couples desiring reproductive life planning.
7. Plan nursing care related to reproductive life planning, such as helping a client select a suitable reproductive planning method.
8. Implement nursing care related to reproductive life planning, such as educating adolescents about the use of condoms as a safer sex practice as well as to prevent unwanted pregnancy.
9. Evaluate expected outcomes for achievement and effectiveness of care.
10. Identify areas related to reproductive life planning that could benefit from additional nursing research or application of evidence-based practice.
11. Integrate knowledge of reproductive life planning with nursing process to achieve quality maternal and child health nursing care.

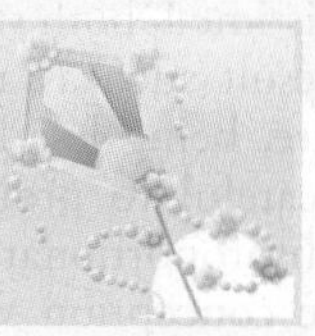

Seventeen-year-old Dana Crews has come to your community health clinic for a pelvic examination and Pap smear. She is sexually active and tells you that her boyfriend "sometimes" uses a condom. She trusts he will "stop in time" when they aren't using one. She doesn't want to take the pill because she can't afford it and she's afraid her parents will find out that she's broken her abstinence pledge.

The previous chapter described the anatomy and physiology of the male and female reproductive systems and the importance of practicing safer sex. This chapter adds information about ways to prevent pregnancy or plan and space children. Such information builds a base for both care and health teaching of families.

What additional health teaching does Dana need to be well informed about reproductive life planning?

Reproductive life planning includes all the decisions an individual or couple make about whether and when to have children, how many children to have, and how they are spaced. Health teaching is necessary because some couples want counseling about how to avoid conception. Others need information on increasing fertility and their ability to conceive. Others need counseling because contraception has failed.

It is important for the health of children that as many pregnancies as possible be intended, because when a pregnancy is unintended or mistimed, both short-term and long-term consequences can result such as a woman being less likely to seek prenatal care, being less likely to breastfeed, and possibly being less careful to protect her fetus from harmful substances. A disproportionate share of women who bear children whose conception was unintended are unmarried; such women are less apt to complete high school or college and more likely to require public assistance and to live in poverty than are their peers who are not mothers. The child of such a pregnancy is at greater risk of low birth weight, dying in the first year, being abused, and not receiving sufficient resources for healthy development (Centers for Disease Control and Prevention [CDC], 2009). Planning for reproductive choices is so important that several National Health Goals speak directly to this area of care (Box 6.1).

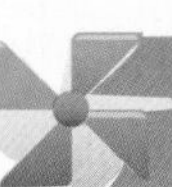

BOX 6.1 * Focus on National Health Goals

Several National Health Goals speak directly to reproductive life planning:

- Reduce the proportion of females experiencing pregnancy despite use of a reversible contraceptive method from a baseline of 13% to a target of 7%.
- Increase the proportion of pregnancies that are intended from a baseline of 51% to a target of 70%.
- Decrease the proportion of births occurring within 24 months of a previous birth from a baseline of 11% to a target of 6%.
- Increase the proportion of females at risk for unintended pregnancy (and their partners) who use contraception from a baseline of 93% to a target of 100%.
- Increase the number of health care providers who provide emergency contraception (new goal; baseline to be determined).
- Increase male involvement in pregnancy prevention and family planning efforts (new goal; baseline to be determined) (http://www.nih.gov).

Nurses can help the nation achieve these objectives by teaching people, especially adolescents, about contraceptive options. This instruction must be done carefully to avoid indirectly encouraging sexual activity among teens. Investigation into which contraceptives adolescents prefer and why they make the choices they do could be an important area of nursing research.

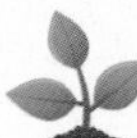

Nursing Process Overview

For Reproductive Health

Assessment

As a result of changing social values and lifestyles, many women are interested in reproductive life planning and so are able to talk easily about types and methods today. Other people are uncomfortable or not interested in using a planning method so may not voice their interest in the subject independently. For this reason, at health assessments, ask clients if they want more information or need any help with reproductive life planning as part of obtaining a basic health history. Before people are begun on a new contraceptive, other information that needs to be obtained is:

- A Pap smear, pregnancy test, gonococcal and chlamydial screening, perhaps hemoglobin for detection of anemia or a mammogram to rule out breast disease
- Obstetric history, including sexually transmitted infections (STIs), past pregnancies, previous elective abortions, failure of previously used methods, and compliance record
- Subjective assessment of the client's desires, needs, feelings, and understanding of conception (teens, for example, may believe that they are too young to get pregnant; many women in the immediate postpartum period may believe that they cannot conceive immediately, especially if they are breastfeeding)
- Sexual practices, such as frequency, number of partners, feelings about sex and body image, or latex allergy

Nursing Diagnosis

Because reproductive life planning touches so many facets of life, nursing diagnoses can differ greatly depending on the circumstances. Examples might include:

- Health-seeking behaviors regarding contraception options related to desire to prevent pregnancy
- Deficient knowledge related to use of diaphragm
- Spiritual distress related to partner's preferences for contraception
- Decisional conflict regarding choice of birth control because of health concerns
- Decisional conflict related to unwanted pregnancy
- Powerlessness related to failure of chosen contraceptive
- Ineffective sexuality pattern related to fear of pregnancy
- Risk for ineffective health maintenance related to lack of knowledge about natural family planning method

Planning and Implementation

When establishing expected outcomes for care in this area, be certain that they are realistic for the individual. Women's decisions are influenced by many factors; a nurse's role is to educate about contraceptives and support a woman about her contraceptive decision. If a woman has a history of poor compliance with medication, for instance, it might not be realistic for her to plan to take an oral contraceptive every day. Be certain to be sensitive to a couple's religious, cultural, and moral beliefs before suggesting possible methods. It is equally important to explore your own beliefs and values. This not only helps develop self-awareness of how these beliefs affect nursing care, but it allows you to become more sensitive to the beliefs of others.

Some couples cannot make realistic plans about contraception because they are uninformed or misinformed about the options. When counseling, be certain to emphasize safer sex practices as well as contraceptive ones (see Box 5.4). For example, although many contraceptive options offer reliable pregnancy prevention, only condoms provide protection against STIs, an important concern if the relationship is not a monogamous one.

Many women update their information on reproductive life planning before birth by using the Internet. Most postpartum services distribute printed information or have DVDs or information classes available for women before discharge. Women are then invited to ask questions as necessary about the material presented. Analyze these materials carefully to see that they are accurate before recommending them, and if suggestions are needed, make them to the correct health care facility committee. Be certain that unlicensed assistive personnel understand that if a woman has a question about the written material, their job is not to answer it but to refer the woman to someone (such as a nurse) who is more knowledgeable about the subject. Otherwise, they may suggest what method works for themselves rather than offering unbiased advice. This can result in a woman's choosing a contraceptive method that is not appropriate for her lifestyle and that may then be ineffective for her.

Clients are required to provide informed consent for surgical contraceptive methods or procedures. The risks, benefits, alternatives, and proper use of the method and the client's understanding of his or her rights and responsibilities should be included in the consent form. If you are helping to obtain a signature for consent for a procedure, always do so in the presence of a witness. Informed consent helps ensure that clients have weighed their options, know that the procedure may be irreversible, and have chosen a method that best meets their needs. An organization that is helpful for referral so people can learn more about reproductive life planning is Planned Parenthood (http://www.plannedparenthood.org).

Outcome Evaluation

Evaluation is important in reproductive life planning, because anything that causes clients to discontinue or misuse a particular method will leave them at risk of pregnancy. Reassess early (within 1 to 3 weeks) after a couple begins a new method of contraception, to prevent such an occurrence. Evaluate not only whether a chosen method is effective but whether the woman and her partner are satisfied with the method. Examples of expected outcomes include:

- Client voices correct technique for using chosen method
- Client voices confidence in chosen method by next visit
- Client expresses satisfaction with chosen method at follow-up visit
- Client consistently uses chosen method without pregnancy for 1 year's time

METHODS OF CONTRACEPTION

Until the 1950s, **contraceptive** products (products to prevent pregnancy) were not very reliable or could not be easily purchased. Today, as many as 40 million women in the United States use some form of contraception, a figure that represents 65% of women of childbearing age (CDC, 2009). Women not only use different methods but use different methods throughout their lifetime. Individuals or couples should choose a contraceptive method carefully, considering the advantages, disadvantages, and side effects of the various options (Box 6.2). Important things to consider when doing this are:

- Personal values
- Ability to use a method correctly
- How the method will affect sexual enjoyment
- Financial factors
- Status of a couple's relationship
- Prior experiences
- Future plans

The widespread use of contraceptives today points to both an increased awareness of responsibility for contraception and the wider range of options available. As nurses' roles are to

Box 6.2 Assessment
Assessing a Client for Possible Contraindications to Contraceptive Use

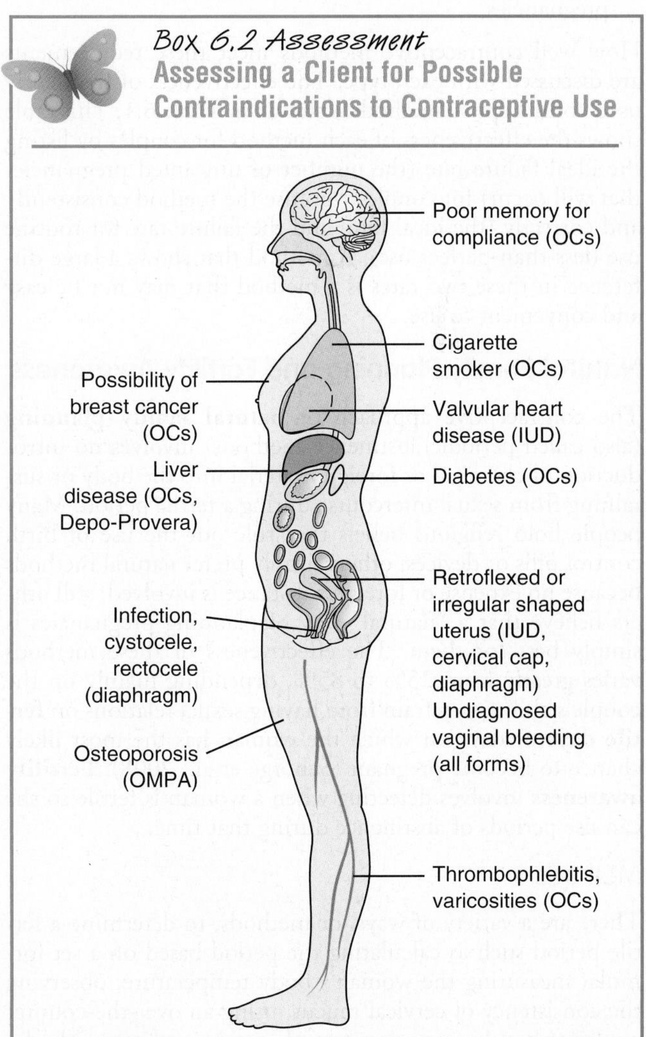

educate couples on what methods are available and how to use methods, understanding how various methods of contraception work and how they compare in terms of benefits and disadvantages is necessary for successful counseling. A major benefit of contraception that has occurred is that there are both fewer adolescent pregnancies today and fewer elective terminations of pregnancy than formerly (CDC, 2009). It is still necessary to be able to answer questions about elective termination of pregnancy with up-to-date knowledge and objectivity for couples whose contraceptive method has failed and are considering this. Legal and ethical issues, such as not allowing the enforced use of contraception for the physically or cognitively challenged, must be considered when counseling clients on the use of contraceptives. With information and the ability to discuss specific concerns, clients can be better prepared to make the decisions that are right for them (Nettleman, Brewer, & Ayoola, 2007).

An ideal contraceptive should be:

- Safe
- One hundred percent effective
- Compatible with religious and cultural beliefs and personal preferences of both the user and sexual partner
- Free of side effects
- Convenient to use and easily obtainable
- Affordable and needing few instructions for effective use
- Free of effects after discontinuation and on future pregnancies

How well contraceptive methods meet these requirements are discussed with each type. The effectiveness of frequently used contraceptive methods is shown in Table 6.1. This table shows the effectiveness of each method for couples by listing the ideal failure rate (the number of unwanted pregnancies that will occur) for couples who use the method consistently and correctly (the ideal rate) and the failure rate for routine use (less-than-perfect use). A method that shows a large difference in these two rates is a method that may not be easy and convenient to use.

Natural Family Planning and Fertility Awareness

The contraceptive approach of **natural family planning** (also called periodic abstinence methods) involves no introduction of chemical or foreign material into the body or sustaining from sexual intercourse during a fertile period. Many people hold religious beliefs that rule out the use of birth control pills or devices; others simply prefer natural methods because no expense or foreign substance is involved; still others believe that a "natural" way of planning pregnancies is simply best for them. The effectiveness of these methods varies greatly from 25% to 85%, depending mainly on the couple's ability to refrain from having sexual relations on **fertile days** or days on which the woman has the most likely chance to become pregnant (Schorge et al., 2008). **Fertility awareness** involves detecting when a woman is fertile so she can use periods of abstinence during that time.

Methods

There are a variety of ways, or methods, to determine a fertile period such as calculating the period based on a set formula, measuring the woman's body temperature, observing the consistency of cervical mucus, using an over-the-counter ovulation test kit, or using a combination of these methods.

Abstinence. **Abstinence,** or refraining from sexual relations, has a theoretical 0% failure rate and is also the most effective way to prevent STIs. However, clients, particularly adolescents, may find it difficult to adhere to abstinence, or they may completely overlook it as an option. Because it fails as an effective birth prevention measure for so many people, use of no contraceptive has a failure rate of 85% (Cunningham et al., 2008). In a moment of passion, many otherwise responsible people are unable to remain abstinent. Only 67% of women still use the method after a year. Many sex education classes advocate abstinence as the only contraceptive measure, so adolescents who take these courses may know little about other options. When discussing abstinence as a contraceptive method, be sure to provide information not only on the method but suggestions of ways to comply with this method (Box 6.3). A worry is that adolescents who make "abstinence pledges" to not have sexual intercourse until they are married may "tune out" not only additional information on contraception but on safer sex practices as well. Then, if they break their pledge (about 50% do), that could leave them more vulnerable to STIs and pregnancy than others (Cherlin, 2008).

Calendar (Rhythm) Method. The calendar method requires a couple to abstain from **coitus** (sexual relations) on the days of a menstrual cycle when the woman is most likely to conceive (3 or 4 days before until 3 or 4 days after ovulation). To plan for this, the woman keeps a diary of six menstrual cycles. To calculate "safe" days, she subtracts 18 from the shortest cycle documented. This number represents her first fertile day. She subtracts 11 from her longest cycle. This represents her last fertile day. If she had six menstrual cycles ranging from 25 to 29 days, her fertile period would be from the 7th day (25 minus 18) to the 18th day (29 minus 11). To avoid pregnancy, she would avoid coitus during those days (Fig. 6.1A).

Basal Body Temperature Method. Just before the day of ovulation, a woman's **basal body temperature (BBT),** or the temperature of her body at rest, falls about 0.5° F. At the time of ovulation, her BBT rises a full degree because of the influence of progesterone. This higher level is then maintained for the rest of her menstrual cycle. This pattern is the basis of the BBT method of contraception.

To use this method, the woman takes her temperature each morning immediately after waking either orally or with an ear thermometer before she undertakes any activity; this is her BBT. As soon as she notices a slight dip in temperature followed by an increase, she knows that she has ovulated. She refrains from having coitus for the next 3 days (the life of the discharged ovum). Because sperm can survive for at least 4 days in the female reproductive tract, it is usually recommended that the couple combine this method with a calendar method, so that they abstain for a few days before ovulation as well. The calendar method has an ideal failure rate of 9%, a typical rate of 25% (MacKay, 2009). For more information on BBT and how its use can aid fertility, see Chapter 8 and Figure 8.2.

A problem with assessing BBT for fertility awareness is that many factors, such as taking an antipyretic, can affect the BBT. For example, a temperature rise caused by illness could be mistaken as the signal of ovulation. If this

TABLE 6.1 ✻ Contraceptive Failure Rates

Type of Contraceptive	Ideal Failure Rate* (%)	Typical Use Failure Rate (%)	% of Women Still Using at 1 Year	Advantages	Disadvantages
Natural Family Planning					
Abstinence	85	85	—	No cost	High motivation needed; highly unreliable
Lactation, amenorrhea	—	—	0	Effective for short term	Temporary measure; not reliable if infant takes supplemental feedings
Calendar	5	25	65	No cost	Requires motivation, cooperation
Ovulation method	3	25	65	No cost	Requires motivation, cooperation
Symptothermal	2	25	65	No cost	Requires motivation, cooperation
Postovulation	1	25	65	Easy to use	Needs funds for monthly kit
Barrier Methods					
Cervical cap (parous woman)	23	35	55	Can use for several days if desired	May be difficult to insert; can irritate cervix
Cervical cap (nulliparous woman)	9	16	57	Can use for several days if desired	May be difficult to insert; can irritate cervix
Sponge (parous woman)	20	35	42	Easy to insert; no prescription	May cause leakage
Sponge (nulliparous woman)	9	18	55	Easy to insert; no prescription	May cause leakage
Diaphragm	6	18	55	Easy to insert	Prescription needed
Female condom	5	15	55	Protection against STIs	Insertion may be difficult
Male condom	2	15	53	Protects against STIs; male responsibility; no prescription necessary	Requires interruption of sexual activity
Hormonal Methods					
Transdermal patch	0.3	5	70	Easy to apply	Irritation at local site
Vaginal ring	0.3	5	65	Easy to insert	May need reminder to insert monthly
IUD (copper T)	0.1	0.1	80	No memory or motivation needed	Cramping, bleeding; expulsion possible; not recommended if risk of STIs
IUD LNG-IUS Mirena	0.1	0.1	80	No memory or motivation needed	Cramping, bleeding; expulsion possible; not recommended if risk of STIs
Combination oral contraceptives (COCs)	0.3	8	70	Coitus independent	Continual cost; possible side effects
Injectable progesterone (Depo-Provera)	0.3	3	55	Coitus independent; dependable for 4 to 12 weeks	Continual cost; continual injections
Intradermal Implants	0.05	0.05	80	Coitus independent; dependable for 5 years	Initial cost; appearance on arm
Surgical Methods					
Female sterilization	0.5	0.5	100	Permanent and highly reliable	Initial cost; irreversible
Male sterilization	0.1	0.15	100	Permanent and highly reliable	Initial cost; irreversible

*Couples who use the method consistently and correctly during 1 year's time.
Modified from Cunningham, F. G., et al. (2008). Contraception. In F. G. Cunningham, et al. (Eds.). *Williams Obstetrics* (22nd ed.). Columbus, OH: McGraw Hill.

Advise all women taking COCs to notify their health care provider if symptoms of myocardial or thromboembolic complications occur. These are:

- Chest pain (pulmonary embolus or myocardial infarction)
- Shortness of breath (pulmonary embolus)
- Severe headache (cerebrovascular accident)
- Severe leg pain (thrombophlebitis)
- Eye problems such as blurred vision (hypertension, cerebrovascular accident)

Early studies of birth control pills found that breastfed infants had lower weight gains when the mother was taking an OC because the estrogen content decreased the woman's milk supply. Although there is less estrogen in today's preparations, it is still not recommended that breastfeeding women take estrogen-based COCs until their milk supply is well established. Women may take progesterone-only pills (mini-pills) during breastfeeding (see later discussion).

COCs can interfere with glucose metabolism. For this reason, women with diabetes mellitus or a history of liver disease, including hepatitis, are evaluated individually before COCs are prescribed. COCs apparently do not increase the risk of breast cancer as was once feared (Stubblefield, Carr-Ellis, & Kapp, 2007).

Typically, COCs increase or strengthen the action of caffeine and corticosteroids. COCs may interact with several drugs such as acetaminophen, anticoagulants, and some anticonvulsants, reducing their therapeutic effect so women may be advised to temporarily change their method of birth control while prescribed these drugs. Several drugs, such as barbiturates, griseofulvin, isoniazid, penicillin, and tetracycline, decrease the effectiveness of COCs, so women might want to change their contraceptive method temporarily while taking these drugs as well (Karch, 2009).

When discussing COCs, be certain to assess both a woman's ability to pay for them and her ability to follow instructions faithfully (Box 6.7). Women using COCs should return for a follow-up visit yearly (for a pelvic examination, Pap smear, and breast examination), as long as they continue to use this form of birth control. Women without risk factors may continue to take low-dose OCs until they reach menopause.

Mini-pills. Oral contraceptives containing only progestins are popularly called mini-pills. The progesterone content thickens cervical mucus and helps prevent sperm entry into the uterine cervix. Ovulation may occur but, because the endometrium does not develop fully, implantation will not take place. Such a pill has advantages for the woman who cannot take an estrogen-based pill because of the danger of thrombophlebitis but who wants high-level contraception assurance (they are as effective as estrogen/progestin pills). They have the disadvantage of causing more breakthrough bleeding than combination pills. They are taken every day, even through the menstrual flow. Because it does not interfere with milk production, they may be taken during breastfeeding.

Effect on Sexual Enjoyment. For the most part, not having to worry about pregnancy because the contraceptive being used is so reliable makes sexual relations more enjoyable for couples. Some women appear to lose interest in coitus after taking the pill for about 18 months, possibly because of the long-term effect of altered hormones in their body. Sexual interest increases again after they change to another form of contraception. Some women experience nausea with the pill and find that this interferes with sexual enjoyment as well as with other activities. If they are having side effects with one brand, they might be able to take another brand that has a different strength of estrogen without problems.

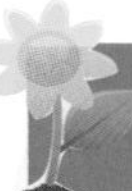

BOX 6.7 *Focus on Communication

You notice that Dana, 17 years old, is reading a pamphlet on oral contraceptives while she waits to be seen by the nurse practitioner.

Less Effective Communication

Nurse: Is that pamphlet helpful? Tell you everything you need to know?

Dana: Not really. I need some way to remind me to take a pill every day.

Nurse: If you're old enough to be sexually active, you should be responsible enough to do that without a separate reminder.

More Effective Communication

Nurse: Is that pamphlet helpful? Tell you everything you need to know?

Dana: Not really. I need some way to remind me to take a pill every day.

Nurse: Will that be a problem?

Dana: I think so.

Nurse: It's good to see you considering your individual lifestyle before making a choice. Some women use a pill dispenser so they have a daily reminder. Or if you'd like, I could help you make out a reminder chart. There are some methods of birth control that don't require reminders at all or more often than once a month. Why don't I discuss all the different types with you?

Reproductive life planning measures must be individualized to fit a person's lifestyle; otherwise, they will be quickly discontinued. Taking the time to help a woman assess how particular measures fit her lifestyle is better than just giving advice with a "one size fits all" philosophy.

Effect on Pregnancy. If a woman taking an estrogen/progestin combination COC suspects that she is pregnant, she should discontinue taking any more pills if she intends to continue the pregnancy. High levels of estrogen or progesterone might be teratogenic to a growing fetus, although the actual risk is thought to be no higher than normally occurs (Burkman, 2007).

Use by the Adolescent. It is usually recommended that adolescent girls have well-established menstrual cycles for at least 2 years before beginning COCs. This reduces the chance that the estrogen content will cause permanent suppression of pituitary-regulating activity. Estrogen has the side effect of causing the epiphyses of long bones to close and growth to halt; therefore, waiting at least 2 years also ensures that the preadolescent growth spurt will not be halted. Because adolescents' compliance with most medications is low, adolescent girls may not take pills reliably enough to make them effective. In addition, the cost of a continuing supply of pills may be prohibitive for teens. COCs have side benefits of improving facial acne in some girls because of the increased estrogen/androgen ratio created and of decreasing dysmenorrhea. These effects are appealing to adolescents so increase the COC compliance rate. The pill may be prescribed to some adolescents specifically to decrease dysmenorrhea, especially if endometriosis is present (see Chapter 47).

Use by the Perimenopausal Woman. As women near menopause, they are likely over age 35 so are less likely to be candidates for COCs than when they were younger. Help women in this age group to find an alternative method that will meet their personal preferences as well as still be maximally effective for them.

Use by the Postpartal Woman. It is not recommended that women who are lactating take estrogen-based contraceptives as a small amount of the hormone will be excreted in breast milk. Women are, therefore, usually prescribed "mini-pills" or OCs that contain only progestin until they are no longer breastfeeding.

Discontinuing Use. After women stop taking COCs, they may not be able to become pregnant for 1 or 2 months, and possibly 6 to 8 months, because the pituitary gland requires a recovery period to begin cyclic gonadotropin stimulation again. If ovulation does not return spontaneously after this time, it can be stimulated by clomiphene citrate (Clomid) therapy to restore fertility.

Emergency Postcoital Contraception. Several regimens, often referred to as "morning-after pills," are available for emergency postcoital contraception (Godding, 2008). The high level of estrogen they contain apparently interferes with the production of progesterone, thereby prohibiting good implantation. The Yuzpe regimen consists of the administration of two fixed-dose combination pills (usually Ovral), taken within 72 hours after unprotected intercourse. This is followed by two additional pills 12 hours later. This high dose of estrogen (200 mcg) almost always causes nausea and vomiting. Pretreatment with an antiemetic, such as 50 mg meclizine (Bonine), is usually recommended to decrease the possibility of vomiting. If vomiting should occur within 2 hours after administration, the pills should be repeated.

A specially designed emergency contraceptive kit (Preven) is a second method available for use after unprotected intercourse, particularly after a sexual assault has occurred. The kit consists of a urine pregnancy test to determine whether pregnancy has occurred and four pills that contain concentrations of estrogen/progestin (the first two taken within 72 hours after intercourse and the next two taken 12 hours later).

A progestin-only method termed "Plan B" is available over the counter or can be purchased from a licensed pharmacist without a prescription by anyone (male or female) over the age of 18 (Shacter, Gee, & Long, 2007). A prescription is required for anyone under age 18. With this plan, two pills containing high doses of levonorgestrel are taken (one pill immediately and one 12 hours later). This plan results in less nausea and may actually prevent more pregnancies than the estrogen-based regimen. Internet drug companies have become a resource for emergency contraception as they provide both privacy protection and competitive prices (Wu et al., 2007).

Overall, the rate of effectiveness for emergency postcoital methods of contraception is between 75% and 85%. These methods should always be used cautiously because of the potential danger that estrogen may be associated with congenital anomalies in the fetus if the pregnancy is not prevented. Mifepristone, discussed later as an abortifacient, or insertion of an intrauterine device (the copper T380) may also be prescribed for emergency postcoital contraception. An ethical question being asked is whether the availability of emergency contraception will encourage risky sexual behavior. This does not seem to be occurring (Wu et al., 2007). Fear of side effects is a major reason limiting the number of these products being used (Rocca, 2007).

Transdermal Route

Transdermal contraception refers to patches that slowly but continuously release a combination of estrogen and progesterone (Fig. 6.3). Patches are applied each week for 3 weeks. No patch is applied the fourth week. During the week on which the woman is patch free, a menstrual flow will occur. After the patch-free week, a new cycle of 3 weeks on/1 week off begins again. The efficiency of transdermal patches is equal to that of COCs, although they may be less effective in women who weigh more than 90 kg (198 lb). Because they contain estrogen, they have the same risk for thromboembolitic symptoms as COCs (Cole et al., 2007).

Patches may be applied to one of following four areas: upper outer arm, upper torso (front or back, excluding the breasts), abdomen, or buttocks. They should not be placed on any area where makeup, lotions, or creams will be applied; at the waist where bending might loosen the patch; or anywhere the skin is red or irritated or has an open lesion.

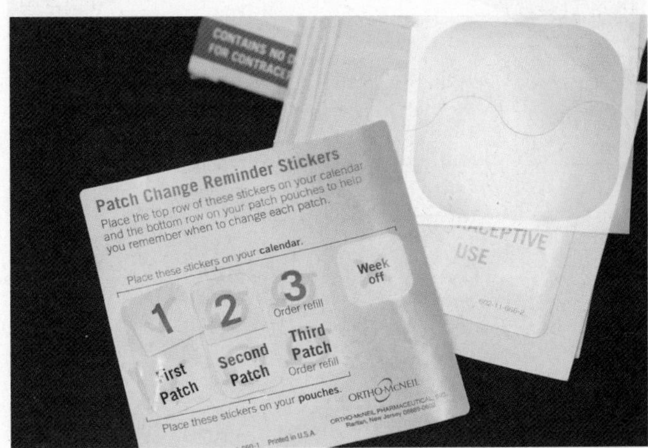

FIGURE 6.3 Estrogen/progesterone-based patches help adherence because they need attention only once a week. They may be applied on arms, the trunk, or buttocks.

Patches can be worn in the shower, while bathing, or while swimming. If a patch comes loose, the woman should remove it and immediately replace it with a new patch. No additional contraception is needed if the woman is sure the patch has been loose for less than 24 hours. If the woman is not sure how long the patch has been loose, she should remove it and apply a new patch, but this will start a new 4-week cycle, with a new day 1 and a new day to change the patch. She also should use a backup contraception method, such as a condom or **spermicide,** a product that is inserted vaginally and kills sperm, for the first week of this new cycle.

Transdermal patches have the potential to increase adherence, because the woman does not need to remember to take a daily pill. Mild breast discomfort and irritation at the application site may occur.

Vaginal Insertion

A **vaginal ring** (NuvaRing) is a silicone ring that surrounds the cervix and continually releases a combination of estrogen and progesterone (Fig. 6.4). The ring was FDA approved in 2001. It is inserted vaginally by the woman and left in place for 3 weeks, then removed for 1 week (Roumen, 2007). Menstrual bleeding occurs during the ring-free week. The hormones released are absorbed directly by the mucous membrane of the vagina, thereby avoiding a "first pass" through the liver, as happens with COCs; this is an advantage for women with liver disease. The effectiveness is equal to that of COCs. Fertility returns immediately after discontinuing using the ring. Women may need to make out a calendar that they post conspicuously to remind themselves to remove and replace the ring. Women may need to be encouraged to use vaginal rings as introducing a ring vaginally may at first seem more complicated than taking a pill every day (Gilliam, Holmquist, & Berlin, 2007). Some women experience vaginal discomfort, which makes a ring not a desirable contraceptive for them. While rings do not need to be removed for intercourse, if a woman senses that a vaginal ring is in place, this could interfere with sexual enjoyment.

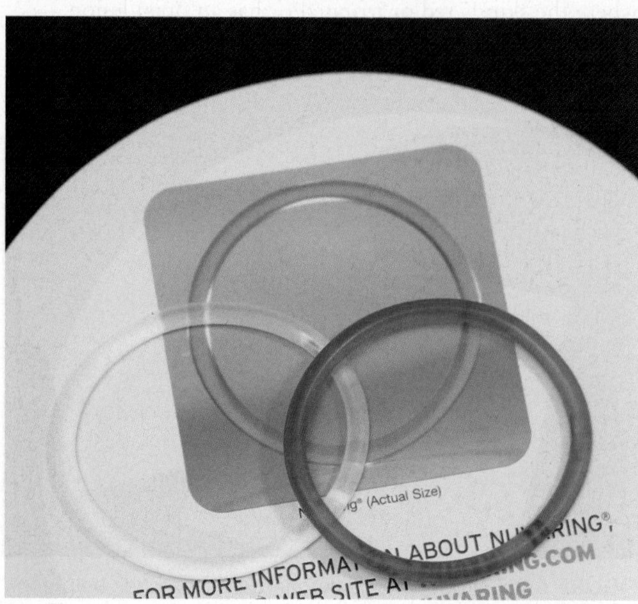

FIGURE 6.4 A vaginal ring. Both estrogen and progesterone are gradually released to be absorbed by the vaginal walls.

✓ Checkpoint Question 6.2

Suppose Dana, 17 years old, chooses to use a combination oral contraceptive (COC) as her family planning method? What is a danger sign of COCs you would ask her to report?

a. A stuffy or runny nose
b. Arthritis-like symptoms
c. Weight gain over 5 lb
d. Severe migraine headache

Implantation

Five subdermal implants, rods the size of pencil lead are embedded just under the skin on the inside of the upper arm, once used extensively by U.S. women are no longer available. One- or two-rod versions (Jadelle, Implanon) have been approved by the FDA and will soon be available and probably back in favor (Stubblefield, Carr-Ellis, & Kapp, 2007). The rods contain etonogestrel, the metabolite of desogestrel, the same progestin that is used in the NuvaRing. Once embedded, the implants appear as irregular lines on the skin, simulating small veins. Over the next 3 to 5 years, the implants slowly release the hormone, suppressing ovulation, stimulating thick cervical mucus, and changing the endometrium so that implantation is difficult.

The implants are inserted with the use of a local anesthetic, during the menses or no later than day 7 of the menstrual cycle, to be certain that the woman is not pregnant at the time of insertion. They can be inserted immediately after an elective termination of pregnancy or 6 weeks after the birth of a baby. The failure rate is less than 1% (Cunningham et al., 2008). At the end of 3 to 5 years, the implants are removed under local anesthesia (a quick minutes-only procedure).

A disadvantage of the implant method is its cost ($500 on average) and side effects such as:

- Weight gain
- Irregular menstrual cycle such as spotting, breakthrough bleeding, amenorrhea, or prolonged periods
- Depression
- Scarring at the insertion site
- Need for removal

A major advantage of this long-term reversible contraceptive is that compliance issues associated with COCs are eliminated. It also offers an effective and reliable alternative to the estrogen-related side effects of COCs. Sexual enjoyment is not inhibited, as may happen with condoms, spermicides, diaphragms, and natural family planning methods. Implants can be used during breastfeeding without an effect on milk production. Also, implants can be used safely in adolescents. The rapid return to fertility (about 3 months after removal) is an advantage for women who wish to have children.

Contraindications to subdermal rods are pregnancy, desire to be pregnant within 1 to 2 years, and undiagnosed uterine bleeding. A complication (rare) that can occur is an infection at the insertion site. If pregnancy does occur with the rods in place, they can be removed to reduce the small possibility of birth defects in a fetus.

Injection

A single intramuscular injection of medroxyprogesterone acetate (Depo-Provera [DMPA]), a progesterone, given every

12 weeks inhibits ovulation, alters the endometrium, and changes the cervical mucus (Box 6.8). The effectiveness rate of this method is almost 100%, making it an increasingly popular contraceptive method (Chrousos, 2008). Do not massage the injection site after administration as you want the drug to absorb slowly from the muscle. Because Depo-Provera contains only progesterone, it can be used during breastfeeding. Advantageous effects are reduction in ectopic pregnancy, endometrial cancer, endometriosis, and, for unknown reasons, reduction in the frequency of sickle cell crises (Burkman, 2007). Potential side effects are similar to those of subdermal implants: irregular menstrual cycle, headache, weight gain, and depression. Depo-Provera may impair glucose tolerance in women at risk for diabetes. Because there also may be an increase in the risk for osteoporosis from loss of bone mineral density, advise women to include an adequate amount of calcium in their diet (up to 1200 mg/day) and to engage in weight-bearing exercise daily to minimize this risk, rules that are good for all women. Depo-Provera is not routinely prescribed to adolescents, to protect their bone mineral density (Glasier, Yan, & Wellings, 2007).

Like subdermal implants, intramuscular injections have the advantage of longer-term reliability without many of the side effects and contraindications associated with COCs. An advantage of intramuscular injections over implants is that there is no visible sign that a birth control measure is being used; this makes them attractive to adolescents (Rickert et al., 2007). Two disadvantages are that a woman must return to a health care provider for a new injection every 4 to 12 weeks for the method to remain reliable, and the return to fertility is often delayed by 6 to 12 months. A reminder system, such as a postcard mailed by the prescribing agency, may be necessary to be certain that women return on time for their next injection. Alternative methods of administration, such as allowing pharmacists to give the injections or selling them over the counter so that women can inject themselves, are being studied.

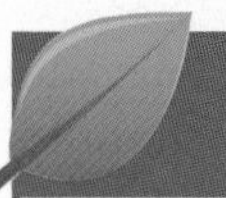

BOX 6.8 ✻ Focus on Pharmacology

Medroxyprogesterone Acetate (Depo-Provera)

Classification: Contraceptive

Action: Medroxyprogesterone acetate (Depo-Provera or DMPA) is a progesterone derivative that inhibits the secretion of pituitary gonadotropins, thereby altering the endometrium and preventing follicular maturation and ovulation (Karch, 2009).

Pregnancy Category: X

Dosage: 150 mg intramuscular injection every 3 months

Possible Adverse Effects: Spotting, breakthrough bleeding, amenorrhea, irregular menstrual flow, headaches, weight fluctuations, fluid retention, edema, rash or acne, abdominal discomfort, glucose intolerance, pain at injection site or osteoporosis (loss of bone density).

Nursing Implications

- Advise client to have an annual physical examination that includes breast examination, pelvic examination, and Pap smear.
- Caution the client that potential side effects may occur.
- Advise client to maintain a high calcium intake to reduce development of osteoporosis.
- Advise the client to report pain or swelling of the legs, acute chest pain or shortness of breath, tingling or numbness in the extremities, loss of vision, sudden severe headaches, dizziness, or fainting; these are signs of potentially serious cardiovascular complications.

✔ Checkpoint Question 6.3

Suppose Dana, 17 years old, chooses intramuscular injections as her method of reproductive life planning. What advice would you give her in regard to this method?

a. Limit cigarette smoking to one pack per day.
b. Drink at least three glasses of milk each day.
c. Do not swim for long periods at a time.
d. Do not expose the injection site to direct sunlight.

Intrauterine Devices

An **intrauterine device (IUD)** is a small plastic object that is inserted into the uterus through the vagina (Postlethwaite et al., 2007). IUDs became popular as a method of birth control in the 1980s, and although still a popular choice worldwide, IUDs are used by only a small number of U.S. women. Few manufacturers continue to provide them since several lawsuits were filed in association with the increased incidence of pelvic inflammatory disease (PID) in women using one particular brand, now no longer available.

Although the insertion of foreign objects into the uterus for contraceptive purposes dates back thousands of years (ancient camel drivers used the technique on their animals), the mechanism of action for the method is still not fully understood. Originally, it was thought that the presence of a foreign substance in the uterus interfered with the ability of an ovum to develop as it traversed the fallopian tube. Today, the IUD is thought to prevent fertilization as well as creating a local sterile inflammatory condition that prevents implantation. When copper is added to the device, sperm mobility appears to be affected as well. This decreases the possibility that sperm will successfully cross the uterine space and reach the ovum.

An IUD must be fitted by a physician, nurse practitioner, or nurse-midwife, who first performs a Pap test and pelvic examination. The device is inserted before a woman has had coitus after a menstrual flow, so the health care provider can be assured that the woman is not pregnant at the time of insertion.

The insertion procedure is performed in an ambulatory setting such as a physician's office or a reproductive planning clinic. The device is inserted in a collapsed position, then enlarged to its final shape in the uterus when the inserter is withdrawn. The woman may feel a sharp cramp as the device is passed through the internal cervical os, but she will not feel the IUD after it is in place. Properly fitted, such devices are contained wholly within the uterus, although the attached string protrudes through the cervix into the vagina (Burkman, 2007).

Two common types of IUDs used in the United States are the Copper T380 (ParaGard), a T-shaped plastic device

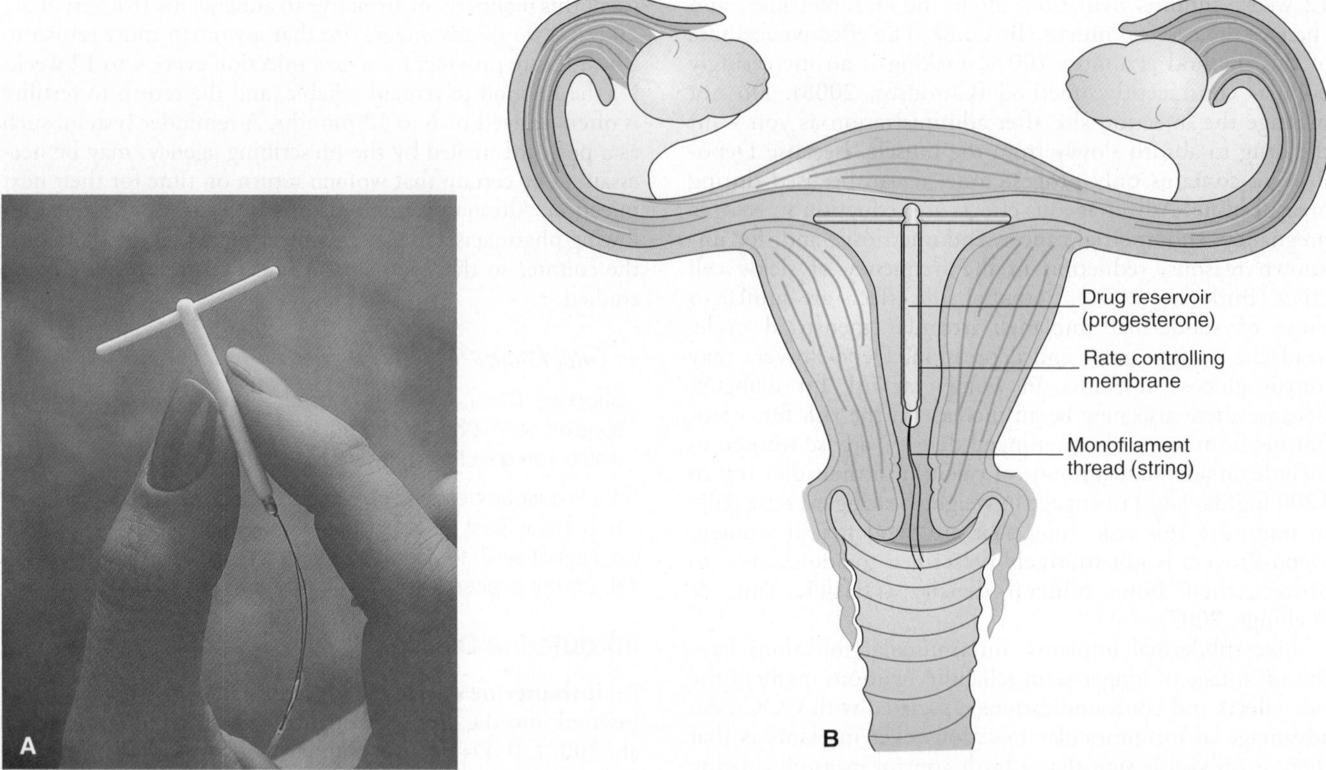

FIGURE 6.5 (**A**) Intrauterine device. (**B**) An IUD in place in the uterus. (Courtesy of ALZA Pharmaceuticals, Palo Alto, CA.)

wound with copper, and LNG-IUS (Mirena), which holds a drug reservoir of progesterone in the stem (Fig. 6.5). The progesterone in the drug reservoir gradually diffuses into the uterus through the plastic; it both prevents endometrium proliferation and thickens cervical mucus. The Mirena type is effective for 5 years (possibly as long as 7 years). It has a failure rate as low as 0.1% to 1.5%. The Copper T380, because of the added copper, has a comparable failure rate (Cunningham et al., 2008). It is effective for 10 years, after which it should be removed and replaced with a new IUD.

IUDs have several advantages over other contraceptives. Only one insertion is necessary, so there is no continuing expense. The device does not require daily attention or interfere with sexual enjoyment. It is appropriate for women who are at risk for complications associated with COCs or who wish to avoid some of the systemic hormonal side effects. They may create lighter or fewer periods. Teach women to regularly check after each menstrual flow, to make sure the IUD string is in place, and to obtain a yearly pelvic examination.

Side Effects and Contraindications

A woman may notice some spotting or uterine cramping the first 2 or 3 weeks after IUD insertion; as long as this is present, she should use an additional form of contraception, such as vaginal foam. Theoretically, a woman with an IUD in place has a higher-than-usual risk for pelvic inflammatory disease (PID), although this does not bear out in practice (Campbell, Cropsey, & Matthews, 2007). This may be because copper wound around the device may help resist infection. Some women have a heavier than usual menstrual flow for 2 or 3 months and experience more dysmenorrhea than other women. Ibuprofen, a prostaglandin inhibitor, is helpful in relieving the pain. Occasionally, a woman continues to have cramping and spotting after insertion; in such instances, she is likely to expel the device spontaneously. Women with IUDs in place should take active steps to avoid toxic shock syndrome (TSS; a staphylococcal infection from the use of tampons), because infection might travel by the IUD string into the uterus to cause uterine infection. TSS is discussed in Chapter 47.

IUDs are not recommended for women with an increased risk of contracting STIs, such as those who have multiple sexual partners, because this combination could lead to pelvic infection (Stubblefield, Carr-Ellis, & Kapp, 2007). They also are not recommended for women who have never been pregnant (their small uterus could be punctured with insertion) or who have a history of having had PID. If PID is suspected, the device should be removed and the woman should receive antibiotic therapy to treat the infection. All women need to know the most common symptoms of PID (fever, lower abdominal tenderness, and pain on intercourse) so they can report these to their health care provider immediately if they occur (see Chapter 47).

IUDs are also contraindicated in the woman whose uterus is distorted in shape (the device might perforate an abnormally shaped uterus). They are not advised for women with severe dysmenorrhea (painful menstruation), menorrhagia (bleeding between menstrual periods), or a history of ectopic (tubal) pregnancy, because their use may increase the symptoms or incidence of these conditions. Women with valvular heart disease may be advised against the use of an IUD because the increased risk of PID could lead to accompanying valve involvement from bacterial endocarditis. Because IUDs can cause a heavier than usual menstrual flow, women with anemia are also not usually considered to be good candidates for IUD use.

Effect on Pregnancy

If a woman with an IUD in place suspects that she is pregnant, she should alert her primary health care provider. Although the IUD may be left in place during the pregnancy, it is usually removed vaginally to prevent the possibility of infection or spontaneous miscarriage during the pregnancy. The woman should receive an early ultrasound to document placement of the IUD. This can also rule out ectopic pregnancy, which has an increased incidence among IUD users who become pregnant with the IUD in place.

Use by the Adolescent

IUDs are rarely prescribed for adolescents, because teens tend to have variable sexual partners and no prior pregnancies, both contraindications to IUD use.

Use by the Perimenopausal Woman

Women who are premenopausal are, overall, good candidates for IUDs unless they have a history of any of the specific contraindications to their use such as multiple sexual partners or a history of pelvic inflammatory disease.

Use by the Postpartal Woman

Although postpartum insertion is usually done at a 6-week postpartal checkup, it can be done immediately after childbirth. An IUD inserted soon after childbirth does not affect uterine involution or its return to a prepregnancy uterine size (Grimes et al., 2009).

Barrier Methods

Barrier methods are forms of birth control that work by the placement of a chemical or other barrier between the cervix and advancing sperm so that sperm cannot enter the uterus or fallopian tubes and fertilize the ovum. A major advantage of barrier methods is that they lack the hormonal side effects associated with COCs. However, compared with COCs, their failure rates are higher and sexual enjoyment may be lessened.

Chemical Barriers

A spermicide is an agent that causes the death of spermatozoa before they can enter the cervix. Such agents are not only actively spermicidal but also change the vaginal pH to a strong acid level, a condition not conducive to sperm survival. They do not protect against STIs. In addition to the general benefits for barrier contraceptives, the advantages of spermicides include:

- They may be purchased without a prescription or an appointment with a health care provider, so they allow for greater independence and lower costs.
- When used in conjunction with another contraceptive, they increase the other method's effectiveness.
- Various preparations are available, including gels, creams, sponges, films, foams, and suppositories.

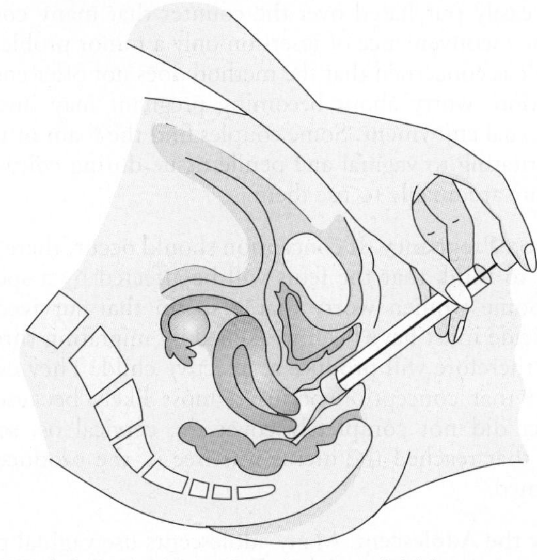

FIGURE 6.6 Vaginal insertion of a spermicidal agent.

Gels or creams are inserted into the vagina before coitus with an applicator (Fig. 6.6). The woman should do this no more than 1 hour before coitus for the most effective results. She should not douche to remove the spermicide for 6 hours after coitus, to ensure that the agent has completed its spermicidal action.

Another form of spermicidal protection is a film of glycerin impregnated with a spermicidal agent that is folded and inserted vaginally. On contact with vaginal secretions or precoital penile emissions, the film dissolves and a carbon dioxide foam forms to protect the cervix against invading spermatozoa.

Still other vaginal products are cocoa butter and glycerin-based vaginal suppositories filled with a spermicide. Inserted vaginally, these dissolve and release the spermicidal ingredients. Because it takes about 15 minutes for a suppository to dissolve, it must be inserted 15 minutes before coitus.

Sponges are foam-impregnated synthetic sponges that are moistened to activate the impregnated spermicide and then inserted vaginally to block sperm access to the cervix. Well liked by most users, they are easy to insert and have an efficiency rate of 80% (ideal) and a typical use failure rate of about 60% (Cunningham et al., 2008). They should remain in place for 6 hours after intercourse to ensure sperm destruction.

Side Effects and Contraindications. Vaginally inserted spermicidal products are contraindicated in women with acute cervicitis, because they might further irritate the cervix. They are generally inappropriate for couples who must prevent conception (perhaps because the woman is taking a drug that would be harmful to a fetus or the couple absolutely does not want the responsibility of children), because the overall failure rate of all forms of these products is about 20%. Some women find the vaginal leakage after use of these products bothersome. Vaginal suppositories, because of the cocoa butter or glycerin base, are the most bothersome in this regard.

Effect on Sexual Enjoyment. Although spermicidal products must be inserted fairly close to the time of coitus, they also are so easily purchased over the counter that many couples find the inconvenience of insertion only a minor problem. If a couple is concerned that the method does not offer enough protection, worry about becoming pregnant may interfere with sexual enjoyment. Some couples find the foam or moisture irritating to vaginal and penile tissue during coitus and therefore are unable to use them.

Effect on Pregnancy. If conception should occur, there is no reason to think that the fetus will be affected by a spermicide. Some women worry that a sperm that survived the spermicide must have been weakened by migrating through it and therefore will produce a defective child. They can be assured that conception occurred most likely because the product did not completely cover the cervical os, so the sperm that reached the uterus was free of the product and unharmed.

Use by the Adolescent. Many adolescents use vaginal products as their chief method of birth control because no parental permission or extensive expense is involved. Caution adolescents that this method has a high failure rate (20%). All women need to be cautioned that preparations labeled "feminine hygiene" products are for vaginal cleanliness and are not spermicidal; therefore, they are not effective contraceptives.

Because of the nontraditional settings in which adolescents may engage in coitus (such as in cars, on couches), some young women find inserting the product awkward and consequently do not use it, even though they have purchased it and intended to be more cautious. Many use a vaginal foam and ask their partner to use a condom, doubling their protection.

Use by the Perimenopausal Woman. The use of vaginal film or suppositories is not recommended for women near menopause as this is a time in life when vaginal secretions are lessening so the film or suppository might not dissolve completely. Spermicide foam can help lubricate the vagina and so increase sexual enjoyment.

Use by the Postpartal Woman. Vaginal spermicides are appealing to postpartal women as these can be purchased over the counter and used in the time period before a postpartal checkup when a more permanent form of contraception will be prescribed. They have no effect on breastfeeding.

Mechanical Barriers

Mechanical barriers, such as a diaphragm, work by blocking the entrance of sperm into the cervix. A **diaphragm** is a circular rubber disk that is placed over the cervix before intercourse (Fig. 6.7). A Lea's Shield, made of silicone rubber and bowl shaped, is a new design. Although use of a spermicide is not required for diaphragms, use of a spermicidal gel with a diaphragm combines a barrier and a chemical method of contraception. With this, the failure rate of the diaphragm is as low as 6% (ideal) to 16% (typical use) (Cunningham et al., 2008).

A diaphragm is prescribed and fitted initially by a physician, nurse practitioner, or nurse-midwife to ensure a correct fit. Because the shape of a woman's cervix changes with pregnancy, miscarriage, cervical surgery (dilatation and curettage [D&C]), or elective termination of pregnancy, teach women to return for a second fitting if any of these circumstances occur. A woman should also have the fit of the diaphragm checked if she gains or loses more than 15 lb, because this could also change her pelvic and vaginal contours. A diaphragm is inserted into the vagina, after first coating the rim and center portion with a spermicide gel, by sliding it along the posterior wall and pressing it up against the cervix so that it is held in place by the vaginal fornices. A woman should check her diaphragm with a finger after insertion to be certain that it is fitted well up over the cervix; she can palpate the cervical os through the diaphragm.

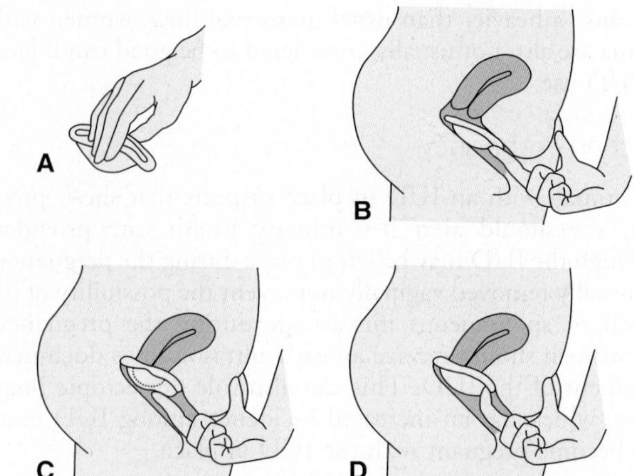

FIGURE 6.7 Proper insertion of a diaphragm. (**A**) After spermicidal jelly or cream is applied to the rim, the diaphragm is pinched between the fingers and thumb. (**B**) The folded diaphragm is then inserted into the vagina and pushed backward as far as it will go. (**C**) To check for proper positioning, the woman should feel the cervix to be certain it is completely covered by the soft rubber dome of the diaphragm. (**D**) To remove the diaphragm, a finger is hooked under the forward rim and the diaphragm is pulled down and out.

A diaphragm should remain in place for at least 6 hours after coitus, because spermatozoa remain viable in the vagina for that length of time. It may be left in place for as long as 24 hours. If it is left in the vagina longer than this, the stasis of fluid may cause cervical inflammation (erosion) or urethral irritation. A diaphragm is removed by inserting a finger into the vagina and loosening the diaphragm by pressing against the anterior rim and then withdrawing it vaginally. A Lea's Shield has an attached rubber loop to grasp for easy removal. After use, a diaphragm should be washed in mild soap and water, dried gently, and stored in its protective case. With this care, a diaphragm will last for 2 to 3 years.

Side Effects and Contraindications. Diaphragms may not be effective if the uterus is prolapsed, retroflexed, or anteflexed to such a degree that the cervix is also displaced in relation to the vagina. Intrusion on the vagina by a cystocele or rectocele, in which the walls of the vagina are displaced by bladder or bowel, may make insertion of a diaphragm difficult. Users of diaphragms may experience a higher number of urinary tract infections (UTIs) than nonusers, probably because of pressure on the urethra. Diaphragms should not be used in the presence of acute cervicitis or a papillomavirus infection, because the close contact of the rubber and the use of a spermicide can cause additional irritation. Other contraindications include:

- History of toxic shock syndrome (TSS; staphylococcal infection introduced through the vagina)
- Allergy to rubber or spermicides
- History of recurrent UTIs

To prevent TSS while using a diaphragm, advise women to:

1. Wash their hands thoroughly with soap and water before insertion or removal.
2. Do not use a diaphragm during a menstrual period.
3. Do not leave a diaphragm in place longer than 24 hours.
4. Be aware of the symptoms of TSS, such as elevated temperature, diarrhea, vomiting, muscle aches, and a sunburn-like rash.
5. If symptoms of TSS should occur, immediately remove the diaphragm and call a health care provider.

Effect on Sexual Enjoyment. Some women dislike using diaphragms because they must be inserted before coitus (although they may be inserted up to 2 hours beforehand, minimizing this problem) and they should be left in place for 6 hours afterward. Use of a vibrator as a part of foreplay, frequent penile insertion, or the woman-superior position during coitus may dislodge a diaphragm; therefore, this may not be the contraceptive of choice for some couples. If coitus is repeated before 6 hours, the diaphragm should not be removed and replaced, but more spermicidal gel should be added. Some couples may find this precaution restricting. An advantage of the diaphragm is that it allows sexual relations during menses (although see the earlier precaution on TSS). It may offer some protection against STIs. If a woman should become pregnant while using a diaphragm, there is no risk of harm to the fetus.

Use by the Adolescent. Adolescents may be fitted for diaphragms. However, because an adolescent girl's vagina will change in size as she matures and begins sexual relations, the device may not remain as effective as it does with older women. Adolescents may need to be reminded that pelvic examinations will be necessary to ensure that a diaphragm continues to fit properly. Some adolescents may not know where their cervix is or how to feel for it when checking the placement of the diaphragm. Use an anatomic diagram or model to show them or give them a mirror to use to view their own cervix during a pelvic examination. Caution them not to accidentally tear the diaphragm with long or sharp fingernails.

What if... Dana, 17 years old, tells you that she and a friend intend to share a diaphragm because they do not have enough money for each to buy one? Is this good planning?

Use by the Perimenopausal Woman. Women over age 35 have a higher incidence of cystocele or rectocele than younger women so diaphragms may not be the ideal contraceptive for them.

Use by the Postpartal Woman. As the cervix changes considerably with childbirth, women must be refitted for diaphragms and cervical caps (see later discussion on cervical caps) after childbirth. This is usually done at a 4- or 6-week checkup.

Cervical Caps

A **cervical cap** is yet another barrier method of contraception. Caps are made of soft rubber, are shaped like a thimble with a thin rim, and fit snugly over the uterine cervix (Fig. 6.8). The failure rate is estimated to be as high as 26% (ideal) to 32% (typical use) (MacKay, 2009). The precautions for use are the same as for diaphragm use except they can be kept in place longer.

Although popular in Europe, many women cannot use cervical caps because their cervix is too short for the cap to fit properly. Also, caps tend to dislodge more readily than diaphragms during coitus. An advantage is that cervical caps can remain in place longer than diaphragms, because they do not put pressure on the vaginal walls or urethra; however, this time period should not exceed 48 hours, to prevent cervical irritation. Cervical caps, like diaphragms, must be fitted individually by a health care provider. They include a small strap, which can be grasped for easy removal. They are contraindicated in any woman who has:

- An abnormally short or long cervix
- A previous abnormal Pap smear
- A history of TSS
- An allergy to latex or spermicide
- A history of pelvic inflammatory disease, cervicitis, or papillomavirus infection
- A history of cervical cancer
- An undiagnosed vaginal bleeding

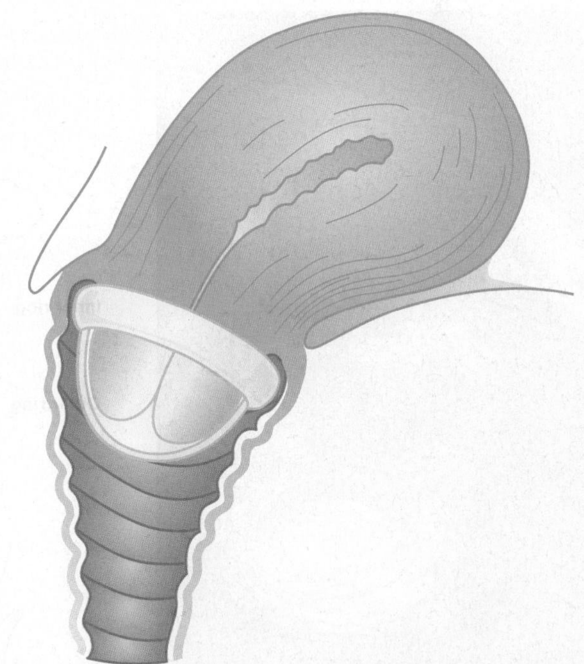

FIGURE 6.8 A cervical cap is placed over the cervix and used with a spermicidal jelly the same as a diaphragm.

Male Condoms

A **condom** is a latex rubber or synthetic sheath that is placed over the erect penis before coitus to trap sperm (Fig. 6.9). Condoms have an ideal failure rate of 2% and a typical failure rate of about 15%, because breakage or spillage occurs in up to 15% of uses (Kaplan & Love-Osborne, 2007). A major advantage of condoms is that they are one of the few "male-responsibility" birth control measures available, and no health care visit or prescription is needed. Latex condoms have the additional potential of preventing the spread of STIs, and their use has become a major part of the fight to prevent infection with human immunodeficiency virus (HIV). Recommend them for any partners who do not maintain a monogamous relationship.

Side Effects and Contraindications. There are no contraindications to the use of condoms except for a sensitivity to latex. If either the male or his partner has a sensitivity to latex, he can use a polyurethrane or natural membrane condom type. Caution him that these types do not give the same level of protection against STIs as does latex.

Effect on Sexual Enjoyment. To be effective, condoms must be applied before any penile-vulvar contact, because even preejaculation fluid may contain some sperm. A condom should be positioned so that it is loose enough at the penis tip to collect the ejaculate without placing undue pressure on the condom. The penis (with the condom held carefully in place) must be withdrawn before it begins to become flaccid after ejaculation. If it is not withdrawn at this time, sperm may leak from the now loosely fitting sheath into the vagina. Some men find that condoms dull their enjoyment of coitus; some couples do not like the fact that the male must withdraw promptly after ejaculation. Concern that the condom may break or slip also may inhibit sexual pleasure.

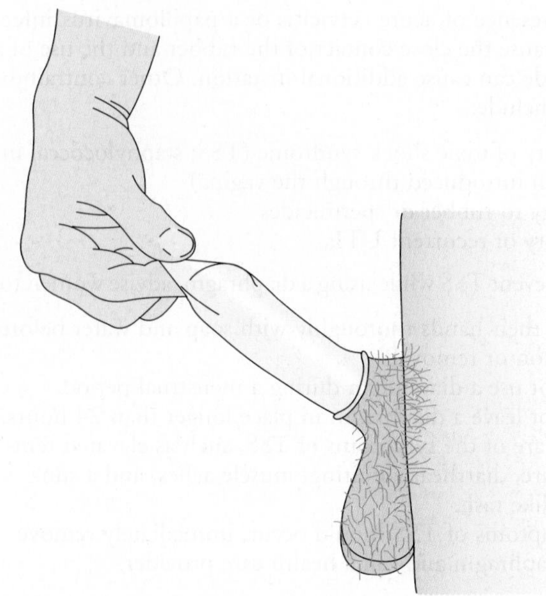

FIGURE 6.9 Male condom. Being certain that space is left at the tip helps to ensure the condom will not break with ejaculation.

Female Condoms

Condoms for females are latex sheaths made of polyurethane and prelubricated with a spermicide. The inner ring (closed end) covers the cervix, and the outer ring (open end) rests against the vaginal opening. The sheath may be inserted any time before sexual activity begins and then removed after ejaculation occurs. Like male condoms, they are intended for one-time use and offer protection against both conception and STIs (Fig. 6.10). Female con-

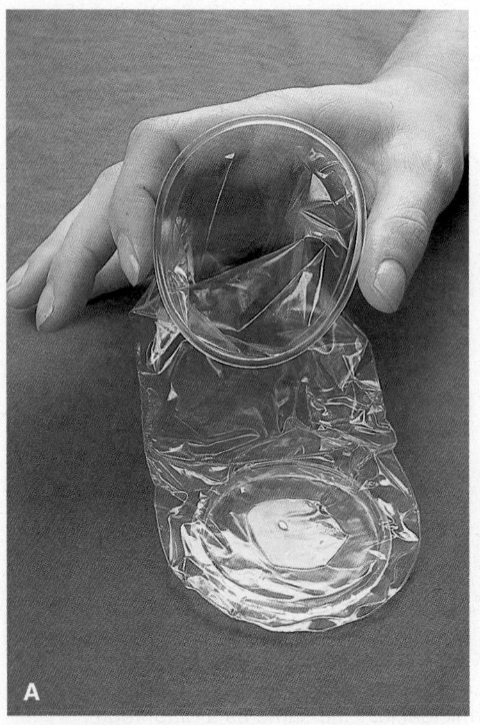

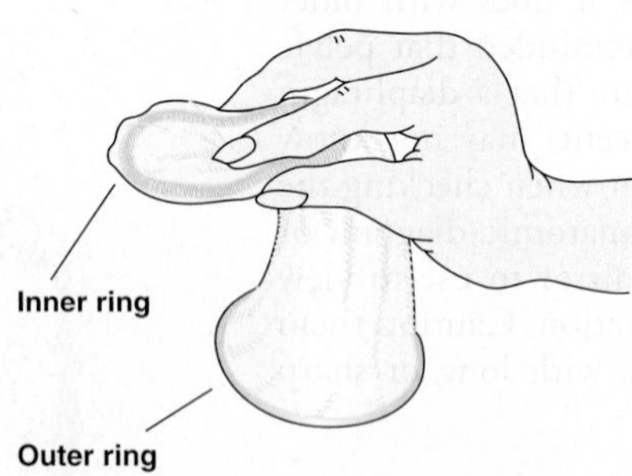

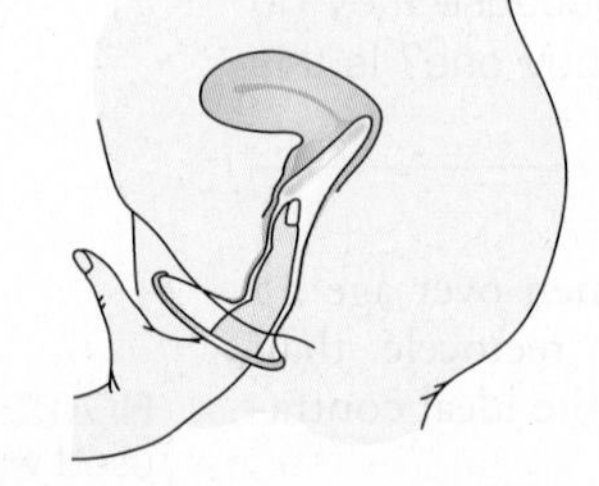

FIGURE 6.10 A female condom. Such a device is effective protection against both STIs and pregnancy. (**A**) The REALITY (WP-333) female condom. (© Barbara Proud.) (**B**) Insertion technique. (Courtesy of Wisconsin Pharmaceutical Company, Inc.)

doms can be purchased without a prescription but are more expensive than male condoms. Male and female condoms should not be used together. The failure rate is somewhat greater than the failure rate for male condoms, 12% to 22%. Most failures occur because of incorrect or inconsistent use. Although female condoms may reduce the risk of acquiring an HIV infection by as much as 90%, they have not gained great popularity, because of their bulk and difficulty in use (Burkman, 2007).

Use of Mechanical Barrier Methods by the Adolescent. Male adolescents are showing an increase in their ability to use condoms responsibly. Adolescents may need to be cautioned that condoms should never be reused, because even a pinpoint hole can allow thousands of sperm to escape. Adolescent boys who have infrequent coitus may use condoms that they have owned and stored for a long time. The effectiveness of these old condoms, especially if they are carried in a warm pocket, is questionable. For many adolescent couples, use of a dual method, such as a vaginally inserted spermicide by the girl and a condom by her partner, is a preferred method of birth control. The effectiveness of these two methods used in conjunction becomes about 95% (Kaplan & Love-Osborne, 2007).

✔ Checkpoint Question 6.4

Dana, 17 years old, wants to try female condoms as her reproductive planning method. Which instruction would you give her?

a. The hormone the condom releases may cause mild weight gain.
b. She should insert the condom before any penile penetration.
c. She should coat the condom with a spermicide before use.
d. Female condoms, unlike male condoms, can be reused.

Surgical Methods of Reproductive Life Planning

Surgical methods of reproductive life planning, often called sterilization, include tubal ligation for women and vasectomy for men. Tubal ligation is chosen by about 28% of all women in the United States of childbearing age as their contraceptive of choice. Vasectomy is the contraceptive method of choice for about 11% of men, making these two procedures the most frequently used methods of contraception in the United States for couples older than 30 years of age (Warehime, Bass, & Pedulla, 2007). Many people choose these surgical methods because they are the most effective methods of contraception besides abstinence, because there are no further costs, and because they have no effect on sexual enjoyment.

Between 6% and 7% of men and women in the United States seek a reversal of the procedure. Although reversal procedures are possible, such techniques are much more complicated and expensive than the sterilization itself, and success rates are only 70% to 80%. For this reason, surgical methods should be chosen with great thought and care and should be considered permanent. Counseling should be especially intensive for men and women younger than 25 years of age, because the possibility of divorce, death of a sexual partner, loss of a child, or remarriage could change a person's philosophy toward childbearing in the future. In addition, sterilization is not recommended for individuals whose fertility is important to their self-esteem.

Vasectomy

In a **vasectomy,** a small incision or puncture wound is made on each side of the scrotum. The vas deferens at that point is then located, cut and tied, cauterized, or plugged, blocking the passage of spermatozoa (Cook et al., 2009) (Fig. 6.11). Vasectomy can be done under local anesthesia in an ambulatory setting, such as a physician's office or a reproductive life planning clinic. The man experiences a small amount of local pain afterward, which can be managed by taking a mild analgesic and applying ice to the site. The procedure is 99.5% effective (MacKay, 2009). Spermatozoa that were present in the vas deferens at the time of surgery can remain viable for as long as 6 months. Therefore, although the man can resume sexual intercourse within 1 week, an additional birth control method should be used until two negative sperm reports have been obtained (proof that all sperm in the vas deferens have been eliminated, usually requiring 10 to 20 ejaculations).

Some men resist the concept of vasectomy because they are not sufficiently aware of their anatomy to know exactly

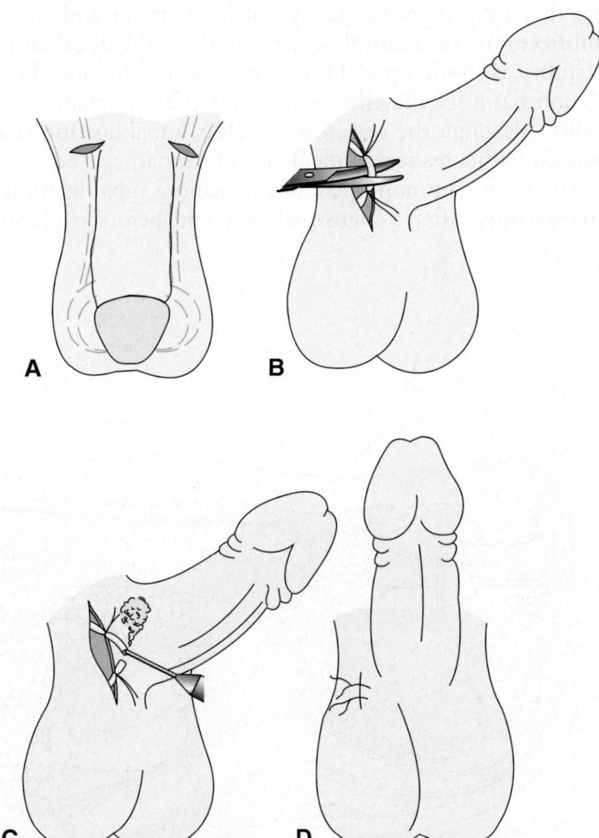

FIGURE 6.11 Vasectomy. (**A**) Site of vasectomy incisions. (**B**) The vas deferens being cut with surgical scissors. (**C**) Cut ends of the vas deferens are cauterized to completely ensure blockage of the passage of sperm. (**D**) Final skin suture.

what the procedure involves. They can be assured that vasectomy does not interfere with the production of sperm; the testes continue to produce sperm as always, but the sperm simply do not pass beyond the severed vas deferens and are absorbed at that point. The man will still have full erection capacity. Because he also continues to form seminal fluid, he will ejaculate seminal fluid—it will just not contain sperm.

There are very few complications associated with vasectomy. A hematoma at the surgical site may occur, although this is seen less frequently with "no scalpel" or puncture incisions (Cook et al., 2009). The procedure may be associated with the development of urolithiasis (kidney stones). A few men develop chronic pain after vasectomy (postvasectomy pain syndrome); having the procedure reversed relieves this pain. Some men develop autoimmunity or form antibodies against sperm, so that even if reconstruction of the vas deferens is successful, the sperm they produce do not have good mobility and are incapable of fertilization. Men who feel a need to have their sperm available for the future can have it stored in a sperm bank before vasectomy.

Tubal Ligation

Sterilization of women could include removal of the uterus or ovaries (hysterectomy), but it usually refers to a minor surgical procedure, such as **tubal ligation,** where the fallopian tubes are occluded by cautery, crushing, clamping, or blocking, thereby preventing passage of both sperm and ova. A fimbriectomy, or removal of the fimbria at the distal end of the tubes, is another possible but little used technique. Tubal ligation has a 99.5% effectiveness rate (Cunningham et al., 2008). Although the reason is not clear, tubal ligation is associated with a decreased incidence of ovarian cancer.

The most common operation to achieve tubal ligation is **laparoscopy.** After a menstrual flow and before ovulation, an incision as small as 1 cm is made just under the woman's umbilicus with the woman under general or local anesthesia. A lighted laparoscope is inserted through the incision. Carbon dioxide is then pumped into the incision to lift the abdominal wall upward and out of the line of vision. The surgeon locates the fallopian tubes by viewing the field through a laparoscope. An electrical current to coagulate tissue is then passed through the instrument for 3 to 5 seconds, or the tubes are clamped by plastic, metal, or rubber rings, then cut or filled with a silicone gel to seal them (Fig. 6.12). The procedure provides immediate contraception.

The procedure can also be done by culdoscopy (a tube inserted through the posterior fornix of the vagina) or colpotomy (incision through the vagina), but the incidence of pelvic infection is higher with these procedures and visualization is less. The woman is discharged from the hospital a few hours after the procedure. She may notice abdominal bloating for the first 24 hours, until the carbon dioxide infused at the beginning of the procedure is absorbed. This can also cause sharp diaphragmatic or shoulder pain if some of the carbon dioxide escapes under the diaphragm and presses on ascending nerves. Complications include bowel perforation, hemorrhage, and the risks of general anesthesia with the procedure (Warehime, Bass, & Pedulla, 2007). A woman may notice a day or two of abdominal discomfort caused by local necrosis if clips were used.

A new system, Essure, consists of a spring-loaded mechanism that, when inserted through the vagina and uterus into the outer end of a fallopian tube (a hysteroscopy procedure), releases a soft micro-insert into the tube that effectively seals the tube (Pavone & Burke, 2007). This can be done as an office procedure. Women must use a second form of contraception afterward until at 3 months, when a hysterosalpingogram is done to confirm that the fallopian tubes are blocked.

A woman may return to having coitus as soon as 2 to 3 days after the procedure. Be certain that they understand

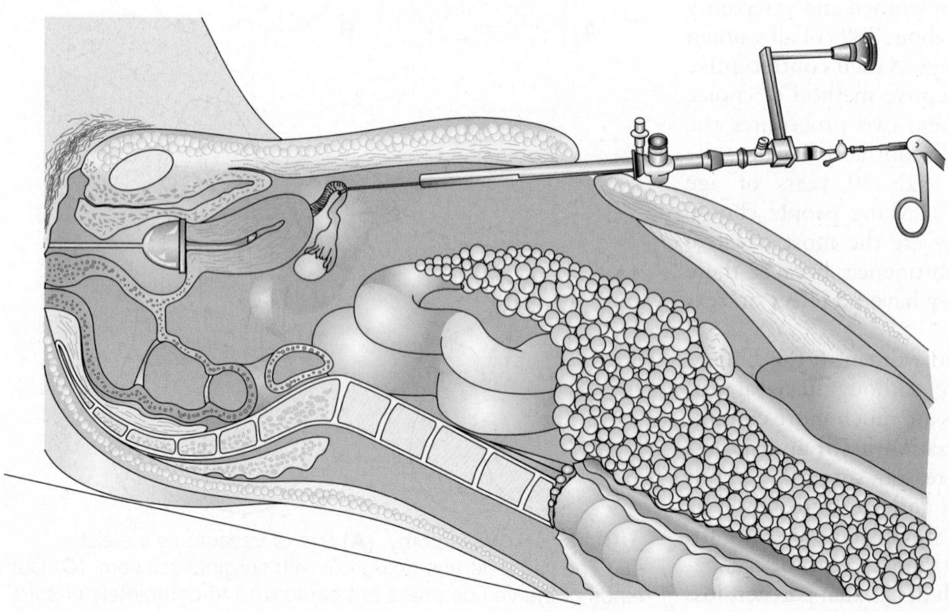

FIGURE 6.12 Laparoscopy for tubal sterilization. (From Richard Wolf Medical Instruments Corporation, with permission).

that tubal ligation, unlike a hysterectomy, does not affect the menstrual cycle, so they will still have a monthly menstrual flow. Be certain that women know to have no unprotected coitus before a tubal ligation (sperm trapped in the tube could fertilize an ovum there and cause an ectopic pregnancy).

Contraindications to tubal ligation surgery if done by laparoscopy are an umbilical hernia, because bowel perforation might result, and extensive obesity, which would probably require a full laparotomy to allow adequate visualization. Some women develop vaginal spotting, intermittent vaginal bleeding, and even severe lower abdominal cramping after tubal ligation; these symptoms are labeled posttubal ligation syndrome. Removal of the fallopian tubes appears to relieve the symptoms.

Not only is it difficult to reconstruct fallopian tubes after they have been cauterized, but there is also a possibility that afterward, the anastomosis site, because of its irregular surface, could cause an ectopic (tubal) pregnancy. If a silicone gel has been instilled into the tubes as a blocking agent, it can be removed at a later date to reverse the procedure. As with vasectomy, however, women should view tubal ligation as a permanent, irreversible procedure. Otherwise, they can regret having the procedure. This happens most in women under age 30 (Pavone & Burke, 2007).

Effect on Sexual Enjoyment. Both tubal ligation and vasectomy may lead to increased sexual enjoyment, because they largely eliminate the possibility of pregnancy. However, if either partner changes his or her mind about having children, the surgery may become an issue between them that interferes not only with sexual enjoyment but also with their entire relationship.

Use by the Adolescent. Counsel adolescents to use more temporary forms of birth control because their future goals may change so drastically that what they think they want at age 16 or 18 years may not be what they want at all at age 30. Later, if they still feel that vasectomy or tubal ligation is the method of reproductive life planning for them, the option will still be available.

Use by the Perimenopausal Woman. When a woman realizes that childbearing for her is complete, vasectomy for her partner or tubal ligation for her are the two most frequently requested forms of contraception.

Use by the Postpartal Woman. Tubal ligation can be done as soon as 4 to 6 hours after the birth of a baby or after an elective termination of a pregnancy, although it is more often done at 12 to 24 hours after birth. The abdominal distention at this time may make locating the tubes difficult, so a mini-laparotomy may be used. Such procedures can be done in an ambulatory surgery department with the patient under local anesthesia. A 2- to 3-cm incision is made transversely just above the pubic hair. The fallopian tubes are pulled to the surface and lifted out of the incision to be visualized. Metal or plastic clips or rubber rings are then used to seal the tubes. Clips cause necrosis at that point in the tubes.

✓ Checkpoint Question 6.5

Dana, 17 years old, asks you how a tubal ligation prevents pregnancy. Which would be the best answer?

a. Sperm can no longer reach the ova, because fallopian tubes are blocked.
b. Sperm cannot enter the uterus, because the cervical entrance is blocked.
c. Prostaglandins released from the cut fallopian tubes effectively kill sperm.
d. The ovary no longer releases ova, as there is nowhere for them to go.

THE COUPLE WITH A PHYSICAL OR COGNITIVE CHALLENGE

Reproductive life planning can be a greater concern than usual for a couple with a physical or cognitive challenge as finding a suitable contraceptive may be more difficult for them than for average couples. For example, a man who has unsteady coordination might not have adequate hand coordination to place a condom effectively. A woman with a similar handicap might have difficulty inserting a diaphragm or vaginal ring, and a woman who is cognitively challenged might not understand the need to take COCs daily. Morbidly obese clients may have difficulty with diaphragm insertion (Cowett, 2007). Women with recurrent convulsions may be unable to take COCs because of the interaction of these with common seizure medications. For these reasons, subdermal implants or surgical intervention may be the ideal contraceptive for many couples with a disability.

What if... Dana, 17 years old, tells you that the reason she wants a birth control method prescribed is to stop menstrual cramps. What advice would you give her?

FUTURE TRENDS IN CONTRACEPTION

Although COCs contain much less estrogen today than originally, because estrogen is responsible for most of the side effects associated with COCs, studies are being conducted using even lower-dose estrogen in pills. Biodegradable implants that do not have to be removed may be used in the future. A progesterone-filled vaginal ring that is permanently implanted is another possibility. A birth control vaccine consisting of antibodies against human chorionic gonadotropin hormone or injections of testosterone for males (which halts sperm production, just as estrogen halts ova production in women) are being tested at major centers. Until some method satisfies all of the criteria for an ideal contraceptive (i.e., completely safe, no side effects, low cost, easy availability, easy reversibility, and user acceptability), research in the field will continue. Both men and women need opportunities to discuss options to find the method that will be right for them (see Focus on Nursing Care Planning Box 6.9).

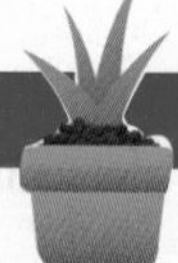

BOX 6.9 ✻ Focus on Nursing Care Planning

A Multidisciplinary Care Map for an Adolescent Seeking Contraceptive Information

Seventeen-year-old Dana Crews has come to your community health clinic for a pelvic examination and Pap smear. She is sexually active and tells you that her boyfriend "sometimes" uses a condom. She trusts he will "stop in time" when they aren't using one. She doesn't want to take the pill because she can't afford it and she's afraid her parents will find out that she's broken her abstinence pledge.

Family Assessment ✻ Client lives at home with parents and younger sister, 12 years old. Father works as Boy Scout Administrator. Mother is stay-at-home mom. Client states family finances are "good; no problem."

Client Assessment ✻ Past medical history is negative for major health problems. Menarche was at age 12. Menstrual cycles range from 28 to 35 days, with a moderately heavy flow lasting 5 to 7 days. She has enough cramping monthly that she "usually has to stay home from school for one day." Last menstrual flow was 1 week ago. Uses contraception inconsistently. Denies any history of sexually transmitted infections or other reproductive problems. Weight is appropriate for her height. Secondary sex characteristics are present. You notice her smoking a cigarette in the hallway. Following her health care visit, she is prescribed Ortho-ovum 7/7/7, a 28-day-cycle triphasic oral contraceptive.

Nursing Diagnosis ✻ Health-seeking behaviors related to knowledge deficit concerning contraception

Outcome Criteria ✻ Client identifies options available to her; states valid reasons for method chosen; demonstrates correct use of and appropriate follow-up care for chosen method; voices satisfaction with method chosen by 1 month's time.

Team Member Responsible	Assessment	Intervention	Rationale	Expected Outcome
		Activities of Daily Living		
Nurse	Assess client's lifestyle.	Discuss when she will take pill and where she will store them. Help make out a reminder sheet. Caution against smoking while taking an estrogen-based pill.	Reviewing lifestyle may provide clues to possible reasons why the method will be ineffective or not continued.	Client describes lifestyle to health care provider and actively participates in devising lifestyle changes that will add to contraceptive's effectiveness.
		Consultations		
Nurse	Consult with M.D., N.P., or nurse-midwife to determine whether method client chooses will be optimal, safe, and effective.	Secure prescription for medication.	Effective health care is a collaborative effort drawing on interdisciplinary expertise.	Consultation reveals that the contraceptive method chosen will be optimal, safe, and effective; client receives prescription.
		Procedures/Medications		
Nurse/nurse practitioner	Assess what form of contraceptive client thinks she could use most effectively.	Complete preprescription procedures such as a Pap test and pelvic exam. Review method of administration with client and steps to take if she forgets to take a pill.	Medication administration invariably requires discussion to help clients comply.	Any procedure necessary for prescription of a contraceptive is carried out safely with optimal respect for client privacy and concern.
Nurse	Determine whether client has any questions regarding pelvic exam or other procedures scheduled.	Assist with procedures such as Pap test; meet with client to answer any questions regarding contraceptive chosen.	Nurses can be instrumental in lending psychological and physical support during procedures.	Client states that she understands the importance of prescription procedures to ensure her safety.

Nutrition				
Nurse/ nutritionist	Determine whether client commonly eats a dietary source of folic acid such as green vegetables.	Discuss with client that oral contraceptive use can lead to folic acid deficiency.	Knowledge of side effects is important to create informed consumers.	Client acknowledges that she needs to be conscious of the need for folic acid; names two good sources of folic acid in food.
Patient/Family Education				
Nurse	Determine whether client has any further questions regarding chosen contraceptive measure.	Instruct client about the method selected. Have client repeat information for return demonstration.	Instruction provides an opportunity for learning to improve compliance.	Client describes the action of oral contraceptives and the need to take them conscientiously.
Psychosocial/Spiritual/Emotional Needs				
Nurse	Assess if client has discussed with boyfriend that contraception is different than safer sex practices.	Review and discuss the need for safer sex practices in addition to contraception.	Safer sex practices promote health, empower the client, and minimize the risk of sexually transmitted infections.	Client acknowledges need for safer sex practices to prevent STIs and states she will ask her partner to use a condom.
Discharge Planning				
Nurse	Assess if client understands she will need continued health supervision while on an oral contraceptive.	Explain the need for routine follow-up in 1 month and yearly pelvic exams.	Follow-up is essential for evaluating adherence and satisfaction and for reducing the risk of possible complications.	Client states that she will return for a follow-up visit in 1 month and every year after that.

ELECTIVE TERMINATION OF PREGNANCY (INDUCED ABORTION)

An **elective termination of pregnancy** is a procedure performed to end a pregnancy before fetal viability. Such procedures are also referred to as therapeutic, medical, or induced abortions. Having such a procedure is a woman's choice; nurses employed in health care agencies where induced abortions are performed are asked to assist with and offer support as a part of their duties. In the United States, although drugs are available, elective termination of pregnancy is still mainly a surgical procedure. Elective termination of pregnancy should not be viewed as a method of reproductive planning but as remediation for failed contraception. It is requested to end a pregnancy:

- That threatens a woman's life such as pregnancy in a woman with class IV heart disease
- That involves a fetus found on amniocentesis to have a chromosomal defect
- That is unwanted because it is the result of rape or incest
- Of a woman who chooses not to have a child at this time in her life for such reasons as being too young, not wanting to be a single parent, wanting no more children, having financial difficulties, or from failed contraception.

The majority of pregnancy terminations are done for these reasons.

Be certain that women who are choosing to have elective terminations are aware of all their options such as adoption or single parenthood before the procedure. Laboratory studies typically performed before the procedure include a pregnancy test, complete blood count, blood typing (including Rh factor), gonococcal smear, serologic test for syphilis, urinalysis, and Pap smear. Pregnancies are confirmed and dated by ultrasound.

In 1973, the U.S. Supreme Court ruled that elective terminations must be legal in all states as long as the pregnancy is less than 12 weeks. Individual states can regulate the termination of second-trimester pregnancies and can prohibit termination of third-trimester pregnancies that are not life-threatening. They can also mandate additional regulations regarding the procedure, such as requiring a 24-hour waiting period for counseling or requiring parental approval for minors. Whether a particular institution or health care provider provides elective termination services depends on the policy and choice of that institution or individual.

About 20 in every 1000 U.S. women will elect to terminate a pregnancy in their lifetime (one half of unintended pregnancies end with elective termination) (CDC, 2009).

women who may have more than one pregnancy termination in their lifetime as the gradual dilation of a cervix by this method helps to safeguard their childbearing potential. Antibiotic prophylaxis may be initiated at the time of the laminaria insertion to protect against infection. The woman is cautioned not to have sexual relations until the process is complete to further reduce the possibility of infection.

After either misoprostol or laminaria dilatation or dilatation by traditional dilators, a narrow suction tip specially designed for the incompletely dilated cervix is introduced into the cervix (see Fig. 6.13C). The negative pressure of a suction pump or vacuum container then gently evacuates the uterine contents over a 15-minute period. The woman will feel pain as the cervical dilatation is performed and some pressure and cramps, similar to menstrual cramps, during suction, but it is not a markedly painful procedure.

Advise the woman to remain flat for at least 15 minutes after the procedure to prevent hypotension. She needs to remain in the hospital or clinic for about 4 hours so she can have careful assessment of vital signs and perineal care. She usually receives oxytocin to ensure firm uterine contraction and minimize bleeding.

Because a rigid cannula is used for the procedure, D&E has the potential for uterine perforation, although this is rare. Because the cervix was dilated, there is a potential, as in all surgical termination procedures, for postprocedure infection. Be sure to teach the danger signals (see Box 6.11).

Prostaglandin or Saline Induction

Prostaglandin or saline induction is used if a pregnancy is between 16 and 24 weeks (see Fig. 6.13D). It is done on an inpatient or ambulatory basis. The woman is given prostaglandin $F_{2\alpha}$ by injection or prostaglandin E_2 by suppository. Both of these prostaglandins cause cervical dilation and uterine cramping, which expels the products of conception.

The woman is admitted to a same-day surgery unit and has oral misoprostol or vaginal laminaria inserted to help prepare the cervix for dilatation. The prostaglandin is then administered. Labor, which takes several hours after the administration of the prostaglandin, may be shortened by administration of a dilute intravenous solution of oxytocin. Because the products of conception are small, the actual expulsion causes only a momentary stinging pain as the perineum is stretched.

During the procedure, the woman needs the same care as any woman in labor:

- Frequent explanations of what is happening
- Medication for discomfort (breathing exercises may be helpful to minimize this)
- Presence of people important to her and health care personnel for support

If large amounts of oxytocin are necessary to induce labor, observe the woman for signs of water intoxication or body fluid accumulating in body tissue such as severe headache, confusion, drowsiness, edema, and decreased urinary output. These are the same symptoms that can occur when oxytocin is used to induce labor with term birth. They occur subtly at first, then grow in severity. If such symptoms occur, stop the oxytocin drip immediately. The symptoms will then decrease as body fluid shifts back to normal compartments. Always infuse oxytocin using a piggyback method during a termination procedure, the same as with a woman in term labor, so the infusion of oxytocin can be stopped quickly this way while still maintaining a fluid line for emergency drugs or fluid.

After expulsion of the products of conception, all the tissue expelled should be examined to determine whether the entire conceptus (fetus and placenta and membranes) has been expelled. If a woman wishes to see the fetus, wrap it as if it were a full-term infant and allow her to do this to begin effective grieving or closure. Observe women conscientiously for vaginal hemorrhage following the procedure, the same as after a term birth. If the procedure was prolonged, the woman may develop disseminated intravascular coagulation from trauma (see Chapter 21); if this occurs, she is very susceptible to hemorrhage, because her blood-clotting mechanism is compromised.

The use of saline for induction is based on the principle that hypertonic (20%) saline causes fluid shifts and sloughing of the placenta and endometrium. For this type of induction, a woman voids to reduce the size of her bladder so it will not be accidentally punctured by the saline injection. A sterile spinal needle is then inserted into the uterus through the anesthetized abdominal wall, and 100 to 200 mL of amniotic fluid is removed by a syringe with amniocentesis technique (see Chapter 19). A 20% hypertonic saline solution of up to 200 mL is then injected by the same needle, through the abdominal wall, into the amniotic fluid. The needle is then withdrawn. Within 12 to 36 hours after the injection, labor contractions begin.

A serious potential complication of saline termination is hypernatremia from accidental injection of the hypertonic saline solution into a blood vessel within the uterine cavity. The presence of such a concentrated salt solution in the bloodstream could cause body fluid to shift into the blood vessels in an attempt to equalize osmotic pressure. Serious dehydration of tissue could result. If an intravascular puncture should occur, the woman immediately experiences an increased pulse rate, a flushed face, and a severe headache. If such symptoms occur, the injection must be stopped immediately and an intravenous solution such as 5% dextrose begun to dilute the saline solution and restore fluid balance.

Hysterotomy

If the gestational age for a pregnancy is more than 16 to 18 weeks, a hysterotomy, or removal of the fetus by surgical intervention similar to a cesarean birth, may be performed. Surgery is necessary at this point, because the uterus becomes resistant to the effect of oxytocin as it reaches this phase of pregnancy and may not respond either to saline induction or prostaglandins, even with the assistance of oxytocin. Furthermore, the chance is great at this gestational age, because the uterus is so enlarged, that it will not respond and contract afterward, leading to hemorrhage. The technique for hysterotomy is identical to that of cesarean birth (see Chapter 24). Because this is so late in pregnancy, fewer than 1% of surgical terminations are done using this technique.

"Partial Birth Abortion"

"Partial birth abortion" was a surgical technique formerly used during the last 3 months of pregnancy if the fetus was discovered to have a congenital anomaly that would be incompatible with life or would result in a severely compromised child such as encephalocele or high spinal meningocele. Labor was induced by a combination of oxytocin and cervical ripening. The fetus was turned so that the breech presented to the birth canal. A clamp was then inserted into the base of the fetal skull and the head contents were destroyed. The head was then collapsed and delivered. "Partial birth abortion" is no longer legal in the United States (Greene, 2007). A cesarean birth or vaginal birth of the infant is scheduled instead.

Isoimmunization

Whenever a placenta is dislodged, either by spontaneous birth or by surgical or medical intervention at any point in pregnancy, blood from the placental villi (the fetal blood) may enter the maternal circulation. This has implications for the Rh-negative woman. If the fetus is Rh-positive, enough Rh-positive blood may enter her circulation to cause isoimmunization or the production by her immunologic system of antibodies against Rh-positive blood. If the fetus in her next pregnancy should also be Rh-positive, those antibodies would attempt to destroy the red blood cells of that infant during the months in utero.

Because the blood type of the conceptus is unknown with either medical or surgical termination, all women with Rh-negative blood should receive Rh_o(D) immune globulin (RhoGAM or RHIG) within 72 hours after the procedure to prevent the buildup of antibodies in the event the conceptus was Rh positive (see Chapter 26 for a full discussion of Rh disease).

Psychological Aspects of Elective Termination of Pregnancy

Women of all ages, married or unmarried, with or without children, request elective terminations. The usual profile of a woman who is having such a procedure

- Is young and unmarried
- Has no previous live births
- Undergoes the procedure to end an unwanted pregnancy
- Has not taken any or adequate protection against becoming pregnant

Adolescents, often blamed for not using responsible contraception, do not appear to have been using a contraceptive any more carelessly than adult women at the time they ask for an elective termination of pregnancy (Harvey & Gaudoin, 2007). Be certain to give women of all ages having elective termination the same kind of explanations and support that women in labor receive (women do not share termination experiences with each other the same way as they share labor experiences, so women usually have received little advance preparation).

Most women feel anxious when they appear at the hospital or clinic for an elective termination procedure. Some of the anxiety comes from having made a difficult decision to reach this step; some comes from having to face the unknown; some may come from feelings of loss or shame and sadness that they had to make a decision with which they are not totally comfortable. Remembering that this is not a decision taken lightly helps in planning nursing care aimed at making an elective termination as nontraumatic as possible.

A few women express sadness and guilt after abortion. These women may need to be referred for professional counseling so they can integrate and accept this event in their lives.

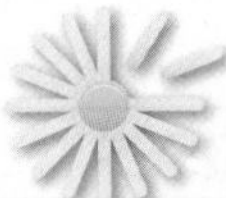

Key Points for Review

- Reproductive life planning involves personal decisions based on each individual's background, experiences, and sociocultural beliefs. It involves thorough planning to be certain that the method chosen is acceptable and can be used effectively.
- Natural family planning (periodic abstinence and fertility awareness) methods are varied but involve determining the fertile period each month and then avoiding sexual relations during that time.
- Oral contraceptives are combinations of estrogen and progesterone. They provide one of the most reliable forms of contraception outside of abstinence. Women older than 40 years of age who smoke are not candidates for OC use because of the danger of cardiovascular complications. They should be counseled to find a form of contraception that is reliable and allows them to remain sexually active.
- Subdermal implants (renewed every 3 to 5 years) and intramuscular injections (renewed every 1 or 3 months), transdermal patches, and vaginal rings are equally effective.
- Intrauterine devices are placed in the uterus to prevent fertilization and implantation. Women with intrauterine devices should limit their number of sexual partners to help prevent sexually transmitted infections, and be aware of the signs and symptoms of pelvic inflammatory disease.
- Barrier methods of contraception include the diaphragm, cervical cap, sponges, vaginal spermicides, and condoms (male and female). Such methods are low in cost but are not as effective as ovulation suppressant methods. Use of diaphragms may be associated with urinary tract infections.
- "Morning-after" or "Plan B" protection involves administration of a high dose of estrogen or progesterone that prevents follicle-stimulating hormone release, preventing ovulation in case unprotected intercourse occurred.
- Surgical methods of contraception are tubal ligation in women and vasectomy in men. Counsel individuals who wish to undergo these procedures that they are largely irreversible.
- Elective termination of pregnancy can be accomplished surgically by menstrual extraction, dilatation and curettage, dilatation and vacuum extraction, or prostaglandin or saline induction, or medically by administration of mifepristone and misoprostol. Counsel women not to think of elective termination of pregnancy as a contraceptive method, but as a recourse to be used only if preventive measures fail. Women who are Rh negative need to receive Rh_o(D) immune globulin after these procedures.

- When counseling clients about reproductive life planning, nurses have a responsibility to teach about safer sex practices as well, such as using a condom during sexual intercourse to avoid HIV infection or other sexually transmitted infections.

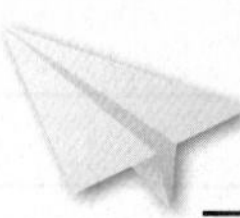

CRITICAL THINKING EXERCISES

1. What patient education information would you provide for Dana Crews, the 17-year-old described at the beginning of this chapter? What method of reproductive life planning would you recommend for her? Would your recommendation be different if she had a guaranteed monogamous relationship?
2. Suppose Dana was 39 years old, had high blood pressure, and smoked? Would your teaching and recommendations differ?
3. Suppose Dana does not follow your advice for reproductive life planning and is admitted to the hospital for a prostaglandin induction to electively terminate a pregnancy. Her mother asks you to give her only a minimum of analgesia so that she will remember the experience as painful and therefore will not get pregnant again. Do you agree with this philosophy of care?
4. Examine the National Health Goals related to reproductive life planning. Most government-sponsored money for nursing research is allotted based on these goals. What would be a possible research topic to explore pertinent to these goals that could advance evidence-based practice in relation to Dana's family?

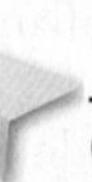

CRITICAL THINKING SCENARIO

Open the accompanying CD-ROM or visit http://thePoint.lww.com and read the Patient Scenario included for this chapter, then answer the questions to further sharpen your skills and grow more familiar with NCLEX types of questions related to reproductive life planning. Confirm your answers are correct by reading the rationales.

REFERENCES

Burkman, R. T. (2007). Contraception & family planning. In A. H. DeCherney & L. Nathan (Eds.). *Current diagnosis & treatment in obstetrics & gynecology* (10th ed.). Columbus, OH: McGraw-Hill.

Campbell, S. J., Cropsey, K. L., & Matthews, C. A. (2007). Intrauterine device use in a high-risk population: experience from an urban university clinic. *American Journal of Obstetrics & Gynecology, 197*(2), 193–197.

Centers for Disease Control and Prevention. (2009). *Adolescent pregnancy.* Washington, DC: Author.

Cherlin, A. J. (2008). *Public and private families.* New York: McGraw-Hill Publishing Company.

Chrousos, G. P. (2008). The gonadal hormones and inhibitors. In P. B. G. Katzung (Ed.). *Basic and clinical pharmacology* (10th ed.). Columbus, OH: McGraw-Hill.

Cole, J. A., et al. (2007). Venous thromboembolism, myocardial infarction, and stroke among transdermal contraceptive system users. *Obstetrics and Gynecology, 109*(2.1), 339–346.

Cook, L., et al. (2009). Vasectomy occlusion techniques for male sterilization. *Cochrane Database of Systematic Reviews, 2009*(1), (CD003991).

Cowett, A. (2007). Contraceptive options for your obese patients. *Contemporary OB/GYN, 52*(3), 52–57.

Cunningham, F. G., et al. (2008). Contraception. In F. G. Cunningham, et al. (Eds.). *Williams obstetrics* (22nd ed.). Columbus, OH: McGraw-Hill.

Fehring, R. J., et al. (2007). Efficacy of cervical mucus observations plus electronic hormonal fertility monitoring as a method of natural family planning. *JOGNN: Journal of Obstetric, Gynecologic, and Neonatal Nursing, 36*(2), 152–160.

Germano E., & Jennings, V. (2007). New approaches to fertility awareness-based methods: incorporating the Standard Days and Two Day Methods into practice. *Journal of Midwifery & Women's Health, 51*(6), 471–477.

Gilliam, M., Holmquist, S., & Berlin, A. (2007). Factors associated with willingness to use the contraceptive vaginal ring. *Contraception, 76*(1), 30–34.

Glasier, A., Yan, Y., & Wellings, K. (2007). How do health care professionals respond to advice on adverse side effects of contraceptive methods? The case of Depo Provera. *Contraception, 76(*1), 18–22.

Godding, J. (2008). Emergency contraception. *Emergency Nurse, 16*(4), 22–24.

Greene, M. F. (2007). The intimidation of American physicians—banning partial-birth abortion. *New England Journal of Medicine, 356(*21), 2128–2129.

Grimes, D. A., et al. (2009). Immediate post-partum insertion of intrauterine devices. *Cochrane Database of Systematic Reviews, 2009*(1), (CD003036).

Harvey, N., & Gaudoin, M. (2007). Teenagers requesting pregnancy termination are no less responsible about contraceptive use at the time of conception than older women. *BJOG: An International Journal of Obstetrics and Gynaecology, 114(*2), 226–229.

Kaplan, D. W., & Love-Osborne, K. A. (2007). Adolescence, In A. H. DeCherney & L. Nathan (Eds.). *Current diagnosis & treatment in obstetrics & gynecology* (10th ed.). Columbus, OH: McGraw-Hill.

Karch, A. M. (2009). *Lippincott's nursing drug guide.* Philadelphia: Lippincott Williams & Wilkins.

Kulier, R., et al. (2009). Medical methods for first trimester abortion. *Cochrane Database of Systematic Reviews, 2009*(1), (CD002855).

MacKay, H. T. (2009). Gynecologic disorders. In S. J. McPhee, et al. (Eds.). *Current medical diagnosis & treatment.* Columbus, OH: McGraw-Hill.

Nettleman, M., Brewer, J., & Ayoola, A. (2007). Reasons for unprotected intercourse in adult women: a qualitative study. *Journal of Midwifery & Women's Health, 52*(2), 148–152.

Noone, J. (2007). Strategies for contraceptive success. *Nurse Practitioner, 32*(6), 29–35.

Pavone, M. E., & Burke, A. (2007). Fertility control: contraception, sterilization, and abortion. In K. B. Fortner, et al. (Eds.). *The Johns Hopkins manual of gynecology and obstetrics* (3rd ed.). Philadelphia: Lippincott Williams & Wilkins.

Postlethwaite, D., et al. (2007). Intrauterine contraception: evaluation of clinician practice patterns in Kaiser Permanente Northern California. *Contraception, 75*(3), 177–184.

Rickert, V. I., et al. (2007). Depo Now: preventing unintended pregnancies among adolescents and young adults. *Journal of Adolescent Health, 40*(1), 22–28.

Rocca, C. H. (2007). Beyond access: acceptability, use and nonuse of emergency contraception among young women. *American Journal of Obstetrics and Gynecology, 196(*1), 29–36.

Roumen, F. J. (2007). The contraceptive vaginal ring compared with the combined oral contraceptive pill: a comprehensive review of randomized controlled trials. *Contraception, 75*(6), 420–429.

Schorge, J. O., et al. (2008). Contraception and sterilization. In J. O. Schorge, et al. (Eds.) *Williams gynecology.* Columbus, OH: McGraw-Hill.

Shacter, H., Gee, R. E., & Long, J. A. (2007). Variation in availability of emergency contraception in pharmacies. *Contraception, 75*(3), 214–217.

Stubblefield, P. G., Carr-Ellis, S., & Kapp, N. (2007). Family planning. In J. S. Berek (Ed.). *Berek & Novak's gynecology.* Philadelphia: Lippincott Williams & Wilkins.

Trego, L. L. (2007). Military women's menstrual experiences and interest in menstrual suppression during deployment. *JOGNN: Journal of Obstetric, Gynecologic, & Neonatal Nursing, 36(4)*, 342–347.

Van der Wijden, C., Brown, J., & Kleijnen, J. (2009). Lactational amenorrhea for family planning. *Cochrane Database of Systematic Reviews, 2009*(1), (CD001329).

Warehime, M. N., Bass, L., & Pedulla, D. (2007). Effects of tubal ligation among American women. *Journal of Reproductive Medicine, 52*(4), 263–272.

Wu, J., et al. (2007). Women seeking emergency contraceptive pills by using the Internet. *Obstetrics & Gynecology, 110*(1), 44–52.

SUGGESTED READINGS

Ahluwalia, I. B., Whitehead, N., & Bensyl, D. (2007). Pregnancy intention and contraceptive use among adult women. *Maternal & Child Health Journal, 11*(4), 347–351.

Cheng, L., et al. (2009). Interventions for emergency contraception. *Cochrane Database of Systematic Reviews, 2009*(1), (CD001324).

Cuffee, J. J., Hallfors, D. D., & Waller, M. W. (2007). Racial and gender differences in adolescent sexual attitudes and longitudinal associations with coital debut. *Journal of Adolescent Health, 41*(1), 19–26.

Edelman, A., et al. (2007). Acceptability of contraceptive-induced amenorrhea in a racially diverse group of US women. *Contraception, 75*(6), 450–453.

Frank-Herrmann, P., et al. (2007). The effectiveness of a fertility awareness based method to avoid pregnancy in relation to a couple's sexual behaviour during the fertile time: a prospective longitudinal study. *Human Reproduction, 22*(5), 1310–1319.

Frost, J. J., Singh, S., & Finer, L. B. (2007). Factors associated with contraceptive use and nonuse, United States. *Perspectives on Sexual & Reproductive Health, 39*(2), 90–99.

Halpern, V., et al. (2009). Strategies to improve adherence and acceptability of hormonal methods of contraception. *Cochrane Database of Systematic Reviews, 2009*(1), (CD004317).

Haynes, K. A. (2007). An update on emergency contraception use in adolescents. *Journal of Pediatric Nursing, 22*(3), 186–195.

Manlove, J., & Terry-Humen, E. (2007). Contraceptive use patterns within females' first sexual relationships: the role of relationships, partners, and methods. *Journal of Sex Research, 44*(1), 3–16.

Nelson, A. L. (2007). Communicating with patients about extended-cycle and continuous use of oral contraceptives. *Journal of Women's Health, 16*(4), 463–470.

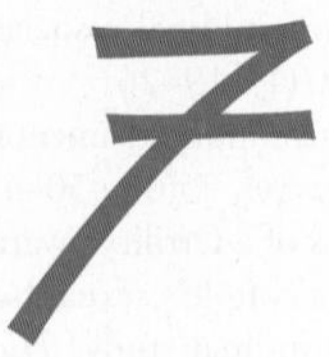

Chapter 7 The Nursing Role in Genetic Assessment and Counseling

KEY TERMS

- alleles
- chromosomes
- cytogenetics
- dermatoglyphics
- genes
- genetics
- genome
- genotype
- heterozygous
- homozygous
- karyotype
- meiosis
- nondisjunction
- phenotype

OBJECTIVES

After mastering the contents of this chapter, you should be able to:

1. Describe the nature of inheritance, patterns of recessive and dominant mendelian inheritance, and common chromosomal aberrations that cause physical or cognitive disorders.
2. Identify National Health Goals related to genetic disorders that nurses can help the nation achieve.
3. Use critical thinking to analyze ways that nurses can make genetic assessment or education more family centered.
4. Assess a family for their adjustment to the probability of inheriting a genetic disorder.
5. Formulate nursing diagnoses related to genetic disorders.
6. Establish expected outcomes that meet the needs of the family undergoing genetic assessment and counseling.
7. Plan nursing care related to a potential alteration in genetic health, such as assisting with an amniocentesis.
8. Implement nursing care such as counseling a family with a genetic disorder.
9. Evaluate expected outcomes for achievement and effectiveness of care.
10. Identify areas related to genetic assessment that could benefit from additional nursing research or application of evidence-based practice.
11. Integrate knowledge of genetic inheritance with nursing process to achieve quality maternal and child health nursing care.

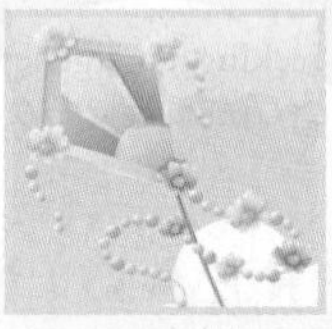

Amy Alvarez, 26 years old, is a woman you meet at a genetic counseling center. She was adopted as a newborn and never felt a need to locate her birth parents because her adoptive parents provided a "close to perfect" childhood for her. After college, she married the most eligible bachelor in her hometown. She is now pregnant with her first child. At 15 weeks into her pregnancy, after serum and ultrasound testing, she has been advised that her child may have translocation Down syndrome. She asks you, "How could this happen? There's no disease like that in either of our families."

Previous chapters described common family types and how they are affected by sociocultural and community influences. This chapter discusses the basic principles by which disorders can be inherited and information about the necessary assessments, care, and guidelines for counseling of families if it is discovered that there is a potential for a genetic disorder in the family. Such information can influence the health of a childbearing or childrearing family for generations to come.

How would you answer Amy?

As many as 1 in 20 newborns inherits a genetic disorder. As many as 70% of pediatric hospital admissions may be for genetic-influenced disorders (Pyeritz, 2009). The possibility that a child could have a genetic disorder crosses the minds of most pregnant women and their partners at some point in a pregnancy, whether or not there is any family history of such disorders. This causes pregnant couples to ask health care providers about their chances of having a child with a genetic disorder and about genetic testing. Due to the Human Genome Project and the determination of the location of specific genes in the human genome, the necessity to improve techniques of screening for genetic disorders has become a national priority (see National Health Goals, Box 7.1).

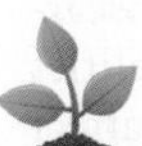

Nursing Process Overview

For Genetic Assessment and Counseling

Assessment

Assessment measures for genetic disorders include a detailed family history, preferably of three generations; physical examination of both the parents and any affected children; and an ever-growing series of laboratory assays of blood, amniotic fluid, and maternal and fetal cells. For example, women are offered routine screening of maternal serum levels of alpha-fetoprotein (MSAFP) early in pregnancy to evaluate for neural tube or chromosomal disorders in the fetus. Chorionic villi sampling (CVS) and amniocentesis are follow-up techniques that may be offered to women who are older than 35 years of age, or to those whose MSAFP level is abnormal, to further screen for genetic disorders. Couples who already know of the existence of a genetic disorder in their family or those who have had a previous child born with a congenital anomaly can have additional, more extensive testing. Nurses serve as members of genetic assessment and counseling teams to help obtain the initial family history, assist with physical examination, obtain blood serum for analysis, and assist with procedures such as amniocentesis in this process.

Certain genetic disorders are more commonly found in some ethnic groups than in others, because people often marry within their own racial or ethnic group. β-Thalassemia, for example, a blood dyscrasia, occurs most frequently in families of Greek or Italian heritage, whereas α-thalassemia occurs most often in persons from the Philippines or Southeast Asia. Sickle cell anemia occurs most often in African Americans. Tay-Sachs disease occurs most often in people of Jewish ancestry.

Identifying which families might be at risk for particular genetic disorders because of their ethnic heritage and being certain they are informed of the incidence of these disorders and that genetic screening is available is a nursing responsibility.

Nursing Diagnosis

Typical nursing diagnoses related to the area of genetic disorders include:

- Decisional conflict related to testing for an untreatable genetic disorder
- Fear related to outcome of genetic screening tests
- Situational low self-esteem related to identified chromosomal abnormality
- Deficient knowledge related to inheritance pattern of the family's inherited disorder
- Health-seeking behaviors related to potential for genetic transmission of disease
- Altered sexuality pattern related to fear of conceiving a child with a genetic disorder

Outcome Identification and Planning

Outcome identification and planning for families undergoing genetic assessment differ according to the types of assessments performed and the results obtained. This may include determining what information the couple needs to know before testing can proceed or helping couples arrange for further assessment measures. Be certain that goals are realistic and consistent with the individual's or couple's lifestyle (not all people want to be totally informed about family illnesses). Helpful websites to use for referral are the March of Dimes Birth Defects Foundation (http://www.marchofdimes.com), the American Association of Klinefelter Syndrome Information and Support (http://www.AAKSIS.org), the National Fragile X Foundation (http://www.NFXF.org), the National Down Syndrome Society (http://www.ndss.org), and the Turner Syndrome Society (http://www.Turner-syndrome-us.org).

Implementation

Parental reactions to the knowledge that their child has a possible genetic disorder or to the birth of a child with a genetically inherited disorder usually involves a grief reaction, similar to that experienced by parents whose child has died at birth (their "perfect" child is gone). Both parents

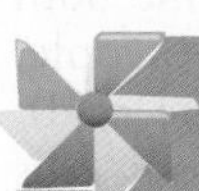

BOX 7.1 ✻ Focus on National Health Goals

A number of National Health Goals speak directly to genetic disease and screening:

- Ensure that all newborns are screened at birth for conditions mandated by their State-sponsored newborn screening programs.
- Ensure that follow-up testing for screened positives is performed.
- Increase the proportion of children with special health care needs who receive their care in family-centered, comprehensive, and coordinated systems from 35% to 100% (http://www.nih.gov).

Nurses can help the nation achieve these goals by being sensitive to the need for genetic screening and counseling in prenatal and birth settings. Questions such as when are people most responsive to genetic counseling or what effect on bonding occurs, if any, when the parents learn about an abnormal alpha-fetoprotein level during pregnancy, are unanswered so would be good topics for nursing research.

may pass through stages of shock and denial ("This cannot be true"), anger ("It's not fair that this happened to us"), and bargaining ("If only this would go away") before they reach reorganization and acceptance ("It has happened to us and it is all right"). For some couples, a genetic disorder is diagnosed during the pregnancy; for others, it may not be discovered until birth, or possibly not even until the child is of school age. For these parents, the reaction will occur at that later point of diagnosis.

As a rule, when parents are under stress, it is most helpful to guide them to concentrate on short-term goals and actions. Help them look first at the immediate needs of their family, the fetus, or the newborn, and later on at what type of continued follow-up will be necessary. For instance, after the birth, will the baby need to be hospitalized for immediate surgical correction of accompanying congenital anomalies, or will the parents be able to take the baby home? These decisions must be made immediately. What kind of special schooling the child will need is a decision that can wait until later.

It is helpful to identify support people who can be helpful to the parents during their time of disorganization. These people may be usual family resources, such as grandparents or other family members. In some families, these people are as disturbed by the diagnosis as the parents and therefore cannot offer their usual support. That makes secondary support sources such as the March of Dimes Foundation necessary.

Not all parents are ready to talk to members of such organizations at the time of diagnosis, however. To contact such an organization may make the diagnosis seem "real" for the first time or move them out of denial before they are ready. Help also to identify health care personnel with whom the parents will need to maintain contact during the next few months such as a surgeon or an orthopedist. Ensuring that the parents have health care providers they know they can turn to, especially when they are moving out of denial, helps them move forward to their next step in accepting their child's diagnosis.

Outcome Evaluation

Examples of expected outcomes for a family with a known genetic disorder might be:

- Couple states they feel capable of coping no matter what the outcome of genetic testing.
- Client accurately states the chances of a genetic disorder occurring in her next child.
- Couple states they have resolved their feelings of low self-esteem related to birth of a child with a genetic disorder.

A couple's decisions about genetic testing and childbearing can change over time. For example, a decision made at age 25 not to have children because of a potential genetic disorder may be difficult to maintain at age 30, as the couple sees many of their friends with growing families. Be certain that such couples have the telephone number of a genetic counselor. Urge them to call periodically for news of recent advances in genetic screening techniques or disease treatments so they can remain current and well informed for future planning.

GENETIC DISORDERS

Inherited or genetic disorders are disorders that can be passed from one generation to the next. They result from some disorder in gene or chromosome structure and occur in 5% to 6% of newborns. **Genetics** is the study of the way such disorders occur. **Cytogenetics** is the study of chromosomes by light microscopy and the method by which chromosomal aberrations are identified.

Genetic disorders may occur at the moment an ovum and sperm fuse or even earlier, in the meiotic division phase of the gametes (ovum and sperm). Some genetic abnormalities are so severe that normal fetal growth cannot continue past that point. This early cell division is so precarious a process, in fact, that up to 50% of first-trimester spontaneous miscarriages may be the result of chromosomal abnormalities (Schorge et al., 2008). Other genetic disorders do not affect life in utero, so the result of the disorder becomes apparent only at the time of fetal testing or after birth. Women having in vitro fertilization (IVF) can have both the egg and sperm examined for genetic disorders of single gene or chromosome concerns before implantation (Van Voorhis, 2007). In the near future, it may be possible not only to identify aberrant genes for disorders this way but also to insert healthy genes in their place using stem cell implantation. Gene replacement therapy this way is encouraging in the treatment of blood, spinal cord, and immunodeficiency syndromes (Cardone, 2007). Women can arrange to have a newborn's cord blood frozen and banked to be available for bone marrow or other cell transplantation procedures in the future (Scott, 2007). As stem cells for replacement therapy can be obtained from menstrual blood, this also may be a future contribution source (Goldman, 2007).

Nature of Inheritance

Genes are the basic units of heredity that determine both the physical and cognitive characteristics of people. Composed of segments of DNA (deoxyribonucleic acid), they are woven into strands in the nucleus of all body cells to form **chromosomes.**

In humans, each cell, with the exception of the sperm and ovum, contains 46 chromosomes (22 pair of autosomes and 1 pair of sex chromosomes). Spermatozoa and ova each carry only half of the chromosome number, or 23 chromosomes. For each chromosome in the sperm cell, there is a like chromosome of similar size and shape and function (autosome, or homologous chromosome) in the ovum. Because genes are always located at fixed positions on chromosomes, two like genes **(alleles)** for every trait are represented in the ovum and sperm on autosomes. The one chromosome in which this does not occur is the chromosome for determining gender. If the sex chromosomes are both type X (large symmetric) in the zygote formed from the union of a sperm and ovum, the individual is female (Fig. 7.1A). If one sex chromosome is an X and one a Y (a smaller type), the individual is a male (Fig. 7.1B).

A person's **phenotype** refers to his or her outward appearance or the expression of genes. A person's **genotype** refers to his or her actual gene composition. It is impossible to predict a person's genotype from the phenotype, or outward appearance.

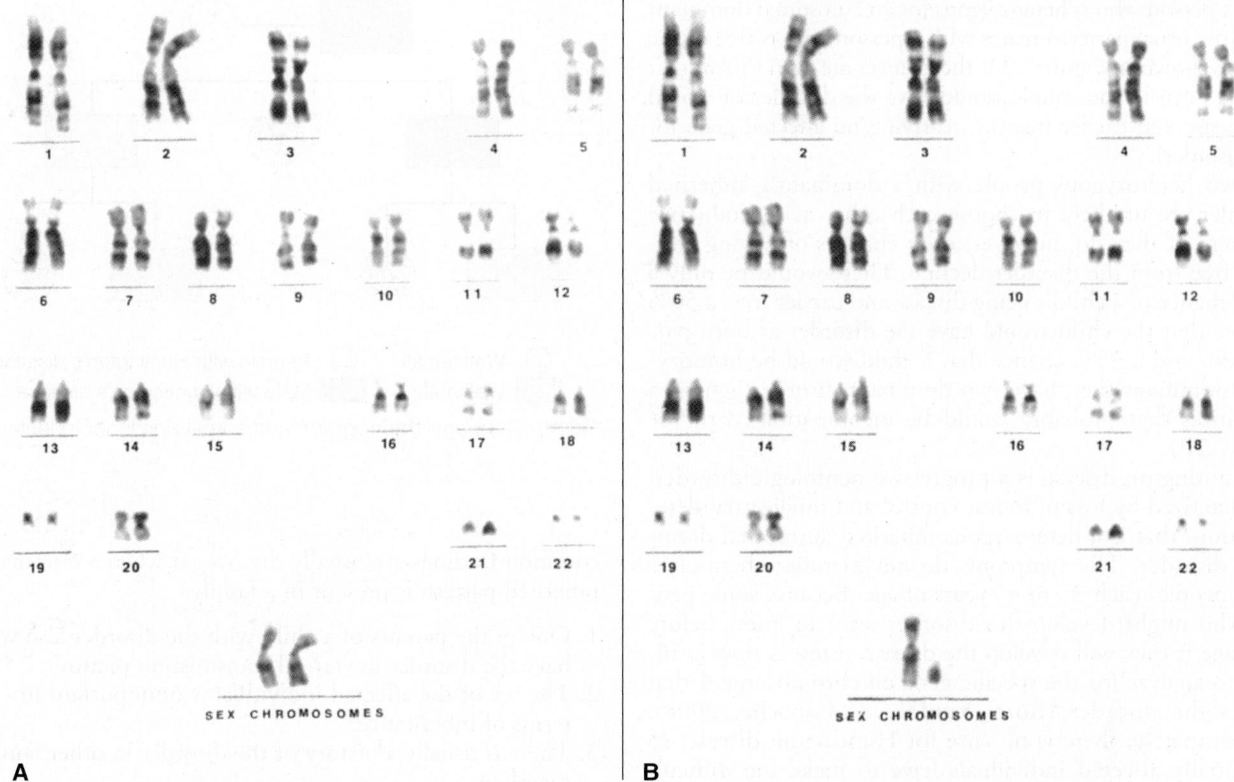

FIGURE 7.1 Photomicrographs of human chromosomes (karyotypes). (**A**) Normal female karyotype. (**B**) Normal male karyotype.

A person's **genome** is the complete set of genes present (about 50,000 to 100,000). A normal genome is abbreviated as 46XX or 46XY (designation of the total number of chromosomes plus a graphic description of the sex chromosomes present). If a chromosomal aberration exists, it is listed after the sex chromosome pattern. In such abbreviations, the letter *p* stands for short arm defects and *q* stands for defects on the long arm of the chromosome. The abbreviation 46XX5p−, for example, is the abbreviation for a female with 46 total chromosomes but with the short arm of chromosome 5 missing (cri-du-chat syndrome). In Down syndrome, the person has an extra chromosome 21, which is abbreviated as 47XX21+ or 47XY21+.

Mendelian Inheritance: Dominant and Recessive Patterns

The principles of genetic inheritance of disease are the same as those that govern genetic inheritance of other physical characteristics, such as eye or hair color. These principles were discovered and described by Gregor Mendel, an Austrian naturalist, in the 1800s and are known as mendelian laws.

A person who has two like genes for a trait—two healthy genes, for example (one from the mother and one from the father)—on two like chromosomes is said to be **homozygous** for that trait. If the genes differ (a healthy gene from the mother and an unhealthy gene from the father, or vice versa), the person is said to be **heterozygous** for that trait. Many genes are dominant in their action over others. When paired with nondominant (recessive) genes, dominant genes are always expressed in preference to the recessive genes. An individual with two homozygous genes for a dominant trait is said to be homozygous dominant; an individual with two genes for a recessive trait is homozygous recessive.

✔ Checkpoint Question 7.1

Amy Alvarez is pregnant with her first child. Her phenotype refers to:

a. Her concept of herself as male or female
b. Whether she has 46 chromosomes
c. Her actual genetic composition
d. Her outward appearance

Inheritance of Disease

Since the entire human genome has been mapped, an increasing number of types of disease inheritance have been identified. (Manipalviratn, Trivax, & Huang, 2007).

Autosomal Dominant Disorders

Although more than 3000 autosomal dominant disorders are known, only a few are commonly seen because the majority of these are not compatible with life after birth. Most of those that do occur cause structural defects. With an autosomal dominant condition, either a person has two unhealthy genes (is homozygous dominant) or is heterozygous, with the gene causing the disease stronger than the corresponding healthy recessive gene for the same trait.

If a person who is heterozygous for an autosomal dominant trait (the usual pattern) mates with a person who is free of the trait, as shown in Figure 7.2A, the chances are even (50%) that a child born to the couple would have the disorder or would be disease and carrier free (i.e., carrying no affected gene for the disorder).

Two heterozygous people with a dominantly inherited disorder are unlikely to choose each other as reproductive partners. If they do, however, their chances of having children free from the disorder decline. There would be only a 25% chance of a child's being disease and carrier free, a 50% chance that the child would have the disorder as both parents do, and a 25% chance that a child would be homozygous dominant (i.e., have two dominant disorder genes), a condition that probably would be incompatible with life (Fig. 7.2B).

Huntington disease is a progressive neurologic disorder, characterized by loss of motor control and intellectual deterioration, that is a heterozygous inherited autosomal dominant disorder. The symptoms do not manifest themselves until people reach 35 to 45 years of age. Because some people who might develop this disorder want to know before that age if they will develop the disease, a test is now available to analyze for the specific gene on chromosome 4 that causes the disorder (Roze, Saudou, & Caboche, 2008). Unfortunately, there is no cure for Huntington disease, so potentially affected individuals have to make the difficult choice to decide to have the analysis or not, as there is nothing but palliative care for this ultimately fatal disorder (Manipalviratn, Trivax, & Huang, 2007).

Other examples of autosomal dominantly inherited disorders include facioscapulohumeral muscular dystrophy (a disorder that results in muscle weakness), a form of osteogenesis imperfecta (a disorder in which bones are exceedingly brittle), Marfan syndrome (a disorder of connective tissue that results in an individual being thinner and taller than usual and perhaps with associated heart disorders (Stuart & Williams, 2007), and breast and breast/ovarian cancer syndrome that accounts for 5% to 10% of breast cancer in women (Weitzel et al., 2007).

In assessing family genograms (maps of family relationships) for the incidence of inherited disorders, a number of common findings are usually discovered when a dominantly inherited pattern is present in a family:

1. One of the parents of a child with the disorder also will have the disorder (a vertical transmission picture).
2. The sex of the affected individual is unimportant in terms of inheritance.
3. There is usually a history of the disorder in other family members.

Figure 7.3 shows a typical genogram of a family with an autosomal dominantly inherited disorder.

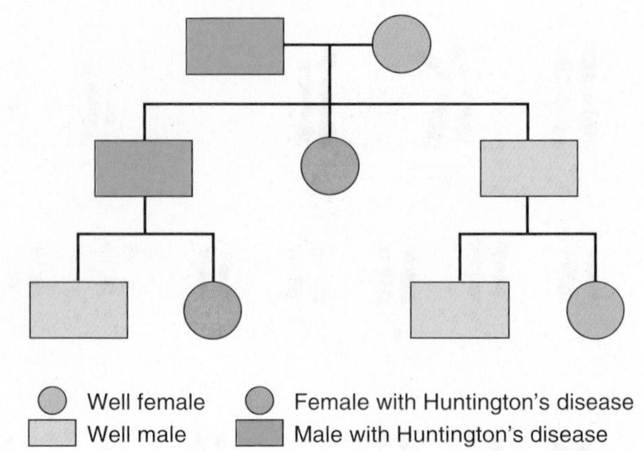

FIGURE 7.3 Family genogram: autosomal dominant inheritance.

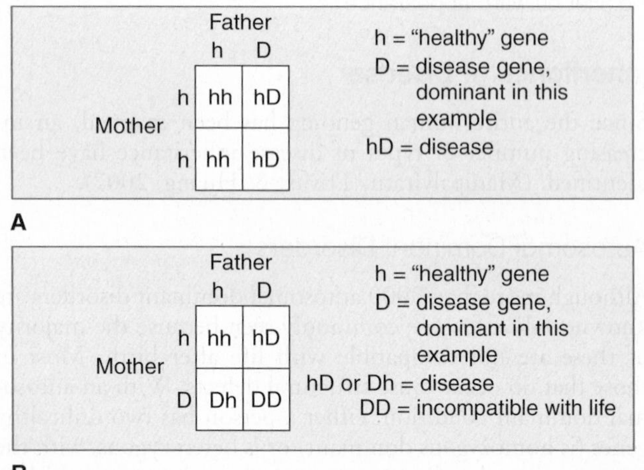

FIGURE 7.2 Autosomal dominant inheritance.

Autosomal Recessive Inheritance

More than 1500 autosomal recessive disorders have been identified. In contrast to structural disorders, these tend to be biochemical or enzymatic. Such diseases do not occur unless two genes for the disease are present (i.e., a homozygous recessive pattern). Examples include cystic fibrosis, adrenogenital syndrome, albinism, Tay-Sachs disease, galactosemia, phenylketonuria, limb-girdle muscular dystrophy, and Rh-factor incompatibility.

An example of autosomal recessive inheritance is shown in Figure 7.4A. Both parents are disease free of cystic fibrosis, but both are heterozygous in genotype, so they carry a recessive gene for cystic fibrosis. When this genetic pattern occurs, there is a 25% chance that a child born to a couple will be disease and carrier free (homozygous dominant for the healthy gene); a 50% chance that the child will be, like the parents, free of disease but carrying the unexpressed disease gene (heterozygous); and a 25% chance that the child will have the disease (homozygous recessive).

Suppose a woman with the heterozygous genotype shown in Figure 7.4A mates with a man who has no trait for cystic fibrosis. There is a 50% chance that a child born to them will be completely disorder and carrier free, like the father. Likewise, there is a 50% chance that their child will be heterozygous (i.e., a carrier), like the mother (see Fig. 7.4B). There is no chance in this instance that any of their children will have the disorder. However, they should be counseled that if a child of theirs who carries the trait has children with a sexual partner who also has a recessive gene for the trait, grandchildren could manifest the disease. Cystic fibrosis is caused by an errant gene on the seventh chromosome. As

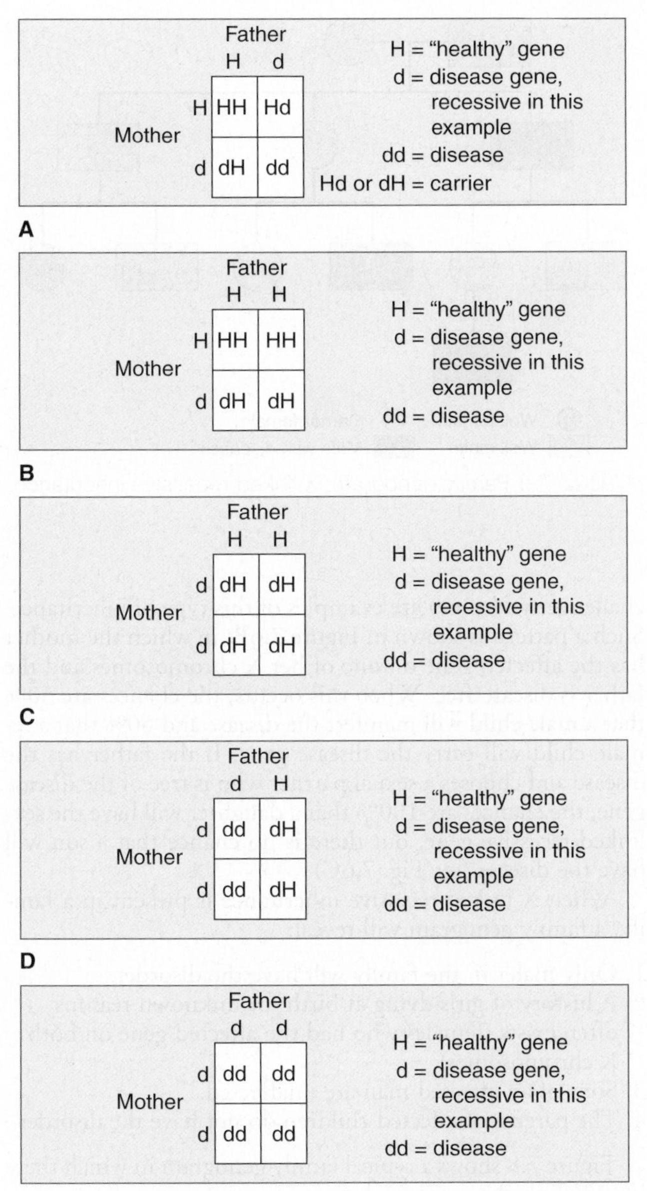

FIGURE 7.4 Autosomal recessive inheritance.

many as 1 in every 29 Caucasian people carries the trait. People who are concerned as to whether they have a recessive gene for the disorder can have a DNA analysis to reveal their status (Gardner, 2007).

Twenty years ago, most children with cystic fibrosis died in early childhood and therefore never reached childbearing age. Today, with good management, such children can live to adulthood and have children of their own. If a person with cystic fibrosis (homozygous recessive) should choose a sexual partner without the trait, none of their children would have the disorder, but all would be carriers of a recessive gene for the disorder (see Fig. 7.4C).

If a person with cystic fibrosis mated with a person with an unexpressed gene for the disease, there would be a 50% chance that a child would have the disorder (homozygous) and a 50% chance that he or she would be heterozygous for the disorder (see Fig. 7.4D). If a person with the disorder mated with a person who also had the disorder, as shown in Figure 7.4E, there is a 100% chance that their child would have the disorder.

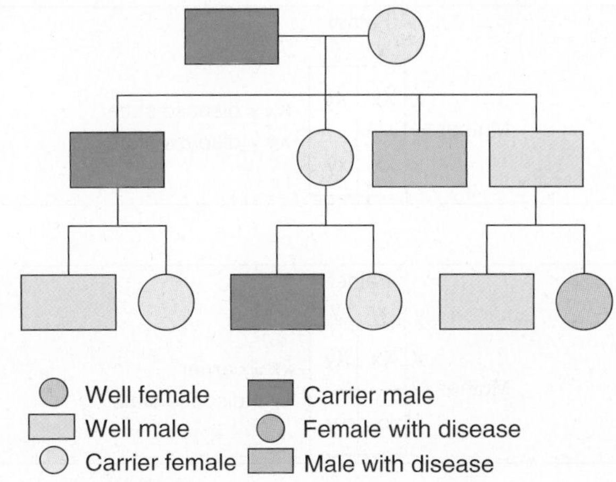

FIGURE 7.5 Family genogram: autosomal recessive inheritance.

When family genograms are assessed for the incidence of inherited disease, situations commonly discovered when a recessively inherited disease is present in the family include:

1. Both parents of a child with the disorder are clinically free of the disorder.
2. The sex of the affected individual is unimportant in terms of inheritance.
3. The family history for the disorder is negative—that is, no one can identify anyone else who had it (a horizontal transmission pattern).
4. A known common ancestor between the parents sometimes exists. This explains how both male and female came to possess a like gene for the disorder.

Figure 7.5 shows a typical genogram of a family with an autosomal recessive inherited disorder.

X-Linked Dominant Inheritance

Some genes for disorders are located on, and therefore transmitted only by, the female sex chromosome (the X chromosome). There are about 300 known disorders associated this way and their transmission is termed X-linked inheritance. If the affected gene is dominant, only one X chromosome with the trait need be present for symptoms of the disorder to be manifested (Fig. 7.6A). Family characteristics seen with this type of inheritance usually include:

1. All individuals with the gene are affected (the gene is dominant).
2. All female children of affected men are affected; all male children of affected men are unaffected.
3. It appears in every generation.
4. All children of homozygous affected women are affected. Fifty percent of the children of heterozygous affected women are affected (Fig. 7.7).

An example of a disease in this group is Alport's syndrome, a progressive kidney failure disorder.

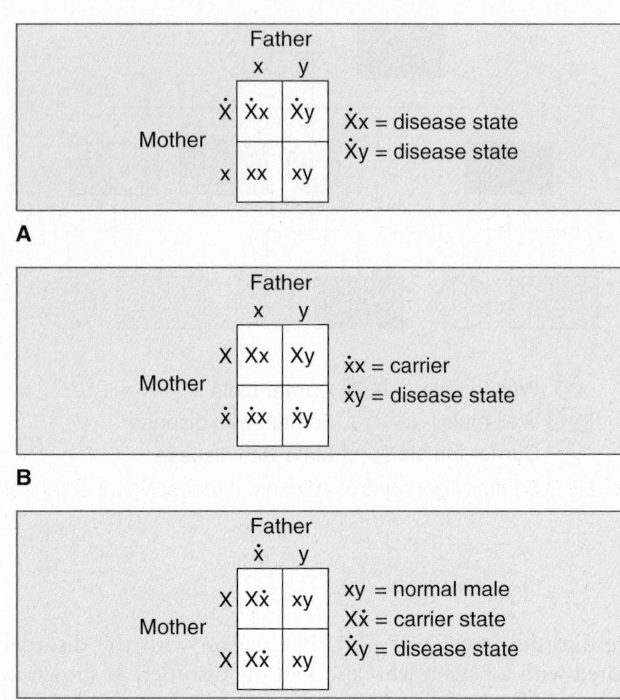

FIGURE 7.6 Sex-linked inheritance: (**A**) sex-linked dominant; (**B, C**) sex-linked recessive.

X-Linked Recessive Inheritance

The majority of X-linked inherited disorders are not dominant, but recessive. When the inheritance of a recessive gene comes from both parents (homozygous recessive) it appears to be incompatible with life. Therefore, females who inherit the affected gene will be heterozygous, and, because a normal gene is also present, the expression of the disease will be blocked. On the other hand, because males have only one X chromosome, the disease will be manifested in any male children who receive the affected gene from their mother.

Hemophilia A and Christmas disease (blood-factor deficiencies), color blindness, Duchenne (pseudohypertrophic) muscular dystrophy, and fragile X syndrome (a cognitive challenge syndrome) are examples of this type of inheritance. Such a pattern is shown in Figure 7.6B, in which the mother has the affected gene on one of her X chromosomes and the father is disease-free. When this occurs, the chances are 50% that a male child will manifest the disease and 50% that a female child will carry the disease gene. If the father has the disease and chooses a sexual partner who is free of the disease gene, the chances are 100% that a daughter will have the sex-linked recessive gene, but there is no chance that a son will have the disease (see Fig. 7.6C).

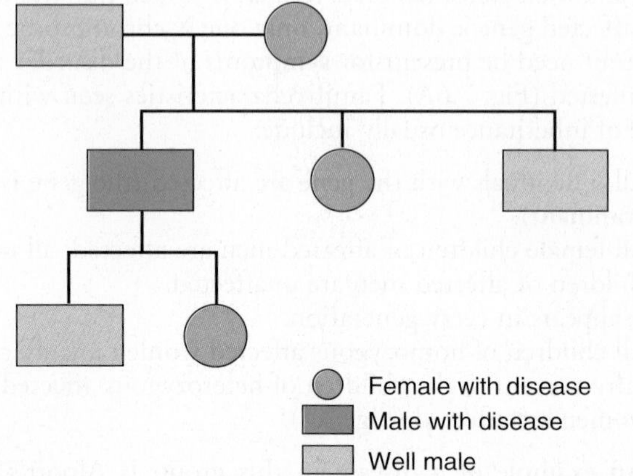

FIGURE 7.7 Family genogram: X-linked dominant inheritance.

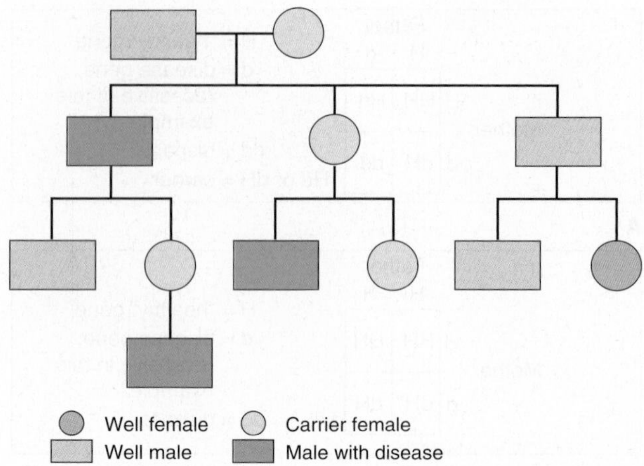

FIGURE 7.8 Family genogram: X-linked recessive inheritance.

When X-linked recessive inheritance is present in a family, a family genogram will reveal:

1. Only males in the family will have the disorder.
2. A history of girls dying at birth for unknown reasons often exists (females who had the affected gene on both X chromosomes).
3. Sons of an affected man are unaffected.
4. The parents of affected children do not have the disorder.

Figure 7.8 shows a typical family genogram in which there is an X-linked recessive inheritance pattern.

Y-Linked Inheritance. Although genes responsible for features such as height and tooth size are found on the Y chromosome, tall stature and perhaps aggressive personality are the only consistent phenotypic features associated with having an extra Y chromosome (karyotype 47XYY) (Pyeritz, 2009).

What if... Amy Alvarez had a recessive X-linked chromosome for a disorder such as, hemophilia, and said that she wanted to have all boys because they would not show symptoms? Would she be well informed?

Multifactorial (Polygenic) Inheritance

Many childhood disorders such as heart disease, diabetes, pyloric stenosis, cleft lip and palate, neural tube disorders, hypertension, and mental illness tend to have a higher-than-usual incidence in some families. They appear to occur from multiple gene combinations possibly combined with environmental factors. Diabetes has been extensively studied in this regard. Certain human lymphocyte antigens (HLAs) inherited from both parents appear to play a role in genetic susceptibility to diabetes mellitus. Children who will develop diabetes mellitus can be shown to have an increased frequency of HLA B8, B15, DR3, and DR4 on chromosome 6. They lack DR2, an HLA that appears to be protective against diabetes mellitus.

Diseases caused by multiple factors this way do not follow Mendelian laws because more than a single gene or HLA is involved. It may be more difficult for parents to understand why these disorders occur because their incidence is so unpredictable. A family history, for instance, may reveal no set pattern. Some of these conditions have a predisposition to occur more frequently in one sex (cleft palate occurs more often in girls than boys), but they can occur in either sex.

Mitochondrial Inheritance. Mitochondria are cell organelles that are found outside the cell nucleus. They are inherited solely from the cytoplasm of the ovum. Male carriers cannot pass a disorder carried in the mitochondria to any of their children. Females, on the other hand, will pass mitochondrial disorders to 100% of their children. A number of rare myopathies (muscle diseases) are inherited in this way (Manipalviratn, Trivax, & Huang, 2007).

Imprinting

Imprinting refers to the differential expression of genetic material and allows researchers to identify whether the chromosomal material has come from the male or female parent. In some instances, such as hydatidiform mole, an embryonic disorder (see Chapter 21), it can be shown that two separate sperm fertilized an ovum (Dorigo, Martinez-Maza, & Berek, 2007). In Prader-Willi syndrome, a chromosome 15 abnormality in which children are severely obese and cognitively challenged, no paternal contribution is present at certain gene points (Benarroch et al., 2007).

Chromosomal Abnormalities (Cytogenic Disorders)

In some instances of genetic disease, the abnormality occurs not because of dominant or recessive gene patterns but through a fault in the number or structure of chromosomes which results in missing or distorted genes. When chromosomes are photographed and displayed, the resulting arrangement is termed a **karyotype.** The number of chromosomes and specific parts of chromosomes can be identified by karyotyping or by a process termed fluorescent in situ hybridization (FISH).

Nondisjunction Abnormalities

Meiosis is the type of cell division in which the number of chromosomes in the cell is reduced to the haploid (half) number for reproduction (i.e., 23 rather than 46 chromosomes). All sperm and ova undergo a meiosis cell division early in formation. During this division, half of the chromosomes are attracted to one pole of the cell and half to the other pole. The cell then divides cleanly, with 23 chromosomes in the first new cell and 23 chromosomes in the second new cell. Chromosomal abnormalities occur if the division is uneven **(nondisjunction).** The result may be that one new sperm cell or ovum has 24 chromosomes and the other has only 22 (Fig. 7.9). If a spermatozoon or ovum

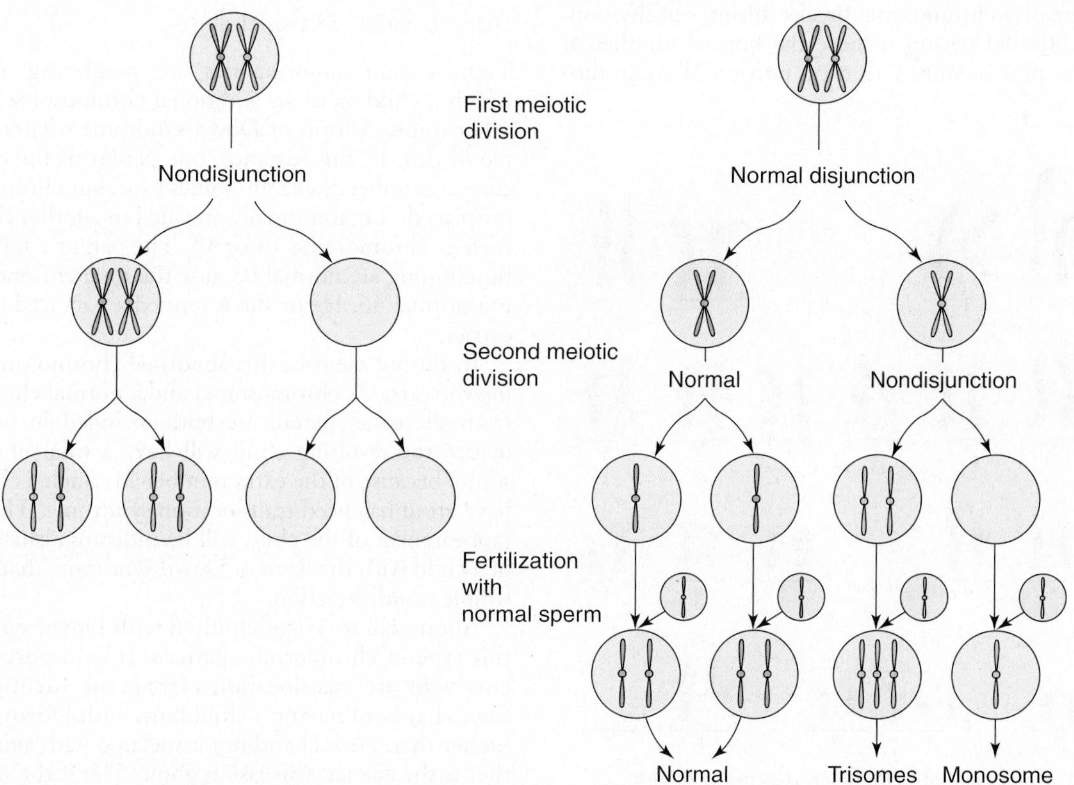

FIGURE 7.9 Process of nondisjunction at the first and second meiotic divisions of the ovum and fertilization with normal sperm.

with 24 or 22 chromosomes fuses with a normal spermatozoon or ovum, the zygote (sperm and ovum combined) will have either 47 or 45 chromosomes, not the normal 46. The presence of 45 chromosomes does not appear to be compatible with life, and the embryo or fetus probably will be aborted. Down syndrome (trisomy 21) (47XX21+ or 47XY21+) is an example of a disease in which the individual has 47 chromosomes. There are three rather than two copies of chromosome 21 (Fig. 7.10).

The incidence of Down syndrome increases with advanced maternal age and is highest if the mother is older than 35 years and the father is older than 55. Thus, aging seems to present an obstacle to clean cell division. The incidence is 1:100 in women older than 40 years, compared with 1:1500 in women younger than 20 years (Dorigo, Martinez-Maza, & Berek, 2007). Other examples of cell nondisjunction include trisomy 13 (Fig. 7.11) and trisomy 18 (cognitively challenged syndromes).

If nondisjunction occurs in the sex chromosomes, other types of abnormalities occur. Turner and Klinefelter syndromes are the most common types. In Turner syndrome (45XO), marked by webbed neck, short stature, sterility, and possibly cognitive challenge, the individual, although female, has only one X chromosome (or has two X chromosomes but one is defective). Her appearance (phenotype) is female because of the one X chromosome. In Klinefelter's syndrome (marked by sterility and possibly cognitive challenge), the individual has male genitals but the sex chromosomal pattern is 47XXY or an extra X chromosome is present.

Deletion Abnormalities

Deletion abnormalities are a form of chromosome disorder in which part of a chromosome breaks during cell division, causing the affected person to have the normal number of chromosomes plus or minus an extra portion of a chromosome, such as 45.75 chromosomes or 47.5. For example, in cri-du-chat syndrome (46XY5q−), one portion of chromosome 5 is missing.

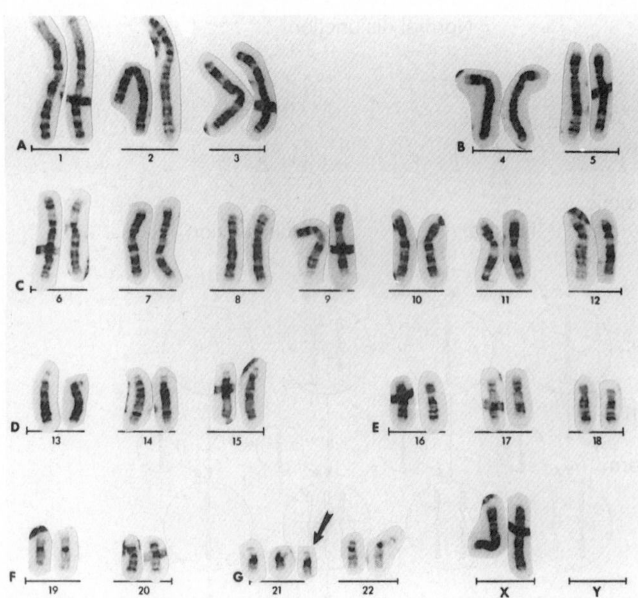

FIGURE 7.10 Karyotype of trisomy 21. (Courtesy of Dr. Kathleen Rao, Department of Pediatrics, University of North Carolina, Chapel Hill, North Carolina.)

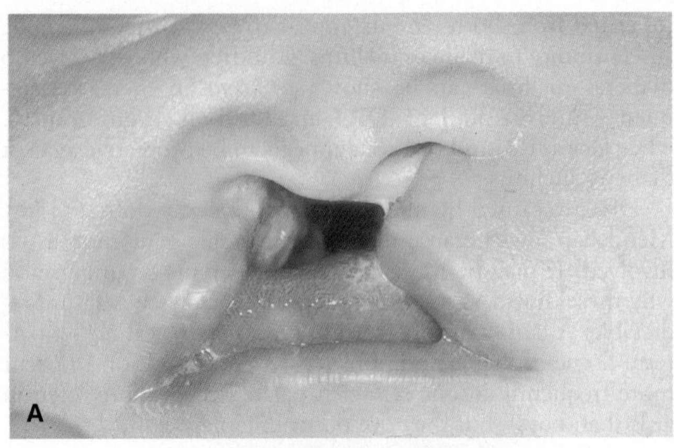

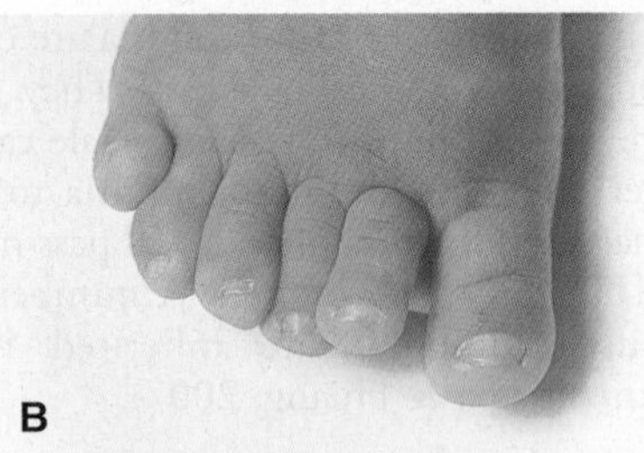

FIGURE 7.11 An infant with trisomy 13 has (**A**) a cleft palate and (**B**) supernumerary digits (polydactyly). (© NMSB/Custom Medical Stock Photograph.)

Translocation Abnormalities

Translocation abnormalities are perplexing situations in which a child gains an additional chromosome through another route. A form of Down syndrome occurs as an example of this. In this instance, one parent of the child has the correct number of chromosomes (46), but chromosome 21 is misplaced; it is abnormally attached to another chromosome, such as chromosome 14 or 15. The parent's appearance and functioning are normal because the total chromosome count is a normal 46. He or she is termed a balanced translocation carrier.

If, during meiosis, this abnormal chromosome 14 (carrying the extra 21 chromosome) and a normal chromosome 21 from the other parent are both included in one sperm or ovum, the resulting child will have a total of 47 chromosomes because of the extra number 21. Such a child is said to have an unbalanced translocation syndrome. The phenotype (appearance) of the child will be indistinguishable from that of a child with the form of Down syndrome that occurs from simple nondisjunction.

About 2% to 5% of children with Down syndrome have this type of chromosome pattern. It is important that parents who are translocation carriers are identified because their chance of having a child born with Down syndrome is higher than normal and not associated with aging. If the father is the carrier, this risk is about 5%; if the mother is the carrier, the risk is about 15%. As many as 15% of couples who have frequent early spontaneous miscarriages may have this type of chromosomal aberration (Manipalviratn, Trivax, & Huang, 2007).

Mosaicism

Usually, a nondisjunction abnormality occurs during the meiosis stage of cell division, when sperm and ova halve their number of chromosomes. Mosaicism is an abnormal condition that is present when the nondisjunction disorder occurs after fertilization of the ovum, as the structure begins mitotic (daughter-cell) division. If this occurs, different cells in the body will have different chromosome counts. The extent of the disorder depends on the proportion of tissue with normal chromosome structure to tissue with abnormal chromosome constitution. Children with Down syndrome who have near-normal intelligence may have this type of pattern. The occurrence of such a phenomenon at this stage of development suggests that a teratogenic (harmful to the fetus) condition, such as x-ray or drug exposure, existed at that point to disturb normal cell division. This genetic pattern in a female with Down syndrome caused by mosaicism would be abbreviated as 46XX/47XX21+ to show that some cells contain 46 and some 47 chromosomes.

Isochromosomes

If a chromosome accidentally divides not by a vertical separation but by a horizontal one, a new chromosome with mismatched long and short arms can result. This is an isochromosome. It has much the same effect as a translocation abnormality when an entire extra chromosome exists. Some instances of Turner syndrome (45XO) may occur because of isochromosome formation.

✔ Checkpoint Question 7.2

Amy Alvarez is a balanced translocation carrier for Down syndrome. This means that:

a. All of her children will be born with some aspect of Down syndrome.
b. All of her female but none of her male children will have Down syndrome.
c. She has a greater than average chance a child will have Down syndrome.
d. It is impossible for any of her children to be born with Down syndrome.

GENETIC COUNSELING

Any individual concerned about the possibility of transmitting a disease to his or her children should have access to genetic counseling for advice on the inheritance of disease. Such counseling can serve to:

- Provide concrete, accurate information about the process of inheritance and inherited disorders
- Reassure people who are concerned that their child may inherit a particular disorder that the disorder will not occur
- Allow people who are affected by inherited disorders to make informed choices about future reproduction
- Offer support to people who are affected by genetic disorders

Genetic counseling can result in making individuals feel "well" or free of guilt for the first time in their lives if they discover that the disorder they were worried about was not an inherited one but was rather a chance occurrence.

In other instances, counseling results in informing individuals that they are carriers of a trait that is responsible for a child's condition. Even when people understand that they have no control over this, knowledge about passing a genetic disorder to a child can cause guilt and self-blame. Marriages and relationships can end unless both partners receive adequate support.

It is essential that information revealed in genetic screening be kept confidential, because such information could be used to damage a person's reputation or harm a future career or relationship. This necessity to maintain confidentiality prevents health care providers from alerting other family members about the inherited characteristic unless the member requesting genetic assessment has given consent for the information to be revealed. In some instances, a genetic history reveals information, such as that a child has been adopted or is the result of artificial insemination, or that a current husband is not the child's father information that a family doesn't want revealed. The member of the family seeking counseling has the right to decide whether this information may be shared with other family members.

The ideal time for counseling is before a first pregnancy. Some couples take this step even before committing themselves to marriage so they can offer not to involve their partner in a marriage if children of the marriage would be subject to a serious inherited disorder. Other couples first become aware of the need for genetic counseling after the birth of a first child with a disorder. It is best if they receive counseling before a second pregnancy. A couple may not be ready for this, however, until the initial shock of their first child's condition and the grief reaction that may accompany it have run their course. Only then are they ready for information and decision making (Box 7.2).

Even if a couple decides not to have any more children, it is important that they know that genetic counseling is available should their decision change. Also be certain that they are aware that as their children reach reproductive age, they, too, may benefit from genetic counseling. Couples who are most apt to benefit from a referral for genetic testing or counseling include:

- *A couple who has a child with a congenital disorder or an inborn error of metabolism.* Many congenital disorders occur because of teratogenic invasion during pregnancy that has gone unrecognized. Learning that the abnormality occurred by chance rather than inheritance is important, because the couple will not have to spend the remainder of their childbearing years in fear that another child may be born with the disorder (although a chance circumstance could occur again). If a definite teratogenic agent, such as a drug a woman took during pregnancy, can be identified, the couple can be advised about preventing this occurrence in a future pregnancy.
- *A couple whose close relatives have a child with a genetic disorder such as a translocation disorder or an inborn error of metabolism.* It is difficult to predict the expected occurrence of many "familial" or multifactorial disorders. In these instances, counseling should be aimed at educating the couple about the disorder, treatment available, and the

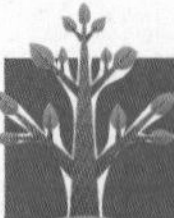

BOX 7.2 ✻ Focus on Family Teaching

Genetic Screening

Q. Amy Alvarez is anxious to have her fetus' health confirmed. She asks you, "Why do I have to wait so late in pregnancy for genetic studies by amniocentesis?"

A. Genetic analysis is done on skin cells obtained from amniotic fluid. The test cannot be scheduled until enough amniotic fluid is present for analysis. Fortunately, this analysis now can be done as early as the 12th week of pregnancy.

Q. Why do laboratories take so long to return karyotyping results?

A. Karyotyping has traditionally (and by necessity) been done on cells at the metaphase (center phase) of division, so the laboratory had to delay testing until the cells had grown to reach this phase. New techniques now allow analysis to be done immediately so that results are available much sooner.

Q. If there are no inherited diseases in a couple's family, should the couple have a karyotype done "just to be sure" before they have their first baby?

A. A genetic analysis is not routinely recommended unless there is evidence or suspicion of genetic disease in the family. Remember that karyotyping reveals only diseases that are present on chromosomes. A "perfect" karyotype does not guarantee that a newborn will not be ill in a noninherited way.

Q. If chorionic villi are part of the placenta, how does testing them reveal the chromosome picture of the fetus?

A. Because the fetus and all accessory structures arise from the same single ovum and sperm, the placenta contains the same cells as the fetus.

prognosis or outcome of the disorder. Based on this information, the couple can make an informed reproductive choice about children.

- *Any individual who is a known balanced translocation carrier.* Understanding of his or her own chromosome structure and the process by which future children could be affected can help such an individual make an informed choice about reproduction or can alert him or her to the importance of fetal karyotyping during any future pregnancy (sees Focus on Nursing Care Planning Box 7.3).
- *Any individual who has an inborn error of metabolism or chromosomal disorder.* Any person with a disease should know the inheritance pattern of the disease and, like those who are balanced translocation carriers, should be aware if prenatal diagnosis is possible for his or her particular disorder.
- *A consanguineous (closely related) couple.* The more closely related are two people, the more genes they have in common, so the more likely it is that a recessively inherited disease will be expressed. A brother and sister, for example, have about 50% of their genes in common; first cousins have about 12% of their genes in common.
- *Any woman older than 35 years and any man older than 55 years.* This is directly related to the association between advanced parental age and the occurrence of Down syndrome.
- *Couples of ethnic backgrounds in which specific illnesses are known to occur.* Mediterranean people, for example, have a high incidence of thalassemia, a blood disorder; those with a Chinese ancestry have a high incidence of glucose-6-phosphate dehydrogenase (G6PD) deficiency, a blood disorder where destruction of red cells can occur (Cappellini & Fiorelli, 2008).

Nursing Responsibilities

Nurses play important roles in assessing for signs and symptoms of genetic disorders, in offering support to individuals who seek genetic counseling, and in helping with reproductive genetic testing procedures by such actions as:

- Explaining to a couple what procedures they can expect to undergo
- Explaining how different genetic screening tests are done and when they are usually offered
- Supporting a couple during the wait for test results
- Assisting couples in values clarification, planning, and decision making based on test results

A great deal of time may need to be spent offering support for a grieving couple confronted with the reality of how tragically the laws of inheritance have affected their lives. Genetic counseling is a role for nurses, however, only if they are adequately prepared in the study of genetics because without this background, genetic counseling can be dangerous and destructive (Box 7.4).

Whether one is acting as a nursing member of a genetic counseling team or as a genetic counselor, some common principles apply. First, the individual or couple being counseled needs a clear understanding of the information provided. People may listen to the statistics of their situation ("Your child has a 25% chance of having this disease") and construe a "25% chance" to mean that if they have one child with the disease, they can then have three other children without any worry. A 25% chance, however, means that with each pregnancy there is a 25% chance that the child will have the disease (chance has no "memory" of what has already happened). It is as if the couple had four cards, all aces, with the ace of spades representing the disease. When a card is drawn from the set of four, the chance of it being the ace of spades is 1 in 4 (25%). When the couple is ready to have a second child, it is as if the card drawn during the first round is returned to the set, so the chance of drawing the ace of spades in the second draw is exactly the same as in the first draw. Similarly, the couple's chances of having a child with the disease remain 1 in 4 in each successive pregnancy.

Second, it is never appropriate for any health care provider to impose his or her own values or opinions on others. Individuals with known inherited diseases in their family must face difficult decisions, such as how much genetic testing to undergo or whether to terminate a pregnancy that will result in a child with a specific genetic disease. Be certain that couples have been made aware of all the options available to them; then leave them to think about the options and make their own decisions by themselves. Help them to understand that nobody is judging their decision because they are the ones who must live with the decision.

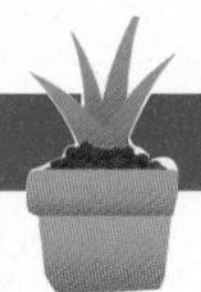

BOX 7.3 ✻ Focus on Nursing Care Planning

A Multidisciplinary Care Map for a Couple Concerned About a Genetic Disorder in Future Children

Amy Alvarez is a woman you meet at a genetic counseling center. She was adopted as a newborn and never felt a need to locate her birth parents because her adoptive parents provided a "close to perfect" childhood for her. After college, she married the most eligible bachelor in her hometown. She is now pregnant with her first child. At 15 weeks into her pregnancy, she has been advised her child may have translocation Down syndrome. She asks you, "Why is this happening? There's no disease like this in either of our families."

Family Assessment ✻ Client's family history is unknown because she was adopted. Husband's family has no history of Down syndrome. Client is presently attending law school. Husband works as a county public defender. Family lives in condo by lakefront. Finances rated as "good."

Client Assessment ✻ Client's and husband's past medical histories show no evidence of major health problems. Pregnancy is at 15 weeks. Maternal serum alpha-fetoprotein showed decreased level.

Nursing Diagnosis ✻ Health-seeking behaviors related to knowledge of possible genetic disorder inheritance

Outcome Criteria ✻ Couple accurately states the cause of this genetic disorder; agrees to further genetic testing; describes range of options open to them so any decision they make regarding the pregnancy is an informed one.

Team Member Responsible	Assessment	Intervention	Rationale	Expected Outcome
		History		
Nurse practitioner/ nurse	Obtain a detailed history and physical examination of the client and spouse, including information about family members and other relatives.	Perform a physical examination to document current health.	A thorough history and physical examination provide baseline information to direct need for follow-up testing.	Couple participates fully in health examination, so family history obtained is as complete as possible.
		Activities of Daily Living		
Nurse	Explore the meaning of genetic testing with the couple and ask how this will affect their everyday life.	Encourage couple to verbalize feelings and concerns. Allow time for questions and answers.	Exploration, verbalization, and active questioning provide a safe outlet for feelings, help to increase the other partner's awareness of needs, and open lines of communication.	Couple describes the effect on their life of needing genetic screening; asks questions as needed.
		Consultations		
Physician/ nurse	Assess whether couple would like to speak to an expert in the field of genetics to clarify their understanding.	Refer client to genetic counselor so she can be made aware of exact inheritance pattern and options available.	Couples cannot make informed choices without being aware of extent of problem.	Couple meets with genetic counselor within 1 week's time

(continued)

BOX 7.3 ✻ Focus on Nursing Care Planning (continued)

Procedures/Medications				
Physician/ nurse	Schedule an amniocentesis for karyotyping. Develop a family genogram for client and spouse.	Be certain couple receives written documentation of chromosome disorder to take to genetic counselor.	Good communication between health care providers helps to ensure a positive outcome. A family genogram may provide additional information about the client's and spouse's family histories.	Couple receives results of tests in a timely and appropriate manner. A family genogram is developed and maintained with health documentation.
Nutrition				
Dietitian/nurse	Assess the couple's nutrition patterns.	Analyze whether couple maintains healthy diet during testing and consultation period.	A healthy diet during pregnancy is important if pregnancy will be continued.	Client confirms that she continues to take prenatal vitamins and adequate protein intake.
Patient/Family Education				
Nurse practitioner/ nurse	Ask couple if they have further questions about their particular inheritance pattern.	Review with the couple the mode of transmission and chances for manifesting Down syndrome in children.	Down syndrome may be inherited at a higher incidence in a balanced translocation carrier than in others.	Couple describes accurately the mode of transmission of Down syndrome.
Spiritual/Psychosocial/Emotional Needs				
Nurse	Assess whether couple would be interested in learning some activities to reduce stress.	Instruct the couple in positive coping mechanisms. Include activities such as information sharing, relaxation and breathing exercises, and physical activity. Provide emotional support and guidance to the couple throughout testing.	Positive coping mechanisms assist in controlling fear and minimizing its intensity, thus promoting effective problem solving. Emotional support from a variety of sources helps to alleviate some of the stress and anxiety associated with genetic testing.	Couple demonstrates positive coping mechanisms. Couple states that the emotional support they received throughout their period of genetic screening and counseling was adequate.
Discharge Planning				
Social worker/ nurse	Assess community for support organizations available.	If the couple chooses to continue the pregnancy, refer them to national support group (Down Syndrome Foundation) and local parents support group.	Additional counseling and support may be necessary as pregnancy progresses or at birth of child. Use of community resources can provide additional support and help reduce feelings of isolation and loneliness.	Couple records the names and telephone numbers of support groups as well as the genetic counseling team and states they will keep numbers available if they should need further future information.

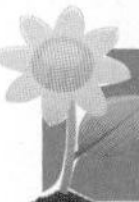

BOX 7.4 * Focus on Communication

Amy Alvarez tells you that her mother has advised her not to have more children, rather than risk having a child with Down syndrome.

Less Effective Communication

Nurse: Hello, Amy. What's the reason you've come to the clinic today?

Amy: I need to know what is the chance that all my children will have Down syndrome.

Nurse: You're only 26, far too young to be worrying about that. Down syndrome only occurs in older women.

Amy: Thanks. It's good to get good information.

More Effective Communication

Nurse: Hello, Amy. What's the reason you've come to the clinic today?

Amy: I need to know what is the chance that all my children will have Down syndrome.

Nurse: That isn't the kind of question I can answer off the top of my head. Let me ask you some questions about your family to get started toward an answer.

Because we live in an age in which information can be obtained quickly, people may believe that predictions about the inheritance of disorders can also be supplied quickly. More important than getting information to people quickly is being certain they are getting it accurately. Because Amy is a balanced translocation carrier, more aspects than her age must be considered.

✔ Checkpoint Question 7.3

Amy Alvarez was told at a genetic counseling session that she is a balanced translocation carrier for Down syndrome. What would be your best action regarding this information?

a. Be certain all of her family members understand what this means.
b. Discuss the cost of various abortion techniques with Amy.
c. Be sure Amy knows that she should not have any more children.
d. Ask Amy if she has any questions that you could answer for her.

Assessment for Genetic Disorders

Genetic assessment begins with careful study of the pattern of inheritance in a family. A history, physical examination of family members, and laboratory analysis, such as karyotyping or DNA analysis, are performed to define the extent of the problem and the chance of inheritance.

History

Taking a health history for a genetic diagnosis is often difficult because the facts detailed may evoke uncomfortable emotions such as sorrow, guilt, or inadequacy in parents. Try, however, to obtain information and document diseases in family members for a minimum of three generations. Remember to include half brothers and sisters or anyone related in any way as family. Document the mother's age because some disorders increase in incidence with age. Document also whether the parents are consanguineous or related to each other.

Documenting the family's ethnic background can reveal risks for certain disorders that occur more commonly in some ethnic groups than others. If the couple seeking counseling is unfamiliar with their family history, ask them to talk to senior family members about other relatives (grandparents, aunts, uncles) before they come for an interview. Have them ask specifically for instances of spontaneous miscarriage or children in the family who died at birth. In many instances, these children died of unknown chromosomal disorders or were miscarried because of one of the 70 or more known chromosomal disorders that are inconsistent with life. Many people have only sketchy information about their families, such as, "The baby had some kind of nervous disease" or "Her heart didn't work right." Attempt to obtain more information by asking the couple to describe the appearance or activities of the affected individual or asking for permission to obtain health records.

An extensive prenatal history of any affected person should be obtained to determine whether environmental conditions could account for the condition. Based on the above information, draw a family genogram (see Fig. 7.7). Such a diagram helps to not only identify the possibility of a chromosomal disorder occurring in a particular couple's children but also helps to identify other family members who might benefit from genetic counseling.

When a child is born dead, parents are advised to have a chromosomal analysis and autopsy performed on the infant. If at some future date they wish genetic counseling, this would allow their genetic counselor to have additional medical information.

Physical Assessment

Because genetic disorders often occur in varying degrees of expression, a careful physical assessment of any family member with a disorder, that child's siblings, and the couple seeking counseling is needed. It is possible for an individual to have a minimal expression of a disorder that has gone previously undiagnosed. During inspection, pay particular attention to certain body areas, such as the space between the eyes; the height, contour, and shape of ears; the number of fingers and toes, and the presence of webbing. **Dermatoglyphics** (the study of surface markings of the skin) can also be helpful. Note any abnormal fingerprints or palmar creases as these are present with some disorders. Abnormal hair whorls or coloring of hair can also be present.

Careful inspection of newborns is often sufficient to identify a child with a potential chromosomal disorder. Infants with multiple congenital anomalies, those born at less than 35 weeks' gestation, and those whose parents have had other children with chromosomal disorders need extremely close assessment. Table 7.1 lists the physical characteristics suggestive of some common inherited syndromes in children.

Diagnostic Testing

Many diagnostic tests are available to provide important clues about possible disorders (Pyeritz, 2009). Before pregnancy, karyotyping of both parents and an already affected

TABLE 7.1 ✻ Common Physical Characteristics of Children With Chromosomal Syndromes

Characteristic	Probable Syndrome
Late closure of fontanelles	Down syndrome
Bossing (prominent forehead)	Fragile X syndrome
Microcephaly	Trisomy 18, trisomy 13
Low-set ears	Trisomy 18, trisomy 13
Slant of eyes	Down syndrome
Epicanthal fold	Down syndrome
Abnormal iris color	Down syndrome
Large tongue	Down syndrome
Prominent jaw	Fragile X syndrome
Low-set hairline	Turner syndrome
Multiple hair whorls	Trisomy 18, trisomy 13
Webbed neck	Turner syndrome
Wide-set nipples	Trisomy 13
Heart abnormalities	Many syndromes
Large hands	Fragile X syndrome
Clinodactyly	Down syndrome
Overriding of fingers	Trisomy 18
Rocker-bottom feet	Trisomy 13
Abnormal dermatoglyphics	Down syndrome
Simian crease on palm	Down syndrome
Absence of secondary sex characteristics	Klinefelter and Turner syndromes

child provides a picture of the chromosome pattern that can be used to predict occurences in future children. Once a woman is pregnant, several other tests may be performed to help in the prenatal diagnosis of a genetic disorder. These include maternal serum alpha-fetoprotein (MSAFP), chronic villi sampling (CVS), amniocentesis, percutaneous umbilical blood sampling (PUBS), ultrasound, and fetoscopy.

Karyotyping. For karyotyping, a sample of peripheral venous blood or a scraping of cells from the buccal membrane is taken. Cells are allowed to grow until they reach metaphase, the most easily observed phase. Cells are then stained, placed under a microscope, and photographed. Chromosomes are identified according to size, shape, and stain; cut from the photograph, and arranged as in Figure 7.1. Any additional, lacking, or abnormal chromosomes can be visualized by this method.

A newer method of staining, FISH, allows karyotyping to be done immediately, rather than waiting for the cells to reach metaphase. This makes it possible for a report to be obtained in only 1 day. Fetal skin cells can be obtained by amniocentesis or CVS. A few fetal cells circulate in the maternal bloodstream, most noticeably trophoblasts, lymphocytes, and granulocytes. They are present but few in number during the first and second trimesters but plentiful during the third trimester. Such cells can be cultured and used for genetic testing for such disorders as the trisomies.

Maternal Serum Screening. Alpha-fetoprotein (AFP) is a glycoprotein produced by the fetal liver that reaches a peak in maternal serum between the 13th and 32nd week of pregnancy. The level is elevated with fetal spinal cord disease (more than twice the value of the mean for that gestational age) and is decreased in a fetal chromosomal disorder such as trisomy 21. Most pregnant women have an MSAFP test done routinely at the 15th week of pregnancy. If the result is abnormal, amniotic fluid is then assessed. Unfortunately, the MSAFP test has a false-positive rate of about 30% if the date of conception is not well documented. Use of a "triple study" (AFP, estriol, and hCG) reduces this false-positive rate, although false-positive reports still occur.

Analysis of a pregnancy-associated plasma protein A, which is also increased with a Down syndrome pregnancy, and measurement of the fetal neck thickness by ultrasound are still other measures used for analysis if an MSAFP test is positive. Women with an elevated serum result need support while they wait for ultrasound or amniocentesis confirmation as they are facing what may be a very grave finding in their infant. Receiving a false-positive report is unfortunate as it can potentially interfere with the mother's bonding with her infant.

Chorionic Villi Sampling. CVS is a diagnostic technique that involves the retrieval and analysis of chorionic villi from the growing placenta for chromosome or DNA analysis (Alfirevic, Mujezinovic, & Sundbert, 2009). The test is highly accurate and yields no more false-positive results than does amniocentesis. Although this procedure may be done as early as week 5 of pregnancy, it is more commonly done at 8 to 10 weeks. With this technique, the chorion cells are located by ultrasound. A thin catheter is then inserted vaginally, or a biopsy needle is inserted abdominally or intravaginally, and a number of chorionic cells are removed for analysis (Fig. 7.12). CVS carries a small risk (less than 1%) of causing excessive bleeding, leading to pregnancy loss. There have been some instances of children being born with missing limbs after the procedure (limb reduction syndrome). This has occurred with a high enough frequency that women need to be well informed of these risks beforehand.

After CVS, instruct a woman to report chills or fever suggestive of infection or symptoms of threatened miscarriage (uterine contractions or vaginal bleeding). Women with an Rh-negative blood type need Rh immune globulin administration after the procedure to guard against isoimmunization in the fetus.

The cells removed in CVS are karyotyped or submitted for DNA analysis to reveal whether the fetus has a genetic disorder. Because chorionic villi cells are rapidly dividing, results are available quickly, perhaps as soon as the next day. If a twin or multiple pregnancy is present, with two or more separate placentas, cells should be removed separately from each placenta. Because fraternal twins are derived from separate ova, one twin could have a chromosomal abnormality while the other does not.

Not all inherited diseases can be detected by CVS. Be certain that parents understand that only those disorders involving abnormal chromosomes or nondisjunction, and those whose specific gene location is known, can be identified by CVS. The test is not apt to reveal the extent of spinal cord abnormalities, for example.

Table 7.2 shows common chromosomal disorders that can be diagnosed prenatally through karyotyping. Additional

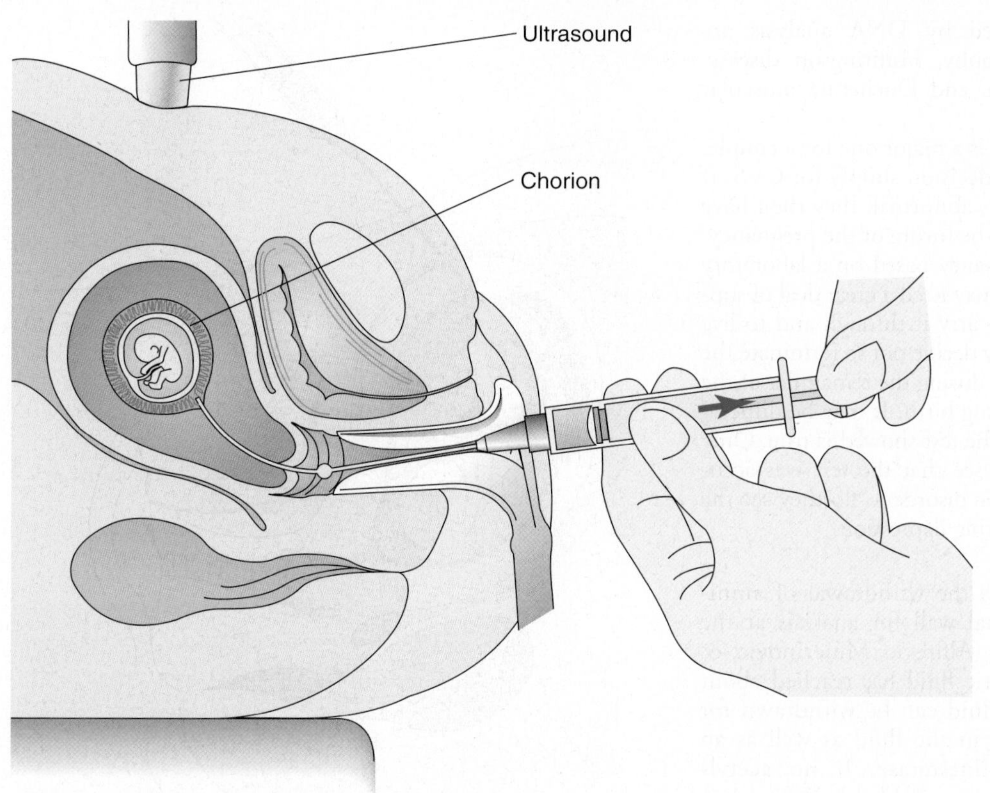

FIGURE 7.12 Chorionic villi sampling. Since the villi arise from trophoblast cells, their chromosome structure is the same as in the fetus.

TABLE 7.2 ❋ Common Genetic Disorders That Can Be Detected by Amniocentesis or Chorionic Villi Sampling

Syndrome	Chromosomal Characteristics	Clinical Signs
Down syndrome	Extra chromosome 21	Cognitively challenged Protruding tongue Epicanthal folds Hypotonia
Translocation Down syndrome	Translocation of a chromosome, perhaps 21/14	Same clinical signs as trisomy 21
Trisomy 18	Extra chromosome 18	Cognitively challenged Congenital malformations
Trisomy 13	Extra chromosome 13	Cognitively challenged Multiple congenital malformations Eye agenesis
Cri-du-chat syndrome	Deletion of short arm of chromosome 5	Cognitively challenged Facial structure anomalies Peculiar cat-like cry
Fragile X syndrome	Distortion of the X chromosome	Cognitively challenged
Philadelphia chromosome	Deletion of one arm of chromosome 21	Chronic granulocytic leukemia
Turner syndrome	Only one X chromosome present	Short stature Streak ovaries Infertility Webbed neck
Klinefelter syndrome	An extra X chromosome present (XXY)	Small testes Gynecomastia Subfertility

disorders that can be identified by DNA analysis are retinoblastoma, myotonic dystrophy, Huntington disease, sickle cell anemia, β-thalassemia, and Duchenne muscular dystrophy.

The decision to undergo CVS is a major one for a couple. As a rule, they are not making a decision simply for CVS. If the CVS reveals that their child is abnormal, they then have to make a second decision about the future of the pregnancy.

Deciding to terminate a pregnancy based on a laboratory finding is rarely easy. The couple may need a great deal of support with their decision, both to carry it through and to live with the decision afterward. If they decide not to terminate the pregnancy, they will need support during the remainder of the pregnancy and in the days following birth. It may be difficult for a couple to believe that what the test showed is true. Only when they inspect the baby and see that the test was accurate—the child does have a genetic disorder—do they see the reality. This can result in long-lasting depression.

Amniocentesis. Amniocentesis is the withdrawal of amniotic fluid through the abdominal wall for analysis at the 14th to 16th week of pregnancy (Alfirevic, Mujezinovic, & Sunberg, 2009). Because amniotic fluid has reached about 200 mL at this point, enough fluid can be withdrawn for karyotyping of skin cells found in the fluid as well as an analysis of AFP or acetylcholinesterase. If no acetylcholinesterase, a breakdown product of blood, is found in the specimen, it confirms that an elevated AFP level is not a false-positive reading caused by blood in the fluid.

For the procedure, a pocket of amniotic fluid is located by ultrasound. Then a needle is inserted transabdominally, and about 20 mL of fluid is aspirated. Skin cells in the fluid are karyotyped for chromosomal number and structure. The level of AFP is analyzed. Some disorders, such as Tay-Sachs disease, can be identified by the lack of a specific enzyme, such as hexosaminidase A, in amniotic fluid.

Amniocentesis has the advantage over CVS of carrying only a 0.5% risk of spontaneous miscarriage. Unfortunately, it usually is not done until the 14th to 16th week of pregnancy. This may prove to be a difficult time because, by this date, a woman is beginning to accept her pregnancy and bond with the fetus. In addition, termination of pregnancy during the second trimester is more difficult than during a first trimester. Support women while they wait for test results and to make a decision about the pregnancy. Women with an Rh-negative blood type need Rh immune globulin administration after the procedure to protect against isoimmunization in the fetus. All women need to be observed for about 30 minutes after the procedure to be certain that labor contractions are not beginning and that the fetal heart rate remains within normal limits. Because amniocentesis is also a common assessment for fetal maturity, it is discussed further in Chapter 9 (see also Fig. 9.14).

Percutaneous Umbilical Blood Sampling. PUBS, or cordocentesis, is the removal of blood from the fetal umbilical cord at about 17 weeks using an amniocentesis technique (Fig. 7.13). This allows analysis of blood components as well as more rapid karyotyping than is possible when only skin cells are removed. PUBS is discussed further in Chapter 9.

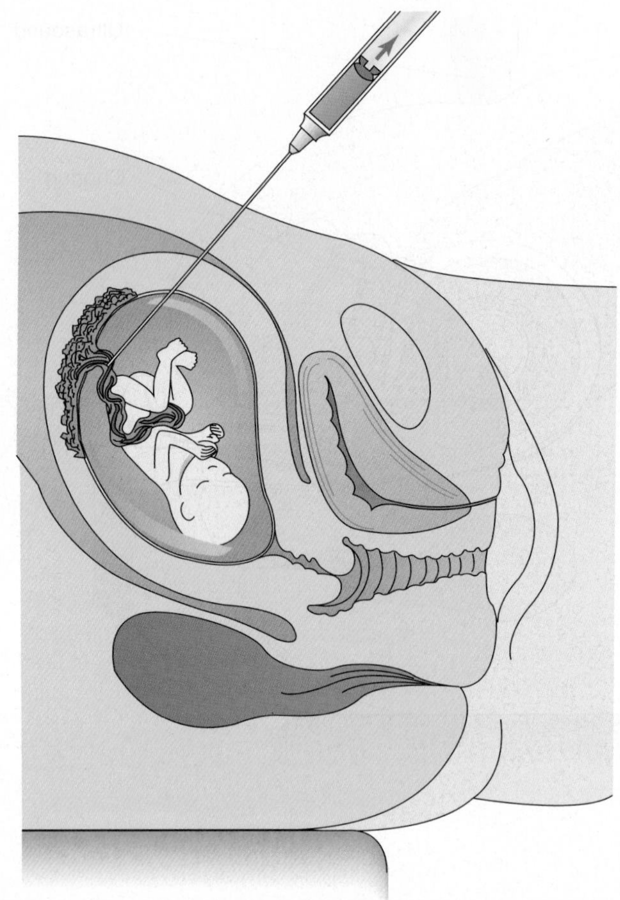

FIGURE 7.13 Percutaneous umbilical blood sampling. Blood is withdrawn from the umbilical cord using amniocentesis technique.

Fetal Imaging. Magnetic resonance imaging (MRI) and ultrasound are diagnostic tools used to assess a fetus for general size and structural disorders of the internal organs, spine, and limbs. Because some genetic disorders are associated with physical appearance, both of these methods may be helpful. Ultrasound is used concurrently with amniocentesis.

Fetoscopy. Fetoscopy is the insertion of a fiberoptic fetoscope through a small incision in the mother's abdomen into the uterus and membranes to visually inspect the fetus for gross abnormalities. It can be used to confirm an ultrasound finding, to remove skin cells for DNA analysis, or to perform surgery for a congenital disorder such as a stenosed urethra.

Preimplantation Diagnosis. Preimplantation diagnosis is possible for in vitro fertilization procedures. It may be possible in the future for a naturally fertilized ovum to be removed from the uterus by lavage before implantation and studied for DNA analysis this same way. The ovum would then be reinserted or not, depending on the findings and the parents' wishes. This would provide genetic information extremely early in a pregnancy.

Reproductive Alternatives

Some couples are reluctant to seek genetic counseling because they are afraid they will be told it would be unwise to have children. Helping them to realize that viable alternatives for having a family exist allows them to seek the help they need.

Artificial insemination by donor (AID) is an option for couples if the genetic disorder is one inherited by the male partner or is a recessively inherited disorder carried by both partners. AID is available in all major communities and can permit the couple to experience the satisfaction and enjoyment of a usual pregnancy (Burney, Schust, & Yao, 2007).

If the inherited problem is one arising from the female partner, surrogate embryo transfer is an assisted reproductive technique that is a possibility (van Berkel, Candido, & Pijffers, 2007). An oocyte donated by a friend or relative or provided by an anonymous donor is fertilized by the husband's sperm in the laboratory and then implanted into a woman's uterus. Like AID, donor embryo transfer offers the couple a chance to experience a normal pregnancy.

Use of a surrogate mother (a woman who agrees to be artificially inseminated, typically by the male partner's sperm, and bear a child for the couple) is still another possibility (Reilly, 2007). All of these procedures are expensive and, depending on individual circumstances, may have disappointing success rates. Assisted reproductive techniques are discussed in more detail in Chapter 8.

Adoption is an alternative many couples can also find rewarding (see Chapter 3). Choosing to remain child-free should not be discounted as a viable option. Many couples who have every reason to think they would have children without a genetic disorder choose this alternative because they believe their existence is full and rewarding without the presence of children.

Diagnosis of a disorder during pregnancy with prompt treatment at birth to minimize the prognosis and outcome of the disorder is another route to explore. Termination of a pregnancy that reveals a chromosomal or metabolic abnormality is a final option.

Help couples decide on an alternative that is correct for them, not one that they sense a counselor feels would be best. They need to consider the ethical philosophy or beliefs of other family members when making their decision, although ultimately they must do what they believe is best for them as a couple. A useful place to start counseling is with values clarification, to be certain a couple understands what is most important to them.

Future Possibilities

Stem cell research is looking at the possibility that immature cells (stem cells) could be implanted into an embryo with a known abnormal genetic makeup, replacing the abnormal cells or righting the affected child's genetic composition (Wiener et al., 2007). Although presently possible, stem cell research is costly and produces some ethical questions (e.g., although stem cells can be harvested from cord blood, adult skin cells or menstrual blood, will these be able to serve as main sources of donor DNA for the new technology?).

Legal and Ethical Aspects of Genetic Screening and Counseling

Nurses can be instrumental in seeing that couples who seek genetic counseling receive results in a timely manner and with compassion about what their results may mean to future childbearing. Always keep in mind several legal responsibilities of genetic testing, counseling, and therapy, including:

- Participation by couples or individuals in genetic screening must be elective.
- People desiring genetic screening must sign an informed consent for the procedure.
- Results must be interpreted correctly yet provided to the individuals as quickly as possible.
- The results must not be withheld from the individuals and must be given only to those persons directly involved.
- After genetic counseling, persons must not be coerced to undergo procedures such as abortion or sterilization. Any procedure must be a free and individual decision.

Failure to heed these guidelines could result in charges of invasion of privacy, breach of confidentiality, or psychological injury caused by "labeling" someone or imparting unwarranted fear and worry about the significance of a disease or carrier state. If couples are identified as being at risk for having a child with a genetic disorder and are not informed of the risk and offered appropriate diagnostic procedures (e.g., amniocentesis) they can bring a "wrongful birth" lawsuit if their child is born with the detected genetic disorder (Box 7.5).

What if... Amy Alvarez was pregnant with twins? One twin fetus is diagnosed as having Down syndrome, and the other is not. How would you counsel her if she wanted to abort the affected child, when the procedure also might endanger the child without the disorder?

COMMON CHROMOSOMAL DISORDERS RESULTING IN PHYSICAL OR COGNITIVE DEVELOPMENTAL DISORDERS

Several chromosomal disorders, particularly nondisjunction disorders, are easily detected at birth on physical examination. Many of these disorders leave children cognitively challenged. Care of the child who is cognitively challenged is discussed in Chapter 54.

Trisomy 13 Syndrome (47XY13+ or 47XX13+)

In trisomy 13 syndrome (Patau syndrome), the child has an extra chromosome 13 and is severely cognitively challenged. The incidence of the syndrome is low, approximately 0.45 per 1000 live births. Midline body disorders such as cleft lip and palate, heart defects, particularly ventricular septal defects, and abnormal genitalia are present (see Fig. 7.11). Other common findings include microcephaly with abnormalities of the forebrain and forehead; eyes that are smaller than normal (microphthalmos) or absent; and low-set ears. Most of these children do not survive beyond early childhood.

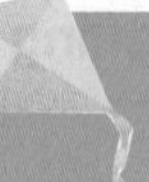

BOX 7.5 ✻ Focus on Evidence-Based Practice

What is the most effective way to present the risk of Down syndrome to pregnant women?

Healthy women under 34 years of age have only a small risk (1 in 100) of having a child with Down syndrome. Explaining what a low risk this is can be difficult, however, if all that women hear is that there is a risk. To find the best way to present this material, researchers recruited 150 pregnant women, all under 32 years of age, and asked them what they perceived a risk of 1 in 100 to mean. They then assigned the woman to three different means of illustrating the risk. In the first group, women viewed a photo showing 99 smiling faces and 1 frowning face. In the second group, women read a paragraph of text describing a room full of 100 people, all dressed alike but 1 person. In a third group, women were shown a plastic box containing 100 ping-pong balls and asked to pull out 1 ball. Women were then re-asked how they perceived their risk of having a child with Down syndrome. Of the visual and written groups, only 37% said they perceived the risk as less than before whereas 66% of the interactive group said they perceived the risk as less than before. The researchers concluded that women worry less when an interactive demonstration is used to illustrate risk. Also, that risk seems less when women are told the chances are 99 to 1 that their child will not have Down syndrome rather than being told that their chance is 1 in 100 of having a child with the syndrome.

Would the above findings be helpful to you when talking to women about their risk of a genetic disorder in pregnancy?

Source: Hinshaw, K., et al. (2007). Randomised controlled trial comparing three methods of presenting risk of Down's syndrome. *European Journal of Obstetrics, Gynecology & Reproductive Biology, 133*(1), 40–46.

Trisomy 18 Syndrome (47XY18+ or 47XX18+)

Children with trisomy 18 syndrome have three copies of chromosome 18. The incidence is approximately 0.23 per 1000 live births. These children are severely cognitively challenged and tend to be small for gestational age at birth, have markedly low-set ears, a small jaw, congenital heart defects, and usually misshapen fingers and toes (the index finger deviates or crosses over other fingers). Also, the soles of their feet are often rounded instead of flat (rocker-bottom feet). As in trisomy 13 syndrome, most of these children do not survive beyond early infancy.

Cri-du-Chat Syndrome (46XX5p− or 46XY5P−)

Cri-du-chat syndrome is the result of a missing portion of chromosome 5. In addition to an abnormal cry, which sounds much more like the sound of a cat than a human infant's cry, children with cri-du-chat syndrome tend to have a small head, wide-set eyes, and a downward slant to the palpebral fissure of the eye. They are severely cognitively challenged.

Turner Syndrome (45X0)

The child with Turner syndrome (gonadal dysgenesis) has only one functional X chromosome. The child is short in stature and has only streak (small and nonfunctional) ovaries. She is sterile and with the exception of pubic hair, secondary sex characteristics do not develop at puberty. The hairline at the nape of the neck is low set, and the neck may appear to be webbed and short. A newborn may have appreciable edema of the hands and feet and a number of congenital anomalies, most frequently coarctation (stricture) of the aorta and kidney disorders. The incidence of the syndrome is approximately 1 per 10,000 live births. The disorder can be identified with an ultrasound during pregnancy because of the increased neck folds.

Although children with Turner syndrome may be severely cognitively challenged, difficulty in this area is more commonly limited to learning disabilities. Socioemotional adjustment problems may accompany the syndrome because of the lack of fertility and if the nuchal folds are prominent.

Human growth hormone administration may help children with Turner syndrome achieve additional height (Baxter et al., 2009). If treatment with estrogen is begun at approximately 13 years of age, secondary sex characteristics will appear, and osteoporosis from lack of estrogen during growing years may be prevented. If females continue taking estrogen for three out of every four weeks, this produces withdrawal bleeding that results in a menstrual flow. This flow, however, does not correct the problem of sterility. Gonadal tissue is scant and inadequate for ovulation because of the basic chromosomal aberration.

Klinefelter Syndrome (47XXY)

Infants with Klinefelter syndrome are males with an extra X chromosome. Characteristics of the syndrome may not be noticeable at birth. At puberty, secondary sex characteristics do not develop; the child has small testes that produce ineffective sperm (Porche, 2007). Affected individuals tend to develop gynecomastia (increased breast size) and have an increased risk of male breast cancer (Pyeritz, 2009). The incidence is about 1 per 1000 live births. Karyotyping can be used to reveal the additional X chromosome.

Fragile X Syndrome (46XY23q−)

Fragile X syndrome is the most common cause of cognitive challenge in males. It is an X-linked disorder in which one long arm of an X chromosome is defective which results in inadequate protein synaptic responses (Bear et al., 2008). The incidence is about 1 in 1000 live births.

Before puberty, boys with fragile X syndrome typically may demonstrate maladaptive behaviors such as hyperactivity and autism. They may have reduced intellectual functioning, with marked deficits in speech and arithmetic (Kornman et al., 2007). They may be identified by the presence of a large head, a long face with a high forehead, a prominent lower jaw, and large protruding ears. Hyperextensive joints and cardiac disorders may also be present. After puberty, enlarged testicles may become evident. Affected individuals are fertile and can reproduce.

Carrier females may show some evidence of the physical and cognitive characteristics. Although intellectual function from the syndrome cannot be improved, both folic acid and an antipsychotic drug such as phenothiazines may improve symptoms of poor concentration and impulsivity.

Down Syndrome (Trisomy 21) (47XY21+ or 47XX21+)

Trisomy 21, the most frequently occurring chromosomal abnormality, occurs in about 1 in 800 pregnancies. The number of children born with the disorder is considerably less as many women choose to end pregnancies when the diagnosis is made (Witters & Fryns, 2008).

The physical features of children with Down syndrome are so marked that fetal diagnosis is possible by ultrasound in utero. The nose is broad and flat. The eyelids have an extra fold of tissue at the inner canthus (an epicanthal fold), and the palpebral fissure (opening between the eyelids) tends to slant laterally upward. The iris of the eye may have white specks, called Brushfield spots. The tongue may protrude from the mouth because the oral cavity is smaller than usual. The back of the head is flat, the neck is short, and an extra pad of fat at the base of the head causes the skin to be so loose it can be lifted easily. The ears may be low-set. Muscle tone is poor, giving the baby a rag-doll appearance. This can be so lax that the child's toe can be touched against the nose (not possible in the average mature newborn). The fingers of many children with Down syndrome are short and thick, and the little finger is often curved inward. There may be a wide space between the first and second toes and between the first and second fingers. The palm of the hand shows a peculiar crease (a simian line), which is a single horizontal palm crease rather than the usual three creases in the palm (Fig. 7.14).

Children with Down syndrome are usually cognitively challenged to some degree. The challenge can range from an intelligence quotient (IQ) of 50 to 70 to a child who is profoundly affected (IQ less than 20). The extent of the cognitive challenge is not evident at birth. The fact that the brain is not developing well is evidenced by a head size that is usually smaller than the 10th or 20th percentile at well-child health care visits.

These children also appear to have altered immune function as they are prone to upper respiratory tract infections. Congenital heart disease, especially atrioventricular defects, is common. Stenosis or atresia of the duodenum, strabismus, and cataract disorders are also common. For as yet undetected reasons, acute lymphocytic leukemia occurs approximately 20 times more frequently in children with Down syndrome than in the general population. Even if children are born without an accompanying disorder such as heart disease, their lifespan usually is only 50 to 60 years, because aging seems to occur faster than normal.

It's important for children with Down syndrome to be enrolled in early educational and play programs (see Chapter 54). Because they are prone to infections, sensible precautions such as using good handwashing technique are important when caring for them. The enlarged tongue may interfere with swallowing and cause choking unless the child is fed slowly. As their neck may not be fully stable, a radiograph to ensure stability is recommended before they engage in strenuous activities such as competitive sports. As with all newborns, these infants need physical examination at birth to enable detection of the genetic disorder and initiation of parental counseling and support.

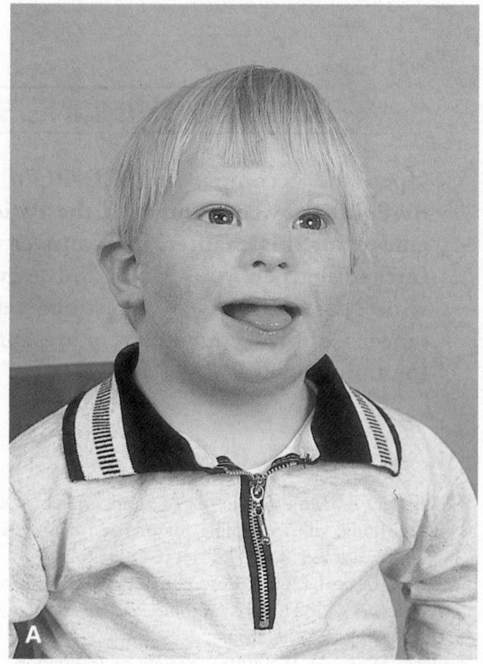

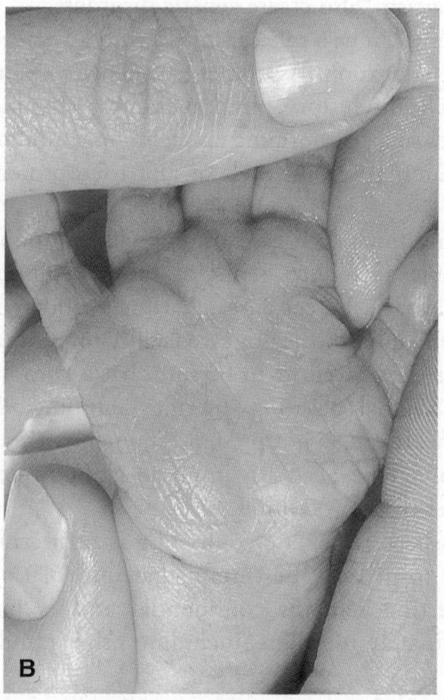

FIGURE 7.14 (**A**) Typical facial features of the child with Down syndrome. (© Barbara Proud.) (**B**) A simian line, a horizontal crease seen in children with Down syndrome. (SPL/Custom Medical Stock Photograph.)

Childhood Tumors

A number of cancers in children are also associated with chromosomal aberrations. Chief among these are retinoblastoma (chromosome 13), Wilms' tumor (chromosome 11) and neuroblastoma (chromosome 1 or 11) (Pyeritz, 2009).

✓ Checkpoint Question 7.4

Amy Alvarez's child is born with Down syndrome. What is a common physical feature of newborns with this disorder?

a. Spastic and stiff muscles
b. Loose skin at back of neck
c. A white lock of forehead hair
d. Wrinkles on the soles of the feet

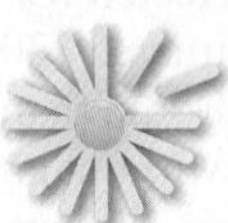

Key Points for Review

- Genetic disorders are disorders resulting from a defect in the structure or number of genes or chromosomes. Genetics is the study of how and why such disorders occur.
- A phenotype is a person's outward appearance. Genotype refers to the actual gene composition. A person's genome is the complete set of genes present. A karyotype is a graphic representation of the chromosomes that are present.
- A person is homozygous if he or she has two like genes for a trait and heterozygous if he or she has two unlike genes for a trait.
- Mendelian laws can predict the likely incidence of recessive or dominant diseases in children. Division disorders, including nondisjunction abnormalities, deletion, translocation, and mosaicism, also create genetic disorders.
- Genetic counseling can be a role for nurses with advanced preparation and education. Assessment of genetic disorders consists of a health history, physical examination, and diagnostic studies such as chorionic villi sampling, amniocentesis, and maternal serum levels of alpha-fetoprotein analysis.
- Some karyotyping tests, such as chorionic villi sampling and amniocentesis, introduce a risk of spontaneous or threatened miscarriage. Be certain that women undergoing these tests remain in the health care facility for at least 30 minutes after the procedure to be sure that a complication such as vaginal bleeding, uterine cramping, or abnormal fetal heart rate is not present. Women with an Rh-negative blood type need Rh immune globulin administration after these procedures.
- An important aspect of genetic counseling is respecting a couple's right to privacy. Be certain that information gained from testing remains confidential and is not given indiscriminately to others, including other family members.
- People who are told that a genetic abnormality does exist in their family may suffer a loss of self-esteem. Offering support to help them deal with the feelings they experience is an important nursing intervention.
- Common nondisjunction genetic disorders include Down syndrome (trisomy 21), trisomy 13, trisomy 18, Turner syndrome, and Klinefelter syndrome. Most of these syndromes include some degree of cognitive challenge.

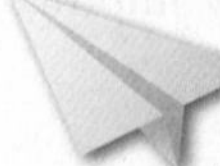

CRITICAL THINKING EXERCISES

1. Amy Alvarez, whom you met at the beginning of the chapter, doesn't know her family history so is unable to answer questions about family members. What questions would you want to ask about her husband's family? Suppose Mr. Alvarez tells you he had two brothers who died at birth. Would that finding be important?
2. Suppose Amy's husband's sister and her husband both carry a gene for a recessively inherited disorder, yet they have had five children and none of the children shows symptoms of the disorder. Is it possible for them to have had five children without any symptoms of the disease? What are the chances that their sixth child will also be disease free?
3. Amy tells you, "My family will be so ashamed if a genetic defect happens in our family." What does her statement tell you about her family's knowledge of genetic disorders?
4. Examine the National Health Goals related to genetic disorders. Most government-sponsored money for nursing research is allotted based on these goals. What would be a possible research topic to explore pertinent to these goals that would be applicable to the Alvarez family and also advance evidence-based practice?

CRITICAL THINKING SCENARIO

Open the accompanying CD-ROM or visit http://thePoint. lww.com and read the Patient Scenario included for this chapter, then answer the questions to further sharpen your skills and grow more familiar with NCLEX types of questions related to inheritance. Confirm your answers are correct by reading the rationales.

REFERENCES

Alfirevic, Z., Mujezinovic, F., & Sundberg, K. (2009). Amniocentesis and chorionic villus sampling for prenatal diagnosis. *Cochrane Database of Systematic Reviews, 2009*(1), (CD003252).

Baxter, L., et al. (2009). Recombinant growth hormone for children and adolescents with Turner syndrome. *Cochrane Database of Systematic Reviews, 2009*(1), (CD003887).

Bear, M. F., et al. (2008). Fragile x: translation in action. *Neuropsychopharmacology, 33*(1), 84–87.

Benarroch, F., et al. (2007). Prader-Willi syndrome: medical prevention and behavioral challenges. *Child & Adolescent Psychiatric Clinics of North America, 16*(3), 695–708.

Burney, R. O., Schust, D. J., & Yao, M. W. M. (2007). Infertility. In J. S. Berek (Ed.). *Berek & Novak's gynecology.* Philadelphia: Lippincott Williams & Wilkins.

Cardone, M. (2007). Prospects for gene therapy in inherited neurodegenerative diseases. *Current Opinion in Neurology, 20*(2), 151–158.

Cappellini, M. D., & Fiorelli, G. (2008). Glucose-6-phosphate dehydrogenase deficiency. *Lancet, 371*(9606), 64–74.

Dorigo, O., Martinez-Maza, O., & Berek, J. S. (2007). Molecular biology and genetics. In Berek, J. S. (Ed.). *Berek & Novak's obstetrics & gynecology.* Philadelphia: Lippincott Williams & Wilkins.

Gardner, J. (2007). What you need to know about cystic fibrosis. *Nursing 2007, 37*(7), 52–55.

Goldman, A. (2007). Stem cells discovered in menstrual blood. *Stem Cell Research News, 9*(21), 1.

Hinshaw, K., et al. (2007). Randomised controlled trial comparing three methods of presenting risk of Down's syndrome. *European Journal of Obstetrics, Gynecology & Reproductive Biology, 133*(1), 40–46.

Kornman, L., et al. (2009). Pre-conception and antenatal screening for the fragile site on the X-chromosome. *Cochrane Database of Systematic Reviews, 2009*(1), (CD001806).

Manipalviratn, S., Trivax, B., & Huang, A. (2007). Genetic disorders & sex chromosome abnormalities. In DeCherney, A. H., & Nathan, L. (Eds.). *Current diagnosis & treatment in obstetrics & gynecology* (10th ed.). Columbus, OH: McGraw-Hill.

Porche, D. J. (2007). Klinefelter syndrome. *Journal for Nurse Practitioners, 3* (7), 443–444.

Pyeritz, R. E. (2009). Basic Genetics. In Mcphee, S. J., Papadakis, M. A., & Tierney, L. M. (Eds.). *Current medical diagnosis & treatment.* Columbus, OH: McGraw-Hill.

Reilly, D. R. (2007). Surrogate pregnancy: a guide for Canadian prenatal health care providers. *Canadian Medical Association Journal, 176* (4), 483–485.

Roze, E., Saudou, F., & Caboche, J. (2008). Pathophysiology of Huntington's disease: from Huntington functions to potential treatments. *Current Opinion in Neurology, 21* (4), 497–503.

Schorge, J. O., et al. (Eds.). (2008). First trimester abortions. In J. O. Schorge, et al. (Eds.). *Williams gynecology.* Columbus, OH: McGraw-Hill.

Scott, A. (2007). Spreading the word: boosting cord blood donations among minorities. *Advance for Nurses, 4* (20), 23–24.

Stuart, A. G., & Williams, A. (2007). Marfan's syndrome and the heart. *Archives of Disease in Childhood, 92* (4), 351–356.

van Berkel, D., Candido, A., & Pijffers, W. H. (2007). Becoming a mother by non-anonymous egg donation: secrecy and the relationship between egg recipient, egg donor and egg donation child. *Journal of Psychosomatic Obstetrics & Gynecology, 28* (2), 97–104.

Van Voorhis, B. J. (2007). In vitro fertilization. *New England Journal of Medicine, 356* (4), 379–386.

Weitzel, J. N., et al. (2007). Limited family structure and BRCA gene mutation status in single cases of breast cancer. *Journal of the American Medical Association, 297* (23), 2587–2595.

Wiener, L. S., et al. (2007). Hematopoietic stem cell donation in children: a review of the sibling donor experience. *Journal of Psychosocial Oncology, 25* (1), 45–66.

Witters, I., & Fryns, J. P. (2008). Prenatal diagnosis of trisomy 21: registration results from a single genetic center. *Genetic Counseling, 19*(2), 157–163.

SUGGESTED READINGS

Ardary, D. A. (2007). Increasing school nurse awareness of Turner syndrome. *Journal of School Nursing, 23*(1), 28–33.

Ball, R. H., et al. (2007). First- and second-trimester evaluation of risk for Down syndrome. *Obstetrics and Gynecology, 110*(1), 10–17.

Calzone, K. A., & Jenkins, J. (2007). Preparing nurses for the future. Where do you fit into the implementation plans for essential genetics and genomics nursing competency? *Nursing Outlook, 55*(2), 114.

Debray, F., Lambert, M., & Mitchell, G. A. (2008). Disorders of mitochondrial function. *Current Opinion in Pediatrics, 20*(4), 471–482.

Jenkins, J., & Calzone, K. A. (2007). Establishing the essential nursing competencies for genetics and genomics. *Journal of Nursing Scholarship, 39*(1), 10–16.

Lea, D. H. (2008). Genetic and genomic healthcare: ethical issues of importance to nurses. *Online Journal of Issues in Nursing, 13*(1), 6.

Oliver, S., et al. (2009). Disclosing to parents newborn carrier status identified by routine blood spot screening. *Cochrane Database of Systematic Reviews, 2009*(1), (CD003859).

Reddy, U. M. (2007). The evolving prenatal screening scene. *Obstetrics and Gynecology, 110*(1), 2–4.

Salvador-Carulla, L., & Bertelli, M. (2008). 'Mental retardation' or 'intellectual disability': time for a conceptual change. *Psychopathology, 41*(1), 10–16.

Williams, P. S. H. (2008). Genetic and genomic public health strategies: imperatives for neonatal nursing genetic competency. *Newborn and Infant Nursing Reviews, 8*(1), 43–50.

Chapter

8 Nursing Care of the Subfertile Couple

KEY TERMS

- anovulation
- cryptorchidism
- endometriosis
- erectile dysfunction
- in vitro fertilization
- pelvic inflammatory disease
- sperm count
- sperm motility
- spermatogenesis
- sterility
- subfertility
- therapeutic insemination
- varicocele

OBJECTIVES

After mastering the contents of this chapter, you should be able to:

1. Describe common causes of subfertility in both men and women.
2. Identify National Health Goals related to subfertility that nurses can help the nation achieve.
3. Use critical thinking to analyze ways that a fertility assessment can be more family centered.
4. Describe common assessments necessary to detect subfertility.
5. Formulate nursing diagnoses related to subfertility.
6. Identify appropriate outcomes for the subfertile couple.
7. Plan nursing interventions to meet the needs of a couple with a diagnosis of subfertility.
8. Implement nursing care associated with the diagnosis of subfertility or measures to promote fertility, such as health teaching.
9. Evaluate outcomes for achievement and effectiveness of care.
10. Identify areas of nursing care related to fertility that could benefit from additional nursing research or application of evidence-based practice.
11. Integrate knowledge about subfertility with the nursing process to achieve quality maternal and child health nursing care.

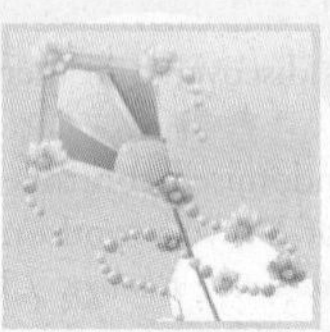

Cheryl and Bob Carl married when they were both 25 and planned to wait 5 years before beginning their family so they could save money for a house. At the end of 5 years, they bought the house. On the day they moved in, Mrs. Carl stopped taking her birth control pills. At the end of a year, however, she still was not pregnant. Three years later, the Carls began fertility testing. They are now undergoing their second cycle of in vitro fertilization and embryo transfer. The Carls have applied for a second mortgage on their house to finance the fertility testing and fertilization procedures. At her last visit, Mrs. Carl stated, "This is my fault because I'm so rigid. I can't relax enough to get pregnant. Look how I had to buy the house before I could even consider getting pregnant, and now we'll probably lose it. Besides that, it feels like our whole life revolves around trying to get pregnant."

Previous chapters described normal anatomy and physiology and ways to prevent pregnancy. This chapter adds information to expand your knowledge base about care of the couple who is unable to conceive.

How could you best help the Carls?

Many marriage customs, such as throwing rice, originate from old rituals to promote fertility. The existence of such common rituals provides evidence about the importance of having children for the average couple and society as a whole.

Infertility is a term used to describe the inability to conceive a child or sustain a pregnancy to birth. Because most couples have the potential to conceive but they are just less able to do this without additional help, the term **subfertility** is more often used today.

Subfertility affects as many as 14% of couples who desire children (Kumar et al., 2007). Couples exploring fertility testing come in all different types: many are married couples who are having trouble conceiving; some are couples who have plans to marry and wonder if they will have trouble conceiving; some desire to remain single or partner with someone of their own sex and bear a child, through an assisted fertility method. Occasionally, people want assurance that they are unable to have children so they can discontinue using a contraceptive.

When a couple first pursues fertility counseling, they usually have fears and anxieties not only about their inability to conceive but also about what this condition will mean to their future lifestyle and family. Without information about the cause of their subfertility, partners can blame themselves or carry unexpressed anger toward a partner. Some couples may strongly desire a child but also feel anxious about impending parenthood, which would bring with it loss of independence and their established lifestyle. For all these reasons, subfertility screening and counseling can be an emotionally difficult and physically demanding process, often creating a high level of strain on a couple's relationship (MacKay, 2009).

Having healthy children is such a priority that a National Health Goal aimed at reducing subfertility has been established (Box 8.1). Because most fertility tests are conducted in ambulatory settings, nurses play key roles in educating couples about the variety of tests and procedures that may be performed. They are important members of fertility health care teams, often assuming responsibility for health assessment, client education, and counseling and helping clients identify and express their feelings about their desire to have a child, express how far they are willing to go in terms of testing and procedures to achieve this desire, and how they might feel if they are not able to have a child. In addition, educating clients about advanced procedures, many of which are complex and demand knowledgeable, ongoing involvement, and participating in the complex planning and implementation of treatment strategies are also important roles. If pregnancy cannot be achieved, nurses can counsel clients about available alternatives, such as adoption or child-free living.

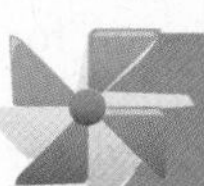

BOX 8.1 ✻ Focus on National Health Goals

One National Health Goal directly addresses the problem of subfertility:

- Reduce the proportion of married couples whose ability to conceive or maintain a pregnancy is impaired from a baseline of 13% to a target of 10% (http://www.nih.gov).

To meet this health goal, nurses need to be active in health promotion and early identification and prevention of problems that could lead to subfertility, playing active roles in teaching clients about safer sex practices (see Chapter 5) to help reduce the incidence of sexually transmitted infections and pelvic inflammatory disease, both of which can contribute to subfertility. Counseling on healthy nutrition can also be important. Good nursing research topics include investigation of how to help women better recognize the symptoms of pelvic inflammatory disease or manage stress when self-esteem is low.

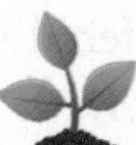

Nursing Process Overview

For the Couple With Subfertility

Assessment

Subfertility assessment used to require many months and many tests, all of which had the potential to interfere with a couple's self-image and self-esteem. Today, a subfertility investigation is usually limited to three assessments: semen analysis, ovulation monitoring, and tubal patency. Even with this more sensible approach to evaluation, nursing assessment often reveals that one or both partners feel inadequate or angry and frustrated by what has happened to them and the need to undergo testing. Questions such as, "How do you feel about what has happened?" or "How do you think your partner feels about not being able to conceive?" may be enough to encourage partners to express these concerns. Talking with both partners together may be advantageous, because they may feel more comfortable speaking about their problem together. On the other hand, it is important to spend some time alone with each client in case there is anything a partner wishes to discuss privately. This might be the only opportunity one of them has to ask that one "silly" question or voice a fear that they believe is too foolish to ask or bring up in front of their partner.

Nursing Diagnosis

Nursing diagnoses related to subfertility are likely to focus on psychosocial issues associated with the inability to conceive and the potentially nerve-wracking process of fertility testing and management. Examples of possible diagnoses include:

- Fear related to possible outcome of subfertility studies
- Situational low self-esteem related to the apparent inability to conceive
- Anxiety related to what the process of fertility testing will entail
- Deficient knowledge related to measures to promote fertility
- Anticipatory grieving related to failure to conceive or sustain a pregnancy
- Powerlessness related to repeated unsuccessful attempts at achieving conception
- Hopelessness related to perception of no viable alternatives to usual conception

If required tests interfere with a couple's relationship (including sexual patterns), "Sexual dysfunction related to command performance of subfertility therapy" might be applicable.

Expected Outcomes and Planning

In establishing expected outcomes with a couple undergoing fertility testing and counseling, be certain that the couple realizes that results may not be instantaneous. A couple may need to change or modify their goals if tests begin to show that what they first wanted—to have a child without medical intervention—is impossible. Participation in a support group may allow a couple to work through the stress that fertility testing places on their lives. Resolve (http://www.resolve.org), a national support group for couples with subfertility, can be helpful in offering referral sources and support that a couple can use in planning. A second helpful organization is the American Society of Reproductive Medicine (htpp://www.asrm.org).

Implementation

Fertility testing can be costly for a couple; however, more and more insurance companies are providing reimbursement for subfertility-related tests and procedures. Couples need to be informed beforehand of specific estimates of the cost of testing or therapy. They also may need help budgeting and planning their resources accordingly.

Suggesting that a couple combine involvement with fertility testing with ongoing activities or that they begin a new activity together (e.g., taking a night school course, planting a garden, learning a new sport or hobby) at the same time they begin fertility testing is a way of helping them reduce the feeling that their entire existence revolves around the testing procedures. It also may help provide them with time for sharing experiences and increasing intimacy, helping to compensate for any decreased enjoyment that comes from "scheduled" sexual relations.

Throughout testing, couples need thorough education about the various procedures. Make sure to review any specific instructions about preprocedural and postprocedural care. Depending on their motivations, a couple's reaction to study results may vary from relief, to stoic acceptance, to grief for children never to be born. Each partner may wonder whether the other will be able to continue the relationship if he or she turns out to be the "subfertile" one. Couples need the active support of health care personnel from the first day they braced themselves to ask, "Exactly why are we childless?" until the end, regardless of the results.

Outcome Evaluation

Examples of expected outcomes in this area include:

- Client rearranges work plans to manage schedule of fertility testing by 1 month's time.
- Couple verbalizes that they understand their individual subfertility problem after preliminary testing.
- Couple demonstrates a high level of self-esteem after fertility studies, even in the face of disappointing study outcomes.

For the couple with the problem of subfertility, evaluation is best if it is ongoing because, as circumstances around them change, so may their goals and desires. Until they can accept an alternative method of having children—adoption or an assisted reproductive technique such as **therapeutic insemination** (deposition of sperm into a woman's cervix or uterus) or **in vitro fertilization** (IVF; the union of sperm and ovum under laboratory conditions)—former plans have been crushed. It is not unusual to see a couple move through steps of denial, anger, bargaining, and depression before they reach a level of acceptance that they are different in this one area of life from others but not limited in their ability to achieve in other areas. Only after acceptance are they able to make adjustments in their wants or plans to feel fulfilled again.

Future evaluation is also important, because a couple who decides at age 20 to choose child-free living may change their minds at a later date. A couple who chooses an assisted reproductive technique may decide after several unsuccessful attempts that they are no longer interested in this method of conception. Keeping evaluation an ongoing process allows such plans to be modified as necessary. Encourage couples seen for subfertility to call or visit their subfertility setting every 6 to 12 months to inquire about new discoveries in the field and how these might apply to their situation.

SUBFERTILITY

Subfertility is said to exist when a pregnancy has not occurred after at least 1 year of engaging in unprotected coitus (Kumar et al., 2007). In *primary subfertility*, there have been no previous conceptions; in *secondary subfertility*, there has been a previous viable pregnancy but the couple is unable to conceive at present. **Sterility** is the inability to conceive because of a known condition, such as the absence of a uterus.

In about 40% of couples with a subfertility problem, the cause of subfertility is multifactorial; in about 30% of couples, it is the man who is subfertile. In women seen for a fertility concern, 20% to 25% experience ovulatory failure; another 20% experience tubal, vaginal, cervical, or uterine problems. In about 10% of couples, no known cause for the subfertility can be discovered despite all the diagnostic tests currently available. Such couples are categorized as having unexplained subfertility (Rybak & Wallach, 2007).

Some couples, because they are unaware of the average length of time it takes to achieve a pregnancy, may worry that they are subfertile when they are not. When engaging in coitus an average of four times per week, 50% of couples will conceive within 6 months, and 85% within 12 months. These periods will be longer if sexual relations are less frequent (Burney, Schust, & Yao, 2007).

Couples who engage in coitus daily, hoping to cause early impregnation, may actually have more difficulty conceiving than those who space coitus to every other day. This is because too-frequent coitus can lower a man's sperm count (number of sperm in a single ejaculation) to a level below optimal fertility. Also, couples who focus their sexual relations on trying to increase sperm/ovum exposure may find their lives governed by temperature charts and "good days" and "bad days" to such an extent that their relationship suffers.

The chance of subfertility increases with age. Because of this gradual decline in fertility, women who defer pregnancy to their late 30s are apt to have more difficulty conceiving than their younger counterparts. Women who are using oral, injectable, or implanted hormones for contraception may have difficulty becoming pregnant for several months after discontinuing these medications, because it takes that long for the body to restore normal functioning.

Male Subfertility Factors

Several factors typically lead to male subfertility:

- Disturbance in **spermatogenesis** (production of sperm cells)
- Obstruction in the seminiferous tubules, ducts, or vessels preventing movement of spermatozoa
- Qualitative or quantitative changes in the seminal fluid preventing **sperm motility** (movement of sperm)
- Development of autoimmunity that immobilizes sperm
- Problems in ejaculation or deposition preventing spermatozoa from being placed close enough to a woman's cervix to allow ready penetration and fertilization

Inadequate Sperm Count

The **sperm count** is the number of sperm in a single ejaculation or in a milliliter of semen (Kumar et al., 2007). The minimum sperm count considered normal is 20 million per milliliter of seminal fluid, or 50 million per ejaculation. At least 50% of sperm should be motile, and 30% should be normal in shape and form. Spermatozoa must be produced and maintained at a temperature slightly lower than body temperature to be fully motile. This is why the testes, in which sperm are produced and stored, are suspended in the scrotal sac away from body heat. Any condition that significantly increases body temperature such as a chronic infection from tuberculosis or recurrent sinusitis can lower a sperm count. Actions that increase scrotal heat, such as working at desk jobs or driving a great deal every day (e.g., salesmen, motorcyclists) may produce lower sperm counts compared with men whose occupations allow them to be ambulatory at least part of each day. Frequent use of hot tubs or saunas may also lower sperm counts appreciably.

Congenital abnormalities such as **cryptorchidism** (undescended testes) may lead to lowered sperm production if surgical repair of this problem was not completed until after puberty or if the spermatic cord became twisted after the surgery.

A worry is that a **varicocele** (varicosity of the spermatic vein) could increase temperature within the testes and slow and disrupt spermatogenesis although whether this actually causes much difference is in doubt (Evers & Collins, 2009). If this is happening, surgery to repair the varicocele has the potential to increase the chance for conception (Davis, Hall, & Kaufmann, 2007).

Other conditions that may inhibit sperm production are trauma to the testes; surgery on or near the testicles that results in impaired testicular circulation; and endocrine imbalances, particularly of the thyroid, pancreas, or pituitary glands. Drug use or excessive alcohol use and environmental factors such as exposure to x-rays or radioactive substances have also been found to negatively affect spermatogenesis. Men who are exposed to radioactive substances in their work environment should be provided adequate protection of the testes. When undergoing pelvic radiography, be certain that men and boys are always furnished with a protective lead testes shield.

Obstruction or Impaired Sperm Motility

Obstruction may occur at any point along the pathway that spermatozoa must travel to reach the outside: the seminiferous tubules, the epididymis, the vas deferens, the ejaculatory duct, or the urethra (see Chapter 5, Figure 5.2). Diseases such as *mumps orchitis* (testicular inflammation and scarring because of the mumps virus), epididymitis (inflammation of the epididymis), and tubal infections such as gonorrhea or ascending urethral infection can result in this type of obstruction because adhesions form and occlude sperm transport (Tracy, Steers, & Costabile, 2008). Congenital stricture of a spermatic duct may occasionally be seen. Benign hypertrophy of the prostate gland occurs in most men beginning at about 50 years of age. Pressure from the enlarged gland on the vas deferens can interfere with sperm transport. Infection of the prostate, through which the seminal fluid must pass, or infection of the seminal vesicles (spread from urinary tract infections) can change the composition of the seminal fluid enough to reduce sperm motility (Parsons, 2007).

A few men who have vasectomies develop an autoimmune reaction or form antibodies that immobilize their own sperm (Burney, Schust, & Yao, 2007). It is also conceivable that men with obstruction in the vas deferens from other causes, such as scarring after an infection, could also develop an autoimmune reaction that immobilizes sperm in the same way.

Anomalies of the penis, such as hypospadias (urethral opening on the ventral surface of the penis) or epispadias (urethral opening on the dorsal surface), can cause sperm to be deposited too far from the sexual partner's cervix to allow optimal cervical penetration. Extreme obesity in a male may also interfere with effective penetration and deposition.

Ejaculation Problems

Psychological problems, diseases such as a cerebrovascular accident, diabetes, or Parkinson's disease, and some medications (e.g., certain antihypertensive agents) may result in **erectile dysfunction** (formerly called impotence or the inability to achieve an erection). This condition is primary if the man has never been able to achieve erection and ejaculation and secondary if the man has been able to achieve ejaculation in the past but now has difficulty. Erectile dysfunction can be a difficult problem to solve if it is associated with stress, because this is not easily relieved. Solutions to the problem can include psychological or sexual counseling as well as use of a drug such as sildenafil (Viagra) (Wessells et al., 2007).

Premature ejaculation (ejaculation before penetration) is another factor that may interfere with the proper deposition of sperm. It is another problem often attributed to psychological causes. Adolescents may experience it until they become more experienced in sexual techniques.

✔ *Checkpoint Question 8.1*

The Carls are a couple undergoing testing for subfertility. Subfertility is said to exist when:

a. A couple has been trying to conceive for 1 year.
b. A woman has no children from a marriage.
c. A woman has no uterus or fallopian tubes.
d. A couple has wanted a child for over 6 months.

Female Subfertility Factors

The factors that cause subfertility in women are analogous to those causing subfertility in men: anovulation (faulty or inadequate production of ova), problems of ova transport through the fallopian tubes to the uterus, uterine factors such as tumors or poor endometrial development, and cervical and vaginal factors that immobilize spermatozoa (Kumar et al., 2007). In addition, nutrition, body weight, and exercise may be responsible.

Anovulation

Anovulation (absence of ovulation), the most common cause of subfertility in women, may occur from a genetic abnormality such as Turner's syndrome (hypogonadism) in which there are no ovaries to produce ova. More often it results from a hormonal imbalance caused by a condition such as hypothyroidism that interferes with hypothalamus-pituitary-ovarian interaction. Ovarian tumors may also produce anovulation because of feedback stimulation on the pituitary. Chronic or excessive exposure to x-rays or radioactive substances, general ill health, poor diet, and stress may all contribute to poor ovarian function.

Nutrition, body weight, and exercise all influence the blood glucose/insulin balance. When either glucose or insulin levels are too high, they can disrupt the production of follicle-stimulating hormone (FSH) and luteinizing hormone (LH) leading to subfertility from ovulation failure.

Women should try to maintain an ideal body weight and height, as represented by a body mass index (BMI) of 20 to 24 (Chavarro et al., 2007). This ideal BMI may also apply to men, as excessive weight may alter testosterone production and sperm production.

For nutrition, eating slowly digested carbohydrate foods such as brown rice, pasta, dark bread, beans, and fiber-rich vegetables rather than food such as white bread and cold breakfast cereals that have easily digested carbohydrates can not only increase fertility but perhaps prevent gestational diabetes when a woman does become pregnant.

Also important may be eating unsaturated fatty acids rather than saturated or trans-fatty acids. Trans-fatty acids are found in foods such as stick margarine, commercial French fries, and doughnuts. Saturated fats are those found in animal products such as cheese, meat, and butter. Unsaturated fats are those derived from plant sources such as corn or olive oil. Although eating adequate protein is important for fertility, excessive intake of protein may be yet another deterrent to fertility. To reduce a heavy protein intake, encourage women to eat plant sources of protein, such as soybeans, tofu, beans, or nuts rather than animal sources.

In addition to healthy eating habits, exercising 30 minutes a day by walking or doing mild aerobics can also help regulate blood glucose levels, thereby providing another way to increase fertility.

Stress reduces hypothalamic secretion of gonadotropin-releasing hormone (GnRH), which then lowers the production of LH and FSH, which leads to anovulation. Decreased body weight or a body/fat ratio of less than 10%, as may occur in female athletes (e.g., competitive runners) or in women who are excessively lean or anorexic, can reduce pituitary hormones such as FSH and LH and halt ovulation (termed hypogonadotrophic hypogonadism).

The most frequent cause, however, is naturally occurring variations in ovulatory patterns or polycystic ovary syndrome, a condition in which the ovaries produce excess testosterone, lowering FSH and LH levels. Polycystic ovary syndrome is associated with the metabolic syndrome (a waist circumference of 35 or above in women, a fasting blood glucose >100 mg/dL, serum triglycerides >150 mg/dL; blood pressure >135/85 mm Hg; and high-density lipoprotein cholesterol <50 mg/dL) (Vignesh & Mohan, 2007). The metabolic syndrome is associated with increased cardiac disease, so efforts to reduce weight and lower triglycerides and cholesterol can improve heart health as well as promote fertility.

Some women ovulate only a few times a year because of polycystic ovary syndrome. The condition can usually be detected by examining the menstrual history, but even if a woman experiences regular monthly menstruation, it does not necessarily indicate that she is ovulating on a regular basis (DuRant & Leslie, 2007).

Tubal Transport Problems

Difficulty with tubal transport usually occurs because scarring has developed in the fallopian tubes. This typically is caused by chronic salpingitis (chronic pelvic inflammatory disease). It can result from a ruptured appendix or from abdominal surgery involving infection that spread to the fallopian tubes and left adhesion formation in the tubes (Walker & Wiesenfeld, 2007). Tubal transport is the chief problem if a woman had a tubal ligation in years past but now wants to become pregnant.

Pelvic inflammatory disease (PID) is infection of the pelvic organs: the uterus, fallopian tubes, ovaries, and their supporting structures. The initial source of the infection is usually a sexually transmitted disease. In some women, infection can spread even further than reproductive organs or involve the pelvis, causing pelvic peritonitis. Many organisms can cause PID, but chlamydia and gonorrhea are among those most frequently seen. PID occurs at a rate of 25 per 100 women; in other words, one fourth of all women will experience this type of infection in a lifetime. About 12% of those who acquire PID are left subfertile (Burney, Schust, & Yao, 2007).

PID invasion of fallopian tubes is most apt to occur at the end of a menstrual period, because menstrual blood provides such an excellent growth medium. There also is loss of the normal cervical mucus barrier at this time, which increases the risk for initial invasion. If left unrecognized and untreated, PID enters a chronic phase, which causes the scarring that can lead to stricture of the fallopian tubes and the resulting fertility problem.

There is apparently a higher incidence of PID among women who use intrauterine devices (IUDs) although this may not bear out in practice (Campbell, Cropsey, & Matthews, 2007). It is good advice for women with IUDs to limit the number of their sexual partners to help reduce the incidence of sexually transmitted infections.

Uterine Problems

Tumors such as fibromas (leiomyomas) may be a rare cause of subfertility if they block the entrance of the fallopian tubes into the uterus or limit the space available on the uterine wall for effective implantation. A congenitally deformed uterine cavity may also limit implantation sites, but this also is rare.

Poor secretion of estrogen or progesterone from the ovary can result in inadequate endometrium formation (overproduction or underproduction), interfering with implantation and embryo growth. Endometriosis also can interfere with uterine fertility.

Endometriosis refers to the implantation of uterine endometrium, or nodules, that have spread from the interior of the uterus to locations outside the uterus (Yap, Furness, & Farquhar, 2007). The most common sites of endometrium spread include Douglas's cul-de-sac, the ovaries, the uterine ligaments, and the outer surface of the uterus and bowel (Fig. 8.1).

Some evidence of endometriosis occurs in as many as 50% of women, most probably from regurgitation through the fallopian tubes at the time of menstruation. Viable particles of endometrium that have been regurgitated in this way begin to proliferate and grow at the new sites, impeding fertility in a variety of ways. If growths occur in the fallopian tubes, tubal obstruction may result or adhesions forming from these growths may displace fallopian tubes away from the ovaries, preventing the entrance of ova into the tubes. Peritoneal macrophages that are drawn to these distant sites when the abnormal tissue is recognized can destroy sperm. The occurrence of endometriosis may indicate that the endometrial tissue has different or more friable qualities than usual (perhaps because of a luteal phase defect) and therefore is a type of endometrium that does not support embryo implantation as well as usual. Symptoms of endometriosis can begin in adolescence. The condition can be treated both medically and surgically (see Chapter 47).

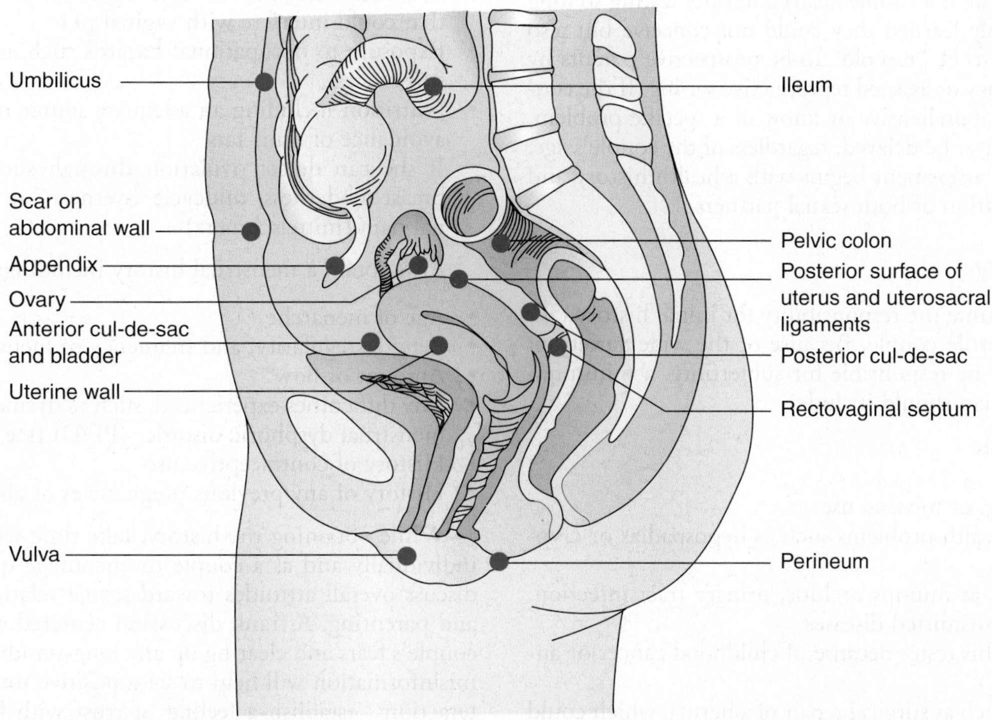

FIGURE 8.1 Common sites of endometriosis formation.

Cervical Problems

At the time of ovulation, the cervical mucus is thin and watery and can be easily penetrated by spermatozoa for a period of 12 to 72 hours. If coitus is not synchronized with this time period, the cervical mucus may be too thick to allow spermatozoa to penetrate the cervix. Infection or inflammation of the cervix (erosion) is another reason that cervical mucus can thicken so much that spermatozoa cannot penetrate it easily or survive in it. A stenotic cervical os or obstruction of the os by a polyp may further compromise sperm penetration. However, this is rarely enough of a problem to be the sole cause of subfertility. A woman who has undergone dilatation and curettage (D&C) procedures several times or cervical conization (cervical surgery) should be evaluated in light of the possibility that scar tissue and tightening of the cervical os has occurred.

Vaginal Problems

Infection of the vagina can cause the pH of the vaginal secretions to become acidotic, limiting or destroying the motility of spermatozoa. Some women appear to have sperm-immobilizing or sperm-agglutinating antibodies in their blood plasma that act to destroy sperm cells in the vagina or cervix. Either of these problems can limit the ability of sperm to survive in the vagina and enter the uterus.

Unexplained Subfertility

In a small proportion of couples, no known cause for subfertility can be discovered. Possibly the problems of either partner alone are not significant, but when these are combined they become sufficient to create subfertility. It is obviously discouraging for couples to complete a fertility evaluation and be told that their inability to conceive cannot be explained. Offer active support to help the couple find alternative solutions, such as continuing to try to conceive, using an assisted reproductive technique, choosing to adopt, or agreeing to a child-free life.

✔ Checkpoint Question 8.2

Cheryl Carl is diagnosed as having endometriosis. This condition interferes with fertility because:

a. The ovaries stop producing adequate estrogen.
b. The uterine cervix becomes inflamed and swollen.
c. Pressure on the pituitary leads to decreased FSH levels.
d. Endometrial implants can block the fallopian tubes.

FERTILITY ASSESSMENT

Not all couples who desire fertility testing want to have children immediately. Some just want to know for their own peace of mind that they are fertile. Others want to know that they are indeed subfertile, so that they can discontinue contraceptive measures (although they need to be cautioned to maintain safer sex practices).

The age of the couple and the degree of apprehension they feel about possible subfertility make a difference in determining when they should be referred for fertility evaluation. Although some health care plans or specific settings set limits on the age range in which fertility testing can be scheduled (e.g., not before age 18 years and not after age 45 years), other settings do not establish such limits, allowing couples of any age to benefit from assessment. As a rule, if a woman is younger than 35 years of age, it is usually suggested that she have an evaluation after 1 year of subfertility; if older than 35 years, after 6 months of subfertility. Referral is recommended sooner for older women because of possible age limitations associated with adoption, assisted reproductive strategies such as in vitro fertilization (IVF), and embryo transfer, common alternatives to natural childbearing. It would be doubly unfortunate if a couple delayed fertility testing so long that they not only learned they could not conceive but also were considered to be "too old" to be prospective parents by an adoption agency or assisted reproductive setting. If the couple is extremely apprehensive or know of a specific problem, studies should never be delayed, regardless of the couple's age.

Basic fertility assessment begins with a health history and physical examination of both sexual partners.

Health History

Nurses often assume the responsibility for initial history taking with a subfertile couple. Because of the wide variety of factors that may be responsible for subfertility, a minimum history for the man should include:

- General health
- Nutrition
- Alcohol, drug, or tobacco use
- Congenital health problems such as hypospadias or cryptorchidism
- Illnesses such as mumps orchitis, urinary tract infection, or sexually transmitted diseases
- Radiation to his testes because of childhood cancer or another cause
- Operations such as surgical repair of a hernia, which could have resulted in a blood compromise to the testes
- Current illnesses, particularly endocrine illnesses or low-grade infections
- Past and current occupation and work habits (e.g., does his job involve sitting at a desk all day or exposure to x-rays or other forms of radiation?)
- Sexual practices such as the frequency of coitus and masturbation, failure to achieve ejaculation, premature ejaculation, coital positions used, and use of lubricants
- Past contraceptive measures, and existence of any children produced from a previous relationship
- Any complementary alternative therapy such as herbal additives the couple is using

Asking about alternative therapy is important because a couple who wants to have a child could be investigating nontraditional as well as traditional methods that they believe will aid in conception. Acupuncture, for example, is an alternative method frequently seen (Anderson et al., 2007). Ask about herbs specifically to be certain that a couple is not using an herb that could possibly be causing subfertility or will interfere with any procedure or medication prescribed for them after their subfertility investigation.

Most couples assume that subfertility is the woman's problem. Many women, even after careful explanation that the problem is their male partner's and not theirs, continue to show low self-esteem, as if the fault did rest with them. For a thorough women's health history, ask about:

- Current or past reproductive tract problems, such as infections
- Overall health, emphasizing endocrine problems such as galactorrhea (breast nipple secretions) or symptoms of thyroid dysfunction
- Abdominal or pelvic operations that could have compromised blood flow to pelvic organs
- Past history of a childhood cancer treated with radiation that might have reduced ovarian function
- The use of douches or intravaginal medications or sprays that could interfere with vaginal pH
- Exposure to occupational hazards such as x-rays or toxic substances
- Nutrition including an adequate source of folic acid and avoidance of trans-fats
- If she can detect ovulation through such symptoms as breast tenderness, midcycle "wetness," or lower abdominal pain (mittelschmerz)

Also obtain a menstrual history including:

- Age of menarche
- Length, regularity, and frequency of menstrual periods
- Amount of flow
- Any difficulties experienced, such as dysmenorrhea or premenstrual dysphoric disorder (PDD) (see Chapter 47)
- History of contraceptive use
- History of any previous pregnancies or abortions

While obtaining the history, take time with each partner individually and as a couple to encourage questions and to discuss overall attitudes toward sexual relations, pregnancy, and parenting. A frank discussion centered on resolving the couple's fears and clearing up any long-standing confusion or misinformation will help to set a positive tone for future interactions, establish a feeling of trust with health care personnel, and increase self-esteem. Talking with both partners

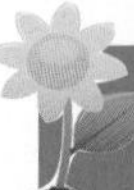

BOX 8.2 * Focus on Communication

Cheryl Carl has been trying to get pregnant for 4 years. She and her husband agreed to in vitro fertilization at a cost of approximately $10,000 per month, even though her religion does not approve of this technique. Every time you see her at the fertility clinic, she seems sadder than the previous time.

Less Effective Communication

Nurse: How is everything going, Mrs. Carl?
Mrs. Carl: Fine. I'm just tired of no results.
Nurse: You know that's partly your fault, Mrs. Carl. You waited 4 years before you came for an evaluation.
Mrs. Carl: I guess I don't make good decisions. I'll probably make a lousy parent if I ever do get pregnant.

More Effective Communication

Nurse: How is everything going, Mrs. Carl?
Mrs. Carl: Fine. I'm just tired of no results.
Nurse: Considering that you have been trying for such a long time, I think you're doing very well. Subfertility management is always difficult.
Mrs. Carl: It is, but practicing to be patient should stand me in good stead the day I do have a child.

Clients may not make the same choices about fertility testing or management that you might make because such decisions are based on individual circumstances and situations. Be careful not to criticize clients for making choices that you think are poor ones. A more effective technique is to support them at that point and help them find ways to continue to feel good about themselves to maintain self-esteem.

can also help them clarify their feelings about subfertility and why they are seeking help in this area (Box 8.2).

Obtaining a sexual history is often difficult because cultural taboos can make couples feel uncomfortable discussing this part of their life. Simple factors, such as how often couples engage in sexual relations, for example, are influenced by culture and religion. According to Orthodox Jewish law, a couple may not engage in sexual relations for 7 days following menstruation (the *nida* period). This practice can result in fertility problems if a woman ovulates within the 7-day period. Some cultures forbid therapeutic insemination because preserving male lineage is so important. Being aware of cultural differences this way can influence how a couple reacts to a diagnosis of subfertility and help you appreciate the meaning of this diagnosis to an individual couple.

Physical Assessment

After a thorough history, both men and women need a complete physical examination. For the man, important aspects of this are detection of the presence of secondary sexual characteristics and genital abnormalities, such as the absence of a vas deferens or the presence of undescended testes or a varicocele (enlargement of a testicular vein). The presence of a hydrocele (collection of fluid in the tunica vaginalis of the scrotum) is rarely associated with subfertility but should be documented if present.

For a woman, a thorough physical assessment including breast and thyroid examination is necessary to rule out current illness. Of particular importance are secondary sex characteristics, which indicate maturity and good pituitary function (see Chapter 33 for a discussion of Tanner stages). A complete pelvic examination including a Pap test (see Chapter 11) is needed to rule out anatomic disorders and infection.

Fertility Testing

Basic fertility testing involves only three tests: semen analysis in the male and ovulation monitoring and tubal patency assessment in the female. Nurses play key roles in preparing couples for these tests, helping them schedule the studies appropriately, and supporting them while they wait for results.

Additional testing for men, if warranted, can include urinalysis; a complete blood count; blood typing, including Rh factor; a serologic test for syphilis; a test for the presence of human immunodeficiency virus (HIV); erythrocyte sedimentation rate (an increased rate indicates inflammation); protein-bound iodine (a test for thyroid function); cholesterol level (arterial plaques could interfere with pelvic blood flow); and gonadotropin and testosterone levels.

Advanced testing for a woman may include a rubella titer, a serologic test for syphilis, and an HIV evaluation. If a woman has symptoms of thyroid dysfunction, a thyroid uptake determination and thyroid-stimulating hormone level may be ordered. If a woman has a history of menstrual irregularities, blood may be assayed for FSH, estrogen, LH, and progesterone levels. If a woman has a history of galactorrhea, a serum prolactin level will be obtained. A pelvic ultrasound may be performed to rule out ovarian, tubal, or uterine structural disorders.

Semen Analysis

For a semen analysis, after 2 to 4 days of sexual abstinence, the man ejaculates by masturbation into a clean, dry specimen jar. The number of sperm in the specimen are counted and then examined under a microscope within 1 hour (Box 8.3). An average ejaculation should produce 2.5 to 5.0 mL of semen and should contain a minimum of 20 million spermatozoa per milliliter of fluid (the average normal sperm count is 50 to 200 million per milliliter). The analysis may need to be repeated after 2 or 3 months, because spermatogenesis is an ongoing process, and 30 to 90 days is needed for new sperm to reach maturity (Anderson & Genadry, 2007). Men can test their sperm motility at home with a self-test kit (Fertell) (Milkin, 2007).

Sperm Penetration Assay and Antisperm Antibody Testing

For impregnation to take place, sperm must be motile enough to navigate the vagina, uterus, and a fallopian tube to reach the ova. Although sperm penetration studies are rarely necessary, they may be scheduled to determine whether a man's sperm, once they reach an ovum, can penetrate it

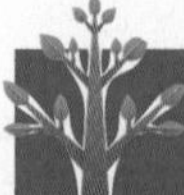

BOX 8.3 ✻ Focus on Family Teaching

Tips for Ensuring an Accurate Semen Analysis

Q. Bob Carl asks you, "What can I do to make sure that the analysis of my semen sample is as accurate as possible?"

A. When obtaining a semen sample for analysis:

- Use a clean, dry plastic or glass container with a secure lid to collect the sample.
- Collect the specimen as close as possible to your usual schedule of sexual activity.
- Avoid using any lubricants when you collect the specimen.
- After you have collected the specimen in the container, close it securely and write down the time you collected it.
- Keep the specimen at body temperature while transporting it. Carrying it next to your chest is one way to do this.
- Take the specimen to the laboratory or health care provider's office immediately so it can be analyzed within 1 hour of collection.

effectively. With the use of an assisted reproductive technique such as IVF, poorly motile sperm or those with poor penetration can be injected directly into a woman's ovum under laboratory conditions (intracytoplasmic sperm injection), bypassing the need for sperm to be fully motile.

Ovulation Monitoring

The least costly way to determine a woman's ovulation pattern is to ask her to record her basal body temperature (BBT) for at least 4 months. To determine this, a woman takes her temperature each morning, before getting out of bed or engaging in any activity, eating, or drinking, using a special BBT or tympanic thermometer. She plots this daily temperature on a monthly graph, noticing conditions that might affect her temperature (e.g., colds, other infections, sleeplessness). At the time of ovulation, the basal temperature can be seen to dip slightly (about 0.5° F); it then rises to a level no higher than normal body temperature and remains at that level until 3 or 4 days before the next menstrual flow. This increase in BBT marks the time of ovulation, because it occurs immediately after ovulation (actually at the beginning of the luteal phase of the menstrual cycle, which can occur only if ovulation occurred). A temperature rise should last approximately 10 days. If it does not, a luteal phase defect is suggested (i.e., progesterone production begins but is not sustained). Typical graphs of BBT are shown in Figure 8.2.

What if... Cheryl Carl tells you that she works nights as a cocktail waitress, goes to bed at 4 AM, then wakes at 6 AM to drive her husband to work? Starting at noon, she sleeps for 4 or 5 hours before getting up to go to work. When during the day should she record her basal body temperature?

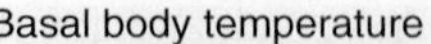

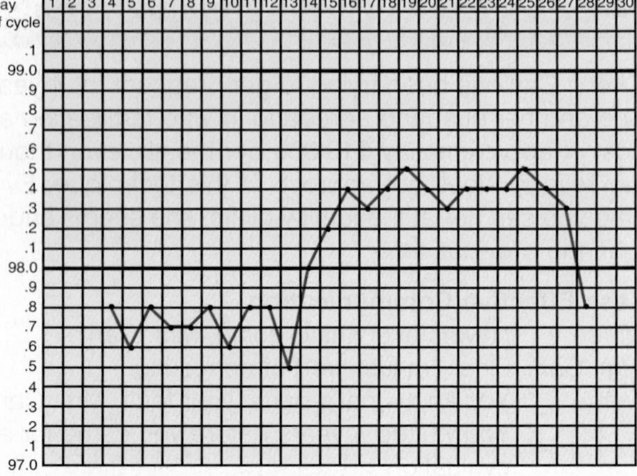

A Ovulation without conception

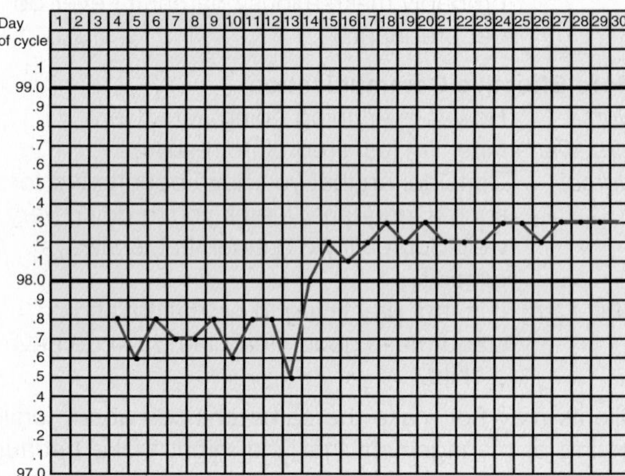

B Ovulation with conception

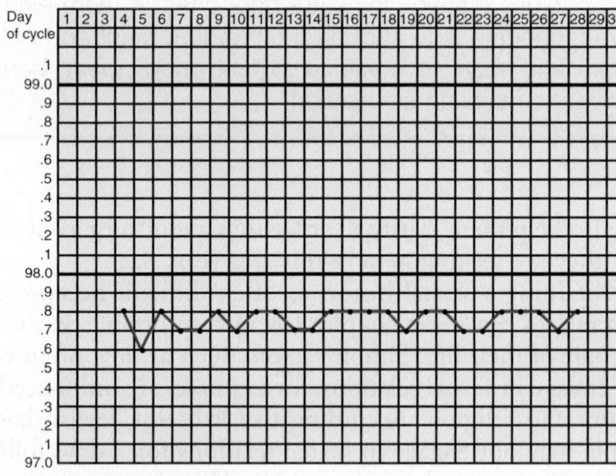

C Anovulatory cycle

FIGURE 8.2 Basal body temperature graph. (**A**) A woman's temperature dips slightly at midpoint in the menstrual cycle, then rises sharply, an indication of ovulation. Toward the end of the cycle (the 24th day), her temperature begins to decline, indicating that progesterone levels are falling or that she did not conceive. (**B**) A woman's temperature rises at the midpoint in the cycle and remains at that elevated level past the time of her normal menstrual flow, suggesting that pregnancy has occurred. (**C**) There is no preovulatory dip, and no rise of temperature anywhere during the cycle. This is the typical pattern of a woman who does not ovulate.

Ovulation Determination by Test Strip

Various brands of commercial kits are available for assessing the upsurge of LH that occurs just before ovulation. These can be used in place of BBT monitoring. A woman dips a test strip into a midmorning urine specimen and then compares it with the kit instructions for a color change. Such kits are purchased over the counter, are easy to use, and have the advantage of marking the point just before ovulation occurs rather than just after ovulation, as is the case with BBT. They are not as economical as simple temperature recording, but they are advantageous for women with irregular work or daily activity schedules (e.g., working the night shift, arising at varying times in the morning), which can make BBT measurements inaccurate.

Another type of testing kit (Fertell) contains both materials to test FSH the third day of a woman's menstrual cycle (an abnormally high level is an indicator that her ovaries are not responding well to ovulation) and a sperm motility test for the male (Milkin, 2007). The woman's result is available in 30 minutes, the man's in 90 minutes. The kits are expensive but can be helpful to a couple as a first step in fertility testing. Be certain a woman realizes this is not a test of her time of ovulation but a test of whether she has adequate FSH to stimulate egg growth, so she does not use the test at the midpoint of her menstrual cycle.

Tubal Patency

Both ultrasound and x-ray imaging can be used to determine the patency of fallopian tubes and assess the depth and consistency of the endometrial lining.

Sonohysterography. Sonohysterography is an ultrasound technique designed for inspecting the uterus. The uterus is filled with sterile saline, introduced through a narrow catheter inserted into the uterine cervix. A transvaginal ultrasound transducer is then inserted into the vagina to inspect the uterus for abnormalities such as septal deviation or the presence of a myoma. Because this is a minimally invasive technique, it can be done at any time during the menstrual cycle.

Hysterosalpingography. Hysterosalpingography (uterosalpingography), a radiologic examination of the fallopian tubes using a radiopaque medium, is a second frequently used technique. The procedure is scheduled immediately after a menstrual flow to avoid reflux of menstrual debris up the tubes and unintentional irradiation of a growing zygote. It is contraindicated if infection of the vagina, cervix, or uterus is present (infectious organisms might be forced into the pelvic cavity). For the procedure, iodine-based radiopaque material is introduced into the cervix under pressure (Fig. 8.3). The radiopaque material outlines the uterus and both tubes, provided that the tubes are patent. Because the medium is thick, it distends the uterus and tubes slightly, causing momentary painful uterine cramping. After the study, the contrast medium drains out through the vagina. The instillation of radiopaque material can be therapeutic as well as diagnostic: the pressure of the solution may actually break up adhesions as it passes through the fallopian tubes, thereby increasing their patency (Johnson et al., 2009). Although extremely rare, the procedure carries a small risk of infection, allergic reaction to the contrast medium, or embolism from dye entering a uterine blood vessel.

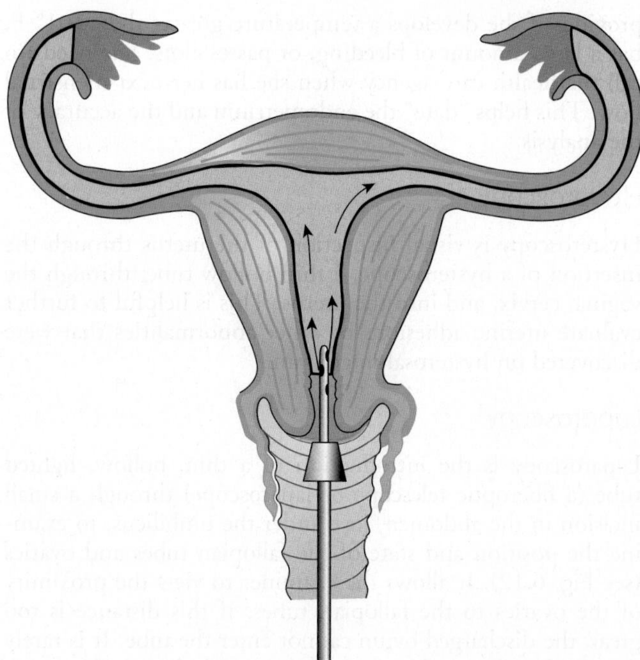

FIGURE 8.3 Insertion of dye for a hysterosalpingogram. The contrast dye outlines the uterus and fallopian tubes on radiographs to demonstrate patency.

Advanced Surgical Procedures

If common assessments do not reveal the cause of subfertility, several surgical procedures may be scheduled.

Uterine Endometrial Biopsy

Uterine endometrial biopsy may be used to reveal an endometrial problem such as a luteal phase defect. If the endometrium removed by biopsy resembles a corkscrew (a typical progesterone-dominated endometrium) in the second half of a menstrual cycle, this suggests that ovulation has occurred. Endometrial biopsies are being performed less commonly than previously, having been replaced with serum progesterone level evaluations that also suggest that ovulation occurred.

Endometrial biopsies are done 2 or 3 days before an expected menstrual flow (day 25 or 26 of a typical 28-day menstrual cycle). After a paracervical block, a thin probe and biopsy forceps are introduced through the cervix. A woman may experience mild to moderate discomfort from the maneuvering of the instruments. There may be a moment of sharp pain as the biopsy specimen is taken from the anterior or posterior uterine wall. Possible complications include pain, excessive bleeding, infection, and uterine perforation. This procedure is contraindicated if pregnancy is suspected (although the chance that it would interfere with a pregnancy is probably less than 10%) or if an infection such as acute PID or cervicitis is present. Caution a woman that she might notice a small amount of vaginal spotting after the procedure. For follow-up, she needs to call her primary care provider if she develops a temperature greater than 101° F, has a large amount of bleeding, or passes clots. She needs to call the health care agency when she has her next menstrual flow. This helps "date" the endometrium and the accuracy of the analysis.

Hysteroscopy

Hysteroscopy is visual inspection of the uterus through the insertion of a hysteroscope, a thin hollow tube, through the vagina, cervix, and into the uterus. This is helpful to further evaluate uterine adhesions or other abnormalities that were discovered on hysterosalpingogram.

Laparoscopy

Laparoscopy is the introduction of a thin, hollow, lighted tube (a fiberoptic telescope or laparoscope) through a small incision in the abdomen, just under the umbilicus, to examine the position and state of the fallopian tubes and ovaries (see Fig. 6.12). It allows the examiner to view the proximity of the ovaries to the fallopian tubes. If this distance is too great, the discharged ovum cannot enter the tube. It is rarely done unless the results of uterosalpingography are abnormal. It is scheduled during the follicular phase of a menstrual period and is done under general anesthesia because of the pain caused by extensive maneuvering. This also allows for good relaxation and a steep Trendelenburg position (which brings the reproductive organs down out of the pelvis). Carbon dioxide is introduced into the abdomen to move the abdominal wall outward and offer better visualization. Women may feel bloating of the abdomen from the infusion of the CO_2 after such a procedure. If some CO_2 escapes under the diaphragm, there may be extremely sharp shoulder pain from pressure.

During the procedure, dye can be injected into the uterus through a polyethylene cannula placed in the cervix to assess tubal patency. Tubes are patent if the dye appears in the abdominal cavity. A scope may be passed directly into a fallopian tube to reveal information about the presence and condition of the fimbria and endometrium lining the tube. If the fimbria have been destroyed by PID, the chance for a normal conception is in doubt, because ova seem to be unable to enter a tube if fimbrial currents are absent.

✓ Checkpoint Question 8.3

Cheryl Carl is scheduled to have a hysterosalpingogram. Which of the following instructions would you give her regarding this procedure?

a. She may feel some mild cramping when the dye is inserted.
b. The ultrasound of the uterus will reveal any tumors present.
c. She will not be able to conceive for 3 months after the procedure.
d. Many women experience mild bleeding as an after effect.

SUBFERTILITY MANAGEMENT

Management of subfertility focuses on correction of any underlying problem that was discovered during assessment. All couples can benefit from some practical information on how to increase the chances of achieving conception on their own (Box 8.4).

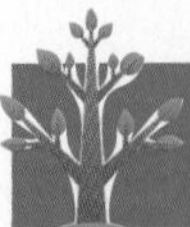

BOX 8.4 ✻ Focus on Family Teaching

Suggestions to Aid Conception

Q. Cheryl Carl asks, "Is there anything we can do to help increase our chances for conception?"

A. The following are time-honored suggestions to help aid conception:

- Determine the time of ovulation through the use of basal body temperature, analysis of cervical secretions, or a commercial ovulation determination kit, then plan sexual relations for every other day around the time of ovulation.
- Although frequent intercourse may stimulate sperm production, men need sperm recovery time after ejaculation to maintain an adequate sperm count. This is why coitus every other day, rather than every day, during the fertile period will probably yield faster results.
- The male-superior position is the best position for intercourse to achieve conception because it places sperm closest to the cervical opening.
- The male should try for deep penetration so ejaculation places sperm as close as possible to the cervix. Elevating a woman's hips on a small pillow can facilitate sperm collection near the opening to the cervix.
- A woman should remain on her back with knees drawn up for at least 20 minutes after ejaculation to help sperm remain near the cervix.
- Do not use douching or lubricants before or after intercourse so vaginal pH is unaltered, which could interfere with sperm motility.
- Eat a diet high in slowly digested carbohydrates, low in saturated or trans-fatty acids, and moderate in protein.
- Maintain a body weight that results in a body mass index between 20 and 24.
- Exercise about 30 minutes a day to help keep blood glucose and insulin levels stabilized.
- Choose a new activity the two of you can do together, such as learning how to bowl or ballroom dance, so you create an activity separate from planning a baby. This can help to pass the time in a positive way and also offer a positive outlook for a month when you do not conceive.

Correction of the Underlying Problem

Such underlying causes as chronic disease, inadequate hormone production, endometriosis, or infection need to be treated. If correction of these problems does not yield success, subfertility management focuses on achieving conception through an assisted reproductive technology such as IVF or sperm donation.

Increasing Sperm Count and Motility

If sperm are not motile because the vas deferens is obstructed, the obstruction is most likely to be extensive and difficult to relieve by surgery. If sperm are present but the total count is low, a man may be advised to abstain from coitus for 7 to 10 days at a time to increase the count.

Ligation of a varicocele (if present) and changes in lifestyle (e.g., wearing looser clothing, avoiding long periods of sitting, avoiding prolonged hot baths) may be helpful to reduce scrotal heat and increase the sperm count.

Sperm can be extracted by syringe from a point proximal to vas deferens blockage and used for intrauterine insemination (Verhulst et al., 2009). If the problem appears to be that sperm are immobilized by vaginal secretions because of an immunologic factor, the response can be reduced by abstinence or condom use for about 6 months. However, to avoid this prolonged time interval, washing of the sperm and intrauterine insemination may be preferred. The administration of corticosteroids to a woman may have some effect in decreasing sperm immobilization because it reduces her immune response and antibody production.

Reducing the Presence of Infection

If a vaginal infection is present, the infection will be treated according to the causative organism based on culture reports (see Chapter 47). Vaginal infections such as trichomoniasis and moniliasis tend to recur, requiring close supervision and follow-up. The possibility that the sexual partner is reinfecting a woman needs to be considered. Caution women who are prescribed metronidazole (Flagyl) for a trichomonal infection that it can be teratogenic early in pregnancy and therefore should not be continued if a pregnancy is suspected (Karch, 2009).

Hormone Therapy

If the problem appears to be a disturbance of ovulation, administration of GnRH is a possibility. Therapy with clomiphene citrate (Clomid, Serophene) may also be used to stimulate ovulation (Box 8.5). In other women, ovarian follicular growth can be stimulated by the administration of human menopausal gonadotropins (Pergonal), combinations of FSH and LH derived from postmenopausal urine in conjunction with administration of human chorionic gonadotropin (hCG) to produce ovulation. If increased prolactin levels are identified, bromocriptine (Parlodel) is added to the medication regimen to reduce prolactin levels and allow for the rise of gonadotropins (Karch, 2009).

Administration of either clomiphene citrate or human menopausal gonadotropins may overstimulate an ovary, causing multiple ova to come to maturity and possibly resulting in multiple births. Counsel women who receive these agents that this is a possibility. If sperm do not appear to survive in vaginal secretions because secretions are too scant or tenacious, a woman may be prescribed low-dose estrogen therapy to increase mucus production during days 5 to 10 of her cycle. Conjugated estrogen (Premarin) is a type of estrogen prescribed for this purpose.

If the problem appears to be a luteal phase defect, this can be corrected by progesterone vaginal suppositories begun on the third day of the temperature rise and continued for the next 6 weeks (if pregnancy occurs) or until a menstrual flow begins.

Surgery

Fallopian tubes that have been ligated can be reopened surgically but the success of the operation is not greater than 70% to 80%. Also, the irregular line left by the surgery may result in an ectopic pregnancy (a tubal pregnancy) if a fertilized ovum is stopped at the irregular point (Ahmad et al., 2009). Intrauterine insemination is more commonly used today and more apt to result in a viable pregnancy.

If a myoma (fibroid tumor) is interfering with fertility, a myomectomy, or surgical removal of the tumor, can be scheduled (Griffiths, D'Angelo, & Amso, 2009). Myomectomy can be done via a hysteroscopic ambulatory procedure if the growth is small. Uterine adhesions may also be lysed by hysteroscopy. After this procedure, a woman is prescribed estrogen for 3 months to prevent adhesions from reforming and an IUD may be inserted to help prevent the uterine sides from touching. This treatment can be difficult for a woman to accept, because preventing pregnancy (using an IUD) is exactly what she does not want to do.

For problems of abnormal uterine formation, such as a septate uterus, surgery is also available. However, these defects are usually related to early pregnancy loss, not subfertility.

BOX 8.5 * Focus on Pharmacology

Clomiphene Citrate (Clomid)

Action: Clomiphene citrate (Clomid) is an estrogen agonist used to stimulate the ovary. The drug binds to estrogen receptors, decreasing the number of available estrogen receptors and falsely signaling the hypothalamus to increase FSH and LH secretion. This results in ovulation (Hughes, 2009).

Pregnancy category: X

Dosage: Initially, 50 mg/day orally for 5 days (started anytime if no uterine bleeding has occurred recently or about the fifth day of the cycle if uterine bleeding occurs). If ovulation does not occur, this can be followed by 100 mg/day for 5 days started as early as 30 days after the initial course of therapy. This second course may be repeated one more time.

Possible adverse effects: Abdominal discomfort, distention, bloating, nausea, vomiting, breast tenderness, vasomotor flushing, ovarian enlargement, ovarian overstimulation, multiple births, visual disturbances.

Nursing Implications

- Ensure that women have had a pelvic examination and baseline hormonal studies before therapy.
- Review medication scheduling. Urge women to use a calendar to mark their treatment schedule and plot ovulation. Remind clients that timing intercourse with ovulation is important for achieving pregnancy.
- Advise clients that 24-hour urine samples may be necessary periodically.
- Caution clients to report any bloating, stomach pain, blurred vision, unusual bleeding, bruising, or visual changes.
- Inform clients that therapy can be repeated for a total of three courses; if no results are obtained, therapy will be discontinued at that point.

If the problem is tubal insufficiency from inflammation, diathermy or steroid administration may be helpful in reducing adhesions. Hysterosalpingography can be repeated to determine whether these produce a therapeutic effect. Canalization of the fallopian tubes and plastic surgical repair (microsurgery) are possible treatments. If peritoneal adhesions or nodules of endometriosis are holding the tubes fixed and away from the ovaries, these can be removed by laparoscopy or laser surgery (Jacobson et al., 2007). Additional hormonal therapy for endometriosis is discussed in Chapter 47.

Assisted Reproductive Techniques

If ovulation, sperm production, or sperm motility problems cannot be corrected, assisted reproductive strategies are the next step.

Therapeutic Insemination

Therapeutic insemination is the instillation of sperm into the female reproductive tract to aid conception (Burney, Schust, & Yao, 2007). The sperm is instilled into the cervix (intracervical insemination) or directly into the uterus (intrauterine insemination). Either the husband's sperm (therapeutic insemination by husband) or donor sperm (therapeutic insemination by donor or therapeutic donor insemination) can be used. Therapeutic insemination is used if the man has an inadequate sperm count or a woman has a vaginal or cervical factor that interferes with sperm motility. Donor insemination can be used if the man has a known genetic disorder that he does not want transmitted to children or if a woman has no male partner. It is a useful procedure for men who, feeling their family was complete, underwent a vasectomy but now wish to have children. In the past, men who underwent chemotherapy or radiation for testicular cancer had to accept being child-free afterward as they were no longer able to produce sperm. Today, sperm can be cryopreserved (frozen) in a sperm bank before radiation or chemotherapy and then used for insemination afterward (Bashore, 2007).

One disadvantage of using frozen sperm is that it tends to have slower motility than unfrozen specimens. However, although the rate of conception may be lower from this source, there appears to be no increase in the incidence of congenital anomalies in children conceived by this method. An advantage of cryopreserved sperm is that it can be used even after years of storage.

What if... Bob Carl has some sperm cryopreserved so that Cheryl could become pregnant, but he and Cheryl divorce before it is used? To whom would the cryopreserved sperm belong at that point?

To prepare for therapeutic insemination, a woman must record her BBT, assess her cervical mucus, or use an ovulation predictor kit to predict her likely day of ovulation. On the day after ovulation, the selected sperm are instilled into her cervix using a device similar to a cervical cap or diaphragm, or they are injected directly into the uterus using a flexible catheter (Fig. 8.4).

If therapeutic donor insemination is selected, the donors are volunteers who have no history of disease and no family history of possible inheritable disorders. The blood type, or at least the Rh factor, can be matched with the woman's to prevent incompatibility. Sperm from sperm banks can be selected according to desired physical or mental characteristics.

Some couples have religious or ethical beliefs that prohibit them from using therapeutic insemination. Some states have specific laws regarding inheritance, child support, and responsibility concerning children conceived by therapeutic insemination. In addition, because therapeutic insemination takes an average of 6 months to achieve conception, it may be a discouraging process for couples to have to wait this long to see results.

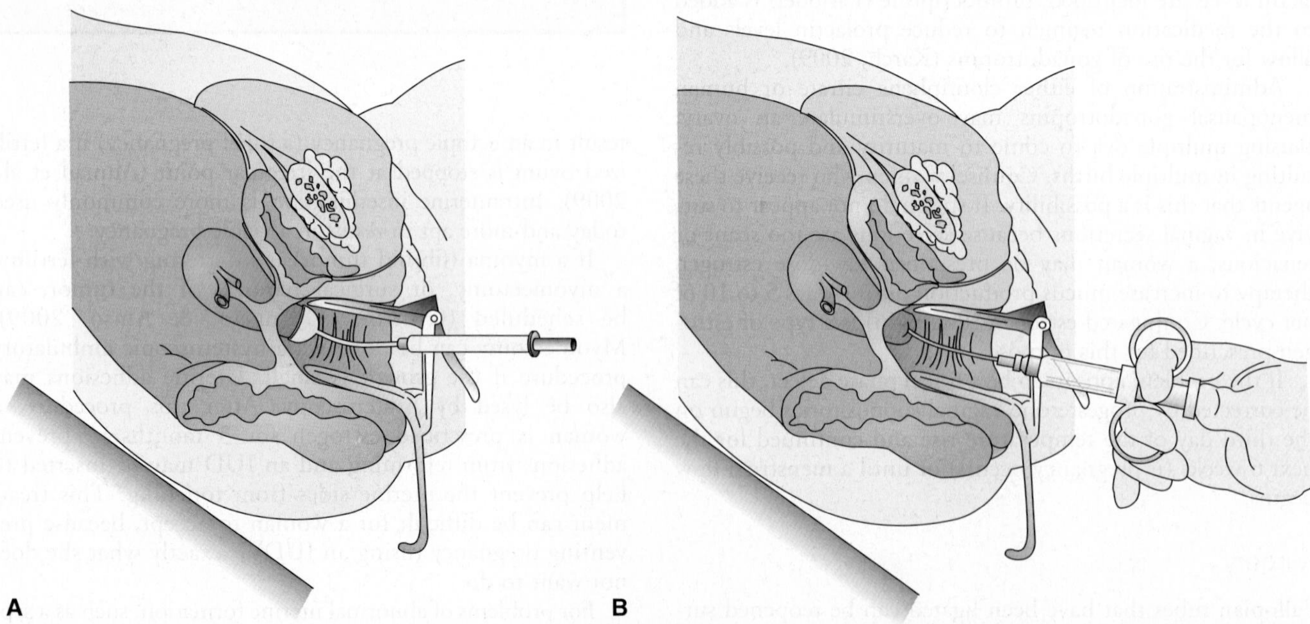

FIGURE 8.4 Therapeutic insemination. Sperm are deposited next to the cervix (**A**) or injected directly into the uterine cavity (**B**).

✔Checkpoint Question 8.4

Bob Carl asks you what therapeutic insemination by donor entails. Which would be your best answer?

a. Therapeutic sperm are injected vaginally to test tubal patency.
b. Donor sperm are introduced vaginally into the uterus or cervix.
c. The husband's sperm is administered intravenously weekly.
d. Donor sperm are injected intra-abdominally into each ovary.

In Vitro Fertilization

In IVF, one or more mature oocytes are removed from a woman's ovary by laparoscopy and fertilized by exposure to sperm under laboratory conditions outside a woman's body. About 40 hours after fertilization, the laboratory-grown fertilized ova are inserted into a woman's uterus, where ideally one or more of them will implant and grow (Van Voorhis, 2007).

IVF is most often used for couples who have not been able to conceive because a woman has blocked or damaged fallopian tubes. It is also used when the man has oligospermia or a very low sperm count, because the controlled, concentrated conditions in the laboratory require only one sperm. IVF may be helpful to couples when an absence of cervical mucus prevents sperm from traveling to or entering the cervix, or antisperm antibodies cause immobilization of sperm. In addition, couples with unexplained subfertility of long duration may be helped by IVF.

A donor ovum, rather than a woman's own ovum, also can be used for a woman who does not ovulate or who carries a sex-linked disease that she does not want to pass on to her children.

Before the procedure, a woman is given an ovulation-stimulating agent such as GnRH, clomiphene citrate (Clomid), or human menopausal gonadotropin (Pergonal). Beginning about the 10th day of the menstrual cycle, the ovaries are examined daily by ultrasound to assess the number and size of developing ovarian follicles. When a follicle appears to be mature, a woman is given an injection of hCG, which causes ovulation in 38 to 42 hours.

A needle is then introduced intravaginally, guided by ultrasound, and the oocyte is aspirated from its follicle. Because of the drugs given to induce ova maturation, many oocytes may ripen at once, and perhaps as many as 3 to 12 can be removed. The oocytes are incubated for at least 8 hours to ensure viability. In the meantime, the husband or donor supplies a fresh semen specimen. The sperm cells and oocytes are mixed and allowed to incubate in a growth medium. Genetic analysis to reveal chromosomal abnormalities or the potential sex can be completed at this point.

In the past, many sperm were necessary even under laboratory conditions to allow sperm to make their way through the resistant zona pellucida surrounding the ovum. Several techniques, such as creating passages through the resistant cells (zona drilling), have been discovered to help sperm cross the zona. In some instances, it has been possible to inject sperm directly under the zona pellucida (intracytoplasmic sperm injection). This is the technique that makes it possible for fertilization to take place with only one sperm. Worry that this technique could lead to an increased number of birth defects is unproven (Van Voorhis, 2007).

After fertilization of the chosen oocytes occurs, the zygotes formed almost immediately begin to divide and grow. By 40 hours after fertilization, they will have undergone their first cell division. In the past, multiple eggs were chosen and implanted to ensure a pregnancy resulted but this technique also resulted in many multiple births. Newborns from multiple births have a much lower chance of surviving the neonatal period than others. For that reason, today, only one or two fertilized eggs are chosen and transferred back to the uterine cavity through the cervix by means of a thin catheter (Van Voorhis, 2007) (Fig. 8.5).

If the couple desires, any eggs not used can be frozen for use at a later time. As with sperm cryopreservation, egg cryopreservation presents a range of ethical and religious dilemmas regarding who would "own" them if the couple should divorce; as well as whether the eggs should be saved, donated, or discarded.

A lack of progesterone can occur if the corpus luteum was injured by the aspiration of the follicle. Therefore, progesterone may be given to a woman if it is believed that she will not produce enough on her own to support implantation. Proof that the zygote has implanted can be demonstrated by a routine serum pregnancy test as early as 11 days after transfer.

In some centers, nurse practitioners are the health care providers who complete oocyte removal and transfer. In all

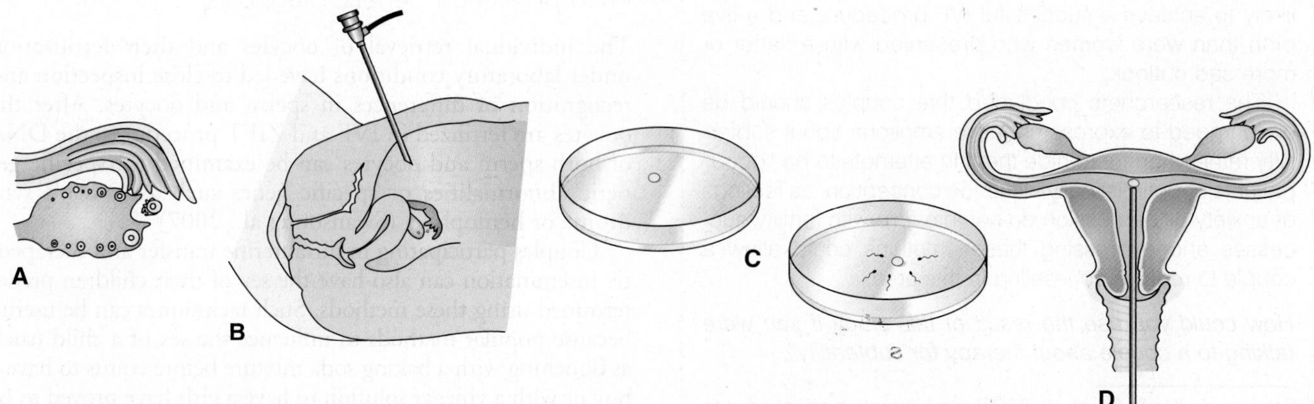

FIGURE 8.5 Steps involved with in vitro fertilization. (**A**) Ovulation. (**B**) Capture of ova (done here intra-abdominally). (**C**) Fertilization of ova and growth in culture medium. (**D**) Insertion of fertilized ova into uterus.

centers, nurses need to supply support and counseling to sustain the couple through the process. The recovery rate for harvesting ripened eggs is high (about 90%), as is the ability to fertilize eggs by sperm in vitro. The overall pregnancy rate by IVF is as low as 38% to 42% per treatment cycle, however (Van Voorhis, 2007). Although IVF programs do not result in an increase in birth defects, about 25% of pregnancies end in spontaneous abortion (the same rate as for natural pregnancies). Once a pregnancy has been successfully established, a woman's prenatal care is the same as that for any pregnancy. Research has shown that, because the couple was so committed to the procedure, they adjust to pregnancy and parenthood well.

If an ultrasound reveals that a multiple pregnancy of more than two zygotes has been achieved, selective termination of gestational sacs until only two are remaining may be recommended. This is done by intra-abdominal injection of potassium chloride into the gestational sacs chosen to be eliminated. Reducing the number of growing embryos to a number a woman can expect to carry to term without difficulty helps to ensure the success of the pregnancy.

IVF is expensive (about $10,000 per cycle) and is available only at specialized centers. There is a risk of maternal infection if bacteria are introduced at any point in the transfer. Waiting to be accepted by a center's program and waiting for the steps of obtaining the oocyte, laboratory growth, and pregnancy success is a major psychological strain (Box 8.6). Couples report a feeling of social isolation during this time and weariness answering friends' and family's questions about the procedure. Supply empathic support through this difficult time (see Focus on Nursing Care Planning Box 8.7).

BOX 8.6 ✻ Focus on Evidence-Based Practice

Does a woman's emotional attitude affect her chance for success with in vitro fertilization?

Because subfertility can lower self-esteem, women may enter an IVF program with anxiety or depression. To determine if a negative (depressed) manner affects the success of IVF, researchers asked 391 women about to undergo the procedure to keep a daily journal documenting their anxiety and depression levels prior to and during the procedure.

In contrast to the expected results, in this study, women with less negative affects (happier) were less likely to achieve a successful IVF procedure and a live birth than were women who presented with a flatter or more sad outlook.

The researchers concluded that couples should be encouraged to express negative emotions about subfertility rather than try to hide them in attempts to be "good" patients or optimistically influence conception, as feelings of anxiety or depression do not interfere with fertility successes and expressing these emotions could allow a couple to receive counseling in this area.

How could you use the result of this study if you were talking to a couple about therapy for subfertility?

Source: de Klerk, C., et al. (2008). Low negative affect prior to treatment is associated with a decreased chance of live birth from a first IVF cycle. *Human Reproduction, 23*(1), 112–116.

Gamete Intrafallopian Transfer

In gamete intrafallopian transfer (GIFT) procedures, ova are obtained from ovaries exactly as in IVF. Instead of waiting for fertilization to occur in the laboratory, however, both ova and sperm are instilled within a matter of hours, using a laparoscopic technique, into the open end of a patent fallopian tube. Fertilization then occurs in the tube, and the zygote moves to the uterus for implantation. This procedure has a pregnancy rate equal to that of IVF. The procedure is contraindicated if a woman's fallopian tubes are blocked, because this could lead to ectopic (tubal) pregnancy.

Zygote Intrafallopian Transfer

Zygote intrafallopian transfer (ZIFT) involves oocyte retrieval by transvaginal, ultrasound-guided aspiration, followed by culture and insemination of the oocytes in the laboratory. Within 24 hours, the fertilized eggs are transferred by laparoscopic technique into the end of a waiting fallopian tube. ZIFT differs from GIFT in that fertilization takes place outside the body, allowing health care providers to be certain that fertilization has occurred before the growing structure is reintroduced. As in GIFT, a woman must have one functioning fallopian tube for the technique to be successful, because the zygotes are implanted into the fimbriated end of a tube rather than into the uterus. This technique allows for genetic analysis the same as IVF.

Surrogate Embryo Transfer

Surrogate embryo transfer is an assisted reproductive technique for a woman who does not ovulate. The process involves use of an oocyte that has been donated by a friend or relative or provided by an anonymous donor (van Berkel, Candido, & Pijffers, 2007). The menstrual cycles of the donor and recipient are synchronized by administration of gonadotropic hormones. At the time of ovulation, the donor's ovum is removed by a transvaginal, ultrasound-guided procedure. The oocyte is then fertilized in the laboratory by the recipient woman's male partner's sperm (or donor sperm) and placed in the recipient woman's uterus by embryonic transfer. Once pregnancy occurs, it progresses the same as an unassisted pregnancy.

Preimplantation Genetic Diagnosis

The individual retrieval of oocytes and their fertilization under laboratory conditions have led to close inspection and recognition of differences in sperm and oocytes. After the oocytes are fertilized in IVF and ZIFT procedures, the DNA of both sperm and oocytes can be examined for specific genetic abnormalities or specific genes such as Down's syndrome or hemophilia (Swanson et al., 2007).

Couples participating in intrauterine transfer and therapeutic insemination can also have the sex of their children predetermined using these methods. Such techniques can be useful, because popular methods to influence the sex of a child (such as douching with a baking soda mixture before coitus to have a boy or with a vinegar solution to have a girl) have proved to be more folklore than scientific fact. Allowing couples to choose the sex of children has ethical concerns because it could result in skewed male/female ratios if used by a majority of couples.

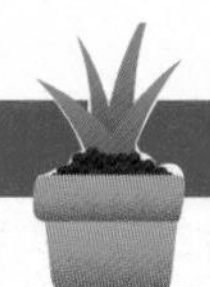

BOX 8.7 * Focus on Nursing Care Planning

A Multidisciplinary Care Map for a Couple Seeking a Fertility Evaluation

Cheryl and Bob Carl married when they were both 25 and planned to wait 5 years before beginning their family so they could save money for a house. At the end of 5 years, they bought the house. On the day they moved in, Mrs. Carl stopped taking her birth control pills. At the end of a year, however, she still was not pregnant. Three years later, the Carls began fertility testing. They are now undergoing their second cycle of in vitro fertilization and embryo transfer. The Carls have applied for a second mortgage on their house to finance the fertility testing and fertilization procedures. At her last visit, Mrs. Carl stated, "This is my fault because I'm so rigid. I can't relax enough to get pregnant. Look how I had to buy the house before I could even consider getting pregnant, and now we'll probably lose it. Besides that, it feels like our whole life revolves around trying to get pregnant."

Family Assessment * Couple lives in three-bedroom middle-income home; husband works as a bank manager; wife works as a receptionist in a medical office. Husband reports finances as "not good." Both appear discouraged about their apparent inability to have children.

Client Assessment * Past medical history negative for any major health problems; wife reports a menstrual cycle of 5 days' duration with moderate flow every 30 to 32 days; moderate dysmenorrhea for the first 2 days of her menses. Oral contraceptive use for 6 years; discontinued 3 years ago. Baseline laboratory studies and vital signs within normal limits.

Nursing Diagnosis * Situational low self-esteem related to seeming inability to conceive

Outcome Criteria * Couple verbalizes feelings about possible subfertility and effect on self-esteem; participates actively in care and treatment decisions; states they feel some control over situation and required treatment.

Team Member Responsible	Assessment	Intervention	Rationale	Expected Outcome
		Activities of Daily Living		
Nurse	Assess couple's lifestyle to identify areas in which they are successful.	Review and reinforce with client activities they have achieved successfully.	Identifying positive attributes can provide a foundation for rebuilding self-esteem.	Couple names at least three positive achievements, such as organizing at work or planting garden.
Nurse	Assess if there is a common interest they could draw on.	Ask couple to propose a new activity that would interest both of them.	Beginning a new activity can eliminate total concentration on fertility management.	Couple names and begins to participate in a new activity by 2 weeks' time.
		Consultations		
Nurse/social worker	Assess the couple's community for available community resources.	Ask couple if they would like a referral to a support group such as Resolve.	A national organization can help supply effective support during a family crisis.	Couple confirms they have contacted an outside support group and have attended at least one meeting or on-line chat group.
		Procedures/Medications		
Nurse/physician/nurse practitioner	Assess whether couple understands what procedures will be scheduled for a basic fertility series.	Encourage clients to ask questions about procedures; if prescribed an ovulation stimulant, review dosage and administration schedule.	Fully informed clients are better able to participate in their own care.	Clients show interest in procedures and medication by asking questions and demonstrating successful medication adherence.

(continued)

BOX 8.7 ✻ Focus on Nursing Care Planning (continued)

		Nutrition		
Nurse/ nutritionist	Assess whether couple ingests a healthy diet in light of busy lifestyle.	Remind client to take prenatal vitamin (because of folic acid content) during fertility studies to be well prepared when pregnancy is achieved.	Folic acid is necessary in early pregnancy to help prevent spinal cord anomalies. Overall health may contribute to fertility.	Client demonstrates that she has filled her prenatal vitamin prescription and confirms that she takes them. Client lists a healthy diet and states that she does not smoke or take recreational drugs.
		Patient/Family Education		
Nurse	Assess whether couple understands why ovulation and conception occur.	Discuss new fertility measures being instituted; include both members of couple in discussion as appropriate.	Discussing conception-related factors helps to provide a baseline for understanding possible procedures and treatments. Including the partners as a couple helps promote family-centered care.	Couple discusses options they need to follow for fertility testing.
		Spiritual/Psychosocial/Emotional Needs		
Nurse	Attempt to identify the meaning of fertility to each client individually and to the couple.	Clarify any misconceptions clients may have about fertility and subfertility.	Misconceptions can negatively affect self-esteem.	Clients accurately describe situation and manifest adequate self-esteem.
		Discharge Planning		
Nurse	Assess whether couple has any further questions about fertility testing and how they are active partners in it.	Stress that waiting for a much-desired pregnancy to come to term can be just as stressful as waiting for fertility measures to be effective.	Identifying stressful situations can help the couple prepare for them.	Couple states they feel well equipped to manage stress following fertility assessment.
Nurse	Determine who the couple has to turn to for support outside of health care providers.	Discuss possible support persons and groups.	Additional support can assist in reinforcing positive attributes, thus enhancing self-esteem.	Clients list appropriate persons or groups to use as support people.

ALTERNATIVES TO CHILDBIRTH

For some couples, even treatments for subfertility with procedures such as IVF are not successful. These couples need to consider still other options.

Surrogate Mothers

A surrogate mother is a woman who agrees to carry a pregnancy to term for a subfertile couple (Reilly, 2007). The surrogate may provide the ova and be impregnated by the man's sperm. In other instances, the ova and sperm both may be donated by the subfertile couple, or donor ova and sperm may be used. Surrogate mothers are often friends or family members who assume the role out of friendship or compassion, or they can be referred to the couple through an agency or attorney and receive monetary reimbursement for their expenses. The subfertile couple can enjoy the pregnancy as they watch it progress in the surrogate.

Several ethical and legal problems arise if the surrogate mother decides at the end of pregnancy that she has formed an attachment to the fetus and wants to keep the baby despite the prepregnancy agreement she signed. Court decisions have been split on whether the surrogate or the subfertile couple has the right to the child. Another potential problem occurs if the child is born imperfect and the subfertile couple then no longer want the child. Who should have responsibility in this instance? For these reasons, the couple and the surrogate mother must be certain they have given adequate thought to the process, and to what will be the outcome should these problems occur, before they attempt surrogate mothering.

Adoption

Adoption, once a ready alternative for subfertile couples, is still a viable alternative, although today there are fewer children available for adoption from official agencies than formerly. Urge couples to consider foreign-born or physically or cognitively challenged children or children of other races to make their family feel complete. The process of adoption is discussed in Chapter 3.

Child-Free Living

Child-free living is an alternative lifestyle available to both fertile and subfertile couples. For many subfertile couples who have been through the rigors and frustrations of subfertility testing and unsuccessful treatment regimens, child-free living may emerge as the option they finally wish to pursue. A couple in the midst of fertility testing may begin to reexamine their motives for pursuing pregnancy and may decide that pregnancy and parenting are not worth the emotional or financial cost of future treatments. They may decide that the additional stress of going through an adoption is not for them, or they may simply decide that children are not necessary for them to complete their family unit. For these couples, child-free living is a positive choice.

Child-free living can be as fulfilling as having children, because it allows a couple more time to help other people and to contribute to society through personal accomplishments. It has advantages for a couple in that it allows time for both members to pursue careers. They can travel more or have more time to pursue hobbies or continue their education. If a couple still wishes to include children in their lives in some way, many opportunities are available to do this through family connections (most parents welcome offers from siblings or other family members to share in childrearing), through volunteer organizations (such as Big Brother or Big Sister programs), or through local schools and town recreational programs.

Many couples who believe that overpopulation is a major concern choose child-free living even if subfertility is not present. Parents who choose child-free living typically rate their marriage as happier than those with children, probably because of decreased expenses involved and more free time that allows them to follow their hearts (Cherlin, 2008).

✔ Checkpoint Question 8.5

Cheryl Carl is having a GIFT procedure. What makes her a good candidate for this procedure?

a. She has patent fallopian tubes, so fertilized ova can be implanted into them.
b. She is Rh negative, a necessary requirement to rule out Rh incompatibility.
c. She has a normal uterus, so sperm can be injected through the cervix into it.
d. Her husband is taking sildenafil (Viagra), so all sperm will be motile.

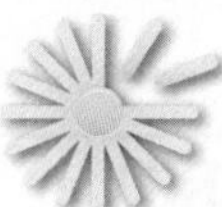

Key Points for Review

- Subfertility is said to exist when a pregnancy has not occurred after 1 year of unprotected coitus. Sterility refers to the inability to conceive because of a known condition.
- About 14% of couples today experience subfertility. The incidence increases with the age of the couple.
- Subfertility testing can be an intense psychological stressor for couples. Help couples not only to persist through the experience but also help them maintain their relationship as a couple.
- Couples who are told that a subfertility problem has been discovered are apt to suffer a loss of self-esteem. Offer support to help them look at other aspects of their lives in which they do achieve and to recognize that they are productive, healthy people in other ways.
- Male factors that contribute to subfertility are inadequate sperm count, obstruction or impaired sperm motility, and problems with ejaculation. Female factors that cause subfertility are problems with ovulation, tubal transport, or impaired implantation.
- Basic subfertility assessment procedures consist of a health history, physical examination, laboratory tests to document general health, and specific tests for semen, ovulation, and tubal patency.
- Measures to induce fertility are aimed at improving sperm number and transport, decreasing infections, stimulating ovulation, improving nutrition, and regulating hormones.
- Therapeutic insemination, donor egg transfer, in vitro fertilization, adoption, surrogate motherhood, and child-free living are all possible solutions for subfertility.

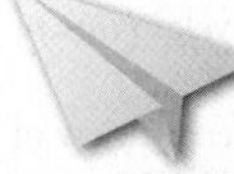

CRITICAL THINKING EXERCISES

1. Cheryl Carl, whom you met at the beginning of the chapter, stated that she believed her subfertility problem was her fault because she was too rigid. She said, “It feels like our whole life revolves around trying to get pregnant.” Does a rigid personality affect subfertility? Does relaxation aid conception?
2. The Carls want to have a child as soon as possible. In addition to their subfertility assessment, what advice would you give them to help increase their chances of conceiving quickly?
3. Cheryl tells you that she eats a lot of “fast foods.” Could this be creating a risk factor for subfertility?
4. Examine the National Health Goal related to subfertility. Most government-sponsored money for nursing research is allotted based on national health goals. What would be a possible research topic to explore pertinent to this goal that would be applicable to the Carl family and also advance evidence-based practice?

CRITICAL THINKING SCENARIO

Open the accompanying CD-ROM or visit http://thePoint.lww.com and read the Patient Scenario included for this chapter, then answer the questions to further sharpen your skills and grow more familiar with NCLEX types of questions related to couples with subfertility. Confirm your answers are correct by reading the rationales.

REFERENCES

Ahmad, G., et al. (2009). Techniques for pelvic surgery in subfertility. *Cochrane Database of Systematic Reviews, 2009*(1), (CD000221).

Anderson, B. J., et al. (2007). In-vitro fertilization and acupuncture: clinical efficacy and mechanistic basis. *Alternative Therapies in Health and Medicine, 13*(3), 38–48.

Anderson, J. R., & Genadry, R. (2007). Anatomy and embryology. In J. S. Berek (Ed.). *Berek & Novak's gynecology.* Philadelphia: Lippincott Williams & Wilkins.

Bashore, L. (2007). Semen preservation in male adolescents and young adults with cancer: one institution's experience. *Clinical Journal of Oncology Nursing, 11*(3), 381–386.

Burney, R. O., Schust, D. J., & Yao, M. W. M. (2007). Infertility. In J. S. Berek (Ed.). *Berek & Novak's gynecology.* Philadelphia: Lippincott Williams & Wilkins.

Campbell, S. J., Cropsey, K. L., & Matthews, C. A. (2007). Intrauterine device use in a high-risk population: experience from an urban university clinic. *American Journal of Obstetrics & Gynecology, 197*(2), 193–197.

Chavarro, J. E., et al. (2007). Dietary fatty acid intakes and the risk of ovulatory infertility. *American Journal of Clinical Nutrition, 85*(1), 231–237.

Cherlin, A. J. (2008). *Public and private families.* New York: McGraw-Hill Publishing Company.

Davis, D. H., Hall, M. N., & Kaufmann, L. (2007). What is the best way to evaluate secondary infertility? *The Journal of Family Practice, 56*(7), 573–575.

de Klerk, C., et al. (2008). Low negative affect prior to treatment is associated with a decreased chance of live birth from a first IVF cycle. *Human Reproduction, 23*(1), 112–116.

DuRant, E., & Leslie, N. S. (2007). Polycystic ovary syndrome: a review of current knowledge. *Journal for Nurse Practitioners, 3*(3), 180–185.

Evers, J. L., & Collins, J. A. (2009). Surgery or embolisation for varicocele in subfertile men. *Cochrane Database of Systematic Reviews, 2009*(1), (CD000479).

Griffiths, A., D'Angelo, A., & Amso, N. (2009). Surgical treatment of fibroids for subfertility. *Cochrane Database of Systematic Reviews, 2009*(1), (CD003857).

Hughes, E., et al. (2009). Clomiphene citrate for unexplained subfertility in women. *Cochrane Database of Systematic Reviews, 2009*(1), (CD000057).

Jacobson, T. Z., et al. (2009). Laparoscopic surgery for subfertility associated with endometriosis. *Cochrane Database of Systematic Reviews, 2009*(1), (CD001398).

Johnson, N., et al. (2009). Tubal flushing for subfertility. *Cochrane Database of Systematic Reviews, 2009*(1), (CD003718).

Karch, A. M. (2009). *Lippincott's nursing drug guide.* Philadelphia: Lippincott Williams & Wilkins.

Kumar, A., et al. (2007). Infertility. In A. H. DeCherney & L. Nathan (Eds.). *Current diagnosis & treatment in obstetrics & gynecology* (10th ed.). Columbus, OH: McGraw-Hill.

MacKay, H. T. (2009). Gynecology. In S. J. McPhee, et al. (Eds.). *Current medical diagnosis & treatment.* Columbus, OH: McGraw-Hill.

Milkin T. (2007). OTC product: Fertell. JAPhA: *Journal of the American Pharmacists Association: JAPhA. 47*(5), e16–17.

Parsons, J. K. (2007). Modifiable risk factors for benign prostatic hyperplasia and lower urinary tract symptoms: new approaches to old problems. *Journal of Urology, 178*(2), 395–401.

Reilly, D. R. (2007). Surrogate pregnancy: a guide for Canadian prenatal health care providers. *Canadian Medical Association Journal, 176*(4), 483–485.

Rybak, E. A., & Wallach, E. E. (2007). Infertility and assisted reproductive technologies. In K. Fortner, et al. (Eds.). *The Johns Hopkins manual of gynecology and obstetrics* (3rd ed.). Philadelphia: Lippincott Williams & Wilkins.

Swanson, A., et al. (2007). Preimplantation genetic diagnosis: technology and clinical applications. *Wisconsin Medical Journal, 106*(3), 145–151.

Tracy, C. R., Steers, W. D., & Costabile, R. (2008). Diagnosis and management of epididymitis. *Urologic Clinics of North America, 35*(1), 101–108.

van Berkel, D., Candido, A., & Pijffers, W. H. (2007). Becoming a mother by non-anonymous egg donation: secrecy and the relationship between egg recipient, egg donor and egg donation child. *Journal of Psychosomatic Obstetrics & Gynecology, 28*(2), 97–104.

Van Voorhis, B. J. (2007). In vitro fertilization. *New England Journal of Medicine, 356*(4), 379–386.

Verhulst, S. M., et al. (2009). Intra-uterine insemination for unexplained subfertility. *Cochrane Database of Systematic Reviews, 2009*(1), (CD001838).

Vignesh, J. P., & Mohan, V. (2007). Polycystic ovary syndrome: a component of metabolic syndrome? *Journal of Postgraduate Medicine, 53*(2), 128–134.

Walker, C. K., & Wiesenfeld, H. C. (2007). Antibiotic therapy for acute pelvic inflammatory disease. *Clinical Infectious Diseases, 44*(Suppl 3), S111–S122.

Wessells, H., et al. (2007). Erectile dysfunction. *Journal of Urology, 177*(5), 1675–1681.

Yap, C., Furness, S., & Farquhar, C. (2009). Pre and post operative medical therapy for endometriosis surgery. *Cochrane Database of Systematic Reviews, 2009*(1), (CD003678).

SUGGESTED READINGS

Adam, G. M. (2007). Assisted human reproduction—legal rights of the unborn in respect of avoidable damage. *Medicine & Law, 26*(2), 325–337.

Agarwal, A., Bragais, F. M., & Sabanegh, E. (2008). Assessing sperm function. *Urologic Clinics of North America, 35*(2), 157–171.

Dodd, J. M., & Crowther, C. A. (2009). Reduction of the number of fetuses for women with triplet and higher order multiple pregnancies. *Cochrane Database of Systematic Reviews, 2009*(1), (CD003932).

Earle, S., & Letherby, G. (2007). Conceiving time? Women who do or do not conceive. *Sociology of Health and Illness, 29*(2), 233–250.

Ficorelli, C. T., & Weeks, B. (2007). Health matters. Untangling the complexities of male infertility. *Nursing, 37*(1), 24–26.

Horwath, D., et al. (2007). Subsequent therapeutic options and outcome in couples who fail to fertilize despite in vitro fertilization (IVF) and intracytoplasmic sperm injection (ICSI). *Clinical & Experimental Obstetrics & Gynecology, 34*(2), 109–110.

McCarthy, M. P. (2008). Women's lived experience of infertility after unsuccessful medical intervention. *Journal of Midwifery & Women's Health, 53*(4), 319–324.

Norcross, S. (2007). Premature menopause: recognition and effects. *Practice Nursing, 18*(6), 281–285.

Oosterhuis, B. E., et al. (2008). Concerns about infertility risks among pediatric oncology patients and their parents. *Pediatric Blood & Cancer, 50*(1), 85–89.

Pandian, Z., et al. (2009). Surgery for tubal infertility. *Cochrane Database of Systematic Reviews, 2009*(1), (CD006415).

Unit 3

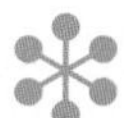

The Nursing Role in Caring for Families During Normal Pregnancy, Birth, the Postpartum, and Newborn Period

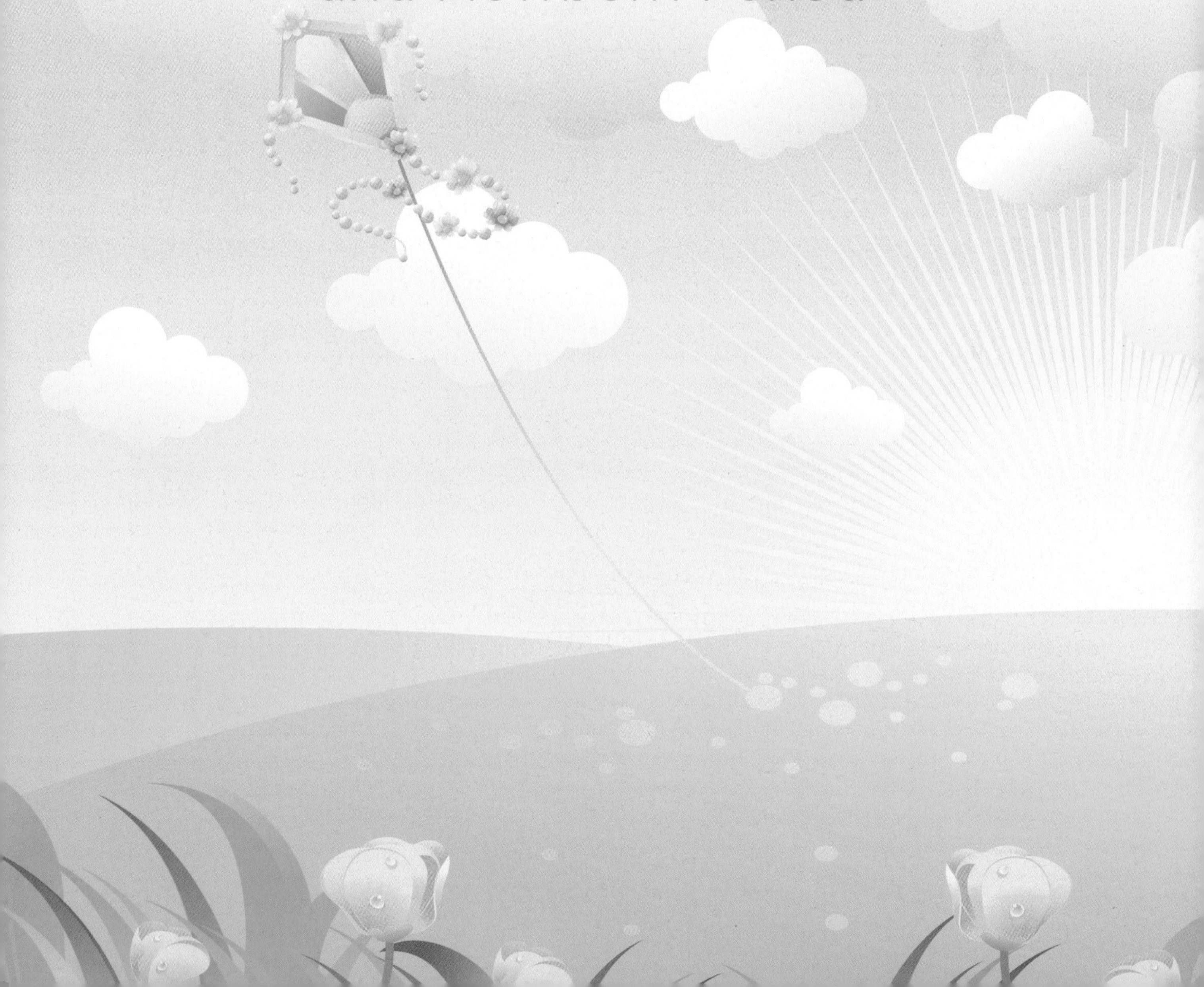

Chapter

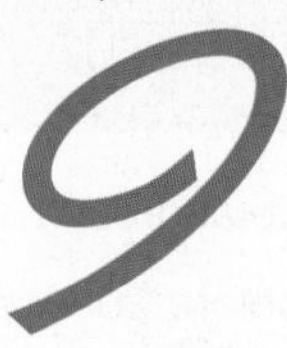

The Growing Fetus

KEY TERMS

- age of viability
- amniocentesis
- amniotic membrane
- cephalocaudal
- chorionic membrane
- chorionic villi
- decidua
- embryo
- estimated date of birth
- fertilization
- fetoscopy
- fetus
- foramen ovale
- hydramnios
- implantation
- McDonald's rule
- meconium
- nonstress test
- oligohydramnios
- rganogenesis
- surfactant
- trophoblast
- umbilical cord
- zygote

OBJECTIVES

After mastering the contents of this chapter, you should be able to:

1. Describe the growth and development of a fetus by gestation week.
2. Identify National Health Goals related to fetal growth that nurses can help the nation achieve.
3. Use critical thinking to analyze ways to make care family centered, even at this early point in life.
4. Assess fetal growth and development through maternal and pregnancy landmarks.
5. Formulate nursing diagnoses related to the needs of a fetus.
6. Establish expected outcomes to meet the needs of a growing fetus.
7. Plan nursing care that promotes healthy fetal growth and development such as nutrition counseling.
8. Implement nursing care to help ensure both a safe fetal environment and a safe pregnancy outcome.
9. Evaluate expected outcomes for achievement and effectiveness of care.
10. Identify areas of fetal health that could benefit from additional nursing research or application of evidence-based practice.
11. Integrate knowledge of fetal growth and development with nursing process to achieve quality maternal and child health nursing care.

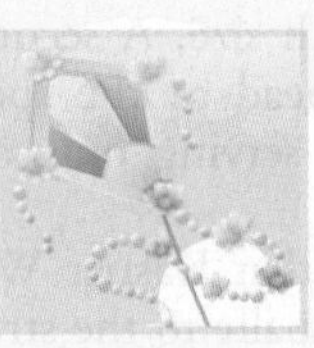

Liz Calhorn, an 18-year-old, is 20 weeks pregnant. Although she says she knows she should have stopped smoking during pregnancy, she has not been able to do this. Twice during the pregnancy (at the 4th and 10th week), she drank beer at summer picnics. Today, at a clinic visit, she tells you she has felt her fetus move. She states, "Feeling the baby move made me realize there's someone inside me, you know what I mean? It made me know it's time I started being more careful with what I do." Her boyfriend (the father of the fetus) is supportive, but the couple has no plans to marry. The client states, "I'm not ready for that big a commitment." Feeling a fetus move is often the trigger that makes having a baby "real" for many women. The more women know about fetal development before and after this event, the easier it is for them to begin to think of the pregnancy not as something interesting happening to them but as an act that is producing a separate life. A previous chapter described reproductive anatomy. This chapter adds information about fetal growth and development and assessment of fetal health.

In light of Liz's realization, how would you modify your health teaching with her?

Throughout history, different societies have held a variety of beliefs and superstitions about the way the **fetus** (the infant during intrauterine life) grows. Medieval artists depicted a fetus as already formed as a miniature man. Leonardo da Vinci, in his notebooks of 1510 to 1512, made several sketches of unborn infants that suggest he believed the fetus was immobile and essentially a part of the mother, sharing her blood and internal organs. During the 17th and 18th centuries, a baby was thought to form to a miniature size in the mother's ovaries; when male cells were introduced, the baby expanded to birth size. A second theory was that the child existed in the head of the sperm cell as a fully formed being, the uterus serving only as an incubator in which it grew.

It was not until 1758 that Kaspar Wolff proposed that both parents contribute equally to the structure of the baby. Because of the work of modern medical researchers and photographers who have been able to capture the process of fertilization and fetal development by high-tech photography, there is now a clear picture of what a fetus looks like from the moment of conception until birth. Surveillance of the fetus by ultrasound documents this growth process.

Because a nation cannot have healthy children without healthy intrauterine growth, several National Health Goals speak to the importance of protecting fetal growth (Box 9.1).

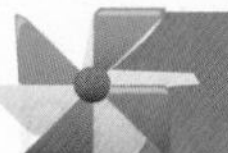

BOX 9.1 ❋ Focus on National Health Goals

Several National Health Goals address fetal growth.

- Reduce the fetal death rate (death before 20 weeks of gestation) to no more than 4.1 per 1000 live births from a baseline of 6.8 per 1000.
- Reduce low birth weight to an incidence of no more than 5% of live births and very low birthweight to no more than 0.9% of live births from baselines of 7.6% and 1.4%.
- Increase the proportion of pregnancies begun with an optimum folic acid level from a baseline of 21% to 80% (http://www.nih.gov).

Nurses can help the nation achieve these goals by urging women to plan their pregnancies so they can enter a pregnancy in good health and with an optimum folic acid level. Educating women about the importance of attending prenatal care is another important role. Nursing research in such areas as the reasons why women avoid prenatal care or how soon women make lifestyle changes during pregnancy could help lead to achievement of these National Health Goals.

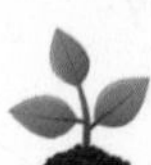

Nursing Process Overview

To Help Ensure Fetal Health

Assessment

Assessing fetal growth throughout pregnancy, by such means as fundal height and fetal heart rate, is important because these predictable signs of fetal development provide guides for determining the well-being of fetuses. For the expectant family, knowledge about fetal growth and development can provide an important frame of reference, helping a mother to understand some of the changes going on in her body and allowing all family members to begin thinking about and accepting the newest member of the family before the baby is actually born. For this reason, convey the findings gained from fetal assessment at prenatal visits in as much detail as the parents request.

Nursing Diagnosis

Common nursing diagnoses related to growth and development of the fetus focus on the mother and family as well as on the fetus. Examples might include:

- Health-seeking behaviors related to knowledge of normal fetal development
- Anxiety related to lack of fetal movement
- Deficient knowledge related to need for good prenatal care for healthy fetal well-being

Outcome Identification and Planning

Be certain that plans for care include ways to educate potential parents about teratogens (any substance that could be harmful to a fetus) that might interfere with fetal health. Be certain that outcome criteria established for teaching about fetal growth are realistic and based on the parents' previous knowledge and desire for information. When additional assessment measures are necessary, such as an amniocentesis or an ultrasound examination, add this information to the teaching plan, explaining why further assessment is necessary and what the parents can expect from the procedure. An interesting web site for parents that shows fetal development in photographs is http://www.paternityangel.com.

Implementation

Most expectant parents are interested in learning about how mature their fetus is at various points in pregnancy because this helps them visualize their coming newborn. This, in turn, helps them to understand the importance of implementing healthy behaviors, such as eating well and avoiding substances that may be dangerous to a fetus such as recreational drugs. Viewing an ultrasound and learning the fetal sex are big steps to help initiate bonding between the parents and the infant.

Outcome Evaluation

Outcome evaluation related to fetal growth and development usually focuses on determining whether a woman or family has made any necessary changes in lifestyle to ensure fetal growth and whether a woman voices confidence that her baby is healthy and growing. Examples of expected outcomes include:

- Parents describe smoke-free living at next prenatal visit.
- Client records number of movements of fetus for 1 hour daily.
- Couple attends all scheduled prenatal visits.
- Client states she is looking forward to the birth of her baby.

STAGES OF FETAL DEVELOPMENT

In just 38 weeks, a fertilized egg (ovum) matures from a single cell to a fully developed fetus ready to be born.

Fetal growth and development are typically divided into three periods: preembryonic (first 2 weeks, beginning with fertilization), embryonic (weeks 3 through 8), and fetal (from week 8 through birth). Table 9.1 lists common terms used to describe the fetus at various stages in this growth.

Fertilization: The Beginning of Pregnancy

Fertilization (also referred to as conception and impregnation) is the union of an ovum and a spermatozoon. This usually occurs in the outer third of a fallopian tube, the ampullar portion (Crombleholme, 2009).

Usually only one of a woman's ova will reach maturity each month. Once the mature ovum is released, fertilization must occur fairly quickly because an ovum is capable of fertilization for only 24 hours (48 hours at the most). After that time, it atrophies and becomes nonfunctional. Because the functional life of a spermatozoon is also about 48 hours, possibly as long as 72 hours, the total critical time span during which sexual relations must occur for fertilization to be successful is about 72 hours (48 hours before ovulation plus 24 hours afterward).

As the ovum is extruded from the graafian follicle of an ovary with ovulation, it is surrounded by a ring of mucopolysaccharide fluid (the zona pellucida) and a circle of cells (the corona radiata). The ovum and these surrounding cells (which increase the bulk of the ovum and serve as protective buffers against injury) are propelled into a nearby fallopian tube by currents initiated by the fimbriae—the fine, hairlike structures that line the openings of the fallopian tubes. A combination of peristaltic action of the tube and movements of the tube cilia help propel the ovum along the length of the tube.

Normally, an ejaculation of semen averages 2.5 mL of fluid containing 50 to 200 million spermatozoa per milliliter, or an average of 400 million sperm per ejaculation. At the time of ovulation, there is a reduction in the viscosity (thickness) of the cervical mucus, which makes it easy for spermatozoa to penetrate it. Sperm transport is so efficient close to ovulation that spermatozoa deposited in the vagina generally reach the cervix within 90 seconds and the outer end of a fallopian tube within 5 minutes after deposition. This is one reason why douching is not an effective contraceptive measure (Burkman, 2007).

The mechanism whereby spermatozoa are drawn toward an ovum is probably a species-specific reaction, similar to an antibody–antigen reaction. Spermatozoa move through the cervix and the body of the uterus and into the fallopian tubes, toward the waiting ovum by the combination of movement by their flagella (tails) and uterine contractions. Capacitation is a final process that sperm must undergo to be ready for fertilization. This process, which happens as the sperm move toward the ovum, consists of changes in the plasma membrane of the sperm head, which reveal the sperm-binding receptor sites.

All of the spermatozoa that achieve capacitation reach the ovum and cluster around the protective layer of corona cells. Hyaluronidase (a proteolytic enzyme) is released by the spermatozoa and dissolves the layer of cells protecting the ovum. One reason that an ejaculation contains such a large number of sperm is probably to provide sufficient enzymes to dissolve the corona cells. Under ordinary circumstances, only one spermatozoon is able to penetrate the cell membrane of the ovum. Once it penetrates the cell, the cell membrane changes composition to become impervious to other spermatozoa. An exception to this is the formation of hydatidiform mole, in which multiple sperm enter an ovum; this leads to abnormal zygote formation (see Chapter 21).

Immediately after penetration of the ovum, the chromosomal material of the ovum and spermatozoon fuse to form a **zygote.** Because the spermatozoon and ovum each carried 23 chromosomes (22 autosomes and 1 sex chromosome), the fertilized ovum has 46 chromosomes. If an X-carrying spermatozoon entered the ovum, the resulting child will have two X chromosomes and will be female (XX). If a Y-carrying spermatozoon fertilized the ovum, the resulting child will have an X and a Y chromosome and will be male (XY).

Fertilization is never a certain occurrence because it depends on at least three separate factors: equal maturation of both sperm and ovum, the ability of the sperm to reach the ovum, and the ability of the sperm to penetrate the zona pellucida and cell membrane and achieve fertilization.

From the fertilized ovum (zygote), both the future child and the accessory structures needed for support during intrauterine life (e.g., placenta, fetal membranes, amniotic fluid, and umbilical cord) are formed.

Implantation

Once fertilization is complete, a zygote migrates over the next 3 to 4 days toward the body of the uterus, aided by the currents initiated by the muscular contractions of the fallopian tubes. During this time, mitotic cell division, or cleavage, begins. The first cleavage occurs at about 24 hours; cleavage divisions continue to occur at a rate of about one every 22 hours. By the time the zygote reaches the body of the uterus, it consists of 16 to 50 cells. At this stage, because of its bumpy outward appearance, it is termed a morula (from the Latin word *morus,* meaning "mulberry").

The morula continues to multiply as it floats free in the uterine cavity for 3 or 4 additional days. Large cells tend to collect at the periphery of the ball, leaving a fluid space surrounding an inner cell mass. At this stage, the structure becomes a blastocyst. It is this structure that attaches to the uterine endometrium. The cells in the outer ring are **trophoblast**

TABLE 9.1 ✻ Terms Used to Denote Fetal Growth

Name	Time Period
Ovum	From ovulation to fertilization
Zygote	From fertilization to implantation
Embryo	From implantation to 5–8 weeks
Fetus	From 5–8 weeks until term
Conceptus	Developing embryo or fetus and placental structures throughout pregnancy
Age of viability	The earliest age at which fetuses could survive if they were born at that time, generally accepted as 24 weeks, or fetuses weighing more than 400 g

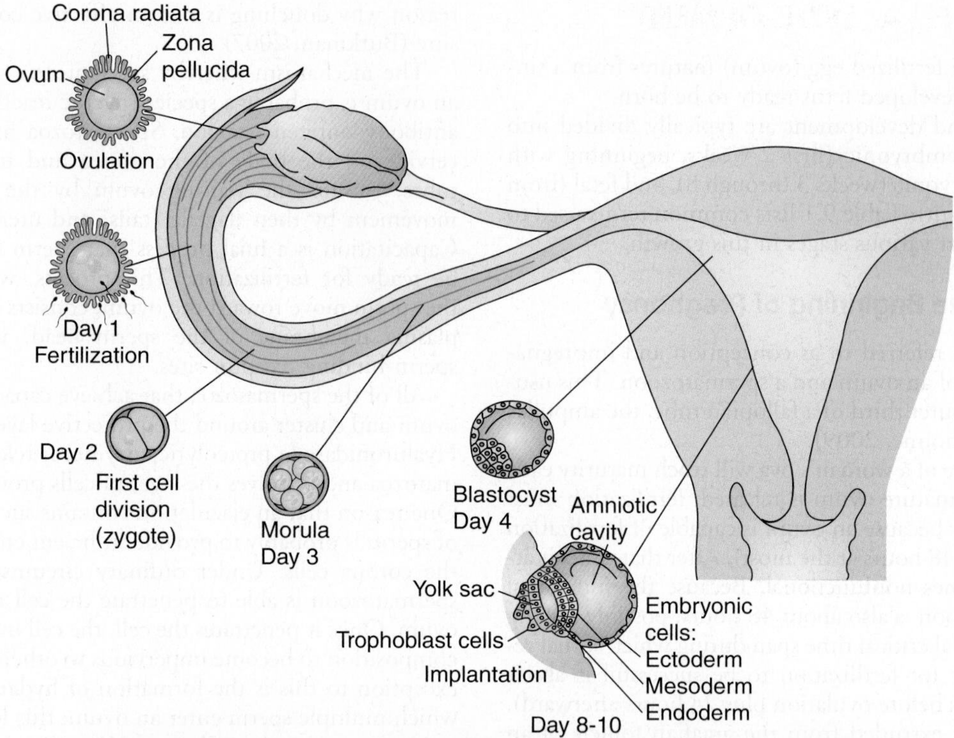

FIGURE 9.1 Ovulation, fertilization, and implantation. The blastocyst is differentiated into three germ layers (ectoderm, mesoderm, and endoderm). Cells at the periphery are trophoblast cells that mature into the placenta.

cells. They are the part of the structure that will later form the placenta and membranes. The inner cell mass (embryoblast cells) is the portion of the structure that will form the embryo.

Implantation, or contact between the growing structure and the uterine endometrium, occurs approximately 8 to 10 days after fertilization. After the third or fourth day of free floating (about 8 days since ovulation), the blastocyst sheds the last residues of the corona and zona pellucida. The structure brushes against the rich uterine endometrium (in the second [secretory] phase of the menstrual cycle), a process termed *apposition.* It attaches to the surface of the endometrium (adhesion) and settles down into its soft folds (invasion). Stages to this point are depicted in Figure 9.1.

The touching or implantation point is usually high in the uterus, on the posterior surface. If the point of implantation is low in the uterus, the growing placenta may occlude the cervix and make birth of the child difficult (placenta previa). The blastocyst is able to invade the endometrium because, as the trophoblast cells on the outside of the structure touch the endometrium, they produce proteolytic enzymes that dissolve any tissue they touch. This action allows the blastocyst to burrow deeply into the endometrium and receive some basic nourishment of glycogen and mucoprotein from the endometrial glands. As invasion continues, the structure establishes an effective communication network with the blood system of the endometrium.

Implantation is an important step in pregnancy, because as many as 50% of zygotes never achieve it (Knuppel, 2007). In these instances, the pregnancy ends as early as 8 to 10 days after conception, often before a woman is even aware she was pregnant. Occasionally, a small amount of vaginal spotting appears on the day of implantation because capillaries are ruptured by the implanting trophoblast cells. A woman who normally has a particularly scant menstrual flow may mistake implantation bleeding for her menstrual period. If this happens, the predicted date of birth of her baby (based on the time of her last menstrual period) will be calculated 4 weeks late. Once implanted, the zygote becomes an **embryo.**

✔ Checkpoint Question 9.1

Liz Calhorn asks how much longer her doctor will refer to the baby inside her as an embryo. The conceptus is an embryo:

a. Until the time of fertilization.
b. Until the placenta forms.
c. From implantation until 20 weeks.
d. From implantation until 5 to 8 weeks.

EMBRYONIC AND FETAL STRUCTURES

The placenta, which will serve as the fetal lungs, kidneys, and digestive tract in utero, begins growth in early pregnancy in coordination with embryo growth.

The Decidua

After fertilization, the corpus luteum in the ovary continues to function rather than atrophying, because of the influence of human chorionic gonadotropin (hCG), a hormone secreted by the trophoblast cells. This causes the uterine endometrium to continue to grow in thickness and vascularity,

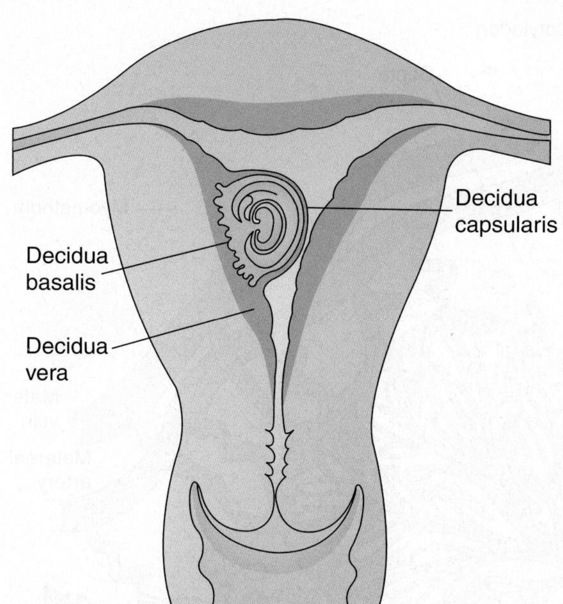

FIGURE 9.2 The three areas of uterine decidua.

instead of sloughing off as in a usual menstrual cycle. The endometrium is now termed the **decidua** (the Latin word for "falling off"), because it will be discarded after the birth of the child. The decidua has three separate areas (Fig. 9.2):

1. *Decidua basalis,* the part of the endometrium that lies directly under the embryo (or the portion where the trophoblast cells establish communication with maternal blood vessels)
2. *Decidua capsularis,* the portion of the endometrium that stretches or encapsulates the surface of the trophoblast
3. *Decidua vera,* the remaining portion of the uterine lining

As the embryo continues to grow, it pushes the decidua capsularis before it like a blanket. Eventually, the embryo enlarges so much that this action brings the decidua capsularis into contact with the opposite uterine wall (the decidua vera). Here, the two decidua areas fuse, which is why, at birth, the entire inner surface of the uterus is stripped away, leaving the organ highly susceptible to hemorrhage and infection.

Chorionic Villi

Once implantation is complete, the trophoblastic layer of cells of the blastocyst begins to mature rapidly. As early as the 11th or 12th day, miniature villi that resemble probing fingers, termed **chorionic villi,** reach out from the single layer of cells into the uterine endometrium to begin formation of the placenta. At term, almost 200 such villi will have formed (Knuppel, 2007).

All chorionic villi have a central core of connective tissue and fetal capillaries. A double layer of trophoblast cells surrounds these. The outer of the two covering layers is the *syncytiotrophoblast,* or the syncytial layer. This layer of cells produces various placental hormones, such as hCG, somatomammotropin (human placental lactogen [hPL]), estrogen, and progesterone. The middle layer, the *cytotrophoblast* or Langhans' layer, is present as early as 12 days' gestation. It appears to function early in pregnancy to protect the growing embryo and fetus from certain infectious organisms such as the spirochete of syphilis. This layer of cells disappears, however, between the 20th and 24th weeks. This is why syphilis is not considered to have a high potential for fetal damage early in pregnancy, only after the point at which cytotrophoblast cells are no longer present (Ainbinder, Ramin, & DeCherney, 2007). The layer appears to offer little protection against viral invasion at any point.

The Placenta

The placenta (Latin for "pancake," which is descriptive of its size and appearance at term) arises out of the continuing growth of trophoblast tissue. Its growth parallels that of the fetus, growing from a few identifiable cells at the beginning of pregnancy to an organ 15 to 20 cm in diameter and 2 to 3 cm in depth, covering about half the surface area of the internal uterus at term.

Circulation

Placental circulation is shown in Figure 9.3. As early as the 12th day of pregnancy, maternal blood begins to collect in the intervillous spaces of the uterine endometrium surrounding the chorionic villi. By the third week, oxygen and other nutrients, such as glucose, amino acids, fatty acids, minerals, vitamins, and water, osmose from the maternal blood through the cell layers of the chorionic villi into the villi capillaries. From there, nutrients are transported to the developing embryo.

Placental osmosis is so effective that all except a few substances are able to cross from the mother into the fetus. Because almost all drugs are able to cross into the fetal circulation, it is important that a woman take no nonessential drugs (including alcohol and nicotine) during pregnancy (Rogers-Adkinson & Stuart, 2007). Alcohol, as an example of a drug which can cause fetal growth disorders, perfuses across the placenta so well that pregnant women are advised to drink no alcohol at all during pregnancy (Crombleholme, 2009). The mechanisms that allow nutrients to cross the placenta are described in Table 9.2. All of these processes are influenced by maternal blood pressure and the pH of the fetal and maternal plasma. A potential complication of twins is that nutrients vessels may fuse in utero, causing one twin to receive more blood than the other (twin-to-twin transfusion) (Norton, 2007). Specific transport of substances and their effects on the fetus are discussed in Chapter 12.

For practical purposes, because the process of osmosis is so effective, there is no direct exchange of blood between the embryo and the mother during pregnancy. Because the outer chorionic villi layer is only one cell thick after the third trimester minute breaks do occur and allow occasional fetal cells to cross into the maternal bloodstream, as well as fetal enzymes such as alpha-fetoprotein (AFP) from the fetal liver.

As the number of chorionic villi increases with pregnancy, the villi form an increasingly complex communication network with the maternal blood. Intervillous spaces grow larger and larger, becoming separated by a series of partitions or septa. In a mature placenta, there are as many as 30 separate segments, or *cotyledons.* These compartments are what make the maternal side of the placenta look rough and uneven.

About 100 maternal uterine arteries supply the mature placenta. To provide enough blood for exchange, the rate of

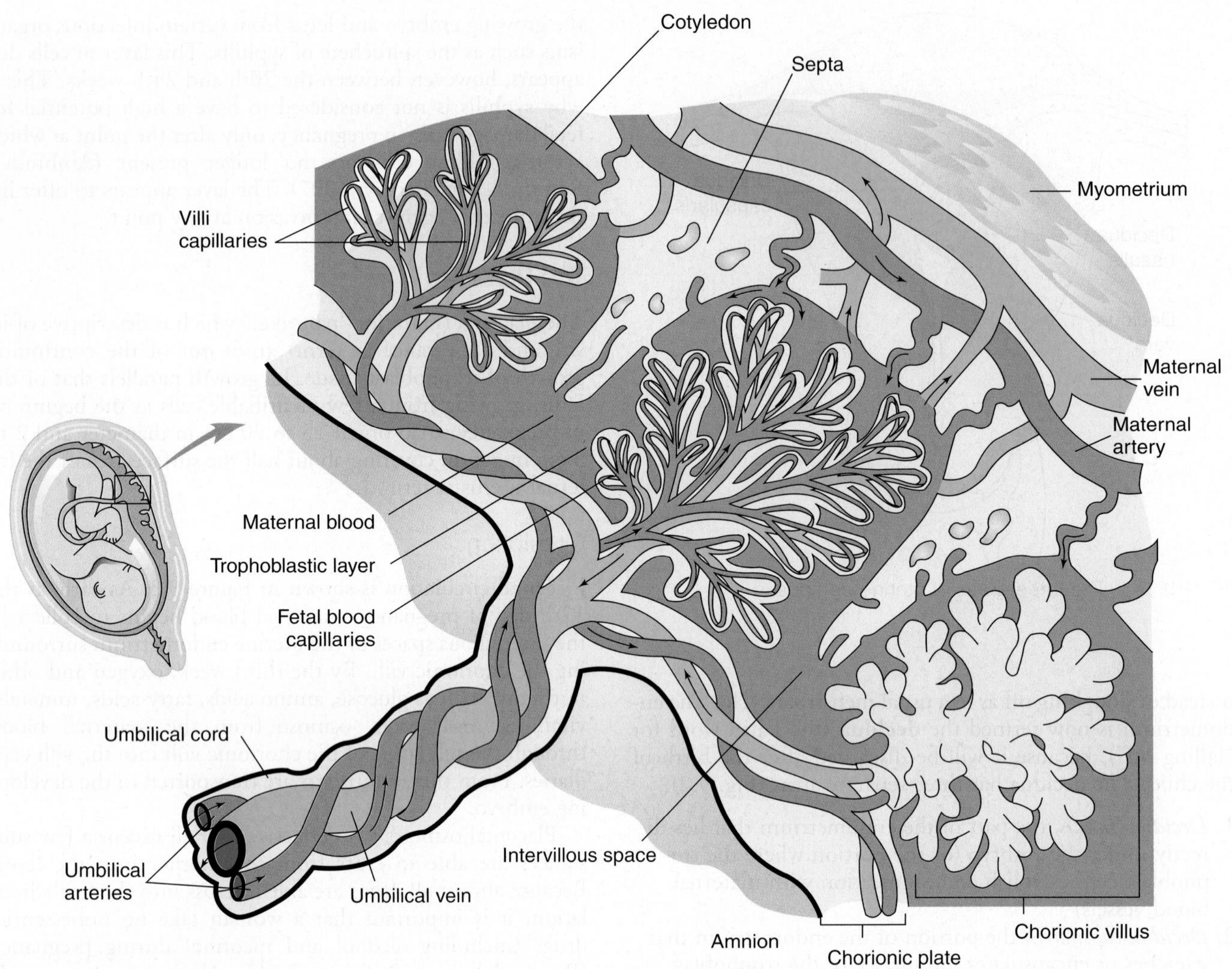

FIGURE 9.3 Placental circulation.

TABLE 9.2 ✲ Mechanisms by Which Nutrients Cross the Placenta

Mechanism	Description
Diffusion	When there is a greater concentration of a substance on one side of a semipermeable membrane than on the other, substances of correct molecular weight cross the membrane from the area of higher concentration to the area of lower concentration. Oxygen, carbon dioxide, sodium, and chloride cross the placenta by this method.
Facilitated diffusion	To ensure that a fetus receives sufficient concentrations of necessary nutrients, some substances cross the placenta guided by a carrier so move more rapidly or easily than would occur if only simple diffusion were operating. Glucose is an example of a substance that crosses by this process.
Active transport	This process requires the action of an enzyme to facilitate transport. Essential amino acids and water-soluble vitamins cross the placenta by this process. The process ensures that a fetus will have adequate amino acid concentrations for fetal growth.
Pinocytosis	This is absorption by the cellular membrane of microdroplets of plasma and dissolved substances. Gamma globulin, lipoproteins, and phospholipids all have molecular structures too large for diffusion so cross in this manner. Unfortunately, viruses that then infect the fetus can also cross in this manner.

uteroplacental blood flow in pregnancy increases from about 50 mL/min at 10 weeks to 500 to 600 mL/min at term. No additional maternal arteries appear after the first 3 months of pregnancy; instead, to accommodate the increased blood flow, the arteries increase in size. The woman's heart rate, total cardiac output, and blood volume increase to supply blood to the placenta.

In the intervillous spaces, maternal blood jets from the coiled or spiral arteries in streams or spurts and then is propelled from compartment to compartment by the currents initiated. As the blood circulates around the villi and nutrients osmose from maternal blood into the villi, the maternal blood gradually loses its momentum and settles to the floor of the cotyledons. From there, it enters the orifices of maternal veins located in the cotyledons and is returned to the maternal circulation. Braxton Hicks contractions, the barely noticeable uterine contractions that are present from about the 12th week of pregnancy, aid in maintaining pressure in the intervillous spaces by closing off the uterine veins momentarily with each contraction.

Uterine perfusion, and thus placental circulation, is most efficient when the woman lies on her left side. This position lifts the uterus away from the inferior vena cava, preventing blood from being trapped in the woman's lower extremities. If the woman lies on her back and the weight of the uterus compresses the vena cava, placental circulation can be so sharply reduced that supine hypotension (very low maternal blood pressure and poor uterine circulation) occurs (Knuppel, 2007).

At term, the placental circulatory network has grown so extensively that a placenta weighs 400 to 600 g (1 lb), one-sixth the weight of the baby. If a placenta is smaller than this, it suggests that circulation to the fetus may have been inadequate. A placenta larger than this may also indicate that circulation to the fetus was threatened, because it suggests that the placenta was forced to spread out in an unusual manner to maintain a sufficient blood supply. The fetus of a woman with diabetes may also develop a larger-than-usual placenta from excess fluid collected between cells.

Endocrine Function

Aside from serving as the conduit for oxygen and nutrients for the fetus, the syncytial (outer) layer of the chorionic villi develops into a separate, important hormone-producing system.

Human Chorionic Gonadotropin. The first placental hormone produced, hCG, can be found in maternal blood and urine as early as the first missed menstrual period (shortly after implantation has occurred) through about the 100th day of pregnancy. Because this is the hormone analyzed by pregnancy tests, a false-negative result from a pregnancy test may be obtained before or after this period. The woman's blood serum will be completely negative for hCG within 1 to 2 weeks after birth. Testing for hCG after birth can be used as proof that placental tissue is no longer present.

The purpose of hCG is to act as a fail-safe measure to ensure that the corpus luteum of the ovary continues to produce progesterone and estrogen. This is important because, if the corpus luteum should fail and the level of progesterone fall, the endometrial lining will slough and the pregnancy will be lost. hCG also may play a role in suppressing the maternal immunologic response so that placental tissue is not detected and rejected as a foreign substance. Because the structure of hCG is similar to that of luteinizing hormone of the pituitary gland, if the fetus is male, it exerts an effect on the fetal testes to begin testosterone production. The presence of testosterone causes maturation of the male reproductive tract.

At about the eighth week of pregnancy, the outer layer of cells of the developing placenta begins to produce progesterone, making the corpus luteum, which was producing progesterone, no longer necessary. In coordination with this, the production of hCG, which sustained the corpus luteum, begins to decrease at this point.

Estrogen. Estrogen (primarily estriol) is produced as a second product of the syncytial cells of the placenta. Estrogen contributes to the woman's mammary gland development in preparation for lactation and stimulates uterine growth to accommodate the developing fetus.

Progesterone. Estrogen is often referred to as the "hormone of women"; progesterone as the "hormone of mothers." This is because, although estrogen influences a female appearance, progesterone is necessary to maintain the endometrial lining of the uterus during pregnancy. It is present in serum as early as the fourth week of pregnancy, as a result of the continuation of the corpus luteum. After placental synthesis begins (at about the 12th week), the level of progesterone rises progressively during the remainder of the pregnancy. This hormone also appears to reduce the contractility of the uterus during pregnancy, preventing premature labor. Such reduced contractility is probably produced by a change in electrolytes (notably potassium and calcium), which decreases the contraction potential of the uterus.

Human Placental Lactogen (Human Chorionic Somatomammotropin). hPL is a hormone with both growth-promoting and lactogenic (milk-producing) properties. It is produced by the placenta beginning as early as the sixth week of pregnancy, increasing to a peak level at term. It can be assayed in both maternal serum and urine. It promotes mammary gland (breast) growth in preparation for lactation in the mother. It also serves the important role of regulating maternal glucose, protein, and fat levels so that adequate amounts of these nutrients are always available to the fetus (Taylor & Lebovic, 2007).

Placental Proteins

The placenta also produces several plasma proteins. The function of these has not been well documented, but it is thought that they may contribute to decreasing the immunologic impact of the growing placenta through being part of the complement cascade (Knuppel, 2007).

The Amniotic Membranes

The chorionic villi on the medial surface of the trophoblast (those that are not involved in implantation, because they do not touch the endometrium) gradually thin, leaving the medial surface of the structure smooth (the chorion laeve, or smooth chorion). The smooth chorion eventually becomes the **chorionic membrane,** the outermost fetal membrane. Its purpose is to form the sac that contains the amniotic fluid. A second membrane lining the chorionic membrane, the **amniotic membrane** or amnion, forms beneath the chorion (Fig. 9.4). Early in pregnancy, these membranes become so adherent that they seem as one at term. At birth they can be

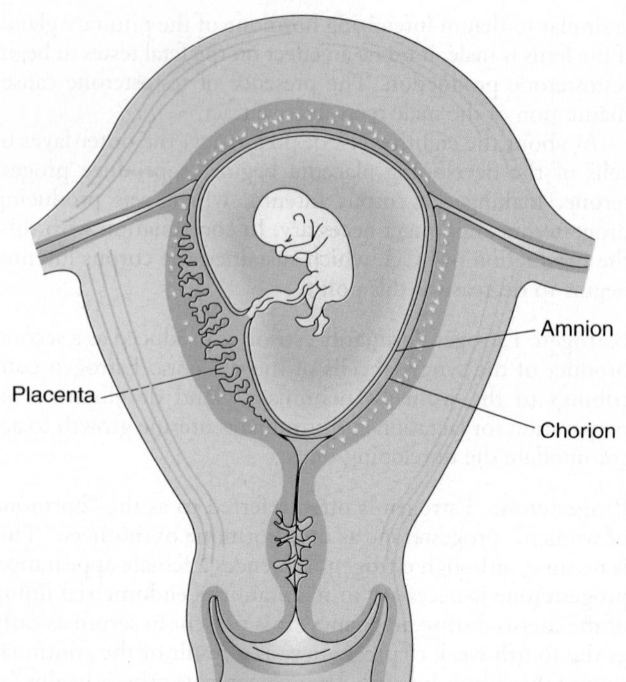

FIGURE 9.4 Membranes, with embryo lying within amniotic sac.

seen covering the fetal surface of the placenta, giving that surface its typically shiny appearance. There is no nerve supply, so when they spontaneously rupture at term or are artificially ruptured, neither woman nor child experiences any pain.

In contrast to the chorionic membrane, the amniotic membrane not only offers support to amniotic fluid but also actually produces the fluid. In addition, it produces a phospholipid that initiates the formation of prostaglandins, which can cause uterine contractions and may be the trigger that initiates labor. Occasionally, fibrous amniotic bands that can constrict an arm or leg of the fetus form in utero. These can close off the blood supply to the distal extremity and cause growth of the extremity to halt at that point (Kumar, Das, & Kumar, 2007).

The Amniotic Fluid

Amniotic fluid is constantly being newly formed and reabsorbed by the amniotic membrane, so it never becomes stagnant. Some of it is absorbed by direct contact with the fetal surface of the placenta. The major method of absorption, however, occurs because the fetus continually swallows the fluid. In the fetal intestine, it is absorbed into the fetal bloodstream. From there, it goes to the umbilical arteries and to the placenta, and it is exchanged across the placenta. At term, the amount of amniotic fluid has increased so much it ranges from 800 to 1200 mL. If for any reason the fetus is unable to swallow (esophageal atresia or anencephaly are the two most common reasons), excessive amniotic fluid, or **hydramnios** (more than 2000 mL in total, or pockets of fluid larger than 8 cm on ultrasound), will result. Hydramnios also tends to occur in women with diabetes, because hyperglycemia causes excessive fluid shifts into the amniotic space (Bush & Pernoll, 2007). Early in fetal life, as soon as the fetal kidneys become active, fetal urine adds to the quantity of the amniotic fluid. A disturbance of kidney function may cause **oligohydramnios,** or a reduction in the amount of amniotic fluid (less than 300 mL in total, or no pocket on ultrasound larger than 1 cm) (Knuppel, 2007).

The most important purpose of amniotic fluid is to shield the fetus against pressure or a blow to the mother's abdomen. Because liquid changes temperature more slowly than air, it also protects the fetus from changes in temperature. As yet another function, it aids in muscular development, because it allows the fetus freedom to move. Finally, it protects the umbilical cord from pressure, protecting the fetal oxygen supply.

Even if the amniotic membranes rupture before birth and the bulk of amniotic fluid is lost, some will always surround the fetus in utero, because new fluid is constantly formed. Amniotic fluid is slightly alkaline, with a pH of about 7.2. Checking the pH of the fluid at the time of rupture helps to differentiate it from urine, which is acidic (pH 5.0–5.5).

The Umbilical Cord

The **umbilical cord** is formed from the fetal membranes (amnion and chorion) and provides a circulatory pathway that connects the embryo to the chorionic villi of the placenta. Its function is to transport oxygen and nutrients to the fetus from the placenta and to return waste products from the fetus to the placenta. It is about 53 cm (21 in) in length at term and about 2 cm (¾ in) thick. The bulk of the cord is a gelatinous mucopolysaccharide called Wharton's jelly, which gives the cord body and prevents pressure on the vein and arteries that pass through it. The outer surface is covered with amniotic membrane.

An umbilical cord contains only one vein (carrying blood from the placental villi to the fetus) but two arteries (carrying blood from the fetus back to the placental villi). The number of veins and arteries in the cord is always assessed and recorded at birth because about 1% to 5% of infants are born with a cord that contains only a single vein and artery. From 15% to 20% of these infants are found to have accompanying chromosomal disorders or congenital anomalies, particularly of the kidney and heart (Lubusky et al., 2007).

The rate of blood flow through an umbilical cord is rapid (350 mL/min at term). The adequacy of blood flow (blood velocity) through the cord, as well as that of both systolic and diastolic cord pressure, can be determined by ultrasound examination during pregnancy. Blood can be withdrawn from the umbilical vein or transfused into the vein during intrauterine life for fetal assessment or treatment (termed percutaneous umbilical blood sampling [PUBS]).

Because the rate of blood flow through the cord is so rapid, it is unlikely that a cord will twist or knot enough to interfere with the fetal oxygen supply. In about 20% of all births, a loose loop of cord is found around the fetal neck (nuchal cord) at birth. If this loop of cord is removed before the newborn's shoulders are born, so that there is no traction on it, the oxygen supply to the fetus remains unimpaired (Jackson, Melvin, & Downe, 2007).

The walls of the umbilical cord arteries are lined with smooth muscle. Constriction of these muscles after birth contributes to hemostasis and helps prevent hemorrhage of the newborn through the cord. Because the umbilical cord contains no nerve supply, it can be cut at birth without discomfort to either the child or woman.

✔ Checkpoint Question 9.2

Liz Calhorn is worried that her baby will be born with a congenital heart disease. What assessment of a fetus at birth is important to help detect congenital heart defects?

a. Assessing whether the Wharton jelly of the cord has a pH higher than 7.2.
b. Assessing whether the umbilical cord has two arteries and one vein.
c. Measuring the length of the cord to be certain that it is longer than 3 feet.
d. Determining that the umbilical cord is not stained green or yellow.

ORIGIN AND DEVELOPMENT OF ORGAN SYSTEMS

Following the moment of fertilization, the zygote, and later the embryo and fetus, continues with active growth.

Stem Cells

During the first 4 days of life, zygote cells are termed *totipotent stem cells,* or cells that are so undifferentiated they have the potential to form a complete human being. In another 4 days, as the structure implants and becomes an embryo, cells begin to show differentiation and lose their ability to become any body cell. Instead, they are now slated to become specific body cells, such as nerve, brain, or skin cells, and are termed *pluripotent stem cells.* In yet another few days, the cells grow so specific that they are termed multipotent or are so specific that they have set a sure course toward the body organ they will create.

If the nucleus is removed from an oocyte and the nucleus of an adult cell is transferred into the oocyte, an embryo has the potential to grow into an infant who is identical to the adult donor (reproductive cloning). If its pluripotent stem cells are removed and allowed to grow in the laboratory, these have the potential to be able to supply a type of body cell needed by the adult donor (therapeutic cloning). Stem cell research has revealed that if stem cells such as these are implanted into an adult with a condition such as spinal cord injury, diabetes, or a blood disorder, they can replace the adult's damaged cells (Firpo & Kikyo, 2007). The majority of embryos used for research today are extra embryos that were removed from the mother's body as part of the process of in vitro fertilization but were not used (see Chapter 8). As exciting as this area of research is, it also carries ethical and costly considerations; for example, if stem cell therapy becomes possible on a large scale, how will enough embryos be available unless they are grown just for this purpose? The ability of researchers to derive stem cells from adult skin cells or menstrual blood should help relieve this concern (Goldman, 2007).

Zygote Growth

From the beginning of fetal growth, development proceeds in a **cephalocaudal** (head-to-tail) direction; that is, head development occurs first and is followed by development of the middle and, finally, the lower body parts. This pattern of development continues after birth as shown by the way infants are able to lift up their heads approximately 1 year before they are able to walk. As a fetus grows, body organ systems develop from specific tissue layers called germ layers.

Primary Germ Layers

At the time of implantation, a blastocyst already has differentiated to a point at which two separate cavities appear in the inner structure: (1) a large one, the amniotic cavity, which is lined with a distinctive layer of cells, the *ectoderm,* and (2) a smaller cavity, the yolk sac, which is lined with *entoderm* cells (see Fig. 9.1).

In chicks, the yolk sac serves as a supply of nourishment for the embryo throughout its development. In humans, the yolk sac appears to supply nourishment only until implantation. After that, its main purpose is to provide a source of red blood cells until the embryo's hematopoietic system is mature enough to perform this function (at about the 12th week of intrauterine life). The yolk sac then atrophies and remains only as a thin white streak discernible in the cord at birth.

Between the amniotic cavity and the yolk sac, a third layer of primary cells, the *mesoderm,* forms. The embryo will begin to develop at the point where the three cell layers (ectoderm, entoderm, and mesoderm) meet, called the embryonic shield. Each of these germ layers of primary tissue

TABLE 9.3 ✻ Origin of Body Tissue

Germ Layer	Body Portions Formed
Ectoderm	Central nervous system (brain and spinal cord) Peripheral nervous system Skin, hair, and nails Sebaceous glands Sense organs Mucous membranes of the anus, mouth, and nose Tooth enamel Mammary glands
Mesoderm	Supporting structures of the body (connective tissue, bones, cartilage, muscle, ligaments, and tendons) Dentin of teeth Upper portion of the urinary system (kidneys and ureters) Reproductive system Heart Circulatory system Blood cells Lymph vessels
Entoderm	Lining of pericardial, pleura, and peritoneal cavities Lining of the gastrointestinal tract, respiratory tract, tonsils, parathyroid, thyroid, thymus glands Lower urinary system (bladder and urethra)

develops into specific body systems (Table 9.3). Knowing which structures arise from each germ layer is important, because coexisting congenital defects found in newborns usually arise from the same layer. For example, a fistula between the trachea and the esophagus (both of which arise from the entoderm) is a common birth anomaly. Heart and kidney defects (which both arise from the mesoderm) are also commonly seen together. In contrast, it is rare to see a newborn with a malformation of the heart (arises from the mesoderm) and a malformation of the lower urinary tract (arises from the entoderm). One reason rubella infection is so serious in pregnancy is because this virus is capable of infecting all three germ layers, or causing congenital anomalies in a myriad of body systems.

Knowing the origins of body structures helps to explain why certain screening procedures are ordered for newborns with congenital malformations. A radiographic examination of the kidney, for example, may be ordered for a child born with a heart defect. A child with a malformation of the urinary tract is often investigated for reproductive abnormalities as well.

All organ systems are complete, at least in a rudimentary form, at 8 weeks' gestation (the end of the embryonic period). During this early time of **organogenesis** (organ formation), the growing structure is most vulnerable to invasion by teratogens (any factor that adversely affects the fertilized ovum, embryo, or fetus, such as cigarette smoking) (Box 9.2). Figure 9.5 illustrates the most critical periods of fetal growth when it is most important for women to minimize their exposure to teratogens (Box 9.3). The effect of individual teratogens is discussed in Chapter 12.

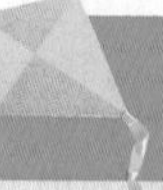

BOX 9.2 * Focus on Evidence-Based Practice

Should a woman who wants to stop cigarette smoking during pregnancy use a nicotine patch?

Every year, a large number of fetuses are exposed to smoking during pregnancy which results in decreased birth weight, fetal morbidity and, perhaps, attention-deficit/hyperactivity disorder (ADHD). Use of nicotine replacement therapy (NRT) or nicotine patches is often considered as an option to help withdrawal from cigarettes.

To see if a nicotine patch could cause fetal harm, the researcher completed a critical review of the literature and, from this, concluded:

1. Maternal smoking causes low birth weight and nicotine seems to play a significant role in reducing fetal weight.
2. Maternal smoking is a risk factor for ADHD, but a causal link between nicotine and hyperactivity is not well established. It is unclear if NRT would have similar long-term effects in children. More research is needed in this area.

Would the results of this literature review influence which nonsmoking method you would advise that pregnant women choose?

Source: Winzer-Serhan, U. H. (2008). Long-term consequences of maternal smoking and developmental chronic nicotine exposure. *Frontiers in Bioscience, 13* (1), 636–649.

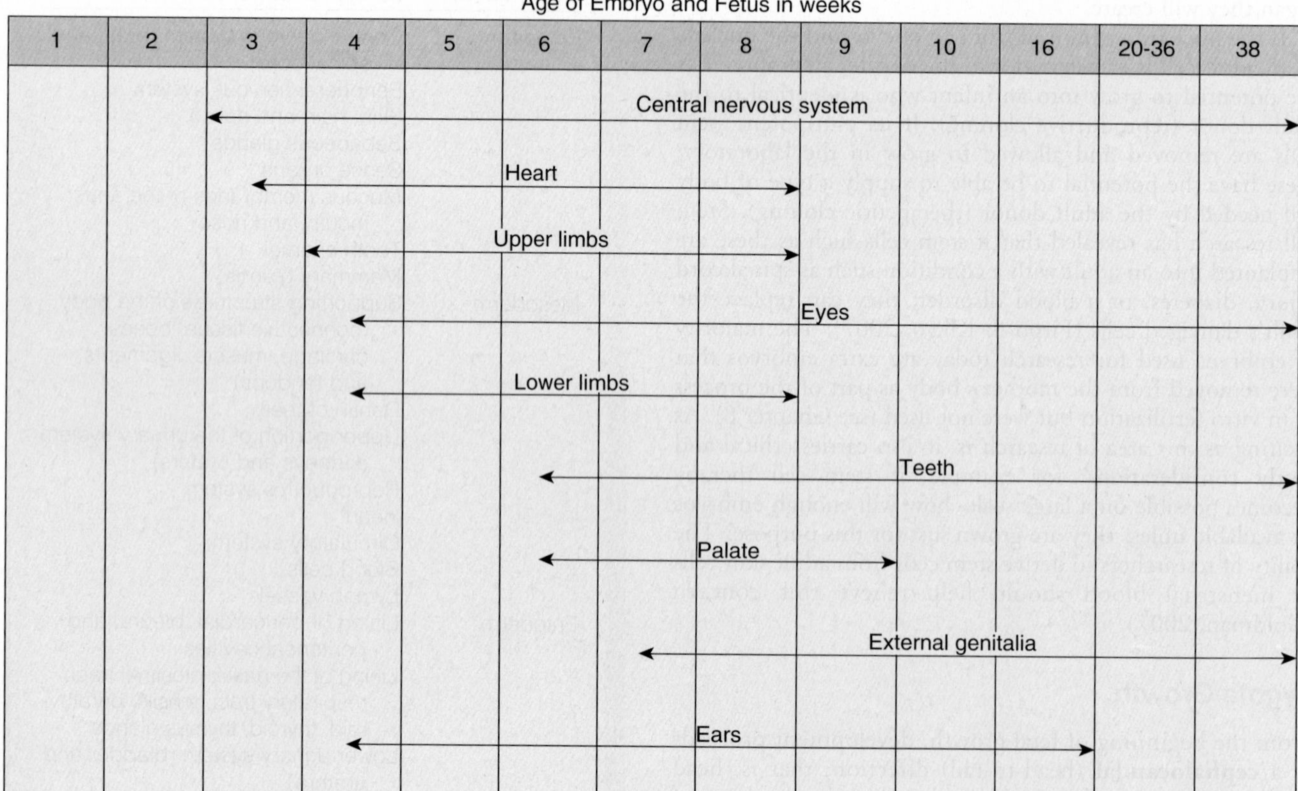

FIGURE 9.5 Critical periods of fetal growth.

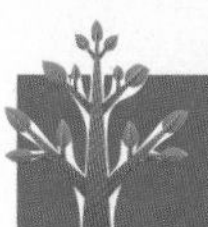

BOX 9.3 ✻ Focus on Family Teaching

Teratogens at Work

Q. Liz Calhom tells you, "I have to work. How can I guard against fetal teratogens at work?"

A. Here are some helpful tips:

- Ask your employer for a statement on hazardous substances at your work site; discuss your need to avoid these substances during pregnancy.
- Ask your employer to maintain a smoke-free site if that is not already a rule.
- Avoid any room, such as a coffee room, where smokers gather.
- Refrain from drinking alcohol, a frequent accompaniment to work lunches or social functions; ask for nonalcoholic drinks to be available at such events.

Cardiovascular System

The cardiovascular system is one of the first systems to become functional in intrauterine life. Simple blood cells joined to the walls of the yolk sac progress to become a network of blood vessels and a single heart tube, which forms as early as the 16th day of life and beats as early as the 24th day. The septum that divides the heart into chambers develops during the sixth or seventh week. Heart valves begin to develop in the seventh week. The heartbeat may be heard with a Doppler instrument as early as the 10th to 12th week of pregnancy. An electrocardiogram (ECG) may be recorded on a fetus as early as the 11th week, although the accuracy of such ECGs is in doubt until about the 20th week of pregnancy, when conduction is more regulated.

The heart rate of a fetus is affected by oxygen level, activity, and circulating blood volume, just as in adult life. After the 28th week of pregnancy, when the sympathetic nervous system has matured, the heart rate begins to show a baseline variability of about 5 beats per minute on a fetal heart rate rhythm strip.

Fetal Circulation

As early as the third week of intrauterine life, fetal blood begins to exchange nutrients with the maternal circulation across the chorionic villi. Fetal circulation (Fig. 9.6) differs from extrauterine circulation because the fetus derives oxygen and excretes carbon dioxide not from gas exchange in the lung but from gas exchange in the placenta.

Blood arriving at the fetus from the placenta is highly oxygenated. This blood enters the fetus through the umbilical vein (called a vein even though it carries oxygenated blood, because the direction of the blood is toward the fetal heart). Specialized structures present in the fetus then shunt blood flow to first supply the most important organs of the body: the brain, liver, heart, and kidneys. Blood flows from the umbilical vein to the *ductus venosus*, an accessory vessel that directs oxygenated blood directly to the fetal liver. Blood then empties into the fetal inferior vena cava so oxygenated blood is directed to the right side of the heart. Because there is no need for the bulk of blood to pass through the lungs, it is shunted, as it enters the right atrium, into the left atrium through an opening in the atrial septum, called the **foramen ovale.** From the left atrium, it follows the course of adult circulation into the left ventricle and into the aorta.

A small amount of blood that returns to the heart via the vena cava does leave the right atrium via the adult circulatory route—that is, through the tricuspid valve into the right ventricle, and then into the pulmonary artery and lungs to service the lung tissue. However, the larger portion of even this blood is shunted away from the lungs through an additional structure, the *ductus arteriosus*, directly into the descending aorta.

Most of the blood flow from the descending aorta is transported by the umbilical arteries (called arteries, even though they are now transporting deoxygenated blood, because they are carrying blood away from the fetal heart) back through the umbilical cord to the placental villi, where new oxygen exchange takes place.

The blood oxygen saturation level of the fetus is about 80% of a newborn's saturation level. The rapid fetal heart rate during pregnancy (120–160 beats per minute) is necessary to supply oxygen to cells, because the red blood cells are never fully saturated. Despite this low blood oxygen saturation level, carbon dioxide does not accumulate in the fetal system because it rapidly diffuses into maternal blood across a favorable placental pressure gradient.

Fetal Hemoglobin

Fetal hemoglobin differs from adult hemoglobin in several ways. It has a different composition (two alpha and two gamma chains, compared with two alpha and two beta chains of adult hemoglobin). It is also more concentrated and has greater oxygen affinity, two features that increase its efficiency. So much hemoglobin is present at birth that a newborn's hemoglobin level is about 17.1 g/100 mL, compared with an adult normal level of 11 g/100 mL; a newborn's hematocrit is about 53%, compared with an adult normal level of 45%.

The change from fetal to adult hemoglobin levels begins before birth and accelerates after birth. The major blood dyscrasias, such as sickle cell anemia, tend to be defects of the beta hemoglobin chain. That is why clinical symptoms do not become apparent until the bulk of fetal hemoglobin has matured to adult hemoglobin composition, at about 6 months of age (Rees, 2007).

Respiratory System

At the third week of intrauterine life, the respiratory and digestive tracts exist as a single tube. Like all body tubes, initially this forms as a solid structure, which then canalizes (hollows out). By the end of the fourth week, a septum begins to divide the esophagus from the trachea. At the same time, lung buds appear on the trachea.

Until the seventh week of life, the diaphragm does not completely divide the thoracic cavity from the abdomen. This causes lung buds to extend down into the abdomen, reentering the chest only as the chest's longitudinal dimension increases and the diaphragm becomes complete (at the end of the seventh week). If the diaphragm fails to close completely, the stomach, spleen, liver, or intestines may be pulled up into the thoracic cavity. This causes the child to be born with a diaphragmatic hernia or with intestine present in the chest, compromising the lungs and perhaps displacing the heart (Moyer et al., 2009).

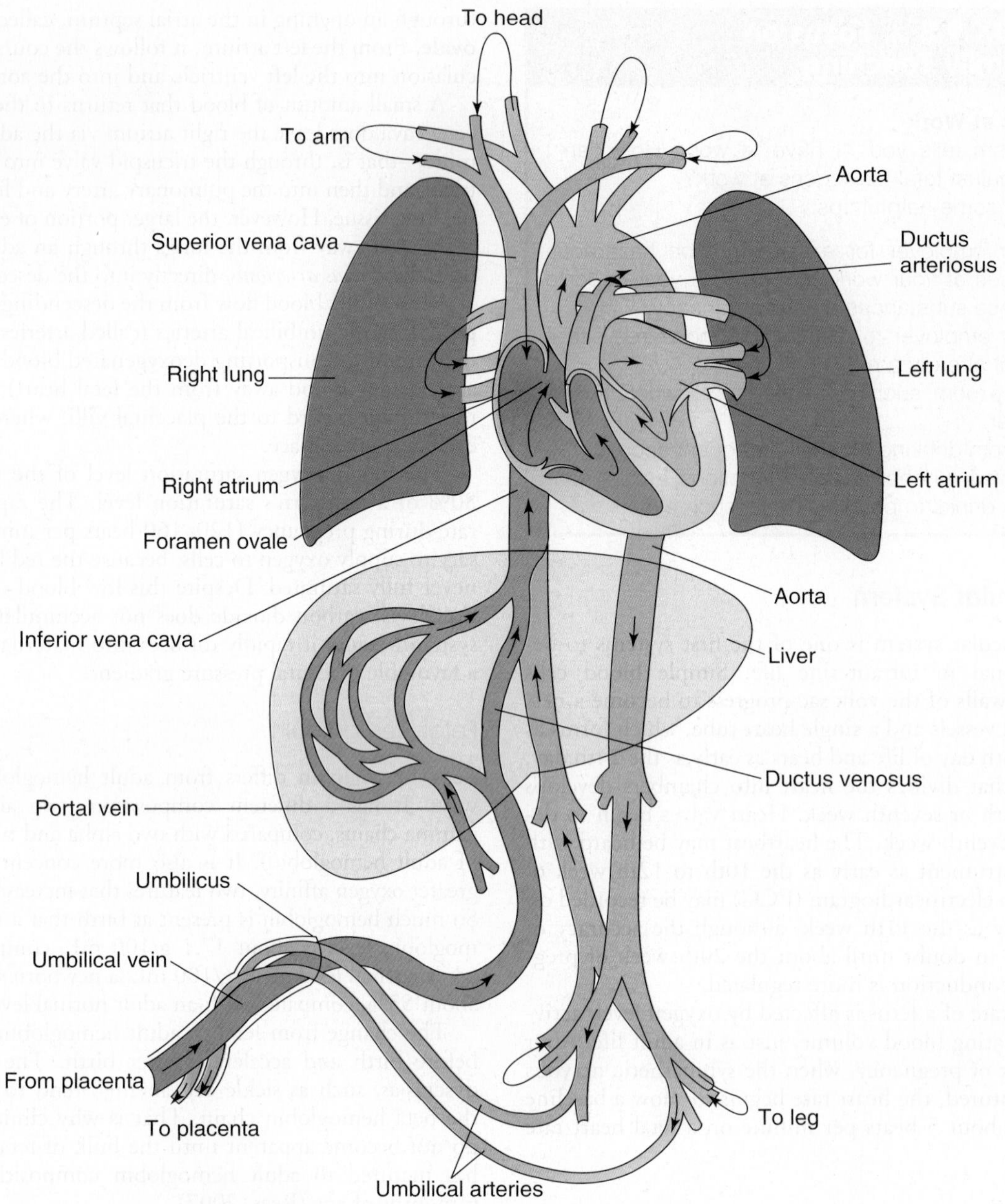

FIGURE 9.6 Fetal circulation.

Other important respiratory developmental milestones include:

- Alveoli and capillaries begin to form between the 24th and 28th weeks. Both capillary and alveoli development must be complete before gas exchange can occur in the fetal lungs.
- Spontaneous respiratory practice movements begin as early as 3 months' gestation and continue throughout pregnancy.
- Specific lung fluid with a low surface tension and low viscosity forms in alveoli to aid in expansion of the alveoli at birth; it is rapidly absorbed after birth.
- **Surfactant,** a phospholipid substance, is formed and excreted by the alveolar cells at about the 24th week of pregnancy. This decreases alveolar surface tension on expiration, preventing alveolar collapse and improving the infant's ability to maintain respirations in the outside environment (Soll, 2009).

Surfactant has two components: lecithin (L) and sphingomyelin (S). Early in the formation of surfactant, sphingomyelin is the chief component. At about 35 weeks, there is a surge in the production of lecithin, which then becomes the chief component by a ratio of 2:1. As a fetus practices breathing movements, surfactant mixes with amniotic fluid. Analysis of the L/S ratio regarding whether lecithin or sphingomyelin is the dominant component by amniocentesis technique is a primary test of fetal maturity. Respiratory distress syndrome, a severe breathing disorder, can develop if there is lack of surfactant or it has not changed to its mature form at birth (see Chapter 26). Any interference with the blood supply to the fetus, such as occurs with placental insufficiency from hypertension, appears to enhance surfactant development. This type of stress probably causes this by increasing steroid levels in the fetus. Although there is little evidence-based information available to document why the phenomenon occurs, synthetically increasing steroid levels in the fetus (the administration of betamethasone to the mother) can hurry alveolar maturation and surfactant production (Roberts & Dalziel, 2009).

✔ Checkpoint Question 9.3

Liz Calhorn asks you why her doctor is so concerned about whether her fetus is producing surfactant. Your best answer would be:

a. Surfactant keeps lungs from collapsing on expiration and so aids newborn breathing.
b. Surfactant is produced by the fetal liver, so its presence reveals liver maturity.
c. Surfactant is the precursor to IgM antibody production, so it prevents infection.
d. Surfactant reveals mature kidney function, as it is produced by kidney glomeruli.

Nervous System

Like the circulatory system, the nervous system begins to develop extremely early in pregnancy. During the third and fourth weeks of intrauterine life, possibly before the woman even realizes she is pregnant, active formation of the nervous system and sense organs has already begun.

- A neural plate (a thickened portion of the ectoderm) is apparent by the third week of gestation. The top portion differentiates into the neural tube, which will form the central nervous system (brain and spinal cord), and the neural crest, which will develop into the peripheral nervous system.
- All parts of the brain (cerebrum, cerebellum, pons, and medulla oblongata) form in utero, although none are completely mature at birth. Growth proceeds rapidly during the first year and continues at high levels until 5 or 6 years of age.
- The eye and inner ear develop as projections of the original neural tube.
- By 24 weeks, the ear is capable of responding to sound; the eyes exhibit a pupillary reaction, indicating that sight is present.
- Brain waves can be detected on an electroencephalogram (EEG) by the eighth week.

The neurologic system seems particularly prone to insult during the early weeks of the embryonic period. Spinal cord disorders such as meningocele (herniation of the meninges) may occur because of lack of folic acid (contained in green leafy vegetables and pregnancy vitamins) (Lumley et al., 2009). All during pregnancy and at birth, the system is vulnerable to damage from anoxia.

Endocrine System

As soon as endocrine organs mature in intrauterine life, function begins.

- The fetal adrenal glands supply a precursor necessary for estrogen synthesis by the placenta.
- The fetal pancreas produces insulin needed by the fetus (insulin is one of the few substances that does not cross the placenta from the mother to the fetus).
- The thyroid and parathyroid glands play vital roles in fetal metabolic function and calcium balance.

Digestive System

The digestive tract separates from the respiratory tract at about the fourth week of intrauterine life and, after that, begins to grow extremely rapidly. Initially solid, the tract canalizes (hollows out) to become patent. Later, the endothelial cells of the gastrointestinal tract proliferate extensively, occluding the lumen once more, and the tract must canalize again. Atresia (blockage) or stenosis (narrowing) can develop if either the first or second canalization does not occur. The proliferation of cells shed in the second recanalization forms the basis for meconium (see below).

Because of this rapid intestinal growth, by the sixth week of intrauterine life, the intestine becomes too large to be contained by the abdomen. A portion of the intestine, guided by the vitelline membrane (a part of the yolk sac), is pushed into the base of the umbilical cord, where it remains until about the 10th week, when the abdominal cavity has grown large enough to accommodate the intestinal mass again. As the intestine returns to the abdominal cavity at this point, it must rotate 180 degrees. Failure to do so can result in inadequate mesentery attachments, possibly leading to volvulus of the intestine in the newborn. If any intestine remains outside the abdomen in the base of the cord, a congenital anomaly, termed *omphalocele*, develops. A similar defect, *gastroschisis*, occurs when the original midline fusion that occurred at the early cell stage is incomplete (Thilo et al., 2008). If the vitelline duct does not atrophy after return of the intestines, a Meckel's diverticulum (a pouch of intestinal tissue) can result (Hol & Kuipers, 2007).

Meconium, a collection of cellular wastes, bile, fats, mucoproteins, mucopolysaccharides, and portions of the vernix caseosa, the lubricating substance that forms on the fetal skin, accumulates in the intestines as early as the 16th week. Meconium is sticky in consistency and appears black or dark green (obtaining its color from bile pigment).

The gastrointestinal tract is sterile before birth. Because vitamin K is synthesized by the action of bacteria in the intestines, vitamin K levels are low in the newborn. Sucking and swallowing reflexes are not mature until the fetus is at about 32 weeks' gestation or weighs 1500 g.

The ability of the gastrointestinal tract to secrete enzymes essential to carbohydrate and protein digestion is mature at 36 weeks. However, amylase, an enzyme found in saliva that is necessary for digestion of complex starches, is not mature until 3 months after birth. Many newborns have not yet developed lipase, an enzyme needed for fat digestion.

The liver is active throughout gestation, functioning as a filter between the incoming blood and the fetal circulation and as a deposit site for fetal stores such as iron and glycogen, but is still immature at birth. This can possibly lead to hypoglycemia and hyperbilirubinemia, two serious problems, in the first 24 hours after birth. The liver does not prevent recreational drugs or alcohol ingested by the mother from entering the fetal circulation.

Musculoskeletal System

During the first 2 weeks of fetal life, cartilage prototypes provide position and support. Ossification of this cartilage into bone begins at about the 12th week. Ossification continues all through fetal life and actually until adulthood. Carpals, tarsals, and sternal bones generally do not ossify until birth is imminent. A fetus can be seen to move on an ultrasound as early as the 11th week, although the woman usually does not feel this movement (*quickening*) until almost 20 weeks of gestation.

Reproductive System

A child's sex is determined at the moment of conception by a spermatozoon carrying an X or a Y chromosome and can be ascertained as early as 8 weeks by chromosomal analysis. At about the sixth week of life, the gonads (ovaries or testes) form. If testes form, testosterone is secreted, apparently influencing the sexually neutral genital duct to form other male organs (maturity of the wolffian, or mesonephric, duct). In the absence of testosterone secretion, female organs will form (maturation of the müllerian, or paramesonephric, duct). This is an important phenomenon, because if a woman should take an androgen or an androgen-like substance during this stage of pregnancy, a child who is chromosomally female could appear more male than female at birth. If deficient testosterone is secreted by the testes, both the müllerian (female) duct and the male (wolffian) duct could develop (pseudo-hermaphroditism, or intersex).

The testes first form in the abdominal cavity and do not descend into the scrotal sac until the 34th to 38th week. Because of this, many male preterm infants are born with undescended testes. These children need follow-up care to be certain that their testes do descend when they reach what would have been the 34th to 38th week of gestational age, because testicular descent does not occur as readily in extrauterine life as it would in utero. Surgery is necessary as undescended testes are associated with poor sperm production and testicular cancer (Zeitler et al., 2008).

Urinary System

Although rudimentary kidneys are present as early as the end of the fourth week of intrauterine life, the presence of kidneys does not appear to be essential for life before birth because the placenta clears the fetus of waste products. Urine is formed by the 12th week and is excreted into the amniotic fluid by the 16th week of gestation. At term, fetal urine is being excreted at the rate of 500 mL/day. An amount of amniotic fluid that is less than normal (oligohydramnios) suggests that fetal kidneys are not secreting adequate urine (Lanni & Loveless, 2007).

The complex structure of the kidneys is gradually developed during intrauterine life and continues for months afterward. The loop of Henle, for example, is not fully differentiated until the child is born. Glomerular filtration and concentration of urine in the newborn are not efficient, because the kidney function is still not mature at birth.

Early in the embryonic stage of urinary system development, the bladder extends as high as the umbilical region. On rare occasions, an open lumen between the urinary bladder and the umbilicus fails to close. Termed a *patent urachus*, this is discovered at birth by the persistent drainage of a clear, acid-pH fluid (urine) from the umbilicus.

Integumentary System

The skin of a fetus appears thin and almost translucent until subcutaneous fat begins to be deposited at about 36 weeks. Skin is covered by soft downy hairs (lanugo) that serve as insulation to preserve warmth in utero and a cream cheese–like substance, vernix caseosa, which is important for lubrication and for keeping the skin from macerating in utero.

Immune System

Immunoglobulin G (IgG) maternal antibodies cross the placenta into the fetus as early as the 20th week and certainly by the 24th week of intrauterine life to give a fetus temporary passive immunity against diseases for which the mother has antibodies. These often include poliomyelitis, rubella (German measles), rubeola (regular measles), diphtheria, tetanus, infectious parotitis (mumps), hepatitis B, and pertussis (whooping cough). Little or no immunity to the herpes virus (the virus of chickenpox, cold sores, and genital herpes) is transferred to the fetus, so the average newborn is potentially susceptible to these diseases. The recommended immunization for teenagers against the virus should reduce the incidence of this in newborns.

Infants born before antibody transfer has taken place have no natural immunity and need more than the usual protection against infectious disease in the newborn period. The level of these acquired passive IgG immunoglobulins peaks at birth and then decreases over the next 8 months as the infant builds up his or her own stores of IgG, as well as IgA and IgM. Because the passive immunity received by the newborn has already declined substantially by about 2 months, immunization against diphtheria, tetanus, pertussis, poliomyelitis, rotovirus, *Haemophilus influenzae,* and pneumococcus is typically started at this time. Passive antibodies to measles have been demonstrated to last for longer than 1 year. Consequently, the immunization for measles is not given until an extrauterine age of 12 months.

A fetus is capable of active antibody production late in pregnancy. Generally this is not necessary, however, because antibodies are manufactured only after stimulation by an invading antigen, and antigens rarely invade the intrauterine space. However, infants whose mothers have had an infection such as rubella during pregnancy typically have active IgM antibodies to rubella in their blood serum at birth. Because IgA and IgM antibodies cannot cross the placenta, their presence in a newborn is proof that the fetus has been exposed to a disease.

Milestones of Fetal Growth and Development

When fetal milestones occur can be confusing, because the life of the fetus is typically measured from the time of ovulation or fertilization (ovulation age), but the length of a pregnancy is more commonly measured from the first day of the last menstrual period (gestational age). Because ovulation and fertilization take place about 2 weeks after the last menstrual period, the ovulation age of the fetus is

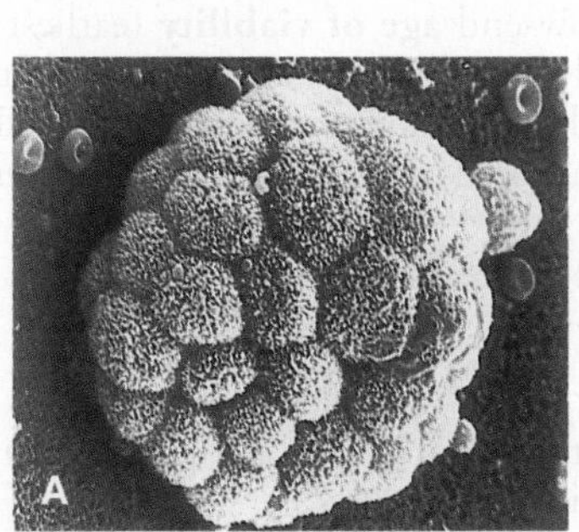

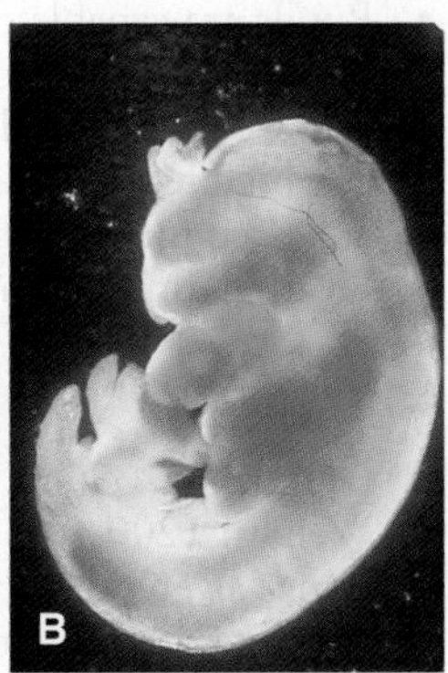

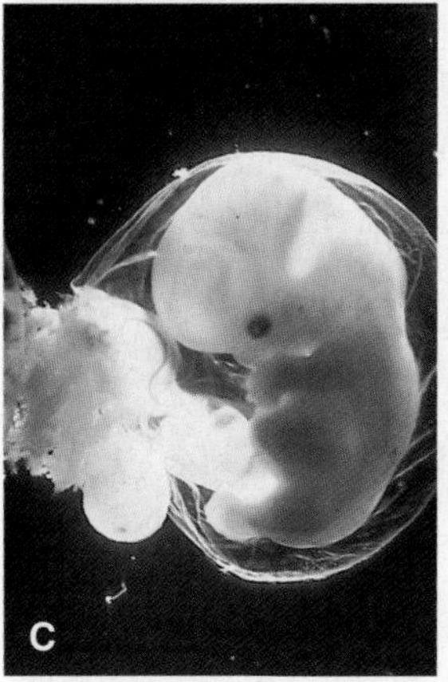

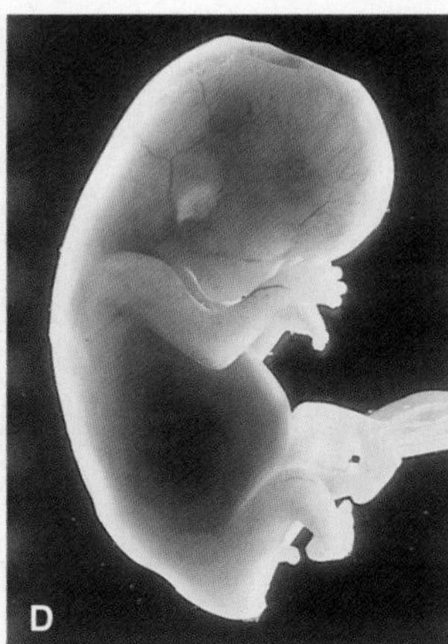

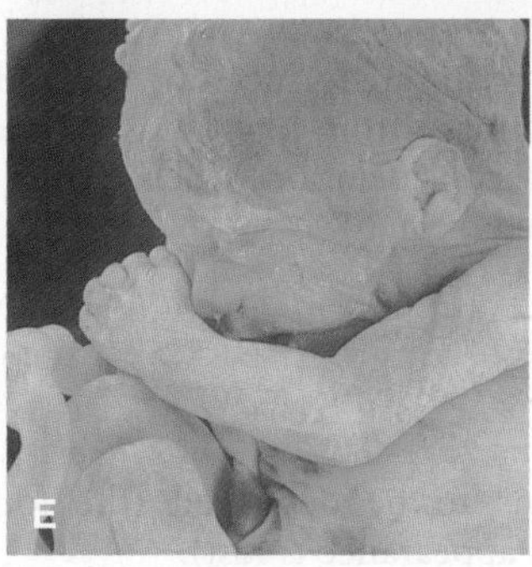

FIGURE 9.7 Human embryos at different stages of life: (**A**) implantation in uterus 7–8 days after conception. (**B**) Embryo at 32 days. (**C**) At 37 days. (**D**) At 41 days. (**E**) Between 12 and 15 weeks. (From Petit Format/Nestle/Science Source/Photo Researchers.)

always 2 weeks less than the length of the pregnancy or the gestational age.

Both ovulation and gestational age are typically reported in lunar months (4-week periods) or in trimesters (3-month periods) rather than in weeks. In lunar months, a pregnancy is 10 months (40 weeks, or 280 days) long; a fetus grows in utero 9.5 lunar months or three full trimesters (38 weeks, or 266 days).

The following discussion of fetal developmental milestones is based on gestational weeks, because it is helpful when talking to expectant parents to be able to correlate fetal development with the way they measure pregnancy—from the first day of the last menstrual period. Figure 9.7 illustrates the comparative size and appearance of human embryos and fetuses at different stages.

End of 4th Gestational Week

At the end of the fourth week of gestation, the human embryo is a group of rapidly growing cells but does not yet resemble a human being.

- Length: 0.75–1 cm
- Weight: 400 mg
- The spinal cord is formed and fused at the midpoint.
- Lateral wings that will form the body are folded forward to fuse at the midline.
- The head folds forward and becomes prominent, representing about one-third of the entire structure.
- The back is bent so that the head almost touches the tip of the tail.
- The rudimentary heart appears as a prominent bulge on the anterior surface.
- Arms and legs are budlike structures.
- Rudimentary eyes, ears, and nose are discernible.

End of 8th Gestational Week

- Length: 2.5 cm (1 in)
- Weight: 20 g
- Organogenesis is complete.
- The heart, with a septum and valves, is beating rhythmically.
- Facial features are definitely discernible.
- Arms and legs have developed.
- External genitalia are forming, but sex is not yet distinguishable by simple observation.
- The primitive tail is regressing.
- The abdomen bulges forward because the fetal intestine is growing so rapidly.
- An ultrasound shows a gestational sac, diagnostic of pregnancy (Fig. 9.8).

End of 12th Gestational Week (First Trimester)

- Length: 7–8 cm
- Weight: 45 g
- Nail beds are forming on fingers and toes.
- Spontaneous movements are possible, although they are usually too faint to be felt by the mother.
- Some reflexes, such as the Babinski reflex, are present.
- Bone ossification centers begin to form.
- Tooth buds are present.
- Sex is distinguishable by outward appearance.
- Urine secretion begins but may not yet be evident in amniotic fluid.
- The heartbeat is audible through Doppler technology.

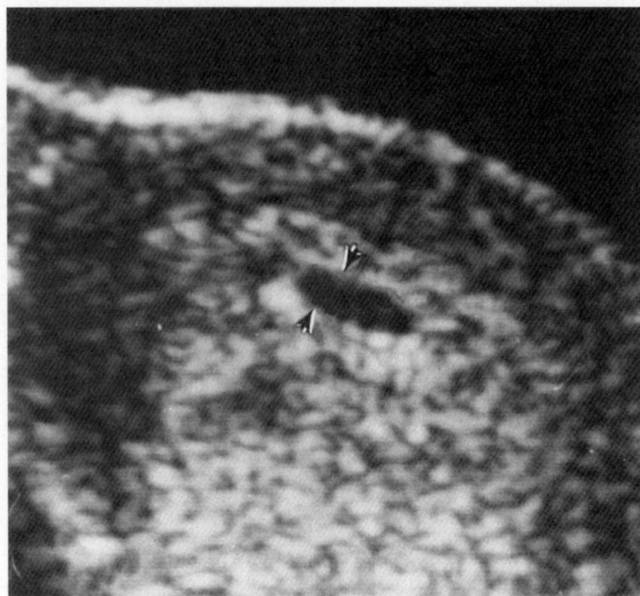

FIGURE 9.8 An ultrasound showing the characteristic circle diagnostic of pregnancy (the gestational sac). (From Benson, C. B., et al. [1988]. *Atlas of obstetrical ultrasound.* Philadelphia: JB Lippincott.)

End of 16th Gestational Week

- Length: 10–17 cm
- Weight: 55–120 g
- Fetal heart sounds are audible by an ordinary stethoscope.
- Lanugo is well formed.
- Liver and pancreas are functioning.
- Fetus actively swallows amniotic fluid, demonstrating an intact but uncoordinated swallowing reflex; urine is present in amniotic fluid.
- Sex can be determined by ultrasound.

End of 20th Gestational Week

- Length: 25 cm
- Weight: 223 g
- Spontaneous fetal movements can be sensed by the mother.
- Antibody production is possible.
- The hair forms on the head, extending to include eyebrows.
- Meconium is present in the upper intestine.
- Brown fat, a special fat that will aid in temperature regulation at birth, begins to be formed behind the kidneys, sternum, and posterior neck.
- Vernix caseosa begins to form and cover the skin.
- Passive antibody transfer from mother to fetus begins.
- Definite sleeping and activity patterns are distinguishable (the fetus has developed biorhythms that will guide sleep/wake patterns throughout life).

End of 24th Gestational Week (Second Trimester)

- Length: 28–36 cm
- Weight: 550 g
- Meconium is present as far as the rectum.
- Active production of lung surfactant begins.
- Eyebrows and eyelashes become well defined.
- Eyelids, previously fused since the 12th week, now open.
- Pupils are capable of reacting to light.
- When fetuses reach 24 weeks, or 601 g, they have achieved a practical low-end **age of viability** (earliest age at which fetuses could survive if born at that time), if they are cared for after birth in a modern intensive care facility.
- Hearing can be demonstrated by response to sudden sound.

End of 28th Gestational Week

- Length: 35–38 cm
- Weight: 1200 g
- Lung alveoli begin to mature, and surfactant can be demonstrated in amniotic fluid.
- Testes begin to descend into the scrotal sac from the lower abdominal cavity.
- The blood vessels of the retina are formed but thin and extremely susceptible to damage from high oxygen concentrations (an important consideration when caring for preterm infants who need oxygen).

End of 32nd Gestational Week

- Length: 38–43 cm
- Weight: 1600 g
- Subcutaneous fat begins to be deposited (the former stringy, "little old man" appearance is lost).
- Fetus responds by movement to sounds outside the mother's body.
- Active Moro reflex is present.
- Iron stores, which provide iron for the time during which the neonate will ingest only milk after birth, are beginning to be developed.
- Fingernails grow to reach the end of fingertips.

End of 36th Gestational Week

- Length: 42–48 cm
- Weight: 1800–2700 g (5–6 lb)
- Body stores of glycogen, iron, carbohydrate, and calcium are deposited.
- Additional amounts of subcutaneous fat are deposited.
- Sole of the foot has only one or two crisscross creases, compared with the full crisscross pattern that will be evident at term.
- Amount of lanugo begins to diminish.
- Most babies turn into a vertex (head down) presentation during this month.

End of 40th Gestational Week (Third Trimester)

- Length: 48–52 cm (crown to rump, 35–37 cm)
- Weight: 3000 g (7–7.5 lb)
- Fetus kicks actively, hard enough to cause the mother considerable discomfort.
- Fetal hemoglobin begins its conversion to adult hemoglobin. The conversion is so rapid that, at birth, about 20% of hemoglobin will be adult in character.
- Vernix caseosa is fully formed.
- Fingernails extend over the fingertips.
- Creases on the soles of the feet cover at least two thirds of the surface.

In primiparas (women having their first baby), the fetus often sinks into the birth canal during the last 2 weeks, giving the mother a feeling that the load she is carrying is less. This event, termed *lightening*, is a fetal announcement that the third trimester of pregnancy has ended and birth is at hand.

Determination of Estimated Birth Date

It is impossible to predict the day an infant will be born with a high degree of accuracy. Traditionally, this date was referred to as the estimated date of confinement (EDC). Because women are no longer "confined" after childbirth, the abbreviation EDB **(estimated date of birth)** or EDD (estimated date of delivery) is more commonly used today.

Fewer than 5% of pregnancies end exactly 280 days from the last menstrual period or exactly on this date; fewer than half end within 1 week of the 280th day.

If fertilization occurred early in a menstrual cycle, the pregnancy will probably end "early"; if ovulation and fertilization occurred later in the cycle, the pregnancy will end "late." Because of these normal variations, a pregnancy ending 2 weeks before or 2 weeks after the calculated EDB is considered well within the normal limit (38–42 weeks). Gestational age wheels or birth date calculators that can be used to predict a birth date are available, but calculation by Nagele's rule is the standard method used to predict the length of a pregnancy (Box 9.4).

What if... Liz Calhorn, the young woman you met at the beginning of the chapter, first came to your prenatal clinic on August 5 and told you that she had her last menstrual period on March 13 to March 18? What would be her estimated date of birth (EDB)?

ASSESSMENT OF FETAL GROWTH AND DEVELOPMENT

Fetal growth and development can be compromised if a fetus has a metabolic or chromosomal disorder that interferes with normal growth, if the supporting structures such as the placenta or cord do not form normally, or if environmental influences such as cigarette smoking (the nicotine in cigarettes causes fetal growth restriction) or alcohol consumption (alcohol causes severe cognitive challenge) interfere with fetal growth. Much information regarding whether a fetus is growing and is healthy can be gathered through a variety of assessment techniques. Nursing responsibilities for these assessment procedures include seeing that a signed consent form has been obtained as needed, scheduling the procedure, explaining the procedure to the woman and her support person including what the procedure will entail and any potential risks, preparing a woman physically and psychologically, providing support during the procedure, assessing both fetal and maternal responses to the procedure, providing any necessary follow-up care, and managing equipment and specimens (see Focus on Nursing Care Planning Box 9.5).

Consent to perform a procedure is necessary if the procedure poses any risk to the mother or fetus that would not otherwise be present.

BOX 9.4 ✻ Nagele's Rule

To calculate the date of birth by this rule, count backward 3 calendar months from the first day of a woman's last menstrual period and add 7 days. For example, if the last menstrual period began May 15, you would count back 3 months (April 15, March 15, February 15) and add 7 days, to arrive at a date of birth of February 22.

Health History

Like all assessments, fetal assessment begins with a health history. Ask specifically about nutritional intake, because, if a woman is not eating a well-balanced diet, she may not be taking in sufficient nutrients for fetal growth. Be certain to also ask about personal habits such as cigarette smoking, recreational drug use, and exercise, because all of these influence glucose/insulin balance and fetal growth. Most women actively protect a fetus growing inside them. Asking if the woman has had any accidents or experienced intimate partner abuse helps reveal whether the fetus could have suffered any trauma (intimate partner abuse tends to increase during pregnancy because of the stress a pregnancy can create) (Records, 2007).

Estimating Fetal Growth

McDonald's rule, a symphysis-fundal height measurement, although not documented to be thoroughly reliable, is an easy method of determining during midpregnancy that a fetus is growing in utero. Typically, the distance from the uterine fundus to the symphysis pubis in centimeters is equal to the week of gestation between the 20th and 31st weeks of pregnancy. Make the measurement from the notch of the symphysis pubis to over the top of the uterine fundus as a woman lies supine (Fig. 9.9). McDonald's rule becomes inaccurate during the third trimester of pregnancy because the fetus is growing more in weight than in height during this time. Until then, a fundal height much greater than this standard suggests multiple pregnancy, a miscalculated due date, a large-for-gestational-age infant, hydramnios (increased amniotic fluid volume), or possibly even hydatidiform mole (see Chapter 21). A fundal measurement much less than this suggests that the fetus is failing to thrive (intrauterine growth restriction), the pregnancy length was miscalculated, or an anomaly, such as anencephaly, has developed.

Determining and recording that the fundus has reached typical milestone measurements, such as over the symphysis pubis at 12 weeks, at the umbilicus at 20 weeks, and at the xiphoid process at 36 weeks, are also helpful.

Assessing Fetal Well-being

Several actions or procedures are helpful in detecting and documenting that the fetus is not only growing but apparently healthy.

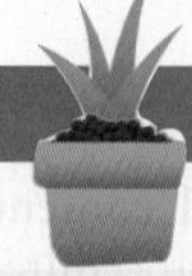

BOX 9.5 ✻ Focus on Nursing Care Planning

A Multidisciplinary Care Map for a Woman Undergoing Fetal Studies

Liz Calhorn, an 18-year-old woman, thinks she is 24 weeks' pregnant. Today, at a clinic visit, she tells you she felt her fetus move for the first time. She states, "Feeling the baby move made me realize for the first time there's someone inside me, you know what I mean? It made me know it's time I started being more careful with what I do."

Family Assessment ✻ Client lives in one-bedroom apartment; supports self with typing position at insurance agency. States, "My parents would help out if I begged them, but I'm not going to do that." Boyfriend (father of fetus) is supportive, but couple has no plans to marry. Client states, "I'm not ready for commitment."

Client Assessment ✻ Client smokes a pack of cigarettes a day. Twice during the pregnancy (at the 4th and 10th week), she drank beer at summer picnics. Takes aspirin, 10 g, for almost-daily sinus headaches. No spotting or falls since last menstrual period. No recreational drugs.

Nutrition:
- Breakfast: None, to help control her weight.
- Lunch: A hotdog and salad. One diet cola.
- Dinner: Macaroni and cheese; applesauce. One cup coffee.
- Snack: ½ bag potato chips and cream-cheese dip

Physical examination: Fundal height is 20 cm. Fetal heart tones by Doppler at 160/min. Has been advised to have an ultrasound done to assess for fetal growth and to date pregnancy.

Nursing Diagnosis ✻ Risk for altered fetal growth related to inadequate nutrition, alcohol and nicotine consumption

Outcome Criteria ✻ Client consents to ultrasound for fetal growth assessment; reports lessened alcohol and cigarette consumption at next visit.

Team Member Responsible	Assessment	Intervention	Rationale	Expected Outcome
Activities of Daily Living				
Nurse	Ask patient to recount a "typical day" to reveal any actions possibly detrimental to fetal growth.	Discuss common actions that are unsafe during pregnancy, such as smoking and drinking alcohol.	Knowing what constitutes unsafe practices during pregnancy is a woman's best safeguard against fetal harm.	Client states that she now knows and will avoid unsafe actions during pregnancy.
Consultations				
Physician/nurse	Determine whether ultrasound department has appointments free in coming week.	Schedule ultrasound 1 week in advance with ultrasound department.	Client believes she is 24 weeks pregnant. Fundal height, recent fetal movements correspond more closely to 20 weeks.	Client reports for scheduled ultrasound in 1 week.
Procedures/Medications				
Nurse	Assess use of over-the-counter and complementary therapies.	Discuss with client inadvisability of taking aspirin during pregnancy; suggest she take acetaminophen (Tylenol) instead.	Acetylsalicylic acid (aspirin) can lead to bleeding or prolonged pregnancy.	Client reports at next prenatal visit that she takes acetaminophen for pain during pregnancy.
Nutrition				
Nurse/ nutritionist	Ask client for a 24-hour recall nutrition history.	Discuss the advisability of eating breakfast while pregnant to help avoid hypoglycemia in fetus.	Knowing what constitutes unsafe practices during pregnancy is a woman's best safeguard against fetal harm.	Client reports at prenatal visits that she eats breakfast before leaving for work in the morning.

		Nutrition		
Nutritionist	Assess and analyze the 24-hour recall history.	Discuss advantages of good pregnancy nutrition with client and define healthy pregnancy nutrition.	Client needs to improve total nutrition, especially intake of protein sources, to better support pregnancy.	Client meets with clinic nutritionist to discuss better nutrition pattern. Reports improved protein sources in diet.
		Patient/Family Education		
Nurse	Determine whether client understands that ultrasound is not x-ray, so is not harmful to fetus.	Instruct client about preparation for ultrasound (drink fluid; avoid emptying bladder).	A well-prepared client is more apt to result in an effective procedure and a satisfied client.	Client will describe accurate preparations for procedure. Receives printed instructions for ambulatory ultrasound.
		Spiritual/Psychosocial/Emotional Needs		
Nurse/ physician	Assess the extent of factors, such as alcohol and cigarette use, that could have led to intrauterine growth restriction.	Review the possibility with client that her pregnancy dating may be wrong, because fundal height is below normal. Alternate cause could be fetal growth restriction.	Understanding contributors to fetal health is necessary for women to make informed choices during pregnancy.	Client states that she understands the discrepancy in fundal height and weeks' gestation following explanation.
		Discharge Planning		
Nurse/ physician	Perform complete assessment to help ensure continuity of care with other services.	Mark chart as high-risk client for intrauterine growth restriction. Stress importance of continuing prenatal care.	Documenting risk factors helps to safeguard the fetus.	The patient chart documents high-risk status. Client continues prenatal care.

Fetal Movement

Fetal movement that can be felt by the mother (quickening) occurs at approximately 18 to 20 weeks of pregnancy and peaks in intensity at 28 to 38 weeks. A healthy fetus moves with a degree of consistency, or at least 10 times a day. In contrast, a fetus not receiving enough nutrients because of placental insufficiency has greatly decreased movements. Based on this, asking a woman to observe and record the number of movements the fetus is making offers a gross assessment of fetal well-being (Chang & Blakemore, 2007).

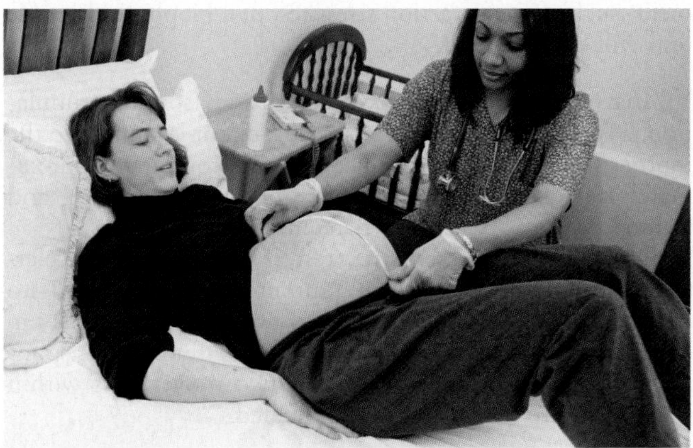

FIGURE 9.9 Measuring fundal height from the superior aspect of the pubis to the fundal crest. The tape is pressed flat against the abdomen for the measurement.

Because of variations in movements among normal, healthy fetuses, as well as variations in different health care providers' level of confidence in the technique, a variety of protocols have been developed by different institutions. One popular way to approach this assessment is to ask the woman to lie in a left recumbent position after a meal and record how many fetal movements she feels over the next hour (the Sandovsky method). In this position, a fetus normally moves a minimum of twice every 10 minutes or an average of 10–12 times an hour. If less than 10 movements occur within an hour, the woman repeats the test for the next hour. She should call her health care provider if she feels fewer than 10 movements (half the normal number) during the chosen 2 hours. Another protocol is "Count-to-Ten" (the Cardiff method). For this, a woman records the time interval it takes for her to feel 10 fetal movements. Usually, this occurs within 60 minutes. Make sure to assure a woman that fetal movements do vary, especially in relation to sleep cycles of the fetus, her activity, and the time since she last ate. Otherwise, she can become unduly worried that her fetus may be in jeopardy when the fetus is just having an inactive time.

What if... You give instructions to Liz Calhorn, the woman described at the beginning of the chapter, to count fetal movements for 1 hour two times a day after meals and she tells you that she snacks all day long rather than eats at regular times? Would you modify your instructions? Which is more important—that she count movements after meals or that she does it two times a day?

Fetal Heart Rate

Fetal hearts beat at 120 to 160 beats per minute throughout pregnancy. Fetal heart sounds can be heard and counted as early as the 10th to 11th week of pregnancy by the use of an ultrasonic Doppler technique (Fig. 9.10).

Rhythm Strip Testing. The term "rhythm strip testing" means assessment of the fetal heart rate for whether a good baseline rate and a degree of variability are present. For this, help a woman into a semi-Fowler's position (either in a comfortable lounge chair or on an examining table or bed with an elevated backrest) to prevent her uterus from compressing the vena cava and causing supine hypotension syndrome during the test. Attach an external fetal heart rate monitor abdominally (Fig. 9.11A). Record the fetal heart rate for 20 minutes.

The baseline reading refers to the average rate of the fetal heartbeat per minute. Variability refers to small changes in rate that occur if the fetal parasympathetic and sympathetic nervous systems are receiving adequate oxygen and nutrients. It is categorized as *absent* (none apparent); *minimal* (extremely small fluctuations); *moderate* (amplitude range of 6–25 beats per minute); and *marked* (amplitude range over 25 beats per minute) (Macones et al., 2008). In the rhythm strip in Figure 9.11B, for example, the baseline (average) of the fetal heartbeat is 130 beats per minute, although over the recorded period, it varies from 120 to 150 beats per minute.

Because the average fetus moves about twice every 10 minutes, and movement causes the heart rate to increase, there will typically be two or more instances of fetal heart rate acceleration in a 20-minute rhythm strip.

Rhythm strip testing requires a woman to remain in a fairly fixed position for 20 minutes. Keep her well informed of the purpose of the test, how it is interpreted, and the meaning of results after the test. The more she understands about the process, the better she can cooperate to make it successful.

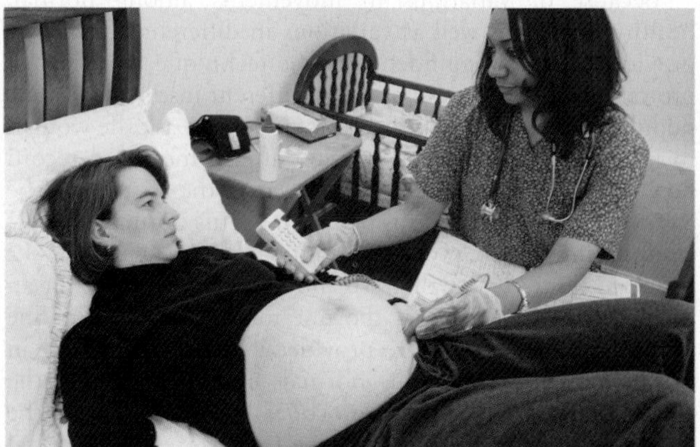

FIGURE 9.10 Measuring fetal heart rate with a Doppler transducer, which detects and broadcasts the fetal heart rate to the parent-to-be as well as to the nurse. (© Barbara Proud.)

Nonstress Testing. A **nonstress test** measures the response of the fetal heart rate to fetal movement. Position a woman and attach both a fetal heart rate and a uterine contraction monitor. Instruct a woman to push a button attached to the monitor (similar to a call bell) whenever she feels the fetus move. This will create a dark mark on the paper tracing at these times.

When the fetus moves, the fetal heart rate should increase about 15 beats per minute and remain elevated for 15 seconds. It should decrease to its average rate again as the fetus quiets (see Fig. 9.11C). If no increase in beats per minute is noticeable on fetal movement, poor oxygen perfusion of the fetus is suggested.

A nonstress test usually is done for 10 to 20 minutes. The test is said to be reactive if two accelerations of fetal heart rate (by 15 beats or more) lasting for 15 seconds occur after movement within the chosen time period. The test is nonreactive if no accelerations occur with the fetal movements. The results also can be interpreted as nonreactive if no fetal movement occurs or if there is low short-term fetal heart rate variability (less than 6 beats per minute) throughout the testing period (Chang & Blakemore, 2007).

If a 20-minute period passes without any fetal movement, it may mean only that the fetus is sleeping. Other reasons for lessened variability are maternal smoking, drug use, or hypoglycemia. If you give the woman an oral carbohydrate snack, such as orange juice, it can cause her blood glucose level to increase enough to cause fetal movement. The fetus also may be stimulated by a loud sound (discussed later) to cause movement.

Because both rhythm strip and nonstress testing are noninvasive procedures and cause no risk to either mother or fetus, they can be used as screening procedures in all pregnancies. They can be done at home daily as part of a home monitoring program for the woman who is having a complication of pregnancy.

If a nonstress test is nonreactive, additional fetal assessment, such as a contraction stress test or a biophysical profile test, will be scheduled.

Vibroacoustic Stimulation. For acoustic (sound) stimulation, a specially designed acoustic stimulator is applied to the mother's abdomen to produce a sharp sound of approximately 80 decibels at a frequency of 80 Hz, startling and waking the fetus (Chang & Blakemore, 2007).

During a standard nonstress test, if a spontaneous acceleration has not occurred within 5 minutes, apply a single 1- to 2-second sound stimulation to the lower abdomen. This can be repeated again at the end of 10 minutes if no further spontaneous movement occurs, so that two movements within the 20-minute window can be evaluated.

Contraction Stress Testing. With contraction stress testing, the fetal heart rate is analyzed in conjunction with contractions. When this test was first developed, contractions were initiated

FIGURE 9.11 Rhythm strip and nonstress testing of fetal heart rate. (**A**) The woman sits in a comfortable chair to avoid supine hypotension. Both a uterine contraction monitor and fetal heart rate monitor are in place on her abdomen. (Photograph by Melissa Olson, with permission of Chestnut Hill Hospital, Philadelphia, PA.) (**B**) A rhythm strip. The upper strip signifies heart rate; the lower strip indicates uterine activity. *Arrows* signal fetal movement. (**C**) Baseline fetal heart rate is 130–132. This strip shows fetal heart rate acceleration in response to fetal movement, shown by *arrows*. (Photograph by Melissa Olson, with permission of Chestnut Hill Hospital, Philadelphia, PA.)

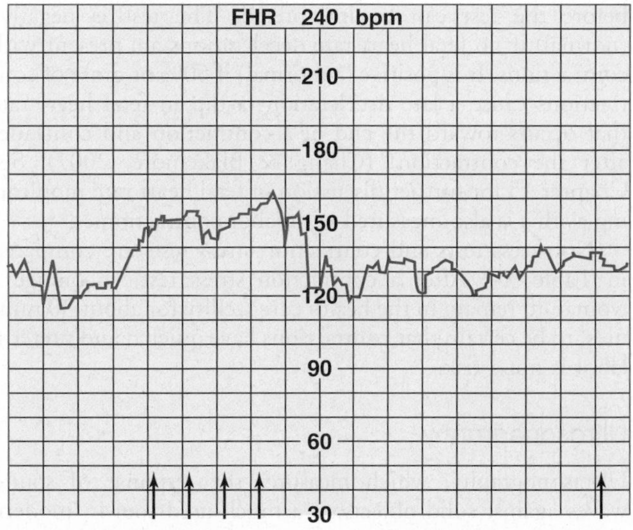

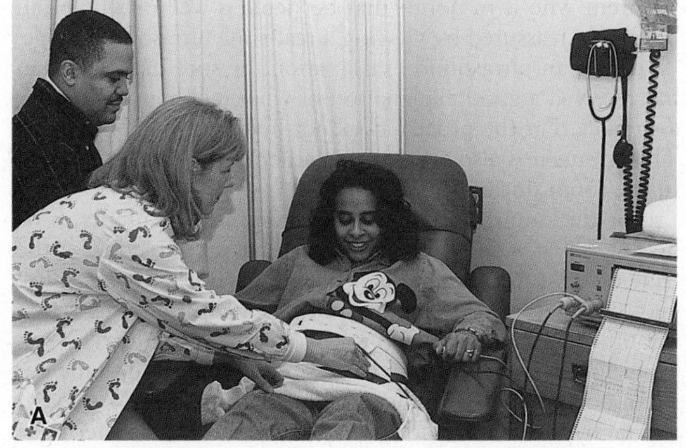

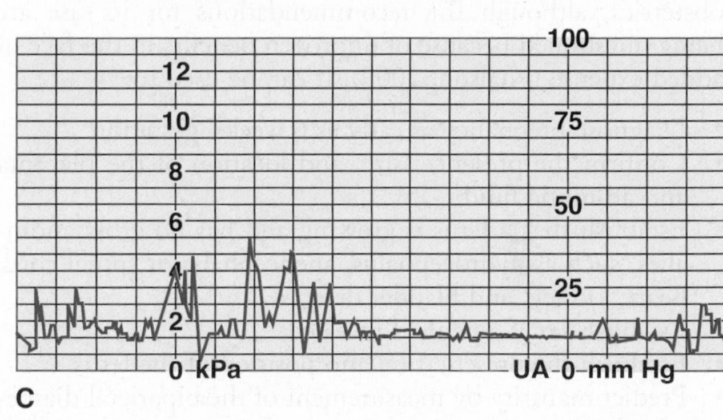

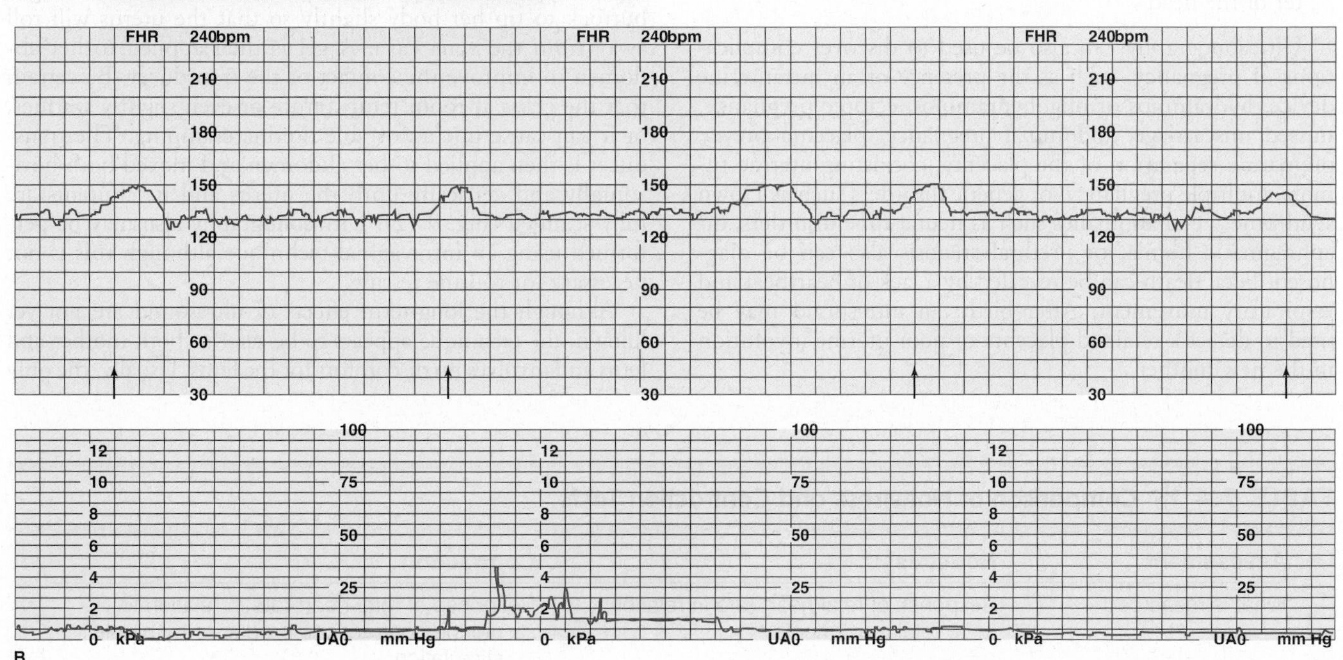

by the intravenous infusion of oxytocin. However, once started, contractions begun this way were sometimes difficult to stop and led to preterm labor. For this reason, a source of oxytocin for contraction stress testing currently is achieved by nipple stimulation. Gentle stimulation of the nipples releases oxytocin in the same way as happens with breastfeeding.

With external uterine contraction and fetal heart rate monitors in place, the baseline fetal heart rate is obtained. Next, the woman rolls a nipple between her finger and thumb until uterine contractions begin, which are recorded by a uterine monitor. Three contractions with a duration of 40 seconds or longer must be present in a 10-minute window before the test can be interpreted. The test is negative (normal) if no fetal heart rate decelerations are present with contractions. It is positive (abnormal) if 50% or more of contractions cause a late deceleration (a dip in fetal heart rate that occurs toward the end of a contraction and continues after the contraction) (Chang & Blakemore, 2007). See Chapter 15 for further discussion of fetal heart rate monitoring as this is also measured with labor contractions.

Nonstress tests and contraction stress tests are compared in Table 9.4. After a contraction stress test, encourage a woman to remain in the health care facility for about 30 minutes, to be certain that contractions have quieted and preterm labor is not a risk.

Ultrasonography

Ultrasonography, which measures the response of sound waves against solid objects, is a much-used tool in modern obstetrics, although the recommendations for its use are being questioned because of unproven benefits in the face of added expense (Neilson, 2009). It can be used to:

- Diagnose pregnancy as early as 6 weeks' gestation
- Confirm the presence, size, and location of the placenta and amniotic fluid
- Establish that a fetus is growing and has no gross anomalies, such as hydrocephalus, anencephaly, or spinal cord, heart, kidney, and bladder defects
- Establish sex if a penis is revealed
- Establish the presentation and position of the fetus
- Predict maturity by measurement of the biparietal diameter of the head

Ultrasonography can also be used to discover complications of pregnancy, such as the presence of an intrauterine device, hydramnios or oligohydramnios, ectopic pregnancy, missed miscarriage, abdominal pregnancy, placenta previa, premature separation of the placenta, coexisting uterine tumors, multiple pregnancy, or genetic disorders such as Down syndrome. Fetal anomalies such as neural tube disorders, diaphragmatic hernia, or urethral stenosis also can be diagnosed. Fetal death can be revealed by a lack of heartbeat and respiratory movement. After birth, an ultrasound may be used to detect a retained placenta or poor uterine involution in the new mother.

For an ultrasound, intermittent sound waves of high frequency (above the audible range) are projected toward the uterus by a transducer placed on the abdomen or in the vagina. The sound frequencies that bounce back can be displayed on an oscilloscope screen as a visual image. The frequencies returning from tissues of various thicknesses and properties present distinct appearances. A permanent record, such as a video or photograph, can be made of the scan.

The intricacy of the image obtained depends on the type or mode of process used. B-mode scanning allows patterns to merge and form a still picture, similar to a black-and-white snapshot (called gray-scale imaging). Real-time mode involves the use of multiple waves that allow the screen picture to move. On this type of ultrasound, the fetal heart can be seen to move, and even movement of the extremities, such as bringing a hand to the mouth to suck a thumb, can be seen. A parent who is in doubt that her fetus is well or whole can be greatly reassured by viewing a real-time ultrasound image.

Before an ultrasound examination, be sure that a woman has received a good explanation of what will happen and reassurance that the process does not involve x-rays (Box 9.6). This means it is also safe for the father of the child to remain in the room during the test.

For the sound waves to reflect best and the uterus to be held stable, it is helpful if the woman has a full bladder at the time of the procedure. To ensure this, have her drink a full glass of water every 15 minutes beginning 90 minutes before the procedure and not void until after the procedure.

Help the woman up to an examining table and drape her for modesty, but with her abdomen exposed. To prevent supine hypotension syndrome, place a towel under her right buttock to tip her body slightly so that the uterus will roll away from the vena cava. A gel is then applied to her abdomen to improve the contact of the transducer. Be certain that the gel is at room temperature or even slightly warmer, or it can cause uncomfortable uterine cramping. The transducer is then applied to her abdomen and moved both horizontally and vertically until the uterus and its contents are fully scanned (Fig. 9.12). Ultrasonography also may be performed using an intravaginal technique although this is not necessary for routine testing.

Although the long-term effects of ultrasound are not yet known, the technique appears to be safe for both mother and fetus and involves no discomfort for the fetus. Usually, the only

TABLE 9.4 * Comparison of Nonstress and Contraction Tests

Assessment	Nonstress	Contraction
What is measured	Response of fetal heart rate in relation to fetal movements	Response of fetal heart rate in relation to uterine contractions produced by nipple stimulation
Normal findings	Two or more accelerations of fetal heart rate of 15 beats/min lasting 15 sec or longer following fetal movements in a 20-min period	No late decelerations with contractions
Safety considerations	Woman should not lie supine to prevent supine hypotension syndrome	In addition to preventing supine hypotension syndrome, observe woman for 30 min afterward to see that contractions are quiet and preterm labor does not begin

BOX 9.6 * Focus on Communication

Liz Calhorn is scheduled for an ultrasound.

Less Effective Communication

Nurse: Do you have any questions about what will happen, Liz?

Liz: I guess. I can't decide if I want to know my baby's sex or not.

Nurse: Most people do these days.. It helps them plan better.

Liz: I think I'd rather be surprised. I know I don't want a boy.

Nurse: If it were me, I'd want to know. How else do you know what color clothes to buy?

Liz: Okay, tell me what the ultrasound shows.

More Effective Communication

Nurse: Do you have any questions about what will happen, Liz?

Liz: I guess. I can't decide if I want to know my baby's sex or not.

Nurse: That's an individual decision. What things are you thinking about?

Liz: I think I'd rather be surprised. I know I don't want a boy.

Nurse: Tell me about that. Why is that?

Liz: A guy got me into this trouble. I don't need another one around the house.

Nurse: Let's talk about what it will mean if you should have a boy.

Becoming so engrossed in sharing her personal feelings, the nurse in the first example forgot to determine the exact information that the client wanted. Taking the time to discover what the client wanted, as was done in the second example, revealed that the sex of the child was only a small part of what the mother was afraid to learn.

discomfort for the woman is that the contact lubricant may be messy and she may experience a strong desire to void before the scan is completed. Taking home a photograph of the ultrasound image can enhance bonding because it is proof that the pregnancy exists and the fetus appears well. As desirable as it is, however, caution women against having ultrasound images done just for the purpose of having "keepsake" photographs, because commercial firms offering these services are not well regulated so their equipment could be outdated and unsafe.

✔ Checkpoint Question 9.4

Liz Calhorn is scheduled to have an ultrasound examination. What instruction would you give her before her examination?

a. "Void immediately before the procedure to reduce your bladder size."
b. "The intravenous fluid infused to dilate your uterus does not hurt the fetus."
c. "You will need to drink at least 3 glasses of fluid before the procedure."
d. "You can have medicine for pain for any contractions caused by the test."

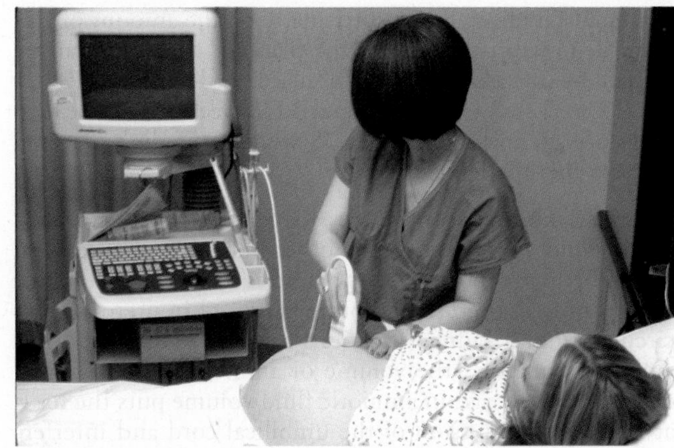

FIGURE 9.12 An ultrasound being recorded. Notice the mother's interest in being able to see her baby's first photograph.

Biparietal Diameter. Ultrasonography may be used to predict fetal maturity by measuring the biparietal diameter (side-to-side measurement) of the fetal head. In 80% of pregnancies in which the biparietal diameter of the fetal head is 8.5 cm or greater, it can be predicted that the infant will weigh more than 2500 g (5.5 lb) or is at a fetal age of 40 weeks. Figure 9.13 is an ultrasound showing the biparietal diameter of a fetus at 24 weeks.

Two other measurements commonly made by ultrasound to predict maturity are head circumference (34.5 cm indicates a 40-week fetus) and femoral length.

Doppler Umbilical Velocimetry. Doppler ultrasonography measures the velocity at which red blood cells in the uterine and fetal vessels travel. Assessment of the blood flow through uterine blood vessels is helpful to determine the vascular resistance present in women with diabetes or hypertension of pregnancy and whether resultant placental insufficiency is occurring. Because it will limit the number of nutrients that can reach the fetus, decreased velocity is an important predictor of poor neonatal outcome (Valcamonico et al., 2007).

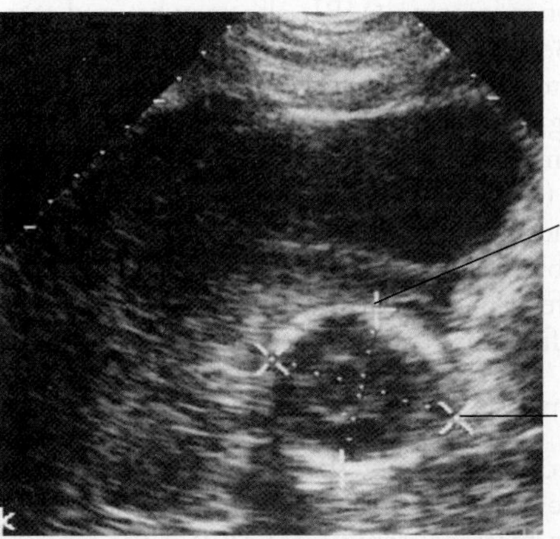

FIGURE 9.13 An ultrasound at 24 weeks' gestation showing measurement of the biparietal diameter. (Courtesy of the Department of Medical Photography, Children's Hospital, Buffalo, NY.)

Placental Grading. Based particularly on the amount of calcium deposits in the base of the placenta, placentas can be graded by ultrasound as 0 (a placenta 12–24 weeks), 1 (30–32 weeks), 2 (36 weeks), and 3 (38 weeks). Because fetal lungs are apt to be mature at 38 weeks, a grade 3 placenta suggests that the fetus is mature.

Amniotic Fluid Volume Assessment. The amount of amniotic fluid present is yet another way to estimate fetal health because a portion of the fluid is formed by fetal kidney output. If a fetus is becoming stressed in utero so that circulatory and kidney functions are failing, urine output and, consequently, the volume of amniotic fluid also will decrease. A decrease in amniotic fluid volume puts the fetus at risk for compression of the umbilical cord and interference with nutrition.

For gestations of less than 20 weeks, the uterus is hypothetically divided along the midpoint (the linea nigra on the woman's abdomen) into two vertical halves. The vertical diameter of the largest pocket of amniotic fluid present on each side is measured in centimeters. The amniotic volume index (AFI) or total is the sum of the two measurements. For gestations of 20 weeks or more, the uterus is divided into four quadrants, using the linea nigra again as the vertical dividing line and the level of the umbilicus as the horizontal dividing line. The vertical diameter of the largest pocket of fluid in each quadrant is obtained, and the four values are then added to produce the amniotic fluid index. The average index is approximately 12–15 cm between 28 and 40 weeks. An index greater than 20–24 cm indicates hydramnios (excessive fluid, perhaps caused by inability of the fetus to swallow); an index less than 5–6 cm indicates oligohydramnios (decreased amniotic fluid, perhaps caused by poor perfusion and kidney failure).

Electrocardiography

Fetal ECGs may be recorded as early as the 11th week of pregnancy. The ECG is inaccurate before the 20th week, however, because until this time fetal electrical conduction is so weak that it is easily masked by the mother's ECG tracing. It is rarely used unless a specific heart anomaly is suspected.

Magnetic Resonance Imaging

Magnetic resonance imaging (MRI) also may be used to assess the fetus. Because the technique apparently causes no harmful effects to the fetus or woman (although extensive long-term testing is not yet available), MRI has the potential to replace or complement ultrasonography as a fetal assessment technique (Laifer-Narin et al,, 2007). It may be most helpful in diagnosing complications such as ectopic pregnancy or trophoblastic disease (see Chapter 21), because later in a pregnancy fetal movement (unless the fetus is sedated) can obscure the findings.

Maternal Serum Alpha-Fetoprotein

AFP is a substance produced by the fetal liver that is present in both amniotic fluid and maternal serum. The level is abnormally high in maternal serum (MSAFP) if the fetus has an open spinal or abdominal defect such as spina bifida or omphalocele, because the open defect allows more AFP to enter the mother's circulation. Although the reason is unclear, the level is low if the fetus has a chromosomal defect such as Down syndrome. MSAFP levels begin to rise at 11 weeks' gestation and then steadily increase until term. Traditionally assessed at the 15th week of pregnancy, between 85% and 90% of neural tube defects and 80% of Down syndrome babies can be detected by this method (Crombleholme, 2009).

Triple Screening

Triple screening, or analysis of three indicators (MSAFP, unconjugated estriol, and hCG), may be performed in place of simple AFP testing to yield even more reliable results. As with the measurement of MSAFP, it requires only a simple venipuncture of the mother.

Chorionic Villi Sampling

Chorionic villi sampling (CVS) is a biopsy and chromosomal analysis of chorionic villi that is done at 10–12 weeks of pregnancy. This procedure is discussed in Chapter 7. Coelocentesis (transvaginal aspiration of fluid from the extraembryonic cavity) is an alternative method to remove cells for fetal analysis.

Amniocentesis

Amniocentesis (from the Greek *amnion* for "sac" and *kentesis* for "puncture") is the aspiration of amniotic fluid from the pregnant uterus for examination. The procedure can be done in a physician's office or in an ambulatory clinic. It is typically scheduled between the 14th and 16th weeks of pregnancy to allow for a generous amount of amniotic fluid to be present. The technique can be used again near term to test for fetal maturity.

Amniocentesis is a technically easy procedure, but it can be frightening to a woman. Because it involves penetration of the integrity of the amniotic sac, there also are risks to the fetus, although the incidence of these is low (less than 0.5%). Fetal complications range from hemorrhage from penetration of the placenta, infection of the amniotic fluid, and puncture of the fetus. If it leads to irritation of the uterus, it can initiate premature labor (Alfirevic, 2009).

In preparation for amniocentesis, ask the woman to void (to reduce the size of the bladder and prevent an inadvertent puncture). Place her in a supine position on an examining table and drape her appropriately, exposing only her abdomen. Place a folded towel under her right buttock to tip her body slightly to the left and move the uterus off the vena cava, to prevent supine hypotension syndrome. Attach fetal heart rate and uterine contraction monitors. Take her blood pressure and measure the fetal heart rate for baseline levels.

An ultrasound is then done to determine the position of the fetus and the location of a pocket of amniotic fluid and the placenta. The abdomen is then washed with an antiseptic solution, and a local anesthetic is injected. Caution the woman that she may feel a sensation of pressure as the needle used for aspiration, a 3- or 4-in, 20- to 22-gauge spinal needle, is introduced. Do not suggest that she take a deep breath and hold it as a distraction against discomfort: this lowers the diaphragm against the uterus and shifts intrauterine contents.

The needle is inserted until it reaches the amniotic cavity and a pool of amniotic fluid, carefully avoiding the fetus and placenta (Fig. 9.14). A syringe is attached, and about 15 mL of amniotic fluid is withdrawn. The needle is then removed, and the woman rests quietly for about 30 minutes. During the procedure and for the 30 minutes afterward, observe the fetal heart rate monitor to be certain the rate remains within normal values and observe the uterine contraction monitor to be sure that no contractions are occurring.

If the woman has Rh-negative blood, Rho(D) immune globulin (RhIG; RhoGAM) is administered after the procedure to prevent fetal isoimmunization. This is to ensure that maternal antibodies will not form against any placental red blood cells that might have accidentally been released during the procedure.

Amniotic fluid is analyzed for:

- **Alpha-Fetoprotein (AFP).** If the fetus has an open body defect, such as anencephaly, myelomeningocele, or omphalocele, increased levels of AFP will be present in the amniotic fluid because of leakage of AFP into the fluid. The level will be decreased in the amniotic fluid of fetuses with chromosomal defects such as Down syndrome. Acetylcholinesterase is another compound that can be obtained from amniotic fluid in high levels if a neural tube defect is present.

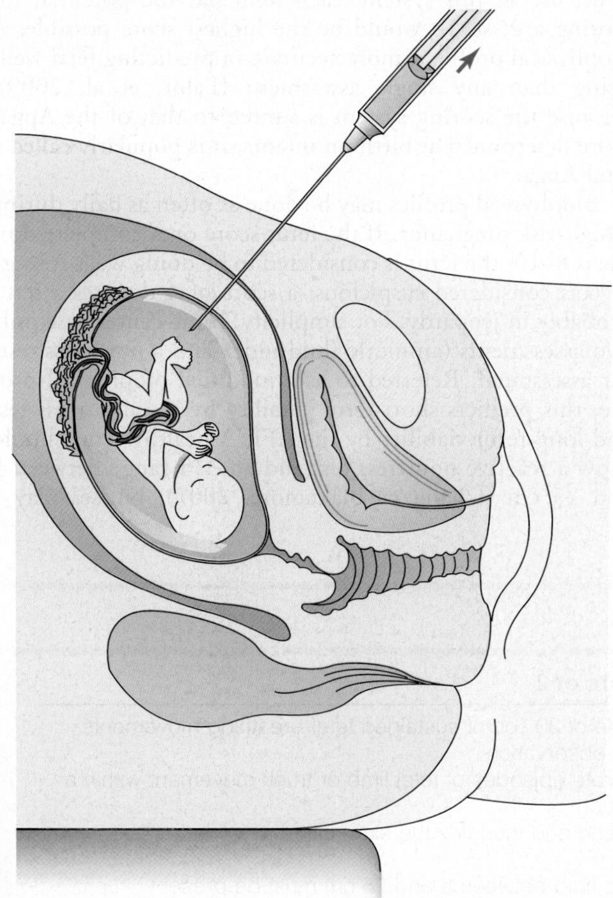

FIGURE 9.14 Amniocentesis. A pocket of amniotic fluid is located by ultrasound. A small amount of fluid is removed by needle aspiration.

- **Bilirubin Determination.** The presence of bilirubin may be analyzed if a blood incompatibility is suspected. If bilirubin is going to be analyzed, the specimen must be free of blood or a false-positive reading will occur.
- **Chromosome Analysis.** A few fetal skin cells are always present in amniotic fluid. These cells may be cultured and stained for karyotyping for genetic analysis. Examples of genetic diseases that can be detected by prenatal amniocentesis and their significance to health are discussed in Chapter 7.
- **Color.** Normal amniotic fluid is the color of water; late in pregnancy, it may have a slightly yellow tinge. A strong yellow color suggests a blood incompatibility (the yellow results from the presence of bilirubin released with the hemolysis of red blood cells). A green color suggests meconium staining, a phenomenon associated with fetal distress.
- **Fetal Fibronectin.** Fibronectin is a glycoprotein that plays a part in helping the placenta attach to the uterine decidua. Early in pregnancy, it can be assessed in the woman's cervical mucus, but the amount then fades until, after 20 weeks of pregnancy, it is no longer present in cervical mucus. As labor approaches and cervical dilatation begins, it can be found again in cervical or vaginal fluid. Damage to fetal membranes from cervical dilatation releases a great deal of the substance, so detection of fibronectin in either the amniotic fluid or in the mother's vagina can serve as an announcement that preterm labor may be beginning.
- **Inborn Errors of Metabolism.** Some inherited diseases that are caused by inborn errors of metabolism can be detected by amniocentesis. For a condition to be identified, an errant enzyme must be present in the amniotic fluid as early as the time of the procedure. Examples of illnesses that can be detected in this way are cystinosis and maple syrup urine disease (amino acid disorders).
- **Lecithin/Sphingomyelin Ratio.** Lecithin and sphingomyelin are the protein components of the lung enzyme surfactant that the alveoli begin to form at the 22nd to 24th weeks of pregnancy. After amniocentesis, the L/S ratio may be determined quickly by a shake test (if bubbles appear in the amniotic fluid after shaking, the ratio is mature) or sent for laboratory analysis. An L/S ratio of 2:1 is traditionally accepted as lung maturity. Infants of mothers with severe diabetes may have false-mature readings of lecithin because the stress to the infant in utero tends to mature lecithin pathways early. This means that fetal values must be considered in light of the presence of maternal diabetes, or the infant may be born with mature lung function but be immature overall (fragile giants) causing them to not do well in postnatal life. Some laboratories interpret a ratio of 2.5:1 or 3:1 as a mature indicator in infants of women with diabetes.
- **Phosphatidyl Glycerol and Desaturated Phosphatidylcholine.** These are additional compounds, in addition to lecithin and sphingomyelin, found in surfactant. Pathways for these compounds mature at 35–36 weeks. Because they are present only with mature lung function, if they are present in the sample of amniotic fluid obtained by amniocentesis, it can be predicted with even greater confidence that respiratory distress syndrome is not likely to occur.

Percutaneous Umbilical Blood Sampling

PUBS (also called cordocentesis or funicentesis) is the aspiration of blood from the umbilical vein for analysis. After the umbilical cord is located by ultrasound, a thin needle is inserted by amniocentesis technique into the uterus and is guided by ultrasound until it pierces the umbilical vein. A sample of blood is then removed for blood studies, such as a complete blood count, direct Coombs' test, blood gases, and karyotyping. To ensure that the blood obtained is fetal blood, it is submitted to a Kleihauer-Betke test which measures the difference between adult and fetal blood. If the test reveals that a fetus is anemic, blood may be transfused using this same technique. Because the umbilical vein continues to ooze for a moment after the procedure, fetal blood could enter the maternal circulation after the procedure, so RhIG is given to Rh-negative women to prevent sensitization. The fetus is monitored by a nonstress test before and after the procedure to be certain that uterine contractions are not present and by ultrasound to see that no bleeding is evident. This procedure carries little additional risk to the fetus or woman over amniocentesis and can yield information not available by any other means, especially about blood dyscrasias.

Amnioscopy

Amnioscopy is the visual inspection of the amniotic fluid through the cervix and membranes with an amnioscope (a small fetoscope). The main use of the technique is to detect meconium staining. It carries some risk of membrane rupture.

Fetoscopy

Fetoscopy, in which the fetus is visualized by inspection through a fetoscope (an extremely narrow, hollow tube inserted by amniocentesis technique), can be helpful to assess fetal well-being (Lopriore et al., 2007). If a photograph is taken through the fetoscope, it can document a problem or reassure parents that their infant is perfectly formed. The procedure is used to:

- Confirm the intactness of the spinal column
- Obtain biopsy samples of fetal tissue and fetal blood samples
- Perform elemental surgery, such as inserting a polyethylene shunt into the fetal ventricles to relieve hydrocephalus or anteriorly into the fetal bladder to relieve a stenosed urethra

The earliest time in pregnancy that fetoscopy can be performed is about the 16th or 17th week. For the procedure, the mother is prepared and draped as for amniocentesis. A local anesthetic is injected into the abdominal skin. The fetoscope is then inserted through a minor abdominal incision. If the fetus is very active, meperidine (Demerol) may be administered to the woman to help sedate the fetus to avoid fetal injury by the scope and to allow better observation.

Fetoscopy carries a small risk of premature labor. Amnionitis (infection of the amniotic fluid) may occur. To avoid this, the woman may be prescribed 10 days of antibiotic therapy after the procedure. The number of procedures performed by fetoscopy is limited because of the manipulation involved and the ethical quandary of the mother's autonomy being compromised by fetal needs if further procedures are necessary (e.g., asking the mother to undergo general anesthesia so that the fetus can have surgery).

Biophysical Profile

A biophysical profile combines five parameters (fetal reactivity, fetal breathing movements, fetal body movement, fetal tone, and amniotic fluid volume) into one assessment. The fetal heart and breathing record measure short-term central nervous system function; the amniotic fluid volume helps measure long-term adequacy of placental function. The scoring for a complete profile is shown in Table 9.5. With use of this system, each item has the potential for scoring a 2, so 10 would be the highest score possible. A biophysical profile is more accurate in predicting fetal well-being than any single assessment (Lalor, et al, 2009). Because the scoring system is similar to that of the Apgar score determined at birth on infants, it is popularly called a fetal Apgar.

Biophysical profiles may be done as often as daily during a high-risk pregnancy. If the fetus score on a complete profile is 8–10, the fetus is considered to be doing well. A score of 6 is considered suspicious; a score of 4 denotes a fetus probably in jeopardy. For simplicity, some centers use only two assessments (amniotic fluid index and a nonstress test) for assessment. Referred to as a modified biophysical profile, this predicts short-term viability by the nonstress test and long-term viability by the AFI. A healthy fetus should show a reactive nonstress test and an AFI range between 5 and 25 cm (Chang & Blakemore, 2007). Nurses play a

TABLE 9.5 ✻ Biophysical Profile Scoring

Assessment	Instrument	Criteria for a Score of 2
Fetal breathing	Ultrasound	At least one episode of 30 sec of sustained fetal breathing movements within 30 min of observation
Fetal movement	Ultrasound	At least three separate episodes of fetal limb or trunk movement within a 30-min observation
Fetal tone	Ultrasound	The fetus must extend and then flex the extremities or spine at least once in 30 min
Amniotic fluid volume	Ultrasound	A range of amniotic fluid between 5 and 25 cm must be present
Fetal heart reactivity	Nonstress test	Two or more fetal heart rate accelerations of at least 15 beats/min above baseline and of 15 sec duration occur with fetal movement over a 20-min time period

large role in obtaining the information for both a modified and a full biophysical profile by obtaining either the nonstress test or the ultrasound reading.

✔ Checkpoint Question 9.5

Liz Calhorn is scheduled to have an amniocentesis to test for fetal maturity. What instruction would you give her before this procedure?

a. "Void immediately before the procedure to reduce your bladder size."
b. "The x-ray used to reveal your fetus's position has no long-term effects."
c. "The intravenous fluid infused to dilate your uterus does not hurt the fetus."
d. "Your fetus will have less amniotic fluid for the remainder of your pregnancy."

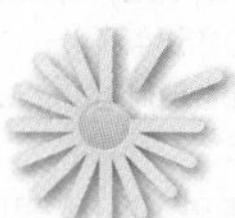

Key Points for Review

- The union of a single sperm and egg (fertilization) signals the beginning of pregnancy.
- The fertilized ovum (zygote) travels by way of a fallopian tube to the uterus, where implantation takes place in about 8 days.
- From implantation to 5 to 8 weeks, the growing structure is called an embryo. The period after 8 weeks until birth is the fetal period.
- Growth of the umbilical cord, amniotic fluid, and amniotic membranes proceeds in concert with fetal growth. The placenta produces several important hormones: estrogen, progesterone, human placental lactogen, and human chorionic gonadotropin.
- Various methods to assess fetal growth and development include fundal height, fetal movement, fetal heart tones, ultrasonography, magnetic resonance imaging, maternal serum alpha-fetoprotein, amniocentesis, percutaneous umbilical blood sampling, amnioscopy, and fetoscopy.
- A biophysical profile is a combination of fetal assessments that predicts fetal well-being better than measuring single parameters.

CRITICAL THINKING EXERCISES

1. Liz Calhorn, whom you met at the beginning of the chapter, has stated that her feelings have changed since she felt her baby move. Would you modify your health teaching with her because of this statement?
2. When Liz is scheduled for an ultrasound examination at 20 weeks' gestation, she tells you she does not want to know the sex of her fetus. Why do some women want to know this, whereas some do not? Is there an advantage to knowing or not knowing?
3. Late in pregnancy, Liz is scheduled for weekly nonstress tests. She invariably comes late for these tests because they are "time-consuming and boring." How could you make such tests more appealing to help increase her cooperation?
4. Examine the National Health Goals related to fetal growth and assessment. Most government-sponsored money for nursing research is allotted based on these goals. What would be a possible research topic to explore pertinent to these goals that would advance evidence-based practice in relation to Liz Calhorn or her family?

CRITICAL THINKING SCENARIO

Open the accompanying CD-ROM or visit http://thePoint.lww.com and read the Patient Scenario included for this chapter, then answer the questions to further sharpen your skills and grow more familiar with NCLEX types of questions related to fetal growth. Confirm your answers are correct by reading the rationales.

REFERENCES

Ainbinder, S. W., Ramin, S. M., & DeCherney, A. H. (2007). Sexually transmitted diseases and pelvic infections. In A. H. DeCherney & L. Nathan (Eds.). *Current diagnosis and treatment in obstetrics and gynecology* (10th ed.). Columbus, OH: McGraw-Hill.

Alfirevic, Z. (2009). Early amniocentesis versus transabdominal chorion villus sampling for prenatal diagnosis. *Cochrane Database of Systematic Reviews, 2009*(1), (CD000077).

Burkman, R. T. (2007). Contraception and family planning. In A. H. DeCherney & L. Nathan (Eds.). *Current diagnosis and treatment in obstetrics and gynecology* (10th ed.). Columbus, OH: McGraw-Hill.

Bush, M. C., & Pernoll, M. L. (2007). Multiple pregnancy. In A. H. DeCherney & L. Nathan (Eds.). *Current diagnosis and treatment in obstetrics and gynecology* (10th ed.). Columbus, OH: McGraw-Hill.

Chang, D., & Blakemore, K. (2007). Fetal assessment. In Fortner, K. B., et al. (Eds). *The Johns Hopkins manual of gynecology and obstetrics.* Philadelphia: Lippincott Williams & Wilkins.

Crombleholme, W. R. (2009). Obstetrics. In McPhee, S. J., & Papadakis, M. A. (Eds.). *Current medical diagnosis and treatment.* Columbus, OH: McGraw-Hill.

Firpo, M., & Kikyo, N. K. (2007). A primer on stem cell research. *Minnesota Medicine, 90*(5), 36–38.

Goldman, A. (2007). Stem cells discovered in menstrual blood. *Stem Cell Research News, 9*(21), 1.

Hol, L., & Kuipers, E. J. (2007). Clinical challenges and images in GI. Meckel's diverticulum. *Gastroenterology, 133*(2), 392–393.

Jackson, H., Melvin, C., & Downe, S. (2007). Midwives and the fetal nuchal cord: a survey of practices and perceptions. *Journal of Midwifery & Women's Health, 52*(1), 49–55.

Knuppel, R. A. (2007). Maternal-placental-fetal unit: fetal and early neonatal physiology. In A. H. DeCherney & L. Nathan (Eds.). *Current diagnosis and treatment in obstetrics and gynecology* (10th ed.). Columbus, OH: McGraw-Hill.

Kumar, M., Das, S., & Kumar, B. (2007). Amniotic band syndrome. *Ultrasound, 15*(2), 96–98.

Laifer-Narin, S., et al. (2007). Fetal magnetic resonance imaging: a review. *Current Opinion in Obstetrics & Gynecology, 19*(2), 151–156.

Lalor, J., et al. (2009). Biophysical profile for fetal assessment in high risk pregnancies. *Cochrane Database of Systematic Reviews, 2009*(1), (CD000038).

Lanni, M. L., & Loveless, E. A. (2007). Oligohydramnios at term: a case report. *Journal of Midwifery & Women's Health, 52*(1), 73–76.

Lopriore, E., et al. (2007). Long-term neurodevelopmental outcome in twin-to-twin transfusion syndrome treated with fetoscopic laser surgery. *American Journal of Obstetrics and Gynecology, 196*(3), 231–234.

Lubusky, M., et al. (2007). Single umbilical artery and its finding in the second trimester of pregnancy: relation to chromosomal defects. *Prenatal Diagnosis, 27*(4), 327–331.

Lumley, J., et al. (2009). Periconceptional supplementation with folate and/or multivitamins for preventing neural tube defects. *Cochrane Database of Systematic Reviews, 2009*(1), (CD001056).

Macones, G. A., et al. (2008). The 2008 National Institute of Child Health and Human Development Workshop Report on Electronic Fetal Monitoring. *JOGNN: Journal of Obstetric, Gynecologic, and Neonatal Nursing, 37*(5), 510–515.

Moyer, V., et al. (2009). Late versus early surgical correction for congenital diaphragmatic hernia in newborn infants. *Cochrane Database of Systematic Reviews, 2009*(1), (CD001695).

Neilson, J. P. (2009). Ultrasound for fetal assessment in early pregnancy. *Cochrane Database of Systematic Reviews, 2009*(1), (CD000182).

Norton, M. E. (2007). Evaluation and management of twin-twin transfusion syndrome: still a challenge. *American Journal of Obstetrics and Gynecology, 196*(5), 419–420.

Rees, D. C. (2007). Neonatal sickle cell disease and thalassaemia. *Infant, 3*(1), 31–35.

Records, K. (2007). A critical review of maternal abuse and infant outcomes: implications for newborn nurses. *Newborn and Infant Nursing Reviews, 7*(1), 7–13.

Roberts, D., & Dalziel, S. (2009). Antenatal corticosteroids for accelerating fetal lung maturation for women at risk of preterm birth. *Cochrane Database of Systematic Reviews, 2009*(1), (CD004454).

Rogers-Adkinson, D. L., & Stuart, S. K. (2007). Collaborative services: children experiencing neglect and the side effects of prenatal alcohol exposure. *Language, Speech, and Hearing Services in Schools, 38*(2), 149–156.

Soll, R. F. (2009). Prophylactic synthetic surfactant for preventing morbidity and mortality in preterm infants. *Cochrane Database of Systematic Reviews, 2009*(1), (CD001079).

Taylor, R. N., & Lebovic, D. I. (2007). The endocrinology of pregnancy. In D. G. Gardner & D. Shoback (Eds.). *Greenspan's basic and clinical endocrinology* (8th ed.). New York: McGraw-Hill.

Thilo, E. H., et al. (2008). The newborn infant. In Hay, W.W., et al. (Eds.). *Current pediatric diagnosis and treatment* (18th ed.). Columbus, OH: McGraw-Hill.

Valcamonico, A., et al. (2007). Mid- and long-term outcome of extremely low birth weight (ELBW) infants: an analysis of prognostic factors. *Journal of Maternal-Fetal & Neonatal Medicine, 20*(6), 465–471.

Winzer-Serhan, U. H. (2008). Long-term consequences of maternal smoking and developmental chronic nicotine exposure. *Frontiers in Bioscience, 13*(1), 636–649.

Zeitler, P. S., et al. (2008). Endocrine disorders. In Hay, W. W., et al. (Eds.). *Current pediatric diagnosis and treatment* (18th ed.). Columbus, OH: McGraw-Hill.

SUGGESTED READINGS

Antony, A. C. (2007). In utero physiology: role of folic acid in nutrient delivery and fetal development. *American Journal of Clinical Nutrition, 85*(2), 598S–603S.

Baschat, A. A., et al. (2007). Predictors of neonatal outcome in early-onset placental dysfunction. *Obstetrics and Gynecology, 109*(2.1), 253–261.

Cleves, M. A., et al. (2007). Association between congenital heart defects and small for gestational age. *Pediatrics, 119*(4), e976–982.

Commare, C. E., & Tappenden, K. A. (2007). Development of the infant intestine: implications for nutrition support. *Nutrition in Clinical Practice, 22*(2), 159–173.

East, C., et al. (2009). Vibroacoustic stimulation for fetal assessment in labour in the presence of a nonreassuring fetal heart rate trace. *Cochrane Database of Systematic Reviews, 2009*(1), (CD004664).

Farrell, J. A. (2007). Fetal treatment center: history, infrastructure, and nursing perspective. *Journal of Perinatal and Neonatal Nursing, 21*(1), 11–21.

Kahn, H. S., et al. (2008). A fingerprint characteristic associated with the early prenatal environment. *American Journal of Human Biology, 20*(1), 59–65.

Perkins, C. C. D., et al. (2007). Physical activity and fetal growth during pregnancy. *Obstetrics and Gynecology, 109*(1), 81–87.

Thompson, J. N. (2007). Fetal nutrition and adult hypertension, diabetes, obesity, and coronary artery disease. *Neonatal Network: The Journal of Neonatal Nursing, 26*(4), 235–240.

Toal, M., et al. (2007). Usefulness of a placental profile in high-risk pregnancies. *American Journal of Obstetrics and Gynecology, 196*(4), 363–365.

Chapter 10

Psychological and Physiologic Changes of Pregnancy

KEY TERMS

- ballottement
- Braxton Hicks contractions
- Chadwick's sign
- couvade syndrome
- diastasis
- Goodell's sign
- Hegar's sign
- lightening
- linia nigra
- melasma
- Montgomery's tubercles
- multipara
- operculum
- polyuria
- primigravida
- quickening
- striae gravidarum

OBJECTIVES

After mastering the contents of this chapter, you should be able to:

1. Describe common psychological and physiologic changes that occur with pregnancy and the relationship of the changes to pregnancy diagnosis.
2. Identify National Health Goals related to preconception counseling and prenatal care that nurses can help the nation achieve.
3. Use critical thinking to analyze how the physiologic and psychological changes of pregnancy affect family functioning, and develop ways to make nursing care more family-centered.
4. Assess a woman for the psychological and physiologic changes that occur with pregnancy.
5. Formulate nursing diagnoses related to the psychological and physiologic changes of pregnancy.
6. Identify expected outcomes for a family's psychological and physical adaptation to pregnancy.
7. Plan nursing care related to the changes and diagnosis of pregnancy, such as helping a woman plan to arrange for adequate rest.
8. Implement nursing care, such as health teaching related to the expected changes of pregnancy.
9. Evaluate outcome criteria for the achievement and effectiveness of care.
10. Identify areas of nursing care related to the psychological and physiologic changes of pregnancy that could benefit from additional nursing research or application of evidence-based practice.
11. Integrate knowledge of the psychological and physiologic changes of pregnancy with nursing process to achieve quality maternal and child health nursing care.

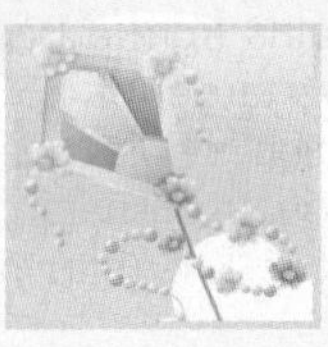

Lauren Maxwell is a part-time model who has come to your clinic for her first prenatal visit. She tells you she missed her period 4 weeks ago and immediately took a home pregnancy test. She's excited that it was positive, because she and her husband have been trying for several months to get pregnant. She is also anxious. "I know there's no turning back now, but I wonder what this will do to my career," she tells you. She adds that her husband, John, doesn't seem a bit scared. "I don't know if that's a good thing or not," she confides. She's also worried about being a good parent. "I'd die," she says, "if I turned into the same kind of parent as my parents."

In addition to the positive home pregnancy test, Lauren presents with amenorrhea, breast tenderness, fatigue, and morning sickness. She is interested in knowing when she will begin to look pregnant and what she can do for the morning sickness.

Previous chapters discussed the anatomy and physiology of women. This chapter adds information about the physical and psychological changes that occur in both a woman and her partner during pregnancy. Knowing such information can help you protect the health of both women and their fetus for the next 9 months.

What psychological development tasks of pregnancy will Lauren need to complete? What suggestions could you make to ease her worry about being a good parent?

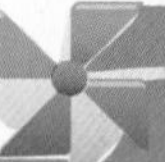

BOX 10.1 * Focus on National Health Goals

Several National Health Goals speak to the physiologic and psychological changes of pregnancy or the care necessary because of these changes:

- Increase abstinence from alcohol, cigarettes, and illicit drugs among pregnant women from baselines of 87%, 90%, and 96% to 95%, 99%, and 100%.
- Reduce maternal deaths from a baseline of 9.9 per 100,000 live births to a target of 4.5 per 100,000.
- Increase the proportion of pregnant women who receive early and adequate prenatal care from a baseline of 74% to a target of 90% (http://www.nih.gov).

Nurses can help the nation achieve these objectives by being certain that women receive counseling in nutrition and safer sex practices before pregnancy so they can enter intended pregnancies in good health. Nursing research to identify the best way to reach women with preconception counseling and effective ways to stop smoking cigarettes are important steps that would help women enter pregnancy in optimum health.

Clients are often interested in learning more about the physical or psychological changes that pregnancy brings, because these changes verify the reality and mark the progress of pregnancy.

Physiologic changes of pregnancy occur gradually but eventually affect all of a woman's organ systems. They are changes that are necessary to allow a woman to be able to provide oxygen and nutrients for her growing fetus as well as extra nutrients for her own increased metabolism during the pregnancy. They also ready her body for labor and birth and for lactation (breastfeeding) once the baby is born. Because the physiologic changes that occur with pregnancy are extensive, women are usually happy to learn that they are also temporary. When pregnancy ends, a woman's body will return virtually to its prepregnant state.

Psychological changes of pregnancy occur in response not only to the physiologic alterations that are happening but also to the increased responsibility associated with welcoming a new and completely dependent person into a family. National Health Goals relevant to these changes of pregnancy are shown in Box 10.1.

Despite the magnitude of some of these changes, they are all extensions of normal physiology and psychology. This makes pregnancy represent a time of wellness, not of illness. A major responsibility of health care personnel caring for pregnant women and their families is to help the family maintain a state of wellness throughout the pregnancy and into early parenthood (Crombleholme, 2009).

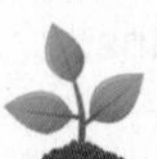

Nursing Process Overview

For Healthy Adaptation to Pregnancy

Assessment

Ideally, assessment for pregnancy begins before the pregnancy with preconception counseling. During a preconception assessment, evaluate a woman's overall health status, nutritional intake (e.g., sufficient intake of folic acid and protein), and lifestyle (e.g., drinking and smoking habits); identify any potential problems (e.g., potential for ectopic pregnancy because of tubal scarring); and identify a woman's understanding and expectations of conception, pregnancy, and parenthood.

In early pregnancy, be certain that you establish a trusting relationship with a woman so she will see you as a person who is capable of counseling her and helping her solve problems, and in whom she is willing to confide as she is about to undergo what could be a stressful 9 month time period. Continue to assess a woman's health and nutritional status, as well as the well-being of her fetus, throughout pregnancy. Document a woman's physiologic adaptations and the family's psychological adaptations to pregnancy, noting any abnormal findings. Physical findings are gained through the health history, physical assessment, and laboratory tests. Assessment in psychological areas is obtained primarily through interviewing and should include societal, cultural, family, and personal influences on a woman's adaptation to pregnancy.

Nursing Diagnosis

Examples of nursing diagnoses involving the changes that occur with pregnancy are:

- Anxiety related to unexpected pregnancy
- Altered breathing pattern related to respiratory system changes of pregnancy
- Disturbed body image related to weight gain with pregnancy
- Deficient knowledge related to normal changes of pregnancy
- Imbalanced nutrition, less than body requirements, related to early morning nausea

Outcome Identification and Planning

Although a woman may have read pamphlets or talked to her friends about the physiologic changes of pregnancy, she is often surprised to see these changes occurring in herself. She may say, "I knew I'd be tired, but I never guessed it would be this bad," or "I've read about dark pigment forming on my abdomen, but is it normal for it to be this dark? Will this go away?"

Planning nursing care in connection with the physiologic and psychological changes of pregnancy should involve a plan to review these types of concerns with a woman as well as a plan to ask about the individual responses she is experiencing. Reliable web sites to help women learn more about prenatal care are

- The March of Dimes (http://www.marchofdimes.com)
- The Department of Health and Human Services (http://Women'sHealth.gov)
- The National Institutes of Health (http://Medlineplus/prenatalcare.html)

Implementation

The changes of pregnancy may appear insignificant if taken one by one, but together they add up to major changes.

Most women of childbearing age have a mental picture of themselves or a good idea of how they will look in a dress before they try it on in a store. They participate in sports or other activities that conform to that self-image. Then, in 9 months, a woman gains 25 to 30 lb and her figure changes so drastically that none of her prepregnancy clothes fit any longer and bicycling is difficult because of her poor balance. At the beginning of pregnancy, she may feel constantly nauseated. Toward the end, the extra weight and the strain of waiting may make her feel tired and short of breath. Endocrine changes can make her feel moody and quick to cry. She may never have been concerned with her health before; now, every month (and toward the end of pregnancy, every week), she reports to a health care provider for a prenatal checkup. She may worry that she will never lose all the weight she has gained, that the stretch marks on her abdomen will remain forever, and that she will always be as tired or as nauseated as she feels during various stages of her pregnancy.

Help women during their prenatal visits to voice their concerns about the changes happening to them so any worry brought on by these does not compound an already potentially stressful situation for them. Women may need suggestions on exercise and nutrition to follow during pregnancy. For many women, a prenatal visit is the first time they have seen a health care provider since childhood. Nursing interventions during these visits can be instrumental in not only guiding a woman safely through a pregnancy but also connecting her back with ongoing health care.

Outcome Evaluation

Evaluation should determine whether a woman has really "heard" your teaching in light of the stress of her pregnancy. People under stress do not always comprehend well, so it is not unusual for a woman to pocket away information, thinking, "I'll concentrate on what that means when it happens to me, not now," then, when a particular change has happened, to realize she has forgotten what you said. Evaluation that reveals learning did not take place confirms that pregnancy is a period of stress more often than it reflects the quality of teaching. Examples of outcome criteria you might strive for are:

- Client states she is able to continue her usual lifestyle throughout pregnancy.
- Family members describe ways they have adjusted their lifestyles to accommodate the mother's fatigue.
- Couple states they accept the physiologic changes of pregnancy as normal.

PSYCHOLOGICAL CHANGES OF PREGNANCY

Pregnancy is such a huge change in a woman's life that it brings about more psychological changes than any other life event besides puberty (Rojas, Wood, & Blakemore, 2007). A woman's attitude toward a pregnancy depends a great deal on psychological aspects such as the environment in which she was raised, the messages about pregnancy her family communicated to her as a child, the society and culture in which she lives as an adult, and whether the pregnancy has come at a good time or less than a good time in her life (Darby, 2007).

Social Influences

Until recently, the heavy emphasis on medical management for women during pregnancy conveyed the idea that pregnancy was a 9-month-long illness. The pregnant woman went alone to a physician's office for care; at the time of birth, she was separated from her family and admitted to a hospital. She was hospitalized in seclusion from visitors and even from the new baby for a week afterward.

Today, health care settings view pregnancy as a time of health. Nurses have played an important role in helping bring about this change by convincing agencies that long-standing protocols that separated women from their families are not appropriate. As a result, instead of coming alone for prenatal care, women now bring their families. Instead of being given general anesthetics so they can "sleep through" labor and birth, they participate actively in the experience.

How well a pregnant woman and her partner feel during pregnancy and childbirth is related to their cultural background, their personal experiences, and the experiences of friends and relatives, as well as that taught by childbirth educators, and the current public philosophy of childbirth. People's opinions about adolescent pregnancies, "late in life" pregnancies, or whether women who have sex with women should have children have changed markedly. By informing women about their new health care options and continuing to work with other health care providers to "demedicalize" childbirth, nurses can help make pregnancy and childbirth even more enjoyable for clients and their families.

Cultural Influences

A woman's cultural background may strongly influence how active a role she wants to take in her pregnancy, because certain beliefs and taboos may place restrictions on her behavior and activities (Andrews & Boyle, 2007). To learn about the beliefs of a particular woman and her partner, ask at prenatal visits if there is anything they believe should or should not be done to make the pregnancy successful and keep the baby healthy. Supporting these beliefs shows respect for the individuality of a woman and her knowledge of good health.

Before evidence-based practice was available to scientifically disprove or prove happenings in pregnancy, every culture circulated explanations about what people thought caused complications of pregnancy, and because these myths are well engrained in cultures, they persist. For example, beliefs that lifting your arms over your head will cause the cord to twist, or that watching a lunar eclipse will cause birth deformities, are typical of this type of myth. Listen to such "tall tales" to show respect for the person's beliefs, but encourage a woman to also respect that physiologically these types of action could not affect a fetus.

Family Influences

The family in which a woman was raised can be influential to her beliefs about pregnancy because it is part of her

for Disease Control and Prevention [CDC], 2009) because no woman can be absolutely confident in advance that she will be able to conceive until it happens. Every pregnancy is a surprise to some extent, either because a woman had not planned on becoming pregnant or because she had been looking forward to being pregnant but the reality of it happening came too quickly. If pregnancy announced itself with more reliable signs than a missed period, slight breast tenderness, or vague nausea and tiredness, women could become more certain how they feel about being pregnant sooner. Home pregnancy test kits have helped women in this regard by confirming pregnancy as early as the first missed menstrual period. Until it is verified by a home test or a health care visit, however, the uncertainty of the symptoms makes pregnancy only a vague theoretical possibility that leaves room for denial. As almost all drugs cross the placenta and many can cause fetal harm, the earlier that a woman realizes that she is pregnant, the sooner she can safeguard fetal health by discontinuing all drugs not specifically prescribed or approved by her physician or nurse-midwife (Cunningham et al., 2008).

Often women immediately experience something less than pleasure and closer to disappointment or anxiety at the news that they are pregnant or a feeling of ambivalence. Ambivalence toward pregnancy does not mean that positive feelings counteract negative feelings so the woman is left feeling nothing toward her pregnancy. Instead, it refers to the interwoven feelings of wanting and not wanting that can exist at high levels. When talking to pregnant women, emphasize that this ambivalence is normal. Otherwise, if a poor outcome should result, a woman may recall her ambivalence and feel guilty.

Fortunately, most women are able to change their attitude toward the pregnancy by the time they feel the child move inside them. Some health care plans provide for a routine ultrasound at 4 months of pregnancy. Seeing a beating heart or a fetal outline on the monitor screen during an ultrasound can be a major step in promoting acceptance (Matsui & Gardiner, 2007).

The Partner

Once partners were forgotten persons in the childbearing process. Unwed fathers, in particular, were dismissed as not interested in the pregnancy or a woman's health. A female partner to a woman was completely ignored. Today, it is recognized that all partners are important and should be encouraged to play an emotional role in the pregnancy. This means that, as a woman adapts to pregnancy, her partner may go through some of the same psychological changes.

For partners, accepting the pregnancy means not only accepting the certainty of the pregnancy and the reality of the child to come but also accepting the woman in her changed state. A partner should try to give a woman emotional support while she is learning to accept the reality of pregnancy, and she should reciprocate when the partner begins to go through the process.

Like women, partners' feelings regarding the pregnancy vary. Often partners are proud and happy about the pregnancy, facilitating acceptance of it. However, partners may experience some feelings that make this task more difficult as it is not unusual for a partner to feel both overwhelmed with what the loss of the woman's salary will mean to the family if she means to quit work and a feeling close to jealousy of the growing baby, who, although not yet physically apparent, seems to be taking up a great deal of the woman's time and thought.

Partners also experience ambivalence, sometimes more so than pregnant women. The feeling of ambivalence can be compounded if partners are afraid to voice their concerns. This happens if they do not want to intensify the pregnant woman's anxieties by appearing anxious themselves. Partners may also feel ambivalent if they are not well prepared for parenthood or have had little experience with children. Often it is harder for partners to resolve their feelings of ambivalence, because they do not personally experience the changes of pregnancy and may not have as strong a support network. To help partners resolve some ambivalence, provide an outlet for them to discuss concerns, and offer parenting information at prenatal visits.

An unwed father may have a great deal of difficulty accepting a pregnancy unless he is actively involved in prenatal care. He tries to picture himself as a father but then realizes that if he does not marry his partner, he may never play a full father role to this child, so the image disappears again. Because the unwed father can relate to the fact that he fathered the child, however, he may feel a deep sense of loss if a woman decides to have an abortion or if the baby is born less than perfect. In addition, he may not have anyone to turn to for support because no one recognizes his loss.

✔ Checkpoint Question 10.1

Lauren sometimes feels ambivalent about being pregnant. What is the psychological task you'd like to see her complete during the first trimester of pregnancy?

a. Explain why morning sickness occurs.
b. Accept the fact that she's pregnant.
c. Accept the fact she's having a baby.
d. Choose a name for her baby.

Second Trimester: Accepting the Baby

As soon as fetal movements can be felt, psychological responses of both partners are apt to change.

The Woman

During the second trimester, the psychological task of a woman is to accept that she is having a baby, a second step from accepting the pregnancy. This change usually happens at **quickening**, or the first moment a woman feels fetal movement. Until a woman experiences for herself this proof of the child's existence, she may think of the life inside her as an integral part of herself rather than as a separate entity. She knows it is there; she eats to meet its needs and takes special vitamins to help it grow, but it seems more like just another part of her body. With quickening, however, the fetus assumes a separate identity. She begins to imagine how she will feel at the birth, when the physician or midwife announces, "It's a boy!" or "It's a girl!" She begins to imagine herself as a mother, perhaps teaching her child the alphabet or how to ride a bicycle. This anticipatory role-playing is an important activity for midpregnancy. It leads her to a larger concept of her condition and helps her realize that not only is she pregnant but also there is a child inside her.

Women often use the term "it" to refer to the child inside them. This does not mean that they have not yet accepted the pregnancy or still consider the baby an inanimate object. Some women believe that referring to the child as "she" or "he" will bring bad luck or disappointment if the child is of the opposite sex. Although an ultrasound can reveal the sex of the child, some women choose not to know because they fear being misled by an inaccurate ultrasound reading or they simply wish to be surprised about the sex of their child at birth.

Most women can pinpoint a moment during each pregnancy when they knew definitely that they wanted their child. For a woman who carefully planned the pregnancy, this moment of awareness may occur as soon as she recovers from the surprise of learning she has actually conceived. For others, it may come when she announces the news to her parents and hears them express their joy or when she sees a look of pride on her partner's face. It might be the moment of quickening, when she realizes that the fetus inside her is not passive but is an active being. Shopping for baby clothes for the first time, setting up the crib, seeing a blurry outline on an ultrasound screen: any of these small actions may suddenly make the coming baby seem real and desired (Fig. 10.1).

On the other hand, accepting the baby as a welcome family addition might not come until labor has begun or after several hours of labor. It might even be the moment a woman first hears her baby's cry or first touches or feeds her newborn. If a woman has a complication of pregnancy, is having financial difficulties, or lacks emotional support, it could take several weeks after the baby is born for her to accept her new reality and come to terms with motherhood. The emotional and physical upheavals brought about by the hormonal changes of pregnancy are so tremendous that they can lead to not only poor acceptance of the child but also postpartum depression or, in rare instances, psychosis (Westdahl et al., 2007).

A good way to measure the level of a woman's acceptance of the coming baby is to measure how well she follows prenatal instructions. Until a woman views the growing structure inside her as something desired, it may be difficult for her to substitute a high-protein food for her favorite coffee drink. After all, watching herself gain weight may be the most certain proof she has that she is pregnant.

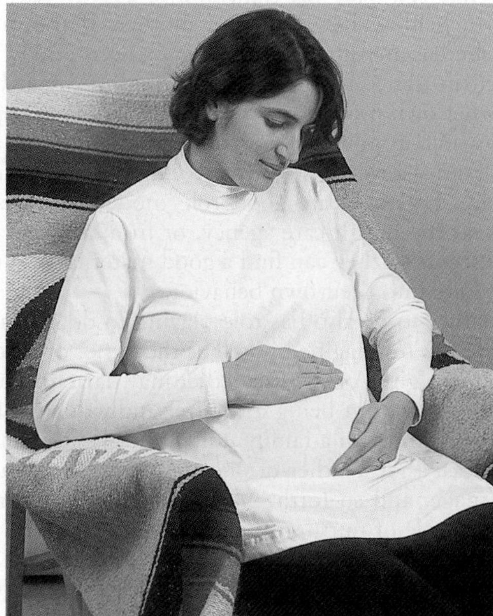

FIGURE 10.1 A growing abdomen and fluttering fetal movements help to make a pregnancy a reality. (© Barbara Proud.)

The Partner

As a woman begins to actively prepare for the coming baby, a partner may feel as if he is left standing in the wings, waiting to be asked to take part in the event. To compensate for this feeling, a partner may become overly absorbed in his work, striving to produce something concrete on the job or to earn enough money to demonstrate that he, too, is capable of creating something. This preoccupation with work may limit the amount of time a partner spends with his family, just when the pregnant woman most needs emotional support.

Some men may have difficulty enjoying the pregnancy because they have been misinformed about sexuality, pregnancy, and women's health. A man might believe, for example, that breastfeeding will make his wife's breasts no longer attractive and so will advise against it. He may believe that childbirth will stretch his wife's vagina so much that sexual relations will no longer be enjoyable and so will advocate for a cesarean birth. Such a man needs education to correct misinformation. Many men comment that the information they receive about childbirth and pregnancy is too concerned with their partner or the child and not enough with how they feel to be relevant to them.

Third Trimester: Preparing for Parenthood

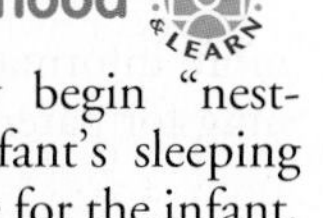

During the third trimester, couples usually begin "nest-building" activities, such as planning the infant's sleeping arrangements, buying clothes, choosing a name for the infant, and "ensuring safe passage" by learning about birth. These preparations are evidence that women are completing the third trimester task of pregnancy or preparing for parenthood.

Couples at this point are interested in attending prenatal classes or preparation for childbirth classes. It is helpful to ask a couple what specifically they are doing to get ready for birth to see if they are interested in taking such a class and to document how well prepared they will be for the baby's arrival.

Certain external life contingencies may slow the mental work of pregnancy on the part of a woman or her partner (Box 10.4). During prenatal visits, ask such questions as, "How does your partner feel about you being pregnant?" or "Has anything changed in your home life since you last came to the clinic?" to reveal if any situation that could interfere with bonding is present. It is unrealistic to believe that one health care professional has all the solutions to the problems that couples reveal when asked these questions. A multidisciplinary approach (e.g., referral to the nutritionist, nurse practitioner, or social services) is often necessary to help solve some of these multifaceted problems.

It is helpful for most couples to attend childbirth education classes or classes on preparing for parenthood as attending these classes can help a couple accept the pregnancy, expose them to other parents as role models, and provide practical information about pregnancy and childcare. It is best if these classes are conducted in small groups so they can meet the individual needs of couples (see Chapter 14 for

BOX 10.4 ✻ Events That Could Contribute to Difficulty Accepting a Pregnancy

- Learning that the pregnancy is a multiple one
- Learning that the fetus has a developmental abnormality
- Pregnancy less than 1 year after a previous one
- Relocation during pregnancy (involves a need to find new support people)
- Moving away from the family or back to the family for economic reasons
- Role reversal (a previously supporting person who becomes dependent, or vice versa)
- Job loss
- Marital infidelity
- Illness in self, husband, or a relative
- Loss of a significant other
- Complications of pregnancy such as severe hypertension
- Having friends or relatives who have had children born with health disorders
- Series of devaluing experiences (e.g., failure in school or work)
- History of previous miscarriages, fertility problems, traumatic births
- Previous fetal or neonatal loss
- History of rape, incest, or domestic violence

more information on childbirth education classes and planning for parenthood).

Reworking Developmental Tasks

Yet another task of pregnancy is working through previous life experiences. Needs and wishes that have been repressed for years may surface to be studied and reworked, often to an extreme extent.

Primary among these life experiences is a woman's relationship with her parents, particularly her mother. For the first time in her life, she finds she can empathize with her mother and the way her mother used to worry when she came home later than expected. The pregnant woman has already begun to worry about her child, to the point that she wonders if something is wrong when she feels no movement for a few hours, even though she is only 5 months into the pregnancy. She may find that her own mother becomes more important to her, and a new, more equal relationship often develops.

For a woman to work through past fears and conflicts of this kind, she needs to think about them when she is alone as well as to discuss them with others. She may throw out comments to her partner, friends, or health care personnel to test their reactions to these thoughts. A typical opening statement is, "I really hated my mother when I was a kid." If the response to this remark is a therapeutic, open-ended one (e.g., "You hated her?"), a woman may feel able to reveal the intensity of her conflict with her mother and how she cannot bear to think of the child inside her feeling that way about her. Teenagers who are pregnant need to resolve the conflict of being both a child and a mother. Unless these feelings are resolved, they can continue to have a negative view about becoming a mother.

Fear of being separated from family or dying are common childhood fears that can be revived during pregnancy. A clue that might signal a woman's distress over this could be, "Am I ever going to make it through this?" This expression might mean simply that she is tired of her backache, but it also might be a plea for reassurance that she will survive this event in her life.

A woman needs to have confidence in those who provide health care for her during pregnancy, so that she can express some of these disturbing thoughts and work through them. As a rule, a woman who is comfortable seeking information experiences less anxiety than one who feels unable to do this.

A pregnant woman's partner needs to do the same reworking of old values and forgotten developmental tasks. A man may rethink his relationship with his father to understand better what kind of father he will be. Some men may have had emotionally distant fathers and wish to be more emotionally available to their own children. These men have to reconcile feelings toward their fathers and learn a new pattern of behavior.

Role-Playing and Fantasizing

Another step in preparing for parenthood is role-playing, or fantasizing about what it will be like to be a parent. Just as a child learns what to do by following her mother as she sets a table or balances her checkbook, a pregnant woman begins to spend time with other pregnant women or mothers of young children to learn how to be a mother. She is drawn into a world of talk about babies and pregnancy with these women. A pregnant woman may offer to babysit for a neighbor or relative so she can "practice" caring for a new baby. As a part of the role-playing process, women's dreams tend to focus on the pregnancy and concerns about keeping herself and her coming child safe.

Although role-playing may be difficult for a pregnant teen who has not yet made the transition to adulthood, it is important in helping her become a mother. If the only role models she has are other girls her age, who typically are not interested in the commitment to mothering—or if her role model is her own mother, who might be unable to cope with problems such as poverty, too many children, or an ineffectual husband—a worry is that the young girl will assume the same role. Try to locate good role models (in classes for mothers, at the health care agency, or from a social agency) for adolescents so they can find a good maternal role to copy and integrate into their own behavior.

The father-to-be also has role-playing to do during pregnancy. He has to imagine himself as the father of a boy or as the father of a girl. A first-time father may have to change his view of himself from being a carefree individual to being a significant member of a family unit. If he already is a father, he has to cast aside a father-of-one identity to accept a father-of-two image, and so forth. Many fathers want or need to take on the role of nurturer but have had little or no experience caring for newborns or infants. Newborn care classes provided before or after the birth can help fathers grow comfortable with this role.

Other support persons who will have an active role in raising the child (e.g., grandparents, close friends) also have to work out their roles in regard to the pregnancy and impending parenthood. This may be particularly difficult, because the roles for these support persons may not be clearly defined, and no role model may be apparent.

Emotional Responses to Pregnancy

Because of all the tasks that need to be worked through during a pregnancy, emotional responses can vary greatly. Common reactions include grief, narcissism, introversion or extroversion, body image and boundary concerns, couvade syndrome (somatic experiences of father during pregnancy simulating those of the pregnant mother), stress, mood swings, and changes in sexual desire. It is helpful to caution a pregnant woman and her partner about common changes they may expect. Otherwise, they can misinterpret the woman's mood swings, decreased sexual interest, introversion, or narcissism not as changes of pregnancy but as a loss of interest in their relationship.

Grief

The thought that grief could be associated with such a positive process as childbirth seems at first incongruent. But before a woman can take on a mothering role, she has to give up or alter her present roles. She will never be a daughter in exactly the same way again. She will never be as irresponsible and carefree as she is now again. She will not even sleep soundly for the next 18 years. She must incorporate her new role as a mother into her other roles as a daughter, wife, or friend. Her partner must incorporate a new role as a father into his other roles of son, husband, or friend.

Narcissism

Self-centeredness (narcissism) is generally an early reaction to pregnancy. A woman who previously was barely conscious of her body, who dressed in the morning with little thought about what to wear, who was unconcerned about her posture or her weight, suddenly begins to concentrate on these aspects of her life. She dresses so her pregnancy will or will not show, making dressing a time-consuming, mirror-studying procedure. She makes a ceremony out of fixing her meals. She may lose interest in her job or community events because the work seems alien to the more important events taking place in her body, events that constantly remind her a new round of life is beginning.

Narcissism may be manifested by a change in activity. A woman may stop playing tennis, for example, even though her physician tells her it will do no harm in moderation. She may criticize her husband's driving, although it never bothered her before. She does these things to unconsciously protect her body and her baby. Men may demonstrate the same behavior by reducing risky activities such as mountain biking, trying to ensure that they will be present to raise their child.

This need of a woman to protect her body has implications for nursing care. It means she may regard unnecessary nudity as a threat to her body (be sure to drape properly for pelvic and abdominal examinations). She may resent casual remarks such as, "Oh my, you've gained weight" (a threat to her appearance) or, "You don't like milk?" (a threat to her judgment).

There is a tendency to organize health instructions during pregnancy around the baby: "Be sure and keep this appointment. You want to have a healthy baby." "You really ought to eat more protein for the baby's sake." This approach may be particularly inappropriate early in pregnancy, before the fetus stirs and before a woman is convinced not only that she is pregnant but also that there is a baby inside her. At early stages, a woman may be much more interested in doing things for herself because it is her body, her tiredness, and her well-being that will be directly affected ("Eat protein because it keeps your fingernails from breaking" or "Protein will give you more energy").

Introversion Versus Extroversion

Introversion, or turning inward to concentrate on oneself and one's body, is a common finding during pregnancy. Some women, however, react in an entirely opposite fashion and become more extroverted. They become more active, appear healthier than ever before and are more outgoing. This tends to occur in women who are finding unexpected fulfillment in pregnancy, perhaps who had seriously doubted that they would be lucky enough or fertile enough to conceive. Such a woman regards her expanding abdomen as proof she is equal to her sisters. Although such a woman may become more varied in her interests during pregnancy, she may be puzzling to those around her who previously regarded her as quiet and self-contained.

Body Image and Boundary

Body image (the way your body appears to yourself) and body boundary (a zone of separation you perceive between yourself and objects or other people) change during pregnancy as a woman begins to envision herself as a mother. In addition to being a daughter or wife, she begins to see herself becoming "bigger" in many different ways. This change in body image is part of the basis for narcissism and introversion. Changes in concept of body boundaries leads to a firmer distinction between objects, yet at the same time her body boundary is perceived as extremely vulnerable, as if her body were delicate and easily harmed. This change in boundary perception is so startling that pregnant women may walk far away from an object such as a table to avoid bumping against it.

Stress

Because pregnancy brings with it such a major role change, it can cause extreme stress in a woman. This stress of pregnancy, like any stress, can make it difficult for a woman to make decisions, be as aware of her surroundings as usual, or maintain time management with her usual degree of skill. Determining whether the twinges she feels in her back are beginning labor contractions or just backache and whether she should call her primary care provider are difficult decisions to make for someone who is stressed. This may cause people who were dependent on a woman before pregnancy to feel neglected, because now that she is pregnant she seems to have strength only for herself. If a woman was in an abusive relationship before the pregnancy, the increased stress of pregnancy is apt to cause even more abuse. Asking whether intimate partner abuse has ever occurred in the past to help predict if it could occur during pregnancy is an important part of prenatal interviewing (Casanueva & Martin, 2007).

To help families keep their perspective for the full length of a pregnancy, remind them that any decrease in the ability to function that happens to a pregnant woman is a reaction to the stress of pregnancy, not the pregnancy itself. Many nonpregnant women and men function at work under just as much stress because of marital discord or a loved one's illness or death and have just as much difficulty with making decisions. Pregnancy may actually be less stressful than those situations because of its predictable 9-month outcome.

A woman with fewer support people around her almost automatically has more difficulty adjusting to and accepting a pregnancy and a new child than do women who have more support. A woman who begins a pregnancy with a strong support person and then loses that person through trauma, illness, separation, or divorce needs special attention in regard to loneliness and depression. Evaluate her carefully regarding how she is managing and give her extra support because her feeling of loss is likely to be extremely acute. A loss of this kind has the potential to interfere not only with her own health but also with parent–child bonding.

Knowing that she has supportive health care providers she can call on when needed is the one thing that may make this pregnancy tolerable.

✓ Checkpoint Question 10.2

Lauren Maxwell is aware that she's been showing some narcissistic tendencies since becoming pregnant. Which of her actions best describes narcissism?

a. She feels pulled in multiple directions.
b. Her thoughts tend to be mainly about herself.
c. She feels a need to sleep a lot more than usual.
d. She often feels "numb" or as if she's taken a narcotic.

Couvade Syndrome

Many men experience physical symptoms such as nausea, vomiting, and backache to the same degree or even more intensely than their partners during a pregnancy. These symptoms apparently result from stress, anxiety, and empathy for the pregnant woman. This is common enough that it has been given a name: **couvade syndrome.** The more the partner is involved in or attuned to the changes of the pregnancy, the more symptoms a woman's partner may experience. As a woman's abdomen begins to grow, the partner may perceive himself as growing larger, too, as if he is experiencing changing boundaries the same as his partner. For the most part, these are healthy happenings and require psychological attention only if the man becomes emotionally stressed or delusional (Brennan et al., 2007).

What If... You were working and found yourself doing twice your normal work because a male coworker whose wife is 5 months' pregnant calls in sick at least 3 days a week because of "nausea"? Could you assume that this symptom is part of couvade syndrome?

Emotional Lability

Mood changes occur frequently in a pregnant woman, partly as a manifestation of narcissism (her feelings are easily hurt by remarks that would have been laughed off before) and partly because of hormonal changes, particularly the sustained increase in estrogen and progesterone. Mood swings may be so common that they make a woman's reaction to her family and to health care routines unpredictable. What she finds acceptable one week she may find intolerable the next. She may cry over her children's bad table manners at one meal and find the situation amusing and even charming at the next. Women and their partners and families need to be cautioned that such mood swings occur, beginning with early pregnancy, so that they can accept them as part of pregnancy (Box 10.5).

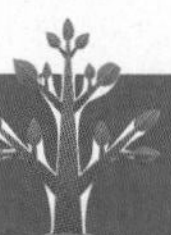

BOX 10.5 ✻ Focus on Family Teaching

Mood Swings During Pregnancy

Q. Lauren Maxwell tells you she has noticed extreme mood swings since she has been pregnant. She asks you how she can reduce them.

A. Try these measures:

- Avoid fatigue, because when you are tired, your normal defenses are most likely to be down.
- Reduce your level of stress by setting priorities. Ask yourself if everything you are doing really needs to be done.
- Do not let little problems grow into big ones; attack them when they first occur.
- Try to view situations from other people's perspective. They are not as involved in your pregnancy as you are. Things that do not seem important to you may be important to them.
- Let others know you are aware that you are having trouble with emotions since you became pregnant. Your family and friends will be more than willing to help you through this time if they realize that your shifting emotions are of concern to you.

Changes in Sexual Desire

Most women report that their sexual desire changes, at least to some degree, during pregnancy. Women who formerly were worried about becoming pregnant may truly enjoy sexual relations for the first time during pregnancy. Others might feel a loss of desire because of their estrogen increase, or they might unconsciously view sexual relations as a threat to the fetus they must protect. Some may worry that having sexual relations could bring on early labor.

During the first trimester, most women report a decrease in libido because of the nausea, fatigue, and breast tenderness that accompany early pregnancy. During the second trimester, as blood flow to the pelvic area increases to supply the placenta, libido, and sexual enjoyment rise markedly. During the third trimester, sexual desire may remain high, or it may decrease because of difficulty finding a comfortable position and increasing abdominal size. When a couple knows early in pregnancy that such changes may occur, they can be interpreted in the correct light (i.e., as a difference, not as loss of interest in the sexual partner). Suggestions for helping women and their partners adjust to these circumstances are discussed in Chapter 12.

Changes in the Expectant Family

Most parents are aware that their older children need preparation when a new baby is on the way; however, knowing that preparation is needed and being prepared to do this are two different things. For this reason, some couples appreciate suggestions from health care personnel regarding how this task can be accomplished.

Both preschool and school-age children may need to be reassured periodically during pregnancy that a new baby will be an addition to the family and will not replace them in their parents' affection. Preparing a child for the birth of a sibling is discussed in Chapters 14 and 31.

THE DIAGNOSIS OF PREGNANCY

The medical diagnosis of pregnancy serves to date when the birth will occur and also helps predict the existence of a high-risk status. If a pregnancy was planned, the diagnosis produces a feeling of intense fulfillment and achievement. If it was not planned or not desired, it can result in an equally extreme crisis state.

From the day the pregnancy is confirmed, most women try to eat a more nutritious diet, give up cigarette smoking and alcohol ingestion, and stop taking nonessential medications. Because a woman may not take these measures before confirmation of her pregnancy, this makes early confirmation of pregnancy important. If a woman does not wish to continue the pregnancy, early diagnosis is also imperative: therapeutic termination of pregnancy always should be carried out at the earliest stage possible for the safest outcome.

If a sexually active woman is scheduled for diagnostic testing that includes a pelvic x-ray study such as an intravenous pyelogram for kidney disease, you might suggest that she first have a rapid serum pregnancy test to rule out pregnancy as a possibility, to avoid exposing a fetus to radiation.

Most women who come to a health care facility for a diagnosis of pregnancy have already guessed that they are pregnant based on a multitude of subjective signs. Most have already used a home pregnancy test to confirm the pregnancy for themselves.

Pregnancy is officially diagnosed on the basis of the symptoms reported by the woman and the signs elicited by a health care provider. These signs and symptoms are traditionally divided into three classifications: presumptive or subjective, probable or objective, and positive or documented (Table 10.2).

Presumptive (Subjective) Signs of Pregnancy

Presumptive signs of pregnancy are those that are least indicative of pregnancy; taken as single entities, they could easily indicate other conditions (Rojas, Wood, & Blakemore, 2007). These findings, discussed in connection with the body system in which they occur, are experienced by the woman but cannot be documented by an examiner (Box 10.6).

Probable Signs of Pregnancy

In contrast to presumptive signs, probable signs of pregnancy are objective so can be documented by an examiner. Although they are more reliable than presumptive signs, they still are not positive or true diagnostic findings (Box 10.7). They are also discussed in connection with the body system in which they occur.

Laboratory Tests

The commonly used laboratory tests for pregnancy are based on detecting the presence of human chorionic gonadotropin (hCG), a hormone created by the chorionic villi of the placenta, in the urine or blood serum of the pregnant woman. Because all laboratory tests for pregnancy are accurate in diagnosing pregnancy only 95% to 98% of the time, positive results from these tests are considered probable rather than positive signs.

These tests are performed by radioimmunoassay (RIA), enzyme-linked immunosorbent assay (ELISA), or radioreceptor assay (RRA) techniques. For these tests, hCG is measured in international units. In the nonpregnant woman, no units are detectable because there are no trophoblast cells producing hCG. In the pregnant woman, trace amounts of hCG appear in the serum as early as 24 to 48 hours after implantation. They reach a measurable level (about 50 mIU/mL) 7 to 9 days after conception. Levels peak at about 100 mIU/mL between the 60th and 80th day of gestation. After that point, the concentration of hCG declines again so that, at term, it is barely detectable in serum or urine.

Urine, formerly used extensively for pregnancy testing, is now used only rarely in health care settings, because blood serum tests give earlier results. Urine tests still form the basis of home pregnancy tests.

Home Pregnancy Tests

Several kits for pregnancy testing based on immunologic reactions are available over the counter. These tests have a high degree of accuracy (about 97%) if the instructions are followed exactly. They are convenient to use, because waiting for a health care appointment to have a pregnancy confirmed can be an anxious, stressful time for many women. For this type of test, a woman dips a reagent strip into her stream of urine. A color change on the strip denotes pregnancy. Home tests can detect as little as 35 mIU/mL of hCG. They take 3 to 5 minutes to perform. Most manufacturers suggest that women wait until the day of the missed menstrual period to test. Advise any woman who thinks she might be pregnant but gets a negative result from a home pregnancy test to repeat the test 1 week later if she is still experiencing amenorrhea. If symptoms persist after two tests, she needs to see a health care provider as she might have a condition such as an ovarian tumor causing the amenorrhea and needs appropriate diagnosis for this condition.

Women taking psychotropic drugs (e.g., antianxiety agents) may have false-positive results on pregnancy tests. Women taking oral contraceptives also may have false-positive results; for such a test to be accurate, oral contraceptives should have been discontinued 5 days before the test. Women who have proteinuria, are postmenopausal, or have hyperthyroid disease also may show false-positive results.

In the past, one of the chief reasons women sought early prenatal care was to obtain an official diagnosis of pregnancy. Now that women can diagnose their pregnancies at home by means of a test kit, they may not seek prenatal care until something seems to be wrong with the pregnancy or until

TABLE 10.2 ✻ Presumptive, Probable, and Positive Signs of Pregnancy

Time From Implantation (Weeks)	Presumptive Finding	Probable Finding	Positive Finding	Description
1		Serum laboratory tests		Tests of blood serum reveal the presence of human chorionic gonadotropin hormone.
2	Breast changes			Feeling of tenderness, fullness, or tingling; enlargement and darkening of areola
2	Nausea, vomiting			Nausea or vomiting on arising
2	Amenorrhea			Absence of menstruation
3	Frequent urination			Sense of having to void more often than usual
6		Chadwick's sign		Color change of the vagina from pink to violet
6		Goodell's sign		Softening of the cervix
6		Hegar's sign		Softening of the lower uterine segment
6		Evidence on ultrasound of gestational sac		Characteristic ring is evident.
8			Evidence on ultrasound of fetal outline	Fetal outline can be seen and measured by ultrasound.
10–12			Fetal heart audible	Doppler ultrasound reveals heartbeat.
12	Fatigue			General feeling of tiredness
12	Uterine enlargement			Uterus can be palpated over symphysis pubis.
16		Ballottement		When lower uterine segment is tapped on a bimanual examination, the fetus can be felt to rise against abdominal wall.
18	Quickening			Fetal movement felt by woman
20			Fetal movement felt by examiner	Fetal movement can be palpated through abdomen.
20		Braxton Hicks contractions		Periodic uterine tightening occurs.
20		Fetal outline felt by examiner		Fetal outline can be palpated through abdomen.
24	Linea nigra			Line of dark pigment on the abdomen
24	Melasma			Dark pigment on face
24	Striae gravidarum			Red streaks on abdomen

they are so far along they feel they should do something about arranging medical coverage for the birth. Caution women that early and regular prenatal care is important to safeguard the pregnancy outcome. After a positive pregnancy test, the first step should be to arrange for prenatal care (Bernstein & Weinstein, 2007).

Positive Signs of Pregnancy

There are only three documented or positive signs of pregnancy:

- Demonstration of a fetal heart separate from the mother's
- Fetal movements felt by an examiner
- Visualization of the fetus by ultrasound

Demonstration of a Fetal Heart Separate From the Mother's Heart

The fetal heart can be shown to be beating on ultrasound as early as the sixth to seventh week of pregnancy. Ultrasonic monitoring systems that convert ultrasonic frequencies to audible frequencies (Doppler technique) can detect fetal heart sounds as early as the 10th to 12th week of gestation. Echocardiography can demonstrate a heartbeat as early as 5 weeks.

Although the fetal heart has been beating since the 24th day after conception, it is audible by auscultation of the abdomen with an ordinary stethoscope only at about 18 to 20 weeks of pregnancy. Fetal heart sounds are difficult to hear if a woman's abdomen has a great deal of subcutaneous fat or if

Box 10.6 Assessment

Assessing the Client for Presumptive Signs of Pregnancy

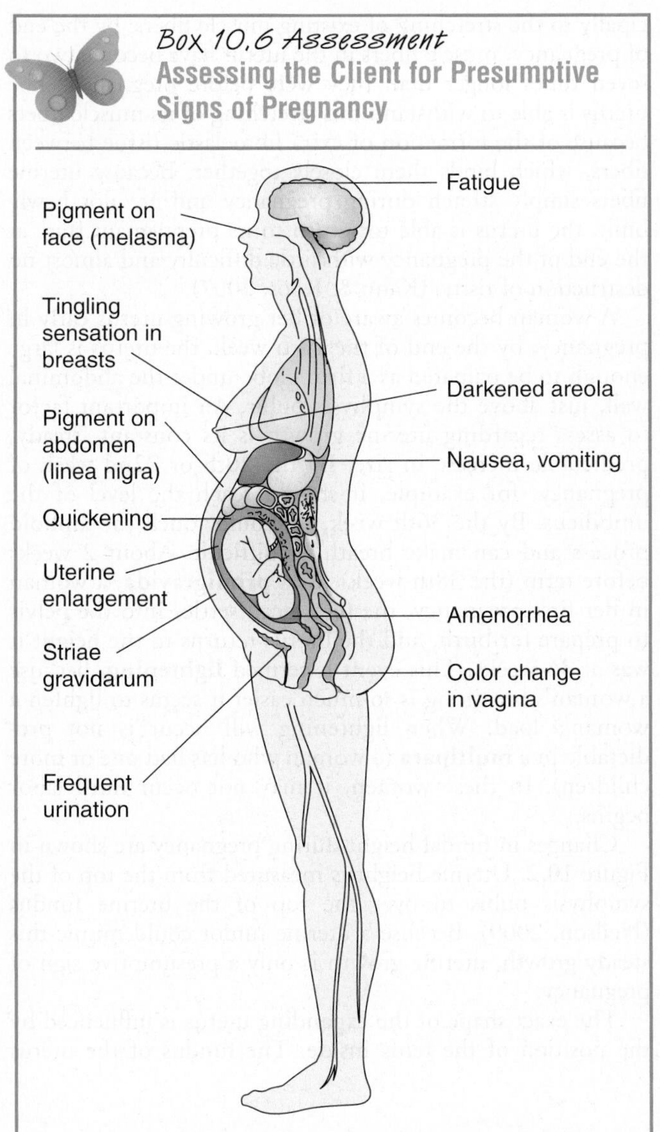

Box 10.7 Assessment

Assessing the Client for Probable Signs of Pregnancy

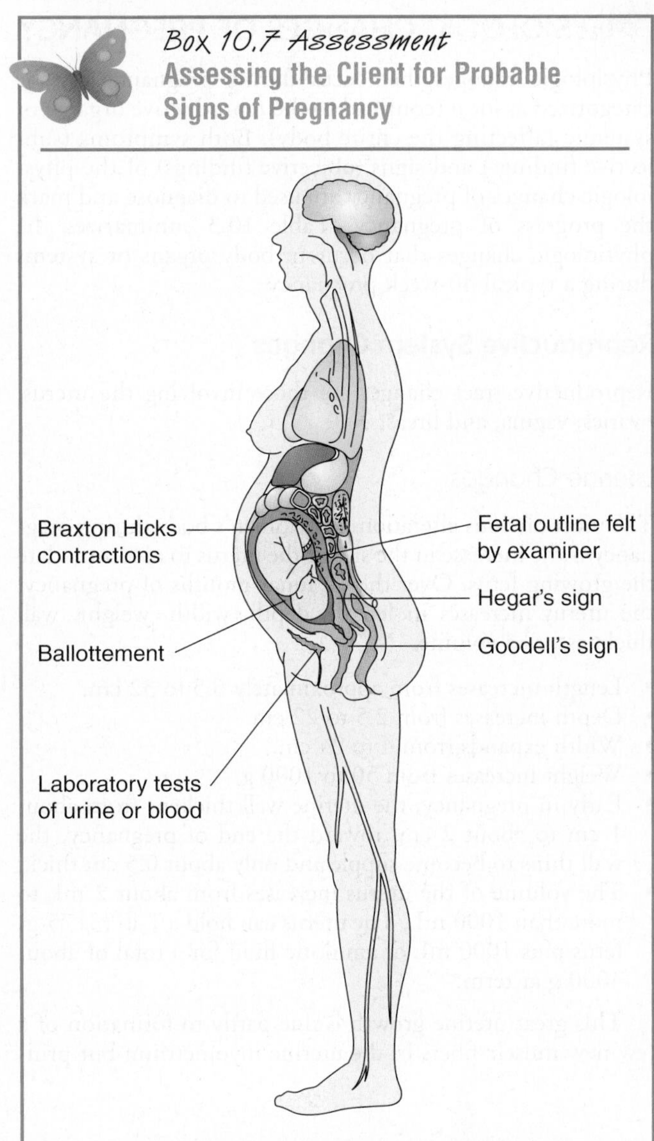

a larger than normal amount of amniotic fluid is present (hydramnios). They are heard best when the position of the fetus is determined by palpation and the stethoscope is placed over the area of the fetus's back. The fetal heart rate usually ranges between 120 and 160 beats per minute.

Fetal Movements Felt by an Examiner

Fetal movements may be felt by a woman as early as 16 to 20 weeks of pregnancy. Those felt by an objective examiner are considered much more reliable because a woman could mistake the movement of gas through her intestines for fetal movement. Fetal movements can be felt by an examiner at the 20th to 24th week of pregnancy unless a woman is extremely obese.

Visualization of Fetus by Ultrasound

High-frequency sound waves projected toward a woman's abdomen are useful in diagnosing pregnancy. If a woman is pregnant, a characteristic ring, indicating the gestational sac, will be revealed on an oscilloscope screen as early as the fourth to sixth week of pregnancy. This method also gives information about the site of implantation and whether a multiple pregnancy exists. By the eighth week, a fetal outline can be seen so clearly within the sac that the crown-to-rump length can be measured to establish the gestational age of the pregnancy. Seeing the fetal outline on an ultrasound is clear proof for a couple that a woman is pregnant if they had any doubt up to that point.

✓ Checkpoint Question 10.3

Lauren Maxwell used a urine pregnancy test but was surprised to learn that a positive result is not a sure sign of pregnancy. She asks you what would be a positive sign. Your best answer would be:

a. She is having consistent uterine growth.
b. She feels the fetus move especially after meals.
c. hCG can be found in her bloodstream.
d. The fetal heart can be seen on ultrasound.

PHYSIOLOGIC CHANGES OF PREGNANCY

Physiologic changes that occur during pregnancy can be categorized as local (confined to the reproductive organs) or systemic (affecting the entire body). Both symptoms (subjective findings) and signs (objective findings) of the physiologic changes of pregnancy are used to diagnose and mark the progress of pregnancy. Table 10.3 summarizes the physiologic changes that occur in body organs or systems during a typical 40-week pregnancy.

Reproductive System Changes

Reproductive tract changes are those involving the uterus, ovaries, vagina, and breasts.

Uterine Changes

The most obvious alteration in a woman's body during pregnancy is the increase in the size of the uterus to accommodate the growing fetus. Over the 10 lunar months of pregnancy, the uterus increases in length, depth, width, weight, wall thickness, and volume.

- Length increases from approximately 6.5 to 32 cm.
- Depth increases from 2.5 to 22 cm.
- Width expands from 4 to 24 cm.
- Weight increases from 50 to 1000 g.
- Early in pregnancy, the uterine wall thickens from about 1 cm to about 2 cm; toward the end of pregnancy, the wall thins to become supple and only about 0.5 cm thick.
- The volume of the uterus increases from about 2 mL to more than 1000 mL. The uterus can hold a 7-lb (3175-g) fetus plus 1000 mL of amniotic fluid for a total of about 4000 g at term.

This great uterine growth is due partly to formation of a few new muscle fibers in the uterine myometrium but principally to the stretching of existing muscle fibers: by the end of pregnancy, muscle fibers in the uterus have become two to seven times longer than they were before pregnancy. The uterus is able to withstand this stretching of its muscle fibers because of the formation of extra fibroelastic tissue between fibers, which binds them closely together. Because uterine fibers simply stretch during pregnancy and are not newly built, the uterus is able to return to its prepregnant state at the end of the pregnancy with little difficulty and almost no destruction of tissue (Kahn & Koos, 2007).

A woman becomes aware of her growing uterus early in pregnancy; by the end of the 12th week, the uterus is large enough to be palpated as a firm globe under the abdominal wall, just above the symphysis pubis. An important factor to assess regarding uterine growth is its constant, steady, predictable increase in size. By the 20th or 22nd week of pregnancy, for example, it should reach the level of the umbilicus. By the 36th week, it should touch the xiphoid process and can make breathing difficult. About 2 weeks before term (the 38th week) for a **primigravida,** a woman in her first pregnancy, the fetal head settles into the pelvis to prepare for birth, and the uterus returns to the height it was at 36 weeks. This event is termed **lightening,** because a woman's breathing is so much easier it seems to lighten a woman's load. When lightening will occur is not predictable in a **multipara** (a woman who has had one or more children). In these women, it may not occur until labor begins.

Changes in fundal height during pregnancy are shown in Figure 10.2. Uterine height is measured from the top of the symphysis pubis to over the top of the uterine fundus (Neilson, 2009). Because a uterine tumor could mimic this steady growth, uterine growth is only a presumptive sign of pregnancy.

The exact shape of the expanding uterus is influenced by the position of the fetus inside. The fundus of the uterus

TABLE 10.3 ✻ Timetable for Physiologic Changes of Pregnancy

Location of Change	1st Trimester	2nd Trimester	3rd Trimester
Circulatory system	Blood volume increasing		
	Pseudoanemia	Blood pressure slightly decreased	Blood pressure returns to prepregnancy levels
	Clotting factors increasing		
Ovary	Corpus luteum active	Corpus luteum fading	
Uterus	Increased growth	Placenta forming estrogen and progesterone	
Cervix	Softening progressive		"Ripe"
Vagina	White discharge present		Increasing
Musculoskeletal system		Progressive cartilage softening	
		Lordosis increasing	
Pigmentation		Progressively increasing	
Kidney	Maternal glomerular filtration rate increasing	Glycosuria	
	Aldosterone increased, retaining sodium and fluid		
Gastrointestinal system		Slowed peristalsis	
Thyroid	Increased metabolic rate		

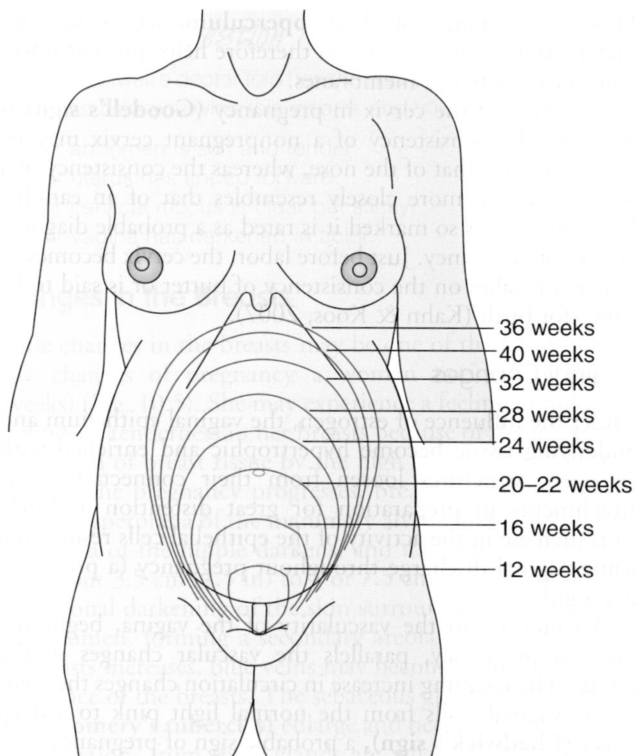

FIGURE 10.2 Fundus height at various weeks of pregnancy.

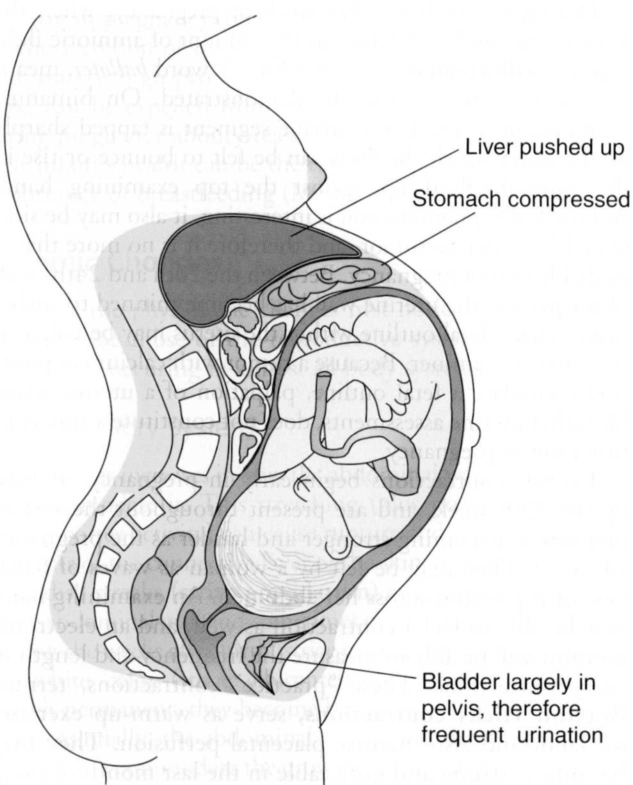

FIGURE 10.3 Crowding of abdominal contents late in pregnancy.

usually remains in the midline during pregnancy, although it may be pushed slightly to the right side because of the larger bulk of the sigmoid colon on the left. As the uterus increases in size, it pushes the intestines to the sides of the abdomen, elevates the diaphragm and liver, compresses the stomach, and puts pressure on the bladder. A woman may worry that there will not be enough room inside her abdomen for this increase in size. You can assure her that the abdominal contents will shift readily to accommodate uterine enlargement (Fig. 10.3).

Uterine blood flow increases during pregnancy as the placenta grows and requires more and more blood for perfusion. Doppler ultrasonography has shown that, before pregnancy, uterine blood flow is 15 to 20 mL/min. By the end of pregnancy, it expands to as much as 500 to 750 mL/min, with 75% of that volume going to the placenta. Measuring that placenta blood volume and velocity is increasing this way is one of the most important gauges of fetal health (Gonzalez et al., 2007).

Toward the end of pregnancy, one-sixth of a woman's blood supply is circulating through the uterus at any given time; therefore, uterine bleeding in pregnancy is always potentially serious because it could result in a major blood loss. Caution women that vaginal blood loss, which suggests uterine bleeding, could pose a major health risk. They should always contact their health care practitioner if such bleeding occurs.

A bimanual examination (one finger of an examiner is placed in the vagina, the other hand on the abdomen) can demonstrate that, with pregnancy, the uterus feels more anteflexed, larger, and softer to the touch than usual. At about the sixth week of pregnancy (at the time of the second missed menstrual period), the lower uterine segment just above the cervix becomes so soft that when it is compressed between examining fingers on bimanual examination, the wall cannot be felt or feels as thin as tissue paper. This extreme softening of the lower uterine segment is known as **Hegar's sign** (Fig. 10.4). It is a probable sign of pregnancy (Rojas, Wood, & Blakemore, 2007).

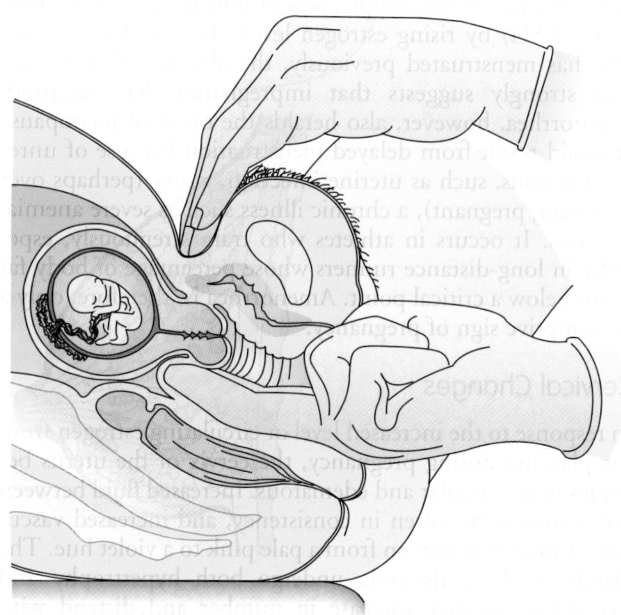

FIGURE 10.4 Examining for Hegar's sign. If the sign is present, the wall of the uterus is softer than usual.

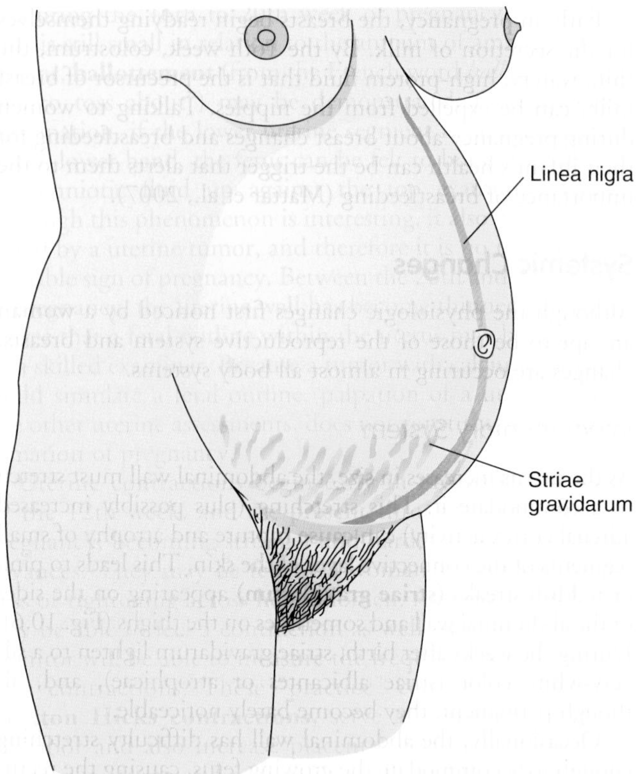

FIGURE 10.6 Skin changes in pregnancy: striae gravidarum and linea nigra.

If this happens, it will appear after pregnancy as a bluish groove at the site of separation.

The umbilicus is stretched by pregnancy to such an extent that by the 28th week, its depression becomes obliterated and smooth because it has been pushed so far outward. In most women, it may appear as if it has turned inside out, protruding as a round bump at the center of the abdominal wall.

Extra pigmentation generally appears on the abdominal wall. A narrow, brown line **(linea nigra)** may form, running from the umbilicus to the symphysis pubis and separating the abdomen into right and left hemispheres (see Fig. 10.6). Darkened areas may appear on the face as well, particularly on the cheeks and across the nose. This is known as **melasma** (chloasma), or the "mask of pregnancy." These increases in pigmentation are caused by melanocyte-stimulating hormone, which is secreted by the pituitary. With the decrease in the level of the hormone after pregnancy, these areas lighten and again disappear.

Vascular spiders or telangiectases (small, fiery-red branching spots) are sometimes seen on the skin of pregnant women, particularly on the thighs. These probably result from the increased level of estrogen in the body. They may fade but not completely disappear after pregnancy. The activity of sweat glands increases throughout the body during pregnancy. Women notice this as an increase in perspiration. Palmar erythema (redness and itching) may occur on the hands from the increased estrogen level. Fewer hairs on the head enter a resting phase because of overall increased metabolism, so scalp hair growth is increased.

Respiratory System

A local change that often occurs in the respiratory system is marked congestion, or "stuffiness," of the nasopharynx, a response to increased estrogen levels. Women may worry that this stuffiness indicates an allergy or a cold. Not realizing that it is happening because they are pregnant, some women take over-the-counter cold medications or antihistamines in an effort to relieve the congestion. Some continue to take the medication after pregnancy is confirmed, not mentioning they are taking this medication to health care providers because they think the stuffiness is a separate problem and not related to the pregnancy. Ask all women at prenatal visits if they are taking any kind of medicine or if they have noticed nasal stuffiness to detect this possibility.

As the uterus enlarges during pregnancy, a great deal of pressure is put on the diaphragm and, ultimately, on the lungs. This can displace the diaphragm by as much as 4 cm upward. This crowding of the chest cavity causes an acute sensation of shortness of breath late in pregnancy, until lightening relieves the pressure.

Even with all this crowding, a woman's vital capacity (the maximum volume exhaled after a maximum inspiration) does not decrease during pregnancy because, although the lungs are crowded in the vertical dimension, they can still expand horizontally. Residual volume (the amount of air remaining in the lungs after expiration) is decreased up to 20% by the pressure of the diaphragm. Tidal volume (the volume of air inspired) is increased up to 40% as a woman draws in extra volume to increase the effectiveness of air exchange. Total oxygen consumption increases by as much as 20%.

The increased level of progesterone during pregnancy appears to set a new level in the hypothalamus for acceptable blood carbon dioxide levels (P_{CO_2}), because, during pregnancy, a woman's body tends to maintain a P_{CO_2} at closer to 32 mm Hg than the normal 40 mm Hg. This low P_{CO_2} level causes a favorable CO_2 gradient at the placenta (the fetal CO_2 level is higher than that in the mother, allowing CO_2 to cross readily from the fetus to the mother).

To keep the mother's pH level from becoming acid because of the load of CO_2 being shifted to her by the fetus, increased ventilation (mild hyperventilation) to blow off excess CO_2 begins early in pregnancy. At full term, a woman's total ventilation capacity may have risen by as much as 40%. This increased ventilation may become so extreme that a woman develops a respiratory alkalosis or exhales more than the usual CO_2. To compensate, kidneys excrete plasma bicarbonate in urine. This results in increased urination or **polyuria,** an early sign of pregnancy. With greater urine output, both additional sodium and additional water are lost.

The slight increase in pH in serum because of the changed expiratory effort is advantageous because it slightly increases the binding capacity of maternal hemoglobin and thereby raises the oxygen content of maternal blood (P_{O_2}), from a normal level of about 92 mm Hg to about 106 mm Hg early in pregnancy. This is advantageous to fetal growth because it allows good placental exchange.

The cumulative effect of these respiratory changes is often experienced by a woman as chronic shortness of breath. Although her breathing rate is more rapid than usual (18–20 breaths per minute), this is normal for pregnancy.

The total respiratory changes and the compensating mechanisms that occur in the respiratory system can be described as

TABLE 10.4 ✻ Respiratory Changes During Pregnancy

Variable	Change
Vital capacity	No change
Tidal volume	Increased by 30% to 40%
Respiratory rate	Increased by 1–2/min
Residual volume	Decreased by 20%
Plasma P_{CO_2}	Decreased to about 27–32 mm Hg
Plasma pH	Increased to 7.40–7.45
Plasma P_{O_2}	Increased to 104–108 mm Hg
Respiratory minute volume	Increased by 40%
Expiratory reserve	Decreased by 20%

a chronic respiratory alkalosis fully compensated by a chronic metabolic acidosis. Changes in respiratory function during pregnancy are summarized in Table 10.4.

Temperature

Early in pregnancy, body temperature increases slightly because of the secretion of progesterone from the corpus luteum (the temperature, which increased at ovulation, remains elevated). As the placenta takes over the function of the corpus luteum at about 16 weeks, the temperature usually decreases to normal.

Some women may mistakenly assume that this slight rise in temperature (99.6° F orally), associated with pregnancy-related nasal congestion, is a sure sign of a cold, and may think they need medication. Explaining the reason for these changes allows a woman to accept them without worrying.

Cardiovascular System

Changes in the circulatory system are extremely significant to the health of the fetus, because they are necessary for adequate placental and fetal circulation. Table 10.5 summarizes these changes.

Blood Volume. To provide for an adequate exchange of nutrients in the placenta and to provide adequate blood to compensate for blood loss at birth, the total circulatory blood volume of a woman's body increases by at least 30% (and possibly as much as 50%) during pregnancy. Blood loss at a normal vaginal birth is about 300 to 400 mL; blood loss from a cesarean birth can be as high as 800 to 1000 mL. The increase in blood volume occurs gradually, beginning at the end of the first trimester. It peaks at about the 28th to the 32nd week and then continues at this high level throughout the third trimester. Because the plasma volume increases faster than red blood cell production, the concentration of hemoglobin and erythrocytes may decline, giving a woman a pseudoanemia early in pregnancy. A woman's body compensates for this change by producing more red blood cells, creating near- normal levels of red blood cells again by the second trimester.

Iron, Folic Acid, and Vitamin Needs. Almost all women need some iron supplementation during pregnancy because of a variety of factors. The fetus requires a total of about 350 to 400 mg of iron to grow. The increases in the mother's circulatory red blood cell mass require an additional 400 mg of iron. This is a total increased need of about 800 mg. Because the average woman's store of iron is less than this amount (about 500 mg), and because iron absorption may be impaired during pregnancy as a result of decreased gastric acidity (iron is absorbed best from an acid medium), additional iron is often prescribed during pregnancy to prevent a true anemia.

Either a hemoglobin concentration of less than 11 g/100 mL or a hematocrit value below 33% in the first or third trimester of pregnancy or a hemoglobin concentration of less than 10.5 g/dL (hematocrit <32%) in the second trimester is considered true anemia, for which iron therapy above normal supplementation is advocated (Arnett & Greenspoon, 2007). Caution women that, like all drugs, a prescribed dose of iron is good for them. Taking excess iron pills over this prescribed amount can cause stomach irritation and possibly iron accumulation in body cells (Pena-Rosas & Viteri, 2009). (See Chapter 20 for additional information on anemia in pregnancy.) The need for folic acid increases even more during pregnancy. If the intake of folic acid is not great enough, megalohemoglobinemia (large, nonfunctioning red blood cells) will result. Inadequate folic acid levels have also been linked to an increased risk for neural tube disorders in fetuses (Lumley et al., 2009).

TABLE 10.5 ✻ Changes in the Cardiovascular System During Pregnancy

Assessment Factor	Prepregnancy	Pregnancy
Cardiac output		25% to 50% increase
Heart rate (bpm)	70–80	80–90
Plasma volume (mL)	2600	3600
Blood volume (mL)	4000	5250
Red blood cell mass (mm^3)	4.2 million	4.65 million
Leukocytes (mm^3)	7000	20,500
Total protein (g/dL)	7.0	5.5–6.0
Fibrinogen (mg/dL)	300	450
Blood pressure		Decreases in second trimester, at prepregnancy level in third trimester

Encourage women to eat foods that are high in folic acid (e.g., spinach, asparagus, legumes) both during the prepregnancy period and during pregnancy. Prenatal vitamins that contain folic acid are routinely prescribed. Unexpectantly, an association between multivitamin supplementation during pregnancy and reduced cancers in children, such as neuroblastoma, leukemia, and brain tumors, can be documented (Goh et al., 2007).

Heart. To handle the increase in blood volume in the circulatory system, a woman's cardiac output increases significantly, by 25% to 50%; the heart rate increases by 10 beats per minute. Like the circulating volume increase, the bulk of the cardiac work increase occurs during the second trimester, with a small increase in the third trimester. An average woman is unaware of the significant circulatory system changes that are occurring inside her to supply adequate blood to the placenta. However, this rise in circulating load has implications for a woman with cardiac disease. Although an average woman's heart is able to adjust to these changes readily, a woman whose heart has difficulty handling her normal circulating load can be overwhelmed by the requirements placed on it when she is pregnant.

Because the diaphragm is pushed upward by the growing uterus late in pregnancy, the heart is shifted to a more transverse position in the chest cavity, a position that may make it appear enlarged on x-ray examination. Some women have audible functional (innocent) heart murmurs during pregnancy, probably because of the altered heart position.

Palpitations of the heart are not uncommon during pregnancy, particularly on quick motion. You can caution women not to feel frightened if palpitations do occur. Palpitations in the early months of pregnancy are probably caused by sympathetic nervous system stimulation; in later months, they may result from increased thoracic pressure caused by the pressure of the uterus against the diaphragm.

Blood Pressure. Despite the hypervolemia of pregnancy, the blood pressure does not normally rise because the increased heart action takes care of the greater amount of circulating blood. Average blood pressures for adult women are shown in Appendix G.

In most women, blood pressure actually decreases slightly during the second trimester because the peripheral resistance to circulation is lowered as the placenta expands rapidly. During the third trimester, the blood pressure rises again to first-trimester levels (Fig. 10.7).

Peripheral Blood Flow. During the third trimester of pregnancy, blood flow to the lower extremities is impaired by the pressure of the expanding uterus on veins and arteries. This resistance to blood flow in the venous system can lead to edema and varicosities of the vulva, rectum, and legs.

Supine Hypotension Syndrome. When a pregnant woman lies supine, the weight of the growing uterus presses the vena cava against the vertebrae, obstructing blood flow from the lower extremities. This causes a decrease in blood return to the heart and, consequently, decreased cardiac output and hypotension (Fig. 10.8). A woman experiences this hypotension as lightheadedness, faintness, and palpitations (Bernstein & Weinstein, 2007).The condition is potentially dangerous because it can cause fetal hypoxia.

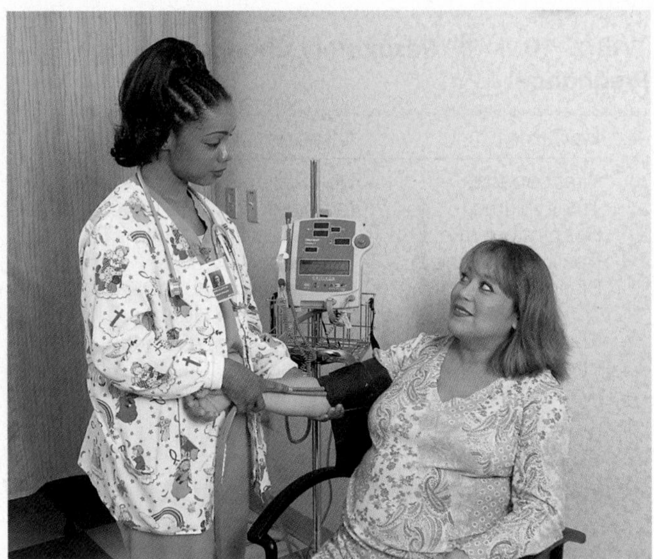

FIGURE 10.7 Blood pressure determination is an important assessment during pregnancy; normally, blood pressure does not elevate during pregnancy.

Supine hypotension syndrome can easily be corrected by having a woman turn onto her side (preferably the left side), so that blood flow through the vena cava increases again. To lessen the possibility of occurrence of this phenomenon, women develop an increase in collateral blood circulation during pregnancy. Teach women always to rest on the left side rather than the back, because even with additional collateral circulation, a supine position tends to lead to hypotension.

Blood Constitution. The level of circulating fibrinogen, a constituent of the blood that is necessary for clotting, increases as much as 50% during pregnancy, probably because of the increased level of estrogen. Other clotting factors, such as factors VII, VIII, IX, and X, and the platelet count also increase. These increases are a safeguard against major bleeding should the placenta be dislodged and the uterine arteries or veins be opened. Total white blood cell count rises slightly, both as a protective mechanism and as a reflection of a woman's increased total blood volume (up to about 20,000 cells/mm^3). The total protein level of blood decreases, perhaps indicating the amount of protein being used by the fetus. Because the circulating system has a lower total protein load and hypervolemia, fluid readily leaves the blood for institial tissue vessels to equalize osmotic and hydrostatic pressure. This causes the common ankle and foot edema of pregnancy (not to be confused with nondependent or generalized edema, which is a symptom of pregnancy-induced hypertension).

Blood lipids increase by one third, and the cholesterol serum level increases by 90% to 100%. These increases provide a ready supply of available energy for the fetus.

Gastrointestinal System

At least 50% of women experience some nausea and vomiting early in pregnancy. This is one of the first sensations a woman may experience with pregnancy (sometimes it is noticed even before the first missed menstrual period). It is most apparent early in the morning, on rising, or if a woman becomes fa-

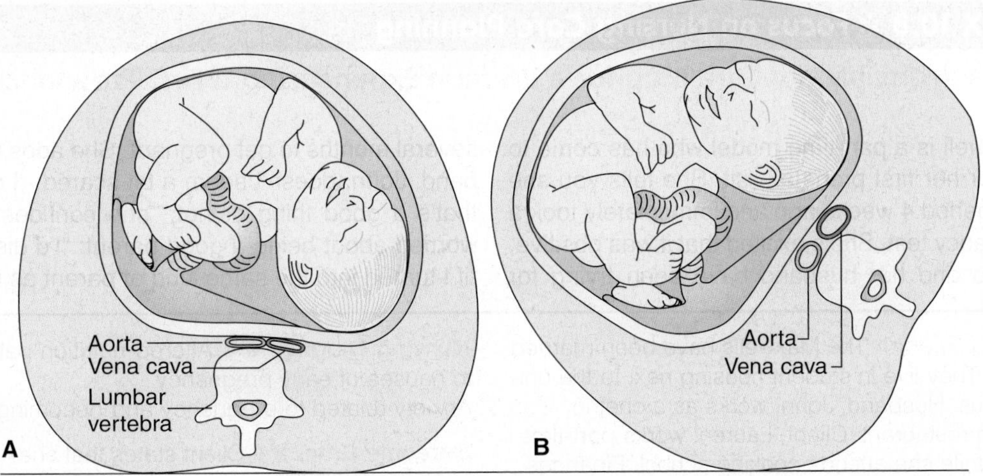

FIGURE 10.8 Supine hypotension can occur if a pregnant woman lies on her back. (**A**) The weight of the uterus compresses the vena cava, trapping blood in the lower extremities. (**B**) If a woman turns on her side, pressure is lifted off of the vena cava.

tigued during the day. It is more frequent in women who smoke cigarettes. Known as morning sickness, nausea and vomiting begin to be noticed at the same time levels of hCG and progesterone begin to rise so these may contribute to its cause. It may occur as a systemic reaction to increased estrogen levels or decreased glucose levels, because glucose is being used in such great quantities by the growing fetus (see Focus on Nursing Care Planning Box 10.8). Many alternative or complementary methods to help reduce nausea with pregnancy are available such as acupuncture or wrist bands, or drinking ginger or peppermint tea. These are discussed in Chapter 13.

This common feeling of nausea usually subsides after the first 3 months, after which time a woman may have a voracious appetite. Although the acidity of stomach secretions decreases during pregnancy, heartburn may result from reflux of stomach contents into the esophagus, caused by upward displacement of the stomach by the uterus, and a relaxed cardioesophageal sphincter, caused by the action of relaxin, an enzyme produced by the ovary. Interventions for heartburn are also discussed in Chapter 13.

As the uterus increases in size, it pushes the stomach and intestines toward the back and sides of the abdomen. At about the midpoint of pregnancy, this pressure may be sufficient to slow intestinal peristalsis and the emptying time of the stomach, leading to increased heartburn, constipation, and flatulence. Relaxin may contribute to decreased gastric motility; this natural slowing can be helpful, because the blood supply may be reduced to the gastrointestinal tract (i.e., blood is drawn to the uterus). Progesterone also has an effect on smooth muscle, such as that in the intestine, making the gastrointestinal tract less active.

Women with chronic gastric reflux usually find their condition improved during pregnancy because the acidity of the stomach is decreased. Because of the gradual slowing of the gastrointestinal tract, decreased emptying of bile from the gallbladder may result. This can lead to reabsorption of bilirubin into the maternal bloodstream, giving rise to a symptom of generalized itching (subclinical jaundice). A woman who has had gallstones may have an increased tendency to stone formation during pregnancy as a result of the increased plasma cholesterol level and additional cholesterol incorporated in bile. Pressure from the uterus on veins returning from the lower extremities can lead to hemorrhoids.

Some pregnant women notice hypertrophy at their gumlines and bleeding of gingival tissue when they brush their teeth. There may be increased saliva formation (hyperptyalism), probably as a local response to increased levels of estrogen. This is an annoying but not serious problem. A lower than normal pH of saliva may lead to increased tooth decay if tooth brushing is not done conscientiously. This can be a problem for homeless women or any other women who do not have frequent access to a place to brush their teeth (Agueda et al., 2008).

What if... Lauren Maxwell, the woman you met at the beginning of this chapter, asks you what to do for morning sickness and fatigue. What if you discovered she was homeless? Would your advice for her be any different?

Urinary System

Like other systems, the urinary system undergoes many physiologic changes during pregnancy. These include alterations in fluid retention and renal, ureter, and bladder function. Changes in the urinary system are summarized in Table 10.6. These changes result from:

- Effects of high estrogen and progesterone levels
- Compression of the bladder and ureters by the growing uterus
- Increased blood volume
- Postural influences

Fluid Retention. To provide sufficient fluid volume for effective placental exchange, total body water increases to 7.5 L; this requires the body to increase its sodium reabsorption in

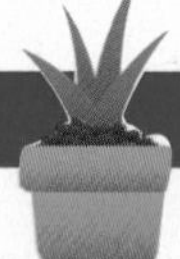

BOX 10.8 ✻ Focus on Nursing Care Planning

A Multidisciplinary Care Map for a Woman Experiencing a First Pregnancy

Lauren Maxwell is a part-time model who has come to your clinic for her first prenatal visit. She tells you she missed her period 4 weeks ago and immediately took a home pregnancy test. She's excited that it was positive, because she and her husband have been trying for several months to get pregnant. She adds that her husband, John, doesn't seem a bit scared: "I don't know if that's a good thing or not," she confides. She's also worried about being a good parent: "I'd die," she says, "if I turned into the same kind of parent as my parents."

Family Assessment ✻ The Maxwells have been married for 3½ years. They live in student housing next to the university campus. Husband, John, works as a chef in nearby Italian restaurant. Client, Lauren, works part-time as a model while she attends cooking school. Finances are listed as "tight" but "okay."

Client Assessment ✻ Lauren presents with amenorrhea, breast tenderness, fatigue, and morning sickness. She is interested in when she will begin to look pregnant and what she can do for the morning sickness (she has eaten almost nothing for 2 days).

Nursing Diagnosis ✻ Altered nutrition pattern related to nausea of early pregnancy
Anxiety related to pregnancy and becoming a parent

Outcome Criteria ✻ Client states that she is able to eat at least one full meal a day even in light of nausea; names two complementary therapies she is using to decrease nausea; states that she is managing anxiety by self-help measures, with support from significant others.

Team Member Responsible	Assessment	Intervention	Rationale	Expected Outcome
		Activities of Daily Living		
Nurse	Determine whether client is able to carry out usual activities (attending work, school, keeping house) by obtaining a health history.	Work with client to see if modifications (reducing work responsibilities, giving more home responsibility to husband) will help alleviate symptoms.	Documenting whether client can complete normal activities helps to document extent of concerns. Nausea can interfere greatly with cooking school.	Client reports that she is able to attend school and work part-time as long into pregnancy as she desires.
		Consultations		
Nurse	Assess if client needs additional suggestions from team expert for dealing with nausea.	Consult with nutritionist if nausea still interferes with eating by 1 week's time.	Nausea in early pregnancy can become extreme if not recognized as potentially serious in early pregnancy.	Client meets with nutritionist if she still describes incapacitating nausea at 1 week telephone follow-up.
		Procedures/Medications		
Physician/ nurse midwife	Assess whether client would like to try a complementary therapy, such as ginger before meals.	Review pros and cons of any alternative therapy chosen by client.	Many alternative therapies are effective at reducing symptoms of nausea during pregnancy.	Client states she is using at least one alternative therapy by 1 week follow-up telephone call.
		Nutrition		
Nurse/team nutritionist	Ask client to list 24-hour recall nutrition history.	Examine 24-hour recall history and analyze for nutrition deficits. Make suggestions for better intake.	Documenting the problem best identifies its extent.	Client gives 24-hour recall history and helps determine any nutritional deficits and possible solutions.

Nurse	Assess whether client feels that anxiety or worry over gaining weight is adding to her nausea.	Discuss with client that anxiety can add to nausea; weight gained during pregnancy can be lost after pregnancy.	Identifying the cause of anxiety is the first step in determining how to best relieve it. Gaining weight means she will lose modeling assignments.	Client states that she recognizes anxiety is normal for her situation. No longer anxious about pregnancy weight gain.
		Patient/Family Education		
Nurse	Determine whether client is aware that nausea and anxiety are both common concerns during pregnancy.	Provide clinic pamphlet, *So You're Pregnant,* to client and discuss early symptoms of pregnancy. Discuss with client how she normally manages anxiety. Offer suggestions as necessary.	Recognizing that a symptom is normal helps client to accept discomfort. Mild anxiety responds to many self-help measures, such as meditation or quiet reflection.	Client reports at 1-week follow-up telephone call that she recognizes nausea as part of early pregnancy. Client reports that she is managing anxiety by suggested self-help measures.
		Psychosocial/Spiritual/Emotional Needs		
Nurse	Determine whether client feels it would be helpful for nurse to meet with husband.	If desired, schedule a time to meet with husband to explain early pregnancy symptoms.	Significant others may be unable to give support if they are not well informed.	Client asks for help as needed by 1-week follow-up telephone call.
Nurse	Assess if client is concerned that differences in husband's and her feelings toward pregnancy will interfere with their relationship.	Urge client to discuss pregnancy fears with husband.	Differences in reactions to pregnancy can potentially interfere with degree of support from significant other.	Client says she has discussed her fears with her husband and will continue to do so as pregnancy progresses.
		Discharge Planning		
Nurse	Assess if client has any further questions before she leaves the clinic.	Meet with client after physical examination to be certain all her questions have been answered.	Unanswered questions can lead to increased anxiety over coming weeks.	Client confirms that her questions have been answered; has telephone number for clinic if further concerns arise.

TABLE 10.6 ✻ Urinary Tract Changes During Pregnancy

Variable	Change
Glomerular filtration rate	Increased by 50%
Renal plasma flow	Increased by 25% to 80%
Blood urea nitrogen	Decreased by 25%
Plasma creatinine level	Decreased by 25%
Renal threshold for sugar	Decreased to allow slight spillage
Bladder capacity	Increased by 1000 mL
Diameter of ureters	Increased by 25%
Frequency of urination	Increased first trimester, last 2 weeks of pregnancy to 10–12 times/day

the tubules to maintain osmolarity. Under the influence of progesterone, there is an increased response of the angiotensin-renin system in the kidney, which leads to an increase in aldosterone production. Aldosterone aids sodium reabsorption. Progesterone appears to be potassium-sparing, so that even with an increased urine output, potassium levels remain adequate.

Water is retained during pregnancy to aid the increase in blood volume and to serve as a ready source of fluid for the fetus. Because nutrients can pass to the fetus only when dissolved in or carried by fluid, this ready fluid supply is a fetal safeguard.

At one time, pregnant women were administered diuretics to help clear this excess fluid from their system. A sodium-restricted diet was also recommended. Today, it is recognized that these practices are actually harmful, because the increased fluid volume provides physiologic benefits for the fetus. In addition, the excess fluid can serve to replenish the mother's own blood volume, should hemorrhage occur.

Renal Function. During pregnancy, a woman's kidneys must excrete not only the waste products from her body but also those of the growing fetus. Also, her kidneys must be able to excrete additional fluid and manage the demands of increased renal blood flow. The kidneys may increase in size, changing their structure and ultimately affecting their function.

During pregnancy, urinary output gradually increases (by about 60% to 80%). The specific gravity of urine decreases. The glomerular filtration rate (GFR) and renal plasma flow begin to increase in early pregnancy to meet the increased needs of the circulatory system. By the second trimester, both the GFR and the renal plasma flow have increased by 30% to 50%, and they remain at these levels for the duration of the pregnancy. This rise is consistent with that of the circulatory system increase, peaking at about 24 weeks. This efficient GFR level leads to a lowered blood urea nitrogen (BUN) and low creatinine levels in maternal plasma. A BUN of 15 mg/100 mL or higher or a serum creatinine concentration greater than 1 mg/100 mL is considered abnormal and reflects the kidneys' difficulty in handling the increased blood load. The higher GFR leads to increased filtration of glucose into the renal tubules. Because reabsorption of glucose by the tubule cells occurs at a fixed rate, there may be some accidental spilling of glucose into the urine during pregnancy. Lactose, which is being produced by the mammary glands but is not used during pregnancy, will also be spilled into the urine. Although minimal spilling of glucose into the urine may occur this way, the finding of more than a trace of glucose in a routine sample of urine from a pregnant woman is considered abnormal until proved otherwise, because this can be a sign of gestational diabetes (see Chapter 20).

Creatinine clearance has become the standard test for renal function during pregnancy, because creatinine is cleared from the body at a steady rate in relation to GFR. A normal pregnancy value is 90 to 180 mL/min. This is analyzed from a 24-hour urine sample.

Ureter and Bladder Function. A pregnant woman may notice an increase in urinary frequency during the first 3 months of pregnancy, until the uterus rises out of the pelvis and relieves pressure on the bladder. Frequency of urination may return at the end of pregnancy, as lightening occurs and the fetal head exerts renewed pressure on the bladder.

Because of the increased level of progesterone during pregnancy, the ureters increase in diameter and the bladder capacity increases to about 1500 mL. The uterus tends to rise on the right side of the abdomen because it is pushed slightly in that direction by the greater bulk of the sigmoid colon. As a result, pressure on the right ureter may lead to urinary stasis and pyelonephritis if not relieved. Pressure on the urethra may lead to poor bladder emptying and bladder infection. Such infections are potentially dangerous to the pregnant woman, because they can ascend to become kidney infections. They are potentially dangerous to the fetus, because urinary tract infections are associated with preterm labor (Cootauco & Althaus, 2007).

Skeletal System

Calcium and phosphorus needs are increased during pregnancy, because the fetal skeleton must be built. As pregnancy advances, there is a gradual softening of a woman's pelvic ligaments and joints to create pliability and to facilitate passage of the baby through the pelvis at birth. This softening is probably caused by the influence of both the ovarian hormone relaxin and placental progesterone. Excessive mobility of the joints can cause discomfort. A wide separation of the symphysis pubis, as much as 3 to 4 mm by 32 weeks of pregnancy, may occur. This makes women walk with difficulty because of pain.

To change her center of gravity and make ambulation easier, a pregnant woman tends to stand straighter and taller than usual. This stance is sometimes referred to as the "pride of pregnancy." Standing this way, with the shoulders back and the abdomen forward, creates a lordosis (forward curve of the lumbar spine), which may lead to backache (Box 10.9).

Endocrine System

Almost all aspects of the endocrine system increase during pregnancy (Table 10.7).

Placenta. The most striking change in the endocrine system during pregnancy is the addition of the placenta as an endocrine organ that produces large amounts of estrogen, progesterone, hCG, human placental lactogen (hPL), relaxin, and prostaglandins. Estrogen causes breast and uterine enlargement. Palmar erythema during early pregnancy may also be a response to the high circulating estrogen levels. Progesterone has a major role in maintaining the endometrium, inhibiting uterine contractility, and aiding in the development of the breasts for lactation. Relaxin, secreted primarily by the corpus luteum, is responsible for helping to inhibit uterine activity and to soften the cervix and the collagen in joints. Softening of the cervix allows for dilatation at birth; softening of collagen allows for laxness in the lower spine and helps enlarge the birth canal. hCG is secreted by the trophoblast cells of the placenta in early pregnancy. It stimulates progesterone and estrogen synthesis in the ovaries until the placenta can assume this role. hPL, also known as human chorionic somatomammotropin, is also produced by the placenta. It serves as an antagonist to insulin, making insulin less effective, which allows more glucose to become available for fetal growth.

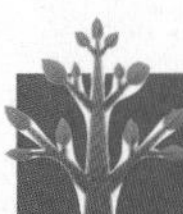

BOX 10.9 ✻ Focus on Family Teaching

Backache During Pregnancy

Q. You notice Lauren Maxwell rubbing her back at a prenatal visit. She asks you how she can keep her backache from becoming worse.

A. Backache is a common symptom of pregnancy because of the strain the extra uterine weight puts on lower vertebrae. It may be serious if

- It is experienced as waves of pain (could be preterm labor).
- There are accompanying urinary symptoms, such as frequency and pain on urination (could be a urinary tract infection).
- The back is tender at the point of backache (could be pyelonephritis or a kidney infection).
- Rest does not relieve it (could be a muscle strain).

Measures to relieve backache in pregnancy are

- Limit the use of high heels, because they add to the natural lordosis of pregnancy.
- Try to rest daily with feet elevated.
- Walk with head high, pelvis straight.
- Pelvic rocking (see Chapter 14) at the end of the day may relieve pain for the night.

In addition to these changes, prostaglandins are found in high concentrations in the female reproductive tract and the decidua during pregnancy. Prostaglandins affect smooth muscle contractility to such an extent they may be the trigger that initiates labor at term.

Pituitary Gland. The pituitary gland is affected by pregnancy, because there is a halt in the production of FSH and LH brought on by the high estrogen and progesterone levels of the placenta. There is increased production of growth hormone and melanocyte-stimulating hormone (which causes skin pigment changes). Late in pregnancy, the posterior pituitary begins to produce oxytocin, which will be needed to aid labor. Prolactin production is also begun late in pregnancy, as the breasts prepare for lactation.

Thyroid and Parathyroid Glands. The thyroid gland enlarges in early pregnancy to such an extent that the basal body metabolic rate increases by about 20%. Levels of protein-bound iodine, butanol-extractable iodine, and thyroxine are all elevated in blood serum. If a sufficient supply of iodine is not present during pregnancy, goiter (thyroid hypertrophy) can occur as the gland intensifies its productive effort.

These thyroid changes, along with emotional lability, tachycardia, palpitations, and increased perspiration, may lead to a mistaken diagnosis of hyperthyroidism if pregnancy has not been determined.

The parathyroid glands, which are necessary for the metabolism of calcium, also increase in size during pregnancy. Because calcium is important for fetal growth, the hypertrophy is probably necessary to satisfy the increased requirement of this.

TABLE 10.7 ✻ Endocrine Gland Changes and Effects During Pregnancy

Gland	Change	Effect
Thyroid gland	Slight enlargement Increased thyroid hormone production	Increased basal metabolism rate Increased oxygen consumption
Parathyroid gland	Slight enlargement Increased parathyroid hormone production	Better utilization of calcium and vitamin D
Pancreas	Early in pregnancy, decreased insulin production because of heavy fetal demand for glucose After first trimester, increased insulin production because of insulin antagonist properties of estrogen, progesterone, and human placental lactogen	Additional glucose is available for fetal growth
Pituitary gland	FSH and LH decrease Prolactin increases Melanocyte-stimulating hormone increases Human growth hormone increases	Anovulation Breasts prepared for lactation Increased skin pigment Aids fetal growth
Placenta	Estrogen and progesterone produced Relaxin increased Human placental lactogen	Uterine and breast enlargement, fat deposits Increased blood coagulation, sodium and water retention Softening of cervix and collagen of joints Increases glucose available for fetus Decreases utilization of protein for energy, increasing availability for fetal growth

Adrenal Glands. Adrenal gland activity increases in pregnancy as increased levels of corticosteroids and aldosterone are produced. It is assumed that these increased levels aid in suppressing an inflammatory reaction or help reduce the possibility of a woman's body rejecting the foreign protein of the fetus, the same as it would a foreign-tissue transplant. They also help to regulate glucose metabolism in a woman. The increased level of aldosterone aids in promoting sodium reabsorption and maintaining osmolarity in the amount of fluid retained. This indirectly helps to safeguard the blood volume and to provide adequate perfusion pressure across the placenta.

Pancreas. The pancreas increases production of insulin in response to the higher levels of glucocorticoid produced by the adrenal glands. Insulin is less effective than normal, however, because estrogen, progesterone, and hPL are all antagonists to insulin. Therefore, a woman who is diabetic and taking insulin before pregnancy will need more insulin during pregnancy. A woman who is prediabetic may develop overt diabetes for the first time during pregnancy. Overall, the effect of diminishing the action of insulin is beneficial because it ensures a ready supply of glucose for fetal growth.

The glucose level of a fetus is about 30 mg/100 mL lower than the maternal glucose level. To prevent fetal hypoglycemia, with resultant cell destruction or lack of fetal growth, the maternal glucose level is usually at a higher than normal level during pregnancy. Several fail-safe physiologic measures are initiated to achieve this.

As mentioned, although the pancreas secretes an increased level of insulin throughout pregnancy, it appears to be not as effective. With insulin that is less effective, fat stores of a woman are utilized, as well as available glucose. This maintains maternal glucose levels at a fairly steady level despite long intervals between meals or days of increased activity. To ensure against hypoglycemia, a pregnant woman should keep her diet high in calories and should never go longer than 12 hours between meals. Because the rapidly developing fetus uses so much glucose in early pregnancy, a fasting blood glucose level at this time is usually low (80–85 mg/100 mL).

Immune System

Immunologic competency during pregnancy apparently decreases, probably to prevent a woman's body from rejecting the fetus as if it were a transplanted organ. Immunoglobulin G (IgG) production is particularly decreased, which can make a woman more prone to infection during pregnancy. A simultaneous increase in the white blood cell count may help to counteract the decrease in IgG response.

✓ Checkpoint Question 10.5

Lauren Maxwell overheard her doctor say that insulin is not as effective during pregnancy as usual. How would you explain how decreased insulin effectiveness safeguards the fetus?

a. Decreased effectiveness prevents the fetus from being hypoglycemic.
b. If insulin is ineffective, it cannot cross the placenta and harm the fetus.
c. The lessened action prevents the fetus from gaining too much weight.
d. The mother, not the fetus, is guarded by this decreased insulin action.

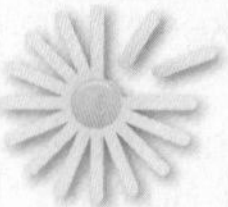

Key Points for Review

- The ability of a woman to accept her pregnancy depends on social, cultural, family, and individual influences.
- The psychological tasks of pregnancy are centered on ensuring safe passage for the fetus. These consist of, in the first trimester, accepting the pregnancy; in the second trimester, accepting the baby; and in the third trimester, preparing for parenthood.
- Common emotional responses that occur with pregnancy include grief, narcissism, introversion or extroversion, stress, couvade syndrome, body image and boundary confusion, emotional lability, and changes in sexual desire.
- Physiologic changes that occur with pregnancy are both local (uterine, ovarian, and vaginal changes) and systemic (respiratory, cardiovascular, urinary, and skin changes).
- Women may have read about the expected psychological and physiologic changes of pregnancy, but once these changes are actually being experienced, they may find them more intense than anticipated.
- The diagnosis of pregnancy is based on three types of findings: presumptive (subjective), probable (objective), and positive (documented).
- The positive signs of pregnancy are demonstration of a fetal heartbeat separate from the mother's, fetal movement felt by an examiner, and visualization of the fetus by ultrasound.
- Although a woman may be in a physician's office or prenatal clinic for only an hour, if her pregnancy was confirmed at that visit, she invariably feels "more pregnant" when she leaves. Early diagnosis is important so that a woman can begin to change unhealthy habits or, if she desires, have adequate time to carry out a therapeutic termination of pregnancy.

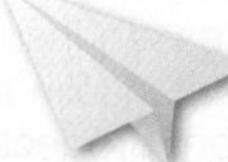

CRITICAL THINKING EXERCISES

1. Lauren Maxwell, the woman described at the beginning of the chapter, said she is worried about being pregnant because she "would die" if she thought she might be the same type of parent as her parents. Is this type of worry a common reaction to learning about a pregnancy? She says her partner is not worried. Would it be better or worse if he felt the same way? Has she completed the psychological development tasks of pregnancy? What suggestions could you make to help her be a better parent?

2. Lauren used a home test kit to determine that she was pregnant. She then did not schedule a prenatal visit, because the most important reason for going would have been to learn whether she was pregnant, and she already knew that. What argument could you use to convince her that prenatal care is important for more than pregnancy diagnosis?
3. You notice that Lauren's husband (35 years old) does not come with her on prenatal visits. He says this is because doing that is only for "young guys." How would you advise him?
4. Examine the National Health Goal related to early prenatal care. Most government-sponsored money for nursing research is allotted based on National Health Goals. What would be a possible research topic to explore pertinent to these goals that would be applicable to the Maxwell family and also advance evidence-based practice?

CRITICAL THINKING SCENARIO

Open the accompanying CD-ROM or visit http://thePoint.lww.com and read the Patient Scenario included for this chapter, then answer the questions to further sharpen your skills and grow more familiar with NCLEX types of questions related to psychological and physiologic changes of pregnancy. Confirm your answers are correct by reading the rationales.

REFERENCES

Agueda, A., et al. (2008). Periodontal disease as a risk factor for adverse pregnancy outcomes: a prospective cohort study. *Journal of Clinical Periodontology, 35*(1), 16–22.

Andrews, M., & Boyle, J. (2007). *Transcultural concepts in nursing care* (5th ed.). Philadelphia: Lippincott Williams & Wilkins.

Arnett, C., & Greenspoon, J. S. (2007). Hematologic disorders in pregnancy. In A. H. DeCherney & L. Nathan (Eds.). *Current diagnosis and treatment in obstetrics and gynecology* (10th ed.). Columbus, OH: McGraw-Hill.

Bernstein, H. B., & Weinstein, M. (2007). Normal pregnancy and prenatal care. In A. H. DeCherney & L. Nathan (Eds.). *Current diagnosis and treatment in obstetrics and gynecology* (10th ed.). Columbus, OH: McGraw-Hill.

Brennan, A., et al. (2007). A qualitative exploration of the Couvade syndrome in expectant fathers. *Journal of Reproductive and Infant Psychology, 25*(1), 18–39.

Casanueva, C. E., & Martin, S. L. (2007). Intimate partner violence during pregnancy and mothers' child abuse potential. *Journal of Interpersonal Violence, 22*(5), 603–622.

Centers for Disease Control and Prevention. (2009). *Unintended pregnancy prevention.* Hyattsville, MD: Department of Health and Human Services.

Cootauco, A. C., & Althaus, J. E. (2007). Preterm labor and premature rupture of membranes. In F. B. Fortner, et al. (Eds.). *The Johns Hopkins manual of gynecology and obstetrics.* Philadelphia: Lippincott Williams & Wilkins.

Crombleholme, W. R. (2009). Obstetrics. In S. J. McPhee & M. A. Papadakis (Eds.). *Current medical diagnosis and treatment.* Columbus, OH: McGraw-Hill.

Cunningham, F. G., et al. (2008). Prenatal care. In F. G. Cunningham, et al. (Eds.). *Williams obstetrics* (22nd ed.). Columbus, OH: McGraw-Hill.

Darby, S. B. (2007). Pre- and perinatal care of Hispanic families: implications for nurses. *Nursing for Women's Health, 11*(2), 160–169.

DiPietro, J. A., et al. (2008). Fetal responses to induced maternal relaxation during pregnancy. *Biological Psychology, 77*(1), 11–19.

Goh, Y. I., et al. (2007). Prenatal multivitamin supplementation and rates of pediatric cancers: a meta-analysis. *Clinical Pharmacology and Therapeutics, 81*(5), 685–691.

Gonzalez, J. M., et al. (2007). Relationship between abnormal fetal testing and adverse perinatal outcomes in intrauterine growth restriction. *American Journal of Obstetrics and Gynecology, 196*(5), e48–e51.

Kahn, D. A., & Koos, B. J. (2007). Maternal physiology during pregnancy. In A. H. DeCherney & L. Nathan (Eds.). *Current diagnosis and treatment in obstetrics and gynecology* (10th ed.). Columbus, OH: McGraw-Hill.

Lumley, J., et al. (2009). Periconceptional supplementation with folate and/or multivitamins for preventing neural tube defects. *Cochrane Database of Systematic Reviews, 2009*(1), (CD001056).

Matsui, H., & Gardiner, H. M. (2007). Examination of the fetal heart: making a diagnosis and avoiding pitfalls. *Ultrasound, 15*(2), 62–67.

Mattar, C. N., et al. (2007). Simple antenatal preparation to improve breastfeeding practice: a randomized controlled trial. *Obstetrics and Gynecology, 109*(1), 73–80.

Neilson, J. P. (2009). Symphysis-fundal height measurement in pregnancy. *Cochrane Database of Systematic Reviews, 2009*(1), (CD000944).

Pena-Rosas, J. P., & Viteri, F. E. (2009). Effects of routine oral iron supplementation with or without folic acid for women during pregnancy. *Cochrane Database of Systematic Reviews, 2009*(1), (CD004736).

Rojas, F., Wood, E., & Blakemore, K. (2007). Preconception counseling and prenatal care. In K. B. Fortner, et al. (Eds.). *The Johns Hopkins manual of gynecology and obstetrics.* Philadelphia: Lippincott Williams & Wilkins.

Savage, C. L., et al. (2007). The culture of pregnancy and infant care in African American women: an ethnographic study. *Journal of Transcultural Nursing, 18*(3), 215–223.

Smeltzer, S. C. (2007). Pregnancy in women with physical disabilities. *JOGNN: Journal of Obstetric, Gynecologic, and Neonatal Nursing, 36*(1), 88–96.

Westdahl, C., et al. (2007). Social support and social conflict as predictors of prenatal depression. *Obstetrics and Gynecology, 110*(1), 134–140.

SUGGESTED READINGS

Friedewald, M. (2007). Facilitating discussion among expectant fathers: is anyone interested? *Journal of Perinatal Education, 16*(2), 16–20.

Furniss, K., et al. (2007). Nurses and barriers to screening for intimate partner violence. *MCN: The American Journal of Maternal/Child Nursing, 32*(4), 238–243.

Mullen, K., et al. (2007). Family-centered maternity care: one hospital's quest for excellence. *Nursing for Women's Health, 11*(3), 282–290.

Ray, K., et al. (2007). Desire for pregnancy and future pregnancy in adolescent females: impact of outside influences. *Journal of Adolescent Health, 40*(2), S20–S21.

Rosich-Medina, A., & Shetty, A. (2007). Paternal experiences of pregnancy and labour. *British Journal of Midwifery, 15*(2), 66–70.

Simkin, P. (2007). Birth plans: after 25 years, women still want to be heard. *Birth, 34*(1), 49–51.

Villar, J., et al. (2009). Patterns of routine antenatal care for low-risk pregnancy. *Cochrane Database of Systematic Reviews, 2009*(1), (CD000934).

Vonderheid, S. C., Norr, K. F., & Handler, A. S. (2007). Prenatal health promotion content and health behaviors. *Western Journal of Nursing Research, 29*(3), 258–276.

Wesley, Y. (2007). Why women want children: defining the meaning of desire for children and the construction of an index. *Journal of National Black Nurses' Association, 18*(1), 14–20.

Xue, F., et al. (2008). Parental characteristics as predictors of birth weight. *Human Reproduction, 23*(1), 168–177.

Chapter 11 Assessing Fetal and Maternal Health: Prenatal Care

KEY TERMS

- chloasma
- conjugate vera
- diagonal conjugate
- erosion
- gravida
- ischial tuberosity
- lithotomy position
- multigravida
- multipara
- nulligravida
- para
- primigravida
- primipara
- speculum
- true conjugate

OBJECTIVES

After mastering the contents of this chapter, you should be able to:

1. Describe the areas of health assessment commonly included in prenatal visits.
2. Identify National Health Goals related to prenatal care that nurses can help the nation achieve.
3. Use critical thinking to analyze ways to ensure that prenatal care is family centered.
4. Assess a pregnant woman's health status and readiness for pregnancy.
5. Formulate nursing diagnoses related to women's health status during pregnancy.
6. Identify expected outcomes to help ensure a safe pregnancy.
7. Plan nursing care such as preparing a woman for a pelvic examination or fundal measurement.
8. Implement nursing care such as establishing a risk score for pregnancy.
9. Evaluate expected outcomes for achievement and effectiveness of care.
10. Identify areas of prenatal care that could benefit from additional nursing research or application of evidence-based practice.
11. Integrate knowledge of pregnancy health assessment with nursing process to achieve quality maternal and child health care.

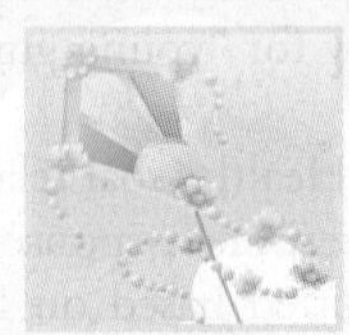

Sandra Czerinski is a 29-year-old woman, 12 weeks' pregnant, who comes for a first prenatal visit. She is concerned because she did not realize she was pregnant until a week ago. Because of this, she has been actively dieting (two diet drinks plus one meal of mainly vegetables daily) plus lifting weights at a health club. She has not had a pelvic examination since she was in high school, when she had a vaginal infection. She remembers that examination as being very painful. She is worried she has a urinary tract infection now because she has to "go all the time." She does not want any blood work done because she does not have health insurance.

Previous chapters described normal anatomy and physiology of the reproductive tract and the psychological and physiologic changes that occur during pregnancy. This chapter adds information about care needed during pregnancy to help ensure a healthy outcome for both a woman and her child.

What type of care does Sandra need? Is Sandra a high-risk or low-risk patient?

Prenatal care, essential for ensuring the overall health of newborns and their mothers, is a major strategy for helping to reduce complications of pregnancy such as the number of low-birth-weight babies born yearly (Crombleholme, 2009). It is so important that several National Health Goals speak directly to it (Box 11.1).

Ideally, prenatal care begins during a woman's childhood. It includes balanced nutrition with adequate intake of calcium and vitamin D during childhood to prevent rickets (which can distort pelvic size); adequate immunizations against contagious diseases so a woman has protection against viral diseases such as rubella during pregnancy; and maintenance of an overall healthy lifestyle to ensure the best state of health possible for a woman and her partner when entering pregnancy.

An overall healthy lifestyle includes a positive attitude about sexuality, womanhood, and childbearing. Once a woman becomes sexually active, preparation for a successful pregnancy includes practicing safer sex, regular pelvic examinations, and prompt treatment of any sexually transmitted infection to prevent complications that could lead to subfertility (Katsufrakis & Workowski, 2008). It includes not smoking or using recreational drugs. Acquisition and use of reproductive life planning information can help to ensure that each pregnancy is planned.

Women who maintain a healthy lifestyle this way come to a first prenatal visit prepared to follow health-promotion strategies. For many women this visit is the first time they have been to a health care facility since their routine health maintenance visits of childhood. It also may be the first time they have had an appointment that focuses more on health promotion than on the diagnosis of a disease. A woman may have a specific reason (her agenda) for coming to a first prenatal visit (e.g., to confirm the diagnosis of pregnancy). A prenatal visit encompasses more than this, though. It is also a time for additional health promotion, pregnancy education, and development of a positive pattern of healthy behaviors for the family to use in the future (your agenda). What and how much is needed vary depending on the lifestyle, age, and parity of a woman and her degree of family support (Bernstein & Weinstein, 2007).

Lack of prenatal care is associated with the birth of preterm infants and various complications for a woman such as hypertension of pregnancy (Cootauco & Athaus, 2007).

BOX 11.1 ✻ Focus on National Health Goals

Several National Health Goals speak directly to the importance of prenatal care:

- Increase the proportion of pregnant women who receive early and adequate prenatal care from a baseline of 74% to a target of 90%.
- Increase the proportion of pregnant women who attend a series of prepared childbirth classes from a baseline of 66% to a target of 77%.
- Increase to at least 90% the proportion of all pregnant women who receive prenatal care in the first trimester of pregnancy from a baseline of 83% (http://www.nih.gov).

Nurses can help the nation achieve these goals by educating women and their families about the importance of prenatal care and by making sites of prenatal care receptive to women and families. Additional nursing research to investigate ways to promote prenatal care or to enlarge the scope of nursing involvement in prenatal care could add a lot to helping the nation meet these goals.

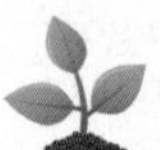

Nursing Process Overview

For Prenatal Care

Assessment

The first prenatal visit is a time to establish baseline data relevant to health assessment and health-promotion strategies that will be important at every prenatal visit. This begins with obtaining a health history, including screening for the presence of teratogens (any factor that may adversely affect the fetus) and any concerns a woman may be experiencing. Explaining why specific assessment data are relevant to the pregnancy is important. For instance, when weighing a woman, discussing what routine weight gain she can expect in the coming months and why monitoring weight gain is important supplies information to a woman as well as allowing you to obtain baseline data. Relating assessment information and health-promotion activities this way throughout the pregnancy helps keep a woman and her family well informed and eager to comply with further health care recommendations.

Nursing Diagnosis

Although most women probably have used a home pregnancy kit to find out if they are pregnant, the first prenatal visit officially confirms this, so nursing diagnoses usually focus on the response of a woman and her family to that information. For example:

- Decisional conflict related to desire to be pregnant
- Risk for ineffective coping related to confirmation of unplanned pregnancy

Nursing diagnoses appropriate to prenatal care include:

- Health-seeking behaviors related to guidelines for nutrition and activity during pregnancy
- Deficient knowledge regarding exposure to teratogens during pregnancy
- Risk for injury to fetus related to current lifestyle behaviors

Outcome Identification and Planning

Be certain to reserve sufficient time at prenatal visits so care can be thorough and there is enough time to set realistic goals and expected outcomes with both a woman and her partner, if desired. Make sure that a woman leaving an initial prenatal visit schedules an appointment for a following visit, as this may not occur to a woman who may be extremely excited or overwhelmed by all the new things that are happening to her and her family; establishing a pattern of regular appointments is crucial to providing effective prenatal care. Although many settings are looking at whether the number of prenatal visits traditionally scheduled is needed during a normal pregnancy, return appointments are usually scheduled every 4 weeks through the 28th week of pregnancy, every 2 weeks through the 36th week, and then every week until birth. Women categorized as high risk are followed more closely.

Reliable Internet sites to use for referral on preconceptual or prenatal care are the National Institute of Health and Human Development (http://www.nichd.nih.gov/health/topics/preconception_care.cfm) and the March of Dimes (http://www.marchofdimes.com).

Implementation

An important nursing intervention at prenatal visits is teaching women and their families about a safe pregnancy lifestyle. It may be helpful to give a woman and her partner pamphlets or books that cover the same topics. Be certain that you have read all the printed material you give families. This helps to ensure that a pamphlet's advice is consistent with what you have said and with the views of a woman's primary care physician or nurse-midwife. A pretty picture on the cover of a pamphlet does not ensure the quality of the advice inside. In addition, reinforce with a woman that she should call, e-mail, or text message the health care setting if she has any problems or questions between visits. Some women may feel reluctant to "bother" a health care provider outside of scheduled visits unless you give them permission to do so.

Outcome Evaluation

Evaluation during prenatal visits should concentrate on a woman's initial progress toward understanding goals of care for pregnancy and assessing outcomes established for specific concerns. Examples of expected outcomes are:

- Couple states they have reached a mutual decision to both stop smoking.
- Client states she feels well informed about the common discomforts of pregnancy and actions to take to relieve them.
- Client lists ways to avoid exposure to teratogens during pregnancy.

HEALTH PROMOTION DURING PREGNANCY

The purposes of prenatal care are to:

- Establish a baseline of present health
- Determine the gestational age of the fetus
- Monitor fetal development and maternal well being
- Identify women at risk for complications
- Minimize the risk of possible complications by anticipating and preventing problems before they occur
- Provide time for education about pregnancy, lactation, and newborn care

If a woman has good health coming into a pregnancy, it helps to ensure a good pregnancy outcome, so care includes both preconceptual and pregnancy timeframes.

The Preconceptual Visit

Ideally, women should schedule an appointment with a physician or nurse-midwife before becoming pregnant to obtain accurate reproductive life planning information, receive reassurance about fertility (as much as can be given based on a health history and a routine physical examination), and detect any problems that may need correction through a thorough health history, and physical and pelvic examinations (Rojas, Wood, & Blakemore, 2007). At this visit, hemoglobin level and blood type (including Rh factor) can be determined; a Papanicolaou (Pap) test can be taken, and minor vaginal infections such as those arising from *Candida* or chlamydia can be corrected to help ensure fertility. A woman can be counseled on the importance of a good protein diet, adequate intake of folic acid and other vitamins, and early prenatal care if she does become pregnant. More often, however, women arriving for their first prenatal visit will not have had a recent health care appointment oriented toward reproduction this way.

Choosing a Health Care Provider for Pregnancy and Childbirth

Once a woman is or suspects that she may be pregnant, her next step is to choose a primary health care provider to care for her throughout the pregnancy and birth. Various options are available, including a prenatal clinic, her health maintenance organization (HMO) or preferred provider (PPO), a certified nurse-midwife, an obstetrician, or a family practitioner. Regardless of the type of health care provider chosen, prenatal care needs to be initiated early and continued throughout pregnancy.

Nurses contribute to the success of prenatal care by listening, counseling, and teaching, three areas of nursing expertise (Box 11.2). Many clinics and group practices provide an initial

BOX 11.2 ✻ Focus on Evidence-Based Practice

Is continuity of care important in a prenatal setting?

In many prenatal settings, women see either one caregiver (usually a midwife) for the majority of their prenatal visits or see a multitude of care providers (midwives, physicians, nurse practitioners). To investigate whether continuity of care with one provider made a difference, researchers reviewed two studies including 1815 women. Women who saw a single care provider for their pregnancy visits were less likely to be admitted to a hospital antenatally. No differences were detected in Apgar scores, low birth weight, and stillbirths or neonatal deaths. They were more likely to be pleased with their antenatal, intrapartum and postnatal care.

Suppose you had the chance to reorganize a prenatal clinic? Would the above study influence the decisions you would make?

Source: Hodnett, E .D. (2009).Continuity of caregivers for care during pregnancy and childbirth. *Cochrane Database of Systematic Reviews, (2009)*(1), (CD000062).

BOX 11.3 ✻ Suggestions for Improving Prenatal Care Services

- Schedule appointments for women within a week after they first call the health care setting. This initial contact can be done through a group orientation session, individually by a health team member or, if risk status warrants, by a physician. Try to schedule further appointments at times convenient for a woman and her support people to encourage attendance.
- Make waiting time educational by providing materials such as pamphlets or videotapes in the waiting room.
- Provide privacy for assessments such as blood pressure and weight.
- Be certain that pregnant women meet health care providers while fully clothed and upright, not exposed or in a lithotomy position on an examining table.
- Encourage women to feel responsible for their health record. If a woman's first language is not English, be sure to record pregnancy information so she can read it.
- Encourage family members and friends to accompany a woman for prenatal care. Allow them to enter the examination room and participate in all aspects of care to the extent they and the woman desire.
- Schedule appointments to provide continuity of care. Be certain that women have a specific person's name as a telephone or e-mail contact for pregnancy-related questions. Without this information, they tend not to call.
- Educate pregnant women about care options and encourage them to participate in making decisions about their care.

educational seminar for women in the early stages of their pregnancy, often led by a nurse or nurse practitioner. Some practices form cohorts of women to meet monthly and discuss their concerns to be certain that women will have support from others all through pregnancy. Box 11.3 summarizes ways that prenatal care can be improved and individualized so that all women can be interested in obtaining it.

HEALTH ASSESSMENT DURING THE FIRST PRENATAL VISIT

The major causes of death during pregnancy today for women are ectopic pregnancy, hypertension, hemorrhage, embolism, infection, and anesthesia-related complications such as intrapartum cardiac arrest (http://www.nih.gov). An important focus of all prenatal visits, therefore, in addition to education about pregnancy, is to screen for danger signs that might reveal any of these conditions (Fig. 11.1).

Screening includes an extensive health history, a complete physical examination, including a pelvic examination, and blood and urine specimens for laboratory work. Manual pelvic measurements can be taken to determine pelvic adequacy.

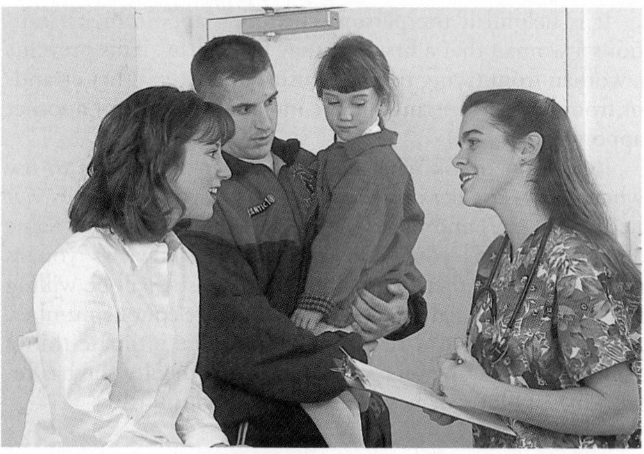

FIGURE 11.1 Include support people in a prenatal visit so that visits are family centered. Here a husband, wife, and child are included in the initial prenatal interview, making all feel a part of the pregnancy. (© Barbara Proud.)

✔ Checkpoint Question 11.1

Sandra Czerinski feels well so she asks you why she needs to come for prenatal care. The best reason for her to receive regular care is:

a. Discovering allergies can help eliminate early birth.
b. It helps document how many pregnancies occur each year.
c. It provides time for education about pregnancy and birth.
d. It will give her something to look forward to every month.

The Initial Interview

Because initial health history taking is often time-consuming, a woman may be asked to complete some of the forms. Good interviewing technique, however, is important to obtain thorough and meaningful health histories. The rapport established by face-to-face interviewing gives a woman a feeling that she is more than just a client number or chart. It may be as much a reason she returns for follow-up care as her desire to be assured that her pregnancy is progressing normally.

Interviewing expectant women often elicits contradictory information. Women are likely to want to talk about their past health and current pregnancy, so interviewing them should go smoothly and be productive. On the other hand, pregnancy symptoms are subtle, so a woman may not regard certain information as important, providing vague answers instead of specific information to questions about these areas. She may be unaware that she is the only person who knows the answers to several vital questions ("How do you feel about being pregnant?" or "Have you been taking anything for your morning nausea?"). Outside pressures, such as having to report for work or older children coming home from school, can limit the length of an interview. Late in pregnancy, a woman may feel uncomfortable sitting for a long interview.

Interviewing is best accomplished in a private, quiet setting. Trying to talk to a woman in a crowded hallway or a full waiting room is rarely effective. Pregnancy is too private an affair to be discussed under these circumstances.

It is helpful if the person scheduling appointments cautions a woman that a first visit may be lengthy. This prevents a woman from trying to fit the visit in between other errands or from having to terminate the interview because of another appointment.

Be certain to ask what name a woman wants you to use when addressing her in a prenatal setting (Mrs? Miss? Ms? Or her first name?) and make certain that she knows your name and understands your role correctly. If she views you as someone only gathering preliminary data, she will be willing to discuss superficial facts (name, address, telephone number, and the like) but will resist discussing more intimate things (her feelings toward this pregnancy, the difficulty she has reworking old fears or how scared she is about birth).

Components of the Health History

An initial interview serves several purposes:

- Establishing rapport
- Gaining information about a woman's physical and psychosocial health
- Obtaining a basis for anticipatory guidance for the pregnancy

If on subsequent visits a symptom is mentioned, establishing a baseline health picture at the initial pregnancy allows you to be able to verify that it is truly a new symptom and a woman is not just becoming more aware of it. General interviewing techniques are discussed in Chapter 34. Included in the following section are the elements pertinent to a pregnancy history.

Demographic Data

Demographic data usually obtained include name, age, address, telephone number, e-mail address, religion, and health insurance information.

Chief Concern

The chief concern is the reason a woman has come to the health care setting—in this instance, the fact that she is or thinks she is pregnant.

To help confirm pregnancy, inquire about the date of her last menstrual period and whether she has had a pregnancy test or used a home test kit. Elicit information about the signs of early pregnancy, such as nausea, vomiting, breast changes, or fatigue. Ask if she has any discomforts of pregnancy, such as constipation, backache, or frequent urination. Also, ask about any danger signs of pregnancy, such as bleeding, continuous headache, visual disturbances, or swelling of the hands and face.

Document if the pregnancy was planned. If you feel uncomfortable asking directly, using a statement such as, "All pregnancies are a bit of a surprise. Is that how it was with this one?" may help her answer this question. Another way to word such a question would be, "Some couples plan on having children right away; some plan on waiting. How was it with you?" If a woman says the pregnancy was not planned, explore to learn if she has reached a decision about whether to continue with the pregnancy. A question such as, "Some women change their mind about wanting a baby once they realize they are pregnant; some don't. How has it been for you?" is an effective way for obtaining this type of information because it says either option is possible and acceptable as an answer. You just want her to tell you which is happening.

Family Profile

In the past, the social history or family setting history (family profile) was left until the end of a health interview. However, obtaining this information early in an interview can help you get to know a woman earlier, identify important support persons, shape the nature and kind of questions to be asked, and evaluate the possible impact of a woman's culture on care. It also lays a foundation for health teaching as before you can begin to offer a woman any more than stereotyped health care instructions, you need to know her age and that of her sexual partner (additional testing such as genetic screening may be necessary if she is over 35), their educational levels (offers an estimation of the level of teaching you will plan), and occupation (does a woman's work involve heavy lifting, long hours of standing in one position, handling of a toxic substance, actions that may need to be modified during pregnancy?).

Be certain to ask about marital status and support people available as part of the information obtained. As a rule, both married and unmarried women want you to know their married status as they want to alert you if they do not have support people readily available.

Ask enough questions about the size of the apartment or house in which a woman lives so you can talk with her in the coming months about a bedroom or space for a baby's bed. It also is important to know whether the essential rooms are on the ground floor or upstairs in case she is restricted from climbing stairs more than once or twice a day during the last part of pregnancy or after birth.

Adaptation to pregnancy is highly individualized. A change in status from independence to dependence because of stopping work, chronic illness at home, the death or loss of a significant person during pregnancy, geographic moves, financial hardship, and lack of support people are examples of situations that can hinder a woman's ability to accept her pregnancy and child. No one in the health care setting will be aware of these potentially harmful situations unless questions of this kind about family profile are asked.

History of Past Illnesses

Questions about a woman's past medical history are an important part of an interview because a past condition can become active during or immediately following pregnancy. Representative diseases that pose potential difficulty during pregnancy include kidney disease, heart disease (coarctation of the aorta and heart valve problems from rheumatic fever cause problems most often), hypertension, sexually transmitted infections (including hepatitis B and human immunodeficiency virus [HIV]), diabetes, thyroid disease, recurrent seizures, gallbladder disease, urinary tract infections, varicosities, phenylketonuria, tuberculosis, and asthma. It is important to find out whether a woman had childhood diseases such as chickenpox (varicella), mumps (epidemic parotitis), measles (rubeola), German measles (rubella), or poliomyelitis and whether she has had immunizations against these. Ask also about HPV (human papillomavirus) vaccine as many women are not yet aware there is a vaccine for this.

The vaccine has the potential to prevent not only HPV infections but the development of cervical cancer (Tanner & Alexander, 2007).

From the information obtained about common infectious diseases and immunizations, you can estimate the degree of antibody protection a woman has against these diseases if she is exposed to them during her pregnancy. While pregnant, she can be immunized against influenza and against poliomyelitis with the Salk (killed virus) vaccine. However, she cannot be immunized against the other diseases because the vaccines against these contain live viruses, as does the oral Sabin poliomyelitis vaccine. Live virus vaccines could be harmful to the fetus if the virus crossed the placenta (Fiore et al., 2007).

Ask also about any allergies, including any drug sensitivities. Although not well proven, encouraging women with allergies of any magnitude to breastfeed rather than bottle-feed may help avoid milk or protein allergy in their infants (Akobeng & Heller, 2007). Any past surgical procedures are also important to know about because adhesions resulting from past abdominal surgery such as appendicitis could interfere with uterine growth.

What if... Sandra Czerinski tells you she has no idea what childhood diseases or immunizations she has had. How would you suggest that she obtain this information?

History of Family Illnesses

A family history documents illnesses that occur frequently in the family and so can help identify potential problems in a woman during pregnancy or in her infant at birth. Ask specifically about cardiovascular and renal disease, cognitive impairment, blood disorders, or any known genetically inherited diseases or congenital anomalies (Dorigo, Martinez-Maza, & Berek, 2007).

Day History/Social Profile

Information about a woman's current nutrition, elimination, sleep, recreation, and interpersonal interactions can be elicited best by asking a woman to describe a typical day of her life. If any of this information is not reported spontaneously as she describes her day, ask for additional details.

Nutrition is an important part of a day history, particularly in light of the number of young adults with eating disorders today. A "24-hour recall" is helpful to obtain accurate nutrition information, because by doing this, a woman tells you what she actually ate, not what she should have eaten (Box 11.4).

Ask about the type, amount, and frequency of exercise to determine a woman's routine pattern and whether it will be consistent with a recommended level for pregnancy as this varies greatly among women (Chasan-Taber et al., 2007). If a woman hikes or camps, for example, this type of exercise is good for her but also can put her at risk for exposure to Lyme disease. Ask if she knows about precautions to prevent this (Chapter 43). Ask also about hobbies. Certain hobbies, such as working with lead-based glazes and ceramics, might not be wise to continue during pregnancy because lead is teratogenic.

BOX 11.4 * Focus on Communication

Sandra Czerinski has come to her obstetrician's office for a first prenatal visit.

Less Effective Communication

Nurse: Tell me what a typical day is like for you.

Ms. Czerinski: I don't usually have typical ones. Or very interesting ones.

Nurse: What about yesterday? Could you describe that to me?

Ms. Czerinski: Okay. I was up at 7:00, was at work by 9:00. A friend picked me up after work and we celebrated his birthday. I was back home and in bed by 10:00. That's pretty much the day.

Nurse: You're right. It doesn't sound too interesting. Next, let me ask you about your family medical history.

More Effective Communication

Nurse: Tell me what a typical day is like for you.

Ms. Czerinski: I don't usually have typical ones. Or very interesting ones.

Nurse: What about yesterday? Could you describe that to me?

Ms. Czerinski: Okay. I was up at 7:00, was at work by 9:00. A friend picked me up after work and we celebrated his birthday. I was back home and in bed by 10:00. That's pretty much the day.

Nurse: What did you have for breakfast?

Ms. Czerinski: Nothing. I was too rushed to eat.

Nurse: Dinner?

Ms. Czerinski: We went to a bar to celebrate. Cheese blintzes, I think. And beer. A lot of beer.

Most people are not aware how much information can be revealed by a day history, so they give only a scant description of their day. Asking additional questions to make them elaborate on various parts often reveals poor nutrition, poor exercise, or risky pregnancy patterns.

As many as 12% of women of childbearing age either smoke cigarettes or are routinely exposed to passive smoke (Venugopalan et al., 2007). As many as 50% of woman drink alcohol (Donnelly et al., 2008). Because smoke, whether first-hand or second-hand, has been shown to be harmful to fetal growth, obtain information about a woman and her family's smoking habits. Excessive alcohol intake can not only lead to poor nutrition but can be directly responsible for fetal alcohol syndrome and preterm birth so also record the amount of alcohol a woman consumes (Pollard, 2007). If a woman answers vaguely about how much she smokes or drinks ("I drink socially" or "I only smoke occasionally"), determine exactly what she means by "socially" or "occasionally" so you can more accurately evaluate the frequency of these events.

Pregnant women, especially adolescents, are at an increased risk for intimate partner abuse (Barlow et al., 2007). Ask enough questions to be certain a woman is not involved in an abusive partnership by questions such as "Have you ever been hurt by someone?" or "Are you afraid of anyone?"

A medication history is also important to obtain. Ask whether a woman takes any medications, prescribed or over-the-counter, because their effect on a growing fetus will have to be evaluated. For example, isotretinoin (Accutane), a vitamin A preparation taken for acne, is associated with spontaneous miscarriage and congenital anomalies (Karch, 2009). Many women use herbal supplements to relieve the nausea of early pregnancy (Evans, 2007), so also ask about any herbal preparations that a woman might be using as even seemingly innocent alternative therapies such as these could be detrimental during pregnancy if they could stimulate uterine contractions or in any other way interfere with fetal health.

Be sure to include the use of recreational drugs, such as marijuana or cocaine, as these also can be deleterious to fetal growth (Pollard, 2007). Include intravenous drug use because of the increased risk for exposure to HIV or hepatitis B that this causes. Although this type of information is not usually readily revealed, most women will answer these questions honestly during pregnancy because they are concerned about protecting the health of their fetus.

Gynecologic History

In the past, most women had children early in their childbearing years, so the number of reproductive tract or women's health problems, such as breast disease, that they had experienced before pregnancy were few. Today, however, women often delay conception of their first child past 30 years of age. That makes it not unusual today to discover a woman who has had a reproductive tract or breast problem. Table 11.1 lists common gynecologic illnesses and their possible significance in pregnancy.

A woman's past experience with her reproductive system may have some influence on how well she accepts a pregnancy so obtain information about her age of menarche (first menstrual period) and how well she was prepared for it as a normal part of life. Ask about her usual cycle, including the interval, duration, amount of menstrual flow, and any discomfort she feels. Ascertain if she has discomfort with periods, including when the discomfort occurs, how long it lasts, and what she does to relieve it. If she describes menstrual cramps as "horrible" and wonders "how I live through them some months," anticipate the need for additional counseling to help her prepare for labor. Some women with severe dysmenorrhea are looking forward to pregnancy as it will mean 9 months without discomfort. Anticipate their need for counseling in the postpartum period about active ways to relieve their menstrual discomfort when their periods resume (see Chapter 47). Also ask if a woman does a monthly perineal self-examination to inspect for lesions or ulcers. Breast self-examination is no longer thought to yield sufficient reliable information to be continued as a self-care routine (Kosters & Gotzsche, 2009), but women should be alerted to continue health care provider exams and begin to have mammograms when they reach 40 years of age (Ruhl, 2007).

Ask about past surgery on the reproductive tract. For example, if a woman has had tubal surgery following an ectopic pregnancy, her statistical risk of another tubal pregnancy is increased because of the tubal scarring present. If she has had uterine surgery, a cesarean birth may be necessary because her uterus may not be able to expand and contract as efficiently as usual because of the surgical scar. If she has undergone frequent dilatation and curettage of the uterus, her cervix may be weakened or unable to remain closed for 9 months. This could lead to premature birth unless she has a surgical procedure (cerclage) for this (see Chapter 21).

Ask also about what reproductive planning methods, if any, have been used. Occasionally, a woman may become pregnant with an intrauterine device (IUD) in place. If this occurs, it will be removed to prevent infection during pregnancy. Another woman, not realizing she is pregnant, may continue to take an oral contraceptive for some time into her pregnancy. Document whether such use occurred, because some evidence suggests that estrogen can harm fetal growth. Be certain to include a sexual history, including the number of sexual partners and use of safer sex practices, to establish a woman's risk for contracting a sexually transmitted infection during pregnancy.

As part of any woman's gynecologic history, assess for the possibility of stress incontinence (incontinence of urine on laughing, coughing, deep inspiration, jogging, or running). With these actions, the diaphragm descends, increasing abdominal pressure, which increases bladder tension and causes emptying. Stress incontinence occurs from lack of strength in the perineal muscles and bladder supports. Commonly, this weakness has occurred from difficult births, the birth of large infants, grand multiparity, and instrumented births. During pregnancy, stress incontinence can become intensified from the increasing abdominal pressure. Some women accept this incontinence as a normal consequence of childbearing and may not report it unless asked.

Women can relieve stress incontinence to some degree by strengthening the perineal muscles with the use of Kegel exercises (periodic tightening of the perineal muscles; see Chapter 12). Surgical correction to increase support to the bladder neck also could be performed following the pregnancy.

Obstetric History

Do not assume that the current pregnancy is a woman's first pregnancy simply because she is very young or says she has only recently been married. She may have had an adolescent pregnancy or this could be a second marriage. For each previous pregnancy, document the child's sex and the place and date of birth. Review the pregnancy briefly for:

- Was it planned?
- Did she have any complications, such as vaginal spotting, swelling of her hands or feet, falls, or surgery?
- Did she take any medication? If so, what and why?
- Did she receive prenatal care? If so, when did she start?
- What was the duration of the pregnancy?
- What was the duration of labor?
- Was labor what she expected? Worse? Better?
- What was the type of birth? Vaginal or cesarean? Vertex or breech? In a hospital or at home?
- What type of anesthesia, if any, was used?
- Did she have perineal stitches following birth?
- Did she have any complications, such as excessive bleeding or infection following the birth?
- What was the infant's birth weight and sex?
- What was the condition of the infant at birth? Did the infant cry right away?
- What was the infant's Apgar score? (Most mothers know this.)
- Was any special care needed for the baby, such as suctioning, oxygen, or an incubator?

TABLE 11.1 ✻ Common Gynecologic Disorders

Disorder	Possible Symptoms	Significance and Suggested Therapy
Vulva		
Cysts of Skene or Bartholin glands	Asymptomatic swelling at the sides of the urinary meatus or vestibule	Such cysts are surgically incised to prevent blockage of gland duct.
Condylomata acuminata	Cauliflower-like lesion on vulva	This lesion tends to occur in women with chronic vaginitis. Caused by the epidermatrophic virus that causes common warts. Removed by cryocautery or knife excision.
Lichen sclerosus	Whitish papules on the vulva; asymptomatic	There is no need for removal; the area is biopsied because leukoplakia, a potentially cancerous condition, has an almost identical appearance.
Leukoplakia	Thick, gray, patchy epithelium that cracks; possibly a premalignant state that infects easily, accompanied by itching and pain	Therapy involves hydrocortisone and frequent return visits to health care personnel (every 6 months) for observation to detect any changes suggestive of carcinoma.
Carcinoma of the vulva	A shallow vulvar ulcer that does not heal	Vulvar cancer occurs most often in postmenopausal women; represents only 3% to 4% of all reproductive tract cancers in women. Therapy is vulvectomy—vagina is left intact, and sexual relations and pregnancy, with cesarean birth to prevent tearing of fibrotic vulvar tissue, may be possible.
Vagina and Cervix		
Adenosis	Asymptomatic vaginal cysts with columnar rather than squamous epithelium present on vaginal walls	This condition is caused by diethylstilbestrol (DES) administration while in utero. Has the potential for becoming malignant (clear cell adenocarcinoma). If adenosis is present, an examination two or three times a year with a Pap test and Lugol's staining is necessary, and a woman should not use estrogen sources such as oral contraceptives. If adenocarcinoma occurs, local destruction of atypical cells can be achieved by excision, cautery, or cryosurgery. This condition is rarely seen today because DES is no longer prescribed during pregnancy.
Cervical polyp	Red, vascular, protruding pedunculated tissue that bleeds readily with trauma	A polyp may be discovered because of vaginal spotting on coitus, tampon insertion, or vaginal examination. Removed vaginally by excision. Often associated with chronic cervical inflammation.
Cervicitis (erosion)	Reddened cervical tissue with whitish exudate	Douching with a vinegar solution aids healing. May be treated with cryosurgery if extensive.
Nabothian cyst	Clear shining circles on cervix from blocked gland ducts	No therapy is necessary.
Cervical carcinoma	Postcoital spotting, unexplained vaginal discharge or spotting between menstrual periods	Cervical cancer is the most frequent type of reproductive tract malignancy; risk factors include coitus with multiple partners or uncircumcised males, herpes simplex 2 infections, or DES use during pregnancy. Diagnosed by Pap test or colposcopy. Therapy is conization, radiation, or surgical excision. Pregnancy is possible following cervical carcinoma; cesarean birth may be necessary because of fibrotic cervical tissue. Can be prevented by HPV vaccine.
Ovaries		
Endometrial cyst	Chocolate-brown cyst on tender enlarged ovary; may cause acute pain if rupture occurs	Endometriosis is the cause; occurs in women aged 20 to 40 years. Therapy is surgical excision; ovary may or may not be removed depending on extent of cyst.
Follicular cyst	Amenorrhea and possibly dyspareunia; ovary tender and enlarged	Cysts typically regress after 1 or 2 months; low-dose oral contraceptive may be prescribed for 6 to 12 weeks to suppress ovarian activity; estrogen may be continued for 6 months.

(continued)

TABLE 11.1 ✻ Common Gynecologic Disorders (continued)

Disorder	Possible Symptoms	Significance and Suggested Therapy
Polycystic ovary syndrome	A syndrome of chronic follicular cysts, anovulation, insulin resistance, and excess testosterone production leading to perimenopausal onset of hirsutism, obesity, subfertility, and elevated triglycerides.	Excess testosterone by ovaries leads to inhibition of FSH and anovulation. Weight loss, reduction in triglycerides and cholesterol, and clomiphene citrate therapy to induce ovulation are used as therapy.
Corpus luteum cyst	Delayed menstrual flow followed by prolonged bleeding; ovary enlarged and tender	A corpus luteum persists rather than atrophies. Most regress in about 2 months; a low-dose oral contraceptive may be prescribed for 6 weeks to suppress ovarian activity.
Dermoid cyst	Asymptomatic; ovary enlarged on examination	Cyst originates from embryonic tissue; may contain hair, cartilage, and fat. Most common ovarian tumor of childhood; also occurs at 30 to 50 years. Therapy is surgical resection.
Serous cystadenoma	Bilateral; asymptomatic except for signs of pelvic pressure	This is the most common type of ovarian cyst; high malignancy rate of 20% to 30%. Therapy is surgical resection.
Carcinoma	Asymptomatic; intermenstrual bleeding	Ovarian cancer originates in epithelial tissue most often in women over 50 years of age. Tendency can be inherited; environmental contamination such as use of talcum powder may play a role in development. Therapy is hysterectomy and salpingo-oophorectomy.
Uterus		
Endometrial polyp	Intermenstrual bleeding	Polyp is removed by dilatation and curettage.
Leiomyomas (fibroids)	Asymptomatic or with increased menstrual flow	Muscle and fibrous connective tissue form in response to estrogen stimulation. May increase in size during pregnancy; may cause interference with cervical dilatation and result in postpartal hemorrhage. Stress to the myometrium by uterine contractions may be the original cause of formation. Therapy is surgical resection (myomectomy) or hysterectomy if childbearing is complete.
Endometrial carcinoma	Vaginal bleeding between menstrual periods	Diagnosis is by endometrial washing, not Pap test. Therapy is hysterectomy.
Uterine prolapse	Vaginal pressure and low back pain	The uterus has descended into the vagina because of overstretching of uterine supports and trauma to the levator ani muscle. Occurs most often in women who had insufficient prenatal care, birth of a large infant, a prolonged second stage of labor, bearing-down efforts or extraction of a baby before full dilatation, instrument birth, and poor healing of perineal tissue postpartally. Therapy is surgery to repair uterine supports or placement of a pessary, a plastic uterine support. Women with pessaries in place need to return for a pelvic examination every 3 months to have the pessary removed, cleaned, and replaced and the vagina inspected; otherwise, vaginal infection or erosion of the vaginal walls can result.

- Was the baby discharged from the health care setting with her?
- What is the child's present state of health?
- How was the pregnancy overall for her?

Ask about any previous miscarriages or therapeutic abortions and whether she had any complications during or following these. If a woman's blood type is Rh negative, ask if she received Rh immune globulin (RhIG [RhoGAM]) after miscarriages or abortions or previous births so you will know whether Rh sensitization could have occurred. Ask if she has ever had a blood transfusion to establish possible risk of hepatitis B or HIV exposure or Rh sensitization from a blood transfusion.

After a history of previous pregnancies is obtained, determine a woman's status with respect to the number of times

TABLE 11.2 ✻ Terms Related to Pregnancy Status

Term	Definition
Para	Number of pregnancies that have reached viability, regardless of whether the infants were born alive
Gravida	Woman who is or has been pregnant
Primigravida	Woman who is pregnant for the first time
Primipara	Woman who has given birth to one child past age of viability
Multigravida	Woman who has been pregnant previously
Multipara	Woman who has carried two or more pregnancies to viability
Nulligravida	Woman who has never been and is not currently pregnant

she has been pregnant, including the present pregnancy (*gravida*), and the number of children above the age of viability she has previously borne (*para*). Table 11.2 explains these terms. For example, a woman who has had two previous pregnancies, has given birth to two term children, and is again pregnant is gravida 3, para 2. A woman who has had two miscarriages at 12 weeks (under the age of viability) and is again pregnant is a gravida 3, para 0.

A more comprehensive system for classifying pregnancy status (GTPAL or GTPALM) provides greater detail on a woman's pregnancy history. By this system, the gravida classification remains the same, but para classification is broken down into:

T: Number of full-term infants born (infants born at 37 weeks or after)
P: Number of preterm infants born (infants born before 37 weeks)
A: Number of spontaneous miscarriages or therapeutic abortions
L: Number of living children
M: Multiple pregnancies

Using this system, a woman in the first example above would be gravida 3, para 2002 (GTPAL) or 320020 (GTPALM). A multigestation pregnancy is considered as one para. For example, a woman who had term twins, then one preterm infant, and is now pregnant again would be a gravida 3, para 21031 (GTPALM).

A pregnant woman who had the following past history—a boy born at 39 weeks' gestation, now alive and well; a girl born at 40 weeks' gestation, now alive and well; a girl born at 33 weeks' gestation, now alive and well—would have her pregnancy information summarized as follows: gravida 4; para 21030 (GTPALM).

Review of Systems

A review of systems completes the subjective information. Use a systematic approach, such as head to toe, and explain what you will be doing by an explanation such as, "I'm going to start at the top of your head and go through to your toes, asking about body parts or systems and any diseases that you may have had." A review of systems helps women recall concerns they forgot to mention earlier, such as a urinary tract infection, a disease that can influence the outcome of pregnancy and so would be important to your history taking.

The following body systems and questions about conditions constitute the minimum information to be addressed in a review of systems for a first prenatal visit:

- *Head:* Headache? Head injury? Seizures? Dizziness? Fainting?
- *Eyes:* Vision? Glasses needed? Diplopia or double vision? Infection? Glaucoma? Cataract? Pain? Recent changes?
- *Ears:* Infection? Discharge? Earache? Hearing loss? Tinnitus? Vertigo?
- *Nose:* Epistaxis (nose bleeds)? Discharge? How many colds a year? Allergies? Postnasal drainage? Sinus pain?
- *Mouth and pharynx:* Dentures? Condition of teeth? Toothaches? Any bleeding of gums? Hoarseness? Difficulty in swallowing? Tonsillectomy? Last dental exam?
- *Neck:* Stiffness? Masses?
- *Breasts:* Lumps? Secretion? Pain? Tenderness?
- *Respiratory system:* Cough? Wheezing? Asthma? Shortness of breath? Pain? Serious chest illness, such as tuberculosis or pneumonia?
- *Cardiovascular system:* History of heart murmur? History of heart disease such as rheumatic fever or Kawasaki disease? Hypertension? Any pain? Palpitations? Anemia? Does she know her blood pressure? Has she ever had a blood transfusion?
- *Gastrointestinal system:* What was her prepregnancy weight? Vomiting? Diarrhea? Constipation? Change in bowel habits? Rectal pruritus? Hemorrhoids? Pain? Ulcer? Gallbladder disease? Hepatitis? Appendicitis?
- *Genitourinary system:* Urinary tract infection? Hematuria? Frequent urination? Sexually transmitted infection? Pelvic inflammatory disease? Hepatitis B? HIV? Was subfertility a concern? Did she have a problem getting pregnant?
- *Extremities:* Varicose veins? Pain or stiffness of joints? Any fractures or dislocations?
- *Skin:* Any rashes? Acne? Psoriasis?

Conclusion

End an interview by asking if there is something you have not covered that a woman wants to discuss. This gives her one more chance to ask any questions she has about this new life experience.

Support Person's Role

Both partners and young children accompany women for prenatal care. Some women bring a female friend or their mother as their best support person. If family members are present, should they be included in an initial interview? As a whole, interviewing is most effective if it is a one-to-one interaction. A woman may be unwilling to mention certain concerns when her family is present for fear of worrying them. A husband may not be the father of her child, for example, and she would be unable to voice

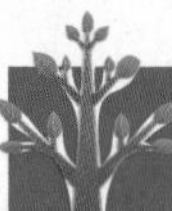

BOX 11.5 ✻ Focus on Family Teaching

Suggestions for Encouraging Partner Participation in Prenatal Visits

Q. Sandra Czerinski asks you, "What can I do to make sure that my boyfriend feels involved with prenatal care?"

A. Here are some suggestions for encouraging your partner's participation:

- Ask for appointments to be scheduled at a time that is convenient for both of you.
- Be certain that your partner reserves enough time so the visit does not become more of an inconvenience than an enjoyable event. A prenatal visit can be lengthy.
- Ask your partner to accompany you into the examining room at visits so you can share progress or decisions.
- Be certain that your partner listens to the fetal heart at visits as soon as it can be heard.
- If an ultrasound is scheduled, ask your partner to view it with you (it is an exciting moment for both of you to see your fetus moving).

her concern over this or alert you to the possibility she is worried about blood incompatibility because another man is the father.

If childbearing is to be a family affair, however, it is important to determine a partner's degree of acceptance of the pregnancy and of assuming a new parenting role. Including siblings in a prenatal visit provides them with an opportunity to involve them with the pregnancy planning and coming baby from the very beginning. Interviewing a woman alone and then inviting the support person and family to join her while you talk about pregnancy symptoms with them as a family is an effective solution. In addition, providing some private interview time with a partner allows the partner to express any concerns or worries. The main areas you should investigate with a partner include current health, feelings and concerns about the pregnancy, and knowledge of pregnancy and childbirth. If a woman wishes, a partner can accompany her during the physical examination. After confirmation of pregnancy, a partner should be included when health care information is given (Box 11.5).

✔ Checkpoint Question 11.2

Why is it important to ask Sandra about past surgery in a pregnancy health history?

a. To test both her recent and long-term memory.
b. Adhesions from surgery could limit uterine growth.
c. To assess whether she could be allergic to any medication.
d. To determine if she has effective health insurance.

Physical Examination

The next step in health assessment is a physical examination. Ask a woman to void for a clean-catch urine specimen before the examination as this can reduce bladder size and make the pelvic examination more comfortable and allow easier identification of pelvic organs, as well as providing a urine specimen for laboratory testing. The urine specimen is sent to the laboratory for evaluation of bacteria, protein, glucose, and ketones, or these can be immediately tested by dipstick analysis. If you are not already familiar with this, Box 11.6 provides instructions on how to obtain a clean-catch urine sample.

A physical examination at a first prenatal visit typically includes inspection of major body systems, with emphasis on the changes that occur with pregnancy or that could signal a developing problem. General techniques of physical examination are discussed in Chapter 34.

Baseline Height/Weight and Vital Sign Measurement

Measure a woman's weight and height at a first prenatal visit to establish a baseline for future comparison. Record this assessment with her prepregnancy weight, if available, to determine how much weight she has already gained or lost (Fig. 11.2). When weighing, be certain to convey an air of "weight gain is healthy" so a woman feels comfortable gaining 30 to 35 lb during pregnancy (many adolescents need to gain 40 lb to ensure a healthy fetus).

Measure vital signs, including blood pressure, respiratory rate, and pulse rate, as well for a baseline level. A sudden increase in blood pressure, the same as a sudden weight gain, is a danger sign of hypertension of pregnancy. A sudden increase in pulse or respirations can suggest bleeding. If close monitoring of vital signs will be necessary during pregnancy, a support person or a woman herself can be taught the techniques of taking and recording these so a woman can continue assessing these at home.

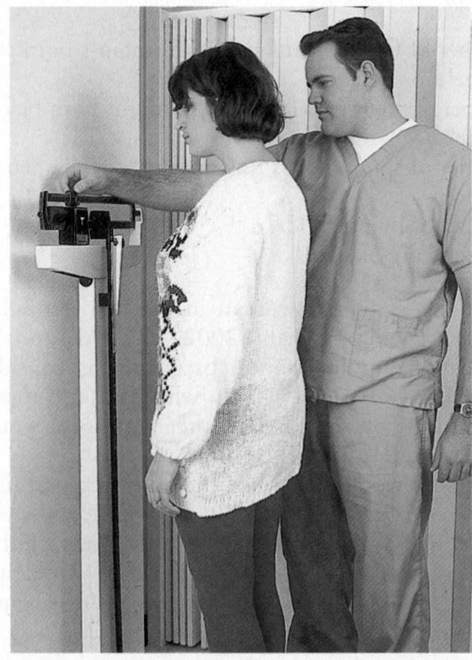

FIGURE 11.2 A woman weighs in at a prenatal visit. Pregnant women may need reassurance that gaining weight aids fetal growth. (© Barbara Proud.)

Box 11.6 Nursing Procedure ✻ Obtaining a clean-catch urine specimen

Purpose: Helping a woman obtain a clean-catch urine specimen

Procedure	Principle
1. Ask the woman to wash her hands.	1. Handwashing helps prevent the spread of microorganisms.
2. Have the woman open the commercial clean-catch urine specimen kit and moisten the cotton balls with the antiseptic solution or open the prepared antiseptic wipes.	2. Preparation enhances efficiency and decreases the possibility of contamination during the procedure.

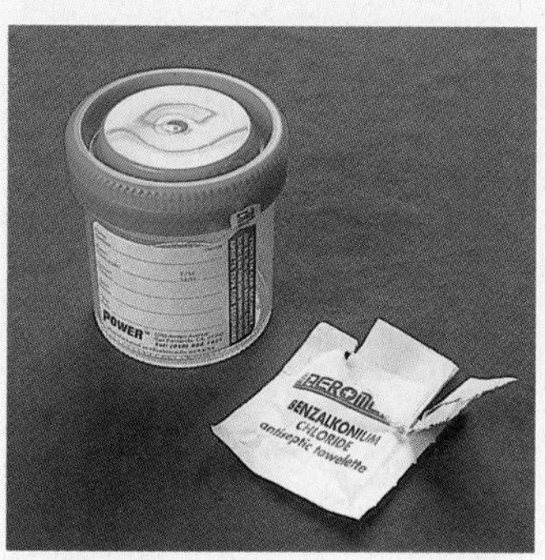

3. a. Ask the woman to sit on the commode and separate her labia with her nondominant hand.

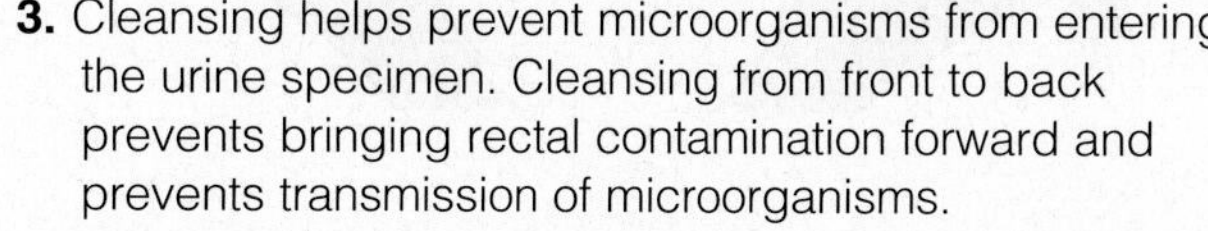

3. Cleansing helps prevent microorganisms from entering the urine specimen. Cleansing from front to back prevents bringing rectal contamination forward and prevents transmission of microorganisms.

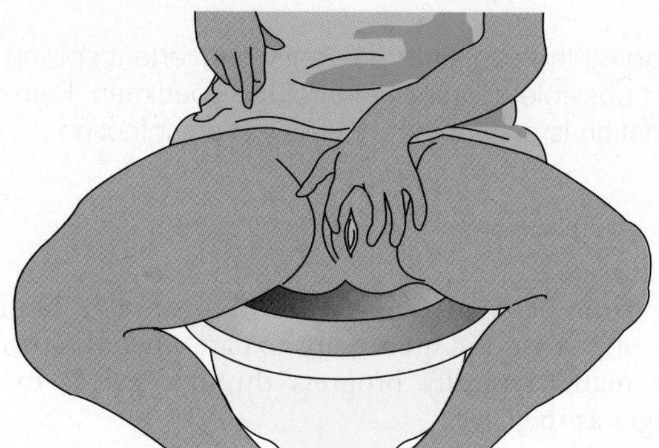

b. Tell her to cleanse the perineum, washing from front to back, using a cotton ball or wipe for only one stroke, then discard it.

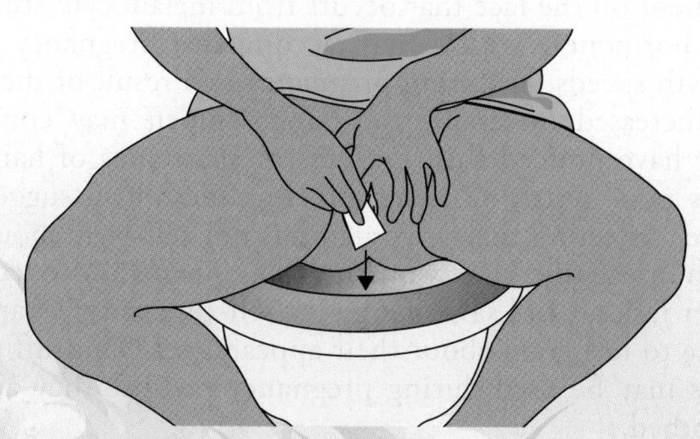

Box 11.6 Nursing Procedure ✻ Obtaining a clean-catch urine specimen (continued)

Procedure	Principle
4. Advise the woman to avoid touching the inside of the container or cap.	**4.** Careful handling of equipment prevents contamination.
5. Ask her to begin urinating, allowing the first urine to flow into the toilet. Then tell her to hold the container under the urine stream to obtain the specimen, removing the container after approximately 10 to 20 mL has been obtained. Once obtained, advise the client to remove the container, release her hand from her labia, and finish voiding into the toilet.	**5.** The first flow of urine washes microorganisms and debris from the urinary meatus. Collecting the specimen midstream helps ensure that a sterile specimen is obtained.

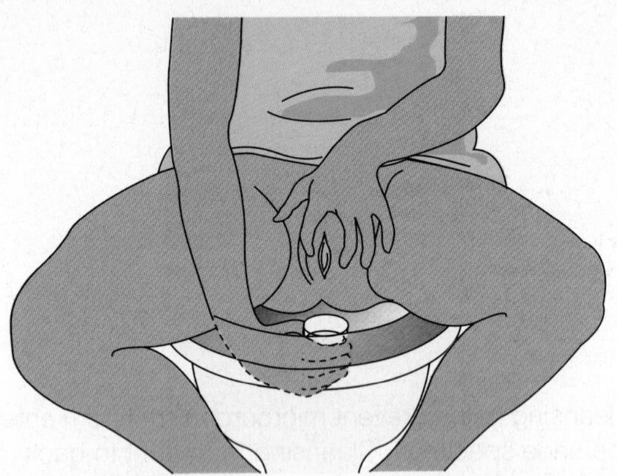

6. Tell the woman to cap the specimen container, wash her hands, and bring it to you. Encourage her to report any pain on urination.	**6.** Capping the container prevents inadvertent spilling and possible contamination of the specimen. Pain on urination is a symptom of urinary tract infection.

Assessment of Systems

General Appearance and Mental Status. Physical examination always begins with an inspection of general appearance to form an overall impression of a woman's health and well-being. General appearance is important because the manner in which people dress, the way they speak, and the body posture they assume all suggest how they feel about themselves. Not all women are happy about being pregnant. Closely inspect for signs such as careless hygiene, unwashed hair, inappropriate or soiled clothing, and sad facial expression that may suggest fatigue or depression about their diagnosis.

If a woman has any bandages or other dressings in place, be sure to remove and replace them because they could hide an important finding such as a malignant melanoma or skin cancer, which are increasing problems in young adults because of excessive sun exposure (Edwards, 2007).

A second increasing problem that bandages could be concealing and one receiving increased recognition is intimate partner abuse, a condition that not only is dangerous to a woman but also may lead to early pregnancy loss (Records, 2007). Ask when and how any skin abnormality, such as an ecchymotic area, occurred. Most marks from battering occur on the face, the ulnar surfaces of the forearms (from a woman raising her arms to defend herself), the abdomen or buttocks (from being kicked), or the upper arms (from being grabbed and held forcefully). Noting the color of ecchymotic spots helps to date when they occurred. Such marks typically progress through purple to yellow changes as they age.

Head and Scalp. Examine a woman's head for symmetry, normal contour, and tenderness and the hair for presence, distribution, thickness, excessive dryness or oiliness, cleanliness, or the use of hair dye (hair dye may be carcinogenic over an extended period of time). Look for **chloasma** (extra pigment on the face that occurs from melanocyte-stimulating hormone), which may accompany pregnancy. Hair growth speeds up during pregnancy as a result of the overall increased metabolic rate, and women may comment they have noticed this. Dryness or sparseness of hair suggests poor nutrition. Lack of cleanliness may suggest fatigue, reflecting that a woman has not felt well enough to wash it recently. Urge women during pregnancy to let some other task go and save energy for self-care so they can continue to feel good about their appearance. Dandruff shampoos may be used during pregnancy because they are not absorbed.

Eyes. Edema of the eyelids combined with a swollen optic disk (identified on ophthalmoscopic examination) suggests edema from pregnancy-induced hypertension, a potentially dangerous condition in pregnancy. On interview, women with pregnancy-induced hypertension also usually report spots before their eyes or diplopia (double vision). Teach pregnant women to recognize symptoms of changing vision as a potential danger sign of pregnancy that should be reported as soon as possible. If they do close desk work, caution them to take a break every hour so they do not confuse sensations of eyestrain with actual danger signs.

Nose. The increased level of estrogen associated with pregnancy may cause nasal congestion or the appearance of swollen nasal membranes. Even topical medicines such as nose drops or nasal sprays used to reduce this are absorbed to some degree. Advise a woman to avoid these during pregnancy without her physician's or nurse-midwife's knowledge and consent.

Ears. The nasal stuffiness that accompanies pregnancy may lead to blocked eustachian tubes and therefore a feeling of "fullness" in the ears or dampening of sound during early pregnancy. Usually this disappears as the body adjusts to the new estrogen level. Normal hearing level and normal tympanic landmarks should be present.

Sinuses. Sinuses should feel nontender. Establishing that tenderness over sinuses does not exist helps to evaluate that a woman's report of headache during pregnancy (a danger sign until ruled otherwise) is probably not sinus related.

Mouth, Teeth, and Throat. Gingival (gum) hypertrophy may result from estrogen stimulation during pregnancy. The gums become slightly swollen and tender to the touch, but not reddened. Pregnant women are prone to vitamin deficiency because of the rapid growth of the fetus. Assess carefully for cracked corners of the mouth, which would reveal vitamin A deficiency. Assess carefully for pinpoint lesions with an erythematous base on the lips; these suggest a herpes infection (a herpes lesion on the gumline is more often a shallow ulcer). Because newborns are susceptible to herpes infection, lesions present at birth may necessitate limiting a woman's contact with her newborn.

Teach all women not to neglect good dental hygiene or yearly dental visits while pregnant. They should maintain thorough toothbrushing (some stop thorough brushing because they notice slightly blood-tinged saliva because of gingival hypertrophy).

If many dental caries are obvious, a woman should be referred to a dentist or dental clinic. Carious teeth are a source of infection and should be treated before abscesses develop and cause more serious problems. Contrary to what many women believe, dental radiographs can be taken during pregnancy as long as a woman reminds her dentist she is pregnant and is given a lead apron to shield her abdomen. Urge her to obtain permission from her primary care provider before consenting to extensive dental work requiring anesthesia.

Neck. Slight thyroid hypertrophy may occur with pregnancy because the overall metabolic rate is increased. Suggest that all women eat a serving of seafood at least once weekly to supply enough iodine for the accompanying increased thyroxine production (eating fish more often than 3 times a week is contraindicated, however, because of potentially high mercury content) (Sunderland, 2007). Encourage a woman who uses iodized salt to continue using this during pregnancy. Without this precaution, some women will view iodine as an unnecessary additive and discontinue using it.

Lymph Nodes. No palpable lymph nodes should be present; however, because pregnant women may develop an increased number of upper respiratory infections because of reduced immunologic resistance, one or two pea-sized cervical lymph nodes may be palpable. If a woman has a tooth abscess from bacterial growth under hypertrophied gingival tissue (periodontal disease), submaxillary lymph nodes will be palpable.

Breasts. Breast changes may be one of the first things women notice in pregnancy:

- Areolae darken.
- Secondary areolae develop.
- Montgomery tubercles (sebaceous glands in the areolae) become prominent.
- Overall breast size increases.
- Breast consistency firms.
- Blue streaking of veins becomes prominent.
- Colostrum may be expelled as early as the 16th week of pregnancy.
- Any supernumerary nipple also may become darker and enlarge in size.

Benign breast lesions that might be discovered on physical examination are discussed in Chapter 47.

Heart. Heart rate typically ranges from 70 to 80 beats per minute in pregnant women, and no accessory sounds or murmurs should be present. Occasionally, a woman may develop an innocent (functional) heart murmur during pregnancy because of her increased vascular volume. If this occurs, she needs further evaluation to ensure that it is only a physiologic change of pregnancy and not a previously undetected heart condition. Many women notice occasional palpitations (heart skipping a beat) during pregnancy, especially when lying supine. Teach pregnant women always to rest or sleep on their side (left side is best) to help avoid this problem.

Lungs. Assess respiratory rate and rhythm. Although lung tissue assumes a more horizontal position during pregnancy, vital capacity is not reduced. Late in pregnancy, diaphragmatic excursion (diaphragm movement) is lessened because the diaphragm cannot descend as fully as usual because of the distended uterus. This causes women to feel short of breath.

Back. The lumbar curve in many pregnant women is accentuated on standing so that they can maintain body posture in the face of increasing abdominal size. This response can cause considerable back pain during pregnancy. Assess a woman's spine for any abnormal curve that would suggest scoliosis. Young women with scoliosis may need a referral to their orthopedist during pregnancy to be certain that the extra abdominal pressure is not worsening the scoliosis.

Rectum. Assess the rectum closely for hemorrhoidal tissue, which commonly occurs from uterine pressure on pelvic

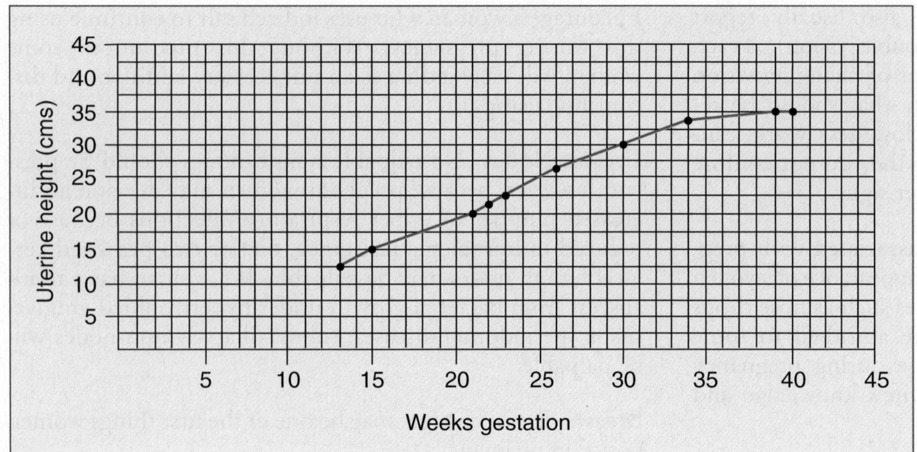

FIGURE 11.3 Plotting uterine height on a uterine height graph at prenatal visits (typically after 12 weeks' gestation) helps to monitor whether fundal height is increasing.

veins. Hemorrhoids can be very uncomfortable for women and worrisome if they are not assured that hemorrhoids are a normal discomfort of pregnancy and will fade afterward.

Extremities and Skin. Many women develop palmar erythema or itching early in pregnancy from a high estrogen level and perhaps subclinical jaundice (jaundice that is not yet apparent by a color change) from reabsorbed bilirubin because of slowed intestinal peristalsis. Assess the lower extremities carefully for varicosities, filling time of the toenails (which should be under 5 seconds), and the presence of edema caused by impaired venous return from the lower extremities. Any edema more than ankle swelling may be a danger sign of pregnancy.

Assess the gait of pregnant women to see that they are keeping their pelvis tucked under the weight of their abdomen. This position prevents them from developing muscle strains from abnormal abdominal muscle tension. Many pregnant women develop a "waddling" gait late in pregnancy from relaxation of the symphysis pubis. This relaxation may cause pain if the cartilage at the joint becomes so unstable that it moves on walking.

Measurement of Fundal Height and Fetal Heart Sounds

At about 12 to 14 weeks of pregnancy, the uterus becomes palpable as a firm globular sphere over the symphysis pubis. It reaches the umbilicus at 20 to 22 weeks and the xiphoid process at 36 weeks, and then often returns to about 4 cm below the xiphoid because of "lightening" at 40 weeks. If a woman is past 12 weeks of a pregnancy, palpate the fundus location, measure the fundal height (from the notch above the symphysis pubis to the superior aspect of the uterine fundus), and plot the height on a graph such as the one shown in Figure 11.3. Plotting uterine growth at each visit this way can help detect any unusual variation in fetal growth. If an abnormality is detected, further investigation with ultrasound can be done to determine the cause of the unusual increase or decrease in growth.

Auscultate for fetal heart sounds (120 to 160 beats per minute). These can be heard at 10 to 12 weeks if a Doppler technique is used but not until 18 to 20 weeks if a regular stethoscope is used. Palpate for fetal outline and position after the 28th week as a further estimation of fetal size and growth.

✔ Checkpoint Question 11.3

Sandra reports that the palms of her hands are always itchy. You notice scratches on them when you do a physical examination. What is the most likely cause of this finding during pregnancy?

a. She must be unduly anxious about her pregnancy.
b. She has an allergy to her fetus and will probably abort.
c. Her weight gain has stretched the skin over her hands.
d. This is a common reaction to increasing estrogen levels.

Pelvic Examination and Estimating Pelvic Size

The pelvis is a bony ring formed by four united bones: the two innominate (flaring hip) bones, which form the anterior and lateral portion of the ring, and the coccyx and sacrum, which form the posterior aspect (Fig. 11.4). It serves both to support and protect the pelvic organs.

Each innominate bone is divided into three parts: *ilium, ischium,* and *pubis*. The ilium forms the upper and lateral portion. The flaring superior border forms the prominence of the hip (the crest of the ilium). The ischium is the inferior portion. At the lowest portion of the ischium are two projections: the ischial tuberosities or the part of the bone on which a person sits. These projections are important markers used to determine lower pelvic width. The ischial spines are small projections that extend from the lateral aspects of the pelvis into the pelvic cavity. The level of the ischial spines marks the midplane or midpoint of the pelvis. This marker is used to assess the level to which the fetus has descended into the birth canal during labor.

The pubis is the anterior portion of the innominate bone. The symphysis pubis is the junction of the innominate bones at the front of the pelvis. The sacrum forms the upper posterior portion of the pelvic ring. There is a marked anterior projection of this bone at the point where it touches the lower lumbar vertebrae (the sacral prominence). This is a landmark to identify when securing pelvic measurements.

The coccyx, just below the sacrum, is composed of five very small bones fused together. Although it is stiff, there is a

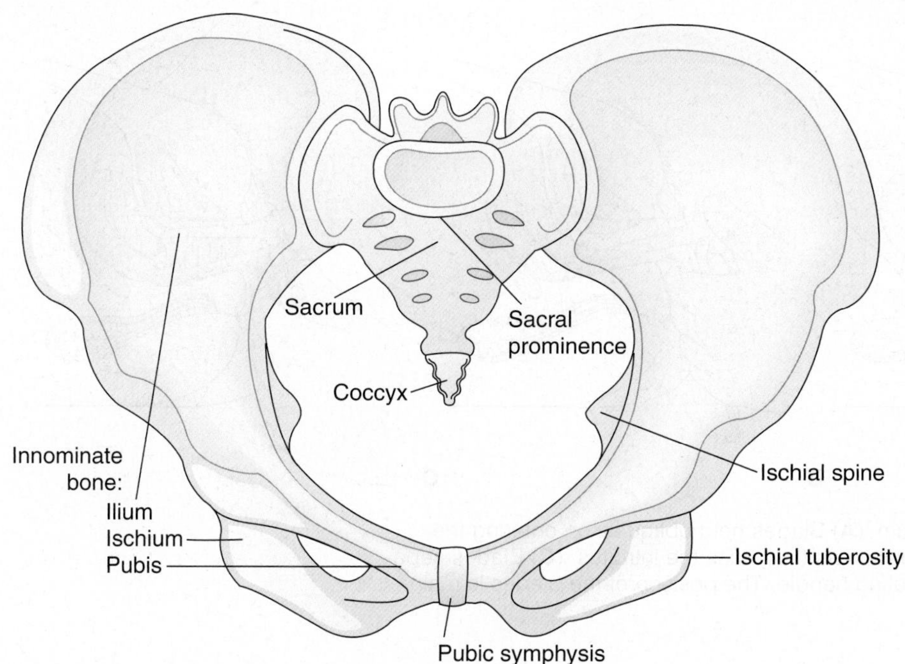

FIGURE 11.4 Structure of the pelvis.

degree of movement possible in the joint between the sacrum and the coccyx (the sacrococcygeal joint). This movement is important because it permits the coccyx to be pressed backward, allowing more room for the fetal head as it passes through the bony pelvic ring at birth.

For obstetric purposes, the pelvis is further divided into the false pelvis (the superior half) and the true pelvis (the inferior half) (Fig. 11.5). The false pelvis supports the uterus during the late months of pregnancy and aids in directing the fetus into the true pelvis for birth. The false pelvis is divided from the true pelvis only by an imaginary line, the linea terminalis. This imaginary line is drawn from the sacral prominence at the back of the pelvis to the superior aspect of the symphysis pubis at the front of the pelvis. The area above the line is the false pelvis and that below it is the true pelvis.

Other important terms in relation to the pelvis are the inlet, the pelvic cavity, and the outlet. The inlet is the entrance to the true pelvis, or the upper ring of bone through which the fetus must pass to be born vaginally. It is at the level of the linea terminalis or is marked by the sacral prominence in the back, the ilium on the sides, and the superior aspect of the symphysis pubis in the front. If you looked down at the pelvic inlet, the passageway would appear heart shaped because of the jutting sacral prominence. It is wider transversely (sideways) than in the anteroposterior dimension.

The outlet is the inferior portion of the pelvis, or that portion bounded in the back by the coccyx, on the sides by the ischial tuberosities, and in the front by the inferior aspect of the symphysis pubis. In contrast to the inlet of the pelvis, the greatest diameter of the outlet is its anteroposterior diameter.

The pelvic cavity is the space between the inlet and the outlet. This space is not a straight but a curved passage that slows and controls the speed of birth and therefore reduces sudden pressure changes in the fetal head, helping prevent ruptured cerebral arteries. The snugness of the cavity compresses the chest of the fetus as he or she passes through, helping to expel lung fluid and mucus and thereby better prepare the lungs for good aeration at birth.

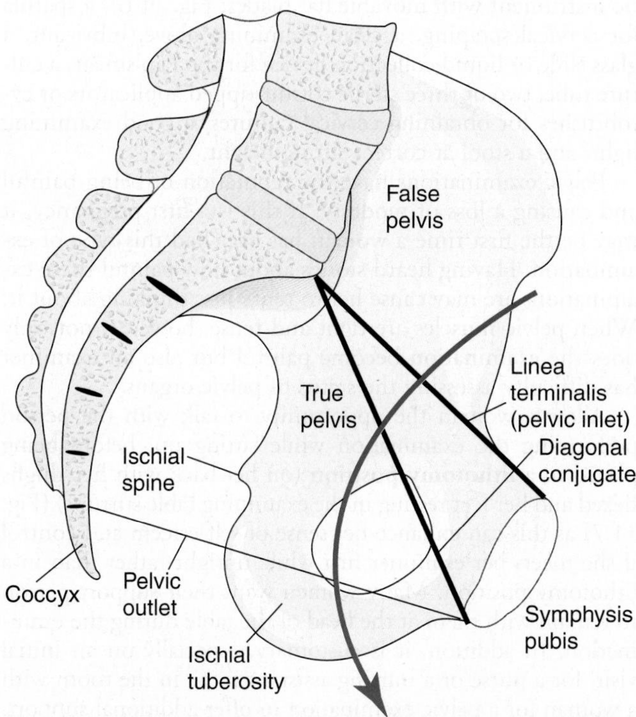

FIGURE 11.5 True and false pelvis. Portion above linea terminalis is false pelvis; portion below is true pelvis. *Arrow* shows "stovepipe" curve that the fetus must follow to be born.

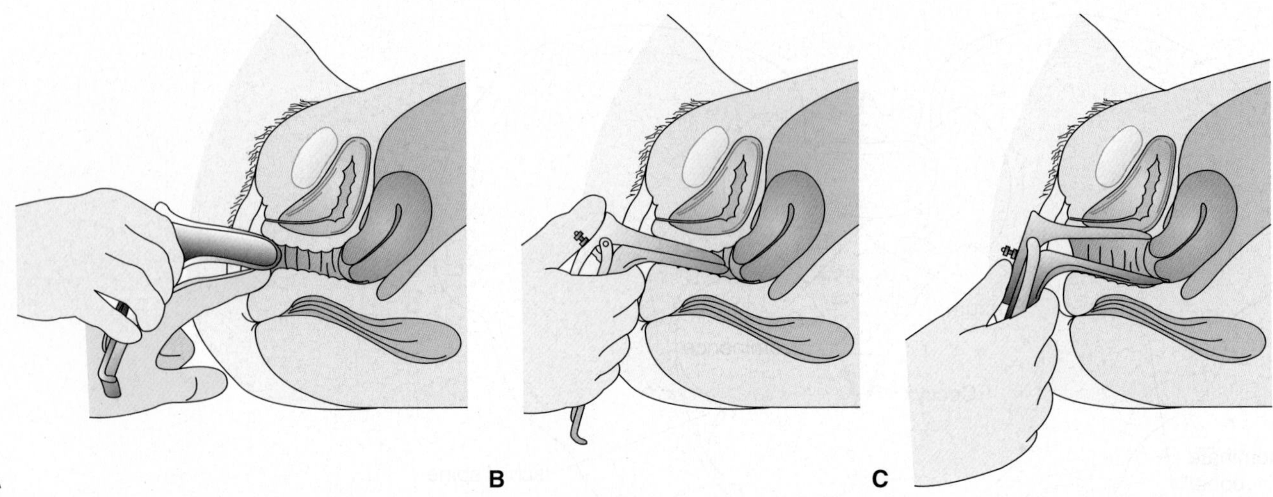

FIGURE 11.6 Insertion of a vaginal speculum. (**A**) Blades held obliquely on entering the vagina. (**B**) Blades rotated to horizontal position as they pass the introitus. (**C**) Blades separated by depressing thumbpiece and elevating handle. The position of the blades is maintained by adjusting a thumbscrew.

For a baby to be born vaginally, he or she must be able to pass through the inlet, the cavity, and the outlet of the pelvic bone. This is not a problem for the average fetus; it may be a problem if the mother is a young adolescent girl who has not yet achieved full pelvic growth (girls younger than 14 years are most prone to this difficulty) or a woman who has had a pelvic injury (e.g., from an automobile accident).

Pelvic Examination. A pelvic examination reveals information on the health of both internal and external reproductive organs. Equipment required is a **speculum** (a metal or plastic instrument with movable flat blades; Fig. 11.6), a spatula for cervical scraping, a clean examining glove, lubricant, a glass slide or liquid collection device for the Pap smear, a culture tube, two or three sterile cotton-tipped applicators or cytobrushes for obtaining cervical cultures, a good examining light, and a stool at correct sitting height.

Pelvic examinations have the reputation of being painful and causing a loss of modesty. If this is a first pregnancy, it may be the first time a woman has ever had this type of examination. Having heard stories about how painful these examinations are may cause her to tense just thinking about it. When pelvic muscles are tight and tense, however, not only does the examination become painful but also an examiner has difficulty assessing the status of pelvic organs.

Allow a woman the opportunity to talk with the person performing the examination while sitting up, before being placed in a **lithotomy position** (on her back with her thighs flexed and her feet resting in the examining table stirrups) (Fig. 11.7) as this can enhance her sense of self-esteem and control if she meets her examiner first while upright rather than in a lithotomy position. Many women want their support person to remain with them at the head of the table during the examination. In addition, it is customary, especially on an initial visit, for a nurse or a nursing assistant to be in the room with a woman for a pelvic examination to offer additional support. This is true whether the examiner is male or female.

Before a pelvic examination, ask a woman to void to reduce her bladder size and then lie in a lithotomy position (see Fig. 11.7). Make sure her buttocks extend slightly beyond the end of the examining table. Place a pillow under her head to help her relax her abdominal muscles.

Properly drape her with a draw sheet over her abdomen that extends over her legs. Be sure pregnant women remain in a lithotomy position for as short a time as possible to help prevent thromboembolism and supine hypotension syndrome or a sudden drop in blood pressure (Rojas, Wood, & Blakemore, 2007).

Recognizing what are the steps included in a pelvic examination helps you to be able to assist with the procedure. When serving as a support person, remember to remain at the head of the table so you can hold a woman's hand or put a hand on her shoulder if she needs the support of physical contact. Give explanations of what is happening or what the examiner is doing as needed. Conversation with the examiner over her head is not helpful. Suggesting that a woman breathe in and out (not hold her breath as she is likely to do) is another technique to help her relax (holding her breath pushes the diaphragm down and makes the pelvic organs tense and unyielding).

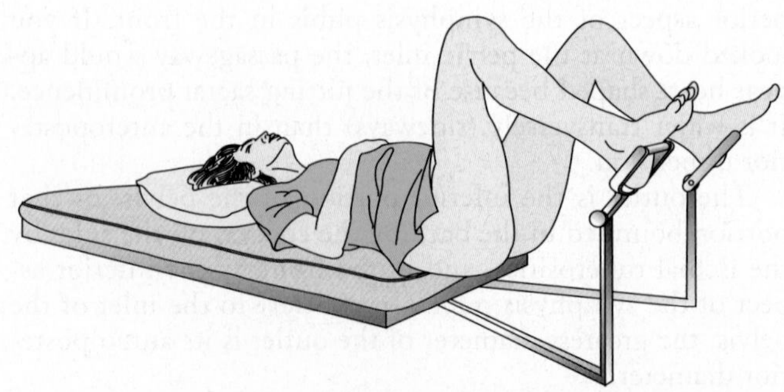

FIGURE 11.7 A lithotomy position used for a pelvic examination. Help position a woman with her buttocks just over the edge of the table. Drape appropriately for modesty.

If desired, a woman may watch the pelvic examination with an overhead mirror or a mirror held by herself or the examiner. Seeing vaginal cervical pathology can help her to understand any kind of problem present and the interventions necessary to improve it. If not already doing so, sexually active women should be taught how to do a monthly perineal examination (holding a mirror) so they can detect perineal lesions such as herpes simplex 2 viral infections so observing their perineum during a pelvic examination is good practice for this.

What if. . . The foot of an examining table in a clinic faces the room door, leaving women to feel exposed if someone should walk in unexpectedly? This saves an examiner steps, but is this the best position for the table?

External Genitalia. A pelvic examination begins with inspection of the external genitalia. Any signs of inflammation, irritation, or infection, such as redness, ulcerations, or vaginal discharge, are noted.

A herpes simplex 2 virus infection appears as clustered, pinpoint vesicles on an erythematous (reddened) base on the vulva. These feel painful when touched or irritated. It is important to detect these during pregnancy as the presence of herpes lesions on the vulva or vagina at the time of birth may necessitate cesarean birth to prevent exposing the fetus to the virus during passage through the birth canal. Note in the record the presence of a herpes infection so a woman receives future follow-up care with cytologic (Pap) smears as there is an association between herpes simplex 2 infections and the development of cervical cancer (American College of Obstetricians and Gynecologists [ACOG], 2007).

Next, the Skene glands that empty into the urethra and the Bartholin glands that empty into the distal vagina are palpated between the vaginal finger and the thumb of the same hand. If a discharge is produced from any of these gland ducts (Skene or Bartholin), a culture is obtained. Infection here could be caused by something as simple as streptococci; often it is gonorrhea.

Problems with vaginal muscle wall support, such as a rectocele (a forward pouching of the rectum into the posterior vaginal wall because of loss of posterior vaginal muscular support) or a cystocele (a pouching of the bladder into the anterior vaginal wall, caused by loss of anterior vaginal muscular support), are also evaluated. To reveal these, while the labia are gently separated to allow a view of the vaginal walls, a woman is asked to bear down as if she were moving her bowels.

Internal Genitalia. To view the cervix, the vagina must be opened with a speculum. When helping prepare for an examination, do not apply any lubricant other than warm water on speculum blades because even a water-soluble lubricant might interfere with the interpretation of the Pap smear that will be taken. Use warm water rather than cold water to warm the blades so a woman does not contract her vaginal muscles when she feels the cold instrument.

A speculum is introduced with the blades in a closed position and directed toward the posterior rather than the anterior vaginal wall because the posterior wall is less sensitive (see Fig. 11.6A). A speculum enters most readily if it is inserted at an oblique angle (the crease of the blades directed to a 4 or 8 o'clock position), then rotated to a horizontal position when fully inserted (the crease of the blades pointing to a 3 or 9 o'clock position) (see Fig. 11.6B). When fully inserted and rotated to a horizontal position, the blades are opened so the cervix is visible and are secured in the open position by tightening the thumb screw at the side (see Fig. 11.6C).

With the speculum in place, the cervix can be inspected for position. Normally it is centered on the vagina; a retroverted uterus has a cervix positioned anteriorly, and an anteverted uterus has its cervix positioned posteriorly. The cervix color (a nonpregnant cervix is light pink; in pregnancy it changes to almost purple) and any lesions, ulcerations, discharge, or otherwise abnormal appearance are documented.

In a nulligravida (a woman who is not or never has been pregnant), the cervical os is round and small. In a woman who has had a previous pregnancy with a vaginal birth, the cervical os has much more of a slitlike appearance. If a woman had a cervical tear during a previous birth, the cervical os may appear as a transverse crease the width of the cervix or a typical starlike (stellate) formation (Fig. 11.8A3). If a cervical infection is present, a mucus discharge may be present. With infection, the epithelium of the cervical canal often enlarges and spreads onto the area surrounding the os, giving the cervix a reddened appearance (**erosion**). This area bleeds readily if it is touched (Fig. 11.8B3).

Trichomoniasis, a protozoal infection, generally causes signs of redness; a profuse, whitish, bubbly discharge; and petechial spots on the vaginal walls. Candidal (*Monilia*) infection typically presents with thick, white vaginal patches that may bleed if scraped away. A gonorrhea infection presents with a thick, greenish-yellow discharge and extreme inflammation. Chlamydia infection, in contrast, shows few symptoms except slight cervical redness.

Carcinoma of the cervix appears as an irregular, granular growth at the os. Cervical polyps (red, soft, pedunculated benign protrusions) also are occasionally seen at the os.

Pap Smear. A Pap smear is taken for early detection and diagnosis of precancerous and cancerous conditions of the uterine cervix, vulva, or vagina; the test also reveals inflammatory and infectious diseases (MacKay, 2009). Although only an endocervical smear (one from inside the cervix) may be taken to be plated for a Pap test in some centers, in others three

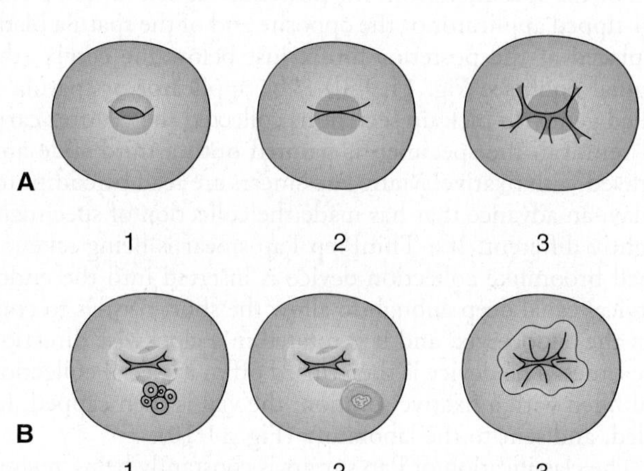

FIGURE 11.8 (**A**) Appearances of the cervix. (1) Nulligravida cervix. (2) Cervix after childbirth. (3) "Stellate" cervix seen after mild cervical tearing. (**B**) Possible cervical lesions. (1) Herpes simplex 2. (2) Chancre of syphilis. (3) Erosion or infection.

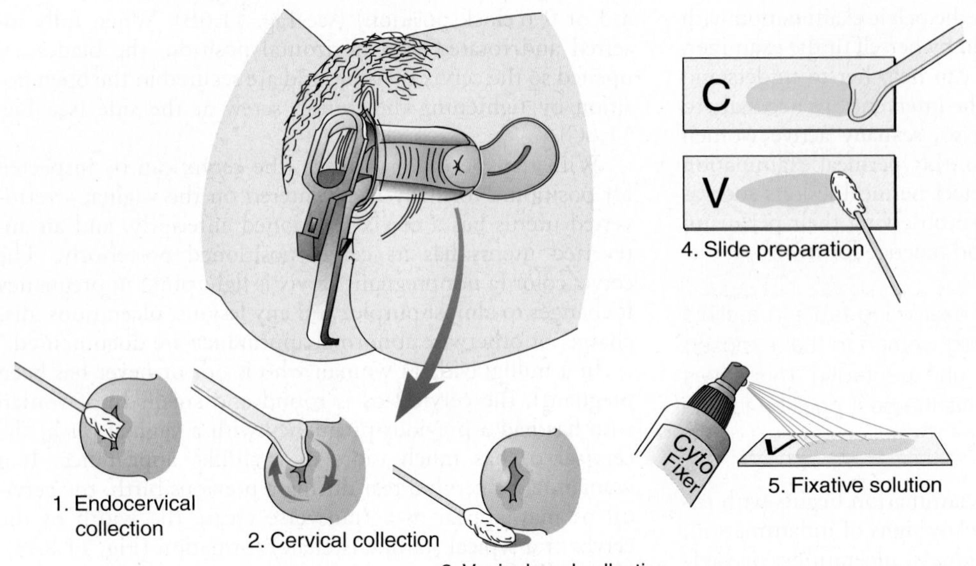

FIGURE 11.9 Obtaining a traditional Pap smear. (**1**) Specimen taken from endocervix. (**2**) Specimen taken from cervix. (**3**) Specimen taken from vaginal pool.

separate specimens—one from the endocervix, one from the cervical os, and one from the posterior vaginal fornix—are obtained (Fig. 11.9). In addition, a cervicogram (a photograph of the cervix) may be taken. Cervicograms serve as complements to Pap smears as a weapon for detecting cervical cancer and documenting that lesions from infections are healing.

To obtain an endocervical specimen for a Pap smear, a sterile cotton applicator, wet with saline, is inserted through the speculum into the os of the cervix and gently rotated, first clockwise, then counterclockwise (see Fig. 11.9[1]). It is then removed without touching the sides of the vagina. The specimen is then gently painted onto a glass slide. The slide is sprayed with a fixative to preserve the cells. Use of cytobrushes for pregnant women is not recommended, because they can cause cervical bleeding because of increased cervical softening.

To take a cervical os specimen, the uneven end of a spatula is inserted through the speculum and pressed on the os of the cervix and rotated to scrape cells in a circle around the os (see Fig. 11.9[2]). After removal, the spatula is then smeared onto a slide and the slide is sprayed with fixative.

For the specimen from the posterior vaginal fornix, a cotton-tipped applicator or the opposite end of the spatula blade is placed at the posterior fornix just below the cervix (the vaginal pool; see Fig. 11.9[3]). The applicator or spatula is rolled gently to pick up secretions collected there. After careful removal, the specimen is painted onto a third slide and sprayed with fixative. Many Pap smears are read by computer today, an advance that has made the collection of specimens slightly different. If a ThinPrep Pap smear is being taken, a small broomlike collection device is inserted into the endocervical canal deep enough to allow the short bristles to contact the endocervix, and it is rotated in a clockwise direction five times. The device is then rinsed off in a special collection vial filled with a fixative solution; the vial is then capped, labeled, and sent to the laboratory (Fig. 11.10).

The classification of Pap smears is constantly being revised as the meaning of abnormal cells is further defined (MacKay, 2009). The Bethesda classification of Pap smears is shown in Table 11.3. Be certain if discussing these reports with women that they do not overinterpret the results. The first category means only normal cells were found. The second category means cells are inflamed probably because infection is present (a woman needs to be treated and re-examined in about 3 months). At the next level (LSIL), cells are moderately suspicious for malignancy. The HSIL category identifies that precancerous cells are present. This level requires a colposcopy examination for further evaluation. Only the last category is indicative that squamous cell carcinoma is present. Therapy at this level will include colposcopy, biopsy, and removal of the affected cells, usually by conization.

Women who engage in anal intercourse may have an anal swab taken as well as vaginal swabs to detect anal squamous neoplasms. The technique for plating anal Pap smears is the same as that for vaginal specimens (a cytobrush is used). Caution the patient that she may have slight rectal bleeding following this procedure.

Many women ask how often repeat Pap smears are necessary. The American Cancer Society recommends women begin to have Pap smears when they turn 21 or 3 years after becoming sexually active (whichever occurs first). After age 30, they then can be done as infrequently as every 2 to 3 years.

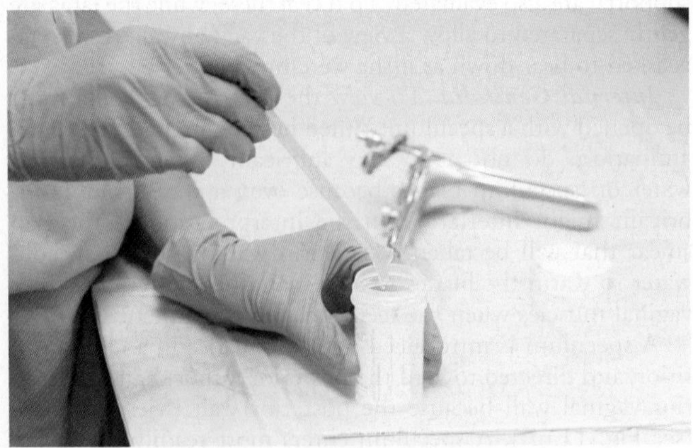

FIGURE 11.10 For liquid Pap tests, the collecting instrument is placed in a commercial vial and capped rather than being smeared onto a slide.

TABLE 11.3 ✻ Interpretation of Pap Smears (CIN and Bethesda Systems)

Number	Dysplasia	CIN: Cervical Intraepithelial Neoplasia	Bethesda System
1	Benign	Benign	Normal
2	Benign with inflammation	Benign with inflammation	Normal but with atypical squamous cells of undetermined significance (ASC-US)
3	Mild dysplasia	CIN I	Low-grade squamous intraepithelial lesion (LSIL).
3a	Low-grade squamous intraepithelial lesion.	CIN II	
3b	Severe dysplasia		
4	Carcinoma in situ	CIN III	High-grade squamous intraepithelial lesion (HSIL).
5	Invasive cancer	Invasive cancer	Invasive cancer

Source: MacKay, H. T. (2009). Gynecology. In S. J. McPhee, et al. (Eds.). *Current medical diagnosis and treatment.* Columbus, OH: McGraw-Hill.

Women who should have them done more frequently are those who have multiple sexual partners, who have a history of human papillomavirus (HPV) infection, who smoke cigarettes, or who were active sexually before age 21. Screening as infrequently as every 3 years could miss pathology in these women.

Vaginal Inspection. Before the vaginal speculum is removed, a culture for gonorrhea, human papillomavirus (HPV), chlamydia, trichomoniasis, or group B streptococci may be taken. After gently swabbing the cervix using a cotton-tipped applicator, the specimen obtained is then plated onto a medium to allow for growth. Treatment to eliminate organisms such as these during pregnancy helps to guard fetal and newborn health (Gulmezoglu, 2007).

A speculum must be unlocked and partially closed before removal; otherwise, pain from excessive stretching could occur. If the speculum is kept partially open as it is removed, however, it should not cause pain, and the sides of the vagina can be inspected as it is withdrawn. In a nonpregnant woman, vaginal walls are light pink; pregnancy turns them dark blue to purple. Any areas of inflammation, ulceration, lesions, or discharge should be noted.

Examination of Pelvic Organs. Following the speculum examination, a bimanual (two-handed) examination is performed to assess the position, contour, consistency, and tenderness of pelvic organs (Fig. 11.11). The index and middle fingers of one gloved hand are lubricated and inserted into the vagina so the walls of the vagina can be palpated for abnormalities. The other hand is then placed on a woman's abdomen and pressed downward toward the hand still in the vagina until the uterus can be felt between them. If a uterus is extremely retroverted, it may not be palpable abdominally. Next, the right and left ovaries are identified by the same method. Ovaries are normally slightly tender, so the pressure caused by palpation may cause a woman some discomfort.

Abnormalities that can be noted by bimanual examination include ovarian cysts, enlarged fallopian tubes (perhaps from pelvic inflammatory disease), and an enlarged uterus (see Table 11.1). An early sign of pregnancy (Hegar's sign) is elicited on bimanual examination as well (see Fig. 10.4).

Rectovaginal Examination. After a bimanual pelvic examination, the hand is withdrawn from the vagina. The index finger is reinserted into the vagina and the middle finger into the rectum. By palpating the tissue between the examining fingers in this way, it is possible to assess the strength and irregularity of the posterior vaginal wall. This maneuver may be slightly uncomfortable for a woman because of the rectal pressure involved. Some examiners use a clean pair of gloves before they perform a vaginal-rectal examination so they will not spread an

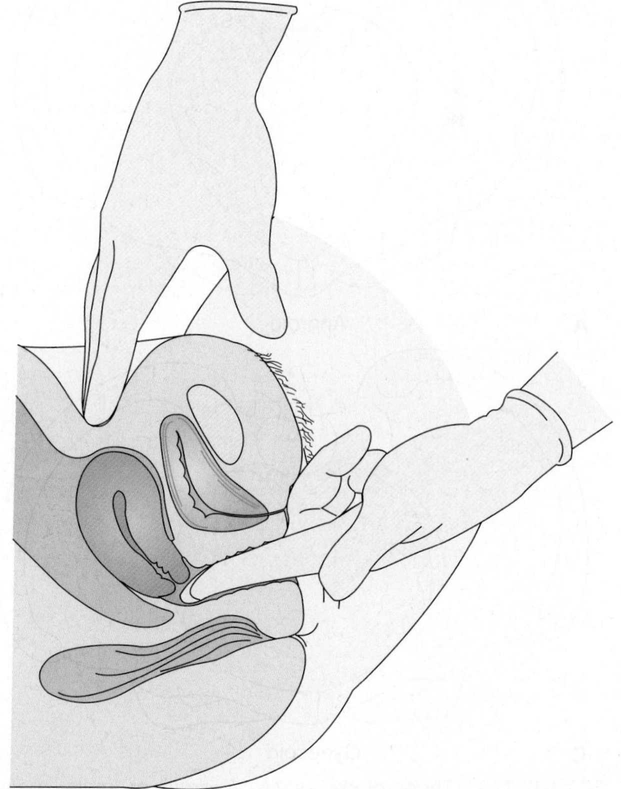

FIGURE 11.11 A bimanual examination to determine uterine size.

infection from the vagina to the rectum. After the rectal examination, if it is necessary to re-examine the vagina for any reason, the glove must be changed to avoid contaminating the vagina with fecal material.

After completing the examination, any excess lubricant is wiped away from the vaginal and rectal openings. It is important to wipe front to back to prevent bringing rectal contamination forward to the vaginal introitus.

✔ Checkpoint Question 11.4

Sandra has not had a pelvic examination since she was in high school. What advice would you give her to help her relax during her first prenatal pelvic examination?

a. Have her take a deep breath and hold it during the examination.
b. Tell her to bear down slightly as the speculum is inserted.
c. Singing out loud helps, because it pushes down the diaphragm.
d. She should breathe slowly and evenly during the examination.

Estimating Pelvic Size. It is impossible to predict from the outward appearance of a woman whether her pelvic ring will be adequate for a fetus to pass through its center. Some women look as if they have a wide pelvis but, in reality, have only wide iliac crests and a normal or even smaller-than-normal internal ring. Other women appear as if their pelvis will be small because the iliac crests are nonflaring, but the internal pelvis, the part that must be sufficiently large for childbirth, is of average size, allowing them to give birth vaginally without difficulty. Differences in pelvic contour and development occur mainly because of hereditary factors, but disease (e.g., rickets, now rarely seen in the United States but still a concern in undeveloped countries, may cause contraction of the pelvis) or injury (inadequate repair following an accident) also may play a role.

If on an initial prenatal visit, the primary care provider establishes that a woman is pregnant, and if she has never given birth vaginally before, pelvic measurements may be taken. Some care providers prefer to take these measurements later in pregnancy, when a woman's pelvic muscles are more relaxed, making measurement easier. Estimation of pelvic adequacy must be done at least by the 24th week of pregnancy, because by this time there is danger that the fetal head will reach a size that will interfere with safe passage and birth if the pelvic measurements are small. If a routine ultrasound is scheduled, estimations of fetal head size may be made by fetal ultrasound.

Once a woman has given birth vaginally, her pelvis has been proven adequate for vaginal birth so it is unnecessary for pelvic measurements to be taken again unless she has an intervening history of trauma to the pelvis.

The types of pelves found in women are categorized into four groups (Fig. 11.12), android, anthropoid, gynecoid, and platypelloid. A *gynecoid,* or "female," pelvis has an inlet that

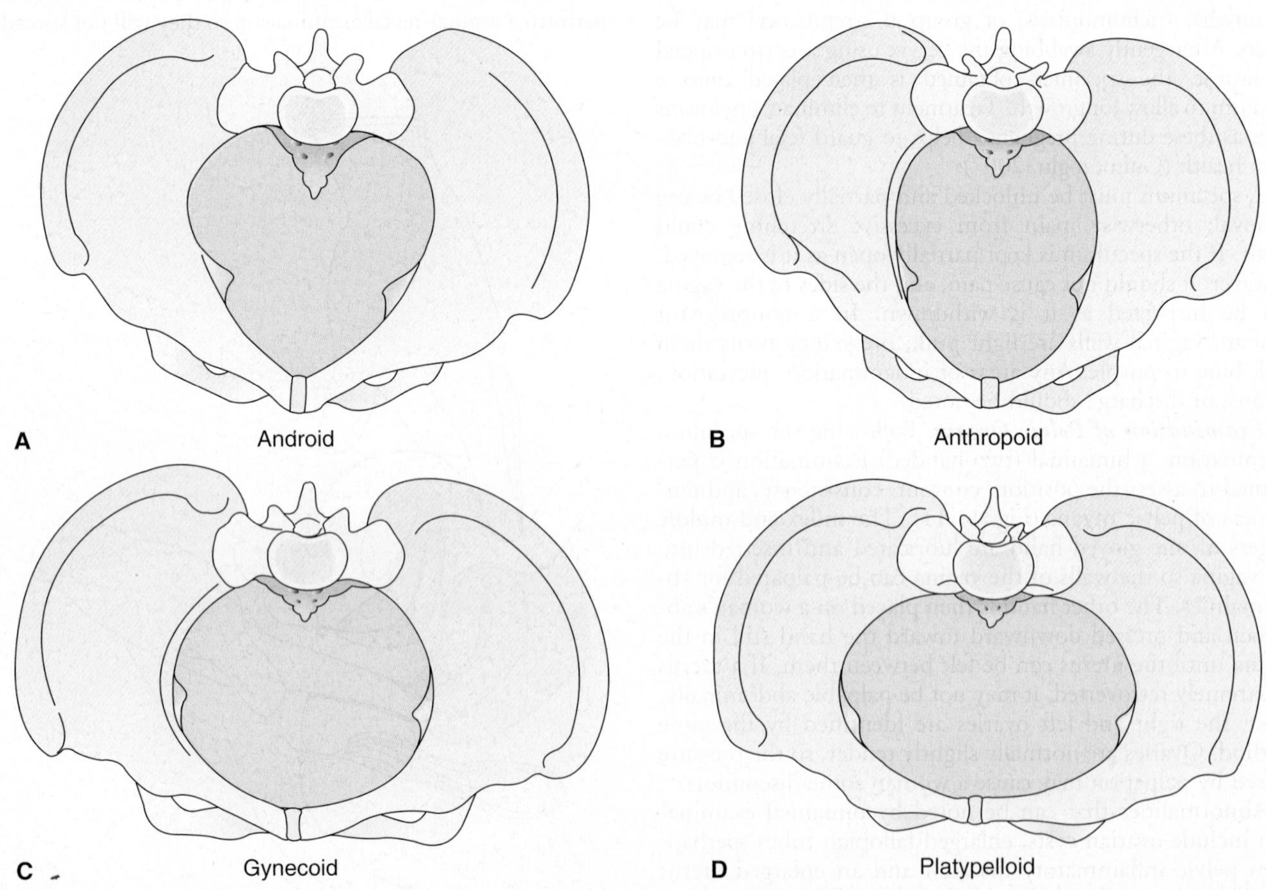

FIGURE 11.12 Types of pelves. (**A**) *Android,* or "male," pelvis. (**B**) *Anthropoid,* or "ape-like," pelvis. (**C**) *Gynecoid,* or "female," pelvis. (**D**) *Platypelloid,* or "flattened," pelvis.

is well rounded forward and backward and a wide pubic arch. This pelvic type is ideal for childbirth. In an *android,* or "male," pelvis, the pubic arch forms an acute angle, making the lower dimensions of the pelvis extremely narrow. A fetus may have difficulty exiting from this type of pelvis. In an *anthropoid,* or "ape-like," pelvis, the transverse diameter is narrow, and the anteroposterior diameter of the inlet is larger than normal. This structure does not accommodate a fetal head as well as a gynecoid pelvis. A *platypelloid,* or "flattened," pelvis has a smoothly curved oval inlet but the anteroposterior diameter is shallow. A fetal head might not be able to rotate to match the curves of the pelvic cavity in this type of pelvis.

Internal pelvic measurements give the actual diameters of the inlet and outlet through which the fetus must pass. The following measurements are made most commonly:

1. The **diagonal conjugate.** This is the distance between the anterior surface of the sacral prominence and the anterior surface of the inferior margin of the symphysis pubis (Fig. 11.13A). The most useful measurement for estimation of pelvic size, it suggests the anteroposterior diameter of the pelvic inlet (the narrower diameter at that level, or the one that is most apt to cause a misfit with the fetal head). The diagonal conjugate is measured while a woman is in a lithotomy position. To measure it, two fingers are introduced vaginally and pressed inward and upward until the middle finger touches the sacral prominence. With the other hand, the part of the examining hand where it touches the symphysis pubis is marked (see Fig. 11.13A). After withdrawing the examining hand, the distance between the tip of the middle finger and the marked point on the glove on that hand is measured by comparing it with a ruler or, for greater accuracy, a pelvimeter. Caution a woman that the measurement may be slightly painful, because she may feel the pressure of the examining finger as it stretches to touch the sacral prominence. If an examiner's hand is small with short fingers, manual pelvic measurements may not be possible, because the fingers may not reach the sacral prominence. If the measurement obtained is more than 12.5 cm, the pelvic inlet is rated as adequate for childbirth (the diameter of the fetal head that must pass that point averages 9 cm in diameter).
2. The **true conjugate** or **conjugate vera** is the measurement between the anterior surface of the sacral prominence and the posterior surface of the inferior margin of the symphysis pubis. This measurement cannot be made directly, but it can be estimated from the measurement made of the diagonal conjugate. To do this, the usual depth of the symphysis pubis (assumed to be 1.5–2 cm) is subtracted from the diagonal conjugate measurement. The distance remaining will be the true conjugate, or the actual diameter of the pelvic inlet through which the fetal head must pass. The average true conjugate diameter is, therefore, 12.5 cm minus 1.5 or 2 cm, or 10.5 to 11 cm.
3. The **ischial tuberosity** diameter. This measurement is the distance between the ischial tuberosities, or the transverse diameter of the outlet (the narrowest diameter at that level, or the one most apt to cause a misfit). It is made at the medial and lowermost aspect of the ischial tuberosities at the level of the anus (see Fig. 11.13B). A pelvimeter is generally used, although the diameter can be measured by a ruler or by comparing it with a known hand span or clenched fist measurement. A diameter of 11 cm is considered adequate because it will allow the diameter of the fetal head, or 9 cm, to pass freely through the outlet.

Laboratory Assessment

Several laboratory studies are included in assessment measures at a first prenatal visit to confirm general health and rule

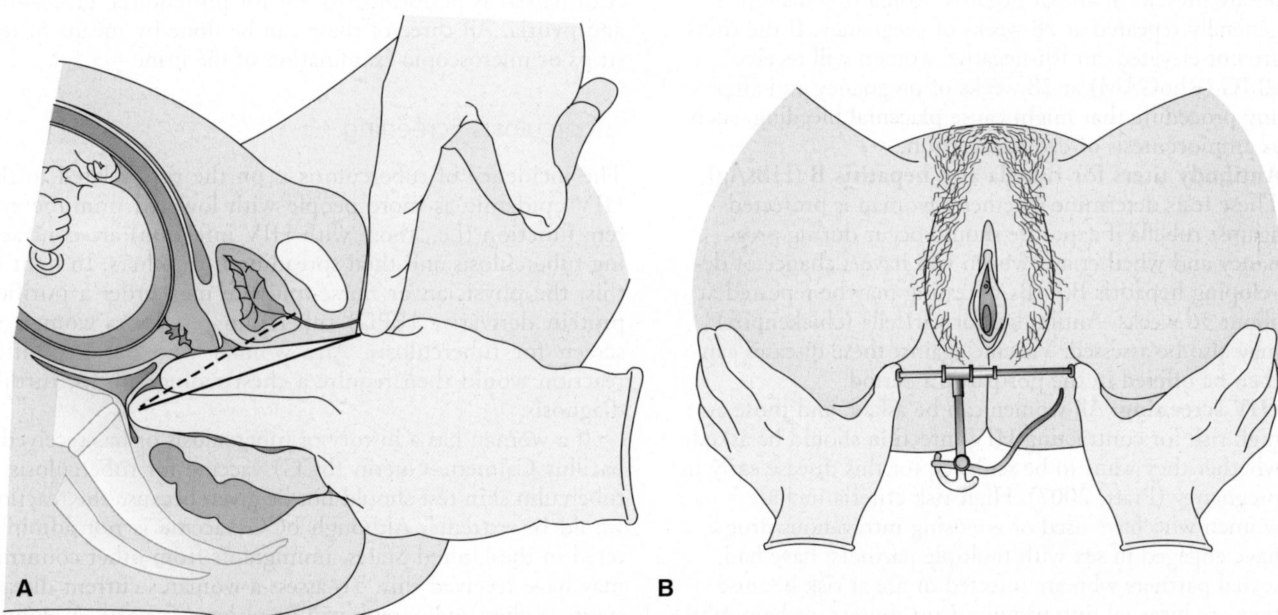

FIGURE 11.13 (**A**) Measurement of diagonal conjugate diameter. *Solid line,* diagonal conjugate; *dotted line,* true conjugate. (**B**) Measurement of ischial tuberosity diameter.

out sexually transmitted infection that could injure the growing fetus. Normal levels for these studies are shown in Appendix F.

Blood Studies

The following blood studies are usually obtained at a first prenatal visit:

1. A **complete blood count,** including hemoglobin or hematocrit and red cell index to determine the presence of anemia, a white blood cell count to determine infection, and a platelet count to estimate clotting ability.
2. A **genetic screen** for common ethnically inherited diseases. African American women, for example, may have a blood sample taken to screen for sickle cell trait or disease and glucose-6-phosphate dehydrogenase (G6PD). Asian and Mediterranean women may have this done for beta-thalassemia; those with Jewish ancestry may have this done for Tay-Sachs disease; and Caucasian women may be tested for cystic fibrosis.
3. A **serologic test for syphilis** (VDRL or rapid plasma reagin test). If syphilis is present, it must be treated early in pregnancy before fetal damage occurs. A blood sample for a serologic test for gonorrhea may be drawn as well.
4. **Blood typing (including Rh factor).** Blood type is documented because blood may have to be made available if a woman has bleeding during pregnancy and to detect the possibility of Rh isoimmunization.
5. **Maternal serum for alpha-fetoprotein (AFP)** (MSAFP). This level will be elevated if a neural tube or abdominal defect is present in the fetus; it may be decreased if a chromosomal anomaly is present. This test is done at 16 to 18 weeks of pregnancy. The level in serum is expressed as "multiples of the mean" (MOM). A normal value is 2.5 MOM. If this is elevated or decreased, an ultrasound or amniocentesis will be ordered to assess for a fetal disorder.
6. An **indirect Coombs' test** (determination if Rh antibodies are present in an Rh-negative woman). This test is generally repeated at 28 weeks of pregnancy. If the titers are not elevated, an Rh-negative woman will receive RhIG (RhoGAM) at 28 weeks of pregnancy and after any procedure that might cause placental bleeding, such as amniocentesis or external version.
7. **Antibody titers for rubella and hepatitis B** (HBsAg). These tests determine whether a woman is protected against rubella if exposure should occur during pregnancy and whether a newborn will have a chance of developing hepatitis B. HBsAg testing may be repeated at about 36 weeks. Antibodies for varicella (chickenpox) may also be assessed. Vaccine against these diseases can then be offered in the postpartum period.
8. **HIV screening.** All women can be asked, and those at high risk for contracting HIV infection should be asked, whether they want to be screened for this disease early in pregnancy (Pratt, 2007). High-risk criteria include women who have used or are using intravenous drugs; have engaged in sex with multiple partners; have had sexual partners who are infected or are at risk because they are bisexual, intravenous drug abusers, or hemophiliacs; or women who received a blood transfusion between 1977 and 1985.

   Screening is done by an enzyme-linked immunosorbent assay (ELISA) on a blood sample. If this is positive, the finding is confirmed by a second test (a Western blot). Testing for HIV early in pregnancy allows a woman who is found to be HIV antibody positive the opportunity to begin therapy with zidovudine (AZT), which can decrease the risk of her infant acquiring the virus. It also allows a woman the option of choosing to terminate a pregnancy to avoid giving birth to an infant who has a high risk of HIV infection.

   As there is still no cure for HIV infection, some women may choose not to have a blood titer taken because they would rather not know that they have the illness. This is their option. Screening cannot be mandatory in prenatal settings. Because HIV testing is controversial, be certain that the information given about test results is accurate (a high blood antibody titer means the person has been exposed to the virus, not that he or she necessarily is infected) and findings are presented with tact and compassion, with respect for the meaning of the results to a woman. Results of HIV testing are kept confidential; be certain not to report this information to anyone other than the woman.
9. If a woman has a history of previously unexplained fetal loss, has a family history of diabetes, has had babies who were large for gestational age (9 lb or more at term), is obese, or has glycosuria, she will need to be scheduled for a 50-g oral 1-hour **glucose loading** or **tolerance test** toward the end of the first trimester to rule out gestational diabetes. If not, she will have this done routinely at the 24th to 28th week to evaluate insulin-antagonistic effects of placental hormones, which can register a noticeable effect at this time. Unless a problem is developing, the plasma glucose level should not exceed 140 mg/dL at 1 hour (see Chapter 20 for a discussion of diabetes in pregnancy).

Urinalysis

A urinalysis is performed to test for proteinuria, glycosuria, and pyuria. All three of these can be done by means of test strips or microscopic examination of the urine.

Tuberculosis Screening

The incidence of tuberculosis is on the rise, related to the HIV epidemic as more people with lowered immune system function (i.e., those with HIV infection) are contracting tuberculosis and then spreading it to others. In light of this, the physician or nurse-midwife may order a purified protein derivative (PPD) tuberculin test for a woman to screen for tuberculosis. Any woman who has a positive reaction would then require a chest radiograph for further diagnosis.

If a woman has a history of tuberculosis or has received a bacillus Calmette-Guérin (bCG) vaccine for tuberculosis, a tuberculin skin test should not be given because the reaction would be extreme. Although bCG vaccine is not administered in the United States, immigrants from other countries may have received this. To assess a woman's current disease status, a chest radiograph will be ordered instead. A woman is often reluctant to have this done because she knows radiation is harmful to a growing fetus. Assure her that she will be given a lead apron to cover her abdomen to protect the fetus, exposing only her chest to radiation.

Screening for tuberculosis early in pregnancy is important because it is a chronic and debilitating disease that increases the risk of miscarriage. Further, the change in the shape of the lung tissue as the growing uterus presses on the lung may reactivate old lesions.

Ultrasonography

If the date of the last menstrual period is unknown, a woman will be scheduled for an ultrasound to confirm the pregnancy length and document healthy fetal growth. Be certain that women know an ultrasound done this early in pregnancy will show only the presence of a gestation sac, not a moving, kicking fetus so their expectations of what they will see are realistic (Lalor & Devane, 2007).

Risk Assessment

Table 11.4 summarizes necessary data assessment for a first prenatal visit. After this assessment, findings are analyzed to determine whether a pregnancy is apt to continue with a good outcome or there is some risk that it will end before term or with an unfavorable fetal or maternal outcome (a high-risk pregnancy).

Table 11.5 lists factors that would identify a pregnancy as being at high risk. A woman identified this way will need close observation during pregnancy to see that the pregnancy is progressing well; the infant born of a woman identified this way needs close observation in the neonatal period until it is confirmed that no anomalies exist.

Risk assessment should be updated at each pregnancy visit, as the failure to identify risk potential in pregnancy leads to increased perinatal mortality. See Chapters 20 through 22 for discussion of high-risk pregnancy and its management.

Following a first prenatal visit, a woman needs to continue with prenatal care. Box 11.7 lists components of assessments and care done during continuing prenatal visits.

BOX 11.7 ✻ Assessments and Care for Continuing Prenatal Visits

Mother's Health

Health Interview

Interim history or new personal or family developments since last visit
Review danger signs of pregnancy
Review symptoms of beginning labor

Physical examination

Blood pressure (every visit)
Clean-catch urine for glucose, protein, and leukocytes (every visit)
Blood serum level for alpha-fetoprotein (MSAFP) (16 weeks)
VDRL test for syphilis if possibility of new exposure
Glucose screen (28 weeks)
Glucose challenge (24–28 weeks) if warranted
Anti-Rh titer (28 weeks)
Group B streptococci (GBS) (35–37 weeks)

Fetal Health

Fetal heart rate
Fundal height
Quickening or fetal movement
Ultrasound dating of pregnancy

TABLE 11.4 ✻ Assessments for a First Pregnancy Visit

Health History	
Demographic data	Name, address, age, telephone number, health insurance
Chief concern	Was pregnancy planned? When was last menstrual period? Any exposure to infectious diseases or ingestion of drugs since a woman thinks she has been pregnant?
Family and social profile	What is family composition? Does the woman have a support person? What is her occupation? Source of income? Level of exercise? Hobbies? Recreational drug use? Living conditions? Nutrition? Sleep pattern?
Past medical history	Any abdominal surgery, kidney, heart, hypertension, sexually transmitted infections, diabetes, allergies? What immunizations has she had?
Gynecologic history	When was menarche? What is length and duration of menstrual cycle?
Obstetric history	Any previous pregnancies? When? Type and outcome of birth? Any history of previous miscarriages?
Review of systems	Brief review of all body systems
Physical Examination	
Baseline data	Height, weight, vital signs, fundal height measurements (after 12 weeks), fetal heart sounds
System assessment	Full physical examination to confirm general health
Pelvic examination	General assessment, Pap smear, cultures for chlamydia, gonorrhea, group B streptococci, pelvic measurements
Laboratory Assessment	
Blood	Complete blood count, serologic test for syphilis, blood type and Rh, alpha-fetoprotein, antibody titer against Rh, hepatitis B, rubella, and possibly varicella and HIV
Urinalysis	Clean catch for glucose, protein, ketones, and culture
Tuberculosis	PPD test
Ultrasound	To date pregnancy or confirm fetal health (if date of last menstrual period is unknown)

TABLE 11.5 ✻ Assessments That Might Categorize a Pregnancy as "at Risk"

Obstetric History	History of subfertility or grand multiparity Previous premature cervical dilatation Existing uterine or cervical anomaly Previous preterm labor or preterm birth or cesarean birth Previous macrosomic infant Two or more spontaneous miscarriages or therapeutic abortions Previous hydatidiform mole/ choriocarcinoma Previous ectopic pregnancy or stillborn/neonatal death Previous multiple gestation Previous prolonged labor Previous low-birth-weight infant Previous midforceps birth Last pregnancy less than 1 year previous Previous infant with neurologic deficit, birth injury, or congenital anomaly		Abnormal fetal surveillance tests Polyhydramnios Placenta previa Abnormal presentation Maternal anemia Maternal weight gain under 10 lb or weight loss Currently over/underweight Fetal or placental malformation Rh sensitization Preterm labor Multiple gestation Premature rupture of membranes Abruptio placentae Postdate pregnancy Fibroid tumors Fetal version Cervical cerclage Sexually transmitted infection Other maternal infection Poor immunization status
Medical History	Cardiac or pulmonary disease, chronic hypertension Metabolic disease such as diabetes mellitus Renal disease, recent urinary tract infection, or bacteriuria Gastrointestinal disorders Seizure disorders Family history of severe inherited disorders Surgery during pregnancy Emotional disorder or cognitive challenge Previous surgeries, particularly involving reproductive organs Endocrine disorders such as hypothyroidism Hemoglobinopathies Sexually transmitted infections Reproductive tract anomalies, history of abnormal Pap smear, malignancy	**Psychosocial Factors**	Inadequate finances Lack of support person Adolescent Poor nutrition More than two children at home; no help Lack of acceptance of pregnancy Attempt or ideation of suicide Inadequate or poor housing Father of baby uninvolved Minority status Dangerous occupation Dysfunctional grieving Psychiatric history
		Demographic Factors	Maternal age under 16 or over 35 Education less than 11 years
		Lifestyle	Cigarette smoking greater than 10 cigarettes a day or living with a person who smokes this much Substance abuse Long amounts of time spent commuting Nonuse of seatbelts Alcohol intake Heavy lifting or long periods of standing Unusual stress No in-home smoke detectors
Current Obstetric Status	Inadequate prenatal care Intrauterine growth-restricted fetus Large-for-gestational-age fetus Pregnancy-induced hypertension or pre-eclampsia		

SIGNS INDICATING COMPLICATIONS OF PREGNANCY

Although most signs indicating complications of pregnancy occur toward the end of pregnancy, women need to know what these are from the beginning (see Focus on Nursing Care Planning Box 11.8). When teaching about these signs, assure a pregnant woman you have every reason to believe she is going to have a normal, uncomplicated pregnancy (assuming that is true) as well as no reason to think that she is going to experience any serious problems, but if any danger signs do occur, she should inform her health care provider by telephone or e-mail immediately. Be certain you give her an alternate contact number to call if the health care facility is closed. Emphasize that if one of these danger signs should occur, it serves merely as a signal of the possibility that something may happen, not that something serious has already happened. It is important for her to report it immediately, though, so it can be dealt with before something harmful does occur.

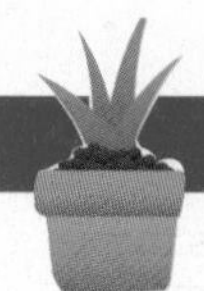

BOX 11.8 ✻ Focus on Nursing Care Planning

A Multidisciplinary Care Map for a Woman's First Prenatal Visit

Sandra Czerinski is a 29-year-old woman, 12 weeks' pregnant, who comes for a first prenatal visit. She is concerned because she did not realize she was pregnant until a week ago. Because of this, she has been actively dieting (two diet drinks plus one meal of mainly vegetables daily) plus lifting weights at a health club. She has not had a pelvic examination since she was in high school, when she had a vaginal infection. She remembers that examination as being very painful. She is worried she has a urinary tract infection now because she has to "go all the time." She does not want any blood work done because she does not have health insurance.

Family Assessment ✻ Single woman; lives by self in one-bedroom apartment. Works at a laundry. Boyfriend is a roofing salesman; out of town 4 days a week.

Client Assessment ✻ Gravida 1, para 0. Last menstrual period 4 months ago. Had nausea last month but thought that was the "flu."

Menarche at age 11; menstrual cycle every 29 days, 6 days' duration with moderate flow and mild cramps. Past history positive for sinusitis; appendectomy at age 12 years. Smokes about ½ pack per day, "more when I'm stressed at work"; denies alcohol use. "I drink club soda with lime or mineral water."

ROS: Height 5 feet 5 inches; prepregnancy weight 160 lb (BMI: 27.5 or overweight). Slight gingival hyperplasia; breasts full and slightly tender.

Pelvic examination by nurse-midwife: cervical os round, clean, and slightly soft; uterus enlarged and soft; + Chadwick's sign, + Hegar's sign, + Goodell's sign. Uterine height palpable at three fingers over symphysis pubis. Fetal heart rate via Doppler at 152 beats per minute.

Remainder of physical examination within normal limits. Weight today: 177 lb.

Nursing Diagnosis ✻ Health-seeking behaviors related to guidelines for pregnancy

Outcome Criteria ✻ Client states the need to stop smoking; identifies measures she will take to reduce number of cigarettes smoked and states she will no longer try to lose weight. Makes appointment for follow-up visits.

Team Member Responsible	Assessment	Intervention	Rationale	Expected Outcome
Activities of Daily Living				
Nurse/nurse-midwife	Assess client's expectations about this pregnancy, including whether she expects to continue to work, continue present lifestyle.	Discuss the effect of pregnancy on her partner and any religious or cultural beliefs that would interfere with her ability to adapt to pregnancy changes.	Assessing expectations is important to assist a woman in identifying areas of need and adaptation necessary for pregnancy to ensure the optimal outcome for the mother, fetus, and partner.	Client describes the likely effect of the pregnancy on herself and partner; identifies areas where she anticipates life changes.
Consultations				
Nurse-midwife	Fully assess symptoms of urinary frequency to rule out urinary tract infection	Consult with primary care provider about further investigation of urinary tract infection if indicated.	Urinary tract infections are associated with preterm birth.	Primary care physician will document urinary tract infection if signs/symptoms warrant and will prescribe appropriate antibiotic.
Procedures/Medications				
Nurse-midwife/nurse	Obtain a gynecologic and obstetrics health history.	Perform initial assessment, including vital signs, height and weight measurement, and history and physical examination.	Initial assessment provides a baseline for future comparison and identification of factors that may place a client at risk for pregnancy concerns.	Client receives a thorough initial assessment, to lay a psychological and physiologic foundation of health care information for pregnancy care.

(continued)

BOX 11.8 ✻ Focus on Nursing Care Planning (continued)

Nurse	Obtain usual weight before pregnancy and weight at each visit. Obtain urine and blood specimens.	Monitor weight at every visit. Explain that blood assessment is not done at every visit.	A baseline weight is necessary for future comparison. Adequate weight gain during pregnancy (typically 25 to 30 lb) is necessary for optimal fetal growth and development.	Client's weight is monitored and compared with previous weights at each prenatal visit. Client states she understands importance of initial blood work, urinalysis, and weight gain during pregnancy.
		Nutrition		
Nurse/ nutritionist	Obtain a 24-hour nutrition recall.	Discuss with client her increased nutritional needs during pregnancy. Provide information about including fresh fruits and vegetables, milk products, and high-protein foods, fluid intake, and prenatal vitamin supplementation.	A well-balanced diet with adequate fluid intake and use of prenatal vitamins helps to ensure an optimal environment for fetal growth and development. Dieting is contraindicated during pregnancy.	Client voices an understanding of the increased nutritional needs during pregnancy and describes her plan to provide for these needs. Voices understanding of why she should discontinue dieting.
		Patient/Family Education		
Nurse	Assess if client is interested in decreasing smoking during pregnancy.	Instruct client in the effects of smoking on the fetus. Assist client with methods to reduce and stop, if possible.	Nicotine in cigarettes has been shown to be teratogenic to a fetus.	Client describes the effect on a fetus of smoking during pregnancy and her plan to stop smoking at least until after the birth and, ideally, long term.
Nurse	Assess if client is aware of the danger signs of pregnancy that she will need to report immediately should they occur.	Instruct client about possible danger signs to report immediately. Emphasize that although these signs are important, they do not necessarily mean that something is wrong.	Knowledge of possible danger signs allows for early detection and prompt intervention should it be necessary.	Client and intimate partner list danger signs of pregnancy to report immediately. They acknowledge that these signs suggest, but do not necessarily mean, that the pregnancy is at risk.
		Psychosocial/Spiritual/Emotional Needs		
Nurse	Assess if client has concerns about success of pregnancy.	Assure client that concern during pregnancy is a normal response. Include information about physiologic and psychological changes of pregnancy.	Anxiety can interfere with client's ability to adjust to pregnancy. Reviewing information reinforces understanding of what is to come and helps to alleviate fears and anxieties related to pregnancy.	Client describes any concerns about pregnancy and receives appropriate assurance.
		Discharge Planning		
Nurse	Assess whether client will have any difficulty continuing with prenatal care.	Assist client with setting up appointments for future visits with respect that she has no health insurance.	Assisting with appointment setting helps to ensure adherence.	Client states plan for expected antepartal care visits and affirms her willingness to adhere to the plan.

Vaginal Bleeding

A woman should report vaginal bleeding, no matter how slight, because some of the serious bleeding complications of pregnancy begin with only slight spotting. When talking with a woman, ask her how she discovered the spotting. If she discovered it on toilet paper following a bowel movement, she is probably reporting spotting from hemorrhoids. Until the bleeding is found to be innocent, however, all women with spotting need further evaluation.

Persistent Vomiting

Once- or twice-daily vomiting is not uncommon during the first trimester of pregnancy. However, persistent, frequent vomiting is not normal. Vomiting that continues past the 12th week of pregnancy is also extended vomiting. Persistent or extended vomiting depletes the nutritional supply available to a fetus so is a danger to the pregnancy. (See Chapter 13 for an in-depth discussion of persistent vomiting [hyperemesis gravidarum].)

Chills and Fever

Chills and fever may be symptoms of a relatively benign gastroenteritis, but they also may indicate an intrauterine infection, a potentially serious complication for both a woman and a fetus. Because a woman cannot make a definite determination about the cause of a fever, further evaluation by a health care provider is necessary.

Sudden Escape of Clear Fluid From the Vagina

When a gush of clear fluid is discharged suddenly from the vagina, it means the membranes have ruptured and mother and fetus are now both threatened, because the uterine cavity is no longer sealed against infection. If a fetus is small so the head does not fit snugly into the cervix, the umbilical cord may prolapse following membrane rupture. If the cord is then compressed by the fetal head, oxygenation is compromised and a fetus will be in immediate and grave danger. Alerting a health care provider to any sudden escape of fluid is crucial so a safe and controlled birth can be planned. Occasionally, a woman confuses stress incontinence (involuntary loss of urine on coughing or sneezing or lifting a heavy object) for this. In this situation, vaginal examination typically reveals that the membranes are still intact.

Abdominal or Chest Pain

Abdominal pain at any time is a signal that something is abnormal, so a woman should report it immediately. Some women may think that this is normal because the growing uterus is deflecting their other organs from their usual alignment, but a pregnant uterus normally expands painlessly. Abdominal pain is therefore a sign of some other problem, such as a tubal (ectopic) pregnancy, separation of the placenta, preterm labor, or something unrelated to the pregnancy but perhaps equally as serious, such as appendicitis, ulcer, or pancreatitis. Chest pain may indicate a pulmonary embolus, a complication that can follow thrombophlebitis.

Pregnancy-Induced Hypertension

Pregnancy-induced hypertension (PIH) refers to a potentially severe and even fatal elevation of blood pressure that occurs during pregnancy. Several symptoms signal that PIH is developing:

- Rapid weight gain (over 2 lb per week in the second trimester, 1 lb per week in the third trimester)
- Swelling of the face or fingers
- Flashes of light or dots before the eyes
- Dimness or blurring of vision
- Severe, continuous headache
- Decreased urine output

One by one, these are vague symptoms so a woman may need some help appreciating that they are important to report during pregnancy. Some edema of the ankles during pregnancy is normal, for example, particularly if it occurs after a woman has been on her feet for a long period. Swelling of the hands (ask if she has noticed if her rings are tight) or face (difficulty opening eyes in the morning because of edema of the eyelids), however, indicates edema that is more extensive than usual. Visual disturbances or a continuous headache may signal cerebral edema or acute hypertension. Be certain a woman is not reporting symptoms she had before she became pregnant. If she had the same visual difficulties and headaches before pregnancy as she is reporting now, she may need to see an ophthalmologist rather than her obstetrician for help with the problem. (See Chapter 21 for more on PIH.)

Increase or Decrease in Fetal Movement

Because a fetus normally moves more or less the same amount every day, an unusual increase or decrease in movement suggests that a fetus is responding to a need for oxygen. Be sure to ask a woman about typical fetal movements and whether she has noticed any increase or decrease in this rate. If there has been a change, she is a candidate for further testing and follow-up. Common tests of fetal movement are discussed in Chapter 9.

✔ Checkpoint Question 11.5

You tell Sandra about the danger signs of pregnancy. Which of the following would you tell her to report if it should occur?

a. Her uterus becomes palpable over the symphysis pubis at 12 weeks.
b. Blue veins can be readily observed on both of her breasts.
c. She gains more weight than 2 lb a week beginning at 20 weeks.
d. Her uterus is growing so slowly the growth is not causing any pain.

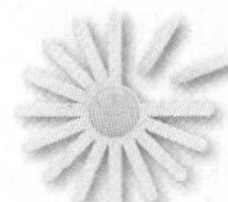

KEY POINTS FOR REVIEW

- Prenatal care has the potential to reduce the incidence of preterm birth and congenital anomalies and the infant mortality rate.

- The purpose of prenatal care is to establish a baseline of present health, determine the gestational age of the fetus, monitor fetal development, identify women at risk for complications, minimize the risk of possible complications by anticipating and preventing problems before they occur, and provide time for education about pregnancy and possible dangers.
- A first prenatal visit confirms a pregnancy, but it is also a time for important assessments such as a health history, physical examination, and laboratory tests. The physical examination includes measurement of fundal height and assessment of fetal heart sounds if the pregnancy is beyond 12 weeks, a pelvic examination (including a Pap test), and possibly an estimation of pelvic size.
- A first prenatal visit sets the tone for visits to follow. Maintaining a supportive manner is helpful to establish rapport and allow a woman to feel comfortable to return for future care.
- Common pelvic types include gynecoid (well-rounded with a wide pubic arch), anthropoid (narrow), platypelloid (flattened), and android (male or with a sharp pubic arch). A gynecoid pelvis is ideal for childbearing.
- The true conjugate (conjugate vera) is the measurement between the anterior surface of the sacral prominence and the posterior surface of the inferior margin of the symphysis pubis (the anterior-posterior diameter of the pelvic inlet). The average is 10.5 to 11 cm. The ischial tuberosity diameter is the distance between the ischial tuberosities or the transverse diameter of the outlet. The average is 11 cm.
- For a pelvic examination, pregnant women should remain in a lithotomy position for as short a time as possible to help prevent thromboembolism and supine hypotension syndrome.
- Danger signs for women to report during pregnancy are vaginal bleeding, persistent vomiting, chills and fever, escape of fluid from the vagina, abdominal or chest pain, swelling of the face and fingers, vision changes or continuous headache, burning with urination, or a pronounced decrease in fetal movement.
- Remember that a family, not a woman alone, is having a baby, and include family members in procedures and health teaching as desired.

CRITICAL THINKING EXERCISES

1. Sandra Czerinski, whom you met at the beginning of the chapter, was worried about having a pelvic examination. How could you help relieve her concern?
2. Sandra works at a commercial laundry ironing sheets. Is this a job that probably keeps her on her feet for long periods? Is she apt to be exposed to toxic substances at work? Is there a greater opportunity than usual for her to develop upper respiratory infections?
3. Sandra's boyfriend rarely comes with her to prenatal visits. Another woman has a supportive husband who always comes. Would your role be different in these two situations?
4. Examine the National Health Goals related to prenatal care. Most government-sponsored money for nursing research is allotted based on these goals. What would be a possible research topic to explore pertinent to these goals that would be applicable to the Czerinski family and also advance evidence-based practice?

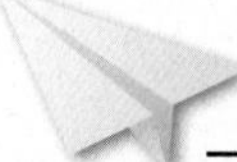

CRITICAL THINKING SCENARIO

Open the accompanying CD-ROM or visit http://thePoint.lww.com and read the Patient Scenario included for this chapter, then answer the questions to further sharpen your skills and grow more familiar with NCLEX types of questions related to prenatal care. Confirm your answers are correct by reading the rationales.

REFERENCES

Akobeng, A. K., & Heller, R. F. (2007). Assessing the population impact of low rates of breast feeding on asthma, coeliac disease and obesity: the use of a new statistical method. *Archives of Disease in Childhood, 92*(6), 483–485.

American College of Obstetricians and Gynecologists (ACOG). (2007). Management of herpes in pregnancy. *Obstetrics and Gynecology, 109*(6), 1489–1498.

Barlow, J., et al. (2007). Role of home visiting in improving parenting and health in families at risk of abuse and neglect: results of a multicentre randomised controlled trial and economic evaluation. *Archives of Disease in Childhood, 92*(3), 229–233.

Bernstein, H. B., & Weinstein, M. (2007). Normal pregnancy and prenatal care. In A. H. DeCherney & L. Nathan (Eds.). *Current diagnosis and treatment in obstetrics and gynecology* (10th ed.). Columbus, OH: McGraw-Hill.

Chasan-Taber, L., et al. (2007). Correlates of physical activity in pregnancy among Latina women. *Maternal and Child Health Journal, 11*(4), 353–363.

Cootauco, A. C., & Althaus, J. E. (2007). Preterm labor and premature rupture of membranes. In K. B. Fortner, et al. (Eds.). *The Johns Hopkins manual of gynecology and obstetrics.* Philadelphia: Lippincott Williams & Wilkins.

Crombleholme, W. R. (2009). Obstetrics. In McPhee, S. J., & Papadakis, M. A. (Eds.). *Current medical diagnosis & treatment.* Columbus, OH: McGraw-Hill.

Donnelly, J. C., et al. (2008). Illegal drug use, smoking and alcohol consumption in a low-risk Irish primigravid population. *Journal of Perinatal Medicine, 36*(1), 70–72.

Dorigo, O., Martinez-Maza, O., & Berek, J. S. (2007). Molecular biology and genetics. In J. S. Berek (Ed.). *Berek & Novak's obstetrics and gynecology.* Philadelphia: Lippincott Williams & Wilkins.

Edwards, M. (2007). Skin cancer. Sun awareness and prevention of skin cancer. *Primary Health Care, 17*(6), 21–24.

Evans, J. M. (2007). Why we need holism in pregnancy care: a review. *Alternative Therapies in Health and Medicine, 13*(3), 60–63.

Fiore, A. E., et al. (2007). Prevention and control of influenza. Recommendations of the Advisory Committee on Immunization Practices (ACIP), 2007. *MMWR: Morbidity and Mortality Weekly Report, 56*(RR-6), 1–53.

Gulmezoglu, A. M. (2009). Interventions for trichomoniasis in pregnancy. *Cochrane Database of Systematic Reviews,* 2009(1), (CD000220).

Hodnett, E. D. (2009). Continuity of caregivers for care during pregnancy and childbirth. *Cochrane Database of Systematic Reviews, 2009*(1), (CD000062).

Karch, A. M. (2009). *Lippincott's nursing drug guide.* Philadelphia: Lippincott Williams & Wilkins.

Katsufrakis, P. J., & Workowski, K. A. (2008). Sexually transmitted diseases. In J. E. South-Paul, S. C. Matheny, & E. L. Lewis (Eds.). *Current diagnosis and treatment in family medicine* (2nd ed.). Columbus, OH: McGraw-Hill.

Kosters, J. P., & Gotzsche, P. C. (2009). Regular self-examination or clinical examination for early detection of breast cancer. *Cochrane Database of Systematic Reviews, 2009*(1), (CD003373).

Lalor, J. G., & Devane, D. (2007). Information, knowledge and expectation of the routine ultrasound scan. *Midwifery, 23*(1), 13–22.

MacKay, H. T. (2009). Gynecology. In S. J. McPhee, & M. A. Papadakis (Eds.). *Current medical diagnosis and treatment.* Columbus, OH: McGraw-Hill.

Pollard, I. (2007). Neuropharmacology of drugs and alcohol in mother and fetus. *Seminars in Fetal and Neonatal Medicine, 12*(2), 106–113.

Pratt, R. J. (2007). Perinatal and infant HIV infection: screening to minimise risk. *Infant, 3*(1), 8–12.

Records, K. (2007). A critical review of maternal abuse and infant outcomes: implications for newborn nurses. *Newborn and Infant Nursing Reviews, 7*(1), 7–13.

Rojas, F., Wood, E., & Blakemore, K. (2007). Preconception counseling and prenatal care. In K. B. Fortner, et al. (Eds.). *The Johns Hopkins manual of gynecology and obstetrics.* Philadelphia: Lippincott Williams & Wilkins.

Ruhl, C. (2007). Well woman. Breast health screening: what all women should know. *Nursing for Women's Health, 11*(3), 326–330.

Sunderland, E. M. (2007). Mercury exposure from domestic and imported estuarine and marine fish in the U.S. seafood market. *Environmental Health Perspectives, 115*(2), 235–242.

Tanner, E., & Alexander, C. J. (2007). Infections of the genital tract. In K. B. Fortner, et al. (Eds.). *The Johns Hopkins manual of gynecology and obstetrics.* Philadelphia: Lippincott Williams & Wilkins.

Venugopalan, L., et al. (2007). Prevalence of smoking during pregnancy in a New York inner city hospital. *Neonatal Intensive Care, 20*(1), 21–23.

SUGGESTED READINGS

Abayomi, J., et al. (2007). Obesity and underweight among first trimester pregnant women. *British Journal of Midwifery, 15*(3), 143–147.

Friedewald, M. (2007). Facilitating discussion among expectant fathers: is anyone interested? *Journal of Perinatal Education, 16*(2), 16–20.

Handley, M. C., & Crow, C. S. (2007). Emotional responses to pregnancy based on geographical classification of residence. *Online Journal of Rural Nursing and Health Care, 6*(2), 1–16.

Maconochie, N., et al. (2007). Risk factors for first trimester miscarriage—results from a UK-population-based case-control study. *BJOG: An International Journal of Obstetrics and Gynaecology, 114*(2), 170–186.

Petrikovsky, B. M., & Egan, J. F. X. (2007). First trimester screening: step by step protocol. *Neonatal Intensive Care, 19*(7), 19–21.

Schmidt, M. D., et al. (2007). Physical activity patterns during pregnancy in a diverse population of women. *Journal of Women's Health, 15*(8), 909–918.

Shankar, K., Ronis, M. J. J., & Badger, T. M. (2007). Effects of pregnancy and nutritional status on alcohol metabolism. *Alcohol Research & Health, 30*(1), 55–59.

Villar J., et al. (2009). Patterns of routine antenatal care for low-risk pregnancy. *Cochrane Database of Systematic Reviews, 2009*(1), (CD000934).

Weissgerber, T. L., & Wolfe, L. A. (2007). Physiological adaptation in early human pregnancy: adaptation to balance maternal-fetal demands. *Applied Physiology, Nutrition, and Metabolism, 31*(1), 1–11.

Xue, F., et al. (2008). Parental characteristics as predictors of birth weight. *Human Reproduction, 23*(1), 168–177.

Chapter 12 Promoting Fetal and Maternal Health

KEY TERMS

- cytomegalovirus
- fetal alcohol syndrome
- leukorrhea
- Sims' position
- teratogen
- toxoplasmosis

OBJECTIVES

After mastering the contents of this chapter, you should be able to:

1. Describe health behaviors important for a healthy pregnancy outcome.
2. Identify National Health Goals related to a healthy pregnancy lifestyle that nurses can help the nation achieve.
3. Use critical thinking to analyze ways to promote both individualized and family-centered prenatal care.
4. Assess a woman for healthy practices and concerns during pregnancy.
5. Formulate nursing diagnoses related to a healthy pregnancy.
6. Identify expected outcomes to promote a healthy pregnancy such as encouraging daily exercise.
7. Plan health-promotion strategies to limit exposure to teratogens or reduce the minor discomforts of pregnancy.
8. Implement nursing care to promote positive health practices during pregnancy.
9. Evaluate outcomes for achievement and effectiveness of care.
10. Identify areas of prenatal care that could benefit from additional nursing research or the application of evidence-based practice.
11. Integrate knowledge of health-promotion strategies with the nursing process to achieve quality maternal and child health nursing care.

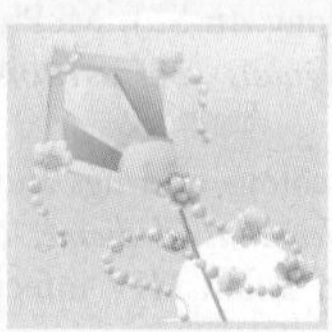

Julberry Adams, a single woman, is 4 months pregnant when you see her in a prenatal clinic. She works as a curator for an art gallery but has missed work this past week because of nausea. She is worried she will not be able to work past 6 months of her pregnancy because her job involves a great deal of walking. She wonders how she will be able to afford her apartment if she has to quit work. She has already stopped volunteer work teaching children's swimming at the YMCA. She wants to travel to see her sister in St. Louis because her sister is very ill but has heard that pregnant women should not drive over 100 miles. She asks you if marijuana would help reduce her early pregnancy nausea. Previous chapters discussed normal anatomy and physiology and the changes that occur with pregnancy. This chapter adds information about the health teaching that women need during pregnancy to ensure a healthy outcome for themselves and their child.

What additional health teaching does Ms. Adams need?

The health of a fetus and the health of the mother are inextricably linked. Generally, a woman who eats well and takes care of her own health during pregnancy provides a healthy environment for fetal growth and development. However, she may need instructions on exactly what constitutes a healthy lifestyle for herself and her baby. Most women have questions regarding how much extra rest they need, what type of exercise they can continue, and whether all the changes going on in their bodies, some of which bring them daily discomfort, are normal. Therefore, a major role in promoting maternal and fetal health is education. Providing empathic advice about ways to alleviate the minor discomforts of pregnancy, alerting a woman to the danger signs of pregnancy, and keeping abreast of the latest evidence-based practice studies done on maternal exposure to **teratogens** (factors detrimental to fetal health) are all part of this role (Knopik, 2009). Because effective prenatal care is vital to healthy fetal growth, National Health Goals have been established to increase the number of women receiving effective prenatal care (Box 12.1).

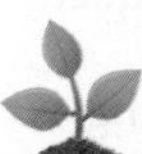

Nursing Process Overview

For Health Promotion of a Fetus and Mother

Assessment

A thorough health history, physical evaluation, and initial laboratory data are obtained at the first prenatal visit. Continuing assessment concentrates on screening for any abnormalities in physical or emotional health that might be occurring and for the possibility of teratogens in the pregnant woman's environment. Encourage a pregnant woman to discuss whatever concerns she is having during all visits. Although some of these concerns may represent minor common discomforts associated with normal pregnancy, others may be early indicators of potential problems (Box 12.2). Early problem identification allows you to provide information and guidance on ways to alleviate the discomforts of pregnancy and also allows you to alert a woman's physician or nurse-midwife of your findings as soon as they appear. Early detection and continued monitoring of conditions such as pregnancy-induced hypertension (PIH) and gestational diabetes reduce the risks of their danger.

Unless women bring problems to their health care provider's attention early in pregnancy, they do not have the opportunity to take the necessary measures to prevent further discomfort during or after the pregnancy. Many women do not mention any concerns or discomforts unless specifically asked because they may not be aware of

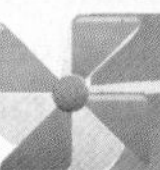

BOX 12.1 * Focus on National Health Goals

Several National Health goals speak to the importance of health promotion during pregnancy.

- Increase the proportion of pregnant women who receive early and adequate prenatal care from a baseline of 74% to a target of 90%.
- Increase to 100% from a baseline of 96% the proportion of pregnant women who abstain from illicit drugs during pregnancy.
- Increase to 99% from a baseline of 87% the proportion of pregnant women who abstain from cigarette smoking during pregnancy.
- Increase to 95% from a baseline of 90% the proportion of pregnant women who abstain from alcohol during pregnancy.
- Increase to 100% from a baseline of 96% the proportion of pregnant women who abstain from binge drinking during pregnancy (http://www.nih.gov).

Because nurses are important members of prenatal health care teams, they play an important role in seeing that services include preconceptual care and that women are aware that early pregnancy care is important. Evidence-based practice and nursing research to answer such questions as what aspects of preconceptual care are most important in reducing pregnancy complications, and what are effective incentives to make women come early for prenatal care, would be important to help the nation meet these goals.

Box 12.2 Assessment: Assessing a Woman for Discomforts of Pregnancy

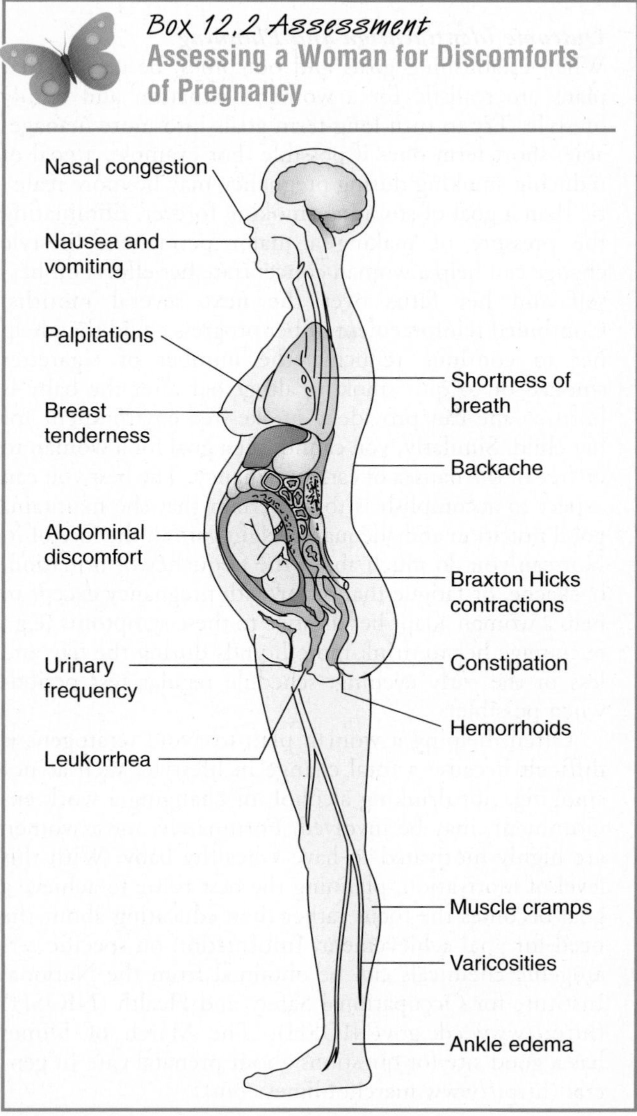

their significance or are reluctant to take up a busy health care provider's time for these things. For example, women experiencing constipation may not take care of the problem early or well enough to prevent the occurrence of hemorrhoids, which can then become a long-term problem not only throughout the pregnancy but afterward as well.

Nursing Diagnosis

Examples of nursing diagnoses related to health promotion of the pregnant woman and fetus are:

- Health-seeking behaviors related to interest in maintaining optimal health during pregnancy
- Anxiety related to minor discomforts of pregnancy
- Risk for deficient fluid volume related to nausea and vomiting of pregnancy
- Disturbed body image related to change of appearance with pregnancy
- Risk for altered sexuality patterns related to fear of harming fetus during pregnancy
- Disturbed sleep pattern related to frequent need to empty bladder during night
- Risk for fetal injury related to maternal cigarette smoking

Outcome Identification and Planning

When establishing goals and outcomes, be certain that plans are realistic for a woman's situation and family lifestyle. Try to turn long-term goals into more manageable, short-term ones if possible. For example, a goal of reducing smoking during pregnancy may be more realistic than a goal of stopping smoking forever. Eliminating the pressure of making a major permanent lifestyle change can help a woman concentrate her efforts on herself and her fetus over the next several months. Continued reinforcement of her progress could then help her to continue reducing the number of cigarettes smoked or to quit smoking altogether after the baby is born so she can provide a smoke-free environment for her child. Similarly, you cannot set a goal for a woman to be free of the nausea of early pregnancy. The best you can expect to accomplish is to be certain that she maintains good nutrition and adequate weight gain in the face of it. Nor can you do much about the frequency of urination, backache, or fatigue that occur with pregnancy except to help a woman adapt her lifestyle to these symptoms (e.g., encourage her to drink more liquids during the day and less in the early evening; schedule regular rest periods when possible).

Often, helping a woman plan to avoid teratogens is difficult because a total change in lifestyle, such as not smoking, not drinking alcohol, or changing a work environment, may be involved. Fortunately, most women are highly motivated to have a healthy baby. With this level of motivation, planning the best route to achieve a goal becomes the focus rather than educating about the need for goal achievement. Information on specific teratogenic chemicals can be obtained from the National Institute for Occupational Safety and Health (NIOSH) (http://www.cdc.gov/NIOSH). The March of Dimes has a good site for questions about prenatal care in general (http://www.marchofdimes.com).

Implementation

The major intervention associated with health promotion during pregnancy is education. Although the average woman is aware that some discomforts may occur, these discomforts may seem extreme when they are happening to her. Often, adolescent girls are uninformed about the common discomforts of pregnancy because they lack a set of peers with pregnancy experience. Even one who knows that it is normal for breast tenderness to occur during pregnancy may not be sure that the amount of breast tenderness she is having is normal. A woman who had a mental image of herself as someone who would not gain much weight during pregnancy may be very concerned because she is, in fact, gaining a great deal of weight.

It is crucial to all teaching to be certain all women understand that they should double-check with their primary care provider before taking any nonessential medication during pregnancy. Other important interventions include good role modeling, such as not smoking in prenatal settings, and exhibiting a healthy lifestyle through adequate nutrition and exercise.

Cultural beliefs play a large role in how teaching is structured. Teaching can be challenging if a woman has limited English proficiency. Women from cultures that view pregnancy as a wellness state may not seek care because they do not view pregnancy as a time when medical intervention is necessary. Other women may be extremely modest and avoid health visits because they find pelvic examinations difficult, intrusive, and embarrassing. Some women may rely on herbs and folk remedies to manage the common discomforts of pregnancy, so they do not feel a need for medical management. This variety of cultural backgrounds makes individualized assessment and education mandatory.

Implementing prenatal care to meet the needs of all of the different cultures represented in the United States may include furnishing interpreters to aid in communication, providing classes in prenatal health, explaining how health-promotion regimens fit with women's cultural belief systems, and maintaining an attitude of advocacy to help women adjust to a formal health care system.

When planning teaching strategies, a woman's receptiveness to instruction is key. Regardless of how excited and pleased a woman is about being pregnant, she can assimilate only so much information at one particular time. Therefore, be selective about the health information you provide and include those points most relevant to the individual woman. For example, you would want to discuss varicosity prevention more for a woman with a history of varicosities in a former pregnancy than for one who is pregnant for the first time and is very athletic. Keep in mind that the health measures being taught must be maintained for an extended time—40 weeks. To help a woman follow changes this long, choose priorities and make health advice meaningful and individualized.

Remember that a basic tenet of teaching and learning is that learning is enhanced when the information has direct application to that person. This principle means that devising a plan that spaces out health-promotion and health-maintenance information based on the changes associated with early and late pregnancy is most helpful. Teach those measures that are immediately applicable first; those that have relevance only toward the end of pregnancy can be taught then.

Outcome Evaluation

Evaluation is an ongoing process at prenatal health care visits. Expected outcomes developed with a woman at one prenatal visit need to be assessed at the next. Examples of outcomes are:

- Client states measures she will use to manage the common discomforts of pregnancy.
- Client reports resting for one half-hour twice a day.
- Client verbalizes positive statements about her appearance.
- Client and her partner both state they have stopped smoking.
- Client documents by use of a pedometer that she walks the length of a city block daily.

HEALTH PROMOTION DURING PREGNANCY

Health promotion during pregnancy begins with reviewing aspects of self-care.

Self-Care Needs

Because pregnancy is not an illness, few special care measures other than common sense about self-care are required. Many women, however, have heard different warnings about what they should or should not do during pregnancy, so they may need some help separating fact from fiction so that they can enjoy their pregnancy unhampered by unnecessary restrictions. In no other area of nursing, except possibly infant feeding, does there seem to be as many misconceptions or inappropriate information available to women.

Bathing

At one time, tub baths were restricted during pregnancy because it was feared that bath water would enter the vagina and cervix and contaminate the uterine contents. Further, it was believed that hot water touching the abdomen might initiate labor. Because the vagina normally is in a closed position, however, the danger of tub bath water entering the cervix is minimal. During pregnancy, sweating tends to increase because a woman excretes waste products for herself and a fetus. She also has an increase in vaginal discharge. For these reasons, daily tub baths or showers are now recommended. Women should not soak for long periods in extremely hot water or hot tubs as heat exposure for a lengthy time could lead to hyperthermia in the fetus (Crombleholme, 2009).

As pregnancy advances, a woman may have difficulty maintaining her balance when getting in and out of a bathtub. If so, she should change to showering or sponge bathing for her own safety. If membranes rupture or vaginal bleeding is present, tub baths are contraindicated because then there might be a danger of contamination of uterine contents. During the last month of pregnancy, when the cervix may begin to dilate, some health care providers restrict tub bathing for the same reason.

Breast Care

A few precautions during pregnancy are helpful to prevent breast discomfort (Graham, 2007). A general rule is for a woman to wear a firm, supportive bra with wide straps to spread breast weight across the shoulders. A woman may need to buy a larger bra halfway through pregnancy to accommodate her increasing breast size. If she plans on breastfeeding her newborn, she might choose bras suitable for breastfeeding so she can continue to use them after the baby's birth.

At about the 16th week of pregnancy, colostrum secretion begins in the breasts. The sensation of a fluid discharge from the breasts can be frightening unless a woman is cautioned that this is a possibility. Teach her to wash her breasts with clear tap water (no soap, because that could be drying and cause nipples to crack) daily to remove the colostrum and reduce the risk of infection. Afterward, she should dry her nipples well by patting them with a soft towel.

If colostrum secretion is profuse, a woman may need to place gauze squares or breast pads inside her bra, changing them frequently to maintain dryness. Constant moisture next to the breast nipple can cause nipple excoriation, pain, and fissuring.

Dental Care

Gingival tissue tends to hypertrophy during pregnancy. Unless a pregnant woman brushes her teeth well, pockets of plaque form readily between the enlarged gumline and teeth. In addition to stressing brushing, encourage pregnant women to see their dentists regularly for routine examination and cleaning because 9 months is a long time to be without preventive dental care. Remind women that x-ray examinations are often included as a part of routine dental health. A pregnant woman may want to consider delaying these until after her baby is born. In the few instances when x-ray examinations are necessary for dental health, they can be done safely as long as a woman's abdomen is shielded with a lead apron.

Tooth decay occurs from the action of bacteria on sugar. This action lowers the pH of the mouth, creating an acid medium that leads to etching or destruction of the enamel of teeth. Encourage women to snack on nutritious foods, such as fresh fruits and vegetables (e.g., apples and carrots), to avoid sugar coming in contact with their teeth. If a woman has trouble avoiding sweet snacks such as candy, suggest eating sweet snacks that dissolve easily (like a chocolate bar) rather than one that remains in the mouth a long time (like chewy candy). This helps to minimize the level of sugar in the mouth and long-term contact with teeth.

Perineal Hygiene

Most women have an increased vaginal discharge during pregnancy and may desire to cleanse with a douche. Douching is contraindicated during pregnancy. The force of the irrigating fluid could cause it to enter the cervix and lead to infection. In addition, douching alters the pH of the vagina, leading to an increased risk of bacterial growth (Bernstein & Weinstein, 2007).

Clothing

Women have a multitude of clothing options to wear during a pregnancy. Recommend loose-fitting, comfortable garments.

Caution women to avoid tight-fitting items such as garters, girdles with panty legs, and knee-high stockings during pregnancy. These items impede lower-extremity circulation. Suggest wearing shoes with a moderate to low heel to minimize pelvic tilt and possible backache. Otherwise, the rules are common sense and comfort.

Sexual Activity

Some women are embarrassed to ask questions about sexual relations during pregnancy. However, most women are concerned about whether sexual intercourse should be restricted. Many need information to refute some of the myths about sexual relations in pregnancy that still exist, such as:

- Coitus on the expected date of her period will initiate labor.
- Orgasm will initiate preterm labor, but participating in sexual relations without orgasm will not.
- Coitus during the fertile days of a cycle will cause a second pregnancy or twins.
- Coitus might cause rupture of the membranes.

None of the above are true. Asking a woman at a prenatal visit if she has any questions about sexual activity allows her to voice such concerns (Box 12.3). By dispelling these myths, you allow a woman to feel more comfortable and secure that coitus is not harming her child.

There are a few situations when sexual relations during a pregnancy are contraindicated. Women with a history of spontaneous miscarriage may be advised to avoid coitus during the time of the pregnancy when a previous miscarriage occurred. Women whose membranes have ruptured or who have vaginal spotting should be advised against coitus until examined to prevent possible infection. Advise caution about male oral–female genital contact, because accidental air embolism has been reported from this act during pregnancy or following birth from air entering open or fragile uterine arteries (Truhlar et al., 2007). Otherwise, there are no sexual restrictions during pregnancy.

Early in pregnancy, a woman may experience a decreased desire for coitus resulting from the increased estrogen level in her body. Breast tenderness may limit a usual pattern of sexual arousal. As pelvic congestion increases from the additional uterine blood supply, most women notice increased clitoral sensation. Some women may experience orgasm for the first time during pregnancy because of this increased pelvic congestion. As pregnancy advances and a woman's abdomen increases in size, she and her sexual partner may need to use new positions for intercourse. A side-by-side position or a woman in a superior position may be more comfortable. As vaginal secretions change, a woman may find a water-soluble lubricant helpful. If she begins to experience discomfort from penile penetration, mutual masturbation or female oral–male genital relations might be satisfying to both partners. Caution women with a nonmonogamous sexual partner that the partner needs to use a condom to prevent transmission of a sexually transmitted infection during pregnancy (Katsufrakis & Workowski, 2008). Women may use female condoms throughout pregnancy.

BOX 12.3 * Focus on Communication

Julberry Adams is 4 months pregnant and no longer lives with the father of her baby.

Less Effective Communication

Nurse: Do you have any questions, Mrs. Adams?
Julberry: I'm not Mrs. Adams.
Nurse: I'm sorry, Ms. Adams. Do you have any questions?
Julberry: How long into pregnancy can I have sex?
Nurse: Well, since you're single, you don't really need that kind of advice. Let's talk about exercise and nutrition instead.

More Effective Communication

Nurse: Do you have any questions, Mrs. Adams?
Julberry: I'm not Mrs. Adams.
Nurse: I'm sorry, Ms. Adams. Do you have any questions?
Julberry: How long into pregnancy can I have sex?
Nurse: Basically, as long as you're comfortable and you don't have any complications.
Julberry: Good. My new boyfriend made me promise to ask today.

Health teaching is an art separate from teaching morality. In the first scenario, the nurse cuts off communication by making a judgment to supply only information that the nurse thinks that her client needs. In the second scenario, the nurse actively listens to the client, focuses on her needs and concerns, and supplies the information the client has requested.

✔ Checkpoint Question 12.1

Which statement by Julberry Adams would alert you that she needs more teaching about self-care practices during pregnancy?

a. "I take either a shower or tub bath, because I know both are safe."
b. "I wash my breasts with clear water, not with soap, every day."
c. "I'm glad I don't have to ask my boyfriend to use condoms anymore."
d. "I'm wearing low-heeled shoes to try to avoid backache."

Exercise

Extreme exercise has been associated with lower birth weight but moderate exercise is healthy during pregnancy. It can help prevent circulatory stasis in the lower extremities. It also can offer a general feeling of well-being. For some women, teaching about exercise focuses on helping them realize the need for exercise and urging them to get enough. Others may need to be cautioned to restrict exercise or participation in contact sports.

The average, well-nourished women should exercise during pregnancy a minimum of 3 times weekly for 30 consecutive minutes (Rojas, Wood, & Blakemore, 2007). An exercise program should consist of 5 minutes of warm-up exercises, an active "stimulus" phase of 20 minutes, and then 5 minutes of cool-down exercises. The type of activity chosen depends on a woman's interests. Exercises that involve large muscle groups rhythmically, such as walking, are best. The intensity of the exercise program depends on a woman's cardiopulmonary fitness. Before she begins any exercise program, make sure a woman has consulted her physician or nurse-midwife. Women who know they have an incompetent cervix or have had cerclage to correct this and women who develop any complication of pregnancy such as bleeding, PIH, preterm rupture of membranes, or preterm labor or whose fetus is growth restricted should check with their primary health care provider before beginning or continuing an exercise program.

Both pregnant and nonpregnant women should exercise at 70% to 85% of their maximum heart rate. The easiest way to calculate this is to subtract a woman's age from 220, then multiply this by 70% or 85%. For example, during exercise a 23-year-old woman should have a pulse range of 137 to 167 (220 minus 23 times 70% and 85%, respectively). For a woman of 35, this target range would be 129 to 157.

Teach women how to assess quickly if they are exercising too strenuously by self-evaluating their ability to continue talking while exercising. If a woman is too short of breath to do this, she is exercising beyond her target heart rate.

In additional to being healthy during pregnancy, a planned exercise program may have long-term benefits such as:

- Lowering cholesterol level
- Reducing risk of osteoporosis
- Increasing energy level
- Maintaining a healthy body weight
- Decreasing risk of heart disease
- Increasing self-esteem and well-being

As a rule, a woman can continue any sport she participated in before pregnancy unless it was one that involved body contact, such as soccer. If a woman is a competent horsewoman, for example, there is little reason for her to discontinue riding until it becomes uncomfortable. Pregnancy is not the time to learn to ride, however, because a beginning rider is at greater risk for being thrown than is an experienced rider. The same principles apply to skiing and bicycling. An accomplished skier or bicyclist may continue the activity in moderation until balance becomes a problem. Pregnancy is not the time to learn to ski or ride a bicycle, however, because the lack of skill could result in many falls.

Walking is the best exercise during pregnancy, and women should be encouraged to take a walk daily unless inclement weather, many levels of stairs, or an unsafe neighborhood are contraindications (Box 12.4). Jogging, in contrast, is questioned because of the strain that the extra weight of pregnancy places on the knees. Late in pregnancy, jogging can cause pelvic pain from relaxed symphysis pubis movement. A high-impact aerobics program is also contraindicated because this can be strenuous on both pelvic and knee joints (Kramer & McDonald, 2007).

Swimming is a good activity for pregnant women and, like bathing, is not contraindicated as long as the membranes are intact. It may help relieve backache during pregnancy (Young & Jewell, 2009). Diving or long-distance swimming or any other activity carried out to a point of extreme fatigue should be avoided. Epidemiologic studies suggest that an elevation of maternal body temperature by 2° C for at least 24 hours can cause a range of developmental defects, but there is little information on thresholds for shorter exposures. Use of hot tubs and saunas after workouts longer than 15 minutes is contraindicated, however, on the chance these could raise the internal fetal temperature. General guidelines for exercise during pregnancy are highlighted in Box 12.5.

BOX 12.4 ✻ Focus on Evidence-Based Practice

Can a telephone call stimulate women to exercise more?

All women need to exercise during pregnancy, but doing this may be more difficult for women living in rural than urban areas as they have less access to classes or facilities for exercise. To investigate whether a simple telephone call could motivate rural adults to increase their activity level, nurse researchers divided into two research groups 86 physically inactive adults living in rural communities who stated that they were ready to increase physical activity during the next 6 months. The first group, or study group, received a pedometer and monthly exercise motivational telephone calls over the next 6 months. The second group, or control group, received an equal number of telephone calls but without exercise motivational content. How much physical activity the participants engaged in was measured by self-reports. Results showed that participants in the study group improved in self-efficacy toward exercise but not in the actual amount of physical exercise they undertook.

Would the results of this study be useful when counseling pregnant women about exercise in pregnancy? Does it suggest that motivating women to exercise is not an easily solved problem?

Source: Bennett, J. A., et al. (2008). A telephone-only motivational intervention to increase physical activity in rural adults: a randomized controlled trial. *Nursing Research, 57*(1), 24–32.

Sleep

The optimal condition for body growth occurs when growth hormone secretion is at its highest level—that is, during sleep. This, plus the overall increased metabolic demand of pregnancy, appears to be the physiologic reason that pregnant women need an increased amount of sleep or at least need rest to build new body cells during pregnancy.

Pregnant women rarely have difficulty falling asleep at night because of this increased physiologic need for sleep. If a woman has trouble falling asleep, drinking a glass of warm milk may help. Relaxation exercises (lying quietly, systematically relaxing neck muscles, shoulder muscles, arm muscles, and so on) also may be effective.

Late in pregnancy, a woman often finds herself awakened from sleep at short, frequent intervals by the activity of her fetus. Frequent waking this way leads to loss of rapid eye movement (REM) sleep. This can cause a woman to feel anxious or not well rested, although she has slept her usual number of hours. Pyrosis (heartburn) or dyspnea (shortness of breath) also can cause her to come awake, especially if she has been lying flat. In this instance, sleeping with two pillows or on a couch with an armrest may be helpful.

To obtain enough sleep and rest during pregnancy, most pregnant women need a rest period during the afternoon as well as a full night of sleep. A good resting or sleeping

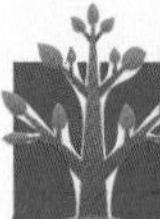

BOX 12.5 ✻ Focus on Family Teaching

Guidelines for Exercise in Pregnancy

Q. Julberry Adams asks you, "Now that I'm pregnant, can I still do aerobic exercises?"

A. Use the following recommendations as guidelines for exercising while you're pregnant:

1. Perform regular exercise (about three times per week) rather than engaging in intermittent activity.
2. Do not perform vigorous exercise in hot, humid weather or if you have a fever to avoid overexerting yourself or developing hyperthermia.
3. Avoid activities that require jumping, jarring motions, or rapid changes in direction such as jogging, because your joints may be unstable.
4. Exercise on a wooden floor or a tightly carpeted surface to reduce shock to the abdomen or knees and provide a sure footing.
5. To avoid muscle cramping, avoid exercises and motions that involve deep flexion or joint extension, such as stretching with the toes extended.
6. Always start your exercise program by warming up for approximately 5 minutes with activities such as slow walking or stationary cycling with low resistance.
7. End your exercise program with a period of gradually declining activity that includes gentle, stationary stretching. Because of the increased risk of joint injury, do not stretch to the point of maximum resistance.
8. Measure your heart rate at times of peak activity. Talk with your primary care provider about target heart rate and limits, and do not exceed them.
9. When getting up from lying on the floor, do so gradually to prevent dramatic blood pressure changes or stretching of the round ligament that can lead to sharp abdominal pain.
10. Drink liquids liberally before and after exercise to prevent dehydration. If necessary, interrupt your activity to replenish fluids.
11. If you were sedentary before pregnancy, begin your exercise program with physical activity of very low intensity and advance your activity level gradually.
12. Stop any activity and contact your primary care provider if any unusual symptoms appear.
13. Perform strenuous activities for no longer than 20 minutes.
14. To prevent supine hypotension do not exercise in the supine position (lying down flat) after the fourth month of pregnancy.
15. Avoid exercises that employ a Valsalva maneuver (holding your breath, bearing down) because these actions decrease blood supply to the fetus.
16. Make sure your caloric intake is adequate to meet not only the extra energy needs of pregnancy but also those of the exercise performed.

position is a modified **Sims' position,** with the top leg forward (Fig. 12.1). This position puts the weight of the fetus on the bed, not on the woman, and allows good circulation in lower extremities.

Be certain a woman knows to avoid resting on her back, as supine hypotension syndrome (faintness, diaphoresis, and hypotension from the pressure of the expanding uterus on the inferior vena cava) can develop in this position. Also be certain she knows not to rest with her knees sharply bent either when sitting or lying down, because of the increased risk of venous stasis this causes below the knee.

Employment

Changes in public assistance laws that encourage women to seek employment have led to more women working during pregnancy than ever before. Unless a woman's job involves exposure to toxic substances, lifting heavy objects, other kinds of excessive physical strain, long periods of standing or sitting, or having to maintain body balance, there are few reasons a woman cannot continue to work throughout pregnancy (Bonzini, Coggon, & Palmer, 2007). Women who are unable to continue work are protected from loss of employment benefits during pregnancy by federal law (Public Law 95-555). However, this law does not cover women who work for companies with fewer than 15 employees.

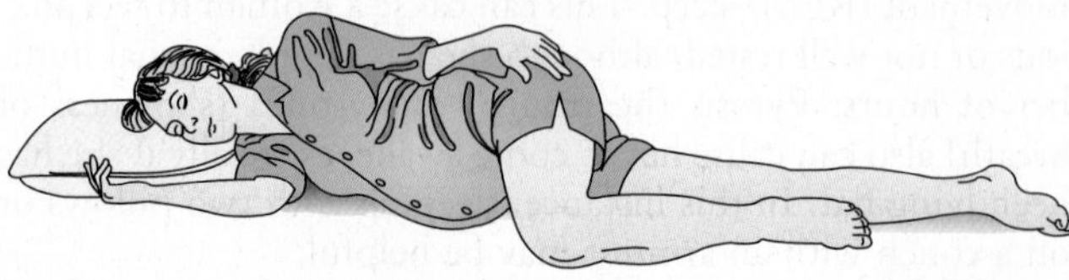

FIGURE 12.1 A modified Sims' position is a good rest position during pregnancy. Notice that the weight of the fetus rests on the bed.

According to this law, an employer cannot:

- Deprive women of seniority rights, in pay or promotion, because they take a maternity leave
- Treat women returning from maternity leave as new hires, starting over on the eligibility period for pension and other benefits
- Force pregnant women to leave if they are able to and want to continue working
- Refuse to hire women just because they are pregnant or fire them for the same reason
- Refuse to cover employees' normal pregnancy and birth expenses in the company health plan or pay less for pregnancy than for other medical conditions
- Refuse to pay sick leave or disability benefits to women whose difficult pregnancies keep them off the job

Passed in 1993, the Family and Medical Leave Act, another federal law, guarantees women the right to 12 weeks of unpaid, job-protected leave for the birth of a child, the adoption of or foster placement of a child, when a woman is needed to care for a parent, spouse, or child with a serious health condition, or because of a serious personal health condition (29 CFR 825.11). Specifically mentioned in this law is any period of incapacity because of pregnancy or for prenatal care. Families need to be educated about this important law because many women are still not aware that they can take time off from work during pregnancy or spend time with a new baby without penalty of losing their job. Additional women may be able to qualify for provisions under the Americans With Disabilities Act.

Some occupations are hazardous during pregnancy and should be discontinued because they bring women into contact with harmful substances. For example, nurses working with anesthetic gases in operating rooms or dental offices are reported to have a higher incidence of spontaneous miscarriage and, possibly, congenital anomalies in children than nurses working in other locales, probably because of exposure to nitrous oxide (National Institute of Occupational Safety and Health, 2007). Nurses working with chemotherapy agents are also at risk. They should wear gloves to protect themselves from exposure to these drugs, which are possibly teratogenic. Ribavirin (Virazole), an antibiotic used to treat respiratory syncytial infections, is also apparently teratogenic if inhaled by health care providers (Karch, 2009).

Other problems that can occur with employment include interference with adequate rest and nutrition. Urge a woman who works outside her home to put her feet up and rest when performing tasks that can be done in that position. Review what she eats at fast-food restaurants or packs for herself to be certain she plans ways to make this type of lunch as nutritious as if she were eating at home.

Remember, most women work to augment or supply the family income, not for fun. Even those who could afford to leave their jobs may not be willing to sacrifice the collegial relationships and sense of fulfillment derived from work, or the lifestyle their income has allowed them to enjoy. Counseling them to reserve periods during the day for rest and to eat a healthy diet is more effective than suggesting they resign from their jobs during pregnancy to get more rest (Box 12.6).

BOX 12.6 * Focus on Family Teaching

Guidelines for Pregnant Women Working Outside their Home

Q. Julberry Adams asks you, "Now that I'm pregnant, can I continue to work at the art gallery?"

A. Use the following suggestions as guidelines for safe pregnancy work practices:

- Plan rest periods during your break periods rather than running errands, etc.
- Try to use at least part of your lunch hour to rest. Lie on your left side in a break room if possible. If this is not possible, then rest sitting with your legs elevated.
- If your job involves long periods of standing, think of times you could stop and elevate your legs (working in a low file drawer, reading time in a classroom, etc.).
- Walk around periodically to avoid prolonged standing or sitting in one position if possible; stretch your back periodically to avoid backache.
- Wear support hose to improve venous return to your lower extremities.
- Avoid excessive overtime or working longer than 8-hour shifts.
- Empty your bladder every 2 hours to help prevent bladder infection.
- Get extra rest on weekends or days off.
- Take great caution when working around equipment that requires good balance. Avoid ladders or climbing late in pregnancy, when balance can be a problem.
- Learn your target heart rate for exercise. If your job involves strenuous exercise, stop and rest at the point your target heart rate is exceeded.
- Be sure you are not relying on fast foods for lunch. Take time to pack or purchase nutritious foods.

✔ Checkpoint Question 12.2

Julberry Adams describes her typical day to you. What would alert you that she may need further pregnancy advice?

a. "I jog rather than walk to get an increased amount of exercise."
b. "I always go to sleep on my side, not on my back."
c. "I pack a lunch every day so I know I won't eat junk food."
d. "I walk around my desk every hour to help leg circulation."

Travel

Because we live in a mobile society, many women have questions about travel during pregnancy (McGovern, Boyce, & Fischer, 2007). Early in a normal pregnancy, there are no restrictions. If a woman is susceptible to motion sickness, advise her not to take any medication for this unless it is specifically prescribed or approved by her physician or nurse-midwife. Suggest that she use a "sea-sick" wrist or acupuncture band instead. Late in pregnancy, travel plans should take into consideration the possibility of early labor, requiring birth at a strange setting where a woman's obstetric history will be unknown.

Regardless of the month of her pregnancy, if a woman plans to spend time at a remote location, such as a campsite, be certain she knows the location of a nearby health care facility should an unexpected complication occur. Caution her not to eat uncooked fruits, vegetables, or meat or drink unpurified water at such sites. If she is going to be away from home for an extended time, she should make arrangements to visit a health care provider in that area so she can keep the schedule of her regular prenatal visits. Encourage her to make these plans far enough in advance so that her records can be copied and sent with her or be forwarded to the interim health care provider with her consent. Also, make sure she has enough of her prescribed vitamin supplement plus adequate prescriptions for refills as necessary.

Advise a woman who is taking a long trip by automobile to plan for frequent rest or stretch periods. Preferably every hour, but at least every 2 hours, she should get out of the car and walk a short distance. This break relieves stiffness and muscle aches and improves lower extremity circulation, helping prevent varicosities, hemorrhoids, and thrombophlebitis.

Pregnant women may drive automobiles as long as they fit comfortably behind the steering wheel. They should use seat belts like everyone else. Occasionally, uterine rupture has been reported from seat belt use, but overall evidence suggests that seat belts reduce mortality among pregnant women in car accidents, as they do for everyone (Rojas, Wood, and Blakemore, 2007). Both shoulder harnesses and lap belts should be used. The lap belt should be worn as snugly as comfortable so that it fits under the abdominal bulge and across the pelvic bones. The shoulder harness should be snug but comfortable, worn across the shoulder, chest, and upper abdomen. A pad may be placed under the shoulder harness at the neck to avoid chafing (Fig. 12.2).

Pregnancy is also a time for a family to think about transportation safety for the newborn. Purchasing a car seat is an investment that not only is legally required for transporting infants but also helps guarantee their safety. Families who cannot afford to purchase an infant car seat may want to ask friends or relatives about the possibility of borrowing one no longer needed. Many hospitals and local Red Cross chapters provide infant seats on a rental or loan basis for families who may find it difficult to obtain one in other ways. The American Academy of Pediatrics (AAP) recommends that when considering using a preowned car seat, parents should be certain that the car seat was not in a previous crash, has not been recalled, is not too old for use according to the manufacturer's instructions, has no cracks in the frame and no missing parts, and has a label from the manufacturer on the car seat along with instructions for use (AAP, 2009). One easy way to determine if a used car seat has been recalled is to check the web site http://www.odi.nhtsa.dotgov/cars/problems/recalls/childseat.cfm.

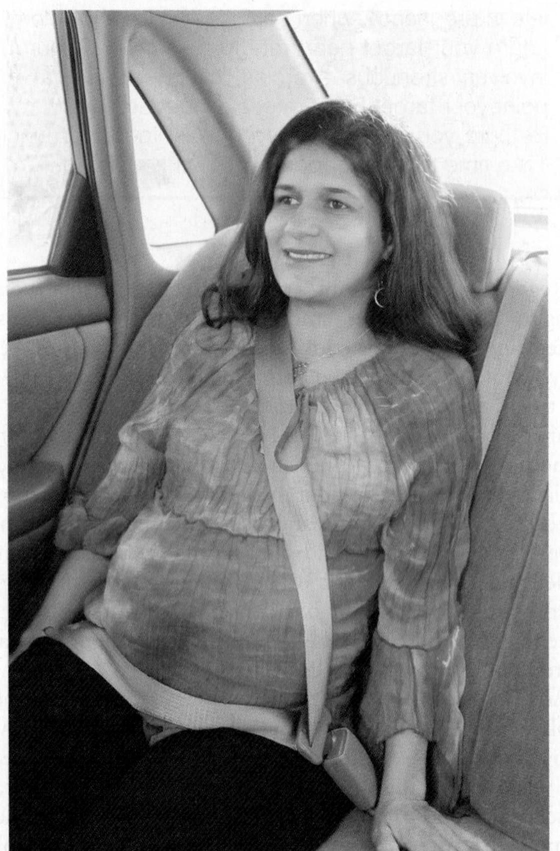

FIGURE 12.2 Encourage women to wear seatbelts during pregnancy. The bottom strap should cross beneath the abdomen.

Traveling by plane for women is not contraindicated during pregnancy as long as the plane has a well-pressurized cabin (true of commercial airlines but not of all small private planes) and a woman walks the length of the plane every hour to help prevent thrombophlebitis. Some airlines do not permit women who are more than 7 months pregnant to board; others require written permission from a woman's primary care provider. Advise a woman to investigate these restrictions by calling the airline or a travel agency before making such travel plans.

With businesses becoming global, more women than ever before are asked to travel internationally. Women who travel abroad may need additional immunizations, such as cholera vaccine, for entry into certain countries (McGovern, Boyce, and Fischer, 2007). All live virus vaccines (measles, mumps, rubella, and yellow fever) are contraindicated during pregnancy and should not be administered unless the risk of the disease outweighs the risk to the pregnancy. Before allowing any immunization during pregnancy, a woman should ask her primary care provider to verify it will be safe. Pregnancy does not alter indications for rabies vaccine because without the vaccine, a fatal disease could occur. Tetanus is also treated the same in pregnant women as in others.

What if... Julberry Adams tells you she usually drives to her parents' house for vacation but cannot this year because she no longer fits behind the wheel of her compact car. She asks you if it would be better for her to take the train or fly. How would you respond?

Discomforts of Early Pregnancy: The First Trimester

Early pregnancy symptoms can often cause discomfort in an expectant woman. Providing empathic and sound advice about measures to relieve these discomforts helps promote overall health and well-being. Although these symptoms are classified as minor, they may not seem minor to a woman who wakes up each morning feeling nauseated, wondering if she will ever feel like herself again. Also, each of these symptoms has the potential to lead to problems that are more serious.

Nursing Diagnoses and Related Interventions

Nursing Diagnosis: Health-seeking behaviors related to learning more about the minor discomforts of early pregnancy such as morning nausea

Outcome Evaluation: Client states she is familiar with early discomforts of pregnancy and will take measures to relieve them such as drinking ginger tea for nausea.

Most women will experience at least one minor discomfort of pregnancy. Because each woman's experience is unique, nursing diagnoses and care must be developed according to each woman's individual needs. Examples of nursing diagnoses that might be developed for women experiencing the discomforts of early pregnancy are:

- Health-seeking behaviors related to interest in using herbal remedies to relieve discomforts of pregnancy
- Constipation related to reduced peristalsis in pregnancy
- Fatigue related to increased physiologic need for sleep and rest during pregnancy
- Acute pain related to frequent muscle cramps secondary to physiologic changes of pregnancy
- Disturbed sleep pattern related to frequent need to empty bladder during night

Breast Tenderness

Breast tenderness is often one of the first symptoms noticed in early pregnancy; it may be most noticeable on exposure to cold air. For most women, the tenderness is minimal and transient, something they are aware of but not something that overly concerns them. If the tenderness is enough to cause discomfort, encourage a woman to wear a bra with a wide shoulder strap for support and to dress warmly to avoid cold drafts if cold increases symptoms. If actual pain exists, the presence of conditions such as nipple fissures or other explanations for the pain, such as breast abscess, need to be ruled out.

Palmar Erythema

Palmar erythema, or palmar pruritus, occurs in early pregnancy and is probably caused by increased estrogen levels. Constant redness or itching of the palms can make a woman believe she has developed an allergy. Explain that this type of itching in early pregnancy is normal before she spends time and effort trying different soaps or detergents or attempting to implicate certain foods she has eaten. Calamine lotion can be soothing. As soon as a woman's body adjusts to the increased level of estrogen, the erythema and pruritus disappear.

Constipation

As peristalsis slows and the weight of a growing uterus presses against the bowel, constipation can occur (Bernstein & Weinstein, 2007). Discuss preventive measures with a woman early in pregnancy to help her avoid this problem. Encourage her to evacuate her bowels regularly (many women neglect this first simple rule); increase the amount of fiber in her diet by eating raw fruits, bran, and vegetables; and to drink at least eight 8-oz glasses of water daily.

Some women find a prescribed oral iron supplement contributes to constipation. Reinforce the need for this supplement to build fetal iron stores. Help a woman find a method to relieve or prevent constipation other than omitting taking the supplement. Iron supplements are more rapidly absorbed on an empty stomach because iron is absorbed best from an acid medium. Women should take iron with juice rather than dairy products for this same reason.

Women should not use mineral oil to relieve constipation as it can absorb fat-soluble vitamins (A, D, K, and E), vitamins that are necessary for both good fetal and maternal health, and flush them out of the body.

Enemas also should be avoided because their action might initiate labor. Over-the-counter laxatives are also contraindicated, as are all nonessential drugs during pregnancy unless specifically prescribed or sanctioned by a woman's physician or nurse-midwife. If dietary measures and attempts at regular bowel evacuation fail, a stool softener, such as docusate sodium (Colace), or evacuation suppositories, such as glycerin, may be prescribed. Some women have extensive flatulence accompanying constipation. Recommend avoiding gas-forming foods, such as cabbage or beans, to help control this problem.

Nausea, Vomiting, and Pyrosis

At least half of pregnant women experience other gastrointestinal symptoms such as nausea, vomiting, and pyrosis (heartburn). Because these symptoms also interfere with nutrition, they are discussed in Chapter 13.

Fatigue

Fatigue is extremely common in early pregnancy, probably because of increased metabolic requirements. Much of it can be relieved by increasing the amount of rest and sleep. Some women, however, are reluctant to take time out of their day for rest. They know that pregnancy is not an illness, and so they proceed as if nothing is happening to them. Rarely is there justification during a normal pregnancy for women to take extra days off from work because of their condition, but it is also unrealistic to proceed as if nothing is different. Fatigue can increase the amount of morning sickness a woman experiences. If she becomes too tired, she may not eat properly and nutrition can suffer. If she remains on her feet without at least one break during a day, the risk for varicosities and the danger of thromboembolic complications increase.

For all these reasons, ask women at prenatal visits whether they manage to have at least one short rest period every day. A woman who works outside her home at a job that requires her to be on her feet most of the day might use part of her lunch hour to sit with her feet elevated, such as on an adjoining chair (Fig. 12.3). After she returns home from work in the evening, she may need to modify her customary routine from typical activities such as cooking dinner or watching a child's soccer game to resting, then cooking dinner and going to the soccer game, or resting while her partner cooks

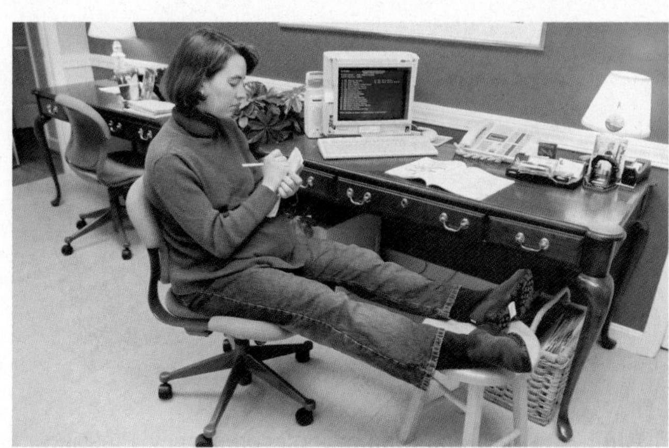

FIGURE 12.3 A "feet-up" break during a workday helps prevent ankle edema. (© Caroline Brown, RNC, MS, DEd.)

dinner (part of "we are having a baby at our house" for a partner who does not usually share in household chores). Women who work at sedentary jobs, inside or outside their home, may, in contrast, need to use this time to increase their activity, such as taking a walk or using a treadmill to ensure healthy lower extremity circulation.

Muscle Cramps

Decreased serum calcium levels, increased serum phosphorus levels, and, possibly, interference with circulation commonly cause muscle cramps of the lower extremities during pregnancy. This problem is best relieved if a woman lies on her back momentarily and extends her involved leg while keeping her knee straight and dorsiflexing the foot until the pain disappears (Fig. 12.4).

If a woman is experiencing frequent leg cramps, she may be advised to take magnesium citrate or aluminum hydroxide gel (Amphojel), which binds phosphorus in the intestinal tract and thereby lowers its circulating level. Lowering milk intake to only 1 pint daily and supplementing this with calcium lactate may also help to reduce the phosphorus level. Elevating lower extremities frequently during the day to improve circulation and avoiding full leg extension, such as stretching with the toes pointed, may also be helpful. Typically, muscle cramps are a minor symptom of pregnancy, but the pain is extreme and the intensity of the contraction can be frightening. Always ask at prenatal visits if this is a problem. Otherwise, women may not realize that cramping is pregnancy related and so fail to report it.

Pregnant women also have a higher incidence of "restless leg syndrome" (waking at night because of spontaneous leg movement) than nonpregnant women. This movement can be so annoying and frequent that women have difficulty sleeping (Smith & Tolson, 2008). Mirapex (pramipexole dihydrochloride), a drug frequently recommended for restless leg syndrome, should not be taken during pregnancy.

Hypotension

Supine hypotension is a symptom that occurs when a woman lies on her back and the uterus presses on the vena cava, impairing blood return to her heart. A woman experiences an irregular heart rate and a feeling of apprehension. The method of relieving the problem is simple: if a woman turns or is turned onto her side, pressure is removed from the vena cava, blood flow is restored, and the symptoms quickly fade. To prevent the syndrome, advise pregnant women to always rest or sleep on their side, not their back. If they can only fall asleep on their back, they should insert a small firm pillow under their right hip to cause the weight of their uterus to shift off their vena cava.

If a woman rises suddenly from a lying or sitting position or stands for an extended time in a warm or crowded area, she may faint from the same phenomenon (blood pooling in the pelvic area or lower extremities). Rising slowly and avoiding extended periods of standing prevent this problem. If a woman should feel faint, sitting with her head lowered—the same action as for any person who feels faint—alleviates the problem.

Varicosities

Varicosities, or the development of tortuous leg veins, are common in pregnancy because the weight of the distended uterus puts pressure on the veins returning blood from the lower extremities. This causes pooling of blood and distention of the vessels. The veins become engorged, inflamed, and painful. Although usually confined to the lower extremities, varicosities can extend up to and include the vulva. They occur most frequently in women with a family history of varicose veins and those who have a large fetus or a multiple pregnancy. Urge such women to take active measures to prevent varicosities beginning in early pregnancy; if left until the second trimester, the best they will be able to accomplish is relief of pain from already formed varicosities.

Resting in a Sims' position or on the back with the legs raised against the wall (a small firm pillow under their right hip) or elevated on a footstool for 15 to 20 minutes twice a day is a good precaution (Fig. 12.5). Caution women not to sit with their legs crossed or their knees bent and to avoid constrictive knee-high hose or garters.

Some women, especially those who developed varicosities during a previous pregnancy, may need elastic support stockings such as T.E.D. stockings for relief of varicosities in a second pregnancy. Urge a woman to put on support stockings before she arises in the morning as once she is on her feet, the

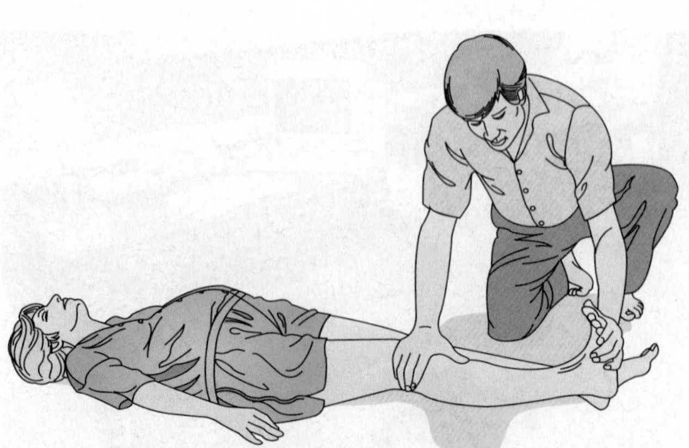

FIGURE 12.4 Relieving a leg cramp in pregnancy. Pressing down on the knee and pressing the toes backward (dorsiflexion) relieves most cramps. Here, a woman's partner helps.

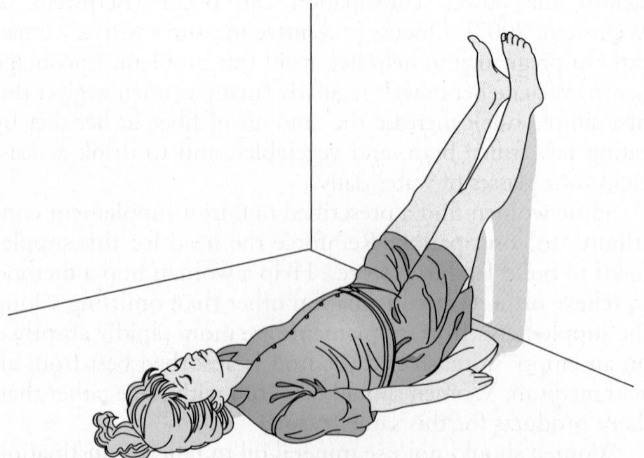

FIGURE 12.5 Position to relieve varicosities. The mother keeps a pad under her right hip to prevent supine hypotensive syndrome.

pooling of blood begins, and the stockings will be less effective. When applied properly, the stockings should reach an area above the point of distention. Be certain that a woman understands the stockings should be labeled "medical support hose." Many pantyhose manufacturers advertise their stockings as giving "firm support," and a woman may assume erroneously this is sufficient for her.

Because it stimulates venous return, exercise is as effective as rest periods for alleviating varicosities. Most women assume they do not need set exercise periods during pregnancy because they work hard at other activities. If they analyze the type of work they do, however, they may realize that a great deal of their work leads to venous stasis of the lower extremities. Women stand in one position to wash dishes, cook dinner, run a copying machine, defend a client in court, process a part on an assembly line, or teach a class. Sitting at a desk for prolonged periods of time with legs dependent also encourages venous stasis. Advise women to break up these long periods of sitting or standing with a "walk break" at least twice a day. As a rule, their families or fellow workers will benefit by accompanying them. Partners, especially, may discover that they, too, walk very little during their workday.

Vitamin C may be helpful in reducing the size of varicosities because it is necessary for the formation of blood vessel collagen and endothelium. Ask at prenatal visits if women include fresh fruit or juice in their diet every day.

Hemorrhoids

Hemorrhoids (varicosities of the rectal veins) occur commonly in pregnancy because of pressure on these veins from the bulk of the growing uterus (Quijano & Abalos, 2009). Daily bowel evacuation to relieve constipation and resting in a modified Sims' position daily are both helpful. At day's end, assuming a knee–chest position (Fig. 12.6) for 10 to 15 minutes is an excellent way to reduce the pressure on rectal veins. A knee–chest position may make a woman feel lightheaded initially. If this happens, she should remain in this position for only a few minutes at first, and then gradually increase the time until she can maintain the position comfortably for about 15 minutes. A stool softener such as docusate sodium (Colace) may be recommended for a woman who already has hemorrhoids. Applying witch hazel or cold compresses to external hemorrhoids can help relieve pain. Replacing hemorrhoids with gentle finger pressure can also be helpful. As with varicosities, think prevention, not just providing help for already established hemorrhoids.

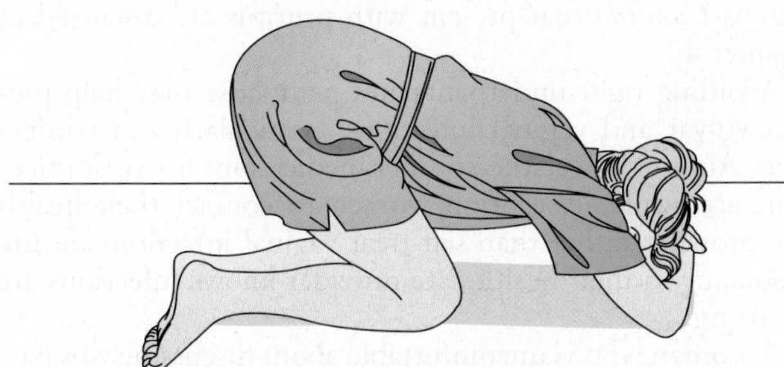

FIGURE 12.6 Knee–chest position. Because the weight of the uterus is shifted forward, this position promotes free flow of urine from the kidneys (preventing urinary tract stasis and infection) and better circulation in the rectal area (preventing hemorrhoids).

✔ Checkpoint Question 12.3

Julberry Adams tells you she is developing painful hemorrhoids. Advice you would give her would be:

a. "Take a tablespoon of mineral oil with each of your meals."
b. "Omit fiber from your diet. This will prevent constipation."
c. "Lie on your stomach daily to drain blood from rectal veins."
d. "Witch hazel pads feel cool against swollen hemorrhoids."

Heart Palpitations

On sudden movement, such as turning over in bed, a pregnant woman may experience a bounding palpitation of the heart. This is probably because of circulatory adjustments necessary to accommodate her increased blood supply during pregnancy. Although only momentary, the sensation can be frightening because the heart seems to skip a beat. It is reassuring for women to know that palpitations are normal and to be expected on occasion. Only if they occur very frequently or continuously or are accompanied by pain are they a concern and should be reported to a physician or nurse midwife. Gradual, slow movements help prevent this from happening so frequently.

Frequent Urination

Frequent urination occurs in early pregnancy because of the pressure of the growing uterus on the anterior bladder. The sensation may last for about 3 months, sometimes beginning as early as the first or second missed menstrual period, disappear in midpregnancy when the uterus rises above the bladder, and return again in late pregnancy as the fetal head presses against the bladder (Fig. 12.7).

When a woman describes frequency of urination, be certain this is the only urinary symptom she is experiencing. Ask her about any burning or pain on urination or whether she has noticed any blood in her urine, signs of urinary tract infection.

Women should not restrict their fluid intake to try to diminish frequency of urination, as fluids are necessary to allow their blood volume to double. Suggesting that a woman reduce the amount of caffeine she is drinking may be helpful. Most importantly, a woman needs to understand that voiding more frequently is a normal phenomenon. Unless a woman is cautioned that the sensation of frequency returns after lightening (the settling of the fetal head into the inlet of the pelvis at pregnancy's end), she may worry at that time that she has a urinary tract infection. Again, unless other symptoms are present, she can be assured this a normal finding.

Occasionally, a woman notices stress incontinence (involuntary loss of urine on coughing or sneezing) during pregnancy. Although this is largely unpreventable, doing Kegel exercises (alternately contracting and relaxing perineal muscles; Box 12.7) helps strengthen urinary control, directly strengthens perineal muscles for birth, and decreases the possibility of stress incontinence (Smith, 2007).

Abdominal Discomfort

Some women experience uncomfortable feelings of abdominal pressure early in pregnancy. Women with a multiple pregnancy may notice this throughout pregnancy. Typically, pregnant women stand with their arms crossed in front of

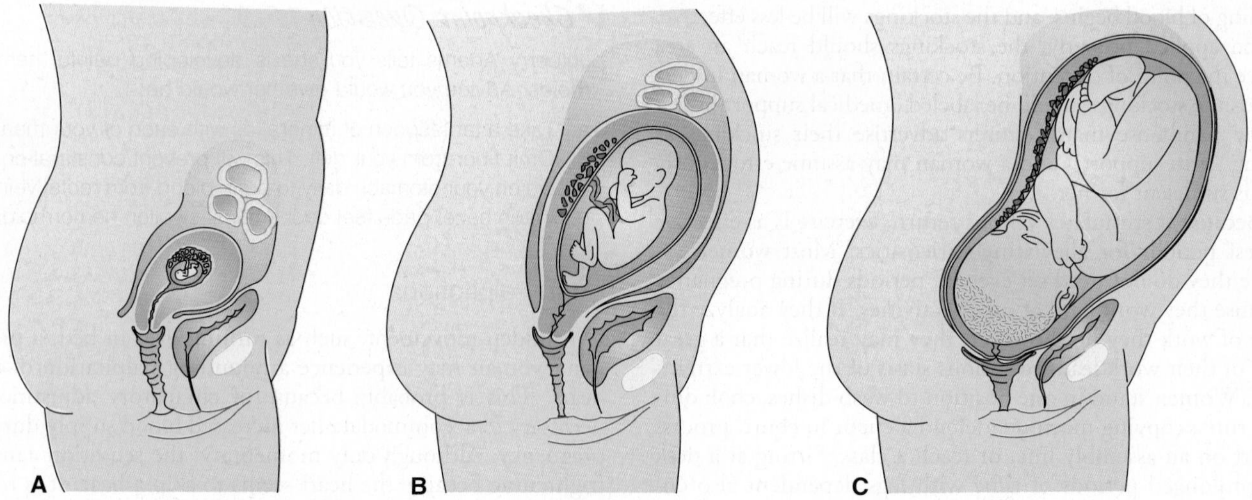

FIGURE 12.7 Bladder changes during pregnancy. (**A**) Early pregnancy: the uterus presses against the bladder, causing frequent urination. (**B**) Middle pregnancy: urinary frequency is relieved. (**C**) Late pregnancy: the uterus is again pressing on the bladder, leading to the recurrence of urinary frequency.

them because the weight of their arms resting on their abdomen relieves this discomfort.

When a woman stands up quickly, she may experience a pulling, sometimes sharp and frightening, pain in the right or left lower abdomen from tension on a round ligament. She can prevent this from happening by always rising slowly from a lying to a sitting, or from a sitting to a standing position.

BOX 12.7 ✻ Kegel Exercises

Kegel exercises are exercises designed to strengthen the pubococcygeal muscles. Each is a separate exercise and should be done about three times a day.

1. Squeeze the muscles surrounding the vagina as if stopping the flow of urine. Hold for 3 seconds. Relax. Repeat this sequence 10 times.
2. Contract and relax the muscles surrounding the vagina as rapidly as possible 10 to 25 times.
3. Imagine that you are sitting in a bathtub of water and squeeze muscles as if sucking water into the vagina. Hold for 3 seconds. Relax. Repeat this action 10 times.
4. Caution: Do not regularly start and stop the flow of urine during urination to try and strengthen muscles as this can lead to incomplete emptying of the bladder.

It may take as long as 6 weeks of exercise before pubococcygeal muscles are strengthened. In addition to strengthening urinary control and preventing stress incontinence, Kegel exercises can lead to increased sexual enjoyment because of the tightened vaginal muscles.

Because round ligament pain may simulate the abrupt pain that occurs with ruptured ectopic pregnancy, a woman's description of the pain must be evaluated carefully.

Leukorrhea

Leukorrhea, a whitish, viscous vaginal discharge or an increase in the amount of normal vaginal secretions, occurs in response to the high estrogen levels and the increased blood supply to the vaginal epithelium and cervix in pregnancy. A daily bath or shower to wash away accumulated secretions and prevent vulvar excoriation usually controls this problem. Wearing cotton underpants and sleeping at night without underwear can be helpful to reduce moisture and possible vulvar excoriation. Some women may need to wear a perineal pad to control the discharge. Caution women not to use tampons because this could lead to stasis of secretions and subsequent infection. Advise women to contact their physician or nurse-midwife if there is a change in the color, odor, or character of this discharge as these suggest infection.

A woman with vulvar pruritus needs evaluation because this strongly indicates infection. Be certain she is describing pruritus-like symptoms and is not describing burning on urination, a sign of an early bladder infection (which also needs therapy, but of a different type). Common vaginal infections such as *Candida* that present with pruritus are discussed in Chapter 47.

Avoiding tight underpants and pantyhose may help prevent vulvar and vaginal infections, particularly yeast infections. Although over-the-counter medications for yeast infections are available, caution women to contact their health care provider rather than self-treat vaginal infections during pregnancy so their health care provider knows infections are occurring.

A woman who is uncomfortable about discussing this part of her body or who associates vaginal infections with poor hygiene or sexually transmitted infection may be reluctant to mention an irritating vaginal discharge. At each prenatal visit, therefore, be sure to ask a woman specifically whether she is experiencing this problem.

What if... Julberry Adams tells you she has urinary frequency. She also reports a white vaginal discharge. How would you go about evaluating whether she is experiencing a normal discomfort of pregnancy or a urinary tract infection?

Discomforts of Middle to Late Pregnancy

At about the 20th to 24th weeks, the midpoint of pregnancy, a woman is usually ready for further health teaching that relates to the new developments that will occur in the latter half of pregnancy. As she starts to view the child within her as a separate person, she becomes interested in discussing and making plans for the signs and symptoms of beginning labor, birth, and the infant's care. The midpoint of a pregnancy is also a good time to describe the new minor symptoms that may occur and to review the precautionary measures to prevent constipation, varicosities, and hemorrhoids, as these increase in intensity late in pregnancy.

Nursing Diagnoses and Related Interventions

Nursing Diagnosis: Health-seeking behaviors related to learning more about the minor discomforts of late pregnancy such as Braxton Hicks contractions.

Outcome Evaluation: Client states that she feels confident in self-managing the minor discomforts of late pregnancy.

Examples of other possible nursing diagnoses associated with the discomforts of middle to late pregnancy are:

- Acute abdominal pain related to sudden postural change in position
- Anxiety related to shortness of breath resulting from expanding uterine pressure on diaphragm
- Deficient knowledge related to beginning signs of labor
- Pain related to almost constant backache

Backache

As pregnancy advances, a lumbar lordosis develops and postural changes necessary to maintain balance lead to backache. Wearing shoes with low to moderate heels reduces the amount of spinal curvature necessary to maintain an upright posture. Encouraging a woman to walk with her pelvis tilted forward (putting pelvic support under the weight of the fetus) is also helpful. In addition, applying local heat may aid in relieving backache.

To avoid back strain, advise women to squat rather than bend over to pick up objects. Also encourage them always to lift objects by holding them close to the body. For some women, a firmer mattress during this time may be required. Sliding a board under the mattress is a cost-effective alternative for achieving a firmer sleeping surface. Pelvic rocking or tilting, an exercise described in Chapter 14, also helps to prevent and relieve backache.

Backache can be an initial sign of a bladder or kidney infection. Obtaining a detailed account of a woman's symptoms is therefore crucial to ensure that she is describing only backache. Too often, women are observed at a prenatal visit only lying in a lithotomy position on an examining table. Always assess the manner in which a woman walks and what type of shoes she wears as she moves from a waiting room to an examining room to evaluate whether her posture or shoes could be a cause of backache.

Generally, acetaminophen (Tylenol) is considered to be safe and effective for relieving this type of pain during pregnancy. Acupuncture can also be effective (Young & Jewell, 2009). Caution women not to take herbal remedies, muscle relaxants, or analgesics (or any other medication) for back pain without first consulting their physician or nurse-midwife.

Headache

Many women experience headache during pregnancy, apparently from their expanding blood volume, which puts pressure on cerebral arteries. Trying to reduce any possible causative situations, such as eye strain or tension, may lessen the number of headaches they experience. Resting with cold towels on their forehead and taking usual adult doses of acetaminophen usually furnishes adequate relief. Although a few women who have migraine headaches find these worsen during pregnancy, most women notice considerable improvement with this type of headache during pregnancy (see Chapter 49). Caution women that if a headache is unusually intense or continuous, they should report it to their primary care provider. A continuous sharp headache may be a danger sign of high blood pressure during pregnancy.

Dyspnea

As the expanding uterus places pressure on the diaphragm, lung compression and shortness of breath result. A woman will notice this primarily at night if she lies flat. She also will definitely notice it on exertion. To relieve nighttime dyspnea, advise her to sleep with her head and chest elevated so the weight of the uterus falls away from her diaphragm. As pregnancy progresses, she may require two or more pillows to sleep at night to avoid the problem. Caution her to limit her activities during the day to prevent exertional dyspnea. Always question women about this important symptom at prenatal visits to be certain the sensation is not continuous, which describes more than usual involvement.

Ankle Edema

Most women experience some swelling of the ankles and feet during late pregnancy, most noticeably at the end of the day. Women are often first conscious of this when they kick off their shoes to rest and then cannot put them on again comfortably.

As long as proteinuria and hypertension are absent, ankle edema of this nature is a normal occurrence of pregnancy. It is probably caused by general fluid retention and reduced blood circulation in the lower extremities because of uterine pressure. This simple edema can be relieved best by resting in a left side-lying position because this increases the kidney's glomerular filtration rate and also allows good venous return. Sitting for half an hour in the afternoon and again in the evening with the legs elevated is also helpful. Caution women to avoid wearing constricting clothing such as panty girdles or knee-high stockings because these impede lower extremity circulation and venous return.

Some women need reassurance that ankle edema is normal during pregnancy. Otherwise, they worry that it is a beginning sign of PIH (Menzies et al., 2007). On the other hand, do not dismiss a report of lower extremity edema lightly until you are certain a woman does not exhibit any signs of proteinuria or edema of other, nondependent parts, or has had a sudden increase in weight indicative of PIH.

Braxton Hicks Contractions

Beginning as early as the 8th to 12th week of pregnancy, the uterus periodically contracts and then relaxes again (Cunningham et al., 2008). Early in pregnancy, these sensations, termed *Braxton Hicks contractions,* are not noticeable. By middle or late pregnancy, the contractions become stronger, and a woman who tenses at the sensation may even experience some minimal pain, similar to a hard menstrual cramp. Although these contractions are not a sign of beginning labor, women should inform their primary care provider about them so that they can be evaluated. A rhythmic pattern of even very light but persistent contractions could be a beginning sign of labor.

✔ Checkpoint Question 12.4

Julberry Adams has ankle edema by the end of each day. Which statement by her would reveal that she understands what causes this?

a. "I know this is a beginning complication; I'll call my doctor tonight."

b. "I understand this is from eating too much salt; I'll restrict that more."

c. "I'll rest in a Sims' position to take pressure off lower extremity veins."

d. "I know this is from gaining too much weight. I'll start to diet tomorrow."

PREVENTING FETAL EXPOSURE TO TERATOGENS

A *teratogen* is any factor, chemical or physical, that adversely affects the fertilized ovum, embryo, or fetus. At one time, it was assumed that a fetus in utero was protected from chemical or physical injury by the presence of the amniotic fluid and by the absence of any direct placental exchange between mother and fetus. When infants were born with disorders, it was attributed to the influence of fate, bad luck, or, in some cultures, evil spirits. Today, it is acknowledged that a fetus is extremely vulnerable to environmental injury. Although the causes of many anomalies occurring in utero are still unknown, many specific teratogenic factors have been isolated.

Effects of Teratogens on a Fetus

Several factors influence the amount of damage a teratogen can cause. The strength of the teratogen is one of these. For example, radiation is a known teratogen. In small amounts (everyone is exposed to some radiation every day, such as from sun rays), it causes no damage. However, in large doses (e.g., the amount of radiation necessary to treat cancer of the cervix), serious fetal defects or death can occur.

The timing of the teratogenic insult makes a significant impact on damage done to the fetus.. If a teratogen is introduced before implantation, either the zygote is destroyed or it appears unaffected. If the insult occurs when the main body systems are being formed (in the second to eighth weeks of embryonic life), a fetus is very vulnerable to injury. During the last trimester, the potential for harm again decreases because all the organs of a fetus are formed and are merely maturing. The times when different anatomic areas of a fetus are most likely to be affected by teratogens are shown in Figure 9.5.

Two exceptions to the rule that deformities usually occur in early embryonic life are the effects caused by the organisms of syphilis and toxoplasmosis. These two infections can cause abnormalities in organs that were originally formed normally.

A third factor determining the effects of a teratogen is the teratogen's affinity for specific tissue. Lead and mercury, for example, attack and disable nervous tissue. Thalidomide, a drug once used to relieve nausea in pregnancy, causes limb defects. Tetracycline, a common antibiotic, causes tooth enamel deficiencies and, possibly, long-bone deformities. The rubella virus can affect many organs: the eyes, ears, heart, and brain are the four most commonly attacked.

Nursing Diagnoses and Related Interventions

Nursing Diagnosis: Health-seeking behaviors related to learning more about teratogens that can affect fetal growth

Outcome Evaluation: Client states that she feels confident in monitoring her environment for the presence of possible teratogens.

Much of the health history information obtained at prenatal visits is taken to help determine if there is a possibility that a woman is being exposed to teratogens during her pregnancy. Examples of nursing diagnoses associated with maternal exposure to teratogens are:

- Health-seeking behavior related to mother's interest in avoiding exposure to substances she could contact at work that would be harmful to a fetus
- Risk for fetal injury related to lack of knowledge about teratogenicity of alcohol, drugs, and cigarettes
- Risk for fetal infection related to maternal transmission of genital herpes

Teratogenic Maternal Infections

Teratogenic maternal infections can involve either sexually transmitted or systemic infections. These organisms that cross the placenta can be viral, bacterial, or protozoan. Most infections important to a healthy pregnancy outcome cause relatively mild, flulike symptoms in a woman but can have much more serious effects on a fetus or newborn. Preventing and predicting fetal injury from infection is complicated because a disease may be subclinical (without any symptoms in the mother) and yet may injure a fetus.

Several diseases that are commonly known to cross the placenta and cause fetal harm are tested for and are described collectively under the umbrella term TORCH, an abbreviation for *to*xoplasmosis, *r*ubella, *c*ytomegalovirus, and *h*erpes simplex virus. Some laboratories spell the test as TORSCH to show that it includes *s*yphilis. Some sources identify the O with "*o*ther infections," which could include hepatitis B virus (HBV) and human immunodeficiency virus (HIV), illnesses discussed in Chapters 20 and 42. However it is spelled, the TORCH screen is an immunologic survey to determine whether common infections exist in either the pregnant woman (to identify fetal risk factors) or the newborn (to detect if antibodies against the common infectious teratogens are present). Although it is now known that many more than these original four or five maternal infections can cause harm to a fetus or newborn (a chlamydial or streptococcal B infection, for example, can cause pneumonia in the newborn [see Chapter 26]), the TORCH screen is still used extensively as it still provides a quick way to assess the potential risk of common teratogenic infections in pregnant women or newborns. In addition to TORCH screening, ask women if it is all right to screen them for human HIV as you must obtain consent for this test (Pratt, 2007).

Toxoplasmosis

Toxoplasmosis, a protozoan infection, is spread most commonly through contact with uncooked meat, although it may also be contracted through handling cat stool in soil or cat litter (Friars, 2007). A woman experiences almost no symptoms of the disease except for a few days of malaise and posterior cervical lymphadenopathy. Even in light of these mild symptoms, if the infection crosses the placenta, the infant may be born with central nervous system damage, hydrocephalus, microcephaly, intracerebral calcification, and retinal deformities. If the diagnosis is established by serum analysis during pregnancy, therapy with sulfonamides may be prescribed. However, the prevention of fetal deformities is uncertain, and sulfa may lead to increased bilirubin levels in the newborn. Pyrimethamine, an antiprotozoal agent, may also be used. This drug is an antifolic acid drug, so it is administered with caution early in pregnancy to prevent reducing folic acid levels.

As many as 1 in 900 pregnancies may be affected by toxoplasmosis. Prepregnancy serum analysis can be done to identify women who have never had the disease and so are susceptible (about 50% of women). Removing a cat from the home during pregnancy as a means of prevention is not necessary as long as the cat is healthy. On the other hand, taking in a new cat is unwise. Instruct pregnant women to avoid undercooked meat and also not to change a cat litter box or work in soil in an area where cats may defecate to avoid exposure to the disease.

Rubella

The rubella virus usually causes only a mild rash and mild systemic illness in a woman, but the teratogenic effects on a fetus can be devastating (Johnson & Ross, 2007). Fetal damage from maternal infection with rubella (German measles) includes hearing impairment, cognitive and motor challenges, cataracts, cardiac defects (most commonly patent ductus arteriosus and pulmonary stenosis), intrauterine growth restriction (IUGR), thrombocytopenic purpura, and dental and facial clefts, such as cleft lip and palate.

Typically, a rubella titer from a pregnant woman is obtained on the first prenatal visit. A titer greater than 1:8 suggests immunity to rubella. A titer of less than 1:8 suggests that a woman is susceptible to viral invasion. A titer that is greatly increased over a previous reading or is initially extremely high suggests that a recent infection has occurred.

A woman who is not immunized before pregnancy cannot be immunized during pregnancy because the vaccine uses a live virus that would have effects similar to those occurring with a subclinical case of rubella. After a rubella immunization, a woman is advised not to become pregnant for 3 months, until the rubella virus is no longer active. Immediately after a pregnancy, assess whether a woman with low rubella titers would like to be immunized to provide protection against rubella in future pregnancies (Johnson & Ross, 2007).

An increasing concern is women who demonstrate antibodies against rubella yet still become reinfected during pregnancy. Because of this, all pregnant women should avoid contact with children with rashes. Infants who are born to mothers who had rubella during pregnancy may be capable of transmitting the disease for a time after birth. Because of this, an infant may be isolated from other newborns during the newborn period. Be certain a woman is aware that her infant might infect others, including pregnant women. Nurses who care for pregnant women or newborns should receive immunization against rubella to ensure that they neither spread nor contract the disease.

Cytomegalovirus

Cytomegalovirus (CMV), a member of the herpes virus family, is another teratogen that can cause extensive damage to a fetus while causing few symptoms in a woman (Lilleri et al., 2007). It is transmitted from person to person by droplet infection such as occurs with sneezing. If a woman acquires a primary CMV infection during pregnancy and the virus crosses the placenta, the infant may be born severely neurologically challenged (hydrocephalus, microcephaly, spasticity) or with eye damage (optic atrophy, chorioretinitis), hearing impairment, or chronic liver disease. The child's skin may be covered with large petechiae ("blueberry-muffin" lesions). Because a woman has almost no symptoms, she may not be aware that she has contracted an infection. However, diagnosis in the mother or infant can be established by the isolation of CMV antibodies in blood serum. Unfortunately, there is no treatment for the infection even if it presents in the mother with enough symptoms to allow detection. Because there is no treatment or vaccine for the disease, routine screening for CMV during pregnancy is not recommended. Women can help prevent exposure by thorough handwashing before eating and avoiding crowds of young children at daycare or nursery settings.

Like herpes simplex, a primary CMV infection may become latent and then reactivate periodically. These recurrences are not thought to have a teratogenic effect on a fetus, but they can cause infection of a newborn during birth from genital secretions or postpartum from exposure to CMV-infected breast milk. CMV infection contracted at or shortly after birth this way is not associated with serious adverse effects except in babies of very low birth weight (1200 g).

Herpes Simplex Virus (Genital Herpes Infection)

The first time a woman contracts a genital herpes infection, systemic involvement occurs. The virus spreads into the bloodstream (viremia) and crosses the placenta to a fetus posing substantial fetal risk (ACOG, 2007).

If the infection takes place in the first trimester, severe congenital anomalies or spontaneous miscarriage may occur. If the infection occurs during the second or third trimester, there is a high incidence of premature birth, intrauterine growth restriction, and continuing infection of the newborn at birth. Unless recognized and treated, the fetal mortality and morbidity rates are as high as 80% (ACOG, 2007).

If a woman has had herpes simplex virus type 1 infections before the genital herpes invasion or if the genital herpes (type 2) infection is a recurrence, antibodies to the virus in her system prevent spread of the virus to a fetus across the placenta. If genital lesions are present at the time of birth, however, a fetus may contract the virus from direct exposure during birth. For women with a history of genital herpes and existing genital lesions, cesarean birth is often advised to reduce the risk of this route of infection. This awareness of the placental spread of herpes simplex virus has increased the importance of obtaining information about exposure to genital herpes or any painful perineal or vaginal lesions that might indicate this infection at prenatal visits.

Intravenous or oral acyclovir (Zovirax) can be administered to women during pregnancy (Karch, 2009). The primary mechanism for protecting a fetus, however, focuses on disease prevention. Urging women to practice safe sex is important to lessen their exposure to this and other sexually transmitted infections. Advising adolescents to obtain a vaccine against HPV (Gardasil) should lessen the incidence of genital herpes infection in the future.

Other Viral Diseases

It is difficult to demonstrate other viral teratogens, but rubeola (measles), coxsackievirus, infectious parotitis (mumps), varicella (chickenpox), poliomyelitis, influenza, and viral hepatitis all may be teratogenic. Parvovirus B19, the causative agent of erythema infectiosum (also called fifth disease), a common viral disease in school age children, if contracted during pregnancy, can cross the placenta and attack the red blood cells of a fetus. Infection with the virus during early pregnancy is associated with fetal death. If the infection occurs late in pregnancy, the infant may be born with severe anemia and congenital heart disease (Barankin, 2008).

Syphilis. Syphilis, a sexually transmitted infection, is of great concern for the maternal–fetal population despite the availability of accurate screening tests and proven medical treatment, as it is growing in incidence and places a fetus at risk for intrauterine or congenital syphilis (Walker, 2009). Early in pregnancy, when the cytotrophoblast layer of the chorionic villi is still intact, the causative spirochete of syphilis, *Treponema pallidum,* cannot cross the placenta and damage the fetus. When this layer atrophies at about the 16th to 18th week of pregnancy, however, the spirochete then can cross and cause extensive damage. If syphilis is detected and treated with an antibiotic such as benzathine penicillin in the first trimester, a fetus is rarely affected. If left untreated beyond the 18th week of gestation, hearing impairment, cognitive challenge, osteochondritis, and fetal death are possible.

For this reason, serologic screening (by either a VDRL or a rapid plasma reagin test) should be done at a first prenatal visit; the test may then be repeated again close to term (the 8th month) if exposure is a concern. Even when a woman has been treated with appropriate antibiotics, the serum titer remains high for more than 200 days; an increasing titer, however, suggests that reinfection has occurred. In an infant born to a woman with syphilis, the serologic test for syphilis may remain positive for up to 3 months even though the disease was treated during pregnancy.

The newborn with congenital syphilis may have congenital anomalies, extreme rhinitis (sniffles), and a characteristic syphilitic rash, all of which identify the baby as high risk at birth (Chakraborty & Luck, 2007). When the baby's primary teeth come in, they are oddly shaped (Hutchinson teeth). As the infant requires long-term follow-up, medical and nursing care of the newborn with congenital syphilis are discussed in Chapter 47.

Lyme Disease. Lyme disease, a multisystem disease caused by the spirochete *Borrelia burgdorferi,* is spread by the bite of a deer tick. The highest incidence occurs in the summer and early fall. The largest outbreaks of the disease are found on the east coast of the United States (Mullen, 2007). After a tick bite, a typical skin rash, *erythema chronicum migrans* (large, macular lesions with a clear center), develops. Pain in large joints such as the knee may develop. Infection in pregnancy can result in spontaneous miscarriage or severe congenital anomalies.

Women anticipating becoming pregnant or who are pregnant should avoid walking in areas such as wooded or tall grassy areas where they are apt to be bitten by ticks. If hiking in these areas, a woman should not use tick repellents containing diethyltoluamide because this ingredient is teratogenic. Instead, she should wear long, light-colored slacks tucked into her socks to prevent her legs from being exposed. To spread the spirochete, the tick must be present on the body possibly as long as 24 hours. After returning home from an outing, therefore, a woman should inspect her body carefully and immediately remove any ticks found. If she has any symptoms that suggest Lyme disease or knows she has been bitten, she should contact her primary health care provider immediately. Treatment of Lyme disease for pregnant women differs from that for nonpregnant women. The drugs used for nonpregnant adults, tetracycline and doxycycline, cannot be used during pregnancy because they cause tooth discoloration and, possibly, long-bone malformation in a fetus. A course of penicillin will be prescribed to reduce symptoms in the pregnant woman.

Because the symptoms of Lyme disease are chronic but not dramatic (a migratory rash and joint pain), women may not report them at a prenatal visit unless they are educated about their importance and are asked at prenatal visits if such symptoms are present.

Infections That Cause Illness at Birth. Several infections are not teratogenic to a fetus during pregnancy but are harmful if they are present at the time of birth. Gonorrhea, candidiasis, *Chlamydia, Streptococcus* B, and hepatitis B infections are examples of these. Chapters 26 and 43 discuss the effects of these infections on maternal, fetal, and neonatal health.

Potentially Teratogenic Vaccines

Live virus vaccines, such as measles, HPV, mumps, rubella, and poliomyelitis (Sabin type), are contraindicated during pregnancy because they may transmit the viral infection to a fetus (Rojas, Wood, & Blakemore, 2007). Care must be taken in routine immunization programs to make sure that adolescents about to be vaccinated are not pregnant. Women who work in biologic laboratories where vaccines are manufactured are well advised not to work with live virus products during pregnancy.

Teratogenic Drugs

Many women, assuming that the rule of being cautious with drugs during pregnancy applies only to prescription drugs, take over-the-counter drugs or herbal supplements freely. Although not all drugs cross the placenta (heparin, for example, does not because of its large molecular size), most do. Also, even though most herbs are safe, ginseng, for example, used to improve general well-being, or senna, used to relieve constipation, may not be safe (Der Marderosian & Beutler, 2007).

To identify drugs that are unsafe during pregnancy, the U.S. Food and Drug Administration (FDA) has established five categories of safety (Table 12.1). Always look for a drug's listed category before administering it to a pregnant woman. In addition, two principles always govern drug intake during pregnancy:

- Any drug or herbal supplement, under certain circumstances, may be detrimental to fetal welfare. Therefore, during pregnancy, women should not take any drug or supplement not specifically prescribed or approved by their physician or nurse-midwife.
- A woman of childbearing age and ability should not take any drug other than one prescribed by a physician or nurse-midwife to avoid exposure to a drug should she become pregnant.

The classic example of a teratogenic drug is thalidomide, once liberally prescribed for morning sickness in Europe. Never approved for use in the United States, thalidomide caused amelia or phocomelia (total or partial absence of extremities) in 100% of instances when taken between the 34th and 45th day of pregnancy. Thalidomide is again available as it is effective as an anticancer drug, particularly with patients with multiple myeloma, so women need to be cautioned again about its detrimental fetal effects (Karch, 2009). Minoxidil (Rogaine), a drug taken by both men and women to restore hair growth, is an example of another drug that is documented to cause fetal deformities and could be readily available in a modern home (Shapiro, 2007). Valproic acid, a common drug prescribed for seizures, is yet another example (Duncan, 2007). Other examples of drugs capable of being teratogenic are shown in Box 12.8.

The use of recreational drugs during pregnancy puts a fetus at risk in two ways: the drug may have a direct teratogenic effect, and intravenous drug use risks exposure to diseases such as HIV and hepatitis B (Donnelly et al., 2008).

Narcotics such as meperidine (Demerol) and heroin have long been implicated as causing intrauterine growth restriction (IUGR). The use of marijuana alone apparently does not, although the long-term effects of marijuana during pregnancy are still unstudied. Cocaine, particularly its crack form, is potentially harmful to a fetus because it causes severe vasoconstriction in the mother, compromising placental blood flow and perhaps dislodging the placenta. Its use is associated with spontaneous miscarriage, preterm labor, meconium staining, and IUGR (Rojas, Wood, & Blakemore, 2007). Whether cocaine causes long-term effects in the infant remains controversial (Bernstein & Weinstein, 2007). See Chapter 22 for more information on the potential hazards of cocaine or heroin use during pregnancy.

An area of recreational drug use that needs to be examined is that of inhalant abuse ("huffing"). Substances frequently used as inhalants include gasoline, butane lighter fluid, Freon, glue, and nitrous oxide (NIOSH, 2007). Although the teratogenic properties of inhalants are not well studied, they all carry the possibility of respiratory distress, which could limit the oxygen supply to a fetus. They are used most often by adolescents.

Teratogenicity of Alcohol

Evidence over the years has shown that when women consume a large quantity of alcohol during pregnancy, their babies show a high incidence of congenital deformities and cognitive impairment. It was assumed in the past that these defects were the result of the mother's poor nutritional status (drinking alcohol rather than eating food), not necessarily the direct result of the alcohol. However, alcohol has now been firmly isolated as a direct teratogen. Fetuses cannot remove the breakdown products of alcohol from their body.

TABLE 12.1 ✻ Pregnancy Risk Categories of Drugs

Category	Description	Example
A	Adequate studies in pregnant women have failed to show a risk to the fetus in the first trimester of pregnancy; there is no evidence of risk in later trimesters.	Thyroid hormone
B	Animal studies have not shown an adverse effect on the fetus, but there are no adequate clinical studies in pregnant women.	Insulin
C	Animal studies have shown an adverse effect on the fetus, but there are no adequate studies on humans, or there are no adequate studies in animals or humans. Pregnancy risk is unknown.	Docusate sodium (Colace)
D	There is evidence of risk to the human fetus, but the potential benefits of use in pregnant women may be acceptable despite potential risks.	Lithium citrate
X	Studies in animals or humans show fetal abnormalities, or adverse reaction reports indicate evidence of fetal risk. The risks involved clearly outweigh potential benefits.	Isotretinoin (Accutane)

From Karch, A. M. (2009). *Lippincott's nursing drug guide.* Philadelphia: Lippincott Williams & Wilkins.

BOX 12.8 * Focus on Pharmacology

Some Potentially or Positively Teratogenic Drugs

Category	***Example***	***Drug Use***	***Teratogenic Effect***
Alcohol (ethanol)	Wine, whiskey	Social use	Fetal alcohol syndrome
Analgesics	Acetylsalicylic acid (aspirin)	Minor pain relief	Prolonged pregnancy; maternal bleeding
	Nonsteroidal anti-inflammatory drugs (NSAIDs)		Patent ductus arteriosus
Antineoplastics	Methotrexate	Chemotherapy	Multiple anomalies
	Cyclophosphamide (Cytoxan)	Chemotherapy	Multiple anomalies
Androgens	Danazol	Endometriosis	Masculinization of female fetus
Anticonvulsants	Phenytoin (Dilantin)	Seizures	Fetal hydantoin syndrome
	Valproic acid		Neural tube defects
	Carbamazepine		Neural tube defects
	Lamotrigine		Possibly fetal anomalies
Anticoagulants	Warfarin (Coumarin)	Anticoagulation	Fetal bleeding or anomalies
Antidepressants	Imipramine (Tofranil)	Elevate mood	Cardiovascular anomalies
Antidiabetic agents	Chlorpropamide	Lower blood glucose	Neonatal hypoglycemia
Antischizophrenic	Lithium	Schizophrenia	Hydramnios
Antithyroid	Methimazole	Hypothyroidism	Hypothyroidism in fetus
Antibiotics	Ribavirin	Respiratory infection	Multiple anomalies
	Sulfonamides	Infection	Hyperbilirubinemia in newborn
	Tetracycline	Infection	Teeth and bone deformities
Antihelmintics	Lindane	Eradication of lice	Manufacturer recommends limiting exposure to 2 doses
Angiotensin-converting enzyme inhibitors	Enalapril (Vasotec) Captopril (Capoten)	Reduce hypertension	Oligohydramnios
Caffeine	Coffee, soft drinks, chocolate	Social use	Low birth weight
Hypoglycemics	Tolbutamide (Orinase)	Type 2 diabetes	Profound hypoglycemia in newborn
Nicotine	Cigarette smoke	Relaxation	Growth restriction
Radiopharmaceuticals	Iodide-131	Diagnostic studies	May destroy thyroid of fetus
Narcotics	Cocaine	Social pleasure	Dysmorphic and CNS anomalies
	Heroin		Growth restriction; narcotic withdrawal in newborn
Tranquilizers	Benzodiazepine (diazepam)	Reduce anxiety	Growth restriction; CNS dysfunction Hypotonia, respiratory depression
Vaccines (live)	Rubella	Provide immunity	Possible infection in fetus
Vitamin A derivatives	Isotretinoin (Accutane)	Acne	Craniofacial, cardiac, CNS anomalies
	Etretinate (Tegison)	Psoriasis	Craniofacial, cardiac, CNS anomalies

CNS, central nervous system.
Source: Koren, G. (2007). Special aspects of perinatal and pediatric pharmacology. In B. G. Katzung (Ed.). *Basic and clinical pharmacology* (10th ed.). Columbus, OH: McGraw-Hill.

The large buildup of this leads to vitamin B deficiency and accompanying neurologic damage.

Women during pregnancy should be screened for alcohol use because an infant born with **fetal alcohol syndrome (FAS)** not only is small for gestational age but can be cognitively challenged (Shankar, Ronis, & Badger, 2007). The infant typically has a characteristic craniofacial deformity including short palpebral fissures, a thin upper lip, and an upturned nose. Because of individual variations in metabolism, it is impossible to define a safe level of alcohol consumption. Women are best advised, therefore, to abstain from alcohol completely. Be certain to ask about binge drinking (consuming more than five alcohol drinks in an evening) as women may refer to this as only "occasional drinking." Refer women with alcohol addiction to an alcohol treatment program as early in pregnancy as possible to help them reduce their alcohol intake (see Focus on Nursing Care Planning Box 12.9).

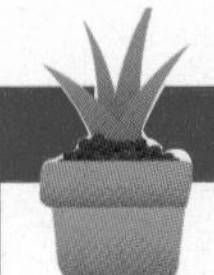

BOX 12.9 ✻ Focus on Nursing Care Planning

A Multidisciplinary Care Map for a Pregnant Woman With Threats to Fetal Health

Julberry Adams, a single woman, is 4 months pregnant when you see her in a prenatal clinic. She works as a curator for an art gallery but has missed work this last week because of nausea. She is worried she will not be able to work past 6 months of her pregnancy because her job involves a great deal of walking. She wonders how she will be able to afford her apartment if she has to quit work. She has already stopped volunteer work teaching children's swimming at the YMCA. She wants to travel to see her sister in St. Louis because her sister is very ill but has heard that pregnant women shouldn't drive over 100 miles. She asks you if marijuana would help reduce her early pregnancy nausea.

Family Assessment ✻ Client lives by herself in one-bedroom apartment. Rates finances as "good, unless I have to quit work because of pregnancy." She asks you, "Will I have to have an ultrasound? I'm worried about that."

Client Assessment ✻ Gravida 1, para 0. Unsure of date of last menstrual period, but it was about 11 weeks ago. Uterine height barely above symphysis. Fetal heart rate at 148 beats per minute by Doppler. History of frequent sinus headaches. "I use Sudafed (pseudoephedrine) at least 3 to 4 times a week; sometimes other things." Smokes one half pack of cigarettes "some days." Drinks 2 to 3 glasses of wine per week at art gallery functions. Denies history of marijuana or other recreational drug use.

Nursing Diagnosis ✻ Risk for fetal injury related to knowledge deficit concerning possible fetal exposure to teratogens.

Outcome Evaluation ✻ Client reports a decrease in smoking to less than 10 cigarettes per day or less and no alcohol consumption.
Verbalizes no use of recreational drugs including marijuana.
States she has contacted health care provider about use of sinus medications and is following advice.

Team Member Responsible	Assessment	Intervention	Rationale	Expected Outcome
		Activities of Daily Living		
Nurse	Assess what activities client wants to participate in during pregnancy.	Discuss desired activities and any modification necessary for pregnancy with client.	Finding a match between desired activities and possible activities will help with adherence.	Client discusses what activities she intends to continue during pregnancy and ways to modify them as necessary.
Physician/nurse	Assess what work or travel plans entail.	Assure client she can continue work, travel to sister's home.	Reassurance helps clients maintain normal lifestyle.	Client states she will continue work, maintain contact with sister.
		Consultations		
Nurse	Assess what medications client is currently taking.	Consult with client's maternal health care provider about safety of over-the-counter (OTC) medications.	Not all OTC medications are safe during pregnancy.	Client states she will follow recommendations of primary health care provider regarding medications.
		Procedures/Medications		
Physician/ nurse-midwife	Anticipate the need for follow-up ultrasound examination for fetal growth evaluation.	Explain the need for ultrasound exam to assess for fetal growth restriction because of alcohol and cigarette smoking habits.	Teratogen exposure may have slowed fetal growth, which will be revealed by ultrasound exam.	Client states that she is aware of purpose of ultrasound exam and will allow exam to be scheduled.

(continued)

BOX 12.9 * Focus on Nursing Care Planning (continued)

		Nutrition		
Nurse	Assess client's lifestyle to see what beverages she could substitute for alcohol, what measures she could use best for nausea.	Suggest client replace alcohol consumption with caffeine-free beverages.	Alcohol consumption during pregnancy is associated with fetal alcohol syndrome.	Client voices intent to replace alcohol consumption with caffeine-free beverages.
	Assess what measures client could use to decrease nausea.	Suggest measures to combat nausea and vomiting, such as dry crackers, acupuncture band.	Decreasing nausea to increase food intake aids fetal growth and development.	Client suggests measures that appeal to her to reduce nausea and vomiting.
		Patient/Family Education		
Nurse/nurse-midwife	Assess whether client has tried any non-medicinal measures to relieve sinus headaches.	Discuss with client possible non-medicinal measures to assist with sinus headache relief, including saline nasal sprays, humidification, and warm compresses to nasal area.	Complementary comfort measures may provide symptomatic relief without danger to a fetus.	Client describes two complementary therapies she will use to relieve sinus congestion.
		Psychosocial/Spiritual/Emotional Needs		
Nurse/social worker	Discuss with client whether her current support system is reliable.	Help client locate at least one person she can depend on if a pregnancy emergency should arise.	Pregnancy can be a very stressful time for a woman who has an insecure support system.	Client telephones or e-mails the health care facility with questions rather than relying on non-experienced friends for information; names one support person.
		Discharge Planning		
Nurse	Assess extent of cigarette smoking.	Encourage the client to decrease smoking and quit if possible. Offer suggestions to accomplish this goal, including use of sugar-free gums or candies, distraction, and activity. Refer to a smoking-cessation group if appropriate.	Cigarette use during pregnancy can lead to fetal growth restriction. Support and suggestions provide concrete measures to assist client with cutting down and quitting.	Client voices intention to decrease smoking and if possible quit smoking during pregnancy.

Teratogenicity of Cigarettes

Cigarette smoking is associated with infertility in women. Cigarette smoking by a pregnant woman has been shown to cause fetal growth restriction (Lawrence & Haslam, 2007). In addition, a fetus may be at greater risk for being stillborn (Hogberg & Cnattingius, 2007) and, after birth, may be at greater risk than others for sudden infant death syndrome. Low birth weight in infants of smoking mothers results from vasoconstriction of the uterine vessels, an effect of nicotine. This limits the blood supply to a fetus. Another contributory effect may be related to inhaled carbon monoxide. Secondary smoke, or inhaling the smoke of another person's cigarettes, may be as harmful as actually smoking the cigarettes. All prenatal health care settings should be smoke-free environments for this reason.

If a woman cannot stop smoking during pregnancy (and, realistically, many women cannot), reducing the number of cigarettes smoked per day should help diminish adverse effects on a fetus as well as also protect a woman's health from long-term illnesses such as chronic respiratory diseases.

The best way to urge women to discontinue smoking is to educate them about the risks to themselves and their fetus at a first prenatal visit. It may be effective to encourage women to sign a contract with a health care provider to try to stop or to join a smoking-cessation program. Be certain pregnant women know that they should not enter a stop-smoking program that uses drug therapy such as nicotine patches, because the substitute drug may be as harmful to a fetus as smoking (Winzer-Serhan, 2008).

Environmental Teratogens

Teratogens from environmental sources can be as damaging to a fetus as those that are directly or deliberately ingested. Women can be exposed through contact at home or at work sites. For example, washing children's hair with a shampoo such as lindane (Kwell) to remove lice should be limited to two exposures because of potential toxicity (Karch, 2009).

Metal and Chemical Hazards

Pesticides and carbon monoxide such as from automobile exhaust should be avoided as these are examples of chemical teratogens. Arsenic, a byproduct of copper and lead smelting, used in pesticides, paints, and leather processing; formaldehyde, used in paper manufacturing; and mercury, used in the manufacture of electrical apparatuses and found in swordfish and tuna fish, are all teratogens that can be contacted at work sites.

Lead poisoning generally is considered a problem of young children eating lead-based paint chips, but it also can be a fetal hazard (Maloney, 2007). Women may ingest lead by drinking water that travels through old pipes that are leaching lead or by "sniffing" lead-based gasoline. Lead ingestion during pregnancy may lead to a newborn who is cognitively or neurologically challenged (Pavone & Hueppchen, 2007).

Radiation

Rapidly growing cells are extremely vulnerable to destruction by radiation. That makes radiation a potent teratogen to unborn children because of their high proportion of rapidly growing cells. Radiation produces a range of malformations depending on the stage of development of the embryo or fetus and the strength and length of exposure. If the exposure occurs before implantation, the growing zygote apparently is killed. If the zygote is not killed, it survives apparently unharmed. The most damaging time for exposure and subsequent damage is from implantation to 6 weeks after conception (when many women are not yet aware that they are pregnant). The nervous system, brain, and retinal innervation are most affected.

As a rule, therefore, all women of childbearing age should be scheduled for pelvic x-ray examinations only in the first 10 days of a menstrual cycle (when pregnancy is unlikely because ovulation has not yet occurred), except in emergency situations. A serum pregnancy test can be done on all women who have reason to believe they might be pregnant before diagnostic tests involving x-rays are scheduled.

Radiation of the pelvis should be avoided all during pregnancy if possible. It should be undertaken only at term if the data obtained are important for birth and cannot be obtained by any other means. Ultrasound and magnetic resonance imaging have replaced x-ray examination for confirmation of situations such as multiple pregnancy because these do not appear to be teratogenic.

In addition to immediate fetal damage, evidence exists that radiation can have long-lasting effects on the health of a child. There appears to be an increased risk of cancer in children who are exposed to radiation in utero. Exposure of the fetal gonads could lead to a genetic mutation that will not be evident until the next generation (Pavone & Hueppchen, 2007).

If a woman needs nonpelvic radiation during pregnancy (e.g., dental x-ray examinations, an arm or leg x-ray examination after a fall), be certain that she is supplied a lead apron to shield her pelvis during the procedure. Even fluoroscopy, which uses lower radiation doses than regular x-ray photography, can cause fetal deformities and should be avoided during pregnancy—again, except in an emergency. Although still being investigated, long-term use of slight radiation sources, such as a word processor, computer, or cellular phone, does not appear to be teratogenic.

Hyperthermia and Hypothermia

Hyperthermia to a fetus can be detrimental to growth because it interferes with cell metabolism. This can occur from the use of saunas, hot tubs, or tanning beds, from a work environment next to a furnace, such as in welding or steel making, or from a high maternal fever early in pregnancy (4–6 weeks). For this reason, after exercise programs, advise pregnant women not to use hot tubs or saunas. Women who use a hot tub at 40° C should not stay in it for longer than about 10 minutes at one time.

The effect of hypothermia on pregnancy is not well known. Because the uterus is an internal organ, a woman's body temperature would have to be lowered significantly before a great deal of fetal temperature change would result.

Teratogenic Maternal Stress

Many myths exist about the effect of being frightened or surprised while pregnant. For example:

- If a woman sees a mouse during pregnancy, her child will be born with a furry or molelike birthmark.
- Eating strawberries causes strawberry birthmarks.
- Looking at a handicapped child while pregnant will cause a child in utero to be handicapped the same way.

Common sense and awareness of fetal–maternal physiology have dispelled these superstitions. There is some evidence, however, that an emotionally disturbed pregnancy, one filled with anxiety and worry beyond the usual amount, could produce physiologic changes through its effect on the sympathetic division of the autonomic nervous system. The primary changes this could cause include constriction of the peripheral blood vessels (a fight-or-flight syndrome). If the anxiety is prolonged, the constriction of uterine vessels (the uterus is a peripheral organ) could interfere with the blood and nutrient supply to a fetus.

These phenomena are characteristic only of long-term, extreme stress, not of the normal anxiety of pregnancy. Illness or death of one's partner, difficulty with relatives, marital discord, and illness or death of another child are examples of stressful situations that might provoke excessive anxiety.

Helping a woman resolve these complex problems during pregnancy is not easy. If maternal stress is severe, however, securing counseling is as important as ensuring good physical care.

PREPARATION FOR LABOR

At about the midpoint of pregnancy, along with cautioning women about discomforts of pregnancy and possible teratogenic situations, it is time to review the events that signal the beginning of labor so that women will not be surprised by these happenings or dismiss them as something other than what they are.

Lightening

Lightening is the settling of the fetal head into the inlet of the true pelvis. It occurs approximately 2 weeks before labor in primiparas but at unpredictable times in multiparas. A woman notices she is not as short of breath as she was before. Her abdominal contour is definitely changed, and on standing she may experience frequency of urination or sciatic pain (pain across a buttock radiating down her leg) from the lowered fetal position.

Show

Show is the common term used to describe the release of the cervical plug (operculum) that formed during pregnancy. It consists of a mucous, often blood-streaked vaginal discharge and indicates the beginning of cervical dilatation.

Rupture of the Membranes

A sudden gush of clear fluid (amniotic fluid) from the vagina indicates rupture of the membranes. A woman should telephone her primary care provider immediately when this occurs as after rupture of the membranes, there is a danger of cord prolapse and uterine infection.

Excess Energy

Feeling extremely energetic is a sign of labor important for women to recognize. It occurs as part of the body's physiologic preparation for labor. If a woman does not recognize the sensation for what it is, she may use this burst of energy to clean her house or finish paperwork at the office and exhaust herself before labor begins. If she can recognize this symptom as an initial sign of labor, she can conserve her energy in preparation for labor.

Uterine Contractions

For most women, labor begins with contractions. True labor contractions usually start in the back and sweep forward across the abdomen like the tightening of a band. They gradually increase in frequency and intensity. Advise a woman to call her primary care provider when contractions begin to alert health care personnel that she is in labor. Inform her at what point in labor her physician or nurse-midwife wants her to come to the health care facility (such as when contractions are 5 minutes apart). Be certain she knows this is not a hard-and-fast rule, however. If she should become exceptionally anxious, will be home alone, or will have a long drive, she should be given the option of using common sense to determine when to leave home.

✓Checkpoint Question 12.5

Julberry Adams makes the following statements. Which one is the safest practice?

a. "My brother takes medicine for heartburn; if I get that, I'll just borrow his."
b. "I'm going to get a measles shot; I don't want measles while I'm pregnant."
c. "There are so many medicines for headache, I have to ask my doctor what to take."
d. "I know all over-the-counter medicine is safe; it's why it's over the counter."

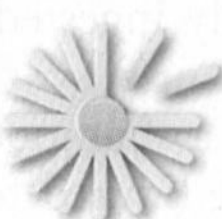

Key Points for Review

- Prenatal education is an important part of prenatal care. The more women know about measures they should take during pregnancy to safeguard their health, the more likely it is that they will avoid substances or activities harmful to fetal growth.
- Urge women to find the best way for them to modify their lifestyle for pregnancy. Pregnancy is 9 months long, so modifications must be agreeable to a woman or she will not maintain them over such a long time span.
- Women need to make provisions for rest periods during their day and to be aware of any potential teratogens at a work site, such as exposure to radiation or heavy metals.
- Women who travel should plan for break periods to avoid congestion in their lower extremities. Seat belts should be used when traveling by car.
- Common discomforts of early pregnancy include breast tenderness, constipation, palmar erythema, nausea and vomiting, fatigue, muscle cramps, pain from varicosities or hemorrhoids, heart palpitations, frequency of urination, and leukorrhea. If women know that these symptoms may occur, they will not interpret them as complications.
- Minor discomforts of middle or late pregnancy include backache, dyspnea, ankle edema, and Braxton Hicks contractions. Caution women that contractions could be a sign of labor.
- Women should take active measures to avoid exposure to infectious diseases such as rubella, HIV, cytomegalovirus, herpes simplex virus, syphilis, Lyme disease, and toxoplasmosis during pregnancy.
- Counsel women about the necessity to avoid the use of any drugs or herbal supplements not specifically approved by their physician or nurse-midwife during pregnancy, as well as alcohol and cigarettes.
- It is almost impossible for a woman to modify a behavior, such as smoking, if her support person does not agree to change also. Including the family in care is an important way of helping support persons understand the need for the modification and increasing cooperation.
- Beginning signs of labor for which the pregnant woman should be alert include lightening, show, excess energy, rupture of membranes, and uterine contractions.

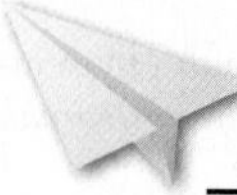

CRITICAL THINKING EXERCISES

1. Julberry Adams, the woman you met at the beginning of the chapter, voiced several concerns, including whether she should stop work and whether it would be safe to take a long trip. What advice would you give her regarding these questions?
2. Although Julberry describes a day she says involves a lot of walking, she also has long periods of sitting with almost no exercise. What would be some recommendations you could make to help her prevent blood clots from the sharp bend in her knee while sitting?
3. Julberry is having trouble remembering to take her prenatal vitamin. What are some suggestions you could make to help her remember to take this daily?
4. Examine the National Health Goals related to prenatal care. Most government-sponsored money for nursing research is allotted based on these goals. What would be a possible research topic to explore pertinent to these goals that would be applicable to Julberry and her family and also advance evidence-based practice?

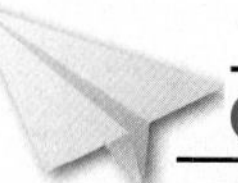

CRITICAL THINKING SCENARIO

Open the accompanying CD-ROM or visit http://thePoint.lww.com and read the Patient Scenario included for this chapter, then answer the questions to further sharpen your skills and grow more familiar with NCLEX style questions related to health promotion in pregnancy. Confirm your answers are correct by reading the rationales.

REFERENCES

American Academy of Pediatrics. (2009). *Car seat checkup.* Washington, DC: Author.

American College of Obstetricians and Gynecologists. (2007). Management of herpes in pregnancy. *Obstetrics and Gynecology, 109*(6), 1489–1498.

Barankin, B. (2008). Parvovirus B19. In F. J. Domino (Ed.). *The 5-minute clinical consult.* Philadelphia: Lippincott Williams & Wilkins.

Bennett, J. A., et al. (2008). A telephone-only motivational intervention to increase physical activity in rural adults: a randomized controlled trial. *Nursing Research 51*(1):24–32.

Bernstein, H. B., & Weinstein, M. (2007). Normal pregnancy and prenatal care. In A. H. DeCherney & L. Nathan (Eds.). *Current diagnosis and treatment in obstetrics and gynecology* (10th ed.). Columbus, OH: McGraw-Hill.

Bonzini, M., Coggon, D., & Palmer, K. T. (2007). Risk of prematurity, low birth weight and pre-eclampsia in relation to working hours and physical activities: a systematic review. *Occupational & Environmental Medicine, 64*(4), 228–243.

Chakraborty, R., & Luck, S. (2007). Managing congenital syphilis again? The more things change... . *Current Opinion in Infectious Diseases, 20*(3), 247–252.

Crombleholme, W. R. (2009). Obstetrics. In S. J. McPhee & M. A. Papadakis (Eds.). *Current medical diagnosis and treatment.* Columbus, OH: McGraw-Hill.

Cunningham, F. G., et al. (2008). Prenatal care. In F. G. Cunningham, et al. (Eds.). *Williams Obstetrics* (22nd ed.). Columbus, OH: McGraw-Hill.

Der Marderosian, A., & Beutler, J.A. (2007). *Review of natural products.* New York: Facts & Comparisons.

Donnelly, J. C., et al. (2008). Illegal drug use, smoking and alcohol consumption in a low-risk Irish primigravid population. *Journal of Perinatal Medicine, 36*(1), 70–72.

Duncan, S. (2007). Teratogenesis of sodium valproate. *Current Opinion in Neurology, 20*(2), 175–180.

Friars, C. (2007). Toxoplasmosis and pregnancy. *Practising Midwife, 10*(4), 20–21.

Graham, H. (2007). Breast health and pregnancy. *British Journal of Midwifery, 15*(3), 137–140.

Hogberg, L., & Cnattingius, S. (2007). The influence of maternal smoking habits on the risk of subsequent stillbirth: is there a causal relation? *BJOG: An International Journal of Obstetrics and Gynaecology, 114*(6), 699–704.

Johnson, A., & Ross, B. (2007). Perinatal infections. In K. B. Fortner, et al. (Eds.). *The Johns Hopkins manual of gynecology and obstetrics.* Philadelphia: Lippincott Williams & Wilkins.

Karch, A. M. (2009). *Lippincott's nursing drug guide.* Philadelphia: Lippincott Williams & Wilkins.

Katsufrakis, P. J., & Workowski, K. A. (2008). Sexually transmitted diseases. In J. E. South-Paul, S. C. Matheny, & E. L. Lewis (Eds.). *Current diagnosis and treatment in family medicine* (2nd ed.). Columbus, OH: McGraw-Hill.

Knopik, V. S. (2009). Maternal smoking during pregnancy and child outcomes: real or spurious effect? *Developmental Neuropsychology, 34*(1):1–36.

Koren, G. (2007). Special aspects of perinatal and pediatric pharmacology. In B. G. Katzung (Ed.). *Basic and clinical pharmacology* (10th ed.). Columbus, OH: McGraw-Hill.

Kramer, M. S., & McDonald, S. W. (2009). Aerobic exercise for women during pregnancy. *Cochrane Database of Systematic Reviews, 2009*(1), (CD000180).

Lawrence, W. T., & Haslam, C. (2007). Smoking during pregnancy: where next for stage-based interventions? *Journal of Health Psychology, 12*(1), 159–169.

Lilleri, D., et al. (2007). Development of human cytomegalovirus-specific T cell immunity during primary infection of pregnant women and its correlation with virus transmission to the fetus. *Journal of Infectious Diseases, 195*(7), 1062–1070.

Maloney, G. (2007). Lead poisoning. In J. Schaider, et al. (Eds.). *Rosen & Barkin's 5-minute emergency medicine consult.* Philadelphia: Lippincott Williams & Wilkins.

McGovern, L. M., Boyce, T. G., & Fischer, P. R. (2007). Congenital infections associated with international travel during pregnancy. *Journal of Travel Medicine, 14*(2), 117–128.

Menzies, J., et al. (2007). Instituting surveillance guidelines and adverse outcomes in preeclampsia. *Obstetrics and Gynecology, 110*(1), 121–127.

Mullen, B. A. (2007). Tick-borne illnesses: beyond Lyme disease. *The American Journal for Nurse Practitioners, 11*(4), 52–61.

National Institute of Occupational Safety and Health (NIOSH). (2007). *Nitrous oxide.* Washington, DC: Department of Health and Human Services (DHHS). DHHS Publication no. 99–105.

Pavone, M. E., & Hueppchen, N. A. (2007). Surgical disease and trauma in pregnancy. In K. B. Fortner, et al. (Eds.). *The Johns Hopkins manual of gynecology and obstetrics.* Philadelphia: Lippincott Williams & Wilkins.

Pratt, R. J. (2007). Perinatal and infant HIV infection: screening to minimize risk. *Infant, 3*(1), 8–12.

Quijano, C. E., & Abalos, E. (2009). Conservative management of symptomatic and/or complicated haemorrhoids in pregnancy and the puerperium. *Cochrane Database of Systematic Reviews, 2009*(1), (CD004077).

Rojas, F., Wood, E., & Blakemore, K. (2007). Preconception counseling and prenatal care. In K. B. Fortner, et al. (Eds.). *The Johns Hopkins manual of gynecology and obstetrics.* Philadelphia: Lippincott Williams & Wilkins.

Shankar, K., Ronis, M. J. J., & Badger, T. M. (2007). Effects of pregnancy and nutritional status on alcohol metabolism. *Alcohol Research & Health, 30*(1), 55–59.

Shapiro, J. (2007). Clinical practice. Hair loss in women. *New England Journal of Medicine, 357*(16), 1620–1623.

Smith, E. (2007). Pregnant? Get moving! *International Journal of Childbirth Education, 22*(2), 35–37.

Smith, J. E., & Tolson, J. M. (2008). Recognition, diagnosis, and treatment of restless legs syndrome. *Journal of the American Academy of Nurse Practitioners, 20*(8), 396–401.

Truhlar, A., et al. (2007). Out-of-hospital cardiac arrest from air embolism during sexual intercourse: case report and review of the literature. *Resuscitation, 73*(3), 475–484.

Walker, G. J. A. (2009). Antibiotics for syphilis diagnosed during pregnancy. *Cochrane Database of Systematic Reviews, 2009*(1), (CD001143).

Winzer-Serhan, U. H. (2008). Long-term consequences of maternal smoking and developmental chronic nicotine exposure. *Frontiers in Bioscience, 13*(1), 636–649.

Young, G. L., & Jewell, D. (2009). Interventions for leg cramps in pregnancy. *Cochrane Database of Systematic Reviews, 2009*(1), (CD000121).

SUGGESTED READINGS

Ciranni, P., & Essex, M. (2007). Better care, better bottom line: the impact of nurse practitioners in OB/GYN triage. *Nursing for Women's Health, 11*(3), 274–281.

Edgerley, L. P., et al. (2007). Use of a community mobile health van to increase early access to prenatal care. *Maternal and Child Health Journal, 11*(3), 235–239.

Fine, P., et al. (2007). Teaching and practicing of pelvic floor muscle exercises in primiparous women during pregnancy and the postpartum period. *American Journal of Obstetrics & Gynecology, 197*(1), 107–113.

Fryer, S. L., et al. (2007). Evaluation of psychopathological conditions in children with heavy prenatal alcohol exposure. *Pediatrics, 119*(3), e733–e741.

Lumley, J., et al. (2009). Interventions for promoting smoking cessation during pregnancy. *Cochrane Database of Systematic Reviews, 2009*(1), (CD001055).

Pennick, V. E., & Young, G. (2009). Interventions for preventing and treating pelvic and back pain in pregnancy. *Cochrane Database of Systematic Reviews, 2009*(1), (CD001139).

Peyron, F., et al. (2009). Treatments for toxoplasmosis in pregnancy. *Cochrane Database of Systematic Reviews, 2009*(1), (CD001684).

Polman, R., Kaiseler, M., & Borkoles, E. (2007). Effect of a single bout of exercise on the mood of pregnant women. *Journal of Sports Medicine & Physical Fitness, 47*(1), 103–111.

Vonderheid, S. C., Norr, K. F., & Handler, A. S. (2007). Prenatal health promotion content and health behaviors. *Western Journal of Nursing Research, 29*(3), 258–276.

Xue, F., et al. (2008). Parental characteristics as predictors of birth weight. *Human Reproduction, 23*(1), 168–177.

Chapter 13

Promoting Nutritional Health During Pregnancy

KEY TERMS

- body mass index
- complete protein
- Hawthorne effect
- heartburn (pyrosis)
- hypercholesterolemia
- hyperplasia
- hypertrophy
- incomplete protein
- lactase
- obese
- overweight
- pica
- underweight

OBJECTIVES

After mastering the contents of this chapter, you should be able to:

1. Discuss the recommendations for healthy nutrition during pregnancy.
2. Identify National Health Goals related to nutrition and pregnancy that nurses can help the nation achieve.
3. Use critical thinking to analyze the effects of different life situations on nutrition patterns to create ways nutritional health can be both improved and family centered.
4. Assess a woman for nutritional adequacy during pregnancy.
5. Formulate nursing diagnoses related to nutritional concerns during pregnancy.
6. Develop expected outcomes to assist a pregnant woman achieve optimal nutrition during pregnancy.
7. Plan health teaching strategies such as ways to increase folic acid and calcium intake to promote optimal nutritional intake during pregnancy.
8. Implement nursing care that encourages healthy nutritional practices during pregnancy.
9. Evaluate expected outcomes for achievement and effectiveness of care.
10. Identify areas related to nutrition and pregnancy that could benefit from additional nursing research or application of evidence-based practice.
11. Integrate nutrition knowledge with nursing process to achieve quality maternal and child health nursing care.

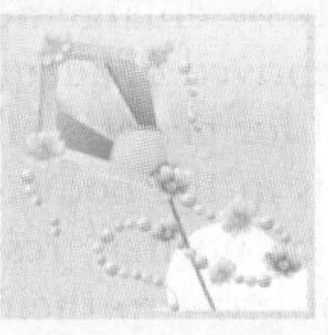

Tori Alarino is 4 months pregnant. She works at a fast-food restaurant and eats her breakfast and lunch at the restaurant at work. Her husband works four evenings a week, so she cooks for herself on those evenings. She dislikes milk, so she drinks milkshakes as a source of calcium. She is concerned because she has already gained 23 lb. She craves oranges, eating six to eight of them a day. She tells you, "I thought pregnant women always craved pickles and ice cream. What's wrong with me?"

Previous chapters described normal anatomy and physiology, the changes associated with pregnancy, and common discomforts and danger signs of pregnancy. This chapter adds information about prenatal nutrition, an important aspect to help ensure a healthy outcome for both a woman and her child. Inadequate nutrition during pregnancy can affect not only fetal health but the child's health for years to come.

What nutritional counseling does Ms. Alarino need?

Although adequate nutrition during pregnancy cannot guarantee a good pregnancy outcome, it does make an important contribution. Both the nutritional state that a woman brings into pregnancy and her nutrition during pregnancy have a direct bearing on her health and on fetal growth and development. A poor diet, such as one deficient in folic acid, for example, is associated with birth anomalies such as neural tube defects.

Early in pregnancy, fetal growth occurs largely by an increase in the number of cells formed **(hyperplasia);** late in pregnancy it occurs mainly by enlargement of existing cells **(hypertrophy).** A fetus deprived of adequate nutrition early in pregnancy can be small for gestational age because of an inadequate number of cells in the body. Later on, although the number of cells may be normal, restricted growth can occur because cells cannot grow to their full potential. To ensure that early pregnancy deficiencies do not occur, encourage women of childbearing age to follow a healthy nutrition plan before pregnancy (preconceptual care) that specifically supplies adequate folic acid (400 μg/day). Otherwise, in the time before a woman recognizes that she is pregnant (about 6 weeks), her poor diet and lack of important nutrient stores could seriously impair fetal growth (Fowles & Murphey, 2009). Good nutrition during pregnancy is so important that the subject is addressed in National Health Goals (Box 13.1).

BOX 13.1 * Focus on National Health Goals

Several National Health Goals speak to nutrition in pregnancy. These are:

- Reduce iron deficiency among young children and females of childbearing age from a baseline of 11% to 7%.
- Reduce anemia among low-income pregnant females in their third trimester of pregnancy from a baseline of 29% to a target of 20%.
- Increase the proportion of pregnancies begun with an optimum folic acid level from a baseline of 21% to a target of 80%.
- Increase the proportion of women who achieve a recommended weight gain during their pregnancies (http://www.nih.gov).

Nurses can help the nation achieve these goals by stressing the importance of balanced nutrition for all people so women enter pregnancy with adequate nutritional stores. They can help pregnant women plan ways to ingest adequate iron daily and to remember to take their prenatal vitamin (which contains an iron and folic acid supplement) daily. Nursing research on such topics as what are effective methods to help people remember to take daily medications, what are the best methods for women who cannot drink milk to obtain adequate calcium during pregnancy, and what are the ways to urge women to eat high-protein, not empty-carbohydrate foods, could add important information in this area of care.

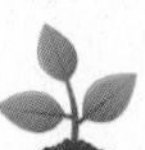

Nursing Process Overview

For Promoting Nutritional Health in a Pregnant Woman

Assessment

Assessment begins with a woman's preconceptual nutrition patterns. From this assessment, determine whether a client is eating healthy food sources as represented by the food pyramid (Fig. 13.1; see also Appendix K) and evaluate any cultural, environmental, or social lifestyles that could affect eating habits. A 24-hour recall history is the best way to secure necessary information, confirm well-balanced nutrition, and identify areas for teaching and learning.

Nursing Diagnosis

Nursing diagnoses related to nutritional status of the pregnant woman consider the desired health and growth of both the fetus and the woman. Both a woman who is eating large amounts of nutritionally inferior food and a woman who has a problem eating because of fatigue or nausea and vomiting may be at risk for the same problem: fetal growth restriction. Being sensitive to a woman's concern about maintaining her own appearance in light of her need to gain sufficient weight helps her keep a healthy perspective on "eating for two." Examples of nursing diagnoses are:

- Imbalanced nutrition, less than body requirements, related to increased physiologic needs
- Imbalanced nutrition, less than body requirements, related to nausea every morning
- Health-seeking behaviors related to determining best food choices in pregnancy
- Imbalanced nutrition, more than body requirements, related to chronic poor eating habits
- Deficient knowledge related to need for increased intake of nutrients and calories during pregnancy

Outcome Identification and Planning

In large health centers, nutritionists are available to meet with women prenatally and help them plan nutrition during pregnancy. In other settings, a nutritionist may be available only for women with special needs, so the responsibility for nutrition advice falls directly on nurses. When helping a woman set expected outcomes for improving nutritional patterns, be certain to consider all the cultural and lifestyle factors that give different meanings to food. Because food is an expensive commodity, consider financial resources as well. Teaching about long-term outcomes such as building iron stores or bone mass is as important as short term goals to eat better for this week. Eating more nutritious foods for a week will probably not make a radical change. However, continuing a healthy eating pattern throughout the pregnancy (and maintaining it throughout life) will bring about important changes and help prepare the woman for feeding her family nutritionally for the years to come. Interesting web sites for pregnant woman to consult about nutrition are the Department of Health and Human Services Women's Health Care site (http://womenshealth.gov/pregnancy/pregnancy/eat.cfm) or the Department of Agriculture MyPyramid site (http://www.mypyramid.gov). Women who need financial or nutritional counseling can

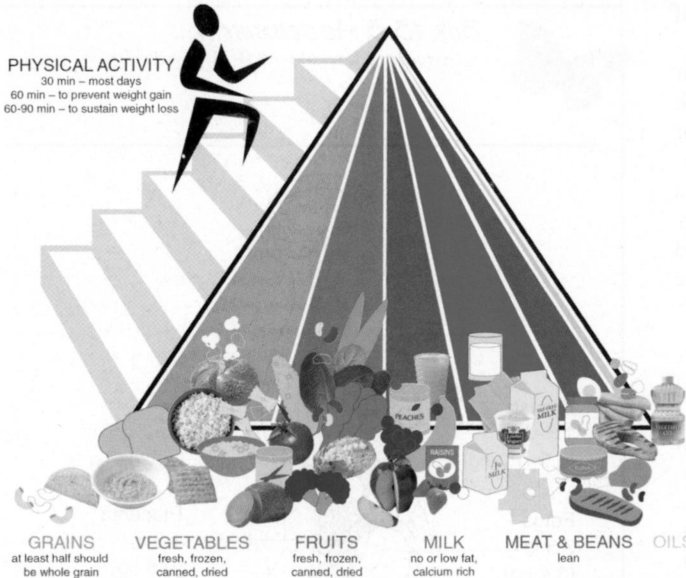
PHYSICAL ACTIVITY
30 min – most days
60 min – to prevent weight gain
60-90 min – to sustain weight loss
GRAINS
at least half should be whole grain
VEGETABLES
fresh, frozen, canned, dried
FRUITS
fresh, frozen, canned, dried
MILK
no or low fat, calcium rich
MEAT & BEANS
lean
OILS

FIGURE 13.1 The food pyramid. (From the Department of Agriculture. [2008]. *Food guide pyramid: a guide to daily food choices.* Washington, DC: Author.)

be referred to the Women, Infants and Children Special Supplemental Food Program (WIC) (http://www.fns.usda.gov/wic).

Implementation

As everyone who has tried to change a nutritional pattern knows, this can be a lonely and seemingly unrewarding endeavor as results occur slowly. Begin by emphasizing the physiologic basis for nutritional needs in pregnancy (a woman is building a whole new person). Based on this, explain what nutritional deficits you have identified, and then show the woman how to change her nutritional pattern to improve this situation. Pregnant women are usually highly motivated to adopt healthy behaviors for the sake of their baby's health, although they still need support and encouragement because this can involve a major life change, such as eating a different lunch than everyone around them is eating; getting up 15 minutes earlier in the morning to prepare breakfast rather than just dashing to work with only coffee; or resisting having a soft drink with dinner and drinking orange juice or milk instead. Asking women to list what foods they eat daily and to bring in a chart to show you at a prenatal visit is an effective motivating technique. In research studies, this is called a **Hawthorne effect,** in which people who are being watched do better than those who are not. With this system, the average woman will eat better than she usually does, so her list looks better when she presents it. As soon as she realizes that these better eating patterns are making her feel better, hopefully, she will continue them indefinitely.

Outcome Evaluation

When evaluating whether a woman's nutritional pattern has been improved, rely on the most important assessments: weight, energy level, general appearance, bowel function, and, when available, hemoglobin and urinalysis findings. Urge women to be honest about whether they are actually following a nutrition plan. If they are not, it probably means that more planning is needed, because the plan did not fit their lifestyle or degree of motivation. Examples of outcomes that would demonstrate improved nutrition are:

- Client plans weekly menus that include three main meals and two snacks per day.
- By next prenatal visit, client demonstrates knowledge of meat and nonmeat sources of protein by providing menus of meals eaten in the last week that include fish, eggs, beans, or peanut butter.
- Client verbalizes correct information about calcium needs during pregnancy.
- Client states she is able to make up later in each day meals missed because of nausea.
- Client's food lists for 1 week include three sources of calcium per day.
- Client describes pattern she is using to increase fluid intake to eight glasses fluid daily.

RELATIONSHIP OF MATERNAL NUTRITION TO INFANT HEALTH

During pregnancy, a woman must eat adequately to supply enough nutrients to the fetus, so it can grow, as well as to support her own nutrition (Crombleholme, 2009). Adequate protein intake is vital because so much is needed by a fetus to build a body framework. Adequate protein may also help prevent complications of pregnancy such as pregnancy-induced hypertension or preterm birth. Either deficiencies or overuse of vitamins may contribute to birth anomalies (Subramanian et al., 2008). Remember that people have some degree of "backsliding," especially at holidays and special events. To prevent this, help a woman make definite, concrete plans for an upcoming holiday or event. Always comment on the things a woman is doing correctly rather than what she is doing wrong. Positive reinforcement, a basic rule of teaching, enhances learning, self-esteem, and compliance more than criticism.

Be careful when nutrition counseling not to make general statements such as, "Eat high-protein foods." Food in the supermarket, after all, is not labeled "high-protein." Instead, provide advice in more specific terms: "Eat three servings of some type of meat or fish every day."

The word "diet" has come to mean a form of unpleasant food denial. Rather than a "pregnancy diet," therefore, talk about "foods that are best for you during pregnancy" or "pregnancy nutrition." These statements sound more positive and refer more closely to what you are encouraging a woman to do. Giving a woman a clearly written list of suggested foods may help. Be sure the list is short, clear, and specific. Complicated lists of foods or a list of don'ts can be overwhelming and, therefore, ignored.

Recommended Weight Gain During Pregnancy

A weight gain of 11.2 to 15.9 kg (25 to 35 lb) is recommended as an average weight gain in pregnancy. If a woman is at high risk for nutritional deficits, a more precise estimation of adequate weight gain can be calculated (Rode et al., 2007). This is done by computing **body mass index** (BMI), the ratio of weight to height (Box 13.2; see also Appendix E). Women who are high or low in weight for their height (BMI below 18.5 or above 25 kg/m^2) need to have their expected outcomes for weight gain adjusted.

BOX 13.2 ✻ Calculating Body Mass Index

Body mass index calculators are available online at the National Heart, Lung, and Blood Institute, National Institutes of Health web site (http://www.nhlbisupport.com/bmi).

BMI also can be calculated using the formula:

1. Convert weight into kilograms (divide weight in pounds by 2.2).
2. Convert height into centimeters (multiply height in inches by 2.5).
3. Convert centimeters into meters (divide result by 100).
4. Square height in meters.
5. Divide weight in kilograms by height in meters squared.

For example: Mrs. Alarino is 5 ft 6 in tall and weighs 150 lb. To determine her BMI:

1. Convert weight into kilograms: 150 lb ÷ 2.2 = 68 kg.
2. Convert height into centimeters: 5′6″ = 66″ (5 × 12 = 60 + 6 = 66 inches) 66 × 2.5 = 165 cm.
3. Convert centimeters into meters: 165 ÷ 100 = 1.65 m.
4. Square height in meters (1.65 × 1.65 = 2.72).
5. Divide weight (kg) by m^2 (68 ÷ 2.72 = 25 BMI).

Normal Prepregnancy BMI

Underweight	Under 18.5
Normal weight	18.5–24.9
Overweight	25.0–29.9
Obese	Above 30.0
Morbidly obese	Above 40.0

With a BMI of 25, Mrs. Alarino enters pregnancy slightly overweight.

Source: Department of Health and Human Services. (2008). *BMI: body mass index.* Hyattsville, MD: Author.

Box 13.3 Assessment
Sources of Maternal Weight Gain

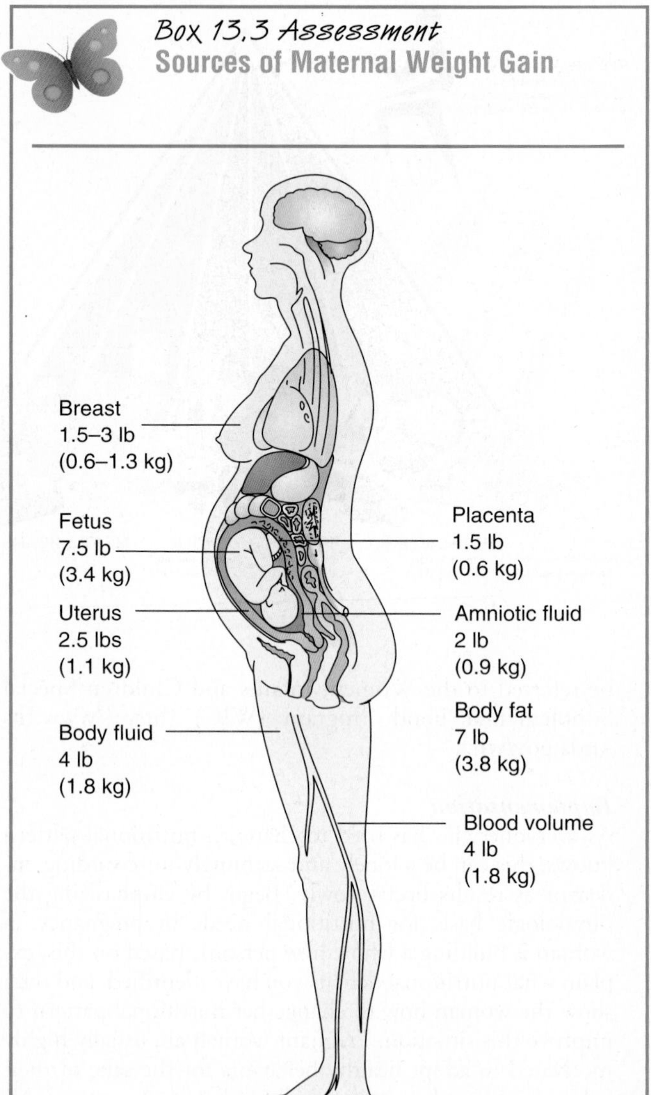

Weight gain in pregnancy occurs from both fetal growth and accumulation of maternal stores (Box 13.3) and occurs at approximately 0.4 kg (1 lb) per month during the first trimester and then 0.4 kg (1 lb) per week during the last two trimesters (a trimester pattern of 3-12-12). As a general rule, in the average woman, weight gain is considered excessive if it is more than 3 kg (6.6 lb) a month during the second and third trimesters; it is less than usual if it is less than 1 kg (2.2 lb) per month during the second and third trimesters. Women can be assured that most of the weight gained with pregnancy will be lost afterward (Bernstein & Weinstein, 2007).

Women who are underweight coming into pregnancy should gain slightly more weight than the average woman (0.5 kg per month or week rather than 0.4, or 30–40 lb). An obese woman might be advised to gain less than average (0.3 kg, or 15–25 lb). However, to ensure adequate fetal nutrition, advise women not to diet to lose weight during pregnancy. Weight gain will be higher for a multiple pregnancy than for a single pregnancy. You can encourage women pregnant with multiple fetuses to gain at least 1 lb per week for a total of 40 to 45 lb (Rolfes, Pinna, & Whitney, 2009). Sudden increases in weight that suggest fluid retention or polyhydramnios (excessive amniotic fluid) or a loss of weight that suggests illness should be carefully evaluated at prenatal visits.

Components of Healthy Nutrition for the Pregnant Woman

The old saying that a pregnant woman must "eat for two" is not a myth; it is a truism. This does not mean, however, that a woman should eat enough for two adults, just enough to provide nutrients for herself and a growing fetus. To do this, many women will not have to increase by much the quantity of food they eat, but they will have to increase the quality of foods.

The Dietary Reference Intake (DRI) values for girls and women and the requirements during pregnancy are shown in Table 13.1. Women should be certain that foods they eat represent the food groups in a food pyramid (see Fig. 13.1). When discussing nutrition, refer to servings of food rather than milligrams or percentages, because this is how women measure amounts.

Energy (Calorie) Needs

The DRI of calories for women of childbearing age is 2200. An additional 300 calories, or a total caloric intake of 2500 calories, is recommended to meet the increased needs of pregnancy. In addition to supplying energy for a fetus, this increase provides calories to sustain an elevated metabolic rate in the woman from increased thyroid function and an increased workload from the extra weight she must carry. An inadequate intake of carbohydrates can lead to protein breakdown for energy, depriving a fetus of essential protein, and possibly resulting in ketoacidosis, a possible cause of fetal and neurologic disorders. Advise women to obtain calories from complex carbohydrates (cereals and grains) rather than simple carbohydrates (sugar and fruits) because these are more slowly digested so help regulate glucose and insulin levels. Do not recommend sugar substitutes for women during pregnancy, because a pregnant woman needs sugar to maintain glucose levels. Even obese women should never consume fewer than 1500 calories per day.

When helping a woman plan an increased caloric intake, consider her lifestyle. For example, many women commonly skip meals, have erratic eating patterns, or rely on fast and convenience foods. For pregnancy, a woman needs to add calories by eating foods rich in protein, iron, and other essential nutrients rather than eating more fast-food, empty-calorie foods such as pretzels and doughnuts. Suggest preparing snacks such as carrot sticks or cheese and crackers early in the day when fatigue is usually less, keeping them readily available in the refrigerator. Otherwise, later in the day when she is tired, a woman may snack on empty-calorie foods simply because they require no preparation.

The easiest method for determining if a woman's caloric intake is adequate is assessing the weight she is gaining. Keep in mind that the weight gain pattern is as important as the total weight gain. Even if a woman has surpassed her target weight before the end of the third trimester, encourage her not to restrict her caloric intake. She should continue to gain weight because a fetus grows rapidly during these final weeks.

Protein Needs

The DRI for protein in women is 46 g/d. During pregnancy, the need for protein increases to 71 g daily. If protein needs are met, overall nutritional needs are likely to be met as well

TABLE 13.1 ✻ Dietary Reference Intakes for Pregnant and Nonpregnant Women

	Nonpregnant Women				Pregnant Women
	Age 11–14	*Age 15–18*	*Age 19–30*	*Age 31–50*	
Calories (kcal)	2,200	2,200	2,200	2,200	2,500
Protein (g/d)	34	46	46	46	71
Fat-Soluble Vitamins					
Vitamin A (μg/d)	600	700	700	700	750
Vitamin D (μg/d)	5	5	5	5	5
Vitamin E (mg/d)	11	15	15	15	15
Water-Soluble Vitamins					
Ascorbic acid (mg/d) (vitamin C)	65	75	75	75	80
Folic acid (μg/d)	300	400	400	400	600
Niacin (mg/d)	12	14	14	14	18
Riboflavin (mg/d)	1.0	1.1	1.1	1.1	1.4
Thiamine (mg/d)(B_1)	1.0	1.1	1.1	1.1	1.4
Vitamin B_{12} (μg/d)	1.8	2.4	2.4	2.4	2.8
Vitamin B_6 (mg/d)	1.3	1.3	1.5	1.5	1.9
Minerals					
Calcium (mg/d)	1,300	1,300	1,000	1,000	1,300
Fluoride (mg/d)	2	3	3	3	3
Iodine (μg/d)	120	150	150	150	220
Iron (mg/d)	8	15	18	18	27
Magnesium (mg/d)	360	360	310	220	400
Phosphorus (mg/d)	1,250	1,250	700	700	700
Zinc (mg/d)	8	9	8	8	12

Institute of Medicine (2008). *Summary tables: dietary reference intakes.* Washington, DC: IOM.

(with the possible exceptions of vitamins C, A, and D) because of the high incorporation of other nutrients with protein foods. If protein intake is inadequate, iron, B vitamins, calcium, and phosphorus also will probably be inadequate. Vitamin B_{12} is found almost exclusively in animal protein, so if animal protein is excluded from the diet, vitamin B_{12} deficiency can occur unless this is supplemented.

Extra protein is best supplied by meat, poultry, fish, yogurt, eggs, and milk, because the protein in these forms contains all nine essential amino acids, or is **complete protein.** The protein in nonanimal sources does not contain all essential amino acids (and so is **incomplete protein).** It is possible to provide all amino acids by combining nonanimal proteins. Proteins that when cooked together provide all essential amino acids are termed *complementary proteins.* Examples are beans and rice, legumes and rice, or beans and wheat.

A woman with a family history of high cholesterol levels **(hypercholesterolemia)** probably should not eat more than two or three eggs per week because of the high cholesterol content of eggs. Encourage such women to eat lean meat, to cook with olive oil instead of lard or butter, and to remove the skin from poultry to reduce its fat content. She also should not eat lunch meats such as bologna or salami as food staples, because their protein content may not be high and their fat content is invariably exceptionally high.

Milk is a rich source of protein. Unfortunately, some women resist drinking it because it can be high in calories as well as fat. Others cannot drink it because of lactose intolerance. Some women find it difficult to drink a quart of milk a day because they simply do not like its taste. Nonfat milk supplies the same protein and half the calories as regular milk and is very low in fat. Buttermilk can be substituted, although it contains a large amount of sodium, or chocolate or another flavoring can be added to make milk palatable. Yogurt or cheese may also be substituted for milk, or milk may be incorporated into custards, eggnogs, or cream soups. Women who are lactose intolerant can add a lactase supplement, buy lactose-free milk, or take a calcium supplement (Bauchner, 2007).

✔Checkpoint Question 13.1

Suppose Tori Alarino has a normal BMI. What would be the recommended weight gain for her during pregnancy?

a. 10 lb
b. 20 lb
c. 30 lb
d. 60 lb

Fat Needs

Only linoleic acid, an essential fatty acid necessary for new cell growth, cannot be manufactured in the body from other sources. Because linoleic acid must be obtained from food, women must be sure to consume a source of this nutrient during pregnancy. Vegetable oils are a good source. In addition, using vegetable oils (e.g., safflower, corn, olive, peanut, and cottonseed) that have a low cholesterol content rather than animal oils (butter) is recommended for all adults as a means of preventing hypercholesterolemia and coronary heart disease. Women should also try and ingest omega-3 oils, found primarily in fish, omega-3–fortified eggs, and the newer omega-3–fortified spreads (Bourre, 2007).

Vitamin Needs

The intake of vitamins as a daily dietary supplement has become so common that their importance may be underestimated by some women. Requirements for both fat-soluble and water-soluble vitamins increase during pregnancy to support the growth of new fetal cells (see Table 13.1).

Vitamin deficiency can result in several common problems. For example, vitamin D, essential for calcium absorption, when lacking, can begin to diminish both fetal and maternal mineral bone density. Lack of vitamin A results in tender gums and poor night vision. For as-yet-unknown reasons, there is an association between multivitamin supplementation during pregnancy and reduced cancers such as neuroblastoma, leukemia, and brain tumors in children (Goh et al., 2007).

Although vitamin needs do increase during pregnancy, most of the vitamin intake requirements (with the exception of folic acid) can be met by eating a healthy, varied diet with plenty of fruits and vegetables plus daily prenatal vitamins. Women who were taking oral contraceptives before they became pregnant should be certain to include good sources of vitamins A and B and folic acid in early pregnancy because oral contraceptives may deplete stores of these vitamins. Counsel women not to use mineral oil as a laxative because it can prevent absorption of fat-soluble vitamins from the gastrointestinal tract, limiting their availability to the body. If a woman is housebound, be certain that she is taking a prenatal vitamin containing vitamin D because she is probably not receiving as much sun exposure as normally (More, 2007).

Commonly, a prenatal vitamin is prescribed during pregnancy to be certain that pregnant women ingest sufficient vitamins (Box 13.4). Caution women to avoid taking megadoses

BOX 13.4 ✻ Focus on Pharmacology

Prenatal Vitamins (Natalins)

Action: Supplements nutrition to ensure adequate intake of vitamins and minerals during pregnancy. The folic acid content helps prevent megaloblastic anemia in the mother and neural tube defects in the fetus (Hale, 2007).

Ingredients: Vitamin A (4000 U), vitamin D (400 U), vitamin E (15 U), vitamin C (80 mg), vitamin B_1 (1.5 mg), vitamin B_2 (2.0 mg), vitamin B_6 (4 mg), vitamin B_{12} (2.5 μg), niacin (17 mg), folic acid (1.0 mg), pantothenic acid (7 mg), calcium (200 mg), iron (54 mg), copper (3 mg), zinc (25 mg), and magnesium (100 mg)

Dosage: One tablet daily

Possible Adverse Effects: None known. Folic acid may mask the signs of pernicious anemia.

Nursing Implications

- Encourage women to take the medication exactly as prescribed; caution women not to exceed the recommended dosage.
- Assist with ways to remind women to take the medication, such as a note on the refrigerator.
- Advise women to keep vitamins, like all medications, out of the reach of small children to prevent accidental poisoning.

of vitamins. The mechanism of placental transfer of water-soluble vitamins makes fetal blood levels regularly higher than maternal blood levels, so a maternal overdosage can cause fetal toxicity. Megadoses of vitamin C may cause withdrawal scurvy in the infant at birth. The fat-soluble vitamins are stored in the body rather than excreted and so can reach toxic levels even more easily. There may be an association between excessive vitamin A intake and fetal malformation. It is well documented that the intake of excessive vitamin A in the form of isotretinoin (Accutane), a medication prescribed for acne, causes congenital anomalies (Karch, 2009).

Although folic acid (folacin) belongs to the B-vitamin group, its importance during pregnancy warrants a separate discussion. Found predominantly in fresh fruits and vegetables, folic acid is necessary for red blood cell formation. As a woman's blood volume doubles during pregnancy, this makes her folic acid needs increase substantially. Without adequate folic acid, a megaloblastic anemia (large but ineffective red blood cells) may develop. If a woman has this blood pattern at the time of birth, the infant may be affected as well.

For this reason, as well as its importance in preventing neural tube defects, women should eat foods high in folic acid such as vegetables and fruit and should take a prenatal vitamin that contains a folic acid supplement of 0.4 to 1.0 mg (Subramanian et al., 2008). When cautioning women about vitamin use, advise them not to leave prenatal vitamins within the reach of small children. The excessive folic acid and iron in them can cause poisoning in small children.

Mineral Needs

Minerals are necessary for new cell building in a fetus. Because they are found in so many foods and because mineral absorption improves during pregnancy, mineral deficiency, with the exceptions of calcium, iodine, and iron, is rare.

Calcium and Phosphorus. The skeleton and teeth constitute a major portion of a fetus. Tooth formation begins as early as 8 weeks in utero. Bones begin to calcify at 12 weeks. To supply adequate calcium and phosphorus for bone formation, pregnant women need to eat foods high in calcium and vitamin D (necessary for calcium to be absorbed from the gastrointestinal tract and to enter bones). The recommended amount of calcium during pregnancy is 1300 mg. If a woman cannot drink milk or eat milk products such as cheese, she can be prescribed a daily calcium supplement. Most foods high in protein are also high in phosphorus, so by eating high-protein foods, women receive enough phosphorus, also important for bone growth.

Before nutrition counseling in pregnancy became common, women expected to lose "a tooth a child"—that is, they believed a fetus, as he or she grew, could drain calcium from their teeth. Although it is unlikely that a woman will lose a tooth with pregnancy today, the concern reflected in this myth about a fetus taking calcium from the mother is well founded. However, the calcium in teeth is not as readily absorbed as that of bone. It is more likely that inadequate calcium intake will result in diminished maternal bone density rather than weakened teeth. With an adequate calcium intake during pregnancy, a fetus will receive the needed calcium for growth and mineralization of the fetal skeleton without taking any away from the maternal bones or teeth.

Iodine. Iodine is essential for the formation of thyroxine and, therefore, for the proper functioning of the thyroid gland. As thyroid function increases during pregnancy, a woman needs to ingest enough iodine during pregnancy to supply this increased need. If iodine deficiency occurs, it can cause hypothyroidism and thyroid enlargement (goiter) in a woman. In extreme instances, it can cause the same symptoms in a fetus. Thyroid enlargement in a fetus at birth is serious because the increased pressure of the enlarged gland on the airway could lead to early respiratory distress. If not discovered at birth, hypothyroidism may lead to the infant's being cognitively challenged. The DRI for iodine is 220 μg daily during pregnancy. Seafood is the best source of iodine.

In areas where the water and soil are known to be deficient in iodine such as the Great Lakes area in the United States, it is suggested that women use iodized salt rather than plain salt to ensure a healthy iodine intake (Marchioni et al., 2008).

Iron. A fetus at term has a hemoglobin level of 17 to 21 g per 100 mL of blood, a level that is necessary to oxygenate the blood during intrauterine life. Iron is needed to build this high level of hemoglobin. In addition, after week 20 of pregnancy, a fetus begins to store iron in the liver to last through the first 3 months of life, when intake will consist mainly of milk, typically low in iron. In addition to supplying these high fetal needs, a woman needs iron to build an increased red cell volume for herself and to protect against iron lost in blood at birth.

The DRI for iron for pregnant women is 27 mg. An average diet supplies about 6 mg of iron per 1000 calories. If a woman eats a 2500-calorie diet daily, her daily intake, therefore, is about 15 mg iron. Because only 10% to 20% of dietary iron is absorbed, she is actually taking in less than this amount (closer to 1.5 to 3 mg). Therefore, dietary supplementation with 15 mg iron per day helps ensure that adequate iron is ingested and absorbed. Stress to women that iron supplementation is intended as a supplement to, not a replacement for, iron-rich foods.

Women with low incomes may find it difficult to eat adequate iron-rich foods, because the foods richest in iron (e.g., organ meats; eggs; green, leafy vegetables; whole grains; enriched breads; dried fruits) are also expensive. Iron absorption increases in an acid environment, so eating iron-rich foods or swallowing iron pills with ascorbic acid (found in orange juice) may increase absorption. Oral iron compounds turn stools black or blackish green. The compounds can be irritating to the stomach or cause constipation in some women. If this happens, urge women not to stop taking the iron compound but to always take the iron pills with food and increase fluid intake or fiber to relieve the constipation. Some women may need a prescribed stool softener such as docusate sodium (Colace); this stool softener is not associated with teratogenic action, so it can be taken safely during pregnancy.

Fluoride. Because fluoride aids in the formation of sound teeth, a pregnant woman should drink fluoridated water. In an area where the water is not fluoridated either naturally or artificially, supplemental fluoride may be recommended. Fluoride in large amounts causes brown-stained teeth, so a woman should not take the supplement more often than prescribed or if tap water in her area is already fluoridated. Many women, worried about added chemicals in their city water supply, switch to bottled water during pregnancy. If they do this, advise them to buy a fluoridated type or alert their health care providers that they may need a supplement.

Sodium. Sodium is the major electrolyte that acts to maintain fluid in the body: when sodium is retained rather than excreted by the kidneys, an equal or balancing amount of fluid is also retained. Retaining enough fluid during pregnancy in the maternal circulation is important to ensure a pressure gradient to allow optimal exchange of nutrients across the placenta.

Unless a woman is hypertensive or has heart disease with required sodium restriction when she enters pregnancy, she should continue to add salt to foods as usual during pregnancy. However, she should use moderation with foods that are extremely salty, such as lunch meats or potato chips, or with additive monosodium glutamate. Too much salt could result in retention of excessive amounts of fluid, putting a strain on her heart as blood volume doubles.

Zinc. Zinc is necessary for the synthesis of DNA and RNA. Although not proved, zinc deficiency may be associated with preterm birth. The DRI for zinc during pregnancy is 12 mg, or an increase of 3 mg over prepregnancy needs. Most people who take in adequate protein also take in adequate zinc because zinc is contained in foods such as meat, liver, eggs, and seafood. It is also a component of prenatal vitamins to help ensure an adequate intake (Rolfes, Pinna, & Whitney, 2009).

Fluid Needs

Extra amounts of water are needed during pregnancy to promote kidney function because a woman must excrete waste products for two. Two or three glasses of fluid daily over and above the three servings of milk recommended by the food pyramid is a common recommendation during pregnancy (a total of six to eight glasses daily).

Fiber Needs

Constipation can occur during pregnancy from slowed peristalsis because of the pressure of the uterus on the intestine. Eating fiber-rich foods, foods consisting of parts of the plant cell wall resistant to normal digestive enzymes such as broccoli and asparagus, are a natural way of preventing constipation, because the bulk of the fiber left in the intestine aids evacuation. Fiber also has the advantage of lowering cholesterol levels and may remove carcinogenic contaminants from the intestine. Therefore, encourage women to eat plenty of fresh fruits and vegetables, especially green, leafy vegetables, to provide fiber. Eating fiber-rich foods this way is a better choice for preventing constipation than taking a fiber laxative. Doing so allows a woman to receive nutrients from the food as well as preventing constipation (Derbyshire, 2007).

Foods to Avoid or Limit in Pregnancy

As discussed in Chapter 12, alcoholic beverages should not be ingested by a pregnant woman because of their potentially teratogenic effects on a fetus. Other foods to be avoided are those that contain food additives, because the effect of many of these is unknown.

Excess Seafood

Women should eat up to 12 ounces (2 to 3 meals) of seafood or shellfish a week for their omega-3 and iodine content. Fish such as shark, swordfish, king mackerel or tilefish are high in mercury contamination, however, so should be avoided (Genuis, 2008). Five types of fish that are low in mercury are shrimp, canned light tuna, salmon, pollock, and catfish. Women should check local advisories about the safety of fish caught by family and friends in local rivers and streams. If no advice is available, women can safely eat up to 6 ounces (one meal) per week of fish from local waters if they don't consume any other fish during that week.

Foods With Caffeine

Caffeine is thought of by many women as just an incidental ingredient in beverages. Actually, it is a central nervous system stimulant capable of increasing heart rate, urine production in the kidney, and secretion of acid in the stomach (Rolfes, Pinna, & Whitney, 2009).

A daily intake of caffeine of two or three cups of coffee has not been associated with low birth weight, but drinking over three cups is associated with an increased rate of early miscarriage (Applebee, 2008). To limit their caffeine intake, women may need to limit not only the amount of coffee they drink but also other sources of caffeine such as chocolate, soft drinks, and tea. If a woman has difficulty omitting these common foods from her diet, she can still reduce the amount of caffeine she ingests. Decaffeinated coffee, as the name implies, contains almost no caffeine.

The longer tea brews, the greater is the caffeine content. Green tea has less caffeine than black tea. Both herbal teas and decaffeinated tea are readily available.

The cocoa bean that is used to make chocolate and cocoa is yet another natural source of caffeine. Chocolate sources tend to be low in caffeine, however, compared with coffee. A cup of coffee contains approximately 120 mg of caffeine, whereas a cup of hot chocolate contains only 10 mg. Baking chocolate, used for cake frostings and glazes, is proportionately higher, containing about 35 mg of caffeine per ounce.

Soft drinks do not naturally contain caffeine; it is added to improve their flavor. To limit the amount of caffeine consumed, encourage pregnant women to choose caffeine-free types.

Artificial Sweeteners

Artificial sweeteners are used to improve the taste and to limit the caloric content of foods. It is probably safest for pregnant women to reduce their intake of these. For instance, although the sweetener aspartame has been approved by the U.S. Food and Drug Administration for consumption and is apparently safe during pregnancy, large amounts of the compound should be avoided by pregnant women until its safety is thoroughly confirmed. The use of saccharine is not recommended during pregnancy because it is eliminated slowly from the fetal bloodstream. In any event, pregnant women need carbohydrates furnished by sugar rather than artificial substances (Rolfes, Pinna, & Whitney, 2009).

What if... Tori Alarino states, "I love coffee. There's always a pot brewing where I work. And I love a cup of cappuccino for lunch." What suggestions could you make to help her reduce her caffeine intake?

Weight Loss Diets

As a rule, weight reduction is not healthy during pregnancy. Liquid reducing diets and/or diets that are combined with weight-reducing drugs are particularly contraindicated during pregnancy because they may lead to fetal ketoacidosis and poor growth. If women have been following such diets before becoming pregnant, they may have few nutritional stores, and additional vitamin supplementation may be necessary.

✔ Checkpoint Question 13.2

Which statement by Tori lets you know she understands how iron is best absorbed?

a. "I always take my iron pills with milk."
b. "I crush my iron pills to disguise the taste."
c. "I take the pills with a carbonated beverage."
d. "I swallow my iron pills with orange juice."

ASSESSMENT OF NUTRITIONAL HEALTH

Women who follow good nutrition practices before pregnancy come into pregnancy in better health and best prepared to avoid pregnancy complications (Box 13.5). The best method for assessing a woman's nutritional intake is to ask for a "typical day" history or a 24-hour nutrition recall to isolate usual patterns and possible nutritional risk factors (Table 13.2). First, ask if yesterday was a typical day. If it was, then ask a woman to list all the food she ate within the past 24 hours, starting with when she awakened until she went to sleep. Be certain she includes all the snack foods she ate, as well as sit-down meals. This method of history taking yields much more accurate information than if a woman is asked how often during the week she eats citrus fruit or how much milk she drinks every day because most people eat automatically with little thought to their food intake (Cohen & Farley, 2008). A woman who knows how much milk she ought to drink a day tends to say she drinks four glasses a day during pregnancy. However, if asked to list the foods she ate the day before, she may report that she drank only one glass of milk all day.

In addition to actual food intake, ask a woman if she thinks she has any problem with nutrition (such as cravings). Also, assess the circumstances of eating, such as cultural preferences, who prepares food in the family, and how many meals are eaten outside the home weekly, as these are important for a total nutrition picture (Table 13.3).

To strengthen history findings, assess a woman's prepregnancy weight and calculate her BMI. People with poor nutrition are typically overweight or underweight and show typical physical signs. Table 13.4 lists important physical examination assessments that suggest a good nutritional intake or evidence of poor nutrition.

BOX 13.5 ✻ Focus on Evidence-Based Practice

Does high-fat nutrition during pregnancy influence the development of gestational diabetes?

What women eat during pregnancy certainly influences their serum glucose levels. Interested in learning if a diet high in total fatty acids, saturated fatty acids, and red meat increases women's risk of developing diabetes during pregnancy, researchers asked 1733 women to record everything they ate during the first trimester of their pregnancies. At 26 to 28 weeks, a glucose tolerance test was done to assess if gestational diabetes had occurred. Of the 1733 women studied, 91 (5%) developed gestational diabetes (a fasting serum glucose over 126 mg/dL) and 206 (11%) developed impaired glucose tolerance or a blood glucose 100 to 125 mg/dL. The types of food women ate, however, did not influence these results, and the type of nutrient or food intake in early pregnancy was not linked to a risk of gestational diabetes. Nutritional status entering pregnancy, as reflected by the women's prepregnancy BMI, appeared to be more predictive than was food eaten during pregnancy.

Would the results of this study be helpful in prepregnancy or adolescent counseling?

Source: Radesky, J. S., et al. (2008). Diet during early pregnancy and development of gestational diabetes. *Paediatric and Perinatal Epidemiology, 22*(1), 47–59.

TABLE 13.2 ✻ Nutritional Risk Factors During Pregnancy

Risk	Rationale
Adolescent (younger than 18 years)	Adolescent growth involves increased nutritional needs.
Short intervals between pregnancies	A woman's body has not had time to replace nutritional stores depleted during a previous pregnancy.
Low income	Family may not have resources to purchase adequate foods to meet pregnancy nutritional needs.
Food fads	Foods eaten may not be those adequate for pregnancy.
Drug use (including cigarettes and alcohol)	Drugs may be ingested in preference to healthy foods.
Existence of a chronic illness requiring a special diet	Intake may be low in an essential substance such as carbohydrate or protein.
Underweight or overweight	Underweight and overweight status may indicate chronic inadequate nutrition patterns.
Multiple pregnancy	A woman must supply enough nutrition for multiple fetal development.
Anemic at conception	A woman has no iron stores for fetal growth.
Lactose intolerance	A woman may not be ingesting adequate calcium for fetal skeletal growth.

TABLE 13.3 ✻ Areas to Be Assessed for a Total Nutrition History

Area of Assessment	Pertinent Questions
Food preparation	Who does the cooking at your house? Do you cook for people besides yourself? How do you usually prepare food (fried or baked)? What spices or condiments do you use commonly? What type of oil do you use for frying (saturated or unsaturated)?
Food pattern	How many meals do you eat on a typical day? Which is your biggest meal? How many snacks do you eat a day? What are they? How many meals do you eat outside your home? Where do you eat them? Cafeteria? Fast-food store? Restaurant? Bagged lunch? Are there any foods that you cannot or will not eat? Why?
Financial concerns	Does your family have enough money for food? Who does the food shopping? Would you eat differently if more money were available? Do you use any supplementary financial programs?
Activity level	Are you normally active or sedentary? (Could increase calorie need.)
Health	Do you have any allergies to food? Do you have any trouble with chewing or digestion? What is your bowel movement frequency? Were you taking oral contraceptives before pregnancy? Do you take supplemental vitamins? What type? How many? Do you drink alcohol? What type? How much? Do you smoke cigarettes? What is your stress level? Does stress affect your appetite?
Personal food preferences	Are there any foods you particularly enjoy or dislike? Are there any foods you feel are harmful or particularly beneficial during pregnancy? Do you have any special cultural or religious preferences?
Family dietary patterns	Is anyone in your family on a special diet? Is anyone obviously overweight or underweight? Does your family eat meals together? Is mealtime a social time?

TABLE 13.4 ✻ Physical Signs and Symptoms of Adequate Pregnancy Nutrition

Assessment Area	Signs of Good Nutrition	Signs of Poor Nutrition
Hair	Shiny; strong with good body	Hair dull and lifeless (possible protein deficit)
Eyes	Good eyesight, particularly at night; conjunctiva moist and pink	Pale and dry conjunctiva (iron and fluid deficit); difficulty with night vision (vitamin A deficit)
Mouth	No cavities in teeth; no swollen or inflamed gingiva; no cracks or fissures at corners of mouth; mucous membrane moist and pink; tongue smooth and nontender	Fissures at corners of mouth; tongue rough and tender (vitamin A deficit); mucous membrane pale (iron deficit)
Neck	Normal contour of thyroid gland	Thyroid gland enlarged (iodine deficit)
Skin	Smooth, with normal color and turgor; no ecchymotic or petechial areas present	Rough texture; poor turgor (fluid deficit) Vitamin K deficiency leads to petechia.
Extremities	Normal muscle mass and circumference; normal strength and mobility; edema limited to slight ankle involvement; normal reflexes	Poor muscle tone; diminished reflexes (protein deficit)
Fingernails and toenails	Smooth; pink; normal contour	Pale; break easily; little growth (protein deficit)
Weight	Within normal limits of ideal weight before pregnancy; following normal pattern of pregnancy weight gain	Overweight or underweight; unusually slow or rapid weight gain (inadequate or excessive carbohydrate).
Blood pressure	Within normal limits for length of pregnancy	Decreased from anemia (iron deficit); increased from hypertension

Hemoglobin or hematocrit determinations (see Appendix F) are also important assessments of good nutrition. These may reveal smoking habits, as cigarette smokers have higher hemoglobin levels than nonsmokers. These values are measured early in pregnancy and then usually repeated close to term and again at birth. A urinalysis can also be important because a finding such as elevated urine specific gravity could suggest a less-than-adequate fluid intake and elevated urine glucose levels suggest gestational diabetes (see Chapter 20).

After obtaining the full nutritional pattern, compare the types and amounts on the list with those shown in Figure 13.1 to see if all food groups and adequate amounts are included. Comparing foods from the person's 24-hour recall with a guide is a helpful way to show clients that what they thought was a "perfect" intake is imperfect or what they thought was a "little" problem actually involves the loss of an entire food group. Once a woman sees that a deficit exists, she may be more motivated to improve her nutrition. Such a picture also offers an instant reward for a woman who is ingesting adequate foods.

PROMOTING NUTRITIONAL HEALTH DURING PREGNANCY

Be certain that plans for improving nutritional patterns take into account a woman's lifestyle, family preferences, financial resources, customs, and cultural desires, because she and her family must follow them for 9 months (Fig. 13.2).

Family Considerations

Meal planning is best if it involves the entire family because even if a woman is receptive to changing her eating habits, she may have difficulty carrying out recommendations if her family resists the change. In families where a member has a special nutritional need, such as restricted sodium, change may be even more difficult. You may need to speak with the person who prepares meals for an adolescent as well as the adolescent to be certain that recommended changes will be carried out.

Financial Considerations

Food is costly, so to provide the extra servings required during pregnancy, a woman must spend more on food for herself per week than she is used to spending. Women generally view this increased expense as an investment in their child's health and do not regard it as a burden. However, a woman on a marginal income, although she may be willing to shoulder the additional cost, may have difficulty actually doing so. If this occurs, review what foods the woman is eating to be certain she is not buying only starchy foods because they are more filling and less expensive than protein foods. Help her secure available financial assistance such as food stamps, or inform her about nutritional aid programs such as WIC.

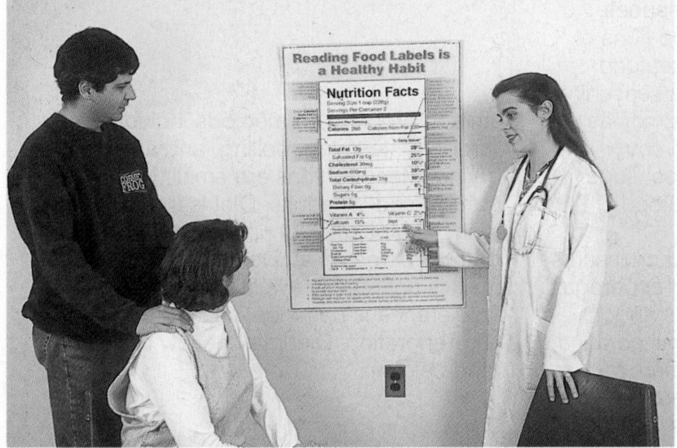

FIGURE 13.2 Encourage pregnant women and their partners to eat a varied diet with a high iron and protein content. This may be difficult for a woman early in pregnancy because of nausea and late in pregnancy because of fatigue. (© Barbara Proud.)

Under the food stamp program, a family with a low income can buy stamps that can be redeemed at grocery stores for any food items except alcohol or pet food. The cost of stamps varies, but the use of food stamps can increase a family's buying power as much as $150 a month.

The advantage of this type of program is that it helps to supplement the cost of food but places almost no restrictions on what foods can be selected and purchased. It can make the difference for a low-income family between being able to eat meat or living on a starchy diet.

WIC is a federal program that provides nutritional support for low-income women and children to reduce not only the risk of low birth weight but also medical costs by preventing costly newborn care. Established in 1972, WIC is funded by the Food and Nutrition Service of the U.S. Department of Agriculture. The program supplies supplemental foods and nutrition education for:

- Pregnant women
- Postpartum women up to 6 months
- Nursing mothers up to 1 year
- Children from birth to age 5

Each state defines the income eligibility level for its citizens, but the eligibility for all programs is based on income level, geographic area, and nutritional risk. To receive food, clients must live in an area that has been designated as a funding area. The nurse or nutritionist in the health care facility determines possible risk and nutritional need. Factors considered that put pregnant women at nutritional risk include age (an adolescent or a woman over 40); poor obstetric history such as previous spontaneous miscarriage, a short period between pregnancies, previous low-birth-weight infant, or gestational diabetes; anemia; poor weight gain; or inadequate consumption of food by nutrition history.

For the pregnant woman, foods typically offered by the program include those with high-quality protein, iron, calcium, and vitamins A and C, such as fruit juice, eggs, milk, and cheese. At predetermined intervals, WIC clients are reevaluated to see if the program supplements are still necessary. WIC has been successful in improving nutrition during pregnancy because not only does it supply additional food to recipients but also the periodic evaluations provide time for nutritional counseling (Watts et al., 2007).

School lunch programs are a way that some pregnant adolescents can receive help with nutrition. Millions of schoolchildren qualify for free or reduced-price school lunches. A school lunch (type A) is designed to provide one third of a child's DRI. For many adolescents, these school lunches may be the most nutritious meal they eat in a day. Although there may be a large selection of foods to choose, children who have a sense of self-efficacy are able to make the wisest choices at school lunches (Thompson et al., 2007).

TABLE 13.5 ✻ Characteristics of Certain Ethnic Diets

Group and Place of Origin	Staple Foods	Common Customs
Hispanic Americans from Puerto Rico	Steamed white rice; many varieties of beans; wheat breads; starchy vegetables such as cassavas, yams, breadfruit, plantains, and green bananas; green peppers; tomatoes; garlic; dried, salted fish; salt pork, bacon; lard; olive oil; sugar; jams and jellies, sweet pastries; sugared fruit juices; cafe con leche (coffee and hot milk)	Milk is rarely consumed as a beverage. Most food is cooked for long periods or fried. Malt beer is believed to be nutritious and may be given to children and breastfeeding mothers.
Hispanic Americans from Mexico, Central America	Many varieties of beans; steamed rice; corn products such as tortillas made from lime-soaked cornmeal; chili peppers, tomatoes; mangoes; prickly pear fruit; potatoes; meat and sausages; fish; poultry; eggs; milk cheeses; milk custards and bread puddings; lard; sweet chocolate and coffee drinks; cakes, pastries	Most vegetables are cooked so long that they lose nutritional value. Diet is high in fiber and starch. Animal fat is frequently added during food preparation. Because milk, green leafy vegetables, and fruit intakes are low, diet may be inadequate in calcium, iron, vitamin A, and vitamin C. Obesity is common.
Hispanic Americans from Cuba	Stews and casseroles flavored with sage, parsley, bay leaf, thyme, cinnamon, curry, capers, onion, cloves, garlic, saffron. Soup is served daily. Fried foods, especially fish, poultry, eggs; rice; many varieties of beans	Fruits and vegetables are not eaten on a regular basis. Main meal is usually served at lunch.
Southern African Americans from West Africa (many generations in United States)	Hominy grits; biscuits; cornmeal and corn bread; rice; legumes; potatoes; onions; tomatoes; hot peppers; green leafy vegetables cooked in fatback or salt pork; okra; sweet potatoes; squashes; corn; cabbage; melons; peaches; pecans; all parts of a pig; fresh meats and poultry; fish; thick stews; butter, shortening, and lard; sugar; bread puddings; pies and sweets	African American food patterns are similar to those of whites in same region. Northern African Americans may be unfamiliar with "soul food." Frying is common; diet tends to be high in fat and salt, low in calcium. High rate of obesity.
Chinese Americans (diets vary sometimes with region)	Rice and rice gruel; wheat noodles; corn; green vegetables, especially from the cabbage family; squashes; cucumbers; eggplant; leafy vegetables; various shoots, including bamboo, mung, and soy; sweet potatoes; radishes; onions; peas and pods; mushrooms; roots; many local, seasonal vegetables; pickled vegetables; sea vegetables; plums; peaches; tangerines; kumquats and other citrus fruits; litchis; longans; mangoes; papayas; pomegranates; soybean products such as tofu (soybean curd), soy sauces, bean noodles, and soy milk; tiny portions of meat, fish with bones, or poultry; seafood; soup or tea as beverage; sugar as seasoning	Yin (feminine)–yang (masculine) concept of balancing intake; moderation is valued. Obesity is rare. Regional differences in food choices exist. Rice symbolizes life and fertility. Raw vegetables are rarely served. Diet is high in fiber and many nutrients, is low in fat, and may be low in protein
Japanese Americans	Rice; vegetables; pickled vegetables; soy as miso (soup), tofu, bean paste, and soy sauce; fruits; salads; fish with bones; sugar as seasoning; sea vegetables; seafood; ginseng; green tea	Common preparation methods include broiling, steaming, boiling, and stir-frying. Meat portions are small. Milk is rarely used by adults. Diet is low in fat, rich in nutrients, high in sodium.
Vietnamese Americans	Rice, rice noodles; French bread and croissants with butter; hot peppers; curries of asparagus and potatoes; salads; tropical fruits and vegetables; lemons and limes; small portions of poultry; eggs; fish parts; *nuoc mam* (a strong, fermented fish sauce added to almost every cooked dish); sweets, candies, sweetened drinks; coffee; tea	Rice may be eaten at every meal. Fresh milk is not readily available; lactose intolerance is common. Little fat is used in preparation. Diet may be low in iron and calcium.

Group and Place of Origin	Staple Foods	Common Customs
Native Americans	Southeast: corn; cornmeal; coontie (flour from a palmlike plant); fried breads; swamp cabbage (now illegal to harvest); pumpkins; squashes; papayas; alligator, snake, wild hog, duck, fish, and shellfish. Northeast: blueberries; cranberries; beans; corn; pumpkins; fish; lobster; wild game; maple syrup. Midwest: bison; beans; corn; melons; squashes; tomatoes. Southwest: corn (many colors and varieties); beans; squash; pumpkins; chili peppers; melons; pinenuts; cactus. Northwest: salmon; caviar; other fish; otter; seal; whale; bear; elk; other game; wild fruits; acorns (and other wild nuts); wild greens	Food has great religious and social significance. Corn is a status food for most tribes. Milk is seldom used; calcium intake is usually low. Diets on some reservations are considered poor. High rate of obesity.

Source: Dudek, S. (2009). *Nutrition handbook for nursing practice* (5th ed.). Philadelphia: Lippincott Williams & Wilkins.

Cultural Considerations

When helping plan nutrition during pregnancy, try to suggest foods that are individually or culturally favored, as these are the foods women tend to enjoy and will eat most consistently. Common cultural differences to be aware of in nutritional counseling are shown in Table 13.5.

✔ Checkpoint Question 13.3

You need to obtain a nutrition history from Tori. What is the best way to do this?

a. Ask her to tell you how much protein she eats daily.
b. Assess if Tori feels satisfied with her nutrition.
c. Ask Tori to describe what she ate in the last 24 hours.
d. Tell Tori to describe her concept of ideal nutrition.

Managing Common Problems Affecting Nutritional Health

Specific nutrition problems may result during pregnancy from several factors or circumstances. Discomforts such as constipation and flatulence that can result from food choices, and possible solutions to these concerns, have been discussed (see Chapter 12).

Nausea and Vomiting

As many as 50% of pregnant women report nausea and vomiting (Rojas, Wood, & Blakemore, 2007). No definite cause has been established for this symptom of early pregnancy, but it may be related to:

- Sensitivity to the high level of chorionic gonadotropin hormone produced by the trophoblast cells
- High estrogen or progesterone levels
- Lowered maternal blood sugar caused by the needs of the developing embryo
- Lack of pyridoxine (vitamin B_6)
- Diminished gastric motility

Nausea is aggravated by fatigue and may be aggravated by emotional disturbance. Most women notice the sensation as early as the first missed menstrual period and experience it throughout the first 3 months of pregnancy. The sensation is usually most intense on arising but may occur while a woman is preparing meals or smelling food. Vomiting at least once a day is common. Women who work nights and sleep days often experience "evening sickness," because that is when they arise.

Methods such as acupressure, anti–motion sickness wrist bands, or avoiding fluid with meals are effective for some women. Mild-flavored ginger tea may be helpful (White, 2007). Increasing carbohydrate intake seems to relieve nausea better than any other nutrition remedy. The traditional solution is for women to keep dry crackers, such as Saltines, by their bedside and eat a few before rising; sourball candies may serve the same purpose. A woman can then eat a light breakfast or delay breakfast until 10 or 11 AM, past the time her nausea seems to persist. To be certain she maintains a good food intake during pregnancy even in the presence of nausea, she should compensate for any missed meals later in the day. If preparing food for others makes her feel queasy, she might try to give this responsibility to another family member, at least through the worst phase of this symptom. Preparing and freezing meals ahead of time, perhaps at night when the nausea is less bothersome, may also help.

It is a good rule for women not to go longer than 12 hours between meals during pregnancy to prevent hypoglycemia. A woman may need to eat a late-evening snack to compensate for a late breakfast. She may be able to tolerate fruit and raw vegetables during the morning before other food. Urge her to experiment with soups or vegetable drinks that she may not usually think of as breakfast foods but that will give her early-morning calories.

Common measures to take to relieve nausea are summarized in Box 13.6. Caution women against self-medicating for nausea by taking antacids. Excessive use of antacids containing sodium bicarbonate may cause fluid retention because of the sodium content.

Fortunately, nausea usually disappears spontaneously as a woman enters her fourth month of pregnancy. If it persists beyond this month or is so extreme in early pregnancy that it interferes with nutrition, it may indicate the development of hyperemesis gravidarum, a serious complication of pregnancy.

Cravings

Cravings for food or aversions to certain foods during pregnancy are so common that they are considered a normal part

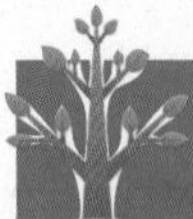

BOX 13.6 * Focus on Family Teaching

Measures to Reduce and Evaluate Nausea During Pregnancy

Q. Tori Alarino tells you, "I've been nauseated ever since I became pregnant. What can I take to make this better?"

A. If nausea and vomiting are causing a fluid imbalance, medications can be prescribed. Common nonpharmacologic measures you can take to reduce nausea are:

- Be aware that at least 50% of women experience nausea during pregnancy, so what you are experiencing is normal.
- Eat a few dry crackers, toast, or a sourball before you get out of bed in the morning to increase your carbohydrate intake.
- Eat small but frequent meals rather than large infrequent ones.
- Avoid greasy or highly seasoned food.
- Delay breakfast until nausea passes (dinner if it is evening nausea).
- Make up missed meals at some other time of the day to maintain nutrition.
- Avoid sudden movements and fatigue because these may increase or cause nausea.
- Eat a snack before bedtime so delaying breakfast will not cause you to go a long time between meals.
- Purchase a wrist acupressure band (purchased in travel stores for motion sickness).

If nausea is present:

- Try sipping a carbonated beverage, water, or an herbal noncaffeinated or ginger tea.
- Try a walk outside in the fresh air or take deep breaths through an open window.

Notify your health care provider if:

- You are losing weight rather than gaining it.
- You have not gained the projected amount of weight for your week of pregnancy.
- You are unable to make up for lost meals some other time of the day.
- You have signs of dehydration such as little urine output.
- Nausea has lasted past 12 weeks of pregnancy.
- You vomit more than once daily.

of adaptation to pregnancy. It was formerly considered that these strange desires for food reflected a woman's need to call attention to a pregnancy or were a reaction to her imposed dependent state. However, cravings are actually more likely the result of a physiologic need for more carbohydrates or particular vitamins and minerals such as iron.

Now that recommended pregnancy nutrition allows for more calories and a greater pregnancy weight gain is encouraged, cravings are seen less often than before. When taking a nutrition history, ask if a woman notices any particular cravings. As long as this is a healthy type of food, help her plan a nutrition intake that includes the food, at least in moderation. This is a positive approach to nutrition counseling: it allows her to enjoy her pregnancy without feeling guilty because she is eating foods she craves.

During pregnancy, some women report an abnormal craving for nonfood substances (termed **pica** from the Latin word for "magpie," a bird that is an indiscriminate eater). The most common form of pica in the past was a craving for laundry starch. Today, women are more apt to report cravings for clay, dirt, cornstarch, or ice cubes (Mills, 2007). Although some of these items can do no harm in themselves, the ingestion of large quantities of nonfood substances can leave a woman deficient in protein, iron, and calcium, nutrients essential for a healthy pregnancy outcome (Box 13.7).

Always ask women at prenatal visits if they crave any nonfood items, as most women do not supply this information unless asked directly. They worry that you will find their behavior odd, or they may not realize their habit is pregnancy related as much as being a nervous habit.

Encouraging a woman to stop eating the nonfood substance may not be effective because the habit may be deeply ingrained. Because pica is a symptom that often accompanies iron deficiency anemia, correcting this underlying problem with an iron supplement may correct the pica. At subsequent visits, be certain to assess if a woman's hemoglobin is increasing and ask if she notices any difference in her cravings.

Heartburn (Pyrosis)

Heartburn (pyrosis) is a burning sensation along the esophagus caused by regurgitation of gastric contents into the lower esophagus. In pregnancy, it may accompany early nausea, but it may persist beyond the resolution of nausea and even increase in severity as pregnancy advances.

Pyrosis is probably caused by decreased gastric motility, which slows gastric emptying, and pressure of the expanding uterus pushing up against the stomach. It is noticed by at least 50% of pregnant women (Orr, 2007). Common suggestions to help prevent reflux into the esophagus are:

- Eat small meals frequently rather than large meals.
- Sleep on the left side with two pillows to elevate the upper torso.
- Do not lie down immediately after eating; try and wait at least 2 hours.
- Avoid fatty and fried foods, coffee, carbonated beverages, tomato products, and citrus juices

Aluminum hydroxide (Amphojel, Alternagel) or a combination of aluminum and magnesium hydroxide (Maalox) may be prescribed for relief. If these do not relieve the discomfort, a histamine antagonist such as cimetidine (Tagamet) or ranitidine (Zantac) may be prescribed (Rojas, Wood, & Blakemore, 2007). Be certain a woman understands that this "chest" pain is from her gastrointestinal tract and that, although it is called heartburn, it has nothing to do with her heart.

Hypercholesterolemia

Women with a family history of hypercholesterolemia may enter pregnancy with an elevated cholesterol level. During pregnancy, increasing progesterone levels cause a further elevation of cholesterol. Combined with intrahepatic cholestasis, this can lead to an increased risk for gallstone formation (cholelithiasis) and cardiovascular disease. Preventing

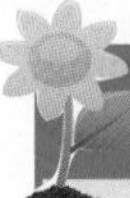

BOX 13.7 * Focus on Communication

Tori comes to your prenatal clinic for her first visit. You want to obtain a nutrition history from her.

Less Effective Communication

Nurse: Hi, Tori. Are you eating a nutritious diet?

Tori: I'm always hungry since I've been pregnant. No problem.

Nurse: Have you ever compared what you eat to a food pyramid to see if you're eating all the different types of food it shows?

Tori: Sure. Grain is on one side; meat is on the other. I eat both of those.

Nurse: It's important to drink at least a quart of milk a day during pregnancy. Are you doing that?

Tori: I'm drinking milkshakes so I not only get calcium but extra calories.

Nurse: That's great. Good nutrition is so important during pregnancy. I'm glad you're so aware of it.

More Effective Communication

Nurse: Hi, Tori. Are you eating a nutritious diet?

Tori: I'm always hungry since I've been pregnant. No problem.

Nurse: Tell me what you ate yesterday.

Tori: A muffin and coffee for breakfast, a milkshake for lunch, a hamburger and fries for supper. A soft drink before bed. And ice cubes. I suck on them all day like candy.

Nurse: Let's talk about ways you might get some fruit and vegetables into your day.

Most people believe they eat well, so if just asked general questions about nutrition, they respond that their nutrition is adequate. Only when they are asked to actually describe what they ate during one day is the truth revealed.

cholelithiasis during pregnancy is important because gallstones can cause extremely sharp pain. Fortunately, surgery to remove gallstones during pregnancy is possible with new ambulatory laparotomy techniques.

A woman who has had difficulty with hypercholesterolemia before pregnancy may need to continue to eat only moderate amounts of fat during pregnancy to prevent any increase in cholesterol. Helpful ways to reduce cholesterol include:

- Exercising daily
- Eating oat cereal
- Broiling meat rather than frying it
- Using a minimum of salad oils
- Substituting new omega-3 products in place of butter
- Eating fish high in omega-3 oil, such as salmon or trout

As discussed earlier, although high in omega-3 oil, current recommendations are that pregnant women limit their intake of tuna, swordfish, King mackerel, and tilefish because of their potentially high mercury content (Sunderland, 2007). Eating raw fish is also not advised because of the danger of parasitic contamination.

Urge women to check with their health care provider about the wisdom of continuing to take cholesterol-lowering drugs during pregnancy, because these drugs may be teratogenic (Karch, 2009). A low-cholesterol diet will automatically be lower in calories than the average diet, because oils and fats add many calories. Therefore, assess these women carefully for adequate weight gain during pregnancy. Make sure that a woman does include some oil daily (perhaps as olive oil on a salad) so she has included a source of linoleic acid in her daily intake.

✔ Checkpoint Question 13.4

Which statement by Tori would best suggest she has pica?

a. "I chew typewriter paper. It helps relieve my heartburn."
b. "I can't eat a thing before 11 o'clock every morning."
c. "I notice I've been eating more sweet stuff than usual."
d. "I crave oranges; can't get enough of them every day."

Promoting Nutritional Health in Women With Special Needs

The Adolescent

A pregnant adolescent needs a high caloric intake (2500 calories per day) to supply energy for her high level of activity and growth. The nutrients most often lacking from a typical adolescent diet tend to be calcium, iron, folic acid, and total calories. Look for sources of these when analyzing a teenager's pregnancy intake.

Good nutrition can be a problem with pregnant teenagers because of the dual demands of consuming enough food to provide for fetal growth and their own continuing growth. Often adolescents, in their search for identity, avoid foods that their parents see as important for them (e.g., milk, warm cereal, vegetables, or fruit) and indulge instead in foods such as soft drinks, potato chips, and French fries. To help an adolescent plan nutritional intake for pregnancy, respect her right to reject traditional foods as long as what she does eat includes sufficient nutrients. A cheese and sausage pizza, a glass of milk, and an apple compose a lunch that provides all basic food groups (meat: sausage; bread: pizza crust; vegetable: tomato sauce; dairy: cheese and milk; fruit: apple). A hamburger "with everything" plus a tangerine and milk provides the same.

Most adolescents snack frequently during the day. Toward the end of pregnancy, when fatigue may be a problem, they may begin to eat more and more "junk food" because preparing nutritious snacks takes more effort. Advise them to prepare nutritious snacks such as carrot sticks or cheese bites early each day when they have more energy so that later in the day, when they are tired, eating a nutritious snack will not involve much effort.

Counseling adolescents about pregnancy nutrition may not be effective, because they often are not responsible for cooking what food they eat. You may need to speak to their parents or support persons (with permission) about certain foods to prepare before you can alter their nutrition pattern. If possible, suggest several foods that would fill a deficit and let the adolescent choose from them to provide a sense of control.

A Woman 40 Years of Age

Today, many women are older than 40 by the time they have their first child, and many more are older than 40 when they have their second or third child (Crombleholme, 2009). The nutritional needs of women in this age group are poorly studied, but it is obvious women in this age group should maintain the same careful pregnancy nutrition as younger women. Because women in this age group may have slightly decreased kidney function, they should be sure to maintain a high fluid intake to remove waste products for themselves and for a fetus. They need adequate calcium to prevent bone density loss. Many women at this point in life are caring for elderly parents, and many have delayed childbearing to establish a career; this means they may eat whatever they are preparing for elderly parents or depend on packed or fast-food lunches for at least part of their nutrition each week. Focus your nutrition counseling on maintaining adequate nutrition during pregnancy, based on these lifestyles.

A Woman With Decreased Nutritional Stores

A woman with high parity or a short interval between pregnancies or one who has been dieting rigorously to lose weight before pregnancy may enter pregnancy with such depleted nutritional reserves that she has little to draw on during the first part of pregnancy. If her folic acid intake has been inadequate, her fetus may be susceptible to neural tube defects (Lumley et al., 2009). This shortage of nutrients may become critical during the time she is unable to eat well because of the normal nausea and vomiting of pregnancy. In addition, nutritional stores may be affected by other variables. Be alert that:

- Women from low-income families may enter pregnancy with anemia.
- Women who used diuretics for a dieting program may be deficient in potassium.
- Women who have been taking oral contraceptives may have decreased folate stores.
- Women who were using intrauterine devices or who have menorrhagia may be deficient in iron from excessive blood loss with menstrual flows.
- Women who drink alcohol excessively may be deficient in thiamine.

Women with these decreased nutritional stores need to be identified early in pregnancy through history taking so they can be referred to a nutritionist for specific nutritional counseling. They may need additional supplements during pregnancy to restore a particular nutrient.

A Woman Who Is Underweight

Today's emphasis on slim, model-like female figures makes it easy to overlook the health problem of a woman who is underweight. A woman who enters a pregnancy underweight, however, needs nutritional counseling just as much as an overweight woman.

Underweight is defined as a state in which a woman's weight is 10% to 15% less than the ideal weight for her height, or a BMI of less than 18.5 kg/m^2. Most women who are underweight tire easily because they have an accompanying iron deficiency anemia. Even when underweight women gain excessive weight during pregnancy, they still tend to have a higher-than-usual incidence of low-birth-weight infants, probably because of depleted nutrient stores at the pregnancy's beginning. This is one reason why preconceptual health care visits and assessments are so important (Bernstein & Weinstein, 2007).

Being underweight may occur for a variety of reasons:

- Dieting for weight loss
- Poverty and the inability to buy adequate food (however, many poor women are obese, not underweight, because starchy foods are less expensive than those that have a higher protein content, such as meat and eggs)
- Excessive worry or stress, emotions that can lead to a loss of appetite
- Depression, which causes a chronic loss of appetite
- An eating disorder, such as anorexia nervosa or bulimia, conditions in which a woman has developed revulsion to food (see Chapter 54)

However, the major reason for being underweight is insufficient intake of food because of chronic poor nutritional habits.

Convincing women who are underweight to eat more may be difficult because you are asking a woman to change lifelong eating habits (Abayomi et al., 2007). Counseling also can be challenging because during the first trimester of pregnancy, when fetal need is greatest and at a time when she has nausea and vomiting, possibly losing all desire to eat, you are asking her to take in additional food.

Begin counseling by asking a woman for a 24-hour nutrition recall. Total daily caloric intake for the underweight woman may need to be as high as 3500 calories (500 to 1000 calories more than the usual specified daily amount). Work with women to develop menus based on well-planned meals rather than on quick take-out foods. Suggest additional calories in the form of a concentrated formula such as an instant liquid breakfast drink. Be certain a woman understands this should not be a high-protein drink used for high-protein dieting regimens. Such diet drinks deliver a concentrated solute load (breakdown products of protein) to the kidney (already working to capacity because of the pregnancy) and provide so little carbohydrate in proportion to protein that they encourage the breakdown of protein for body energy, a process that results in acidosis. High-protein diets of this nature are not recommended for long-term use by anyone, but they should be totally avoided by women during pregnancy.

A 500-calorie increase over normal requirements should result in a weight gain of an additional pound per week. Be certain to plan for this additional gain when the total weight gain during pregnancy is calculated at each office visit. Otherwise, the total weight gain of a woman may seem excessive when it is actually healthy.

If a lack of nutritional stores makes a woman feel tired, urge her to schedule adequate rest periods daily so she can feel sufficiently energetic to prepare nutritious meals. Be certain she is taking her prescribed vitamin and iron supplements. Additional nutritional counseling in the postpartum period may be necessary so she can maintain better nutrition throughout her life and can enter a subsequent pregnancy (if she desires one) in a state of nutritional health.

A Woman Who Is Overweight

A woman is considered **overweight** if she is 20% above ideal weight or has a BMI over 25 kg/m^2. She is considered **obese** if she weighs more than 200 lb, she is 50% above ideal body weight for height, or her BMI is above 30 kg/m^2. As many as 10% of pregnant women in the United States are overweight. Less-educated women and those living in poverty tend to be more overweight than others. Obesity in pregnancy is serious because it is associated with an increased incidence of gestational diabetes and pregnancy-induced hypertension (Rode et al., 2007).

Although obesity may occur from hypothyroidism, it most often occurs as a result of excessive caloric intake and decreased energy expenditure. Obesity becomes a problem during pregnancy for a variety of reasons:

- Pregnancy causes circulatory volume to increase 20% to 50% and metabolism to increase to meet the demands of the pregnancy, placing additional stress on a possibly already overworked body. Hypertension and thrombophlebitis are more likely to occur.
- It is often difficult to hear fetal heart tones in an obese woman; palpating for position and size of a fetus at birth is also difficult.
- Obese women are at an increased risk for giving birth to infants with *macrosomia* (excessive fetal growth); this increases the incidence of cesarean births in this population.
- Performing a cesarean birth, if necessary, may be difficult because of the excessive adipose tissue that must be incised to reach the uterus.
- Gestational diabetes is more apt to develop; the pregnancies of obese women are more apt to be prolonged, leading to postmature infants.
- Ambulating during pregnancy and immediately afterward is more difficult because of the increased energy expenditure necessary, increasing the risk for complications such as thrombophlebitis and pneumonia.

Most obesity is caused by overeating but the habit of overeating has many causes. For some women, this is a coping mechanism for stress; whenever they feel tense or worried, they help themselves to something "comforting" to eat. Because pregnancy is stressful, it may be a particularly difficult time for a woman to change her food intake pattern. Other women overeat because their parents did and they were raised to always "clean their plate." If a woman has been serving her family an excessive intake of calories as well as herself, then the entire family may have to change their eating pattern to bring about a change in a woman's intake.

Dieting to reduce weight is not recommended during pregnancy because if carbohydrates are reduced too much, the body will use protein and fat for energy. This could deprive a fetus of essential nutrients. It could lead to ketoacidosis. Although the long-term effects of mild ketoacidosis on a fetus are not well studied, it can be avoided if the daily caloric intake, even in the most obese woman, does not go below 1500 to 1800 per day.

Overweight women tend to exercise less than do women of normal weight. Exercising is more awkward and more tiring, and they may feel self-conscious wearing exercise clothing. Try to encourage them to engage in at least a minimum activity program, such as walking around the block once a day, in conjunction with lessened carbohydrate intake.

Helping a woman look at her nutrition in terms of empty-calorie versus nutritious foods may help her to eat more sensibly. Early in pregnancy, when she is eager to appear pregnant, she may resist limiting her intake. Stress that a fetus grows best on nutritious foods, not necessarily those with the most calories. Provide additional nutritional counseling in the postpartum period so she can prepare more nutritious meals in the future for herself and her growing family. If successful, she will not enter another pregnancy severely overweight.

A Woman Who Is Morbidly Obese

When a women weighs over 300 lb or has a BMI over 40 kg/m^2, she is classified as *morbidly obese*. During a pregnancy, she presents with a series of special care problems as she is even more prone to complications of pregnancy such as gestational or type 2 diabetes, hypertension, back pain, and thrombophlebitis than obese women. She is prone to sleep apnea so may feel tired over and above normal pregnancy fatigue. Hearing fetal heart sounds and palpating for fetal position can be difficult. Because exercise is difficult, a woman may be prescribed support hose to aid lower leg circulation and help avoid thromboembolitic complications. Pregnancies tend to be prolonged with a high rate of cesarean birth (Mahlmeister, 2007).

In addition, morbidly obese women may need special care equipment furnished for them such as a larger hospital bed, examining gown, wheelchair, and straps for fetal monitoring equipment than usual. Be discreet when arranging for this type of equipment for a woman as she may be sensitive to her appearance and weight.

Although women with morbid obesity generally eat large amounts of food, take a nutrition history to be assured that their large intake includes protein-rich, not empty-calorie, foods. Some women who are morbidly obese have had bariatric surgery for weight reduction (either a gastric bypass that causes weight loss by decreasing stomach space and promoting malabsorption or stomach banding that encourages weight loss by simple food restriction). Gastric bypass surgery results in a 60% to 80% loss in weight; banding is less effective, resulting in a 45% to 50% weight loss (Landsberger & Gurewitsch, 2007). Although still uncommon in adolescents, the proportion of older adolescents who are having this type of surgery is also increasing (Tsai, Inge, & Burd, 2007). Both women and adolescents are advised to not become pregnant for at least a year after bariatric surgery, during their period of greatest weight loss.

All women who have had bariatric surgery are unable to eat large meals or a meal rich in calories as this causes a "dumping syndrome" or sudden symptoms of nausea, bloating, and diarrhea. Mark their chart as someone who has had bariatric surgery so they are not scheduled for a routine 50 or 100 g glucose tolerance test because this will stimulate acute dumping symptoms. Because their overall intake will be small during pregnancy, their weight gain will be less than others and they are prone to develop iron, protein, folic acid, and vitamin B_{12} deficiencies. Women who have had a gastric bypass are also prone to fat-soluble vitamin deficiencies as fat is no longer well absorbed.

A Woman Who Is a Vegetarian

More women of childbearing age are turning to vegetarianism to maintain healthy nutrition and avoid excess fat and food contaminants. Vegetarian diets are consistent with Dietary Guidelines for Americans. Most women vegetarians are closer to their ideal weight and have lower serum cholesterol levels and lower blood pressure levels than women who eat a more typical American diet. Nurses may find that many pregnant women, therefore, plan to exclude meat from their diets (Cox, 2008). There are many different types of vegetarians: lacto-ovo-vegetarians (no animal flesh or fish is eaten, but dairy products and eggs are), lactovegetarians (no meat, fish, or eggs are eaten, but dairy products are), and vegans (nothing derived from an animal is eaten). Most vegetarians are knowledgeable about their diets and can discuss what foods are high in various nutrients and how they incorporate such foods into their daily intake (Rifkin, 2007).

A vegetarian food pyramid is identical to a usual one, except it contains no meat (shows fish and eggs). Women should try to eat three or more servings a day of both fruits and vegetables, six or more servings per day of grains, and two or more servings per day of legumes such as kidney, black, or lima beans.

Special concerns for pregnant vegetarians include lack of vitamin B_{12} (meat is the chief source of this) and an inadequate intake of calcium (recommend dark-green vegetables as sources) and vitamin D (fortified milk and sunlight are the main sources of this). Urge women who are vegetarians to take a daily prenatal supplement, like all women, to ensure adequate iron and folic acid. Vegetarian nutrition for their new infant is discussed in Chapter 29.

A Woman With Phenylketonuria

Phenylketonuria (PKU), named for the breakdown product of phenylalanine, is an essential amino acid that is excreted in the urine in this form. It is an inherited disorder in which a person cannot convert phenylalanine into tyrosine, the form used for cell growth. Without conversion, phenylalanine accumulates in the person's blood serum, eventually leaving the bloodstream to invade body cells. When brain cells are invaded, severe cognitive challenge and accompanying neurologic damage, such as recurrent seizures, develop (see Chapter 48). A fetus of a woman with uncontrolled PKU can develop microcephaly, intrauterine growth restriction, and neurologic damage (Poustie, Wildgoose, & Rutherford, 2009).

Foods high in phenylalanine are those high in protein; examples of foods low in phenylalanine are fruits and vegetables such as orange juice, bananas, squash, spinach, and peas. Children with PKU follow a diet with restricted phenylalanine intake until at least past adolescence. A woman with PKU should consult her internist when she is planning to become pregnant and should plan to return to a low-phenylalanine diet for at least 3 months before she becomes pregnant. A woman typically follows this low-phenylalanine diet during the pregnancy and afterward as long as she is breastfeeding.

A woman with PKU needs support during pregnancy to adhere to these nutritional restrictions. It is particularly disappointing if she does not become pregnant immediately after starting the restricted diet, because each month she is "prepregnant" extends the period she must follow the restrictions. A woman with PKU is usually well informed about her particular nutritional needs. She is aware that phenylalanine is destructive to developing brain cells and that not following her restricted plan could leave her future child severely cognitively challenged.

A Woman With a Multiple Pregnancy

A woman with a multiple pregnancy gains more weight overall and at a greater pace than a woman carrying a single child because of the increased fetal weight (a total weight gain of 40–45 lb). To sustain her own nutrition stores, she must ingest high levels of protein and carbohydrate. In particular, there is an increased burden on maternal iron and folic acid stores. For this reason, multiple pregnancy needs to be recognized early so nutrition supplements can be added as needed (Bernstein & Weinstein, 2007).

What if... Tori Alarino was pregnant with a multiple pregnancy and told you she was "eating for three"? You notice she takes three desserts every day for lunch. Will this hurt her or just add a few extra pounds?

A Woman Who Smokes or Uses Drugs or Alcohol

The specific effects of alcohol, cigarette smoking, and recreational drug use on fetal growth are discussed in Chapter 12. In addition to specific teratogenic fetal effects, these substances can lead to general nutrition problems because a woman is ingesting these substances rather than eating nutritious foods.

A Woman With Concurrent Health Problems

Any health concern that requires rigid salt, protein, or carbohydrate restriction poses a potential threat to fetal nutrition during pregnancy. Women who have medical problems such as kidney disease, diabetes, tuberculosis, bulimia, inflammatory bowel disease, celiac disease, or anorexia nervosa should consult their primary care provider before pregnancy because of the specific metabolic disorders that occur with these illnesses. Nursing interventions and nutrition concerns for women with health problems such as these are discussed in Chapter 20.

A Woman Who Eats Many Fast-Food Meals

As many as 90% of women of childbearing age work at least part-time outside their homes. This means that nutritional counseling must involve helping women who rely on packed lunches or fast-food meals to maintain adequate pregnancy nutrition. The difficulty with fast-food restaurants is the limited choice of food available. This can cause a woman to grow tired of the same thing and so eat little. Unless there is a salad bar, there is likely to be a limited menu of fruits and vegetables. Fast-food restaurants have also been associated with outbreaks of infection because of undercooked hamburger or contaminated salad bars. Caution women to order hamburgers well done to help prevent *Escherichia coli* contamination and severe diarrhea, which could lead to a fluid and electrolyte imbalance (Todd, 2007).

A packed lunch poses few problems in pregnancy as long as a woman uses some creativity in preparation so she does not grow so tired of packed lunches that she reduces her noontime intake. Packing her lunch at bedtime rather than in the morning, when she may feel nauseated (and therefore packs little because nothing looks good), is a good recommendation early in pregnancy. Late in pregnancy, a woman may feel too tired at bedtime to do this and should change to preparing it in the morning, when she has more energy. Including a thermos with a cream soup is a good way to add milk and calcium to her diet. Packing carrot sticks or sliced cucumbers, tomatoes, or apples helps to make a lunch nutritious and also provides a mid-morning or mid-afternoon snack. Having these snacks available prevents her from having long stretches of time without eating or eating empty-calorie foods from vending machines (see Focus on Nursing Care Planning Box 13.8).

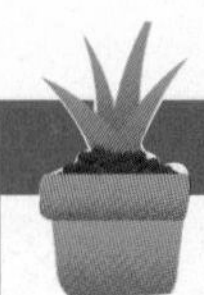

BOX 13.8 ✻ Focus on Nursing Care Planning

Multidisciplinary Care Map for a Pregnant Woman With an Inadequate Nutritional Pattern

Tori Alarino, 28, is 4 months pregnant and works at a fast-food restaurant during the day. She eats her breakfast and lunch at work. Her husband works four evenings a week, so she cooks for herself on those evenings. She dislikes milk, so she drinks milkshakes as a source of calcium. She is concerned because she has already gained 23 lb. She craves oranges, eating six to eight of them a day. She tells you, "I thought pregnant women always craved pickles and ice cream. What's wrong with me?"

Family Assessment ✻ Client lives with husband in four-bedroom home; husband works as an electrician. Client's father (aged 58) lives with them since recent divorce.

Client Assessment ✻ Primigravida; LMP 16 weeks ago. Height 5 ft 6 in. Prepregnancy weight: 150 lb (1–2 lbs over desirable weight for height); BMI 25.0.

Weight today: 133 lb. History of weight problem during adolescence; currently controls weight by eating only one main meal per day. 24-hour dietary recall: Breakfast—1 cup coffee with muffin; lunch—1 milkshake; dinner—1 hamburger with French fries, 1 milkshake; snacks—8-ounce soft drink. Reports feeling tired and "run-down".

Nursing Diagnosis ✻ Imbalanced nutrition, less than body requirements, related to desire to control weight

Outcome Criteria ✻ Client reports intake of foods adequate in calories, high in iron, calcium, and protein by next prenatal visit.
Demonstrates weight gain appropriate for stage of pregnancy and prepregnancy weight.

Team Member Responsible	Assessment	Intervention	Rationale	Expected Outcome
		Activities of Daily Living		
Nurse	Assess if the fatigue client reports is interfering with adequate food preparation.	If fatigue is a problem, recommend preparing nutritious lunch early in day when less fatigued.	Fatigue can increase nausea/vomiting in early pregnancy; interfere with food preparation all through pregnancy.	Client states she is able to cook and realizes eating all fast foods may not be her best action.
		Consultations		
Nurse/physician/women's health practitioner	Assess nutrition requirements based on client's BMI and individual preferences.	Consult with nutritionist about recommended caloric and mineral requirements.	Caloric recommendations may need to be attached in light of client's BMI and prepregnancy and current weight.	An ideal nutrition plan is created and presented to client.
		Procedures/Medications		
Nurse	Assess if client has experience with keeping a journal.	Instruct client to keep a journal recording all food and fluid intake for 1 week, and review with client on next visit.	Keeping a journal provides concrete evidence of client's adherence to nutritional plan.	Client brings log to next prenatal visit and reviews it with prenatal staff.
		Nutrition		
Nutritionist	Assess the nutritional requirements based on client's BMI, present weight, and individual choices.	Provide client with food suggestions. Provide written information as needed.	Assistance from a dietitian ensures a nutritionally sound diet with culturally acceptable food choices. Printed information enhances learning.	Client lists an "ideal" nutrition plan for healthy pregnancy nutrition.

(continued)

BOX 13.8 ✻ Focus on Nursing Care Planning (continued)

Patient/Family Education				
Nurse/ nutritionist	Assess if client is aware of the importance of healthy nutrition for pregnancy.	Review healthy pregnancy nutrition with client.	Knowledgeable clients can best follow a nutritious meal plan.	Client lists foods she will include for healthy pregnancy nutrition.
Psychosocial/Spiritual/Emotional Needs				
Nurse	Question client about food likes and dislikes. Investigate any cultural influences on food choices.	Ask client to list foods in each food group that are her favorites and she enjoys cooking.	Ascertaining food preferences and cultural influences provides a baseline for future food selections and suggestions.	Client lists foods she prefers and knows she can eat consistently.
Discharge Planning				
Nurse	Assess best times for client to return for prenatal appointments based on work/family obligations.	Schedule a follow-up appointment in 1 week.	Changing nutritional habits and behaviors can be difficult. Scheduling close follow-up provides an opportunity for evaluation and instruction.	Client states she will return for follow-up nutritional counseling.

A Woman With Lactose Intolerance

The sugar in milk is lactose. In the intestine, lactose is broken down into glucose and galactose by the enzyme **lactase.** Most of the world's population has sufficient lactase as an infant but the amount of lactase available fades by school age. After this point, people have difficulty digesting lactose or are lactose intolerant. African Americans, Native Americans, and Asians tend to have the highest percentage of lactose intolerance (approximately 70% of African American adults cannot drink milk). Those most able to tolerate milk are northern Europeans and their descendants.

When people who are lactose-intolerant drink milk, they experience nausea, diarrhea, cramps, gas, and a general feeling of bloating. The intestinal slowing that accompanies pregnancy does not change the intensity of symptoms (Bauchner, 2007).

Women who cannot drink milk because of lactose intolerance may be able to eat cheese because the processing of cheese changes the lactose content; yogurt may also be tolerated. Fortified soy milk is another possible substitute. Lactase tablets can be prescribed to supplement absent lactase. Typically, a woman chews these before ingesting milk products. Even with this, however, a calcium supplement (1200 mg daily) and a vitamin D supplement (400 IU) may be necessary. This is because the amount of cheese or yogurt needed to replace the calcium of milk is too great to be practical. Because milk is also a good source of protein, be sure to assess whether, without milk, a woman's intake of protein is adequate.

Many baby magazines, television advertisements, and government pamphlets on pregnancy mention repeatedly that it is important to drink milk during pregnancy. You may need to explain that as long as a woman ingests the same nutrients from other foods, the actual drinking of milk is not important.

A Woman With Hyperemesis Gravidarum

Hyperemesis gravidarum (sometimes called *pernicious* or *persistent vomiting*) is nausea and vomiting of pregnancy that is prolonged past week 12 of pregnancy or is so severe that dehydration, ketonuria, and significant weight loss occur within the first 12 weeks of pregnancy (Alalade, Khan, & Dawlatly, 2007). It occurs at an incidence of 1 in 200 to 300 women. The cause is unknown, but women with the disorder may have increased thyroid function because of the thyroid-stimulating properties of human chorionic gonadotropin. Some studies reveal that it is associated with *Helicobacter pylori,* the same bacteria that cause peptic ulcers (Golberg, Szilagyi, & Graves, 2007).

Assessment. With hyperemesis gravidarum, a woman's nausea and vomiting are so severe that she cannot maintain her usual nutrition. She may show an elevated hematocrit concentration at her monthly prenatal visit because her inability to retain fluid has resulted in hemoconcentration. Concentrations of sodium, potassium, and chloride may be reduced because of her low intake, and hypokalemic alkalosis may result if vomiting is severe. In some women, polyneuritis, because of a deficiency of B vitamins, develops. Weight loss can be severe. Urine may test positive for ketones, evidence that a woman's body is breaking down stored fat and protein for cell growth. If left untreated, the condition is associated with intrauterine growth restriction or preterm birth if a woman becomes dehydrated and can no longer provide a fetus with essential nutrients for growth.

Always try to determine exactly how much nausea and vomiting women are having during pregnancy. Ask a woman to describe the events of the day before if she says it was a typical day. How late into the day did the nausea last? How many times did she vomit, and how much? What was the total amount of food she was able to eat?

Therapeutic Management. Women with hyperemesis gravidarum usually need to be hospitalized for about 24 hours to monitor intake, output, and blood chemistries and to restore hydration.

All oral food and fluids are usually withheld. Intravenous fluid (3000 mL of Ringer's lactate with added vitamin B, for example) may be administered to increase hydration. An antiemetic, such as metoclopramide (Reglan), may be prescribed to control vomiting. Throughout this period, carefully measure intake and output, including the amount of vomitus.

If there is no vomiting after the first 24 hours of oral restriction, small amounts of clear fluid may be begun and the woman may be discharged home, usually with a referral for home care. If she can continue to take clear fluid, small quantities of dry toast, crackers, or cereal may be added every 2 or 3 hours, then she can be gradually advanced to a soft diet, then to a normal diet. If vomiting returns at any point, enteral or total parenteral nutrition may be prescribed. Home care follow-up provides further information about the client's status after hospital discharge (see Chapter 4).

Nursing Diagnoses and Related Interventions

A woman with hyperemesis gravidarum needs the opportunity to express how she feels about this strange thing that is happening to her or how it feels to live with ever-present nausea. Some women are under such psychosocial stress that they appreciate counseling to help them decide whether to terminate a pregnancy or allow it to go to completion. An appropriate nursing diagnosis may be "ineffective coping related to stress of pregnancy or concurrent life events." Be certain that the outcomes established are realistic. It may not be possible to stop vomiting completely, but enough supplemental fluid to counteract the loss of fluid with vomiting can be supplied.

Nursing Diagnosis: Risk for deficient fluid volume related to vomiting secondary to hyperemesis gravidarum

Outcome Evaluation: Client remains free of signs and symptoms of dehydration (i.e., poor skin turgor or dry skin or mucous membranes); urine output is greater than 30 mL/h; urine specific gravity ranges between 1.003 and 1.030; no further episodes of vomiting occur.

Like the typical nausea and vomiting of pregnancy, the vomiting of hyperemesis gravidarum may be precipitated by fatigue and the smell of cooking. Encourage a woman to serve herself small portions so the amount on her plate does not appear overwhelming. It is best if foods are presented attractively. Hot foods should be hot, and cold foods should be cold. Remember not to talk about food while you give care (e.g., "What's the soup of the day in the cafeteria?") or to urge a woman to "Eat just a little more. You're starving your baby." Urging women with hyperemesis gravidarum to eat this way can cause them to feel guilty on top of feeling so nauseated that they cannot eat.

An emesis basin is an important piece of equipment for a woman who is vomiting. While she is hospitalized, put it out of sight and not on the bedside table, however, so she is not constantly reminded of vomiting. Try to limit her exposure to food odors. Be sure that food carts with smells of food such as fish, bacon, or coffee are not parked outside her door at mealtimes. Be sure to reinforce these instructions with other health care providers.

Nursing Diagnosis: Imbalanced nutrition, less than body requirements, related to prolonged vomiting

Outcome Evaluation: Client eats at least 2500 calories daily or receives supplemental nutrition intravenously or enterally.

Some women have such extreme symptoms that vomiting recurs with the introduction of food. To maintain adequate nutrition to support fetal growth, a woman may need to be maintained on total parenteral nutrition or enteral feedings. While she is receiving total parenteral nutrition at home, instruct her to check her urine for glucose and ketones twice daily. If there is glucose in the urine, this suggests that the infusion solution contains more glucose than her body's metabolism can use. Ketones in the urine mean that her body is not receiving enough nutrients and it is breaking down protein. If either of these findings is positive, she should call her health care provider because she needs a nutrition reassessment.

Fortunately, despite its extreme symptoms, excessive vomiting during pregnancy rarely leads to pregnancy loss or low-birth-weight newborns when it is properly treated.

✓ Checkpoint Question 13.5

Suppose Tori is a vegetarian. What is apt to be her greatest nutritional risk?

a. Lack of iron
b. Lack of vitamin C
c. Lack of folic acid
d. Lack of vitamin B_{12}

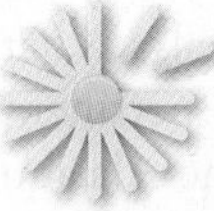

Key Points for Review

- Assessment of nutritional health should include a health history (24-hour recall) and physical examination.
- Nutrition during pregnancy should include about 300 additional calories daily to provide energy, spare protein, and provide for fetal growth requirements.
- Important minerals necessary for pregnancy include iron, iodine, calcium, fluoride, sodium, and zinc. Most women need to take an iron supplement to prevent iron deficiency anemia.
- Women should monitor their intake of caffeine, fish, and artificial sweeteners during pregnancy.
- Prenatal vitamins contain additional folic acid supplements and iron, so these should be used instead of over-

the-counter vitamins during pregnancy. Be certain that women regard pregnancy vitamins as medication and follow the medication rule: take nothing other than medications specifically recommended by their primary care providers, or else toxicity could result.

- Advise pregnant women not to go longer than 12 hours between meals, to avoid hypoglycemia.
- Women who are at high risk for inadequate nutrition include those who are adolescent or over age 40; those who have decreased nutrition stores; those with a multiple pregnancy; those who are lactose intolerant; those who are underweight or overweight; those on a special diet; those using recreational drugs, including alcohol or cigarettes; and those with hyperemesis gravidarum (extreme nausea and vomiting).
- Common nutrition concerns associated with pregnancy include nausea and vomiting, constipation, cravings (including pica), and pyrosis.
- Hyperemesis gravidarum is nausea and vomiting of pregnancy that extends past 12 weeks of pregnancy or is too extreme to allow for adequate nutrition. Women with this condition may need their nutrition supplemented by total parenteral nutrition or enteral feedings.

CRITICAL THINKING EXERCISES

1. Tori Alarino, whom you met at the beginning of the chapter, drinks milkshakes as a source of calcium. Is this a wise choice? Why do you think she craves oranges?
2. Tori works at a fast-food restaurant. She states she is too nauseated in the morning to eat before she leaves for work, and she is too tired of seeing food go by her to prepare a good meal after work. What suggestions could you give to help her increase her food intake?
3. Tori rarely eats vegetables; when she does, she fries them in butter. How would you use a food pyramid to explain better pregnancy nutrition to her?
4. Examine the National Health Goals related to nutrition and pregnancy. Most government-sponsored money for nursing research is allotted based on these goals. What would be a possible research topic to explore pertinent to these goals that would be applicable to the Alarino family and also advance evidence-based practice?

CRITICAL THINKING SCENARIO

Open the accompanying CD-ROM or visit http://thePoint.lww.com and read the Patient Scenario included for this chapter, then answer the questions to further sharpen your skills and grow more familiar with NCLEX style questions related to nutrition and pregnancy. Confirm your answers are correct by reading the rationales.

REFERENCES

Applebee, B. K. (2008). The deleterious effects of caffeine on pregnancy. *Nutritional Perspectives, 3*(3), 23–25.

Abayomi, J., et al. (2007). Obesity and underweight among first trimester pregnant women. *British Journal of Midwifery, 15*(3), 143–147.

Alalade, A. O., Khan, R., & Dawlatly, B. (2007). Day-case management of hyperemesis gravidarum: feasibility and clinical efficacy. *Journal of Obstetrics & Gynaecology, 27*(4), 363–364.

Bauchner, H. (2007). Lactose intolerance: a common problem. *Archives of Disease in Childhood, 92*(5), 464–465.

Bernstein, H. B., & Weinstein, M. (2007). Normal pregnancy and prenatal care. In A. H. DeCherney & L. Nathan (Eds.). *Current diagnosis and treatment in obstetrics and gynecology* (10th ed.). Columbus, OH: McGraw-Hill.

Bourre, J. M. (2007). Dietary omega-3 fatty acids for women. *Biomedicine & Pharmacotherapy, 61*(2–3), 105–112.

Cohen, D., & Farley, T. A. (2008). Eating as an automatic behavior. *Preventing Chronic Disease, 5*(1), A23.

Cox, S. R. (2008). Staying healthy on a vegetarian diet during pregnancy. *Journal of Midwifery & Women's Health, 53*(1), 91–92.

Crombleholme, W. R. (2009). Obstetrics. In S. J. Mcphee & M. A. Papadakis (Eds.). *Current medical diagnosis and treatment.* Columbus, OH: McGraw-Hill.

Derbyshire, E. (2007). The importance of adequate fluid and fibre intake during pregnancy. *Nursing Standard, 21*(24), 40–43.

Dudek, S. (2009). *Nutrition handbook for nursing practice* (5th ed.). Philadelphia: Lippincott Williams & Wilson.

Fowles, E. R., & Murphey, C. (2009). Nutrition and mental health in early pregnancy: a pilot study. *Journal of Midwifery & Women's Health, 54*(1), 73–77.

Genuis, S. J. (2008). To sea or not to sea: benefits and risks of gestational fish consumption. *Reproductive Toxicology, 26*(2), 81–85.

Goh, Y. I., et al. (2007). Prenatal multivitamin supplementation and rates of pediatric cancers: a meta-analysis. *Clinical Pharmacology and Therapeutics, 81*(5), 685–691.

Golberg, D., Szilagyi, A., & Graves, L. (2007). Hyperemesis gravidarum and *Helicobacter pylori* infection: a systematic review. *Obstetrics & Gynecology, 110*(3), 695–703.

Hale, R. (2007). Maternal nutrition during pregnancy and folic acid. *British Journal of Midwifery, 15*(3), 167–170.

Institute of Medicine. (2008). *Summary tables: dietary reference intakes.* Washington, DC: Author.

Karch, A. M. (2009). *Lippincott's nursing drug guide.* Philadelphia: Lippincott Williams & Wilkins.

Landsberger, E. J., & Gurewitsch, E. D. (2007). Reproductive implications of bariatric surgery: pre- and postoperative considerations for extremely obese women of childbearing age. *Current Diabetes Reports, 7*(4), 281–288.

Lumley, J., et al. (2009). Periconceptional supplementation with folate and/or multivitamins for preventing neural tube defects. *Cochrane Database of Systematic Reviews, 2009*(1), (CD001056).

Mahlmeister, L. R. (2007). Best practices in perinatal nursing: improving outcomes for obese and morbidly obese women during the intrapartum and postpartum periods. *Journal of Perinatal and Neonatal Nursing, 21*(2), 86–88.

Marchioni, E., et al. (2008). Iodine deficiency in pregnant women residing in an area with adequate iodine intake. *Nutrition, 24*(5), 458–461.

Mills, M. E. (2007). Craving more than food: the implications of pica in pregnancy. *Nursing for Women's Health, 11*(3), 266–273.

More, J. (2007). Who needs vitamin supplements? *The Journal of Family Health Care, 17*(2), 57–60.

Orr, W. C. (2007). Consequences of nighttime heartburn: quality of life and sleep disturbances *Sleep Medicine, 11*(2), 1–5.

Poustie, V. J., Wildgoose, J., & Rutherford, P. (2009). Dietary interventions for phenylketonuria. *Cochrane Database of Systematic Reviews, 2009*(1), (CD001304).

Radesky, J. S., et al. Diet during early pregnancy and development of gestational diabetes. *Paediatric and Perinatal Epidemiology, 22*(1), 47–59.

Rifkin, M. (2007). 10 Ways to improve your vegetarian lifestyle. *Vegetarian Journal, 26*(1), 27–29.

Rode, L., et al. (2007). Association between maternal weight gain and birth weight. *Obstetrics and Gynecology, 109*(6), 1309–1315.

Rojas, F., Wood, E., & Blakemore, K. (2007). Preconception counseling and prenatal care. In K. B. Fortner, et al. (Eds.). *The Johns Hopkins manual of gynecology and obstetrics.* Philadelphia: Lippincott Williams & Wilkins.

Rolfes, S. R., Pinna, K., & Whitney, E. (2009). *Understanding normal and clinical nutrition* (8th ed.). New York: Wadsworth/Cengage Learning.

Subramanian, A., et al. (2008). *Drug facts and comparisons.* St. Louis: Wolters Kluwer Health.

Sunderland, E. M. (2007). Mercury exposure from domestic and imported estuarine and marine fish in the U.S. seafood market. *Environmental Health Perspectives, 115*(2), 235–242.

Todd, B. (2007). Emerging infections. Outbreak: *E. coli* O157:H7. *American Journal of Nursing, 107*(2), 29–32.

Tsai, W. S., Inge, T. H., & Burd, R. S. (2007). Bariatric surgery in adolescents: recent national trends in use and in-hospital outcome. *Archives of Pediatric Adolescent Medicine, 161,* 217–221.

Thompson, V. J., et al. (2007). Self-efficacy and norm measures for lunch fruit and vegetable consumption are reliable and valid among fifth grade students. *Journal of Nutrition Education and Behavior, 39*(1), 2–7.

Watts, V., et al. (2007). Assessing diet quality in a population of low-income pregnant women: a comparison between Native Americans and Whites. *Maternal and Child Health Journal, 11*(2), 127–136.

White, B. (2007). Ginger: an overview. *American Family Physician, 75*(11), 1689–1691.

SUGGESTED READINGS

Clemmens, D. A., & Kerr, A. R. (2008). Improving oral health in women: nurses' call to action. *MCN, American Journal of Maternal Child Nursing. 33*(1), 10–14.

Georgieff, M. K. (2007). Nutrition and the developing brain: nutrient priorities and measurement. *American Journal of Clinical Nutrition, 85*(2), 614S–620S.

Greenfield, R. H. (2007). Smarting from fish? Seafood consumption and pregnancy. *Alternative Therapies in Women's Health, 9*(5), 37–39.

Hodnett, E. D., & Fredericks, S. (2009). Support during pregnancy for women at increased risk of low birthweight babies. *Cochrane Database of Systematic Reviews, 2009*(1), (CD000198).

Kramer, M. S., & Kakuma, R. (2009). Maternal dietary antigen avoidance during pregnancy or lactation, or both, for preventing or treating atopic disease in the child. *Cochrane Database of Systematic Reviews, 2009*(1), (CD000133).

Maillot, F., et al. (2007). A practical approach to maternal phenylketonuria management. *Journal of Inherited Metabolic Disease, 30*(2), 198–201.

Neher, J. O. (2007). Transforming practice. New evidence challenges IOM gestational weight gain goals. *Evidence-Based Practice, 10*(8), 1–3.

Salsberry, P. J., & Reagan, P. B. (2007). Taking the long view: the prenatal environment and early adolescent overweight. *Research in Nursing & Health, 30*(3), 297–307.

Say, L., Gulmezoglu, A. M., & Hofmeyr, G. J. (2009). Maternal nutrient supplementation for suspected impaired fetal growth. *Cochrane Database of Systematic Reviews, 2009*(1), (CD000148).

Theobald, H. E. (2007). Encouraging healthier lifestyles: Eating for pregnancy and breast-feeding. *The Journal of Family Health Care, 17*(2), 45–49.

Chapter 14 Preparing a Family for Childbirth and Parenting

KEY TERMS

- alternative birthing centers (ABCs)
- birthing bed
- birthing chairs
- birthing room
- cleansing breath
- conditioned reflexes
- consciously controlled breathing
- conscious relaxation
- distraction
- doula
- effleurage
- gating control theory of pain perception
- labor-delivery-recovery-postpartum room (LDRP)
- Leboyer method
- psychoprophylactic
- vaginal birth after cesarean birth (VBAC)

OBJECTIVES

After mastering the contents of this chapter, you should be able to:

1. Describe common preparations for childbirth and parenting including common settings for birth.
2. Identify National Health Goals related to preparation for parenthood that nurses can help the nation achieve.
3. Use critical thinking to analyze ways that birth can be made more family centered through the use of prepared childbirth classes and alternative birth settings.
4. Assess a couple for readiness for childbirth in regard to choice of birth attendant, preparation for labor, and setting.
5. Formulate nursing diagnoses related to preparation for childbirth and parenting.
6. Identify expected outcomes for a couple preparing for childbirth and parenting.
7. Plan nursing care such as teaching exercises for strengthening abdominal and perineal muscles for childbirth.
8. Implement nursing care such as supporting a woman during labor by the Lamaze method of childbirth or helping a couple select and prepare for an alternative birth setting such as the home.
9. Evaluate outcome criteria for achievement and effectiveness of care.
10. Identify areas related to preparation for childbirth that could benefit from additional nursing research or application of evidence-based practice.
11. Integrate the principles of prepared childbirth with nursing process to achieve quality maternal and child health nursing care.

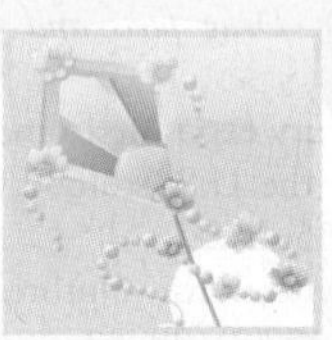

Julia Marco is pregnant with her second child. During her first pregnancy, she did not attend any childbirth classes and received an epidural for the birth. During a prenatal visit for this pregnancy, Julia tells you that she would now like to have a natural birth in a birthing center. She asks you for information on childbirth education classes. Her husband, Joe, wants Julia to go to the hospital and have an epidural like the last time. He insists, "The doctors know what they're doing. We should just let them do their job." After speaking further with Joe, you discover he does not want Julia to go through the pain of natural childbirth because he fears he will not be able to help her during labor.

Previous chapters discussed normal anatomy, physiology, and nursing care necessary during pregnancy. This chapter adds information about ways that couples can make labor and birth a more satisfying experience. Such information helps protect the mental as well as physical health of both women and children throughout the continuum of pregnancy, birth, and childrearing.

How can you help alleviate some of Joe's concerns and best advise the Marcos on preparations for childbirth?

As active consumers of health care, expectant families can find themselves faced with a wide array of choices about a childbirth experience and preparation for parenting. Three of the most important decisions they need to make involve the choice of birth attendant and setting and how much or what type of analgesic they want to use in labor. For example, a woman may elect to have her family physician, obstetrician, or nurse-midwife attend the birth and to be supported by her husband, partner, family member, friend, or **doula** (a woman who is experienced in childbirth and provides continuous emotional and physical support). Most women choose to give birth in a birthing center or a hospital. Birthing centers and birthing rooms within hospitals both provide environments for families who desire a childbirth experience that is relaxed, "homey," and "family centered" yet close to medical sources should any complication arise during the birth or early postpartum period. Families who are rated as low risk have yet another option or may plan a home birth (Olsen & Jewell, 2009).

No matter what setting a woman or couple chooses, expectant parents are well advised to be as prepared as possible for the physical and emotional aspects of childbirth and nonpharmacologic methods of pain relief during labor such as aromatherapy (Burns et al., 2007). Preparation for childbirth courses that teach this material can be individualized to meet parents' needs by being structured for women with special needs such as adolescents, career women, women who are physically challenged, or those experiencing a high-risk pregnancy. Also available are classes to help prepare siblings or grandparents to learn more about their role. Women having a **vaginal birth after cesarean birth (VBAC)** or women who know they will have a cesarean birth also can attend specially designed classes for this.

Most childbirth preparation classes are sponsored by community health care agencies but some work sites also offer such classes. Classes benefit employers as much as employees, because prenatal care and guidance correlate with healthier pregnancy outcomes and fewer lost workdays. National Health Goals related to preparation for parenting or childbirth are shown in Box 14.1.

BOX 14.1 ✻ Focus on National Health Goals

Preparation-for-childbirth classes supply information not only on how to prepare for childbirth but also on how to parent. Several National Health Goals speak directly to such classes:

- Increase the proportion of pregnant women who attend a series of prepared childbirth classes from a baseline of 66% to 77%.
- Increase the proportion of pregnant women who receive early and adequate prenatal care from a baseline of 74% to a target of 90%.
- Increase the proportion of pregnant women who receive early and adequate prenatal care beginning in the first trimester of pregnancy from a baseline of 83% to a target of 90%. (http://www.nih.gov).

Nurses participate as instructors in preparation for childbirth and parenting classes and help supervise prenatal care, so they have direct roles in helping the nation achieve these objectives. Issues such as what is the best timing during pregnancy for education about birth, what teaching techniques help parents retain information best, and what support parents want most from nurses during labor would be helpful research areas to better identify the needs for preparation for labor.

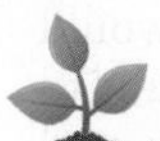

Nursing Process Overview

For Childbirth and Parenting Education

Assessment

Some couples have a clear idea of where and how they wish their child's birth to occur from the moment they realize they are pregnant. Others cannot even consider the actual birth until they have adjusted to the idea of pregnancy. Assessing each woman's or couple's readiness for decision making, as well as providing information early in the process, can help a woman or couple make this kind of decision. Whether women want or are able to take a childbirth and parenting preparation course depends a great deal on cultural and socioeconomic factors and individual choices (Greene, 2007). In some cultures, for example, the advice of a friend or family member carries more weight than the advice of a professional health care practitioner. Asking each woman separately whether she is interested in a course and being certain that women are fully informed about the options available to them are two ways to be certain all women receive as much advice and knowledge as they wish about childbirth.

Childbirth education is not just for primiparas because if a woman expecting her second or third child has waited several years between children, she usually appreciates refresher information as much as a primipara hungers for new information. Always, therefore, whether a woman is a primipara or multipara, ask whether either she or her support person wants to attend childbirth or parenting courses. Provide appropriate information on what classes are available and how and when they could enroll.

Nursing Diagnosis

Nursing diagnoses tend to cluster around whether a couple is sure of their decision about a birth setting or preparation. An example is:

- Health-seeking behaviors related to learning more about childbirth and newborn care

If there is a lack of a support person, diagnoses that might apply are:

- Ineffective coping related to lack of a support person
- Anxiety related to absence of significant other

For a couple unable to make a decision about a childbirth setting, an appropriate diagnosis might be:

- Decisional conflict related to lack of information about advantages and disadvantages of childbirth settings

If there are older children in the family, a nursing diagnosis might be:

- Anxiety related to role in pending birth event and ability to welcome a sibling

Outcome Identification and Planning

Be certain when planning with couples for labor and birth that the goals they set not only seem realistic but also flexible. Not all women want to go through labor without any analgesia, so setting a goal to do so would not be realistic for such a woman. Most women want to participate as fully as possible, however, so setting a goal for them to do that would be very realistic. Some women may be reluctant to attend a childbirth preparation course because they fear that would mean they are committing themselves to a medication-free birth. You can assure them that learning about methods to make childbirth easier does not preclude their learning about what medications are available for pain relief and using those medications if desired. At the same time a couple is planning goals for childbirth, encourage them to be flexible in their expectations. A woman who has decided ahead of time that she absolutely does not want any medication during labor and birth may find the intensity or duration of labor to be so severe that she will need an analgesic or epidural block to make the experience tolerable. If she and her support person have made the goal of medication-free labor too strict, they may believe they have failed when medication becomes necessary. A birth plan (discussed later) that includes information regarding a woman's or couple's preferences for labor, birth, immediate care of the newborn, and actions to be taken if complications should arise can help a woman and her support person set realistic expected outcomes.

Finally, talk to a woman or couple about the ultimate goal of childbirth: a healthy baby and healthy parents. This discussion can prevent them from concentrating on limited goals such as not having fetal monitoring or using a particular birthing position and concentrate instead on doing whatever is required to make the birth safest for both them and the baby.

Culture is a major determinant of the plans that women make for childbirth. A woman from a culture in which modesty is stressed, for example, may not want to have a mirror positioned over a birthing bed. A very old cross-cultural belief is that a knife placed under the mattress will "cut the pain" better than a Lamaze program. Whom women choose as a support person or coach in labor can also differ, depending on their cultural background. Some women would not think of choosing anyone but their male partner; others choose a female relative or friend. Assess each couple individually to be certain that cultural preferences such as these are respected.

Helpful Internet referral sources for couples are Childbirth Connection (http://www.childbirthconnection.org); Lamaze International (http://www.lamaze.org); International Childbirth Education Association (http://www.icea.org); La Leche League International (http://www.lalecheleague.org), and The Coalition for Improving Maternity Services (http://www.motherfriendly.org).

Implementation

It is important to provide a woman and her partner with information on the benefits and drawbacks of birthing options, without influencing them in a particular direction. To remain objective, examine your own attitudes, cultural influences, and values related to childbirth and explore how these beliefs might differ from those of your clients. Referring couples to a childbirth preparation course can answer many questions for them in a sympathetic group setting, where feelings and anxieties can be shared as well. Be familiar with the content of courses in your community so you can be certain that the courses you suggest present adequate and accurate information and are appropriate for individual couples.

Review the arrangements a woman needs to make for labor and birth at a midpoint in pregnancy. No matter how calm a woman seems when discussing these details, many women have some fear that at the last minute they will forget what they need to do when labor begins. Be certain that a woman has thought through arrangements for transportation to the hospital or birthing center and has arranged for child care if she has other children at home. Be certain that a woman who anticipates a home birth has organized her home and purchased supplies for birth well in advance of her expected due date.

Outcome Evaluation

Evaluate whether expected outcomes for childbirth education have been achieved during the last few prenatal visits. By this time, a woman or couple should know where the baby will be born and should have worked out transportation and child care details. Encourage women who will be coached through childbirth by their husbands or another support person to continue practicing breathing and relaxation techniques together up to the time of birth so they do not lose these skills. Final evaluation regarding whether the couple was satisfied with their birth setting or preparation choices takes place after the birth. Examples of expected outcomes that would demonstrate the success of interventions are:

- Couple states they feel prepared for childbirth.
- Client states she feels confident she can use breathing exercises for contractions as long as 70 seconds.
- Client has made preparations for a doula to support her during labor.
- Sibling states she is ready to welcome a new brother or sister into the family.
- Couple states they were well enough prepared for birth that it was a satisfying and growth experience for them

CHILDBIRTH EDUCATION

Although parenting is unarguably an important occupation, it is one of the few that requires no formal education, no examination to test a person's ability to take on such a role, and no refresher course to ensure that a parent is following healthy standards of childrearing. Assessing whether couples need a preparation for childbirth or parenting class or encouraging them to take one, therefore, can be extremely important to make childbirth a satisfying experience, help a

Box 14.2 Assessment
Assessing a Woman's Preparation for Labor

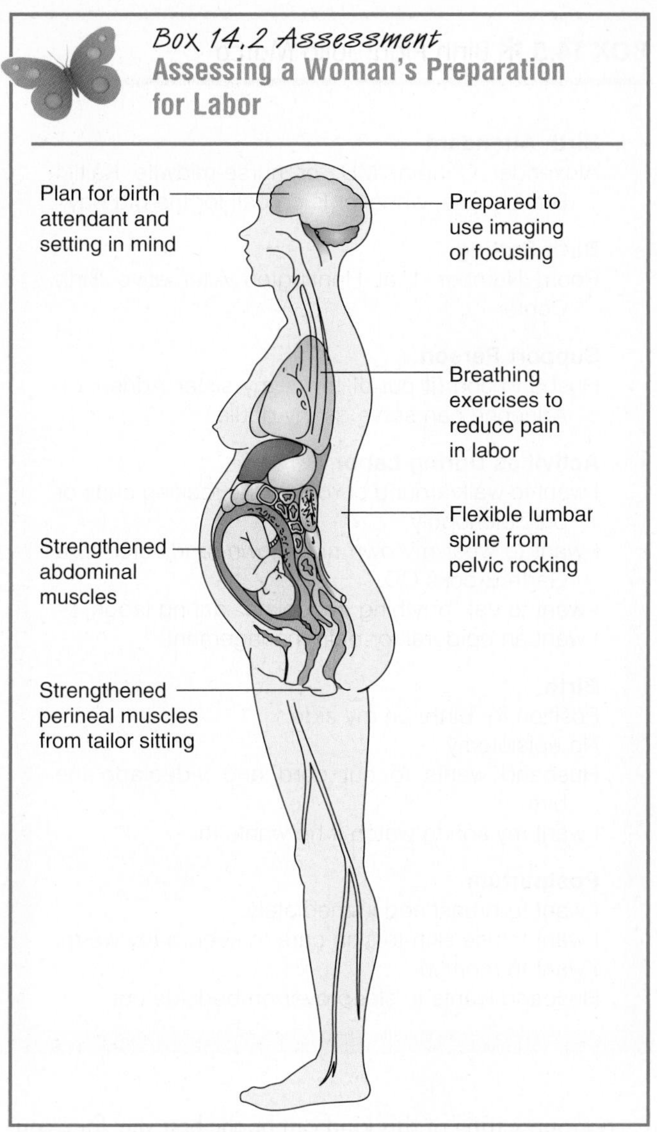

family bond with its new member, and become effective parents (Box 14.2).

As many as 7% of women voice that they are afraid of what will happen in labor. Those who are young, have a low educational level, low self-rated health, and lack a social network express this most (Laursen, 2008).

Preparation for childbirth courses began initially in the early 1900s to encourage women to come for prenatal care. They continue because, with all the birth choices available today, they fulfill the important second need for education about labor and childbirth. The overall goals of childbirth education are to prepare expectant parents emotionally and physically for childbirth while promoting wellness behaviors that can be used by parents and families for life. Women enjoy such classes because they offer them a sense of empowerment and confirm that they can have direct input into their labor experience (Box 14.3).

Childbirth Educators and Methods of Teaching

Childbirth educators are health care providers who usually have a professional degree in the helping professions as well as a certificate from a course specifically about childbirth education. They teach expectant parents about the physical and emotional aspects of pregnancy, childbirth, and early parenthood and present coping skills and labor support techniques. Although childbirth education is an interdisciplinary field, it has historically been associated with nursing and nurses play a major role in designing and teaching such courses. Most classes are taught in a group format; most incorporate a variety of teaching techniques such as videotapes and slides, lecture, and demonstration (especially for content on relaxation and breathing techniques). One of the most important aspects of these courses, however, is group interaction. Women and their partners enjoy the opportunity to share their fears and hopes about their pregnancy and upcoming birth with others as they learn together (Box 14.4).

Efficacy of Childbirth Education Courses

Many studies have been done to determine just how effective childbirth courses are in reducing the pain of childbirth, shortening the length of labor, decreasing the amount of medication used, and increasing overall enjoyment of the experience. Because of the variability in courses offered, however, it is often difficult to compare results of attending childbirth classes versus not attending classes. This is partly because people who volunteer to attend classes already have a high degree

BOX 14.3 ✻ Focus on Communication

You care for Julia Marco at a prenatal clinic visit. She is in the 24th week of an uncomplicated pregnancy.

Less Effective Communication

Nurse: Have you signed up for a childbirth preparation class yet, Julia?
Julia: No.
Nurse: Don't wait too much longer. You're already in your sixth month.
Julia: I don't really need to go to one.
Nurse: Okay. You know best.

More Effective Communication

Nurse: Have you signed up for a childbirth preparation class yet, Julia?
Julia: No.
Nurse: Don't wait too much longer. You're already in your sixth month.
Julia: I don't really need to go to one.
Nurse: Why is that?
Julia: Classes are all at the wrong time. And cost too much.
Nurse: Let's work together to find a course that's right for you. We can use the Internet to find out what options are available.

It is important for couples to attend preparation for labor classes but, also, is easy to ignore the reasons clients present for not wanting to attend them. Careful listening often reveals that time or money concerns are reasons why couples choose not to attend a course. Helping to investigate the many options is the beginning of problem solving.

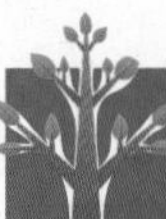

BOX 14.4 ❋ Focus on Family Teaching

Choosing a Birth Setting

Q. Julia and her husband Joe ask you, "There are so many options available for a birth setting. How do we decide which one to choose?"

A. Choosing a birth setting is a personal decision. Some questions to ask yourself to help with the decision are:

- What type of caregiver do I want to supervise my prenatal care and labor and birth? Nurse-midwife? Family doctor? Obstetrician?
- What settings does a particular childbirth provider let me choose from? A birthing room? An alternative birthing center? My home?
- Will the same person be present at prenatal visits as for birth? Does the setting offer preparation for childbirth or childrearing classes?
- Will I be allowed to choose a birth position? Will I have input into the amount of anesthesia used? Can administration of ophthalmic ointment for the baby be delayed? Can I begin breastfeeding immediately? Will nurses who are supportive and informed about breastfeeding be available? Can I use a doula?
- Will the setting allow my partner to participate? Will he or she be allowed to be with me throughout labor and birth? Could he or she cut the cord or help with the birth? Can older children participate? Can I record the birth on videotape or by photograph?
- Is early discharge available? Will a follow-up home visit be included in care?
- If I should have a complication during labor or birth, is there adequate equipment and personnel available for emergency care? If our baby should have a complication, is there provision for immediate emergency care or transport to a high-risk facility?

of positive motivation, which may skew the results. Despite these difficulties with measurement, it is generally accepted that preparation courses can increase satisfaction, reduce the amount of reported pain, and increase feelings of control (Lauzon & Hodnett, 2009). It is documented that by discussion of breastfeeding, classes can increase the proportion of new mothers who breastfeed (American College of Obstetrics and Gynecology [ACOG], 2007).

THE CHILDBIRTH PLAN

Most classes for expectant parents urge couples to make a written childbirth plan or spell out their choice of setting, birth attendant, special needs such as the extent of family participation they wish during labor, birthing positions, medication options, plans for the immediate postpartum period and baby care, and family visitation (Simkin, 2007). Urge couples to make decisions about these issues before the day of birth to avoid feeling stressed by last minute decisions.

BOX 14.5 ❋ Birth Plan: Julia Marco

Birth Attendant

Alexander Coppin, MD, or nurse-midwife Kaitlin Brandywine, whoever is on call for the big day.

Birth Setting

Room Number 1 at Huntington Alternative Birth Center

Support Person

Husband Joe (if out of town, my sister Adrienne). Adrienne can serve as my doula.

Activities During Labor

I want to walk around or rock in the rocking chair or play Monopoly.

I want to wear my own nightgown, and listen to a Garth Brooks CD.

I want to eat "anything chocolate" during labor.

I want an epidural for pain management.

Birth

Position for birth: on my side.

No episiotomy

Husband wants to cut cord and videotape the birth.

I want my son to watch if he wants to.

Postpartum

I want to breastfeed immediately.

I want to use skin-to-skin care to keep baby warm.

I want to room in.

Husband wants to sleep over on bedside cot.

A group setting of this kind can be the best way for a couple to sort out their questions and feelings about what they want to consider in a birth plan as they share information with others. If the expectant family has a strong desire in a certain area, planning ahead will allow them to communicate this so their wish can be accommodated if possible. Be certain all couples understand, however, that the birth plan should be flexible in case a complication or change of plans arises. For example, in the event of a complication of labor or birth that requires an emergency cesarean birth, a preference to have the baby without anesthesia will need to be modified. Box 14.5 is a sample birth plan.

PRECONCEPTION CLASSES

Preconception classes are held for couples who are planning to get pregnant within a short time and want to know more about what they can expect a pregnancy to be like and what are birth setting/procedure choices. These classes stress that pregnancy brings with it psychological as well as physical changes and include recommended preconception nutrition modifications such as a good intake of folic acid (green leafy vegetables) and protein (meat, tofu, beans) during the time waiting to get pregnant, to ensure a healthy fetus (Lu, 2007).

BOX 14.6 ✻ Focus on Evidence-Based Practice

Is periodontal disease a factor that can lead to preterm birth?

An important health care practice to remind women about during pregnancy is to continue care of their teeth through thorough toothbrushing and routine dental assessments. To study whether periodontal disease in pregnant women could be a factor that leads to preterm birth or restricted fetal growth, researchers assessed the oral health of 1635 pregnant women; 3.8% of these (62 women) had peridontal disease. Those women with periodontal disease had a significantly higher outcome of preterm or fetal growth restriction.

When writing out a curriculum for a preparation for childbirth class, would this information be important to include?

Source: Pitiphat, W., et al. (2008). Maternal periodontitis and adverse pregnancy outcomes. *Community Dentistry & Oral Epidemiology, 36*(1), 3–11.

EXPECTANT PARENTING CLASSES

Expectant parenting classes are designed for couples who are already pregnant. They focus on family health during a pregnancy, covering such topics as the psychological and physical changes of pregnancy, pregnancy nutrition, routine health care such as dental checkups, and newborn care (Box 14.6). A typical course plan for 8 weeks is shown in Box 14.7.

Most preparation-for-parenthood programs last 4 to 8 hours over a 4- to 8-week period. Both women and their support people are invited, and the curriculum is individualized for the group and its needs such as women in the military, sibling preparation, refresher classes for grandparents, classes for expectant adoptive parents, pregnant adolescents, or women with physical disabilities (Smeltzer, 2007). If all the women in the group already have children, for example, they may not need a tour of a maternity unit as part of the program; instead, they may want to learn what is new in baby food or child care. If all the women in the class work at least part-time, discussion of "brown bag nutrition" and how to include rest periods during work hours might be most useful. If all the women are teenagers, they may be most interested in what is going to happen to their bodies during pregnancy or what sports are safe to continue during pregnancy. They also need information on how to care for a newborn. They probably will want a tour of the maternity unit (Fig. 14.1).

Sibling Education Classes

Sibling classes are organized to acquaint older brothers and sisters with what happens during birth and what they can expect a newborn to look and act like. The classes review how babies grow and things children can do to help their mother during a pregnancy, such as eating healthy foods with her and not leaving toys on the floor she could trip over and fall.

BOX 14.7 ✻ Sample Content for Expectant Parents Class

- **Lesson 1** Review of Physiologic Changes of Pregnancy and Fetal Growth
- **Lesson 2** Personal Care During Pregnancy
  Nutrition
  Hygiene such as bathing, dental care
  Exercise
  Rest
- **Lesson 3** Emotional Changes During Pregnancy
- **Lesson 4** Labor and Birth
  The process of birth
  Exercises and breathing techniques
  Medication in labor
- **Lesson 5** Plans for Birth
  Birth settings available
  Supplies to take to birth settings
  Tour or film of a typical setting
- **Lesson 6** The Postpartum Period
- **Lesson 7** Infant Care
  Nutrition
  Hygiene
- **Lesson 8** Reproductive Life Planning

If the classes are held at a hospital, a tour of a newborn nursery is included so children can see how small their new sibling will be. A hospital room like the one their mother will occupy may also be visited.

To be certain that sibling classes will be successful, be sure that the information presented is age-appropriate. Chapters 29 to 33 discuss growth and development expectations by age group. Younger children may need reassurance that their parents will continue to love them after the new baby arrives. Older children may be interested in learning about newborn care and receiving assurance that their life will not be totally changed after this new family member's birth.

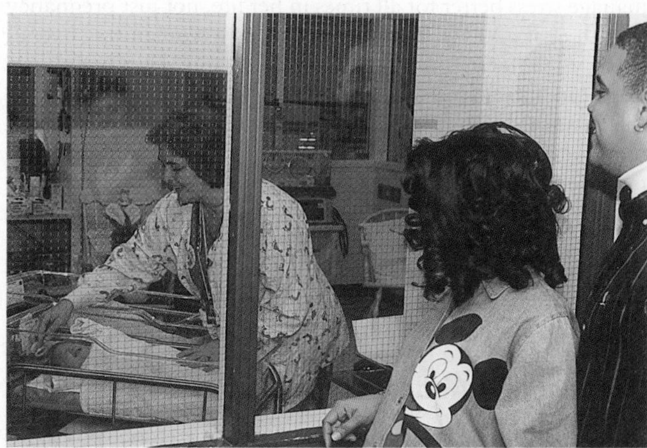

FIGURE 14.1 An enjoyable part of a preparation-for-parenthood class is touring a maternity service. Here, parents-to-be view a newborn nursery. (Photograph by Melissa Olson, with permission of Chestnut Hill Hospital, Philadelphia, PA.)

Breastfeeding Classes

Breastfeeding classes are designed to help women learn more about breastfeeding so they can appreciate the advantages of breastfeeding over formula feeding. Such classes cover the physiology of breastfeeding as well as psychological aspects. They stress that women should try to breastfeed exclusively for the first 6 months and ways to fit breastfeeding into busy schedules so they can continue it for the full first year (American Academy of Pediatrics [AAP], 2008). They are often taught by a certified La Leche League instructor who is an expert on what problems new mothers are apt to encounter (see Chapter 19 for breastfeeding techniques).

What if... Julia Marco tells you her husband won't be coming to class with her because he won't be able to be with her during labor. She asks you if it is really important to have someone with her. How would you advise her?

Preparation for Childbirth Classes

Preparation for childbirth classes focus mainly on explaining the birth process rather than pregnancy and ways to prevent or reduce the pain of childbirth. Common goals of preparation are to:

- Prepare an expectant woman and her support person for the childbirth experience
- Create clients who are knowledgeable consumers of obstetric care
- Help women reduce and manage pain with both pharmacologic and nonpharmacologic methods
- Help increase a couple's overall enjoyment of and satisfaction with the childbirth experience

In addition to teaching about normal labor, they include several exercises to ready the body for labor, as well as methods of pain prevention or pain relief in labor.

Prenatal Yoga

Prenatal yoga classes are aimed at helping a woman relax and manage stress better for all times in her life, not just pregnancy (Smith et al., 2007). Yoga exercises help a woman stay overall fit by their focus on gentle stretching and deep breathing. Yoga can also help a woman feel a high level of self-esteem as she masters difficult levels or positions. Yoga breathing techniques can be used in labor to help both relaxation and pain management.

Caution women, as pregnancy progresses, that it will become difficult to maintain difficult yoga positions. Women should use a chair or a wall for stabilization. They should avoid twisting exercises late in pregnancy because when joints soften in preparation for labor, muscle or joint strain could occur.

Perineal and Abdominal Exercises

In addition to encouraging an overall exercise program, childbirth preparation classes teach women specific exercises to strengthen pelvic and abdominal muscles and make these muscles stronger and more supple. Supple perineal muscles allow for stretching during birth, reduce discomfort, and help muscles revert more quickly to their normal condition and function more efficiently after childbirth (Hay-Smith & Dumoulin, 2009).

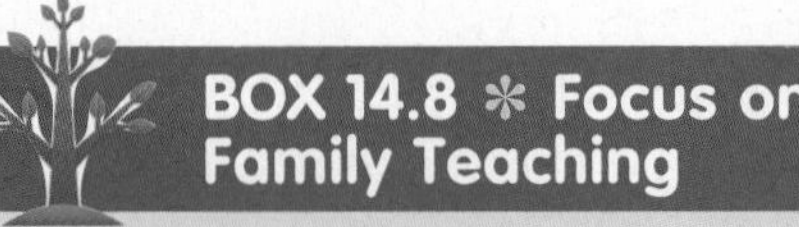

BOX 14.8 * Focus on Family Teaching

Exercise Guidelines for Labor Preparation

Q. Julia asks you, "How can I be sure the exercises I'm doing to be ready for birth won't hurt me or my baby?"

A. Good rules to follow are:

- Never exercise to a point of fatigue.
- Always rise from the floor slowly, to prevent feeling dizzy from orthostatic hypotension.
- To rise from the floor, roll over to the side first and then push up to avoid strain on the abdominal muscles or round ligaments as this can cause intense pain.
- To prevent leg cramps when doing leg exercises, never point the toes (extend the heel instead).
- To prevent back pain, do not attempt exercises that hyperextend the lower back.
- Do not hold your breath while exercising, because this increases intra-abdominal and intrauterine pressure.
- Do not continue with exercises if any danger signal of pregnancy occurs.
- Never practice second-stage pushing. Pushing increases intrauterine pressure and could rupture membranes.

A woman may begin exercises as early in pregnancy as she likes. Many exercises to strengthen abdominal or perineal muscles can be incorporated into daily activities so they take little time from a woman's day. It is best, however, for a woman to set aside a specific time each day for practicing exercises; otherwise, her participation is apt to be sporadic. Initially, women should do each exercise only a few times, gradually increasing the number at each session.

In addition to specific exercises, encourage women to maintain an overall active exercise program during pregnancy, as being in good physical condition can help prevent the need for cesarean birth. Women should not enroll or participate in a formal exercise program without their physician's or nurse-midwife's approval. They should not attempt to exercise if any of the danger signs of pregnancy are present, and they should never exercise to a point of fatigue. Common safety precautions for preparation for childbirth exercises in pregnancy are summarized in Box 14.8.

Tailor Sitting

Although many women may be familiar with tailor sitting, they may have to be re-taught the position so it is done in a way that stretches perineal muscles without occluding blood supply to the lower legs. A woman should not put one ankle on top of the other but should place one leg in front of the other (Fig. 14.2). As she sits in this position, she should gently push on her knees toward the floor until she feels her perineum stretch. This is a good position to use to watch television, read, or talk to friends on the telephone or file papers in a lower cabinet at work. It is good to plan on sitting in this position for at least 15 minutes every day. If she does this, by the end of pregnancy,

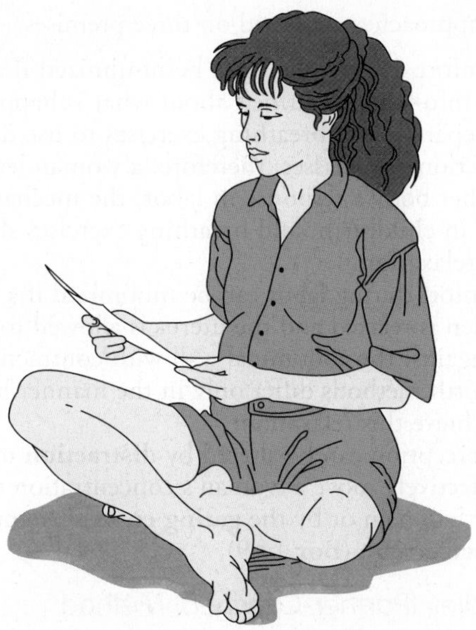

FIGURE 14.2 Tailor sitting stretches perineal muscles to make them more supple. Notice that the legs are parallel so that one does not compress the other. A woman could use this position for television watching, telephone conversations, or playing with an older child.

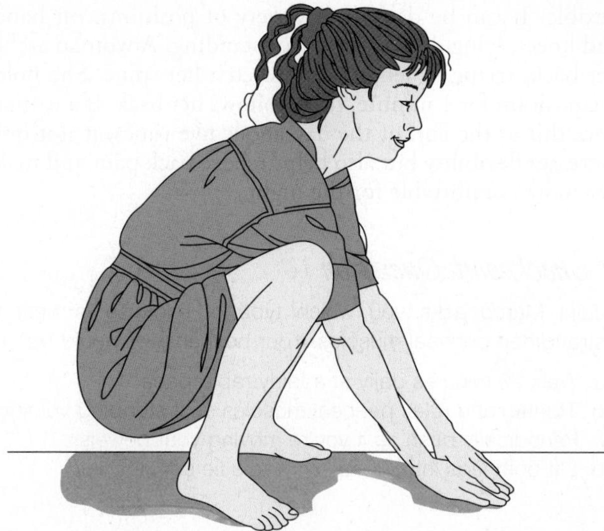

FIGURE 14.3 Squatting helps to stretch the muscles of the pelvic floor. Notice that the feet are flat on the floor for optimal perineal stretching.

a woman's perineum should be so supple that when she tailor-sits, her knees will almost touch the floor if pushed.

Squatting

Squatting (Fig. 14.3) also stretches perineal muscles and can be a useful position for second-stage labor, so a woman should also practice this position for about 15 minutes a day. Most women need a demonstration of effective squatting; otherwise, they tend to squat on their tiptoes. For pelvic muscles to stretch, a woman should keep her feet flat on the floor. Incorporating squatting into daily activities such as picking up toys from the floor reduces the amount of time a woman must devote to daily exercises.

Pelvic Floor Contractions (Kegel Exercises)

Pelvic floor contractions can be done easily during daily activities. While sitting at her desk or working around the house, a woman can tighten the muscles of her perineum by doing Kegel exercises (see Chapter 12, Box 12.7). Such perineal muscle-strengthening exercises are helpful in the postpartum period to reduce pain and promote perineal healing. They have long-term effects of increasing sexual responsiveness and helping prevent stress incontinence (Hay-Smith & Dumoulin, 2009).

Abdominal Muscle Contractions

Abdominal muscle contractions help strengthen abdominal muscles during pregnancy and therefore may help prevent constipation as well as help restore abdominal tone after pregnancy. Strong abdominal muscles can also contribute to effective second-stage pushing during labor. Abdominal contractions can be done in a standing or lying position along with pelvic floor contractions. A woman merely tightens her abdominal muscles, then relaxes them. She can repeat the exercise as often as she wishes during the day.

Another way to do the same thing is to practice "blowing out a candle." A woman takes a fairly deep inspiration, then exhales normally. Holding her finger about 6 inches in front of herself, as if it were a candle, she then exhales forcibly, pushing out residual air from her lungs as if her finger were a lit candle. She can feel her abdominal muscles contract as she reaches the end of a forcible exhalation.

Pelvic Rocking

Pelvic rocking (Fig. 14.4) helps relieve backache during pregnancy and early labor by making the lumbar spine more

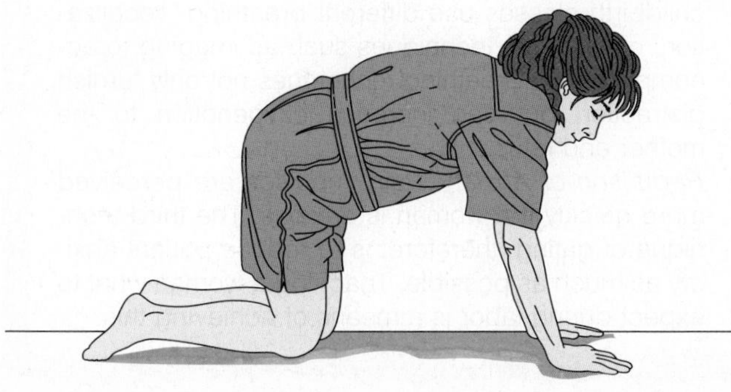

FIGURE 14.4 Pelvic rocking is helpful in relieving backache during pregnancy and labor. To do this, a woman first hollows her back and then arches it.

flexible. It can be done in a variety of positions: on hands and knees, lying down, sitting, or standing. A woman arches her back, trying to lengthen or stretch her spine. She holds the position for 1 minute, then hollows her back. If a woman does this at the end of the day about five times, it not only increases flexibility but also helps relieve back pain and make her more comfortable for the night.

✔ Checkpoint Question 14.1

Julia Marco asks you which type of exercise is best to strengthen perineal muscles. Your best answer would be:

a. Walk 20 minutes daily at a fairly rapid pace.
b. Tighten and relax perineal muscles as if stopping voiding.
c. Periodically push as if you're moving your bowels.
d. Lift both legs into the air while you lie supine.

Methods for Managing Pain in Childbirth

Beginning in the late 1950s, many specific methods for nonpharmacologic pain reduction during labor were developed. These included the Lamaze, Dick-Read, and Bradley methods, all named after the professionals who developed them. More recently, childbirth education has moved away from these strict method approaches to more eclectic ones. Ongoing research is being done to verify the effectiveness of each of these many techniques, and in practice many educators are teaching a variety of approaches including the use of complementary or herbal therapies (Smith, et al, 2009).

Most approaches are based on three premises:

1. Discomfort during labor can be minimized if a woman comes into labor informed about what is happening and prepared with breathing exercises to use during contractions. In classes, therefore, a woman learns about her body's response in labor, the mechanisms involved in childbirth, and breathing exercises she can use to aid relaxation.
2. Discomfort during labor can be minimized if a woman's abdomen is relaxed and the uterus is allowed to rise freely against the abdominal wall with contractions. Childbirth methods differ only in the manner by which they achieve this relaxation.
3. Pain perception can be altered by **distraction** techniques that effectively move a woman's concentration to other things than pain or by the **gating control theory of pain perception** (Box 14.9).

The Bradley (Partner-Coached) Method

The Bradley method of childbirth, originated by Robert Bradley, is based on the premises that pregnancy and childbirth are joyful natural processes and that a woman's partner should play an important role during pregnancy, labor, and the early newborn period. During pregnancy, a woman performs muscle-toning exercises and limits or omits foods that contain preservatives, animal fat, or a high salt content. She reduces pain in labor by abdominal breathing. In addition, she is encouraged to walk during labor and to use an internal focus point as a disassociation technique. The method is used

BOX 14.9 ✻ Gate Control Mechanisms to Reduce Pain

Pain Flows Through Pathways Because:

1. The endings of small peripheral nerve fibers detect a stimulus.
2. They transmit it to cells in the dorsal horn of the spinal cord.
3. Impulses pass through a dense, interfacing network of cells in the spinal cord (the substantia gelatinosa).
4. Immediately, a synapse occurs that returns the transmission to the peripheral site through a motor nerve. For example, a person touches a candle flame; the impulse travels to the spinal cord and back, and the person jerks his or her hand away from the flame.
5. After this short-circuit synapse, the impulse then continues in the spinal cord to reach the hypothalamus and cortex of the brain.
6. The impulse is interpreted (the candle is hot) and perceived as pain.

Gating Theory of Pain Control

The gating theory of pain refers to gate control mechanisms in the substantia gelatinosa that are capable of halting an impulse at the level of the spinal cord so the impulse is never perceived at the brain level as pain: a process similar to closing a gate.

Techniques to Assist Gating Mechanisms

- *Cutaneous Stimulation.* If large peripheral nerves next to an injury site are stimulated, the ability of the small nerve fibers at the injury site to transmit pain impulses appears to decrease. Therefore, rubbing an injured part or applying transcutaneous electrical nerve stimulation (TENS) or heat or cold to the site (cutaneous stimulation) are effective maneuvers to suppress pain. Effleurage, or light massage used in the Lamaze method, also accomplishes this.
- *Distraction.* If the cells of the brain stem that will register an impulse as pain are preoccupied with other stimuli, a pain impulse cannot register. Different childbirth classes use different breathing, vocalization, or focusing techniques such as imaging to accomplish this. Breathing techniques not only furnish distraction but can increase oxygenation to the mother and fetus.
- *Reduction of Anxiety.* Pain impulses are perceived more quickly if a woman is anxious. The third technique of gating, therefore, is to reduce patient anxiety as much as possible. Teaching a woman what to expect during labor is a means of achieving this.

widely in some areas of the United States and at specific centers (Bradley, 1996).

The Psychosexual Method

The psychosexual method of childbirth was developed by Sheila Kitzinger in England during the 1950s. The method stresses that pregnancy, labor and birth, and the early newborn period are some of the most important points in a woman's life. It includes a program of conscious relaxation and levels of progressive breathing that encourage a woman to "flow with" rather than struggle against contractions (Kitzinger, 1990).

The Dick-Read Method

The Dick-Read method is based on an approach proposed by Grantly Dick-Read, an English physician. The premise is that fear leads to tension, which leads to pain. If a woman can prevent fear from occurring, or break the chain between fear and tension or tension and pain, then she can reduce the pain of labor contractions. A woman achieves lack of fear through education about childbirth and relaxation and reduced pain by focusing on abdominal breathing during contractions (Dick-Read, 1987).

The Lamaze Philosophy

The Lamaze method of prepared childbirth, a philosophy based on the gating control theory of pain relief, is the one most often taught in the United States today (Amis & Green, 2007). The method is based on the theory that through stimulus-response conditioning, women can learn to use controlled breathing to reduce pain during labor. It was originally termed the **psychoprophylactic** method, as it focuses on preventing pain in labor (prophylaxis) by use of the mind (psyche).

The method was developed in Russia based on Pavlov's conditioning studies but was popularized by a French physician, Ferdinand Lamaze. Formal classes are organized by Lamaze International or the International Childbirth Education Association.

Lamaze preparation is not so much a method to help a woman cope with labor but rather a total philosophy of how to enjoy a safe and satisfying childbirth experience. Information to guide a woman and her coach through pregnancy such as prenatal nutrition, exercises, and common discomforts of pregnancy are discussed as well as information to prepare couples for unexpected circumstances of birth (e.g., malpresentation, cesarean birth, or the need for analgesia or anesthesia) is provided. Suggestions for supplies that a woman or couple might want to pack in advance and bring to the hospital for a Lamaze birth are shown in Table 14.1.

Throughout the program, six major concepts are stressed:

1. Labor should begin on its own, not be artificially induced.
2. Women should be able to move about freely during labor, not be confined to bed.
3. Women should receive continuous support during labor.
4. No routine interventions such as intravenous fluid are needed.
5. Women should be allowed to assume a nonsupine (e.g., upright or side-lying) position for birth.
6. Mother and baby should be housed together following birth, with unlimited opportunity for breastfeeding (Amis & Green, 2007).

TABLE 14.1 ✻ Supplies to Use During Labor

Item	Purpose
Lip balm	To prevent dry lips
Mouthwash	For rinsing dry mouth
Toothbrush and toothpaste	To prevent dry mouth
Warm socks	Comfort
Small rolling pin covered with soft cloth	Back massage
Focal point	To increase concentration
Busy work (e.g., book or laptop computer)	To pass time
Paper bag	To correct hyperventilation
Extra pillow	For semi-Fowler's position in labor
Wristwatch	For timing contractions
Baby powder	For reducing friction of effleurage
Lollipops	For energy and dry mouth
Snacks (e.g., apples or potato chips)	For coach's comfort
Tapes or compact discs and player	To increase relaxation

Three main premises are taught in the prenatal period related to the gating control method of pain relief:

1. Women learn in class about reproductive anatomy and physiology and the process of labor and birth in the belief that if women are familiar with what will happen in labor and the nature of contractions, the couple can enter labor with decreased tension.
2. A woman is taught to concentrate on breathing patterns and to use imagery or focusing (concentrating) on a specified object to block incoming pain sensations. The effectiveness of focusing can be observed in athletes who hurt themselves in basketball or football games but do not feel the pain until after the game because they are so focused on winning.
3. **Conditioned reflexes,** or reflexes that automatically occur in response to a stimulus, can also be used to displace pain during labor. For example, a woman is conditioned to relax automatically on hearing a command ("contraction beginning") or at the feel of a contraction beginning. The responses to contractions must be recently conditioned to be effective (because conditioned responses fade if not reinforced). This is the reason it is generally recommended that women attend Lamaze classes in the last trimester of pregnancy. A disadvantage of enrolling so late is that it limits the total amount of time directed to perineal exercises. If labor begins early, a woman may have had little or no practice with this type of exercise.

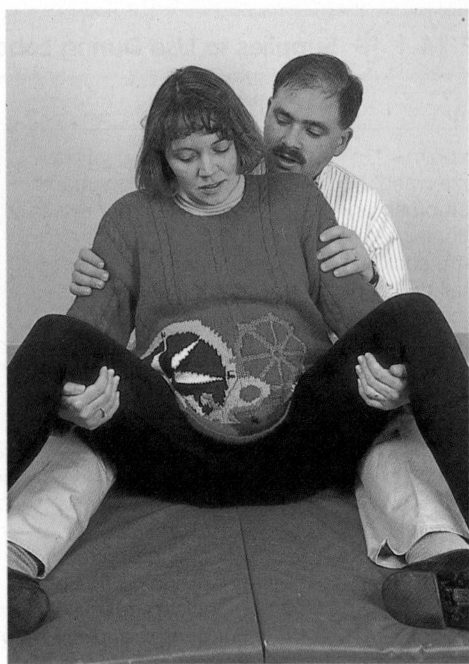

FIGURE 14.5 Every woman needs to be well prepared for birth. Here a couple practices positions for pushing in a childbirth preparation class. Caution women not to actually push.

Lamaze classes are kept small so that there is time for individual instruction and attention to each couple (Fig. 14.5). Advise a woman to bring a support person with her to class to practice breathing exercises. This person will then act as her coach in labor. Exercises taught in class vary from teacher to teacher, especially in terms of complexity, but have common features.

Conscious Relaxation. **Conscious relaxation** is learning to relax body parts so that, unknowingly, a woman does not remain tense and cause unnecessary muscle strain and fatigue during labor. She practices this during pregnancy by deliberately relaxing one set of muscles, then another and another until her body is completely relaxed. Her support person concentrates on noticing symptoms of tension such as a wrinkled brow, clenched fists, or a stiffly held arm. By either placing a comforting hand on the tense body area or telling a woman to relax that area, the support person helps her to achieve complete relaxation.

The Cleansing Breath. To begin all breathing exercises, a woman breathes in deeply and then exhales deeply (a **cleansing breath**). To end each exercise, she repeats this step. It is an important step to take because it limits the possibility of either hyperventilation (blowing off too much carbon dioxide) or hypoventilation (not exhaling enough carbon dioxide), both of which could happen with rapid breathing patterns, and so it helps ensure an adequate fetal oxygen supply. If women do become light-headed during labor from hyperventilation (develop respiratory alkalosis), breathing into a paper bag can help, as it causes rebreathing of exhaled carbon dioxide.

Consciously Controlled Breathing. Using **consciously controlled breathing,** or set breathing patterns at specific rates, provides distraction as well as prevents the diaphragm from descending fully and putting pressure on the expanding uterus. To practice, a woman inhales comfortably but fully, then exhales, with her exhalation a little stronger than her inhalation (to help prevent hypoventilation). She practices breathing in this manner at a controlled pace, depending on the intensity of contractions. Various levels of breathing are:

Level 1. Slow chest breathing of comfortable but full respirations at a rate of 6 to 12 breaths per minute. The level is used for early contractions.

Level 2. Lighter and more rapid breathing than level 1. The rib cage should expand but be so light the diaphragm barely moves. The rate of respirations is up to 40 per minute. This is a good level of breathing for contractions when cervical dilation is between 4 and 6 cm.

Level 3. Even more shallow and more rapid breathing. The rate is 50 to 70 breaths per minute. As the respirations become faster, the exhalation must be a little stronger than the inhalation to allow good air exchange and to prevent hypoventilation. If a woman practices saying "out" with each exhalation, she almost inevitably will make exhalation stronger than inhalation. A woman uses this level for transition contractions. Keeping the tip of her tongue against the roof of her mouth helps prevent her oral mucosa from drying out during such rapid breathing.

Level 4. A "pant-blow" pattern, or taking three or four quick breaths (in and out), then a forceful exhalation. Because this type of breathing sounds like a train (breath-breath-breath-huff), it is sometimes referred to as "choo-choo" or "hee-hee-hee-hoo" breathing.

Level 5. Quiet, continuous, very shallow panting at about 60 breaths per minute. This can be used during strong contractions or during the second stage of labor to prevent a woman from pushing before full dilatation.

Some courses stop teaching at the point a woman has mastered these levels of breathing; others have her learn to shift from one level to the other on command or at the point she feels a need for more pain relief.

Figure 14.6 illustrates the use of levels of breathing. An early labor contraction is mild. When the contraction begins, her coach says, "Contraction beginning." A woman takes a cleansing breath, then breathes at level 1; she feels no bite from the contraction and so does not need to change to a more involved breathing pattern. Later in labor, contractions are stronger and longer. Now, at the sound of "Contraction beginning," a woman takes a cleansing breath, then begins level 1 breathing (3 breaths); shifts to level 2 (4 to 6 breaths); then shifts to level 3 (10 breaths). The contraction is lessening. She shifts down to level 2 (4 to 6 breaths), then to level 1 (3 or 4 breaths). The contraction is gone. She takes a final cleansing breath. During actual labor, her coach can tell the strength of contractions by resting a hand on her abdomen or observing a uterine contraction monitor. A coach can tell a woman when to shift breathing levels depending on the coach's estimation of the strength of the contraction with words such as, "contraction beginning, getting stronger, now getting weaker, gone." In the time before transition to the second stage of labor, when contractions are longest and strongest, a woman may need to use her level 4 breathing or continuous light panting as well. A woman who can perform

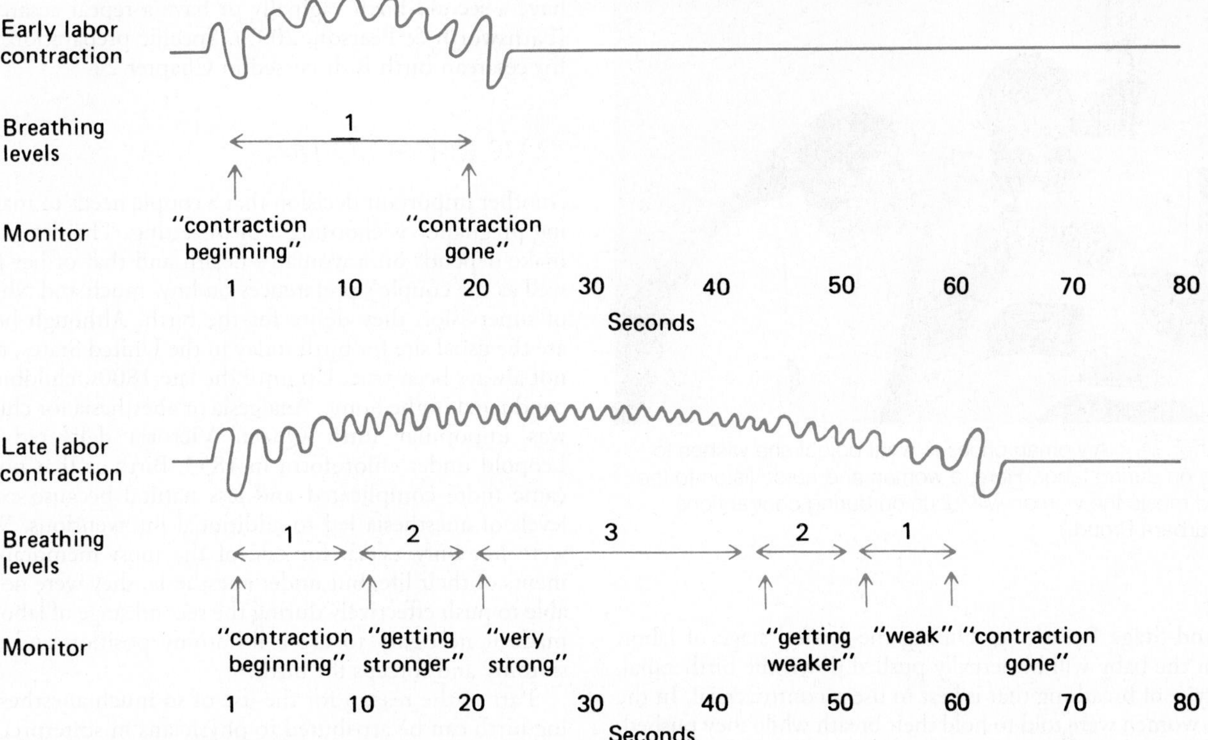

FIGURE 14.6 An example of differing breathing patterns during a single contraction; 1, 2, and 3 are levels of breathing. A cleansing breath is taken at the beginning and end of the contraction.

the various levels of breathing and maintain relaxation can be assured that she is prepared to handle all labor contractions up to the second stage of labor.

Effleurage. One additional technique to encourage relaxation and displace pain in the Lamaze method is **effleurage**, which is French for "light abdominal massage," done with just enough pressure to avoid tickling. To do this, a woman traces a pattern on her abdomen with her fingertips (Fig. 14.7). The rate of effleurage should remain constant even though breathing rates change. Effleurage serves as a distraction technique and decreases sensory stimuli transmission from the abdominal wall, helping limit local discomfort. If an external electronic monitor is in place on the abdomen, effleurage can be done superior or inferior to it or even on the thighs. Effleurage can also be done by the support person.

Focusing or Imagery. Focusing intently on an object (sometimes called "sensate focus") is another method of keeping sensory input from reaching the cortex of the brain. A woman brings into labor a photograph of her partner or children, a graphic design, or just something that appeals to her (Fig. 14.8). She concentrates on it during contractions. Be careful not to step into a woman's line of vision during a contraction and break this focused concentration. Other women use imagery by imagining they are in a calm place such as on a beach watching waves rolling in to them or relaxing on a porch swing (Stein, 2007). Try not to ask questions or talk to women using this technique or you will break their concentration.

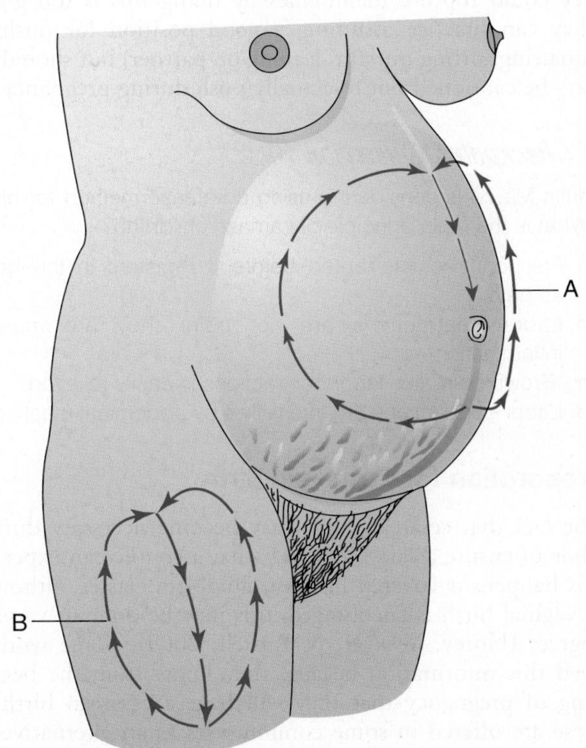

FIGURE 14.7 Effleurage patterns. (**A**) During uterine contractions, a woman traces a pattern on her bare abdomen with her fingers. (**B**) If electronic fetal monitoring is being used, effleurage may be performed on the thigh.

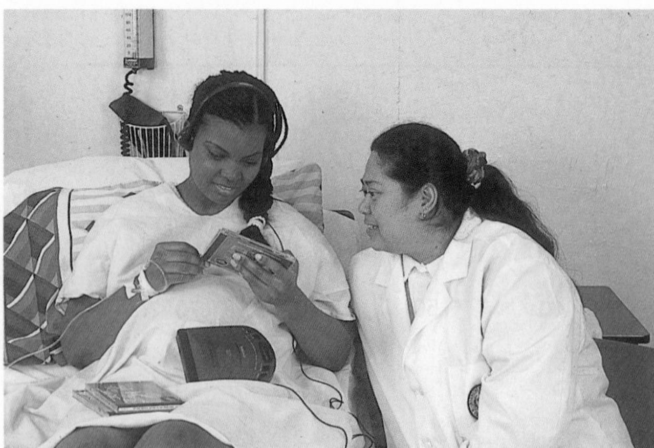

FIGURE 14.8 A woman chooses what object she wishes to focus on during labor. Here, a woman and nurse listen to the taped music the woman will focus on during contractions. (© Barbara Proud.)

Second-Stage Breathing. During the second stage of labor, when the baby will be actually pushed down the birth canal, the type of breathing that is best to use is controversial. In the past, women were told to hold their breath while they pushed. Now it is believed that holding the breath for a prolonged time impairs blood return from the vena cava (a Valsalva maneuver), so this is now discouraged. Based on this, most classes suggest that women breathe any way that is natural for them, except holding their breath during this stage of labor.

Women should not practice pushing. The possibility that they could rupture membranes by doing this is too great. They can practice assuming a good position for pushing (squatting, sitting upright, leaning on partner) but should always be cautioned not to actually push during pregnancy.

✔ Checkpoint Question 14.2

Julia Marco is considering using a Lamaze method for birth. What is the main principle of Lamaze childbirth?

a. Pain can be interrupted before it registers in the brain as pain.
b. Labor contractions are not pain; they are muscle inflammation.
c. "Brown pain" like labor contractions is easily relieved.
d. Labor contractions are intensified by abdominal massage.

Preparation for Cesarean Birth

The fact that cesarean birth may become necessary during labor to ensure a safe birth and what a couple can expect if this happens is covered in most childbirth classes, although as vaginal birth is encouraged, this may be done to varying degrees (Horey, Weaver, & Russell, 2009). Some women need this information because they know from the beginning of pregnancy that they will have a cesarean birth as these are offered in some communities as an alternative to vaginal birth to help prevent uterine prolapse or urinary incontinence in later years or to be more convenient for the family, although this policy is controversial (McCourt et al., 2007). Still other women had a cesarean birth for a first pregnancy and now need information on whether they should have a second birth vaginally or have a repeat cesarean one (Farnsworth & Pearson, 2007). Specific preparation needed for cesarean birth is discussed in Chapter 24.

THE BIRTH SETTING

Another important decision that a couple needs to make during pregnancy is choosing a birth setting. The decision they make depends on a woman's health and that of her fetus as well as the couple's preferences on how much and what kind of supervision they desire for the birth. Although hospitals are the usual site for birth today in the United States, that has not always been true. Up until the late 1800s, childbirth was conducted in the home. Analgesia or anesthesia for childbirth was unpopular until Queen Victoria delivered Prince Leopold under chloroform in 1853. Birth at that point became more complicated and less natural because extensive levels of anesthesia led to additional interventions. Women were not only asleep for one of the most memorable moments of their life, but under anesthesia, they were no longer able to push effectively during the second stage of labor. That made it necessary to use a lithotomy position and an episiotomy and forceps for birth.

Part of the reason for the use of so much anesthesia during birth can be attributed to physicians misinterpreting the type of pain of childbirth. It was assumed that the moment of birth was the major time of discomfort. As a result, women were allowed to labor without any pain medication and then were given anesthesia or analgesia right before the baby was born. Although the pain felt at birth is intense, it is also over quickly, unlike the hours of labor that precede it, so in reality, women may not be as uncomfortable during the actual birth as they are during labor. Birth is also such an exhilarating time that the excitement of the moment can mask pain.

Fortunately, birthing practices have changed to better meet women's needs based on their descriptions of the pain of childbirth. If women choose physicians or hospitals who subscribe to more progressive birth practices over the services of more traditional facilities, the overall standard of care in communities leans toward the more progressive settings. The addition of birthing rooms to hospitals in the past 20 years is an example of this. Nurses are in a strong position to advocate for making childbirth a "natural" process in the least restrictive setting possible. At the same time, nurses have a strong responsibility to encourage parents to maintain enough restrictions that birth remains safe.

Choosing the Appropriate Setting

Women having uncomplicated pregnancies may choose hospitals, birthing centers, or their homes as settings for birth. Women with high-risk pregnancies have less choice; women with potential complications are advised to give birth at hospitals where immediate emergency care will be available.

Choosing a Birth Attendant and Support Person

In the United States, most births are supervised by an obstetrician, a physician specializing in labor and birth. As the tendency for specialized physician practice declines, however, it is becoming more common for family practitioners to serve as birth attendants. It is also becoming more common for certified nurse-midwives to attend births, especially at alternative birth centers.

In addition to selecting who will medically supervise her baby's birth, a woman needs to choose who will support her in labor. In years past, this support was offered by experienced women in the community. In the 1960s, the role was given to the father of the baby. Today, many different family members offer this type of support. In addition to having the father of their baby present, many women choose a doula, or a person specially prepared to assist with birth. Doulas can be helpful as fathers may find it hard to provide doula-type support during labor when they are so emotionally involved themselves in the birth. Having such a person present frees the father to enjoy the birth rather than feeling occupied with coaching instructions. Although research in the subject is not extensive, there are suggestions that rates of oxytocin augmentation, epidural anesthesia, and cesarean birth can all be reduced with doula support (McGrath & Kennell, 2008).

Hospital Birth

Maternity services of hospitals have changed a great deal in recent years, influenced by the First Consensus Initiative of the Coalition for Improving Maternity Services (CIMS). This organization rates hospitals regarding whether they are mother friendly based on, through its practices, if the hospital respects that birth is a normal, natural, and healthy process and a woman has the opportunity to:

- Experience a healthy and joyous birth experience, regardless of her age or circumstances
- Give birth as she wishes in an environment in which she feels nurtured and secure
- Have access to the full range of options for pregnancy, birth, and nurturing her baby
- Receive accurate and up-to-date information about the benefits and risks of all procedures, drugs, and tests suggested for use during pregnancy, birth, and the postpartum period, with the rights to informed consent and informed refusal
- Receive support for making informed choices about what is best for her and her baby based on her individual values and beliefs (CIMS, 1996)

Based on the above criteria, 10 steps to a mother-friendly hospital climate have been identified (Box 14.10). Urge women to ask hospitals in their community if they are rated as mother-friendly as this should influence their choice of a hospital or birth attendant.

BOX 14.10 ✻ Characteristics of a Mother-Friendly Hospital

A mother-friendly hospital:

1. Offers a birthing mother:
   - Unrestricted access to the birth companions of her choice, including fathers, partners, children, family members, and friends
   - Unrestricted access to continuous emotional and physical support from a skilled woman—for example, a doula or labor-support professional
   - Access to professional midwifery care.
2. Provides accurate descriptive and statistical information to the public about its practices and procedures for birth care, including measures of interventions and outcomes.
3. Provides culturally competent care—that is, care that is sensitive and responsive to the specific beliefs, values, and customs of the mother's ethnicity and religion.
4. Provides a birthing woman with the freedom to walk, move about, and assume the positions of her choice during labor and birth (unless restriction is specifically required to correct a complication), and discourages the use of the lithotomy position.
5. Has clearly defined policies and procedures for:
   - Collaborating and consulting throughout the perinatal period with other maternity services, including communicating with the original caregiver when transfer from one birth site to another is necessary
   - Linking the mother and baby to appropriate community resources, including prenatal and post-discharge follow-up and breastfeeding support
   - Does not routinely employ practices and procedures that are unsupported by scientific evidence such as routine perineal shaving
6. Educates staff in nondrug methods of pain relief and does not promote the use of analgesic or anesthetic drugs not specifically required to correct a complication.
7. Encourages all mothers and families, including those with sick or premature newborns or infants with congenital problems, to touch, hold, breastfeed, and care for their babies to the extent compatible with their conditions.
8. Discourages nonreligious circumcision of the newborn.
9. Promotes successful breastfeeding by:
   - Having a written breastfeeding policy that is routinely communicated to all health care staff
   - Educating all health care staff in skills necessary to implement this policy
   - Informing all pregnant women about the benefits and management of breastfeeding
   - Helping mothers initiate breastfeeding within a half-hour of birth
   - Showing mothers how to breastfeed and how to maintain lactation even if they should be separated from their infants
   - Giving newborn infants no food or drink other than breast milk unless medically indicated
   - Practicing rooming in to allow mothers and infants to remain together 24 hours a day
   - Encouraging breastfeeding on demand
   - Giving no pacifiers to breastfeeding infants
   - Fostering the establishment of breastfeeding support groups and referring others to them on discharge from hospitals or clinics (Hotelling, 2007).

Advantages and disadvantages of hospital birth are summarized in Box 14.11. The major advantage of a hospital is that equipment and expert personnel are readily available if the mother or fetus or newborn should have a complication.

In evaluating studies that compare the complications of birthing centers or home births with those of hospitals, women who gave birth in hospitals invariably have more complications than those who give birth in other settings but that happens because high-risk mothers give birth at hospitals so the number of complications in hospital settings is bound to be higher than in other settings.

A woman usually comes to the hospital when her contractions are approximately 5 minutes apart and regular in pattern. If she has preregistered at the hospital, she is admitted to a **birthing room** without any separation time from her support person. Birthing rooms are also called labor-delivery-recovery rooms (LDRs) or **labor-delivery-recovery-postpartum rooms (LDRPs)**. Such rooms are decorated in a homelike way; couples can bring favorite music or reading materials with them to use during labor; and the bed can be used as a labor bed until birth, when it converts into a **birthing bed** or a lithotomy position bed (Fig. 14.9). Women are expected to use a prepared method of childbirth with a minimum of analgesia and anesthesia (although an advantage of a hospital birth is that anesthesia such as an epidural is readily available if needed). An important aspect of birthing rooms is that the support person and often other family members can stay with a woman throughout labor and birth, allowing a couple and their families to feel that they have control over their birth experience. Women report greater satisfaction with birth when they use a more homelike setting than a bare, functional labor room for birth (Hodnett et al., 2009).

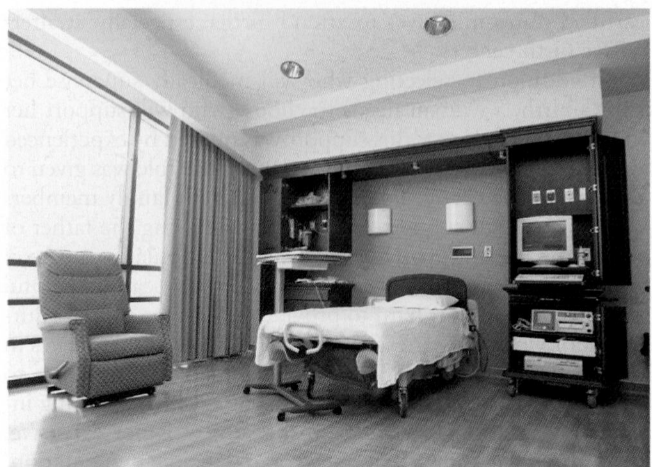

FIGURE 14.9 A birthing (labor-birth-recovery) room designed to maintain a homelike atmosphere in a hospital setting.

BOX 14.11 ✻ Advantages and Disadvantages of Hospital Birth

Advantages

- A woman is encouraged to be prepared to control the discomfort of labor through nonmedication measures such as controlled breathing although anesthesia such as an epidural is readily available.
- A woman is encouraged to be knowledgeable about the labor process and make decisions about procedures performed.
- A woman is encouraged to consider breastfeeding to aid uterine contraction and infant bonding after birth.
- Labor, birth, and immediate postpartal care can all be scheduled in a single room.
- A woman is attended by skilled professionals during labor and birth and the postpartal period.
- Emergency care and extended high-risk care are immediately available.

Disadvantages

- Separation of the family for at least one night
- Mother may not feel as much in control of the childbirth experience as she may wish.
- Care may be fragmented, particularly if a woman's physician is not present during the entire labor and birth, or if labor nurses change shifts in the middle of labor. (Many nurse-midwives and physicians make it a point, however, to remain with their client throughout the entire childbirth experience.)

At the time of birth, additional cabinets in the room are opened and converted into a space for baby care. Women can choose a birthing position: lithotomy, squatting, supine recumbent, or side-lying. A support person remains with a woman during birth and in some settings can cut the umbilical cord if desired.

Most hospitals screen women in early labor with an external monitor for both fetal heart rate and uterine contractions. If the fetal heart rate is good, such a monitor can usually be removed and used again only for periodic screening as labor progresses. A woman may have intravenous access started as a prophylactic measure. If this is done, be sure to insert the needle into a dorsal vein of her nondominant hand so it causes little discomfort and she will be able to hold her newborn with little inconvenience.

Birthing chairs (Fig. 14.10) are comfortable reclining chairs with a slide-away seat that allows a woman to assume a comfortable position during labor and also furnishes perineal exposure so a birth attendant can assist with the birth. The semi-Fowler's position acts with gravity and so may speed the second stage of labor.

If a woman chooses to use a supine recumbent position (on her back with knees flexed) or a side-lying position rather than a lithotomy position (legs elevated into stirrups) for birth, she uses a birthing bed. Such positions reduce tension on the perineum and may result in fewer perineal tears than a lithotomy position.

Postpartum Care

Women giving birth in LDRPs remain in the room with their families for the rest of their hospital stay. Women giving birth in birthing rooms may be transferred to a postpartum unit after birth; they remain there for the length of their hospital stay. Both LDRPs and postpartum units serve as "rooming-in" units in which the infant remains in the

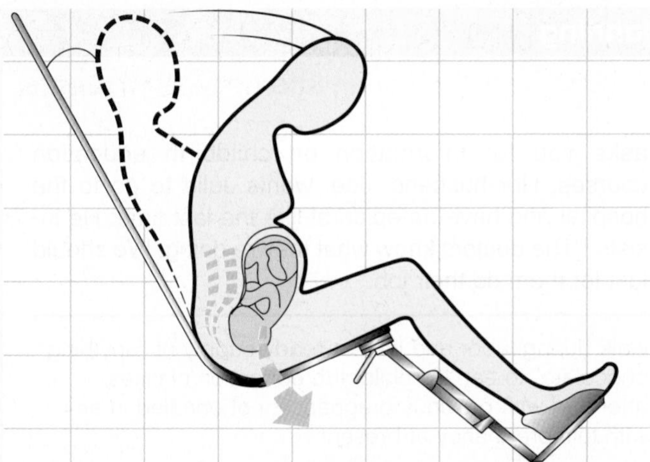
A

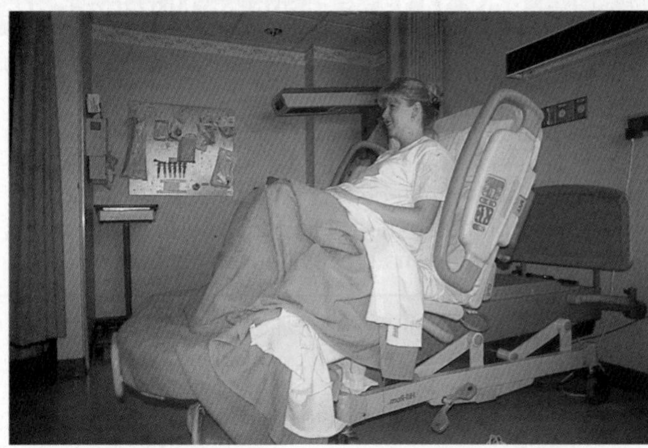
B

FIGURE 14.10 (A) A birthing chair allows a woman to maintain a semi-Fowler's position. (B) A birthing chair used during labor. (© Caroline Brown, RNC, MS, DEd.)

mother's room for most of the day. After birth, encourage mothers to breastfeed immediately. Urge a couple to keep their newborn with them in their hospital room so they have ample time to become acquainted. Breastfeeding on demand for infants should be the rule. There should be no restrictions on visiting for the primary support person; in many institutions, a rollaway bed is provided so he or she can remain constantly. Siblings of the newborn should be allowed to visit at least once and touch and become acquainted with the newborn.

Alternative Birthing Centers

Alternative birthing centers (ABCs) are wellness-oriented childbirth facilities designed to remove childbirth from the acute care hospital setting while still providing enough medical resources for emergency care should a complication of labor or birth arise. Such a setting is established within, or at least within an easy distance of a hospital. Because it is located outside an acute care setting, where infections abound, the risk of hospital-acquired infection to a woman is thought to be reduced. The birth attendants tend to be nurse-midwives. Women who deliver in ABCs are screened for complications before being admitted. Because women are carefully screened, the mortality rate of mothers and infants is no higher and may be lower in these out-of-hospital settings than in hospital settings.

Like hospitals, ABCs have LDRP rooms where a woman and her support person can invite friends and siblings to participate in the birth. In some centers, a central play area for siblings and cooking facilities are also available. ABCs encourage a woman to express her own needs and wishes during the labor process. A minimum of analgesia and anesthesia is provided, and she can choose a birth position. She can bring her own music or distraction objects, and the partner can perform such tasks as cutting the umbilical cord if he or she chooses. Advantages and disadvantages of ABCs are summarized in Box 14.12.

Women remain in an ABC from 4 to 24 hours after birth. Because a minimum of analgesia or anesthesia is used, a woman recovers quickly after birth and is ready to be discharged this early. The Nursing Care Plan (Box 14.13) summaries preparation for birth in such an alternative setting.

Home Birth

Home birth is the usual mode of birth in developing countries. It is also a popular choice for birth in Europe, but only about 1% of women in the United States choose this method. Home birth may be supervised by a physician, but nurse-midwives are the more likely choice as birth attendants in this setting (Vedam, Goff, & Marnin, 2007). The Frontier Nursing Service of Kentucky is an example of an organization in the United States that maintains an active and well-accepted program of home birth.

BOX 14.12 ❋ Advantages and Disadvantages of ABCs

Advantages

- A woman is encouraged to be prepared to control the discomfort of labor through nonmedication measures such as controlled breathing.
- A woman is encouraged to be knowledgeable about the labor process and to help care providers with decision making.
- A woman is encouraged to breastfeed to aid uterine contraction and infant bonding after birth.
- Family integrity can be maintained because family members may accompany a woman to the birthing center.
- A woman is attended by skilled professionals during labor and birth.
- Emergency care is immediately available. Extended high-risk care is easily arranged.

Disadvantages

- Extended high-risk care is not immediately available.
- A woman may be fatigued after birth because of brief health care setting stay.
- She must independently monitor her postpartal status because of brief health care setting stay.

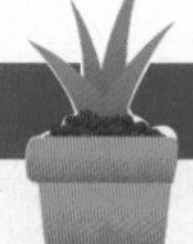

BOX 14.13 ✻ Focus on Nursing Care Planning

A Multidisciplinary Care Map for a Family Who Desires Birth at an Alternative Birth Center

Julia Marco is pregnant with her second child. During her first pregnancy, she did not attend childbirth classes and she received an epidural for the birth. During a prenatal visit, Julia tells you that she would now like to have a natural birth in a birthing center. She asks you for information on childbirth education courses. Her husband, Joe, wants Julia to go to the hospital and have an epidural like the last time. He insists, "The doctors know what they're doing. We should just let them do their job."

Family Assessment ✻ Family lives with 4-year-old Josh in apartment in central downtown. Julia is a stay-at-home mom; Joe works as a parking garage attendant. Family has limited financial resources, with no medical insurance.

Client Assessment ✻ Pregnancy progressing without evidence of problems or complications. Gravida 2, para 1, 24 weeks' gestation. Client states that she wants to use alternative birth center (ABC); reports concern over previous hospital birth of son. Wants son Josh, now 4 years old, to be a part of new baby's birth. Wants a doula but doesn't know how to contact one. Wants to walk during labor and have a ready supply of "anything chocolate" to eat. No childbirth education classes attended with previous pregnancy; not enrolled in any with this pregnancy at present.

Nursing Diagnosis ✻ Decisional conflict related to choice of birth setting and birth process

Outcome Criteria ✻ Client and partner state advantages and disadvantages of birth setting options; plans for birth and birth setting chosen by 3 weeks time.

Client and partner verbalize goal of healthy mother and baby as motivation for choice of birth setting.

Team Member Responsible	Assessment	Intervention	Rationale	Expected Outcome
		Activities of Daily Living		
Nurse	Assess the family to see what plans they want to make for child care during labor.	Suggest the couple ask a family member to be caretaker for son during the birth.	A caretaker can enhance the experience for the older child promoting a positive, family-centered event.	Couple states they have located a suitable caretaker for son.
		Consultations		
Nurse/nurse-midwife	Assess what family expects of a doula for labor.	Give couple list of available doulas in community and help arrange for meeting.	Doulas can offer strong support in labor; prearrangements help meet mutual goals.	Couple confirms they have arranged for a doula to help offer support in labor.
		Consultations		
Nurse/social worker	Investigate the type of birth facilities available in local area in regard to wishes for labor.	Review the requirements, advantages, and disadvantages for birth setting choices available.	Review of options allows the couple to make an informed decision appropriate for their needs.	Client and partner state they have reviewed and understand options available to them.
		Procedures/Medications		
Physician/nurse	Determine if there are any contraindications to walking during labor.	Educate client about the few situations, such as placenta previa, that would contradict walking in labor.	Walking during labor has the potential to decrease the time of labor unless contraindicated.	Client states that she will be flexible in regard to wishes in labor based on her own and fetal safety.

		Nutrition		
Nurse	Assess whether client knows if her chosen food options during labor are approved by local facilities.	Help client modify her goals for nutrition during labor as appropriate based on facility requirements.	As many choices for food exist, coordinating plans with facility should result in least stress during labor.	Client confirms that she has agreed on food type agreeable with chosen agency.
		Patient/Family Education		
Nurse	Obtain information about local childbirth education classes available.	Assist couple as necessary with selecting class that fits their resources.	Education can enhance the chances of a positive childbirth experience. Choosing a program that fits the couple's resources helps to promote adherence.	Client attends the chosen preparation for childbirth class before the 38th week of pregnancy.
Nurse	Assess if any classes for sibling preparation for birth are available in community.	Help couple plan for mother and son to attend class on sibling preparation for birth or meet with nurse for instruction.	Adequate preparation for all involved improves the chances of a positive experience.	Couple states that they will either attend a class for sibling preparation or meet with nurse for information.
		Psychosocial/Spiritual/Emotional Needs		
Nurse/nurse-midwife	Explore with client and partner past experiences with childbirth and current expectations and beliefs.	Encourage couple to verbalize feelings, concerns, and needs.	Verbalization of feelings permits a safe outlet for emotions and assists in increasing the other person's awareness.	Couple states their overall goal for childbirth is a safe one for mother and new child.
		Discharge Planning		
Nurse	Assess if couple has any further questions about birth centers.	Ascertain couple has phone number and directions to chosen birthing center.	Advance planning can help avoid increased stress at time of birth.	Couple states they are happy with birth setting decision and prepared to follow through on plans.
Social worker	Assess the finances the couple will need to complete birth at their chosen setting.	Review financing options with couple.	Advance planning can help avoid increased stress at time of birth.	Couple states they have a plan for financial arrangements.

Most women who choose home birth in the United States are well educated and from middle-income families. They choose home birth so they can have their baby close by after birth, can have more control over the childbirth experience, and can give birth in familiar, low-cost surroundings.

The main advantage of a home birth is that it encourages family integrity: a woman and her family are not separated so the baby can be immediately integrated into the family. On the other hand, it puts responsibility on a woman to prepare her home for the birth (which is difficult if she is exhausted toward the end of pregnancy) and to take care of the infant after birth. Some people, however willing, may be unable to take on these roles in a crisis situation such as childbirth. Many women passing through their first postpartum or "taking-in" phase may be happier maintaining a dependent passive role than immediately taking responsibility for the infant's care.

To be a candidate for a home birth, a woman must be in good health, must be able to adjust to changing circumstances, and must have adequate support people who will sustain her during labor and assist her for the first few days after birth. Women with any complication of pregnancy are not candidates for home birth. Advantages and disadvantages of home birth are summarized in Box 14.14.

Freebirthing

Freebirthing refers to women giving birth without any health care provider supervision (Cooper & Clarke, 2008). Women may also refer to it as unassisted birth or couples birth. It differs from home birth because using this technique, a woman learns pregnancy care from reading articles on the Internet and then arranges to have her child at home, perhaps accompanied by her family or friends and support person, but without health care supervision.

Freebirthing is potentially dangerous because if a complication of birth should occur, the woman may not recognize that the complication is occurring until damage to her child or herself results. Even after she recognizes that a problem is occurring, there is a space of time before emergency help can arrive to assist her. Freebirthing is particularly dangerous if a woman avoids prenatal care or depends solely on Internet information. Educating women that not all Internet information is reliable and that supervised birth does not mean that they have no choice in their care such as whether they want pain relief or to use a special position for birth are effective ways to help women make safer choices about birth.

What if... Julia and her husband have a serious disagreement about whether to plan for a home birth or hospital birth? What issues would you suggest they explore? If they cannot agree, how could they compromise?

Children Attending the Birth

Most birthing centers and some hospitals allow children to view the birth of a sibling. Attendance at sibling classes designed to prepare children to witness the birth is often required. If children will be present, a person separate from the main support person needs to be designated to provide entertainment, explanations, food, and a place for them to sleep. A child who is without supervision during this time could remember the experience as a time of rejection rather than an exciting, happy experience. The mother should not be expected to provide such supervision during labor as she will want to concentrate on distraction or breathing techniques.

BOX 14.14 ✻ Advantages and Disadvantages of Home Birth

Advantages

- A woman is encouraged to become knowledgeable about the birth process and be an active participant in independently reducing the discomfort of labor.
- A woman has the greatest freedom for expressing her individuality.
- There is no separation of the family at birth.
- A skilled professional can attend the birth.

Disadvantages

- Adequate equipment other than first-line emergency equipment is unavailable.
- An abrupt change of goals is necessary if hospitalization is required.
- A woman and support person may become exhausted because of the responsibility placed on them.
- Interference with the "taking-in phase" may occur postpartally because a woman must "take hold."
- A woman must independently monitor her postpartal status.

Help couples consider whether the birth experience will be a positive and enjoyable one for the child based on the child's developmental level. Allowing a child to witness the birth of kittens or puppies might be a more appropriate way to expose a child to birth.

ALTERNATIVE METHODS OF BIRTH

In addition to varied settings, several different methods of childbirth have become popular in the past 15 to 20 years. These include alternative birth methods such as the Leboyer method and birth under water.

Leboyer Method

Frederick Leboyer was a French obstetrician who postulated that moving from a warm, fluid-filled intrauterine environment to a noisy, air-filled, brightly lit birth room creates a major shock for a newborn (Leboyer, 1975). With the **Leboyer method,** the birthing room is darkened so there is no sudden contrast in light; it is kept pleasantly warm, not chilled. Soft music is played, or at least harsh noises are kept to a minimum. The infant is handled gently; the cord is cut late; and the infant is placed immediately after birth into a warm-water bath.

Some neonatologists question the wisdom of a warm bath because it could reduce spontaneous respirations and allow a high level of acidosis to occur. Late cutting of a cord can lead to excess blood viscosity in a newborn. Certainly, soft music, gentle handling, and a welcoming atmosphere are important ingredients for all birth attendants to try to incorporate into birth. Providing dim lights (or at least not bright, glaring ones) and providing a warm temperature could be given more consideration in most institutions.

Hydrotherapy and Water Birth

Reclining or sitting in warm water during labor can be soothing; the feeling of weightlessness that occurs under water as well as the relaxation from the warm water both can contribute to reducing discomfort in labor. Using this principle, many birthing centers allow women to labor in warm showers or give birth in spa tubs of warm water (Maude & Foureur, 2007). The baby is born underwater and then immediately brought to the surface for a first breath. Most women who choose underwater birth are very pleased that they chose this method. A potential difficulty is contamination of the bath water with feces expelled with pushing efforts during the second stage of labor. This could lead to uterine infection in the mother or aspiration of contaminated bath water by a newborn, which could lead to pneumonia. Maternal chilling when a woman leaves the water is another factor to consider and prevent.

✔ Checkpoint Question 14.3

Suppose Julia Marco decides on a hospital birth. What is an advantage of hospital birth over other settings?

a. Women can use breathing exercises.
b. Labor and childbirth can be pain free.
c. Extended high-risk care is available.
d. The cost of a hospital stay is low.

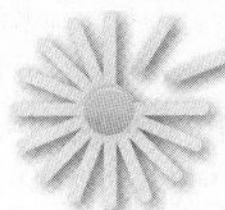

Key Points for Review

- Couples should be encouraged to make a childbirth plan early in pregnancy that includes birth attendant, setting, desired method of pain management, and any special wishes.
- Common exercises taught in pregnancy to strengthen perineal muscles are tailor sitting, squatting, and Kegel exercises. Abdominal muscle-contraction and pelvic rocking exercises strengthen the abdominal muscles and help relieve backache.
- Types of childbirth preparation include the Bradley (partner-coached), psychosexual (Kitzinger), Dick-Read, yoga, and Lamaze methods. Lamaze is the most common method used in the United States.
- Commonly used nonpharmacologic techniques for pain relief in labor are conscious relaxation, consciously controlled breathing, effleurage, focusing, imagery, and hydrotherapy.
- Classes for expectant parents provide information on pregnancy, birth, and childcare.
- Common sites for childbirth include hospitals, alternative birthing centers, and homes.
- Couples should ask birth settings if they are rated as mother-friendly before choosing them as a birth site.

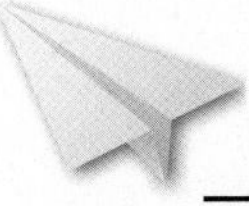

CRITICAL THINKING EXERCISES

1. Joe Marco, the husband you met at the beginning of the chapter, wants his wife to have their baby at a hospital and have epidural anesthesia for pain relief. He insists, "The doctors know what they're doing. We should just let them do their job." After further speaking with Joe, you discover he does not want Julia to go through the pain of natural childbirth because he fears he will not be able to help her during labor. How would you convey to Joe that natural childbirth can be a positive experience for him and his wife? How would you assure him that he and Julia can have a safe and active part in the birth of their child?
2. Suppose Julia told you she does not intend to take a preparation for labor class because she wants to have epidural anesthesia as soon as she is admitted to the hospital in labor. Would you advise her to attend a class?
3. Suppose Julia wants to have a Leboyer birth. How would you prepare her birthing room?
4. Examine the National Health Goals related to childbirth education. Most government-sponsored money for nursing research is allotted based on these goals. What would be a possible research topic to explore pertinent to these goals that would be applicable to Julia and her husband and also advance evidence-based practice?

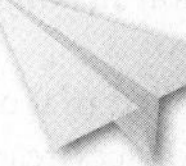

CRITICAL THINKING SCENARIO

Open the accompanying CD-ROM or visit http://thePoint.lww.com and read the Patient Scenario included for this chapter, then answer the questions to further sharpen your skills and grow more familiar with NCLEX style questions related to preparation for childbirth and parenting. Confirm your answers are correct by reading the rationales.

REFERENCES

American Academy of Pediatrics (AAP). (2008). *Breastfeeding and the use of human milk.* Elk Grove Village, IL: Author.

American College of Obstetrics and Gynecology (ACOG). (2007). Breastfeeding: maternal and infant aspects. *ACOG Clinical Review, 12*(1), 1S–16S.

Amis, D., & Green, J. (2007). *Prepared childbirth: the family way.* New York: Lamaze International.

Bradley, R. (1996). *Husband-coached childbirth* (4th ed.). New York: Bantam Books.

Burns, E., et al. (2007). Aromatherapy in childbirth: a pilot randomized controlled trial. *BJOG: An International Journal of Obstetrics & Gynaecology, 114*(7), 838–844.

Coalition for Improving Maternity Services. (1996). *The mother-friendly childbirth initiative.* Ponte Vedra Beach, FL: CIMS.

Cooper, T., & Clarke, P. (2008). Freebirthing. Birthing alone: a concern for midwives? *Midwives, 11*(4), 34–35.

Dick-Read, G. (1987). *Childbirth without fear: the original approach to natural childbirth* (5th ed.). New York: HarperCollins.

Farnsworth, A., & Pearson, P. H. (2007). Choosing mode of delivery after previous caesarean birth. *British Journal of Midwifery, 15*(4), 188–194.

Greene, M. J. (2007). Strategies for incorporating cultural competence into childbirth education curriculum. *Journal of Perinatal Education, 16*(2), 33–37.

Hay-Smith, E. J. C., & Dumoulin, C. (2009). Pelvic floor muscle training versus no treatment, or inactive control treatments, for urinary incontinence in women. *Cochrane Database of Systematic Reviews, 2009*(1), (CD005654).

Hodnett, E. D., et al. (2009). Home-like versus conventional institutional settings for birth. *Cochrane Database of Systematic Reviews, 2009*(1), (CD000012).

Horey, D., Weaver, J., & Russell, H. (2009). Information for pregnant women about caesarean birth. *Cochrane Database of Systematic Reviews, 2009*(1), (CD003858).

Hotelling, B. A. (2007).The coalition for improving maternity services: evidence basis for the ten steps of mother-friendly care. *Journal of Perinatal Education, 16*(2), 38–43.

Kitzinger, S. (1990). *The experience of childbirth.* New York: Viking Penguin.

Laursen, M., et al. (2008). Fear of childbirth: predictors and temporal changes among nulliparous women in the Danish National Birth Cohort. *BJOG: An International Journal of Obstetrics & Gynaecology, 115*(3), 354–360.

Lauzon, L., & Hodnett, E. D. (2009). Antenatal education for self-diagnosis of the onset of active labour at term. *Cochrane Database of Systematic Reviews, 2009*(1), (CD000935).

Leboyer, F. (1975). *Birth without violence.* New York: Alfred A. Knopf.

Lu, M. C. (2007). Recommendations for preconception care. *American Family Physician, 76*(3), 397–400.

Maude, R. M., & Foureur, M. J. (2007). It's beyond water: stories of women's experience of using water for labour and birth. *Women and Birth, 20*(1), 17–24.

McCourt, C., et al. (2007). Elective cesarean section and decision making: a critical review of the literature. *Birth, 34*(1), 65–79.

McGrath, S. K., & Kennell, J. H. (2008). A randomized controlled trial of continuous labor support for middle-class couples: effect on cesarean delivery rates. *Birth, 35*(2), 92–97.

Olsen, O., & Jewell, M. D. (2009). Home versus hospital birth. *Cochrane Database of Systematic Reviews, 2009*(1), (CD000352).

Pitiphat, W., et al. (2008). Maternal periodontitis and adverse pregnancy outcomes. *Community Dentistry & Oral Epidemiology, 36*(1), 3–11.

Simkin, P. (2007). Birth plans: after 25 years, women still want to be heard. *Birth, 34*(1), 49–51.

Smeltzer, S. C. (2007). Pregnancy in women with physical disabilities. *JOGNN: Journal of Obstetric, Gynecologic, and Neonatal Nursing, 36*(1), 88–96.

Smith, C., et al. (2007). A randomized comparative trial of yoga and relaxation to reduce stress and anxiety. *Complementary Therapies in Medicine, 15*(2), 77–83.

Smith, C. A., et al. (2009). Complementary and alternative therapies for pain management in labour. *Cochrane Database of Systematic Reviews, 2009*(1), (CD003521).

Stein, H. (2007). Patient-centered imagery in obstetrics. *International Journal of Childbirth Education, 22*(3), 13–15.

Vedam, S., Goff, M., & Marnin, V. N. (2007). Closing the theory-practice gap: intrapartum midwifery management of planned homebirths. *Journal of Midwifery & Women's Health, 52*(3), 291–312.

SUGGESTED READINGS

Allen, L., & Fountain, L. (2007). Addressing sexuality and pregnancy in childbirth education classes. *Journal of Perinatal Education, 16*(1), 32–36.

Cluett, E. R., et al. (2009). Immersion in water in pregnancy, labour and birth. *Cochrane Database of Systematic Reviews, 2009*(1), (CD000111).

DeVito, J. (2007). Self-perceptions of parenting among adolescent mothers. *Journal of Perinatal Education, 16*(1), 16–23.

Friedewald, M. (2007). Facilitating discussion among expectant fathers: is anyone interested? *Journal of Perinatal Education, 16*(2), 16–20.

Gagnon, A. J., & Sandall, J. (2009). Individual or group antenatal education for childbirth/parenthood. *Cochrane Database of Systematic Reviews, 2009*(1), (CD002869).

Kaufman, T. (2007). Evolution of the birth plan. *Journal of Perinatal Education, 16*(3), 47–52.

Lothian, J. A. (2007). Selling normal birth: six ways to make birth easier. *Journal of Perinatal Education, 16*(3), 44–46.

Nichols, M. R., Roux, G. M., & Harris, N. R. (2007). Primigravid and multigravid women: prenatal perspectives. *Journal of Perinatal Education, 16*(2), 21–32.

Polomeno, V. (2007). Relationship or content? Which is more important in perinatal education? *International Journal of Childbirth Education, 22*(1), 4–11.

Stark, M. A., & Jones, M. (2006). Advanced preparation and positive labor support create an optimal experience for normal birth. *Journal of Perinatal Education, 15*(2), 4–7.

Chapter 15

Nursing Care of a Family During Labor and Birth

KEY TERMS

- attitude
- breech presentation
- cardinal movements of labor
- cephalic presentation
- crowning
- dilatation
- effacement
- engagement
- episiotomy
- fetal descent
- Leopold's maneuvers
- lie
- molding
- pathologic retraction ring
- physiologic retraction ring
- position
- ripening of the cervix
- station
- transition

OBJECTIVES

After mastering the contents of this chapter, you should be able to:

1. Describe common theories explaining the onset of labor and the role of passenger, passage, and powers in labor.
2. Identify National Health Goals related to safe labor and birth that nurses can help the nation achieve.
3. Use critical thinking to analyze ways that nurses can make labor and birth more family centered.
4. Assess a family in labor, identifying the woman's readiness, stage, and progression.
5. Formulate nursing diagnoses related to the physiologic and psychological aspects of labor and birth.
6. Establish expected outcomes to meet the needs of a family throughout the labor process.
7. Plan nursing interventions to meet the needs and promote optimal outcomes for a woman and her family during labor and birth.
8. Implement nursing care for a family during labor such as teaching about the stages of labor.
9. Evaluate expected outcomes for achievement and effectiveness of care.
10. Identify areas related to labor and birth that could benefit from additional nursing research or application of evidence-based practice.
11. Integrate knowledge of nursing care in labor with nursing process to achieve quality maternal and child health nursing care.

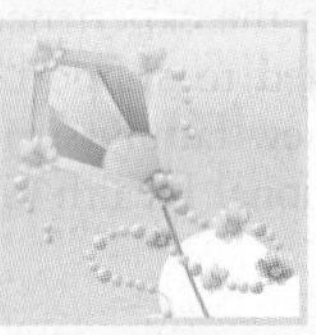

Celeste Bailey is a 26-year-old woman you admit to a birthing room. She has been having labor contractions 45 seconds long and 3 minutes apart for the last 6 hours. She tells you she wants to have her baby "naturally" without any analgesia or anesthesia. Her husband is in the Army and assigned overseas, so he is not with her. Although her sister lives only two blocks from the hospital, Celeste does not want her called. She asks if she can talk to her mother on the telephone instead. As you finish assessing contractions, she screams with pain and shouts, "I'm doing everything I'm supposed to do! How much longer does this go on?"

Previous chapters described the anatomic and physiologic changes that occur in pregnancy as well as effective steps women can take to prepare for labor. This chapter adds information about the actual labor process and how to offer effective support and education to a woman in labor. Without adequate support, labor can be a frightening rather than an enjoyable event.

What additional teaching does Celeste need about labor and birth?

Labor is the series of events by which uterine contractions and abdominal pressure expel a fetus and placenta from a woman's body. Regular contractions cause progressive dilatation (enlargement or widening of the cervical canal) and create sufficient muscular force to allow a baby to be pushed from the birth canal (or vagina). It is a time of change, both an ending and a beginning, for a woman, a fetus, and her family.

Labor and birth require a woman to use all the psychological and physical coping methods she has available. Regardless of the amount of childbirth preparation or the number of times she has been through the experience before, family-focused nursing care is needed to support the family as they mark the beginning of a new family structure. This need is further emphasized by National Health Goals (Box 15.1).

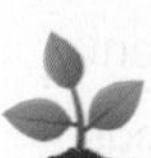

Nursing Process Overview

For a Woman in Labor

Assessment

Assessment of a woman in labor must be done quickly yet thoroughly and gently. A woman is keenly aware of words spoken around her and the manner with which procedures are carried out. Because of this sensitivity, she may have difficulty relaxing for a vaginal examination if she fears that pressure on the fetal head will cause her pain. Remember that pain is a subjective symptom. Only the woman can evaluate how much she is experiencing or how much she wants to endure.

Assess how much discomfort a woman in labor is having, not only by what she scores on a pain scale but also by subtle signs of pain such as facial tenseness, flushing or paleness of the face, hands clenched in a fist, rapid breathing, or rapid pulse rate. Knowing the extent of a woman's discomfort helps guide the choice of comfort interventions she may need.

Nursing Diagnosis

Common nursing diagnoses pertinent to labor include:

- Pain related to labor contractions
- Anxiety related to process of labor and birth
- Health-seeking behaviors related to management of discomfort of labor
- Situational low self-esteem related to inability to use prepared childbirth method

Although the discomfort of labor is commonly referred to as "contractions" rather than "pain," do not omit the word "pain" from a nursing diagnosis, because the term strengthens an understanding of the problem.

Outcome Identification and Planning

When establishing expected outcomes for a woman in labor and her partner, be certain they are realistic. Because labor usually takes place over a relatively short timeframe (average, 12 hours), outcomes must be met within this period. On the other hand, it is important not to project a definite time limit for labor to be completed, because the length of labor can vary from woman to woman and still be within normal limits. It is necessary also to appreciate the magnitude of labor. It is unlikely that all the fear or anxiety experienced during a woman's labor can be alleviated. Often, because it is such an unusual and significant experience, an average couple may need assistance with using additional coping measures.

Be certain to incorporate both the woman and her support person in planning, so that the experience is a shared one. Planning may include review and education about the normal labor process. Although a couple may have learned this information during pregnancy, the reality of labor may seem much different from what they imagined. Planning also must be flexible, changing with the progress of labor, and individualized, allowing a woman to experience the significance of the event for herself. Good web sites to use for referral are The National Women's Health Information Center (http://www.womenshealth.gov) and The American Pregnancy Association (http://www.americanpregnancy.org).

Comfort promotion is a vital part of care. A plan that addresses the discomforts of labor includes planning for education, validation, and response to a woman's pain to help her maintain realistic perceptions about it. Be certain to include nonpharmacologic comfort measures such as changing a wet sheet or offering a moisturizing cream for dry lips.

Implementation

Interventions in labor must always be carried out between contractions if possible, so that a woman is free to use a

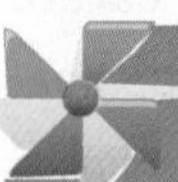

BOX 15.1 * Focus on National Health Goals

Because labor and birth are high-risk times for both a fetus and a mother, several National Health Goals speak directly to them:

- Reduce the rate of maternal deaths to no more than 3.3 per 100,000 live births, from a baseline of 7.1 per 100,000.
- Reduce the rate of fetal deaths at 20 or more weeks' gestation to no more than 4.1 per 1000 live births, from a baseline of 6.8 per 1000.
- Reduce the rate of fetal and infant deaths during the perinatal period (28 weeks' gestation to 7 days after birth) to no more than 4.5 per 1000 live births, from a baseline of 7.5 per 1000 live births (http://www.nih.gov).

Nurses can help the nation achieve these goals by closely monitoring women during labor and birth and by teaching women as much as possible about labor, so that they are able to use as little analgesia and anesthesia as possible. The less anesthesia and analgesia used, the fewer are the complications that can result in fetal or maternal death.

Topics that could benefit from additional nursing research in this area are what women feel are advantages and disadvantages of various birthing settings, the best way to teach unprepared women a breathing pattern in labor, how support people can best be prepared for their role, and advantages and disadvantages of various birthing or labor positions.

prepared childbirth technique to limit the discomfort of contractions. This calls for good coordination of care among health care providers and planning with the woman and her support person. The person a woman chooses to stay with her during childbirth can be a husband, the father of the child, a sister or parent, or a close friend. Which of these persons a woman chooses is somewhat culturally determined.

It is important for women to be able to understand what is happening to them during labor. If the woman is not proficient in English, make arrangements to locate an interpreter. If she is hearing challenged, it is the hospital's responsibility to provide an interpreter for her so that she can receive adequate explanations of her progress. Remember that whether a woman enjoys being touched or not during labor is in part culturally determined. Assess early in a woman's labor whether she might benefit from such caring measures as having her hand held or her back rubbed.

Outcome Evaluation

During labor, evaluation must be ongoing to preserve the safety of a woman and her new child. After birth, evaluation helps to determine a woman's opinion of her experience with labor and birth. Ideally, the experience should be not only one that she was able to endure but one that allowed her self-esteem to grow and the family to grow through a shared experience. It is advantageous to talk to women in the early postpartum period about their labor experience. Doing so serves as a means of evaluating nursing care during labor. It also provides a woman the chance to "work through" this experience and incorporate it into her self-image. Examples of possible outcome criteria include:

- Client states that pain during labor was tolerable because of her advance preparation.
- Client verbalizes that her need for additional comfort measures was met.
- Client and family members state that the labor and birth experience was a positive growth experience for them, both individually and as a family.

THEORIES OF LABOR ONSET

Labor normally begins when a fetus is sufficiently mature to cope with extrauterine life yet not too large to cause mechanical difficulty with birth. Although in animals it has been shown that progesterone withdrawal is the trigger that simulates labor, the association that converts the random, painless Braxton Hicks contractions of pregnancy into strong, coordinated, productive labor contractions in women is still largely undocumented (Crombleholme, 2009). In some instances, labor begins before a fetus is mature (preterm birth). In others, labor is delayed until the fetus and the placenta have both passed beyond the optimal point for birth (postterm birth).

Several theories including a combination of factors originating from both the woman and fetus have been proposed to explain why progesterone withdrawal begins:

- Uterine muscle stretching, which results in release of prostaglandins
- Pressure on the cervix, which stimulates the release of oxytocin from the posterior pituitary
- Oxytocin stimulation, which works together with prostaglandins to initiate contractions
- Change in the ratio of estrogen to progesterone (increasing estrogen in relation to progesterone, which is interpreted as progesterone withdrawal)
- Placental age, which triggers contractions at a set point
- Rising fetal cortisol levels, which reduces progesterone formation and increases prostaglandin formation
- Fetal membrane production of prostaglandin, which stimulates contractions

SIGNS OF LABOR

A common concern of women as they near the end of pregnancy is how they will know if they are beginning labor.

Preliminary Signs of Labor

Before labor, a woman often experiences subtle signs that signal labor is imminent. It is important to review these with women during the last trimester of pregnancy so they can more easily recognize beginning signs.

Lightening

In primiparas, *lightening*, or descent of the fetal presenting part into the pelvis, occurs approximately 10 to 14 days before labor begins. This **fetal descent** changes a woman's abdominal contour, because it positions the uterus lower and more anterior in the abdomen. Lightening gives a woman relief from the diaphragmatic pressure and shortness of breath that she has been experiencing and in this way "lightens" her load. Lightening probably occurs early in primiparas because of tight abdominal muscles. In multiparas, it is not as dramatic and usually occurs on the day of labor or even after labor has begun. As the fetus sinks lower into the pelvis, a woman may experience shooting leg pains from the increased pressure on her sciatic nerve, increased amounts of vaginal discharge, and urinary frequency from pressure on her bladder.

Increase in Level of Activity

A woman may awaken on the morning of labor full of energy, in contrast to the feeling of chronic fatigue she felt during the previous month. This increase in activity is related to an increase in epinephrine release initiated by a decrease in progesterone produced by the placenta. This additional epinephrine prepares a woman's body for the work of labor ahead.

Slight Loss of Weight

As progesterone level falls, body fluid is more easily excreted from the body. This increase in urine production can lead to a weight loss between 1 and 3 pounds.

Braxton Hicks Contractions

In the last week or days before labor begins, a woman usually notices extremely strong Braxton Hicks contractions. Women having their first child may have great difficulty distinguishing between these and true contractions. A woman may come

TABLE 15.1 ✻ Differentiation Between True and False Labor Contractions

False Contractions	True Contractions
Begin and remain irregular.	Begin irregularly but become regular and predictable.
Felt first abdominally and remain confined to the abdomen and groin.	Felt first in lower back and sweep around to the abdomen in a wave.
Often disappear with ambulation or sleep.	Continue no matter what the woman's level of activity.
Do not increase in duration, frequency, or intensity.	Increase in duration, frequency, and intensity.
Do not achieve cervical dilatation.	Achieve cervical dilatation.

to the labor unit of a hospital or birthing center because false contractions so closely simulate true labor. It is discouraging for a woman who is having what seem like contractions (and strong Braxton Hicks contractions cause true discomfort) to be told she is not in true labor and should return home. When this happens, you can assure a woman that misinterpreting labor signals is common. Remind her that if false contractions have become strong enough to be mistaken for true labor, true labor is not far away. Table 15.1 summarizes the ways in which false contractions can be differentiated from true labor.

Ripening of the Cervix

Ripening of the cervix is an internal sign seen only on pelvic examination. Throughout pregnancy, the cervix feels softer than normal to palpation, similar to the consistency of an earlobe (Goodell's sign). At term, the cervix becomes still softer (described as "butter-soft"), and it tips forward. Cervical ripening this way is an internal announcement that labor is very close at hand.

Signs of True Labor

Signs of true labor involve uterine and cervical changes. The more a woman knows about these labor signs, the better she will be able to recognize them. This is helpful both to prevent preterm birth and for the woman to feel secure knowing what will happen during labor.

Uterine Contractions

The surest sign that labor has begun is productive uterine contractions. Because contractions are involuntary and come without warning, their intensity can be frightening in early labor. Helping a woman appreciate that she can predict when her next one will occur and therefore can control the degree of discomfort she feels by using breathing exercises offers her a sense of well-being.

Show

As the cervix softens and ripens, the mucus plug that filled the cervical canal during pregnancy (operculum) is expelled. The exposed cervical capillaries seep blood as a result of pressure exerted by the fetus. This blood, mixed with mucus, takes on a pink tinge and is referred to as "show" or "bloody show." Women need to be aware of this event so that they do not think they are bleeding abnormally.

Rupture of the Membranes

Labor may begin with rupture of the membranes, experienced either as a sudden gush or as scanty, slow seeping of clear fluid from the vagina. Some women may worry if their labor begins with rupture of the membranes, because they have heard that labor will then be "dry" and that this will cause it to be difficult and long. Actually, amniotic fluid continues to be produced until delivery of the membranes after the birth of a fetus, so no labor is ever "dry." Early rupture of the membranes can be advantageous as it can cause the fetal head to settle snugly into the pelvis, actually shortening labor.

Two risks associated with ruptured membranes are intrauterine infection and prolapse of the umbilical cord, which could cut off the oxygen supply to the fetus (Lewis et al., 2007). In most instances, if labor has not spontaneously occurred by 24 hours after membrane rupture and the pregnancy is at term, labor will be induced to help reduce these risks.

✔ Checkpoint Question 15.1

Celeste Bailey did not recognize for over an hour that she was in labor. A sign of true labor is:

a. Sudden increased energy from epinephrine release.
b. "Nagging" but constant pain in the lower back.
c. Urinary urgency from increased bladder pressure.
d. "Show" or release of the cervical mucus plug.

COMPONENTS OF LABOR

A successful labor depends on four integrated concepts:

1. A woman's pelvis (the *passage*) is of adequate size and contour.
2. The *passenger* (the fetus) is of appropriate size and in an advantageous position and presentation.
3. The *powers* of labor (uterine factors) are adequate. (The powers of labor are strongly influenced by the woman's position during labor.)
4. A woman's *psychological outlook* is preserved, so that afterward labor can be viewed as a positive experience.

Passage

The passage refers to the route a fetus must travel from the uterus through the cervix and vagina to the external perineum. Because the cervix and vagina are contained inside the pelvis, a fetus must also pass through the bony pelvic ring. (Pelvic anatomy is discussed in Chapter 11; see Figs. 11.4 and 11.5.) Two pelvic measurements are important to determine

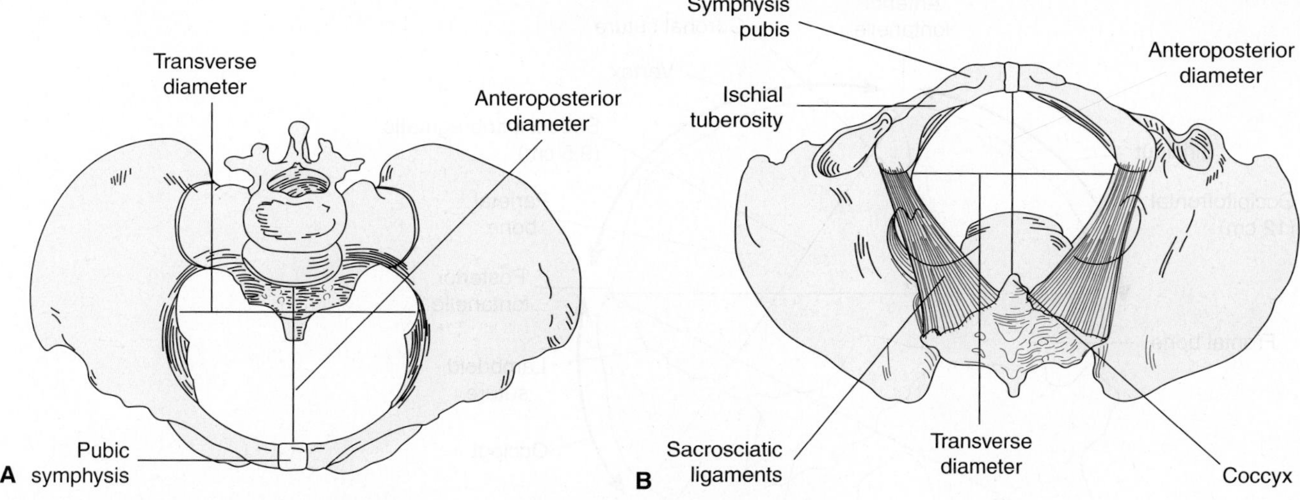

FIGURE 15.1 Views of the pelvic inlet and outlet. (**A**) Pelvic inlet. (**B**) Pelvic outlet.

the adequacy of the pelvic size: the diagonal conjugate (the anteroposterior diameter of the inlet) and the transverse diameter of the outlet. At the pelvic inlet, the anteroposterior diameter is the narrowest diameter; at the outlet, the transverse diameter is the narrowest (Fig. 15.1).

In most instances, if a disproportion between fetus and pelvis occurs, the pelvis is the structure at fault. If the fetus is the cause of the disproportion, it is often because the fetal head is presented to the birth canal at less than its narrowest diameter, not because the fetal head is actually too large. Keep this in mind when discussing with parents why an infant cannot be born vaginally. In this situation, emphasize that it is the pelvis that is too small, not that the head is too big. When parents learn that a child cannot be born vaginally because the mother's pelvis is too small, it can be upsetting. It can be much more upsetting, however, to think that their infant's head is too large, because it implies that something may be seriously wrong with their baby (which usually is not true). Avoiding this type of negative thought helps promote good parent–child bonding.

Passenger

The passenger is the fetus. The body part of the fetus that has the widest diameter is the head, so this is the part least likely to be able to pass through the pelvic ring. Whether a fetal skull can pass depends on both its structure (bones, fontanelles, and suture lines) and its alignment with the pelvis.

Structure of the Fetal Skull

The cranium, the uppermost portion of the skull, is composed of eight bones. The four superior bones—the frontal (actually two fused bones), the two parietal, and the occipital—are the bones that are important in childbirth. The other four bones of the skull (sphenoid, ethmoid, and two temporal bones) lie at the base of the cranium so are of little significance in childbirth because they are never presenting parts. The chin, referred to by its Latin name *mentum,* can be a presenting part.

The bones of the skull meet at suture lines. The sagittal suture joins the two parietal bones of the skull. The coronal suture is the line of juncture of the frontal bones and the two parietal bones. The lambdoid suture is the line of juncture of the occipital bone and the two parietal bones. The suture lines are important in birth because, as membranous interspaces, they allow the cranial bones to move and overlap, molding or diminishing the size of the skull so that it can pass through the birth canal more readily.

Significant membrane-covered spaces called the fontanelles are found at the junction of the main suture lines. The anterior fontanelle (sometimes referred to as the bregma) lies at the junction of the coronal and sagittal sutures. Because the frontal bone consists of two fused bones, four bones (counting the two parietal bones) are actually involved at this junction so the anterior fontanelle is diamond shaped. Its anteroposterior diameter measures approximately 3 to 4 cm; its transverse diameter, 2 to 3 cm. It closes when the infant is 12 to 18 months of age.

The posterior fontanelle lies at the junction of the lambdoidal and sagittal sutures. Because three bones—the two parietal bones and the occipital bone—are involved at this junction, the posterior fontanelle is triangular shaped. It is smaller than the anterior fontanelle, measuring approximately 2 cm across its widest part. Because of its small size, it closes when an infant is about 2 months of age.

Fontanelle spaces compress during birth to aid in molding of the fetal head. Their presence can be assessed manually through the cervix after the cervix has dilated during labor. Palpating for them during a pelvic examination helps to establish the position of the fetal head and whether it is in a favorable position for birth. The space between the two fontanelles is referred to as the vertex. The area over the frontal bone is referred to as the sinciput. The area over the occipital bone is referred to as the occiput (Fig. 15.2).

Diameters of the Fetal Skull

The shape of a fetal skull causes it to be wider in its anteroposterior diameter than in its transverse diameter. To best fit through the birth canal, a fetus must present the smaller

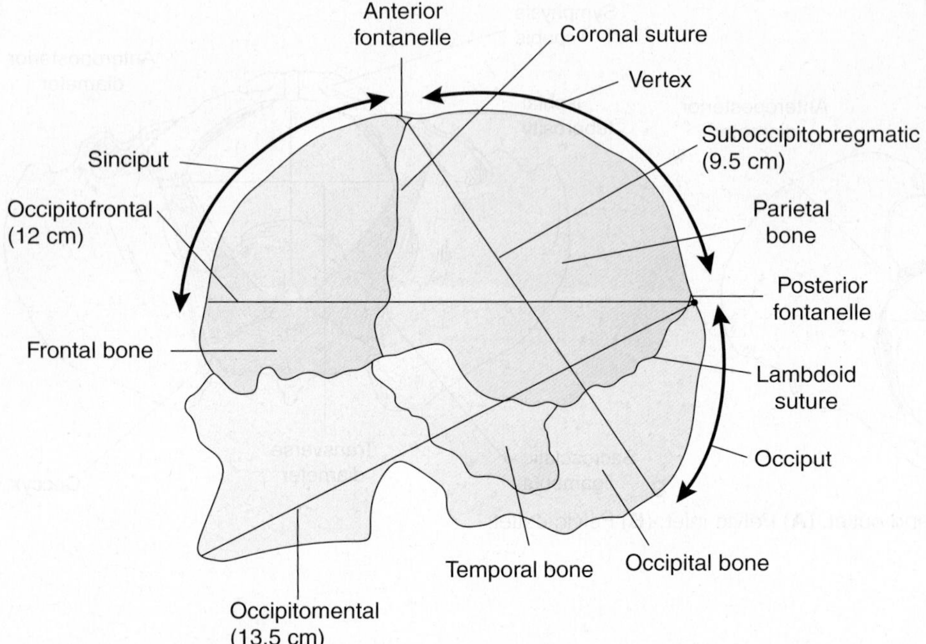

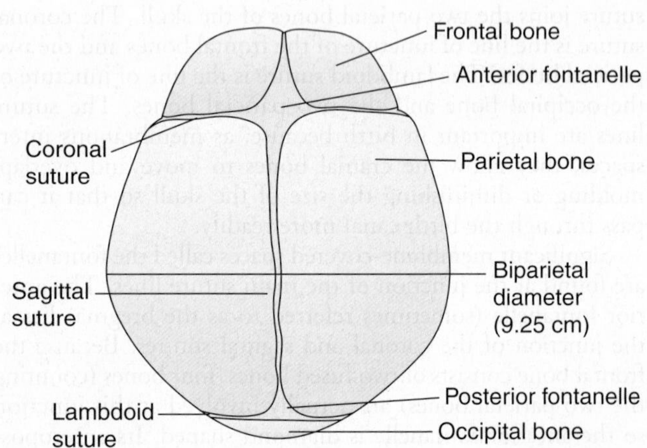

FIGURE 15.2 The fetal skull. (**A**) Lateral view. (**B**) Vertex view.

diameter (the transverse diameter) to the smaller diameter of the maternal pelvis; otherwise, progress can be halted and birth may not be accomplished.

The diameter of the anteroposterior fetal skull depends on where the measurement is taken. The narrowest diameter (approximately 9.5 cm) is from the inferior aspect of the occiput to the center of the anterior fontanelle (the suboccipitobregmatic diameter). The occipitofrontal diameter, measured from the occipital prominence to the bridge of the nose, is approximately 12 cm. The occipitomental diameter, which is the widest anteroposterior diameter (approximately 13.5 cm), is measured from the posterior fontanelle to the chin.

The anteroposterior diameter of the pelvis, a space approximately 11 cm wide, is the narrowest diameter at the pelvic inlet so to be born most easily, a fetus must present a biparietal diameter, the narrowest fetal head diameter (approximately 9.25 cm) to this (see Fig. 15.2A). At the outlet, the fetus must rotate to present the narrowest fetal head diameter to the maternal transverse diameter, a space approximately 11 cm wide. If a fetus presents the anteroposterior diameter of the skull (a measurement wider than the biparietal diameter) to the anteroposterior diameter of the inlet, **engagement,** or the settling of the fetal head into the pelvis, may not occur. If the fetus does not rotate so the anteroposterior diameter of the skull is presented to the transverse diameter of the outlet, arrest of progress may occur.

Which anteroposterior diameter that presents to the birth canal is determined not only by rotation but by the degree of flexion of the fetal head (Fig. 15.3). In full flexion, a fetal head flexes so sharply the chin rests on the chest, and the smallest anteroposterior diameter, the suboccipitobregmatic, is presented to the birth canal. If the head is held in moderate flexion, the occipitofrontal diameter will be presented. In poor flexion (the head hyperextended), the largest diameter (the occipitomental) will present. It follows

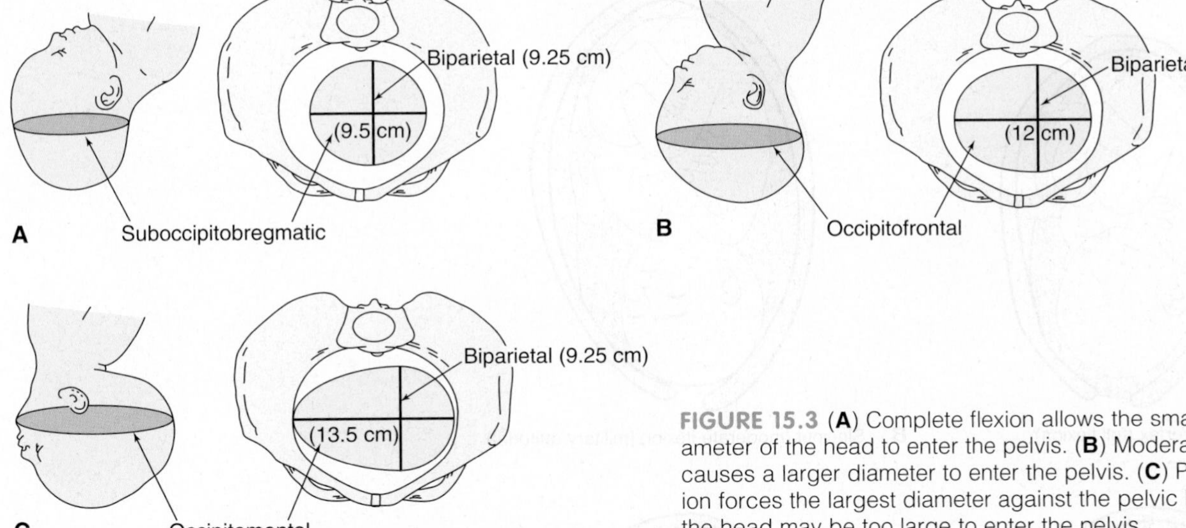

FIGURE 15.3 (**A**) Complete flexion allows the smallest diameter of the head to enter the pelvis. (**B**) Moderate flexion causes a larger diameter to enter the pelvis. (**C**) Poor flexion forces the largest diameter against the pelvic brim, so the head may be too large to enter the pelvis.

that a fetal head presenting a diameter of 9.5 cm will fit through a pelvis much more readily than if the diameter is 12.0 or 13.5 cm.

Molding

Molding is a change in the shape of the fetal skull produced by the force of uterine contractions pressing the vertex of the head against the not-yet-dilated cervix. Because the bones of the fetal skull are not yet completely ossified and therefore do not form a rigid structure, pressure causes them to overlap and molds the head into a narrower and longer shape, a shape that facilitates passage through the rigid pelvis. Molding is commonly seen in infants just after birth. The overlapping of the sagittal suture line and, generally, the coronal suture line can be easily palpated in the newborn skull. Parents can be reassured that molding only lasts a day or two and is not a permanent condition. There is little molding when the brow is the presenting part (described later), because frontal bones are fused. No skull molding occurs when a fetus is breech, because the buttocks, not the head, are presented first.

Fetal Presentation and Position

Two other factors play a part in whether a fetus is lined up in the best position to be born: fetal presentation and position.

Attitude. **Attitude** describes the degree of flexion a fetus assumes during labor or the relation of the fetal parts to each other (Fig. 15.4). A fetus in *good* attitude is in complete flexion: the spinal column is bowed forward, the head is flexed forward so much that the chin touches the sternum, the arms are flexed and folded on the chest, the thighs are flexed onto the abdomen, and the calves are pressed against the posterior aspect of the thighs (see Fig. 15.4A). This normal "fetal position" is advantageous for birth because it helps a fetus present the smallest anteroposterior diameter of the skull to the pelvis and also because it puts the whole body into an ovoid shape, occupying the smallest space possible.

A fetus is in moderate flexion if the chin is not touching the chest but is in an alert or "military position" (see Fig. 15.4B). This position causes the next-widest anteroposterior diameter, the occipital frontal diameter, to present to the birth canal. A fair number of fetuses assume a military position during the early part of labor. This does not usually interfere with labor, because later mechanisms of labor (descent and flexion) force the fetal head to fully flex.

A fetus in partial extension presents the "brow" of the head to the birth canal (see Fig. 15.4C). If a fetus is in complete extension, the back is arched, and the neck is extended, presenting the occipitomental diameter of the head to the birth canal (a face presentation; see Fig. 15.4D). This unusual position presents too wide a skull diameter to the birth canal for normal birth. Such a position may occur if there is less than the normal amount of amniotic fluid present (*oligohydramnios*), which does not allow a fetus adequate movement. It also may reflect a neurologic abnormality in the fetus causing spasticity.

Engagement. Engagement refers to the settling of the presenting part of a fetus far enough into the pelvis to be at the level of the ischial spines, a midpoint of the pelvis. Descent to this point means that the widest part of the fetus (the biparietal diameter in a cephalic presentation; the intertrochanteric diameter in a breech presentation) has passed through the pelvis inlet or the pelvic inlet has been proved adequate for birth. In a primipara, nonengagement of the head at the beginning of labor indicates a possible complication, such as an abnormal presentation or position, abnormality of the fetal head, or cephalopelvic disproportion. In multiparas, engagement may or may not be present at the beginning of labor. The degree of engagement is assessed by vaginal and cervical examination. A presenting part that is not engaged is said to be "floating." One that is descending but has not yet reached the ischial spines is said to be "dipping."

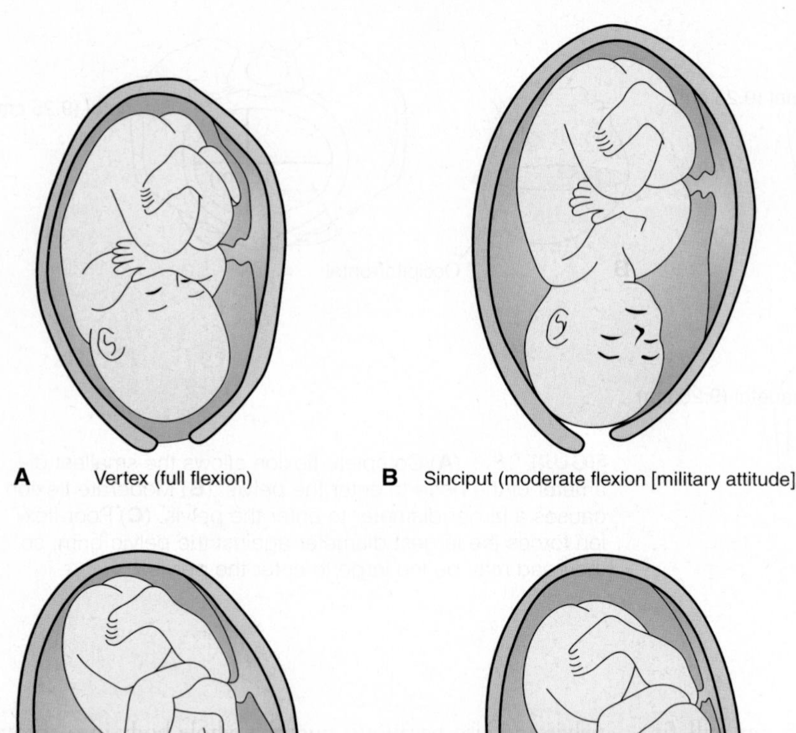

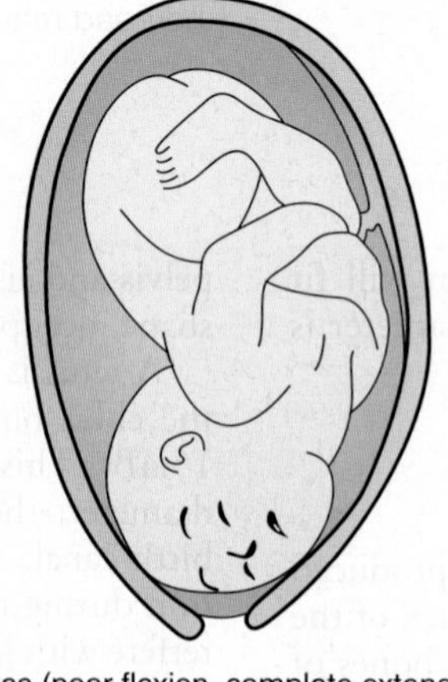

FIGURE 15.4 Fetal attitude. (**A**) Fetus in full flexion presents smallest (suboccipitobregmatic) anteroposterior diameter of skull to inlet in this good attitude (vertex presentation). (**B**) Fetus is not as well flexed (military attitude) as in **A** and presents occipitofrontal diameter to inlet (sinciput presentation). (**C**) Fetus in partial extension (brow presentation). (**D**) Fetus in complete extension presents wide (occipitomental) diameter (face presentation).

Station. **Station** refers to the relationship of the presenting part of a fetus to the level of the ischial spines (Fig. 15.5). When the presenting fetal part is at the level of the ischial spines, it is at a 0 station (synonymous with engagement). If the presenting part is above the spines, the distance is measured and described as minus stations, which range from −1 to −4 cm. If the presenting part is below the ischial spines, the distance is stated as plus stations (+1 to +4 cm). At a +3 or +4 station, the presenting part is at the perineum and can be seen if the vulva is separated (i.e., it is crowning).

FIGURE 15.5 Station (anteroposterior view). Station, or degree of engagement, of the fetal head is designated by centimeters above or below the ischial spines. At −4 station, head is "floating." At 0 station, head is "engaged." At +4 station, head is "at outlet."

Fetal Lie. **Lie** is the relationship between the long (cephalocaudal) axis of the fetal body and the long (cephalocaudal) axis of a woman's body; in other words, whether the fetus is lying in a horizontal (transverse) or a vertical (longitudinal) position. Approximately 99% of fetuses assume a longitudinal lie (with their long axis parallel to the long axis of the woman). Longitudinal lies are further classified as cephalic, which means the head will be the first part to contact the cervix, or breech, with the breech, or buttocks, as the first portion to contact the cervix.

Types of Fetal Presentation

Fetal presentation denotes the body part that will first contact the cervix or be born first. This is determined by a combination of fetal lie and the degree of fetal flexion (attitude).

Cephalic Presentation. A **cephalic presentation** is the most frequent type of presentation, occurring as often as

TABLE 15.2 ✻ Types of Cephalic Presentation

Type	Lie	Attitude	Description
Vertex	Longitudinal	Good (full flexion)	The head is sharply flexed, making the parietal bones or the space between the fontanelles (the vertex) the presenting part. This is the most common presentation and allows the suboccipitobregmatic diameter to present to the cervix.
Brow	Longitudinal	Moderate (military)	Because the head is only moderately flexed, the brow or sinciput becomes the presenting part.
Face	Longitudinal	Poor	The fetus has extended the head to make the face the presenting part. From this position, extreme edema and distortion of the face may occur. The presenting diameter is so wide that birth may be impossible.
Mentum	Longitudinal	Very poor	The fetus has completely hyperextended the head to present the chin. The widest diameter (occipitomental) is presenting. As a rule, a fetus cannot enter the pelvis in this presentation.

95% of the time. With this type of presentation, the fetal head is the body part that will first contact the cervix. The four types of cephalic presentation (vertex, brow, face, and mentum) are described in Table 15.2. The vertex is the ideal presenting part, because the skull bones are capable of effectively molding to accommodate the cervix. This may actually aid in cervical dilatation and prevents complications such as a prolapsed cord (i.e., a portion of the cord passing between the presenting part and the cervix and entering the vagina before the fetus) (Kish & Collea, 2007). During labor, the area of the fetal skull that contacts the cervix often becomes edematous from the continued pressure against it. This edema is called a *caput succedaneum*. In the newborn, the point of presentation can be analyzed from the location of the caput.

Breech Presentation. A **breech presentation** means that either the buttocks or the feet are the first body parts that will contact the cervix. Breech presentations occur in approximately 3% of births and are affected by fetal attitude. A good attitude brings the fetal knees up against the fetal abdomen; a poor attitude means that the knees are extended. Breech presentations can be difficult births, with the presenting point influencing the degree of difficulty. Three types of breech presentation (complete, frank, and footling) are possible (Table 15.3).

Shoulder Presentation. In a transverse lie, a fetus lies horizontally in the pelvis so that the longest fetal axis is perpendicular to that of the mother. The presenting part is usually one of the shoulders (acromion process), an iliac crest, a hand, or an elbow (Fig. 15.6).

Fewer than 1% of fetuses lie transversely. This presentation may be caused by relaxed abdominal walls from grand multiparity, which allow the unsupported uterus to fall forward. Another cause is pelvic contraction, in which the horizontal space is greater than the vertical space. Placenta previa (in which the placenta is located low in the uterus, obscuring some of the vertical space) may also limit a fetus's ability to turn, resulting in a transverse lie. With a transverse lie, the usual contour of the abdomen at term is distorted or is fuller side to side rather than top to bottom.

If an infant is preterm and smaller than usual, an attempt to turn the fetus to a horizontal lie may be made. Most infants in a transverse lie must be born by cesarean birth, however, because they cannot be turned and cannot be born vaginally from this "wedged" position. Discovering a shoulder presentation is an important assessment, because it almost always identifies a birth position that puts both mother and child in jeopardy unless skilled health care personnel are available to complete a cesarean birth.

Types of Fetal Position

Position is the relationship of the presenting part to a specific quadrant of a woman's pelvis. For convenience, the maternal pelvis is divided into four quadrants according to the mother's right and left: (a) right anterior, (b) left anterior, (c) right posterior, and (d) left posterior.

Four parts of a fetus have been chosen as landmarks to describe the relationship of the presenting part to one of the pelvic quadrants. In a vertex presentation, the occiput is the chosen point; in a face presentation, it is the chin (mentum); in a breech presentation, it is the sacrum; and in a shoulder presentation, it is the scapula or the acromion process.

Position is indicated by an abbreviation of three letters. The middle letter denotes the fetal landmark (O for occiput, M for mentum or chin, Sa for sacrum, and A for acromion process). The first letter defines whether the landmark is pointing to the mother's right (R) or left (L). The last letter defines whether the landmark points anteriorly (A), posteriorly (P), or transversely (T).

If the occiput of a fetus points to the left anterior quadrant in a vertex position, for example, this is a left occipitoanterior (LOA) position. If the occiput points to the right posterior quadrant, the position is right occipitoposterior (ROP). LOA is the most common fetal position, and right occipitoanterior (ROA) the second most frequent. Box 15.2

TABLE 15.3 ✻ Types of Breech Presentation

Type	Lie	Attitude	Description
Complete	Longitudinal	Good (full flexion)	The fetus has thighs tightly flexed on the abdomen; both the buttocks and the tightly flexed feet present to the cervix.
Frank 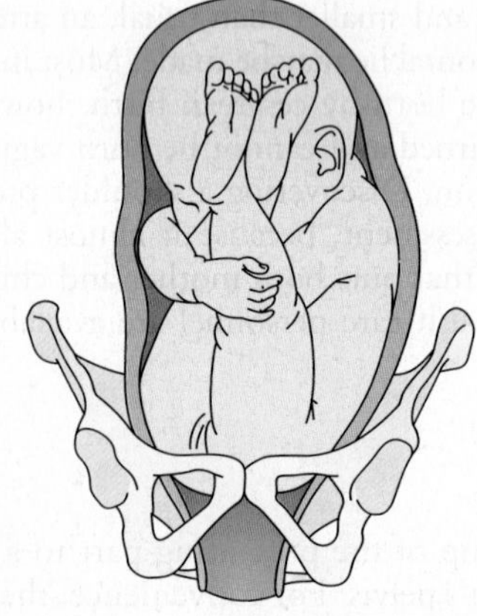	Longitudinal	Moderate	Attitude is moderate because the hips are flexed but the knees are extended to rest on the chest. The buttocks alone present to the cervix.
Footling 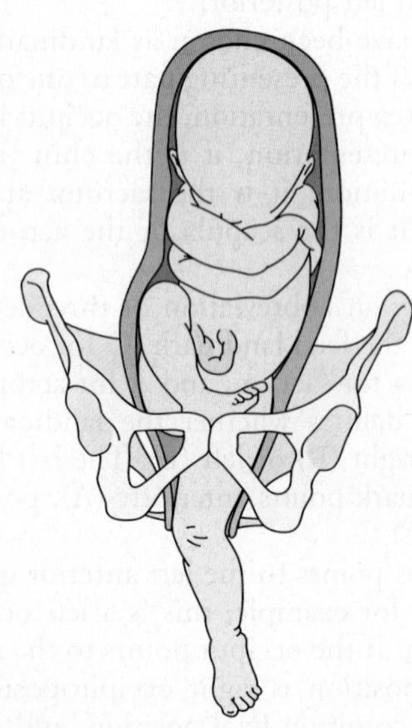	Longitudinal	Poor	Neither the thighs nor lower legs are flexed. If one foot presents, it is a single-footling breech; if both present, it is a double-footling breech.

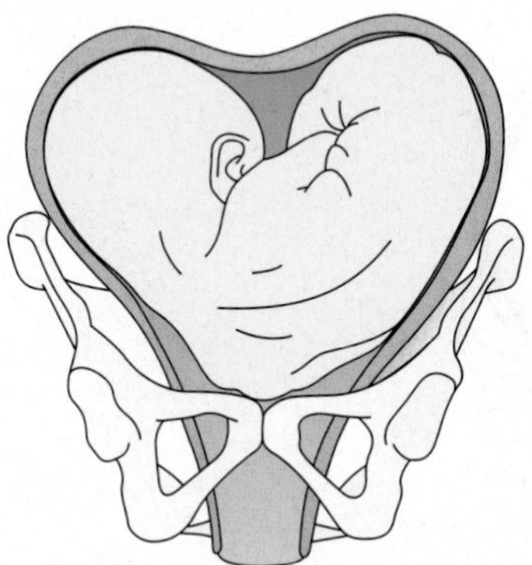

FIGURE 15.6 Transverse or shoulder presentation.

summarizes the possible positions. Six common positions in cephalic presentations are illustrated in Figure 15.7.

Position is important, because it can influence the process and efficiency of labor. Typically, a fetus is born fastest from an ROA or LOA position. Labor is considerably extended if the position is posterior (ROP or LOP). Posterior positions may also be more painful for a woman, because the rotation of the fetal head puts pressure on sacral nerves, causing sharp back pain. Encouraging a woman to rest in a Sims' position on the same side as the fetal spine may encourage rotation from an occipitoposterior to an occipitoanterior position before and during labor (Ridley, 2007).

BOX 15.2 ✻ Possible Fetal Positions

Vertex Presentation (occiput)
LOA, left occipitoanterior
LOP, left occipitoposterior
LOT, left occipitotransverse
ROA, right occipitoanterior
ROP, right occipitoposterior
ROT, right occipitotransverse

Breech Presentation (sacrum)
LSaA, left sacroanterior
LSaP, left sacroposterior
LSaT, left sacrotransverse
RSaA, right sacroanterior
RSaP, right sacroposterior
RSaT, right sacrotransverse

Face Presentation (mentum)
LMA, left mentoanterior
LMP, left mentoposterior
LMT, left mentotransverse
RMA, right mentoanterior
RMP, right mentoposterior
RMT, right mentotransverse

Shoulder Presentation (acromion process)
LAA, left scapuloanterior
LAP, left scapuloposterior
RAA, right scapuloanterior
RAP, right scapuloposterior

✔ Checkpoint Question 15.2

Celeste's obstetrician asks you which fetal position and presentation are ideal. Your best answer would be:

a. Right occipitoanterior with full flexion.
b. Left transverse anterior in moderate flexion.
c. Right occipitoposterior with no flexion.
d. Left sacroanterior with full flexion.

Mechanisms (Cardinal Movements) of Labor

Passage of a fetus through the birth canal involves several different position changes to keep the smallest diameter of the fetal head (in cephalic presentations) always presenting to the smallest diameter of the pelvis. These position changes are termed the **cardinal movements of labor:** descent, flexion, internal rotation, extension, external rotation, and expulsion (Fig. 15.8).

Descent. Descent is the downward movement of the biparietal diameter of the fetal head to within the pelvic inlet. Full descent occurs when the fetal head extrudes beyond the dilated cervix and touches the posterior vaginal floor. Descent occurs because of pressure on the fetus by the uterine fundus. The pressure of the fetal head on the sacral nerves at the pelvic floor causes the mother to experience a pushing sensation. Full descent may be aided by abdominal muscle contraction as the woman pushes.

Flexion. As descent occurs and the fetal head reaches the pelvic floor, the head bends forward onto the chest, making the smallest anteroposterior diameter (the suboccipitobregmatic diameter) present to the birth canal. Flexion is also aided by abdominal muscle contraction during pushing.

Internal Rotation. During descent, the head enters the pelvis with the fetal anteroposterior head diameter (suboccipitobregmatic, occipitomental, or occipitofrontal, depending on the amount of flexion) in a diagonal or transverse position. The head flexes as it touches the pelvic floor, and the occiput rotates to bring the head into the best relationship to the outlet of the pelvis (the anteroposterior diameter is now in the anteroposterior plane of the pelvis). This movement brings the shoulders, coming next, into the optimal position to enter the inlet, putting the widest diameter of the shoulders (a transverse one) in line with the wide transverse diameter of the inlet.

Extension. As the occiput is born, the back of the neck stops beneath the pubic arch and acts as a pivot for the rest of the head. The head extends, and the foremost parts of the head, the face and chin, are born.

External Rotation. In external rotation, almost immediately after the head of the infant is born, the head rotates (from the anteroposterior position it assumed to enter the outlet) back to the diagonal or transverse position of the early part of labor. This brings the aftercoming shoulders into an anteroposterior position, which is best for entering the outlet. The

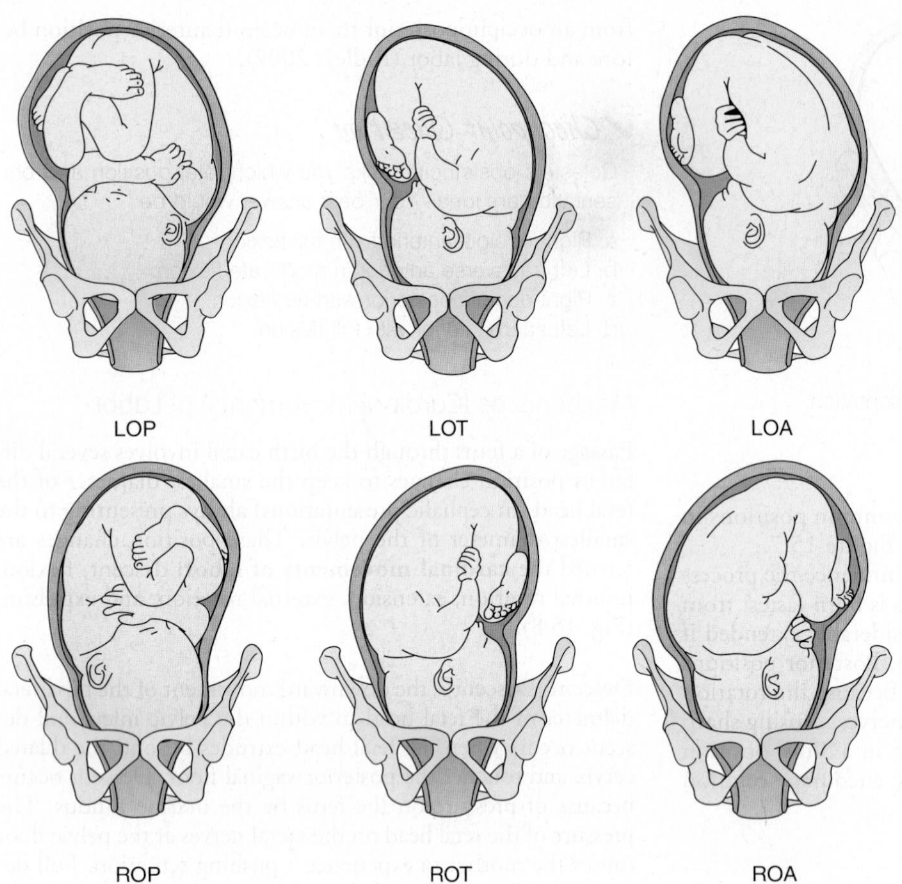

FIGURE 15.7 Fetal position. All are vertex presentations. A = anterior; L = left; O = occiput; P = posterior; R = right; T = transverse.

anterior shoulder is born first, assisted perhaps by downward flexion of the infant's head.

Expulsion. Once the shoulders are born, the rest of the baby is born easily and smoothly because of its smaller size. This movement, called expulsion, is the end of the pelvic division of labor. For a view of the complete birth sequence, see Figure 15.9.

Importance of Determining Fetal Presentation and Position

It is important to document fetal presentation and position, because these help predict if the presentation of a body part other than the vertex could be putting a fetus at risk. If a body part other than the vertex presents to the cervix, labor is invariably longer because of ineffective descent of the fetus, ineffective dilatation of the cervix, or irregular and weak uterine contractions.

It may also lead to early rupture of membranes, increasing the possibility of infection, fetal anoxia, and meconium staining, complications that lead to respiratory distress at birth and may require cesarean birth.

When labor is ineffective for any reason, the longer it extends, the more it tires both a woman and her fetus, as well as reducing the excitement of the experience. If a cesarean birth is necessary and postoperative complications occur, a woman may require a longer hospital stay and have more pain and disability after the birth. If a fetus is born vaginally after a complicated labor, there is an increased risk for perineal tears or cervical lacerations, which may also increase a woman's disability and possibly interfere with her future childbearing (Fitzgerald et al., 2007). If labor is threatening and unsatisfactory, it can also interfere with maternal–child bonding.

Four methods are used to determine fetal position, presentation, and lie: (a) combined abdominal inspection and palpation, called Leopold's maneuvers; (b) vaginal examination; (c) auscultation of fetal heart tones; and (d) ultrasound.

Powers of Labor

The second important requirements for a successful labor are effective powers of labor. This is the force supplied by the fundus of the uterus, implemented by uterine contractions, a natural process that causes cervical dilatation and then expulsion of the fetus from the uterus. After full dilatation of the cervix, the primary power is supplemented by use of the abdominal muscles. It is important for women to understand they should not bear down with their abdominal muscles until the cervix is fully dilated. Doing so impedes the primary force and could cause fetal and cervical damage.

Uterine Contractions

The mark of effective uterine contractions is rhythmicity and progressive lengthening and intensity.

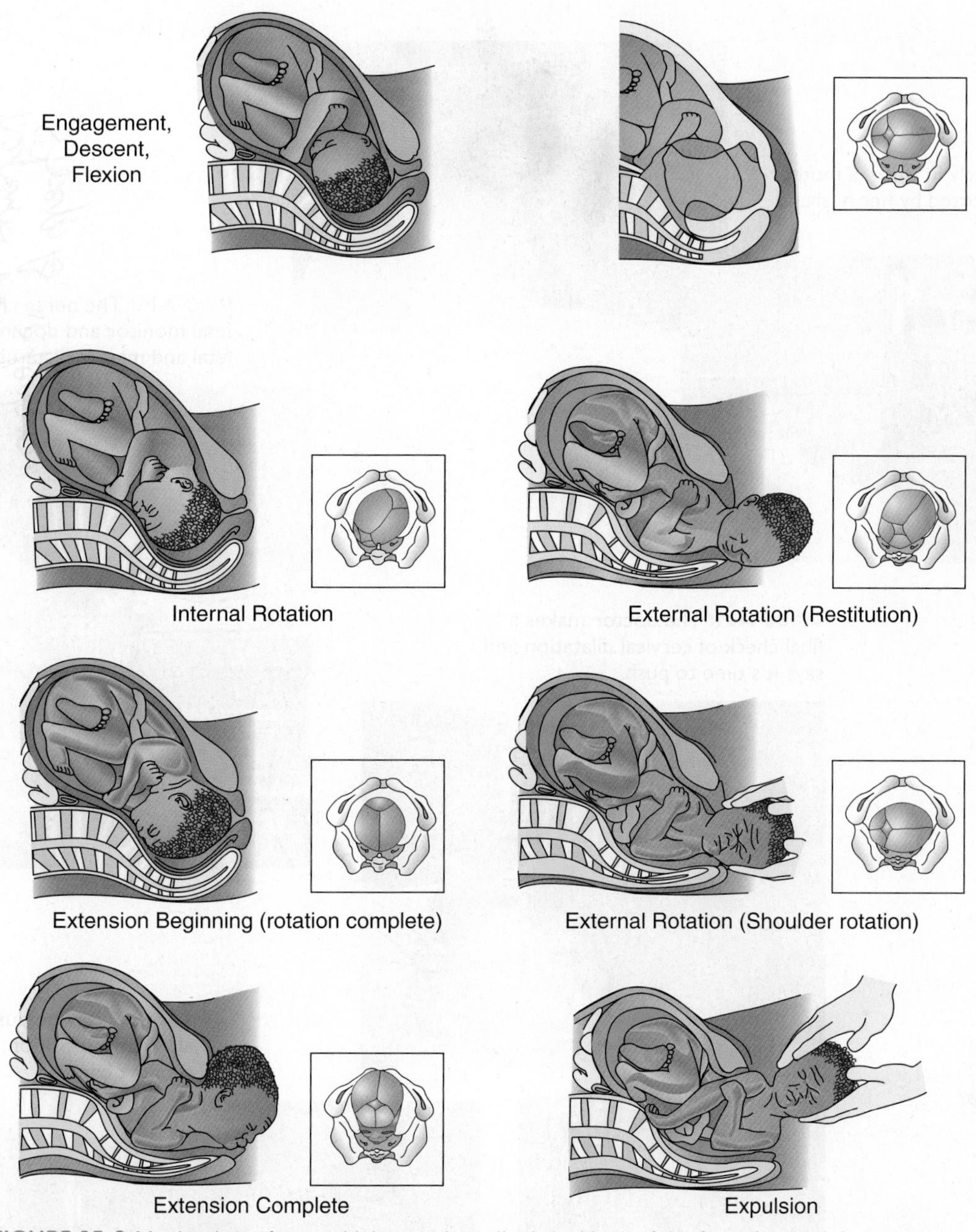

FIGURE 15.8 Mechanism of normal labor and cardinal positions of the fetus from a left occipitoanterior position.

Origins. Like cardiac contractions, labor contractions begin at a "pacemaker" point located in the uterine myometrium near one of the uterotubal junctions. Each contraction begins at that point and then sweeps down over the uterus as a wave. After a short rest period, another contraction is initiated and the downward sweep begins again.

In early labor, the uterotubal pacemaker may not be working in a synchronous manner. This makes contractions sometimes strong, sometimes weak, and perhaps irregular. This mild incoordination of early labor improves after a few hours as the pacemaker becomes more attuned to calcium concentrations in the myometrium and begins to function smoothly.

In some women, contractions appear to originate in the lower uterine segment rather than in the fundus. These are reverse, ineffective contractions, and they may actually cause tightening rather than dilatation of the cervix. That contractions are being initiated in a reverse pattern is difficult to tell from palpation. It can be suspected if the woman tells you she feels pain in her lower abdomen before the contraction is readily palpated at the fundus. It is truly revealed only when cervical dilatation does not occur.

Some women seem to have additional pacemaker sites in other portions of the uterus. If so, contractions can be unco-

(text continues on page 358)

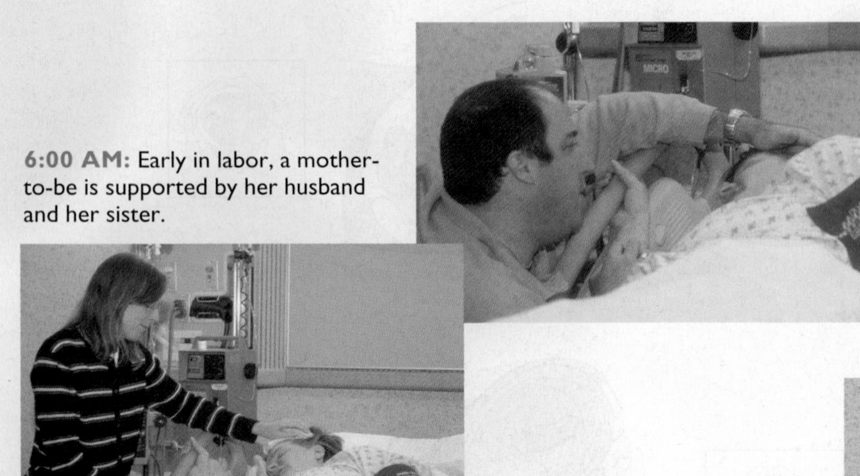

6:00 AM: Early in labor, a mother-to-be is supported by her husband and her sister.

9:00 AM: The nurse checks the fetal monitor and documents fetal and maternal status.

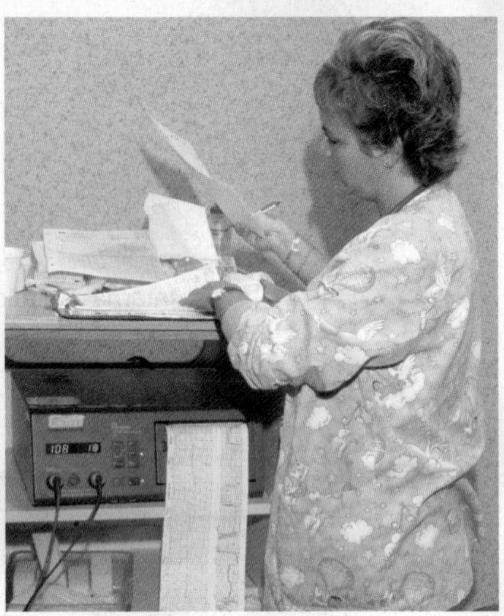

10:00 AM: The doctor makes a final check of cervical dilatation and says it's time to push.

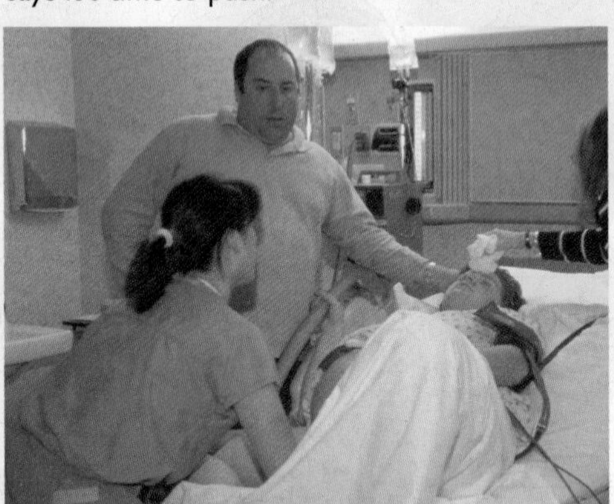

11:15 AM: She pushes from an alternative position, using a support bar.

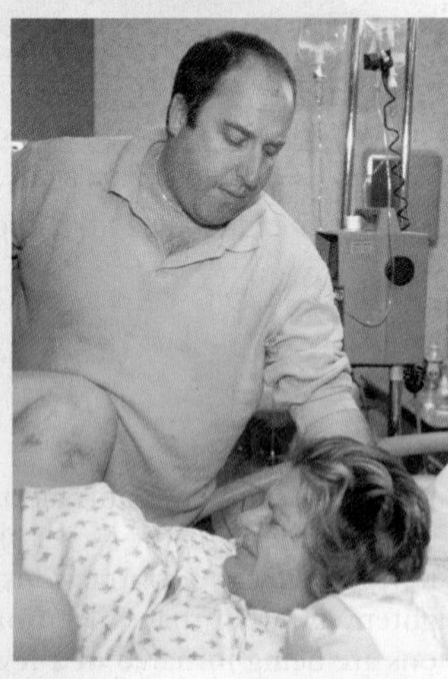

10:30 AM: The mother pushes in the lithotomy position, with her coach.

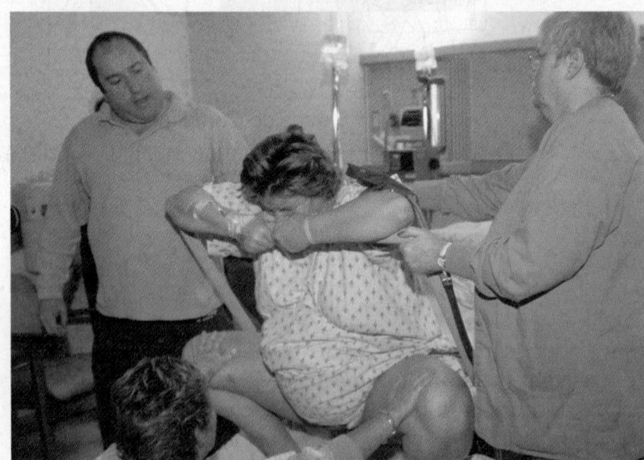

FIGURE 15.9 A day in the life of a new family.

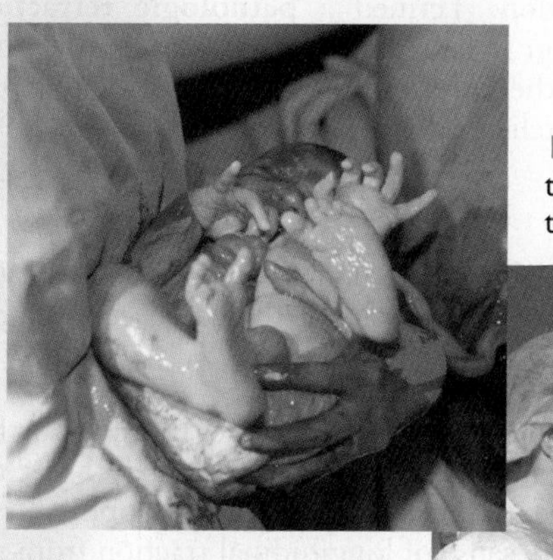

12:12 PM: Welcome to the world! Dad cuts the cord.

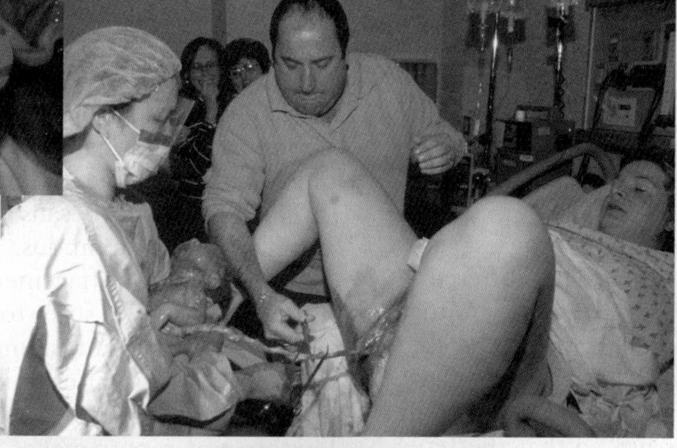

12:15 PM: Mom holds her son for the first time. Her mother and sister (now a grand-mother and aunt!) look on.

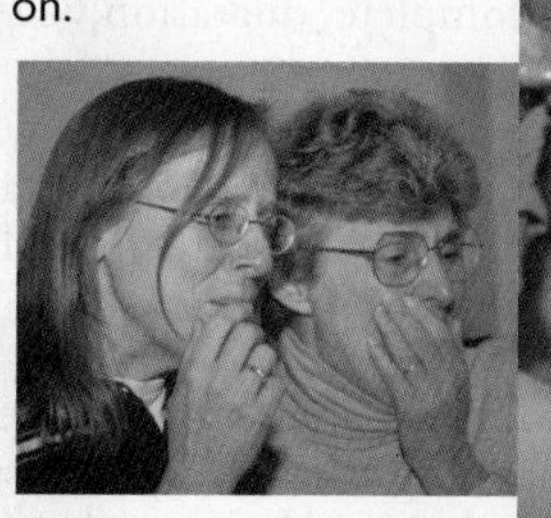

12:30 PM: The nurse suctions to clear the airway and takes the baby's footprints.

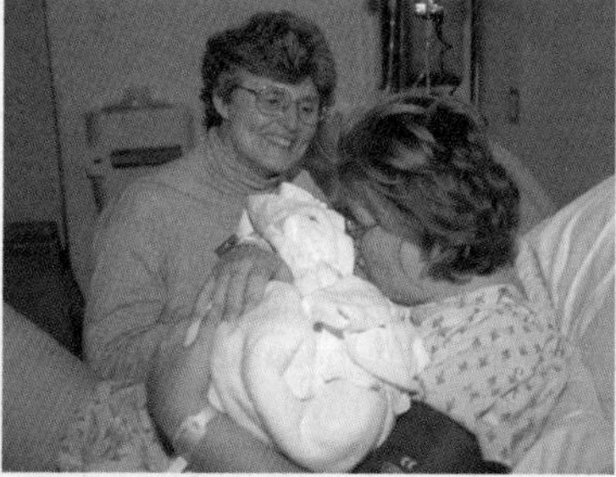

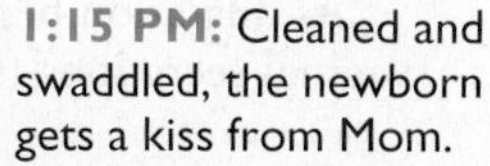

1:15 PM: Cleaned and swaddled, the newborn gets a kiss from Mom.

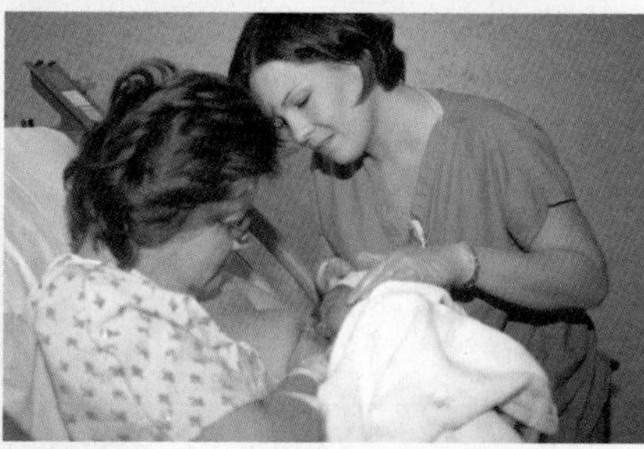

3:00 PM: The new mom gives Stephen his first feeding, with support from the nurse.

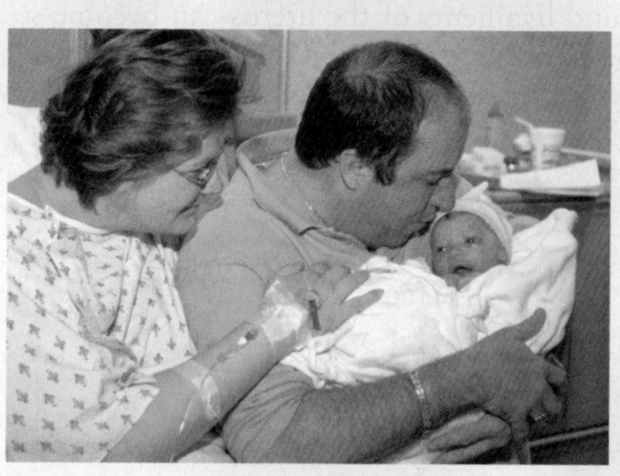

5:00 PM: New parents bond with the new member of their family.

FIGURE 15.9 *(continued)*

ordinated. Uncoordinated contractions may slow labor and can lead to failure to progress and fetal distress as they may not allow for adequate placental filling. All of these possibilities make evaluating the rate, intensity, and pattern of uterine contractions an important nursing responsibility.

Phases. A contraction consists of three phases: the increment, when the intensity of the contraction increases; the acme, when the contraction is at its strongest; and the decrement, when the intensity decreases (Fig. 15.10). Between contractions, the uterus relaxes. As labor progresses, the relaxation intervals decrease from 10 minutes early in labor to only 2 to 3 minutes. The duration of contractions also changes, increasing from 20 to 30 seconds to a range of 60 to 90 seconds.

Contour Changes. As labor contractions progress and become regular and strong, the uterus gradually differentiates itself into two distinct functioning areas. The upper portion becomes thicker and active, preparing it to be able to exert the strength necessary to expel the fetus when the expulsion phase of labor is reached. The lower segment becomes thin walled, supple, and passive, so that the fetus can be easily pushed out of the uterus. As these events occur, the boundary between the two portions becomes marked by a ridge on the inner uterine surface, the **physiologic retraction ring.**

The contour of the overall uterus also changes from a round, ovoid structure to an elongated one whose vertical diameter is markedly greater than its horizontal diameter. This lengthening serves to straighten the body of the fetus, placing it in better alignment with the cervix and pelvis. As the uterus contracts, the round ligaments tighten, keeping the fundus forward, again to assist in placing the fetus in good alignment with the cervix. The elongation of the uterus exerts pressure against the diaphragm and causes the often-expressed sensation that a uterus is "taking control" of a woman's body.

Although rarely seen today because abnormal contractions or fetal response to contractions is detected, in a difficult labor, particularly if the fetus is larger than the birth canal, the round ligaments of the uterus can become so tense they may be palpable on the abdomen. The normal physiologic retraction ring may become prominent and observable as an abdominal indentation. Termed a **pathologic retraction ring** or Bandl's ring, it is a danger sign that signifies impending rupture of the lower uterine segment if the obstruction to labor is not relieved.

Cervical Changes

Even more marked than the changes in the body of the uterus are two changes that occur in the cervix: effacement and dilatation.

Effacement. Effacement is shortening and thinning of the cervical canal. Normally, the canal is approximately 1 to 2 cm long. With effacement, the canal virtually disappears (Fig. 15.11). This occurs because of longitudinal traction from the contracting uterine fundus.

In primiparas, effacement is accomplished before dilatation begins. Be sure to inform women of this fact. Otherwise, they can become discouraged if, for example, at noon after a cervical examination a woman is told she is 2 cm dilated and then at 4 PM is told she is still 2 cm dilated. This type of report makes it seem as if absolutely nothing has happened in 4 hours. However, effacement will have been occurring, and when it is complete, dilatation will then progress rapidly.

In multiparas, dilatation may proceed before effacement is complete. Effacement must occur at the end of dilatation, however, before the fetus can be safely pushed through the cervical canal; otherwise, cervical tearing could result.

Dilatation. Dilatation refers to the enlargement or widening of the cervical canal from an opening a few millimeters wide to one large enough (approximately 10 cm) to permit passage of a fetus (see Fig. 15.11).

Dilatation occurs for two reasons. First, uterine contractions gradually increase the diameter of the cervical canal lumen by pulling the cervix up over the presenting part of the fetus. Second, the fluid-filled membranes press against the cervix. If the membranes are intact, they push ahead of the fetus and serve as an opening wedge. If they are ruptured, the presenting part serves this same function.

As dilatation begins, there is an increase in the amount of vaginal secretions (show), because the last of the operculum

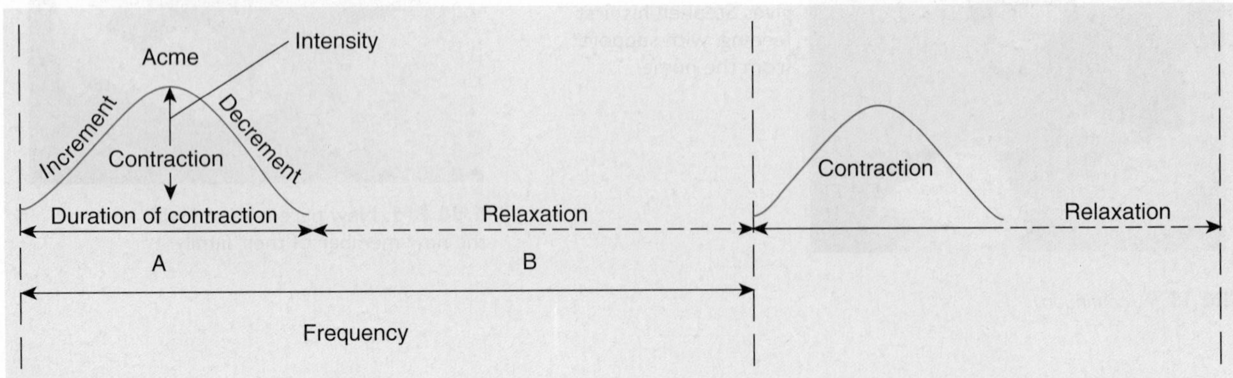

FIGURE 15.10 The interval and duration of uterine contractions. The frequency of contractions is the time from the beginning of one contraction to the beginning of the next contraction. It consists of two parts: (**A**) the duration of the contraction and (**B**) the period of relaxation. The broken line indicates an indeterminate period because the relaxation time (**B**) is usually of longer duration than the actual contraction (**A**).

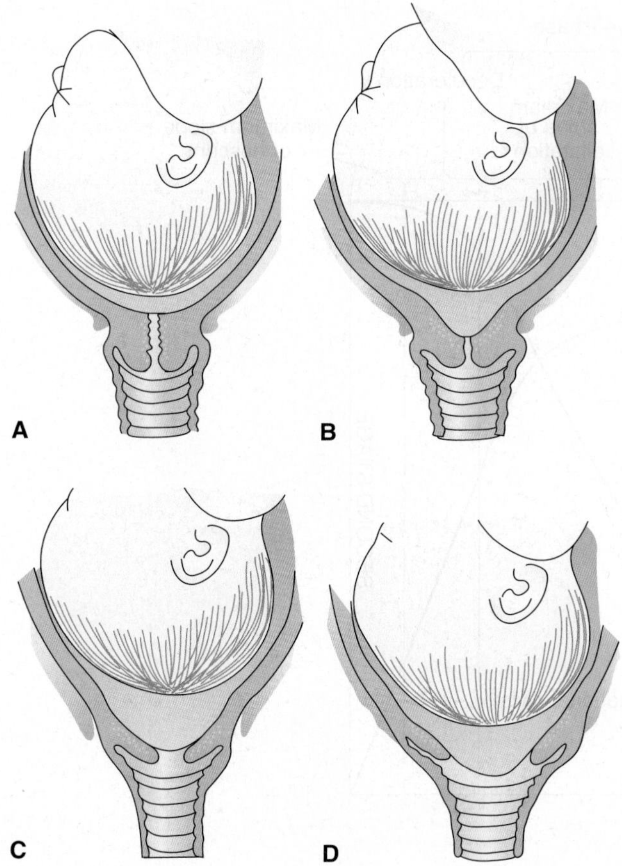

FIGURE 15.11 Effacement and dilatation of cervix. (**A**) Beginning labor. (**B**) Effacement is beginning; dilatation is not apparent yet. (**C**) Effacement is almost complete. (**D**) After complete effacement, dilatation proceeds rapidly.

or mucus plug in the cervix is dislodged and minute capillaries in the cervix rupture.

Psyche

The fourth "P," or a woman's psychological outlook, refers to the psychological state or feelings that a woman brings into labor. For many women, this is a feeling of apprehension or fright. For almost everyone, it includes a sense of excitement or awe.

Women who manage best in labor typically are those who have a strong sense of self-esteem and a meaningful support person with them. These factors allow women to feel in control of sensations and circumstances that they have not experienced previously and that may not be at all what they pictured as happening. Women without adequate support can have an experience so frightening and stressful they can develop a post-traumatic stress syndrome (Tam & Chung, 2007).

Encouraging women to ask questions at prenatal visits and to attend preparation for childbirth classes helps prepare them for labor. Encouraging them to share their experience after labor serves as "debriefing time" and helps them integrate the experience into their total life.

STAGES OF LABOR

Labor is traditionally divided into three stages: a first stage of dilatation, which begins with the initiation of true labor contractions and ends when the cervix is fully dilated; a second stage, extending from the time of full dilatation until the infant is born; and a third or placental stage, lasting from the time the infant is born until after the delivery of the placenta. The first 1 to 4 hours after birth of the placenta is sometimes termed the "fourth stage" to emphasize the importance of the close maternal observation needed at this time. These designations are helpful in planning nursing interventions to ensure the safety of both a woman and her fetus.

Friedman (1978), a physician who studied the process of labor extensively, used data to divide the first two stages of labor into phases: latent and active labor. Table 15.4 lists clinical features of these divisions of labor. When plotted in graph form, these divisions are useful in monitoring an individual woman's labor progress (Fig. 15.12). How much and what type of analgesia a woman receives in labor can influence the length of labor. Because "norms" refer to averages, an individual woman's labor can vary greatly from the ideal projected course of labor and still be normal for that woman.

Typically, a labor progress graph is labeled as:

- Left side numbered from 1 to 10 (representing the centimeters of cervical dilatation)

TABLE 15.4 ✻ Principal Clinical Features of the Divisions of Labor

	First Stage		Second Stage
Feature	***Preparatory Division***	***Dilatational Division***	***Pelvic Division***
Functions	Contractions coordinated, cervix prepared	Cervix actively dilating	Pelvis negotiated; mechanisms of labor; fetal descent; birth
Interval	Latent phase	Acceleration and phase of maximum slope	Deceleration phase and maximum descent
Measurement	Elapsed duration	Linear rate of dilatation	Linear rate of descent
Diagnosable disorders	Prolonged latent phase	Protracted dilatation; protracted descent	Prolonged deceleration; secondary arrest of dilatation; arrest of descent; failure of descent

Source: Friedman, E. (1978). *Labor, clinical evaluation and management* (2nd ed.). New York: Appleton-Century-Crofts.

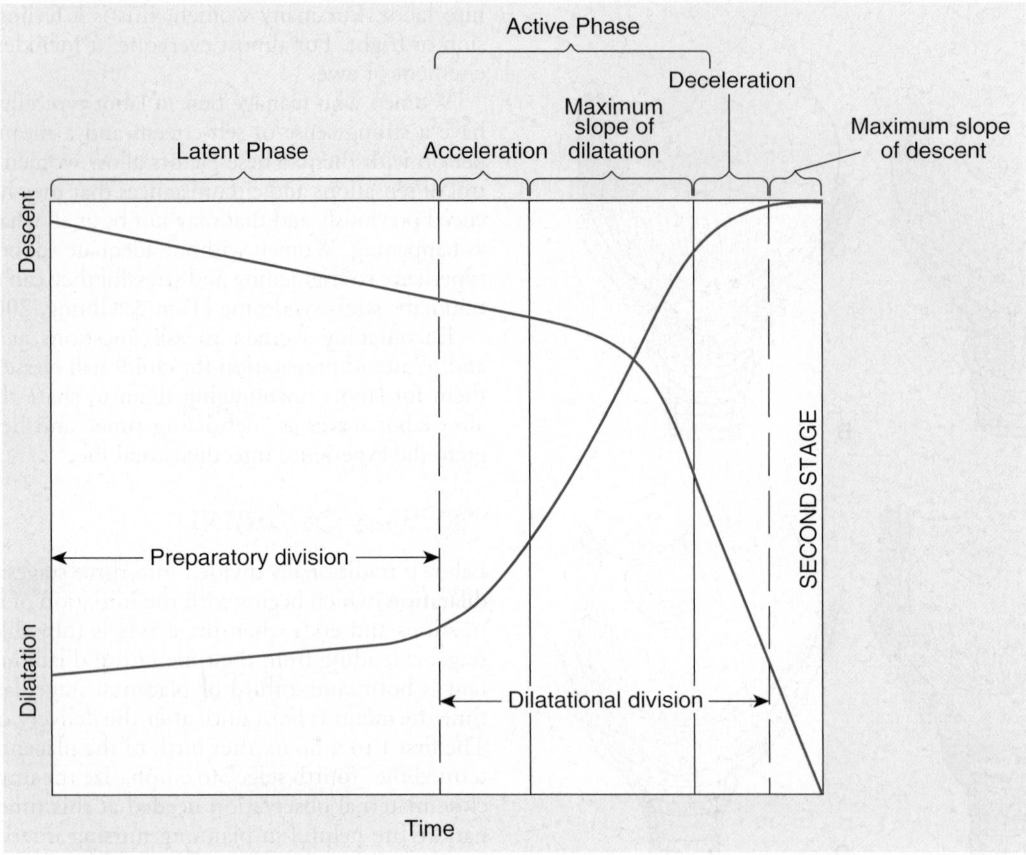

FIGURE 15.12 Divisions of labor.

- Bottom line numbered to represent the number of hours of labor
- Right side numbered from −4 to +4 (representing the station of the presenting part)

After each cervical examination, cervical dilatation and fetal descent are plotted on the graph. The pattern of cervical dilatation usually plots as an S-shaped curve. The fetal descent pattern forms a downward curve. Both lines cross at the point of maximum cervical dilatation. A typical labor graph is shown in Figure 15.13. You may need to remind women that assessments of cervical dilation are subjective so one examiner may report a different finding from another (Buchmann & Libhaber, 2007).

First Stage

Three separate divisions mark the first stage of labor: the latent, the active, and the transition phase.

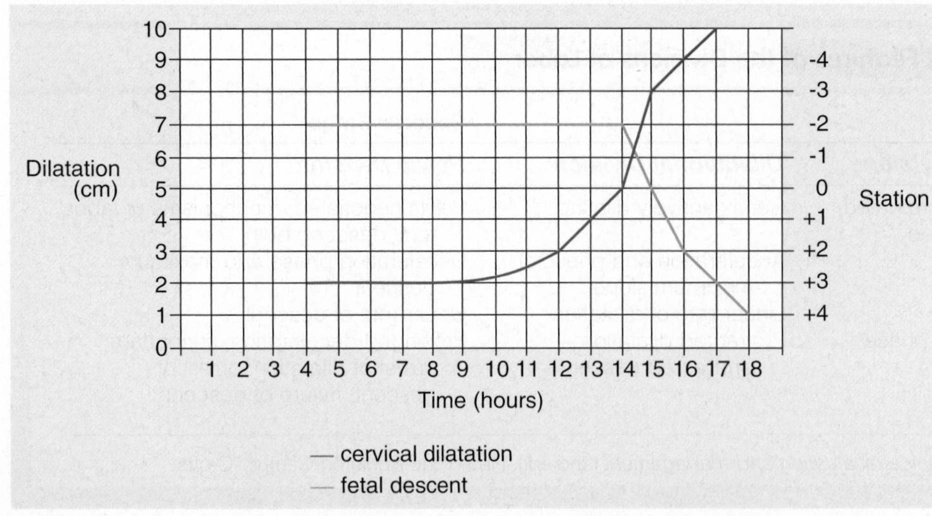

FIGURE 15.13 Normal labor graph. Fetal descent and cervical dilatation are occurring at the same time.

Latent Phase

The latent or preparatory phase begins at the onset of regularly perceived uterine contractions and ends when rapid cervical dilatation begins. Contractions during this phase are mild and short, lasting 20 to 40 seconds. Cervical effacement occurs, and the cervix dilates from 0 to 3 cm. The phase lasts approximately 6 hours in a nullipara and 4.5 hours in a multipara. A woman who enters labor with a "nonripe" cervix will have a longer than usual latent phase. Although women should not be denied analgesia at this point, analgesia given too early may prolong this phase. Measuring the length of the latent phase is important because a reason for a prolonged latent phase is cephalopelvic disproportion (a disproportion between the fetal head and pelvis) that could require a cesarean birth.

In a woman who is psychologically prepared for labor and who does not tense at each tightening sensation in her abdomen, latent phase contractions cause only minimal discomfort. A woman can (and should) continue to walk about and make preparations for birth, such as doing last-minute packing for her stay at the hospital or birthing center, preparing older children for her departure and the upcoming birth, or giving instructions to the person who will take care of them while she is away. In a birth setting, allow her to continue to be active (Greulich & Tarrant, 2007). Encourage her to continue or begin alternative methods of pain relief such as aromatherapy or distraction (Smith et al., 2007).

Active Phase

During the active phase of labor, cervical dilatation occurs more rapidly, increasing from 4 to 7 cm. Contractions grow stronger, lasting 40 to 60 seconds, and occur approximately every 3 to 5 minutes. This phase lasts approximately 3 hours in a nullipara and 2 hours in a multipara. Show (increased vaginal secretions) and perhaps spontaneous rupture of the membranes may occur during this time. This phase can be a difficult time for a woman because contractions grow strong, last longer, and begin to cause true discomfort. It is also an exciting time, because something dramatic is suddenly happening. It can be a frightening time as a woman realizes labor is truly progressing and her life is about to change forever.

The active stage of labor in a Friedman graph can be subdivided into the following periods: acceleration (4 to 5 cm) and maximum slope (5 to 9 cm). During the period of maximum slope, cervical dilatation proceeds at its most rapid pace, averaging 3.5 cm per hour in nulliparas and 5 to 9 cm per hour in multiparas. Encourage women to remain active participants in labor by assuming what position is most comfortable for them during this time (Albers, 2007).

Transition Phase

During the **transition** phase, contractions reach their peak of intensity, occurring every 2 to 3 minutes with a duration of 60 to 90 seconds and causing maximum cervical dilatation of 8 to 10 cm. If the membranes have not previously ruptured or been ruptured by amniotomy, they will rupture as a rule at full dilatation (10 cm). If it has not previously occurred, show occurs as the last of the mucus plug from the cervix is released. By the end of this phase, both full dilatation (10 cm) and complete cervical effacement (obliteration of the cervix) have occurred.

During this phase, a woman may experience intense discomfort, so strong that it is accompanied by nausea and vomiting. Because of the intensity and duration of the contractions, a woman may also experience a feeling of loss of control, anxiety, panic, or irritability. Sensations may be so intense it may seem as though labor has taken charge of her. A few minutes before, she enjoyed having her forehead wiped with a cool cloth. Now she may knock a husband's hand away. A moment before, she enjoyed having her partner rub her back. Now she may resist being touched and push that person away. Her focus is entirely inward on the task of birthing her baby.

The peak of the transition phase can be identified by a slight slowing in the rate of cervical dilatation when 9 cm is reached (termed deceleration on a labor graph). As a woman reaches the end of this stage at 10 cm of dilatation, a new sensation (i.e., an irresistible urge to push) occurs.

Second Stage

The second stage of labor is the period from full dilatation and cervical effacement to birth of the infant; with uncomplicated birth, this stage takes about 1 hour (Archie, 2007). A woman feels contractions change from the characteristic crescendo–decrescendo pattern to an overwhelming, uncontrollable urge to push or bear down with each contraction as if to move her bowels. She may experience momentary nausea or vomiting because pressure is no longer exerted on her stomach as the fetus descends into the pelvis. She pushes with such force that she perspires and the blood vessels in her neck may become distended.

As the fetal head touches the internal side of the perineum, the perineum begins to bulge and appears tense. The anus may become everted, and stool may be expelled. As the fetal head pushes against the perineum, the vaginal introitus opens and the fetal scalp appears at the opening to the vagina. At first, the opening is slitlike, then becomes oval, and then circular. The circle enlarges from the size of a dime, then a quarter, then a half-dollar. This is called **crowning**.

It takes a few contractions of this new type for a woman to realize everything is still all right, just different, and to appreciate that it feels good, not frightening, to push with contractions. In fact, the need to push becomes so intense that she cannot stop herself. She barely hears the conversation in the room around her. All of her energy, her thoughts, her being are directed toward giving birth. As she pushes, using her abdominal muscles to aid the involuntary uterine contractions, the fetus is pushed out of the birth canal.

Third Stage

The third stage of labor, the placental stage, begins with the birth of the infant and ends with the delivery of the placenta. Two separate phases are involved: placental separation and placental expulsion.

After the birth of an infant, a uterus can be palpated as a firm, round mass just inferior to the level of the umbilicus. After a few minutes of rest, uterine contractions begin again, and the organ assumes a discoid shape. It retains this new shape until the placenta has separated, approximately 5 minutes after the birth of the infant.

Placental Separation

As the uterus contracts down on an almost empty interior, there is such a disproportion between the placenta and the contracting wall of the uterus that folding and separation of the placenta occur. Active bleeding on the maternal surface of the placenta begins with separation; this bleeding helps to separate the placenta still farther by pushing it away from its attachment site. As separation is completed, the placenta sinks to the lower uterine segment or the upper vagina.

The following signs indicate that the placenta has loosened and is ready to deliver:

- Lengthening of the umbilical cord
- Sudden gush of vaginal blood
- Change in the shape of the uterus
- Firm contraction of the uterus
- Appearance of the placenta at the vaginal opening

If the placenta separates first at its center and last at its edges, it tends to fold onto itself like an umbrella and presents at the vaginal opening with the fetal surface evident. Appearing shiny and glistening from the fetal membranes, this is called a *Schultze* presentation. Approximately 80% of placentas separate and present in this way. If, however, the placenta separates first at its edges, it slides along the uterine surface and presents at the vagina with the maternal surface evident. It looks raw, red, and irregular, with the ridges or cotyledons that separate blood collection spaces showing; this is called a *Duncan* presentation. A simple trick of remembering the presentations is associating "shiny" with Schultze (the fetal membrane surface) and "dirty" with Duncan (the irregular maternal surface) (Fig. 15.14).

Bleeding occurs as part of the normal consequence of placental separation, before the uterus contracts sufficiently to seal maternal sinuses. The normal blood loss is 300 to 500 mL.

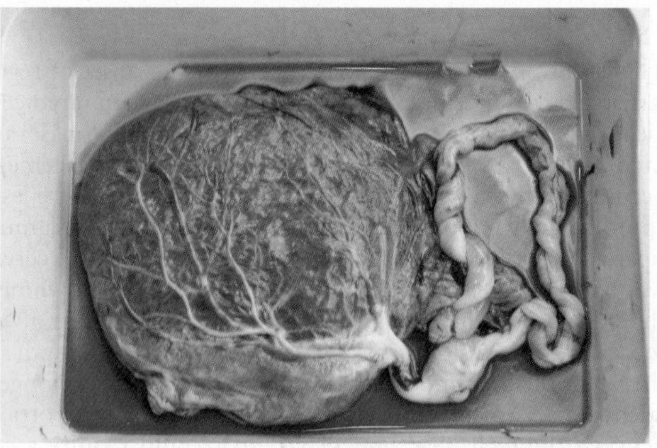

A

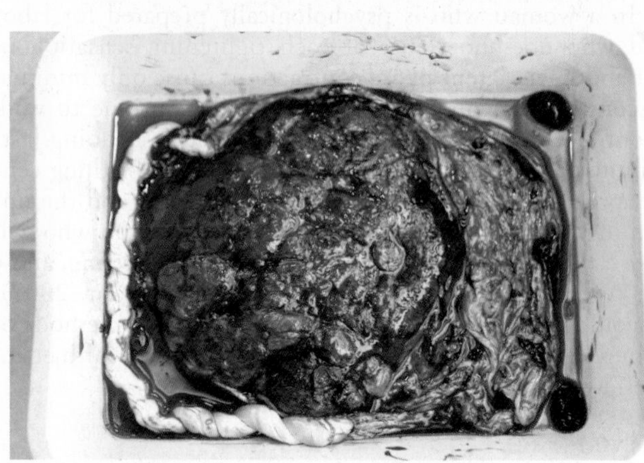

B

FIGURE 15.14 Fetal (**A**) and maternal (**B**) surface of the placenta. (Photographs by Joe Mitchell.)

Placental Expulsion

After separation, the placenta is delivered either by the natural bearing-down effort of the mother or by gentle pressure on the contracted uterine fundus by a physician or nurse-midwife (Credé's maneuver). Pressure must never be applied to a uterus in a noncontracted state, because doing so may cause the uterus to evert and hemorrhage. This is a grave complication of birth, because the maternal blood sinuses are open and gross hemorrhage could occur (Poggi, 2007). If the placenta does not deliver spontaneously, it can be removed manually. With delivery of the placenta, the third stage of labor is complete.

For most health care providers in the United States, a placenta has little importance or meaning after its work of oxygenation is done and it is delivered. For many women, however, the placenta has continuing importance. For this reason, women may ask if they can take it home with them. In several Asian and Native American cultures, women bury the placenta to ensure that the child will continue to be healthy. In some parts of China, the placenta is cooked and eaten to ensure the continued health of the mother. Ask parents whether saving the placenta is important to them before it is destroyed. Be certain when supplying placentas to women to take home with them that you respect standard infection precautions and hospital policy.

In major health centers, women may be asked to donate their newborn's placenta so blood can be removed and banked to be available for bone marrow or stem cell transplantation (Scott, 2007). Placental membranes can be salvaged to be used as temporary coverings for burns.

MATERNAL AND FETAL RESPONSES TO LABOR

Because labor is such an intense process, it has systemic physiologic effects on both a woman and her fetus.

Physiologic Effects of Labor on a Woman

Labor is a local process that involves the abdomen and reproductive organs, but its intensity is so great that almost all body systems are affected by it.

Cardiovascular System

Labor involves strenuous work and effort and requires a response from the cardiovascular system.

Cardiac Output. Each contraction greatly decreases blood flow to the uterus because the contracting uterine wall puts pressure on the uterine arteries. This increases the amount of blood that remains in a woman's general circulation, leading to an increase in peripheral resistance, which in turn results in an increase in systolic and diastolic blood pressure. In addition, the work of pushing during labor may increase cardiac output by as much as 40% to 50% above the prelabor level.

The average blood loss with birth (300 to 500 mL) is not detrimental to most women because of the blood volume increase that occurred during pregnancy and may actually play an advantageous role by reducing blood volume to prepregnancy levels. Immediately after birth, with the weight and pressure removed from the pelvis, blood from the peripheral circulation floods into the pelvic vasculature, momentarily dropping blood pressure in the vena cava. The body quickly compensates for this by sending a heavy bolus of blood to the heart, raising cardiac output to about 80% above prelabor levels. Cardiac output then gradually decreases from this high level, within the first hour after birth, by about 50%. An average woman's heart adjusts well to these sudden changes. If she has a cardiac problem, however, these sudden hemodynamic changes can have implications for her health (see Chapter 25).

Blood Pressure. With the increased cardiac output caused by contractions during labor, systolic blood pressure rises an average of 15 mm Hg with each contraction. Higher increases could be a sign of pathology. When a woman lies in a supine position and pushes during the second stage of labor, pressure of the uterus on the vena cava causes her blood pressure to drop precipitously, leading to hypotension. An upright or side-lying position during the second stage of labor not only makes pushing more effective but also can help avoid such a problem (Gupta, Hofmeyr, & Smyth, 2009).

Hemopoietic System

The major change in the blood-forming system that occurs during labor is the development of leukocytosis, or a sharp increase in the number of circulating white blood cells, possibly as a result of stress and heavy exertion. At the end of labor, the average woman has a white blood cell count of 25,000 to 30,000 cells/mm^3, compared with a normal count of 5000 to 10,000 cells/mm^3.

Respiratory System

Whenever there is an increase in cardiovascular parameters, the body responds by increasing the respiratory rate to supply additional oxygen. Total oxygen consumption increases by about 100% during the second stage of labor. Women adjust well to this change, which is comparable to that of a person performing a strenuous exercise such as running. It can result in hyperventilation. Using appropriate breathing patterns during labor can help avoid severe hyperventilation.

Temperature Regulation

The increased muscular activity associated with labor can result in a slight elevation (1° F) in temperature. Diaphoresis occurs with accompanying evaporation to cool and limit excessive warming.

Fluid Balance

Because of the increase in rate and depth of respirations (which causes moisture to be lost with each breath) and diaphoresis, insensible water loss increases during labor. Fluid balance is further affected if a woman eats nothing but sips of fluid or ice cubes or hard candy. Although not a concern in usual labor, the combination of increased fluid losses and decreased oral intake may make intravenous fluid replacement necessary if labor becomes prolonged.

Urinary System

With a decrease in fluid intake during labor and the increased insensible water loss, the kidneys begin to concentrate urine to preserve both fluid and electrolytes. Specific gravity may rise to a high normal level of 1.020 to 1.030. It is not unusual for protein (trace to 1+) to be evident in urine because of the breakdown of protein caused by the increased muscle activity. Pressure of the fetal head as it descends in the birth canal against the anterior bladder reduces bladder tone or the ability of the bladder to sense filling. Therefore, unless the woman is asked to void approximately every 2 hours during labor, overfilling may occur, possibly decreasing bladder tone in the postpartal period.

Musculoskeletal System

All during pregnancy, relaxin, an ovarian-released hormone, has acted to soften the cartilage between bones. In the week before labor, considerable additional softening causes the symphysis pubis and the sacral/coccyx joints to become even more relaxed and movable, allowing them to stretch apart to increase the size of the pelvic ring by as much as 2 cm. A woman may report this increased pubic flexibility as increased back pain or irritating, nagging pain at the pubis as she walks or turns in labor.

Gastrointestinal System

The gastrointestinal system becomes fairly inactive during labor, probably because of the shunting of blood to more life-sustaining organs and also because of pressure on the stomach and intestines from the contracting uterus. Digestive and emptying time of the stomach become prolonged. Some women experience a loose bowel movement as contractions grow strong, similar to what they may experience with menstrual cramps.

Neurologic and Sensory Responses

The neurologic responses that occur during labor are responses related to pain (increased pulse and respiratory rate). Early in labor, the contraction of the uterus and dilatation of the cervix cause the discomfort. This pain is registered at uterine and cervical nerve plexuses (at the level of the 11th and 12th thoracic nerves). At the moment of birth, the pain is centered on the perineum as it stretches to allow the fetus to move past it. Perineal pain is registered at S2 to S4 nerves.

Psychological Responses of a Woman to Labor

Labor can lead to emotional distress because it represents the beginning of a major life change for a woman and her partner.

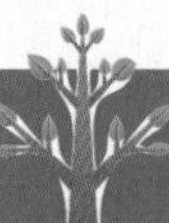

BOX 15.3 * Focus on Family Teaching

Admission Procedures for a Woman in Labor

Q. Celeste Bailey asks you, "What will happen when I arrive at a birthing center?"

A. Every setting differs, but actions you can expect include:

- Orientation to a birthing room
- Baseline assessment of your temperature, pulse, respirations, and blood pressure
- Interview to obtain your pregnancy history
- Brief physical examination
- Assessment of fetal heart rate
- Vaginal examination
- Urine and necessary blood samples obtained
- Explanation of fetal or uterine monitoring equipment if this will be used and connection of this equipment

Even for the most patient woman, pain reduces the ability to cope and may make her short-tempered or quick to criticize things around her. Admitting her quickly to a birthing room, an environment free from outside interference, can help her begin to control her breathing patterns and reduce the pain of early contractions, as well as begin to organize coping strategies (Box 15.3).

Fatigue

By the time a date of birth approaches, a woman is generally tired from the burden of carrying so much extra weight. In addition, most women do not sleep well during the last month of pregnancy (Beebe & Lee, 2007). They have a backache in a side-lying position; they turn on their back and a fetus kicks and wakens them; they turn to their side and their back aches again; and so on. Sleep hunger from this discomfort can make it difficult for them to perceive situations clearly or to adjust rapidly to new situations. It can make a little deficiency such as a wrinkled sheet appear as a threatening discrepancy in their care. It can make the process of labor loom as an overwhelming, unendurable experience unless they have competent support people with them.

Fear

Women appreciate a review of the labor process early in labor as a reminder that childbirth is not a strange, bewildering event but a predictable and well-documented one.

Being taken by surprise—labor moving faster or slower than the woman thought it would or contractions harder and longer than she remembers from last time—can lead a woman to feel out of control and increase the pain she experiences (Box 15.4). It may make her begin to worry that her infant may die or be born with an abnormality; it may make her afraid that she will not meet her own behavioral expectations. Explain that labor is predictable, but also variable, to limit this kind of fear. Be sure to explain that contractions last a certain length and reach a certain firmness but always have a pain-free rest period in between.

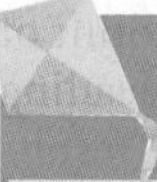

BOX 15.4 * Focus on Evidence-Based Practice

Is the average woman worried or fearful of labor and birth?

Even though a woman attends a preparation for childbirth class, a first labor and birth are still unknown experiences for her. To discover how many women fear beginning labor, researchers asked women attending a prenatal clinic if they were fearful of labor and birth early in pregnancy (about 16 weeks) and again late in pregnancy (about 32 weeks). In this study, 7.6% of women said they feared childbirth early in pregnancy; 7.4% feared this late in pregnancy. Those most apt to feel fearful were those without solid support people around them (Laursen et al., 2008).

In a second but similar study, women attending a prenatal clinic were asked to fill out a questionnaire at 37 to 38 weeks of pregnancy and then again 6 weeks after birth that asked them to report their reaction to anticipating birth or their impressions of their labor and birth.

Women who were well prepared anticipated *"quick," "easy," "smooth,"* or *"short" labors.* When labor and birth went as planned or anticipated, women reported the experience as *"wonderful," "like a dream," "perfect," "enjoyable and fulfilling," "incredibly empowering,"* and *"amazing."* In contrast, women who were not that well prepared anticipated labor and birth as being scary, potentially dangerous, and stressful. When labor did not go as planned, respondents wrote of feeling *"worried about being harmed," "nervous at the thought of having no control,"* and *"fearful for my safety."* An important factor in making labor and birth a positive experience was laboring in a relaxed setting and being supported by a knowledgeable health care professional (Baves, Fenwick, & Hauck, 2008).

Could you use these studies to guide actions when caring for women during labor and birth?

Sources: Laursen, M., et al. (2008). Fear of childbirth: predictors and temporal changes among nulliparous women in the Danish National Birth Cohort. *BJOG: An International Journal of Obstetrics and Gynaecology, 115*(3), 354–360; and Baves, S., Fenwick, J., & Hauck, Y. A. (2008). Qualitative analysis of women's short accounts of labour and birth in a Western Australian public tertiary hospital. *Journal of Midwifery and Women's Health, 53*(1), 53–61.

Cultural Influences

Cultural factors can strongly influence a woman's experience of labor. In the past, American women were accustomed to following hospital procedures and the medical model of care; therefore, they followed instructions during labor with few questions. Today, women are educated to help plan their care. In addition, every woman responds to cultural cues in some way. This makes her response to pain, her choice of nourishment, her preferred birthing position, the proximity and involvement of a support person, and customs related to the immediate postpartal period individualized (Price, Noseworthy, & Thornton, 2007).

To make labor a positive experience, be prepared to adapt your care to the woman's specific circumstances. A woman may have traditions that run counter to American hospital protocols. Address these differences, and make arrangements to accommodate her beliefs or customs if possible (e.g., providing warm food or fluids during labor, saving the placenta for the mother to take home). If the woman is not proficient in English, arranging for an interpreter or working closely with a family member who can interpret is important.

Physiologic Effects of Labor to a Fetus

Although a fetus is basically a passive participant in labor, the pressure and circulatory changes that occur with contractions cause detectable physiologic changes.

Neurologic System

Uterine contractions exert pressure on the fetal head, so the same response that is involved with any instance of increased intracranial pressure occurs. The fetal heart rate (FHR) decreases by as much as 5 beats per minute (bpm) during a contraction, as soon as contraction strength reaches 40 mm Hg. This decrease appears on a fetal heart monitor as a normal or early deceleration pattern.

Cardiovascular System

The ability to respond to cardiovascular changes is usually mature enough that the fetus is unaffected by the continual variations of heart rate that occur with labor—a slight slowing and then a return to normal (baseline) levels. During a contraction, the arteries of the uterus are sharply constricted and the filling of cotyledons almost completely halts. The amount of nutrients, including oxygen, exchanged during this time is reduced, causing a slight but inconsequential fetal hypoxia. Increased intracranial pressure caused by uterine pressure on the fetal head serves to keep circulation from falling below normal during the duration of a contraction.

Integumentary System

The pressure involved in the birth process is often reflected in minimal petechiae or ecchymotic areas on a fetus (particularly the presenting part). There may also be edema of the presenting part (caput succedaneum).

Musculoskeletal System

The force of uterine contractions tends to push a fetus into a position of full flexion, the most advantageous position for birth.

Respiratory System

The process of labor appears to aid in the maturation of surfactant production by alveoli in the fetal lung. The pressure applied to the chest from contractions and passage through the birth canal helps to clear it of lung fluid. For this reason, an infant born vaginally is usually able to establish respirations more easily than a fetus born by cesarean birth.

Box 15.5 Assessment
Assessing for Danger Signs of Labor

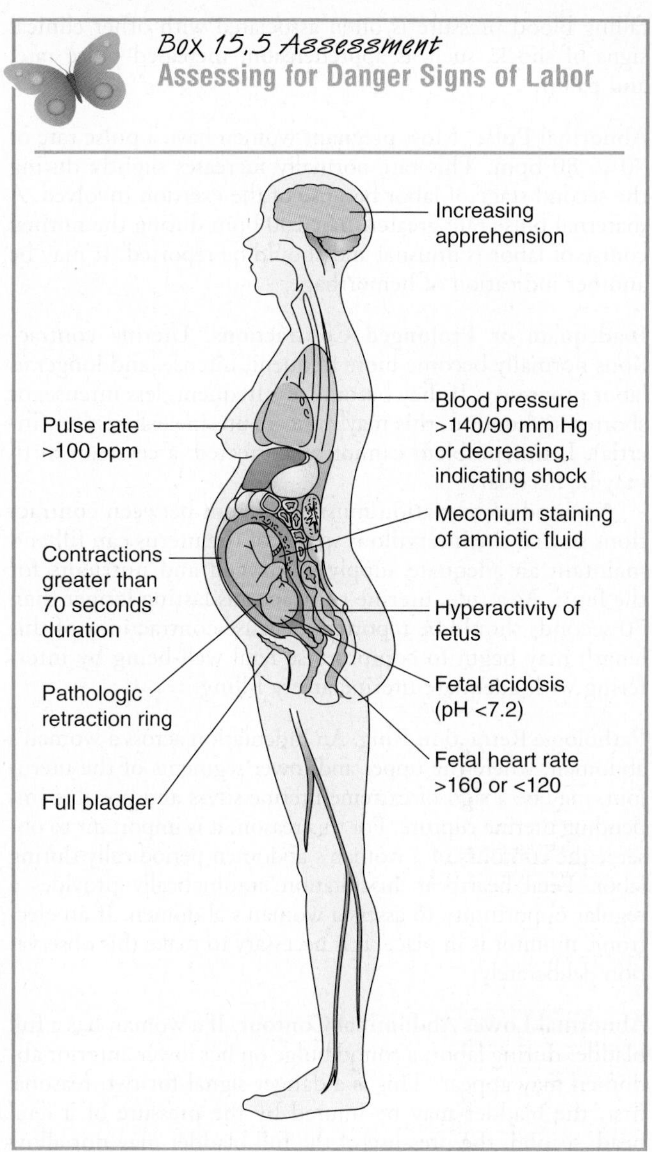

Danger Signs of Labor

Wide variation exists among individuals in their patterns of labor contractions and in maternal responses to labor and birth. Certain signs, however, indicate that the course of events is deviating from normal. These signs, both fetal and maternal, are described in Box 15.5. Nursing care of a woman who is experiencing these signs or has developed a complication during labor or birth is addressed in Chapter 23.

Maternal Danger Signs

High or Low Blood Pressure. Normally, a woman's blood pressure rises slightly in the second (pelvic) stage of labor because of her pushing effort. A systolic pressure greater than 140 mm Hg and a diastolic pressure greater than 90 mm Hg, or an increase in the systolic pressure of more than 30 mm Hg or in diastolic pressure of more than 15 mm Hg (the basic criteria for pregnancy-induced hypertension), should be reported. Just as important to report is a falling blood pressure, because it may be the first sign of intrauterine hemorrhage. A falling blood pressure is often associated with other clinical signs of shock, such as apprehension, increased pulse rate, and pallor.

Abnormal Pulse. Most pregnant women have a pulse rate of 70 to 80 bpm. This rate normally increases slightly during the second stage of labor because of the exertion involved. A maternal pulse rate greater than 100 bpm during the normal course of labor is unusual and should be reported. It may be another indication of hemorrhage.

Inadequate or Prolonged Contractions. Uterine contractions normally become more frequent, intense, and longer as labor progresses. If they become less frequent, less intense, or shorter in duration, this may indicate uterine exhaustion (inertia). If this problem cannot be corrected, a cesarean birth may be necessary.

A period of relaxation must be present between contractions so that the intervillous spaces of the uterus can fill and maintain an adequate supply of oxygen and nutrients for the fetus. As a rule, uterine contractions lasting longer than 70 seconds should be reported, because contractions of this length may begin to compromise fetal well-being by interfering with adequate uterine artery filling.

Pathologic Retraction Ring. An indentation across a woman's abdomen, where the upper and lower segments of the uterus join, may be a sign of extreme uterine stress and possible impending uterine rupture. For this reason, it is important to observe the contours of a woman's abdomen periodically during labor. Fetal heartbeat auscultation automatically provides a regular opportunity to assess a woman's abdomen. If an electronic monitor is in place, it is necessary to make this observation deliberately.

Abnormal Lower Abdominal Contour. If a woman has a full bladder during labor, a round bulge on her lower anterior abdomen may appear. This is a danger signal for two reasons: first, the bladder may be injured by the pressure of a fetal head; second, the pressure of the full bladder may not allow the fetal head to descend. To avoid a full bladder, women need to try to void about every 2 hours during labor.

Increasing Apprehension. Warnings of psychological danger during labor are as important to consider in assessing maternal well-being as are physical signs. A woman who is becoming increasingly apprehensive despite clear explanations of unfolding events may only be approaching the second stage of labor. She may, however, not be "hearing" because she has a concern that has not been met. Using an approach such as, "You seem more and more concerned. Could you tell me what is worrying you?" may be helpful. Increasing apprehension also needs to be investigated for physical reasons, because it can be a sign of oxygen deprivation or internal hemorrhage.

Fetal Danger Signs

High or Low Fetal Heart Rate. As a rule, an FHR of more than 160 bpm (fetal tachycardia) or less than 110 bpm (fetal bradycardia) is a sign of possible fetal distress. An equally important sign is a late or variable deceleration pattern (described later) on a fetal monitor. The FHR may return to a normal range in between these irregular patterns, giving a false sense of security if FHR is assessed only between contractions.

Meconium Staining. Meconium staining, a green color in the amniotic fluid, is not always a sign of fetal distress but is highly correlated with its occurrence. It reveals that the fetus has had loss of rectal sphincter control, allowing meconium to pass into the amniotic fluid. It may indicate that a fetus has or is experiencing hypoxia, which stimulates the vagal reflex and leads to increased bowel motility. Although meconium staining may be normal in a breech presentation, because pressure on the buttocks causes meconium loss, it should always be reported immediately so that its cause can be investigated.

Hyperactivity. Ordinarily, a fetus is quiet and barely moves during labor. Fetal hyperactivity may be a sign that hypoxia is occurring, because frantic motion is a common reaction to the need for oxygen.

Oxygen Saturation. If a fetus is assessed for oxygen saturation level by a catheter inserted next to the cheek, a low oxygen saturation level (under 40%) or if fetal blood was obtained by scalp puncture, the finding of acidosis (blood pH <7.2) suggests that fetal well-being is becoming compromised. Oxygen saturation in a fetus is normally 40% to 70%.

✔ *Checkpoint Question 15.3*

Suppose Celeste is having long and hard uterine contractions. What length of contraction would you report as abnormal?

a. Any length over 30 seconds.
b. A contraction over 70 seconds in length.
c. A contraction that peaks at 20 seconds.
d. A contraction shorter than 60 seconds.

MATERNAL AND FETAL ASSESSMENT DURING LABOR

Nursing assessment is instrumental to keep women safe during labor.

Immediate Assessment of a Woman in Stage 1

Several immediate assessment measures are necessary to safeguard maternal and fetal health when a woman first arrives at a birthing facility. Encourage every woman to bring a support person with her into labor (Hodnett et al., 2009). After she and her support person are oriented to the area, focus on obtaining vital assessment data.

Initial Interview and Physical Examination

Important data that need to be obtained include a description of labor thus far, the woman's general physical condition, and her preparedness for labor and birth.

Ask about the following areas:

- Expected date of birth
- Frequency, duration, and intensity of contractions
- Amount and character of show

- Whether rupture of membranes has occurred
- Time the woman last ate
- Any known drug allergies
- Past pregnancy and previous pregnancy history
- Her birth plan or what individualized measures she has planned, such as no analgesia or who will cut the umbilical cord

Assess:

- Vital signs—temperature, pulse, respirations, and blood pressure (assessed between contractions)
- Contractions (frequency, duration and intensity)
- Her preparedness and readiness for labor

This amount of information is scant but helps to establish whether the woman is in active labor and needs immediate preparation for birth or whether she has arrived at the birthing setting at an early stage of labor and therefore can benefit most from paced interventions.

Detailed Assessment During the First Stage of Labor

If the woman is in active labor, the history taken on arrival may be the only history obtained until after her baby is born. If birth is not imminent, obtain a more extensive history and physical examination.

History

The full history should include a review of a woman's pregnancy, including both physical and psychological events, and a review of past pregnancies, her general health, and family medical information—all data necessary to plan nursing care.

Performing a detailed interview of a woman in labor can be difficult because of the constant interruptions caused by labor contractions. Be patient. Remember that the longest contraction is rarely more than 60 seconds. If a woman concentrates so intently on a breathing exercise she completely forgets a question asked just before a contraction, repeat the question as the contraction subsides, as if it had not been asked before, or as if it is no trouble to ask it again.

Current Pregnancy History. Important information needed for a complete history includes documentation of gravida and para status; a description of this pregnancy (planned or not, pattern and place of prenatal care, adequacy of nutrition, whether any complication such as spotting, falls, hypertension of pregnancy, infection, or alcohol or drug ingestion has occurred); plans for labor (does she want medication for pain, will she use breathing exercises, will she have a support person with her); and future child care (will she breastfeed or formula feed, has she chosen a pediatrician).

Past Pregnancy History. Document prior pregnancies, including number, dates, types of birth, any complications, and outcomes, including sex and birth weights of children. What is the current health status of the children?

Past Health History. Document any previous surgeries (surgical adhesions might interfere with free fetal passage); heart disease or diabetes (special precautions are required during labor and birth); anemia (blood loss at birth may be more important than it is usual); tuberculosis (lung lesions may be reactivated at birth by changes in lung contour); kidney disease or hypertension (blood pressure must be monitored even more carefully than usual); or if she has ever had a sexually transmitted infection such as herpes (the infant may be exposed to the disease by vaginal contact if the disease is still active). Determine also whether a woman's lifestyle places her at high risk for prescription or nonprescription drug use or human immunodeficiency virus (HIV) exposure.

Family Medical History. Ask if any family member is cognitively challenged or has a condition such as heart disease, a blood dyscrasia, diabetes, kidney disease, cancer, allergies, seizures, or a congenital disorder. Adequate preparation can then be made for a child who might have special needs.

Physical Examination

After history taking, a woman receives a thorough physical examination, including a pelvic examination, to confirm the presentation and position of the fetus and the stage of cervical dilatation.

Physical assessment during labor begins, as does all physical assessment, with the woman's overall appearance: Does she appear tired? Pale? Ill? Frightened? Is there obvious edema or dehydration? Does she have open lesions anywhere? Be prepared to adapt further examination techniques to a woman's stage of labor, frequency of contraction, and labor progression.

Palpate for enlargement of lymph nodes to detect the possibility of infection. Inspect the mucous membrane of the mouth and the conjunctiva of the eyes for color. Does the color (paleness) suggest anemia? What is the condition of the woman's teeth? Are there any caries? Do any teeth appear abscessed (such a condition needs to be documented because it might account for a postpartal fever)? Examine the outer and inner surfaces of her lips carefully. Does she have herpes lesions (pinpoint vesicles on an erythematous base)? Mothers with active lesions, regardless of the lesion site, should use care when handling their infants, such as ensuring that they wash their hands before touching the infant. Either the woman or family members with oral herpetic lesions should avoid kissing the newborn. Breastfeeding is encouraged even if the woman is taking an antiviral drug as long as there are no lesions on the breasts (Aziz & Cohen, 2007).

Assess lungs to be certain they are clear to auscultation. Listen for normal heart sounds and rhythms. Many pregnant women at term have a grade II to III systolic ejection murmur because of the extra volume of blood that must cross the heart valves. Inspect and palpate her breasts. Are they free of cysts and lumps? Mark the chart of a woman who has a palpable mass in her breasts for re-examination after labor and birth. This is probably an enlarged milk gland but needs further evaluation.

Abdominal Assessment. Assessing a woman's abdomen is important to estimate fetal size by fundal height (should be at the level of the xiphoid process at term). Palpate and percuss the bladder area (over the symphysis pubis) to detect a full bladder. Assess for abdominal scars to reveal previous abdominal or pelvic surgery that could have left adhesions.

Finally, inspect lower extremities for skin turgor to assess hydration, and also for edema and varicose veins. Women with large varicosities are more prone to thrombophlebitis after birth than other women. Severe edema suggests hypertension of pregnancy. A blood pressure of 140/90 mm Hg or higher confirms this.

Leopold's Maneuvers

Leopold's maneuvers are a systematic method of observation and palpation to determine fetal presentation and position. Steps for this are described in Box 15.6.

Assessing Rupture of Membranes

One of every four labors begins with spontaneous rupture of the fetal membranes. When this occurs, a woman feels a sudden gush of amniotic fluid from her vagina. This is a startling sensation because it feels as if she has lost bladder control. She may feel embarrassed before she realizes the warm fluid on her perineum and legs is not urine but a sudden announcement that labor is beginning. In other women, rupture of membranes is subtle, occurring as a slow loss of fluid. When this happens, there may be a question of whether the membranes have ruptured.

A vaginal examination using a sterile speculum usually reveals whether amniotic fluid is present in the vagina. After vaginal secretions are obtained (usually with the use of a sterile, cotton-tipped applicator), test them with a strip of Nitrazine paper. Vaginal secretions are usually acid; amniotic fluid, in contrast, is alkaline. If amniotic fluid has passed through the vagina recently, the pH of the vaginal fluid will probably be alkaline (>6.5) when tested by Nitrazine paper (appears blue-green or gray to deep blue). A false reading may occur in a woman with intact membranes who has a heavy, bloody show, because blood is also alkaline. An additional test is a fern test (examination of vaginal secretions under a microscope). Because of its high estrogen content, amniotic fluid will show a fern pattern (see Chapter 5, Fig. 5.14) when dried and examined in this way; urine will not.

If the woman's membranes ruptured at home, ask her to describe the color of the amniotic fluid. It should be as clear as water. Yellow-stained fluid may indicate a blood incompatibility between mother and fetus (the amniotic fluid is bilirubin stained from the breakdown of red blood cells). Green fluid suggests meconium staining. Although meconium staining is normal in breech births because of buttocks compression, in a vertex presentation it may indicate fetal anoxia. Either way, a fetus with meconium staining needs immediate assessment to safeguard well-being. The infant will need continuing close assessment after birth to rule out possible meconium aspiration.

Vaginal Examination

A vaginal examination is necessary to determine the extent of cervical effacement and dilatation and to confirm the fetal presentation, position, and degree of descent. The technique for a vaginal examination during labor is shown in Box 15.7.

Vaginal examinations may be done either between contractions or during contractions. More of the fetal skull may be palpated during a contraction, because the cervix retracts more at that time. However, examination during a contraction is more painful and rarely is justified by the additional amount of information gained. Palpation of membranes during a contraction, when they are under pressure, may cause them to rupture.

Women are anxious to have frequent progress reports during labor, to reassure them everything is progressing well. Tell a woman immediately after an examination, therefore, about her progress. Most women are aware of dilatation but not the word "effacement." Just saying, "no further dilatation" is a depressing report. "You're not dilated a lot more, but a lot of thinning is happening and that's just as important" is the same report given in a positive manner. After finishing a vaginal examination, plot the new degree of dilatation and descent of the presenting part on a labor progress graph, as described earlier.

Do not conduct vaginal examinations in the presence of fresh bleeding, because this may indicate a placenta previa (implantation of the placenta so low in the uterus that it encroaches on the cervical os) is present. Performing a vaginal examination in this instance might tear the placenta and cause hemorrhage, resulting in danger to both mother and fetus. If in doubt, err on the side of postponing a vaginal examination.

Assessment of Pelvic Adequacy

Evaluating pelvic adequacy using internal conjugate and ischial tuberosity diameters is generally done during pregnancy, so that, by weeks 32 to 36 of pregnancy, the nurse-midwife or physician is alerted that a cephalopelvic disproportion could occur. Women with this potential problem are cautioned not to attempt a home birth or use a birthing center without nearby hospital facilities available.

Whether the pelvis is wide enough to allow the fetus to pass through the internal diameters can be reassessed during early labor. Because these procedures involve vaginal manipulation and discomfort (and the diameters obtained during pregnancy have not changed), they are not retaken if already obtained. However, if the woman did not receive prenatal care, they need to be estimated at this time. (These procedures are described in Chapter 11.)

The suprapubic angle may be estimated early in labor to determine how readily the fetal head will be born (if the angle is too steep, the fetal head can lock behind it and perineal tissue may tear during birth as the fetal head is pushed posteriorly). To estimate this angle, place the fingers vaginally and press up against the pubic arch. If the fingers cannot be separated in this position, the angle is unusually steep (less than 90 degrees).

Ultrasound

Although not routine, an ultrasound may be used at term to determine the diameters of the fetal skull and to determine presentation, presenting part, position, flexion, and degree of descent of a fetus. If a woman is going to be transported to another department to have this done, be sure someone accompanies her, so that, if labor should become more active, she can be returned quickly to the labor and birth service.

Vital Signs

Vital signs are taken at the beginning and then periodically during labor, as summarized in Table 15.5.

(text continues on page 372)

Box 15.6 Nursing Procedure 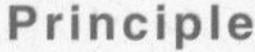 Leopold's Maneuvers

Purpose: Systematically observing and palpating the abdomen to determine fetal presentation and position

Procedure	Principle
1. Prepare the client.	
a. Explain the procedure.	**a.** Explanation reduces anxiety and enhances cooperation.
b. Instruct the client to empty her bladder.	**b.** Doing so promotes comfort and allows for more productive palpation because fetal contour will not be obscured by a distended bladder.
c. Position the woman supine with knees slightly flexed. Place a small pillow or rolled towel under one side.	**c.** Flexing the knees relaxes the abdominal muscles. Using a pillow or towel tilts the uterus off the vena cava, thus preventing supine hypotension syndrome.
d. Wash your hands using warm water.	**d.** Handwashing prevents the spread of possible infection. Using warm water aids in client comfort and prevents tightening of abdominal muscles.
e. Observe the woman's abdomen for longest diameter and where fetal movement is apparent.	**e.** The longest diameter (axis) is the length of the fetus. The location of activity most likely reflects the position of the feet.
2. Perform the first maneuver.	**2.** This maneuver determines whether fetal head or breech is in the fundus.
a. Stand at the foot of the client, facing her, and place both hands flat on her abdomen.	**a.** Proper positioning of hands ensures accurate findings.
b. Palpate the superior surface of the fundus. Determine consistency, shape, and mobility.	**b.** When palpating, a head feels more firm than a breech. A head is round and hard; the breech is less well defined. A head moves independently of the body; the breech moves only in conjunction with the body.

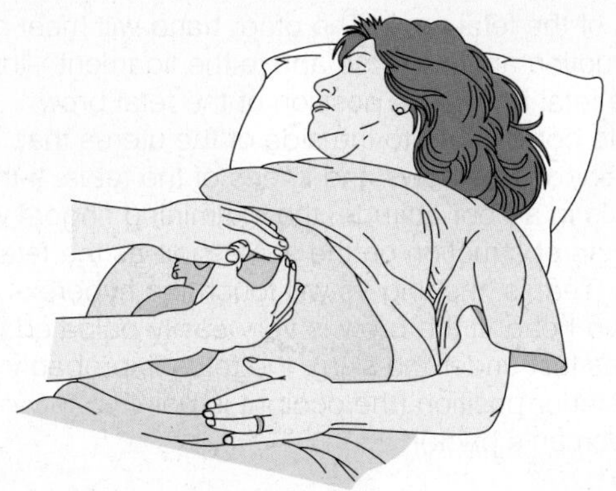

Procedure	Principle
3. Perform the second maneuver.	**3.** This maneuver locates the back of the fetus.
a. Face the client and place the palms of each hand on either side of the abdomen.	**a.** Proper positioning of hands ensures accurate findings.
b. Palpate the sides of the uterus. Hold the left hand stationary on the left side of the uterus while the right hand palpates the opposite side of the uterus from top to bottom. Then hold the right hand steady, and repeat palpation using the left hand on the left side.	**b.** This method is most successful to determine the direction the fetal back is facing. One hand will feel a smooth, hard, resistant surface (the back), while on the opposite side, a number of angular nodulations (the knees and elbows of the fetus) will be felt.

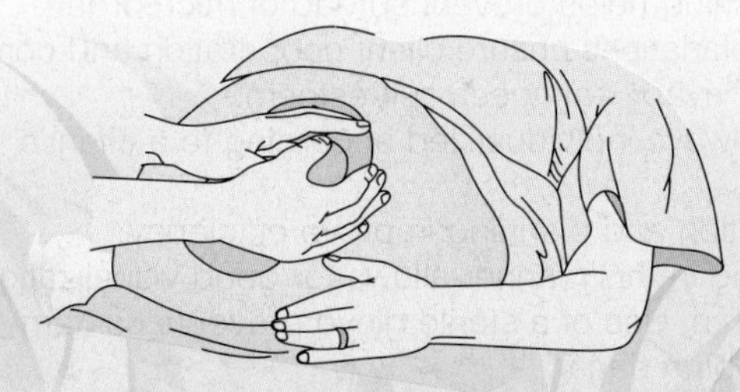

Box 15.6 Nursing Procedure ✻ Leopold's Maneuvers (continued)

Procedure	Principle
4. Perform the third maneuver.	**4.** This maneuver determines the part of the fetus at the inlet and its mobility.
a. Gently grasp the lower portion of the abdomen just above the symphysis pubis between the thumb and index finger and try to press the thumb and finger together. Determine any movement and whether the part is firm or soft.	**a.** If the presenting part moves upward so an examiner's hands can be pressed together, the presenting part is not engaged (not firmly settled into the pelvis). If the part is firm, it is the head; if soft, then it is the breech.
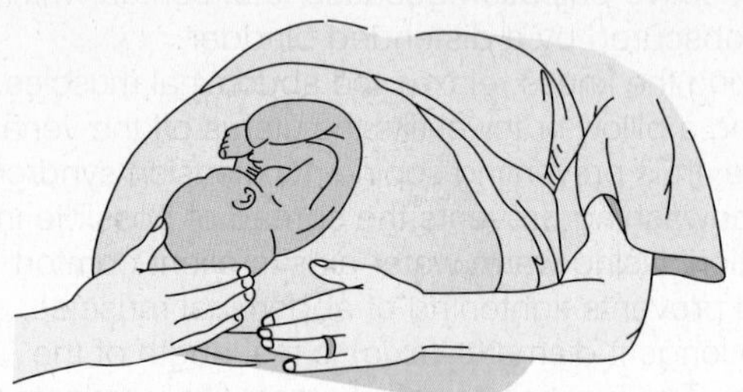	
5. Perform the fourth maneuver.	**5.** This maneuver determines fetal attitude and degree of fetal extension into the pelvis; it should be done only if the fetus is in a cephalic presentation. Information about the infant's anteroposterior position may also be gained from this final maneuver.
a. Place fingers on both sides of the uterus approximately 2 inches above the inguinal ligaments, pressing downward and inward in the direction of the birth canal. Allow fingers to be carried downward.	**a.** The fingers of one hand will slide along the uterine contour and meet no obstruction, indicating the back of the fetal neck. The other hand will meet an obstruction an inch or so above the ligament—this is the fetal brow. The position of the fetal brow should correspond to the side of the uterus that contained the elbows and knees of the fetus. If the fetus is in a poor attitude, the examining fingers will meet an obstruction on the same side as the fetal back. That is, the fingers will touch the hyperextended head. If the brow is very easily palpated (as if it lies just under the skin), the fetus is probably in a posterior position (the occiput is pointing toward the woman's back).
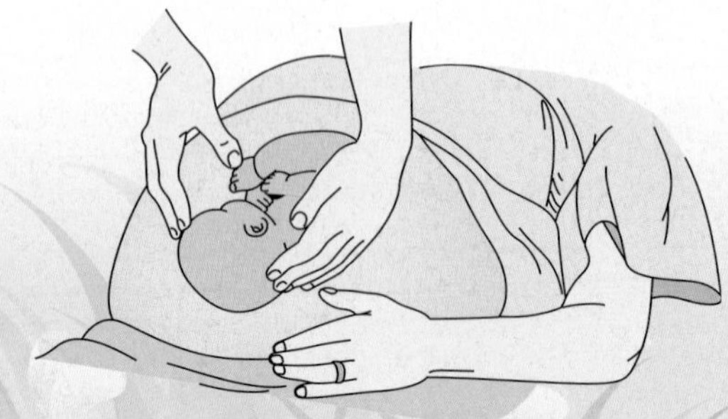	

Box 15.7 Nursing Procedure ✻ Vaginal Examination

Purpose: Determine cervical readiness and fetal position and presentation.

Procedure	Principle
1. Wash your hands; explain procedure to client. Provide privacy.	**1.** Handwashing helps prevent spread of microorganisms; explanations ensure client cooperation and compliance. Privacy enhances self-esteem.
2. Assess client status and adjust plan to individual client need.	**2.** Care is always individualized according to a client's needs.
3. Assemble equipment: sterile examining gloves, sterile lubricant, antiseptic solution. Ask the woman to turn onto her back with knees flexed (a dorsal recumbent position). Put on sterile examining gloves.	**3.** Organization and planning improve efficiency. Positioning in this manner allows for good visualization of perineum. Use of a sterile glove prevents contamination of birth canal.

Box 15.7 Nursing Procedure ✻ Vaginal Examination

Procedure	Principle
4. Discard one drop of clean lubricating solution and drop an ample supply on tips of gloved fingers.	**4.** Discarding the first drop ensures that quantity used will not be contaminated.
5. Pour antiseptic solution over vulva using nondominant hand.	**5.** This prevents the spread of organisms from perineum to birth canal.
6. Place nondominant hand on the outer edges of the woman's vulva and spread her labia while inspecting the external genitalia for lesions. Look for red, irritated mucous membranes; open, ulcerated sores; clustered, pinpoint vesicles.	**6.** Positioning hands in this way allows for good perineal visualization. Presence of any lesions may indicate an infection and possibly preclude vaginal birth.
7. Look for escaping amniotic fluid or the presence of umbilical cord or bleeding.	**7.** Amniotic fluid implies membranes have ruptured and umbilical cord may have prolapsed. Bleeding may be a sign of placenta previa. *Do not do a vaginal examination if a possible placenta previa is present.*
8. If there is no bleeding or cord visible, introduce your index and middle fingers of dominant hand gently into the vagina, directing them toward the posterior vaginal wall.	**8.** The posterior vaginal wall is less sensitive than the anterior wall. Stabilize the uterus by placing your nondominant hand on the woman's abdomen.
9. Touch the cervix with your gloved examining fingers.	**9.** The cervix feels like a circular rim of tissue around a center depression.
a. Palpate for cervical consistency and rate if *firm* or *soft.*	**a.** Firm is similar to the tip of a nose; soft is as pliable as an earlobe. The anterior rim is usually the last portion to thin.
b. Measure the extent of dilatation; palpate for an anterior rim or lip of cervix. 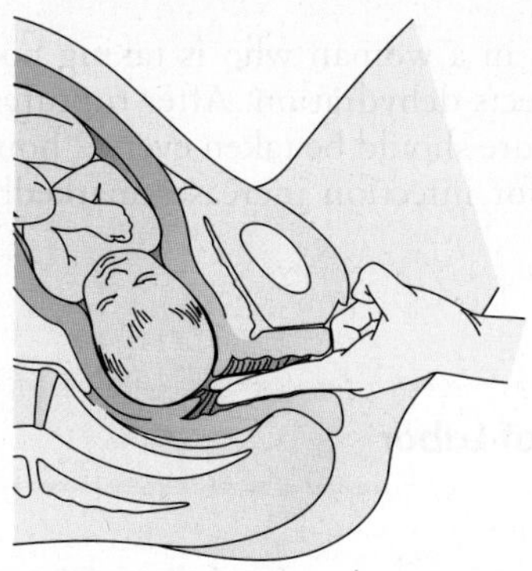	**b.** The width of the fingertip helps to estimate the degree of dilatation. An index finger averages about 1 cm; a middle finger about 1½ cm. If they can both enter the cervix, the cervix is dilated 2½ to 3 cm. If there would be room for double the width of your examining fingers in the cervix, the dilatation is about 5 to 6 cm. When the space is four times the width of your fingertips, dilatation is complete—10 cm. Measure the width of your fingertips on a centimeter scale if you are going to do a vaginal examination, so you know how wide your index and middle fingers are at the tip.
10. Estimate the degree of effacement.	**10.** Effacement is estimated in percentage depending on thickness. A cervix before labor is 2 to 2½ cm thick. If it is only 1 cm thick now, it is 50% effaced. If it is tissue paper thin, it is 100% effaced. With a 100% effaced cervix, dilatation is difficult to feel because the edges of the cervix are so thin.
11. Estimate whether membranes are intact.	**11.** The membranes (with a slight amount of amniotic fluid in front of the presenting part) are the shape of a watch crystal. With a contraction, they bulge forward and become prominent and can be felt much more readily.
12. Locate the ischial spines. Rate the station of the presenting part. Identify the presenting part.	**12.** Ischial spines are palpated as notches at the 4 and 8 o'clock positions at the pelvic outlet. Station is the number of centimeters above or below the spines where the presenting part is. Identifying the presenting part confirms findings obtained with Leopold's maneuvers. Differentiating a vertex from a breech may be more difficult than would first appear. A vertex has a hard, smooth surface. Fetal hair may be palpable but massed together and wet; it may be difficult to appreciate through gloves. Palpating the two fontanelles, one

Box 15.7 Nursing Procedure ✻ Vaginal Examination (continued)

Procedure	Principle
	diamond-shaped and one triangular, helps the identification. Buttocks feel softer and give under fingertip pressure. Identifying the anus may be possible because the sphincter action will "trap" the index finger.
13. Establish the fetal position.	**13.** The fontanelle palpated is invariably the posterior one because the fetus maintains a flexed position, presenting the posterior not the anterior fontanelle. In an ROA position, the triangular fontanelle will point toward the right anterior pelvic quadrant. In an LOA position, the posterior fontanelle will point toward the left anterior pelvis. In a breech presentation, the anus can serve as a marker for position. When the anus is pointing toward the left anterior quadrant of the woman's pelvis, the position is LSA.
14. Withdraw your hand. Wipe the perineum front to back to remove secretions or examining solution. Leave client comfortable and turned to side.	**14.** Use as gentle a technique with withdrawal as with insertion. Wiping front to back prevents moving rectal contamination forward to the vagina. Side-lying is the best position to prevent supine hypotension syndrome in labor.
15. Document procedure and assessment findings and how client tolerated procedure.	**15.** Documentation provides a means for communication and evaluation of care and client outcomes.

Temperature. Temperature is usually obtained every 4 hours during labor. Report a temperature greater than 37.2° C (99° F) to the attending physician or nurse-midwife, because it may indicate the development of infection. Unless there are accompanying symptoms, however, temperature elevation in a woman who is taking no fluids by mouth usually reflects dehydration. After rupture of the membranes, temperature should be taken every 2 hours, because the possibility for infection increases markedly after this time.

TABLE 15.5 ✻ Time Intervals for Nursing Interventions During First Stage of Labor

Intervention	Assessment on Admission	Latent Phase (0–3 cm)	Active Phase (4–7 cm)	Transition Phase (8–10 cm)
Assess and Record				
Temperature	X	q4hr (unless membranes are ruptured, then q2hr)	q4hr (unless membranes are ruptured, then q2hr)	q4hr (unless membranes are ruptured, then q2hr)
Pulse	X	q30–60 min	q30–60 min	q15–30 min
Respirations	X	q30–60 min	q30–60 min	q15–30 min
Blood pressure	X	q30–60 min	q30–60 min	q15–30 min
Voiding	X	q2hr	q2hr	q2hr
Fetal heart rate	X	Continuously by monitor or q30–60 min	Continuously by monitor or q15–30 min	Continuously by monitor or q15–30 min
Contractions	X	Continuously by monitor or q30–60 min	Continuously by monitor or q15–30 min	Continuously by monitor or q10–15 min
Perineum	X	q30–60 min	q30 min	q15 min
Provide				
Ambulation	X	Until membranes rupture	Until membranes rupture	
Support	X	Continuously	Continuously	Continuously

Pulse and Respiration. Pulse and respiration rate should be measured and recorded every 4 hours during labor. A woman's pulse may be rapid on admission because she is nervous and anxious. After she has become better acquainted with her surroundings and has been assured that everything is going well, her pulse usually ranges between 70 and 80 bpm. A persistent pulse rate of more than 100 bpm suggests tachycardia from dehydration or hemorrhage. Respiratory rate during labor is usually 18 to 20 breaths per minute. Do not count respirations during contractions, because women tend to breathe rapidly from pain. Conversely, if a woman is using controlled breathing to decrease pain in labor, her respirations could be abnormally slow.

Observe for hyperventilation (rapid, deep respirations). Prolonged hyperventilation leads to the "blowing off" of carbon dioxide and accompanying symptoms of dizziness and tingling of hands and feet. Rebreathing into a paper bag and reassurance help to reverse this process.

Blood Pressure. Blood pressure is usually measured and recorded every 4 hours during labor. Always measure this between contractions, both for a woman's comfort and for accuracy, because blood pressure tends to rise 5 to 15 mm Hg during a contraction. An increase in blood pressure may indicate the development of pregnancy-induced hypertension. A decrease in blood pressure or a decrease in the pulse pressure (the difference between the systolic and diastolic pressures) may indicate hemorrhage. If a woman receives an analgesic agent (such as meperidine) that tends to be hypotensive, check her blood pressure approximately 15 minutes after administration to be certain that extreme hypotension is not occurring.

Laboratory Analysis

Most women have some preliminary laboratory studies done in early labor.

Blood. Blood is drawn for hemoglobin and hematocrit, a serologic test for syphilis (VDRL), hepatitis B antibodies, and blood typing to determine a woman's baseline level of health. These findings can be used to alert the laboratory that a woman with a certain blood type is in labor and to help predict whether a blood incompatibility is likely to exist in the newborn. If a woman gives permission for human immunodeficiency (HIV) testing, blood for this will be drawn as well.

Urine. Obtain a clean-catch urine specimen and test it at the point of care for protein and glucose; then send it to the laboratory for a complete urinalysis. If a woman reports any symptoms that suggest a urinary tract infection (e.g., burning on urination, blood in urine, extreme frequency, flank pain), obtain a clean-catch specimen for culture. A woman in labor is able to void most easily if she is allowed to use a bathroom. However, if a woman has ruptured membranes, check whether she should ambulate to a bathroom until it is confirmed that the fetal head is engaged, so that gravity will not cause a prolapsed cord. A bedpan or receptacle placed on a commode allows for collection of any material passed from the vagina.

Assessment of Uterine Contractions

Uterine contractions may be monitored intermittently by a hand or continuously by an internal or external system. Most women are monitored for a short period in early labor to screen for fetal well-being. Continuing to monitor the duration, strength, and interval between contractions can aid in tracking the progress of labor, although use of extensive monitoring with low-risk women may lead to an increase in cesarean birth (Gourounti & Sandall, 2007).

Length of Contractions. To determine the length of a contraction with a monitor in place, simply observe the rhythm strip and count the time interval of the contraction. To determine the beginning of a contraction without a monitor, rest a hand on a woman's abdomen at the fundus of the uterus very gently to sense the gradual tensing and upward rising of the fundus that accompanies a contraction (Fig. 15.15). It is possible to palpate this tensing approximately 5 seconds before the woman is able to feel the contraction. (Contractions are palpable when the intrauterine pressure reaches approximately 20 mm Hg. The pain of a contraction is not usually felt until pressure reaches approximately 25 mm Hg.). Time the duration of a contraction from the moment the uterus first tenses until it has relaxed again.

Intensity of Contractions. In addition to observing the duration of contractions, estimate the intensity or strength. On a monitor, this is the height of the waveform. If you are assessing manually, rate a contraction as mild if the uterus does not feel more than minimally tense, as moderate if the uterus feels firm, and as strong if the uterus feels as hard as a wooden board at the peak of the contraction. With a strong contraction, you will also not be able to indent the uterus with your fingertips.

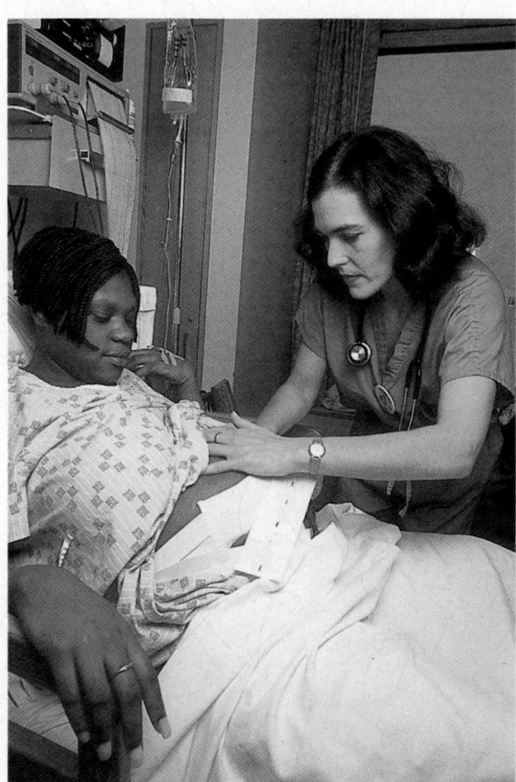

FIGURE 15.15 Contractions can be assessed by very gently placing the hand over the fundus of the uterus.

After estimating the intensity and duration of a contraction, recheck the fundus at the conclusion of the contraction, to be certain that it is relaxing and becoming soft to the touch again. This demonstrates that the uterus is not in continuous contraction but is providing a relaxation time during which blood vessels can fill to supply the fetus with adequate oxygen.

Frequency of Contractions. Next, time the frequency of contractions. The frequency is timed from the beginning of one contraction to the beginning of the next (see Fig. 15.10).

Use as light a touch as possible on a woman's abdomen while timing contractions or estimating their strength manually. The fundus of the uterus becomes tender if it has to push against the extra weight of a hand with each contraction. This is an unnecessary discomfort for a woman in labor.

Initial Fetal Assessment

Although passive in labor, a fetus is subjected to extreme pressure by uterine contractions and passage through the birth canal, so it is important to ascertain that the FHR remains within normal limits despite these pressures.

Auscultation of Fetal Heart Sounds

Fetal heart sounds are transmitted best through the convex portion of a fetus, because that is the part that lies in closest contact with the uterine wall. This means that in a vertex or breech presentation, fetal heart sounds are usually best heard through the fetal back; in a face presentation, the back becomes concave so the sounds are best heard through the more convex thorax. In breech presentations, fetal heart

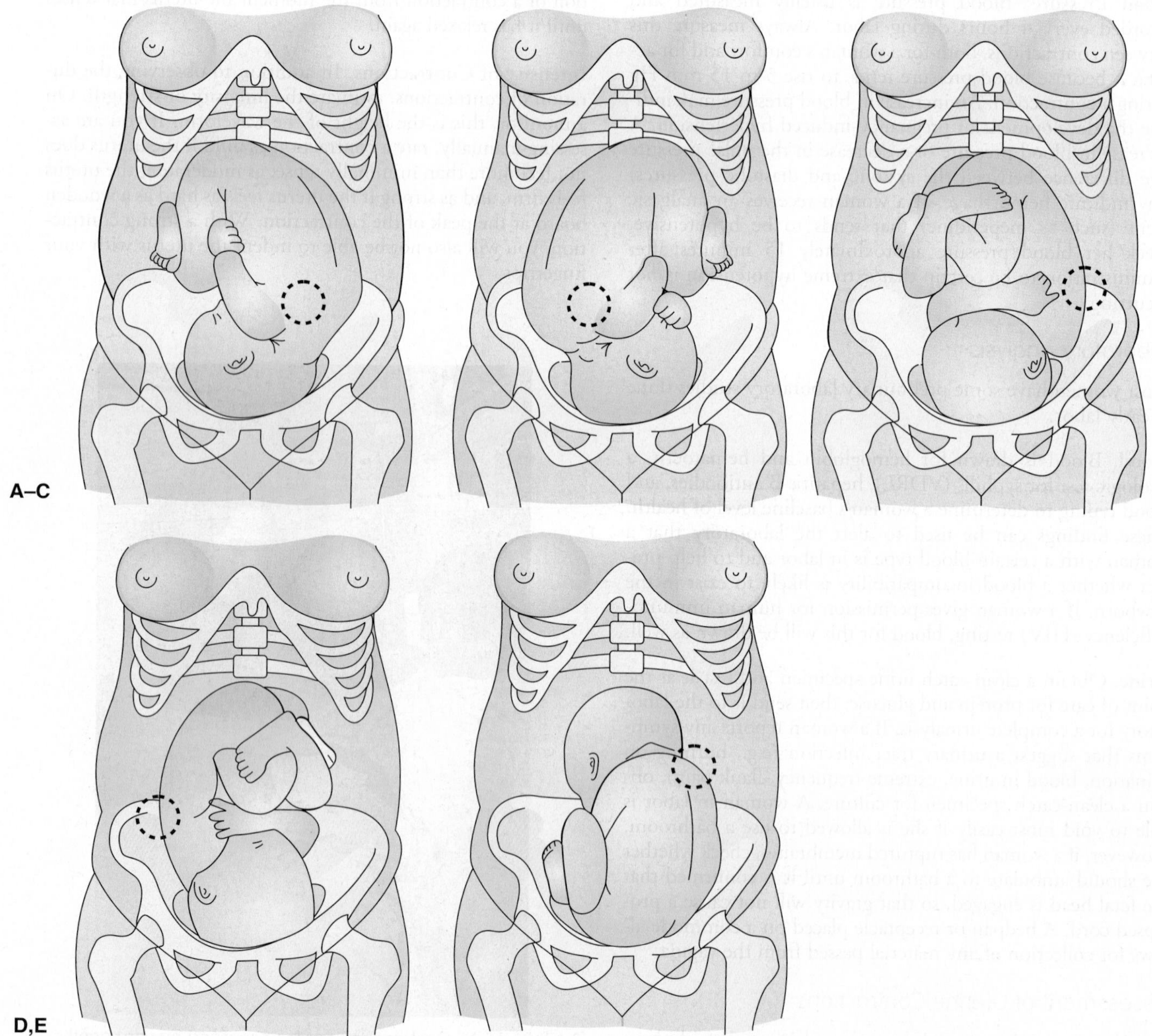

FIGURE 15.16 Locating fetal heart sounds by fetal position. (**A**) LOA. (**B**) ROA. (**C**) LOP. (**D**) ROP. (**E**) LSA.

sounds are heard most clearly high in the uterus, at a woman's umbilicus or above. In cephalic presentations, they are heard loudest low in the abdomen. In an ROA position, the sounds are heard best in the right lower quadrant; in an LOA position, in the left lower quadrant. In posterior positions (LOP or ROP), heart sounds are loudest at a woman's side. Figure 15.16 shows how to locate heart sounds for various fetal positions.

Hearing fetal heart sounds in these positions provides confirmatory information about fetal position. Conversely, recognizing fetal position aids in locating fetal heart sounds.

Determine the FHR every 30 minutes during beginning labor, every 15 minutes during active labor, and every 5 minutes during the second stage of labor. This can be done by viewing the FHR monitoring strip or by periodic auscultation.

To auscultate fetal heart sounds, use either a stethoscope or a fetoscope (a modified stethoscope attached to a headpiece), or obtain them with a Doppler unit, which uses ultrasound waves that bounce off the fetal heart to produce echoes or clicking noises (Fig. 15.17). Each click reflects the fetal heartbeat.

Electronic Monitoring

In most settings, FHR is screened at least for a short time in early labor by an external electronic monitoring system. The monitor is left in place for continuous monitoring on women who are categorized as high risk for any reason or who have oxytocin stimulation.

The use of fetal monitors has provoked one of the biggest controversies in modern obstetric health care. Monitors were widely adopted in the mid-1970s as a means of immediately detecting variations in FHR. However, prepared childbirth advocates have long criticized the overuse of monitoring devices, arguing that they intrude on the childbirth experience, causing needless discomfort and distraction to the mother. The medical profession readily admits that monitors contribute to the growing number of cesarean births (National Center for Health Statistics, 2009). Advocates of monitoring would say that the prevention of complications in even one baby is worth this increase. However, others believe that monitors often point to a problem where none exists, resulting in unnecessary cesarean births (which carries its own set of risks) and unnecessary frightening of parents (which could adversely affect early parent–infant bonding).

Monitoring does offer many advantages from a health care provider's standpoint. Observing the FHR on a monitor is easier than listening with a stethoscope, fetoscope, or Doppler. In addition, most health care providers have grown accustomed to monitors and may feel insecure without them. Few people advocate a return to the use of stethoscopes for total assessment; use of monitors for periodic assessment rather than continuous monitoring is a compromise solution.

Be certain to tell parents that the FHR can vary greatly during labor and that the monitor is only an aid and should not be the focus of their attention. Parents can become so focused on what is happening on the monitor that they can lose the ability to concentrate on previously learned relaxation and breathing techniques.

External Electronic Monitoring

External electronic monitoring is useful for monitoring both uterine contractions and FHR continuously or intermittently. The information is obtained from sensors strapped to the woman's abdomen (Fig. 15.18).

Contractions are monitored by means of a pressure transducer or tocodynamometer (*toko* is the Greek word for "contraction"). Place the transducer over the uterine fundus or the area of greatest contractility. Verify that it is securely held in

A

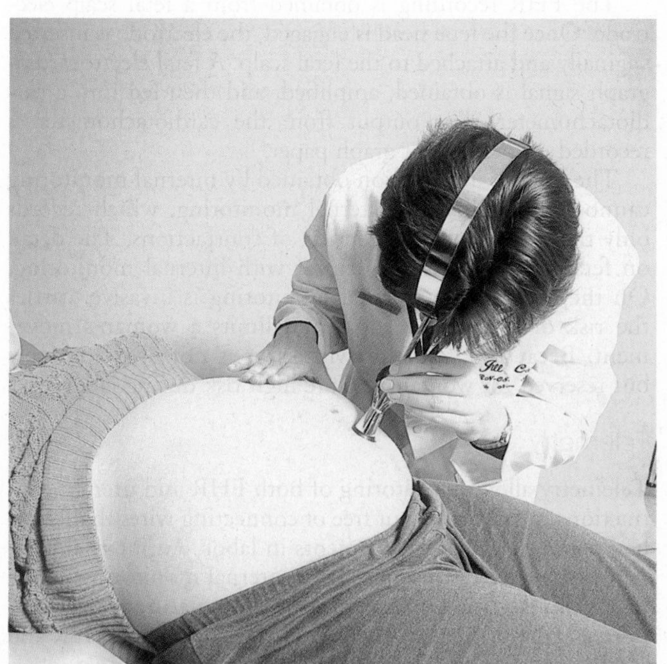

B

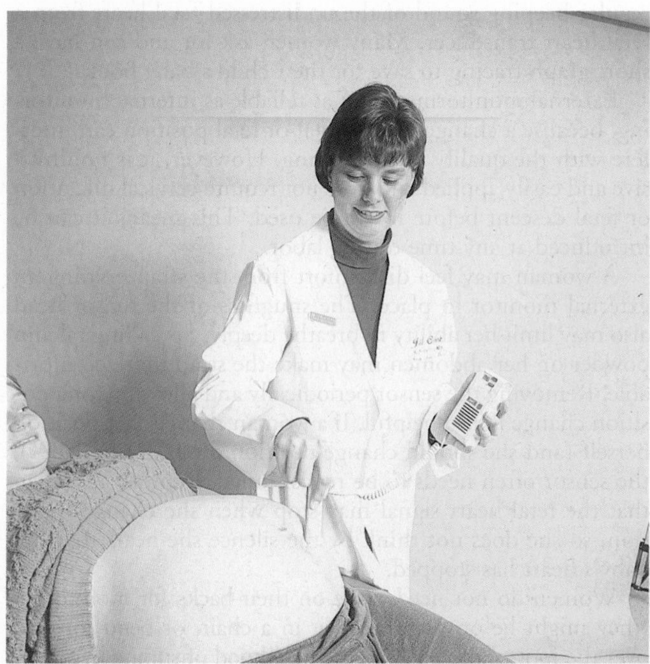

FIGURE 15.17 (**A**) Auscultation of the fetal heartbeat using a fetoscope. (**B**) A Doppler ultrasound device can be used to monitor fetal heart rate intermittently in low-risk labor. (Photographs by Keith Cotton.)

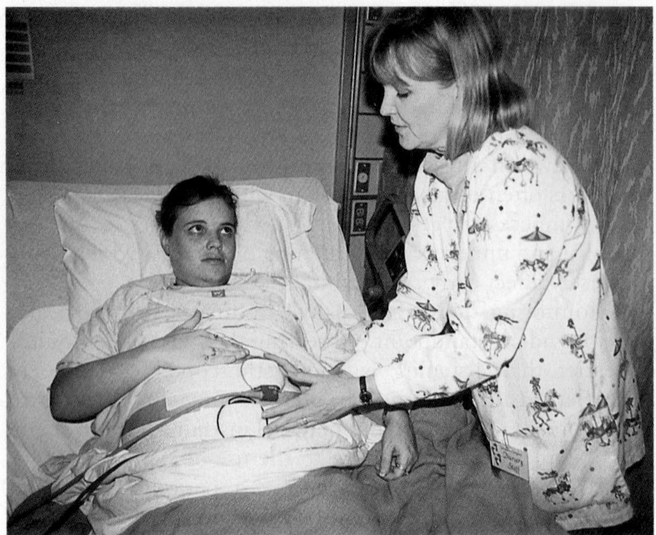

FIGURE 15.18 External electronic monitoring in place. Two devices (a transducer for the uterus and an ultrasound sensor for the fetus) are strapped to the woman's abdomen. (© Caroline Brown, RNC, MS, DEd.)

place by an adjustable strap or stockinette girdle (Fig. 15.19A). The transducer converts the pressure registered by the contraction into an electronic signal that is recorded on graph paper. These may be difficult to apply to morbidly obese women and the readings may not be as accurate (Euliano et al., 2007).

The FHR is monitored with the use of an ultrasonic sensor or monitor (see Fig. 15.19A), also strapped against a woman's abdomen at the level of the fetal chest. The small Doppler unit converts fetal heart movements into audible beeping sounds and also records them on graph paper.

A woman who is worried that something will happen to her child during labor can find it reassuring to listen to the regular beeping sound of the undistressed fetal heart from a fetal heart transducer. Many women ask for and can have a short graph tracing to save for their child's baby book.

External monitoring is not as reliable as internal monitoring, because a change in maternal or fetal position can interfere with the quality of the tracing. However, it is noninvasive and easily applied and does not require cervical dilatation or fetal descent before it can be used. This means it can be introduced at any time during labor.

A woman may feel discomfort from the strap holding an external monitor in place. The snugness of the sensor head also may limit her ability to breathe deeply. Spreading talcum powder on her abdomen may make the strap more comfortable. Removing the sensor periodically and allowing for a position change is also helpful. If a woman changes her position herself (and she should change position often during labor), the sensor often needs to be repositioned. Remind a woman that the fetal heart signal may stop when she changes position, so she does not think by the silence she hears that her baby's heart has stopped.

Women do not need to lie on their backs for monitoring (they might lie on their side, sit in a chair, or bend forward over the foot of the bed), so the likelihood of supine hypotension syndrome is not increased. When giving care, be sure not to focus solely on the equipment; continue to communicate and offer support to the woman and her partner as needed. Although not well studied, if a fetus shows an unresponsive heartbeat during labor, vibroacoustic stimulation can be used the same as is done for nonstress tests during pregnancy to be certain that a fetus is responding well (East et al., 2009).

What if... You enter Celeste Bailey's room while she has an electronic monitor in place and discover that she is lying on her back, seemingly frozen in one position? Would you urge her to turn or let her lie in that position because the monitor strip is recording so well?

Internal Electronic Monitoring

Internal electronic monitoring is the most precise method for assessing FHR and uterine contractions. A pressure-sensing catheter is passed through the vagina, into the uterine cavity, and alongside the fetus, after the membranes have ruptured and the cervix has dilated to at least 3 cm (see Fig. 15.19B). The end of the catheter extending from the vagina is attached to a pressure recorder. As each contraction puts pressure on the uterine contents, the pressure exerted on the catheter is recorded. When uterine contractions are monitored by an internal pressure gauge in this way, the frequency, duration, baseline strength, and peak strength of contractions can all be evaluated. Strength of contractions is evaluated by the height of the peak of the contraction on the tracing. Equally important to evaluate is the return of the uterine tone to baseline strength between contractions. This ensures placental filling between contractions.

With contractions during the latent phase, the baseline level is usually less than 5 mm Hg; with active contractions, it is about 12 mm Hg. During the second stage of labor, the baseline may be as high as 20 mm Hg. Baseline readings that do not return to 20 mm Hg or less suggest uterine hypertonia and a possible compromise of fetal well-being.

The FHR recording is obtained from a fetal scalp electrode. Once the fetal head is engaged, the electrode is inserted vaginally and attached to the fetal scalp. A fetal electrocardiograph signal is obtained, amplified, and then fed into a cardiotachometer. The output from the cardiotachometer is recorded on permanent graph paper.

The level of information obtained by internal monitoring cannot be matched by external monitoring, which records only the frequency and duration of contractions. The detail on fetal heartbeats is also clearer with internal monitoring. On the other hand, internal monitoring is invasive, carries the risk of uterine infection, and limits a woman's movement. Because of these drawbacks, it is not used routinely but reserved for women who are high risk during labor.

Telemetry

Telemetry allows monitoring of both FHR and uterine contractions to be carried out free of connecting wires that could hamper the woman's movements in labor. An internal pressure uterine lead is inserted, as in internal monitoring, and a fetal scalp electrode is also attached. A miniature radio transmitter is then placed in the vagina to transmit the FHR and uterine contraction signals to a distant monitor.

Nurses and physicians view the distant monitor located at a nursing station to track fetal status instead of visiting

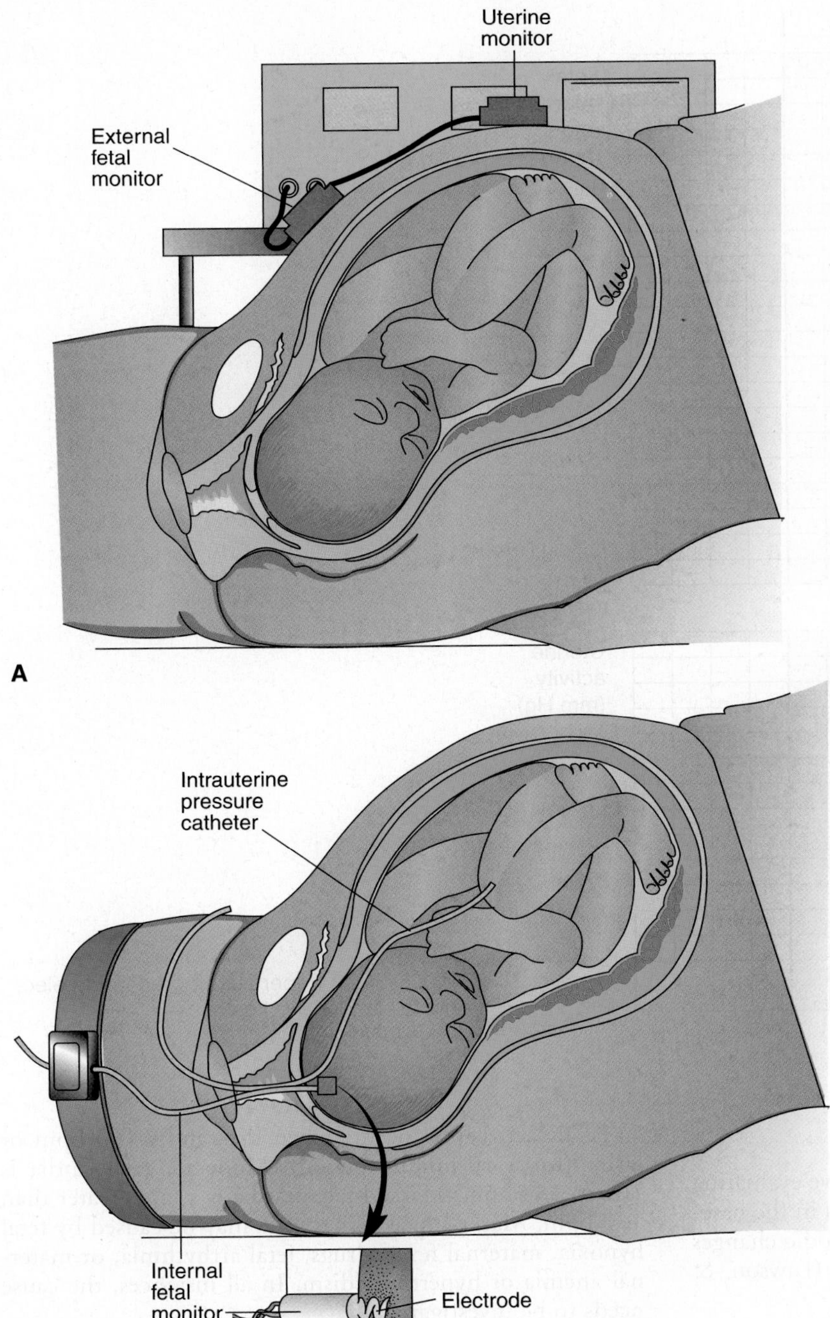

FIGURE 15.19 Placement of electronic monitoring leads. (**A**) External leads to monitor for FHR and uterine contractions. (**B**) An internal fetal heart rate lead in place on the fetal scalp. Uterine contractions are monitored by the intrauterine catheter.

individual birthing rooms. The major advantage of telemetry is that it allows a woman to ambulate while being internally monitored. Although central monitoring of this type has been used effectively in intensive care units for years and has the advantage of saving footsteps, because it reduces bedside contact, a worry is that its use can isolate laboring women, fragment their care, and reduce supportive care during labor. It also does not appear to make a difference in the cesarean birth rate or newborn outcomes (Devoe, 2008). Because it is more expensive than other equipment, not all birth settings have telemetry capability.

FETAL HEART RATE AND UTERINE CONTRACTION RECORDS

Labor monitors trace both the FHR and the duration and interval of uterine contractions onto an oscilloscope screen and produce a permanent record on paper rolls (Fig. 15.20). Uterine contraction information is recorded on the bottom half of the paper, FHR on the top half. Time can be calculated by counting the number of bold vertical lines on the paper (the space between two bold lines represents 60 seconds).

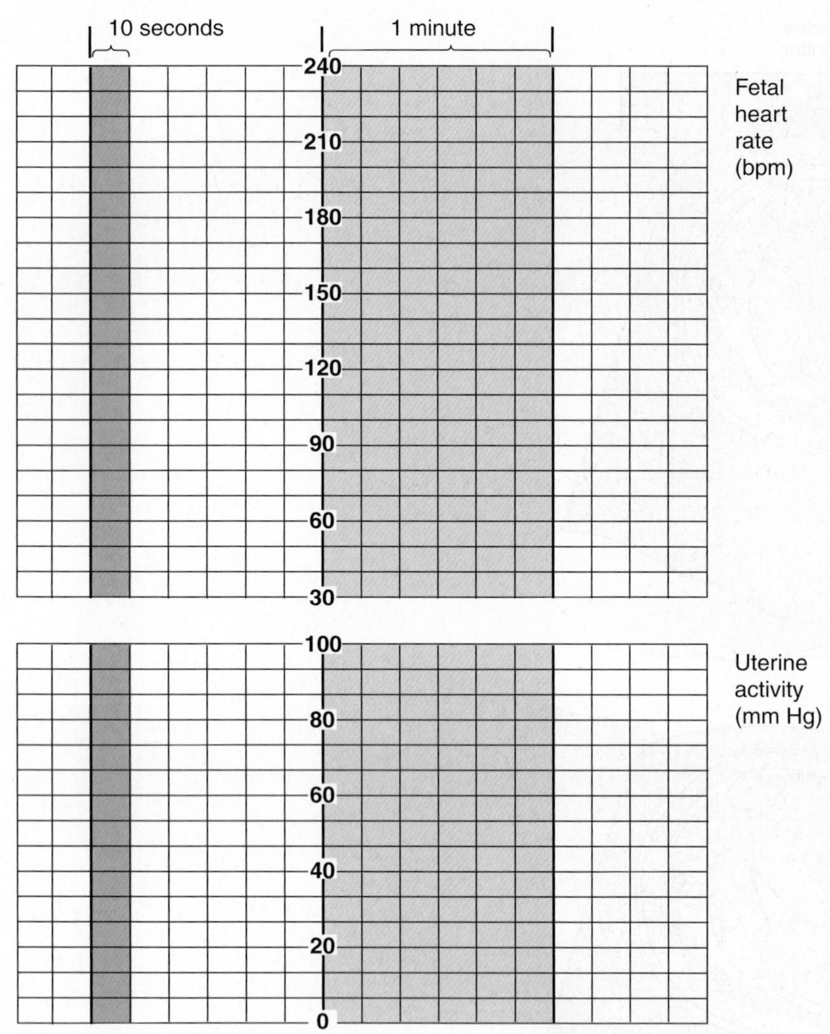

FIGURE 15.20 Paper strip for recording electronic fetal monitoring data.

Fetal Heart Rate Patterns

Assessing and interpreting FHR patterns involve evaluating three parameters: the baseline rate, variabilities in the baseline rate (long term and short term), and periodic changes in the rate (acceleration and deceleration) (Lawson & Bienstock, 2007).

Baseline Fetal Heart Rate

A baseline FHR is determined by analyzing the range of fetal heartbeats recorded on a 10-minute tracing that was obtained between contractions. A normal rate is 120 to 160 bpm. The rate fluctuates slightly (5 to 15 bpm) when a fetus moves or sleeps. If an increase or decrease occurs and is sustained for a 10-minute period, then a new baseline or a baseline change is established. Abnormal patterns in the baseline rate include fetal bradycardia and fetal tachycardia.

Fetal bradycardia occurs when the FHR is lower than 120 bpm for 10 minutes. A moderate bradycardia of 100 to 119 bpm is not considered serious and is probably because of a vagal response elicited by compression of the fetal head during labor. Marked bradycardia (less than 100 bpm) is a sign of possible hypoxia and is potentially dangerous.

Fetal tachycardia occurs when the rate is 160 bpm or faster (for a 10-minute period). Moderate tachycardia is 161 to 180 bpm. Marked tachycardia is a rate greater than 180 bpm. Marked fetal tachycardia may be caused by fetal hypoxia, maternal fever, drugs, fetal arrhythmia, or maternal anemia or hyperthyroidism. In all instances, the cause needs to be investigated.

Variability

FHR variability is one of the most reliable indicators of fetal well-being. Baseline variability is the variation or differing rhythmicity in the heart rate over time and is reflected on the FHR tracing as a slight irregularity or "jitter" to the wave. The degree of baseline variability increases when the fetus is stimulated and slows when the fetus sleeps. If no variability is present, it indicates that the natural pacemaker activity of the fetal heart (effects of the sympathetic and parasympathetic nervous systems) has been affected. This may occur as a response to narcotics or barbiturates administered to a woman in labor, but the possibility of fetal hypoxia and acidosis must be investigated. Very immature fetuses show diminished baseline variability because of reduced nervous system response to stimulation and immature cardiac node function.

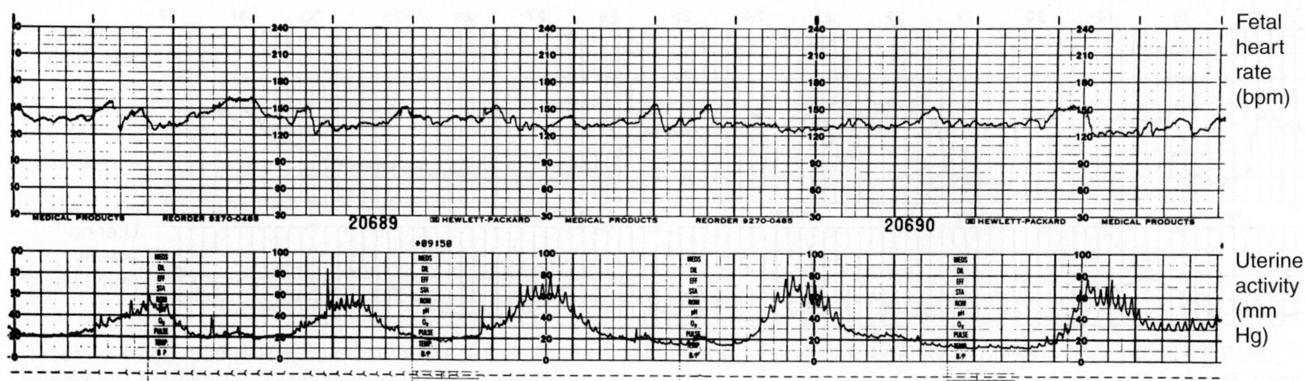

FIGURE 15.21 Fetal monitoring strip showing both long-term and short-term (beat-to-beat) variability.

Baseline variability is defined as being either long term or short term (beat-to-beat) (Fig. 15.21). Long-term variability is seen on a broad view of the recording and results from fluctuations in the FHR, of 6 to 10 bpm, that occur 3 to 10 times per minute. Short-term or beat-to-beat variability refers to the difference between successive heartbeats, usually about 3 to 5 bpm. These changes are very subtle and can be picked up only with internal electronic monitoring. Beat-to-beat variability can be rated as "present," "decreased," or "absent." Decreasing variability indicates the development of fetal distress. Absent variability is considered a severe sign, indicating that serious fetal compromise must be present.

Periodic Changes

Periodic changes or fluctuations in FHR occur in response to contractions and fetal movement and are described in terms of accelerations or decelerations. Periodic changes are short-term changes in rate rather than baseline; they last from a few seconds to 1 or 2 minutes. Four such responses are acceleration, early deceleration, late deceleration, and variable deceleration.

Accelerations. Nonperiodic accelerations are temporary normal increases in FHR caused by fetal movement, a change in maternal position, or administration of an analgesic. They are innocent findings.

Early Decelerations. Early decelerations are normal periodic decreases in FHR resulting from pressure on the fetal head during contractions. Parasympathetic stimulation in response to vagal nerve compression brings about a slowing of FHR. Early deceleration follows the pattern of the contraction, beginning when the contraction begins and ending when the contraction ends. However, the waveform of the FHR change is the inverse of the contraction waveform, with the lowest point of the deceleration occurring with the peak of the contraction. In this way, it serves as a mirror image of the contraction. The rate rarely falls below 100 bpm, and it returns quickly to between 120 and 160 beats at the end of the contraction (Fig. 15.22).

Early decelerations normally occur late in labor, when the head has descended fairly low. As such, they are viewed as a normal pattern. However, if they occur early in labor, before the head has fully descended, the head compression causing the waveform change could be the result of cephalopelvic disproportion and is a cause to investigate.

Late Decelerations. Late decelerations are those that are delayed until 30 to 40 seconds after the onset of a contraction

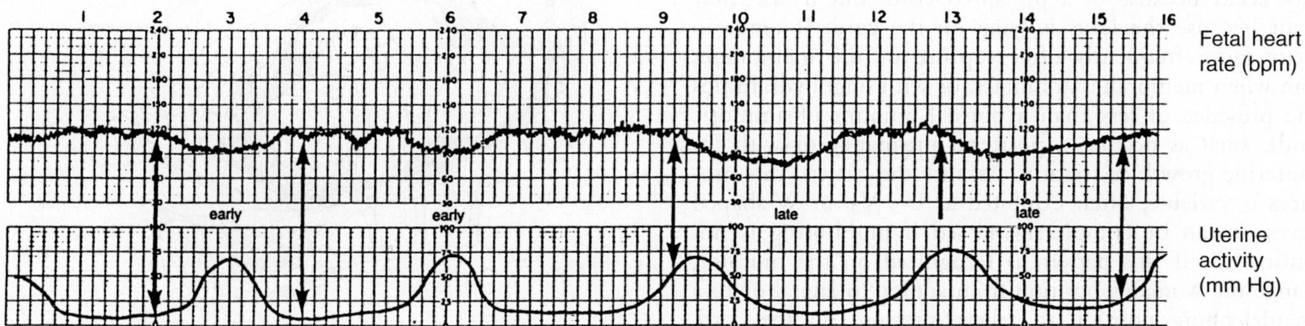

FIGURE 15.22 Schematic drawing of periodic FHR changes. Although the shape and depth of early and late decelerations are similar, note the differences in the onset of the decelerations and the recovery time to the baseline rate.

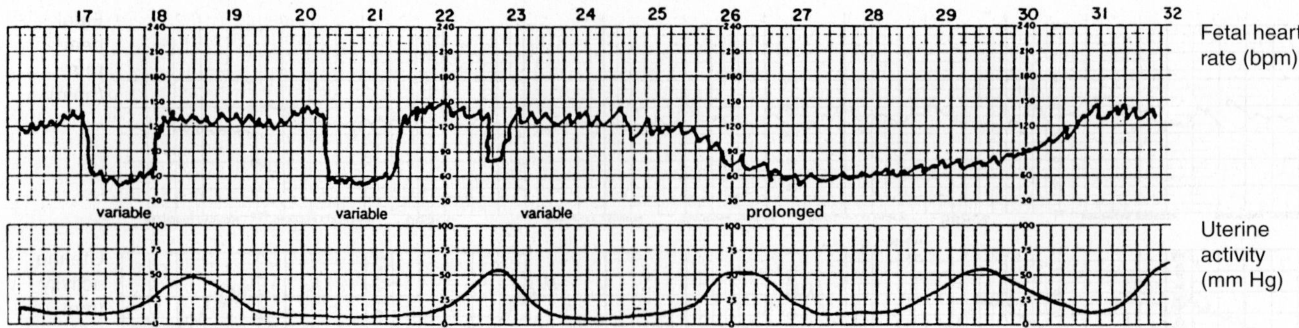

FIGURE 15.23 Schematic drawing of variable and prolonged decelerations. Note the abrupt drop in FHR in both types of decelerations. The variable decelerations return to baseline more quickly than the prolonged deceleration at 26–31 minutes, however.

and continue beyond the end of a contraction (see Fig. 15.22). This is an ominous pattern in labor, because it suggests uteroplacental insufficiency or decreased blood flow through the intervillous spaces of the uterus during uterine contractions. The lowest point of the deceleration (nadir) occurs near the end of the contraction instead of at its peak. This pattern may occur with marked hypertonia or increased uterine tone caused by the administration of oxytocin. Immediate steps to correct the situation must be initiated. If oxytocin is being used, stop or slow the rate of administration. Change the woman's position from supine to lateral (to relieve pressure on the vena cava and supply more blood to the uterus and fetus). Administer intravenous fluids or oxygen as prescribed. Prepare for possible prompt birth of the infant if the late decelerations persist or if FHR variability becomes abnormal (absent or decreased).

Prolonged Decelerations. Prolonged decelerations are decelerations that last longer than 2 to 3 minutes but less than 10 minutes. They generally reflect an isolated occurrence, but they may signify a significant event, such as cord compression or maternal hypotension. For this reason, they must be reported and documented.

Variable Decelerations. The pattern of variable decelerations refers to decelerations that occur at unpredictable times in relation to contractions. They indicate compression of the cord, which can be an ominous development in terms of fetal well-being (Fig. 15.23). Cord compression may occur because of a prolapsed cord, but it also may occur because the fetus is lying on the cord. It tends to occur more frequently after rupture of the membranes than when membranes are intact, or with oligohydramnios (the presence of less than a normal amount of amniotic fluid), such as occurs in postterm pregnancy or with intrauterine growth restriction. Because the pattern this produces is variable, often exhibited as U-, V-, or W-shaped waves, it can be completely missed if monitoring is not continuous. If this pattern is recognized on the monitor, change the woman's position from supine to lateral or to a Trendelenburg position to relieve pressure on the cord. Administer fluids and oxygen as prescribed. If variable decelerations are not relieved by these measures, amnioinfusion (addition of a sterile fluid into the uterus to supplement the amniotic fluid) may be prescribed to lift the uterine wall away from the cord (see Chapter 23).

Sinusoidal Fetal Heart Rate Pattern

In a fetus who is severely anemic or hypoxic, central nervous system control of heart pacing may be so impaired that the FHR pattern resembles a frequently undulating wave. Long-term variability consists of 5 to 15 bpm every 3 to 5 minutes; beat-to-beat variability is minimal or absent; and there is a lack of specific responses to contractions. Although the cause of this pattern is poorly understood, it is recognized to be as ominous as a late deceleration or variable deceleration pattern.

Other Assessment Techniques

Scalp Stimulation

If FHR variability is depressed, the welfare of a fetus can be further assessed by scalp stimulation. This is done by applying pressure with the fingers to the fetal scalp through the dilated cervix (Fig. 15.24). This causes a tactile response in

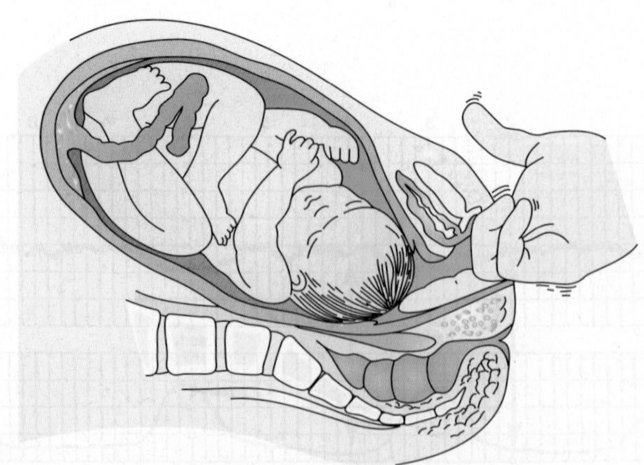

FIGURE 15.24 Technique for scalp stimulation. (Redrawn from *Journal of Perinatal and Neonatal Nursing, (1)*16; with permission from Aspen Publishers, Inc.)

the fetus that momentarily increases the FHR. If the fetus is in distress and becoming acidotic, FHR acceleration will not occur. Scalp stimulation, therefore, is an assessment of acid–base balance in a fetus.

Fetal Oxygen Saturation Level

Fetal oxygen saturation may be measured by an oxygen saturation sensor that is introduced into the uterus and placed beside the fetus's cheek after membranes have ruptured. Although oxygen saturation may be important to measure in some women, it is generally reserved for women who have an internal contraction or fetal monitor already in place (Potera, 2007).

Fetal Blood Sampling

Monitoring of the fetal blood composition may reveal hypoxia in a fetus before it becomes apparent on an electrocardiogram or external monitoring system. As this is invasive, it is reserved only for a fetus at high risk (see Chapter 23).

✓ Checkpoint Question 15.4

You assess Celeste Bailey's uterine contractions. In relation to a contraction, when does a late deceleration begin?

a. Forty-five seconds after the contraction is over.
b. Thirty seconds after the start of a contraction.
c. After every 10th or more contraction.
d. Totally unrelated to a contraction.

CARE OF A WOMAN DURING THE FIRST STAGE OF LABOR

Labor is a natural process and nurses can be instrumental in keeping labor as free of unnecessary interventions as possible (Sleutel, Schultz, & Wyble, 2007). Six major concepts to make labor and birth as natural as possible are:

1. Labor should begin on its own, not be artificially induced.
2. Women should be able to move about freely throughout labor, not be confined to bed.
3. Women should receive continuous support during labor.
4. No interventions such as intravenous fluid should be used routinely.
5. Women should be allowed to assume a nonsupine (e.g., upright, side-lying) position for birth.
6. Mother and baby should be together after the birth, with unlimited opportunity for breastfeeding (Amis & Green, 2007).

The first stage of labor begins with the beginning of uterine contractions and ends when the cervix has reached full dilatation. Most women have had labor contractions for hours before they arrive at a birthing center, because they deliberately stay at home until they are well into the first stage. This means that most likely, they have been experiencing pain and relying on their own judgment that everything is going well for a long time. One of their chief needs when they arrive at a birthing center, therefore, is to be reassured that everything is going well. For a woman who has been unable to manage pain by breathing exercises, pain relief may be her priority need.

Nursing Diagnoses and Related Interventions

Nursing Diagnosis: Powerlessness related to duration of labor

Outcome Evaluation: Client expresses preferences for position and techniques to control pain; asks questions about her progress and states feelings about what is happening.

Care during the first stage of labor centers on helping a woman feel confident in her ability to control the pain and progress of labor and maintain physiologic stability. At first, it is exciting for a woman to feel labor contractions. They are little more than menstrual cramps and project a "this-is-really-happening" sensation. Soon, however, if a woman is not concentrating on controlled breathing exercises, the contractions become biting in their intensity. Despite the fact that she is becoming more and more uncomfortable, however, nothing seems to be happening. A couple can begin to worry that something is going wrong; they may think that because the 9 months are over, victory is near, yet it is eluding them. Give couples frequent progress reports during labor so they do not become discouraged or fearful at this seeming lack of progress (Box 15.8).

BOX 15.8 ✻ Focus on Communication

Celeste Bailey's baby is in an occipitoposterior position, so she has had extensive back pain since labor began.

Less Effective Communication

Nurse: You don't look very comfortable, Celeste. Would you feel better if you sat in the rocking chair rather than stay in bed?
Celeste: Can I do that?
Nurse: I told you on admission. You can do whatever is most comfortable for you.
Celeste: Can I walk over to the window?
Nurse: I told you on admission. Do whatever is most comfortable for you.
Celeste: I guess I'm not being a very good patient.

More Effective Communication

Nurse: You don't look very comfortable, Celeste. Would you feel better if you sat in the rocking chair rather than stay in bed?
Celeste: Can I do that?
Nurse: You can use any position that is comfortable for you.
Celeste: Can I walk over to the window?
Nurse: Whatever is most comfortable for you.
Celeste: Thank you. You're very understanding.

Women in labor may be enduring so much pain and are under so much stress they do not "hear" or process instructions well. Reminding them that they have not processed information well is not therapeutic, because it can lower their self-esteem and sense of self-control.

A woman needs to feel that she has some control over her situation during labor to face this big event in her life. Most women accomplish this by stating their preferences, breathing with contractions, and changing their position to the one that makes them most comfortable. In contrast, some women handle the stress of labor by becoming extremely quiet and passive. Others feel most comfortable when they can show their emotions by shouting or crying. Help a woman express her feelings in her own way, one that works the best for her.

Respect Contraction Time. Do not interrupt a woman who is in the middle of breathing exercises during labor because, once her concentration is disrupted, she will feel the extent of the contraction. If she has been successfully using breathing exercises to reduce pain, suddenly feeling the full force of a contraction can be frightening. She tenses, the pain becomes worse, and she may doubt her ability to breathe constructively in the face of such sharp pain with the next contraction. Instead of interrupting, allow her to finish breathing with her contraction, then ask questions or announce what procedure needs to be done next, or ask the question but wait patiently for the answer. (See Chapter 16 for a discussion of pain management techniques during labor.)

Promote Change of Positions. Because the bed is the main piece of furniture in a birthing room, many women assume that they are expected to lie quietly in bed during labor. In early labor, however, a woman may be out of bed walking or sitting up in bed or in a chair, kneeling, squatting, or in whatever position she prefers (Fig. 15.25). Reassure a woman that she may move about as she wants.

A woman whose membranes have ruptured should lie on her side until a fetal monitor shows good baseline variability and no variable decelerations or until she has been checked by a physician or nurse-midwife, because, unless the head of the fetus is well engaged (firmly fitting into the pelvic inlet), the umbilical cord may prolapse into the vagina if she walks.

If medication such as a narcotic is given, educate a woman to remain in bed for approximately 15 minutes afterward to avoid a fall if she should become dizzy from the medication. While a woman is in bed, encourage her to lie on her side, preferably the left side. This position causes the heavy uterus to tip forward, away from the vena cava, allowing free blood return from the lower extremities and adequate placental filling and circulation. Most women are comfortable in this position and adjust to it readily. Position the chair for the support person facing the laboring woman. Otherwise, she will keep turning to her back to talk.

Some women have learned to do breathing exercises in a supine position and may need additional coaching to do them in a side-lying position. If a woman must turn to her back during a contraction to make her breathing exercises effective, help her to remember to return to her side between contractions. A squatting position is very effective for birth because it helps to align the fetal presenting part with the cervix and also uses the fetal weight to help bring about cervical dilatation.

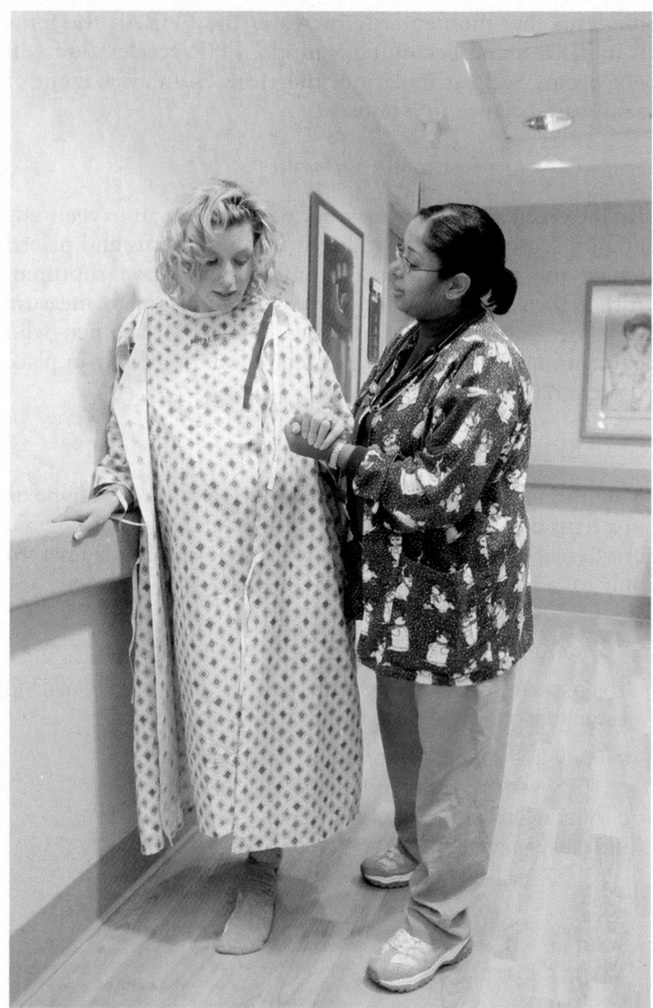

FIGURE 15.25 Finding a comfortable position during early labor is important. Here, a nurse assists a woman with walking during labor.

Promote Voiding and Provide Bladder Care. A full bladder or bowel can impede fetal descent, so encourage a woman to void, if possible, at least every 2 to 4 hours. The way a full bladder can impede descent of a fetus is illustrated in Figure 15.26. You need to remind a woman to void during labor, because she may mistakenly interpret the discomfort of a full bladder as part of the sensations of labor. Assess for a full bladder by percussion (an empty bladder sounds dull; a full one sounds resonant). If she cannot void and the bladder becomes distended, she may need to be catheterized. Catheterizing a woman in labor is uncomfortable for her and difficult for you: the vulva is edematous from the pressure of the fetal presenting part, stretching the urethral canal downward and making the urethra difficult to locate. For best results, use a small catheter (no. 12F–14F), and insert it between contractions. Use extremely careful aseptic technique

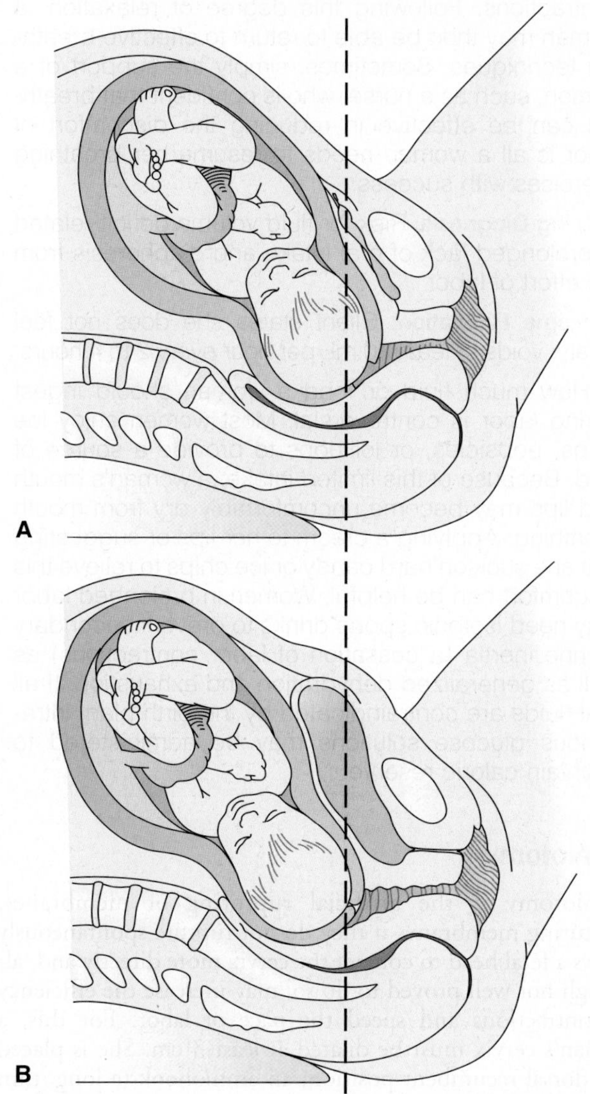

FIGURE 15.26 Effect of a full bladder on fetal descent. (**A**) Bladder is empty. (**B**) A full bladder impedes fetal progress.

to avoid introducing any microorganisms that might then result in a urinary tract infection.

Nursing Diagnosis: Risk for ineffective breathing pattern related to breathing exercises

Outcome Evaluation: Client's respiratory rate is within normal limits; skin is normal color, cool, and dry. No reports of lightheadedness or tingling/numbness in extremities.

Hyperventilation (an accelerated rate of respiration) occurs when a woman exhales more deeply than she inhales. As a result, extra carbon dioxide is blown off and respiratory alkalosis results. This can occur when a woman is practicing breathing exercises in preparation for labor, but it is most apt to occur during actual labor. The woman feels lightheaded and may have tingling or numbness in her toes and fingertips. If allowed to progress, hyperventilation can lead to coma.

To halt hyperventilation, urge a woman to keep a paper bag nearby when doing breathing exercises. Breathing in and out into the paper bag causes her to rebreathe the carbon dioxide she has exhaled, replacing the carbon dioxide lost. If a paper bag is unavailable, she can use her cupped hands instead.

The best way to handle hyperventilation is to prevent it. Be certain when a woman is breathing rapidly that she is not hyperventilating and that she ends all breathing sessions with a long cleansing breath to help restore carbon dioxide balance.

Nursing Diagnosis: Anxiety related to stress of labor

Outcome Evaluation: Client states she feels in control of her situation; she and her support person express confidence in themselves and in health care personnel.

Labor is such an intense process that it creates a high level of emotional stress for both a woman and her support person. Ability to tolerate stress (to cope adequately) depends on a person's perception of the event, the support people available, and past experience in using coping mechanisms. Ways to reduce stress in labor, therefore, center on helping a woman to perceive labor clearly and providing the opportunity for her partner to provide support.

Offer Support. There is no substitute for personal touch and contact as a way to provide support during labor. Patting a woman's arm while telling her that she is progressing in labor, brushing a wisp of hair off her forehead, wiping her forehead with a cool cloth—these are indispensable methods of conveying concern. This caring attitude has several benefits. First, it may make the difference in helping a woman feel safe and able to continue in control. In addition, a woman who is touched, who experiences the warmth and friendliness of human contact during labor—a time when she is physically dependent—may handle her newborn (who is also physically dependent and undergoing an adjustment not unlike the one she has just gone through) more warmly and affectionately. On the other hand, not all women care for physical contact during labor, as enjoyment of touch is culturally determined.

Respect and Promote the Support Person. Admit a woman's support person to the birthing area and allow him or her to remain with a woman throughout the birth. Having someone with her during labor is important, because everything is new and unexpected. Acquaint the woman and her support person with the physical facilities, and point out where supplies such as towels, washcloths, and ice chips are stored, so the support person can get them when necessary. Review procedures and reassure the support person early in labor that he or she is welcome there. Also, be sure that all health care personnel are aware of who the support person is and make him or her feel welcome.

Often the support person will be acting as a labor coach. Ask both the woman and the support person whether they have been to prepared childbirth classes and whether the support person plans to help the woman with her breathing. If so, support this person's

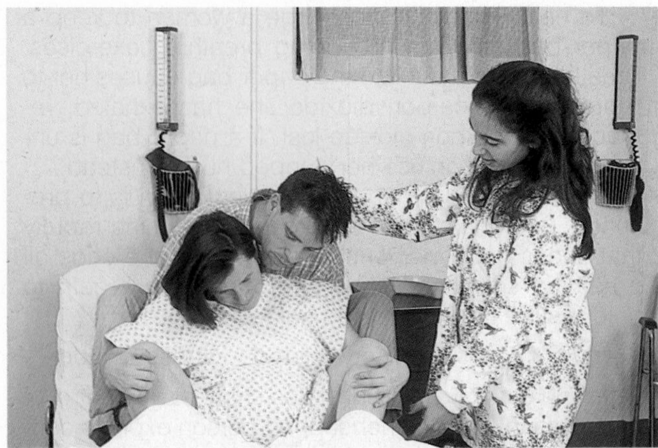

FIGURE 15.27 Encouraging a support person, so he can continue to give support, is an important nursing role. (© Barbara Proud.)

role. If he or she is hesitant, it is better to review techniques than to take over. Offer praise not only for the woman but for the support person as well because watching a birth is apt to be as totally a new experience for this person as for the mother (Rosich-Medina & Shetty, 2007). Relieve the support person as necessary, so that he or she can take a break and get something to eat or visit with older children (Fig. 15.27). If older children will view the birth, be certain that they are oriented and have a child care provider.

In addition to having the father of their baby present, many women choose a doula or another woman to be with them in labor. This is because fathers may find it hard to provide doula-type support during labor because of their own emotional involvement in the birth. Having such a person present frees the father to enjoy the birth rather than feel occupied with coaching instructions. Although research in the subject is not extensive, there are suggestions that rates of oxytocin augmentation, epidural anesthesia, and cesarean birth can be reduced by doula support (McGrath & Kennell, 2008).

What if... A doula and Celeste Bailey's mother disagree on whether Celeste needs additional medication for pain while in labor? Whose suggestion would you pay most attention to? How could you resolve the issue?

Support a Woman's Pain Management Needs. Many women plan on using nonpharmacologic pain relief measures such as aromatherapy during labor; ask what the woman has planned and what your role should be (Burns et al., 2007). Some women believe that using a prepared childbirth method will create a pain-free, effortless labor. When this does not happen, they may panic and lose the ability to use prepared breathing. Some support people are more nervous than they anticipated and have difficulty being supportive, leaving the woman to manage her anxiety on her own. In these instances, accepting an analgesic might be a way to reduce anxiety or take the edge off contractions. Following this degree of relaxation, a woman may then be able to return to effective breathing techniques. Sometimes, simply the support of a person, such as a nurse, who is confident that breathing can be effective in reducing the discomfort of labor is all a woman needs to resume her breathing exercises with success.

Nursing Diagnosis: Risk for fluid volume deficit related to prolonged lack of oral intake and diaphoresis from the effort of labor

Outcome Evaluation: Client states she does not feel thirsty; voids at least 30 mL per hour every 2 to 4 hours.

How much fluid or food a woman should ingest during labor is controversial. Most women enjoy ice chips, popsicles, or lollipops to provide a source of fluid. Because of this limited intake, a woman's mouth and lips may become uncomfortably dry from mouth breathing. Applying a cream to her lips or suggesting that she suck on hard candy or ice chips to relieve this discomfort can be helpful. Women in prolonged labor may need isotonic sports drinks to prevent secondary uterine inertia (a cessation of labor contractions) as well as generalized dehydration and exhaustion. If all oral fluids are contraindicated by the birth plan, intravenous glucose solutions may be administered to maintain caloric reserve.

Amniotomy

Amniotomy is the artificial rupturing of membranes. Rupturing membranes if they do not rupture spontaneously allows a fetal head to contact the cervix more directly and, although not well proved to do so, may increase the efficiency of contractions and speed the pace of labor. For this, a woman's cervix must be dilated at least 3 cm. She is placed in a dorsal recumbent position; an amniohook (a long, thin instrument) or a hemostat is passed vaginally. The membranes are torn, and amniotic fluid is allowed to escape. This puts a fetus momentarily at risk for cord prolapse, because there is a possibility that a loop of cord will escape with the fluid. Always measure the FHR immediately after the rupture of membranes to determine that this did not happen (Szymanski & Bienstock, 2007).

CARE OF A WOMAN DURING THE SECOND STAGE OF LABOR

The second stage of labor is the time from full cervical dilatation to birth of the newborn. Even women who have taken childbirth education classes are surprised at the intensity of the contractions in this phase of labor. Because the feeling to push is so strong, some women react to this change in contractions by growing increasingly argumentative and angry or by crying and screaming. Other women react by tensing their abdominal muscles and trying to resist, making the sensation even more painful and frightening. In the past, women were told to hold their breath while they pushed. Now it is believed that holding the breath for a prolonged time impairs blood return from the vena cava (a Valsalva maneuver), so this is now discouraged. Encourage women to assume any position, which is comfortable for them and breathe any way that is natural for them, except holding their breath (Roberts & Hanson, 2007).

A support person plays a vital role during this time, because all of the preparations done up to this point may still not be enough to sustain a woman during these final contractions unless she feels well supported. This participation also creates an important sharing time, after the birth, that gives a couple a sense of family for the first time.

Women need to have an experienced health care person with them as well as they enter this stage of labor, to reassure them that the change in contractions is normal and to give knowledgeable support that everything is all right (see Focus on Nursing Care Planning Box 15.9).

Assess fetal heart sounds at the beginning of the second stage of labor to be certain that the start of the baby's passage into the birth canal is not occluding the cord and interfering with fetal circulation. A general timetable for second-stage interventions is shown in Table 15.6. Prolonged second stages of labor are associated with chorioamionitis (uterine infection) and an increased rate of cesarean birth (Cheng et al., 2007).

Preparing the Place of Birth

For a multipara, convert a birthing room into a birth room by opening the sterile packs of supplies on waiting tables when the cervix has dilated to 9 to 10 cm. For a primipara, this can be delayed until the head has crowned to the size of a quarter or half-dollar (full dilatation and descent). A table set with equipment such as sponges, drapes, scissors, basins, clamps, bulb syringe, vaginal packing, and sterile gowns, gloves, and towels can be left, covered, for up to 8 hours. Be certain that drapes and materials used for birth are sterile, so that no microorganisms can be accidentally introduced into the uterus.

To provide for baby care, open the partition at the end of the room to reveal the "baby island," or newborn care area. Such areas include a radiant heat warmer, equipment for suction and resuscitation, and supplies for eye care and identification of the newborn. Turn on the radiant heat warmer in advance, so that the bottom mattress is pleasantly warm to the touch at the time of birth. Place sterile towels and a blanket on the warmer, so that they will also be warm to use to dry and cover the infant.

Positioning for Birth

Women can choose a variety of positions for birth. At one time, the lithotomy position was the major position for birth, but it is no longer the position of choice in birthing rooms or alternative birth centers—although the labor beds in these locales have attached stirrups to allow birth in a lithotomy position. Alternative birth positions include the lateral or Sims' position, the dorsal recumbent position (on the back with knees flexed), semi-sitting, and squatting.

Nurse-midwives tend to favor these alternative birth positions for their clients because they place less tension on the perineum, resulting in fewer perineal tears (Hastings-Tolsma, 2007).

If a physician prefers a lithotomy position for birth, position the woman into the bed stirrups while the physician is scrubbing and donning a sterile mask, gown, and gloves. Raise both of the woman's legs at the same time to prevent strain on her back and lower abdominal muscles. The strap holding the leg in the stirrups should be secured snugly but not so tightly that it causes constriction. Many women perceive stirrups as an unnatural position for birth, but they provide the best position for performing an episiotomy or a forceps-assisted birth or for viewing the perineum to detect lacerations or other problems at birth, and they are generally not uncomfortable. Pad the stirrups with abdominal pads if a woman has ankle edema; to prevent thrombophlebitis, be certain that there is no pressure on her calves.

Because pushing becomes less effective in a lithotomy position, the top portion of the table should be raised to a 30- to 60-degree angle, so that the woman can continue to push effectively. Lying for longer than 1 hour in a lithotomy position leads to intense pelvic congestion, because blood flow to the lower extremities is impeded. Pelvic congestion may lead to an increase in thrombophlebitis in the postpartal period. It may also contribute to excessive blood loss with birth and placental loosening. For these reasons, place the woman's legs in a lithotomy position only at the last moment.

Once a woman is in a lithotomy position, the bed's lower half is folded downward ("broken") so the physician can be in close proximity to the birth outlet. Make sure there is always someone at the foot of a broken birthing bed so that, if birth should occur precipitously, the infant will not fall and be injured.

Promoting Effective Second-Stage Pushing

For the most effective pushing during the second stage of labor, a woman should wait to feel the urge to push even though a pelvic examination has revealed that she is fully dilated. She should push with contractions and rest between them. Pushing is usually best done from a semi-Fowler's, squatting, or "all-fours" position rather than lying flat, to allow gravity to aid the effort (Fig. 15.28). A woman can use short pushes or long, sustained ones, whichever are more comfortable. Holding the breath during a contraction could cause a Valsalva maneuver or temporarily impede blood return to the heart because of increased intrathoracic pressure. This could also interfere with blood supply to the uterus. To prevent her from holding her breath during pushing, urge her to breathe out during a pushing effort.

In a multipara, to keep the second stage of labor from moving too fast, it may be necessary to prevent the woman from pushing. To accomplish this, ask her to pant with contractions. Because it is difficult to push effectively when she is using her diaphragm for panting, this limits pushing. Remember that pushing is involuntary. Regardless of how much a woman wants to cooperate, stopping this overwhelming urge to push is almost beyond her power. Demonstrating "panting like a puppy" and panting with her may be most effective. Be sure she is inhaling adequately. Otherwise, she might hyperventilate and become lightheaded while panting. Have her take deep cleansing breaths between contractions to prevent this.

Perineal Cleaning

To remove vaginal or rectal secretions and prepare the cleanest environment for the birth of the baby, clean the perineum

(text continues on page 388)

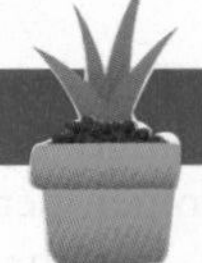

BOX 15.9 * Focus on Nursing Care Planning

A Multidisciplinary Care Map for a Woman During Labor and Birth

Celeste Bailey is a 26-year-old you admit to a birthing room. She tells you she wants to have her baby "naturally" without any analgesia or anesthesia. Her husband is in the Marines and is assigned overseas, so he is not with her. Although her sister lives only two blocks from the hospital, Celeste does not want her called. She asks if she can talk to her mother on the telephone instead. As you finish assessing contractions, she screams with pain and shouts, "I'm doing everything I'm supposed to! How much longer does this go on?"

Family Assessment * Client lives with husband in Marine base apartment. Husband currently assigned overseas. Finances rated as "horrible. If you want to be rich, don't marry a Marine." Both her mother and her married sister live nearby.

Client Assessment * Gravida 1, para 0. Contractions of moderate intensity, 45 seconds' duration, 3 minutes apart. Cervix dilated 3 cm, 60% effaced. Membranes intact. FHR 148; fetus in ROA position. Attended childbirth education classes, but is using breathing exercises ineffectively without coach. Brought a red rose to use as a focusing object.

Nursing Diagnosis * Pain related to uterine contractions and pressure on pelvic structures during labor

Outcome Criteria * Client manages her discomfort in labor with nonpharmacologic methods; identifies need for additional pain relief measures if needed; responds to questions and instructions; states labor and birth were a positive experience for her.

Team Member Responsible	Assessment	Intervention	Rationale	Expected Outcome
		Activities of Daily Living		
Nurse	Inspect the client's suprapubic area and palpate for bladder distention.	Encourage client to void every 2 hours.	A full bladder contributes to the client's discomfort and impedes fetal descent, possibly prolonging labor.	Client has no signs of bladder distention; voids every 2 hours during labor.
Nurse	Assess level of pain from uterine contractions and pelvic pressure by both verbal and nonverbal indicators; use 1 to 10 pain score.	Review and observe Lamaze breathing patterns with client to be certain she is obtaining maximum relief. Inform client about possible pharmacologic relief methods available to her if she should need them.	Pain is a subjective symptom, so only the client can determine her degree of pain or need for analgesia.	Client rates her level of pain from labor contractions as good to tolerable.
		Consultations		
Physician/ Nurse	Determine what personnel are available to prescribe or administer pharmacologic pain relief during labor, such as an epidural block if she voices a need for this.	Consult with nurse anesthetist about client's wish to not receive any pharmacologic pain relief.	Respecting client's wishes is a prime mode of encouraging self-efficacy.	Pain management team supports client's wish for no pharmacologic interventions, but will be prepared to administer pain relief if client's wishes change or an emergency should change the client's goal.

		Procedures/Medications		
Nurse	Assess what particular care measures, if any, client desires during labor (e.g., walking or not, birth position).	Establish a birth plan with client so all staff members can be aware of her individual preferences.	Respecting a client's choice helps to maintain self-esteem and a feeling of control.	Client expresses her preferences during labor.
		Nutrition		
Nurse	Assess when client last ate. Ask about preferences for fluid during labor.	Provide client with ice chips, hard candy, or other fluid as desired.	Ice chips or hard candy can relieve mouth dryness from breathing exercises.	Client states she has no mouth discomfort and does not feel hungry.
		Patient/Family Education		
Nurse	Assess what client knows about the usual process and time intervals of labor.	Provide information to supplement client's knowledge of labor; update client frequently on labor progress.	Teaching is most efficient if it is based on prior knowledge. Frequent updates about client's progress help to alleviate anxiety.	Client states that she understands the process of usual labor; indicates progress reports are helpful.
		Psychosocial/Spiritual/Emotional Needs		
Nurse	Assess if physical environment seems conducive to labor without pharmacologic support.	Provide a comfortable environment (e.g., change sheets frequently, adjust room temperature, offer cool washcloths to forehead).	A comfortable environment aids in relaxation and minimizes distractions, promoting effective coping to manage discomfort.	Client reports that environment is comfortable and she feels secure.
		Encourage client to assume different positions and to change them regularly. Allow client to walk or sit in chair, if desired.	Position changes promote comfort, reduce muscle tension, relieve pressure, and promote fetal descent.	Client assumes a variety of positions during labor as desired.
		Respect the need for focusing during contractions. Refrain from intervening with client during a contraction.	Interrupting client's focusing can be distracting, making the technique ineffective as a pain relief measure.	Client expresses that she is able to focus during contractions unimpaired by health care providers.
Nurse	Assess if client would like to have a support person with her.	Help client locate a suitable support person (mother?). If none is available, serve as primary support person.	A support person can play a major role in making labor a tolerable experience.	Client names a person she wants as her support person. Person or nurse serves as a support person during labor.
		Discharge Planning		
Nurse	Assess how client evaluates her labor experience.	Help client voice her satisfaction or dissatisfaction with her labor experience.	Reviewing a possibly traumatic experience helps debrief (put it into perspective among life events).	Client states that labor and birth was at worst a tolerable experience; at best, a highlight of her life.

TABLE 15.6 ✻ Time Intervals for Nursing Interventions During Second Stage of Labor

Intervention	Beginning of Second Stage	Continued Frequency	After Birth of Infant	After Delivery of Placenta
Assess and Record				
Temperature	X	q2hr		q1hr
Pulse	X	q1hr	X	q15 min
Respirations	X	q5–30 min	X	q15 min
Blood pressure	X	q5–30 min	X	X
Fetal heart rate	X	Continuously by monitor or q5 min		
Contractions	X	Continuously by monitor or q5 min		
Perineum	X	q15 min		q15 min
Provide				
Support	X	Continuously	Continuously	Continuously

with a warmed antiseptic such as Iodophor (cold solution causes cramping) and then rinse it with a designated solution before birth, according to the policy of the physician, nurse-midwife, or agency. Always clean from the vagina outward (so that microorganisms are moved away from the vagina, not toward it), using a clean compress for each stroke. Be sure and include a wide area (vulva, upper inner thighs, pubis, and anus). Figure 15.29 shows a typical pattern for cleaning. If a physician or nurse-midwife plans to use sterile drapes, help place them around the perineum.

As the woman pushes, the pressure of the fetal head on the bowel may cause fecal material to be expelled from the rectum. The physician or nurse-midwife will sponge this away as it occurs, to prevent contamination of the birth canal.

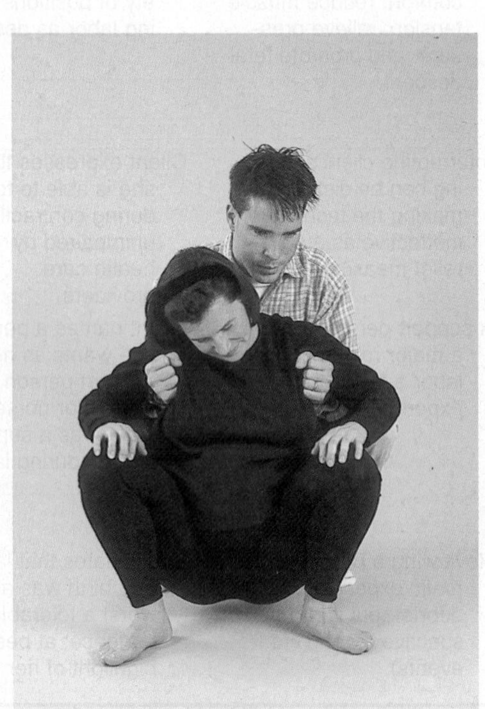
A

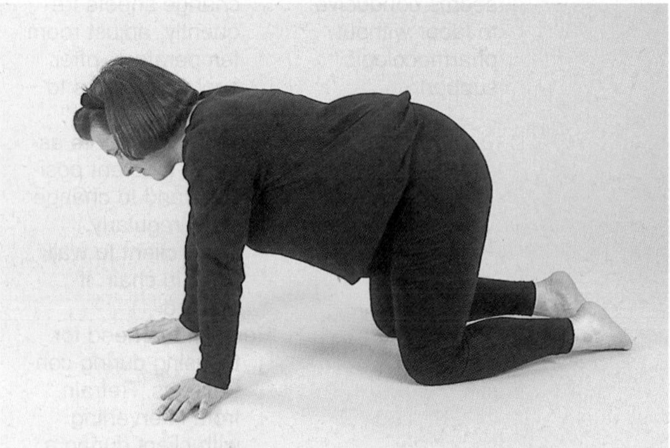
B

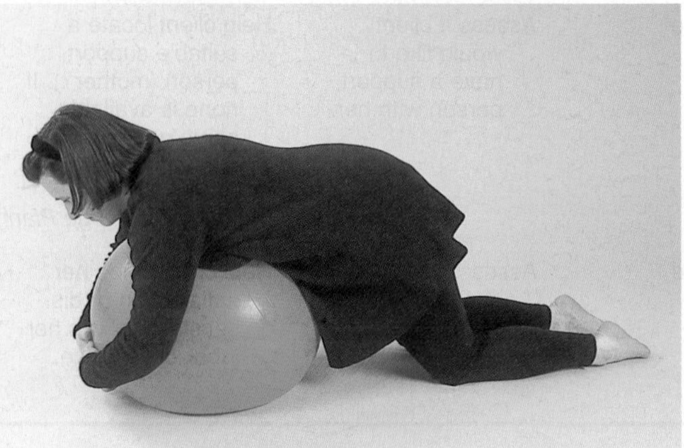
C

FIGURE 15.28 Positions for pushing during second stage labor. (**A**) Squatting with support person. (**B**) All-fours. (**C**) All-fours with chest support. (© Barbara Proud.)

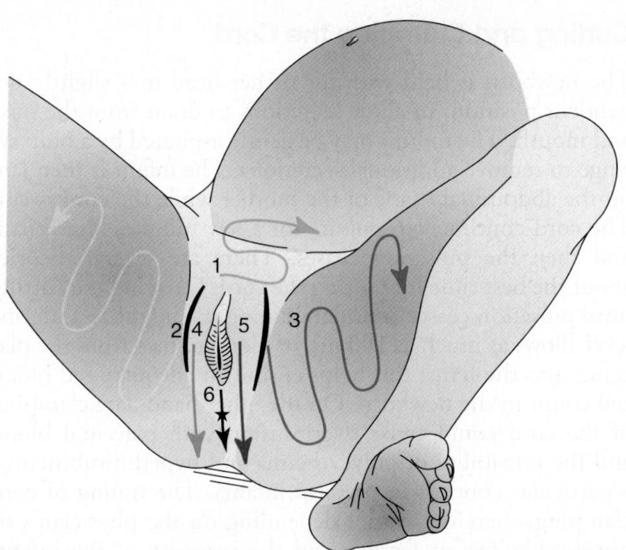

FIGURE 15.29 Pattern for cleaning perineum before birth. Cleaning from the birth canal outward moves bacteria away from, not into, the vagina. Numbers refer to steps of the procedure.

Episiotomy

An **episiotomy** is a surgical incision of the perineum that is made both to prevent tearing of the perineum and to release pressure on the fetal head with birth (Lawson & Bienstock, 2007).

Rarely used today, an episiotomy incision is made with blunt-tipped scissors in the midline of the perineum (a midline episiotomy) or is begun in the midline but directed laterally away from the rectum (a mediolateral episiotomy) (Fig. 15.30). Mediolateral episiotomies have the advantage over midline cuts in that, if tearing occurs beyond the incision, it will be away from the rectum, creating less danger of complication from rectal mucosal tears (de Leeuw et al., 2008). Anal sphincter tears can lead to fecal incontinence later in life (Mous, Muller, & de Leeuw, 2008). Midline episiotomies, however, heal more easily, cause less blood loss, and result in less postpartal discomfort.

Obstetric practice varies regarding which type of episiotomy is done and how it is done. At one time this procedure was done only if tearing seemed imminent; later, it was considered routine with a normal birth; and now it is rarely used again. The advantage of an episiotomy is that it substitutes a clean cut for a ragged tear, minimizes pressure on the fetal head, and may shorten the last portion of the second stage of labor (Incerpi, 2007).

The pressure of the fetal presenting part against the perineum is so intense that the nerve endings in the perineum are momentarily deadened. This lack of sensation allows an episiotomy to be done without anesthesia. For some women, a pudendal block may be done beforehand to ensure that there is no pain; for this, lidocaine is injected via a long needle through the vaginal wall near the ischial spine, numbing the lower vaginal area and the perineum.

At the time of an episiotomy incision, there is a slight loss of blood, but the pressure of the presenting part immediately seals the cut edges and minimizes bleeding. The fetal head usually moves forward considerably once the tension on the perineum is relieved.

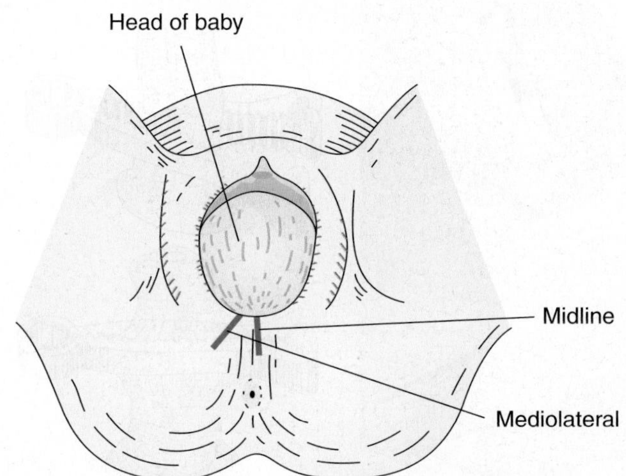

FIGURE 15.30 Position of episiotomy incision in a woman during second stage of labor. Baby's head is presenting to vagina outlet (crowning).

Birth

As soon as the head of a fetus is prominent (approximately 8 cm across) at the vaginal opening, the physician or nurse-midwife may place a sterile towel over the rectum and press forward on the fetal chin while the other hand is pressed downward on the occiput (a Ritgen maneuver) (Fig. 15.31). This helps a fetus achieve extension, so that the head is born with the smallest diameter presenting. This also controls the rate at which the head is born. Pressure should never be applied to the fundus of the uterus to effect birth, because uterine rupture could occur.

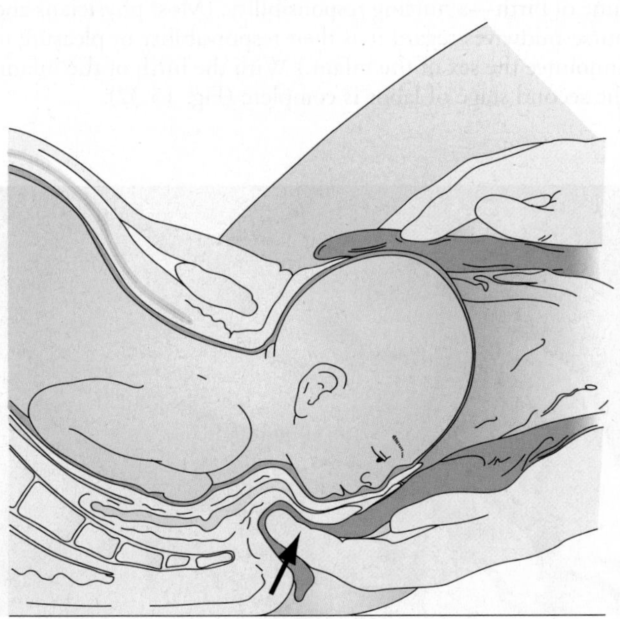
FIGURE 15.31 Ritgen's maneuver. The *arrow* shows direction of pressure.

A woman is asked to continue pushing until the occiput of the fetal head is firmly at the pubic arch. Then the head is born between contractions. This helps to prevent the head from being expelled too rapidly. It also helps to avoid perineal tears and a rapid change in pressure in the infant's head (which could rupture cerebral blood vessels). The woman may be asked to pant deliberately, so that she does not push during a contraction. She may be asked to push again without a contraction present to deliver the shoulders. Instructions should be repeated as necessary, because often a woman is so involved with the coming birth that she does not hear. Offer guidance and support to the partner as well, because he or she may be almost as overwhelmed by the birth process as the woman.

A woman who has not had anesthesia experiences the birth of the head as a flash of pain or a burning sensation, as if someone had momentarily poured hot water on her perineum. It is a fleeting sensation and is not particularly uncomfortable.

Immediately after birth of the baby's head, the physician or nurse-midwife suctions the infant's mouth with a bulb syringe and then passes his or her fingers along the occiput to the newborn's neck, to determine whether a loop of umbilical cord is encircling the neck. It is not uncommon for a single loop of cord to be positioned this way (termed a nuchal cord). If such a loop is felt, it is gently loosened and drawn down over the fetal head. If it is too tightly coiled to allow this, it is clamped and cut before the shoulders are born. Otherwise, it could tear and interfere with the fetal oxygen supply.

After expulsion of the fetal head, external rotation occurs. Gentle pressure is exerted downward on the side of the infant's head, and the anterior shoulder is born. Slight upward pressure on the side of the head allows the anterior shoulder to nestle against the symphysis as the posterior shoulder is born. The remainder of the body then slides free without any further difficulty.

A child is considered born when the whole body is born. This is the time that should be noted and recorded as the time of birth—a nursing responsibility. (Most physicians and nurse-midwives regard it as their responsibility or pleasure to announce the sex of the infant.) With the birth of the infant, the second stage of labor is complete (Fig. 15.32).

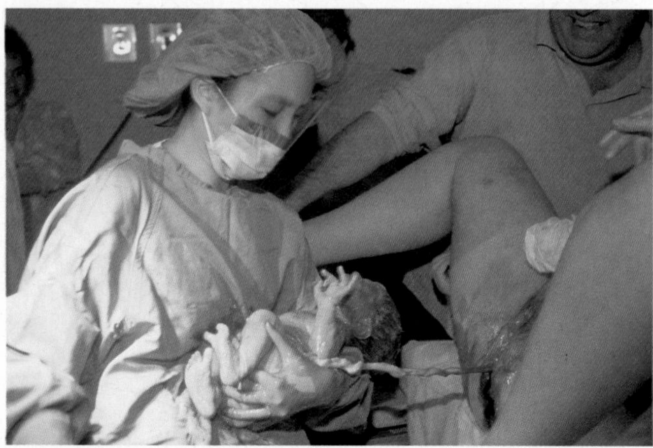

FIGURE 15.32 A child is considered born when the whole body is delivered. (© Barbara Proud.)

Cutting and Clamping the Cord

The newborn is held with his or her head in a slightly dependent position, to allow secretions to drain from the nose and mouth. The mouth may be gently aspirated by a bulb syringe to remove additional secretions. The infant is then laid on the abdominal drape of the mother while the cord is cut. The cord continues to pulsate for a few minutes after birth, and then the pulsation ceases. There are several theories about the best time for cutting the cord. Delaying the cutting until pulsation ceases and maintaining the infant at a uterine level allows as much as 100 mL of blood to pass from the placenta into the fetus; this helps ensure an adequate red blood cell count in the newborn. On the other hand, late clamping of the cord could cause overinfusion with placental blood and the possibility of polycythemia and hyperbilirubinemia, a particular concern in preterm infants. The timing of cord clamping, therefore, varies depending on the physician's or nurse-midwife's preference and the maturity of the infant. Placing the infant on the mother's abdomen may modify the amount of blood infused as well as allowing the parents a free, unobstructed view of their new child.

The cord is clamped with two Kelly hemostats placed 8 to 10 inches from the infant's umbilicus and then is cut between them. A cord blood sample is obtained to provide a ready source of infant blood if blood typing or other emergency measures such as establishing whether fetal acidosis was present need to be done. Blood may also be taken for cord blood banking so the family has stem cells available if needed in the future. An umbilical clamp is then applied (Fig. 15.33). Some umbilical clamps have an alarm attached that will ring if the infant is taken farther than set hospital boundaries, a precaution against newborn kidnapping. The vessels in the cord are then counted to be certain that three are present. In most births, the woman's partner may have the privilege of cutting the cord.

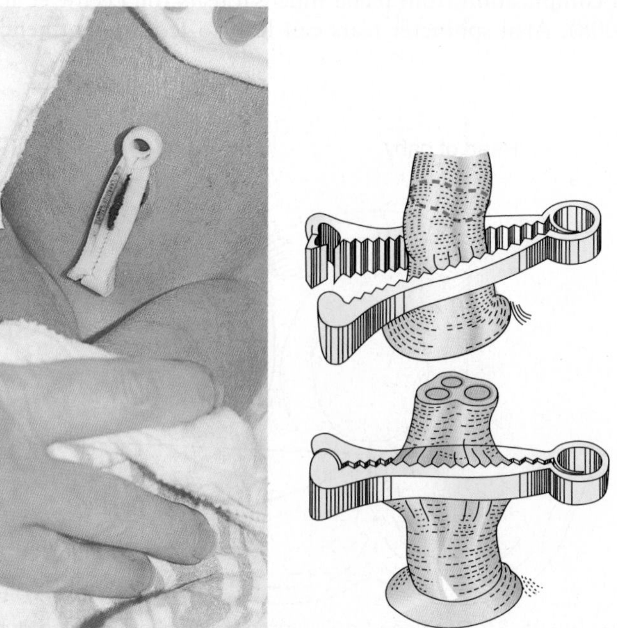

FIGURE 15.33 (**A**) Umbilical clamp applied to cord. (© Caroline Brown, RNC, MC, DEd.) (**B**) Placing clamp; locking clamp.

Cutting the cord is part of the stimulus that initiates a first breath. With this, the infant's most important transition to the outside world, the establishment of independent respirations, has begun.

Introducing the Infant

After the cord is cut, it is time for the new parents to spend some time with their newborn. Take the infant from the physician or nurse-midwife and wrap the infant in a sterile blanket. Be sure to hold newborns firmly, because they are covered with slippery amniotic fluid and vernix. Lay the infant on a radiant heat warmer and dry him or her well with a warmed towel. Rewrap the infant snugly and cover the head with a wrapped towel or cap. Assuming that the newborn's respirations are good, take the infant to the head of the table to visit with the new parents.

Both the mother and her partner usually want to see and touch their newborn immediately; this assures them the baby is well and is an important step in establishing a parent–child relationship. Do not administer prophylactic eye ointment to the infant until after the parents have had this chance to see their infant (and the infant has had a chance to see them). (See Chapter 18 for infant care after birth.) If the woman wishes to breastfeed, this is an optimal time for her to begin. An infant sucking at the breast stimulates the release of endogenous oxytocin, encouraging uterine contraction and involution, or the return of the uterus to its prepregnant state.

CARE OF A WOMAN DURING THE THIRD AND FOURTH STAGES OF LABOR

The third stage of labor is the time from the birth of the baby until the placenta is delivered. For most women, this is a time of excitement, because the infant has safely been born, but also a time of feeling anticlimactic, because the infant has finally arrived after being expected for so long. The fourth stage includes the first few hours after birth. It signals the beginning of dramatic changes because it marks the beginning of a new family.

Placenta Delivery

If the placenta does not deliver spontaneously, the physician or nurse-midwife will ask the new mother to bear down gently or else apply gentle pressure on the contracted uterine fundus or gentle traction on the umbilical cord. If these measures are not successful, the placenta can be removed manually to limit the amount of postpartum bleeding (Bair & Williams, 2007). After delivery, the placenta is inspected to be certain that it is intact and normal in appearance and weight. Normally, a placenta is one-sixth the weight of the infant. If it is unusually large or small, you may be asked to weigh it.

Oxytocin

Once the placenta is delivered, oxytocin is usually ordered to be administered intramuscularly or intravenously to the mother. Such medication increases uterine contractions and thereby minimizes uterine bleeding (Bair & Williams, 2007).

> **BOX 15.10 ✻ Focus on Pharmacology**
>
> **Oxytocin (Pitocin)**
>
> ***Action:*** A synthetic form of the hormone produced by the hypothalamus and stored in the posterior pituitary. An oxytocic, it stimulates the uterus to contract to control postpartum hemorrhage (Karch, 2009).
>
> ***Pregnancy Category:*** X
>
> ***Dosage:*** Add 10–40 units to 1000 mL of a nonhydrating intravenous solution, or administer 10 units intramuscularly after delivery of the placenta.
>
> ***Possible Adverse Effects:*** Hypertension, excessive uterine contractility.
>
> **Nursing Implications**
>
> - Do not administer after delivery of the placenta until the physician or nurse-midwife approves the drug's use.
> - Monitor the woman for blood pressure, because hypertension can occur.

Oxytocin (Pitocin) may be added to an existing intravenous line (10 to 40 U/L in intravenous fluid) or given as 10 U intramuscularly (Karch, 2009) (Box 15.10). Carboprost tromethamine (Hemabate) may be administered if the woman has excess bleeding with poor uterine contraction.

The administration of oxytocin is a nursing responsibility in most health care facilities. Do not administer it until the physician or nurse-midwife indicates it is appropriate. Although the agent may be given as early as the birth of the fetal anterior shoulder, the physician or nurse-midwife may want to inspect the placenta first to ensure that it is intact and without gross abnormalities and that none of its cotyledons remain in the uterus. Because oxytocin causes hypertension by vasoconstriction, be sure to obtain a baseline blood pressure measurement before administration. Question the use of such a drug with women who have elevated blood pressure.

If a uterus is resistant to contraction, intravenous administration of oxytocin may be continued for up to 8 hours after birth to ensure uterine contraction. Continue to monitor blood pressure during this time.

Perineal Repair

After delivery of the placenta, if an episiotomy was performed, the woman needs perineal stitches put into place. This process can be a tedious one from the mother's perspective. She must lie on her back and wait for the procedure to be completed, while the attention of others is riveted on the newborn lying in the warmer off to one side. It is important to be sensitive to the mother's needs at this time. Be certain to include her in explanations and appreciate how anticlimactic she may feel at this time.

Theoretically, if suturing of an episiotomy is done immediately after the birth of the placenta, a woman who gave birth without anesthesia will still have so much natural-pressure anesthesia of the perineum that she will not require an anesthetic. In actuality, by the time the placenta is delivered (approximately 5 minutes), enough sensation has returned to the perineum that the woman will probably need some type of medication for comfort. Women who received a regional anesthetic during labor (e.g., pudendal block) and those who have had epidural anesthesia will probably not need additional medication during episiotomy repair.

Immediate Postpartum Assessment and Nursing Care

Following placenta delivery, lower both of a woman's legs from stirrups, if they were used, at the same time to prevent back injury.

Obtain vital signs (i.e., pulse, respirations, and blood pressure) every 15 minutes for the first hour and then according to agency policy. Pulse and respirations may be fairly rapid immediately after birth (80 to 90 bpm and 20 to 24 respirations per minute) and blood pressure slightly elevated because of the excitement of the moment and recent oxytocin administration. Palpate a woman's fundus for size, consistency, and position and observe the amount and characteristics of lochia. Perform perineal care, and apply a perineal pad.

If the birth was in a birthing room, return the birthing bed to its original position. Offer a clean gown and a warmed blanket, because a woman often experiences a chill and shaking sensation 10 to 15 minutes after birth. This may be because of the low temperature of the birthing room but may also be a result of the sudden release of pressure on pelvic nerves or of excess epinephrine production during labor. In any event, it is a normal phenomenon but it can be frightening to the mother. She may associate the shaking chill with fever or infection and worry she will be ill at a time when she most wants to be well to care for her new child. You can reassure her that this is a normal, transitory sensation.

Aftercare

This is the beginning of the postpartal period or the fourth stage of labor. Because the uterus may be so exhausted from labor that it cannot maintain contraction, there is a high risk for hemorrhage during this time. In addition, a woman often is so exhausted that she may be unable to assess her own condition or report any changes. Specific assessments done during this time are continued throughout the postpartal period. These assessments are discussed in Chapter 17.

UNIQUE CONCERNS OF A WOMAN IN LABOR

A Woman Without a Support Person

Some women have chosen to reject or want to labor without the infant's father, who is the usual support person during labor. Such women may appreciate having a family member or close friend act as their support person. A woman who has no support person needs a supportive nurse to be with her.

A woman whose acceptance of her pregnancy was slow to develop because of lack of adequate support people may not have completed the psychological tasks of pregnancy by the time she is in labor. This could make her more apprehensive about a new life role and calls for increased assessment of parent–child bonding in the immediate postpartal period.

A Woman Who Will Be Placing Her Baby for Adoption

If a woman has decided to place her baby for adoption, she needs to be an active participant in her labor and birth experience and be allowed to hold her child as desired. Each state has a set number of days in which a mother must decide whether to keep her baby. Although this decision may have seemed easy to make during pregnancy, once she holds the baby in her arms, the prospect of giving up the child may be more painful than she realized. She needs support no matter what decision she eventually makes. Be certain you do not offer influencing advice, because the woman is the only person who knows whether keeping this child is right for her.

Vaginal Birth After Cesarean Birth

Women who have had a previous cesarean birth that involved a low transverse uterine incision are usually candidates for vaginal birth with their next pregnancy (Landon, 2008). The length of labor for vaginal birth after cesarean birth (VBAC) is usually comparable to that of primiparas, not multiparas, because it is the first vaginal birth. Most women are anxious for vaginal birth to be successful so that they do not have to undergo surgery again. At the same time, they may be surprised and dismayed at the length and discomfort of labor and wish that they could have another cesarean. Keep the woman well informed, and urge her to breathe with contractions and to push effectively to make the experience a positive one for her. Afterward, many women are relieved to realize that, although they did have more discomfort before birth, they have appreciably less pain afterward.

If during the previous labor a complication occurred that necessitated the cesarean birth, a woman cannot help but worry that this will happen again. She needs a support person with her and health care providers who are aware of her possible level of apprehension. Women having a VBAC usually have external electronic monitoring because of the risk for uterine rupture. The outcome of VBAC is usually without complication. If necessary, oxytocin augmentation (see Chapter 23) can be used to strengthen uterine contractions; vacuum extraction and forceps birth can be used as necessary.

✓Checkpoint Question 15.5

Celeste has an amniotomy (artificial rupture of the membranes). After this procedure, which of the following would be an important nursing assessment?

a. Ask her if her pain level is tolerable postprocedure.
b. Assess maternal heart rate to detect possible bleeding.
c. Assess FHR to detect possible cord prolapse.
d. Document the amount of amniotic fluid that has been lost.

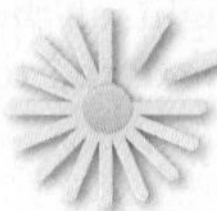

Key Points for Review

- Labor is the series of events by which uterine contractions expel a fetus and placenta from a woman's body.
- The exact reason why labor begins is unknown. It most likely occurs because of an interplay between fetal and uterine factors that registers as progesterone withdrawal.

- Effective labor depends on interactions between the passage, the passenger, the power of contractions, and a woman's psychological readiness.
- Labor is an almost overwhelming experience because it involves such intense sensations and emotions. Women enjoy having a support person with them to help them cope with the experience.
- Fetal presentation (the fetal body part that will initially contact the cervix) and position (the relationship of the fetal presenting part to a specific quadrant of the woman's pelvis) are both important in determining the success of labor.
- The first stage of labor lasts from the onset of cervical dilatation until dilatation is complete (10 cm). The second stage extends from the time of full dilatation until the infant is born. A third or placental stage lasts from the time the infant is born until after delivery of the placenta. A fourth stage comprises the first few hours after birth.
- Danger signs of labor include an abnormal FHR, meconium staining of amniotic fluid, abnormal maternal pulse or blood pressure, inadequate or prolonged contractions, formation of a pathologic retraction ring (development of an abnormal lower abdomen contour), and increasing apprehension.
- Monitoring of uterine contractions and FHR is an important nursing responsibility. Fetal bradycardia, tachycardia, and late and variable decelerations are important observations to make. Interventions such as keeping the woman on her left side and promoting voiding help to prevent fetal distress. Offering psychological support is crucial to maternal well-being.
- Pushing during the second stage of labor should be guided by the woman's need to push. Urge her to breathe out while pushing, if possible.
- The placental stage follows birth and consists of placental separation and expulsion. Observe for excessive bleeding during this time. Do not pull on the cord to hasten separation, because this can lead to uterine inversion.
- A fetus is in potential danger when the membranes rupture, because of the possibility of cord prolapse. Always assess FHR at this point to safeguard the fetus.
- A woman is at potential risk for hemorrhage throughout labor because of the possibility that the placenta could be dislodged. Assess for vaginal bleeding and vital signs to be certain this is not occurring.

CRITICAL THINKING EXERCISES

1. Celeste Bailey, the woman you met at the beginning of the chapter, was certain her labor was not normal because it had lasted for 6 hours. Is this an unusually long time for a first stage of labor? Do you think she would have been more comfortable knowing the usual length?
2. Suppose that, when Celeste is admitted to a birthing room, she states she has read nothing during her pregnancy about labor and so has no idea what to expect. What would you want to teach her early in labor? Midway in labor? Why might a woman enter labor without having learned anything about it?
3. Most women today accept fetal monitoring equipment as an expected part of labor care. What would you do if Celeste Bailey absolutely refuses to have this type of fetal monitoring?
4. Examine the National Health Goals related to labor. Most government-sponsored funds for nursing research are allotted based on these goals. What would be a possible research topic to explore pertinent to these goals that would be applicable to the Bailey family and also advance evidence-based practice?

CRITICAL THINKING SCENARIO

Open the accompanying CD-ROM or visit http://thePoint.lww.com and read the Patient Scenario included for this chapter, then answer the questions to further sharpen your skills and grow more familiar with NCLEX style questions related to care of families in labor. Confirm your answers are correct by reading the rationales.

REFERENCES

Albers, L. L. (2007). The evidence for physiologic management of the active phase of the first stage of labor. *Journal of Midwifery and Women's Health, 52*(3), 207–215.

Amis, D., & Green, J. (2007). *Prepared childbirth: the family way.* New York: Lamaze International.

Archie, C. L. (2007). The course and conduct of normal labor and delivery. In A. H. DeCherney & L. Nathan (Eds.). *Current diagnosis and treatment in obstetrics and gynecology* (10th ed.). Columbus, OH: McGraw-Hill.

Aziz, N., & Cohen, C. R. (2007). Sexually transmitted diseases in pregnancy. In J. D. Klausner & E. W. Hook III (Eds.). *Current diagnosis and treatment of sexually transmitted diseases.* Columbus, OH: McGraw-Hill.

Bair, M. E., & Williams, J. (2007). Management of the third stage of labor. *Journal of Midwifery and Women's Health, 52*(4), 412–414.

Baves, S., Fenwick, J., & Hauck, Y. A. (2008). Qualitative analysis of women's short accounts of labour and birth in a Western Australian public tertiary hospital. *Journal of Midwifery and Women's Health,* 53(1), 53–61.

Beebe, K. R., & Lee, K. A. (2007). Sleep disturbance in late pregnancy and early labor. *Journal of Perinatal and Neonatal Nursing, 21*(2), 103–108.

Buchmann, E. J., & Libhaber, E. (2007). Accuracy of cervical assessment in the active phase of labour. *BJOG: An International Journal of Obstetrics and Gynaecology, 114*(7), 833–837.

Burns, E., et al. (2007). Aromatherapy in childbirth: a pilot randomised controlled trial. *BJOG: An International Journal of Obstetrics and Gynaecology, 114*(7), 838–844.

Cheng, Y. W., et al. (2007). Duration of the second stage of labor in multiparous women: maternal and neonatal outcomes. *American Journal of Obstetrics and Gynecology, 196*(6), 585–591.

Crombleholme, W. R. (2009). Obstetrics. In McPhee, S. J., & Papadakis, M. A. *Current medical diagnosis and treatment.* Columbus, OH: McGraw-Hill.

de Leeuw, J. W., et al. (2008). Mediolateral episiotomy reduces the risk for anal sphincter injury during operative vaginal delivery. *BJOG: An International Journal of Obstetrics and Gynaecology, 115*(1), 104–108.

Devoe, L. D. (2008). Antenatal fetal assessment: contraction stress test, nonstress test, vibroacoustic stimulation, amniotic fluid volume, biophysical profile, and modified biophysical profile—an overview. *Seminars in Perinatology, 32*(4), 247–252.

East, C. E., et al. (2009). Vibroacoustic stimulation for fetal assessment in labour in the presence of a nonreassuring fetal heart rate trace. *Cochrane Database of Systematic Reviews, 2009*(1), (CD004664).

Euliano, T. Y., et al. (2007). Monitoring contractions in obese parturients: electrohysterography compared with traditional monitoring. *Obstetrics and Gynecology, 109*(5), 1136–1140.

Fitzgerald, M. P., et al. (2007). Risk factors for anal sphincter tear during vaginal delivery. *Obstetrics and Gynecology, 109*(1), 29–34.

Friedman, E. (1978). *Labor, clinical evaluation and management* (2nd ed.). New York: Appleton-Century-Crofts.

Gourounti, K., & Sandall, J. (2007). Admission cardiotocography versus intermittent auscultation of fetal heart rate: effects on neonatal Apgar score, on the rate of caesarean sections and on the rate of instrumental delivery—a systematic review. *International Journal of Nursing Studies, 44*(6), 1029–1035.

Greulich, B., & Tarrant, B. (2007). The latent phase of labor: diagnosis and management. *Journal of Midwifery and Women's Health, 52*(3), 190–198.

Gupta, J. K., Hofmeyr, G. J., & Smyth, R. (2009). Position in the second stage of labour for women without epidural anaesthesia. *Cochrane Database of Systematic Reviews, 2009*(1), (CD002006).

Hastings-Tolsma, M., et al. (2007). Getting through birth in one piece: protecting the perineum. *MCN: American Journal of Maternal Child Nursing, 32*(3), 158–164.

Hodnett, E. D., et al. (2009). Continuous support for women during childbirth. *Cochrane Database of Systematic Reviews, 2009*(1), (CD003766).

Incerpi, M. H. (2007). Operative delivery. In A. H. DeCherney & L. Nathan (Eds.). *Current diagnosis and treatment in obstetrics and gynecology* (10th ed.). Columbus, OH: McGraw-Hill.

Karch, A. M. (2009). *Lippincott's nursing drug guide.* Philadelphia: Lippincott Williams & Wilkins.

Kiss, K., & Collea, J. V. (2007). Malpresentation and cord prolapse. In A. H. DeCherney & L. Nathan (Eds.). *Current diagnosis and treatment in obstetrics and gynecology* (10th ed.). Columbus, OH: McGraw-Hill.

Landon, M. B. (2008). Vaginal birth after cesarean delivery. *Clinics in Perinatology, 35*(3), 491–504.

Laursen, M., et al. (2008). Fear of childbirth: predictors and temporal changes among nulliparous women in the Danish National Birth Cohort. *BJOG: An International Journal of Obstetrics and Gynaecology, 115*(3), 354–360.

Lawson, S. M., & Bienstock, J. L. (2007). Normal labor and delivery, operative delivery and malpresentations. In K. B. Fortner, et al. (Eds.). *The Johns Hopkins manual of gynecology and obstetrics.* Philadelphia: Lippincott Williams & Wilkins.

Lewis, D. F., et al. (2007). Expectant management of preterm premature rupture of membranes and nonvertex presentation: what are the risks? *American Journal of Obstetrics and Gynecology, 196*(6), 566–572.

McGrath, S. K., & Kennell, J. H. (2008). A randomized controlled trial of continuous labor support for middle-class couples: effect on cesarean delivery rates. *Birth, 35*(2), 92–97.

Mous, M., Muller, S. A., & de Leeuw, J. W. (2008). Long-term effects of anal sphincter rupture during vaginal delivery: faecal incontinence and sexual complaints. *BJOG: An International Journal of Obstetrics and Gynaecology, 115*(2), 234–238.

National Center for Health Statistics. (2009). *Trends in the health of Americans.* Hyattsville, MD: Author.

Poggi, S. B. H. (2007). Postpartum hemorrhage and the abnormal puerperium. In A. H. DeCherney & L. Nathan (Eds.). *Current diagnosis and treatment in obstetrics and gynecology* (10th ed.). Columbus, OH: McGraw-Hill.

Potera, C. (2007). In search of evidence supporting electronic fetal monitoring: recent studies fail to show benefits. *American Journal of Nursing, 107*(6), 22.

Price, S., Noseworthy, J., & Thornton, J. (2007). Women's experience with social presence during childbirth. *MCN: The American Journal of Maternal/Child Nursing, 32*(3), 184–191.

Ridley, R. T. (2007). Diagnosis and intervention for occiput posterior malposition. *JOGNN: Journal of Obstetric, Gynecologic, and Neonatal Nursing, 36*(2), 135–143.

Roberts, J., & Hanson, L. (2007). Best practices in second stage labor care: maternal bearing down and positioning. *Journal of Midwifery and Women's Health, 52*(3), 238–245.

Rosich-Medina, A., & Shetty, A. (2007). Paternal experiences of pregnancy and labour. *British Journal of Midwifery, 15*(2), 66–70.

Scott, A. (2007). Spreading the word: boosting cord blood donations among minorities. *Advance for Nurses, 4*(20), 23–24.

Sleutel, M., Schultz, S., & Wyble, K. (2007). Nurses' views of factors that help and hinder their intrapartum care. *JOGNN: Journal of Obstetric, Gynecologic, and Neonatal Nursing, 36*(3), 203–211.

Smith, C. A., et al. (2009). Complementary and alternative therapies for pain management in labour. *Cochrane Database of Systematic Reviews, 2009*(1), (CD003521).

Szymanski, L. M., & Bienstock, J. L. (2007). Complications of labor and delivery. In K. B. Fortner, et al. (Eds.). *The Johns Hopkins manual of gynecology and obstetrics.* Philadelphia: Lippincott Williams & Wilkins.

Tam, W. H., & Chung, T. (2007). Psychosomatic disorders in pregnancy. *Current Opinion in Obstetrics and Gynecology, 19*(2), 126–132.

SUGGESTED READINGS

Calvert, J., & Steen, M. (2007). Homeopathic remedies for self-administration during childbirth. *British Journal of Midwifery, 15*(3), 159–165.

Forster, D. A., & McLachlan, H. L. (2007). Breastfeeding initiation and birth setting practices: a review of the literature. *Journal of Midwifery and Women's Health, 52*(3), 273–280.

Grobman, W. A. (2007). Elective induction: When? Ever? *Clinical Obstetrics and Gynecology, 50*(2), 537–546.

Hodnett, E. D., et al. (2009). Home-like versus conventional institutional settings for birth. *Cochrane Database of Systematic Reviews, 2009*(1), (CD000012).

Jordan, P. L. (2007). Enhancing understanding of the transition to fatherhood. *International Journal of Childbirth Education, 22*(2), 4–6.

Mullen, K., et al. (2007). Family-centered maternity care: one hospital's quest for excellence. *Nursing for Women's Health, 11*(3), 282–290.

Parer, J. T., & Ikeda, T. (2007). A framework for standardized management of intrapartum fetal heart rate patterns. *American Journal of Obstetrics and Gynecology, 197*(1), 26–32.

Roberts, J. M., Gonzalez, C. B., & Sampselle, C. (2007). Why do supportive birth attendants become directive of maternal bearing-down efforts in second-stage labor? *Journal of Midwifery and Women's Health, 52*(2), 134–141.

Sauls, D. J. (2007). Nurses' attitudes toward provision of care and related health outcomes. *Nursing Research, 56*(2), 117–123.

Wedig, K. E., & Whitsett, J. A. (2008). Down the primrose path: petechiae in a neonate exposed to herbal remedy for parturition. *Journal of Pediatrics, 152*(1), 140–141.

Chapter 16 Providing Comfort During Labor and Birth

KEY TERMS

- analgesia
- anesthesia
- doula
- endorphins
- epidural anesthesia
- pain
- pressure anesthesia
- pudendal nerve block
- transcutaneous electrical nerve stimulation (TENS)

OBJECTIVES

After mastering the contents of this chapter, you should be able to:

1. Describe the physiologic basis of contractions during labor and how analgesia, anesthesia, and alternative therapies can be used to promote a woman's comfort during labor and birth.
2. Identify National Health Goals related to analgesia, anesthesia, and childbirth that nurses can help the nation achieve.
3. Use critical thinking to analyze ways to maintain family-centered care when analgesia and anesthesia are used in childbirth.
4. Assess the degree and type of discomfort a woman is experiencing during labor and birth, including her ability to cope with it effectively.
5. Formulate nursing diagnoses related to the effect of pain or pain management during labor and birth.
6. Establish expected outcomes to meet the needs of a woman experiencing discomfort during labor and birth.
7. Plan nursing interventions to promote comfort during labor and birth such as teaching about relaxation or breathing exercises.
8. Implement common complementary and pharmacologic measures for pain management during labor and birth.
9. Evaluate expected outcomes for effectiveness and achievement of care.
10. Identify areas related to promoting comfort during labor that could benefit from additional nursing research or application of evidence-based practice.
11. Integrate knowledge of pain management during labor and birth with the nursing process to achieve quality maternal and child health nursing care.

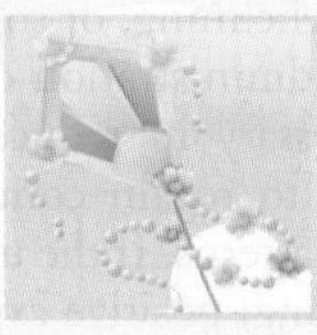

Susan Baranca is a primipara in early labor whom you admit to a birthing unit. Her cervix is dilated 3 cm. She tells you her sister had epidural anesthesia that completely obliterated her pain in labor for the birth of her baby 3 months ago. Based on her sister's experience, Susan expected to be given epidural anesthesia as soon as she arrived at the hospital. As she is barely in labor, however, her physician asked her to wait until she is 4 cm dilated. When you enter her room, you find her lying on her back in a birthing bed, crying from pain. Her husband shouts that his wife deserves better care than this.

The previous chapter discussed the process of labor and care for a woman in labor. This chapter adds information to your knowledge base about how to promote comfort during labor. Pain management in labor can help change labor from an experience so negative that it can result in posttraumatic stress syndrome to a positive, forward-moving experience.

Was the advice Susan received from her sister realistic?

What are some immediate interventions you could do to help Susan better manage her pain?

Concerns about the discomfort and pain that accompany labor and birth can dominate a pregnant woman's or couple's thoughts about childbirth during pregnancy and particularly as the baby's due date approaches. Providing information during prenatal visits about the numerous methods of comfort promotion and pain control available to women can help allay some of these fears. As discussed in Chapter 14, prepared childbirth classes can provide couples with an opportunity to learn and practice a variety of techniques, such as breathing patterns, to help reduce the pain of labor. Often, however, the labor experience is so overwhelming, or so much greater than the couple expected, that administration of an analgesic or a regional anesthetic is necessary to reduce discomfort sufficiently to allow a woman to regain control over her labor process and use breathing patterns. If the use of regional anesthesia makes labor a satisfying, positive experience, the intervention can ultimately promote the entire family's health. Using or not using medication only reflects different routes to becoming new parents (Carlton et al., 2009).

Much has been written in nursing literature about using the neutral term *contractions* instead of *labor pains,* to keep from reminding a woman how painful contractions can be. The theory is a sound one, not only because a woman is experiencing a *contracting* sensation but also because calling it *pain* could magnify her fear and tension. Tension, in turn, magnifies pain. Remember, however, that renaming it will not change its basic nature. By any name, discomfort accompanies labor. Fortunately, many nursing interventions can help reduce pain, so that labor is as fulfilling and rewarding an experience as a woman hoped it would be.

Making labor and birth a memorable experience for families is so important that National Health Goals have been established to address this topic. These are shown in Box 16.1.

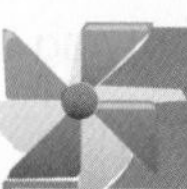

BOX 16.1 ✻ Focus on National Health Goals

Because administration of either analgesia and anesthesia during labor can increase both maternal and fetal mortality, several National Health Goals are related to the types of pain relief used in labor. Examples include:

- Reduce the maternal mortality rate to no more than 3.3 per 100,000 live births, from a baseline of 7.1 per 100,000.
- Reduce the fetal death rate during the perinatal period (28 weeks of gestation to 7 days after birth) to no more than 4.5 per 1000 live births, from a baseline of 7.5 per 1000 (http://www.nih.gov).

Nurses can help the nation achieve these goals by educating women about the advantages of preparing for childbirth, helping them to use breathing patterns or other complementary and alternative therapies and techniques during labor so that they need a minimum of analgesia and anesthesia, and conscientiously monitoring women who receive analgesics and anesthesia during labor and birth.

Areas that could benefit from additional nursing research include women's satisfaction with complementary or alternative therapy comfort measures, women's satisfaction with regional anesthesia in labor, and reasons that childbirth methods women prepare are not adequate for pain relief.

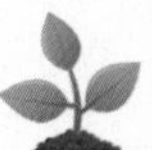

Nursing Process Overview

For Pain Relief During Childbirth

Assessment

Pain, the sensation of discomfort, is a subjective, personal symptom; it is what the person says it is and present when the person says it is (Cho & Penning, 2007). It is unique to each individual, so a woman is the only person who can describe or know the extent of her pain. To assess the amount of discomfort a woman is having in labor, listen carefully to what she is saying as well as how she rates her discomfort level on a pain assessment scale. Also look for subtle signs such as facial tenseness, flushing or paleness, hands clenched in fists, rapid breathing, or rapid pulse rate.

Nursing Diagnosis

Although pain related to labor contractions is the most obvious nursing diagnosis applicable to labor, it is not the only relevant one during this time. Pain can create other problems for the laboring woman that can negatively affect the childbirth experience. If not resolved, these problems can intensify pain. Some women may become more concerned with their reaction to the pain than to the pain itself. Because of this, applicable nursing diagnoses might include:

- Pain related to labor contractions
- Powerlessness related to the unexpected duration and intensity of labor
- Anxiety related to lack of knowledge about "normal" labor process
- Risk for situational low self-esteem related to ineffectiveness of prepared childbirth breathing exercises
- Decisional conflict related to use of analgesia or anesthesia during labor

Outcome Identification and Planning

When developing outcomes and planning interventions to manage discomfort during labor, consider the woman's perceptions about childbirth, her past childbirth experiences (if any), and the amount and type of childbirth preparation she and her partner made so the expected outcomes are realistic. For example, an expectation that no medication will be used might be inappropriate.

Be aware that pharmacologic agents used during labor and birth may pose risks for both the woman (e.g., hypotension) and the fetus (e.g., bradycardia). Therefore, their use must always be weighed against the alternative risk of having labor become an unbearable experience. The decision may also affect family functioning if the method chosen limits the partner's participation in the birth. A good Internet site for referral is the American Pain Society web page (http://www.ampainsoc.org).

Implementation

Keeping a woman and her support person informed about their options and how they differ as labor progresses is important. Simply knowing that birth is getting even a little closer can make the next few contractions easier to withstand. Supporting and encouraging a woman to use methods of complementary and alternative therapies for pain management (e.g., relaxation) also are helpful. Offering analgesia or assisting with anesthesia administration during labor or birth requires nursing judgment and a caring presence to help one woman accept analgesia when she needs it and to encourage another to experience childbirth without heavy sedation.

Outcome Evaluation

Evaluation is ongoing and typically must occur within a short timeframe. Examples of expected outcomes that would indicate successful achievement of outcomes are:

- Client states that pain during labor was within a tolerable level for her.
- Couple report that they felt in control throughout the labor process.
- Client states that she does not feel intimidated by degree of pain during labor.

Long-term evaluation should reveal that the woman found labor and birth to be an experience that was not only endurable but allowed her to grow in self-esteem and the family to grow through a shared experience. Asking a woman to describe her labor experience afterward in relation to pain not only aids evaluation of whether pain management was adequate but helps her work through this emotional period of life and integrate it into her previous experiences.

Box 16.2 Assessment
Assessing Pain Level for a Woman in Labor

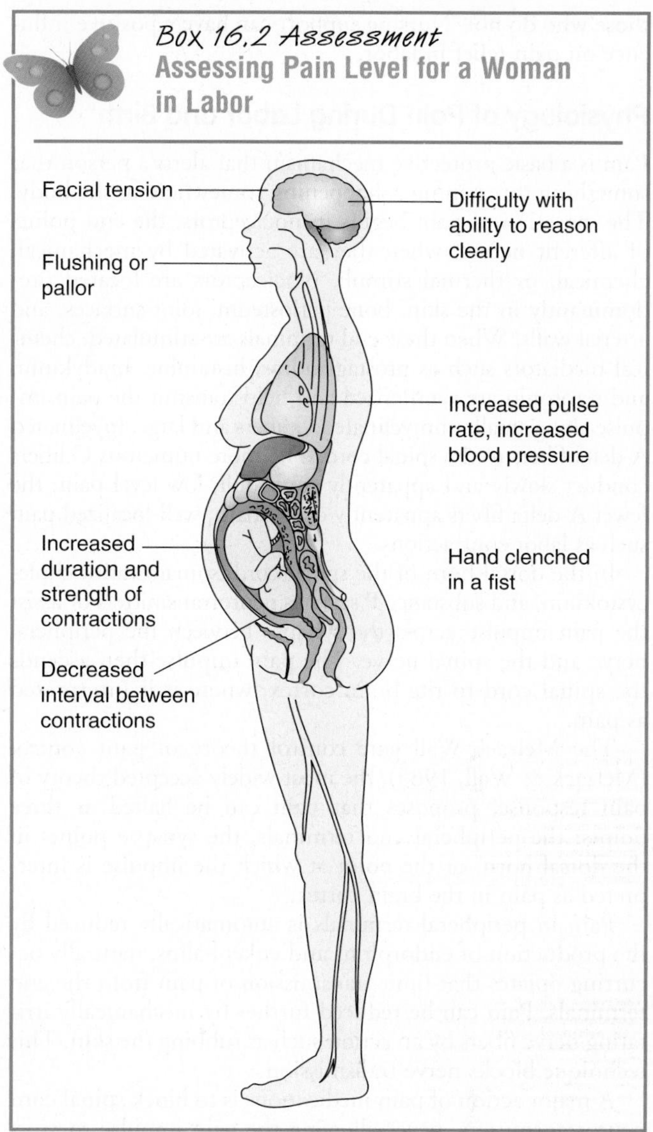

EXPERIENCE OF PAIN DURING CHILDBIRTH

Pain accompanies labor contractions for several different reasons and is manifested in different ways in individual women (Box 16.2).

Etiology of Pain During Labor and Birth

Normally, contractions of involuntary muscles, such as the heart, stomach, and intestine, do not cause pain. This concept makes uterine contractions unique because they do cause pain. Several explanations exist for why this happens. During contractions, blood vessels constrict, reducing the blood supply to uterine and cervical cells, resulting in anoxia to muscle fibers. This anoxia can cause pain in the same way that blockage of the cardiac arteries causes the pain of a heart attack. As labor progresses and contractions become longer and harder, the ischemia to cells increases, the anoxia increases, and the pain intensifies.

Pain also probably results from stretching of the cervix and perineum. This phenomenon is the same as that causing intestinal pain when accumulating gas stretches the intestines. At the end of the transitional phase in labor, when stretching of the cervix is complete and the woman feels she has to push, pain from the contractions often disappears as long as the woman is pushing, until the fetal presenting part causes the final stretching of the perineum.

Additional discomfort in labor may stem from the pressure of the fetal presenting part on tissues, including pressure on surrounding organs, such as the bladder, the urethra, and the lower colon. Pain at birth largely results from stretching of the perineal tissue.

In addition, the perception of pain is, in part, culturally determined. Some women believe that being stoic and nonverbal is what is expected of them. Others believe that expressing their discomfort by screaming or verbalizing their feelings will best reduce pain. If a woman is not proficient in English, it may be particularly difficult for her to describe her level of discomfort. Assess each woman individually to determine not only what level of comfort she feels is right for her during labor but also the manner in which she feels most able to express discomfort (Herr et al., 2007).

The amount of analgesia that women desire or will accept is both situationally and culturally determined. In a culture in which birth is seen as a "natural" process, less analgesia is generally desired. Women who have an effective support person with them may need less pharmacologic pain relief than those who do not. Nursing support can have a positive influence on pain relief in labor.

Physiology of Pain During Labor and Birth

Pain is a basic protective mechanism that alerts a person that something threatening is happening somewhere in the body. The sensation of pain begins in nociceptors, the end points of afferent nerves, when they are activated by mechanical, chemical, or thermal stimuli. Nociceptors are located predominantly in the skin, bone periosteum, joint surfaces, and arterial walls. When these end terminals are stimulated, chemical mediators such as prostaglandins, histamine, bradykinin, and serotonin are synthesized and help transmit the pain impulse along small, unmyelinated C fibers and large, myelinated A-delta fibers to the spinal cord. The more numerous C fibers conduct slowly and apparently carry dull, low-level pain; the fewer A-delta fibers apparently carry sharp, well-localized pain such as labor contractions.

In the dorsal horn of the spinal cord, somatostatin, cholecystokinin, and substance P serve as neurotransmitters or assist the pain impulse across the synapse between the peripheral nerve and the spinal nerve. The pain impulse then ascends the spinal cord to the brain cortex, where it is interpreted as pain.

The Melzack-Wall gate control theory of pain control (Melzack & Wall, 1965), the most widely accepted theory of pain response, proposes that pain can be halted at three points: the peripheral end terminals, the synapse points in the dorsal horn, or the point at which the impulse is interpreted as pain in the brain cortex.

Pain in peripheral terminals is automatically reduced by the production of endorphins and enkephalins, naturally occurring opiates that limit transmission of pain from the end terminals. Pain can be reduced further by mechanically irritating nerve fibers by an action such as rubbing the skin. This technique blocks nerve transmission.

A major action of pain medications is to block spinal cord neurotransmitters, never allowing the pain impulse to cross to a spinal nerve. The brain cortex can be distracted from sensing impulses as pain by the use of such techniques as imagery, thought stopping, aromatherapy, or yoga.

Sensory impulses from the uterus and cervix synapse at the spinal column at the level of T10 through L1. Pain relief measures for the first stage of labor, therefore, must block these upper synapse sites. For the elimination of pain during cesarean birth, higher receptors at the level of T6 through T8 must also be blocked, so that both the upper and lower uterus receptors are blocked.

Sensory impulses from the perineum are carried by the pudendal nerve to join the spinal column at S2, S3, and S4. When the perineum is initiating the pain, pain relief must block these lower receptor sites. This is an important point to remember when talking to a woman in labor about pain relief. Some interventions relieve pain for both the first and second stages of labor, whereas others work for one stage but not both.

Perception of Pain

The amount of discomfort a woman experiences during contractions differs according to her expectations of and preparation for labor; the length of her labor; the position of her fetus; the presence of fear, anxiety, or worry; body image; self-efficacy; and the availability of support people around her (Fig. 16.1). Women who believe that they can control their situation (have self-efficacy) are more apt to report a satisfactory birth experience than are those who do not feel in control.

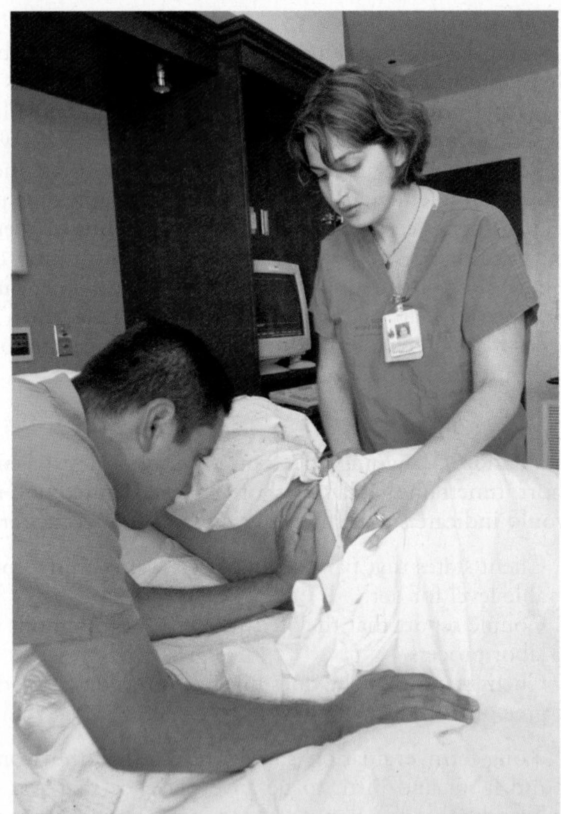

FIGURE 16.1 The discomfort a woman experiences during childbirth may be related to the amount of support she receives from her family or health care providers. Here, the woman's support person uses the palm of his hand to apply counterpressure to her lower back, helping to ease back pain, while the nurse assists.

Fetal position is a physical variable that can influence the degree of pain a woman experiences. If the fetus is in an occiput posterior position, for example, the woman often reports intense or nagging back pain, even between contractions.

Pain is perceived differently by different individuals because of psychosocial, physiologic, and cultural responses. The body's ability to produce and maintain **endorphins** (naturally occurring opiate-like substances) may influence a person's overall pain threshold and the amount of pain a person perceives at any given time. Women who come into labor believing the pain will be horrible are usually surprised afterward to realize that the agony they expected never materialized. On the other hand, women who thought that pain would be minimal can be overwhelmed by its intensity. Unreal expectations of pain this way can make a woman so tense during labor that her pain is worse than it would have been if she had been relaxed. A woman cannot relax simply because she is instructed to do so by another person, however. Some additional interventions must be used.

COMFORT AND PAIN RELIEF MEASURES

The pattern of interventions to promote comfort and manage pain in labor has swung from a philosophy of no intervention (none given because pain in labor was a "woman's lot"), to a philosophy that drug intervention was required (too much given), to a modern approach of empowering women and their partners with information so that they can choose how to best relieve pain during labor, within the limits of medical safety. For centuries, in Western civilization, offering pain relief in labor was thought to be amoral because, according to the Biblical account, God commanded Eve, "I will greatly multiply thy sorrow and thy conception; in sorrow thou shalt bring forth children..." (Genesis 3:16).

With the discovery of ether and chloroform in the 1800s, it became apparent that childbirth could be managed relatively pain free. Unfortunately, this goal was achieved by means of complete anesthesia or unconsciousness during labor and birth. Women, afterward, had difficulty realizing that the birth was over and they were a new parent.

This led to an era in which women refused pharmacologic pain relief in labor, depending entirely on prepared childbirth measures. Since the advent of epidural anesthesia (anesthetic agent placed just inside the ligamentum flavum in the epidural space), women have become more agreeable to accepting interventions for pain management (Green & Baston, 2007). Nurses play a key role in educating women and their support persons about the numerous comfort and pain relief strategies available and making sure couples understand the choices available to them along with the benefits and risks. Throughout their decision-making process, couples need support for their choices so that they can feel confidence in the method chosen.

Support From a Doula or Coach

A woman's husband or the father of her child has traditionally served as the chief support person in labor. However, some husbands or fathers find it difficult to provide effective coaching or support in labor because of their emotional involvement in the birth. Women who are aware that they may not have effective one-to-one support in labor from their baby's father should be encouraged to identify an additional person who could come with them and provide this support. A **doula** is a woman who is experienced in childbirth, but without professional credentials, who guides and assists women in labor (McGrath & Kennell, 2008). Having a doula can increase a woman's self-esteem as well as decrease rates of oxytocin augmentation, epidural anesthesia, and cesarean birth.

✔ Checkpoint Question 16.1

Susan asks you what is the purpose of a doula in labor. Your best answer would be:

a. "She can time contractions to keep them from becoming too long."
b. "She can cook you something to keep you from becoming dehydrated."
c. "She can serve as a support person and coach during your labor."
d. "She replaces your husband as your support person during labor."

Complementary and Alternative Therapies for Pain Relief

Complementary and alternative therapies for pain relief involve nonpharmacologic measures that may be used either as a woman's total pain management program or to complement pharmacologic interventions. Most of these interventions are based on the gate control theory concept that distraction can be effective in preventing the brain from processing pain sensations coming into the cortex.

Relaxation

The technique of relaxation, as discussed in Chapter 14, is taught in most preparation for childbirth classes. Relaxation keeps the abdominal wall from becoming tense, allowing the uterus to rise with contractions without pressing against the hard abdominal wall. It also serves as a distraction technique because, while concentrating on relaxing, a woman cannot concentrate on pain. In addition to conscious relaxation, having a woman shift position or find the position in labor that is most comfortable for her can be helpful. Asking a woman to bring favorite music tapes or aromatherapy with her to enjoy in the birthing room is a good way to aid relaxation (Burns et al., 2007).

Focusing and Imagery

Concentrating intently on an object is another method of distraction, or another method of keeping sensory input from reaching the cortex of the brain. For this technique, a woman uses a photograph of someone important to her or some image she finds appealing. She concentrates on it during contractions (focusing). Other women concentrate on a mental image, such as waves rolling onto a beach (imagery). Do not ask questions or talk to a woman while she is using imagery or focusing, because it breaks her concentration.

Prayer

For many women, any time they are facing a stressful situation, prayer is the first measure that they use to relieve stress. Women may bring helpful worship objects such as a Bible or cross into a hospital with them to use during prayer. These are sacred objects so be careful when changing sheets during labor that you do not accidentally throw away such important objects.

Breathing Techniques

Breathing patterns are also taught in most preparation for childbirth classes (see Chapter 14). They are advantageous because they help to relax a woman's abdomen. They are largely distraction techniques, because a woman concentrating on slow-paced breathing cannot concentrate on pain. Breathing strategies can be taught to a woman in labor if she is not familiar with their advantages before labor.

Herbal Preparations

Several herbal preparations have traditionally been used to reduce pain with dysmenorrhea or labor, although there is little factual support for their effectiveness. Examples include raspberry leaves, fennel, and life root. Blue cohosh (squaw root), an herb that induces uterine contractions, is not recommended because of the risk of acute toxic effects (e.g., cerebrovascular accident) to the mother or fetus (DerMarderosian & Beutler, 2007).

Aromatherapy and Essential Oils

Aromatherapy is the use of aromatic oils to complement emotional and physical well-being. Their use is based on the principle that the sense of smell plays a significant role in overall health. When an essential oil is inhaled, its molecules are transported via the olfactory system to the limbic system in the brain. The brain responds to particular aromas with emotional responses. When applied externally, they are absorbed by the skin and then carried throughout the body. The oils used may be able to penetrate cell walls and transport nutrients or oxygen to the inside of cells. Jasmine and lavender are oils thought to be responsible for an easier labor. When a drop of oil, such as lavender, is placed on the skin, a woman is able to taste it within 15 seconds.

Heat or Cold Application

Heat and cold have always been used for pain relief after injuries such as minor burns or strained muscles. It is only lately that they have been investigated as effective ways to help relieve the pain of labor contractions. Women who are having back pain may find application of heat to the lower back by a heating pad or a moist compress comforting.

Women who become warm from the exertion of labor find a cool washcloth to the forehead comforting. Ice chips to suck on to relieve mouth dryness are also refreshing.

Bathing or Hydrotherapy

Standing under a warm shower or soaking in a tub of warm water, jet hydrotherapy tub, or whirlpool is another way to apply heat to help reduce the pain of labor (Maude & Foureur, 2007). The temperature of water used should be between 95° and 100° F (35.0° and 37.8° C) to prevent hyperthermia. Soaking in a tub is not usually recommended for women at the beginning of labor because the heat and relaxations may slow contractions and not in women whose membranes have ruptured because of the risk of infection.

Therapeutic Touch and Massage

Therapeutic touch is the use of touch to comfort and relieve pain (Engebretson & Wardell, 2007). It is based on the concept that the body contains energy fields that, when plentiful, lead to health and, when in lesser supply, result in ill health. Krieger (1990), in a classic work, defined therapeutic touch as the laying on of hands to redirect the energy fields that lead to pain. Although the action is not well documented, touch and massage probably work to relieve pain by increasing the release of endorphins. Massage, especially, can be helpful in the first and second stages of labor (Kimber, 2007). Both these techniques also serve as forms of distraction. Effleurage, the technique of gentle abdominal massage often taught with Lamaze preparation for childbirth classes, is a form of therapeutic touch (see Fig. 14.7).

Yoga and Meditation

Yoga, a term derived from the Sanskrit word for "union," describes a series of exercises that were originally designed to bring people closer to their God. It offers a significant variety of proven health benefits, including increasing the efficiency of the heart, slowing the respiratory rate, improving fitness, lowering blood pressure, promoting relaxation, reducing stress, and allaying anxiety. Exercises consist of deep breathing exercises, body postures to stretch and strengthen muscles, and meditation to focus the mind and relax the body. It may be helpful in reducing the pain of labor through its ability to relax the body and possibly through the release of endorphins that may occur (Smith, 2009).

Meditation is a self-directed practice for relaxing the body and calming the mind (Gaudet, 2007). Mindfulness-based stress reduction (MBSR), based on Vipassana meditation from India, is based on the cultivation of intentional awareness of experiences in the present moment. Transcendental meditation (TM) is a simple, natural, effortless effort while resting comfortably with the eyes closed. Using this technique, an individual experiences a state of deep rest that can change physical and emotional responses to stress.

Reflexology

Reflexology is the practice of stimulating the hands, feet, and ears as a form of therapy (O'Mathuna, 2007). Professional reflexologists apply pressure to specific areas of the hands, feet, and ears to alleviate common ailments such as headaches, back pain, sinus colds, and stress. The theory behind reflexology is that each of the body's organs and glands are linked to corresponding areas of the hands and feet. The body is divided into 10 zones that run in longitudinal lines from the top of the head to the tips of the toes. Application of pressure to the specific area aims to restore energy to the body and improve the overall condition.

Crystal or Gemstone Therapy

Some gemstones or crystals are thought to have healing powers, and women may bring these into a birthing room to have with them during labor. A woman who uses crystals or gemstones may believe that their healing power is magnified when they are positioned around her body. Be especially careful when changing bedding or rearranging equipment in a birthing room to respect the position of these crystals. A woman may feel that they do not work their healing powers in an altered position.

Hypnosis

Hypnosis is yet another method of pain relief for labor. A woman who wants to use this modality needs to meet with her hypnotherapist during pregnancy. At these visits, she is evaluated for and further conditioned for susceptibility to hypnotic suggestion. At the last prenatal visit, she is given the posthypnotic suggestion that she will experience reduced pain or absence of pain during labor. For a woman who is susceptible to hypnotic suggestion, the method can provide a very satisfactory drug-free method of pain relief (Stephenson, 2007).

Biofeedback

Biofeedback is based on the belief that people have control and can regulate internal events such as heart rate and pain responses (Smith, 2009). Women who are interested in using biofeedback for pain relief in labor must attend several sessions during pregnancy to condition themselves to regulate their pain response. During these sessions, a biofeedback apparatus is used to measure muscle tone or the woman's ability to relax.

Transcutaneous Electrical Nerve Stimulation

Transcutaneous electrical nerve stimulation (TENS) relieves pain by counterirritation on nociceptors (Halls, 2008). With two pairs of electrodes attached to a woman's back to coincide with the T10–L1 nerve pathways, low-intensity electrical stimulation is given continuously or is applied by the woman herself as a contraction begins. This stimulation blocks the afferent fibers, preventing pain from traveling to the spinal cord synapses from the uterus. As labor progresses and the pelvic division begins, the electrodes are moved to stimulate the S2–4 level. High-intensity stimulation is generally needed to control the pain at this stage.

TENS can be as effective as epidural anesthesia for pain relief in labor, but some women may object to being "tied down" to the equipment. Women with extreme back pain during labor may benefit the most from a TENS unit, because this type of pain is difficult to relieve with controlled breathing exercises. TENS is also discussed in Chapter 24 as it is helpful for the postoperative pain of a cesarean birth.

Acupressure and Acupuncture

Acupuncture is based on the concept that illness results from an imbalance of energy. To correct the imbalance, needles are inserted into the skin at designated susceptible body points (*tsubos*) located along meridians that course throughout the body to supply the organs of the body with energy. These points are not necessarily near the affected organ. Activation of these points apparently results in release of endorphins, so the system can be helpful, especially in the first stage of labor (Rosen, 2007).

Acupressure, in contrast, is the application of pressure or massage at these points. A common point used for a woman in labor is Co4 (Hoku or Hegu point) located between the first finger and thumb on the back of the hand. When a support person holds and squeezes a woman's hand in labor, he or she may be accidentally triggering this point.

Intracutaneous Nerve Stimulation

Intracutaneous nerve stimulation (INS) is a technique of counterirritation involving the intradermal injection of sterile water or saline along the borders of the sacrum to relieve low back pain during labor. Some women find the technique helpful; others prefer to bear back pain rather than submit to injections.

✔ Checkpoint Question 16.2

Susan asks you if she could use warm-water tub bathing during labor. Your best answer would be:

a. "No. No one is allowed to tub bathe during labor."
b. "Yes, as long as your membranes are not ruptured."
c. "No, because warm water can cause uterine infections."
d. "Yes, as long as you know that warm water has no effect."

Pharmacologic Measures for Pain Relief During Labor

Pharmacologic management of pain during labor and birth includes **analgesia,** which reduces or decreases awareness of pain, and **anesthesia,** which causes partial or compete loss of sensation. For the best results, be sure women are included in a selection that is right for them.

Virtually all medication given during labor crosses the placenta and has some effect on the fetus, which makes it important for a woman to receive as little systemic medication as possible. On the other hand, labor should not test a woman to the limit of her endurance, especially since local anesthesia is available. Be sure to caution women not to take acetylsalicylic acid (aspirin) for pain in labor. Aspirin interferes with blood coagulation, increasing the risk for bleeding in the newborn or mother.

Goals of Pharmacologic Management of Pain During Labor

Medication effectively used during labor must relax a woman and relieve her discomfort, yet have minimal systemic effects on her uterine contractions, her pushing effort, or her fetus. Whether a drug affects a fetus depends on its ability to cross the placenta. Drugs with a molecular weight of greater than 1000 cross poorly, whereas those with a molecular weight of less than 600 cross very readily. Drugs with highly charged molecules or molecules strongly bound to protein cross more slowly than others. Fat-soluble drugs cross most easily. A preterm fetus, which has an immature liver and is unable to metabolize or inactivate drugs, is generally more affected by drugs than a term fetus. If a drug causes a systemic response, such as hypotension, in a woman, it can result in a decreased oxygen (PO_2) gradient across the placenta and fetal hypoxia. If it causes confusion or disorientation, a woman may be unable to work effectively with contractions, prolonging labor. If a medication causes changes in a fetus, such as a decreased heart rate or central nervous system (CNS) depression, it may be difficult for the newborn infant to initiate respirations at birth, severely compromising the infant in the important first minutes of life.

For all these reasons, there is no perfect medicine to use to reduce the pain of labor. Because pain is a subjective sensation, some women are most aware of pain early in labor, whereas some report the second stage of labor as the most difficult. The point at which pain medication is needed, therefore, differs from one individual to another. It should be given as early in labor as an individual woman needs it. Once labor is well under way, medication to relieve discomfort can speed its progress: with pain gone, a woman can relax and work with, not against, her contractions. Unfortunately, no perfect analgesic agent exists for labor or birth that has no effect on labor, the mother, and the fetus.

Preparation for Medication Administration

The type of medication used during labor varies among different health care agencies and also changes based on new research as the effectiveness and safety of new drugs for use during labor are tested. To be safe, remember the criteria that a drug must fulfill to be used in pregnancy, or expand the rule of basic medication administration from "Never give any drug unless you know it is safe for your individual client" to "Never give a drug during labor unless you know it is safe for both of your clients: the mother and the fetus."

Medicines commonly used in labor and birth are shown in Table 16.1. Prepare a woman for the type of agent prescribed,

TABLE 16.1 ✻ Analgesics and Anesthetics Commonly Used in Labor and Birth

Type	Drug	Usual Dosage/Route	Effect on Mother	Effect on Labor Progress	Effect on Fetus or Newborn
Narcotic analgesic	Meperidine (Demerol)	25 mg IV, 50–100 mg IM q3–4 hr; also epidurally	Effective analgesic; feeling of well-being	Relaxation, possibly aiding progress during cervical relaxation. Slows labor contractions if given early.	Should be given 3 hr before birth to avoid respiratory depression in newborn. Decreases beat-to-beat variability in FHR.
	Nalbuphine (Nubain)	10–20 mg IM q3–6 hr, 0.3–3 mg/kg over 10–15 min IV	Slowing of respiratory rate; effective analgesic	Mild maternal sedation	Results in some respiratory depression
	Butorphanol (Stadol)	1–2 mg IM or IV q3–4 hr	Withdrawal symptoms if woman is opiate dependent	Possible slowing of labor if given early	Results in some respiratory depression
	Morphine sulfate	Intrathecally 0.2–1 mg; 5 mg epidurally	Pruritus; effective analgesia	Possible slowing of labor contractions.	Some respiratory depression
	Fentanyl (Sublimaze)	50–100 μg IM or 25–50 μg IV; also epidurally	Hypotension; respiratory depression	Slowing of labor if given early	May result in respiratory depression
Lumbar epidural block	Local anesthetic bupivacaine (Marcaine), ropivacaine (Naropin)	Administered for first stage of labor; with continuous block, anesthesia will last through birth; injected at L3–4; fentanyl or morphine possibly added	Rapid onset, in minutes; lasting 60–90 min; loss of pain perception for labor contractions and birth; possible maternal hypotension	Slowing of labor if given early; pushing feeling obliterated, resulting in possible prolonged second stage	May be some differences in response in first few days of life
Pudendal block	Local anesthetic lidocaine (Xylocaine)	Administered just before birth for perineal anesthesia; injected through vagina	Rapid anesthesia of perineum	None apparent	None apparent
Local infiltration of perineum	Local anesthetic lidocaine (Xylocaine)	Injected just before episiotomy incision	Anesthesia of perineum almost immediately	None apparent	None apparent
General intravenous anesthetic	Thiopental	Administered IV by anesthesiologist or nurse-anesthetist	Rapid anesthesia; also rapid recovery	Forceps required because abdominal pushing is no longer possible	Results in infant being born with CNS depression

Source: Karch, A. M. (2009). *Lippincott's nursing drug guide.* Philadelphia: Lippincott Williams & Wilkins.

how it will be administered (e.g., "You'll need to lie on your side"), and what she can expect to happen after administration (e.g., "I'll be taking your blood pressure frequently"). Women in labor are under stress. Experiencing surprising body sensations from a drug without preparation can be so frightening that it can defeat their individual coping abilities and any relaxation potential associated with it. When a woman struggles this way against medication administration because she does not understand the strange feeling it is causing, the risk of inadvertent problems increases.

What if... Susan tells you she wants epidural anesthesia for pain in labor but also wants to be wide awake? How would you advise her? You notice that Susan's husband grips her hand very tightly during contractions. What possible pain relief measure is her husband's tight pressure providing for her?

Narcotic Analgesics

Narcotics may be given during labor because of their potent analgesic effect, but all drugs in this category cause fetal CNS depression to some extent so are used cautiously (McDonald & Yarnell, 2007). Be sure to question an order for a narcotic if a woman is in preterm labor. Because of possible lung immaturity, a preterm infant may have extreme difficulty coping with the added insult of respiratory depression at birth.

Narcotic analgesics commonly used include meperidine hydrochloride (Demerol), nalbuphine (Nubain), fentanyl (Sublimaze), and butorphanol tartrate (Stadol). *Meperidine* is advantageous as an analgesic in labor because it has additional sedative and antispasmodic actions; these make it effective not only for relieving pain but also for helping to relax the cervix and provide a feeling of euphoria and well-being. It may be given either intramuscularly or intravenously. The dose is 25 to 100 mg, depending on a woman's weight and the route of administration. The drug begins to act about 30 minutes after intramuscular (IM) injection and about 5 minutes after intravenous (IV) administration. Its duration of action is 2 to 3 hours (Karch, 2009).

Meperidine also may be self-administered by a patient-controlled analgesic (PCA) pump for low-dose but frequent administration during labor. Intrathecal administration (injection into the cerebrospinal fluid [CSF]) is used less frequently.

Because meperidine crosses the placenta, it can cause respiratory depression in a fetus. The drug crosses the placenta minutes after either IV or IM administration to the woman. However, because the fetal liver takes 2 to 3 hours to activate the drug into the fetal system, the effect will not be registered in the fetus for 2 to 3 hours after maternal administration. For this reason, meperidine is given when the mother is more than 3 hours away from birth. This allows the peak action of the drug in the fetus to have passed by the time of birth.

It may be puzzling to see a sleepy baby delivered to a woman who was given meperidine 2 hours before birth and an alert baby delivered to a woman who had received meperidine within 1 hour of birth. In the second instance, the peak action or peak effect has not yet occurred in the infant. This newborn needs careful assessment for the next 4 hours until the drug reaches its peak.

Nalbuphine hydrochloride (Nubain) and *butorphanol tartrate* (Stadol) are both synthetic narcotic analgesics. The action of these agents is comparable to that of meperidine. Like meperidine, they may also leave a degree of respiratory depression in the newborn.

BOX 16.3 * Focus on Pharmacology

Naloxone Hydrochloride (Narcan)

Action: Naloxone hydrochloride is a narcotic antagonist that counteracts the effect of narcotic analgesics (Karch, 2009). It is used to counteract newborn respiratory depression when a mother has received a narcotic analgesic during labor.

Pregnancy category: B

Dosage: 0.01 mg/kg, administered either IV via umbilical vein, SC, or IM; repeated at 2- to 3-minute intervals until response is obtained.

Possible adverse effects: Hypotension, hypertension, tachycardia, diaphoresis, tremulousness

Nursing Implications

- Anticipate the need for newborn resuscitative measures; have resuscitative equipment and emergency drugs readily available.
- If no IV access is available, prepare for possible administration via endotracheal tube.
- If no response is seen after two or three doses, question whether respiratory depression is caused by narcotics or another reason.
- Continuously monitor all vital signs for changes.
- Remember that the pain-relieving effect of narcotics will be reversed; assess for pain in the neonate.

Whenever a narcotic is given during labor, a narcotic antagonist such as *naloxone* (Narcan) should be available for administration to the infant at birth (Box 16.3). Carefully observe an infant who receives naloxone in the immediate postpartum period, because the infant's respirations may become severely depressed again when the drug's effect wears off. If severe infant respiratory depression is anticipated, naloxone can be given to a woman just before birth. It readily crosses the placenta and, because it interferes with or competes for narcotic binding sites, may increase the chance for spontaneous respiratory activity in the newborn.

What if... Susan receives no narcotics during labor, yet her newborn is born very sleepy. Would you administer naloxone? Would asking Susan if she used recreational drugs be warranted?

Intrathecal Narcotics. *Intrathecal* administration refers to injection into the spinal cord. With intrathecal narcotic injection, a catheter is introduced into the spinal canal (the subarachnoid space), and a narcotic such as morphine or fentanyl citrate is injected into the canal by way of the catheter. Both drugs provide excellent pain relief for labor pain. They take effect in 15 to 30 minutes, and pain relief lasts 4 to 7 hours. A woman is able to feel the urge to push at the second stage of labor, allowing her to actively participate in the birth. Because intrathecal injections are not as effective in reducing the pain of the actual birth, they may be supplemented with a pudendal block in late labor.

Possible side effects of intrathecal morphine are intense pruritus, nausea, and vomiting. The pruritus can be treated with IV diphenhydramine (Benadryl) if it becomes too uncomfortable.

Additional Drugs

Additional drugs, such as tranquilizers, may be administered during labor to reduce anxiety or potentiate the action of a narcotic. Examples include hydroxyzine hydrochloride (Vistaril) or a short-acting benzodiazepine such as midazolam (Versed). These drugs do not relieve pain, so the woman in labor needs pain management measures in addition to these drugs.

Regional Anesthesia

Regional anesthesia is the injection of a local anesthetic such as tetracaine (Pontacaine) or bupivacaine (Marcaine) to block specific nerve pathways (Cho & Penning, 2007). This achieves pain relief by blocking sodium and potassium transport in the nerve membrane, thereby stabilizing the nerve in a polarized resting state, so that it is unable to conduct sensations.

Various regional anesthetic injection sites are shown in Figure 16.2. Women with pre-eclampsia may have associated bleeding defects and need to be assessed carefully before regional anesthesia is administered.

Because regional anesthetics are not introduced into the maternal circulation, it was once believed that they had no effect on a fetus. However, research has demonstrated that there is some uptake of these drugs by a fetus, possibly resulting in fetal heart rate (FHR) decelerations and symptoms of flaccidity, bradycardia, and hypotension in the newborn (Subramanian, 2008). Effects are minimal compared with those of systemic anesthetic agents, however. Most important, regional anesthesia allows a woman to be completely awake and aware of what is happening during birth. They do not depress uterine tone, so the uterus remains capable of optimal contraction after birth, thereby helping to prevent postpartal hemorrhage.

It is rare that an infant is born with symptoms of toxicity from a regional anesthetic. If this should occur, an exchange transfusion at birth will remove the anesthetic from the infant's bloodstream. Gastric lavage also will remove a great deal of anesthetic, because anesthetics have a strong affinity for acid media such as stomach acid.

Epidural Anesthesia. The nerves in the spinal cord are protected by several tissue layers. The pia mater is the membrane adhering to the nerve fibers. Surrounding this is the *cerebrospinal fluid.* Next comes the arachnoid membrane and outside that, the *dura mater.* Outside the dura mater is a vacant space (the *epidural space*). Beyond it is the *ligamentum flavum,* yet another protective shield for the vulnerable spinal cord (see Fig. 16.2).

An anesthetic agent introduced into the CSF in the subarachnoid space is called a *spinal injection* or *spinal anesthesia.* An anesthetic agent placed just inside the ligamentum flavum in the epidural space is **epidural anesthesia.** Anesthetic agents placed in the epidural space at the L4–5, L3–4, or L2–3 interspace block not only spinal nerve roots in the space but also the sympathetic nerve fibers that travel with them. Therefore, these blocks provide pain relief for both labor and birth. Such a block may actually increase contraction strength and blood flow to the uterus. Because a woman no longer experiences pain, the release of catecholamines (epinephrine) with a β-blocking effect from a pain response is decreased, making this a very effective pain relief measure for labor (Anim-Somuah, Smyth, & Howell, 2009).

Women worry if they will experience a "spinal headache" after receiving anesthesia. These headaches are apparently caused by leakage of CSF or instillation of air into the CSF. With epidural anesthesia, the CSF space is not entered, so this problem should not occur (Box 16.4). Because the

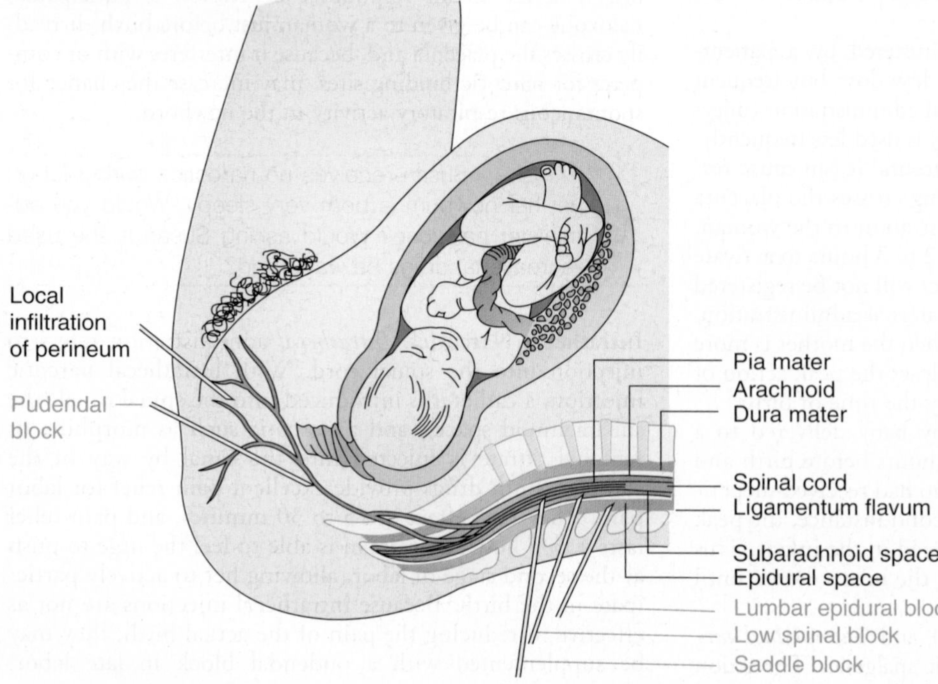

FIGURE 16.2 Anatomy of the spinal canal and sites of injection for regional anesthesia.

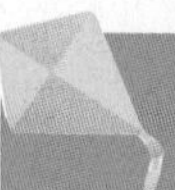

BOX 16.4 ✻ Focus on Evidence-Based Practice

How often do postepidural headaches occur?

Theoretically, epidural anesthesia does not result in a postprocedure headache because such headaches are caused by loss of spinal fluid and with epidural anesthesia, the spinal fluid or subarachnoid space is not entered. A few women do report frontal or occipital headaches accompanied by photophobia, nausea, and vomiting following epidural anesthesia. To investigate the incidence of epidural postprocedure headaches, researchers reviewed the labor and birth charts of 18,337 women who received epidural anesthesia for labor or birth. Of these women, 167, or 0.91%, were identified as women who had had an accidental dural puncture. Of these women, 88% developed a postprocedure headache (147 women), or the overall incidence of headache following routine epidural administration to women in labor was 0.8%.

If a woman is worried about developing a "spinal headache," would you use the above study to assure her she will not develop a headache?

Sprigge, J. S., & Harper, S. J. (2008). Accidental dural puncture and post dural puncture headache in obstetric anaesthesia: presentation and management: a 23-year survey in a district general hospital. *Anaesthesia, 63*(1), 36–43.

injection technique is potentially frightening, however, women need continuous support during the process.

Epidural blocks, administered by an anesthesiologist or nurse-anesthetist, are suitable for almost all women. They are advantageous for women with heart disease, pulmonary disease, diabetes, and sometimes severe pregnancy-induced hypertension, because they make labor virtually pain free and thereby reduce stress from the discomfort of labor to a minimum. Because the woman does not feel contractions, her physical energy is preserved. Epidural blocks are acceptable for use in preterm labor because the drug has scant effect on a fetus and allows for a controlled and gentle birth with less trauma to an immature fetal skull. Because the woman receives no systemic medication, the infant responds more quickly after birth than if systemic narcotic analgesics were used.

The chief concern with epidural anesthesia is its tendency to cause hypotension because of its blocking effect on the sympathetic nerve fibers in the epidural space. This blocking leads to decreased peripheral resistance in the woman's circulatory system. Decreased peripheral resistance causes blood to flow freely into peripheral vessels, and a pseudohypovolemia develops, registering as hypotension. The combined use of fentanyl and bupivacaine can lower the risk for hypotension. In addition, the risk also can be reduced by being sure a woman is well hydrated with 500 to 1000 mL of IV fluid, such as Ringer's lactate, before the anesthetic is given. Ringer's lactate is preferable to a glucose solution, because too much maternal glucose can cause hyperglycemia with rebound hypoglycemia in the newborn. Be certain that a woman does not lie supine but remains on her side after an epidural block, to help prevent supine hypotension syndrome.

If hypotension should occur, raising the woman's legs and administering oxygen and additional IV fluid, along with an agent such as ephedrine to elevate blood pressure, may be necessary to stabilize cardiovascular status.

The use of an epidural block may prolong the second stage of labor, but whether this leads to an increase in cesarean births is controversial (Cho & Penning, 2007). Descent can slow, for example, taking 3 hours rather than 2 hours, but if there is no indication that this is detrimental to the fetus, it should not lead to a greater need for vacuum extraction or cesarean birth (Crombleholme, 2009). Relaxation of the levator ani muscle may impede internal rotation of the fetal head, further slowing labor or making the use of forceps necessary to effect rotation. This occurs primarily when the fetus is in an occipitoposterior position. Oxytocin may be given to shorten labor. Allowing an epidural to wear off by the second stage of labor, so that a woman can push with contractions, is another option. However, experiencing contractions at this point can be overwhelming for a woman and counteracts the original reason for giving the anesthetic: to reduce pain in labor.

In rare instances, the anesthetic enters the blood circulation. This occurrence is manifested as drowsiness, a metallic taste on the tongue, slurred speech, blurred vision, unconsciousness, and seizure leading to cardiac arrest. If such symptoms occur, it is an emergency situation. The woman needs oxygen and an anticonvulsant such as diazepam (Valium) or thiopental (Pentothal) IV, followed by prompt birth of the fetus.

Technique for Administration. Epidural anesthesia is begun when the cervix is dilated 3 to 5 cm. An IV infusion and equipment for blood pressure monitoring should be in place. Help position the woman on her side. Her back should not be flexed, because this increases the possibility of puncturing the dura and accidentally giving the anesthetic as a spinal, not epidural, injection. The lumbar area of the back is cleaned with an antiseptic solution. A local anesthetic is injected into the skin to form a wheal over the L3 and L4 vertebrae. A special 3- to 5-inch needle is then passed through the L3–4 interspace into the epidural space. After needle placement, a polyethylene catheter is passed through the needle into the space, and the needle is then withdrawn, leaving the catheter to be taped in place. A closed system (a syringe is attached) is established to prevent infection through the catheter (Fig. 16.3).

The anesthetist then injects a small test dose of a local anesthetic solution into the catheter. Five minutes later, the woman's legs are inspected for flushing and warmness, evidence that the anesthetic is in the epidural space (peripheral dilatation is beginning). Assess a woman's pulse and blood pressure at this time. If the anesthetic was accidentally placed in a blood vessel, toxic symptoms of hypotension, slurred speech, and rapid pulse will be present. After assurance that the anesthetic is epidural, the initial dose of anesthetic is given through the catheter. This produces anesthesia up to the level of the umbilicus in 10 to 15 minutes. The effect of epidural anesthesia is short lived (40 minutes to 2 hours). To keep a woman free from discomfort during the duration of labor, another dose of anesthetic, termed a "top-up," must be added, or anesthetic must be continually infused by an infusion pump. A nurse should be in continuous attendance while an epidural anesthetic is given. Be certain to review agency policy regarding nursing responsibility for catheter care before caring for a woman with a catheter in place (Pasero et al., 2007).

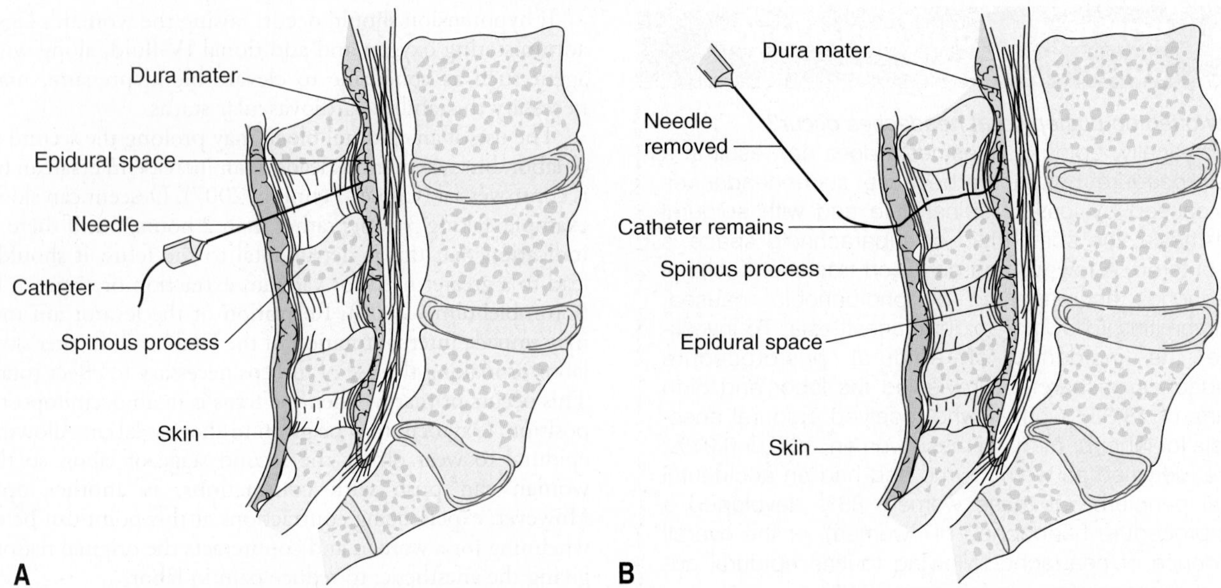

FIGURE 16.3 Epidural anesthesia. (**A**) A needle is inserted into the epidural space. (**B**) A catheter is threaded into the epidural space; the needle is then removed. The catheter allows medication to be administered intermittently or continuously to relieve pain during labor and childbirth.

Before an additional top-up dose is administered, ask the woman to both write and say out loud a phrase such as "I can do it" three times. If she is unable to do this, question the dose: lack of fine motor coordination and slurred speech indicate a slowly occurring toxic reaction.

Yet another technique used with epidural anesthesia is self-administered or patient-controlled epidural analgesia (PCEA). With this technique, an epidural catheter delivers an analgesic mixture whenever the client presses a button on a special pump (Topcu et al., 2007). A lockout period follows each self-administration, to avoid overdosage. This method of administration is advantageous because less anesthetic is required, compared with continuous epidural infusion (CEI), and gives a woman a feeling of empowerment as she controls her own pain management (Marshall & Baker, 2007). Epidural anesthesia can cause a temporary elevation in temperature although this is not serious (Goetzl et al., 2007). Keep in mind this may occur when evaluating a woman's temperature. To detect hypotension, continuously monitor blood pressure for the first 20 minutes after each new injection of anesthetic. Continue to monitor blood pressure throughout the time the anesthetic is in effect, to be certain that the systolic pressure does not fall to less than 100 mm Hg or decrease by 20 mm Hg or more in a hypertensive woman. A drop greater than this could be life-threatening to a fetus unless prompt, effective corrective measures are taken, such as repositioning and administering an antihypotensive agent. If such measures are instituted quickly, fetal outcome will not be compromised.

Epidural anesthesia may also be given in a "segmented" fashion. With this technique, after the test dose, only a small dose (about 4 mL) is given. This provides anesthesia for uterine contractions but not perineal relaxation. Close to birth, if the woman sits up and an additional dose is given, perineal anesthesia will result. Leaving the lower anesthesia for late in labor in this way allows for better internal rotation of the fetal head, because the perineal muscle is not lax and there is less chance that forceps for rotation will be necessary.

With an epidural block, a woman loses sensation of her bladder filling. Remind her to void every 2 hours, monitor intake and output, and observe and palpate for bladder distention to avoid overfilling. To assess after birth whether the anesthesia is wearing off, touch a woman's legs and ask if she feels your touch. Ask her to raise her knees and observe whether she can do this. Even after feeling in legs returns, walking may be difficult. Be certain to stay with a woman the first time she is out of bed following regional block anesthesia.

Spinal (Subarachnoid) Anesthesia. Spinal anesthesia is used less frequently today, in preference to lumbar epidural blocks. It may be used in an emergency, however, because the administration technique is simpler than that of an epidural and can be accomplished more rapidly.

For spinal anesthesia, a local anesthetic agent such as bupivacaine (Marcaine) or ropivacaine (Naropin) is injected using lumbar puncture technique into the subarachnoid space (into the CSF) at the third or fourth lumbar interspace. A narcotic agonist such as morphine or fentanyl may be added for additional pain relief. For administration, the woman is placed in a sitting position on the side of the birthing bed, with legs dangling and head bent. She is asked to bend her head forward so that her back curves and the intravertebral spaces open. Be sure to support her in this position, because she is "front-heavy" as a result of her pregnancy and could easily fall forward if not well supported.

After injection, the anesthetic normally rises to the level of T10. Anesthesia up to the umbilicus and including both legs will be achieved. Spinal anesthetic agents may be "loaded" or "weighted" with glucose to make them heavier than CSF. This helps prevent them from rising too high in the spinal canal and interfering with the motor control of the uterus or with respiratory muscles.

After injection of the anesthetic, the anesthesiologist asks the woman to lie down again. It is important that she does lie down at this time, because if she sits up too long, the anesthetic will not rise high enough in the canal to achieve pain relief. On the other hand, she must not lie down before this time, or the anesthetic will rise too high in the canal. Lying with a pillow under the head also helps ensure that the anesthesia will be confined to the lower spinal canal.

Hypotension from sympathetic blockage in the lower extremities can occur immediately after administration. This leads to vasodilation and a decrease in central blood pressure. If hypotension occurs, placental blood perfusion could be compromised. Turn the woman to her left side to reduce vena cava compression. The anesthesiologist will quickly increase the rate of IV fluid administration to increase blood volume. A vasopressor (e.g., ephedrine) to increase blood pressure and oxygen also may be administered. Never place a woman in a Trendelenburg position to help restore blood pressure after spinal anesthesia. This could make the anesthetic rise high in her spinal column, causing uterine or respiratory function to cease.

To guard against hypotension, IV fluids such as lactated Ringer's solution are usually given before the injection to ensure hydration. Be certain the fluid is infusing well before the anesthesia is administered.

A late complication of spinal anesthesia is a postpartal dural puncture headache (PDPH) or "spinal headache." This occurs because of continuous leakage of CSF from the needle insertion site and possibly from the irritation of a small amount of air that enters at the injection site. The shift in pressure of the CSF causes strain on the cerebral meninges, initiating the pain. The incidence of such headaches is reduced if a small-gauge needle is used for the injection and the woman drinks a quantity of fluid afterward, because a high fluid intake rapidly provides replacement of spinal fluid. Although it is usually encouraged, asking a woman to remain flat may not be necessary because of the routine use of small needles in most settings.

If a headache does occur, it can be relieved by having the woman lie flat and administering an analgesic. Some women find a cold cloth applied to the forehead helpful. If a headache is incapacitating, it can be treated with a blood patch technique. For this, 10 mL of blood is withdrawn from an accessible vein and then immediately injected into the epidural space over the spinal injection site. The injected blood clots and seals off any further leakage of CSF.

✔ Checkpoint Question 16.3

Susan chooses to have epidural anesthesia. What are two risks associated with this?

a. Hypotension and prolonged second stage of labor.
b. Severe headache and coldness of all extremities.
c. Continued back pain and short first stage of labor.
d. Hypertension and a reduced red blood cell count.

Combined Spinal Epidural Technique. Spinal anesthesia has an advantage over epidural anesthesia in that the pain control is immediate after injection of the anesthetic. A disadvantage of spinal anesthesia is that the woman cannot ambulate afterward. To take advantage of the rapid onset of pain control but also allow for ambulation, combined spinal epidural (CSE) technique was originated (Simmons et al., 2009). To administer this, the anesthesiologist first inserts an epidural needle using usual epidural technique. A catheter is inserted into the epidural needle and taped in place. The anesthesiologist then inserts a very fine spinal needle into the subarachnoid space and the CSF. It is confirmed that the second needle is into the CSF if a drop of fluid falls from the end of the needle. A small dose of narcotic (e.g., fentanyl) is then added to the CSF, and the spinal needle is withdrawn.

The advantage of a CSE administration is immediate pain relief, whereas an epidural block alone would take 15 to 30 minutes to accomplish this. In addition, it allows the woman to be ambulatory, because the drug added to the CSF is a narcotic, not a local anesthetic. Possible complications that can occur from the CSE method include hypotension, pruritus, urinary retention, nausea and vomiting, and a PDPH (although all of these are rare). Additional anesthesia for the duration of labor is achieved by the epidural route.

Medication for Pain Relief During Birth

Stretching of the perineum causes the pain during birth. The simplest form of pain relief for birth is the natural **pressure anesthesia** that results from the fetal head pressing against the stretched perineum. This natural anesthesia is often adequate to allow an episiotomy to be performed without a woman feeling the cut. The pain she experiences as the fetal head is born, although intense and hot, occurs suddenly and is over quickly. Often, after the hours of hard contractions a woman has come through, this flash of pain seems almost nothing. For some women, however, additional medication is needed to reduce the pain of birth.

Local Anesthetics

Local anesthesia reduces the ability of local nerve fibers to conduct pain.

Local Infiltration. Local infiltration is the injection of an anesthetic such as lidocaine (Xylocaine) into the superficial nerves of the perineum. It is used when the fetal head is too low to allow for a pudendal block. The anesthetic is placed along the borders of the vulva. The effect lasts for approximately 1 hour, allowing for a pain-free birth and suturing of an episiotomy without additional anesthetic.

Pudendal Nerve Block. A **pudendal nerve block** (Fig. 16.4) is the injection of a local anesthetic such as bupivacaine (Marcaine) near the right and left pudendal nerves at the level of the ischial spine. The injection, made through the vagina with the woman in a lithotomy or dorsal recumbent position, provides relief of perineal pain in 2 to 10 minutes that lasts for approximately 1 hour. Anesthesia achieved with this method is sufficiently deep to allow the use of low forceps during birth and an episiotomy repair. Although the injection is only local, the FHR and the mother's blood pressure should be checked immediately after the injection, in case maternal hypotension occurs.

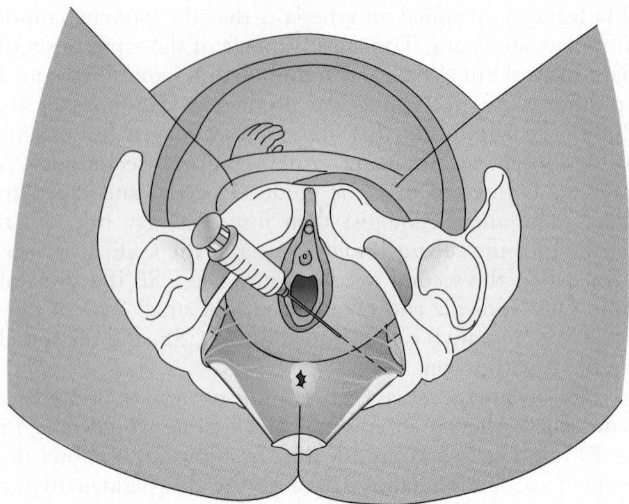

FIGURE 16.4 Pudendal nerve block.

General Anesthesia

General anesthesia is never preferred for childbirth, because it carries the dangers of hypoxia and possible inhalation of vomitus during administration. Pregnant women are particularly prone to gastric reflux and aspiration because of increased stomach pressure from the weight of the full uterus beneath it. The gastroesophageal valve also may be displaced and possibly functioning improperly. Despite these risks, general anesthesia may be necessary in emergency situations (e.g., premature separation of the placenta) when an immediate cesarean birth is required.

For complete and rapid anesthesia during childbirth, thiopental sodium (Pentothal), a short-acting barbiturate, is usually the drug of choice. It causes rapid induction of anesthesia and, because it has a short half-life, allows for good uterine contraction afterward, with minimal postpartal bleeding. After intravenous induction with thiopental sodium, the woman is intubated, and anesthesia is then maintained by administration of nitrous oxide and oxygen. Thiopental sodium crosses the placenta rapidly. Infants born of a woman anesthetized by this method may be slow to respond at birth and may need resuscitation. However, in view of the degree of barbiturate intoxication demonstrable in these infants, their ability to respond and alertness at birth are always surprising.

All women who receive a general anesthetic must be observed closely in the postpartal period, because most gases used for general anesthesia cause uterine relaxation, opening the possibility of uterine atony and postpartal hemorrhage. Some women comment that their throat feels raw or sore afterward from insertion of the endotracheal tube. Using an anesthetic throat spray or gargle, sipping cold liquids, or sucking on ice chips (as soon as this is safe after general anesthesia) may help to relieve the discomfort.

Preparation for the Safe Administration of General Anesthesia. To ensure safe anesthesia administration, an anesthesiologist or nurse anesthetist needs a minimum of six drugs readily available: (a) ephedrine, to use in the event blood pressure falls; (b) atropine sulfate, to dry oral and respiratory secretions to prevent aspiration; (c) thiopental sodium (Pentothal), for rapid induction of a general anesthetic; (d) succinylcholine (Anectine), to achieve laryngeal relaxation for intubation; (e) diazepam (Valium), to control seizures, a possible reaction to anesthetics; and (f) isoproterenol (Isuprel), to reduce bronchospasm should aspiration occur. In addition to these medications, an adult laryngoscope, an endotracheal tube, a breathing bag with a source of 100% oxygen, and a suction catheter and suction source should be at hand.

Aspiration of Vomitus. Inhalation of vomitus from pressure of the uterus on the stomach can be fatal if a woman's airway becomes occluded by the foreign matter. In addition, stomach contents have an acid pH that can cause chemical pneumonitis and secondary infection of the respiratory tract.

Some anesthesiologists may order IV ranitidine (Zantac) or an oral antacid such as cimetidine to be given before general anesthesia is administered, to reduce the level of acid in stomach contents should aspiration occur. Metoclopramide (Reglan) increases gastric emptying and may also be prescribed.

For general anesthesia administration, a woman should be placed on her back with a wedge under her right hip to displace the uterus from the vena cava. To reduce the occurrence of hypotension and to establish a line for emergency medications, IV fluid administration is begun. The woman is given a rapid-induction IV agent and is then intubated with a cuffed endotracheal tube. To prevent gastric reflux and aspiration before intubation is achieved, cricoid pressure (which seals off the esophagus by compressing it between the cricoid cartilage and the cervical vertebrae) must be applied as soon as the IV agent is begun until the cuff on the tube is in place.

The moments of induction of general anesthesia before the endotracheal tube is safely in place are critical ones for the anesthesiologist. Respect his or her need to concentrate until the task is achieved.

If aspiration of vomitus should occur in a birthing room, prompt attention is essential. The anesthesiologist suctions the woman's trachea to remove as much foreign material as possible. The woman is intubated, if she was not previously, and given 100% oxygen. IV isoproterenol to reduce bronchospasm and a corticosteroid to reduce inflammation may be given. Positive-pressure ventilation may be started. Blood gas analysis and a chest radiograph usually are obtained to determine the degree of aeration of which the woman is still capable.

Usually, the woman will receive mechanical ventilation until her overall clinical condition improves, as shown by the x-ray films and blood gas concentrations. She is critically ill at the time of aspiration and often will be transferred to an intensive care unit for the special care she needs to survive this emergency.

✔ Checkpoint Question 16.4

There is no reason to think that Susan will need a general anesthetic. If she did, what type of drug is usually prescribed to minimize the risk of aspiration of vomitus?

a. An anticonvulsant such as diazepam (Valium).
b. A nerve relaxant such as phenobarbital.
c. Metoclopramide (Reglan) to speed gastric emptying.
d. Oxytocin to increase the effectiveness of labor.

NURSING CARE TO PROMOTE THE COMFORT OF A WOMAN DURING LABOR

The best approach to pain management for women in labor is to always complement any pharmacologic intervention with a complementary or alternative therapy measure.

Nursing Diagnoses and Related Interventions

Nursing Diagnosis: Anxiety related to fear of pain from labor contractions

Outcome Evaluation: Client identifies beginning and ending of contractions; expresses confidence rather than confusion about ongoing process; states she feels less anxious.

In addition to causing local discomfort, pain can evoke a general stress response (fight-or-flight syndrome). This releases epinephrine, which causes peripheral and uterine vasoconstriction. This can increase the degree of pain experienced because of the resulting increase in tissue anoxia. Reducing anxiety through relaxation techniques such as planned breathing exercises, or through administration of medication to reduce anxiety, can reduce vasoconstriction and help reduce pain.

Reduce Anxiety With Explanations of the Labor Process. Planning with women about their options for pain relief during labor should begin prenatally (Box 16.5). During labor, use a standard method of pain assessment, such as a scale of 1 to 10, so that a woman can rate her pain. Evaluate whether pain relief is adequate—not only whether pain relief was offered, but whether it was effective.

Help women use natural methods based on the gate control theory (see Chapter 14) as well as pharmacology relief. Be sure to offer careful explanations of what is happening or what will happen during labor, because this can help alleviate anxiety and thereby reduce some discomfort.

Be sure to explain the characteristics of contractions and reinstruct as necessary (e.g., that labor contractions are rhythmic in nature and come and go repeatedly). Do not assume that a woman is aware of this simply because she is experiencing the contractions. Her pain may be so intense that she is unaware of any relief between contractions (Box 16.6). She may fear that things will worsen as labor progresses and that the pain will become continuous.

This on–off effect differentiates the pain of labor contractions from that of a toothache or headache, which is continuous. Sometimes, just knowing this can help a woman tolerate the pain even as it increases in intensity.

Do not assume everyone knows that the rupturing of membranes is painless, that a pink-stained show is normal, or that contractions change in character during the pelvic division of labor. A woman having her first child probably does not know these things. A woman having her second child may not remember, or she may find this time so different from the last time (even if it is well within normal limits) that she is frightened. Be certain to give explanations to a woman's husband or support person, as well; otherwise, he or she may start to convey anxiety back to the woman in labor.

Nursing Diagnosis: Ineffective coping related to combination of uterine contractions and anxiety

Outcome Evaluation: Client expresses confidence in her ability to maintain active participation during labor; demonstrates continued breathing techniques; expresses need to change position; and expresses confidence in the labor nurse and other health care providers.

BOX 16.5 * Focus on Family Teaching

Learning More About Options for Pain Relief During Labor

Q. Susan tells you, "My friends have told me horrible stories about pain during labor. What can I do so I won't hurt so much?"

A. Here are some suggestions to help with pain relief:

- Ask your obstetrician or nurse-midwife early in pregnancy about pain management options. The options your care provider suggests may actually influence your decision as to whether this is the optimal care provider for you.
- Attend childbirth preparation classes during pregnancy, and conscientiously practice breathing or other relaxation exercises. These measures can be adequate all by themselves; if not, they complement pharmacologic methods of pain relief.
- Make a birth plan detailing what position you choose for labor and other options you want to use. This helps give you a greater sense of control.
- Be certain a support person will be with you during labor. Name a second person or investigate using a doula if you are uncertain whether your usual support person can fill this role.
- Late in pregnancy, if you are still concerned, let your primary care provider know. In addition to medication for pain relief during labor, medication to reduce anxiety is also available.
- On admission to the hospital, let the medical and nursing staff know that you are concerned. The most commonly used options today are oral, intramuscular, or intravenous administration of narcotics and injection of regional anesthesia by epidural block. Ask questions about any method suggested that you do not understand.
- Be aware that the choice of receiving analgesia or anesthesia is yours. On the other hand, if a complication occurs, be ready to compromise in the interest of safety for yourself or your child.

BOX 16.6 * Focus on Communication

Suppose Susan stated early in labor that she did not want to use any medication for pain relief. As soon as her contractions became 30 seconds in length, however, she requested some analgesia. Her physician prescribed intramuscular meperidine. Her contractions are now 40 seconds in duration and only moderately strong. She looks increasingly uncomfortable with each contraction.

Less Effective Communication

Nurse: How are you feeling, Susan? Is there anything I can do for you?

Susan: I need something else for pain. I can't stand this any longer.

Nurse: Didn't the medicine I gave you work at all?

Susan: It's working for now, but it won't be enough by another half hour. I'll need something else by then.

Nurse: You won't be able to get anything for another 2 hours. I'm sorry.

More Effective Communication

Nurse: How are you feeling, Susan? Is there anything I can do for you?

Susan: I need something else for pain. I can't stand this any longer.

Nurse: On a scale of 0 to 10, with 0 being no pain and 10 being the worst pain ever, how would you rate your pain now?

Susan: It's about a 2 now, but it'll be a 10 in another half-hour when my contractions start to be constant. How will I be able to stand them when they don't let up at all.

Nurse: I'm sorry. I must not have explained that contractions always have a space in between them. Let's talk about that.

Because women in labor are under stress, they may not hear instructions as well as they normally would. First, assess the pain. Asking a woman to rate her pain on a scale of 0 to 10 is an effective method for pain assessment. Also, be certain to assess whether the woman has a clear understanding of the nature of labor contractions so that she is well prepared to manage them.

Help the Woman Identify Coping Strategies. Because pain is not a new phenomenon for a woman of childbearing age, it can be helpful to ask a woman to recall methods she usually uses to combat pain or anxiety such as meditation or applying a cool cloth. This can go a long way toward helping her collect her resources and decide on a pain relief strategy (see Focus on Nursing Care Planning Box 16.7).

Provide Comfort Measures. Usually, anyone can tolerate a little discomfort from a backache, being thirsty, having dry lips, or having a leg cramp. However, few people can tolerate having all of these discomforts simultaneously or feeling even one of them while experiencing labor contractions.

Assist a woman's support person to provide the usual comfort measures that are helpful for anyone with pain, such as reassurance or a change in position. For dry lips, ice chips to suck on, moistening the lips with a wet cloth, or using a moisturizing jelly may be helpful. A cool cloth to wipe perspiration from her forehead can prevent her from feeling overheated.

Be aware of what is happening to a woman's bedclothes and clothing, which will wrinkle rapidly and stick to her skin because she is perspiring. If a waterproof pad is used under her buttocks, it will become soiled with vaginal secretions and feel hot and sticky. However, never apply sanitary pads in labor. Although they absorb vaginal secretions well, they tend to slip out of place, possibly carrying pathogens from the rectal area forward to the vaginal opening. Instead, change the waterproof pad frequently. At least halfway through the first stage of labor, or more frequently as indicated by the woman's condition, change the sheets and give her a clean gown. She could bathe or take a shower if that would be helpful. These measures can help her feel clean and refreshed, with a ready-to-go-again feeling.

Think of comfort measures for the woman's support person as well. Is the chair by the side of the bed comfortable? Does he or she need to stretch or take a beverage or bathroom break? It is difficult for the support person to comfort a woman if he or she is uncomfortable because of spending hours sitting still in one position.

Nursing Diagnosis: Pain related to labor contractions

Outcome Evaluation: Client states pain is reduced to a tolerable level with techniques used and is able to handle or "work with" contractions; demonstrates ability to listen and respond to questions and instructions.

Encourage Comfortable Positioning. An upright, sitting, or walking position may be most comfortable for a woman in early labor. Contractions also are most efficient in this position. Before membranes have ruptured, therefore, a woman may be most comfortable either sitting in a chair or ambulating. After the membranes have ruptured and if the fetal head is not engaged, there may be danger in walking about, because the cord might prolapse and impede fetal circulation. If this is so, a woman should remain in bed at this time. Urge her not to lie on her back, to avoid supine hypotension syndrome.

Encouraging position changes from time to time is important. Assist a woman to find a satisfying position by moving bedclothes or monitor leads, if any are attached. If she wishes to walk and has no support person, walk with her. Pelvic rocking between contractions may relieve tense back muscles.

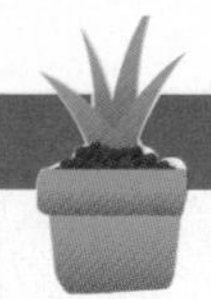

BOX 16.7 ✻ Focus on Nursing Care Planning

A Multidisciplinary Care Map for a Woman Requiring Comfort Measures During Labor and Birth

Susan Baranca is a primipara in early labor whom you admit to a birthing unit. She tells you her sister had epidural anesthesia for the birth of her baby 3 months ago. She told Susan that preparation for labor really was not necessary because an epidural block completely obliterated her pain in labor. Based on her sister's experience, Susan expected to be given epidural anesthesia as soon as she arrived at the hospital. As she is barely in labor, however, her physician asked her to wait until she is 4 cm dilated. When you enter her room, you find her lying on her back in a birthing bed, crying. Her husband is standing outside in the hallway at the nursing desk, shouting that his wife deserves better care than this.

Family Assessment ✻ Gravida 1, para 0; accompanied by husband who will act as support person and coach. Client works as clerk in clothing store; husband is law student at local university.

Client Assessment ✻ Contractions are of moderate intensity, every 6 to 7 minutes, 35 seconds' duration. Cervix dilated 3 cm, 60% effaced. Membranes intact. FHR 148; fetus in ROA position. Attended childbirth education classes but did not practice breathing exercises.

Nursing Diagnosis ✻ Pain related to effects of uterine contractions and pressure on pelvic structures

Outcome Criteria ✻ Client confirms that discomfort is controlled with either nonpharmacologic or pharmacologic methods; responds to questions and instructions; identifies need for additional pain relief measures if required during labor.

Team Member Responsible	Assessment	Intervention	Rationale	Expected Outcome
Activities of Daily Living				
Nurse	Assess what birth plan the woman wants to follow. Inspect the client's suprapubic area and palpate for bladder distention.	Remind client she does not need to remain in bed. Encourage client to void every 2 hours.	Ambulation can increase comfort. A full bladder contributes to the client's discomfort and may impede fetal descent, possibly prolonging labor.	Client ambulates in early labor. Has no signs of bladder distention; voids every 2 hours during labor.
Consultations				
Physician/nurse	Locate which health care provider is on call to provide anesthetic pain relief in labor.	Notify nurse-anesthetist concerning client's wish to receive an epidural block as soon as possible.	Respecting client's wishes is a prime mode of encouraging self-efficacy.	Pain management team supports client's wish for pharmacologic intervention; encourages nonpharmacologic measures until epidural anesthetic is appropriate.
Procedures/Medications				
Nurse	Assess how client's husband views his role in labor.	Allow client's husband to take occasional breaks. Stay with the client during this time to provide support.	Occasional relief breaks allow a support person to conserve energy and provide continued support throughout labor.	Client allows health care providers to substitute for husband so husband can take occasional breaks.

(continued)

BOX 16.7 ✻ Focus on Nursing Care Planning (continued)

Team Member Responsible	Assessment	Intervention	Rationale	Expected Outcome
		Nutrition		
Nurse	Determine when patient last ate.	Provide client with ice chips as desired.	Ice chips or hard candy can relieve mouth dryness from breathing exercises.	Client states she has no mouth discomfort.
		Patient/Family Education		
Nurse	Assess what couple learned in preparation for childbirth classes about pain control in labor.	Provide information on epidural anesthesia; update the couple on labor progress.	An epidural is the pain control method chosen; frequent updates on progress help alleviate anxiety and fears that may exacerbate pain.	Couple confirm that they are certain epidural anesthesia is their method of choice; receive frequent updates on labor progress.
		Psychosocial/Spiritual/Emotional Needs		
Nurse	Assess level of client's pain by both verbal and nonverbal indicators. Use 1-to-10 scale and evaluate response to techniques used.	Teach breathing exercises for use during early labor until client receives epidural relief.	Pain is a subjective experience, so only the woman can know her level of pain. Breathing exercises can be an effective way to reduce the pain of labor.	Client rates her level of pain from labor contractions not above 3 on a 1-to-10 scale.
Nurse	Assess what nonpharmacologic measures (e.g., music, room temperature) client thinks would help complement epidural block and aid comfort.	Provide a comfortable environment: clean sheets, comfortable room temperature, cool washcloth to forehead, closed room door. Refrain from intervening with client during a contraction.	A comfortable environment aids in relaxation, promoting effective coping. Interrupting the client's breathing can make the technique ineffective as a pain relief measure.	Client reports she feels environment is comfortable and complements other pain relief measures.
		Discharge Planning		
Nurse	Ask client and husband to evaluate their labor experience.	Review with client pain relief measures used and determine which were most effective.	Reviewing a possibly traumatic experience helps to put it into perspective among life events.	Client and support person state that labor and birth was at worst a tolerable experience; at best, a highlight of their lives.

Position changes are also essential in the second stage of labor. Depending on medical protocols and barring any medical contraindications, a woman might prefer to sit, stand, kneel on hands and knees, lie in dorsal recumbent or lateral recumbent positions, or squat (see Chapter 15). Keep in mind that maintaining these positions often requires assistance from one or two support people.

Assist the Woman With Prepared Childbirth Method. Depending on the type of childbirth preparation a woman and her support person have had, the method used may include breathing exercises, distraction by focusing on an external object, acupressure, therapeutic touch, music therapy, guided imagery, self-hypnosis, or a combination of these methods (see Chapter 14). Biofeedback is not well documented in labor but also may be effective.

Often, with the discomfort and stress of labor, it is easy for a woman to forget what was learned in the relaxed, fun setting of an antepartal class. As necessary, review previously learned breathing techniques with the woman. Urge her to begin these early in labor, even before contractions become strong. It is not essential for women to use complex breathing patterns in labor; even a woman who has had no prior training in breathing exercises can use a simple breathing pattern to alleviate discomfort with just a little guidance from a nurse.

Massage is another pain relief method that can be taught to a woman and her support person during labor. It may be especially useful if a woman is experiencing back pain from labor, because rubbing or massaging the sacral area often alleviates back pain. Firm counterpressure on the lower back, thighs, feet, hands, or shoulders can provide a relaxing distraction from the sensation of internal pressure and pain.

Provide Pharmacologic Pain Relief. Helping a woman decide if and when medication for pain relief should be given requires an in-depth understanding of the available drugs, their effects on the mother and the fetus, and their mechanism and duration of action. It also requires sympathetic listening and counseling skills. Many women come into labor wishing to avoid drugs entirely. Once in labor, they may change their minds but hesitate to say so, especially if their partners also believe that a birth without the use of drugs is ideal. Other women come into labor asking to receive something immediately to avoid experiencing any pain. In both instances, provide information about the use of drugs and their ultimate effects. Maintain a supportive presence to help a woman make the best decision for herself and her baby. Some women require analgesia or anesthesia because of a complication. Helping these women and their support persons understand why the medication is necessary calls for equal care and skill. As a rule, record a baseline FHR and maternal blood pressure and pulse before administering medication; reassess 15 minutes later for fetal and maternal safety.

✓ Checkpoint Question 16.5

Susan, still in early labor, tells you that she is not having much pain. You assess that her contractions are also not strong. What position usually promotes efficient uterine contractions in early labor?

a. Sitting or standing.
b. Lying supine.
c. Lying prone.
d. Side-lying.

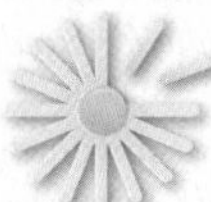

Key Points for Review

- Pain in labor occurs because of anoxia to uterine cells, stretching of the cervix and perineum, and pressure of the presenting part of the fetus on maternal tissues.
- Each person perceives pain differently. Only a woman herself can describe the extent of her pain.
- Usually, the better prepared a woman is for childbirth, the less analgesia and anesthesia is necessary.
- Encourage complementary and alternative therapies such as reducing anxiety, providing changes in position, increasing knowledge, and supporting prepared childbirth exercises in conjunction with prescribed analgesics.
- Be certain to ask about allergy to a medication before administering it during labor. Women under stress may omit mentioning this unless directly asked.
- Women may lose their ability to use controlled breathing after systemic narcotic administration because of a "lightheaded" feeling. They may need additional support during this time to be able to continue with a breathing technique until the analgesic agent begins to have an effect.
- Regional anesthesia (e.g., epidural anesthesia) is extremely effective in relieving labor pain. Be certain the woman is well hydrated with IV fluid and that her blood pressure is within normal limits before administration of the anesthetic agent.
- During regional or general anesthesia administration, if a woman must lie supine, she should have a wedge positioned under her right buttock to help prevent supine hypotension syndrome. If hypotension should occur after epidural anesthesia administration, elevating a woman's legs is an emergency measure to help relieve hypotension.
- If a narcotic analgesic is used, naloxone (Narcan) must be available for possible newborn resuscitation.
- General anesthesia is not administered for an uncomplicated labor, because it has risks for both the mother and the infant, but may still be used in an emergency.

CRITICAL THINKING EXERCISES

1. Susan, the patient you met at the beginning of the chapter, did not attend any preparation for childbirth classes because she planned to rely totally on a regional block for pain relief. If you had met her during pregnancy, instead of when she was beginning labor, would you have supported this plan? Are there any complementary and alternative therapies that she could have planned for in addition to relying on a regional block?
2. Suppose Susan says she wants a general anesthetic for labor or she will leave the hospital. Her physician has said that he cannot justify a general anesthetic for uncomplicated labor. You find Susan crying because her doctor will not give her anything for pain. How would you handle this situation?
3. Suppose Susan seems well prepared for labor but, after an injection of meperidine early in labor, grows angry with her husband and refuses to use breathing exercises because she feels "so lightheaded" from the medicine. How would you help her at this point?
4. Examine the National Health Goals related to comfort in labor. Most government-sponsored funds for nursing research are allotted based on these goals. What would be a possible research topic to explore pertinent to these goals that would be applicable to the Baranca family and also advance evidence-based practice?

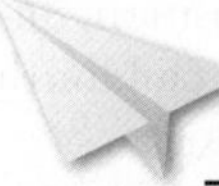

CRITICAL THINKING SCENARIO

Open the accompanying CD-ROM or visit http://thePoint.lww.com and read the Patient Scenario included for this chapter, then answer the questions to further sharpen your skills and grow more familiar with NCLEX style questions related to comfort measures for labor and birth. Confirm your answers are correct by reading the rationales.

REFERENCES

Anim-Somuah, M., Smyth, R. & Howell, C. (2009). Epidural versus non-epidural or no analgesia in labour. *Cochrane Database of Systematic Reviews, 2009*(1), (CD000331).

Burns, E., et al. (2007). Aromatherapy in childbirth: a pilot randomised controlled trial. *BJOG: An International Journal of Obstetrics and Gynaecology, 114*(7), 838–844.

Carlton, T., et al. (2009). Labor and delivery nurses' perceptions of caring for childbearing women in nurse-managed birthing units. *MCN: American Journal of Maternal Child Nursing, 34*(1), 50–56.

Cho, J. E., & Penning, D. H. (2007). Obstetric anesthesia. In K. B. Fortner, et al. (Eds.). *The Johns Hopkins manual of gynecology and obstetrics.* Philadelphia: Lippincott Williams & Wilkins.

Crombleholme, W. R. (2009). Obstetrics. In S. J. McPhee & M. A. Papadakis (Eds.). *Current medical diagnosis and treatment.* Columbus, OH: McGraw-Hill.

DerMarderosian, A., & Beutler, J. A. (2007). *The review of natural products facts and comparisons.* St. Louis: Wolters Kluwer.

Engebretson, J., & Wardell, D. W. (2007). Energy-based modalities. *Nursing Clinics of North America, 42*(2), 243–259.

Gaudet, T. W. (2007). Complementary therapy. In J. S. Berek (Ed.). *Berek & Novak's gynecology.* Philadelphia: Lippincott Williams & Wilkins.

Goetzl, L., et al. (2007). Intrapartum epidural analgesia and maternal temperature regulation. *Obstetrics & Gynecology, 109*(3), 687–690.

Green, J. M., & Baston, H. A. (2007). Have women become more willing to accept obstetric interventions and does this relate to mode of birth? Data from a prospective study. *Birth, 34*(1), 6–13.

Halls, K. L. (2008). Maternal satisfaction regarding anesthetic services during childbirth. *British Journal of Midwifery, 16*(5), 296–301.

Herr, K., et al. (2007). Pain assessment in the nonverbal patient: position statement with clinical practice recommendations. *Pain Management Nursing, 7*(2), 44–52.

Karch, A. M. (2009). *Lippincott's nursing drug guide.* Philadelphia: Lippincott Williams & Wilkins.

Kimber, L. (2007). Massage techniques in labour. *Practicing Midwife, 10*(9), 54–56.

Krieger, D. (1990). Therapeutic touch: two decades of research, teaching, and clinical practice. *Imprint, 37*(3), 83–89.

Marshall, K. M., & Baker, J. (2007). Doing it better: putting research into practice. Are patients in labor satisfied with PCEA? *Nursing, 36*(6), 18–19.

Maude, R. M., & Foureur, M. J. (2007). It's beyond water: stories of women's experience of using water for labour and birth. *Women and Birth, 20*(1), 17–24.

McDonald, J. S., & Yarnell, R. W. (2007). Obstetric analgesia and anesthesia. A. H. DeCherney & L. Nathan (Eds.). *Current diagnosis and treatment in obstetrics and gynecology* (10th ed.). Columbus, OH: McGraw-Hill.

McGrath, S. K., & Kennell, J. H. (2008). A randomized controlled trial of continuous labor support for middle-class couples: effect on cesarean delivery rates. *Birth, 35*(2), 92–97.

Melzack, R., & Wall, P. (1965). Pain mechanisms: a new theory. *Science, 150*(2), 971–982.

O'Mathuna, D. P. (2007). Reflexology for relaxation. *Alternative Therapies in Women's Health, 9*(3), 17–21.

Pasero, C., et al. (2007). Registered nurse management and monitoring of analgesia by catheter techniques: position statement. *Pain Management Nursing, 8*(2), 48–54.

Rosen, J. (2007). Health matters. Acupuncture delivers. *Alternative Medicine, 97*(5), 22.

Simmons, S. W., et al. (2009). Combined spinal-epidural versus epidural analgesia in labour. *Cochrane Database of Systematic Reviews, 2009*(1), (CD003401).

Smith, C. A., et al. (2009). Complementary and alternative therapies for pain management in labour. *Cochrane Database of Systematic Reviews, 2009*(1), (CD003521).

Sprigge, J. S., & Harper, S. J. (2008). Accidental dural puncture and post dural puncture headache in obstetric anaesthesia: presentation and management: a 23-year survey in a district general hospital. *Anaesthesia, 63*(1), 36–43.

Stephenson, K. (2007). The benefits of self-hypnosis for childbirth. *Positive Health, 137*(1), 9–12.

Subramanian, A., et al. (Eds.). (2008). *Drug Facts and Comparisons.* St. Louis: Wolters Kluwer Health.

Topcu, I., et al. (2007). The comparison of efficiency of ropivacaine and addition of fentanyl or clonidine in patient controlled epidural analgesia for labour. *Internet Journal of Anesthesiology, 11*(2), 1–15.

SUGGESTED READINGS

Abushaikha, L. A. (2007). Methods of coping with labor pain used by Jordanian women. *Journal of Transcultural Nursing, 18*(1), 35–40.

Albers, L. L. (2007). The evidence for physiologic management of the active phase of the first stage of labor. *Journal of Midwifery and Women's Health, 52*(3), 207–215.

Ayers, S., McKenzie-McHarg, K., & Eagle, A. (2007). Cognitive behaviour therapy for postnatal post-traumatic stress disorder: case studies. *Journal of Psychosomatic Obstetrics and Gynecology, 28*(3), 177–184.

Beebe, K. R., et al. (2007). The effects of childbirth self-efficacy and anxiety during pregnancy on prehospitalization labor. *JOGNN: Journal of Obstetric, Gynecologic, and Neonatal Nursing, 36*(5), 410–418.

Christiaens, W., & Bracke, P. (2007). Assessment of social psychological determinants of satisfaction with childbirth in a cross-national perspective. *BMC: Pregnancy and Childbirth, 7*(3), 26.

Cluett, E. R., et al. (2009). Immersion in water in pregnancy, labour and birth. *Cochrane Database of Systematic Reviews, 2009*(1), (CD000111).

Greulich, B., & Tarrant, B. (2007). The latent phase of labor: diagnosis and management. *Journal of Midwifery and Women's Health, 52*(3), 190–198.

Jacobson, P., & Turner, L. (2008). Management of the second stage of labor in women with epidural analgesia. *Journal of Midwifery and Women's Health, 53*(1), 82–85.

Meyer, M., et al. (2007). Intrapartum and postpartum analgesia for women maintained on methadone during pregnancy. *Obstetrics and Gynecology, 110*(2.1), 261–266.

Ohel, I., et al. (2007). A rise in pain threshold during labor: a prospective clinical trial. *Pain, 132*(Suppl 1), S104–S108.

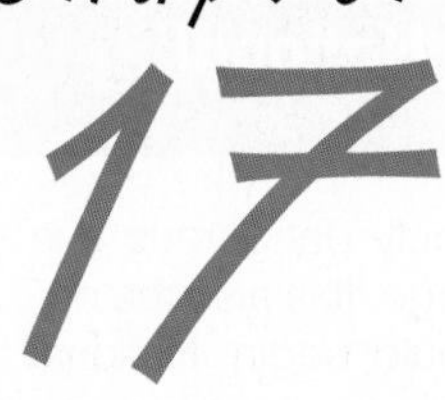

Nursing Care of a Postpartal Family

KEY TERMS

- afterpains
- diastasis recti
- en face position
- engorgement
- engrossment
- Homans' sign
- involution
- letting-go phase
- lochia
- postpartal depression
- rooming-in
- sitz bath
- taking-hold phase
- taking-in phase
- uterine atony

OBJECTIVES

After mastering the contents of this chapter, you should be able to:

1. Describe the psychological and physiologic changes that occur in a postpartal woman.
2. Identify National Health Goals related to the postpartal period that nurses can help the nation achieve.
3. Use critical thinking to analyze ways that postpartum nursing care can be more family centered.
4. Assess a woman and her family for physiologic and psychological changes after childbirth.
5. Formulate nursing diagnoses related to physiologic and psychological transitions of the postpartal period.
6. Identify expected outcomes for a postpartal woman and family related to the changes during this period.
7. Plan nursing care such as measures to aid uterine involution or encourage bonding.
8. Implement nursing care to aid the progression of physiologic and psychological transitions occurring in a postpartal woman and family such as teaching about breastfeeding.
9. Evaluate outcome criteria for the achievement and effectiveness of care.
10. Identify areas related to care of the postpartal family that could benefit from additional nursing research or application of evidence-based practice.
11. Integrate knowledge of the physiologic and psychological changes of the postpartal period with the nursing process to achieve quality maternal and child health nursing care.

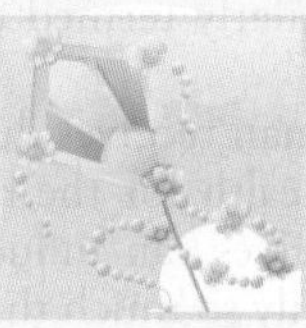

As the nurse working in a postpartum unit, you care for Mike and Joan Cooper, who have just become parents of an 8-lb 2-oz baby girl. Joan is on maternity leave from her job as a court reporter. Mike plans to take off a week from work to spend time with Joan and the new baby.

As you prepare them for discharge, you notice they seem overwhelmed with the amount of information they have been provided. Joan says, trying to get the baby to nurse, "He's so big and my breasts are so small, will he get enough milk? I was hoping by breastfeeding I wouldn't have to worry about birth control for a while, but I'm having so much trouble maybe that won't work out." Mike pulls you aside and says, "Sometimes, I see my wife crying for no reason. Why isn't she as happy as I am?"

Previous chapters discussed caring for the pregnant woman and her family during the antepartal and intrapartal periods. This chapter adds information about caring for a postpartal woman and family. Nurses are able to play major roles in assessment, comfort promotion, and education during this period as they help a new family adjust to the many physiologic and psychological changes that occur during this period.

What additional postpartal teaching does the Cooper family need?

The postpartal period, or *puerperium* (from the Latin *puer,* for "child," and *parere,* for "to bring forth"), refers to the 6-week period after childbirth. It is a time of maternal changes that are both retrogressive (involution of the uterus and vagina) and progressive (production of milk for lactation, restoration of the normal menstrual cycle, and beginning of a parenting role). Protecting a woman's health as these changes occur is important for preserving her future childbearing function and for ensuring that she is physically well enough to incorporate her new child into her family. The period is popularly termed the *fourth trimester of pregnancy*.

The physical care a woman receives during the postpartal period can influence her health for the rest of her life. The emotional support she receives can influence the emotional health of her child and family so much that it can be felt into the next generation (McGarry et al., 2009). National Health Goals related to the postpartal period that nurses can help the nation achieve are shown in Box 17.1.

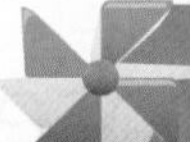

BOX 17.1 * Focus on National Health Goals

The first hour after birth is an extremely dangerous one because of the possibility of hemorrhage. It is also the optimal period when breastfeeding should begin. National Health Goals that involve this time period include:

- Reduce the maternal mortality rate to no more than 3.3/100,000 live births from a baseline of 7.1/100,000.
- Reduce the proportion of births occurring within 24 months of a previous birth to 6% from a baseline of 11%.
- Increase to at least 75% the proportion of mothers who breastfeed their babies in the early postpartum period from a baseline of 64% and increase the proportion of mothers who still breastfeed at 6 months to 29% from a baseline of 50% (http://www.nih.gov).

Nurses can help the nation achieve these goals by maintaining close observation in the immediate postpartal period to detect maternal hemorrhage, encouraging and supporting women who breastfeed, and ensuring that women receive reproductive life planning information if desired.

Areas that could benefit from additional nursing research include discovering effective means to encourage women to maintain breastfeeding and effective ways to teach women to monitor their own health in the postpartal period, particularly because, with early discharge, they may be at home when uterine hemorrhage occurs.

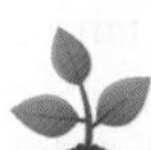

Nursing Process Overview

For a Postpartal Woman and Family

Assessment

During the puerperium, assessment of a woman is accomplished by health interview, physical examination, and analysis of laboratory data. It is important to ensure that physical changes, such as uterine involution, are occurring by evaluating uterine size and consistency and lochia flow amount.

Assessment of a woman's psychological adjustment begins with her reaction at birth (Was she disappointed or happy with the appearance of her baby? Is she glad to be through with the pregnancy or still longing to be back in it?) and continues with every contact made with the family during and after a hospital stay. Assess the extent and quality of the woman's interaction with her child (Does she hold the infant and talk to him or her?), her overall mood (Do you observe her crying? Does she have long periods of staring into space or not talking?), and her ability to begin infant care. Observe also for self-care. A woman who feels good about herself, even though she is exhausted from childbirth, usually will try to maintain her appearance. On the other hand, if she is depressed, she probably has little energy to do things such as comb her hair or worry about her appearance.

Nursing Diagnosis

Nursing diagnoses during the postpartal period usually are concerned either with a family's inability to accept and bond with a new child or with physiologic considerations. Examples might include:

- Health-seeking behaviors related to care of newborn
- Risk for impaired parenting related to disappointment in the sex of the child
- Fear related to lack of preparation for child care
- Risk for deficient fluid volume related to postpartal hemorrhage

Outcome Identification and Planning

Be certain that outcomes established during this time are realistic in light of a woman's changed life pattern. Most postpartal families remain in the hospital for a relatively short time, only 48 to 72 hours. The postpartum stay in an alternative birth center can be as short as 4 hours. That means outcomes must be devised that can be accomplished and evaluated during this short period of client contact. If an outcome cannot be evaluated within this short timeframe, follow-up home care or ambulatory visits may be necessary.

When planning care in the postpartal period, try to arrange procedures to allow optimal time for family infant–interaction and yet provide adequate time for a woman to rest, to prevent exhaustion. Prevention of exhaustion can improve coping ability and plans for self-care. After adequate instruction, a woman should be prepared to monitor her own health after she returns home.

Planning should also include ample time for health teaching. An important part of teaching related to care of the newborn is preparation for the unexpected and the need for flexibility, because parents do not yet know what their new life will be like (whether their child will sleep deeply or fitfully at night, whether their child will become hungry at long or short intervals) or how tired they will become after being awakened frequently during the night.

Brainstorming—practicing to produce at least three different methods of reaching a particular goal—is excellent practice for parenting. A helpful Internet site to recommend to parents who feel a need for additional knowledge or support during this time is the Postpartal Support International web site (http://www.postpartum.net).

Implementation

All interventions in the postpartal period should be family centered, to enhance family functioning and bonding.

Interventions also should be geared toward increasing a woman's self-esteem and allowing her to view herself as a new mother and her new infant as part of her family. Teaching new mothers is important, but it is also important to explore what they already know about child care and what they think would be a sensible solution to a problem. Giving advice only solves an immediate problem; helping a woman learn good problem-solving technique improves her ability to handle the many challenges that will arise with childrearing.

Outcome Evaluation

If a woman fails to make an adequate adjustment to her new life changes, she may have difficulty integrating an infant into the family. This could affect a child's mental health, self-esteem, and ability to form a sense of trust.

Evaluation in the postpartal period involves being certain not only that a woman and her baby are safe but also that the woman knows how to maintain her own health. Such follow-up evaluation can be done by telephone, during home visits, or during postpartal and well-child assessments.

Examples of expected outcomes include:

- Parents spontaneously make at least one positive comment about their child's characteristics before hospital discharge.
- Client states that she believes she will be able to manage newborn care with the support of her significant other.
- Client's lochial flow is no more than one saturated perineal pad (50 mL) every 3 hours.
- Client states she is tired but feels able to manage her newborn and family care.

PSYCHOLOGICAL CHANGES OF THE POSTPARTAL PERIOD

A transition is a movement or passage from one position or concept to another or a pause between what was and what is to be. It represents the internal process experienced by people when change occurs. In a classic presentation of what transition entails, Bridges (1994) stated that change is something that happens to people, and transition is how they respond to that change.

People move through several predictable stages during transition: first is the act of ending old ways of thinking or believing (letting go); next, there is a neutral zone, during which the old way is gone but the new way is not yet comfortable; and finally, there is a new beginning, during which new ideas and concepts are put into action (Bridges, 1994). The postpartum period is a time of transition, during which a couple gives up concepts such as "childless" or "parents of one" and moves to the beginning of new parenthood. The immediate postpartal period is a neutral time during which a couple tries out the new role and attempts to "fit" their expectations for that role. Nurses can help couples acknowledge the extent of the change, so that they can gain closure on their previous lifestyle. Opening channels for communication, anticipating new needs, and highlighting potential gains that will occur because of the change are important actions.

Phases of the Puerperium

In her classic work on maternal behavior, Reva Rubin, a nurse, divided the puerperium into three separate phases (Rubin, 1977). She viewed the first of these as a **taking-in phase,** or a time when the new parents review their pregnancy and the labor and birth. The subsequent phases, called the **taking-hold phase** and the **letting-go phase,** are times of renewed action and forward movement. At the time these phases of the puerperium were identified, women were hospitalized for 5 to 7 days after childbirth and moved in a paced manner from one step to the next. Today, with hospitalization as short as a few hours, women appear to move through these phases much more quickly and may even be experiencing two different phases at once.

Taking-In Phase

The taking-in phase, the first phase experienced, is a time of reflection. During this 2- to 3-day period, a woman is largely passive. She prefers having a nurse minister to her (such as bringing her a bath towel or a clean nightgown) and make decisions for her, rather than do these things herself. This dependence results partly from her physical discomfort because of afterpains or hemorrhoids; partly from her uncertainty in caring for her newborn; and partly from the extreme exhaustion that follows childbirth.

As a part of thinking and pondering about her new role, the woman usually wants to talk about her pregnancy, especially about her labor and birth. She holds her new child with a sense of wonder and asks: Is birth really over? Could this child really have been inside me? Could I be this lucky? During the taking-in phase, she rests to regain her physical strength and to calm and contain her swirling thoughts. Encouraging her to talk about the birth helps her integrate it into her life experiences (Box 17.2).

Taking-Hold Phase

After a time of passive dependence, a woman begins to initiate action. She prefers to get her own washcloth and to make her own decisions. Women who give birth without any anesthesia may reach this second phase in a matter of hours after birth.

During the taking-in period, a woman may have expressed little interest in caring for her child. Now, she begins to take a strong interest. As a rule, therefore, it is always best to give a woman brief demonstrations of baby care and then allow her to care for her child herself—with watchful guidance.

Although a woman's actions suggest strong independence during this time, she often still feels insecure about her ability

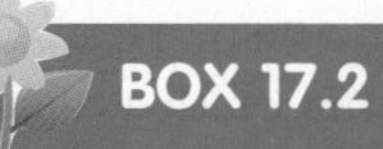

BOX 17.2 ✻ Focus on Communication

Joan Cooper gave birth 6 hours ago. You want to assess her for postpartal pain, so you enter her hospital room. She is wearing a hospital gown and sitting in the chair by her bed.

Less Effective Communication

Nurse: How are you feeling, Mrs. Cooper?

Mrs. Cooper: Like I'm still rushing around. I called my husband as soon as my water broke. He hit a truck on the way home, though, so he couldn't get here in time. I tried to call—

Nurse: Do you have any pain?

Mrs. Cooper: It's not bad. I tried to call my mother, but she couldn't come over because she didn't have a car. Our neighbor—

Nurse: Okay, then let me check your stitches.

More Effective Communication

Nurse: How are you feeling, Mrs. Cooper?

Mrs. Cooper: Like I'm still rushing around. I called my husband as soon as my water broke. He hit a truck on the way home, though, so he couldn't get here in time. I tried to call—

Nurse: Do you have any pain?

Mrs. Cooper: It's not bad. I tried to call my mother, but she couldn't come over because she didn't have a car. Our neighbor—

Nurse: Go on. I didn't mean to interrupt.

Mrs. Cooper: Our neighbor said he'd drive me but then discovered his wife had his car keys. It was a three-ring circus of problems.

Nurse: A three-ring circus?

Mrs. Cooper: Finally, my husband made it home, but then there was such a bad accident on the freeway we had to drive all the way around the lake. I thought I'd have the baby in the middle of the bridge!

Nurse: That must have been terrifying for you.

Most women are interested in discussing their labor and birth experience in the days immediately after birth as a part of a "taking-in" phase. Repeating the story of how worried they were when labor started, how much pain they had, or how scared they were when their membranes broke helps them put these sensations into perspective and integrate them into their life experiences. Communication that encourages women to elaborate on a story is therapeutic; communication that discourages story-telling is not. Once you have talked about what concerned her most, returning to a discussion and assessment of her pain would be appropriate.

to care for her new child. She needs praise for the things she does well such as supporting the baby's head or beginning breastfeeding to give her confidence. This positive reinforcement begins in the health care facility and continues after discharge, at home, and at postpartum and well-baby visits.

Do not rush a woman through the phase of taking-in or prevent her from taking hold when she reaches this point. For many young mothers, learning to make decisions about their child's welfare is one of the most difficult phases of motherhood. It helps if a woman has practice in making such decisions in a sheltered setting, such as a hospital, rather than first taking on that level of responsibility after she is home alone.

Letting-Go Phase

In the third phase, called letting-go, a woman finally redefines her new role. She gives up the fantasized image of her child and accepts the real one; she gives up her old role of being childless or the mother of only one or two (or however many children she had before this birth). This process requires some grief work and readjustment of relationships, similar to what occurred during pregnancy. It is extended and continues during the child's growing years. A woman who has reached this phase is well into her new role.

✔ Checkpoint Question 17.1

Which of the following actions would alert you that Joan Cooper, 2 days postpartum, is entering a postpartal taking-hold phase?

a. She tells you she has painful contractions for 8 hours.
b. She sleeps as if exhausted from the effort of her labor.
c. She urges her baby to stay awake so that she can breastfeed.
d. She says that she has not selected a name for her baby as yet.

Development of Parental Love and Positive Family Relationships

During pregnancy, almost every woman worries about her ability to be a "good" mother, and this concern does not evaporate as soon as the baby is born. Some women seem able to recognize a newborn's needs immediately and to give care with confident understanding right from the start. More often, however, a woman enters into a relationship with her newborn tentatively and with qualms and conflicts that must be addressed before the relationship can be meaningful. This is because parental love is only partly instinctive. A major portion develops gradually, in stages such as planning the pregnancy, hearing the pregnancy confirmed, feeling the child move in utero, birthing, seeing the baby, touching the baby, and, finally, giving total care to the child. Factors such as a difficult labor or transport and separation from the newborn may lead to symptoms of a traumatic stress disorder that slows the process or interferes with the ability to bond warmly (Tam & Chung, 2007).

Many women may not experience maternal feelings for their infants until days or even weeks after giving birth. Some fathers admit they have difficulty "claiming" or bonding with an infant (feeling fatherly toward the new child) until as late as 3 months after the birth, when the child begins to smile or coo and interact more directly with them. The ability of both parents to reach out to their child can be strengthened by allowing them to touch and spend as much time as possible with the new child during the first few hours of life.

Forming a strong bond with a child is not a problem only for first-time parents. Experienced parents can have just as much difficulty—they know they love 4-year-old Johnny and 2-year-old Sue at home, but worry that their hearts may not be big enough to love a third child, too.

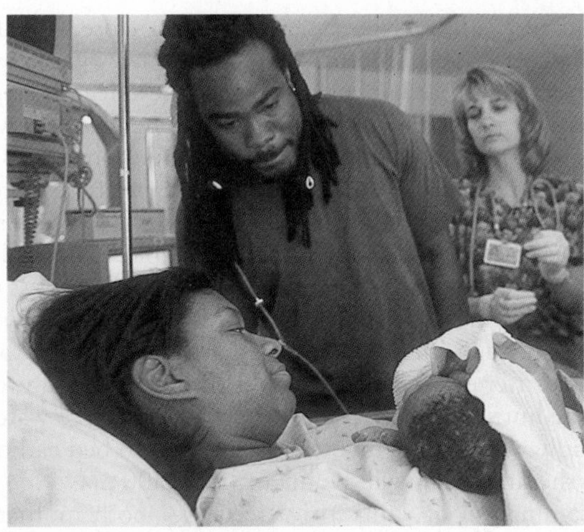

FIGURE 17.1 A mom and dad begin interaction with their newborn immediately after birth: a very special moment in their life. (© Kathy Sloane.)

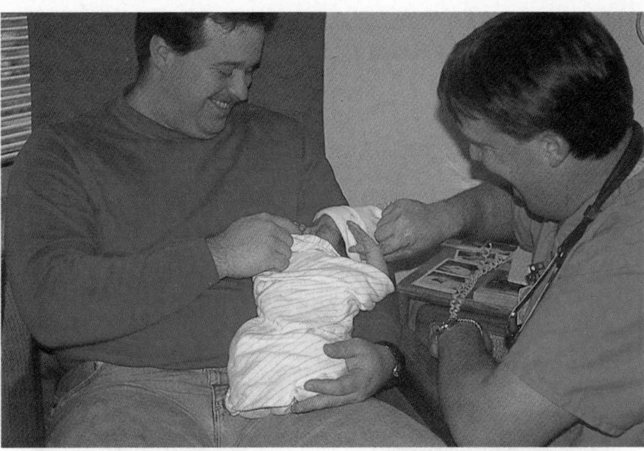

FIGURE 17.2 A nurse encourages a father as he interacts and bonds with his newborn. (© Caroline Brown, RNC, MS, DEd.)

Because of these mixed feelings, parents may not show genuine warmth the first time they hold their infant. Although a woman carried the child inside her for 9 months, she now approaches her newborn as she would a stranger. The first time she holds the infant, she may touch only the blanket and never make close physical contact. If she unfolds the blanket to examine the baby or count the fingers or toes, she may use only her fingertips for touch (Fig. 17.1).

Gradually, as a woman holds her child more, she begins to express more warmth, touching the child with the palm of her hand rather than with her fingertips. She smoothes the baby's hair, brushes a cheek, plays with toes, and lets the baby's fingers clasp hers. Soon, she feels comfortable enough to press her cheek against the baby's or kiss the infant's nose or mouth; she has become a mother tending to her child. This identification process is termed *claiming* or *bonding*. Looking directly at her newborn's face, with direct eye contact (termed an **en face position**), is a sign a woman is beginning effective interaction. Many fathers can be observed staring at a newborn for long intervals in this same way. Often termed **engrossment,** this action alerts caregivers to how actively the father, as well as the mother, is beginning bonding (Fig. 17.2). The length of time parents take to bond with a child depends on the circumstances of the pregnancy and birth, the wellness and ability of the child to meet the parent's expectations, reciprocal actions by the newborn, and the opportunities the parents have to interact with the child. Freedom from stringent health agency rules helps good parent–child relationships to develop. To help parents sort out their feelings about being a mother or father and about their new responsibility, provide a supportive presence and offer anticipatory guidance as necessary.

✔ Checkpoint Question 17.2

You observe Joan Cooper holding her newborn. Which position would best reassure you that she is relating well to her newborn?

a. She looks directly at her infant's face and talks to him.
b. She holds the infant over her shoulder to burp him.
c. She sits in a rocking chair and rocks the new infant.
d. She lies in bed and places the infant on her stomach.

Rooming-In

The more time a woman has to spend with her baby, the sooner she may feel competent in child care, and the more likely she may be to form a sound mother–child relationship (Moore, Anderson, & Bergman, 2009). If her infant stays in the birthing room with her (called **rooming-in**) rather than in a central nursery, she can become better acquainted with her child and begin to feel more confident in her ability to care for him or her after discharge (Fink, 2007). In many settings, the father can stay overnight in the room, or room-in, as well.

There are two types of rooming-in: complete, in which the mother and child are together 24 hours a day, and partial, in which the infant remains in the woman's room for most of the time, perhaps from 8:00 AM to 9:00 PM, but then the infant is taken to a small nursery near the woman's room or returned to a central nursery for the night. With both complete and partial rooming-in, the father and siblings can hold and feed the infant when they visit.

Sibling Visitation

Separation from children is often as painful for a mother as it is for her children. Waiting at home, separated from their mother and listening only to telephone reports of what a new brother or sister looks like, can be very difficult for older children. They may picture the new baby as much older than he or she actually is. "He is eating well" may produce an image of a child sitting at a table using a fork and spoon. "He weighs 8 pounds" can be meaningless information. A chance to visit the hospital and see the new baby and their mother reduces feelings that their mother cares more about the new baby than about them. It can help to relieve some of the impact of separation. It helps to make the baby a part of the family (Fig. 17.3).

Assess to be sure that siblings are free of contagious diseases such as upper respiratory tract illnesses or recent exposure to chickenpox before they visit. Then, have them wash their hands and, if they choose, hold or touch the newborn with parental assistance.

You may need to caution a woman that the opinions of a new brother or sister expressed by her older children may not

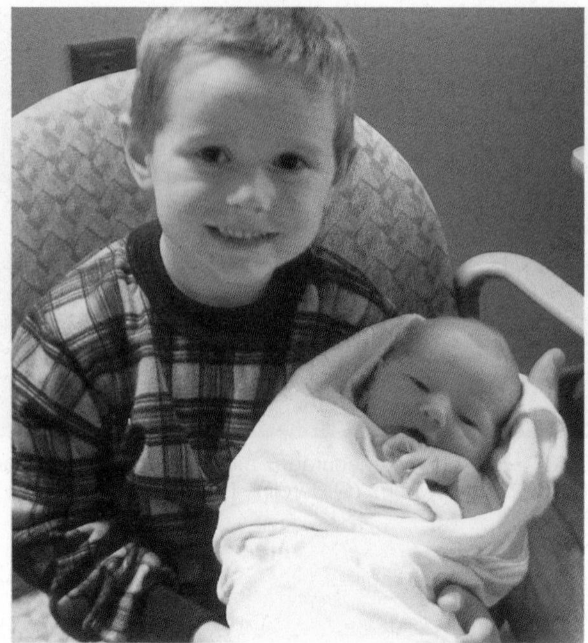

FIGURE 17.3 Sibling visiting is important to bring a family together.

be complimentary. This baby with little hair is not their idea of a "pretty baby." If they thought the new baby would be big enough to play with, they may not believe that he is a "big baby." However, seeing the baby, even if the baby's appearance is not what the other children expected, is helpful in establishing strong relationships and should be encouraged.

Maternal Concerns and Feelings in the Postpartal Period

Traditionally, it is assumed that the bulk of a woman's concerns in the postpartal period center on the care of her new infant. Based on this, classes in the postpartal period have traditionally focused on teaching how to breastfeed and bathe infants. Although these acts are concerns for many mothers, they are not necessarily every new mother's chief concern. A woman has come through a tremendous psychological experience during pregnancy and the birth of a child. She is in the middle of a complete role change. It can be expected, therefore, that some of her attention and interest during this time will be directed inward as she tries to view herself in this new role.

Typical issues identified by postpartal women include breast soreness; regaining their figure; regulating the demands of housework, their partner, and their children; coping with emotional tension and sibling jealousy; and fatigue.

Abandonment

Many mothers, if given the opportunity, admit to feeling abandoned and less important after giving birth than they did during pregnancy or labor. Only hours before, they were the center of attention, with everyone asking about their health and well-being. Now, suddenly, the baby seems to be everyone's chief interest. Relatives ask about the baby; the gifts are all for the baby. Even a woman's obstetrician, who has made her feel so important for the last 9 months, may ask during a visit, "How's that healthy 8-pound boy?" It can make a woman feel confused by a sensation very close to jealousy. And how can a good mother be jealous of her own baby?

You can help a woman move past these feelings by verbalizing the problem: "How things have changed! Everyone's asking about the baby today and not about you, aren't they? How does that make you feel?" These are welcome words for a woman to hear. It is reassuring to know that the sensation she is experiencing, although uncomfortable, is normal.

When a newborn comes home, a father may express much the same feelings. He may become resentful of the time the mother spends with the infant. Perhaps the two used to sit at the table after dinner and discuss their day or the future, and now she hurries away to feed the baby. She used to watch the late show with him at night; now she goes to bed earlier, because she knows she will be up again at 2:00 AM.

Examination of competitive feelings—both motherhood and fatherhood involve some compromise in favor of the baby's interests—should start during the pregnancy or early in the postpartal period. Making infant care a shared responsibility can help alleviate these feelings and make both partners feel equally involved in the baby's care.

Disappointment

Another common feeling parents may experience is disappointment in the baby. All during pregnancy, they pictured a chubby-cheeked, curly-haired, smiling girl or boy. They have instead a skinny baby, without any hair, who seems to cry constantly. It can be difficult for parents to feel positive immediately about a child who does not meet their expectations in this way. It can cause parents to remember their adolescence, when they felt gangly and unattractive, or to experience feelings of inadequacy all over again.

You can never change the sex, size, or look of a child, but in the short time you care for a postpartal family, you can help to change the feelings of a mother or father about their infant. Handle the child warmly, to show that you find the infant satisfactory or even special. Comment on the child's good points, such as long fingers, lovely eyes, and good appetite. During periods of crisis such as childbearing, it is possible for a key person such as a nurse to offer support to tip a scale toward acceptance or at least help a person involved to take a clearer look at his or her situation and begin to cope with the new circumstances.

Postpartal Blues

During the postpartal period, as many as 50% of women experience some feelings of overwhelming sadness (Buultjens & Liamputtong, 2007). They may burst into tears easily or feel let down or irritable. This temporary feeling after birth has long been known as the "baby blues." This phenomenon may be caused by hormonal changes, particularly the decrease in estrogen and progesterone that occurs with delivery of the placenta. For some women, it may be a response to dependence and low self-esteem caused by exhaustion, being away from home, physical discomfort, and the tension engendered by assuming a new role, especially if a woman is not receiving support from her partner. The syndrome is evidenced by tearfulness, feelings of inadequacy, mood lability, anorexia, and sleep disturbance.

Anticipatory guidance and individualized support from health care personnel are important to help the parents understand that this response is normal. You can assure a woman that sudden crying episodes may occur; otherwise, she may have difficulty understanding what is happening to her. Her support person also needs assurance, or he can think the woman is unhappy with him or their new baby or is keeping some terrible secret about the baby from him.

It is also important to give the woman a chance to verbalize her feelings: "I know there's absolutely no reason for me to be crying, but I cannot stop." Allowing her to make as many decisions as possible can help give her a sense of control over her life and help her move past these strange postpartal emotions.

Remember, however, that not all postpartal women cry because they have baby blues. A woman sometimes has other reasons to feel sad during this time. Perhaps problems at home have become overwhelming. Her husband may have been laid off from his job just when they most need the money. One of her parents may be ill, or her house may have been damaged by a disaster such as a flood. Keeping lines of communication open is important to help differentiate between problems that can be handled best with discussion and concerned understanding and those that should be referred to a social service department or a community health agency.

Thirty percent of women experience a more serious level of sadness after birth or **postpartal depression** (Lipscomb & Novy, 2007). Serious depression requiring formal counseling or psychiatric care also can occur in women during this time (Engqvist et al., 2007). Because these are deeper level concerns, postpartal depression and psychosis are discussed in Chapter 25.

PHYSIOLOGIC CHANGES OF THE POSTPARTAL PERIOD

Retrogressive physiologic changes that occur during the postpartal period include those related specifically to the reproductive system as well as other systemic changes (Box 17.3).

Reproductive System Changes

Involution is the process whereby the reproductive organs return to their nonpregnant state. A woman is in danger of hemorrhage from the denuded surface of the uterus until involution is complete (Poggi, 2007).

The Uterus

Involution of the uterus involves two main processes. First, the area where the placenta was implanted is sealed off to prevent bleeding. Second, the organ is reduced to its approximate pregestational size.

The sealing of the placenta site is accomplished by rapid contraction of the uterus immediately after delivery of the placenta. This contraction pinches the blood vessels entering the 7-cm-wide area left denuded by the placenta and stops bleeding. With time, thrombi form within the uterine sinuses and permanently seal the area. Eventually, endometrial tissue undermines the site and obliterates the organized thrombi, covering and healing the area so completely that the process leaves no scar tissue within the uterus and does not compromise future implantation sites.

Box 17.3 Assessment
Assessing the Postpartal Woman

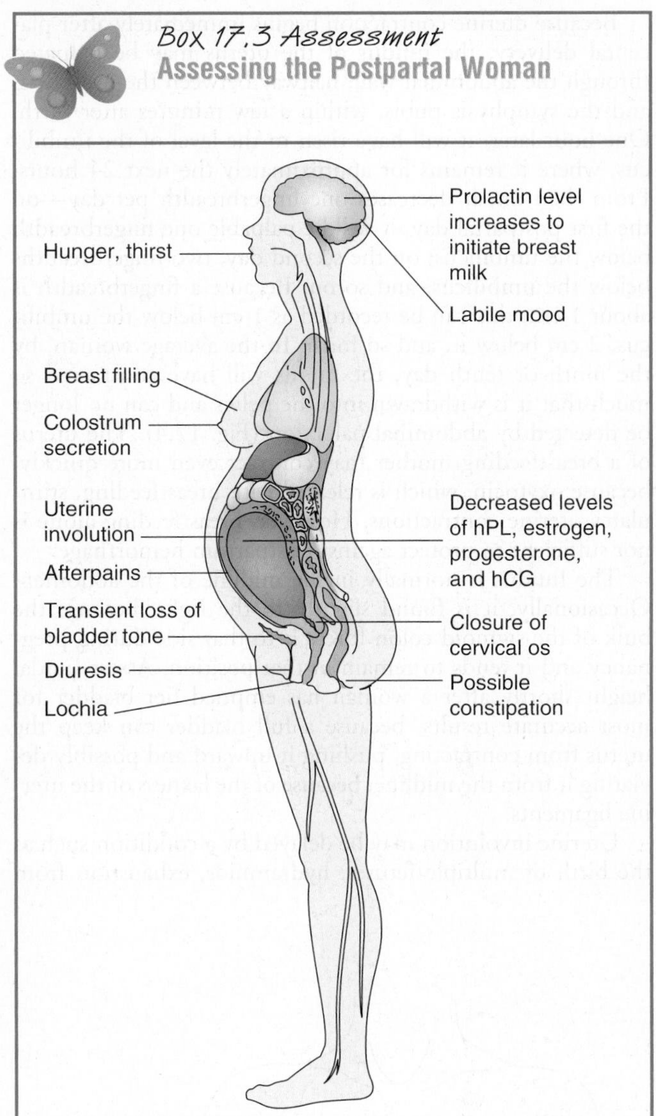

The same contraction process reduces the bulk of the uterus. Devoid of the placenta and the membranes, the walls of the uterus thicken and contract, gradually reducing the uterus from a container large enough to hold a full-term fetus to one the size of a grapefruit. A few cells of the uterine wall are broken down into their protein components by an autolytic process. These components are then absorbed by the bloodstream and excreted by the body in urine. The main mechanism that reduces the bulk of the uterus, however, is contraction, a phenomenon that can be compared with a rubber band which has been stretched for many months and now is regaining its normal contour. None of the rubber band is destroyed; the shape is simply altered. For this reason, the postpartal period, like pregnancy, is not a period of illness, of necrosing cells being evacuated, but primarily a period of healthy change (Pavone, Purinton, & Petersen, 2007).

Although the uterus will never completely return to its prepregnancy state, its reduction in size is dramatic. Immediately after birth, the uterus weighs about 1000 g. At the end of the first week, it weighs 500 g. By the time involution is complete (6 weeks), it weighs approximately 50 g, similar to its prepregnancy weight.

Because uterine contraction begins immediately after placental delivery, the fundus of the uterus may be palpated through the abdominal wall, halfway between the umbilicus and the symphysis pubis, within a few minutes after birth. One hour later, it will have risen to the level of the umbilicus, where it remains for approximately the next 24 hours. From then on, it decreases one fingerbreadth per day—on the first postpartal day, it will be palpable one fingerbreadth below the umbilicus; on the second day, two fingerbreadths below the umbilicus; and so on. Because a fingerbreadth is about 1 cm, this can be recorded as 1 cm below the umbilicus, 2 cm below it, and so forth. In the average woman, by the ninth or tenth day, the uterus will have contracted so much that it is withdrawn into the pelvis and can no longer be detected by abdominal palpation (Fig. 17.4). The uterus of a breastfeeding mother may contract even more quickly, because oxytocin, which is released with breastfeeding, stimulates uterine contractions. However, breastfeeding alone is not sufficient to protect against postpartum hemorrhage.

The fundus is normally in the midline of the abdomen. Occasionally, it is found slightly to the right, because the bulk of the sigmoid colon forces it to that side during pregnancy and it tends to remain in that position. Assess fundal height shortly after a woman has emptied her bladder for most accurate results, because a full bladder can keep the uterus from contracting, pushing it upward and possibly deviating it from the midline, because of the laxness of the uterine ligaments.

Uterine involution may be delayed by a condition such as the birth of multiple fetuses, hydramnios, exhaustion from prolonged labor or a difficult birth, grand multiparity, or physiologic effects of excessive analgesia. Contraction may be difficult if there is retained placenta or membranes. Involution will occur most dependably in a woman who is well nourished and who ambulates early after birth (gravity may play a role).

An estimation of the consistency of the postpartal uterus is as important as measurement of its height. A well-contracted fundus feels firm. It can be compared with a grapefruit in both size and tenseness. Whenever the fundus feels boggy (soft or flabby), it is not as contracted as it should be, despite its position in the abdomen.

The first hour after birth is potentially the most dangerous time for a woman. If her uterus should become relaxed during this time **(uterine atony),** she will lose blood very rapidly, because no permanent thrombi have yet formed at the placental site.

In some women, contraction of the uterus after birth causes intermittent cramping termed **afterpains,** similar to that accompanying a menstrual period. Afterpains tend to be noticed most by multiparas rather than primiparas and by women who have given birth to large babies or multiple births. In these situations, the uterus must contract more forcefully to regain its prepregnancy size and has difficulty maintaining a steady contracted state. These sensations are noticed most intensely with breastfeeding, when the infant's sucking causes a release of oxytocin from the posterior pituitary, increasing the strength of the contractions.

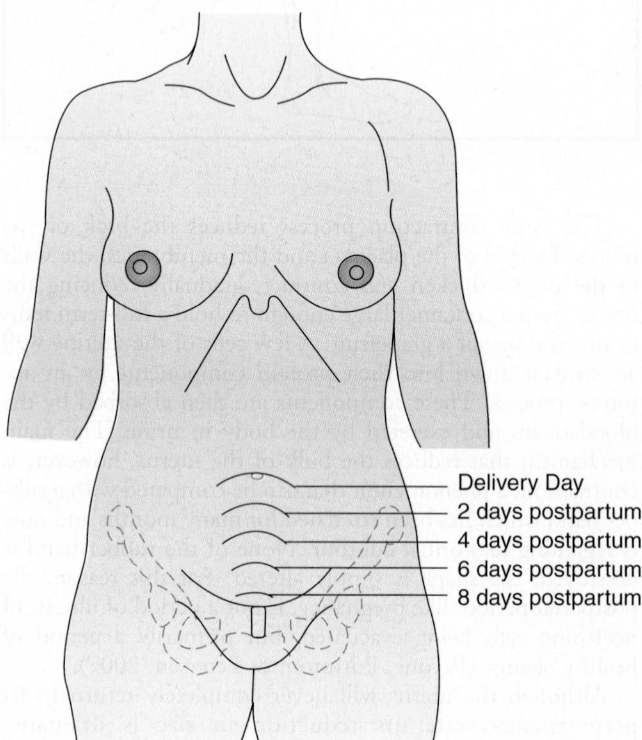

FIGURE 17.4 Uterine involution. The uterus decreases in size at a predictable rate during the postpartal period. After 10 days, it recedes under the pubic bone and is no longer palpable.

Lochia

The separation of the placenta and membranes occurs in the spongy layer or outer portion of the decidua basalis of the uterus. By the second day after birth, the layer of decidua remaining under the placental site (an area 7 cm wide) and throughout the uterus differentiates into two distinct layers. The inner layer attached to the muscular wall of the uterus remains, serving as the foundation from which a new layer of endometrium will be formed. The layer adjacent to the uterine cavity becomes necrotic and is cast off as a uterine discharge similar to a menstrual flow. This uterine flow, consisting of blood, fragments of decidua, white blood cells, mucus, and some bacteria, is known as **lochia.**

The portion of the uterus where the placenta was not attached is so fully cleansed by this sloughing process that it will be in a reproductive state in about 3 weeks' time. It takes approximately 6 weeks (the entire postpartal period) for the placental implantation site to be healed.

For the first 3 days after birth, a lochia discharge consists almost entirely of blood, with only small particles of decidua and mucus. Because of its mainly red color, it is termed *lochia rubra.* As the amount of blood involved in the cast-off tissue decreases (about the fourth day) and leukocytes begin to invade the area, as they do with any healing surface, the flow becomes pink or brownish (*lochia serosa*). On about the 10th day, the amount of the flow decreases and becomes colorless or white (*lochia alba*). Lochia alba is present in most women until the third week after birth, although it is not unusual for a lochia flow to last the entire 6 weeks of the puerperium. Characteristics of lochia are summarized in Table 17.1. Several rules for judging whether lochia flow is normal are summarized in Box 17.4.

TABLE 17.1 ✻ Characteristics of Lochia

Type of Lochia	Color	Postpartal Day	Composition
Lochia rubra	Red	1–3	Blood, fragments of decidua, and mucus
Lochia serosa	Pink	3–10	Blood, mucus, and invading leukocytes
Lochia alba	White	10–14 (may last 6 weeks)	Largely mucus; leukocyte count high

The Cervix

Immediately after birth, a uterine cervix is soft and malleable. Both the internal and external os are open. Like contraction of the uterus, contraction of the cervix toward its prepregnant state begins at once. By the end of 7 days, the external os has narrowed to the size of a pencil opening; the cervix feels firm and nongravid again.

In contrast to the process of uterine involution, in which the changes consist primarily of old cells being returned to their former position by contraction, the process in the cervix involves the formation of new muscle cells. Like the fundus, the cervix does not return exactly to its prepregnancy state. The internal os closes as before, but after a vaginal birth the external os usually remains slightly open and appears slitlike or stellate (star shaped), whereas previously it was round. Finding this pattern on pelvic examination suggests that childbearing has taken place.

The Vagina

After a vaginal birth, the vagina is soft, with few rugae, and its diameter is considerably greater than normal. The hymen is permanently torn and heals with small, separate tags of tissue. It takes the entire postpartal period for the vagina to involute (by contraction, as with the uterus) until it gradually returns to its approximate prepregnancy state. Thickening of the walls also appears to depend on renewed estrogen stimulation from the ovaries. Because a woman who is breastfeeding may have delayed ovulation, she may continue to have thin-walled or fragile vaginal cells that cause slight vaginal bleeding during sexual intercourse until about 6 weeks' time. Like the cervix, the vaginal outlet remains slightly more distended than before. If a woman practices Kegel exercises, the strength and tone of the vagina will increase more rapidly (see Chapter 12). This may be important for the sexual enjoyment of both a woman and her partner.

The Perineum

Because of the great amount of pressure experienced during birth, the perineum feels edematous and tender immediately after birth. Ecchymosis from ruptured capillaries may show on the surface. The labia majora and labia minora typically remain atrophic and softened after birth, never returning to their prepregnancy state.

Systemic Changes

The same body systems that were involved in pregnancy are also involved in postpartal changes as the body returns to its prepregnancy state.

The Hormonal System

Pregnancy hormones begin to decrease as soon as the placenta is no longer present. Levels of human chorionic gonadotropin (hCG) and human placental lactogen (hPL) are almost negligible by 24 hours. By week 1, progestin, estrone,

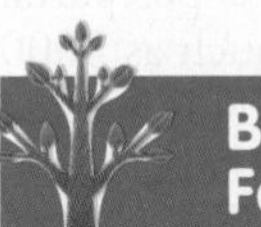

BOX 17.4 ✻ Focus on Family Teaching

Evaluating Lochia Flow

Q. Joan Cooper asks you, "How do I know if my lochia is normal?"

A. Several guidelines are helpful for evaluating lochia flow:

Evaluate the Amount: Lochia amount will vary from woman to woman. Mothers who breastfeed tend to have less lochial discharge than those who do not, because the natural release of the hormone oxytocin during breastfeeding strengthens uterine contractions. Conservation of fluid for lactation also may be a factor. Lochial flow increases on exertion, especially the first few times a woman is out of bed, but decreases again with rest. The increase in amount that occurs with ambulation is the result of vaginal discharge of pooled lochia, not a true increase in amount. However, lochia amount truly does increase with strenuous exercise, such as lifting a heavy weight or walking up stairs. Saturating a perineal pad in less than 1 hour is considered an abnormally heavy flow and should be reported.

Check the Consistency: Lochia should contain no large clots. Clots may indicate that a portion of the placenta has been retained and is preventing closure of the maternal uterine blood sinuses. In any event, large clots denote poor uterine contraction, which needs to be corrected.

Observe the Pattern: Lochia is red for the first 1 to 3 days (lochia rubra), pinkish-brown from days 4 to 10 (lochia serosa), and then white (lochia alba) for as long as 6 weeks after birth. The pattern of lochia (rubra to serosa to alba) should not reverse. A red flow after a pink or white flow may indicate that placental fragments have been retained or that uterine contraction is decreasing and new bleeding is beginning.

Assess the Odor: Lochia should not have an offensive odor. Lochia has the same odor as menstrual blood. An offensive odor usually indicates that the uterus has become infected. Immediate intervention is needed to halt postpartal infection.

Watch for Absence: Lochia should never be absent during the first 1 to 3 weeks. Absence of lochia, like presence of an offensive odor, may indicate postpartal infection. Lochia may be scant in amount after cesarean birth, but it is never altogether absent.

and estradiol are all at prepregnancy levels. Estrol may be elevated for an additional week before it reaches prepregnancy levels. Follicle-stimulating hormone (FSH) remains low for about 12 days and then begins to rise as a new menstrual cycle is initiated.

The Urinary System

During pregnancy, as much as 2000 to 3000 mL excess fluid accumulates in the body. An extensive diuresis begins to take place almost immediately after birth to rid the body of this fluid. This easily increases the daily output of a postpartal woman from a normal level of 1500 mL to as much as 3000 mL/day during the second to fifth day after birth. This marked increase in urine production causes the bladder to fill rapidly.

During a vaginal birth, the fetal head exerts a great deal of pressure on the bladder and urethra as it passes on the bladder's underside. This pressure may leave the bladder with a transient loss of tone that, together with the edema surrounding the urethra, decreases a woman's ability to sense when she has to void. A woman who has undergone epidural or spinal anesthesia can feel no sensation in the bladder area until the anesthetic has worn off.

To prevent permanent damage to the bladder from overdistention, assess a woman's abdomen frequently in the immediate postpartal period. On palpation, a full bladder is felt as a hard or firm area just above the symphysis pubis. On percussion (placing one finger flat on the woman's abdomen over the bladder and tapping it with the middle finger of the other hand), a full bladder sounds resonant, in contrast to the dull, thudding sound of non–fluid-filled tissue. Pressure on this area may make a woman feel as if she has to void, but she is then unable to do so. As the bladder fills, it displaces the uterus; uterine position is therefore a good gauge of whether a bladder is full or empty. If the uterus is becoming uncontracted or feels soft on palpation and is pushed to the side, the usual cause is an overfilled bladder.

The hydronephrosis or increased size of ureters that occurred during pregnancy remains present for about 4 weeks after birth. The increased size of these structures, in conjunction with reduced bladder sensitivity, increases the possibility of urinary stasis and urinary tract infection in the postpartal period.

During the entire postpartal period, urine tends to contain more nitrogen than normal. This is probably due in part to a woman's increased muscle activity during labor and in part to the breakdown of protein in a portion of the uterine muscle that occurs during involution. Lactose levels in the urine are slightly elevated the same as during pregnancy, as the body prepares for breastfeeding. Diaphoresis (excessive sweating) is another way by which the body rids itself of excess fluid. This is noticeable in women soon after birth.

The Circulatory System

The diuresis that is evident between the second and fifth days after birth, as well as the blood loss at birth, acts to reduce the added blood volume a woman accumulated during pregnancy. This reduction occurs so rapidly, in fact, that the blood volume returns to its normal prepregnancy level by the first or second week after birth.

The usual blood loss with a vaginal birth is 300 to 500 mL. With a cesarean birth, it is 500 to 1000 mL. A 4-point decrease in hematocrit (proportion of red blood cells to circulating plasma) and a 1-g decrease in hemoglobin value occur with each 250 mL of blood lost. For example, if an average woman enters labor with a hematocrit of 37%, it will be about 33% on the first postpartal day, and hemoglobin will fall from 11 to 10 g/dL. If the woman was anemic during pregnancy, she can expect to continue to be anemic afterward. As excess fluid is excreted, the hematocrit gradually rises (because of hemoconcentration), reaching prepregnancy levels by 6 weeks after birth.

Women usually continue to have the same high level of plasma fibrinogen during the first postpartal weeks as they did during pregnancy. This is a protective measure against hemorrhage. However, this high level also increases the risk of thrombus formation. There is also an increase in the number of leukocytes in the blood. The white blood cell count may be as high as 30,000 cells/mm^3 (mainly granulocytes) compared to a normal level of 5000 to 10,000 cells/mm^3, particularly if labor was long or difficult. This, too, is part of the body's defense system, a defense against infection and an aid to healing.

Any varicosities that are present will recede, but they rarely return to a completely prepregnant appearance. Although vascular blemishes, such as spider angiomas, fade slightly, they may not disappear completely either.

The Gastrointestinal System

Digestion and absorption begin to be active again soon after birth unless a woman has had a cesarean birth. Almost immediately, the woman feels hungry and thirsty and she can eat without difficulty from nausea or vomiting during this time.

Hemorrhoids (distended rectal veins) that have been pushed out of the rectum because of the effort of pelvic-stage pushing often are present. Bowel sounds are active, but passage of stool through the bowel may be slow because of the still-present effect of relaxin on the bowel. Bowel evacuation may be difficult because of the pain of episiotomy sutures or hemorrhoids.

The Integumentary System

After birth, the stretch marks on a woman's abdomen (striae gravidarum) still appear reddened and may be even more prominent than during pregnancy, when they were tightly stretched. Typically, in a Caucasian woman, these will fade to a pale white over the next 3 to 6 months; in an African American woman, they may remain as areas of slightly darker pigment. Excessive pigment on the face and neck (chloasma) and on the abdomen (linea nigra) will become barely detectable in 6 weeks' time. If **diastasis recti** (overstretching and separation of the abdominal musculature) is present, the area will appear slightly indented. If the separation is large, it will appear as a bluish area in the abdominal midline. Modified sit-ups help to strengthen abdominal muscles and return abdominal support to its prepregnant level. Both the abdominal wall and the ligaments that support the uterus, which were obviously stretched during pregnancy, usually require the full 6 weeks of the puerperium to return to their former state.

Effects of Retrogressive Changes

The overall effects of postpartal retrogressive changes are exhaustion and weight loss.

Exhaustion

As soon as birth is completed, a woman experiences total exhaustion. For the last several months of pregnancy, she probably has experienced some difficulty sleeping. Near the end of pregnancy, she probably was unable to find a comfortable position to sleep because of the fetus' activity or the presence of back or leg pain. All during labor, she worked hard with little or no sleep. Now she has "sleep hunger," which may make it difficult for her to cope with new experiences and stressful situations until she has enjoyed a sustained period of sleep.

Weight Loss

The rapid diuresis and diaphoresis during the second to fifth days after birth usually result in a weight loss of 5 lb (2 to 4 kg), in addition to the approximately 12 lb (5.8 kg) lost at birth. Lochia flow causes an additional 2- to 3-lb (1-kg) loss, for a total weight loss of about 19 lb. Additional weight loss is most dependent on the amount of pregnancy weight gain and on whether a woman takes active measures to lose weight. It is also influenced by nutrition, exercise, and breastfeeding. The weight a woman reaches at 6 weeks after birth becomes her baseline postpartal weight unless she takes active measures to lose the weight (Box 17.5). In many women, this baseline is higher than their prepregnancy weight and one of the reasons that obesity has become a national health concern (Ebbeling et al., 2007).

BOX 17.5 ✻ Focus on Evidence-Based Practice

What is an effective action for women to do to lose the additional weight they gained during pregnancy?

Women are usually interested in losing the weight they gained during pregnancy. It is not always easy to lose those extra pounds they gained, though, because they are exhausted from labor and their days are filled with new baby care. To investigate whether lack of sleep, a common postpartal concern, is linked to obesity, researchers selected 940 participants who were enrolled in prenatal care and assessed them for their sleep pattern and whether they lost their pregnancy weight during their postpartal period. Of the 940 women, 124 (13%) developed postpartum weight retention or were 5 kg or more above pregravid weight at 1 year postpartum. Of these 940 women, 114 (12%) women slept 5 hours or less per day, 280 (30%) slept 6 hours per day, 321 (34%) slept 7 hours per day, and 225 (24%) slept more than 8 hours per day. The women who slept the most (8 hours) were most apt to have lost their pregnancy weight gain at 1 years time; those who slept the least (under 5 hours) were most apt to retain their additional pregnancy weight.

The researchers suggest that interventions to prevent postpartum obesity should consider strategies to obtain optimal maternal sleep during the year after birth.

Would this study be helpful when talking to postpartum women about their need to rest to prevent exhaustion?

Source: Gunderson, E. P., et al. (2008). Association of fewer hours of sleep at 6 months postpartum with substantial weight retention at 1 year postpartum. *American Journal of Epidemiology, 167*(2), 178–187.

Vital Sign Changes

Vital sign changes in the postpartum period reflect the internal adjustments that occur as a woman's body returns to its prepregnant state.

Temperature

Temperature is always taken orally or tympanically (never rectally) during the puerperium, because of the danger of vaginal contamination and the discomfort involved in rectal intrusion.

A woman may show a slight increase in temperature during the first 24 hours after birth because of dehydration that occurred during labor. If she receives adequate fluid during the first 24 hours, this temperature elevation will return to normal. Most women are thirsty immediately after birth and are eager to take in fluid. This makes drinking a large quantity of fluid not a problem unless the woman is nauseated from a birth anesthetic.

Any woman whose oral temperature rises above 100.4° F (38° C), excluding the first 24-hour period, is considered by criteria of the Joint Commission on Maternal Welfare to be febrile. In such women, a postpartal infection may be present (Poggi, 2007).

Occasionally, when a woman's breasts fill with milk on the third or fourth postpartum day, her temperature rises for a period of hours because of the increased vascular activity involved. If the elevation in temperature lasts longer than a few hours, however, infection is a more likely reason. Infection is a major cause of postpartal mortality and morbidity. Because nurses play a major role in assessing postpartum temperature, they have the important role of being the health care providers who may first detect the problem.

Pulse

A woman's pulse rate during the postpartal period is usually slightly slower than normal. During pregnancy, the distended uterus obstructed the amount of venous blood returning to the heart; after birth, to accommodate the increased blood volume returning to the heart, stroke volume increases. This increased stroke volume reduces the pulse rate to between 60 and 70 beats per minute. As diuresis diminishes the blood volume and causes blood pressure to fall, the pulse rate increases accordingly. By the end of the first week, the pulse rate will have returned to normal.

Evaluate pulse rate conscientiously in the postpartal period, because a rapid and thready pulse during this time could be a sign of hemorrhage. Be certain to compare a woman's pulse rate with the slower range expected in the postpartal period, not with the normal pulse rate in the general population. Otherwise, this important finding of hemorrhage may be missed.

Blood Pressure

Blood pressure should also be monitored carefully during the postpartal period, because a decrease in this can indicate bleeding. In contrast, an elevation above 140 mm Hg systolic or 90 mm Hg diastolic may indicate the development of postpartal pregnancy-induced hypertension, an unusual but serious complication of the puerperium (Bailis & Witter, 2007) (see Chapter 21).

To evaluate blood pressure, compare a woman's pressure with her prepregnancy level if possible, rather than with standard blood pressure ranges; otherwise, if her blood pressure rose during pregnancy, a significant postpartal decrease in pressure could be missed.

Oxytocics, drugs frequently administered during the postpartal period to achieve uterine contraction, cause contraction of all smooth muscle, including blood vessels (Subramanian et al., 2008). Consequently, these drugs can increase blood pressure. To prevent blood pressure from rising too high, always measure it before administering one of these agents. If the blood pressure is greater than 140/90 mm Hg, withhold the agent and notify the woman's physician or nurse-midwife to prevent hypertension and, possibly, a cerebrovascular accident.

A major complication in women who have lost an appreciable amount of blood with birth is orthostatic hypotension, or dizziness that occurs on standing because of the lack of adequate blood volume to maintain nourishment of brain cells. To test whether a woman will be susceptible to orthostatic hypotension, assess her blood pressure and pulse while she is lying supine. Next, raise the head of the bed fully upright, wait 2 or 3 minutes, and reassess these values. If the pulse rate is increased by more than 20 beats per minute and blood pressure is 15 to 20 mm Hg lower than formerly, the woman might be susceptible to dizziness and fainting when she ambulates. Advise her to always sit up slowly and "dangle" on the side of her bed before attempting to walk. If she notices obvious dizziness on sitting upright, support her during ambulation to avoid the possibility of a fall. Caution her not to attempt to walk carrying her newborn until her cardiovascular status adjusts better to her blood loss. Inform the woman's physician or nurse-midwife of these findings.

What if... Joan Cooper, now 12 hours postpartum, has an oral temperature of 99° F (37.2° C) and is uncomfortable from profuse diaphoresis and extreme fatigue. What actions would you take?

Progressive Changes

Two physiologic changes that occur during the puerperium involve progressive changes, or the building of new tissue. Because building new tissue requires good nutrition, caution women against strict dieting that would limit cell-building ability during the first 6 weeks after childbirth (Rolfes, Pinna, & Whitney, 2009).

Lactation

The formation of breast milk (lactation) begins in a postpartal woman whether or not she plans to breastfeed (Pavone, Purinton, & Petersen, 2007). Early in pregnancy, the increased estrogen level produced by the placenta stimulates the growth of milk glands; breasts increase in size because of the larger glands, accumulated fluid, and some extra adipose tissue. For the first 2 days after birth, an average woman notices little change in her breasts from the way they were during pregnancy. Since midway through pregnancy, she has been secreting colostrum, a thin, watery, prelactation secretion. She continues to excrete this fluid the first 2 postpartum days. On the third day, her breasts become full and feel tense or tender as milk forms within breast ducts.

Breast milk forms in response to the decrease in estrogen and progesterone levels that follows delivery of the placenta (which stimulates prolactin production and, consequently, milk production). When breast milk first begins to form, the milk ducts become distended. The nipple secretion changes from the clear colostrum to bluish white, the typical color of breast milk. A woman's breasts become fuller, larger, and firmer. In many women, breast distention becomes marked, and this often is accompanied by a feeling of heat or throbbing pain. Breast tissue may appear reddened, simulating an acute inflammatory or infectious process. The distention is not limited to the milk ducts but occurs in the surrounding tissue as well, because blood and lymph enter the area to contribute fluid to the formation of milk. This feeling of tension in the breasts on the third or fourth day after birth is termed primary **engorgement.** It fades as the infant begins effective sucking and empties the breasts of milk. Whether milk production continues depends on the sucking of the infant at the breasts as this releases oxytocin and causes new milk to form. Whether women continue to breastfeed after hospital discharge is influenced by such factors as employment, personal habits, and how important they view breastfeeding to be (Abdulwadud & Snow, 2009). They must be certain to drink adequate fluid daily, eat a nutritious diet, and check with their health care provider before ingesting alternative therapies such as herbs as most of these can be found in breast milk and could be toxic to a newborn (Seely et al., 2008). Techniques of breastfeeding are discussed in Chapter 19.

Return of Menstrual Flow

With the delivery of the placenta, the production of placental estrogen and progesterone ends. The resulting decrease in hormone concentrations causes a rise in production of FSH by the pituitary, which leads, with only a slight delay, to the return of ovulation. This initiates the return of normal menstrual cycles.

A woman who is not breastfeeding can expect her menstrual flow to return in 6 to 10 weeks after birth. If she is breastfeeding, a menstrual flow may not return for 3 or 4 months (lactational amenorrhea) or, in some women, for the entire lactation period. However, the absence of a menstrual flow does not guarantee that a woman will not conceive during this time, because she may ovulate well before menstruation returns (Van der Wijden, Kleijnen, & Van den Berk, 2009).

NURSING CARE OF A WOMAN AND FAMILY DURING THE FIRST 24 HOURS AFTER BIRTH

A woman remains in a birthing room for at least the first hour after birth so she has time to become acquainted with her newborn and to provide for careful health care team observation. After this initial hour, teach perineal care and encourage a woman to shower. She then remains in the room as a postpartal patient or is transferred to a separate postpartal room. The most dangerous hour in childbearing—the first hour after birth—has passed.

Hemorrhage is still a possibility for the first 2 or 3 days after birth, until the myometrial vessels have sclerosed. One of the worries for a woman giving birth at home is that she will not appreciate how dangerous a time this is. With attention focused more on the newborn than on her, postpartal hemorrhage could occur. In the hospital, various health care personnel may be involved in caring for a woman: be sure all members of the health care team are knowledgeable about this danger.

Assessment

Assessment of a postpartal woman includes history, physical examination, and analysis of laboratory findings.

Health History

The technical aspects of a woman's pregnancy, labor, and birth can be learned from her pregnancy, labor, and birth charts. Most of this information is best obtained from a woman herself, however, because this supplies not only information on the events of her pregnancy and labor but also her emotions and impressions about them. If you previously cared for a woman during labor and birth and gained this information, then it is unnecessary to do so again.

Family Profile. Information for a family profile includes age, support persons, other children, type of housing and community setting, occupation, education level, and socioeconomic level or the information necessary to evaluate the impact a new child will have on the woman and her family. This information also lays a foundation for teaching self-care and child care specific to the woman's knowledge level and needs.

Pregnancy History. Information for a pregnancy history includes para and gravida status (and the reason for any discrepancy), expected date of birth, whether the pregnancy was planned, and any problems or complications such as spotting or pregnancy-induced hypertension that occurred. This information helps you to gauge a woman's potential for bonding, because an unplanned pregnancy or complications arising during pregnancy can interfere greatly with bonding.

Labor and Birth History. It is important to gather information on the length of labor, position of the fetus, type of birth, any analgesia or anesthesia used, problems during labor such as fetal distress, supine hypotension syndrome, and the presence of perineal sutures. This information helps in planning for necessary procedures.

Infant Data. The sex and weight of the infant, any difficulty at birth such as the need for resuscitation, plans to breastfeed or formula feed, and any congenital anomalies present are the major facts to obtain. This information helps in planning care for the infant and promoting bonding with the parents.

Postpartal Course. Ask about a woman's general health; her activity level since the birth; a description of lochia; the presence of perineal, abdominal, or breast pain; difficulty with elimination; success with infant feeding; and response of her support person to parenting. This information helps in planning what anticipatory guidance will be needed for home care.

Laboratory Data

Women routinely have their hemoglobin and hematocrit levels measured 12 to 24 hours after birth, to determine whether blood loss at birth has left them anemic. If the hemoglobin finding is lower than 10 g/100 mL, supplementary iron is usually prescribed. Take note of the laboratory reports on a postpartal woman, and make certain that any abnormal finding, such as low hemoglobin, is brought to the attention of the woman's physician or nurse-midwife. The responsibilities of being a new mother, coupled with the additional burden of an undetected low hemoglobin level, can severely tax a woman's energy levels (Dodd, Dare, & Middleton, 2009).

If a woman required catheterization during labor or had a urinary tract infection during pregnancy, a urinalysis or urine culture may be ordered in the postpartal period. Obtain the urine specimen with a clean-catch technique, using a sterile cotton ball tucked in the vaginal introitus to prevent lochia from contaminating the specimen. In some women, it may be necessary to obtain a specimen by urinary catheterization to rule out urinary infection.

Physical Assessment

During early labor, a woman is given a fairly complete physical examination. During the immediate postpartal period, therefore, repetition of a complete examination is not necessary. Crucial assessments examining particular aspects of health, such as an estimation of nutrition and fluid state, energy level, presence or absence of pain, breast health, fundal height and consistency, lochia amount and character, perineal integrity, and circulatory adequacy, are required.

General Appearance. A woman's general appearance in the postpartal period reveals a great deal about her energy level, her self-esteem, and whether she is moving into the taking-hold phase of recovery. Before beginning assessment, ask a woman to void so that she has an empty bladder. Observe how much energy she uses when reaching for her robe or walking to the bathroom—does she struggle or move listlessly, or does she accomplish this task quickly? Observe for a cringing expression or hand pressure against her abdomen that suggests pain on movement. Observe whether she has combed her hair, applied makeup, and put on her own clothing or an agency gown. Many women choose to sleep in an agency gown to prevent lochia stains on their own clothing, but a woman who is pleased with herself, her pregnancy, and her birth experience is usually anxious to wear her own clothing and "fuss" with her appearance within an hour after birth. A woman who is extremely exhausted or depressed probably will not bother with her appearance this way. Keep in mind that a woman whose labor progressed so rapidly that she came to a health care agency as an emergency admission may not have had time to pack a comb and brush or her own clothing. Cultural variations also affect appearance and actions.

In the United States, the postpartal period is generally regarded as a time of wellness; early ambulation and eating a varied diet are encouraged. In other cultures, the period after childbirth may be regarded primarily as a time of rest. Cultural differences include restricting certain foods, reducing activity levels, or both; taboos and rituals are not uncommon. Assessing women in the postpartal period for cultural variations of these types is important, because such variations explain why a woman might be reluctant to ambulate or why she leaves a lunch of food she views as unacceptable uneaten although she said she was hungry.

Hair. Palpate the woman's hair to determine its firmness and strength. Whenever a diet is deficient in nutrients, hair becomes listless and "stringy." A woman who had good nutritional intake during pregnancy has firm, crisp hair. Many women begin to lose a quantity of hair in the postpartal period. This is because, during pregnancy, metabolism was increased and hair growth was rapid, so many hairs reached maturity at the same time. As the woman's body returns to a normal metabolism level, this hair is lost. You may need to reassure a woman that hair loss is not a sign of illness but just another aspect of return to her prepregnant state.

Face. Assess the woman's face for evidence of edema such as puffy eyelids or a prominent fold of tissue inferior to the lower eyelid. Normally, this is negligible. However, in a woman who had pregnancy-induced hypertension and accumulated excessive fluid, it may be evident. It also will become evident in a woman who is developing postpartal pregnancy-induced hypertension, although this condition is rare. Facial edema is most apparent early in the morning if a woman has been lying supine with her head level during the night.

Eyes. Inspect the color and texture of the inner conjunctiva. If a woman is dehydrated, the area appears dry. A woman who is anemic from poor pregnancy nutrition or excessive blood loss at birth has pale conjunctiva. Be alert to possible variations because of skin color, however. The conjunctiva always appears lightly shaded in fair-skinned women. Dark-skinned women may have a ruddy conjunctiva appearance even with anemia. Check the hemoglobin level of any woman with paler than usual conjunctivae to determine whether anemia is present.

Breasts. Breast tissue increases in size as breast milk forms, so a bra that was adequate during pregnancy may no longer be adequate by the second or third postpartal day. Use of a bra supports breast tissue that feels heavy because of increased fluid accumulation and aids comfort. Advise a woman to buy a nursing bra for the postpartal period that is one to two sizes larger than her pregnancy size to allow for this increase. Properly fitted, a bra should fit firmly and snugly. The straps of a bra should not leave erythematic marks on a woman's shoulders.

To assess breasts, ask a woman to remove her bra and cover her breasts with a towel or folded sheet to protect modesty. Ask her to raise her hands over her head and then tuck them under her head, because this stretches and thins breast tissue. Inspect and then palpate for breast size, shape, and color.

Breast tissue should feel soft on palpation on the first and second postpartal day. On the third day, it should begin to feel firm and warm (described as *filling*). On the third or fourth day, breasts appear large and reddened, with taut, shiny skin (engorgement). On palpation, they feel hard and tense and are painful. Normally, engorgement causes the entire breast to feel warm or appear reddened. If only one portion of a breast is warm or reddened, mastitis or inflammation or, possibly, infection of glands or milk ducts is suggested (Deshpande, 2007).

Occasionally, a firm nodule is detected on palpation. Usually, this is only a temporarily blocked milk duct or milk contained in a gland that is not flowing forward to the nipple. However, the location of the nodule should be noted and reported to the woman's physician or nurse-midwife, so that it can be reassessed before discharge from the hospital. Such blocking of breast milk usually is relieved by the infant's sucking. Nevertheless, any nodule needs reassessment, because a fibrocystic or malignant growth unrelated to the pregnancy could be present.

Note whether the breast nipples are normally erect and not inverted. Assess for any cracks, fissures, or the presence of caked milk. Avoid squeezing the nipples, because this can be painful. Unnecessary nipple manipulation also may increase the risk of mastitis by providing a portal for infection.

Uterus. For uterine assessment, position the woman supine so that the height of the uterus is not influenced by an elevated position. Observe her abdomen for contour, to detect distention, and for the appearance of striae or a diastasis. If a diastasis is present (a slightly indented, possibly bluish-tinged groove in the midline of the abdomen), measure the width and length by fingerbreadths.

Palpate the fundus of the uterus by placing one hand on the base of the uterus, just above the symphysis pubis, and the other at the umbilicus. Press in and downward with the hand at the umbilicus until you "bump" against a firm globular mass in the abdomen: the uterine fundus (Fig. 17.5). Assess consistency (firm, soft, or boggy), location (midline), and height. For the first hour after birth, the height of the fundus is at the umbilicus or even slightly above it. It decreases one fingerbreadth in size daily. Measure the height in fingerbreadths, such as "2 F↓ umbilicus" (2 cm beneath the umbilicus). Although this measurement seems less scientific than a measurement of the height of the uterus from the pubis might be, it is the most useful measurement because it shows the gradual decline in size or distance from the umbilicus.

Never palpate a uterus without supporting the lower segment, because the uterus potentially could invert if not stabilized (resulting in a massive hemorrhage).

Palpation of a fundus should not cause pain as long as the action is done gently. If the uterus is not firm on palpation, massage it gently with the examining hand. This usually causes the uterus to contract and become firm immediately. Use a gentle rotating motion, never a hard or forceful touch, so that you do not cause pain or cause the uterus to expend excess energy in contracting. If the uterine fundus does not grow firm with massage, extreme atony, possibly retained placenta fragments, or an excess amount of blood loss may be occurring. Notify the woman's physician or nurse-midwife. Administer PRN oxytocin as ordered. In addition, placing the woman's infant at breast will cause endogenous release of oxytocin and achieve the same effect as oxytocin administration.

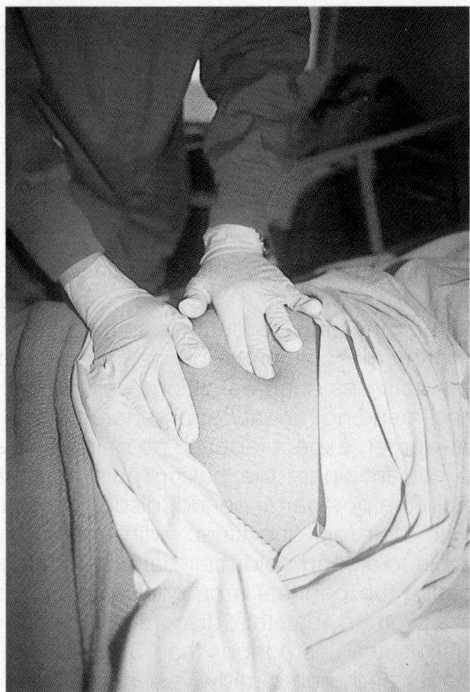

FIGURE 17.5 To palpate a uterus, be certain to place one hand at the base of the uterus. This fundus measures about two fingerbreadths below the umbilicus.

If massage appears ineffective, a clot may be present in the cavity of the uterus. The clot may be expressed from the uterus by gentle pressure on the fundus, but only after the uterus has been massaged. If the uterus is totally relaxed, fundal pressure could cause inversion of the uterus, an extremely serious complication that leads to rapid hemorrhage. Another reason the uterus may not be well contracted is that a rapidly filling bladder is preventing contraction. If contraction remains inadequate, a uterine ultrasound may be ordered to help detect any abnormalities.

A woman who received no oxytocin after birth to help her uterus contract is at greater risk for poor uterine contraction than is a woman who did receive this. If no oxytocin was given, assess the woman's uterine fundus every 10 to 15 minutes immediately after birth, to evaluate and assist the fundus to contract should it become soft or relaxed.

Once the first hour after birth has passed, a woman's uterus may be evaluated for height and consistency less frequently, depending on institutional policy. By the ninth or tenth day after delivery, the uterus will have become so small it is no longer palpable above the symphysis pubis.

Lochia. A woman can expect to have lochia for 2 to 6 weeks. Characteristics of normal lochia and the change in pattern from red to pink to white were described in Table 17.1.

During the first hour after birth, when the fundus is checked every 15 minutes, also remove the mother's perineal pad and evaluate lochia character, amount, color (rubra, serosa, or alba), odor, and presence of any clots. Be certain that a pad is not adhering to perineal stitches before removing it.

When you ask a woman to turn so you can inspect her perineum, be sure to check under her buttocks to observe any blood that may be pooling beneath her. If you observe a constant trickle of vaginal flow or a woman is soaking through a pad every 60 minutes, she is losing more than the average amount of blood. She needs to be checked by a physician or nurse-midwife to be certain that there is no cervical or vaginal tear causing excessive bleeding.

While a woman is at the health care facility, inspect her lochia discharge once every 15 minutes for the first hour, and then according to the institution's policy. Make certain a woman understands that she must wash her hands after handling pads and must use only her own personal care equipment so that she does not contract or spread infection. Demonstrate good role modeling for handwashing and equipment use. Encourage a woman to change perineal pads frequently as she begins self-care, because lochia is an excellent medium for bacterial growth that could spread through the vagina to the uterus. The presence of constantly wet pads against an episiotomy suture line also slows healing. Changing pads frequently is not a problem for a woman while she is at the health care facility, but if she is trying to save money, she may try to conserve on the number of pads she uses at home. Be certain she knows not to use tampons until after she returns for her postpartal checkup, to diminish the risk for infection and toxic shock syndrome (see Chapter 47). Ensure that women know the criteria for judging the amount and type of normal lochia (see Box 17.4), so they can do this accurately.

Perineum. While evaluating lochia, also inspect the perineum. Ask a woman to turn on her side, into a Sims' position with her back toward you. If a midline episiotomy was performed, position the mother on either side. If a mediolateral incision is present, turning her so that the incision is on the bottom buttock often causes less pain and offers better visibility. Gently lift the upper buttock and inspect the perineum. Observe for ecchymosis, hematoma, erythema, edema, intactness, and presence of drainage or bleeding from any episiotomy stitches.

An episiotomy is usually 1 or 2 inches long. However, if a laceration was involved, stitches may extend from the vagina back to the rectum. Rarely, they extend forward toward the urethra. An episiotomy incision is usually fused (edges sealed) by 24 hours after birth; if it is a midline incision, it may be almost invisible because the perineal fold obscures it. A hematoma (blood-filled, protruding sphere) could be present if surface capillaries were broken during the pressure of birth; this should be noted as a potential complication. If there is clotted lochia along the incision line, review postpartal perineal care so that this does not continue to occur. Before discharge, teach a woman who has episiotomy stitches how to lie on her back and view her perineum with a handheld mirror, so that, once a day while at home, she can inspect her perineum for redness, sloughing of sutures, pus formation, or drainage at the suture line.

After perineal assessment, assess the rectal area for the presence of hemorrhoids. If any are present, document their number, appearance, and size in centimeters.

What if... Joan Cooper, at 18 hours postpartum, states that she has had to change her perineal pads twice in the last 30 minutes because they were saturated. She noticed two large clots on the last pad. What assessment should you first perform on her, and why?

Nursing Diagnoses and Related Interventions

Nursing Diagnosis: Pain related to uterine cramping (afterpains)

Outcome Evaluation: Client states degree of pain is tolerable; demonstrates knowledge of measures for adequate pain relief.

Provide Pain Relief for Afterpains. Pain from uterine contractions can be intense, but you can assure a woman that this type of discomfort is normal and rarely lasts longer than 3 days. If necessary, either ibuprofen (such as Motrin), which has anti-inflammatory properties, or a common analgesic such as acetaminophen (such as Tylenol) is effective for pain relief. As with any abdominal pain, heat to the abdomen should be avoided, because it could cause relaxation of the uterus and subsequent uterine bleeding.

Relieve Muscular Aches. Many women feel sore and aching after labor and birth because of the excessive energy they used for pushing during the pelvic division of labor. They describe feeling as if they have "run for miles." A woman may need a mild analgesic such as acetaminophen for the pain. A backrub is effective for relieving an aching back or shoulders. Carefully assess a woman who states that she has pain on standing. Pain in the calf of the leg on standing (a position that dorsiflexes the foot) is a sign similar to Homans' sign suggesting thrombophlebitis may be present (see later discussion).

Administer Cold and Hot Therapy. Applying an ice or cold pack to the perineum during the first 24 hours reduces perineal edema and the possibility of hematoma formation, thereby reducing pain and promoting healing and comfort. Be certain not to place ice or plastic directly on the woman's perineum. Wrap an ice bag first in a towel or disposable pad, to decrease the chance of a thermal burn (risk of injury increases because the perineum has decreased sensation from edema after birth). Commercial cold packs combined with perineal pads also are available. For a low-cost alternative, a rubber glove may be partially filled with ice chips, provided latex allergy is not a concern.

Ice to the perineum after the first 24 hours is no longer therapeutic. After this time, healing increases best if circulation to the area is encouraged by the use of heat. Dry heat in the form of a perineal hot pack or moist heat with a sitz bath is an effective way to increase circulation to the perineum, provide comfort, reduce edema, and promote healing.

Commercial hot packs are available, which grow warm after they are "cracked" and the chemicals in them combine. Caution women to use a washcloth or gauze square between the pack and their skin, to prevent a possible burn.

Promote Perineal Exercises. Some women find that carrying out perineal exercises three or four times a day can greatly relieve perineal edema. The exercise consists of contracting and relaxing the muscles of the perineum 5 to 10 times in succession, as if trying to stop voiding (Kegel exercises). This aids comfort by improving circulation to the area and decreasing edema. When repeated frequently, Kegel exercises also help a woman regain her prepregnant muscle tone and help prevent urinary incontinence (Hay-Smith & Dumoulin, 2009).

Give Episiotomy Care. Although relatively small in size, episiotomy sutures can cause considerable discomfort, because the perineum is an extremely tender area and the muscles of the perineum are involved in so many activities such as sitting, walking, stooping, squatting, bending, urinating, and defecating.

Most women expect labor to be painful. They usually do not anticipate the pulling pain from perineal stitches in the postpartal period, discomfort that interferes with their rest and sleep, with eating, and with being able to sit and hold their baby comfortably.

Because the perineal area heals rapidly, you can assure a woman that this discomfort is normal and does not usually last longer than 5 or 6 days. Many physicians and nurse-midwives order a soothing cream or anesthetic spray to be applied to the suture line to reduce discomfort. A cortisone-based cream or sitz bath helps to decrease inflammation and relieve tension in the area. Because of their cooling effect, witch hazel preparations are a mainstay for relief of both perineal and hemorrhoidal discomfort. A woman may worry that she will experience additional discomfort when the episiotomy sutures are removed. Explain that these sutures are made of an absorbable material so will not need to be removed. Sutures usually dissolve within 10 days.

Administer Sitz Baths. A **sitz bath** is a portable basin that fits on a toilet seat. A reservoir filled with water provides a constant supply of swirling water to the basin. The movement of water soothes healing tissue, decreases inflammation by causing vasodilation in the area, and thereby effectively reduces discomfort and promotes healing.

Sitz baths usually use water that is maintained at 100° to 105° F (38° to 41° C). Be certain that the water in a sitz bath is not too hot before you help a woman to use it; it should feel pleasantly warm, not hot. The woman may not be sensitive to the temperature herself, because healing surfaces are not good indicators of temperature. This caution applies particularly to a woman who is using an analgesic cream or spray on her perineum or who has a great deal of generalized perineal edema. Both situations make her prone to burns from scalding water unless you act to protect her (Box 17.6).

Women should use a sitz bath three to four times a day for a maximum of 20 minutes each time. Because of the soothing effect of the warm water and the sitting position, alert a woman that she may feel extremely tired and unsteady on her feet after using a sitz bath and may need help in getting back to bed.

Provide Pain Management. Several topical medications with lidocaine (Xylocaine) bases, such as gels or

Box 17.6 Nursing Procedure ✻ Sitz baths

Purpose: To aid healing of the perineum through application of moist heat

Procedure	Principle
1. Wash your hands; identify client and explain procedure.	**1.** Handwashing prevents the spread of infection; identification ensures that procedure is performed on correct client, thereby promoting safety; explanation assists in alleviating any anxiety.
2. Assess client's condition; ascertain whether client is able to ambulate to bathroom; assist and modify as necessary.	**2.** A sitz bath can make a woman feel lightheaded, increasing her risk of injury. Fatigue and exhaustion may interfere with client's ability to ambulate or tolerate procedure, also increasing her risk for injury.
3. Assemble equipment, including sitz bath, clean towel, perineal pad.	**3.** Organization of equipment increases efficiency of the procedure.
4. Place sitz bath on toilet seat. Fill collecting bag with warm water at a temperature of 100° F to 105° F (38° C to 41° C). Hang the bag overhead so a steady stream of water will flow from the bag, through the tubing, and into the basin.	**4.** Using correct temperature of water (pleasantly warm) eliminates risk of thermal injury. Adequate flow of warm water increases circulation to the perineum, thereby reducing inflammation and aiding healing.

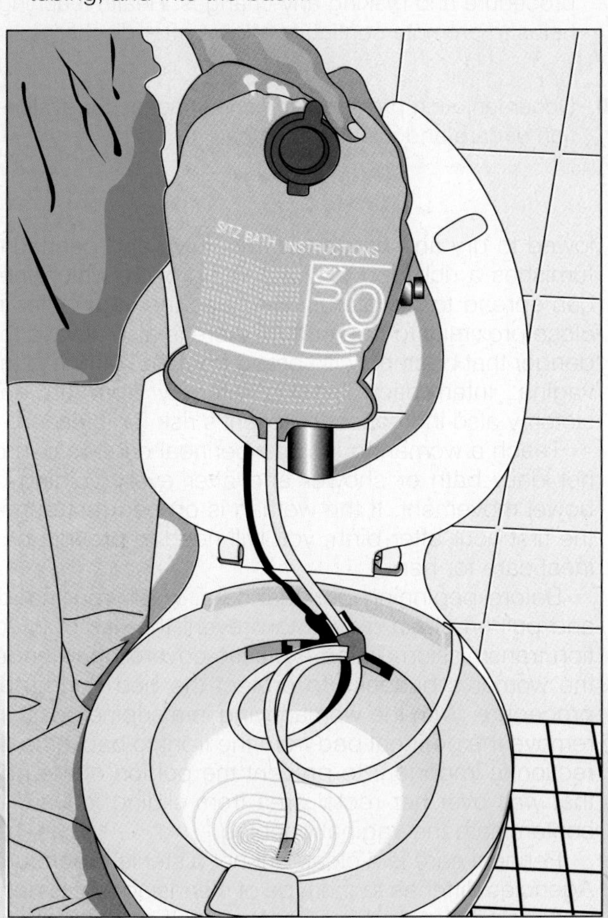

Box 17.6 Nursing Procedure ✻ Sitz baths (continued)

Procedure	Principle
5. Assist client with ambulating to bathroom; help with removal of perineal pad from front to back. Assist client to sit in basin.	5. Assisting ambulation minimizes risk of injury. Removing pad from front to back minimizes risk of infection transmission. Proper placement ensures effectiveness of treatment.
6. Instruct client to use clamp on tubing to regulate water flow; use robe or blankets to prevent chilling and provide for privacy. Have call bell within reach.	6. Continuous swirling water aids in reducing edema and promoting comfort. Privacy enhances self-esteem. Quick, easy access to call bell allows for prompt intervention should problems arise.
7. After 20 minutes, assist client with drying perineum and applying clean pad (holding pad by the bottom side or ends).	7. After 20 minutes, heat is no longer therapeutic because vasoconstriction occurs. Proper handling of pad prevents contamination and possible risk of infection.
8. Assist client with ambulating back to room.	8. Client may become fatigued from the procedure or lightheaded from the warm water, increasing her risk of falling.
9. Evaluate client's tolerance and response to procedure; ask client to report how she feels. Institute health teaching, such as continuing sitz baths when at home.	9. Evaluation assists with determining effectiveness of procedure and making any changes. Health teaching helps to promote continuity of care after discharge.
10. Record completion of procedure, condition of perineum, and client's condition and response.	10. Documentation provides additional means for evaluation of care and client outcomes.

sprays, are available to relieve perineal pain. These are applied to the incision line with a clean gauze square or via a spray. Because of their anesthetic action, they instantly reduce incision line pain. Tucks, a commercial form of soft pad impregnated with witch hazel that can be tucked between the perineum and a sanitary pad, also are effective in relieving perineal pain. Some women doubt the efficacy of suture-line medications or worry that applying the cream will hurt more than not applying it. They may need extra encouragement to try these helpful aids.

In addition to local perineum creams or sprays, many women require an oral or parenteral analgesic to relieve their episiotomy discomfort. Most physicians and nurse-midwives order a moderate-strength analgesic such as propoxyphene/acetaminophen (Darvocet) or codeine for the first 24 hours, then a milder one such as acetaminophen for the remainder of the first week. Ibuprofen also is widely prescribed. Advise a woman not to use aspirin for pain relief during the postpartal period, because it interferes with blood clotting and may increase her risk for hemorrhage from the denuded placental site (Karch, 2009).

Nursing Diagnosis: Risk for infection (uterine) related to lochia and denuded uterine surface

Outcome Evaluation: Client's temperature remains below 100.4° F; lochia is present and without foul odor.

Provide Perineal Care. Postpartal women are particularly prone to perineal infection because lochia, if allowed to dry and harden on the vulva and perineum, furnishes a rich bed for bacterial growth, which then can spread to the uterus. Because the vagina lies in close proximity to the rectum, there is also always the danger that bacteria will spread from the rectum to the vagina. Interruption in skin integrity from an episiotomy also increases the client's risk for infection.

Teach a woman to include perineal care as part of her daily bath or shower and after every voiding or bowel movement. If the woman is on bed rest during the first hour after birth, you will need to provide perineal care for her.

Before beginning perineal care, wash your hands and pull on clean gloves to prevent the risk of infection transmission. Place a plastic-covered pad under the woman's buttocks to protect the bed during the procedure. With the woman lying in a supine position, remove the perineal pad from the front to back; the direction is important to prevent the portion of the pad that was over her rectal area from sliding forward to contaminate the vaginal opening.

Perineal care is a clean but not a sterile procedure. Agencies differ as to the type of cleansing that is done and the articles and solutions used. If actual washing is to be done, use a clean gauze square or a clean portion of a washcloth with soap and water for each stroke, always washing from front to back, from the pubis toward the rectum. Rinse the area in the same manner, and dry it.

A second common method is to spray the perineum with clear tap water from a spray bottle. Direct the spray toward the front of the perineum, and allow it to flow from front to back. Be certain that none of the solution enters the vagina, as it could be a source of contamination. The labia have a tendency to close and cover the vaginal opening, which normally prevents solution from entering the vagina. Do not separate the labia; instead, allow them to perform this protective function. Spray gently to avoid splashing any blood-tinged solution on yourself (to guard against contacting body secretions).

It may be advantageous to have a woman turn on her side in a Sims' position, to permit better visualization of an episiotomy area. In some women, better cleaning of this area can also be done in this position.

Promote Perineal Self-Care. As soon as a woman is allowed to get up to go to the bathroom (if her infant was born without an anesthetic, this is within the first hour after birth), teach her how to carry out her own perineal care.

The bathroom should have an area close to the toilet where a woman can place the equipment she needs for care: a spray bottle, sponges to dry, clean pads, and so forth. Instruct her how to remove the soiled perineal pad and where to dispose of it. Remind her of the importance of using any cream or medication that has been prescribed. Caution her not to flush the toilet until she is standing upright. Otherwise, the flushing water might spray her perineum and cause infection.

If women are given a clear explanation as to why perineal care is important, they perform it well. However, self-care does not eliminate a nurse's responsibility for checking a woman's perineum to assess its condition and the amount and type of lochia flow present. By continuing with these assessments, a nurse remains a woman's first line of defense against postpartal complications such as infection and hemorrhage.

Nursing Diagnosis: Disturbed sleep pattern related to exhaustion from and excitement of childbirth

Outcome Evaluation: Client states she is able to sleep and feels rested during postpartal period.

After birth, a woman is a paradox. She is excited. She has a baby and she wants to hold and be with this new person in her life. She wants to talk to her support person about the experience, their child, and their future. At the same time, she is so exhausted that she falls asleep easily.

Allow a woman to have time with her expanded family in the birthing room immediately after the baby's birth so she can then enjoy sound rest.

Promote Rest in the Early Postpartal Period. Few women are prepared for the degree of fatigue they experience after childbirth. Try to do all procedures swiftly yet gently, to allow as much time for sleep as possible. If a woman has discomfort from hemorrhoids, perineal stitches, or afterpains, be sure she has pain relief so that she can rest comfortably or sleep. Urge her not to fall asleep in a narrow hospital bed with her new infant. Sharing bed space is controversial even in a large bed (Horsley et al., 2007). A newborn in a narrow bed could easily fall and be injured.

Some women experience shaking chills immediately or within a half-hour after birth. This is caused in part by the pressure changes in the abdomen that occur with reduction in the bulk of the uterus and temperature readjustment in response to the diaphoresis of labor. It also may result from the exhilaration the woman is feeling, combined with exhaustion. In any event, shaking chills at this point are common. Reassure the woman that chills are common, so that she will not attribute them to a developing cold or infection. Cover her with a warm blanket, offer her a warm drink, and assure her the occurrence is normal. These actions are usually enough to make the chill transient and allow the woman to fall into a sound, much-needed sleep of about an hour.

Although a woman may choose any position to sleep, she may enjoy being able to sleep on her stomach, something she was not able to do during pregnancy.

Promote Rest Throughout the Puerperium. The importance of rest throughout the entire puerperium cannot be stressed enough. As long as a woman is in the health care facility, reserve time for naps. Include suggestions for getting adequate rest while at home in discharge instructions, because rest may prove difficult. The newborn will wake at least twice a night, and relatives and friends will be coming to see the baby during the day.

Many women do not realize how long it will take to fully return to their previous level of functioning. When families were closely knit and neighborhoods were smaller, a new mother had someone in her family or neighborhood to look after the baby while she napped. Today, many couples do not have family or close friends nearby. If the parents have not thought through this problem before birth, you can help them look at their situation and see what is available to them. Perhaps the woman's mother, a sister, her partner's mother, or another relative could come and stay with them for the first week. Perhaps the father could take a week off from work or school to help out at home; many employment benefit programs provide for this time. If none of these solutions seems appropriate, the couple might appreciate being given the name of a community service agency that supplies homemakers on a short-term basis. A referral to a community health agency for an early home visit is yet another suggestion.

A woman without support has many demands for her new role—being a mother instead of a daughter; a mother as well as a wife; a mother of three, not two. If she is overcome by sleep hunger, her judgment and sense of balance can be blurred. Although it is not the only contributing factor, extreme fatigue is associated with the development of postpartal depression (Corwin & Arbour, 2007).

Nursing Diagnosis: Risk for bathing/hygiene self-care deficit related to exhaustion from childbirth

Outcome Evaluation: Client takes daily responsibility for own hygiene. Client appears clean, dressed, and well groomed.

After childbirth, women often report that their hospital or birthing center room is being kept too warm; to prove it, they point out how heavily they are perspiring. Postpartal rooms often are kept warm so that newborns will be comfortable, but the profuse perspiration a woman is experiencing normally comes from her body's attempt to regulate fluid, not from the heat of the environment.

You can assure a woman that sweating is a normal postpartal event that helps to bring her body back to its prepregnant state. If she has profuse diaphoresis, particularly at night, she usually prefers to wear a hospital gown rather than one of her own. She may need frequent gown changes during the day to be comfortable and not become chilled.

A daily shower is refreshing. Be certain to accompany a woman for a shower on her first postpartal day, because she often is more fatigued than she realizes. Standing under warm water may also make her dizzy, and she may need help to walk safely back to bed.

Formerly, women were not allowed to take tub baths after birth, for fear that bacteria from the bath water would enter the vagina and cause infection. There appears to be little evidence that this is a real danger, however, so if a woman wants to bathe instead of shower, she may do so.

Nursing Diagnosis: Imbalanced nutrition, less than body requirements, related to lack of knowledge about postpartal needs

Outcome Evaluation: Client ingests a 2200- to 2700-kcal diet and drinks 6 to 8 glasses of fluid daily.

Postpartal menu planning should include a diet of between 2200 and 2300 calories daily. Foods should be high in protein and in the vitamins and minerals needed for good tissue repair. An adequate supply of roughage is important to help restore the peristaltic action of the bowel. A woman who is breastfeeding needs an additional 500 calories (i.e., a 2700-kcal diet) and an additional 500 mL of fluid (these may be from the same source) each day to encourage the production of high-quality breast milk. Most mothers are hungry during the immediate postpartal period and consume an adequate diet without urging.

Teach a woman to continue to eat a nutritious diet after she returns home. This can be a problem, because some women become so fatigued during their first weeks at home that they feel unable to prepare adequate meals. Neglecting to eat properly leads to more fatigue and, ultimately, to an even less nutritious diet.

If a woman has any prenatal vitamins or supplementary iron preparations left over from pregnancy, she should, as a rule, continue to take them until her supply is used. If she needs further supplements, her physician or nurse-midwife will prescribe them for her, either on discharge or when she returns for her postpartum checkup (Lipscomb & Novy, 2007).

Promote Adequate Fluid Intake. The rapid diuresis and diaphoresis that occur during the second to fifth postpartal days ordinarily result in a weight loss of 5 lb in addition to the approximately 12 lb lost at childbirth.

Women often feel thirsty during this period of rapid fluid loss and want additional fluid. It seems a paradox that while the body is ridding itself of unwanted fluid, it should also demand fluid. Part of this paradox stems from a woman's having had little to drink during labor. She may say immediately after the birth, "I don't think I'll ever get enough to drink again." Part of the need for fluid stems from the increased amount of nitrogen being released from catabolized uterine cells. A woman needs to increase her fluid intake to rid her body of these wastes.

You may need to encourage some women to drink adequate fluid during the first few postpartum days because they are restricting fluid in the hope of preventing their breasts from becoming engorged. Other mothers are beginning diets that they hope will bring their bodies more quickly back to their nonpregnant slim state. However, fluid restriction does little to deter breast engorgement, and overall, this is not a good time for dieting. The postpartal period is a time of rebuilding and readjusting, for which a woman needs both ample nourishment and adequate fluid intake. Encourage her to drink at least three to four 8-oz glasses of fluid each day (six to eight glasses if breastfeeding).

Nursing Diagnosis: Risk for impaired urinary elimination or constipation related to loss of bladder and bowel sensation after childbirth

Outcome Evaluation: Client voids more than 30 mL/hr without urinary retention, beginning 1 hour after birth, and has a bowel movement by postpartum day 4. No urinary incontinence is noted.

Promote Urinary Elimination. Because the diuresis of the postpartal period begins almost immediately after birth, a woman's bladder begins filling almost immediately. A full bladder puts pressure on the uterus and causes difficulty with uterine contraction. An overdistended bladder may also damage bladder function. Women who have had epidural anesthesia are particularly prone to developing urinary retention (Musselwhite et al., 2007).

Professional judgment is necessary here to assess what is adequate voiding. A woman may report that she is out of bed and using the bathroom to void. However, only a person with knowledge of the extent of the diuresis being accomplished and the amount that should be voided during this time is able to estimate whether bladder function is adequate.

Encourage a woman to walk to the bathroom and void at the end of the first hour after birth, to help prevent bladder distention. Some women have too much perineal edema to be able to void this early. A woman with an episiotomy may be reluctant to void because she knows that acid urine against her sutures will sting. However, many women have enough residual effect of epidural or pudendal anesthesia at this time that voiding is painless. Assist by providing privacy (but remain in close proximity in case a woman becomes dizzy if this is her first time out of bed), running water at the sink, or offering the woman a drink of water. Pouring warm tap water over the vulva, if consistent with the agency's policy for perineal care, also may help.

If the woman still has not been able to void by 4 to 8 hours after birth, and bladder distention is present, she will need to be catheterized. Because the perineum is edematous after birth, the vulva in a postpartal woman appears out of proportion. This makes it difficult to locate the urethra for urinary catheterization. Be certain that, during catheterization, you do not invade the vagina by mistake and thereby carry contamination to the denuded uterus. Occasionally, because of poor tone, the bladder retains large amounts of residual urine after voiding. This urine harbors bacteria, which can cause bladder infection.

To detect whether urinary retention is occurring, be certain to measure the first voiding after birth. Whether the bladder is emptying also may be judged by measuring fundal height and position or by palpating or percussing bladder prominence in the lower abdomen. If a woman is voiding less than 100 mL at a time or has a displaced uterus or a palpable bladder, her physician or nurse-midwife may order catheterization for residual urine after a voiding. As a rule, if the residual urine is more than 150 mL, the catheter is left in place for 12 to 24 hours to give the bladder time to regain its normal tone and to begin to function efficiently.

Fortunately for most women who must be catheterized, the procedure needs to be done only once after birth. Usually, after another 6 to 8 hours has passed and the bladder has filled again, some of the perineal edema has subsided, the bladder has achieved better tone, and the woman is able to void by herself if helped to the bathroom.

Because catheterization can lead to urinary infection, it should not be used indiscriminately in the postpartal period. On the other hand, it should be done before the woman's bladder is injured or the uterus is displaced and uncontracted, resulting in bleeding.

Some women report urinary incontinence during the postpartal period, resulting from poor perineal tone and sensation. Kegel exercises are helpful to strengthen perineal muscles and eliminate incontinence in the future.

Prevent Constipation. Many women have difficulty moving their bowels during the first week of the puerperium, a condition that can be worrisome and uncomfortable. Constipation occurs because of relaxation of the abdominal wall and the intestine, now that they are no longer compressed by the bulky uterus. For a bowel movement, the abdominal wall must exert pressure. In its relaxed state, the pressure is not strong enough to be effective. Also, if hemorrhoids or perineal stitches are present, a woman may decline to try to move her bowels for fear of pain.

To prevent constipation, many women are prescribed a stool softener such as docusate sodium, beginning with the first day after birth (Box 17.7). If a woman has not moved her bowels by the third postpartum day, a mild laxative or cathartic may be prescribed. There is danger in giving cathartics before the third day, because the resulting increase in intestinal activity could cause uterine irritation and lead to insufficient contraction.

Early ambulation, a good diet with adequate roughage, and an adequate fluid intake all aid in preventing the problem of constipation.

BOX 17.7 * Focus on Pharmacology

Docusate Sodium (Colace, Surfak)

Classification: Docusate sodium is a stool softener.

Action: Used in the postpartal period to prevent constipation. It works by lowering the surface tension of feces, allowing water and lipids to penetrate the stool and soften it (Karch, 2009).

Pregnancy Risk Category: C

Dosage: 50–100 mg PO daily.

Possible Adverse Effects: Occasional abdominal pain and diarrhea

Nursing Implications

- Encourage a woman to swallow the medication with a full glass of water or juice.
- Instruct a woman to consume high-fiber foods to encourage elimination.
- Encourage activity to promote intestinal motility.

Prevent Development of Hemorrhoids. The pressure of the fetal head on the rectal veins during birth tends to aggravate or produce hemorrhoids (swollen rectal veins) to such an extent that some women find hemorrhoidal discomfort to be their chief discomfort in the first few days after birth (Quijano & Abalos, 2009). This discomfort can be relieved by sitz baths, anesthetic sprays, witch hazel or astringent preparations, or preparations such as hydrocortisone acetate (Proctofoam). Gentle manual replacement of hemorrhoidal tissue may also give relief. Assuming a Sims' position several times a day aids in good venous return to the rectal area and also reduces discomfort. Increased fluid and the administration of a stool softener prevent the development of hardened stool, which can irritate hemorrhoids.

Nursing Diagnosis: Risk for ineffective peripheral tissue perfusion related to immobility and increased estrogen level

Outcome Evaluation: Client demonstrates negative Homans' sign and absence of erythema or pain in calves of legs.

Assess Peripheral Circulation. To determine whether peripheral circulation is adequate, assess a woman's thigh for skin turgor. Assess for edema at the ankle and over the tibia on the lower leg. Although this technique is not totally reliable, assess for thrombophlebitis by dorsiflexing a woman's ankle and asking her if she notices pain in her calf on that motion (**Homans' sign**). Assess also for redness in the calf area, because thrombophlebitis can be present even with a negative Homans' sign. Continue to assess for adequate peripheral circulation once every 8 hours during the woman's stay in a health care facility. If you suspect thrombophlebitis, do not massage the area—doing so could cause an embolus.

Be certain to allow a woman to dangle her legs on the edge of the bed for a few minutes to prevent

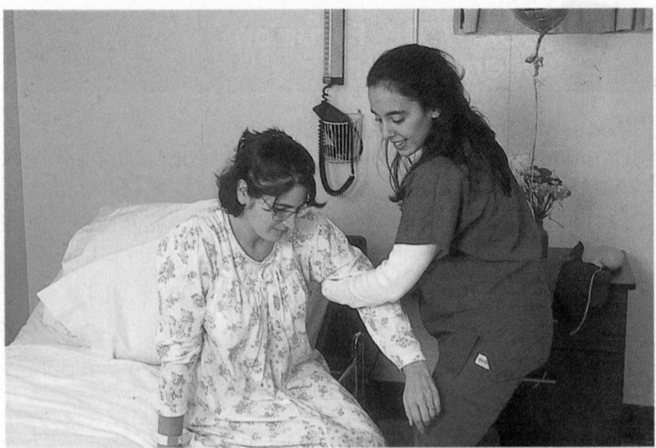

FIGURE 17.6 Ambulating postpartally is not always easy but helps to prevent complications.

dizziness before she gets up for the first time. Then, assist her as needed to take the few steps to a nearby bathroom. Remain with her to be certain that dizziness does not occur. After this, she may be up on her own as she wishes.

As a rule, women who ambulate quickly feel stronger and healthier by the end of their first week and have fewer bowel, bladder, and circulatory complications than those who do not (Fig. 17.6).

Nursing Diagnosis: Pain related to primary breast engorgement

Outcome Evaluation: Client states pain from breast engorgement is at a tolerable level.

Prevent/Alleviate Breast Engorgement. If a woman is breastfeeding, encouraging her newborn to suck at the breast is the main treatment for relief of the tenderness and soreness of primary breast engorgement (techniques of breastfeeding are discussed in Chapter 19).

Many women find the application of warm compresses or standing under a warm shower beneficial to relieve engorgement discomfort. Good support from a bra also offers relief because it prevents unnecessary strain on the supporting muscles of the breasts, positions the breasts in good alignment, and diminishes the amount of engorgement caused by blocked milk ducts. If the woman has not packed a bra in her suitcase, ask her to arrange to have one brought from home.

A woman who is not breastfeeding may experience even stronger discomfort. However, when little or no milk is removed from the breasts, the accumulation of milk inhibits further milk formation, and engorgement subsides in about 2 days. Cold compresses, applied to the breasts three or four times a day during the period of engorgement, or an oral analgesic, or both, provide relief. Wearing a snug-fitting bra and avoiding nipple stimulation may help. Restricting fluid and pumping milk from the breasts are not effective measures and are to some degree harmful, so these actions should be avoided.

Promote Breast Hygiene. Breast care during the postpartal period includes cleanliness and support. These issues are the same whether or not a woman is breastfeeding.

Teach a woman to wash her breasts daily with clear water at the time of her bath or shower and then dry them with a soft towel. She should avoid using soap, because it tends to dry and crack the nipples, possibly leading to fissures and breast abscess. It is not necessary for women to wash their breasts more often than daily, because excessive washing means unnecessary manipulation.

A woman who has a considerable discharge of colostrum or milk from her breasts (whether breastfeeding or not) should insert clean gauze squares or commercial nursing pads into her bra to absorb the moisture, changing them as often as necessary to keep the nipples dry. If the nipples remain wet for any length of time, fissures may form and lead to infection.

Nursing Diagnosis: Health-seeking behaviors related to future breast health

Outcome Evaluation: Client states the importance of once-yearly breast examination by a health care provider (or a yearly mammogram, if appropriate for her age) and her intention to schedule this examination yearly.

Because breast tumors are a major type of neoplasm in women, all women of childbearing age should know the importance of yearly breast assessment (Calhoun & Giuliano, 2007). Many women are not interested in hearing about cancer prevention measures during pregnancy; the possibility of developing cancer is too far removed from what they are doing during pregnancy—creating life. In the postpartal period they become conscious of the need to remain well to raise this new child to maturity. This makes them receptive to having you review with them or teach them the necessity for regular breast assessment at health care visits.

A breastfeeding woman will, of course, have a milk discharge from her nipples. She may occasionally discover a distended milk gland that feels very much like a cyst or tumor. You can assure her she should not worry about such distended glands unless they persist beyond two breastfeedings. Also, remind her that, if she does notice a lump or have an abnormal nipple discharge in a breast, she should call her health care provider about the finding but be aware that most lumps found in breasts are not cancerous. Also, breast carcinoma, if discovered early and treated promptly (often without removal of more than the local lesion), has a good cure rate.

Nursing Diagnosis: Health-seeking behaviors related to client's desire to return to prepregnant weight and appearance

Outcome Evaluation: Client states realistic goals for return to former appearance; is able to demonstrate appropriate exercises.

After childbirth, the abdominal wall and the uterine ligaments are stretched. The abdomen pouches forward.

Wearing a girdle may help a woman feel more comfortable during the first few weeks after birth, but it does not aid, and may actually hinder, strengthening the tone of the abdominal wall.

A woman can best help her abdominal wall to return to good tone by using proper body mechanics and posture, getting adequate rest, and performing prescribed exercises. Exercises to strengthen the abdominal and pelvic muscles may be started, with the consent of the woman's physician or nurse-midwife, as early as the first day after birth. She should continue these exercises until the end of the puerperium to derive the maximum benefit from them. Common abdominal and perineal strengthening exercises are described in Table 17.2. Many women find commercial abdominal exercisers helpful to fully strengthen their abdominal wall.

Teach Methods to Promote Uterine Involution. All during the postpartal period, lying on the abdomen gives support to abdominal muscles and may aid involution, because it tips the uterus into its natural forward position. If this puts too much pressure on sore breasts, placement of a small pillow under the abdomen usually solves the problem.

It may be dangerous for a woman to assume a knee–chest position until at least the third week after birth. In a knee–chest position, the vagina tends to open. Because the cervical os remains open to some extent until the third week, there is a danger that air will enter the vagina and the open cervix, penetrate the open blood sinuses inside the uterus, enter the circulatory system, and cause an air embolism.

Although this would be a rare occurrence, it is good practice for a woman to avoid this position until she returns for a postpartal examination and is assured that her cervix has closed. Women who have used a knee–chest position during pregnancy to relieve the pressure of hemorrhoids need to be cautioned that a modified Sims' position, such as they used for a rest position during pregnancy, is better for them now.

Nursing Diagnosis: Risk for ineffective sexuality patterns related to physiologic changes of postpartal period

Outcome Evaluation: Client states she has a satisfactory sexual relationship with her partner; demonstrates understanding of both coital and noncoital methods of sexual expression.

At one time, women were cautioned not to resume sexual relations after the birth of a baby until after their medical checkup at 6 weeks. However, there is no apparent physiologic reason to delay sexual relations this long. For most couples, coitus may be resumed as soon as lochia serosa has stopped—about 1 to 2 weeks after birth.

Caution women, however, that sex may be somewhat uncomfortable if it is begun this early. Tissue at an episiotomy site may be sensitive. Because the vaginal epithelium is still thin, vaginal tenderness may be noticed. Use of a lubricant will help any mucosal dryness. A female-superior position can be suggested because it allows the woman to control the depth of penile penetration.

A woman who is breastfeeding may notice that milk is released from her nipples with sexual arousal.

TABLE 17.2 ✻ Muscle-Strengthening Exercises

Exercise	Description
Abdominal breathing	Abdominal breathing may be started on the first day after birth, because it is a relatively easy exercise. Lying flat on her back or sitting, a woman should breathe slowly and deeply in and out 5 times, using her abdominal muscles. Check by watching her abdominal wall rise that she is actually using these muscles.
Chin-to-chest	The chin-to-chest exercise is excellent for the second day. Lying on her back with no pillow, a woman raises her head and bends her chin forward on her chest without moving any other part of her body while exhaling. She should start this gradually, repeating it no more than 5 times the first time and then increasing it to 10–15 times in succession. The exercise can be done 3 or 4 times a day. She will feel her abdominal muscles pull and tighten if she is doing it correctly.
Perineal contraction	If a woman is not already using this exercise as a means of alleviating perineal discomfort, it is a good one to add on the third day. She should tighten and relax her perineal muscles 10–25 times in succession as if she were trying to stop voiding (Kegel exercises). She will feel her perineal muscles working if she is doing it correctly.
Arm raising	Arm raising helps both the breasts and the abdomen return to good tone and is a good exercise to add on the fourth day. Lying on her back, arms at her sides, a woman moves her arms out from her sides until they are perpendicular to her body. She then raises them over her body until her hands touch and lowers them slowly to her sides. She should rest a moment, then repeat the exercise 5 times.
Abdominal crunches	It is advisable to wait until the 10th or 12th day after birth before attempting abdominal crunches. Lying flat on her back with knees bent, a woman folds her arms across her chest and raises herself to a sitting position. This exercise expends a great deal of effort and tires a postpartal woman easily. Caution her to begin very gradually and work up slowly to doing it 10 times in a row.

BOX 17.8 ✻ Signs of Good Parent–Child Adaptation

Good parent–child adaptation is demonstrated when a parent:

- Speaks of infant as desirable and attractive
- Is not upset by vomiting, drooling, and the like
- Holds the baby warmly
- Makes eye contact with the infant
- Plays with and soothes the infant
- Talks or sings to the baby
- Expresses confidence that the infant is well
- Finds physical or psychological attributes to admire about the baby
- Is able to discriminate between the baby's signs of hunger, sleep, and so on

Women may already be aware that their degree of exhaustion can make them less receptive to sexual arousal than before. Be sure that women receive adequate reproductive planning information, if desired, before they resume sexual relations (see Chapter 6).

Nursing Diagnosis: Risk for impaired parenting related to inadequate bonding behavior after childbirth

Outcome Evaluation: Parents hold and comfort their infant appropriately and voice positive characteristics of child.

To assess that bonding is occurring, listen to what parents say about their newborn in the immediate postpartal period. Do they make positive statements such as, "I'm glad he's a boy" or "She's cute," or negative ones such as, "I really hoped it would be a girl" or "She looks like a circus clown with no hair"? First impressions may not be lasting ones. However, negative comments need to be identified, so that extra discussion about things such as what it feels like to have four boys, or not to have the prettiest child in the nursery, can take place. Although brief hospital stays are advantageous in many ways, if such discussion does not occur, a family may be discharged from the health care agency with their needs unmet (Brown et al., 2009). At home, away from health care personnel who are attuned to how disappointment can interfere with parent–child interaction, parents may have great difficulty adjusting to and relating to this new child. Typical signs of good parent–child adaptation are shown in Box 17.8.

NURSING CARE OF A WOMAN AND FAMILY IN PREPARATION FOR DISCHARGE

The greatest need of a postpartal woman before discharge from a health care agency is education to prepare her to care for herself and her newborn at home (see Focus on Nursing Care Planning Box 17.9). She must be aware of danger signs to look for and know whom to call if she notices any of them. She must understand safe baby care. Because of shortened lengths of stay, every contact with a woman during a health agency stay should include some teaching information. At the same time, be aware that learning does not take place if the learner is overwhelmed and hurried. Use common sense to determine when it is time to teach and when it is time to observe or listen. Observation of mother–child or parent–child interactions and evaluation of a woman's support system at home are the basis for much of the teaching.

Most women attend classes in newborn care during their pregnancies. They remember many points from these classes, but when they actually have a newborn they can become worried that they do not remember enough. Many mothers say that child care did not seem real during pregnancy. The postpartal period is a time for teaching, reteaching, and offering anticipatory guidance to help in the new situations a family can expect when they go home.

During the taking-in phase of the puerperium, a woman may not show much interest in learning; she is more in need of the comfort of being taken care of. As she enters her taking-hold period, she grows increasingly receptive to advice and looks to nurses for the information she needs. Some nurses assume that multiparas will react negatively to child care suggestions. They are, after all, veterans of child care. If you listen carefully, however, you may discover that a mother of two girls feels insecure about the care of her new baby boy. A woman whose next youngest child is 5 years old may admit that in 5 years she has completely forgotten how small newborns are. She yearns to have a nurse who is comfortable with such small human beings reassure her that she is holding her new baby correctly and giving proper care. All mothers, whether primiparas or multiparas, need to be evaluated individually and helped whenever they ask or you find that they need guidance.

Group Classes

Providing group classes on bathing infants, breastfeeding techniques, minimizing jealousy in older children, and maintaining health in the newborn can be helpful to mothers and fathers, because in these settings they can learn not only from the instructor but also from other parents. Brain-storming this way is helpful to women who envision jealousy problems with older children or who plan to return to a full-time job and also breastfeed (Abdulwadud & Snow, 2009). Be certain that a time for questions and answers is planned at these sessions, so parents can apply what is being taught to their individual circumstances. Urging fathers to attend classes is helpful, because many fathers give direct child care for at least part of every day. Including the father in teaching is also important, because the problems that arise with newborn care are, by their nature, family problems, and every effort should be made by nursing personnel to help both parents prepare to deal with them.

Individual Instruction

Every family needs some individual instruction in how to care for their infant and how the woman can care for herself after discharge. How to bathe and feed the baby, how to care for the infant's cord and circumcision if the infant has this, a review of how much infants sleep during 24 hours, and how to fit a newborn into the family's pattern of living are topics

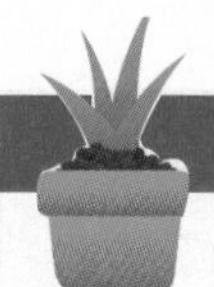

BOX 17.9 ✻ Focus on Nursing Care Planning

A Multidisciplinary Care Map for a Postpartal Woman

Joan Cooper is 6 hours postpartum after birth of an 8-lb 2-oz baby girl. She states, "I haven't urinated since before the birth. What kind of mother am I going to be if I can't even manage my own care?" Her husband Mike pulls you aside and says, "Sometimes, I see my wife crying for no reason. Why isn't she as happy as I am?"

Family Assessment ✻ Couple has been married for 3 years. Husband works as a pharmacist. Will be taking a week off from work to spend time with Joan and the new baby. Joan is on maternity leave from her job as a court reporter.

Client Assessment ✻ Labor and birth were without incident. Abdomen soft. Uterus ½ fingerbreadth above umbilicus, soft, and displaced to the right. Moderate lochia rubra. Bladder firm on palpation above symphysis pubis. Resonant on percussion. Vital signs within acceptable parameters.

Nursing Diagnosis ✻ Altered urinary elimination related to perineal edema and decreased bladder tone from fetal head pressure during labor and birth.

Outcome Criteria ✻ Client attempts common measures to initiate voiding; voids more than 100 mL within 2 hours' time. Voices that she understands that crying is a common reaction postbirth.

Team Member Responsible	Assessment	Intervention	Rationale	Expected Outcome
		Activities of Daily Living		
Nurse	Assess amount of urine voided during labor, and reassess fundal height and position.	Discuss importance of continuing to drink to help initiate bladder reflex. Also discuss importance of emptying bladder.	Assessing fundal height and position provides evidence about the degree of bladder filling. Retention of urine in the bladder predisposes to infection.	Client voids a minimum of 100 mL by 2 hours' time, and fundal height returns to 1 fingerbreadth below umbilicus after voiding.
		Consultations		
Nurse	Determine which member of client's primary care team is on call.	If client has not voided by 8 hours after birth, notify team member on call and keep her or him informed.	Bladder distention can interfere with uterine involution and, if allowed to persist, may result in permanent loss of bladder tone.	Primary health care provider is notified of client's inability to void.
		Procedures/Medications		
Nurse	Assess what measures client thinks would help her to void.	Instigate measures client suggests, such as ambulating to bathroom or hearing water running. Respect privacy while staying nearby for support.	Respecting client's preferences helps her to maintain feeling of control. Remaining nearby ensures client safety.	Client ambulates to the bathroom to void with assistance from health care provider.
		Nutrition		
Nurse	Assess whether intake, both intravenous and oral, has been adequate since birth.	Stress importance of drinking extra water during the postpartum period.	Women should drink ample fluid during the postpartum period, to counteract normal diuresis and ensure good urine output.	Client confirms she has been drinking 1 glass of fluid an hour. Knows to drink 6 to 8 glasses of fluid daily.

(continued)

BOX 17.9 ✻ Focus on Nursing Care Planning (continued)

Team Member Responsible	Assessment	Intervention	Rationale	Expected Outcome
		Patient/Family Education		
Nurse	Assess client's knowledge of postpartal care measures.	Teach normal physiologic changes that occur after birth and the importance of preventing complications such as urinary retention or thrombophlebitis.	The more informed clients are, the more they can participate in self-care.	Client states that she understands the importance of a good fluid output to help prevent urinary tract infection.
		Psychosocial/Spiritual/Emotional Needs		
Nurse	Assess whether client can explain why she has episodes of crying.	Emphasize that "baby blues" are common during the postpartal period. Most difficulties are transitory and will not interfere with parenting.	Feeling of sadness is common. The change to being a parent is a major role change.	Client states that she views inability to void as a temporary setback and one that will not interfere with her success as she moves into a parenting role.
		Discharge Planning		
Nurse/nurse midwife	Assess client to see whether she understands the importance of monitoring voiding at home, maintaining perineal tone.	Once voiding pattern is re-established, instruct client in Kegel exercises.	Kegel exercises help strengthen perineal muscles.	Client describes Kegel exercises that she will continue to use to strengthen perineal muscles.

parents like to discuss. Teaching does not have to be formal. You can teach without lecturing by making a comment such as, "Notice how large all newborns' heads seem" while you are showing the parents how to bathe the baby, or "Babies like to be bundled firmly" while you are helping dress the child, or "Notice how uneven newborn respirations are." This kind of instruction saves parents many anxious moments when they are at home. Techniques for home care of the newborn are discussed in Chapter 18.

Discharge Planning

Before a postpartal family is discharged from the health care agency, a woman will be given instructions by her physician or nurse-midwife concerning her care at home. These instructions differ among health care providers but have common points that are summarized in Table 17.3.

Before discharge, make sure a woman is aware that she must return for an examination 4 to 6 weeks after birth, and that she should make an appointment to take her baby to a primary care provider for an examination at 2 to 4 weeks of age. If a woman does not have an adequate rubella antibody titer and anticipates further pregnancies, she may receive a rubella immunization before discharge. Women who are Rh negative and who have had an Rh-positive infant will receive RhiG or Rh antibodies to prevent problems in a future pregnancy (Crowther & Middleton, 2009).

Be certain that discharge instructions for the family are given both verbally and in writing. Getting ready to go home, dressing the baby, seeing him or her in new clothes for the first time, and experiencing the thrill of realizing the baby is really theirs to take home is so exciting that oral instructions may go unheard. On the other hand, parents should not simply be handed a list of printed material. Review the instructions with the parents to be sure they understand them.

Many health care agencies have a community liaison person, ideally a nurse, who calls or makes a home visit to mothers after discharge. This person helps the new mother assess her own health and that of her baby and answers questions from families who lose their instructions or are unable to interpret them after they have returned home.

Making a telephone call to or visiting a family 24 hours after discharge is the most helpful way to evaluate whether the family is able to continue self-evaluation and infant care and is able to integrate the new infant into the family. Such calls or visits may also reduce the number of acute care visits and rehospitalizations for newborns.

TABLE 17.3 ✻ Postpartal Discharge Instructions

Area	Instructions
Work	All women should avoid heavy work (lifting or straining) for at least the first 3 weeks after birth. Women differ in their concept of heavy work, so it is a good idea to explore what a woman considers heavy work. If she plans to do too much, you can perhaps help her to modify her plans. It is usually advised that a woman not return to an outside job for at least 3 weeks (or better, 6 weeks), not only for her own health but also for enjoyment of the early weeks with her newborn.
Rest	A woman should plan at least one rest period each day and try to get a good night's sleep. She can rest during the day when her newborn is sleeping, unless she has other children or an aged parent to care for. If she has others dependent on her, explore the possibility of having a neighbor, another family member, or a person from a community health agency relieve her.
Exercise	A woman should limit the number of stairs she climbs to one flight/day for the first week at home. Beginning the second week, if her lochial discharge is normal, she may start to increase this activity. This limitation will involve some planning on her part, especially if her washing machine is in the basement and she must wash diapers every day, or if she must go up and down stairs to check on her baby. It is probably better to arrange for a place for the baby to sleep downstairs as well as upstairs, so the baby must be taken upstairs only at bedtime. She should continue with muscle-strengthening exercises, such as abdominal crunches.
Hygiene	A woman may take either tub baths or showers. She should continue to apply any cream or ointment as ordered for the perineal area and cleanse her perineum from front to back. Any perineal stitches will be absorbed within 10 days. She should not use vaginal douches until she returns for her postpartal checkup.
Coitus	Coitus is safe as soon as a woman's lochia has turned to alba and, if present, the episiotomy is healed (usually about the first week after birth). Vaginal cells may not be as thick as formerly because prepregnancy hormone balance has not yet completely returned. Use of a contraceptive foam or lubricating jelly will aid comfort. Be certain she knows safer sex precautions.
Contraception	If desired, a woman should begin a contraception measure with the initiation of coitus. If she wishes an IUD, this may be fitted immediately after birth or at her first postpartal checkup. Oral contraceptives are begun about 2–3 weeks after birth. A diaphragm must be refitted at a 6-week checkup. Until she returns for this checkup, an over-the-counter spermicidal jelly and condoms can provide protection.
Follow-up	A woman should notify her physician or nurse-midwife if she notices an increase, not a decrease, in lochial discharge, or if lochia serosa or lochia alba becomes lochia rubra. Delayed postpartal hemorrhage can occur in women who become extremely fatigued. Getting adequate rest during her first weeks at home will do much to prevent the possibility of this complication. Four to 6 weeks after birth, a woman should return to her physician or nurse-midwife for an examination. This visit is important to ensure that involution is complete, immunization against the virus associated with cervical cancer (HPV), and reproductive life planning (if desired) can be discussed.

NURSING CARE OF A WOMAN AND FAMILY AFTER DISCHARGE

Postpartal Home Visits

In today's health care climate of cost containment, most women are discharged from a health care facility 2 to 3 days after childbirth. Such a practice has the advantage of allowing the family unit to be interrupted as little as possible. A new mother may rest better at home than in a strange setting, and she may eat better if she has cultural preferences for specific foods. The infant can be more quickly exposed to family routines rather than a superficial facility schedule. However, early discharge has the disadvantage of not allowing a new family to have the ready support of health care personnel if they have questions about their newborn or about the woman's condition. Although home visits are helpful for everyone, they should especially be planned for high-risk newborns, including newborns who are preterm, those born with a congenital anomaly, infants of adolescent mothers, and infants of mothers who have abused drugs during pregnancy.

The purposes of a home visit for the well postpartum woman and her newborn are to help integrate the infant into the family and to provide the family with additional information on newborn care that they may not have been able to learn during a brief hospital stay. Such a visit also allows for physical examination of the woman and newborn and for newborn screening procedures or bilirubin testing, if these were not done before hospital discharge.

Because women need to preserve their energy during the postpartal period, try to arrange a home visit at the woman's convenience. Preparation for home visiting is discussed in Chapter 4, with other aspects of home care. Important assessments to make at a postpartal home visit include:

Pregnancy History: Were there physical factors that could have interfered with pregnancy bonding, such as painful varicose veins or gestational diabetes? Were there psychosocial factors such as an unwelcome move or loss of an important support person? Ask the woman to describe her labor and birth, both to determine whether any complications were present and to evaluate her reaction to the event.

Newborn History: Has the baby had a return visit for a physical examination, and what were the findings? Is there anything about her infant for which a woman is concerned? Is the baby eating well? Sleeping at spaced intervals? Constantly fretful? Is the baby voiding?

Postpartal Course: Does a woman still have pain? Are there any concerns about her health? Is she managing to obtain adequate rest? A woman may be unprepared for feelings of postpartal depression ("baby blues") that she is experiencing. Ask whether she feels "blue" or extremely fatigued.

Future Plans: Will the woman be returning to work outside her home? If so, what plans has she made for child care?

Family Assessment: How are other children adapting? Does the client have adequate help with the new baby? How are her finances?

Physical Examination of the Mother: Assess temperature, pulse, and respiratory rate to detect possible infection or excessive blood loss. Assess uterine height and consistency (by the 10th day after delivery, the uterus should no longer be palpable as an abdominal organ). Assess the perineum to be certain there are no signs of infection in episiotomy stitches and that lochia color and odor are normal. Assess breasts for engorgement or any sign of infection.

Physical Examination of the Infant: Assess temperature, pulse, respiratory rate, and skin turgor. Assess the abdomen for distention. Inspect for any ecchymotic marks. Assess for full range of motion of extremities and that the child follows a moving light. Assess for jaundice. Inspect for possible diaper rash. Check that the skin around the cord is not reddened. (Full assessment of a newborn is discussed in Chapter 18.)

Follow-up Information: Be certain the family has made plans (or knows how to make plans) for continued care for both the infant and the mother. Be certain that they have the telephone number of a health care provider they can call if they have a concern before their next follow-up appointment.

Visiting a new family a few days after a hospital discharge this way is enjoyable, because most families have at least one question about their newborn that they are pleased to have answered. They are always pleased to be reassured that they are parenting well.

Postpartal Examination

Every newborn should have a health maintenance visit 2 to 4 weeks after birth (see Chapter 18). Every woman should have a checkup by her physician or nurse-midwife at 4 to 6 weeks after birth (the end of the postpartal period), to assure herself and her health care provider that she is in good health and has no residual problems from childbearing.

During this examination, the woman's abdominal wall is inspected for tone. Her breasts are inspected to see whether they have returned to their nonpregnant state if she is not breastfeeding or to see that they are unfissured and free of complications if she is breastfeeding. Most important, a thorough internal examination is performed to be certain that involution is complete, the ligaments and the pelvic muscle supports have returned to good functional alignment, and any lacerations sustained during birth have healed (Table 17.4). Ask about the possibility of intimate partner abuse, because it can increase during the postpartal period because of the added stress of forming a new family.

If a woman has hemorrhoids or varicosities as a result of the pregnancy, her physician or nurse-midwife will discuss with her whether further management of these conditions is necessary. You should review the necessity of having a breast examination, Papanicolaou (Pap) smear, and pelvic examination every year as a means of screening for breast, cervical, and uterine cancer. If a woman is older than 40 years, include a discussion about the need for mammogram examinations at least every other year. Encourage women who have stopped smoking during pregnancy to continue to be smoke free as yet another good health measure.

The postpartal examination should be a time for a woman to discuss any problems she had with childbearing and any she now has with childrearing, because these are a continuum. If reproductive life planning was not discussed immediately after birth, this visit is an opportune time for such a discussion. If a woman desires to use a diaphragm or a cervical cap, they can be fitted during this examination. Subcutaneous implanted hormonal contraception also can be inserted at this time. Women who are breastfeeding can begin on progesterone-only birth control pills (Truitt et al., 2009).

NURSING CARE OF A POSTPARTAL WOMAN AND FAMILY WITH UNIQUE NEEDS

A Woman Who Chooses Not to Keep Her Child

Although the availability of birth control information and the ability of women to secure abortions have reduced the number of unwanted or unplanned children, some women still may complete a pregnancy and then give up their child for adoption (Fontenot, 2007). There are numerous reasons for this decision: a woman may be unmarried, or her marriage may be failing, and she does not want to raise a child alone. She may feel that her family is already complete. She may want to finish school before having a child, or she may want to pursue a career.

During pregnancy, most women decide whether they will keep their child. During labor, they express confidence in their decision, but with the actual birth of their child, they may find that their resolve wavers. A woman who was certain she was going to surrender her child for adoption may realize she wants to keep the child. A woman who was certain she was going to keep her child could become aware for the first time of the responsibility involved and decide that the best course for the child is adoption. In either event, a woman's feelings can become confused.

For a woman who chooses not to keep her child, the wait in the birthing room for preparations to transfer the baby to a nursery may seem unusually long. She may also be alone, with no partner or support person with her during this time. Every woman has a right to see, hold, and feed her child if she wishes. A woman who is not going to keep her child may feel proud that she has produced a healthy baby. The realization that the baby is well can provide a foundation on which to build a sounder future so she does not have to make this choice again.

Do not attempt to change a woman's mind about keeping her child or placing the child for adoption during the post-

TABLE 17.4 ✻ Six-Week Physical Assessment

Area of Assessment	Data Collection
History	Assess chief concern, family profile (support system, bonding, self-esteem, family integrity), interval history, and review of systems (urinary system for pain, frequency, or stress incontinence along with gastrointestinal tract and reproductive tract in particular). Assess maternal intake. Some new mothers are too fatigued to eat well, so they eat mainly carbohydrate snack foods or, at least, not a balanced diet.
Physical Examination	Expected Findings
General appearance	Alert; positive mood. If not, woman is probably still extremely fatigued
Weight	Achievement of prepregnant weight; if not, this will be her baseline postpregnant weight
Hair	Healthy, firm hair; excess loss of hair from early postpartal period has halted
Eyes	Pink and moist conjunctiva; if pallor persists, diet may be inadequate because of fatigue
Breasts	
Nursing woman	Full and firm to palpation; blue veins prominent under skin; only slightly tender. No palpable nodules or lumps. If erythematous or tender, mastitis may be present. If fissures on nipples are present, the woman may need to expose her nipples to air or to apply additional cream. An occasional filled milk gland may present as a lump; re-examine after breastfeeding
Non-nursing woman	Return to prepregnant size; no palpable nodules or lumps
Abdomen	Striae less prominent; linea nigra fading, muscle tone improving. No distended bowel from constipation. No distended bladder from retention. No history of pain, frequency, or blood on urination. (If lax abdominal muscle tone is present, women need to increase abdominal exercises. For constipation, increase fluid and fiber. Urinary symptoms probably reflect urinary infection that needs specific treatment.)
Perineum and uterus	No lochia; cervix closed; uterus has returned to prepregnant size. Pap test is normal. Ask woman to bear down during pelvic examination to observe for uterine prolapse, rectocele, or cystocele. If involution is not complete, reason for subinvolution must be investigated
Lower extremities	Varicosities barely noticeable
Rectum	Hemorrhoids receded to prepregnant size or are no longer observable
Laboratory Report	
Laboratory values	Hct: 37%; Hgb: 11–12 g/100 mL. If these are low, reassess diet; possibly iron supplement may be needed
	Rubella antibody titer: 1:8; if low, additional immunization is recommended before a second pregnancy
Immunization status	Assess need for human papillomavirus (HPV) [Gardasil], or rubella vaccine

Hct, hematocrit; Hgb, hemoglobin.

partal period. She is extremely vulnerable to suggestion at this time, and such decisions are too long range and too important to be made at such an emotional time. Her earlier conclusions may be the sound ones. Instead, offer nonjudgmental support. Be especially aware of your own feelings about this issue, to avoid influencing a woman's decision making unnecessarily.

During the taking-in phase of the puerperium, be especially careful that you do not "lead" the woman's thinking. Women enjoy having decisions made for them during this time and may ask what you think is best. An answer such as, "You're the one who has to make this decision. What are your thoughts about it?" can help her begin to think through the problem.

It is not uncommon for women who surrender their infants for adoption to experience grief reactions, the same as those of women whose children have died. If a woman decides to surrender her child for adoption, refer her to an official adoption agency, if she has not contacted one already. An official agency gives a woman the best assurance that the parents chosen for her child will be appropriate. This assurance helps to relieve any misgivings or guilt she may have about surrendering the child and should reduce the moments of doubt that can come in future years, such as wondering whether the child is well cared for and is getting everything the mother could have given her.

Some women do not openly voice a wish to give up their child, but their actions demonstrate that they feel little attachment to their newborn. A woman who wants to keep her baby has a tentative but eager approach to her newborn, whereas a woman who has doubts is slow to make contact, barely touching the baby even by the time of discharge, and asking few questions about newborn care. When this happens, the hospital social service department can be of assistance in helping the woman plan the child's future. Either a single mother or a married couple may place an infant for adoption or into a foster home, although for some couples family counseling may be a greater need.

It is a fallacy to assume that everything will work out once the woman and infant arrive home. The number of abused children seen in hospital emergency departments is proof of the harm that can follow when assessment to detect poor parent–child bonding is inadequate in the first few days of life (Hicks & Stolfi, 2007).

A Woman Who Is Discharged but Whose Child Remains Hospitalized

Newborns who are ill at birth often are transported to a regional center or to a neonatal intensive care nursery for care, a move that automatically separates them from their parents. Many transport teams take an instant photograph of the baby and leave it with the mother. They also leave the nursery telephone number and the name of a nurse or physician to contact for questions or information. Most transport teams call the mother after they arrive at the distant hospital to assure her that her infant managed the stress of transport well.

Maintaining communication with the nursery is important so that parents can begin to bond with their child. Urge them to call the nursery at least once daily to ask about their infant. If the infant is hospitalized in the same hospital, help the mother arrange visiting time with the infant. Transport her to the nursery, so that she can see and, ideally, hold her child. Without this assistance, some women will not call or visit, because they are afraid that this is an imposition or inconvenience for the nursery. Assure the mother that her telephone calls and visits are expected (the nursery wants to encourage bonding). Visiting in an intensive care nursery is further discussed in Chapter 26.

It is easy for a woman who is separated from her newborn to feel despondent (Amankwaa, Pickler, & Boonmee, 2007). Some mothers whose infants are ill at birth feel uncomfortable sharing a hospital room with a postpartal roommate who is caring for a well baby. This is often a good time to arrange for a visit to the nursery or to suggest that you and the woman take a walk in the hallway to increase her amount of ambulation.

A Family Who Is Adopting a Child

A family who is adopting an infant may come into the hospital or birthing center to meet their new infant for the first time. Such a couple needs the same introduction to newborn care as biologic parents. Additional needs of adopting parents are discussed in Chapter 3.

✔Checkpoint Question 17.3

You care for Joan Cooper at a 6-week postpartum visit. What should her fundal height be at this time?

a. Six fingerbreadths below the umbilicus.
b. No longer palpable on her abdomen.
c. One centimeter above the symphysis pubis.
d. Inverted and palpable at the cervix.

Key Points for Review

- The postpartal period (puerperium) is the 6-week period after childbirth. This is an important period, because it marks the child's introduction to the family. Women move through an initial "taking-in" phase, in which they are dependent; a "taking-hold" phase, in which they manifest independence; and a "letting-go" phase, in which the mother role is finally defined.
- Rooming-in is the preferred health care agency arrangement for postpartal families, because it allows a new family the best chance for quality interaction. The more time new parents spend with a newborn, the more likely it is that effective bonding will occur. Help parents to feel comfortable with their newborn by offering anticipatory guidance and role modeling infant care.
- "Postpartal blues" are a normal accompaniment to childbirth. You can assure a woman that her feelings are normal and offer supportive care until the emotion passes.
- Uterine involution is the process whereby the uterus returns to its prepregnant state. A uterus decreases in size one fingerbreadth a day until it disappears under the pubic bone at about day 10. Lochia is the name of the vaginal flow after childbirth: the flow is lochia rubra (red) for the first 1 to 3 days; lochia serosa (pink to brown) on days 4 through 10; and lochia alba (white) until 2 to 6 weeks after the birth.
- A woman is at great risk for hemorrhage in the postpartal period, so assessments done during this time are some of the most critical assessments made in nursing. Do not discount the importance of these assessments because the overall content of the postpartal period is so focused on wellness.
- Lactation is the production of breast milk. Colostrum is present immediately after birth; milk forms on the third to fourth postpartal day. A feeling of fullness and firmness on this day is termed *filling;* if warmth and discomfort occur, it is termed *engorgement.*
- Women may need various comfort measures to alleviate pain from sutures, uterine pain (afterpains), and breast tenderness. Application of cold or heat and administration of analgesics are important nursing interventions.
- Women need to learn about self-care before health care agency discharge, so that they can maintain self-care at home. A follow-up telephone call or home visit is helpful. All women should conscientiously return for a visit at 6 weeks after childbirth, to be certain their reproductive organs have returned to their nonpregnant state. A menstrual flow should return within 6 to 10 weeks in the non-breastfeeding mother, or 3 to 4 months in the breastfeeding mother.

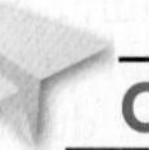

CRITICAL THINKING EXERCISES

1. As the nurse working in a postpartum unit, you care for Mike and Joan Cooper, who have just become parents of an 8-lb 2-oz baby girl. Joan is on maternity leave from her job as a court reporter. Mike plans to take off a week from work to spend time with Joan and the new baby. As you prepare them for discharge, you notice they seem overwhelmed with the amount of information they have been provided. Joan says, trying to get the baby to nurse, "He's so big and my breasts are so small, will he get enough milk? I was hoping by breast-

feeding I wouldn't have to worry about birth control for a while, but I'm having so much trouble maybe that won't work out." Mike pulls you aside and says, "Sometimes, I see my wife crying for no reason. Why isn't she as happy as I am?" What additional postpartal teaching does the Cooper family need?

2. Suppose because Joan Cooper does not have an episiotomy incision, you expect her to have little perineal discomfort. Instead, she states that her perineal pain is excruciating. You notice she has hemorrhoids. You overhear her tell her husband that he is acting selfishly for paying more attention to their new daughter than to her. You observe her handing her baby roughly to her husband. What could you suggest to make her more comfortable?
3. Suppose you are present at Joan's 6-week postpartal checkup. What would you include in an assessment plan to ensure that she has physically and emotionally adjusted well to childbirth?
4. Examine the National Health Goals related to the postpartal period. Most government-sponsored funds for nursing research are allotted based on these goals. What would be a possible research topic to explore pertinent to these goals that would be applicable to the Cooper family and also advance evidence-based practice?

CRITICAL THINKING SCENARIO

Open the accompanying CD-ROM or visit http://thePoint.lww.com and read the Patient Scenario included for this chapter, then answer the questions to further sharpen your skills and grow more familiar with NCLEX style questions related to nursing care of the postpartal family. Confirm your answers are correct by reading the rationales.

REFERENCES

Abdulwadud, O. A., & Snow, M. E. (2009). Interventions in the workplace to support breastfeeding for women in employment. *Cochrane Database of Systematic Reviews, 2009*(1), (CD006177).

Amankwaa L. C., Pickler, R. H., & Boonmee, J. (2007). Maternal responsiveness in mothers of preterm infants. *Newborn and Infant Nursing Reviews, 7*(1), 25–30.

Bailis, A., & Witter, F. R. (2007). Hypertensive disorders of pregnancy. In K. B. Fortner, et al. (Eds.). *The Johns Hopkins manual of gynecology and obstetrics.* Philadelphia: Lippincott Williams & Wilkins.

Bridges, W. (1994). *Job shift: how to prosper in a workplace without jobs.* Menlo Park, CA: Addison-Wesley.

Brown, S., et al. (2009). Early postnatal discharge from hospital for healthy mothers and term infants. *Cochrane Database of Systematic Reviews, 2009*(1), (CD002958).

Buultjens, M., & Liamputtong, P. (2007). When giving life starts to take the life out of you: women's experiences of depression after childbirth. *Midwifery, 23*(1), 77–91.

Calhoun, K. E., & Giuliano, A. E. (2007). Breast cancer. In J. S. Berek (Ed.). *Berek & Novak's gynecology* (14th ed.). Philadelphia: Lippincott Williams & Wilkins.

Corwin, E. J., & Arbour, M. (2007). Postpartum fatigue and evidence-based interventions *MCN: The American Journal of Maternal/Child Nursing, 32*(4), 215–222.

Crowther, C., & Middleton, P. (2009). Anti-D administration after childbirth for preventing Rhesus alloimmunisation. *Cochrane Database of Systematic Reviews, 2009*(1), (CD000021).

Deshpande, W. (2007). Mastitis. *Community Practitioner, 80*(5), 44–45.

Dodd, J., Dare, M. R., & Middleton, P. (2009). Treatment for women with postpartum iron deficiency anaemia. *Cochrane Database of Systematic Reviews, 2009*(1), (CD004222).

Ebbeling, C. B., et al. (2007). Conceptualization and development of a theory-based healthful eating and physical activity intervention for postpartum women who are low income. *Health Promotion Practice, 8*(1), 50–59.

Engqvist, I., et al. (2007). Strategies in caring for women with postpartum psychosis—an interview study with psychiatric nurses. *Journal of Clinical Nursing, 16*(7), 1333–1342.

Fink, J. L. W. (2007). Clinical tips. Rooming-in isn't sleeping-in. *RN, 70*(1), 49–50.

Fontenot, H. B. (2007). Transition and adaptation to adoptive motherhood. *JOGNN: Journal of Obstetric, Gynecologic, and Neonatal Nursing, 36*(2), 175–182.

Gunderson, E. P., et al. (2008). Association of fewer hours of sleep at 6 months postpartum with substantial weight retention at 1 year postpartum. *American Journal of Epidemiology, 167*(2), 178–187.

Hay-Smith, E. J. C., & Dumoulin, C. (2009). Pelvic floor muscle training versus no treatment, or inactive control treatments, for urinary incontinence in women. *Cochrane Database of Systematic Reviews, 2009*(1), (CD005654).

Hicks, R. A., & Stolfi A. (2007). Skeletal surveys in children with burns caused by child abuse. *Pediatric Emergency Care, 23*(5), 308–313.

Horsley, T., et al. (2007). Benefits and harms associated with the practice of bed sharing. *Archives of Pediatric Adolescent Medicine, 161*(2), 237–245.

Karch, A. M. (2009). *Lippincott's nursing drug guide.* Philadelphia: Lippincott Williams & Wilkins.

Lipscomb, K., & Novy, M. J. (2007). The normal puerperium. In A. H. DeCherney & L. Nathan (Eds.). *Current diagnosis and treatment in obstetrics and gynecology* (10th ed.). Columbus, OH: McGraw-Hill.

McGarry, J., et al. (2009). Postpartum depression and help-seeking behavior. *Journal of Widwifery & Women's Health, 54*(1), 50–56.

Moore, E. R., Anderson, G. C., & Bergman, N. (2009). Early skin-to-skin contact for mothers and their healthy newborn infants. *Cochrane Database of Systematic Reviews, 2009*(1), (CD003519).

Musselwhite, K. L., et al. (2007). Use of epidural anesthesia and the risk of acute postpartum urinary retention. *American Journal of Obstetrics and Gynecology, 196*(5), 472–473.

Pavone, M. E., Purinton, S. C., & Petersen, S. M. (2007). Postpartum care and breast-feeding. In K. B. Fortner, et al. (Eds.). *The Johns Hopkins manual of gynecology and obstetrics.* Philadelphia: Lippincott Williams & Wilkins.

Poggi, S. B. H. (2007). Postpartum hemorrhage and the abnormal puerperium. In A. H. DeCherney & L. Nathan (Eds.). *Current diagnosis and treatment in obstetrics and gynecology* (10th ed.). Columbus, OH: McGraw-Hill.

Quijano, C. E., & Abalos, E. (2009). Conservative management of symptomatic and/or complicated haemorrhoids in pregnancy and the puerperium. *Cochrane Database of Systematic Reviews, 2009*(1), (CD004077).

Rolfes, S. R., Pinna, K., & Whitney, E. (2009). Life cycle nutrition: pregnancy and lactation. In S. R. Rolfes, K. Pinna, & E. Whitney (Eds.). *Understanding normal and clinical nutrition* (8th ed.). Columbus, OH: McGraw-Hill.

Rubin, R. (1977). Binding-in in the postpartum period. *Maternal Child Nursing Journal, 6*(2), 67–69.

Seely, D., et al. (2008). Safety and efficacy of panax ginseng during pregnancy and lactation. *Canadian Journal of Clinical Pharmacology, 15*(1), e87–e94.

Subramanian, A., et al. (Eds.) (2008). *Drug facts and comparisons.* St. Louis, MO: Wolters Kluwer Health.

Tam, W. H., & Chung, T. (2007). Psychosomatic disorders in pregnancy. *Current Opinion in Obstetrics & Gynecology, 19*(2), 126–132.

Truitt, S. T., et al. (2009). Combined hormonal versus nonhormonal versus progestin-only contraception in lactation. *Cochrane Database of Systematic Reviews, 2009*(1), (CD003988).

Van der Wijden, C., Kleijnen, J., & Van den Berk, T. (2009). Lactational amenorrhea for family planning. *Cochrane Database of Systematic Reviews, 2009*(1), (CD001329).

SUGGESTED READINGS

Conde, A. A., et al. (2008). Perception of the childbirth experience: continuity and changes over the postpartum period. *Journal of Reproductive and Infant Psychology, 26*(2), 139–154.

Herman, D. R., et al. (2008). Effect of a targeted subsidy on intake of fruits and vegetables among low-income women in the special supplemental nutrition program for women, infants, and children. *American Journal of Public Health, 98*(1), 98–105.

Hill, P. D., & Aldag, J. C. (2007). Maternal perceived quality of life following childbirth. *JOGNN: Journal of Obstetric, Gynecologic, and Neonatal Nursing, 36*(4), 328–334.

Kabir, K., Sheeder, J., & Kelly, L. S. (2008). Identifying postpartum depression: are 3 questions as good as 10? *Pediatrics, 122*(3), e696–e702.

Keister, D., Roberts, K. T., & Werner, S. L. (2008). Strategies for breastfeeding success. *American Family Physician, 78*(2), 225–232.

Kramer, M. S., & Kakuma, R. (2009). Optimal duration of exclusive breastfeeding. *Cochrane Database of Systematic Reviews, 2009*(1), (CD003517).

Leeds, L., & Hargreaves, I. (2008). The psychological consequences of childbirth. *Journal of Reproductive and Infant Psychology, 26*(2), 108–122.

Schumacher, M., Zubaran, C., & White, G. (2008). Bringing birth-related paternal depression to the fore. *Women and Birth, 21*(2), 65–70.

St. Pierre, C. M. (2007). The taboo of motherhood: postpartum depression. *International Journal for Human Caring, 11*(2), 22–31.

Webb, D. A., et al. (2008). Postpartum physical symptoms in new mothers: their relationship to functional limitations and emotional well-being. *Birth, 35*(3), 179–187.

Chapter

18 Nursing Care of a Family With a Newborn

KEY TERMS

- acrocyanosis
- caput succedaneum
- cavernous hemangioma
- central cyanosis
- cephalhematoma
- conduction
- convection
- erythema toxicum
- evaporation
- hemangiomas
- jaundice
- kernicterus
- lanugo
- meconium
- milia
- mongolian spot
- natal teeth
- neonatal period
- neonate
- nevus flammeus
- physiologic jaundice
- pseudomenstruation
- radiation
- strawberry hemangioma
- subconjunctival hemorrhage
- thrush
- transitional stool
- vernix caseosa

OBJECTIVES

After mastering the contents of this chapter, you should be able to:

1. Describe the normal characteristics of a term newborn.
2. Identify National Health Goals related to newborn care that nurses could help the nation achieve.
3. Use critical thinking to analyze ways that the care of a term newborn can be more family centered.
4. Assess a newborn for normal growth and development.
5. Formulate nursing diagnoses related to a newborn or the family of a newborn.
6. Identify expected outcomes for a newborn and family during the first 4 weeks of life.
7. Plan nursing care to augment normal development of a newborn, such as ways to aid parent–child bonding.
8. Implement nursing care of a normal newborn, such as instructing parents on how to care for their newborn.
9. Evaluate outcome criteria for the achievement and effectiveness of care.
10. Identify areas related to newborn assessment and care that could benefit from additional nursing research or application of evidence-based practice.
11. Integrate knowledge of newborn growth and development and immediate care needs with the nursing process to achieve quality maternal and child health nursing care.

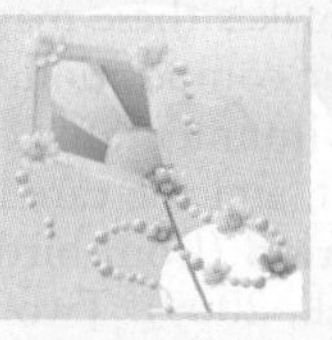

Carlotta Ruiz has just given birth to her second child, a 6-lb 5-oz baby girl she named Beth. Apgar scores at 1 and 5 minutes were 6 and 8. Vital signs are temperature (axillary), 98.2° F (36.8° C); heart rate, 136 beats per minute; and respirations, 74 breaths per minute. She is 18.5 inches long, with a head circumference of 34 cm and a chest circumference of 32 cm. She has a small port-wine birthmark on her right thigh.

While Jose, Carlotta's husband, is in the room, Carlotta tells you she is a "veteran" at baby care. Jose adds, "Little Joe [their 3-year-old] will be so excited to see his new sister. That's all he's been talking about lately."

When Carlotta is alone, you notice she seems a little apprehensive about caring for her new daughter. She tells you, "She's so much smaller than Joe was. And why does it sound like she has a cold? And what is this rash all over her? Isn't it bad enough she has a birthmark?"

Previous chapters described the care of a pregnant woman and family during the antepartal, intrapartal, and postpartal periods. This chapter adds information about caring for a newborn and family. The newborn period is important to a family's well-being because it lays the foundation for the rest of the family's childrearing years.

Does Carlotta know as much about newborns as she thought? What additional teaching does this family need?

Newborns undergo profound physiologic changes at the moment of birth (and, probably, psychological changes as well), as they are released from a warm, snug, dark, liquid-filled environment that has met all of their basic needs into a chilly, unbounded, brightly lit, gravity-based, outside world. Within minutes after being plunged into this strange environment, a newborn has to initiate respirations and adapt a circulatory system to extrauterine oxygenation. Within 24 hours, neurologic, renal, endocrine, gastrointestinal, and metabolic functions must be operating competently for life to be sustained.

How well a newborn makes these major adjustments depends on his or her genetic composition, the competency of the recent intrauterine environment, the care received during the labor and birth period, and the care received during the newborn or **neonatal period** (from birth through the first 28 days of life) (Ruiz et al., 2009). Two thirds of all deaths that occur during the first year of life occur in the neonatal period. More than half occur in the first 24 hours after birth—an indication of how hazardous a time this is for an infant.

BOX 18.1 * Focus on National Health Goals

Several National Health Goals deal directly with the newborn period:

- Increase to at least 75% the proportion of mothers who breastfeed their babies in the early postpartal period from a baseline of 64%.
- Increase to at least 50% the proportion of women who continue breastfeeding until their babies are 5 to 6 months old from a baseline of 29%.
- Increase to 70% the percentage of healthy full-term infants who are put to sleep on their backs from a baseline of 35%.
- Increase to 60% from a baseline of 43% the number of women who breastfeed exclusively until their infant is 3 months of age; from 13% to 25% for those who breastfeed exclusively until 6 months.
- Increase to at least 75% the proportion of parents and caregivers who use feeding practices that prevent baby-bottle tooth decay.
- Reduce the neonatal mortality rate to no more than 2.9 per 1000 live births from a baseline of 4.8 per 1000 live births (http://www.nih.gov).

Nurses can help the nation achieve these goals, by encouraging women not only to begin breastfeeding but also to continue it through the first 6 months of life; by advising parents on the advantage of placing infants on their backs to sleep and on the danger of tooth decay from letting a baby drink from a bottle of milk or juice while falling asleep; and by discussing with parents who use formula the proper methods for preparation so that gastrointestinal illness does not occur.

Areas that could benefit from additional nursing research include identifying the reasons why some women end breastfeeding shortly after discharge from a health care agency and investigating common methods of encouraging sleep in infants other than by bottle feeding or offering solid food.

Newborn health is so important that National Health Goals related to the first days of life have been devised. These are shown in Box 18.1. Nurses play a major role in achieving these goals because nurses are the people who provide newborn care and give newborn instructions to new parents.

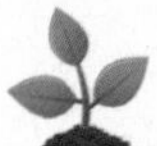

Nursing Process Overview

For Health Promotion of the Term Newborn

Assessment

Assessment of a newborn or **neonate** (a baby in the neonatal period) includes a review of the mother's pregnancy history; physical examination of the infant; analysis of laboratory reports such as hematocrit and blood type, if indicated; and assessment of parent–child interaction for the beginning of bonding. Assessment begins immediately after birth and is continued at every contact during a newborn's hospital or birthing center stay, early home visits, and well-baby visits. Teaching parents to make assessments concerning their infant's temperature, respiratory rate, and overall health is crucial so that they can continue to monitor their infant's health at home (Box 18.2).

Nursing Diagnosis

Nursing diagnoses associated with a newborn often center on the problems of establishing respirations, beginning nutrition, and assisting with parent–newborn bonding. Examples are:

- Ineffective airway clearance related to mucus in airway
- Ineffective thermoregulation related to heat loss from exposure in birthing room
- Imbalanced nutrition, less than body requirements, related to poor sucking reflex

Box 18.2 Assessment: Assessing the Average Newborn

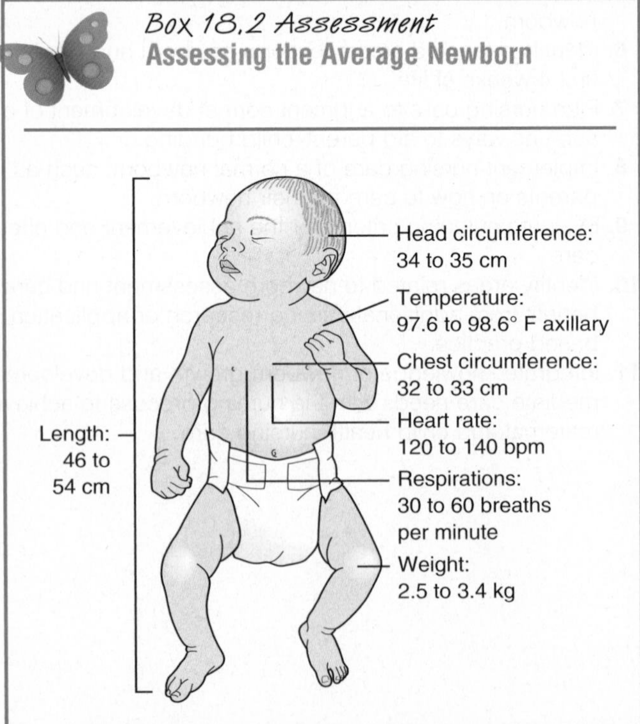

- Readiness for enhanced family coping related to birth of planned infant
- Health-seeking behaviors related to newborn needs

If a minor deviation from the normal is present, such as a hemangioma, a diagnosis such as "Parental fear related to hemangioma on left thigh of newborn" might be relevant.

Outcome Identification and Planning

Planning nursing care should take into account both the newborn's needs during this transition period and a mother's need for adequate rest during the postpartal period. Try to adapt teaching time to the schedules of the mother and her newborn. Although the woman must learn as much as possible about newborn care, she also must go home from the health care setting with enough energy to practice what she has learned. Important planning measures for newborns include helping them regulate their temperature and helping them grow accustomed to breastfeeding or bottle feeding. A helpful Internet site to recommend to parents is the Yale/New Haven Children's Hospital web site (http://www.ynhh.org).

Implementation

A major portion of implementation in the newborn period is role modeling to help new parents grow confident with their newborn. Be aware how closely parents observe you for guidance in newborn care. Conserving newborn warmth and energy, to help prevent hypoglycemia and respiratory distress, should be an important consideration to accompany all interventions.

Outcome Evaluation

Evaluation of expected outcomes should reveal that parents are able to give beginning newborn care with confidence. Be certain parents make arrangements for continued health supervision for their newborn, so that evaluation can be continued and the family's long-term health needs can be met. Examples indicating achievement of outcomes concerning newborns are:

- Infant establishes respirations of 30 to 60 per minute.
- Infant maintains temperature at 97.8° to 98.6° F (36.5° to 37° C).
- Infant bottle feeds or breastfeeds well with a strong sucking reflex.

PROFILE OF A NEWBORN

It is not unusual to hear the comment "all newborns look alike" from people viewing a nursery full of babies. In actuality, every child is born with individual physical and personality characteristics that make him or her unique right from the start (Fig. 18.1).

Some newborns are born stocky and short, some large and bony, some thin and rangy. Some have a temperament that causes them to feed greedily, protest procedures loudly, and respond to their parent's inexperienced handling with restlessness and spitting up. Other newborns sleep soundly, make no protest over procedures or diaper changes, and seem passive in accepting this new step in life. With experience in working with newborns, it becomes easier to differentiate newborns who are merely demonstrating these extremes of normal behavior from those whose behavior or appearance indicates a need for more skilled care as their adjustment to independent life is not progressing smoothly.

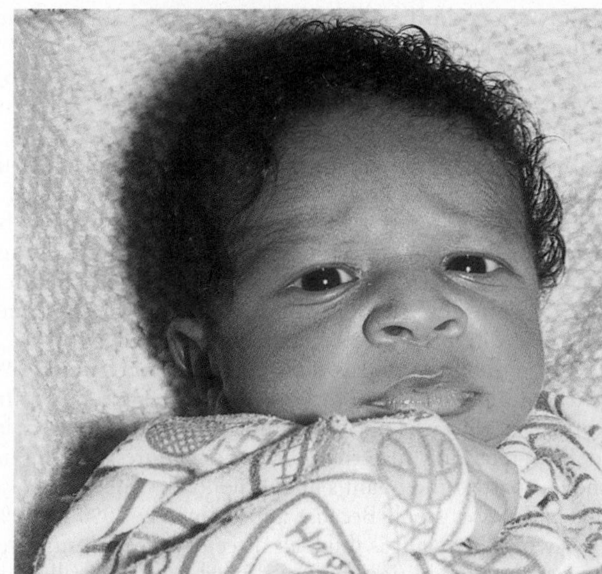

FIGURE 18.1 Personality is apparent in a newborn from the start. Note the alert, searching interest.

Vital Statistics

Vital statistics measured in a newborn are weight, length, and head and chest circumference. The technique for obtaining these is shown in Chapter 34, along with other aspects of health assessment. Be sure all health care providers involved with newborns are aware of safety issues specific to newborn care when taking these measurements such as not leaving a newborn unattended on a bed or scale.

Weight

The birth weight of newborns varies depending on the racial, nutritional, intrauterine, and genetic factors that were present during conception and pregnancy. The weight in relation to the gestational age should be plotted on a standard neonatal graph, such as the one shown in Appendix E. Plotting weight this way helps identify newborns who are at risk because of their small size. This information also separates those who are small for their gestational age (newborns who have suffered intrauterine growth restriction) from preterm infants (infants who are healthy but small only because they were born early). These first measurements also establish a baseline for future evaluation.

Plotting weight in conjunction with height and head circumference is also helpful because it highlights disproportionate measurements (see Appendix E). All three of these measurements should fall near the same percentile in an individual child. For example, a newborn who falls within the 50th percentile for height and weight but whose head circumference is in the 90th percentile may have abnormal head growth. A newborn who is in the 50th percentile for weight and head circumference but in the 3rd percentile for height may have a growth problem.

The average birth weight (50th percentile) for a white, mature female newborn in the United States is 3.4 kg (7.5 lb); for a white, mature male newborn, it is 3.5 kg (7.7 lb). Newborns of other races weigh approximately 0.5 lb less. The arbitrary lower limit of normal for all races is 2.5 kg (5.5 lb). Birth weight exceeding 4.7 kg (10 lb) is unusual, but weights as high as 7.7 kg (17 lb) have been documented. If a newborn weighs more than 4.7 kg, the baby is said to be macrosomic and a maternal illness, such as diabetes mellitus, must be suspected (Kwik et al., 2007). Second-born children usually weigh more than first-born. Birth weight continues to increase with each succeeding child in a family.

During the first few days after birth, a newborn loses 5% to 10% of birth weight (6 to 10 oz). This weight loss occurs because a newborn is no longer under the influence of salt- and fluid-retaining maternal hormones. Diuresis begins to remove a part of the infant's high fluid load. A newborn also voids and passes stool. Because approximately 75% to 90% of a newborn's weight is fluid, all three of these measures reduce weight. In addition, breastfed newborns have a limited intake until about the third day of life because of the relatively low caloric content and amount of colostrum they ingest. If newborns are formula-fed, their intake during this time is also limited because of the time needed to establish effective sucking.

After this initial loss of weight, a newborn has 1 day of stable weight, then begins to gain weight. The breastfed newborn recaptures birth weight within 10 days; a formula-fed infant accomplishes this gain within 7 days. After this, a newborn begins to gain about 2 lb per month (6 to 8 oz per week) for the first 6 months of life.

Length

The average birth length (50th percentile) of a mature female neonate is 53 cm (20.9 in). For mature males, the average birth length is 54 cm (21.3 in). The lower limit of normal length is arbitrarily set at 46 cm (18 in). Although rare, babies with lengths as great as 57.5 cm (24 in) have been reported.

Head Circumference

In a mature newborn, the head circumference is usually 34 to 35 cm (13.5 to 14 in). A mature newborn with a head circumference greater than 37 cm (14.8 in) or less than 33 cm (13.2 in) should be carefully assessed for neurologic involvement, although occasionally a well newborn falls within these limits. Head circumference is measured with a tape measure drawn across the center of the forehead and around the most prominent portion of the posterior head (the occiput; see Fig. 34.6 in Chapter 34).

Chest Circumference

The chest circumference in a term newborn is about 2 cm (0.75 to 1 in) less than the head circumference. This is measured at the level of the nipples. If a large amount of breast tissue or edema of breasts is present, this measurement will not be accurate until the edema has subsided.

Vital Signs

Vital sign measurements begin to change from those present in intrauterine life at the moment of birth.

Temperature

The temperature of newborns is about 99° F (37.2° C) at birth because they have been confined in an internal body organ. The temperature falls almost immediately to below normal because of heat loss and immature temperature-regulating mechanisms. The temperature of birthing rooms, approximately 68° to 72° F (21° to 22° C), can add to this loss of heat.

Newborns lose heat by four separate mechanisms: convection, conduction, radiation, and evaporation (Fig. 18.2).

Convection is the flow of heat from the newborn's body surface to cooler surrounding air. The effectiveness of convection depends on the velocity of the flow (a current of air cools faster than nonmoving air). Eliminating drafts from windows or air conditioners reduces convection heat loss.

Conduction is the transfer of body heat to a cooler solid object in contact with a baby. For example, a baby placed on a cold counter or on the cold base of a warming unit quickly loses heat to the colder metal surface. Covering surfaces with a warmed blanket or towel helps to minimize conduction heat loss.

Radiation is the transfer of body heat to a cooler solid object not in contact with the baby, such as a cold window or air conditioner. Moving an infant as far from the cold surface as possible helps reduce this type of heat loss.

Evaporation is loss of heat through conversion of a liquid to a vapor. Newborns are wet, so they lose a great deal of heat as the amniotic fluid on their skin evaporates. To prevent this heat loss, dry newborns as soon as possible, especially their face and hair as the head, a large surface area in a newborn, can be responsible for a great amount of heat loss. Covering the hair with a cap after drying it further reduces the possibility of evaporation cooling. Be certain to remove any wet blankets used to dry the infant immediately and place the infant on a warm, dry blanket.

A newborn not only loses heat easily by the means just described but also has difficulty conserving heat under any circumstance. Insulation, an efficient means of conserving heat in adults, is not effective in newborns because they have little subcutaneous fat to provide insulation. Shivering, a means of increasing metabolism and thereby providing heat in adults, is rarely seen in newborns.

Newborns can conserve heat by constricting blood vessels and moving blood away from the skin. *Brown fat,* a special tissue found in mature newborns, apparently helps to conserve or produce body heat by increasing metabolism. The greatest amounts of brown fat are found in the intrascapular region, thorax, and perirenal area. Brown fat is thought to aid in controlling newborn temperature similar to temperature control in a hibernating animal. In later life, it may influence the proportion of body fat retained.

Newborns exposed to cool air tend to kick and cry to increase their metabolic rate and produce more heat. This reaction, however, also increases their need for oxygen and their respiratory rate increases. An immature newborn with poor lung development has trouble making such an adjustment. Newborns who cannot increase their respiratory rate in response to increased needs will be unable to deliver sufficient oxygen to their systems. In addition, a newborn becomes fatigued by rapid breathing, placing additional strain on an already stressed cardiovascular system. The resultant anaerobic catabolism of body cells releases acid. Every newborn is born

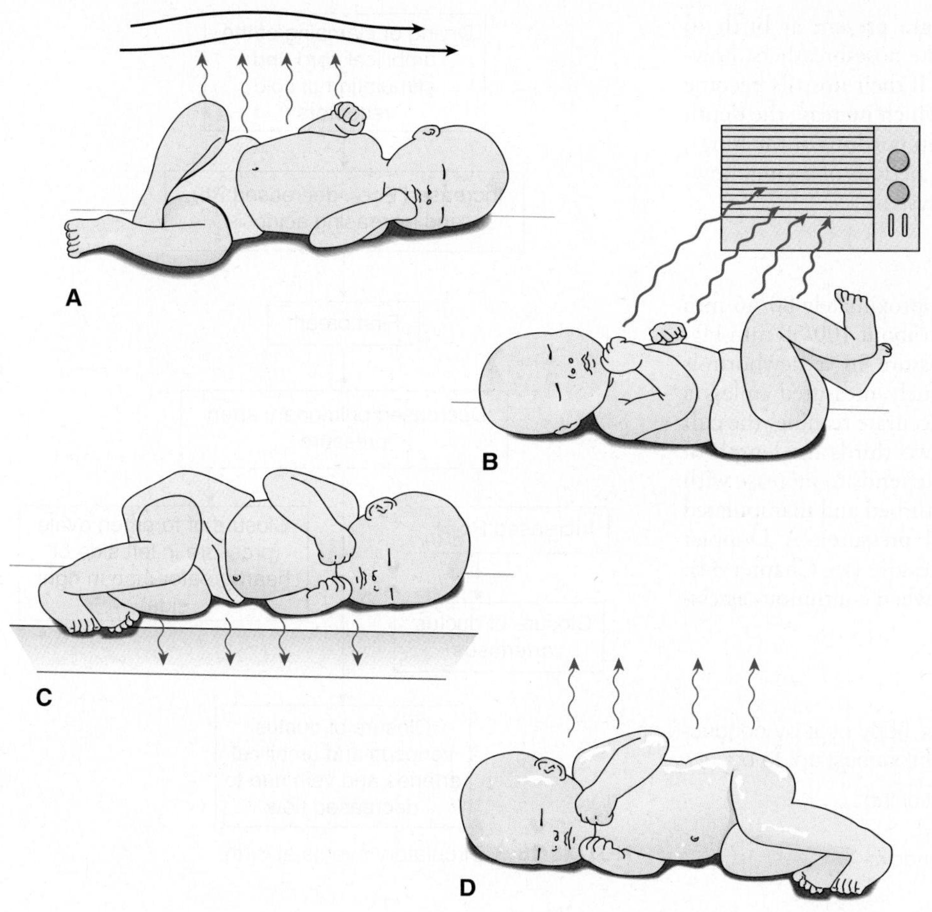

FIGURE 18.2 Heat loss in the newborn. (**A**) Convection. (**B**) Radiation. (**C**) Conduction. (**D**) Evaporation.

slightly acidotic. Any new buildup of acid may lead to severe, life-threatening acidosis.

Drying and wrapping newborns and placing them in warmed cribs, or drying them and placing them under a radiant heat source, are excellent mechanical measures to help conserve heat. In addition, placing a newborn against the mother's skin and then covering the newborn with a blanket helps to transfer heat from the mother to the newborn; this is termed skin-to-skin care (Moore, Anderson, & Bergman, 2009).

All early care of newborns should be done speedily to avoid exposing the newborn to cool air unnecessarily. Any procedure during which a newborn must be uncovered such as resuscitation or circumcision should be done under a radiant heat source to prevent damaging heat loss. If chilling is prevented, a newborn's temperature stabilizes at 98.6° F (37° C) within 4 hours after birth.

In contrast to an adult, a newborn with a bacterial infection may run a subnormal temperature. Therefore, if a newborn's temperature does not stabilize shortly after birth, the cause must be investigated to rule out infection.

Pulse

The heart rate of a fetus in utero averages 120 to 160 beats per minute (bpm). Immediately after birth, as the newborn struggles to initiate respirations, the heart rate may be as rapid as 180 bpm. Within 1 hour after birth, as the newborn settles down to sleep, the heart rate stabilizes to an average of 120 to 140 bpm.

The heart rate of a newborn often remains slightly irregular because of immaturity of the cardiac regulatory center in the medulla. Transient murmurs may result from the incomplete closure of fetal circulation shunts. During crying, the rate may rise again to 180 bpm. In addition, heart rate can decrease during sleep, ranging from 90 to 110 bpm.

You should be able to palpate brachial and femoral pulses in a newborn, but the radial and temporal pulses are more difficult to palpate with any degree of accuracy. Therefore, a newborn's heart rate is always determined by listening for an apical heartbeat for a full minute, rather than assessing a pulse in an extremity. Always palpate for femoral pulses, however, because their absence suggests possible coarctation (narrowing) of the aorta, a common cardiovascular abnormality.

Respiration

The respiratory rate of a newborn in the first few minutes of life may be as high as 80 breaths per minute. As respiratory activity is established and maintained, this rate settles to an average of 30 to 60 breaths per minute when the newborn is at rest. Respiratory depth, rate, and rhythm are likely to be irregular, and short periods of apnea (without cyanosis) which last less than 15 seconds, sometimes called *periodic respirations,* are normal. Respiratory rate can be observed most easily by watching the movement of a newborn's abdomen, because breathing primarily involves the use of the diaphragm and abdominal muscles.

Coughing and sneezing reflexes are present at birth to clear the airway. Newborns are obligate nose-breathers, however, and show signs of acute distress if their nostrils become obstructed. Short periods of crying, which increase the depth of respirations and aid in aerating deep portions of the lungs, may be beneficial to a newborn. Long periods of crying, however, can exhaust the cardiovascular system.

Blood Pressure

The blood pressure of a newborn is approximately 80/46 mm Hg at birth. By the 10th day, it rises to about 100/50 mm Hg. Because measurement of blood pressure in a newborn is somewhat inaccurate, it is not routinely measured unless a cardiac anomaly is suspected. For an accurate reading, the cuff width used must be no more than two thirds the length of the upper arm or thigh. Blood pressure tends to increase with crying (and a newborn cries when disturbed and manipulated by such procedures as taking blood pressure). A Doppler method may be used to take blood pressure (see Chapter 34). Hemodynamic monitoring is helpful when continuous assessment is necessary.

✔ Checkpoint Question 18.1

Beth Ruiz, like all newborns, can lose body heat by conduction. Under which condition is conduction most apt to occur?

a. The nursery is cooled by air conditioning.
b. The infant is wet from amniotic fluid.
c. There is a breeze from an open window.
d. Beth is placed in a cold bassinet.

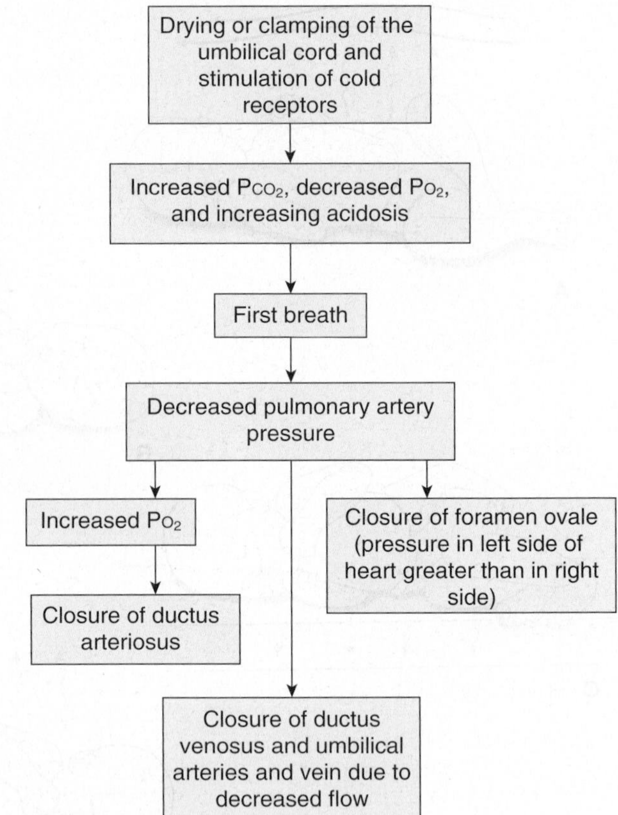

FIGURE 18.3 Circulatory events at birth.

Physiologic Function

Just as changes occur in vital signs after birth, so do changes occur in all the major body systems.

Cardiovascular System

Changes in the cardiovascular system are necessary after birth because now the lungs must oxygenate the blood that was formerly oxygenated by the placenta. When the cord is clamped, a neonate is forced to take in oxygen through the lungs. As the lungs inflate for the first time, pressure decreases in the pulmonary artery (the artery leading from the heart to the lungs). This decrease in pressure plays a role in promoting closure of the ductus arteriosus, a fetal shunt. As pressure increases in the left side of the heart from increased blood volume, the foramen ovale between the two atria closes because of the pressure against the lip of the structure (permanent closure does not occur for weeks). With the remaining fetal circulatory structures (umbilical vein, two umbilical arteries, and ductus venosus) no longer receiving blood, the blood within them clots, and the vessels atrophy over the next few weeks.

Figure 18.3 shows the respiratory and cardiovascular changes that occur at birth, beginning with the first breath. The peripheral circulation of a newborn remains sluggish for at least the first 24 hours. It is common to observe cyanosis in the infant's feet and hands **(acrocyanosis)** and for the feet to feel cold to the touch at this time.

Blood Values. A newborn's blood volume is 80 to 110 mL per kilogram of body weight, or about 300 mL total. The oxygen dissociation curve is shifted to the left; that is, the quantity of oxygen bound to hemoglobin and the partial pressure of oxygen are greater in newborn blood than in an adult's blood, or a newborn's hemoglobin carries a greater proportion of oxygen than adult hemoglobin.

Hemoglobin level averages 17 to 18 g/100 mL of blood. The hematocrit is between 45% and 50%. A newborn also has an elevated red blood cell count, about 6 million cells per cubic millimeter. Capillary heel-sticks may reveal a falsely high hematocrit or hemoglobin value because of sluggish peripheral circulation. Before obtaining a blood specimen from a heel, warm the foot by wrapping it in a warm cloth. This increases circulation and improves the accuracy of this value.

Once proper lung oxygenation has been established, the need for the high red cell count diminishes. Therefore, within a matter of days, a newborn's red cells begin to deteriorate. Bilirubin is a byproduct of the breakdown of red blood cells. An indirect bilirubin level at birth is 1 to 4 mg/100 mL. Any increase over this amount reflects the release of bilirubin as excessive red blood cells begin their breakdown (Chetham, 2007).

A newborn has an equally high white blood cell count at birth, about 15,000 to 30,000 cells/mm^3. Values as high as 40,000 cells/mm^3 may be seen if the birth was stressful. Polymorphonuclear cells (neutrophils) account for a large part of this leukocytosis, but by the end of the first month, lymphocytes become the predominant cell type. This leukocytosis is a response to the trauma of birth and is nonpathogenic; an increased white blood cell count should not be taken as evidence of infection. On the other hand, although the high white blood cell count makes infection difficult to prove in a newborn, infection must not be dismissed as a possibility if other signs of infection such as pallor, respiratory difficulty, or cyanosis are present. Usual blood values in a newborn are summarized in Appendix F.

Blood Coagulation. Because most newborns are born with a lower than normal level of vitamin K, they have a prolonged coagulation or prothrombin time. Vitamin K, synthesized through the action of intestinal flora, is necessary for the formation of factor II (prothrombin), factor VII (proconvertin), factor IX (plasma thromboplastin component), and factor X (Stuart-Prower factor). Because a newborn's intestine is sterile at birth unless membranes were ruptured more than 24 hours before birth, it takes about 24 hours for flora to accumulate and for vitamin K to be synthesized. Because almost all newborns can be predicted to have this diminished blood coagulation ability, vitamin K (AquaMEPHYTON) is usually administered intramuscularly into the lateral anterior thigh, the preferred site for all injections in a newborn, immediately after birth.

Respiratory System

A first breath is a major undertaking because it requires a tremendous amount of pressure (about 40 to 70 cm H_2O). It is initiated by a combination of cold receptors; a lowered partial pressure of oxygen (PO_2), which falls from 80 to as low as 15 mm Hg before a first breath; and an increased partial carbon dioxide pressure (PCO_2), which rises as high as 70 mm Hg before a first breath. All newborns have some fluid in their lungs from intrauterine life that will ease the surface tension on alveolar walls and allows alveoli to inflate more easily than if the lung walls were dry. About a third of this fluid is forced out of the lungs by the pressure of vaginal birth. Additional fluid is quickly absorbed by lung blood vessels and lymphatics after the first breath.

Once the alveoli have been inflated with a first breath, breathing becomes much easier for a baby, requiring only about 6 to 8 cm H_2O pressure. Within 10 minutes after birth, most newborns have established a good residual volume. By 10 to 12 hours of age, vital capacity is established at newborn proportions. The heart in a newborn takes up proportionately more space than in an adult, so the amount of lung expansion space available is proportionately limited.

A baby born by cesarean birth does not have as much lung fluid expelled at birth as one born vaginally and so may have more difficulty establishing effective respirations, because excessive fluid blocks air exchange space. Newborns who are immature and whose alveoli collapse each time they exhale (because of the lack of pulmonary surfactant) have difficulty establishing effective residual capacity and respirations. If the alveoli do not open well, a newborn's cardiac system becomes compromised, because closure of the foramen ovale and ductus arteriosus depends on free blood flow through the pulmonary artery and good oxygenation of blood. Therefore, a newborn who has difficulty establishing respirations at birth should be examined closely in the postpartal period for a cardiac murmur or other indication that he or she still has patent fetal cardiac structures, especially a patent ductus arteriosus.

Gastrointestinal System

Although the gastrointestinal tract is usually sterile at birth, bacteria may be cultured from the intestinal tract in most babies within 5 hours after birth and from all babies at 24 hours of life. Most of these bacteria enter the tract through the newborn's mouth from airborne sources. Others may come from vaginal secretions at birth, from hospital bedding, and from contact at the breast. Accumulation of bacteria in the gastrointestinal tract is necessary for digestion and for the synthesis of vitamin K.

Although a newborn's stomach holds about 60 to 90 mL, a newborn has limited ability to digest fat and starch because the pancreatic enzymes, lipase and amylase, remain deficient for the first few months of life. A newborn regurgitates easily because of an immature cardiac sphincter between the stomach and esophagus. Immature liver functions may lead to lowered glucose and protein serum levels.

Stools. The first stool of a newborn is usually passed within 24 hours after birth. It consists of **meconium,** a sticky, tarlike, blackish-green, odorless material formed from mucus, vernix, lanugo, hormones, and carbohydrates that accumulated during intrauterine life. If a newborn does not pass a meconium stool by 24 to 48 hours after birth, the possibility of some factor such as meconium ileus, imperforate anus, or volvulus should be suspected.

About the second or third day of life, newborn stool changes in color and consistency, becoming green and loose. This is termed **transitional stool,** and it may resemble diarrhea to the untrained eye. By the fourth day of life, breastfed babies pass three or four yellow stools per day. They are sweet-smelling, because breast milk is high in lactic acid, which reduces the amount of putrefactive organisms in the stool. A newborn who receives formula usually passes two or three yellow stools a day. These have a slightly more noticeable odor, compared with the stools of breastfed babies.

A newborn placed under phototherapy lights as a treatment for jaundice has bright green stools because of increased bilirubin excretion. Newborns with bile duct obstruction have clay-colored (gray) stools, because bile pigments are not entering the intestinal tract. Blood-flecked stools usually indicate an anal fissure. Occasionally, a newborn has swallowed some maternal blood during birth and either vomits fresh blood immediately after birth or passes a black tarry stool after 2 or more days. Maternal blood may be differentiated from fetal blood by a dipstick Apt test. If the stools remain black or tarry, intestinal bleeding should be suspected. If mucus is mixed with stool or the stool is watery and loose, a milk allergy, lactose intolerance, or some other condition interfering with digestion or absorption should be suspected.

Urinary System

The average newborn voids within 24 hours after birth. A newborn who does not take in much fluid for the first 24 hours may void later than this, but the 24-hour point is a good general rule. Newborns who do not void within this time should be examined for the possibility of urethral stenosis or absent kidneys or ureters.

The possibility of obstruction in the urinary tract can be assessed by observing the force of the urinary stream in both male and female infants. Males should void with enough force to produce a small projected arc; females should produce a steady stream, not just continuous dribbling. Projecting urine farther than normal may signal urethral obstruction, because it indicates that urine is being forced through a narrow channel.

The kidneys of newborns do not concentrate urine well, making newborn urine usually light-colored and odorless. The infant is about 6 weeks of age before much control over reabsorption of fluid in tubules and concentration of urine becomes evident.

A single voiding in a newborn is only about 15 mL and may be easily missed in a thick diaper. Specific gravity ranges from 1.008 to 1.010. The daily urinary output for the first 1 or 2 days is about 30 to 60 mL total. By week 1, total daily volume rises to about 300 mL. The first voiding may be pink or dusky because of uric acid crystals that were formed in the bladder in utero; this is an innocent finding. A small amount of protein may be normally present in voidings for the first few days of life, until the kidney glomeruli are more fully mature. Diapers can be weighed to determine the amount of urine output.

Immune System

Because they have difficulty forming antibodies against invading antigens until about 2 months of age, newborns are prone to infection. This inability to form antibodies is the reason that most immunizations against childhood diseases are not given to infants younger than 2 months of age. Newborns do have some immunologic protection, because they are born with passive antibodies (immunoglobulin G) from their mother that crossed the placenta. In most instances, these include antibodies against poliomyelitis, measles, diphtheria, pertussis, chickenpox, rubella, and tetanus. Newborns are routinely administered hepatitis B vaccine during the first 12 hours after birth to protect against this disease (American Academy of Pediatrics [AAP], 2009). Little natural immunity is transmitted against herpes simplex. Any health care personnel with herpes simplex eruptions (cold sores) should not care for newborns until the lesions have crusted. Without antibody protection, herpes simplex infections can become systemic or create a rapidly fatal form of the disease in a newborn.

Neuromuscular System

Mature newborns demonstrate neuromuscular function by moving their extremities, attempting to control head movement, exhibiting a strong cry, and demonstrating newborn reflexes. Limpness or total absence of a muscular response to manipulation is never normal and suggests narcosis, shock, or cerebral injury. A newborn occasionally makes twitching or flailing movements of the extremities in the absence of a stimulus because of the immaturity of the nervous system. Newborn reflexes can be tested with consistency by using simple maneuvers.

Blink Reflex. A blink reflex in a newborn serves the same purpose as it does in an adult—to protect the eye from any object coming near it by rapid eyelid closure. It may be elicited by shining a strong light such as a flashlight or an otoscope light on an eye. A sudden movement toward the eye sometimes can elicit the blink reflex.

Rooting Reflex. If the cheek is brushed or stroked near the corner of the mouth, a newborn infant will turn the head in that direction. This reflex serves to help a newborn find food: when a mother holds the child and allows her breast to brush the newborn's cheek, the reflex makes the baby turn toward the breast. The reflex disappears at about the sixth week of life. At about this time, newborn eyes focus steadily, so a food source can be seen, and the reflex is no longer needed.

Sucking Reflex. When a newborn's lips are touched, the baby makes a sucking motion. The reflex helps a newborn find food: when the newborn's lips touch the mother's breast or a bottle, the baby sucks and so takes in food. The sucking reflex begins to diminish at about 6 months of age. It disappears immediately if it is never stimulated such as in a newborn with a tracheoesophageal fistula who cannot take in oral fluids. It can be maintained in such an infant by offering the child a non-nutritive sucking object such as a pacifier (after the fistula has been corrected by surgery and until oral feedings can be given).

Swallowing Reflex. The swallowing reflex in a newborn is the same as in the adult. Food that reaches the posterior portion of the tongue is automatically swallowed. Gag, cough, and sneeze reflexes also are present in newborns to maintain a clear airway in the event that normal swallowing does not keep the pharynx free of obstructing mucus.

Extrusion Reflex. A newborn extrudes any substance that is placed on the anterior portion of the tongue. This protective reflex prevents the swallowing of inedible substances. It disappears at about 4 months of age. Until then, the infant may seem to be spitting out or refusing solid food placed in the mouth.

Palmar Grasp Reflex. Newborns grasp an object placed in their palm by closing their fingers on it (Fig. 18.4). Mature

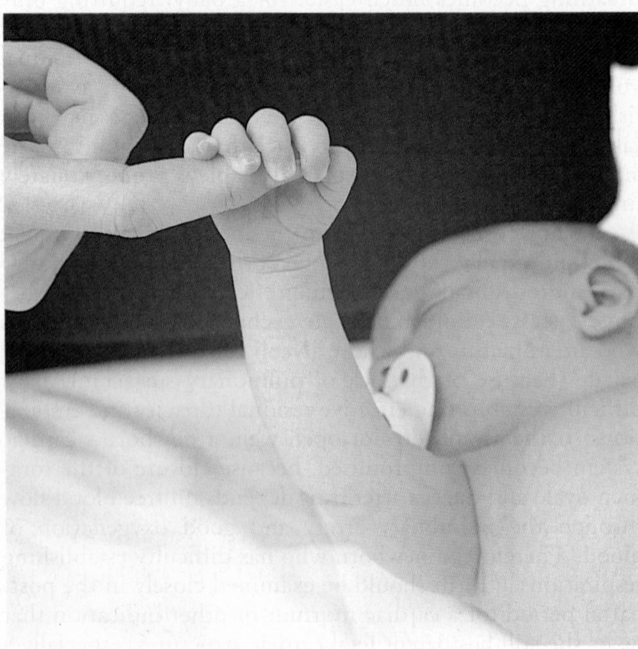

FIGURE 18.4 Palmar grasp reflex.

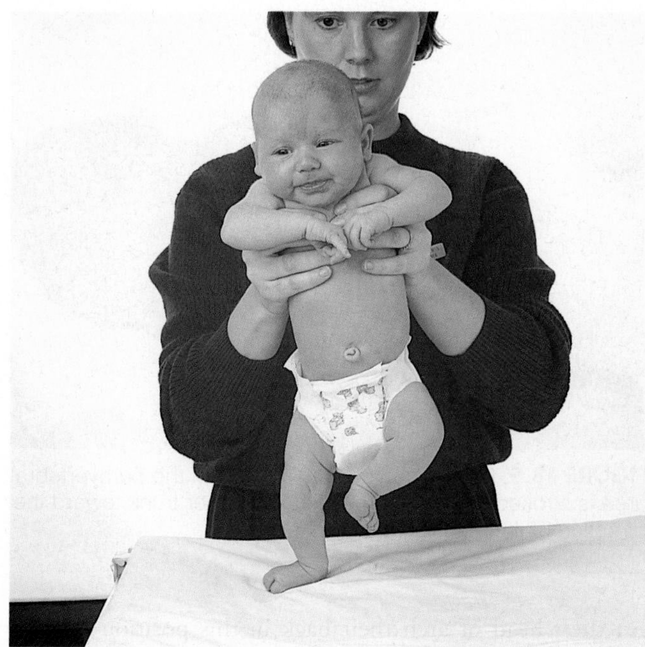

FIGURE 18.5 Step-in-place reflex.

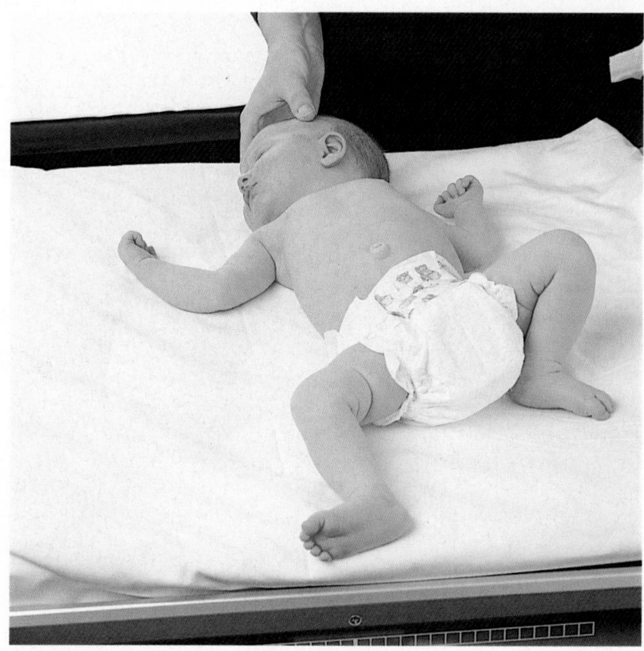

FIGURE 18.6 Tonic neck reflex.

newborns grasp so strongly that they can be raised from a supine position and suspended momentarily from an examiner's fingers. This reflex disappears at about 6 weeks to 3 months of age. A baby begins to grasp meaningfully at about 3 months of age.

Step (Walk)-in-Place Reflex. Newborns who are held in a vertical position with their feet touching a hard surface will take a few quick, alternating steps (Fig. 18.5). This reflex disappears by 3 months of age. By 4 months, babies can bear a good portion of their weight unhindered by this reflex.

Placing Reflex. The placing reflex is similar to the step-in-place reflex, except that it is elicited by touching the anterior surface of the lower part of a newborn's leg against a hard surface such as the edge of a bassinet or table. The newborn makes a few quick lifting motions, as if to step onto the table, because of the reflex.

Plantar Grasp Reflex. When an object touches the sole of a newborn's foot at the base of the toes, the toes grasp in the same manner as do the fingers. This reflex disappears at about 8 to 9 months of age in preparation for walking. However, it may be present during sleep for a longer period.

Tonic Neck Reflex. When newborns lie on their backs, their heads usually turn to one side or the other. The arm and the leg on the side toward which the head turns extend, and the opposite arm and leg contract (Fig. 18.6). The movement is most evident in the arms but may also be observed in the legs. If you turn a newborn's head to the opposite side, he or she will often change the extension and contraction of legs and arms accordingly. This is also called a boxer or fencing reflex, because the position simulates that of someone preparing to box or fence. Unlike many other reflexes, the tonic neck reflex does not appear to have a function. It does stimulate eye coordination, because the extended arm moves in front of the face. It may signify handedness. The reflex disappears between the second and third months of life.

Moro Reflex. A Moro (startle) reflex (Fig. 18.7) can be initiated by startling a newborn with a loud noise or by jarring the bassinet. The most accurate method of eliciting the reflex is to hold newborns in a supine position and allow their heads to drop backward about 1 inch. In response to this sudden head movement, they abduct and extend their arms and legs. Their fingers assume a typical "C" position. Finally,

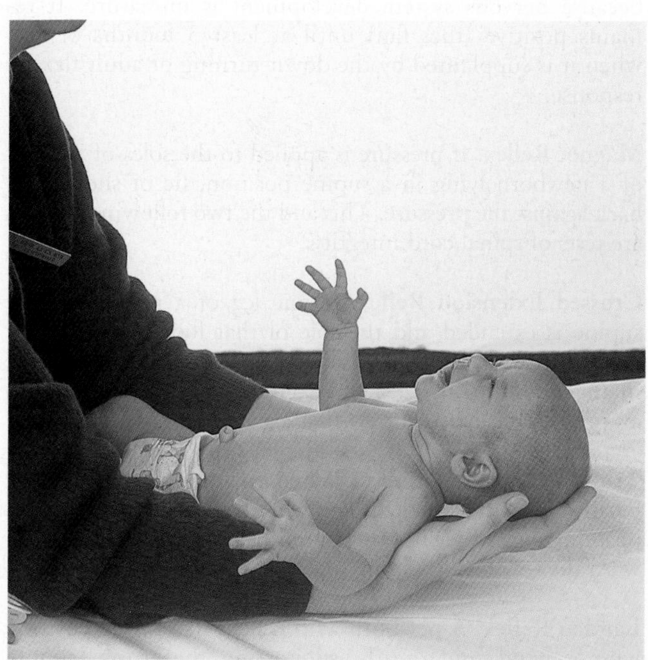

FIGURE 18.7 Moro reflex.

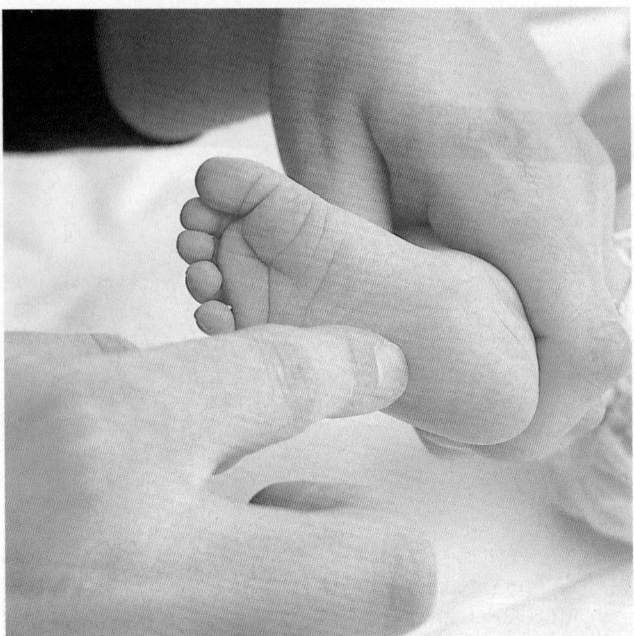

FIGURE 18.8 Babinski reflex. When the examiner moves her finger upward, the newborn's toes will fan outward.

they swing their arms into an embrace position and pull up their legs against their abdomen (adduction). The reflex simulates the action of someone trying to ward off an attacker, then covering up to protect himself. It is strong for the first 8 weeks of life and then fades by the end of the fourth or fifth month, at the same time an infant can roll away from danger.

Babinski Reflex. When the sole of the foot is stroked in an inverted "J" curve from the heel upward, a newborn fans the toes (positive Babinski sign) (Fig. 18.8). This is in contrast to the adult, who flexes the toes. This reaction occurs because nervous system development is immature. It remains positive (toes fan) until at least 3 months of age, when it is supplanted by the down-turning or adult flexion response.

Magnet Reflex. If pressure is applied to the soles of the feet of a newborn lying in a supine position, he or she pushes back against the pressure. This and the two following reflexes are tests of spinal cord integrity.

Crossed Extension Reflex. If one leg of a newborn lying supine is extended and the sole of that foot is irritated by being rubbed with a sharp object, such as a thumbnail, the infant raises the other leg and extends it, as if trying to push away the hand irritating the first leg.

Trunk Incurvation Reflex. When newborns lie in a prone position and are touched along the paravertebral area by a probing finger, they flex their trunk and swing their pelvis toward the touch (Fig. 18.9).

Landau Reflex. A newborn who is held in a prone position with a hand underneath, supporting the trunk, should demonstrate some muscle tone. Babies may not be able to lift their head or arch their back in this position (as they will at 3 months of age), but neither should they sag into an inverted "U" position. The latter response indicates extremely poor muscle tone, the cause of which should be investigated.

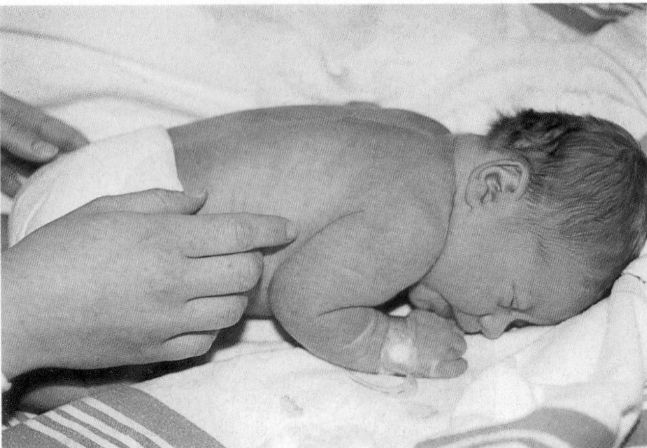

FIGURE 18.9 Trunk incurvation reflex. When the paravertebral area is stroked, the newborn flexes his or her trunk toward the direction of the stimulation.

Deep Tendon Reflexes. A patellar reflex can be elicited in a newborn by tapping the patellar tendon with the tip of the finger. The lower leg moves perceptibly if the infant has an intact reflex. To elicit a biceps reflex, place the thumb of your left hand on the tendon of the biceps muscle on the inner surface of the elbow. Tap the thumb as it rests on the tendon. You are more likely to feel the tendon contract than to observe movement. A biceps reflex is a test for spinal nerves C5 and C6; a patellar reflex is a test for spinal nerves L2–L4.

✔ Checkpoint Question 18.2

A Moro reflex is the single best assessment of neurologic ability in a newborn. What is the best way to test this reflex?

a. Observe the infant while she is on her abdomen to see whether she can turn her head.
b. Lift the infant's head while she is supine and allow it to fall back 1 inch.
c. Shake the infant's crib until the infant responds by flailing her arms.
d. Make a sharp noise, such as clapping your hands, to wake the infant.

The Senses

The senses in newborns are already developed at birth.

Hearing. A fetus is able to hear in utero even before birth. As soon as amniotic fluid drains or is absorbed from the middle ear by way of the eustachian tube—within hours after birth—hearing becomes acute. Newborns appear to have difficulty locating sound, however, and so do not turn toward it consistently. Perhaps they must learn to interpret small differences among sounds arriving at their ears at different times. They respond with generalized activity to a sound such as a bell ringing a short distance from their ear. A newborn who is actively crying when a bell is rung stops crying and seems to attend. Similarly, newborns calm in response to a soothing voice and startle at loud noises. They recognize their mother's voice almost immediately, as if they have heard it in utero.

Vision. Newborns see as soon as they are born and possibly have been "seeing" light and dark in utero for the last few months of pregnancy, as the uterus and the abdominal wall were stretched thin. Newborns demonstrate sight at birth by blinking at a strong light (blink reflex) or by following a bright light or toy a short distance with their eyes. Because they cannot follow past the midline of vision, they lose track of objects easily. This is why parents sometimes think and report that their newborn does not see. Newborns focus best on black and white objects at a distance of 9 to 12 in. A pupillary reflex or ability to contract the pupil is present from birth.

Touch. The sense of touch is also well developed at birth. Newborns demonstrate this by quieting at a soothing touch and by sucking and rooting reflexes, which are elicited by touch. They also react to painful stimuli.

Taste. A newborn has the ability to discriminate taste, because taste buds are developed and functioning even before birth. A fetus in utero, for example, will swallow amniotic fluid more rapidly than usual if glucose is added to sweeten its taste. The swallowing decreases if a bitter flavor is added. A newborn turns away from a bitter taste such as salt but readily accepts the sweet taste of milk or glucose water.

Smell. The sense of smell is present in newborns as soon as the nose is clear of lung and amniotic fluid. Newborns turn toward their mothers' breast partly out of recognition of the smell of breast milk and partly as a manifestation of the rooting reflex. Their ability to respond to odors can be used to document alertness.

Physiologic Adjustment to Extrauterine Life

All newborns seem to move through periods of irregular adjustment in the first 6 hours of life, before their body systems stabilize. These periods were first described by Desmond in 1963 and are termed periods of reactivity (Desmond, 1963). The first phase lasts about half an hour. During this time, the baby is alert and exhibits exploring, searching activity, often making sucking sounds. Heart beat and respiratory rate are rapid. This is called the *first period of reactivity.*

Next comes a quiet *resting period.* Heartbeat and respiratory rates slow, and the newborn typically sleeps for about 90 minutes. The *second period of reactivity,* between 2 and 6 hours of life, occurs when the baby wakes again, often gagging and choking on mucus that has accumulated in the mouth. He or she is again alert and responsive and interested in surroundings.

These three periods are summarized in Table 18.1. Newborns who are ill or who had difficulty at birth may not pass through these typical stages; they may never have periods of alertness or periods of quiet. Their vital signs may not fall and rise again but remain rapid; their temperature may remain subnormal. Demonstration of this typical reactivity pattern, therefore, is an indication that a newborn is healthy and adjusting well to extrauterine life. The ability to transition from one period to another is an important indicator of neurologic status.

TABLE 18.1 ✻ Periods of Reactivity: Normal Adjustment to Extrauterine Life

Assessment	First Period (First 15–30 min)	Resting Period (30–120 min)	Second Period (2–6 hr)
Color	Acrocyanosis	Color stabilizing	Quick color changes occur with movement or crying
Temperature	Temperature begins to fall from intrauterine temperature of about 100.6° F (38.1° C)	Temperature stabilizes at about 99° F (37.2° C)	Temperature increases to 99.8° F (37.6° C)
Heart rate	Rapid, as much as 180 bpm while crying	Slowing to 120–140 bpm	Wide swings in rate with activity
Respirations	Irregular; 30–90 breaths per min while crying; some nasal flaring, occasional retraction may be present	Slowing to 30–50 breaths per min; barreling of chest occurs	Becoming irregular again with activity
Activity	Alert; watching	Sleeping	Awakening
Ability to respond to stimulation	Vigorous reaction	Difficult to arouse	Becoming responsive again
Mucus	Visible in mouth	Small amount present while sleeping	Mouth full of mucus, causing gagging
Bowel sounds	Can be heard after first 15 min	Present	Often passage of first meconium stool

Source: Desmond, M. N., et al. (1963). The clinical behavior of the newly born: the term infant. *Journal of Pediatrics, 62*(3), 307–309.

APPEARANCE OF A NEWBORN

Although all newborns have similar physical findings, there are individual differences.

Skin

General inspection of a newborn's skin reveals many characteristic findings.

Color

Most term newborns have a ruddy complexion because of the increased concentration of red blood cells in blood vessels and a decrease in the amount of subcutaneous fat, which makes the blood vessels more visible. This ruddiness fades slightly over the first month. Infants with poor central nervous system control may appear pale and cyanotic. A gray color in newborns generally indicates infection. Twins may be born with a twin transfusion phenomenon, in which one twin is larger and has good color and the smaller twin has pallor (Roberts, Neilson, & Weindling, 2009).

Cyanosis. Generalized mottling of the skin is common. A newborn's lips, hands, and feet are likely to appear blue from immature peripheral circulation. Acrocyanosis (blueness of hands and feet) is so prominent in some newborns that it appears as if some stricture were cutting off circulation, with usual skin color on one side and blue on the other. Acrocyanosis is a normal phenomenon in the first 24 to 48 hours after birth; however, **central cyanosis,** or cyanosis of the trunk, is always a cause for concern. Central cyanosis indicates decreased oxygenation. It may be the result of a temporary respiratory obstruction or an underlying disease state.

Mucus obstructing a newborn's respiratory tract causes sudden cyanosis and apnea. Suctioning of the mucus relieves this. Always suction the mouth of a newborn before the nose, because suctioning the nose first may trigger a reflex gasp, possibly leading to aspiration if there is mucus in the posterior throat. Follow mouth suctioning with suction to the nose, because the nose is the chief conduit for air in a newborn.

What if... Ms. Ruiz inspects her new baby and says to you, "Her hands are cold and blue. Is something wrong with her hands?" How should you answer?

Hyperbilirubinemia. Hyperbilirubinemia leads to **jaundice,** or yellowing of the skin (Beachy, 2007). This occurs on the second or third day of life in about 50% of all newborns, as a result of a breakdown of fetal red blood cells **(physiologic jaundice).** The infant's skin and the sclera of the eyes appear noticeably yellow. This happens because the high red blood cell count built up in utero is destroyed, and heme and globin are released. Globin is a protein component that is reused by the body and is not a factor in the developing jaundice. Heme is further broken down into iron (which is also reused and not involved in the jaundice) and protoporphyrin. Protoporphyrin is further broken down into indirect bilirubin. Indirect bilirubin is fat soluble and cannot be excreted by the kidneys in this state. For removal from the body, it is converted by the liver enzyme glucuronyl transferase into direct bilirubin, which is water soluble. This is incorporated into stool and then excreted in feces. Many newborns have such immature liver function that indirect bilirubin cannot be converted to the direct form; it therefore remains indirect. As long as the buildup of indirect bilirubin remains in the circulatory system, the red coloring of the blood cells covers the yellow tint of the bilirubin. After the level of this indirect bilirubin has risen to more than 7 mg/100 mL, however, bilirubin permeates the tissue outside the circulatory system and causes the infant to appear jaundiced.

Observe infants who are prone to extensive bruising (large, breech, or immature babies) carefully for jaundice, because bruising leads to hemorrhage of blood into the subcutaneous tissue or skin. A **cephalhematoma** is a collection of blood under the periosteum of the skull bone. As the bruising in these locations heals and the red blood cells are hemolyzed, additional indirect bilirubin is released and can be another cause of jaundice (Nicholson, 2007).

If intestinal obstruction is present and stool cannot be evacuated, intestinal flora may break down bile into its basic components, leading to the release of indirect bilirubin into the bloodstream again. Early feeding of newborns promotes intestinal movement and excretion of meconium and helps prevent indirect bilirubin buildup from this source.

The level of jaundice in newborns may be judged grossly by estimating the extent to which it has progressed on the surface of the infant's body, as it is noticed first in the head and then spreads to the rest of the body.

Various commercial devices (transcutaneous bilirubinometry devices) are available to measure skin tone for jaundice and help in estimating jaundice levels. Although use of these devices rarely replaces serum measurements, they can be used to identify infants who need serum bilirubin determinations. The technique for obtaining a serum bilirubin specimen by heel puncture is shown in Chapter 37.

Treatment for physiologic jaundice or the routine rise in bilirubin in newborns is rarely necessary, except for measures such as early feeding to speed passage of feces through the intestine and prevent reabsorption of bilirubin from the bowel.

Above-normal indirect bilirubin levels are potentially dangerous because, if enough indirect bilirubin (about 20 mg/100 mL) leaves the bloodstream, it can interfere with the chemical synthesis of brain cells, resulting in permanent cell damage, a condition termed **kernicterus.** If this occurs, permanent neurologic damage, including cognitive challenge, may result.

There is no set level at which indirect serum bilirubin requires treatment, because other factors, such as age, maturity, and breastfeeding status, affect this determination. If the level rises to more than 10 to 12 mg/100 mL, treatment is usually considered. Phototherapy (exposure of the infant to light to initiate maturation of liver enzymes) is a common therapy (see Chapter 26). If this is necessary, the incubator and light source can be moved to the mother's room so that the mother is not separated from her baby. Some infants need continued therapy after discharge and receive phototherapy at home (Mills & Tudehope, 2009).

Compared with formula-fed babies, a small proportion of breastfed babies may have more difficulty converting indirect bilirubin to direct bilirubin, because breast milk contains pregnanediol (a metabolite of progesterone), which depresses the action of glucuronyl transferase. However, breastfeeding alone rarely causes enough jaundice to warrant therapy (Thilo

& Rosenberg, 2008). The decision to stop nursing in the first 2 weeks of life must never be made lightly, because it could interfere with breast filling and a breast milk supply.

Pallor. Pallor in newborns is usually the result of anemia. This may be caused by (a) excessive blood loss when the cord was cut, (b) inadequate flow of blood from the cord into the infant at birth, (c) fetal–maternal transfusion, (d) low iron stores caused by poor maternal nutrition during pregnancy, or (e) blood incompatibility in which a large number of red blood cells were hemolyzed in utero. It also may be the result of internal bleeding. A baby who appears pale should be watched closely for signs of blood in stool or vomitus.

Harlequin Sign. Occasionally, because of immature circulation, a newborn who has been lying on his or her side appears red on the dependent side of the body and pale on the upper side, as if a line had been drawn down the center of the body. This is a transient phenomenon; although startling, it is of no clinical significance. The odd coloring fades immediately if the infant's position is changed or the baby kicks or cries vigorously.

Birthmarks

Several common types of birthmarks occur in newborns. Most will fade by school age, although an association between children with birthmarks and the development of childhood cancer exists (Johnson et al., 2007). It is important to be able to differentiate the various types of hemangiomas that occur, so that you neither give false reassurance to parents nor worry them unnecessarily about these lesions.

Hemangiomas. The **hemangiomas** are vascular tumors of the skin. Three types occur.

Nevus Flammeus. **Nevus flammeus** (Fig. 18.10A) is a macular purple or dark-red lesion (sometimes called a *port-wine stain* because of its deep color) that is present at birth. These lesions typically appear on the face, although they are often found on the thighs as well. Those above the bridge of

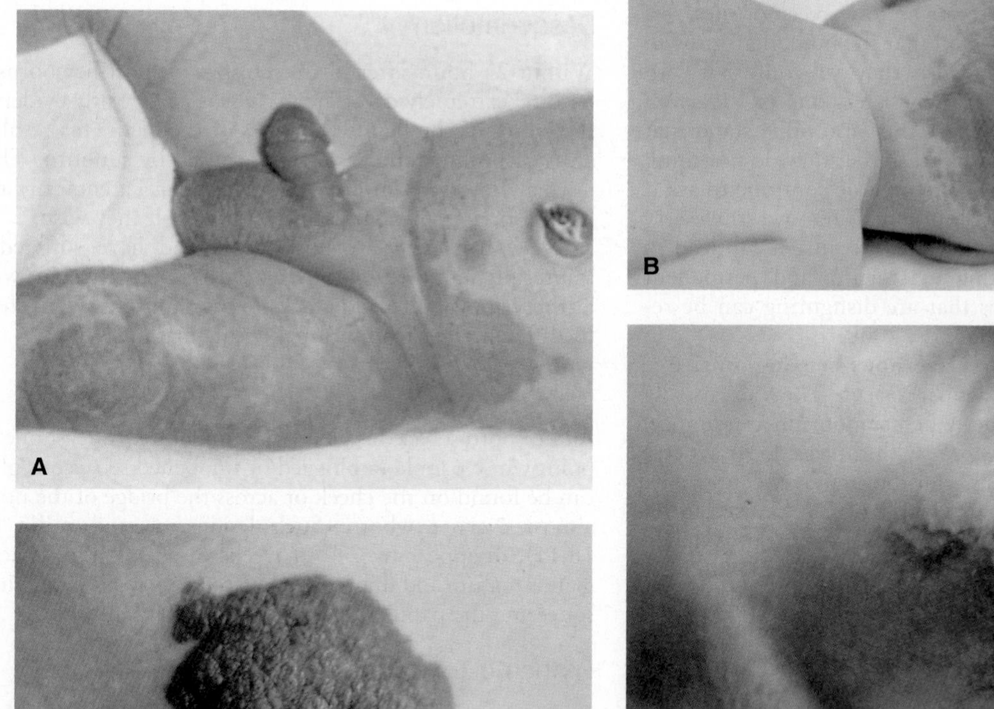

FIGURE 18.10 Types of hemangiomas found on a newborn. (**A**) Nevus flammeus (port-wine stain) formed of a plexus of newly formed capillaries in the papillary layer of the corium. It is deep red to purple, does not blanch on pressure, and does not fade with age. (**B**) A telangectasia or stork's beak mark, commonly occurring on the nape of the neck. It blanches on pressure; although it does not fade, it is not noticeable as it becomes covered by hair. (**C**) Strawberry hemangiomas consist of dilated capillaries in entire dermal and subdermal layers. They continue to enlarge after birth but usually disappear by age 10 years. (**D**) Cavernous hemangiomas consist of a communicating network of venules in subcutaneous tissue and do not fade with age.

the nose tend to fade; the others are less likely to fade. Because they are level with the skin surface (macular), they can be covered by a cosmetic preparation later in life or removed by laser therapy, although lesions may reappear after treatment (Berger, 2009).

Nevus flammeus lesions also occur as lighter, pink patches at the nape of the neck, known as *stork's beak marks* or telangiectasia (see Fig. 18.10B). These do not fade, but they are covered by the hairline and therefore are of no consequence. They occur more often in females than in males.

Strawberry Hemangioma. **Strawberry hemangioma** refers to elevated areas formed by immature capillaries and endothelial cells (see Fig. 18.10C). Most are present at birth in the term neonate, although they may appear up to 2 weeks after birth. Typically, they are not present in the preterm infant because of the immaturity of the epidermis. Formation is associated with the high estrogen levels of pregnancy. They may continue to enlarge from their original size up to 1 year of age. After the first year, they tend to be absorbed and shrink in size. By the time the child is 7 years old, 50% to 75% of these lesions have disappeared. A child may be 10 years old before the absorption is complete. Application of hydrocortisone ointment may speed the disappearance of these lesions by interfering with the binding of estrogen to its receptor sites.

Be certain parents understand that the mark may grow in their child's early years. Otherwise, they can confuse it with cancer (a skin lesion increasing in size is one of the seven danger signals of cancer). Be sure they also understand that the mark will eventually disappear, so that they do not think of their child as imperfect or disfigured or continue to ask if the baby should have surgery. Surgery to remove strawberry hemangiomas is rarely recommended because it can lead to secondary infection, resulting in scarring and permanent disfigurement. Large lesions that are disfiguring can be removed by laser therapy (Edmonds, 2008).

Cavernous Hemangioma. **Cavernous hemangiomas** (see Fig. 18.10D) are dilated vascular spaces. They are usually raised and resemble a strawberry hemangioma in appearance. However, they do not d isappear with time as do strawberry hemangiomas. Such lesions can be removed surgically. Steroids, interferon-alfa-2a, or vincristine can be used to reduce these lesions in size, although their use must be weighed in light of side effects (Edmonds, 2008). Children who have a skin lesion may have additional ones on internal organs. Blows to the abdomen, such as those from childhood games, can cause bleeding from an internal hemangioma. For this reason, children with cavernous hemangiomas usually have their hematocrit levels assessed at health maintenance visits, to evaluate for possible internal blood loss.

Mongolian Spots. **Mongolian spots** are collections of pigment cells (melanocytes) that appear as slate-gray patches across the sacrum or buttocks and possibly on the arms and legs. They tend to occur in children of Asian, southern European, or African ethnicity (Thilo & Rosenberg, 2008). They disappear by school age without treatment. Be sure to inform parents that these are not bruises; otherwise, they may worry their baby sustained a birth injury.

Vernix Caseosa

Vernix caseosa is a white, cream cheese–like substance that serves as a skin lubricant in utero. Usually, it is noticeable on a term newborn's skin, at least in the skin folds, at birth. Document the color of vernix, because it takes on the color of the amniotic fluid. For example, a yellow vernix implies that the amniotic fluid was yellow from bilirubin; green vernix indicates that meconium was present in the amniotic fluid.

Until the first bath, when vernix is washed away, handle newborns with gloves to protect yourself from exposure to this body fluid. Never use harsh rubbing to wash away vernix. A newborn's skin is tender, and breaks in the skin caused by too vigorous attempts at removal may open portals of entry for bacteria.

Lanugo

Lanugo is the fine, downy hair that covers a newborn's shoulders, back, and upper arms. It may be found also on the forehead and ears. A baby born between 37 to 39 weeks of gestation has more lanugo than a newborn of 40 weeks' gestational age. Postmature infants (more than 42 weeks of gestation) rarely have lanugo. Lanugo is rubbed away by the friction of bedding and clothes against the newborn's skin. By 2 weeks of age, it has disappeared.

Desquamation

Within 24 hours after birth, the skin of most newborns has become extremely dry. The dryness is particularly evident on the palms of the hands and soles of the feet. This results in areas of peeling similar to those caused by sunburn. This is normal, however, and needs no treatment. Parents may apply hand lotion to prevent excessive dryness if they wish.

Newborns who are postmature and have suffered intrauterine malnutrition may have extremely dry skin, with a leathery appearance and cracks in the skin folds. This should be differentiated from normal desquamation.

Milia

All newborn sebaceous glands are immature. At least one pinpoint white papule (a plugged or unopened sebaceous gland) can be found on the cheek or across the bridge of the nose of almost every newborn. Such lesions, termed **milia** (Fig. 18.11), disappear by 2 to 4 weeks of age, as the sebaceous glands mature and drain. Teach parents to avoid scratching or squeezing the papules, to prevent secondary infections.

Erythema Toxicum

In most normal mature infants, a newborn rash called **erythema toxicum** can be observed (Fig. 18.12). This usually appears in the first to fourth day of life but may appear up to 2 weeks of age. It begins with a papule, increases in severity to become erythema by the second day, and then disappears by the third day. It is sometimes called a *flea-bite rash* because the lesions are so minuscule. One of the chief characteristics of the rash is its lack of pattern. It occurs sporadically and unpredictably and may last hours rather than days. It is caused by a newborn's eosinophils reacting to the environment as the immune system matures. It requires no treatment.

Forceps Marks

Forceps are rarely used for birth today but if they are used, they may leave a circular or linear contusion matching the rim of

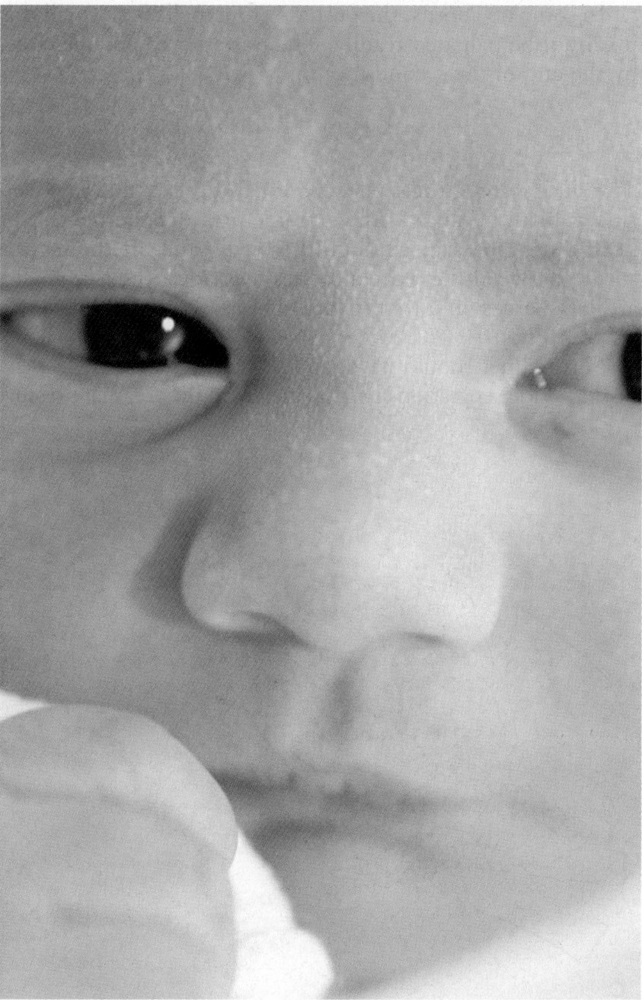

FIGURE 18.11 Milia are unopened sebaceous glands frequently found on the nose, chin, or cheeks of a newborn.

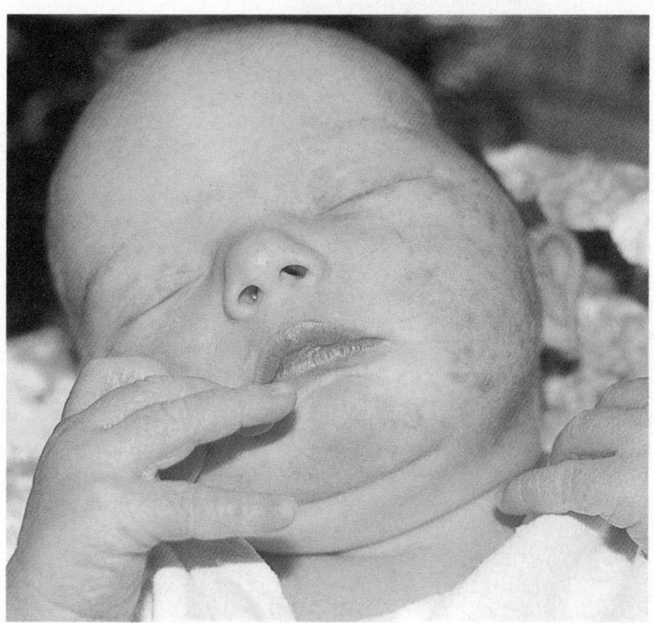

FIGURE 18.12 Erythema toxicum is found on almost all newborns. The reddish rash consists of sporadic pinpoint papules on an erythematous base. It fades spontaneously in a few days.

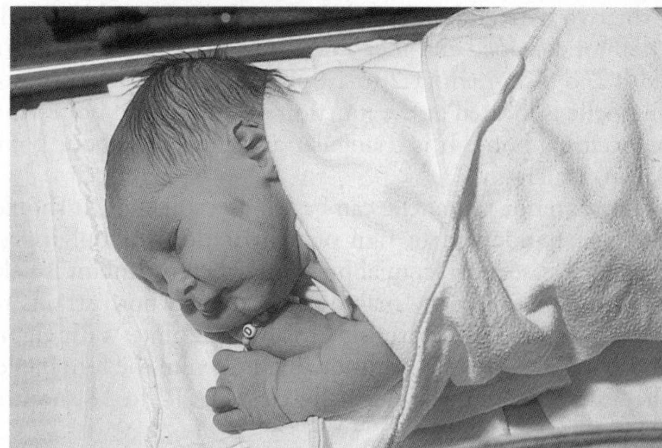

FIGURE 18.13 Forceps marks are commonly found in newborns born by forceps. Such marks are transient and disappear in a day or two.

the blade of the forceps on the infant's cheek (Fig. 18.13). This mark disappears in 1 to 2 days, along with the edema that accompanies it. The mark is the result of normal forceps use and does not denote unskilled or too vigorous application of forceps. Closely assess the facial nerve while a newborn is at rest and during crying episodes, to detect any potential facial nerve compression requiring further evaluation.

Skin Turgor

Newborn skin should feel resilient if the underlying tissue is well hydrated. If a fold of the skin is grasped between the thumb and fingers, it should feel elastic. When it is released, it should fall back to form a smooth surface. If severe dehydration is present, the skin will not smooth out again but will remain in an elevated ridge. Poor turgor is seen in newborns who suffered malnutrition in utero, who have difficulty sucking at birth, or who have certain metabolic disorders such as adrenocortical insufficiency.

✔ Checkpoint Question 18.3

Beth Ruiz has milia on her nose. What is the necessary therapy for this?

a. Ice packs to reduce inflammation.
b. Warm heat to increase circulation.
c. No therapy is necessary for milia.
d. Lancing the lesions so they drain.

Head

A newborn's head appears disproportionately large because it is about one fourth of the total body length; in an adult, a head is one eighth of total height. The forehead of a newborn is large and prominent. The chin appears to be receding, and it quivers easily if an infant is startled or cries. Well-nourished newborns have full-bodied hair; poorly nourished and preterm infants have thin, lifeless hair. If internal fetal monitoring was used during labor, a newborn may exhibit a pinpoint ulcer at the point where the monitor was attached.

Fontanelles

The fontanelles are the spaces or openings where the skull bones join. The anterior fontanelle is located at the junction of the two parietal bones and the two fused frontal bones. It is diamond shaped and measures 2 to 3 cm (0.8 to 1.2 in) in width and 3 to 4 cm (1.2 to 1.6 in) in length. The posterior fontanelle is located at the junction of the parietal bones and the occipital bone. It is triangular and measures about 1 cm (0.4 in) in length.

The anterior fontanelle can be felt as a soft spot. It should not appear indented (a sign of dehydration) or bulging (a sign of increased intracranial pressure) when the infant is held upright. The fontanelle may bulge if the newborn strains to pass a stool or cries vigorously or is lying supine. With vigorous crying, a pulse may additionally be seen in the fontanelle. The anterior fontanelle normally closes at 12 to 18 months of age.

In some newborns, the posterior fontanelle is so small that it cannot be palpated readily. The posterior fontanelle closes by the end of the second month.

Sutures

The skull *sutures,* the separating lines of the skull, may override at birth because of the extreme pressure exerted on the head during passage through the birth canal. If the sagittal suture between the parietal bones overrides, the fontanelles are less perceptible than usual. The overriding subsides in 24 to 48 hours.

Suture lines should never appear widely separated in newborns. Wide separation suggests increased intracranial pressure

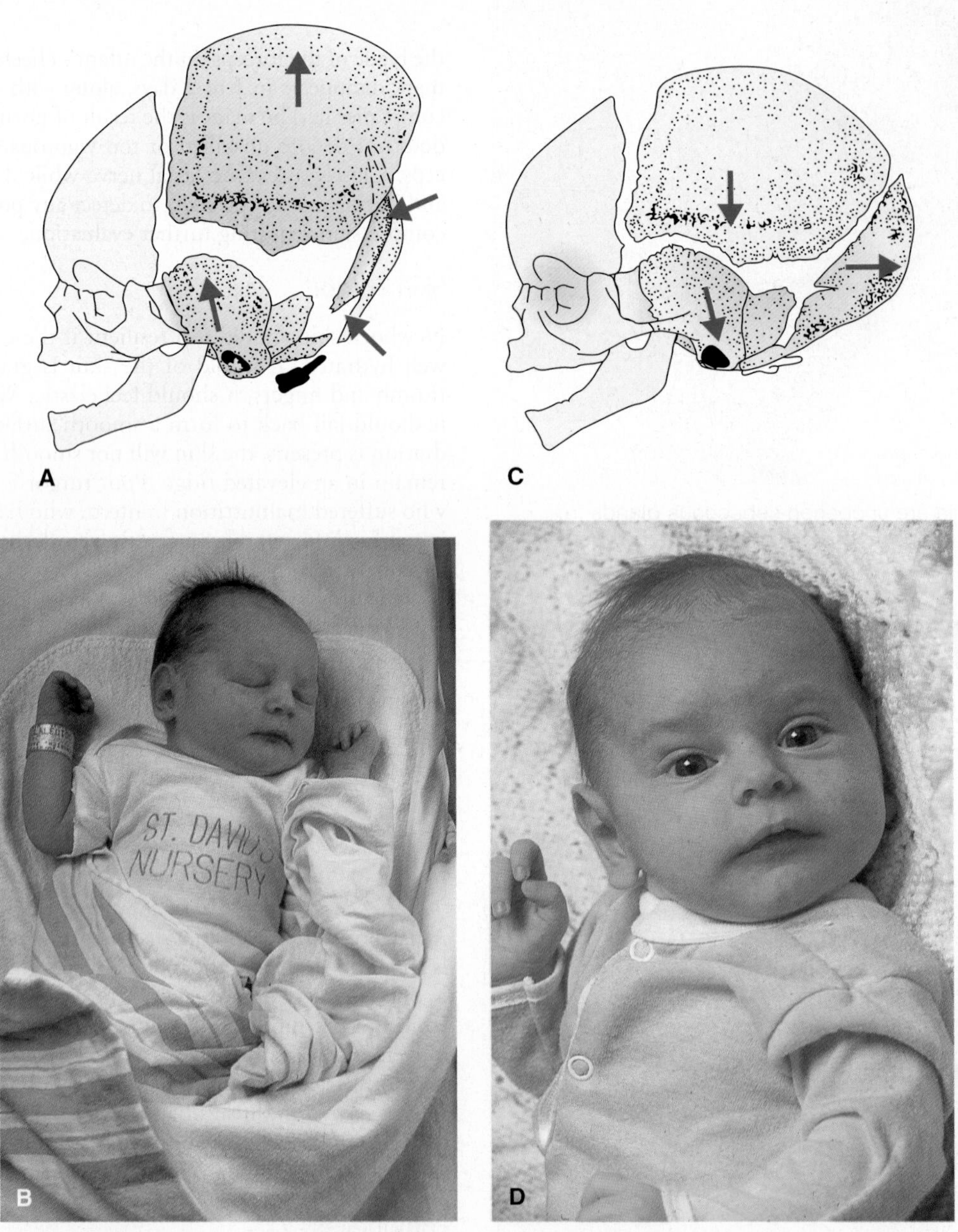

FIGURE 18.14 Molding. (**A, B**) The infant head molds to fit the birth canal more easily. On palpation, the skull sutures will be felt to be overriding. (**C, D**) The head shape returns to normal within 1 week.

because of abnormal brain formation, abnormal accumulation of cerebrospinal fluid in the cranium (hydrocephalus), or an accumulation of blood from a birth injury such as subdural hemorrhage. Fused suture lines also are abnormal; they require radiographic confirmation and further evaluation, because they will prevent the head from expanding with brain growth.

Molding

The part of the infant's head that engaged the cervix (usually the vertex) molds to fit the cervix contours during labor. After birth, this area appears prominent and asymmetric. Molding may be so extreme in the baby of a primiparous woman that the baby's head appears as a dunce cap (Fig. 18.14). The head will restore to its normal shape within a few days after birth.

Caput Succedaneum

Caput succedaneum (Fig. 18.15A) is edema of the scalp at the presenting part of the head. It may involve wide areas of the head, or it may resemble a large egg. The edema, which crosses the suture lines, is gradually absorbed and disappears at about the third day of life. It needs no treatment (Nicholson, 2007).

Cephalhematoma

A *cephalhematoma,* a collection of blood between the periosteum of a skull bone and the bone itself, is caused by rupture of a periosteal capillary because of the pressure of birth (see Fig. 18.15B). Swelling usually appears 24 hours after birth. Although the blood loss is negligible, the swelling is usually severe and is well outlined as an egg shape. It may be discolored (black and blue) because of the presence of coagulated blood. A cephalhematoma is confined to an individual bone, so the associated swelling stops at the bone's suture line.

It often takes weeks for a cephalhematoma to be absorbed. It might be supposed that the blood could be aspirated to relieve the condition. However, such a procedure would introduce the risk of infection and is unnecessary, because the condition will subside by itself. As the blood captured in the space is broken down, a great amount of indirect bilirubin may be released, leading to jaundice.

Craniotabes

Craniotabes is a localized softening of the cranial bones that is probably caused by pressure of the fetal skull against the mother's pelvic bone in utero. It is more common in first-born infants than in infants born later, because of the lower position of the fetal head in the pelvis during the last 2 weeks of pregnancy in primiparous women. With craniotabes, the skull is so soft that the pressure of an examining finger can indent it. The bone returns to its normal contour after the pressure is removed. The condition corrects itself without treatment after a few months, as the infant takes in calcium in milk. It is an example of a condition that is normal in a newborn but would be pathologic in an older child or adult (in whom it probably would be the result of faulty metabolism or kidney dysfunction).

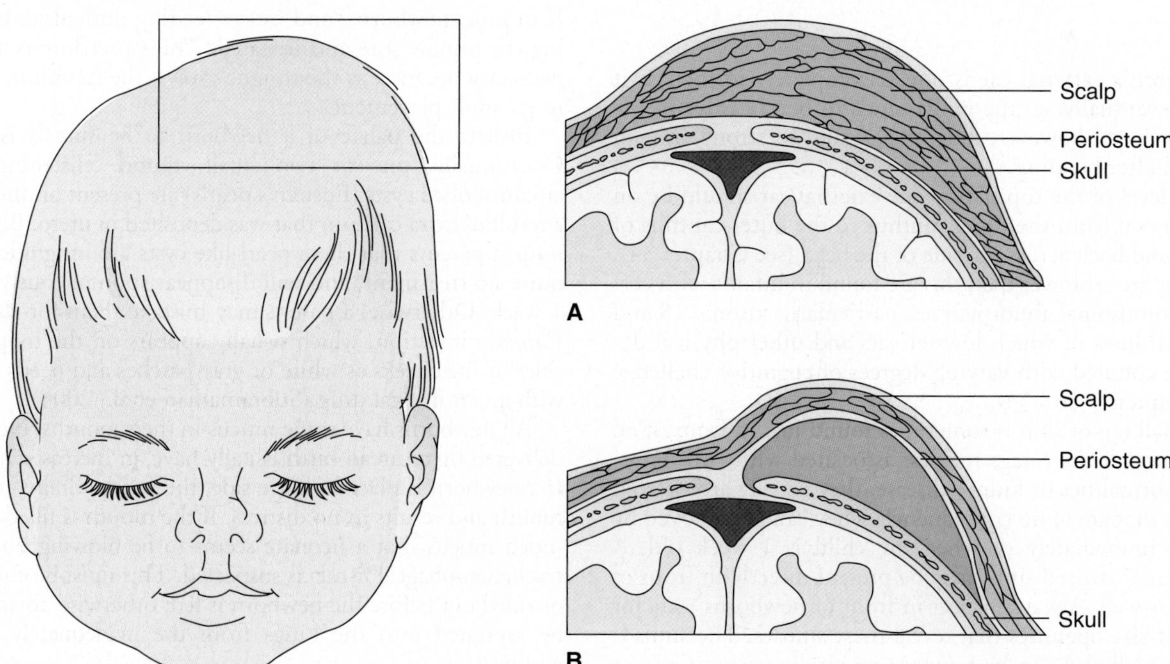

FIGURE 18.15 (**A**) Caput succedaneum. From pressure of the birth canal, an edematous area is present beneath the scalp. Note how it crosses the midline of the skull. (**B**) Cephalhematoma. A small capillary beneath the periosteum of the skull bone has ruptured, and blood has collected under the periosteum of the bone. Note how the swelling now stops at the midline. Because the blood is contained under the periosteum, it is necessarily stopped by a suture line.

Eyes

Newborns usually cry tearlessly, because their lacrimal ducts do not fully mature until about 3 months of age. Almost without exception, the irises of the eyes of newborns are gray or blue; the sclera may be blue because of its thinness. Infant eyes assume their permanent color between 3 and 12 months of age.

To inspect the eyes, lay the newborn in a supine position and lift the head. This maneuver causes the baby to open the eyes. A newborn's eyes should appear clear, without redness or purulent discharge. Occasionally, the administration of an antibiotic ointment such as erythromycin given at birth, to protect against *Chlamydia* infection and ophthalmia neonatorum (gonorrheal conjunctivitis), has caused a purulent discharge that lasts for the first 24 hours of life.

Pressure during birth sometimes ruptures a conjunctival capillary of the eye, resulting in a small **subconjunctival hemorrhage.** This appears as a red spot on the sclera, usually on the inner aspect of the eye, or as a red ring around the cornea. The bleeding is slight, requires no treatment, and is completely absorbed within 2 or 3 weeks. You can assure parents that these hemorrhages are normal variations. Otherwise, they may assume that their baby is bleeding from within the eye and that vision will be impaired.

Edema is often present around the orbit or on the eyelids. This remains for the first 2 or 3 days, until the newborn's kidneys are capable of evacuating fluid more efficiently.

The cornea of the eye should appear round and proportionate in size to that of an adult eye. A cornea that appears larger than usual may be the result of congenital glaucoma. An irregularly shaped pupil or discolored iris may denote disease such as a coloboma (see Chapter 50). The pupil should be dark. A white pupil suggests the presence of a congenital cataract.

Ears

A newborn's external ear is not as completely formed as it will be eventually, so the pinna tends to bend easily. In the term newborn, however, the pinna should be strong enough to recoil after bending.

The level of the top part of the external ear should be on a line drawn from the inner canthus to the outer canthus of the eye and back across the side of the head (see Chapter 34). Ears that are set lower than this are found in infants with certain chromosomal abnormalities, particularly trisomy 18 and 13, syndromes in which low-set ears and other physical defects are coupled with varying degrees of cognitive challenge (see Chapters 7 and 54).

A small tag of skin is sometimes found just in front of an ear. Although these tags may be associated with chromosomal abnormalities or kidney disease, they usually are isolated findings that are of no consequence. They can be removed by ligation immediately or when the child is 1 week old. A preauricular dermal sinus may be present directly in front of the ear as well. Always inspect in front of newborns' ears for pinpoint-size openings that reveal these sinuses. The sinus is usually small and can be removed surgically without consequence when the child is near school age.

Visualization of the tympanic membrane of the ear in a newborn is difficult and usually is not attempted, because amniotic fluid and flecks of vernix still fill the canal, obliterating the drum and its accompanying landmarks.

A good practice is to test a newborn's hearing by ringing a bell held about 6 inches from each ear. A hearing infant who is crying will stop momentarily at the sound. If quiet, a newborn who can hear will blink the eyes, appear to attend to the sound, and possibly startle. Although this method of testing is not highly accurate, a negative response (lack of response) is unusual. Infants with negative responses should be retested later. In many health care facilities, all newborns are tested by a commercial standardized response to sound before discharge (AAP, 2007; MacNeil et al., 2007).

Nose

A newborn's nose tends to appear large for the face. As the infant grows, the rest of the face grows more than the nose does, and this discrepancy disappears.

Test for choanal atresia (blockage at the rear of the nose) by closing the newborn's mouth and compressing one naris at a time with your fingers. Note any discomfort or distress while breathing this way. Nasal flaring upon inspiration is another indication of respiratory distress and should be further evaluated. Also record any evidence of milia on the nose.

Mouth

A newborn's mouth should open evenly when he or she cries. If one side of the mouth moves more than the other, cranial nerve injury is suggested. A newborn's tongue appears large and prominent in the mouth. Because the tongue is short, the frenulum membrane is attached close to the tip of the tongue, creating the impression that the infant is "tongue tied." At one time, it was almost routine to snip a newborn's frenulum membrane to lengthen it. Now this procedure is regarded as harmful, because it leaves a portal of entry for infection, risks hemorrhage because of the low level of vitamin K in most newborns, and causes feeding difficulties by making the tongue sore and irritated. This procedure is also unnecessary because, as the tongue grows, the frenulum recedes to its adult placement.

Inspect the palate of a newborn to be sure it is intact. Occasionally, one or two small, round, glistening, well-circumscribed cysts (Epstein's pearls) are present on the palate, a result of extra calcium that was deposited in utero. Be sure to inform parents that these pearl-like cysts are insignificant, require no treatment, and will disappear spontaneously within 1 week. Otherwise, a parent may mistake them for **thrush,** a *Candida* infection, which usually appears on the tongue and sides of the cheeks as white or gray patches and needs therapy with an antifungal drug (Subramanian et al., 2008).

All newborns have some mucus in their mouths. Newborns delivered by cesarean birth usually have an increased amount. If a newborn is placed on the side, the mucus drains from the mouth and results in no distress. If the mouth is filled with so much mucus that a neonate seems to be blowing bubbles, a tracheoesophageal fistula is suspected. This must be confirmed or ruled out before the newborn is fed; otherwise, formula can be aspirated into the lungs from the inadequately formed esophagus.

Small, white epithelial pearls (benign inclusion cysts) may be present on the gum margins. No therapy is necessary for these. It is unusual for a newborn to have teeth, but sometimes one or two (called **natal teeth**) will have erupted. Any teeth that are present must be evaluated for stability. If loose, they should be extracted to prevent possible aspiration during feeding.

Neck

The neck of a newborn is short and often chubby, with creased skin folds. The head should rotate freely on it. If there is rigidity of the neck, congenital torticollis, caused by injury to the sternocleidomastoid muscle during birth, might be present (see Chapter 27). In newborns whose membranes were ruptured more than 24 hours before birth, nuchal rigidity suggests meningitis.

The neck of a newborn is not strong enough to support the total weight of the head but in a sitting position, a newborn should make a momentary effort at head control. When lying prone, newborns can raise the head slightly, usually enough to lift the nose out of mucus or spit-up formula. If they are pulled into a sitting position from a supine position, the head will lag behind considerably. Again, however, they should make some effort to control and steady the head as they reach a sitting position.

The trachea may be prominent on the front of the neck, and the thymus gland may be enlarged because of the rapid growth of glandular tissue (in comparison with other body tissues) early in life. The thymus gland will triple in size by 3 years of age; it remains at that size until the child is about 10 years old, and then shrinks. Although the thymus may appear to be bulging in a newborn, it is rarely a cause of respiratory difficulty, as was once believed.

Chest

The chest in some newborns looks small because the head is large in proportion. It is actually approximately 2 inches smaller in circumference and as wide in the anteroposterior diameter as it is across. Not until a child is 2 years of age does the chest measurement exceed that of the head. The clavicles should be straight. A crepitus or actual separation on one or the other clavicle may indicate that a fracture occurred during birth and calcium is now being deposited at that point. As the area heals, it may be possible to palpate a lump on the clavicle caused by temporary calcium overgrowth. Overall, a newborn's chest should appear symmetric side to side. Respirations are normally rapid (30 to 60 breaths per minute) but not distressed. A supernumerary nipple (usually found below and in line with the normal nipples) may be present. If so, it may be removed later for cosmetic purposes although this is not necessary.

In both female and male infants, the breasts may be engorged. Occasionally, the breasts of newborn babies secrete a thin, watery fluid popularly termed *witch's milk.* Engorgement develops in utero as a result of the influence of the mother's hormones. As soon as the hormones are cleared from the infant's system (about 1 week), the engorgement and any fluid that is present subside. Fluid should never be expressed from infants' breasts, because the manipulation could introduce bacteria and lead to mastitis.

Retraction (drawing in of the chest wall with inspiration) should not be present. An infant with retractions (Fig. 18.16) is using such strong force to pull air into the respiratory tract that he or she is pulling in the anterior chest muscle.

Because a newborn's lung alveoli open slowly over the first 24 to 48 hours and the baby invariably has mucus in the back of the throat, listening to lung sounds often reveals the sounds of rhonchi—the harsh, innocent sound of air passing over mucus. An abnormal sound, such as grunting, suggests respiratory distress syndrome; a high, crowing sound on inspiration suggests stridor or immature tracheal development.

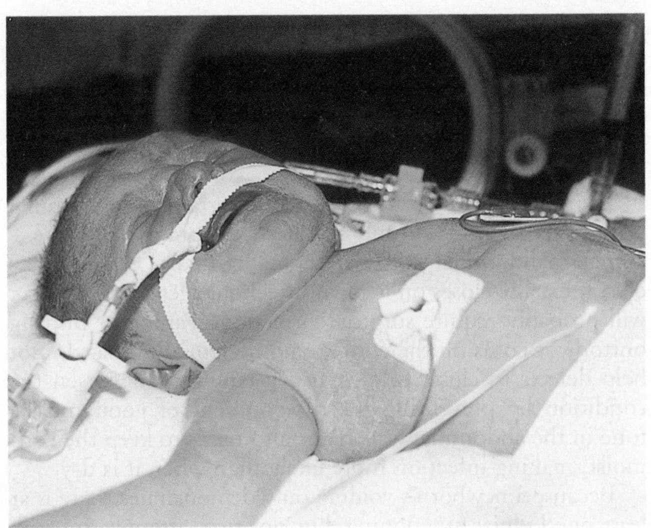

FIGURE 18.16 Sternal retractions are a sign of respiratory distress requiring immediate intervention, such as mechanical ventilation or increased oxygen.

Abdomen

The contour of a newborn abdomen looks slightly protuberant. A scaphoid or sunken appearance may indicate missing abdominal contents or a diaphragmatic hernia (bowel positioned in the chest instead of the abdomen). Bowel sounds should be present within 1 hour after birth. The edge of the liver is usually palpable 1 to 2 cm below the right costal margin. The edge of the spleen may be palpable 1 to 2 cm below the left costal margin. Tenderness is difficult to determine in a newborn. If it is extreme, however, palpation will cause the infant to cry, thrash about, or tense the abdominal muscles to protect the abdomen.

For the first hour after birth, the stump of the umbilical cord appears as a white, gelatinous structure marked with the blue and red streaks of the umbilical vein and arteries. When the cord is first cut, the vessels are counted to be certain that one vein and two arteries are present. In 0.5% of births (3.5% of twin births), there is only a single umbilical artery, and in one-third of such infants, this single artery is associated with a congenital heart or renal abnormality. Because these heart and kidney anomalies may not be readily apparent, any child with a single umbilical artery needs close observation and assessment until anomalies are ruled out.

Inspect the cord clamp to be certain it is secure. After the first hour of life, the cord begins to dry and shrink, and it turns brown like the dead end of a vine. By the second or third day, it has turned black. It breaks free by day 6 to 10, leaving a granulating area a few centimeters wide that heals during the following week.

There should be no bleeding at the cord site. Bleeding suggests that the cord clamp has become loosened or the cord has been tugged loose by the friction of bedclothes. The base of the cord should appear dry. A moist or odorous cord suggests infection. If present, infection should receive immediate treatment or it may enter a newborn's bloodstream and cause septicemia. Moistness at the base of the cord also may indicate a patent urachus (a canal that connects the bladder and the umbilicus), which will drain urine at the cord site until it is surgically repaired.

Inspect the base of the cord to be certain no abdominal wall defect such as an umbilical hernia is present. If there is a fascial (abdominal wall) defect smaller than 2 cm in diameter, it usually closes on its own by school age; a larger defect will probably require surgical correction. Taping or putting buttons or coins on the cord are home remedies that do not help defects to close. In fact, heavy taping may worsen the condition by preventing the development of good muscle tone in the abdominal wall. Tape also tends to keep the cord moist, making infection more likely than when it is dry.

Because a newborn's voiding only demonstrates there is at least one kidney functioning, but not two, attempt to verify the presence of kidneys by deep palpation of the right and left abdomen within the first few hours after birth. After this time, the intestines fill with air, making palpation more difficult. The right kidney (at least its lower pole) can usually be palpated readily, because it is located lower than the left; the left kidney is more difficult to locate, because the intestine is bulkier on the left side and the kidney is higher in the retroperitoneal space. Nonetheless, try to locate both of them. Placing one hand behind the infant while you palpate offers a firmer base and helps when evaluating kidney size (newborn kidneys are about the size of a walnut). An enlarged kidney suggests a polycystic kidney or pooling of urine from a urethral obstruction.

To finish the abdominal assessment, elicit an abdominal reflex. Stroking each quadrant of the abdomen will cause the umbilicus to move or "wink" in that direction. This superficial abdominal reflex is a test of spinal nerves T8–T10. The reflex may not be demonstrable in newborns until the 10th day of life.

Anogenital Area

Inspect the anus of a newborn to be certain it is present, patent, and not covered by a membrane (imperforate anus). Test for anal patency by gently inserting the tip of your gloved and lubricated little finger. Also note the time after birth at which the infant first passes meconium. If a newborn does not do so in the first 24 hours, suspect imperforate anus or meconium ileus.

Male Genitalia

The scrotum in most male newborns is edematous and has rugae (folds in the skin). It may be deeply pigmented in African American or dark-skinned newborns. Make a practice of pressing your nondominant hand against the inguinal ring before palpating for testes, so they do not slip upward and out of the scrotal sac as you palpate (Fig. 18.17).

Both testes should be present in the scrotum. If one or both testicles are not present (cryptorchidism), referral is needed to establish the extent of the problem. This condition could be caused by agenesis (absence of an organ), ectopic testes (the testes cannot enter the scrotum because the opening to the scrotal sac is closed), or undescended testes (the vas deferens or artery is too short to allow the testes to descend).

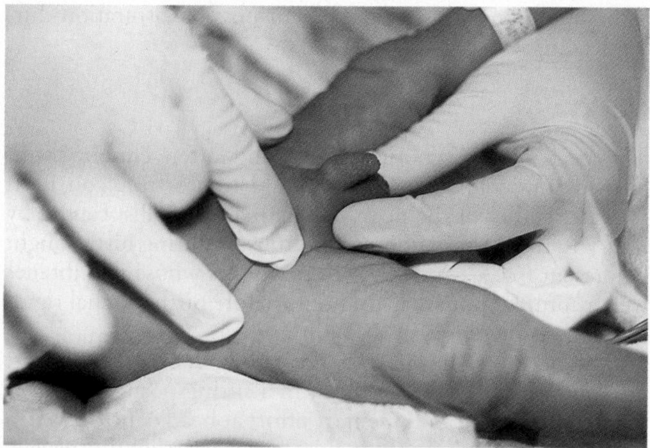

FIGURE 18.17 Press the nondominant hand against the inguinal ring when palpating testes.

Newborns with agenesis of the testes are usually referred for investigation of kidney anomalies, because the testes arise from the same germ tissue as the kidneys.

Elicit a cremasteric reflex by stroking the internal side of the thigh. As the skin is stroked, the testis on that side moves perceptibly upward. This is a test for the integrity of spinal nerves T8–T10. The response may be absent in newborns who are younger than 10 days.

The penis of newborns appears small, approximately 2 cm long. If it is less than this, the newborn should be referred for evaluation by an endocrinologist. Inspect the tip of the penis to see that the urethral opening is at the tip of the glans, not on the dorsal surface (epispadias) or on the ventral surface (hypospadias).

In most newborns, the prepuce (foreskin) slides back poorly from the meatal opening, so this should not be done. Although today most male newborns are circumcised, the necessity for this operation can be questioned unless it is for religious reasons, because it is rare to find an infant who physically requires it (i.e., has a foreskin so constricted that it interferes with voiding or circulation). In addition, surgery this early in life poses the risk of hemorrhage and infection. Circumcision should not be done if hypospadias or epispadias is present, because the surgeon may want to use the foreskin as tissue when repairing these conditions (see Chapter 46).

Female Genitalia

The vulva in female newborns may be swollen because of the effect of maternal hormones. Some female newborns have a mucus vaginal secretion, which is sometimes blood-tinged **(pseudomenstruation).** Again, this is caused by the action of maternal hormones. The discharge disappears as soon as the infant's system has cleared the hormones. The discharge should not be mistaken for an infection or taken as an indication that trauma has occurred.

Back

The spine of a newborn typically appears flat in the lumbar and sacral areas. The curves seen in an adult appear only after a child is able to sit and walk. Inspect the base of a newborn's spine carefully to be sure there is no pinpoint opening, dimpling, or sinus tract in the skin, which would suggest a dermal sinus or spinal bifida occulta. True neural tube defects in newborns are greatly decreased in incidence because of the recognition that lack of folic acid during pregnancy leads to these (De Wals et al., 2007).

A newborn normally assumes the position maintained in utero, with the back rounded and the arms and legs flexed on the abdomen and chest. A child who was born in a frank breech position tends to straighten the legs at the knee and bring their feet up next to the face. The position of a baby with a face presentation sometimes simulates opisthotonos for the first week, because the curve of the back is deeply concave.

Extremities

The arms and legs of a newborn appear short. The hands are plump and clenched into fists. Newborn fingernails are soft and smooth, and usually long enough to extend over the fingertips. Test the upper extremities for muscle tone by unflexing the arms for approximately 5 seconds. If tone is good, an arm should return immediately to its flexed position after being released. Hold the arms down by the sides and note their length. The fingertips should reach the proximal thigh. Unusually short arms may signify achondroplastic dwarfism. Observe for unusual curvature of the little finger, and inspect the palm for a simian crease (a single palmar crease, in contrast to the three creases normally seen in a palm). Although curved fingers and simian creases can occur normally, they are commonly associated with Down syndrome (Elias, Chun-Hui, & Manchester, 2008).

A newborn's arms and legs should move symmetrically (unless the infant is demonstrating a tonic neck reflex). An arm that hangs limp and unmoving suggests possible birth injury, such as injury to a clavicle or to the brachial or cervical plexus or fracture of a long bone. Assess for webbing (syndactyly), extra toes or fingers (polydactyly), or unusual spacing of toes, particularly between the big toes and the others (this finding is present in certain chromosomal disorders, although it is also a normal finding in some families). Test to see whether the toenails fill immediately after blanching from pressure.

Normally, newborn legs are bowed as well as short. The sole of the foot appears flat because of an extra pad of fat in the longitudinal arch. The foot of a term newborn has many crisscrossed lines on the sole, covering approximately two-thirds of the foot. If these creases cover less than two-thirds of the foot or are absent, suspect immaturity.

Move the ankle through a range of motion to evaluate whether the heel cord is unusually tight. Check for ankle clonus by supporting the lower leg in one hand and dorsiflexing the foot sharply two or three times by pressure on the sole of the foot with the other hand. After the dorsiflexion, one or two continued movements are normal. Rapid alternating contraction and relaxation (clonus) is abnormal, suggesting neurologic involvement. The feet of many newborns turn in (varus deviation) because of their former intrauterine position. This simple deviation needs no correction if the feet can be brought into the midline position by easy manipulation. When the infant begins to bear weight, the feet will align themselves. If a foot does not align readily (will not turn to a definite midline position), a talipes deformity (clubfoot) may be present. This condition needs further investigation, because congenital problems of this kind are best treated in the immediate newborn period.

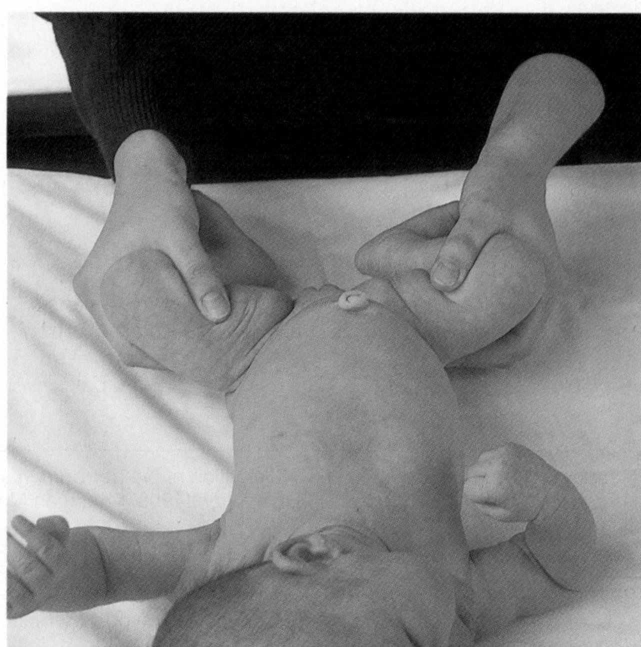

FIGURE 18.18 Hip abduction in a newborn—both hips should abduct so completely they lie almost flat against the mattress (180 degrees).

With a newborn in a supine position, both hips can be flexed and abducted to such an extent (180 degrees) that the knees touch or nearly touch the surface of the bed (Fig. 18.18). If the hip joint seems to lock short of this distance (160 to 170 degrees), hip subluxation (a shallow and poorly formed acetabulum) is suggested (McCarthy & MacEwen, 2007). A further test for subluxation can be elicited by holding the infant's leg with the fingers on the greater and lesser trochanter and then abducting the hip; if subluxation is present, a "clunk" of the femur head striking the shallow acetabulum can be heard (Ortolani's sign). If the hip can be felt to actually slip in the socket, this is Barlow's sign. Subluxated hip may be bilateral but is usually unilateral. It is important that hip subluxation be discovered as early as possible, because correction is most successful if it is initiated early.

When lying on the abdomen, newborns are capable of bringing their arms and legs underneath them and raising their stomach off the bed high enough for a hand to be slipped underneath. This ability helps to prevent pressure or rubbing at the cord site, because the cord does not actually touch the bedding when in this position. The preterm newborn does not have this ability, so it is an indication of maturity.

ASSESSMENT FOR WELL-BEING

There are several traditional standardized assessments to evaluate a newborn quickly at birth.

Apgar Scoring

At 1 minute and 5 minutes after birth, newborns are observed and rated according to an Apgar score, an assessment scale used as a standard since 1958 (Apgar et al., 1958). As shown in Table 18.2, heart rate, respiratory effort, muscle

TABLE 18.2 ✻ Apgar Scoring Chart

Sign	Score 0	1	2
Heart rate	Absent	Slow (<100)	>100
Respiratory effort	Absent	Slow, irregular; weak cry	Good; strong cry
Muscle tone	Flaccid	Some flexion of extremities	Well flexed
Reflex irritability:			
Response to catheter in nostril, *or*	No response	Grimace	Cough or sneeze
Slap to sole of foot	No response	Grimace	Cry and withdrawal of foot
Color	Blue, pale	Body normal pigment, extremities blue	Normal skin coloring

Source: Apgar, V., et al. (1958). Evaluation of the newborn infant: Second report. *JAMA: Journal of the American Medical Association, 16*(82), 1985–1988. Copyright 1958, American Medical Association.

tone, reflex irritability, and color of the infant are each rated 0, 1, or 2; the five scores are then added. A newborn whose total score is less than 4 is in serious danger of respiratory or cardiovascular failure and needs resuscitation. A score of 4 to 6 means that the infant's condition is guarded and the baby may need clearing of the airway and supplementary oxygen. A score of 7 to 10 indicates that the infant scored as high as 70% to 90% of all infants at 1 to 5 minutes after birth or is adjusting well to extrauterine life (10 is the highest score possible). The Apgar score is repeated every additional 5 minutes, until a minimum score of 7 is reached.

The Apgar score standardizes infant assessment at birth and serves as a baseline for future evaluations. There is a high correlation between low 5-minute Apgar scores and neurologic illness (Harrington et al., 2007). The following points should be considered in obtaining an Apgar rating.

Heart Rate

Auscultating a newborn heart with a stethoscope is the best way to determine heart rate; however, heart rate also may be obtained by observing and counting the pulsations of the cord at the abdomen if the cord is still uncut. Once the cord has been cut and clamped, a pulse may often be palpated by placing an index finger and thumb at the base of the cord.

Respiratory Effort

Respirations are counted by watching respiratory movements. A mature newborn usually cries and aerates the lungs spontaneously at about 30 seconds after birth. By 1 minute, he or she is maintaining regular, although rapid, respirations. A depressed respiratory effort might be anticipated in a newborn whose mother received large amounts of analgesia or a general anesthetic during labor or birth.

Muscle Tone

Mature newborns hold their extremities tightly flexed, simulating their intrauterine position. Muscle tone is tested by observing their resistance to any effort to extend their extremities. Poor muscle tone is observed when the infant shows no flexion of the arms and legs and extremities "flop" back to the mattress when manipulated or flexed.

Reflex Irritability

One of two possible cues is used to evaluate reflex irritability in a newborn: response to a suction catheter in the nostrils or response to having the soles of the feet slapped. A good response to these actions would be vigorous crying or a strong facial grimace. A baby whose mother was heavily sedated will probably demonstrate a low score in this category.

Color

All infants appear cyanotic at the moment of birth. They grow pink with or shortly after the first breath, which makes the color of newborns correspond to how well they are breathing. Acrocyanosis (cyanosis of the hands and feet) is so common in newborns that a score of 1 in this category can be thought of as normal.

Respiratory Evaluation

Good respiratory function obviously has the highest priority in newborn care, so assessment for it is ongoing at every newborn contact. The Silverman and Andersen index, originally devised in 1956 (Silverman & Andersen, 1956), can be used to estimate degrees of respiratory distress in newborns. For this assessment, a newborn is observed and then scored on each of five criteria (Fig. 18.19). Each item is given a value of 0, 1, or 2; the values are then added. A total score of 0 indicates no respiratory distress. Scores of 4 to 6 indicate moderate distress. Scores of 7 to 10 indicate severe distress. Notice that the scores of this index run opposite to those of the Apgar: an Apgar score of 7 to 10 would indicate a well infant.

✔ Checkpoint Question 18.4

Beth Ruiz had Apgar scores of 6 and 8. The five areas assessed with Apgar scoring are:

a. Heart rate, respiratory effort, muscle tone, reflex irritability, and color.
b. Respiratory rate, abdominal tone, reflex irritability, color, and head circumference.
c. Color, breathing rate, cry, amount of brown fat, and response to an adult voice.
d. Abdominal tone, persistence, gastric acidity, arterial pressure, and response to pain.

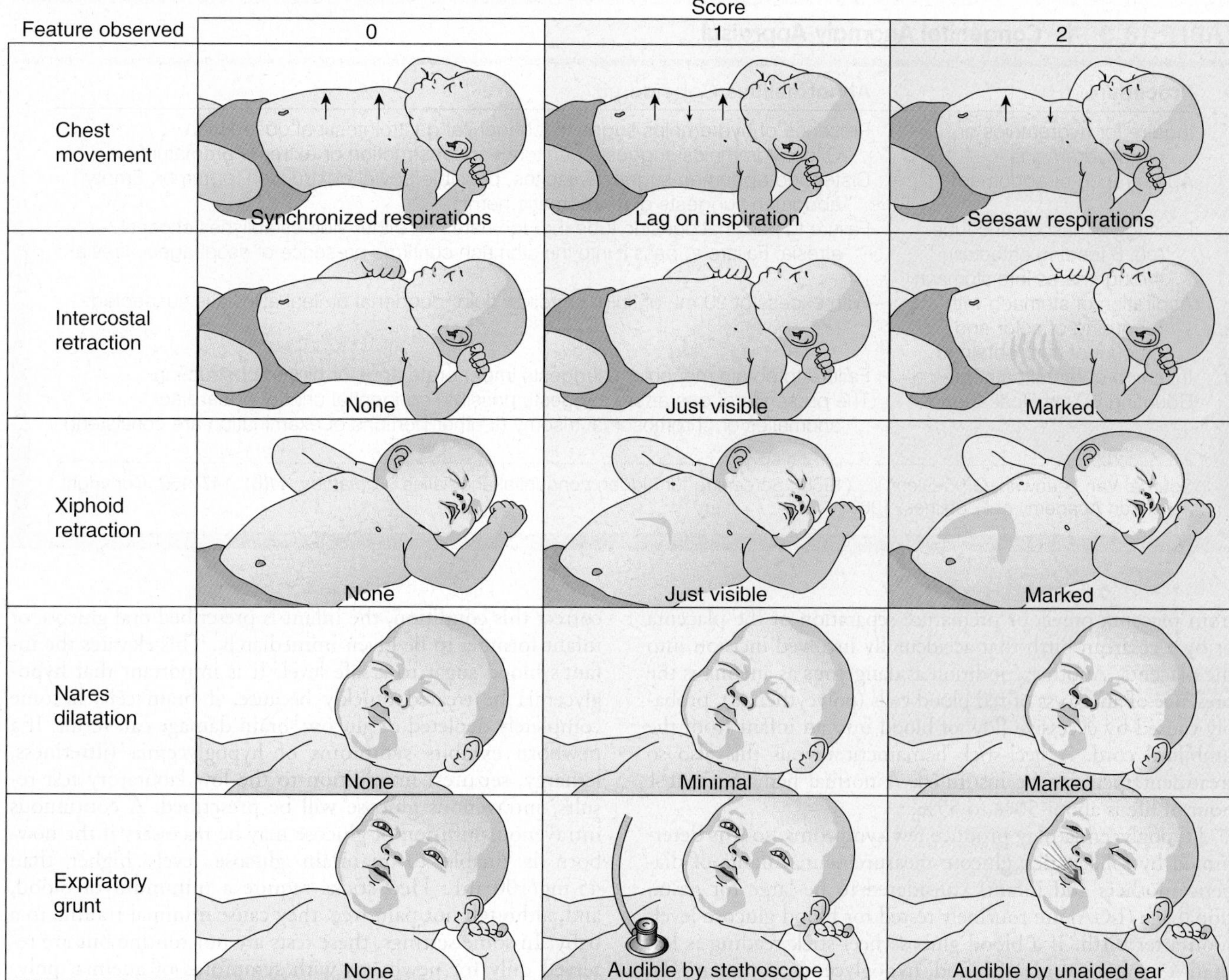

FIGURE 18.19 Grading of neonatal respiratory distress based on Silverman-Andersen index. (Silverman, W. A., & Andersen, D. H. [1956]. A controlled clinical trial of effects of water mist on obstructive respiratory signs, death rate and necroscopy findings among premature infants. *Pediatrics, 17*[4], 1–9.)

Physical Examination

A newborn is given a preliminary physical examination immediately after birth, to establish gestational age and to detect any observable condition such as difficulty breathing, a congenital heart anomaly, meningocele, cleft lip or palate, hydrocephalus, a birthmark, imperforate anus, tracheoesophageal atresia, or bowel obstruction (Table 18.3). This assessment may be the responsibility of the delivering physician, nurse practitioner, nurse-midwife, pediatrician, or nurse. This health assessment is done quickly, to prevent overexposing a newborn, yet not so swiftly that important findings are overlooked.

Height and Weight

Assuming newborns are breathing well, they are weighed nude and without a blanket soon after birth in the birthing room (Fig. 18.20). Measurements such as body length and head, chest, and abdominal circumferences can be obtained later. Performing these measurements while an infant is still damp only exposes the newborn unnecessarily to chilling.

A newborn's weight is important because it helps to determine maturity as well as establish a baseline against which all other weights can be compared. Following this initial weight, an infant is weighed nude once a day, at approximately the same time every day, during a hospital or birthing center stay. Compare the weight obtained each day with that of the preceding day to be certain an infant is not losing more than the normal physiologic amount (5% to 10% of birth weight). Abnormal loss of weight may be the first indication that a newborn has an inborn error of metabolism, such as adrenocortical insufficiency (salt-dumping type), or is becoming dehydrated.

Laboratory Studies

After the first hour of undisturbed rest, depending on health agency policy, newborns may have heel-stick tests for hematocrit, hemoglobin, and hypoglycemia determinations. Hematocrit and hemoglobin are assessed to detect newborn anemia that can be caused by hypovolemia because of bleeding

TABLE 18.3 ✻ Congenital Anomaly Appraisal

Procedure	Abnormalities Considered
Inquire for hydramnios or oligohydramnios	Presence of hydramnios suggests congenital gastrointestinal obstruction. Oligohydramnios suggests genitourinary obstruction or extreme prematurity.
Appearance of abdomen	Distended abdomen suggests ascites, possible bowel obstruction, or tumor. Empty abdomen suggests diaphragmatic hernia.
Passage of nasogastric tube (no. 8 feeding catheter) through nares into stomach	Failure to pass nasogastric tube through nares on either side establishes choanal atresia. Failure to pass it into the stomach confirms presence of esophageal atresia.
Aspiration of stomach with recording of color and amount of fluid obtained	With excess of 20 mL of fluid, or yellow fluid, duodenal or ileal atresia is suspected.
Insertion of rectal catheter	Failure to obtain meconium suggests imperforate anus or higher obstruction.
Counting of umbilical arteries	The presence of one artery suggests possible congenital urinary or cardiac anomalies or chromosomal trisomy (if other portions of examination are consistent).

Source: Van Leeuwen, G., & Glenn, L. (1968). Screening for hidden congenital anomalies. *Pediatrics, 41*(6), 147–152. Copyright American Academy of Pediatrics, 1968.

from placenta previa or premature separation of the placenta or by a cesarean birth that accidentally involved incision into the placenta. Another condition as dangerous as anemia is the presence of an excess of red blood cells (polycythemia), probably caused by excessive flow of blood into an infant from the umbilical cord. A heel-stick hematocrit reveals this also so treatment then can be instituted. A normal hematocrit at 1 hour of life is about 50% to 55%.

Hypoglycemia may produce few symptoms, so it is determined by a heel-stick glucose measurement. Infants of diabetic mothers and infants considered to be large for gestational age (LGA) are routinely tested for blood glucose levels soon after birth. If a blood glucose heel-stick reading is less than 45 mg/100 mL of blood, hypoglycemia is present. To correct this condition, the infant is prescribed oral glucose or infant formula to be given immediately. This elevates the infant's blood sugar to a safe level. It is important that hypoglycemia be treated quickly because, if brain cells become completely depleted of glucose, brain damage can result. If a newborn exhibits symptoms of hypoglycemia (jitteriness, lethargy, seizures) in addition to the low laboratory test results, intravenous glucose will be prescribed. A continuous intravenous infusion of glucose may be necessary if the newborn is unable to maintain glucose levels higher than 45 mg/100 mL. Heel-sticks require a minimum of blood, and, although not pain free, they cause minimal trauma to a baby. In some settings, these tests are not routine but are reserved only for newborns with symptoms of anemia, polycythemia, or hypoglycemia.

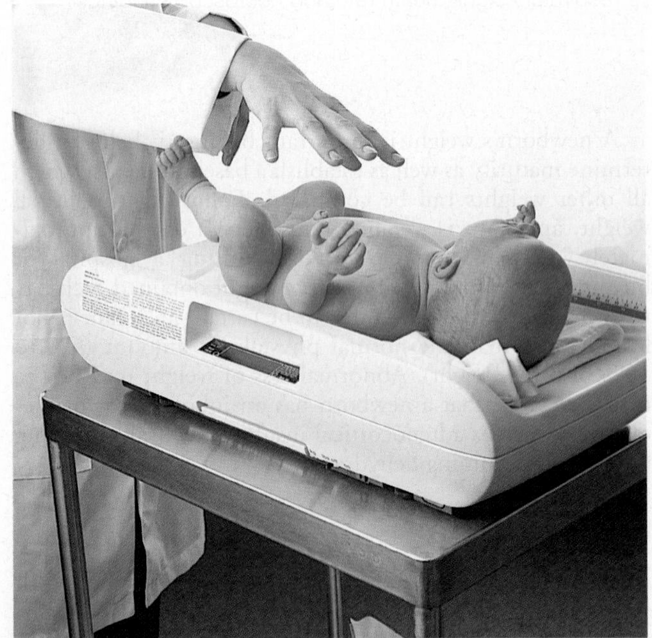

FIGURE 18.20 Weighing a newborn. Notice the protective hand held over the infant.

Assessment of Gestational Age

Specific findings on physical assessment provide clues to a newborn's gestational age. As early as 1966, Usher and colleagues (1966) proposed five criteria to evaluate gestational maturity (Table 18.4). These quick criteria can be used for assessment of all newborns.

Dubowitz Maturity Scale

Dubowitz and colleagues (1970) devised a gestational rating scale that uses more extensive criteria. All newborns appearing to be immature by Usher's criteria or who are light in weight at birth or early by dates should be assessed by means of these more definitive criteria. Although completing a Dubowitz assessment takes practice, it can yield important results; it can help determine whether a newborn needs immediate high-risk nursery intervention.

During the 1970s and again in the 1990s, Ballard modified the Dubowitz scale (Ballard et al., 1991) to an assessment scale that can be completed in 3 to 4 minutes. The assessment consists of two portions: physical maturity and neuromuscular maturity (Fig. 18.21). The first is a series of observations about skin texture, color, lanugo, foot creases, genitalia, ear, and breast maturity. Each designated body part is inspected and

TABLE 18.4 ✻ Clinical Criteria for Gestational Assessment

	Gestation Age (wk)		
Finding	***0–36***	***37–38***	***39 and Over***
Sole creases	Anterior transverse crease only	Occasional creases in anterior two thirds	Sole covered with creases
Breast nodule diameter (mm)	2	4	7
Scalp hair	Fine and fuzzy	Fine and fuzzy	Coarse and silky
Ear lobe	Pliable; no cartilage	Some cartilage	Stiffened by thick cartilage
Testes and scrotum	Testes in lower canal; scrotum small; few rugae	Intermediate	Testes pendulous, scrotum full; extensive rugae

Source: Usher, R., et al. (1966). Judgment of fetal age. *Pediatric Clinics of North America, 13*(4), 835–840.

A

	0	1	2	3	4	5
SKIN	gelatinous red, transparent	smooth pink, visible veins	superficial peeling &/or rash, few veins	cracking pale area, rare veins	parchment, deep cracking, no vessels	leathery, cracked, wrinkled
LANUGO	none	abundant	thinning	bald areas	mostly bald	
PLANTAR CREASES	no crease	faint red marks	anterior transverse crease only	creases ant. 2/3	creases cover entire sole	
BREAST	barely percept.	flat areola, no bud	stippled areola, 1–2 mm bud	raised areola, 3–4 mm bud	full areola, 5–10 mm bud	
EAR	pinna flat, stays folded	sl. curved pinna, soft with slow recoil	well-curv. pinna, soft but ready recoil	formed & firm with instant recoil	thick cartilage, ear stiff	
GENITALS Male	scrotum empty, no rugae		testes descending, few rugae	testes down, good rugae	testes pendulous, deep rugae	
GENITALS Female	prominent clitoris & labia minora		majora & minora equally prominent	majora large, minora small	clitoris & minora completely covered	

B

	0	1	2	3	4	5
Posture						
Square Window (Wrist)	90°	60°	45°	30°	0°	
Arm Recoil	180°		100°-180°	90°-100°	<90°	
Popliteal Angle	180°	160°	130°	110°	90°	<90°
Scarf Sign						
Heel to Ear						

C

Score	Wks
5	26
10	28
15	30
20	32
25	34
30	36
35	38
40	40
45	42
50	44

FIGURE 18.21 Ballard's assessment of gestational age criteria. (**A**) Physical maturity assessment criteria. (**B**) Neuromuscular maturity assessment criteria. *Posture:* With infant supine and quiet, score as follows: arms and legs extended = 0; slight or moderate flexion of hips and knees = 2; legs flexed and abducted, arms slightly flexed = 3; full flexion of arms and legs = 4. *Square Window:* Flex hand at the wrist. Exert pressure sufficient to get as much flexion as possible. The angle between hypothenar eminence and anterior aspect of forearm is measured and scored. Do not rotate wrist. *Arm Recoil:* With infant supine, fully flex forearm for 5 sec, then fully extend by pulling the hands and release. Score as follows: remain extended or random movements = 0; incomplete or partial flexion = 2; brisk return to full flexion = 4. *Popliteal Angle:* With infant supine and pelvis flat on examining surface, flex leg on thigh and fully flex thigh with one hand. With the other hand, extend leg and score the angle attained according to the chart. *Scarf Sign:* With infant supine, draw infant's hand across the neck and as far across the opposite shoulder as possible. Assistance to elbow is permissible by lifting it across the body. Score according to location of the elbow: elbow reaches opposite anterior axillary line = 0; elbow between opposite anterior axillary line and midline of the thorax = 1; elbow at midline of thorax = 2; elbow does not reach midline of thorax = 3; elbow at proximal axillary line = 4. *Heel to Ear:* With infant supine, hold infant's foot with one hand and move it as near to the head as possible without forcing it. Keep pelvis flat on examining surface. (**C**) Scoring for a Ballard assessment scale. The point total from assessment is compared to the left column. The matching number in the right column reveals the infant's age in gestation weeks. (From Ballard, J. L. [1991]. New Ballard score expanded to include extremely premature infants. *Journal of Pediatrics, 119*[3], 417–424.)

given a score of 0 to 5, as described in Figure 18.21A. This observational scoring should be done as soon as possible after birth, because skin assessment becomes much less reliable after 24 hours. Illustrations of mature and immature body features for Ballard scale use are shown in Chapter 26 as part of the discussion of the preterm infant.

To complete the second half of the gestational examination, observe or position a newborn as shown in Figure 18.21B. Again, score the child's response numerically from 0 to 5.

To establish a baby's gestational age, the total score obtained (on both sections) is compared with the rating scale in Figure 18.21C. An infant with a total score of 5 is at 26 weeks' gestational age; a total score of 10 reveals a gestational age of about 28 weeks; a total score of 40 points is found in infants at term or 40 weeks' gestation.

Using such a standard method to rate maturity is helpful in detecting infants who are small for gestational age (they are light in weight, but the neuromuscular and physical observation scales are adequate for their weeks in utero) and differentiating them from newborns who are immature because of a miscalculated due date. An infant who is found to be less than 35 weeks' gestation requires close observation, usually in a special care nursery.

Assessment of Behavioral Capacity

Term newborns are physically active and emotionally prepared to interact with the people around them. They are people oriented from the beginning—how much so can be demonstrated by the way they immediately attune to human voices or concentrate on their mother's face (Fig. 18.22).

Brazelton Neonatal Behavioral Assessment Scale

The *Brazelton Neonatal Behavioral Assessment Scale* is a rating scale devised by Brazelton in the early 1970s (Brazelton, 1973) to evaluate a newborn's behavioral capacity or ability to respond to set stimuli. Six major categories of behavior—habituation, orientation, motor maturity, variation, self-quieting ability, and social behavior—are assessed.

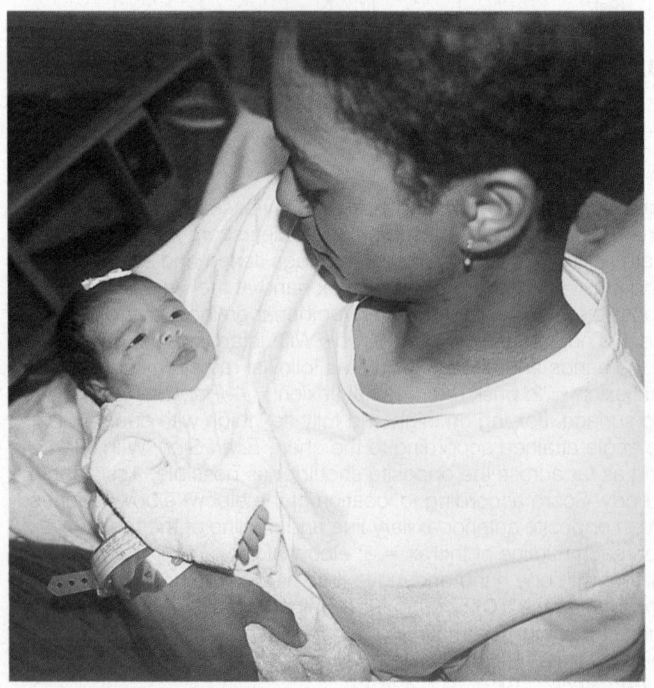

FIGURE 18.22 A newborn recognizes her parent's face.

To perform an assessment using the scale requires training to ensure that it is used consistently from one individual to another. Unlike many assessment scales, the infant is scored on best performance rather than on average performance. A total evaluation takes 20 to 30 minutes to complete. It is useful for comparing different groups of infants, such as those exposed or not exposed to cocaine in utero (Richardson, Goldschmidt, & Larkby, 2007).

The information supplied by this scale has provided concrete evidence that newborns are not passive, nonhearing, unseeing, unresponsive, or even all alike. An important finding from the scale is that newborns are able to quiet themselves after crying. Many of the items tested on the scale, such as how infants alert (eyes widen, head held as if listening) or orient to sound (turn toward the direction of the parent's voice or appear to listen to the sound of a voice) and how they naturally cuddle when held next to their parent, are excellent examples of newborn behavior to point out to parents. If parents perceive a newborn as passive and unresponsive, they are likely to talk to or look at their newborn very little. The more they know about their baby, the more they will be able to understand the baby's cues and determine and meet the baby's needs. Performing a Brazelton assessment and pointing out positive infant behavior can lead to improved parenting ability.

CARE OF A NEWBORN AT BIRTH

Birthing rooms provide an island for newborn care separate from the supplies needed for the mother's care. Necessary equipment includes a radiant heat table or warmed bassinet; a warm, soft blanket; and equipment for oxygen administration, resuscitation, suction, eye care, identification, and weighing of a newborn.

The philosophy of health care providers has always been that newborns should be handled as gently at birth as they are at any other time. The image of an obstetrician holding a newborn up by the heels and spanking to stimulate breathing has existed only in movies. It has long been accepted that holding a baby by the feet and letting the back extend fully is probably painful after the months spent in a flexed position in utero; in addition, a measure such as spanking is not as effective in helping a newborn breathe as is gentle stimulation, such as rubbing the back.

Newborn Identification and Registration

Infant identification is important, because there always exists the possibility that a newborn may be handed to the wrong parents or be switched or kidnapped from a health care facility, although these events are rare. The profile of a newborn kidnapper is a woman who has recently lost a pregnancy or had an infant stillborn and therefore desires an infant very much. She often is someone familiar with hospitals; she pretends to be a volunteer or an unlicensed health care worker and says she needs to take a baby out of the nursery or the mother's room for a procedure. Health care agency personnel need to be alert to the potential danger of kidnapping, and not only take measures to prevent this from happening but also alert parents to the danger (Box 18.3).

BOX 18.3 * Focus on Family Teaching

Measures to Help Prevent Kidnapping From a Hospital Unit

Q. Beth's mother tells you, "I've heard babies are being kidnapped from hospitals. How can we make sure this doesn't happen to us?"

A. Although kidnapping is rare, it can happen. To minimize the risk, use the following guidelines:

- Review the hospital's newborn identification procedure with a nurse so you are familiar with it and can feel comfortable with the safeguards being taken.
- Check that identification bands are in place on your infant as you care for her. These can slide off easily over small newborn hands and feet. If a band or necklace is missing, ask a nurse to replace it immediately.
- Do not allow any person without proper hospital identification to remove your baby from your room.
- Do not leave your baby unattended in your room. Either return the baby to the nursery or take your baby with you if you are leaving your room to walk in the hall, for example.
- Report the presence of any suspicious person in the unit.
- Be aware that some hospitals use a microchip system embedded in identification bands, similar to the tag used to thwart shoplifting in department stores, that sounds an alarm if a baby is removed from the unit. If this type of band is used, be certain it is removed before hospital discharge, or it will set off the alarm.

Identification Band

One traditional form of identification used with newborns is a plastic bracelet with permanent locks that require cutting to be removed. A number that corresponds to the mother's hospital number, the mother's full name, and the sex, date, and time of the infant's birth are printed on the band. If an identification band is attached to a newborn's arm or leg, two bands should be used. This is because a newborn's wrist and hand, as well as the ankle and foot, are not very different in width, and bands can slide off easily. A newer form of identification band has a built-in sensor unit that sounds an alarm, similar to those attached to clothing in department stores to stop shoplifting, if a baby is transported beyond set hospital boundaries (Fig. 18.23).

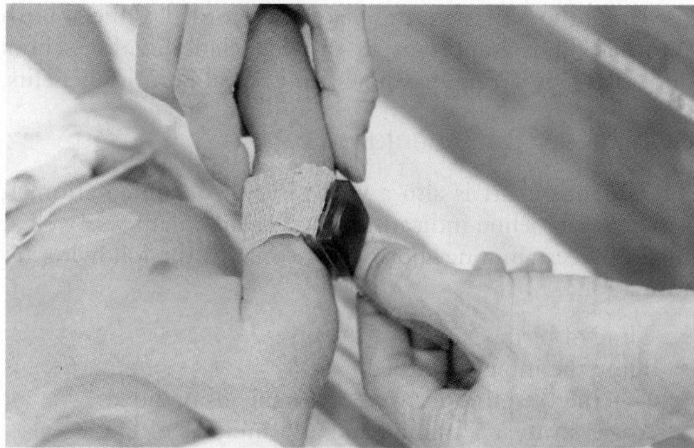

FIGURE 18.23 This newborn is wearing a security band, which sets off an alarm and locks exits if an infant is taken off the unit.

After identification bands are attached, an infant's footprints may be taken (Fig. 18.24A) and thereafter kept with the baby's chart for permanent identification (see Fig. 18.24B). Babies who are born elsewhere and then admitted to the hospital should have their footprints taken and identification band secured on admission.

Birth Registration

The physician or nurse-midwife who supervised the birth of an infant has the responsibility to see that a birth registration is filed with the Bureau of Vital Statistics of the state in which the infant was born. The infant's name, the mother's name, the father's name (if the mother chooses to reveal

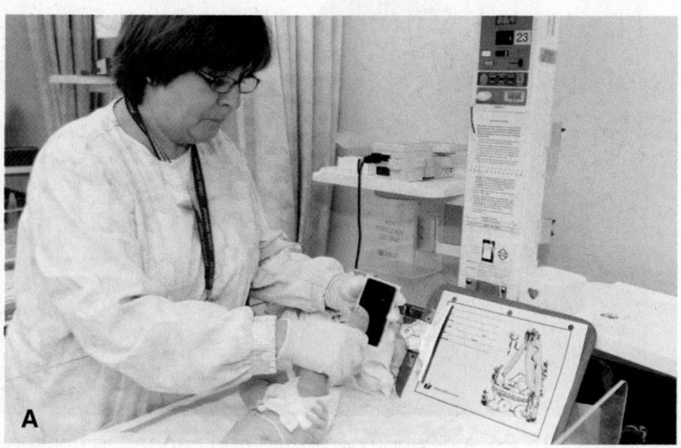

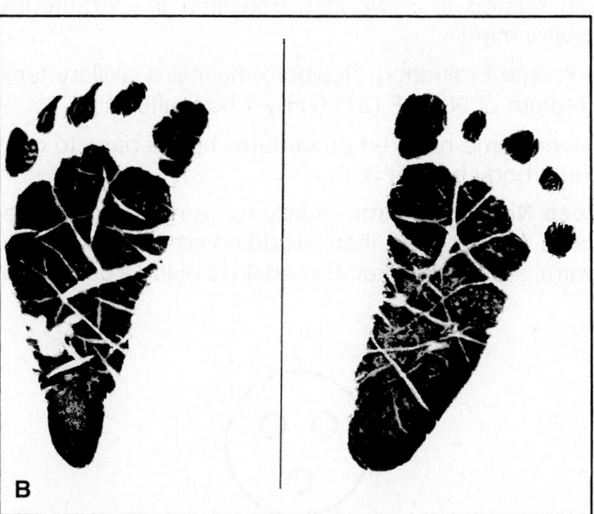

FIGURE 18.24 (**A**) Footprinting a newborn for identification. (**B**) Newborn footprints.

this), and the birth date and place are recorded. Official birth information is important in proving eligibility for school and, later, for voting, passports, and Social Security benefits.

Birth Record Documentation

The infant's chart is also a vital piece of documentation. It serves as a baseline indicating whether the infant was well at birth. Be certain a newborn chart contains the following information:

- Time of birth
- Time the infant breathed
- Whether respirations were spontaneous or aided
- Apgar score at 1 minute and at 5 minutes of life
- Whether eye prophylaxis was given
- Whether vitamin K was administered
- General condition of the infant
- Number of vessels in the umbilical cord
- Whether cultures were taken (they are taken if at some point sterile birth technique was broken or the mother has a history of vaginal or uterine infection)
- Whether the infant voided and whether he or she passed a stool (this information is helpful if, later on, the diagnosis of bowel obstruction or absence of a kidney is considered)

Many nurses indicate a three-vessel cord with the symbol shown in Figure 18.25. Do not mistake this drawing for a "smiling face" and assume that it is not important.

Nursing Diagnoses and Related Interventions

In most health care facilities, the physician or nurse-midwife hands the newborn to a nurse moments after birth to begin care. Be certain to adhere to standard infection precautions when caring for newborns. To avoid touching the vernix caseosa, wear gloves. Hold a warm, sterile blanket and grasp the infant through the blanket by placing one hand under the back and the other around a leg. Newborns are slippery because they are wet from amniotic fluid and the vernix.

Nursing Diagnosis: Risk for ineffective thermoregulation related to newborn's transition to extrauterine environment

Outcome Evaluation: Newborn maintains axillary temperature of 98.6° F (37° C) by 1 hour after birth.

Several time-honored procedures help a baby to conserve body heat at birth.

Keep Newborn Warm. Gently rub a newborn dry, remove the wet linen, then swaddle loosely with a clean, warm, and dry blanket. Be certain to place a cap on the infant's head (Fig. 18.26). These actions all help to prevent heat loss. Swaddling helps to mimic the tight confines of the uterus and appears to offer a sense of security as swaddled infants sleep for longer periods (Bregje et al., 2007).

Ask which parent wants to hold the child, and place the infant in the parent's arms as this not only helps conserve heat but also encourages bonding. The period immediately after birth is an important time for parents to begin interaction with their child. Newborns are alert (first period of activity) and respond well to the parents' first tentative touches or interactions with them. Although the temperature of newborns who are dried, wrapped, and then held by their parents immediately after birth apparently falls slightly lower than that of infants placed in heated cribs, their core temperature does not fall below safe limits. Any extensive procedures, such as resuscitation, should be done under a radiant heat source to reduce heat loss.

At the end of the first hour of life, reassess the newborn's temperature. Axillary rather than rectal temperatures are recommended for newborns, to prevent accidental bowel perforation. If the temperature is subnormal and the baby is in a bassinet, he or she should be placed in a heated bassinet or under a radiant warmer for additional heat. If the temperature is normal, a newborn can be bathed quickly to remove excess vernix caseosa and blood, then dressed in a shirt and diaper, reswaddled in a snug blanket (to give the baby a familiar feeling of the tight confines of the uterus), and placed in a bassinet or returned to the mother's side.

During the first day of life, a newborn's temperature is usually taken every 4 to 8 hours. Thereafter, unless the temperature is elevated or subnormal, or the infant appears to be in distress, measurement once a day while in the health care facility is enough.

Nursing Diagnosis: Risk for ineffective airway clearance related to presence of mucus in mouth and nose at birth

Outcome Evaluation: Neonate maintains a respiratory rate of 30 to 60 breaths per minute without evidence of retraction or grunting by 5 minutes after birth.

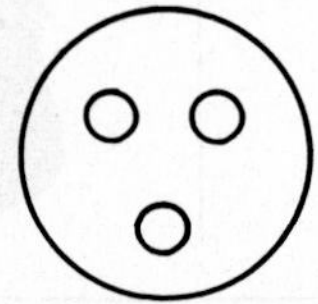

FIGURE 18.25 A chart abbreviation for a three-vessel cord.

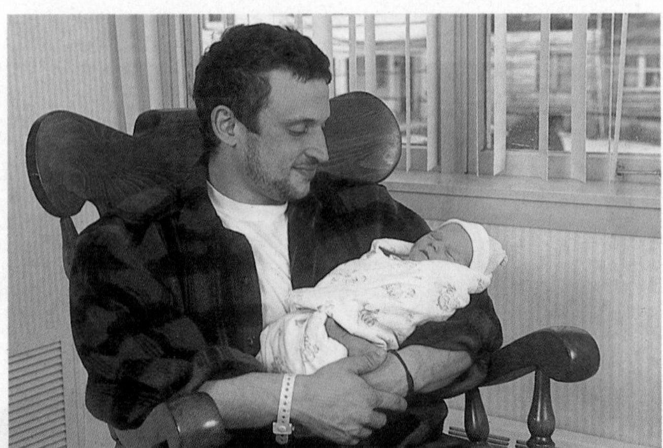

FIGURE 18.26 A newborn wrapped and capped to conserve body heat.

Record the First Cry. A crying infant is a breathing infant, because the sound of crying is made by a current of air passing over the larynx. The more lusty the cry, the greater the assurance the newborn is breathing deeply and forcefully. Vigorous crying also helps blow off the extra carbon dioxide that makes all newborns slightly acidotic, so helps to correct this condition. Although gentleness is necessary to make an infant's transition from intrauterine life to extrauterine life as untraumatic as possible, there is no need to completely halt the initial crying of a newborn.

A newborn who does not breathe spontaneously or who takes a few quick, gasping breaths but is unable to maintain respirations needs resuscitation as an emergency measure. An infant with grunting respirations needs careful observation for respiratory distress syndrome (see Chapter 26).

Promote Adequate Breathing Pattern and Prevent Aspiration. Mucus is suctioned from a newborn's mouth by a bulb syringe as soon as the head is born. As soon as the body is born, the baby should be held for a few seconds with the head slightly dependent, for further drainage of secretions. It is important that mucus be removed from the mouth and pharynx before the first breath this way to prevent aspiration of the secretions. If the infant continues to have an accumulation of mucus in the mouth or nose after these first steps, you may need to suction further after the baby is placed under a warmer (Fig. 18.27). Use a bulb syringe or a soft, small (no. 10 or 12) catheter to suction. Never suction vigorously, because this irritates the mucous membrane and could leave a portal of entry for infection. Brisk suctioning also has been associated with bradycardia in newborns because of vagal nerve stimulation. If you use a bulb syringe, decompress the bulb before inserting it into the infant's mouth or nose; otherwise, the force of decompression will push secretions back into the pharynx or bronchi rather than remove them. Although the effectiveness of the procedure is not well documented, when an infant is born with meconium-stained amniotic fluid, intubation may be performed so that deep tracheal suction can be accomplished before the first breath, to help prevent meconium aspiration (Halliday & Sweet, 2009). Administration of surfactant may also be helpful to assist breathing (El Shahed et al., 2009).

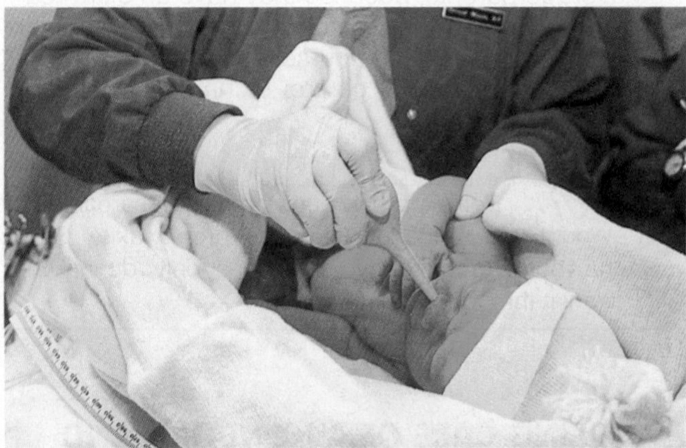

FIGURE 18.27 A newborn is suctioned by means of a bulb syringe to remove mucus from the mouth and nose. The head-down-and-to-the-side position facilitates drainage. Care is given with the infant under a radiant heat source.

Nursing Diagnosis: Risk for infection related to newly clamped umbilical cord and exposure of eyes to vaginal secretions

Outcome Evaluation: Area around cord is dry and free of erythema. Eyes are free of inflammation and drainage. Axillary temperature is maintained between 97.6° and 98.6° F (36.5° and 37° C).

Inspect and Care for Umbilical Cord. The umbilical cord pulsates for a moment after an infant is born as a last flow of blood passes from the placenta into the infant. Two clamps are then applied to the cord about 8 inches from the infant's abdomen, and the cord is cut between the clamps. Some fathers choose to do this as their responsibility. The infant cord is then clamped again by a permanent cord clamp, such as a Hazeltine or a Kane clamp. The clamp on the maternal end of the cord should not be released after the cord is cut, to prevent blood still remaining in the placenta from leaking out. This loss is not important, because the mother's circulation does not connect to the placenta. It is messy, however, and that is why the clamp is left in place.

Every time you handle a newborn, inspect the cord to be certain it is clamped securely. If a clamp loosens before thrombosis obliterates the umbilical vessels, hemorrhage could result. As previously mentioned, the number of cord vessels should be counted and noted immediately after the cord is cut. Cords begin to dry almost immediately, and the vessels may be obscured by the time of the infant's first thorough physical examination in the nursery. Wiping the cord with alcohol at each diaper change helps to hurry drying and possibly reduce the development of infection.

Until the cord falls off, at about day 7 to 10 of life, a newborn should receive sponge baths rather than be immersed in a tub of water to keep the cord dry. Be certain that diapers are folded below the level of the umbilical cord, so that, when the diaper becomes wet, the cord does not become wet also.

Remind parents to continue to keep the cord dry until it falls off after they return home. The use of creams, lotions, and oils near the cord should be discouraged, because they tend to slow drying of the cord and invite infection. Some health care agencies recommend applying rubbing alcohol to the cord site once or twice a day to hasten drying. Others prefer the cord be left strictly alone, because manipulation could invite infection.

After the cord falls off, a small, pink, granulating area about a quarter of an inch in diameter may remain. This should also be left clean and dry until it has healed (about 24 to 48 additional hours). If the ulcerous area has remained as long as 1 week, it may require cautery with silver nitrate to speed healing.

Administer Eye Care. Although the practice may shortly become obsolete (as it is in Europe), every U.S. state still requires that newborns receive prophylactic eye treatment against gonorrheal conjunctivitis (Raab, 2007). Such infections are usually acquired from the mother as the infant passes through the birth canal. Formerly, eye prophylaxis was applied immediately after birth. Many parents today prefer to visit with their infant before the procedure, to be certain their newborn can focus on them without blurry vision caused by ointment or drops. Parents who know that they are free of a gonococcal or chlamydial infection can ask to have eye prophylaxis omitted entirely. Silver nitrate was exclusively used for prophylaxis in the past; today, erythromycin ointment is the drug of choice. Erythromycin ointment has the advantage of eliminating not only the organism of gonorrhea but that of *Chlamydia* as well (Box 18.4).

Always use a single-use tube or package of ointment, to avoid transmitting infection from one newborn to another. To instill the ointment, first dry the face of the newborn with a soft gauze square so that the skin is not slippery. The best procedure to open a newborn's eyes is to shade them from the overhead light and open one eye at a time by pressure on the lower and upper lids. Squeeze a line of ointment along the lower conjunctival sac, from the inner canthus outward, and then close the eye to allow the ointment to spread across the conjunctiva.

Credé, a German gynecologist, first proposed silver nitrate prophylaxis against gonorrheal conjunctivitis in 1884. For this reason, it is often referred to as the *Credé treatment* and may be listed that way on a health care agency form even though silver nitrate is no longer used. Babies born outside hospitals, in homes or in less orthodox settings such as a car or taxi, have the prophylactic treatment administered on admission to the hospital.

BOX 18.4 ✻ Focus on Pharmacology

Erythromycin Ophthalmic Ointment

Classification: Erythromycin ointment is a topical antibiotic.

Action: Erythromycin is effective against gonorrhea and chlamydia organisms, making it the drug of choice for eye prophylaxis at birth (Karch, 2009).

Pregnancy Risk Category: B

Dosage: 0.5–1 cm each eye

Possible Adverse Effects: Mild irritation to conjunctiva; slight blurring of vision.

Nursing Implications

- Use a single-dose application tube.
- After gently pulling down on a newborn's lower eyelid, extrude a line of ointment the length of the lower eyelid from the inner canthus outward.
- Discard any remaining ointment to prevent its being used again.
- Close the child's eyes and count to about 5.
- Wipe away any excess ointment from the child's face.
- If desired, delay application for an hour after birth to allow the infant to view his or her parents clearly.

General Infection Precautions. Each newborn should have his or her own bassinet. Compartments in the bassinet should hold a supply of diapers, shirts, gowns, and individual equipment for bathing and temperature taking. Avoid sharing of these items, which could lead to the spread of infection.

Health care workers, parents, or siblings caring for newborns should wash their hands and arms to the elbows thoroughly with an antiseptic soap before handling an infant. Although not proved to reduce infections, agency personnel are usually required to wear cover gowns or nursery uniforms (Webster & Pritchard, 2009).

Staff members with infections (sore throats, upper respiratory tract infections, skin lesions, or gastrointestinal upsets) should be excluded from caring for mothers or infants until the condition is completely cleared. If a mother could have a contagious illness, her newborn should be excluded from her room until there is no longer a possibility of contagion. An instant photograph can be taken of the baby and shown to the mother so that she can follow the baby's progress. If the infant is breastfed, the mother could manually express milk during the time the infant is excluded, to maintain her milk supply. The mother can resume breastfeeding as soon as it is both possible and safe for her infant.

Any baby born outside a hospital or under circumstances conducive to infection such as rupture of membranes more than 24 hours before birth should be kept in a closed bassinet or in the mother's room until negative cultures show that the newborn is free of infection. Any newborn in whom symptoms of infection develop such as skin lesions or fever should be removed to an isolation nursery or housed in the mother's room to prevent the spread of infection to other babies. There is no reason for parents not to visit a baby housed in isolation care. In fact, they may have more need to hold a baby who is isolated than do average parents, because they have an extra reason to be worried that something is wrong with their child. To visit in isolation nurseries, teach parents to use the same infection control techniques that staff members use.

What if... Beth Ruiz had been born by cesarean birth? Would you still administer eye prophylaxis? Or do newborns acquire eye infections only during their transit through the birth canal?

NURSING CARE OF A NEWBORN AND FAMILY IN THE POSTPARTAL PERIOD

Newborns are usually kept in either a birthing room or a transitional nursery for optimal safety in the first few hours of life.

Newborn care is not universal but varies among cultures. For example, although it is usually a sound policy to point out the positive aspects of a child to parents to aid parent–child bonding, in some areas of the world, such as traditional Cambodia and Laos, newborns are not given compliments this way. It is believed that compliments will leave them vulnerable to evil spirits.

In the traditional Haitian culture, infants are not named immediately, but only after a full month. In some cultures, it is important for newborns to have an amulet (good-luck charm) tied around their neck or wrist. Respect these and leave them in place when bathing the infant. Oiling the infant's body and placing a belly band over the umbilical cord also are common care procedures. Being aware of cultural variations in newborn care such as these helps you plan care that is specific and meaningful to individual parents and can aid parent–child bonding. During this period of close observation, certain principles of care always apply.

Initial Feeding

A term newborn who is to be breastfed may be fed immediately after birth. A baby who is to be formula-fed may receive a first feeding at about 2 to 4 hours of age. Both formula-fed and breastfed infants do best on a demand schedule; many need to be fed as often as every 2 hours in the first few days of life. Chapter 19 covers the elements of breastfeeding and formula feeding in detail. Encouraging women to not only begin breastfeeding but also to continue for a minimum of 6 months is important (Box 18.5).

BOX 18.5 * Focus on Evidence-Based Practice

Does self-efficacy influence whether women continue breastfeeding until 6 months' time?

Many women try breastfeeding in the hospital, then stop breastfeeding shortly after they return home; others continue for the minimum time recommended or until 6 months of age. To discover if a feeling of self-efficacy (the belief that one can bring about positive results) is important in determining whether women will continue breastfeeding, researchers assessed general self-efficacy in 27,753 pregnant women at 17 and 30 weeks during their pregnancy as well as by a questionnaire on infant feeding at 6 months postpartum. Analysis of the results of the study showed that high self-efficacy decreases the chance that mothers bottle feed. It helps them use predominantly breastfeeding. The researchers recommend that discussions of women about breastfeeding during pregnancy and the early postpartum period should include efforts to strengthen self-efficacy as this may be a prime reason why some women continue with breastfeeding.

Based on this study, would you include efforts to increase a mother's self-efficacy when helping her begin breastfeeding?

Source: Ystrom, E., et al. (2008). The impact of maternal negative affectivity and general self-efficacy on breastfeeding. *Journal of Pediatrics, 152*(1), 68–72.

Bathing

In most hospitals, newborns receive a complete bath to wash away vernix caseosa within an hour after birth. Thereafter, they are bathed once a day, although the procedure may be limited to washing only the baby's face, diaper area, and skin folds. Wear gloves when handling newborns until the first bath, to avoid exposing your hands to body secretions; babies of mothers with human immunodeficiency virus (HIV) infection should have a thorough bath immediately, to decrease the possibility of HIV transmission.

Bathing of an infant is best done by the parents under a nurse's supervision. Be sure the room is warm (about 75° F [24° C]), to prevent chilling. Bath water should be approximately 98° to 100° F (37° to 38° C), a temperature that feels pleasantly warm to the elbow or wrist. If soap is used, it should be mild and without a hexachlorophene base. Bathing should take place before, not after, a feeding, to prevent spitting up or vomiting and possible aspiration.

Equipment necessary for an infant's bath consists of a basin of water, soap, washcloth, towel, comb, and clean diaper and shirt. Assemble these items beforehand, so the baby is not left exposed or unattended while you go for more equipment.

Bathing should proceed from the cleanest to the most soiled areas of the body—that is, from the eyes and face to the trunk and extremities and, last, to the diaper area. Wipe a newborn's eyes with clear water from the inner canthus outward, using a clean portion of the washcloth for each eye to prevent spread of infection to the other eye. Wash the face with clear water only (no soap) to avoid skin irritation; soap may be used on the rest of the body.

Teach parents to wash the infant's hair with each bath. The easiest way to do this is to first soap the hair with the baby lying in the bassinet. Then, hold the infant in one arm over the basin of water, as you would a football (Fig. 18.28). Splash water from the basin against the head to rinse the hair. Dry the hair well to prevent chilling.

Wash each area of the baby's body, rinse so no soap is left on the skin (soap is drying and newborns are susceptible to desquamation), and then dry the body part. When you wash the skin around the cord, take care not to soak the cord. Give

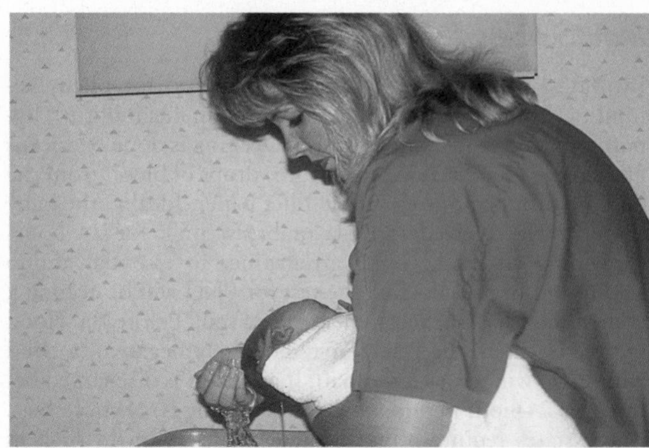

FIGURE 18.28 A football hold. Such a position supports the infant's head and back and leaves the nurse's or mother's other hand free for assembling or using equipment.

particular care to the creases of skin, where milk tends to collect if the child spits up after feedings.

In male infants, the foreskin of the uncircumcised penis should not be forced back, or constriction of the penis may result. Wash the vulva of a female infant, wiping from front to back to prevent contamination of the vagina or urethra by rectal bacteria.

Most health care agencies do not apply powder or lotion to newborns, because some infants are allergic to these products. In addition, many adult talcum powders contain zinc stearate, which is irritating to the respiratory tract; such preparations should always be avoided. If a newborn's skin seems extremely dry and portals for infection are becoming apparent, a lubricant such as Nivea oil, added to the bath water or applied directly to the baby's skin, should relieve the condition.

Sleeping Position

Stress to parents that a newborn should be positioned on the back for sleep. Sudden infant death syndrome (SIDS) is the sudden, unexplained death of an infant younger than 1 year of age. Although the specific cause of SIDS cannot be explained, placing infants to sleep in a supine position with a pacifier has been shown to decrease the incidence of the syndrome (Damato, 2007). As one of the reasons that SIDS may occur is the infant rebreathing expired carbon dioxide–rich air, using a fan in the room during sleep or opening a window so there is a breeze in the room may be yet another way the incidence of SIDS can be reduced (Coleman-Phox, Odouli, & Li, 2008).

Diaper Area Care

Preventing diaper dermatitis is a practice that parents need to start from the very beginning with their newborns. With each diaper change, the area should be washed with clear water and dried well, to prevent the ammonia in urine from irritating the infant's skin and causing a diaper rash. After cleaning, a mild ointment such as petroleum jelly or A+D Ointment may be applied to the buttocks. The ointment keeps ammonia away from the skin and also facilitates the removal of meconium, which is sticky and tarry. Wear gloves for diaper care as part of standard precautions.

Metabolic Screening Tests

By state law, every infant must be screened for phenylketonuria (PKU; a disease of defective protein metabolism), hypothyroidism, and cystic fibrosis. Screening is done by means of a simple blood test in which three drops of blood from the heel are dropped onto a special filter paper. Ideally, the baby should have received formula or breast milk for 24 hours (providing an intake of phenylalanine, an essential amino acid found in milk) before the test for PKU will be accurate. If the infant has not received adequate milk before the blood sample is taken, the results may be falsely negative (a child with PKU will test as if normal). If an infant is discharged before this 24-hour period, a second screening test is necessary. Many states require other metabolic tests at birth, such as screening for galactosemia, cystic fibrosis, and maple syrup urine disease (Kayton, 2007). These also require filter paper blood tests.

If blood testing is not done before discharge, alert the parents that they must schedule the tests to be done at a home health visit or at an ambulatory visit in 2 to 3 days' time. Always assess at the first newborn health supervision visit whether these procedures were done. As with any heel-stick for blood, sampling of this nature is done best by a spring-activated lancet rather than a regular lancet, so that the skin incision is made as quickly and painlessly as possible. Allowing a newborn to suck on a pacifier during painful procedures may be helpful.

Hepatitis B Vaccination

All newborns receive a first vaccination against hepatitis B within 12 hours after birth; a second dose is administered at 1 month and a third at 6 months. Infants whose mothers are positive for the hepatitis B surface antigen (HBsAg) also receive hepatitis B immune globulin (HBIG) at birth (APA, 2009).

Vitamin K Administration

Newborns are at risk for bleeding disorders during the first week of life because their gastrointestinal tract is sterile at birth and unable to produce vitamin K, which is necessary for blood coagulation. A single dose of 0.5 to 1.0 mg of vitamin K is administered intramuscularly within the first hour of life to prevent such problems (Box 18.6). Infants

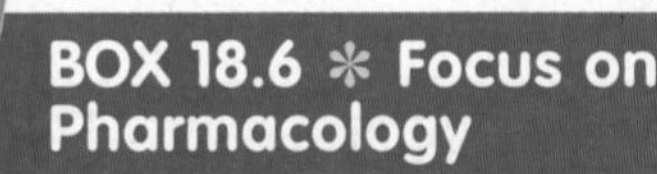

BOX 18.6 ✻ Focus on Pharmacology

Vitamin K (Phytonadione, AquaMEPHYTON)

Action: Vitamin K is used to prevent and treat hemorrhagic disease in newborns. It is a necessary component for the production of certain coagulation factors (II, VII, IX, and X) and is produced by microorganisms in the intestinal tract (Karch, 2009).

Pregnancy risk category: C

Dosage: Prophylaxis—0.5 to 1.0 mg IM one time immediately after birth; treatment of hemorrhagic disease—1 to 2 mg IM or SC daily.

Possible adverse reactions: Local irritation, such as pain and swelling at the site of injection.

Nursing Implications

- Anticipate the need for injection immediately after birth.
- Administer IM injection into large muscle, such as the anterolateral muscle of a newborn's thigh.
- If giving for treatment, obtain prothrombin time before administration (the single best indicator of vitamin K–dependent clotting factors).
- Assess for signs of bleeding, such as black, tarry stools (different from meconium stools, which have a greenish shade), hematuria, decreased hemoglobin and hematocrit levels, and bleeding from any open wounds or base of the cord. (These signs would indicate that more vitamin K is necessary, because bleeding control has not been achieved.)

born outside a hospital also should receive this important protection.

Circumcision

Circumcision is the surgical removal of the foreskin of the penis. In only a few babies, constriction (phimosis) of the foreskin is so severe that it obstructs the urinary meatal opening; otherwise, there are few medical indications for circumcision of a male newborn. Circumcision is performed on Jewish boys on the eighth day of life as part of a religious rite, in a ceremony called a *bris.* In the United States, from the 1920s to the 1960s, circumcision became so popular for aesthetic reasons that most male infants were routinely circumcised at birth. The reasons supporting circumcision include easier hygiene because the foreskin does not have to be retracted during bathing, and possibly fewer urinary tract infections develop. There also may be an increased incidence of penile cancer in uncircumcised men, as well as increased cervical cancer in their sexual partners. However, because the procedure is not essential and does carry some risk, parents need to be well informed about the procedure so they can evaluate carefully whether they wish to have it performed on their son.

Contraindications for circumcision include congenital abnormalities such as hypospadias or epispadias, because the prepuce skin may be needed when a plastic surgeon repairs these defects. Another contradiction is a history of a bleeding tendency in the family.

The procedure is not done immediately after birth, because at that time a newborn's level of vitamin K, which is necessary to prevent hemorrhage, is at a low point and the child would be exposed to unnecessary cold. It is best performed during the first or second day of life, after the baby has synthesized enough vitamin K to reduce the chance of faulty blood coagulation. If parents elect early discharge, they may be asked to return the infant to the hospital or to an ambulatory setting for the surgery. Parents should check that their health insurance plan will reimburse for the procedure if it is done on a return visit, after their newborn has been discharged from the hospital.

For the procedure, an infant is placed in a supine position and restrained either manually or with a commercial swaddling board. In the past the procedure was done without anesthesia, but today use of local or regional block anesthesia to reduce the pain as much as possible is used. Application of EMLA cream (a *e*utectic *m*ixture of *l*ocal *a*nesthetics) is a popular choice for local anesthesia (Taddio, Ohlsson, & Ohlsson, 2009).

For the procedure, a metal clamp (Gomco) or a specially designed plastic bell (Plastibell) is used. If the Gomco clamp is used, the infant's foreskin is stretched over the bell-shaped attachment of the clamp. The foreskin is then cut away with a scalpel. Petrolatum gauze is then wound around the penis to keep the surgical area from sticking to a diaper and to reduce bleeding and the threat of infection.

If a Plastibell is used, it is fitted over the end of the penis. A suture is then tied around the rim of the bell and a circle of the prepuce is cut away so that the foreskin can be easily retracted and the glans will be fully exposed (Fig. 18.29). The rim of the bell, which remains in place for about 1 week and then falls off by itself, protects the healing penis from sticking to a diaper, and helps protect against infection and bleeding. Although not necessary with the bell rim in place, petrolatum ointment may be applied if desired.

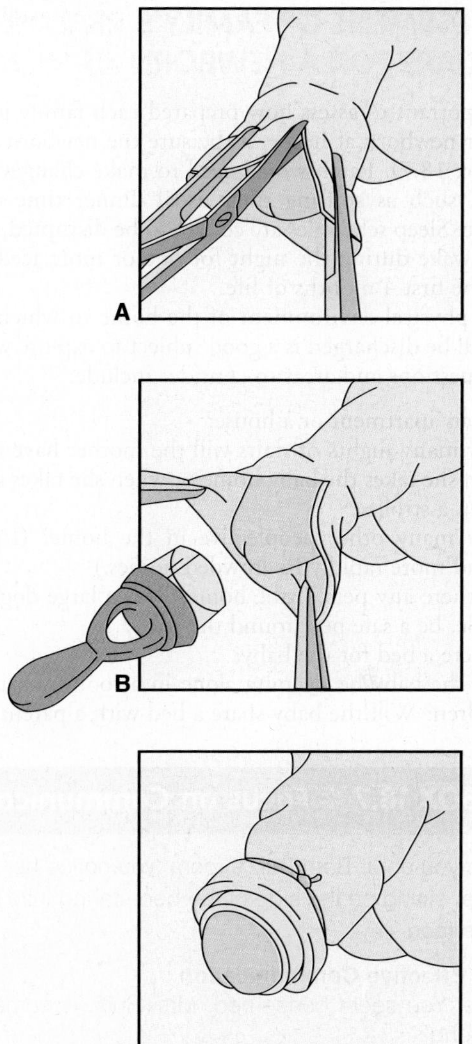

FIGURE 18.29 Technique for performing circumcision using a Plastibell. (**A**) An incision is made in the top of the foreskin. (**B**) The Plastibell is placed over the head of the penis, and the foreskin is pulled over the Plastibell. (**C**) A suture is tied around the foreskin over the tying groove in the Plastibell. Excess skin beyond the suture is trimmed away. The Plastibell falls off in 3 to 7 days. (Courtesy of Hollister Inc., Libertyville, IL.)

Complications that can occur from circumcision include hemorrhage, infection, and urethral fistula formation. To keep the risk of these complications to a minimum, observe infants closely for the first 2 hours after circumcision. Check the infant for bleeding every 15 minutes for the first hour. Also, document that the infant is voiding after the procedure.

Parents should keep the area clean and covered with petrolatum (if used) for about 24 hours. If they see any redness or tenderness, or if the baby cries as if in constant pain, they should report it by telephone. Circumcision sites appear red but should never have a strong odor or discharge. A film of yellowish mucus often covers the glans (similar to a scab) by the second day after surgery. This should not be washed away. The yellow color is from accumulated serum, an innocent finding, and should not be mistaken for the yellow of a purulent exudate.

ASSESSMENT OF FAMILY'S READINESS TO CARE FOR A NEWBORN AT HOME

It is important to assess how prepared each family is to care for their newborn at home, to be sure the newborn remains safe (Box 18.7). Parents may need to make changes in their routine, such as shifting their usual dinner time or work schedule. Sleep schedules are certain to be disrupted, because infants wake during the night for one or more feedings for about the first 4 months of life.

The physical environment of the home to which a newborn will be discharged is a good subject to explore with parents. Questions and areas to consider include:

- Is it an apartment or a house?
- How many flights of stairs will the mother have to climb when she takes the baby home or when she takes the baby out in a stroller?
- How many other people live in the home? (Infections spread more rapidly in crowded homes.)
- Are there any pets in the home? Will a large dog, for example, be a safe pet around the baby?
- Is there a bed for the baby?
- Will the baby be sleeping alone in a room or with older children? Will the baby share a bed with a parent?
- Who will be the primary caregiver?
- Will grandparents or other persons offer support by visiting or helping with care of the child?
- Do the parents have anyone to turn to if they have questions about the baby?
- Is there a refrigerator in which formula or breast milk can be stored?
- Is there adequate heat? An infant needs a temperature of 70° to 75° F during the day and 60° to 65° F at night.
- Are the windows draft free and screened to keep out insects?
- If housing is in poor condition, is there a danger that rodents might attack the baby?
- Is there a danger of lead poisoning?
- Does the mother or do the parents have a source of income? If not, what sort of referral should be made so that money can be provided to care for this child?

These are not prying questions but means of determining whether the home will be adequate and safe. Good prenatal and postnatal care is wasted if an infant contracts pneumonia during the first week at home because no one at a hospital or a birthing center took the time to ask the right questions about the home environment. If the home environment is found to be unsafe, a referral to social services may be necessary before the newborn is discharged.

BOX 18.7 ✻ Focus on Communication

When you enter Beth Ruiz's room, you notice her mother sitting on the side of the bed staring into Beth's face.

Less Effective Communication

Nurse: You seem concerned, Mrs. Ruiz. Is something wrong?

Mrs. Ruiz: Do you think she can tell how little I remember about babies?

Nurse: You're doing a great job. That's the important thing.

Mrs. Ruiz: How long will it take for me to feel like a great mother?

Nurse: You're worrying too much. Relax and enjoy your new baby.

More Effective Communication

Nurse: You seem concerned, Mrs. Ruiz. Is something wrong?

Mrs. Ruiz: Do you think she can tell how little I remember about babies?

Nurse: Is there something special you feel you don't know?

Mrs. Ruiz: My big problem is, I don't feel anything toward her yet. Why do I keep wondering if this whole thing is real?

Nurse: Let's talk about how maternal love develops. It isn't automatic.

Most new mothers have so many questions, it is easy to dismiss a very serious question as "just another question." Resist assuring women that they will be good mothers until you are certain their concern isn't something that could interfere with good mothering.

Nursing Diagnoses and Related Interventions

Nursing Diagnosis: Health-seeking behaviors related to needs of a normal newborn after discharge from the health care facility

Outcome Evaluation: Parents state ways in which they have already altered their home and lifestyle to accommodate their newborn and indicate that they are prepared for other changes; parents voice relative confidence in their ability to care for the newborn and state names of individuals within their family or community who can be resources to them when needed.

Before discharge, the parents should think through how they are going to care for their child at home. Many parents have been mulling over these concerns throughout the pregnancy, whereas others may not yet have addressed some or any of these important issues (see Focus on Nursing Care Planning Box 18.8).

Young mothers without family support and mothers who did not seek regular prenatal care in particular may be unprepared for newborn care. With all parents, try to anticipate problems that may be relevant to them. If there are other children at home, discuss whether the parents are aware that sibling jealousy may occur. Pets in the home can cause similar problems with jealousy. Discuss with a mother who is not going to breastfeed what she will use to feed her baby until she has time to buy formula. Most hospitals sell a discharge formula kit to help parents through the first day at home. Be sure the parents have decided when and where they will take their newborn for health supervision. Check the child's identification band against the mother's one final

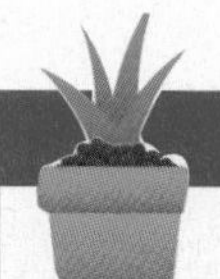

BOX 18.8 ✻ Focus on Nursing Care Planning

A Multidisciplinary Care Map for a Term Newborn

Carlotta Ruiz has just given birth to her second child, a 6-lb 5-oz baby girl. While Jose, Carlotta's husband, is in the room, Carlotta tells you she is a "veteran" at baby care. Jose adds, "Little Joe [their 3-year-old] will be so excited to see his new sister. That's all he's been talking about lately." When Carlotta is alone, you notice she seems a little apprehensive about caring for her new daughter. She tells you, "She's so much smaller than Joe was. And why does it sound like she has a cold? And what is this rash all over her? Isn't it bad enough she has a birthmark?"

Family Assessment ✻ Family is composed of two parents, a 3-year-old sibling, and newborn. They live in a three-bedroom flat over a dry cleaning store. Father clerks in a grocery store; mother works as a school bus driver. Finances rated as "hanging in there."

Client Assessment ✻ Apgar score: 6 at 1 minute; 8 at 5 minutes. Birth from LOA position. Breathed at 30 seconds after birth after administration of blow-by oxygen. Respiratory rate, 74 breaths per minute with mild substernal retractions; rhonchi in upper lobes bilaterally; no grunting or nasal flaring present. Vital signs: temperature (axillary), 98.2° F (36.8° C); heart rate, 136 bpm. Length, 18.5 in; head circumference, 34 cm; chest circumference, 32 cm. She has a 2 × 3 cm red pigmented area on outer right thigh. Mother attempted breastfeeding in birthing room, but newborn had difficulty sucking because of rapid respirations. Remainder of physical examination within acceptable parameters.

Nursing Diagnosis ✻ Risk for ineffective parenting related to infant's smaller than expected size, continuing rapid respirations, and birthmark.

Outcome Criteria ✻ Respiratory rate is decreased to 30 to 50 breaths per minute; retractions, nasal flaring, and grunting are absent; lungs are clear to auscultation. Infant sucks well at breast q2 to 3 hours; mother responds to infant's clues as if bonding with infant.

Team Member Responsible	Assessment	Intervention	Rationale	Expected Outcome
		Activities of Daily Living		
Nurse	Assess respiratory rate every 15 min for 1 hr.	Report increase in rate, retractions, or development of nasal flaring or grunting.	Increases in respiratory rate and retractions, accompanied by nasal flaring and grunting, may indicate respiratory distress.	Infant gradually decreases respiratory rate to 30–50/min by 24 hr.
Nurse	Monitor newborn's temperature every hour.	Keep infant warm via radiant warmer or swaddled and held by parent; place a cap on her head.	Newborns have difficulty conserving body heat. Exposure to cold increases metabolic rate, increasing need for oxygen and a higher respiratory rate.	Infant's temperature remains at 98.2° F axillary.
		Consultations		
Nurse/ physician	Assess whether parents would like a dermatology consultation for child's birthmark.	Refer parents to dermatology consultant if desired.	A second opinion can help assure parents birthmark is no more than a birthmark.	Parents visit with consultant if desired; state they understand the prognosis for port-wine lesions.

(continued)

BOX 18.8 ✻ Focus on Nursing Care Planning (continued)

Team Member Responsible	Assessment	Intervention	Rationale	Expected Outcome
		Procedures/Medications		
Nurse	Assess whether infant's lung sounds reveal fluid.	Position newborn on her side with head slightly lower than body; suction mouth and then nose with bulb syringe as indicated.	Positioning facilitates drainage of secretions from airway. Gentle suctioning removes secretions. Suctioning mouth before nose prevents possible aspiration of oral secretions.	Infant appears comfortable in chosen position; need for suctioning becomes infrequent.
		Nutrition		
Nurse	Assess mother's knowledge of breastfeeding techniques.	Assist mother with breastfeeding as needed; remind her that rapid respirations make sucking difficult.	Breast milk is the preferred milk for human newborns; a mother may need assistance if an infant sucks poorly.	Infant and mother establish mutually enjoyable breastfeeding by hospital discharge.
		Patient/Family Education		
Nurse/ physician	Review with parents what were their expectations of new child (bigger? prettier? more relaxed?)	Inform parents that a rapid respiratory rate is common in newborns because of unabsorbed lung fluid. Help them mold expectations with reality.	Providing information helps to allay parents' anxieties and fears.	Parents state they understand their infant's condition.
		Psychosocial/Spiritual/Emotional Needs		
Nurse	Assess what is parents' greatest concern about taking newborn home.	Explain that the presence of a birthmark, rapid respirations, and smaller than expected size are normal variations of newborns.	Explanation of normal range of infant variation provides information to help allay parents' fears and concerns.	Parents state they were initially surprised by baby's appearance, but are adjusting to new image.
Nurse	Assess infant for general physical condition.	Point out positive attributes of newborn, such as pretty eyes, alert expression.	Pointing out positive areas helps parents focus attention on the unique and special qualities of their child.	Parents state they appreciate learning more about their newborn from health care professionals.
		Discharge Planning		
Nurse	Assess whether parents have made plans for hospital discharge.	Remind parents about importance of car seat, sleeping on back, and aspiration.	Safety awareness plays a big role in preventing early-age accidents.	Parents state they feel ready to begin parenting their new infant.

time before discharge, to help prevent the possibility of wrong identification of the infant.

Daily Home Care. Newborns thrive on a gentle rhythm of care, a sense of being able to anticipate what is to come next. Based on this, parents can decide what is the best daily at-home routine for them and their new child. There are no fixed rules. There is no set time at which an infant must be bathed, nor even a rule that requires a bath every day. All infants do not have to be in bed for the night by 8:00 PM. If the father works evenings, it may be important to have the baby awake at midnight so that he has time to spend with his child.

Your aim in helping parents plan their schedule of care is to arrive at one that:

- Offers a degree of consistency (a mother cannot expect an infant to stay awake until midnight 5 nights a week, then go to sleep at 7:00 PM on the sixth night)
- Appears to satisfy the infant
- Gives the parents a sense of well-being and contentment with their child

Sleep Patterns. A newborn sleeps an average of 16 of every 24 hours during the first week home, an average of 4 hours at a time. By 4 months of age, an infant sleeps an average of 15 hours of every 24 and through the night.

It is exhausting for a parent who is already tired from labor and birth to have to awaken during the night to feed a newborn. For this reason, parents may try various methods to induce a baby to sleep through the night much earlier than 4 months. One approach is to introduce solid food (particularly cereal) in the first weeks of life, on the theory that the bulk will fill the infant's stomach so that he or she will not wake up crying to be fed. In practice, there is no correlation between the age at which solid food is introduced and a baby's capability for sustained sleep. Also, a newborn is not developmentally ready to deal with nonliquid food until about the end of the third month. There are also other reasons not to introduce solid food early: large protein molecules from solid foods can pass through a newborn's immature gastrointestinal tract, becoming antigens that may sensitize the newborn for possible allergic reactions. In breastfed infants, too-early introduction of solid foods may interfere with the desire for breast milk, decrease the newborn's sucking, and subsequently decrease the mother's milk supply.

A baby probably wakes every 4, 5, 6, or 8 hours because of a physiologic need for fluid. Advise parents that, because of this fluid need, they should not try to eliminate night feedings. Knowing their baby is not sick, that you are concerned and willing to listen to their questions, and that every other parent of a newborn is also up at night does not solve the difficulty of interrupted sleep, but it is a help.

They should be certain their infant does not sleep on the stomach, because there is an association between this sleeping position and SIDS (Richardson, Walker, & Horne, 2008. They also need to use an approved crib with a firm mattress that is free of stuffed animals and toys. Placing a fan in the room and sucking on a pacifier may also reduce the possibility of SIDS as the infant stirs and sucks periodically and does not fall as deeply asleep.

Crying. Many new parents are not prepared for the amount of time a newborn spends crying. Infants, however, typically cry an average of 2 of every 24 hours during the first 7 weeks of life. The frequency seems to peak at age 6 or 7 weeks and then tapers off.

Almost all infants have a period during the day when they are wide awake and invariably fussy. New parents need to recognize this as normal and not worry that it means their child is ill. Parents might use this fussy time for bathing or playing with the infant, arranging their schedules accordingly. It is important to learn the infant's cues and to help the infant learn to self-quiet. The most typical time for wakefulness is between 6:00 and 11:00 PM, which, unfortunately, is when parents may be tired and least able to tolerate crying.

Whether to use pacifiers to reduce crying is a question parents must decide for themselves, depending on how they feel about them and their infant's needs. It is rare that infants have such a need for sucking they must have a pacifier in their mouth constantly. Discussing a few pros and cons with parents helps clarify the subject.

An infant who completes a feeding and still seems restless and discontented, who actively searches for something to put into the mouth, and who sucks on hands and clothes may need the increased sucking activity a pacifier provides. The major drawback of pacifiers is the problem of cleanliness. They tend to fall on the floor or sidewalk and are then put back into the infant's mouth. Clipping the pacifier onto the infant's shirt prevents this problem. If parents use pacifiers, be certain they are of one-piece construction, so that loose parts cannot be aspirated.

Parental Concerns Related to Breathing. Some parents report that their newborns have stuffy noses or make snoring noises in their sleep and that they sneeze frequently. This occurs because most newborns continue to have some mucus in the upper respiratory tract and posterior pharynx for up to 2 weeks after birth. The snoring noise is a result of this mucus, not a cold. In addition, infants continue to breathe irregularly for about the first month. A new parent may wake at night, notice this breathing pattern, and grow alarmed that the baby is in respiratory distress. If these are the only symptoms, this is a normal newborn respiratory pattern. If the child has rhinitis (nasal discharge) or a fever, he or she needs to be seen by a health care provider, because these symptoms suggest an upper respiratory tract infection.

Continued Health Maintenance for a Newborn. Parents do not need to continue to weigh a newborn or take the temperature at home. These practices only cause worry, because weight fluctuates day by day, and infant activity and clothing can influence temperature. Teach parents to judge their infant's state of health by overall appearance, eagerness to eat, general activity, and disposition, as well as weight gain (Box 18.9).

Make certain that parents make and keep a health care appointment for a first newborn assessment according to their primary care provider's schedule (2 to 6 weeks). The mother was conscientious throughout pregnancy to bring a well child into the world. Parents must now begin a health care program to keep the child well.

Car Safety. Automobile accidents are a safety problem all during childhood. For protection while in automobiles, newborns should always be transported in car seats (Decina & Lococo, 2007). Without this protection, if a car stops suddenly, an infant can be thrown onto the floor or, in a collision, thrown out of the car or through the windshield. In an accident, centrifugal force on an infant can be as much as 450 lb,

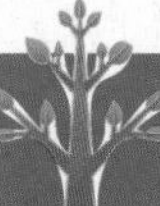

BOX 18.9 * Focus on Family Teaching

Determining If a Newborn Is Well

Q. Ms. Ruiz asks you, "Could you review with me how to know if a newborn is well?"

A. The following items are helpful to determine your newborn is well:

- Sucks as if she is hungry
- Possibly spits up a slight amount after feeding, but has no vomiting
- Moves bowels approximately three to four times per day (may be more often if breastfed), with stools that are loose or semiformed but not runny and watery
- Appears happy overall (despite a fussy period during the day) and sleeps for 2 to 3 hours at a time
- Has a normal temperature
- Breathes more rapidly than an adult, but breathing is easy and not stressed
- Skin is neither yellow nor blue in tone.

making it impossible for a passenger to hold onto a child. At a speed of only 30 mph, an infant may hit the dashboard with a force equal to a fall from a three-story building. If an adult holding the infant is not wearing a seat belt, the adult can be thrown against the infant, killing the child.

When purchasing a car seat, parents should look at the label to be sure the seat meets federal guidelines. Local health departments or Red Cross chapters have lists of all the approved car seats available in a particular area as well as details of their comparable features and cost. The AAP web site (http://www.aap.org) lists these as well. Some hospitals and Red Cross chapters loan infant car seats for temporary use, such as when visiting out of state with grandparents or when first coming home from the hospital. New cars are mandated to be equipped with lower anchors and tethers for car seats.

The best location for a car seat is the back seat of the car; this is especially true if the car has a passenger seat air bag, because the force of an air bag expanding could kill an infant in the front seat. While the infant is less than 21 lb or 26 in long, the best type of car seat is an "infant-only" seat that, when properly positioned, faces the back of the car (Fig. 18.30). The ideal model has a five-point harness with broad straps, which help spread the force of a collision over the chest and hips, and a shield, which cushions the head. A mirror can be positioned in the back seat so the parent can observe the infant from the front seat or while driving.

Parents should dress an infant in clothing with pant legs if the infant is to be placed in a car seat, because the harness crotch strap must pass between the legs for a snug and correct fit. Advise parents not to use a sack sleeper or papoose bunting; nor should they wrap the baby in a bulky blanket so that the straps do not fit securely while the baby is in the seat. To support the baby's head, parents can use a rolled-up receiving blanket, towel, or diaper on each side of the head. The AAP recommends to only use a manufactured head rest if it comes packaged with the car seat. To provide extra warmth, they can cut holes in a blanket for the harness and crotch straps to pass through, place the baby in the seat, fasten the buckles, and then fold the blanket over the child for warmth. A second blanket can be draped over the seat if needed.

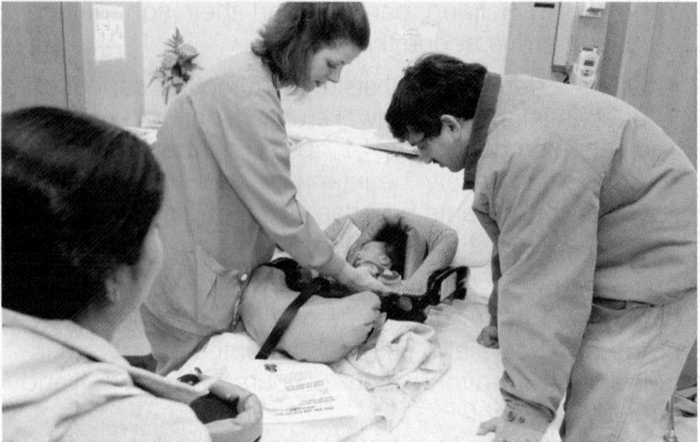

FIGURE 18.30 Newborns should ride in a supportive car seat. Be certain every parent planning to drive a child home from the health care facility is properly equipped.

Infants should sit in a backward-facing seat until they are able to sit up without support, usually when they weigh about 21 lb. At that point, they are old enough for a forward-facing toddler seat. Caution parents that plastic car seats grow extremely hot in the summer, so they need to test the temperature of the surface before placing an infant in one. Stress also that it is dangerous to use a car seat improperly, such as not fastening the harness or not securing the seat belt. To ensure proper car seat installation, an inspection may be performed by a certified CPS (Child Passenger Safety) technician at a local inspection station. These may be located at http://www.seatcheck.org.

✔ Checkpoint Question 18.5

Ms. Ruiz is preparing to take her new daughter home. On about what day of life can she expect her baby's umbilical cord to fall off?

a. Day 1.
b. Days 2 to 3.
c. Days 6 to 10.
d. Day 30.

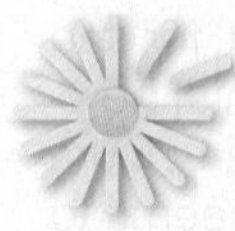

Key Points for Review

- Converting from fetal to adult respiratory function is a major step in adaptation to extrauterine life. Newborns need particularly close observation during the first few hours of life to determine that this adaptation has been made.
- Maintaining body heat is a second major problem of newborns. The temperature of the term baby's environment

should be about 75° F (24° C). When procedures that require undressing an infant for an extended period are being carried out such as circumcision, a radiant heat source should be used.

- Newborns may suffer hypoglycemia in the first few hours of life because they use energy to establish respirations and maintain heat. Signs of jitteriness and a blood glucose level of less than 45 mg/100 mL by heel-stick help to identify hypoglycemia.
- Identification bands should be attached securely to newborns; assess these bands carefully before hospital discharge. To help prevent the possibility of kidnapping, be certain of the identification of anyone to whom you give a newborn.
- To feel confident with newborn care, parents need to hold and give care in the hospital. Encouraging them to spend as much time as possible with a newborn is a major nursing role. Be certain parents have a car seat to use at discharge and know to schedule a well child visit for their newborn at 2 to 6 weeks.

CRITICAL THINKING EXERCISES

1. Beth Ruiz is the newborn described at the beginning of the chapter. Her mother is concerned because Beth seems small, is covered by erythema toxicum, and has noisy respirations. You discover that the family has no car seat to transport the baby home. What would you teach the mother to make her feel more comfortable with her newborn? What would you do about the car seat—ask that they stay until they can arrange to rent or borrow one, or discharge them?
2. When you are assessing Beth in her mother's room, what newborn reflexes would you assess? Suppose it is cold in the room, so that you have time to test only one reflex. Which one would you test, and why?
3. Beth has a port-wine stain on her left thigh. Her father tells you he is not concerned about this because he knows that all birthmarks fade by school age. How would you respond to him?
4. Examine the National Health Goals related to newborn care. Most government-sponsored money for nursing research is allotted based on these goals. What would be a possible research topic to explore pertinent to these goals that would be applicable to the Ruiz family and also advance evidence-based practice?

CRITICAL THINKING SCENARIO

Open the accompanying CD-ROM or visit http://thePoint.lww.com and read the Patient Scenario included for this chapter, then answer the questions to further sharpen your skills and grow more familiar with NCLEX style questions related to nursing care of a newborn. Confirm your answers are correct by reading the rationales.

REFERENCES

American Academy of Pediatrics. (2007). Year 2007 position statement: principles and guidelines for early hearing detection and intervention programs. *Pediatrics, 120*(10), 898–921.

American Academy of Pediatrics. (2009). *2009 Immunization schedule.* Washington, DC: Author.

Apgar, V., et al. (1958). Evaluation of a newborn infant: second report. *JAMA: Journal of the American Medical Association, 16*(82), 1985–1988.

Ballard, J. L., et al. (1991). The new Ballard Scale. *Journal of Pediatrics, 119*(3), 417–424.

Beachy, J. M. (2007). Lab values. Investigating jaundice in the newborn. *Neonatal Network: The Journal of Neonatal Nursing, 26*(5), 327–333.

Berger, T. G. (2009). Dermatologic disorders. In S. J. McPhee & M. A. Papadakis (Eds.). *Current medical diagnosis and treatment.* Columbus, OH: McGraw-Hill.

Brazelton, T. B. (1973). Neonatal behavior assessment scale. *Clinics in Developmental Medicine, 50*(5), 1–15.

Bregje, E., et al. (2007). Swaddling: a systematic review. *Pediatrics, 120*(10), e1097–e1106.

Chetham, M. (2007). Neonatal jaundice. In S. R. Hayden, et al. (Eds.). *Rosen & Barkin's 5-minute emergency medicine consult.* Philadelphia: Lippincott Williams & Wilkins.

Coleman-Phox, K., Odouli, R., & Li, D. K. (2008). Use of a fan during sleep and the risk of sudden infant death syndrome. *Archives of Pediatrics and Adolescent Medicine, 162*(10), 963–968.

Damato, E. G. (2007). 28 days. Safe sleep: can pacifiers reduce SIDS risk? *Nursing for Women's Health, 11*(1), 72–76.

Decina, L. E., & Lococo, K. H. (2007). Observed LATCH use and misuse characteristics of child restraint systems in seven states. *Journal of Safety Research, 38*(3), 273–281.

Desmond, M. N., et al. (1963). The clinical behavior of the newly born: the term infant. *Journal of Pediatrics, 62*(3), 307–309.

De Wals, P., et al. (2007). Reduction in neural-tube defects after folic acid fortification in Canada. *New England Journal of Medicine, 357*(2), 135–142.

Dubowitz, L., et al. (1970). Clinical assessment of gestational age in a newborn infant. *Journal of Pediatrics, 77*(10), 1–12.

Edmonds, J. L. (2008). Hemangiomas of infancy and vascular malformations. In A. K. Lalwani (Ed.). *Current diagnosis & treatment in otolaryngology* (2nd Ed.). Columbus, OH: McGraw-Hill.

Elias, E. R., Chun-Hui, A., & Manchester, D. K. (2008). Genetics and dysmorphology. In W. W. Hay, et al. (Eds.). *Current pediatric diagnosis and treatment* (18th ed.). Columbus, OH: McGraw-Hill.

El Shahed, A. I., et al. (2009). Surfactant for meconium aspiration syndrome in full term/near term infants. *Cochrane Database of Systematic Reviews, 2009*(1), (CD002054).

Halliday, H. L., & Sweet, D. (2009). Endotracheal intubation at birth for preventing morbidity and mortality in vigorous, meconium-stained infants born at term. *Cochrane Database of Systematic Reviews, 2009*(1), (CD000500).

Harrington, D. J., et al. (2007). Long-term outcome in surviving infants with Apgar zero at 10 minutes: a systematic review of the literature and hospital-based cohort. *American Journal of Obstetrics and Gynecology, 196*(5), 463–464.

Johnson, K. J., et al. (2007). Childhood cancer and birthmarks in the Collaborative Perinatal Project. *Pediatrics, 119*(5), e1088–e1093.

Karch, A. M. (2009). *Lippincott's nursing drug guide* (11th ed.). Philadelphia: Lippincott Williams & Wilkins.

Kayton, A. (2007). Newborn screening: a literature review. *Neonatal Network: The Journal of Neonatal Nursing, 26*(2), 85–95.

Kwik, M., et al. (2007). Outcomes of pregnancies affected by impaired glucose tolerance. *Diabetes Research and Clinical Practice, 77*(2), 263–268.

MacNeil, J. R., et al. (2007). Evaluating families' satisfaction with early hearing detection and intervention services in Massachusetts. *American Journal of Audiology, 16*(1), 29–56.

McCarthy, J. J., & MacEwen, G. D. (2007). Hip arthroscopy for the treatment of children with hip dysplasia: a preliminary report. *Orthopedics, 30*(4), 262–264.

Mills, J. F., & Tudehope, D. (2009). Fibreoptic phototherapy for neonatal jaundice. *Cochrane Database of Systematic Reviews, 2007, 2009*(1), (CD002060).

Moore, E. R., Anderson, G. C., & Bergman, N. (2009). Early skin-to-skin contact for mothers and their healthy newborn infants. *Cochrane Database of Systematic Reviews, 2009*(1), (CD003519).

Nicholson, L. (2007). Caput succedaneum and cephalohematoma: the Cs that leaves bumps on the head. *Neonatal Network: The Journal of Neonatal Nursing, 26*(5), 277–281.

Raab, E. L. (2007). Essentials of normal newborn assessment and care. In A. H. DeCherney & L. Nathan (Eds.). *Current diagnosis and treatment in obstetrics and gynecology* (10th ed.). Columbus, OH: McGraw-Hill.

Richardson, G. A., Goldschmidt, L., & Larkby, C. (2007). Effects of prenatal cocaine exposure on growth: a longitudinal analysis. *Pediatrics, 120*(10), e1017–e1027.

Richardson, H. L., Walker, A. M., & Horne, R. S. (2008). Sleep position alters arousal processes maximally at the high-risk age for sudden infant death syndrome. *Journal of Sleep Research, 17*(4), 450–457.

Roberts, D., Neilson, J. P., & Weindling, A. M. (2009). Interventions for the treatment of twin-to-twin transfusion syndrome. *Cochrane Database of Systematic Reviews, 2009*(1), (CD002073).

Ruiz, M. J., et al. (2009). Neonatal outcomes associated with intestinal abnormalities diagnosed by fetal ultrasound. *Journal of Pediatric Surgery, 44*(1), 71–74.

Silverman, W. A., & Anderson, H. (1956). A controlled clinical trial of effects of water mist on obstructive respiratory signs, death rate and necroscopy findings among premature infants. *Pediatrics, 17*(4), 1–9.

Subramanian, A., et al. (Eds.). (2008). *Drug facts and comparisons.* St. Louis: Wolters Kluwer Health.

Taddio, A., Ohlsson, K., & Ohlsson, A. (2009). Lidocaine-prilocaine cream for analgesia during circumcision in newborn boys. *Cochrane Database of Systematic Reviews, 2009*(1), (CD000496).

Thilo, E. H., & Rosenberg, A. A. (2008). The newborn infant. In W. W. Hay, et al. (Eds.). *Current pediatric diagnosis and treatment* (18th ed.). Columbus, OH: McGraw-Hill.

Usher, R., et al. (1966). Judgment of fetal age. *Pediatric Clinics of North America, 13*(4), 835–840.

Van Leeuwen, G., & Glenn, L. (1968). Screening for hidden congenital anomalies. *Pediatrics, 41*(6), 147–152.

Webster, J., & Pritchard, M. A. (2009). Gowning by attendants and visitors in newborn nurseries for prevention of neonatal morbidity and mortality. *Cochrane Database of Systematic Reviews, 2009*(1), (CD003670).

Ystrom, E., et al. (2008). The impact of maternal negative affectivity and general self-efficacy on breastfeeding. *Journal of Pediatrics, 152*(1), 68–72.

SUGGESTED READINGS

Brown, S., et al. (2009). Early postnatal discharge from hospital for healthy mothers and term infants. *Cochrane Database of Systematic Reviews, 2009*(1), (CD002958).

Eronen, R., Pincombe, J., & Calabretto, H. (2007). Support for stressed parents of young infants. *Neonatal, Paediatric and Child Health Nursing, 10*(2), 20–27.

Forster, D. A., & McLachlan, H. L. (2007). Breastfeeding initiation and birth setting practices: a review of the literature. *Journal of Midwifery and Women's Health, 52*(3), 273–280.

Fowlie, P. W., & Jackson, A. (2007). Communicating with parents on the neonatal unit: should we be doing more than just talking? *BMJ: British Medical Journal, 33*(7583), 1.

Hale, R. (2007). Protecting neonates' delicate skin. *British Journal of Midwifery, 15*(4), 231–235.

Holsti, L., et al. (2008). Is it painful or not? Discriminant validity of the Behavioral Indicators of Infant Pain (BIIP) scale. *Clinical Journal of Pain, 24*(1), 83–88.

Jacknowitz, A. (2007). Increasing breastfeeding rate: do changing demographics explain them? *Women's Health Issues, 17*(2), 84–92.

Jennissen, C. (2007). Evaluating fever in neonates and infants. *Emergency Medicine, 39*(6), 41–48.

Kuo, A. A., & Inkelas, M. (2007). The changing role of pediatric well-child care. *Zero to Three, 27*(3), 5–11.

Thomas, K. (2007). Physiology. Biorhythms in the nursery. *Journal of Perinatal and Neonatal Nursing, 21*(2), 89–90.

Chapter 19 Nutritional Needs of a Newborn

KEY TERMS

- areola
- bifidus factor
- colostrum
- engorgement
- fore milk
- hind milk
- interferon
- lactiferous sinuses
- lactoferrin
- let-down reflex
- lysozyme
- prolactin

OBJECTIVES

After mastering the contents of this chapter, you should be able to:

1. Describe nutritional requirements for a term newborn.
2. Identify National Health Goals related to newborn nutrition that nurses can help the nation achieve.
3. Use critical thinking to assist parents with nutritional problem solving and be sure newborn nutrition is family centered.
4. Assess nutritional intake and feeding method of a newborn to determine adequate nutritional status.
5. Formulate nursing diagnoses related to newborn nutrition.
6. Identify outcomes for a newborn and parents related to nutrition.
7. Plan nursing care such as helping a mother decide on a type of infant feeding that will be satisfying for both her and her infant.
8. Implement nursing care such as supporting a new mother while breastfeeding.
9. Evaluate expected outcomes for achievement and effectiveness of care.
10. Identify areas related to nutrition and newborns that could benefit from additional nursing research or application of evidence-based practice.
11. Integrate knowledge of normal newborn nutrition with nursing process to achieve quality maternal and child health nursing care.

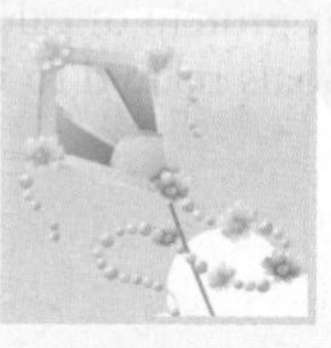

Linda Satir is a new mother of a term baby girl. During the pregnancy, she and her husband, Paul, both agreed Linda would breastfeed. Linda will be returning to work as an executive assistant after her 6-week maternity leave. She attempted to breastfeed her newborn in the birthing room with minimal success. As you offer to help her feed her baby for the second time, she says, "Do you think I made the right choice? Maybe I should formula feed her. Paul could help that way and I won't have to worry about what to do when I go back to work."

Previous chapters described the care of a woman and family during the antepartal, intrapartal, postpartal, and newborn periods. This chapter adds information about the nutritional needs of a newborn. A newborn's nutritional needs are high during this time because of a rapid rate of growth and development. Knowing these needs fortifies you to play a key role in educating parents about how to provide adequate nutrition to meet both physiologic and psychological needs of their newborn.

How would you answer Linda?

Proper nutrition is essential for optimal growth and development, especially in the first few months of life, because brain growth proceeds at such a rapid rate during this time. Providing adequate nutrition for a newborn extends beyond physiologic need, however; it also fulfills important psychological needs. During feeding, a parent is close to the infant, and a baby is apt to be particularly sensitive to the parent's demonstration of affection or lack of warmth. An infant who does not experience a warm relationship with a mother or primary caregiver may fail to thrive as surely as one who is denied sufficient protein or calories (Britton et al., 2009). National Health Goals related to newborn nutrition are shown in Box 19.1.

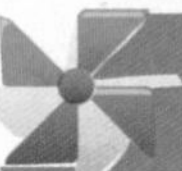

BOX 19.1 ✻ Focus on National Health Goals

The number of National Health Goals that address nutrition of a newborn was increased in the midcourse review to include two that speak to exclusive breastfeeding.

- Increase to at least 75% the proportion of mothers who breastfeed their babies in the early postpartum period from a baseline of 64%.
- Increase to at least 50% the proportion of mothers who continue breastfeeding until their babies are 5 to 6 months old from a baseline of 29%.
- Increase to 25% the proportion of mothers who continue breastfeeding until 1 year of age from a baseline of 16%.
- Increase to at least 60% the proportion of mothers who breastfeed exclusively through 3 months from a baseline of 43%.
- Increase to 25% the proportion of mothers who breastfeed exclusively through 6 months from a baseline of 13%.
- Decrease the proportion of children with untreated dental decay in primary or permanent teeth to 21% from a baseline of 29% (http://www.nih.gov).

Nurses can help the nation achieve these goals by educating women about breastfeeding during pregnancy and supporting a family during the postpartal period while a woman is breastfeeding. Home visits with postpartal families and well-child health assessments provide opportunities to advocate for continued and exclusive breastfeeding. For the woman who will formula feed her infant, education during pregnancy should include the fact that putting an infant to bed with a bottle of milk or juice is associated with tooth decay and should be avoided.

Areas that could benefit from additional nursing research include techniques parents could use to initiate sleep without using a bedtime bottle; reasons women discontinue breastfeeding early in the postpartal period; and legislation or education necessary in the workplace to encourage women to continue breastfeeding after they return to work.

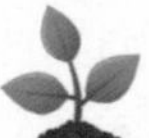

Nursing Process Overview

For Promoting Nutritional Health in a Newborn

Assessment

Assessment of infant nutrition begins during pregnancy with assessment of the mother's and father's attitudes and choices about infant feeding. Breastfeeding is widely accepted as the preferred method of human newborn nutrition. However, if a mother chooses not to breastfeed because of her individual circumstances, it is important that she not be made to feel guilty for her choice, because formula feeding can be substituted. Most important, parents need to feel comfortable with and confident about the feeding method they choose.

Teach parents how to recognize signs of hunger in a newborn such as restlessness, tense body posture, smacking lips, and tongue thrusting. Otherwise, they may wait for their infant to cry, and this is actually a late sign of newborn hunger. Once infant feeding begins, teach parents to assess whether the amount the infant is receiving is adequate—not by how long the newborn breastfeeds at a time or by how much formula is taken at a feeding, but by a larger measure, such as whether the newborn is voiding, growing, and alert (Box 19.2). A formula-fed newborn regains birth weight at about 10 days, a breastfed infant at about 14 days.

Nursing Diagnosis

Nursing diagnoses in relation to nutrition usually center on a woman's choice regarding method of feeding or a newborn's nutritional intake and feeding patterns. It may be difficult to establish diagnoses during the first part of the

Box 19.2 Assessment
Assessing the Newborn for Adequate Nutrition

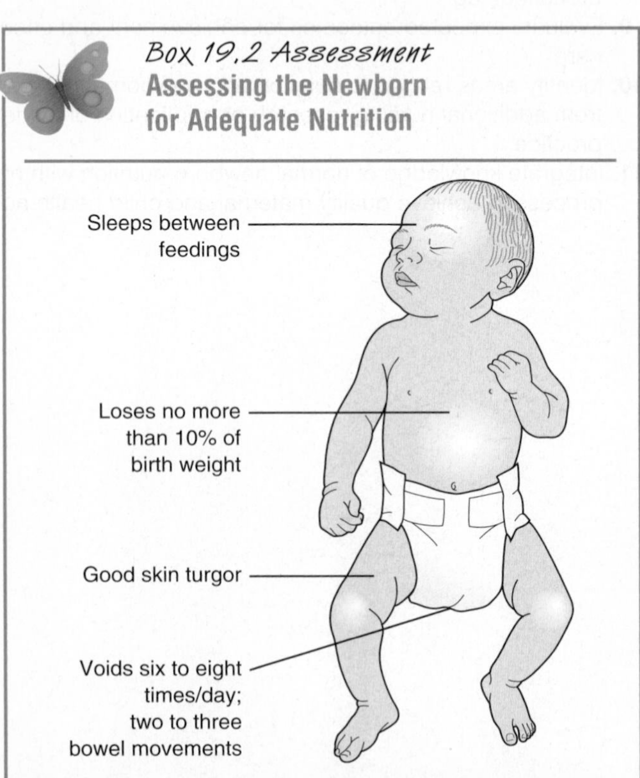

newborn period, because the mother and infant are still getting used to each other. Examples of nursing diagnoses are:

- Effective breastfeeding related to well-prepared mother and healthy newborn
- Risk for ineffective breastfeeding related to nipple soreness
- Imbalanced nutrition, less than body requirements, related to poor newborn sucking response
- Risk for impaired parenting related to need to formula feed newborn

Outcome Identification and Planning

As breastfeeding is best for newborns, planning begins while a woman is still pregnant, focusing on providing her with the information necessary to allow her to become familiar and comfortable with breastfeeding. After birth, a teaching plan addressing the nutritional needs of both the woman and her newborn can be developed. Helpful Internet sites for referral are La Leche League International (http://www.llli.org) and the International Lactation Consultant Association (http://www.ilca.org). Despite the advantages of breastfeeding, some parents still choose formula feeding because of their individual preferences. Parents who choose formula feeding need to plan ways to make feeding time special for both themselves and the baby. An Internet site that discusses formula feeding is a pediatrician's site, http://www.askdrsears.com.

Implementation

A major intervention related to newborn nutrition is supporting a mother's choice of feeding method and helping her to trust her judgment as to whether her infant is full and content and the feeding method is as natural as possible. In addition to sponsoring classes on breastfeeding, a helpful service of La Leche League is its hotline, through which a breastfeeding woman who is discouraged or is having difficulty can contact a member and ask for advice. *The Womanly Art of Breastfeeding*, published by the League (2004), is a comprehensive and informative book to recommend for both new mothers and fathers.

When assisting a new mother with breastfeeding, remember that breast milk can carry the human immunodeficiency virus (HIV). Adhere to standard infection precautions, therefore, when helping with manual expression of milk or disposing of soiled breast pads.

Outcome Evaluation

Evaluation is an important final step to ensure that a newborn receives adequate nutrition, because unforeseen circumstances, such as an unsuspected milk allergy or mastitis (breast infection), may interfere and require drastic changes to reach desired outcomes. Help parents appreciate that newborns are very adaptive and can adjust to another feeding method if necessary. Examples suggesting successful expected outcomes related to newborn feeding are:

- Infant breastfeeds every 2 to 3 hours; is content and sleeps between feedings.
- Newborn ingests a total of 12 oz of formula with iron every 24 hours.
- Mother states she feels satisfied with chosen method of infant feeding.
- Infant voids six times daily as a measure of adequate hydration by 1 week.

NUTRITIONAL ALLOWANCES FOR A NEWBORN

Nutritional allowances for a newborn need to take into account total calories, protein, vitamins, minerals, and fluid. Dietary reference intake for calories, protein, vitamins, and minerals for newborns are shown in Table 19.1.

Calories

Growth in the neonatal period and early infancy is more rapid than at any other period of life (Raab, 2007). Therefore, the caloric requirements exceed those at any other age. An infant up to 2 months of age requires 110 to 120 calories per kilogram of body weight (50 to 55 kcal/lb) every 24 hours to provide an adequate amount for maintenance and growth. After 2 months of age, this amount gradually declines until the requirement at 1 year is 100 kcal/kg (45 kcal/lb) per day. In contrast, the adult requirement is 42 kcal/kg (20 kcal/lb) per day.

The actual caloric requirement, of course, depends on an infant's individual activity level and growth rate. For example, an active infant, one who cries frequently and squirms constantly, needs more calories than one who is more passive, content to spend long hours playing quietly or just studying the environment. During growth spurts, more calories are needed to supply additional energy.

TABLE 19.1 ✻ Dietary Reference Intakes For Newborns And Infants

Nutrient	Recommended Dietary Allowance	
	Birth to 6 Mo	*6 Mo to 1 Yr*
Calories	kg × 110	kg × 100
Protein (g)	kg × 2.2	kg × 1.6
Vitamin A (μg, RE)	400	500
Vitamin D (μg, cholecalciferol)	5	5
Vitamin E (mg, TE)	4	5
Vitamin C (mg)	40	50
Folate (μg)	65	80
Niacin (mg, NE)	2	4
Riboflavin (mg)	0.3	0.4
Thiamine (mg)	0.2	0.3
Vitamin B_6 (mg)	0.1	0.3
Vitamin B_{12} (μg)	0.4	0.5
Calcium (mg)	210	270
Phosphorus (mg)	100	275
Iodine (μg)	110	130
Magnesium (mg)	30	75
Zinc (mg)	2	3
Iron (mg)	0.27	11

RE, retinol equivalents; TE, tocopherol equivalents; NE, niacin equivalents.

Adapted from Department of Agriculture. (2005). *2005 dietary guidelines for Americans.* Washington, DC: Author.

Commercial infant formulas simulate breast milk. They contain about 9% to 12% of their calories as protein and 45% to 55% of calories as lactose carbohydrate. The balance is fat, of which about 10% (4% of the calories) is linoleic acid.

Protein

Protein, necessary for the formation of new cells, has a high requirement during the newborn and infancy periods to provide for rapid growth of new cells as well as maintenance of existing cells. The nutritional allowance of protein for the first 2 months of life is 2.2 g per kilogram of body weight. Both human milk and commercial formulas provide all the essential amino acids necessary to form protein. Histidine, an amino acid that appears to be essential for infant growth but is not necessary for adult growth, is found in both milk forms.

Unaltered cow's milk is not recommended for newborns, because it contains about 16% of its calories as protein, whereas human milk contains about 8%. This means that cow's milk can create such a rich solute load (the amount of urea and electrolytes that must be excreted in the urine) that a newborn's kidneys could be overwhelmed. In addition, the protein in cow's milk, casein, differs from that in human milk, lactalbumin, both in composition and in amount. The amount of casein present in milk determines its curd tension. The curd in cow's milk is large, tough, and difficult to digest, whereas in human milk the curd is softer and easier to digest. This is the rationale for formula-fed infants to be given a commercial formula containing albumin rather than cow's milk. Cow's milk products, such as yogurt and cottage cheese, should not be introduced until 9 to 12 months of age for the same reason.

Fat

Linoleic acid, an essential fatty acid necessary for growth and skin integrity in infants, is found in both human milk and commercial formulas. Use of fat-free milk for long periods (when other sources of food are not being offered) can result in linoleic acid deficiency. Therefore, parents should not feed fat-free milk as a means of preventing obesity in a young infant. In addition, fat-free milk does not contain sufficient calories for a newborn; it has only about half as many calories as commercial formulas or breast milk.

Carbohydrate

Lactose, the disaccharide found in human milk and added to commercial formulas, appears to be the most easily digested of the carbohydrates. Lactose also improves calcium absorption and aids in nitrogen retention. It produces stools consisting predominantly of gram-positive rather than gram-negative bacteria and therefore decreases the possibility of gastrointestinal illness (which usually results from gram-negative organisms). Adequate lactose also allows protein to be used for building new cells rather than for calories, encouraging normal water balance and preventing abnormal metabolism of fat. Lactose intolerance, which can occur in older children, is rarely present in newborns; they typically use the calories provided by lactose well.

Fluid

It is important to maintain a sufficient fluid intake in newborns because their metabolic rate is so high (and metabolism requires water). In addition, a newborn's body surface area is large in relation to body mass. This means that a baby loses water by evaporation much more readily than does an adult. Because the kidneys of a newborn are not yet capable of fully concentrating urine, a newborn cannot conserve body water by this mechanism to prevent dehydration.

Another difference between newborns and adults is that body water is distributed differently. In a newborn, 30% to 35% of body weight is extracellular fluid; in an adult, this proportion is only 20%. Consequently, if a newborn's extracellular fluid store is depleted through loss of fluid or inadequate fluid intake, as much as 35% of a newborn's fluid component may be lost.

Because of all these factors, a newborn needs 150 to 200 mL/kg (2.5 to 3.0 oz/lb) of water intake every 24 hours (adults require 2400 mL/day or less than 1 oz/lb). This requirement can be supplied completely by breastfeeding or formula feeding. Fruit juice is not recommended as a supplemental fluid because it supplies no protein and, if not pasteurized, can carry infectious organisms (American Academy of Pediatrics [AAP] Committee on Nutrition, 2001).

Minerals

A number of minerals are particularly important to early growth.

Calcium

Calcium is an important mineral in the newborn period because a newborn's skeleton is growing so rapidly. Because milk is high in calcium, tetany resulting from a low calcium level seldom occurs in infants who suck well, regardless of whether they are fed human milk or commercial formula.

Iron

The term newborn of a mother who had an adequate iron intake during pregnancy will be born with iron stores that, theoretically, last for the first 3 months of life, until the newborn begins to produce adult hemoglobin. Because not all mothers eat an iron-rich diet during pregnancy (and socioeconomic level is not a good criterion for judging the quality of a diet), the AAP recommends that infants who are formula fed ingest an iron enriched formula for the entire first year of life (AAP Committee on Nutrition, 1999). It is unnecessary to provide iron supplementation for breastfed infants, because breast milk usually provides an adequate amount of iron.

Fluoride

Fluoride is essential for building sound teeth and for preventing tooth decay. Because teeth grow into their primary form during pregnancy, it is important for women to drink fluoridated water during pregnancy. A lactating mother should continue drinking fluoridated water (although only a small amount of fluoride passes into breast milk), and formulas should be prepared with fluoridated water. This is an essential point to remember, because a mother may think she is helping her child by using bottled, "natural" water in formula rather than chlorinated (and fluoridated) water from a tap.

If a mother is breastfeeding and a source of fluoridated water is not available (the family drinks well, spring, or bottled water, or the tap water is not fluoridated), a fluoride supplement, 0.25 mg daily, may be given to the infant beginning at 6 months of age. Remind parents that too much fluoride can be detrimental or cause staining of the teeth, to prevent them from giving infants unnecessary fluoride supplements.

Vitamins

Vitamin additives are unnecessary for a formula-fed infant because vitamins A, C, and D are incorporated into commercial formula. Because vitamins are naturally included in breast milk, supplementation is not necessary for breastfed infants either. If a newborn will not be exposed to sunlight for some reason, 400 U of vitamin D daily may be prescribed for the breastfeeding mother, to increase the level of the vitamin in breast milk, or given to the formula-fed infant. Additional vitamins are not usually begun until the infant approaches 6 months of age.

BREASTFEEDING

WATCH LEARN

It is universally agreed that breast milk is the preferred method of feeding a newborn, because it provides numerous health benefits to both a mother and an infant; it remains the ideal nutritional source for infants through the first year of life (American College of Obstetricians & Gynecologists [ACOG], 2007). Nurses are prime people to teach women about the benefits of breastfeeding and provide anticipatory guidance for problems that may occur (Li, Rock, & Grummer-Strawn, 2007). You can also help create an atmosphere conducive to breastfeeding success in health care facilities by implementing steps such as:

- Educating all pregnant women about the benefits and management of breastfeeding
- Helping women initiate breastfeeding within half an hour after birth
- Assisting mothers to breastfeed and maintain lactation even if they should be separated from their infant
- Not giving newborns food or drink other than breast milk unless medically indicated, so they are hungry to breastfeed
- Supporting rooming-in (such as allowing mothers and infants to remain together) 24 hours a day
- Encouraging breastfeeding on demand
- Fostering the establishment of breastfeeding support groups and referring mothers to them on discharge from the birthing center or hospital

Women are recognized as the "keepers of the culture," or the main people who transmit customs to the next generation. Chief among these customs is the method for feeding newborns. The rate of breastfeeding varies in communities from almost 70% to a low of 13% as this is culturally influenced (Singh, Kogan, & Dee, 2007). If a woman comes from a family where no one has ever breastfed, she may be very interested in being a "pioneer" in her family. On the other hand, she may be more interested in following her family's tradition of formula feeding.

How soon women want to begin breastfeeding after birth is also culturally determined. Although it is the usual practice in hospitals to begin immediately after birth, some cultures believe that colostrum is not appropriate for newborns and have a cultural preference not to begin breastfeeding until milk is present, at about 3 days of age. It is necessary to assess each family individually to recognize cultural preferences such as these.

Physiology of Breast Milk Production

Breast milk is formed in the acinar or alveolar cells of the mammary glands (Fig. 19.1). With the delivery of the placenta, the level of progesterone in a woman's body falls dramatically, stimulating the production of **prolactin,** an anterior pituitary hormone. Prolactin acts on the acinar cells of the mammary glands to stimulate the production of milk. In addition, when an infant sucks at a breast, nerve impulses travel from the nipple to the hypothalamus to stimulate the production of prolactin-releasing factor. This factor stimulates further active production of prolactin. Other anterior pituitary hormones, such as adrenocorticotropic hormone, thyroid-stimulating hormone, and growth hormone, probably also play a role in growth of the mammary glands and their ability to secrete milk.

Colostrum, a thin, watery, yellow fluid composed of protein, sugar, fat, water, minerals, vitamins, and maternal antibodies, is secreted by the acinar breast cells starting in the fourth month of pregnancy. For the first 3 or 4 days after birth, colostrum production continues. Because it is high in protein and fairly low in sugar and fat, colostrum is easy to digest and capable of providing adequate nutrition for a newborn until it is replaced by transitional breast milk on the second to fourth day. True or mature breast milk is produced by the 10th day.

Milk flows from the alveolar cells, where it is produced, through small tubules to reservoirs for milk, the **lactiferous sinuses,** located behind the nipple. This constantly forming milk is called **fore milk.** Its availability depends very little on the infant's sucking at the breast. As the infant sucks at the breast, oxytocin, released from the posterior pituitary, causes the collecting sinuses of the mammary glands to contract,

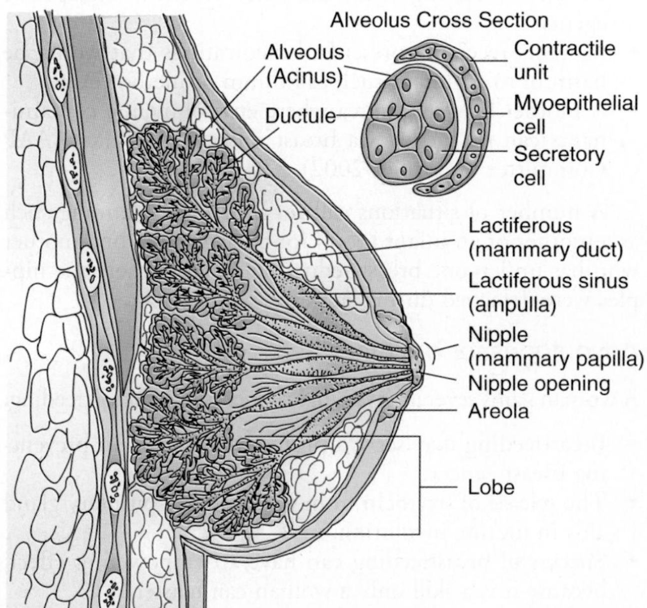

FIGURE 19.1 Anatomy of the breast.

forcing milk forward through the nipples, making it available for the baby. This action is called a **let-down reflex.** A let-down reflex may also be triggered by the sound of a baby crying or by thinking about the baby. New milk, called **hind milk,** is formed after the let-down reflex. Hind milk, higher in fat than fore milk, is the milk that makes a breastfed infant grow most rapidly. Release of oxytocin has a second advantage in that, by causing smooth muscle contraction, it helps contract the uterus. As a result, a woman may feel a small tugging or cramping in her lower pelvis during the first few days of breastfeeding (afterpains) (Pavone & Purinton, 2007).

Advantages of Breastfeeding

Little controversy exists about breastfeeding as the best nutrition for human infants, but the ultimate decision to breastfeed should depend on what would please a woman and her infant most. If she is pleased with what she is doing, her infant will be comfortable and pleased, will enjoy being fed, and will thrive.

Breastfeeding is contraindicated in only a few circumstances, such as:

- An infant with galactosemia (such infants cannot digest the lactose in milk)
- Herpes lesions on a mother's nipples
- Maternal diet is nutrient restricted, preventing quality milk production
- Maternal exposure to radioactive compounds (e.g., during thyroid testing)
- Breast cancer
- Maternal active, untreated tuberculosis, hepatitis B or C, cytomegalovirus, or human immunodeficiency syndrome
- Maternal active, untreated varicella. Once the infant has been given varicella zoster immunoglobulin, the infant can receive expressed breast milk if there are no lesions on the breast. Within 5 days of the appearance of the rash, maternal antibodies are produced, and thus breastfeeding could be beneficial in providing passive immunity against varicella (Sadeharju et al., 2007)
- Mothers receiving antimetabolites or chemotherapeutic agents
- Mothers receiving prescribed medications that would be harmful to an infant such as lithium or methotrexate
- A mother lives in an area where environmental contaminants can be carried via breast milk to the infant (AAP Committee on Drugs, 2002)

A number of situations call for individual planning such as a mother or an infant too ill for breastfeeding or a mother who has undergone breast-reduction surgery where the nipples were detached during surgery.

Advantages for a Mother

A woman gains several physiologic benefits from breastfeeding:

- Breastfeeding may serve a protective function in preventing breast cancer.
- The release of oxytocin from the posterior pituitary gland aids in uterine involution.
- Successful breastfeeding can have an empowering effect, because it is a skill only a woman can master.
- Breastfeeding reduces the cost of feeding and preparation time.
- Breastfeeding provides an excellent opportunity to enhance a true symbiotic bond between mother and child. Although this does occur readily with breastfeeding, a woman who holds her baby to formula feed can form this bond as well.

Common reasons that women give for not exclusive breastfeeding are (a) they want to provide the "best of both" or ensure that their babies get both the healthy aspects of breast milk and "vitamins" in formula, (b) breastfeeding can be embarrassing in public places, and (c) relatives give messages that supplementation is good for babies who are crying or not chubby (Deshpande, 2008).

Some women believe that breastfeeding, because it causes a delay in menstruation (lactational amenorrhea), is a foolproof contraceptive technique. It is not: 50% of women resume ovulating by the fourth week after delivery, even while breastfeeding (Van der Wijden, Kleijnen, & van den Berk, 2009).

Some women believe that breastfeeding will help them lose weight gained during pregnancy. This also is not true, and women who are breastfeeding need to concentrate on eating a well-balanced diet to ensure their milk will be rich in nutrients. Some women are reluctant to breastfeed because they fear that having to be available to feed the baby every 3 or 4 hours will tie them down. Like mothers who formula feed, however, they can leave a bottle (with expressed breast milk) with the baby's father or a caregiver if they need to be away from their baby at the time of a feeding.

Advantages for an Infant

Breastfeeding has major physiologic advantages for an infant as well. Breast milk contains secretory immunoglobulin A (IgA), which binds large molecules of foreign proteins, including viruses and bacteria, keeping them from being absorbed from the gastrointestinal tract into the infant. **Lactoferrin** is an iron-binding protein in breast milk that interferes with the growth of pathogenic bacteria. The enzyme **lysozyme** in breast milk apparently actively destroys bacteria by lysing (dissolving) their cell membranes, possibly increasing the effectiveness of antibodies. Leukocytes in breast milk provide protection against common respiratory infectious invaders. Macrophages, responsible for producing **interferon** (a protein that protects against viruses), help interfere with virus growth. The **bifidus factor** is a specific growth-promoting factor for the beneficial bacteria *Lactobacillus bifidus.* The presence of *L. bifidus* in breast milk interferes with the colonization of pathogenic bacteria in the gastrointestinal tract, reducing the incidence of diarrhea.

In addition to these anti-infective properties, breast milk contains the ideal electrolyte and mineral composition for human infant growth. It is high in lactose, an easily digested sugar that provides ready glucose for rapid brain growth. The protein in breast milk is easily digested, and the ratio of cysteine to methionine (two amino acids) in breast milk favors rapid brain growth in the early months. It contains nitrogen in compounds other than protein, so that an infant can receive cell-building materials from sources other than just protein.

Breast milk contains more linoleic acid, an essential fatty acid for skin integrity, and less sodium, potassium, calcium, and phosphorus than do many formulas. Breast milk also has a better balance of trace elements, such as zinc. These levels of nutrients are enough to supply the infant's needs, yet they spare the infant's kidneys from having to process a high renal solute load of unused nutrients. Women who have a familial history of allergy are usually encouraged to breastfeed to try and eliminate the possibility of exposing their infant to cow's milk protein, which could be allergenic this early in life (Hampton, 2008).

Yet another advantage is that breastfed newborns appear to be able to regulate their calcium/phosphorus levels better than infants who are formula fed. Decreased calcium levels in a newborn can lead to tetany (muscle spasm). The increased concentration of fatty acid in commercial formulas may bind calcium in the gastrointestinal tract, increasing the danger of tetany. Breastfeeding may also help prevent excessive weight gain in infants (Box 19.3).

A great deal of discussion about the benefits of breastfeeding has centered on the effects of breastfeeding on the formation of the dental arch, because babies suck differently from a breast than from a bottle (Fig. 19.2). Babies pull their tongue backward as they suck from a breast. They thrust their tongue forward to suck from a rubber nipple. That may make breastfeeding the best preparation for forming common speech sounds (Ferguson & Molfese, 2007).

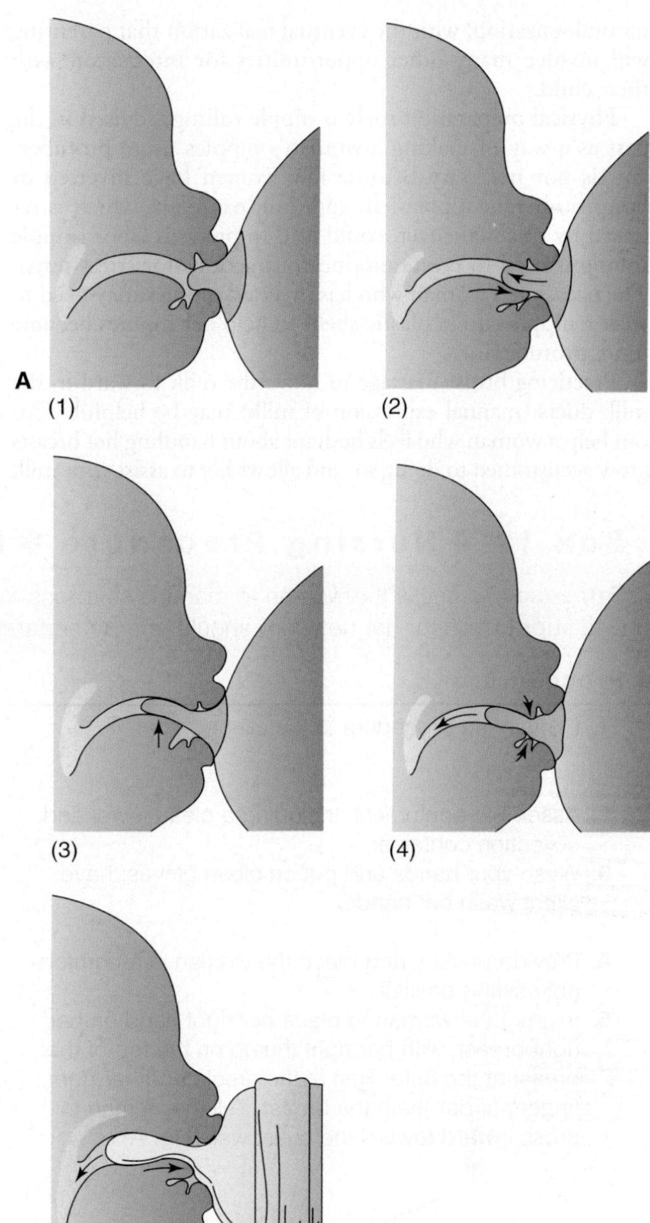

FIGURE 19.2 Differences in sucking mechanism. (**A**) The breast. (**1**) Lips of the infant clamp in a C-shape. The cheek muscles contract. (**2**) The tongue thrusts forward to grasp nipple and areola. (**3**) The nipple is brought against the hard palate as the tongue pulls backward, bringing the areola into the mouth. (**4**) The gums compress the areola, squeezing milk into the back of the throat. (**B**) Formula feeding. The large rubber nipple of a bottle strikes the soft palate and interferes with the action of the tongue. The tongue moves forward against the gums to control the overflow of milk into the esophagus.

✔ Checkpoint Question 19.1

Newborns need more fluid than adults, because their extracellular fluid component differs from that of adults. How much of a newborn's body weight is extracellular fluid?

a. 20%, compared with 35% in an adult.
b. 35%, compared with 20% in an adult.
c. 50%, compared with 70% in an adult.
d. 70%, compared with 40% in an adult.

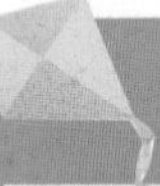

BOX 19.3 ✻ Focus on Evidence-Based Practice

Can breastfeeding help reduce the epidemic of obesity in children?

To answer this question, researchers studied the health records of 3692 children at 4 years of age to determine whether they were overweight and whether they had been breastfed.

Overweight was defined as body mass index for age at the 95th percentile and above. Results of the study showed that the longer the period of breastfeeding, the more apt a child was less likely to be overweight, or breastfeeding offered a significant protective association against childhood obesity for non-Hispanic children.

Would this study be helpful when discussing an advantage of breastfeeding?

Source: Procter, S. B., & Holcomb, C. A. (2008). Breastfeeding duration and childhood overweight among low-income children in Kansas, 1998–2002. *American Journal of Public Health, 98*(1), 106–110.

Techniques of Breastfeeding

Ask all women during pregnancy whether they plan to breastfeed or formula feed their newborn as thinking about feeding in advance allows couples to make informed choices. Some fathers experience jealousy at the thought of breastfeeding. Early discussion can help them work through this natural sensation, with the eventual realization that parenting will involve many other opportunities for interaction with their child.

Physical preparation such as nipple rolling, advised in the past as a way of making a woman's nipples more protuberant, is not necessary because few women have inverted or nonprotuberant nipples. In addition, oxytocin, which is released by this maneuver, could lead to preterm labor (nipple rolling is used to create uterine contractions for stress tests). The occasional woman who has inverted nipples may need to wear a nipple cup (a plastic shell) to help her nipples become more protuberant.

Practicing breast massage to move the milk forward in the milk ducts (manual expression of milk) may be helpful. This can help a woman who feels hesitant about handling her breasts grow accustomed to doing so, and allows her to assist with milk production in the first few days after birth. Manual expression consists of supporting the breast firmly, then placing the thumb and forefinger on the opposite sides of the breast, just behind the areolar margin, first pushing backward toward the chest wall and then downward until secretions begins to flow (Box 19.4). During the last months of pregnancy and immediately after birth, the fluid obtained will be colostrum. By the third day of infant life, milk will be obtained.

Teach women to wash their breasts with clear water because soap tends to dry and crack nipples.

Beginning Breastfeeding

Breastfeeding should begin as soon after birth as possible, ideally while the woman is still in the birthing room and while the infant is in the first reactivity period (Forster & McLachlan,

Box 19.4 Nursing Procedure ✻ Manual Breast Milk Expression

Purpose: To assist the woman to manually express milk so she can strengthen her milk supply and supply milk for her newborn should she be separated from the newborn

Procedure	Principle
1. Explain the procedure to the client.	1. Explanations help decrease anxiety and enhance learning; they also provide information for the client to carry out the procedure on her own.
2. Assemble equipment, including a clean towel and collection container.	2. Assembling equipment aids in organization and efficiency.
3. Wash your hands and put on clean gloves; have client wash her hands.	3. Handwashing prevents the transmission of infection; use of gloves protects self and client from possible infection.
4. Provide privacy and place the woman in a comfortable sitting position.	4. The let-down reflex may not occur readily if the woman is tense or nervous.
5. Instruct the woman to place her right hand on her right breast, with her right thumb on the top of the breast at the outer limit of the areola and her right fingers underneath the breast. Tell the woman to press inward toward the chest wall (Fig. A).	5. Milk is expressed by pressure on the collecting ducts, not the nipple.

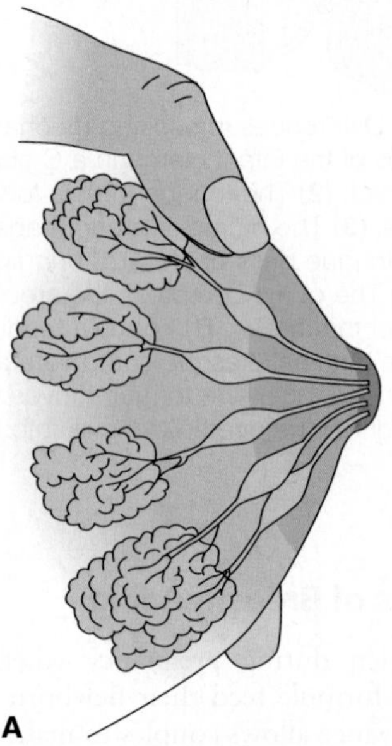

Box 19.4 Nursing Procedure ✻ Manual Breast Milk Expression

6. Help the woman hold the collecting jar just under her nipple.

6. Collecting bottles should be made of plastic to preserve antibodies found in milk; having the container close by prevents waste of any breast milk that is expressed.

7. Have the woman slide her hand forward in a milking motion, causing the milk to be expressed from the nipple into the container (Fig. B).

7. Pressure on the lactiferous sinuses pushes milk forward.

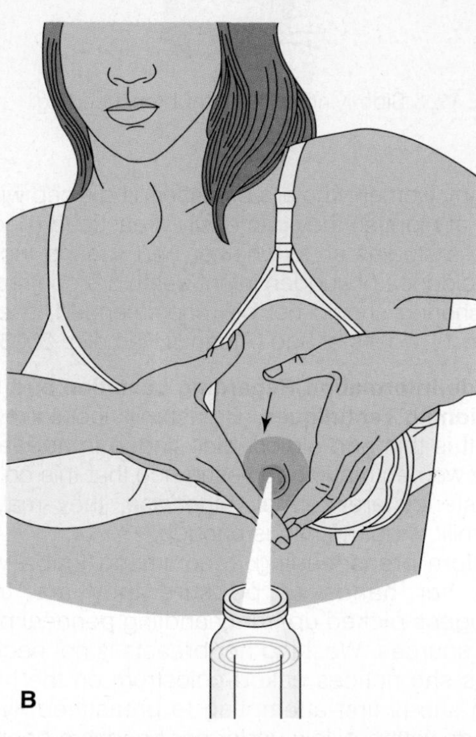

8. Have the woman move her thumb and fingers around her breast, repeating the technique.

8. Repeating the technique ensures that all milk sinuses are emptied.

9. Caution the woman not to use excess force.

9. Excess force will damage sensitive breast tissue.

10. After collection, refrigerate milk if it will be used within 24 hours; freeze if this time is longer.

10. Breast milk spoils in the same manner as cow's milk if not protected.

11. Reinforce the woman's success with this maneuver, regardless of the amount of breast milk expressed.

11. Manual breast milk expression is an easy technique to carry out once it is learned, but it can be difficult to grasp at first. Positive reinforcement enhances progress and self-esteem.

2007). The release of oxytocin by breastfeeding at this time begins the let-down of milk and also stimulates uterine contraction. However, if the woman is overly fatigued or extremely modest, trying to learn this new skill at this time may only convince her that breastfeeding is not for her.

Most women enjoy having an experienced nurse with them for a first feeding to offer suggestions. It is important that infants open their mouths wide enough to grasp both the nipple and the **areola** (the pigmented circle surrounding the nipple) when sucking. This gives them effective sucking action and helps to empty the collecting sinuses completely.

Milk forms in response to being used. If breasts are completely emptied, they completely fill again. If half emptied, they only half fill, and, after a time, milk production will be insufficient for proper nourishment. A woman should always place her infant first at the breast at which the infant fed last in the previous feeding, to help ensure that each breast is completely emptied at every other feeding.

Because it takes less energy for an infant to suck at a bottle, urge parents not to offer bottles of breast milk until 4 to 6 weeks of age, after they are thoroughly accustomed to breastfeeding. The American Academy of Pediatrics (2008) recommends the use of pacifiers when placing infants to sleep for the first year of life to help prevent sudden infant death syndrome (SIDS) but delaying this practice until 1 month of age in breastfed infants. As one of the reasons that SIDS may occur is the infant rebreathing expired carbon dioxide–rich air, using a fan in the room during sleep or opening a window so there is a breeze in the room may be yet another way the incidence of SIDS can be reduced (Coleman-Phox, Odouli, & Li, 2008).

What if... Linda told you that she doesn't want to breastfeed but her husband is insisting that she do so? What would you do?

Prolonged Jaundice in Breastfed Infants

Jaundice occurs in as many as 15% of breastfed infants. This is because pregnanediol (a breakdown product of progesterone) in breast milk depresses the action of glucuronyl transferase, the enzyme that converts indirect bilirubin to the direct form, which is then readily excreted in bile (Huether, & McCance, 2008). To prevent hyperbilirubinemia in their infant, women should feed frequently in the immediate birth period, because colostrum is a natural laxative and helps promote passage of meconium and bile. Newborns who are discharged early need to be observed for jaundice while at home. However, breastfeeding rarely results in a serum bilirubin level high enough to warrant therapy or to require discontinuation of breastfeeding, because pregnanediol remains in breast milk for only 24 to 48 hours (Thilo & Rosenberg, 2008).

Nursing Diagnoses and Related Interventions

Nursing Diagnosis: Health-seeking behaviors related to lack of knowledge about lactation and breastfeeding techniques

Outcome Evaluation: Woman states correct information as to how lactation begins and is maintained in adequate supply; demonstrates effective positioning for baby and herself by 24 hours.

In cultures where breastfeeding is practiced by almost all mothers, the technique is learned early in life by observation. In the United States, women may have had few, if any, opportunities to observe breastfeeding. Lactation consultants are health care professionals especially educated to assist women with breastfeeding. Making a referral to such a person can be extremely helpful. With managed care, however, fewer such specialists may be available, so all nurses need to be well prepared to assist with breastfeeding.

When a woman first begins breastfeeding, help her learn to reserve a special part of her day for this so she can relax to do it. If she is tense and anxious, she may have difficulty achieving a let-down reflex, and her infant may have difficulty obtaining adequate milk. This can lead to increasing tension and anxiety because the infant does not seem content. As a result, the infant becomes hungrier and is left even more unsatisfied, creating a vicious circle of events. Support, adequate instruction, and reassurance from health care personnel are important in helping a woman feel secure enough to be able to relax (Furber & Thomson, 2007). Rooming-in is ideal for breastfeeding, because it allows a woman to sense when her infant is hungry and feed before the infant grows fatigued from crying or her breasts grow uncomfortable from filling.

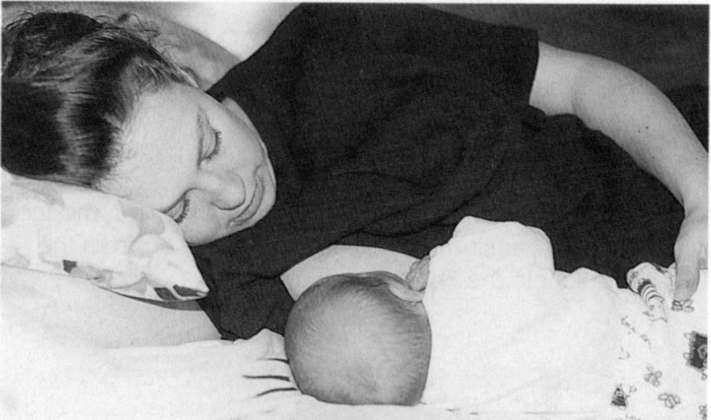

FIGURE 19.3 Side-lying position for breastfeeding.

Many women who are breastfeeding sleep with their infant at night so they can easily breastfeed (bed sharing). As studies as to whether bed sharing increases the incidence of sudden infant death are contradictory, bed sharing should not be recommended, especially before 11 weeks of age (Ateah & Hamelin, 2008).

Provide Information Regarding Lactation and Proper Positioning Techniques. Breast milk looks like nonfat milk. It is thin and almost blue-tinged in appearance. Some women may need assurance that this color and consistency are normal; otherwise, they may think their milk is not nutritious enough.

Before breastfeeding, recommend that a woman wash her hands to be sure they are free of pathogens picked up from handling perineal pads or other sources. Washing her breasts is not necessary unless she notices caked colostrum on the nipples. When she is first attempting to breastfeed, lying on her side with a pillow under her head is a good position to use (Fig. 19.3). This relieves fatigue because it allows her infant to rest on the bed. Figure 19.4

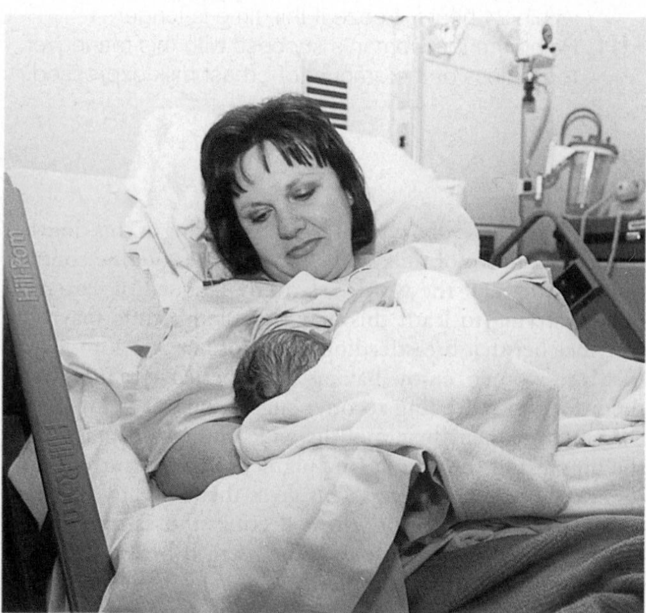

FIGURE 19.4 Sitting position for breastfeeding.

shows a sitting position with a pillow under the baby. Using a football hold with the baby supported on a pillow also may be helpful, especially if a mother had a cesarean birth.

Brushing the infant's cheek with a breast nipple stimulates a newborn's rooting reflex. The baby then turns toward the breast. Do not try to initiate a rooting reflex by pressing a baby's face against the mother's breast; this will cause the child to turn away from the mother and toward your hand. Although not well documented as to efficiency or reliable results, an assessment tool such as the LATCH assessment (Table 19.2) can provide measures to help evaluate a newborn's breastfeeding effectiveness (Howe et al., 2008).

If a woman has large breasts, the infant may have trouble breathing while nursing because breast tissue presses against the nose. A woman can prevent this happening by grasping the areolar margin of her breast between her thumb and forefinger, holding the bulk of the breast supported while her infant feeds. This also makes the nipple more protuberant.

During the first few days of life, because they are receiving only colostrum and need the nutrients and fluid obtained by frequent sucking, babies should be fed as often as they seem hungry (every 2 to 3 hours). Frequent feeding also is advantageous to sustain a milk supply, because the more often breasts are emptied, the more efficiently they fill and continue to maintain a good supply of milk.

As important as making certain that infants grasp the breast areola is helping them to break away from the breast when they are through feeding. Teach a woman to insert a finger in the corner of the infant's mouth or pull down the infant's chin to release suction. Otherwise, the baby may pull too hard on the nipple, causing cracking or soreness.

Promote Adequate Sucking. Often, a newborn being breastfed drops off to sleep during the first few feedings. To both stimulate milk production effectively and ensure adequate fluid intake, a woman may need to keep the infant awake and urge him or her to suck. Advise mothers to be sure to awaken newborns fully before feeding by handling them, stroking their backs, changing their position, rubbing their arms and chest, or changing their diaper. Gently tickling the bottom of a baby's feet will also wake a baby effectively. Many women are unwilling to cause their newborns discomfort in these ways. This reaction is a positive one, because it may be one of the first signs that a woman is transferring the protectiveness toward her own body that she felt during pregnancy to her newborn.

If an infant is not sucking well, a woman can use breast massage after a feeding to empty her breasts manually. This helps ensure good milk production for the time when the infant is ready to suck.

Provide Immediate Support If Problems Arise. When handled intelligently by health care personnel, the common problems that arise with breastfeeding usually pass and seem unimportant to a woman. Handled otherwise, they can complicate breastfeeding and discourage a woman from continuing. It is unfortunate when complications deter a woman from using the most natural and least complicated of all infant feeding methods.

Provide Information Regarding Techniques for Burping the Breastfed Baby. Some infants seem to swallow little air when they breastfeed, whereas others swallow a great deal. As a rule, it is helpful to bubble (burp) newborns after they have emptied the first breast and again after the total feeding.

TABLE 19.2 ✻ Latch Breastfeeding Charting System

	0	1	2
L Latch	Too sleepy or reluctant; no latch achieved	Repeated attempts; hold nipple in mouth; stimulate to suck	Grasps breast; tongue down; lips flanged; rhythmic sucking
A Audible Swallowing	None	A few with stimulation	Spontaneous and intermittent under 24 hr old; spontaneous and frequent over 24 hr old
T Type of Nipple	Inverted	Flat	Everted (after stimulation)
C Comfort (Breast/Nipple)	Engorged; cracked, bleeding, large blisters or bruises; severe discomfort	Filling; reddened/small blisters or bruises; mild/moderate discomfort	Soft, nontender
H Hold (Positioning)	Full assist (staff holds infant at breast)	Minimal assist (i.e., place pillows for support, elevate head of bed); teach one side, mother does other; staff holds and then mother takes over	No assist from staff; mother able to position/hold baby by self

Source: Jensen, D., Wallace, S., & Kelsey, P. (1994). LATCH: a breastfeeding charting system and documentation tool. *Journal of Obstetric, Gynecologic, and Neonatal Nursing, 23*(1), 27–32.

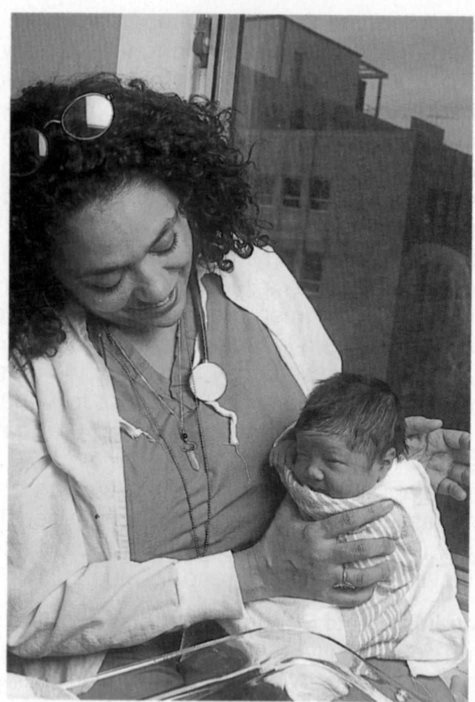

FIGURE 19.5 A nurse burps a newborn using a sitting position. The infant's head is supported by the nurse's hand.

Placing the baby over one shoulder and gently patting or stroking the back is an acceptable position. However, this position is not always satisfactory for a small infant, who has poor head control. In addition, a parent may have difficulty supporting the baby's head and patting the back at the same time.

Holding the baby in a sitting position on the lap, then leaning the child forward against one hand, with the index finger and thumb supporting the head, is often the best position to use. This position provides head support but leaves the other hand free to pat the baby's back (Fig. 19.5). Parents usually need to be shown this method, because it does not seem as natural as placing a baby against the shoulder. Laying the baby prone across the lap is another alternative position.

Support for a Mother Who Is Breastfeeding Multiple Infants. Because of in vitro fertilization, many more women today than previously give birth to twins or multiple infants. You can assure women that the average woman can easily produce enough milk to feed multiple infants. Because of the time involved, however, many fewer women with multiple infants choose to breastfeed than do mothers of single infants (Moore, 2007). Support those who want to breastfeed multiple infants by being sure they drink adequate fluid and help them to organize their time.

Nursing Diagnosis: Pain related to breast engorgement or sore nipples

Outcome Evaluation: Client states she is experiencing little or no discomfort; can breastfeed without undue discomfort; infant grasps nipple firmly.

On the third or fourth day after birth, when breast milk forms, some women may notice breast distention, accompanied by hardness, tenderness, and perhaps heat in their breasts. The skin appears red, tense, and shiny. This is primary **engorgement,** caused by vascular and lymphatic congestion arising from an increase in the blood and lymph supply to the breasts. Infants have difficulty sucking on engorged breasts, because the areola is too hard to grasp (Fig. 19.6). A woman also may have difficulty breastfeeding her infant, because her breasts feel so tender.

Prevent or Relieve Engorgement. The primary method for relieving engorgement is emptying the breasts of milk by having the infant suck more often, or at least continue to suck as much as before. Unfortunately, a woman's breasts are sometimes so painful that it is difficult for her to continue to breastfeed unless she is given something for pain relief. Good breast support from a firm-fitting bra helps prevent a pulling, heavy feeling.

If an infant cannot grasp a nipple to suck strongly because of engorgement, warm packs applied to both breasts or standing under a warm shower for a few minutes before feeding, combined with massage to begin milk flow, often promotes breast softness so an infant can suck. Manual expression or the use of a breast pump to complete emptying of the breasts after the baby has nursed can help maintain or promote a good milk supply during a period of engorgement (Fig. 19.7).

Fortunately, engorgement is a transient problem. Unfortunately, it occurs just as women are beginning to feel skilled at breastfeeding. Suddenly their breasts are swollen, hot, and tender. They may worry that an infection has developed or their baby will not get enough milk. Assure a mother that symptoms of engorgement are healthy; it is an announcement her breasts are producing milk. Assure her that engorgement is only temporary and should begin to subside 24 hours after it first becomes apparent.

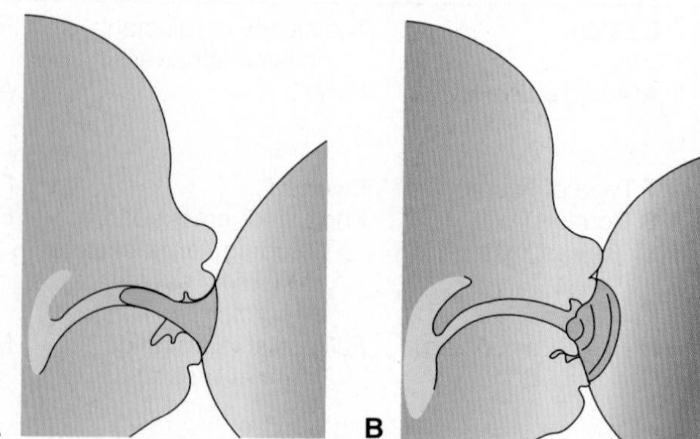

FIGURE 19.6 The problem that breast engorgement causes to breastfeeding. (**A**) When sucking at a normal breast, the infant's lips compress the areola and fit neatly against the sides of the nipple. The infant also has adequate room to breathe. (**B**) When a breast is engorged, the infant has difficulty grasping the nipple. Breathing ability is compromised.

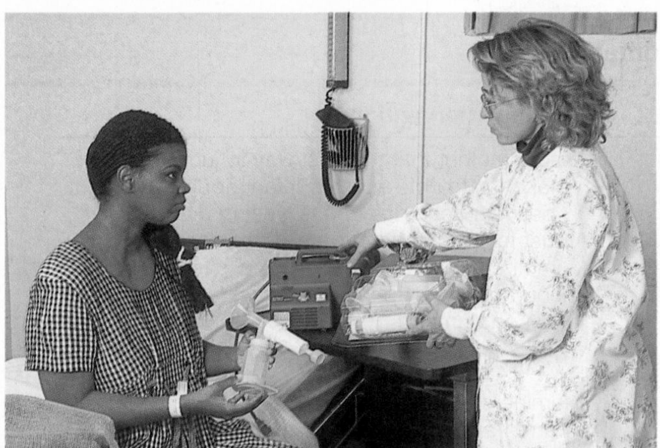

FIGURE 19.7 A nurse and mother discuss the advantages and disadvantages of an electric breast pump (shown on the table) and a manual pump (shown in the mother's hands).

Promote Healing of Sore Nipples. Painful nipples result from the strong sucking action of a newborn. This may be worsened by:

- Improper positioning of an infant (failure to grasp the areola as well as the nipple)
- Forcefully pulling an infant from a breast
- Allowing an infant to suck too long at a breast after the breast is emptied
- Permitting a nipple to remain wet from leaking milk

Normally, nipples are kept supple from the secretions of the Montgomery tubercles in the areola. They can become sore when they are excessively dry or wet, which makes them crack or fissure. To help prevent soreness, encourage a mother to position her baby slightly differently for each feeding. This helps prevent the same area of the nipple from receiving the majority of pressure. Advise her to expose her nipples to air by leaving her bra unsnapped for 10 to 15 minutes after feeding. Some mothers use a hair dryer set on low to aid drying. Discourage the use of plastic liners that come with nursing bras; it is preferable to have air always circulating around the breasts. Applying vitamin E lotion after air exposure may toughen the nipples and prevent further irritation. Applying a few drops of breast milk to the nipples after feeding and gently massaging it into the areola is also recommended.

Advise women not to use a hand pump with sore nipples, because the pressure may cause fissures to worsen. An electric or battery-operated pump (standard equipment in most maternity or pediatric hospitals) usually can be used; these devices exert less pressure on the nipples.

Sore nipples, like engorgement, are not a contraindication to breastfeeding. If steps to prevent sore nipples are followed, the problem is unlikely to become acute again.

Nursing Diagnosis: Anxiety related to inability to measure amount of milk taken by the baby

Outcome Evaluation: Client states the baby seems satisfied after feeding and voices confidence that the baby is getting enough milk; baby voids six to eight times per day after the first week.

Some breastfeeding mothers wonder whether their infant is getting enough to eat. They watch a woman formula feed and listen to her report, "He took 3 ounces this feeding," and wish they could tell as surely whether their infant's intake is adequate. Assure them that the ultimate test with either breastfeeding or formula feeding is not how much an infant swallows at one time but whether the infant seems content between feedings. Acceptable criteria during the first week of life are wetting six to eight diapers within 24 hours or losing no more than 10% of birth weight. After the first week, weight gain and voiding six to eight times each 24 hours are good criteria. Although the formula-feeding mother measures the amount of formula as a way of determining adequate feeding in the early weeks, soon she, too, begins to use the alternative criteria: her baby is happy, voids an adequate number of times, and is gaining weight. Helping a woman use these criteria allows her to develop confidence in her judgment to evaluate her child's health, a role that will be hers for the next 18 or more years.

Nursing Diagnosis: Deficient knowledge related to potential harm to baby from drugs taken by breastfeeding mother

Outcome Evaluation: Client states she is aware almost all drugs taken may be excreted in her breast milk; voices importance of consulting physician or nurse practitioner before taking any medication.

For years, it was believed that a placental barrier protected a fetus from exposure to drugs taken by a woman during pregnancy; a similar protection was postulated for breast milk. However, it is clear a fetus is extremely susceptible to drugs ingested by a woman, and the same is true of breastfed infants. Almost any drug may cross into the acinar cells and be secreted in breast milk. Drugs that should be avoided by breastfeeding mothers because of their documented harmful effects on infants are shown in Appendix C. The rule a woman followed all during pregnancy, that she should take no drug unless prescribed or approved by her primary care provider, continues to apply during lactation.

Nursing Diagnosis: Effective breastfeeding related to mother's desire to provide the best nutrition for her child

Outcome Evaluation: Client states she intends to continue breastfeeding at home; voices confidence in her ability to provide adequate milk for infant; names resources for help if needed; infant exhibits adequate weight gain and elimination pattern for age.

Anticipate Potential Problems and Suggest Methods for Resolving Them. Common problems that can arise with breastfeeding once a mother returns home are summarized in Table 19.3. Women who do not remember to begin nursing the baby at the breast the infant finished on the last time may find their milk supply decreasing in one breast. Although changing breasts may be easy to remember in the hospital,

TABLE 19.3 ✻ Common Concerns of Breastfeeding Mothers

Concern	Cause	Nursing Interventions
Mother worries about amount of milk being taken	Mother cannot see the amount taken	Assure mother that the best way to judge amount taken is to note whether infant appears content between feedings and is wetting diapers.
Infant does not suck well	Possible effect of analgesia from labor	Adjust feeding pattern to child's needs; assure mother that effect of analgesia is temporary.
	Infant brought to mother when not hungry	Encourage rooming-in. Encourage feeding on cue, not on demand.
	Infant exhausted by crying from hunger	
Mother reports infant's stools are loose and thin	Stools normally looser and lighter in color than in formula-fed babies	Examine stools; explain normal stool pattern and transitions.
Father feels shut out of parent–child relationship	Father does not participate in infant feeding	Show other ways of interacting with infant than through feeding.
Sore nipples	Infant not gripping entire areola	Help infant to grasp nipple correctly; expose nipple to air between feedings; aloe vera or vitamin E applied to nipples helps heal tissue.
	Nipple kept wet	
Engorgement	Lymphatic filling as milk production begins	Encourage infant to suck (engorgement subsides best if infant can be encouraged to suck); apply warm packs to breasts or have mother take a warm shower before feeding to help soften breast tissue.
Breastfeeding in public	Some people make a woman feel uncomfortable breastfeeding at work or other public places.	Encourage a woman to use discretion to avoid confrontation (unless she wants to make a point that breastfeeding is a natural action) and to speak to work site administrator about comfortable arrangements.

distractions at home can make the sequence difficult to remember. Pinning a safety pin to the bra strap on the side to start with at the next feeding is a useful way to help remember this.

Fatigue can be another problem on returning home if a woman does not take adequate measures to conserve her energy. Sitting relaxed in a comfortable chair with her feet elevated, feeding her baby, and enjoying this time is an excellent way to rest.

Remind women that adequate maternal fluid intake is necessary to maintain an adequate milk supply. Women who are breastfeeding should drink at least four 8-oz glasses of fluid a day, and many need to drink six glasses. They need to increase their calorie intake by about 500 calories a day (Table 19.4). A daily diet plan for a lactating woman is given in Table 19.5.

At one time, women were given a list of foods not to eat while they were breastfeeding because it was thought they caused diarrhea, constipation, or colic in infants. Today, there are no rules other than to use common sense. A woman can eat anything that agrees with her, is taken in moderation, and to which she is not allergic.

Some women stop breastfeeding because they have no one to talk to about a problem or to give them support. A nurse working as a hospital community liaison person, community health nurse, or lactation consultant can be a valuable resource to provide answers and support while a woman is at home (see Focus on Nursing Care Planning Box 19.5).

TABLE 19.4 ✻ Daily Reference Intakes for Women During Lactation

Nutrient	During Lactation
Calories (kcal)	+500
Protein (g)	71
Vitamin A	1300
Vitamin D (μg)	5.0
Vitamin E (mg)	19
Vitamin K (μg)	75–90
Vitamin C (mg)	120
Folate (μg)	500
Niacin (mg)	17
Riboflavin (mg)	1.6
Thiamine (mg)	1.4
Vitamin B_6 (mg)	2.0
Calcium (mg)	1000–1300
Vitamin B_{12} (μg)	2.8
Phosphorus (mg)	700–1250
Iodine (μg)	290
Iron (mg)	9–10
Magnesium (mg)	320–360
Zinc (mg)	12–13

Source: U.S. Department of Health and Human Services and U.S. Department of Agriculture. (2005). *Dietary guidelines for Americans, 2005.* (6th ed). Washington, DC: U.S. Government Printing Office.

TABLE 19.5 ✻ Daily Quantities of Food Necessary for a Woman During Lactation

Food Group	Quantities for Active Nonpregnant Woman	Quantities for Lactating Woman
Meat, fowl, or fish	2 servings daily	2–3 servings daily
Vegetables	3–5 servings daily	4 servings daily
Fruits	2–4 servings daily	4 servings daily
Breads, cereals, rice, pasta	6–11 servings daily	6–12 servings daily
Milk	2 glasses (8-oz) daily	4–6 glasses (8-oz) daily
Fats, oils, sweets	Use sparingly	1 serving daily
Additional fluid	As desired	4–6 glasses daily

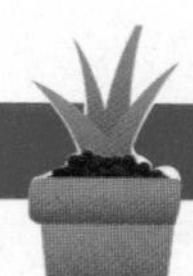

BOX 19.5 ✻ Focus on Nursing Care Planning

A Multidisciplinary Care Map for a Woman Who Is Breastfeeding for the First Time

Linda Satir is a new mother of a term baby girl. During the pregnancy, she and her husband, Paul, both agreed Linda would breastfeed. She attempted to breastfeed her newborn in the birthing room, with minimal success. As you offer to help her feed her baby for the second time, she says, "Do you think I made the right choice? Maybe I should formula-feed her. Paul could help that way and I won't have to worry about what to do when I go back to work."

Family Assessment ✻ Client lives with husband in two-bedroom trailer in suburban trailer park. Husband works as an interpreter for local Chamber of Commerce. Linda will be returning to work as an executive assistant at an advertising agency after her 6-week maternity leave.

Client Assessment ✻ Mother is 2 hours postpartum. Newborn had difficulty latching onto breasts immediately after birth. Nipples without signs of redness or irritation. Breasts slightly firm. Colostrum present. Client discouraged with first breastfeeding attempt.

Nursing Diagnosis ✻ Risk for ineffective breastfeeding related to anxiety and inexperience

Outcome Criteria ✻ Client describes ways to properly position a newborn at the breast; states that newborn is latching on and sucking; verbalizes satisfaction and confidence with each feeding session.

Team Member Responsible	Assessment	Intervention	Rationale	Expected Outcome
		Activities of Daily Living		
Nurse	Assess client's usual daily activity pattern.	Review with client how she intends to adjust activities to accommodate breastfeeding.	Preplanning can help to avoid problems with breastfeeding.	Client describes her daily routines and identifies adjustments she can predict will need to be made for breastfeeding.
		Consultations		
Nurse	Investigate whether client would like consultation from a lactation consultant; determine which lactation consultant is available.	If client agrees, initiate a referral to a lactation consultant.	Lactation consultants can provide an additional source of support, encouragement, and information.	Client meets with consultant if desired.

(continued)

BOX 19.5 ✻ Focus on Nursing Care Planning (continued)

Team Member Responsible	Assessment	Intervention	Rationale	Expected Outcome
		Procedures/Medications		
Nurse	Observe client breastfeeding to determine techniques she uses.	Make suggestions as necessary regarding breastfeeding techniques such as how to break suction, remove newborn from breast, or begin next feeding on breast newborn used most recently.	Additional suggestions can help make breastfeeding successful by encouraging client to relax during feedings.	Client states she is willing to try additional suggestions to help improve breastfeeding success.
		Nutrition		
Nurse	Assess client's present daily fluid intake.	Advise client to drink at least four to six 8-oz glasses of fluid per day.	Adequate fluid intake is essential to maintain an adequate milk supply.	Client confirms she drinks suggested fluid every day and will continue to do this at home.
		Patient/Family Education		
Nurse/ lactation consultant	Assess client's knowledge about breastfeeding. Allow time for questions.	Educate client regarding any gaps in knowledge.	The better informed women are about breastfeeding, the more apt they are to feel comfortable with the process.	Client asks questions regarding areas of breastfeeding of which she is unsure.
		Psychosocial/Spiritual/Emotional Needs		
Nurse/ lactation consultant	Assess what client thought breastfeeding would be like.	Acknowledge that breastfeeding involves newly learned skills and is not as easy as it looks.	Assurance can increase self-esteem when a person is learning a new skill.	Client states she is willing to try for a longer time than a few feedings to see if she can be successful at breastfeeding.
		Discharge Planning		
Nurse	Assess steps client intends to take to ensure breastfeeding success after return home or returning to work.	Provide feedback and suggestions, reinforcing accomplishments and assisting with any difficulties.	Feedback and positive reinforcement promote self-confidence and learning, enhancing the success of teaching and effectiveness of breastfeeding.	Client describes well-thought-out plans for continuing breastfeeding and integrating it into her lifestyle.
Nurse	Assess if local support organization is available for referral.	Suggest client keep telephone numbers of support group and lactation consultant available if she needs additional help while at home or work.	Support can go a long way toward preventing a client from becoming discouraged once she returns home.	Client states she will contact support people as necessary if she has questions after discharge.

Provide Information on Supplemental Feedings. A breastfeeding woman may leave her child during the day or evening in the care of a babysitter or another care provider, just as a formula-feeding woman may. She can express breast milk manually and leave it in a bottle in the refrigerator or prepare a single bottle of formula for the time she is away.

Bottles used for storage should be washed using normal dishwashing practice. Breast milk then may be refrigerated for 24 hours, frozen for 30 days, or placed in a deep freezer for 6 months. Use of commercially prepared formula or powder formula is appropriate and convenient to replace a single feeding because one bottle at a time can be prepared. The bottle used should be glass or opaque, nonshiny plastic as shiny types may contain polycarbonate, a compound that can leech into stored milk and is associated with chromosomal aberrations (Raloff, 2007).

Once breastfeeding has been established (after about 6 weeks), missing one feeding will not affect milk production enough to make a difference at the next feeding. There is no need for a mother to express milk manually to safeguard a supply while the infant takes a supplemental feeding, although she may prefer to do so to reduce tension and discomfort.

Provide Information for a Mother Who Works Outside the Home. Many women return to work while continuing to breastfeed by bringing their infant with them to their workplace. Others express breast milk for a caregiver to give by bottle while they work. As there are many considerations to think about, women should review with an employer the best way for them to continue breastfeeding at their worksite (Abdulwadud & Snow, 2009) (Box 19.6).

Provide Information on Weaning. It is best for infants if they are exclusively breastfed for at least 6 months (Kramer & Kakuma, 2009). Women breastfeed for varying lengths of time, however. Some do it for 1, 2, or 3 months and then wean their children from breast to formula. Others continue until their children are 6 to 12 months of age and then wean directly to a small cup or glass. Some continue to breastfeed until the child is of toddler or preschool age (Fig. 19.8). The AAP recommends that infants be breastfed for a full year; the World Health Organization (2002) recommends exclusive breastfeeding for 6 months and continuation for 2 years. Discontinuing breastfeeding may make infants more susceptible to infection as infants are no longer receiving immune protection (Akus & Bartick, 2007). Too lengthy a time of breastfeeding, however, may lead to nutritional deficiencies if the child is taking in a large quantity of milk at the expense of other foods (Ambruso, Hays, & Goldenberg, 2008).

At any age, breastfeeding should be discontinued gradually to prevent engorgement and pain in a mother's breasts while still providing satisfaction for the infant. To do this, a woman could first omit one breastfeeding a day, substituting a formula feeding or milk from a glass or cup. Then she could omit two breastfeedings, then three, and so on, until her infant is feeding entirely from a bottle, glass, or cup. If breasts are not emptied by regular feedings, the resulting pressure leads to milk suppression and natural, gradual discontinuance of milk secretion. If weaned before 12 months, infants should be weaned to formula, not whole milk, so that they continue to receive the added vitamins and the low solute load of commercial formulas.

Urge women who have discontinued breastfeeding to explore whether there is a breast milk bank in their community that would appreciate breast milk donors. Such milk is used to feed hospitalized infants, especially preterm infants. Being fed breast milk can help prevent necrotizing enterocolitis, a possibly fatal bowel infection (see Chapter 45) (Boyd, Quigley, & Brocklehurst, 2007).

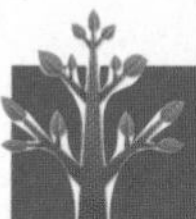

BOX 19.6 ✻ Focus on Family Teaching

Suggestions for Returning to Work While Breastfeeding

Q. Linda Satir tells you, "I'm going to be returning to work in 6 weeks. How can I continue to breastfeed my baby?"

A. Here are some suggestions for returning to work while breastfeeding:

- Some women are able to arrange for child care near or at their worksite so they can breastfeed at lunch or during a morning or afternoon break. Discuss with your employer or your immediate work supervisor whether this would be a possibility for you.
- Breastfeeding can be done in a public place, such as a lounge area, without undue exposure if you wear a smock-type or buttoned blouse that you lift or unfasten only as far as necessary; covering any bared breast with a shawl or towel ensures modesty.
- If you are not able to breastfeed during work hours, you will need to express milk manually at least once during the day to maintain a milk supply. You might want to rent an electric pump to keep at work. Expressed breast milk can be safely stored in the refrigerator or in an iced container for 24 to 48 hours and used by your caregiver to feed the infant the next day.
- Plastic is the best type of storage container for breast milk, because antibodies apparently cling to glass and may therefore be lost to the milk.
- Any reminder of a baby may cause leaking of milk from breasts. Wear gauze pads inside your bra to prevent stains on your clothing, and keep an extra change of clothing at work. Pressing against your breasts with the heel of your hands may be helpful in halting leakage.
- Drink four to six 8-oz glasses of fluid during the day to ensure a high fluid intake.
- Try to arrive early at your day care center or sitter so you can breastfeed just before leaving the baby.
- Fatigue can interfere with breastfeeding. Relax and enjoy your baby during the time you are home.

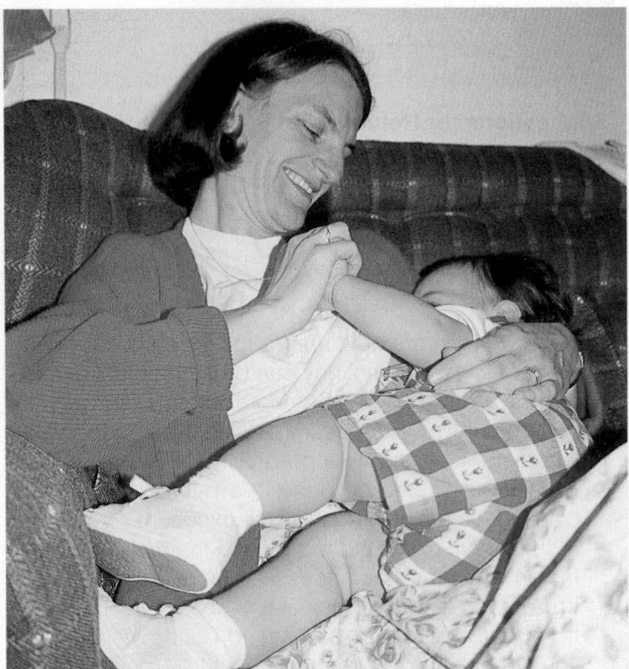

FIGURE 19.8 Some women choose to breastfeed their child beyond 1 year. Accepting various preferences is important in care planning.

BOX 19.7 * Focus On Communication

Mrs. Morgan, Linda 's roommate in the hospital, is a new mother who has chosen to formula feed her newborn. You notice on the second day after birth that she is studying her baby closely.

Less Effective Communication

Nurse: Is everything all right? You look worried.
Mrs. Morgan: I feel guilty I'm not breastfeeding.
Nurse: Breastfeeding would be better for your baby.
Mrs. Morgan: I can't. I'm going back to work next week.
Nurse: You really should breastfeed. It's so much better for the baby.
Mrs. Morgan: I guess I'm not going to be a very good mother.

More Effective Communication

Nurse: Is everything all right? You look worried.
Mrs. Morgan: I feel guilty I'm not breastfeeding.
Nurse: What made you decide not to do that?
Mrs. Morgan: I work as an electrician at a construction site. I can't breastfeed on a scaffold a hundred feet in the air in freezing weather.
Nurse: Your work situation definitely sounds like an exception to the rule. Infant formula may be the best option for you.
Mrs. Morgan: I'm trying to be a good mother. Thanks for the support.

Imposing your opinions on someone is not therapeutic. Allowing a woman to explain her individual situation permits a nurse to understand the woman's decision and support her in it.

✔ Checkpoint Question 19.2

How does breast milk help prevent infection in a newborn?

a. It is rich in fatty acid, so bacteria are destroyed by it.
b. It is always flowing forward in the breast, so it is not static.
c. It contains maternal antibodies and viral binding factors.
d. It is low in lactose, so it becomes a poor culture medium.

FORMULA FEEDING

There is little opposition to the concept that breastfeeding is the best method for feeding human infants unless it is contraindicated. Women who develop a breast abscess may be advised not to breastfeed. Some women who are uncomfortable with the thought of exposing their breasts may not be able to hold a baby warmly and enjoy breastfeeding. Others who plan to return to work outside their home or who have older children to care for may choose not to breastfeed (Box 19.7). Fortunately, formulas that closely resemble human milk are available for infants who will be formula fed, and formula feeding still allows women to establish a close bond with their infant. Support a woman's choice by helping her adjust to formula feeding (Gomella & Haist, 2007).

Preparing for Formula Feeding

Women should use commercial formulas for formula feeding because they so closely mimic human milk. Occasionally, an infant is allergic to the protein in infant formulas. This can lead to such severe intestinal inflammation, diarrhea, and vomiting that the infant becomes anemic and dehydrated from loss of blood and inability to absorb nutrients. In these instances, the infant needs to be switched to a specially designed prescription formula.

Commercial Formulas

The contents of commercial formulas are supervised by the U.S. Food and Drug Administration. Formulas are available in three types: milk based, soy based, and elemental (fat, protein, and carbohydrate content is modified, such as in lactose-free formula). Milk-based formulas are used for the average newborn; lactose-free formulas are used for infants with lactose intolerance or galactosemia (inability to use sugar). Soy formulas were devised for infants who are allergic to cow's milk protein. Today, such infants may be given casein hydrolysate formulas, which have protein particles too small to be recognized by the immune system, rather than soy formulas. Elemental formulas are used for infants with protein allergies or fat malnutrition. Milk-based, soy-based, and lactose-free formulas are all designed to simulate the nutritional content of breast milk. They all contain supplemental vitamins. Parents should be advised to purchase types with added iron to ensure that their newborn receives enough of this element to prevent iron-deficiency anemia (Marotz,

2009). Formulas for term newborns contain 20 cal/oz when diluted according to directions (the same number of calories as breast milk). Common brands are shown in Appendix B. Parents should plan on using formula for the first full year of their infant's life. Participation in a supplemental food program such as the Special Supplemental Nutrition Program for Women, Infants, and Children (WIC) can help low-income parents afford formula.

Four separate forms of commercial formulas are available:

- Powder that is combined with water
- Condensed liquid that is diluted with an equal amount of water
- Ready-to-pour type, which requires no dilution
- Individually prepackaged and prepared bottles of formula

The powder is the least expensive. A single bottle at a time is easy to prepare by vigorous shaking. The prepackaged type does not need refrigeration or preparation (simply remove the bottle cap and it is ready), but it is the most expensive type. Cost should not be the only basis for a parent's choice, however. Tolerance of the formula by the infant and convenience for the parents also are important.

Calculating a Formula's Adequacy

To calculate the adequacy of a formula, remember these two rules of thumb:

1. The total fluid ingested for 24 hours must be sufficient to meet the infant's fluid needs: 75 to 90 mL (2.5 to 3 oz) of fluid per pound of body weight (150 to 200 mL/kg) per day.
2. The number of calories required per day is 50 to 55 per pound of body weight (100 to 120 kcal/kg).

If an infant is taking a commercial formula, only total fluid needs to be calculated. For example, a 7-lb infant needs 17.5 to 21 oz (7 lb × 2.5 to 3 oz) per day. Commercial formula contains 20 cal/oz, so this amount supplies 350 to 420 cal/day. The total volume can be divided into six feedings of 3 to 3.5 oz each. A 9-lb infant would need 22.5 to 27 oz of fluid per day, supplying 450 to 540 cal/day as well as adequate protein, minerals, and vitamins.

A quick rule of thumb to estimate how much an infant will drink at a feeding is to add 2 or 3 to the infant's age in months. After initially taking 0.5 to 1 oz for the first 2 days, a newborn (0 age) will take 2 to 3 oz each feeding; a 3-month-old child, 5 to 6 oz; and a 6-month-old child, 8 oz. As infants change from six to five feedings a day (at about 4 months of age, when they begin to sleep through the night), they begin to take more at each feeding, keeping their total intake the same. Knowing the minimum requirements for fluid and calories per day, being able to calculate whether formula is adequate, and remembering to assess an infant's intake over 24 hours allow evaluation of the adequacy of an infant's intake.

Nursing Diagnoses and Related Interventions

Nursing Diagnosis: Health-seeking behaviors related to techniques of formula feeding

Outcome Identification: Client verbalizes knowledge of techniques of formula feeding by hospital discharge.

Provide Information Regarding Supplies Needed. Most parents today do not prepare a full day's supply of formula at once but prepare it bottle by bottle, as needed. Caution parents to keep opened cans of liquid formula covered and refrigerated, discarding any unused formula within 24 hours. They should use glass or nonshiny plastic bottles as these do not contain polycarbonate, a chemical that is capable of leeching into stored milk and possibly causing chromosomal aberrations (Raloff, 2007). A baby who develops colic (abdominal pain after feeding) may be pulling in too much air and would benefit from an angled or disposable liner bottle.

Nipples for bottles should be firm enough so an infant sucks vigorously. A soft, flabby nipple allows a baby to suck in milk so rapidly that the need for sucking may not be satisfied. A way to judge a nipple's adequacy is to hold a bottle of milk with nipple attached upside down. The milk should drip from it at a rate of about one drop a second. Bottle caps to cover nipples are helpful to keep nipples clean when outdoors or during transport.

Provide Information Regarding Formula Preparation. Infant formula of any type must be prepared with careful attention to cleanliness to prevent pathogenic microorganisms from growing in it.

When using presterilized formula, the parent need only do the following to prepare a full day's supply of formula:

- Wash off the top of the can with warm, soapy water and rinse.
- Open the can and pour the desired amount of formula and water into each previously cleaned bottle (cleaning in a dishwasher is best).
- Put on the nipples, taking care not to handle the nipple projection.
- Place the bottle caps over the nipples and refrigerate.

To prepare a single bottle, the parent simply combines clean water and liquid or powdered formula in a previously cleaned bottle, caps the bottle, and shakes it to mix the ingredients.

Provide Information Regarding Feeding Techniques. Whether to warm formula or not is a parental decision: infants who are fed cooled formula directly from the refrigerator thrive as well as those who are fed warmed formula. The best method to warm formula is to stand the bottle in a bowl of warm water or hold it under a faucet of running hot water for a few minutes. Caution parents not to use a pan on the stove to warm formula because if the pan boils dry, the bottle of milk will burst. Disposable bottles with plastic liners should definitely not be heated on the stove; the liner tends to melt and then leak during feeding.

It also is not recommended to warm bottles in a microwave oven, because the milk in the center of the bottle can become hotter than that near the sides. If

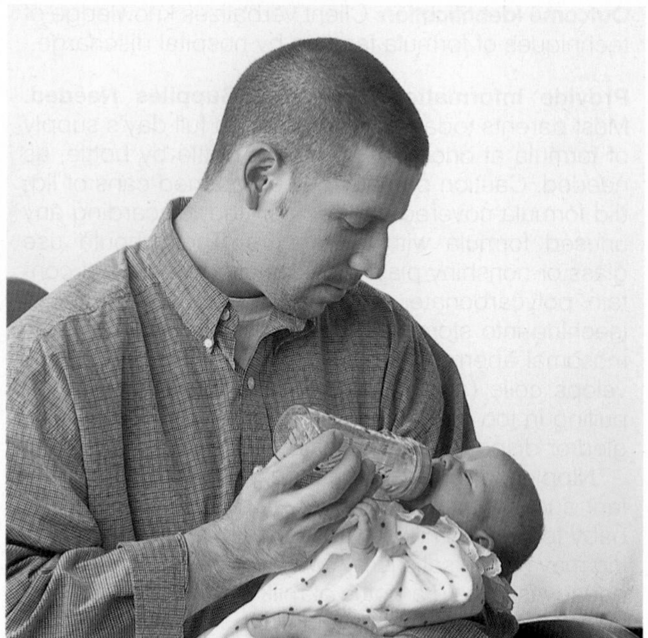

FIGURE 19.9 A newborn receives a bottle feeding from her father. Notice the en face position.

parents do not follow this recommendation, caution them to heat no longer than 30 seconds for a 4-oz bottle and 45 seconds for an 8-oz bottle (Goldenring, 2007). After warming, they should add the nipple and shake the bottle well to mix the cool and warm portions. Finally, with all warming methods. parents should test the temperature of the formula by allowing a drop or two to fall onto the inside of a wrist, to make sure it is not hot enough to burn the baby's mouth.

With any type of bottle, any contents remaining after a feeding should be thrown away, not stored and reused. When sucking, an infant exchanges a small amount of saliva for milk. Because milk is a good growth medium for bacteria and the baby's mouth harbors many bacteria, the bacterial content in reused formula is likely to be high.

Like breastfeeding, formula feeding an infant is a skill that must be learned. A parent needs a comfortable chair (as does a nurse who feeds babies) and adequate time (at least half an hour) to enjoy the process and not rush the baby (Fig. 19.9). Holding the baby with the head slightly elevated reduces the danger of aspiration and retention of air bubbles. A parent should be sure the nipple is kept filled so that the baby is sucking milk, not air. He or she can be assured a baby is sucking effectively if small bubbles rise in the bottle. Babies in the early weeks should be bubbled (burped) after every ounce of milk taken. The technique is the same as that used for breastfed infants.

Remind parents not to prop up bottles, because babies are in danger of aspiration if a bottle is propped. In addition, an increased incidence of otitis media has been associated with bottle-propping, because the infant's head is not upright and formula may enter the eustachian tube. Propping also can limit the amount of parent–child interaction. Also remind parents not to put a baby to bed with a bottle of formula, because this can lead to "baby-bottle syndrome," or cavities of the lower teeth (see Chapter 29). Some common problems that can arise with formula feeding are summarized in Table 19.6.

What if... Linda tells you she is going to give her baby one supplemental bottle of formula daily in addition to breastfeeding while she works? She does not plan to refrigerate this bottle during the day. What questions would you want to ask her to be certain this approach is safe for her baby?

DISCHARGE PLANNING

Mothers only remain in a hospital or birthing center a short time so teaching a mother and her family about either breastfeeding or formula feeding is crucial. Be certain to review a

TABLE 19.6 ✻ Common Concerns of Formula-Feeding Mothers

Concern	Possible Causes	Nursing Interventions
Infant sucks for a few minutes, then stops and cries	Either nipple is blocked and infant is unable to get milk or flow is too fast and baby has choking sensation.	Show parent how to test flow of milk from the nipple (hold bottle upside down); milk should flow from nipple at rate of about 1 drop/sec.
Infant does not burp well after feeding	Some infants swallow little air with feeding. Parent may be handling infant too tentatively or not burping effectively.	Observe baby feeding and parent's technique of handling; rubbing newborn's back may be more effective than patting it.
Parent reports constipation	Bowel movements from formula-fed infants are not as loose as those from breastfed infants, so parents may be concerned.	Examine stools; assure parent and explain normal stool pattern and that straining to pass stool is normal.

mother's plans for feeding her baby just before discharge, so there is time to answer any remaining questions. If needed, check to see that a home care referral or visit has been scheduled and that the new mother has a telephone number she can call if she has a question before the home visit occurs.

Review with a mother the criteria for adequate nutrition (wetting a diaper six to eight times a day, sleeping between feedings, no excessive crying). Supply the telephone number of the local La Leche League or Association of Lactation Consultants or another local support group as needed.

Be certain a woman has an appointment with a primary care provider for her infant or the telephone number of this person to call for an appointment. Remind her that infant nutrition is an important topic and one she should always feel free to discuss at health care visits. Babies experience growth spurts during the first year at about 3 months, 6 months, and 9 months; during these times, they need to be fed more frequently to meet their nutritional needs. No one can anticipate all of the questions or problems regarding feeding that will arise in the next few months. Empowering women to learn to make decisions regarding feeding and not be reluctant to ask for help when they need it will go a long way toward solving these problems.

✔ Checkpoint Question 19.3

Linda 's husband will offer their baby bottled breast milk once a day when Linda returns to work. Which of the following would you teach him?

a. He should stop feeding bottled milk if the baby has loose yellow stools.
b. He should microwave the milk for a full minute to be certain it is sterile.
c. He should prop the bottle so the baby continues to enjoy breastfeeding.
d. After the baby drinks from a bottle, discard any milk still in the bottle.

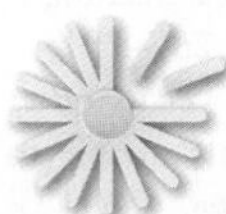

Key Points for Review

- Breastfeeding is the preferred feeding method for newborns, because it supplies antibodies as well as nutrients. Urge all women at least to try breastfeeding unless they are taking a drug that would be a contraindication or there is a potential for spreading a microorganism through the breast milk.
- Linoleic acid is an essential fatty acid that is necessary for growth and skin integrity and cannot be manufactured by the body. It is supplied by both infant formula and human milk but not by nonfat milk.
- Both breast milk and commercial formulas contain 20 kcal/oz. A term newborn requires 120 kcal/kg/day and 150 to 200 mL/kg of fluid.
- Encourage mothers who are breastfeeding to drink fluoridated water and formula-feeding mothers to prepare formula using fluoridated water to help build strong teeth in the infant. If a newborn will not have exposure to sunlight, the breastfeeding mother may need to take a supplement of vitamin D; formula-fed infants may need supplemental oral vitamin D.
- Almost all drugs pass into breast milk. A breastfeeding mother must be certain not to take any medication without contacting her primary care provider to be certain it is compatible with breastfeeding.
- If a baby will be formula fed, be certain the parents understand the potential danger of warming bottles in a microwave oven (the inner core of milk may grow very hot).
- Caution parents not to prop bottles, because it increases the risk for aspiration and otitis media. It also deprives infants of the pleasure of being held for feedings.
- To avoid nursing bottle syndrome (cavities of the lower teeth), infants should not be put to bed with a bottle.

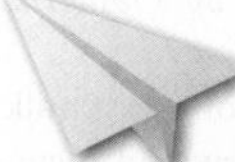

CRITICAL THINKING EXERCISES

1. Linda Satir is the new mother you met at the beginning of the chapter. She is unsure whether she wants to breastfeed, especially because she does not know how she will manage breastfeeding when she returns to work. How would you advise her?
2. Linda worries that her 1-day-old newborn is not receiving enough milk. How could you assure her that her baby is receiving enough?
3. Linda's grandmother tells you that she always changed her babies to fat-free milk at 3 months to keep them from gaining too much weight. Would you support this practice?
4. Examine the National Health Goals related to newborn nutrition. Most government-sponsored money for nursing research is allotted based on these goals. What would be a possible research topic to explore pertinent to these goals that would be applicable to the Satir family and also advance evidence-based practice?

CRITICAL THINKING SCENARIO

Open the accompanying CD-ROM or visit http://thePoint.lww.com and read the Patient Scenario included for this chapter, then answer the questions to further sharpen your skills and grow more familiar with NCLEX style questions related to nutritional needs of newborns. Confirm your answers are correct by reading the rationales.

REFERENCES

Abdulwadud, O. A., & Snow, M. E. (2009). Interventions in the workplace to support breastfeeding for women in employment. *Cochrane Database of Systematic Reviews, 2009*(1), (CD006177).

Akus, M., & Bartick, M. (2007). Lactation safety recommendations and reliability compared in 10 medication resources. *Annals of Pharmacotherapy, 41*(9), 1352–1360.

Ambruso, D. R., Hays, T., & Goldenberg, N. (2008). Hematologic disorders. In W. W. Hay, et al. (Eds.). *Current pediatric diagnosis and treatment* (18th ed.). Columbus, OH: McGraw-Hill.

American Academy of Pediatrics. (1999). Iron fortification of infant formulas. *Pediatrics, 104*(1), 119–123.

American Academy of Pediatrics Committee on Drugs. (2002). Transfer of drugs and other chemicals into human milk. *Pediatrics, 108*(3), 776–789.

American Academy of Pediatrics Committee on Nutrition. (2001). The use and misuse of fruit juice in pediatrics. *Pediatrics, 107*(5), 1210–1213.

American Academy of Pediatrics. (2008). *Breastfeeding your baby.* Elk Grove, IL: Author.

American College of Obstetricians and Gynecologists (ACOG). (2007). Special report from ACOG: breastfeeding: maternal and infant aspects. *ACOG Clinical Review, 12*(1), 1S-16S.

Ateah, C. A., & Hamelin, K. J. (2008). Maternal bedsharing practices, experiences, and awareness of risks. *JOGNN: Journal of Obstetric, Gynecologic, and Neonatal Nursing, 37*(3), 274–281.

Boyd, C. A., Quigley, M. A., & Brocklehurst, P. (2007). Donor breast milk versus infant formula for preterm infants: systematic review and meta-analysis. *Archives of Disease in Childhood Fetal and Neonatal Edition, 92*(3), F169–F175.

Britton, C., et al. (2009). Support for breastfeeding mothers. *Cochrane Database of Systematic Reviews, 2009*(1), (CD001141).

Coleman-Phox, K., Odouli, R., & Li, D. K. (2008). Use of a fan during sleep and the risk of sudden infant death syndrome. *Archives of Pediatrics & Adolescent Medicine, 162*(10), 963–968.

Deshpande, W. (2008). Exclusive breastfeeding for the first six months. *Community Practitioner, 81*(5), 34–36.

Ferguson, M., & Molfese, P. J. (2007). Breastfed infants process speech differently from formula-fed infants: evidence from neuroelectrophysiology. *Developmental Neuropsychology, 31*(3), 337–347.

Forster, D. A., & McLachlan, H. L. (2007). Breastfeeding initiation and birth setting practices: a review of the literature. *Journal of Midwifery and Women's Health, 52*(3), 273–280.

Furber, C. M., & Thomson, A. M. (2007). Midwives in the UK: an exploratory study of providing newborn feeding support for postpartum mothers in the hospital. *Journal of Midwifery & Women's Health, 52*(2), 142–147.

Goldenring, J. M. (2007). What to tell parents before they leave the hospital. *Contemporary Pediatrics, 24*(4), 74–79.

Gomella, L. G., & Haist, S. A. (2007). *Clinician's pocket reference* (11th ed.). Columbus, OH: McGraw-Hill.

Hampton, T. (2008). Report assesses effects of early nutrition options on atopic diseases. *Journal of the American Medical Association, 299*(6), 621.

Howe, T., et al. (2008). A review of psychometric properties of feeding assessment tools used in neonates. *JOGNN: Journal of Obstetric, Gynecologic, and Neonatal Nursing, 37*(3), 338–349.

Huether, S. E., & McCance, K. L. (2008). *Understanding pathophysiology.* (4th ed.). New York: Elsevier.

Jensen, D., Wallace, S., & Kelsey, P. (1994). LATCH: A breastfeeding charting system and documentation tool. *Journal of Obstetric, Gynecologic, and Neonatal Nursing, 23*(1), 27–32.

Kramer, M. S., & Kakuma, R. (2009). Optimal duration of exclusive breastfeeding. *Cochrane Database of Systematic Reviews, 2009*(1), (CD003517).

La Leche League International. (2004). *The womanly art of breastfeeding* (6th ed.). Schaumberg, IL: Author.

Li, R., Rock, V. J., & Grummer-Strawn, L. (2007). Changes in public attitudes toward breastfeeding in the United States, 1999–2003. *Journal of the American Dietetic Association, 107*(1), 122–127.

Marotz, L. R. (2009). Infant feeding. In L. R. Marotz (Ed.). *Health, safety and nutrition for the young child.* Clifton Park, NY: Delmar/Cengage Learning.

Moore, J. E. (2007). Multiple births: the art and science of caring for twins, triplets, and more. *Pediatrics in Review, 28*(3), e9–e15.

Pavone, M. E., & Purinton, S. C. (2007). Postpartum care and breastfeeding. In A. H. DeCherney & L. Nathan (Eds.). *Current diagnosis and treatment in obstetrics and gynecology* (10th ed.). Columbus, OH: McGraw-Hill.

Procter, S. B., & Holcomb, C. A. (2008). Breastfeeding duration and childhood overweight among low-income children in Kansas, 1998–2002. *American Journal of Public Health, 98*(1), 106–110.

Raab, E. L. (2007). Essentials of normal newborn assessment and care. In A. H. DeCherney & L. Nathan (Eds.). *Current diagnosis and treatment in obstetrics and gynecology* (10th ed.). Columbus, OH: McGraw-Hill.

Raloff, J. (2007). Bad for baby: new risks found for plastic constituent. *Science News,* (7) 11.

Sadeharju, K., et al. (2007). Maternal antibodies in breast milk protect the child from enterovirus infections. *Pediatrics, 119*(5), 941–946.

Singh, G. K., Kogan, M. D., & Dee, D. L. (2007). Nativity/immigrant status, race/ethnicity, and socioeconomic determinants of breastfeeding initiation and duration in the United States, 2003. *Pediatrics, 119* (Supplement 1), S38–S46.

Thilo, E. H., & Rosenberg, A. A. (2008). The newborn infant. In W. W. Hay, et al. (Eds.). *Current Pediatric Diagnosis and Treatment* (18th ed.). Columbus, OH: McGraw-Hill.

U.S. Department of Health and Human Services and U.S. Department of Agriculture. (2005). *Dietary guidelines for Americans, 2005* (6th ed.). Washington, DC: U.S. Government Printing Office.

Van der Wijden, C., Kleijnen, J., & Van den Berk, T. (2009). Lactational amenorrhea for family planning. *Cochrane Database of Systematic Reviews, 2009*(1), (CD001329).

World Health Organization. (2002). *The optional duration of exclusive breast feeding.* Geneva: Author.

SUGGESTED READINGS

Adair, L. S., & Daniels, M. (2007). Early nutrition and the development of cardiovascular disease risk. *Nutrition Today, 42*(1), 6–15.

Britton, C., et al. (2009). Support for breastfeeding mothers. *Cochrane Database of Systematic Reviews, 2009*(1), (CD001141).

Cairney, P., & Barbour, R. (2007). A research study of sources of support for bottle feeding in new mothers. *Community Practitioner, 80*(6), 30–34.

Dorea, J. G. (2007). Maternal smoking and infant feeding: breastfeeding is better and safer. *Maternal and Child Health Journal, 11*(3), 287–291.

Flint, A., New, K., & Davies, M. W. (2009). Cup feeding versus other forms of supplemental enteral feeding for newborn infants unable to fully breastfeed. *Cochrane Database of Systematic Reviews, 2009*(1), CD005092.

Glenn, L. L., & Quillin, S. I. (2007). Opposing effects of maternal and paternal socioeconomic status on neonatal feeding method, place of sleep, and maternal sleep time. *Journal of Perinatal & Neonatal Nursing, 21*(1), 165–172.

Hall Moran, V., et al. (2007) A systematic review of the nature of support for breastfeeding adolescent mothers. *Midwifery, 23*(2), 157–171.

Law, C. S. (2007). The impact of changing parenting styles on the advancement of pediatric oral health. *Journal of the California Dental Association, 35*(3), 192–197.

Johnson, T. S., Mulder, P. J., & Strube, K. (2007). Mother-infant breastfeeding progress tool: a guide for education and support of the breastfeeding dyad. *JOGNN: Journal of Obstetric, Gynecologic, and Neonatal Nursing, 36*(4), 319–327.

Rosetta, L., & Baldi, A. (2008). On the role of breastfeeding in health promotion and the prevention of allergic diseases. *Advances in Experimental Medicine & Biology, 606*(2), 467–483.

Unit 4

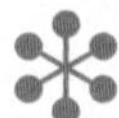

The Nursing Role in Caring for a Family During a Complication of Pregnancy, Birth, or the Postpartal Period

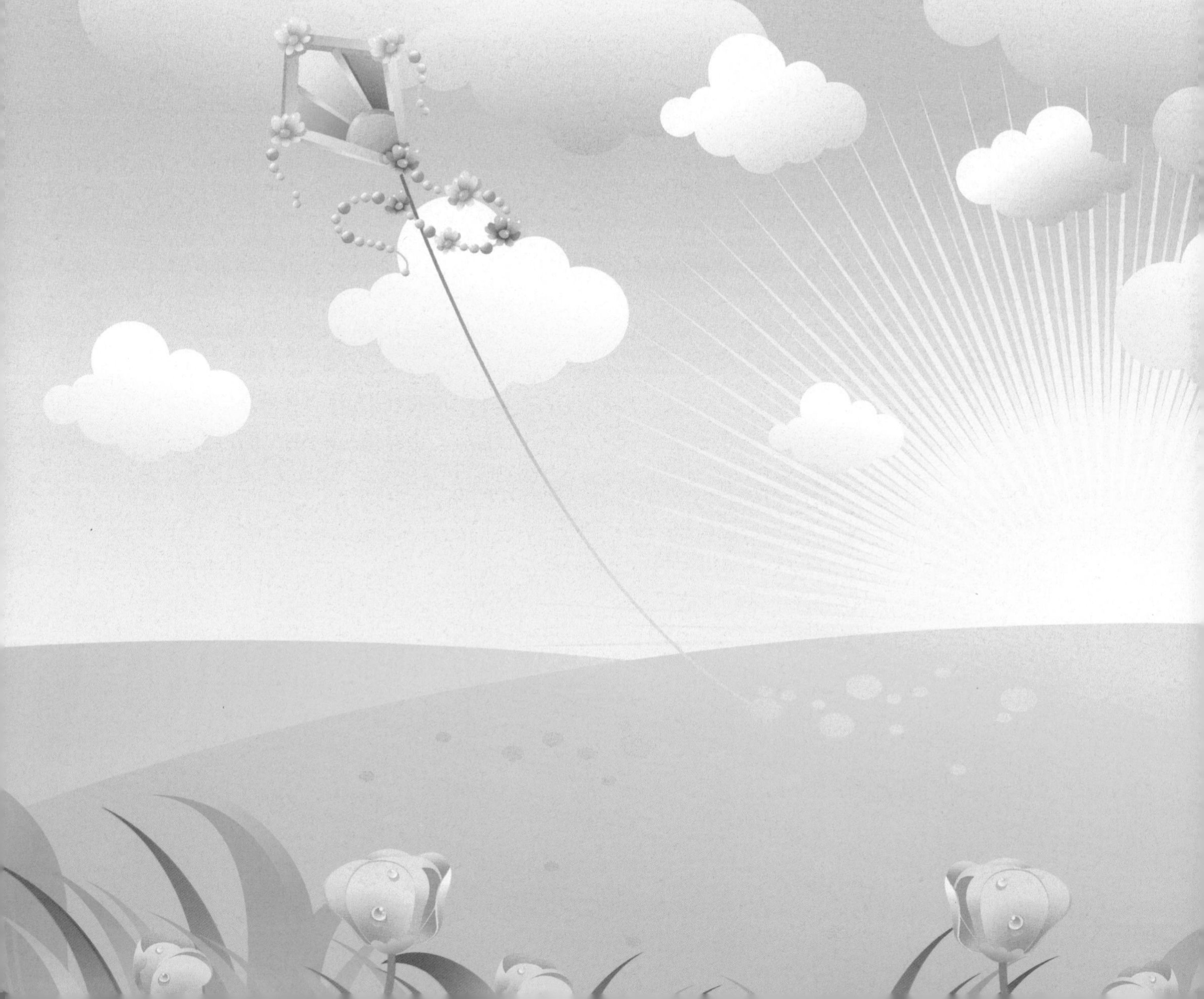

Chapter 20 Nursing Care of a Family Experiencing a Pregnancy Complication From a Pre-existing or Newly Acquired Illness

KEY TERMS

- deep vein thrombosis
- glucose tolerance test
- glycosuria
- glycosylated hemoglobin
- high-risk pregnancy
- hyperglycemia
- hypoglycemia
- megaloblastic anemia
- orthopnea
- paroxysmal nocturnal dyspnea
- peripartal cardiomyopathy
- proteinuria

OBJECTIVES

After mastering the contents of this chapter, you should be able to:

1. Define *high-risk pregnancy,* including pre-existing factors that contribute to its development.
2. Describe common illnesses such as cardiovascular disease, diabetes mellitus, or renal and blood disorders that can result in complications when they exist with pregnancy.
3. Identify National Health Goals related to complications of pregnancy that nurses can help the nation achieve.
4. Use critical thinking to analyze ways that nursing care can remain family centered when a pre-existing or newly acquired illness develops during pregnancy.
5. Assess a woman with an illness during pregnancy for changes occurring in the illness because of the pregnancy or the pregnancy because of the illness.
6. Formulate nursing diagnoses related to the effect of a pre-existing or newly acquired illness on pregnancy.
7. Identify expected outcomes that will contribute to a safe pregnancy outcome when illness occurs with pregnancy.
8. Plan nursing care for a woman with an illness during pregnancy such as how a woman with heart disease could manage to get more rest.
9. Implement nursing care for a woman when illness complicates pregnancy such as teaching how to measure blood glucose.
10. Evaluate expected outcomes for achievement and effectiveness of care.
11. Identify areas related to illness and pregnancy that could benefit from additional nursing research or application of evidence-based practice.
12. Integrate knowledge of high-risk pregnancy and nursing process to achieve quality maternal and child health nursing care.

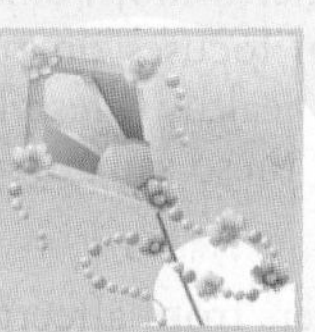

Angelina Gomez, 22, is pregnant with her first child. She had rheumatic fever with mitral stenosis as a child. She developed gestational diabetes early in her pregnancy. By the 34th week, she has already been hospitalized twice for hyperglycemia. She fainted this afternoon while participating in her weekly hour-long aerobic class. When seen in the emergency department, her serum glucose is 207 mg/dL. Her blood pressure is 90/40 mm Hg; her pulse is 130/min; the fetal heart rate is 180/min. An abdominal monitor shows moderate-strength uterine contractions 7 minutes apart. The emergency physician asks for an echocardiogram to see if her mitral stenosis is contributing to her low blood pressure. Angelina says to you, "If exercise is supposed to be good for you, why did this happen?"

Previous chapters discussed normal pregnancy and the minor discomforts that may occur. This chapter adds information about illnesses and other events that can complicate pregnancy when they occur prior to or during pregnancy. As more women wait until they are over 30 to have their first child, more and more women enter pregnancy with a pre-existing disorder such as cardiac or respiratory illness that can complicate pregnancy.

How would you answer Angelina? Do you think she realizes that pregnancy often becomes high risk not because of any one factor, but an accumulation of them?

When a woman enters pregnancy with a chronic condition such as cardiovascular or kidney disease, both she and the fetus can be at risk for complications because either the pregnancy can complicate the disease or the disease can complicate the pregnancy, affecting the baby or leaving a woman less equipped to function in the future or undergo a future pregnancy. Nursing care for a woman with a pre-existing illness focuses on close observation of maternal health and fetal well-being, education of a woman and her family about special danger signs to watch for during pregnancy, and actions to minimize complications whenever possible.

In addition to pre-existing illnesses, the pregnant woman, like any person, may develop a new illness during a pregnancy. When this occurs, the illness can adversely affect not only the woman but also her unborn child. Nursing care for the well, pregnant woman focuses on preventing illness by promoting an especially healthy lifestyle. When accidents and illness occurs despite these safeguards, nursing care focuses on:

- Preventing such disorders from affecting the health of the fetus
- Helping a woman regain her health as quickly as possible so she can continue a healthy pregnancy and prepare herself psychologically and physically for labor and birth and the arrival of her newborn
- Helping a woman learn more about her chronic illness so she can continue to safeguard her health during her childrearing years

Conditions that cause severe symptoms such as a marked change in fluid and electrolyte balance, altered cardiovascular or respiratory function, or severe blood loss are especially dangerous to a fetus. Because of this danger, National Health Goals related to complications of pregnancy have been established (Box 20.1).

Although pregnancy can be a stressful time, generally women experience overall good health during their pregnancies, perhaps in part because of their extra care and concern in keeping healthy for two. This extra motivation also encourages a woman with a high-risk pregnancy to carefully follow a therapeutic regimen established for her to keep her and her fetus safe.

BOX 20.1 * Focus on National Health Goals

Several National Health Goals are aimed at reducing complications of pregnancy that arise from existing or newly acquired disorders. These goals are:

- Reduce the rate of fetal deaths to 4.1 per 1000 live births from a baseline of 6.8 per 1000.
- Reduce the rate of maternal deaths to 3.3 per 100,000 live births from a baseline of 7.1 per 100,000.
- Reduce the rate of maternal illness and complications during pregnancy to 24 per 100 births from a baseline of 31.2 per 100 (http://www.nih.gov).

Nurses can help the nation reach these goals by educating women about the importance of entering pregnancy in the best state of health possible. Helping women who have diabetes mellitus understand the importance of prepregnancy care so they enter pregnancy without hyperglycemia is an important step toward reducing congenital anomalies in newborns. Supporting women with kidney, heart, or respiratory disease during pregnancy to continue to follow their medical regimen is yet another way.

Evidence-based practice and nursing research in specific effects of illnesses on pregnancy or the fetus and how women can best deal with these are needed.

Nursing Process Overview

For Care of a Woman With a Pre-existing or Newly Acquired Illness

Assessment

Accurate prenatal assessment of a woman with a pre-existing or newly acquired illness requires a thorough understanding of the signs and symptoms of illnesses, such as cardiovascular disease or diabetes mellitus, in addition to an understanding of the course of a normal pregnancy. Assessment techniques include objective measures such as establishing baseline vital signs as well as subjective factors such as the extent of edema or level of exhaustion a woman is experiencing (Fig. 20.1). Such assessment is best made by health care personnel who care for a woman consistently throughout the pregnancy so that subtle changes in data can be recognized. In the absence of a consistent care provider, teach a woman to assess her own health in relation to objective parameters. She could report exhaustion, for example, in relation to daily activity such as, "Two weeks ago I could walk a block without being short of breath. Today I could walk only half a block"; "The last time I was in for a checkup, edema didn't occur until bedtime. Now I notice it every afternoon by the time my son comes home from school."

Nursing Diagnosis

Nursing diagnoses developed for a woman with a high-risk pregnancy address her specific, disease-related condition as

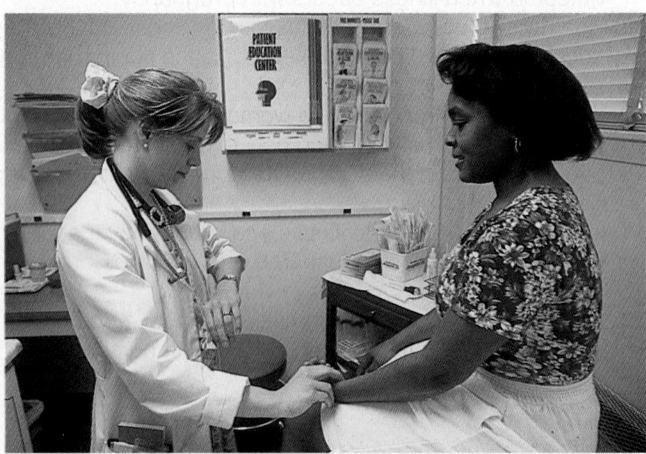

FIGURE 20.1 It is important to establish baseline vital signs to later identify a complication related to a pre-existing condition. (© Bob Kramer.)

well as any therapeutic restrictions her condition might require. Examples of possible nursing diagnoses are:

- Ineffective tissue perfusion (cardiopulmonary) related to poor heart function secondary to mitral valve prolapse during pregnancy
- Pain related to pyelonephritis secondary to pressure on ureters
- Social isolation related to prescribed bed rest during pregnancy secondary to concurrent illness
- Ineffective role performance related to increasing level of daily restrictions secondary to chronic illness and pregnancy
- Knowledge deficit related to normal changes of pregnancy versus illness complications
- Fear regarding pregnancy outcome related to chronic illness
- Health-seeking behaviors related to the effects of illness on pregnancy
- Situational low self-esteem related to illness during pregnancy

Outcome Identification and Planning

Be certain that expected outcomes established are realistic in light of a woman's pregnancy and the restrictions placed on her by her health. One family member with illness affects all family members; therefore, outcomes should relate to the entire family's health.

Try to make plans with a woman who has a pre-existing medical condition based on the pattern of her life before the pregnancy. For example, to ensure that a pregnant woman receives adequate rest during pregnancy, planning for an afternoon rest period a day is usually adequate. However, for a woman with cardiac disease who took two rest periods a day before pregnancy, this would be ineffective because now she probably needs four rest periods. Remember that the additional health supervision needed during pregnancy may involve increased expenses for a family, so a family may need to develop new ways to meet these expenses. A primary goal for a woman with a severe chronic condition might be to maintain her health during pregnancy, so she can remain at home as long as possible, thereby minimizing hospitalization and family disruptions.

Planning for a new illness may be difficult for a woman because of the shock of the diagnosis. Be careful, however, not to make plans for her such as, "Your best plan would be to begin strict bedrest." Instead, give a woman the available alternatives such as, "As the doctor explained, there are two separate therapies possible; let me review with you the advantages and disadvantages of each therapy." Allowing a woman to choose among alternatives this way helps her to participate in her own care and also maintain self-esteem, helping her move a step toward parenthood and assuming care for her family. Web sties that can be helpful to recommend to families are those of The American Heart Association (http://www.americanheart.org), The National Kidney Foundation (http://www.kidney.org), The American Diabetes Association (http://www.diabetes.org), and The Sickle Cell Association of America (http://www.sickle celldiseaseorg).

Implementation

Nursing interventions for the pregnant woman with a chronic illness may focus on teaching her new or additional measures to maintain health because of the pregnancy. Imaginative solutions to problems may need to be created because a woman may be unable to adjust to the extent of changes she must make.

An illness during pregnancy can complicate not only a pregnancy but also a woman's entire lifestyle and that of her family. Women who think of pregnancy as a time of wellness may have a great deal of difficulty accepting a medical regimen such as daily blood glucose monitoring because this is contradictory to their primary belief about pregnancy. Women in extended families may have an easier time accepting hospitalization during pregnancy than those living in nuclear families, because more people are available to take over their role at home. Conversely, women in extended families may have more difficulty with hospitalization because more people are depending on them to be at home.

Provide a pregnant woman who develops a new illness with an opportunity to talk about the event after her initial care is complete. She may feel guilty that she was not more careful to avoid infection or failed to recognize beginning signs of the illness. Her partner may feel equally guilty that he or she wasn't more alert to what was happening.

A woman and her partner can usually work through these emotions if the pregnancy progresses normally after this point and the fetus is uninjured. If the fetus is injured or the pregnancy disrupted, the event may cause a great deal of stress, and a woman and her partner may need counseling to overcome feelings of guilt and anger. Assessing all families individually and asking about the effect on the entire family of an illness during pregnancy helps to identify concerns and can lead to timely timely solving.

Outcome Evaluation

If evaluation of outcomes at health care visits reveals that an expected outcome is not being met, new assessment, analysis, and planning need to be done. In some instances, an outcome is not met because a woman did not understand the need for an additional pregnancy measure. In another instance, a woman may need better psychological support to continue to follow a health care routine consistently. Nine months is a long time to adhere to restrictions. Make evaluation ongoing to ensure that you know throughout the pregnancy whether interventions are successful. Some examples of outcomes that might be established are:

- Client states she rests for 2 hours morning and afternoon; dependent edema remains at 1+ or less at next prenatal visit.
- Family members state they are all participating in an exercise program since mother developed gestational diabetes.
- Client reports no burning on urination or flank pain at next prenatal visit.
- Client states she understands the importance of taking daily thyroid medicine for total length of pregnancy.

IDENTIFYING A HIGH-RISK PREGNANCY

A **high-risk pregnancy** is one in which a concurrent disorder, pregnancy-related complication, or external factor jeopardizes the health of the woman, the fetus, or both.

Some women enter pregnancy with a chronic illness that, when superimposed on the pregnancy, makes it high risk. Other women enter pregnancy in good health but then develop a complication of pregnancy that causes it to become high risk. In some instances, a combination of particular circumstances—poverty, lack of support people, poor coping mechanisms, genetic inheritance, or past history of pregnancy complications—can cause a pregnancy to be categorized as high risk.

In most instances, more than one factor contributes to the classification of a pregnancy this way. The pregnancy of a woman who is diabetic, for example, is automatically termed one with greater than normal risk because it forces a fetus to grow in an environment in which **hyperglycemia** (increased serum glucose levels) becomes the rule. During such a pregnancy, a woman, worrying that something will happen to her baby, may fail to begin the "pregnancy work" that she must do so bonding can take place. At birth, her child is in double jeopardy: not only is the baby born with altered glucose metabolism, but he or she also is at high risk for poor maternal–child attachment.

A preterm infant born to a teenage girl, likewise, could have this double problem. Not only is the infant immature (and at risk for all the complications that accompany immaturity), but also he or she may have a mother who is immature as well (see Chapter 22 for discussion of the special needs of the pregnant adolescent).

Table 20.1 lists psychological, social, and physical factors that commonly cause a pregnancy to be categorized as high risk. Categorizing risks as minimal, moderate, or extensive differs with each woman because of her individual coping mechanisms and level of support. A woman living in extreme poverty who does not have access to community support, for example, would be at high risk for poor nutritional intake during pregnancy, whereas a woman with a similar income who could depend on a nutritional assistance program such as WIC and counseling from a community health nurse might be only at minimal risk.

Remembering that the term "high risk" rarely refers to just one causative factor helps in the planning of holistic and ultimately effective nursing care. Pre-existing or newly acquired maternal illnesses that can make a pregnancy high risk are discussed in this chapter. Chapter 21 discusses conditions specific to pregnancy that can make a pregnancy high risk. Chapter 22 covers populations that are at high risk because of age (younger than 18 years or older than 40 years), the presence of a disability or trauma, or drug abuse.

CARDIOVASCULAR DISORDERS AND PREGNANCY

The number of women of childbearing age who have heart disease is diminishing as more and more congenital heart anomalies (discussed in Chapter 41) are corrected in early infancy. Also, rheumatic fever is being more actively prevented and treated so that cardiac damage from this disorder is also reduced. For these reasons, even with hypertension included, once a major threat to pregnancy, cardiovascular disease now complicates only approximately 1% of all pregnancies (Cunningham et al., 2008). Cardiovascular disease is still a concern in pregnancy, however, because it can lead to serious complications: it is responsible for 5% of maternal deaths during pregnancy (Crombleholme, 2009). Because of improved management of women with cardiac disorders, women who might never have risked pregnancy in the past are able to complete pregnancies successfully today.

The cardiovascular disorders that most commonly cause difficulty during pregnancy are valve damage caused by rheumatic fever or Kawasaki disease and congenital anomalies such as atrial septal defect or uncorrected coarctation of the aorta. Aortic dilatation may occur from Marfan's syndrome and also be a concern (Chaffins, 2007). As the number of women delaying their first pregnancy until later in life is increasing, there is a corresponding increase in the incidence of coronary artery disease and varicosities during pregnancy. In contrast, heart disease that occurs specifically with pregnancy (peripartum heart disease) still only rarely occurs as it is apparently unrelated to age.

A woman with cardiovascular disease needs a team approach to care during pregnancy, combining the talents of an internist, obstetrician, and nurse. Ideally, a woman should visit her obstetrician or family physician before conception so the health care team can become familiar with her state of health when she is not pregnant and establish baseline evaluations of her heart function, such as with an echocardiogram (Hameed & Akhter, 2007). A woman should begin prenatal care as soon as she suspects she is pregnant (1 week after the first missed menstrual period) so that her general condition and circulatory system can be monitored (Mooney, 2007).

Pregnancy taxes the circulatory system of every woman, even without cardiac disease, because both the blood volume and cardiac output increase approximately 30% (perhaps as much as 50%). Half of this increase occurs by 8 weeks; it is maximized by mid pregnancy.

Because of the increased blood flow past valves, functional (innocent) or transient murmurs can be heard in many women during a usual pregnancy. Heart palpitations on sudden exertion are also normal in pregnancy. Neither of these symptoms is a sign of cardiovascular disease, but merely an indication of the normal physiologic adjustment to pregnancy. These symptoms disappear after pregnancy. Women who had Kawasaki disease or rheumatic fever as a child may have both valvular and aortic artery constrictions that lead to true valve dysfunction and organic murmurs (Hibbard, Fajardo, & Briller, 2007).

The danger of pregnancy in a woman with cardiac disease occurs primarily because of the increase in circulatory volume. The most dangerous time for a woman is in weeks 28 to 32, just after the blood volume peaks. However, if heart disease is severe, symptoms can occur as early as the beginning of pregnancy. A woman's heart may become so overwhelmed by the increase in blood volume toward the end of pregnancy that her cardiac output falls to the point that vital organs (including the placenta) are no longer perfused adequately. When this happens, neither the oxygen nor nutritional requirements of her cells or those of the fetus can be met.

The estimation of whether a woman with cardiovascular disease can complete a pregnancy successfully or not depends

TABLE 20.1 ✻ Factors That Categorize a Pregnancy as High Risk

Psychological	Social	Physical
Prepregnancy		
History of drug dependence (including alcohol) History of intimate partner abuse History of mental illness History of poor coping mechanisms Cognitively challenged Survivor of childhood sexual abuse	Occupation involving handling of toxic substances (including radiation and anesthesia gases) Environmental contaminants at home Isolated Lower economic level Poor access to transportation for care High altitude Highly mobile lifestyle Poor housing Lack of support people	Visual or hearing challenges Pelvic inadequacy or misshape Uterine incompetency, position, or structure Secondary major illness (heart disease, diabetes mellitus, kidney disease, hypertension, chronic infection such as tuberculosis, hemopoietic or blood disorder, malignancy) Poor gynecologic or obstetric history History of previous poor pregnancy outcome (miscarriage, stillbirth, intrauterine fetal death) History of child with congenital anomalies Obesity (BMI >30) Underweight (BMI <18.5) Pelvic inflammatory disease History of inherited disorder Small stature Potential of blood incompatibility Younger than age 18 years or older than 35 years Cigarette smoker Substance abuser
Pregnancy		
Loss of support person Illness of a family member Decrease in self-esteem Drug abuse (including alcohol and cigarette smoking) Poor acceptance of pregnancy	Refusal of or neglected prenatal care Exposure to environmental teratogens Disruptive family incident Decreased economic support Conception less than 1 year after last pregnancy	Subject to trauma Fluid or electrolyte imbalance Intake of teratogen such as a drug Multiple gestation A bleeding disruption Poor placental formation or position Gestational diabetes Nutritional deficiency of iron, folic acid, or protein Poor weight gain Pregnancy-induced hypertension Infection Amniotic fluid abnormality Postmaturity
Labor and Birth		
Severely frightened by labor and birth experience Inability to participate because of anesthesia Separation of infant at birth Lack of preparation for labor Birth of infant who is disappointing in some way (such as sex, appearance, or congenital anomalies) Illness in newborn	Lack of support person Inadequate home for infant care Unplanned cesarean birth Lack of access to continued health care Lack of access to emergency personnel or equipment	Hemorrhage Infection Fluid and electrolyte imbalance Dystocia Precipitous birth Lacerations of cervix or vagina Cephalopelvic disproportion Internal fetal monitoring Retained placenta

on the type and extent of her disease. As a rule, a woman with artificial but well-functioning heart valves can be expected to complete a pregnancy without difficulty as long as she has consistent prenatal and postpartum care. A woman with a pacemaker implant can also expect to complete pregnancy successfully. Even women who have had heart transplants can be expected to have successful pregnancies (Sibanda et al., 2007).

To predict pregnancy outcome, heart disease is divided into four categories based on criteria established by the New York State Heart Association (Table 20.2). A woman with class I or II heart disease can expect to experience a normal pregnancy and birth. Women with class III can complete a pregnancy by maintaining almost complete bed rest. Women with class IV heart disease are poor candidates for pregnancy because they are in cardiac failure even at rest and when they are not pregnant. They are usually advised to avoid pregnancy.

A Woman With Cardiac Disease

Cardiac disease affects either the left or right side of the heart.

TABLE 20.2 ✻ Classification of Heart Disease

Class	Description
I	Uncompromised. Ordinary physical activity causes no discomfort. No symptoms of cardiac insufficiency and no anginal pain.
II	Slightly compromised. Ordinary physical activity causes excessive fatigue, palpitation, and dyspnea or anginal pain.
III	Markedly compromised. During less than ordinary activity, woman experiences excessive fatigue, palpitations, dyspnea, or anginal pain.
IV	Severely compromised. Woman is unable to carry out any physical activity without experiencing discomfort. Even at rest symptoms of cardiac insufficiency or anginal pain are present.

Source: Criteria Committee of the New York Heart Association. (1994). *Nomenclature and criteria for diagnosis of diseases of the heart and great vessels* (9th ed.). Boston: Little, Brown & Co.

A Woman With Left-Sided Heart Failure

Left-sided heart failure occurs in conditions such as mitral stenosis, mitral insufficiency, and aortic coarctation. In these instances, the left ventricle cannot move the volume of blood forward that it has received by the left atrium from the pulmonary circulation. The heart becomes so overwhelmed it fails to function. The reason for the failure is most often at the level of the mitral valve. The normal physiologic tachycardia of pregnancy shortens diastole (atrial contraction) and decreases the time available for blood to flow across this valve. The inability of the mitral valve to push blood forward causes back-pressure on the pulmonary circulation, causing it to become distended; systemic blood pressure decreases in the face of lowered cardiac output, and pulmonary hypertension occurs. When pressure in the pulmonary vein reaches a point of about 25 mm Hg, fluid begins to pass from the pulmonary capillary membranes into the interstitial spaces surrounding the alveoli and then into the alveoli themselves (pulmonary edema). Pulmonary edema produces profound dyspnea as it interferes with oxygen–carbon dioxide exchange as the fluid coats the alveolar exchange space (Bashore & Granger, 2009). If pulmonary capillaries rupture under the pressure, small amounts of blood leak into the alveoli and a productive cough of blood-speckled sputum develops. Because of the limited oxygen exchange, women with pulmonary hypertension are at extremely high risk for spontaneous miscarriage, preterm labor, or maternal death.

As the oxygen saturation of the blood decreases from dysfunction of the alveoli, chemoreceptors stimulate the respiratory center to increase respiratory rate. At first this is noticeable only on exertion, then finally with rest also. A woman experiences increased fatigue, weakness, and dizziness (specifically from lack of oxygen in brain cells). As the systemic decrease in blood pressure registers on the pressoreceptors in the aorta, the heart rate increases and peripheral vasoconstriction occurs in an attempt to increase the systemic blood pressure. As the fall in blood pressure is registered with the renal-angiotensin system, retention of both sodium and water occurs. The placenta may not receive adequate blood because of the decreased peripheral circulation.

As pulmonary edema becomes severe, a woman cannot sleep in any position except with her chest and head elevated (**orthopnea**). Elevating her chest allows fluid to settle to the bottom of her lungs and frees space for gas exchange. She may also notice **paroxysmal nocturnal dyspnea**—suddenly waking at night short of breath. This occurs because heart action is more effective when she is at rest. With the more effective heart action, interstitial fluid returns to the circulation. This overburdens the circulation, causing increased left-side failure and increased pulmonary edema.

If mitral stenosis is present, it is so difficult for blood to leave the left atrium that a secondary problem of thrombus formation can occur from noncirculating blood. A woman may need to be prescribed an anticoagulant to prevent this. If coarctation of the aorta is causing the difficulty, dissection of the aorta from high blood pressure from trying to push blood past the constriction can occur. In this instance, a woman may be prescribed antihypertensives to control blood pressure, diuretics to reduce blood volume, and beta-blockers to improve ventricular filling (Hameed & Akhter, 2007). If these complications result in impaired blood flow to the uterus, poor placental perfusion, intrauterine growth restriction, and fetal mortality can occur. A woman needs serial ultrasound and nonstress tests done after weeks 30 to 32 of pregnancy to monitor fetal health. Balloon valve angioplasty to loosen mitral valve adhesions can be performed safely during pregnancy (Davidson & Graham, 2007).

If an anticoagulant is required, heparin is the drug of choice for early pregnancy because it does not have teratogenic effects, as does sodium warfarin (Coumadin). Warfarin can be used after week 12 but a woman will then be returned to heparin therapy during the last month of pregnancy so the fetus will not develop a coagulation disorder at birth (heparin does not cross the placenta and enter the fetus).

A Woman With Right-Sided Heart Failure

Congenital heart defects such as pulmonary valve stenosis and atrial and ventricular septal defects can result in right-sided heart failure. Right-sided failure occurs when the output of the right ventricle is less than the blood volume received by the right atrium from the vena cava. Back-pressure from this results in congestion of the systemic venous circulation and decreased cardiac output to the lungs. Blood pressure decreases in the aorta because less blood is reaching it; pressure is high in the vena cava from back-pressure of blood; both jugular venous distention and increased portal circulation occur. The liver and spleen become distended. Liver enlargement can cause extreme dyspnea and pain in a pregnant woman because the enlarged liver, as it is pressed upward by the enlarged uterus, puts extreme pressure on the diaphragm. Distention of abdominal vessels can lead to exudate of fluid from the vessels into the peritoneal cavity (ascites). Fluid also moves from the systemic circulation into lower extremity interstitial spaces (peripheral edema).

The congenital anomaly most apt to cause right-sided heart failure in women of reproductive age is Eisenmenger syndrome, a right-to-left atrial or ventricular septal defect with an accompanying pulmonary stenosis (Davidson & Graham, 2007).

Women who have an uncorrected anomaly of this type may be advised not to become pregnant. If they do become pregnant, they can expect to be hospitalized for the last part of pregnancy. They need oxygen administration and frequent arterial blood gas assessments to ensure fetal growth. During labor, they may need a pulmonary artery catheter inserted to monitor pulmonary pressure. They need extremely close monitoring after epidural anesthesia to minimize the risk of hypotension.

✔ Checkpoint Question 20.1

Angelina Gomez is the 22-year-old woman you met at the beginning of the chapter. Suppose she develops a deep vein thrombosis while in the hospital on bed rest and is prescribed low-molecular-weight heparin subcutaneous. What education will she need in relation to this?

a. Her infant will be born with scattered petechiae on his trunk.
b. Heparin can cause darkened or nonflexible skin in newborns.
c. Heparin does not cross the placenta and so does not affect a fetus.
d. Some infants will be born with allergic symptoms to heparin.

A Woman With Peripartum Heart Disease

An extremely rare condition, **peripartal cardiomyopathy** can originate in pregnancy in women with no previous history of heart disease (American College of Obstetrics and Gynecology [ACOG], 2007). Although the cause is unknown, it is apparently because of the effect of the pregnancy on the circulatory system. The mortality rate can be as high as 50%. In many instances, it occurs from previously undetected heart disease, although it occurs most often in African American multiparas in conjunction with hypertension of pregnancy. A woman develops signs of myocardial failure such as shortness of breath, chest pain, and edema. Her heart begins to increase in size (cardiomegaly). If cardiomegaly occurs, she must sharply reduce her physical activity. Many women need a diuretic, an arrhythmia agent, and digitalis therapy to maintain heart action. Low-molecular-weight heparin may be administered to decrease the risk of thromboembolism. Immunosuppressive therapy may improve the symptoms.

If the cardiomegaly persists past the postpartum period, it is generally suggested that a woman not attempt any further pregnancies because the condition tends to recur in additional pregnancies. Oral contraceptives are contraindicated because of the danger of thromboembolism they could create. The disease may progress to the point that following pregnancy, a woman may need a heart transplant (McAnulty, Metcalfe, & Ueland, 2008).

Assessment of a Woman With Cardiac Disease

Nurses play a major role in the care of a pregnant woman with cardiovascular disease because continuous assessment of a woman's health status, health education, and health-promotion activities are so essential. Assessment of a woman with cardiac disease begins with a thorough health history to document her prepregnancy cardiac status (Box 20.2). Ask about her level of exercise performance (what level she can do before growing short of breath and what physical symptoms she experiences, such as cyanosis of the lips or nail beds). Ask if she normally has a cough or edema. Instruct women with cardiac disease always to report coughing during pregnancy, because pulmonary edema from heart failure may first manifest itself as a simple cough.

Never assess edema in women with heart disease lightly as the normal edema of pregnancy (innocent) must be distinguished from the beginning of pregnancy-induced hypertension (serious) or the edema of heart failure (also serious). The normal edema of pregnancy involves only the feet and ankles, but edema of either pregnancy-induced hypertension or heart failure also begins this way. Edema of pregnancy-induced hypertension usually begins after week 20. If the edema is a sign of heart failure, it can begin at any time and other symptoms will probably also be present: irregular pulse, rapid or difficult respirations, and perhaps chest pain on exertion. Record a baseline blood pressure, pulse rate, and

Box 20.2 Assessment
Assessing a Pregnant Woman With Cardiac Disease

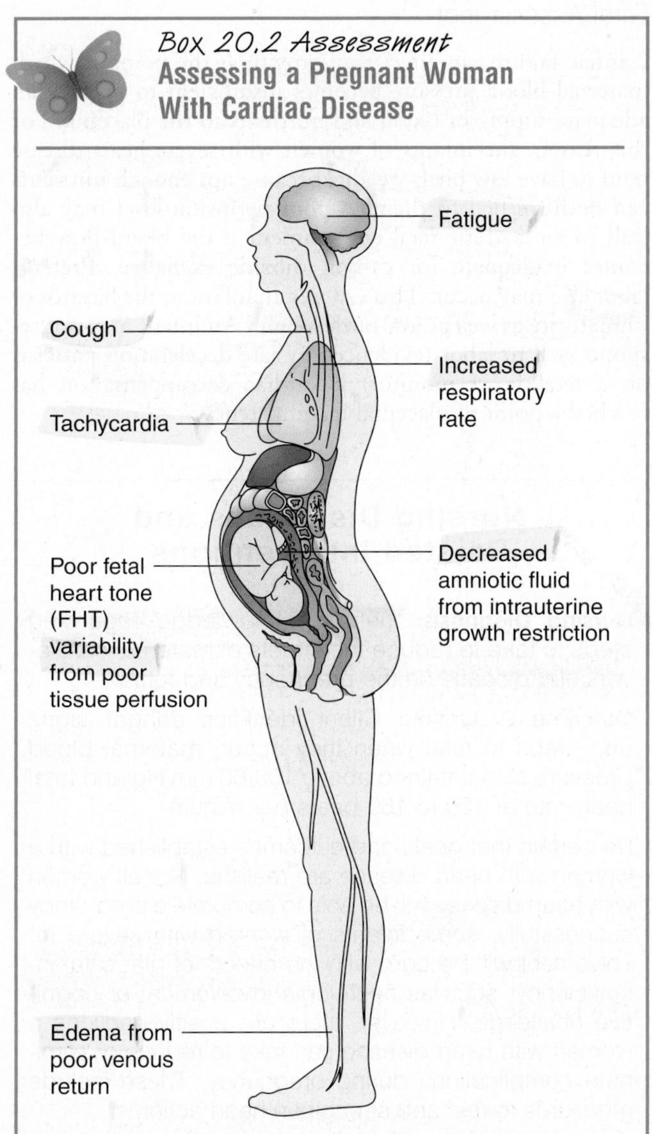

respiratory rate in either a sitting or lying position at the first prenatal visit; then, at future health visits, always take these in the same position for the most accurate comparison. Making comparison assessments for nail bed filling (should be <5 seconds) and jugular venous distention is also helpful throughout pregnancy. If a woman's heart disease involves right-sided heart failure, assessment of liver size is helpful. Keep in mind that liver assessment becomes difficult and probably inaccurate late in pregnancy because the enlarged uterus presses the liver upward under the ribs and makes it difficult to palpate.

For additional cardiac status assessment, a woman may need an electrocardiogram (ECG), chest radiograph, or echocardiogram done at periodic points in pregnancy. Assure her that an ECG merely measures cardiac electrical discharge and so cannot harm her fetus in any way. Echocardiography uses ultrasound and so will also not harm her fetus. Chest radiography is considered safe as long as a woman's abdomen is covered by a lead apron during the exposure. An ECG may become less accurate late in pregnancy (demonstrates left axis deviation) because the enlarged uterus presses upward on the diaphragm and displaces the heart laterally.

Fetal Assessment

Cardiac failure can affect fetal growth at the point at which maternal blood pressure becomes insufficient to provide an adequate supply of blood and nutrients to the placenta. For this reason, the infants of women with severe heart disease tend to have low birth weights because not enough nutrients can be furnished to them. A poor perfusion level may also lead to an acidotic fetal environment if the blood flow becomes inadequate for carbon dioxide exchange. Preterm labor also may occur. This exposes an infant to the hazards of immaturity as well as low birth weight. An infant may not respond well to labor (evidenced by late deceleration patterns on a fetal heart monitor) if cardiac decompensation has reached a point of placental incompetency.

Nursing Diagnoses and Related Interventions

Nursing Diagnosis: Deficient knowledge regarding steps to take to reduce the effects of maternal cardiovascular disease on the pregnancy and fetus

Outcome Evaluation: Client identifies danger signs and steps to take when they occur; maternal blood pressure is maintained above 100/60 mm Hg and fetal heart rate at 120 to 160 beats per minute.

Be certain that goals and outcomes established with a woman with heart disease are realistic. Not all women with heart disease will be able to complete a pregnancy successfully; some infants of women with severe involvement will be born with the effects of placental insufficiency, such as neurologic involvement or cognitive challenge. However, there are positive actions a woman with heart disease can take to reduce or eliminate complications during pregnancy. These include measures to rest and strengthen heart action.

Promote Rest. As a rule, women with cardiac disease need two rest periods a day (fully resting, not getting up frequently to answer the door or telephone) and a full night's sleep (not tossing and turning because of excess noise or heat in the room) to obtain adequate rest. Rest should be in the left lateral recumbent position to prevent supine hypotension syndrome and increased heart effort.

Remember that when cardiac output is not enough to meet systemic body demands, peripheral vasoconstriction occurs. Because the uterus is a peripheral organ, this causes uterine/placental constriction. Therefore, a rest program must be carefully designed so a woman stops exercising before this point is reached. Exactly how much rest she is to have should be carefully detailed for her. She may need to discontinue employment early in pregnancy rather than work until the end of pregnancy, as the average woman usually plans to do. Exactly how much work she will be allowed to do at home should be detailed as well. Allowing "normally heavy" housework may mean nothing more strenuous than dusting to some women. To others, it may mean washing windows, turning mattresses, and shoveling snow. Make certain a woman's definition of "heavy work" is the same as yours and her physician's or nurse-midwife's.

Promote Healthy Nutrition. A woman with cardiac disease may need closer supervision of nutrition during pregnancy than the average woman because she must gain enough weight to ensure a healthy pregnancy and a healthy baby, but she must not gain so much weight that she has to supply additional cells with nutrients. This could overburden her heart and circulatory system.

Be certain she is taking her prenatal vitamins. These contain an iron supplement to help prevent anemia. Anemia places an extra burden on the heart because it requires the body to circulate blood more vigorously to distribute oxygen to all body cells. If a woman was following a sodium-restricted diet before pregnancy, this may be continued during pregnancy, although typically a woman's sodium intake is only limited, not severely restricted, during pregnancy. Sodium is necessary for maintaining fluid volume and balance and thus is necessary to allow a woman's body to retain enough blood volume to supply blood to the placenta.

Educate Regarding Medication. Women taking cardiac medication before pregnancy may need to increase their maintenance dose because of their expanded blood volume during pregnancy. A woman who needed digoxin before pregnancy for heart action will continue to require it (and can take it safely) during pregnancy. A woman who was not digoxin dependent before pregnancy may need such therapy prescribed as pregnancy advances and her cardiac output has to be increased or strengthened. To aid a woman in continuing to think of herself as basically a well person, help her to understand that this does not mean her heart function is weakening, but rather that it is only being stressed further by the increased circulatory load of pregnancy. Digoxin is sometimes administered to a woman during pregnancy to slow the fetal heart if fetal tachycardia is present. An arrhythmia agent such as adenosine, beta-blockers, and angiotensin-converting enzyme (ACE) inhibitors to reduce hypertension are safe to use during pregnancy. Nitroglycerin, a compound often prescribed for angina, is not well studied during pregnancy (a category C drug) but is apparently safe (Karch, 2009).

A woman who was taking penicillin prophylactically because she had rheumatic fever as a child to prevent a recurrence (often taken for 10 years after the occurrence of rheumatic fever, or at least until age 18 years) should continue to take this drug during pregnancy because penicillin is not known to be a fetal teratogen (a category B drug). Close to the anticipated day of birth, some physicians begin a course of an antibiotic for women with heart disease such as penicillin. This is because the postpartum period always involves some mild invasion of bacteria from the denuded placental site on the uterus into the bloodstream. Since this invading bacteria may be streptococci, the bacteria often responsible for subacute bacterial endocarditis, a course of ampicillin, amoxicillin (Amoxil), or clindamycin (Cleocin) at this time offers women needed protection against bacterial endocarditis developing (Chambers, 2009).

It is often difficult to keep healthy women from taking over-the-counter medicines during pregnancy; conversely, it can be just as difficult to encourage women to take the medicine they need to take during pregnancy. Help women with heart disease to understand that there are valid exceptions to the rule of "no medicine during pregnancy."

Educate Regarding Avoidance of Infection. A systemic infection almost automatically increases body temperature, causing a woman to have to expend more energy and increase her cardiac output as her metabolism increases, an insult that could be too extreme for a woman with heart disease to withstand. Caution a woman with heart disease, therefore, to avoid visiting or being visited by people with infections. She should alert health care personnel at the first indication of an upper respiratory tract infection or urinary tract infection so that, if warranted, antibiotic therapy can be begun early in the course of the infection. Monthly screening for bacteriuria with a clean-catch urine test may be recommended.

Be Prepared for Emergency Actions. Women with heart disease may need supplemental oxygen if they overexert as could happen during a prenatal visit. Cardiac resuscitation in women who are pregnant does not differ from usual instructions (Box 20.3).

BOX 20.3 Nursing Procedure ✻ CPR During Pregnancy

Purpose: To restore respiratory and cardiac function.

Plan	Principle
1. Shake the woman's shoulders and shout.	**1.** Shaking the shoulders and shouting are an attempt to determine unconsciousness and to rouse a woman who may have fainted or be asleep.
2. Phone or call for help.	**2.** The woman may need more than simple resuscitation.
3. Place a rolled or folded towel under the woman's right hip.	**3.** A towel placed under one hip helps to prevent urterine compression on the vena cava or helps prevent supine hypotension syndrome.
4. Lift the chin to position the airway.	**4.** Lifting the chin aids in straightening the airway to ensure that it is patent.
5. Establish lack of respirations by listening and feeling for air movement.	**5.** Listening and feeling for air movement provides evidence of breathing.
6. Begin rescue breathing with administration of two quick breathing-bag breaths.	**6.** Rescue breathing introduces oxygen for gas exchange.
7. Assess carotid pulse.	**7.** Presence of carotid pulse indicates cardiac function.
8. Begin chest compressions if there is no carotid pulse. Place both hands on the lower sternum just above xiphoid process and deliver 15 chest compressions followed by 2 rescue breaths (1 second each) until cardiopulmonary function returns.	**8.** External chest compressions stimulate the action of the heart to maintain tissue perfusion. They should be at a rate of 100 bpm and allow the chest to rise in between compressions.
9. If an automated external defibrillator (AED) is necessary, remove any fetal or uterine monitors if these are in place. Follow standard application and procedure according to agency protocol.	**9.** AED is effective in stimulating heart action and is not detrimental to pregnancy or a fetus.

What if... Angelina tells you she has abruptly discontinued the daily penicillin she has been taking for her heart disease since childhood? As it has been a long time since she had rheumatic fever, what would you recommend she do?

Nursing Interventions During Labor and Birth

Monitor fetal heart rate and uterine contractions during labor in all women with heart disease. Assess a woman's blood pressure, pulse, and respirations frequently. A rapidly increasing pulse rate (>100 beats per minute) is an indication that a heart is pumping ineffectively and has increased its rate in an effort to compensate. Advise a woman to assume a side-lying position to reduce the possibility of supine hypotension syndrome. If she has some pulmonary edema, it may be necessary for her to have her chest and head elevated (semi-Fowler's position) to ease the work of breathing. Remember, fatigue is a symptom of heart decompensation. If this occurs in labor, evaluate a woman carefully to determine whether the fatigue is heart or labor related.

Women with extreme heart disease need oxygen administered during labor to compensate for the added oxygen required because of the increased exertion needed for labor as well as continuous hemodynamic monitoring such as by a Swan-Ganz catheter to monitor heart function. The anesthetic of choice during labor for women with heart disease is an epidural, because this can make both labor and birth less taxing. Many women with heart disease should not push with contractions; pushing requires more effort than they should expend. If an epidural anesthetic is used, low forceps or a vacuum extractor can be used for birth. A woman may be disappointed that her birth is not more "natural." Stress that these measures can help her achieve her ultimate goals, which are a healthy newborn and a mother able to care for her new baby.

Postpartum Nursing Interventions

The period immediately after birth may be a critical time for a woman with heart disease. With delivery of the placenta, the blood that supplied the placenta is now released into her general circulation, subsequently increasing her blood volume 20% to 40%. During pregnancy, the increase in blood volume occurred over a 6-month period, so the heart had time to adjust to this change gradually. After birth, the increase in pressure takes place within 5 minutes, so the heart must make a rapid and major adjustment (Davidson & Graham, 2007).

If a woman is in severe congestive heart failure after birth, she needs a program of decreased activity and possibly anticoagulant and digoxin therapy until her circulation stabilizes. Antiembolic stockings and ambulation may be needed to increase venous return from the legs. If prophylactic antibiotics had not been started prior to birth, they will be started immediately after birth to discourage subacute bacterial endocarditis caused by introduction of microorganisms through the placental site.

A woman with heart disease is often interested in close inspection of her baby immediately after birth because she wants to know her infant does not have a heart defect or was not harmed by any medication she took. Be sure to point out that acrocyanosis is normal in newborns, so she does not interpret her baby's severe peripheral cyanosis as cardiac inadequacy.

In the postpartum period, agents to encourage uterine involution such as oxytocin (Pitocin) must be used with caution because they tend to increase blood pressure, and this necessitates increased heart action. As a rule, a woman with heart disease can breastfeed without difficulty. Kegel exercises are acceptable for perineal strengthening immediately, but the woman should not begin postpartum exercises to improve abdominal tone until her physician or nurse-midwife approves them. A stool softener can be prescribed to prevent straining with bowel movements.

Before discharge, be certain a woman has thought through what help she will need at home so she can continue getting periods of rest. Also ensure that she schedules a return appointment for a postpartum checkup for both her gynecologic health and her cardiac status.

What if... Angelina tells you she tries to eat absolutely no salt in an attempt to limit ankle edema and to keep her heart symptoms to a minimum? What would you do?

A Woman With an Artificial Valve Prosthesis

Once, women with heart valve prostheses were advised not to become pregnant for fear the increased blood volume gained during pregnancy would overwhelm the artificial valve. Today, women with a valve prosthesis complete pregnancy safely (Davidson & Graham, 2007). One potential problem involves the use of oral anticoagulants that a woman takes to prevent the formation of clots at the valve site. Because sodium warfarin (Coumadin) may increase the risk of congenital anomalies in infants (pregnancy risk category D), women are usually placed on low-molecular-weight heparin therapy before becoming pregnant to reduce this risk. Heparin does not cross the placenta and so does not interfere with fetal development or fetal coagulation (category C). Subclinical bleeding from the anticoagulant in the mother can cause placental dislodgement. Observe a woman who is taking an anticoagulant for signs of petechiae and signs of premature separation of the placenta during pregnancy and labor.

A Woman With Chronic Hypertensive Vascular Disease

Women with chronic hypertensive disease come into pregnancy with an elevated blood pressure (140/90 mm Hg or above). Hypertension of this kind is usually associated with arteriosclerosis or renal disease, making it a problem of the older pregnant woman. Chronic hypertension places both the woman and fetus at high risk because fetal well-being can be compromised by poor placental perfusion during the pregnancy (Schulenburg, 2007). Management is prescription of beta-blockers and ACE inhibitors to reduce blood pressure by peripheral dilation to a safe level but not reduce it below the threshold that allows for good placenta circulation. Methyldopa (Aldomet) is a typical drug that is prescribed.

A Woman With Venous Thromboembolic Disease

The incidence of venous thromboembolic disease increases during pregnancy because of a combination of stasis of blood in the lower extremities from uterine pressure and hypercoagulability (the effect of elevated estrogen; Box 20.4). When the pressure of the fetal head at birth puts additional pressure on lower extremity veins, damage can occur to the walls of the veins. When this triad of effects is in place (stasis, vessel damage, and hypercoagulation), the stage is set for thrombus formation in the lower extremities. The likelihood of **deep vein thrombosis (DVT)** leading to pulmonary emboli increases for women 30 years of age or older because increased age is yet another risk factor for thrombosis formation (Segal et al., 2007).

A woman notices pain and redness usually in the calf of a leg. The risk of thrombus formation can be reduced through common-sense measures such as avoiding the use of constrictive knee-high stockings, not sitting with legs crossed at the knee, and avoiding standing in one position for a long period. If a thrombus does occur during pregnancy, it is diagnosed by a woman's history and Doppler ultrasonography. A woman will be treated with bed rest and intravenous heparin for 24 to 48 hours. After this, she may be prescribed subcutaneous heparin every 12 or 24 hours for the duration of the pregnancy. It is generally recommended that the lower abdomen be used for rotating sites for subcutaneous heparin administration. With pregnancy, however, this site is usually avoided and the injection sites are limited to the arms and thighs. Heparin dosage is regulated by frequent partial thromboplastin time (PTT) determinations. Additional measures of care for a woman with DVT, such as heat, elevation, and bed rest, are discussed in Chapter 25, because 50% of thromboses that occur with pregnancy occur in the postpartum period.

Women taking heparin during pregnancy should not take any additional injections once labor begins to help reduce the possibility of hemorrhage at birth; they are not candidates for routine episiotomy or epidural anesthesia for this same reason unless at least 4 hours has passed since the last heparin dose was given. PTT determinations should be continued during labor. Either heparin or sodium warfarin (Coumadin) can be prescribed after birth if a woman is not breastfeeding; Coumadin should be used cautiously wih breastfeeding.

A particular group of women has been identified as being more susceptible to thrombi formation, spontaneous miscarriage, fetal death, and hypertension of pregnancy: women with antiphospholipid antibodies (aPLA) (Mavragani et al., 2007). It is not known why aPLA occur in some women and not in others, but these antibodies probably represent an autoimmune process. Women who are identified as aPLA positive may be started on a prophylactic program of aspirin or subcutaneous heparin during pregnancy that is continued postpartum to reduce the possibility of DVT. Administration of a corticosteroid may help to reduce the formation of additional antibodies and so may also be prescribed. After pregnancy, such women should not begin an oral contraceptive because it can increase blood coagulation and the possibility of thrombi formation.

The chief danger of thrombophlebitis is pulmonary embolism or a clot lodging in the pulmonary artery and blocking circulation to the lungs and heart. Symptoms of pulmonary embolism include:

- Chest pain
- Sudden onset of dyspnea
- Cough with hemoptysis
- Tachycardia or missed beats
- Severe dizziness or fainting from lowered blood pressure

Pulmonary embolism needs to be recognized as it is an immediate emergency (Cansino & Lipsett, 2007). Care measures for this are discussed in Chapter 25.

Box 20.4 Assessment

Assessing a Pregnant Woman With Venous Thromboembolic Disease

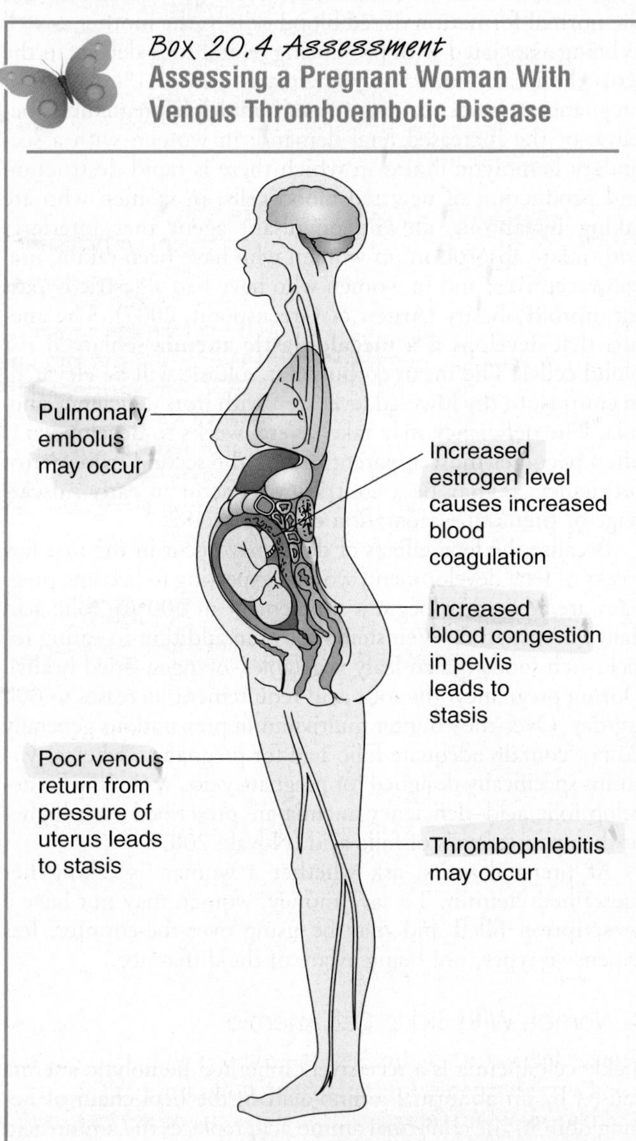

HEMATOLOGIC DISORDERS AND PREGNANCY

Hematologic disorders during pregnancy involve either blood formation or coagulation disorders.

Anemia and Pregnancy

Because the blood volume expands during pregnancy slightly ahead of the red cell count, most women have a pseudo-anemia of early pregnancy. This condition is normal and should not be confused with true types of anemia that can occur as complications of pregnancy. True anemia is present when a woman's hemoglobin concentration is less than 11 g/dL (hematocrit <33%) in the first or third trimester of pregnancy or hemoglobin concentration is less than 10.5 g/dL (hematocrit <32%) in the second trimester (Arnett & Greenspoon, 2007).

Nursing Diagnoses and Related Interventions

Nursing Diagnosis: Risk for ineffective tissue perfusion related to maternal anemia during pregnancy.

Outcome Evaluation: Client's hemoglobin is above 11 mg/dL; fetal heart rate is 120 to 160 beats per minute; client takes prenatal supplement daily.

A Woman With Iron-Deficiency Anemia

Iron-deficiency anemia is the most common anemia of pregnancy, complicating as many as 15% to 25% of all pregnancies (Reveiz, Gyte, & Cuervo, 2009). Many women enter pregnancy with a deficiency of iron stores resulting from a diet low in iron, heavy menstrual periods, or unwise weight-reducing programs. Iron stores are apt to be low in women who were pregnant less than 2 years before the current pregnancy or those from low socioeconomic levels who have not had iron-rich diets. When the hemoglobin level is below 12 mg/dL (hematocrit <33%), iron deficiency is suspected. It is confirmed by a corresponding low serum iron level and an increased iron-binding capacity.

Iron is made available to the body by absorption from the duodenum into the bloodstream after it is ingested. In the bloodstream, it is bound to transferrin for transport to the liver, spleen, and bone marrow. At these sites, it is incorporated into hemoglobin or stored as ferritin.

Iron-deficiency anemia is characteristically a microcytic (small red blood cell), hypochromic (less hemoglobin than the average red cell) anemia because when an inadequate supply of iron is ingested, iron is unavailable for incorporation into red blood cells. Both hematocrit and hemoglobin will be reduced (<33% and <12 mg/dL, respectively). The serum transferrin level will be under 100 mg/dL, the transferrin saturation level will be under 5%, the serum iron level will be under 30 μg/dL, and the mean corpuscular hemoglobin concentration will be under 30; iron-binding capacity, in contrast, will be increased (>400 μg/dL). Iron-deficiency anemia is mildly associated with low birth weight and preterm birth. Because the body recognizes that it needs increased nutrients, some women with this develop pica, or the craving and eating of substances such as ice or starch (Mills, 2007). A woman experiences extreme fatigue and poor exercise tolerance because she cannot transport oxygen effectively.

To prevent this common anemia, women should take prenatal vitamins containing an iron supplement of 60 mg elemental iron as prophylactic therapy during pregnancy. In addition, they need to eat a diet high in iron and vitamins (green leafy vegetables, meat, legumes, fruit). Women who develop iron-deficiency anemia will be prescribed therapeutic levels of medication (120 to 200 mg elemental iron/day), usually in the form of ferrous sulfate or ferrous gluconate.

Iron is best absorbed from an acid medium. Therefore, advise women to take iron supplements with orange juice or a vitamin C supplement, which supplies ascorbic acid. If they are not already enrolled in the Special Supplemental Nutrition Program for Women, Infants, and Children (WIC) but are eligible, making a referral could help ensure a better diet. When women begin to take a prescribed iron supplement, new red blood cells should begin to increase, or their reticulocyte counts should rise from a normal range (0.5% to 1.5%) to 3% to 4% by 2 weeks' time. Some women report constipation or gastric irritation when taking oral iron supplements. Increasing roughage in the diet and always taking the pills with food help reduce these symptoms. Ferrous sulfate turns stools black so caution women about this to prevent them worrying that they are bleeding internally. If iron-deficiency anemia is severe and a woman has difficulty with oral iron therapy, intramuscular or intravenous iron dextran can be prescribed.

A Woman With Folic Acid–Deficiency Anemia

Folic acid, or folacin, one of the B vitamins, is necessary for the normal formation of red blood cells in the mother as well as being associated with preventing neural tube defects in the fetus. Folic acid–deficiency anemia is seen in 1% to 5% of pregnancies. It occurs most often in multiple pregnancies because of the increased fetal demand; in women with a secondary hemolytic illness in which there is rapid destruction and production of new red blood cells; in women who are taking hydantoin, an anticonvulsant agent that interferes with folate absorption; in women who have been taking oral contraceptives; and in women who have had a gastric bypass for morbid obesity (Arnett & Greenspoon, 2007). The anemia that develops is a **megaloblastic anemia** (enlarged red blood cells). The mean corpuscular volume will be elevated, in contrast to the lowered level seen with iron-deficiency anemia. The deficiency may take several weeks to develop, so it often becomes most apparent during the second trimester of pregnancy. It may be a contributory factor in early miscarriage or premature separation of the placenta.

Because the fetal effects of deficiency occur in the first few weeks of fetal development, women expecting to become pregnant are advised to begin a supplement of 400 μg folic acid daily (Bernstein & Weinstein, 2007) in addition to eating folacin-rich foods (green leafy vegetables, oranges, dried beans). During pregnancy, the folic acid requirement increases to 600 μg/day. Over-the-counter multivitamin preparations generally do not contain adequate folic acid for pregnancy, whereas vitamins specifically designed for pregnancy do. Women who develop folic acid–deficiency anemia are prescribed even higher or therapeutic levels of folic acid (Novak, 2007).

At prenatal visits, ask whether a woman is taking her prescribed vitamin. To save money, women may not have a prescription filled and may be using over-the-counter, less expensive types, not being aware of the difference.

A Woman With Sickle Cell Anemia

Sickle cell anemia is a recessively inherited hemolytic anemia caused by an abnormal amino acid in the beta chain of hemoglobin. If the abnormal amino acid replaces the amino acid valine, sickle hemoglobin (HbS) results; if it is substituted for the amino acid lysine, nonsickling hemoglobin (HbC) results. An individual who is heterozygous (has only one gene in which the abnormal substitution has occurred) has the sickle cell trait (HbAS). If the person is homozygous (has two genes in which the substitution has occurred), sickle cell disease (HbSS) results.

With the disease, the majority of red blood cells are irregular or sickle shaped so they cannot carry as much hemoglobin as can normally shaped red blood cells. When oxygen tension becomes reduced, as occurs at high altitudes, or blood becomes more viscid than usual (dehydration), the cells tend to clump because of the irregular shape. This clumping can result in vessel blockage with reduced blood flow to organs. The cells then will hemolyse, reducing the number available and causing a severe anemia.

Approximately 1 in every 10 African Americans has the sickle cell trait (i.e., carries a recessive gene for S hemoglobin but is asymptomatic); theoretically, 1 in every 400 African Americans has the disease, although with interracial marriages increasing, the disease is no longer confined to one ethnic group (Zack-Williams, 2007).

Although the sickle cell trait does not appear to influence the course of pregnancy, prematurity, miscarriage, or perinatal mortality rates of these may be higher for women with the homozygous disease. Women with the trait seem to have an increased incidence of asymptomatic bacteriuria, resulting in an increased incidence of pyelonephritis.

At any time in life, sickle cell anemia is a threat to life if vital blood vessels such as those to the liver, kidneys, heart, lungs, or brain become blocked. In pregnancy, blockage to the placental circulation can directly compromise the fetus, causing low birth weight and possibly fetal death.

Assessment. All African American women who have not been previously tested should be screened for sickle cell anemia at a first prenatal visit. Hemoglobin levels for all women with sickle cell disease should be obtained throughout pregnancy. A woman with sickle cell disease may normally have a hemoglobin level of 6 to 8 mg/100 mL. Unless she receives active interventions to raise this level, she will maintain it during pregnancy, reducing oxygen to the fetus. Hemolysis in a sickle cell crisis may occur so rapidly that a woman's hemoglobin level can fall to 5 or 6 mg/100 mL in a few hours. There is an accompanying rise in her indirect bilirubin level because she cannot conjugate the bilirubin released from so many red blood cells so quickly destroyed.

Because a pregnant woman with sickle cell anemia is more susceptible to bacteriuria than other women, a clean-catch urine sample is collected periodically during pregnancy to detect developing bacteriuria while a woman is still asymptomatic.

Throughout pregnancy, monitor a woman's diet to be certain she is consuming sufficient amounts of folic acid and possibly an additional folic acid supplement, which may be necessary to build new red blood cells. Her fluid intake should also be carefully monitored. She should consume at least eight glasses of fluids daily. Early in pregnancy, when she may be nauseated, her fluid intake can easily decrease, and dehydration and a subsequent sickle cell crisis may occur.

Assess a woman's lower extremities at prenatal visits for varicosities or pooling of blood in leg veins, which are apt to occur from uterine pressure as pregnancy advances. Such pooling and pressure can lead to red cell destruction. Standing for long periods during the day increases this pressure, whereas sitting on a chair with the legs elevated or lying on the side in a modified Sims' position encourages venous return from the lower extremities. Help a woman plan her day so she has limited long periods of standing and adequate rest periods.

Fetal health is usually monitored during pregnancy by an ultrasound examination at 16 to 24 weeks to assess for intrauterine growth restriction and by weekly nonstress or ultrasound examinations beginning at about 30 weeks. Blood flow through the uterus and placenta may be measured by blood flow velocity. If blood flow velocity is reduced, the chance of intrauterine growth restriction is increased.

Therapeutic Management. Interventions to prevent sickle cell crisis can include periodic exchange transfusions throughout pregnancy to replace sickled cells with non-sickled cells. An exchange transfusion serves a secondary purpose of removing a quantity of the increased bilirubin resulting from the breakdown of red blood cells as well as restoring the hemoglobin level (Linker, 2009). If a crisis occurs, controlling pain, administering oxygen as needed, and increasing the fluid volume of the circulatory system to lower viscosity are important interventions (see Chapter 44 for a discussion of therapy of sickle cell anemia in children). The fluid administered is often hypotonic (0.45 saline) to keep plasma tension low because of the difficulty a woman has concentrating urine to remove large amounts of fluid. As a rule, women with sickle cell disease are not given an iron supplement during pregnancy. Sickled cells cannot incorporate iron in the same manner as non-sickled cells can, so excessive iron buildup may result. Women do need a folic acid supplement to keep the new cells produced from being megaloblastic.

If a woman develops an infection that raises her temperature and causes her to perspire more than normally (creates dehydration) or contracts a respiratory infection that compromises air exchange so that her PO_2 is lowered, hospitalization for observation may be necessary to rule out the development of a sickle cell crisis and subsequent hemolysis of crowded cells (Szymanski & Aina-Mumuney, 2007).

When the fetus is mature, the time and method of birth are individualized. Keep a woman well hydrated in labor. If an operative birth is necessary, she generally receives epidural anesthesia as general anesthesia poses a possible risk of hypoxia. In the postpartal period, early ambulation and wearing pressure stockings can help reduce the risk of thromboembolism from stasis in lower extremities.

Women generally are interested in determining at birth whether their child has inherited the disease. Because the disorder is recessively inherited, if one of the parents has the disease and the other is free of the disease and trait, the chances that the child will inherit the disease are zero. If a woman has the disease and her partner has the trait, the chances that the child will be born with the disease are 50% (see Chapter 7). If both parents have the disease, all their children will also have the disease.

Symptoms of sickle cell disease do not become clinically apparent until an infant's fetal hemoglobin converts to a largely adult pattern (in 3 to 6 months). Fetal hemoglobin is composed of two alpha and two gamma chains; adult hemoglobin is composed of two alpha and two beta chains. Because the sickle cell trait is carried on the beta chain, symptoms will not be manifested clinically until this chain appears. Electrophoresis of red blood cells obtained during fetal life by percutaneous umbilical blood sampling or amniocentesis, however, can reveal the presence of the disease on the few beta chains already present in utero. Newborns have approximately 15% adult hemoglobin at birth, so electrophoresis testing at birth can also reveal if the disease is present. Screening is routine in some settings. Nursing care of the child with sickle cell disease is discussed in Chapter 44.

The Woman with Thalassemia

The thalassemias are a group of autosomal recessively inherited blood disorders that lead to poor hemoglobin formation and severe anemia. They occur most frequently in Mediterranean, African, and Asian populations (Waterbury, 2007). Symptoms first appear in childhood. Treatment focuses on combating anemia through such measures as folic acid supplementation and perhaps blood transfusion to infuse hemoglobin rich red blood cells. Women do not usually take an iron supplement during pregnancy or they could receive an iron overload because of the iron also infused by blood transfusions. Care of a child with both forms of thalassemia, alpha and beta, is discussed in Chapter 44.

The Woman with Malaria

Malaria is a protozoan infection that is transmitted to people by *Anopheles* mosquitoes (Garner & Gulmezoglu, 2009). The infection causes red blood cells to stick to the surface of capillaries causing obstruction of these vessels. This can result in end organ anoxia when blood can not reach organs effectively.

Although the disorder does not have a high incidence in the United States, newly immigrated women may be infected with it. It is important to consider during pregnancy as it can be transmitted to a fetus by mother-to-fetus transmission.

The incubation period for the most frequently occurring type is 12 to 14 days. The most noticeable symptoms are elevated liver function tests accompanying fever, malaise, and headache. If not treated, thrombocytopenia, anemia, and renal failure can develop.

Malaria can be prevented by wearing clothing that covers most of the body and using an insect repellent when in an area infested with mosquitoes, sleeping at night with mosquito nets, or keeping windows closed to prevent mosquitoes from entering. As further prevention, urge women to delay travel to endemic areas until after pregnancy if possible.

Treatment is with several antimalaria drugs. Chloroquine is safe to administer during all trimesters of pregnancy so it is the drug of choice (Wiltz et al., 2008). Sulfadoxine-pyrimethamine may be administered during the last trimester. Quinine, malarone, or tetracyclines should not be used at any point in pregnancy or with women who are breastfeeding. Antimalarial therapy may also reduce the incidence of low birth weight and preterm birth.

Coagulation Disorders and Pregnancy

Most coagulation disorders are sex linked or occur only in males and so have little effect on pregnancies. However, von Willebrand disease is a coagulation disorder inherited as an autosomal dominant trait that does occur in women (Linker, 2009). From the time she was a child, a woman would have noticed menorrhagia or frequent episodes of epistaxis. If these symptoms were not severe, though, the condition may go undiagnosed until pregnancy, when a woman experiences a spontaneous miscarriage or postpartum hemorrhage.

Women with the disorder have normal platelet counts, but bleeding time is prolonged. Levels of factor VIII–related antigen (VIII-R) and factor VIII coagulation activity (VIII-C) are both reduced. Replacement of these factors by infusion of cryoprecipitate or fresh-frozen plasma may be necessary before labor to prevent excessive bleeding.

Hemophilia B (Christmas disease, factor IX deficiency) is a sex-linked disorder, so the actual disease occurs only in males. However, female carriers may have such a reduced level of factor IX (only 33% of normal) that hemorrhage with labor or a spontaneous miscarriage can be a serious complication in these women. Carriers of the disorder need to be identified before pregnancy. Restoration of factor IX levels can be done by infusion of factor IX concentrate or fresh-frozen plasma.

Percutaneous umbilical blood sampling can be used to detect whether a male fetus has hemophilia. If there is a family history of hemophilia, before an internal fetal heart rate monitor is attached or fetal scalp blood sampling is done during labor, the fetal status needs to be determined. If the fetus has a coagulation disorder, these procedures would be contraindicated because they could result in extensive fetal blood loss.

Idiopathic thrombocytopenic purpura (ITP), a decreased number of platelets, can occur at any time in life and so occasionally occurs during pregnancy. The cause of the condition is unknown, but it is assumed to be an autoimmune illness (an antiplatelet antibody that destroys platelets is apparently released). Symptoms of the illness usually occur shortly after a viral invasion such as an upper respiratory infection (McMillan, 2007).

Without an adequate level of platelets, minute petechiae or large ecchymoses appear on a woman's body. Frequent nosebleeds may occur. Laboratory studies reveal a marked thrombocytopenia (platelet count may be as low as $20{,}000/mm^3$ from a usual count of $150{,}000\ mm^3$).

The illness typically runs a 1- to 3-month limited course, but because the symptoms are similar to pregnancy-induced hypertension with HELLP syndrome, a serious complication of pregnancy (see Chapter 21), they are frightening when they occur during pregnancy. A platelet transfusion or plasmapheresis may be administered to temporarily increase the platelet count. Oral prednisone is also effective. Women with the phenomenon need to be identified during pregnancy because the decreased platelet count can lead to increased bleeding at birth. In addition, the antiplatelet factor can cross the placenta and cause accompanying platelet destruction in the newborn, or allow a newborn to be born with the illness (see Chapter 44 for care of the child with ITP).

✔ Checkpoint Question 20.2

Which statement by a woman with sickle cell anemia would alert you she may need further instruction on prenatal care?

a. "I understand why folic acid is important for red cell formation."

b. "I'm careful to drink at least eight glasses of fluid every day."
c. "I take an iron pill every day to help grow new red blood cells."
d. "I've stopped jogging so I don't risk becoming dehydrated."

RENAL AND URINARY DISORDERS AND PREGNANCY

Adequate kidney function is important to a successful pregnancy outcome because a woman is excreting waste products not only for herself but also for the fetus. This dual function makes any condition that interferes with kidney or urinary function potentially serious.

A Woman With a Urinary Tract Infection

As many as 4% to 10% of nonpregnant women have asymptomatic bacteriuria (organisms are present in the urine without symptoms of infection). In a pregnant woman, because the ureters dilate from the effect of progesterone, stasis of urine occurs. The minimal glucosuria that occurs with pregnancy allows more than the usual number of organisms to grow. This causes asymptomatic urinary tract infections (UTIs) in as many as 10% to 15% of pregnant women (Vazquez & Villar, 2009). Asymptomatic infections are potentially dangerous because they can progress to pyelonephritis (infection of the pelvis of the kidney) and are associated with preterm labor and premature rupture of membranes. Women with known vesicoureteral reflux (backflow of urine into the ureters) tend to develop UTIs or pyelonephritis more often than others. The organism most commonly responsible for UTI is *Escherichia coli* from an ascending infection. A UTI can also occur as a descending infection, or begin in the kidneys from the filtration of organisms present from other body infections. If the infectious organism is determined to be *Streptococcus* B, vaginal cultures should be obtained because streptococcal B infection of the genital tract is associated with pneumonia in newborns.

Assessment

A UTI typically is manifested by frequency and pain on urination. With pyelonephritis, a woman develops pain in the lumbar region (usually on the right side) that radiates downward. The area feels tender to palpation. She may have accompanying nausea and vomiting, malaise, pain, and frequency of urination. Her temperature may be elevated only slightly or may be as high as 103° to 104° F (39° to 40° C). The infection usually occurs on the right side because there is greater compression and urinary stasis on the right ureter from the uterus being pushed that way by the large bulk of the intestine on the left side. A urine culture will reveal over 100,000 organisms per milliliter of urine, a level diagnostic of infection.

Therapeutic Management

Obtain a clean-catch urine sample for culture and sensitivity from women with possible symptoms of UTI (see Chapter 11). Many health care agencies ask women for clean-catch urine specimens at intervals during pregnancy (tested by a rapid dipstick method) to detect infection before it becomes symptomatic. A sensitivity test after a culture will determine which antibiotic will best combat the infection. Amoxicillin, ampicillin, and cephalosporins are effective against most organisms causing UTIs and are safe antibiotics during pregnancy. The sulfonamides can be used early in pregnancy but not near term because they can interfere with protein binding of bilirubin, which then leads to hyperbilirubinemia in the newborn. Tetracyclines are contraindicated in pregnancy as they cause retardation of bone growth and staining of the fetal teeth (Subramanian et al., 2008).

Nursing Diagnoses and Related Interventions

Nursing Diagnosis: Risk for infection related to stasis of urine with pregnancy

Outcome Evaluation: Oral temperature is below 100.4° F (38° C), and a clean-catch urine specimen has a bacteria count below 100,000 colonies per milliliter.

All women during pregnancy can be reminded of common measures to prevent UTIs, such as:

- Voiding frequently (at least every 2 hours)
- Wiping front to back after voiding and bowel movements
- Wearing cotton, not synthetic fiber, underwear
- Voiding immediately after sexual intercourse

The pregnant woman with a UTI needs to take the additional measure of drinking an increased amount of fluid to flush out the infection from the urinary tract. Do not merely tell her to "push fluids" or "drink lots of water." Give her a specific amount to drink every day (up to 3 to 4 L per 24 hours) to make certain she does increase her fluid intake sufficiently.

A woman can promote urine drainage by assuming a knee–chest position for 15 minutes morning and evening. In this position, the weight of the uterus is shifted forward, releasing the pressure on the ureters and allowing urine to drain more freely.

If a woman has one UTI during pregnancy, the chances are high that she will develop another late in pregnancy, when urinary stasis tends to be even greater. She may, therefore, be kept on prophylactic antibiotics throughout the remainder of the pregnancy. Ask at prenatal visits whether she is continuing to take this type of prophylactic medicine. When women have pain and symptoms of urinary frequency, they take medication well. When they no longer have any clinical evidence that they are sick, their compliance rate, like any other adult's, begins to fall dramatically. A woman may need to post a chart on her refrigerator door or in her bathroom to remind herself to take the medication. Leaving the medicine on a counter to remind herself to take it is not a good habit to develop because soon she will have a new baby in the house; encourage her to keep medicine out of sight and reach to get into the habit of "childproofing" even at this early stage.

Pyelonephritis occurs as an extension of a urinary tract infection or infection that originated in or spread to the kidney (Nguyen & Witter, 2007). If this develops, a woman may be hospitalized for 24 to 48 hours while she is treated with intravenous antibiotics. After this acute episode, she will be maintained on a drug such as oral nitrofurantoin (Macrodantin) for the remainder of the pregnancy. Acidifying urine by the use of ascorbic acid (vitamin C), which is often recommended in nonpregnant women, is not usually recommended during pregnancy because a newborn can develop scurvy in the immediate neonatal period from withdrawal.

After birth, a woman who developed more than one UTI may have an intravenous pyelogram or ultrasound scheduled to help detect any urinary tract abnormality that might be present, such as vesicoureteral reflux, to help prevent future infections.

A Woman With Chronic Renal Disease

In the past, females with chronic renal disease did not reach childbearing age or were advised not to have children because of their high risk status during pregnancy. Today, women with chronic renal disease can have children because pregnancy does not appear to cause progressive deterioration of kidney lesions. With conscientious prenatal care, even women who have had renal transplants can expect to have healthy pregnancies and healthy children (Fischer, 2007).

Women with chronic renal disease may develop severe anemia during pregnancy because their diseased kidneys do not produce erythropoietin, which is necessary for red cell formation. Fortunately, synthetic erythropoietin is now available and is safe to take during pregnancy (Masters, 2007).

Because the glomerular filtration rate normally increases during pregnancy, a woman's serum creatinine level (a measure of kidney function that elevates when kidneys are under stress) may be actually slightly below normal during pregnancy. A usual serum creatinine level is 0.7 mg/100 mL; during pregnancy, it falls to about 0.5 mg/100 mL. Women with kidney disease who normally have a serum creatinine level of more than 2.0 mg/dL may be advised not to undertake a pregnancy in case the increased strain on already damaged kidneys leads to kidney failure.

In many women, it is difficult to interpret kidney function during pregnancy based on nonpregnant values (Box 20.5). Trace amounts of glucose and protein in the urine are common during pregnancy because of increased glomerular permeability, so **proteinuria** (protein in urine) must be compared to a woman's individualized prepregnancy level to be meaningful. If a woman is told proteinuria may occur during pregnancy, she will understand it is an expected change of pregnancy, not a forecast of changing kidney function. Many women with renal disease have elevated blood pressure. To be meaningful, their blood pressure levels during pregnancy must also be compared with prepregnancy levels (Williams & Davison, 2008).

Many women with renal disease routinely take a corticosteroid such as oral prednisone at a maintenance level. This drug therapy typically is continued throughout pregnancy. Although animal studies have shown an increased incidence of cleft palate from corticosteroid use during pregnancy, this does not appear to be true in humans. The infant may be hyperglycemic at birth because of the suppression of insulin activity by the corticosteroid.

Box 20.5 Assessment
Assessing a Pregnant Woman With Renal Disease

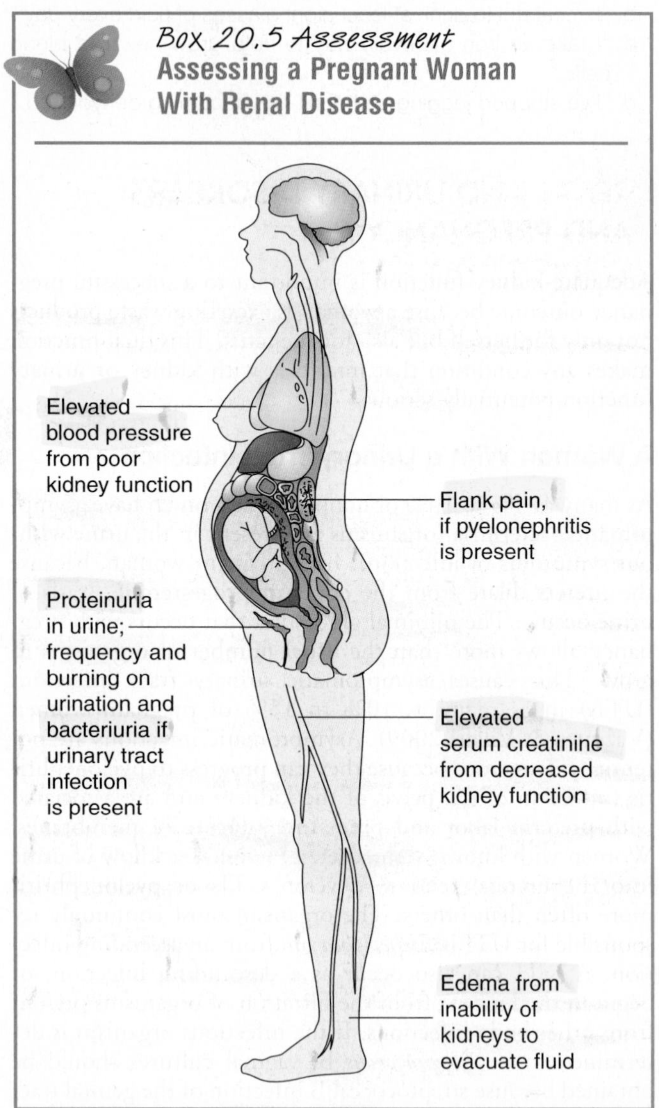

Although successful pregnancy in women with kidney transplants is to be expected, women should be considered individually to determine whether they will be able to carry a pregnancy to term before a pregnancy is initiated (del Mar Colon & Hibbard, 2007). Criteria to be evaluated include:

- A woman's general health and the time since the transplant (preferably >2 years)
- Serum creatinine level
- The presence of proteinuria or hypertension or signs of graft rejection
- Medications taken to reduce graft rejection

It is helpful if the drugs a woman is taking are limited to prednisone and azathioprine (an antimetabolite [Imuran], but with no reports of fetal compromise from its use). Women with severe renal disease may require dialysis to aid kidney function during pregnancy (Gomez et al., 2007). With dialysis, there is a risk of preterm labor, perhaps because progesterone is removed with the dialysis. To prevent this complication, progesterone may be administered intramuscularly before the procedure. If hemodialysis is used, it should be scheduled frequently and for short durations to avoid acute fluid shifts. The heparin administered in connection with hemodialysis is safe during pregnancy because it does not cross the placenta. Even in light of the expanding uterine size, peritoneal dialysis is actually preferred over hemodialysis because it normally causes less drastic fluid shifts. This can be accomplished on an ambulatory basis (continuous ambulatory peritoneal dialysis) throughout pregnancy.

Women with renal disease may need a nutrition consultation during pregnancy if they are on a low potassium diet to avoid a buildup of potassium that accumulates because their diseased kidneys do not evacuate this well (Stover, 2007). They also may need a great deal of emotional support during pregnancy. They are aware that kidneys are vital for life and that the stress of pregnancy on damaged kidneys may cause them to fail. They are aware that by being pregnant they are risking not only the life of the child growing inside them but also their own life. They may need extra support and information to know how their fetus is doing. They may need extra time with their infant at birth for bonding because they may have been too concerned during pregnancy to begin this process.

RESPIRATORY DISORDERS AND PREGNANCY

Respiratory diseases range from mild (the common cold) to severe (pneumonia) to chronic (tuberculosis or chronic obstructive pulmonary disease [COPD]). Any respiratory condition can worsen in pregnancy because the rising uterus compresses the diaphragm, reducing the size of the thoracic cavity and available lung space. Any respiratory disorder can pose serious hazards to the fetus if allowed to progress to the point where the mother's oxygen–carbon dioxide exchange is altered or the mother or fetus cannot receive enough oxygen.

Nursing Diagnoses and Related Interventions

Nursing Diagnosis: Risk for ineffective breathing pattern related to respiratory changes during pregnancy

Outcome Evaluation: Respiratory rate is 16 to 20 per minute, Po_2 is above 80 mm Hg, Pco_2 is below 40 mm Hg, and fetal heart rate is 120 to 160 beats per minute with good variability.

A Woman With Acute Nasopharyngitis

Acute nasopharyngitis (common cold) tends to be more severe during pregnancy than at other times because during pregnancy, estrogen stimulation normally causes some degree of nasal congestion. This means that even with a minor cold, a woman can find it difficult to breathe. Aspirin should be avoided as a cold remedy during pregnancy because of possible interference with blood clotting in both mother and fetus and the possibility of prolonged pregnancy at term (Karch, 2009). Because common colds are invariably caused by a virus, antibiotic therapy is unnecessary except to prevent a secondary infection. Although most simple cough syrups contain no ingredients that would make them unsafe for use during pregnancy, women should check with their health care provider before taking any over-the-counter medication for a cold (Box 20.6).

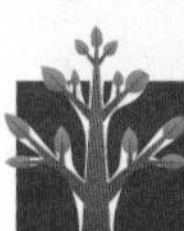

BOX 20.6 * Focus on Family Teaching

Relieving Upper Respiratory Symptoms During Pregnancy

Q. Angelina tells you, "I get a lot of colds. What should I do to keep symptoms under control during pregnancy?"

A. Use the following guidelines to help combat common cold symptoms during pregnancy:

- Be sure to get extra rest and sleep and eat a diet high in vitamin C (orange juice and fruit) to help boost the immune system.
- If you experience any aches and pains, take acetaminophen (Tylenol) every 4 hours. Do not take acetosalicylic acid (aspirin) during pregnancy.
- Use a room humidifier, especially at night, to moisten nasal secretions and help mucus drain.
- Use only over-the-counter cough drops or syrups that contain natural ingredients such as honey and lemon to help reduce coughing.
- Apply a medicated vapor rub to your chest if you prefer to help relieve nasal congestion.
- Use cool or warm compresses to relieve sinus headaches. Check with your health care provider regarding the use of over-the-counter cough drops, syrups, or decongestants to be certain that any drug you take is safe during pregnancy.

A Woman With Influenza

Influenza is caused by a virus, identified as type A, B, or C. The disease spreads in epidemic form and is accompanied by high fever, extreme prostration, aching pains in the back and extremities, and generally a sore, raw throat. Contrary to early reports, influenza infection has not been clearly correlated with congenital anomalies in children although it can be a cause of preterm labor. For unknown reasons, some studies have shown a link between influenza during pregnancy and schizophrenia in children born of that pregnancy (Venables et al., 2007). Treatment includes an antipyretic such as acetaminophen (Tylenol) to control fever. Oseltamivir (TamiFlu), an oral antiviral drug that is category C, should be used cautiously until its long-term effects are known (Subramanian et al., 2008). Because influenza vaccines are made from killed virus, women may be immunized safely against influenza during pregnancy (Fiore et al., 2007).

A Woman With Pneumonia

Pneumonia is the bacterial or viral invasion of lung tissue by pathogens such as *S. pneumoniae, Haemophilus influenzae,* and *Mycoplasma pneumoniae.* After the invasion, an acute inflammatory response occurs in the lung alveoli with exudate of red blood cells, fibrin, and polymorphonuclear leukocytes into the alveoli. This process confines the bacteria or virus within segments of the lobes of the lungs but also fills alveoli with fluid, blocking off breathing space. If the collection of fluid is extreme, it can limit the oxygen available to the fetus. Therapy involves the use of an appropriate antibiotic and perhaps oxygen administration (Cansino & Lipsett, 2007). With severe disease, ventilation support may be necessary. There is a tendency for women with pneumonia late in pregnancy to begin preterm labor because of the oxygen deficit. If pneumonia is present during labor, oxygen should be administered so the fetus has adequate oxygen resources during contractions.

A Woman With Severe Acute Respiratory Syndrome

Severe acute respiratory syndrome (SARS) is a newly emerged infectious disease with the clinical symptoms of persistent fever, chills, muscle aches, malaise, dry cough, headache, and dyspnea. Common laboratory findings are decreased lymphocyte and platelet counts. A coronavirus has been identified as the pathogen responsible for the illness, which appears to have originated in southern China and has spread to become a potentially worldwide pandemic (Longman & Johnson, 2007). SARS spreads by close person-to-person contact via droplet transmission. The incubation period is 2 to 10 days. Therapy is vigorous, with intravenous antibiotics. Many women need respiratory support to survive. SARS during pregnancy creates such an acute illness that it is associated with high incidences of spontaneous miscarriage, preterm birth, and intrauterine growth restriction. There is no evidence of perinatal SARS infection among infants born to these mothers.

A Woman With Asthma

Asthma is a disorder marked by reversible airflow obstruction, airway hyperreactivity, and airway inflammation. It complicates about 5% to 9% of pregnancies and is potentially associated with an increased risk of perinatal complications. Women who have had asthma since childhood so know how to manage their asthma well are most apt to have successful pregnancies (Tata et al., 2007). Symptoms are often triggered by an inhaled allergen such as pollen or cigarette smoke. With inhalation of the allergen, there is an immediate release of bioactive mediators such as histamine and leukotrienes from an IgE/immunoglobulin interaction. This results in constriction of the bronchial smooth muscle, marked mucosal inflammation and swelling, and the production of thick bronchial secretions. These three processes cause a marked reduction in the size of the lumen of air passages. This causes a woman to have difficulty pulling in air; on exhalation, she has so much difficulty releasing air that she makes a high-pitched whistling sound (bronchial wheezing) from air being pushed past the bronchial narrowing. Asthma has the potential of reducing the oxygen supply to a fetus leading to preterm birth or fetal growth restriction if a major attack should occur during pregnancy, although this is not likely with well-managed asthma. Many women find that their asthma improves during pregnancy because of the high circulating levels of corticosteroids that are present. A woman should check with her physician or nurse-midwife about the safety of the medications she routinely takes for this disorder before pregnancy to be certain it will be safe to continue using them during pregnancy and breastfeeding.

The inhaled corticosteroids beclomethasone (Beclovent, Vancenase) and budesonide (Pulmicort, Rhinocort) are commonly used by women with persistent asthma and are also good choices for pregnant women and those who might become pregnant. Women who have been taking a corticosteroid during pregnancy may need parenteral administration of hydrocortisone during labor because of the added stress during this time. Beta-adrenergic agonists such as terbutaline and albuterol may be taken safely during pregnancy, but because they have the potential to reduce labor contractions the dosage is tapered close to term if possible (Boushey, 2007).

Many women use cromolyn sodium (Intal), a mast cell stabilizer, to help prevent symptoms. Many adolescents with asthma are prescribed leukotriene receptor antagonists such as montelukast sodium (Singulair) or zafirlukast (Accolate). All of these are pregnancy category B drugs and so may be continued during pregnancy (Montoro, 2007).

A Woman With Tuberculosis

Tuberculosis is a disease that should have been eradicated in view of the effective treatment available. However, in highly populated areas, the incidence has actually increased and in some areas is at epidemic proportions. Worldwide, it is still one of the leading causes of death.

With tuberculosis, lung tissue is invaded by *Mycobacterium tuberculosis,* an acid-fast bacillus. Macrophages and T lymphocytes surround the invading bacillus, but rather than actually killing it they merely surround and confine it. Fibrosis, calcification, and a final ring of collagenous scar tissue develop, effectively sealing off the organisms from the body and any further invasion or spread. The antibodies produced will thereafter cause a woman to have a positive response to a Mantoux (purified protein derivative [PPD]) test.

Assessment

In high-risk areas, women should undergo skin testing (a PPD test) at their first prenatal visit. Women need to be cautioned that a positive reaction does not necessarily mean they have the disease; it can mean they have at some time been exposed to tuberculosis and so have antibodies in their system. If a woman has a positive reaction, a chest radiograph to confirm the diagnosis will be scheduled. This can be done safely during pregnancy if the woman's abdomen is shielded. Symptoms of tuberculosis include:

- Chronic cough
- Weight loss
- Hemoptysis (coughing blood)
- Night sweats
- Low-grade fever
- Chronic fatigue

Therapeutic Management

Women with active tuberculosis need treatment during pregnancy (Cox, 2007). Isoniazid (INH) and ethambutol hydrochloride (Myambutol), the drugs of choice for tuberculosis, may be given without apparent teratogenic effects during pregnancy. INH may result in a peripheral neuritis if a woman does not take supplemental pyridoxine (vitamin B_6) as well. Ethambutol may cause optic nerve involvement (optic atrophy and loss of green color recognition) in the mother. To detect this, test a woman monthly using the color section of a Snellen (eye test) chart. If symptoms develop, advise her to check with her health provider about discontinuing the drug.

A woman who had tuberculosis earlier in life must be especially careful to maintain an adequate level of calcium during pregnancy to ensure that tuberculosis pockets are not broken down. With tuberculosis, a woman is usually advised to wait 1 to 2 years after the infection becomes inactive before attempting to conceive. This is because recent inactive tuberculosis is more apt to become active during pregnancy than well-calcified lesions. Pressure on the diaphragm from below changes the shape of the lung, and an incompletely sealed pocket could be broken in this process. Pushing during labor may increase intrapulmonary pressure and cause the same phenomenon. Recent inactive tuberculosis may also become active during the postpartum period as the lung suddenly returns to its more vertical prepregnant position following birth, allowing calcium deposits to break open.

Although tuberculosis can be spread by the placenta to the fetus, it usually is spread to the infant after birth. A woman with a recent history of tuberculosis should have three negative sputum cultures before she holds or cares for her infant. If these are negative, there is no need to isolate the infant from the mother; she can even breastfeed. If active tuberculosis is in the home, the infant is generally discharged on prophylactic INH to prevent infection, with follow-up skin testing at 3-month intervals. If the infant is to be placed on INH, a mother also taking INH should not breastfeed (or the infant's dosage should be reduced). Otherwise, the combined dosage the infant receives (INH is found in breast milk) could be toxic to the infant.

A Woman with Chronic Obstructive Pulmonary Disease

COPD is constriction of the airway associated most often with long-term cigarette smoking. When women had their children between 20 and 30 years of age, COPD was rarely associated with pregnancy. Now that more and more women are waiting until age 35 to 40 to have children, the condition can be seen with pregnancy. Constrictive air disease limits the amount of oxygen that can reach the lungs so women may need additional rest because of fatigue and continuous supplemental oxygen for oxygen want. Some women have such severe symptoms while nonpregnant that they will be advised to avoid pregnancy (Wexler et al., 2007).

A Woman With Cystic Fibrosis

Cystic fibrosis is a recessively inherited disease in which there is generalized dysfunction of the exocrine glands (Uppalapati & Landry, 2007). This dysfunction leads to mucous secretions, particularly in the pancreas and lungs, becoming so viscid or thick that normal lung and pancreatic function is compromised.

Many men with cystic fibrosis are sterile because their semen is so thick that sperm cannot be motile. Fertility may be lessened in women with the disorder because sperm cannot migrate through viscid cervical mucus. This can make conception a concern. Reproductive technologies such as artificial insemination or in vitro fertilization may be necessary for conception so sperm are not obstructed by cervical mucus or fallopian tubal transport is not impaired.

Persons with the disease typically develop symptoms of chronic respiratory infection and overinflation of their lungs from the thickened mucus as well as an inability to digest fat and protein because the pancreas cannot release amylase. Because of poor pulmonary function that results in inadequate oxygen supply to the fetus, there is an increased risk for preterm labor and perinatal death during pregnancy. The presence of cystic fibrosis in the fetus may be identified by chorionic villi sampling or amniocentesis and identification of the abnormal gene on chromosome 7 during pregnancy or immediately after birth. Screening for the disorder is included in routine neonatal screening programs after birth.

Therapy for the illness consists of pancrelipase (Pancrease) to supplement pancreatic enzymes. Caution women to continue to take this even with nausea of early pregnancy. Although pancrelipase is a pregnancy risk category C drug (teratogenic effects are unknown), it does not appear to affect the fetus. Women are often also prescribed a bronchodilator or antibiotic to reduce pulmonary symptoms. In addition to pharmacologic measures, women with cystic fibrosis must perform chest physiotherapy daily to reduce the buildup of lung secretions. As women with the disorder excrete a higher level of sodium in persperation than others, they need to be carefully monitored during labor to be certain that they do not become dehydrated. Although pregnancy is a strain on an already stressed respiratory system, pregnancy does not appear to shorten the life span of women with the disorder.

Modifications for Pregnancy

Because pancrelipase may interfere with iron absorption, a woman is at greater risk for iron-deficiency anemia during pregnancy than other women. Therefore, an iron supplement usually is prescribed. Persons with cystic fibrosis have a higher-than-usual incidence of developing diabetes mellitus because of pancreas involvement; therefore, women need close monitoring of serum glucose levels at prenatal visits to detect the development of gestational diabetes.

Chest physiotherapy becomes difficult late in pregnancy because the process is exhausting. Moving to new positions is difficult, and lying prone, a position used frequently in postural drainage, is contraindicated in late pregnancy. A woman may need to plan more frequent and shorter sessions in modified positions (other than prone) to prevent exhaustion (Fig. 20.2). Fetal health will be monitored by ultrasound and nonstress tests to identify intrauterine growth restriction.

Modifications for the Postpartum Period

Help a woman plan how to conserve her energy for infant care in the immediate postpartum period so she does not become exhausted and can enjoy her newborn. The milk of a nursing mother with cystic fibrosis is high in sodium, and potentially places the infant at risk for hypernatremia, so

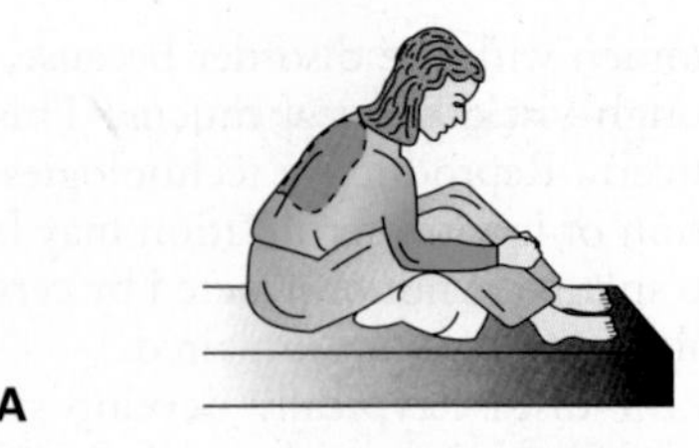

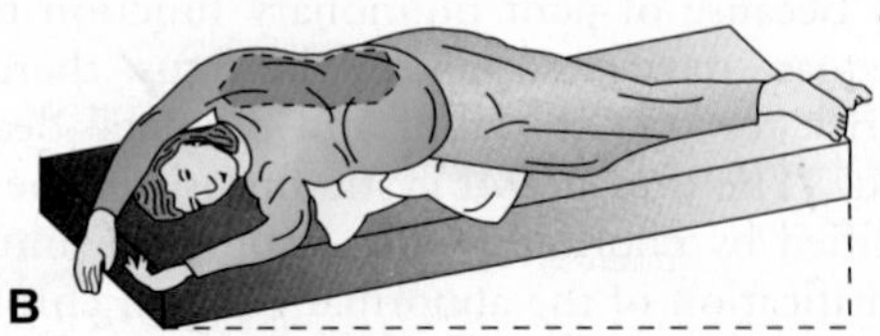

FIGURE 20.2 Modified positions for chest physiotherapy during pregnancy: (**A**) chest physiotherapy for the upper lobes; (**B**) chest physiotherapy for the lower lobes.

women with cystic fibrosis are usually advised not to breastfeed (Lipscomb & Novy, 2007). Breastfeeding could also be more tiring for the mother.

✔Checkpoint Question 20.3

Suppose Angelina Gomez had tuberculosis as a teenager. What is a danger of this during pregnancy?

a. Calcium deposits that wall off old tuberculosis lesions can break down.
b. Tuberculosis can turn to pneumonia if a woman has a folic acid deficit.
c. PPD tests are always negative during pregnancy so TB goes undetected.
d. If tuberculosis spreads to the stomach, it can cause serious stomach ulcers.

RHEUMATIC DISORDERS AND PREGNANCY

Several rheumatic disorders occur in young adult women and so are seen during pregnancy. Because most of these illnesses result in discomfort, potential or actual pain related to disease pathology is the primary nursing diagnosis used. Women may not achieve a pain-free outcome during pregnancy because of the nature of these illnesses, but outcomes should center on a woman stating that her pain level is tolerable.

Nursing Diagnoses and Related Interventions

*

Nursing Diagnosis: Pain related to rheumatic disorder during pregnancy

Outcome Evaluation: Client states she is moderately comfortable and able to maintain her usual level of daily activity.

A Woman With Rheumatoid Arthritis

Juvenile rheumatoid arthritis (sometimes referred to as chronic rheumatoid arthritis), a disease of connective tissue with joint inflammation and contracture, is most likely the result of an autoimmune response (Golding, Haque, & Giles, 2007). The disease pathology involves synovial membrane destruction. Inflammation with effusion, swelling, erythema, and painful motion of the joints occurs. Over time, formation of granulation tissue can fill the joint space, resulting in permanent disfigurement and loss of joint motion.

Women with juvenile rheumatoid arthritis frequently take corticosteroids and nonsteroidal anti-inflammatory drugs (NSAIDs) to prevent joint pain and loss of mobility. Some women may be taking oral aspirin therapy. Although they should continue to take these medications during pregnancy to prevent joint damage, large amounts of salicylates may lead to increased bleeding at birth or prolonged pregnancy (salicylate interferes with prostaglandin synthesis, so labor contractions are not initiated) (Karch, 2009). The infant may be born with a bleeding defect and may also experience premature closure of the ductus arteriosus because of the drug's effects. For this reason, a woman is asked to decrease her intake of salicylates approximately 2 weeks before term. A few women may be taking low-dose methotrexate, a carcinogen (pregnancy risk category X). They should consult their health care practitioner before becoming pregnant about the advisability of continuing this drug during pregnancy.

Symptoms of the disease may improve during pregnancy because of the naturally increased circulating level of corticosteroids in the maternal bloodstream during pregnancy. During the postpartum period, when a woman's corticosteroid levels fall to prepregnancy levels again, arthritis symptoms will probably recur.

In the postpartum period, the determination as to the safety of breastfeeding must be individualized based on the medication that each woman is taking. Those taking an NSAID such as ibuprofen can breastfeed. Those taking large doses of aspirin may be advised not to breastfeed because of the danger of increased bleeding in the infant.

A Woman With Systemic Lupus Erythematosus

Systemic lupus erythematosus (SLE) is a multisystem chronic disease of connective tissue that can occur in women of childbearing age: its highest incidence is in women aged 20 to 40 years (Petri, 2007). It affects about 1 in every 2000 to 3000 pregnancies. Widespread degeneration of connective tissue (especially of the heart, kidneys, blood vessels, spleen, skin, and retroperitoneal tissue) occurs with onset of the illness. The most marked skin change is a characteristic erythematous butterfly-shaped rash on the face. In the kidneys, fibrin deposits develop, plugging and blocking the glomeruli and leading to necrosis and scarring. The thickening of collagen tissue in the blood vessels causes vessel obstruction. This can be life-threatening to a woman if blood flow to vital organs becomes compromised and life-threatening to a fetus if blood flow to the placenta is obstructed. Many women with SLE have antiphospholipid antibodies, which increase the tendency for thrombi to form (Mavragani et al., 2007). In contrast, marked thrombocytopenia (decreased platelet count) is present, so clotting may be deficient. A woman may be taking a corticosteroid, NSAIDs, heparin, and salicylates to reduce disease symptoms.

The naturally increased circulation of corticosteroids during pregnancy may lessen symptoms in some women. In others, the chief complication of the disorder—acute nephritis with glomerular destruction—may occur for the first time during pregnancy.

With associated nephritis, a woman's blood pressure will rise. She will develop hematuria and decreased urine output. Proteinuria and edema may begin. It is difficult to differentiate these symptoms from the symptoms of pregnancy-induced hypertension, except that with pregnancy-induced hypertension there is no hematuria. Frequent monitoring of serum creatinine levels is necessary to assess kidney function. If this value is over 1.5 mg/dL and proteinuria and a decreased creatinine clearance value are also present, the fetus is seriously threatened. Dialysis to remove excess creatinine or plasmapheresis to replace platelets may be necessary to guard against hemorrhage at birth.

Women are asked to decrease salicylate use about 2 weeks prior to their anticipated birth to reduce the possibility of bleeding in the newborn. Intravenous hydrocortisone may be administered during labor to help a woman adjust to the stress at this time. During the postpartum period, there may be an acute exacerbation of symptoms in a woman as corticosteroid levels again fall to normal. Infants of women with SLE tend to be small for gestational age because of a decreased blood flow to the placenta. There is a greater-than-usual incidence of spontaneous miscarriage and preterm birth (Witter, 2007). Infants may be born with a lupus-like rash, anemia, thrombocytopenia (low platelet count), and neonatal heart block. Newborn symptoms last about 6 months and then fade. If congenital heart block occurs, a newborn pacemaker may be necessary. Screening for the exact type of autoantibodies present may be helpful in predicting which newborns are susceptible to this.

✔ Checkpoint Question 20.4

Suppose Angelina Gomez routinely takes acetylsalicylic acid (aspirin) for sinus headaches. Why should she limit or discontinue this toward the end of pregnancy?

a. Salicylates can lead to increased maternal bleeding at childbirth.
b. Newborns develop withdrawal headaches from salicylates.
c. Aspirin can lead to deep vein thrombosis following birth.
d. Newborns develop a red rash from salicylate toxicity.

GASTROINTESTINAL DISORDERS AND PREGNANCY

Although minor gastrointestinal discomforts (such as nausea, heartburn, constipation) are common during pregnancy, acute abdominal pain and protracted vomiting are causes for concern. Pregnancy complications such as premature separation of the placenta or ectopic pregnancy often manifest with acute abdominal pain, so differentiating the cause of abdominal pain is important. In other instances, abdominal pain is associated with a condition completely unrelated to the pregnancy such as ulcerative colitis, hepatitis, hiatal hernia, or cholecystitis. These conditions may be known to a woman before she becomes pregnant, or they may develop or be discovered during her pregnancy. Women who have colostomies can complete pregnancy without difficulty. Even a previous liver transplant is not a contraindication to pregnancy (Pan et al., 2007).

Nursing Diagnoses and Related Interventions

Nursing Diagnosis: Imbalanced nutrition, less than body requirements, related to a gastrointestinal disorder during pregnancy

Outcome Evaluation: Client's weight gain amounts to 25 to 30 lb during pregnancy; hemoglobin is above 11 mg/dL; specific gravity of urine is below 1.030.

A Woman With Appendicitis

Appendicitis is inflammation of the appendix. Its incidence is high in young adults so occurs as frequently as 1 in 1500 to 2000 pregnancies (Parangi et al., 2007).

Assessment

History taking is important. Appendicitis usually begins with a few hours of nausea, and then an hour or two of generalized abdominal discomfort. A woman may have vomiting during this time. Then comes the typical sharp, peristaltic, lower right quadrant pain of acute appendicitis.

The pain associated with appendicitis is different from the pain that occurs suddenly from an overstretched round ligament during pregnancy. Pain from an overstretched ligament may cause sharp lower quadrant pain if a woman stands up suddenly, but the pain fades again almost instantly. Appendicitis pain not only continues but grows more intense. Appendicitis pain is also different from that of ectopic pregnancy. With ectopic pregnancy, a woman may have morning sickness because she is pregnant; the nausea and vomiting of appendicitis is much more intense. The pain of ectopic pregnancy may be either diffuse or sharp. In the nonpregnant woman, the pain of appendicitis becomes sharp and localized at McBurney's point (a point halfway between the umbilicus and the iliac crest on the lower right abdomen). In the pregnant woman, the appendix is often displaced so far up in the abdomen that the localized pain may resemble the pain of gallbladder disease (Fig. 20.3). A complete blood count will reveal leukocytosis. However, because pregnant women have an elevated white blood cell count anyway, this finding is not as helpful in pregnancy as it might be otherwise. A woman's temperature may be elevated. There are typically ketones in the urine. An ultrasound will reveal the inflamed appendix.

Advise a woman not to take food, liquid, or laxatives while she is waiting to be evaluated for possible appendicitis, because increasing peristalsis could cause an inflamed appendix to rupture.

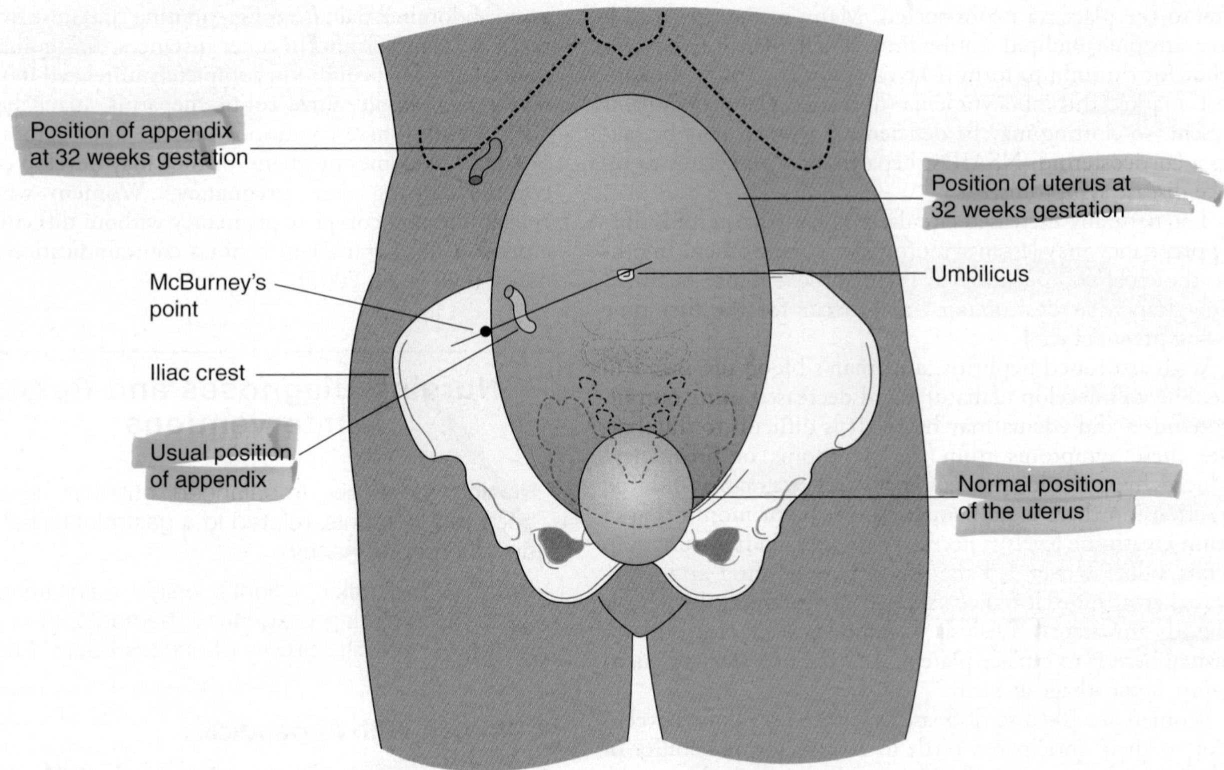

FIGURE 20.3 Change in position of appendix during pregnancy.

Therapeutic Management

If a woman is near term (past 36 weeks) and the fetus is believed to be mature, a cesarean birth may be done to birth the baby and then remove the inflamed appendix at the same time. If appendicitis occurs early in pregnancy, the inflamed appendix is removed by laparoscopy. As long as the anesthesiologist is aware that a woman is pregnant and carefully controls oxygen levels during anesthesia administration, the outcome of both the surgery and the pregnancy will be good.

If the appendix ruptures before surgery, the risk to both mother and fetus increases dramatically. This is because with rupture, infected fecal material escapes into the peritoneum and could spread by the fallopian tubes to the fetus. Also generalized peritonitis is such an overwhelming infection that it is difficult for a woman's body to combat it effectively and also maintain the pregnancy. As a third concern, peritoneal adhesions may develop after an appendix ruptures, resulting in future subfertility because of changes in the placement of fallopian tubes.

A Woman With Gastroesophageal Reflux Disease or Hiatal Hernia

Gastroesophageal reflux disease (GERD) refers to the reflux of acid stomach secretions into the esophagus. Hiatal hernia is a condition in which a portion of the stomach extends and protrudes up through the diaphragm into the chest cavity, trapping stomach acid and causing it to reflux into the esophagus. Although these conditions can be present constantly, symptoms most often occur only sporadically after increased peristaltic action. Both conditions may generate symptoms for the first time during pregnancy as the uterus pushes the stomach up against the esophageal valve and increases the reflux of acid or the extent of the hernia. Symptoms include:

- Heartburn, which is particularly extreme when lying supine after a full meal
- Gastric regurgitation
- Dysphagia (difficulty swallowing)
- Possible weight loss because of the inability to eat
- Hematemesis (vomiting of blood) if extreme esophageal irritation occurs from the reflux of hydrochloric acid from the stomach

During pregnancy, these conditions are usually diagnosed by direct endoscopy or ultrasound to avoid exposing a woman to barium x-rays. In most women, antacids will relieve pain. A histamine receptor antagonist, such as ranitidine, can be prescribed to inhibit gastric acid production and help minimize pain. Proton pump inhibitors such as esomeprazole magnesium (Nexium) are also safe during pregnancy (pregnancy category B) (Subramanian et al., 2008). Advise a woman to wear loose clothing and sleep with her head elevated to help confine stomach secretions. After pregnancy, as the uterine pressure is decreased, the symptoms generally become less noticeable or disappear. Some women may need to continue to take esomeprazole magnesium for several months until their esophagus is completely healed.

A Woman With Cholecystitis and Cholelithiasis

Cholecystitis (gallbladder inflammation) and cholelithiasis (gallstone formation) are most frequently associated with women older than 40 years, obesity, multiparity, and ingestion of a high-fat diet. Symptoms (constant aching and pressure in the right epigastrium, perhaps accompanied by jaundice), therefore, are more apt to occur in the older pregnant woman. Gallstones are formed from cholesterol. It is debated whether the hypercholesterolemia that naturally occurs during pregnancy leads to an increased incidence of cholecystitis or cholelithiasis, but both these conditions are seen with pregnancy.

Medical therapy for both conditions is to lower fat intake. A woman should eat a low-fat but not a fat-free diet during pregnancy because of the importance of linoleic acid for fetal growth. Cholecystitis can be diagnosed by ultrasound. If an acute episode occurs during pregnancy, it can generally be managed by halting oral intake to rest the gastrointestinal tract, administering intravenous fluids to provide fluid and nutrients as well as analgesics for pain. Surgery for gallbladder removal by laparoscopic technique may be done during pregnancy if a woman's symptoms cannot be controlled by conservative management (Augustin & Majerovic, 2007).

A Woman With Pancreatitis

Pancreatitis, inflammation of the pancreas, tends to occur in young adults and so is also seen during pregnancy (Parangi et al., 2007). Diagnosis may be difficult as serum amylase, which rises with pancreatitis, is also normally elevated during pregnancy. Only if this is greater than 2 times above normal is pancreatitis suspected. Pancreatitis is treated the same in pregnancy as in nonpregnant women: nasogastric suction, bowel rest, analgesia (pancreatic pain is sharp), and intravenous hydration through parenteral nutritional supplementation. Pancreatic inflammation usually subsides within a week. Pregnancy loss can occur from acidosis, hypovolemia, and fetal hypoxia.

A Woman With Hepatitis

Hepatitis is a liver disease that may occur from invasion of the A, B, C, D, or E virus. Hepatitis A is spread mainly by fecal–oral contact (children in day-care settings have a high incidence) or by ingestion of fecally contaminated water or shellfish. It has an incubation period of 2 to 6 weeks. Pregnant women exposed to hepatitis A may be given prophylactic gamma globulin to try to prevent the disease after exposure. This form follows a rather benign course and is not known to be transmitted to the fetus.

Hepatitis B and C are spread by exposure to contaminated blood or blood products. These two types also can be spread by contact with contaminated semen or vaginal secretions and so are considered STIs. Maternal/fetal transmission is now one of the most important modes of transmission. Hepatitis D and E are apparently spread by the same methods as hepatitis B but are rarely seen in pregnant women.

Hepatitis C demonstrates few symptoms, and these may not be present for 12 months after exposure. It is, however, the most common cause of chronic liver disease and liver transplantation in the United States (Jain et al., 2007).

Hepatitis B occurs about 1 in every 2000 pregnancies (Johnson & Ross, 2007). It has an incubation period of 6 weeks to 6 months. It occurs in both an acute and chronic form, leading to liver cell necrosis with scarring and inability to convert indirect to direct bilirubin or excrete direct bilirubin. Women exposed to the virus receive immune globulin for prophylaxis; hepatitis B vaccine may be administered to those who are at high risk, such as women who handle blood products to prevent the illness.

Assessment

With all forms of hepatitis, a woman experiences nausea and vomiting. Her liver area may feel tender to palpation. Urine will be dark yellow from excretion of bilirubin; stools will be light-colored from lack of bilirubin. Jaundice occurs as a late symptom. On physical examination, hepatomegaly (enlargement of the liver) is noted. The bilirubin level is elevated. Levels of liver enzymes such as transaminase are increased. Specific antibodies against the virus can be detected in the blood serum, so women at high risk may be routinely screened for this during pregnancy. If a liver biopsy is necessary for diagnosis, this can be performed safely during pregnancy.

Therapeutic Management

A woman is usually prescribed bed rest and encouraged to eat a high-calorie diet because her liver has difficulty converting stored glycogen into glucose in its diseased state so hypoglycemia could result. Cesarean birth may be planned to reduce the possibility of blood exchange between mother and fetus. Follow standard infection precautions when you give care to avoid contact with body fluids.

Hepatitis during pregnancy may lead to spontaneous miscarriage or preterm labor. Unlike other diseases, the later in pregnancy the mother contracts hepatitis B infection, the greater the risk the infant will be affected or develop hepatitis B. When this occurs, it is a serious consequence because a proportion of HB Ag-positive infants will develop liver cirrhosis or carcinoma later in life (Johnson & Ross, 2007). If the mother has anti-HB antibodies present (antibodies toward a virus subgroup), the incidence of this appears to be less. After birth, the infant should be washed well to remove any maternal blood, and hepatitis B immune globulin (HBIG) and immunization against hepatitis B should be administered (see Chapter 18 for additional newborn care). A mother may breastfeed. The infant needs to be observed carefully for symptoms of infection during the first few months of life and chronic liver disease as he or she grows older.

A Woman With Inflammatory Bowel Disease

Crohn's disease (inflammation of the terminal ileus) and ulcerative colitis (inflammation of the distal colon) occur most often in young adults between ages 12 and 30 years (childbearing years) and so are seen in pregnancy. The cause of these diseases is unknown, but an autoimmune process is thought to be responsible. They are associated with passive and active smoking (Mahid et al., 2007). In both diseases, the bowel develops shallow ulcers. A woman experiences chronic diarrhea, weight loss, occult blood in stool, and nausea and vomiting. If extreme, obstruction and fistula formation with peritonitis can occur. With Crohn's disease, malabsorption, particularly of vitamin B (a substance whose absorption occurs almost entirely in the ileum), occurs. Because of the potential difficulty with absorbing nutrients, women with both disorders need careful monitoring for weight gain during pregnancy (Bortoli et al., 2007).

These diseases obviously have the potential for interfering with fetal growth if extreme malabsorption occurs. Therapy for the disorders is total rest for the gastrointestinal tract by administration of total parenteral nutrition. Although it is possible to sustain a pregnancy by this route, it is obviously not a desirable nutrition pattern. Sulfasalazine (Azulfidine), an anti-inflammatory and a mainstay of therapy, may be continued during pregnancy without fetal injury. Close to birth, the dosage of sulfasalazine, because of its sulfa base, is reduced because it may interfere with bilirubin binding sites and cause neonatal jaundice (Karch, 2009).

NEUROLOGIC DISORDERS AND PREGNANCY

Neurologic illness, as a whole, does not occur at a high incidence in women of childbearing age. However, any neurologic disease with symptoms of seizures must be carefully managed during pregnancy because the anoxia that could be caused by severe seizures could deprive a fetus of oxygen.

Nursing Diagnoses and Related Interventions

Nursing Diagnosis: Risk for injury (maternal) related to recurrent seizures

Outcome Evaluation: Client states she is seizure free, with no signs and symptoms of injury; no automobile or other accidents are documented.

A Woman With a Seizure Disorder

Recurrent seizures have several causes, such as head trauma or meningitis. The causes of most recurrent seizures, however, are unknown (idiopathic).

Recurrent seizures were at one time so incapacitating and it was believed that seizure control medications caused such a high risk of congenital anomaly that women with seizures were advised not to have children. Today, however, no contraindication to pregnancy exists for women with seizures as long as the medication they take is at the lowest dose possible and serum levels are carefully monitored.

Therapeutic Management

Because seizure medications as a group are mildly teratogenic, women with recurrent seizures need to meet with their obstetrician and primary care provider before pregnancy to be certain the medications they are taking are the least teratogenic ones possible and the dosage they are taking is the lowest possible to control seizures (Adab et al., 2009). In the early months of pregnancy, you may need to remind women to continue to take their antiseizure medications despite the nausea or vomiting of early pregnancy. Be certain they understand that the rule "Do not take medication during pregnancy" does not apply to their antiseizure medications. Recurrent seizures put a woman into the difficult position of having to take a drug to safeguard her own health, but by taking them may not be safeguarding the health of her fetus. The risk of adverse maternal or fetal outcome from seizures during pregnancy, however, is greater than the risk of teratogenicity from taking anticonvulsant drugs (Karch, 2009).

All women should have an evaluation of serum drug levels before pregnancy or early in pregnancy to establish that their medication is being prescribed at a therapeutic level (Adab et al., 2009). As blood volume increases with pregnancy, some women may need their dosage increased or their serum level will be diluted. Common drugs prescribed to control seizures are:

- Trimethadione (Tridione) (pregnancy risk category D)
- Valproic acid (sodium valproate and divalproex sodium) (pregnancy risk category D)
- Carbamazepine (Tegretol) (pregnancy risk category C)
- Ethosuximide (Zarontin), a drug often used to control absence seizures (pregnancy risk category C)
- Phenytoin sodium (Dilantin) (pregnancy risk category D). Dilantin can cause a syndrome involving fetal cognitive impairment and a peculiar facial proportion not unlike that of fetal alcohol syndrome. This may occur because of competition for folic acid binding sites. Some infants have an increased danger of neural tube disorders as a result of this folic acid displacement. An ultrasound can rule out the possibility of this.

Infants are also prone to hemorrhagic disease of the newborn because of decreased levels of vitamin K coagulation factors at birth from phenytoin. To counteract this, women may be prescribed vitamin K during labor or the last 4 weeks of gestation. Women who have been taking phenytoin (Dilantin) may have developed chronic hypertension. For these women, a baseline blood pressure should be established early in pregnancy so that changes can be interpreted correctly.

Nursing Diagnoses and Related Interventions

Nursing Diagnosis: Risk for ineffective tissue (placental) perfusion related to hypoxia resulting from maternal seizure

Outcome Evaluation: Client informs health care personnel about history of seizures; states importance of immediate care and oxygen therapy should she begin a seizure. Apgar score of infant is 7 to 10, with no apparent birth anomalies.

Absence seizures (often just a rapid fluttering of the eyelids or a moment's staring into space) should have no effect on a woman or fetus. Tonic-clonic seizures (sustained, full-body involvement) could affect a fetus because spasm of the chest muscles could lead to hypoxia. If a seizure should occur, a woman must be evaluated to ascertain that the cause of the seizure was the underlying disease, not beginning hypertension of pregnancy. Nonpregnant women experiencing tonic-clonic seizures do not need oxygen during a seizure, but in pregnancy, administering oxygen by mask is good prophylaxis to ensure adequate fetal oxygenation.

Urge a woman to alert hospital personnel at the time of labor that she has recurrent seizures and to report the type of medication she is taking. She should continue to take the medication during labor. If a general anesthetic should be necessary, the anesthesiologist needs to know about her condition before administering anesthesia; otherwise, during the excitement phase of anesthesia induction, a seizure could occur.

Nursing Diagnosis: Risk for impaired parenting related to maternal low self-esteem

Outcome Evaluation: Client accurately states the nature of her disorder (acquired or idiopathic) and the statistical chances of her child inheriting the disorder. After her child is born, client identifies sudden jerking movements in her newborn (such as Moro reflex) as healthy newborn characteristics.

A woman who has recurrent seizures may worry that her child will develop seizures as the child grows older. If a woman's seizures are the result of an acquired disorder such as meningitis or head trauma, a woman can be assured that her child's risk for seizures is no greater than that for any other child. If the etiology of her seizures is unknown, the chance that her child also will have them is slightly higher than in the normal population. This prediction is only theoretical, however, and cannot be made without a thorough review of the onset and nature of a woman's disorder. Be certain a woman has her newborn with her for long periods so she can become acquainted with the sudden jerking motions that occur such as when a newborn is startled (Moro reflex) or quivering of the jaw with prolonged crying. Otherwise she could interpret these normal movements as seizure activity.

A Woman With Myasthenia Gravis

Myasthenia gravis is an autoimmune disorder characterized by the presence of an IgG antibody against acetylcholine receptors in striated muscle. This causes failure of the striated muscles to contract, particularly those of the oropharyngeal, facial, and extraocular groups (Kalidindi et al., 2007).

Myasthenia gravis is treated with anticholinesterase drugs such as pyridostigmine (Mestinon) or neostigmine (Prostigmin) and possibly a corticosteroid such as prednisone. These medications may be continued during pregnancy, as the fetus will experience no effects from these drugs. Plasmapheresis (removal of and replacement of plasma) to remove immune complexes from the bloodstream may be prescribed to reduce symptoms. Plasmapheresis must be carried out gradually during pregnancy to reduce the risk of fluid overload or hypotension. Because smooth muscle is not affected by the disease, labor should occur normally. Magnesium sulfate should be avoided because it can diminish the acetylcholine effect and therefore increase disease symptoms.

An infant born to a woman with myasthenia gravis may demonstrate disease symptoms at birth because of the transfer of antibodies. This is further discussed in Chapter 51.

A Woman With Multiple Sclerosis

Multiple sclerosis (MS) occurs predominantly in women of childbearing age, usually between 20 and 40 years of age (Saraste et al., 2007). With MS, nerve fibers become demyelinated and therefore lose function. Women develop symptoms of fatigue, numbness, blurred vision, and loss of coordination. ACTH or a corticosteroid is commonly given to strengthen nerve conduction. These both can be administered safely during pregnancy. In contrast, cyclosporine (Sandimmune), azathioprine (Imuran), and cyclophosphamide (Cytoxan), drugs also frequently administered, are not safe for use during pregnancy. The pregnancy safety of interferon has not been tested; as such, it is classified as a pregnancy category C drug. Women may continue with plasmapheresis (withdrawal and replacement of plasma), another treatment regimen, during pregnancy as long as the volume of exchange is well controlled. Although women with the disorder may grow increasingly fatigued as pregnancy progresses, pregnancy does not affect the long-term course of MS. MS may actually improve with pregnancy because of the increased circulating corticosteroid levels. UTIs tend to occur as a poorly defined consequence of the illness.

MUSCULOSKELETAL DISORDERS AND PREGNANCY

Women of childbearing age have falls or other accidents that lead to bone fractures or muscle sprains. These are discussed in Chapter 22. A chronic musculoskeletal disorder that may be seen with pregnancy is scoliosis.

A Woman With Scoliosis

Scoliosis (lateral curvature of the spine) begins to be noticed first in girls between 12 and 14 years of age. If it is uncorrected at this time, the curvature progresses until it causes deformity, interfering with respiration and heart action because of chest compression. Pelvic distortion can interfere with childbirth, especially at the pelvic inlet. If a woman's spine is extremely curved, spinal or epidural anesthesia may be difficult to administer for pain management in labor.

Girls with scoliosis may wear a body brace during their adolescent years to maintain an erect posture. Although these braces are not as bulky as they once were, unless they are modified, they cannot be worn during the last half of pregnancy. Other girls have stainless-steel rods surgically implanted on both sides of their vertebrae to strengthen and straighten their spine. Such rod implantations do not interfere with pregnancy; a woman will notice some back pain from tension on the back muscles similar to that experienced by the average pregnant woman. If a woman's pelvis is distorted, a cesarean birth may be necessary to ensure a safe birth. Vaginal birth, if permitted, requires the same management as for any woman. Plot the course of labor on a labor graph so an unusually long first stage, suggesting cephalopelvic disproportion, can be recognized. Chapter 51 discusses in detail the nursing care of adolescents with scoliosis.

ENDOCRINE DISORDERS AND PREGNANCY

Endocrine disorders have the potential to be serious complications of pregnancy because enzymes or hormones control so many specific body functions.

A Woman With a Thyroid Dysfunction

As a normal effect of pregnancy, the thyroid gland enlarges (hypertrophies) slightly because of increased vascularity and blood flow. A woman with pre-existing thyroid problems may have difficulty making this pregnancy transition.

Nursing Diagnoses and Related Interventions

Nursing Diagnosis: Risk for maternal and fetal injury related to pre-existing thyroid disorder during pregnancy

Outcome Evaluation: No congenital anomalies are present in infant at birth; Apgar score is 7 to 10. Mother can continue prepregnancy level of activities.

A Woman With Hypothyroidism

Hypothyroidism is a rare condition in young adults and especially in pregnancy, because women with symptoms of untreated hypothyroidism are often anovulatory and unable to conceive. A woman who does conceive can have difficulty increasing thyroid functioning to a necessary pregnancy level. This can lead to early spontaneous miscarriage. Women with hypothyroidism fatigue easily and tend to be obese; their skin is dry (myxedema), and they have little tolerance for cold. It may be associated with an increased incidence of extreme nausea and vomiting (hyperemesis gravidarum).

Most women with hypothyroidism take levothyroxine (Synthroid) to supplement their lack of thyroid hormone. A woman who is taking levothyroxine needs to consult with her obstetrician and internist when she is planning on becoming pregnant. She needs to come for early diagnosis and close follow-up as soon as she suspects she is pregnant (1 week past her missed menstrual period). As a rule, her dose of levothyroxine will need to be increased as much as 20% to 30% for the duration of the pregnancy to simulate the increase that would normally occur in pregnancy (Neto et al., 2007). Be certain that a woman realizes the importance of taking this increased dose. Women should separate thyroxine ingestion from any medication containing iron, calcium, or soy products by about 4 hours to be sure that there is no problem with the absorption of thyroxine (Kyriazopoulou et al., 2008).

After the pregnancy, the dose of levothyroxine prescribed for pregnancy must be gradually tapered back to the prepregnancy level. Be certain a woman does not continue to take her pregnancy dose (trying to be economical and use up her higher-dose pills), or she could pass beyond normal thyroid function and develop hyperthyroidism.

A Woman With Hyperthyroidism

Hyperthyroidism, or overproduction of thyroid hormone, causes symptoms such as:

- Rapid heart rate
- Exophthalmos (protruding eyeballs)
- Heat intolerance
- Nervousness
- Heart palpitations
- Weight loss

Hyperthyroidism (Graves' disease) is more apt to be seen in pregnancy than hypothyroidism. If undiagnosed, a woman may develop heart failure during pregnancy because her heart rate, already high at the beginning of pregnancy, cannot increase enough to handle the increasing blood volume that occurs with pregnancy. She is more prone to symptoms of hypertension of pregnancy, fetal growth restriction, and preterm labor than the average woman.

Hyperthyroidism is normally diagnosed by a nuclear medicine imaging study involving the radioactive uptake of ^{131}I subtype. This diagnostic procedure should not be used during pregnancy because the fetal thyroid will also incorporate this drug, possibly resulting in destruction of the fetal thyroid.

Treatment for hyperthyroidism is with thioamides (methimazole [Tapazole] or propylthiouracil [PTU]), which reduce thyroid activity. These drugs are, unfortunately, teratogens. They cross the placenta and can lead to congenital hypothyroidism and consequently an enlarged thyroid gland (a goiter) in the fetus. If this abnormal neck growth enlarges enough, it can obstruct the airway and make resuscitation difficult for the infant at birth. Methimazole is the preferred drug for pregnant women as it appears to cross the placenta less easily (Chattaway & Klepser, 2007).

If hyperthyroidism is not regulated during pregnancy, an infant may be born with symptoms of hyperthyroidism because of the excess stimulation he or she receives in utero. The infant may appear jittery, and tachypnea and tachycardia may be present. An assay of fetal cord blood will reveal the level of T_4 and thyroid-stimulating hormone and the need for therapy in the infant. Women receiving smaller or minimal doses of antithyroid drugs may breastfeed, although women receiving large doses of these drugs may be advised not to breastfeed because these drugs are excreted in breast milk (Greenspan & Dong, 2007).

A woman should be regulated on the lowest possible dose of drug and cautioned to keep a careful record of doses taken so she does not forget or accidentally duplicate a dose. Surgical treatment to reduce the functioning of the maternal thyroid gland can be accomplished, but this is generally not the treatment of choice during pregnancy because of the need for general anesthesia. After a pregnancy, if a woman desires other children, the procedure might be suggested as an interpregnancy procedure so she does not enter a second pregnancy hyperthyroid.

A Woman With Diabetes Mellitus

Diabetes mellitus is an endocrine disorder in which the pancreas cannot produce adequate insulin to regulate body glucose levels. The disorder affects 3% to 5% of all pregnancies and is the most frequently seen medical condition in pregnancy (Strehlow et al., 2007). Before insulin was produced synthetically in 1921, women with type 1 diabetes, or diabetes acquired in childhood, died before reaching childbearing age, were infertile, or had spontaneous miscarriages early in pregnancy. Now that diabetes can be well managed and type 2 diabetes is occurring more frequently in young adults, four new problems have developed:

- How to care for women with both type 1 and type 2 diabetes during pregnancy

- How to bring a woman with type 1, type 2, and gestational diabetes through a pregnancy with good glucose and insulin control
- How to protect an infant in utero from the adverse effects of the increased glucose levels
- How to care for the infant in the first 24 hours after birth until the infant's insulin-glucose regulatory mechanism stabilizes

Reproductive planning may be a fifth concern as women with diabetes may not be good candidates for oral contraceptives because progesterone interferes with insulin activity and therefore increases blood glucose levels. The estrogen in contraceptives also has the potential for increasing lipid and cholesterol levels and blood coagulation. Intrauterine devices have been associated with higher-than-usual rates of pelvic inflammatory disease; because women with diabetes have difficulty fighting infections, these are not usually advised either. Subcutaneous implanted or intramuscular injections of progestin may be good choices (see Chapter 6).

Pathophysiology and Clinical Manifestations

The possible etiology and pathology of diabetes mellitus are discussed in detail in Chapter 48. The primary problem of any woman with this disorder is controlling the balance between insulin and blood glucose levels to prevent hyperglycemia or hypoglycemia. Both of these conditions are dangerous during pregnancy because they can become threats to normal fetal growth. Infants of diabetic women are five times more apt to be born with heart anomalies than others because of this threat (Strehlow et al., 2007).

If a woman's insulin level is insufficient, glucose cannot be used by body cells. The cells register their glucose want, and the liver quickly converts stored glycogen to glucose to increase the serum glucose level. Because of the insulin insufficiency, however, the body cells still cannot use the glucose, so the serum glucose levels continue to rise (hyperglycemia). When the level of blood sugar rises to 150 mg/100 mL (normal is 80 to 120 mg/dL), the kidneys begin to excrete quantities of glucose in the urine **(glycosuria)** in an attempt to lower the level. During pregnancy, the point at which this happens may be even lower than 150 mg/100 mL. Because of osmotic action, the increased amount of glucose in the urine reduces fluid absorption in the kidney, and large quantities of fluid are lost in urine (polyuria).

Dehydration begins to occur; the blood serum becomes concentrated and the blood volume may fall. With the reduced blood flow, cells do not receive adequate oxygen, and anaerobic metabolic reactions cause large stores of lactic acid to pour out of muscles into the bloodstream. Fat is mobilized from fat stores and metabolized for energy, pouring large amounts of ketone bodies into the bloodstream. Ketone bodies are acidic (the best example is acetone). These two acid sources lower the pH of the blood, and a metabolic acidosis develops.

Next, protein stores are tapped by the body as it attempts to find a source of energy. Protein breakdown reduces the supply of protein to body cells. As cells die, they release potassium and sodium, and this is lost from the body in the extensive polyuria. Long-term effects of diabetes mellitus are vascular narrowing that leads to kidney, heart, and retinal dysfunction.

Diabetes During Pregnancy

Diabetes often occurs as type 1 or diabetes which occurs in childhood and represents failure of the pancreas to produce adequate insulin for body requirements. Although not proved, it probably represents an autoimmune disorder as marker antibodies are present (Masharani, 2009). Type 2 diabetes traditionally has occurred in older adults and represents gradual failure of insulin production that occurs with aging. The incidence of type 2 diabetes in adolescents has increased dramatically in the last decade related to obesity in adolescents, so now, both type 1 and type 2 diabetes are seen during pregnancy.

Even a woman with type 1 or type 2 diabetes who has successful regulation of glucose and insulin metabolism before pregnancy is apt to develop less-than-optimal control during pregnancy, because all women experience several changes in the glucose-insulin regulatory system as pregnancy progresses. Glomerular filtration of glucose is increased (the glomerular excretion threshold is lowered), causing slight glycosuria. The rate of insulin secretion is increased, and the fasting blood sugar level is lowered. All women appear to develop an insulin resistance as pregnancy progresses or insulin does not seem as effective during pregnancy, a phenomenon that is probably caused by the presence of the hormone human placental lactogen (chorionic somatomammotropin) and high levels of cortisol, estrogen, progesterone, and catecholamines. Placental insulinase may cause increased breakdown or degradation of insulin. This resistance to or destruction of insulin is helpful in a usual pregnancy because it prevents the blood glucose from falling to dangerous limits, despite the increased insulin secretion that occurs. It causes difficulty for a pregnant woman with diabetes in that she must increase her insulin dosage beginning at about week 24 of pregnancy to prevent hyperglycemia.

At the same time, the continued use of glucose by the fetus may lead to **hypoglycemia** (lowered serum glucose levels) for the mother between meals; this is most apt to occur overnight. A low maternal level of glucogenic amino acids (used by the liver to produce glucose) compounds this. A woman may become ketoacidotic from the breakdown of stored fat between meals, most likely during the second and third trimesters. An increase in the amount of amniotic fluid occurs in at least 25% of diabetic women, probably because of hyperglycemia in the fetus that causes increased urine production. If this becomes extreme, amniocentesis may need to be done to decrease the level of amniotic fluid. Unfortunately, this exposes a woman to infection and possible preterm labor and is only a temporary measure because amniotic fluid is continually produced. If a woman has preexisting kidney disease (revealed by proteinuria, decreased creatinine clearance, and hypertension), the risk of fetal growth restriction, asphyxia, stillbirth, and maternal pregnancy-induced hypertension rises markedly (Masharani, 2009).

When glucose regulation is poor, a woman is at greater risk for pregnancy-induced hypertension and infection (particularly monilial infection) than other women. Infants of women with poorly controlled diabetes tend to be large (>10 lb) because the increased insulin the fetus must produce to counteract the overload of glucose he or she receives acts as a growth stimulant (Campaigne & Conway, 2007). The increased glucose adds subcutaneous fat deposits.

Box 20.7 Assessment

Assessing a Pregnant Woman With Diabetes Mellitus

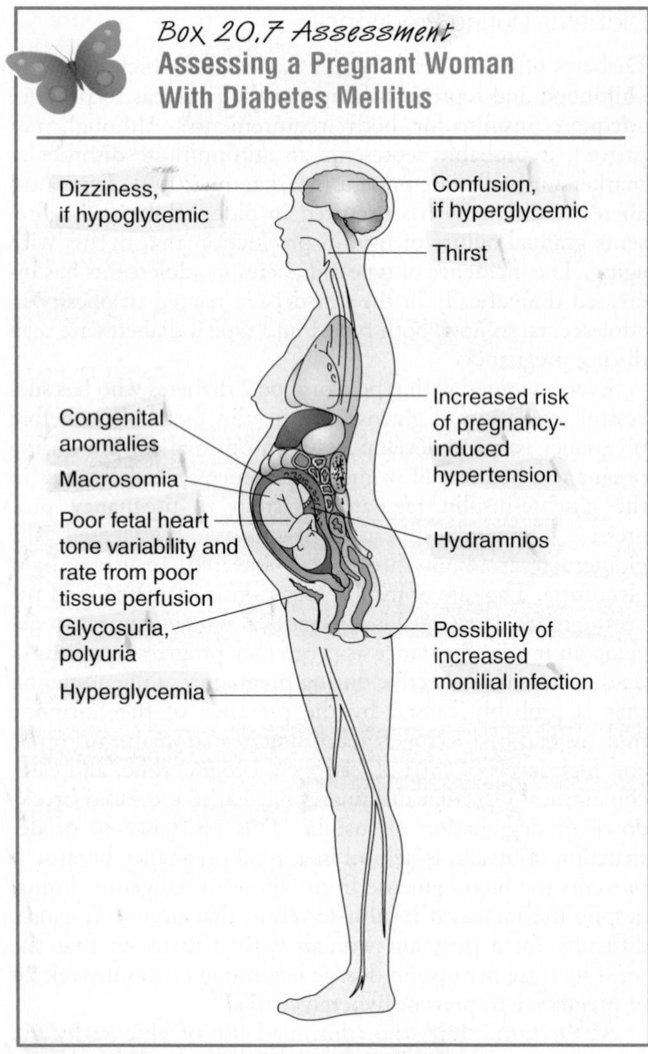

A macrosomic infant may create birth problems at the end of the pregnancy because of cephalopelvic disproportion. This, combined with an increased risk for shoulder dystocia, may make it necessary for infants of women with diabetes to be born by cesarean birth.

There is a high incidence of congenital anomaly, especially caudal regression syndrome (failure of the lower extremities to develop), spontaneous miscarriage, and stillbirth in infants of women with uncontrolled diabetes. At birth, the neonates are more prone to hypoglycemia, respiratory distress syndrome, hypocalcemia, and hyperbilirubinemia. The first trimester of pregnancy is the most important time for fetal development; if a woman can be kept from becoming hyperglycemic during this time, the chances of a congenital anomaly are greatly lessened (Box 20.7) (Barnes-Powell, 2007).

Classification of Diabetes Mellitus

Diabetes is divided into various categories that can be used to predict pregnancy outcome (Table 20.3).

Approximately 2% to 3% of all women who do not begin a pregnancy with diabetes become diabetic during pregnancy, usually at the midpoint of pregnancy when insulin resistance becomes most noticeable. This is termed gestational diabetes mellitus (Ferrara, 2007). The symptoms fade again at the completion of pregnancy, but the risk of developing type 2 diabetes later in life may be as high as 50% to 60% (Box 20.8). It is unknown whether gestational diabetes results from inadequate insulin response to carbohydrate or from excessive resistance to insulin; a combination of both may occur. Risk factors for gestational diabetes include:

- Obesity
- Age over 25 years
- History of large babies (10 lb or more)
- History of unexplained fetal or perinatal loss
- History of congenital anomalies in previous pregnancies
- History of polycystic ovary syndrome
- Family history of diabetes (one close relative or two distant ones)
- Member of a population with a high risk for diabetes (Native American, Hispanic, Asian)

Assessment

Because diabetes is such a serious complication in pregnancy, all women should be screened during pregnancy for gestational diabetes. A fasting plasma glucose of 126 mg/dl or above or a nonfasting plasma glucose of 200 mg/dl or above meets the threshold for the diagnosis of diabetes and needs to be confirmed on a subsequent day as soon as possible. This is usually done using a 50-g oral glucose challenge test.

After the oral 50-g glucose load is ingested, a venous blood sample is taken for glucose determination 60 minutes later. If the serum glucose level at 1 hour is more than 140 mg/dL, the woman is scheduled for a 100-g, 3-hour fasting **glucose tolerance test.** If two of the four blood samples collected for this test are abnormal or the fasting value is above 95 mg/dL, a diagnosis of diabetes is made. The values that confirm diabetes are shown in Table 20.4.

Monitoring a Woman With Diabetes

A woman who is diabetic (type 1 or type 2) should meet with her obstetrician before she becomes pregnant; during this period, her condition can be well regulated so that hyperglycemia does not develop during the early weeks of pregnancy, when the tendency for congenital anomalies in the fetus is highest. A woman should use a home test kit to determine she is pregnant so she knows this at the earliest possible time. The best insulin control program for her during pregnancy can then be determined. The measurement of **glycosylated hemoglobin** is used to detect the degree of hyperglycemia present. This is a measure of the amount of glucose attached to hemoglobin. As glucose circulates in the bloodstream, it binds to a portion of the total hemoglobin in the blood. The amount of glucose that attaches to hemoglobin in this way will be high if the hemoglobin has been exposed to a greater level of glucose than normally present. Measuring glycosylated hemoglobin is advantageous because it reflects the average blood glucose level over the past 4 to 6 weeks (the time the red blood cells were picking up the glucose) not just the level on the day of testing. The upper normal level of HbA is 6% of total hemoglobin.

Ophthalmic examination should be done once during pregnancy for a woman with gestational diabetes and at each trimester for women with known diabetes. Background retinal

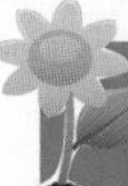

BOX 20.8 * Focus on Communication

Angelina Gomez has developed gestational diabetes. You notice in her history she moved from Guadalajara, Mexico, only 2 years ago.

Less Effective Communication

Nurse: Buenos dias, Ms. Gomez. *Como esta usted?*
Ms. Gomez: Bien, gracias.
Nurse: Oh, that was fun. I love practicing Spanish with patients. I don't understand much, though. If you'd said anything other than a one-word answer, I wouldn't have known what you meant. How's your diet going? Are you having any trouble following the diet the nutritionist gave you?
Ms. Gomez: No.
Nurse: Do you get out for a walk every day?
Ms. Gomez: Si.
Nurse: Any trouble doing your blood sugar? Your *azucar de sangre?*
Ms. Gomez: No.
Nurse: Good. Glad you're doing well. It was fun talking to you.

More Effective Communication

Nurse: Buenos dias, Ms. Gomez. *Como esta usted?*
Ms. Gomez: Bien, gracias.
Nurse: Oh, that was fun. I love practicing Spanish with patients. I've noticed that sometimes when people answer that question with "Bien, gracias," though, they're only being polite. Do you really feel well?
Ms. Gomez: I'm tired all the time.
Nurse: Tell me more about that.
Ms. Gomez: I'm so tired by evening, I can't cook. So I haven't been eating much.

Women who develop a complication of pregnancy have an added stress to their life. In the example above, the nurse made an admirable attempt to communicate with a patient in the patient's primary language. She forgot, however, that people under stress do not necessarily process new information well, and if she was having trouble interpreting Spanish, a patient might have equal trouble interpreting her English. This patient interpreted the instruction that she could not understand more than a one-word answer to mean she shouldn't answer with more than one word. Learning a second language can be important in inner-city communities. This nurse would have communicated better, however, if she had remembered that the purpose of a nurse–patient exchange was not for her to have fun but for effective assessment.

TABLE 20.3 * Classification of Diabetes Mellitus

Class	Description
Type 1	Formerly known as insulin-dependent diabetes mellitus. A state characterized by the destruction of the beta cells in the pancreas that usually leads to absolute insulin deficiency. a. Immune-mediated diabetes mellitus results from autoimmune destruction of the beta cells. b. Idiopathic type 1 refers to forms that have no known cause.
Type 2	Formerly known as non-insulin-dependent diabetes mellitus. A state that usually arises because of insulin resistance combined with a relative deficiency in the production of insulin.
Gestational diabetes	A condition of abnormal glucose metabolism that arises during pregnancy. Possible signal of an increased risk for type 2 diabetes later in life.
Impaired glucose homeostasis	A state between "normal" and "diabetes" in which the body is no longer using and/or secreting insulin properly. a. Impaired fasting glucose: A state when fasting plasma glucose is at least 110 but under 126 mg/dL. b. Impaired glucose tolerance: A state when results of the oral glucose tolerance test are at least 140 but under 200 mg/dL in the 2-hour sample.

Source: American Diabetes Association. (2005). *New classifications and recommendations for diabetes mellitus.* New York: Author.

TABLE 20.4 ✻ Oral Glucose Challenge Test Values (Fasting Plasma Glucose Values) for Pregnancy

Test Type	Pregnant Glucose Level (mg/dL)*
Fasting	95
1 hour	180
2 hours	155
3 hours	140

*Following a 100-g glucose load. Rate is abnormal if two values are exceeded.

changes, such as increased exudate (Fig. 20.4), dot hemorrhage, and macular edema, can progress or originate during pregnancy. If proliferation retinopathy was present before pregnancy, this also progresses and can lead to blindness. Laser therapy to halt these changes can be done during pregnancy without risk to the fetus. A urine culture may be done each trimester to detect asymptomatic UTI as the increased glucose concentration in urine leads to increased infection.

Nursing Diagnoses and Related Interventions

✻

Because diabetes is such a complex disorder, associated nursing diagnoses are many and varied. They include:

- Risk for ineffective tissue perfusion related to reduced vascular flow
- Imbalanced nutrition, less than body requirements, related to inability to use glucose
- Risk for ineffective coping related to required change in lifestyle
- Risk for infection related to impaired healing accompanying condition
- Deficient fluid volume related to polyuria accompanying disorder

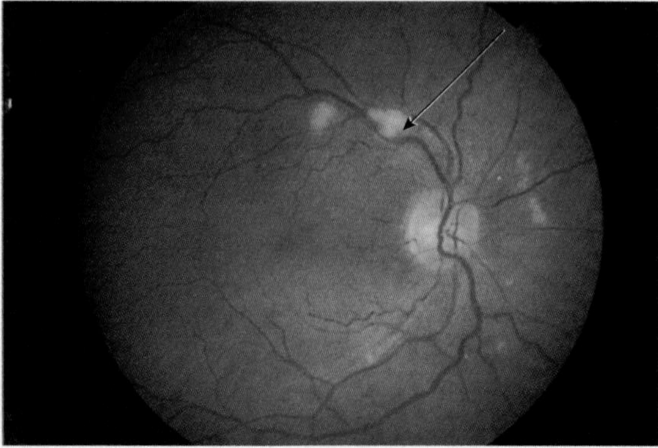

FIGURE 20.4 Increased exudate in the retina can occur with progressing diabetes during pregnancy. It appears as a "cloud-like" finding obscuring a retinal vessel.

- Deficient knowledge related to complex health problem
- Health-seeking behaviors related to voiced need to learn home glucose monitoring

The following nursing diagnosis and related interventions illustrate one of the most important facets of the nurse's role in caring for the pregnant woman with diabetes: health teaching.

Nurses can be instrumental in teaching women with diabetes how to change their therapeutic regimen during pregnancy (or begin one if newly diagnosed). Important topics include nutrition, exercise, insulin administration, blood glucose monitoring, and explanations of the various fetal assessment tests that will be done (see Focus on Nursing Care Planning Box 20.9).

Nursing Diagnosis: Deficient knowledge related to therapeutic regimen necessary during pregnancy

Outcome Evaluation: Client states importance of careful attention to nutrition, exercise, and home monitoring of glucose levels during pregnancy; describes nutrition and exercise program; states intention to keep nutrition and exercise constant.

Education Regarding Nutrition During Pregnancy. Many women of childbearing age who have had diabetes since early childhood do not follow a strict diabetic diet but eat sensibly, covering any excess food eaten with the administration of additional insulin. This type of regimen is apt to require excessive insulin administration during pregnancy as a woman begins to "eat for two." Therefore, a woman is well advised to begin a stricter diabetic diet before she becomes pregnant. Women who develop gestational diabetes are advised to begin a diabetic diet complemented by an exercise program as soon as they are diagnosed (Box 20.10).

Dietary control, or maintaining an adequate glucose intake so hypoglycemia does not occur, may be extremely difficult early in pregnancy because of nausea and vomiting. A 1800- to 2400-calorie diet (or one calculated at 30 Kcal per kg of ideal weight), divided into three meals and three snacks, is a usual regimen for a woman with diabetes during pregnancy. Keeping calories evenly distributed this way helps to keep the serum glucose level constant.

In addition, her diet should include a reduced amount of saturated fats and cholesterol and an increased amount of dietary fiber. Increasing fiber decreases postprandial hyperglycemia and so lowers insulin requirements. Of dietary calories, 20% should be from protein, 40% to 50% from carbohydrate, and up to 30% from fat (Strehlow et al., 2007).

If a woman cannot eat because of vomiting or nausea early in pregnancy or heartburn in later pregnancy, she should notify her health care provider. She may need temporary intravenous fluid supplementation. Women are extremely vulnerable to hypoglycemia at night during pregnancy because of the continuous fetal use of glucose during the time they sleep. Urge a woman to make her final snack of the day one of protein and complex carbohydrate to allow slow digestion during the night.

No woman should reduce her intake to below 1800 calories during pregnancy. A diet this low in carbohydrates causes fat breakdown, which produces acidosis. In a woman with

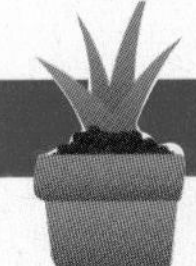

BOX 20.9 ✻ Focus on Nursing Care Planning

A Multidisciplinary Care Map for a Woman With Multiple Threats to Pregnancy

Angelina Gomez, 22, is pregnant with her first child. She fainted this afternoon while participating in an aerobic class.

Family Assessment ✻ Client lives with 30-year-old Josh, the father of her child. Angelina works as a fundraiser for a movie producer. Josh works as an animation artist. Finances are rated as "workable." She fainted this afternoon while participating in her weekly hour-long aerobic class.

Client Assessment ✻ Client had rheumatic fever with mitral stenosis as a child. She developed gestational diabetes early in this pregnancy. By the 34th week, she has already been hospitalized twice for hyperglycemia. In the emergency department, her serum glucose level is 207 mg/dL. Her blood pressure is 90/40 mm Hg; her pulse is 130/min; the fetal heart rate is 180/min. An abdominal monitor shows moderate-strength uterine contractions 7 minutes apart. The emergency physician asks for an echocardiogram to see if mitral stenosis is contributing to low blood pressure. Angelina says to you, "If exercise is supposed to be good for you, why did this happen?"

Nursing Diagnosis ✻ Risk for ineffective tissue perfusion (peripheral) related to lowered blood pressure secondary to mitral stenosis and gestational diabetes.

Outcome Criteria ✻ Blood pressure returns to 100/70; pulse rate at 70–90; fetal heart rate at 120–160 bpm. Serum glucose is less than 126 mg/dl; labor is halted.

Team Member Responsible	Assessment	Intervention	Rationale	Expected Outcome
		Activities of Daily Living		
Nurse/ physician	Assess whether client understands need for consistent exercise in light of cardiac and diabetes restrictions.	Review with client the need to regulate glucose during pregnancy by consistent diet and exercise.	Exercise increases energy expenditure, metabolic rate, and cardiac output, placing additional workload on the heart and reducing plasma glucose.	Client describes a more consistent exercise program to use during pregnancy rather than an aerobic class once a week.
		Consultations		
Physician/ nurse	Telephone pregnancy and cardiac care providers and alert them to client's admission.	Coordinate care with pregnancy and cardiac health care providers who know her best.	Collaboration with pregnancy and cardiac health care providers helps to ensure a healthy outcome for the woman and fetus.	Both pregnancy and cardiac care providers contact emergency staff to coordinate care.
		Procedures/Medications		
Physician/ nurse-midwife	Monitor client BP, pulse, fetal heart rate, and uterine contractions by continuous monitors.	Determine client progress by monitor and physical exam reports. Inform client of potential fetal distress and possibility of beginning labor	Increased fetal heart rate (tachycardia) is a sign of possible fetal distress. Uterine contractions could mark the beginning of preterm labor.	Client voices an understanding that excessive exercise could have compromised her infant's health.
Cardiac ultrasound technician/ physician	Record an echocardiogram to document mitral valve function.	Determine if heart disorder is complicating condition; assure client that procedure is safe during pregnancy.	Mitral stenosis can lower blood pressure by not allowing adequate blood flow to aorta.	Echocardiogram is recorded in an expedient manner.

(continued)

BOX 20.9 ✻ Focus on Nursing Care Planning (continued)

Nutrition				
Nurse	Assess serum glucose q 15 minutes by finger stick.	Keep client NPO. Document pattern of blood glucose. Administer IV fluid, insulin additive as prescribed.	Client's serum glucose was above normal on admission. Correcting this is vital to both maternal and fetal well-being. NPO is necessary in light of possible cesarean birth.	Client's serum glucose is within normal level within 45 minutes.
Patient/Family Education				
Nurse	Assess client's understanding that her complex situation (both cardiac and diabetes disorders) could be compromising her pregnancy.	Educate client about need for rest until condition is stabilized. Encourage client to rest in lateral recumbent position.	Activity restriction can help prevent uteroplacental insufficiency. Lateral recumbent position prevents supine hypotension syndrome.	Client voices she understands need for continuous monitoring and rest. Complies with position for rest.
Psychosocial/Spiritual/Emotional Needs				
Nurse	Assess who is client's main support person and ask if she would like him notified.	Locate support person and invite him to join client in emergency department.	Anxiety and stressors can increase the workload of the heart. Support person can be instrumental in reducing stress.	Support person arrives and works with staff to alleviate anxiety.
Discharge Planning				
Nurse/ physician	Assess if client is aware of need to admit to hospital for continuing monitoring and possible problems related to incident.	Assist client in transfer to hospital unit.	Continuous monitoring is necessary to detect if uterine contractions and preterm birth were halted.	Client is transferred to hospital unit for further monitoring and care.

BOX 20.10 ✻ Focus on Evidence-Based Practice

Should women who develop gestational diabetes limit any further pregnancies to reduce their risk of developing diabetes mellitus type 2 later in life?

The occurrence of gestational diabetes makes it more likely that a woman will develop diabetes mellitus type 2 later in life. If the chance of developing diabetes mellitus type 2 increases in women who have more than one pregnancy in which gestational diabetes occurred compared to women who have only one pregnancy marked by gestational diabetes, women might be well advised to limit their number of future pregnancies after one marked by gestational diabetes.

To investigate what are the risk factors for developing diabetes mellitus type 2, researchers followed the health course of 1401 nulliparous women with gestational diabetes for 13 years. Of the 1401 women, 251 (17.9%) developed diabetes during this follow-up period. Factors significantly associated with an increased risk of developing diabetes mellitus included a prepregnancy weight over 86 kg, the need for insulin therapy during the index pregnancy, hypoglycemia in their newborn, and a subsequent pregnancy when gestational diabetes again developed. A subsequent pregnancy where gestational diabetes did not develop did not increase the risk of developing diabetes mellitus type 2.

Would the above study be helpful when discussing the future risk of developing diabetes mellitus type 2 following a pregnancy with gestational diabetes?

Source: Russell, C., et al. (2008). Diabetes mellitus following gestational diabetes: role of subsequent pregnancy. *BJOG: An International Journal of Obstetrics and Gynaecology, 115*(2), 253–259.

diabetes, the weight of the infant is directly correlated with how much she gains during pregnancy (which directly correlates with her disease control). She must be extremely nutrition-conscious to maintain good control and keep her weight gain to a suitable amount (approximately 25 to 30 lb) in the hope of limiting the size of her infant and making a vaginal birth possible.

Education Regarding Exercise During Pregnancy. Exercise is another mechanism that lowers the serum glucose level and thereby the need for insulin. If a woman begins an exercise program for the first time during pregnancy, she may notice excessive glucose fluctuations at first. Therefore, she should begin her exercise program before pregnancy, when glucose fluctuation can be evaluated and food and snacks adjusted accordingly before a fetus is involved.

With exercise, the blood glucose level decreases because the muscles increase their need for glucose. This effect lasts for at least 12 hours after exercise. If the arm in which a woman injected insulin is actively exercised, the insulin is released so quickly that it can cause hypoglycemia. To avoid this phenomenon, a woman should eat a snack consisting of protein or complex carbohydrate before exercise and should maintain a consistent exercise program (she should not do aerobic exercises one day and then none the next, but rather 30 minutes of walking every day). In a woman with poor blood glucose control, extreme exercise will cause hyperglycemia and ketoacidosis as the liver both releases glucose and breaks down fatty acids in an attempt to supply enough energy for the exercise (yet the body cannot use them because of inadequate insulin) so exercise should be consistent day to day.

Therapeutic Management

As keeping blood glucose levels near normal helps minimize the risk of maternal and fetal complications, both women with gestational diabetes and those with overt diabetes need more frequent prenatal visits than usual to ensure close monitoring of their condition and that of the fetus.

Insulin. Early in pregnancy, a woman with diabetes may need less insulin than before pregnancy because the fetus is using so much glucose for rapid cell growth. Later in pregnancy, she will need an increased amount because her metabolic rate and need increase. If she has been taking one particular kind of insulin and a specified dosage for a long time before the pregnancy, changing the type and dosage may be unnerving for her. Be certain she understands that re-regulation is a necessity because of the changes in her metabolism. Women with gestational diabetes will be started on insulin therapy if diet alone is unsuccessful in regulating glucose values.

The type of insulin chosen is usually a short-acting insulin (regular) combined with an intermediate type. Two thirds of the total amount of the day's insulin is given in the morning; the other third is given in the evening. This is self-administered 30 minutes before breakfast in a ratio of 2:1 (intermediate to regular) and again just before dinner in a ratio of 1:1. Human insulin is recommended because it has the potential for provoking a lesser antibody response than beef or pork insulins. Use of a very-short-acting insulin such as Lispro or insulin aspart, which have a 1-hour peak time, can lead to more fluctuations in blood glucose levels than regular insulin but are ideal for some women. Women should eat almost immediately after injecting these short-acting insulins to prevent hypoglycemia before mealtimes. Oral hypoglycemia agents are not used for regulation during pregnancy because, unlike insulin, they cross the placenta and are potentially teratogenic to a fetus.

Help a woman plan her day based on the time interval her insulin takes to reach its peak. For example, an intermediate insulin given before breakfast reaches its peak after lunch or late in the afternoon just before dinner. Regular insulin given before breakfast reaches its peak just after breakfast. An intermediate insulin given in the evening reaches its peak into the next day before breakfast; the evening regular insulin injection peaks after dinner or at bedtime. Knowing when insulin reaches its peak level makes serum glucose monitoring meaningful and alerts women to the time of the day when they are most apt to be hypoglycemic (see Chapter 48).

Be certain a woman is using an injection technique for insulin of stretching the skin taut and injecting at a 90-degree angle. Although this is normally intramuscular injection technique, insulin syringes have such short needles (5/8 in) that this places the insulin in the subcutaneous tissue. Most women prefer not to use abdominal sites during pregnancy. Because insulin is absorbed more slowly from the thigh than the upper arm, a woman should maintain a consistent rotating injection routine (such as using all sites in one limb before using another or rotating limbs) to maintain as consistent a level of absorption as possible. Insulin is adjusted to keep a fasting blood glucose level below 95 to 100 mg/dL and a 2-hour postprandial level below 120 mg/dL.

Blood Glucose Monitoring. All women with diabetes need to do blood glucose monitoring to determine whether hyperglycemia or hypoglycemia exists. For this, a woman typically uses a fingerstick technique, using one of her fingertips as the site of lancet puncture. She places a drop of blood on a test strip. The strip is then inserted into a glucose meter that determines the glucose level. A fasting blood glucose level below 95 to 100 mg/dL and a 2-hour postprandial level below 120 mg/dL are well-adjusted values.

When a woman discovers that hypoglycemia is present, she should ingest some form of sustained carbohydrate such as a glass of milk and some crackers. Taking a less-concentrated fluid such as milk rather than orange juice and including a complex carbohydrate helps prevent a rebound phenomenon in which a high glucose level is created that produces even more pronounced hypoglycemia.

If a woman discovers an elevated blood glucose level, she should assess her urine for ketones. She should inform her health care provider if she finds ketones in two separate specimens. Acidosis during pregnancy must be prevented because maternal acidosis leads to fetal anoxia because of fetal inability to use oxygen when body cells are acidotic. The most common time during pregnancy for hypoglycemia is the second and third months, before insulin resistance peaks; for hyperglycemia, it is the 6th month, or the time insulin resistance is becoming most pronounced.

Insulin Pump Therapy (Continuous Subcutaneous Insulin Infusion). Because a woman will have some periods of relative hyperglycemia and hypoglycemia no matter how carefully she maintains her diet and balances her exercise level, an effective method to keep serum glucose constant is to administer insulin by a continuous pump during pregnancy (Strehlow et al., 2007). An insulin pump is an automatic pump about the size of an mp3 player. A syringe of regular insulin is placed in the pump chamber and a small-gauge needle is attached to a length of thin polyethylene tubing and implanted into the subcutaneous tissue of a woman's abdomen or thigh (Fig. 20.5). Day and night, at a continuous rate of about 1 U per hour, the pump edges the syringe barrel forward, infusing insulin continually into the subcutaneous tissue. Depending on the individual prescription, before a snack and before a meal, a woman can dial or press a button on the pump; the pump then pushes the syringe barrel forward to administer the bolus. The site of the pump insertion is cleaned daily and covered with sterile gauze; the site is changed every 24 to 48 hours to ensure that absorption remains optimal.

Several restrictions are necessary when using an insulin pump. The pump must not be allowed to become wet; therefore, a woman should remove the pump (not the syringe and tubing) when showering and remove the complete apparatus (pump, syringe, and tubing) to bathe or swim (caution her not to leave it disconnected for more than 1 hour). A woman might prefer to wear clothing that hides the pump's outline (it can either be held against her abdomen by an over-the-shoulder sling or hung from a belt around her waist). To assess whether the pump is delivering insulin at the designated rate, a woman must do blood glucose determinations about four times throughout the day (fasting and 1 hour after each meal). When pump therapy first begins, she must wake at night and do a 2:00 AM blood glucose determination because this is a time when she is most vulnerable for hypoglycemia.

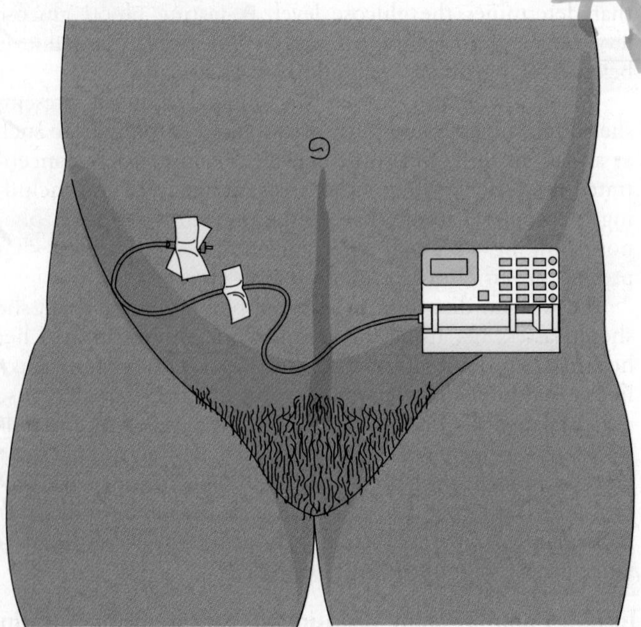

FIGURE 20.5 Using an insulin pump during pregnancy is the best assurance that insulin levels will remain constant.

Tests for Placental Function and Fetal Well-Being. Monitoring of fetal well-being is individualized depending on the woman's overall health. Because women with diabetes tend to have infants with a higher-than-normal incidence of birth anomalies, a woman will have a serum alpha-fetoprotein level obtained at 15 to 17 weeks to assess for a neural tube defect and an ultrasound examination performed at approximately 18 to 20 weeks to detect gross abnormalities. A creatinine clearance test may be ordered each trimester. A normal creatinine clearance rate suggests that a woman's vascular system is intact because kidney function is normal. This implies that uterine perfusion is also adequate. Placental functioning may also be assessed by a weekly nonstress test or biophysical profile during the last trimester (see Chapter 9) if a woman is in good control, or a daily nonstress test if her regulation is poor.

A woman may be asked to self-monitor fetal well-being by recording how many movements occur an hour. Be certain she knows that fetal activity varies depending on her activity and meal patterns to prevent her from becoming frightened by normal variations. The healthy fetus makes approximately 10 movements per hour (see Chapter 9). Ultrasounds may be taken at week 28 and then again at week 36 to 38 to determine fetal growth, amniotic fluid volume, placental location, and biparietal diameter. Oligohydramnios (a small amount of amniotic fluid) may indicate fetal growth restriction or fetal renal abnormality, whereas hydramnios (an excessive amount of amniotic fluid) may indicate gastrointestinal malformation or poorly controlled disease. The lecithin–sphingomyelin ratio by amniocentesis is performed by week 36 of pregnancy to assess fetal maturity. In pregnancies complicated by diabetes, this ratio tends not to show maturity as early as in other pregnancies because the synthesis of phosphatidylglycerol, the compound that stabilizes surfactant, is delayed in a diabetes-complicated pregnancy.

Because lung surfactant does not appear to form as early in these fetuses as others (because of the decreased level of cortisone present because of high serum glucose levels), the presence of phosphatidylglycerol at amniocentesis is used to indicate lung maturity. Although it is known that administering corticosteroids to the mother during the last week of pregnancy can hasten lung maturity, corticosteroids may also impair fetal insulin release and perhaps fetal pancreatic islet development. Therefore, with a fetus who already has a risk at birth from poor glucose control, corticosteroid use to improve lung maturity is not usually recommended.

Fetal surveillance is difficult for a woman. Having to wait during each weekly test to hear how her fetus is doing is emotionally draining especially for a woman who believes it is somehow her fault (it is, after all, her diabetes) this has happened and if the monitoring equipment shows fetal distress. She needs health care personnel with her who support her to minimize the feeling that she is alone.

Timing for Birth. Before women with diabetes were managed with maximum control during pregnancy, the timing of birth was a chief concern. Among the most hazardous times for a fetus are weeks 36 to 40 of pregnancy (when the fetus is drawing large stores of maternal nutrients because of its large size). In the past, many pregnancies were terminated early enough to prevent fetal loss from placental insufficiency because of poor perfusion during these weeks; it was hoped that this was not so early that immaturity posed further complications.

To accomplish these early births, cesarean birth was routinely performed in pregnant diabetic women at 37 weeks' gestation. Cesarean birth had to be chosen as it is difficult to induce labor this early in pregnancy because the cervix is not yet ripe or responsive to labor contractions. Further, babies of diabetic women were large, making vaginal birth difficult. Moreover, a fetus suffering placental dysfunction or insufficiency did not do well in labor. Early cesarean births, however, often resulted in immature infants who died in the neonatal period because of respiratory distress syndrome (infants of diabetic women may be more prone to this than usual because surfactant is not mature).

Today, when accurate assessment of fetal age is available and the pregnancy can be maintained within safe limits by the use of nonstress testing for a longer period, the last weeks of pregnancy are not as hazardous as before, and the timing and type of birth is much more individualized.

Vaginal birth is preferred if at all possible. Cesarean birth always presents a higher risk than vaginal birth for a fetus, and because of the difficulty of glucose regulation, the fetus of a diabetic mother is already under stress. Labor may be induced by rupture of the membranes or an oxytocin infusion after measures to induce cervical ripening (see Chapter 23). Both labor contractions and fetal heart sounds should be monitored continuously during labor to ensure early detection of placental dysfunction. An internal fetal monitor may be used with pH monitoring. A woman's glucose level is regulated during labor by an intravenous infusion of regular insulin, with a blood glucose assay every hour. Regulating the glucose level carefully during labor reduces the possibility of rebound hypoglycemia in the newborn (see Chapter 26 for care of the infant of a diabetic woman at birth).

If a woman will be given an epidural anesthetic, use of an intravenous glucose solution as a plasma volume expander should be avoided to prevent hyperglycemia from developing; Ringer's lactate is infused instead.

Postpartum Adjustment. During the postpartum period, a woman who came into pregnancy with diabetes must undergo yet another readjustment to insulin regulation. With insulin resistance gone, often she needs no insulin during the immediate postpartum period; in another few days, however, she will return to her prepregnant insulin diabetic requirements. One- or 2-hour postprandial blood glucose determinations help to regulate how much insulin she needs. A woman with gestational diabetes usually demonstrates normal glucose values by 24 hours after birth and needs no further diet or insulin therapy. She requires careful observation, however, during the immediate postpartum period because if hydramnios was present during pregnancy, she is at risk of hemorrhage from poor uterine contraction. Women with diabetes may breastfeed because insulin is one of the few substances that does not pass into breast milk from the bloodstream (Koren, 2007).

Because a woman who has had gestational diabetes is at risk for developing type 2 diabetes later in life, she should have glucose testing done during health maintenance visits throughout life. Be certain women receive contraceptive information as appropriate. Remind women with diabetes that before they plan a second pregnancy, they will need to be certain their disease is stabilized and in good control.

CANCER AND PREGNANCY

Cancer occurs in about 1 in 1000 pregnancies (Cunningham, 2008b). The malignancies most commonly seen with pregnancy are those that occur most frequently in women during childbearing years:

- Cervical
- Breast
- Ovarian
- Thyroid
- Leukemia
- Melanoma
- Lymphomas

As so many women delay having their first child until they are past 30, the incidence of malignancy during pregnancy, especially breast cancer, which tends to occur in women over 40, is increasing. Although immunologic mechanisms are altered during pregnancy, there is no proof that pregnant women are more prone to cancer than other women or that pregnancy changes the course of existing disease.

If a woman is in the first trimester of pregnancy when a malignancy is diagnosed, she and her partner are asked to make a difficult decision: to delay treatment to avoid teratogenic risks to a fetus from treatment (possibly increasing a woman's risk); to end the pregnancy to allow chemotherapy or radiation treatment to be initiated; or to choose chemotherapy or radiation treatment with the knowledge that they may cause birth anomalies in the fetus (Latimer, 2007).

As a rule, women can receive chemotherapy in the second and third trimesters without adverse fetal effects. Radiation therapy, in contrast, another modality that is a mainstay of cancer therapy, puts the fetus at risk throughout pregnancy if the fetus is directly exposed.

Surgery to remove a tumor can be completed during pregnancy with the understanding that the fetus is at risk for anoxia during anesthesia. A woman is at more than the usual risk of thrombus formation postoperatively because of the increased coagulation process accompanying pregnancy. Cervical conization for cervical cancer has a particularly high fetal risk because the surgery may directly disrupt the pregnancy. With a vaccine against HPV now available, cervical cancer incidence should be seen much less in the future (Wysocki, Reiter, & Berman, 2007).

Cancer in a woman does not appear to metastasize to the fetus. This is because the placenta serves as a barrier against this spread and also because the fetus may be capable of resisting the invasion of the foreign cells. Melanoma is the only type of cancer that seems capable of spreading to the fetus (Leachman et al., 2007).

MENTAL ILLNESS AND PREGNANCY

Mental illness may precede or occur with pregnancy. Schizophrenia tends to have its highest incidence in adolescents and young adults and so occurs in young pregnant women. Depression occurs almost four times more commonly in women than in men, and often in young adults. It is the most common mental illness seen in pregnant women.

Even normal levels of stress make it difficult to use effective coping mechanisms so pregnancy or childbirth may be the additional stress that reveals mental illness for the first time. A woman with a psychiatric disorder should be cared for by both a psychiatric care team and a prenatal care group to ensure that the stress of pregnancy is not exacerbating the mental illness, and distorted perceptions or depression do not complicate the pregnancy. Any psychotropic medication taken by a pregnant woman should be evaluated for possible fetal harm (Louik et al., 2007). For example, lithium, a mainstay of therapy for mood disorders such as bipolar disorder (manic depression), and serotonin-reuptake inhibitors used to counteract depression, are potentially teratogenic (Karch, 2009).

Mental illness may also occur in the postpartum period (postpartum depression or psychosis; see Chapter 25).

✔Checkpoint Question 20.5

Angelina uses an insulin pump to administer insulin for gestational diabetes. Why is nighttime a particularly hazardous time for her fetus with pump therapy?

a. The fetus can develop hyperglycemia from excessive insulin administration.
b. Continuous insulin administration with no food can lead to hypoglycemia.
c. The mother's lack of exercise at night tends to lead to hypercalcemia.
d. The pump's needle can migrate inward and possibly pierce the fetus.

Key Points for Review

- A high-risk pregnancy is one in which a concurrent disorder, pregnancy-related complication, or external factor jeopardizes the health of the mother, the fetus, or both.
- Pregnancy is a stress to any family because it involves financial expenses plus changes in family roles. If a complication of pregnancy develops, this stress is almost automatically intensified. Families need support to be able to cope with the increased burden.
- When women with a pre-existing disease become pregnant, a thorough history and physical examination are crucial to obtain at the first prenatal visit to establish a baseline of information on the condition. Documentation of any medication being taken for a secondary condition is important to protect against adverse drug interactions and the possibility of teratogenic action on the fetus.
- Teaching is an important nursing intervention because a woman with a pre-existing illness must make modifications in her usual therapy to adjust to pregnancy. Pregnancy often stimulates women to learn more about their primary disease as well.
- Women who have a complication early in pregnancy may continue to worry about the health of their fetus all during pregnancy. They need to be assured (appropriately) that the episode was temporary and that, with continued monitoring, their fetus should not suffer harm. After giving birth, women may need to spend additional time with their newborns to convince themselves that their infants are healthy so bonding can begin.
- Because blood volume increases by as much as 50% during pregnancy, cardiac function may become inadequate if cardiovascular disease is present. Illnesses that cause difficulty can be either acquired disorders such as Kawasaki disease and rheumatic fever or congenital disorders such as mitral valve stenosis and coarctation of the aorta.
- Various forms of anemia can cause complications of pregnancy; iron-deficiency anemia, sickle cell anemia, and folic acid–deficiency anemia are examples. All these anemias can result in fetal distress because of inadequate oxygen transport.
- Urinary tract disorders can lead to pregnancy complications because pregnancy increases the workload of the kidneys. UTIs and chronic renal disease are two disorders that may lead to early pregnancy loss.
- Acute nasopharyngitis, asthma, pneumonia, influenza, and tuberculosis are common respiratory disorders seen in pregnancy. The incidence of tuberculosis is on the increase and these patients need special assessment and care.
- Juvenile rheumatoid arthritis and systemic lupus erythematosus are examples of rheumatic disorders seen in pregnancy. These disorders generally require large doses of NSAIDs for therapy. Women taking salicylates are advised to decrease use 2 weeks before birth to avoid bleeding disorders in the newborn.
- Some gastrointestinal illnesses that occur with pregnancy are hiatal hernia, cholecystitis, viral hepatitis, inflammatory bowel disease, and appendicitis. If surgery is necessary for conditions such as cholecystitis or appendicitis, it can be performed by laparoscopic technique during pregnancy, but this may result in preterm labor.
- Recurrent seizures are the most frequently seen neurologic condition during pregnancy. Many drugs used to control seizures are teratogenic; women need to have their medical regimen evaluated before pregnancy to be certain they are regulated on the fewest medications and the lowest dosages possible.
- The major endocrine disorder seen during pregnancy is diabetes mellitus. Gestational diabetes is diabetes that occurs during pregnancy and fades after it.

CRITICAL THINKING EXERCISES

1. Angelina Gomez, the woman you met at the beginning of the chapter, has developed congestive heart failure. She works at a job where she is on her feet almost all day. What suggestions could you make to her to help her incorporate some rest periods into her day?
2. Angelina has also developed gestational diabetes. She's resistant to learning about her condition, though, because she knows her symptoms are only temporary and

will fade at the end of pregnancy. What type of teaching plan would you devise to help her learn in the face of this attitude?

3. Angelina is prone to urinary tract infections during pregnancy because of her gestational diabetes. What are common measures you can suggest to women to help avoid UTIs during pregnancy?
4. Examine the National Health Goals related to complications of pregnancy. Most government-sponsored money for nursing research is allotted based on these goals. What would be a possible research topic to explore pertinent to these goals that would be applicable to the Gomez family and also advance evidence-based practice?

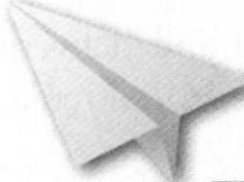

CRITICAL THINKING SCENARIO

Open the accompanying CD-ROM or visit http://thePoint.lww.com and read the Patient Scenario included for this chapter, then answer the questions to further sharpen your skills and grow more familiar with NCLEX style questions related to nursing care of families during a high-risk pregnancy. Confirm your answers are correct by reading the rationales.

REFERENCES

Adab, N., et al. (2009). Common antiepileptic drugs in pregnancy in women with epilepsy. *Cochrane Database of Systematic Reviews, 2009*(1), (CD004848).

American College of Obstetrics and Gynecology (ACOG). (2007). Peripartum cardiomyopathy. *ACOG Clinical Review, 12*(2), 3.

Arnett, C., & Greenspoon, J. S. (2007). Hematologic disorders in pregnancy. In A. H. DeCherney & L. Nathan (Eds.). *Current diagnosis and treatment in obstetrics and gynecology* (10th ed.). Columbus, OH: McGraw-Hill.

Augustin, G., & Majerovic, M. (2007). Non-obstetrical acute abdomen during pregnancy. *European Journal of Obstetrics, Gynecology, & Reproductive Biology, 131*(1), 4–12.

Barnes-Powell, L. L. (2007). Infants of diabetic mothers: the effects of hyperglycemia on the fetus and neonate. *Neonatal Network: The Journal of Neonatal Nursing, 26*(5), 283–290.

Bashore, T. M., & Granger, C. B. (2009). Cardiology. In S. J. McPhee & M. A. Papadakis (Eds.). *Current medical diagnosis and treatment.* Columbus, OH: McGraw-Hill.

Bernstein, H. B., & Weinstein, M. (2007). Normal pregnancy and prenatal care. In A. H. DeCherney & L. Nathan (Eds.). *Current diagnosis and treatment in obstetrics and gynecology* (10th ed.). Columbus, OH: McGraw-Hill.

Bortoli, A., et al. (2007). Pregnancy before and after the diagnosis of inflammatory bowel diseases: retrospective case-control study. *Journal of Gastroenterology & Hepatology, 22*(4), 542–549.

Boushey, H. A. (2007). Drugs used in asthma. In B. G. Katzung (Ed.). *Basic and clinical pharmacology* (10th ed.). Columbus, OH: McGraw-Hill.

Campaigne, A. L., & Conway, D. L. (2007). Detection and prevention of macrosomia. *Obstetrics and Gynecology Clinics of North America, 34*(2), 309–322.

Cansino, C. D., & Lipsett, P. (2007). Critical care. In K. B. Fortner, et al. (Eds.). *The Johns Hopkins manual of gynecology and obstetrics.* Philadelphia: Lippincott Williams & Wilkins.

Chaffins, J. A. (2007). Marfan syndrome. *Radiologic Technology, 78*(3), 222–239.

Chambers, H. F. (2009). Infectious diseases: bacterial & chlamydial. In S. J. McPhee & M. A. Papadakis (Eds.). *Current medical diagnosis and treatment.* Columbus, OH: McGraw-Hill.

Chattaway, J. M., & Klepser, T. B. (2007). Propylthiouracil versus methimazole in treatment of Graves' disease during pregnancy. *Annals of Pharmacotherapy, 41*(6), 1018–1022.

Cox, S. R. (2007). Tuberculosis and pregnancy. *Journal of Midwifery & Women's Health, 52*(4), 415–416.

Crombleholme, W. R. (2009). Obstetrics. In S. J. McPhee & M. A. Papadakis (Eds.). *Current medical diagnosis and treatment.* Columbus, OH: McGraw-Hill.

Cunningham, F. G., et al. (2008a). Cardiovascular disease. In Cunningham, F. G., et al. (Eds.). *William's obstetrics* (22nd ed.). Columbus, OH: McGraw-Hill.

Cunningham, F. G., et al. (2008b). Neoplasms and Pregnancy. *William's obstetrics* (22nd ed.). Columbus, OH: McGraw-Hill.

Davidson, S., & Graham, E. M. (2007). Cardiopulmonary disorders of pregnancy. In K. B. Fortner, et al. (Eds.). *The Johns Hopkins manual of gynecology and obstetrics.* Philadelphia: Lippincott Williams & Wilkins.

del Mar Colon, M., & Hibbard, J. U. (2007). Obstetric considerations in the management of pregnancy in kidney transplant recipients. *Advances in Chronic Kidney Disease, 14*(2), 168–177.

Ferrara, A. (2007). Increasing prevalence of gestational diabetes mellitus: a public health perspective. *Diabetes Care, 30*(Suppl 2), S141–S146.

Fiore, A. E., et al. (2007). Prevention and control of influenza. Recommendations of the Advisory Committee on Immunization Practices (ACIP). *MMWR: Morbidity and Mortality Weekly Report, 56*(RR-6), 1–53.

Fischer, M. J. (2007). Chronic kidney disease and pregnancy: maternal and fetal outcomes. *Advances in Chronic Kidney Disease, 14*(2), 132–145.

Garner, P., & Gulmezoglu, A. M. (2009). Drugs for preventing malaria in pregnant women. *Cochrane Database of Systematic Reviews, 2009*(1), (CD000169).

Golding, A., Haque, U. J., & Giles, J. T. (2007). Rheumatoid arthritis and reproduction. *Rheumatic Disease Clinics of North America, 33*(2), 319–343.

Gomez, V. J. A., et al. (2007). Pregnancy in end-stage renal disease patients and treatment with peritoneal dialysis: report of two cases. *Peritoneal Dialysis International, 27*(3), 353–358.

Greenspan, F. S., & Dong, B. J. (2007). Thyroid and antithyroid drugs. In B. G. Katzung (Ed.). *Basic and clinical pharmacology* (10th ed.). Columbus, OH: McGraw-Hill.

Hameed, A. B., & Akhter, M. W. (2007). Cardiac disorders. In A. H. DeCherney & L. Nathan (Eds.). *Current diagnosis and treatment in obstetrics and gynecology* (10th ed.). Columbus, OH: McGraw-Hill.

Hibbard, J. U., Fajardo, J.E., & Briller, J. (2007). Kawasaki disease with coronary artery sequelae. *Obstetrics and Gynecology, 109*(2 Part 2), 517–519.

Jain, S., et al. (2007). Hepatitis C in pregnancy. *American Journal of Perinatology, 24*(4), 251–256.

Johnson, A., & Ross, B. (2007). Perinatal infections. In K. B. Fortner, et al. (Eds.). *The Johns Hopkins manual of gynecology and obstetrics.* Philadelphia: Lippincott Williams & Wilkins.

Kalidindi, M., et al. (2007). Myasthenia gravis and pregnancy. *Journal of Obstetrics & Gynaecology, 27*(1), 30–32.

Karch, A. M. (2009). *Lippincott's nursing drug guide.* Philadelphia: Lippincott Williams & Wilkins.

Koren, G. (2007). Special aspects of perinatal and pediatric pharmacology. In B. G. Katzung (Ed.). *Basic and clinical pharmacology* (10th ed.). Columbus, OH: McGraw-Hill.

Kyriazopoulou, V., et al. (2008). Recommendations for thyroxin therapy during pregnancy. *Expert Opinion on Pharmacotherapy, 9*(3), 421–427.

Larsen, C. P., Ejiofor, M. C., & Walker, P. D. (2009). Acute kidney failure in the third trimester of pregnancy. *American Journal of Kidney Diseases, 53*(1), 175–179.

Latimer, J. (2007). Gynaecological malignancies in pregnancy. *Current Opinion in Obstetrics and Gynecology, 19*(2), 140–144.

Leachman, S. A., et al. (2007). Management of melanoma during pregnancy. *Dermatology Nursing, 19*(2), 145–152.

Linker, C. A. (2009). Hematology. In S. J. McPhee & M. A. Papadakis (Eds.). *Current medical diagnosis and treatment.* Columbus, OH: McGraw-Hill.

Lipscomb, K., & Novy, M. J. (2007). The normal puerperium. In A. H. DeCherney & L. Nathan (Eds.). *Current diagnosis and treatment in obstetrics and gynecology* (10th ed.). Columbus, OH: McGraw-Hill.

Longman, R. E., & Johnson, T. R. B. (2007). Viral respiratory disease in pregnancy. *Current Opinion in Obstetrics and Gynecology, 19*(2), 120–125.

Louik, C., et al. (2007). First-trimester use of selective serotonin-reuptake inhibitors and the risk of birth defects. *New England Journal of Medicine, 356*(26), 2675–2683.

Mahid, S. S., et al. (2007). Active and passive smoking in childhood is related to the development of inflammatory bowel disease. *Inflammatory Bowel Diseases, 13*(4), 431–438.

Masharani, U. (2009). Diabetes mellitus & hypoglycemia. In McPhee, S. J., & Papadakis, M. A. (Eds.). *Current Medical Diagnosis and Treatment.* Columbus, OH: McGraw-Hill.

Masters, S. B. (2007). Agents used in anemias; hematopoietic growth factors. In B. G. Katzung (Ed.). *Basic and clinical pharmacology* (10th ed.). Columbus, OH: McGraw-Hill.

Mavragani, C. P., et al. (2007). Antiphospholipid syndrome: current diagnostic and therapeutic issues. *Journal of Musculoskeletal Medicine, 24*(4), 148–161.

McAnulty, J. H., Metcalfe, J., & Ueland, K. (2008). Heart disease and pregnancy. In V. Fuster, et al. (Eds.). *Hurst's the heart* (12th ed.). Columbus, OH: McGraw-Hill.

McMillan, R. (2007). The pathogenesis of chronic immune thrombocytopenic purpura. *Seminars in Hematology, 44*(4 Suppl 5), S3–S11.

Mills, M. E. (2007). Craving more than food: the implications of pica in pregnancy. *Nursing for Women's Health, 11*(3), 266–273.

Montoro, M. N. (2007). Pulmonary disorders in pregnancy. In A. H. DeCherney & L. Nathan (Eds.). *Current diagnosis and treatment in obstetrics and gynecology* (10th ed.). Columbus, OH: McGraw-Hill..

Mooney, M. (2007). Managing cardiac disease in pregnancy. *British Journal of Midwifery, 15*(2), 76–78.

Neto, L. V., et al. (2007). Prospective evaluation of pregnant women with hypothyroidism: implications for treatment. *Gynecological Endocrinology, 23*(3), 138–141.

Nguyen, T., & Witter, F. R. (2007). Renal, hepatic, and gastrointestinal disorders and systemic lupus erythematosus in pregnancy. In K. B. Fortner, et al. (Eds.). *The Johns Hopkins manual of gynecology and obstetrics.* Philadelphia: Lippincott Williams & Wilkins.

Novak, B. (2007). Health benefits of folic acid. *Nurse Prescribing, 5*(5), 215–220.

Pan, G. D., et al. (2007). A successful pregnancy following liver transplantation. *Hepatobiliary and Pancreatic Diseases International, 6*(1), 98–100.

Parangi, S., et al. (2007). Surgical gastrointestinal disorders during pregnancy. *American Journal of Surgery, 193*(2), 223–232.

Petri, M. (2007). The Hopkins Lupus Pregnancy Center: ten key issues in management. *Rheumatic Disease Clinics of North America, 33*(2), 227–235.

Reveiz, L., Gyte, G. M. L., & Cuervo, L. G. (2009). Treatments for iron-deficiency anaemia in pregnancy. *Cochrane Database of Systematic Reviews, 2009*(1), (CD003094).

Russell, C., et al. (2008). Diabetes mellitus following gestational diabetes: role of subsequent pregnancy. *BJOG: An International Journal of Obstetrics & Gynaecology, 115*(2), 253–259.

Saraste, M., et al. (2007). Clinical and immunologic evaluation of women with multiple sclerosis during and after pregnancy. *Gender Medicine, 4*(1), 45–55.

Schulenburg, M. (2007). Management of hypertensive emergencies: implications for the critical care nurse. *Critical Care Nursing Quarterly, 30*(2), 86–93.

Segal, J. B., et al. (2007). Management of venous thromboembolism: a systematic review for a practice guideline. *Annals of Internal Medicine, 146*(3), 211–222.

Sibanda, N., et al. (2007). Pregnancy after organ transplantation: a report from the UK Transplant pregnancy registry. *Transplantation, 83*(10), 1301–1307.

Stover, J. (2007). Nutritional management of pregnancy in chronic kidney disease. *Advances in Chronic Kidney Disease, 14*(2), 212–214.

Strehlow, S., et al. (2007). Diabetes mellitus and pregnancy. In A. H. DeCherney & L. Nathan (Eds.). *Current diagnosis and treatment in obstetrics and gynecology* (10th ed.). Columbus, OH: McGraw-Hill.

Subramanian, A., et al. (Eds.) (2008). *Drug facts and comparisons.* St. Louis: Wolters Kluwer Health.

Szymanski, L. M., & Aina-Mumuney, A. (2007). Hematologic disorders of pregnancy. In K. B. Fortner, et al. (Eds.). *The Johns Hopkins manual of gynecology and obstetrics.* Philadelphia: Lippincott Williams & Wilkins.

Tata, L. J., et al. (2007). Comprehensive analysis of adverse obstetric and pediatric complications in women with asthma. *American Journal of Respiratory and Critical Care Medicine, 175*(10), 991–997.

Uppalapati, R., & Landry, M. S. (2007). S.O.S! I'm short of breath! *Obstetrics and Gynecology, 109*(6), 1443–1460.

Vazquez, J. C., & Villar, J. (2009). Treatments for symptomatic urinary tract infections during pregnancy. *Cochrane Database of Systematic Reviews, 2009*(1), (CD002256).

Venables, P. H., et al. (2007). Prenatal influenza exposure and delivery complications: implications for the development of schizophrenia. *Family and Community Health, 30*(2), 151–159.

Waterbury, L. (2007). Anemia. In N. H. Fiebach, et al. (Eds.). *Principles of ambulatory medicine* (7th ed.). Philadelphia: Lippincott Williams & Wilkins.

Wexler, I. D., et al. (2007). Pregnancy and chronic progressive pulmonary disease. *American Journal of Respiratory and Critical Care Medicine, 175*(4), 300–305.

Williams, D., & Davison, J. (2008). Chronic kidney disease in pregnancy. *BMJ: British Medical Journl, 336*(7637), 211–215.

Wiltz, S. A., et al. (2008). What is the most effective and safe malaria prophylaxis during pregnancy? *Journal of Family Practice, 57*(1), 51–53.

Witter, F. R. (2007). Management of the high-risk lupus pregnant patient. *Rheumatic Disease Clinics of North America, 33*(2), 253–265.

Wysocki, S., Reiter, S., & Berman, N. R. (2007). Strategies for preventing cervical cancer and HPV-related disease: the role of vaccination. *Women's Health Care, 6*(1), 6–22.

Zack-Williams, D. (2007). Sickle cell anaemia in pregnancy and the neonates: ethical issues. *British Journal of Midwifery, 15*(4), 205–209.

SUGGESTED READINGS

Beigi, R. H. (2007). Pandemic influenza and pregnancy: a call for preparedness planning. *Obstetrics and Gynecology, 109*(5), 1193–1196.

Blowey, D. L., & Warady, B. A. (2007). Outcome of infants born to women with chronic kidney disease. *Advances in Chronic Kidney Disease, 14*(2), 199–205.

Clark, C. A., et al. (2007). Incidence of postpartum thrombosis and preterm delivery in women with antiphospholipid antibodies and recurrent pregnancy loss. *Journal of Rheumatology, 34*(5), 992–996.

Dean, A. (2007). Pregnancy and breast cancer. *Practice Nurse, 33*(8), 45–48.

Kilpatrick, K., & Purden, M. (2007). Using reflective nursing practice to improve care of women with congenital heart disease: considering pregnancy. *MCN: The American Journal of Maternal/Child Nursing, 32*(3), 140–147.

Laurberg, P., et al. (2009). Management of Graves' hyperthyroidism in pregnancy. *European Journal of Endocrinology, 160*(1), 1–8.

Martens, T. Z., & Emed, J. D. (2007). The experiences and challenges of pregnant women coping with thrombophilia. *JOGNN: Journal of Obstetric, Gynecologic, and Neonatal Nursing, 36*(1), 55–62.

Matzo, M. (2007). Evidence for excellence. Screening recommendations for iron deficiency anemia: benefits of routinely screening pregnant women outweigh risks. *American Journal of Nursing, 107*(8), 51.

Reece, E. A. (2008). Perspectives on obesity, pregnancy and birth outcomes in the United States: the scope of the problem. *American Journal of Obstetrics and Gynecology, 198*(1), 23–27.

Shapiro-Mendoza, C. K., et al. (2008). Effect of late-preterm birth and maternal medical conditions on newborn morbidity risk. *Pediatrics, 121*(2), e223–e232.

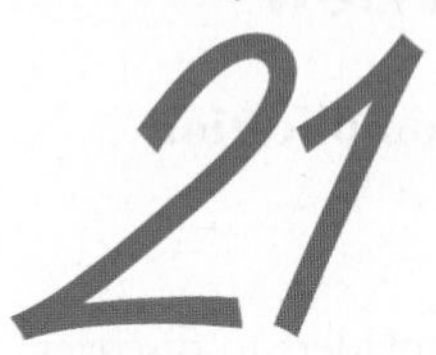

Chapter 21 Nursing Care of a Family Experiencing a Sudden Pregnancy Complication

KEY TERMS

- abortion
- ankle clonus
- cervical cerclage
- chorioamnionitis
- Couvelaire uterus
- early pregnancy failure
- eclampsia
- ectopic pregnancy
- erythroblastosis fetalis
- gestational trophoblastic disease
- HELLP syndrome
- hemolytic disease of the newborn
- hydramnios
- isoimmunization
- miscarriage
- oligohydramnios
- placenta previa
- post term pregnancy
- pre-eclampsia
- premature cervical dilatation
- premature separation of the placenta
- preterm labor
- preterm rupture of membranes
- pseudocyesis
- recurrent pregnancy loss
- Rh incompatibility
- tocolytic agent

OBJECTIVES

After mastering the contents of this chapter, you should be able to:

1. Describe complications of pregnancy that place a pregnant woman and her fetus at high risk.
2. Identify National Health Goals related to complications of pregnancy and specific measures nurses can take to help the nation achieve these goals.
3. Use critical thinking to analyze ways that nurses can help prevent complications of pregnancy while keeping care family centered.
4. Assess a woman who is experiencing a complication of pregnancy.
5. Formulate nursing diagnoses that address the needs of a woman and her family experiencing a complication of pregnancy.
6. Identify expected outcomes to minimize the risks to a pregnant woman and her fetus when a complication of pregnancy occurs.
7. Plan nursing interventions to meet the needs and promote optimal outcomes for a woman and her family during a complication of pregnancy.
8. Implement nursing care specific to a woman who has developed a complication of pregnancy such as teaching her how to recognize the symptoms of preterm labor.
9. Evaluate expected outcomes for effectiveness and achievement of care.
10. Identify areas of nursing care related to high-risk pregnancy that could benefit from additional nursing research or the application of evidence-based practice.
11. Integrate knowledge of complications of pregnancy with nursing process to achieve quality maternal and child health nursing care.

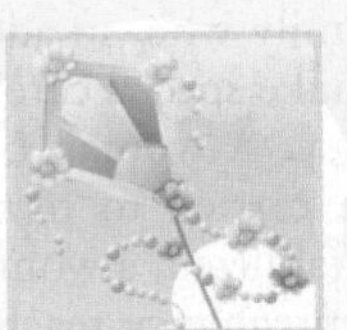

Beverly Muzuki is a 20-year-old gravida 2, para 0, 30 weeks pregnant, whom you see in a prenatal clinic. She has had symptoms of a urinary tract infection for the past few days but did not call the clinic because she knew she had an appointment today and thought getting some help for it could wait until she came in. Yesterday she noticed some mild abdominal pain but thought it was irritation from the bladder infection. During the night, she woke twice because of a nagging backache. This morning, she has intermittent sharp uterine contractions. "Why am I starting labor so early?" she asks you. "I didn't do anything wrong."

Previous chapters described normal pregnancy and pre-existing and newly acquired conditions that can complicate pregnancy. This chapter adds knowledge about complications directly related to the pregnancy. Such complications can cause as much concern and worry for women as illnesses brought into a pregnancy.

Were Beverly's actions as informed as they could have been?

What additional health teaching might have prevented her from starting labor so early?

The majority of women who enter pregnancy in good health expect to complete a pregnancy and birth without complications. In a few women, however, for reasons that usually are unclear, unexpected deviations or complications from the course of normal pregnancy occur. When this happens, it places a severe burden on a woman and her family as well as her health care providers. All families benefit from the support and skill of a professional nurse who helps them work through the stages of pregnancy and prepare them to become new parents. The support and skills of a professional nurse are essential to a family who, in addition to the usual tasks of pregnancy, must take special care to ensure the continuation of the pregnancy. A woman becomes concerned that her baby cannot be carried to term. Hospitalization may be necessary. Once stabilized, a woman has to be monitored carefully until the pregnancy reaches term. As this is done on an ambulatory basis, nurses continue to be instrumental in care (Skouteris et al., 2009).

The leading complications related directly to the pregnancy are thromboembolism, hemorrhage, infection, pregnancy-induced hypertension, and ectopic pregnancy (Fortner, Althaus, & Gurewitsch, 2007). All of these have the potential to threaten the life of the mother and the fetus. National Health Goals established to help reduce complications of pregnancy such as these are shown in Box 21.1.

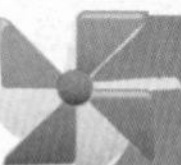

BOX 21.1 Focus on National Health Goals

Preventing complications of pregnancy is viewed as so important by most people that this issue is included in the National Health Goals. Four of these goals are:

- Reduce the rate of maternal deaths from pregnancy-related causes to 3.3 per 100,000 live births from a baseline of 7.1 per 100,000.
- Reduce the rate of maternal illness and complications because of pregnancy to 24 per 100 births from a baseline of 31 per 100 births.
- Reduce the proportion of preterm births to 7.6% from a baseline of 11.6%.
- Reduce the incidence of low birthweight to no more than 5% of live births from a baseline of 7.6%, and of very low birth weight to no more than 0.9% of live births from a baseline of 1.4% (http://www.nih.gov).

Nurses working in prenatal settings can help to ensure that women are well informed about the normal course of pregnancy so they can recognize and alert health care providers when a complication is occurring. They can actively participate in risk assessment at prenatal visits. Nursing research is needed in areas such as what is the best way to determine each woman's individual needs so prenatal instructions can be specifically planned, and whether increasing the number of prenatal visits for high-risk women could reduce complications during pregnancy.

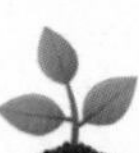

Nursing Process Overview

For a Woman Who Develops a Complication of Pregnancy

Assessment

Nurses often are the first health care providers to discover that a complication of pregnancy is beginning because they are the people who talk to clients first at prenatal visits. Always ask women at such visits about any symptoms that might indicate a complication such as pain or bleeding. Provide enough time for a thorough health history so more subtle problems such as headache, blurred vision, or vaginal spotting can be discovered and investigated thoroughly.

In addition, at the close of a visit, review the danger signs of pregnancy with a woman so she can recognize potential problems and contact the health care center if a problem should occur. Assure women that they are free to call whenever they are concerned. Otherwise, they may wait until a symptom is acute rather than call when they first notice it.

Nursing Diagnosis

Nursing diagnoses pertaining to a woman with a pregnancy complication should reflect both the physical problem and the family's concern. Some examples are:

- Anxiety related to guarded pregnancy outcome
- Deficient fluid volume related to third-trimester bleeding
- Risk for infection related to incomplete miscarriage
- Risk for ineffective tissue perfusion related to pregnancy-induced hypertension
- Deficient knowledge related to signs and symptoms of possible complications
- Fear of preterm labor ending the pregnancy

Outcome Identification and Planning

Complications of pregnancy produce emergency situations, so outcomes usually focus on a short timeframe. Be sure that outcomes address both fetal and maternal welfare and often total family welfare. Treatment protocols, such as those related to bleeding, preterm labor, and pregnancy-induced hypertension, should be regularly updated and maintained so they remain current. Be certain that they reflect a current nursing management level so nurses can act swiftly and independently as needed with life-saving measures. Once a woman's condition stabilizes, outcome identification can then focus on long-term objectives.

Many women who develop a pregnancy complication spend a few days in the hospital for therapy and monitoring followed by discharge to their homes. Waiting for a pregnancy that has been threatened this way to come to term can be difficult and anxious. Readmission to the health care facility, especially when a new complication occurs, compounds these feelings. Be certain that planning considers the many feelings this experience can cause. Offer referrals for counseling and/or community support groups. An Internet site that discusses complications of pregnancy that can be helpful to women is The American Pregnancy Association (http://www.americanpregnancy.org).

Implementation

Interventions for a woman experiencing a complication of pregnancy include measures to maintain several different areas:

- Continued healthy fetal growth
- Continued maternal physical health
- A woman's and family's psychological health
- Continuation of the pregnancy as long as possible

Maintaining an optimistic attitude of fetal progress is important so a woman does not begin anticipatory grieving for her fetus and halt the growth of bonding. If the complication can be contained and the pregnancy continues uninterrupted, this will help protect the mental health of the whole family. If the pregnancy cannot be continued, be available to offer support to a family who grieves for the loss of an unborn child and, in rare instances, loss of future childbearing potential or the woman herself.

After a pregnancy with complications, a woman has reason to be especially worried about her infant's health at the time of birth. The infant may be hospitalized in a special care nursery. Help her spend enough time with her child to see that although, perhaps born before term, her infant is well and healthy. This may be difficult because she still may be ill herself. It is helpful to assess the infant for such things as ability to follow a light and respond to a voice while the woman is present. This helps to demonstrate that the infant is well.

Outcome Evaluation

Although the success or failure of some nursing interventions cannot be fully evaluated until a child is born or even into the postnatal period, outcomes should be evaluated throughout the pregnancy if possible. Be aware that after a complication of early pregnancy, a woman cannot help but worry for the remainder of the pregnancy that the complication will recur or that the original insult to the fetus was severe enough to cause long-term effects. Evaluate a woman's attitude and physical status at each health care visit to be certain she is coping with the situation and the fear and strain she lives under until the child is born.

Unfortunately, even with sustained care, not all fetal outcomes will be optimal. Evaluation will then include the ability of the family to care for an ill infant or grieve because a newborn dies. Examples of expected outcomes are:

- Client's blood pressure is maintained within acceptable parameters.
- Couple state they feel able to cope with anxiety associated with the pregnancy complication.
- Client's signs and symptoms of pregnancy-induced hypertension do not progress to eclampsia.
- Client accurately verbalizes crucial signs and symptoms she should immediately report to her primary health care provider.
- Couple expresses feelings of sadness over pregnancy loss

BLEEDING DURING PREGNANCY

Vaginal bleeding during pregnancy is always a deviation from the normal, may occur at any point during pregnancy, and is always frightening. It must always be carefully investigated because if it occurs in sufficient amount or for sufficient cause, it can impair both the outcome of the pregnancy and a woman's life or health. The primary causes of bleeding during pregnancy are summarized in Table 21.1.

TABLE 21.1 * Summary of Primary Causes of Bleeding During Pregnancy

Time	Type	Cause	Assessment	Cautions
First trimester	Threatened miscarriage (early—under 16 weeks; late—16 to 24 weeks)	Unknown; possibly chromosomal, uterine abnormalities	Vaginal spotting, perhaps slight cramping	
	Imminent (inevitable) miscarriage		Vaginal spotting, cramping, cervical dilatation	
	Missed miscarriage		Vaginal spotting, perhaps slight cramping; no apparent loss of pregnancy	Disseminated intravascular coagulation associated with missed miscarriage
	Incomplete miscarriage		Vaginal spotting, cramping, cervical dilatation, but incomplete expulsion of uterine contents	
	Complete miscarriage		Vaginal spotting, cramping, cervical dilatation, and complete expulsion of uterine contents	

(continued)

TABLE 21.1 ✻ Summary of Primary Causes of Bleeding During Pregnancy (continued)

Time	Type	Cause	Assessment	Cautions
	Ectopic (tubal) pregnancy	Implantation of zygote at site other than in uterus; tubal constricture, adhesions associated	Sudden unilateral lower abdominal quadrant pain; minimal vaginal bleeding, possible signs of shock or hemorrhage	May have repeat ectopic pregnancy in future if tubal scarring is bilateral
Second trimester	Hydatidiform mole (gestational trophoblastic disease)	Abnormal proliferation of trophoblast cells; fertilization or division defect	Overgrowth of uterus; highly positive human chorionic gonadotropin (hCG) test; no fetus present on ultrasound; bleeding from vagina of old or fresh blood accompanied by cyst formation	Retained trophoblast tissue may become malignant (choriocarcinoma); follow for 6 months to 1 year with hCG testing
	Premature cervical dilatation	Cervix begins to dilate and pregnancy is lost at about 20 weeks; unknown cause, but cervical trauma from dilatation and curettage (D&C) may be associated	Painless bleeding leading to expulsion of fetus	Can have cervical sutures placed to ensure a second pregnancy
Third trimester	Placenta previa	Low implantation of placenta possibly because of uterine abnormality	Painless bleeding at beginning of cervical dilatation	No vaginal examinations to minimize placental trauma
	Premature separation of the placenta (abruptio placentae)	Unknown cause; associated with hypertension; placenta separates from uterus	Sharp abdominal pain followed by uterine tenderness; vaginal bleeding; signs of maternal shock, fetal distress	Disseminated intravascular coagulation associated with condition
	Preterm labor	Many possible etiologic factors such as trauma, substance abuse, pregnancy-induced hypertension or cervicitis; increased chance in multiple gestation, maternal illness	Show (pink-stained vaginal discharge) accompanied by uterine contractions becoming regular and effective	Preterm labor may be halted if the cervix is less than 4 cm dilated and the membranes are intact. Corticosteroids are administered to aid fetal lung maturity.

Although vaginal bleeding may be innocent, any degree of this during pregnancy is potentially serious because it may mean that the placenta has loosened, cutting off nourishment to the fetus. Also, the amount visualized may be only a fraction of the blood actually being lost. This happens because an undilated cervix and intact membranes can contain blood within the uterus. A woman with any degree of bleeding, therefore, needs to be evaluated for the possibility that she is experiencing a significant blood loss or is developing hypovolemic shock.

The process of shock because of blood loss is shown in Figure 21.1. Because the uterus is a nonessential body organ, danger to the fetal blood supply occurs when a woman's body begins to decrease blood flow to peripheral organs (although the increased blood volume of pregnancy allows more than normal blood loss before

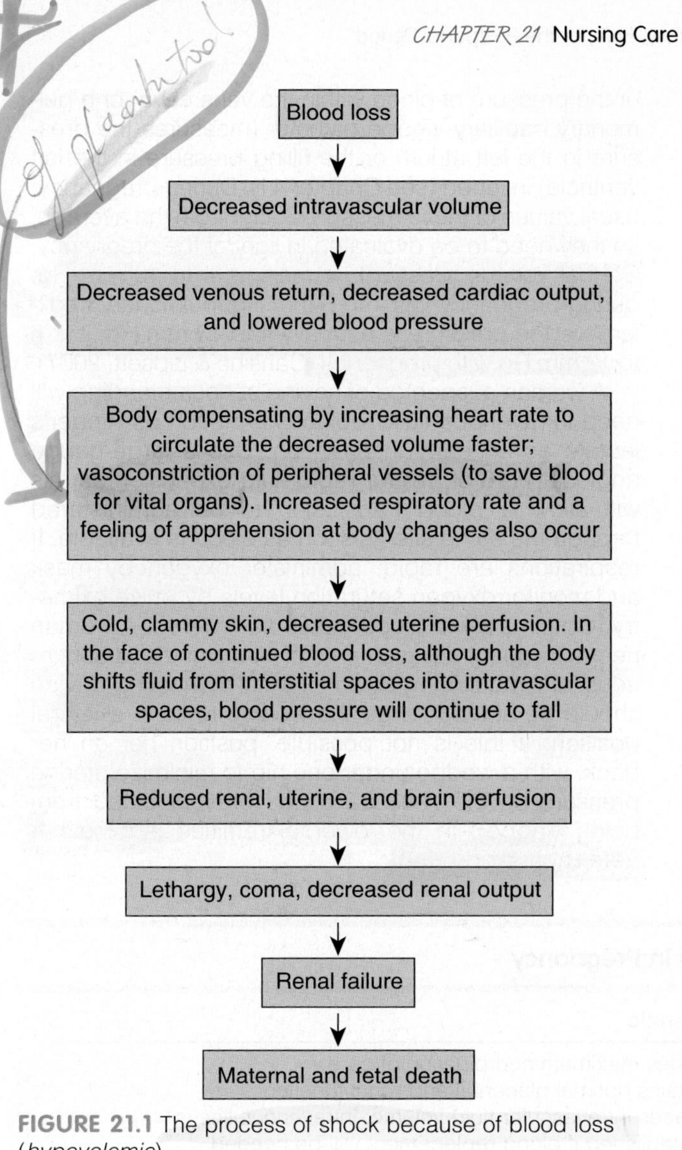

FIGURE 21.1 The process of shock because of blood loss (*hypovolemia*).

Box 21.2 Assessment
Assessing a Pregnant Woman With Hypovolemic Shock

Confusion
Pallor
Increased pulse
Tachypnea
Decreased blood pressure
Decreased cardiac output
Fetal bradycardia
Peripheral vasoconstriction (placenta reacts as a peripheral organ)
Decreased urinary output
Cold extremities

hypovolemic shock processes begin). Signs of hypovolemic shock (Table 21.2) occur when 10% of blood volume, or approximately 2 units of blood, have been lost; fetal distress occurs when 25% of blood volume is lost (Box 21.2). Because "normal" blood pressure varies from woman to woman, it is important to know the baseline blood pressure for a pregnant woman when evaluating for shock. Inform women of their blood pressure at prenatal visits; for example, "Your blood pressure is 110 over 70—that's normal," not just "Your pressure is normal." Then if blood loss should occur, a woman can supply her baseline pressure.

TABLE 21.2 ✻ Signs and Symptoms of Hypovolemic Shock

Assessment	Significance
Increased pulse rate	Heart is attempting to circulate decreased blood volume
Decreased blood pressure	Less peripheral resistance because of decreased blood volume
Increased respiratory rate	Increases gas exchange to better oxygenate decreased red blood cell volume
Cold, clammy skin	Vasoconstriction occurs to maintain blood volume in central body core
Decreased urine output	Inadequate blood is entering kidneys because of decreased blood volume
Dizziness or decreased level of consciousness	Inadequate blood is reaching cerebrum because of decreased blood volume
Decreased central venous pressure	Decreased blood is returning to heart because of reduced blood volume

Nursing Diagnoses and Related Interventions

Nursing Diagnosis: Risk for deficient fluid volume related to bleeding during pregnancy

Outcome Evaluation: Client's blood pressure is maintained at above 100/60 mm Hg; pulse rate is below 100 beats per minute (bpm); only minimal bleeding is apparent; fetal heart rate is maintained at 120 to 160 bpm, with adequate short-term and long-term variability; urine output is greater than 30 mL/hr.

Therapy for hypovolemic shock is aimed at restoring blood volume and halting the source of hemorrhage (Table 21.3). Monitoring urine output is a good gauge of blood loss because kidneys need sufficient arterial blood flow and pressure to function. If they are not producing urine, it suggests that they are not obtaining adequate blood. If the blood deficit continues so blood cannot reach other major organs, multiorgan failure can result (Dambro, 2008). Obtaining hemoglobin and hematocrit levels and securing a blood sample for typing or cross-matching are essential to help not only predict the extent of blood loss but prepare for blood replacement. A woman may have a central venous pressure catheter (measurement of right atrial pressure or the pressure of blood within the vena cava) or a pulmonary capillary wedge catheter (measures the pressure in the left atrium or the filling pressure in the left ventricle) inserted (see Chapter 41). During pregnancy, usual values of these measures differ from the average, so they need to be evaluated in light of the pregnancy. Central venous pressure normally is 4 to 10 mm Hg; during pregnancy it is 1 to 6 mm Hg; pulmonary capillary wedge pressure is normally 4 to 12 mm Hg; it is 6 to 12 mm Hg with pregnancy (Cansino & Lipsett, 2007).

A woman suspected of having serious bleeding will need intravenous fluid replacement such as Ringer's lactate as an early intervention. Use a large-gauge angiocath (16 or 18) for rapid fluid expansion as this will allow a blood transfusion to be administered through the same site as soon as blood is available. If respirations are rapid, administer oxygen by mask and monitor oxygen saturation levels by pulse oximetry. Obtain arterial blood gases as ordered. A woman needs frequent assessments of vital signs and continuous fetal monitoring by an external monitoring device should be started. Urge the woman to lie in a lateral position. If this is not possible, position her on her back, with a wedge under one hip to minimize uterine pressure on the vena cava and prevent blood from being trapped in the lower extremities (supine hypotension syndrome).

TABLE 21.3 * Emergency Interventions for Bleeding in Pregnancy

Intervention	Rationale
Alert health care team of emergency situation.	Provides maximum coordination of care
Place woman flat in bed on her side.	Maintains optimal placental and renal function
Begin intravenous fluid such as lactated Ringer's with a 16- or 18-gauge angiocath.	Replaces intravascular fluid volume; intravenous line is established if blood replacement will be needed
Administer oxygen as necessary at 6–10 L/min by face mask.	Provides adequate fetal oxygenation despite lowered maternal circulating blood volume
Monitor uterine contractions and fetal heart rate by external monitor.	Assesses whether labor is present and fetal status; external system avoids cervical trauma
Omit vaginal examination.	Prevents tearing of placenta if placenta previa is cause of bleeding
Withhold oral fluid.	Anticipates need for emergency surgery
Order type and cross-match of 2 units whole blood.	Allows for restoring circulating maternal blood volume if needed
Measure intake and output.	Enables assessment of renal function (will decrease to under 30 mL/hour with massive circulating volume loss)
Assess vital signs (pulse, respirations, and blood pressure every 15 min; apply pulse oximeter and automatic blood pressure cuff as necessary).	Provides baseline data on maternal response to blood loss
Assist with placement of central venous pressure or pulmonary artery catheter and blood determinations.	Provides more accurate data on maternal hemodynamic state
Measure maternal blood loss by weighing perineal pads; save any tissue passed.	Provides objective evidence of amount of bleeding. Saturating a sanitary pad in less than 1 hour is heavy blood loss; tissue may be abnormal trophoblast tissue.
Set aside 5 mL of blood drawn intravenously in a clean test tube; observe in 5 min for clot formation.	Tests for possible blood coagulation problem (disseminated intravascular coagulation; suspect this if no clot forms within time limit)
Assist with ultrasound examination.	Supplies information on placental and fetal well-being
Maintain a positive attitude about fetal outcome.	Supports mother–child bonding
Support woman's self-esteem; provide emotional support to woman and her support person.	Assists problem solving, which is lessened by poor self-esteem.

Spontaneous Miscarriage

Abortion is the medical term for any interruption of a pregnancy before a fetus is viable (able to survive outside the uterus if born at that time). A viable fetus is usually defined as a fetus of more than 20 to 24 weeks of gestation or one that weighs at least 500 g. A fetus born before this point is considered a miscarriage or premature or immature birth (Cootauco & Althaus, 2007).

Elective abortion, discussed in Chapter 6, is the planned medical termination of a pregnancy. When the interruption occurs spontaneously, it is clearer to refer to it as a **miscarriage.**

Spontaneous miscarriage occurs in 15% to 30% of all pregnancies and arises from natural causes (Uzelac & Garmel, 2007). A spontaneous miscarriage is an early miscarriage if it occurs before week 16 of pregnancy and a late miscarriage if it occurs between weeks 16 and 24. For the first 6 weeks of pregnancy, the developing placenta is tentatively attached to the decidua of the uterus; during weeks 6 to 12, a moderate degree of attachment to the myometrium is present. After week 12, the attachment is penetrating and deep. Because of the degrees of attachment achieved at different weeks of pregnancy, it is important to attempt to establish the week of the pregnancy at which bleeding has become apparent. Bleeding before week 6 is rarely severe; bleeding after week 12 can be profuse because the placenta is implanted so deeply. Fortunately, at this time, with such deep placental implantation, the fetus tends to be expelled as in natural childbirth before the placenta separates. Uterine contractions then help to control placental bleeding as it does postpartally. For some women, then, the stage of attachment between weeks 6 and 12 can lead to the most severe, even life-threatening, bleeding.

Causes of Spontaneous Miscarriage

The most frequent cause of miscarriage in the first trimester of pregnancy is abnormal fetal development, due either to a teratogenic factor or to a chromosomal aberration. Between 50% and 80% of fetuses aborted early have structural abnormalities (Crombleholme, 2009). In other miscarriages, immunologic factors may be present or rejection of the embryo through an immune response may occur.

Another common cause of early miscarriage involves implantation abnormalities, as up to 50% of zygotes probably never implant securely because of inadequate endometrial formation or from an inappropriate site of implantation. With inadequate implantation, the placental circulation does not develop adequately, leading to poor fetal nutrition.

Miscarriage may also occur if the corpus luteum on the ovary fails to produce enough progesterone to maintain the decidua basalis. Progesterone therapy may be attempted to prevent this if this cause is documented (Ruis & Altman, 2007).

Systemic infection in a woman may be yet another cause of miscarriage. Rubella, syphilis, poliomyelitis, cytomegalovirus, and toxoplasmosis infections readily cross the placenta. Urinary tract infections are also associated with miscarriage. With an infection, if the fetus fails to grow, estrogen and progesterone production by the placenta falls. This leads to endometrial sloughing. With the sloughing, prostaglandins are released, leading to uterine contraction and cervical dilatation along with expulsion of the products of the pregnancy.

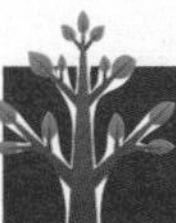

BOX 21.3 * Focus on Family Teaching

Coping With a Spontaneous Miscarriage

Q. Beverly Muzuki tells you, "I had a miscarriage when I was younger, but my doctor called it an abortion. What is the difference?"

A. *Abortion* is the medical term for any pregnancy loss before a fetus is mature enough to live outside the uterus. Think of the word as interchangeable with *miscarriage.*

Q. Did I do something wrong to cause the miscarriage?

A. Early miscarriage is largely not preventable, because it is caused by such things as abnormal chromosome formation or poor uterine implantation—things over which you have no control. Eating a nutritious diet, so you enter a pregnancy in good health, and avoiding cigarette smoking or drinking alcohol are sensible recommendations to reduce your risk of miscarriage. If you had extensive blood loss with your miscarriage, be certain to eat iron-rich foods (such as meat and green vegetables) to help restore red blood cells for a second pregnancy.

Ingestion of a teratogenic drug is still another cause. For example, isotretinoin (Accutane), a drug commonly prescribed for adolescent acne, if taken early in pregnancy, can lead to miscarriage or fetal abnormality (Karch, 2009). Ingestion of alcohol at the time of conception may also be linked to early pregnancy loss from abnormal fetal growth (Thilo & Rosenberg, 2008).

Because miscarriage can occur from so many causes and because the cause is unlikely to be determined with an early miscarriage, couples may have difficulty understanding why it happened to them (Box 21.3).

Assessment

The presenting symptom of spontaneous miscarriage is almost always vaginal spotting. At the first indication of this, a woman should telephone her health care provider and describe what is happening. Because a nurse often takes this initial call, nurses need to be aware of guidelines for assessing vaginal bleeding quickly during pregnancy (Table 21.4).

The history of the episode is important to help a physician or nurse-midwife diagnose the cause. Knowledge of a woman's actions is important to ensure she did not attempt to self-abort. She may prefer not to mention such an attempt but usually will if asked directly. Ask what she has done about the bleeding to be certain that she has not inserted a tampon to stop vaginal bleeding. If she has, although reporting only slight spotting, she actually has an unknown amount of blood loss and might be bleeding much more heavily than she first reports.

TABLE 21.4 ✻ Immediate Assessment of Vaginal Bleeding During Pregnancy

Assessment Factor	Specific Questions to Ask
Confirmation of pregnancy	Does the woman know for certain that she is pregnant (positive pregnancy test or physician/nurse-midwife confirmation)? A woman who has been pregnant before and states that she is sure she is pregnant is probably right, even if she has not yet had this confirmed.
Pregnancy length	What is the length of the pregnancy in weeks?
Duration	How long did the bleeding episode last? Is it continuing?
Intensity	How much bleeding occurred? (Ask the woman to compare it to a common measure [e.g., a tablespoon, a cup].)
Description	Was blood mixed with amniotic fluid or mucus? Was it bright red (fresh blood) or dark (old blood)? Was it accompanied by tissue fragments? Was it odorous?
Frequency	Steady spotting? A single episode?
Associated symptoms	Cramping? Sharp pain? Dull pain? Has she ever had cervical surgery?
Action	What was happening when the bleeding started? What has she done (if anything) to control bleeding?
Blood type	Does she know this? (Rh-negative women will need Rh immune globulin to prevent Rh isoimmunization.)

Therapeutic Management

Depending on the symptoms and the description of the bleeding a woman gives, the physician or nurse-midwife will decide whether she needs to be seen by a health care provider and, if so, whether she should be seen in an ambulatory setting or the hospital.

Threatened Miscarriage

Symptoms of a *threatened miscarriage* begin as vaginal bleeding, initially only scant and usually bright red. A woman may notice slight cramping, but no cervical dilatation is present on vaginal examination. A woman with an apparent threatened miscarriage may be asked to come to the clinic or office to have fetal heart sounds assessed or an ultrasound performed to evaluate the viability of the fetus. Blood for human chorionic gonadotropin hormone (hCG) may be drawn at the start of bleeding and again in 48 hours (if the placenta is still intact, the level in the bloodstream should double in this time). If it does not double, poor placental function is suspected. Avoidance of strenuous activity for 24 to 48 hours is the key intervention, assuming the threatened miscarriage involves a live fetus and presumed placental bleeding. Complete bed rest is usually not necessary. Bed rest may stop the vaginal bleeding but only because blood is pooling vaginally. When a woman does ambulate again, the vaginal blood collection will drain and bleeding will recur.

Women are apt to be extremely worried at the sight of bleeding. They need to talk with a sympathetic, supportive person about how distressed they feel. Be certain to convey concerned assurance that miscarriages happen spontaneously, not because of anything a woman did. Women with threatened miscarriages look for reasons why this could have happened, such as running up a flight of stairs, forgetting to take an iron pill, or getting angry with an older child. Being told that none of these events causes miscarriage can help to minimize the guilt that many women feel.

Most women are disappointed to learn that there is no cure to "hold the pregnancy." In the past, estrogen in the form of diethylstilbestrol (DES) was prescribed for this purpose, but there is no conclusive evidence that this helped, and because DES could be teratogenic, this practice is no longer advocated.

If the spotting with threatened miscarriage is going to stop, it usually does so within 24 to 48 hours after a woman reduces her activity. Once bleeding stops, she can gradually resume normal activities. Coitus is usually restricted for 2 weeks after the bleeding episode to prevent infection and to avoid inducing further bleeding.

As many as 50% of women with a threatened miscarriage continue the pregnancy; for the other 50%, unfortunately, the threatened miscarriage changes to imminent or inevitable miscarriage.

Imminent (Inevitable) Miscarriage

A threatened miscarriage becomes an imminent (inevitable) miscarriage if uterine contractions and cervical dilation occur. With cervical dilation, the loss of the products of conception cannot be halted. A woman who reports cramping or uterine contractions is usually asked to come to the hospital or office, where she is examined. She should save any tissue fragments she has passed and bring them with her so they can be examined. If no fetal heart sounds are detected and an ultrasound reveals an empty uterus or nonviable fetus, a physician may perform a vacuum extraction (dilation and evacuation [D&E]) to ensure that all the products of conception are removed (Uzelac & Garmel, 2007). Be certain the woman has been told that the pregnancy was already lost and that all procedures, such as suction curettage, are to clean the uterus and prevent further complications such as infection, not to end the pregnancy. Save any tissue fragments passed in the labor room, along with any brought from home, so they can be examined for an abnormality such as gestational trophoblastic disease (hydatidiform mole; see later) or for assurance that all the products of conception have been removed from the uterus. After a woman is discharged following the D&E, a woman should assess vaginal bleeding by recording the number of pads she uses. Saturating more than one pad per hour is abnormally heavy bleeding.

Complete Miscarriage

In a complete miscarriage, the entire products of conception (fetus, membranes, and placenta) are expelled spontaneously without any assistance. The bleeding usually slows within 2 hours and then ceases within a few days after passage of the products of conception.

Incomplete Miscarriage

In an incomplete miscarriage, part of the conceptus (usually the fetus) is expelled, but the membrane or placenta is retained in the uterus. The term "incomplete" can be confusing for women. They may interpret it to mean that because the miscarriage is incomplete, the pregnancy will continue. Be careful not to encourage false hopes by also misinterpreting this term.

In an incomplete miscarriage, there is a danger of maternal hemorrhage as long as part of the conceptus is retained in the uterus because the uterus cannot contract effectively under this condition. The physician will usually perform a dilation and curettage (D&C) or suction curettage to evacuate the remainder of the pregnancy from the uterus. Be certain a woman knows that the pregnancy is already lost and that this procedure is being done only to protect her from hemorrhage and infection, not to end the pregnancy.

Missed Miscarriage

In a missed miscarriage, also commonly referred to as **early pregnancy failure,** the fetus dies in utero but is not expelled. Women may also find this term misleading because it suggests that if a miscarriage is "missed," then the pregnancy can continue. A missed miscarriage is usually discovered at a prenatal examination when the fundal height is measured and no increase in size can be demonstrated or when previously heard fetal heart sounds cannot be heard. A woman may have had symptoms of a threatened miscarriage (painless vaginal bleeding), or she may have had no prior clinical symptoms.

An ultrasound can establish the fetus has died. Often the embryo actually died 4 to 6 weeks before the onset of miscarriage symptoms or failure of growth was noted. After the ultrasound, most commonly a D&E will be done. If the pregnancy is over 14 weeks, labor may be induced by a prostaglandin suppository or misoprostol (Cytotec) to dilate the cervix, followed by oxytocin stimulation or administration of mifepristone techniques used for elective termination of pregnancy (Uzelac & Garmel, 2007). If the pregnancy is not actively terminated, miscarriage usually occurs spontaneously within 2 weeks. There is a danger of allowing this normal course to happen, however, because disseminated intravascular coagulation (DIC), a coagulation defect, may develop if the dead (and possibly toxic) fetus remains too long in utero (Linker, 2009).

Most women hope, until the moment the ultrasound shows that their fetus is dead, that their baby is alive. They may need support in accepting the reality of the situation (Box 21.4) and need counseling to accept a future pregnancy because of fears that they may never be able to carry a baby to full term.

Box 21.4 * Focus on Communication

Beverly's neighbor noticed some vaginal spotting at 10 weeks into her pregnancy. The bleeding stopped spontaneously but her doctor was unable to hear fetal heart tones. An ultrasound revealed a missed miscarriage. You talk to her neighbor after she has received this news.

Less Effective Communication

Nurse: Hello, Vivian. All right if I take your temperature and pulse?

Vivian: I'm sure they're fine. I feel fine.

Nurse: I'm sorry that this happened. It must be upsetting.

Vivian: The bleeding was scary. Made me really nervous that something was wrong with the baby.

Nurse: Bleeding is always scary. I hate to see it.

Vivian: All I want to do now is get this surgery over with so I can get on with having a baby.

Nurse: That's the advantage of being young. There's lots of time for babies. Both temperature and pulse are good. You were right—you are fine.

More Effective Communication

Nurse: Hello, Vivian. All right if I take your temperature and pulse?

Vivian: I'm sure they're fine. I feel fine.

Nurse: I'm sorry this happened. It must be upsetting.

Vivian: The bleeding was scary. Made me really nervous that something was wrong with the baby.

Nurse: Did the doctor talk to you about what she thought the bleeding meant? Or what the ultrasound showed?

Vivian: She said I missed having a miscarriage. I feel really lucky for that.

Nurse: I'll ask your doctor to re-explain what she meant by a missed miscarriage. That term can be confusing.

Because many women want so badly to be pregnant, it can be easy for them to "miss" bad news about a pregnancy. In the above scenario, the nurse was so intent on chatting that she failed to realize her client was misinformed. Better listening skills in the second example revealed a serious misunderstanding of what "missed miscarriage" means.

Recurrent Pregnancy Loss

In the past, women who had three spontaneous miscarriages that occurred at the same gestational age were called "habitual aborters." They were advised they were apparently too "nervous" or that something was so wrong with their hormones that childbearing was not for them. Today, the term **recurrent pregnancy loss** is used to describe this miscarriage pattern, and a thorough investigation is done to discover the cause of the loss and help ensure the outcome of a future pregnancy. Recurrent pregnancy loss occurs in about 1% of women who want to be pregnant. Although many losses occur for unknown reasons, possible causes include:

- Defective spermatozoa or ova
- Endocrine factors such as lowered levels of protein-bound iodine (PBI), butanol-extractable iodine (BEI), and globulin-bound iodine (GBI); poor thyroid function; or luteal phase defect
- Deviations of the uterus, such as septate or bicornuate uterus

- Resistance to uterine artery blood flow
- Chorioamnionitis or uterine infection
- Autoimmune disorders such as those involving lupus anticoagulant and antiphospholipid antibodies (Ruis & Altman, 2007)

Complications of Miscarriage

As with full-term childbirth, hemorrhage and infection are two of the most likely complications after miscarriage. The risk for Rh isoimmunization and a woman's psychological state also need to be considered.

Hemorrhage. With a complete spontaneous miscarriage, serious or fatal hemorrhage is rare. With an incomplete miscarriage or in a woman who develops an accompanying coagulation defect (usually DIC), major hemorrhage is a possibility. Monitor vital signs for changes to detect possible hypovolemic shock. If excessive vaginal bleeding is occurring, immediately position a woman flat and massage the uterine fundus to try to aid contraction (see Chapter 17). This may be impossible with an early pregnancy because the small uterus is not palpable above the symphysis pubis. A woman may need a D&C or suction curettage to empty the uterus of the material that is preventing it from contracting and achieving hemostasis. A transfusion may be necessary to replace blood loss. Direct replacement of fibrinogen or another clotting factor may be used to increase coagulation ability.

After a self-limiting complete miscarriage, a woman needs clear instructions on how much bleeding is abnormal (more than one sanitary pad per hour is excessive) and what color changes she should expect in bleeding (gradually changing to a dark color and then to the color of serous fluid as it does with the postpartum woman). She should know that any unusual odor or passing of large clots is also abnormal. If her physician has prescribed an oral medication such as oral methylergonovine maleate (Methergine) to aid uterine contraction, be certain she understands why it is being prescribed and the importance of taking it. Some women repress their feelings, anxious to forget the experience as quickly as possible. Repression helps them to handle their anger or grief at the loss of the pregnancy. Be careful that in repressing the experience, however, a woman does not also repress the memory of her medication and leave herself open to hemorrhage.

Infection. The possibility of infection is minimal when pregnancy loss occurs over a short time, bleeding is self-limiting, and instrumentation is limited. However, there is always a possibility it may occur.

Infection tends to develop in women who have lost appreciable amounts of blood. Such women need especially close observation to rule out this second and possibly fatal complication.

After a miscarriage, be certain a woman knows the danger signs of infection, such as fever, abdominal pain or tenderness, and a foul vaginal discharge. Fever can be a transient reaction to a period of decreased fluid intake that preceded the miscarriage. In other instances, the fever may be a systemic reaction to the miscarriage process. All temperatures higher than 100.4° F (38.0° C) require careful evaluation of avoid overlooking the possibility that infection is developing.

The organism responsible for infection after miscarriage is usually *Escherichia coli* (spread from the rectum forward into the vagina). Caution a woman to wipe her perineal area from front to back after voiding and particularly after defecation to prevent the spread of bacteria from the rectal area. Caution her not to use tampons to control vaginal discharge, because stasis of any body fluid increases the risk of infection. Be careful about using statements such as, "You'll have some vaginal flow now, almost exactly like a menstrual flow." Otherwise, a woman might treat it as a menstrual period and use tampons.

If infection occurs, endometritis (infection of the uterine lining) is the type that usually occurs. It may be more extensive, however, and parametritis, peritonitis, thrombophlebitis, and septicemia can develop. The management of these infections is the same as if they were occurring after the safe birth of a child, so they are discussed in Chapter 25.

Septic Abortion. A septic abortion is an abortion that is complicated by infection (Uzelac & Garmel, 2007). Infection can occur after a spontaneous miscarriage, but more frequently it occurs in women who have tried to self-abort or were aborted illegally using a nonsterile instrument such as a knitting needle. Because the uterus is a warm, moist, dark cavity, infectious organisms, once introduced, grow rapidly in this environment, particularly if products of conception such as necrotic membranes are still present.

A woman has symptoms of fever and crampy abdominal pain, and her uterus feels tender to palpation. Left untreated, such an infection can lead to toxic shock syndrome, septicemia, kidney failure, and death (Vasquez et al., 2007).

Women with septic abortion need immediate, intensive assessment and treatment. Typically, complete blood count, serum electrolytes, serum creatinine, blood type and crossmatch, and cervical, vaginal, and urine cultures are obtained. An indwelling urinary (Foley) catheter may be inserted to monitor urine output hourly to assess kidney function. Intravenous fluid to restore fluid volume and to provide a route for high-dose, broad-spectrum antibiotic therapy is started. A combination of penicillin (gram-positive coverage), gentamicin (gram-negative aerobic coverage), and clindamycin (gram-negative anaerobic coverage) is commonly used.

A central venous pressure or pulmonary artery catheter may be inserted to monitor left atrial filling pressure and hemodynamic status. The removal of all infected or necrotic tissue from the uterus is important, so a D&C or D&E will be performed. Tetanus toxoid given subcutaneously or tetanus immune globulin given intramuscularly will be prescribed for prophylaxis against tetanus.

Infection following a septic abortion can be so severe that a woman needs to be admitted to an intensive care setting for continuing care. Dopamine and digitalis may be necessary to maintain sufficient cardiac output. Oxygen and perhaps ventilatory support may be necessary to maintain respiratory function.

Assuming a woman recovers from such an intense episode, septic abortion may lead to infertility because of uterine scarring or fibrotic scarring of the fallopian tubes. If a woman caused the infection by trying to self-abort, she needs follow-up counseling to assist her to learn better problem-solving methods for the future.

Isoimmunization. Whenever a placenta is dislodged, either by spontaneous birth or by a D&C at any point in pregnancy, some blood from the placental villi (the fetal blood) may enter the maternal circulation. If the fetus was Rh positive and the woman is Rh negative, enough Rh-positive fetal blood may enter the maternal circulation to cause **isoimmunization**—the production of antibodies against Rh-positive blood. If the woman's next child should have Rh-positive blood, these antibodies would attempt to destroy the red blood cells of this infant during the months that infant is in utero (Crowther & Middleton, 2009).

After a miscarriage, because the blood type of the conceptus is unknown, all women with Rh-negative blood should receive Rh (D antigen) immune globulin (RhIG) to prevent the buildup of antibodies in the event the conceptus was Rh positive.

Powerlessness or Anxiety. As with pregnancy loss for any reason, assess a woman's adjustment to a spontaneous miscarriage. Sadness and grief over the loss or a feeling that a woman has lost control of her life is to be expected. Do not forget to assess a partner's feelings as well, or that person's grief over the pregnancy loss can be missed.

Spontaneous miscarriage can be particularly heartbreaking for an older woman, because she realizes that her window of childbearing is limited.

✔ Checkpoint Question 21.1

Beverly Muzuki, the woman you met at the beginning of the chapter, had a miscarriage when she was younger. What would be the best advice to give a woman who tells you she is miscarrying?

a. Lie down and do not move for 24 hours to stop the bleeding.
b. Do not do anything special; early miscarriages happen all the time.
c. Save any clots or material passed for your health care provider.
d. Use a tight tampon to put pressure on your cervix and stop the bleeding.

Ectopic Pregnancy

An **ectopic pregnancy** is one in which implantation occurs outside the uterine cavity. The implantation may occur on the surface of the ovary or in the cervix. The most common site (in approximately 95% of such pregnancies) is in a fallopian tube (Fig. 21.2). Of these fallopian tube sites, approximately 80% occur in the ampullar portion, 12% occur in the isthmus, and 8% are interstitial or fimbrial (Yates & King, 2007).

With ectopic pregnancy, fertilization occurs as usual in the distal third of the fallopian tube. Immediately after the union of ovum and spermatozoon, the zygote begins to divide and grow. Unfortunately, because an obstruction is present, such as an adhesion of the fallopian tube from a previous infection (chronic salpingitis or pelvic inflammatory disease), congenital malformations, scars from tubal surgery, or a uterine tumor pressing on the proximal end of the tube, the zygote cannot travel the length of the tube. It lodges at a strictured site along the tube and implants there instead of in the uterus.

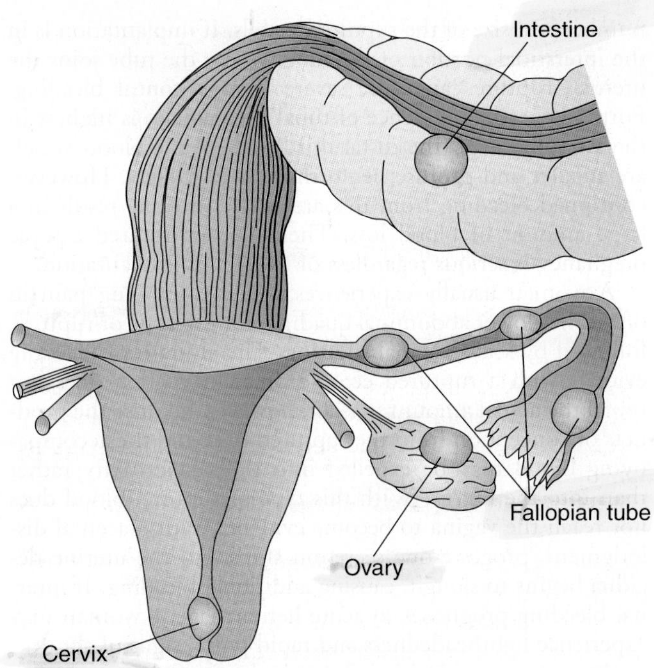

FIGURE 21.2 Sites at which an ectopic pregnancy may occur.

Approximately 2% of pregnancies are ectopic; it is the second most frequent cause of bleeding early in pregnancy. The incidence is increasing because of the increasing rate of pelvic inflammatory disease, which leads to tubal scarring. It occurs more frequently in women who smoke compared with those who do not. There is some evidence that intrauterine devices (IUDs) used for contraception may slow the transport of the zygote and lead to an increased incidence of tubal or ovarian implantation. The incidence also increases following in vitro fertilization. Women who have one ectopic pregnancy have a 10% to 20% chance that a subsequent pregnancy will also be ectopic. This is because salpingitis that leaves scarring is usually bilateral. Congenital anomalies such as webbing (fibrous bands) that block a fallopian tube may also be bilateral. For unknown reasons, oral contraceptives used before pregnancy reduce the incidence of ectopic pregnancy (Burkman, 2007).

Assessment

With ectopic pregnancy, there are no unusual symptoms at the time of implantation. The corpus luteum of the ovary continues to function as if the implantation were in the uterus. No menstrual flow occurs. A woman may experience the nausea and vomiting of early pregnancy, and a pregnancy test for hCG will be positive. Many ectopic pregnancies are diagnosed by an early pregnancy ultrasound. Magnetic resonance imaging (MRI) is also effective to use for this.

If not revealed by an ultrasound, at weeks 6 to 12 of pregnancy (2 to 8 weeks after a missed menstrual period), the zygote grows large enough to rupture the slender fallopian tube or the trophoblast cells actually break through the narrow base. Tearing and destruction of the blood vessels in the tube result. The extent of the bleeding that occurs depends on the number and size of the ruptured vessels. If implantation is in the interstitial portion of the tube (where the tube joins the uterus), rupture can cause severe intraperitoneal bleeding. Fortunately, the incidence of tubal pregnancies is highest in the ampullar area (the distal third), where the blood vessels are smaller and profuse hemorrhage is less likely. However, continued bleeding from this area may, in time, result in a large amount of blood loss. Therefore, a ruptured ectopic pregnancy is serious regardless of the site of implantation.

A woman usually experiences a sharp, stabbing pain in one of her lower abdominal quadrants at the time of rupture, followed by scant vaginal spotting. The amount of bleeding evident with a ruptured ectopic pregnancy often does not reveal the actual amount present, however, because the products of conception from the ruptured tube and the accompanying blood may be expelled into the pelvic cavity rather than into the uterus. With this type of rupture, blood does not reach the vagina to become evident. With placental dislodgment, progesterone secretion stops and the uterine decidua begins to slough, causing additional bleeding. If internal bleeding progresses to acute hemorrhage, a woman may experience lightheadedness and rapid pulse, signs of shock.

Any woman with sharp abdominal pain and vaginal spotting needs to be evaluated by her health care provider to rule out the possibility of ectopic pregnancy. When helping determine the possibility of an ectopic pregnancy, ask a woman whether she has pain or vaginal bleeding. Occasionally, a woman will move suddenly and pull one of her round ligaments, the anterior uterine supports. This can cause a sharp, but momentary and innocent, lower quadrant pain. However, it would be rare for this phenomenon to be reported in connection with vaginal spotting.

By the time a woman with a ruptured ectopic pregnancy arrives at the hospital or physician's office, she may already be in severe shock, as evidenced by a rapid, thready pulse, rapid respirations, and falling blood pressure. Leukocytosis may be present, not from infection but from the trauma. Temperature is usually normal. A transvaginal ultrasound will demonstrate the ruptured tube and blood collecting in the peritoneum. Either a falling hCG or serum progesterone level suggests that the pregnancy has ended. If the diagnosis of ectopic pregnancy is in doubt, a physician may insert a needle through the posterior vaginal fornix into the cul-de-sac under sterile conditions to see whether blood can be aspirated. A laparoscopy or culdoscopy can be used to visualize the fallopian tube if the symptoms alone do not reveal a clear picture of what has happened. However, ultrasonography alone usually reveals a clear-cut diagnostic picture (Yates & King, 2007).

If a woman waits for a time before seeking help, gradually her abdomen becomes rigid from peritoneal irritation. Her umbilicus may develop a bluish tinge (Cullen's sign). A woman may have continuing extensive or dull vaginal and abdominal pain; movement of the cervix on pelvic examination may cause excruciating pain. There may be pain in her shoulders from blood in the peritoneal cavity causing irritation to the phrenic nerve. A tender mass is usually palpable in Douglas' cul-de-sac on vaginal examination.

Therapeutic Management

Some ectopic pregnancies spontaneously end before they rupture and are reabsorbed over the next few days, requiring no treatment. It is difficult to predict when this will happen, so when an ectopic pregnancy is revealed by an early ultrasound, some action is taken. An unruptured ectopic pregnancy can be treated medically by the oral administration of methotrexate followed by leucovorin (Hajenius et al., 2009). Methotrexate, a folic acid antagonist chemotherapeutic agent, attacks and destroys fast-growing cells. Because trophoblast and zygote growth is so rapid, the drug is drawn to the site of the ectopic pregnancy (see Chapter 53 for a general discussion of chemotherapy agents of this type). Women are treated until a negative hCG titer is achieved. A hysterosalpingogram or ultrasound is usually performed after the chemotherapy to assess whether the tube is fully patent. Mifepristone, an abortifacient, is also effective at causing sloughing of the tubal implantation site. The advantage of these therapies is that the tube is left intact, with no surgical scarring that could cause a second ectopic implantation.

If an ectopic pregnancy ruptures, it is an emergency situation (Stevens & Gilbert-Cohen, 2007). Keep in mind the amount of blood evident is a poor estimate of the actual blood loss. A blood sample needs to be drawn immediately for hemoglobin level, typing and cross-matching, and possibly hCG level for immediate pregnancy testing, if pregnancy has not yet been confirmed. Intravenous fluid using a large-gauge catheter to restore intravascular volume is begun. Blood then can be administered through this same line when matched.

The therapy for a ruptured ectopic pregnancy is laparoscopy to ligate the bleeding vessels and to remove or repair the damaged fallopian tube. A rough suture line on a fallopian tube may lead to another tubal pregnancy, so either the tube will be removed or suturing on the tube is done with microsurgical technique.

If a tube is removed, a woman is theoretically only 50% fertile, because every other month, when she ovulates from the ovary next to the removed tube, sperm cannot reach the ovum on that side. However, this is not a reliable contraceptive measure. Research in rabbits has shown that translocation of ova can occur—that is, an ovum released from the right ovary can pass through the pelvic cavity to the opposite (left) fallopian tube and become fertilized, and vice versa.

As with miscarriage, women with Rh-negative blood should receive Rh (D) immune globulin (RhIG) after an ectopic pregnancy for isoimmunization protection in future childbearing.

Nursing Diagnoses and Related Interventions

Nursing Diagnosis: Powerlessness related to early loss of pregnancy secondary to ectopic pregnancy

Outcome Evaluation: Client states she feels sad at pregnancy loss but is able to deal with situation; has returned to previous level of activities and has forward-thinking plans.

A woman who has had an ectopic pregnancy not only has grief stages to work through (she has lost a child) but also may have problems of diminished self-image and a sense of powerlessness to resolve if surgery included removal of a fallopian tube. She may believe that she is now "half a woman" if she equated reproductive structures and childbearing with being feminine. Encourage her to verbalize her concerns about this and future childbearing. The process of working through grief and role images takes weeks to months. It should begin in the hospital, however, where a woman has professional people to help her through the first days and to determine whether she will need further counseling.

Abdominal Pregnancy

Very rarely after an ectopic pregnancy ruptures—so rarely that the instances are difficult to document—the products of conception are expelled into the pelvic cavity with a minimum of bleeding. The placenta continues to grow in the fallopian tube, spreading perhaps into the uterus for a better blood supply; or it may escape into the pelvic cavity and implant on an organ such as an intestine. The fetus will grow in the pelvic cavity (an abdominal pregnancy). This can also occur if a uterus ruptures because an old uterine scar ruptures during pregnancy (Teng, Kumar, & Ramli, 2007).

In an abdominal pregnancy, the fetal outline is easily palpable through the abdomen because it is directly below the abdominal wall, not inside the uterus. A woman may not be as aware of movements as she would be normally, or she may experience painful fetal movements and abdominal cramping with fetal movements.

A woman may report she noticed sudden lower quadrant pain earlier in the pregnancy. An ultrasound or MRI will reveal the fetus outside the uterus.

The danger of abdominal pregnancy is that the placenta will infiltrate and erode a major blood vessel in the abdomen, leading to hemorrhage. If implanted on the intestine, it may erode so deeply that it causes bowel perforation and peritonitis. The fetus is also at high risk because without a good uterine blood supply, nutrients may not reach the fetus in adequate amounts. The survival rate in an abdominal pregnancy is only approximately 60% because of poor nutrient supply. In infants who do survive, there is an increased threat of fetal deformity or growth restriction from an inadequate nutrient supply.

At term, the infant must be born through laparotomy. The placenta is often difficult to remove after birth if it has implanted onto an abdominal organ such as the intestine. It may be left in place, therefore, and allowed to absorb spontaneously in 2 or 3 months. A follow-up ultrasound can be used to detect whether this has occurred, or a woman can be treated with methotrexate to help the placenta absorb. This therapy may not be effective because the remaining trophoblasts are no longer fast-growing.

✓ Checkpoint Question 21.2

Suppose Beverly Muzuki was discovered to have an ectopic pregnancy. What advice would you give her?

a. Most ectopic pregnancies go to completion, although the newborn is small.
b. If she must have a fallopian tube removed, she will be sterile afterward.
c. She will have a continuous nagging pain through the rest of pregnancy.
d. Ectopic pregnancy can be either medically or surgically treated.

Gestational Trophoblastic Disease (Hydatidiform Mole)

Gestational trophoblastic disease is abnormal proliferation and then degeneration of the trophoblastic villi (Garg & Giuntoli, 2007). As the cells degenerate, they become filled with fluid and appear as clear fluid-filled, grape-sized vesicles. The embryo fails to develop beyond a primitive start. Abnormal trophoblast cells must be identified because they are associated with choriocarcinoma, a rapidly metastasizing malignancy (Fig. 21.3).

The incidence of gestational trophoblastic disease is approximately 1 in every 1500 pregnancies. The condition tends to occur most often in women who have a low protein intake, in women older than age 35 years, in women of Asian heritage, and in blood group A women who marry blood group O men (Aghajanian, 2007).

Two types of molar growth can be identified by chromosome analysis. With a *complete mole,* all trophoblastic villi swell and become cystic. If an embryo forms, it dies early at only 1 to 2 mm in size, with no fetal blood present in the villi. On chromosomal analysis, although the karyotype is a normal 46XX or 46XY, this chromosome component was contributed only by the father or an "empty ovum" was fertilized and the chromosome material was duplicated (Fig. 21.4A).

With a *partial mole,* some of the villi form normally. The syncytiotrophoblastic layer of villi, however, is swollen and misshapen. A macerated embryo of approximately 9 weeks' gestation may be present and fetal blood may be present in the villi. A partial mole has 69 chromosomes (a triploid formation in which there are three chromosomes instead of two for every pair, one set supplied by an ovum that apparently was fertilized by two sperm or an ovum fertilized by one sperm in which meiosis or reduction division did not occur). This could also occur if one set of 23 chromosomes was supplied by one sperm and an ovum that did not undergo reduction division supplied 46 (see Fig. 21.4B).

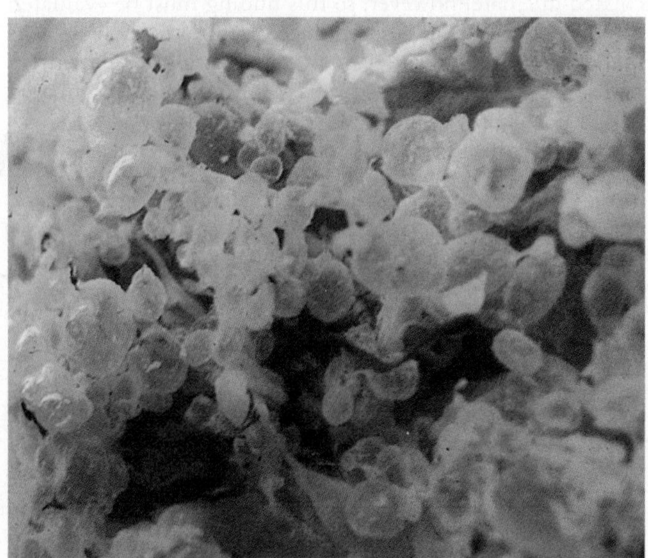

FIGURE 21.3 Gestational trophoblastic disease (hydatidiform mole). (From Rubin, E., & Farber, J. L. [1994]. Pathology [2nd ed.]. Philadelphia: JB Lippincott.)

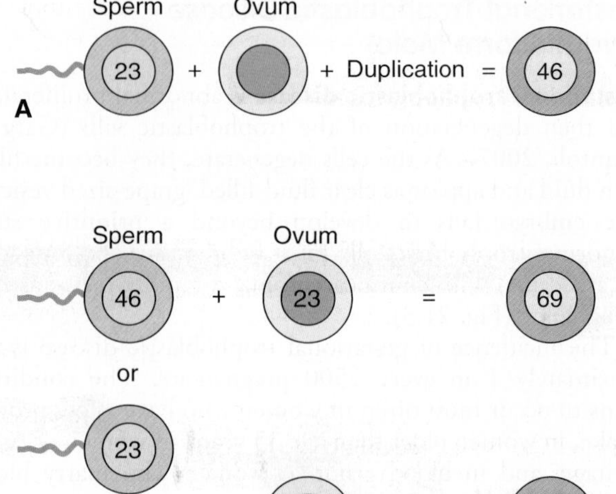

FIGURE 21.4 Formation of gestational trophoblastic disease (hydatidiform mole). (**A**) Complete mole. (**B**) Partial mole.

In contrast to complete moles, partial moles rarely lead to choriocarcinoma. Although still above average, hCG titers are lower in partial than in complete moles; titers also return to normal faster after mole evacuation.

Assessment

Because proliferation of the trophoblast cells occurs so rapidly with this condition, the uterus tends to expand faster than normally. This causes the uterus to reach its landmarks (just over the symphysis brim at 12 weeks, at the umbilicus at 20 to 24 weeks) before the usual time. This rapid development is also diagnostic of multiple pregnancy or a miscalculated due date, however, so this finding must be evaluated carefully. Because hCG is produced by the trophoblast cells that are overgrowing, a serum or urine test of hCG for pregnancy will be strongly positive (1 to 2 million IU compared with a normal pregnancy level of 400,000 IU).

Results continue to be strongly positive after day 100 of pregnancy, when the level of hCG normally would begin to decline. This fact must be evaluated carefully also, however, because highly positive test results can be characteristic of multiple pregnancies with more than one placenta. The nausea and vomiting of early pregnancy is usually marked, probably because of the high hCG level present. Symptoms of pregnancy-induced hypertension such as hypertension, edema, and proteinuria are ordinarily not present before week 20 of pregnancy. With gestational trophoblastic disease, they may appear before this time. An ultrasound will show dense growth (typically a snowflake pattern) but no fetal growth in the uterus. No fetal heart sounds are heard because there is no viable fetus.

At approximately week 16 of pregnancy, if the structure was not identified earlier by ultrasound, it will identify itself with vaginal bleeding. This may begin as spotting of dark-brown blood or as a profuse fresh flow. As the bleeding progresses, it is accompanied by discharge of the clear fluid-filled vesicles. This is why it is important for any woman who begins to miscarry at home to bring any clots or tissue passed to the hospital with her. The presence of clear fluid-filled cysts changes the diagnosis from miscarriage to gestational trophoblastic disease.

Therapeutic Management

Therapy for gestational trophoblastic disease is suction curettage to evacuate the mole.

Following mole extraction, women should have a baseline pelvic examination, a chest radiograph, and a serum test for the beta subunit of hCG. After surgery, hCG levels remain high. Half of women still have a positive reading at 3 weeks; one-fourth still have a positive test result at 40 days. The hCG is then analyzed every 2 weeks until levels are again normal. After that, serum hCG levels are assessed every 4 weeks for the next 6 to 12 months. Gradually declining hCG titers suggest no complication is developing. Levels that plateau for three times or increase suggest that a malignant transformation is occurring. A woman should use a reliable contraceptive method such as an oral contraceptive agent for 12 months so that a positive pregnancy test (the presence of hCG) resulting from a new pregnancy will not be confused with increasing levels and a developing malignancy. After 6 months, if hCG levels are still negative, a woman is theoretically free of the risk of a malignancy developing. By 12 months, she could plan a second pregnancy. Although the development of gestational trophoblastic disease means that a pregnancy never materialized and that a fetus never formed, a woman may experience the same feeling of loss after its evacuation that she would have experienced after the loss of a true pregnancy: she did, after all, believe she was pregnant. In addition, she is faced with the possibility that a malignancy may develop. She also must delay her childbearing plans for a year. If she had already put off having a child for some time, this may seem to be an unbearably long time.

Some physicians give women who have had gestational trophoblastic disease a prophylactic course of methotrexate, the drug of choice for choriocarcinoma. However, because the drug interferes with white blood cell formation (leukopenia), prophylactic use must be weighed carefully. If malignancy should occur, it can be treated effectively in most instances with methotrexate at that time (Garg & Giuntoli, 2007). Dactinomycin is added to the regimen if metastasis occurs.

Women need the opportunity to express their anger and sense of unfairness at this type of event. They may feel inadequate because something went wrong with the pregnancy. They may wonder whether it will happen again or whether they will ever be able to have children. Unfortunately, women who have one incidence of gestational trophoblastic disease have an increased risk of a second molar pregnancy (Aghajanian, 2007). They need early screening with ultrasound during a second pregnancy to be certain this is not happening again.

What if... Beverly Muzuki told you, after having had a gestational trophoblastic disorder, that she did not believe in birth control so she did not intend to take the oral contraceptives prescribed following her mole evacuation? How would you advise her?

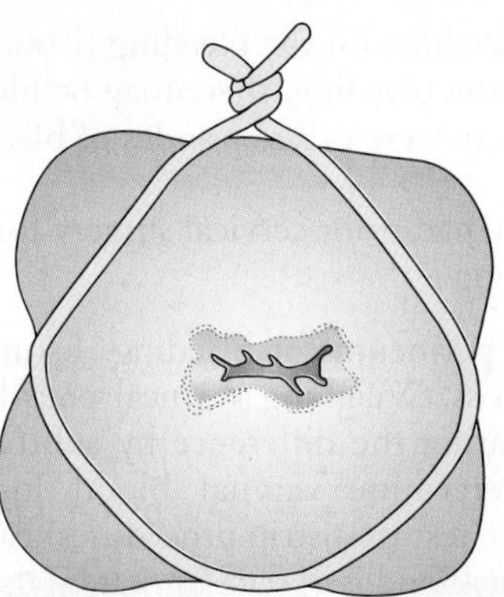

FIGURE 21.5 Shirodkar suture for cervical cerclage.

Premature Cervical Dilatation

Premature cervical dilatation, previously termed an *incompetent cervix,* refers to a cervix that dilates prematurely and therefore cannot hold a fetus until term (Kogan, Ben-Shushan, & Pernoll, 2007). It occurs in about 1% of women. The dilatation is usually painless. Often the first symptom is show (a pink-stained vaginal discharge) or increased pelvic pressure, which may be followed by rupture of the membranes and discharge of the amniotic fluid. Uterine contractions begin, and after a short labor the fetus is born. Unfortunately, this commonly occurs at approximately week 20 of pregnancy, when the fetus is still too immature to survive.

It is often difficult to explain in a particular instance what causes premature dilatation. It is associated with increased maternal age, congenital structural defects, and trauma to the cervix, such as might have occurred with a cone biopsy or repeated D&Cs. Although it may be diagnosed by an early ultrasound before symptoms occur, it is usually diagnosed only after the pregnancy is lost.

After the loss of one child because of premature cervical dilatation, a surgical operation termed **cervical cerclage** can be performed to prevent this from happening in a second pregnancy (Fox & Chervenak, 2008). As soon as an ultrasound confirms that the fetus of a second pregnancy is healthy, at approximately weeks 12 to 14, purse-string sutures are placed in the cervix by the vaginal route under regional anesthesia. This procedure is called a McDonald or a Shirodkar procedure after the surgeons who perfected the technique. The sutures serve to strengthen the cervix and prevent it from dilating (Fig. 21.5).

In a McDonald procedure, nylon sutures are placed horizontally and vertically across the cervix and pulled tight to reduce the cervical canal to a few millimeters in diameter. With a Shirodkar technique, sterile tape is threaded in a purse-string manner under the submucous layer of the cervix and sutured in place to achieve a closed cervix. Although routinely accomplished by a vaginal route, sutures may be placed by a transabdominal route.

With these procedures, the sutures are then removed at weeks 37 to 38 of pregnancy so the fetus can be born vaginally. When a transabdominal approach is used, the sutures may be left in place and a cesarean birth performed.

Women who are discovered to have cervical dilatation but with membranes still intact at a prenatal visit may have emergent cerclage sutures placed in the cervix even at that point as prophylaxis against preterm birth. The success of this procedure is limited, however, compared to preventive suturing. Still newer techniques allow purse-string sutures to be set before a woman becomes pregnant, providing added assurance that she will not begin miscarrying before week 14 of pregnancy.

Be certain to ask women who are reporting painless bleeding (the symptoms of spontaneous miscarriage also) whether they have had past cervical operations, to remind them they may have sutures in place.

Currently, the prognosis for a successful pregnancy after surgical correction for premature cervical dilatation is very favorable. The success rate with both types of cerclage techniques is 80% to 90%. After cerclage surgery, women remain on bed rest (perhaps in a slight or modified Trendelenburg position) for a few days to decrease pressure on the new sutures. Usual activity and sexual relations can be resumed in most instances after this rest period.

Placenta Previa

Placenta previa (Fig. 21.6) is a condition of pregnancy in which the placenta is implanted abnormally in the uterus. It is the most common cause of painless bleeding in the third trimester of pregnancy (Scearce & Uzelac, 2007). It occurs in

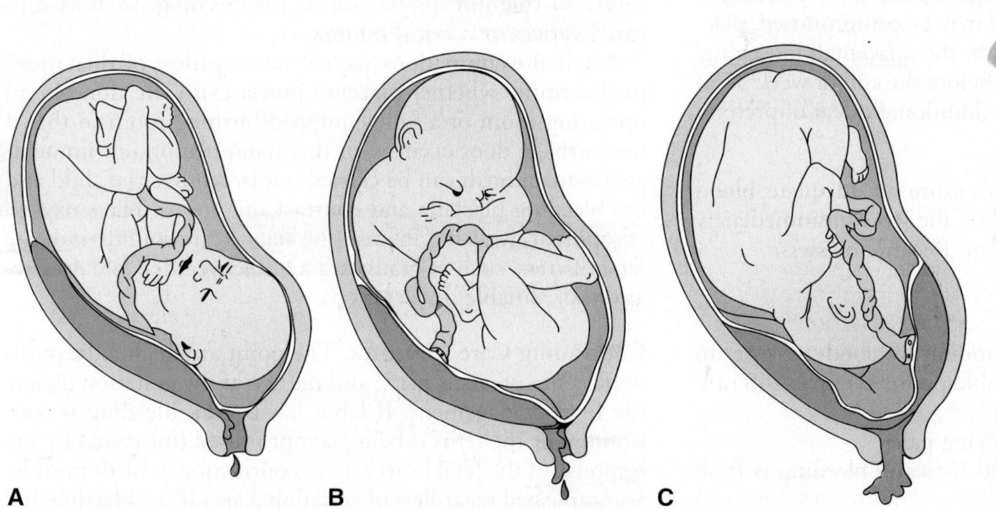

FIGURE 21.6 Degrees of placenta previa: **(A)** low implantation; **(B)** partial placenta previa; **(C)** total placenta previa.

four degrees: implantation in the lower rather than in the upper portion of the uterus (low-lying placenta); marginal implantation (the placenta edge approaches that of the cervical os); implantation that occludes a portion of the cervical os (partial placenta previa); and implantation that totally obstructs the cervical os (total placenta previa). The degree to which the placenta covers the internal cervical os is generally estimated in percentages: 100%, 75%, 30%, and so forth.

Increased parity, advanced maternal age, past cesarean births, past uterine curettage, multiple gestation, and perhaps a male fetus are all associated with placenta previa. The incidence is approximately 5 per 1000 pregnancies. It is thought to occur whenever the placenta is forced to spread to find an adequate exchange surface. An increase in congenital fetal anomalies may occur if the low implantation does not allow optimal fetal nutrition or oxygenation (Arquette & Holcroft, 2007).

Assessment

Because routine ultrasounds are performed so frequently during pregnancy, most instances of placenta previa are diagnosed today before any symptoms occur. Although many low-lying placentas detected on early ultrasounds migrate upward to a noncervical position, the condition is explained to a woman and she is cautioned to avoid coitus, to get adequate rest, and to call her health care provider at any sign of vaginal bleeding. Bleeding with placenta previa begins when the lower uterine segment starts to differentiate from the upper segment late in pregnancy (approximately week 30) and the cervix begins to dilate. The bleeding results from the placenta's inability to stretch to accommodate the differing shape of the lower uterine segment or the cervix. The bleeding that occurs is usually abrupt, painless, bright red, and sudden enough to frighten a woman. It is not associated with increased activity or participation in sports. It may stop as abruptly as it began, so that by the time a woman is seen at the health care site she is no longer bleeding, or it may slow after the initial hemorrhage but continue as continuous spotting.

Therapeutic Management

The bleeding of placenta previa, like that of ectopic pregnancy, is an emergency situation. The site of bleeding, the open vessels of the uterine decidua (maternal blood), places the mother at risk for hemorrhage. Because the placenta is loosened, the fetal oxygen supply may be compromised, placing the fetus at risk also. With the placental loosening, preterm labor (labor that occurs before the end of week 37 of gestation) may begin, posing the additional threat of preterm birth to the fetus.

Immediate Care Measures. To ensure an adequate blood supply to a woman and fetus, place the woman immediately on bed rest in a side-lying position. Be sure to assess:

- Duration of the pregnancy
- Time the bleeding began
- Woman's estimation of the amount of blood—ask her to estimate in terms of cups or tablespoons (a cup is 240 mL; a tablespoon is 15 mL)
- Whether there was accompanying pain
- Color of the blood (red blood indicates bleeding is fresh or is continuing)
- What she has done for the bleeding (if she inserted a tampon to halt the bleeding, there may be hidden bleeding)
- Whether there were prior episodes of bleeding during the pregnancy
- Whether she had prior cervical surgery for premature cervical dilatation

Inspect the perineum for bleeding. Estimate the present rate of blood loss. Weighing perineal pads before and after use and calculating the difference by subtraction is a good method to determine vaginal blood loss. An Apt or Kleihauer-Betke test (test strip procedures) can be used to detect whether the blood is of fetal or maternal origin. *Never* attempt a pelvic or rectal examination with painless bleeding late in pregnancy because any agitation of the cervix when there is a placenta previa may initiate massive hemorrhage, possibly fatal to both mother and child. Obtain baseline vital signs to determine whether symptoms of shock are present. Continue to assess blood pressure every 5 to 15 minutes or continuously with an electronic cuff. Other necessary actions are intravenous fluid therapy using a large-gauge catheter and monitoring urine output frequently, as often as every hour, as an indicator of blood volume adequacy. Attach external monitoring equipment to record fetal heart sounds and uterine contractions. An internal monitor for either fetal or uterine assessment that requires invasion of the cervix, is contraindicated. Hemoglobin, hematocrit, prothrombin time, partial thromboplastin time, fibrinogen, platelet count, type and cross-match, and antibody screen will be assessed to establish baselines, detect a possible clotting disorder, and ready blood for replacement if necessary. Vaginal birth is always safest for an infant. Therefore, it is essential to determine the placenta's location as accurately as possible in the hope that its position will make vaginal birth feasible. If the previa is under 30% by ultrasound, it may be possible for the fetus to be born past it. If over 30%, and the fetus is mature, the safest birth method for both mother and baby is often a cesarean birth (Arquette & Holcroft, 2007).

An abdominal examination may reveal that the fetal head is not engaged because of the interfering placenta. However, this finding gives little indication of how much of the placenta is obscuring the os and preventing the head from engaging. Anticipate the order for a transvaginal ultrasound to detect this. If no previa is detected, the physician may attempt a careful speculum examination of the vagina and cervix to rule out another cause for bleeding, such as ruptured varices or cervical trauma.

Vaginal examinations (actual investigation of dilatation) to determine whether placenta previa exists are done in an operating room or a fully equipped birthing room so that if hemorrhage does occur with the manipulation, an immediate cesarean birth can be carried out to remove the child and the bleeding placenta and contract the uterus. Have oxygen equipment available in case the fetal heart sounds indicate fetal distress, such as bradycardia or tachycardia, late deceleration, or variable decelerations.

Continuing Care Measures. The point at which a diagnosis of placenta previa is made and the age of the gestation dictate the final management. If labor has begun, bleeding is continuing, or the fetus is being compromised (measured by the response of the fetal heart rate to contractions), birth must be accomplished regardless of gestational age. If the bleeding has stopped, the fetal heart sounds are of good quality, maternal vital signs are good, and the fetus is not yet 36 weeks of age, a woman is usually managed by expectant watching. As many as half of all women with bleeding from placenta previa are managed this way.

Typically, a woman remains in the hospital on bed rest for close observation for 48 hours. If the bleeding stops, she can be sent home with a referral for bed rest and home care. Careful assessment of fetal heart sounds is made and laboratory tests, such as hemoglobin or hematocrit, are frequently obtained. Betamethasone, a steroid that hastens fetal lung maturity, may be prescribed for the mother to encourage the maturity of fetal lungs if the fetus is less than 34 weeks' gestation (Box 21.5).

Nursing Diagnoses and Related Interventions

Because the diagnosis of placenta previa with bleeding is an emergency, all goals should reflect the short timeframe of the emergency condition.

Nursing Diagnosis: Fear related to outcome of pregnancy after episode of placenta previa bleeding

Outcome Evaluation: Client discusses concerns with nurse and other health care providers; states hearing fetal heartbeat helps to reassure her about baby's health.

Often it is difficult for a woman who has experienced bleeding late in a pregnancy to wait for the baby to come to term, wondering whether her infant will be all right. Regardless of her outward appearance, most likely she is experiencing severe emotional stress. She cannot help but wonder if the next bleeding she experiences will kill her, the infant, or both. She may become so worried about the safety of her child that she begins to think of her baby as already dead. If this happens, she might begin to neglect her diet or her supplementary vitamins because "it doesn't matter any more." Listening to fetal heart sounds and being reassured that they are in a healthy range is helpful. She also needs to be able to talk to someone about her fears so she does not feel alone with her concerns.

Birth

As soon as the fetus reaches 37 weeks of age (2500 g), an amniocentesis analysis for lung maturity shows a positive result (a favorable lecithin–sphingomyelin ratio), bleeding occurs again, labor begins, or the fetus shows symptoms of distress, the fetus needs to be born (Scearce & Uzelac, 2007).

On the day of birth, a woman needs a great deal of support. It is one thing to talk about being ready for surgery; it is another to be truly ready. She may be as frightened as she was the evening her bleeding first began. If the pregnancy is past 36 weeks at the time of the initial bleeding, a birth decision will generally be made immediately. If the placenta previa is found to be total, birth through the placenta is impossible and the baby must be born by cesarean birth. If the placenta previa is partial, the amount of the blood loss, the condition of the fetus, and a woman's parity will influence the birth decision. With a cesarean birth for placenta previa, although the skin incision is still a transverse (bikini) one, the uterine cut must be made high, possibly vertically above the low implantation site of the placenta. If an ultrasound clearly reveals the placental location, a transverse uterine incision may be possible.

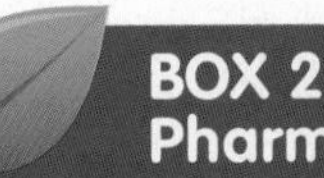

BOX 21.5 ✻ Focus on Pharmacology

Betamethasone (Celestone)

Action: Betamethasone is a corticosteroid that acts as an anti-inflammatory and immunosuppressive agent. It is given to pregnant women 12 to 24 hours before birth to hasten fetal lung maturity if a fetus is less than 34 weeks' gestation and help prevent respiratory distress syndrome in the newborn (Karch, 2009).

Pregnancy Risk Category: C

Dosage: 12–12.5 mg IM initially; may be repeated in 24 hours and again in 1 to 2 weeks

Possible Adverse Effects: Burning, itching, and irritation at the injection site; swelling, tachycardia, headache, dizziness, weight gain, sodium and fluid retention; increased risk of infection if used long term

Nursing Implications

- Explain the purpose of the drug to the client.
- Administer the initial dose IM. Anticipate the need for repeat dosing within 24 hours and again in 1 to 2 weeks.
- Assist with measures to halt preterm labor if indicated.
- Continue to monitor client's vital signs and fetal heart rate for changes.
- If client is also receiving a tocolytic agent, be alert for possible cardiac decompensation as a result of a drug–drug interaction. Observe for signs such as increased pulse, decreased blood pressure, and presence of edema.
- Assess for signs and symptoms of possible infection with long-term use.
- Instruct client about the possibility that a repeat dose may be necessary.

After birth, most women inspect their child carefully. A woman may worry that because of the problem with placental implantation, there might be something wrong with her child. During the postpartum period, she needs adequate time with her child to be certain he or she is all right.

Any woman who has had a placenta previa is more prone than normal to postpartum hemorrhage because the placental site is in the lower uterine segment, which does not contract as efficiently as the upper segment. Also, because the uterine blood supply is less in the lower segment, the placenta tends to grow larger than it would normally, leaving a larger denuded surface area when it is removed. As a second complication, a woman is more likely to develop endometritis because the placental site is close to the cervix, the portal of entry for pathogens.

Premature Separation of the Placenta (Abruptio Placentae)

Unlike placenta previa, in **premature separation of the placenta** (also called *abruptio placentae;* Fig. 21.7), the placenta

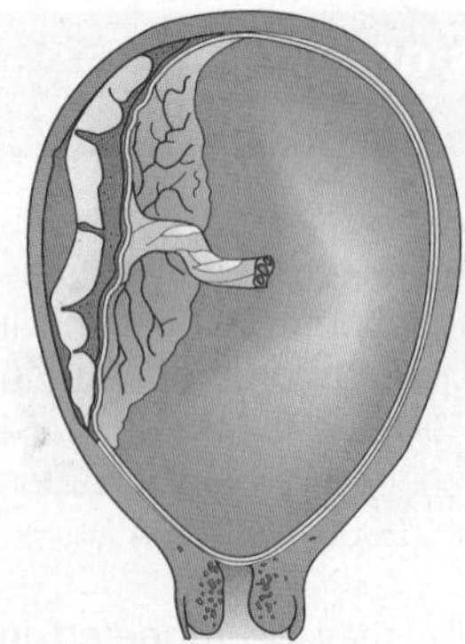

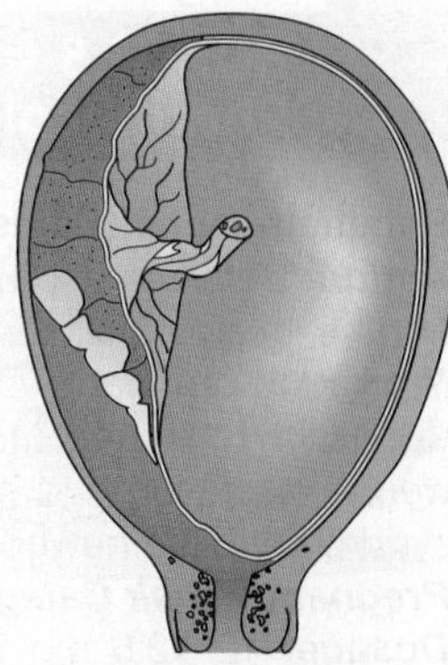

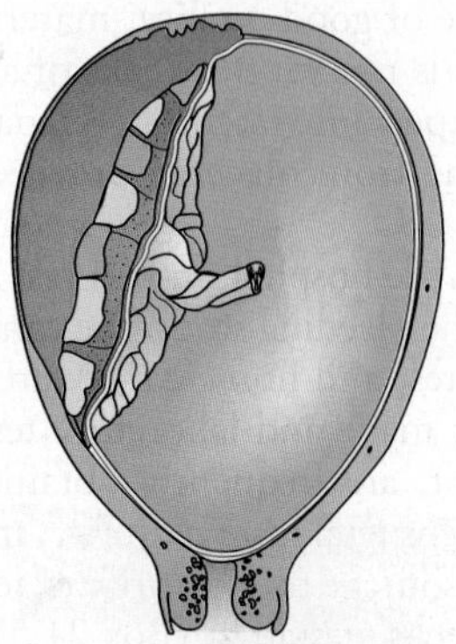

FIGURE 21.7 Premature separation of the placenta.

appears to have been implanted correctly. Suddenly, however, it begins to separate and bleeding results. Premature separation of the placenta occurs in about 10% of pregnancies and is the most frequent cause of perinatal death (Arquette & Holcroft, 2007). The separation generally occurs late in pregnancy; it may occur as late as during the first or second stage of labor. Because premature separation of the placenta may occur during an otherwise normal labor, it is important always to be alert to the amount and kind of vaginal bleeding a woman is having in labor. Listen to her description of the kind of pain she is experiencing to help detect this grave complication.

The primary cause of premature separation is unknown, but certain predisposing factors have been identified, including high parity, advanced maternal age, a short umbilical cord, chronic hypertensive disease, pregnancy-induced hypertension, direct trauma (as from an automobile accident or intimate partner abuse), vasoconstriction from cocaine or cigarette use, and thrombophilitic conditions that lead to thrombosis such as autoimmune antibodies, protein C, and factor V Leiden (a common inherited thrombophilia that occurs in 5% of whites and 1% of blacks [Szymanski & Aina-Mumuney, 2007]). It may be caused by **chorioamnionitis,** which is an infection of the fetal membranes and fluid (Nath et al., 2007).

Premature separation of the placenta may also follow a rapid decrease in uterine volume, such as occurs with sudden release of amniotic fluid. Usually the fetal head is low enough in the pelvis that it prevents loss of the total volume of the amniotic fluid at one time, so normally a rapid reduction in amniotic fluid does not occur when membranes rupture.

Assessment

A woman experiences a sharp, stabbing pain high in the uterine fundus as the initial separation occurs. If labor begins with the separation, each contraction will be accompanied by pain over and above the pain of the contraction. In some women, additional pain is not evident with contractions but tenderness can be felt on uterine palpation.

Heavy bleeding usually accompanies premature separation of the placenta, like placenta previa, although it may not be readily apparent. There will be external bleeding only if the placenta separates first at the edges and blood escapes freely from the cervix. If the center of the placenta separates first, blood can pool under the placenta, and although bleeding is intense, it is hidden from view. Whether blood is evident or not, signs of shock usually follow quickly because of the blood loss. The uterus becomes tense and feels rigid to the touch. If blood infiltrates the uterine musculature, **Couvelaire uterus** or uteroplacental apoplexy, forming a hard, boardlike uterus with no apparent, or minimally apparent, bleeding present occurs. As bleeding progresses, a woman's reserve of blood fibrinogen may be used up in her body's attempt to accomplish effective clot formation, and disseminated intravascular coagulation (DIC syndrome) can occur (see later).

If a woman is being admitted to the hospital after experiencing symptoms at home, assess the time the bleeding began, whether pain accompanied it, the amount and kind of bleeding, and her actions to detect if trauma could have led to the placental separation. Initial blood work should include hemoglobin level, typing and cross-matching, and a fibrinogen level and fibrin breakdown products to detect DIC. For a quick assessment of blood clotting ability, draw 5 mL and place it in a clean, dry test tube. Stand it aside untouched for 5 minutes. At the end of this time, if a clot has not formed, suspect an interference with blood coagulation.

Therapeutic Management

Separation of the placenta is an emergency situation (Neilson, 2009). A woman needs a large-gauge intravenous catheter inserted for fluid replacement and oxygen by mask to limit fetal anoxia. Monitor fetal heart sounds externally and record maternal vital signs every 5 to 15 minutes to establish baselines and observe progress. The baseline fibrinogen determination is followed by additional determinations up to the time of birth. Keep a woman in a lateral, not supine, position to prevent pressure on the vena cava and additional interference with fetal circulation. It is important not to disturb the injured placenta any further. Therefore, do not perform any abdominal, vaginal, or pelvic examination on a woman with a diagnosed or suspected placental separation.

For better prediction of fetal and maternal outcome, the degrees of placental separation can be graded (Table 21.5). Unless the separation is minimal (grades 0 and 1), the pregnancy must be terminated because the fetus cannot obtain

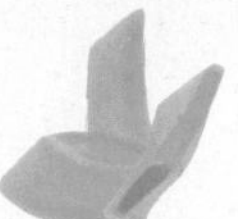

TABLE 21.5 ✻ Premature Separation of the Placenta: Degrees of Separation

Grade	Criteria
0	No symptoms of separation were apparent from maternal or fetal signs; the diagnosis that a slight separation did occur is made after birth, when the placenta is examined and a segment of the placenta shows a recent adherent clot on the maternal surface.
1	Minimal separation, but enough to cause vaginal bleeding and changes in the maternal vital signs; no fetal distress or hemorrhagic shock occurs, however.
2	Moderate separation; there is evidence of fetal distress; the uterus is tense and painful on palpation.
3	Extreme separation; without immediate interventions, maternal shock and fetal death will result.

adequate oxygen and nutrients. If vaginal birth does not seem imminent, cesarean birth is the birth method of choice.

If DIC has developed, cesarean surgery may pose a grave risk because of the possibility of hemorrhage during the surgery and later from the surgical incision. Intravenous administration of fibrinogen or cryoprecipitate (which contains fibrinogen) may be used to elevate a woman's fibrinogen level prior to and concurrently with surgery. With the worst outcome, a hysterectomy might be necessary to prevent exsanguination.

Fetal prognosis depends on the extent of the placental separation and the degree of fetal hypoxia. Maternal prognosis depends on how promptly treatment can be instituted. Death can occur from massive hemorrhage leading to shock and circulatory collapse or renal failure from the circulatory collapse. These factors cause premature separation of the placenta to be a significant cause of both maternal and fetal mortality.

Any woman who has had bleeding before birth is more prone to infection after birth than the average woman. A woman with a history of premature separation of the placenta, therefore, needs to be observed closely for the development of infection in the postpartum period.

✔ Checkpoint Question 21.3

Suppose Beverly Muzuki develops a placenta previa. What would be an important assessment to make with her after her baby's birth?

a. Whether she recognizes that this is inherited and will probably happen again.
b. Assessment of vaginal bleeding, as she is prone to have more than usual.
c. Whether she appears "jittery" or nervous from the prebirth drugs she received.
d. Whether she understands that her uterus has a scar and so will be always weakened.

Disseminated Intravascular Coagulation

DIC is an acquired disorder of blood clotting in which the fibrinogen level falls to below effective limits. Early symptoms include easy bruising or bleeding from an intravenous site. Conditions such as premature separation of the placenta, pregnancy-induced hypertension, amniotic fluid embolism, placental retention, septic abortion, and retention of a dead fetus are all associated with its development (Goldberg & Smith, 2007). Normally, platelets quickly form a seal over a point of bleeding to prevent further loss of blood. Intrinsic and extrinsic clotting pathways then activate and strengthen this plug by fibrin threads to produce a firm, fixed structure. To prevent too much clotting from occurring, at the same time the clot is being formed, thrombin activates fibrinolysin, a proteolytic enzyme, to begin to digest excess fibrin threads (anticoagulation). This lysis results in the release of fibrin degradation products.

DIC occurs when there is such extreme bleeding and so many platelets and fibrin from the general circulation rush to the site that not enough are left in the rest of the body. This results in a paradox: at one point in the circulatory system, the person has increased coagulation, but throughout the rest of the system, a bleeding defect exists. DIC is an emergency because it can result in extreme blood loss. Goals should reflect the presence of the emergency.

Testing clotting time can be done by placing a small amount of blood in a test tube. After 30 minutes, a clot should not only form but retract and the volume of serum in the tube should exceed the size of the clot. If this does not occur, a low fibrinogen level is suggested. For a definite diagnosis, blood needs to be drawn for platelets (will be decreased to $\leq$100,000/μL), prothrombin (will be low because it depends on the conversion of fibrinogen to fibrin), thrombin time (will be elevated because it measures the time necessary for conversion of fibrinogen to fibrin), fibrinogen (will be decreased to $<$150 mg/dL because fibrinogen has been used up), and fibrin split products (will be $>$40 μg/mL reflecting the destruction of fibrinogen or fibrin). A D-dimer is specific for fibrin (not fibrinogen) degradation products and will be abnormal in 90% of patients with DIC (Goldberg & Smith, 2007).

To stop the process of DIC, the underlying insult that began the phenomenon must be halted. When the insult was a complication of pregnancy such as premature separation of the placenta, ending the pregnancy by birthing the fetus and delivering the placenta is part of the solution. Next, the marked coagulation must be stopped so that coagulation factors can be freed and normal clotting function can be restored. This is accomplished by the intravenous administration of heparin to halt the clotting cascade. Heparin must be given cautiously close to birth or postpartum hemorrhage could occur from poor clotting after delivery of the placenta. If bleeding during pregnancy was the stimulus for DIC, a blood or platelet transfusion may be necessary to replace blood or platelet loss. This administration may be delayed, however, until after heparin therapy so the new blood factors are also not consumed by the coagulation process. Antithrombin III factor, fibrinogen, or cryoprecipitate (which contains fibrinogen) can all be used to restore blood clotting. If these are not available, fresh-frozen plasma or platelets can also aid in restoring clotting function.

It can be confusing for a woman with a disorder such as premature separation of the placenta to have her physician tell her one minute that bleeding is what he or she is worried about and to hear the next minute that an anticoagulant such as heparin has been ordered. If a woman understands the action of heparin—to discourage blood coagulation—it seems as if the physician has ordered exactly the wrong medication. Be certain a woman and her support person have a full explanation of what is happening (she has an increased risk of hemorrhage because part of her system has tied up coagulation factors; by releasing them, coagulation can be restored throughout the rest of her body). This helps to instill and maintain confidence in her caregivers.

Evaluation focuses on determining whether a woman's blood coagulation studies are returning to normal and if any anoxia has occurred, particularly in renal or brain cells from occluded coagulated capillaries. Fetal and newborn assessment is important to evaluate the efficiency of the placental circulation in light of increased clotting.

What if... A pregnant client is receiving subcutaneous heparin and asks why she cannot take this drug orally? How would you answer? Would you need to assess her infant after birth for blood coagulation ability?

PRETERM LABOR

Preterm labor is labor that occurs before the end of week 37 of gestation. It occurs in approximately 9% to 11% of all pregnancies. It is responsible for almost two-thirds of all infant deaths in the neonatal period (Cootauco & Althaus, 2007). Any woman having persistent uterine contractions (four every 20 minutes) should be considered to be in labor. A woman is documented as being in actual labor rather than having false labor contractions if she is having uterine contractions that cause cervical effacement over 80% or dilation over 1 cm. Preterm labor is always serious because if it results in the infant's birth, the infant will be immature.

Some women wait before they seek help for preterm labor, unwilling to face the fact that labor contractions have started. Some diagnose their contractions as nothing more than extremely hard Braxton Hicks contractions and think they are innocent. Currently, when there is treatment available to delay labor until a fetus reaches a level of maturity that will allow a newborn to survive in the outside environment, evaluation and the institution of therapy before membranes rupture are vital, as ruptured membranes make it that much more difficult to halt labor.

Why labor begins before a fetus is mature is unclear in most instances. It can happen for unknown reasons, but it is associated with dehydration, urinary tract infection, periodontal disease, and chorioamnionitis. African American women, adolescents, and those who receive inadequate prenatal care are most susceptible (Goldenberg et al., 2008). Women who continue to work at strenuous jobs during pregnancy or perform shift work that leads to extreme fatigue may have a higher incidence than others (Whelan et al., 2007). It tends to occur in pregnancies of women who were born small but the father of their child is overweight, as if the fetus growing faster than its mother can accommodate might trigger preterm birth (Klebanoff, 2008). Intimate partner abuse may be yet another cause (Rodrigues, Rocha, & Barros, 2008). Participating in mild leisure sports activities such as walking may help prevent preterm birth (Box 21.6).

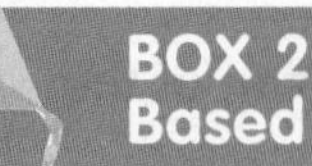

BOX 21.6 * Focus on Evidence-Based Practice

Do leisure sports cause preterm birth?

Most women today participate in some form of leisure sport. To investigate if there is an association between sports participation in the first and second trimesters of pregnancy and preterm birth, researchers assessed the sports histories of 5749 healthy pregnant women seen for prenatal care. The results of the research showed that women who practiced more than one type of sport had a significantly reduced risk of preterm birth compared with women who participated in no sports activities. Women who engaged in light leisure time physical activity had a 24% reduced risk of preterm labor, and those engaged in moderate-to-heavy leisure time activity had a 66% reduced risk. Participation in leisure sports activities, therefore, does not add to the incidence of preterm birth, but may actually help to prevent it beginning.

Could you use the above study to help women judge if they should continue to participate in leisure sports activities during pregnancy?

Source: Hegaard, H. K., et al. (2008). Leisure time physical activity is associated with a reduced risk of preterm delivery. *American Journal of Obstetrics and Gynecology, 198*(2), 180–185.

Common symptoms of early preterm labor include a persistent, dull, low backache; vaginal spotting; a feeling of pelvic pressure or abdominal tightening; menstrual-like cramping; increased vaginal discharge; uterine contractions; and intestinal cramping. Listen carefully to any woman who has these symptoms or believes she is in preterm labor because beginning symptoms of labor are subtle and best recognized by a woman herself. Be certain all women receive information on the signs and symptoms of preterm labor so they do not overlook the more subtle signs.

Therapeutic Management

It is possible to predict which pregnancies will end early by analyzing changes in vaginal mucus, such as the presence of fetal fibronectin, a protein produced by trophoblast cells (Mateus et al., 2007). If this is present in vaginal mucus, it predicts that preterm contractions are ready to occur; absence of the protein predicts that labor will not occur for at least 14 days. A shortened cervix, revealed by ultrasound, may be just as predictive (Cootauco & Althaus, 2007).

Medical attempts can be made to stop labor if the fetal membranes are intact, fetal distress is absent, there is no evidence that bleeding is occurring, the cervix is not dilated more than 4 to 5 cm, and effacement is not more than 50%.

A woman who is in preterm labor is usually first admitted to the hospital and placed on bed rest to relieve the pressure of the fetus on the cervix. Intravenous fluid therapy to keep her well hydrated is begun because hydration may help stop contractions. If a woman is dehydrated, the pituitary gland is activated to secrete antidiuretic hormone, and this may cause it to release oxytocin as well. Oxytocin strengthens uterine contractions. By keeping a woman well hydrated, therefore, the release of oxytocin may be minimized.

Vaginal and cervical cultures and a clean-catch urine sample are obtained to rule out infection. If a urinary tract infection is present the woman will be started on an antibiotic (Smaill & Vazquez, 2009). She may also receive an antibiotic for group B streptococcus prophylaxis as an infection with this could be fatal in a newborn. A **tocolytic agent,** an agent to halt labor, such as terbutaline may be prescribed. Following this initial therapy, women in preterm labor can be safely cared for at home as long as they can dependably drink enough fluid to remain well hydrated and continue to take an oral tocolytic agent (Box 21.7). Although there is little evidence to show that strict bed rest prevents preterm labor (Sosa et al., 2009), a woman should limit strenuous activities (see Chapter 4 for a discussion of home care). It is important that women also maintain adequate nutrition and do not smoke cigarettes as both poor nutrition and smoking put them at high risk for preterm birth (Dew, 2007).

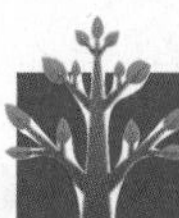

BOX 21.7 * Focus on Family Teaching

Measures to Help Prevent a Recurrence of Preterm Labor for Women on Bed Rest

Q. Beverly Muzuki has started preterm labor and so is put on bed rest. She asks you, "What else can I do to help prevent having this baby early?"

A. Several actions can be helpful to prevent a recurrence of preterm labor:

- Remain on bed rest except to use the bathroom (lie in a bed or put feet up on a couch or lounge).
- Drink 8 to 10 glasses of fluids daily (keep a pitcher by your bed so you do not have to get up).
- Take your prescribed tocolytic medication on time to maintain a constant blood level. Set an alarm clock as necessary, especially at night.
- Keep mentally active by reading or working on a project to prevent boredom.
- Avoid activities that could stimulate labor, such as nipple stimulation.
- Consult your primary care provider regarding whether sexual relations should be restricted.
- Immediately report signs of ruptured membranes (sudden gush of vaginal fluid) or vaginal bleeding.
- Report signs of urinary tract or vaginal infection (burning or frequency of urination; vaginal itching or pain).
- Report symptoms of pulmonary congestion (cough and difficulty breathing unless upright), which can be effects of tocolytic drugs.
- Keep appointments for prenatal care.

If uterine contractions recur:

- Empty your bladder to relieve pressure on the uterus.
- Lie down on your left or right side to encourage blood return to the uterus.
- Drink two or three glasses of fluid to increase hydration.
- Telephone your health care provider to report the incident and ask for further care measures.

Drug Administration

For reasons not clearly understood, the administration of a corticosteroid to the fetus appears to accelerate the formation of lung surfactant. During the time labor is being chemically halted, therefore, if the pregnancy is under 34 weeks, a woman may be given a steroid (betamethasone) to attempt to hasten fetal lung maturity (two doses of 12 mg betamethasone given intramuscularly 24 hours apart, or four doses of 6 mg dexamethasone given intramuscularly 12 hours apart). Betamethasone is preferred as it leads to lower rates of respiratory distress syndrome or bronchopulmonary dysplasia in newborns (Feldman et al., 2007).

It takes about 24 hours for betamethasone to have an effect, so it is important labor be halted for at least this long. The effect lasts approximately 7 days. If the fetus is not born within that time span, the dose of betamethasone may be repeated, but this is controversial because any corticosteroid can interfere with glucose regulation.

Although calcium channel blockers such as nifedipine (Procardia) or a prostaglandin antagonist such as indomethacin (Indocin) can be used as tocolytic agents, these are not drugs of choice because of their side effects. Although not as serious a concern as once believed, decreased fetal urine output, resulting in oligohydramnios (a pregnancy with less than the average amount of amniotic fluid; refer to discussion later) and premature closure of the fetal ductus arteriosus with resultant fetal pulmonary hypertension can occur, after indomethacin administration (Karch, 2009). Magnesium sulfate, once a popular drug to halt contractions, is no longer recommended because of its many side effects (Simhan & Caritis, 2007).

Beta-sympathomimetic drugs are yet another tocolytic option. Beta-1 receptor sites are found in adipose tissue, heart, liver, pancreatic islet cells, and gastrointestinal smooth muscle. Beta-2 receptor sites are found in uterine smooth muscle, bronchial smooth muscle, and blood vessels. All of these drugs act to halt contractions by coupling with adrenergic receptors on the outer surface of the membrane of myometrial cells. This releases adenylcyclase, which triggers the conversion of adenosine triphosphate into cyclic adenosine monophosphate. This substance is responsible for reducing the intracellular concentration of calcium through protein binding. With a lowered intracellular calcium concentration, muscle contraction is ineffective and uterine contractions halt. An ideal tocolytic drug is one that acts entirely on beta-2 receptor sites and so does not cause any cardiac or gastrointestinal symptoms.

Ritodrine hydrochloride (Yutopar) and terbutaline (Brethine) are examples of drugs that act almost entirely on beta-2 receptor sites and so have only mild hypotensive and tachycardiac effects. Of these two drugs, terbutaline is more frequently used. As a beta-2 receptor, it causes blood vessels and bronchi to relax along with the uterine muscle. As a result, hypotension can occur. This causes the heart rate to increase to move blood more effectively. Hypokalemia may also occur from a shift of potassium into cells, and blood glucose and accompanying plasma insulin levels may increase. Pulmonary edema may occur. Headache, because of the dilatation of cerebral blood vessels, is a common side effect; nausea and emesis also may occur. These are side effects to be observed for but are not reasons to discontinue therapy. Terbutaline should be used cautiously in women with diabetes mellitus and thyroid dysfunction. In a woman who is predisposed to develop gestational diabetes, terbutaline can raise her blood sugar glucose so much that she becomes overtly diabetic, which further complicates her pregnancy.

Before a tocolytic drug is administered, obtain baseline blood data (hematocrit, serum glucose, potassium, sodium chloride, and PCO_2). An electrocardiogram may be scheduled. An external uterine and fetal monitor should be in place.

When administering terbutaline, mix the drug with Ringer's lactate rather than a dextrose solution to prevent any unnecessary hyperglycemia. Administer it as a piggyback connected to a main intravenous solution so that it can be stopped immediately if effects such as tachycardia or arrhythmias occur. Use microdrip tubing and an infusion pump to ensure a consistent, accurate flow rate.

After an initial flow rate is calculated and started, this rate may be increased every 10 minutes until uterine activity halts or side effects become extreme. Assess pulse and blood pressure approximately every 15 minutes while the flow rate is being increased and thereafter every 30 minutes until contractions halt. Assess for chest pain and dyspnea. Auscultate the lungs for rales to detect signs of pulmonary edema. Promptly report a pulse rate of more than 120 beats per minute, blood pressure below 90/60 mm Hg, chest pain, dyspnea, rales, or cardiac arrhythmias. Obtain hematocrit and serum electrolyte levels every 4 hours or as ordered during administration. Be certain to assess the total parenteral intake, because an excess can lead to pulmonary edema. Measure intake and output and obtain daily weights to rule out retention of fluid or edema. Observe the fetal heart rate closely for tachycardia (heart rate over 160 beats per minute), late decelerations, or variable decelerations that suggest possible uterine bleeding or the need for emergency birth of the fetus rather than continuation of the pregnancy.

After contractions halt, a tocolytic infusion usually is continued for 12 to 24 hours, and then oral administration of terbutaline is begun. The first oral dose is given 30 minutes before the intravenous infusion is discontinued to prevent any drop in the serum concentration. After this initial stabilization, a woman will continue to take an oral tocolytic until 37 weeks' gestation or until fetal lung maturity is established by amniocentesis. Before hospital discharge, teach a woman how to take her pulse before each dose of medication and to call if her pulse rate is more than 120 beats per minute or if she experiences palpitations or extreme nervousness.

Women must set their alarm clocks so they awaken at night to take the around-the-clock dose prescribed. Otherwise, their serum level of medication in the morning could be too low to be effective. Caution them that if they forget a dose, they must take a pill as soon as they remember and then space their doses accordingly from that time. They should not double the dose to make up for the missed pill because extreme tachycardia could result.

Terbutaline may also be administered subcutaneously by continuous pump. This allows for home drug administration using lower doses of medicine. Oral terbutaline therapy has the potential of prolonging labor an average of 2 weeks. With subcutaneous pump infusions, labor can be delayed an average of 8 to 9 weeks. Similar to an insulin pump, a terbutaline pump contains a syringe filled with the drug. A small polyethylene catheter leads from the pump to a subcutaneous needle. When the needle is inserted into the subcutaneous tissue of the abdomen or the thigh, the pump automatically injects a continuous low dose of medication subcutaneously. The pump can be set to "bolus" an injection of the drug at the time of day when contractions tend to occur the most. A woman could manually trigger the pump to inject extra medicine (within set limits) if she should begin to feel contractions. Like insulin pumps, the pump can be carried in a sash around the waist or kept in a pocket of clothing. Pumps should never get wet, so the syringe should be removed from the pump while a woman showers. For tub bathing, she should remove both the pump and needle and replace the needle immediately afterward.

Fetal Assessment

In addition to supervising tocolytic therapy, be certain to assess overall fetal welfare daily in a woman trying to delay preterm labor (see Focus on Nursing Care Planning Box 21.8). A woman may be instructed to use a daily fetal movement count or "count to 10" test. Teach her how to do this before hospital discharge so she can continue it when she is at home. The typical fetus moves 10 times in an hour. To evaluate fetal movement, a woman lies down on her left side and times the number of minutes it takes for her to feel 10 fetal movements (about an hour) or counts the number of fetal movements she feels in 1 hour (the average is 10 to 12). If the time it takes to feel 10 fetal movements is twice what it was the day before or if she feels fewer than 5 movements during an hour (half of what she should feel), she monitors again for a second hour. If at the end of this second hour fetal activity is still under 10 per hour, she should report it immediately. Because of the variation of movements among normal, healthy fetuses, different perinatal centers use different protocols for counting fetal movements. What standard is accepted as normal also varies.

Labor That Cannot Be Halted

In some women, preterm labor is too far advanced when they are first seen in a health care facility for it to be halted. Usually, if membranes have ruptured or the cervix is more than 50% effaced and more than 3 to 4 cm dilated, it is unlikely labor can be halted. The rupturing of membranes, especially, can be thought of as a "point of no return" in stopping or delaying labor because of the increased risk of infection that begins from that point.

If the fetus is very immature at the time labor cannot be halted, a cesarean birth may be planned to reduce pressure on the fetal head and reduce the possibility of subdural or intraventricular hemorrhage from a vaginal birth.

Most women assume that if a fetus is preterm, labor will be shorter than normal because the infant is still so small. This is not necessarily true because the first stage of labor, the longest stage, proceeds exactly as it would with a term pregnancy. The second stage of labor may be shorter because a

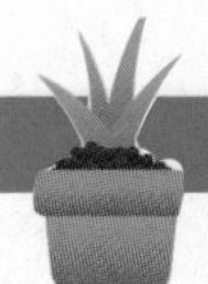

BOX 21.8 ✻ Focus on Nursing Care Planning

A Multidisciplinary Care Map for a Woman in Preterm Labor

Beverly Muzuki is a 20-year-old primipara, 30 weeks pregnant, whom you see in a prenatal clinic. She has had symptoms of a urinary tract infection for the past few days but did not call the clinic because she knew she had an appointment today and thought getting some help for it could wait until she came in. Yesterday she noticed some mild abdominal pain but thought it was irritation from the bladder infection. During the night, she woke twice because of a nagging backache. This morning, she has intermittent sharp uterine contractions. "Why did this happen?" she asks you. "I didn't do anything wrong."

Family Assessment ✻ Client, 20, lives in two-bedroom third-floor university housing. Undeclared major and works as a secretary in Personnel; husband (26) is a campus groundskeeper. Finances rated as, "Who couldn't use more money?"

Client Assessment ✻ Gravida 2, para 0, 30 week pregnancy. Heart rate 88 bpm; respirations 22; blood pressure 130/78. Fetal heart rate 142 bpm; reports positive fetal movements. Uterine contractions every 7 minutes lasting 40 seconds. Intravenous tocolytic therapy with terbutaline prescribed.

Nursing Diagnosis ✻ Risk for injury (maternal and fetal) related to preterm labor and tocolytic therapy

Outcome Criteria ✻ Contractions halt after treatment with tocolytic; fetal heart rate remains within acceptable parameters; fetal lung maturity improves as evidenced by rising lecithin–sphingomyelin ratio; client remains free of signs and symptoms of adverse effects of tocolytic therapy. Client verbalizes concerns and fears; participates in decision making and relaxation measures.

Team Member Responsible	Assessment	Intervention	Rationale	Expected Outcome
		Activities of Daily Living		
Physician/ nurse	Attach contraction and fetal heart rate monitors for continuous evaluation of contractions and fetal response.	Institute bed rest with client in side-lying position.	Bed rest relieves pressure of the fetus on the cervix. Side-lying position enhances uterine perfusion. Uterine and fetal monitoring provides evidence of fetal well-being.	Client will remain on bed rest until labor contractions halt or further action becomes necessary.
		Consultations		
Physician	Contact ultrasound personnel.	Obtain client consent for ultrasound. Arrange for ultrasound to establish fetal health.	An ultrasound can document fetal health and cervical dilation.	Client agrees to procedure. Completes preprocedure readiness actions.
		Procedures/Medications		
Nurse/ certified nurse's aide	Assess vital signs of client. Obtain history of events leading up to beginning of labor.	Obtain laboratory studies, including complete blood count, hemoglobin and hematocrit, serum electrolytes. Obtain clean-catch urine for culture, vaginal and cervical cultures, and fibronectin as ordered.	Assessment provides a baseline for future comparisons. Urine, vaginal, and cervical cultures help to rule out infection as a causative factor for preterm labor. Fibronectin can help predict whether labor can be halted.	Specimens are sent to lab promptly to ensure rapid assessment.

(continued)

BOX 21.8 ✻ Focus on Nursing Care Planning (continued)

		Procedures/Medications		
Physician/ nurse	Assess for contraindications to betamethasone administration. Obtain reports of urine and cervical cultures and fibronectin.	Administer betamethasone to aid fetal lung maturity and an antibiotic for urinary tract infection as prescribed.	Betamethasone, a steroid, helps to decrease the risk of respiratory distress syndrome should birth of the fetus become necessary. An antibiotic decreases urinary tract infection.	Client agrees to betamethasone and antibiotic administration.
Nurse	Establish strength, duration, and frequency of baseline uterine contractions.	Administer terbutaline as ordered, as an IV piggyback. Use microdrip tubing and an infusion pump. Continue infusion for 12–24 hours after cessation of contractions.	Terbutaline is a beta-2 selective agonist that acts as a uterine relaxant, helping to halt preterm contractions.	Uterine contractions halt within 1 hour of terbutaline therapy.
Nurse	Continue maternal and fetal vital sign assessment.	Monitor client's vital signs closely, every 15 minutes during adjustment of flow rate and then every 30 minutes until contractions cease. Auscultate lungs for changes in breath sounds. Assess for chest pain and dyspnea. Monitor fetal heart rates and patterns every 15 to 30 minutes.	Maternal pulse over 120 beats per minute or persistent tachycardia or tachypnea, chest pain, dyspnea, or adventitious breath sounds may indicate impending pulmonary edema. Fetal tachycardia or late or variable decelerations indicate possible uterine bleeding or fetal distress, which requires emergency birth.	Client's and fetal vital signs remain within normal parameters during infusion.
		Nutrition		
Nurse	Obtain hematocrit and serum electrolyte levels every 4 hours or as ordered. Monitor IV fluid total every hour during infusion, keeping intake to 100 mL/hour or less.	Assist with or insert an IV line. Begin IV fluid therapy as ordered.	Hematocrit, electrolyte levels, and IV intake measures the client's fluid volume status. If fluid intake is greater than 100 mL/hour, overload may occur, placing the client at risk for pulmonary edema.	IV fluid improves hydration, which may help to minimize contractions.
		Patient/Family Education		
Nurse	Assess client's knowledge of preterm labor.	Instruct client about preterm labor and about steps to be taken to counteract the process.	A well-informed client can participate more fully in her own care.	Client states the cause of preterm labor cannot always be identified; describes the part she can play in halting process.

Psychosocial/Spiritual/Emotional Needs				
Nurse	Assess anxiety level of client over preterm labor. Assess for possible feelings of guilt related to cause of preterm labor.	Assist client with using relaxation techniques, such as muscle relaxation, breathing, and music. Provide frequent updates about progress. Allow client to verbalize feelings and concerns.	Relaxation techniques help to decrease anxiety and fear, enhancing feelings of control. Frequent updates about progress help to minimize fear about the unknown. Client may feel responsible for preterm labor because of UTI.	Client verbalizes her feelings about this crisis in her life. Demonstrates anxiety but at a level that allows her to cooperate with caregivers.
Nurse	Determine whether client wants a support person to be with her.	Contact support person as necessary.	The presence of a support person can offer additional comfort to a client.	Client names a support person she wants notified about hospital admission.
Discharge Planning				
Nurse	Assess client's home surroundings to determine whether they are appropriate for bed rest and continuing monitoring at home.	Change tocolytic therapy to oral form as prescribed, administering first oral dose 30 minutes before discontinuing IV infusion. Contact home care nurse service to provide monitoring at home.	Administering oral dose prior to discontinuation of IV infusion maintains consistent serum drug concentrations for effective control. Home monitoring requires professional supervision.	Client states that she feels her home and support system will be adequate for home care with self-monitoring. Agrees on appointment for first home visit with home care nurse service.

small infant can be pushed through the dilated cervix and the birth canal more easily. Because the second stage takes at most 1 hour, however, this means the difference will not be more than 30 minutes to 1 hour. Unless a woman is given this explanation, she may worry not only that her labor is preterm but also that something is going wrong because it is lasting so long.

Because of the increased risk for prolapse of the cord around a small head, artificial rupture of the membranes is not done as a rule in preterm labor until the fetal head is firmly engaged. Delaying rupture of the membranes is another factor that may prolong the first stage of labor.

Analgesic agents are administered with caution during preterm labor because of the immaturity of the fetus. The immature infant will have enough difficulty breathing at birth without the additional burden of being sedated from a drug such as meperidine (Demerol). If a woman wants pain relief, an epidural is preferable.

Continuously monitor uterine contractions and fetal heart sounds during preterm labor. A woman can feel reassured by the evidence of the monitor screen or graph or the projected sound that although her infant is likely to be small, heart tones seem to be of good quality and the infant is reacting well to labor.

A woman may assume that because her infant's head is small, an episiotomy will not be needed for birth, and she will be able to avoid the discomfort of postpartum stitches. Although the head of a preterm infant is smaller than that of a mature infant, it is also more fragile. Excessive pressure could result in a subdural or intraventricular hemorrhage that could be fatal. That means a woman may actually need an episiotomy incision larger than usual. Forceps are another measure that may be used at birth to reduce pressure on the fetal head.

Following birth, the cord of the preterm infant is usually clamped immediately rather than waiting for pulsations to stop. This is because an immature infant has a difficult time excreting the large amount of bilirubin that will be formed if this extra blood is added to the circulation. The extra amount of blood could also overburden the circulatory system.

Nursing Diagnoses and Related Interventions

Examples of nursing diagnoses for a woman with preterm labor that cannot be halted include:

- Fear related to uncertain outcome of pregnancy
- Pain related to labor contractions
- Situational low self-esteem related to inability to carry pregnancy to term
- Risk for fetal injury related to preterm birth

Be certain that the outcomes established for care are realistic. Although many measures are available to help the preterm baby adjust to birth, a baby born preterm will be at risk for a variety of health problems, especially difficulty with respirations (see Chapter 26).

Nursing Diagnosis: Situational low self-esteem related to feelings of responsibility for preterm labor

Outcome Evaluation: Client expresses feelings and worries to nurse; states it is unknown why labor began, but she knows she is not responsible for her labor beginning prematurely.

A woman in preterm labor is undergoing an extreme crisis situation. She cannot help asking herself, "What did I do to cause this?" Time spent taking the initial history or timing contractions presents an opportunity to bring the concern out in the open: "Did Dr. Smith explain to you labor sometimes begins early this way without any reason? Some women worry they did something to bring on preterm labor. Have you had any thoughts like that?"

A woman in preterm labor that cannot be halted needs a support person with her because she is apt to be more concerned than the average woman about labor. She needs frequent assurance during labor that she is breathing well with contractions or just that she is "doing well." She may not be mentally prepared for labor because it has come unexpectedly. During the postpartum period, she may need continued reassurance. Helping rebuild self-esteem this way can better prepare her to be a parent to her preterm infant.

✔Checkpoint Question 21.4

Beverly Muzuki is in preterm labor. When you see her in the emergency department, what should be your first action?

a. Keep her walking so the fetal head puts harder pressure on the cervix.
b. Ask her to lie down in a side-lying position and assess her contractions.
c. Obtain blood for a human chorionic gonadotropin hormone assessment.
d. Caution her to not allow anyone to start IV fluid; dehydration halts contractions.

PRETERM RUPTURE OF MEMBRANES

Preterm rupture of membranes is rupture of fetal membranes with loss of amniotic fluid during pregnancy before 37 weeks (Mercer et al., 2007). The cause of preterm rupture is unknown, but it is associated with infection of the membranes (chorioamnionitis). It occurs in 5% to 10% of pregnancies. If rupture occurs early in pregnancy, it poses a major threat to the fetus as, after rupture, the seal to the fetus is lost and uterine and fetal infection may occur. A second complication that can result from preterm membrane rupture is increased pressure on the umbilical cord from the loss of amniotic fluid, inhibiting the fetal nutrient supply, or cord prolapse (extension of the cord out of the uterine cavity into the vagina), a condition that could also interfere with fetal circulation. Cord prolapse is most apt to occur when the fetal head is still too small to fit the cervix firmly. Yet another risk to the fetus of remaining in a non-fluid-filled environment is the development of a Potter-like syndrome or distorted facial features and pulmonary hypoplasia from pressure (Hofmeyr, 2009). Preterm labor may follow rupture of the membranes and end the pregnancy.

Assessment

Rupture of the membranes is suggested by the history. A woman usually describes a sudden gush of clear fluid from her vagina, with continued minimal leakage. Occasionally, a woman mistakes urinary incontinence caused by exertion for rupture of membranes. Amniotic fluid cannot be differentiated from urine by appearance, so a sterile vaginal speculum examination is done to observe for vaginal pooling of fluid. If the fluid is tested with Nitrazine paper, amniotic fluid causes an alkaline reaction on the paper (appears blue) and urine causes an acidic reaction (remains yellow). The fluid can also be tested for ferning, or the typical appearance of a high-estrogen fluid on microscopic examination (amniotic fluid shows this; urine does not). The presence of a high level of alpha-fetoprotein (AFP) in the vagina is also diagnostic (Shahin & Raslan, 2007). If there is still a question regarding whether the membranes have ruptured, an ultrasound may be ordered to assess the amniotic fluid index. Because preterm rupture of membranes is associated with vaginal infection, cultures for *Neisseria gonorrhoeae, Streptococcus* B, and *Chlamydia* are usually taken. Blood is drawn for white blood count and C-reactive protein, which increase with membrane rupture. Avoid doing routine vaginal examinations because the risk of infection rises significantly when digital examinations are performed after preterm rupture of membranes.

If a fetus is estimated to be mature enough to survive in an extrauterine environment at the time of rupture and labor does not begin within 24 hours, labor contractions are usually induced by intravenous administration of oxytocin so the infant is born before infection can occur.

Therapeutic Management

If labor does not begin and the fetus is not at a point of viability, a woman is placed on bed rest either in the hospital or at home and administered a corticosteroid to hasten fetal lung maturity. Prophylactic administration of broad-spectrum antibiotics during this period may both delay the onset of labor and reduce the risk of infection in the newborn sufficiently to allow the corticosteroid to have its effect. Women positive for *Streptococcus* B need intravenous administration of penicillin or ampicillin to reduce the possibility of this infection in the newborn. A woman with no signs of infection may be administered a tocolytic agent if labor contractions begin (Mercer, 2007). Although its effectiveness is not well documented, a woman might be given an amnioinfusion (see Chapter 23) to reduce pressure on the fetus or cord and allow a term birth (Hofmeyr, 2009).

Following endoscopic intrauterine procedures, membranes can be resealed by use of a fibrin-based commercial sealant so they are again intact. This is a future possibility for premature rupture of the membranes also.

Nursing Diagnoses and Related Interventions

*

Nursing Diagnosis: Risk for infection related to preterm rupture of membranes without accompanying labor

Outcome Evaluation: Maternal white blood cell count remains below 20,000/mm^3; maternal temperature is less than 100.4° F (38.0° C) while awaiting fetal maturity.

An infection can be dangerous for both the mother and fetus. If at home, a woman is asked to take her temperature twice a day and to report a fever (a temperature greater than 100.4° F [38.0° C]), uterine tenderness, or odorous vaginal discharge. She should refrain from tub bathing, douching, and coitus because of the danger of introducing infection. The white cell count will need to be assessed frequently, perhaps as often as daily. A count of more than 18,000 to 20,000/mm^3 suggests infection.

Before a woman is discharged to home care, be certain she knows how to read a thermometer, she has specific instructions regarding what degree of temperature she should report, and she understands what degree of bed rest is expected of her. Help her make arrangements for a daily white blood cell count through a laboratory service or home care nurse.

Many misconceptions about the difficulty of labor after preterm rupture of the membranes (dry labor) exist. Every day, a woman hopes the fetus is ready to be born, ending the long wait, yet she is also afraid to begin labor because of these stories. You can assure her that because amniotic fluid is always being formed, there is no such thing as a "dry labor."

PREGNANCY-INDUCED HYPERTENSION

Pregnancy-induced hypertension (PIH) is a condition in which vasospasm occurs during pregnancy in both small and large arteries. Signs of hypertension, proteinuria, and edema develop. It is unique to pregnancy and occurs in 5% to 7% of pregnancies (Bailis & Witter, 2007). Despite years of research, the cause of the disorder is still unknown although it is highly correlated with the antiphospholipid syndrome or the presence of antiphospholipid antibodies (Clark, Silver, & Branch, 2007). Originally it was called toxemia because researchers pictured a toxin of some kind being produced by a woman in response to the foreign protein of the growing fetus, the toxin leading to the typical symptoms.

A condition separate from chronic hypertension, PIH tends to occur most frequently in women of color or with a multiple pregnancy, primiparas younger than 20 years or older than 40 years, women from low socioeconomic backgrounds (perhaps because of poor nutrition), those who have had five or more pregnancies, those who have hydramnios (overproduction of amniotic fluid; refer to discussion later), or those who have an underlying disease such as heart disease, diabetes with vessel or renal involvement, and essential hypertension.

Pathophysiologic Events

The symptoms of PIH affect almost all organs. The vascular spasm may be caused by the increased cardiac output that occurs with pregnancy and injures the endothelial cells of the arteries or the action of prostaglandins (notably decreased prostacyclin, a vasodilator, and excessive production of thromboxane, a vasoconstrictor and stimulant of platelet aggregation). Normally, blood vessels during pregnancy are resistant to the effects of pressor substances such as angiotensin and norepinephrine, so blood pressure remains normal during pregnancy. With PIH, this reduced responsiveness to blood pressure changes appears to be lost. Vasoconstriction occurs and blood pressure increases dramatically.

With hypertension, the cardiac system can become overwhelmed because the heart is forced to pump against rising peripheral resistance. This reduces the blood supply to organs, most markedly the kidney, pancreas, liver, brain, and placenta. Poor placental perfusion may reduce the fetal nutrient and oxygen supply. Ischemia in the pancreas may result in epigastric pain and an elevated amylase–creatinine ratio. Spasm of the arteries in the retina leads to vision changes. If retinal hemorrhages occur, blindness can result.

Vasospasm in the kidney increases blood flow resistance. Degenerative changes develop in kidney glomeruli because of back-pressure. This leads to increased permeability of the glomerular membrane, allowing the serum proteins albumin and globulin to escape into the urine (proteinuria). The degenerative changes also result in decreased glomerular filtration, so there is lowered urine output and clearance of creatinine. Increased kidney tubular reabsorption of sodium occurs. Because sodium retains fluid, edema results. Edema is further increased because as more protein is lost, the osmotic pressure of the circulating blood falls and fluid diffuses from the circulatory system into the denser interstitial spaces to equalize the pressure (Fig. 21.8). Extreme edema can lead to cerebral and pulmonary edema and seizures **(eclampsia).**

Yet another effect is that arterial spasm causes the bulk of the blood volume in the maternal circulation to be pooled in the venous circulation, so a woman has a deceptively low arterial intravascular volume. In addition, thrombocytopenia or a lowered platelet count occurs as platelets cluster at the sites of endothelial damage. Measuring hematocrit levels helps to assess the extent of plasma loss to the interstitial space or the extent of the edema (the higher the hematocrit, the more is being lost). A hematocrit level above 40% suggests significant fluid loss into interstitial spaces.

Assessment

Although women may have additional symptoms such as vision changes, typically hypertension, proteinuria, and edema are considered the classic signs of PIH. Of the three, hypertension and proteinuria are the most significant as extensive edema occurs only after the other two are present. Symptoms rarely occur before 20 weeks of pregnancy (Box 21.9).

PIH is classified as gestational hypertension, mild pre-eclampsia, severe pre-eclampsia, and eclampsia, depending on how far development of the syndrome has advanced (Table 21.6). Any woman with a high risk for PIH should be observed carefully for symptoms at prenatal visits. She needs instructions about what further symptoms to watch for so she can alert her clinician if additional symptoms occur between visits.

Gestational Hypertension

A woman is said to have gestational hypertension when she develops an elevated blood pressure (140/90 mm Hg) but has no proteinuria or edema. Perinatal mortality is not increased with simple gestational hypertension, so no drug therapy is necessary.

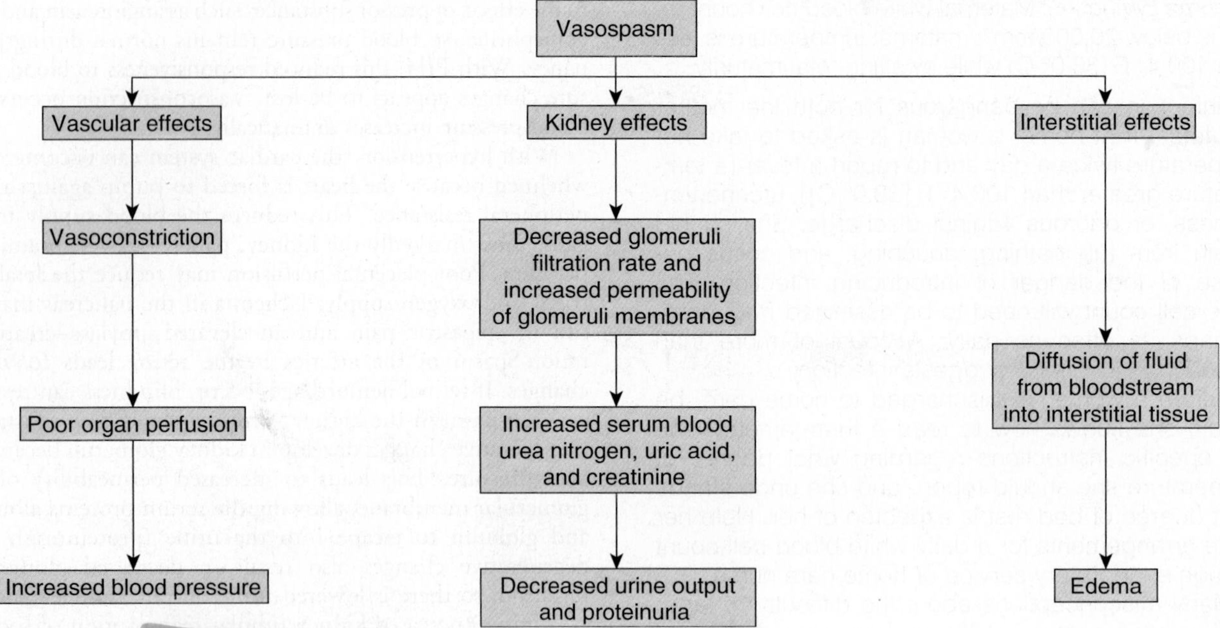

FIGURE 21.8 Physiologic changes with pregnancy-induced hypertension.

Mild Pre-eclampsia

If a seizure from PIH occurs, a woman has eclampsia, but any status above gestational hypertension and below a point of seizures is **pre-eclampsia.** A woman is said to be mildly pre-eclamptic when she has proteinuria and blood pressure rises to 140/90 mm Hg, taken on two occasions at least 6 hours apart. The diastolic value of blood pressure is extremely important to document because it is this pressure that best indicates the degree of peripheral arterial spasm present.

A second criterion for evaluating blood pressure is a systolic blood pressure greater than 30 mm Hg and a diastolic pressure greater than 15 mm Hg above prepregnancy values. This rule is helpful, but the value of 140/90 mm Hg is a more useful cutoff point when there are no baseline data available, such as when a woman seeks prenatal care late in pregnancy.

Average blood pressures in American women are shown in Appendix G. According to these averages, a woman younger than age 20 could have a blood pressure of 98/61 mm Hg and still be within normal limits. If her blood pressure were elevated 30 mm Hg systolic and 15 mm Hg diastolic, it would be only 128/76 mm Hg. This is well beneath the traditional warning point of 140/90 but would represent hypertension for her.

With mild pre-eclampsia, in addition to the hypertension a woman has proteinuria (1+ or 2+ on a reagent test strip on a random sample). Many women show a trace of protein during pregnancy. Actual proteinuria is said to exist when it registers as 1+ or more (this represents a loss of 1 g/L).

Occasionally women have orthostatic proteinuria (on long periods of standing, they excrete protein; at bed rest, they do not). If proteinuria is present without other signs of PIH (no hypertension and no edema), check to see when the specimen was obtained. Ask her to bring in a first morning urine sample. This may reveal that orthostatic proteinuria, not pre-eclampsia, may be the cause of protein in her urine.

Edema develops, as mentioned, because of the protein loss, sodium retention, and lowered glomerular filtration rate. The edema is not just the typical ankle edema of pregnancy but begins to accumulate in the upper part of the body. A weight gain of more than 2 lb/wk in the second trimester or 1 lb/wk in the third trimester usually indicates abnormal tissue fluid retention. This is likely to be the first symptom a woman notices, or it may be discovered when a woman is weighed at a prenatal visit. Noticeable edema may or may not be present when this sudden increase in weight first occurs.

Severe Pre-eclampsia

A woman has passed from mild to severe pre-eclampsia when her blood pressure rises to 160 mm Hg systolic and 110 mm Hg diastolic or above on at least two occasions 6 hours apart at bed rest (the position in which blood pressure is lowest) or her diastolic pressure is 30 mm Hg above her prepregnancy level. Marked proteinuria, 3+ or 4+ on a random urine sample or more than 5 g in a 24-hour sample, and extensive edema are also present.

With severe pre-eclampsia, the extreme edema is most readily palpated over bony surfaces, such as over the tibia on the anterior leg, the ulnar surface of the forearm, and the cheekbones, where the sponginess of fluid-filled tissue can be palpated against bone. If there is swelling or puffiness at these points to a palpating finger but the swelling cannot be indented with finger pressure, the edema is nonpitting. If the tissue can be indented slightly, this is 1+ pitting edema; moderate indentation is 2+; deep indentation is 3+; and

Box 21.9 Assessment
Assessing the Woman With Pregnancy-Induced Hypertension

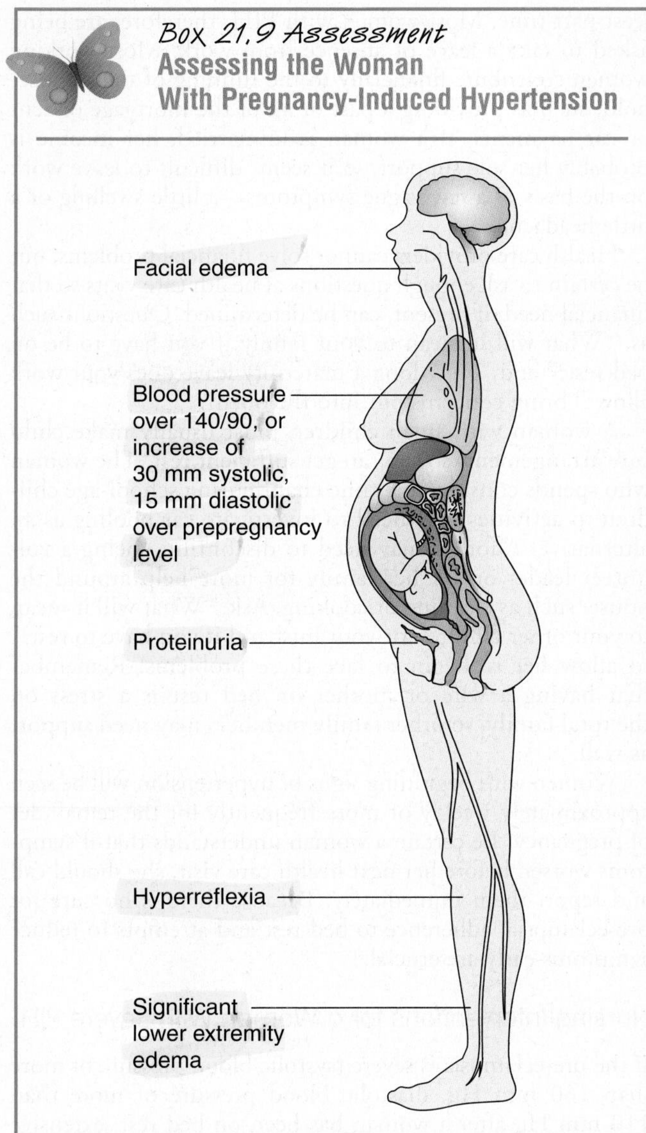

indentation so deep it remains after removal of the finger is 4+ pitting edema.

Further assess edema by asking a woman if she has noticed any swelling anywhere in her body. Most women at the end of pregnancy have edema of the feet at the end of the day. They report this as difficulty fitting into their bedroom slippers, or kicking off their shoes at dinnertime and then not being able to put them back on again. This is a normal discomfort of pregnancy. However, edema that has progressed to the upper extremities or the face is abnormal. Women report upper extremity edema as "my rings are so tight I can't get them off" and facial edema as "when I wake in the morning, my eyes are swollen shut" or "I can't talk until I walk around awhile." This accumulating edema will reduce their urine output to approximately 400 to 600 mL per 24 hours.

Some women have severe epigastric pain and nausea and vomiting, possibly because of abdominal edema or ischemia to the pancreas and liver. If pulmonary edema develops, a woman may report feeling short of breath. If cerebral edema occurs, reports may be voiced of visual disturbances such as blurred vision or seeing spots before the eyes. Cerebral edema also produces symptoms of severe headache and marked hyperreflexia and perhaps **ankle clonus** (a continued motion of the foot).

Eclampsia

This is the most severe classification of PIH. A woman has passed into this stage when cerebral edema is so acute that a grand-mal seizure (tonic-clonic) or coma occurs. With eclampsia, the maternal mortality rate is as high as 20% from causes such as cerebral hemorrhage, circulatory collapse, or renal failure (Bailis & Witter, 2007).

The fetal prognosis with eclampsia is also poor because of hypoxia and consequent fetal acidosis. If premature separation of the placenta from vasospasm occurs, the fetal prognosis is even graver. If a fetus must be born before term, all the risks of immaturity will be faced. In pre-eclampsia, the fetal mortality rate is approximately 10%. If eclampsia develops, the mortality rate increases to as high as 20% (Bailis & Witter, 2007).

TABLE 21.6 ✻ Symptoms of Pregnancy-Induced Hypertension

Hypertension Type	Symptoms
Gestational hypertension	Blood pressure 140/90 or systolic pressure elevated 30 mm Hg or diastolic pressure elevated 15 mm Hg above prepregnancy level; no proteinuria or edema; blood pressure returns to normal after birth
Mild pre-eclampsia	Blood pressure 140/90 or systolic pressure elevated 30 mm Hg or diastolic pressure elevated 15 mm Hg above prepregnancy level; proteinuria of 1–2+ on a random sample; weight gain over 2 lb per wk in second trimester and 1 lb per wk in third trimester; mild edema in upper extremities or face
Severe pre-eclampsia	Blood pressure of 160/110; proteinuria 3–4+ on a random sample and 5 g on a 24-hour sample; oliguria (500 mL or less in 24 hours or altered renal function tests; elevated serum creatinine more than 1.2 mg/dL); cerebral or visual disturbances (headache, blurred vision); pulmonary or cardiac involvement; extensive peripheral edema; hepatic dysfunction; thrombocytopenia; epigastric pain
Eclampsia	Seizure or coma accompanied by signs and symptoms of pre-eclampsia

Nursing Diagnoses and Related Interventions

The nursing diagnoses used with PIH are numerous because the disease has such wide-ranging effects. Some possible nursing diagnoses are:

- Ineffective tissue perfusion related to vasoconstriction of blood vessels
- Deficient fluid volume related to fluid loss to subcutaneous tissue
- Risk for fetal injury related to reduced placental perfusion secondary to vasospasm
- Social isolation related to prescribed bed rest

Nursing Interventions for a Woman With Mild PIH

Clients with mild pre-eclampsia can be managed at home with frequent follow-up care. Regardless of the setting, the care is similar.

Monitor Antiplatelet Therapy. Because of the increased tendency for platelets to cluster along arterial walls, a mild antiplatelet agent, such as low-dose aspirin, may prevent or delay development of pre-eclampsia (Duley et al., 2009). Because aspirin is such a common, over-the-counter drug, women may not appreciate that this is a serious drug prescription for them. Be certain they are taking low-dose aspirin (50–150 mg) as excessive salicylic levels can cause maternal bleeding at the time of birth.

Promote Bed Rest. When the body is in a recumbent position, sodium tends to be excreted at a faster rate than during activity. Bed rest, therefore, is the best method of aiding increased evacuation of sodium and encouraging diuresis. Rest should always be in a lateral recumbent position to avoid uterine pressure on the vena cava and prevent supine hypotension syndrome.

Promote Good Nutrition. A woman needs to continue her usual pregnancy nutrition. At one time, stringent restriction of salt was advised to reduce edema. This is no longer true because stringent sodium restriction may activate the renin-angiotensin-aldosterone system and result in increased blood pressure, compounding the problem.

Provide Emotional Support. It is difficult for a woman with pre-eclampsia to appreciate the potential seriousness of symptoms because they are so vague. Neither high blood pressure nor protein in urine is something she can see or feel. She may be aware that edema is present, but it seems unrelated to the pregnancy: it is her hands that are swollen, not a body area near her growing child.

Women are also used to having severe disorders treated with some form of medication. With mild pre-eclampsia, no medication other than low-dose aspirin is prescribed. This can make a woman underestimate the severity of her situation. She may take instructions such as getting rest lightly. In addition, it is not always easy to comply with an instruction such as to get additional rest during the day. Ninety percent of women of childbearing age work outside their home at least part time. Most women with PIH, therefore, are being asked to take a leave of absence from work. Most working women contribute financially to the running of their household, such as providing a part or all of the mortgage or rent or car payments. If a woman is unmarried, her income is probably her sole support, so it seems difficult to leave work on the basis of a few vague symptoms—a little swelling or a little headache.

Health care providers cannot solve financial problems, but be certain to ask enough questions at health care visits so that financial need, if present, can be determined. Questions such as, "What will it mean to your family if you have to be on bed rest?" and "How long a maternity leave does your work allow?" bring concerns out into the open.

A woman with small children must usually make child care arrangements so she can get sufficient rest. The woman who spends considerable time chauffeuring school-age children to activities may need to investigate car pooling as an alternative. Another may need to discontinue being a volunteer leader or ask her family for more help around the house, such as cleaning or cooking. Ask, "What will it mean to your other children or your husband if you have to rest?" to allow her to begin to face these problems. Remember that having a wife or mother on bed rest is a stress on the total family, so other family members may need support as well.

Women with beginning signs of hypertension will be seen approximately weekly or more frequently for the remainder of pregnancy. Be certain a woman understands that if symptoms worsen before her next health care visit, she should call and report them immediately. Because there is no cure for pre-eclampsia, adherence to bed rest and attempts to reduce symptoms early are crucial.

Nursing Interventions for a Woman With Severe PIH

If the pre-eclampsia is severe (systolic blood pressure of more than 160 mm Hg, diastolic blood pressure of more than 110 mm Hg after a woman has been on bed rest; extensive edema; marked proteinuria [3+ to 4+]; cerebral or visual disturbances; marked hyperreflexia; or oliguria [500 mL per 24 hours or less]), a woman may be admitted to a health care facility. If the pregnancy is 36 weeks or further along or fetal lung maturity can be confirmed by amniocentesis, labor can be induced or a cesarean birth performed to end the pregnancy at this point. If the pregnancy is less than 36 weeks or amniocentesis reveals immature lung function, interventions will be instituted to attempt to alleviate the severe symptoms and allow the fetus to come to term.

Support Bed Rest. With severe pre-eclampsia, most women are hospitalized so that bed rest can be enforced and a woman can be observed more closely than she can be on home care. Visitors are usually restricted to support people such as a husband, father of the child, mother, or older children. Because a loud noise such as a crying baby or a dropped tray of equipment can be sufficient to trigger a seizure initiating eclampsia, a woman with severe pre-eclampsia is admitted to a private room so she can rest as undisturbed as possible. Raise side rails to help prevent injury if a seizure should occur.

Darken the room if possible because a bright light can also trigger seizures. However, the room should not be so dark that caregivers need to use a flashlight to make assessments. Shining a flashlight beam into a woman's eyes is the kind of sudden stimulation to be avoided.

Stress is another stimulus capable of increasing blood pressure and evoking seizures in a woman with severe pre-eclampsia. Be certain the woman receives clear explanations of what is happening and what is planned. Clear explanations help her accept the need for visitor restrictions and not to "cheat" on bed rest. Allow her opportunities to express her feelings about what is happening or how bewildered she is because the few simple symptoms she noticed 2 weeks ago (increase in weight or increasing edema) have now developed into a syndrome that may be lethal to her baby and possibly to herself.

Monitor Maternal Well-being. Take blood pressure frequently (at least every 4 hours) or with a continuous monitoring device to detect any increase, which is a warning that a woman's condition is worsening. Obtain blood studies such as a complete blood count, platelet count, liver function, blood urea nitrogen, and creatine and fibrin degradation products as ordered to assess renal and liver function and the development of DIC, which often accompanies severe vasospasm. Because a woman is at high risk for premature separation of the placenta and resulting hemorrhage, a blood sample for type and cross-match is usually also obtained.

Daily hematocrit levels are used to monitor blood concentration. This level will rise if increased fluid is leaving the bloodstream for interstitial tissue (edema). Also, anticipate the need for frequent plasma estriol levels (a test of placenta function) and electrolyte levels. A woman's optic fundus is assessed daily for signs of arterial spasm, edema, or hemorrhage.

Obtain daily weights at the same time each day as another evaluation of fluid retention. Ensure that a woman is wearing the same amount of clothing at each weighing so any change in weight is not influenced by a change in the weight of her clothing.

An indwelling urinary catheter may be inserted to allow accurate recording of output and comparison with intake. Urinary output should be more than 600 mL per 24 hours (more than 30 mL/hr); an output lower than this suggests oliguria. Urinary proteins and specific gravity are measured and recorded with voiding or hourly if an indwelling catheter is present. A 24-hour urine sample may be collected for protein and creatinine clearance determinations to evaluate kidney function. A woman with mild pre-eclampsia spills between 0.5 g and 1 g of protein every 24 hours (1+ on a random sample); a woman with severe pre-eclampsia spills approximately 5 g per 24 hours (3+ to 4+ on an individual specimen).

Monitor Fetal Well-being. Generally, single Doppler auscultation at approximately 4-hour intervals is sufficient at this stage of management. However, the fetal heart rate may be assessed continuously with an external fetal monitor. A woman may have a nonstress test or biophysical profile done daily to assess uteroplacental sufficiency (see Chapter 9). Oxygen administration to the mother may be necessary to maintain adequate fetal oxygenation and prevent fetal bradycardia.

Support a Nutritious Diet. A woman needs a diet moderate to high in protein and moderate in sodium to compensate for the protein she is losing in urine. An intravenous fluid line is usually initiated and maintained to serve as an emergency route for drug administration as well as to administer fluid to reduce hemoconcentration and hypovolemia.

Administer Medications to Prevent Eclampsia. A hypotensive drug such as hydralazine (Apresoline), labetalol (Normodyne), or nifedipine may be prescribed to reduce hypertension. These drugs act to lower blood pressure by peripheral dilatation and thus do not interfere with placental circulation. They can cause maternal tachycardia. Therefore, assess pulse and blood pressure before and after administration. Diastolic pressure should not be lowered below 80 to 90 mm Hg or inadequate placental perfusion could occur. Even with these new drugs, magnesium sulfate (Table 21.7), however, still remains the drug of choice to prevent eclampsia (Shilva, Kalra, & Prasad, 2007).

This drug, classified as a cathartic, reduces edema by causing a shift in fluid from the extracellular spaces into the intestine. It also has a central nervous system depressant action (it blocks peripheral neuromuscular transmissions), which lessens the possibility of seizures (Karch, 2009).

To achieve immediate reduction of the blood pressure, magnesium sulfate is first given intravenously in a loading or bolus dose. Given intravenously over 15 minutes, the drug acts almost immediately; unfortunately, the effect lasts only 30 to 60 minutes, so administration must be continuous.

For magnesium sulfate to act as an anticonvulsant, blood serum levels must be maintained at 5 to 8 mg/100 mL. If the blood serum level rises above this, respiratory depression, cardiac arrhythmias, and cardiac arrest can occur. The importance of different serum levels is shown in Box 21.10.

The most evident symptoms of overdose from magnesium sulfate administration include decreased urine output, depressed respirations, reduced consciousness, and decreased deep tendon reflexes (Subramanian, 2008). Because magnesium is excreted from the body almost entirely through the urine, urine output must be monitored closely to ensure adequate elimination. If severe oliguria should occur (less than 100 mL in 4 hours), excessively high serum levels of magnesium can result. Before you administer further magnesium sulfate, therefore, ensure that urine output is above 25 to 30 mL/hr, with a specific gravity of 1.010 or lower. Respirations should be above 12 per minute, a woman should be able to answer questions asked of her such as her name or address, ankle clonus (a continued motion of the foot) should be minimal, and deep tendon reflexes should be present. Make these assessments every hour if a continuous intravenous infusion is being used.

The easiest deep tendon reflex to assess is the patellar reflex (knee jerk). Instructions for initiating this reflex and ankle clonus are shown in Box 21.11. If an epidural block has been given for labor anesthesia, assess the biceps or triceps reflex (see Chapter 34).

In addition to making the above assessments when magnesium sulfate is being given, a solution of 10 mL of a 10% calcium gluconate solution (1 g) should be kept ready nearby for immediate intravenous administration should a woman develop signs and symptoms of magnesium toxicity, as calcium is the specific antidote for magnesium toxicity.

TABLE 21.7 ✻ Drugs Used in Pregnancy-Induced Hypertension

Drug	Indication	Dosage	Comments
Magnesium sulfate Pregnancy risk category B	Muscle relaxant; prevents seizures	Loading dose 4–6 g Maintenance dose 1–2 g/h IV	Infuse loading dose slowly over 15–30 min. Always administer as a piggyback infusion Assess respiratory rate, urine output, deep tendon reflexes, and clonus every hour. Urine output should be over 30 mL/hour and respiratory rate over 12/min. Serum magnesium level should remain below 7.5 mEq/L. Observe for CNS depression and hypotonia in infant at birth and calcium deficit in the mother.
Hydralazine (Apresoline) Pregnancy risk category C	Antihypertensive (peripheral vasodilator); used to decrease hypertension	5–10 mg/IV	Administer slowly to avoid sudden fall in blood pressure. Maintain diastolic pressure over 90 mm Hg to ensure adequate placental filling.
Diazepam (Valium) Pregnancy risk category D	Halt seizures	5–10 mg/IV	Administer slowly. Dose may be repeated q 5–10 min (up to 30 mg/hour). Observe for respiratory depression or hypotension in mother and respiratory depression and hypotonia in infant at birth.
Calcium gluconate Pregnancy risk category C	Antidote for magnesium intoxication	1 g/IV (10 mL of a 10% solution)	Have prepared at bedside when administering magnesium sulfate. Administer at 5 mL/min.

Source: Karch, A. M. (2009). *Lippincott's nursing drug guide.* Philadelphia: Lippincott Williams & Wilkins.

Severe oliguria may be treated by the intravenous infusion of salt-poor albumin. This high-colloid solution will call fluid into the bloodstream from interstitial tissue by osmotic pressure; the kidneys will then excrete the extra fluid along with magnesium sulfate levels.

On the planned day of birth, a pediatrician should be alerted that the woman has been receiving magnesium sulfate. This is because if magnesium sulfate is given intravenously within 2 hours of a baby's birth, the baby may be born with respiratory depression because the drug crosses the placenta. A fetal heart rate monitor may show loss of variability of heartbeat immediately after magnesium therapy; an ultrasound may reveal reduced fetal breathing movements. Observe carefully for other signs of fetal effects, such as late deceleration with labor contractions. Magnesium sulfate is continued for 12 to 24 hours after birth in the woman to prevent eclampsia during this period. The dose is then tapered and discontinued. Breastfeeding usually is delayed until the medication is discontinued. A long-term effect of magnesium sulfate therapy is osteoporosis. A woman may be started on a course of calcium postpartally to decrease this problem.

Nursing Interventions for a Woman With Eclampsia

Degeneration of a woman's condition from severe preeclampsia to eclampsia occurs when cerebral irritation from increasing cerebral edema becomes so acute that a seizure occurs. This usually happens late in pregnancy but can happen up to 48 hours after childbirth. Immediately before a seizure, a woman's blood pressure rises suddenly from additional vasospasm. Her temperature rises sharply to 103° to 104° F (39.4° to 40° C) from increased cerebral pressure. She notices blurring of vision or severe headache (from the increased cerebral edema) and her reflexes become hyperactive. She may experience a premonition that "something is happening." Vascular congestion of the liver or pancreas can lead to severe epigastric pain and nausea. Urinary output may decrease abruptly to less than 30 mL/hour. Eclampsia has actually occurred, however, only when a woman experiences a seizure.

Tonic-Clonic Seizures. An eclamptic seizure is a tonic-clonic type that occurs in stages. After the preliminary signal or aura that something is happening, all the muscles of the woman's body contract. Her back arches, her arms and legs stiffen, and her jaw closes abruptly. She may bite her tongue from the rapid closing of her jaw. Respirations halt because her thoracic muscles are held in contraction. This phase of the seizure, called the tonic phase, lasts approximately 20 seconds. It may seem longer because a woman may grow slightly cyanotic from the cessation of respirations.

During the second (clonic) stage, the woman's bladder and bowel muscles contract and relax; incontinence of urine and feces may occur. Although a woman begins to breathe during this stage, the breathing is not entirely effective. She

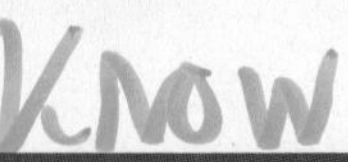

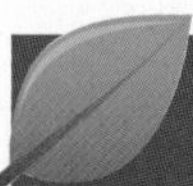

BOX 21.10 ✻ Focus on Pharmacology

Magnesium Sulfate

Action: Magnesium sulfate is a central nervous system depressant that acts to block neuromuscular transmission of acetylcholine to halt convulsions. It also halts premature labor, as it relaxes smooth muscle (Karch, 2009).

Pregnancy Risk Category: A

Dosage: Initially, 2–6 g IV administered in a 250-mL solution over a 20-minute period, followed by individually calculated IV infusion at a rate to maintain designated serum levels

- Therapeutic range: 5.0–8.0 mg/100 mL
- Patellar reflex disappears: 8–10 mg/100 mL
- Respiratory depression occurs: 15–20 mg/100 mL
- Cardiac conduction defects occur: More than 20 mg/100 mL

Possible Adverse Effects: Flushing, thirst; with toxicity, absence of deep tendon reflexes, respiratory depression, cardiac arrhythmias, cardiac arrest, and decreased urine output

Nursing Implications

- Administer continuous infusion piggybacked into a main IV line so it can be discontinued immediately without interfering with fluid administration.
- Always use an infusion control device to maintain a regular flow rate.
- Assess maternal blood pressure and fetal heart rate continuously with bolus IV administration.
- Assess deep tendon reflexes every 1–4 hours during continuous infusion. Use patellar reflex. If patient has received epidural anesthesia, use biceps reflex.
- Monitor intake and output every hour during continuous infusion. Urine output should be 30 mL/hr or greater.
- Assess client's level of consciousness, including ability to respond to questions, every hour.
- Obtain serum magnesium levels as indicated, usually every 6 to 8 hours.
- Keep calcium gluconate, the antidote for toxicity, readily available at the bedside.
- Maintain serum blood levels (for anticonvulsant use) at 5–8 mg/100 mL. If blood serum levels rise above this, respiratory depression, cardiac arrhythmias, and cardiac arrest can occur.
- Do not administer additional doses and stop infusion if deep tendon reflexes are absent or if respiratory rate is less than 14 or urine output is less than 30 mL/hr.
- This drug may cause respiratory depression in the newborn if administered close to birth. Alert neonatal care personnel about this possibility.
- Magnesium sulfate may cause osteoporosis in the mother if given over a long time. Supplemental calcium can prevent this outcome.

BOX 21.11 ✻ Eliciting A Patellar Reflex And Ankle Clonus

Patellar Reflex

With the woman in a supine position, ask her to bend her knee slightly. Place your hand under her knee to support the leg. Locate the patellar tendon in the midline just below the kneecap. Strike it firmly and quickly with a reflex hammer or the side of your hand. If the leg and foot move, a patellar reflex is present. The reflex is scored as:

0 = No response; hypoactive; abnormal
1+ = Somewhat diminished response but not abnormal
2+ = Average response
3+ = Brisker than average but not abnormal
4+ = Hyperactive; very brisk; abnormal

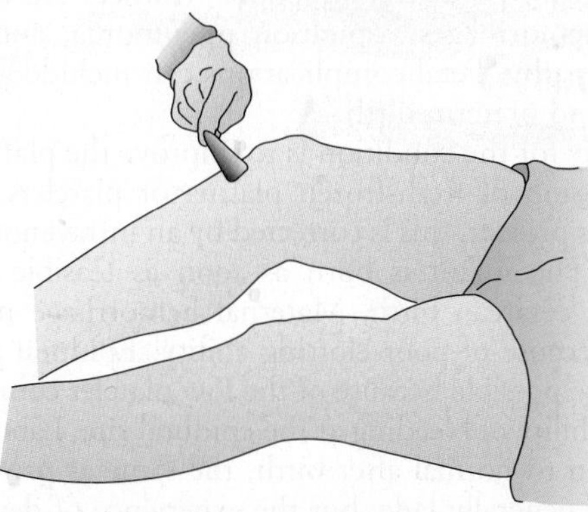

Ankle Clonus

To elicit ankle clonus, dorsiflex the woman's foot three times in rapid succession. As you take your hand away, observe the foot. If no further motion is present, no ankle clonus is present. If the foot continues to move involuntarily, clonus is present. Although usually just rated as present or absent, it can be rated as:

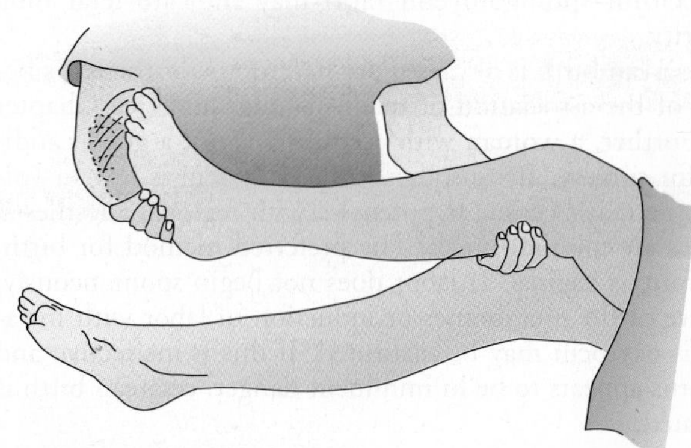

Mild (2 movements)
Moderate (3–5 movements)
Severe (over 6 movements)

may remain cyanotic. The clonic stage of a seizure lasts up to 1 minute.

The priority care for a woman with a tonic-clonic seizure is to maintain a patent airway. Administer oxygen by face mask to protect the fetus. To prevent aspiration, turn a woman on her side to allow secretions to drain from her mouth. Magnesium sulfate or diazepam (Valium) may be administered intravenously as an emergency measure. Assess oxygen saturation via a pulse oximeter. Apply an external fetal heart monitor if one is not already in place to assess the condition of the fetus. As labor may progress despite the seizure activity, continuously assess fetal heart sounds and uterine contractions. Check for vaginal bleeding to detect placental separation. Evidence that placental separation has occurred will appear first on the fetal heart record; vaginal bleeding will strengthen the presumption.

The third stage of the seizure is the postictal state. During this stage, a woman is semicomatose and cannot be roused except by painful stimuli for 1 to 4 hours. Extremely close observation is as important during the postictal stage as it was during the first two stages, because if the seizure caused premature separation of the placenta, labor may begin during this period but a woman will be unable to report the sensation of contractions. Also, the painful stimulus of contractions may initiate another seizure. Keep a woman on her side so secretions can drain from her mouth. Give her nothing to eat or drink. Remember that with coma, hearing is the last sense lost and the first one regained, so limit conversation as she may be able to hear even though she does not respond. Continuously assess fetal heart sounds and uterine contractions. Continue to check for vaginal bleeding every 15 minutes.

Birth. If the pregnancy is more than 24 weeks along, a decision about birth will be made as soon as a woman's condition stabilizes, usually 12 to 24 hours after the seizure. There is some evidence that a fetus does not continue to grow after eclampsia occurs, so terminating the pregnancy at this point is appropriate for both mother and child. For an unexplained reason, fetal lung maturity appears to advance rapidly with PIH (possibly from the intrauterine stress), so even though the fetus is younger than 36 weeks, the lecithin–sphingomyelin ratio may indicate fetal lung maturity.

Cesarean birth is always more hazardous for the fetus because of the association of retained lung fluid (see Chapter 26). Further, a woman with eclampsia is not a good candidate for surgery. Because her vascular system is low in volume, she may become hypotensive with regional anesthesia, such as an epidural block. The preferred method for birth, therefore, is vaginal. If labor does not begin spontaneously, rupture of the membranes or induction of labor with intravenous oxytocin may be instituted. If this is ineffective and the fetus appears to be in imminent danger, cesarean birth is indicated.

Nursing Interventions During the Postpartum Period

Postpartum hypertension may occur up to 10 to 14 days after birth, although it usually occurs no more than 48 hours after birth. Monitoring blood pressure in the postpartum period and being alert that eclampsia can occur as late as 2 to 3 weeks post birth is essential to detect residual hypertensive or renal disease (Cantey, Tecklenburg, & Titus, 2007). Urge women who had an elevation of blood pressure during pregnancy to return for a postpartum checkup to have their blood pressure evaluated to be certain it has returned to normal.

✓ Checkpoint Question 21.5

If Beverly Muzuki had developed severe pre-eclampsia, what would be the drug you would expect to administer?

a. Magnesium sulfate.
b. Ranitidine (Zantac).
c. A nonsteroidal anti-inflammatory agent.
d. A loop diuretic.

HELLP SYNDROME

HELLP syndrome is a variation of PIH named for the common symptoms that occur: *h*emolysis that leads to anemia, *e*levated *l*iver enzymes that lead to epigastric pain, and *l*ow *p*latelets that lead to abnormal bleeding/clotting and petechia (Guberman, Greenspon, & Goodwin, 2007).

The syndrome occurs in 4% to 12% of patients with PIH. It is a serious syndrome because it results in a maternal mortality rate as high as 24% and an infant mortality rate as high as 35%.

Why some women with severe pre-eclampsia also develop the HELLP syndrome is unknown. It occurs in both primigravidas and multigravidas. It may be associated with antiphospholipid syndrome or the presence of antiphopholipid antibodies (Clark, Silver, & Branch, 2007). In addition to proteinuria, edema and increased blood pressure, additional symptoms of nausea, epigastric pain, general malaise, and right upper quadrant tenderness from liver inflammation occur. Laboratory studies reveal hemolysis of red blood cells (they appear fragmented on a peripheral blood smear), thrombocytopenia (a platelet count $<100,000/mm^3$), and elevated liver enzyme levels (alanine aminotransferase [ALT] and serum aspartate aminotransferase [AST]). The liver enzyme levels are elevated from hemorrhage and necrosis of the liver. Because of the low platelet count, women with the HELLP syndrome need close observation for bleeding, in addition to the observations necessary for pre-eclampsia. Complications associated with the syndrome are subcapsular liver hematoma, hyponatremia, renal failure, and hypoglycemia from poor liver function. Mothers are at risk for cerebral hemorrhages, aspiration pneumonia, and hypoxic encephalopathy. Fetal complications can include growth restriction and preterm birth.

Therapy for the condition is to improve the platelet count by transfusion of fresh-frozen plasma or platelets. If hypoglycemia is present, this is corrected by an intravenous glucose infusion. The infant is born as soon as feasible by either vaginal or cesarean birth. Maternal hemorrhage may occur at birth because of poor clotting ability. Epidural anesthesia may not be possible because of the low platelet count and the high possibility of bleeding at the epidural site. Laboratory results return to normal after birth, the same as pre-eclamptic symptoms generally fade, but the experience of developing a

HELLP syndrome is frightening. Women need assurance afterward that symptoms were pregnancy related so will completely fade.

MULTIPLE PREGNANCY

Multiple gestation is considered a complication of pregnancy because a woman's body must adjust to the effects of more than one fetus. The incidence of multiple births has increased dramatically because of the use of in vitro fertilization but still only occurs in 2% to 3% of all births. The rate of twinning in the United States is about 1 in 80 births; triplets, 1 in 8000 (Bush & Pernoll, 2007).

Identical (monozygotic) twins begin with a single ovum and spermatozoon. In the process of fusion, or in one of the first cell divisions, the zygote divides into two identical individuals. Single-ovum twins usually have one placenta, one chorion, two amnions, and two umbilical cords. The twins are always of the same sex. Two thirds of twins are fraternal (dizygotic, nonidentical), the result of the fertilization of two separate ova by two separate spermatozoa (possibly not from the same sexual partner). Double-ova twins have two placentas, two chorions, two amnions, and two umbilical cords. The twins may be of the same or different sex (Fig. 21.9). It is sometimes difficult to determine by ultrasound or at birth whether twins are identical or fraternal because the two fraternal placentas may fuse and appear as one large placenta.

Multiple pregnancies of two to eight children may be single-ovum conceptions, multiple-ova conceptions, or a combination of the two types. Most today occur from multiple ova being implanted as an in vitro fertility process. Naturally occurring multiple pregnancies are more frequent in nonwhites than in whites. The higher a woman's parity and age, the more likely she is to have a multiple gestation. Inheritance appears to play a role in natural dizygotic twinning; this has a familial maternal pattern of occurrence (Bush & Pernoll, 2007).

Assessment

Multiple gestation is suspected early in pregnancy, when the uterus begins to increase in size at a rate faster than usual. Alpha-fetoprotein levels are elevated. At the time of quickening, a woman may report flurries of action at different portions of her abdomen rather than at one consistent spot (where the feet are located). On auscultation of the abdomen, multiple sets of fetal heart sounds are heard, but if one or more fetus has his or her back positioned toward a woman's back, only one fetal heart sound may be heard.

An ultrasound can reveal multiple gestation sacs early in pregnancy. In some instances, early ultrasound examinations reveal multiple amniotic sacs but then later in pregnancy, in as many as 30% of women, only one fetus remains (vanishing twin syndrome) (Anand, Platt, & Pharoah, 2007). Women may grieve for a vanished twin as much as if the baby had died at birth, a feeling that could disrupt pregnancy bonding work.

Therapeutic Management

Women with a multiple gestation are more susceptible to complications of pregnancy such as PIH, hydramnios, placenta previa, preterm labor, and anemia than are women carrying one fetus. They also are more prone to postpartum bleeding because of the additional uterine stretching that must occur. Because a multiple pregnancy usually ends before the normal term, 25% of low-birth-weight babies are from multiple pregnancies. There is a higher risk of congenital anomalies in twins, such as spinal cord defect, than with single births. There is a higher incidence of velamentous cord insertion (the cord inserted into the fetal membranes) with twins than with single births, so the risk of

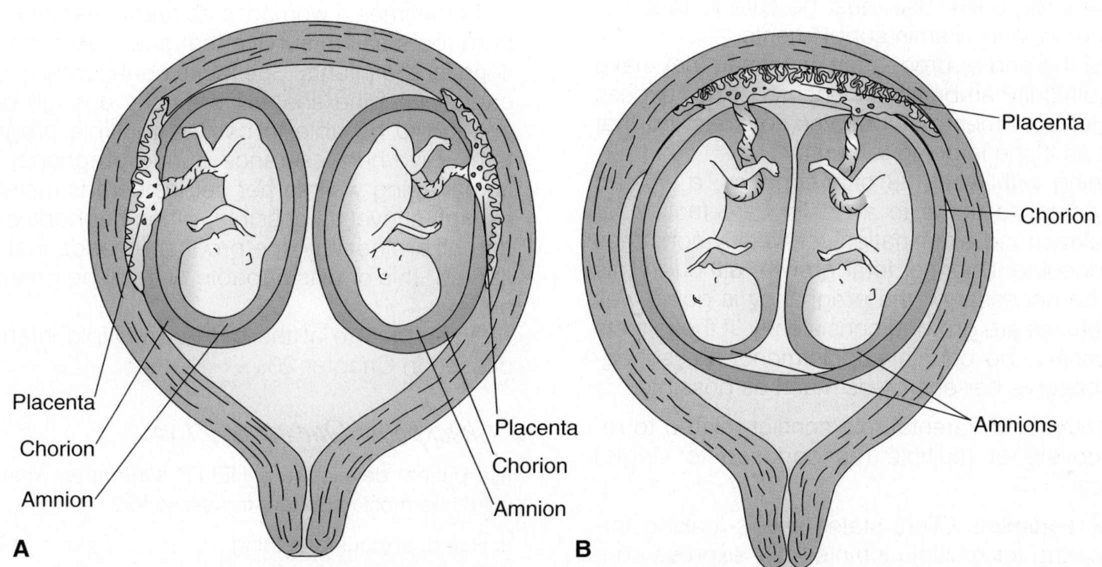

FIGURE 21.9 Multiple gestations. (**A**) Dizygotic twins showing two placentas, two chorions, and two amnions. (**B**) Monozygotic twins with one placenta, one chorion, and two amnions.

bleeding at the time of birth from a torn cord is increased. With monozygotic twins, the fetuses can share vascular communication, possibly leading to overgrowth of one fetus and undergrowth of the second (a twin-to-twin transfusion), resulting in discordant infants (Norton, 2007) (see Chapter 26). If a single amnion is present, there can be knotting and twisting of umbilical cords, causing fetal distress or difficulty with birth. Because of the possibility of these complications, a woman with a twin pregnancy needs closer prenatal supervision than a woman with a single gestation to detect these problems as early as possible. A woman carrying more than two fetuses is at greatest risk (Bush & Pernoll, 2007).

Nursing Diagnoses and Related Interventions

Nursing Diagnosis: Fatigue related to increased stress on body functioning secondary to multiple gestation

Outcome Evaluation: Client states she is tired but identifies steps she has taken to minimize fatigue.

Although there is little evidence that strict bed rest helps prolong multiple pregnancies (Crowther, 2009), spend time at health care visits reviewing with a woman with a multiple pregnancy her need for extra rest, especially in a side-lying position during the day, to increase placental perfusion.

Because a woman is carrying a double weight during pregnancy, she may notice extreme fatigue and backache late in each day. She may have more difficulty resting or sleeping than the average woman because of this greater discomfort and increased fetal activity. As the growing uterus compresses her stomach, she may find her appetite decreasing and her intake falling. To compensate and maintain nutrition, a woman may need to eat six small meals a day rather than three large ones. She must be sure to take her iron, folic acid, and vitamin supplements.

Toward the end of pregnancy, a woman may have extreme difficulty ambulating because of her excess weight. Her abdomen may become so stretched that she feels as if she is going to burst.

Beginning with week 28 of pregnancy, a woman may be asked to come to a health care facility for monthly ultrasound examinations or weekly nonstress tests to document normal fetal growth, although this may not be necessary if the pregnancy is going well and the fetuses are growing consistently. If these tests are necessary, be certain appointments are scheduled to conserve her energy as much as possible.

Nursing Diagnosis: Parental role conflict related to recent discovery of multiple (as opposed to single) pregnancy

Outcome Evaluation: Client states she is looking forward to caring for multiple infants (may express concern about her ability to manage their arrival); client identifies changes she is making in preparation now that more than one baby is expected.

A woman with a multiple pregnancy has to work through an additional role change during pregnancy. First, she completes the work to accept she is pregnant, then the work to accept she is having a baby. Then suddenly, at a routine office visit, two or more gestational sacs are seen on ultrasound or two or more sets of heart sounds are heard on auscultation. She is told she is going to have more than one child. Now she has to work through a second role change—for example, becoming a mother of two, not of one, or a mother of four or five. This role change may be difficult to complete, especially if the pregnancy ends early. Because of this, a woman may need extra help after birth to form a close mother–child relationship with her newborns.

Nursing Diagnosis: Fear concerning her own and the babies' health related to risks of multiple pregnancy

Outcome Evaluation: Client accurately states risks of multiple pregnancy; expresses confidence in health care team's ability to care for her and her babies through pregnancy and birth.

In addition to having to work through a role change, a woman with a multiple pregnancy has more reason to fear for her life and the life of her babies than does the average woman. Every woman has heard stories about twins being born so prematurely they did not survive, and about the special danger for the last infant born. If she has not already heard these stories, someone will mention them to her before her due date. Unfortunately, all these risks cannot simply be filed away under the heading of untrue stories: both prematurity and high risk to the last-born infant are real hazards in multiple gestation. Help a woman deal with her fears as positively as possible. It is helpful to tell her there is no indication so far that her babies are in any danger, so right now it is best to continue doing the things that have to be done; if any problems should arise, the health care team and a woman's family will be there to support her.

Sometimes a woman is so fearful her infants will be born too small to survive that she makes no preparations for the infants. She lacks confidence in herself or cannot imagine she will be lucky enough or "good" enough to be able to carry a multiple pregnancy to term. Give her assurance during pregnancy that she is managing well so her self-esteem is maintained at as high a level as possible. When her babies are born and all are healthy, the proof she needs that she "deserved" this or was capable of it will be present in her arms.

Nursing care at the birth of multiple infants is discussed in Chapter 23.

✔ Checkpoint Question 21.6

If a patient developed a HELLP syndrome, what symptoms would be most important to assess for?

a. Rapid, anxious breathing.
b. Ecchymosis or petechiae.
c. Blink reflex.
d. Enlarged thyroid.

HYDRAMNIOS

Usually the amniotic fluid volume during pregnancy is 500 to 1000 mL at term. Excess fluid more than 2000 mL or an amniotic fluid index above 24 cm is considered **hydramnios** (Fortner, Althaus, & Gurewitsch, 2007). Too much amniotic fluid can cause fetal malpresentation because the additional uterine space can allow the fetus to turn to a transverse lie. It also can lead to premature rupture of the membranes from the increased pressure with possible prostaglandin release. Preterm rupture of the membranes adds the additional risks of infection, prolapsed cord, and preterm birth.

Assessment

Amniotic fluid is formed by a combination of the cells of the amniotic membrane and from fetal urine. It is evacuated by being swallowed by the fetus, absorbed across the intestinal membrane into the fetal bloodstream, and transferred across the placenta. Although hydramnios can occur separate from fetal involvement, accumulation of amniotic fluid suggests difficulty with the fetus's ability to swallow or absorb or else excessive urine production. Inability to swallow occurs in infants who are anencephalic or who have tracheoesophageal fistula with stenosis or intestinal obstruction (Smith & Henderson, 2007). Excessive urine output occurs in the fetuses of diabetic women (hyperglycemia in the fetus causes increased urine production).

The first sign of hydramnios may be unusually rapid enlargement of the uterus. The small parts of the fetus are difficult to palpate because the uterus is unusually tense. Auscultating the fetal heart rate is difficult because of the increased amount of fluid surrounding the fetus.

A woman may begin to notice extreme shortness of breath as the overly distended uterus pushes up against her diaphragm. She may develop lower extremity varicosities and hemorrhoids because of poor venous return from the extensive uterine pressure. She will have increased weight gain. Generally, an ultrasound is ordered to document the presence of hydramnios and to discover a reason for the excessive amount of fluid.

Therapeutic Management

Women with severe hydramnios may be admitted to a hospital for bed rest and further evaluation or may be cared for at home. Regardless of the setting, maintaining bed rest helps to increase uteroplacental circulation and reduces pressure on the cervix, which may help prevent preterm labor. Teach a woman to report any sign of ruptured membranes or uterine contractions. Although not common, there is a possibility that straining to defecate could increase uterine pressure and cause rupture of membranes. Help her avoid constipation, therefore, by encouraging her to eat a high-fiber diet. Suggest a stool softener be prescribed if diet alone is ineffective.

Assess vital signs and lower extremity edema frequently, because the extremely tense uterus puts unusual pressure on both the diaphragm and the vessels of the pelvis.

A regimen of a nonsteroidal anti-inflammatory agent may be started to reduce inflammation (Rode et al., 2007). Amniocentesis can be performed to remove some of the extra amniotic fluid. Because amniotic fluid is replaced rapidly, however, this has to be repeated almost daily. If contractions begin, tocolysis may be begun to prevent or halt preterm labor.

Even with these precautions, in most instances of hydramnios, there will be preterm rupture of the membranes because of excessive pressure, followed by preterm birth. To prevent the sudden loss of fluid and the accompanying danger of a prolapsed cord, membranes can be "needled" (a thin needle is inserted vaginally to pierce them) to allow a slow, controlled release of fluid. After birth, the infant must be assessed carefully for factors that may have interfered with the ability to swallow in utero (Touboul et al., 2007).

OLIGOHYDRAMNIOS

Oligohydramnios refers to a pregnancy with less than the average amount of amniotic fluid (Chauhan et al., 2007). As part of the volume of amniotic fluid is formed by the addition of fetal urine, this is usually caused by a bladder or renal disorder in the fetus that interferes with voiding. It can occur from severe growth restriction. Because the fetus is so cramped for space, muscles are left weak at birth, lungs fail to develop (hypoplastic lungs), leading to severe difficulty breathing after birth, and features of the face become distorted (termed Potter's syndrome).

The condition is suspected during pregnancy when the uterus fails to meet its expected growth rate. It is confirmed by ultrasound when the pockets of amniotic fluid are less than average. Amniotransfusion or instillation of fluid into the uterus by amniocentesis procedure can help relieve this concern (Chhabra, Dargan, & Nasare, 2007). Infants need careful inspection at birth to rule out kidney disease and compromised lung development.

POST TERM PREGNANCY

A term pregnancy is 38 to 42 weeks long. A pregnancy that exceeds these limits is prolonged (**post term pregnancy,** *postmature,* or *postdate*). The infant of such a pregnancy is considered postmature, or dysmature, if there is evidence that placental insufficiency has interfered with fetal growth. Post term pregnancy occurs in 3% to 12% of all pregnancies (Fortner, Althaus, & Gurewitsch, 2007).

Included in this group are some pregnancies that appear to extend beyond the due date set for them because of a faulty due date. Women who have long menstrual cycles (40 to 45 days, for example) do not ovulate on day 14 as in a typical menstrual cycle. Because they ovulate 14 days from the end of their cycle, or on day 26 or 31, their children will be "late" by 12 to 17 days.

In other instances, the pregnancy is truly overdue. For some reason, the trigger that initiates labor did not turn on. Prolonged pregnancy can occur in a woman receiving a high dose of salicylates (for severe sinus headaches or rheumatoid arthritis) because salicylate interferes with the synthesis of prostaglandins, which may be responsible for the initiation of labor. It is also associated with myometrial quiescence, or a uterus that does not respond to normal labor stimulation.

Remaining in utero for longer than 2 weeks beyond term creates a danger to a fetus for several reasons. Meconium aspiration is more apt to occur as fetal intestinal contents are more likely to reach the rectum. If the fetus continues to grow, macrosomia could create a birth problem. However, the usual effect of being post term is lack of growth. A placenta seems to have adequate functioning ability for only 40 to 42 weeks. After that time, it acquires calcium deposits (becomes grade 3). This exposes a fetus to decreased blood perfusion. Such a fetus may suffer from a lack of oxygen, fluid, and nutrients (Neilson, 2007). Oligohydramnios (a decreased amount of amniotic fluid from lessened urine production in the fetus) can lead to variable decelerations from cord compression.

If labor has not begun by 41 weeks, a maternal vaginal fibronectin level, a nonstress test, and/or a biophysical profile may be ordered to document the state of placental perfusion and the amount of amniotic fluid present. If these are normal, it suggests the due date was miscalculated. If the test results are abnormal or the physical examination or biparietal diameter measured on ultrasound suggests the fetus is term size, labor will be induced (Norwitz, Snegovskikh, & Caughey, 2007). Prostaglandin gel or misoprostol (Cytotec) applied to the cervix to initiate ripening, or stripping of membranes followed by an oxytocin infusion are common methods used to begin labor. If oxytocin is ineffective, cesarean birth will be necessary. Monitor the fetal heart rate closely during labor to be certain placental insufficiency is not occurring from aging of the placenta. Nursing care for the post term infant at birth is discussed in Chapter 26.

PSEUDOCYESIS

In **pseudocyesis** (false pregnancy), nausea and vomiting, amenorrhea, and enlargement of the abdomen occur in either a nonpregnant woman or a man (Ayakannu et al., 2007). There are several theories regarding why the phenomenon occurs: wish-fulfillment theory suggests a woman's desire to be pregnant actually causes physiologic changes to occur; conflict theory suggests a desire for and fear of pregnancy create an internal conflict leading to physiologic changes; and depression theory attributes the cause to major depression. In any event, a woman's body responds with physiologic symptoms such as breast tenderness and an enlarging abdomen. Her abdomen can become so enlarged that she appears to be 7 or 8 months pregnant. On physical examination, however, it is obvious only the abdomen, not the uterus, is enlarged. Ultrasound imaging will rule out pregnancy. Both men and women with the disorder need psychological counseling to help them better handle their needs.

ISOIMMUNIZATION (RH INCOMPATIBILITY)

Approximately 15% of white and 10% of African Americans in the United States are missing the Rh (D) factor in their blood or have an Rh-negative blood type. **Rh incompatibility** occurs when an Rh-negative mother (one negative for a *D* antigen or one with a *dd* genotype) carries a fetus with an Rh-positive blood type (*DD* or *Dd* genotype). For such a situation to occur, the father of the child must either be homozygous (*DD*) or heterozygous (*Dd*) Rh-positive. If the father of the child is homozygous (*DD*) for the factor, 100% of the couple's children will be Rh-positive (*Dd*). If the father is heterozygous for the trait, 50% of their children can be expected to be Rh-positive (*Dd*). Although this is basically a problem that affects the fetus, it causes such concern and apprehension in a woman during pregnancy that it becomes a maternal problem as well.

Because people who have Rh-positive blood have a protein factor (the *D* antigen) that Rh-negative people do not, when an Rh-positive fetus begins to grow inside an Rh-negative mother who is sensitized, it is as though her body is being invaded by a foreign agent. Her body reacts in the same manner it would if the invading factor were a substance such as a virus: she forms antibodies against the invading substance. The Rh factor exists as a portion of the red blood cell, so these maternal antibodies cross the placenta and cause red blood cell destruction (hemolysis) of fetal red blood cells (Fig. 21.10). A fetus can become so deficient in red blood cells that sufficient oxygen transport to body cells cannot be maintained. This condition is termed **hemolytic disease of the newborn** or **erythroblastosis fetalis.** Management of the infant born with this condition is discussed in Chapter 26.

Theoretically, there is no connection between fetal blood and maternal blood during pregnancy, so the mother should

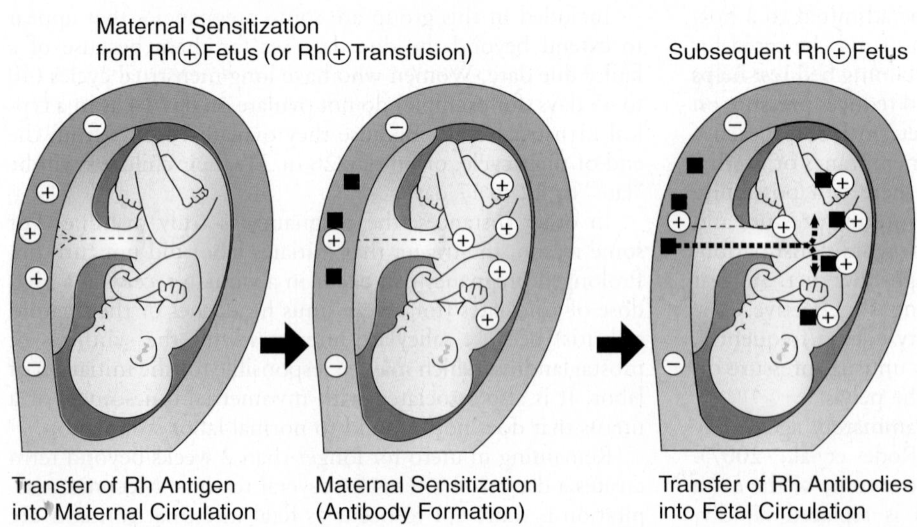

FIGURE 21.10 Maternal antibody formation against the Rh antigen.

not be exposed to fetal blood. It is well documented, however, that an occasional villus ruptures, allowing a drop or two of fetal blood to enter the maternal circulation. Procedures such as amniocentesis or percutaneous umbilical blood sampling can also cause this. During a first pregnancy this effect is small. As the placenta separates after birth of the first child, there is an active exchange of fetal and maternal blood from damaged villi. Therefore, most of the maternal antibodies formed against the Rh-positive blood are not formed during pregnancy but in the first 72 hours after birth, making them a threat to a second pregnancy.

Assessment

All women with Rh-negative blood should have an anti-D antibody titer done at a first pregnancy visit. If the results are normal or the titer is minimal (normal is 0; a ratio below 1:8 is minimal), the test will be repeated at week 28 of pregnancy. If this is also normal, no therapy is needed.

If a woman's anti-D antibody titer is elevated at a first assessment (1:16 or greater), showing Rh sensitization, the well-being of the fetus in this potentially toxic environment will be monitored every 2 weeks (or more often) by Doppler velocity of the fetal middle cerebral artery, a technique that can predict when anemia is present or fetal red cells are being destroyed (Valcamonico et al., 2007).

If the artery velocity remains high, a fetus is not developing anemia and most likely is an Rh-negative fetus. If the reading is low, it means a fetus is in danger, and immediate birth will be carried out providing the fetus is near term. If not near term, efforts to reduce the number of antibodies in the woman or replace damaged red cells in the fetus are begun.

Therapeutic Management

To reduce the number of maternal Rh (D) antibodies being formed, Rh (D) immune globulin (RhIG), a commercial preparation of passive Rh (D) antibodies against the Rh factor, is administered to women who are Rh-negative at 28 weeks of pregnancy. These cannot cross the placenta and destroy fetal red blood cells because the antibodies are not the IgG class, the only type that crosses the placenta. RhIG is given again by injection to the mother in the first 72 hours after birth of an Rh-positive child to further prevent the woman from forming natural antibodies. Because RhIG is passive antibody protection, it is transient, and in 2 weeks to 2 months, the passive antibodies are destroyed. Only those few antibodies that were formed during pregnancy are left. For this reason, every pregnancy is like a first pregnancy in terms of the number of antibodies present, ensuring a safe intrauterine environment for any future pregnancies.

After birth, the infant's blood type will be determined from a sample of the cord blood. If it is Rh-positive—Coombs' negative, indicating that a large number of antibodies are not present in the mother—the mother will receive the RhIG injection. If the newborn's blood type is Rh-negative, no antibodies have been formed in the mother's circulation during pregnancy and none will form, so passive antibody injection is unnecessary.

Although in future years the problem of Rh sensitization will be greatly reduced, it currently remains a complication of pregnancy, particularly in women who gave birth to a first child in an undeveloped nation where they did not receive passive anti-D antibodies. Any woman who does not receive a RhIG injection after an induced abortion, miscarriage, ectopic pregnancy, or amniocentesis can also have antibody formation begin.

Intrauterine Transfusion

To restore fetal red blood cells, blood transfusion can be performed on the fetus in utero. This is done by injecting red blood cells, by amniocentesis technique, directly into a vessel in the fetal cord or depositing them in the fetal abdomen where they migrate into the fetal circulation.

Blood used for transfusion in utero is either the fetus's own type (determined by percutaneous blood sampling) or group O negative if the fetal blood type is unknown. From 75 to 150 mL of washed red cells are used, depending on the age of the fetus. After deposition of the blood in the cord or abdomen, the cannula is withdrawn and a woman is urged to rest for approximately 30 minutes while fetal heart sounds and uterine activity are monitored.

Obviously, intrauterine transfusion is not without risk. A cord blood vessel could be lacerated by the needle, or the uterus may be so irritated by the invasive procedure that labor contractions begin. For the fetus who is severely affected by isoimmunization, however, such a risk is no greater than that of leaving the fetus untreated in a destructive intrauterine environment. The mother receives an RhIG injection after the transfusion to help reduce increased sensitization from any blood that might have been exchanged. Transfusion is sometimes done only once during pregnancy, or it may be repeated as often as every 2 weeks. As soon as fetal maturity is reached, as shown by a mature lecithin–sphingomyelin ratio, birth will be induced.

After birth, the infant may require an exchange transfusion to remove hemolyzed red blood cells and replace them with healthy blood cells (see Chapter 26). A woman needs to discuss her plans for further childbearing and should be provided with contraceptive information if she believes the strain of this pregnancy, the constant feeling of wishing that everything was all right but never being certain that it was, is more than she wants to endure again.

FETAL DEATH

Obviously, one of the most severe complications of pregnancy is fetal death. The most likely causes include chromosomal abnormalities, congenital malformations, infections such as hepatitis B, immunologic causes, and complications of maternal disease. If fetal death occurs before the time of quickening, a woman will not be aware the fetus has died because she is not able to feel fetal movements. This type of fetal death may be discovered at a routine prenatal visit when no fetal heartbeat can be heard. A real-time ultrasound will reveal no fetal heartbeat is present.

That a fetus has died early in intrauterine life may first be revealed by the natural miscarriage that occurs. A woman begins painless spotting, gradually accompanied by uterine contractions with cervical effacement and dilatation. The fetus is born lifeless and emaciated. Carefully observe all women who give birth to a dead fetus for excess bleeding because if the fetus has been dead in utero for any length of time, the risk for the development of DIC increases.

If a fetus dies in utero past the point of quickening, a woman becomes aware that fetal movements are suddenly absent. She may lie down or sit in a position that she knows usually causes fetal movement. Unable to believe that something could have happened, she may attribute the lack of movement to "sleeping" or "saving enough strength to be born." Because she is denying what is happening, it may be a full 24 hours before she calls the health care facility to report the apparent lack of fetal movement. On assessment, no fetal heartbeat can be heard. An ultrasound will confirm the absence of a fetal heartbeat.

If labor does not begin spontaneously, it will be induced through a combination of prostaglandin gel such as misoprostol (Cytotec) applied to the cervix to effect cervical ripening and oxytocin administration to begin uterine contractions (Neilson, Hickey, & Vazquez, 2009). Blood for coagulation studies to detect DIC should be obtained.

Nursing Diagnoses and Related Interventions

Nursing Diagnosis: Powerlessness related to fetal death

Outcome Evaluation: Client and support person express meaning of pregnancy loss; identify support people/family with whom they can share grief.

Going through labor knowing a fetus is dead is difficult. A woman grieves for both her dead child and her inability to carry a pregnancy to term. She may wonder what she could have done to cause this such as forget to take an iron supplement or paint a crib or may worry she is not as good a woman as others. Give her opportunities to express how she feels about this loss. "This must be a very difficult day for you" is the kind of statement that opens up the topic for discussion. If there are older children, it might be a help to explore how a woman plans to explain the fetal death to them.

Ask a couple about their desire for clergy or religious rites, such as baptism. Encourage a support person to remain with a woman during labor, but remember the support person is grieving, too. Although this is a difficult time, expressing grief makes the birth real, ends the pregnancy, and allows the couple to begin rebuilding their life.

Labor involving a dead fetus is the same as for a live fetus because every fetus is basically a passive participant during labor. It may be difficult for a woman to use controlled breathing exercises, although encouraging her to use them is helpful in making the experience one of controllable pain. If a woman wishes a high level of analgesia or an epidural, she may have it because there is no fetus to protect from narcotic effects, although too much may lead to poor uterine involution in the postpartum period.

Ask if the parents wish to see the child. If they do, wash away obvious blood, swaddle the baby as if he or she were a well newborn, and bring the baby to them. Point out particularly endearing features of the child that may provide a focus for memories. Some parents want to keep a lock of the child's hair. Others want to keep the hospital identification bracelet or to take a photograph. Parents may want to name the child. All of these measures help to make the death real to parents and let them begin the healthy process of grieving (Chambers & Chan, 2009).

If the child has a congenital anomaly that led to the death, prepare them for this before bringing the child to them, and explain how the anomaly affected the child. Explain hospital procedures such as when the body will be released or what additional permission for autopsy is needed. Different communities have different laws concerning whether burial for an immature fetus is necessary. Consult local health department regulations so you can serve as a resource person for parents concerning this.

A woman needs to remain for only a short stay in the hospital, assuming no complications with labor developed. Many couples ask how soon it will be safe for them to have another child. For the answer to this, they need to consult with their obstetrician or nurse-midwife about why this fetal death occurred. For some couples, beginning a second pregnancy immediately is a good recommendation. For others, waiting for an interval of time (perhaps 6 months) is better as this gives them more time to work through their grief before starting a new pregnancy. This helps prevent the new baby from becoming a "replacement baby" or someone to take the place of the dead infant rather than a unique individual in his or her own right. This is important in years to come because replacement children are rarely able to live up to the image of what the dead baby would have been if only that baby had lived.

Prepare the couple for the possibility that they may feel sad on the day the infant would have been born if the pregnancy had been carried to term, or if they visit a friend's child of the age their child would have been. Be certain before a woman is discharged from the hospital that she has a support person she can rely on during the following week or month, when the full impact of the fetal loss registers. Be certain she has a return appointment for a gynecologic checkup so her physiologic and psychological health can be evaluated at that time.

✓ Checkpoint Question 21.7

Suppose Beverly Muzuki is Rh negative. Under what circumstance would she be eligible for Rh (D) immune globulin (RhIG) following her child's birth?

a. If she had a multiple pregnancy.
b. If her fetus was found to be Rh negative.
c. If her fetus's heartbeat was tachycardic.
d. If her fetus's blood type was Rh positive.

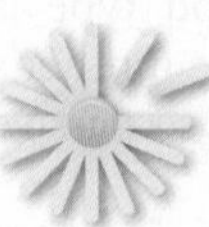

Key Points for Review

- Vaginal bleeding during pregnancy is always serious until ruled otherwise because it has the potential to diminish the blood supply of both the mother and fetus.

- The amount of bleeding which is evident may not be truly indicative of the amount of bleeding occurring as hidden, internal bleeding may also be happening. As a rule, women with bleeding during pregnancy should be positioned on their side to improve placental circulation.
- Spontaneous miscarriage is the loss of a pregnancy before viability of the fetus (20 to 24 weeks). The majority of these early pregnancy losses are attributed to chromosomal abnormalities. Miscarriages are classified as threatened, imminent, complete, incomplete, missed, or recurrent pregnancy loss. Women who have a spontaneous miscarriage at home should bring any tissue passed to the hospital for an analysis for gestational trophoblastic disease.
- Ectopic pregnancy is pregnancy implantation outside the uterus, usually in a fallopian tube. If discovered before the tube ruptures, methotrexate or mifepristone can be administered to cause the conceptus to be reabsorbed. If not discovered early, sharp lower quadrant pain occurs at about 6 to 12 weeks as the tube ruptures. Surgery is done to remove the conceptus and repair the tube to halt bleeding.
- Gestational trophoblastic disease is abnormal overgrowth of trophoblast cells. If not discovered by an ultrasound early in pregnancy, bleeding and expulsion of the abnormal growth occur at about the 16th week of pregnancy. Women need close follow-up after this because it can lead to choriocarcinoma, a malignancy.
- Premature cervical dilatation occurs when the cervix dilates early in pregnancy, before viability of the fetus. Sutures (cervical cerclage) can be placed to prevent the cervix from dilating prematurely this way again in a second pregnancy.
- Placenta previa is low implantation of the placenta so that it crosses the cervical os. If this is not discovered before labor, cervical dilatation may cause the placenta to tear, causing severe blood loss. Women who have symptoms of placenta previa (painless vaginal bleeding in the third trimester) should not have vaginal examinations done to prevent disruption of the low-implanted placenta.
- Premature separation of the placenta (abruptio placentae), placental separation from the uterus before the fetus is born, usually occurs late in pregnancy. This separation immediately cuts off blood supply to the fetus. Women with increased parity, those with previous uterine surgery, and those who use cocaine are at highest risk for this. Often it is manifested by sudden, sharp fundal pain, then a continuing dull pain and vaginal bleeding.
- Disseminated intravascular coagulation is a blood disorder that may occur with any trauma, so it can accompany such conditions as premature separation of the placenta and pregnancy-induced hypertension. Blood coagulation is so extreme at one point in the circulatory system that clotting factors are used up, resulting in their absence in the remainder of the system. Beginning symptoms of this include easy bruising, petechiae, and oozing from intravenous sites. Heparin is used to stop the local coagulation and free up clotting factors for systemic use.
- Preterm labor is labor that occurs after 20 weeks and before the end of the 37th week of pregnancy. A woman is said to be in preterm labor when she has had uterine contractions every 10 minutes for 1 hour and cervical dilatation begins. Common tocolytics, drugs that can halt labor, are beta-sympathomimetic agents such as terbutaline (Brethine).
- Preterm rupture of the membranes is tearing of the fetal membranes with loss of amniotic fluid before the pregnancy is at term. After rupture, there is a high risk of fetal and uterine infection (chorioamnionitis) and preterm birth.
- Pregnancy-induced hypertension is a unique disorder that occurs with pregnancy with three classic symptoms: hypertension, edema, and proteinuria. It is categorized as pre-eclampsia or eclampsia. If mild (blood pressure not over 140/90), treatment is bed rest and perhaps low-dose aspirin. If severe (blood pressure over 160/110), bed rest plus administration of magnesium sulfate is necessary. If a seizure occurs, the condition becomes eclampsia. Helping prevent the disease from progressing to this stage is an important nursing responsibility.
- The HELLP syndrome is a unique form of pregnancy-induced hypertension marked by hemolysis of red blood cells, elevated liver enzymes, and a low platelet count.
- Multiple gestation puts an additional strain on a woman's physical resources and may lead to preterm birth with immaturity of her infants. Helping a woman plan adequate nutrition and rest during pregnancy are nursing responsibilities.
- Post term pregnancy is pregnancy that extends beyond 42 weeks. As the placenta deteriorates at this time, it can cause a fetus to receive decreased nutrients.
- Hydramnios is overproduction of amniotic fluid (above 2000 mL), a condition that can lead to ruptured membranes and premature birth because of increased intrauterine pressure. Oligohydramnios is the lessened amount of fluid and suggests a renal disorder exists in the fetus.
- Isoimmunization (Rh incompatibility) is a possibility when a woman who is Rh negative is sensitized and carries a fetus who is Rh positive. Maternal antibodies form and destroy fetal red blood cells, leading to anemia, edema, and jaundice in the newborn. Being certain women are screened for blood type and antibody titer early in pregnancy is a nursing responsibility.

CRITICAL THINKING EXERCISES

1. Beverly Muzuki is the woman you met at the beginning of the chapter who was in preterm labor at 30 weeks of pregnancy. Beverly discounted the symptoms she was having because she did not think they could be early labor. What are the signs of early labor that you would have liked her to have been more aware of?
2. Suppose Beverly is bleeding because of placenta previa; everyone else on the unit is at lunch, and you are alone.

You know you should not do a pelvic examination with a placenta previa. How would you estimate the amount of blood she has lost? How would you determine that blood loss was not affecting the fetus?

3. Suppose Beverly is placed on home care after preterm rupture of membranes at 30 weeks of pregnancy. What assessments would you want to do to ensure she is not developing chorioamnionitis? Suppose she tells you she is too busy to stay on bed rest at home? What suggestions would you give her so she could best achieve bed rest? Does she have an ethical obligation to her fetus to rest? What about a legal obligation?
4. Examine the National Health Goals related to complications of pregnancy. Most government-sponsored money for nursing research is allotted based on these goals. What would be a possible research topic to explore pertinent to these goals that would be applicable to the Muzuki family and also advance evidence-based practice?

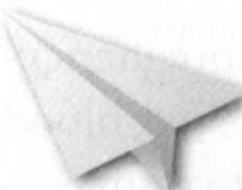

CRITICAL THINKING SCENARIO

Open the accompanying CD-ROM or visit http://thePoint.lww.com and read the Patient Scenario included for this chapter, then answer the questions to further sharpen your skills and grow more familiar with NCLEX style questions related to sudden pregnancy complications. Confirm your answers are correct by reading the rationales.

REFERENCES

Aghajanian, P. (2007). Gestational trophoblastic diseases. In A. H. DeCherney & L. Nathan (Eds.). *Current diagnosis and treatment in obstetrics and gynecology* (10th ed.). Columbus, OH: McGraw-Hill.

Anand, D., Platt, M. J., & Pharoah, P. O. (2007). Comparative development of surviving co-twins of vanishing twin conceptions, twins and singletons. *Twin Research and Human Genetics: the Official Journal of the International Society for Twin Studies, 10*(1), 210–215.

Arquette, N., & Holcroft, C. J. (2007). Third-trimester bleeding. In K. B. Fortner, et al. (Eds.). *The Johns Hopkins manual of gynecology and obstetrics.* Philadelphia: Lippincott Williams & Wilkins.

Ayakannu, T., et al. (2007). Pseudocyesis in a teenager using long-term contraception. *Journal of Obstetrics and Gynaecology, 27*(3), 322–323.

Bailis, A., & Witter, F. R. (2007). Hypertensive disorders of pregnancy. In K. B. Fortner, et al. (Eds.). *The Johns Hopkins manual of gynecology and obstetrics.* Philadelphia: Lippincott Williams & Wilkins.

Burkman, R. T. (2007). Contraception and family planning. In A. H. DeCherney & L. Nathan (Eds.). *Current diagnosis and treatment in obstetrics and gynecology* (10th ed.). Columbus, OH: McGraw-Hill.

Bush, M. C., & Pernoll, M. L. (2007). Multiple pregnancy. In A. H. DeCherney & L. Nathan (Eds.). *Current diagnosis and treatment in obstetrics and gynecology* (10th ed.). Columbus, OH: McGraw-Hill.

Cansino, C. D., & Lipsett, P. (2007). Critical care. In K. B. Fortner, et al. (Eds.). *The Johns Hopkins manual of gynecology and obstetrics.* Philadelphia: Lippincott Williams & Wilkins.

Cantey, J. B., Tecklenburg, F. W., & Titus, M. O. (2007). Late postpartum eclampsia in adolescents. *Pediatric Emergency Care, 23*(6), 401–403.

Chambers, H. M., & Chan, F. Y. (2009). Support for women/families after perinatal death. *Cochrane Database of Systematic Reviews, 2009*(1), (CD000452).

Chhabra, S., Dargan, R., & Nasare, M. (2007). Antepartum transabdominal amnioinfusion. *International Journal of Gynaecology and Obstetrics, 97*(2), 95–99.

Chauhan, S. P., et al. (2007). Intrauterine growth restriction and oligohydramnios among high-risk patients. *American Journal of Perinatology, 24*(4), 215–221.

Clark, E. A. S., Silver, R. M., & Branch, D. W. (2007). Do antiphospholipid antibodies cause preeclampsia and HELLP syndrome? *Current Rheumatology Reports, 9*(3), 219–225.

Crombleholme, W. R. (2009). Obstetrics. In S. J. McPhee & M. A. Papadakis (Eds.). *Current medical diagnosis and treatment.* Columbus, OH: McGraw-Hill.

Cootauco, A. C., & Althaus, J. E. (2007). Preterm labor and premature rupture of membranes. In K. B. Fortner, et al. (Eds.). *The Johns Hopkins manual of gynecology and obstetrics.* Philadelphia: Lippincott Williams & Wilkins.

Crowther, C. A. (2009). Hospitalisation and bed rest for multiple pregnancy. *Cochrane Database of Systematic Reviews, 2009*(1), (CD000110).

Crowther, C., & Middleton, P. (2009). Anti-D administration after childbirth for preventing Rhesus alloimmunisation. *Cochrane Database of Systematic Reviews, 2009*(1), (CD000021).

Dambro, M. R. (2008). Shock, circulatory. In F. J. Domino (Ed.). *The 5-minute clinical consult.* Philadelphia: Lippincott Williams & Wilkins.

Dew, P. C., et al. (2007). The effect of health compromising behaviors on preterm births. *Maternal and Child Health Journal, 11*(3), 227–233.

Duley, L., et al. (2009). Antiplatelet agents for preventing pre-eclampsia and its complications. *Cochrane Database of Systematic Reviews, 2009*(1), (CD004659).

Feldman, D. M., et al. (2007). Betamethasone vs dexamethasone for the prevention of morbidity in very-low-birthweight neonates. *American Journal of Obstetrics and Gynecology, 197*(3), 284–288.

Fortner, K. B., Althaus, J. E., & Gurewitsch, E. D. (2007). Gestational complications. In K. B. Fortner, et al. (Eds.). *The Johns Hopkins manual of gynecology and obstetrics.* Philadelphia: Lippincott Williams & Wilkins.

Fox, N. S., & Chervenak, F. A. (2008). Cervical cerclage: a review of the evidence. *Obstetrical and Gynecological Survey, 63*(1), 58–65.

Garg, R., & Giuntoli, R. L. (2007). Gestational trophoblastic disease. In K. B. Fortner, et al. (Eds.). *The Johns Hopkins manual of gynecology and obstetrics.* Philadelphia: Lippincott Williams & Wilkins.

Goldberg, J. W., & Smith, R. S. (2007). Critical care obstetrics. In A. H. DeCherney & L. Nathan (Eds.). *Current diagnosis and treatment in obstetrics and gynecology* (10th ed.). Columbus, OH: McGraw-Hill.

Goldenberg, R. L., et al. (2008). Epidemiology and causes of preterm birth. *Lancet, 371*(9606), 75–84.

Guberman, C., Greenspon, J., & Goodwin, M. (2007). Renal, urinary tract, gastrointestinal, and dermatologic disorders in pregnancy. In A. H. DeCherney & L. Nathan (Eds.). *Current diagnosis and treatment in obstetrics and gynecology* (10th ed.). Columbus, OH: McGraw-Hill.

Hajenius, P. J., et al. (2009). Interventions for tubal ectopic pregnancy. *Cochrane Database of Systematic Reviews, 2009*(1), (CD000324).

Hegaard, H. K., et al. (2008). Leisure time physical activity is associated with a reduced risk of preterm delivery. *American Journal of Obstetrics and Gynecology, 198*(2), 180–185.

Hofmeyr, G. J. (2009). Amnioinfusion for preterm rupture of membranes. *Cochrane Database of Systematic Reviews, 2009*(1), (CD000942).

Karch, A. M. (2009). *Lippincott's nursing drug guide.* Philadelphia: Lippincott Williams & Wilkins.

Klebanoff, M. A. (2008). Paternal and maternal birthweights and the risk of infant preterm birth. *American Journal of Obstetrics and Gynecology, 198*(1), 58–59.

Kogan, A., Ben-Shushan, A., & Pernoll, M. L. (2007). Benign disorders of the uterine cervix. In A. H. DeCherney & L. Nathan (Eds.). *Current diagnosis and treatment in obstetrics and gynecology* (10th ed.). Columbus, OH: McGraw-Hill.

Linker, C. A. (2009). Hematology. In S. J. McPhee & M. A. Papadakis (Eds.). *Current medical diagnosis and treatment.* Columbus, OH: McGraw-Hill.

Mateus. J., et al. (2007). Effectiveness of fetal fibronectin testing compared with digital cervical assessment of women with preterm contractions. *American Journal of Perinatology, 24*(6), 381–385.

Mercer, B. M. (2007). Is there a role for tocolytic therapy during conservative management of preterm premature rupture of the membranes? *Clinical Obstetrics and Gynecology, 50*(2), 487–496.

Nath, C. A., et al. (2007). Histologic evidence of inflammation and risk of placental abruption. *American Journal of Obstetrics and Gynecology, 197*(3), 319–322.

Neilson, J. P., Hickey, M., & Vazquez, J. (2009). Medical treatment for early fetal death (less than 24 weeks). *Cochrane Database of Systematic Reviews, 2009*(1), (CD002253).

Neilson, J. P. (2009). Interventions for treating placental abruption. *Cochrane Database of Systematic Reviews, 2009*(1), (CD003247).

Neilson, J. P. (2007). Induction of labour for improving birth outcomes for women at or beyond term. *Obstetrics and Gynecology, 109*(3), 753–754.

Norton, M. E. (2007). Evaluation and management of twin-twin transfusion syndrome: still a challenge. *American Journal of Obstetrics and Gynecology, 196*(5), 419–420.

Norwitz, E. R., Snegovskikh, V. V., & Caughey, A. B. (2007). Prolonged pregnancy: when should we intervene? *Clinical Obstetrics and Gynecology, 50*(2), 547–557.

Rode, L., et al. (2007). Acute recurrent polyhydramnios: a combination of amniocenteses and NSAID may be curative rather than palliative. *Fetal Diagnosis and Therapy, 22*(3), 186–189.

Rodrigues, T., Rocha, L., & Barros, H. (2008). Physical abuse during pregnancy and preterm delivery. *American Journal of Obstetrics and Gynecology, 198*(2), 171–177.

Ruis, K., & Altman, K. (2007). Recurrent pregnancy loss. In K. B. Fortner, et al. (Eds.). *The Johns Hopkins manual of gynecology and obstetrics.* Philadelphia: Lippincott Williams & Wilkins.

Scearce, J., & Uzelac, P. S. (2007). Third-trimester vaginal bleeding. In A. H. DeCherney & L. Nathan (Eds.). *Current diagnosis and treatment in obstetrics and gynecology* (10th ed.). Columbus, OH: McGraw-Hill.

Shahin, M., & Raslan, H. (2007). Comparative study of three amniotic fluid markers in premature rupture of membranes: prolactin, beta subunit of human chorionic gonadotropin, and alpha-fetoprotein. *Gynecologic and Obstetric Investigation, 63*(4), 195–199.

Shilva, S. C., Kalra, J., & Prasad, R. (2007). Safety and efficacy of low-dose $MgSO_4$ in the treatment of eclampsia. *International Journal of Gynaecology and Obstetrics, 97*(2), 150–151.

Simhan, H. N., & Caritis, S. N. (2007). Prevention of preterm delivery. *New England Journal of Medicine, 357*(5), 477–487.

Skouteris, H., et al. (2009). Depression and anxiety through pregnancy and the early postpartum: an examination of prospective relationships. *Journal of Affective Disorders, 113*(3), 303–308.

Smaill, F., & Vazquez, J. C. (2009). Antibiotics for asymptomatic bacteriuria in pregnancy. *Cochrane Database of Systematic Reviews, 2009*(1), (CD000490).

Smith, M. H., & Henderson, J. L. (2007). Congenital anomalies. In K. B. Fortner, et al. (Eds.). *The Johns Hopkins manual of gynecology and obstetrics.* Philadelphia: Lippincott Williams & Wilkins.

Sosa, C., et al. (2009). Bed rest in singleton pregnancies for preventing preterm birth. *Cochrane Database of Systematic Reviews, 2009*(1), (CD003581).

Stevens, E., & Gilbert-Cohen, J. (2007). Surgical considerations in early pregnancy: ectopic pregnancy and ovarian torsion. *Journal of Perinatal and Neonatal Nursing, 21*(1), 22–29.

Subramanian, A., et al. (Eds.) (2008). *Drug facts and comparisons.* St. Louis: Wolters Kluwer Health.

Szymanski, L. M., & Aina-Mumuney, A. (2007). Hematologic disorders of pregnancy. In K. B. Fortner, et al. (Eds.). *The Johns Hopkins manual of gynecology and obstetrics.* Philadelphia: Lippincott Williams & Wilkins.

Teng, H. C., Kumar, G., & Ramli, N. M. (2007). A viable secondary intra-abdominal pregnancy resulting from rupture of uterine scar: role of MRI. *British Journal of Radiology, 80*(955), e134–136.

Thilo, E. H., & Rosenberg, A. A. (2008). The newborn infant. In W. W. Hay, et al. (Eds.). *Current pediatric diagnosis and treatment* (18th ed.). Columbus, OH: McGraw-Hill.

Touboul, C., et al. (2007). Outcome of children born out of pregnancies complicated by unexplained polyhydramnios. *BJOG: An International Journal of Obstetrics and Gynaecology, 114*(4), 489–492.

Uzelac, P. S., & Garmel, S. H. (2007). Early pregnancy risks. In A. H. DeCherney & L. Nathan (Eds.). *Current diagnosis and treatment in obstetrics and gynecology* (10th ed.). Columbus, OH: McGraw-Hill.

Valcamonico, A., et al. (2007). Mid- and long-term outcome of extremely low birth weight (ELBW) infants: an analysis of prognostic factors. *Journal of Maternal-Fetal and Neonatal Medicine, 20*(6), 465–471.

Vasquez, D. N., et al. (2007). Clinical characteristics and outcomes of obstetric patients requiring ICU admission. *Chest, 131*(3), 718–724.

Whelan, E. A., et al. (2007). Work schedule during pregnancy and spontaneous abortion. *Epidemiology, 18*(3), 350–355.

Yates, M., & King, J. (2007). Ectopic pregnancy. In K. B. Fortner, et al. (Eds.). *The Johns Hopkins manual of gynecology and obstetrics.* Philadelphia: Lippincott Williams & Wilkins.

SUGGESTED READINGS

Bodnar, L. M., Catov, J. M., & Roberts, J. M. (2007). Racial/ethnic differences in the monthly variation of preeclampsia incidence. *American Journal of Obstetrics and Gynecology, 196*(4), 324–326.

Fertl, K. I., et al. (2009). Levels and effects of different forms of anxiety during pregnancy after a prior miscarriage. *European Journal of Obstetrics, Gynecology, & Reproductive Biology, 142*(1), 23–29.

Ganzevoort, W. (2007). Dynamics and incidence patterns of maternal complications in early-onset hypertension of pregnancy. *BJOG: An International Journal of Obstetrics and Gynaecology, 114*(6), 741–750.

Iams, J. D., et al. (2008). Primary, secondary, and tertiary interventions to reduce the morbidity and mortality of preterm birth. *Lancet, 371*(9607), 164–175.

Lyerly, A. D., et al. (2007). Risks, values, and decision making surrounding pregnancy. *Obstetrics and Gynecology, 109*(4), 979–984.

Marowitz, A., & Jordan, R. (2007). Midwifery management of prelabor rupture of membranes at term. *Journal of Midwifery and Women's Health, 52*(3), 199–206.

Reedy, N. J. (2007). Born too soon: the continuing challenge of preterm labor and birth in the United States. *Journal of Midwifery and Women's Health, 52*(3), 281–290.

Roy, D. J. (2007). When newborn babies have to die... perinatal palliative care? *Journal of Palliative Care, 23*(2), 67–68.

Smith, L. K., et al. (2007). Socioeconomic inequalities in very preterm birth rates. *Archives of Disease in Childhood Fetal and Neonatal Edition, 92*(1), F11-F14.

Toal, M., et al. (2007). Usefulness of a placental profile in high-risk pregnancies. *American Journal of Obstetrics and Gynecology, 196*(4), 363–365.

Chapter

22 Nursing Care of a Pregnant Family With Special Needs

KEY TERMS

- autonomic dysreflexia
- emancipated minor
- substance dependent

OBJECTIVES

After mastering the contents of this chapter, you should be able to:

1. Identify the characteristics and the risks of pregnancy of a pregnant woman who has special needs such as one who has been injured, an adolescent, a woman over age 40, one who is physically or cognitively challenged, or a woman who is drug dependent.
2. Identify National Health Goals related to women with special needs that nurses can be instrumental in helping the nation achieve.
3. Use critical thinking to analyze ways that nursing care of a pregnant woman with a special need can be optimally family centered.
4. Assess a woman with special needs during pregnancy.
5. Formulate nursing diagnoses related to pregnancy for a woman with special needs.
6. Identify expected outcomes for a pregnant woman with special needs.
7. Plan nursing care to address the special needs of women at the extremes of the childbearing spectrum, have a physical or cognitive challenge, have been injured, or are substance dependent.
8. Implement nursing care for a woman with special needs such as encouraging her to remain ambulatory during pregnancy.
9. Evaluate outcomes for effectiveness and achievement of care.
10. Identify areas related to care of a pregnant woman with special needs that would benefit from additional nursing research or application of evidence-based practice.
11. Integrate knowledge of the risks of pregnancy for women with special needs with nursing process to achieve quality maternal and child health nursing care.

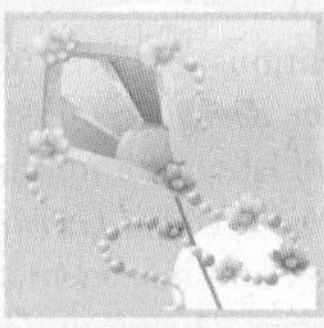

Mindy Carson, 16 years old and 15 weeks pregnant, was in an automobile accident on her way into prenatal clinic this morning. She received a 4-inch laceration on one leg. The father of Mindy's baby is a college student. He does not want Mindy to keep her baby after the birth because he does not want to get married until he finishes graduate school. Mindy insists she is old enough to be a parent and wants to keep her baby. Mindy's mother accuses the father of sharing methamphetamines with Mindy. She is worried Mindy has been working as a prostitute to support her drug habit. Mindy turns to you and asks you what you would recommend she do.

Previous chapters discussed high-risk pregnancies for women who are ill when they become pregnant and for those who develop an illness while pregnant. This chapter presents information about women who do not fit the description of the average pregnant woman—a well young adult who maintains a healthy lifestyle. Representative of such women are very young adolescents, women who have waited until midlife to have their first child, those who are physically or cognitively challenged, those who are accidentally injured, and those who are drug dependent.

What type of immediate assessment does Mindy need? Is she old enough to be a parent? What qualities would you look for in her to decide if she is ready to parent?

The United States has a high teenage birth rate, although this has decreased in recent years from a high of 71 per 1000 to about 41 per 1000 teenagers (National Center for Health Statistics [NCHS], 2009). In contrast, as more and more women delay beginning a family until their 30s, the birth rate for women over age 40 is steadily increasing. It is currently as high as 17 per 1000 (NCHS, 2009). Adolescents require special consideration during pregnancy because they are physically and psychosocially immature. Women over age 40 may need special consideration also because they can have difficulty adjusting psychosocially to a first pregnancy and the physical changes that are required.

The pregnancy rate also is increasing among women who are physically or cognitively challenged, including those with conditions such as cerebral palsy that might have precluded pregnancy a few years ago. Physical and cognitive conditions present a challenge to childbearing and childrearing but do not necessarily prevent women from establishing their own families. Supportive nursing care that considers the limitations imposed by a particular disability, while focusing on the normal aspects of childbearing and childrearing and a woman's strengths, helps to make these pregnancies successful.

Women who are drug dependent or who are injured are other categories of high-risk women who require a great deal of nursing support and care. Ideally, a woman would give up substance abuse for the health of a fetus, but that may not be possible. When this does not happen, every effort must be made to provide enough prenatal care and attention to protect the fetus in other ways. Women who are injured in automobile accidents or from intimate partner abuse can have substantial blood loss that threatens the health of the fetus. They need rapid emergency department assessment and care to be certain that fetal health is protected.

Women with special needs have become such a large number of pregnant women that National Health Goals related to them have been established (Box 22.1).

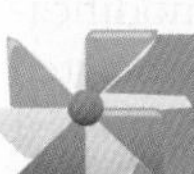

BOX 22.1 * Focus on National Health Goals

Several National Health Goals have been formulated to improve the health of women with special needs during pregnancy. These are:

- Reduce the pregnancy rate among adolescent females to no more than 43 per 1000 adolescents from a baseline of 68 per 1000.
- Increase abstinence from alcohol, cigarettes, and illicit drugs among pregnant women to 100% from baselines of 90% (alcohol), 87% (cigarette smoking), 96% (binge drinking), and 96% (illicit drugs) (http://www.nih.gov).

Nurses can help the nation achieve these goals by teaching accident prevention and the dangers of substance abuse and the complications, both psychological and physical, of teenage pregnancy.

Topics for possible research investigation might include the most effective way to impress adolescents about the dangers of substance abuse, and the ideal birth control measure for adolescents (i.e., one that would actually be used). As more and more women over age 40 are becoming pregnant, the effects of pregnancy on this age group and their adjustment to it also need to be investigated.

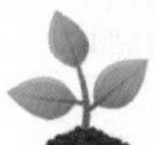

Nursing Process Overview

For Care of a Pregnant Woman With Special Needs

Assessment

Assessing the strengths and weaknesses of individual women is always crucial to establish an accurate nursing diagnosis and realistic outcomes as well as planning effective nursing care. When a woman has a special need, assessment becomes even more important. Establishing as thorough a database as possible early in pregnancy helps to predict the risks a woman may be exposed to when pregnancy is affected by age extremes, physical or cognitive challenges, an accidental injury, or an unhealthy lifestyle.

When caring for a woman who is physically challenged, keep in mind that physical disabilities occur in degrees; therefore, first establish the impact of the disability on a woman's lifestyle before offering any guidance for care measures during pregnancy. The capacity of a woman with special needs to adapt to pregnancy depends both on her physical capabilities and on her ability to persevere against odds to overcome obstacles. Be certain to assess physical strengths as well as limitations and psychosocial strengths as well as challenges. A woman with a spinal cord injury, for example, is likely to have developed ways of coping in daily life that may never occur to someone who has not experienced that disability.

For some drug-dependent women, pregnancy may be the impetus they need to break a drug habit. All that other women can accomplish is to reduce their drug use. In both instances, encourage a woman to keep coming for prenatal care. As long as a woman feels comfortable with you during regular visits, you may be able to establish a trusting relationship that will eventually provide her with the confidence to try a more healthful pattern of living.

Nursing Diagnosis

Nursing diagnoses established for pregnant women with special needs differ in degree, but not in substance, from the nursing diagnoses established for all pregnant women. For example, if a pregnant adolescent is still growing, nutrition is an important issue for both her and her fetus. Examples of nursing diagnoses for women with special needs are:

- Risk for imbalanced nutrition related to combined needs of adolescence and pregnancy
- Risk for fetal injury related to drug and alcohol use
- Impaired physical mobility related to physical disability
- Risk for injury related to unstable balance
- Impaired verbal communication related to spastic muscle functioning
- Impaired home maintenance related to a sensory challenge
- Readiness for enhanced family coping, related to commitment to have a child in the face of a disabling condition

Outcome Identification and Planning

Be especially careful to establish realistic outcomes given a woman's particular condition or situation. An adolescent, for instance, cannot achieve independent decision making if she is not mature enough to do this. A woman who is visually challenged may not be able to read a digital display on a glucometer or use a wall clock to time contractions no matter how much she would like to.

Often, a pregnant woman with a special need already has significant stressors to deal with in her life. Adolescence, for example, is a period of growth and change that can be stressful for both the teenager and her family. The physically challenged woman constantly copes with a condition that must be considered in all activities, even if she has adjusted completely to the limitations the disability imposes. The drug-dependent woman is confined by a life-threatening habit. A woman who has been injured in an accident may have to temporarily restructure her life to accommodate a hospital admission.

Pregnancy brings with it a whole new set of stressors that can be overwhelming if a woman has no outside support. Planning for a pregnant woman with a special need, therefore, often involves identifying support people to help with this added stress. This support can come from family, friends, a professional organization, or health care providers. If a woman is not totally independent in her care, some planning may be required with her support person, who may be the person who actually carries out the proposed action. At the same time, be sure not to ignore a woman and plan around her. Only if she approves of the plan can pregnancy be the enjoyable experience she had planned it would be. This principle applies to any woman, but especially one with special needs.

A major problem encountered when planning with a pregnant adolescent is that she may have difficulty accepting the reality of her pregnancy, and so she may not be interested in attending prenatal care. Some primiparas older than 40 years may have delayed pregnancy to pursue further education or a career. Remember that a woman who has been submerged in a career instead of the world of babies and homemaking may, like the adolescent, be less informed about normal pregnancy findings or healthful pregnancy practices than a younger woman. Be certain you do not equate a woman's knowledge in one field, such as chemistry or law, with her knowledge of good prenatal care.

Plans should include ways to strengthen confidence and self-esteem, crucial attributes for a new mother. These also are areas in which a woman with a special need, especially one who perceives herself as too young or too old or who has experienced physical dysfunction, may not have developed fully. Drug dependence may also be related to feelings of lowered self-worth, which may have been intensified if the drug-dependent woman has tried unsuccessfully to limit her drug intake in the past.

Being certain that plans are established in a wide range of areas helps to ensure that planning is comprehensive. Remember to include safe care of the newborn in plans as well, as once an infant is born, it may be too late to make these plans in a comprehensive manner. The Department of Health and Human Services (DHHS) has initiated a special program to help reduce teenage pregnancy (http://www.girlpower.gov) that is helpful to use for referral as is The Substance Abuse & Mental Health Services Internet site (http://www.SAMHSA.gov). The Narcotics Anonymous site can be helpful to women who are drug dependent (http://www.NA.org). Alcoholics Anonymous is the standby for women with alcohol dependence (http://www.AA.org). Women who feel they will be injured by an intimate partner can locate shelters for abused women by calling their local police department or using the Salvation Army Web site (http://www.shelterforwomen.net).

Implementation

Interventions for the high-risk pregnant woman include promoting a healthy pregnancy and preventing pregnancy complications. Care focuses on teaching and encouraging a woman with any special need to determine how best to manage her pregnancy according to her particular situation.

A high proportion of adolescents do not seek prenatal care early in pregnancy because they deny they are pregnant. Others may not feel comfortable in a health care facility at which mainly adults are seen. The same may be true of a woman with drug dependency who fears reprisals from health care providers regarding her drug use. An ultrasound following an injury may first reveal that a woman is pregnant. She needs to be scheduled for prenatal care. A nonjudgmental, welcoming attitude that focuses on the pregnancy and the baby, while avoiding recriminations about a woman's youth or circumstances, is essential to attracting such women to prenatal care and keeping them coming for regular visits. They hear from a friend that the staff members at the clinic are helpful, not judgmental, and then take the first step into the facility.

For women who are physically challenged, modifications may be necessary for some interventions associated with typical pregnancy-related procedures. For example, it may be necessary to modify a pelvic examination when a woman cannot place her legs in table stirrups. Modifying procedures promotes individualized care for all women, improving overall nursing care.

Outcome Evaluation

Evaluation of nursing interventions for the care of a pregnant woman with a special need often focuses on a woman's physical and emotional readiness for childbearing, maintenance of fetal health, and a woman's ability to provide a safe and healthy environment for her newborn. The following are examples:

- Client states she will use walker to maintain balance during pregnancy.
- Adolescent lists a weekly intake of adequate calories, even with frequent meals at fast-food restaurants.
- Family members state they have been able to adjust to changing demands of pregnancy in mother who is physically challenged.
- Client reports to methadone maintenance clinic daily and reports no other drug use.
- Client states that she is able to manage a rest period daily even in light of busy work and travel schedule.
- Client states she is able to carry out usual lifestyle activities in spite of cast on injured arm.

THE PREGNANT ADOLESCENT

Adolescent pregnancy is not a new phenomenon. Historically, it was common for women to marry as early as age 12 or 13 and have their first baby at age 15. In today's society, however, marriage and childbearing are life situations that are thought of as belonging to later years. Teenage pregnancies still continue, however. Reasons for the high number of them include:

- Earlier age of menarche in girls (the average age is 12.4 years; many girls begin menstruating at age 10 and so are ovulating and able to conceive by age 11)
- Increase in the rate of sexual activity among teenagers
- Lack of knowledge about (or failure to use) contraceptives or abstinence
- Desire by young girls to have a child

Having an equally young sexual partner can contribute to pregnancy incidence as in this situation, neither partner may be well versed in contraceptive options (Buston, Williamson, & Hart, 2007). In addition, some adolescents become pregnant as the result of rape or incest (Kandakai & Smith, 2007).

Failure of adolescents to obtain adequate knowledge of contraceptive measures or abstinence is an issue that can be addressed by health care providers. As protective measures are easy to use, the average adolescent should not have difficulty following instructions. Adolescents are also capable of using emergency contraceptive measures correctly and safely. Access to emergency contraception is not associated with increased rates of unprotected intercourse or with higher rates of pregnancy or sexually transmitted infections (Haynes, 2007). Unfortunately, providing this type of information does not always resolve the problem because adolescents may lack money to purchase protection such as birth control pills or a diaphragm. In addition, the egocentric phenomenon of adolescence makes a sexually active teenager believe she will not become pregnant: "It won't happen to me." On the other hand, some adolescent girls actually plan pregnancy. They believe being pregnant will free them from an intolerable school or home situation and give them someone to love and someone to love them. This puts a tremendous responsibility on a newborn to furnish love and change a girl's life, and child abuse can occur when the newborn cannot meet such expectations (Records, 2007).

At one time, pregnant unmarried girls were sent to a "secret" home or shelter where they would stay throughout their pregnancy, give birth, place the child for adoption, and return home as if nothing had happened to them. Today, pregnant teenagers remain at home, attend prenatal clinics, or come to physicians' offices just as older women. They give birth in birthing rooms at hospitals, and as many as 90% keep their babies (NCHS, 2009). Few give birth in alternative birth centers because the risk of cephalopelvic disproportion makes adolescent pregnancies high risk. Home birth is not recommended for the same reason. Offering increased guidance during pregnancy and for child care during the following years can be an important nursing role.

Developmental Tasks of Adolescence

Adolescence is a vulnerable time for pregnancy because the developmental tasks of pregnancy are superimposed on those of adolescence. The developmental tasks of the average adolescent are fourfold: to establish a sense of self-worth or a value system, to emancipate from parents, to adjust to a new body image, and to choose a vocation (Erikson, 1963). A girl in the process of separating from her parents may be devastated by the reality of someone else being dependent on her. She may need her parents' financial help more than ever to obtain prenatal care and buy clothing for her new baby. If she must depend on her parents' health insurance, she may feel virtually trapped into dependence. Helping adolescents to make their own health care decisions at health care visits helps to foster a sense of independence in the middle of this forced dependency. Consider, for example, the decision that the adolescent must make about where to place a medication reminder chart: if it hangs in the kitchen, her mother may monitor it; in her bedroom or in her school locker, she alone will monitor it. An adolescent may not be able to choose when she comes for care (her mother has the car to drive her only on Tuesday afternoons), but during a visit she can do many things to feel independent, such as weigh herself, hold a mirror to view her pelvic examination, or be interviewed apart from her parent.

Parents may have difficulty allowing a daughter to make her own health care decisions this way. You may need to remind them that a pregnant adolescent is regarded as an **emancipated minor** or a *mature minor*—a person capable of making health care decisions—and so may sign permission for her own care. Soon she will be caring for an infant, so she needs this practice in independence and responsibility.

Pregnancy may interfere with the development of a healthy sexual relationship and cause difficulty in establishing future intimate relationships if a girl realizes that her current relationship has led to a situation detrimental to her. To prevent this, it is useful to help her view the pregnancy as a growth-producing experience. Most people can point to a day in their life when they "grew up" (perhaps a day a parent became ill or the day they left home for college). This pregnancy can be that "growing-up" revelation or a growth-producing experience for her.

Establishing a value system or sense of identity can be difficult if health care personnel treat a pregnant adolescent as though she is irresponsible. Encouraging her to continue school is crucial to her self-esteem and to her future, as well as to the future of her unborn child. Many schools have special programs for pregnant adolescents that include aspects of prenatal care.

Prenatal Assessment

Adolescents are considered high-risk clients because they have a high incidence of pregnancy-induced hypertension, iron-deficiency anemia, and premature labor (Box 22.2). They also have a higher incidence of low-birth-weight infants, a disproportion between fetal and pelvic size, and a high rate of intimate partner abuse (Datner et al., 2007). Early and consistent prenatal care is essential to their health and the health of their baby.

Unfortunately, many adolescents do not seek prenatal care until late in their pregnancies as not seeking prenatal care is a way of protecting the pregnancy—if she doesn't tell anyone, no one can suggest she terminate the pregnancy. After the sixth month, abortion is no longer a possibility, so she can feel free to come for care without being subjected to this pressure.

Box 22.2 Assessment

Assessing the Pregnant Adolescent for Complication Risk

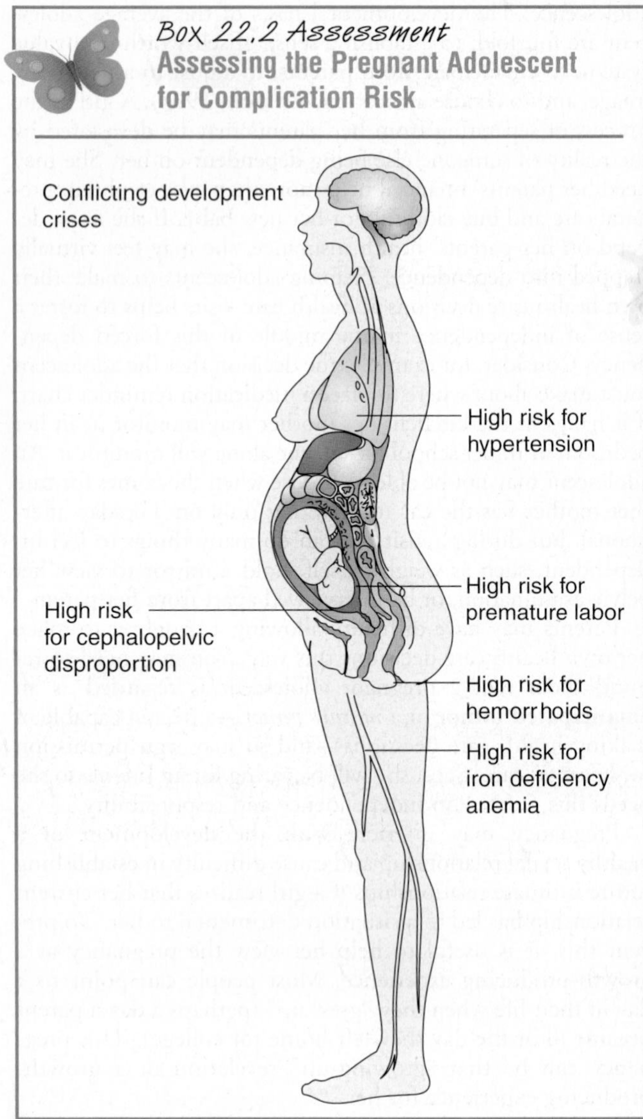

Other factors contributing to the lack of prenatal care include:

- Denial she is pregnant
- Lack of knowledge of the importance of prenatal care
- Dependence on others for transportation
- Feeling awkward in a prenatal setting (an adult setting)
- Fear of a first pelvic examination
- Difficulty relating to authority figures

A primary nursing or case management approach that minimizes the number of health care providers a teenager is exposed to may be the most effective method for providing care during the prenatal period. Some adolescents do well in group prenatal care because it allows them to interact with a peer group. If a community does not have a facility designed especially for adolescents, all settings should accommodate adolescents' needs, eliminating this reason for poor prenatal care.

Health History

Take a detailed health history at the first prenatal visit of an adolescent to establish individual risks. This is best done without the girl's parents present. The girl needs practice in being responsible for her own health, and having to account for her health practices helps her do this. It also helps prevent her from fabricating an answer to please a parent.

Some adolescents come to a facility with concerns such as "weight gain" or "feeling tired all the time" rather than saying they are pregnant, hoping health care providers will think of pregnancy as a possible reason for their symptoms. This is part denial and part pregnancy protection. Always be alert to the possibility of pregnancy when an adolescent describes symptoms that are vague and hard to define. If the importance of what she is saying when she mentions feeling "tired" or "nauseated" is missed, she may ask if someone will feel her stomach. If told this is not necessary for any of the symptoms she has mentioned, she may describe bigger symptoms, such as "terrible stomach pain." Think of possible pregnancy when you hear such a "growing" history.

Many adolescents want to keep their world totally separate from the adult world and, to keep it separate, they do not voluntarily share information with adults. When interviewing adolescents, be certain to press for the responses needed to assess safely. Do not accept statements such as "I eat okay" as a nutrition history or "I'm a very active person" as a history of rest and activity. Ask for details.

If an adolescent delayed seeking health care, ask for the reason for this at her first prenatal visit. Acknowledge that "protecting" the pregnancy is a desirable motive, but that continuing with prenatal care is much more beneficial.

If a parent does accompany a girl, ask the parent separately what, if any, concerns he or she wishes to discuss. A young adolescent is still a daughter, and a parent may be as concerned about her health during this pregnancy as the parent was at health visits when the girl was being seen for a cold or a sports injury.

A baby's father may accompany a teenage girl into the clinic or office to have the pregnancy diagnosis established. Because he is not married to her, he does not have a legal right to participate in her decision concerning pregnancy, abortion, or adoption, but he may not be devoid of feelings for the girl or the baby. If he is an adolescent, he may feel sorrow that because of his age he cannot provide adequately for the girl and baby. If a complication occurs, he may feel genuine grief. Allowing him to offer support in the current pregnancy helps him to learn more about himself and better define his role (Parra-Cardona, Sharp, & Wampler, 2008). Be sure he receives compassionate education on preventing further pregnancies until he is more mature.

Often, adolescent girls have not talked much to many pregnant women, so they may need extra teaching to help them become aware of common pregnancy symptoms such as urinary frequency, fatigue, and breast tenderness. Asking what symptoms an adolescent is having, and reassuring her they are part of a normal pregnancy, can help prevent her from attempting to treat them with potentially teratogenic over-the-counter medications.

As pregnancy progresses, listen for signs of "nest-building" behavior during a pregnancy history. An adolescent girl may not have the financial resources to buy clothing or a baby bed. She may reveal nest-building feelings by asking an increasing number of questions about newborns. Offer suggestions, such as making one article of clothing for the baby or saving her own money for one article—activities that promote active involvement in the pregnancy and provide a measure of nest-building behavior (the girl who, week after week, spends her money on something else is probably not as involved in the pregnancy as the girl who puts away even 1 dollar each week toward a pair of baby shoes).

Some adolescents have difficulty telling their parents about the pregnancy. Role-playing or simulation may be an effective technique to help them prepare to do this. Some girls report on a second visit that their parents were not nearly as angry as they had anticipated. Instead, their parents reacted as if they had been waiting to hear this news, having accepted it as inevitable months before.

Family Profile. Adolescents may leave home if their family disapproves of their pregnancy, joining the ranks of homeless or adolescent runaways. Others do not leave home but separate themselves emotionally from their family. Trying to manage by themselves leaves adolescents with tremendous financial strain and a devastating sense of loneliness. Be sure to ask a girl at prenatal visits where she is living, what is the source of her income, and whom she would call if she suddenly became ill.

Asking about home life may reveal a dysfunctional family or an incest relationship as the cause of the pregnancy. If the girl is under legal age, incest is considered child abuse. Know your local and state laws on this topic and make the necessary report.

Because of family relationship problems, a girl may need help in making arrangements for the next few months of her pregnancy and for child care afterward. Will her parents allow her to live at home during the pregnancy? If not, is there a relative she may go to? What kind of financial support does she need? Family and social supports for pregnant adolescents have been shown to be important influences on the maintenance of a healthy pregnancy lifestyle and help prevent low birth weight in their children (Kaplan & Love-Osborne, 2008).

Be certain to ask if the girl is planning to continue with school. Pregnancy is an egocentric time when outside interests do not always seem important. Help her to see that the months of pregnancy will go by faster if she is busy. Remaining in school is a way of helping her stay busy. It also is important in preparing for the future, because a high school education will be necessary to obtain marketable skills to support herself and her baby. Once she has given birth, returning to school may be difficult because she may have child care problems and because she may feel she is more mature than the other girls (or the other girls may make her feel this way). Any school that obtains federal money cannot discriminate against students because they are physically challenged. Many states interpret pregnancy as physically challenging, so in those states a girl cannot be forced to leave school (or even asked to go to an alternate school) because of pregnancy. You may need to advocate for a girl with a school committee for a proper school placement.

Day History. Adolescents may be unwilling to provide a detailed day history unless its purpose is well explained. Tell a pregnant teenager the purpose of the history is to learn more about her as a whole person, not to discover if she is doing things during the day she should not do. Adolescents are private people; to allow you to walk through their adolescent world for a day is a breach of adolescent philosophy. Ask in particular about nutritional practices, sleep, daily activity, use of drugs, and whether she has friends who can support her through this experience.

Be certain to include questions about her medication history. Ask if she is taking anything over the counter. Some adolescents take acne medication that is potentially teratogenic, such as tetracycline or isotretinoin (Accutane) (Karch, 2009). Some take frequent doses of over-the-counter cold remedies or herbal supplements. Impress upon adolescents the importance of not taking any medication—even nonprescription—without prior approval from their physicians or nurse-midwives during pregnancy. Pregnancy can become an important growth experience if it provides the motivation some adolescents need to withdraw from recreational drug use.

Physical Examination

Physical examination procedures with pertinent adolescent findings are discussed in Chapter 34. Be certain to explain procedures as you do the examination. A statement such as "Oh, you're starting to have colostrum," a positive finding of pregnancy, may be frightening to an adolescent who does not know what colostrum is. A better way to phrase such a finding might be, "Your breasts are healthy. You're already beginning to produce early breast milk. Later on we'll talk about the importance of breast milk for newborns." This kind of feedback makes a health examination a learning experience and relieves anxiety for adolescents, who tend to be very concerned about body appearance. It is an effective way to encourage healthy behavior patterns.

Adolescents are at an increased risk for pregnancy-induced hypertension, probably because of immature blood vessels or an immune response to the foreign protein of their fetus (Clark, Silver, & Branch, 2007). Few adolescents are told the results of blood pressure determinations at health maintenance visits, so they do not know what is their typical finding. Obtain a baseline blood pressure at the first prenatal visit and make a point of informing the girl of her blood pressure reading to encourage active health care participation in the future. Adolescents are often active in a waiting room—walking to get a magazine, returning it, or looking out the window; be certain that the girl has 15 minutes of rest before you take a blood pressure or the recording will be falsely high.

Use a Doppler technique to obtain fetal heart tones, if possible, because hearing the fetal heart helps an adolescent acknowledge the reality of her pregnancy. For the same reason, make a point of assessing fundal height from visit to visit to show the baby is growing.

Adolescents who use drugs may be reluctant to supply a urine specimen for testing because they are afraid you are secretly looking for evidence of drug use. In this instance, you may receive a cupful of water in place of a urine specimen. If in doubt regarding the substance you are testing, check the specific gravity. The specific gravity of water is 1.000, whereas urine specific gravity ranges from 1.003 to 1.030.

Many adolescents like to weigh themselves at prenatal visits as weight gain in early pregnancy is proof they are pregnant. It is good practice to make a note of the clothing a girl is wearing the first time she is weighed (e.g., jeans, T-shirt) so later weight determinations can be compared accurately. Be certain she knows a healthy weight gain is important for fetal growth and that this weight can be lost afterward.

✔ Checkpoint Question 22.1

Mindy Carson is still an adolescent. What is a task of adolescence, according to Erikson, that she needs to complete to be ready to become a mother?

a. Establish a value system.
b. Grow to her final height.
c. Prepare clothes for the baby.
d. Finish her education.

Nursing Diagnoses and Related Interventions

Nursing Diagnosis: Health-seeking behaviors related to special care necessary for healthy adolescent pregnancy

Outcome Evaluation: Client states she feels confident in her ability to take care of herself and avoid pregnancy complications, and asks questions about her pregnancy.

Pregnancy Education

Adolescents need a great deal of health teaching during pregnancy because they do not know many common measures of care that an older woman has learned from experience. They are also often unwilling to follow health care advice that makes them different in any way from their peers. On the other hand, adolescents often do not have well-established health practices, so they are adaptable.

Adolescent girls may respond to health teaching that is directed to their own health more than to that of a fetus inside them: "Eat a high-protein diet because protein makes your hair shiny (or prevents split fingernails)" often leads to better adherence than a statement such as "Protein is good for your baby." "Taking the iron supplement should make you feel less tired" is better than "It will help build the baby's blood supply," for the same reason. These are truthful statements and they appeal to an adolescent's preoccupation with self. In addition, this type of health teaching is the only form to which an adolescent who is denying her pregnancy can respond.

Adolescents also need instructions about possible discomforts and changes associated with pregnancy, and measures to relieve them. (See Chapter 12 for a complete discussion.) Many adolescents develop hemorrhoids during pregnancy because the disproportion of their body size to a fetus puts extra pressure on pelvic vessels, causing blood to pool in rectal veins. Assure girls that this is a pregnancy-related phenomenon that will resolve when the pregnancy is over.

Adolescents may also develop many striae across the sides of their abdomens because so much stretching of the abdominal skin occurs. Assure them again that, because of skin elasticity, these marks will probably fade after pregnancy. Chloasma, excess pigment deposition on the face and neck, appears at the same rate in adolescents as in older women. Adolescents, however, may be more conscious of this pigment because overall they are more conscious and concerned about their facial appearance. Suggesting a cover makeup and offering reassurance the pigmentation will fade after pregnancy can help.

Nutrition

Good nutrition can be a major problem during an adolescent pregnancy because many girls enter pregnancy with poor nutritional stores from years of eating a less-than-optimal diet. Lack of good nutrition can result in preterm birth and low-birth-weight newborns. The younger the girl is, the more likely she is to have a low-birth-weight infant. To prevent these complications, a girl should eat a sufficient diet to allow for the growth of a fetus and also provide for the needs of her own growing body. Otherwise, protein, iron, folic acid, and vitamin A and C deficiencies may become acute. She may need to gain more weight than does the mature woman to supply adequate nutrients.

As more and more children are obese today than ever before because of overeating and lack of exercise, many adolescents enter pregnancy overweight or obese. This can lead to macrosomia or overgrowth in a fetus, a situation that leads to an increase in the number of cesarean births (Zhang et al., 2008). Such adolescents should not actively restrict nutrients during pregnancy, however, because although they are obese, their body may be deficient in protein and vitamins.

Many adolescent girls eat poorly during pregnancy because they simply do not know what constitutes good nutrition. Some girls have little choice in what foods are prepared at home. To change a dietary pattern, you may have to talk to the person who does the cooking in the family.

Besides eating the right amount of food, a pregnant adolescent should be sure to eat proper foods, possibly abandoning a food fad she has been following. Some girls are so peer-oriented they balk at substituting a glass of orange juice for a cola beverage because no one else they know drinks orange juice. The best you may be able to accomplish is to secure her agreement to switch to noncaffeinated soft drinks.

Many adolescents eat at least one meal a week at a fast-food restaurant. Remember that if the girl is attending school, she eats at least one meal away from home each day. If she travels by school bus, she may have to leave by 6:00 or 7:00 in the morning, so she needs suggestions on how to construct a quick but healthy breakfast. If she leaves home this early, she will have a long wait until lunchtime. Suggest midmorning snacks, such as fruit, that also supply vitamins, not just empty calories. Be certain nutrition education includes how to "brown-bag" or buy a nutritious cafeteria lunch (type A school lunches are discussed in Chapter 32).

Adolescents traditionally do not take medicine conscientiously, so they may need frequent reminders that vitamin and iron supplements intended to complement nutrition during pregnancy must not only be purchased but also must be taken. Be sure a girl posts a medication reminder chart at home or in her school locker to help increase adherence.

What if... Mindy Carson tells you her daily nutrition consists of a liquid diet beverage for breakfast and lunch and then she has pizza for dinner? Will this typical teenage diet be adequate for her during pregnancy?

Activity and Rest

Adolescents vary greatly in their level of activity. Assess a girl's participation in sports and determine which ones (if any) may have to be discontinued during pregnancy (e.g., diving, gymnastics, touch football). Many girls practice sports not for the enjoyment of the sport but for the feeling of "team" or companionship. You may need to suggest alternative activities (joining the drama or language club, inviting friends over once a week to watch a movie) so they do not suffer from the loss of companionship.

Adolescent girls may not plan enough rest time during pregnancy, especially if they are acting as if nothing is happening to them (Box 22.3). It may help to explore a typical day and suggest ways to rest without compromising social relationships (sitting, talking after school rather than walking through the park).

Physiologic Changes

A young girl may have distorted beliefs about her body. All adolescent girls need substantial education on the physiologic changes that occur during pregnancy. Despite all the health information given to children in school, it is not uncommon to find an adolescent who thinks her baby is growing in her stomach. Such a girl may be unwilling to eat large meals during pregnancy for fear of suffocating or drowning her fetus. In addition, specific information about labor and delivery is essential to counteract all the "scare stories" girls may be hearing from their peers. Gaining this type of knowledge is another way that pregnancy can be a growth experience. At the end of the pregnancy, this adolescent will know a great deal more about her body and her ability to monitor her health than her average classmate.

BOX 22.3 ✻ Focus on Communication

Mindy Carson is 16 years old and pregnant. You talk to her at a prenatal clinic.

Less Effective Communication

Nurse: Hello, Mindy. How are you feeling?
Mindy: Good, but always tired. You know.
Nurse: You should try and rest more.
Mindy: Right.
Nurse: Why don't you ask your boyfriend to help you more?
Mindy: I'll do that.
Nurse: Or stop working at the fast food restaurant. That'll leave you time to rest more.
Mindy: Right. Great solution.
Nurse: Glad I could be of help.

More Effective Communication

Nurse: Hello, Mindy. How are you feeling?
Mindy: Good, but always tired. You know.
Nurse: Are you getting enough sleep?
Mindy: How can I? I work every day after school.
Nurse: Is there anyone who could help you out more? Your boyfriend? A friend?
Mindy: I'm pretty much alone since I got pregnant.
Nurse: As long as you're coming to this clinic, you're not alone. Tell me about a typical day and let's investigate together what could be done.

In the first scenario, the nurse was so intent on problem solving she forgot the first step of effective problem solving—identify the exact problem that needs solving. In the second scenario, when the nurse continues to assess rather than offer advice, she is able to identify the problem.

Childbirth Preparation

Adolescents have a strong need for peer companionship. When they become pregnant, they often are cut off from fellow adolescents. This makes them "ripe," therefore, to join a class of adolescents in preparation for childbirth. They are excellent students because being a student is age-appropriate for them. They have enough childish magical belief operating that they are not skeptical about whether prepared childbirth will work. In fact, believing that prepared childbirth will work is an important component in a successful prepared childbirth experience, so this becomes a self-fulfilling prophecy.

Birth Decisions

Pelvic measurements should be taken early and carefully in adolescent girls as cephalopelvic disproportion is a real possibility because of the girl's incomplete pelvic growth (Shields et al., 2007). Most girls who are told their baby will have to be born by cesarean birth respond well to the news, and many are relieved, because surgery seems controlled and simple compared with the agonies of labor they imagine. When a cesarean birth must be scheduled because of cephalopelvic disproportion or poor fetal growth, the information should be shared with the girl and her parents as soon as possible. Adolescents want to know the truth. They tend to regard the withholding of information not as protection but as an indication they are being treated as children.

Plans for the Baby

Adolescents may need additional time at prenatal visits to talk to a good listener about how they feel about being pregnant and becoming a mother. Scared? Bewildered? Numb? Happy? Be certain they know all the options available to them: keeping the baby, placing the baby in a temporary foster home or adoption. Adolescents, like all women, should be encouraged to breastfeed (Britton et al., 2009). Breast tissue matures with pregnancy, so even the very young adolescent is physically capable of breastfeeding.

Complications of Adolescent Pregnancy

As mentioned earlier, adolescent pregnancy carries the increased incidence of pregnancy-induced hypertension, iron-deficiency anemia, preterm labor, and cephalopelvic disproportion (see Box 22.2). Fortunately, with conscientious prenatal care, these complications can be minimized.

Pregnancy-Induced Hypertension

Because adolescents are more prone to pregnancy-induced hypertension than the average woman, establishing a baseline blood pressure is important (see Chapter 21). It is particularly important if an adolescent has not had her blood pressure measured since a preschool or school-age checkup as long as 10 years earlier.

The best intervention for reducing an increasing blood pressure during pregnancy is bed rest, preferably in a side-lying position. Bed rest may be difficult for a teenager to achieve because she easily grows bored and being confined to bed limits her interactions with peers and school activities. Many girls on bed rest at home may rest better if they are lying on the living room couch, where they can be aware of household activity, rather than in an upstairs bedroom, where they have to get up time and again to see what is happening. Also, it is easier for a parent to encourage bed rest if a girl is within eyesight. If called too many times to the distant bedroom for small tasks, a parent tends to say, "Get up and get it yourself this time."

Help to establish a specific routine of bed rest—does it mean being strictly confined to bed or sitting up part of the day in a lounge chair with legs elevated? Can she take a shower? Use the bathroom? Knowing the exact rules from the beginning helps prevent misunderstandings and hurt feelings.

Girls on bed rest need activities to keep them busy. These can include homework or listening to music. If the end of the pregnancy is near, a girl may be able to have a friend bring her homework assignments. If the bed rest period will be longer than 2 weeks, however, she may need to make arrangements for home tutoring. You may need to advocate for her with her school system for this service (remembering that only rarely can it be denied on the basis of pregnancy). "Assignments" from the health care agency, such as reading about appropriate toys and games for infants, is also a way to occupy time. Frequent telephone calls from the health care facility show concern and offer an opportunity to enforce health teaching points. Be certain a girl does not interpret being placed on bed rest as being ill. This can cause her to reduce her nutritional intake or to curtail body hygiene.

Although its effect is controversial, low-dose aspirin therapy may be prescribed to help reduce symptoms of hypertension of pregnancy (Barton & Sibai, 2008). Keep in mind adolescents often are not reliable at taking daily medicine, particularly if it seems as unimportant as aspirin. Help a girl make a medicine reminder chart to promote adherence to this aspect of care.

If the hypertension continues after a period of bed rest at home (or if the symptoms of pregnancy-induced hypertension are advanced when they are first discovered), a girl may be admitted to the hospital so bed rest can be better enforced. As soon as the fetus is mature, labor will be induced or a cesarean birth scheduled.

Iron-Deficiency Anemia

Many adolescent girls are deficient in iron because their low protein intake cannot balance the amount of iron lost with menstrual flows. Deficiency is revealed by chronic fatigue, pale mucous membranes, and a hemoglobin level less than 11 g/dL. As if the girl's body has identified a mineral lack, iron-deficiency anemia is associated with pica, or the ingestion of inedible substances (Mills, 2007). Cravings for ice cubes or blackboard chalk may develop because of this.

A pregnancy compounds iron-deficiency anemia because a girl must now supply enough iron for fetal growth and her increasing blood volume. All pregnant women should take an iron and folic acid supplement (folic acid is important for red blood cell growth and prevention of neural tube defects) and these are especially important for the adolescent (Bernstein & Weinstein, 2007).

Help an adolescent plan a daily time for taking her iron supplement. Review with her how many iron-rich foods she needs to eat daily in addition to this. An iron supplement is not a supplement until her dietary intake is already strong in iron-rich foods.

As soon as the body has iron, it will begin forming immature red blood cells (reticulocytes) rapidly. A reticulocyte count may be obtained in 2 weeks to evaluate these levels and provide evidence that the iron supplement is being taken. If the reticulocyte count is not elevated by 2 weeks, it implies a girl did not take the supplement. Taking a stool swab and assessing it for the black tinge of an iron supplement or reassessing her serum iron level are other methods of assessing for adherence.

Preterm Labor

Adolescents are at high risk for preterm labor, probably because their uteruses are not fully grown (Muram, 2007). Review the signs of labor with them by the third month of pregnancy. Stress that labor contractions begin as only a sweeping contraction no more intense than menstrual cramps. Also, any vaginal bleeding is suspicious of labor and should be reported. Adolescent girls have gained much of their knowledge of labor from television (where a woman suddenly announces she is in labor and within 15 minutes gives birth). Therefore, they may dismiss light contractions as simple discomfort, not realizing they might be the start of labor. Adolescents who recognize labor contractions early can seek care to have premature labor halted.

Complications of Adolescent Labor, Birth, and the Postpartum Period

Cephalopelvic Disproportion

Cephalopelvic disproportion is suggested by lack of engagement at the beginning of labor, a prolonged first stage of labor, and poor fetal descent. Adolescent labor does not differ from labor in the older woman if cephalopelvic disproportion is absent. Graphing labor progress is a good way to detect labor that is becoming abnormal. Be certain an adolescent has a support person with her in labor so she can relax and breathe effectively with contractions. If this person is also an adolescent, you may need to serve as the true support person, or at least spend considerable time coaching so this person can support the girl in labor.

Postpartum Hemorrhage

Young adolescents are more prone to postpartum hemorrhage than the average woman because if a girl's uterus is not yet fully developed, it becomes overdistended by pregnancy. An overdistended uterus does not contract as readily as a normally distended uterus in the postpartum period, allowing bleeding to occur (Poggi, 2007). Adolescents also may have more frequent or deeper perineal and cervical lacerations than older women because of the size of the infant in relation to their body. On the other hand, young adolescents are generally healthy and have supple body tissue that allows for adequate perineal stretching. If a laceration does occur, it usually heals readily without complication.

Inability to Adapt Postpartally

The immediate postpartum period may be an almost unreal time for an adolescent (Holub et al., 2007). Giving birth is such a stress and a major crisis that all women have difficulty integrating it into their life. It may be particularly difficult for the adolescent. The girl may "block out" the hours of labor as if they did not happen. If she was particularly frightened by labor, she may have received a narcotic, so her memory of the labor hours may not be clear. Urge her to talk about labor and birth to make the happening real to her; otherwise, postpartum depression is more apt to occur (Haessler & Rosenthal, 2007).

Lack of Knowledge About Infant Care

Adolescents show the same positive bonding behavior with their infants as their more mature counterparts (Fig. 22.1). They may, however, lack knowledge of infant care. Although they may consider themselves to be knowledgeable in child care because they have babysat for a neighbor's child or a younger sibling, they can be overwhelmed in the postpartum period to realize that when the baby is their own, child care is not as simple as it once seemed. When the child cries, they cannot hand it to someone else; at the end of 4 hours, when they are tired of caring for the baby, they cannot leave and walk away. Although these things were most likely discussed with an adolescent during pregnancy, these feelings may not become prominent until the child is actually born. Spend time with a girl observing how she handles her infant. Demonstrate bathing and changing the baby as appropriate. Model good parenting behaviors whenever possible by being aware of how you hold and care for the child.

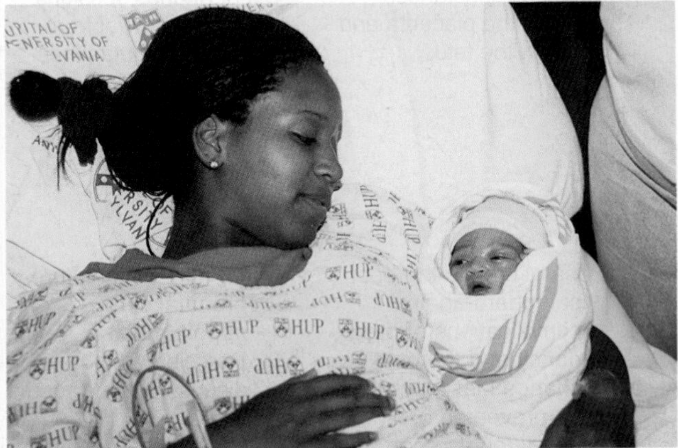

FIGURE 22.1 A new adolescent mother begins to bond with her infant. (Photograph by John Gallagher, with permission of University of Pennsylvania Medical Center, Philadelphia, PA.)

Unfortunately, most adolescent mothers do not breastfeed. This is related to their perception of breastfeeding as something that will "tie me down" and the reality (in many instances) that they will be returning to school full-time soon after birth. Education about the importance of breastfeeding and tips for how to incorporate it into a busy lifestyle can increase the number of adolescents who breastfeed (see Chapter 19). Help young mothers who do not choose to breastfeed to find a feeding method that is satisfying to them and safe for the infant as part of the process of becoming a young, but effective, new mother (see Focus on Nursing Care Planning Box 22.4).

✓ Checkpoint Question 22.2

Mindy Carson was placed on an iron supplement because her hemoglobin level was below normal. What is a common test to demonstrate adherence to an iron supplement?

a. Assessing if her skin appears darker.
b. Assessing her blood reticulocyte count.
c. Analyzing her urine for iron deposits.
d. Measuring if she has grown in height.

THE PREGNANT WOMAN OVER AGE 40

The incidence of women delaying their first pregnancy until their late 30s or early 40s is increasing. Twelve percent of births in the United States today are to women over age 35; 2% to 4% are to women over age 40 (NCHS, 2009). In the past, it was assumed a woman of this age was past the optimal age for childbearing and was at risk for many complications. Today, with the exception of a greater incidence of chromosomal abnormality, there is little evidence of serious complications in women older than age 40 as long as prenatal care is begun early in the pregnancy.

A woman over age 40 is more likely than a younger woman to have a previously diagnosed condition, such as hypertension, varicosities, or hemorrhoids. In addition, by age 40, a woman usually has a major role change to undertake during pregnancy, because she often is well established in a career or has an accustomed routine at home or in her community. She needs to think through how this pregnancy and childrearing are going to fit into and change her life. Although she may feel rich in the number of support people she perceives around her, she may discover she has few "pregnancy support" people because she does not have many friends her age who are also having babies—some may be close to becoming grandparents. The only things these friends remember of pregnancy and labor are their particular highs and lows, and the care they received may not reflect current practice. This may leave a woman without access to the daily "shop talk" of other pregnant women, or someone to turn to with questions such as whether the backache she is experiencing or frequent need to urinate is normal. On the other hand, because many women delay childbearing today, she may be one of a sizable group of women in her community experiencing pregnancy at this stage of life.

Developmental Tasks and Pregnancy

The developmental challenge of the over-40 age group is to expand their awareness or develop generativity—that is, a sense

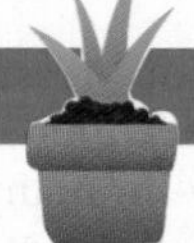

BOX 22.4 ✻ Focus on Nursing Care Planning

A Multidisciplinary Care Map for a Pregnant Adolescent

Mindy Carson, 16 years old and 15 weeks pregnant, was in an automobile accident on her way into prenatal clinic this morning. She received a 4-inch laceration on one leg. The father of Mindy's baby is a college student. He does not want Mindy to keep her baby after the birth because he does not want to get married until he finishes graduate school. Mindy insists she is old enough to be a parent and wants to keep her baby. Mindy's mother accuses the father of sharing methamphetamines with Mindy. She's worried Mindy has been working as a prostitute to support her drug habit.

Family Assessment ✻ Lives with family in second-floor apartment above convenience store, which parents own and run. Attends school but is "ready to drop out." Cares for 5-year-old sister after school while parents work downstairs.

Client Assessment ✻ Pale, tired-appearing adolescent female. Failed to come for two previous appointments. Admits to methamphetamine use since becoming pregnant. Hinted she might be using prostitution as income source. Parents want her to end pregnancy; client wants to continue pregnancy because "Now I can eat anything I want since I'm eating for two." Unhappy with arguing that is happening between parents and boyfriend. Says, "I'm coming apart at the seams."

Nursing Diagnosis ✻ Altered family processes related to the stress of adolescent pregnancy

Outcome Criteria ✻ Client and family members demonstrate positive coping mechanisms by communicating effectively; client identifies plans for self and infant; clarifies relationship desired with father of child. Baby's father participates in pregnancy activities as desired; client halts unhealthful practices.

Team Member Responsible	Assessment	Intervention	Rationale	Expected Outcome
		Activities of Daily Living		
Nurse	Assess the reason client states she is ready to drop out of school.	Discuss with client advantages of staying in school during pregnancy.	It is difficult for young women to support themselves and an infant without at least a high school education.	Client contracts to stay in school through graduation if possible.
		Consultations		
Social worker/ nurse	Investigate client's options for schooling if she no longer feels comfortable in her local public school.	Contact the client's school (with her permission) to explore options for her for continued school attendance.	Discussion promotes active problem solving and positive adaptation.	Client and school personnel agree on a course of action that will optimally benefit the client.
Social worker/ nurse	Assess what community resources are available for withdrawal for methamphetamine users.	Discuss the advantages of a withdrawal program during pregnancy.	Almost all substances cross the placenta and reach the fetus.	Client attends sessions for withdrawal from methamphetamines.
		Procedures/Medications		
Nurse	Assess what client expects from prenatal care and if she understands the importance of regular attendance.	Discuss importance of prenatal care for adolescents, who are prone to complications because of immature body development.	Prenatal care is the best safeguard against complications of pregnancy and the best chance that they will be prevented or alleviated as soon as they appear.	Client attends all future prenatal care appointments; Participates in discussions at these times.

Nurse	Assess what drugs client is taking.	List for medical personnel the possible drugs to which the fetus has been exposed.	Recreational drugs can lead to fetal growth restriction or birth defect.	Client agrees to a drug therapy program during pregnancy to reduce recreational drug use.
		Nutrition		
Nutritionist/nurse	Assess 24-hour dietary recall with client.	Examine diet to see if it contains all essential nutrients for pregnancy.	"Eating for two" does not mean eating more: it means eating more nutritious foods.	Client's 24-hour recall history at next visit shows improvement in necessary nutrients for healthy pregnancy.
		Patient/Family Education		
Nurse	Assess what client means by "I'm coming apart at the seams" in reference to her lack of support.	Reinforce understanding of those involved about the client's need for support. Instruct them in ways to offer support.	Additional help may be required to cope with the added demands of pregnancy.	Client states she is receiving adequate support from her family or boyfriend or health care providers to sustain her throughout the pregnancy.
		Psychosocial/Spiritual/Emotional Needs		
Nurse	Assess if client's disagreement with family over continuing pregnancy is a major stressor.	Assist client with ways to adapt to changes of pregnancy and responsibility for fetal safety. Support client's decision to continue pregnancy.	Adolescence is a highly stressful time, especially without parental support, so change can be difficult if not anticipated.	Client states she is open to changes she knows will occur with pregnancy; will ask health care providers for additional suggestions as needed.
		Discharge Planning		
Nurse	Assess what would be the best days for client and boyfriend to attend prenatal care.	Set up follow-up visits with client and support person; plan teaching strategies and discussion of all parties' needs and concerns as appropriate.	Prenatal care can help detect and prevent complications of pregnancy.	Client attends prenatal care regularly during remainder of pregnancy.

of moving away from themselves and becoming involved with the world or community (Erikson, 1963). Some people assume that once they reach adulthood, the way they are is the way they will always be. They are amazed to find that their bodies change (e.g., men may lose their hair; women and men both gain weight) and so do their interests. They find themselves joining committees and clubs, coaching Little League teams, or organizing fundraising or community events.

A woman in this age group who is pregnant may begin to feel ambivalent during pregnancy, because she may want to continue with community activities, yet also wants to concentrate on the baby inside her. You may need to help her balance her life so she can manage crossing two life phases this way.

What is perceived as the best time in life to have children is culturally influenced. In developing countries, many people believe having children while young allows parents to grow with children. In other cultures, such as the United States, many believe delaying childbirth until a family is financially secure is best. Delaying childbirth too long, however, is not approved. Because of these various beliefs, what you believe may not be the belief of a family for whom you provide care. What may be a catastrophe to you may seem like a blessing to someone else (and vice versa). Assess couples by history and observation to determine if childbearing appears to be timed correctly for them. If not, they may need extra time to accept a pregnancy and adapt to becoming parents.

Women who have a child after age 40 fall into one of two groups: those who are having their final child and those who have delayed childbearing because of education or a career and are having their first child. Many adults over the age of 40 care for aging parents. This additional responsibility may make it difficult for a woman to complete the psychological work of pregnancy. It also may create extra strain on her finances and time (creates a "sandwich generation," or one pressured by responsibilities by both older and younger family members). Worries also include having enough energy, arranging for child care, and financial strain.

Prenatal Assessment

A woman over age 40, like all women, should begin prenatal care early in pregnancy. Fortunately, most women of this age group are well informed about the advisability of early prenatal care and have adequate health insurance, so they do seek an early appointment. A few mistakenly believe their lack of menstruation is the result of early menopause so do not seek an early health care consultation.

Health History

Ask women in this age group about their present symptoms of pregnancy, how they feel about the pregnancy, and how it fits into their lifestyle. If a woman did not realize she was pregnant, she may have self-medicated. Ask if she has been taking any medication or herbal remedies to relieve reported symptoms, such as nausea or fatigue. Because a woman is functioning well in a business world does not mean she has a healthy pregnancy lifestyle. Do not accept answers such as "I drink socially" or "I take the usual drugs" without exploring what those phrases mean specifically.

Family Profile. Some women over age 40 who are pregnant for the first time have recently changed their life pattern (married or became involved in a long-term sexual relationship) or have decided to have a child, perhaps through in vitro fertilization, without a spouse before they are no longer able to conceive. Whereas a younger woman often waits a while after marrying to become pregnant, a woman over age 40 often plans to become pregnant immediately after marriage because she senses her reproductive time clock ticking. Because of this, she may find herself making many adjustments at once (not only to a new life partner, house or apartment, and perhaps community, but also to a pregnancy).

Identify a woman's source of income. If she has a well-paying job, stopping work because of a pregnancy complication may greatly reduce her family's income. Also evaluate how many people are financially or emotionally dependent on her (such as children from a former marriage, elderly parents, an elderly neighbor, or fellow workers who count on her). During pregnancy, when a woman often needs extra emotional support, feeling responsible for so many people can be difficult.

Day History. Ask specifically about a woman's job and estimate the amount of walking or back strain it entails. Ask about recent diet or exercise programs. If a woman belongs to a health club, remind her that the use of saunas and hot tubs for longer than 10 minutes at a time is contraindicated during pregnancy because of possible hyperthermia and teratogenic effects of extreme heat on a developing fetus. Identify personal habits, such as cigarette smoking and alcohol consumption, that may be detrimental to a fetus to determine if counseling to halt or decrease these habits could be effective.

Physical Examination

A woman over age 40 needs a thorough physical examination at her first prenatal visit to establish her general health and to identify any problems, particularly circulatory disturbances she may have. Inspect her lower extremities thoroughly for varicosities, because these are more common in women over age 40 (Box 22.5). Obtain a urine specimen and test it for specific gravity, glucose, and protein to evaluate overall renal function and the possibility of gestational or type 2 diabetes, because older women are more prone than younger women to develop these conditions.

Assess a woman's breasts for any abnormalities, as women over age 40 are in a higher-risk group for breast cancer than are younger women. Ask if she has had yearly mammograms. In addition, assess for fetal heart sounds and fetal movement at prenatal visits because gestational trophoblastic disease (hydatidiform mole) is also more common in women over age 40 (see Chapter 21).

Chromosomal Assessment

Women over 35 are offered a triple-screen (alpha-fetoprotein [AFP], human chorionic gonadotropin, and unconjugated estriol levels) drawn on blood serum at the 15th week of pregnancy to detect whether an open spinal cord or chromosomal

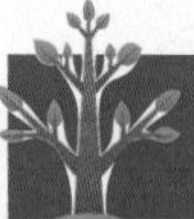

BOX 22.5 ✻ Focus on Family Teaching

Tips on Preventing Varicose Veins

Q. Mindy says to you, "My mother was old when she had me so developed terrible varicose veins. How can I stop that from happening to me?

A. Although the following activities are not foolproof, incorporating them into your day helps prevent the development of varicose veins:

- Find opportunities during the day, such as a coffee or lunch break, to elevate your legs.
- Be certain your diet includes vitamin C, because this is important to strengthen vein walls.
- Rest in a side-lying position with your body tipped slightly forward (Sims' position). This allows leg veins to drain and empty.
- Avoid long periods of standing in one place by taking "walk breaks"; active muscle contraction helps venous return.
- Avoid sitting with your legs crossed.
- Do not wear anything constricting, such as knee-high stockings, on your lower legs.
- If you wear support hose, put them on before you get out of bed in the morning, before veins become swollen, for best results.

defect could be present in the fetus, because their risk for Down syndrome is so much higher than it is in younger women, an incidence of about 1 in 1000 compared to 1 in 1500 in younger women (Ball et al., 2007). If this test is positive, an amniocentesis will be scheduled at the 16th week of pregnancy. Be certain a woman is prepared for these studies and receives support during them. Alert her that false-positive results can occur with AFP testing, which is why amniocentesis is important. Many women of this age group do not begin nest-building until these tests confirm that their child will be healthy.

Nursing Diagnoses and Related Interventions

Nursing Diagnosis: Health-seeking behaviors related to special care necessary for healthy pregnancy

Outcome Evaluation: Client states she feels confident in self-care and her ability to decrease possible complications of pregnancy.

Be certain to adapt prenatal teaching to fit an older woman's lifestyle. If she had not planned on ever being pregnant, she may have isolated herself through the years from "mothering" activities and so, despite her years, may know little about pregnancy and newborn care. In terms of knowledge, this puts her at the same level as the adolescent. Others have read so extensively that they may know more theoretical information than a woman who has already given birth. Be certain to review information about possible discomforts of pregnancy (see Chapter 12). A pregnant woman over age 40 is prone to hemorrhoids because she may have some rectal varicosities present at the beginning of pregnancy. Pain from rectal distention may, in fact, be one of the primary symptoms she reports at a first visit. Review measures to increase comfort.

Varicosities, like hemorrhoids, develop readily in a woman over age 40 because she may have had some tendency toward them even before the pregnancy. As with hemorrhoids, her best approach during pregnancy is to prevent varicosities.

Record on a woman's chart any degree of varicosity formation during pregnancy so nurses caring for her during the postpartum period can take special precautions to prevent thrombophlebitis as with venous stasis present after birth, a woman is even more prone to develop this complication immediately postpartum.

Pregnancy Education

Childbirth education classes oriented toward the older woman provide important information on pregnancy and bring these women and their support people together. A woman over age 40, like any other pregnant woman, needs access to health care personnel who can supply her with factual information during a pregnancy. She also needs additional support while she works through this role change in her life.

Nutrition

Assess the number of meals a woman eats outside her home each week, including those she packs for lunch or eats in restaurants. She may need tips on how to adjust pregnancy nutrition so she can obtain the same nutrition whether she prepares meals at home or eats them at an office or community function. Urge her to substitute a caffeine-free soft drink in place of an alcoholic beverage. In some offices, large amounts of coffee are consumed. Urge her to substitute milk or juice or decaffeinated coffee. Many women this age normally drink little milk. Rather than getting used to milk again, a woman may appreciate suggestions on other ways to ingest calcium, such as puddings or yogurt.

Prenatal Classes

Because a pregnant woman over age 40 may be unique in her circle of friends, she may feel shut out of her usual group because of the pregnancy. This makes her ready, therefore, to join a childbirth preparation or prenatal exercise class where she is "one of the group" (Fig. 22.2).

Be certain a woman plans (or the couple plans together) to set aside a specific time every day to do breathing exercises in preparation for labor. Otherwise, a busy woman may never find time to get to them and will be unprepared in labor.

Complications of Pregnancy for a Woman Over Age 40

The complications of pregnancy most likely to occur in a woman over age 40—hypertension of pregnancy, preterm or post term birth, and cesarean birth—are related to the fact that the woman's circulatory system may not be as competent as when she was younger or her body tissues may not be as elastic as they were once (Box 22.6).

Pregnancy-Induced Hypertension

A woman over age 40 may have a higher incidence of pregnancy-induced hypertension than a younger woman, possibly related to blood vessel inelasticity or because hypertension tends to occur more frequently in nulliparas than in

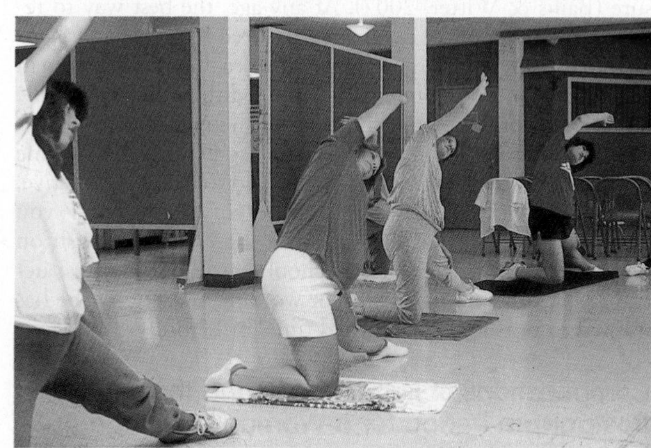

FIGURE 22.2 Exercise classes during pregnancy provide women with an opportunity to interact with other pregnant women while benefiting from a carefully monitored workout. (© Kathy Sloane.)

Box 22.6 Assessment

Assessing the Pregnant Woman Over 40 for Complications

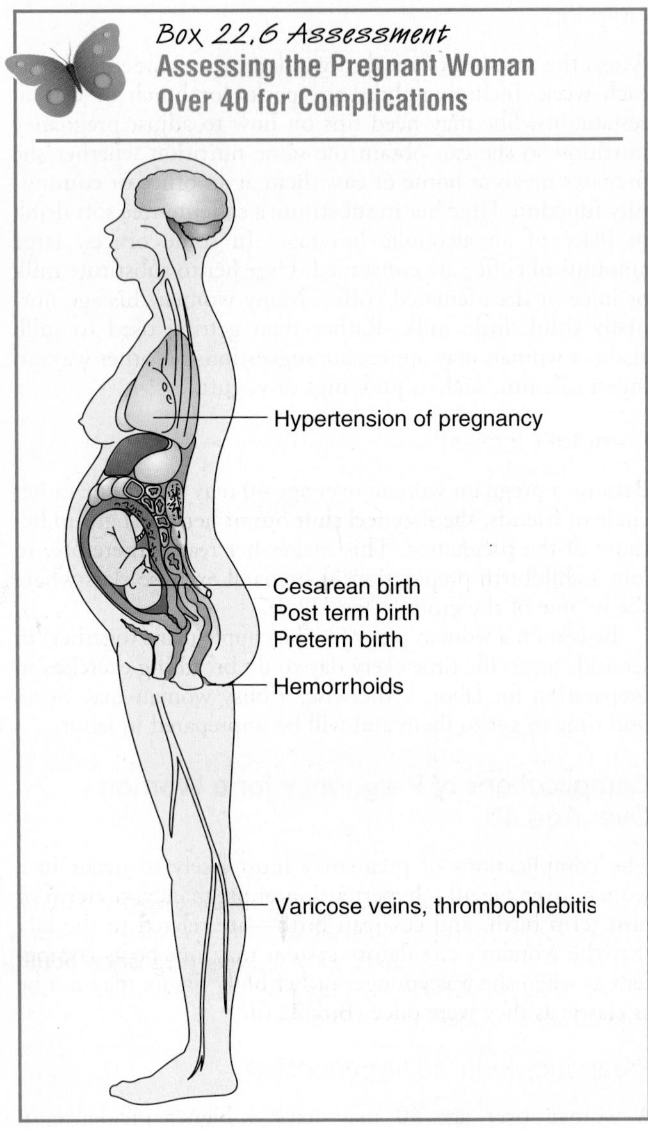

multiparas as well as those with already elevated blood pressure (Bailis & Witter, 2007). At any age, the best way to reduce the symptoms of pregnancy-induced hypertension is for a woman to rest for a good portion of each day. If a woman works full-time, stopping work may be difficult or impossible for her, not only because she believes she may miss out on a promotion or risk losing her job, but also because her income is important to her family and she is used to being productive, not merely resting all day. To allow her to rest effectively, you may need to help her plan activities she can accomplish on bed rest, such as reworking a school course outline, restructuring her office filing system, or working at a hobby she has wanted to pursue but never had time for before.

Complications of Labor, Birth, and the Postpartum Period for a Woman Over Age 40

Complications that occur with a woman over age 40 related to birth or the immediate period after birth also are the results of a body that may not be as elastic as it was when the woman was younger.

Failure to Progress in Labor

Labor in an older primipara may be prolonged because cervical dilatation may not occur as spontaneously as in a younger woman. Graphing labor progress is a good method to use to determine when labor is becoming prolonged. Many women this age may need a cesarean birth if labor is overly prolonged and places a fetus at risk. Encourage a woman to verbalize how she is feeling about her progress throughout labor to allow for reassurance and prompt intervention should problems arise. Urge her support person to be present for the birth to offer needed support. Keep in mind that some older men may not be as comfortable in a birthing room as their younger counterparts would be because when they were younger, men were excluded from watching births.

Difficulty Accepting the Event

Women over age 40 may begin to have second thoughts about childbearing this late in life as the reality of a new baby registers with them during the intrapartal and postpartum periods. Although they may have read a great deal about babies during pregnancy, they may wish they had read more or were as confident with this phase of their life as they are about other areas such as their home, office, or classroom. Review plans for child care and postpartum rest, with an emphasis on helping women learn to balance their lives, especially if they are planning on returning to work soon after the birth. They might appreciate help making child care arrangements. You can assure them that day care for preschool children has positive socialization results (Zoritch, Roberts, & Oakley, 2009).

Postpartum Hemorrhage

Just as the cervix may not dilate as readily during an older woman's labor, the uterus may not contract as readily in the postpartum period because of inelasticity. Therefore, an older woman may be at higher risk for postpartum hemorrhage (Poggi, 2007). She may be more prone to perineal-anal tears because her perineum is less subtle (Fitzgerald et al., 2007). Close observation is essential. Because a woman over age 40 may be an independent woman who is interested in self-care, she may ask for little help. Be sure to assess the amount of her lochial flow to detect this complication.

✔ Checkpoint Question 22.3

Women over 40 are at increased risk for developing pregnancy-induced hypertension. The reason for this is:

a. Many are overweight before they enter pregnancy.
b. They drink more fluids daily than younger women.
c. They do not exercise much, so edema fluid accumulates.
d. Their blood vessels are not as elastic as those of younger women.

THE PREGNANT WOMAN WHO IS PHYSICALLY OR COGNITIVELY CHALLENGED

In the past, women with conditions such as vision, hearing, cognitive, neurologic, or orthopedic challenges were sheltered by their families to such an extent that women with

TABLE 22.1 ✻ Areas of Planning With Physically or Cognitively Challenged Women During Pregnancy

Area	Assessment and Planning Guidelines
Transportation	Ask if a woman has transportation for prenatal care and for emergencies.
Pregnancy counseling	Assess the special modifications of care that will need to be made depending on a woman's special challenge. Use additional visual or auditory aids to make your teaching points clear.
Support person	Determine who is the woman's support person. In some instances, a woman's condition requires so much assistance during pregnancy that one support person will not be enough. If necessary, contact community agencies to lend additional support, with her consent.
Health	Do not lose track of a woman's primary health problem. For example, a woman with cerebral palsy may need to continue an active muscle exercise program during pregnancy for her primary illness.
Work	Assess whether a woman works outside her home and, if work is discontinued during pregnancy, what she could substitute for a social contact activity. Women with physical or cognitive challenges may be lonely because they do not have a wide range of friends or social contacts.
Recreation	Assess whether her level of activity is adequate, and make concrete suggestions within her limitations for increasing it. Many women with a physically challenging condition lead a rather sedentary life (partly because they do not have many social contacts).
Self-esteem	Assess a woman's level of self-esteem: it may be low because of repeated failures in her life. Give praise at prenatal visits and help her make pregnancy a growth experience.

even moderately physically challenging conditions could not meet potential sexual or marriage partners and so did not become pregnant. In addition, most people believed these individuals should not become pregnant. Today, women with varying degrees of disability attend public schools, work in offices, join community organizations, establish sexual relationships, marry, and plan pregnancies just like everyone else. Urge women with a physical or cognitive disability or illness to come for preconceptual care so medicines they are taking can be evaluated and careful planning for safe pregnancy care can be started early (Thierry, 2007). Because these women (and in some instances also their support persons) face special problems related to their conditions, nursing care during pregnancy must be designed with these special concerns in mind so the woman's and her family's problems and needs can be addressed and met (Piotrowski & Snell, 2007).

Table 22.1 lists general areas of care that are important in planning for the physically or cognitively challenged woman who is pregnant.

Rights of the Physically or Cognitively Challenged Person

There are ethical and legal considerations related to women with disabilities and pregnancy. By federal law, physically disabled persons must have freedom of access to public buildings by means of ramps or handrails. All public health care facilities must be in compliance with these laws both in terms of physical facilities and in the true spirit of the law: that is, people should be made to feel psychologically welcome as well as physically able to reach the inside of the building. Under the same law, a hospital cannot deny care to a person with a disability even though the disabling condition complicates treatment considerably, possibly requiring extra personnel and time. A woman with a disability has full rights to her child, so the baby cannot be taken from her at birth without her full consent. Likewise, she cannot be forced to terminate a pregnancy or undergo sterilization unless that is her informed decision.

Modifications for Pregnancy

Explore with women at a first prenatal visit the exact nature of their disability and their general self-image to identify what modifications they may need in care during pregnancy. Some women who are physically or cognitively challenged maintain high self-esteem despite severe limitations and are able to modify, grow, and learn with a pregnancy, whereas others have a poor sense of self-esteem that will make this particularly difficult for them. For many of them, pregnancy will become a special event, a 9-month announcement to everyone that, despite their seeming limitations, they are equal to other women and capable of participating in one of life's miracles. If a woman is housebound, be certain that she is taking a prenatal vitamin containing vitamin D as she is probably not receiving as much sun exposure as usual (More, 2007).

Safety Measures to Explore

Safety is a key area of concern when caring for a pregnant woman who is physically or cognitively challenged. Be sure to assess areas such as emergency contact persons, suppliers of transportation, and individual considerations such as mobility, elimination, and possible autonomic responses. Be certain that a woman reviews any medicine she is taking for her primary condition with her primary care provider to be certain that this will continue to be safe during pregnancy. Women with recurrent seizures, for example, may need to have their dose of antiseizure medicine reduced during pregnancy because these may be teratogenic (Adab et al., 2009).

Emergency Contacts. Evaluate the client's ability to contact someone in case of pregnancy-related emergency. Does a woman have a telephone she can reach readily? Does she know how to activate the emergency medical system (911) in her community? If a woman's speech is not clear, evaluate whether she will be understood while using a telephone to call for help in an emergency. Some women with limited mobility, such as those with spinal cord injury or cerebral palsy, have a specially designed telephone contact system in their home that connects to a paramedic or hospital emergency service through a beeper system. Check that they intend to maintain this throughout pregnancy. Women who are hearing challenged use a specially equipped telephone (a TDD device) that prints out messages for them.

Transportation. Assess a client's ability to come for prenatal care. If a woman depends on a support person for transportation to a health care facility, appointments may have to be arranged according to that person's schedule to prevent missed appointments. If a woman does not drive, who would transport her if a pregnancy emergency should occur? Women with cognitive or vision challenges, for example, may not qualify for a driver's license and so may need someone, such as a family member or friend, to drive. Women with spinal cord injury may have difficulty transferring into the specially equipped, hand-controlled car they usually drive as pregnancy progresses.

Mobility. All women who use wheelchairs are taught to press with their hands against the armrests and lift their buttocks up off the wheelchair seat for 5 seconds every hour. This prevents the formation of pressure ulcers on the buttocks and posterior thighs. Encourage a pregnant woman to continue to perform this maneuver during pregnancy as the increased weight of a fetus increases her risk for pressure ulcer formation from compression. In addition, severe hip flexion from sitting in a wheelchair limits venous return from the lower extremities. For at least 1 hour every morning and afternoon, encourage women who ambulate by wheelchair to decrease the sharp bend at their knees that results from sitting in the chair, to promote venous return and help prevent varicosities and thrombi formation. Adjusting the footrests of the wheelchair so a woman's legs are not sharply bent at the knees accomplishes this.

If balance is a problem, a woman may need re-evaluation at the midpoint of pregnancy as the weight of her abdomen increases. She may need to use crutches if she did not use them before, or use a wheelchair if she was ambulatory with crutches or a walker before pregnancy. Keep in mind that a woman who is physically challenged achieved the degree of ambulation that she first presents with usually after years of physical therapy and strengthening of leg and arm muscles. Help her see that reducing her degree of independence during pregnancy is not a step backward for her but a step forward, allowing her to have a safe pregnancy without the danger of falling (Fig. 22.3).

Elimination. When mobility is an effort, a woman may not drink as much as usual or use a bathroom as frequently as she would if those actions were effortless. Encourage a high fluid intake and frequent voiding, however, to prevent urinary tract infections. Women with spinal cord injury who use an indwelling catheter are at especially high risk for contracting urinary tract infections during pregnancy. Women who perform self-catheterization or change their own indwelling catheter may be unable to continue to do this late in pregnancy because the increasing size of their abdomen interferes with their ability to see or reach their perineum comfortably. If this happens, it may be necessary for a woman to arrange for a support person, a home care nurse, or a home health aide to do this for her.

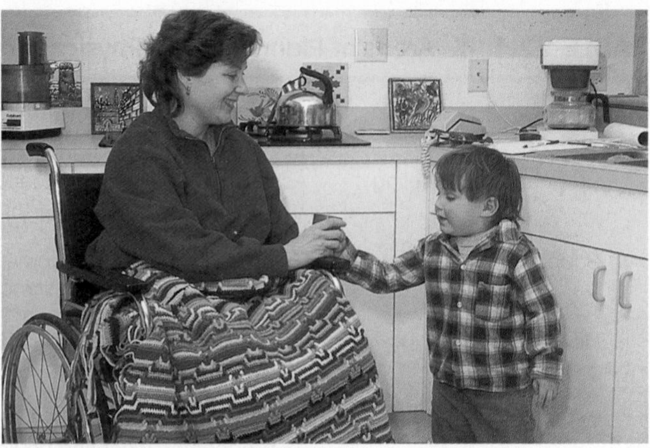

FIGURE 22.3 During pregnancy, a woman who is physically challenged may need to use a wheelchair to help safeguard herself against injury. Assure her that she may still enjoy her independence and daily activities, such as caring for an older child. (© Keith/Custom Medical Stock Photograph.)

Autonomic Responses. In a woman who has a high spinal cord injury (cervical or high thoracic), observe for **autonomic dysreflexia** during pregnancy, labor, and the immediate postpartum period. This is an exaggerated autonomic response to stimuli. Any irritating condition, such as a distended bladder, increasing uterine size, labor contractions, or breastfeeding, may initiate the response (Smeltzer, 2007). Without upper motor neuron control to reverse the phenomenon, extreme symptoms such as severe hypertension (300/160 mm Hg), throbbing headache, flushing of the skin and profuse diaphoresis above the level of the spinal lesion, nausea, and bradycardia may occur. Immediate action is necessary to protect against cerebrovascular accident or intraocular damage. Elevate a woman's head to reduce cerebral pressure and locate the irritating stimulus (usually a distended bladder or bowel). If bladder distention is the cause, the woman needs bladder pressure relieved by catheterization if an indwelling catheter is not in place. If a catheter is in place, check to see why it is not draining, then encourage it to drain by unkinking or flushing to allow urine to flow freely again. Anticipate the need for an antihypertensive agent to alleviate the extreme hypertension, although as soon as the source of irritation is removed, symptoms typically fade quickly.

Prenatal Care Modifications to Meet Specific Needs

Physical examination may need to be modified depending on individual circumstances for women with disabilities (Richman, 2007). Although women with disabilities have been followed by health care providers most of their life, they may never have had a pelvic examination before and so need clear instructions about why it is needed and what it will consist of. Many obstetric examining tables are built for the comfort of the examiner and are too high for a woman to transfer to from a wheelchair by simply sliding onto the table.

To help a woman move to the table, a ramp from the physical therapy department may be necessary so the wheelchair can be elevated to the level of the table. Woman with spinal cord injury or cerebral palsy may be unable to maintain their legs in a lithotomy position because of either hip flexion contracture or laxness of leg support. This means a dorsal recumbent, rather than a lithotomy, position may be required for a pelvic examination.

Women who are cognitively challenged may not be aware how they became pregnant. If a woman became pregnant because she was taken advantage of sexually, she may need some time to talk and work through this experience before she can allow a pelvic examination.

If a visually challenged woman brings a guide dog with her to a health care visit, remember that although the dog's chief function is to offer direction, its instinct causes it to become a woman's protector. In this role, the dog may feel threatened by people who try to pet it. Petting a guide dog also distracts it from safeguarding its owner.

When interviewing or teaching visually challenged women, be certain not to use your hands to illustrate points ("I'll need a urine sample of at least this much urine [measured with your fingers]"). Do not use colors as descriptions of objects ("put on the blue gown"). Use demonstration aids that allow a woman to feel or touch instead. When helping with or performing physical assessment, let a woman know you are closing the door or drawing a curtain to ensure privacy. Always alert a woman when you are going to touch her, so as not to startle her. Otherwise, you may find yourself facing a growling guide dog that rises to protect her.

If a woman is hearing impaired, she may not be able to see the examiner's face during a pelvic examination. This means any question asked of her during this time will not be understood because she cannot see the examiner's lips to lip read (O'Hearn, 2007).

Pregnancy Education

Modify health teaching to meet each woman's specific needs. For a woman who is cognitively challenged, for example, instructions about pregnancy may need to be limited to those few items crucial for safety, such as "do not drink alcohol or take any medicine."

If a woman and her support person are both visually challenged, pamphlets about pregnancy care will not be useful. If the support person can see, offer the pamphlets to him or her, suggesting the support person read them to the pregnant woman as a shared activity. This will not only be helpful to her but also make the partner a more informed support person. Many visually challenged women have tape recorders supplied by Recording for the Blind and Dyslexic (http://www.rfbd.org), a national, nonprofit, voluntary organization. Call the local association and ask if they have any material already recorded on pregnancy or breastfeeding that they can supply. If not, make a tape recording of any information you particularly want a woman to remember or she seems concerned about. Supply the health care facility telephone number at the beginning of the tape for an easy reminder in an emergency, and perhaps the date of her next visit as well.

Nutritional education is another area that should be designed based on each client's specific challenges and usual routine. A visually challenged woman or one who ambulates by wheelchair, for example, may prepare her own breakfast and lunch, meals that do not require a stove. The one hot meal a woman eats is one a support person cooks in the evening. Nutrition counseling for two meals daily, therefore, needs to center on foods that can be prepared without cooking.

Activity and exercise, important for any pregnant woman, are crucial for a woman who is physically challenged. If mobility is a concern, exercise can be very reduced in bad weather. In this case, be sure a woman understands that walking around her home or apartment can provide the same level of exercise as if she were walking around the block or exercising at a health club.

Although labor and her child's birth may be modified somewhat because of a woman's physical condition, gaining general knowledge about labor and birth and participating in a shared experience with her partner are still valuable. Urge women to attend childbirth preparation classes if at all possible. If a woman is not working outside her home, she may have more time than others to practice breathing exercises and enter labor more adept at using such a method to control pain in labor than other women.

If a woman is severely hearing challenged, she may not have heard the many spot television announcements on not smoking or drinking alcohol during pregnancy; she may need more time at prenatal visits so this can be discussed. In addition, lip reading is a difficult skill to learn, so many hearing-challenged persons cannot do this with ease. Even if a woman is skilled at this, she may not be able to decipher new words such as amniotic, gestation, or edema. Show her the printed words so she can see what your lip motion represents when presenting new pregnancy terms. If a woman uses sign language, she may bring an interpreter with her to translate. Be certain to talk to her, not the interpreter, when interviewing.

Modifications for Labor and Birth

Women who are physically or cognitively challenged will need adaptations in preparation for labor and birth. Helpful suggestions are:

- A woman with a spinal cord injury may not be able to feel uterine contractions. Late in pregnancy, she will need to palpate her abdomen periodically for tightening or the presence of contractions so she is aware of beginning labor.
- Women with muscle spasticity or spinal cord injury may not be able to push effectively for the second stage of labor and so may need cesarean or forceps birth.
- If a woman cannot assume a lithotomy position because of hip contracture, vaginal delivery from a Sims' or dorsal recumbent position is best.
- Braille watches used by visually challenged persons may not have second hands. They may need to time the length of contractions by counting rather than timing them by a watch.
- During labor, the hearing-challenged woman cannot hear information on how she is progressing if you are not directly facing her. If she needs to communicate with her support person in sign language, act as an advocate to keep her hands unencumbered by equipment such as intravenous lines. Remember she cannot hear her infant cry at birth. Hand the infant to her as soon as possible after birth so she can see and feel the baby is crying and breathing well.

- Be certain to identify the usual sounds of birthing rooms (the beeping of a monitor, the swish of a central supply routing system, and so forth) for the visually challenged woman. Hearing sounds and not being able to identify them can be frightening.

Modifications for Postpartum Care

After birth, be sure to assess and teach:

- Whether a woman desires contraceptive information.
- Whether she needs additional support to be successful at breastfeeding.
- Whether she has a return appointment for both herself and her infant for follow-up care and that the arrangements are within her capabilities, transportation, and understanding.

Women with disabilities generally feel a need to space pregnancies so be certain that they receive information on their contraceptive choices as these may be different than for nonhandicapped women (Frost & Darroch, 2008). A woman with poor hand control, for example, might not be able to effectively insert a diaphragm; a woman who is cognitively challenged might not understand the importance of taking an oral contraceptive every day.

Modifications for Planning Child Care

Allow for extra time during the first days after birth for mother–child interaction. For example, after birth, a woman who is cognitively challenged may need extra time to understand the transition from "being pregnant" to "having a baby." She may have difficulty learning to judge when her infant is hungry. She may need extra supervision to be certain she does not leave the baby unprotected on a bed. A woman with a spinal cord disability may be particularly interested in inspecting her baby's back. A visually challenged woman will probably want to reassure herself her baby can see. Be sure to give her baby to her as soon as possible after birth so she can touch the baby and feel for intact body parts. If the birthing room is cold, explain to her that you want to rewrap the baby to prevent chilling, not because her touching is wrong or because you are trying to hide an imperfection in the baby.

Breastfeeding has special advantages for women who are physically or cognitively challenged because it is the method of feeding that is not only best for the baby, but also requires the least preparation effort on the mother's part. For a woman who is visually challenged and unable to read printed instructions, breastfeeding eliminates formula errors. For a woman who uses a wheelchair, it eliminates trips to the refrigerator. However, breastfeeding may not be possible for a woman with muscle spasticity because the let-down reflex, which depends on muscle relaxation, may not occur. Be certain that women who are cognitively challenged understand they need to feed until the infant is satisfied, not until they are tired of feeding.

Encourage women to think through what baby care equipment will be best for them. Some infant crib rails lower by pressure on a foot pedal. Others use a waist-high lever. A woman who ambulates by wheelchair usually finds the waist-high lever most convenient because she can reach this most easily. Some women will need a referral for home care follow-up and possibly the use of a home health aide to ensure safe child care.

If a woman has difficulty with mobility, ask how she anticipates carrying her infant. Using an anterior baby sling is usually effective with a wheelchair. Women who are mobile by crutches or a walker can place the baby in a small wagon and pull it. Some women lie on their back on the floor, place the baby on their chest, and scoot across the floor. The important point is not how a woman carries her baby but that she has thought through a safe and comfortable way to do this.

Urge a visually challenged woman to make eye contact when talking to her infant. Many visually challenged people do not turn on lights in their home because they do not perceive the difference between light and dark. Encourage a woman to develop a habit of turning on lights after dinner because her infant will need light to develop vision. If her support person also is visually challenged, suggest she check with a close friend or neighbor monthly to see that light bulbs have not burned out.

One of the biggest worries for the hearing-impaired woman is that she will not be able to hear her baby crying. Help her plan to bring the infant's crib or bassinet close to her bed so she can feel the vibration of the baby's stirring and waking. Urge her to talk to her infant as she gives care so the infant is introduced to sounds and words. Some women whose speech is severely affected by their hearing disorder are reluctant to speak to strangers. Assure her that her infant is not a stranger and will quiet readily to the sound of her voice. The child may develop her speech pattern because of this. Being spoken to and sung to during the first year is important for overall development, however, so this is still preferable to living in a world of silence.

Some women who are cognitively challenged may have been raised in a group home and only recently moved to their own apartment. Unlike those raised at home, these women may have unusual difficulty making plans for child care because they have never seen the care of young children. You have a legal obligation to investigate whether a newborn will receive safe care before hospital discharge. Be certain to ask enough questions so that you are sure a woman who is severely cognitively challenged, for example, has a responsible friend or partner to help her with child care.

✔ Checkpoint Question 22.4

Women with high thoracic spinal cord injury can develop autonomic dysreflexia during labor. The best action to take for this would be:

a. Ask her to lie flat and take deep breaths.
b. Elevate her legs to restore her blood pressure.
c. Give a prescribed hypotensive medicine.
d. Talk to her calmly to reduce her anxiety.

A WOMAN WHO IS SUBSTANCE DEPENDENT

Substance dependence is a growing health problem in women of childbearing age, so its incidence during pregnancy is increasing. As many as 10% to 20% of pregnant women use illegal drugs during pregnancy (NCHS, 2009). The use of cocaine, amphetamines, and multiple drugs has increased dramatically in recent years. Adolescents have an increased rate of inhalant abuse and binge drinking.

Substance abuse is defined as the inability to meet major role obligations, an increase in legal problems or risk-taking behavior, or exposure to hazardous situations because of an addicting substance. A person is **substance dependent** when he or she has withdrawal symptoms following discontinuation of the substance, combined with abandonment of important activities, spending increased time in activities related to substance use, using substances for a longer time than planned, or continued use despite worsening problems because of substance use.

Typically, substance-dependent women are thought to be in the younger age group, as the overall incidence of drug use is highest in this group. However, any woman could be substance dependent so all pregnant women need to be assessed for the possibility of this.

A mark of a woman with a substance abuse problem is that she may come late in the pregnancy for prenatal care because she is afraid her drug use will be discovered and she will be reported to authorities. If she is using a drug that sustains her for only a few hours, she cannot wait long at a health care facility to be seen for an appointment. She may have difficulty following prenatal instructions for proper nutrition because although she may desire to eat well, she may lack sufficient money to buy both drugs and nutritious food, and choosing drugs over food makes her nutrition inadequate. She may not have money for supplemental vitamins or iron preparations for the same reason.

Illicit drugs tend to be of small molecular weight, so they readily cross the placenta. As a result, a fetus of an addicted mother has a drug concentration of about 50% that of the mother. Because this can lead to fetal effects, drug abuse can account for fetal abnormalities or preterm birth (Dew, 2007). If a woman uses injected drugs, the risk for hepatitis B or human immunodeficiency virus (HIV) infection increases. Additionally, a woman may earn money to buy drugs through prostitution, which increases the risk for sexually transmitted infection and poses an additional threat to a fetus.

Nursing Diagnoses and Related Interventions

Nursing Diagnosis: Risk for injury to self and fetus related to chronic substance abuse

Outcome Evaluation: Client states she has enrolled in a substance abuse treatment program and consequently has reduced or is no longer abusing drugs.

Women who are substance dependent need anticipatory guidance and nursing support all during pregnancy, as this is a long time to change and then maintain a new lifestyle. Often, women who abuse substances have few effective support people with whom they feel free to discuss their problems or concerns or who can answer their questions about pregnancy. Because of their numerous needs, they require a multidisciplinary team approach not only from pregnancy health care providers but substance abuse treatment providers as well. Fortunately, with good support and active participation in a treatment program, pregnancy can become a stimulus for drug withdrawal and a maturing and growth experience for a woman.

If a woman is still abusing a drug by the time she begins labor, her infant may experience drug withdrawal symptoms after birth (usually nervousness, irritability or lethargy, and possibly seizures; see Chapter 26). Breastfeeding is usually not encouraged for women with substance abuse because just as all drugs cross the placenta to some extent, they also are all excreted into breast milk. Women receiving methadone as part of their drug treatment can breastfeed as only a small amount of this drug is excreted in breast milk (Jansson et al., 2008). In some states, women who test positive for drug abuse, either during pregnancy or at the time of birth, are reported to state child protective agencies; they may be accused of child abuse and jailed, and their infant may be placed in foster care. Be certain you are familiar with agency and state policy concerning these directives (Wright & Walker, 2007).

What if... Mindy Carson tells you she is not using drugs during pregnancy, but when she opens her purse, you notice several packets of white powder inside? What would you do?

Common Substances Abused During Pregnancy

Recreational drugs commonly used in pregnancy are those commonly used by women in their childbearing years: cocaine, amphetamines, marijuana, phencyclidine, inhalants, opiates, and alcohol.

Cocaine

Cocaine is derived from *Erythroxylum coca,* a plant grown almost exclusively in South America. When sniffed into the nose or smoked in a pipe, cocaine is absorbed across the mucous membranes to affect the central nervous system. As a result, sudden vasoconstriction occurs. Respiratory and cardiac rates and blood pressure increase rapidly in response to the vasoconstriction. Immediate death may result from cardiac failure. Alkaloidal cocaine (crack), a concentrated mixture, produces an even more rapid and intense "high" when inhaled.

Cocaine has become one of the most frequently abused drugs during pregnancy, and its use is exceptionally harmful during pregnancy because the extreme vasoconstriction that occurs can severely compromise placental circulation, leading to premature separation of the placenta, which then results in preterm labor or fetal death (Box 22.7). Infants born to cocaine-dependent women may suffer the immediate effects of intracranial hemorrhage and a withdrawal syndrome of tremulousness, irritability, and muscle rigidity. Long-term effects are not well documented, but learning defects are suspected (Accornero et al., 2007).

Counseling women to discontinue cocaine use during pregnancy is often disappointing. The effects of the drug are so intense that it is difficult for addicted women to withdraw. Cocaine use can be detected by urinalysis because the metabolites of cocaine can be detected in urine up to 1 week after use.

Box 22.7 Assessment
Assessing the Pregnant Cocaine-Abusing Woman

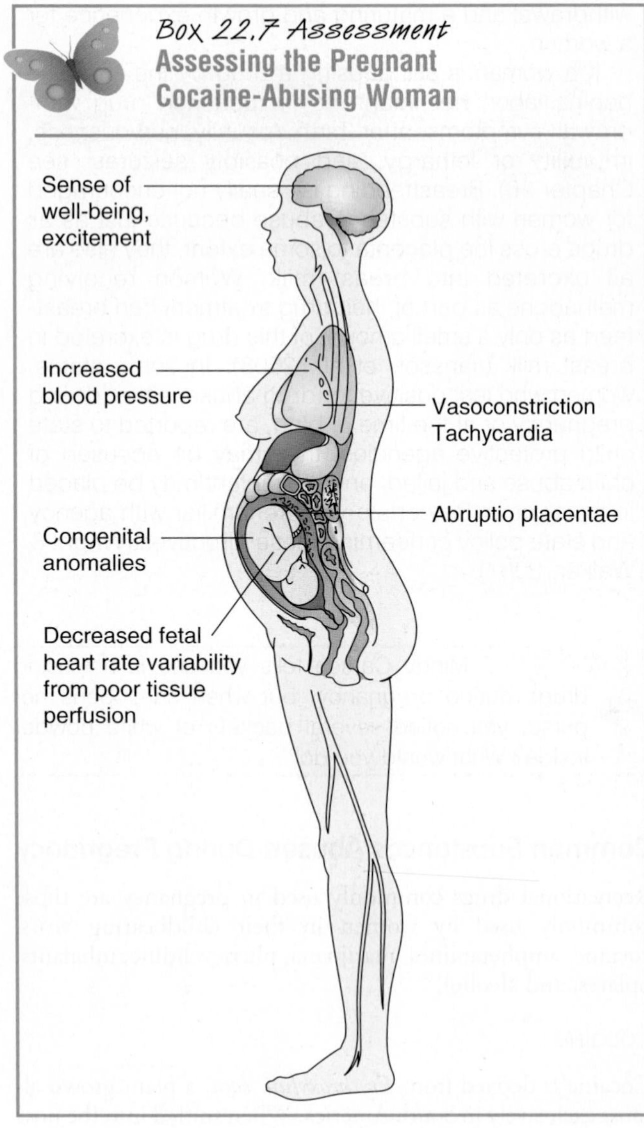

Amphetamines

Methamphetamine (speed) has a pharmacologic effect similar to cocaine. Its use is becoming more common because it is easily and cheaply manufactured (Wu, 2007). Ice, a rock type of methamphetamine that is smoked, can produce high concentrations of drug in the maternal circulation. Newborns whose mothers used the drug show jitteriness and poor feeding at birth and may be growth restricted.

Marijuana and Hashish

Both marijuana and hashish are obtained from the hemp plant, cannabis. When smoked, they produce tachycardia and a sense of well-being. Although not advised, some women use marijuana to counteract nausea in early pregnancy. These drugs are frequently part of polydrug abuse, so their effects on fetal development are not well documented (Bernstein & Weinstein, 2007). They are associated with loss of short-term memory and an increased incidence of respiratory infection in adults. A frequent user may not be able to breastfeed because of reduced milk production and the risk to the newborn from excretion of the drug in the milk.

Phencyclidine

Phencyclidine (PCP) is an animal tranquilizer that is a frequently used street drug in polydrug abuse. It causes increased cardiac output and a sense of euphoria. It has the potential for causing long-term hallucinations (flashback episodes). PCP tends to leave the maternal circulation and concentrate in fetal cells, so it may be particularly injurious to a fetus.

Narcotic Agonists

Narcotic agonists, used for the treatment of pain (e.g., morphine or meperidine [Demerol]) and cough suppression (codeine), are also widely abused because of their potent analgesic and euphoric effect. Heroin, a raw opiate, is the main opiate used recreationally to the point of dependence, and its use is increasing in incidence in young adults. A short-acting narcotic, heroin is inactive until it crosses the blood–brain barrier (which it does more quickly than morphine). It may be administered intradermally ("skin popping"), through inhalation ("snorting"), or intravenously ("shooting"). It produces an immediate and short-lived feeling of euphoria followed by sedation. Pregnancy complications related to its use include pregnancy-induced hypertension and, because narcotics are often injected with shared needles, phlebitis, subacute bacterial endocarditis, and hepatitis B and HIV infection.

Withdrawal symptoms include nausea, vomiting, diarrhea, abdominal pain, hypertension, restlessness, shivering, insomnia, body aches, and muscle jerks. Withdrawal symptoms may begin as soon as 6 hours after the last drug dose and can continue for several days. Their severity and duration depend on the amount of drug used daily and the length of the dependence period.

Heroin abuse in the pregnant woman can result in fetal opiate dependence and severe withdrawal symptoms in the infant after birth. Infants of opiate-abusing women tend to be small for gestational age and have an increased incidence of fetal distress and meconium aspiration. They will have the same withdrawal symptoms after birth as the mother would if she abruptly stopped taking the drug.

Because the fetus is exposed to drugs that must be processed by the liver during pregnancy, the fetal liver is forced to mature faster than normally. For this reason, newborns of substance-abusing women seem better able to cope with bilirubin at birth than other babies; hyperbilirubinemia is therefore rarely a problem. Fetal lung tissue also appears to mature more rapidly than usual, apparently from the stress of the intrauterine drug exposure. Therefore, although an infant is born preterm, the chance that he or she will develop a condition such as respiratory distress syndrome is less than average.

If possible, an opiate-dependent woman should be enrolled in a methadone maintenance program during pregnancy (Goff & O'Connor, 2007). As this is an analgesic, women receiving methadone may need stronger prescriptions for pain relief in labor or postpartum than others (Meyer et al., 2007). Infants of women taking methadone do not escape withdrawal symptoms at birth, and some infants appear to have more severe reactions to methadone withdrawal than to heroin withdrawal. Because a woman is being provided an oral drug legally, however, a fetus is at least ensured better nutrition, better prenatal care, and less exposure to pathogens such as hepatitis B and HIV. If a methadone program is not available, women may be treated with buprenorphine. Suboxone is a combination of naloxone and buprenorphine, an analgesic similar to morphine in action (Mattick et al., 2009). Drug withdrawal symptoms for this in the newborn and accompanying nursing care are discussed in Chapter 26.

Inhalants

Inhalant abuse refers to the "sniffing" or "huffing" of aerosol drugs. Frequently abused substances include airplane glue, cooking sprays, and computer keyboard cleaner. Most of these substances contain freon as a propellant and can lead to severe respiratory and cardiac irregularities. The effect of these drugs during pregnancy is not well documented, but they appear to have effects similar to alcohol abuse (Elias, Chun-Hui Tsai, & Manchester, 2008). The respiratory depression they can cause could be enough to limit the fetal oxygen supply to a serious level.

Alcohol

Although alcohol can be legally purchased and is served generously at social functions, it is just as detrimental to fetal growth as illegal drugs. Excessive use tends to occur in women with impulsive personalities (Magnusson, Goransson, & Heilig, 2007). There is little documentation regarding how much alcohol must be ingested before fetal alcohol syndrome, a syndrome with significant facial features, possible cognitive challenges and memory deficits, occurs, so women are advised to drink no alcohol during pregnancy (Crombleholme, 2009). When discussing alcohol ingestion with young adults, be certain to talk about binge drinking (five or more alcohol drinks on one occasion) to be certain a woman does not believe this type of occasional drinking is safe during pregnancy.

✔ Checkpoint Question 22.5

Mindy Carson tells you she takes methamphetamine almost daily. A fetus of a drug-addicted mother receives approximately what percentage of the mother's drug concentration?

a. 20%.
b. 50%.
c. 70%.
d. 100%.

TRAUMA AND PREGNANCY

Trauma (injury by force) is a phenomenon that seems remote from pregnancy because pregnant women usually take extra safety precautions to protect their body. However, trauma in women occurs at a high incidence during the childbearing years because, for this age group, automobile accidents, homicide, and suicide are among the leading causes of death. During pregnancy, the incidence of trauma is 6% to 7% (as many as 250,000 pregnant women experience trauma per year). A high incidence occurs during the last trimester because of poor balance and fainting from hyperventilation. Orthopedic injuries such as broken wrists or sprained ankles occur because a pregnant woman's sense of balance is altered (Box 22.8). In an automobile accident, a pregnant woman is often the front-seat passenger, and this is the passenger who, in an accident, often receives the most severe injury. Other women seen in emergency departments have suffered intimate partner abuse (Rodrigues, Rocha, & Barros, 2008).

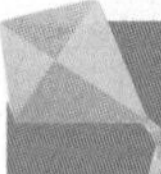

BOX 22.8 * Focus on Evidence-Based Practice

What are the most common types of injuries seen in pregnant women?

Women become high risk for tripping and falling in late pregnancy because their balance becomes unstable. They also can be so busy reworking pregnancy tasks that they are responsible for automobile accidents. To investigate what are the common types of injuries which occur, nurse researchers analyzed the records of 100,051 women seen for injuries during pregnancy. Overall, of the 100,000 women, one in seven sought hospital care for pregnancy-associated injuries at some point in pregnancy, and rates were as high as one in four for some subgroups. Most women (91%) were seen in emergency departments.

More than 4% of women had a motor vehicle collision, the leading cause of injury. The risk for injury was significantly higher among women who were adolescents, black non-Hispanic, and those who had less than a high school education than with other groups. The researchers recommend that preparation for childbirth classes include information on accident prevention.

Would the above study be helpful to mention when discussing accident prevention with pregnant women?

Source: Nannini, A., et al. (2008). Injury: a major cause of pregnancy-associated morbidity in Massachusetts. *Journal of Midwifery and Women's Health, 53*(1), 3–10.

Preventing Accidents

Accidents occur more frequently in people under stress than in those with little stress in their lives because, under stress, people concentrate on the stressor, not their immediate surroundings. Because pregnancy is a life event that may cause stress in a family's life, a woman and her family should take extra precautions for safety during this time. Pregnancy counseling should include education about ways to avoid accidents and trauma such as automobile seat belt use (Pavone & Hueppchen, 2007) (Box 22.9).

Physiologic Changes in Pregnancy That Affect Trauma Care

In an emergency situation, for physical assessment to be meaningful you must consider the physiologic changes that normally occur with pregnancy. A primary rule to remember is that after a traumatic injury, a woman's body will maintain her own homeostasis at the expense of the fetus. To maintain blood pressure in the face of hemorrhage, for example, a woman's body will use peripheral vasoconstriction. As the uterus is a peripheral organ in a shock response, the blood supply to the uterus can be greatly diminished and

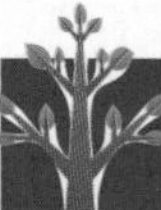

BOX 22.9 ✻ Focus on Family Teaching

Preventive Measures to Reduce Accidents During Pregnancy

Q. Mindy tells you, "I feel so clumsy since I'm pregnant. What can I do to make sure I don't hurt my baby?"

A. To help reduce your risk for accidental injury during pregnancy, follow these guidelines:

- Do not stand on stepstools or stepladders (it is difficult to maintain balance on a narrow base).
- Keep small items such as footstools out of pathways (a pregnant woman has difficulty seeing her feet).
- Avoid throw rugs without a nonskid backing.
- Use caution stepping in and out of a bathtub.
- Do not overload electrical circuits (it is difficult for a pregnant woman to escape a fire because of poor mobility).
- Do not smoke, so falling asleep with a cigarette will not be a problem.
- Do not take medicine in the dark, so you can clearly read the label.
- Avoid working to a point of fatigue, because this lowers judgment.
- Avoid long periods of standing, because this can lead to a drop in your blood pressure, causing you to feel dizzy and faint.
- Always use a seat belt while driving or as a passenger in an automobile.
- Refuse to ride with anyone in an automobile who has been drinking alcohol or whose judgment might be impaired.

the nutrient supply to the fetus greatly compromised (see Fig. 21.1, Chapter 21).

A woman's total plasma volume increases during pregnancy from approximately 2600 mL to 4000 mL at term. This increase serves as a safeguard to a woman if trauma with bleeding should occur because a woman can lose more blood than normally (up to 30% of her blood volume) before hypovolemia is clinically evident. This also means, however, that fluid replacement volume will undoubtedly have to be higher because a pregnant woman needs more fluid than a nonpregnant woman to restore her circulatory volume. Central venous pressure (normal is 0 to 5 cm H_2O in a nonpregnant state) is increased to 2 to 7 cm H_2O. Although a woman needs a large amount of replacement fluid, this means her circulation can also be overwhelmed more easily than normal by intravenous fluid infusion.

To accommodate the increased vascular load of pregnancy, cardiac output increases from 1 L/min early in pregnancy to 6 to 7 L/min in the second trimester. This volume circulates through the placenta at a rapid rate: approximately one-sixth of the total blood volume is present in the placenta at all times. This fact makes a uterine laceration always potentially serious, because up to one-sixth of blood volume can be quickly lost.

To move this increased blood volume adequately through the circulation, a woman's heart rate increases 15 to 20 beats above normal, so a pulse rate of 80 to 95 is not unusual. Based on this, following an accident during pregnancy, do not assume a rapid pulse rate indicates hemorrhage. In addition, since the heart is displaced by the elevated diaphragm, an electrocardiogram taken after an accident will show a left-axis deviation or the pattern may look distorted from the usual while this is normal during pregnancy.

Peripheral venous pressure in the pregnant woman is unchanged. However, it tends to be higher in the lower extremities because of compression by the uterus on the vena cava that causes back-pressure. As a result, lacerations of the legs or perineum bleed much more profusely than usual. Peripheral blood flow in general is increased because of decreased peripheral vascular resistance (the effect of estrogen and decreased sympathetic activity all through pregnancy). As a result, the pregnant woman can be in severe shock, yet her extremities will still not feel cold and clammy.

During pregnancy, the leukocyte count rises (to 20,000 mm^3 at term), so using this measure as a sign of infection after an open wound is problematic. The serum albumin level decreases during pregnancy, making the large loss that normally occurs with burns a more serious response than usual. Serum liver enzyme levels (i.e., serum glutamic-oxaloacetic transaminase, serum glutamate pyruvate transaminase, and lactate dehydrogenase) remain the same during pregnancy. This means, if these are elevated after trauma, liver trauma can still be detected. Since levels of alkaline phosphatase, a substance also usually helpful in detecting liver trauma, are three to four times greater in the pregnant woman at term than normally (from placental origin), this marker loses its importance. Pancreatic amylase levels remain unchanged during pregnancy, so the pancreas can be evaluated as usual.

Abdominal pain is difficult to localize during pregnancy because organs are pushed aside by the growing uterus. The abdomen often feels tense during pregnancy, so the important findings of guarding and rigidity of the abdominal wall may be lost. Bleeding into the abdominal cavity with an abdominal injury is apt to be forceful and extreme because of the increased pressure in the pelvic vessels. A procedure such as a needle paracentesis to assess for bleeding into the abdominal cavity is potentially dangerous because the bowel, dislocated from its usual position, can be easily punctured. Culdocentesis, or needle aspiration through the posterior vaginal fornix into the peritoneal cavity, may be done instead. Peritoneal lavage (the process of inserting a peritoneal dialysis catheter into the abdominal cavity, adding a quantity of an isotonic solution, aspirating it again, and analyzing it for blood or urine) may reveal bleeding or bladder rupture best.

The bladder of a pregnant woman is extremely susceptible to rupture because it is the most anterior organ and is elevated abnormally. After abdominal trauma, an indwelling bladder catheter is often inserted to assess for blood in the urine (Box 22.10).

Psychosocial Considerations

When a pregnant woman is seen at a health care facility after an accident, she is apt to be apprehensive and frightened, both for herself and for her fetus. She is worried not only about what has happened but also about what could have

Box 22.10 Assessment
Assessing the Effects of Trauma in the Pregnant Woman

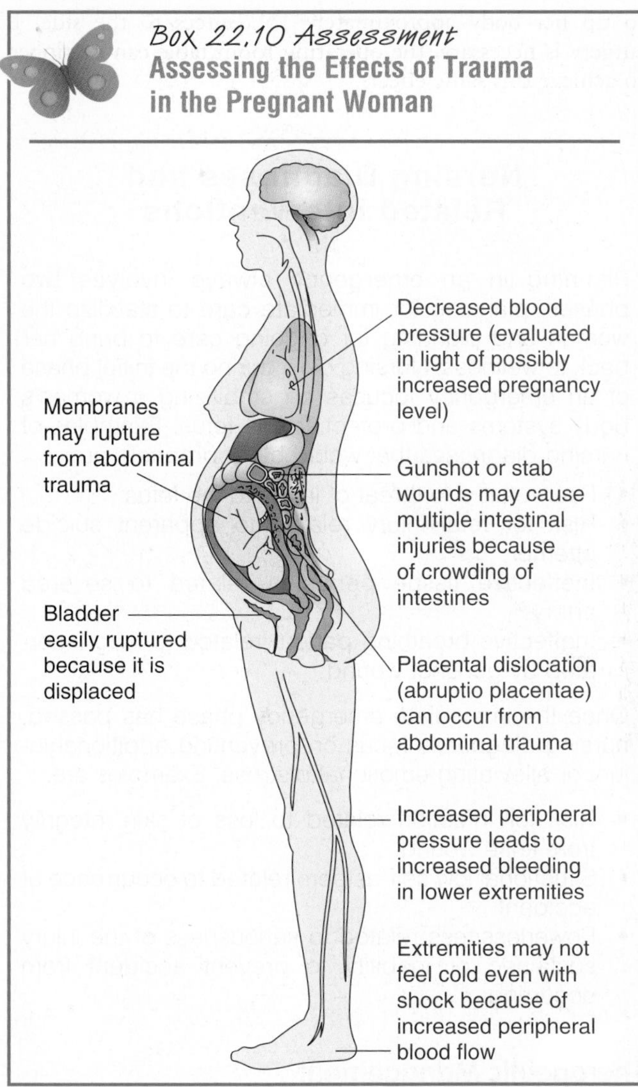

happened (if the knife had slipped an inch farther, if the automobile had been moving faster, if she had fallen from further up the stepladder) and about what medical care will be required (Does she need a radiograph? If she does, will this be safe for the fetus?). She may feel guilty about her carelessness (if she were really a good mother, she would have had her seat belt fastened or would not have tried to stand on a stepladder to hang drapes alone). A feeling of guilt lowers her self-esteem and can increase her level of stress. Remember, people under stress do not process information well and may not perceive correctly the information given to them. Always try to review information with a woman before discharge from an emergency department to be certain she has the facts of her injury and understands the follow-up care necessary.

Assessment

Assessment of an injured pregnant woman must be done quickly yet thoroughly and should include both her psychological and physical status. A pregnant woman may be so concerned with her fetus' health that she does not realize she is injured. Another woman might not even consider the possibility that her fetus could be injured until someone asks if she has felt the fetus move since the accident (not realizing that a loss of blood from her leg would affect uterine blood flow). Assessment, therefore, should be done concurrently with supportive reassurance ("Your blood pressure is low, but the fetal heartbeat sounds good") to try to relieve her fear of fetal damage. Use a Doppler to assess fetal heart tones if possible to demonstrate to a woman as well as yourself that the fetus still appears to be well. External monitoring of fetal heart rate and uterine contractions best rules out fetal distress and preterm labor.

In an emergency situation, a woman needs her support people around her. Locate them as necessary and also assess their reaction to the trauma.

Health History

In an emergency situation, a few minutes spent attempting to calm a woman and move her past her initial fright is time well spent unless symptoms of major body system disturbances require immediate efforts to be directed elsewhere. Reducing a woman's level of anxiety can enhance her ability to cooperate with the history and physical assessment.

Take a brief pregnancy history as well as a trauma history (i.e., length of pregnancy or any complications). Ask specifically if fetal heart tones have been heard by an examiner during the pregnancy, if she has felt the fetus move since the accident, if she has any sensation of tightening or pain in her abdomen or back that could be uterine contractions, and if she knows what her prepregnancy and pregnancy blood pressures have been to help evaluate the extent of blood loss from the trauma.

Document the circumstances of the trauma: what happened, the time of the injury, signs and symptoms of injury she is experiencing, and actions she has taken to counteract these.

If a woman fell, for example, how far did she fall? (A fall from the top of a stepladder is more likely to be serious than a fall from a low rung.) What body part did she land on? (Landing on her abdomen may be very serious, although she may be in less pain than if she injured a wrist in the fall.) For an automobile accident, ask how fast the car was traveling, if she was thrown from the car, or if the windshield broke (generally in automobile accidents, windshields are broken from the impact of a head striking the windshield; a woman will need to be assessed for a head injury).

As a final measure, evaluate whether a woman's degree of injury is in proportion to the history. Injuries out of proportion to the history (a woman states she tripped on her front steps, but you notice all her extremities are ecchymotic and her jaw is broken) suggest intimate partner abuse rather than a simple accident (Records, 2007). It is important to identify such women as they can have an increased incidence of postpartal depression and perhaps an increased risk of wanting to harm themselves (Tiwari et al., 2008). See Chapter 55 for care of an abused woman. Analyze also whether a woman seemed to be using a sensible degree of caution for the circumstances. If not, assess her awareness of common safety measures. In rare situations, this may reveal a woman who self-inflicted an injury in an attempt to end an unwanted pregnancy. A naive adolescent, for example, may attempt to end a pregnancy by a deliberate fall or poisoning, which she then reports as an accident.

Physical Examination

Accidents become fatal when lung, heart, kidney, or brain function becomes inadequate; fetal health is in jeopardy when uteroplacental function is impaired. Following trauma, therefore, it is important to evaluate these body systems first (Table 22.2). All women who receive a blow to their abdomen need to be evaluated for complications such as premature separation of the placenta, although the incidence of this occurring is actually small (Cahill et al., 2008).

With multiple trauma, a nasogastric tube is usually passed to empty the stomach. A Foley catheter is inserted to assess urine output and to rule out a ruptured bladder (blood would return or urine would be blood-tinged if bleeding were occurring).

To prevent supine hypotension syndrome, be certain a woman does not lie supine for an examination. If she must lie on her back, manually displace the uterus from the vena cava by placing a rolled towel or blanket under her right side to tip her body approximately 15 degrees to the side. If surgery is necessary, the operating room table can be tipped to achieve this same effect.

TABLE 22.2 ✻ Initial Assessments After Trauma During Pregnancy

Body System	Assessment
Respiratory system	Quality of respirations (labored or even?) Rate of respirations Sounds of obstruction (wheezing, retractions, coughing?) Color (cyanotic?) Oxygen hunger (inability to lie flat, nasal flaring?)
Cardiovascular system	Color (pallor from hemorrhage?) Gross bleeding Pulse rate (increases with hemorrhage) Blood pressure (decreases with hemorrhage) Feeling of apprehension from altered vascular pressure?
Nervous system	Level of consciousness (woman answers questions coherently?) Pupils (equal and reacting to light?) Bruises or bump on head or spinal column Loss of motion or sensory function in a body part
Renal system	Bruising on anterior abdominal wall over bladder or on back over kidneys Blood in urine
Uterine-fetal system	Bradycardia, tachycardia, or absence of fetal heart tones or loss of variability on fetal monitor Vaginal bleeding Clear (amniotic) fluid leaking from vagina Bruising on abdomen over uterus

Nursing Diagnoses and Related Interventions

✻

Planning in an emergency always involves two phases: planning for immediate care to stabilize the woman and planning for ongoing care to bring her back to wellness. Nursing care during the initial phase of an emergency focuses on stabilizing a woman's body systems and protecting the fetus. Examples of nursing diagnoses that would be appropriate are:

- Fear related to threat of injury to the fetus
- Risk for fetal injury related to apparent suicide attempt
- Ineffective tissue perfusion related to severed artery
- Ineffective breathing pattern related to lung lacerated by gunshot wound

Once the immediate emergency phase has passed, nursing diagnoses focus on preventing additional injury or alleviating emotional distress. Examples are:

- Risk for infection related to loss of skin integrity from knife wound
- Situational low self-esteem related to occurrence of accident
- Powerlessness related to seriousness of the injury sustained or inability to prevent accident from occurring

Therapeutic Management

Implementations in emergency situations must be done quickly yet it must always be remembered that a woman's primary health condition is that she is pregnant. If respirations are not present or are ineffective, cardiopulmonary resuscitation (CPR) should begin, the same as with any person (see Box 20.3, Chapter 20). To be certain a woman has not just fainted, try to rouse her by calling her name or shaking her shoulders. If she does not respond, assess whether her airway is obstructed by holding your cheek next to her nostrils and assessing for air exchange. Look in her mouth for a foreign object. If she is not breathing, pull her chin forward and, using a resuscitation bag, administer two breaths. Although an enlarged uterus puts considerable pressure on the diaphragm and consequently the lungs, only normal pressure is necessary to inflate the lungs fully in a resuscitation attempt. Assess cardiovascular function by palpating the carotid pulse. If this is not palpable or the pupils are fixed, heart function must also be supplemented. Begin external heart massage at a rate of two breaths to every 15 heart compressions (one rescuer) or one breath to every 5 heart compressions for two rescuers (the same as for all adults). Cardiac massage may be awkward late in pregnancy because of the size of the uterus, but undue pressure should not be necessary to create heart action. Cardioversion is done according to usual agency protocol.

After assessment of the level of consciousness and cardiovascular and respiratory status, if there has been blood loss, a central line may be inserted and lactated Ringer's or another isotonic solution infused to restore fluid volume or provide an open line for emergency medication.

If hypotension is present, it must be corrected quickly to maintain a pressure gradient across the placenta. However, any antihypotensive agent that achieves increased blood pressure by causing peripheral vasoconstriction is contraindicated (vessels in the uterus would constrict and cut off the fetal blood supply). Ephedrine is the drug of choice with a pregnant woman to restore blood pressure in an emergency situation because it has a minimal peripheral vasoconstrictive effect. Dopamine in low doses is a second drug that can be used. After emergency interventions, care depends on the specific injury or trauma present.

Nursing Diagnoses and Related Interventions

Nursing Diagnosis: Risk for ineffective tissue perfusion related to blood loss from trauma

Outcome Evaluation: Client's blood pressure remains above 100/60 mm Hg; pulse below 100 beats per minute; no signs of labor are present; fetal heart rate is 120 to 160 beats per minute; nonstress test shows good variability.

Open Wounds

Several types of open wounds occur with trauma. Because the white blood cell count is normally elevated during pregnancy, a single count is a poor indicator of the presence or extent of infection in wounds. However, serial measurements can be used to assess if infection is occurring.

Lacerations. A laceration (a jagged cut) may involve only the skin layer or may penetrate to deeper subcutaneous tissue or tendons. Lacerations generally bleed profusely. Halt bleeding by putting pressure on the edges of the laceration (this is difficult to achieve in the lower extremities because venous pressure is greatly increased in pregnancy). After cleaning, the area is sutured through each layer of tissue involved to approximate the edges. For sutures to be used, a local anesthetic such as lidocaine (Xylocaine) is necessary. Because this has only a local effect, it is safe to use during pregnancy. If the laceration is superficial and a woman is nervous about the use of an anesthetic, the edges can be approximated with a butterfly strip. This will allow it to heal, although with a slightly more noticeable scar.

Puncture Wounds. A puncture wound results from penetration of a sharp object such as a nail, splinter, nail file, or knife. Puncture wounds bleed little—an advantage in terms of minimizing blood loss but not in terms of wound cleaning. A puncture wound is usually not sutured because suturing would create a sealed, unoxygenated cavity below the sutures with a space where tetanus bacilli could grow. If a woman has had a tetanus immunization within the past 10 years, tetanus toxoid is administered. If a woman has not had a tetanus immunization within 10 years (the usual condition), tetanus toxoid plus immune tetanus globulin are administered. These are both safe to administer during pregnancy.

Puncture wounds are frightening because the average woman knows they can cause internal harm. Stab wounds usually occur with the added association of violence.

Knife wounds cause deep penetration and are often directed into the abdomen. They may easily reach the depth of the uterus, possibly directly cutting the fetus. Most stab wounds of the abdomen, however, occur in the upper quadrants of the abdomen, above the uterus, and are more apt to strike the liver or pancreas. To determine the depth and extent of a wound, a fistulogram may be done. This involves inserting a thin catheter into the wound; the wound is then filled with a radiopaque solution. A radiograph of the area filled by the solution reveals the extent of the puncture. If the peritoneal cavity was perforated, dye will outline the intestines. If there is a suspicion of bleeding into the abdominal cavity, a celiotomy or an exploratory surgical procedure into the abdominal cavity may be performed. Surgery this close to the uterus usually does not result in disruption of the pregnancy. If the diaphragm was cut, the intestines may herniate into the chest cavity (diaphragmatic hernia) because of the increased abdominal pressure from the enlarged uterus, causing acute shortness of breath. After surgical repair of an injured diaphragm, cesarean birth may be planned to avoid strain on the newly repaired diaphragm during labor. The uterus appears to have a natural resistance to infection, so even if it is punctured, infection in the uterus rarely occurs.

Animal or Snake Bites. Pregnant women are occasionally bitten by venomous snakes but rarely are bitten by any animal but a dog. Animal bites produce a form of puncture wound, so if the rabies immunization status of the dog is known, the wound is washed and treated as a puncture wound. If the dog cannot be located or is proved to be rabid after 48 hours of observation, a woman must be administered rabies immune globulin and vaccine. Pregnancy is not a contraindication to rabies immunization because contracting the disease would be fatal (Bernstein & Weinstein, 2007). The same is true of anti-venom serum for snake bites (Olson, 2009).

Caution pregnant women to avoid contact with unfamiliar dogs to prevent bites. If a woman is camping in a remote location, caution her to avoid feeding any wild animals such as squirrels and raccoons for the same reason.

Blunt Abdominal Trauma

Blunt trauma occurs generally from automobile accidents, when a woman's abdomen strikes the steering wheel or dashboard, or from someone kicking or punching her abdomen. No visible break is present in the skin. After the injury, the underlying tissue becomes edematous; broken underlying blood vessels ooze and form ecchymoses or a hematoma at the site. To assess if there is abdominal bleeding, a diagnostic peritoneal lavage may be done by introducing a small amount of normal saline by a syringe into the peritoneum and then withdrawing it to see if blood is evident. Ultrasound may also be used.

Careful assessment that the pregnancy has not been harmed must be made because a traumatic blow to the abdomen could cause dislodgement of the placenta (abruptio placentae) or preterm labor. Palpate the uterus for any abnormal contours that would suggest edema or internal bleeding, and listen for fetal heart tones. Use Doppler to help assure a woman that her fetus is unharmed. Real-time ultrasound may also be helpful in showing that the uterus and placenta are intact. A pelvic examination is usually performed to assess for vaginal bleeding or seepage of clear fluid that would suggest rupture of the amniotic membranes. If a woman reports uterine contractions, attach uterine and fetal monitors to estimate the strength and effect of contractions on the fetal heart rate and also determine if preterm labor has begun. A tocolytic such as terbulaline can be administered to halt preterm labor if it has been demonstrated that the uterine environment is still intact (see Chapter 21 for a full discussion of tocolysis).

The possibility that placental blood will enter the maternal circulation with uterine trauma is a threat to an Rh-negative woman. Rh-negative women are therefore typically administered Rh immune globulin after abdominal trauma. The presence of fetal blood cells in the maternal bloodstream can be documented by a Kleihauer-Betke test (on staining, maternal cells remain colorless; fetal cells turn purple-pink).

Gunshot Wounds

A woman may receive a gunshot wound because she was an intended victim or because she was an innocent bystander. Occasionally, a woman attempts suicide by a gunshot wound. Assessment of the wound includes inspection for the point where the bullet entered the body and the point where it exited (the entry wound is small but the exit wound is large because as a bullet slows, it begins to tumble, enlarging the space it occupies). The uterine wall is so thick during pregnancy that it may trap a bullet, so there may be no exit point from a woman's body if the uterus was punctured. If the bullet entered high in the abdomen, the intestines will surely be injured because so many loops of these are compressed above the uterus.

Gunshot wounds are surgically cleaned and débrided, and a woman is treated with a high-dose antibiotic. Ampicillin, a drug that is safe to administer during pregnancy, is frequently prescribed. If a bullet enters the uterus, the incidence of fetal mortality is high, especially if the placenta is torn by the bullet. After providing emergency care to a woman for the injury, it is important to investigate carefully the circumstances of the injury. Since President Lincoln's assassination, gunshot wounds must be reported to the police. Stay with a woman as necessary while she recounts her history of the incident again for law enforcement officers.

Poisoning

Pregnant women are not apt to swallow a poison, although this can occur accidentally, especially if a woman wakes at night and attempts to take medicine in the dark. Food poisoning from inadequately refrigerated or undercooked foods can occur. Some women poison themselves as a suicide attempt.

Poisoning in the pregnant woman is managed the same as in any other person. A woman should telephone a local poison control center, state she is pregnant and what she accidentally swallowed, and follow the specific recommendation of personnel at the poison control center. In an emergency department, activated charcoal is the drug of choice to neutralize stomach poison.

After a woman has been treated and the emergency of the poisoning is over, investigate carefully the circumstances of the poisoning to help a woman learn about safety with medications or food or to discover possible suicidal intent.

Choking

If a pregnant woman chokes on a piece of meat or any foreign object blocks her airway, attempting to dislodge the object with a sudden upward thrust to the upper abdomen is difficult. This is because of a lack of space between the uterus and the end of the sternum and because the average person cannot reach from the rear around a woman's enlarged abdomen. Late in pregnancy, therefore, a rescuer might use successive chest thrusts instead. Box 22.11 describes how to perform chest thrusts for a pregnant woman.

Orthopedic Injuries

Because a woman has poor balance late in pregnancy, it is easy for her to trip; when she falls, she automatically reaches out a hand to cushion the fall and to prevent landing on her abdomen. Because of her extra weight, this can cause a serious wrist injury (a Colles fracture). Apply ice to the area to decrease swelling as an immediate first-aid measure. If she has limited motion, a radiograph may be necessary to determine whether a fracture is present. Assure a woman that a radiograph of an extremity is safe during pregnancy as long as her abdomen is shielded during the radiation exposure. Delegate someone to accompany her to the radiography department and remain with her (outside the actual x-ray room) to ensure that lead protection is offered. Also caution this person to be alert for signs of preterm labor that could suddenly develop as a result of an undetected injury.

Because women of childbearing age are usually healthy, healing of fractures or torn ligaments generally occurs quickly and without complications. Be certain a woman can identify good calcium food sources if she has a fracture so both she and the fetus can have adequate calcium for new bone growth.

Because many more adolescent girls and young adult women participate in sports today than ever before, an increasing number of women of childbearing age have weakened knee cartilage or ligaments (formerly thought of only as a football injury). During pregnancy, when all body cartilage softens, combined with the excessive abdominal weight a woman carries, a woman may dislocate her knee or strain a knee ligament again.

Any woman who has had a previous knee injury should have it re-evaluated early in pregnancy. A support device such as a knee immobilizer may be required for the last 3 months of pregnancy to keep the joint from dislocating or the ligament from tearing again. Discuss with her the advantage of prevention because if a ligament cannot sustain her added weight and tears again, she will fall. She can be assured that having a knee immobilizer in place at the time of birth will not interfere with birth; if a lithotomy position and stirrups for birth are necessary, a modified stirrups position can be devised for her.

The laxness of body cartilage may also cause separation of the symphysis pubis if a woman falls with her legs outspread. Many women experience some nagging suprapubic joint pain during pregnancy. A suture separation this way, however, is very painful, especially on walking or turning. To avoid pain and allow the cartilage to heal, a woman needs to remain on bed rest at home for 4 to 6 weeks. If separation of

Box 22.11 Nursing Procedure ✻ Chest Thrusts for the Pregnant Woman

Purpose: To relieve tracheal aspiration

Plan	Principle
For Conscious Victim in Standing Position	***For Conscious Victim in Standing Position***
1. Stand behind the woman and encircle her chest with your arms.	**1.** Proper positioning ensures proper placement of chest pressure and prevents inadvertent injury to underlying body structures.

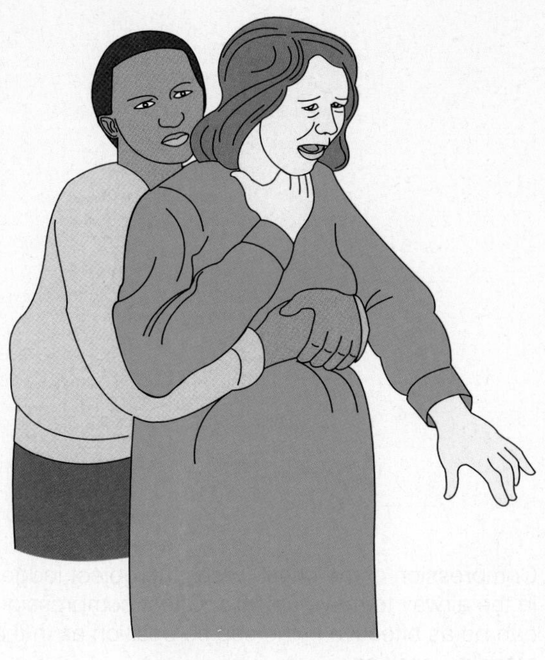

Plan	Principle
2. Place the thumb side of your fist on the middle of the woman's sternum.	**2.** Placement of fist against the chest ensures a solid structure for compression.
3. Grab the fist with the other hand and perform backward thrusts until the foreign body is expelled.	**3.** Pressure on the chest compresses the ribs, increasing chest and lung pressure. This increased pressure forces an object lodged in the airway to move upward.

(continued)

Box 22.11 Nursing Procedure ✻ Chest Thrusts for the Pregnant Woman (continued)

Plan	Principle
For Unconscious Victim in Supine Position	***For Unconscious Victim in Supine Position***
1. Place the woman in the same position as for external heart compressions (heel of the hand on the lower sternum).	**1.** Loss of consciousness interferes with the woman's ability to maintain an upright position.
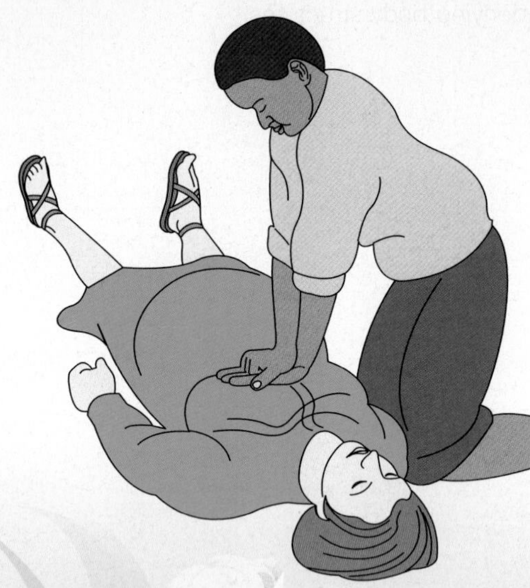	
2. Follow Steps 2 and 3 as with standing victim.	**2.** Compression of the chest forces the object lodged in the airway to move upward. Chest compression can be as effective in the supine position as in the standing position.

the symphysis pubis is present at the time of birth, this will make labor very painful, especially the pelvic division of labor as the fetus is pushed through the pelvic ring.

Burns

Burns are dangerous in the pregnant woman not only because of the thermal injury that occurs but because of inhalation of carbon monoxide gases from the fire, which could lead to extreme fetal hypoxia as carbon monoxide crosses the placenta in place of oxygen.

In addition, smoke is irritating to lung tissue and can result in extensive lung edema; this can cause additional fetal hypoxia because of the lack of oxygen–carbon dioxide exchange space in the mother. Because fluid and electrolyte losses can be great with burns, hypotension from hypovolemia or an electrolyte imbalance can occur. In response to a severe trauma such as a burn, prostaglandins are produced, possibly causing preterm labor. Both maternal and fetal prognoses are poor if burns cover more than 50% of body surface area. Fortunately, few women of childbearing age experience this degree of burn in the United States.

Interestingly, burn tissue heals more quickly than normal during pregnancy. This is probably related to the overall increased metabolism and possibly to the increased corticosteroid serum level that prevents inflammation and damage to tissue from the pressure of edema.

Postmortem Cesarean Birth

If a pregnant woman does not survive serious trauma, it may still be possible for her child to be born safely by a postmortem cesarean birth (Phelan, Roller, & Minei, 2008). This is usually attempted if the fetus is past 24 weeks and less than 20 minutes has passed since the mother died. Infant survival is best in these circumstances if no more than 5 minutes has passed. By general practice, no consent is necessary for this procedure because the fetus is assumed to want to live but cannot give consent. A classic cesarean incision is used. Personnel should be available to resuscitate the newborn immediately.

✔ Checkpoint Question 22.6

Mindy received a laceration on her leg from an automobile accident. Why are lacerations of lower extremities potentially more serious in pregnant women than in others?

a. A woman is less able to keep the laceration clean because of her fatigue.
b. Increased bleeding can occur from uterine pressure on lower extremity veins.
c. Lacerations can provoke allergic responses because of gonadotropic hormone.
d. Healing is limited during pregnancy, so these will not heal until after birth.

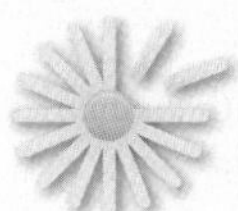

Key Points for Review

- Adolescent pregnancy is a major concern, because although it is decreasing in incidence, it still occurs at a high rate and can interfere with the development of both an adolescent and fetus. Nursing care needs to be individualized to meet the prepartal, intrapartal, and postpartum needs of this age group. Helping adolescents view a pregnancy as a growth experience can help them mature in their ability to parent.
- Women who delay childbearing until age 40 may need additional discussion time at prenatal visits to help them incorporate a pregnancy into their lifestyle. They may need reminders to save time during the day for rest, particularly if at risk for pregnancy-induced hypertension or varicosities.
- Women who are physically, cognitively, visually, or hearing challenged or who have a spinal cord injury are apt to have special needs during pregnancy that must be addressed by health care providers. Providing time for discussion early in pregnancy so these needs can be identified and anticipated is an important role for nurses.
- Women who are physically or cognitively challenged may need help in adjusting their usual regimen to pregnancy. Be certain they are aware of how to contact help in an emergency. Ensure that all medications they are taking for their primary disorder are safe for use during pregnancy.
- A woman who is substance dependent presents a unique challenge during pregnancy. Encouraging her to decrease or halt her drug intake to safeguard the health of a fetus is a short-term goal. Addressing her need to decrease drug intake for the remainder of her life so she can be a quality parent is a long-term goal.
- A fetus of a woman who is substance dependent is at high risk because of the direct effects of the drug and the indirect effects of an unhealthy lifestyle. Women should be encouraged to join drug reduction maintenance programs if possible to reduce fetal risk.
- Trauma in pregnancy results from sources such as violence, automobile accidents, and falls. Women with traumatic injuries need to be carefully assessed to determine if intimate partner abuse was the cause of the trauma.

CRITICAL THINKING EXERCISES

1. Mindy, the 16-year-old girl you met at the beginning of the chapter who is 15 weeks pregnant, tells you she is old enough to be a responsible parent and plans to keep her baby. What clues would you look for to see if her self-evaluation is correct?
2. Mindy makes friends with Clara, a 44-year-old woman, at the prenatal clinic. Clara works at a desk job as a stockbroker. She eats most of her meals at restaurants. Mindy lives at home and attends school. Both have inactive lifestyles. Mindy "experiments" with methamphetamine. Clara takes no drugs but acetaminophen (Tylenol). How would what you teach to prevent pregnancy complications differ for these two clients?
3. Mindy was seen in an emergency department after an automobile accident. Following a severe injury of this kind, what body systems would you assess first?
5. Examine the National Health Goals related to women with special needs. Most government-sponsored funds for nursing research is allotted based on these goals. What would be a possible research topic to explore pertinent to these goals that would be applicable to the Carson family and also advance evidence-based practice?

CRITICAL THINKING SCENARIO

Open the accompanying CD-ROM or visit http://thePoint.lww.com and read the Patient Scenario included for this chapter, then answer the questions to further sharpen your skills and grow more familiar with NCLEX style questions related to pregnant families with special needs. Confirm your answers are correct by reading the rationales.

REFERENCES

Accornero, V. H., et al. (2007). Impact of prenatal cocaine exposure on attention and response inhibition as assessed by continuous performance tests. *Journal of Developmental and Behavioral Pediatrics, 28*(3), 195–205.

Adab, N., et al. (2009). Common antiepileptic drugs in pregnancy in women with epilepsy. *Cochrane Database of Systematic Reviews, 2009*(1), (CD004848).

Ball, R. H., et al. (2007). First- and second-trimester evaluation of risk for Down syndrome. *Obstetrics and Gynecology, 110*(1), 10–17.

Bailis, A., & Witter, F. R. (2007). Hypertensive disorders of pregnancy. In Fortner, K. B., et al. (Eds.). *The Johns Hopkins manual of gynecology and obstetrics.* Philadelphia: Lippincott Williams & Wilkins.

Barton, J. R., & Sibai, B. M. (2008). Prediction and prevention of recurrent preeclampsia. *Obstetrics and Gynecology, 112*(2.1), 359–372.

Bernstein, H. B., & Weinstein, M. (2007). Normal pregnancy and prenatal care. In A. H. DeCherney & L. Nathan (Eds.). *Current diagnosis and treatment in obstetrics and gynecology* (10th ed.). Columbus, OH: McGraw-Hill.

Britton, C., et al. (2009). Support for breastfeeding mothers. *Cochrane Database of Systematic Reviews, 2009*(1), (CD001141).

Buston, K., Williamson, L., & Hart, G. (2007). Young women under 16 years with experience of sexual intercourse: who becomes pregnant? *Journal of Epidemiology and Community Health, 61*(3), 221–225.

Cahill, A. G., et al. (2008). Minor trauma in pregnancy—is the evaluation unwarranted? *American Journal of Obstetrics and Gynecology, 198*(2), 208–213.

Clark, E. A. S., Silver, R. M., & Branch, D. W. (2007). Do antiphospholipid antibodies cause preeclampsia and HELLP syndrome? *Current Rheumatology Reports, 9*(3), 219–225.

Crombleholme, W. R. (2009). Obstetrics. In McPhee, S. J., & Papadakis, M. A. *Current medical diagnosis & treatment.* Columbus, OH: McGraw-Hill.

Datner, E. M., et al. (2007). Identifying pregnant women experiencing domestic violence in an urban emergency department. *Journal of Interpersonal Violence, 22*(1), 124–135.

Dew, P. C., et al. (2007). The effect of health compromising behaviors on preterm births. *Maternal & Child Health Journal, 11*(3), 227–233.

Elias, E. R., Chun-Hui Tsai, A., & Manchester, D. K. (2008). Genetics and dysmorphology. In W. W. Hay, et al. (Eds.). *Current pediatric diagnosis and treatment* (18th ed.). Columbus, OH: McGraw-Hill.

Erikson, E. (1963). *Childhood and society.* New York: Norton.

Fitzgerald, M. P., et al. (2007). Risk factors for anal sphincter tear during vaginal delivery. *Obstetrics and Gynecology, 109*(1), 29–34.

Frost, J. J., & Darroch, J. E. (2008). Factors associated with contraceptive choice and inconsistent method use. *Perspectives on Sexual and Reproductive Health, 40*(2), 94–104.

Goff, M., & O'Connor, M. (2007). Perinatal care of women maintained on methadone. *Journal of Midwifery and Women's Health, 52*(3), e23–e26.

Haessler, A., & Rosenthal, M. B. (2007). Psychological aspects of obstetrics and gynecology. In A. H. DeCherney & L. Nathan (Eds.). *Current diagnosis and treatment in obstetrics and gynecology* (10th ed.). Columbus, OH: McGraw-Hill.

Haynes, K. A. (2007). An update on emergency contraception use in adolescents. *Journal of Pediatric Nursing: Nursing Care of Children and Families, 22(*3), 186–196.

Holub, C. K., et al. (2007). Prenatal and parenting stress on adolescent maternal adjustment: identifying a high-risk subgroup. *Maternal and Child Health Journal, 11*(2), 153–159.

Jansson, L. M., et al. (2008). Methadone maintenance and breastfeeding in the neonatal period. *Pediatrics, 121*(1), 106–114.

Kandakai, T. L., & Smith, L. C. (2007). Denormalizing a historical problem: teen pregnancy, policy, and public health action. *American Journal of Health Behavior, 31*(2), 170–180.

Kaplan, D. W., & Love-Osborne, K. (2008). Adolescence. In W. W. Hay, et al. (Eds.). *Current Pediatric Diagnosis and Treatment* (18th ed.). Columbus, OH: McGraw-Hill.

Karch, A. M. (2009). *Lippincott's nursing drug guide.* Philadelphia: Lippincott Williams & Wilkins.

Magnusson, A., Goransson, M., & Heilig, M. (2007). Hazardous alcohol users during pregnancy: psychiatric health and personality traits. *Drug and Alcohol Dependence, 89*(2–3), 275–281.

Mattick, R. P., et al. (2009). Buprenorphine maintenance versus placebo or methadone maintenance for opioid dependence. *Cochrane Database of Systematic Reviews, 2009*(1), (CD002207).

Meyer, M., et al. (2007). Intrapartum and postpartum analgesia for women maintained on methadone during pregnancy. *Obstetrics and Gynecology, 110*(2.1), 261–266.

Mills, M. E. (2007). Craving more than food: the implications of pica in pregnancy. *Nursing for Women's Health, 11*(3), 266–273.

More, J. (2007). Who needs vitamin supplements? *The Journal of Family Health Care, 17*(2), 57–60.

Muram, D. (2007). Pediatric and adolescent gynecology. In A. H. DeCherney & L. Nathan (Eds.). *Current diagnosis and treatment in obstetrics and gynecology* (10th ed.). Columbus, OH: McGraw-Hill.

Nannini, A., et al. (2008). Injury: a major cause of pregnancy-associated morbidity in Massachusetts. *Journal of Midwifery and Women's Health, 53*(1), 3–10.

National Center for Health Statistics (NCHS). (2009). *Trends in the health of Americans.* Hyattsville, MD: Author.

O'Hearn, A. (2007). Deaf women's experiences and satisfaction with prenatal care: a comparative study. *Family Medicine, 38*(10), 712–716.

Olson, K. R. (2009). Poisoning. In S. J. McPhee & M. A. Papadakis (Eds.). *Current medical diagnosis and treatment.* Columbus, OH: McGraw-Hill.

Parra-Cardona, J. R., Sharp, E. A., & Wampler, R. S. (2008). "Changing for my kid": fatherhood experiences of Mexican-origin teen fathers involved in the justice system. *Journal of Marital & Family Therapy, 34*(3), 369–387.

Pavone, M. E., & Hueppchen, N. A. (2007). Surgical disease and trauma in pregnancy. In K. B. Fortner, et al. (Eds.). *The Johns Hopkins manual of gynecology and obstetrics.* Philadelphia: Lippincott Williams & Wilkins.

Phelan, H. A., Roller, J., & Minei, J. P. (2008). Perimortem cesarean section after utilization of surgeon-performed trauma ultrasound. *Journal of Trauma-Injury Infection and Critical Care, 64*(1), e12–e14.

Piotrowski, K., & Snell, L. (2007). Health needs of women with disabilities across the lifespan. *JOGNN: Journal of Obstetric, Gynecologic, and Neonatal Nursing, 36*(1), 79–87.

Poggi, S. B. H. (2007). Postpartum hemorrhage and the abnormal puerperium. In A. H. DeCherney & L. Nathan (Eds.). *Current diagnosis and treatment in obstetrics and gynecology* (10th ed.). Columbus, OH: McGraw-Hill.

Records, K. (2007). A critical review of maternal abuse and infant outcomes: implications for newborn nurses. *Newborn and Infant Nursing Reviews, 7*(1), 7–13.

Richman, S. (2007). Gynecologic care of women with physical disabilities. *Obstetrical and Gynecological Survey, 62*(7), 421–423.

Rodrigues, T., Rocha, L., & Barros, H. (2008). Physical abuse during pregnancy and preterm delivery. *American Journal of Obstetrics and Gynecology, 198*(2), 171–177.

Shields, S. G., et al. (2007). Dystocia in nulliparous women. *American Family Physician, 75*(11), 1671–1678.

Smeltzer, S. C. (2007). Pregnancy in women with physical disabilities. *JOGNN: Journal of Obstetric, Gynecologic, and Neonatal Nursing, 36*(1), 88–96.

Thierry, J. M. (2007). The importance of preconception care for women with disabilities. *Maternal and Child Health Journal, 10*(5), S175–S176.

Tiwari, A., et al. (2008). The impact of psychological abuse by an intimate partner on the mental health of pregnant women. *BJOG: An International Journal of Obstetrics and Gynaecology, 115*(3), 377–384.

Wright, A., & Walker, J. (2007). Management of women who use drugs during pregnancy. *Seminars in Fetal and Neonatal Medicine, 12*(2), 114–118.

Wu, L., et al. (2007). Misuse of methamphetamine and prescription stimulants among youths and young adults in the community. *Drug and Alcohol Dependence, 89*(2–3), 195–205.

Zhang, X., et al. (2008). How big is too big? The perinatal consequences of fetal macrosomia. *American Journal of Obstetrics and Gynecology, 198*(5), 517–523.

Zoritch, B., Roberts, I., & Oakley, A. (2009). Day care for pre-school children. *Cochrane Database of Systematic Reviews, 2009*(1), (CD000564).

SUGGESTED READINGS

Burns, L., et al. (2007). Methadone in pregnancy: treatment retention and neonatal outcomes. *Addiction, 102*(2), 264–270.

Garwick, A. W., et al. (2007). Native Teen Voices: adolescent pregnancy prevention recommendations. *Journal of Adolescent Health, 42*(1), 81–88.

Gearing, R. E., et al. (2008). Perspectives of mothers with substance use problems on father involvement. *Canadian Journal of Clinical Pharmacology, 15*(1), e99–e107.

Goodman, D. C., et al. (2007). Geographic access to family planning facilities and the risk of unintended and teenage pregnancy. *Maternal and Child Health Journal, 11*(2), 145–152.

Kissin, D. M., et al. (2007). Is there a trend of increased unwanted childbearing among teenagers? *Journal of Adolescent Health, 40*(2), S2.

Kristjansson, A. L., et al. (2009). Adolescent health behavior, contentment in school, and academic achievement. *American Journal of Health Behavior, 33*(1), 69–79.

Pei, J. R., et al. (2008). Memory patterns of acquisition and retention of verbal and nonverbal information in children with fetal alcohol spectrum disorders. *Canadian Journal of Clinical Pharmacology, 15*(1), e44–e56.

Steinhausen, H.C., Blattmann, B., & Pfund, F. (2007). Developmental outcome in children with intrauterine exposure to substances. *European Addiction Research, 13*(2), 94–100.

VanLenten, B. (2007). Today's pregnant teen: how can healthcare professionals combat this prevalent pandemic? *International Journal of Childbirth Education, 22*(1), 12–15.

Wilkinson, S., & Walker, A. (2007). Healthy Start: improving maternal, infant and child health. *Nursing Standard, 21*(20), 48–56.

Chapter

23 Nursing Care of a Family Experiencing a Complication of Labor or Birth

KEY TERMS

- amnioinfusion
- amniotic fluid embolism
- augmentation of labor
- battledore placenta
- dysfunctional labor
- dystocia
- external cephalic version
- forceps birth
- hypertonic uterine contractions
- hypotonic uterine contractions
- induction of labor
- oxytocin
- pathologic retraction ring
- placenta accreta
- placenta circumvallata
- placenta marginata
- placenta succenturiata
- precipitate labor
- umbilical cord prolapse
- uterine inversion
- vacuum extraction

OBJECTIVES

After mastering the contents of this chapter, you should be able to:

1. Define the terms *dystocia* and *dysfunctional labor* and how common deviations in the power (force of labor), the passage, or the passenger can cause dystocia or dysfunctional labor.
2. Identify National Health Goals related to complications of labor that nurses could help the nation achieve.
3. Use critical thinking to analyze ways to maintain family-centered nursing care when deviations from the normal in labor or birth occur.
4. Assess a woman in labor and during birth for deviations from the normal labor process.
5. Formulate nursing diagnoses related to deviations from normal in labor and birth.
6. Identify expected outcomes associated with deviations from normal labor and birth and resultant complications.
7. Plan nursing interventions to help the family meet expected outcomes when complications of labor occur.
8. Implement nursing care related to complications of labor or birth such as preparing the family for a cesarean birth.
9. Evaluate expected outcomes for achievement and effectiveness of care.
10. Identify areas related to complications of labor that could benefit from additional nursing research or application of evidence-based practice.
11. Integrate the knowledge of deviations of normal in labor and birth with nursing process to achieve quality maternal and child health nursing care.

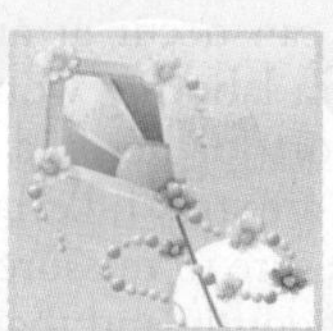

Roseann Bigalow, a 28-year-old woman about to give birth to her first baby, is admitted to a birthing room. Her contractions have been 5 minutes apart for 10 hours. She feels more pain in her back than in her abdomen, "like my spine is tearing apart." A contraction monitor shows contractions are hypotonic. An ultrasound shows the fetus is above average in weight and in an occipitoposterior position. Her husband asks you if the reason Roseann's labor is taking so long is because she's overweight.

Previous chapters discussed pregnancy and normal labor and birth. This chapter adds information about what happens when complications of labor occur. Nurses play a vital role in making labor safe. The sooner a complication in labor is recognized, the better is the chance the situation can be corrected and both fetal and maternal health can be protected.

How would you answer Mr. Bigalow?

Although labor often proceeds without any deviation from the normal, many potential complications can occur. A difficult labor—**dystocia**—can arise from any of the four main components of the labor process: (a) the power, or the force that propels the fetus (uterine contractions), (b) the passenger (the fetus), (c) the passageway (the birth canal), or (d) the psyche (the woman's and family's perception of the event). The earlier in labor that a complication is recognized, the better is the chance that it can be resolved (Buhimschi, 2009).

Because complications can occur at any point in labor, continuous monitoring of a laboring woman and fetus and providing emotional support for her and her family are essential. The hours of labor are stressful even when everything is proceeding normally. Be sure to reassure a woman in labor that everything is going smoothly and that both she and her fetus appear to be doing well. If a complication arises and assurances cannot be given as freely, a woman needs someone who is knowledgeable about the deviation and its treatment as well as a person who understands her feelings of helplessness. Nurses play a key role in providing this type of skilled physical and emotional care.

National Health Goals related to attempts to decrease maternal complications and prevent infant injury are shown in Box 23.1.

BOX 23.1 ✻ Focus on National Health Goals

A number of National Health Goals speak directly to complications of labor.

- Reduce the number of cesarean births among low-risk women to no more than 15 per 100 births from a baseline of 18 per 100.
- Reduce the maternal mortality rate to no more than 3.3 per 100,000 live births from a baseline of 7.1 per 100,000.
- Reduce the rate of maternal complications during hospitalized labor and birth to no more than 24 per 100 births from a baseline of 31.2 per 100 births (http://www.nih.gov).

Nurses can help the nation achieve these goals by helping identify women in labor who are developing a complication; by assisting with cesarean births and uterine monitoring; and by being alert to the preliminary symptoms of uterine rupture, which accounts for a substantial number of maternal deaths during labor. Further nursing research is needed to explore whether breech and occipitoposterior positions can be effectively prevented by position changes during pregnancy.

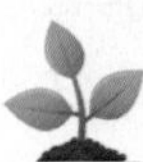

Nursing Process Overview

For a Woman With a Labor or Birth Complication

Assessment

One of the major assessments used to detect deviations from normal in labor and birth is fetal and uterine monitoring. Working with such apparatus involves explaining its importance to a woman and her partner, winning their cooperation, and using judgment in reading the various patterns. Typically, monitoring women in labor entails problems not found in other high-risk areas such as an intensive care unit (ICU). In an ICU, the person being monitored has been admitted to the unit because he or she is seriously ill. The person lies still to prevent artifacts on the tracing. However, a woman in labor, who is well except for the complication of labor, may be less accepting of technologic or pharmacologic intervention. She moves about rather than lying still, because she is in pain. Her movement causes artifacts on tracings, requiring frequent adjustment of equipment to achieve a clear tracing. Understanding that this is a normal consequence of labor is essential for effective assessment and continued care.

Nursing Diagnosis

Common nursing diagnoses specific to a woman experiencing a complication during labor or birth refer to specific problems. Some examples might include:

- Fear related to uncertainty of pregnancy outcome
- Anxiety related to medical procedures and apparatus necessary to ensure health of woman and fetus
- Fatigue related to loss of glucose stores through work and duration of labor
- Risk for ineffective tissue perfusion related to excessive loss of blood with complication of labor
- Risk for injury (maternal or fetal) related to effect on woman and fetus of a labor complication and treatment required
- Risk for injury (maternal or fetal) related to labor involving a multiple-gestation pregnancy
- Anticipatory grieving related to nonviable monitoring pattern of fetus

Outcome Identification and Planning

If a complication of labor or childbirth occurs, identification of expected outcomes can be difficult because an outcome that must be included in planning is not what the woman desires. Encouraging a couple to clarify their priorities when a complication occurs is helpful. For example, early in labor, a woman might say that her chief goal is to avoid monitoring equipment or any surgical intervention. If fetal bradycardia occurs, however, monitoring and a cesarean birth may become necessary. If this happens, reminding the woman that her primary goal is really to have a healthy baby can help her accept the change, including whatever interventions are necessary to achieve her ultimate objective. A helpful Internet site for referral about complications in childbirth is The Childbirth Organization (http://www.childbirth.org).

Implementation

If a woman develops a complication of labor or birth, actions to increase the fetal heart rate or strengthen uterine contractions are a priority, possibly an emergency. Interventions must be planned and performed efficiently and effectively, based on the individual circumstances. Be certain to provide psychological reassurance to accompany actions to fully safeguard both the woman and her fetus.

Outcome Evaluation

Evaluation of proposed outcomes may reveal unhappiness, because not every woman who experiences a deviation from the normal in labor and birth will be able to give birth to a healthy child. Some deviations will be too great. Some interventions will not be maximally effective because of individual circumstances. Some infants will die; a few women may be left unable to bear future children. Evaluation may lead to a new analysis that the couple's chief need at that point is to grieve for the child or for a lifestyle that can no longer be theirs. If the outcome is more positive, evaluate the couple for signs that they are able to begin interaction with their child after their harrowing experience.

Examples of outcome achievement might include:

- Client voices confidence that she can cope with the fear she feels about her fetus' welfare.
- Client demonstrates adequate energy during course of labor to maintain effective breathing patterns.
- Client's blood pressure remains higher than 110/60 mm Hg despite excessive blood loss with delivery of the placenta.
- Client begins positive grieving behaviors in response to loss of newborn.

COMPLICATIONS WITH THE POWER (THE FORCE OF LABOR)

Inertia is a time-honored term to denote that sluggishness of contractions, or the force of labor, has occurred. A more current term used is **dysfunctional labor** (Strehlow & Uzelac, 2007). Dysfunction can occur at any point in labor, but it is generally classified as primary (occurring at the onset of labor) or secondary (occurring later in labor). The risk of maternal postpartal infection, hemorrhage, and infant mortality is higher in women who have a prolonged labor than in those who do not. Therefore, it is vital to recognize and prevent dysfunctional labor to the extent possible (Shields et al., 2007).

Prolonged labor appears to result from several factors. It is most likely to occur if a fetus is large. Hypotonic, hypertonic, and uncoordinated contractions all play additional roles (Box 23.2).

BOX 23.2 ✻ Common Causes of Dysfunctional Labor

- Inappropriate use of analgesia (excessive or too early administration)
- Pelvic bone contraction that has narrowed the pelvic diameter so that a fetus cannot pass such as could occur in a woman with rickets
- Poor fetal position (posterior rather than anterior position)
- Extension rather than flexion of the fetal head
- Overdistention of the uterus, as with multiple pregnancy, hydramnios, or an excessively oversized fetus
- Cervical rigidity (unripe)
- Presence of a full rectum or urinary bladder that impedes fetal descent
- Woman becoming exhausted from labor
- Primigravida status

Ineffective Uterine Force

Uterine contractions are the basic force moving the fetus through the birth canal. They occur because of the interplay of the contractile enzyme adenosine triphosphate and the influence of major electrolytes such as calcium, sodium, and potassium, specific contractile proteins (actin and myosin), epinephrine and norepinephrine, oxytocin (a posterior pituitary hormone), estrogen, progesterone, and prostaglandins. About 95% of labors are completed with contractions that follow a predictable, normal course. When they become abnormal or ineffective, ineffective labor occurs.

Hypotonic Contractions

Figure 23.1A illustrates the appearance of normal uterine contractions. With **hypotonic uterine contractions,** the number of contractions is unusually low or infrequent (not more two or three occurring in a 10-minute period). The resting tone of the uterus remains less than 10 mm Hg, and the strength of contractions does not rise above 25 mm Hg (Fig. 23.1B). Hypotonic contractions are most apt to occur during the active phase of labor. They may occur after the administration of analgesia, especially if the cervix is not dilatated to 3 to 4 cm or if bowel or bladder distention prevents descent or firm engagement. They may occur in a uterus that is overstretched by a multiple gestation, a larger-than-usual single fetus, hydramnios, or in a uterus that is lax from grand multiparity. Such contractions are not exceedingly painful, because of their lack of intensity. Keep in mind, however, that the strength of a contraction is a subjective symptom. Some women may interpret these contractions as very painful.

Hypotonic contractions increase the length of labor, because more of them are necessary to achieve cervical dilatation. This can cause the uterus to not contract as effectively during the postpartal period because of exhaustion, increasing a woman's chance for postpartal hemorrhage. In the first hour after birth following a labor of hypotonic contractions, palpate the uterus and assess lochia every 15 minutes to ensure that postpartal contractions are not also hypotonic and therefore inadequate to halt bleeding.

Hypertonic Contractions

Hypertonic uterine contractions are marked by an increase in resting tone to more than 15 mm Hg (see Fig. 23.1C). However, the intensity of the contraction may be no stronger than that associated with hypotonic contractions. In contrast to hypotonic contractions, hypertonic ones tend to occur frequently and are most commonly seen in the latent phase of labor. This type of contraction occurs because the muscle fibers of the myometrium do not repolarize or relax after a contraction, thereby "wiping it clean" to accept a new pacemaker stimulus. They may occur because more than one pacemaker is stimulating contractions. They tend to be more painful than usual, because the myometrium becomes tender from constant lack of relaxation and the anoxia of uterine cells that results. A woman may become frustrated or disappointed with her

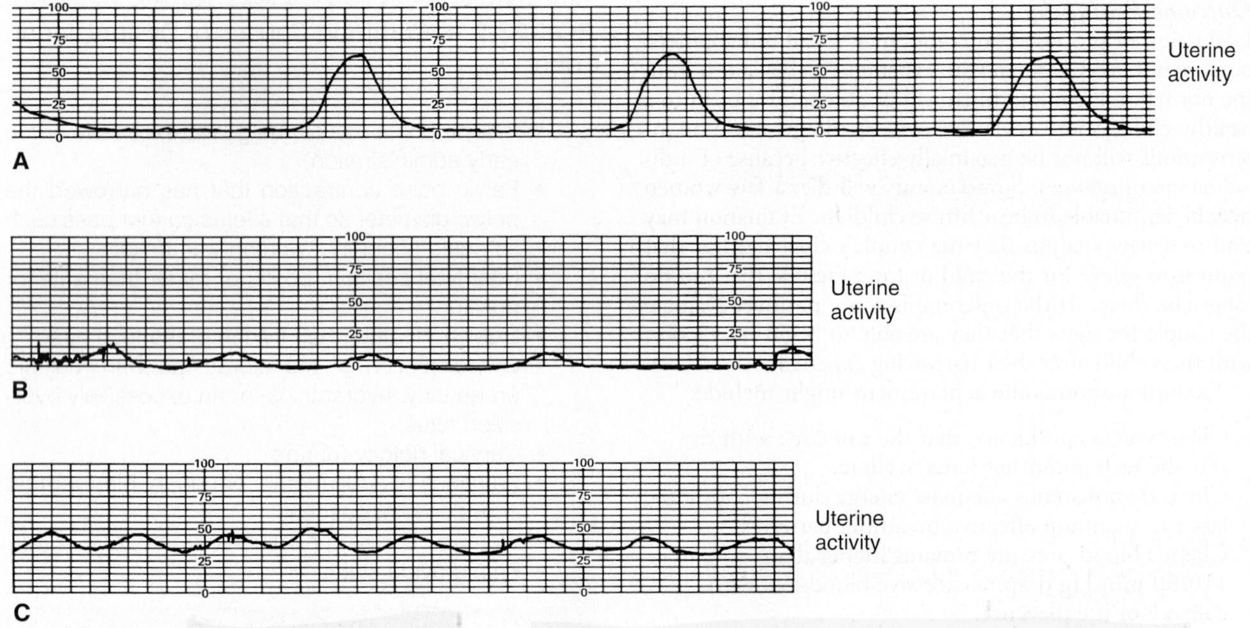

FIGURE 23.1 (**A**) Normal uterine contractions. (**B**) Hypotonic contractions; notice rise in pressure no more than 10 mm Hg. (**C**) Hypertonic contractions; notice the high resting pressure (35–40 mm Hg).

breathing exercises for childbirth, because such techniques are ineffective with this type of contraction.

A danger of hypertonic contractions is that the lack of relaxation between contractions may not allow optimal uterine artery filling; this could lead to fetal anoxia early in the latent phase of labor. Any woman whose pain seems out of proportion to the quality of her contractions should have both a uterine and a fetal external monitor applied for at least 15 minutes to ensure that the resting phase of the contractions is adequate and that the fetal pattern is not showing late deceleration.

If deceleration in the fetal heart rate (FHR) or an abnormally long first stage of labor or lack of progress with pushing ("second-stage arrest") occurs, cesarean birth may be necessary. Both the woman and her support person need to understand that, although the contractions are strong, they are ineffective and are not achieving cervical dilatation. To help identify the difference, hypotonic and hypertonic contractions are compared in Table 23.1.

TABLE 23.1 ✻ Comparison of Hypotonic and Hypertonic Contractions

Criteria	Hypertonic	Hypotonic
Phase of labor	Latent	Active
Symptoms	Painful	Limited pain
Medications used:		
Oxytocin	Unfavorable reaction	Favorable reaction
Sedation	Helpful	Little value

Uncoordinated Contractions

Normally, all contractions are initiated at one pacemaker point high in the uterus. A contraction sweeps down over the organ, encircling it; repolarization occurs; relaxation or a low resting tone is achieved; and another pacemaker-activated contraction begins. With uncoordinated contractions, more than one pacemaker may be initiating contractions, or receptor points in the myometrium may be acting independently of the pacemaker. Uncoordinated contractions may occur so closely together that they do not allow good cotyledon (one of the visible segments on the maternal surface of the placenta) filling. Because they occur so erratically such as one on top of another and then a long period without any, it may be difficult for a woman to rest between contractions or to use breathing exercises with contractions.

Applying a fetal and a uterine external monitor and assessing the rate, pattern, resting tone, and fetal response to contractions for at least 15 minutes (or longer if necessary in early labor) reveals the abnormal pattern. Oxytocin administration may be helpful in uncoordinated labor to stimulate a more effective and consistent pattern of contractions with a better, lower resting tone.

Dysfunctional Labor and Associated Stages of Labor

For a graphic illustration of the most frequent times dysfunctional labor is apt to occur, see Figure 23.2. Regardless of when dysfunctional labor occurs, the effect on a woman and her support person will be the same: anxiety, fear, or discouragement. A woman needs good explanations of what is happening: "We're going to take an ultrasound to check the

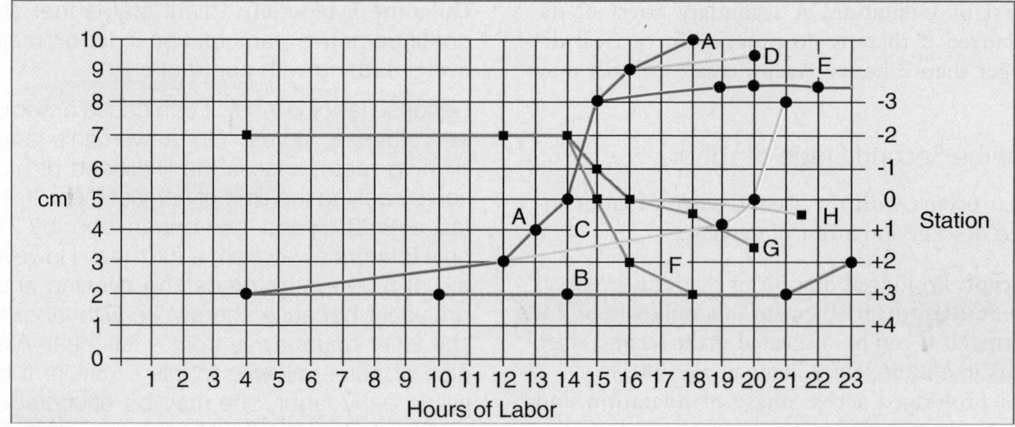

FIGURE 23.2 Graph showing types of abnormal labor. (**A**) Normal labor curve. (**B**) Prolonged latent phase. (**C**) Protracted active-phase dilatation. (**D**) Prolonged deceleration phase. (**E**) Secondary arrest of dilatation. (**F**) Normal descent. (**G**) Prolonged descent. (**H**) Arrest of descent.

baby's position." "This is a drug to make your contractions stronger." "I know resting is the last thing you feel like doing, but that is what I want you to try to do."

Dysfunction at the First Stage of Labor

Dysfunction that occurs with the first stage of labor involves a prolonged latent phase, protracted active phase, prolonged deceleration phase, and secondary arrest of dilatation.

Prolonged Latent Phase. When contractions become ineffective during the first stage of labor, a prolonged latent phase can develop. The normal parameters for the stages of labor are highlighted in Table 23.2. A prolonged latent phase, as defined by Friedman (1978), is a latent phase that is longer than 20 hours in a nullipara or 14 hours in a multipara. This may occur if the cervix is not "ripe" at the beginning of labor and time must be spent getting truly ready for labor. It may occur if there is excessive use of an analgesic early in labor. With a prolonged latent phase, the uterus tends to be in a hypertonic state. Relaxation between contractions is inadequate, and the contractions are only mild (less than 15 mm Hg on a monitor printout) and therefore ineffective. One segment of the uterus may be contracting with more force than another segment.

TABLE 23.2 ✻ Lengths of Phases and Stages of Normal Labor in Hours

	Nullipara		Multipara	
Phase	***Average***	***Upper Normal***	***Average***	***Upper Normal***
Latent phase	8.6	20.0	5.3	14.0
Active phase	5.8	12.0	2.5	6.0
Second stage	1	1.5	0.25	—*

*There is no limit to the length of the second stage as long as progress is being made and fetal distress is not present.

Management of a prolonged latent phase in labor that has been caused by hypertonic contractions involves helping the uterus to rest, providing adequate fluid for hydration, and pain relief with a drug such as morphine sulfate. Changing the linen and the woman's gown, darkening room lights, and decreasing noise and stimulation can also be helpful. These measures usually combine to allow labor to become effective and begin to progress. If it does not, a cesarean birth or amniotomy (artificial rupture of membranes) and oxytocin infusion to assist labor may be necessary. Because amniotomy is also used in uncomplicated labor, it is discussed in Chapter 15.

Protracted Active Phase. A protracted active phase is usually associated with cephalopelvic disproportion (CPD) or fetal malposition, although it may reflect ineffective myometrial activity. This phase is prolonged if cervical dilatation does not occur at a rate of at least 1.2 cm/hr in a nullipara or 1.5 cm/hr in a multipara, or if the active phase lasts longer than 12 hours in a primigravida or 6 hours in a multigravida (see Fig. 23.2). If the cause of the delay in dilatation is fetal malposition or CPD, cesarean birth may be necessary. Dysfunctional labor during the dilatational division of labor tends to be hypotonic, in contrast to the hypertonic action at the beginning of labor. After an ultrasound to show that CPD is not present, oxytocin may be prescribed to augment labor (see later discussion on augmentation by oxytocin).

Prolonged Deceleration Phase. A deceleration phase has become prolonged when it extends beyond 3 hours in a nullipara or 1 hour in a multipara. Prolonged deceleration phase most often results from abnormal fetal head position. A cesarean birth is frequently required.

Secondary Arrest of Dilatation. A secondary arrest of dilatation has occurred if there is no progress in cervical dilatation for longer than 2 hours. Again, cesarean birth may be necessary.

Dysfunction at the Second Stage of Labor

Dysfunction that occurs with the second stage of labor involves prolonged descent and arrest of descent.

Prolonged Descent. Prolonged descent of the fetus occurs if the rate of descent is less than 1.0 cm/hr in a nullipara or 2.0 cm/hr in a multipara. It can be suspected if the second stage lasts over 3 hours in a multipara (Cheng et al., 2007).

With both a prolonged active phase of dilatation and prolonged descent, contractions have been of good quality and proper duration, and effacement and beginning dilatation have occurred, but then the contractions become infrequent and of poor quality and dilatation stops. If everything is normal except for the suddenly faulty contractions and CPD and poor fetal presentation have been ruled out by ultrasound, then rest and fluid intake, as advocated for hypertonic contractions, also apply. If the membranes have not ruptured, rupturing them at this point may be helpful. Intravenous (IV) oxytocin may be used to induce the uterus to contract effectively (see later discussion on induction of labor by oxytocin). A semi-Fowler's position, squatting, kneeling, or more effective pushing may speed descent.

Arrest of Descent. Arrest of descent results when no descent has occurred for 1 hour in a multipara or 2 hours in a nullipara. Failure of descent has occurred when expected descent of the fetus does not begin or engagement or movement beyond 0 station has not occurred. The most likely cause for arrest of descent during the second stage is CPD. Cesarean birth usually is necessary. If there is no contraindication to vaginal birth, oxytocin may be used to assist labor.

✔ Checkpoint Question 23.1

Roseann Bigalow has prolonged labor. What is the most common cause for arrest of descent during the second stage of labor?

a. Cephalopelvic disproportion (CPD).
b. Maternal calcium deficiency.
c. The fetus is asleep during labor.
d. The maternal outlet is narrow.

Nursing Diagnoses and Related Interventions for Dysfunctional Labor

It is impossible to prevent all dysfunctional labor, just as it is impossible to predict the functioning of any woman's hormonal system or individual response to labor. However, a number of nursing interventions can contribute to the progression of normal labor and help change a dysfunctional labor to a functional one.

Nursing Diagnosis: Fatigue and anxiety related to prolonged labor

Outcome Evaluation: Client states that she is able to continue active participation in labor; maintains effective breathing with contractions.

Because labor is work, it can cause a woman to deplete her glucose stores. On a woman's admission to a birthing room, assess the likelihood of glucose depletion by asking the time of her last meal. If she ate breakfast at 8:00 AM and then began labor by 2:00 PM, she is only 6 hours away from a full meal. However, if she last ate at 5:00 PM the preceding evening and did not eat breakfast because she awoke with labor this morning, she is 11 hours away from a full meal. Alert her physician or nurse-midwife to this situation. If the woman is still in early labor, she may be encouraged to drink a high-carbohydrate fluid such as a sports drink or to eat a light meal. IV fluid therapy also may be initiated to provide glucose for energy. Sucking on a lollipop or hard candy during labor can also supply additional glucose.

Although the effect of emotion on labor is difficult to document, it seems that the cervix dilates more rapidly and therefore normal labor is shortened if a woman is neither tense nor frightened. Manage stress by making the transfer from home to the health care facility as untraumatic as possible. Ask directly whether a woman has any concerns. Offer explanations of all procedures. Help the support person feel just as welcome and comfortable as the woman herself. Asking a question such as, "Is labor what you thought it would be?" of both the woman and her support person often helps them to express their concerns. Allow the woman and her support person as many choices as possible to give them a sense of control.

Remember that pain is an exhausting phenomenon. Encourage the use of nonpharmacologic comfort measures such as breathing with the woman, giving back rubs, changing sheets, using cool washcloths, and so forth. Complementary therapies such as aromatherapy or music are also helpful (Smith, 2009).

To increase the blood supply to the uterus and prevent hypotension, urge a woman when she is in bed to lie on her side so that the uterus is lifted off the vena cava. If a woman insists on lying supine, place a hip roll under one or the other of her buttocks to cause her pelvis to "tip" and, at least to some extent, move the uterus to the side.

A full bladder prevents descent of the fetus and may impede uterine contractions. Urge a woman in labor to void every 2 hours to keep the bladder empty and to aid progress.

Nursing Diagnosis: Risk for deficient fluid volume related to length and work of labor

Outcome Evaluation: Urine is free of ketones; specific gravity is between 1.003 and 1.030; skin turgor and serum electrolyte levels are within acceptable parameters.

Low levels of serum electrolytes or body fluid can occur in labor for the same reason as a decreased glucose level—a long interval between eating and the end of labor. Additionally, vomiting and diarrhea occasionally accompany labor so can increase fluid and electrolyte losses. Ask if a woman has had any vomiting or

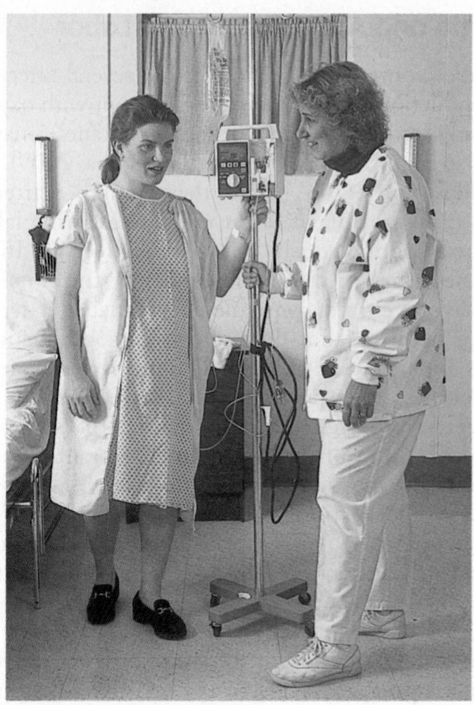

FIGURE 23.3 If intravenous fluid is used for women in labor, it does not need to limit mobility.

diarrhea to determine the possible extent of the problem. One episode of a small amount of diarrhea or vomiting is probably not serious; extended vomiting or diarrhea could lead to serious dehydration. Profuse diaphoresis and hyperventilation that occur with labor can further increase fluid and electrolyte losses through insensible water loss.

Test voidings frequently during labor for glucose, protein, ketones, and specific gravity. Ketones in the urine suggest starvation ketosis. A concentrated specific gravity suggests a lack of fluid. Extreme dehydration not only may slow labor but can lead to increased blood viscosity, possibly increasing the risk for thrombophlebitis during the postpartal period.

Many women react negatively to the idea of IV fluid therapy during labor to restore body fluid, possibly perceiving it as loss of control over their bodies or removal of the "naturalness" of labor and birth. Introduce the idea that IV fluid therapy will be helpful because of her particular complication before arriving with the bag of fluid and tubing. When inserting the IV catheter, try to use an insertion site in a woman's nondominant hand and, if necessary, only a small "reminder" handboard. Assure a woman that she can be out of bed and walking, can turn freely, squat, sit, or use whatever position she prefers during labor with the IV line in place. None of these acts will interfere with the infusion (Fig. 23.3).

Contraction Rings

A contraction ring is a hard band that forms across the uterus at the junction of the upper and lower uterine segments and interferes with fetal descent. The most frequent type seen is termed a **pathologic retraction ring** (Bandl's ring). The ring usually appears during the second stage of labor and can be palpated as a horizontal indentation across the abdomen (Fig. 23.4). It is a warning sign that severe dysfunctional

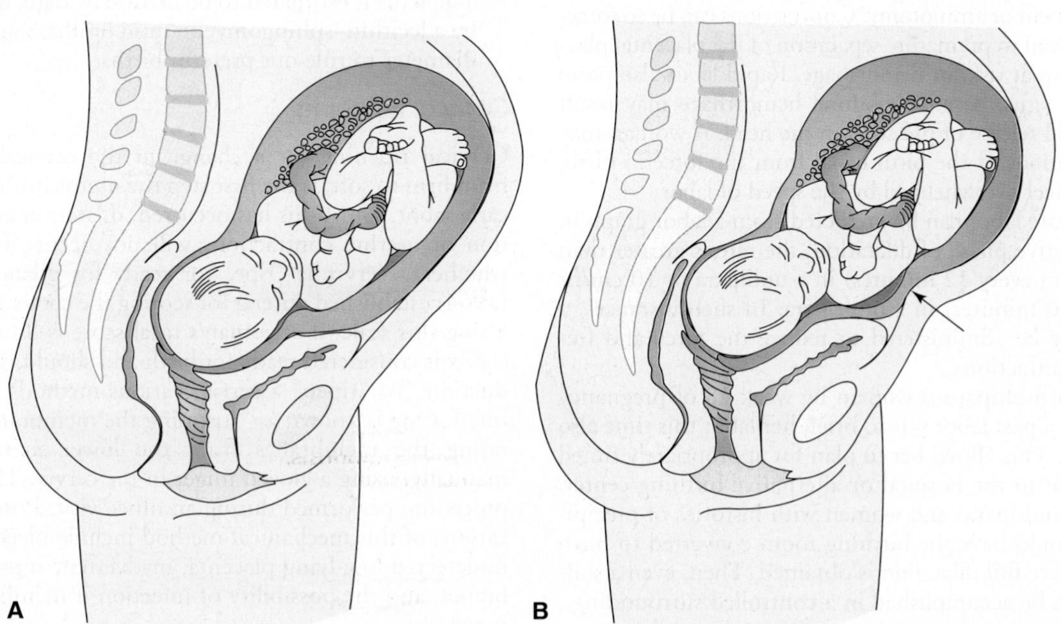

FIGURE 23.4 Pathologic retraction ring. (**A**) Uterus in the normal second stage of labor. Notice how the upper uterine segment is becoming thicker and the lower uterine segment is thinning. A physiologic retraction ring is normally formed at the division of the upper and lower uterine segments. (**B**) Uterus with a pathologic retraction ring (Bandl's ring). The wall below the ring is thin and the abdomen shows an indentation. This constriction is caused by obstructed labor and is a warning sign that if the obstruction is not relieved, the lower segment may rupture.

labor is occurring as it is formed by excessive retraction of the upper uterine segment; the uterine myometrium is much thicker above than below the ring.

When a pathologic retraction ring occurs in early labor, it is usually caused by uncoordinated contractions. In the pelvic division of labor, it is usually caused by obstetric manipulation or by the administration of oxytocin. In either event, the fetus is gripped by the retraction ring and cannot advance beyond that point. The undelivered placenta will also be held at that point.

Contraction rings often can be identified by ultrasound. Such a finding is extremely serious and should be reported promptly. Administration of IV morphine sulfate or the inhalation of amyl nitrite may relieve a retraction ring. A tocolytic can also be administered to halt contractions. If the situation is not relieved, uterine rupture and neurologic damage to the fetus may occur (Lauria et al., 2007). In the placental stage, massive maternal hemorrhage may result, because the placenta is loosened but then cannot deliver, preventing the uterus from contracting.

Most likely, a cesarean birth will be necessary to ensure safe birth of the fetus. Manual removal of the placenta under general anesthesia may be required if the retraction ring does not allow the placenta to be delivered.

Precipitate Labor

Precipitate labor and birth occur when uterine contractions are so strong that a woman gives birth with only a few, rapidly occurring contractions. It is often defined as a labor that is completed in fewer than 3 hours. *Precipitate dilatation* is cervical dilatation that occurs at a rate of 5 cm or more per hour in a primipara or 10 cm or more per hour in a multipara (Strehlow & Uzelac, 2007). Such rapid labor is likely to occur with grand multiparity, or it may occur after induction of labor by oxytocin or amniotomy. Contractions can be so forceful that they lead to premature separation of the placenta, placing the woman at risk for hemorrhage. Rapid labor also poses a risk to the fetus, because subdural hemorrhage may result from the rapid release of pressure on the head. A woman may sustain lacerations of the birth canal from the forceful birth. She also can feel overwhelmed by the speed of labor.

A precipitate labor can be predicted from a labor graph if, during the active phase of dilatation, the rate is greater than 5 cm/hr (1 cm every 12 minutes) in a nullipara or 10 cm/hr (1 cm every 6 minutes) in a multipara. In such instances, a tocolytic may be administered to reduce the force and frequency of contractions.

Caution a multiparous woman by week 28 of pregnancy that, because a past labor was so brief, her labor this time also may be brief. This allows her to plan for appropriately timed transportation to the hospital or alternative birthing center. Both grand multiparas and women with histories of precipitate labor should have the birthing room converted to birth readiness before full dilatation is obtained. Then, even a sudden birth can be accomplished in a controlled surrounding.

What if... Roseann tells you that her sister was only in labor 1 hour when she had her baby, but Roseann is planning to spend the last days of this pregnancy in a mountain cabin 60 miles from the hospital? What would you do?

Induction and Augmentation of Labor

When labor contractions are ineffective, several interventions, such as induction and augmentation of labor with oxytocin or amniotomy (artificial rupture of the membranes), may be initiated to strengthen them (Howarth & Botha, 2009).

Induction of labor means that labor is started artificially. **Augmentation of labor** refers to assisting labor that has started spontaneously but is not effective. Induction may be necessary to initiate labor before the time when it would have occurred spontaneously because a fetus is in danger or because labor does not occur spontaneously and the fetus appears to be at term. The primary reasons for inducing labor include the presence of pre-eclampsia; eclampsia; severe hypertension; diabetes; Rh sensitization; prolonged rupture of the membranes; intrauterine growth restriction; and postmaturity (a pregnancy lasting beyond 42 weeks)—all situations that increase the risk for a fetus to remain in utero. Augmentation of labor or assistance to make uterine contractions stronger may be necessary if the contractions are hypotonic or too weak or infrequent to be effective.

Because augmentation or initiation of labor carries a risk of uterine rupture, decrease in the fetal blood supply from poor cotyledon filling, or premature separation of the placenta, it is used cautiously with women with a multiple gestation, hydramnios, grand parity, maternal age older than 40 years, or previous uterine scars.

Before induction of labor is begun, the following conditions should be present:

- The fetus is in a longitudinal lie.
- The cervix is ripe, or ready for birth.
- A presenting part is engaged.
- There is no CPD.
- The fetus is estimated to be mature by date, demonstrated by a lecithin–sphingomyelin ratio or ultrasound biparietal diameter to rule out preterm birth.

Cervical Ripening

Cervical ripening, or a change in the cervical consistency from firm to soft, is the first step the uterus must complete in early labor. Until this has occurred, dilatation and coordination of uterine contractions will not occur. To determine whether a cervix is "ripe," or ready for dilatation, Bishop (1964) established criteria for scoring the cervix (Table 23.3). Using this scale, if a woman's total score is 8 or greater, the cervix is considered ready for birth and should respond to induction. To "ripen" a cervix, various methods can be instituted. One is known as "stripping the membranes," or separating the membranes from the lower uterine segment manually, using a gloved finger in the cervix. This is an easy procedure performed during an office visit. Possible complications of this mechanical method include bleeding from an undetected low-lying placenta, inadvertent rupture of membranes, and the possibility of infection if membranes should rupture.

The use of hygroscopic suppositories (suppositories of seaweed that swell on contact with cervical secretions) is also a time-honored method. These suppositories can be inserted to gradually and gently urge dilatation (laminaria technique). They are held in place by gauze sponges saturated with povidone-iodine or an antifungal cream. Documentation of how

TABLE 23.3 ✻ Scoring of the Cervix for Readiness for Elective Induction

	Score			
Scoring Factor	*0*	*1*	*2*	*3*
Dilatation (cm)	0	1–2	3–4	3–4
Effacement (%)	0–30	40–50	60–70	80
Station	−3	−2	−1–0	+1–+2
Consistency	Firm	Medium	Soft	
Position	Posterior	Mid-position	Anterior	

Adapted with permission from Bishop, E. H. (1964). Pelvic scoring for elective induction. *Obstetrics and Gynecology, 24*(2), 266.

many dilators and sponges were placed is important, so it can be documented afterward that none remain.

A more commonly used method of speeding cervical ripening is the application of a prostaglandin gel, such as misoprostol, to the interior surface of the cervix by a catheter or suppository, or to the external surface by applying it to a diaphragm and then placing the diaphragm against the cervix (Alfirevic & Weeks 2009). Additional doses may be applied every 6 hours. Two or three doses are usually adequate to cause ripening. Women should remain in bed in a side-lying position to prevent leakage of the medication, and the FHR should be monitored continuously for at least 30 minutes after each application (perhaps up to 2 hours after vaginal insertion). Side effects are vomiting, fever, diarrhea, and hypertension, so these should also be monitored. Oxytocin induction may be started 6 to 12 hours after the last prostaglandin dose (beginning it sooner might lead to hyperstimulation of the uterus [Karch, 2009]). Even with their side effects, prostaglandins are well accepted by women (Hofmeyr & Gulmezoglu, 2009). As a rule, they should be used with caution in women with asthma, renal or cardiovascular disease, or glaucoma (Box 23.3). They are contraindicated for women who have had past cesarean births (Lawson & Bienstock, 2007).

Induction of Labor by Oxytocin

Administration of **oxytocin** (synthetic form of naturally occurring pituitary hormone) initiates contractions in a uterus at pregnancy term (Archie, 2007). Oxytocin is always administered intravenously, so that, if hyperstimulation should occur, it can be quickly discontinued. Because the half-life of oxytocin is approximately 3 minutes, the falling serum level and effects are apparent almost immediately after discontinuation of IV administration.

Usually a form of oxytocin, such as Pitocin, is mixed in the proportion of 10 IU in 1000 mL of Ringer's lactate. Ten international units of oxytocin is the same as 10,000 milliunits (mU), so each milliliter of this solution contains 10 mU of oxytocin. An alternative dilution method is to add 15 IU of oxytocin to 250 mL of an IV solution; this yields a concentration of 60 mU/1 mL. Physician's orders for administration of oxytocin for induction usually designate the number of milliunits to be administered per minute. Be sure to know the dilution prescribed and recognize the concentration in each milliliter (Box 23.4).

When administering the infusion, "piggyback" the oxytocin solution to a maintenance IV solution such as Ringer's lactate. Then, if the oxytocin needs to be discontinued quickly during the induction, the main IV line can still be maintained. Always attach the oxytocin solution to the infusion port closest to the woman. This way, if it is stopped, little solution remains in the tubing to still infuse. Use an infusion pump to regulate the infusion rate, so that the rate will not change even if a woman changes position. A physician should be immediately available during the entire procedure to ensure safety.

Infusions are usually begun at a rate of 0.5 to 1 mU/min. If there is no response, the infusion is gradually increased every 15 to 60 minutes by small increments of 1 to 2 mU/min until contractions begin. Many women respond with as little as 4 mU/min; most women respond at 16 mU/min. Do not

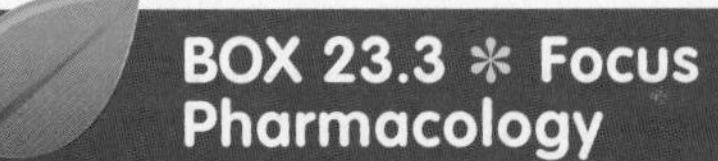

BOX 23.3 ✻ Focus on Pharmacology

Misoprostol (Cytotec)

Classification: Misoprostol is a synthetic prostaglandin (PGE1 analog).

Action: Produces cervical dilatation

Pregnancy Risk Category: X

Dosage: 50 to 100 μg orally or 25 to 50 μg placed intravaginally in the posterior fornix

Possible Adverse Effects: Uterine hyperstimulation, nonreassuring fetal heart rate pattern, nausea, diarrhea, flatulence, headache

Nursing Implications

- Ensure that the woman's condition is rated as safe for cervical dilatation and vaginal birth (absence of placenta previa, vasa previa, or cephalopelvic disproportion and the fetus is mature) before administration.
- Anticipate the need for a nonstress test to ensure fetal health before the drug is used.
- Continuously monitor uterine activity and fetal heart rate.
- Have an intravenous fluid line and a tocolytic readily available should uterine hyperstimulation occur (Karch, 2009).

BOX 23.4 * Focus on Pharmacology

Oxytocin for Labor Induction

Classification: Oxytocin is a synthetic form of the naturally occurring posterior pituitary hormone.

Action: Used to initiate uterine contractions in a term pregnancy

Pregnancy Risk Category: C

Dosage: Initially 1 to 2 mU/min by intravenous (IV) infusion, increased at a rate no more than 1 to 2 U/min at 15- to 30-minute intervals until a contraction pattern similar to normal labor is achieved

Possible Adverse Effects: Nausea, vomiting, cardiac arrhythmias, uterine hypertonicity, tetanic contractions, uterine rupture (with excessive dosages), severe water intoxication, and fetal bradycardia

Nursing Implications

- Prepare IV solution by adding 1 mL (10 IU) to 1000 mL of designated intravenous fluid (resulting solution contains 10 mU/mL).
- Use an infusion pump to ensure accurate control of infusion rate.
- Regulate infusion rate to establish uterine contractions similar to a normal labor pattern.
- Monitor frequency, duration, and strength of contractions.
- Assess maternal pulse and blood pressure, and watch for possible hypertension. If hypertension occurs, discontinue drug and notify physician.
- Continuously monitor fetal heart rate for signs of fetal distress.
- Monitor intake and output and watch for signs of possible water intoxication, such as headache or vomiting. Limit IV fluids to 150 mL/hr.
- Prepare the woman for birth (Karch, 2009)

Box 23.5 Assessment
Assessing the Pregnant Woman for Danger Signs of Oxytocin Administration

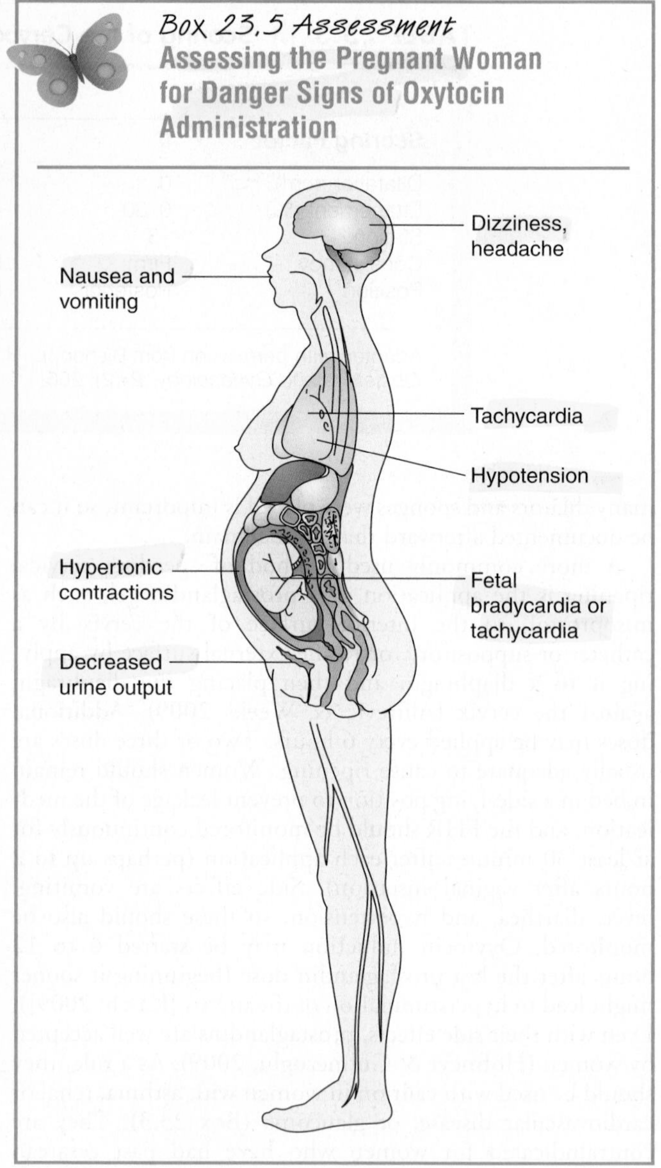

increase the rate to more than 20 mU/min without checking for further instructions, because an administration rate greater than this is likely to cause tetanic contractions. Aggressive induction (an increment of 6 mU/min instead of the usual 1 to 2 mU/min) has been suggested as a way to shorten labor and may be used in some research facilities.

After cervical dilatation reaches 4 cm, artificial rupture of the membranes may be performed to further induce labor, and the infusion may be discontinued at that point. For other women, the infusion is continued through full dilatation.

Peripheral vessel dilatation, a side effect of oxytocin, may cause extreme hypotension. To ensure safe induction, take the woman's pulse and blood pressure every 15 minutes. Monitor uterine contractions and FHR conscientiously. (See Box 23.5 for additional assessments for danger signs of oxytocin administration.)

Contractions should occur no more often than every 2 minutes, should not be stronger than 50 mm Hg pressure, and should last no longer than 70 seconds. The resting pressure between contractions should not exceed 15 mm Hg by monitor (Fig. 23.5). If contractions become more frequent or longer in duration than these safe limits, or if signs of fetal distress occur, stop the IV infusion and seek help immediately. Anticipate the need for oxygen administration. Excessive stimulation of the uterus by oxytocin may lead to tonic uterine contractions with fetal death or rupture of the uterus.

If stopping the oxytocin infusion does not stop the hyperstimulation, a beta-adrenergic receptor drug such as terbutaline sulfate (Brethine) or magnesium sulfate may be prescribed to decrease myometrial activity.

Oxytocin has an antidiuretic side effect that can result in decreased urine flow, possibly leading to water intoxication. Water intoxication is first manifested by headache and vomiting. If you observe these danger signs in a woman during induction of labor, report them immediately and halt the infusion. Water intoxication in its most severe form can lead to seizures, coma, and death because of the large shift in interstitial tissue fluid. Keep an accurate intake and output record, and test and record urine specific gravity throughout oxytocin administration to detect fluid retention. Limit the amount of IV fluid being given to 150 mL/hr by ensuring that the main IV fluid line is infusing at a rate not greater than 2.5 mL/min.

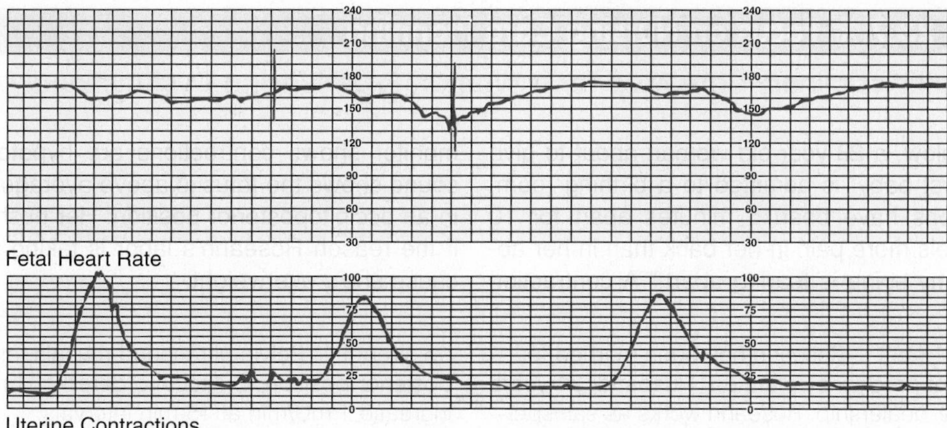

FIGURE 23.5 Hypertonic uterine contractions caused by an oxytocin infusion. Contractions are as high as 100 mm Hg in intensity. Late decelerations and an FHR of 170 beats per minute baseline are present.

Women may worry that induced labor will be more painful or "so different" from normal labor that breathing exercises will be worthless, or that it will progress so fast it will be harmful to the fetus. Induced labors do tend to have a slightly shorter first stage than the average unassisted labor. However, this is an advantage to a woman, not a disadvantage. Once contractions begin by this method, they are basically normal uterine contractions. You can assure the woman of this, so that she does not fight the contractions or become unnecessarily tense, which could prevent her from using her breathing techniques effectively. Induction of labor with oxytocin can predispose a newborn to hyperbilirubinemia and jaundice. Observe the infant closely for these conditions during the first few days of life.

Augmentation by Oxytocin

Augmentation of labor is required if labor contractions begin spontaneously but then become so weak, irregular, or ineffective (hypotonic) that assistance is needed to strengthen them (Box 23.6).

Precautions regarding oxytocin augmentation are the same as for primary induction of labor. A uterus may be very responsive or respond very effectively to oxytocin used as augmentation (see the Focus on Nursing Care Planning Box 23.7). Be certain that the drug is increased in small increments only and that fetal heart sounds are well monitored during the procedure.

Active Management of Labor

A technique of active management of labor began in Europe and has spread to some centers in the United States. It includes the aggressive administration of oxytocin (increases of 6 mU/min rather than 1 or 2 mU/min) to shorten labor to 12 hours, which presumably reduces the incidence of cesarean birth and postpartal infection. The maximum dosage of oxytocin used may be as high as 36 to 40 mU/min. Active management is controversial because it violates the tradition of birth as a normal, procedure-free process. Because it can shorten labor, it has the potential to reduce the number of postpartal fevers that occur from infection or dehydration.

BOX 23.6 * Focus on Family Teaching

Understanding Augmentation of Labor

Q. Roseann Bigalow says to you, "My doctor said she's going to augment my labor. What did she mean by that?"

A. Augmentation of labor is used when labor contractions are ineffective. It can shorten labor and avoid the necessity of cesarean birth. The drug used is oxytocin, a synthetic form of the hormone naturally released by your body during labor. It is administered intravenously. Once labor contractions begin by this method, they are the same as naturally occurring contractions. You will be able to use your prepared breathing exercises with them.

Uterine Rupture

Rupture of the uterus during labor, although rare, is always a possibility (Scearce & Uzelac, 2007). It is always serious, because it accounts for as many as 5% of all maternal deaths. Uterine rupture occurs when a uterus undergoes more strain than it is capable of sustaining. Rupture occurs most commonly when a vertical scar from a previous cesarean birth or hysterotomy repair tears (it occurs in less than 1% of women who have a low transverse cesarean scar from a previous pregnancy; about 4% to 8% of women who have a classic cesarean incision) (Szymanski & Bienstock, 2007). Contributing factors may include prolonged labor, abnormal presentation, multiple gestation, unwise use of oxytocin, obstructed labor, and traumatic maneuvers of forceps or traction. When uterine rupture occurs, fetal death will follow unless immediate cesarean birth can be accomplished. In these instances, fetal outcome can be optimal.

Impending rupture may be preceded by a pathologic retraction ring (see earlier discussion) and by strong uterine contractions without any cervical dilatation. To prevent rupture when these symptoms are present, anticipate the need for an immediate cesarean birth. If a uterus should rupture, the woman experiences a sudden, severe pain during a strong labor contraction, which she may report as a "tearing" sensation.

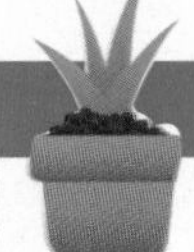

BOX 23.7 * Focus on Nursing Care Planning

A Multidisciplinary Care Map for a Woman Experiencing Dysfunctional Labor

Roseann Bigalow, a 28-year-old woman about to give birth to her first baby, is admitted to a birthing room. Her contractions have been 5 minutes apart for 10 hours. She feels more pain in her back than in her abdomen, "like my spine is tearing apart." A contraction monitor shows contractions are hypotonic. An ultrasound shows the fetus is above average in weight and in an occipitoposterior position. Her husband asks you if the reason Roseann's labor is taking so long is because she's overweight.

Family Assessment * Roseann has been married for 2 years. Present pregnancy planned. Husband, 34 years old, owns a car dealership. Roseann works as salesperson in dealership. Finances rated as "no problem."

Client Assessment * Client G1P0 in latent stage of labor. Membranes artificially ruptured approximately 1 hour ago. Cervix dilatated 4 cm, 80% effaced. Internal electronic fetal monitor in place. Contractions every 5 minutes, with peak strength at 20–25 mm Hg and a duration of 10 seconds. FHR at 130 to 140 bpm with beat-to-beat variability present. Client and partner visibly apprehensive, watching monitor intensely.

Client vital signs within normal parameters. Ringer's lactate IV solution infusing at 150 mL/hr via infusion pump. Client NPO, asking for something to eat "to keep up strength." Pelvic ultrasound reveals fetus in occipitoposterior position. Oxytocin ordered at 1 mU/min; increase 1 mU/min at 15-min intervals.

Nursing Diagnosis * Risk for injury (maternal and fetal) related to prolonged labor with ineffective contractions and requiring oxytocin

Outcome Criteria * Client's vital signs remain within acceptable parameters; FHR and fetal heart patterns within acceptable limits; contractions increase after oxytocin administration without becoming hypertonic; labor progresses without signs and symptoms of maternal or fetal distress. Urine output is at least 30 mL/hr; urine specific gravity 1.010–1.030.

Team Member Responsible	Assessment	Intervention	Rationale	Expected Outcome
		Activities of Daily Living		
Nurse	Assess what position allows client the most comfort with a occipitoposterior fetal position.	Encourage client to lie on her side or on hands and knees as much as possible. Encourage partner to apply back massage.	A side-lying position enhances placental perfusion. Back massage can aid comfort. A hands and knees position may encourage fetal rotation.	Client determines position of comfort. Requests massage if helpful with contractions.
		Consultations		
Physician	Assess whether resident physician coverage will be available for oxytocin administration.	Discuss need for oxytocin administration because of prolonged labor.	Oxytocin administration requires a physician's presence.	Resident physician will be available during oxytocin infusion time.
		Procedures/Medications		
Nurse/ Physician/ Nurse-Midwife	Assess client's vital signs, fetal heart rate, contraction strength and frequency.	Begin piggybacked IV oxytocin administration as ordered, using an infusion control device.	Oxytocin stimulates uterine contractions. Piggybacking the solution with an infusion control device allows for accurate dosing. Should an emergency arise, the infusion can be stopped immediately.	Oxytocin solution infuses at prescribed rate. Client's blood pressure remains <150/90 mm Hg; FHR is 120–160 bpm; no late decelerations occur.

		Nutrition		
Nurse	Assess intake and output and test urine for specific gravity.	Monitor the IV fluid infusion and adjust rate as ordered.	Intake and output and urine specific gravity are reliable indicators of fluid volume status. Inadvertent administration of too rapid a rate or too great an amount of IV fluid can increase the risk of fluid overload.	Client shows no symptoms of water intoxication: headache, lethargy, confusion, or a change in level of consciousness.
Nurse	Assess what measure client feels would relieve dry mouth best in light of NPO status.	Suggest hard candy or ice chips.	Fluid restrictions may be necessary to minimize the risk for increased fluid overload.	Client states she is comfortable while minimizing fluid intake.
		Patient/Family Education		
Nurse	Explore the meaning of prolonged labor with the couple. Assess for possible feelings related to "cause" of prolonged labor.	Encourage couple to verbalize feelings and concerns. Allow time for questions and answers.	Exploration, verbalization, and active questioning provide a safe outlet for feelings, help to increase the partner's awareness of needs, and open lines of communication.	Client and partner are able to discuss their feelings with caregivers. They state that they understand prolonged labor is not anyone's fault.
		Psychosocial/Spiritual/Emotional Needs		
Nurse	Assess what the couple thought labor would be like.	Include couple in the treatment process; provide frequent updates about labor progress.	Frequent updates about progress help to minimize the feelings of fear about the unknown.	Couple state they feel well informed about progress in labor.
		Discharge Planning		
Nurse	Assess whether labor experience was tolerable for couple in light of a complication.	Provide time for couple to "debrief" their labor experience.	Discussing or "putting a fence around" an experience helps to integrate it into other life events.	Couple state they feel comfortable with labor outcome.

Rupture can be complete, going through the endometrium, myometrium, and peritoneum layers, or incomplete, leaving the peritoneum intact. With a complete rupture, uterine contractions will immediately stop. Two distinct swellings will be visible on the woman's abdomen: the retracted uterus and the extrauterine fetus. Hemorrhage from the torn uterine arteries floods into the abdominal cavity and possibly into the vagina. Signs of shock begin, including rapid, weak pulse; falling blood pressure; cold and clammy skin; and dilatation of the nostrils from air hunger. Fetal heart sounds fade and then are absent.

If the rupture is incomplete, the signs of rupture are less evident. With an incomplete rupture, a woman may experience only a localized tenderness and a persistent aching pain over the area of the lower uterine segment. However, fetal heart sounds, a lack of contractions, and the changes in the woman's vital signs will gradually reveal fetal and maternal distress (Box 23.8). Uterine rupture can be confirmed by ultrasound (Has et al., 2008).

Because the uterus at the end of pregnancy is such a vascular organ, uterine rupture is an immediate emergency situation, comparable to splenic or hepatic rupture. Administer emergency fluid replacement therapy as ordered. Anticipate use of IV oxytocin to attempt to contract the uterus and minimize bleeding. Prepare the woman for a possible laparotomy as an emergency measure to control bleeding and achieve a repair. The viability of the fetus depends on the extent of the rupture and the time elapsed between rupture and abdominal extraction. A woman's prognosis depends on the extent of the rupture and the blood loss.

Most women are advised not to conceive again after a rupture of the uterus, unless the rupture occurred in the inactive lower segment. The physician, with consent, may perform a cesarean hysterectomy (removal of the damaged uterus) or

Box 23.8 Assessment
Assessing the Pregnant Woman With Complete Uterine Rupture

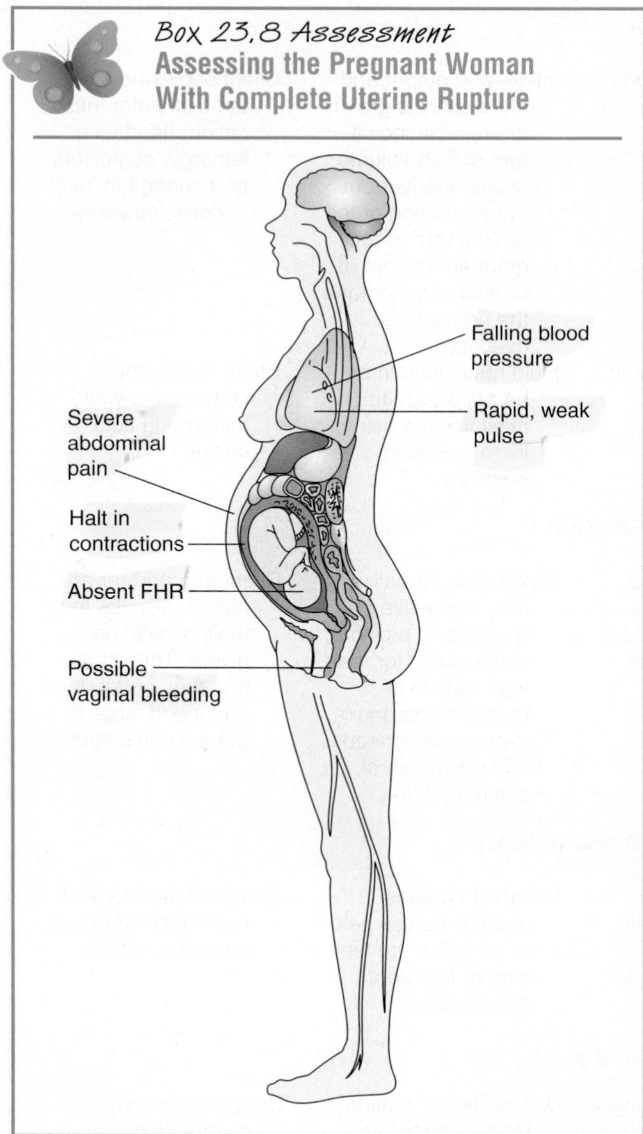

tubal ligation at the time of the laparotomy; both procedures result in loss of childbearing ability. A woman may have difficulty giving her consent at this time, because it is unknown whether her present baby will live. If blood loss was acute, she may be nonresponsive because of decreased cerebral perfusion from hypotension. If this has happened, the woman's support person must be the one who gives this consent, relying on the information provided by the operating surgeon to decide whether a functioning uterus can be saved.

Be prepared to offer information to the support person and to inform him or her about fetal outcome, the extent of the surgery, and the woman's safety as soon as possible. Initially, a woman and her support person will probably be thankful that her life was saved. However, they may become almost immediately angry that the rupture occurred, especially if the fetus died and the woman will no longer be able to have children. Allow them time to express these emotions without feeling threatened. Explaining to them about the death of the fetus is very difficult; utilize clergy or counselors as needed to help begin the coping process. The parents may want to plan a funeral, as oftentimes the babies are full term. They are grieving for the loss of both the child and their fertility as a couple. The couple is also dealing with an unexpected surgery to the mother, causing stressors that they did not plan for both financially and emotionally.

Inversion of the Uterus

Uterine inversion refers to the uterus turning inside out with either birth of the fetus or delivery of the placenta. It is a rare phenomenon, occurring in about 1 in 20,000 births (Poggi, 2007). It may occur if traction is applied to the umbilical cord to remove the placenta or if pressure is applied to the uterine fundus when the uterus is not contracted. It may also occur if the placenta is attached at the fundus so that, during birth, the passage of the fetus pulls the fundus down.

Inversion occurs in various degrees. The inverted fundus may lie within the uterine cavity or the vagina, or, in total inversion, it may protrude from the vagina. When an inversion occurs, a large amount of blood suddenly gushes from the vagina. The fundus is not palpable in the abdomen. If the loss of blood continues unchecked for longer than a few minutes, the woman will show signs of blood loss: hypotension, dizziness, paleness, or diaphoresis. Because the uterus is not contracted in this position, bleeding continues, and exsanguination could occur within a period as short as 10 minutes.

Never attempt to replace an inversion, because handling of the uterus may increase the bleeding. Never attempt to remove the placenta if it is still attached, because this only creates a larger surface area for bleeding. In addition, administration of an oxytocic drug only compounds the inversion or makes the uterus more tense and difficult to replace. An IV fluid line needs to be started, if one is not already present (use a large-gauge needle, because blood will need to be replaced). If a line is already in place, open it to achieve optimal flow of fluid to restore fluid volume. Administer oxygen by mask, and assess vital signs. Be prepared to perform cardiopulmonary resuscitation (CPR) if the woman's heart should fail from the sudden blood loss. The woman will immediately be given general anesthesia or possibly nitroglycerin or a tocolytic drug intravenously, to relax the uterus. The physician or nurse-midwife then replaces the fundus manually. Administration of oxytocin after manual replacement helps the uterus to contract and remain in its natural place. Because the uterine endometrium was exposed, a woman will need antibiotic therapy to prevent infection. She needs to be informed that cesarean birth will probably be necessary in any future pregnancy, to prevent the possibility of repeat inversion.

✔ Checkpoint Question 23.2

Suppose a woman experiences a uterine inversion and the placenta is still attached. What would be your best action?

a. Remove the placenta manually so that the uterus contracts.
b. Attempt to replace the uterus so that it becomes compressed.
c. Increase the woman's intravenous fluid to help restore blood loss.
d. Give an emergency bolus of an oxytocin such as Pitocin IV.

Amniotic Fluid Embolism

Amniotic fluid embolism occurs when amniotic fluid is forced into an open maternal uterine blood sinus through some defect in the membranes or after membrane rupture or partial premature separation of the placenta (Schoening, 2007). Previously, it was thought that particles such as meconium or shed fetal skin cells in the amniotic fluid entered the maternal circulation and reached the lungs as small emboli. Now, it is recognized that a humoral or anaphylactoid response is the more likely cause. This condition may occur during labor or in the postpartal period. The incidence is about 1 in 20,000 births; it accounts for at least 10% of maternal deaths in the United States (Szymanski & Bienstock, 2007). It is not preventable because it cannot be predicted. Possible risk factors include oxytocin administration, abruptio placentae, and hydramnios.

The clinical picture is dramatic. A woman, in strong labor, sits up suddenly and grasps her chest because of sharp pain and inability to breathe as she experiences pulmonary artery constriction. She becomes pale and then turns the typical bluish gray associated with pulmonary embolism and lack of blood flow to the lungs. The immediate management is oxygen administration by face mask or cannula. Within minutes, she will need CPR. CPR may be ineffective, however, because these procedures (inflating the lungs and massaging the heart) do not relieve the pulmonary constriction. Therefore, blood still cannot circulate to the lungs. Death may occur within minutes.

A woman's prognosis depends on the size of the embolism, the speed with which the emergency condition was detected, and the skill and speed of emergency interventions. Even if the woman survives the initial insult, the risk for disseminated intravascular coagulation (DIC) is high, further compounding her condition. In this event, she will need continued management that includes endotracheal intubation to maintain pulmonary function and therapy with fibrinogen to counteract DIC. Most likely, she will be transferred to an ICU. The prognosis for the fetus is guarded, because reduced placental perfusion results from the severe drop in maternal blood pressure. Labor often begins or the fetus is born immediately by cesarean birth.

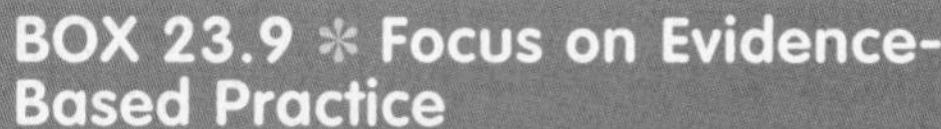

BOX 23.9 * Focus on Evidence-Based Practice

Is human papillomavirus (HPV) associated with preterm birth?

It is well documented that HPV is associated with the development of cervical cancer. To analyze whether it also could be responsible for some preterm births, researchers inspected placenta cells for the presence of HPV in placentas from three groups of women: those who had had a spontaneous preterm delivery, those who had had severe pre-eclampsia requiring early birth of their child, and, as a control group, those who had had an uncomplicated term birth. Results showed that HPV was present more frequently in placentas from spontaneous preterm births than in placentas from term births ($p = 0.03$). Identification of HPV in placentas from women with pre-eclampsia was not significantly different than placentas from term births. Researchers found that HPV infection caused cell death of placental trophoblast cells which reduce the ability of the placenta to invade into the uterine wall for firm attachment. Thus, HPV infection may cause placental dysfunction. and is associated with adverse pregnancy outcomes, including spontaneous preterm birth.

Would the above study suggest another reason to advise adolescent girls to have an HPV vaccine (Gardasil)?

Source: Gomez, L. M., et al. (2008). Placental infection with human papillomavirus is associated with spontaneous preterm delivery. *Human Reproduction, 23*(3), 709–715.

PROBLEMS WITH THE PASSENGER

Birth complications may arise if an infant is immature or preterm (Box 23.9). Complications may also occur if the maternal pelvis is so undersized, such as occurs in early adolescence or in women with altered bone growth from a disease such as rickets that its diameters are smaller than the fetal skull diameters. It also can occur if the umbilical cord prolapses, if more than one fetus is present, or if a fetus is malpositioned or too large for the birth canal.

Prolapse of the Umbilical Cord

In **umbilical cord prolapse,** a loop of the umbilical cord slips down in front of the presenting fetal part (Fig. 23.6).

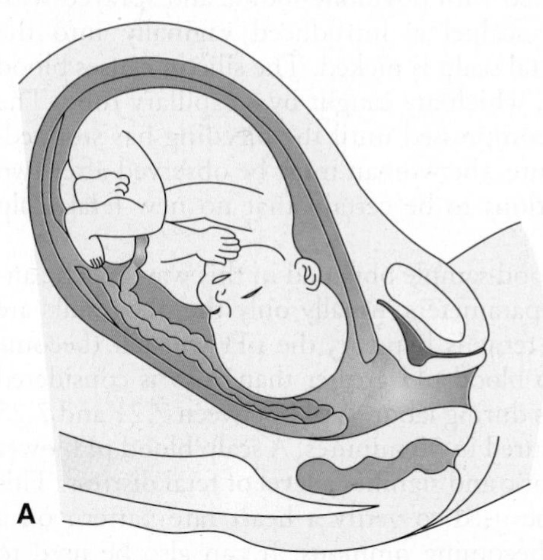

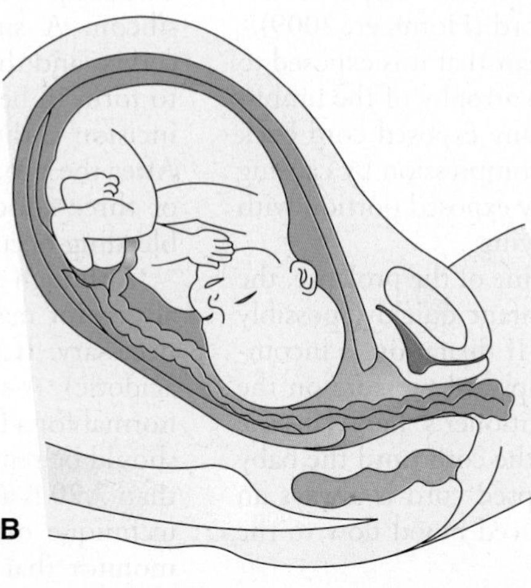

FIGURE 23.6 Prolapse of the umbilical cord. (**A**) The cord is prolapsed but still within the uterus. (**B**) The cord is visible at the vulva. In both instances the fetal nutrient supply is being compromised, although only a cord such as that shown in B would be visible. Both prolapses could be detected by fetal monitoring.

Prolapse may occur at any time after the membranes rupture if the presenting fetal part is not fitted firmly into the cervix. It tends to occur most often with:

- Premature rupture of membranes
- Fetal presentation other than cephalic
- Placenta previa
- Intrauterine tumors preventing the presenting part from engaging
- A small fetus
- Cephalopelvic disproportion preventing firm engagement
- Hydramnios
- Multiple gestation

The incidence is about 0.5% of cephalic births; this rises as high as 15% to 20% with breech or transverse lies (Kish & Collea, 2007).

Assessment

In rare instances, the cord may be felt as the presenting part on an initial vaginal examination during labor. It may also be identified in this position on an ultrasound. When this happens, cesarean birth is necessary before rupture of the membranes occurs. Otherwise, membrane rupture would cause the cord to slide down into the vagina from the pressure exerted by the amniotic fluid. More often, however, cord prolapse is first discovered only after the membranes have ruptured, when a variable deceleration FHR pattern suddenly becomes apparent. The cord may be visible at the vulva.

To rule out cord prolapse, always assess fetal heart sounds immediately after rupture of the membranes whether this occurs spontaneously or by amniotomy.

Therapeutic Management

Cord prolapse automatically leads to cord compression, because the fetal presenting part presses against the cord at the pelvic brim. Management is aimed at relieving pressure on the cord, thereby relieving the compression and the resulting fetal anoxia. This may be done by placing a gloved hand in the vagina and manually elevating the fetal head off the cord, or by placing the woman in a knee–chest or Trendelenburg position, which causes the fetal head to fall back from the cord. Administering oxygen at 10 L/min by face mask to the woman is also helpful to improve oxygenation to the fetus. A tocolytic agent may be prescribed to reduce uterine activity and pressure on the fetus. Amnioinfusion (see later) is yet another way to relieve pressure on the cord (Hofmeyr, 2009).

If the cord has prolapsed to the extent that it is exposed to room air, drying will begin, leading to atrophy of the umbilical vessels. Do not attempt to push any exposed cord back into the vagina. This may add to the compression by causing knotting or kinking. Instead, cover any exposed portion with a sterile saline compress to prevent drying.

If the cervix is fully dilated at the time of the prolapse, the physician may choose to birth the infant quickly, possibly with forceps, to prevent fetal anoxia. If dilatation is incomplete, the birth method of choice is upward pressure on the presenting part, applied by a practitioner's hand in the woman's vagina, to keep pressure off the cord until the baby can be born by cesarean birth. Prolapsed cord is always an emergency situation, because the reduced blood flow to the fetus can quickly cause fetal harm.

Amnioinfusion. **Amnioinfusion** is the addition of a sterile fluid into the uterus to supplement the amniotic fluid (Chhabra, Dargan, & Nasare, 2007). The technique neither shortens nor prolongs labor; it just prevents additional cord compression. For this, a sterile catheter is introduced through the cervix into the uterus after rupture of the membranes. It is attached to intravenous tubing, and a solution of warmed normal saline or lactated Ringer's solution is rapidly infused. Initially, approximately 500 mL is infused, and then the rate is adjusted to infuse the least amount necessary to maintain a monitor pattern without variable decelerations. Throughout the procedure, urge a woman to lie in a lateral recumbent position to prevent supine hypotension syndrome.

Help maintain strict aseptic technique during insertion and while caring for the catheter. Continuously monitor FHR and uterine contractions internally during the infusion. Record maternal temperature hourly to detect infection. Be sure the solution is warmed to body temperature before the infusion, to prevent chilling of the woman and fetus. This can be done by placing the bag of fluid on a radiant heat warmer or by using a blood/fluid warmer before administration.

Because there will be a continuous flow of the infusing solution out of the woman's vagina during the procedure, change her bed frequently. Also assess that there is constant drainage. If vaginal leakage should stop, it usually means that the fetal head is firmly engaged and all fluid being infused is being held in the uterus. This is dangerous because it could lead to hydramnios (presence of excessive amniotic fluid) and possibly uterine rupture.

Fetal Blood Sampling. Although obtaining a fetal oxygen saturation level by inserting a fetal oximeter into the uterus to rest next to the fetal cheek or obtaining a positive response to scalp stimulation usually supplies the information as to whether a fetus is becoming acidotic (see Chapter 15), this information can also be obtained by scalp blood or fetal blood sampling (Lawson & Bienstock, 2007).

The oxygen saturation, partial pressures of oxygen (PO_2) and carbon dioxide (PCO_2), pH, bicarbonate excess, and hematocrit of fetal blood may all be determined during labor if a sample of capillary blood is taken from the fetal scalp as it presents at the dilated cervix. After cervical dilatation of 3 to 4 cm and rupture of the membranes, the fetal head is visualized by the use of an amnioscope—a small, cone-shaped instrument with a light source at the far end. The scalp is cleaned with povidone-iodine and sprayed with silicon. A small scalpel is introduced vaginally into the cervix, and the fetal scalp is nicked. The silicon causes blood to form in beads, which are caught by a capillary tube. The incision is then compressed until the bleeding has stopped. After the procedure, the woman must be observed after two or three contractions to be certain that no new fetal scalp bleeding occurs.

Although a blood sample obtained in this way may be analyzed for many parameters, usually only the pH results are necessary. If the fetus is hypoxic, the pH will fall (become acidotic). A scalp blood pH greater than 7.25 is considered normal for a fetus during labor. A pH between 7.21 and 7.25 should be remeasured in 30 minutes. A scalp blood pH lower than 7.20 is acidotic and signifies a level of fetal distress. This technique may be used to verify a heart rate pattern on a monitor that is becoming ominous. It can also be used to verify that no acidosis is occurring, even if a monitor rate is showing decreased variability.

Fetal blood sampling involves no pain for the woman, but it may involve an uncomfortable sensation of pressure because of the examining hand in the vagina. Infants who have had internal scalp blood samples taken should not be born by vacuum extraction, because this procedure can lead to renewed bleeding at the puncture site.

Multiple Gestation

A woman with a multiple gestation usually causes a flurry of excitement in a birthing room. Additional personnel are needed for the birth (as many nurses to attend to possibly immature infants as there are infants, plus additional pediatricians or neonatal nurse practitioners). In the middle of all the preparatory activity, it is easy to forget that a woman having a multiple birth may be more frightened than excited. Be sure to focus on her needs as well as those of her babies. Twins may be born by cesarean birth to decrease the risk that the second fetus will experience anoxia; this also is often the situation in multiple gestations of three or more, because of the increased incidence of cord entanglement and premature separation of the placenta (Fortner, Althaus, & Gurewitsch, 2007).

Anemia and pregnancy-induced hypertension occur at higher-than-usual incidences during multiple gestations. To detect these, be certain to assess the woman's hematocrit level and blood pressure closely during labor or while waiting for cesarean surgery.

If a woman with a multiple gestation will be giving birth vaginally, she is usually instructed to come to the hospital early in labor. The first stage of labor does not differ greatly from that of a woman with a single-gestation pregnancy. Coming to a hospital this early in labor, however, will make labor seem long. Urge the woman to spend the early hours of labor engaged in an activity such as playing cards or reading, to make the time pass more quickly. Multiple pregnancies often end before full term, so the woman may not yet have practiced breathing exercises. The early hours of labor can be used for this as well. During labor, support the woman's breathing exercises to minimize the need for analgesia or anesthesia; this helps to minimize any respiratory difficulties the infants may have at birth because of their immaturity.

If possible, monitor each FHR by a separate fetal monitor during labor. Because the babies are usually small, firm head engagement may not occur, increasing the risk for cord prolapse after rupture of the membranes. Because of the multiple fetuses, abnormal fetal presentation may occur. Uterine dysfunction from a long labor, an overstretched uterus, unusual presentation, and premature separation of the placenta after the birth of the first child may also be more common.

Most twin pregnancies present with both twins vertex. This is followed in frequency by vertex and breech, breech and vertex, and then breech and breech (Fig. 23.7). Multiple gestations of three or more fetuses have extremely varied presentations. After the first infant is born, both ends of the baby's cord are tied or clamped permanently, rather than with cord clamps, which could slip. This prevents hemorrhage

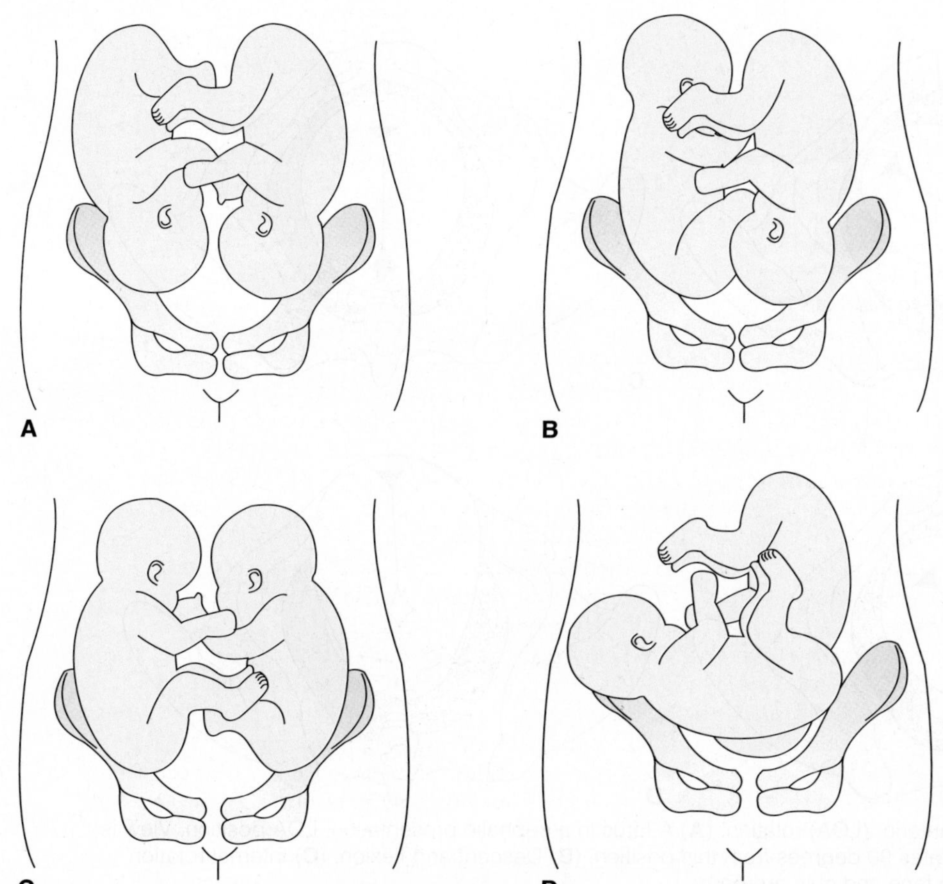

FIGURE 23.7 Four different twin presentations. (**A**) Both infants vertex. (**B**) One infant vertex and one breech. (**C**) Both infants breech. (**D**) One infant vertex and one in a transverse lie.

through an open cord end if additional infants have shared the placenta. The first infant is identified as *A*, and newborn care is started. In singleton pregnancies oxytocin usually is given immediately to contract the uterus and minimize bleeding after an infant is born; with this woman, however, it will not be given, to avoid compromising the circulation of the infants not yet born.

After the birth of the first child, the lie of the second fetus is determined by external abdominal palpation or ultrasound. If the presentation is not vertex, external version may be attempted to make it so (Longo & Hankins, 2007). If this is not successful, a decision for a breech birth or cesarean birth must be made (Cruikshank, 2007). If the infant will be born vaginally, an oxytocin infusion may be begun at this point to assist uterine contractions, thereby shortening the time span between births. If uterine relaxation is needed, nitroglycerin, an uterine relaxant, may be administered.

Occasionally, the placenta of the first infant separates before the second fetus is born, and there is sudden, profuse bleeding at the vagina. This creates a risk for the woman. The uterus cannot contract as it normally would, because it is still full with the second twin, so it is difficult to halt the bleeding. If the separation of the first placenta caused loosening of additional placentas, or if a common placenta is involved, the fetal heart sounds of the other fetuses will register distress immediately. They need to be born at once if they are to survive. For this reason, with most multiple gestations today, if all of the fetuses are not vertex presentations, they will be born by cesarean birth.

Parents usually want to inspect multiple-gestation infants thoroughly after birth. The time allowed for this inspection depends on the infants' weights and conditions. Some parents worry that the hospital will confuse their infants through improper identification. Review with them the measures used to ensure correct identification.

Even though women have known for months that they are having multiple infants, many have difficulty believing that this has really happened. They feel a need to recount over and over their surprise and to view all their infants together to prove to themselves that it is true. If parents are unable to inspect their infants thoroughly immediately after birth because of the infants' low birthweights and the danger of chilling, they need the opportunity to do so as soon as possible, to dispel any fears they had throughout pregnancy that the babies would be born less than perfect.

Assess the woman carefully in the immediate postpartal period, because the uterus that has been overly distended owing to the multiple gestation may have more difficulty contracting than usual, placing her at risk for hemorrhage from uterine atony (lacking normal tone). In addition, the risk for uterine infection increases if labor or birth was prolonged. The infants need careful assessment to determine their true gestational age and whether a phenomenon such as twin-to-twin transfusion could have occurred (see Chapter 26).

Problems With Fetal Position, Presentation, or Size

Occipitoposterior Position

In approximately one tenth of all labors, the fetal position is posterior rather than anterior. That is, the occiput (assuming

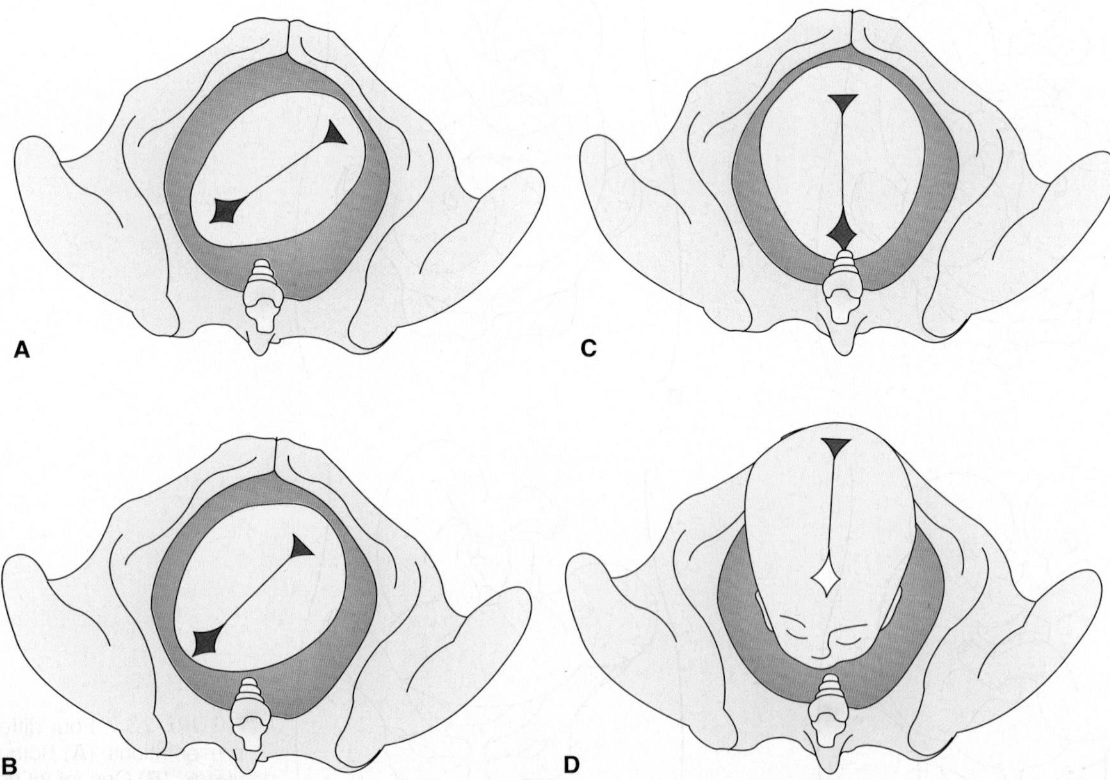

FIGURE 23.8 Left occipitoanterior (LOA) rotation. (**A**) A fetus in a cephalic presentation, LOA position. View is from the outlet. The fetus rotates 90 degrees from this position. (**B**) Descent and flexion. (**C**) Internal rotation complete. (**D**) Extension; the face and chin are born.

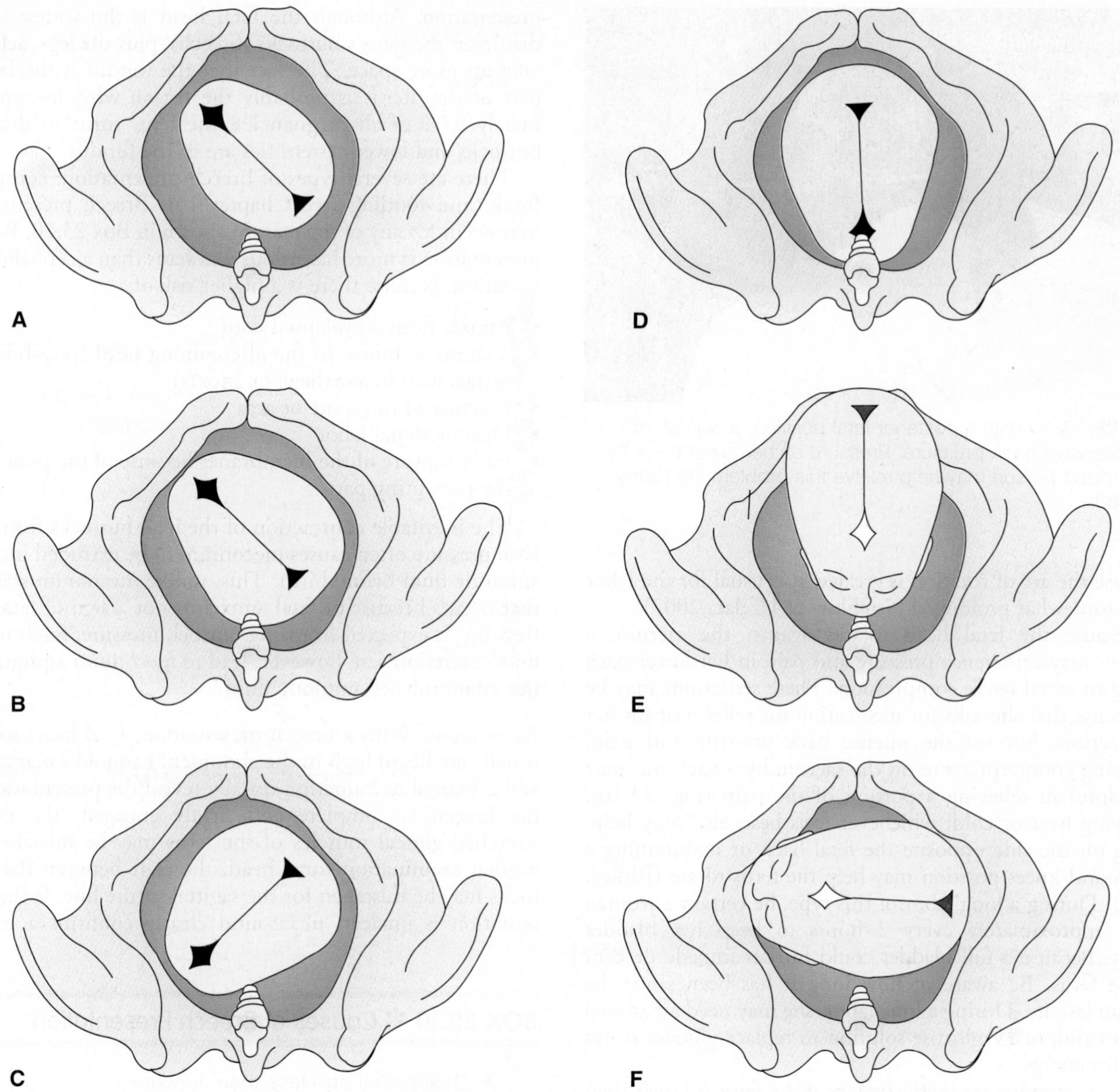

FIGURE 23.9 Left occipitoposterior (LOP) rotation. (**A**) Fetus in a cephalic presentation, LOP position. View is from outlet. The fetus rotates 135 degrees from this position. (**B**) Descent and flexion. (**C**) Internal rotation beginning. Because of the posterior position, the head will rotate in a longer arc than if it were in an anterior position. (**D**) Internal rotation complete. (**E**) Extension; the face and chin are born. (**F**) External rotation; the fetus rotates to place the shoulders in an anteroposterior position.

the presentation is vertex) is directed diagonally and posteriorly, either to the right (ROP) or to the left (LOP). In these positions, during internal rotation, the fetal head must rotate, not through a 90-degree arc (Fig. 23.8), but through an arc of approximately 135 degrees (Fig. 23.9). Rotation from a posterior position can be aided by having the woman assume a hands and knees position, squatting, or lying on her side (on her left side if the fetus is right occiput posterior; on her right side if the fetus is left occiput posterior). Theoretically, shifting the weight from right to left or "lunging" or swinging her body right to left while elevating her left foot on a chair widens the pelvic path and makes fetal rotation easier. This is unproved, however, and is tiring for women in labor.

Posterior positions tend to occur in women with android, anthropoid, or contracted pelves. A posterior position is suggested by a dysfunctional labor pattern such as a prolonged active phase, arrested descent, or fetal heart sounds heard best at the lateral sides of the abdomen.

A posteriorly presenting head does not fit the cervix as snugly as one in an anterior position. Because this increases the risk of umbilical cord prolapse, the position of the fetus is confirmed by vaginal examination or by ultrasound. The majority of fetuses presenting in posterior positions, if they are of average size and in good flexion and aided by forceful uterine contractions, rotate through the large arc, arrive at a good birth position for the pelvic outlet, and are born satisfactorily with only increased molding and caput formation.

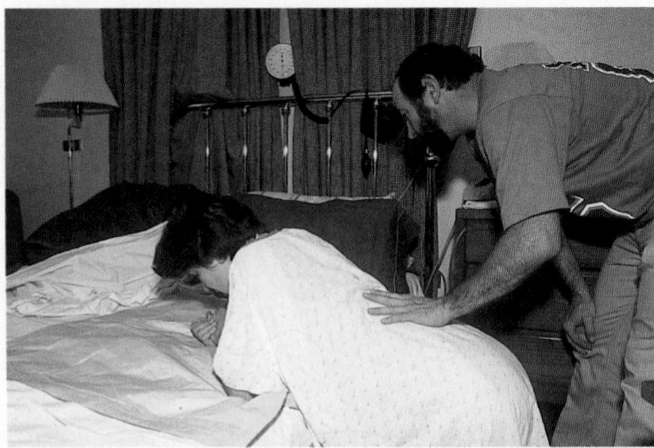

FIGURE 23.10 With a posterior fetal position, a woman may feel extensive back pressure. Pressure on her lower back by her support person may help relieve this problem. (© Kathy Sloane.)

Because the arc of rotation is greater, it is usual for the labor to be somewhat prolonged (Strehlow & Uzelac, 2007).

Because the fetal head rotates against the sacrum, a woman may experience pressure and pain in her lower back owing to sacral nerve compression. These sensations may be so intense that she asks for medication for relief, not for her contractions but for the intense back pressure and pain. Applying counterpressure on the sacrum by a back rub may be helpful in relieving a portion of the pain (Fig. 23.10). Applying heat or cold, whichever feels best, also may help. Lying on the side opposite the fetal back or maintaining a hands-and-knees position may help the fetus rotate (Ridley, 2007). During a long labor of this type, be certain a woman voids approximately every 2 hours to keep her bladder empty, because a full bladder could further impede descent of the fetus. Be aware of how long it has been since the woman last ate. During a long labor, she may need an an oral sports drink or IV glucose solution to replace glucose stores used for energy.

If contractions are ineffective, or if the fetus is larger than average or not in good flexion, rotation through the 135-degree arc may not be possible. Uterine dysfunction may result from maternal exhaustion. The fetal head may arrest in the transverse position (transverse arrest), or rotation may not occur at all (persistent occipitoposterior position). In these instances, the fetus must be born by cesarean birth.

During labor, a woman needs a great deal of support to prevent her from becoming panicked about the length of the labor. Paradoxically, women who are best prepared for labor are often most frightened when deviations occur, because things are not going "by the book"—not happening just as described by the instructor of the course they attended or the book they read. Provide frequent reassurance that, although their pattern of labor is not "textbook," it is within safe, controlled limits. If forceps are used to help the fetus rotate, this places a woman at risk for cervical lacerations, hemorrhage, and infection in the postpartum period.

Breech Presentation

Most fetuses are in a breech presentation early in pregnancy. However, by week 38, a fetus normally turns to a cephalic presentation. Although the fetal head is the widest single diameter, the fetus's buttocks (breech), plus the legs, actually take up more space. The fact that the fundus is the largest part of the uterus is probably the reason why, in approximately 97% of all pregnancies, the fetus turns so that the buttocks and lower extremities are in the fundus.

There are several types of breech presentation: complete, frank, and footling (see Chapter 15). Breech presentation may occur for any of the reasons shown in Box 23.10. Breech presentation is more hazardous to a fetus than a cephalic presentation, because there is a higher risk of:

- Anoxia from a prolapsed cord
- Traumatic injury to the aftercoming head (possibility of intracranial hemorrhage or anoxia)
- Fracture of the spine or arm
- Dysfunctional labor
- Early rupture of the membranes because of the poor fit of the presenting part

The inevitable contraction of the fetal buttocks from cervical pressure often causes meconium to be extruded into the amniotic fluid before birth. This, unlike meconium staining that occurs because of fetal anoxia, is not a sign of fetal distress but is expected from the buttock pressure. Such meconium excretion can, however, lead to meconium aspiration if the infant inhales amniotic fluid.

Assessment. With a breech presentation, fetal heart sounds usually are heard high in the abdomen. Leopold's maneuvers and a vaginal examination usually reveal the presentation. If the breech is complete and firmly engaged, the tightly stretched gluteal muscles of the fetus may be mistaken on vaginal examination for a head; the cleft between the buttocks may be mistaken for the sagittal suture line. If the presentation is unclear, ultrasound clearly confirms a breech

BOX 23.10 ✻ Causes of Breech Presentation

- Gestational age less than 40 weeks
- Abnormality in a fetus, such as anencephaly, hydrocephalus, or meningocele. (In a fetus with hydrocephalus, the widest fetal diameter is the head, so it retains the most "comfortable" position.)
- Hydramnios that allows for free fetal movement, so that the fetus fits within the uterus in any position
- Congenital anomaly of the uterus, such as a mid-septum, that traps the fetus in a breech position
- Any space-occupying mass in the pelvis, such as a fibroid tumor of the uterus or a placenta previa, that does not allow the head to present
- Pendulous abdomen. If the abdominal muscles are lax, the uterus may fall so far forward that the fetal head comes to lie outside the pelvic brim, causing a breech presentation.
- Multiple gestation. The presenting infant cannot turn to a vertex position.
- Unknown factors

presentation. Such a study also gives information on pelvic diameters, fetal skull diameters, and evidence of possible placenta previa causing the breech presentation.

In a breech birth, the same stages of flexion, descent, internal rotation, expulsion, and external rotation occur as in a vertex birth. Always monitor FHR and uterine contractions continuously, if possible, during this time. This allows early detection of fetal distress from a complication such as prolapsed cord and allows for prompt intervention.

Birth Technique. If the infant will be born vaginally, a woman is allowed to push after full dilatation is achieved, and the breech, trunk, and shoulders are born (Fig. 23.11). As the breech spontaneously emerges from the birth canal, it is steadied and supported by a sterile towel held against the infant's inferior surface (see Fig. 23.11C). The shoulders present to the outlet with their widest diameter anteroposterior. If they are not born readily, the arm of the posterior shoulder may be drawn down by passing two fingers over the infant's shoulder and down the arm to the elbow, then sweeping the flexed arm across the infant's face and chest and out. The other arm is delivered in the same way. External rotation is allowed to occur, to bring the head into the best outlet diameter.

Birth of the head is the most hazardous part of a breech birth. Because the umbilicus precedes the head, a loop of cord passes down alongside the head. The pressure of the head against the pelvic brim automatically compresses this loop of cord.

A second danger of a breech birth is intracranial hemorrhage. With a cephalic presentation, molding to the confines of the birth canal occurs over hours. With a breech birth, pressure changes occur instantaneously. Tentorial tears, which can cause gross motor and mental incapacity or lethal damage to the fetus, may result. The infant who is born suddenly to reduce the duration of cord compression may suffer an intracranial hemorrhage. In contrast, the infant who is born gradually to reduce the possibility of intracranial injury may suffer hypoxia.

To aid in birth of the head, the trunk of the infant is usually straddled over the physician's right forearm (see Fig. 23.11D). Two fingers of the physician's right hand are placed in the infant's mouth. The left hand is slid into the woman's vagina, palm down, along the infant's back. Pressure is applied to the occiput to flex the head fully.

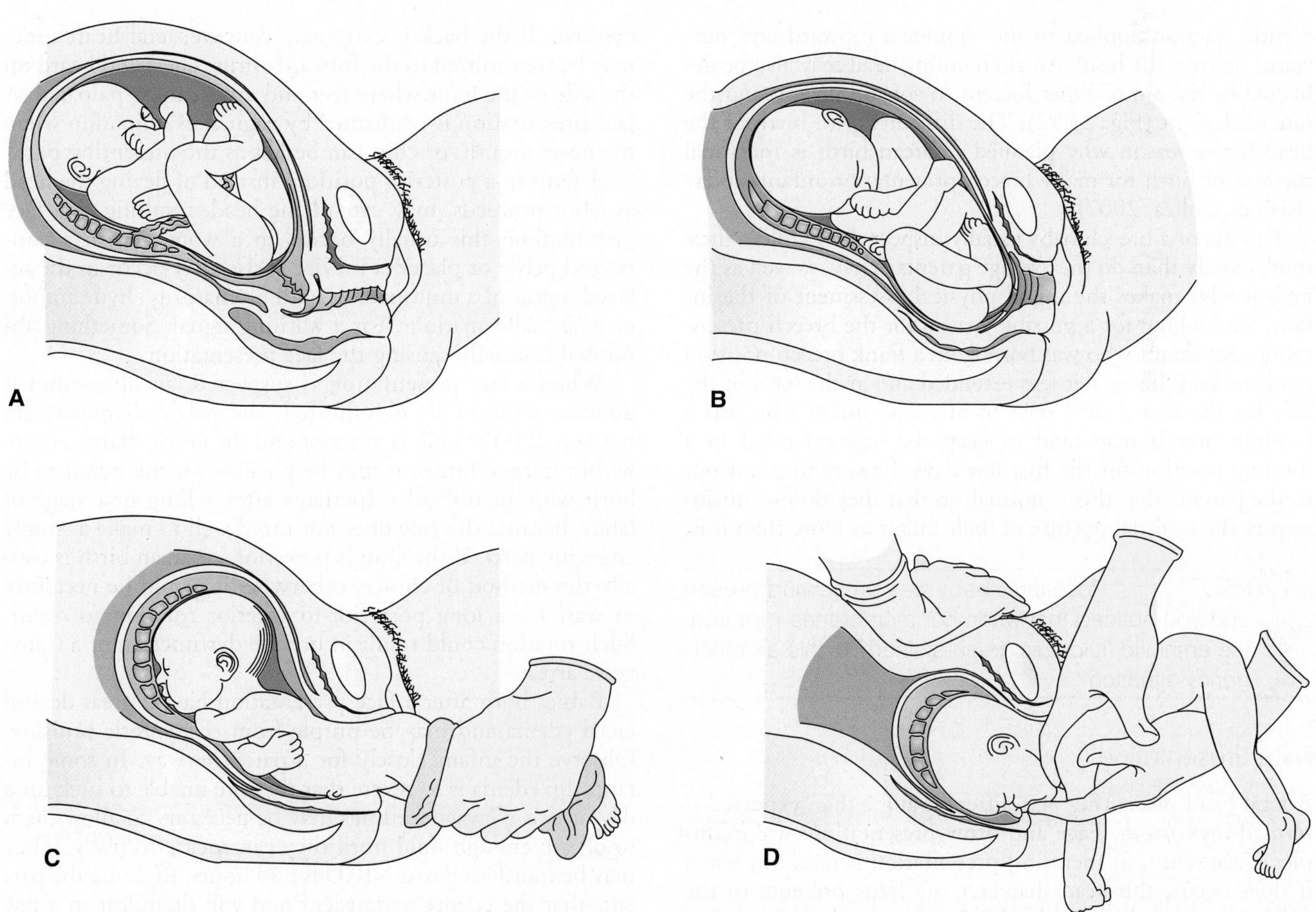

FIGURE 23.11 Breech birth. (**A**) Position before labor; left sacroposterior. (**B**) Descent and internal rotation. (**C**) Legs being born; the shoulders turn to present to the anteroposterior diameter. (**D**) The head is born. External rotation has put the anteroposterior diameter of the head in line with the anteroposterior diameter of the woman's pelvis. The head is born by gentle pressure to flex the head fully and by gentle traction to the shoulders upward and outward. Additional pressure might be applied by an assistant to the abdominal wall to ensure head flexion.

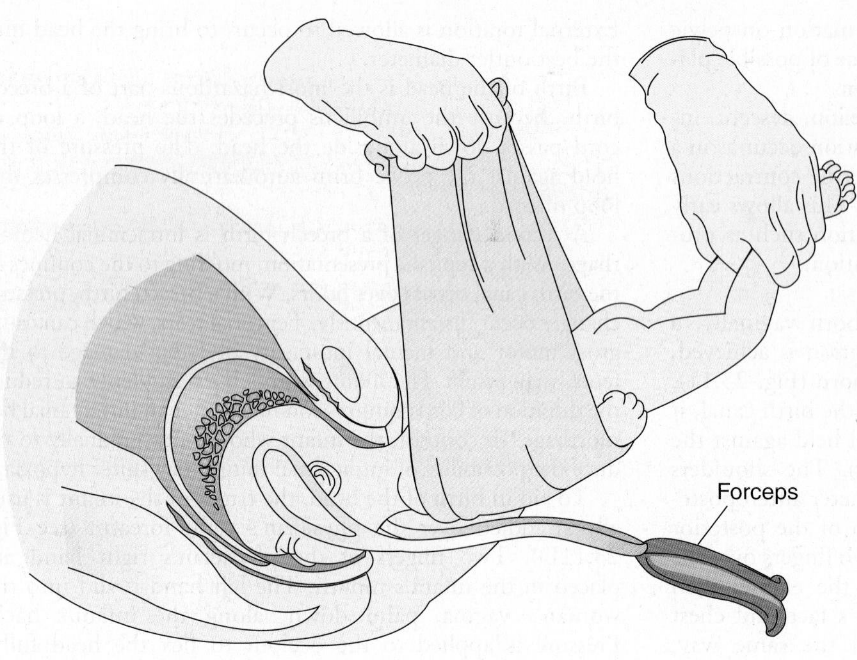

FIGURE 23.12 With Piper forceps used for a breech birth, traction is applied directly to the head, so damage to the infant's neck is avoided.

Gentle traction applied to the shoulders (upward and outward) delivers the head. An aftercoming head may also be delivered by the aid of Piper forceps to control flexion and the rate of descent (Fig. 23.12). The difficulty with birth of the head is the reason why planned cesarean birth is the usual method of birth for many breech-presentation infants today (Kish & Collea, 2007).

Parents of a breech baby usually inspect their child a little more closely than do the average parents. They, as well as the person who makes the initial physical assessment of the infant, are looking for a possible reason for the breech presentation. An infant who was born from a frank breech position tends to keep his or her legs extended and at the level of the face for the first 2 or 3 days of life. The infant who was a footling breech may tend to keep the legs extended in a footling position for the first few days. Be sure to point out to the parents that this is normal, so that they do not misinterpret the unusual posture of their infant as more than it is.

What if . . . Roseann's baby was presenting breech and you noticed that when her membranes ruptured, the amniotic fluid was green-stained? Is this an emergency situation?

Face Presentation

A fetal head presenting at a different angle than expected is termed *asynclitism.* Face and brow presentations are examples. Face (chin, or mentum) presentation is rare, but when it does occur, the head diameter the fetus presents to the pelvis is often too large for birth to proceed. A head that feels more prominent than normal, with no engagement apparent on Leopold's maneuvers, suggests a face presentation. It is also suggested when the head and back are both felt on the same side of the uterus with Leopold's maneuvers. The back is difficult to outline in this presentation because it is concave. If the back is extremely concave, fetal heart tones may be transmitted to the forward-thrust chest and heard on the side of the fetus where feet and arms can be palpated. A face presentation is confirmed by vaginal examination when the nose, mouth, or chin can be felt as the presenting part.

A fetus in a posterior position, instead of flexing the head as labor proceeds, may extend the head, resulting in a face presentation; this usually occurs in a woman with a contracted pelvis or placenta previa. It also may occur in the relaxed uterus of a multipara or with prematurity, hydramnios, or fetal malformation. It is a warning signal. Something abnormal is usually causing the face presentation.

When a face presentation is suspected, an ultrasound is done to confirm it; if indicated, the pelvic diameters are measured. If the chin is anterior and the pelvic diameters are within normal limits, it may be possible for the infant to be born without difficulty (perhaps after a long first stage of labor, because the face does not mold well to make a snugly engaging part). If the chin is posterior, cesarean birth is usually the method of choice; otherwise, it would be necessary to wait for a long posterior-to-anterior rotation to occur. Such rotation could result in uterine dysfunction or a transverse arrest.

Babies born after a face presentation have a great deal of facial edema and may be purple from ecchymotic bruising. Observe the infant closely for a patent airway. In some infants, lip edema is so severe that they are unable to suck for a day or two. Gavage feedings may be necessary to allow them to obtain enough fluid until they can suck effectively. They may be transferred to a NICU for 24 hours. Reassure the parents that the edema is transient and will disappear in a few days, with no aftermath.

Brow Presentation

A brow presentation is the rarest of the presentations. It occurs in a multipara or a woman with relaxed abdominal muscles.

It almost invariably results in obstructed labor, because the head becomes jammed in the brim of the pelvis as the occipitomental diameter presents. Unless the presentation spontaneously corrects, cesarean birth will be necessary to birth the infant safely. Brow presentations also leave an infant with extreme ecchymotic bruising on the face. On seeing this bruising over the same area as the anterior fontanelle, or "soft spot," parents may need additional reassurance that the child is well after birth.

Transverse Lie

Transverse lie occurs in women with pendulous abdomens, with uterine fibroid tumors that obstruct the lower uterine segment, with contraction of the pelvic brim, with congenital abnormalities of the uterus, or with hydramnios. It may occur in infants with hydrocephalus or another abnormality that prevents the head from engaging. It may also occur in prematurity if the infant has room for free movement, in multiple gestation (particularly in a second twin), or if there is a short umbilical cord.

A transverse lie usually is obvious on inspection, because the ovoid of the uterus is found to be more horizontal than vertical. The abnormal presentation can be confirmed by Leopold's maneuvers. An ultrasound may be taken to further confirm the abnormal lie and to provide information on pelvic size.

A mature fetus cannot be delivered vaginally from this presentation. Often, the membranes rupture at the beginning of labor. Because there is no firm presenting part, the cord or an arm may prolapse, or the shoulder may obstruct the cervix. Cesarean birth is necessary.

Oversized Fetus (Macrosomia)

Size may become a problem in a fetus who weighs more than 4000 to 4500 g (approximately 9 to 10 lb). Babies of this size complicate up to 10% of all births and are most frequently born to women who enter pregnancy with diabetes or develop gestational diabetes (Campaigne & Conway, 2007). Large babies are also associated with multiparity, because each infant born to a woman tends to be slightly heavier and larger than the one born just before.

An oversized infant may cause uterine dysfunction during labor or at birth because of overstretching of the fibers of the myometrium. The wide shoulders may pose a problem at birth, because they can cause fetal pelvic disproportion or even uterine rupture from obstruction. If the infant is so oversized that he or she cannot be born vaginally, cesarean birth becomes the birth method of choice. The large size of a fetus may be missed in an obese woman, because the fetal contours are difficult to palpate and obesity does not necessarily indicate a larger-than-usual pelvis. Pelvimetry or ultrasound can be used to compare the size of the fetus with the woman's pelvic capacity.

The perinatal mortality rate of larger infants is substantially increased to about 15%, compared with the normal 4%. In addition, a large infant born vaginally has a higher-than-normal risk of cervical nerve palsy, diaphragmatic nerve injury, or fractured clavicle because of shoulder dystocia. Postpartally, the woman has an increased risk of hemorrhage, because the overdistended uterus may not contract as readily as usual.

Shoulder Dystocia

Shoulder dystocia is a birth problem that is increasing in incidence along with the increasing average weight of newborns (Strehlow & Uzelac, 2007). The problem occurs at the second stage of labor, when the fetal head is born but the shoulders are too broad to enter and be born through the pelvic outlet. This is hazardous to the woman because it can result in vaginal or cervical tears. It is hazardous to the fetus if the cord is compressed between the fetal body and the bony pelvis. The force of birth can result in a fractured clavicle or a brachial plexus injury for the fetus.

Shoulder dystocia is most apt to occur in women with diabetes, in multiparas, and in post-date pregnancies. The problem often is not identified until the head has already been born and the wide anterior shoulder locks beneath the symphysis pubis. The condition may be suspected earlier if the second stage of labor is prolonged, if there is arrest of descent, or if, when the head appears on the perineum (crowning), it retracts instead of protruding with each contraction (a turtle sign).

Although there is no evidence-based data, asking a woman to flex her thighs sharply on her abdomen (McRobert's maneuver) may widen the pelvic outlet and allow the anterior shoulder to be born. Applying suprapubic pressure may also help the shoulder escape from beneath the symphysis pubis and be born (Athukorala, Middleton, & Crowther, 2009).

Fetal Anomalies

Fetal anomalies of the head such as hydrocephalus (fluid-filled ventricles) or anencephaly (absence of the cranium) can also complicate birth because the fetal presenting part does not engage the cervix well (see Chapter 27 for a discussion of these).

PROBLEMS WITH THE PASSAGE

Still another reason that dystocia can occur is a contraction or narrowing of the passageway or birth canal. This can happen at the inlet, at the midpelvis, or at the outlet. The narrowing causes CPD, or a disproportion between the size of the fetal head and the pelvic diameters. This results in failure to progress in labor.

Inlet Contraction

Inlet contraction is narrowing of the anteroposterior diameter to less than 11 cm, or of the transverse diameter to 12 cm or less. It usually is caused by rickets in early life or by an inherited small pelvis. Rickets is rare in developed countries but can occur among immigrants who were raised in an undeveloped country where milk supplies were not plentiful. In primigravidas, the fetal head normally engages between weeks 36 to 38 of pregnancy. If this occurs before labor begins, it is proof that the pelvic inlet is adequate. Following the general rule that "what goes in, comes out," a head that engages or proves it fits into the pelvic brim will probably also be able to pass through the midpelvis and through the outlet.

If engagement does not occur in a primigravida, then either a fetal abnormality (larger-than-usual head) or a pelvic abnormality (smaller-than-usual pelvis) should be suspected.

As a rule, engagement does not occur in multigravidas until labor begins. For these women, previous birth of a full-term infant vaginally without problems is proof that their birth canals are adequate.

Every primigravida should have pelvic measurements taken and recorded before week 24 of pregnancy. Based on these measurements and the assumption the fetus will be of average size, a birth decision can be made.

With CPD, because the fetus does not engage but remains "floating," malposition may occur, further complicating an already difficult situation. Should the membranes rupture, the possibility of cord prolapse increases greatly.

Outlet Contraction

Outlet contraction is narrowing of the transverse diameter at the outlet to less than 11 cm. This is the distance between the ischial tuberosities, a measurement that is easy to make during a prenatal visit, so the narrow diameter can be anticipated before labor begins. It is also easily reassessed during labor (see Chapter 15).

Trial Labor

If a woman has a borderline (just adequate) inlet measurement and the fetal lie and position are good, her physician or nurse-midwife may allow her a "trial" labor to determine whether labor can progress normally. A trial labor continues as long as descent of the presenting part and dilatation of the cervix continue to occur. Monitor fetal heart sounds and uterine contractions continuously, if possible, during this time. Urge the woman to void every 2 hours so that her urinary bladder is as empty as possible, allowing the fetal head to use all the space available. After rupture of the membranes, assess FHR carefully; if the fetal head is still high, there is an increased danger of prolapsed cord and anoxia to the fetus. If after a definite period (6 to 12 hours) adequate progress in labor cannot be documented, or if at any time fetal distress occurs, the woman will be scheduled for a cesarean birth.

It may be difficult for women to undertake labor they know they may be unable to complete, because the effort subjects them needlessly to pain. Emphasize, but do not overstress, that it is best for their baby to be born vaginally. If the trial labor fails and cesarean birth is scheduled, provide an explanation about why cesarean birth is necessary and now is the best route for the birth of their baby (Box 23.11).

Some women undergoing a trial labor feel as if they themselves are on trial. When dilatation does not occur, they feel discouraged and inadequate, as if they are somehow at fault or have failed. A woman may not be aware of how much she wanted the trial labor to work until she is told it is not working. The support person also may be as frightened and feel as helpless as the woman when a deviation occurs in labor. You can assure a woman and her support person that a cesarean birth will be an alternative, not an inferior, method of birth for them. Because labor is not progressing, it is the best method of choice to allow them to achieve their goal of a healthy mother and healthy child.

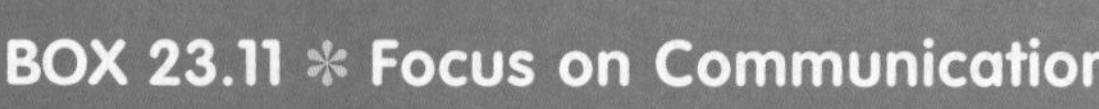

BOX 23.11 ✻ Focus on Communication

Roseann Bigalow is having her first baby. Her physician has told her she has a borderline pelvis but he wants her to try a trial labor.

Less Effective Communication

Nurse: Hello, Roseann. Is it all right if I attach a fetal heart rate and uterine contraction monitor so we can observe you closely during labor?

Roseann: Sure. Although I should have this baby any minute. It's already been 10 hours.

Nurse: I thought I heard your doctor say he's thinking of this as a trial labor.

Roseann: Whatever. I told him anything but surgery would be all right.

Nurse: I'm glad you have a positive outlook. That always makes labor seem to go faster.

More Effective Communication

Nurse: Hello, Roseann. Is it all right if I attach a fetal heart rate and uterine contraction monitor so we can observe you closely during labor?

Roseann: Sure. Although I should have this baby any minute. It's already been 10 hours.

Nurse: I thought I heard your doctor say he's thinking of this as a trial labor.

Roseann: Whatever. I told him anything but surgery would be all right.

Nurse: Let's talk about what a trial labor means.

If a woman develops a complication of pregnancy that is referred to by a strange name, it is generally expected that the couple will not understand the term and will need to have it thoroughly explained. If a condition has a common name, such as protracted pelvis or trial labor, however, it is easy to assume that little explanation of the condition is necessary. In reality, couples need explanations about all conditions, because what is common to health care personnel is not common to everyone. In the first scenario, the nurse assumed that she and the woman were talking about the same thing. In the second scenario, the nurse explored a little further and discovered that Roseann was not aware a trial labor might mean she would need surgery.

External Cephalic Version

External cephalic version is the turning of a fetus from a breech to a cephalic position before birth. It may be done as early as 34 to 35 weeks, although the usual time is 37 to 38 weeks of pregnancy (Hofmeyr & Gyte, 2009). For the procedure, FHR and possibly ultrasound are recorded continuously. A tocolytic agent may be administered to help relax the uterus. The breech and vertex of the fetus are located and grasped transabdominally by the examiner's hands on the woman's abdomen. Gentle pressure is then exerted to rotate the fetus in a forward direction to a cephalic lie (Fig. 23.13). Although not always successful, the use of external version can decrease the number of cesarean births necessary from breech presentations (Kish & Collea, 2007). Contraindications to the procedure include multiple gestation, severe oligohydramnios, contraindications to vaginal birth, a cord that wraps around the fetal neck, and unexplained third-trimester bleeding, which might

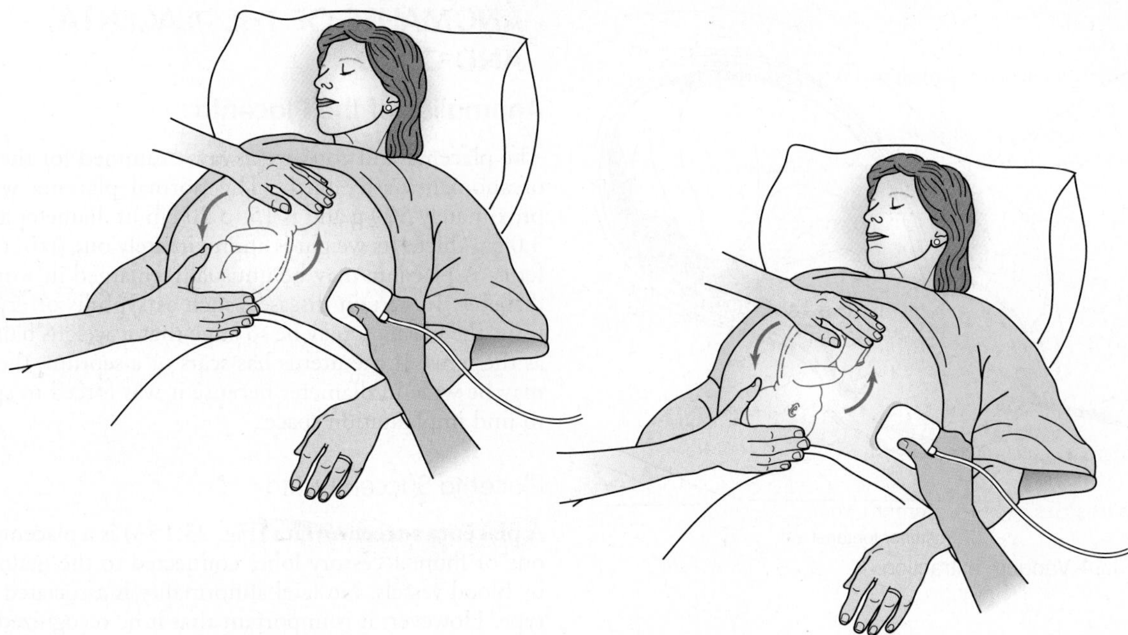

FIGURE 23.13 External cephalic version. The fetus is rotated by external pressure to a cephalic lie. An ultrasound helps guide a safe result.

be a placenta previa. External version can be uncomfortable for a woman because of the feeling of pressure. Women who are Rh negative should receive Rh immunoglobulin after the procedure in case minimal bleeding occurs.

Forceps Birth

Obstetrical forceps are steel instruments constructed of two blades that slide together at their shaft to form a handle. One blade is slipped into the woman's vagina next to the fetal head, and then the other is slipped into place on the other side of the head. Next, the shafts of the instrument are brought together in the midline to form the handle. The physician then applies pressure on the handle to manually extract the fetus from the birth canal.

In years past, babies were routinely born with forceps. Today, the technique is rarely used (about 4% to 8% of births) because it can lead to rectal sphincter tears in the woman which lead to dyspareunia, anal incontinence, or increased urinary stress incontinence in women (Mous, Muller, & De Leeuw, 2008). Forceps may be necessary, however, if any of the following conditions occur:

- A woman is unable to push with contractions in the pelvic division of labor such as might happen with a woman who receives regional anesthesia or has a spinal cord injury.
- Cessation of descent in the second stage of labor occurs.
- A fetus is in an abnormal position or is immature.
- A fetus is in distress from a complication such as a prolapsed cord.

Although forceps appear as if they would put forceful pressure on the fetal head, the pressure registers on the steel blades rather than the head so they actually reduce pressure. Reducing pressure in this way can avoid subdural hemorrhage in a fetus as the fetal head reaches the perineum, which is why forceps may be used with preterm birth (Incerpi, 2007).

A **forceps birth** is a forceps outlet procedure in which the forceps are applied after the fetal head reaches the perineum. The term *low forceps birth* may be used to indicate that the fetal head is at a +2 station or more. If the fetal head is engaged but at less than +2 station, the procedure is called a *midforceps birth*. This type of forceps extraction is rarely justified, because it has been associated with birth trauma to both the woman and the fetus, and cesarean birth involves less risk. Some anesthesia, at least a pudendal block, is necessary for forceps application to achieve pelvic relaxation and reduce pain. Usually, an episiotomy is performed to prevent perineal tearing due to pressure on the perineum.

Before forceps are applied,

- Membranes must be ruptured.
- CPD must not be present.
- The cervix must be fully dilated.
- The woman's bladder must be empty.

Record FHR before forceps application. Because there is a danger that the cord could be compressed between the forceps blade and the fetal head, assess FHR again immediately after application. The woman's cervix needs to be carefully assessed after forceps birth to be certain that no laceration has occurred. To rule out bladder injury, record the time and amount of the first voiding. In addition, assess the newborn to be certain that no facial palsy or subdural hematoma exists. A forceps birth may leave a transient erythematous mark on the newborn's cheek (see Chapter 18). This mark will fade in 1 to 2 days with no long-term effects.

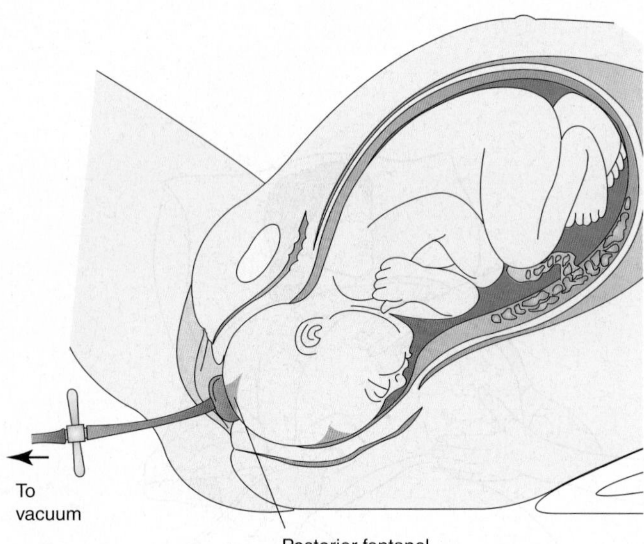

FIGURE 23.14 Vacuum extraction.

Vacuum Extraction

A fetus, if positioned far enough down the birth canal, may be born by **vacuum extraction** (Incerpi, 2007). With the fetal head at the perineum, a disk-shaped cup is pressed against the fetal scalp, over the posterior fontanelle. When vacuum pressure is applied, air beneath the cup is suctioned out and the cup then adheres so tightly to the fetal scalp that traction on the cord leading to the cup extracts the fetus (Fig. 23.14).

Vacuum extraction has advantages over forceps birth in that little anesthesia is necessary (leaving the fetus with less respiratory depression at birth) and fewer lacerations of the birth canal occur (Johanson & Menon, 2009). Its major disadvantage is that it causes a marked caput on the newborn head that may be noticeable as long as 7 days after birth. Tentorial tears from extreme pressure also have occurred. A woman may need reassurance that the caput swelling is harmless to her infant and will decrease rapidly. Vacuum extraction should not be used as a method of birth if fetal scalp blood sampling was used, because the suction pressure can cause severe bleeding at the sampling site. Moreover, vacuum extraction is not advantageous for preterm infants because of the softness of the preterm skull.

ANOMALIES OF THE PLACENTA AND CORD

Anomalies of the Placenta

The placenta and cord are always examined for the presence of anomalies after birth. The normal placenta weighs approximately 500 g and is 15 to 20 cm in diameter and 1.5 to 3.0 cm thick. Its weight is approximately one sixth that of the fetus. A placenta may be unusually enlarged in women with diabetes. In certain diseases, such as syphilis or erythroblastosis, the placenta may be so large that it weighs half as much as the fetus. If the uterus has scars or a septum, the placenta may be wide in diameter because it was forced to spread out to find implantation space.

Placenta Succenturiata

A **placenta succenturiata** (Fig. 23.15A) is a placenta that has one or more accessory lobes connected to the main placenta by blood vessels. No fetal abnormality is associated with this type. However, it is important that it be recognized, because the small lobes may be retained in the uterus after birth, leading to severe maternal hemorrhage. On inspection, the placenta appears torn at the edge, or torn blood vessels extend beyond the edge of the placenta. The remaining lobes are removed from the uterus manually to prevent maternal hemorrhage from poor uterine contraction.

Placenta Circumvallata

Ordinarily, the chorion membrane begins at the edge of the placenta and spreads to envelop the fetus; no chorion covers the fetal side of the placenta. In **placenta circumvallata,** the fetal side of the placenta is covered to some extent with chorion (see Fig. 23.15B). The umbilical cord enters the placenta at the usual midpoint, and large vessels spread out from there. They end abruptly at the point where the chorion folds back onto the surface, however. (In **placenta marginata,** the fold of chorion reaches just to the edge of the placenta.) Although no abnormalities are associated with this type of placenta, its presence should be noted.

Battledore Placenta

In a **battledore placenta,** the cord is inserted marginally rather than centrally (see Fig. 23.15C). This anomaly is rare and has no known clinical significance either.

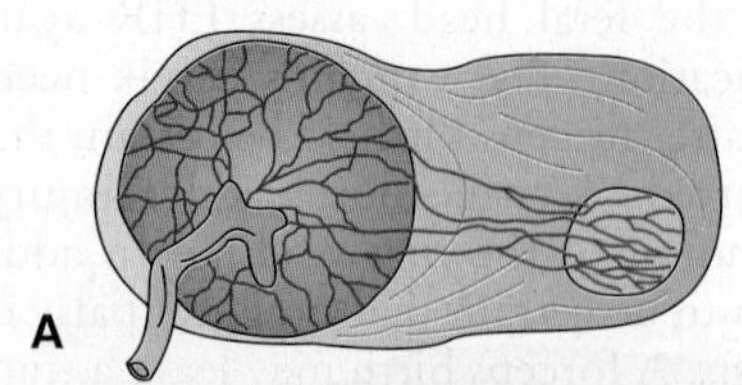

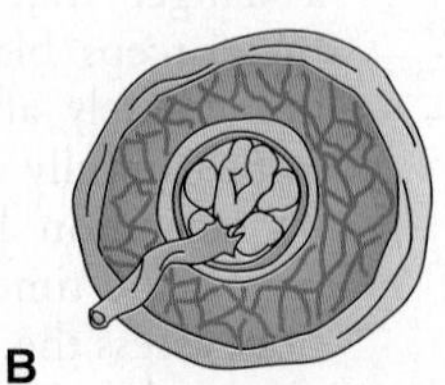

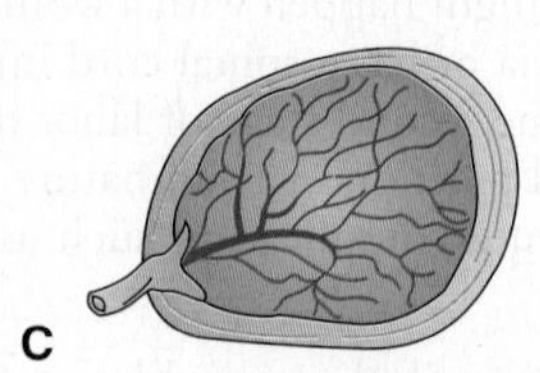

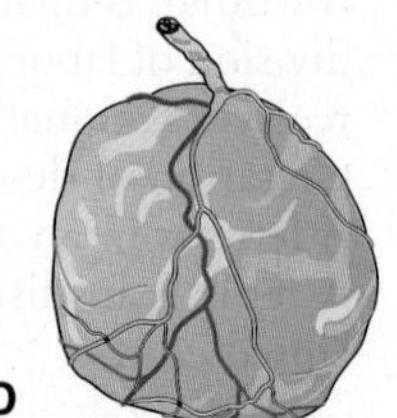

FIGURE 23.15 Abnormal placental formation. (**A**) Placenta succenturiata. (**B**) Placenta circumvallata. (**C**) Battledore placenta. (**D**) Velamentous cord insertion.

Velamentous Insertion of the Cord

Velamentous insertion of the cord is a situation in which the cord, instead of entering the placenta directly, separates into small vessels that reach the placenta by spreading across a fold of amnion (see Fig. 23.15D). This form of cord insertion is most frequently found with multiple gestation. Because it may be associated with fetal anomalies, an infant born with this type of placenta should be examined carefully.

Vasa Previa

In vasa previa, the umbilical vessels of a velamentous cord insertion cross the cervical os and therefore deliver before the fetus (Strehlow & Uzelac, 2007). The vessels may tear with cervical dilatation, just as a placenta previa may tear. Before inserting any instrument such as an internal fetal monitor, be certain to identify structures to prevent accidental tearing of a vasa previa as tearing would result in sudden fetal blood loss. If sudden, painless bleeding occurs with the beginning of cervical dilatation, either placenta previa or vasa previa is suspected. It can be confirmed by ultrasound. If vasa previa is identified, the infant needs to be born by cesarean birth.

Placenta Accreta

Placenta accreta is an unusually deep attachment of the placenta to the uterine myometrium so deeply the placenta will not loosen and deliver (Poggi, 2007). Attempts to remove it manually may lead to extreme hemorrhage because of the deep attachment. Hysterectomy or treatment with methotrexate to destroy the still-attached tissue may be necessary.

Anomalies of the Cord

Two-Vessel Cord

A normal cord contains one vein and two arteries. The absence of one of the umbilical arteries is associated with congenital heart and kidney anomalies, because the insult that caused the loss of the vessel may have affected other mesoderm germ layer structures as well. Inspection of the cord as to how many vessels are present must be made immediately after birth, before the cord begins to dry, because drying distorts the appearance of the vessels. Document the number of vessels present conscientiously. An infant with only two vessels needs to be observed carefully for other anomalies during the newborn period.

Unusual Cord Length

Although the length of the umbilical cord rarely varies, some abnormal lengths may occur. An unusually short umbilical cord can result in premature separation of the placenta or an abnormal fetal lie. An unusually long cord may be easily compromised because of its tendency to twist or knot. Occasionally, a cord actually forms a knot, but the natural pulsations of the blood through the vessels and the muscular vessel walls usually keep the blood flow adequate. It is not unusual for a cord to wrap once around the fetal neck (nuchal cord) but, again, with no interference to fetal circulation (Reed, 2007).

✓ Checkpoint Question 23.3

Oxytocin is administered to Roseann to augment labor. What are the first symptoms of water intoxication to observe for during this procedure?

a. A high, choking voice.
b. Headache and vomiting.
c. A swollen, tender tongue.
d. Abdominal bloating and pain.

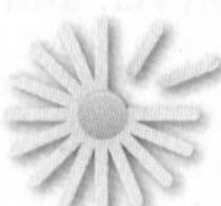

Key Points for Review

- Complications of labor can arise from problems with the force of labor, the passage, the passenger, or the woman's reaction to the experience (the psyche). Hypotonic, hypertonic, and uncoordinated contractions all can occur, resulting in ineffective first or second stages of labor.
- Precipitate labor is birth that is completed in less than 3 hours. It can be responsible for subdural hemorrhage in the fetus and cervical lacerations in the woman.
- Uterine rupture, although rare, is usually preceded by a pathologic retraction ring (shown by an indentation across the abdomen over the uterus).
- Uterine inversion is a grave complication. If the situation is not immediately corrected, emergency hysterectomy is necessary to save the woman's life. Almost all occurrences of uterine inversion can be avoided by two axioms of care: (a) *do not put pressure on an uncontracted fundus immediately after birth* (massage it first to cause it to contract); and (b) *do not exert pressure on an umbilical cord to achieve placental delivery.*
- Amniotic fluid embolism occurs when amniotic fluid is forced into an open maternal uterine blood sinus. A woman notices chest pain and dyspnea. Administer oxygen and notify the woman's primary care provider of this emergency.
- Prolapse of the umbilical cord is an emergency situation that requires prompt action. Position a woman quickly into either a Trendelenburg or a knee–chest position to relieve cord compression, or apply manual pressure vaginally to lift the fetal head away from the cord. Notify the woman's primary caregiver of the emergency.
- Multiple gestation can complicate birth. Many infants of multiple gestations are born by cesarean birth.
- Abnormal position, presentation, or size of the fetus (such as occipitoposterior position; breech, face, or brow presentation; transverse lie), as well as problems of the passage such as inlet and outlet contraction, can lead to labor complications.
- Be certain a woman meets the criteria for labor induction before preparing an oxytocin solution. These criteria include engagement of the fetal head, a "ripe" cervix, and absence of CPD. Question an order if these criteria are not met.
- Always prepare oxytocin as a "piggyback" solution, being extremely careful of the dose used. Both a uterine

monitor and an FHR monitor should be used continuously during labor induction. Observe that contractions occur no less than 2 minutes apart and are no longer than 70 seconds in duration.

- Vacuum extraction and forceps are methods to assist birth. The woman as well as the infant needs special observation after these procedures to detect head trauma or cervical or vaginal tearing.
- Anomalies of the placenta and cord (such as placenta succenturiata, velamentous cord insertion, vasi a previa, and two-vessel cord) can lead to birth complications.

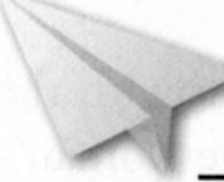

CRITICAL THINKING EXERCISES

1. Roseann Bigalow is the woman you met at the beginning of the chapter. Her fetus is in a posterior position, and she has severe back pain. What actions could her husband take to help relieve his wife's pain caused by this posterior fetal position?
2. Suppose that, after rupture of Roseann's membranes, the fetal monitor shows variable decelerations. On inspection, you are able to see the umbilical cord at the vaginal opening. You are aware that this is a fetal emergency. In order of priority, what would be your best actions?
3. Roseann is scheduled for augmentation of labor with oxytocin. What factors would you ensure are in place before augmentation is begun?
4. Examine the National Health Goals related to complications of labor. Most government-sponsored funds for nursing research are allotted based on these goals. What would be a possible research topic to explore pertinent to these goals that would be applicable to the Bigalow family and also advance evidence-based practice?

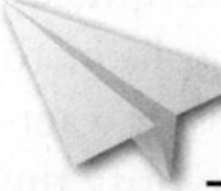

CRITICAL THINKING SCENARIO

Open the accompanying CD-ROM or visit http://thePoint.lww.com and read the Patient Scenario included for this chapter, then answer the questions to further sharpen your skills and grow more familiar with NCLEX style questions related to nursing care of a family with a complication of labor. Confirm your answers are correct by reading the rationales.

REFERENCES

Alfirevic, Z., & Weeks, A. (2009). Oral misoprostol for induction of labour. *Cochrane Database of Systematic Reviews, 2009*(1), (CD001338).

Archie, C. L. (2007). The course and conduct of normal labor and delivery. In A. H. DeCherney & L. Nathan (Eds.). *Current diagnosis and treatment in obstetrics and gynecology* (10th ed.). Columbus, OH: McGraw-Hill.

Athukorala, C., Middleton, P., & Crowther, C. A. (2009). Intrapartum interventions for preventing shoulder dystocia. *Cochrane Database of Systematic Reviews, 2009*(1), (CD005543).

Bishop, E. H. (1964). Pelvic scoring for elective induction. *Obstetrics and Gynecology, 24*(2), 266.

Buhimschi, C .S. (2009). Spatiotemporal electromyography during human labor to monitor propagation of the uterine contraction wave and diagnose dystocia. *American Journal of Obstetrics & Gynecology, 2009*(1), 1–3.

Campaigne, A. L., & Conway, D. L. (2007). Detection and prevention of macrosomia. *Obstetrics and Gynecology Clinics of North America, 34*(2), 309–322.

Cheng, Y. W., et al. (2007). Duration of the second stage of labor in multiparous women: maternal and neonatal outcomes. *American Journal of Obstetrics and Gynecology, 196*(6), 585–590.

Chhabra, S., Dargan R., & Nasare, M. (2007). Antepartum transabdominal amnioinfusion. *International Journal of Gynaecology and Obstetrics, 97*(2), 95–99.

Cruikshank, D. P. (2007). Intrapartum management of twin gestations. *Obstetrics and Gynecology, 109*(5), 1167–1176.

Fortner, K. B., Althaus, J. E., & Gurewitsch, E. D. (2007). Gestational complications. In K. B. Fortner, et al. (Eds.). *The Johns Hopkins manual of gynecology and obstetrics*. Philadelphia: Lippincott Williams & Wilkins.

Friedman, E. A. (1978). *Labor: clinical evaluation and management* (2nd ed.). New York: Appleton.

Gomez, L. M., et al. (2008). Placental infection with human papillomavirus is associated with spontaneous preterm delivery. *Human Reproduction, 23*(3), 709–715.

Has, R., et al. (2008). Imaging features of postpartum uterine rupture: a case report. *Abdominal Imaging, 33*(1), 101–103.

Hofmeyr, G. J. (2009). Amnioinfusion for potential or suspected umbilical cord compression in labour. *Cochrane Database of Systematic Reviews, 2009*(1), (CD000013).

Hofmeyr, G. J., & Gulmezoglu, A. M. (2009). Vaginal misoprostol for cervical ripening and induction of labour. *Cochrane Database of Systematic Reviews, 2009*(1), (CD000941).

Hofmeyr, G. J., & Gyte, G. (2009). Interventions to help external cephalic version for breech presentation at term. *Cochrane Database of Systematic Reviews, 2009*(1), (CD000184).

Howarth, G. R., & Botha, D. J. (2009). Amniotomy plus intravenous oxytocin for induction of labour. *Cochrane Database of Systematic Reviews, 2009*(1), (CD003250).

Incerpi, M. H. (2007). Operative delivery. In A. H. DeCherney & L. Nathan (Eds.). *Current diagnosis and treatment in obstetrics and gynecology* (10th ed.). Columbus, OH: McGraw-Hill.

Johanson, R. B., & Menon, V. (2009).Vacuum extraction versus forceps for assisted vaginal delivery. *Cochrane Database of Systematic Reviews, 2009*(1), (CD000224).

Karch, A. M. (2009). *Lippincott's nursing drug guide* (11th ed.). Philadelphia: Lippincott Williams & Wilkins.

Kish, K., & Collea, J. V. (2007). Malpresentation and cord prolapse. In A. H. DeCherney & L. Nathan (Eds.). *Current diagnosis and treatment in obstetrics and gynecology* (10th ed.). Columbus, OH: McGraw-Hill.

Lauria, M. R., et al. (2007). Pathologic uterine ring associated with fetal head trauma and subsequent cerebral palsy. *Obstetrics and Gynecology, 109*(2.2), 495–497.

Lawson, S. M., & Bienstock, J. L. (2007). Normal labor and delivery, operative delivery, and malpresentations. In K. B. Fortner, et al. (Eds.). *The Johns Hopkins manual of gynecology and obstetrics*. Philadelphia: Lippincott Williams & Wilkins.

Longo, M., & Hankins, G. D. V. (2007). External cephalic version. *Contemporary OB/GYN, 52*(5), 64–69.

Mous, M., Muller, S. A., & de Leeuw, J. W. (2008). Long-term effects of anal sphincter rupture during vaginal delivery: faecal incontinence and sexual complaints. *BJOG: An International Journal of Obstetrics and Gynaecology, 115*(2), 234–238.

Poggi, S. B. H. (2007). Postpartum hemorrhage and the abnormal puerperium. In A. H. DeCherney & L. Nathan (Eds.). *Current diagnosis and treatment in obstetrics and gynecology* (10th ed.). Columbus, OH: McGraw-Hill.

Reed, R. (2007). Nuchal cords: think before you check. *Practising Midwife, 10*(5), 18–20.

Ridley, R. T. (2007). Diagnosis and intervention for occiput posterior malposition. *JOGNN: Journal of Obstetric, Gynecologic, and Neonatal Nursing, 36*(2), 135–143.

Scearce, J., & Uzelac, P. S. (2007). Third-trimester vaginal bleeding. In A. H. DeCherney & L. Nathan (Eds.). *Current diagnosis and treatment in obstetrics and gynecology* (10th ed.). Columbus, OH: McGraw-Hill.

Schoening, A. M. (2007). Amniotic fluid embolism: recognizing trouble. *Nursing, 37*(1), 1–3.

Shields, S. G., et al. (2007). Dystocia in nulliparous women. *American Family Physician, 75*(11), 1671–1678.

Smith, C. A. (2009). Homoeopathy for induction of labour. *Cochrane Database of Systematic Reviews, 2009*(1), (CD003399).

Strehlow, S., & Uzelac, P. (2007). Complications of labor and delivery. In A. H. DeCherney & L. Nathan (Eds.). *Current diagnosis and treatment in obstetrics and gynecology* (10th ed.). Columbus, OH: McGraw-Hill.

Szymanski, L. M., & Bienstock, J. L. (2007). Complications of labor and delivery. In K. B. Fortner, et al. (Eds.). *The Johns Hopkins manual of gynecology and obstetrics*. Philadelphia: Lippincott Williams & Wilkins.

SUGGESTED READINGS

Bailit, J. L., et al. (2008). Maternal-Fetal Medicine Units Network cesarean registry: impact of shift change on cesarean complications. *American Journal of Obstetrics and Gynecology, 198*(2), 173–178.

Bricker, L., & Luckas, M. (2009). Amniotomy alone for induction of labour. *Cochrane Database of Systematic Reviews, 2009*(1), (CD002862).

Getahun, D., Ananth, C. V., & Kinzler, W. L. (2007). Risk factors for antepartum and intrapartum stillbirth: a population-based study. *American Journal of Obstetrics and Gynecology, 196*(6), 499–507.

Greulich, B., & Tarrant, B. (2007). The latent phase of labor: diagnosis and management. *Journal of Midwifery and Women's Health, 52*(3), 190–198.

Hill, P. D., & Aldag, J. C. (2007). Maternal perceived quality of life following childbirth. *JOGNN: Journal of Obstetric, Gynecologic, and Neonatal Nursing, 36*(4), 328–334.

Lowe, N. K. (2007). A review of factors associated with dystocia and cesarean section in nulliparous women. *Journal of Midwifery and Women's Health, 52*(3), 216–228.

Lydon-Rochelle, M. T., et al. (2007). Induction of labor in the absence of standard medical indications: incidence and correlates. *Medical Care, 45*(6), 505–512.

McDonald, S. (2007). Management of the third stage of labor. *Journal of Midwifery and Women's Health, 52*(3), 254–261.

Prendiville, W. J., Elbourne, D., & McDonald, S. (2009). Active versus expectant management in the third stage of labour. *Cochrane Database of Systematic Reviews, 2009*(1), (CD000007).

Williams, A., Herron-Marx, S., & Knibb, R. (2007). The prevalence of enduring postnatal perineal morbidity and its relationship to type of birth and birth risk factors. *Journal of Clinical Nursing, 16*(3), 549–561.

Chapter 24 Nursing Care of a Family During Cesarean Birth

KEY TERMS

- cesarean birth
- classic cesarean incision
- dehiscence
- low segment incision

OBJECTIVES

After mastering the contents of this chapter, you should be able to:

1. Describe the usual indications for cesarean birth.
2. Identify National Health Goals related to cesarean birth that nurses can help the nation achieve.
3. Use critical thinking to analyze how to keep birth family centered when a cesarean birth is scheduled.
4. Assess a woman scheduled for cesarean birth for effective preoperative, intraoperative, and postoperative needs.
5. Formulate nursing diagnoses related to the family experiencing a cesarean birth.
6. Establish outcomes that meet the needs of a woman requiring a cesarean birth.
7. Plan appropriate nursing care for the family experiencing a cesarean birth.
8. Implement common preoperative and postoperative care measures for cesarean birth.
9. Evaluate expected outcomes for achievement and effectiveness of care.
10. Identify areas related to cesarean birth that could benefit from additional nursing research or application of evidence-based practice.
11. Integrate knowledge of cesarean birth with the nursing process to achieve quality maternal and child health nursing care.

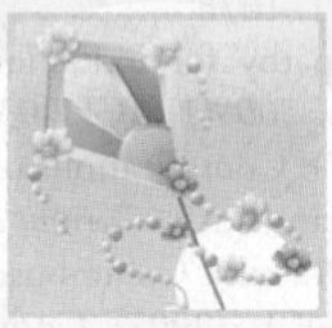

Moja Hamma is a 29-year-old woman pregnant with her first baby. Her labor began with ruptured membranes and dark green meconium-stained amniotic fluid. Moja called her nurse-midwife, who asked her to come to the hospital immediately. Moja drove herself and arrived in 20 minutes. Fetal heart rate was 100 beats per minute. An obstetrician was consulted, and she scheduled Moja for an immediate cesarean birth. Moja reacted calmly to the news that she needed surgery until she realized her boyfriend would not be able to get to the hospital until her surgery was over. At that point she refused to sign for permission, saying, "I can't. I just can't go through this alone."

Previous chapters described the physiology of labor and the sequence of usual birth. This chapter adds information about cesarean birth for those women who choose to have cesarean birth or must have a cesarean birth to ensure a safe outcome for themselves or their child.

Is Moja's response typical of a woman who is told she needs a surgical procedure for the birth of her baby?

What would be your best action to help her accept this procedure?

Cesarean birth, or birth accomplished through an abdominal incision into the uterus, is one of the oldest types of surgical procedures known. It is always slightly more hazardous than vaginal birth, but compared with other surgical procedures, it is one of the safest types of surgeries and one with few complications (Lavender et al., 2009).

The word "cesarean" is derived from the Latin word *caedore,* which means "to cut." At one time, there was a popular belief that Julius Caesar was born by a cesarean birth and the procedure was named for him. However, because Caesar was born before antibiotics and sterile surgical technique, it seems unlikely that his mother (who is known to have been alive in his adult years) would have survived such a procedure.

The term *cesarean birth,* rather than *cesarean delivery,* is used to accentuate that this is a birth more than a surgical procedure. National Health Goals related to cesarean birth are shown in Box 24.1.

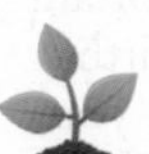

Nursing Process Overview

For a Woman Having a Cesarean Birth

Assessment

Some women elect cesarean rather than vaginal birth. Some women with smaller-than-usual pelvic diameters are told during pregnancy that a cesarean birth may be necessary. Others learn only during labor that a cesarean birth is necessary because a complication is developing. Assessment as to whether a woman will be a good candidate for surgery is sometimes done throughout pregnancy and sometimes done very quickly in an emergency. Either way, assessment must include both physiologic and psychological status and preparedness.

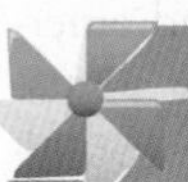

BOX 24.1 ✻ Focus on National Health Goals

Two National Health Goals speak directly to cesarean birth:

- Reduce the rate of cesarean births among low-risk (full-term, singleton, vertex presentation) women having their first child to 15% of live births from a baseline of 18%.
- Reduce the rate of cesarean births among women who have had a prior cesarean birth to 63% of live births from a baseline of 72% (http://www.nih.gov).

Nurses can help the nation achieve these goals by encouraging women who fulfill the criteria for vaginal birth after cesarean (VBAC) to attempt a vaginal birth with a second child.

Additional nursing research in this area could include studies and application of evidence-based practice on the effect of nursing practice and the cesarean birth rate, effective pain management for cesarean birth, and measures to help the family adjust smoothly from the hospital to the home setting after a cesarean birth.

Nursing Diagnosis

Nursing diagnoses specific to cesarean birth are often related to prevention of common complications from surgery or patient/family concerns about surgical birth. Specific examples might include:

- Risk for infection related to a surgical incision
- Fear related to impending surgery
- Pain related to a surgical incision
- Deficient fluid volume related to blood loss from surgery
- Powerlessness related to medical need for cesarean birth

Outcome Identification and Planning

The same important outcome applies to a woman giving birth by cesarean as a woman giving birth vaginally: a healthy mother and a healthy child. Because cesarean birth decisions can be made suddenly, planning can be limited to only a few minutes. This means you have only a very short time to organize presurgical steps such as gastrointestinal or anesthesia preparation (and run through the presurgical checklist when it is an emergency). Plans must include discharge instructions and home care, because a woman will remain in the health care facility only 2 or 3 days. For a woman who knows in advance that she will have a cesarean birth, helpful Web sites to use for referral are the March of Dimes (http://www.marchofdimes.com) and the International Cesarean Awareness Network (http://www.ICAN-ONLINE.org).

Implementation

Every woman is aware that childbirth poses some risk to her health. When major surgery is superimposed on top of this, it is imperative that a woman and her support person feel confidence in the health care personnel who will care for them. Otherwise, they could have difficulty coping with the additional insult of surgery. When giving care to any woman during labor, be certain to establish early on a helping relationship with both the woman and her support person. This relationship becomes especially advantageous should the birth method need to be altered.

An important intervention includes coordination of health care team members such as an anesthesiologist, surgeon, pediatrician or neonatologist, and recovery room or nursery personnel (Box 24.2). This is particularly important if the surgery will be performed in a hospital surgery department rather than in a labor and birthing suite, or if the infant will be transferred to an intensive care nursery or a distant site for intensive care after the birth.

Many interventions focus on teaching and support, because the more a woman understands about what is happening, the more she can accept and cooperate with procedures. During surgery, sterile technique is essential. A postpartal infection can be devastating to a woman who already has made many other physical adaptations. After surgery, be sure to provide adequate "talk time" to allow a woman time to review what has happened and integrate it into what she and her partner expected.

Outcome Evaluation

Evaluation of expected outcomes is important in the care of a woman after cesarean birth to ensure she is not

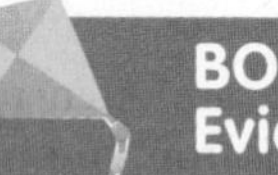

BOX 24.2 * Focus on Evidence-Based Practice

Is cesarean birth less safe at health care personnel shift changes than at other times?

To answer this question, researchers reviewed the charts of 17,996 women who underwent an unscheduled cesarean birth. They examined the outcomes of their surgery and their newborns' well-being at both the times of physician change of shift (6 AM–8 AM, 5 PM–7 PM) and the time of nursing change of shift (6 AM–8 AM, 2 PM–4 PM, 10 PM–12 AM) and compared surgical outcome at these times to all other times. Results showed that physician change of shift made no measurable effect on maternal and neonatal outcomes. Surprisingly, neonatal facial nerve palsies and hysterectomies were significantly increased in incidence during nursing change of shift times. The researchers were unable to explain why this incidence occurred and suggested further research would be helpful to determine why this happened.

Suppose you were asked to plan an inservice program to help nurses on an obstetrical unit be more thorough in their reports at shift changes. Would the above study influence what you would include in your class?

Source: Bailit, J., et al. (2008). Maternal-Fetal Medicine Units Network cesarean registry: impact of shift change on cesarean complications. *American Journal of Obstetrics and Gynecology, 198*(2),173–177.

developing a complication. It is especially important to consider the overall goals of a healthy baby and a healthy mother and the development of a positive mother–infant (or parent– or family–infant) relationship. The following are examples that would demonstrate successful achievement of outcomes:

- Patient states that she understands the reason for a cesarean birth.
- Patient states that she felt well prepared for cesarean birth even in light of an emergency.
- Couple states that they feel able to cope with newborn care even with mother recovering from surgery.
- Patient remains free of signs and symptoms of infection after cesarean birth.
- Patient states that incisional pain is controlled and tolerable.
- Patient states birth was a fulfilling experience for her even in light of the unplanned cesarean birth.

CESAREAN BIRTH

Currently, cesarean birth is used most often as a prophylactic measure, to alleviate problems of birth such as cephalopelvic disproportion or failure to progress in labor.

A major concern in maternal and child health nursing is the increasing number of cesarean births being performed annually (Clark et al., 2007). In 1970, only 5.5% of women in the United States had infants born by cesarean birth. Currently, the incidence of primary cesarean births is about 30.2% or one-third of births (National Vital Statistics System [NVSS], 2008). This increased rate results from a combination of the increasing safety of cesarean birth, the use of fetal monitors (which provide for early detection of fetal problems), an increased incidence in obese women (Bhattacharva et al., 2007), and elective cesarean births chosen by women for convenience or to prevent potential urinary or anal incontinence later in life (Gourounti & Sandall, 2007; Lavender et al., 2009).

The increase in rate may also be related to physicians' fears of malpractice suits should a fetus be allowed to be born vaginally and then be discovered to have suffered anoxia. Although this present incidence of cesarean births is a concern, this concern must be weighed against the potential for the procedure to reduce the incidence of infants who are born cognitively or physically challenged or who die at birth. Few parents insist that giving birth vaginally is more important than ensuring the birth of a healthy baby by cesarean birth.

Several legal and ethical issues have arisen in recent years when women have refused to undergo cesarean birth after being advised that they need one. Because women do have a right to decide whether they will undergo surgery, the right to refuse the procedure is respected. In some instances, however, a court order for the procedure has been obtained to save a fetus. Most circumstances do not come to this point of conflict with health care providers. Maternal child care nurses should be aware of the opinion of their agency's ethics committee on this issue. As a rule, nurse-midwifery birthing services have a lower incidence of cesarean births than hospital services because of the higher incidence of low-risk women in these settings. Continuous support during labor appears to decrease the incidence (Hodnett et al., 2009).

Scheduled Cesarean Birth

There are two types of cesarean birth: scheduled and emergent. In the first instance, there is time for thorough preparation for the experience throughout the antepartal period. Some women even take a childbirth preparation class specifically for cesarean birth. With the second type of cesarean birth, preparation must be done much more rapidly but with the same concern for fully informing a woman and her support person about what circumstances created the need for a cesarean birth and how the birth will proceed. Cesarean birth is mentioned in most childbirth classes, so any woman who has taken such a class may at least understand that cesarean births are sometimes necessary.

In the 1950s, cesarean birth became a status symbol when Hollywood stars asked to have cesarean births to save themselves the strain of labor and in some instances to schedule the birth conveniently between movie contracts. The average woman came to think of cesarean birth not as a surgical procedure but as an easy method of painless childbirth. Because the risk of injury from cesarean birth is higher than that from vaginal birth, this philosophy put both women and fetuses at greater risk than necessary. Scheduling cesarean births this freely also resulted in preterm births.

Although many cesarean births are done because the woman had a past cesarean birth, with new surgical techniques, particularly the use of a low cervical incision, "once a cesarean, always a cesarean" no longer applies. Most women who have had a cesarean birth within the past 10 years are eligible to give birth vaginally in subsequent pregnancies if the circumstances otherwise are appropriate for vaginal birth (Dodd et al., 2009). The incidence of women electing a vaginal birth after a previous cesarean birth (VBAC) ranges from about 11% to 13% of women (NVSS, 2008). For more information on VBAC, see Chapter 15.

Cesarean birth is mandatory when there is a physical indication such as a transverse presentation, genital herpes, or cephalopelvic disproportion. Other indications for cesarean birth are shown in Box 24.3. Cesarean birth may reduce the transfer of the human immunodeficiency virus (HIV), hepatitis C, or herpes type 2 from mother to newborn, so it is recommended for women who have these infections (Read & Newell, 2009; McIntyre, Tosh, & McGuire, 2009). It can reduce mortality among infants presenting breech (Hofmeyr & Hannah, 2009). It may be advantageous for a preterm birth to avoid pressure on the fetal head (Robilio et al., 2007) or to avoid postprocedure stress incontinence but whether this last procedure helps is controversial (Dietz, 2007). It is generally contraindicated when there is a documented dead fetus (labor can be induced to avoid a surgical procedure).

Emergent Cesarean Birth

Emergent cesarean births are done for reasons such as placenta previa, premature separation of the placenta, fetal distress, or failure to progress in labor. An emergent cesarean birth carries with it the risk of any emergent surgery: the woman may not be a prime candidate for anesthesia and is psychologically unprepared for the experience. In addition, the woman may have a fluid and electrolyte imbalance and be both physically and emotionally exhausted from a long labor.

BOX 24.3 ✻ Selected Indications for Cesarean Birth

Maternal Factors
- Active genital herpes or perhaps human papillomavirus
- AIDS or HIV-positive status
- Cephalopelvic disproportion
- Cervical cerclage
- Disabling conditions, such as severe hypertension of pregnancy, that prevent pushing to accomplish the pelvic division of labor
- Failed induction or failure to progress in labor
- Obstructive benign or malignant tumor
- Previous cesarean birth by classic incision
- Elective—no indicated risks

Placenta Factors
- Placenta previa
- Premature separation of the placenta
- Umbilical cord prolapse

Fetal Factors
- Compound conditions such as macrosomic fetus in a breech lie
- Extreme low birth weight
- Fetal distress
- Major fetal anomalies, such as hydrocephalus
- Multigestation or conjoined twins
- Transverse fetal lie

Effects of Surgery on a Woman

Like any surgical procedure, cesarean birth has systemic effects.

Stress Response

Whenever the body is subjected to stress, either physical or psychosocial, it responds with measures to preserve the function of major body systems. This results in release of epinephrine and norepinephrine from the adrenal medulla. Epinephrine causes an increased heart rate, bronchial dilatation, and elevation of the blood glucose level. It also leads to peripheral vasoconstriction, which forces blood to the central circulation and increases blood pressure. These normally positive responses (the person is tensed or ready for action with good heart and lung function and glucose for energy) may antagonize anesthetic action, which is aimed at minimizing body activity. In the pregnant woman, such responses may minimize blood supply to the lower extremities. The woman is already prone to thrombophlebitis from stasis of blood flow, so these responses compound or greatly increase the risk of thrombophlebitis. Combined with interferences to major body systems, these effects can add to the risks of surgery.

Interference With Body Defenses

The skin serves as the primary line of defense against bacterial invasion. When skin is incised for a surgical procedure, this important line of defense is lost. Strict adherence to aseptic technique during surgery and in the days following the procedure are necessary to compensate for this impaired defense. If cesarean birth is performed hours after the membranes ruptured, a woman's risk for infection will be higher than if the membranes were intact. Many women receive prophylactic antibiotics, such as ampicillin (Omnipen), or a cephalosporin such as Ancef to ensure protection against postsurgical endometritis, even if the membranes were intact (Hopkins & Smaill, 2009).

Interference With Circulatory Function

Although vessels that must be cut for surgery are immediately clamped and ligated, some blood loss always occurs with surgery. Extensive blood loss can lead to hypovolemia and lowered blood pressure. This could lead to ineffective perfusion of all body tissues if the problem is not quickly recognized and corrected. The amount of blood lost in cesarean birth is comparatively high, because pelvic vessels are congested with blood waiting to supply the placenta. During a vaginal birth, a woman loses 300 to 500 mL of blood. This loss increases to 500 to 1000 mL with a cesarean birth.

Interference With Body Organ Function

When any body organ is handled, cut, or repaired in surgery, it may respond with a temporary disruption in function. Pressure from edema or inflammation as fluid moves into the injured area further impairs function of the primary organ involved, as well as that of surrounding organs. If blood vessels become compressed as a result of edema, distant organs may be deprived of blood flow, leading to reduced function in those organs. Postoperatively, close assessment, not only of the primary organ involved but of total body function, is necessary, therefore, to determine the total degree of disruption.

Because the uterus is handled during cesarean birth, it may not contract well afterward, which can lead to postpartum hemorrhage. For a surgeon to reach the uterus, the bladder must be displaced anteriorly. As a result of this handling, the bladder may not sense filling as well as usual after the procedure (Datta & Gutman, 2007). During surgery, pressure is also felt by the intestine, so a paralytic ileus or halting of intestinal function may occur (Gates, Brocklehurst, & Davis, 2009). Thrombopheblitis from impaired lower extremity blood flow is yet another possibility. After a cesarean birth, therefore, uterine, bladder, intestinal, and lower extremity circulatory function must all be carefully assessed.

Interference With Self-Image or Self-Esteem

Surgery always leaves an incisional scar that will be noticeable to some extent afterward. Fortunately, the scar resulting from cesarean birth (a horizontal one across the lower abdomen) is not overly noticeable, but its appearance may cause a woman to feel self-conscious later. Although most women accept cesarean birth well, a woman may feel a loss of self-esteem if she believes it marks her as a woman less than others because she was unable to give vaginal birth (Wiklund et al., 2008).

✔ Checkpoint Question 24.1

Moja Hamma is concerned she may lose an excessive amount of blood with cesarean surgery. What is the usual amount of blood lost with cesarean birth?

a. 100–220 mL
b. 250–350 mL
c. 300–500 mL
d. 500–1000 mL

NURSING CARE OF A WOMAN ANTICIPATING A CESAREAN BIRTH

A woman who is admitted to the hospital for an anticipated cesarean birth may be more worried about the procedure, because she has had more time to worry, than a woman who is told during labor that an emergent cesarean is necessary. After the woman is admitted to the health care facility, allow her time to talk about any fears she has. Encourage her to do as much as possible for herself preoperatively, to help her feel in control and diminish her fear (Lobel & DeLuca, 2007).

A woman undergoing surgery cannot begin to relax as long as her support person is nervous and worried. Make a point of including this person in all explanations and admission routines, to keep his or her anxiety under control as well.

Preoperative Interview

Both the physician and the anesthesiologist or nurse-anesthetist will interview a woman preoperatively to obtain a health history and make an assessment and decision for safe use of anesthesia. A nursing assessment is also essential. Be sure to ask about any past surgeries, secondary illnesses, allergies to foods or drugs, reactions to anesthesia, bleeding problems, and current medications to help establish surgical risk and if a woman has any piercing that needs to be removed because of the use of the bovie or arterial cauterizing machine. In addition, include questions to discover:

- The woman's knowledge about the procedure
- The length of hospitalization anticipated
- If she knows about any postsurgical equipment to be used, such as an indwelling catheter or intravenous fluid line
- Any special precautions that will be necessary for her infant

Operative Risk for a Woman

For any surgery to be performed safely, a woman must be in the best possible physical and psychological state. Women who are in less than optimal physical or psychological health are at risk for a complicated surgical outcome unless the risk factor is identified and special precautions are taken.

Poor Nutritional Status

A woman who is obese because of poor nutrition is at risk because such a condition interferes with wound healing. Tissue that contains an abundance of fatty cells is difficult to suture, so the incision may take longer to heal. A prolonged healing period increases the risk for infection and rupture of the incision (**dehiscence**). The woman's heart may also have an increased workload. Therefore, the physiologic shock of surgery may place greater stress on the already overworked organ. In addition, an obese woman often has more difficulty turning and ambulating postoperatively than does a woman of normal weight and therefore has an increased risk for development of respiratory or circulatory complications such as pneumonia or thrombophlebitis (Datta & Gutman, 2007).

A woman with a protein or vitamin deficiency is also at risk for poorer healing, because protein and vitamins C and D are necessary for new cell formation at the incision site. In addition, vitamin K is necessary for blood clotting after surgery. Although most pregnant women follow sound nutritional practices and take iron supplements, some may still be iron deficient (particularly women with a multiple gestation or women who have not taken supplements). This places them at high risk for extreme fatigue after surgery, which could interfere with parent–child bonding.

Age Variations

Age affects surgical risk because it can cause decreased circulatory and renal function. Fortunately, most pregnant women fall within the young adult age group, so they are excellent candidates for surgery. A woman older than 40 years falls into a category of slightly higher risk.

Altered General Health

A woman who has a secondary illness such as cardiac disease, diabetes mellitus, anemia, or kidney or liver disease is at greater than usual surgical risk, depending on the extent of disease, because the pathology from the secondary illness may interfere with her ability to adjust physically to the demands

TABLE 24.1 ✻ Drugs That May Result in Complications of Surgery

Type of Drug	Action
Antibiotics	Specific antibiotics may predispose to renal insufficiency or increase neuromuscular blockage; can lead to opportunistic infections
Anticoagulants	May cause hemorrhage due to lack of hemostasis during surgery
Anticonvulsants	May increase liver action and metabolism of anesthetic agent
Antihypertensives	May result in hypotension after anesthesia
Corticosteroids	May block body's response to shock and lead to lack of adrenal function
Insulin	May lead to hypoglycemia during labor or hyperglycemia if a dextrose solution is administered
Antianxiety agents	May cause hypotension after anesthesia

of surgery. A woman with a secondary illness may also have an accompanying nutritional or electrolyte imbalance caused by her primary illness.

Therefore, asking about any secondary illnesses is an essential component of a preoperative nursing history. While waiting for surgery, people are under stress, a condition that can limit their reasoning and decision-making abilities. For example, it is not unusual for people admitted for any type of surgery to state that they are generally healthy and, minutes later, ask if they should take insulin on the day of surgery because they are diabetic.

A general medication history also is important, because some drugs increase surgical risk by interfering with the effect of an anesthetic or with healing of tissue. Examples of drugs that pregnant women might be taking and their potential complications are shown in Table 24.1.

Fluid and Electrolyte Imbalance

A woman who enters surgery with a lower than normal blood volume will feel the effect of surgical blood loss more than a woman who has a normal blood volume. A woman who began labor and later was told that she is to have a cesarean birth may fall into this category, because she may have had nothing to eat or drink for almost 24 hours. Recent vomiting, diarrhea, or a chronic poor fluid intake can compound her risk. Intravenous fluid replacement usually is initiated preoperatively and continued postoperatively to prevent fluid and electrolyte imbalances.

Fear

Women who are extremely worried need a very detailed explanation of the procedure before they can enter surgery without intense fear. Most cesarean births currently are performed under epidural anesthesia, so they are less frightening for women than when general anesthesia was used. With all anesthesia, a woman who is frightened is at a greater risk for cardiac arrest during anesthesia administration than a woman who is calm and relaxed.

In many instances, just helping a woman acknowledge that her fear of surgery is normal can be helpful. This does not make the procedure any less traumatic, but the woman can view her feelings as "normal" and expected, which helps to enhance her self-esteem and lower anxiety (Barnes, 2007).

Operative Risk to the Newborn

Cesarean birth places a newborn at a greater risk than does a vaginal birth for a number of reasons. When a fetus is pushed through the birth canal, pressure on the chest helps to rid the newborn's lungs of fluid. This makes respirations more likely to be adequate at birth than if a fetus had not been subjected to this pressure. For this reason, more infants born by cesarean birth develop some degree of respiratory difficulty for a day or two after birth than those born vaginally (Hansen et al., 2008). See Chapter 26 for a discussion of this condition, which is often referred to as transient tachypnea of the newborn.

Preoperative Diagnostic Procedures

Preoperative diagnostic procedures for a woman who is to have a cesarean birth include assessments of circulatory and renal function and fetal heart rate including:

- Vital sign determination
- Urinalysis
- Complete blood count
- Coagulation profile (prothrombin time [PT], partial thromboplastin time [PTT])
- Serum electrolytes and pH
- Blood typing and cross-matching
- Ultrasound to determine fetal presentation and maturity

During pregnancy, a woman, and particularly one who was in prolonged labor, may have an elevated leukocyte count (up to 20,000/mm^3), so this finding is not as helpful an indicator for the presence of infection in the pregnant woman as it is in others.

Preoperative Teaching

Fear of the unknown is one of the hardest fears to conquer. Preoperative teaching is aimed at acquainting a woman with cesarean procedure and any special equipment to be used, to make her as informed as possible. Activities that help maintain respiratory and skeletal muscle function, to prevent postsurgical complications, should also be included in teaching.

Before beginning teaching, assess how much a woman already knows about the surgery. A woman who has had a cesarean birth for her first child and now is being admitted for a second procedure already knows many details. Even so, she will undoubtedly appreciate having her memory refreshed and recall confirmed. Answer all specific questions, and fill in gaps in knowledge. Ensure that all information offered is accurate. It is confusing and potentially frightening for a woman to be told, for instance, that she will not have intravenous fluid after the surgery and then discover that an intravenous line will be placed. Be certain not to use hospital jargon such as "NPO." People under stress do not process new information well. They cannot process information at all if they do not understand the terminology. Ask a woman to return-demonstrate activities, such as deep breathing, to show that she understands the information and can do this well.

Be certain to explain the preoperative measures that will be necessary, such as surgical skin preparation, eating nothing before the time of surgery, premedication (if this will be used), and method of transport to surgery. Review the necessity for an indwelling catheter, intravenous fluid administration, placement of an epidural catheter (if used for postprocedural pain relief), and the advantage of early ambulation afterward.

Throughout teaching, use visual aids as necessary. Draw pictures or show illustrations of anatomy, if necessary. Be careful not to leave textbooks about cesarean procedure techniques with a woman. Typically, these books also describe complications, and, although knowledge of possible complications is necessary for informed consent, reading about complications complete with color illustrations can be overwhelming.

Teaching to Prevent Complications

Women who practice exercises to maintain good respiratory and circulatory function postoperatively will tend to experience fewer postoperative respiratory and circulatory complications than those who do not. These preventive exercises are best taught during the preoperative period, when the woman is free of pain and can concentrate on learning. Such teaching also gives a woman a positive outlook about surgery and a sense of control over her situation. By teaching about postoperative care, you are saying, "I'll see you and your new child safely back here in your room afterward"—a communication with a comforting subliminal message for a woman who has serious doubts that there will be an afterward, or at least not one with a healthy newborn.

Deep Breathing. Periodic deep breathing exercises fully aerate the lungs and help to prevent the stasis of lung mucus from the prolonged time spent in the supine position during surgery. Because stasis always has the potential to cause infection, preventing this helps prevent lung infection such as pneumonia.

A typical exercise is to take 5 to 10 deep breaths every hour. Teach a woman to do this simply by inhaling as deeply as possible, holding her breath for a second or two, and then exhaling as deeply as possible. Be certain she inhales and exhales fully. Otherwise, she might experience lightheadedness from hyperventilation.

Incentive Spirometry. A common device used postoperatively to encourage deep breathing is an incentive spirometer. These devices which cause a small ping-pong-like ball to rise in a narrow tube or cause lights to flash, are not only easy and fun to operate but give a woman a sense of reward for her effort. The initial impression of most people is that the device works by blowing into it. Because its purpose is to fully aerate lung spaces, though, most models are triggered by *inhalation,* not exhalation. There is a gauge to monitor levels and tabs to set goals.

Turning. Women do not need to practice turning side to side before surgery, because this activity is tiring for them to do while pregnant. They should understand, however, that turning postoperatively is important to prevent both respiratory and circulatory stasis.

Ambulation. The most effective way to stimulate lower-extremity circulation after a cesarean birth is by early ambulation. For this reason, most surgeons prefer a woman to be out of bed and walking by 4 hours after surgery (as soon as the effect of the epidural anesthesia has worn off). Helping a woman ambulate this early can be difficult, because she is both fatigued and in pain. Help her to understand that ambulation is extremely important after cesarean birth, because the edema of the low pelvic surgery compresses circulation to the lower extremities, increasing the risk for lower-extremity circulatory stasis. Some women may be prescribed antiembolic stockings (TEDS) to support and encourage venous return in addition to ambulation.

Immediate Preoperative Care Measures

A number of measures must be taken immediately before surgery to ensure a safe outcome.

Informed Consent

Obtaining operative consent is the surgeon's responsibility, but seeing that it is obtained is everyone's responsibility. You may be asked to witness a woman's signature on such a form. Before signing as a witness, be certain that it was *informed* consent, or one in which the risks and benefits of the procedure were explained in terms the woman could easily understand.

The law differs from state to state regarding emancipated minors or mature minors (girls under legal age who are pregnant or already the mother of a previous child). Emancipated minors can sign their own surgical permission, even though they are legally underage.

Overall Hygiene

Most women who are having a planned cesarean birth are admitted to the facility on the morning of surgery and have showered or bathed at home. On admission, provide a clean hospital gown. If a woman's hair is long, encourage her to braid it or put it into a ponytail so that it will more easily fit under the surgical cap she will wear. Hair contained by a cap that way is less likely to spread microorganisms during surgery. Follow institutional procedure about removing nail polish, jewelry, contact lenses, piercings, or hair ornaments before surgery. A growing number of women wear acrylic fingernails and are reluctant to remove them for surgery. If this is so, ensure that the woman's toenails are free of polish so toenails can be used to assess capillary refill if this is needed.

What if... Moja Hamma, who is going to have epidural anesthesia, refuses to remove her contact lenses for surgery even though it is hospital policy for anyone receiving anesthesia? She says, "Without them, I won't be able to see my baby being born." Would you ask the nurse anesthetist whether removing them is absolutely necessary, or would you insist that she follow procedure without question?

Gastrointestinal Tract Preparation

A gastric emptying agent such as metoclopramide (Reglan) to speed stomach emptying or a histamine blocker such as ranitidine (Zantac) to decrease stomach secretions may be prescribed prior to surgery. Yet another possibility is an oral antacid such as sodium citrate (Bicitra), which acts to neutralize acid stomach secretions. These precautions are necessary because the woman will be lying on her back during the procedure, making esophageal reflux and aspiration highly possible.

Baseline Intake and Output Determinations

To reduce bladder size and keep the bladder away from the surgical field, an indwelling urinary catheter may be prescribed before transport for surgery or after arrival in the surgical suite. Catheterizing a pregnant woman is more difficult than catheterizing a nonpregnant woman, because the pressure of the fetal head puts pressure on the urethra and distorts anatomic landmarks. In addition, the vulva may be swollen and distorted from vulval varicosities or edema. Use good lighting so that the perineum is clearly revealed and save a sample for culture to rule out a urinary tract infection. After catheter insertion, be certain that urine is draining freely, because fetal pressure on the urethra may reduce the flow of urine considerably. During transport, keep the drainage bag below the level of the woman's bladder, to prevent urine backflow and the possible introduction of microorganisms into the bladder.

If catheterization is difficult before surgery, do not traumatize the urethra by repeated attempts. Catheterization can be done in the birthing or delivery room after the anesthetic agent is given. If there is a delay between the catheter insertion time and surgery, mark the drainage bag just before surgery with the amount in the bag, or empty it, so that presurgery urine output can be differentiated from postsurgery urine output. One of the gravest dangers of any surgical procedure is kidney failure from the physiologic stress of surgery or lack of blood flow to the kidneys due to decreased blood pressure. All reproductive tract surgery puts ureter flow as well as kidney function at risk, because edema that collects in the surgery area can press on the ureters.

Hydration

Most women have an intravenous fluid line begun before surgery with a fluid such as lactated Ringer's solution. Doing so helps to ensure that a woman is fully hydrated and will not experience hypotension from epidural anesthesia administration, temporary use of a supine position, or blood loss at birth. Be certain that this line is started in the woman's nondominant hand, so that she can hold her newborn after surgery without interference. Use a large-size catheter or needle (18 or 20 gauge), so that blood replacement therapy can be administered, if needed, by the same line.

Preoperative Medication

A minimum of preoperative medication is used with a woman having a cesarean birth, to prevent compromising the fetal blood supply and to ensure that the newborn is wide awake at birth and can initiate respirations spontaneously.

Patient Chart and Presurgery Checklist

Documentation of nursing care up until the time a woman leaves the nursing care unit or labor room must be completed before a woman leaves for the surgical suite. Many hospitals use a preoperative checklist, such as that shown in Figure 24.1, as a reminder of all necessary measures to be taken. Checking and signing such a form indicates that the specific measures were completed.

Patient concerns — Completed

- Skin preparation ______ ______
- Identification in place ______
- Temperature, pulse, respiration ______ ______
- Blood pressure ______ ______
- Height ______ Weight ______ ______
- Voided ______ Time ______ Amount ______ ______
- NPO after ______ ______
- Hospital gown ______
- Hairpins removed ______
- Nail polish removed ______
- Jewelry removed ______
- Preoperative medication ______ ______
- Dentures removed ______ In place ______ ______
- Contact lenses removed ______ ______
- Prosthetic devices removed ______ ______
- Abdominal piercing removed ______ ______

Chart concerns

- Addressograph plate attached ______
- Operative permit obtained ______
- Urinalysis ______
- Hematocrit or CBC ______
- Blood order of ______ ______

Signature ______ R.N.

FIGURE 24.1 Preoperative checklist for cesarean birth. Checklists vary from hospital to hospital.

Transport to Surgery

A woman may be transferred to surgery in her bed, or she may be helped to move to a stretcher. If a stretcher is used, be certain to hold it tightly against the side of the woman's bed or use a slide board for safe transfer. A woman is awkward in her movements at term and could easily slip and fall if the stretcher moved. Urge her to lie on her left side during transport, to prevent supine hypotension syndrome. Ensure additional safety by raising the side rails on the bed or stretcher. Cover her with a blanket or sheet to avoid her feeling chilled. Check that her identification is secure before she leaves the patient unit. Make sure that her chart with the surgical checklist accompanies her.

Role of the Support Person

In most instances, a woman's family can be as involved in a cesarean birth as they would be for a vaginal birth. A support person may need more encouragement to watch a cesarean birth than a vaginal one, because he or she may believe that the surgery will be much bloodier than it actually is. Helping family members realize that cesarean birth is little different from vaginal birth not only allows them to watch the procedure but helps them progress to bonding with the infant and incorporating a new member into the family more easily.

✔ Checkpoint Question 24.2

What is an important measure to reduce the size of the bladder and keep it away from the surgical field during a cesarean birth?

a. Restrict fluids in the woman for 4 hours before surgery.
b. Insert a urinary catheter to drain the bladder and decrease its size.
c. Administer an oxytocic to contract the bladder.
d. Give a diuretic to reduce the bladder to its smallest size.

NURSING CARE OF A WOMAN HAVING AN EMERGENT CESAREAN BIRTH

Many women who will have a cesarean birth have no warning during pregnancy that this will be necessary. Suddenly, during labor, they develop a complication such as prolapsed cord or fetal distress, and it becomes necessary.

A woman who was having severe pain with labor and is told an emergent procedure is necessary actually may be relieved that surgery has been suggested, because the surgery will alleviate the pain. In contrast, another woman might feel great disappointment when told her baby must be born by cesarean birth. In many women, both emotions are present.

Surgical risk in an emergent situation is determined from the baseline history and physical examination information previously obtained at the beginning of labor. Preoperative preparation measures such as vital signs, urinalysis, and blood work have also been obtained. Immediate preparation concerns such as informed consent, application of elastic stockings (if appropriate), gastrointestinal tract preparation, bladder catheterization, and establishment of an intravenous line will be the same. Because most cesarean births are completed within 30 minutes of the time one is documented to be necessary, teaching about postoperative measures needs to be delayed until after surgery (Simpson, 2007).

Available time must be spent explaining the immediate procedures to the woman such as transfer, abdominal preparation, and anesthesia. Document carefully what was taught, so that the nurse caring for the woman postoperatively will be aware of the need for additional teaching. At birth, at least one person whose sole responsibility is neonatal resuscitation should be present to care for the baby. Approximately 10% of babies born by cesarean birth need assistance to begin breathing at birth; about 1% of babies need extensive resuscitation to survive (Simpson, 2007).

INTRAOPERATIVE CARE MEASURES

Cesarean birth is most similar to vaginal birth if the woman is awake during the surgery; therefore, after discussion with a woman, the anesthesia of choice is usually a regional block (Box 24.4).

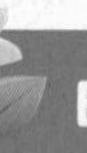

BOX 24.4 * Focus on Communication

Moja Hamma has been told she will need a cesarean birth because of fetal distress that has led to meconium staining.

Less Effective Communication

Nurse: Moja. Can I answer any questions for you?
Moja: I want something to put me to sleep so I won't know what's happening.
Nurse: Most women want an epidural.
Moja: I have to be so sound asleep I won't know what's happening.
Nurse: Most people . . .
Moja: . . . don't have cesarean births, so what applies to them doesn't apply to me.
Nurse: I'll tell the anesthesiologist you want general anesthesia.

More Effective Communication

Nurse: Moja. Can I answer any questions for you?
Moja: I want something to put me to sleep so I won't know what's happening.
Nurse: Most women want an epidural.
Moja: I have to be so sound asleep I won't know what's happening.
Nurse: You're not interested in seeing your baby born?
Moja: I'm not interested in seeing him born dead.
Nurse: Let me find your doctor to explain to you again that you need surgery to prevent something going wrong, not because something is wrong.

Most women appreciate that cesarean births are done to prevent their infant from being harmed. Others interpret a cesarean birth as being done because the harm has already occurred. Some women interpret a cesarean birth as an announcement they are somehow not as competent as other women. Still others are relieved that labor is being interrupted. Be certain to ask enough questions so that you can learn the importance or meaning of the event to an individual woman.

Administration of Anesthesia

A surgical nurse will assist a woman to move from the transport stretcher or bed to the operating room table and will remain with her while anesthesia is administered. If the woman has an epidural catheter in place from labor, be careful not to dislodge it while she is being moved. During transport or in surgery, encourage the woman to remain on her side, or insert a pillow under her right hip to keep her body slightly tilted to the side, to prevent supine hypotension syndrome. If a spinal anesthetic (which may be used in an emergency) is to be administered, the anesthesiologist usually will do this with the woman sitting up. The anesthesiologist may ask you to help the woman curve her back to separate the vertebrae and facilitate entry of the spinal needle. It is difficult for a woman having uterine contractions to remain in this position for long. Talking to her while gently restraining her and letting her lean against you is the most effective means of helping her maintain this position. Epidural anesthesia is usually administered with the woman lying on her side. Duramorph is a form of morphine commonly used in epidurals. Its effect lasts up to 24 hours but because it can cause late occurring respiratory depression, continuous pulse oximetry must be used for 24 hours postsurgery (Ng et al., 2009).

Skin Preparation

Reducing the number of bacteria on the skin before surgery automatically reduces the possibility of bacteria entering the incision at the time of surgery. Shaving away abdominal hair, if indicated, and washing the skin area over the incision site with soap and water accomplishes this.

The skin preparation area for a cesarean birth varies among agencies. Some require extensive skin preparation, from above the umbilicus to below the pubic hair, whereas others require only a limited preparation of the immediate incisional area.

Surgical Incision

After anesthetic administration, a woman is positioned with a towel under her right hip to move abdominal contents away from the surgical field and to lift her uterus off the vena cava. A screen may be placed at her shoulder level and covered with a sterile drape to block the flow of bacteria from her respiratory tract to the incision site. This also helps block the woman's and support person's lines of vision, preventing additional anxiety caused by the sight of the incision. Be sure the support person is positioned at the woman's head to provide support.

The incision area on the woman's abdomen is then scrubbed with an antiseptic such as iodine, and appropriate drapes are placed around the area of incision, so that only a small area of skin is left exposed. Watching a cesarean birth is usually the first time a father or support person has ever witnessed surgery. Because of this, the person may be too overwhelmed by and interested in the procedure to be of optimum support. He or she may become concerned about the amount of manipulation and cutting that occurs before the uterus itself is cut (assuming fetal distress is not extreme). Prepare the woman and support person for the sights they might see, or help talk them through them as they occur. Sponge and instrument counts are simplified by the use of prepackaged cesarean birth components.

Types of Cesarean Incision

There are two types of cesarean incision. The type chosen depends on the presentation of the fetus and the speed with which the procedure will be performed (Fig. 24.2).

In a **classic cesarean incision,** the incision is made vertically through both the abdominal skin and the uterus. It is made high on the uterus so that it can be used with a placenta previa, to avoid cutting the placenta. A disadvantage of this type of incision is that it leaves a wide skin scar and also runs through the active contractile portion of the uterus. Because this type of scar could rupture during labor, it is likely, if this type of incision is used, that a woman will not be able to have a subsequent vaginal birth.

A **low segment incision** (commonly referred to as a low transverse incision) is one made horizontally across the abdomen just over the symphysis pubis and also horizontally across the uterus just over the cervix. This is the most common type of cesarean incision. It is also referred to as a Pfannenstiel incision or a "bikini" incision, because even a low-cut bathing suit will cover the scar. Because this type of incision is through the nonactive portion of the uterus (the part that contracts minimally with labor), it is less likely to rupture in subsequent labors, making it possible for a woman to have a VBAC with a future pregnancy (Lawson &

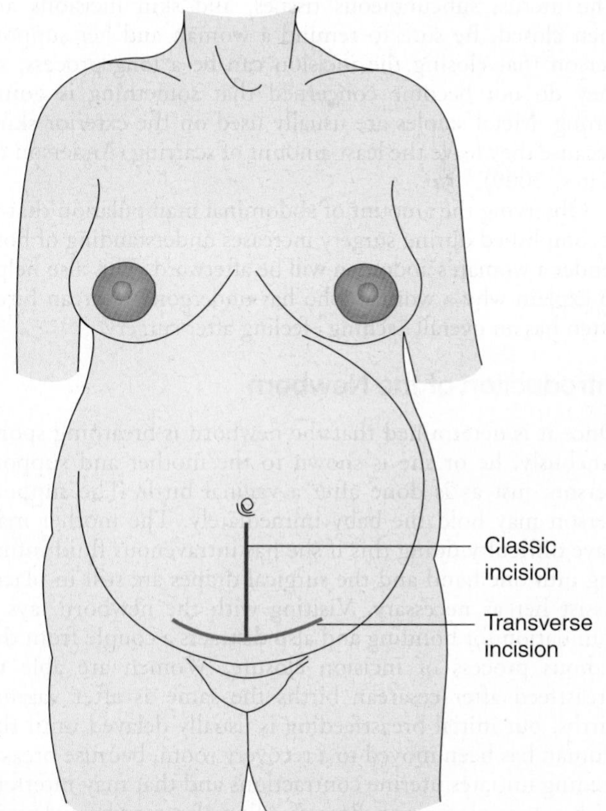

FIGURE 24.2 Types of cesarean incisions.

Bienstock, 2007). It also results in less blood loss, is easier to suture, decreases postpartal uterine infections, and is less likely to cause postpartum gastrointestinal complications (Incerpi, 2007). The major disadvantage of this incision is that it takes longer to perform, possibly making it impractical for an emergent cesarean birth. In a few instances, the skin incision is made horizontally and then the uterine incision is made vertically, or vice versa. For this reason, during a future pregnancy, do not assume that a woman who has a small skin incision also has had a small uterine incision.

Birth of the Infant

Once the surgical incision is complete, retractors (long, curved, metal instruments) are slipped into the incision. Gentle traction on the handles by an assistant keeps the incision spread apart, allowing good visualization of the uterus and the internal incision. Sterile towels may be placed in the incision to separate the uterus from other organs. The uterus is then cut, and the child's head is born manually or by the application of forceps (Fig. 24.3). The mouth and nose of the baby are suctioned by a bulb syringe, the same as in a vaginal birth, before the remainder of the child is born. Oxytocin is administered intravenously by the anesthesiologist as the child or placenta is delivered, to increase uterine contraction and reduce blood loss. In many instances, a woman's partner may be allowed to cut the umbilical cord. After full birth, the uterus is pulled forward onto the abdomen and covered with moist gauze. The internal cavity of the uterus is then inspected, and the membranes and placenta are manually removed. If the woman wishes to have a tubal ligation, it can be done at this time. The uterus, subcutaneous tissues, and skin incisions are then closed. Be sure to remind a woman and her support person that closing the incision can be a long process, so they do not become concerned that something is going wrong. Metal staples are usually used on the exterior skin, because they leave the least amount of scarring (Anderson & Gates, 2009).

Observing the amount of abdominal manipulation that is accomplished during surgery increases understanding of how tender a woman's abdomen will be afterward. This also helps to explain why a woman who has undergone cesarean birth often has an overall "aching" feeling after surgery.

Introduction of the Newborn

Once it is determined that the newborn is breathing spontaneously, he or she is shown to the mother and support person, just as is done after a vaginal birth. The support person may hold the baby immediately. The mother may have difficulty doing this if she has intravenous fluid infusing into one hand and the surgical drapes are still in place. Assist her as necessary. Visiting with the newborn lays a foundation for bonding and also distracts a couple from the tedious process of incision closure. Women are able to breastfeed after cesarean births the same as after vaginal births, but initial breastfeeding is usually delayed until the woman has been moved to a recovery room, because breastfeeding initiates uterine contractions and that may interfere with suture placement. Breastfeeding also may be awkward with the anesthesia screen in place and because of the lack of privacy.

✔ Checkpoint Question 24.3

Moja Hamma asks you how big her scar will be after cesarean birth. Your best answer would be:

a. The incision is big and runs vertically across your abdomen.
b. The incision is made through the vagina so it does not leave a scar.
c. Most cesarean-birth incisions are so low they do not show over a bikini.
d. It is so large that it will always show, but think of it as a mark of pride.

POSTPARTAL CARE MEASURES

Women who have infants by cesarean birth develop an additional care concern in the immediate postpartal period because they are not only postpartal patients but postsurgical ones as well. Due to the strain of the unexpected procedure, they may have increased difficulty bonding with their new infant. They have postsurgical pain in additional to afterpains. As with all postpartal women, the postpartal phase for a woman who has her child by cesarean birth can be divided into an immediate recovery period (the so-called fourth stage of labor) and an extended postpartal period.

Nursing Diagnoses and Related Interventions During the Immediate Postpartal Period

Immediately after surgery, a woman is transferred by stretcher from the operating room table to the postanesthesia care unit (PACU) or postpartal room. If spinal anesthesia was used, remember that her legs are fully anesthetized and she will not be able to help move them.

Nursing Diagnosis: Pain related to surgical incision

Outcome Evaluation: Patient verbalizes extent of pain (from 1 to 10) and need for relief; states that level of pain is tolerable.

In the past, pain control was a major problem after cesarean birth. Pain was so intense from the uterine or abdominal incision that it interfered with a woman's ability to move and deep breathe. This led to surgical complications such as pneumonia or thrombophlebitis. It also impaired a woman's ability to bond with her newborn, because holding her infant was so painful. Today, a number of effective types of pain management are available. Use a pain rating scale to allow a woman to rate her pain. Without the use of a specific tool, assessment can be unreliable, because a woman's overall excitement at having a new child may interfere with the accuracy of the assessment.

A woman who is concerned about her infant may experience more pain than a woman who feels confident that her infant is doing well, because anxiety and fear heighten a pain response, and a tense body posture causes pressure on sutures. Be certain a woman understands that her infant has survived the surgical

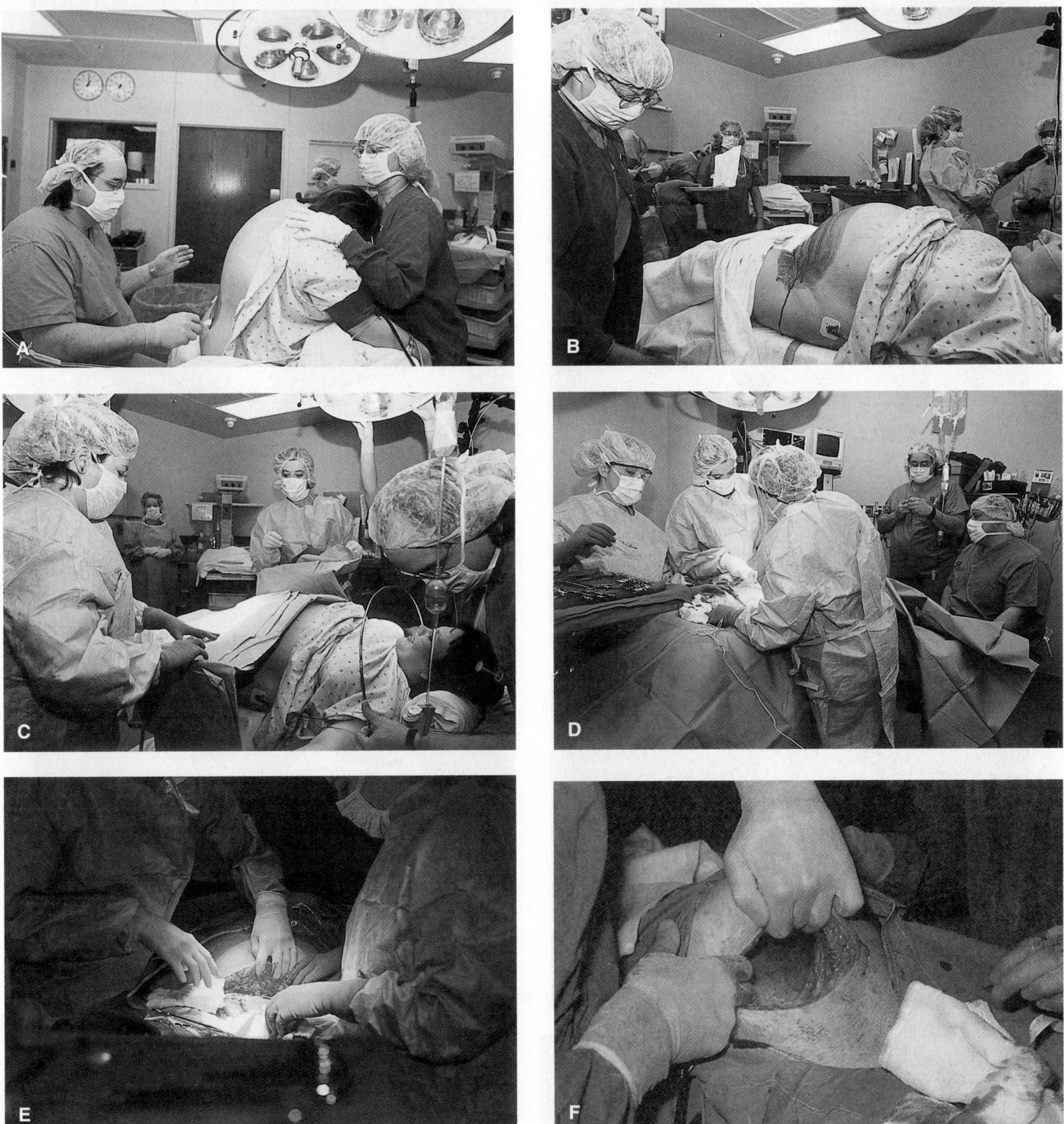

FIGURE 24.3 Cesarean birth. (**A**) Preparation for anesthesia. (**B**) Abdominal skin preparation. (**C**) Draping of operative site. (**D**) Preparation for initial incision. (**E**) Initial incision. (**F**) Opening of the peritoneum. *(continued)*

birth well (assuming this is true) or what steps are being taken to make the infant well.

Women who had a long-action morphine epidural for labor have good pain relief up to 24 hours. Others, who give birth without analgesia or received a shorter acting drug for birth, need analgesia to be comfortable. Patient-controlled analgesia (PCA) or continued epidural injections give maximum pain relief. No matter what system of pain relief is used, when administering analgesics after surgery, be sure to supplement them with other comfort measures, such as change of position or straightening of bed linen. Always ask a woman what type of pain she is experiencing before administering a new dose of analgesia, to be certain that she is describing incisional or uterine pain and not pain in a leg or some other body part that would suggest a complication of surgery. Check for abdominal distention, which suggests the pain may be

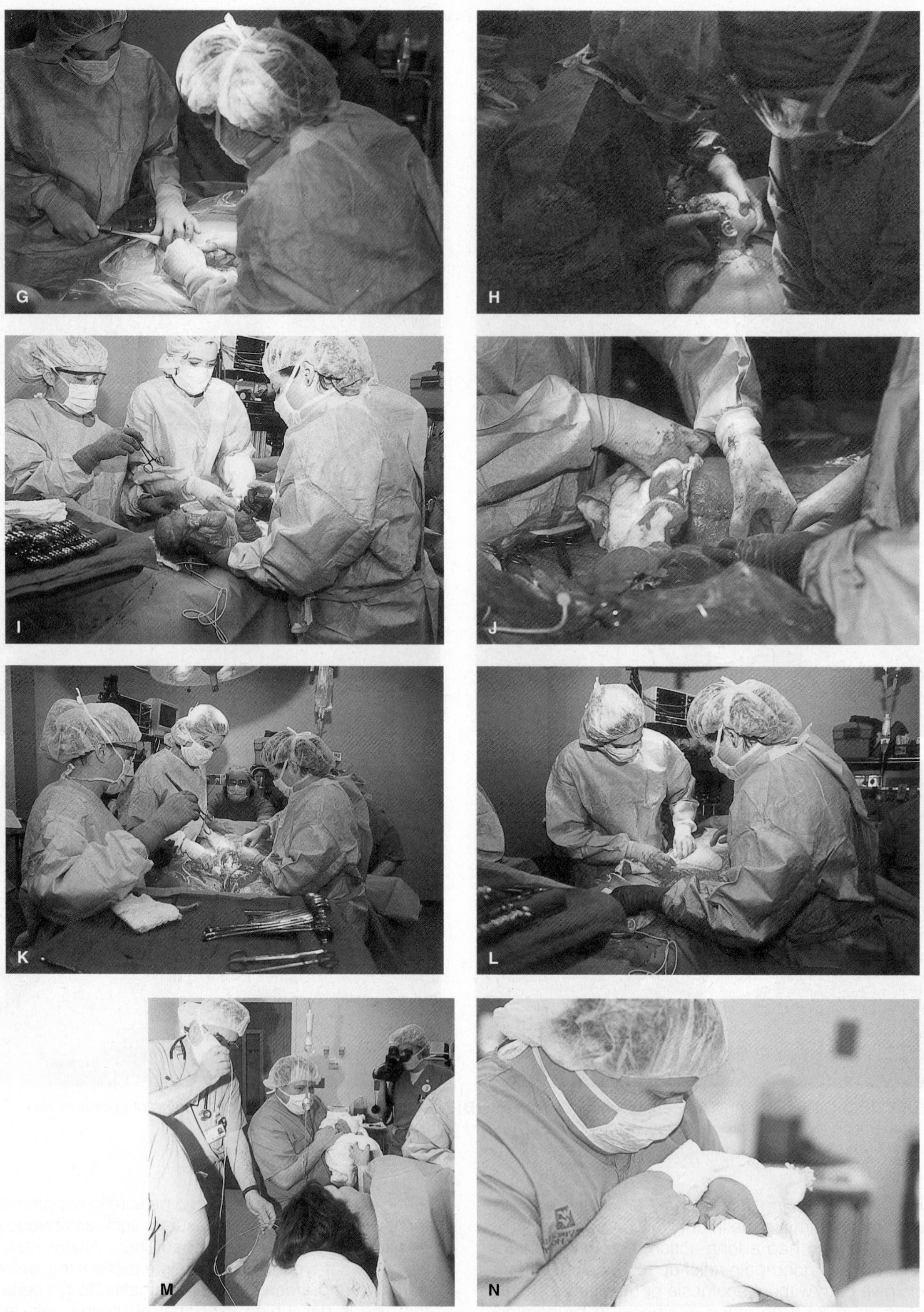

FIGURE 24.3 *(continued)* (**G**) Retractors in place. (**H**) Birth of head and posterior shoulder. (**I**) Infant born. (**J**) Suturing of uterus complete. (**K**) Suturing of abdominal layers. (**L**) Skin closure. (**M**) Family bonding with mother's first touch. (**N**) Father bonding with newborn. (© Caroline Brown, RNC, MS, DEd.)

caused by intestinal gas rather than incision pain. If so, ambulation is often the most effective method to relieve this type of pain.

Urge a woman to continue to take adequate analgesia to effectively manage her pain after she returns home, so she is not so distressed that she cannot nurse her infant. Be certain she understands not to use acetylsalicylic acid (aspirin), because this can interfere with blood clotting and healing. Many women who are breastfeeding are reluctant to accept any type of analgesic, especially just before breastfeeding, for fear that it will pass in breast milk to the infant. Although it is true that most analgesics do pass in breast milk, the infant takes such a small amount of breast milk (mainly colostrum) during the first days after surgery that the amount of analgesia received would be negligible. Also, without the analgesic, the woman may be so uncomfortable that she is unable to hold her infant comfortably and enjoy having the infant with her. Placing a pillow over her lap while she feeds can deflect the weight of the infant from her suture line and lessen pain. Encourage the football hold for breastfeeding as another way to keep the infant's weight off the mother's incision.

Patient-Controlled Analgesia. PCA is a method of pain control in which women administer doses of intravenous narcotic analgesia such as morphine to themselves as needed. Although the technique may be used during labor, it is most frequently used to control postsurgical pain. With a solution such as Ringer's lactate infusing intravenously, a PCA pump containing a locked syringe of narcotic (meperidine or morphine) is attached to the intravenous line at a port close to the woman. To receive a dose of analgesia, the woman pushes a button similar to a call bell. This alerts the automatic pump to deliver a set amount of narcotic into the intravenous line. The pump has a "lock-out" setting that prevents a woman from administering a larger dose or doses more frequently than would be safe such as every 8 minutes (Fig. 24.4).

With PCA, a fairly constant level of pain relief can be maintained, and the pain and fear of injections are eliminated. PCA works well with postcesarean women because they feel well enough to be interested in self-care and self-administration of analgesia. Overall, women tend to use less analgesia with a PCA system than they would with intramuscular injections.

Epidural Analgesia. Today, women who have epidural anesthesia for cesarean birth can have morphine (Duramorph) or fentanyl added to the epidural catheter immediately after surgery, a technique that keeps them pain free for the next 24 hours (see Chapter 16). Although epidural analgesia provides effective pain relief after cesarean birth, side effects of epidural morphine administration, such as intense itching and nausea and vomiting, can occur. An antihistamine such as diphenhydramine (Benadryl) may be given to reduce pruritus; an antiemetic such as metoclopramide (Reglan) may be administered to counteract nausea. The use of fentanyl reduces the risk for these side effects. Even with these annoying side effects, however, epidural analgesia with morphine can be a very effective means of pain control after cesarean birth (Marshall & Baker, 2007).

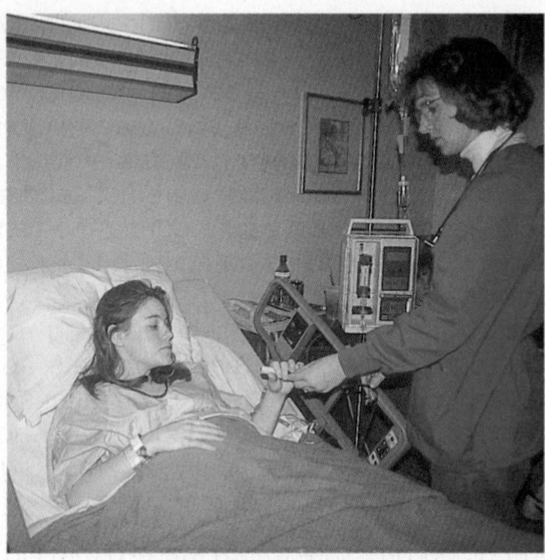

FIGURE 24.4 Patient-controlled analgesia (PCA) pump. By pushing the button, a client delivers a bolus of narcotic to herself. (© Caroline Brown, RNC, MS, DEd.)

On the postpartal unit, an infusion pump is connected to the woman's epidural catheter and the woman can infuse a bolus of narcotic as additional pain relief is needed. This patient-controlled epidural anesthesia (PCEA) not only is an effective means of relieving pain but omits the problem of infiltration of an intravenous infusion, which can occur with intravenous PCA (Cho & Penning, 2007).

Transcutaneous Electrical Nerve Stimulation. Transcutaneous electrical nerve stimulation (TENS) is, as the name implies, the transmission of an electrical current across the skin. Small electrodes are attached to the woman's skin near her incision; when she feels pain, she pushes a transformer button. Irritation or stimulation of large afferent nerve fibers by the electrical stimulation block the ability of the smaller, pain-carrying nerve fibers to transmit impulses (as predicted by gating control theory). This is the same phenomenon that rubbing or scratching skin at the point of pain achieves (see also Chapter 16). The use of TENS can provide important pain relief after a cesarean birth, because it gives a woman a sense of control over her situation, as does PCA or PCEA (Halls, 2008).

What if... Moja Hamma refuses to allow you to assess her fundal height after her cesarean birth because she has so much pain? How would you approach this situation?

Nursing Diagnosis: Risk for deficient fluid volume related to blood loss during surgery

Outcome Evaluation: Patient's blood pressure is 100/60 mm Hg or higher; pulse remains between 60 and 100 beats per minute; scant to no bleeding on surgical dressing is apparent.

The potential always exists for deficient fluid volume because of blood loss from surgery until all blood vessels that were cut and ligated during surgery have thrombosed, sclerosed, and permanently sealed closed. The risk of heavy bleeding doubles for the postpartum woman, because she may hemorrhage vaginally from an uncontracted uterus as well as internally from blood vessels that were not securely ligated. This danger is most acute during the first hour after surgery, but it remains an acute problem for the first 24 hours.

To detect the earliest signs of bleeding, monitor blood pressure, pulse, and respiratory rate approximately every 15 minutes for the first hour after surgery, every 30 minutes for the next 2 hours, every hour for the next 4 hours, or as specifically ordered. Signs indicative of possible hemorrhage include:

- Falling blood pressure (more than 20 mm Hg), or a systolic blood pressure less than 80 mm Hg, or a drop of 5 to 10 mm Hg over several readings
- A change in pulse rate (greater than 110 beats per minute or less than 60 beats per minute)
- Rapid respirations
- Restlessness and a sense of thirst

Inspect the dressing over the surgical incision for blood staining each time vital signs are assessed. Observe the perineal pad for lochia flow, and palpate the fundal height each time as well. Lochial discharge may be decreased in a woman after a cesarean birth because the uterus was cleaned during surgery, but some lochia will always be present, and it follows a typical rubra, serosa, alba pattern. Be certain to help a woman turn so you can look under her body for bleeding. Blood oozing from a surgical wound or vaginally can pool considerably under a woman before it is visible.

Oxytocin may be ordered to be added to the first 1 or 2 L of intravenous fluid after surgery to ensure firm uterine contraction. If the rate of fluid administration gets behind, be careful about "catch-up" administration. Oxytocin can elevate blood pressure by causing vasoconstriction. It may be safer to allow the fluid to remain behind for a time, rather than risk causing blood pressure to elevate. Be aware that a woman is very prone to hemorrhage at the point the oxytocin is discontinued, because this is the first time her uterus is being asked to maintain contraction on its own. Notify her care provider of any changes in vital signs that might indicate hemorrhage, so that prompt action can be taken. Remember that a minimal but continued change in vital signs (pulse steadily increasing, blood pressure steadily declining) is as ominous a sign of hemorrhage as is a sudden alteration in these measurements.

A woman who has had either spinal or epidural anesthesia usually will not experience pain on uterine palpation until the anesthesia has worn off, approximately 4 to 24 hours. Therefore, uterine palpation should not increase her pain. Once the effect of the anesthesia or analgesia has decreased, palpate gently to not cause increased pain but thoroughly enough to determine uterine consistency.

At the same time you assess a woman's uterus for firmness, assess the remainder of her abdomen for softness. A hard, "guarded" abdomen is one of the first signs of peritonitis (peritoneal infection), a complication that may occur with any abdominal surgical procedure.

Nursing Diagnoses and Related Interventions During the Extended Postpartal Period

The average woman whose child is born by cesarean birth remains in the hospital from 48 hours to 4 days, depending on her preferences and the regulations of her insurance carrier. During this period and until she returns to have her sutures or staples removed, several interventions are necessary to promote healing, prevent postoperative complications, and help the woman and her family establish bonding with the new child. Common concerns of women include pain, fatigue, interference with gastrointestinal function, and reduced activity level.

Nursing Diagnosis: Risk for deficient fluid volume related to postsurgical fluid restriction

Outcome Evaluation: Patient's urine specific gravity remains between 1.003 and 1.030; weight loss is not more than 5 to 10 lb; fluid intake equals 2 to 3 L/day.

Adequate fluid intake is important after surgery, to replace blood loss from surgery and to maintain blood pressure and renal function. Because the intestine is handled during surgery, it takes approximately 24 to 48 hours before full peristaltic function is restored and oral intake is possible. It is important that intravenous fluids be infused during this time, at a rate that is not too rapid (which could lead to cardiac overload) or too slow (which could lead to inadequate circulatory compensation). Keep an accurate intake and output record for at least the first 24 hours, to be certain an adequate fluid balance has been achieved.

Teach a woman to "guard" her intravenous fluid line, because she needs a high proportion of fluid during this time (all postpartal women undergo diuresis as a physiologic postpartal change). At the same time, do not urge such caution that she is afraid to turn or ambulate. Her risk for thrombophlebitis is high, so she must turn frequently when in bed and ambulate early in the postpartal period to reduce this risk.

Women are kept NPO for a time after surgery to avoid paralytic ileum that occurs from bowel handling during surgery. Because the bowel is not actually handled, however, there is probably little reason to withhold food and fluid as long as common protocols require (Mangesi & Hofmeyr, 2009; Izbizky et al., 2008).

To establish that bowel function has returned, assess a woman's abdomen at least once every 8 hours for bowel sounds, small "pinging" sounds heard on auscultation at a rate of 5 to 10 per minute, which demonstrate that air and fluid are moving through the intestines. Passage of flatus is another indication that intestinal function is again active. As soon as these signs are present, intravenous fluid therapy is usually discontinued and the woman is allowed sips of fluid. After she begins oral intake, wait 1 hour before removing the intravenous line. Doing so ensures that a woman is not experiencing nausea and vomiting, which might require restarting intravenous therapy. Introduce oral fluid slowly—for example, ice chips for the first hour, then sips of clear fluid such as ginger ale, Jello, tea, or flavored frozen ice. Gradually advance her diet to a soft and then a regular diet as prescribed. Some women assume that they will not be allowed to eat for a long time and are surprised (and suspicious) to learn that they can have ice chips only hours after surgery. This is possible because ice chips dissolve so slowly that the woman receives little fluid from them; they feel cool, however, and quickly take away the dry, "cottony" feeling in her mouth caused by lack of fluid.

Teach women to continue to drink large quantities of fluid after they return home (at least six glasses daily), so that they have adequate body fluid to make breastfeeding successful.

Nursing Diagnosis: Constipation related to effects of abdominal surgery and anesthesia

Outcome Evaluation: Woman voices she has a bowel movement every 2 to 3 days or her usual pattern.

Note carefully the time of a woman's first bowel movement after surgery. If there has been no bowel movement by the time of hospital discharge, her physician may order a stool softener, a suppository, or an enema to facilitate stool evacuation. Reassure a woman who is not receiving much food yet that it is normal not to have bowel movements for 3 or 4 days postoperatively, especially if an enema was administered before surgery.

Teach women to eat a diet high in roughage and fluid and to attempt to move their bowels at least every other day to avoid constipation after they return home. Some women need a stool softener prescribed, because incisional pain interferes with their ability to use their abdominal muscles effectively. Caution them not to strain to pass stools, because this puts pressure on their incision. Keep their water pitcher full to remind them to drink fluids.

Nursing Diagnosis: Risk for impaired urinary elimination related to surgical procedure

Outcome Evaluation: Urinary output is more than 30 mL/h; patient reports no pain, frequency, burning, or hesitancy on voiding.

Voiding after surgery provides evidence of adequate renal and circulatory function, because the kidneys must have adequate blood flow through them to function. Because the bladder was handled and displaced during surgery, its tone or ability to sense filling may be inadequate to initiate voiding. For this reason, the indwelling catheter placed before surgery is usually left in place for 4 to 24 hours to ensure good urine drainage. Assess that the catheter is draining (a postpartal woman has a urine output of 3000 to 5000 mL per 24 hours). Bladder distention will occur rapidly if the catheter becomes blocked.

Before catheter removal, a urine culture may be ordered to check for the possibility of a urinary tract infection. After removal of the catheter, the average woman voids in 4 to 8 hours. Assess for bladder filling at the end of this time by palpation, pressing lightly over the symphysis pubis to assess fullness (Fig. 24.5A), and by percussion. On percussion, an empty bladder sounds dull; a full bladder, resonant; and an extended bladder, hyperresonant (Fig. 24.5B). If a bladder has filled to capacity but cannot empty properly, the woman may have "retention with overflow," or

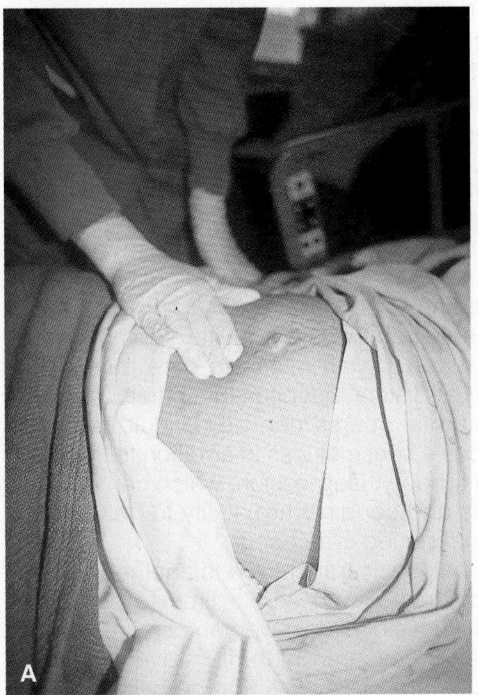

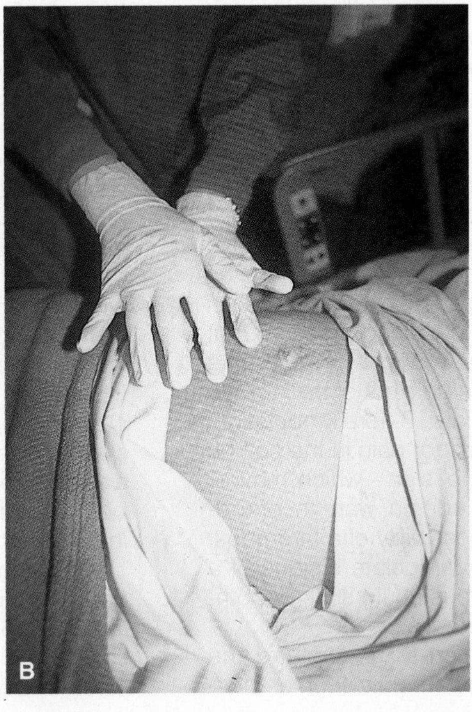

FIGURE 24.5 (**A**) Assessing bladder filling by palpation. (**B**) Assessing bladder filling by percussion. (© Caroline Brown, RNC, MS, DEd.)

voiding 30 to 60 mL of urine every 15 to 20 minutes. This voiding pattern is potentially dangerous because it means that the woman's bladder is held continuously under tension. This can result in permanent bladder damage if the condition goes undetected. In addition, the constantly full bladder may prevent the uterus from contracting, possibly increasing the risk of postpartal hemorrhage.

To help a woman void, suggest she take her prescribed analgesic to help relax abdominal musculature. In addition, provide privacy for voiding, and assist the woman to walk to the bathroom at least every 2 hours. Other measures that might be effective include pouring warm water over her vulva (measure the amount of water used, so that it can be differentiated from urine) or running water from a tap within hearing distance.

Teach women to continue to drink adequate fluid (at least five to six glasses daily) to ensure an adequate fluid output and help prevent urinary tract infection after they return home. Be certain they know to telephone their primary care provider if they should develop symptoms of a urinary tract infection, such as pain or frequency with voiding or blood in urine.

Nursing Diagnosis: Risk for ineffective peripheral tissue perfusion related to immobility during and after surgery

Outcome Evaluation: Capillary refill is less than 5 seconds; there is absence of calf pain, redness, edema, or areas of warmth on lower extremities.

Because a woman's abdominal muscles are lax from the stretching that occurred during pregnancy, abdominal contents tend to shift forward and put pressure on the suture line when she is sitting or standing, causing pain and an uncomfortable feeling often described as "everything falling out." A woman may feel more comfortable turning and sitting up if she supports her abdomen with one hand or splints the incision with a pillow.

Leg exercises such as flexing and extending her knees and early ambulation are a woman's best safeguards against lower-extremity circulatory problems. Thrombohemolytic stockings may be prescribed to help promote venous return and prevent venous stasis. Teach a woman to apply these before arising, while she is supine and venous distention is minimal. Always allow her to sit on the edge of the bed for a few minutes before helping her to a standing position, to prevent orthostatic hypotension (sudden low blood pressure that occurs with sudden position changes). Assessing blood pressure before a woman gets out of bed for the first time is an additional safeguard. Before ambulation, also assess the lower extremities for pain in the calf on dorsiflexion of the foot (Homans' sign—which may or may not be reliable) or for pain, edema, warmth, or redness in the calf, to detect the possibility of a thrombus. It is dangerous for a woman to ambulate if signs of a thrombus are present. A thrombus could shift, becoming an embolus, a potentially lethal situation.

Often, it is difficult for women to understand the importance of turning and ambulating as soon as possible after surgery (Fig. 24.6). Still experiencing the "taking in" postpartal phase, a woman may prefer to spend the first days after surgery just resting quietly in bed. Encourage her to use adequate analgesia during this time, to enable her to move and ambulate with the least amount of pain. Reinforce the need for continued activity balanced with rest after discharge. Be certain she understands the signs and symptoms of complications, such as thrombophlebitis.

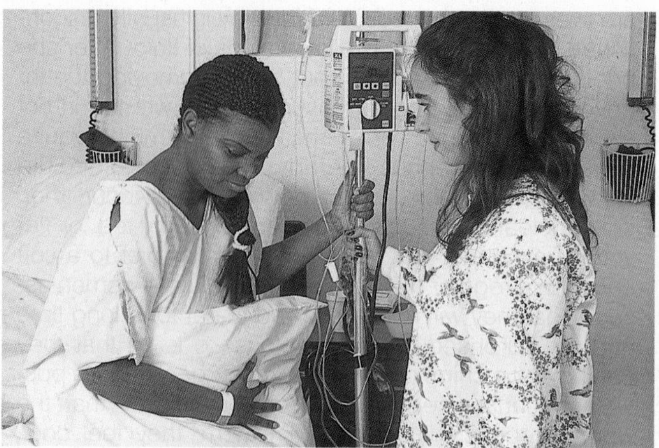

FIGURE 24.6 Encouraging women to be out of bed will help prevent complications from a cesarean birth. It is important to splint the incision area while getting up and ambulating. (© Barbara Proud.)

Nursing Diagnosis: Risk for impaired parenting related to the emergent nature of birth or discomfort from surgery

Outcome Evaluation: Parents hold and feed child and voice positive comments about the infant.

When a cesarean birth is unscheduled, a woman does not have much time preoperatively to think about how she will feel after surgery. Most women are surprised to realize how well they feel overall but also how quickly they become fatigued and how painful a simple surgical incision can be. Being reassured they are recovering well but that surgery is a physiologic shock to their system helps them to accept temporary discomforts. It can help them bond with their newborn after a cesarean birth, just as women who give birth vaginally. Encourage women to breastfeed even if this causes temporary uterine pain as the uterus contracts with breastfeeding.

If the woman's baby was born with a complication or has been placed in an intensive care nursery or transferred to a distant hospital for tertiary care, a woman's postpartal course can be difficult because she experiences a sense of loss in addition to the pain and fatigue of surgery. Depression, which can slow all body functions and certainly her ability to "take hold" in the postpartal period, can occur.

Unless her baby was transferred to another site, be certain to provide her with ample time to hold and feed her child if possible. Most women can breastfeed satisfactorily after cesarean birth. If intravenous lines or other devices are present, assist her with holding

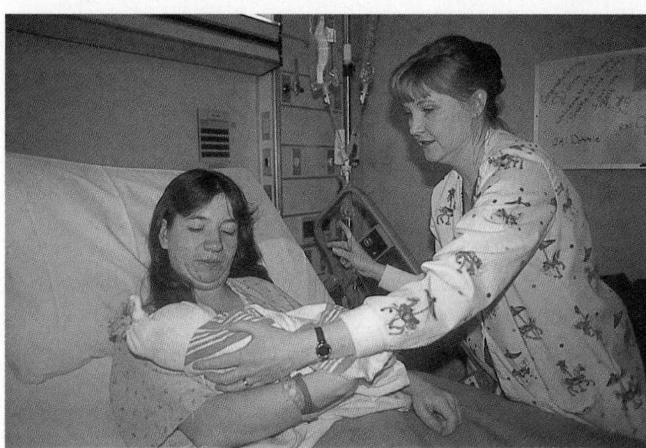

FIGURE 24.7 A nurse assists with holding the newborn and positioning the equipment so that the intravenous line does not interfere with mother–child interactions. (© Caroline Brown, RNC, MS, DEd.)

her newborn, so that equipment does not interfere with her time spent with her infant. She may have some reason to think her baby is not quite perfect—after all, the baby was not born "perfectly"—so she may need additional time to inspect her baby and feel comfortable with him or her (Fig. 24.7).

Nursing Diagnosis: Fatigue related to effects of surgery

Outcome Evaluation: Patient states she is pleased with level of self-care; ambulates well by 24 hours, and sleeps restfully at night.

Although a woman needs activity and movement after surgery, she also needs adequate rest. Many women attempt to handle their own and their newborn's needs immediately after surgery, because their excitement over their baby and their new role makes them unaware of their underlying fatigue. Extreme fatigue interferes with healing and possibly increases the risk for infection, however. It also can eventually interfere with bonding. Help a woman plan a day that includes care of her new child as well as periods of rest for herself. Be certain she has adequate analgesic medication at bedtime to allow her to be pain free for the night. Provide a time in the middle of the morning and again in the afternoon for uninterrupted rest. Explore her plans for care at home to be certain that her plans for rest seem realistic for a postsurgical-postpartal woman (Box 24.5).

Once a woman returns home, rest is often best accomplished if it is scheduled for every time her newborn sleeps. Without adequate rest this way, she can notice increased uterine bleeding, which has the potential to lead to excessive loss of fluid and iron stores.

Nursing Diagnosis: Impaired skin integrity related to surgical incision

Outcome Evaluation: Incision line is clean, dry, and intact without erythema; oral temperature is less than 38° C.

Surgical incisions heal by primary intention, or by the gradual removal and replacement of dead or damaged cells at the wound site with new cells produced by the surrounding tissue. Assess the surgical incision once during each nursing shift while a woman is hospitalized, to ensure that the wound edges are approximated and there are no signs of infection, such as erythema. As soon as she can walk steadily, a woman can take a shower (after first removing the dressing), because warm, clean water on the incision is soothing. After this point, she can make a decision about whether to continue to wear a dressing. Lack of a dressing prevents moisture accumulation at the incision site and decreases the possibility of infection.

Teach women to continue to observe their incision daily at home. Instruct them in signs and symptoms of possible infection, including redness or the presence of a discharge, and to report any of these signs to their primary care provider. With a cesarean birth, healing will be adequate enough by day 3 that skin sutures or clamps can be removed, although many are left in place until the woman returns for a follow-up appointment in 2 weeks.

Discharge Planning

A woman being discharged after cesarean birth takes home not only her new baby but a fair amount of pain and discomfort. Be certain to discuss home care arrangements, emphasizing the need for adequate help with her newborn and other responsibilities at home, before discharge. Be sure a woman is aware of any restrictions on exercise or activity

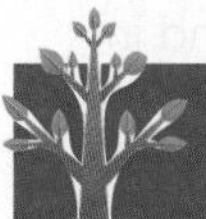

BOX 24.5 ✻ Focus on Family Teaching

Measures to Regain Energy After a Cesarean Birth

Q. Moja Hamma tells you, "I feel so tired after my cesarean. What can I do to feel stronger again?"

A. After a cesarean birth, women usually regain energy rapidly. This is because, unlike most people who have had surgery, you did not have it because you were ill, but because it was an alternative method to have a healthy baby. Good suggestions to help regain your energy rapidly are:

- Drink adequate fluid daily (at least six glasses). This helps prevent a urinary tract infection and also helps supply all the cells in your body with adequate fluid.
- Rest twice a day for at least one-half hour each time. This helps because your baby will probably wake you at least once during the night.
- Do not hesitate to accept help from family and friends for tasks such as house cleaning or grocery shopping.
- Limit the number of stairs that you climb daily to one flight once a day. Also limit the amount of weight you lift to the weight of your new baby.
- Do not attempt to be the "perfect" new mom. Relax and enjoy your new baby.

that she needs to follow (common restrictions are not to lift any object heavier than 10 lb or walk upstairs more than once a day for the first 2 weeks). Also teach her to recognize signs of possible complications directly related to the surgery, such as:

- Redness or drainage at the incision line
- Lochia heavier than a normal menstrual period
- Abdominal pain (other than suture line or afterpain discomfort)
- Temperature greater than 38° C (100.4° F)
- Frequency or burning on urination

A woman can plan on resuming coitus as soon as the act is comfortable for her, possibly as early as 1 week after discharge. Cesarean birth does not interfere with future fertility so be sure that she has contraceptive information, if desired (Oral & Elter, 2007). Also ensure that she has an appointment for a return visit with her health care provider (usually in 2 weeks), for both herself and her newborn.

Unless the reason for the cesarean birth was cephalopelvic disproportion, a woman can probably have her next child vaginally (see Chapter 15). Being certain the woman is aware of this not only makes her an informed consumer of health care but also can influence whether she plans an additional pregnancy (see Focus on Nursing Care Planning Box 24.6).

✔ Checkpoint Question 24.4

Moja Hamma wonders if she can breastfeed following a cesarean birth. Your best answer would be:

a. You do not recommend she try to breastfeed because she will feel so ill.
b. It is difficult for a woman with an abdominal incision to hold a newborn.
c. She will need too much analgesia postoperatively to make breastfeeding safe.
d. Women can breastfeed without difficulty following a cesarean birth.

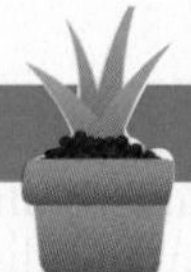

BOX 24.6 * Focus on Nursing Care Planning

A Multidisciplinary Care Map for a Woman Following an Emergent Cesarean Birth

Moja Hamma is a 29-year-old primigravida who underwent an emergent cesarean birth with combined spinal-epidural anesthesia for fetal distress. Moja gave birth to a healthy 8-lb 2-oz baby girl. She tells you, "I'm thirsty, and it hurts so much I can't move. Take the baby away. I can't hold her right now."

Family Assessment * Client lives with boyfriend in west-side apartment. Works as a clerk in a bridal salon. Boyfriend is currently unemployed. Borrowed money from a friend for hospital bill.

Client Assessment * Post-cesarean birth 4 hours ago. Estimated blood loss of 700 mL. Abdomen soft but tender with low transverse incision. No bowel sounds present. Incisional dressing clean, dry, and intact. Uterus firm, 1 fingerbreadth below umbilicus. Minimal lochia rubra vaginal drainage. Urine output 100 mL in last hour. Skin pink, warm, and dry. Skin turgor good. Ringer's lactate infusing at 100 mL/hr. Intravenous site clean, dry, without signs of infiltration. Vital signs: temperature, 98.4° F; pulse, 78 beats per minute; respirations, 23 per minute; blood pressure, 130/76 mm Hg. Pulse, respirations, and blood pressure slightly elevated above baseline. Respirations shallow. States she has abdominal pain, especially at incisional area. Holding hands over abdomen; barely moving in bed. Client's mother at bedside holding her hand and stroking her forehead. PCEA pump in place but not being used by client. When asked why she wasn't using the PCEA pump, she answered, "I don't want to take the chance of being paralyzed forever."

Nursing Diagnosis * Pain related to tissue trauma from abdominal incision of cesarean birth

Outcome Criteria * Client identifies pain management measure of choice; reports a decrease in pain with analgesic administration; pulse, respirations, and blood pressure return to baseline.
Client holds infant warmly; maintains eye contact with infant; makes positive statements about the newborn prior to discharge.

Team Member Responsible	Assessment	Intervention	Rationale	Expected Outcome
		Activities of Daily Living		
Nurse	Assess client's ability to move in bed and breastfeed infant.	Stress the importance of getting out of bed and caring for infant.	Early ambulation helps prevent thrombophlebitis; early breastfeeding helps establish adequate milk supply.	Client feels well enough to be out of bed and feeding infant by 4 hours' time due to chosen pain relief method.

Consultations				
Nurse	Investigate whether pain management team is available for consultation.	Ask pain management team to consult on more appropriate pain relief measures.	Client states she is afraid to use PCEA for pain relief.	Pain management team discusses options for pain relief with client and they agree on a suitable procedure by 2 hours.
Procedures/Medications				
Nurse	Assess what measures client feels would make her most comfortable.	Institute additional comfort measures, such as changing position, splinting incision, using pillows and blankets for support. Institute different pain management system if one is employed or assist with present system if client agrees with system.	Comfort measures reduce stress and anxiety, elevate mood, and raise the pain threshold, enhancing the therapeutic effectiveness of analgesics and the client's control over and ability to tolerate pain.	Client reports additional comfort measures aid pain relief. Client reports pain management system is operating effectively.
Nurse	Assess what measures client thinks would help her be more successful with breastfeeding.	Assist client with handling newborn. Support breastfeeding efforts.	Breastfeeding is a new skill for a first time mother.	Client breastfeeds the infant successfully with support from health care providers.
Nutrition				
Nurse	Assess bowel sounds to determine when oral fluid can be offered.	Offer ice cubes for dry mouth as soon as bowel sounds are present.	Client cannot drink full liquids until bowel sounds return.	Client states mouth discomfort is reduced by 1 hour after first fluid.
Patient/Family Education				
Pain management Team/ nurse	Assess client's expectations of pain relief measures.	Review PCEA pump and technique with client.	Client cannot have realistic expectations unless she understands technique.	Client states that she will use PCEA pump on trial basis for 4 hours or choose an alternative method of pain management.
Psychosocial/Spiritual/Emotional Needs				
Nurse	Assess what additional measures client feels she needs to feel secure after frightening experience of emergent cesarean birth.	Provide reinforcement for positive coping mechanisms that client demonstrates.	Positive reinforcement enhances self-esteem and control. Praise promotes self-esteem and confidence to manage new situations.	Client states she feels her coping measures are reinforced by health care providers. Client states she feels health care providers provide her support equal to her level of pain and fatigue.
Nurse	Assess client's expectations of a newborn.	Praise client for positive behaviors and interactions with the child in light of pain and fatigue level. Encourage client to keep newborn in the room with her for extended periods as she is able.	Extended contact within the client's ability to tolerate the activity encourages bonding while minimizing the risk for additional fatigue.	Client keeps newborn with her in room for the majority of daylight hours. Interacts actively with child.

(continued)

BOX 24.6 * Focus on Nursing Care Planning (continued)

Discharge Planning				
Nurse	Assess the level of support client will have after she returns home.	Review with client importance of maintaining a level of pain relief at home so she can ambulate and care for new child.	Ambulation and child care are important for both maternal and child health. Keeping pain to a minimum helps the client achieve these activities.	Client states she will take enough pain relief at home to allow her to be active and care for newborn. She names at least one person to serve as support person.
Nurse	Assess whether client understands signs and symptoms such as pain on urination she will need to report after discharge.	Teach signs of complications she should report to her health care provider.	Knowing signs and symptoms of complications adds to client's base of knowledge.	Client repeats danger signs that she will report to her health care provider.

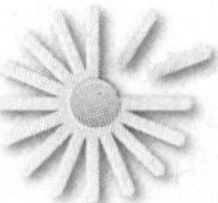

Key Points for Review

- The term *cesarean birth* is preferred to *cesarean section* or *delivery,* because it puts the focus on the childbirth rather than surgical elements of the procedure.
- Cesarean birth may be either a scheduled or an emergent procedure. Because it carries more risk for the woman and infant than does vaginal birth, it is usually undertaken only when medically necessary, although a current trend allows for elective procedures.
- Establishing surgical risk includes assessment of nutritional status, age, general health, fluid and electrolyte balance, and psychological condition.
- Assessment measures before surgery usually include vital sign determination; urinalysis; blood studies such as complete blood count, electrolytes, blood typing, and cross-matching; and ultrasound.
- The skin incision may be vertical (a classic incision), although it is usually a horizontal one just above the pubic hair. The internal incision into the uterus is also usually a horizontal incision into the lower uterine segment.
- The old saying, "Once a cesarean, always a cesarean," is no longer true, as long as cephalopelvic disproportion does not exist and the previous incision was a low transverse one.
- Support people can lose a great deal of their ability to support if they feel intimidated and out of place in an operating room; offer them support as needed to make this a positive experience for them as well.
- Cesarean birth is one of the safest types of surgery performed. To keep a woman safe after the procedure, remember that she is both a postsurgical and a postpartum patient. Make assessments to ensure that neither postpartum nor postsurgical complications occur.
- Adequate pain management is important to allow a woman a sense of control and comfort and bonding with her newborn.
- Women are physically exhausted after cesarean birth and may be psychologically exhausted because of the emergent nature of the experience. Provide rest time to relieve the physical strain and a chance to verbalize the experience to help relieve the psychological strain.
- A major intervention after cesarean birth is early ambulation to prevent complications. Incisional pain may make this difficult, so strong nursing support and adequate pain management are necessary.

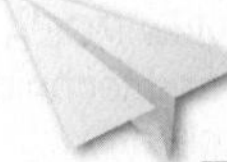

CRITICAL THINKING EXERCISES

1. Moja, the woman you met at the beginning of this chapter, was afraid to have a cesarean birth because she did not want to be alone. What actions could you take to make her situation easier to accept?
2. Suppose Moja is receiving PCEA after her cesarean birth. She tells you that she is not interested in PCEA and would rather have injections for pain. Describe and explain the action you might take. Would you advocate for use of PCEA or advocate with her physician for a changed order?
3. Moja's boyfriend tells you that he cannot possibly stay with her in the operating room while she has a cesarean birth. He's sure he'll feel nauseated and probably faint. How would you intervene to promote family-centered care and meet the couple's needs?
4. Examine the National Health Goals related to cesarean birth. Most government-sponsored funds for nursing research are allotted based on these goals. What would be a possible research topic to explore pertinent to these goals that would be applicable to the Hamma family and also advance evidence-based practice?

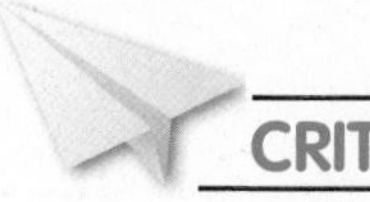

CRITICAL THINKING SCENARIO

Open the accompanying CD-ROM or visit http://thePoint.lww.com and read the Patient Scenario included for this chapter, then answer the questions to further sharpen your skills and grow more familiar with NCLEX style questions related to cesarean birth. Confirm your answers are correct by reading the rationales.

REFERENCES

Anderson, E. R., & Gates, S. (2009). Techniques and materials for closure of the abdominal wall in caesarean section. *Cochrane Database of Systematic Reviews, 2009*(1), (CD004663).

Bailit, J., et al. (2008). Maternal-Fetal Medicine Units Network cesarean registry: impact of shift change on cesarean complications. *American Journal of Obstetrics and Gynecology, 198*(2), 173–177.

Barnes, M. (2007). PTSD after childbirth. *AIMS Journal, 19*(1), 9–10.

Bhattacharya, S., et al. (2007). Effect of Body Mass Index on pregnancy outcomes in nulliparous women delivering singleton babies. *BMC Public Health, 7*(1), 168.

Cho, J. E., & Penning, D. H. (2007). Obstetric anesthesia. In K. B. Fortner, et al. (Eds.). *The Johns Hopkins manual of gynecology and obstetrics.* Philadelphia: Lippincott Williams & Wilkins.

Clark, S. L., et al.(2007). Variation in the rates of operative delivery in the United States. *American Journal of Obstetrics and Gynecology, 196*(6), 526–531.

Datta, M. S., & Gutman, R. E. (2007). Perioperative care and complications of gynecologic surgery. In K. B. Fortner, et al. (Eds.). *The Johns Hopkins manual of gynecology and obstetrics.* Philadelphia: Lippincott Williams & Wilkins.

Dietz, H. P. (2007). Pelvic floor trauma following vaginal delivery. *Current Opinion in Obstetrics and Gynecology, 18*(5), 528–537.

Dodd, J. M., et al. (2009). Planned elective repeat caesarean section versus planned vaginal birth for women with a previous caesarean birth. *Cochrane Database of Systematic Reviews, 2009*(1), (CD004224).

Gates, S., Brocklehurst, P., & Davis, L. J. (2009). Prophylaxis for venous thromboembolic disease in pregnancy and the early postnatal period. *Cochrane Database of Systematic Reviews, 2009*(1), (CD001689).

Gourounti, K., & Sandall, J. (2007). Admission cardiotocography versus intermittent auscultation of fetal heart rate: effects on neonatal Apgar score, on the rate of caesarean sections and on the rate of instrumental delivery—a systematic review. *International Journal of Nursing Studies, 44*(6), 1029–1035.

Halls, K. L. (2008). Maternal satisfaction regarding anaesthetic services during childbirth. *British Journal of Midwifery, 16*(5), 296–301.

Hansen, A. K., et al. (2008). Risk of respiratory morbidity in term infants delivered by elective caesarean section: cohort study. *BMJ: British Medical Journal, 336*(7635), 85–87.

Hodnett, E. D., et al. (2009). Continuous support for women during childbirth. *Cochrane Database of Systematic Reviews, 2009*(1), (CD003766).

Hofmeyr, G. J., & Hannah, M. E. (2009). Planned caesarean section for term breech delivery. *Cochrane Database of Systematic Reviews, 2009*(1), (CD000166).

Hopkins, L., & Smaill, F. (2009). Antibiotic prophylaxis regimens and drugs for cesarean section. *Cochrane Database of Systematic Reviews, 2009*(1), (CD001136).

Incerpi, M.H. (2007). Operative delivery. In A. H. DeCherney & L. Nathan (Eds.). *Current diagnosis and treatment in obstetrics and gynecology* (10th ed.). Columbus, OH: McGraw-Hill.

Izbizky, G. H., et al. (2008). The effect of early versus delayed postcaesarean feeding on women's satisfaction: a randomised controlled trial. *BJOG: An International Journal of Obstetrics and Gynaecology, 115*(3), 332–338.

Lavender, T., et al. (2009). Caesarean section for non-medical reasons at term. *Cochrane Database of Systematic Reviews, 2009*(1), (CD004660).

Lawson, S. M., & Bienstock, J. L. (2007). Normal labor and delivery, operative delivery, and malpresentations. In K. B. Fortner, et al. (Eds.). *The Johns Hopkins manual of gynecology and obstetrics.* Philadelphia: Lippincott Williams & Wilkins.

Lobel, M., & DeLuca, R. S. (2007). Psychosocial sequelae of cesarean delivery: review and analysis of their causes and implications. *Social Science and Medicine, 64*(11), 2272–2284.

Mangesi, L., & Hofmeyr, G. J. (2009). Early compared with delayed oral fluids and food after caesarean section. *Cochrane Database of Systematic Reviews, 2009*(1), (CD003516).

Marshall, K. M., & Baker, J. (2007). Doing it better: putting research into practice. Are patients in labor satisfied with PCEA? *Nursing, 36*(6), 18–19.

McIntyre, P. G., Tosh, K., & McGuire, W. (2009). Caesarean section versus vaginal delivery for preventing mother to infant hepatitis C virus transmission. *Cochrane Database of Systematic Reviews, 2009*(1), (CD005546).

National Vital Statistics System (NVSS). (2008). *National vital statistics reports. Birth data.* Hyattsville, MD: Author.

Ng, K., et al. (2009). Spinal versus epidural anaesthesia for caesarean section. *Cochrane Database of Systematic Reviews, 2009*(1), (CD003765).

Oral, E., & Elter, K. (2007). The impact of cesarean birth on subsequent fertility. *Current Opinion in Obstetrics and Gynecology, 19*(3), 238–243.

Read, J. S., & Newell, M. L. (2007). Efficacy and safety of cesarean delivery for prevention of mother-to-child transmission of HIV-1. *Cochrane Database of Systematic Reviews, 2009*(1), (CD005479).

Robilio, P., et al. (2007). Vaginal vs. cesarean delivery for preterm breech presentation of singleton infants in California: a population-based study. *Journal of Reproductive Medicine, 52*(6), 473–479.

Simpson, K. R. (2007). Perinatal patient safety. Emergent cesarean birth preparedness. *MCN: The American Journal of Maternal/Child Nursing, 32*(4), 264.

Wiklund, I., et al. (2008). Expectation and experiences of childbirth in primiparae with caesarean section. *BJOG: An International Journal of Obstetrics and Gynaecology, 115*(3), 324–331.

SUGGESTED READINGS

Clarkson, C., Derrick, D. C., & Newburn, M. (2007). Vaginal birth after caesarean. *Practising Midwife, 9*(11), 34–37.

Clements, C. J., et al. (2007). Priority #1: safety. OB team stat: rapid response to obstetrical emergencies. *Nursing for Women's Health, 11*(2), 194–199.

Declercq, E., et al. (2007). Maternal outcomes associated with planned primary cesarean births compared with planned vaginal births. *Obstetrics and Gynecology, 109*(3), 669–677.

Horey, D., Weaver, J., & Russell, H. (2009). Information for pregnant women about caesarean birth. *Cochrane Database of Systematic Reviews, 2009*(1), (CD003858).

Montgomery, A. A., et al. (2007). Two decision aids for mode of delivery among women with previous caesarean section: randomised controlled trial. *BMJ: British Medical Journal: 334*(7607), 1305–1309.

Regan, M., & Liaschenko, J. (2007). In the mind of the beholder: hypothesized effect of intrapartum nurses' cognitive frames of childbirth cesarean section rates. *Qualitative Health Research, 17*(5), 612–624.

Simpson, K. R. (2007). Surgical safety: minimizing risk of retained foreign bodies during cesarean birth. *MCN: The American Journal of Maternal/Child Nursing, 32*(3), 200.

Sorensen, S. S. (2007). Emergency drills in obstetrics: reducing risk of perinatal death or permanent injury. *JONA's Healthcare Law, Ethics, and Regulation, 9*(1), 9–18.

Tita, A. T., et al. (2008). Decreasing incidence of postcesarean endometritis with extended-spectrum antibiotic prophylaxis. *Obstetrics and Gynecology, 111*(1), 51–56.

Waldenstrom, U., Hildingsson, I., & Ryding, E. (2007). Antenatal fear of childbirth and its association with subsequent caesarean section and experience of childbirth. *BJOG: An International Journal of Obstetrics and Gynaecology, 113*(6), 638–646.

Chapter 25 Nursing Care of a Family Experiencing a Postpartal Complication

KEY TERMS

- endometritis
- mastitis
- peritonitis
- postpartal depression
- postpartal psychosis
- thrombophlebitis
- uterine inversion

OBJECTIVES

After mastering the contents of this chapter, you should be able to:

1. Describe common deviations from the normal that can occur during the puerperium.
2. Identify National Health Goals related to postpartal complications that nurses can help the nation achieve.
3. Use critical thinking to analyze ways that promote family-centered nursing care when a postpartal complication occurs.
4. Assess a woman and her family for deviations from the normal during the puerperium.
5. Formulate nursing diagnoses related to deviations from the normal during the puerperium.
6. Identify expected outcomes for a postpartal woman experiencing a complication.
7. Plan nursing interventions that meet the special needs of a family with a postpartal complication, such as planning for an extended hospitalization.
8. Implement nursing care when a postpartal complication such as hemorrhage, infection, pregnancy-induced hypertension, or postpartal psychosis develops.
9. Evaluate expected outcomes for achievement and effectiveness of care.
10. Identify areas related to care of women with postpartal complications that could benefit from additional nursing research or application of evidence-based practice.
11. Integrate knowledge of postpartal complications with the nursing process to achieve quality maternal and child health nursing care.

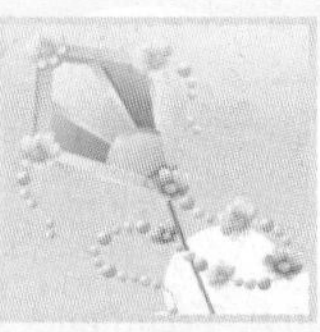

Mary Blackhawk is a 30-year-old woman who had a "textbook-perfect" pregnancy. You enter her room 4 hours after she gave birth to an 8-lb girl, but, because she is sleeping and appears comfortable, you hesitate to awaken her. When you observe her more closely, however, you realize she appears abnormally pale. You obtain her vital signs and document her pulse as 90 beats per minute and her blood pressure as 96/50 mm Hg. When you fold back her bedclothes, you discover her bed is soaked with blood. You suspect she is experiencing one of the most serious complications of pregnancy: postpartum hemorrhage. Yet because she was sleeping, she was totally unaware of it.

In an earlier chapter, you learned about caring for a woman during the usual postpartal period. This chapter adds information about how to care for a woman and her family when there is a complication during this time. Conscientious nursing care is important when a postpartal complication develops because it plays a major role in protecting the health of both women and their families.

What immediate measures does Ms. Blackhawk need? What would be your first action?

Although the puerperium is usually a period of health, complications can occur. When they do, immediate intervention is essential to prevent long-term disability and interference with parent–child relationships. Box 25.1 describes National Health Goals related to this period.

A woman with a postpartal complication is at risk from three points of view: her own health, her future childbearing potential, and her ability to bond with her new infant. Her family may be disrupted because of an extended hospital stay that removes her from other family members. Financial difficulties may arise because of the need for additional child and health care. Fortunately, most postpartal complications are preventable, and if they do occur, the majority can be treated effectively without long-term complications.

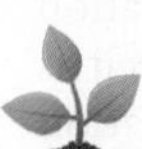

Nursing Process Overview

For a Woman Experiencing a Postpartal Complication

Assessment

Women who assume that they will immediately return to an active lifestyle after birth of their child may view hospitalization for a postpartal complication as more upsetting than do women who view the postpartal period as one in which they are expected to rest. Assessing each woman individually is necessary to establish the personal impact of a postpartal complication.

Assessment findings associated with a postpartal complication may be extremely subtle, such as tenderness in the calf of a leg, a slight increase in uterine or perineal pain, a slight elevation in temperature, or a slight increase in the amount of lochia flow (Box 25.2). Because the average woman usually has no postpartal complications and the length of stay in a hospital is short, it is easy to overlook these subtle signs. It is important to be alert to any findings that are "different from usual," because they may be the beginning of a problem. To be certain, do not rely solely on a woman's report of perineal healing or amount of lochia. Always inspect her perineum yourself, because the report of "I feel fine" may be deceptive because she expected to have pain and so reports extreme pain as nothing out of the norm; she has no knowledge of "normal" lochia or fundal height against which to accurately compare her own condition.

An increased temperature during the first 24 hours after birth is an extremely serious finding. Women may try to "explain away" an increased temperature, because they know that if they have an elevated temperature they

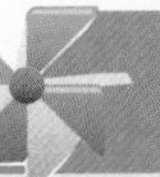

BOX 25.1 * Focus on National Health Goals

The postpartal period is a time when women are very susceptible to hemorrhage and thrombophlebitis, and with a complication women after childbirth may choose not to breastfeed. Three National Health Goals directly relate to this period:

- Reduce the maternal mortality rate to no more than 3.3 per 100,000 live births from a baseline of 7.1 per 100,000.
- Increase to at least 75% the proportion of mothers who breastfeed their babies in the early postpartal period from a baseline of 64%.
- Increase to at least 60% the proportion of mothers who breastfeed exclusively through 3 months from a baseline of 43% (http://www.nih.gov).

Nurses can help the nation achieve these goals by careful monitoring of uterine involution in the postpartal period and by encouraging women to breastfeed even in the face of a postpartal complication.

Areas related to complications of the postpartal period that could benefit from additional nursing research include methods to better identify risk factors for mastitis and endometritis; identifiable differences between women who stop breastfeeding and those who continue when a complication is present; and health teaching that is effective in preventing mastitis.

Box 25.2 Assessment: Assessing the Postpartal Woman With Complications

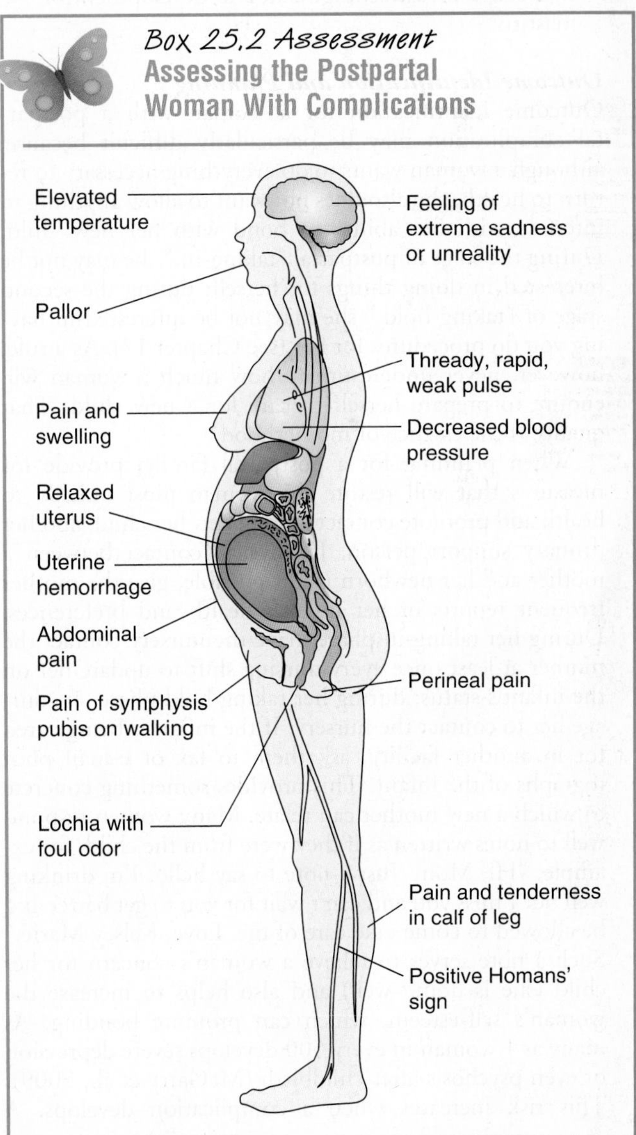

may not be allowed to go home or feed their infant. Do not be tempted to rationalize such a finding with explanations such as, "The room was warm," or "She just drank some hot coffee." Although these factors may make a slight difference (part of 1°) in temperature level, they do not affect it enough to account for an oral temperature greater than 100.4° F (38.0° C).

Nursing Diagnosis

Nursing diagnoses during this time vary depending on the postpartal complication. Some examples are:

- Deficient fluid volume related to increased lochia flow
- Risk for infection related to microorganism invasion of episiotomy
- Ineffective peripheral tissue perfusion related to interference with circulation from thrombophlebitis
- Situational low self-esteem related to postpartal infection and inability to feed infant
- Social isolation related to precautions necessary to protect infant and others from infection transmission
- Risk for impaired parenting related to postpartal depression
- Ineffective breastfeeding related to development of mastitis

Outcome Identification and Planning

Outcome identification for a woman with a postpartal complication may be particularly difficult because, although a woman wants to do everything necessary to return to health, she also does not want to allow anything to interfere with her ability to bond with her new child. During the stage of postpartal "taking-in," she may not be interested in doing things for herself; during the second stage of "taking-hold," she may not be interested in having you do procedures for her (see Chapter 17). As a rule, however, never underestimate how much a woman will endure to prepare herself to care for a new child. That quality is the essence of motherhood.

When planning for a postpartal family, provide for measures that will restore the woman most quickly to health and promote contact among her, her child, and her primary support person. If physical contact between a mother and her newborn is not possible, give the mother frequent reports of her infant's health and preferences. During her taking-in phase, have the nursery contact the mother at least once every nursing shift to update her on the infant's status; during her taking-hold phase, encourage her to contact the nursery. If the infant is being cared for in another facility, ask them to fax or e-mail photographs of the infant. This provides something concrete to which a new mother can relate. Many women respond well to notes written as if they were from the child, for example, "Hi, Mom. Just a note to say hello. I'm drinking well but I miss you and can't wait for you to get better and be allowed to come take care of me. Love, Kelsey Marie." Such a note serves to relieve a woman's concern for her child (she is doing well) and also helps to increase the woman's self-esteem, which can promote bonding. As many as 1 woman in every 500 develops severe depression or even psychosis after childbirth (McGarry et al., 2009). This risk increases when a complication develops. A helpful national volunteer support group for women who are depressed after childbirth is Depression After Delivery (http://www.depressionafterdelivery.com).

Implementation

Interventions for a woman with a postpartal complication should include instruction for both self-care and child care (if appropriate), emphasizing the transitory nature of the complication. Continuing to review well-child care in this way helps a woman accept her situation as temporary, reinforcing the idea she will be able to care for her infant when she is healthy again.

Outcome Evaluation

Evaluation of a woman with a postpartal complication should address both her and her family's health as well as her family's ability to bond with the new child. Evaluation may suggest the need for home care follow-up to assist a woman in coping with the responsibility of child care and integrating a new child into the family in the face of reduced energy from illness.

Examples of expected outcomes might include:

- Oral temperature decreases to less than 100.4° F (38.0° C).
- Lochia is free of foul odor.
- Client maintains blood pressure higher than 110/60 mm Hg.
- Client demonstrates bonding behaviors with infant despite separation.
- Client demonstrates warm contact with her child while maintaining required bed rest.

POSTPARTAL HEMORRHAGE

Hemorrhage, one of the most important causes of maternal mortality associated with childbearing, poses a possible threat throughout pregnancy and is also a major potential danger in the immediate postpartal period. Significant hemorrhage occurs in 5% to 8% of women postpartally (Poggi, 2007). Traditionally, postpartal hemorrhage has been defined as any blood loss from the uterus greater than 500 mL within a 24-hour period (Pavone, Purinton, & Petersen, 2007). In specific agencies, the loss may not be considered hemorrhage until it reaches 1000 mL. Hemorrhage may occur either early (within the first 24 hours) or late (anytime after the first 24 hours during the remaining days of the 6-week puerperium). The greatest danger of hemorrhage is in the first 24 hours because of the grossly denuded and unprotected uterine area left after detachment of the placenta.

There are five main causes for postpartal hemorrhage: uterine atony, lacerations, retained placental fragments, uterine inversion, and disseminated intravascular coagulation (Fig. 25.1).

Uterine Atony

Uterine atony, or relaxation of the uterus, is the most frequent cause of postpartal hemorrhage (Poggi, 2007). The uterus must remain in a contracted state after birth to keep the open vessels at the placental site from bleeding. Factors that predis-

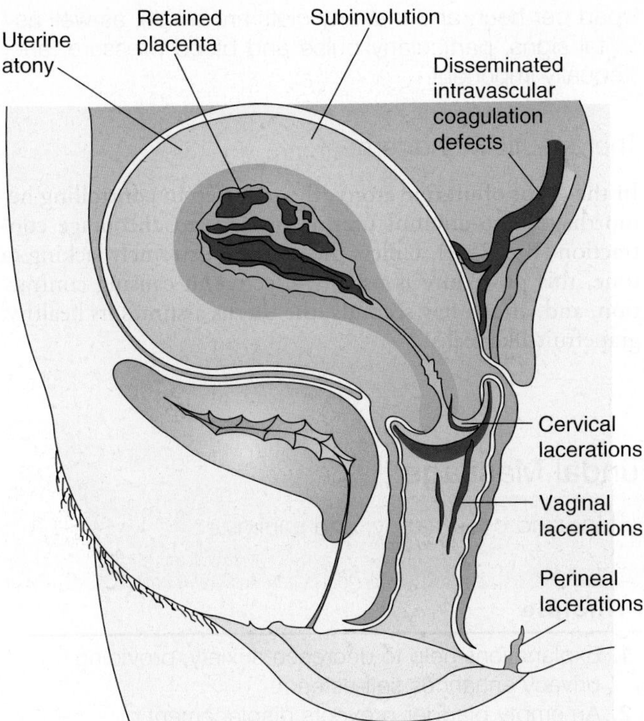

FIGURE 25.1 Common causes of postpartal hemorrhage.

pose to poor uterine tone or any inability to maintain a contracted state are summarized in Box 25.3. When caring for a woman in whom any of these conditions are present, be especially cautious in your observations and be on guard for signs of uterine bleeding. This is especially important because many postpartal women are discharged within 48 hours after birth.

BOX 25.3 ✻ Conditions That Increase a Woman's Risk for Postpartal Hemorrhage

Conditions That Distend the Uterus Beyond Average Capacity

Multiple gestation
Hydramnios (excessive amount of amniotic fluid)
Large baby (>9 lb)
Presence of uterine myomas (fibroid tumors)

Conditions That Could Have Caused Cervical or Uterine Lacerations

Operative birth
Rapid birth

Conditions With Varied Placental Site or Attachment

Placenta previa
Placenta accreta
Premature separation of the placenta
Retained placental fragments

Conditions That Leave the Uterus Unable to Contract Readily

Deep anesthesia or analgesia
Labor initiated or assisted with an oxytocin agent
Maternal age greater than 35 years
High parity
Previous uterine surgery
Prolonged and difficult labor
Possible chorioamnionitis
Secondary maternal illness (e.g., anemia)
Prior history of postpartum hemorrhage
Endometritis
Prolonged use of magnesium sulfate or other tocolytic therapy

Conditions That Lead to Inadequate Blood Coagulation

Fetal death
Disseminated intravascular coagulation

Nursing Diagnosis and Related Interventions

✻

Nursing Diagnosis: Deficient fluid volume related to excessive blood loss after birth.

Outcome Evaluation: Client's blood pressure remains higher than 100/60 mm Hg; pulse remains between 70 and 90 beats per minute; lochia flow is less than one saturated perineal pad per hour.

If the uterus suddenly relaxes, there will be an abrupt gush of blood vaginally from the placental site. If the vaginal bleeding is extremely copious, a woman will exhibit symptoms of shock and blood loss. This can occur immediately after birth or more gradually, over the first postpartum hour, as the uterus slowly becomes uncontracted. When the vaginal bleeding occurs gradually, it results in seepage, not a gush of blood. Over a period of hours, however, continued seepage can be as lethal as a sudden release of blood.

It is difficult to estimate the amount of blood a postpartal woman has lost, because it is difficult to estimate the amount of blood it takes to saturate a perineal pad. The amount is between 25 and 50 mL. By counting the number of perineal pads saturated in given lengths of time such as half-hour intervals, you can form a rough estimate of blood loss. Five pads saturated in half an hour is obviously a different situation from five pads saturated in 8 hours. In either situation, however, a woman will have lost approximately 250 mL of blood, and if either scenario is allowed to continue unattended, she will be in grave danger. Be sure you differentiate between *saturated* and *used* when counting pads. Weighing perineal pads before and after use and then subtracting the difference is an accurate way to measure vaginal discharge: 1 g of weight is comparable to 1 mL of blood volume. Always be sure to turn a woman on her side when inspecting for blood loss, to be certain that a large amount of blood is not pooling undetected beneath her.

Palpate a woman's fundus at frequent intervals postpartally to be certain that her uterus is remaining in a state of contraction. This is the best measure for preventing early hemorrhage. When palpating a uterine fundus, if you are unsure whether you have located it, the uterus is probably in a state of relaxation. Under normal circumstances, a well-contracted uterus is firm and easily recognized because it feels like no other abdominal organ. Frequent assessments of lochia (to be certain that the amount of the flow is under a saturated pad per hour, and that any clots are small), as well as vital signs, particularly pulse and blood pressure, are equally important.

Therapeutic Management

In the event of uterine atony, the first step in controlling hemorrhage is to attempt uterine massage to encourage contraction (Box 25.4). Unless the uterus is extremely lacking in tone, this procedure is usually effective in causing contraction, and, after a few seconds, the uterus assumes its healthy, grapefruit-like feel.

Box 25.4 Nursing Procedure ✻ Fundal Massage

Purpose: To stimulate uterine contraction, promote uterine tone and consistency, and minimize the risk of hemorrhage.

Procedure	Principle
1. Explain the procedure to the client and provide privacy.	**1.** Explanations help to decrease anxiety; providing privacy enhances self-esteem.
2. Ask the client to void (unless bleeding is extensive and more rapid action seems necessary).	**2.** An empty bladder prevents displacement of the uterus and ensures accurate assessment of uterine tone.
3. Place the client supine with her knees flexed and feet together.	**3.** Proper positioning enhances visualization and effectiveness of procedure.
4. a. Put on gloves. Place one hand on the abdomen just above the symphysis pubis.	**4. a.** This location anchors the lower uterine segment.
b. Place the other hand around the top of the fundus.	**b.** This location helps to assess and locate the fundus and determine height.

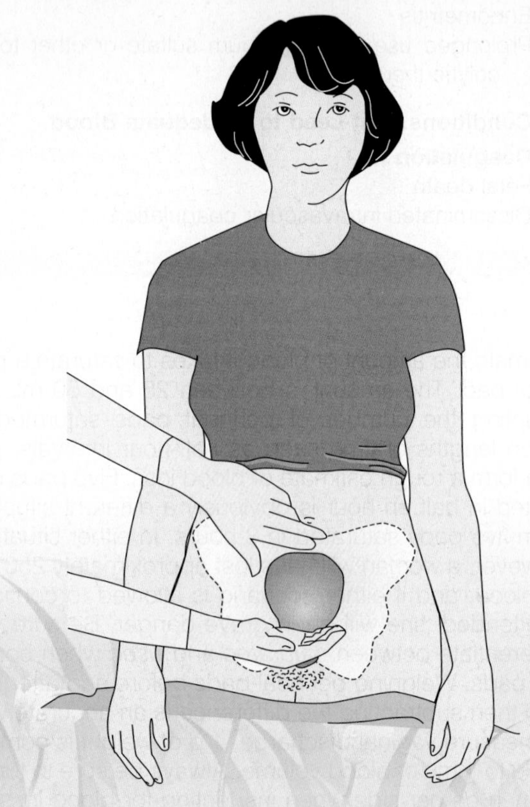

Procedure	Principle
5. Rotate the upper hand to massage the uterus until it is firm, being careful not to overmassage the uterus.	**5.** Massage should be done only when uterus is not firm; otherwise muscle fatigue and uterine relaxation may occur. Aggressive massage may lead to partial or complete uterine prolapse.

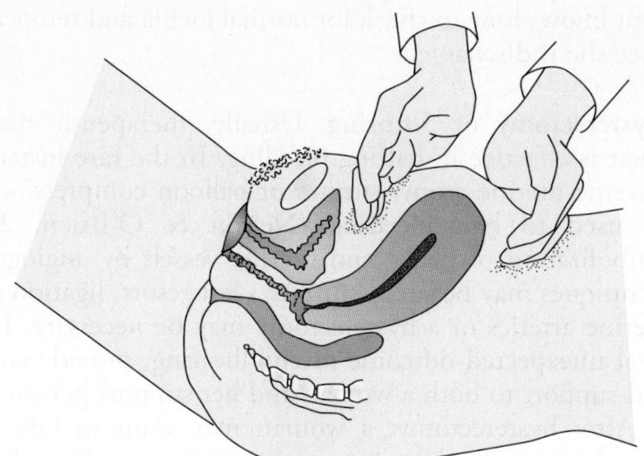

Procedure	Principle
6. When the uterus is firm, gently press the fundus between the hands using slight downward pressure against the lower hand.	**6.** Gently squeezing with downward pressure helps to expel blood or clots collected in the uterine cavity.
7. Remove the perineal pad. Observe the perineum for passage of clots and amount of bleeding.	**7.** This helps to assess the degree of bleeding.
8. When the uterus is again firm, cleanse the perineum and apply a clean perineal pad. Discard gloves and soiled pads according to agency policy.	**8.** This helps to promote comfort and hygiene while reducing the risk for infection.
9. Document results of procedure. Continue to assess fundus and lochia according to agency policy. Notify physician or nurse-midwife if fundus does not remain firm or bleeding continues.	**9.** Documentation provides a means for evaluation. Continued assessment allows for early identification and prompt intervention with additional measures, such as oxytocin, to prevent hemorrhage.

With uterine atony, even if the uterus responds well to massage, the problem may not be completely resolved. After you remove your hand from the fundus, the uterus may relax and the lethal seepage may begin again. Therefore, remain with the woman after massaging her fundus, to be certain the uterus is not relaxing again. Observe carefully, including fundal height and consistency and lochia, for the next 4 hours.

If a uterus cannot remain contracted, her physician or nurse-midwife probably will order a dilute intravenous infusion of oxytocin (Pitocin) to help the uterus maintain tone (see Box 15.10 in Chapter 15). Carboprost tromethamine (Hemabate), a prostaglandin F_{2a} derivative, or methylergonovine maleate (Methergine), an ergot compound, given intramuscularly, are second possibilities. Rectal misoprostol, a prostaglandin E_1 analogue, may be administered rectally. Hemabate may be repeated every 15 to 90 minutes up to 8 doses; methylergonovine may be repeated every 2 to 4 hours up to 5 doses. All these drugs should be readily available for use on a hospital unit in the event of postpartal hemorrhage. Because prostaglandins tend to cause diarrhea as a side effect, assess for this frequently.

The usual dosage of oxytocin is 10 to 40 U per 1000 mL of a Ringer's lactate solution. When oxytocin is given intravenously, its action is immediate. However, be aware that oxytocin has a short duration of action, approximately 1 hour, so symptoms of uterine atony can recur quickly after administration of only a single dose. Methylergonovine causes increased blood pressure so it is contraindicated with a woman with hypertension (generally a blood pressure over 140 mm Hg systolic).

Additional measures that can be helpful:

- Offer a bedpan or assist the woman with ambulating to the bathroom at least every 4 hours to be certain her bladder is empty. A full bladder pushes an uncontracted uterus into an even more uncontracted state. To reduce bladder pressure, insertion of a urinary catheter may be ordered.
- If a woman is experiencing respiratory distress from decreasing blood volume, administer oxygen by face mask at a rate of about 4 L/min. Position her supine to allow adequate blood flow to her brain and kidneys.
- Obtain vital signs frequently and make sure to interpret them accurately, looking for trends. For example, a continuously rising pulse rate is an ominous pattern.

If a woman is losing enough blood to affect her systemic circulation, she will develop signs of shock, such as an increased, thready, and weak pulse; decreased blood pressure; increased and shallow respirations; pale, clammy skin; and increasing anxiety.

In the event of slow bleeding, there is little change in pulse and blood pressure at first because of circulatory compensation. Suddenly, however, the system can compensate no more, and then the pulse rate rises rapidly. The pulse becomes weak and thready, and the blood pressure drops abruptly. The woman's skin becomes cold and clammy, and she shows obvious signs of shock. Consistent frequent assessments of uterine tone and vital signs and laboratory assessments such as hemoglobin and hematocrit levels help to detect blood loss before this point is ever reached.

When planning continuing care after sudden blood loss, understand that a woman may be so exhausted that she resents frequent uterine and blood pressure assessments. Explain that these measures, although disturbing, are important for her welfare. Obtain vital signs as quickly and gently as possible, so that a woman feels a minimum of discomfort and disruption, allowing her time to rest.

Bimanual Massage. If fundal massage and administration of oxytocin or methylergonovine are not effective in stopping uterine bleeding, a sonogram may be done to detect possible retained placental fragments. The woman's physician or nurse-midwife may attempt bimanual compression. With this procedure, the physician or nurse-midwife inserts one hand into a woman's vagina while pushing against the fundus through the abdominal wall with the other hand. The woman may be returned to the delivery or birthing room so that her uterine cavity can be explored manually. Uterine packing may be inserted during this procedure to help halt bleeding. Uterine manipulation is painful; anticipate the need for analgesia or anesthesia to provide comfort. If uterine packing is used, be certain this is documented in a woman's chart so it can be removed before agency discharge. Retained packing serves as a growth medium for microorganism invasion that could lead to a postpartal infection (Begley & Barnes, 2007).

Prostaglandin Administration. Prostaglandins promote strong, sustained uterine contractions. Intramuscular injection of prostaglandin F_{22} is another way to initiate uterine contractions. Observe for nausea, diarrhea, tachycardia, and hypertension, all of which are possible adverse effects of prostaglandin administration (Karch, 2009).

Blood Replacement. Blood transfusion to replace blood loss with postpartal hemorrhage may be necessary. Make certain that blood typing and cross-matching were done when the woman was admitted and that blood is available. Some women donate blood during pregnancy so that they can be autotransfused if hemorrhage should occur postpartally.

The average woman takes the full postpartal period to regain her strength. Women who experience postpartal hemorrhage tend to have a longer than average recovery period, because the physiologic exhaustion of body systems can interfere with their recovery. Iron therapy may be prescribed to ensure good hemoglobin formation. Activity level, exertion, and postpartal exercise may be restricted somewhat. Discuss with a woman the possibility of having someone stay with her at home, at least for the first week, to help with the care of her new baby and to prevent exhaustion from turning childbearing into a less-than-satisfying event.

Extensive blood loss is one of the precursors of postpartal infection because of the general debilitation that results. For any woman who has experienced more than a normal loss of blood, observe for changes in lochia discharge. Also, monitor her temperature closely in the postpartal period, to detect the earliest signs of developing infection. Make certain the patient knows how to check for normal lochia and temperature once she is discharged.

Hysterectomy or Suturing. Usually, therapeutic management is effective in halting bleeding. In the rare instance of extreme uterine atony, sutures or balloon compression may be used to halt bleeding (Nelson & O'Brien, 2007). Embolization of pelvic and uterine vessels by angiographic techniques may be successful. As a last resort, ligation of the uterine arteries or a hysterectomy may be necessary. In this total unexpected outcome of childbearing, provide comfort and support to both a woman and her support person.

After hysterectomy, a woman may want to talk about what happened, why surgery was necessary, or how she feels now that she can no longer bear children. She needs to discuss her feelings with a person who will listen quietly and help her sort through her feelings of "Why me?" She may have ambiguous feelings: she wanted to have more children (or at least have the ability to have more), but she also wants to live. She is thankful that her life was saved, but she may feel resentful that she has been left incapable of future childbearing. She may grieve for children who will not be born. If this child was born outside the hospital and the woman was brought there under emergency circumstances, she may have a need to talk about her choice of location for childbirth. She may feel guilty that she did not choose a more controlled place for childbirth.

Open lines of communication between the couple and health care providers that allow a family to vent its feelings are most helpful to a couple in this crisis. Referral to a grief counselor may be necessary as grieving for future children who will not be born can interfere with bonding with the present child.

Lacerations

Small lacerations or tears of the birth canal are common and may be considered a normal consequence of childbearing. Large lacerations, however, can cause complications. They occur most often:

- With difficult or precipitate births
- In primigravidas
- With the birth of a large infant (>9 lb)
- With the use of a lithotomy position and instruments

Either cervical, vaginal, or perineal lacerations may occur. After birth, any time a uterus feels firm but bleeding persists, suspect a laceration of one of these three sites.

Cervical Lacerations

Lacerations of the cervix are usually found on the sides of the cervix, near the branches of the uterine artery. If the artery is torn, the blood loss may be so great that blood gushes from the vaginal opening. Because this is arterial bleeding, it is brighter red than the venous blood lost with uterine atony. Fortunately, this bleeding ordinarily occurs immediately after delivery of the placenta, when the physician or nurse-midwife is still in attendance.

Therapeutic Management. Repair of a cervical laceration is difficult, because the bleeding can be so intense that it obstructs visualization of the area. Be certain that a physician or nurse-midwife has adequate space to work, adequate sponges and suture supplies, and a good light source. The woman is not always aware of what is happening at this point, but she senses quickly that something is seriously wrong. Try to maintain an air of calm and, if possible, stand beside the woman, at the head of the table. She may be worried that the extra activity in the room has something to do with her baby. Assure her about her baby's condition and inform her about the need to stay in the birthing room a little longer than expected while the physician or nurse-midwife places additional sutures. Remember that the protective attitude a woman has felt toward her body all during pregnancy is now turned toward her baby, so she usually is relieved to learn that any problem that may be occurring is hers, not her infant's.

If the cervical laceration appears to be extensive or difficult to repair, it may be necessary for the woman to be given a regional anesthetic to relax the uterine muscle and to prevent pain. Explain the need for an anesthetic and the procedures being carried out.

Vaginal Lacerations

Although they are rare, lacerations can also occur in the vagina. They are easier to assess than cervical lacerations, because they are easier to view.

Therapeutic Management. Because vaginal tissue is friable, vaginal lacerations are also hard to repair. Some oozing often occurs after a repair, so the vagina may be packed to maintain pressure on the suture line. An indwelling urinary catheter (Foley catheter) may be placed at the same time, because the packing causes pressure on the urethra and can interfere with voiding. If packing is inserted, document in a woman's nursing care plan when and where it was placed, so you can be certain it will be removed after 24 to 48 hours or before discharge. Packing that is left in place too long leads to stasis and infection similar to toxic shock syndrome, a form of septic shock (Begley & Barnes, 2007).

Perineal Lacerations

Lacerations of the perineum usually occur when a woman is placed in a lithotomy position for birth, because this position increases tension on the perineum. Perineal lacerations are classified by four categories, depending on the extent and depth of the tissue involved. These categories are shown in Table 25.1.

Therapeutic Management. Perineal lacerations are sutured and treated as an episiotomy repair. Make certain that the degree of the laceration is documented, because women with fourth-degree lacerations need extra precautions to avoid having repair sutures loosened or infected. Both lacerations and episiotomy incisions tend to heal in the same length of time. A diet high in fluid and a stool softener may be prescribed for the first week after birth to prevent constipation and hard stools, which could break the sutures.

TABLE 25.1 ✻ Classification of Perineal Lacerations

Classification	Description of Involvement
First degree	Vaginal mucous membrane and skin of the perineum to the fourchette
Second degree	Vagina, perineal skin, fascia, levator ani muscle, and perineal body
Third degree	Entire perineum, extending to reach the external sphincter of the rectum
Fourth degree	Entire perineum, rectal sphincter, and some of the mucous membrane of the rectum

Any woman who has a third- or fourth-degree laceration should not have an enema or a rectal suppository prescribed or have her temperature taken rectally, because the hard tips of equipment could open sutures near to or including those of the rectal sphincter. Be sure that ancillary caregivers such as nurses' aides are informed of this, so that they understand these measures. Although fourth-degree lacerations can lead to long-term dyspareunia, rectal incontinence, or sexual dissatisfaction, they usually heal without further complications.

Retained Placental Fragments

Occasionally, a placenta does not deliver in its entirety; fragments of it separate and are left behind. Because the portion retained keeps the uterus from contracting fully, uterine bleeding occurs. Although this is most likely to happen with a succenturiate placenta—a placenta with an accessory lobe (see Chapter 23)—it can happen in any instance. Placenta accreta—a placenta that fuses with the myometrium because of an abnormal decidua basalis layer—may also be retained. This occurs at an incidence of about 1 in 3000 births (Poggi, 2007). To detect the complication of retained placenta, every placenta should be inspected carefully after birth to see that it is complete. Retained placental fragments may also be detected by ultrasound. A blood serum sample that contains human chorionic gonadotropin hormone (hCG) also reveals that part of a placenta is still present.

Assessment

If an undetected retained fragment is large, bleeding will be apparent in the immediate postpartal period, because the uterus cannot contract with the fragment in place. If the fragment is small, bleeding may not be detected until postpartum day 6 to 10, when the woman notices an abrupt discharge and a large amount of blood. On examination, usually the uterus is not fully contracted.

Therapeutic Management

Removal of the retained placental fragment is necessary to stop the bleeding. Usually, a dilatation and curettage (D&C) is performed to remove the placental fragment. In some instances, placenta accreta is so deeply attached that it cannot be surgically removed. Balloon occlusion and embolization of the internal iliac arteries may minimize blood loss. Methotrexate may be prescribed to destroy the retained placental tissue (Szymanski & Bienstock, 2007). Because the hemorrhage from retained fragments may be delayed until after a woman is at home, be certain a woman knows to continue to observe the color of lochia discharge and to report any tendency for the discharge to change from lochia serosa or alba back to rubra.

✔ Checkpoint Question 25.1

Suppose Mary Blackhawk has a retained placental fragment that is causing extensive postpartal bleeding. What hormone test would you anticipate being ordered to detect whether placenta is still present?

a. Placental and cord blood estrogen.
b. Progesterone from the placenta.
c. Human chorionic gonadotropin hormone.
d. Systemic prolactin (a pituitary hormone).

Uterine Inversion

Uterine inversion is prolapse of the fundus of the uterus through the cervix so that the uterus turns inside out. This usually occurs immediately after birth so is discussed in Chapter 23.

Disseminated Intravascular Coagulation

Disseminated intravascular coagulation (DIC) is a deficiency in clotting ability caused by vascular injury. It may occur in any woman in the postpartal period, but it is usually associated with premature separation of the placenta, a missed early miscarriage, or fetal death in utero. DIC is discussed in Chapter 21 along with these disorders.

Subinvolution

Subinvolution is incomplete return of the uterus to its prepregnant size and shape. With subinvolution, at a 4- or 6-week postpartal visit, the uterus is still enlarged and soft. Lochial discharge usually is still present. Subinvolution may result from a small retained placental fragment, a mild **endometritis** (infection of the endometrium), or an accompanying problem such as a uterine myoma that is interfering with complete contraction.

Therapeutic Management

Oral administration of methylergonovine, 0.2 mg four times daily, usually is prescribed to improve uterine tone and complete involution. If the uterus is tender to palpation, suggesting endometritis, an oral antibiotic also will be prescribed. Being certain that women are able to recognize the normal process of involution and lochial discharge before hospital discharge helps women to be able to identify subinvolution and seek early health care if it occurs. A chronic loss of blood from subinvolution will result in infection or anemia and lack of energy, conditions that possibly could interfere with infant bonding.

Perineal Hematomas

A perineal hematoma is a collection of blood in the subcutaneous layer of tissue of the perineum. The overlying skin, as a rule, is intact with no noticeable trauma. Such blood collections can be caused by injury to blood vessels in the perineum during birth. They are most likely to occur after rapid, spontaneous births and in women who have perineal varicosities. They may occur at the site of an episiotomy or laceration repair if a vein was punctured during repair. Although they can cause a woman acute discomfort and concern, they usually represent only minor bleeding.

Assessment

Perineal sutures almost always give a postpartal woman some discomfort. If a woman reports severe pain in the perineal area or a feeling of pressure between her legs, inspect the perineal area for a hematoma. If one is present, it appears as an area of purplish discoloration with obvious swelling. It may be as small as 2 cm or as large as 8 cm in diameter (Fig. 25.2). The area is tender to palpation. At first it may feel fluctuant, but as seepage into the area continues and tissue is drawn taut, it palpates as a firm globe.

Therapeutic Management

Report the presence of a hematoma, its size, and the degree of the woman's discomfort to her primary care provider. Assess the size by measuring it in centimeters with each inspection. Describing a hematoma as "large" or "small" gives little information about the actual size. Describing a lesion as 5 cm across or the size of a quarter or a half dollar is more meaningful because it establishes a basis for comparison.

Administer a mild analgesic as ordered for pain relief. Applying an ice pack (covered with a towel to prevent thermal injury to the skin) may prevent further bleeding. Usually the hematoma is absorbed over the next 3 or 4 days. If the hematoma is large when discovered or continues to increase in size, the woman may have to be returned to the delivery or birthing room to have the site incised and the bleeding vessel ligated under local anesthesia.

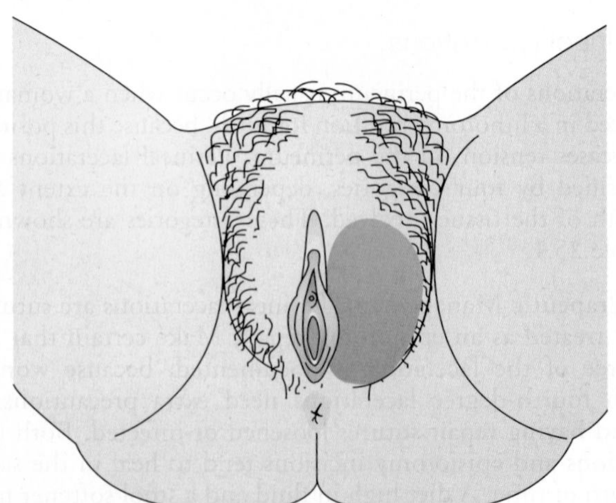

FIGURE 25.2 Appearance of a perineal hematoma from a bleeding subcutaneous vessel.

You can reassure a woman that, even though the hematoma is causing her considerable discomfort, her hospital stay probably will not be lengthened by its occurrence (unless it is extremely extensive). In most women, hematomas absorb over the next 6 weeks, causing no further difficulty. If an episiotomy incision line is opened to drain a hematoma, it may be left open and packed with gauze rather than resutured. Packing is usually removed within 24 to 48 hours. Be certain to record that this packing was placed, so it can be removed before discharge or when the woman returns to an ambulatory setting. A suture line opened in this way heals by tertiary intention, more slowly than a first-degree intention suture line. Be certain the woman has clear instructions before discharge regarding necessary suture line care that she needs to do at home such as keeping it clean and dry and perhaps using a sitz bath once or twice a day.

PUERPERAL INFECTION

Infection of the reproductive tract is another leading cause of maternal mortality (Pavone, Purinton, & Petersen, 2007). Factors that predispose women to infection in the postpartal period are shown in Box 25.5. When caring for a woman who has any of these circumstances, be aware that the risk for postpartal infection is greatly increased.

Theoretically, the uterus is sterile during pregnancy and until the membranes rupture. After rupture, pathogens can invade. The risk of infection is even greater if tissue edema and trauma are present. If infection occurs, the prognosis for complete recovery depends on:

- Virulence of the invading organism
- The woman's general health
- Portal of entry
- Degree of uterine involution at the time of the microorganism invasion
- Presence of lacerations in the reproductive tract

A puerperal infection is always potentially serious, because, although it usually begins as only a local infection, it can spread to involve the peritoneum (peritonitis) or the circulatory system (septicemia). These conditions can be fatal in a woman whose body is already stressed from childbirth.

Management for puerperal infection focuses on the use of an appropriate antibiotic after culture and sensitivity testing of the isolated organism. Organisms commonly cultured postpartally include group B streptococci and aerobic gram-negative bacilli such as *Escherichia coli.* Staphylococcal infections also are becoming more common. Staphylococcal infections are the cause of toxic shock syndrome, an infection similar to puerperal infection in its ability to cause death and morbidity (see Chapter 47).

BOX 25.5 ✻ Conditions That Increase a Woman's Risk for Postpartal Infection

1. Rupture of the membranes more than 24 hours before birth (bacteria may have started to invade the uterus while the fetus was still in utero)
2. Placental fragments retained within the uterus (the tissue necroses and serves as an excellent bed for bacterial growth)
3. Postpartal hemorrhage (the woman's general condition is weakened)
4. Pre-existing anemia (the body's defense against infection is lowered)
5. Prolonged and difficult labor, particularly instrument births (trauma to the tissue may leave lacerations or fissures for easy portals of entry for infection)
6. Internal fetal heart monitoring (contamination may have been introduced with placement of the scalp electrode)
7. Local vaginal infection was present at the time of birth (direct spread of infection has occurred)
8. The uterus was explored after birth for a retained placenta or abnormal bleeding site (infection was introduced with exploration)

Nursing Diagnoses and Related Interventions

Nursing Diagnosis: Risk for infection related to loss of uterine sterility with childbirth

Outcome Evaluation: Client's temperature remains below 100.4° F or 38° C orally, excluding the first 24 hours after birth; lochia is present without foul odor.

To help prevent infection, any articles such as gloves or instruments that are introduced into the birth canal during labor, birth, and the postpartal period should be sterile. In addition, adherence to standard infection precautions is essential.

Instruct a postpartal woman in proper perineal care, including wiping from front to back so that she does not bring *E. coli* organisms forward from the rectum. Use good handwashing technique before, during, and after any client care, to prevent cross-contamination. When giving perineal care, both wash your hands and wear gloves. Each postpartal woman should have her own bedpan and perineal supplies and should not share them, to prevent transfer of pathogens from one woman to another.

Intravenous antibiotics usually are prescribed for a postpartal infection. Frequently used antibiotics include ampicillin, gentamicin, and third-generation cephalosporins such as cefixime (Suprax). If the woman will be continuing drug therapy at home, stress that she must take the full course to prevent the infection from recurring. Be certain that women who are breastfeeding are not prescribed antibiotics incompatible with breastfeeding. Alert them to observe for problems in their infant, such as white plaques or thrush (oral *Candida*) in their infant's mouth. This occurs because a portion of the maternal antibiotic passes into breast milk and can cause an overgrowth of fungal organisms (opportunistic infection) in the infant. The infant also should be assessed for easy bruising. A decrease of microorganisms in the bowel caused by an antibiotic passed in breast milk may lead to insufficient vitamin K formation and, consequently, decreased blood-clotting ability.

Nursing Diagnosis: Social isolation related to precautions necessary to protect baby and others from exposure to infectious microorganisms

Outcome Evaluation: Client describes agency policy regarding precautions and states plans for diversional activities to pass time; demonstrates bonding behaviors, such as asking about newborn and expressing desire to see infant.

Most hospitals have well-defined guidelines on whether a woman who has an infection should be separated from other women or allowed to feed and care for her baby (Box 25.6). It is difficult for many women to accomplish their new role change even when things are going well. If a woman is segregated from others, frightened by her condition, and denied the pleasure of holding and feeding her baby, her situation may seem overwhelming. Women who are isolated this way need friendly, understanding support from hospital personnel who give them care. Fortunately, because modern antibiotics work quickly to reduce the possibility of contagion, the required period of separation may be as short as 24 hours. Encourage women who are breastfeeding to pump their breasts to maintain their milk supply during this time.

Often, the choice to breastfeed is culturally influenced. If a postpartal complication interferes with breastfeeding, a woman who feels that breastfeeding is very important can be expected to react less favorably than a woman from a culture in which formula feeding is preferred.

Endometritis

Endometritis is an infection of the endometrium, the lining of the uterus. Bacteria gain access to the uterus through the vagina and enter the uterus either at the time of birth or during the postpartal period. This may occur with any birth, but the infection is usually associated with chorioamnionitis and cesarean birth (Szymanski & Bienstock, 2007).

Assessment

A benign temperature elevation may occur on the first postpartal day, particularly if a woman is not drinking enough fluid. The fever of endometritis usually manifests on the third

BOX 25.6 * Common Guidelines for the Woman With a Postpartal Infection

1. As a rule, the baby of a mother with an increased temperature (100.4° F [38° C]) for two consecutive 24-hour periods exclusive of the first 24 hours is kept in an isolation nursery until the cause of the infection is determined. The mother may have an upper respiratory tract or gastrointestinal infection that is unrelated to childbearing but transmittable to a newborn.
2. If the cause of the fever is found to be related to childbirth but involves a closed infection, such as thrombophlebitis, with no danger of the baby contracting the disease, the woman may care for her child as long as she maintains bed rest in the prescribed position while doing so.
3. If the infection involves drainage such as can occur with endometritis or a perineal abscess, newborn visiting may be contraindicated. If rooming-in is continued, the mother should wash her hands thoroughly before holding her infant. She should never place her baby on the bottom bed sheet, where there may be some infected drainage from her perineal pad (furnish a clean sheet to spread over the covers).
4. Most hospitals are reluctant to return a baby to a central nursery after a baby has visited in a room where there is an infection. The hospital should provide a small nursery that may be used as an isolation nursery for these situations, or the baby can be placed in a closed Isolette in a central nursery or continue to be cared for in the woman's room.
5. If the woman has a high fever, breast milk may be deficient. With modern antimicrobial therapy, puerperal infections are limited, and the period of high fever usually is transient. If the mother is too ill to nurse her baby during this time or if she is receiving an anticoagulant or antibiotic that is passed in breast milk and would be harmful to the baby, the infant should be fed by a supplementary milk formula. The woman's breast milk can be manually expressed or pumped to maintain the production of milk so it will be available when she is again able to nurse. You may need to assist her with this, because she fatigues easily and her energy level may not be enough to support her good intentions. If it appears that the course of the infection will be long, a woman may choose to discontinue breastfeeding.
6. If it is necessary for a woman to discontinue breastfeeding, she needs to be assured that she can meet the needs of the child through bottle feeding.
7. If a woman is going to be hospitalized beyond the usual time, she may have to make arrangements for the discharge and care of her baby. She may be interested in a homemaker service or temporary foster care if she has no close friends or family. If she has older children at home, she needs to keep in close contact with them, calling them on the telephone or writing them short notes if possible. If the infant is housed in a high-risk nursery, she needs to see a photograph of the newborn (a Polaroid or digital camera should be a piece of equipment on every postpartal unit) and hear daily reports of his or her progress and well-being.

or fourth postpartal day, suggesting that much of the invasion occurred during labor or birth (consistent with the time it takes for infectious organisms to grow).

Normally, the white blood cell count of a postpartal woman is increased to 20,000 to 30,000 cells/mm^3. Because of this increase, the conventional method of detecting infection (elevated white blood cell count) is not of great value in the puerperium. An increase in oral temperature to more than 100.4° F (38° C) for two consecutive 24-hour periods, excluding the first 24-hour period after birth, is defined by the Joint Committee on Maternal Welfare as a febrile condition suggesting infection (Crombleholme, 2009). Infection should be suspected in all postpartal women with temperatures in this range, until proved otherwise. Because many women are at home when this elevated temperature occurs, any woman who feels as if she has an increased temperature should measure her temperature to be certain.

A rise in temperature that occurs on the third or fourth day postpartum occurs at the same time during which breast filling occurs. Do not be led astray by attributing an elevated temperature at this time to breast filling. Suspect fever on the third or fourth day postpartum as possible endometritis until proved otherwise.

Depending on the severity of the infection, a woman may have accompanying chills, loss of appetite, and general malaise. Her uterus usually is not well contracted and is painful to the touch. She may feel strong afterpains. Lochia usually is dark brown and has a foul odor. It may be increased in amount because of poor uterine involution, but if the infection is accompanied by high fever, lochia may be scant or absent. Ultrasound may be ordered to confirm the presence of placental fragments that are a possible cause of the infection.

Therapeutic Management

Treatment of endometritis consists of the administration of an appropriate antibiotic, such as clindamycin (Cleocin), as determined by a culture of the lochia. Be sure to obtain the culture from the vagina, using a sterile swab, rather than from a perineal pad, to ensure that you are culturing the endometrial infectious organism and not an unrelated one from the pad. An oxytocic agent such as methylergonovine, may be prescribed to encourage uterine contraction. The woman requires additional fluid to combat the fever. If strong afterpains and abdominal discomfort are present, she needs an analgesic for pain relief.

Sitting in a Fowler's position or walking encourages lochia drainage by gravity and helps prevent pooling of infected secretions. Because this drainage is contaminated, be certain to wear gloves when helping a woman change her perineal pads. In addition, both you and the woman must use good handwashing techniques before and after handling these pads.

As with any infection, endometritis can be controlled best if it is discovered early. If you can interpret the normal color, quantity, and odor of lochia discharge and the size, consistency, and tenderness of a normal postpartal uterus, you may be the first person to recognize that infection is present. Because a woman may be at home when signs of infection occur, teaching about the signs and symptoms of endometritis is essential. In addition, follow-up by a home care nurse can help with early detection.

If the infection is limited to the endometrium, the course of infection is about 7 to 10 days. If this occurs while a woman is hospitalized, she may have to make arrangements for her baby's discharge before her own, or for help with newborn care, if her hospital stay is extended for a few days. Or, she may be discharged home on intravenous antibiotic therapy with follow-up by a home care nurse.

An added danger of endometritis is that it can lead to tubal scarring and interference with future fertility. At a future time, if the woman desires more children, she may need a fertility assessment (including a hysterosalpingogram) to determine tubal patency. With mild endometritis this is usually not a problem, but a woman should be forewarned that it could occur.

What if... Mary Blackhawk tells you she has developed chills and a fever of 101.5° F (41.6° C) on her second postpartal day? Her lochia is dark brown and foul smelling. On palpation, you notice her abdomen is very tender. What should you do next?

Infection of the Perineum

If a woman has a suture line on her perineum from an episiotomy or a laceration repair, a portal of entry exists for bacterial invasion.

Assessment

Infections of the perineum usually remain localized. They are revealed by symptoms similar to those of any suture-line infection, such as pain, heat, and a feeling of pressure. The woman may or may not have an elevated temperature, depending on the systemic effect and spread of the infection.

Inspection of the suture line reveals the inflammation. One or two stitches may be sloughed away, or an area of the suture line may be open with purulent drainage present (Fig. 25.3). Notify the woman's physician or nurse-midwife of the localized symptoms, and culture the discharge using a sterile cotton-tipped applicator touched to the secretions.

Therapeutic Management

A woman's physician or nurse-midwife may choose to remove perineal sutures, to open the area and allow for drainage. Packing, such as iodoform gauze, may be placed in the open lesion to keep it open and allow drainage. Be sure the woman is aware that the packing is in place, so she knows not to dislodge it as she changes her perineal pad.

Typically, a systemic or topical antibiotic is ordered even before the culture report is returned. An analgesic may be prescribed to alleviate discomfort. Sitz baths, moist warm compresses, or Hubbard tank treatments may be ordered to hasten drainage and cleanse the area. Remind the woman to change perineal pads frequently, because they are contaminated by drainage. If they are left in place too long, they might cause vaginal contamination or reinfection. Be certain a woman wipes front to back after a bowel movement, to prevent bringing feces forward onto the healing area.

With a local infection of this nature, a woman is usually discharged with a referral for home care follow-up, because

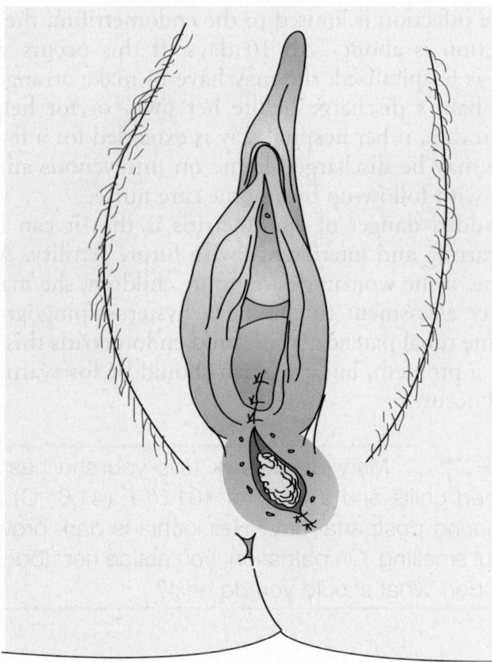

FIGURE 25.3 An infected suture line appears reddened and edematous and often contains infected secretions.

the incision site, once opened, must heal by tertiary rather than primary intention. Infections of this nature are annoying and painful, but fortunately, with improved techniques during parturition and the puerperium, perineal infections occur only rarely. Because they are localized, there is no need to restrict the woman from caring for her infant, as long as she washes her hands well before holding her newborn. Be certain not to place the infant on the bottom bed sheet of the woman's bed, where the baby could contact pathogenic bacteria. Encourage the woman to ambulate and ask for analgesia as needed. Often the pain from an infected suture line is severe, and the woman may decrease ambulation unless she is urged to continue.

Peritonitis

Peritonitis, or infection of the peritoneal cavity, usually occurs as an extension of endometritis. It is one of the gravest complications of childbearing and is a major cause of death from puerperal infection. The infection spreads through the lymphatic system or directly through the fallopian tubes or uterine wall to the peritoneal cavity. An abscess may form in the cul-de-sac of Douglas, because this is the lowest point of the peritoneal cavity and gravity causes infected material to localize there.

Assessment

Symptoms are the same as those of a surgical patient in whom a peritoneal infection develops: rigid abdomen, abdominal pain, high fever, rapid pulse, vomiting, and the appearance of being acutely ill. When assessing the abdomen of a postpartal woman, be sure to note not only that her uterus is well contracted but also that the remainder of her abdomen is soft. The occurrence of a rigid abdomen (guarding) is one of the first symptoms of peritonitis.

Therapeutic Management

Peritonitis is often accompanied by paralytic ileus (blockage of inflamed intestines). This requires insertion of a nasogastric tube to prevent vomiting and rest the bowel. Intravenous fluid or total parenteral nutrition may be necessary. A woman will need analgesics for pain relief. She will be administered large doses of antibiotics to treat the infection. Her hospital stay will be extended, but with effective antibiotic therapy, the outcome usually is good. Peritonitis can interfere with future fertility, because it leaves scarring and adhesions in the peritoneum. Adhesions formed this way may separate the fallopian tubes from the ovaries to the extent that ova can no longer easily enter the tubes.

✔ Checkpoint Question 25.2

Mary Blackhawk develops endometritis. What would be the best activity for her?

a. Lying in bed with a cold cloth on her forehead.
b. Walking around her room listening to music.
c. Reading while resting in a Trendelenburg position.
d. Sitting with her feet elevated while playing cards.

THROMBOPHLEBITIS

Phlebitis is inflammation of the lining of a blood vessel. **Thrombophlebitis** is inflammation with the formation of blood clots. When thrombophlebitis occurs in the postpartal period, it is usually an extension of an endometrial infection. It tends to occur because:

- A woman's fibrinogen level is still elevated from pregnancy, leading to increased blood clotting.
- Dilatation of lower extremity veins is still present as a result of pressure of the fetal head during pregnancy and birth.
- The relative inactivity of the period or a prolonged time spent in delivery or birthing room stirrups leads to pooling, stasis, and clotting of blood in the lower extremities.
- Obesity from increased weight before pregnany and pregnancy weight gain can lead to relative inactivity and lack of exercise.
- The woman smokes cigarettes.

Thrombophlebitis is classified as superficial vein disease (SVD) or deep vein thrombosis (DVT). Women most prone to thrombophlebitis are those who are obese, have varicose veins, have had a previous thrombophlebitis, are older than 35 years of age with increased parity, or have a high incidence of thrombophlebitis in their family (Gates, Brocklehurst, & Davis, 2009).

Prevention of endometritis by the use of good aseptic technique during birth helps to prevent thrombophlebitis. Ambulation and limiting the time a woman remains in obstetric stirrups encourages circulation in the lower extremities, promotes venous return, and decreases the possibility of clot formation, also helping to prevent thrombophlebitis. If stirrups of examining or delivery tables are used, be certain they are well padded, to prevent any sharp pressure against the calves of the legs. If a woman had varicose veins during pregnancy, wearing support stockings for the first 2 weeks after birth can help increase venous circulation and prevent stasis. If these are prescribed, be certain a woman knows to put them on before she rises in the morning. If she waits until she is already up and walking, venous congestion has already occurred and the stockings are less effective. Urge her to remove the support stockings twice daily and assess her skin underneath for mottling or inflammation that would suggest inflammation of her veins. Beginning such activities as walking can also be important. An exercise program will also be important in helping women lose their pregnancy weight (Keller et al., 2008). Additional measures for preventing thrombophlebitis are summarized in Box 25.7.

Femoral Thrombophlebitis

With femoral thrombophlebitis, the femoral, saphenous, or popliteal veins are involved. Although the inflammation site in thrombophlebitis is a vein, an accompanying arterial spasm often occurs, diminishing arterial circulation to a leg as well. This decreased circulation, along with edema, gives the leg a white or drained appearance. It was formerly believed that breast milk drained into the leg, giving it its white appearance. The condition was, therefore, formerly called *milk leg* or *phlegmasia alba dolens* ("white inflammation").

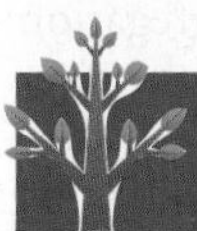

BOX 25.7 ✻ Focus on Family Teaching

Preventing Thrombophlebitis

Q. Mary Blackhawk tells you, "My sister got thrombophlebitis after the birth of her first baby. How can I prevent that from happening to me?"

A. Here are a few helpful hints for preventing thrombophlebitis:

- Ask your primary care provider if you can use a side-lying or back-lying (supine recumbent) position for birth, rather than a lithotomy position (lithotomy position can increase the tendency for pooling of blood in the lower extremities).
- If you will be using a lithotomy position, ask for padding on the stirrups to prevent calf pressure.
- Drink adequate fluids to be certain you're not dehydrated (6–8 glasses of fluid/day).
- Do not sit with your knees bent sharply, and avoid wearing constricting clothing such as knee-high stockings.
- Ambulate as soon after birth as you are able. Early ambulation is the best preventive measure. When resting in bed, wiggle your toes or do leg lifts to improve venous return.
- Ask your primary care provider if he or she recommends support stockings in the immediate postpartal period. Be certain to put these on before ambulating in the morning, before leg veins fill.
- Quit smoking as this is associated with the development of thrombophlebitis.

Assessment

If femoral thrombophlebitis develops, a woman notices an elevated temperature, chills, pain, and redness in the affected leg about 10 days after birth. Her leg begins to swell below the lesion at the point at which venous circulation is blocked. Her skin becomes so stretched from swelling that it appears shiny and white. Homans' sign (pain in the calf of the leg on dorsiflexion of the foot) may be positive; however, a negative Homans' sign does not rule out obstruction. The diameter of the leg at thigh or calf level may be increased compared with the other leg. Doppler ultrasound or contrast venography usually is ordered to confirm the diagnosis.

Therapeutic Management

Treatment consists of bed rest with the affected leg elevated, administration of anticoagulants, and application of moist heat. Women who have been discharged from the hospital may be cared for at home or may return to the hospital so that strict bed rest can be enforced. A bed cradle keeps pressure of the bedclothes off the affected leg, both to decrease the sensitivity of the leg and to improve circulation. Provide good back, buttocks, and heel care. Check for bed wrinkles so that a woman does not develop the secondary problem of a pressure ulcer while on bed rest.

Never massage the skin over the clot; this could loosen the clot, causing a pulmonary or cerebral embolism. Heat supplied by a moist, warm compress can help decrease inflammation. Although simple in theory, unfortunately, this is one of the most technically difficult treatments to carry out, because dressings invariably dry or become cold after only a short time. Compresses and water used in this way do not have to be sterile because, with thrombophlebitis, there is no break in the skin. Be certain to test water temperature by dipping your inner wrist in it before soaking a dressing, to be sure it is not too warm (because edema decreases sensation in a woman's leg, she can burn easily). Always cover wet, warm dressings with a plastic pad to hold in heat and moisture. In addition, a commercial pad with circulating heating coils or chemical hot packs may be positioned over the plastic to ensure that soaks stay warm. Be certain the weight of a hot pack or pad does not rest on the leg, causing an obstruction to flow of blood.

Check a woman's bed frequently when moist compresses are used, to be certain the mattress does not become wet from seeping water. For soaks to stay in place, a woman must keep her leg fairly immobile. However, be certain she does not interpret this as meaning that she cannot turn or move about. Provide her with appropriate activities to exercise the other parts of her body and stimulate her mind. One way of helping a woman use her time on bed rest is to offer reading material about newborns. This activity helps her maintain bed rest and also educates her about infant care.

The pain of thrombophlebitis is usually severe enough to require administration of an analgesic. An appropriate antibiotic to reduce the initial infection is prescribed. Often, an anticoagulant (coumarin derivative or heparin) or a thrombolytic agent such as streptokinase or urokinase is prescribed to dissolve the clot through the activation of fibrinolytic precursors and prevent further clot formation. Blood coagulation levels to determine the effectiveness of the drug therapy are measured daily before administration of the anticoagulant. Depending on the drug prescribed, a baseline activated partial thromboplastin time (aPTT) or prothrombin time (PT) is obtained.

Heparin, an anticoagulant, can be administered by continuous intravenous infusion or intermittently by intravenous or subcutaneous injection (Box 25.8). If a woman will be discharged on subcutaneous therapy, be certain she has demonstrated good injection technique before discharge and understands the importance of required blood work (coagulation studies) so that she schedules these appropriately. Protamine sulfate, the antagonist for heparin, should be readily available any time heparin is administered.

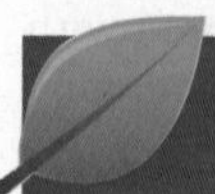

BOX 25.8 * Focus on Pharmacology

Heparin Calcium Injection (Hepalean, Liquamin Sodium) or Dalteparin (low-molecular-weight heparin)

Classification: Heparin is an anticoagulant.

Action: Heparin blocks the conversion of prothrombin to thrombin and of fibrinogen to fibrin, decreasing clotting ability and resulting in the inhibition of thrombus and clot formation. It is used to prevent and treat thrombosis and pulmonary embolism (Karch, 2009).

Pregnancy risk category: B

Dosage: Dosage is dependent on coagulation studies. Dosage is considered therapeutic when the activated partial thromboplastin time (aPTT) is 1.5 to 3 times the control value. The drug can be given by continuous intravenous (IV) infusion or by intermittent direct IV or subcutaneous injection.

Possible adverse effects: Hemorrhage, bruising, thrombocytopenia, urticaria

Nursing Implications

- Obtain baseline coagulation studies as ordered.
- Continue to monitor aPTT results and adjust dosage as ordered. Obtain aPTT results 30 minutes before intermittent dosage administration or every 4 hours for continuous IV infusion.
- Anticipate use of an intermittent infusion device to minimize the number of intravenous injections.
- Avoid any intramuscular injection of other medications, because a hematoma may form at injection site.
- When administering an IV infusion, do not add heparin to existing IV solutions or piggyback other drugs into a heparin infusion. Use an infusion pump.
- When administering heparin subcutaneously, inject deeply, and rotate injection sites. Do not aspirate for blood return or massage the injection site afterward. Apply direct pressure to the injection site after administration. Inspect the injection site for signs of hematoma formation.
- Assess a woman for signs and symptoms of bleeding, such as oozing from the gums, nosebleeds, hematuria, or frank or occult blood in stool.
- Closely monitor client's lochia, including amount and color. Assess pad count to determine extent of vaginal bleeding.
- Keep protamine sulfate, the antidote, readily available in case of overdose.
- Instruct a woman about antibleeding precautions such as using a soft toothbrush to minimize the risk of bleeding.

A woman can continue to breastfeed while receiving heparin. If she does not wish to breastfeed, she can be switched to warfarin (an oral coumarin derivative) before hospital discharge. The antidote to warfarin is vitamin K. A woman has to discontinue breastfeeding during therapy with coumarin, because coumarin-derived anticoagulants are passed in breast milk. If the thrombophlebitis does not seem to be severe and the woman wants to restart breastfeeding after the course of anticoagulant (about 10 days), encourage her to manually express breast milk at the time of normal feedings, to maintain a good milk supply.

Lochia usually increases in amount in a woman who is receiving an anticoagulant. Be sure to keep a meaningful record of the amount of this discharge so that it can be estimated. "Lochia serosa with scattered pinpoint clots; three perineal pads saturated in 8 hours" is far more meaningful than "large amount of lochia." Also assess for other possible signs of bleeding, such as bleeding gums, ecchymotic spots on the skin, or oozing from an episiotomy suture line.

Women taking anticoagulants are not normally prescribed salicylic acid (aspirin) for pain, because salicylic acid prevents blood clotting by preventing platelet aggregation and clot formation. However, some women may be prescribed aspirin every 4 hours as a preventive measure if they are at high risk for recurrent thrombophlebitis. If this is so, be certain you do not interpret aspirin used this way as a PRN analgesic order and withhold it depending on the woman's level of pain.

With proper treatment, the acute symptoms of femoral thrombophlebitis last only a few days, but the full course of the disease takes 4 to 6 weeks before it is resolved. Anticoagulant therapy may need to be continued for 3 to 6 months. The affected leg may never return to its former size and may always cause discomfort after long periods of standing.

Pelvic Thrombophlebitis

Pelvic thrombophlebitis involves the ovarian, uterine, or hypogastric veins. It usually follows a mild endometritis and occurs later than femoral thrombophlebitis, often around the 14th or 15th day of the puerperium.. Risk factors are the same as for femoral thrombophlebitis.

Assessment

With pelvic thrombophlebitis, a woman suddenly becomes extremely ill, with high fever, chills, and general malaise. Her infection can be so severe it necroses the vein and results in a pelvic abscess. It can become systemic and result in a lung, kidney, or heart valve abscess.

Therapeutic Management

As with femoral thrombophlebitis, therapy involves total bed rest and administration of antibiotics and anticoagulants.

The disease runs a long course of 6 to 8 weeks. If an abscess forms, it can be located by sonogram and incised by laparotomy, if necessary. Formation of an abscess is associated with a high mortality rate. An inflammation of this extent may leave tubal scarring and interfere with future fertility. A woman may need surgery to remove the affected vessel before she attempts to become pregnant again.

Regardless of the type of thrombophlebitis, teach women preventive measures to reduce the risk of recurrence with future pregnancies. These measures include not wearing constricting clothing such as garters or tight stockings on the lower extremities, resting with the feet elevated, and ambulating daily during pregnancy. Caution a woman to tell her physician or nurse-midwife before her next pregnancy of the difficulty she experienced this time, so that extra prophylactic precautions can be taken to prevent thrombophlebitis.

Pulmonary Embolus

A pulmonary embolus is obstruction of the pulmonary artery by a blood clot; it usually occurs as a complication of thrombophlebitis. The signs of pulmonary embolus are sudden, sharp chest pain; tachypnea; tachycardia; orthopnea (inability to breathe except in an upright position); and cyanosis (the blood clot is obstructing the pulmonary artery, blocking blood flow to the lungs and return to the heart). It is an emergency. A woman needs oxygen administered immediately and is at high risk for cardiopulmonary arrest. Her condition is extremely guarded until the clot is lysed or adheres to the pulmonary artery wall and is reabsorbed. Because of the seriousness of this condition, a woman with a pulmonary embolism commonly is transferred to an intensive care unit for continuing care (Cansino & Lipsett, 2007).

MASTITIS

Mastitis (infection of the breast) may occur as early as the seventh postpartal day or not until the baby is weeks or months old (Reddy et al., 2007).

The organism causing the infection usually enters through cracked and fissured nipples. Therefore, measures that prevent cracked and fissured nipples also help prevent mastitis. These measures include:

- Making certain the baby is positioned correctly and grasps the nipple properly, including both nipple and areola
- Releasing a baby's grasp on the nipple before removing the baby from the breast
- Washing hands between handling perineal pads and touching the breasts
- Exposing nipples to air for at least part of every day
- Using a vitamin E ointment to soften nipples daily
- If a woman has one cracked and one well nipple, encourage her to begin breastfeeding (when the infant sucks most forcefully) on the unaffected nipple.

Occasionally, the organism that causes mastitis comes from the nasal–oral cavity of the infant. In these instances, the infant has usually acquired a *Staphylococcus aureus* infection while in the hospital. Candidiasis can also be spread this way. By sucking on a nipple, the infant introduces the organisms into the milk ducts, where they proliferate (breast milk is an excellent medium for bacterial growth). This is an epidemic breast abscess. When it occurs, it is usually discovered that several women discharged from the hospital at the same time have similar infections.

Assessment

Mastitis is usually unilateral, although epidemic mastitis, because it originates with the infant, may be bilateral. The affected breast is painful, swollen, and reddened. Fever accompanies these first symptoms within hours, and breast milk becomes scant.

Therapeutic Management

Treatment consists of antibiotics effective against penicillin-resistant staphylococci such as dicloxacillin or a cephalosporin (Crombleholme, 2009). Breastfeeding is continued, because keeping the breast emptied of milk helps to prevent growth of bacteria. Some women find an infected breast too painful to allow their infant to suck and prefer to express milk manually from the affected breast until their antibiotic has taken effect and the mastitis has diminished (about 3 days). Cold or ice compresses and a good supportive bra help with pain relief until the process improves. Warm, wet compresses may be ordered to reduce inflammation and edema.

If therapy is started as soon as symptoms are apparent, the condition runs a short course of about 2 or 3 days. If left untreated, a breast infection can become a localized abscess. This may involve a large portion of the breast and rupture through the skin, with thick, purulent drainage, necessitating incision and drainage of the abscess. If an abscess forms, breastfeeding on that breast is discontinued. However, a woman is encouraged to continue to pump breast milk until the abscess has resolved, to preserve breastfeeding. Some women find that the infected breast is too tender to do this. They can be reassured that formula feeding will be an acceptable alternative for their child.

Neither mastitis nor breast abscess leaves any permanent breast disease. A woman can be assured that such an incident is not associated with development of breast cancer and does not interfere with future breastfeeding potential (see Focus on Nursing Care Planning Box 25.9).

URINARY SYSTEM DISORDERS

Because a woman's bladder is compressed by the infant's head during birth, several urinary tract disorders can occur.

Urinary Retention

Urinary retention occurs as a result of inadequate bladder emptying. After childbirth, bladder sensation for voiding is decreased because of bladder edema caused by the pressure of birth. Unable to empty, the bladder fills to overdistention. When the woman does void, instead of emptying completely, the bladder empties only a small portion of its contents (retention with overflow). As a result, it becomes overdistended again. Bladder overdistention is potentially serious. If it is allowed to continue, permanent damage may occur from loss of bladder tone, leading to permanent incontinence (Chelmow, Aronson, & Wosu, 2007).

Assessment

Urinary retention is associated with the use of anesthesia, especially epidural anesthesia (Musselwhite et al., 2007). In a postpartal woman, urinary retention with overflow

BOX 25.9 ✻ Focus on Nursing Care Planning

A Multidisciplinary Care Map for a Woman With Mastitis

Mary Blackhawk calls your clinic 3 weeks after childbirth because she has a fever and swelling and pain in her right breast. She comes to the clinic for an evaluation.

Family Assessment ✻ Client lives in three-bedroom apartment with boyfriend. Worked as a card dealer in casino before birth; has not returned to work. Describes finances as "good—I'm on maternity leave." Boyfriend is a short-order cook but is currently unemployed. Wants her to stop breastfeeding because of her infection.

Client Assessment ✻ A 30-year-old primipara woman who gave birth vaginally 3 weeks ago and is breastfeeding. Temperature 101.1° F (38.4° C). Other vital signs within acceptable parameters. Right breast reddened and edematous, tender and warm to touch. Slight fissure noted on right nipple. States, "I hurt too much to breastfeed any longer. How can I be a good mother if I don't breastfeed my baby?"

Nursing Diagnosis ✻ Pain related to development of mastitis

Outcome Criteria ✻ Client states that pain is decreasing with treatment; demonstrates measures to promote comfort. Breast swelling, redness, fever, and tenderness decrease.

Team Member Responsible	Assessment	Intervention	Rationale	Expected Outcome
		Activities of Daily Living		
Physician/ nurse	Assess whether client could continue breastfeeding with additional support.	Encourage client to continue breastfeeding on left breast to keep breast empty of milk. Pump right breast if too tender for nursing.	Milk provides a good medium for bacterial growth. Complete emptying of breasts prevents stasis of milk and engorgement and aids in reducing the risk of further infection and pain.	Client states she will try to continue breastfeeding even though infection is present.
		Consultations		
Nurse	Assess whether client has a support person she uses for breastfeeding advice or would like one.	Suggest client contact local La Leche League chapter hot line for consultation and support.	Support from experts in the technique of breastfeeding can offer helpful tips to ensure success.	Client states she will contact a support service for additional information within 2 days.
		Procedures/Medications		
Nurse/ physician	Assess what actions client feels will help relieve her pain best.	Apply warm compresses to right breast at visit. Instruct in ways to apply warm moist heat, such as with a shower or warm packs, at home.	Moist heat promotes comfort and increases circulation to the area, decreasing inflammation and edema.	Client states she understands purpose and techniques of warm moist heat.
Nurse	Review good breastfeeding strategies with client.	Encourage client to nurse every 2–3 hr, to wear a support bra, and to start each infant feeding on the unaffected breast.	Beginning a feeding on the unaffected breast reduces discomfort, because infant will not suck as hard on affected breast. Breast care promotes integrity of breasts, reducing risk of cracked or fissured nipples and future mastitis.	Client states she will try suggested techniques.

Procedures/Medications				
Nurse	Assess whether client has health insurance and can afford antibiotic prescribed.	Review necessity of taking antibiotic for full 7-day course.	The antibiotic must be taken for a full course or the infective organisms could regrow.	Client states she has means to purchase medicine and will take it conscientiously.
Nutrition				
Nurse	Assess whether client understands importance of a good fluid intake for breastfeeding success.	Advise client to be certain to drink at least 8 glasses of fluid daily.	Fluid is important for breast milk formation and to prevent dehydration with fever.	Client states she has access to fluid and understands the importance of fluid intake.
Patient/Family Education				
Nurse/nurse-midwife	Assess client's knowledge of mastitis and how microorganisms enter and infect a breast.	Clarify any misconceptions client may have about mastitis. Inform client that mastitis does not result in permanent breast disease or interfere with continued breastfeeding.	Misconceptions can negatively affect self-esteem. Providing information helps to alleviate possible anxiety related to any misconceptions and lack of knowledge.	Client states she realizes the infection is not her fault; she is not a "bad mother" because of it.
Psychosocial/Spiritual/Emotional Needs				
Nurse	Attempt to identify the meaning of breastfeeding to client.	Encourage client to express feelings and thoughts about herself, breastfeeding, and mastitis. Review and reinforce with client positive attributes about herself.	Identifying the meaning of breastfeeding assists in determining the effect that a diagnosis of mastitis may have on client.	Client states that she views this event as only a minor setback to her childrearing plans.
Discharge Planning				
Nurse	Determine whether client has appointment for follow-up care.	Encourage active participation in decision making to foster self-esteem. Urge boyfriend to provide breastfeeding support.	Adequate self-esteem is important to make effective childrearing decisions.	Client will discuss apparent lack of breastfeeding support with boyfriend. Will keep follow-up appointment.

may be more difficult to detect than primary or simple overdistention.

With primary overdistention, a woman does not void at all. A longer-than-usual time (>8 hours) passes after the birth or between voids. Assessment by percussion or palpation of the bladder reveals the bladder distention.

With urinary retention and overflow, a woman is able to void. Voiding is very frequent, however, and in small amounts; her overall output is inadequate. Always measure the amount of a woman's first voiding after birth. As a rule, if this voiding is less than 100 mL, suspect urinary retention.

Urinary retention is confirmed by catheterizing a woman immediately after she voids. If the amount of urine left in the bladder after voiding (termed *residual*) is greater than 100 mL, the woman has retention of more than the normal amount. Typically, her physician or nurse-midwife writes an order such as, "Catheterize for residual urine. If this is greater than 100 mL, leave indwelling catheter in place." Always use strict antiseptic technique to prevent introducing pathogenic bacteria into the sterile urinary tract and causing a urinary tract infection. Always use an indwelling (Foley) catheter rather than a temporary one (straight catheter) to catheterize for residual urine. This helps to minimize the risk of introducing pathogens with a second catheterization, should an indwelling catheter be needed.

Catheterizing a woman during the early postpartal period can be difficult. Vulvar edema often distorts the position and appearance of the urinary meatus. Use a gentle technique, remembering that a woman's perineum is apt to feel tender to touch.

Therapeutic Management

The amount of urine to remove from an overdistended bladder is controversial. There is a suggestion that removing more than 750 to 1000 mL of urine at any one time may create extreme pressure changes in the bladder and lower abdomen. Decreased pressure may cause blood to flow into the area, creating supine hypotension. There are few documented occurrences of this happening, however. Particularly in the postpartal period, when a bladder is easily distended and the uterus is larger than normal, this shift in pressure may not be as important as usual. Follow your health care agency's policy concerning how much urine to remove from a full bladder at catheterization.

If an indwelling catheter will be left in place, be certain to explain the rationale for its insertion and how it works. Explain how the balloon is inflated to hold it in place. This prevents a woman from limiting her activity to try and keep it in place. Activity and ambulation help to prevent other complications, such as thrombophlebitis.

Catheterization is a procedure that has a reputation as being extremely painful. Assure a woman that, as a rule, it involves only a momentary discomfort, such as a pinprick, as the catheter is inserted. Because the pain sensation of edematous tissue is decreased, a woman with extreme vulvar edema may experience only slight discomfort.

After 24 hours, the physician or nurse-midwife may order the indwelling catheter to be clamped for a short time and then removed. Encourage the woman to void by the end of 6 hours after removal of the catheter by offering fluid, administering an analgesic so she can relax, assisting her to the bathroom as necessary, and trying time-tested solutions such as running water at the sink or letting her hold her hand under warm running water. In most women, bladder and vulvar edema have decreased significantly by this time, so they are able to void without further difficulty. You may be asked to assess for residual urine again. If a woman has not voided by 8 hours after catheter removal, the physician or nurse-midwife may order reinsertion of the indwelling catheter for an additional 24 hours.

Difficulty with bladder function after childbirth is becoming less of a problem as less anesthesia and fewer forceps are used at birth, decreasing bladder and vulvar pressure. If problems do arise, they may be difficult for a woman to accept, because bladder elimination is a basic step of self-care. Bladder problems can be disappointing and discouraging to a woman who wants not only to be able to care for herself but also to care for a new infant. Reassure a woman that bladder complications are not uncommon after childbirth. Usually they are present for no longer than 48 hours, and most likely they will not recur.

Urinary Tract Infection

A woman who is catheterized at the time of childbirth or during the postpartal period is prone to development of a urinary tract infection, because bacteria may be introduced into the bladder at the time of catheterization.

Assessment

If a urinary tract infection develops, a woman notices symptoms of burning on urination, possibly blood in the urine (hematuria), and a feeling of frequency or that she always has to void. The pain is so sharp on voiding that she may resist voiding, further compounding the problem of urinary stasis. She may also have a low-grade fever and discomfort from lower abdominal pain.

Obtain a clean-catch urine specimen from any woman with symptoms of urinary tract infection (see Nursing Procedure Box 11.6 in Chapter 11). This can be done as an independent nursing action. So that lochial discharge does not contaminate the specimen, provide a sterile cotton ball for the woman to tuck into her vagina after perineal cleansing. Be certain to ask if she removed the cotton ball after the procedure; otherwise, it could cause stasis of vaginal secretions and increase the possibility of endometritis. Mark the specimen "possibly contaminated by lochia," so that any blood in the specimen will not be overly interpreted by the laboratory technician.

Therapeutic Management

Although sulfa drugs are normally prescribed for urinary tract infection, they are contraindicated for breastfeeding women because they can cause neonatal jaundice. Typically, therefore, a broad-spectrum antibiotic such as amoxicillin or ampicillin will be prescribed to treat a postpartal urinary tract infection. If an antibiotic contraindicated by breastfeeding is prescribed, check with a woman's physician about possibly changing the antibiotic to one that is safe for breastfeeding. Otherwise, once she is home, the woman may decide to breastfeed and not take the prescribed antibiotic.

Encourage a woman to drink large amounts of fluid (a glass every hour) to help flush the infection from her bladder. She may need an oral analgesic, such as acetaminophen (Tylenol), to reduce the pain of urination for the next few times she voids until the antibiotic begins to have an effect and the burning sensation disappears. Otherwise, because voiding is painful, she may not drink the fluid you suggest, knowing that it will increase the number of times she needs to void.

Although symptoms of urinary tract infection decrease quickly, be certain a woman understands the importance of continuing to take the prescribed antibiotic for the full 5 to 7 days to eradicate the infection completely. Women often stop taking medicine after the symptoms disappear, especially if they are busy—and women at home with new babies are busy. Make a chart for a woman to post on her refrigerator door as a reminder to continue to take the medication. If she stops the antibiotic, bacteria in the urine will begin to multiply again, and in another week symptoms and the active infection will recur. Be certain a woman is aware of common methods all women should use to prevent urinary tract infections (see Chapter 46).

What if... It has been approximately 7 hours since Mary Blackhawk gave birth and she still has not voided? What should you do next?

CARDIOVASCULAR SYSTEM DISORDERS

Because pregnancy requires major changes in the volume of blood and blood pressure, some excess volume and pressure can still be present in the postpartal period.

Postpartal Pregnancy-Induced Hypertension

Because pregnancy-induced hypertension (PIH) usually develops during pregnancy, it is discussed in Chapter 21. Mild pre-existing hypertension may increase in severity during the first few hours or days after birth. Rarely, PIH develops for the first time in a woman who has had no prenatal or intranatal symptoms. When this happens, the cardinal symptoms are the same as those of prenatal PIH: proteinuria, edema, and hypertension (Bailis & Witter, 2007).

The treatment measures for postpartal PIH are also the same as for antepartal PIH: bed rest, a quiet atmosphere, frequent monitoring of vital signs and urine output, and administration of magnesium sulfate or an antihypertensive agent. Antihypertensive therapy can be administered in higher doses than during pregnancy, because there is no longer any risk of injury to a fetus. The reason the condition occurs is usually retention of some placental material. The woman may be taken to surgery to have a D&C to be certain that all placental fragments have been removed from her uterus. After the D&C, blood pressure often falls dramatically to normal.

Seizures, if they occur postpartally as a symptom of PIH, typically develop 6 to 24 hours after birth. Seizures occurring more than 72 hours after birth are probably not the result of PIH but the result of some cause unrelated to childbearing.

Women in whom postpartal PIH develops are bewildered by what is happening to them. If seizures occur, they are frightened to discover how little control they have over their body. They worry that they will have a seizure after they are at home, while holding their baby. You can assure them that PIH, although it appears late, is a condition of pregnancy, so the symptoms will now fade quickly. Women with chronic hypertension need frequent monitoring during a future pregnancy to prevent PIH symptoms from occurring again (Miller, 2007).

REPRODUCTIVE SYSTEM DISORDERS

Pregnancy may leave reproductive system organs weakened or displaced.

Reproductive Tract Displacement

If the support systems of the uterus are weakened because of pregnancy, the ligaments may no longer be able to maintain the uterus in its usual position or level after pregnancy. Problems of retroflexion, anteflexion, retroversion, and anteversion or prolapse of the uterus may occur. These uterine displacement disorders may interfere with future childbearing and fertility and may cause continued pain or a feeling of lower abdominal heaviness or discomfort.

If the walls of the vagina are weakened, a cystocele (outpouching of the bladder into the vaginal wall) or a rectocele (outpouching of the rectum into the vaginal wall) may occur. These problems tend to develop most frequently in women with a high parity and after a forceps birth (see Figure 5.8 in Chapter 5). Surgery to repair such conditions may be necessary. If stress incontinence (involuntary voiding on exertion) occurs, Kegel exercises to strengthen perineal muscles may be helpful (Hay-Smith & Dumoulin, 2009).

Separation of the Symphysis Pubis

During pregnancy, many women feel some discomfort at the symphysis pubis because of relaxation of the joint preparatory to birth. If a fetus is unusually large or fetal position is not optimal, the ligaments of the symphysis pubis may be so stretched by birth that they actually tear. After birth, the woman experiences acute pain on turning or walking; her legs tend to rotate externally, giving her a waddling gait. A defect over the symphysis pubis can be palpated; the area is swollen and tender to touch.

Bed rest and the application of a snug pelvic binder to immobilize the joint are necessary to relieve pain and allow healing. As with all ligament injuries, a 4- to 6-week period is necessary for healing to take place. During this time, a woman may need to arrange for a person to help her with child care at home. She should avoid heavy lifting for an extended period, until healing in the pubic ligaments is complete. She may be advised to consider cesarean birth for any future pregnancy.

EMOTIONAL AND PSYCHOLOGICAL COMPLICATIONS OF THE PUERPERIUM

Any woman who is extremely stressed or who gives birth to an infant who in any way does not meet her expectations such as being the wrong sex, being physically or cognitively challenged, or being ill may have difficulty bonding with her infant. Inability to bond is a postpartal complication with far-reaching implications, possibly affecting the future health of the entire family.

A Woman Whose Child Is Born With an Illness or Is Physically Challenged

The average woman often has difficulty immediately after birth believing that her pregnancy is over and her child has been born. This difficulty is further compounded for a woman whose child is challenged in some way. She must not only grasp the fact that her baby has been born but also understand that her actual baby is different from her wished-for one.

Most women say during pregnancy they do not care about the sex of their child so long as the child is born healthy. This can make them feel cheated when this one requirement is not met. They can feel angry, hurt, and disappointed. They may feel a loss of self-esteem: they have given birth to an imperfect child, and so they see themselves as imperfect. A woman sometimes responds with a grief reaction, as if her child had died. The image of the "perfect" child she thought she was carrying *has* died.

In most instances, parents are shown their child moments after birth, so if a condition or problem exists, it can be immediately explained to them. Although this is a shock to couples, it allows them to face the problem with support people readily available. The physician or nurse-midwife usually makes it her or his responsibility to tell the parents about the defect. Be prepared to reinforce this information or review the problem. People who are under stress are not good listeners and may need repeated explanations before they completely understand the problem.

If possible, it is important for the parents to care for the child during the postpartal period, so that they can touch, relate to, and "claim" the infant in as nearly normal a manner as possible. Many women wait until their support person is present to visit an intensive care nursery, so that visiting with their newborn is a family activity.

Open lines of communication between the parents and the hospital staff that allow for free discussion of feelings and fears will do much to strengthen parent–child relationships and prepare for future hospitalizations or care of the child.

A Woman Whose Newborn Has Died

A woman whose newborn dies at birth always has questions about what happened. She is likely to feel bewildered, perhaps bitter, and perhaps resentful that the hospital staff could not save her child. "Why me? Of all the women here, why did my baby die?" She needs concerned support from health care personnel to help her cope with such a devastating loss.

Most women are interested in seeing the baby. This is generally therapeutic because it helps them begin grieving. Clean the baby, wrap the baby in an infant blanket, and bring him or her to the parents. Remain with them, but give them time to handle and inspect the child as they wish. Parents may want to take a photograph of the baby for a memory book. Be familiar with the forms the mother or father have to sign when a baby dies or is born dead. Know whether your state requires stillborn infants to be given a name and a funeral.

Other women on the unit tend to stay away from a woman whose child has died, as if what happened to her baby was contagious. Friends and relatives may be equally unable to talk about the situation. Most women, therefore, want a nurse to approach them and say, "Do you want to talk about what's happened?" or "How do you feel?" Be careful not to use trite sympathy phrases such as, "One door closes, another one opens" or "God must have another purpose for you." These may be your beliefs but they may not be the woman's.

Do not place a woman whose child has died in a hospital room with a woman who has a healthy baby. Provide a private room, to allow the woman an opportunity to grieve. Allow her family to visit freely. She needs them with her to fill a portion of the void left by her loss. The process of grieving and the support a woman requires at this time is further discussed in Chapter 56.

Postpartal Depression

Almost every woman notices some immediate (1 to 10 days postpartum) feelings of sadness (postpartal "blues") after childbirth. This probably occurs as a response to the anticlimactic feeling after birth and also probably is related to hormonal shifts as the levels of estrogen, progesterone, and gonadotropin-releasing hormone in her body decline or rise (Baker, 2008).

In as many as 20% of women, these normal feelings continue beyond the immediate postpartal period and may even be present for longer than 1 year (Box 25.10). The sensations of overwhelming sadness can interfere with breastfeeding, child care, and returning to work (Box 25.11). In addition to an overall feeling of sadness, a woman may notice extreme fatigue, an inability to stop crying, increased anxiety about her own or her infant's health, insecurity (unwillingness to be left alone or inability to make decisions), psychosomatic symptoms (nausea and vomiting, diarrhea), and either depressive or manic mood fluctuations. Depression of this kind is termed **postpartal depression** and reflects a more serious problem than normal "baby blues" (Schatzberg, Cole, & DeBattista, 2007) (Table 25.2). Risk factors for postpartal depression include a history of depression, a troubled childhood, low self-esteem, stress in the home or at work, and lack of effective support people. Different expectations between partners (if a woman wants a child and her partner does not,

BOX 25.10 * Focus on Communication

Mary Blackhawk is about to be discharged from the hospital, 72 hours after childbirth. You notice that, although her boyfriend visited with her, left some baby clothes, and then went downstairs to complete the discharge papers, Mary has made no attempt to change to street clothes or dress her new baby girl. The baby clothes her boyfriend left include a baseball-type shirt.

Less Effective Communication

Nurse: Mary? Do you need some help with the baby?
Mary: Are you sure I can't stay? I feel too tired to go home.
Nurse: Your insurance won't pay if you stay. [Mary starts to cry.]
Mary: This isn't right. I am just too tired to go home.
Nurse: It's the baby blues. If you change your mind and do need help with the baby, let me know. I'll be glad to dress her for you.

More Effective Communication

Nurse: Mary? Do you need some help with the baby?
Mary: Are you sure I can't stay? I feel just too tired to go home.
Nurse: Tell me more about that. [Mary starts to cry.]
Mary: I'm tired all over. It would be easier for me to kill myself than go home, try and take care of this baby myself, work full-time, and still finish school.
Nurse: Is that different from how you thought things would be after you had the baby?
Mary: I thought he'd ask me to marry him. I bet he would have if I'd had a boy instead of a girl.
Nurse: I'm worried about you going home, too.

Almost all women experience some fatigue after childbirth. As many as 70% experience a temporary feeling of sadness (baby blues). About 10%, however, develop depression severe enough to need therapy. Be sure to ask enough questions to be certain that a woman's crying is not something more serious than simple "baby blues" before she is discharged from the health care facility. In this way, a woman who has more serious problems can be referred to the proper professionals for help and support.

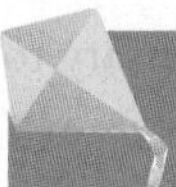

BOX 25.11 ✻ Focus on Evidence-Based Practice

What is the effect of postpartum depression on breastfeeding success?

To investigate this concern, researchers asked 163 women to complete an Edinburgh Postnatal Depression Scale questionnaire and to submit hand-expressed breast milk for sodium and potassium analysis between the 2nd and 12th weeks after birth. Of these women, 40 (24.5%) were rated as having a high risk for a depressive episode; 63 (41%) did not feel confident about breastfeeding. Women who have symptoms of depression or lack of confidence in their ability to breastfeed tend to supplement breastfeeding more than women without depression or lack of confidence. It is well documented that sodium levels rise in the breast milk of women who produce a limited supply of breast milk. Women who supplement breastfeeding with formula feeding produce less breast milk and so have higher sodium levels in milk. In this study, supplementation increased the risk of high sodium in relation to potassium in breast milk by as much as 209%. The researchers suggest that any measures to help women avoid postpartal depression and to feel confident in their ability to breastfeed can be instrumental in ensuring healthy breast milk for newborns.

What interventions could you use with postpartal women to help them feel confident at breastfeeding?

Source: Flores-Quijano, M. E., et al. (2008). Risk for postpartum depression, breastfeeding practices, and mammary gland permeability. *Journal of Human Lactation, 24*(1), 50–57.

for example) or disappointment in the child (a boy instead of a girl, for example) could play major roles.

It is difficult to predict which women will develop postpartal depression before birth, because childbirth can result in so many varied reactions; if factors could be identified, pregnancy counseling might be able to prevent symptoms (Haessler & Rosenthal, 2007). In the postpartal period, discovery of the problem as soon as symptoms develop is a

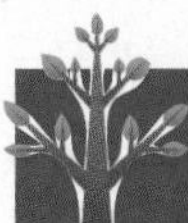

BOX 25.12 ✻ Focus on Family Teaching

Q. Mary asks you, "How can I avoid becoming depressed after I return home with my new baby?"

A. Some helpful guidelines are:

- Plan a balanced program of nutrition, exercise, and sleep. Plan meals that are easy to prepare; sleep whenever your baby sleeps; begin a program of walking daily with your baby.
- Share your feelings with a support person. Many communities have postpartum support groups to help with this.
- Take some time every day to do something for yourself (work on a scrapbook, go shopping, for example) so you have a break from baby care.
- Do not try to be perfect. Analyze what are the important things to do and get them done. Let unimportant things go for another day.
- Do not let yourself be isolated by baby care. Use the Internet or telephone to keep in contact with your friends so you are not lonely.

nursing priority. A number of depression scales to help detect postpartum depression are available but conscientious observation and discussion with women can reveal symptoms just as well. A woman may need counseling and possibly antidepressant therapy to integrate the experience of childbirth into her life (Leahy-Warren & McCarthy, 2007). This is crucial to development of a healthy maternal–infant bond, to the health of any other children in the family, and to overall family functioning. Ask at postpartal return visits and well-child visits about symptoms that would suggest depression, and recommend an appropriate referral. Measures to help prevent depression are shown in Box 25.12.

Postpartal Psychosis

As many as 1 woman in 500 has enough symptoms during the year after the birth of a child to be considered psychiatrically ill. This statistic represents the current rate of overall mental

TABLE 25.2 ✻ Comparing Postpartal Blues, Depression, and Psychosis

	Postpartal Blues	Postpartal Depression	Postpartal Psychosis
Onset	1–10 days after birth	1–12 months after birth	Within first year after birth
Symptoms	Sadness, tears	Anxiety, feeling of loss, sadness	Delusions or hallucinations of harming infant or self
Incidence	70% of all births	10% of all births	1%–2% of all births
Etiology (possible)	Probable hormonal changes, stress of life changes	History of previous depression, hormonal response, lack of social support	Possible activation of previous mental illness, hormonal changes, family history of bipolar disorder
Therapy	Support, empathy	Counseling, drug therapy	Psychotherapy, drug therapy
Nursing role	Offer compassion and understanding	Refer to counseling	Refer to psychiatric care, safeguarding mother from injury to self or to newborn

illness (American Psychiatric Association [APA], 2000). When the illness coincides with the postpartal period, it is called **postpartal psychosis** (Haessler & Rosenthal, 2007). Rather than being a response to the physical aspects of childbearing, however, it is probably a response to the crisis of childbearing. The majority of these women have had symptoms of mental illness before pregnancy. If the pregnancy had not precipitated the illness, a death in the family, loss of a job or income, divorce, or some other major life crisis would probably have precipitated the same recurrence.

A woman with postpartal psychosis usually appears exceptionally sad. By definition, psychosis exists when a person has lost contact with reality. A woman with a postpartal psychosis may deny that she has had a child and, when the child is brought to her, insist that she was never pregnant. She may voice thoughts of infanticide or that her infant is possessed. If observation tells you that a woman is not functioning in reality, you cannot improve her concept of reality by a simple measure such as explaining what a correct perception is. Her sensory input is too disturbed to comprehend this. In addition, she may interpret your attempt as threatening. She may respond with anger or become equally threatening. A psychosis is a severe mental illness that requires referral to a professional psychiatric counselor and antipsychotic medication.

While waiting for such a skilled professional to arrive, do not leave the woman alone, because her distorted perception might lead her to harm herself. Nor should you leave her alone with her infant.

Always keep in mind that postpartum psychosis does exist, although it is rare. Remembering that childbearing can lead to this degree of mental illness helps you to put childbearing into perspective. For some people, childbearing is such a crisis in their lives that it triggers mental illness. Certainly, it cannot be considered an everyday incident in anyone's life.

✔ Checkpoint Question 25.3

Which statement by Mary Blackhawk is most suggestive of a woman developing postpartal psychosis?

a. "I wish my baby had more hair."
b. "My baby has the devil's eyes."
c. "I feel exhausted since birth."
d. "Breastfeeding is harder than I thought."

Key Points for Review

- Establishing a firm family–newborn relationship may be difficult when a woman has a postpartal complication. Investigate ways that will allow a woman to care for her baby, or offer necessary support to family members so that they can fulfill this role.
- Hemorrhage (defined as a loss of blood greater than 500 mL within a 24-hour period) is a major potential danger in the immediate postpartal period. The most frequent cause of postpartal hemorrhage is uterine atony. Continuous limited blood loss can be as important over time as sudden, intense bleeding. With hemorrhage, administration of oxytocin may be necessary to initiate uterine tone and halt the bleeding.
- Other causes of hemorrhage include lacerations (vaginal, cervical, or perineal) and retained placental fragments. Lacerations are most apt to occur with forceps birth or with the birth of a large infant. Disseminated intravascular coagulation can also cause postpartum hemorrhage.
- Puerperal infection (a temperature greater than 100.4° F or 38.0° C) is a potential complication after any birth until the denuded placental surface has healed. Retained placental fragments and the use of internal fetal heart monitoring leads are potential sources of infection.
- Thrombophlebitis, an inflammation of the lining of a blood vessel, occurs most often as an extension of an endometrial infection. Therapy includes bed rest with moist heat applications and anticoagulant therapy. *Never massage the leg of a woman with thrombophlebitis;* doing so can cause the clot to move and become a pulmonary embolus, a possibly fatal complication.
- Mastitis is infection of the breast. The symptoms include pain, swelling, and redness. Antibiotic therapy is necessary.
- A woman whose child is born with a physical or cognitive challenge needs special consideration after birth. This is obviously a time of stress, and a woman needs supportive nursing care.
- Postpartal "blues" are a normal accompaniment to birth. Postpartal depression (a feeling of extreme sadness) and postpartal psychosis (an actual separation from reality) are not normal and need accurate assessment so a woman can receive adequate therapy for these conditions.

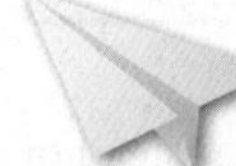

CRITICAL THINKING EXERCISES

1. Mary Blackhawk, whom you met at the beginning of the chapter, was having heavy vaginal bleeding at 4 hours after birth. Because she was sleeping, however, she was totally unaware of it. What action on your part would have prevented so much blood loss? What action would be most appropriate now?
2. Eight hours after birth, Mary Blackhawk tells you that she has frequency and burning on urination. She had a urinary tract infection during pregnancy, so she recognizes the symptoms. She has some medicine left from pregnancy and tells you that she will take it to cure the infection. What advice would you give her?
3. When Mary returns for a postpartal checkup, you notice red streaks on both legs along the course of her veins, and she has pain on dorsiflexion of her foot. You are concerned that she is developing thrombophlebitis. Describe a plan of care that could have reduced this risk during labor and in the immediate postpartal period.
4. Examine the National Health Goals related to complications of the puerperium. Most government-sponsored funds for nursing research are allotted based on these goals. What would be a possible research topic to ex-

plore pertinent to these goals that would be applicable to the Blackhawk family and also advance evidence-based practice?

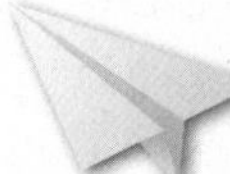

CRITICAL THINKING SCENARIO

Open the accompanying CD-ROM or visit http://thePoint.lww.com and read the Patient Scenario included for this chapter, then answer the questions to further sharpen your skills and grow more familiar with NCLEX style questions related to postpartal complications. Confirm your answers are correct by reading the rationales.

REFERENCES

American Psychiatric Association (APA). (2000). *Diagnostic and statistical manual (DSM-IV).* Washington, D.C.: Author.

Bailis, A., & Witter, F. R. (2007). Hypertensive disorders of pregnancy. In K. B. Fortner, et al. (Eds.). *The Johns Hopkins manual of gynecology and obstetrics.* Philadelphia: Lippincott Williams & Wilkins.

Baker, E. G. (2008). Beyond the blues: a guide to understanding and treating prenatal and postpartum depression. *Journal of Midwifery and Women's Health, 53*(1), 9.

Begley, J. S., & Barnes, R. C. (2007). Group B streptococcus toxic shock-like syndrome in a healthy woman: a case report. *Journal of Reproductive Medicine, 52*(4), 323–325.

Cansino, C. D., & Lipsett, P. (2007). Critical care. In K. B. Fortner, et al. (Eds.). *The Johns Hopkins manual of gynecology and obstetrics.* Philadelphia: Lippincott Williams & Wilkins.

Chelmow, D., Aronson, M. P., & Wosu, U. (2007). Intraoperative and postoperative complications of gynecologic surgery. In A. H. DeCherney & L. Nathan (Eds.). *Current diagnosis and treatment in obstetrics and gynecology* (10th ed.). Columbus, OH: McGraw-Hill.

Crombleholme, W. R. (2009). Obstetrics. In S. J. McPhee & M. A. Papadakis (Eds.). *Current medical diagnosis and treatment.* Columbus, OH: McGraw-Hill.

Flores-Quijano, M. E., et al. (2008). Risk for postpartum depression, breastfeeding practices, and mammary gland permeability. *Journal of Human Lactation, 24*(1), 50–57.

Gates, S., Brocklehurst, P., & Davis, L. J. (2009). Prophylaxis for venous thromboembolic disease in pregnancy and the early postnatal period. *Cochrane Database of Systematic Reviews, 2009*(1), (CD001689).

Haessler, A., & Rosenthal, M. B. (2007). Psychological aspects of obstetrics and gynecology. In A. H. DeCherney & L. Nathan (Eds.). *Current diagnosis and treatment in obstetrics and gynecology* (10th ed.). Columbus, OH: McGraw-Hill.

Hay-Smith, E. J. C., & Dumoulin, C. (2009). Pelvic floor muscle training versus no treatment, or inactive control treatments, for urinary incontinence in women. *Cochrane Database of Systematic Reviews, 2009*(1), (CD005654).

Karch, A. M. (2009). *Lippincott's nursing drug guide.* Philadelphia: Lippincott Williams & Wilkins.

Keller, C., et al. (2008). Interventions for weight management in postpartum women. *JOGNN: Journal of Obstetric, Gynecologic, and Neonatal Nursing, 37*(1), 71–79.

Miller, D. A. (2007). Hypertension in pregnancy. In A. H. DeCherney & L. Nathan (Eds.). *Current diagnosis and treatment in obstetrics and gynecology* (10th ed.). Columbus, OH: McGraw-Hill.

Leahy-Warren, P., & McCarthy, G. (2007). Postnatal depression: prevalence, mothers' perspectives, and treatments. *Archives of Psychiatric Nursing, 21*(2), 91–100.

McGarry, J., et al. (2009). Postpartum depression and help-seeking behavior. *Journal of Midwifery & Women's Health, 54*(1), 50–56.

Musselwhite, K. L., et al. (2007). Use of epidural anesthesia and the risk of acute postpartum urinary retention. *American Journal of Obstetrics and Gynecology, 196*(5), 472–473.

Nelson, W. L., & O'Brien, J. M. (2007). The uterine sandwich for persistent uterine atony: combining the B-Lynch compression suture and an intrauterine Bakri balloon. *American Journal of Obstetrics and Gynecology, 196*(5), e9–e10.

Pavone, M. E., Purinton, S. C., & Petersen, S. M. (2007). Postpartum care and breast-feeding. In K. B. Fortner, et al. (Eds.). *The Johns Hopkins manual of gynecology and obstetrics.* Philadelphia: Lippincott Williams & Wilkins.

Poggi, S. B. H. (2007). Postpartum hemorrhage and the abnormal puerperium. In A. H. DeCherney & L. Nathan (Eds.). *Current diagnosis and treatment in obstetrics and gynecology* (10th ed.). Columbus, OH: McGraw-Hill.

Reddy, P., et al. (2007). Postpartum mastitis and community-acquired methicillin-resistant *Staphylococcus aureus. Emerging Infectious Diseases, 13*(2), 298–301.

Schatzberg, A. F., Cole, J. O., & DeBattista, C. (2007). *Manual of clinical psychopharmacology* (6th ed.). Columbus, OH: McGraw-Hill.

Szymanski, L. M., & Bienstock, J. L. (2007). Complications of labor and delivery. In K. B. Fortner, et al. (Eds.). *The Johns Hopkins manual of gynecology and obstetrics.* Philadelphia: Lippincott Williams & Wilkins.

SUGGESTED READINGS

Cuijpers, P., Brannmark, J. G., & van Straten, A. (2008). Psychological treatment of postpartum depression: a meta-analysis. *Journal of Clinical Psychology, 64*(1), 103–118.

Krummel, D. A. (2007). Postpartum weight control: a vicious cycle. *Journal of the American Dietetic Association, 107*(1), 37–40.

Porter, S. (2007). Blood loss, replacement and belief. *RCM Midwives, 10*(2), 72–75.

Mahlmeister, L. R. (2007). Legal issues and risk management. Best practices in perinatal nursing: improving outcomes for obese and morbidly obese women during the intrapartum and postpartum periods. *Journal of Perinatal and Neonatal Nursing, 21*(2), 86–88.

Mousa, H. A., & Alfirevic, Z. (2009). Treatment for primary postpartum haemorrhage. *Cochrane Database of Systematic Reviews, 2009*(1) (CD003249).

Rowan, C., Bick, D., & Bastos, M. H. S. (2007). Postnatal debriefing interventions to prevent maternal mental health problems after birth: exploring the gap between the evidence and UK policy and practice. *Worldviews on Evidence-Based Nursing, 4*(2), 97–105.

Runquist, J. (2007). Persevering through postpartum fatigue. *JOGNN: Journal of Obstetric, Gynecologic, and Neonatal Nursing, 36*(1), 28–37.

Rychnovsky, J. D. (2007). Postpartum fatigue in the active-duty military woman. *JOGNN: Journal of Obstetric, Gynecologic, and Neonatal Nursing, 36*(1), 38–46.

Walker, L. O., & Sterling, B. S. (2007).The structure of thriving/distress among low-income women at 3 months after giving birth. *Family and Community Health, 30*(1S), S95–S103.

Williams, A., Herron-Marx, S., & Knibb, R. (2007). The prevalence of enduring postnatal perineal morbidity and its relationship to type of birth and birth risk factors. *Journal of Clinical Nursing, 16*(3), 549–561.

Chapter 26 Nursing Care of a Family With a High-Risk Newborn

KEY TERMS

- apnea
- apparent life-threatening event
- appropriate for gestational age (AGA)
- brown fat
- caudal regression syndrome
- developmental care
- dysmature
- extracorporeal membrane oxygenation (ECMO)
- fetal alcohol syndrome
- gestational age
- hemorrhagic disease of the newborn
- hydrops fetalis
- hyperbilirubinemia
- intrauterine growth restriction
- large for gestational age (LGA)
- low-birth-weight infant
- macrosomia
- ophthalmia neonatorum
- periodic respirations
- periventricular leukomalacia
- postterm syndrome
- preterm infants
- retinopathy of prematurity
- shoulder dystocia
- small for gestational age (SGA)

OBJECTIVES

After mastering the contents of this chapter, you should be able to:

1. Define the following terms—*small-for-gestational-age infant, term infant, large-for-gestational-age infant, preterm infant,* and *postterm infant*—and describe common illnesses that occur in these and other high-risk newborns.
2. Identify National Health Goals related to high-risk newborns nurses can be instrumental in helping the nation achieve.
3. Use critical thinking to analyze the special crisis imposed on families when alterations of newborn development or neonatal illness occur to make nursing family centered.
4. Assess a high-risk newborn to determine whether safe transition to extrauterine life has occurred.
5. Formulate nursing diagnoses related to a high-risk newborn.
6. Identify expected outcomes for a high-risk newborn and family.
7. Plan nursing care focused on priorities to stabilize a high-risk newborn's body systems.
8. Implement nursing care for a high-risk newborn such as monitoring body temperature.
9. Evaluate expected outcomes for achievement and effectiveness of care.
10. Identify areas related to the care of high-risk newborns that could benefit from additional nursing research or application of evidence-based practice.
11. Integrate knowledge of the needs of a high-risk newborn with nursing process to achieve quality maternal and child health nursing care.

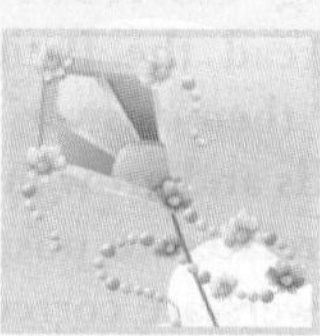

Mr. and Mrs. Atkins are the parents of a 34-week-gestation, 2-lb baby boy born last night after a short, 4-hour labor. Their baby took a few gasping respirations at birth but then stopped breathing. He was resuscitated by the neonatal nurse practitioner and respiratory therapist and then transported to the intensive care nursery. Mr. Atkins was not present for the birth because he was out of town on business. You notice Mrs. Atkins has not visited the intensive care nursery to see her son. She also refused to sign the birth certificate because she could not decide on a name. She said, "I don't want to give him our favorite name because he might die." Mr. Atkins called early this morning and acted more upset the baby was born than relieved the baby was receiving intensive care. You hear him ask his wife, "What did you do to cause this?" Previous chapters described the birth of well newborns and care of newborns who are well at birth. This chapter adds information on care of newborns who are ill or have a significant variation in gestational age or weight. Learning to recognize these infants at birth and organizing care for them can be instrumental in helping protect both their present and future health.

What type of help do the Atkinses need to better accept what has happened to them?

During pregnancy, screening women for risk factors that could lead to illness in a newborn such as younger or older than average maternal age, concurrent disease conditions such as diabetes or human immunodeficiency virus (HIV) infection, pregnancy complications such as placenta previa, or an unhealthy maternal lifestyle such as drug abuse is essential to identify infants who may need greater-than-usual care at birth (Pinheiro, 2007). Unfortunately, not all instances of high risk can be predicted. Even a newborn from a "perfect" pregnancy may require specialized care or develop a problem over the first few days of life necessitating special interventions. Any infant who is born **dysmature** (before term or postterm, or who is underweight or overweight for gestational age) is also at risk for complications at birth or in the first few days of life. Parents need thorough education about their baby's health because these problems may require rehospitalization or additional follow-up at home. National Health Goals related to the high-risk newborn are shown in Box 26.1.

Being able to predict an infant is at high risk allows for advanced preparation so that specialized, skilled health care personnel can be present at the child's birth to perform necessary interventions, such as resuscitating a newborn who has difficulty establishing respirations. Immediate, skilled handling of any problems that occur may help to save the newborn's life and also prevent future problems, such as neurologic disorders (Saigal & Doyle, 2008).

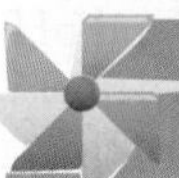

BOX 26.1 ✻ Focus on National Health Goals

Preterm birth has the potential for leading to so many complications in newborns that National Health Goals were written specifically concerning preterm birth:

- Reduce low birth weight (LBW) to an incidence of no more than 5% of live births and very low birth weight (VLBW) to an incidence of no more than 0.9% of live births from baselines of 7.6% and 1.4%, respectively.
- Increase the proportion of very low birth weight (VLBW) infants born at level III hospitals or subspecialty perinatal centers from a baseline of 73% to a target level of 90%.
- Reduce the rate of fetal and infant deaths during the perinatal period (28 weeks of gestation to 7 days or more after birth) to 4.4 per 1000 live births from a baseline of 7.3 per 1000 live births.
- Reduce the rate of deaths from sudden infant death syndrome (SIDS) to 0.23 per 1000 live births from a baseline of 0.67 per 1000 live births (http://www.nih.gov).

Nurses can help the nation achieve these goals by teaching women the symptoms of preterm labor so that, ideally, birth can be delayed until infants reach term. Nurses also need to be prepared for resuscitation at birth of preterm infants and to plan developmental care that can help prevent conditions such as apnea, intraventricular hemorrhage, and periventricular leukomalacia.

Further research is needed regarding how best to position infants to promote development and prevent fatigue, what measures can best prevent conditions such as intraventricular hemorrhage, and what measures can make parents feel most comfortable and allow them to best interact with their infants in neonatal intensive care units.

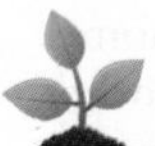

Nursing Process Overview

For the Family of a High-Risk Newborn

Assessment

All infants need to be assessed at birth for obvious congenital anomalies and **gestational age** (number of weeks they remained in utero). Both determinations can be done by the nurse who first examines an infant. Be certain these assessments are made with an infant under a prewarmed radiant heat warmer to guard against heat loss.

Continuing assessment of high-risk infants involves the use of instrumentation such as cardiac, apnea, and blood pressure monitoring. However, no matter how many monitors are used, they never replace the role of frequent, close, common-sense observation. Carefully evaluate comments from fellow nurses that an infant "isn't himself" or "breathes oddly." These comments, although not scientific, are the same observations that parents who know their baby well report at health visits. A nurse who knows an infant well from having cared for a baby consistently over time often senses changes before a monitor or other equipment begins to put a quantitative measurement on the factor.

Nursing Diagnosis

To establish nursing diagnoses for high-risk infants, it is important to be aware of the normal assessment parameters of newborns. Nursing diagnoses generally center on the nine priority areas of care for any newborn:

- Ineffective airway clearance related to presence of mucus or amniotic fluid in airway
- Ineffective cardiovascular tissue perfusion related to breathing difficulty
- Risk for deficient fluid volume related to insensible water loss
- Ineffective thermoregulation related to newborn status and stress from birth weight variation
- Risk for imbalanced nutrition, less than body requirements related to lack of energy for sucking
- Risk for infection related to lowered immune response in newborn
- Risk for impaired parenting related to illness in newborn at birth
- Deficient diversional activity (lack of stimulation) related to illness at birth
- Readiness for developmental care to decrease overstimulation easily caused by necessary life-saving procedures

Outcome Identification and Planning

Be certain when establishing expected outcomes that they are consistent with a newborn's potential. A goal that implies complete recovery from a major illness, for example, may be unrealistic for one newborn but completely appropriate for another. Plan care that is individualized considering a newborn's developmental as well as physiologic strengths, weaknesses, and needs. This helps to ensure that parents as well as the health care team understand the newborn's particular care priorities and potential. Many families of high-risk newborns will need continued support to care for their infants at home. They may need referral to a home health care or other agency. Helpful Internet sites to use for referring parents are the Web sites of the March of Dimes (http://www.marchofdimes.com), American Sudden Infant Death Syndrome Institute (http://www.sids.org), and Newborn Individualized Developmental Care and Assistance Program (http://www.nidcap.org).

Implementation

Interventions for any high-risk newborn are best carried out by a consistent caregiver and should focus on conserving the baby's energy and providing a thermoneutral environment to prevent exhaustion and chilling. Painful procedures should be kept to a minimum to help the infant achieve a sense of comfort and balance. Assisting parents to participate in care such as bathing or feeding their infant may help make the child real to them for the first time and start the bonding process.

Outcome Evaluation

High-risk newborns need long-term follow-up so any consequences of their birth status, such as minimal neurologic injury, can be identified and arrangements for special schooling or counseling can be made. Examples of expected outcomes include:

- Infant maintains a patent airway.
- Infant tolerates all procedures without accompanying apnea.
- Infant demonstrates growth and development appropriate for gestational age, birth weight, and condition.
- Infant maintains body temperature at 98.6° F (37.0° C) in open crib with one added blanket.
- Parents visit at least once and make three telephone calls to neonatal nursery weekly.
- Parents demonstrate positive coping skills and behaviors in response to newborn's condition.

NEWBORN PRIORITIES IN FIRST DAYS OF LIFE

All newborns have eight priority needs in the first few days of life:

1. Initiation and maintenance of respirations
2. Establishment of extrauterine circulation
3. Control of body temperature
4. Intake of adequate nourishment
5. Establishment of waste elimination
6. Prevention of infection
7. Establishment of an infant–parent relationship
8. Developmental care, or care that balances physiologic needs and stimulation for best development

These are also the priority needs of high-risk newborns. Because of small size or immaturity or illness, fulfilling these needs, however, may require special equipment or care measures. Not all newborns will be able to achieve full wellness because of extreme insults to their health at birth or difficulty adjusting to extrauterine life. Indications that a newborn is having difficulty making the transition from intrauterine to extrauterine life may be apparent during the intrapartum period, at birth, or at initial assessment because of a low Apgar score (see Chapter 18).

Initiating and Maintaining Respirations

Ultimately, the prognosis of a high-risk newborn depends primarily on how the first moments of life are managed. Most deaths occurring during the first 48 hours after birth result from the newborn's inability to establish or maintain adequate respirations (National Vital Statistics System [NVSS], 2009). An infant who has difficulty accomplishing effective respiratory action in the first hours of life and yet survives may experience residual neurologic difficulties because of cerebral hypoxia. Prompt, thorough care is necessary for effective intervention.

Most infants are born with some degree of respiratory acidosis. However, this is rapidly corrected by the spontaneous onset of respirations. If respiratory activity does not begin immediately, respiratory acidosis will increase. The blood pH and bicarbonate buffer system will fail. Newborn defense mechanisms are inadequate to reverse the process. Therefore, the effort to establish respirations must be started immediately after birth. By 2 minutes, the development of severe acidosis is already well under way (Thilo & Rosenberg, 2008).

Any infant who sustains some degree of asphyxia in utero, such as could occur from cord compression, maternal anesthesia, placenta previa, or preterm separation of the placenta, may already be experiencing acidosis at birth and may have difficulty before the first 2 minutes of life.

Resuscitation

Factors that commonly predispose infants to respiratory difficulty and so may require resuscitation are shown in Box 26.2. If breathing is ineffective, circulatory shunts, particularly the

BOX 26.2 ✻ Factors Predisposing Infants to Respiratory Difficulty in the First Few Days of Life

- Low birth weight
- Maternal history of diabetes
- Premature rupture of membranes
- Maternal use of barbiturates or narcotics close to birth
- Meconium staining
- Irregularities detected by fetal heart monitor during labor
- Cord prolapse
- Lowered Apgar score (<7) at 1 or 5 minutes
- Postmaturity
- Small for gestational age
- Breech birth
- Multiple birth
- Chest, heart, or respiratory tract anomalies

ductus arteriosus, can fail to close. Because left-side heart pressure is stronger than right-side pressure, blood circulates through a patent ductus arteriosus left to right or from the aorta to the pulmonary artery, creating ineffective pump action in the heart. Struggling to breathe and circulate blood, an infant uses available serum glucose quickly and may become hypoglycemic, compounding the initial problem.

For all these reasons, resuscitation becomes important for infants who fail to take a first breath or have difficulty maintaining adequate respiratory movements on their own.

Resuscitation follows an organized process: (a) establish and maintain an airway, (b) expand the lungs, and (c) initiate and maintain effective ventilation. If respiratory depression becomes severe, a newborn's heart will fail. Resuscitation then must also include cardiac massage (American Heart Association [AHA], 2008).

Airway

For a well term newborn, usually bulb syringe suction, which removes mucus and prevents aspiration of any mucus and amniotic fluid present in the mouth or nose with the first breath, is all that is necessary to help establish a clear airway (see Chapter 18).

If a newborn does not draw in a first breath spontaneously, suction the infant's mouth and nose with a bulb syringe again and rub the back to see if skin stimulation initiates respirations. Be certain an infant is dry, including the hair and head, to prevent chilling. If a newborn has to attempt to raise body temperature because of chilling, this will increase the need for oxygen, which the baby cannot supply because breathing has not yet been initiated. Warmed, blow-by oxygen by face mask or positive-pressure mask may be administered.

If a newborn's amniotic fluid was meconium stained, do not stimulate an infant to breathe by rubbing the back or administering air or oxygen under pressure as doing so could push meconium down into an infant's airway, further compromising respirations. Give oxygen by mask without pressure. Wait for a laryngoscope to be passed and the trachea to be deep suctioned before giving oxygen under pressure.

If deeper suctioning than by a bulb syringe is required, place an infant on the back and slide a folded towel or pad under the shoulders to raise them slightly so the head is in a neutral position. Slide a catheter (8F to 12F) over the infant's tongue to the back of the throat (Fig. 26.1). Do not suction for longer than 10 seconds at a time (count seconds as you suction) to avoid removing excessive air from an infant's lungs. Use a gentle touch. Bradycardia or cardiac arrhythmias can occur because of vagus stimulation (at the posterior oropharynx) from vigorous suctioning. In most newborns, this degree of resuscitation will initiate responsive respirations and a strong heartbeat. Color, muscle response, and reflexes will improve.

An infant who still makes no effort at spontaneous respirations requires immediate laryngoscopy to open the airway. Once a laryngoscope has been inserted, deep tracheal suctioning can be performed. After deep suctioning, an endotracheal tube can be inserted and oxygen administered by a positive-pressure bag and mask with 100% oxygen at 40 to 60 breaths per minute.

In the first few seconds of life, a newborn this severely depressed may take several weak gasps of air and then almost immediately stop breathing; the heart rate begins to fall.

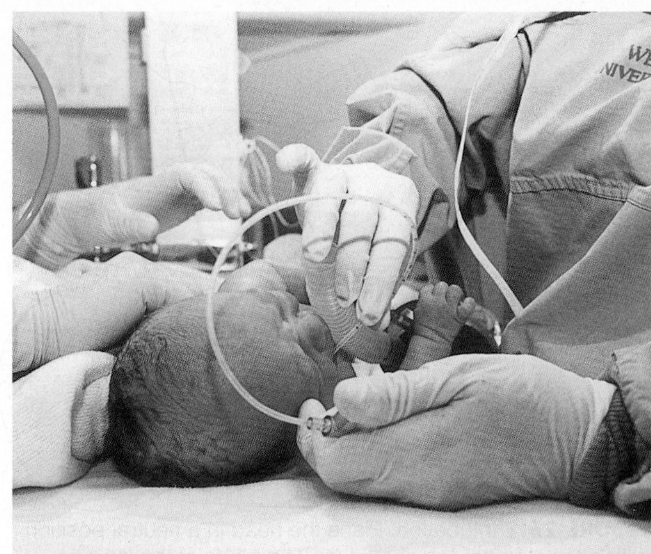

FIGURE 26.1 Suctioning a newborn with mechanical suction controlled by a finger valve. Suction is applied as the catheter is withdrawn. If the catheter is rotated as it is withdrawn, the risk of traumatizing membrane is reduced.

This period of halted respirations is termed *primary apnea*. After 1 or 2 minutes of apnea (a pause in respirations longer than 20 seconds with accompanying bradycardia), an infant again tries to initiate respirations with a few strong gasps. However, a newborn cannot maintain this effort longer than 4 or 5 minutes. After this, the respiratory effort will become weaker again and the heart rate will fall further until the newborn stops the gasping effort altogether. The infant then enters a period of *secondary apnea*. Although usually a phenomenon that occurs after birth, both types of apnea may occur in utero.

During the period of first gasps, resuscitation attempts are generally successful. Once a newborn is allowed to enter a secondary apnea period, however, resuscitation measures become difficult and may be ineffective. Because it is impossible to distinguish between the two periods simply by observation, resuscitation must always be started as if secondary apnea were occurring.

An obstetrician, pediatrician, neonatologist, anesthesiologist, or neonatal nurse practitioner skilled in laryngoscope and endotracheal tube insertion should be present at the birth of all infants identified as high risk so a laryngoscope can be quickly passed (Raab, 2007). Laryngoscope insertion is easy in theory; in practice, the wide variation in the size of infants' posterior pharynx and trachea and the emergency conditions present make it difficult (Fig. 26.2).

Laryngoscopes are equipped with different-size blades. Size 0 or 1 is used with newborns. The endotracheal tube fits inside the laryngoscope. Infants under 1000 g need a 2.5-mm endotracheal tube; those over 3000 g need a 4.0-mm tube. Because preterm infants are prone to hemorrhage because of capillary fragility, gentle care during insertion is crucial.

Lung Expansion

Once an airway has been established, a newborn's lungs need to be expanded. Well newborns inflate their lungs adequately

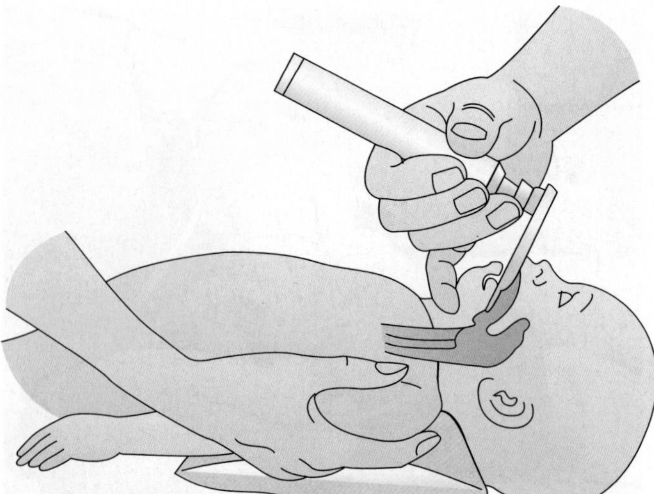

FIGURE 26.2 Intubation. Place the head in a neutral position with a towel under the shoulders. The blade of the laryngoscope is inserted to reveal the vocal cords. An endotracheal tube for ventilation is then passed into the trachea, past the laryngoscope.

with a first breath. The sound of the baby crying is proof that lung expansion is good because the vocal sounds are produced by a free flow of air over the vocal cords.

An infant who breathes spontaneously but then cannot sustain effective respirations may need oxygen by bag and mask to aid lung expansion. The mask should cover both the mouth and the nose to be effective. It should not cover the eyes, because it can cause eye injury mechanically from the mask or drying of the cornea from oxygen administration. Administer 100% oxygen by face mask and pressure bag at a rate of 40 to 60 compressions per minute. To prevent cooling, oxygen should be administered both warmed (between 89.6° and 93.2° F, or 32° and 34° C) and humidified (60%–80%).

The pressure needed to open lung alveoli for the first time is approximately 40 cm H_2O. After that, pressures of 15 to 20 cm H_2O are generally adequate to continue inflating alveoli (Thilo & Rosenberg, 2008). The pressure from anesthesia bags is controlled solely by the pressure of a hand against the bag. Other types of bags such as the Ambu-bag can be set with a blow-off valve that limits the pressure in the apparatus (Fig. 26.3).

It is important not to let oxygen levels in a newborn fluctuate, as fluctuation can cause bleeding from immature cranial vessels. In addition, no pressure above what is necessary should be used because excessive force can rupture lung alveoli. On the other hand, if adequate insufflation is not achieved, a newborn stands little chance of survival. To be certain oxygen is reaching the lungs with resuscitation, monitor the newborn's oxygen level with pulse oximetry in addition to auscultating the chest for the sound of breathing (Shiao & Ou, 2007).

Be certain to listen to both lungs to be sure both lungs are being aerated. If air can be heard on only one side or sounds are not symmetric, the endotracheal tube is probably at the bifurcation of the trachea and blocking one of the main-stem bronchi. Drawing it back half a centimeter will usually free it and allow oxygen to flow to both lungs.

When oxygen is given under pressure to a newborn this way, the stomach also quickly fills with oxygen. If the resuscitation continues for over 2 minutes, inserting an orogastric tube and leaving the distal end open will help deflate the stomach and decrease the possibility that vomiting and aspiration of stomach contents from overdistention will occur.

Drug Therapy

Stimulants have little place in newborn resuscitation unless an infant's respiratory depression appears to be related to the

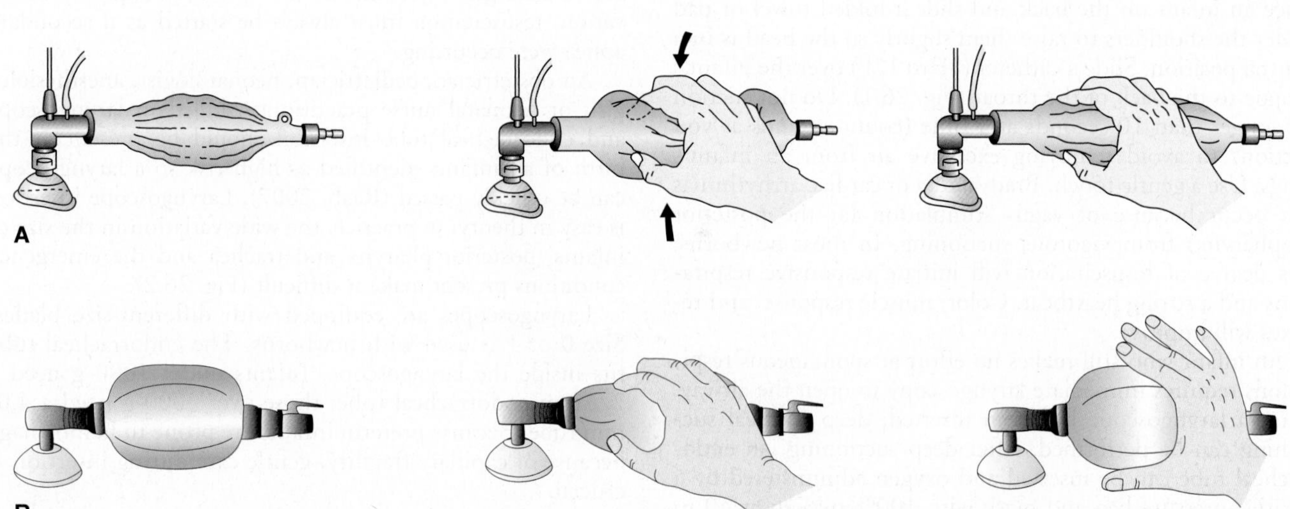

FIGURE 26.3 Types of ventilation bags used in neonatal resuscitation. (**A**) The flow-inflating (anesthesia) bag requires a compressed gas source for inflation but is able to deliver 100% oxygen. (**B**) The self-inflating (Ambu) bag remains inflated at all times and is not dependent on a compressed gas source. It is limited to delivering oxygen concentration of 40%, which may be inadequate for resuscitation at birth.

BOX 26.3 * Focus on Pharmacology

Naloxone (Narcan)

Classification: Naloxone is a pure narcotic antagonist.

Action: Administered parenterally to reverse the effects, such as respiratory depression, that may occur with opioid narcotic agents (Karch, 2009).

Pregnancy risk category: B

Dosage: Initially 0.01 mg/kg IV. Dosage may be repeated at 2- to 3-minute intervals.

Possible adverse effects: Hypertension, irritability, tachycardia

Nursing Implications

- Assess respiratory status carefully, including rate, depth, and character of respirations.
- Anticipate the need for repeat doses.
- Maintain a patent airway at all times.
- Have emergency resuscitation equipment readily available and prepare to resuscitate if necessary.

administration of a narcotic such as morphine or meperidine (Demerol) to the mother during labor. In these instances, a narcotic antagonist such as naloxone (Narcan) injected into an umbilical vessel or intramuscularly into a thigh will relieve the depression (Box 26.3). The dose of naloxone is determined by institutional policy but is usually 0.01 to 0.1 mg/kg body weight (Karch, 2009). If there is suspicion of maternal drug abuse, naloxone is used cautiously because it might cause acute withdrawal in the neonate. Other drug therapies in addition to naloxone are shown in Boxes 26.4 and 26.5.

BOX 26.5 * Focus on Pharmacology

Surfactant (Survanta)

Action: Surfactant restores naturally occurring lung surfactant to improve lung compliance.

Pregnancy risk category: X

Dosage: 4 mL/kg intratracheally; four doses in first 48 hours of life

Possible adverse effects: Transient bradycardia, rales

Nursing Implications

- Suction infant before administration.
- Assess infant's respiratory rate, rhythm, arterial blood gases, and color before administration.
- Ensure proper endotracheal tube placement before dosing.
- Change infant's position during administration to encourage drug to flow to both lungs.
- Assess infant's respiratory rate, color, and arterial blood gases after administration.
- Do not suction endotracheal tube for 1 hour after administration, to avoid removing drug.

Ventilation Maintenance

To allow a newborn to adjust to and maintain cardiovascular changes, effective ventilation (continued respirations) must be maintained. Healthy newborns accomplish this task on their own. All infants, especially those who had difficulty establishing respirations at birth, should be carefully observed in the next few hours to be certain respirations are maintained.

BOX 26.4 * Focus on Pharmacology

Drugs Used in Resuscitation

Drugs commonly used in newborn resuscitation include:

Atropine: Reduces bronchial secretions, keeping the airway clear during resuscitation. Reduces vagus nerve effects, relieving bradycardia.

Calcium chloride: Increases heart contractility.

Dopamine: Increases systemic blood perfusion by increasing blood pressure through beta-agonist action.

Epinephrine: Strengthens or initiates cardiac contractions; increases heart rate and blood pressure.

Lidocaine: Counteracts ventricular arrhythmias by decreasing automaticity of ventricular cells.

Sodium bicarbonate ($NaHCO_3$) or tromethamine: Corrects metabolic acidosis. **Caution:** Do not give these agents unless ventilation is adequate or acidosis can be increased by retained CO_2.

Many preterm infants have such respiratory distress at birth that they need continued therapy, including:

Surfactant: All preterm infants weighing less than 1500 g receive surfactant administered by endotracheal tube at birth (see Box 26.5). Some newborns need administration of additional surfactant to prevent symptoms of respiratory distress syndrome.

Nitric oxide: Nitric oxide is a potent vascular dilator. Because it dilates the capillaries next to alveoli, it reduces the pulmonary resistance and therefore increases oxygenation and lung function (Barrington & Finer, 2009).

Liquid ventilation: Liquid ventilation is the instillation of liquid fluorocarbon (Perflubron) into the lungs. It fills and clings to alveoli. Perflubron is not absorbed by the body but instead leaves the lungs by evaporation. Although studies in young infants are few in number, liquid ventilation has the potential to reduce lung disease (Davies & Sargent, 2009). It acts as an anti-inflammatory and reduces oxygen toxicity and perhaps infection because bacteria cannot live in the medium. Adverse effects may be pneumothorax and mucus plugging.

An increasing respiratory rate in a newborn is often the first sign of obstruction or respiratory compromise. If the respiratory rate is increased, undress the baby's chest and look for retractions (inward sucking of the anterior chest wall on inspiration). Retractions of this type reflect the difficulty the newborn is having in drawing in air (tugging so hard to inflate the lungs that the anterior chest muscles are drawn inward).

A newborn who is having difficulty with maintaining respirations should be placed under an infant warmer and have the weight of clothing removed from the chest. Keeping the infant warm is important to prevent acidosis. Positioning an infant on the back with the head of the mattress elevated approximately 15 degrees allows the abdominal contents to fall away from the diaphragm, offering additional breathing space.

If secretions are accumulating in the respiratory tract, they must be suctioned. If the newborn has an endotracheal tube in place, perform tracheal suctioning. "Bagging" an infant for a minute before suctioning can improve the infant's oxygen level and prevent it from dropping to dangerous levels during suctioning. Use pulse oximetry or transcutaneous oxygen monitoring to monitor oxygen level if available (see Chapter 40). The cause of the respiratory distress must be determined and appropriate interventions undertaken to correct the difficulty (see Chapter 40).

Establishing Extrauterine Circulation

Although establishing respirations is the usual priority at a high-risk infant's birth, lack of cardiac function may be present concurrently or may develop if respiratory function cannot be quickly initiated and maintained. If an infant has no audible heartbeat, or if the cardiac rate is below 80 beats per minute, closed-chest massage should be started. Hold an infant with fingers supporting the back and depress the sternum with two fingers (see Chapter 41). Depress the sternum approximately one third of its depth (1 or 2 cm) at a rate of 100 times per minute (AHA, 2008). Lung ventilation at a rate of 30 times per minute should be continued and interspersed with the cardiac massage at a ratio of 1:3.

Continue to monitor transcutaneous oxygen or pulse oximetry to evaluate respiratory function and cardiac efficiency. If the pressure and the rate of massage are adequate, it should be possible, in addition, to palpate a femoral pulse. If heart sounds are not resumed above 80 beats per minute after 30 seconds of combined positive-pressure ventilation and cardiac compressions, 0.1 to 0.3 mL/kg epinephrine (1:10,000) may be sprayed into the endotracheal tube to stimulate cardiac function (AHA, 2008). Newborns who have difficulty maintaining cardiac function need to be transferred to a transitional or high-risk nursery for continuous cardiac surveillance.

Maintaining Fluid and Electrolyte Balance

After an initial resuscitation attempt, hypoglycemia (decreased blood glucose) may result from the effort the newborn expended to begin breathing. Dehydration may result from increased insensible water loss from rapid respirations. Infants with hypoglycemia are treated initially with 10% dextrose in water to restore their blood glucose level. Fluids such as Ringer's lactate or 5% dextrose in water are commonly used to maintain fluid and electrolyte levels. Electrolytes (particularly sodium and potassium) and glucose are added as necessary, depending on electrolyte analysis.

The rate of fluid administration must be carefully monitored because a high fluid intake can lead to patent ductus arteriosus or heart failure. When using a radiant warmer, there is an increase in water loss from convection and radiation. A newborn on a warmer, therefore, will require more fluid than if he or she were placed in a double-walled incubator.

Dehydration may be monitored by urine output and urine specific gravity measures. An output less than 2 mL/kg/hr or a specific gravity greater than 1.015 to 1.020 suggests inadequate fluid intake. Elevated specific gravity may also be caused by inappropriate antidiuretic hormone secretion or kidney failure because of a primary illness.

If an infant has hypotension without hypovolemia, a vasopressor such as dopamine may be given to increase blood pressure and improve cell perfusion. If hypovolemia is present, the cause is usually fetal blood loss from a condition such as placenta previa (see Chapter 21) or twin-to-twin transfusion. With hypovolemia, typically tachypnea, pallor, tachycardia, decreased arterial blood pressure, decreased central venous pressure, and decreased tissue perfusion of peripheral tissue, with a progressively developing metabolic acidosis, will be present. The hematocrit may be normal for some time after acute blood loss because blood cells present are in proportion to plasma. Normal saline or Ringer's lactate may be administered to increase blood volume. Control the rate carefully to prevent heart failure, patent ductus arteriosus, or intracranial hemorrhage from fluid pressure overload.

✓ Checkpoint Question 26.1

Baby Atkins was given a drug at birth to reverse the effects of a narcotic given to his mother in labor. What drug is commonly used for this?

a. Sodium chloride
b. Morphine sulfate
c. Penicillin G
d. Naloxone (Narcan)

Regulating Temperature

All high-risk infants may have difficulty maintaining a normal temperature. This is because, in addition to stress from an illness or immaturity, the infant's body is often exposed during procedures such as resuscitation and blood drawing.

It is important to keep newborns in a neutral-temperature environment, one that is neither too hot nor too cold, as doing so places less demand on them to maintain a minimal metabolic rate necessary for effective body functioning. If the environment is too hot, they must decrease metabolism to cool their body. If it is too cold, they must increase metabolism to warm body cells. The increased metabolism required calls for increased oxygen; without this oxygen available, body cells become hypoxic. To save oxygen for essential body functions, vasoconstriction of blood vessels occurs. If this process continues for too long, pulmonary vessels become affected and pulmonary perfusion becomes decreased. An infant's PO_2 level falls and PCO_2 increases. The decreased PO_2 level may open fetal right-to-left shunts again. Surfactant production may halt, which may further interfere with lung function. To supply glucose to maintain increased metabolism, an infant begins anaerobic glycolysis, which pours acid into the bloodstream. An infant becomes acidotic, and with acidosis comes the increased risk of kernicterus (invasion of brain cells with unconjugated bilirubin) as more bilirubin-binding sites are lost and more bilirubin is free to pass out of the bloodstream into brain cells. In short, because of becoming chilled, heart action, breathing, and electrolytic balance are all affected.

To prevent a newborn from becoming chilled after birth, wipe an infant dry, cover the head with a cap, and place the baby immediately under a prewarmed radiant warmer or in a warmed incubator (Fig. 26.4) or skin-to-skin against the mother. Additional measures are the use of plastic wrap, plastic shields, or warmed mattresses. Air, incubator, or radiant warmer temperatures should be kept regulated to maintain an infant's axillary temperature at 97.8° F (36.5° C). Be certain that during procedures an infant is placed on a radiant heat warmer or a chemical warming pad, not placed directly on cool x-ray tables, scales, or an unheated radiant warmer to prevent heat loss (Box 26.6).

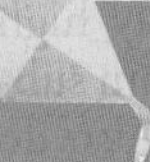

BOX 26.6 * Focus on Evidence-Based Practice

Does placing a cap on a low-birth-weight infant guard against hypothermia?

It is critical to guard against hypothermia in low-birth-weight infants because they are unable to increase their metabolism rate to warm themselves again. To investigate whether the simple act of covering the infant's head with a cap prevents enough evaporation and heat loss to prevent hypothermia, researchers reviewed six studies with a total of 304 infants comparing different methods of guarding against newborn cooling. Conclusions of this meta-analysis revealed that plastic wraps or bags, skin-to-skin care, and warmed mattresses all keep preterm infants warmer, leading to higher temperatures on admission to neonatal units. Stockinette caps alone do not provide this same protection.

Based on this study, at the birth of a low-birth-weight infant, would you omit a cap or use it in addition to other measures?

Source: McCall, E. M., et al. (2009). Interventions to prevent hypothermia at birth in preterm and/or low birth weight infants. *Cochrane Database of Systematic Reviews, 2009*(1), (CD004210).

Radiant Heat Sources

Radiant heat warmers are open beds that have an overhead radiant heat source. Such units have servocontrol probes, which when placed on an infant's skin continually monitor his or her temperature. Abdominal skin temperature, when measured this way, should be 95.9° to 97.7° F (35.5° to 36.5° C). If an infant's temperature falls below this level, an alarm will sound. Be certain to tape the probe or disk onto the infant's abdomen between the umbilicus and the xiphoid process. Do

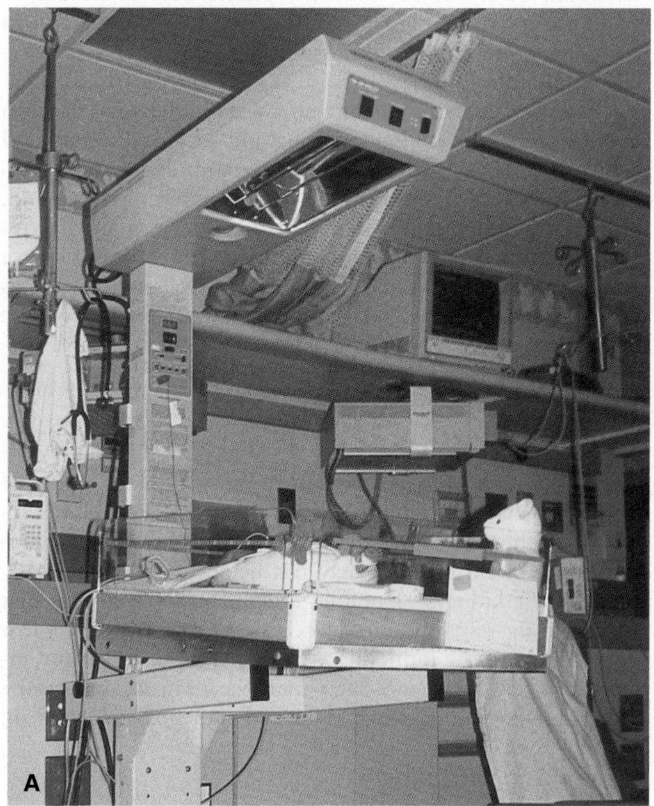

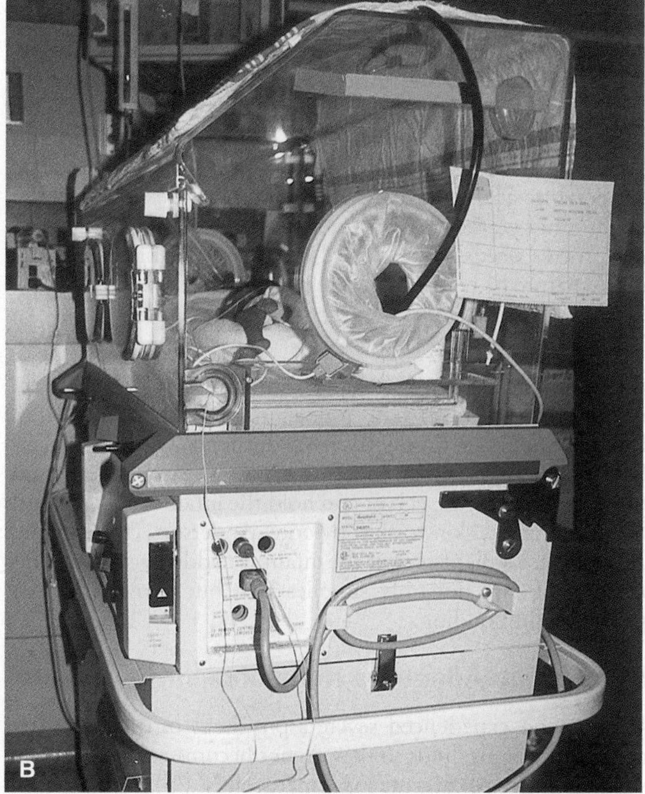

FIGURE 26.4 Neutral thermal environment. (**A**) A neonate in the intensive care bed with overhead radiant warmer can be examined periodically with ease. (**B**) Use of an incubator allows maintenance of a neutral thermal environment for neonates not requiring minute-to-minute intervention.

not tape it under an infant or it will register a falsely high reading. Be sure it is not over the rib cage, where the thin subcutaneous tissue will not allow an accurate reading. Also do not place it over the liver, because increased metabolism may lead to falsely high readings. A plastic bridge or shield placed over the child will better preserve heat by reducing convection and radiation losses; plastic wrap placed over an infant will produce this same effect. When performing care or leaning over an infant, be careful your head does not block the heat from an overhead source and keep it from reaching the baby. An additional warming pad placed under an infant may be necessary for very preterm infants or for lengthy procedures to maintain body heat.

Incubators

After an initial resuscitation attempt, newborns may be cared for in incubators. The temperature of incubators varies with the amount of time portholes remain open and the temperature of the area in which the incubator is placed. Placing it in direct sunlight or near a warm radiator can increase the internal temperature markedly. For this reason, a newborn's temperature must be checked at frequent intervals when in an incubator to be certain the temperature level designated is being maintained. Use of an additional acrylic shield inside the incubator helps prevent radiation and convection heat loss when portholes are opened for care.

Similar to radiant warmers, some incubators have servocontrol mechanism units that monitor the infant's temperature and automatically change the temperature of the incubator as needed. Portholes must remain closed to keep the servocontrol operating efficiently.

As infants' conditions improve, they can be weaned from an incubator. Dress the infant as if he or she were going to be in a bassinet, then set the incubator about 2° F (1.2° C) below the infant's temperature. After a half-hour, assess whether the infant is able to maintain body temperature. If so, lower the incubator temperature another 2° F and continue until room temperature is reached. If an infant cannot maintain adequate temperature as the incubator temperature level is lowered, the infant is not yet ready for room-temperature air, and the weaning process needs to be slowed or stopped until the baby is more mature or better able to self-regulate temperature.

Skin-to-Skin Care

Originally referred to as kangaroo care, skin-to-skin care is the use of skin-to-skin contact to maintain body heat. Provide a quiet setting with lights dimmed. Undress the infant except for a diaper and perhaps a cap. Assist the parent to sit comfortably in a chair and hold the infant snugly against his or her chest, skin to skin (Moore, Anderson, & Bergman, 2009). Place a blanket over the infant for added warmth. This method of care not only supplies heat but also encourages parent–child bonding.

Establishing Adequate Nutritional Intake

Infants who experienced severe asphyxia at birth usually receive intravenous fluids so they do not become exhausted from sucking or until necrotizing enterocolitis (NEC) has been ruled out, as this could result from the temporary reduction in oxygen to the bowel (see Chapter 45 for a discussion of NEC). If an infant's respiratory rate remains rapid and NEC has been ruled out, gavage feeding may be introduced (Fig. 26.5). Preterm infants should be breastfed if possible because of the immune protection this offers. If breastfeeding is not possible because the infant is too immature to suck effectively, a mother can manually express breast milk or use a breast pump to initiate and continue her milk supply until the time the infant is mature enough or otherwise ready for effective sucking. Her expressed breast milk can be used in the infant's gavage feeding (Jones & Spencer, 2007). Be sure when bottled breast milk is supplied by parents that it is well marked with the infant's name or breast milk errors can occur the same as medication errors (Drenckpohl, Bowers, & Cooper, 2007). It should be stored in nonshiny plastic bags or bottles to avoid the infant being exposed to polycarbonate, which can leech into stored milk and possibly cause chromosomal aberrations (Raloff, 2007).

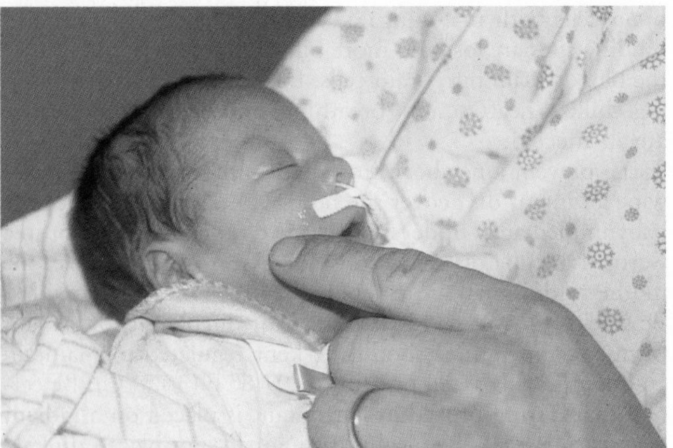

FIGURE 26.5 Infants who are ill at birth often need supplemental feedings by nasogastric or gastrostomy tube.

Preterm infants reveal hunger by the same signs as term infants, such as rooting and crying and sucking motions. All babies who are gavage fed and need oral stimulation from nonnutritive sucking seem to enjoy a pacifier at feeding times and, in immature infants, this may help them develop an effective sucking reflex. Exceptions are infants too immature to have a sucking reflex and infants who must not swallow air, such as those with a tracheoesophageal fistula awaiting surgery. The techniques of gavage feeding, intravenous feeding, and gastrostomy feeding are discussed in Chapter 37.

Establishing Waste Elimination

Although most immature infants void within 24 hours of birth, they may void later than term newborns because, as a result of all the procedures that may be necessary for resuscitation, their blood pressure may not be adequate to optimally supply their kidneys. Carefully document any voidings that occur during resuscitation. This is proof that hypotension is improving and the kidneys are being perfused. Immature infants also may pass stool later than the term infant because meconium has not yet reached the end of the intestine at birth.

Preventing Infection

Contracting an infection could drastically complicate a high-risk newborn's ability to adjust to extrauterine life. Infection, like chilling, increases metabolic oxygen demands, which the stressed newborn may not be able to meet. In addition, infection stresses the immature immune system and already stressed defense mechanisms of a high-risk newborn. Infections may have prenatal, perinatal, or postnatal causes. In some instances, such as preterm rupture of the membranes, it is an infection such as pneumonia or skin lesions that place the infant in a high-risk category (Herbst & Kallen, 2007).

Common viruses that affect infants in utero are cytomegalovirus and toxoplasmosis virus. An infant with either of these infections may be born with congenital anomalies from the virus invasion (see Chapter 12). The most prevalent perinatal infections are those contracted from the vagina during birth. Early-onset sepsis is most commonly caused by group B streptococcus, *E. coli, Kelbsiella*, and *Listeria monocytogenes*. Late-onset, or nosocomial, infections are more commonly caused by *Staphylococcus aureus, Enterobacter*, and *Candida*. These late-onset infections are probably most commonly spread to newborns from health care personnel. For this reason, all persons coming in contact with or caring for infants must observe good handwashing technique and standard precautions to reduce the risk of infection transmission. Health care personnel with infections have a professional and moral obligation to refrain from caring for newborns.

Establishing Parent–Infant Bonding

It is helpful if all women who are diagnosed as having a high-risk pregnancy are offered a tour of a neonatal intensive care unit (NICU) during pregnancy so if their infant should be admitted to a NICU, they will be more comfortable in the high-tech environment.

Be certain that the parents of a high-risk newborn are kept informed of what is happening during resuscitation at birth. They should be able to visit the special nursing unit to which the child is admitted as often as they choose, and, after washing and gowning, hold and touch their child. This helps to make the child's birth real to them. Should a child not survive an initial illness, these interactions can help make the death more real. Only when both birth and death seem real can parents begin to work through their feelings and accept these events.

All parents handle newborn babies tentatively until they have "claimed" them or have become better acquainted. It may be months before the parents of a child who has been ill since birth can handle their baby comfortably and confidently. Urge parents to spend time with their infant in the intensive care nursery as the infant improves. Be certain that parents have access to health care personnel after discharge to help them care confidently for the child at home.

If an infant dies despite newborn resuscitation attempts, parents need to see the infant without being covered by a myriad of equipment. This is a time for parents to reassure themselves their newborn was a perfect baby in every other way except lung function or whatever was the infant's fatal disorder. Thinking this way can give them confidence to plan for other children or simply to continue their lives after such a stressful experience.

Anticipating Developmental Needs

High-risk newborns need special care to ensure that the amount of pain they experience during procedures is limited to the least amount possible and that they receive adequate stimulation for growth. Most high-risk infants enjoy "catch-up" growth once they stabilize from the trauma of birth or whatever caused them to be classified as high risk. They quickly move to playing with age-appropriate toys. Some parents may need support before and after their infants are discharged home to begin to view them as well and capable of doing all the things they are now capable of doing. Anticipatory guidance helps them to be ready for the next developmental step.

Follow-up of High-Risk Infants at Home

Each time parents visit a high-risk nursery, assess their level of knowledge about their child's condition and development. Thorough education and referral to a home care agency may be necessary to help parents continue with the level of care that is required when their infant is discharged home (see Chapter 4). Before discharge, the safety of their home for the care of such a small infant needs to be evaluated. Transporting a preterm infant in a car requires special care, including a blanket or commercial head support, because a very small infant does not fit securely in a standard infant car seat.

Although not well documented regarding when or why it occurs, some preterm infants experience episodes of oxygen desaturation, apnea, or bradycardia when seated in standard car safety seats (DeGrazia, 2007). To detect if this will occur, the American Academy of Pediatrics (AAP, 2009) recommends that all preterm infants be assessed for cardiorespiratory stability in their car seat prior to discharge—the "car seat challenge."

High-Risk Infants and Child Abuse

When a child is ill or born preterm, the expected reaction of the parents would be to protect the child even more than the average child so no further harm can result. In reality, particularly in reference to preterm children, the opposite may occur. Preterm children are at high risk for abuse (Sirotnak & Krugman, 2008). This is probably because of the separation of the child from the family at birth, which interferes with bonding. Child abuse is discussed in Chapter 55.

What if... Mrs. Atkins is about to visit her preterm newborn for the first time and states, "I'm so scared. He's so tiny and frail. How can I even hold him?" How should you respond to this new mother to make her visit easier?

THE NEWBORN AT RISK BECAUSE OF ALTERED GESTATIONAL AGE OR BIRTH WEIGHT

Infants need to be evaluated as soon as possible after birth to determine their weight and gestational age as classification by growth charts and gestational history is important to determine immediate health care needs and to help anticipate possible problems. Birth weight is normally plotted on a growth chart such as the Colorado (Lubchenco) Intrauterine Growth Chart (see Appendix E). Infants born after the beginning of week 38 and before week 42 of pregnancy (calculated from the first day of the last menstrual period) are classified as *term infants*. Approximately 90% of all live births are term. Infants born before term (less than the full 37th week of pregnancy) account for approximately 7% to 19% of all births and are classified as **preterm infants,** regardless of their birth weight. Infants born after the onset of week 43 of pregnancy are classified as postterm, dysmature, or postmature (Fortner, Althaus, & Gurewitsch, 2007).

Normally, birth weight varies for each gestational week of age. Infants who fall between the 10th and 90th percentiles of weight for their age regardless of gestational age are considered **appropriate for gestational age (AGA).** Infants who fall below the 10th percentile of weight for their age are considered **small for gestational age (SGA).** Those who fall above the 90th percentile in weight are considered **large for gestational age (LGA).** Infants weighing under 2500 g are **low-birth-weight infants.** Those weighing 1000 to 1500 g are *very-low-birth-weight infants* (VLB). Those born weighing 500 to 1000 g are considered *extremely very-low-birth-weight infants* (EVLB). Preterm infants may be AGA, SGA, LGA, low birth weight, VLB, or EVLB.

All such infants have immediate needs that are different from or more pronounced than the needs of term newborns. Each of these categories carries its own set of potential risks.

The Small-for-Gestational-Age Infant

An infant is SGA if the birth weight is below the 10th percentile on an intrauterine growth curve for that age. SGA infants may be born preterm (before week 38 of gestation), term (between weeks 38 and 42), or postterm (past 42 weeks). SGA infants are small for their age because they have experienced **intrauterine growth restriction (IUGR)** or failed to grow at the expected rate in utero (Rahimian & Varner, 2007). This characteristic makes them distinctly different from infants whose weight is low but who are average for gestational age.

Etiology

A woman's nutrition during pregnancy plays a major role in fetal growth, so lack of adequate nutrition may be a major contributor to IUGR. Pregnant adolescents have a high incidence of SGA infants. Because adolescents must meet their own nutritional and growth needs, needs of a growing fetus can be compromised. However, the most common cause of IUGR is a placental anomaly: either the placenta did not obtain sufficient nutrients from the uterine arteries or it was inefficient at transporting nutrients to the fetus. Placental damage, such as partial placental separation with bleeding, limits placental function because the area of placenta that separated becomes infarcted and fibrosed, reducing the placental surface available for nutrient exchange. A developmental defect in the placenta can also prevent it from functioning properly. Women with systemic diseases that decrease blood flow to the placenta, such as severe diabetes mellitus or pregnancy-induced hypertension (both are diseases in which blood vessel lumens are narrowed), are at higher risk for delivering SGA babies than others. Women who smoke heavily or use narcotics also tend to have SGA infants (Rahimian & Varner, 2007).

In other instances, the placental supply of nutrients is adequate but an infant cannot use them because the infant has contracted an intrauterine infection such as rubella or toxoplasmosis or has a chromosomal abnormality.

Assessment

The SGA infant may be detected in utero when fundal height during pregnancy becomes progressively less than expected. However, if a woman is unsure of the date of her last menstrual period, this discrepancy can be hard to substantiate. A sonogram can then demonstrate the decreased size. A biophysical profile including a nonstress test, placental grading, amniotic fluid amount, and ultrasound examination can provide additional information on placental function. If poor placental function is apparent from such determinations, it can be predicted the infant will do poorly during labor because of periods of relative hypoxia during contractions may result. Cesarean birth is the birth method of choice in such circumstances.

Appearance. Generally, an infant who suffers nutritional deprivation early in pregnancy, when fetal growth consists primarily of an increase in the number of body cells, is below average in weight, length, and head circumference. An infant who suffers deprivation late in pregnancy, when growth consists primarily of an increase in cell size, may have only a reduction in weight. Regardless of when deprivation occurs, an infant tends to have an overall wasted appearance. The child may have a small liver, which can cause difficulty regulating glucose, protein, and bilirubin levels after birth. The infant also may have poor skin turgor and generally appear to have a large head because the rest of the body is so small. Skull sutures may be widely separated from lack of normal bone growth. Hair is dull and lusterless. The abdomen may be sunken. The umbilical cord often appears dry and may be stained yellow.

In contrast, because an infant's age is more advanced than the weight implies, a child may have better-developed neurologic responses, sole creases, and ear cartilage than expected for a baby of that weight. The skull may be firmer, and the infant may seem unusually alert and active for that weight. The SGA infant needs careful assessment for possible congenital anomalies occurring as a result of the poor nutritional intrauterine environment.

Laboratory Findings. Blood studies at birth usually show a high hematocrit level (less than normal amounts of plasma in proportion to red blood cells are present because of a lack of fluid in utero) and an increase in the total number of red blood cells (polycythemia). The increase in red blood cells occurs because anoxia during intrauterine life stimulates the development of red blood cells. The polycythemia that results causes increased blood viscosity, a condition that puts extra work on the infant's heart because it is more difficult to effectively circulate thick blood. As a consequence, acrocyanosis (blueness of the hands and feet) may be prolonged and persistently more marked than usual. If the polycythemia is extreme, vessels may actually become blocked and thrombus formation can result. If the hematocrit level is more than 65% to 70%, an exchange transfusion to dilute the blood may be necessary.

Because SGA infants have decreased glycogen stores, one of the most common problems is hypoglycemia (decreased blood glucose, or a level below 45 mg/dL). Such infants may need intravenous glucose to sustain blood sugar until they are able to suck vigorously enough to take sufficient oral feedings.

Nursing Diagnoses and Related Interventions

*

Nursing Diagnosis: Ineffective breathing pattern related to underdeveloped body systems at birth

Outcome Evaluation: Newborn maintains respirations at a rate of 30 to 60 breaths per minute after resuscitation at birth.

Birth asphyxia is a common problem for SGA infants, both because they have underdeveloped chest muscles and because they are at risk for developing meconium aspiration syndrome as a result of anoxia during labor. Fetal hypoxia causes a reflex relaxation of the anal sphincter and increased intestinal movement. When gasping for breath in utero, the fetus draws meconium that was discharged from the intestine into the amniotic fluid down into the trachea and bronchi. Acting as a foreign substance, this blocks airflow into the alveoli, leading to hypoxemia, acidosis, and hypercapnia. For this reason, many SGA infants require resuscitation at birth. Closely observe both respiratory rate and character in the first few hours of life. Underdeveloped chest muscles can make SGA infants unable to sustain the rapid respiratory rate of a normal newborn.

Nursing Diagnosis: Risk for ineffective thermoregulation related to lack of subcutaneous fat

Outcome Evaluation: Infant's temperature is maintained at 36.5° C (97.8° F) axillary.

SGA infants are less able to control body temperature than other newborns because they lack subcutaneous fat. A carefully controlled environment is essential to keep the infant's body temperature in a neutral zone (see Chapter 18).

Nursing Diagnosis: Risk for impaired parenting related to child's high-risk status and possible cognitive or neurologic impairment from lack of nutrients in utero

Outcome Evaluation: Parents express interest in infant and ask questions about what the child's care needs will be at home.

Although SGA infants may gain weight and appear to thrive in the first few days of life, their cognitive development may have been impaired because of lack of oxygen and nourishment in utero. Babies who were growing normally in utero but whose gestation was interrupted preterm (true preterm babies) usually gain weight and height so rapidly that by the end of the first year of life they are near the 50th percentile on growth charts. SGA infants, in contrast, may always be below usual on standard growth charts. This inability to reach normal levels of growth and development may interfere with bonding because a child does not meet the parents' expectations. Eventually, it can interfere with the child's self-esteem if the child is never able to meet parental expectations or reach full height.

An SGA infant needs adequate stimulation during the infant period to reach normal growth and developmental milestones. Encourage parents to provide toys suitable for their child's chronologic age, not physical size. Because an infant tires easily in the first few weeks of life, urge them to space play periods with rest periods or hypoglycemia or apnea can occur. All infants with IUGR need continued follow-up after hospital discharge as they may have neurologic deficits that will interfere with learning at school age (Leitner et al., 2007).

✔ Checkpoint Question 26.2

Why are small-for-gestational-age newborns at risk for difficulty maintaining body temperature?

a. They are preterm so they are born relatively small in size.
b. They are more active than usual so they throw off covers.
c. They do not have as much fat stores as do other infants.
d. Their skin is more susceptible to conduction of cold.

The Large-for-Gestational-Age Infant

An infant is LGA (also termed **macrosomia**) if the birth weight is above the 90th percentile on an intrauterine growth chart for that gestational age. Such a baby appears deceptively healthy at birth because of the weight, but a gestational age examination will reveal immature development. It is important that LGA infants be identified immediately so that they can be given care appropriate to their gestational age rather than being treated as term newborns (Lawrence, 2007).

Etiology

Infants who are LGA have been subjected to an overproduction of growth hormone in utero. This happens most often to infants of women with diabetes mellitus or women who are obese (Strehlow et al., 2007). Extreme macrosomia occurs in fetuses of diabetic women whose symptoms are poorly controlled, because these fetuses are exposed to high glucose levels. Multiparous women are also prone to have large babies because with each succeeding pregnancy, babies tend to grow larger. Other conditions associated with LGA infants include transposition of the great vessels, Beckwith syndrome (a rare condition characterized by overgrowth), and congenital anomalies such as omphalocele.

Assessment

A fetus is suspected of being LGA when a woman's uterus is unusually large for the date of pregnancy. Abdominal size can be deceptive, however—because a fetus lies in a flexed fetal position, he or she does not occupy significantly more space at 10 lb than at 7 lb. If a fetus does seem to be growing at an abnormally rapid rate, a sonogram can confirm the suspicion. A nonstress test to assess the placenta's ability to sustain a large fetus during labor may be performed. To see if an LGA fetus is mature, lung maturity may be assessed by amniocentesis.

If an infant's large size was not detected during pregnancy, it may be first recognized during labor when the baby cannot descend through the pelvic rim. If this happens, cesarean birth may be necessary to avoid **shoulder dystocia** (the wide fetal shoulders cannot pass through the outlet of the pelvis).

Appearance. At birth, LGA infants may show immature reflexes and low scores on gestational age examinations in relation to their size. They may have extensive bruising or a birth injury such as a broken clavicle or Erb-Duchenne paralysis from trauma to the cervical nerves if they were born vaginally (see Chapter 51). Because the head is large, it may have been exposed to more than the usual amount of pressure during birth, causing a prominent caput succedaneum, cephalhematoma, or molding.

An LGA newborn requires the same cautious care necessary for a preterm infant. Specific criteria for initial or continuing assessment are shown in Table 26.1.

Cardiovascular Dysfunction. Observe LGA infants closely for signs of hyperbilirubinemia (increased serum bilirubin level), which may result from absorption of blood from bruising and polycythemia. Polycythemia has been caused by an infant's system attempting to fully oxygenate all body tissues. This effort puts extra stress on the heart, so the heart rate of LGA infants should be carefully observed. If cyanosis is present, it may be a sign of transposition of the great vessels, a serious heart anomaly associated with macrosomia (see Chapter 41).

Hypoglycemia. LGA infants also need to be carefully assessed for hypoglycemia in the early hours of life because infants require large amounts of nutritional stores to sustain their weight. If the mother had diabetes that was poorly controlled, the infant will have had an increased blood glucose level in utero causing the infant to produce elevated levels of insulin. After birth, these increased insulin levels will continue for up to 24 hours of life, possibly causing rebound hypoglycemia.

Nursing Diagnoses and Related Interventions

Nursing Diagnosis: Ineffective breathing pattern related to possible birth trauma in LGA newborn

Outcome Evaluation: Newborn initiates breathing at birth; maintains normal newborn respiratory rate of 30 to 60 breaths per minute.

Some LGA infants have difficulty establishing respirations at birth because of birth trauma. Increased intracranial pressure from birth of the larger-than-usual head could have led to pressure on the respiratory center. This, in turn, can cause a decrease in respiratory function. A diaphragmatic paralysis may occur because of cervical nerve trauma as the head is bent sideways to allow for birth of the large shoulders. This prevents active lung motion on the affected side. If an infant was born by cesarean birth, transient fluid can remain in the lungs and interfere with effective gas exchange. Careful observation is needed to detect these conditions. Care of an infant with transient lung fluid is discussed later in this chapter.

Nursing Diagnosis: Risk for imbalanced nutrition, less than body requirements, related to additional nutrients needed to maintain weight and prevent hypoglycemia

Outcome Evaluation: Infant's weight follows percentile growth curve; skin turgor is good; specific gravity of urine is 1.003 to 1.030; serum glucose is above 45 mg/dL.

As a rule, an LGA infant needs to be breastfed immediately to prevent hypoglycemia. The infant may need supplemental formula feedings after breastfeeding to supply enough fluid and glucose for the larger-than-normal size for the first few days. Newborns who are offered bottles often have more difficulty than do others learning to breastfeed. Offer both the mother and baby support to overcome this hurdle.

Do not overestimate LGA infants' ability to suck effectively at birth. Such infants may seem as if they should be able to suck well because they are already the size of a 2-month-old. However, the infant is an inexperienced newborn, so sucking may not be effective enough to obtain the larger-than-usual amount of milk needed.

Nursing Diagnosis: Risk for impaired parenting related to high-risk status of large-for-gestational-age infant

TABLE 26.1 ✻ Important Assessment Criteria for a Large-for-Gestational-Age Infant

Assessment	Rationale
Skin color for ecchymosis, jaundice, and erythema	Bruising occurs with vaginal birth; jaundice may occur from breakdown of ecchymotic collections of blood; polycythemia causes ruddiness of skin.
Motion of extremities on spontaneous movement and in response to a Moro's reflex to detect clavicle fracture (crepitus or swelling may then be palpated at the fracture site) or Erb's palsy because of edema of the cervical nerve plexus	Clavicle or cervical nerve injuries may occur because of problem at birth of wider-than-normal shoulders.
Asymmetry of the anterior chest or unilateral lack of movement to detect diaphragmatic paralysis from edema of the phrenic nerve	This cervical nerve may be stretched by birth of wide shoulders.
Eyes for evidence of unresponsive or dilated pupils; vomiting, bulging fontanelles, and a high-pitched cry suggestive of increased intracranial pressure	Compression of third, fourth, and sixth cranial nerves by increased pressure limits eye response; other signs of increased intracranial pressure may occur.
Activities such as jitteriness, lethargy, and uncoordinated eye movements that suggest seizure activity	Seizures may be caused by increased intracranial pressure; hypoglycemia seizures in newborns often produce only vague symptoms.

Outcome Evaluation: Parents hold infant; speak of the child in positive terms; state accurately why their infant needs to be closely observed in postnatal period.

Parents may underestimate this infant's needs because of the child's large size. He or she seems so big and healthy; parents may be confused about why their infant needs careful watching. They may read more into the child's condition than is present (he or she must be sick in some way they are not being told about), and so bonding does not happen as instinctively as it might. If a woman sustained a cervical or perineal tear or required a cesarean birth, she may need some time to air any resentment she may feel toward the infant for causing her extra pain. Otherwise, her perception that her infant is the cause of her additional distress may interfere with her ability to bond with the child.

An LGA infant needs the same developmental care as all infants. Singing or talking to the baby, stroking the child's back, and rocking the baby are all important for the large infant's development. Encourage parents to treat their baby as a fragile newborn who needs warm nurturing of this type, not as a tough big infant who has grown past that stage. Also remind parents an infant's birth weight is not a correlation of the child's projected adult size. Otherwise, parents may fear their infant may grow to be a larger-than-usual adult.

A Preterm Infant

A preterm infant is traditionally defined as a live-born infant born before the end of week 37 of gestation; another criterion used is a weight of less than 2500 g (5 lb 8 oz) at birth. Preterm birth occurs in approximately 7% of live births of white infants. In African American infants, the rate is doubled to approximately 14% (Thilo & Rosenberg, 2008). When a preterm infant is recognized by a gestational age assessment, observe closely for the specific problems of prematurity, such as respiratory distress syndrome, hypoglycemia, and intracranial hemorrhage.

All preterm infants need intensive care from the moment of birth to give them their best chance of survival without neurologic after-effects. A lack of lung surfactant makes them extremely vulnerable to respiratory distress syndrome (Thilo & Rosenberg, 2008).

The maturity of a newborn is determined by physical findings such as sole creases, skull firmness, ear cartilage, and neurologic findings that reveal gestational age, as well as the mother's report of the date of her last menstrual period and sonographic estimations of gestational age.

Preterm babies, regardless of their weight, need to be differentiated at birth from SGA babies (who also may have a low birth weight). The two conditions result from different situations and therefore will cause different problems in adjustment to extrauterine life. A preterm infant is immature and small but well proportioned for age. Unlike the SGA infant, this baby appears to have been doing well in utero. For an unexplained reason, however, the trigger that initiates labor was activated too early and birth resulted, even though the baby is immature. Preterm infants are invariably low-birth-weight infants. Characteristics of SGA and preterm infants are compared in Table 26.2.

Etiology

Preterm infant deaths account for 80% to 90% of infant mortality in the first year of life (NVSS, 2009). Infant mortality could be reduced dramatically if the causes of preterm birth could be discovered and corrected and all pregnancies brought to term. However, the exact cause of premature labor and early birth is rarely known.

There is a high correlation between low socioeconomic level and early termination of pregnancy. In women from middle and upper socioeconomic groups, only 4% to 8% of pregnancies are terminated early. However, in women from low socioeconomic levels, as many as 10% to 20% end before term. The major influencing factor in these instances appears to be inadequate nutrition before and during pregnancy, as a result of either lack of money for or lack of knowledge about good nutrition. Additional factors that seem to be related to preterm birth are shown in Box 26.7. Iatrogenic (health care–caused) issues, such as elective cesarean birth and inducing labor according to dates rather

TABLE 26.2 ✻ Differences Between Small-for-Gestational-Age and Preterm Infants

Characteristic	Small-for-Gestational-Age Infant	Preterm Infant
Gestational age	24–44 wk	<37 wk
Birth weight	<10th percentile	Normal for age
Congenital malformations	Strong possibility	Possibility
Pulmonary problems	Meconium aspiration, pulmonary hemorrhage, pneumothorax	Respiratory distress syndrome
Hyperbilirubinemia	Possibility	Very strong possibility
Hypoglycemia	Very strong possibility	Possibility
Intracranial hemorrhage	Strong possibility	Possibility
Apnea episodes	Possibility	Very strong possibility
Feeding problems	Most likely because of accompanying problem such as hypoglycemia	Small stomach capacity; immature sucking reflex
Weight gain in nursery	Rapid	Slow
Future restricted growth	Possibly always be <10th percentile because of poor organ development	Not likely to be restricted in growth as "catch-up" growth occurs

BOX 26.7 ✻ Common Factors Associated With Preterm Birth

- Low socioeconomic level
- Poor nutritional status
- Lack of prenatal care
- Multiple pregnancy
- Previous early birth
- Race (nonwhites have a higher incidence of prematurity than whites)
- Cigarette smoking
- Age of the mother (highest incidence is in mothers younger than age 20)
- Order of birth (early termination is highest in first pregnancies and in those beyond the fourth pregnancy)
- Closely spaced pregnancies
- Abnormalities of the mother's reproductive system, such as intrauterine septum
- Infections (especially urinary tract infection)
- Obstetric complications, such as premature rupture of membranes or premature separation of the placenta
- Early induction of labor
- Elective cesarean birth

than fetal maturity, also result in preterm births. Testing fetal maturity by amniocentesis or ultrasound is used to avoid these problems. The increasing use of assisted fertility methods such as in vitro fertilization that results in multiple births leads to an increased preterm rate as more multiple pregnancies result in preterm birth than term pregnancies (Goldenberg et al., 2008).

Assessment

Although a detailed pregnancy history may sometimes reveal the reason for a preterm birth, the pregnancy history is often normal up to the beginning of labor.

When interviewing parents of a preterm infant, be careful not to convey disapproval of reported pregnancy behaviors such as cigarette smoking or working a 12-hour shift that may have contributed to preterm birth. Once an infant is born, a new mother needs a high level of self-esteem and all of her inner resources to sustain her through the crisis. Being overburdened by guilt may be detrimental to her attempts to bond with her infant. A good answer to her direct inquiries about causes is, "No one really knows what causes prematurity." Teaching about better pregnancy practices can wait until she is ready for a second pregnancy.

In many instances, preterm labor might have been halted had a woman been able to recognize she was in true labor and not having Braxton Hicks contractions. In a first labor, this can easily occur because a woman does not know how true labor feels. Television shows often depict women in labor as having agonizingly painful contractions or the opposite, simply announcing, "This is it," and then proceeding to give birth within the 30-minute show. In reality, a first-time

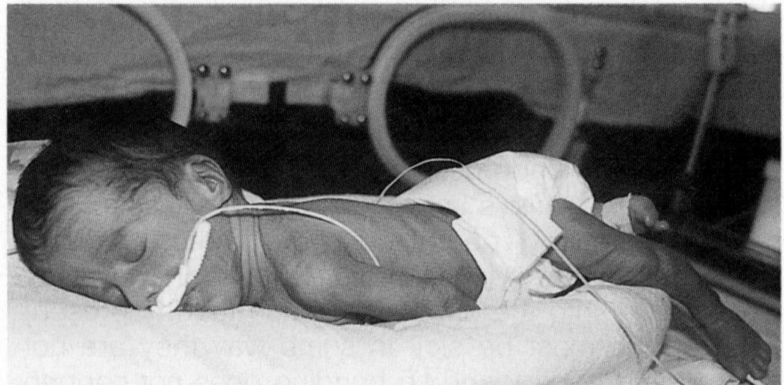

FIGURE 26.6 An immature infant. Notice the lax position of limbs because of immature muscle development.

mother does not realize that labor usually begins with subtle signs and mild contractions, not with a dramatic announcement. With preterm labor, often a woman reports that she thought she was having intestinal cramps. Because each labor proceeds differently, even a multipara may miss the signs of early labor until it is too far advanced to be reversed. Reassure a woman it is understandable she did not realize what was happening until cervical dilatation had occurred and labor could not be reversed.

On gross inspection, a preterm infant appears small and underdeveloped (Fig. 26.6). The head is disproportionately large (≥3 cm greater than chest size). The skin is generally unusually ruddy because there is little subcutaneous fat beneath it; veins are easily noticeable, and a high degree of acrocyanosis may be present. The preterm neonate, 24 to 36 weeks, typically is covered with vernix caseosa. However, in very preterm newborns (less than 25 weeks' gestation), vernix is absent because it is not formed this early in pregnancy. Lanugo is usually extensive, covering the back, forearms, forehead, and sides of the face, because this amount is present until late in pregnancy. Both anterior and posterior fontanelles are small. There are few or no creases on the soles of the feet.

Physical findings and reflex testing are used to differentiate between term and preterm newborns (Fig. 26.7). The eyes of most preterm infants appear small. Although difficult to elicit, pupillary reaction is present. Ophthalmoscopic examination is extremely difficult and often uninformative because the vitreous humor may be hazy. A preterm infant has varying degrees of myopia (nearsightedness) because of lack of eye globe depth.

The ears appear large in relation to the head. The cartilage of the ear is immature and allows the pinna to fall forward. The level of the ears should be carefully inspected to rule out chromosomal abnormalities (see Chapter 7).

Neurologic function in the preterm infant is often difficult to evaluate as the neurologic system is still so immature. The observation of spontaneous or provoked movements may yield findings as important as reflex testing. If tested, reflexes such as sucking and swallowing will be absent if an infant's age is below 33 weeks; deep tendon reflexes such as the Achilles tendon reflex are also markedly diminished. During an examination, a preterm infant is much less active than a mature infant and rarely cries. If the infant does cry, the cry is weak and high-pitched.

Laboratory values for a preterm infant are compared with those of the term infant in Appendix F.

Potential Complications

Because of immaturity, preterm infants are prone to several specific conditions.

Anemia of Prematurity. Many preterm infants develop a normochromic, normocytic anemia (normal cells, just few in number). The reticulocyte count is low because the bone marrow does not increase its production until approximately 32 weeks. The infant will appear pale and may be lethargic and anorectic. The fault appears to be immaturity of the hematopoietic system combined with destruction of red blood cells because of low levels of vitamin E, which normally protects red blood cells against oxidation. Excessive blood drawing for electrolyte or blood gas analysis can potentiate the problem. For this reason, keep a record of the amount of blood drawn for analysis.

Red blood cell production can be stimulated by the administration of DNA recombinant erythropoietin. In addition, an infant may need blood transfusions to supply needed red blood cells and vitamin E and iron, which can be supplemented (Thilo & Rosenberg, 2008).

Kernicterus. Kernicterus is destruction of brain cells by invasion of indirect bilirubin (Symons & Mahoney, 2008). This invasion results from the high concentrations of indirect bilirubin in the blood from excessive breakdown of red blood cells. Preterm infants are more prone to the condition than term infants because with the acidosis that occurs from poor respiratory exchange, brain cells are more susceptible to the effect of indirect bilirubin than usually. Preterm infants also have less serum albumin available to bind indirect bilirubin and inactivate its effect. Because of this, kernicterus may occur at lower levels (as low as

A

Premature Infant

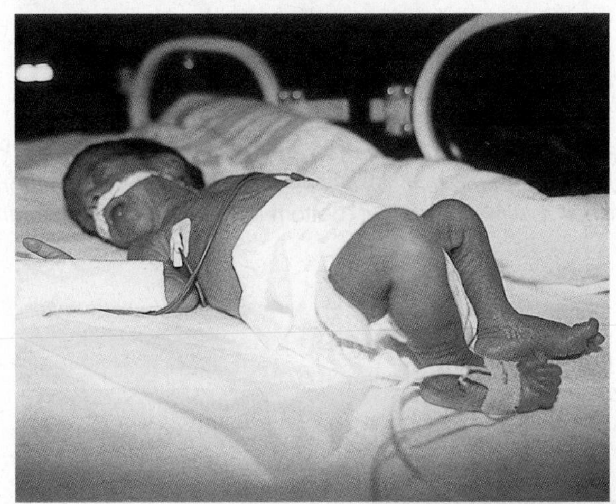

Full-term Infant

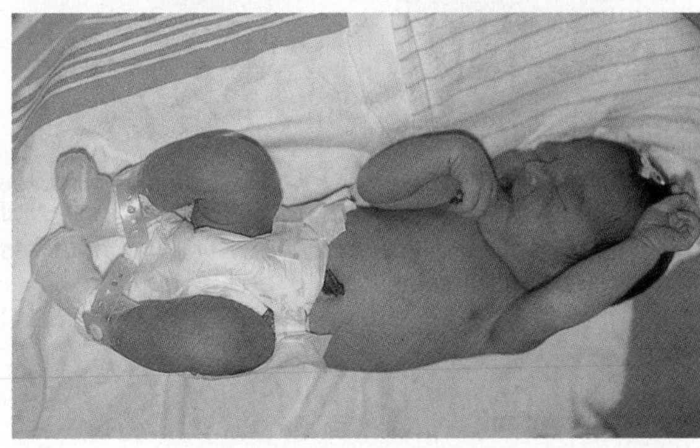

RESTING POSTURE *The premature infant is characterized by very little, if any, flexion in the upper extremities and only partial flexion of the lower extremities. The full-term infant exhibits flexion in all four extremities.*

B

Premature Infant, 28–32 Weeks

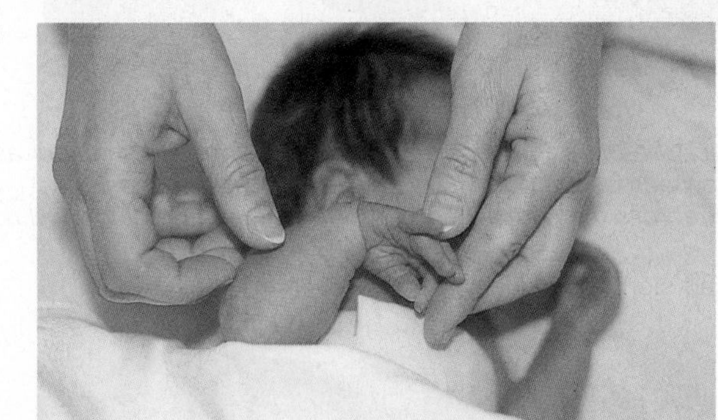

Full-term Infant

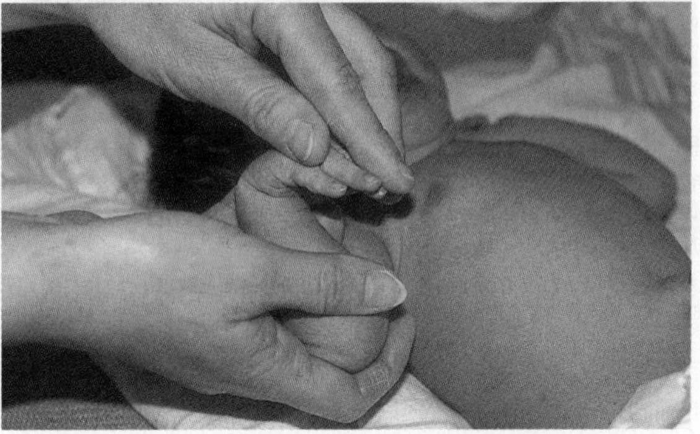

WRIST FLEXION *The wrist is flexed, applying enough pressure to get the hand as close to the forearm as possible. The angle between the hypothenar eminence and the ventral aspect of the forearm is measured. (Care must be taken not to rotate an infant's wrist.) The premature infant at 28–32 weeks' gestation will exhibit a 90-degree angle. With the full-term infant it is possible to flex the hand onto the arm.*

FIGURE 26.7 Examples of physical examination findings and reflex tests used to judge gestational age. (**A**) Resting posture. (**B**) Wrist flexion. *(continued)*

C

Premature Infant

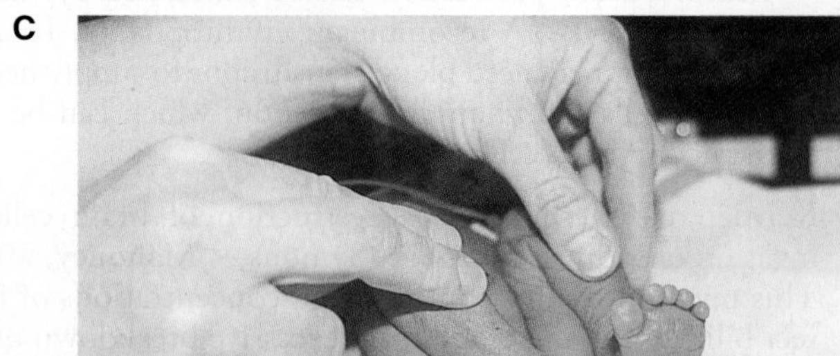

Full-term Infant

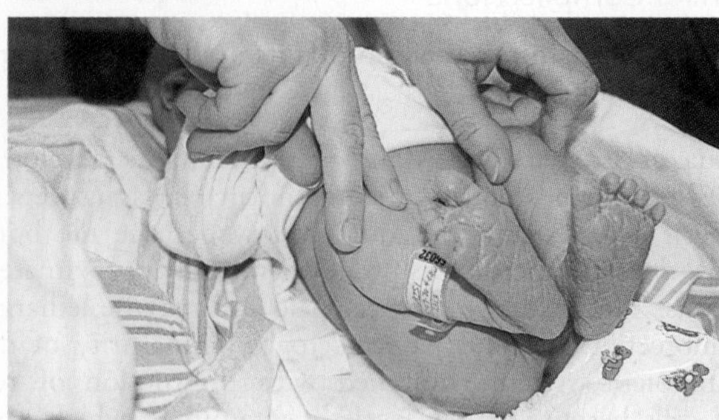

Response in Premature Infant

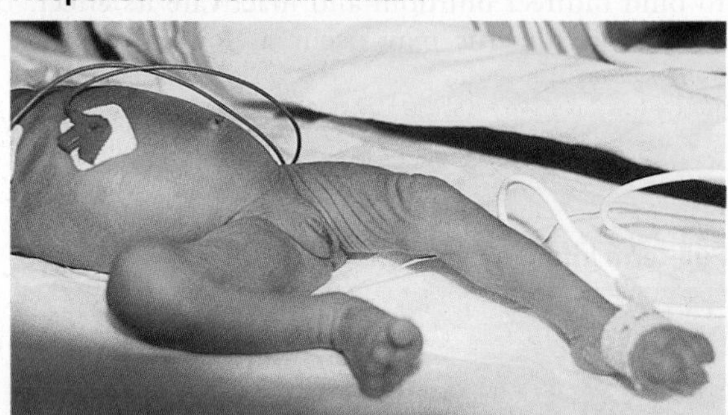

Response in Full-term Infant

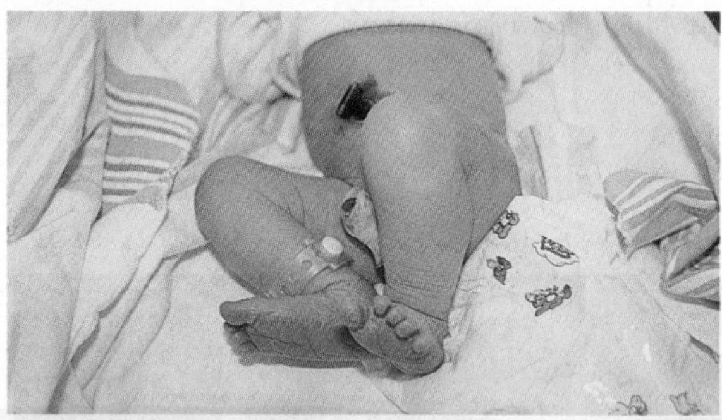

RECOIL OF EXTREMITIES *Place an infant supine. To test recoil of the legs (1) flex the legs and knees fully and hold for 5 seconds (shown in top photographs), (2) extend the legs fully by pulling on the feet, (3) release. To test the arms, flex forearms and follow same procedure. In the premature infant response is minimal or absent* (bottom left); *in the full-term infant extremities return briskly to full flexion* (bottom right).

D

Premature Infant

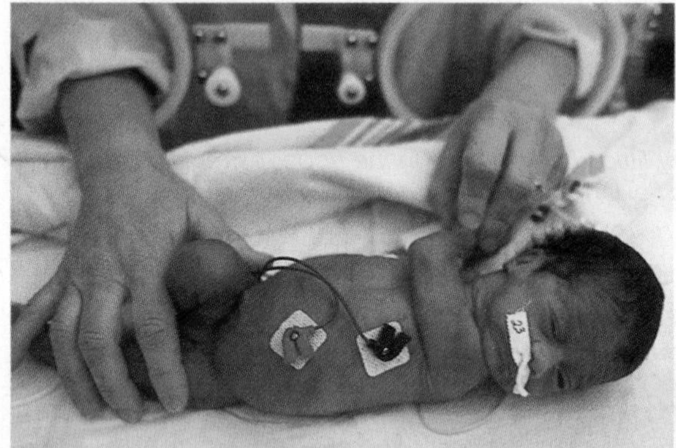

Full-term Infant

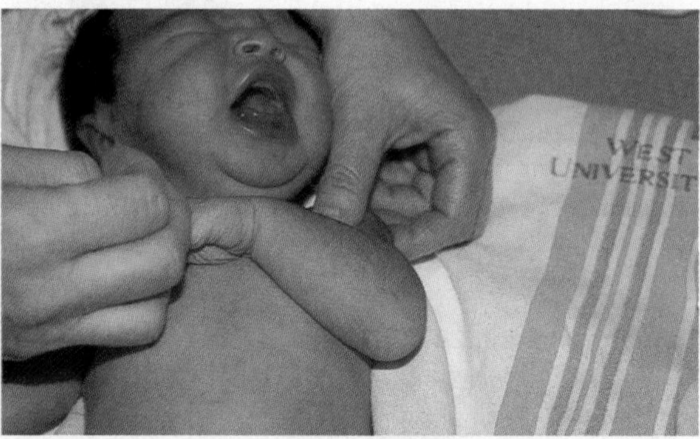

SCARF SIGN *Hold the baby supine, take the hand, and try to place it around the neck and above the opposite shoulder as far posteriorly as possible. Assist this maneuver by lifting the elbow across the body. See how far across the chest the elbow will go. In the premature infant the elbow will reach near or across the midline. In the full-term infant the elbow will not reach the midline.*

FIGURE 26.7 *(continued)* (**C**) Recoil of extremities (legs). (**D**) Scarf sign. *(continued)*

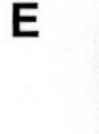

Premature Infant

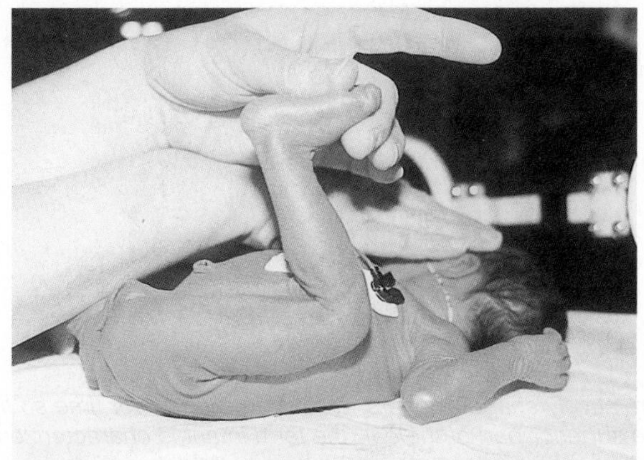

Full-term Infant

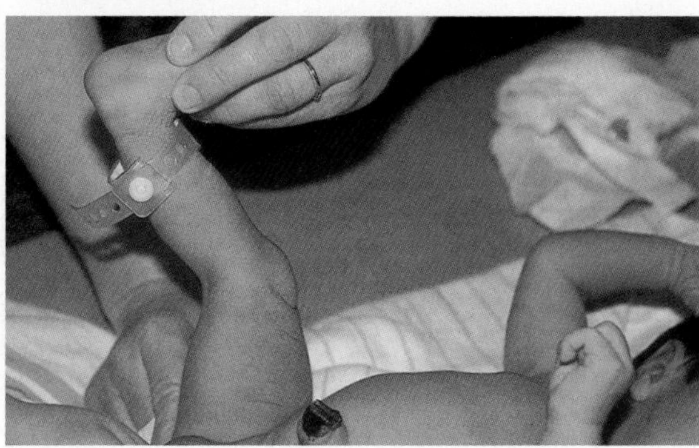

HEEL TO EAR *With the baby supine and the hips positioned flat on the bed, draw the baby's foot as near to the ear as it will go without forcing it. Observe the distance between the foot and head as well as the degree of extension at the knee. In the premature infant very little resistance will be met. In the full-term infant there will be marked resistance; it will be impossible to draw the baby's foot to the ear.*

Premature Infant

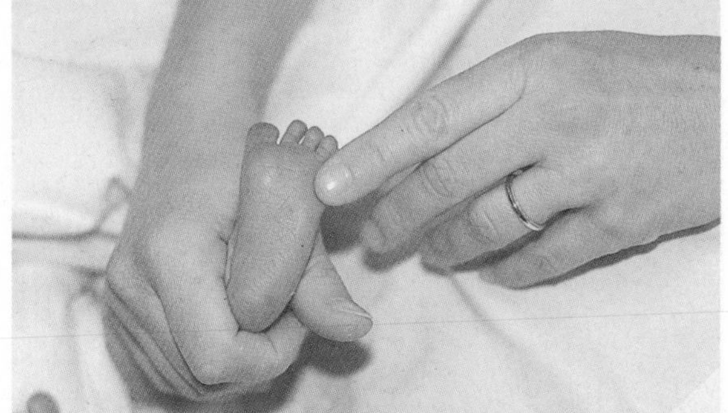

Full-term Infant

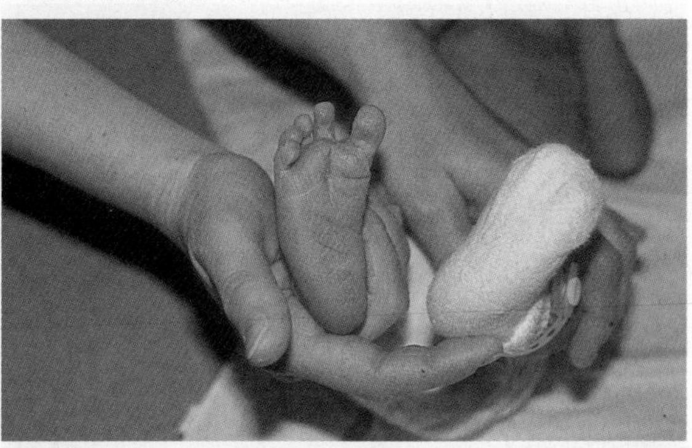

SOLE (PLANTAR) CREASES *The sole of the premature infant has very few or no creases. With the increasing gestation age, the number and depth of sole creases multiply, so that the full-term baby has creases involving the heel. (Wrinkles that occur after 24 hours of age can sometimes be confused with true creases.)*

Premature Infant

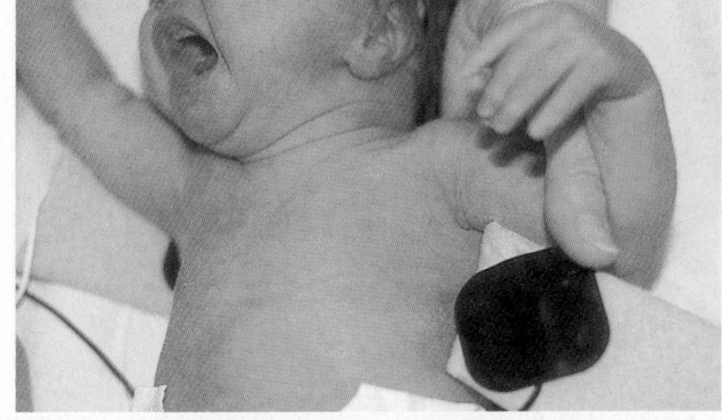

Full-term Infant

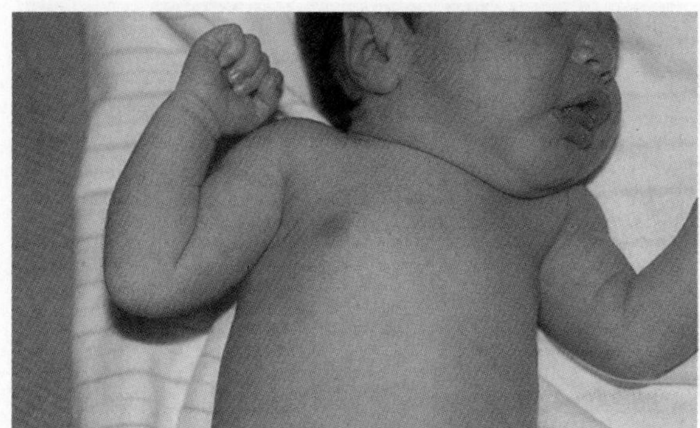

BREAST TISSUE *In infants younger than 34 weeks' gestation the areola and nipple are barely visible. After 34 weeks the areola becomes raised. Also, an infant of less than 36 weeks' gestation has no breast tissue. Breast tissue arises with increasing gestational age because of maternal hormonal stimulation. Thus, an infant of 39–40 weeks will have 5–6 mm of breast tissue, and this amount will increase with age.*

FIGURE 26.7 *(continued)* (**E**) Heel to ear. (**F**) Plantar creases. (**G**) Breast tissue. *(continued)*

H

Premature Infant, 34–36 Weeks

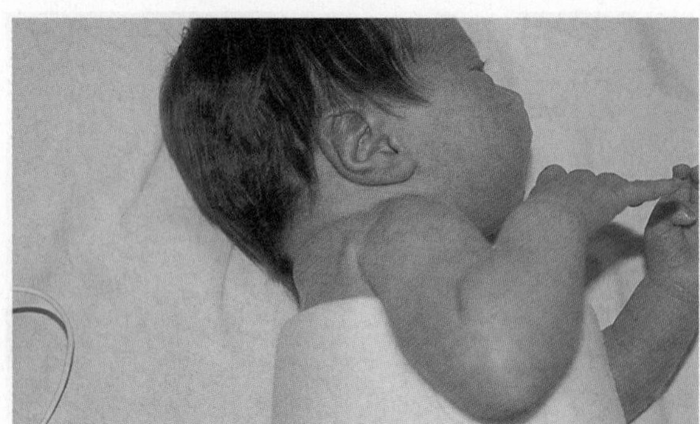

Full-term Infant

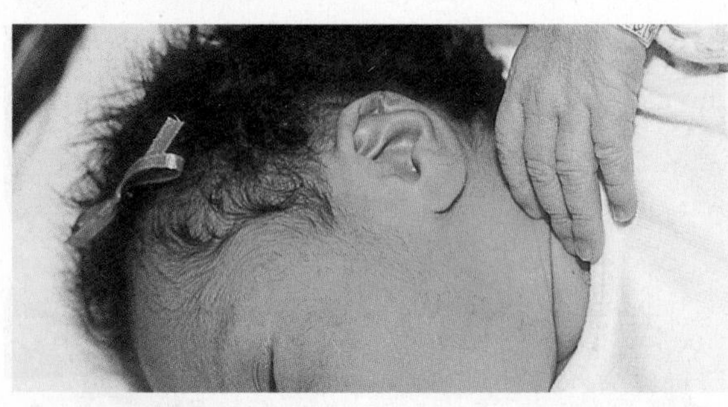

EARS *At fewer than 34 weeks' gestation infants have very flat, relatively shapeless ears. Shape develops over time so that an infant between 34 and 36 weeks has a slight incurving of the superior part of the ear; the term infant is characterized by incurving of two thirds of the pinna; and in an infant older than 39 weeks the incurving continues to the lobe. If the extremely premature infant's ear is folded over, it will stay folded. Cartilage begins to appear at approximately 32 weeks so that the ear returns slowly to its original position. In an infant of more than 40 weeks' gestation, there is enough ear cartilage so that the ear stands erect away from the head and returns quickly when folded. (When folding the ear over during examination, be certain that the surrounding area is wiped clean or the ear may adhere to the vernix.)*

I

Premature Male

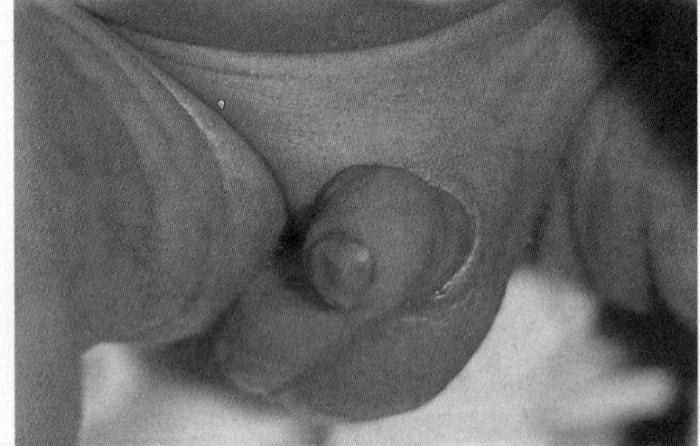

Full-term Male

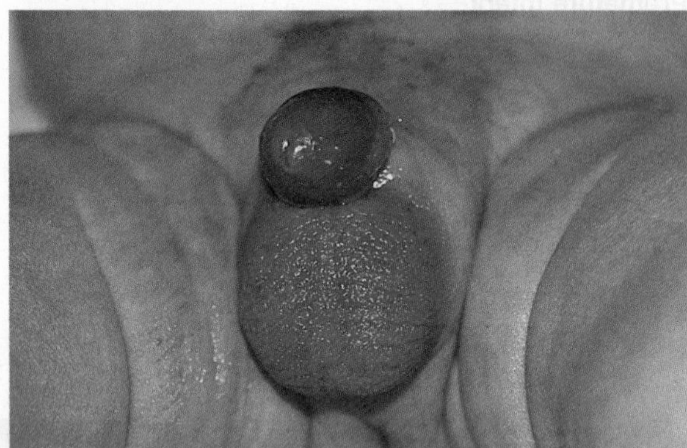

MALE GENITALIA *In the premature male the testes are very high in the inguinal canal and there are very few rugae on the scrotum. The full-term infant's testes are lower in the scrotum and many rugae have developed.*

J

Premature Female

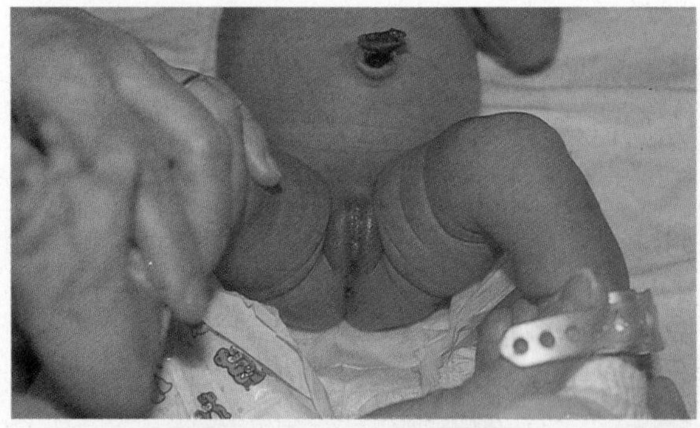

Full-term Female

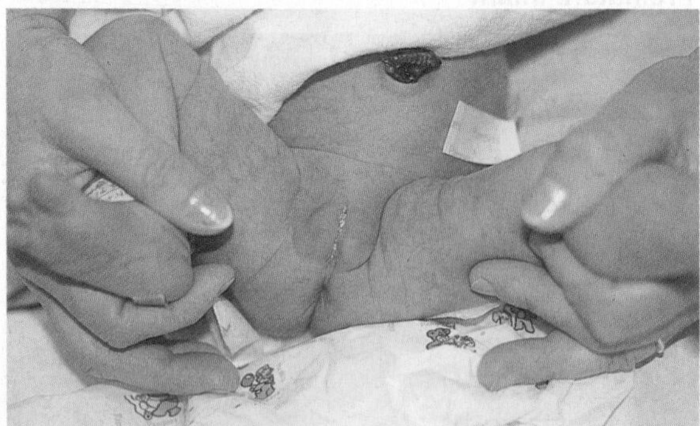

FEMALE GENITALIA *When the premature female is positioned on her back with hips abducted, the clitoris is very prominent and the labia majora are very small and widely separated. The labia minora and the clitoris are covered by the labia majora in the full-term infant.*

FIGURE 26.7 *(continued)* (**H**) Ears. (**I**) Male genitalia. (**J**) Female genitalia. (© Caroline Brown, RNC, MS, DEd.)

12 mg per 100 mL of indirect bilirubin) in these infants. If jaundice occurs, phototherapy or exchange transfusion can be initiated to prevent excessively high indirect bilirubin levels.

Persistent Patent Ductus Arteriosus. Because preterm infants lack surfactant, their lungs are noncompliant, so it is more difficult for them to move blood from the pulmonary artery into the lungs. This condition leads to pulmonary artery hypertension, which may interfere with closure of the ductus arteriosus. Administer intravenous therapy cautiously to preterm infants to avoid increasing blood pressure and further compounding this problem. Either indomethacin or ibuprofen may be administered to close the patent ductus arteriosus (Donze, Smith, & Bryowsky, 2007). A side effect of indomethacin is oliguria, so urine output needs to be monitored closely if this is used.

Periventricular/Intraventricular Hemorrhage. Preterm infants are prone to periventricular hemorrhage (bleeding into the tissue surrounding the ventricles) or intraventricular hemorrhage (bleeding into the ventricles); these conditions occur in as many as 50% of infants of very low birth weight (Thilo & Rosenberg, 2008). This occurs because preterm infants have both fragile capillaries and immature cerebral vascular development. When there is a rapid change in cerebral blood pressure, such as with hypoxia, intravenous infusion, ventilation, or pneumothorax, capillaries rupture. An infant experiences brain anoxia distal to the rupture. Hydrocephalus may occur from bleeding into the aqueduct of Sylvius with resulting clotting and obstruction of the aqueduct. Preterm infants often have a cranial ultrasound performed after the first few days of life to detect if a hemorrhage has occurred. An infant's prognosis is guarded until it can be shown that development in an infant is progressing normally after an intracranial bleed.

Other Potential Complications. Preterm infants are particularly susceptible to several illnesses in the early postnatal period, including respiratory distress syndrome, apnea, retinopathy of prematurity (all discussed later in this chapter), and necrotizing enterocolitis (discussed in Chapter 45).

Nursing Diagnoses and Related Interventions

Because a preterm infant has few body resources, both physiologic and psychological stress must be reduced as much as possible and interventions initiated gently to prevent depletion of resources. Close observation and analysis of findings are essential to managing problems quickly.

Nursing Diagnosis: Impaired gas exchange related to immature pulmonary functioning

Outcome Evaluation: Newborn initiates breathing at birth after resuscitation; maintains normal newborn respirations of 30 to 60 breaths per minute free of assisted ventilation; exhibits oxygen saturation levels of at least 90% as evidenced by arterial blood gases (ABGs).

Many preterm babies, particularly those under 32 weeks of age, have an irregular respiratory pattern (a few quick breaths, a period of 5 to 10 seconds without respiratory effort, a few quick breaths again, and so on). There is no bradycardia with this irregular pattern (sometimes termed **periodic respirations**). Although the pattern is seen in term infants as well, it seems to be intensified by immaturity. With true apnea, the pause in respirations is more than 20 seconds and bradycardia does occur. True apnea is discussed in more detail later in this chapter.

Preterm infants have great difficulty initiating respirations at birth because pulmonary capillaries are still so immature. Lung surfactant does not form in adequate amounts until about the 34th to 35th week of pregnancy. Inadequate lung surfactant leads to alveolar collapse with each expiration. This condition forces an infant to use maximum strength to inflate lung alveoli each time. It is very difficult for infants to maintain effective expirations under these conditions. In addition, because a fetus usually turns to a vertex presentation late in pregnancy, a preterm infant may still be in a breech position at birth. Breech-born infants are apt to expel meconium into the amniotic fluid. If the fetus aspirates either vaginal secretions or meconium, the respiratory problem can be aggravated by inflammation or pneumonia.

Cesarean birth, although it has the advantage of reducing pressure on the immature head, may lead to additional respiratory complications because of retained lung fluid. Giving the mother oxygen by mask during the birth can help provide a preterm infant with optimal oxygen saturation at birth (85%–90%). Keeping maternal analgesia and anesthesia to a minimum also offers an infant the best chance of initiating effective respirations.

Even term infants experience temporary respiratory acidosis until they take a first breath. Once respirations are established, however, this condition quickly clears. Because preterm infants cannot initiate effective respirations as quickly as mature infants, they are susceptible to irreversible acidosis. Birthing room teams need to be prepared with preterm-size laryngoscopes, endotracheal tubes, suction catheters, and synthetic surfactant to be administered by the endotracheal tube so resuscitation can be accomplished within 2 minutes. Infants must be kept warm during resuscitation procedures so they are not expending extra energy to increase metabolic rate to maintain body temperature. All procedures must be carried out gently; a preterm infant's tissues are extremely sensitive to trauma and can be damaged or bruised easily by an oxygen mask. When blood from bruising is reabsorbed, this could lead to hyperbilirubinemia, yet another problem.

Giving 100% oxygen to preterm infants during resuscitation or to maintain respirations presents two additional dangers: pulmonary edema and retinopathy of prematurity (blindness of prematurity; see discussion later in this chapter) may develop. The development of both of these conditions depends on saturation of the blood with oxygen (Po_2 of more than 100 mm Hg, which usually occurs when oxygen is administered at a concentration over 70%). Although a newborn's oxygen saturation level should be continually monitored, as long as an infant is cyanotic, the blood saturation level of oxygen is likely to be low or well beneath this level.

The soft rib cartilage of a preterm infant tends to create respiratory problems because it collapses on expiration. The accessory muscles of respiration may be underdeveloped as well, leaving preterm infants with no backup muscles to use when they become fatigued from trying to maintain respirations. Because of this, preterm infants may need continued oxygen administration after resuscitation to allow them to effectively maintain respirations.

Nursing Diagnosis: Risk for deficient fluid volume related to insensible water loss at birth and small stomach capacity

Outcome Evaluation: Plasma glucose is between 40 and 60 mg per 100 mL; specific gravity of urine is maintained at 1.003 to 1.030; urine output is maintained at a minimum of 1 mL/kg/hr; electrolyte levels are within normal limits.

A preterm newborn experiences a high insensible water loss because of a large body surface relative to total body weight. Preterm infants also cannot concentrate urine well because of immature kidney function. Because of this, a high proportion of body fluid is excreted. All these factors make it important for a preterm baby to receive up to 160 to 200 mL of fluid per kilogram of body weight daily (higher than the term infant).

Intravenous fluid administration typically begins within hours after birth to fulfill this fluid requirement and provide glucose to prevent hypoglycemia. Intravenous fluid should be given via a continuous infusion pump to ensure a constant infusion rate and prevent accidental overload. Intravenous sites must be checked conscientiously because if infiltration should occur, the lack of subcutaneous tissue places a preterm newborn at risk for damaged tissue. Specially designed 27-gauge needles are available for use on small veins. However, many preterm infants lack adequately sized peripheral veins for even this small a needle. Therefore, they need to receive intravenous fluid by an umbilical venous catheter.

Monitor the baby's weight, urine output and specific gravity, and serum electrolytes to ensure adequate fluid intake. Too little fluid and calories can lead to dehydration and starvation, acidosis, and weight loss. Overhydration may lead to nonnutritional weight gain, pulmonary edema, and heart failure.

Most preterm infants void and pass meconium within 24 hours after birth, although this is delayed in very small infants. Measure urine output by weighing diapers rather than using urine collection bags, as disposable collection bags can lead to skin irritation and breakdown from frequent changing and leaking.

The amount of urine output for the first few days of life in preterm babies is high in comparison with that of the term baby because of poor urine concentration: 40 to 100 mL per kg per 24 hours, compared with 10 to 20 mL per kg per 24 hours. The specific gravity is low, rarely more than 1.012 (normal term babies may concentrate urine up to 1.030). Also, test urine for glucose and ketones. Hyperglycemia caused by the glucose infusion may lead to glucose spillage into the urine and an accompanying diuresis. If too little glucose is being supplied and body cells are using protein for metabolism, ketone bodies will appear in urine.

Blood glucose determinations every 4 to 6 hours help to determine hypoglycemia or hyperglycemia (increased serum glucose). Blood glucose should range between 40 and 60 mg/dL. Because of the numerous blood tests performed, be certain to keep a record of all blood drawn so an infant does not become hypovolemic from the amount removed. Check for blood in stools to evaluate possible bleeding from the intestinal tract. This is helpful in determining the possible cause of hypovolemia if it occurs.

Nursing Diagnosis: Risk for imbalanced nutrition, less than body requirements, related to additional nutrients needed for maintenance of rapid growth, possible sucking difficulty, and small stomach

Outcome Evaluation: Infant's weight follows percentile growth curve; skin turgor is good; specific gravity of urine is maintained between 1.003 and 1.030; infant has no more than 15% weight loss in first 3 days of life and continues to gain weight after this point.

Nutrition problems can arise with a preterm infant because the infant's body is attempting to continue to maintain the rapid rate of intrauterine growth. Because of this, a preterm newborn requires a larger amount of nutrients than the mature infant. If these nutrients are not supplied, an infant can develop hypocalcemia (decreased serum calcium) or azotemia (low protein level in blood). Delayed feeding and a resultant decrease in intestinal motility may also add to hyperbilirubinemia, a problem an infant already is at high risk of developing when fetal red blood cells begin to be destroyed.

Digestion and absorption of nutrients in a preterm infant's stomach and intestine may be immature. Nutrition problems are further compounded by a preterm infant's immature reflexes, which make swallowing and sucking difficult. Increased activity that occurs from ineffective sucking may increase the metabolic rate and oxygen requirements. This increases the caloric requirements even more. In addition, the preterm infant's stomach capacity is small, possibly limiting adequate intake. If a small stomach is distended from a full feeding, this puts pressure on the diaphragm and can lead to respiratory distress. An immature cardiac sphincter (between the stomach and esophagus) allows regurgitation to occur readily. The lack of a cough reflex may lead an infant to aspirate regurgitated formula.

Feeding Schedule. With the early administration of intravenous fluid to prevent hypoglycemia and supply fluid, feedings may be safely delayed until an infant has stabilized his or her respiratory effort from birth. Preterm infants may be fed by total parenteral nutrition until they are stable enough for other means. Breast, gavage, or bottle feedings are begun as soon as an infant is able to tolerate them to prevent deterioration of the intestinal villi. Most preterm infants have a chest radiograph taken before a first feeding. The presence of air in the stomach shows that the route to the stomach is clear.

A preterm infant needs 115 to 140 calories per kilogram of body weight per day, compared with 100 to 110 needed by a term infant. Protein requirements are 3 to 3.5 g per kilogram of body weight, compared with 2.0 to 2.5 for a term newborn. Because preterm infants have a smaller stomach capacity than term neonates, they cannot take large feedings and so must be fed more frequently with smaller amounts. Feedings may be as small as 1 or 2 mL every 2 to 3 hours.

Gavage Feeding. A gag reflex is not intact until 32 weeks' gestation. Although a sucking reflex is present earlier, the ability to coordinate sucking and swallowing is inconsistent until approximately 34 weeks' gestation. Infants who are born before 32 to 34 weeks' gestation and those who are ill or experiencing respiratory distress are usually started on gavage feedings. Bottle feeding or breastfeeding is gradually introduced as an infant matures and begins to demonstrate feeding behaviors such as being awake, moving or fussing as if hungry (Fig. 26.8). To avoid tiring, preterm nipples that are softer than regular nipples are used.

Observe preterm infants closely after both oral and gavage feeding to be certain their filled stomach is not causing respiratory distress. Offering a pacifier during gavage feeding can help strengthen the sucking reflex, better prepare an infant for bottle feeding or breastfeeding, and provide oral satisfaction. In addition, initiating and maintaining nonnutritive sucking can help a newborn remember how to suck.

Gavage feedings may be given intermittently every few hours or continuously via tubes passed into the stomach or intestine through the mouth or nose. Infants may be fed by continuous drip feedings at about 1 mL/hr. This can be helpful for infants on ventilators or those who experience oxygen deprivation with handling. If feedings are given intermittently, stomach secretions are usually aspirated, measured, and replaced before each feeding. An infant who has a stomach content of more than 2 mL just before a feeding is receiving more formula than he or she can digest in the time allowed. Feedings should not be increased and possibly even cut back to ensure better digestion and to decrease the possibility of regurgitation and aspiration. Inability to digest this way is also a sign that necrotizing enterocolitis, a destructive intestinal disorder that often occurs in preterm babies, may be developing (Raab, 2007) (see Chapter 45).

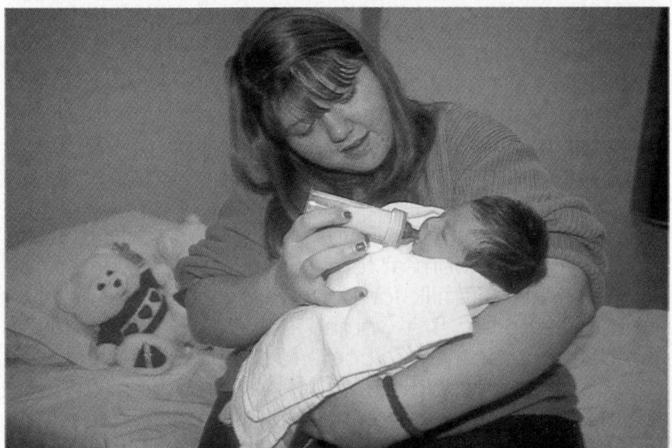

FIGURE 26.8 Feeding a preterm infant. Notice the small bottle used. (© Caroline Brown, RNC, MS, DEd.)

Formula. The caloric concentration of formulas used for preterm infants is usually 24 cal/oz, compared with 20 cal/oz for a term baby. Supplementing additional minerals such as iron, calcium, and phosphorus and electrolytes such as sodium, potassium, and chloride may be necessary, depending on the newborn's blood studies. As with a term neonate, vitamin K should be administered at birth. However, the amount administered is more often 0.5 mL instead of 1 mL because of the infant's small size. Vitamin A is important in improving healing and possibly reducing the incidence of lung disease (Wiswell, Tin, & Ohler, 2007). Vitamin E seems to be important in preventing hemolytic anemia in preterm infants.

Breast Milk. There is increasing evidence that although preterm infants grow well on the increased caloric distribution of commercial formulas, the best milk for them, the same as with term infants, is breast milk (Sisk et al., 2007). The immunologic properties of breast milk apparently play a major role in preventing neonatal necrotizing enterocolitis, as well as increase immune defenses (Conti, 2007).

The mother who wants to breastfeed can manually express breast milk for her infant's gavage feedings. If she cannot bring this in daily, expressed breast milk can be frozen for safe transport and storage. The sodium content of breast milk in a mother whose infant has been born preterm is higher than that of milk in a mother whose infant has been born at term. Therefore, it is better for infants to receive their own mother's breast milk rather than banked milk. This high level of sodium is necessary for fluid retention in the preterm infant. Breast milk is 20 cal/oz, so parents may be advised to add a human milk fortifier to supplemental bottles of breast milk to supply additional calories, protein, vitamins, and minerals (Conti, 2007). Mothers should continue to breastfeed their preterm infants after hospital discharge (Greer, 2007).

Nursing Diagnosis: Ineffective thermoregulation related to immaturity

Outcome Evaluation: Infant's temperature is maintained at 97.6° F (36.5° C) axillary.

Preterm newborns have a great deal of difficulty maintaining body temperature because they have a relatively large surface area per kilogram of body weight. In addition, because they do not flex their body well but remain in an extended position, rapid cooling from evaporation is more likely to occur (Knobel & Holditch-Davis, 2007).

A preterm infant has little subcutaneous fat for insulation and poor muscular development and so cannot move as actively as an older infant to produce body heat. A preterm infant also has a limited amount of **brown fat,** the special tissue present in newborns to maintain body temperature. Preterm infants also cannot shiver, a useful mechanism to increase body temperature; at the same time, they cannot sweat and thereby reduce body temperature because of an immature central nervous system and hypothalamic control. This makes preterm infants dependent on the environmental temperature provided to keep warm. In a birthing room, typically kept at 62° to 68° F (16.6° to 20° C), preterm infants should be kept under radiant heat warmers or warmed by skin-to-skin contact. A 1500-g infant exposed to this low a temperature loses 1° C of body heat every 3 minutes if left unprotected.

Be certain that a radiant heat warmer is warmed before the infant is born. Unless there are obvious abnormalities noted when the child is born, physical assessment of a preterm infant, even weighing, can be delayed until the infant can be placed in the warmth of an incubator or under a radiant warmer with a servo-control.

If an infant is going to be transported to a department within the hospital, such as the x-ray department, or to a regional center for specialized care, keeping the newborn warm during transport is crucial. Remember infants lose heat by radiation as well as conduction. If a warmed incubator is placed near a cold window or air conditioner or in a cold transport ambulance, the infant will lose heat to the distant source. An additional heat shield or plastic wrap may be placed over an infant on a radiant warmer to help conserve heat during transport.

Nursing Diagnosis: Risk for infection related to immature immune defenses in preterm infant

Outcome Evaluation: Temperature is maintained at 97.6° F (36.5° C) axillary; further signs and symptoms of infection such as poor growth or a reduced temperature are absent.

The skin of a preterm baby is easily traumatized and therefore offers less resistance to infection than the skin and mucous membrane of a mature baby. In addition, preterm infants have a lowered resistance to infection. They have difficulty producing phagocytes to localize infection and have a deficiency of IgM antibodies because of insufficient production. To help prevent infection, linen and equipment used with preterm infants must not be shared with other infants. Staff members must be free of infection, and handwashing and gowning regulations should be strictly enforced.

Nursing Diagnosis: Risk for impaired parenting related to interference with parent–infant attachment resulting from hospitalization of infant at birth

Outcome Evaluation: Parents visit frequently and hold infant; speak of him or her in positive terms.

In a preterm infant, the first and second periods of reactivity normally observed in newborns at 1 hour and 4 hours of life (see Chapter 18) may be delayed. In some infants, no period of increased activity or tachycardia may appear until 12 to 18 hours of age. If the purpose of a period of reactivity is to stimulate respiratory function, this places a preterm infant at an even greater threat of respiratory failure, because respiratory efforts may not be stimulated. A second consequence of a delayed period of reactivity is the loss of an opportunity for interaction between parents and the newborn in the early postpartum period.

At one time, a preterm infant was handled as little as possible by hospital staff to conserve the infant's energy. Parents were strictly isolated from the nursery to prevent the introduction of infection. When the child reached a "magic" weight of 4.5 or 5.5 lb, the parents were called and told their child was ready to be discharged. Some nursery personnel offered to allow the mother to feed her infant once under supervision before the day of discharge. In other nurseries, the mother was simply handed the smallest infant she had ever seen and told to take the child home and "mother" this stranger.

Although it is extremely important to conserve a preterm infant's strength by reducing sensory stimulation as much as possible and handling an infant gently, it is now recognized that preterm infants need as much loving attention as term newborns. Rocking, singing, and talking to them and gentle holding are measures to help preterm infants develop a sense of trust in people, which will enable them to relate satisfactorily to people in the future. Encourage parents to begin interacting with their infant in as normal a manner as possible as soon as possible to strengthen bonding (Box 26.8). Holding an infant with skin-to-skin contact is an effective way to begin this (Moore, Anderson, & Bergman, 2009).

Before effective bonding can be established, parents may need time to come to terms with their feelings of disappointment that the infant is so small or guilt that they were not able to stop the preterm birth. A nurse can be instrumental in helping them air these feelings and develop a more positive attitude toward their preterm infant.

If an infant cannot be removed from an incubator or a radiant heat warmer, parents can still handle and stroke the infant in the incubator or warmer. Because parents may not be psychologically ready for birth when a preterm baby is born, it may be more difficult for them to believe they have a child than if the baby were born at term. Encourage a woman to express breast milk for her infant if the child is too young to nurse. If a woman decides not to breastfeed, encourage her to come to the hospital and hold the baby before and after gavage feedings or to give bottle feedings. By feeding her baby or expressing milk for the feedings, she is directly participating in the care and taking on responsibility for the infant's welfare.

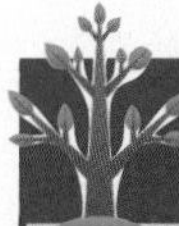

BOX 26.8 * Focus on Family Teaching

Guidelines for Parents of a Newborn in Intensive Care

Q. Mrs. Atkins tells you, "I'm always afraid I'll touch the wrong thing when I visit our son in the neonatal intensive care unit. What can I do to feel more comfortable there?"

A. Here are some guidelines that should be helpful:

- Learn the name of your child's primary nurse or care manager and physician. Make a point of talking to them when you visit, so the information you receive is consistent, and these people can get to know you.
- Discuss with your child's care manager or primary nurse the time you will usually visit, so she or he can reserve this time for you. It helps them to schedule the baby's procedures and rest times so there is time during your visits for you to hold your child and interact with him.
- Ask for explanations of any equipment or medications being used with your child, so you understand the plan of care. Insist on being included in care decisions.
- If you cannot visit on any day, call the nursery and ask to talk to your child's primary care nurse or physician. Such telephone calls are not viewed as a bother but are welcomed as the mark of a concerned parent.
- If you planned to breastfeed, ask if you can supply expressed breast milk for your infant as soon as feedings are started. This contribution may help to give you a feeling of having a greater part in your baby's care.
- Supply a tape recording of your voice, so your baby can learn to recognize it, and a small toy for your baby's bed. These actions not only supply auditory and visual stimulation for your child but also help to give you a more "normal" feeling toward infant care.
- Use your baby's name when you talk about him (not "the baby") to help you gain a firm feeling that this is your baby, not the nursery's.
- If your child is hospitalized a distance from home, ask if transfer to a local hospital in a less technical environment will be possible at a later date.

If the baby is transferred to a regional center, make sure the parents have an opportunity to see the baby before the transfer. A photograph of the baby for them to keep is helpful in making the birth more real. Encourage them to visit the distant site as often as possible. Notes to convey messages from the baby to them can be taped to the incubator or warmer.

On the days they cannot visit, parents can still stay in touch by telephone or nursery e-mail. By the time a baby is ready for discharge, the parents should be able to feel they are taking home "their" baby, one whom they know and have already begun to love.

Parents visiting a high-risk nursery often need a great deal of support from nursing personnel (Box 26.9). Remember that although radiant warmers, incubators, ventilators, and monitors become familiar equipment to nurses, they are unusual and frightening to parents. A parent may want very much to touch an infant but be so

BOX 26.9 * Focus on Communication

Mrs. Atkins gave birth to a 2-lb boy at 34 weeks of pregnancy, 2 days ago. The infant has been classified as a small-for-gestational-age preterm infant. Although you have told Mrs. Atkins twice that she is welcome to visit the neonatal intensive care unit (NICU), you notice that her chart indicates that she has not yet done so.

Less Effective Communication

Nurse: Mrs. Atkins, I've noticed you haven't been to the nursery to see your son yet.
Mrs. Atkins: I'm waiting for my husband to come in.
Nurse: Will that be today?
Mrs. Atkins: Tomorrow. He's out of town on business.
Nurse: Have you called the nursery to ask about your son?
Mrs. Atkins: No. I'm waiting for my husband. We'll do it together.
Nurse: Okay. Let me know if there is anything else you need.

More Effective Communication

Nurse: Mrs. Atkins, I've noticed you haven't been to the nursery to see your son yet.
Mrs. Atkins: I'm waiting for my husband to come in.
Nurse: Will that be today?
Mrs. Atkins: Tomorrow. He's out of town on business.
Nurse: Have you called the nursery to ask about your son?
Mrs. Atkins: No. I'm waiting for my husband. We'll do it together.
Nurse: Often it's intimidating to visit or telephone a high-risk nursery. I know it's important to you to go as a family, but I hate to see you miss these first few days with your son. What if I go with you?
Mrs. Atkins: Could you? I don't want to go alone.

Visiting an NICU is intimidating for parents, not only because of the high-tech equipment that surrounds their baby but also because their baby often appears much smaller or sicker than they imagined. In the first scenario, the nurse assumed that waiting for the husband to come to the hospital was what was important to the mother. In the second scenario, the nurse asked enough questions to realize that having another person accompany her to the nursery was the mother's need, a need the nurse could meet.

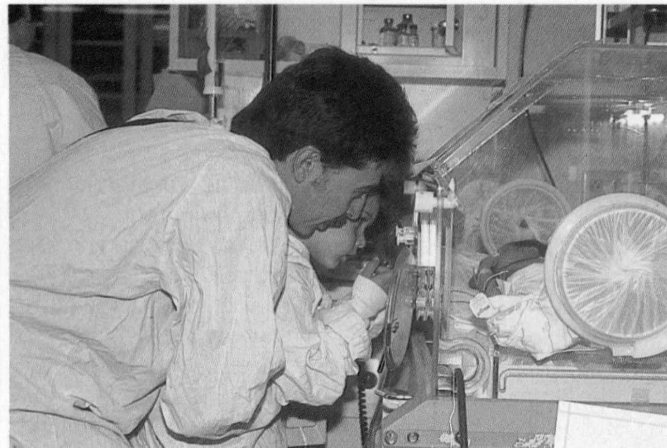

FIGURE 26.9 Encourage families to visit with immature infants to establish bonding. (© Caroline Brown, RNC, MS, DEd.)

afraid touching might set off an alarm that he or she stands back with arms folded instead (Fig. 26.9).

Because preterm infants are hospitalized for long periods, parents can be baffled by receiving information from a parade of different health care professionals or a different person every time they visit. Primary nursing or case management with one nurse as the consistent caregiver helps to reduce the number of people who contact the parents and who communicate the baby's nursing needs to the rest of the staff.

Making the baby's siblings as welcome in a high-risk nursery as the baby's parents is yet another major role for a nurse of high-risk infants. Check to be certain that siblings do not have an upper respiratory infection or fever. Their immunizations should be up to date and they should not have been recently exposed to a communicable disease, such as chickenpox.

Nursing Diagnosis: Deficient diversional activity (lack of stimulation) related to preterm infant's rest needs

Outcome Evaluation: Infant demonstrates interaction with caregivers by attuning to faces or voices.

Preterm infants need rest to conserve energy for growth and respiratory function, to combat hypoglycemia and infection, to stabilize temperature, and to develop inner balance and attentiveness. To allow for this, procedures should be organized to maximize the amount of rest available to an infant. If this is not a coordinated effort, an infant may be awakened constantly for procedures. Preterm infants may have more difficulty blocking out stimuli than term infants do because their nervous systems are immature. They may react negatively by such behaviors as gagging, crying, splaying fingers and toes, or going limp when exposed to bright lights, noise, or overly strenuous handling. Because these infants have little strength to move away from an unwanted stimulus, it is a caregiver's responsibility to be sensitive to these cues and move the object or noise away from the infant (Thomas & Uran, 2007). Until ready to take in stimuli, the infant may need to be shielded from noise and light as much as possible. Likewise, pain should be kept to a minimum.

At the same time as a preterm infant needs rest, he or she needs planned periods of pleasing sensory stimulation. Like all newborns, preterm infants respond best to stimulation that appeals to their senses—sight, sound, and touch. A passive face, picture, or decal may be appealing for only short periods.

The view from inside an incubator can be distorted by the acrylic dome. Most people view an infant in an incubator from the side. This means an infant's face is rarely in the same line of vision as the adult's (an en face position). It is important to look directly at an infant in the straightforward position so the infant is provided with the stimulation of a human face. As infants mature, they should have mobiles (perhaps black and white) or bright objects placed in view. As an infant's position is changed from side to stomach to opposite side, the object should be moved to be in line with the child's vision.

Infants in closed incubators may be able to hear nothing but the sound of the incubator motor. They may see people looking or nodding at them and may see their mouths moving, but they cannot benefit from the sound of their voices because this is obscured by the continuous hum of the motor. Provide some "talk time"—words spoken softly but clearly to an infant's ear—during each nursing shift to offer normal contact.

Even an infant who cannot be removed from an incubator should not suffer from lack of touch. Gently stroking an infant's back or smoothing the back of the head should not be tiring. Transcutaneous oxygen determinations allow you to recognize when an infant is comforted by handling (oxygen saturation remains steady or increases) and when the child is growing tired (oxygen saturation falls). There should be time during every nursing shift for this interaction, particularly if clinical interventions with an infant include uncomfortable procedures such as suctioning or blood drawing. As soon as infants can be out of incubators or removed from warmers, they need special time just to be rocked and held.

Nursing Diagnosis: Risk for disorganized infant behavior related to prematurity and environmental overstimulation

Outcome Evaluation: Newborn's vital signs remain within normal limits; infant demonstrates increasing ability to adapt to stimuli; demonstrates decreasing levels of irritability, crying, respiratory pauses, tachypnea, and color changes.

The amount of rest and stimulation required by preterm infants for healthy development is best individualized. **Developmental care** (care designed to meet the specific needs of each infant) can lead to increased weight gain and decreased crying and apnea spells in preterm infants (Symington & Pinelli, 2009) (Box 26.10). Because preterm infants have immature central nervous systems, their reactions or adjustments to stimuli may be different from those of term infants. The environment of an intensive care unit is also totally different from what infants would have experienced if they had remained in utero until term. Based on these two premises, nursing care must be geared toward making the environment of infants as

BOX 26.10 ✻ Developmental Care

Developmental care is individually designed care based on a preterm infant's behavioral cues to meet the special needs of a preterm infant. Common measures included are:

Parent Welcoming Procedures

- Welcoming parents to the intensive care environment by both words and actions.
- Providing room around incubators or warmers for rocking chairs so parents can hold their baby comfortably.
- Encouraging parent participation in feeding or supplying nonnutritive sucking experiences.
- Demonstrating the infant's capabilities and how, although immature, these are correct for the age or weight.
- Keeping parents informed of the baby's progress and rationale for therapies.
- Asking parents for input into the baby's rhythm of care that will best suit them and the infant after they return home.

Infant Developmental Procedures

- Providing a consistent routine to help infant develop sleep/wake cycles.
- Timing infant care and feeding based on the sleep/wake cycle of the infant.
- Clustering aspects of care so the infant enjoys the longest possible sleep intervals to conserve energy.
- Providing a "nest" with blankets to offer a sense of boundaries or security.
- Providing "quiet or rest times" by covering an incubator and limiting sound.
- Providing tactile stimulation by back stroking or massage.
- Providing audio and visual stimulation by the use of mobiles or music or a parent's voice.
- Halting procedures when the infant evidences stress.

atraumatic as possible while helping them adjust to new experiences within their limited ability.

The usual sound level of nurseries has been documented to be about 40 to 50 dB; a radio playing raises this to 60 to 65 dB. The closing of portholes or tapping on the sides of incubators raises the sound level inside them to 80 dB or more, or a sound level that can be painful. Other abnormal stimuli are bright lights for 24 hours a day, frequent handling, and painful procedures.

When a preterm infant is stressed, behaviors such as respiratory pauses, tachypnea, color changes, tremors, sighing, flaccidity, finger splaying, and gaze averting occur. Such behaviors are alerts that the environment has become too stimulating and needs to be modified. Activities such as dimming the lights or covering an incubator, turning an infant to the side and containing his body with rolled towels, offering nonnutritive sucking, and maintaining a "quiet hour" to reduce sound are all ways to reduce stimuli (Symington & Pinelli, 2009).

Nursing Diagnosis: Parental health-seeking behaviors related to preterm infant's needs for health maintenance

Outcome Evaluation: Parents describe schedule for basic immunizations and health assessments and state who will provide ongoing health care.

Discharge from an NICU is a major transition for parents as well as their infant. Before discharge, the parents of a preterm infant need to learn and practice any special methods of care necessary for their infant and interventions to help maximize their child's development. Some parents tend to overprotect preterm infants, such as not allowing visitors or not taking an infant outside. Let parents know their concern is normal, but overprotection is not necessary.

Ongoing health maintenance of a preterm infant follows the usual pattern of well-child care. Basic immunizations are given according to the chronologic age of an infant. In many communities, NICUs maintain their own well-child settings for infants who were hospitalized there. This allows for long-term follow-up studies on the effect of oxygen or drug therapy and continuity of care. Many parents prefer bringing their infant back to such a facility rather than establishing a new network of health care because they have already established trust and confidence in that health care team. This often also increases their self-esteem because they hear the staff's delight in the progress made by their child. However, preterm infants can be followed by any health care provider for well-child care.

When plotting the height and weight of preterm infants at well-child visits, remember to account for early birth on the growth chart by double charting—that is, plotting the child's weight and height according to the chronologic age (a pattern that probably in the early months places the child below the 10th percentile). Then, in another color, plot the height and weight according to an infant's "setback" or adjusted age, or the age an infant would be if he or she had been born at term. A preterm baby typically gains "catch-up" weight in the first 6 months of life, so by 1 year of age a baby plots over the 10th percentile on a growth chart without accounting for a setback age.

Evaluate growth and development of a preterm infant by the same manner. A preterm infant can be expected to meet first-year milestones not at the chronologic age but at the setback age.

To evaluate the parents' transition to having so small an infant at home, ask at health promotion visits if the parents are:

- Beginning to feel more comfortable with their infant
- Able to allow the child to stay with a babysitter or another family member
- Beginning to incorporate their infant normally into their family life
- Making plans for the infant beyond the immediate newborn period

The Postterm Infant

A postterm infant is one born after the 42nd week of a pregnancy (Fortner, Althaus, & Gurewitsch, 2007). Most nurse-midwives and obstetricians recommend inducing labor at 2 weeks postterm to avoid postmature births. However, when gestational age has been miscalculated or if for some other reason labor is not induced until week 43 of pregnancy or after, the pregnancy may result in a postterm infant.

An infant who stays in utero past week 42 of pregnancy is at special risk because a placenta appears to function effectively for only 40 weeks. After that time, it seems to lose its ability to carry nutrients effectively to the fetus. A fetus who remains in utero with a failing placenta may die or develop **postterm syndrome.** Infants with this syndrome have many of the characteristics of the SGA infant: dry, cracked, almost leather-like skin from lack of fluid, and absence of vernix. They may be lightweight from a recent weight loss that occurred because of the poor placental function. The amount of amniotic fluid may be less at birth than normal, and it may be meconium stained. Fingernails will have grown well beyond the end of the fingertips. Such infants may demonstrate an alertness much more like a 2-week-old baby than a newborn.

When a pregnancy becomes postterm, a sonogram is usually obtained to measure the biparietal diameter of the fetus. A nonstress test or complete biophysical profile (see Chapter 9) may be done to establish whether the placenta is still functioning adequately. Cesarean birth may be indicated if a nonstress test reveals that compromised placental functioning may occur during labor.

At birth, the postterm baby is likely to have difficulty establishing respirations, especially if meconium aspiration occurred. In the first hours of life, hypoglycemia may develop because the fetus had to use stores of glycogen for nourishment in the last weeks of intrauterine life. Subcutaneous fat levels may also be low, having been used in utero. This can make temperature regulation difficult, making it important to prevent a postterm infant from becoming chilled at birth or during transport. Polycythemia may have developed from decreased oxygenation in the final weeks. The hematocrit may be elevated because the polycythemia and dehydration have lowered the circulating plasma level.

Any woman is anxious when she does not have her baby on her due date. She is apt to become extremely anxious and perhaps angry when it is determined her baby is postterm or should have been born earlier. It may seem that if a baby stayed so long in utero, the baby should be extra healthy and strong. Why, then, she asks, is her baby being transferred for special care? A mother may also feel guilty for not providing well for her infant in the last few weeks of pregnancy.

Make sure a woman spends enough time with her newborn to assure herself that although birth did not occur at the predicted time, the baby should do well with appropriate interventions to control possible hypoglycemia or meconium aspiration. All postterm infants need follow-up care until at least school age to track their developmental abilities. The lack of nutrients and oxygen in utero may have left them with neurologic symptoms that will not become apparent until they attempt fine-motor tasks.

ILLNESS IN THE NEWBORN

A number of illnesses occur specifically in newborns. These automatically cause the infant to become high risk.

Respiratory Distress Syndrome

Respiratory distress syndrome (RDS) of the newborn, formerly termed *hyaline membrane disease,* most often occurs in preterm infants, infants of diabetic mothers, infants born by cesarean birth, or those who for any reason have decreased blood perfusion of the lungs, such as occurs with meconium aspiration (Raab, 2007). The pathologic feature of RDS is a hyaline-like (fibrous) membrane formed from an exudate of an infant's blood that begins to line the terminal bronchioles, alveolar ducts, and alveoli. This membrane prevents exchange of oxygen and carbon dioxide at the alveolar–capillary membrane. The cause of RDS is a low level or absence of surfactant, the phospholipid that normally lines the alveoli and reduces surface tension to keep the alveoli from collapsing on expiration.

Because surfactant does not form until the 34th week of gestation, as many as 30% of low-birth-weight infants and as many as 50% of very-low-birth-weight infants are susceptible to this complication.

Pathophysiology

High pressure is required to fill the lungs with air for the first time and overcome the pressure of lung fluid. For example, it takes a pressure between 40 and 70 cm H_2O to inspire a first breath but only 15 to 20 cm H_2O to maintain quiet, continued breathing. If alveoli collapse with each expiration, as happens when surfactant is deficient, forceful inspirations requiring optimum pressure are still required to inflate them.

Even very immature infants release a bolus of surfactant at birth into their lungs from the stress of birth. However, with deficient surfactant, areas of hypoinflation begin to occur and pulmonary resistance increases. Blood then shunts through the foramen ovale and the ductus arteriosus as it did during fetal life. The lungs are poorly perfused, affecting gas exchange. As a result, the production of surfactant decreases even further.

The poor oxygen exchange that results leads to tissue hypoxia, which causes the release of lactic acid. This, combined with the increasing carbon dioxide level resulting from the formation of the hyaline membrane on the alveolar surface, leads to severe acidosis. Acidosis causes vasoconstriction, and decreased pulmonary perfusion from vasoconstriction further limits surfactant production. With decreased surfactant production, the ability to stop alveoli from collapsing with each expiration becomes impaired. This vicious cycle continues until the oxygen–carbon dioxide exchange in the alveoli is no longer adequate to sustain life without ventilator support.

Assessment

Most infants who develop RDS have difficulty initiating respirations at birth. After resuscitation, they appear to have a period of hours or a day when they are free of symptoms because of an initial release of surfactant. During this time, however, subtle signs may appear:

- Low body temperature
- Nasal flaring

- Sternal and subcostal retractions
- Tachypnea (more than 60 respirations per minute)
- Cyanotic mucous membranes

Within several hours, expiratory grunting, caused by closure of the glottis to create a prolonged expiratory time, can be heard. A partially closed glottis this way is helpful as it increases the pressure in the alveoli on expiration, helps to keep the alveoli from collapsing, and makes oxygen exchange more complete. Even with this attempt at better oxygen exchange, however, as the disease progresses, infants become cyanotic and their PO_2 and oxygen saturation levels fall in room air. On auscultation, there may be fine rales and diminished breath sounds because of poor air entry. As distress increases, an infant may exhibit:

- Seesaw respirations (on inspiration, the anterior chest wall retracts and the abdomen protrudes; on expiration, the sternum rises)
- Heart failure, evidenced by decreased urine output and edema of the extremities
- Pale gray skin
- Periods of apnea
- Bradycardia
- Pneumothorax

The diagnosis of RDS is made on the clinical signs of grunting, central cyanosis in room air, tachypnea, nasal flaring, retractions, and shock. A chest radiograph will reveal a diffuse pattern of radiopaque areas that look like ground glass (haziness). Blood gas studies (taken from an umbilical vessel catheter) will reveal respiratory acidosis. A β-hemolytic, group B streptococcal infection may mimic RDS, as this infection is so severe in newborns that the insult to the lungs is enough to stop surfactant production. Cultures of blood, cerebrospinal fluid, and skin may be obtained to rule out this condition. An antibiotic (penicillin or ampicillin) and an aminoglycoside (gentamicin or kanamycin) may be started while culture reports are pending.

Therapeutic Management

RDS can be largely prevented by the administration of surfactant through an endotracheal tube at birth for an infant at risk because of low gestational age.

Surfactant Replacement. As a preventive measure, synthetic surfactant is sprayed into the lungs by a syringe or catheter through an endotracheal tube at birth while an infant is first positioned with the head held upright and then tilted downward. It is important an infant's airway not be suctioned for as long a period as possible after administration of surfactant to avoid suctioning the drug away. Although there are almost no unfavorable reactions to surfactant administration, some, such as mucus plugging from the solution, do occur. An infant who is receiving surfactant and then is placed on a ventilator needs close observation because lung expansion can improve rapidly. Anticipate the need to adjust ventilator settings to prevent excessive lung pressure.

Oxygen Administration. Administration of oxygen is necessary to maintain correct PO_2 and pH levels. Continuous positive airway pressure (CPAP) or assisted ventilation with positive end-expiratory pressure (PEEP) will exert pressure on the alveoli at the end of expiration and keep the alveoli from collapsing (Ho et al., 2009). This greatly improves oxygen exchange. A possible complication of oxygen therapy in the very immature or very ill infant is retinopathy of prematurity (see discussion later in chapter) or bronchopulmonary dysplasia (see Chapter 40).

Ventilation. Normally, on a ventilator, inspiration is shorter than expiration, or there is an inspiratory/expiratory ratio (I/E ratio) of 1:2. It is difficult to deliver enough oxygen to stiff, noncompliant lungs in this usual ratio, however, without forcing the air into the lungs at such a high pressure and rapid rate that a pneumothorax becomes a constant concern (Snow & Brandon, 2007). Infant ventilators are therefore available with a reversed I/E ratio (2:1). These are pressure-cycled to control the force with which air is delivered. High-frequency, oscillatory, and jet ventilation are other methods of introducing oxygen to infants with noncompliant lungs. These systems maintain airway pressure and then intermittently "jet" or oscillate at a rapid rate (400–600 times a minute) an additional amount of air to inflate alveoli.

Complications of any type of ventilation are possible, such as pneumothorax and impaired cardiac output because of decreased blood flow through the pulmonary artery from lung pressure. There is also a possible risk of increased intracranial and arterial pressure and hemorrhage from changing blood pressure. Being certain that infants are not overhydrated is important to help prevent increased blood pressure and increased pulmonary artery pressure.

Indomethacin or ibuprofen may be used to cause closure of a patent ductus arteriosus, making ventilation more efficient (Donze, Smith, & Bryowsky, 2007). Indomethacin has been associated with adverse effects such as decreased renal function, decreased platelet count, and gastric irritation. Carefully monitor urine output and observe for bleeding, especially at puncture sites, if this is prescribed.

Additional Therapy. Yet another method of increasing pulmonary blood flow is by using muscle relaxants. Pancuronium (Pavulon) can be administered intravenously to the point of abolishing spontaneous respiratory action. Doing so allows mechanical ventilation to be accomplished at lower pressures because there is no normal muscle resistance to overcome. The possibility of pneumothorax is reduced while PO_2 is increased. Obviously infants who have no spontaneous respiratory function because of drug administration need critical observation and frequent ABG analysis because they totally depend on caregivers at this point (Playfor et al., 2007).

The effect of pancuronium decreases as the life of the drug expires; its effect can be interrupted by the administration of atropine or injectable neostigmine methylsulfate (Prostigmin Methylsulfate Injectable). For this reason, when pancuronium is being administered, both atropine and Prostigmin should be immediately available. An infant's plan of care should be specially marked to show that pancuronium therapy is being used so in the event of a power failure, manual ventilatory assistance can be begun immediately.

Some infants are maintained on **extracorporeal membrane oxygenation** (ECMO) to ensure adequate oxygenation (Maclaren & Butt, 2007). Other therapies include liquid ventilation or administration of perfluorocarbons and inhalation of nitric oxide (Stephens & Fawcett, 2007).

Extracorporeal Membrane Oxygenation. ECMO was first developed as a means of oxygenating blood during cardiac surgery. Its current use has expanded to the management of chronic severe hypoxemia in newborns with illnesses such as meconium aspiration, RDS, pneumonia, and diaphragmatic hernia. It is used also for near-drowning victims or infants with severe lung infection. With ECMO, blood is removed from the baby by gravity using a venous catheter advanced into the right atrium of the heart. The blood circulates from the catheter to the ECMO machine, where it is oxygenated and rewarmed. It is then returned to an infant's aortic arch by a catheter advanced through the carotid artery. ECMO is typically used for 4 to 7 days. It has many potential complications, chief of which is intracranial hemorrhage, possibly from the anticoagulation therapy necessary to prevent thromboembolism. Constant nursing care is required for a child receiving ECMO to ensure that the child's blood volume remains adequate, bleeding does not occur, and adequate oxygen is being supplied to body tissues.

Liquid Ventilation. Liquid ventilation involves the use of perfluorocarbons, substances used in industry to assess for leakage in pipes. When oxygen is bubbled through it, perfluorocarbons pick up and carry the oxygen with them. When perfluorocarbons are introduced into lungs that inflate poorly because they are deficient in surfactant, or in lungs damaged by trauma or disease, the weight of the fluid, which is heavy compared with air, helps to distend the lungs. As the liquid moves into a lung, oxygen is carried along with it; as the liquid spreads over all lung surfaces, an exchange of oxygen occurs (Lindemann et al., 2007). The administration of liquid ventilation can also be used to deliver surfactant to a newborn's lungs.

Nitric Oxide. An additional measure that can help to oxygenate a newborn's lungs is the administration of nitric oxide. This causes pulmonary vasodilation, which can be helpful to increase blood flow to the alveoli when persistent pulmonary hypertension is present (Kumar et al., 2007).

What if... While you were caring for Baby Atkins, who is ventilator dependent and receiving pancuronium, a power failure occurred? What would be your first actions?

Supportive Care. An infant with RDS must be kept warm because cooling increases acidosis in all newborns, and for the newborn with RDS it may increase to lethal levels. Keeping an infant warm also reduces the metabolic oxygen demand. Provide hydration and nutrition with intravenous fluids, glucose, or gavage feeding because the respiratory effort makes an infant too exhausted to suck (see Focus on Nursing Care Planning Box 26.11).

Prevention

RDS rarely occurs in mature infants. Dating a pregnancy by sonogram and by documenting that the level of lecithin in surfactant obtained from amniotic fluid exceeds that of sphingomyelin by 2:1 are important ways to be certain an in-

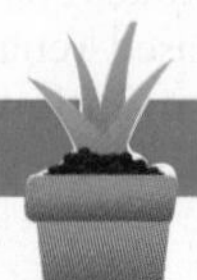

BOX 26.11 ✻ Focus on Nursing Care Planning

A Multidisciplinary Care Map for a Newborn With Respiratory Distress Syndrome

Mr. and Mrs. Atkins are the parents of a 34-week-old, 2-lb baby boy, born last night after a short, 4-hour labor.

Family Assessment ✻ Family consists of two parents. Mr. Atkins works as a consulting engineer; Mrs. Atkins worked before pregnancy as a home decorator. Mr. Atkins was out of town on business so was not present for the infant's birth. Mrs. Atkins has not visited the intensive care nursery. She refused to sign the birth certificate because she could not decide on a name. She said, "I don't want to give him our favorite name because he might die." Mr. Atkins telephoned early this morning and acted more upset the baby was born than relieved the baby was receiving intensive care. He asked his wife, "What did you do to cause this?"

Client Assessment ✻ Newborn, 5 hours old, delivered vaginally. Difficulty establishing respirations at birth. Resuscitated by the neonatal nurse practitioner and respiratory therapist and then transported to the intensive care nursery. Temperature 97.2° F (36.2° C). Bradycardic and tachypneic with grunting respirations. Sternal and subcostal retractions present. Skin pale and somewhat cyanotic. Chest x-ray with ground-glass appearance. Arterial blood gases (ABGs) reveal respiratory acidosis. Endotracheal (ET) intubation, mechanical ventilation, supplemental oxygen, and intravenous fluid therapy initiated.

Nursing Diagnosis ✻ Impaired gas exchange related to immaturity of newborn's lungs and lack of surfactant

Outcome Criteria ✻ Vital signs within acceptable parameters. Temperature maintained at 97.7° F (36.5° C). Absence of cyanosis; diminished retractions; ABG values within acceptable parameters; no sound of grunting respirations.

Activities of Daily Living				
Nurse/ neonatal nurse practitioner	Assess respiratory rate, depth, and rhythm; auscultate lung sounds; evaluate ABG results and skin color.	Maintain respiratory program as prescribed, such as oxygen by ET tube or ventilator.	Signs of increasing respiratory distress may denote lessening air exchange.	Infant maintains a stable respiratory rate and depth with assistive respiratory aids in place.
Nurse	Assess infant's axillary temperature every hour.	Maintain a neutral thermal environment so infant's temperature remains stable.	Neutral thermal environment minimizes the risk of cold stress, which increases metabolic demands for oxygen.	Infant's temperature is maintained at 36.5° C (97.7° F) axillary.
Consultations				
Nurse	Determine what developmental care resources will be available for infant care.	Consult with developmental care coordinator regarding specific developmental care measures for infant.	Developmental care or trying to reduce infant stress can improve infant's outcome.	Developmental care coordinator establishes an individualized program for infant care.
Procedures/Medications				
Nurse/ neonatal nurse practitioner; physician	Assess infant's response to respiratory support. Assess oxygen saturation levels via pulse oximetry.	Maintain ET tube, mechanical ventilation, and supplemental warm humidified oxygen. Anticipate the need for CPAP or PEEP.	The ET tube protects a patent airway. Mechanical ventilation assists with delivering necessary air to the lungs. Using warm, humidified oxygen prevents cold stress and drying of mucous membranes. Oxygen saturation levels provide information about tissue oxygenation. CPAP and PEEP exert pressure on alveoli at end-expiration, preventing alveolar collapse.	Respiratory support measures are in place, and infant's respiratory rate remains within designated parameters.
Physician/nurse	Assess availability of surfactant for administration.	Administer surfactant via ET tube as per protocol. Refrain from suctioning for 1 hour if possible.	Surfactant restores the naturally occurring lung surfactant to improve lung compliance. Suctioning would remove the drug from its intended site.	Surfactant is administered.
Nutrition				
Nurse/ nutritionist/ physician	Assess infant's need for nourishment based on gestational age and exhaustion from rapid breathing.	Administer nutrition via enteral feedings: breast milk supplemented with high-calorie formula. Anticipate the need for total parenteral nutrition if weight gain is not sufficient.	Additional nutrients are necessary because stress of RDS requires increased caloric expenditure. Total parenteral nutrition may be necessary to meet these additional needs.	Infant tolerates enteral feedings without difficulty. Mother supplies breast milk for feedings.

(continued)

BOX 26.11 ✻ Focus on Nursing Care Planning (continued)

		Nutrition		
Nurse	Assess blood glucose levels every 4 hours by heel stick.	Report hypoglycemia (blood glucose level <45 mg/dL).	Glucose is a source of energy. Monitoring glucose levels helps to determine if sufficient energy is available to meet the newborn's metabolic needs.	Infant maintains a glucose level >45 mg/dL.
		Patient/Family Education		
Nurse	Assess what parents know about the cause of preterm labor.	Teach parents that the cause of preterm birth often cannot be identified.	Parents will need to work together to arrange for best care for preterm infant.	Parents state they are adjusting to shock of preterm birth based on better knowledge of cause.
		Psychosocial/Spiritual/Emotional Needs		
Nurse	Assess what activities parents think their very small infant can accomplish.	Invite parents to see, touch, and spend as much time as possible with newborn. Guide them in activities such as skin-to-skin contact and basic caregiving.	Seeing, touching, and caring promote attachment. Guidance in activities helps to alleviate anxiety.	Parents visit in nursery or telephone at least every other day; touch and talk to newborn.
		Psychosocial/Spiritual/Emotional Needs		
Nurse	Assess if parents have worked through shock of preterm birth.	Suggest parents bring in a mobile or toy to keep near newborn.	A mobile or toy provides visual stimulation and promotes feelings of participation in the newborn's care.	Parents state they know preterm birth is no one's fault; express interest in parenting.
		Discharge Planning		
Nurse	Assess what community organizations will be available to family for continued support.	Refer parents to Web sites helpful for preterm information; suggest they join local Parents of Preemies organization.	Parents may need continued support after they return home with a small infant.	Parents give examples of how they are making active plans for infant's discharge and care.

fant born by cesarean birth or has labor induced is mature enough that RDS is not likely to occur.

Using a tocolytic agent such as terbutaline can help to prevent preterm birth for a few days. Because steroids appear to quicken the formation of lecithin, it may be possible to prevent RDS in infants by administering two injections of a glucocorticosteroid, such as betamethasone, to the mother at 12 and 24 hours during this time. This is most effective when given between weeks 24 and 34 of pregnancy. Unfortunately, there is often no warning that preterm birth is imminent until hours before birth. Because the steroid does not take effect before 24 to 48 hours, some labors and births will progress too rapidly for this preventive measure to be effective.

✔Checkpoint Question 26.3

Baby Atkins has surfactant administered at birth. The purpose of surfactant is to:

a. Help raise lung secretions by relaxing the airway.
b. Prevent alveoli from collapsing on expiration.
c. Paralyze respiratory muscles to synchronize breathing.
d. Reduce gastric secretions by action on the pancreas.

Transient Tachypnea of the Newborn (TTN)

At birth, a newborn may have a rapid rate of respirations, up to 80 breaths per minute when crying, caused by retained lung fluid (Raab, 2007). Within 1 hour, however, this rapid rate slows to between 30 and 60 breaths per minute. In about 10 in 1000 live births, the respiratory rate remains at a high level, between 80 and 120 breaths per minute. The infant does not appear to be in a great deal of distress, aside from the tiring effort of breathing so rapidly. Mild retractions but not marked cyanosis, mild hypoxia, and hypercapnia may be present. Feeding is difficult because the child cannot suck and breathe this rapidly at the same time. A chest radiograph will reveal some fluid in the central lung, but aeration is, overall, adequate. An ultrasound may show like findings (Copetti & Cattarossi, 2007).

Transient tachypnea may reflect a slight decrease in production of phosphatidyl glycerol or mature surfactant but is a direct result of retained lung fluid. Retained lung fluid limits the amount of alveolar surface that is available for oxygen exchange. This limitation requires an infant to increase respiratory rate and depth of respirations to better use the surface available. Transient tachypnea occurs more often in infants who are born by cesarean birth, in infants whose mothers received extensive fluid administration during labor, and in preterm infants. Infants born by cesarean birth are probably more prone to develop this form of respiratory distress because the thoracic cavity is not compressed as it is in vaginal birth, so less lung fluid is expelled than normally.

Close observation of such a newborn is a priority. Watch carefully to be certain the increased effort is not tiring. Also watch for beginning signs of a more serious disorder, because a rapid respiratory rate is often the first sign of respiratory obstruction. Oxygen administration may be necessary. Transient tachypnea of the newborn peaks in intensity at approximately 36 hours of life and then begins to fade. Typically, by 72 hours of life, it spontaneously fades as the lung fluid is absorbed and respiratory activity becomes effective.

Meconium Aspiration Syndrome

Meconium is present in the fetal bowel as early as 10 weeks' gestation. If hypoxia occurs, a vagal reflex is stimulated, resulting in relaxation of the rectal sphincter. This releases meconium into the amniotic fluid. Babies born breech may expel meconium into the amniotic fluid from pressure on the buttocks. In both instances, the appearance of the fluid at birth is green to greenish black from the staining. Meconium staining occurs in approximately 10% to 12% of all pregnancies; in 2% to 9% of these pregnancies, infants will aspirate the meconium (Szymanski & Bienstock, 2007). Meconium aspiration does not tend to occur in extremely-low-birth-weight infants because the substance has not passed far enough in the bowel for it to be at the rectum in these infants.

An infant may aspirate meconium either in utero or with the first breath at birth. Meconium can cause severe respiratory distress in three ways: it causes inflammation of bronchioles because it is a foreign substance; it can block small bronchioles by mechanical plugging; and it can cause a decrease in surfactant production through lung trauma. Hypoxemia, carbon dioxide retention, and intrapulmonary and extrapulmonary shunting occur. A secondary infection of injured tissue may lead to pneumonia.

Assessment

Infants with meconium-stained amniotic fluid can have difficulty establishing respirations at birth (those who were not born breech have had a hypoxic episode in utero to cause the meconium to be in the amniotic fluid). The Apgar score is apt to be low. Almost immediately, tachypnea, retractions, and cyanosis occur.

With meconium-stained amniotic fluid, an infant should be suctioned with a bulb syringe or catheter while at the perineum, before the birth of the shoulders, to avoid meconium aspiration. Although there is some dispute regarding whether all infants with meconium staining need intubation, those with severe staining are intubated and meconium is suctioned from their trachea and bronchi (Halliday & Sweet, 2009). Do not administer oxygen under pressure (bag and mask) until an infant has been intubated and suctioned, so that the pressure of the oxygen does not drive small plugs of meconium farther down into the lungs, worsening the irritation and obstruction.

After the initiation of respirations, an infant's respiratory rate may remain elevated (tachypnea) and coarse bronchial sounds may be heard on auscultation. An infant may continue to have retractions because the inflammation of bronchi tends to trap air in the alveoli, limiting the entrance of oxygen. This air trapping may also cause enlargement of the anteroposterior diameter of the chest (barrel chest). Blood gases will reveal a poor gas exchange, evidenced by a decreased PO_2 and an increased PCO_2. A chest radiograph will show bilateral coarse infiltrates in the lungs, with spaces of hyperaeration (a peculiar honeycomb effect). The diaphragm will be pushed downward by the overexpanded lungs.

Therapeutic Management

Amnioinfusion can be used to dilute the amount of meconium in amniotic fluid and reduce the risk of aspiration although this is usually reserved for instances where the fetus shows distress (Szymanski & Bienstock, 2007). Some infants are scheduled to be born by cesarean birth after deeply meconium-stained amniotic fluid becomes evident during labor. After birth and tracheal suction, infants may need to be treated with oxygen administration and assisted ventilation. Antibiotic therapy may be used to forestall the development of pneumonia as a secondary problem. Surfactant may be administered to increase lung compliance (El Shahed et al., 2009). Lung tissue is fairly noncompliant after meconium aspiration, which may necessitate high inspiratory pressure. This can cause pneumothorax or pneumomediastinum. Infants must be observed closely for signs of trapping air in the alveoli, because the alveoli can expand only so far and then will rupture, sending air into the pleural space (pneumothorax).

Because of increased pulmonary resistance, the ductus arteriosus may remain open, causing blood to shunt from the pulmonary artery into the aorta, compromising cardiac efficiency and increasing hypoxia. Observe an infant closely for signs of heart failure such as increased heart rate or respiratory distress. Maintain a temperature-neutral environment to prevent increasing metabolic oxygen demands. Chest physiotherapy with clapping and vibration may be helpful to encourage removal of remnants of meconium from the lungs (see Chapter 40). Some infants will be maintained on ECMO to ensure adequate oxygenation (Radhakrishnan et al., 2007).

Although meconium aspiration is a serious insult to a newborn, with therapeutic interventions, the symptoms of this will begin to fade by a week's time with no long-term results.

Apnea

Apnea is a pause in respirations longer than 20 seconds with accompanying bradycardia. Beginning cyanosis also may be present. Many preterm infants have periods of apnea as a result of fatigue or the immaturity of their respiratory mechanisms. Babies with secondary stresses, such as infection, hyperbilirubinemia, hypoglycemia, or hypothermia, tend to have a high incidence of apnea (Thilo & Rosenberg, 2008).

Gently shaking an infant or flicking the sole of the foot often stimulates the baby to breathe again, almost as if the child needed to be reminded to maintain this function. If an infant does not respond to these simple measures, resuscitation is necessary.

Closely observe all newborns, but especially preterm ones, to detect these apneic episodes. Apnea monitors that record respiratory movements are invaluable tools to detect failing respiration and sound a warning an infant needs attention. Infants with frequent or difficult-to-correct episodes may be placed on ventilators to provide respiratory coordination until they are more mature.

To help prevent episodes of apnea, maintain a neutral thermal environment and use gentle handling to avoid excessive fatigue. Always suction gently to minimize nasopharyngeal irritation, which can cause bradycardia because of vagal stimulation. Using indwelling nasogastric tubes rather than intermittent ones can also reduce the amount of vagal stimulation. After feeding, observe an infant carefully because a full stomach can put pressure on the diaphragm and potentially compromise respirations. Careful burping also helps to reduce this effect. Never take rectal temperatures in infants prone to apnea; the resulting vagal stimulation can reduce the heart rate (bradycardia), which can lead to apnea. Theophylline or caffeine sodium benzoate may be administered to stimulate respirations. The mechanism by which these drugs reduce the incidence of apneic episodes is unclear, but they appear to increase an infant's sensitivity to carbon dioxide, ensuring better respiratory function. Infants who have had an apneic episode severe enough to require resuscitation are at a high risk for sudden infant death syndrome (SIDS). Such infants may be discharged home with a monitoring device to be used for 2 to 6 months.

Sudden Infant Death Syndrome (SIDS)

SIDS is sudden unexplained death in infancy. It tends to occur at a higher-than-usual rate in infants of adolescent mothers, infants of closely spaced pregnancies, and underweight and preterm infants. Also prone to SIDS are infants with bronchopulmonary dysplasia, twins, Native American infants, Alaskan Native infants, economically disadvantaged black infants, and infants of narcotic-dependent mothers. The peak age of incidence is 2 to 4 months of age (Barkin & James, 2007).

Although the cause of SIDS is unknown, in addition to prolonged but unexplained apnea, other possible contributing factors include:

- Viral respiratory or botulism infection
- Pulmonary edema
- Brain stem abnormalities
- Neurotransmitter deficiencies
- Heart rate abnormalities
- Distorted familial breathing patterns
- Decreased arousal responses
- Possible lack of surfactant in alveoli
- Sleeping in a room without moving air currents (the infant rebreathes expired carbon dioxide)

Typically, affected infants are well nourished. Parents report that an infant may have had a slight head cold. After being put to bed at night or for a nap, the infant is found dead a few hours later. Infants who die this way do not appear to make any sound as they die, which indicates they die with laryngospasm. Although many infants are found with blood-flecked sputum or vomitus in their mouths or on the bedclothes, this seems to occur as the result of death, not as its cause. An autopsy often reveals petechiae in the lungs and mild inflammation and congestion in the respiratory tract. However, these symptoms are not severe enough to cause sudden death. It is clear these children do not suffocate from bedclothes or choke from overfeeding, underfeeding, or crying. Since the American Academy of Pediatrics made its recommendation to put newborns to sleep on their back and with a pacifier, the incidence of SIDS has declined almost 50% (Damato, 2007). With the recommendation that infants sleep with a fan in their room to keep air moving, the incidence is expected to decrease further (Coleman-Phox, Odouli, & Li, 2008).

Parents have a difficult time accepting the death of any child. This can be especially difficult when it happens so suddenly. In discussing the child, they often use both the past and present tense as if they are not yet aware of the death. Many parents experience a period of somatic symptoms that occur with acute grief, such as nausea, stomach pain, or vertigo. Parents should be counseled by a nurse or someone else trained in counseling at the time of the infant's death; it helps if they can talk to this same person periodically for however long it takes to resolve their grief. The American Sudden Infant Death Institute, listed at the beginning of the chapter, offers suggestions for counseling.

Autopsy reports should be given to parents as soon as they are available (if toxicology tests are included in the autopsy, results will not be available for weeks). Reading that their child's death was unexplained can help to reassure parents the death was not their fault. They need this assurance if they are to plan for other children. If there are older children in the family, they also need assurance that SIDS is a disease of infants and that the strange phenomenon that invaded their home and killed a younger brother or sister will not also kill them. If they wished the infant dead, as all children wish siblings were dead on some days, they need reassurance that their wishes did not cause the baby's death.

When another child is born, parents can be expected to become extremely frightened at any sign of illness in their child. They need support to see them through the first few months of the second child's life, particularly past the point at which the first child died. Some parents may need support to view a second child as an individual child and not as a replacement for the one who died.

Often a new baby born to a family in which a SIDS infant died is screened using a sleep assessment as a precaution within the first 2 weeks of life. Depending on the parents' level of anxiety, the new baby may receive this screening before hospital discharge. The baby may then be placed on continuous apnea monitoring pending the results of the sleep assessment.

Apparent Life-Threatening Event

Some infants have been discovered cyanotic and limp in their beds but have survived after mouth-to-mouth resuscitation by parents. An episode of this kind is called an **apparent life-threatening event** (Shah & Sharieff, 2007). For these infants as well as for preterm infants with a tendency toward apnea or new babies born to a family whose child died from SIDS, apnea monitoring is available. With apnea monitoring in place, an alarm sounds when the neonate experiences a period of apnea of 20 seconds or longer or a decreased heart rate below 80 beats per minute (Fig. 26.10). If parents are going to use an apnea monitor at home, make certain they will be able to hear it in all parts of the house or apartment. Usually the alarm is not loud enough to be heard in the basement from an upstairs bedroom. Caution them about household noises such as a loud television, radio, vacuum cleaner, or hair dryer that may interfere with hearing the alarm. Be certain they know how to apply and reposition the apnea leads and that they are comfortable enough with the monitor to see past it to the child. In addition, parents should be taught cardiopulmonary resuscitation before their infant is discharged from the hospital (Fig. 26.11).

Caring for a child at home on an apnea monitor may be extremely stressful for the parents and their relationship. They often have difficulty finding a competent babysitter. These parents can benefit from a community or home care referral so they have a second opinion regarding how well they are managing, as well as a listening ear to discuss the strain of having to be constantly alert for a sound that means their infant has stopped breathing. Having someone periodically review with them what steps to take should the alarm sound (jiggle the baby, begin mouth-to-mouth resuscitation, call the emergency response personnel) can be very comforting. Because SIDS is a baffling disease, these parents will live in fear of SIDS until their child reaches at least 1 year of age.

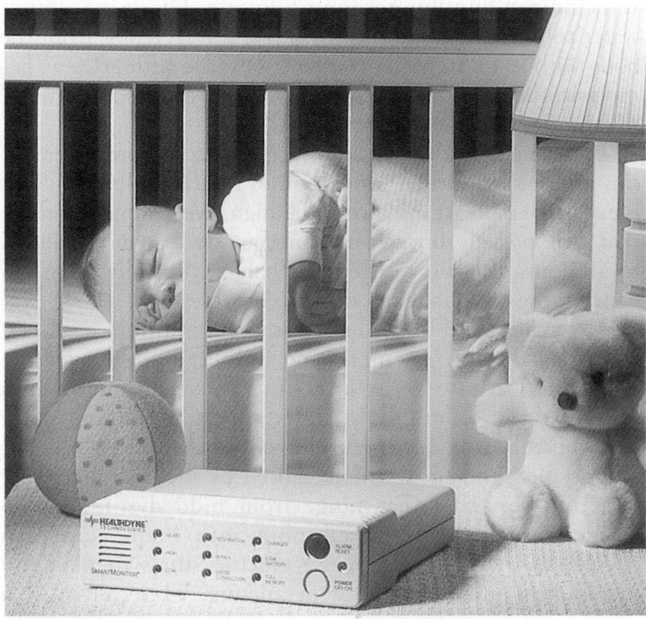

FIGURE 26.10 An apnea monitor for home monitoring. (Photograph courtesy of Respironics/Healthdyne Technologies, Marietta, GA.)

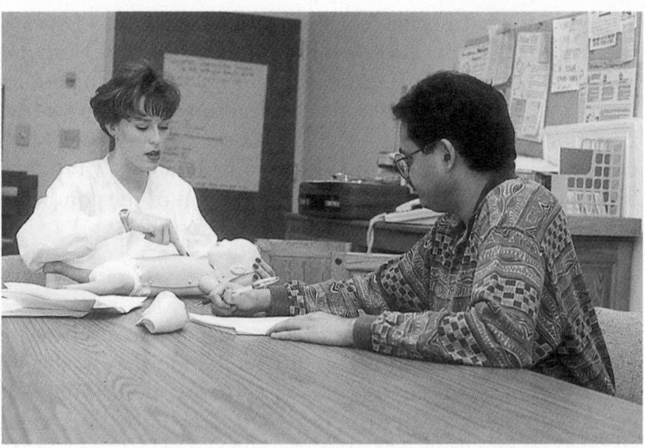

FIGURE 26.11 Parents of infants with respiratory disorders need to learn cardiac resuscitation before their infant is discharged from the hospital. Here a nurse teaches the technique using a doll.

Periventricular Leukomalacia

Periventricular leukomalacia (PVL) is abnormal formation of the white matter of the brain (Tsukimori et al., 2007). It is caused by an ischemic episode that interferes with circulation to a portion of the brain. Phagocytes and macrophages invade the area to clear away necrotic tissue. What is left is an abnormality in the white matter of the brain (revealed on a sonogram as a hollow space). PVL occurs most frequently in preterm infants who experience cerebral ischemia. Once the condition has occurred, there is no therapy. Infants may die of the original insult; they may be left with long-term effects such as learning disabilities. Any action to reduce environmental stimuli or sudden shifts in cerebral blood flow, such as avoiding rapid fluid infusions or sudden noises, is important in preventing PVL and limiting the long-term effects of prematurity (Brunssen & Harry, 2007).

Hemolytic Disease of the Newborn

The term "hemolytic" is derived from the Latin word for "destruction" (lysis) of red blood cells. Lysis of red blood cells in the newborn leads to **hyperbilirubinemia** (an elevated level of bilirubin in the blood). This can result from destruction of red blood cells by a normal physiologic process (see Chapter 18). When abnormal destruction of red blood cells occurs, it is termed hemolytic disease. In the past, hemolytic disease of the newborn was most often caused by an Rh blood type incompatibility. Because prevention of Rh antibody formation has been available for almost 40 years, the disorder is now most often caused by an ABO incompatibility. In both instances, the mother builds antibodies against an infant's red blood cells, leading to hemolysis (destruction) of the cells. The destruction of red blood cells causes severe anemia and hyperbilirubinemia from the bilirubin released from red cells. Prevention of the condition begins in pregnancy, as discussed in Chapter 21.

Rh Incompatibility

Theoretically, no direct connection exists between the fetal and maternal circulation, so no fetal blood cells should enter the maternal circulation. In actuality, occasional placental villi break and a drop or two of fetal blood does enter the maternal circulation. If the mother's blood type is Rh (D) negative and the fetal blood type is Rh positive (contains the D antigen), the introduction of fetal blood causes sensitization to occur, and the woman begins to form antibodies against the D antigen. Few antibodies form this way, however. Most form in the woman's bloodstream in the first 72 hours after birth because there is an active exchange of fetal–maternal blood as placental villi loosen and the placenta is delivered. After this sensitization, in a second pregnancy there will be a high level of antibody D circulating in the woman's bloodstream, which will then act to destroy the fetal red blood cells early in the pregnancy if the new fetus is Rh positive. By the end of pregnancy, a fetus can be severely compromised by the action of these antibodies crossing the placenta and destroying red blood cells. Some infants require intrauterine transfusions to combat red cell destruction. Preterm labor may be induced to remove the fetus from the destructive maternal environment. Administering phenobarbital to women during their last weeks of pregnancy has been tried to reduce symptoms in newborns as it speeds liver maturity so that the infant liver better converts indirect to direct bilirubin. This, unfortunately, also carries the risk of fetal sedation (Thomas, Muller, & Wilkinson, 2009).

ABO Incompatibility

In most instances of ABO incompatibility, the maternal blood type is O and the fetal blood type is A; it may also occur when the fetus has type B or AB blood. A reaction in an infant with type B blood is often the most serious.

Hemolysis can become a problem with a first pregnancy in which there is an ABO incompatibility as the antibodies to A and B cell types are naturally occurring antibodies or are present from birth in individuals whose red cells lack these antigens. Unlike the antibodies formed against the Rh D factor, these antibodies are of the large (IgM) class and do not cross the placenta. An infant of an ABO incompatibility, therefore, is not born anemic, as is the Rh-sensitized child. Hemolysis of the blood begins with birth, when blood and antibodies are exchanged during the mixing of maternal and fetal blood as the placenta is loosened; destruction of red cells may continue for up to 2 weeks of age. Interestingly, preterm infants do not seem to be affected by ABO incompatibility. This may be because the receptor sites for anti-A or anti-B antibodies do not appear on red cells until late in fetal life. Even in the mature newborn, a direct Coombs' test may be only weakly positive because of the few anti-A or anti-B sites present. The reticulocyte count (immature or newly formed red blood cells) is usually elevated as the infant attempts to replace destroyed cells.

Assessment

Rh incompatibility of the newborn can be predicted by finding a rising anti-Rh titer or a rising level of antibodies (indirect Coombs' test) in a woman during pregnancy. It can be confirmed by detecting antibodies on the fetal erythrocytes in cord blood (positive direct Coombs' test) by percutaneous umbilical blood sampling (see Chapter 9) or at birth. The mother in this situation will always have Rh-negative blood (*dd*), and the baby will be Rh positive (*DD* or *Dd*).

With Rh incompatibility, an infant may not appear pale at birth despite the red cell destruction that has occurred in utero. This is because the accelerated production of red cells during the last few months in utero compensates to some degree for the destruction. The liver and spleen may be enlarged from an attempt to destroy damaged blood cells. If the number of red cells has significantly decreased, the blood in the vascular circulation may be hypotonic to interstitial fluid; fluid will shift from the lower to higher isotonic pressure by the law of osmosis, causing extreme edema. Finally, the severe anemia can result in heart failure as the heart has to beat so fast to push the dilute blood forward. **Hydrops fetalis** is an old term for the appearance of a severely involved infant at birth. Hydrops refers to the edema, and fetalis refers to the lethal state.

Most infants do not appear jaundiced at birth because the maternal circulation has evacuated the rising indirect bilirubin level. With birth, progressive jaundice, usually occurring within the first 24 hours of life, will begin, indicating in both Rh and ABO incompatibility that a hemolytic process is at work. The jaundice occurs because as red blood cells are destroyed, indirect bilirubin is released. Indirect bilirubin is fat soluble and cannot be excreted from the body. Under normal circumstances, the liver enzyme glucuronyl transferase converts indirect bilirubin to direct bilirubin. Direct bilirubin is water soluble and combines with bile for excretion from the body with feces. In preterm infants or those with extreme hemolysis, the liver cannot convert indirect to direct bilirubin, so jaundice becomes extreme.

Pregnanediol, the breakdown product of progesterone, can interfere with the conjugation of indirect bilirubin. This is excreted in breast milk until the high levels of progesterone that were present during pregnancy are decreased, usually 24 to 48 hours after birth. Breastfed babies, therefore, may evidence more jaundice than bottle-fed babies.

Normally, cord blood has an indirect bilirubin level of 0 to 3 mg/100 mL. An increasing indirect bilirubin level is dangerous because if the level rises above 20 mg/dL in a term infant or 12 mg/dL in a preterm infant, brain damage from bilirubin-induced neurologic dysfunction (BIND) or a wide spectrum of disorders caused by increasingly severe hyperbilirubinemia that range from mild dysfunction to kernicterus (invasion of bilirubin into brain cells) can occur. An infant needs to use glucose stores to maintain metabolism in the presence of anemia. This can cause a progressive hypoglycemia, compounding the initial problem. A decrease in hemoglobin during the first week of life to a level less than that of cord blood is a later indication of blood loss or hemolysis.

Therapeutic Management

Initiation of early feeding, use of phototherapy, and exchange transfusion all may be immediate measures necessary to reduce indirect bilirubin levels in an infant affected by ABO or Rh incompatibility. In infants with severe hemolytic disease, the hemoglobin concentration may continue to drop during the first 6 months of life, or their bone marrow may fail to increase production of erythrocytes in response to continuing hemolysis. If this occurs, an infant may need an additional blood transfusion to correct this late anemia. Therapy with erythropoietin to stimulate red blood cell production is also possible.

Initiation of Early Feeding. Bilirubin is removed from the body by being incorporated into feces. Therefore, the sooner bowel elimination begins, the sooner bilirubin removal begins. Early feeding (either breast milk or formula), therefore, stimulates bowel peristalsis and accomplishes this.

Phototherapy. An infant's liver processes little bilirubin in utero because the mother's circulation does this for an infant. With birth, exposure to light apparently triggers the liver to assume this function. Additional light supplied by phototherapy appears to speed the conversion potential of the liver. In phototherapy, an infant is continuously exposed to specialized light such as quartz halogen, cool white daylight, or special blue fluorescent light. The lights are placed 12 to 30 inches above the newborn's bassinet or incubator. Specialized fiberoptic light systems incorporated into a fiberoptic blanket also have been developed and are ideal for home care. The infant is undressed except for a diaper so as much skin surface as possible is exposed to the light (Fig. 26.12).

Term newborns are generally scheduled for phototherapy when the total serum bilirubin level rises to 10 to 12 mg/dL at 24 hours of age; preterm infants may have treatment begun at levels lower than this (Symons & Mahoney, 2008).

Continuous exposure to bright lights this way may be harmful to a newborn's retina, so the infant's eyes must always be covered while under bilirubin lights. Eye dressings or cotton balls can be firmly secured in place by an infant mask.

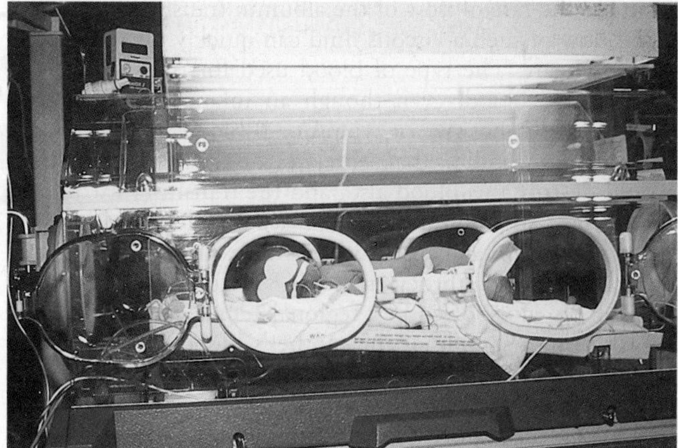

FIGURE 26.12 A newborn receiving phototherapy is undressed except for a diaper so he receives maximum exposure to the lights. His eyes are covered snugly to protect them from the bright light.

Check the dressings frequently to be certain they have not slipped or are causing corneal irritation. A constant concern is that suffocation from eye patches could occur.

The stools of an infant under bilirubin lights are often bright green because of the excessive bilirubin that is excreted as the result of the therapy. They are also frequently loose and may be irritating to skin. Urine may be dark-colored from urobilinogen formation. Monitor axillary temperature to prevent an infant from overheating under the bright lights. Assess skin turgor and intake and output to ensure that dehydration is not occurring from the warm environment.

Infants receiving phototherapy should be removed from under the lights for feeding so that they continue to have interaction with their mother. In addition, supplemental feedings with additional formula may be recommended to prevent dehydration. Remove the eye patches while the infant is with the mother to give an infant a period of visual stimulation. To prevent a lengthy hospital stay, infants may be discharged and continue therapy at home.

Parents need an explanation of the rationale for phototherapy. Incubators are automatically associated with seriously ill infants, but the use of lights does not seem scientific (almost a home remedy). Parents can easily be confused by the two interventions, one seemingly serious and the other seemingly not serious at all. Although the long-term effects have not yet been studied, there appears to be minimal risk to an infant from phototherapy, provided the infant's eyes remain covered and dehydration from increased insensitive water loss does not occur. It is too early to predict if all infants who receive phototherapy need follow-up in coming years to detect skin cancer that possibly could occur from the therapy (Newman & Maisels, 2007).

Home Phototherapy. Home phototherapy is primarily used for decreasing physiologic jaundice rather than that associated with blood incompatibility. It has the advantage of allowing for uninterrupted contact between the parents and a newborn and therefore has the potential to aid bonding. Parents must understand the importance of the therapy; the lights must be a full 12 inches away from an infant to prevent burning; an infant must continuously wear eye patches and a diaper during phototherapy to protect the retinas and the ovaries or testes; and bilirubin levels should be assessed approximately every 12 hours.

An infant should have the eye patches removed when away from the lights for feeding for a period of visual stimulation and interaction. The point at which infants are most apt to dislodge eye patches is when they cry as they wake for a feeding. Urge parents not to allow an infant under bilirubin lights to cry for a sustained period to avoid having this happen.

An infant's progress can be measured daily by a transcutaneous bilirubinometer, a hand-held fiberoptic light placed against an infant's skin. The intensity of the yellow color of the skin is measured by the meter, and a numeric level of bilirubin is calculated.

A newer innovation for hyperbilirubinemia management is the phototherapy blanket, a fiberoptic blanket that is wrapped around the baby. Light generated by the blanket has the same effect on bilirubin levels as banks of overhead lights. The advantages of a blanket are that an infant can be held for long periods without interrupting the phototherapy, and eye patches are unnecessary (Box 26.12).

Exchange Transfusion. Intensive phototherapy in conjunction with hydration and close monitoring of serum bilirubin levels is the preferred method of treatment of neonatal jaundice. Despite these measures, if bilirubin levels continue to rise, exchange transfusion may be necessary. Before the procedure, the baby's stomach is aspirated to minimize the risk of aspiration from the manipulation involved. The umbilical vein is catheterized as the site for transfusion. The procedure involves alternatively withdrawing small amounts (2–10 mL) of the infant's blood and then replacing it with equal amounts of donor blood. The blood is exchanged slowly this way to prevent alternating hypovolemia and hypervolemia. This can make an exchange transfusion a lengthy procedure of 1 to 3 hours. Automatic pumps are helpful to perform the exhausting repeated ritual. At the end of the procedure, using the last specimen of blood withdrawn, hematocrit, bilirubin, electrolytes (especially calcium), glucose determination, and blood culture are taken. Exchange transfusion may need to be repeated because additional unconjugated bilirubin from tissue moves into the circulation after the exchange.

The therapy may be used for any condition that leads to hyperbilirubinemia or polycythemia. When used as therapy for blood incompatibility, it removes approximately 85% of sensitized red cells. It reduces the serum concentration of indirect bilirubin and often prevents heart failure in infants. Because indirect bilirubin levels rise at relatively predictable levels, standards for performing exchange transfusion depend on the indirect bilirubin concentration, and transfusion is used when this level exceeds:

- 5 mg/100 mL at birth
- 10 mg/100 mL at age 8 hours
- 12 mg/100 mL at age 16 hours
- 15 mg/100 mL at 24 hours

It also may be used if the serum bilirubin level is rising more than 0.5 mg/hr in infants with Rh incompatibility or 1.0 mg/hr in infants with ABO incompatibility.

Keep a newborn warm during the procedure to prevent energy expenditure from having to maintain body temperature. Maintain the blood being given at room temperature, or shock from the cold insult can result. Use only commercial blood warmers to warm blood, not hot towels or a radiant heat warmer, to avoid destroying red cells.

Albumin may be administered 1 to 2 hours before the procedure to increase the number of bilirubin binding sites and to increase the efficiency of the transfusion. Be careful to monitor the rate of flow of the albumin transfusion, because rapid flow of such a viscous fluid can quickly overburden an infant's heart. The type of blood used for transfusion is O Rh-negative blood, even though an infant's blood type is positive; if Rh-positive or type A or B blood were given, the maternal antibodies that entered the infant's circulation would destroy this blood also, and the transfusion would be ineffective. An amount equal to twice the blood volume (average is 86 mL/kg) is used because this quantity will ensure an exchange of erythrocytes that is 85% to 90% effective. If the baby is transported to a regional center for the exchange transfusion, a sample of the mother's blood should accompany the infant, so cross-matching on the mother's serum can be done there.

During the transfusion, carefully monitor the newborn's heart rate, respirations, and blood pressure. Because blood stored for transfusion contains acid-citrate-dextrose (ACD), added to blood as an anticoagulant, which can lower blood calcium levels and cause acidosis, calcium gluconate is given

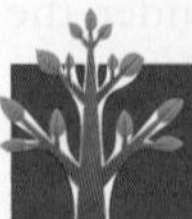

BOX 26.12 ✻ Focus on Family Teaching

Home Phototherapy Blanket

Q. Mrs. Atkins' doctor has ordered a phototherapy blanket for her to use at home to help reduce her son's jaundice. She asks you, "What are the rules for using the blanket effectively?"

A. Use the guidelines below to ensure the effectiveness of a home phototherapy blanket:

- Be aware that a home care nurse will assist you in setting up and using the equipment. The nurse will also obtain daily blood specimens to check your infant's bilirubin levels.
- Take your infant's temperature every 8 hours throughout the course of therapy. Because the blanket being used does not provide heat, changes in temperature may indicate a problem, such as an infection.
- Monitor your infant's urine output. Keep track of the number of diapers he wets.
- Also monitor your infant's bowel movements. He may have loose, green-tinged bowel movements as the bilirubin begins to break down. Keep the skin clean and dry to prevent irritation.
- Keep track of the amount (if bottle feeding) or duration (if breastfeeding) of feeding and the frequency of feedings. Usually, an infant receiving phototherapy should be fed approximately every 3 hours to prevent dehydration.
- Supplement formula or breast milk with glucose water unless you are told otherwise. An infant needs additional fluids during this time.
- When placing the child in the blanket device, be sure the fabric side goes against the infant's skin, with the lower portion on the outside of the baby's diaper. Be sure to fold the diaper down below the baby's navel in front and as far as possible in back so as much of the skin as possible is exposed to the light.
- Do not wrap the baby too tightly. Leave a space about the size of two fingers between the panel and the baby's skin.
- Do not be afraid to pick up the baby at any time and hold him. You can rock, cuddle, or feed him. Be careful not to walk around with the baby wrapped in the blanket, because you could trip on the cord and fall, injuring yourself or the baby.
- Call your pediatric care provider if you find any of the following: refusal of feedings, persistent temperature control problems, fewer than five wet diapers in 24 hours, pronounced change in the child's level of activity, or vomiting of entire feedings.

through the exchange catheter after each 100 mL of blood. If citrate-phosphate-dextrose was used as a preservative, hyperglycemia may occur during the transfusion from the dextrose in the preservative. This may be followed by overproduction of insulin and hypoglycemia in the infant. If heparinized blood is used, the heparin content may interfere with clotting after the transfusion. In addition, because of its relatively low glucose concentration, heparinized blood may also lead to hypoglycemia. Administering protamine sulfate aids in the metabolism of heparin and restoration of clotting ability.

After the transfusion, closely observe the infant for umbilical vessel bleeding. Redness or inflammation of the cord suggests infection. Report any changes in vital signs. Take and record a blood glucose determination at 1 hour after the procedure. Monitor bilirubin levels for 2 or 3 days after the transfusion to ensure the level of bilirubin is not rising again and that no further transfusion is necessary. Erythropoietin may be administered to increase new blood cell growth and prevent extended anemia.

Hemorrhagic Disease of the Newborn

Hemorrhagic disease of the newborn results from a deficiency of vitamin K (McNinch, Busfield, & Tripp, 2007). Vitamin K is essential for the formation of prothrombin by the liver. Lack of it causes decreased prothrombin function and impaired blood coagulation. Vitamin K is formed by the action of bacteria in the intestine. Because the intestinal tract of a newborn is sterile at birth, an infant forms minimal amounts of vitamin K until normal intestinal tract flora are established at about 24 hours of age. Babies born to women receiving anticonvulsive medication are at high risk for the condition because many of these medications interfere with vitamin K formation. Administering vitamin K intramuscularly to these women before birth can help to protect the newborn.

Newborns with vitamin K deficiency show petechiae from superficial bleeding into the skin. They may have conjunctival, mucous membrane, or retinal hemorrhage. They may vomit fresh blood or pass black, tarry stools because of bleeding into the gastrointestinal tract.

Distinguishing between tarry stools and normal meconium stools can be difficult in the first 1 or 2 days of life by simple observation. However, if an infant's stool does not change as it should from greenish-black (meconium) to the yellow color of a bottle-fed or breastfed baby, or if the stool color changes normally and then becomes black again, gastrointestinal bleeding should be suspected. You can check for the presence of blood in the stool by a dipstick guaiac test.

Vitamin K deficiency bleeding usually occurs on day 2 to day 5 of life, when the available prothrombin is at its lowest level. The prothrombin time will be prolonged; the coagulation time may be normal or prolonged.

Hemorrhagic disease of the newborn can be prevented by the intramuscular administration of 1 mg of vitamin K to all newborns immediately after birth. Make certain infants who were born in unusual circumstances, such as those born outside the hospital, are given vitamin K on their admission to the hospital nursery. Also double-check that infants whose birth involved an emergency, such as maternal hemorrhage or failure of the newborn to breathe spontaneously, have received it.

An infant who develops hemorrhagic disease of the newborn is treated with vitamin K, given intravenously or intramuscularly. If bleeding is severe, an infant may need a transfusion of fresh, whole blood to increase the prothrombin level immediately.

Handle infants with this disease extremely gently to prevent further bleeding, because they bruise easily from heavy pressure. Subdural hemorrhage may occur, making hemorrhagic disease a serious and potentially fatal disorder.

Twin-to-Twin Transfusion

Twin-to-twin transfusion is a phenomenon that can occur if twins are monozygotic (identical; share the same placenta) or if abnormal arteriovenous shunts occur that direct more blood to one twin than the other (Norton, 2007). The process occurs in as many as one third of all identical twin pregnancies. Enough blood is exchanged to be clinically important in only about 15% of such pregnancies. The result of this shift of blood leads to anemia in the donor twin and polycythemia in the receiving twin. The anemic twin may also be SGA because of the lack of nutrients or oxygen for growth. This same SGA twin will be prone to hypoglycemia from lack of glucose stores. The hypovolemic twin will appear pale next to the polycythemic twin; the polycythemic twin is prone to hyperbilirubinemia as the excessive red blood cell level is broken down.

Twin-to-twin transfusion can be identified in utero by a sonogram because one twin is noticeably larger than the other. All identical twins should have hemoglobin determinations done at birth and the results compared. A difference of more than 5.0 g per 100 mL is enough to suggest a transfusion has occurred. Each twin needs therapy as indicated by the extent of the blood distribution. The donor twin may need a transfusion to establish a functioning blood level; the recipient twin may need an exchange transfusion to reduce the polycythemia and viscosity of the blood.

✔ Checkpoint Question 26.4

Baby Atkins develops hyperbilirubinemia. What is a method used to treat hyperbilirubinemia in a newborn?

a. Keeping infants in a warm and dark environment.
b. Early feeding to speed passage of meconium.
c. Gentle exercise to stop muscle breakdown.
d. Administration of a cardiovascular stimulant.

Necrotizing Enterocolitis

Necrotizing enterocolitis (NEC) develops in approximately 5% of all infants in intensive care nurseries (Carter, 2007). The bowel develops necrotic patches, interfering with digestion and possibly leading to a paralytic ileus. Perforation and peritonitis may follow. NEC may occur as a complication of exchange transfusion. The disorder is discussed in Chapter 45.

Retinopathy of Prematurity

Retinopathy of prematurity (ROP), an acquired ocular disease that leads to partial or total blindness in children, is caused by vasoconstriction of immature retinal blood vessels. It was first recognized as an eye disorder in 1942, but only later was a high concentration of oxygen established as the causative agent (Askie & Henderson-Smart, 2009). Immature retinal blood vessels constrict when exposed to high oxygen concentrations. In addition, endothelial cells in the layer of nerve fibers in the periphery of the retina proliferate, leading to retinal detachment and blindness. Infants who are most immature and most ill (and consequently receive the most oxygen) are at highest risk.

A preterm infant who is receiving oxygen must have blood Po_2 levels monitored by pulse oximeter, transcutaneous oxygen saturation, or blood gas monitoring. Keeping blood Po_2 levels within normal limits lowers the risk. When blood Po_2 levels rise to higher than 100 mm Hg, the risk of the disease increases greatly.

In the past, once ROP occurred, there was no reversing it. Today, cryosurgery or laser therapy may be effective in preserving sight. A person experienced in recognizing ROP should examine the eyes of all low-birth-weight newborns and those who have received oxygen therapy before discharge from a hospital nursery and again at age 4 to 6 weeks of age to detect any occurrence of the syndrome. Nurses can be instrumental in limiting the occurrence of ROP by conscientious oxygen management (Coe, 2007).

THE NEWBORN AT RISK BECAUSE OF MATERNAL INFECTION OR ILLNESS

Maternal Infection

Newborns are susceptible to infection at birth because their ability to produce antibodies is immature. A number of infections in newborns, such as toxoplasmosis, rubella, syphilis, and cytomegalovirus infections, are spread to the fetus across the placenta in utero. The effect on the woman of these disorders is discussed in Chapter 12. Other infections are contracted from exposure to vaginal secretions at birth. Those infections are described next.

β-Hemolytic, Group B Streptococcal Infection

The major cause of infection in newborns is the β-hemolytic, group B streptococcal organism (GBS). This gram-positive bacterium is a natural inhabitant of the female genital tract. Between 50 and 300 infants in every 1000 live births display a positive culture for the organism (Heath & Schuchat, 2007). It may be spread from baby to baby if good handwashing technique is not used in handling newborns. If a woman is found to be positive for GBS during late pregnancy (see Chapter 21), ampicillin administered intravenously at 28 weeks and again during labor helps to reduce the possibility of newborn exposure.

Assessment. Typically, a newborn at risk, such as one born after prolonged rupture of membranes or if the woman's vaginal culture is positive for GBS, will be screened for infection with a blood culture.

Colonization by GBS can result in an early-onset or a late-onset illness. With the early-onset form, signs of pneumonia become apparent within the first day of life, as well as tachypnea, apnea, and signs of shock such as decreased urine output, extreme paleness, or hypotonia. A chest radiograph is almost indistinguishable from that of RDS (a ground-glass appearance). Pneumonia may develop so rapidly that as many as 20% of infants who contract the infection die within 24 hours of birth.

A late-onset type occurs at 2 to 4 weeks of age. With this, instead of pneumonia being the infection focus, meningitis tends to occur. Typical signs include lethargy, fever, loss of appetite, and bulging fontanelles from increased intracranial pressure as meningitis develops. Mortality from the late-onset type is not as high as that from the early-onset form (15% versus 20%), but neurologic consequences can occur in up to 50% of infants who survive.

Therapeutic Management. If a newborn displays signs or a blood screening test is positive, antibiotics are administered. Gentamicin, ampicillin, and penicillin are all effective against GBS infections.

Parents may have difficulty understanding how their infant could suddenly become this ill and may need a great deal of support in caring for their infant. This is even more important if the newborn survives the infection but is left neurologically challenged. In the future, immunization of all women of childbearing age against streptococcal B organisms could decrease the incidence of newborns infected at birth.

Ophthalmia Neonatorum

Ophthalmia neonatorum is an eye infection that occurs at birth or during the first month (MacDonald, Mailman, & Desai, 2008). The most common causative organisms are *Neisseria gonorrhoeae* and *Chlamydia trachomatis*. An infant contracts the organism during birth, from vaginal secretions. *N. gonorrhoeae* infection is an extremely serious form of conjunctivitis because, if left untreated, the infection progresses to corneal ulceration and destruction, resulting in opacity of the cornea and severe vision impairment.

Assessment. Ophthalmia neonatorum is generally bilateral. The conjunctivae become fiery red, with thick pus. The eyelids are edematous. Although this usually occurs on day 1 to day 4 of life, it should be considered as a possibility when conjunctivitis occurs in any infant younger than 30 days.

Prevention. The prophylactic instillation of erythromycin ointment into the eyes of newborns prevents both gonococcal and chlamydial conjunctivitis. In the past, eye prophylaxis was given immediately after birth so it was never forgotten. Now it is customary to delay administration of the ointment until after the first reactivity period so the newborn can clearly see the parents during this important attachment period. This makes it easy for administration to be forgotten, so use some type of a checklist as a reminder of this important prophylaxis. Infants born outside the hospital also need prophylaxis to prevent ophthalmia neonatorum, the same as infants born in a birthing room.

Therapeutic Management. Therapy is individualized depending on the organism cultured from the exudate. If gonococci are identified, intravenous ceftriaxone (Rocephin) and penicillin are effective drugs. If chlamydia is identified, an ophthalmic solution of erythromycin is used.

Use standard and contact infection precautions when caring for this newborn. In addition to systemic antibiotic therapy, the eyes are irrigated with sterile saline solution to clear the copious discharge. When irrigating eyes, use a sterile medicine dropper or bulb syringe, and use barrier protection, including goggles to avoid splashing any solution into your own eye. The solution should be at room temperature. Direct the stream of the irrigation fluid laterally so it does not enter and contaminate the other eye.

The mother of the infected infant needs treatment for gonorrhea or chlamydia, before fallopian tube sterility or pelvic inflammatory disease results. Sexual contacts of the mother should be treated also, so the spread of the disease can be halted. With either infection, parents can be assured that with early diagnosis and treatment the prognosis for normal eyesight in their child is good.

Hepatitis B Virus Infection

Hepatitis B virus (HBV) can be transmitted to the newborn through contact with infected vaginal blood at birth when the mother is positive for the virus (HBsAg+). Hepatitis B is a destructive illness: 70% to 90% of infected infants become chronic carriers of the virus. As many as 15% of these will develop liver cancer later in life (McKinlay & Matheny, 2007).

To reduce the possibility of HBsAg being spread to newborns in the future, infants are now routinely vaccinated at birth (Lee et al., 2009). If the mother is identified as HBsAg+, an infant is also administered immune serum globulin (HBIG) within 12 hours of birth to decrease the possibility of infection. The infant should be bathed as soon as possible after birth to remove HBV-infected blood and secretions. Gentle suctioning is necessary to avoid trauma to the mucous membrane, which could allow HBV invasion. Although the virus is transmitted in breast milk, once immune globulin has been administered, women may breastfeed without risk to an infant. Hepatitis B is further discussed in Chapter 45, because it also occurs in older children.

Generalized Herpesvirus Infection

A herpes simplex virus type 2 (HSV-2) infection, most prevalent among women with multiple sexual partners, can be contracted by a fetus across the placenta if the mother has a primary infection during pregnancy. More often, however, the virus is contracted from the vaginal secretions of a mother who has active herpetic vulvovaginitis at the time of birth. Between 15% and 30% of women of childbearing age demonstrate antibodies to this virus or have the potential to have active lesions during labor (American College of Obstetricians and Gynecologists [ACOG], 2007).

Assessment. If the infection was acquired during pregnancy, an infant may be born with vesicles covering the skin. The long-term prognosis of the child is guarded, because severe neurologic damage may have occurred simultaneously. If infants acquire the infection at birth, at approximately day 4 to day 7 of life they show a loss of appetite, perhaps a low-grade fever, and lethargy. Stomatitis (ulcers of the mouth) or a few vesicles on the skin appear. Herpes vesicles are always clustered, pinpoint in size, and surrounded by a reddened base. After the vesicles appear, infants become extremely ill. They develop dyspnea, jaundice, purpura, convulsions, and shock. Death may occur within hours or days. Between 25% and 70% of newborns who survive generalized herpesvirus infections have permanent central nervous system sequelae.

To confirm the diagnosis, cultures are obtained from representative vesicles as well as the nose, throat, anus, and umbilical cord. Blood serum is analyzed for IgM antibodies.

Therapeutic Management. An antiviral drug such as Acyclovir (Zovirax), a drug that inhibits viral deoxyribonucleic acid synthesis, is effective in combating this overwhelming infection. Prevention, however, is the newborn's best protection. Women with active herpetic vulvar lesions are advised to have cesarean birth rather than vaginal birth to minimize the newborn's exposure. Antenatal antiviral prophylaxis reduces viral shedding and recurrences at birth and reduces the need for cesarean birth (Hollier & Wendel, 2009). Infants with an infection should be separated from other infants. Although transmission from this source is rare, women with herpes lesions on their face (herpes simplex or cold sores) should not feed or hold their newborns until lesions are crusted and no longer contagious. Health care personnel who have herpes simplex infections should not care for newborns until the lesions are crusted. Although facial herpes simplex lesions are probably caused by herpesvirus type 1, limiting contact does not seem excessive in light of the severity of HSV-2 disease. Urge a woman who is separated from her newborn at birth to view her infant from the nursery window and participate in planning care to aid bonding.

Human Immunodeficiency Virus Infection

HIV infection and acquired immunodeficiency syndrome (AIDS) can be caused by placental transfer or direct contact with maternal blood during birth. As older children are also exposed to this, the care of children with this infection is discussed in Chapter 42.

An Infant of a Woman Who Has Diabetes Mellitus

An infant of a woman who has diabetes mellitus whose illness was poorly controlled during pregnancy is typically longer and weighs more than other babies (macrosomia). The baby also has a greater chance of having a congenital anomaly such as a cardiac anomaly, as if hyperglycemia is teratogenic to a rapidly growing fetus. **Caudal regression syndrome** (hypoplasia of the lower extremities) is a syndrome that occurs almost exclusively in such infants (Strehlow et al., 2007).

Most such babies have a cushingoid (fat and puffy) appearance. They tend to be lethargic or limp in the first days of life as a result of hyperglycemia. The macrosomia results from overstimulation of pituitary growth hormone and extra fat deposits created by high levels of insulin during pregnancy. The infant's large size is deceptive, however: such babies are often immature. RDS occurs frequently in these infants because they may be born preterm or, even at term, lecithin pathways may not mature as rapidly in them. High fetal insulin secretion during pregnancy to counteract the hyperglycemia may interfere with cortisol release. This could block the formation of lecithin and prevent lung maturity. A term frequently used for these infants is "fragile giant."

An infant of a diabetic woman loses a greater proportion of weight in the first few days of life than does the average newborn because of the loss of the extra fluid accumulated. Observe an infant closely to be certain that this large weight loss actually represents a loss of extra fluid and that dehydration is not occurring.

Complications

A macrosomic infant has a greater chance of birth injury, especially shoulder and neck injury. Cesarean birth may be necessary to avoid cephalopelvic disproportion. Immediately after birth, the infant tends to be hyperglycemic because the mother was at least slightly hyperglycemic during pregnancy and excess glucose transfused across the placenta. During pregnancy, the fetal pancreas responds to this high glucose level with islet cell hypertrophy, resulting in matching high insulin levels. After birth, as an infant's glucose level begins to fall because the mother's circulation is no longer supplying glucose, the overproduction of insulin will cause the development of severe hypoglycemia. Hyperbilirubinemia also may occur in these infants because, if immature, they cannot effectively clear bilirubin from their system. Hypocalcemia also frequently develops because parathyroid hormone levels are lower in these infants because of hypomagnesemia from excessive renal losses of magnesium.

Although infants of diabetic women are usually LGA, an infant born to a woman with extensive blood vessel involvement may be SGA because of poor placental perfusion. The problems of hypoglycemia, hypocalcemia, and hyperbilirubinemia remain the same.

Therapeutic Management

In a newborn, hypoglycemia is defined as a serum glucose level of less than 45 mg/dL. To avoid a serum glucose level from falling this low, infants of diabetic women are fed early with formula or administered a continuous infusion of glucose. It is important the infant not be given only a bolus of glucose; otherwise, rebound hypoglycemia (accentuating the problem) may occur. Some infants of diabetic women have a smaller-than-usual left colon, apparently another effect of intrauterine hyperglycemia, which limits the amount of oral feedings they can take in their first days of life. Signs of an inadequate colon include vomiting or abdominal distention after the first few feedings. Careful monitoring for normal bowel movements is important.

An Infant of a Drug-Dependent Mother

Infants of drug-dependent women tend to be SGA. If the woman is dependent on a drug, an infant will show withdrawal symptoms (neonatal abstinence syndrome) shortly after birth (Box 26.13). These include such signs as:

- Irritability
- Disturbed sleep pattern
- Constant movement, possibly leading to abrasions on the elbows, knees, or nose
- Tremors
- Frequent sneezing
- Shrill, high-pitched cry

Box 26.13 Assessment
Assessing the Newborn of a Drug-Addicted Mother

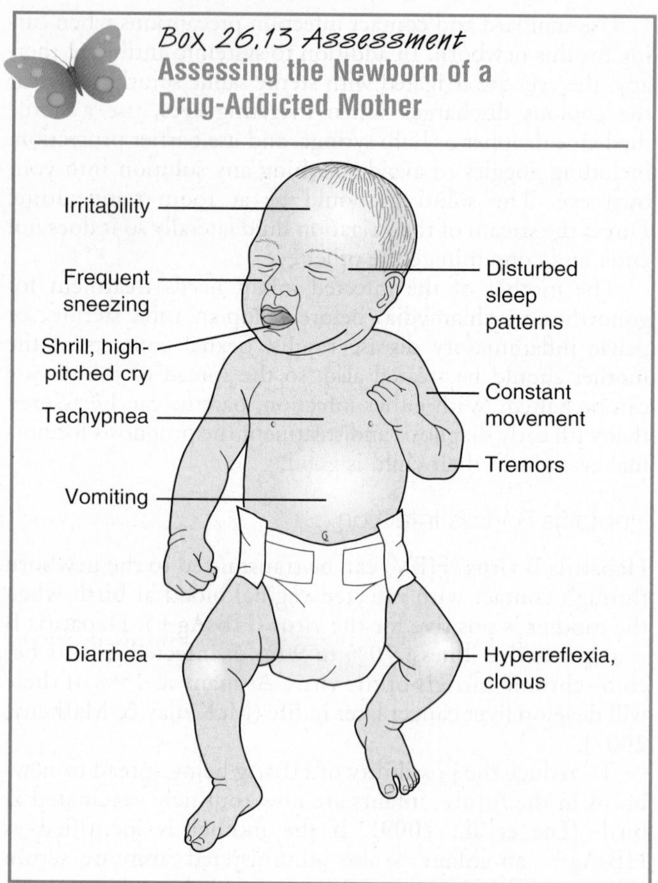

- Possible hyperreflexia and clonus (neuromuscular irritability)
- Convulsions
- Tachypnea (rapid respirations), possibly so severe that it leads to hyperventilation and alkalosis
- Vomiting and diarrhea, leading to large fluid losses and secondary dehydration

Specific neonatal abstinence scoring tools may be used to quantify and assess an infant's status. In newborns experiencing opiate withdrawal, signs usually begin 24 to 48 hours after birth, but in some infants they may not appear for up to 10 days. Generally signs last approximately 2 weeks, but mild signs may appear for up to 6 months. In heroin-addicted neonates, the signs begin within the first 2 weeks of life, with an average onset of approximately 72 hours. The signs may last 8 to 16 weeks or longer. In methadone-addicted newborns, withdrawal begins later and lasts longer than heroin withdrawal. The onset varies. A newborn may exhibit signs beginning at 24 to 28 hours, or these early signs may improve, then reappear at 2 to 4 weeks of age. Other newborns exhibit no signs until they are 2 to 3 weeks old.

There is no predictable withdrawal sequence noted for the cocaine-addicted neonate. Whether cocaine causes long-term effects varies with different studies, but factors such as maladaptive coping behaviors may be present in such newborns (Bernstein & Weinstein, 2007).

Narcotic metabolites or quinine (heroin is often mixed with quinine) may be obtained from an infant's urine or meconium in the first hour after birth. These products are quickly cleared from the body, however, so by the time symptoms become severe, detection of narcotic substances may no longer be possible. Cocaine may be detected in infants' hair samples for an extended time.

Infants of drug-dependent women usually seem most comfortable when firmly swaddled. Keep them in an environment free from excessive stimuli (a small isolation nursery, not a large, noisy one). Some quiet best if the room is darkened. Many infants of heroin-addicted women suck vigorously and continuously and seem to find comfort and quiet if given a pacifier. Infants of methadone- and cocaine-addicted women may have extremely poor sucking ability and may have difficulty achieving sufficient fluid intake unless gavage fed.

Specific therapy for an infant is individualized according to the nature and severity of the signs. Maintenance of electrolyte and fluid balance is essential. If an infant has vomiting or diarrhea, intravenous administration of fluid may be indicated. The drugs used to counteract withdrawal symptoms include paregoric, phenobarbital, methadone, chlorpromazine (Thorazine), and diazepam (Valium). These are typically used if the neonatal abstinence scoring system average score is elevated on three successive occasions and nursing interventions do not reduce the score. An infant should not be breastfed to avoid passing narcotics in breast milk to the child.

Once an infant has been identified as having been exposed to drugs in utero, the mother needs treatment for withdrawal symptoms and follow-up care as much as the infant. In addition, evaluation is necessary to determine before discharge whether an environment that allowed for drug abuse will be safe for an infant at home (Sun, Freese, & Fitzgerald, 2007). Infants who are exposed to drugs in utero may have long-term neurologic problems (Pulsifer et al., 2008).

An Infant With Fetal Alcohol Exposure

Alcohol crosses the placenta in the same concentration as is present in the maternal bloodstream. This results in fetal alcohol exposure and **fetal alcohol syndrome** (Elias, Tsai, & Manchester, 2008). The syndrome appears in about 2 per 1000 newborns and is often more difficult to document than recreational drug exposure. Alcohol has deteriorating effects on the placenta (Burd et al., 1007). Because it is unknown if there is a safe threshold of alcohol ingestion during pregnancy, all pregnant women are advised to avoid alcohol intake to prevent any teratogenic effects on their newborn (Welch & Mullins, 2007).

The newborn with fetal alcohol syndrome has several possible problems at birth. Characteristics that mark the syndrome include prenatal and postnatal growth restriction; central nervous system involvement such as cognitive challenge, microcephaly, and cerebral palsy; and a distinctive facial feature of a short palpebral fissure and thin upper lip. During the neonatal period, an infant may be tremulous, fidgety, and irritable and may demonstrate a weak sucking reflex. Sleep disturbances are common, with the baby tending to be either always awake or always asleep, depending on the mother's alcohol level close to birth.

The most serious long-term effect is cognitive challenge. Behavior problems such as hyperactivity may occur in school-age children. Growth deficiencies may remain throughout life. An infant needs follow-up so any future problems can be discovered. The mother needs follow-up to see if she can reduce her alcohol intake for better overall health.

✔ Checkpoint Question 26.5

Why is it important for infants of diabetic women to be fed early?

a. Their stomachs are empty at birth.
b. To help prevent hypoglycemia.
c. Their mothers could not eat during labor.
d. To clear mucus from their intestinal tracts.

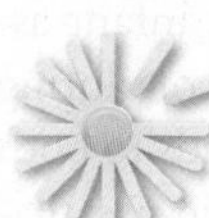

Key Points for Review

- Priorities for infants born with special needs, such as preterm or postterm infants, are the same as for term infants: initiation and maintenance of respirations, establishment of extrauterine circulation, control of body temperature, intake of adequate nourishment, establishment of waste elimination, establishment of an infant–parent relationship, prevention of infection, and provision of developmental care for mental and social development.
- Many high-risk infants need resuscitation at birth. Prompt action with such measures as warmth, oxygen, intubation, and suctioning are needed.
- A small-for-gestational-age infant is one whose birth weight is below the 10th percentile on an intrauterine growth curve for that age infant. An infant could be preterm, term, or postterm.
- Small-for-gestational-age infants have difficulty maintaining body warmth because of low fat stores and may develop hypoglycemia from low glucose stores.
- A large-for-gestational-age infant is one whose birth weight is above the 90th percentile on an intrauterine growth chart for that gestational age. The infant could be born preterm, term, or postterm.
- Large-for-gestational-age infants tend to be infants of diabetic women; they are particularly prone to hypoglycemia or birth trauma.
- A preterm infant is one born before 37 weeks of gestation. Preterm infants have particular problems with respiratory function, anemia, jaundice, persistent patent ductus arteriosus, and intracranial hemorrhage. Infants who are born weighing 1500 to 2500 g are also termed low-birth-weight infants; those born weighing 1000 to 1500 g are very-low-birth-weight infants; those born weighing between 500 and 1000 g are extremely very-low-birth-weight infants. All such infants need intensive care from the moment of birth to give them their best chance of survival without neurologic aftereffects caused by their being so close to the age of viability.
- A postterm infant is one who has remained in utero past week 42 of pregnancy. Postterm infants have particular problems with establishing respirations, meconium aspiration, hypoglycemia, temperature regulation, and polycythemia.
- Respiratory distress syndrome commonly occurs in preterm infants from a deficiency or lack of surfactant in the alveoli. Without surfactant, the alveoli collapse on ex-

piration and require extreme force for reinflation. Primary therapy is synthetic surfactant replacement at birth by endotracheal tube insufflation, followed by oxygen and ventilatory support.

- Transient tachypnea of the newborn is a temporary condition caused by slow absorption of lung fluid at birth. Close observation of the infant is necessary until the fluid is absorbed and respirations slow to a normal rate.
- Meconium aspiration syndrome occurs when an infant aspirates meconium-stained amniotic fluid before or during birth. Meconium is irritating to the airway and leads to both airway spasm and pneumonia. Infants need oxygen, ventilatory support, and possibly an antibiotic until the effects of the insult to the airway subside. Infants should be suctioned before oxygen administration under pressure to prevent meconium from being forced further into their lungs.
- Apnea is a pause in respirations longer than 20 seconds, with accompanying bradycardia. It tends to occur in preterm infants who have secondary stresses such as infection, hyperbilirubinemia, hypoglycemia, or hypothermia. Apnea monitors are used to detect this, and infants who are at high risk for apnea may be discharged home on a home monitoring program.
- Sudden infant death syndrome is the sudden, unexplained death of an infant. It is associated with infants sleeping on their stomachs (prone) and preterm birth. An important preventive measure is advising parents to position their infant on the back for sleeping.
- Hyperbilirubinemia results from the destruction of red blood cells, owing either to a normal physiologic response or an abnormal destruction of red blood cells. Hemolytic disease of the newborn is destruction of red blood cells from Rh or ABO incompatibility. The administration of RHIG (Rh antibodies) to Rh-negative mothers during pregnancy and after the birth of an Rh-positive infant to an Rh-negative mother has greatly reduced the incidence of the condition. Affected infants are jaundiced from release of bilirubin from injured red blood cells. Phototherapy and exchange transfusion are used to prevent kernicterus (deposition of bilirubin in brain cells, causing destruction of the cells).
- Hemorrhagic disease of the newborn is a lack of clotting ability resulting from a deficiency of vitamin K at birth. This disorder is prevented by administering vitamin K to infants at birth.
- Retinopathy of prematurity is destruction of the retina caused by exposure of immature retinal capillaries to high levels of oxygen. Monitoring oxygen saturation via arterial blood gases is an important preventive measure.
- Severe infections acquired at birth that may be seen in newborns include streptococcal group B pneumonia, hepatitis B infection, ophthalmia neonatorum (gonococcal and chlamydial conjunctivitis), and herpesvirus infection. Assessing newborns for symptoms of these infections is an important nursing responsibility.
- Infants of women with diabetes and those of drug-abusing women are at high risk at birth for further complications. Both need careful assessment for respiratory distress and hypoglycemia.

CRITICAL THINKING EXERCISES

1. The Atkinses are the family you met at the beginning of the chapter. Mrs. Atkins does not want to visit or "waste her favorite name" on her new baby because the baby might die. How would you advise her?
2. Infants who are cared for in neonatal nurseries may need either reduced stimulation because they fatigue so easily or increased stimulation because their stay in the nursery will be so extended. What are examples of developmental care you might use with Baby Atkins?
3. Retinopathy of prematurity is an example of a disease caused by the therapy given an infant. What measures would you take to safeguard Baby Atkins against this disorder?
4. Examine the National Health Goals related to high-risk newborns. Most government-sponsored funds for nursing research are allotted based on these goals. What would be a possible research topic to explore pertinent to these goals that would be applicable to the Atkins family and also advance evidence-based practice?

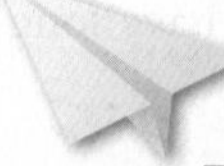

CRITICAL THINKING SCENARIO

Open the accompanying CD-ROM or visit http://thePoint.lww.com and read the Patient Scenario included for this chapter, then answer the questions to further sharpen your skills and grow more familiar with NCLEX style questions related to care of a family with a high-risk newborn. Confirm your answers are correct by reading the rationales.

REFERENCES

American Academy of Pediatrics. (2009). Car safety seats: a guide for families. http://www.aap.org/family/carseatguide.htm.

American College of Obstetricians and Gynecologists (ACOG). (2007). Management of herpes in pregnancy. *Obstetrics and Gynecology, 109*(6), 1489–1498.

American Heart Association. (2008). *Pediatric advanced life support.* Dallas, TX: Author.

Askie, L. M., & Henderson-Smart, D. J. (2009). Restricted versus liberal oxygen exposure for preventing morbidity and mortality in preterm or low birth weight infants. *Cochrane Database of Systematic Reviews, 2009*(1), (CD001077).

Barkin, R., & James, T. (2007). Sudden infant death syndrome (SIDS). In J. Schaider, et al. (Eds.). *Rosen & Barkin's 5-minute emergency medicine consult.* Philadelphia: Lippincott Williams & Wilkins.

Bernstein, H. B., & Weinstein, M. (2007). Normal pregnancy & prenatal care. In A. H. DeCherney & L. Nathan (Eds.). *Current diagnosis and treatment in obstetrics and gynecology* (10th ed.). Columbus, OH: McGraw-Hill.

Barrington, K. J., & Finer, N. N. (2009). Inhaled nitric oxide for respiratory failure in preterm infants. *Cochrane Database of Systematic Reviews, 2009*(1), (CD000509).

Brunssen, S. H., & Harry, G. J. (2007). Diffuse white matter injury and neurologic outcomes of infants born very preterm in the 1990s. *Journal of Obstetric, Gynecologic, and Neonatal Nursing, 36*(4), 386–395.

Burd, L., et al. (2007). Ethanol and the placenta: a review. *Journal of Maternal-Fetal and Neonatal Medicine, 20*(5), 361–375.

Carter, B. M. (2007). Treatment outcomes of necrotizing enterocolitis for preterm infants. *JOGNN: Journal of Obstetric, Gynecologic, and Neonatal Nursing, 36*(4), 377–385.

Coe, K. (2007). Nursing update on retinopathy of prematurity. *JOGNN: Journal of Obstetric, Gynecologic, and Neonatal Nursing, 36*(3), 288–292.

Coleman-Phox, K., Odouli, R., & Li, D. K. (2008). Use of a fan during sleep and the risk of sudden infant death syndrome. *Archives of Pediatrics and Adolescent Medicine, 162*(10), 963–968.

Conti, T. D. (2008). Breastfeeding and infant nutrition. In J. E. South-Paul, S. C. Matheny, & E. L. Lewis (Eds.). *Current diagnosis and treatment in family medicine* (2nd ed.). Columbus, OH: McGraw-Hill.

Copetti, R., & Cattarossi, L. (2007). The 'double lung point': an ultrasound sign diagnostic of transient tachypnea of the newborn. *Neonatology, 91*(3), 203–209.

Damato, E. G. (2007). 28 days. Safe sleep: can pacifiers reduce SIDS risk? *Nursing for Women's Health, 11*(1), 72–76.

Davies, M. W., & Sargent, P. H. (2009). Partial liquid ventilation for the prevention of mortality and morbidity in paediatric acute lung injury and acute respiratory distress syndrome. *Cochrane Database of Systematic Reviews, 2009*(1), (CD003845).

DeGrazia, M. (2007). Stability of the infant car seat challenge and risk factors for oxygen desaturation events. *JOGNN: Journal of Obstetric, Gynecologic, and Neonatal Nursing, 36*(4), 300–307.

Drenckpohl, D., Bowers, L., & Cooper, H. (2007). Use of the six sigma methodology to reduce incidence of breast milk administration errors in the NICU. *Neonatal Network: Journal of Neonatal Nursing, 26*(3), 161–166.

Donze, A., Smith, J. R., & Bryowsky, K. (2007). Safety and efficacy of ibuprofen versus indomethacin for the treatment of patent ductus arteriosus in the preterm infant: reviewing the evidence. *Neonatal Network: Journal of Neonatal Nursing, 26*(3), 187–195.

Elias, E. R., Tsai, A., & Manchester, D. K. (2008). Genetics and dysmorphology. In W. W. Hay, et al. (Eds.). *Current pediatric diagnosis and treatment* (18th ed.). Columbus, OH: McGraw-Hill.

El Shahed, A. I., et al. (2009). Surfactant for meconium aspiration syndrome in full term/near term infants. *Cochrane Database of Systematic Reviews, 2009*(1), (CD002054).

Fortner, K. B., Althaus, J.E., & Gurewitsch, E.D. (2007). Gestational complications. In K. B. Fortner, et al. (Eds.). *The Johns Hopkins manual of gynecology and obstetrics.* Philadelphia: Lippincott Williams & Wilkins.

Goldenberg, R. L., et al. (2008). Epidemiology and causes of preterm birth. *Lancet, 371*(9606), 75–84.

Greer, F. R. (2007). Post-discharge nutrition: what does the evidence support? *Seminars in Perinatology, 31*(2), 89–95.

Halliday, H. L., & Sweet, D. (2009). Endotracheal intubation at birth for preventing morbidity and mortality in vigorous, meconium-stained infants born at term. *Cochrane Database of Systematic Reviews, 2009*(1), (CD000500).

Heath, P. T., & Schuchat, A. (2007). Perinatal group B streptococcal disease. *Practice and Research in Clinical Obstetrics and Gynaecology, 21*(3), 411–424.

Herbst, A., & Kallen, K. (2007). Time between membrane rupture and delivery and septicemia in term neonates. *Obstetrics and Gynecology, 110*(3), 612–618.

Ho, J. J., et al. (2009). Continuous distending pressure for respiratory distress syndrome in preterm infants. *Cochrane Database of Systematic Reviews, 2009*(1), (CD002271).

Hollier, L. M., & Wendel, G. D. (2009). Third trimester antiviral prophylaxis for preventing maternal genital herpes simplex virus (HSV) recurrences and neonatal infection. *Cochrane Database of Systematic Reviews, 2009*(1), (CD004946).

Jones, E., & Spencer, S. A. (2007). Optimising the provision of human milk for preterm infants. *Archives of Disease in Childhood Fetal and Neonatal Edition, 92*(4), F236–F238.

Karch, A. M. (2009). *Lippincott's nursing drug guide.* Philadelphia: Lippincott Williams & Wilkins.

Knobel, R., & Holditch-Davis, D. (2007). Thermoregulation and heat loss prevention after birth and during neonatal intensive-care unit stabilization of extremely low-birth weight infants. *JOGNN: Journal of Obstetric, Gynecologic, and Neonatal Nursing, 36*(3), 280–287.

Kumar, V. H., et al. (2007). Characteristics of pulmonary hypertension in preterm neonates. *Journal of Perinatology, 27*(4), 214–219.

Lawrence, E. J. (2007). A matter of size: evaluating the large-for-gestational-age neonate. *Advances in Neonatal Care, 7*(4), 187–197.

Lee, C., et al. (2009). Hepatitis B immunisation for newborn infants of hepatitis B surface antigen-positive mothers. *Cochrane Database of Systematic Reviews, 2009*(1), (CD004790).

Leitner, Y., et al. (2007). Neurodevelopmental outcome of children with intrauterine growth retardation: a longitudinal, 10-year prospective study. *Journal of Child Neurology, 22*(5), 580–587.

Lindemann, R., et al. (2007). Bronchioalveolar lavage with perfluorochemical liquid during conventional ventilation. *Pediatric Critical Care Medicine, 8*(5), 486–488.

Maclaren, G., & Butt, W. (2007). Extracorporeal membrane oxygenation and sepsis. *Critical Care & Resuscitation, 9*(1), 76–80.

MacDonald, N., Mailman, T., & Desai, S. (2008). Gonococcal infections in newborns and in adolescents. *Advances in Experimental Medicine and Biology, 609*(5), 108–130.

McCall, E. M., et al. (2009). Interventions to prevent hypothermia at birth in preterm and/or low birth weight infants. *Cochrane Database of Systematic Reviews, 2009*(1), (CD004210).

McKinlay, R., & Matheny, S. C. (2008). Hepatobiliary disorders. In J. E. South-Paul, S. C. Matheny, & E. L. Lewis (Eds.). *Current diagnosis and treatment in family medicine* (2nd ed.). Columbus, OH: McGraw-Hill.

McNinch, A., Busfield, A., & Tripp, J. (2007). Vitamin K deficiency bleeding in Great Britain and Ireland. *Archives of Disease in Childhood, 92*(9), 759–766.

Moore, E. R., Anderson, G. C., & Bergman, N. (2009). Early skin-to-skin contact for mothers and their healthy newborn infants. *Cochrane Database of Systematic Reviews, 2009*(1), (CD003519).

National Vital Statistics System (NVSS), National Center for Vital Statistics. (2009). *Trends in the health of Americans.* Hyattsville, MD: Author.

Newman, T. B., & Maisels, M. J. (2007). Evidence insufficient to recommend melanoma surveillance following phototherapy for jaundice. *Archives of Dermatology, 143*(9), 1216.

Norton, M. E. (2007). Evaluation and management of twin-twin transfusion syndrome: still a challenge. *American Journal of Obstetrics and Gynecology, 196*(5), 419–420.

Pinheiro, J. M. (2009). The Apgar cycle: a new view of a familiar scoring system. *Archives of Disease in Childhood Fetal & Neonatal Edition, 94*(1), F70–72.

Playfor, S., et al. (2007). Consensus guidelines for sustained neuromuscular blockade in critically ill children. *Paediatric Anaesthesia, 17*(9), 881–887.

Pulsifer, M. B., et al. (2008). Prenatal drug exposure: effects on cognitive functioning at 5 years of age. *Clinical Pediatrics, 47*(1), 58–65.

Raab, E. L. (2007). The resuscitation and care of the newborn at risk In A. H. DeCherney & L. Nathan (Eds.). *Current diagnosis and treatment in obstetrics and gynecology* (10th ed.). Columbus, OH: McGraw-Hill.

Radhakrishnan, R. S., et al. (2007). ECMO for meconium aspiration syndrome: support for relaxed entry criteria. *ASAIO: American Society for Artificial Internal Organs Journal, 53*(4), 489–491.

Rahimian, J., & Varner, M. W. (2007). Disproportionate fetal growth. In A. H. DeCherney & L. Nathan (Eds.). *Current diagnosis and treatment in obstetrics and gynecology* (10th ed.). Columbus, OH: McGraw-Hill.

Raloff, J. (2007). Bad for baby: new risks found for plastic constituent. *Science News,* (7) 11.

Saigal, S., & Doyle, L. W. (2008). An overview of mortality and sequelae of preterm birth from infancy to adulthood. *Lancet, 371*(9608), 261–269.

Shah, S., & Sharieff, G. Q. (2007). An update on the approach to apparent life-threatening events. *Current Opinion in Pediatrics, 19*(3), 288–294.

Shiao, S., & Ou, C. N. (2007).Validation of oxygen saturation monitoring in neonates. *American Journal of Critical Care, 16*(2), 168–178.

Sirotnak, A. P., & Krugman, R. D. (2008). Child abuse and neglect. In W. W. Hay, et al. (Eds.). *Current pediatric diagnosis and treatment* (18th ed.). Columbus, OH: McGraw-Hill.

Sisk, P. M., et al. (2007). Early human milk feeding is associated with a lower risk of necrotizing enterocolitis in very low birth weight infants. *Journal of Perinatology, 27*(7), 428–433.

Snow, T., & Brandon, D. (2007). A nurse's guide to common mechanical ventilation techniques and modes used in infants: nursing implications. *Advances in Neonatal Care, 7*(1), 8–21.

Strehlow, S. L., et al. (2007). Diabetes mellitus and pregnancy. In A. H. DeCherney & L. Nathan (Eds.). *Current diagnosis and treatment in obstetrics and gynecology* (10th ed.). Columbus, OH: McGraw-Hill.

Stephens, C., & Fawcett, T. N. (2007). Nitric oxide and nursing: a review. *Journal of Clinical Nursing, 16*(1), 67–76.

Sun, A., Freese, M. P., & Fitzgerald, M. (2007). An exploratory study of drug-exposed infants: case substantiation and subsequent child maltreatment. *Child Welfare, 86*(3), 33–50.

Symington, A., & Pinelli, J. (2009). Developmental care for promoting development and preventing morbidity in preterm infants. *Cochrane Database of Systematic Reviews, 2009*(1), (CD001814).

Szymanski, L. M., & Bienstock, J. L. (2007). Complications of labor and delivery. In K. B. Fortner, et al. (Eds.). *The Johns Hopkins manual of gynecology and obstetrics.* Philadelphia: Lippincott Williams & Wilkins.

Symons, A. B., & Mahoney, M. C. (2008). Neonatal hyperbilirubinemia. In J. E. South-Paul, S. C. Matheny, & E. L. Lewis (Eds.). *Current diagnosis and treatment in family medicine* (2nd ed.). Columbus, OH: McGraw-Hill.

Thilo, E. H., & Rosenberg, A. A. (2008). The newborn. In W. W. Hay, et al. (Eds.). *Current pediatric diagnosis and treatment* (18th ed.). Columbus, OH: McGraw-Hill.

Thomas, J. T., Muller, P., & Wilkinson, C. (2009). Antenatal phenobarbital for reducing neonatal jaundice after red cell isoimmunization. *Cochrane Database of Systematic Reviews, 2009*(1), (CD005541).

Thomas, K. A., & Uran, A. (2007). How the NICU environment sounds to a preterm infant. *MCN: The American Journal of Maternal/Child Nursing, 32*(4), 250–253.

Tsukimori, K., et al. (2007). Increased inflammatory markers are associated with early periventricular leukomalacia. *Developmental Medicine and Child Neurology, 49*(8), 587–590.

Welch, G. L., & Mullins, S. M. (2007). Special issues in child care: supporting infants prenatally exposed to drugs and alcohol. *Zero to Three, 27*(4), 26–33.

Wiswell, T. E., Tin, W., & Ohler, K. (2007). Evidence-based use of adjunctive therapies to ventilation. *Clinics in Perinatology, 34*(1), 191–204.

SUGGESTED READINGS

Claudius, I., & Keens, T. (2007). Do all infants with apparent life-threatening events need to be admitted? *Pediatrics, 119*(4), 679–683.

Hamilton, K. E. S., Redshaw, M. E., & Tarnow-Mordi, W. (2007). Nurse staffing in relation to risk-adjusted mortality in neonatal care. *Neonatal Intensive Care, 20*(4), 37–42.

Iams, J. D., et al. (2008). Primary, secondary, and tertiary interventions to reduce the morbidity and mortality of preterm birth. *Lancet, 371*(9607), 164–175.

Klebanoff, M. A. (2008). Paternal and maternal birth weights and the risk of infant preterm birth. *American Journal of Obstetrics and Gynecology, 198*(1), 58–59.

Shaker, C. S., & Woida, A. M. (2007). An evidence-based approach to nipple feeding in a level III NICU: nurse autonomy, developmental care, and teamwork. *Neonatal Network: Journal of Neonatal Nursing, 26*(2), 77–83.

Taylor, A. K., Cousins, R., & Butt, W. W. (2007).The long-term outcome of children managed with extracorporeal life support: an institutional experience. *Critical Care and Resuscitation, 9*(2), 172–177.

Thoyre, S. M. (2007). Feeding outcomes of extremely premature infants after neonatal care. *Journal of Obstetric, Gynecologic, and Neonatal Nursing, 36*(4), 366–376.

Tsai, J., et al. (2007). Patterns and average volume of alcohol use among women of childbearing age. *Maternal and Child Health Journal, 11*(5), 437–445.

Valcamonico, A., et al. (2007). Mid- and long-term outcome of extremely low birth weight (ELBW) infants: an analysis of prognostic factors. *Journal of Maternal-Fetal and Neonatal Medicine, 20*(6), 465–471.

Wilkinson, A. R., et al. (2009). Management of babies born extremely preterm at less than 26 weeks of gestation. *Archives of Disease in Childhood Fetal & Neonatal Edition, 94*(1), F2–5.

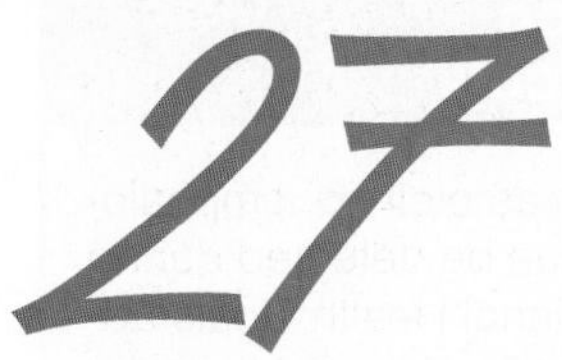

Chapter 27 Nursing Care of the Child Born With a Physical or Developmental Challenge

KEY TERMS

- ankyloglossia
- atresia
- cleft lip
- cleft palate
- developmental hip dysplasia
- fistula
- frenulum
- hydrocephalus
- meconium plug
- omphalocele
- polydactyly
- spina bifida
- stenosis
- syndactyly
- transillumination
- volvulus

OBJECTIVES

After mastering the contents of this chapter, you should be able to:

1. Describe common physical and developmental birth disorders.
2. Identify National Health Goals related to children born physically or developmentally challenged that nurses can help the nation achieve.
3. Use critical thinking to analyze the effect of a physically or developmentally challenged child on a family and propose ways to make care more family centered.
4. Assess a child who is born physically or developmentally challenged.
5. Formulate nursing diagnoses for children born with a physical or developmental challenge.
6. Establish expected outcomes to meet the needs of a child with a physical or developmental challenge.
7. Plan nursing care to meet the needs of a child born with a physical or developmental challenge such as encouraging mobility.
8. Implement nursing interventions for care of children born with physical or developmental challenges, such as preventing infection in a child with a neural tube disorder.
9. Evaluate expected outcomes to determine achievement and effectiveness of care.
10. Identify areas related to physically or developmentally challenged infants that could benefit by additional nursing research or application of evidence-based practice.
11. Integrate knowledge of congenital physical or developmental challenges with the nursing process to achieve quality maternal and child health nursing care.

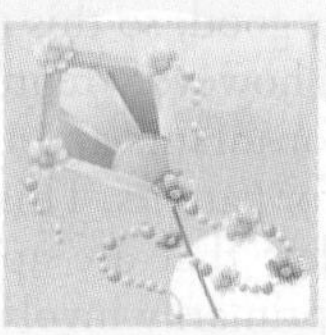

Bobby Jo Sparrow, age 16, is a new mother whose child has been admitted to the neonatal intensive care unit because of a neural tube disorder and congenital hip dysplasia. Ms. Sparrow is obviously upset over the diagnosis. She says, "I'm a good person. The only thing I did wrong during pregnancy was to take some cough medicine, so how could this have happened?"

Previous chapters described the importance of assessing all infants at birth. This chapter adds information about common congenital anomalies or structural disturbances that may occur in newborns. This information can serve as a basis for newborn assessment and for health teaching for parents.

How would you answer this mother? What type of advice would be most helpful to her?

Few things can change the usually joyous tone of a birthing room faster than the birth of a baby with a physical or developmental challenge. Physicians or nurse-midwives, who are used to saying "perfect boy" or "beautiful girl" and holding up the infant for the parents' first glance, are suddenly without words. Words of congratulations hang unsaid in the air.

When a child is born with an apparent physical or developmental challenge, nurses must play a major role in supporting and educating the parents to help them move forward from this point. Some congenital disorders require surgery but the prognosis is good, so this is only a temporary concern. Other disorders, however, represent serious, even life-threatening concerns for infants and financially draining long-term responsibilities for parents. This chapter covers the physical congenital disorders that are apparent at birth or soon after. Such disorders primarily involve the gastrointestinal, neurologic, and skeletal systems. Congenital disorders of the cardiovascular system, which also represent life-threatening problems for an infant, are addressed in Chapter 41. National Health Goals related to children with congenital anomalies are shown in Box 27.1.

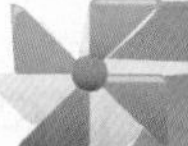

BOX 27.1 * Focus on National Health Goals

Many congenital anomalies, such as cleft lip, omphalocele, and neural tube disorders, can be detected during intrauterine life. The following National Health Goals address the importance of early identification and therapy:

- Reduce the occurrence of developmental disabilities by 5% (actual rate varies with condition).
- Reduce the occurrence of spina bifida and other neural tube disorders by 50% from a baseline of 6 per 10,000 births to 3 per 10,000 births.
- Increase the proportion of pregnancies begun with an optimal folic acid level from a baseline of 21% to a target level of 80%.
- Increase the proportion of territories and states that have service systems for children with special health care needs to 100% from a baseline of 15% (http://www.nih.gov).

Nurses can help the nation achieve these goals by ensuring that women obtain prenatal care and receive comprehensive advice after diagnosis of a fetal disorder.

Additional nursing research in this area is needed concerning factors that determine which women will continue their pregnancies after a congenital anomaly is discovered in the fetus; how far it is reasonable to ask parents to travel for follow-up care for a newborn; the measures parents feel were most helpful to them at the time that a fetal or newborn anomaly was diagnosed; and the most effective way to inform all women about the importance of folic acid during pregnancy.

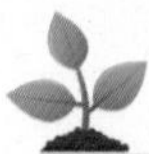

Nursing Process Overview

For Care of a Physically or Developmentally Challenged Child

Assessment

Nursing assessment of a physically or developmentally challenged newborn focuses on determining an infant's immediate physiologic needs required to sustain life and the parents' immediate emotional needs to promote bonding between the child and parents. Assess how the anomaly affects the infant's eight primary needs:

- Establishment and maintenance of adequate respiration
- Establishment of extrauterine circulation
- Establishment of normal body temperature
- Ability to take in adequate nourishment
- Establishment of waste elimination
- Prevention of infection
- Development of an infant–parent bond
- Exposure to adequate stimulation

The parents' response to the diagnosis of a congenital challenge must also be assessed. Anomalies that affect a child's appearance may have the most immediate effect on the parents' ability to establish a positive feeling about their child. It is important, however, not to jump to conclusions about parents' responses. Assessment of the family's verbal and nonverbal responses may reveal parents ready to meet this infant's special needs.

Nursing Diagnosis

Many nursing diagnoses established for children who are physically or developmentally challenged address the effect of the disorder on body function, including the child's primary needs, and also on family interaction. Examples of possible diagnoses are:

- Imbalanced nutrition, less than body requirements, related to inability to take in adequate nutrition secondary to physical challenge
- Impaired physical mobility related to congenital anomaly
- Risk for impaired parenting related to birth of child with congenital anomaly
- Anticipatory grieving (parental) related to loss of "perfect" child

Outcome Identification and Planning

Nurses play an important role in providing care to high-risk infants at birth and guarding their health until a child care team arrives to transport the infant to a high-risk nursery. When establishing expected outcomes and planning care, be certain to consider both the short- and long-term needs of the newborn and how these needs may affect the family. Also consider the family's resources, both emotional and financial, and devise a plan of care with these in mind. Parents with supportive family members nearby may be able to accept the limits of a child's challenge and turn their attention to the planned treatment regimen or care priorities sooner than those without close friends or relatives to whom they can turn for comfort and support. For the latter, you may need to act not only as a source of information and support but also as a sounding board and advocate until the parents can begin to develop positive coping mechanisms that will help them come to terms with this unexpected event. Referrals for support groups may be beneficial, allowing parents to learn they are not alone in this situation. The following organizations can be helpful sources of support for parents: National Easter Seal Society (http://www.easterseals.com), Spina Bifida Association of America (http://www.sbaa.org), March of Dimes Birth Foundation (http://www.marchofdimes.com), and American Cleft Palate Foundation (http://www.cleftline.org).

Implementation

Nursing interventions for a baby born physically challenged include immediate life-sustaining measures such as providing for adequate intake of nutrients when a disorder prevents the infant from sucking. Educating the parents about pretreatment and posttreatment procedures and encouraging them to hold, touch, and talk with their baby are especially important to the future emotional well-being of the child and family.

Parents may suffer a loss of self-esteem with the child's birth, feeling as if the baby is proof that something in the combination of their genes or the prenatal environment they provided was inadequate. They may need to hear positive comments about themselves and need to be given support until they can realize that by caring for the child they are accomplishing more, not less, than other couples.

You can expect parents to move through the same stages of grief as those whose child has died at birth. Chapter 56 describes those stages and helpful nursing interventions in more detail.

Parents are acutely aware of what people think of their child. They watch closely how nurses and other health care providers handle their baby to see if they are giving as much attention to their baby as to other babies. To encourage parents to accept the child, be certain to treat the child in the same manner as any other—for example, rocking the baby after feeding or cooing and talking to the baby as much as with other babies. Otherwise, parents may think that if a professional finds their child distasteful, how will they dare show the child to their family and friends? If you are able to look past the anomaly to the whole child, however, they begin to do so, too. Through positive role modeling, you can set the stage for healthy parent–child interaction every time you handle an infant born with a physical or developmental challenge.

Outcome Evaluation

Evaluation should focus on expected outcomes established for a child's physical health and developmental needs, as well as the family's ability to cope with whatever special care and growth needs the child may have in the future. Be sure parents have numbers to call for questions, follow-up care, and support.

Evidence suggesting achievement of expected outcomes may include:

- Parent describes positive features of child by 2 weeks.
- Parents state they understand talipes anomaly is a correctable condition by 1 month.
- Child is ambulatory with walker by 2 years of age.

IMMEDIATE CARE AT THE BIRTH OF AN INFANT BORN PHYSICALLY OR DEVELOPMENTALLY CHALLENGED

Most physicians and nurse-midwives believe that relating the news of congenital physical or developmental anomalies to parents is their responsibility. However, because the physician or nurse-midwife must deliver the placenta and suture the perineum if an episiotomy was used for birth, if a neonatal specialist is not immediately available, many minutes may pass before this person is ready to make a second inspection of the baby, assess the extent of the disorder from the physical symptoms present, and tell the parents about the baby's condition and prognosis. This delay affects the parents in two ways: It leaves them believing they have just given birth to a perfect child among people who do not share their enthusiasm, or they have just given birth to a child so deformed all the professionals in the room find it too horrible to even talk to them. Because parents are aware of the atmosphere in a birthing room, the second response is by far more likely. In terms of parent–child interaction, this response is unhealthy. Parents may begin anticipatory grieving for what they believe is a severely deformed child. Even when they are told later the disorder is not extensive and is easily correctable, and that as soon as the correction is made the child will be fine, the anticipatory grief reaction may be hard to stop. They may continue to cut themselves off emotionally from their child.

For this reason, nurses need to be familiar with the most frequently encountered physical or developmental anomalies so that as the person who at that moment in the birth process is most available for patient education, they can explain the problem to parents. In other instances, nurses must be ready to serve as back-up informants to answer parents' questions after they have been told by a primary care provider their child has been born less than perfect (Glenny et al., 2009).

The causes of most congenital anomalies are unknown, although they probably arise from a combination of environmental and genetic factors. Still, many people persist in believing that infants with congenital anomalies are born to people less deserving than others or to those who have sinned or have been looked on by someone with envy during pregnancy. That eating raisins during pregnancy causes brown spots, and that strawberries cause hemangiomas, are common beliefs that are still prevalent.

New parents need explanation of their child's disorder and a chance to talk about why they believe their child's disorder occurred, to relieve their guilt that they were the cause and to allow them to regain sufficient self-esteem to be able to raise a child with a congenital disorder.

It is probably best to explain to parents what the disorder consists of and what the usual prognosis is before showing the baby to them. Parents may find it hard to look at an infant with a cleft lip or palate or exposed abdominal contents, for example, and also listen. Their minds are so consumed with the sight, so unlike the child they had imagined, that they cannot hear. A typical explanation would be: "Your baby's upper lip isn't completely formed. That's called a cleft lip. Your doctor will call one of the plastic surgeons here to look at your baby. This is a problem that can be repaired so well surgically you'll barely be able to tell your baby had this problem. I'll bring the baby over so you can see her. Remember when you look at her this can be repaired. She seems perfect in every other way."

These statements define and limit the problem for the parents. They also give them direction about where and how they should proceed in beginning to seek help for their child. As most congenital abnormalities involve surgery, be certain to plan for adequate pain assessment and management postoperatively to make the experience of surgery this early in life not an unbearable procedure for a neonate (American Academy of Pediatrics [AAP], 2007).

PHYSICAL AND DEVELOPMENTAL DISORDERS OF THE GASTROINTESTINAL SYSTEM

Many of the most common congenital anomalies involve the gastrointestinal system because the gastrointestinal tract forms first as a solid tube, then undergoes canalization. If this canalization does not occur, a partial or complete blockage or obstruction can occur. Other disorders of the tract, such as cleft lip and cleft palate, are the result of midline closure failure extremely early in intrauterine life. All of these disorders can interfere with an infant's ability to take in nourishment at birth. You may need to reinforce a mother's resolve to breastfeed as appropriate to aid in her success with this method of feeding.

Ankyloglossia (Tongue-Tie)

Ankyloglossia is an abnormal restriction of the tongue caused by an abnormally tight **frenulum,** the membrane attached to the lower anterior tip of the tongue (Kelley et al., 2008). Normally, in newborns, the frenulum appears short and is positioned near the tip of the tongue. As the anterior portion of the infant's tongue grows, the frenulum becomes located farther back. In most instances, therefore, an infant suspected of being tongue-tied has a normal tongue at birth; it just seems short to parents who are unaware of a newborn's appearance. This condition rarely causes speech difficulty or destructive pressure on gingival tissue. If it does, then surgical release can be performed, but this is rare.

Showing parents other newborns or photographs of normal tongues is helpful in convincing them a short frenulum is normal. Explore with them why they are concerned. Is there a child in the family with a speech disorder or a cleft lip and palate? Do the parents need assurance in any other way that their child is all right?

Thyroglossal Cyst

A thyroglossal cyst arises from an embryogenic fault that leaves a cyst formed at the base of the tongue, which then drains through a **fistula** (opening) to the anterior surface of the neck (Lin & Deschler, 2008). This condition may occur as a dominantly inherited trait. The cyst may involve the hyoid bone (the bone at the anterior surface of the neck at the root of the tongue) or may contain aberrant thyroid gland tissue. As the cyst fills with fluid, swelling and obstruction can lead to respiratory difficulty from pressure on the trachea. If infected, the cyst appears swollen and reddened, with drainage of mucus or pus from the anterior neck.

The cyst is surgically removed to avoid future infection of the space or, if thyroid tissue is present, the possibility of developing thyroid carcinoma later in life. Observe infants closely in the immediate postoperative period for respiratory distress, because the operative area will develop some edema from surgical trauma. Position infants on their sides so secretions drain freely from their mouths. Intravenous fluid therapy is given after surgery until the edema at the incision recedes somewhat and swallowing is safe once more (approximately 24 hours). If the mother is breastfeeding but the infant is NPO, encourage her to express her milk manually to preserve her milk supply. Observe infants closely the first time they take fluid orally to be certain they do not aspirate. Be certain parents feed their infant before the infant is discharged from the surgical unit so they can see that the infant is swallowing safely. This is important to help them develop confidence in themselves as parents and their ability to feed the infant at home in a relaxed and comfortable way.

Cleft Lip and Palate

The maxillary and median nasal processes normally fuse between weeks 5 and 8 of intrauterine life. In infants with **cleft lip,** the fusion fails to occur in varying degrees, causing this disorder to range from a small notch in the upper lip to total separation of the lip and facial structure up into the floor of the nose, with even the upper teeth and gingiva absent. The deviation may be unilateral or bilateral. The nose is generally flattened because the incomplete fusion of the upper lip has allowed it to expand in a horizontal dimension (see Fig. 7.12). Cleft lip is more prevalent among boys than girls. It occurs at a rate of approximately 1 in every 750 live births. This incidence is significantly higher in the Asian population, 1 in 300, and significantly lower in the black population, 1 in 2000. About 46% of children have combined cleft lip and palate, 21% only a cleft lip, and 33% only a cleft palate. Almost 30% of children with cleft lip and palate deformity have associated birth defects or the cleft palate occurs as only a portion of a larger syndrome (Hoffman, 2008).

Cleft lip occurs as a familial tendency or most likely occurs from the transmission of multiple genes. Formation may be aided by teratogenic factors present during weeks 5 to 8 of intrauterine life, such as a viral infection or possibly a

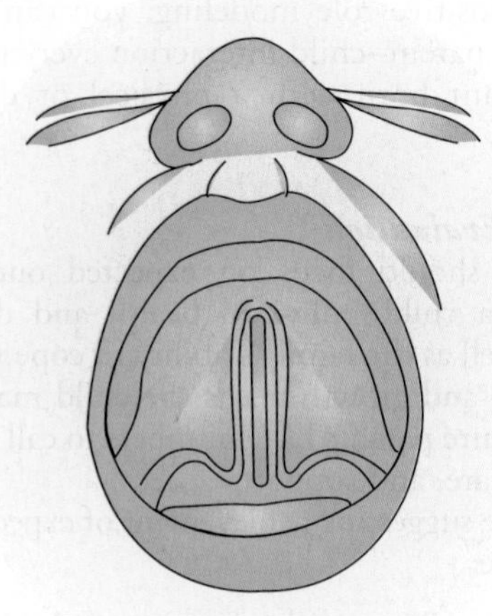

FIGURE 27.1 Appearance of a cleft palate. Both the hard and soft palate are involved.

deficiency of folic acid (Novak, 2007). Parents of a child with a cleft lip should be referred for genetic counseling to ensure they understand that they have about a 4% chance of having another child with a cleft lip or palate or future children are at a greater risk than usual for this problem.

The palatal process closes at approximately weeks 9 to 12 of intrauterine life. A **cleft palate,** an opening of the palate, is usually on the midline and may involve the anterior hard palate, the posterior soft palate, or both (Fig. 27.1). It may be a separate anomaly, but as a rule it occurs in conjunction with a cleft lip. As a single entity, it tends to occur more frequently in girls than boys. Like cleft lip, it appears to be the result of polygenic inheritance or environmental influences. In connection with cleft lip, the incidence is approximately 1 in every 1000 births. As a single entity, it occurs in approximately 1 in every 2000 births (Hoffman, 2008).

Assessment

Cleft lip may be detected by a sonogram while an infant is in utero. If not detected then, it is readily apparent on inspection at birth. Cleft palate can be determined by depressing the newborn's tongue with a tongue blade. This reveals the total palate and the extent of any cleft present. Be sure to have good lighting to visualize the palate clearly. Because cleft palate is a component of many syndromes, a child with a cleft palate must be assessed for other congenital anomalies.

Therapeutic Management

If a cleft lip is discovered while the infant is still in utero, fetal surgery can repair the condition, although this procedure is not usually attempted. If the disorder is not discovered until birth, a cleft lip is repaired surgically shortly thereafter, often at the time of the initial hospital stay or between 2 and 10 weeks of age. Some infants may have a nasal mold apparatus applied before surgery to shape a better nostril (Ezzat et al., 2007). Because the deviation of the lip interferes with nutrition, infants may be a better surgical risk at birth than they are after a month or more of poor nourishment. Early repair also helps infants experience the pleasure of sucking as soon as possible. It is equally important from a psychological standpoint that these disorders be repaired early. Parents can find it extremely difficult to bond with an infant whose face is deformed in this way. This is not a sign of a "bad" parent, but it is reality and a problem that requires intervention. Because facial contours change as a child grows, a revision of the original repair or a nasal rhinoplasty to straighten a deviated nasal septum may be necessary when the child reaches 4 to 6 years of age.

The optimal time for repair of cleft palate is controversial as early repair increases speech development but may result in a necessary second-stage repair as the child's palate arch grows. A two-stage palate repair, with soft palate repair at 3 to 6 months of age and hard palate repair at 15 to 18 months of age, may be recommended (van Aalst, Kolappa, & Sadove, 2008).

Currently, the results of surgical repair of cleft lip and cleft palate are excellent (Fig. 27.2). It is helpful to show parents photographs of babies with good repairs to assure them that their child's outcome can also be this successful. Do not use the older term for this condition, *harelip,* when talking with parents about the problem. Before modern surgical techniques were available, children were left with large lip scars, gross speech impediments, and a poor appearance after surgery. The word "harelip" tends to be associated with these negative outcomes rather than with the current positive outlook.

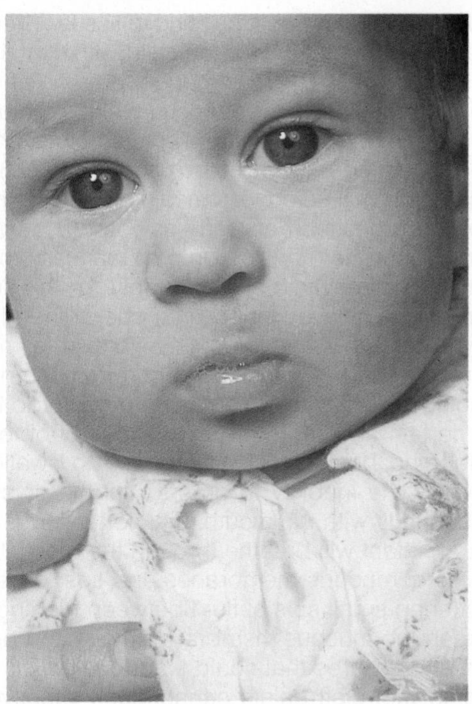

FIGURE 27.2 Infant showing surgical repair of cleft lip. Parents can be encouraged that the results of cleft lip repair are generally excellent. (Photo Researchers, Inc.)

Because palate repair narrows the upper dental arch, there may be less space in the upper jaw for the eruption of teeth, causing poor teeth alignment. All children born with a cleft palate need follow-up treatment by a pedodontist, or a dentist skilled in children's dental problems, so that as the child grows, extractions or realignment of teeth can be done as indicated (Cheng, Moor, & Ho, 2007). They also need follow-up to detect if speech or hearing difficulty occurs.

Nursing Diagnoses and Related Interventions

Nursing Diagnosis: Risk for imbalanced nutrition, less than body requirements, related to feeding problem caused by cleft lip or palate

Outcome Evaluation: Newborn ingests an adequate diet of 50 kcal/lb (110 kcal/kg) in 24 hours; weight is maintained within 10% of birth weight.

Preoperative Period. Before a cleft lip or palate is repaired, feeding the infant is a problem because the infant has difficulty maintaining suction (Glenny et al., 2009). In addition, it is important that the child does not aspirate.

It may be possible for an infant with a cleft lip to breastfeed because the bulk of the mother's breast tends to form a seal against the incomplete upper lip. Although the baby needs the enjoyment of sucking, some surgeons do not want a baby to breastfeed or suck on a nipple before surgical correction of the disorder to avoid any local bruising of tissue. Therefore, the best feeding method for the child with cleft lip may be to support the baby in an upright position and feed the infant gently using a commercial cleft lip nipple. A Breck feeder, an apparatus similar to a bulb syringe, or a Haberman feeder may also be used (Fig. 27.3). If the surgical repair will be done immediately, the mother will be able to breastfeed as early as 7 to 10 days after surgery. Teach her how to pump or manually express breast milk to maintain a milk supply for this time. If surgery will be delayed for 1 month, she will need to decide whether she wants to continue to express milk for this long a period; continuing support from the nursing staff could be important to encourage her to do this.

Be certain an infant with a cleft lip is bubbled well after feeding because of a tendency to swallow air caused by the inability to grasp a nipple or syringe edge securely with the mouth. If a cleft extends to the nares, an infant will breathe through the mouth, causing the oral mucous membranes and lips to become dry. Offering small sips of fluid between feedings can help keep the mucous membranes moist and prevent cracks and fissures that could lead to infection.

Infants with cleft palate cannot suck effectively either, because pressing their tongue or a nipple against the roof of their mouth would force milk up into their pharynx, leading to aspiration. The most successful method for feeding this infant, like the child with cleft lip, therefore, is to use a commercial cleft palate nipple that has an extra flange of rubber to close the roof of the mouth. The nipple can be used with a plastic bottle that can be squeezed gently to increase the flow of the feeding to compensate for poor sucking. A Breck feeder may also be used.

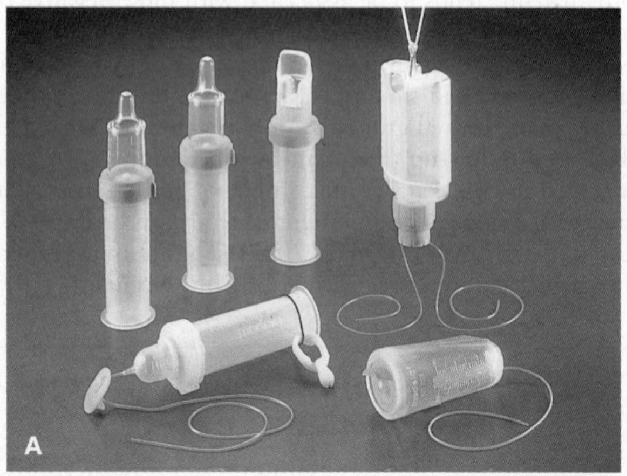

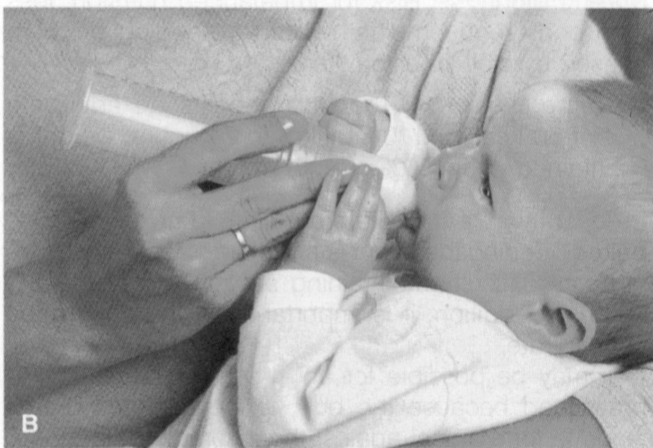

FIGURE 27.3 (**A**) Specialty feeding devices used for infants with cleft lip and cleft palate. (**B**) An infant uses a Haberman Feeder™.

If surgery is delayed beyond 6 months of age or the time solid food would be introduced, teach parents to be certain any food offered is soft. Particles of coarse food could invade the nasopharynx and cause aspiration. Infants whose surgery is delayed to this point can be fitted with a plastic palate guard to form a synthetic palate and help prevent this.

Postoperative Period. After surgery for cleft lip or palate, an infant is kept NPO for approximately 4 hours. The infant is then introduced to liquids (plain water). Begin the process with only a small amount to prevent vomiting.

It is important that no tension is placed on a lip suture line; avoiding tension helps keep the sutures from pulling apart and leaving a large scar. During this immediate postoperative period, the infant is usually fed using a specialized feeder because this causes less suture line tension than bottle feeding or breastfeeding.

After palate surgery, liquids are generally continued for the first 3 or 4 days, and then a soft diet is followed until healing is complete. Ask parents what fluids the child prefers so they can be available after surgery.

After a cleft palate repair, when children begin eating soft food, they should not use a spoon, because they will invariably push it against the roof of the mouth and possibly disrupt sutures. If being fed rather than being allowed to use a spoon himself evokes an intense reaction, it is better to leave a child on a liquid diet until the sutures are removed. Be certain milk is not included in the first fluids offered because milk curds tend to adhere to the suture line. After a feeding, offer the child clear water to rinse the suture line and keep it as clean as possible.

Nursing Diagnosis: Risk for ineffective airway clearance related to oral surgery

Outcome Evaluation: Child's respiratory rate remains between 20 to 30 respirations per minute without retractions or obvious distress.

Because of the local edema that occurs after cleft lip or palate surgery, observe children closely in the immediate postoperative period for respiratory distress. Before surgery, the infant with a cleft lip breathed through the mouth. After surgery, the infant now has to learn to breathe through the nose, possibly adding to respiratory difficulty. Generally, however, this is not a problem because newborns normally are strict nose-breathers.

Infants may need suction to remove mucus, blood, and unswallowed saliva. When performing suctioning, be gentle and do not touch the suture line with the catheter. After cleft lip surgery, place infants on their side to allow mouth secretions to drain. Support them well so they do not turn onto their abdomen, as this could put pressure on the suture line, possibly tearing it. Placing them in an infant bouncy chair is another possibility.

Nursing Diagnosis: Impaired tissue integrity at incision line related to cleft lip or cleft palate surgery

Outcome Evaluation: Incision line appears clean and intact and free of erythema or drainage during postoperative period.

After cleft lip surgery, the suture line is held in close approximation by a Logan bar (a wire bow taped to both cheeks; Fig. 27.4) or an adhesive bandage such as a Band-Aid simulating a bar that brings together the incision line but does not cover the incision. Assess the Logan bar or Band-Aid–simulated bar after each feeding or cleaning of the suture line to be certain it is secure and continues to protect the suture line from tension. Furnish adequate pain relief so, if possible, the infant does not cry, because crying increases tension on the sutures. To help avoid crying, try to anticipate the infant's needs. Have formula ready to feed on demand—do not wait until after the infant is awake and crying. Help the parents use whatever measures, such as rocking, carrying, or holding, that are necessary to make the infant feel secure and comfortable. The baby also will need to be bubbled well after a feeding because there is a tendency to swallow more air than the average infant.

Nothing hard or sharp must come in contact with a recent cleft suture line. Observe infants after palate repair carefully to be certain they do not put toys with sharp edges into their mouths. They should not use a straw to drink, nor should they brush their own teeth—they will certainly brush the suture line accidentally. Keep elbow restraints in place as necessary when no one is with them so they do not put their fingers in their mouth and poke or pull at the sutures. Most children run their tongue over their sutures because of the odd feeling in the roof of their mouth, and most children this age do not respond to a caution not to do this. Because this often occurs when children have nothing to think about, help the parents provide diversional activities such as reading or singing to them.

If parents will be continuing to give an analgesic such as acetaminophen (Tylenol) after they return home, be certain they are aware of the correct dosage and time schedule for administration. Be sure they can demonstrate measures to protect the suture line at home until healing is complete.

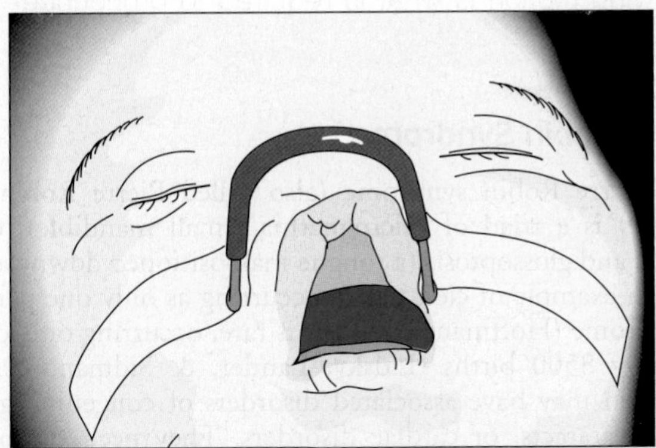
FIGURE 27.4 A Logan bar is an apparatus that may be used to protect the surgical incision for a cleft lip repair.

Nursing Diagnosis: Risk for infection related to surgical incision

Outcome Evaluation: Infant's temperature is below 98.6° F (37° C) axillary; incision site is clean, dry, and intact without erythema or foul drainage.

Infection, and subsequent scarring, may result if crusts from serous drainage are allowed to form on a cleft lip suture line. Most surgeons prescribe cleaning the suture line with sterile water, sterile saline, or 50% hydrogen peroxide in sterile water used with sterile cotton-tipped applicators after every feeding or whenever the normal serum that forms on suture lines accumulates. Use a smooth, gentle, rolling motion to apply the solution. Do not rub, because this can loosen sutures. If hydrogen peroxide is used, it will foam as it reacts with the protein particles at the suture line. Rinse the area with sterile water afterward. Gently dry the suture line with a dry sterile cotton-tipped applicator. Remember that an infant has sutures on the inside of the lip that need the same meticulous care as those visible on the outside.

Nursing Diagnosis: Risk for impaired parenting related to the birth of an infant who is physically challenged

Outcome Evaluation: Parents state a belief in a positive outcome for child; demonstrate positive coping behaviors, evidenced by holding and helping with infant care.

To promote bonding, parents need to hold and interact with their infant during both the preoperative and postoperative periods. Caution them the incision line will appear swollen in the immediate postoperative period. Reassure them this appearance will improve over time. As soon as the child's sutures have been removed, the infant may be bottle fed (with an ordinary bottle) or breastfed. Caution both the breastfeeding mother (who has been maintaining her milk supply through expression) and the formula-feeding mother that because the infant has never sucked before, time will be needed to learn, just as does a newborn.

Notice whether the parents look at their baby's face while feeding the baby. Help them to understand that any negative feelings directed toward the child or themselves, such as sadness or anger their baby was born this way, are normal. This does not instantly make them feel better about what has happened, but the knowledge that what they are experiencing is normal can help them begin to deal with such emotions. Many communities have support groups for parents of children born with a cleft lip or palate. Referral to these groups can be helpful (Box 27.2).

Nursing Diagnosis: Risk for situational low self-esteem related to facial surgery

Outcome Evaluation: Child participates in normal childhood activities that involve contact with other people; states activities he or she enjoys at health care visits; demonstrates age-appropriate developmental milestones.

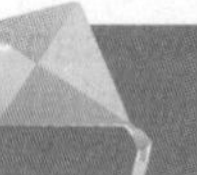

BOX 27.2 * Focus on Evidence-Based Practice

Does the timing of a cleft lip repair make a difference in mother–child interaction?

To answer this question, researchers compared mother–infant attachment in 94 infants who were born with a cleft lip and 96 nonaffected infants at 2, 6, and 12 months. They then compared cognitive development and infant behavior at 18 months. The infants who were born with cleft lips received either early (immediate) repair or late repair (3–4 months). Results of the study revealed that both the infants with cleft lip and control infants scored equally well on measures of behavior problems or attachment regardless of the timing of the surgical repair. Those infants who had a late surgical repair, however, scored lower on cognitive functioning (measured by the Bayley Scale of Mental Development) at 18 months than those infants with an early surgical repair. As parent–child interaction is important in gaining early cognitive development, this difference could reflect difficulties with parent–child interaction.

Based on the above, what type of role modeling would you demonstrate when caring for a newborn with a cleft lip?

Source: Murray, L., et al. (2008). The effect of cleft lip and palate, and the timing of lip repair on mother–infant interactions and infant development. *Journal of Child Psychology and Psychiatry and Allied Disciplines, 49*(2), 115–123.

If a scar remains after cleft lip surgery, children may need some help adjusting to it until a cosmetic repair can be completed later in life. Reinforce children's positive attributes, stressing that the scar is only one small aspect of who they are. As children reach adolescence, you may need to review a familial inheritance pattern of cleft lip so they are informed of the possible risk of transmission to their own children.

Nursing Diagnosis: Risk for infection (ear) related to altered slope of eustachian tube with cleft palate surgery

Outcome Evaluation: Parents state possible signs and symptoms of ear infection and state importance of early treatment; parents list signs of diminished hearing and appropriate agencies for support and guidance.

Changing the contour of the palate when it is repaired also changes the slope of the eustachian tube to the middle ear. This can lead to a high incidence of middle ear infection (otitis media) because organisms are more readily able to reach this area from the oral cavity. Review the signs of infection such as fever, pain, pulling on the ear, or discharge from the ear with parents. Also remind them of the importance of reporting pharyngeal infection to their primary care provider promptly so it can be treated before the infection spreads to the middle ear. Because the eustachian tube may remain partially closed because of its changed position, serous otitis media (accumulation of fluid in the middle ear) also tends to occur more frequently in these children than in others. If this happens, myringotomy tubes may be inserted to drain middle ear fluid and help protect hearing (see Chapter 50). Be certain that parents understand the need for routine screening for hearing loss during childhood, because this is a common early sign of serous otitis media.

Nursing Diagnosis: Risk for impaired verbal communication related to cleft palate

Outcome Evaluation: Family members voice satisfaction with child's speech; developmental milestone of clearly articulated two-word sentences by age 2 years is met.

Infants with a cleft palate will begin to make speech sounds at the normal time (age 2 months), although their speech may be guttural and harsh. By 9 months, when other infants begin to say meaningful words ("bye-bye," "mama," "dada"), assuming the cleft palate is still unrepaired, speech sounds will be unclear. Some parents try to discourage their baby from talking, thinking if the child does not talk until after the cleft palate repair is made, a speech impediment will not develop. Speech occurs at a specified developmental time, however, and despite the unfused palate it should be encouraged at these age-appropriate times. A child with a cleft palate can enunciate vowel sounds with the most clarity, so these are the sounds a parent should encourage the child to voice. Words such as "me," "they," "no," "mama," "home," "moon," "rain," "yell," and "row" are words consisting largely of vowel sounds and can be enunciated most clearly by the child before a cleft palate repair.

Almost all children who have had cleft palates continue to have accompanying speech problems after the repair (Brunnegard & Lohmander, 2007). The soft palate must function for the child to pronounce "p" and "b" sounds. If cleft palate surgery is going to be delayed much past age 2 years (as might happen if the child has other congenital anomalies, such as heart disease), a plastic prosthesis to cover the incomplete palate may be prescribed. This allows the child to articulate more normally.

Children do not spontaneously outgrow faulty speech patterns, so training by a speech therapist may be necessary. Commonly used exercises children are asked to perform include blowing games, such as blowing a feather or a table tennis ball (a blowing motion is what is required to pronounce "p" and "b").

Pierre Robin Syndrome

The Pierre Robin syndrome (also called Pierre Robin sequence) is a triad of micrognathia (small mandible), cleft palate, and glossoptosis (a tongue malpositioned downward). It is an example of cleft palate occurring as only one part of a syndrome (Hoffman, 2008). It is rare, occurring only once in every 8500 births (Lidsky, Lander, & Sidman, 2008). Children may have associated disorders of congenital glaucoma, cataracts, or cardiac disorders. They need thorough physical and genetic assessments to be certain that none of these associated disorders are present.

Observe all infants with Pierre Robin syndrome carefully to be certain they are not developing an airway obstruction. They may need frequent nasopharyngeal suctioning to remove unswallowed saliva. Beginning at birth, children with this syndrome are apt to have episodes in which they have difficulty breathing because, as a result of their small jaws, their tongues are too large for their mouths. This discrepancy causes the tongue to drop backward and obstruct the airway. Obstruction is most likely to occur when the child is in a supine position. Unlike well infants, no infant with this syndrome should be placed in a supine position to sleep; they are in grave danger of anoxia if left in this position. Use a side-lying position instead. Occasionally, infants have such extensive airway obstruction that attaching a suture to the anterior aspect of the tongue and pulling it forward is used to provide relief. The suture is attached to the mucous membrane of the lower lip, creating an artificial tongue-tied condition.

Parents need instructions to feed these infants with the same care and concern given all children with cleft palate. A gastrostomy tube or button may be inserted to relieve feeding difficulty (see Chapter 37). As the child grows older, the jaw will grow somewhat, although the mandible will always be small. Growth, coupled with a repair of the cleft palate, will decrease the respiratory problems.

Parents of the child with Pierre Robin syndrome take on a great deal of responsibility when they assume their infant's care. Be certain they have the name and number of a health care provider they can call when they have questions. Many of these parents grow exhausted during the first few weeks of their child's life, afraid they may fall soundly asleep at night and miss their child having respiratory difficulty. Using a respiratory monitor at night can be helpful to give assurance that the infant is breathing. As parents' confidence grows in their ability to provide care, this problem lessens, but it may be months or even years before a high level of confidence is achieved.

Tracheoesophageal Atresia and Fistula

Between weeks 4 and 8 of intrauterine life, the laryngotracheal groove develops into the larynx, trachea, and beginning lung tissue. The esophageal lumen forms parallel to this. A number of anomalies may occur if the trachea and esophagus are affected by some teratogen that does not allow the two organs to separate but remain connected.

Esophageal atresia is obstruction of the esophagus. Often a fistula (opening) occurs between the closed esophagus and the trachea. The five usual types of esophageal atresia that occur are:

1. The esophagus ends in a blind pouch; there is a tracheoesophageal fistula between the distal part of the esophagus and the trachea (see Fig. 27.5A).
2. The esophagus ends in a blind pouch; there is no connection to the trachea (see Fig. 27.5B).
3. A fistula is present between an otherwise normal esophagus and trachea (see Fig. 27.5C).
4. The esophagus ends in a blind pouch. A fistula connects the blind pouch of the proximal esophagus to the trachea (see Fig. 27.5D).
5. There is a blind end portion of the esophagus. Fistulas are present between both widely spaced segments of the esophagus and the trachea (see Fig. 27.5E).

These are all serious disorders because during a feeding, milk can fill the blind esophagus and overflow into the trachea, or a fistula can allow milk to enter the trachea, resulting in aspiration. The incidence of tracheoesophageal fistula is approximately 1 in 3000 live births (Fowler & Lee, 2008).

Assessment

Tracheoesophageal atresia must be ruled out in any infant born to a woman with hydramnios (excessive amniotic fluid). Hydramnios occurs because normally a fetus swallows amniotic fluid during intrauterine life. A fetus with a tracheoesophageal atresia cannot swallow, so the amount of amniotic fluid can grow abnormally large. Many infants with tracheoesophageal fistula are born preterm because of the accompanying hydramnios, compounding their original problem with immaturity. The infant needs to be examined carefully for other congenital anomalies that could have occurred from the

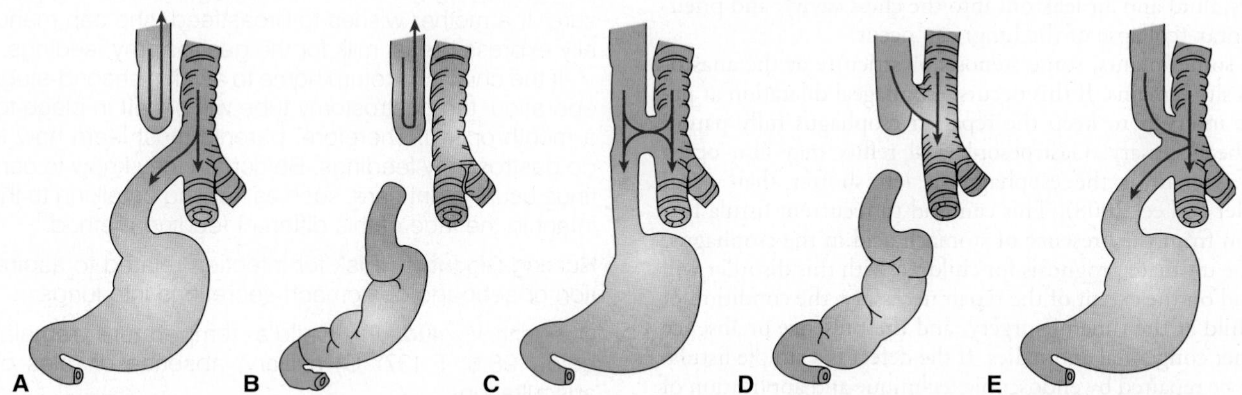

FIGURE 27.5 Esophageal atresia and tracheoesophageal fistula. (**A**) In the most common type of esophageal atresia, the esophagus ends in a blind pouch. The trachea communicates by a fistula with the lower esophagus and stomach (approximately 90% of infants with the defect have this type). (**B**) Both upper and lower segments end in blind pouches (5%–8% of infants with the defect have this type). (**C**) Both upper and lower segments communicate with the trachea (2%–3% of infants with the defect have this type). (**D**) Very rarely, the upper segment ends in a blind pouch and communicates by a fistula to the trachea, or (**E**) a fistula connects to both upper and lower segments of the esophagus.

teratogenic effect at the same week in gestation, such as *v*ertebral, *a*nal, *c*ardiac, *t*racheo*e*sophageal, *r*enal, and *l*imb anomalies (a VACTERL syndrome) (Pelluard-Nehme et al., 2007).

If not diagnosed in utero, diagnosing a child who has a tracheoesophageal fistula before the infant is first fed is important. Otherwise, the infant will cough, become cyanotic, and have obvious difficulty breathing as fluid is aspirated. Newborns who have so much mucus in their mouths that they appear to be blowing bubbles should be suspected of having tracheoesophageal fistula. The condition can be diagnosed with certainty if a catheter cannot be passed through the infant's esophagus to the stomach or the stomach contents cannot be aspirated. If doing this, use a firm catheter because a soft one will curl in a blind-end esophagus and appear to have passed. If a radiopaque catheter is used, it can be demonstrated coiled in the blind end of the esophagus on radiography. A flat-plate radiograph of the abdomen or ultrasound also may reveal a stomach distended with the air that is passing from the trachea into the esophagus and stomach. Either a barium swallow or a bronchial endoscopy examination can also reveal the blind-end esophagus and fistula.

Therapeutic Management

Emergency surgery for the infant with tracheoesophageal fistula is essential to prevent the development of pneumonia from leakage of stomach secretions into the lungs or dehydration or an electrolyte imbalance from lack of oral intake. Antibiotics may be prescribed to help prevent infection. A gastrostomy may be performed (under local anesthesia) and the tube allowed to drain by gravity to keep the stomach empty of secretions and prevent reflux into the lungs. Upper right lobe pneumonia from aspiration is one of the major complications of this disorder.

Surgery consists of closing the fistula and anastomosing the esophageal segments. It may be necessary to complete the surgery in different stages and to use a portion of the colon to complete the anastomosis if the esophageal segments are far apart from each other. Observe infants closely at postoperative days 7 to 10, when sutures dissolve, because leaks occurring at anastomosis sites can occur at this time. If this occurs, fluid and air leak out into the chest cavity, and pneumothorax (collapse of the lung) can occur.

In some infants, some stenosis or stricture at the anastomosis site remains. If this occurs, esophageal dilatation at periodic intervals to keep the repaired esophagus fully patent may be necessary. Gastroesophageal reflux may also occur after a repair if the esophagus is left shorter than usual (Fowler & Lee, 2008). This can lead to recurrent fistula formation from the presence of stomach acid in the esophagus.

The ultimate prognosis for children with this disorder will depend on the extent of the repair necessary, the condition of the child at the time of surgery, and the presence or absence of other congenital anomalies. If the defect is a simple fistula, it can be repaired by endoscopic technique and application of fibrin glue to seal the fistula (Richter et al., 2008). Even with larger disorders, if surgery can be performed before pneumonia develops, the prognosis is good. However, the mortality rate for the condition remains high because of the presence of other congenital disorders and low birth weight that often accompanies the tracheal abnormality.

Nursing Diagnoses and Related Interventions

Outcomes established for the child with tracheoesophageal fistula must be realistic in terms of the extent of the disorder, the timing of anticipated surgery, and the stage of grief or readiness for decision making and planning the parents have reached.

Nursing Diagnosis: Risk for imbalanced nutrition, less than body requirements, related to inability to take in oral feedings

Outcome Evaluation: Child maintains weight within 10% of birth weight; maintains weight in same percentile on growth curve.

Before surgery, because oral fluid cannot be given until the esophagus is repaired, intravenous therapy or total parenteral nutrition can supply fluid and calories. This is continued for a time after surgery until the possibility of vomiting from the anesthetic is decreased. Then the infant may be fed orally, may be continued on total parenteral nutrition, or may be started on gastrostomy feedings, depending on whether the surgery could be completed in one stage or not. Early introduction of oral fluid may help to ensure patency of the esophagus because it helps to decrease adhesion formation at the anastomosis site and also allows the infant the enjoyment and practice of sucking. If formula is given by gastrostomy feedings, introduce it into the tube slowly and allow it to run by gravity pressure only to prevent fluid from entering the esophagus and putting pressure on the suture line. After the feeding, the end of the tube should be elevated, covered by sterile gauze, and kept in the elevated position. Do not clamp it closed. In this way, any air introduced during the feeding will bubble from the tube and not enter the esophagus and pass the fresh suture line. This also helps to ensure that if the infant should vomit the feeding, the vomitus will be projected into the gastrostomy tube and will not contaminate the fresh sutures. Most newborns enjoy sucking a pacifier during gastrostomy feedings for sucking pleasure. If a mother wishes to breastfeed, she can manually express breast milk for the gastrostomy feedings.

If the child is to return home to await a second-stage operation, the gastrostomy tube will be left in place for a month or two. Therefore, parents must learn how to do gastrostomy feedings. Be certain they know to continue usual infant care, such as holding or talking to the infant in the face of this different feeding method.

Nursing Diagnosis: Risk for infection related to aspiration or seepage of stomach secretions into lungs

Outcome Evaluation: Child's temperature remains below 98.6° F (37° C) axillary; absence of rales on auscultation.

Preoperative Care. Before surgery, position the infant upright in an infant chair or on the right side to prevent gastric fluid from entering the lungs from the fistula. Because the infant cannot swallow mucus, frequent oropharyngeal suctioning is necessary. A catheter may be passed into the blind-end esophagus and attached to low continuous or intermittent suction to keep this segment of the esophagus from filling with swallowed saliva and causing aspiration from overflow. Irrigation of the catheter may be necessary to keep it patent, because mucus tends to dry and plug it.

If surgery will be delayed, the infant may have a cervical esophagostomy (the distal end of the blind esophagus is brought to the surface just over the sternum so that mucus can drain). Apply a protective ointment liberally to protect skin. Use absorbent gauze around the opening to absorb moisture and prevent excoriation of the skin. A consult by a wound, ostomy, and continence therapy nurse may be needed to prevent further skin irritation.

Keeping the infant under a radiant heat warmer with a high-humidity oxygen source helps to maintain body heat and liquefy bronchial secretions while awaiting surgery. Try to keep the infant from crying; with crying, air enters the stomach from the trachea, distending the stomach and possibly causing vomiting with aspiration into the lungs. A pacifier may help relax a baby and also satisfy a sucking need.

Postoperative Care. After surgery, the infant will have one or two chest tubes in place because the chest cavity was entered for the repair. The posterior tube drains collecting fluid; the anterior tube allows air to leave the chest space, re-expanding the lungs. Care of the child with chest tubes is discussed in Chapter 41.

In the first few days after surgery, observe the infant closely for respiratory distress. Continue to suction saliva from the mouth as ordered because mucus tends to accumulate in the pharynx from surgical trauma. Suctioning must be done only shallowly, however, to prevent the suction catheter from touching the suture line in the esophagus. Turn the child frequently to discourage fluid from accumulating in the lungs. Humidified oxygen helps to keep respiratory secretions moist. Keep an infant laryngoscope and endotracheal tube readily available at the bedside in case extreme edema develops, increasing the infant's risk for airway obstruction.

Nursing Diagnosis: Risk for impaired skin integrity related to gastrostomy tube insertion site

Outcome Evaluation: Skin surrounding gastrostomy tube remains clean and dry, without erythema.

Gastric secretions, which are highly acidic, may leak onto the skin from the gastrostomy site, leading to skin irritation. Protect the skin by using a cream or commercial skin protection system. Consulting with a wound, ostomy, and continence therapy nurse can be helpful to reduce the possibility of skin irritation.

Omphalocele

An **omphalocele** is a protrusion of abdominal contents through the abdominal wall at the point of the junction of the umbilical cord and abdomen (Fig. 27.6). The herniated organs are usually the intestines, but they may include stomach and liver. They are usually covered and contained by a thin transparent layer of amnion and chorion with the umbilical cord protruding from the exposed sac. When the defect is less than 4 cm, it is termed a hernia of the umbilical cord; when greater than 10 cm, it is a true omphalocele. This condition occurs because at approximately weeks 6 to 8 of intrauterine life, the fetal abdominal contents, growing faster than the fetal abdomen, are extruded from the abdomen into the base of the umbilical cord. At 7 to 10 weeks, when the abdomen has enlarged sufficiently, the intestine returns to the abdomen. Omphalocele occurs when the abdominal contents fail to return in the usual way. The occurrence is associated with chromosomal aberrations. A previous association between serotonin-reuptake ingestion during pregnancy has proven to be false (Louik et al., 2007).

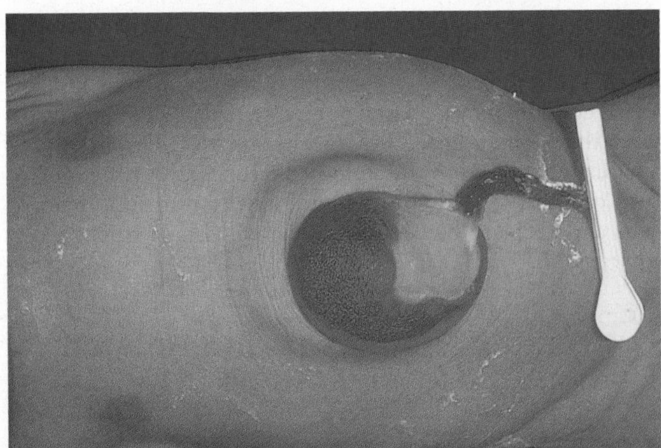

FIGURE 27.6 Omphalocele. This large example seen at birth contains intestine and liver. (Ansary/Custom Medical Stock Photograph.)

Assessment

The incidence of omphalocele is about 1 in 5000 live births. Many omphaloceles are diagnosed by prenatal sonogram. It may also be revealed by an elevated maternal serum α-fetoprotein (MSAFP) examination (see Chapter 11) during pregnancy (Smith & Henderson, 2007). If not, the presence of omphalocele is obvious on inspection at birth. When an omphalocele is identified in utero, cesarean birth may be performed to protect the exposed intestine. If this is the only disorder identified, however, vaginal birth can be allowed to proceed. Be sure to document the omphalocele's general appearance and its size in centimeters at birth.

Therapeutic Management

Most infants will have surgery within 24 hours to replace the bowel before the thin membrane surrounding it ruptures or becomes infected. It is often difficult to replace the entire bowel with immediate surgery because the infant's abdomen, which did not need to grow to accommodate the abdominal contents, is smaller than usual. If the total bowel were replaced into this small abdomen, respiratory distress could result from the pressure of the visceral bulk on the diaphragm and lungs. Also, the bowel might not have room for effective peristalsis. If the omphalocele is small, a one-stage repair may be possible (van Eijck et al., 2008). If large, one surgical approach is the use of a prosthetic patch repair that bridges the unformed gap on the abdomen with a synthetic material with the skin drawn tight and closed over the patch. A second approach is to replace only a portion of the bowel. The remainder is contained by a Silastic pouch termed a "silo" suspended over the infant's bed. Over the next 5 to 7 days, bowel is gradually returned to the abdomen. During this time, the infant can be fed by total parenteral nutrition to supply nutrients and keep the bowel from filling with air or stool.

Nursing Diagnoses and Related Interventions

Outcomes established for the infant with omphalocele must be realistic in terms of the extent of the disorder, the timing of anticipated surgery, and the stage of grief or readiness for decision making and planning that the parents have reached. Omphalocele is a shock to parents; it is a condition that is obviously severe yet one that is generally unknown.

Nursing Diagnosis: Risk for infection related to exposed abdominal contents

Outcome Evaluation: Child's temperature remains below 98.6° F (37° C) axillary; skin surrounding omphalocele remains clean, dry, and intact, without erythema or foul drainage.

Before surgery, it is important that the lining of peritoneum covering the omphalocele not be ruptured or allowed to dry out and crack; if this happens, infection and malrotation of the uncontained intestine can occur, complicating the surgical repair. Exposure of intestine to air also causes a rapid loss of body heat. Therefore, immediately place the baby in a warmed incubator. Do not leave the infant under a radiant heat source because this will quickly dry the exposed bowel. To keep the sac moist, cover it with either sterile saline-soaked gauze or a sterile plastic bowel bag until surgery. Because of the large amount of exposed intestinal surface, the saline used must be at body temperature to prevent lowering body temperature. If the omphalocele is large, infants may be prescribed a topical application of a solution such as silver sulfadiazine to prevent infection of the sac.

The prognosis for a final successful surgical repair is good. Except for a large abdominal scar, the child who had an omphalocele will be the child originally envisioned by parents. If the size of the scar is a problem for the child in later life, cosmetic surgery can reduce its appearance.

Nursing Diagnosis: Risk for imbalanced nutrition, less than body requirements, related to exposed abdominal contents

Outcome Evaluation: Child's weight remains within 10% of birth weight; skin turgor is good; specific gravity of urine is 1.003 to 1.030.

A nasogastric tube is inserted at birth to prevent intestinal distention, which would enlarge the bowel lumen, making it even more difficult to replace. Do not feed the infant orally or allow the infant to suck on a pacifier until the bowel repair is complete, as doing so would distend the exposed bowel with food or air and also make its return to the abdomen more difficult. Some infants have an accompanying **volvulus** (a twisting of the bowel causing obstruction), which is another reason to omit oral feedings. After surgery, the infant is maintained on total parenteral nutrition. Once the final stage of bowel repair is completed, a normal infant diet can be introduced gradually. Observe infants carefully for signs of obstruction such as abdominal distention, constipation, diarrhea, or vomiting when they begin oral feedings.

Infants with omphalocele can be hospitalized or receive home care for a long time (a minimum of 1 or 2 months) waiting for a second-stage or even a third-stage operation, depending on the extent of bowel involved. If the infant is hospitalized, encourage parents to visit frequently. Be sure the infant has age-appropriate toys available for stimulation.

Parents can become distressed that their child's operation is being done in such small stages. Offer support to help them accept that this treatment method is the best way to manage this type of intestinal disorder.

Gastroschisis

Gastroschisis is a condition similar to omphalocele, except that the abdominal wall disorder is a distance from the umbilicus, usually to the right, and abdominal organs are not contained by a membrane but rather spill freely from the abdomen (Thilo & Rosenberg, 2008). Also, a greater amount of intestinal content tends to herniate, increasing the potential for volvulus and obstruction. The condition occurs because of ischemia to blood vessels that supply the abdominal wall during the first trimester of pregnancy. For unknown reasons, it is increasing in incidence from about 2 in 10,000 births to 4.5 per 10,000 births, particularly in young mothers (Lund, Bauer, & Berrios, 2007). The care and surgical procedure are the same as those for omphalocele. Children with gastroschisis often have decreased bowel motility, and even after surgical correction may have difficulty with absorption of nutrients and passage of stool. Long-term follow-up may be necessary to ensure that nutrition and elimination are adequate (Raab, 2007).

✔ Checkpoint Question 27.1

What is the most important consideration in the care of the child with an omphalocele at birth?

a. Position the infant on his stomach to contain the intestine.
b. Wrap the omphalocele in cold icy gauze to prevent fever.
c. Keep the infant seated upright under a radiant warmer.
d. Contain the intestine in a sterile saline–lined bowel bag.

Intestinal Obstruction

If canalization of the intestine does not occur in utero at some point in the bowel, an **atresia** (complete closure) or **stenosis** (narrowing) of the fetal bowel can develop. The most common site of this occurrence is in the duodenum.

Obstruction may occur because the mesentery of the bowel twisted as the bowel re-entered the abdomen (after being contained in the base of the umbilical cord early in intrauterine life) or from looseness of the intestine in the abdomen after it has returned (Ingoe & Lange, 2007). This twisting pattern is termed a volvulus and continues to be a problem for the first 6 months of life until the infant develops firmer intestinal supports. Obstruction also can occur because of thicker-than-usual meconium formation, blocking the lumen (meconium plug or meconium ileus).

Assessment

Intestinal obstruction may be anticipated if the mother had hydramnios during pregnancy (swallowed amniotic fluid could not be absorbed effectively by the fetus) or if more than 30 mL of stomach contents can be aspirated from the newborn stomach by catheter and syringe at birth (fluid is not passing freely through the tract). If the obstruction is not revealed by either of these findings, then symptoms of intestinal obstruction in the neonate are the same as at any other time in life: the infant passes no meconium or may pass one stool (meconium that formed below the obstruction) and then not pass any more; the abdomen becomes distended and tender. As the effect of the obstruction progresses, the infant will vomit. Remember that many neonates spit up feedings when burped. This rapid ejection of milk smells barely sour. True vomiting is usually sour-smelling (stomach acid has acted on it) and occurs spontaneously without coughing or back-patting.

Obstructions are rare above the ampulla of Vater, the junction of the bile duct with the duodenum, so vomitus will be bile stained (greenish). Because meconium is black, vomitus may also be dark. Bowel sounds increase with obstruction because of the increase in peristaltic action that occurs as the intestine attempts to push stool pass the point of obstruction. Waves of peristalsis may be apparent across the abdomen. The infant may evidence pain by crying—hard, forceful, indignant crying—and by pulling the legs up against the abdomen. The child's respiratory rate will increase as the intestine fills and the diaphragm is pushed up against the lungs and lung capacity decreases. An abdominal flat-plate radiograph or sonogram will reveal no air below the level of obstruction in the intestines. A barium swallow or barium enema x-ray film may be used to reveal the position of the obstruction.

Therapeutic Management

When bowel obstruction is confirmed, an orogastric or a nasogastric tube is inserted and then attached to low suction or left open to the air to prevent further gastrointestinal distention from swallowed air (see Chapter 37). Always use low intermittent suction with decompression tubes in neonates. Pressure greater than this can irritate and ulcerate their stomach lining.

Intravenous therapy is necessary to restore fluid, and immediate surgery is scheduled because bowel obstruction is an emergency that must be treated before dehydration, electrolyte imbalance, or aspiration of vomitus occurs (Ingoe & Lange, 2007).

Repair of the obstruction (with the exception of meconium plug syndrome) is accomplished by laparoscopy or through an abdominal incision. The area of stenosis or atresia is removed, and the bowel is anastomosed. If the repair is anatomically difficult or the infant has other anomalies that interfere with overall health, a temporary colostomy may be constructed and the infant discharged to home care, with surgery rescheduled at about 3 to 6 months of age. Care of the child with a colostomy is discussed in Chapter 37. A final surgical procedure will restore the child to full health unless a large portion of the bowel had to be removed, which would have an impact on nutrient absorption (short bowel syndrome).

Nursing Diagnoses and Related Interventions

Nursing Diagnosis: Risk for deficient fluid volume related to vomiting

Outcome Evaluation: Child's skin turgor is good; pulse rate is 100 to 120 beats per minute; no further vomiting occurs; urine output is at least 30 mL/hr.

Once an obstruction is suspected, keep an infant NPO to prevent the bowel from filling, and compounding the problem, and to prevent vomiting and aspiration. Vomiting in neonates is always serious, not only because aspiration may occur but also because infants lose fluid rapidly, which results in dehydration. They also lose chloride (a component of the hydrochloric acid found in stomach contents), and this leads to metabolic alkalosis. The body attempts to compensate for the loss of chloride by excreting potassium, which can cause infants to become hypokalemic quickly. Keeping an infant NPO, restoring fluid by intravenous therapy, and monitoring laboratory values for electrolyte balance until surgery can be scheduled are crucial.

Meconium Plug Syndrome

A **meconium plug** is an extremely hard portion of meconium that has completely blocked the intestinal lumen, causing bowel obstruction. The cause is unknown but probably reflects normal variations of meconium consistency. Meconium plugs usually form in the lower end of the bowel because this meconium formed early in intrauterine life and has the best chance to become dry and obstruct the bowel lumen. It may be associated with Hirschsprung's disease and is strongly associated with cystic fibrosis (Balfour-Lynn, 2008).

Assessment

Because the obstruction is low in the intestinal tract, signs of obstruction such as abdominal distention and vomiting may not occur for at least 24 hours. Typically, the infant will be identified first as an infant who has had no meconium passage and is past 24 hours of age. A gentle rectal examination may reveal the presence of hardened stool, although the plug may be too high up in the bowel to be palpated. A radiograph or sonogram may reveal distended air-filled loops of bowel up to the point of obstruction. A slightly hypertonic water-soluble contrast agent enema not only may reveal the level of obstruction but also may be therapeutic in loosening the plug.

Therapeutic Management

The administration of saline enemas (never use tap water in newborns because it can lead to water intoxication) may cause enough peristalsis to expel the plug. Instillation of acetylcysteine (Mucomyst) with diatrizoate (Hypaque) rectally may also be prescribed to dissolve the plug. Gastrografin, a highly osmotic radiographic substance, can be administered as an enema. The substance pulls fluid into the bowel because of its low osmotic pressure, allowing the stool to soften and the plug to pass. Infants need to be well hydrated before and after the procedure or they can become hypovolemic from the effect of the contrast medium.

Once the thickened portion of meconium has been passed, the infant should have no further difficulty and, over the next several hours, may pass a great amount of stool. Observe the infant for further passage of meconium (should occur at least once daily) over the next 3 days, however, to be certain that additional plugs do not exist farther up in the bowel. If an infant is going to be discharged before this time, instruct parents on the importance of observing for meconium and also about phoning their primary care provider should the infant have no further bowel movements while at home.

Occasionally, a neonate passes a small plug of hardened meconium—hard enough it would have caused an obstruction except that it is so small—in the first 1 or 2 days of life. Be certain to record and report such a finding, because the infant will need close observation for continued defecation, the same as for the infant who actually had an obstruction, to be certain that there is not a larger and truly obstructing plug higher in the bowel.

Assess the family history of a newborn who has a meconium plug for cystic fibrosis, a recessively inherited disorder (see Chapter 40), or aganglionic megacolon (Hirschsprung's disease), a polygenic inherited disorder (see Chapter 45), as these disorders may be the cause of the hardened meconium. Hypothyroidism is yet another disorder that may present with constipation or hardened stool in newborns. Additional signs of hypothyroidism include a large protruding tongue, lethargy, and subnormal body temperature. Both hypothyroid and cystic fibrosis screening is done along with phenylketonuria screening. Be certain this blood test is obtained in any newborn with a meconium plug.

Meconium Ileus

Meconium ileus (obstruction of the intestinal lumen by hardened meconium) is a specific phenomenon that occurs almost exclusively in infants with cystic fibrosis (Kerby et al., 2008). It reflects extreme meconium plugging. A genetically recessive disease, with cystic fibrosis, the enzyme that moistens and makes all body fluids free-flowing is absent. All body fluids are therefore thick and tenacious. Cystic fibrosis (see Chapter 40) is most often thought of as a lung disorder, because the most severe manifestation of tenacious secretions is in the lung; tenacious lung fluid leads to stasis and infection and alveolar obstruction that reduces air exchange. Intestinal and pancreatic secretions are affected also, however, and this may be signaled at birth by hardened obstructive meconium at the ileus level from lack of pancreatic trypsin secretion (meconium ileus). This will lead to the usual symptoms of bowel obstruction: no meconium passage, abdominal distention, and vomiting of bile-stained fluid. If the obstruction is too high for enemas to reduce it, the bowel must be incised and the hardened meconium removed by laparotomy. The infant must be further assessed for cystic fibrosis in the following months.

What if... On the second day of life you notice Baby Sparrow, who was born with meconium staining, is spitting up green mucus? Would it be safe to assume this is meconium-stained mucus? Is there a possibility the baby is vomiting bile-stained vomitus?

Diaphragmatic Hernia

A diaphragmatic hernia is a protrusion of an abdominal organ (usually the stomach or intestine) through a defect in the diaphragm into the chest cavity. This usually occurs on the left side, causing cardiac displacement to the right side of the chest and collapse of the left lung. It occurs in approximately 1 in 2000 to 4000 live births. There is no difference between male and female incidence (Warner, 2007).

It occurs because early in intrauterine life, the chest and abdominal cavity are one; at approximately week 8 of growth, the diaphragm forms to divide them. If the diaphragm does not form completely, the intestines can herniate through the diaphragm opening into the chest cavity (Fig. 27.7).

Assessment

Diaphragmatic hernia is occasionally detected in utero by a sonogram. If extreme, surgery to remove the bowel from the chest can be attempted by fetoscopy while the fetus is still in utero. More often, however, the condition is diagnosed at birth. Newborns with a diaphragmatic hernia will have respiratory difficulty from the moment of birth, because at least one of the lobes of their lungs cannot expand completely (and may not have fully formed). Their abdomen generally appears sunken because it is not as filled with intestine as in the normal newborn. Breath sounds will be absent on the affected side of the chest cavity. There may be cyanosis and intercostal or subcostal retractions. These infants have a potential for developing persistent pulmonary hypertension because blood cannot perfuse readily through the unexpanded lung. This leads to right-to-left shunting through the foramen ovale in the heart and also causes the ductus arteriosus to remain patent. One condition, then, has led to another,

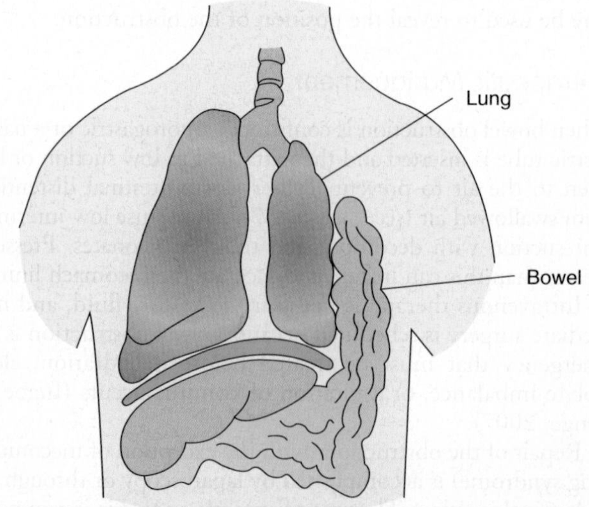

FIGURE 27.7 Diaphragmatic hernia. The bowel loop in the chest compresses the heart and lung on that side.

and heart involvement complicates an already complicated lung picture. The mechanics of right-to-left heart shunts are further discussed in Chapter 41.

Therapeutic Management

Although surgical repair may be delayed until an infant is better stabilized, treatment is usually an emergency surgical repair of the diaphragm and replacement of the herniated intestine back into the abdomen (Moyer et al., 2009). A surgical repair can be accomplished by laparoscopy, a helpful technique for newborns as it requires less anesthesia and cold exposure (Harres, 2007). Difficult repairs may require a thoracic incision and the placement of chest tubes. If the disorder of the diaphragm is large, an insoluble polymer (Teflon) patch may be used in reconstruction. The repair is complicated if there is not enough room in the abdomen for the intestine to be returned. In these infants, the abdominal incision may not be closed but left open to allow the intestine to protrude abdominally. It is covered by silicone elastomer (Silastic) and left to be closed at a later date after the abdomen has grown.

Over the next week, the compressed lung (if it is normal) will gradually expand and begin to function. If it is hypoplastic from the pressure of the intestine in utero, it will not expand; it will be removed at the time of surgery. Because of poor lung compliance, the infant's postoperative course is often complicated by severe pulmonary hypertension, perhaps requiring therapy with high-frequency oscillatory ventilation, inhaled nitric oxide, or extracorporeal membrane oxygenation (ECMO). The mortality rate of children with diaphragmatic hernia ranges from 25% to 40%, with death often because of associated anomalies of the heart, lung, and intestine (Thilo & Rosenberg, 2008).

Nursing Diagnoses and Related Interventions

Nursing Diagnosis: Risk for ineffective airway clearance related to displaced bowel

Outcome Evaluation: Child's respiration rate is 30 to 50 breaths per minute; Po_2 is 60 to 100 mm Hg; Pco_2 is 30 to 35 mm Hg; lungs are clear to auscultation.

The infant with a diaphragmatic hernia breathes better with the head elevated, as this allows the herniated intestine to fall back as far as possible into the abdomen, providing a maximum amount of respiratory space in the chest. Positioning the infant so the compressed lung is down also allows the unaffected lung to expand most completely. A nasogastric tube or a gastrostomy tube is inserted immediately to prevent distention of the herniated intestine, which would cause further respiratory difficulty. Be certain only low intermittent suction is used to avoid injuring the lining of the stomach. Keep the infant NPO, again, to prevent the bowel from filling and becoming distended.

After surgery, continue to maintain the infant in a semi-Fowler's position in an infant chair to keep the pressure of the replaced intestine off the repaired diaphragm. Keep the infant in a warmed humidified environment to encourage lung fluid drainage from the now uncompromised lungs. Suction the airway as necessary. Chest physiotherapy may be ordered to ensure that lung secretions do not pool and to prevent pneumonia. Positive-pressure ventilation may be ordered to increase lung expansion, although this pressure is kept to a minimum to prevent tearing the undeveloped or previously unopened lung tissue. Maintaining arterial oxygen (Po_2) at a high level of 100 mm Hg and the Pco_2 at a low level of 30 to 35 mm Hg may help to prevent arterial vasoconstriction of the hypoplastic lung, thereby improving lung function.

Nursing Diagnosis: Risk for imbalanced nutrition, less than body requirements, related to NPO status

Outcome Evaluation: Child's skin turgor remains good; weight is maintained within 10% of birth weight or between a percentile curve on growth chart.

After surgery, to prevent pressure on the suture line in the diaphragm by a full stomach and bowel, nutrition will be supplied intravenously, such as with total parenteral nutrition. When starting oral feedings, be certain to bubble the infant well after feeding to reduce the amount of swallowed air and limit bowel pressure against the diaphragm.

Umbilical Hernia

An umbilical hernia is a protrusion of a portion of the intestine through the umbilical ring, muscle, and fascia surrounding the umbilical cord (Skandalakis et al., 2007). This creates a bulging protrusion under the skin at the umbilicus. It is rarely noticeable at birth while the cord is still present but becomes increasingly noticeable at health care visits during the first year.

Umbilical hernias occur most frequently in African American children and more often in girls than in boys. The structure is generally 1 to 2 cm (0.5 to 1 in) in diameter but may be as large as an orange when children cry or strain. The size of the protruding mass is not as important as the size of the fascial ring through which the intestine protrudes. If this fascial ring is less than 2 cm, closure will usually occur spontaneously and no repair of the disorder will be necessary. If the disorder is more than 2 cm, surgery for repair will generally be indicated to prevent herniation and intestinal obstruction or bowel strangulation. This usually is done when the child is 1 to 2 years of age.

Some parents believe that holding an umbilical hernia in place by using "belly bands" or taping a silver dollar over the area will help to reduce the hernia. These actions can actually lead to bowel strangulation and should be avoided.

Surgery is generally accomplished on an ambulatory outpatient basis. The child returns from surgery with a pressure dressing, which remains in place until the sutures are well healed. Remind parents to sponge-bathe the child until they return for a postoperative visit and the dressing is removed. If the child is not yet toilet-trained, they need to keep diapers folded down below the dressing to prevent contaminating the suture line with stool.

Imperforate Anus

Imperforate anus (Fig. 27.8) is stricture of the anus (Vick et al., 2007). In week 7 of intrauterine life, the upper bowel elongates

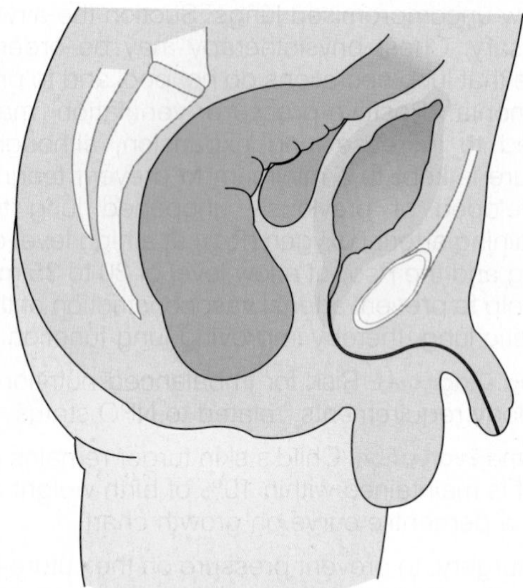

FIGURE 27.8 Imperforate anus. The lower bowel ends in a blind pouch.

to pouch and combine with a pouch invaginating from the perineum. These two sections of bowel meet, the membranes between them are absorbed, and the bowel is then patent to the outside. If this motion toward each other does not occur or if the membrane between the two surfaces does not dissolve, imperforate anus occurs. The disorder can be relatively minor, requiring just surgical incision of the persistent membrane, or much more severe, involving sections of the bowel that are many inches apart with no anus. There may be an accompanying fistula to the bladder in boys and to the vagina in girls, further complicating a surgical repair. The problem occurs in approximately 1 in 5000 live births, more commonly in boys than in girls. Imperforate anus may occur as an additional complication of spinal cord disorders, because both the external anal canal and the spinal cord arise from the same germ tissue layer.

Assessment

The condition may be detected by a prenatal sonogram. It is definitely discovered at birth when inspection of a newborn's anal region reveals that no anus is present, although this observation may not be helpful, because the anus can appear normal and the condition can still exist far inside, so that it is missed on simple inspection. Occasionally, the condition may be revealed because a membrane filled with black meconium can be seen protruding from the anus. A "wink" reflex (touching the skin near the rectum should make it contract) will not be present if sensory nerve endings in the rectum are not intact. If these methods fail to detect the condition, it can be discovered in a newborn by the inability to insert a rubber catheter into the rectum. No stool will be passed, and abdominal distention will become evident. A radiograph or sonogram will reveal the disorder if the infant is held in a head-down position to allow swallowed air to rise to the end of the blind pouch of the bowel. This method is also helpful to estimate the distance the intestine is separated from the perineum or the extent of the correction that will be necessary.

Formerly, when all newborns stayed in the hospital 3 to 4 days after birth, imperforate anus was always discovered. When infants failed to pass stools after the first 24 hours, the reason was investigated. Currently, because newborns are discharged at 2 or 3 days or even a few hours after birth, possibly no one will notice that an infant has not passed a stool in that time. For an infant born in a birthing center or at home, follow-up, therefore, must include assessment of whether the infant is defecating. Collect a urine specimen on infants with imperforate anus so it can be examined for the presence of meconium to help determine whether the child has a rectal–bladder fistula. Placing a urine collector bag over the vagina in girls may reveal a meconium-stained discharge or a rectovaginal fistula.

Therapeutic Management

The degree of difficulty in repairing an imperforate anus depends on the extent of the problem. If the rectum ends close to the perineum (below or at the level of the levator ani muscle) and the anal sphincter is formed, repair involves simple anastomosis of the separated bowel segments. The repair becomes complicated if the end of the rectum is at a distance from the perineum (above the levator ani muscle) or the anal sphincter exists only in an underdeveloped form. All repairs are complicated if a fistula to the bladder or vagina is present. If the repair will be extensive, the surgeon may create a temporary colostomy, anticipating final repair when the infant is somewhat older (6 to 12 months). For a successful repair, it is unnecessary for an internal rectal sphincter to be present as long as the subrectal muscle is judged to be intact.

Nursing Diagnoses and Related Interventions

*

Nursing Diagnosis: Imbalanced nutrition, less than body requirements, related to bowel obstruction and inability for oral intake

Outcome Evaluation: Child's weight remains within 10% of birth weight or is maintained on a percentile curve on a growth chart; skin turgor is good.

Preoperative Care. Before surgery, keep the infant NPO to avoid further bowel distention. A nasogastric tube attached to low intermittent suction for decompression will be inserted to relieve vomiting and prevent pressure on other abdominal organs or the diaphragm from the distended intestine. Intravenous therapy or total parenteral nutrition will be started to maintain fluid and electrolyte balance.

Postoperative Care. The newborn will return from surgery with a nasogastric tube still in place. When bowel sounds are present and the nasogastric tube is removed, small oral feedings of glucose water, formula, or breast milk can be begun.

Some infants, who are scheduled for repair in a second-stage operation and who have a temporary colostomy, are not permitted high-residue foods to lessen the bulk of stools. Although this is rarely a problem with infants because their diet naturally is a low-residue one, do not assume that parents know what low residue means. Examples include rice cereal and strained fruits and vegetables. They should avoid unrefined rice and grains, vegetables with fibers, or fruits with peels.

Nursing Diagnosis: Impaired tissue integrity at rectum related to surgical incision

Outcome Evaluation: Incision line remains free of erythema or drainage until it heals by about day 7 after surgery.

If a rectal repair was completed, remember there is a fresh suture line at the rectum. Take axillary or tympanic temperatures rather than rectal temperatures to avoid loosening a suture. Infants should also have no enemas, suppositories, or any other intrusive rectal procedures. It might be helpful to hang a sign above the infant's crib cautioning against any intrusive rectal procedure. Infants may be given a stool softener daily to keep the stool from becoming hard and tearing the healing suture line. Clean the suture line well after bowel movements by irrigating it with normal saline. Placing a diaper under, not on, the infant may be helpful so bowel movements can be cleansed away as soon as they occur. Do not place the infant on the abdomen because, in this position, newborns tend to pull their knees under them, causing tension in the perineal area. A side-lying position is best.

An infant may need rectal dilatation done once or twice a day for a few months after surgery to ensure proper patency of the rectal sphincter. Review this technique (gently inserting a lubricated cot-covered finger into the rectum) with the parents and document that they are able to perform this procedure before the child is discharged. Be certain they also understand the importance of the procedure. The best surgical repair could end in failure if constriction occurs because the parents do not follow up with this procedure. If infants are to be discharged with a prescription for a daily stool softener, be certain parents understand why this is also important and have a plan for remembering the correct times and dosage.

Nursing Diagnosis: Risk for impaired parenting related to difficulty in bonding with infant ill from birth

Outcome Evaluation: Parents hold and comfort infant; describe positive characteristics of infant.

An imperforate anus may be a difficult anomaly for a parent to accept because it deals with a body area that they may not feel comfortable discussing. If it involves a temporary (or permanent) colostomy, learning to care for their infant may be difficult. For these reasons, parents need a great deal of support following the diagnosis. If a final surgical repair can be completed, they can be assured their child will have normal bowel function thereafter. If a final repair could not be surgically achieved, they have the even harder task of caring for a child with a permanent ostomy. They can be assured that children who always have ostomies accept these well as they grow older because they have never known any other method of defecation (see Chapter 37 for a discussion of care priorities for the child with an ostomy).

✔ Checkpoint Question 27.2

What is an important nursing measure for a newborn with a diaphragmatic hernia?

a. Feed the infant immediately to decrease air in the intestine.
b. Keep the infant positioned head down so the intestine can expand.
c. Wrap the infant's abdomen tightly to better contain intestine.
d. Position the infant in an infant chair to contain intestine in abdomen.

PHYSICAL AND DEVELOPMENTAL DISORDERS OF THE NERVOUS SYSTEM

The most common developmental disorders of the nervous system at birth include abnormal accumulation of cerebrospinal fluid (CSF) (hydrocephalus), which has several causes, and abnormalities associated with neural tube closure (meningocele or spinal dysraphism). All these are the result of multifactoral inheritance as well as nutritional deficits (Donahue, 2008).

Hydrocephalus

CSF is formed in the first and second ventricles of the brain and then passes through the aqueduct of Sylvius and the fourth ventricle to empty into the subarachnoid space of the spinal cord, where it is absorbed. **Hydrocephalus** is an excess of CSF in the ventricles or the subarachnoid space (Moe, Benke, & Bernard, 2008). In the infant whose cranial sutures are not firmly knitted, this excess fluid causes enlargement of the skull. If fluid can reach the spinal cord, the disorder is called communicating hydrocephalus or extraventricular hydrocephalus. If there is a block to such passage of fluid, the disorder is an obstructive hydrocephalus or intraventricular hydrocephalus. Hydrocephalus is also classified regarding whether it occurs at birth (congenital) or from an incident later in life (acquired). The cause of congenital hydrocephalus is unknown, although maternal infection such as toxoplasmosis or infant meningitis may be factors (Smith & Henderson, 2007).

An excess of CSF in the newborn occurs for one of three main reasons:

- Overproduction of fluid by a choroid plexus in the first or second ventricle, as could occur from a growing tumor (rare).
- Obstruction of the passage of fluid in the narrow aqueduct of Sylvius (the most common cause). Other common sites of obstruction include the foramina of Magendie and Luschka, the openings that allow fluid to leave the fourth ventricle. Obstruction occurs because infections such as meningitis or encephalitis may leave adhesions behind that block fluid flow. Hemorrhage from trauma or a growing tumor also may obstruct the passage of CSF. An Arnold-Chiari disorder (elongation of the lower brain stem and displacement of the fourth ventricle into the upper cervical canal) is yet another cause.
- An interference with the absorption of CSF from the subarachnoid space if a portion of the subarachnoid membrane is removed, as occurs with surgery for meningocele, or after extensive subarachnoid hemorrhage, when portions of the membrane absorption surface become obscured.

Assessment

Hydrocephalus occurs in approximately 3 to 4 per 1000 live births (Moe, Benke, & Bernard, 2008). With an obstruction present, excessive fluid accumulates and dilates the system above the point of obstruction. If the atresia is in the aqueduct of Sylvius, the first, second, and third ventricles will dilate. If it is at the exit from the fourth ventricle, all ventricles will dilate. Symptoms may develop rapidly or slowly, depending on the extent of the atresia.

If hydrocephalus is present prenatally, it can sometimes be detected on a prenatal sonogram and can even be shunted in utero. The condition is generally not evident during pregnancy or even at birth, however, because of the effect of intrauterine pressure. It becomes evident in the first few weeks or months of life. The infant's fontanelles widen and appear tense, the suture lines on the skull separate, and the head diameter enlarges. As the fluid accumulation continues, the scalp becomes shiny and scalp veins become prominent. The brow bulges forward (bossing), and the eyes become "sunset eyes" (the sclera shows above the iris because of upper lid retraction). Infants show symptoms of increased intracranial pressure, such as decreased pulse and respirations, increased temperature and blood pressure, hyperactive reflexes, strabismus, and optic atrophy. They may become either irritable or lethargic, and they fail to thrive. They may have a typical shrill, high-pitched cry (Box 27.3).

Treatment is most effective when the disorder is recognized early, because once intracranial pressure becomes so acute that brain tissue is damaged and motor or mental deterioration results, even the best shunting procedure cannot replace and repair this damage to the brain cells. Assisting with detection of hydrocephalus is an important role for nurses in ambulatory child health settings. All children under age 2 years should have their head circumference recorded and plotted on an appropriate growth chart at health care visits, so a child whose head is growing abnormally can be detected (Zahl & Wester, 2008).

Measure the head circumference of all infants within an hour of birth and again before discharge from the health care facility to establish a baseline. Older children who have suffered head trauma severe enough to be seen in a medical facility should have their head circumference noted at the time of the accident; then, if other symptoms of increased intracranial pressure appear, this head circumference measurement may be a meaningful part of the store of information available concerning the child's condition.

In addition to the general enlargement of the head, note any asymmetry that is occurring, because this may suggest the point of obstruction. A skull that is enlarging anteriorly with a shallow posterior fossa, for example, suggests the obstruction is in the aqueduct or third ventricle.

The infant's motor function becomes impaired as the head enlarges, because of both neurologic impairment and atrophy caused by the inability to move such a heavy head. However, as long as a child has more than 1 cm of cerebral tissue present, motor function often is not impaired. Even with an extremely enlarged head, children's intelligence may remain normal, although fine motor development may be affected.

That hydrocephalus is present can be demonstrated by ultrasound, computed tomography (CT), or magnetic resonance imaging (MRI). A skull x-ray film will reveal the separating sutures and thinning of the skull. **Transillumination** (holding a bright light such as a flashlight or a specialized light [a Chun gun] against the skull with the child in a darkened room) will reveal the skull is filled with fluid rather than solid brain (Fig. 27.9). If the hydrocephalus is a noncommunicating type, dye inserted into a ventricle through the anterior fontanelle will not appear in CSF obtained from a lumbar puncture.

Box 27.3 Assessment
Assessing an Infant With Hydrocephalus

Enlarged fontanelles
Separated suture line
Prominent scalp veins
"Bossing" of forehead
Increased head circumference
"Sunset" eyes
Lethargy or irritability
Shrill cry
Signs of increased cranial pressure
↓ pulse
↑ temperature
↓ respirations
↑ blood pressure
Hyperactive reflexes

Therapeutic Management

The treatment of hydrocephalus depends on its cause and extent. If it is caused by overproduction of fluid, acetazolamide (Diamox), a diuretic, may be prescribed to promote the excretion of this excess fluid. Destruction of a portion of the choroid plexus may be attempted by ventricular endoscopy, or if a tumor in that area is responsible for the overproduc-

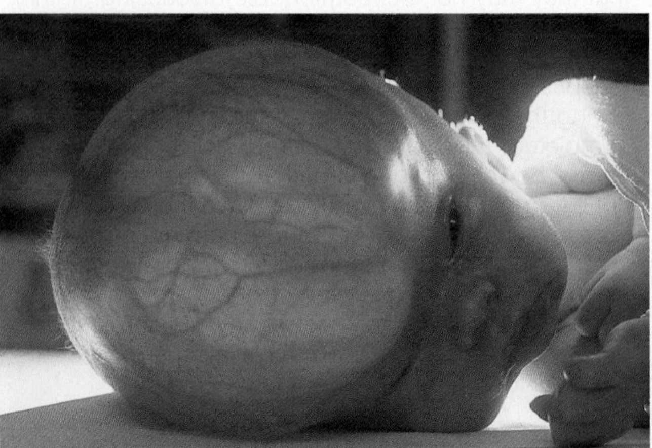

FIGURE 27.9 An infant with hydrocephalus. Transillumination reveals a fluid-filled skull. (Southern Illinois University/Photo Researchers, Inc.)

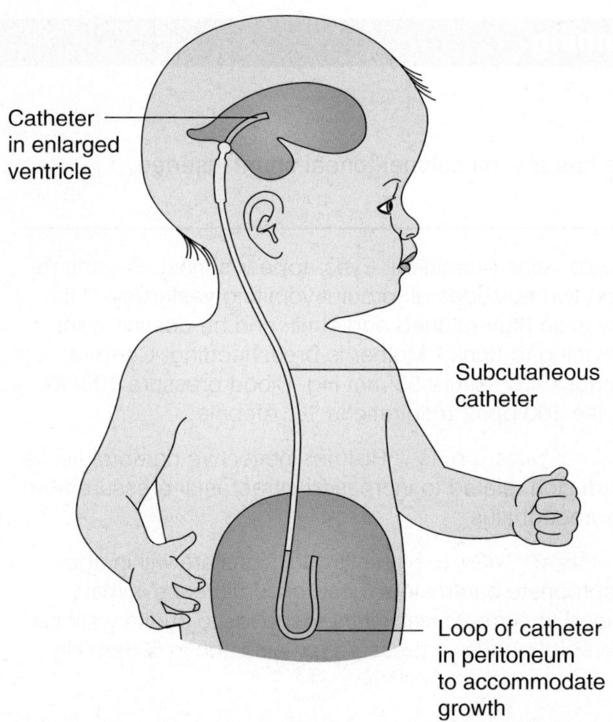

FIGURE 27.10 A ventriculoperitoneal shunt removes excessive cerebrospinal fluid from the ventricles and shunts it to the peritoneum. A one-way valve is present in the tubing behind the ear.

tion of fluid, removal of the tumor should provide a solution. Hydrocephalus is usually caused by obstruction, however, so the treatment usually involves laser surgery to reopen the route of flow or bypassing the point of obstruction by shunting the fluid to another point of absorption.

As ventricular endoscopy is perfected and obstructions in the third or fourth ventricle can be relieved, the next generation of children with hydrocephalus may not need artificial shunting. Children today may still undergo a shunting procedure, however, and you may care for many older children or adults who have shunts in place (Komolafe, Adeolu, & Komolafe, 2008). A shunting procedure involves threading a thin polyethylene catheter under the skin from the ventricles to the peritoneum (Fig. 27.10). Fluid drains via this route into the peritoneum and is absorbed across the peritoneal membrane into the body circulation. This type of shunt usually has to be replaced as the child grows or it will become too short. As another complication, it could become enclosed in a fold of peritoneum and become obstructed or it could become infected (Box 27.4).

The ultimate prognosis for a child with hydrocephalus depends on whether brain damage occurred before shunting and, if a shunt is in place, whether the parents can recognize when it needs to be replaced to prevent increased intracranial pressure.

BOX 27.4 ✻ Focus on Communication

Baby Sparrow is scheduled to have a ventriculoperitoneal shunt inserted this afternoon. You talk to his mother before surgery.

Less Effective Communication

Nurse: Is there anything I can explain to you about your son's surgery, Ms. Sparrow?

Ms. Sparrow: No. I just want to see him back here with a smaller head.

Nurse: The shunt won't actually make his head smaller. Its purpose is to keep his head from growing any larger.

Ms. Sparrow: What is the chance that he'll die in surgery?

Nurse: All surgery has a risk, certainly, but he should do well.

Ms. Sparrow: But there is a chance he'll die in surgery?

Nurse: You're worrying over nothing. Why don't you relax and go get something to drink until he gets back?

More Effective Communication

Nurse: Is there anything I can explain to you about your son's surgery, Ms. Sparrow?

Ms. Sparrow: No. I just want to see him back here with a smaller head.

Nurse: The shunt won't actually make his head smaller. Its purpose is to keep his head from growing any larger.

Ms. Sparrow: What is the chance that he'll die in surgery?

Nurse: All surgery has a risk, certainly, but he should do well.

Ms. Sparrow: But there is a chance he'll die in surgery?

Nurse: You sound more worried than I'd expect. Is there something specific you're worried about?

Ms. Sparrow: I'd like him to die in surgery. How am I going to take care of a child with such a deformed head?

Nurse: Let's sit down and talk about this some more.

Because surgical procedures are so safe today and the results of surgery for newborns are so successful, it is easy to begin to think of these disorders as more inconvenient than serious: the infant, after all, will grow up with only a few minor problems. To a parent, however, the difference between a child born with one of these conditions and the "perfect" child the parent envisioned can be great. Careful listening is necessary to appreciate the extent of a parent's understanding of the problem. Handling a problem by giving quick reassurance, as in the first scenario here, can lead to missing a parent's concern. Better listening, as in the second scenario, revealed the true problem.

Nursing Diagnoses and Related Interventions

✻

Nutrition and parent–child bonding are two major concerns for the infant with hydrocephalus. Box 27.5 on nursing care planning illustrates these and other concerns.

Nursing Diagnosis: Risk for ineffective cerebral tissue perfusion related to increased intracranial pressure

Outcome Evaluation: Child shows no increased temperature or blood pressure, or decreased pulse rate, decreased respiratory rate, or decreased level of consciousness; PERLA (pupils equal and reactive to light

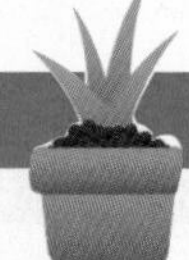

BOX 27.5 ✻ Focus on Nursing Care Planning

A Multidisciplinary Care Map for a Child With Hydrocephalus

At 3 months of age, Baby Sparrow develops hydrocephalus after repair of his neural tube disorder. He has a ventriculoperitoneal shunt inserted.

Family Assessment ✻ Child lives with 16-year-old mother and her parents and four of mother's siblings. Child's father works as motorcycle mechanic; visits infant frequently. Mother no longer attending school because of child care. Has not named child as yet. Mother asking many questions about the surgery. "This'll fix everything, right? I want a healthy baby."

Client Assessment ✻ A 3-month-old infant whose head circumference has continued to increase since myelomeningocele surgery at birth. Head circumference at birth was 40th percentile, at 60th percentile at 6 weeks of age and now at 80th percentile. Mother noted infant had increasing irritability and lethargy over the last few weeks.

Anterior fontanelle 4 cm × 4 cm; posterior fontanelle 3 cm × 1 cm. Sagittal suture line separated ¼ inch. Scalp veins prominent. Eyes appear sunset. Parents report two episodes of forceful vomiting yesterday. "His cry is so high-pitched and shrill, and he doesn't want anything to drink." Mother is breastfeeding. Cerebral perfusion pressure 55 mm Hg. Blood pressure 100/40; pulse 100 bpm; respirations 16. Afebrile.

Nursing Diagnosis ✻ Risk for ineffective cerebral tissue perfusion related to increased intracranial pressure from hydrocephalus

Outcome Criteria ✻ Infant's vital signs are within age-appropriate parameters; head circumference is maintained at current level; infant responds to auditory stimuli. Cerebral perfusion pressure remains above 50 mm Hg.

Team Member Responsible	Assessment	Intervention	Rationale	Expected Outcome
Activities of Daily Living				
Nurse	Assess if infant is able to turn because of increased head size.	Provide an environment for child that is stimulating yet not tiring (mobile, soft toys in crib). Urge parent to interact with child.	Lack of mobility can lead to pressure ulcers on head as well as insufficient 3-month development.	Child's parent plays with infant. Infant appears interested in age-appropriate toys. No irritated areas on head.
Consultations				
Nurse/ physician	Assess if neurosurgeon is available for consultation.	Arrange for consultation for mother with neurosurgeon to discuss surgery and child's prognosis.	Viewing a child as totally disabled can cause a parent to not appreciate the child's capabilities.	Neurosurgeon meets with mother to discuss that child's IQ appears normal; shunting will halt head growth.
Procedures/Medications				
Nurse	Assess infant's neurologic status postoperatively, including response to sound, pupillary response, increasing irritability or lethargy.	Position the infant with the head of the bed elevated 15 degrees and prevent hyperextension, flexion, or rotation of the head. Record cerebral perfusion pressure.	Elevating head of bed aids shunt functioning, helping reduce intracranial pressure. Cerebral perfusion pressure reveals extent of intracranial pressure.	Child's cerebral perfusion pressure remains greater than established parameter. Responds to sound; no increasing irritability or lethargy.
Nurse	Measure and record head circumference every 4 hours. Assess anterior fontanelle for tenseness and bulging.	Document head circumference and appearance of anterior fontanelle.	Head circumference, if increasing, or a tense, bulging fontanelle indicates accumulating CSF.	Child's head circumference does not increase in size; fontanelles no longer feel tense.

		Nutrition		
Nurse/ nutritionist	Observe mother breastfeeding infant.	Encourage mother to breastfeed infant; assist mother with positioning the infant properly, supporting the head without flexion or hyperextension during feeding.	Breast milk is the optimal nutrition for an infant. Proper positioning is important to avoid neck vein compression, which could increase intracranial pressure.	Mother breastfeeds successfully following surgery.
Nurse	Monitor intake and output closely.	Administer osmotic diuretic and corticosteroids as ordered.	Adequate hydration is necessary to ensure renal function. Osmotic diuretics decrease intracranial pressure. Corticosteroids reduce inflammation.	Child's output remains over set parameter. Diuretic and corticosteroids administered as necessary.
		Patient/Family Education		
Nurse/nurse practitioner	Assess the parents' understanding of hydrocephalus and treatment measures.	Review the structure and function of the brain and explain how hydrocephalus develops. Clarify any misconceptions.	Reviewing and clarifying aid in learning and strengthen understanding.	Mother states she understands purpose of shunt to relieve excess CSF.
		Psychosocial/Spiritual/Emotional Needs		
Nurse/nurse practitioner	Assess mother's acceptance of child in light of many congenital disorders and no name for baby as yet.	Observe mother's interaction with infant; remind her that congenital disorders occur in a proportion of all births.	Young mother may have had little experience with life crises. Needs support from health care providers for this crisis.	Mother states she understands child's condition is neither her nor the child's fault; states she can handle the present crisis.
		Discharge Planning		
Nurse	Assess if child's parents have questions about care he will need for future shunt care; if they understand postsurgery appointment is important.	Assist parents with caring for the child as much as possible; offer positive reinforcement frequently.	Caring for the child promotes active participation and parent–infant bonding. Positive reinforcement enhances self-esteem and aids in coping.	Mother and grandmother state they understand future care necessary for shunt; will contact neurosurgeon if any questions regarding child's progress. Mother keeps postsurgery appointment.
Nurse	Assess if home care follow-up will be necessary.	Make referral for home care if needed. Refer parents to support group of other parents of children with hydrocephalus.	Support groups can decrease feelings of isolation, provide opportunities for further learning. Follow-up home care provides continuing support, guidance, and education.	Mother and grandmother state they will attend a support group at least once to evaluate benefit for them. Agree to at least one home visit for follow-up care.

and accommodation); muscle strength equal and strong bilaterally; head circumference is maintained at age-appropriate level.

After a shunt is inserted, the infant's bed is usually left flat or raised only about 30 degrees so the child's head remains level with the body. This is because if the child's head is raised excessively, CSF may flow too rapidly and decompression can then occur too rapidly, leading to possible tearing of cerebral arteries.

A one-way valve is inserted in the shunt that opens when CSF has accumulated to the extent that pressure has increased. It closes when enough fluid has drained to reduce the pressure. The surgeon who performs the shunting procedure writes specific orders about how often the infant is to be turned and to what side after surgery. Often infants are not turned to lie on the side with the shunt to prevent putting pressure on the valve, which might cause it to open and rapidly decompress CSF.

Assess for signs of increased intracranial pressure after surgery such as tense fontanelles, increasing head circumference, irritability or lethargy, decreased level of consciousness, poor sucking ability, vomiting, an increase in blood pressure (difficult to measure accurately in infants unless arterial or umbilical lines are used with Doppler instrumentation), increasing temperature, and a decrease in pulse and respiratory rates (see Chapter 49 for tips on a complete neurologic assessment). Also assess for symptoms of infection such as increased temperature, increased pulse rate, general malaise, and signs of meningitis such as a stiff neck and marked irritability (Box 27.6). Be certain a child receives adequate pain management, because crying elevates CSF pressure.

Nursing Diagnosis: Risk for imbalanced nutrition, less than body requirements, related to increased intracranial pressure

Outcome Evaluation: Child's weight remains within 5th to 95th percentile on height and weight chart; no vomiting occurs.

Because an abdominal incision is involved to thread the catheter into the peritoneum, most children have a nasogastric tube placed during surgery. Keep them NPO until bowel sounds return and the tube can be removed. Introduce fluid gradually in small quantities after removal of the tube as vomiting that results from the introduction of fluid too soon after any surgery causes increased intracranial pressure.

Like other infants, infants with hydrocephalus should be held when being fed if possible. Be certain to support their heads well when moving them to avoid strain on their neck from their heavier than usual head. Hold their head with the whole palm, not just the fingertips, because the skull can thin to such a degree that it can actually be punctured with a stiff, forceful touch. Urge parents to use a rocking chair with an armrest to provide support for their arm while feeding the infant. Otherwise, the infant's head can be so heavy that they cannot spend as much time holding the infant after a feeding as they might otherwise. No contraindications for breastfeeding exist.

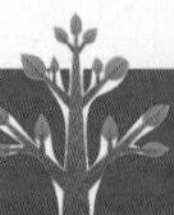

BOX 27.6 * Focus on Family Teaching

Caring for a Child With a Ventriculoperitoneal Shunt

Q. Following ventriculoperitoneal shunt surgery, Baby Sparrow's mother asks you, "What do I need to do to care for him?"

A. Here are some helpful things to remember:

- Observe for signs of increased intracranial pressure, such as drowsiness, vomiting, headache, irritability, and anorexia.
- Observe the pump site daily for any sign of swelling or redness.
- Have your child sleep with his head slightly elevated at night to help ensure fluid flow through the tube. Do not allow your child to fall asleep with his head hanging over the side of a couch or bed.
- Do not allow your child to become constipated, because hard stool might press against the shunt in the abdomen and obstruct the flow of fluid. Encourage fruit, vegetables, cereal, and a generous amount of fluid in his diet.
- Do not call attention to the pump behind your child's ear; teach him not to touch the pump when he's nervous or as an attention-getting action.
- Be certain your child wears a helmet for tricycle and bicycle riding (as should all children) to avoid injury to the shunt. Otherwise, there are no special precautions that need to be taken for normal play.
- If your child develops signs of infection such as an increased temperature, phone your primary care provider. Also remind the person that your child has a shunt in place. This is probably a simple infection of childhood but could indicate an infected shunt.
- Be certain to keep your regularly scheduled health assessment visits. As your child grows taller, the shunt will eventually need to be replaced for proper functioning.

Help breastfeeding mothers to find a comfortable position for feeding so that they can be successful with this.

Note how the child sucks. Increased intracranial pressure may be noted first because of poor or ineffective sucking. Vomiting after feeding, without nausea (difficult to detect in a small infant), is also a common first sign of increased intracranial pressure.

Observe for constipation, because straining while passing stool causes increased intracranial pressure. This is not usually a problem with infants who are totally breastfed or formula fed. However, it can be a problem when children return for shunt replacement at an older age. Urge parents to offer adequate fluid and roughage in their child's diet as a preventive measure.

Nursing Diagnosis: Risk for impaired skin integrity related to extra weight and immobility of head

Outcome Evaluation: Child's skin remains clean, dry, and intact, without signs of erythema or ulceration.

The head of an infant with hydrocephalus can become so heavy the infant cannot move it freely. As the skin of the head stretches thin, skin breakdown can occur at the pressure points. Wash the child's head daily and change the position of the head approximately every 2 hours so that no portion of the head rests against the mattress for a long period. A synthetic sheepskin or silicon pad or an air, water, or alternating air mattress may help to relieve pressure points. If a Kling or stockinette bandage is used to hold a surgical head dressing in place, place a piece of gauze or cotton behind the child's ear before the bandage is applied to prevent skin surfaces from touching and becoming excoriated. Make sure the bandage does not become wet from backward-draining oral secretions or shunt leakage.

Nursing Diagnosis: Deficient knowledge related to home care needs of child with hydrocephalus

Outcome Evaluation: Parents state fears regarding ability to provide care but are able to manage this; state signs of increased intracranial pressure for which they should watch; demonstrate competence in shunt care.

Caring for a child with a shunt in place is an ongoing responsibility for parents. If parents do not seem to be asking many questions about the child's care after surgery, do not assume this is because they are taking the child's care in stride. They may be too frightened or not understand neuroanatomy enough to know what questions to ask. An opening such as, "Most parents are a little nervous when they think about taking a child home with a shunt in place; do you feel that way?" gives them an opportunity to admit how they feel. Talking about how nervous they feel about the responsibility will not immediately make them more comfortable with the child's care. However, it can provide them with a starting point to bring their anxiety down to a manageable size. Assure them the health care providers caring for their child are interested in helping and supporting them.

If a valve has been inserted in the shunt, it can be palpated underneath the skin just behind the ear. Remind parents to stress to their child that this strange object is not to be felt continually. A child nervously fidgeting with a pressure pump can inadvertently evacuate CSF from the ventricles at a dangerously rapid rate.

Before an infant is discharged after surgery, be certain the parents have ample opportunity to feed and provide care so they can be comfortable and feel they "know" their infant. Because irritability, lethargy, vomiting, and a change in the baby's cry are signs of increased intracranial pressure, be certain parents know to report these immediately to their primary care provider. Before parents can report a change in the infant's disposition in this way, they must know the infant well, why it is important that they give care while their infant is hospitalized. A referral for home care follow-up may be appropriate to offer further support.

Nursing Diagnosis: Risk for delayed growth and development related to potential neurologic challenge

Outcome Evaluation: Child demonstrates regular observable growth and achieves age-appropriate developmental milestones.

Like all children, children with hydrocephalus need intellectual and emotional stimulation: they need to be talked to, smiled at, and played with. If the child's head is enlarged, turning it to look at things can be difficult. It may be necessary to reposition mobiles or pictures so the child receives adequate visual stimulation. Role-model talking and singing to the child to help parents include these actions in their care.

At the time of hospital discharge, be certain parents have the telephone number of the person they should call if they have a question or concern about their child's condition or care, and a referral for home care follow-up, if appropriate. They also need an appointment for the child's first checkup. Be sure they understand that infection of the shunt is a possibility and a severe complication because it can lead to meningitis. If this should occur, the infant will show signs of increased intracranial pressure as well as an increased temperature. In addition to being hospitalized, receiving the usual treatment for meningitis (see Chapter 49), and receiving intravenous antibiotics, the child may have an extraventricular shunt placed to promote drainage during this time. This allows antibiotics to be administered directly to the CSF and ensures that infected CSF is not draining to the peritoneal cavity, where it could cause peritonitis.

As the child reaches preschool and school age, parents need to confer with the school nurse to make the nurse aware that the child has a shunt in place and that the child may need special head protection for sports activities.

✓ Checkpoint Question 27.3

Baby Sparrow may be developing increased intracranial pressure. What vital sign changes occur with this?

a. Decreased temperature; increased blood pressure.
b. Increased respirations; decreased pulse rate.
c. Increased temperature; decreased pulse rate.
d. Decreased blood pressure; increased temperature.

Neural Tube Disorders

Because the neural tube forms in utero first as a flat plate and then molds to form the brain and spinal cord, it is susceptible to malformation. The term **spina bifida** (Latin for "divided spine") is most often used as a collective term for all spinal cord disorders, but there are well-defined degrees of spina bifida involvement, and not all neural tube disorders involve the spinal cord. All of these disorders, however, occur because of lack of fusion of the posterior surface of the embryo in early intrauterine life. They can be compared with cleft palate or cleft lip—these are also midline closure disorders.

The incidence of neural tube disorders has fallen dramatically in recent years, from 3 to 0.6 per 1000. Such disorders may occur as a polygenic inheritance pattern, but poor nutrition, especially a diet deficient in folic acid, appears to be a major contributing factor (Lumley et al., 2009). As a result, pregnant women are advised to ingest 600 micrograms of folic acid daily to help prevent these disorders. The risk of bearing a second child with a neural tube disorder once one child is born with such a disorder increases to as much as 1 in 20. For this reason, women who have had one child with a spinal cord disorder are advised to have a maternal serum assay or amniocentesis for AFP levels to determine if such a disorder is present in a second pregnancy (levels will be abnormally increased if there is an open spinal lesion). Serum assessment of MSAFP is done at week 15 of pregnancy, when AFP reaches its peak concentration. If the result is elevated, an amniocentesis is then done to assess the level of AFP in amniotic fluid. A prenatal sonogram is also helpful to determine the presence of the disorder (see Chapter 11 for further discussion of these prenatal assessments).

Types of Disorders

Anencephaly. Anencephaly is absence of the cerebral hemispheres. It occurs when the upper end of the neural tube fails to close in early intrauterine life. It is revealed by an elevated level of AFP in the maternal serum or on amniocentesis and confirmed by a prenatal sonogram.

Infants with anencephaly may have difficulty in labor because the underdeveloped head does not engage the cervix well. Many such infants present in a breech position. On visual inspection at birth, the disorder is obvious (Fig. 27.11). Children cannot survive with this disorder because they have no cerebral function. Because the respiratory and cardiac centers are located in the intact medulla, however, they may survive for several days after birth.

When the condition is discovered prenatally, parents are offered the option of abortion. An ethical problem has arisen in several instances when parents, aware that the child cannot survive, elect to carry the infant to term so the organs can be used for transplant. Nurses need to think through their feelings about caring for such infants, because it can be difficult to give care to a child who will most likely die or who has been born only to help others live.

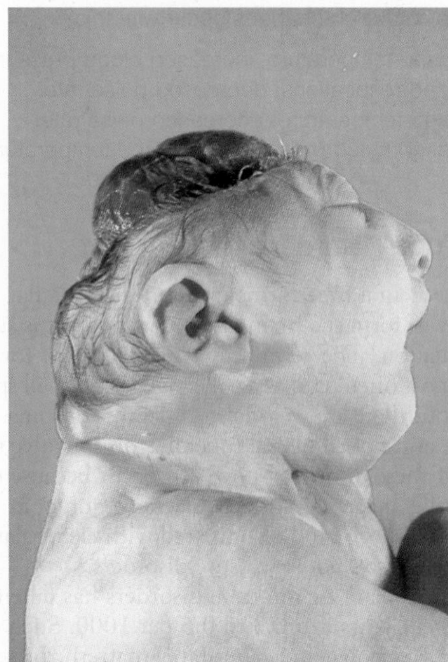

FIGURE 27.11 An infant with anencephaly. (Joseph R. Siebert, PhD/Custom Medical Stock Photograph.)

Microcephaly. Microcephaly is a disorder in which brain growth is so slow that it falls more than three standard deviations below normal on growth charts. The cause might be a disorder in brain development associated with an intrauterine infection such as rubella, cytomegalovirus, or toxoplasmosis. Microcephaly may also result from severe malnutrition or anoxia in early infancy.

The prognosis for a normal life is guarded in children with microcephaly and depends on the extent of restriction of brain growth and on the cause. Generally the infant is cognitively challenged because of the lack of functioning brain tissue. True microcephaly must be differentiated from *craniosynostosis* (normal brain growth but premature fusion of the cranial sutures), which also causes decreased head circumference. Infants with craniosynostosis have abnormally closed fontanelles and often show bossing of the forehead and signs of increased intracranial pressure similar to infants with hydrocephalus. With surgery, craniosynostosis can be relieved and brain growth will be normal.

Spina Bifida Occulta. Spina bifida occulta occurs when the posterior laminae of the vertebrae fail to fuse. This occurs most commonly at the fifth lumbar or first sacral level but may occur at any point along the spinal canal. The normal spinal cord is shown in Figure 27.12A. Spina bifida occulta may be noticeable as a dimpling at the point of poor fusion; abnormal tufts of hair or discolored skin may be present (Sponseller, 2007). Simple spina bifida occulta is a benign disorder; it occurs as frequently as in one of every four children (see Fig. 27.12B).

The term "spina bifida" is often used to denote all spinal cord anomalies. Because of this usage, parents, when told that their child has a spina bifida occulta, may interpret this as meaning their child has an extremely serious disorder. Help clarify the degree of defect for them.

Meningocele. If the meninges covering the spinal cord herniate through unformed vertebrae, a meningocele occurs. The anomaly appears as a protruding mass, usually approximately the size of an orange, at the center of the back (see Fig. 27.12C). It generally occurs in the lumbar region, although it might be present anywhere along the spinal canal. The protrusion may be covered by a layer of skin or only the clear dura mater.

Myelomeningocele. In a myelomeningocele, the spinal cord and the meninges protrude through the vertebrae the same as with a meningocele. The difference is that the spinal cord ends at the point, so motor and sensory function is absent beyond this point (see Fig. 27.12D). Because this results in lower motor neuron damage, the child will have flaccidity and lack of sensation of the lower extremities and loss of bowel and bladder control. Infants' legs are lax, and they do not move them; urine and stools continually dribble because of lack of sphincter control. Children often have accompanying talipes (clubfoot) disorders and developmental hip dysplasia. Hydrocephalus accompanies myelomeningocele in as many as 80% of infants because of the lack of an adequate subarach-

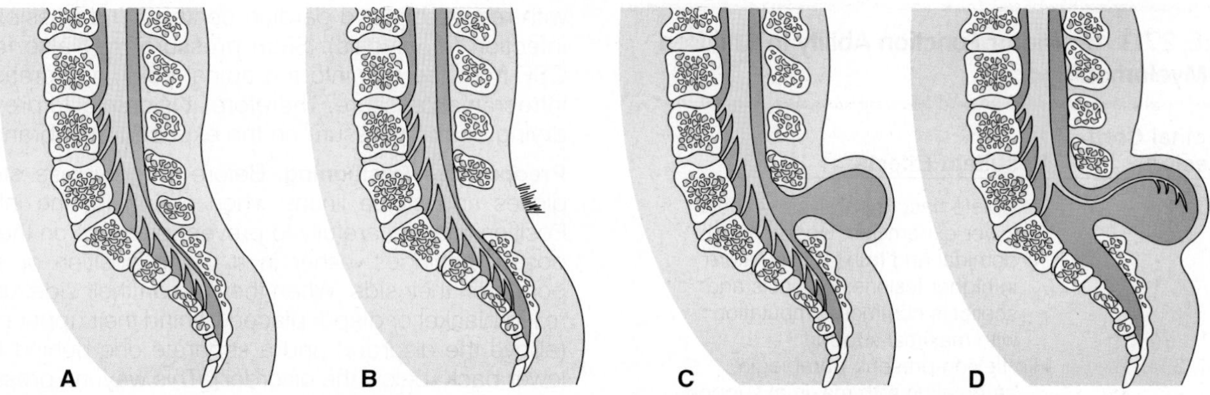

FIGURE 27.12 Degrees of spinal cord anomalies. (**A**) Normal spinal cord. (**B**) Spina bifida occulta. (**C**) Meningocele. (**D**) Myelomeningocele.

noid membrane for CSF absorption; the higher the myelomeningocele occurs on the cord, the more likely it is that hydrocephalus will accompany it. It is generally difficult to tell from visual appearance whether the disorder is myelomeningocele or the simpler meningocele (Fig. 27.13). A CT or ultrasound scan or MRI will reveal this.

Encephalocele. An encephalocele is a cranial meningocele or myelomeningocele. The disorder occurs most often in the occipital area of the skull but may occur as a nasal or nasopharyngeal disorder. Encephaloceles generally are covered fully by skin, but they may be open or covered only by the dura. It is difficult to tell from the size of the encephalocele if only CSF is trapped in the protruding meninges or whether brain tissue could also be involved. Transillumination of the sac will reveal solid substance or fluid in the sac. CT, MRI, or ultrasound will reveal the size of the skull disorder.

Assessment

Neural tube disorders may be discovered during intrauterine life by prenatal ultrasound, fetoscopy, amniocentesis (discovery of increased AFP in amniotic fluid), or analysis of AFP in the maternal serum. If the condition is discovered in utero, it may be possible to close the lesion by fetoscopic surgery. Infants may be born by cesarean birth to avoid pressure and injury to the spinal cord. Observe and record whether an infant born with a neural tube disorder has spontaneous movement of the lower extremities to assess if the child has lower motor function. Also assess the nature and pattern of voiding and defecation. A normal infant appears to be "always wet" from voiding but actually voids in amounts of approximately 30 mL and then is dry for 2 or 3 hours before voiding again. An infant without motor or sphincter control voids continually. This pattern is the same for defecation. Observing these features aids in differentiating between meningocele and myelomeningocele. Differentiation will be further established by ultrasound or MRI.

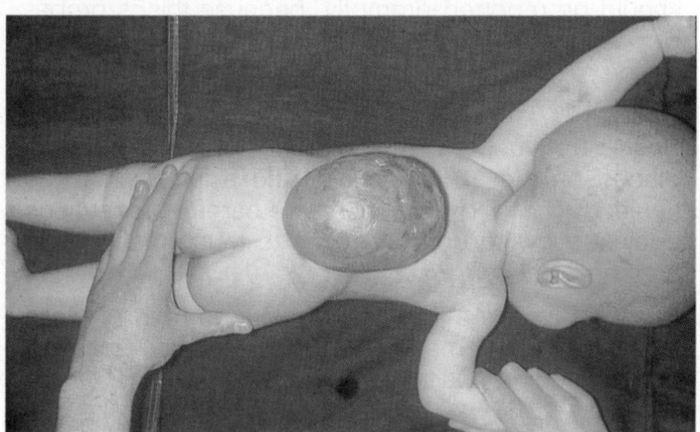

FIGURE 27.13 A myelomeningocele. The infant also has hydrocephaly and a subluxated hip. (NMSB/Custom Medical Stock Photograph.)

Therapeutic Management

Children with spina bifida occulta need no immediate surgical correction. The parents should be made aware of the defect, however, so they are not surprised if it is revealed on a spinal x-ray taken for some reason later in life. Some children may eventually need surgery to prevent vertebral deterioration because of the unbalanced spinal column.

Treatment for a meningocele, myelomeningocele, or encephalocele involves immediate surgery to replace the contents that are replaceable and to close the skin disorder to prevent infection. In the past, surgery for neural tube disorders was done only after the infant had survived the newborn period. Currently, it is done as soon after birth as possible (usually within 24 to 48 hours) so infection through the exposed meninges does not occur.

Surgery for repair of a meningocele or myelomeningocele is not without risk, and brain disorders accompanying an encephalocele may limit the child's cognitive potential. The loss of meninges removed by surgery may limit the rate of absorption of CSF. This may lead to a buildup of CSF, resulting in hydrocephalus. Parents need a great deal of support to care for a child with a myelomeningocele because their child has multiple challenges. The child with myelomeningocele will continue to have paralysis of the lower extremities and loss of bowel and bladder function after surgery because the absent lower cord cannot be replaced. Table 27.1 provides a classification of motor function ability according to the location of spinal cord disruptions.

TABLE 27.1 ✻ Motor Function Ability in Children With Myelomeningocele

Spinal Cord Lesion	Resultant Effects
T6–12	Complete flaccid paralysis of the lower extremities; weakened abdominal and trunk musculature in higher lesions; kyphosis and scoliosis common; ambulation with maximal support
L1–2	Hip flexion present; paraplegia, ambulation with maximal support
L3–4	Hip flexion, adduction, and knee extension present; hip dislocation common; some control of hip and knee movement possible; ambulation with moderate support
L5	Hip flexion, adduction, and varying degrees of abduction; knee extension and weak knee flexion; paralysis of the lower legs and feet; ambulation with moderate support
S1–2	As above, with preservation of some foot and ankle movement; ambulation with minimal support
S3	Mild loss of intrinsic foot muscular function possible; ambulation without support

Nursing Diagnoses and Related Interventions: Immediate Concerns

✻

Although parents of an infant with a myelomeningocele were told before surgery that their child's spinal disorder is a type that means motor and sensory function are absent in the child's lower extremities, the parents do not necessarily "hear" this information. Only after surgery do they begin to comprehend the extent of the condition. When the child is discharged from the hospital, be certain the parents understand what is the next step they need to follow for further care. This prevents them from feeling deserted when they most need support—the time when they first begin to appreciate what this problem will mean to them in the coming years, and what it will mean to their child throughout life.

Nursing Diagnosis: Risk for infection related to rupture or bacterial invasion of the neural tube sac

Outcome Evaluation: Neural tube sac remains intact; axillary temperature remains below 98.6° F (37° C).

If the exposed meningeal sac is allowed to dry, it can crack, allowing CSF to drain and microorganisms to enter. Pressure on the protruding mass is a prime reason why the sac ruptures, leading to quick decompression of the CSF (which can lead to herniation of the brainstem into the spinal cord and interference with respiratory and cardiac centers) and possibly to infection (meningitis). Such pressure may also force CSF from the sac into the spinal column, increasing intracranial pressure. Therefore, it is crucial to prevent drying of and pressure on the exposed membrane.

Preoperative Positioning. Before surgery, use sterile gloves and sterile linens when caring for the infant. Position infants carefully to prevent pressure on the exposed meninges, either in a prone position or supported on their side. When they are on their side, use a rolled blanket or diaper placed behind their upper back (above the disorder) and a separate one behind their lower back (below the disorder). This way, no pressure will be exerted on the lesion, and the infant will be protected from rolling backward onto it. Placing infants on their abdomen has the added advantage of keeping the flow of feces and urine away from the spinal defect as well as keeping it free from pressure. A folded towel under the abdomen helps to flex the infant's hips, reduce pressure on the sac, and ensure good leg position. If an infant is lying on a side, putting a folded diaper between the legs prevents skin surfaces from touching and rubbing (and also helps to keep the hips from internally rotating). Always notice the position of the infant's legs. If they are paralyzed because of lack of motor control, the infant cannot move and straighten them to a more comfortable position.

Placing a piece of plastic or sturdy plastic wrap below the meningocele on the child's back like an apron and taping it in place is another method of preventing feces from touching the open lesion. A sterile wet compress of saline, antiseptic, or antibiotic gauze over the lesion may be used to keep the sac moist. Rather than remove this to wet it again and risk rupturing the sac, merely add additional fluid.

Although no pressure should be exerted on the open lesion by a top sheet, make certain that the child is adequately warm. The presence of the sac adds to the amount of body surface area exposed, thereby increasing heat loss. The infant may need to be kept in an incubator to maintain body heat if a large area of the back cannot be covered. Use caution when placing the infant under a radiant heat source for warmth because radiant heat can dry the lesion and cause cracking. Any seepage of clear fluid from the defect should be reported promptly, because this is probably escaping CSF. Checking any leakage for evidence of glucose will confirm the fluid is CSF (urine or mucus will not test positive for glucose).

Postoperative Care. After surgery, a child is again placed on the abdomen until the skin incision has healed (about 7 days). The same careful precautions against allowing urine or feces to touch the incision area are necessary.

Nursing Diagnosis: Risk for imbalanced nutrition, less than body requirements, related to difficulty assuming normal feeding position.

Outcome Evaluation: Child's skin turgor is good; weight is maintained within 10% of birth weight; specific gravity of urine remains between 1.003 and 1.030.

To maintain nutrition, help parents hold the infant in as normal a feeding position as possible. Make certain that a supporting arm does not press against the lesion. Remind the parents that when bubbling the infant, they should not pat the back over the defect. If the defect is large and the risk in picking up the infant is too great, the infant may be fed while lying on the side in bed or prone on a specialized bed frame. Raise the infant's head slightly by slipping a folded diaper under it. Stroke the head, arms, or upper back while the infant sucks to give the child the same comfort and assurance at feeding time as a baby receives while being held. Infants may enjoy a pacifier after feeding, because they do not experience the same enjoyment of sucking while feeding that would be experienced if they could be held and cuddled. All new parents have some difficulty getting comfortable with feeding an infant. Parents who must feed their child in an unusual position or with an infant on a support frame will have even more difficulty. Role-model a warm, comforting parental role so parents can begin to form a positive parent–child interaction.

Children with increased intracranial pressure tend to suck poorly. If this complication develops after surgery, breastfeeding may be difficult. Parents need a realistic explanation of the treatment planned for the child so they can decide whether to continue breastfeeding. If it is necessary to forgo breastfeeding for this child, you can assure parents that the child will thrive on commercial formula.

Nursing Diagnosis: Risk for ineffective cerebral tissue perfusion related to increased intracranial pressure.

Outcome Evaluation: Child's head circumference remains within present percentile on growth chart; signs and symptoms of increased intracranial pressure are absent.

Preoperative Care. Increasing head size from poor absorption of CSF (hydrocephalus) is a common complication of neural tube disorders. To detect increased head size (development of hydrocephalus), measure head circumference once daily (or more frequently if ordered) in the preoperative period. Head circumference measurements are accurate only if the tape measure is placed on the same points of the child's head each time. Placing an indelible or ballpoint pen mark on the forehead just above the eyebrows and at the most prominent point of the occiput allows different people to measure the head during the day and yet be sure that they all measure at the same point.

Postoperative Care. Children may develop hydrocephalus after surgery as well, probably because of interference with subarachnoid absorption of CSF. The shortening of the meninges can create an Arnold-Chiari disorder (see later) or can cause traction of the hindbrain into the spinal cord. Observe the child frequently for signs of increased intracranial pressure such as changes in vital signs, neurologic signs such as pupillary changes, or an increase in head circumference or bulging fontanelles, as well as behavioral changes such as irritability or lethargy to help detect if this is happening.

Nursing Diagnosis: Risk for impaired skin integrity related to required prone positioning.

Outcome Evaluation: Infant's skin remains intact, without erythema or ulceration.

Preserving skin integrity is a major problem before surgery because the constant prone position puts pressure on the infant's knees and elbows. Laying the infant on a synthetic sheepskin helps reduce friction; after surgery, use paper tape or stockinette for dressing changes or place protective dressings such as Stomahesive on the skin under the area where the tape will touch. Change diapers frequently to prevent excessive contact of acid urine with skin. If hydrocephalus has developed, the head will be heavy and pressure areas at the temples can occur if the head is not repositioned about every 2 hours.

Nursing Diagnoses and Related Interventions: Long-term Concerns

Nursing Diagnosis: Impaired physical mobility related to neural tube disorder

Outcome Evaluation: Child ambulates with the least amount of accessory equipment possible.

Help parents begin to plan stimulation activities their infant can accomplish with limited mobility. Encourage them to take the infant to the places children normally accompany parents—relatives' homes, shopping, the zoo, and so forth as encouraging children to be independent helps them lead as active a life as possible (Davis et al., 2007). (Fig. 27.14).

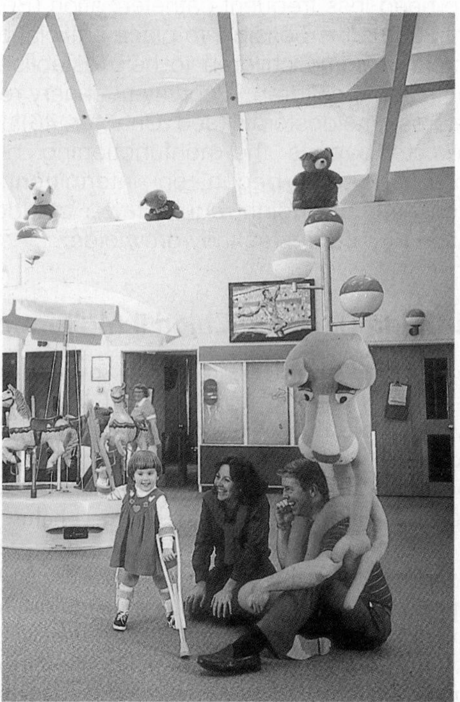

FIGURE 27.14 A child born with a neural tube disorder demonstrates her ability to walk using braces and a crutch. (Alexander Tsiara/Photo Researchers, Inc.)

Parents will need to perform passive exercises to prevent muscle atrophy and formation of contractures if a child has impaired lower extremity motor control. The child may need leg braces to help maintain good alignment and enable walking with crutches. Parents are generally anxious to do something for their child and follow routines of passive exercises well if they are given sufficient support for their accomplishments at health care visits. As the child grows older, tendon transplants or osteotomy may be necessary to prevent contractures and poor bone alignment. Because children with myelomeningocele have no sensation in their lower extremities, parents should make a routine of inspecting the child's lower extremities and buttocks daily for any area of irritation or possible infection. Teach children as they grow older to do this themselves. When children are using a wheelchair, be certain they press with their arms on the armrests to raise their buttocks off the wheelchair seat at least once every hour to help provide adequate circulation to lower extremities.

Nursing Diagnosis: Risk for impaired elimination related to neural tube disorder

Outcome Evaluation: Child demonstrates ability to independently manage bowel and bladder elimination by school age.

To ensure bladder emptying, an intermittent clean urinary catheterization technique may be taught to parents (inserting a clean catheter through the urethra into the bladder every 4 hours to drain urine from the bladder; Box 27.7). As children reach early school age, they can learn this technique for themselves. Prescription of a drug such as oxybutynin chloride (Ditropan) may improve bladder capacity and allow a child to need less frequent catheterization (Box 27.8) (Karch, 2009). It is possible to place artificial bladder sphincters in some children to help establish continence. In some children, a continent urinary reservoir or ureterosigmoidostomy (see Chapter 46) is constructed to bypass the nonfunctioning bladder. Children who are begun on intermittent clean catheterization from birth require fewer bladder augmentation procedures as they grow older.

Arnold-Chiari Disorder (Chiari II Malformation)

An Arnold-Chiari disorder is caused by overgrowth of the neural tube in weeks 16 to 20 of fetal life. The specific anomaly is a projection of the cerebellum, medulla oblongata, and fourth ventricle into the cervical canal. This causes the upper cervical spinal cord to jackknife backward, obstructing CSF flow and causing hydrocephalus. A lumbosacral myelomeningocele is also present in approximately 50% of children with this anomaly (Donahue, 2008).

The prognosis for the child with an Arnold-Chiari malformation depends on the extent of the disorder and the surgical procedure possible. Because of the upper motor neuron involvement, gagging and swallowing reflexes may be absent, increasing the risk for tracheal aspiration. Serious levels of sleep apnea may occur that also require surgical intervention (Tubbs et al., 2007).

BOX 27.7 * Focus on Family Teaching

Instructions for Clean Intermittent Catheterization

Q. Baby Sparrow's mother needs to learn clean intermittent catheterization for her son. She asks you, "How do I do this?"

A. Here are some helpful guidelines to follow:

1. Remember that the purpose of intermittent catheterization is to keep the bladder empty by using clean technique and frequent emptying so microorganisms do not have time to grow in urine in the bladder. Always use clean equipment and catheterize at least every 4 hours.
2. Always carry catheterization equipment with you when away from home (a plastic bag containing a clean catheter and water-soluble lubricant). This enables you to stay longer away from home if you wish. If you will be using a public lavatory, you might want to include a presoaped washcloth rather than have to use rough paper towels.
3. To begin catheterization, wash your hands in warm, soapy water. This reduces the chance you will introduce germs from your hands into your child's bladder.
4. Next wash around your child's urinary meatus with a clean washcloth or paper towel and warm, soapy water. Rinse the washcloth and wash again with clear water. This reduces the chance that germs on the child's skin will be pushed into the bladder.
5. Coat the tip of a clean catheter with water-soluble lubricant. This reduces friction and makes the catheter slide into the bladder easily.
6. Quickly but gently insert the catheter into the urinary meatus approximately 3 inches. Urine should begin to flow immediately through the catheter. Let this drain into a collecting basin.
7. When urine stops flowing, gently remove the catheter. To reuse the catheter, clean it with soap and water, rinse with clear water, and replace in the plastic bag with the lubricant or replace with a new cathether.
8. Be certain that on special days such as family celebrations or vacation you do not forget the importance of catheterization.
9. As your child reaches school age, you can teach him how to do this himself. He will need to insert the catheter about 6 inches. Be certain he will be able to have access to a school bathroom every 4 hours during the day.
10. Phone your health care provider if urine is blood-tinged, smells foul, or is cloudy rather than clear or if your child appears to have pain in his abdomen or lower back or has an elevated temperature. These may be symptoms of a urinary tract infection.

PHYSICAL AND DEVELOPMENTAL DISORDERS OF THE SKELETAL SYSTEM

Either genetic or environmental factors can compromise fetal physical growth to such an extent they result in skeletal disorders in the newborn.

BOX 27.8 ✻ Focus on Pharmacology

Oxybutynin Chloride (Ditropan)

Classification: Oxybutynin is an anticholinergic, urinary antispasmodic.

Action: Relaxes smooth muscle to relieve symptoms of bladder instability associated with neurogenic bladder (Karch, 2009).

Pregnancy Risk Category: C

Dosage: 5 mg orally twice daily

Possible Adverse Effects: Drowsiness, dizziness, blurred vision, decreased sweating

Nursing Implications

- Advise the parents to give or have the child take the medication exactly as prescribed.
- Alert the parents about the need for frequent bladder examinations during treatment to document the drug's effect.
- Ask the child to report drowsiness or blurred vision. Caution the child not to attempt activities that require balance while taking the drug.
- Caution the child and parents that with decreased sweating, body temperature can rise. Encourage the parents to keep the child's environment cool and avoid high temperatures.

Absent or Malformed Extremities

Congenital skeletal disorders may result from reasons such as maternal drug ingestion, virus invasion during pregnancy, or amniotic band formation in utero. In most instances, however, the cause of the anomaly cannot be established. Children born without an extremity or with a malformed extremity can be fitted with a prosthesis early in life. In most instances, children will have better function if the malformed portion of an extremity is amputated before a prosthesis is fitted. This is a difficult decision for parents to make, however, because it is one that they cannot undo later. They need assurance that hands with malformed fingers, for example, will not later grow to become normal. A well-fitted prosthesis that a child learns to use at an early age will provide more function and allow a more normal childhood and adult life than if the original disorder is left unchanged (Fig. 27.15). Lower extremity prostheses are fitted as early as age 6 months (so an infant will learn to stand at the normal time). Upper extremity prostheses are fitted this early also, so an infant can handle and explore objects readily.

Introducing a prosthesis early also prevents a child from adjusting to a missing extremity, such as writing with the feet or sliding across a floor rather than walking. Children can become so proficient at these adjustments that later in life they do not see the advantage of a prosthesis and refuse to use one. Although these self-adjustments may be cute in infants, in the long run they greatly limit a child's potential.

Learning to use a hand prosthesis takes weeks to months. Help parents think of interesting activities when introducing the prosthesis so the child can see immediately how useful it will be to use. Gait training for use of lower extremity

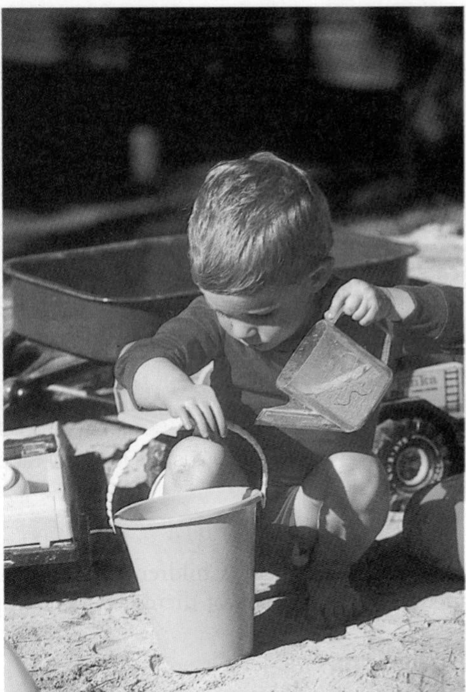

FIGURE 27.15 A young child learns to use a hand prosthesis during play. (M. Grecco/Stock Boston.)

prostheses begins with the use of parallel bars and proceeds to independent walking and mastery of steps.

Children who are born with an absent extremity may need help in mastering not only the use of a prosthesis but also a positive body image of themselves as whole. If possible, in the newborn period, introduce parents to the rehabilitation team who will be following their child. Further steps then will be outlined for them to help them move past the helplessness they may feel to more positive action. Visiting with a child who uses a prosthesis well can be a great help in convincing parents that their child can lead a normal life. Children with a congenital extremity loss do not grieve over the lost extremity as do adults or older children, which means they are often better prepared to move on quickly to rehabilitation.

Finger and Toe Conditions

Finger or hand deformities occur in about 3% of all births. **Polydactyly** is the presence of one or more additional fingers or toes. When an entire extra finger or toe forms, the supernumerary digit is usually amputated in infancy or early childhood. These extra fingers are often just cartilage or skin tags, and removal is simple and cosmetically sound. In **syndactyly** (two fingers or toes are fused), the fusion is usually caused by a simple webbing (Fig. 27.16); separation of the digits into two sound and cosmetically appealing ones is usually successful. In other instances, the bones of the fingers or toes are also fused, and cosmetic appearance and function cannot be fully reconstructed.

These hand anomalies are always upsetting to parents (one of the first things that new parents do is count the fingers and toes of newborns). They may need time to air their feelings and concerns. They may need reassurance at health maintenance visits throughout their child's development that the child is normal in other ways so they can accept and help

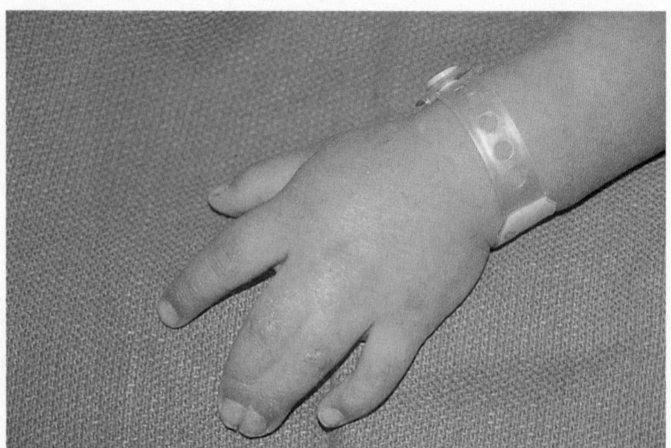

FIGURE 27.16 Syndactyly. (JPD/Custom Medical Stock Photograph.)

the child develop self-esteem. Children need this same type of assurance so they can think of themselves as well people.

Chest Deviations

Pectus excavatum is an indentation of the lower portion of the sternum (Mavanur & Hight, 2008). Children usually are born with this condition, but they may also develop it after chronic obstructive lung disease or rickets. As a result, lung volume decreases and the heart is displaced to the left. This condition can be repaired, either for cosmetic reasons or to expand lung volume. With pectus carinatum, the sternum is displaced anteriorly, increasing the anterior-posterior diameter of the chest. This condition also can be repaired for physiologic or cosmetic reasons.

Torticollis (Wry Neck)

Torticollis is a term derived from *tortus* (twisted) and *collum* (neck). Torticollis (wry neck) occurs as a congenital anomaly when the sternocleidomastoid muscle is injured and bleeds during birth (Waldman & Manista, 2007). This tends to occur in newborns with wide shoulders when pressure is exerted on the head to deliver the shoulder. The infant holds the head tilted to the side of the muscle involved; the chin rotates to the opposite side. The injury may not be noticeable in the newborn and may become evident only as the original hemorrhage recedes and fibrous contraction occurs at 1 to 2 months of age. A thick mass over the muscle can usually be palpated at this time.

To relieve torticollis, parents need to begin a program of passive stretching exercises, lying the infant on a flat surface and rotating the head through a full range of motion. In addition, parents should always encourage the infant to look in the direction of the affected muscle. They can encourage this by holding the child to feed in such a position that the child must look in the desired direction. Placing a mobile on the child's crib to encourage the child to look toward the affected side also is helpful. Speaking to and handing the child objects from the affected side to make the child look that way are also helpful exercises.

If manual stretching is begun early and consistently by the parents, further treatment usually is not necessary. Help parents understand that these actions are important therapy and not just games. Otherwise, the exercises seem so simple parents may not take them seriously. In the few instances in which simple exercises are not effective and the condition still exists at 1 year of age, surgical correction followed by a neck immobilizer will be necessary. If extreme injury to the muscle occurred, torticollis can lead to the continued elevation of one shoulder. Although a rare complication, this has the potential to lead to scoliosis later in life.

Parents may ask about the use of botulism (Botox) injections, because adults who develop spastic torticollis may receive this type of treatment (Benecke & Dressler, 2007). It is not recommended or necessary for most infants.

✓ Checkpoint Question 27.4

What is an important care measure to teach parents of a child with torticollis?

a. Encourage the infant to turn his head to stretch the neck.
b. Wrap the infant's neck in a warm towel twice daily.
c. Massage the infant's shoulders and torso at bedtime.
d. Administer 1 grain of aspirin with each bottle feeding.

Craniosynostosis

Craniosynostosis is premature closure of the sutures of the skull. This may occur in utero or early in infancy because of rickets or irregularities of calcium or phosphate metabolism; it also occurs as a dominantly inherited trait (Elias, Tsai, & Manchester, 2008). It occurs more often in boys than in girls.

This condition needs to be detected early because premature closure of the suture line will seal the skull closed and compromise brain growth. When the sagittal suture line closes prematurely, the child's head tends to grow anteriorly and posteriorly. If the coronal suture line fuses early, the orbits of the eyes become misshapen, and the increased intracranial pressure may lead to exophthalmos, nystagmus, papilledema, strabismus, and atrophy of the optic nerve with consequent loss of vision. Premature closure of the coronal suture line is associated with syndactyly. Therefore, closely observe all infants with syndactyly for head circumference. Conversely, assess all infants with craniosynostosis for syndactyly. Cardiac anomalies, choanal atresias, or disorders of elbows and knee joints are also associated with craniosynostosis.

Measure head circumference on all children age 2 years or younger at health maintenance visits and compare these measurements with normal head circumference charts. The posterior fontanelle normally closes at 2 months of age, the anterior fontanelle at 12 to 18 months. Children whose fontanelles close before these typical times need continued assessment to ensure that craniosynostosis is not developing.

Craniosynostosis is diagnosed by radiography or ultrasound, which reveals the fused suture line. If the suture line is the sagittal one, treatment may involve only careful observation; if the coronal suture line is involved, it will need to be surgically opened to prevent brain compression and an abnormally shaped head (Elias, Tsai, & Manchester, 2008).

Achondroplasia

Achondroplasia (chondrodystrophia) is a failure of bone growth inherited as a dominant trait. It causes a disorder in cartilage production in utero. The epiphyseal plate of long bones cannot produce adequate cartilage for longitudinal bone growth, which results in both arms and legs becoming stunted.

Because the bones of the cranium are of membranous origin, they continue to grow normally. Children's heads will therefore appear unusually large in contrast to their extremities. The forehead is prominent and the bridge of the nose is flattened. Because this is a cartilage, not a brain, problem, intelligence proceeds normally. Children's trunks are of near-normal size, but a thoracic kyphosis (outward curve) and lumbar lordosis (inward curve) of the spine may develop.

Achondroplasia can be diagnosed in utero or at birth by comparing the length of extremities to the normal length (in the average child, the arms can be extended to the distance of the midthigh) or by radiography, which will reveal characteristic abnormally flaring epiphyseal lines. People with achondroplasia rarely reach a height of more than 4 feet 6 inches (140 cm). Women with this condition will have difficulty with childbearing because of a small pelvis, generally necessitating a cesarean birth.

Children with achondroplasia become aware of their appearance as early as the preschool years. They are apt to become acutely aware of their appearance during school age, when they realize they look different from other children. Children may be prescribed growth hormone to increase their ultimate height or, although controversial, leg lengthening may be possible (Horton, Hall, & Hecht, 2007). Ideally, such children have parents who have adjusted well to their own short stature and therefore have developed good self-esteem and can implant these qualities in their child.

Children should be informed that, as with all dominantly inherited disorders, there is a high probability that their children will inherit the disorder. Adolescence may be a particularly difficult time for these children as they realize that occupational and reproductive options may be limited for them. Continued guidance or counseling can help them to emerge from this period with feelings of high self-esteem in themselves as adults.

What if... Baby Sparrow's mother tells you she wants to let her newborn die rather than undergo palliative surgery to close the neural tube disorder? Whose rights should be honored, the parent's or the child's, and how should these rights be determined? What would be your role?

Talipes Disorders

Talipes is a word formed from the Latin words *talus* ("ankle") and *pes* ("foot"). The talipes deformities are ankle–foot disorders, popularly called clubfoot (Forster & Fraser, 2007). The term "clubfoot" implies permanent crippling to many people, so avoid using this term when discussing talipes disorders with parents. With the orthopedic correction techniques currently available, correction should leave the child with normal foot position. However, shoe size may vary as much as two shoe sizes, and the child may have asymmetry of leg length.

Approximately 1 in every 1000 children is born with a talipes disorder, occurring more often in boys than in girls. It probably is inherited as a polygenic pattern. It usually occurs as a unilateral problem (Eilert, 2008).

Some newborns have a pseudo-talipes disorder that has developed because of their intrauterine position. In these infants, the foot looks to be turned in but can be brought into a straight position by manipulation. In a true disorder, the foot cannot be properly aligned without further intervention. Be certain to demonstrate to parents that if a pseudo-disorder is present, the foot can easily be brought into line or is not deformed. Otherwise, the first time parents fit booties or shoes on the infant, they will notice this and worry that the foot is misshapen.

A true talipes disorder can be one of four separate types: plantarflexion (an equinus or "horsefoot" position, with the forefoot lower than the heel); dorsiflexion (the heel is held lower than the forefoot or the anterior foot is flexed toward the anterior leg); varus deviation (the foot turns in); or valgus deviation (the foot turns out). Most children with talipes deformities have a combination of these conditions or have an equinovarus (Fig. 27.17A) or a calcaneovalgus disorder (a child walks on the heel with the foot everted).

Assessment

The earlier a true disorder is recognized, the better will be the correction. Make a habit of straightening all newborn feet to the midline as part of initial assessment to detect this disorder.

Therapeutic Management

Correction is achieved best if it is begun in the newborn period. A cast is applied while the foot is placed in an

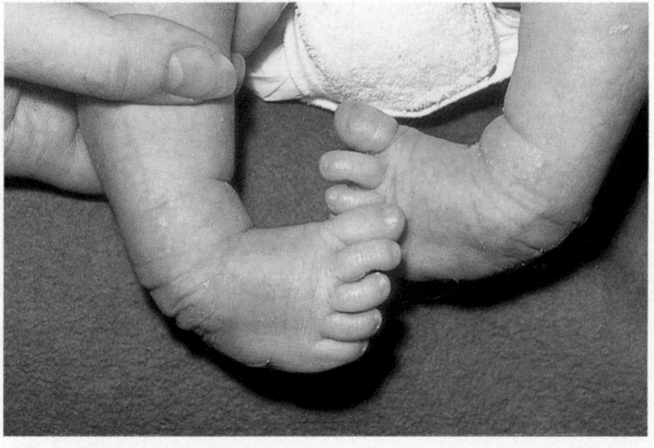

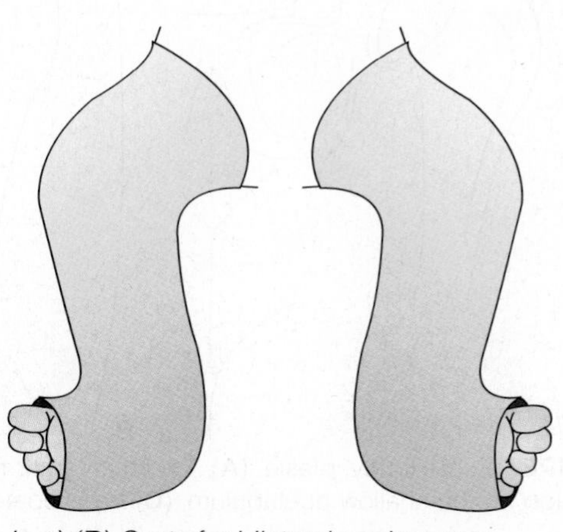

FIGURE 27.17 (**A**) Talipes equinovarus. (SPL/Photo Researchers, Inc.) (**B**) Casts for bilateral equinovarus.

overcorrected position. Although the disorder involves the ankle, the cast extends above the knee to ensure firm correction (see Fig. 27.17B). (Care of the child in a cast is discussed in Chapter 51.) Because talipes casts are high on the leg, change diapers frequently to prevent a wet diaper from touching the cast and causing it to become soaked with urine or meconium. Review with parents how to check the infant's toes for coldness or blueness and how to blanch a toenail bed and watch it turn pink to assess for good circulation. Because a newborn cannot report pain except by generalized crying, crying episodes in the infant must be evaluated carefully. Such crying may be because of colic, hunger, or wet diapers; it might also be because of the tingling feeling of circulatory compression (as when a foot is "asleep") from too tight a cast.

Infants grow so rapidly in the neonatal period that casts for talipes deformities must be changed almost every 1 or 2 weeks. If a mother has a complication of childbirth or is exhausted from childbirth (depression because of the child having been born congenitally challenged may manifest itself as exhaustion), be certain she knows to make arrangements for another family member to bring the infant to the hospital for cast changes.

After approximately 6 weeks (the time varies depending on the extent of the problem), the final cast is removed. After this, parents may need to perform passive foot exercises such as putting the infant's foot and ankle through a full range of motion several times a day for several months. These seem like simple maneuvers, so be sure to stress their importance to the parents; otherwise, they are easy exercises to omit when people's lives are busy. The infant may have to sleep in Denis Browne splints (shoes attached to a metal bar to maintain position; see Chapter 51) or high-top shoes at night for a few more months.

Although a successful correction cannot be guaranteed, the prognosis for a full correction is good. For children who do not achieve correction by casting, surgery is yet another option to achieve a final correction.

Developmental Hip Dysplasia

Developmental hip dysplasia (often referred to as congenital hip dysplasia) is improper formation and function of the hip socket (Eilert, 2008). The disorder occurs in 1 in 1000 births. It may be evident as subluxation or dislocation of the head of the femur (Fig. 27.18).

With this disorder, the acetabulum of the pelvis is flattened or shallow. This prevents the head of the femur from remaining in the acetabulum and rotating adequately. In a subluxated hip, the femur "rides up" because of the flat acetabulum; in a dislocated hip, the femur rides so far up that it actually leaves the acetabulum. Why the disorder occurs is unknown, but it may be from a polygenic inheritance pattern. It may also occur from a uterine position that causes less-than-usual pressure of the femur head on the acetabulum.

Developmental hip dysplasia occurs most often in children of Mediterranean ancestry. It is found six times more frequently in girls than in boys, possibly because the hips are normally more flaring in females and possibly because the maternal hormone relaxin causes the pelvic ligaments to be more relaxed. Therefore, the femur does not press as effectively into the acetabulum during intrauterine life, deepening

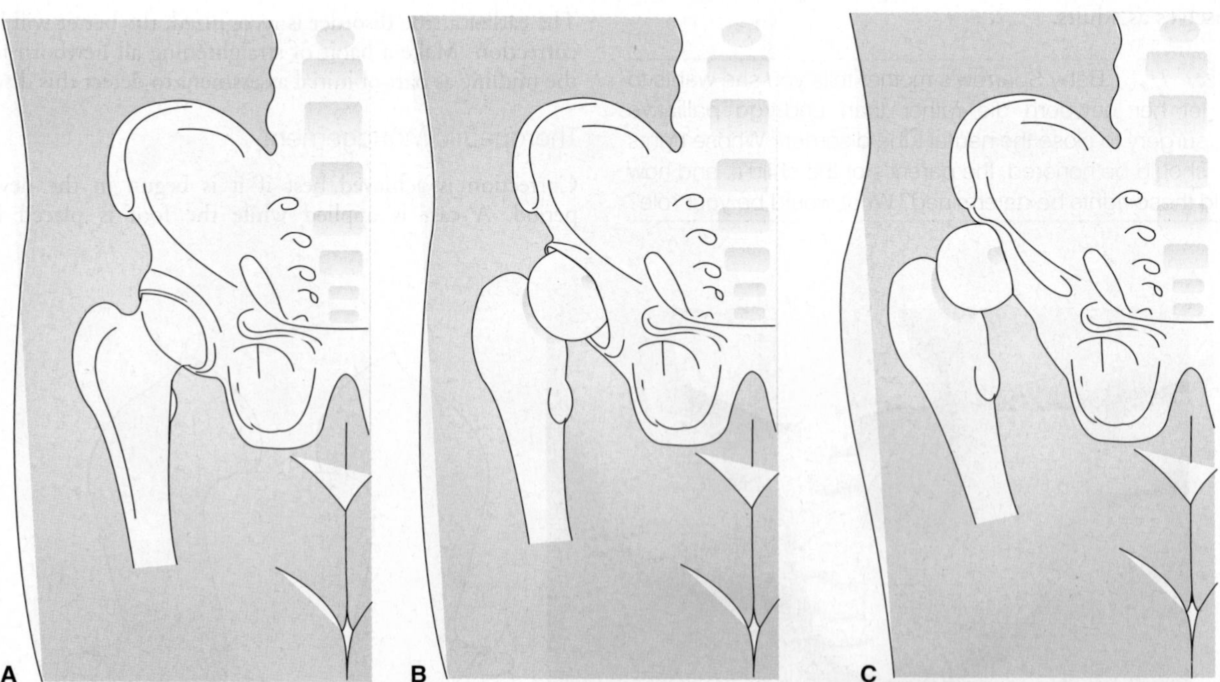

FIGURE 27.18 Hip dysplasia. (**A**) A normal femur head and acetabulum. (**B**) A subluxated hip. The femur head is "riding high" in the shallow acetabulum. (**C**) A dislocated hip. The femur head is not engaged in the shallow acetabulum.

the space. Involvement usually is unilateral. Sociocultural methods of childrearing, such as the way infants are carried, may promote or decrease the extent of the involvement.

Assessment

Detecting developmental hip dysplasia in the newborn is important because the longer the condition goes undetected, the more difficult it is to correct. Sometimes the affected leg may appear slightly shorter than the other one because the femur head rides so high in the socket. This is most noticeable when the child is lying supine and the thighs are flexed to a 90-degree angle toward the abdomen. One knee will appear to be lower than the other (a Galeazzi sign (Fig. 27.19A). An unequal number of skin folds may be present on the posterior thighs (see Fig. 27.19B). This finding is unreliable, however, because some infants with normal hips have an uneven number of posterior thigh skin folds. Subluxated or dislocated hips are best assessed by noting whether the hips abduct (Box 27.9).

In some infants, the hip abducts properly at a newborn assessment, but at the time of a health maintenance visit at 4 to 6 weeks, a secondary shortening of the adductor muscles will have occurred, and the disorder will be evident. Hip dysplasia is difficult to detect at birth in an infant who was born from a footling or frank breech presentation because the knees are stiff and do not flex readily. Always assess hip function in these infants at each health maintenance visit. Tight adductor muscles occur in children with cerebral palsy, so this disorder must be ruled out. Radiography, ultrasound, or MRI will reveal the shallow acetabulum and a more lateral placement of the femur head than is ordinarily seen.

Therapeutic Management

Correction of subluxated and dislocated hips involves positioning the hip into a flexed, abducted (externally rotated) position to press the femur head against the acetabulum and cause it to deepen its contour by the pressure. Splints, halters, or casts may be used. The small number of children who do not achieve correction by these methods will have surgery and a pin inserted to stabilize the hip.

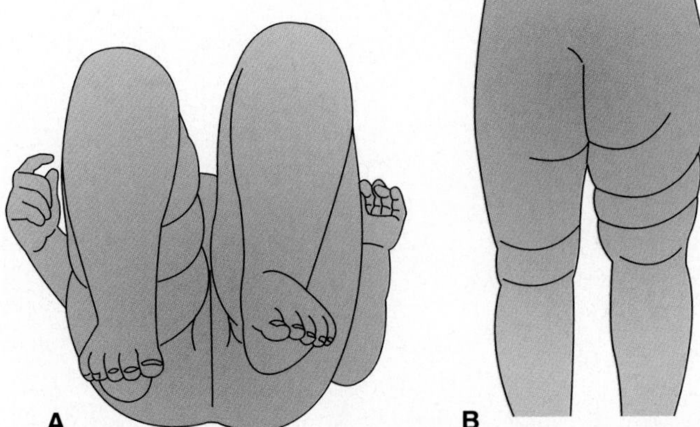

FIGURE 27.19 Signs of developmental hip dysplasia. (**A**) With child in a supine position, the right knee on the side of the subluxation appears lower than the left because of malposition of the femur head. (**B**) Asymmetry of skin folds and prominence of the trochanter on the right side.

Nursing Diagnoses and Related Interventions

Nursing Diagnosis: Deficient parental knowledge related to splint, halter, or cast correction for hip dysplasia

Outcome Evaluation: Parents verbalize correct technique for and correctly demonstrate application and removal of splint or halter device and care of device or cast.

Multiple Diapers or Splints. Often splint correction (to hold the legs in a frog-leg, or abducted, externally rotated position) is begun during the newborn's initial hospital stay by placing two or three diapers on the infant. The extra bulk of cloth between the child's legs effectively separates and spreads them. Many brands of disposable diapers are cut narrow between the legs so they do not offer this much bulk and will not work as well as cloth diapers.

The way that parents carry infants may contribute to the formation of hip dysplasia. Infants who are carried straddled on their parents' hips, the way Latin American mothers carry their infants, may have less hip dysplasia than those carried with their legs consistently brought together, such as Native American infants carried on swaddling boards. Swaddling babies is comforting. Be certain, however, these parents understand that bringing this child's legs together with a tight swaddling blanket will not be good for this infant.

Pavlik Harness. A Pavlik harness is an adjustable chest halter that abducts the legs. It is the method of choice for long-term therapy because it reduces the time interval for therapy to 3 to 4 weeks and simplifies care (see Fig. 27.20B). Soft plastic stirrups (booties) with quick-fastening closures such as Velcro attach to leg extension straps and hold the hips flexed, abducted, and externally rotated. Instruct parents to lay the infant supine, grasp the infant's thighs and abduct them to place the femoral head into the acetabulum, and then apply the harness. The harness is then worn continually except for bathing. Advise parents to assess the skin under the straps daily for irritation or redness.

A Pavlik harness does not show under a shirt and long trousers and promotes gentle reduction of the hip. However, if a hip is completely dislocated, a Pavlik harness may not be firm enough to hold the hips in the proper position. In addition, the harness will be ineffective if parents remove it too frequently.

Spica Cast. If a hip is fully dislocated or the subluxation is severe, an infant may be placed immediately in a frog-leg, A-line cast or a spica cast to maintain an externally rotated hip position (see Fig. 27.20C). These casts are heavy and are so wide that dressing infants or sitting them in an infant car seat or bassinet can be

Box 27.9 Nursing Procedure ✻ Assessing Ortolani's and Barlow's Signs

Purpose: To assist in detecting developmental hip dysplasia

Procedure	Principle
1. Lay the infant supine and flex the knees to 90° at the hips.	**1.** Proper positioning ensures accurate results.
2. Place your middle fingers over the greater trochanter of the femur and your thumb on the internal side of the thigh over the lesser trochanter.	**2.** Placing your fingers in this way allows for abduction of the hips.

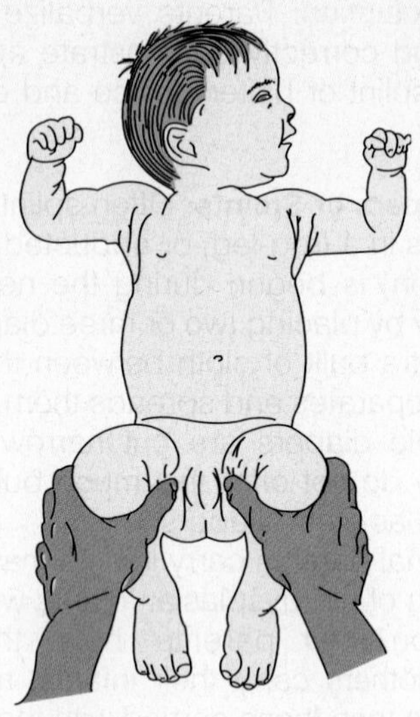

Procedure	Principle
3. Abduct the hips while applying upward pressure over the greater trochanter, and listen for a clicking sound.	**3.** Normally, no sound is heard. A clicking or clunking sound is a positive Ortolani's sign and occurs when the femoral head re-enters the acetabulum.
4. Next, with your fingers in the same position, and holding the hips and knees at 90° flexion, apply a backward pressure (down and laterally) and adduct the hips. Note any feeling of the femoral head slipping.	**4.** Normally, the hip joint is stable. A feeling of the femur head slipping out of the socket posterolaterally is a positive Barlow's sign indicative of hip instability associated with developmental hip dysplasia.

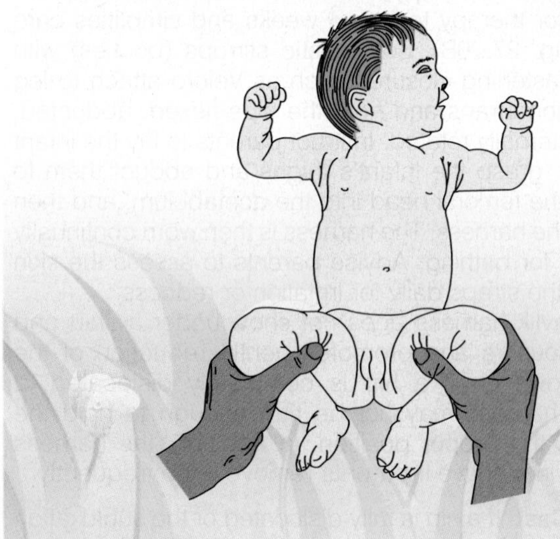

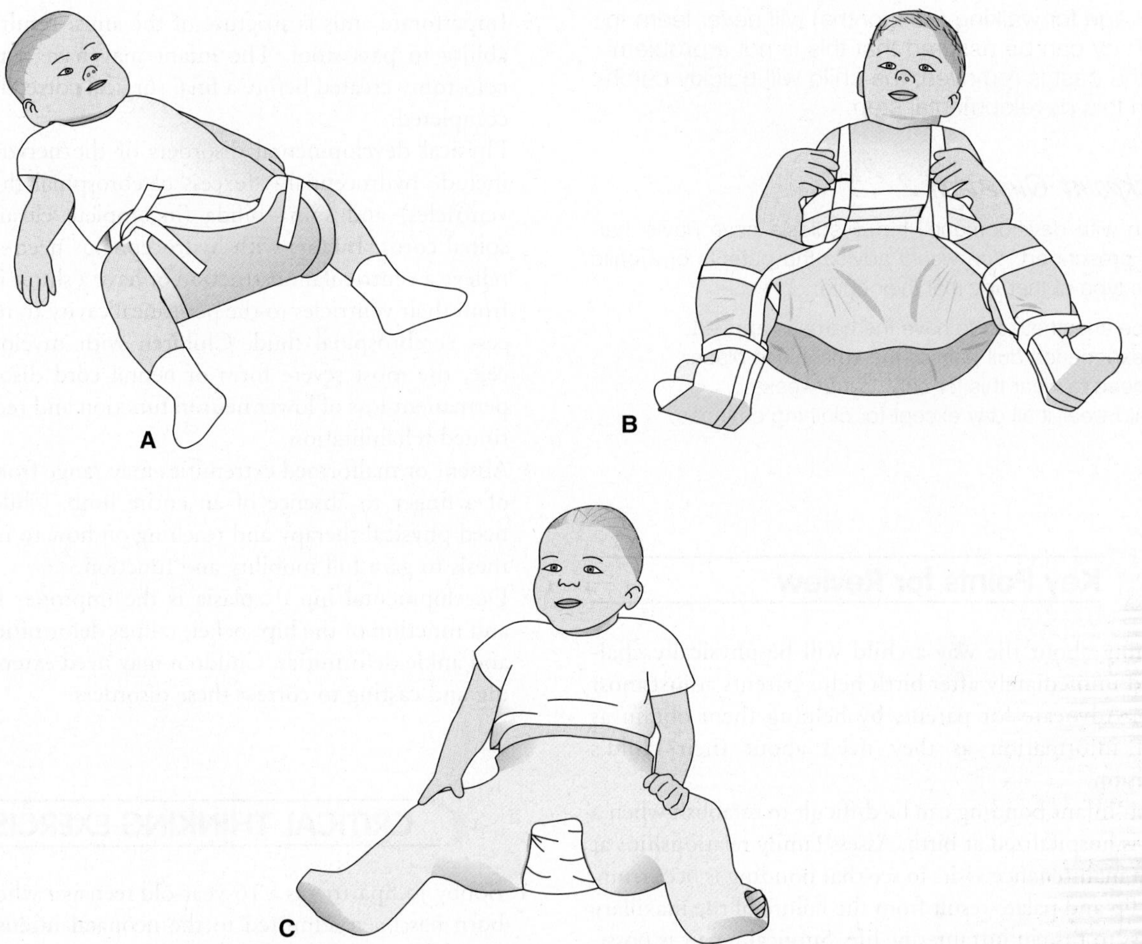

FIGURE 27.20 (**A**) Hip abduction splint (Frejka splint) holds the hips in an abduction position, forcing the femur head into the acetabulum. (**B**) A Pavlik harness. (**C**) A hip abduction cast for correction of subluxation of the hip.

difficult. Be certain parents have a car seat that can be modified to accommodate a large cast. Newborns are unable to report that a cast is causing circulatory constriction, so they need to be assessed hourly for circulation to the extremities for the first 24 hours the cast is in place and daily thereafter. Teach parents how to do this type of neurovascular assessment (check temperature and circulation in toes) before they take an infant home from the hospital so they can prevent circulatory compression from a rapidly growing leg outgrowing a cast. Casts will be changed periodically but maintained for 6 to 9 months. If a reduction maneuver for congenital dislocated hip was forceful, causing tension in the soft tissues around the hip, the resulting compression of the joint may cause transient blockage of the blood supply to the femoral head or avascular necrosis. In its severest form, this can lead to femoral head death and loss of future growth at the proximal growth plate causing unequal leg lengths (Eilert, 2008).

General Care Guidelines. No matter what type of therapy is used—double-diapering, harness, or cast—surgery may still be necessary for a final correction. Making parents aware of this from the start prevents them from thinking their child's condition is so serious that the usual methods of treatment failed. It helps them from becoming discouraged or dissatisfied with health care. It also helps them to accept from the beginning that this condition will be a long-term care concern. Some children will be 2 years old before the final cast or harness is removed.

The child and parents will be visiting their orthopedist frequently during these early years. Assess that parents also schedule general health maintenance visits for routine immunizations and overall growth and development assessment. Spend time during health maintenance visits talking with them about infant stimulation. Because the child is not fully mobile, special adaptations are necessary. Teach parents to hold their child for feeding and to rock and cuddle the infant, even though a large cast or a brace may be bulky and awkward. They need to bring experiences to the infant because the child cannot crawl and walk toward interesting objects in the environment. A child's wagon can supply convenient and fun transportation. The child may also be able to lie prone and move about on a large skateboard. Many parents worry that the child who is still in a large cast at the normal age for walking (12 months) will never learn to walk. They can be assured that this is not a problem; when the cast is removed, the child will quickly catch up with this developmental step.

✔ Checkpoint Question 27.5

Children with developmental hip dysplasia have Pavlik harnesses prescribed. You would advise the parents of a child with this type of therapy that their child:

a. Will be anesthetized to have the harness applied.
b. Will experience dull pain all the time it is in place.
c. Will need to wear this for only 1 or 2 weeks.
d. Should wear it all day except for clothing changes.

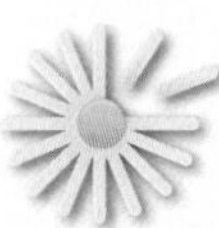

Key Points for Review

- Learning about the way a child will be physically challenged immediately after birth helps parents adjust most easily. Advocate for parents by helping them obtain as much information as they need about their child's condition.
- Parent–infant bonding can be difficult to establish when a child is hospitalized at birth. Assess family relationships at health maintenance visits to see that bonding is occurring.
- Cleft lip and palate result from the failure of the maxillary process to fuse in intrauterine life. Surgical repair is possible early in life, with a good prognosis for both these conditions.
- Tracheoesophageal atresia and fistula occur from failure of the trachea and esophagus to divide appropriately in intrauterine life. Surgical intervention often needs to be performed in several stages.
- Omphalocele is the protrusion of abdominal contents through the abdominal wall at birth, protected only by a peritoneal membrane. When the membrane is not present, this is called gastroschisis. Although several stages of repair are often necessary, surgical correction has a good outcome.
- Intestinal obstruction can result from atresia (complete closure) or stenosis (narrowing) of a part of the bowel. Correction is surgical removal of the narrowed bowel portion.
- A meconium plug occurs when an extremely hard portion of meconium blocks the lumen of the intestine. Infants with meconium plug syndrome need to be observed for continuing bowel function and need to be assessed for cystic fibrosis, because a meconium plug is often a symptom of this.
- Diaphragmatic hernia occurs when the abdominal organs protrude through a defect in the diaphragm into the chest cavity. This prevents the lungs from fully expanding at birth. These infants are critically ill at birth and need extensive surgical correction.
- Imperforate anus is stricture of the anus, resulting in inability to pass stool. The infant may have a temporary colostomy created before a final surgical correction can be completed.
- Physical developmental disorders of the nervous system include hydrocephalus (excess cerebrospinal fluid in the ventricles) and spina bifida (incomplete closure of the spinal cord). Infants with hydrocephalus need surgery to relieve a ventricular obstruction or have a shunt implanted from their ventricles to the peritoneal cavity to remove excess cerebrospinal fluid. Children with myelomeningocele, the most severe form of neural cord disorder, face permanent loss of lower neuron function and require continued rehabilitation.
- Absent or malformed extremities may range from absence of a finger to absence of an entire limb. Children may need physical therapy and teaching on how to use a prosthesis to gain full mobility and function.
- Developmental hip dysplasia is the improper formation and function of the hip socket; talipes deformities are foot and ankle deformities. Children may need extensive bracing and casting to correct these disorders.

CRITICAL THINKING EXERCISES

1. Bobby Jo Sparrow is a 16-year-old teenager whose newborn has been admitted to the neonatal intensive care unit because of a neural tube disorder and congenital hip dysplasia. Ms. Sparrow is obviously upset over the diagnosis. She says, "I'm a good person. The only thing I did wrong during pregnancy was to take some cough medicine, so how could this have happened?" How would you answer her? What type of advice would be most helpful to her?
2. Baby Sparrow has developmental hip dysplasia and will be placed in a Pavlik harness. What suggestions could you make to his mother to help her instill a strong sense of trust in her child? A sense of autonomy?
3. You notice Baby Sparrow's mother is obviously upset at her child's appearance. She does not want to feed the baby and voices the thought of placing him for adoption. In contrast, the child's father, age 22, handles the baby warmly and asks questions about surgery. No grandparents visit. What interventions would you want to begin with this family?
4. Examine the National Health Goals related to children born with physical or developmental disorders. Most government-sponsored funds for nursing research are allotted based on these goals. What would be a possible research topic to explore pertinent to these goals that would be applicable to the Sparrow family and also advance evidence-based practice?

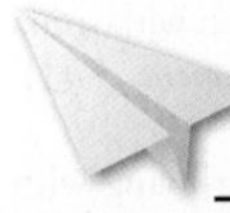

CRITICAL THINKING SCENARIO

Open the accompanying CD-ROM or visit http://thePoint.lww.com and read the Patient Scenario included for this chapter, then answer the questions to further sharpen your skills and grow more familiar with NCLEX style questions related to families with an infant who has a physiologic or developmental challenge. Confirm your answers are correct by reading the rationales.

REFERENCES

American Academy of Pediatrics (AAP); Committee on Fetus and Newborn; Canadian Paediatric Society; Fetus and Newborn Committee. (2007). Prevention and management of pain in the neonate: an update. *Advances in Neonatal Care, 7*(3), 151–160.

Balfour-Lynn, I. M. (2008). Newborn screening for cystic fibrosis: evidence for benefit. *Archives of Disease in Childhood, 93*(1), 7–10.

Benecke, R., & Dressler, D. (2007). Botulinum toxin treatment of axial and cervical dystonia. *Disability & Rehabilitation, 29*(23), 1769–1777.

Brunnegard, K., & Lohmander, A. (2007). A cross-sectional study of speech in 10-year-old children with cleft palate: results and issues of rater reliability. *Cleft Palate-Craniofacial Journal, 44*(1), 33–44.

Cheng, L. L., Moor, S. L., & Ho, C. T. C. (2007). Predisposing factors to dental caries in children with cleft lip and palate: a review and strategies for early prevention. *Cleft Palate-Craniofacial Journal, 44*(1), 67–72.

Davis, B. E., et al. (2007). Acquisition of autonomy skills in adolescents with myelomeningocele. *Developmental Medicine and Child Neurology, 48*(4), 253–258.

Donahue, D. (2008). Meningomyelocele. In F. J. Domino (Ed.). *The 5-minute clinical consult.* Philadelphia: Lippincott Williams & Wilkins.

Eilert, R. E. (2008). Orthopedics. In W. W. Hay, et al. (Eds.). *Current pediatric diagnosis and treatment* (18th ed.). Columbus, OH: McGraw-Hill.

Elias, E. R., Tsai, A., & Manchester, D. K. (2008). Genetics and dysmorphology. In W. W. Hay, et al. (Eds.). *Current pediatric diagnosis and treatment* (18th ed.). Columbus, OH: McGraw-Hill.

Ezzat, C. F., et al. (2007). Presurgical nasoalveolar molding therapy for the treatment of unilateral cleft lip and palate: a preliminary study. *Cleft Palate-Craniofacial Journal, 44*(1), 8–12.

Forster, E., & Fraser, J. (2007). Turning around talipes: nursing considerations. *Neonatal, Paediatric and Child Health Nursing, 10*(1), 27–32.

Fowler, S. F., & Lee, H. (2008). Congenital disorders of the trachea and esophagus. In A. K. Lalwani (Ed.). *Current diagnosis and treatment in otolaryngology—head and neck surgery* (2nd ed.). Columbus, OH: McGraw-Hill.

Glenny, A. M., et al. (2009). Feeding interventions for growth and development in infants with cleft lip, cleft palate or cleft lip and palate. *Cochrane Database of Systematic Reviews, 2009*(1), (CD003315).

Harres, A. E. (2007). Minimally invasive neonatal surgery. *Journal of Perinatal and Neonatal Nursing, 21*(1), 39–49.

Hoffman, W. Y. (2008). Cleft lip and palate. In A. K. Lalwani (Ed.). *Current diagnosis and treatment in otolaryngology—head and neck surgery* (2nd ed.). Columbus, OH: McGraw-Hill.

Horton, W. A., Hall, J. G., & Hecht, J. T. (2007). Achondroplasia. *Lancet, 370*(9582), 162–172.

Ingoe, R., & Lange, P. (2007). The Ladd's procedure for correction of intestinal malrotation with volvulus in children. *AORN: Association of Perioperative Registered Nurses Journal, 85*(2), 300–312.

Karch, A. M. (2009). *Lippincott's nursing drug guide.* Philadelphia: Lippincott Williams & Wilkins.

Kelley, P. E., et al. (2008). Ear, nose and throat. In W. W. Hay, et al. (Eds.). *Current pediatric diagnosis and treatment* (18th ed.). Columbus, OH: McGraw-Hill.

Kerby, G. S., et al. (2008). Respiratory tract and mediastinum. In W. W. Hay, et al. (Eds.). *Current pediatric diagnosis and treatment* (18th ed.). Columbus, OH: McGraw-Hill.

Komolafe, E. O., Adeolu, A. A., & Komolafe, M. A. (2008). Treatment of cerebrospinal fluid shunting complications in a Nigerian neurosurgery programme. *Pediatric Neurosurgery, 44*(1), 36–42.

Lidsky, M. E., Lander, T. A., & Sidman, J. D. (2008). Resolving feeding difficulties with early airway intervention in Pierre Robin Sequence. *Laryngoscope, 118*(1), 120–123.

Lin, D. T., & Deschler, D. G. (2008). Neck masses. In A. K. Lalwani (Ed.). *Current diagnosis and treatment in otolaryngology—head and neck surgery* (2nd ed.). Columbus, OH: McGraw-Hill.

Louik, C., et al. (2007). First-trimester use of selective serotonin-reuptake inhibitors and the risk of birth defects. *New England Journal of Medicine, 356*(26), 2675–2683.

Lumley, J., et al. (2009). Periconceptional supplementation with folate and/or multivitamins for preventing neural tube defects. *Cochrane Database of Systematic Reviews, 2009*(1), (CD001056).

Lund, C. H., Bauer, K., & Berrios, M. (2007). Gastroschisis: incidence, complications, and clinical management in the neonatal intensive care unit. *Journal of Perinatal and Neonatal Nursing, 21*(1), 63–68.

Mavanur, A., & Hight, D. W. (2008). Pectus excavatum and carinatum: new concepts in the correction of congenital chest wall deformities in the pediatric age group. *Connecticut Medicine, 72*(1), 5–11.

Moe, P. G., Benke, T. A., & Bernard, T. J. (2008). Neurologic and muscular disorders. In W. W. Hay, et al. (Eds.). *Current pediatric diagnosis and treatment* (18th ed.). Columbus, OH: McGraw-Hill.

Moyer, V., et al. (2009). Late versus early surgical correction for congenital diaphragmatic hernia in newborn infants. *Cochrane Database of Systematic Reviews, 2009*(1), (CD001695).

Murray, L., et al. (2008). The effect of cleft lip and palate, and the timing of lip repair on mother-infant interactions and infant development. *Journal of Child Psychology and Psychiatry and Allied Disciplines, 49*(2), 115–123.

Novak, B. (2007). Health benefits of folic acid. *Nurse Prescribing, 5*(5), 215–220.

Pelluard-Nehme, F., et al. (2007). A new case of VACTERL association with unilateral amelia of upper limb. *Clinical Dysmorphology, 16*(3), 185–187.

Raab, E. L. (2007). The resuscitation and care of the newborn at risk. In A. H. DeCherney & L. Nathan (Eds.). *Current diagnosis and treatment in obstetrics and gynecology* (10th ed.). Columbus, OH: McGraw-Hill.

Richter, G. T., et al. (2008). Endoscopic management of recurrent tracheoesophageal fistula. *Journal of Pediatric Surgery, 43*(1), 238–245.

Skandalakis, J. E., et al. (2007). Surgical anatomy of the hernial rings. In J. E. Fischer (Ed.). *Mastery of surgery.* Philadelphia: Lippincott Williams & Wilkins.

Smith, M. H., & Henderson, J. L. (2007). Congenital anomalies. In K. B. Fortner, et al. (Eds.). *The Johns Hopkins manual of gynecology and obstetrics.* Philadelphia: Lippincott Williams & Wilkins.

Sponseller, P. D. (2007). Spina bifida. In F. J. Frassica, P. D. Sponseller, & J. H. Wilckens (Eds.). *5-minute orthopaedic consult.* Philadelphia: Lippincott Williams & Wilkins.

Thilo, E. H., & Rosenberg, A. A. (2008). The newborn. In W. W. Hay, et al. (Eds.). *Current pediatric diagnosis and treatment* (18th ed.). Columbus, OH: McGraw-Hill.

Tubbs, R. S., et al. (2007). The pediatric Chiari I malformation: a review. *Childs Nervous System, 23*(11), 1239–1250.

van Aalst, J. A., Kolappa, K. K., & Sadove, M. (2008). Nonsyndromic cleft palate. *Plastic and Reconstructive Surgery, 121*(1 Suppl), 1–14.

van Eijck, F. C., et al. (2008). Closure of giant omphaloceles by the abdominal wall component separation technique in infants. *Journal of Pediatric Surgery, 43*(1), 246–250.

Vick, L. R., et al. (2007). Primary laparoscopic repair of high imperforate anus in neonatal males. *Journal of Pediatric Surgery, 42*(11), 1877–1881.

Waldman, B., & Manista, A. P. (2007). Torticollis. In F. J. Frassica, P. D. Sponseller, & J. H. Wilckens (Eds.). *5-minute orthopaedic consult.* Philadelphia: Lippincott Williams & Wilkins.

Warner, B. W. (2007). Congenital diaphragmatic hernia. In J. E. Fischer (Ed.). *Mastery of surgery.* Philadelphia: Lippincott Williams & Wilkins.

Zahl, S. M., & Wester, K. (2008). Routine measurement of head circumference as a tool for detecting intracranial expansion in infants: what is the gain? *Pediatrics, 121*(3), e416–e420.

SUGGESTED READINGS

Kain, V. J. (2007). Moral distress and providing care to dying babies in neonatal nursing. *International Journal of Palliative Nursing, 13*(5), 243–248.

Mahan, S. T., & Kasser, J. R. (2008). Does swaddling influence developmental dysplasia of the hip? *Pediatrics, 121*(1), 177–178.

Moore, K. N., Fader, M., & Getliffe, K. (2009). Long-term bladder management by intermittent catheterisation in adults and children. *Cochrane Database of Systematic Reviews, 2009*(1), (CD006008).

Murphy, K. M . (2008). Managing skin health in obese children with spina bifida: an overview and case study. *Ostomy/Wound Management, 54*(1), 34–43.

Roux, G., et al. (2007). The experience of adolescent women living with spina bifida part II: peer relationships. *Rehabilitation Nursing, 32*(3), 112–119.

Schlatter, D., et al. (2008). Severe fetal hydrocephalus with and without neural tube defect: a comparative study. *Fetal Diagnosis and Therapy, 23*(1), 23–29.

Tam, P. K. (2008). Towards predictive, preventive, and personalized paediatric surgery. *Journal of Pediatric Surgery, 43*(2), 267–273.

Tobias, N., et al. (2008). Management principles of organic causes of childhood constipation. *Journal of Pediatric Health Care, 22*(1), 12–23.

Twycross, A. (2007). Children's nurses' post-operative pain management practices: an observational study. *International Journal of Nursing Studies, 44*(6), 869–881.

Yang, J., et al. (2008). Socioeconomic status in relation to selected birth defects in a large multicentered US case-control study. *American Journal of Epidemiology, 167*(2), 145–154.

Unit 5

The Nursing Role in Health Promotion for a Childrearing Family

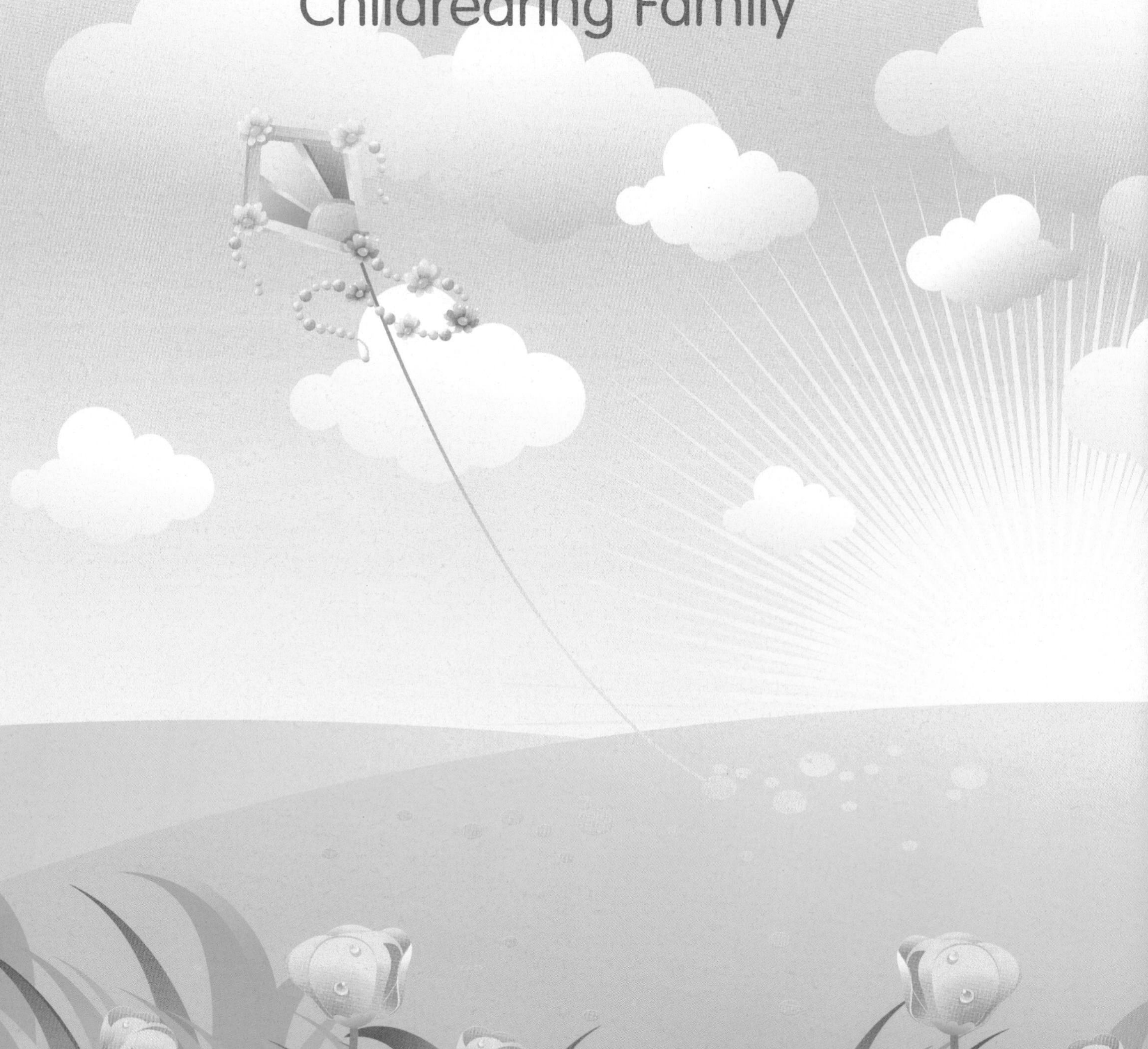

Chapter 28 Principles of Growth and Development

KEY TERMS

- abstract thought
- accommodation
- assimilation
- autonomy versus shame or doubt
- centering
- cognitive development
- conservation
- development
- developmental milestones
- developmental task
- egocentrism
- growth
- identity versus role confusion
- industry versus inferiority
- initiative versus guilt
- integrity versus despair
- maturation
- permanence
- reversibility
- role fantasy
- schemas
- sensorimotor stage
- temperament
- trust versus mistrust

OBJECTIVES

After mastering the contents of this chapter, you should be able to:

1. Describe principles of growth and development and developmental stages according to major theorists.
2. Identify National Health Goals related to growth and development that nurses can help the nation achieve.
3. Use critical thinking to analyze ways that paths to achieving a new developmental stage remain family centered.
4. Assess a child to determine the stage of development that has been achieved.
5. Formulate nursing diagnoses that address wellness as well as both a potential for and an actual delay in growth and development.
6. Identify expected outcomes for nursing goals for a growing child.
6. Plan nursing interventions to assist a child in achieving and maintaining normal growth and development such as encouraging a parent to read to a child.
7. Implement nursing care such as suggesting age-appropriate play materials to support normal growth and development.
8. Evaluate outcome criteria for achievement and effectiveness of care.
9. Identify areas of nursing care related to growth and development that could benefit from additional nursing research or application of evidence-based practice.
11. Integrate knowledge of growth and development with nursing process to achieve quality maternal and child health nursing care.

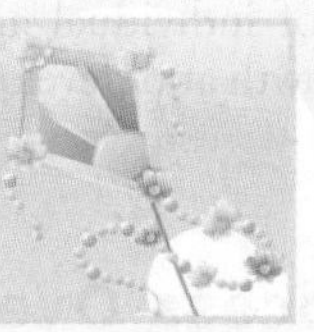

John Olson is a 6-year-old boy you see in an emergency department because he has a broken leg from a bicycle accident. At 4 months of age, John was taken away from his mother because she was not caring for him adequately. He was then moved back and forth among 12 different foster homes until he was finally adopted at age 3½. His adoptive parents have 3-year-old twins of their own. They tell you although John has lived with them for 3 years, they find him cold and unloving. They ask you what they can do to change this. Nurses are directly responsible for assessing the growth and development of children in many health care settings. Previous chapters discussed childbearing and what an important time the first weeks after birth can be in a child's life. This chapter adds information about growth and development that is important for all the continuing years of a child's life.

How has John's background contributed to his behavior? What stage of psychosocial development does he not seem to have achieved? How could his adoptive parents help him at this point?

All children pass through predictable stages of growth and development as they mature. Parents often ask what to expect from their children regarding their developmental progress at health care visits. Such visits provide opportunities for you not only to assess present growth and development but also to supply anticipatory guidance on the topic.

For these reasons, including growth and development is essential in the establishment of complete and effective nursing care plans for children. This chapter addresses the most important factors to assess for each age group. Later chapters supply detailed descriptions of individual age groups. National Health Goals related to growth and development are presented in Box 28.1.

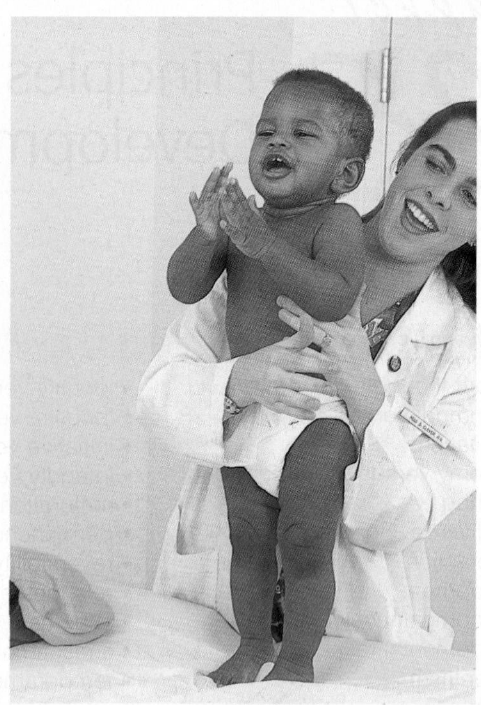

FIGURE 28.1 Growth and development are assessed by both observation and specific testing. Here a 12-month-old demonstrates mastery of well-coordinated and intentional hand movements.

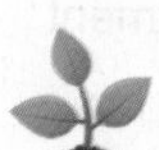

Nursing Process Overview

For Promotion of Normal Growth and Development

Assessment

Measure and plot height and weight on a standard growth chart for children at all health care visits to document growth is occurring and the child's growth remains within a constant percentile. Take a health history from both parents and the child and observe what specific activities the child can accomplish to establish whether **developmental milestones** (major markers of normal development) are being met (Fig. 28.1). Document a 24-hour recall history for nutritional intake, sleep, and a description of school and play behaviors. Periodic screening tests (i.e., the Denver II, vision tests, and audiometry screening) should be scheduled at standard times, as discussed in Chapter 34. For the most accurate assessments, be certain to account for illness, sleepiness, fatigue, or "bad days" (a day on which a child did not test well).

Nursing Diagnosis

When assessment is completed, a child profile can be devised and needs and problems identified. Examples of nursing diagnoses applicable to this area include:

- Risk for delayed growth and development related to lack of age-appropriate toys and activities
- Delayed growth and development related to prolonged illness
- Readiness for enhanced family coping related to parent's seeking information about child's growth and development
- Health-seeking behaviors related to appropriate stimulation for infants
- Imbalanced nutrition, less than body requirements, related to parental knowledge deficit regarding child's protein need
- Deficient knowledge related to potential long-term effects of obesity in school-age child

Outcome Identification and Planning

To provide holistic nursing care, consider all aspects of a child's health (physical, emotional, cultural, cognitive,

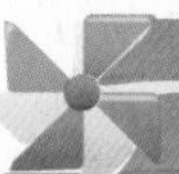

BOX 28.1 * Focus on National Health Goals

National Health Goals that address growth or development of children include:

- Reduce the prevalence of growth restriction among low-income children aged 5 and younger to less than 5% from a baseline of 8%. Growth restriction is defined as height-for-age below the fifth percentile on a standard growth chart.
- Reduce the occurrence of developmental disabilities in children such as cognitive challenge from a baseline of 131 per 100,000 to a target of 124 per 100,000
- Reduce the identification of autism from a baseline of 50 months to 48 months of age.
- Reduce the proportion of children and adolescents who are overweight or obese from a baseline of 11% to 5% (http://www.nih.gov).

Recognizing normal growth and development patterns for children helps to determine if children are following normal development and when referrals are needed. Nursing research topics that could add information in this area are: Are there differences between urban and rural children in the way they approach childhood problems? How do characteristics of temperament affect the way children respond to hospitalization? What are specific ways the environment of children influences health? What can nurses do to help reduce the obesity epidemic in children?

spiritual, nutritional, and social), remembering that each child's developmental progress is unique. Children cannot be forced to achieve milestones faster than their own timetable will allow. However, through anticipatory guidance, children can be encouraged to reach maximum developmental potential. Nurses can play important roles in suggesting expected outcomes and guidance to both a child and family on ways to encourage child development and preparing children for new experiences.

Not all nations foster the growth and development of children in the same manner, in part because of cultural variations. Childhood in the United States covers a relatively long period. In other countries, childhood is short because girls are asked to assume domestic responsibilities early in life and outside or farm work is required early for boys. In some countries, the predominant theory of childrearing is protective nurturing. Children are not rushed into new experiences like toilet training or beginning school. In others, it is customary to treat children in a harsh, strict manner, using shame or corporal punishment for discipline. Praising children for learning a new skill may be viewed as unnecessary or actually harmful, because this could result in a child being subject to evil forces. In some Asian cultures, an infant's personality is thought to depend not so much on genetic or environmental influences but on the year and time of birth.

What foods children receive depends very much on culture also. Vegetables such as jicama and chayote, for example, may not even be recognized by children in the northeast United States but are popular with those in the southwest.

Asking a parent questions such as, "What do you do when your baby cries?" "What kind of things do you think a 2-year-old should be able to do?" "What do you do when your 4-year-old misbehaves?" can help you to isolate and better understand cultural differences. Recognizing cultural variations this way helps to plan care that is specific to a particular child and family.

Planning should include a child's family as growth and development proceed within a family context. To develop psychosocially, children continue to need emotional support from loved ones, just as they need nutritional support to grow physically. Parents of a child with a developmental delay may use denial as a protective mechanism for a long time. This means that planning may have to be centered first on helping parents accept what is happening; plans for a child may have to be delayed until the parents are convinced a problem exists. Helpful Web sites to use for parent referral are the Sutter Health Network (http://www.Kids.Sutterhealth.org) and the Learning Place (http://www.Learningplaceonline.com).

Implementation

Interventions to foster growth and development include encouraging age-appropriate self-care in a child and suggesting age-appropriate toys or activities to parents. It may be necessary to help parents accept a child's delayed growth or motivate a child to reach anticipated upper limits. Role modeling is an important ongoing intervention with both children and families. Modeling, for example, can demonstrate that problem solving is a more effective approach to life's challenges than "acting out" behaviors.

Outcome Evaluation

Evaluation for specific growth and developmental milestones (see Chapters 29 through 33) must be ongoing to be accurate and useful, because many children do not test well on any given day. Ongoing evaluation is necessary also because it provides an opportunity for early detection of various problems. If a child has difficulty achieving one developmental task, for example, the next one may be difficult to achieve as well. Evaluation must also be comprehensive. If a developmental task involves only gross motor function, it may not be apparent that something is wrong with a child's fine motor function until the child is asked to perform fine motor tasks in school. Examples of expected outcomes are:

- Child, 5 years of age, expresses less negativism at next clinic visit.
- At 9-month checkup, parents describe how they have made a safe space in their home for their infant to crawl so that he is not confined to a playpen.
- Parents list household tasks they believe are appropriate for a 6-year-old child by next office visit.
- Parents state the pattern they are using to phase out high-carbohydrate, nonnutritive snacks for their preschooler.

GROWTH AND DEVELOPMENT AND THE ROLE OF THE NURSE

Information about growth and development is important in all phases of childcare.

Health Promotion and Illness Prevention

Determining a child's developmental stage is often the primary focus of a health interview. For instance, during her child's 24-month checkup, a mother might ask if it is normal that her child cannot yet pedal a tricycle. This question, or any other questions about a child's developmental progress, cannot be answered without a full understanding of the average ranges of motor coordination.

Parenting style and competence are major influences on the behavioral and mental health of children (Coren & Barlow, 2009). In addition to reassurance that their child is doing well, parents also need periodic anticipatory guidance regarding their child's development. For example, it would be important to discuss additional home safety with a parent when a child is approaching the age for creeping. Parents should be cautioned to think about fencing open stairways and clearing cleaning compounds out of bottom cupboards. Parents of a child who is almost 1 year old will appreciate being cautioned that their child's appetite may decrease during the coming year; armed with this knowledge, they will not interpret a child's rejection of food as the beginning of a feeding problem but will see it as a usual step in development. The parent of a child approaching puberty generally welcomes a discussion on how to prepare a child for this challenging growth phase.

If anticipatory guidance is not offered at appropriate times, it can be useless. Information given too early is forgotten by the time it is needed. Given too late, parents may have already addressed (or ignored) the issue, possibly not in the most growth-enhancing way for their child. To be able to supply anticipatory guidance this way at the appropriate time or to plan nursing care to meet the needs of children and families, you must be able to recognize the predictable stages of growth and development, from newborn to young adult, through which each child passes (Goldson & Reynolds, 2008).

Health Restoration and Maintenance

It is equally essential to consider developmental stages when caring for a sick child or one having surgery. Preparing a 5-year-old child for surgery, for example, would be ineffective unless you know how much a 5-year-old child can be expected to comprehend. You would need to assess if a child will understand things such as an anesthetic is a gas, what a surgeon is, and what stitches are or how to best explain what these are. It is just as important to keep developmental stages in mind when teaching parents; for example, you need to evaluate whether an oral form of medicine is appropriate for a child or if a child is too young to coordinate tongue and throat muscles.

Physical growth is another important factor to consider, because disease affects children differently at various stages of growth. A 12-year-old child who has fractured a long bone, for example, has a potentially more serious fracture than an 8-year-old child who fractures the identical bone. The 8-year-old child must metabolize enough calcium to meet two major needs: healing the fracture site and maintaining healthy bone cells. The 12-year-old child, who is undergoing a period of rapid growth, must meet three needs: calcium for healing and maintaining existing healthy bone cells and an additional amount for rapid bone growth. If a child does not take in adequate calcium during the healing period to supply the extra amount for growth, the affected limb could be left shorter than its mate. Recommending extra calcium could help ensure no permanent disability results.

PRINCIPLES OF GROWTH AND DEVELOPMENT

Growing up is a complex phenomenon because of the many interrelated facets involved. Children do not merely grow taller and heavier as they get older; maturing also involves growth in their ability to perform skills, to think, to relate to people, and to trust or have confidence in themselves.

The terms "growth" and "development" are occasionally used interchangeably, but they are different. **Growth** is generally used to denote an increase in physical size or a quantitative change. Growth in weight is measured in pounds or kilograms; growth in height is measured in inches or centimeters. **Development** is used to indicate an increase in skill or the ability to function (a qualitative change). Development can be measured by observing a child's ability to perform specific tasks such as how well a child picks up small objects such as raisins, by recording the parent's description of a child's progress, or by using standardized tests such as the Denver II. **Maturation** is a synonym for development.

Psychosexual development is a specific type of development that refers to developing instincts or sensual pleasure (Freudian theory). Psychosocial development refers to Erikson's stages of personality development. Moral development is the ability to know right from wrong and to apply these to real-life situations. Kohlberg is a theorist who studied this.

Cognitive development refers to the ability to learn or understand from experience, to acquire and retain knowledge, to respond to a new situation, and to solve problems (see the section below on Piaget's theory of cognitive development). It is measured by intelligence tests and by observing children's ability to function effectively in their environment.

Patterns

Neither physical growth nor aspects of maturation occur haphazardly; several principles govern this process (Box 28.2). As shown in Figure 28.2, general growth, such as growth of respiratory, digestive, renal, musculoskeletal, and circulatory tissue, proceeds fairly smoothly during childhood. Certain body tissues, however, mature more rapidly than others. Neurologic tissue (spinal cord and brain) grows so rapidly the first 2 years that the brain reaches mature proportions by 2 to 5 years. Lymphoid tissue (spleen, thymus, lymph nodes, and tonsillar tissue) also grows rapidly during infancy and childhood so children are protected against infection. Although the spleen is not usually palpable in adults, the spleen is palpable 1 or 2 cm below the left ribs in preschool children because of this rapid growth. In 5-year-olds, tonsillar tissue has already reached its peak size (about twice that of an adult). On assessment, young school-age children appear to have large tonsils (the back of their throat seems to be "all tonsils"). In contrast, reproductive organs (genital tissue) show little growth until puberty.

✔ Checkpoint Question 28.1

John is 6 years old. What body system is reaching its peak point of development at this time?

a. Neurologic system.
b. Lymphatic system.
c. Reproductive system.
d. Musculoskeletal system.

FACTORS INFLUENCING GROWTH AND DEVELOPMENT

Genetic inheritance, or whether a child receives healthy genes or genes that will lead to an illness, and environmental influences, such as whether the family a child is born into has sufficient funds to supply adequate food, are two primary factors that determine a child's pattern of growth and development. Temperament (the typical way a child reacts to situations) is an example of genetic influence. Whether a fetus enjoyed a healthy uterine existence is an example of environmental influence (Barnes-Powell, 2007). Whether a child receives good nutrition, beginning with being breastfed, is another (Hale, 2007). A unique combination of these factors determines how each child grows and matures (Shulruf et al., 2007).

Genetics

From the moment of conception when a sperm and ovum fuse, the basic genetic makeup of an individual is cast.

BOX 28.2 ✻ Principles of Growth and Development

Growth and development are continuous processes from conception until death. Although there are highs and lows in terms of the rate at which growth and development proceed, at all times a child is growing new cells and learning new skills. An example of how the rate of growth changes is a comparison between that of the first year and later in life. An infant triples birth weight and increases height by 50% during the first year of life. If this tremendous growth rate were to continue, the 5-yr-old child, ready to begin school, would weigh 1600 lb and be 12 ft 6 in tall.

Growth and development proceed in an orderly sequence. Growth in height occurs in only one sequence—from smaller to larger. Development also proceeds in a predictable order. For example, the majority of children sit before they creep, creep before they stand, stand before they walk, and walk before they run. Occasionally, a child will skip a stage (or pass through it so quickly that the parents do not observe the stage). Occasionally, a child will progress in a different order, but most children follow a predictable sequence of growth and development.

Different children pass through the predictable stages at different rates. All stages of development have a range of time rather than a certain point at which they are usually accomplished. Two children may pass through the motor sequence at such different rates, for example, that one begins walking at 9 mo, another only at 14 mo. Both are developing normally. They are both following the predictable sequence; they are merely developing at different rates.

All body systems do not develop at the same rate. Certain body tissues mature more rapidly than others. For example, neurologic tissue experiences its peak growth during the first year of life, whereas genital tissue grows little until puberty.

Development is cephalocaudal. *Cephalo* is a Greek word meaning "head"; *caudal* means "tail." Development proceeds from head to tail. Newborns can lift only their head off the bed when they lie in a prone position. By age 2 mo, infants can lift both the head and chest off the bed; by 4 mo, the head, chest, and part of the abdomen; by 5 mo, infants have enough control to turn over; by 9 mo, they can control legs enough to crawl; and by 1 yr, children can stand upright and perhaps walk. Motor development has proceeded in a cephalocaudal order—from the head to the lower extremities.

Development proceeds from proximal to distal body parts. This principle is closely related to cephalocaudal development. It can best be illustrated by tracing the progress of upper extremity development. A newborn makes little use of the arms or hands. Any movement, except to put a thumb in the mouth, is a flailing motion. By age 3 or 4 mo, the infant has enough arm control to support the upper body weight on the forearms, and the infant can coordinate the hand to scoop up objects. By 10 mo, the infant can coordinate the arm and thumb and index fingers sufficiently well to use a pincerlike grasp or be able to pick up an object as fine as a piece of breakfast cereal on a highchair tray.

Development proceeds from gross to refined skills. This principle parallels the preceding one. Once children are able to control distal body parts such as fingers, they are able to perform fine motor skills (a 3-yr-old colors best with a large crayon; a 12-yr-old can write with a fine pen).

There is an optimum time for initiation of experiences or learning. Children cannot learn tasks until their nervous system is mature enough to allow that particular learning. A child cannot learn to sit, for example, no matter how much the child's parents have him or her practice, until the nervous system has matured enough to allow back control. Children who are not given the opportunity to learn developmental tasks at the appropriate or "target" times for that task may have more difficulty than the usual child learning the task later on. A child who is confined to a body cast at 12 mo, the time the child would normally learn to walk, may take a long time to learn this skill once free of the cast at, say, age 2 yr. The child has passed the time of optimal learning for that particular skill.

Neonatal reflexes must be lost before development can proceed. An infant cannot grasp with skill until the grasp reflex has faded nor stand steadily until the walking reflex has faded. Neonatal reflexes are replaced by purposeful movements.

A great deal of skill and behavior is learned by practice. Infants practice over and over taking a first step before they accomplish this securely. If children fall behind in growth and development because of illness, they are capable of "catch-up" growth to bring them equal again with their age group

Although each child is unique, certain gender-related characteristics will influence growth and development. In addition to physical characteristics such as eye color and height potential, inheritance determines other characteristics such as learning style and temperament. An individual may also inherit a genetic abnormality, which could result in disability or illness at birth or later in life.

Gender

On average, girls are born lighter (by an ounce or two) and shorter (by an inch or two) than boys. Boys tend to keep this height and weight advantage until prepuberty, at which time girls surge ahead because they begin their puberty growth spurt 6 months to 1 year earlier than boys. By the end of pu-

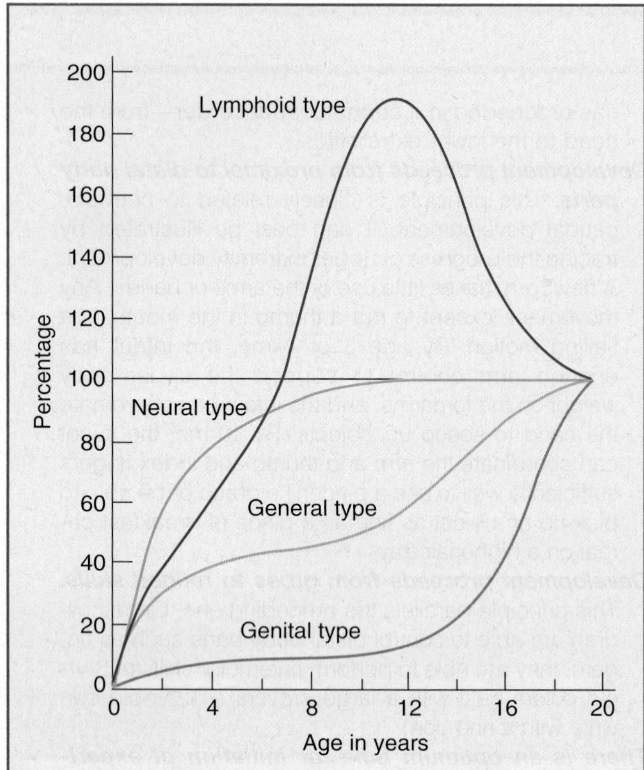

FIGURE 28.2 Main types of postnatal growth of various body tissue types. (Redrawn from Scammon, R. E. [1930]. The measurement of the body in childhood. In Harris, J. A., et al. [Eds.]. *The measurement of man* [pp. 214–226]. Minneapolis: University of Minnesota Press, with permission.)

berty (14 to 16 years), boys again tend to be taller and heavier than girls. This difference in growth patterns is reflected in the different growth charts used for boys and girls (see Appendix E).

Health

A child who inherits a genetically transmitted disease may not grow as rapidly or develop as fully as a healthy child, depending on the type of illness and the therapy or care available for the disease. Before insulin was discovered in 1922, for example, many children with type 1 diabetes mellitus died in early childhood; those who lived were left physically challenged. Currently, with good health supervision and insulin therapy, the effects of type 1 disease can be so minimized that children with diabetes both thrive and grow. Diabetes is still a major factor in the health of children, however. As more and more children in developed countries become obese, type 2 diabetes now has begun to occur in children as young as school-age (Hussain et al., 2007).

Intelligence

Children with high intelligence do not generally grow faster physically than other children, but they do tend to advance faster in skills. Occasionally, children of high intelligence fall behind in physical skills because they spend their time with books or mental games rather than with games that develop motor skills and so do not receive practice in these areas.

Temperament

Temperament is the usual reaction pattern of an individual, or an individual's characteristic manner of thinking, behaving, or reacting to stimuli in the environment (Chess & Thomas, 1995). Unlike cognitive or moral development, temperament is not developed by stages but is an inborn characteristic set at birth. Understanding that children are not all alike—some adapt quickly to new situations and others adapt slowly, and some react intensely and some passively—can help parents better understand why their children are different from each other and help them care for each child more constructively.

Reaction Patterns

Chess and Thomas (1995) identified nine separate characteristics that define temperament or how children react to situations. Each child's pattern is made up of a combination of these individual elements.

Activity Level. The level of activity among children differs widely. Some babies are constantly on the go and rarely quiet. They wiggle and squirm in their crib as early as 2 weeks of age. Parents put such children to sleep in one end of a crib and find them in the other end an hour later; such children will not stay seated in bathtubs and refuse to be confined in playpens. Other babies, by contrast, move little, stay where they are placed, and appear to take in their environment in a quieter, more docile way. Both patterns are normal; they merely reflect two extremes of *motor activity,* one characteristic of temperament.

Rhythmicity. A child who has *rhythmicity* manifests a regular rhythm in physiologic functions. Even as infants, such children tend to wake up at the same time each morning, are hungry at regular 4-hour periods, nap the same time every day, and have a bowel movement at the same time every day. They are predictable and easy to care for because their parents learn early on what to expect from them. On the other end of the scale are infants with an irregular rhythmicity. They rarely awaken at the same time 2 days in a row. They may go a long time without eating one day and the next day appear hungry almost immediately after a feeding. Such children may be more difficult to care for because it is difficult to plan a schedule for them. Parents must constantly adapt their own routine to the child's routine.

Approach. *Approach* refers to a child's response on initial contact with a new stimulus. Some children approach new situations in an unruffled manner. They smile and "talk" to strangers and accept a first feeding or a new food without spitting up or fussing. They explore new toys without apprehension. Other children demonstrate withdrawal rather than approach to new situations. They cry at the sight of strangers, new toys, and new foods; they fuss the first time they are placed in a bathtub. They are difficult to take on vacation or to meet a new childcare provider because they react so fearfully to new situations.

Adaptability. *Adaptability* is the ability to change one's reaction to stimuli over time. Infants who are adaptable can change their first reaction to a situation without exhibiting extreme distress. The first time such children are placed in a bathtub they might protest loudly, for example, but by the third time they sit splashing happily. This is in contrast to infants who cry for months whenever they are put into a bathtub or who cannot seem to accustom themselves to a new bed, new car seat, or new caregiver.

Intensity of Reaction. Some children react to situations with their whole being. They cry loudly, thrash their arms, and begin temper tantrums when their diapers are wet, when they are hungry, and when their parents leave them. Others rarely demonstrate such overt symptoms of anger or have a mild or low-intensity *reaction to stress.*

Distractibility. Children who are easily distracted or who can easily shift their attention to a new situation (*distractibility*) are easy to care for. If they are crying over the loss of a toy, they can be appeased by the offer of a different one. Other children cannot be distracted in this way; their parents may describe them as stubborn, willful, or unwilling to compromise because they persistently return to an activity or refuse to adapt or change.

Attention Span and Persistence. *Attention span* is the ability to remain interested in a project or activity. Like other aspects of temperament, this varies among children. Some play by themselves with one toy for an hour; others spend no more than 1 or 2 minutes with each toy. The degree of *persistence* also varies. Some infants keep trying to perform an activity even when they fail time after time; others stop trying after one unsuccessful attempt.

Threshold of Response. The *threshold of response* is the intensity level of stimulation that is necessary to evoke a reaction. Children with a low threshold need little stimulation; those with a high threshold need intense stimulation before they become upset over a situation.

Mood Quality. A child who is always happy and laughing has a positive *mood quality.* Obviously, this can make a major difference in the parents' enjoyment of a child. Parents are bound to spend more time with a child who is always happy than with a child who has a negative mood quality.

Nursing Implications Regarding Temperament

Three categories of temperament are shown in Box 28.3. Children who have a normal activity level and regular rhythmicity, who approach and adapt to new situations easily, and who have a long attention span, a high level of persistence, and a positive mood quality are "ideal" or "easy" children to care for, from a parent's point of view. Highly active infants are much more difficult for parents to care for, especially if they demonstrate irregular physiologic rhythms, withdrawal rather than approach, and little ability to adapt. Such children require more planning and creative distraction measures.

It is useful to talk to parents about their child's reactivity patterns at health maintenance visits because these patterns tend to persist: the way a child will react in the future depends a great deal on the way a child reacts today. A child who withdraws from rather than approaches a first toy, for example, may react the same way to toilet training or starting day care. The parents of such a child will need to focus on extra preparation for new activities more than will the parents of a child who approaches new situations easily. Parents who are aware their baby shies away from new experiences such as baths and new foods will be able to take it in stride when their child is slow to adapt to a Head Start program at age 4; they will know it is simply their child's method of coping.

Bringing these characteristics to parents' attention helps them better understand their child and lays the foundation for beginning to accept and respect the child as an individual. It is essential for successful childrearing (Foley, 2007).

Noticing children's temperamental characteristics as they are admitted to a hospital can help you anticipate children's probable reactions to procedures or pain. For example, a child with a mild reactivity pattern may not show a great deal of response to even acute pain, but a child with an intense pattern may react as strongly to minor discomfort as to major pain, making it difficult to evaluate the true level of pain the child is experiencing.

One instrument that is helpful in evaluating temperament is the Carey-McDevitt Infant Temperament Questionnaire (Carey & McDevitt, 1978). This consists of 95 responses and can be answered by a parent in approximately 25 minutes. General categories center on the child's responses to feeding, sleeping, soiling and wetting, dressing, bathing, and diapering, as well as to people and new situations.

Parents fill out the questionnaire when their infant is between 4 and 8 months of age (before this, temperament is not developed enough to be evident). The parent reads each

BOX 28.3 ✻ Categories of Temperament

The Easy Child
Children are rated as "easy to care for" if they have a predictable rhythmicity, approach and adapt to new situations readily, have a mild to moderate intensity of reaction, and have an overall positive mood quality. Most children are rated by their parents as being in this category.

The Difficult Child
Children are "difficult" if they are irregular in habits, have a negative mood quality, and withdraw rather than approach new situations. Only about 10% of children fall into this category.

Slow-to-Warm-Up Child
Children fall into this category if they are overall fairly inactive; respond only mildly and adapt slowly to new situations, and have a general negative mood. About 15% of children display this pattern. When discussing this temperament with parents, try to use positive terms such as "ways to find a healthy fit for your child" rather than stressing ways the child is hard to manage.

behavioral description and then selects the option that most accurately describes the child. If an item does not apply at all, the parent crosses it out. Finally, parents are asked to describe general impressions of the child's temperament, activity level, positive and negative moods, and distractibility.

Although individual children show characteristics from all groups, most children can be categorized into one of four groups:

1. Difficult: arrhythmic, withdrawing, low in adaptability, intense, and negative in mood
2. Slow to warm up: inactive, low in approach and adaptability, and negative in mood
3. Intermediate: some characteristics of both groups
4. Easy: rhythmic, approaching, adaptable, mild, and positive in mood

Environment

Although children cannot grow taller than their genetically programmed height potential allows, their adult height may be considerably less than genetic potential if their environment hinders their growth in some way. For example, a child could receive inadequate nutrition because of a family's low socioeconomic status; a parent could lack childcare skills or not give a child enough attention; or a child could have a chronic illness (O'Shea et al., 2007). Many illnesses lower children's appetite; others, such as certain endocrine disorders, directly alter their growth rate. Having a parent who abuses alcohol or other substances can cause such inconsistency in care it affects mental health (Fitzgerald & Das Edien, 2007; Motz, Leslie, & DeMarchi, 2007).

Environmental influences, however, are not always detrimental (Dooley & Stewart, 2007). For example, children with phenylketonuria, an inherited metabolic disease, can achieve normal growth and development in spite of their genetic makeup if their diet (a part of the environment) is properly regulated. The following environmental influences are those most likely to affect growth and development.

Socioeconomic Level

Because health care and good nutrition both cost money, children born into families of low socioeconomic means may not receive adequate health supervision or good nutrition. Poor health supervision can leave them without immunization against measles or other childhood illnesses and therefore vulnerable to diseases that could cause permanent neurologic damage if complications occur (Demicheli et al., 2009). Poor nutrition can also leave them vulnerable to disease as antibody formation depends on a good protein intake (Rolfes, Pinna, & Whitney, 2009).

Parent–Child Relationship

Cultural norms within a family play a role in determining when a child is expected to achieve particular developmental milestones. Children who are loved thrive better than those who are not. Either parent or a nonparent caregiver may serve as the primary caregiver or form a primary parent–child love relationship. It is the quality of time spent with children, not the amount of time, that is important. Loss of love from a primary caregiver, as might occur with the death of a parent, or interruption of parental contact through hospitalization, imprisonment, divorce, or inadequate parental love, can interfere with a child's desire to eat, improve, and advance. Helping parents feel involved in their child's care is important in both health care and childcare settings (Knitzer, 2008).

Ordinal Position in the Family

The position of a child in the family (first-born child, middle child, youngest child, only child) and the size of the family have some bearing on a child's growth and development. An only child or the oldest child in a family, for example, generally excels in language development because conversations are mainly with adults. Youngest children may develop language more slowly, especially if older children talk "baby talk" with them. Children learn by watching other children, however, so a youngest child who has many examples to watch may excel in other skills, such as toilet training at an early age.

Health

Diseases that come from environmental sources can have as strong an influence on growth and development as genetically inherited diseases. Infants cared for in neonatal intensive care units, for example, may develop some decrease in hearing because of the overstimulation of sound, an example of health being directly influenced by the environment (Thomas & Uran, 2007). Children who have residual heart impairment as a result of contracting rheumatic fever might be limited in their ability to play an active sport. The eventual degree of disability will depend not only on the damage caused by the actual disease but also on the attitudes of the people around the child—how disabled they believe the child to be (Ulrich, 2007).

Treating children as if they were sick or vulnerable to sickness is referred to as "vulnerable child syndrome" (Green & Solnit, 1964). Fortunately, if an illness does not last long, most children achieve "catch-up" growth afterward.

Nutrition

In the past 20 years, nutrition has become a major focus of health promotion and disease prevention in the United States because the quality of a child's nutrition during the growing years (including prenatally) has a major influence on health and stature (Rolfes, Pinna, & Whitney, 2009). Poor maternal nutrition may limit the growth and intelligence potential of a child from the moment of birth. Children whose diets lack essential nutrients show inadequate physical growth. A lack of energy and stamina prevents children from learning at their best intellectual level. In some communities, as many as 50% of American children are obese today (Kline, 2008). Children who eat too many carbohydrates and become obese may develop motor skills more slowly than other children because physical movement is more tiring for them. Obese children are sometimes taunted by their playmates and may become loners or have difficulty relating to their peers because of behavior problems or depression about their weight.

Nutrition also plays a vital role in the body's susceptibility to disease because poor nutrition limits the body's ability to resist infection. Lack of calcium could leave a child prone to rickets, a disease that affects growth by causing shortening or bowing of long bones. Lack of vitamins can lead to visual impairments, poor healing, and poor bone growth (Ondrak & Morgan, 2007).

Poor nutrition also plays a major role in the development of chronic illness. Of the eight leading causes of death in adults, six have been linked to dietary excesses: heart disease, cancer, cerebrovascular disease, diabetes mellitus, cirrhosis, and arteriosclerosis. It is clear, too, that dietary habits have a cumulative effect; for instance, although heart disease is not one of the top causes of death in children, the arterial changes that cause cardiovascular disease begin in childhood. Increased consumption of food and alcohol, decreased levels of exercise, and smoking all lead to a greater incidence of these diet-related diseases in adult life. Establishing healthy eating patterns early in life, therefore, can contribute to better health in adult years.

Food Guide Pyramid Guidelines for a Healthy Diet

Basic guidelines for a healthy diet have been outlined by a variety of governmental groups, including the U.S. Department of Agriculture (USDA) and the U.S. Department of Health and Human Services. In 1992, a food guide pyramid was developed by the USDA to illustrate these guidelines. It was updated in 2005 to emphasize variety, moderation, and balance and suggest a range of daily servings from each major food group (USDA, 2005). Table 28.1 lists recommended servings for children from the five pyramid food groups. In addition, good nutrition in children should follow a number of "healthy eating" guidelines:

Eat a Variety of Foods. Choices from all food pyramid groups—dairy, meat and poultry, fruits, vegetables, cereals and grains—should be included in meals every day (vegetarians omit meat and poultry but supplement this with vegetable protein). It is also important to vary choices within each food group, as not all foods within a group are nutritionally equivalent.

Balance the Food You Eat With Physical Activity—Maintain or Improve Your Weight. Although the tendency for obesity may be inherited, being overweight in early life also appears to play a role. Urge parents to be certain their infants receive all the nutrients they need for the substantial growth they are undergoing (including a percentage of fat, because this is important for myelination of nerves); at the same time, it is important that infants not be overfed so they do not become obese. Balancing a lifestyle of physical activity with sound nutrition, such as omitting sugar-heavy soft drinks, helps to do this (Vartanian, Schwartz, & Brownell, 2007). Physical activity, balanced with calcium intake, is the secret to strong bones and reduction of osteoporosis later in life (Ondrak & Morgan, 2007).

Choose a Diet With Plenty of Grain Products, Vegetables, and Fruits. Foods with starch and fiber are more beneficial for gastrointestinal function than more processed foods. Fiber, in particular, has been linked to the lowered incidence of a variety of illnesses such as constipation and perhaps colon cancer in later life. Fiber can be included as early as during preschool years in the form of whole-grain cereals and raw fruits such as apples.

Choose a Diet Low in Fat, Saturated Fat, and Cholesterol. The American diet has changed substantially over the past 10 years to reflect this important goal. Many adults now consume low-fat diets, substituting nonfat milk for whole milk,

TABLE 28.1 ✻ Servings of the Five Pyramid Food Groups for Children

		Recommended Daily Amounts		
Group	**Foods**	***Children 2–6 yr***	***Older Children***	**Major Nutrients Provided**
Bread, cereals, rice, pasta	Whole-grain and enriched	6 servings	6–11 servings	Thiamine, niacin, riboflavin (if enriched); iron (if enriched); incomplete protein, carbohydrates
Vegetables	Vegetables (yellow and green)	3 servings	3–5 servings	Vitamin A, iron, calcium, carbohydrates (include vitamin A source at least every other day)
Fruit	Fruit	2 servings	2–4 servings	Vitamin C (include vitamin C daily); carbohydrates
Milk, yogurt, cheese	Whole milk and other milk products except butter	2 servings	2–3 servings	Calcium, phosphorus, complete protein, riboflavin, niacin, vitamin D (if vitamin D–fortified milk used), fats
Meat, poultry, fish	Muscle meats (veal, beef, pork) dry beans, eggs; fish; poultry	2 servings	2–3 servings	Complete protein, iron, thiamine, riboflavin, niacin, vitamin B_{12}, fats
Fats, oils, sweets	Candy, cake, fried foods	Use sparingly	Use sparingly	Essential fatty acids, carbohydrates

Data from U.S. Department of Agriculture (USDA). (2005). *Dietary guidelines for Americans.* Washington, DC: USDA.

decreasing their consumption of eggs and other high-cholesterol sources, and reducing their consumption of red meat. For children, fat intake does not need to be restricted for the first 2 years of life. Thereafter, fat intake can be tailored to meet the guidelines of 30% total intake for both children and adults. Some foods now contain Olestra, a synthetic fat. Do not recommend this for children (or urge parents to offer this sparingly) until further study is completed because of the danger of fat-soluble vitamins being excreted and lost with the product.

Choose a Diet Moderate in Sugars. Too much sugar in a diet can contribute to both dental caries and obesity. In addition, refined sugar such as that used in soft drinks, prepared foods, candy, and chocolate represents "empty" calories: it is high in calories yet provides no essential nutrients. Although children need adequate carbohydrates for energy, parents can give their children a good start by preventing excessive sugar intake.

Choose a Diet Moderate in Salt and Sodium. The taste for salt is acquired. If unsalted or only lightly salted solid food is offered to infants, they do not develop a desire for heavily salted foods. It is helpful to assess the diet of school-age children and check whether they are eating a diet heavier in salt than necessary because of many salty after-school snacks.

If Drinking Alcoholic Beverages, do so in Moderation. Adolescents are at increased risk for establishing unhealthy patterns of alcohol use, particularly binge drinking. Educating them about the long-term consequences of alcohol use is as important as educating them on the importance of healthy nutrition for growth (see Chapter 33).

Components of a Healthy Diet

Eating a variety of foods from all five pyramid food groups in moderation is a way of guaranteeing the intake of a balanced diet of proteins, carbohydrates, fats, vitamins, and minerals (Fig. 28.3).

Protein. Protein is the major component of bones, skin, hair, and muscle and is responsible for a wide variety of essential functions in the body. Because it is essential for growth, protein intake is crucial for children. Complete proteins contain all amino acids; incomplete proteins do not. Mixing these two types of incomplete protein (pasta and beans, for example) common dietary staples, furnishes complete protein.

Carbohydrate. Carbohydrates are the main and preferred fuel of the body to supply energy, so they are essential to the functioning of most body systems, the neurologic system in particular. This is why carbohydrates are so important to infants and toddlers, whose brain cells are actively growing. Sugar supplies an immediate but short-term source of energy; starches, as a rule, supply sustained energy.

Fat. Dietary fat is also a source of energy to the body. It can be an immediate energy source or can be stored if not used, then released when energy is required. Some fat deposits also serve as insulating material for subcutaneous tissues; in infants, fats are necessary to ensure myelination of nerve fibers.

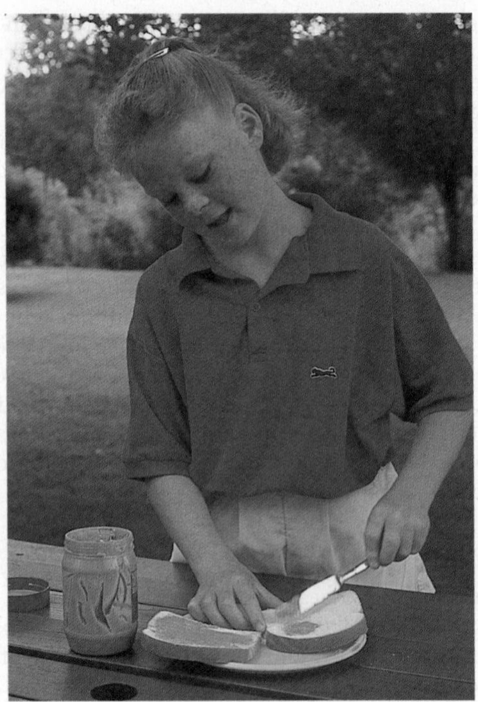

FIGURE 28.3 Good nutritional habits developed early in life provide a child with a health advantage.

Vitamins. Vitamins are organic compounds that are essential for specific metabolic actions in cells. They do not produce energy but are needed by cells to produce energy. For children, fat-soluble vitamins (A, D, K, and E) are mainly supplied by fortified dairy products, fortified cereals, and plant oils or fish oils. Such vitamins can leave the gastrointestinal tract and be used by the body only by being absorbed along with fat molecules. Once absorbed, they are used by the cells for growth and function or are stored in the liver and fat cells for later use. Because fat-soluble vitamins can be stored by the body, an infant or child can ingest too many of them, although overdosing usually occurs from supplements rather than dietary sources. Water-soluble vitamins (B complex and C) do not need fat for absorption but are not stored well in the body, so they must be taken daily to maintain effective levels in the body. Sources and functions of essential vitamins and results of their deficiencies are summarized in Table 28.2.

Minerals. Minerals are necessary to build new cells and regulate body processes such as fluid and electrolyte balance, nerve transmission, and muscle contraction, so they are vital to the health of a growing infant or child. Deficiency in a mineral such as potassium can lead to poor heart function and childhood growth. Minerals are classified according to the amounts needed daily or their importance for body functioning. If more than 100 mg is needed daily, a mineral is a *macronutrient*, or major mineral. If the amount needed is less than 100 mg, it is a *micronutrient*, or minor mineral. Trace minerals refer to those needed in only extremely small amounts. Sources and functions of various minerals and results of their deficiencies are listed in Table 28.3.

TABLE 28.2 ✻ Vitamins Essential for Health

Vitamin	Selected Dietary Sources	Function in Body	Results of Deficiency
Fat-Soluble*			
A (retinol)	Liver, carrots, spinach	Important for night vision and corneal integrity and growth	Keratinization of the eye (xerophthalmia) and blindness
D	Egg yolk, margarine, salmon, fortified milk, fortified cereals	Regulates absorption of calcium and phosphorus for bone growth	Rickets (bone deformity) in growing children
E	Margarine, corn oil, peanuts	An antioxidant that protects red blood cells from destruction by oxygen	In immature infants, severe anemia from destruction of red blood cells
K	Cabbage, spinach, pork. Best source: Green leafy vegetables	Aids blood clotting (synthesis of prothrombin)	Bleeding from lack of sufficient clotting action
Water-Soluble			
B complex:			
Thiamine	Wheat germ, yeast, pork	Important for use of glucose in cells	Beriberi, a disease that causes nerve paralysis
Riboflavin	Beef, chicken, liver, avocados, milk	Breaks down fatty acids and amino acids for energy	Red swollen tongue, inflamed eyes, fissures of lips
Niacin	Peanuts, rice bran, liver	Converts glucose to energy, involved in carbohydrate, protein, and fat metabolism	Pellagra (diarrhea, mental confusion, dermatitis, death)
B_6 (pyridoxine)	Liver, herring, salmon, chicken, fish, pork, eggs	Metabolizes amino acids and glucose	Neuritis, depression, nausea, vomiting
B_{12} (cobalamin)	Lamb, beef kidney, egg yolk, animal products	Blood formation; DNA and RNA synthesis; myelin formation; carbohydrate, protein, and fat metabolism	Macrocytic, megaloblastic anemia (large, nonfunctioning red blood cells)
Folic acid (folacin)	Liver, asparagus, bran	Red and white blood cell structure	Poor red cell formation
C (ascorbic acid)	Broccoli, collards, citrus fruit	Collagen structure, antioxidant	Scurvy (weakness, easy bleeding, joint pain)

*All fat-soluble vitamins can be absorbed only in the presence of lipids and can be transported only in the presence of protein.

Promoting Adequate Nutritional Intake in Vegetarian Diets

Families may select vegetarian diets for many reasons:

- Economic: Vegetables and grains are less expensive than animal-based food.
- Ecologic: If everyone ate lower on the food chain, world hunger could be reduced.
- Medical or health-related: Avoiding animal foods stops the ingestion of hormones and chemicals used in meat and poultry production and lowers serum cholesterol, thereby reducing the frequency of atherosclerosis and obesity; avoiding red meat may reduce the likelihood of developing colon cancer as well. Because of the association between saturated fat and bowel cancer and atherosclerosis, the number of families avoiding red meat will probably increase in the future.
- Philosophical: A belief that killing animals for food is unnecessary.
- Religious: Religions such as Hindu and Seventh-Day Adventist promote a vegetarian lifestyle.

Increasing numbers of adults of childrearing age are vegetarians; therefore, many women during pregnancy and children during their years of most rapid growth eat such diets (Cox, 2008). Although a balanced vegetarian diet can be sufficient during childhood, careful assessment and family education are necessary to ensure that it is adequate for growth. Urge parents to become knowledgeable about good nutrition so they are aware of ways to include essential nutrients for growing children in vegetarian diets, particularly if their children participate in active sports.

Four main types of vegetarian diets are usually seen:

- A lacto-ovo-vegetarian diet includes dairy products ("lacto"), eggs ("ovo"), and plants (vegetables, fruits, and grains).
- An ovovegetarian diet includes eggs but excludes dairy products.

TABLE 28.3 ✻ Minerals Essential for Health

Mineral	Selected Dietary Sources	Function in Body	Results of Deficiency or Excess
Macronutrients			
Calcium	Milk, hard cheese	Formation of bone and teeth; muscle contractility	Improper bone growth and maintenance shown by diseases such as rickets in children
Phosphorus	Milk, meats	Formation of bone and teeth; used in cell structure; aids use of glucose	Deficiency unlikely as long as calcium and protein needs are met
Sodium	Table salt	Regulates fluid volume and pH	Deficiency rare but excess leads to hypertension in genetically determined individuals
Chloride	Table salt	Formation of hydrochloric acid; regulates body fluid with sodium	Deficiency rare except with vomiting, which causes loss of hydrochloric acid
Potassium	Meats, dried fruits	Major cation of cells; essential for electrical conduction in muscle and therefore in heart action	Deficiency leading to muscle weakness and heart irritability; occurs in people taking diuretics, because potassium is excreted with urine
Sulfur	Milk, meat, eggs	Essential for protein formation and cell growth	Deficiency rare as long as protein intake is adequate
Magnesium	Cocoa, nuts, green leafy vegetables	Relaxation of muscles after contraction	Deficiency leads to muscle contraction
Micronutrients			
Iodine	Seafood, dairy, iodized salt	Formation of thyroxine and regulation of metabolic rate	Reduced basal metabolic rate and goiter (enlarged thyroid gland)
Iron	Meats, fish, dried fruits, nuts, fortified cereals	Formation of hemoglobin; transport of oxygen to body cells	Deficiency leads to microcytic (small) and hypochromic (pale) red blood cells (iron-deficiency anemia); excess leads to infiltration of tissue (hemosiderosis)
Copper	Nuts, raisins, legumes	Formation of collagen and nerve fiber	Anemia, neutropenia, and severe bone demineralization
Fluoride	Fluoridated water	Reduces dental caries and demineralization from bone	Dental caries
Zinc	Meat, eggs, seafood	Formation of eyes, male reproductive organs, insulin, and taste sensation	Diabetes-like symptoms because of decreased insulin production; poor taste sensation leading to poor food intake
Manganese	Nuts, grains, legumes	Formation of enzymes	Deficiency unlikely
Molybdenum	Organ meats, grains	Mobilizes iron in body	Deficiency apparently unknown
Cobalt	Many sources	Formation of red blood cells in bone marrow	Deficiency rare as long as animal food sources are ingested
Selenium	Seafood, kidney, liver	Immunoglobulin formation and prevention of oxidation of cells	Deficiency unknown
Chromium	Meat, cheese, grains	Glucose metabolism	Deficiency seen only in severe malnutrition
Silicon	Many sources	Aids growth of connective tissue and bone	Retarded growth and bone deformity
Nickel	Many sources	Duplication of growth of cells	Has not been determined to be essential for health in humans
Vanadium	Many sources	Lipid metabolism	Has not been determined to be essential for health in humans
Tin	Many sources	Blood formation	Has not been determined to be essential for health in humans

- A lactovegetarian diet includes dairy products but excludes eggs.
- A vegan diet excludes all animal products and consists of only vegetables, fruits, and grains.

The vegan diet is most restrictive, so it is usually recommended that parents consult with a dietitian or nutritionist to ensure their children receive adequate nutrients on this diet. A fifth type of vegetarian diet is a macrobiotic diet, which falls between vegetarian and vegan diets. Its main sources of protein are grains, seeds, and nuts, but small quantities of egg, fish, and wild game can be added. All families who eat vegetarian diets need to ensure that their children receive adequate amounts of several specific nutrients.

Protein. Lacto-ovo-vegetarian, ovovegetarian, and lactovegetarian diets provide all of the essential amino acids for growth (both eggs and dairy products provide complete proteins). Vegan diets can also supply essential amino acids by cereal and legume combinations such as peanut butter and wheat bread, corn and lima beans, pasta and beans, corn tortillas and beans, or chickpeas and sesame seeds. Complementary proteins do not have to be eaten at the same meal to be effective, as long as varied plant proteins are consumed over the course of a day.

Calcium. Dairy products such as milk and cheese supply calcium as well as protein. When these are not eaten, calcium must be obtained from other sources, by eating green leafy vegetables such as broccoli or spinach or grain products such as calcium-fortified tofu or soy flour.

Iron. As there may be an association between iron-deficiency anemia and learning deficits, children need to consume good sources of iron (McCann & Ames, 2007). Meat is the best source of iron. With meat omitted from a diet, parents should include this from foods such as legumes, whole grains, fortified cereals, dark-green leafy vegetables, or dried fruits. Vitamin C enhances the duodenal absorption of iron found in plants, so eating fruits and vegetables rich in vitamin C such as oranges or broccoli aids iron absorption.

Vitamins. Vitamin B_{12} is unique among vitamins because it is present only in animal products (Rolfes, Pinna, & Whitney, 2009). This includes eggs and milk. Children who totally omit animal sources, therefore, need to have this vitamin supplemented daily. Reliable supplements of B_{12} include vitamin B_{12} tablets or fortified foods such as commercial breakfast cereals, soy beverages, and some brands of nutritional yeast.

Riboflavin is normally supplied by fortified milk. However, it may be supplied by soy milk, vegetables, or brewer's yeast, all of which contain all the B vitamins except B_{12}, so riboflavin is usually adequate in a vegetarian diet daily without additional supplementation. Good sources of riboflavin in vegan diets are whole and enriched grains and cereals, nuts, and dark-green leafy vegetables.

Vitamin D is necessary for calcium and phosphorus metabolism and is normally supplied in fortified milk. It is not present in plant foods and therefore must be supplemented in a vegan or ovovegetarian diet by vitamin D drops or tablets. Exposure to sunshine is generally an inadequate source (Rolfes, Pinna, & Whitney, 2009).

Minerals. Zinc is present primarily in animal foods but is also present in brewer's yeast, nuts, and wheat germ. Iodine is supplied normally by seafood. In a vegan or vegetarian diet, it can be supplied by seaweed and iodized table salt. Many families add a small amount of powdered kelp (a seaweed) to food two or three times a week to ensure an adequate iodine intake.

Total Calories. Plant foods have fewer total calories than meats. Therefore, one serving of nuts and one serving of legumes are recommended in place of two meat servings. All other recommended serving sizes for various caloric level patterns are the same as those presented in the usual food guide pyramid (see Appendix K).

What if... John's mother tells you she cannot afford to buy meat, explaining she can get more food for the family if she purchases mostly pasta and cereals? How would you help her plan meals that are low in cost but high in nutritional value?

THEORIES OF DEVELOPMENT

A *theory* is a systematic statement of principles that provides a framework for explaining some phenomenon. Developmental theories provide road maps for explaining human development.

A **developmental task** is a skill or a growth responsibility arising at a particular time in an individual's life, the achievement of which will provide a foundation for the accomplishment of future tasks. It is not so much chronologic age as the completion of developmental tasks that defines whether a child has passed from one developmental stage of childhood to another. For example, children are not toddlers just because they are 1 year plus 1 day old; they become toddlers when they have passed through the developmental stage of infancy. For reference, however, childhood is generally divided into the age periods shown in Table 28.4.

A number of theories have been proposed to describe how children grow emotionally, psychologically, and intellectually as they pass through these different periods. Sociocultural theories stress the importance of environment on growth and development. Learning theory proposes children are like blank pages that can be shaped by learning (Horowitz, 1994). Epigenetic theories stress that genes are the true basis for growth and development. Previously discounted as too simplistic, epigenetic theories are being revised and given new credence based on new knowledge about genes now available through the National Genome Project or the mapping of all the body's genes (Fisler & Warden, 2007). Still other theories deal mainly with negative aspects of childrearing that can cause mental illness in children, either immediately or later, when a child reaches adulthood (see discussion on Freud that follows). Erikson discusses positive aspects necessary for normal growth and for development of a mentally healthy and productive adult (Coles, 2001).

TABLE 28.4 ✻ Basic Divisions of Childhood

Stage	Age Period
Neonate	First 28 days of life
Infant	1 mo–1 yr
Toddler	1–3 yr
Preschooler	3–5 yr
School-age child	6–12 yr
Adolescent	13–21 yr

Freud's Psychoanalytic Theory

Sigmund Freud (1856–1939), an Austrian neurologist and the founder of psychoanalysis, offered the first real theory of personality development (Edmundson, 2007). Freud based his theory on his observations of mentally disturbed adults. He described adult behavior as being the result of instinctual drives that have a primarily sexual nature (*libido*) that arise from within the person and the conflicts that develop between these instincts (represented in the individual as the *id*), reality (the *ego*), and society (the *superego*). He described child development as being a series of psychosexual stages in which a child's sexual gratification becomes focused on a particular body part. Freud's stages of childhood are summarized in Table 28.5.

Infant

Freud termed the infant period the "oral phase" because infants are so interested in oral stimulation or pleasure during this time. According to this theory, infants suck for enjoyment or relief of tension, as well as for nourishment.

Toddler

Freud described the toddler period as an "anal phase" because during this time, children's interests focus on the anal region as they begin toilet training. Elimination takes on new importance for them. Children find pleasure in both the retention of feces and defecation. This anal interest is part of toddlers' self-discovery, a way of exerting independence, and probably accounts for some of the difficulties parents may experience in toilet-training children of this age.

Preschooler

During the preschool period, children's pleasure zone appears to shift from the anal to the genital area. Freud called this period the "phallic phase." Masturbation is common during this phase. Children may also show exhibitionism, suggesting they hope this will lead to increased knowledge of the two sexes.

School-Age Child

Freud saw the school-age period as a "latent phase," a time in which children's libido appears to be diverted into concrete thinking. He saw no developments as obvious as those in earlier periods appearing during this time.

Adolescent

Freud termed the adolescent period the "genital phase." Freudian theory considers the main events of this period to be the establishment of new sexual aims and the finding of new love objects.

Criticisms of Freud's Theory

To construct his theory, Freud relied on his knowledge of people with mental illness or looked at circumstances that led to mental illness. This "looking at illness" rather than "looking at wellness" perspective limits the applicability of the theory as a health promotion measure, although the behaviors he discussed are as observable as ever.

Erikson's Theory of Psychosocial Development

Erik Erikson (1902–1996) was trained in psychoanalytic theory but later developed his own theory of psychosocial development, a theory that stresses the importance of culture and society in development of the personality (Erikson, 1993). One of the main tenets of his theory, that a person's social view of self is more important than instinctual drives in determining behavior, allows for a more optimistic view of the possibilities for human growth. While Freud looked at ways mental illness develops, Erikson looked at actions that lead to mental health. Erikson describes eight developmental stages covering the entire life span. At each stage, there is a conflict between two opposing forces. The resolution of each conflict, or accomplishment of the developmental task of that stage, allows the individual to go on to the next phase of development. Table 28.5 shows Erikson's developmental stages through adolescence compared to Freud's.

The Infant

According to Erikson, the developmental task for infants is learning **trust versus mistrust** (other terms are "learning confidence" or "learning to love"). Infants whose needs are met when those needs arise, whose discomforts are quickly removed, who are cuddled, played with, and talked to, come to view the world as a safe place and people as helpful and dependable. However, when their care is inconsistent, inadequate, or rejecting, this fosters a basic mistrust: infants become fearful and suspicious of the world and of people. Like a burned child who avoids fire, emotionally burned children may shun the potential pain of further emotional involvement and carry this attitude through later stages of development. Such children can be "stuck" emotionally at this stage, although they continue to grow and develop in other ways.

Fortunately, because not all children achieve developmental tasks readily, each task need not be resolved once and for all the first time it arises. The problem of trust versus mistrust, for example, is not resolved forever during the first year of life but arises again at each successive stage of development. Children who enter school with a sense of mistrust may come to trust a teacher with whom they form a close relationship; given this second chance, children may overcome early mistrust. On the other hand, children who come through infancy with a vital sense of trust intact may still have a sense of mistrust activated at a later stage if their parents are divorced or separate under unpleasant circumstances.

TABLE 28.5 ✻ Summary of Freud's and Erikson's Theories of Personality Development

	Freud's Stages of Childhood		Erikson's Stages of Childhood	
	Psychosexual Stage	*Nursing Implications*	*Developmental Task*	*Nursing Implications*
Infant	Oral stage: Child explores the world by using mouth, especially the tongue.	Provide oral stimulation by giving pacifiers; do not discourage thumb-sucking. Breastfeeding may provide more stimulation than formula feeding because it requires the infant to expend more energy.	Developmental task is to form a sense of trust versus mistrust. Child learns to love and be loved.	Provide a primary caregiver. Provide experiences that add to security, such as soft sounds and touch. Provide visual stimulation for active child involvement.
Toddler	Anal stage: Child learns to control urination and defecation.	Help children achieve bowel and bladder control without undue emphasis on its importance. If at all possible, continue bowel and bladder training while child is hospitalized.	Developmental task is to form a sense of autonomy versus shame. Child learns to be independent and make decisions for self.	Provide opportunities for decision making, such as offering choices of clothes to wear or toys to play with. Praise for ability to make decisions rather than judging correctness of any one decision.
Preschooler	Phallic stage: Child learns sexual identity through awareness of genital area.	Accept children's sexual interest, such as fondling their own genitals, as a normal area of exploration. Help parents answer child's questions about birth or sexual differences.	Developmental task is to form a sense of initiative versus guilt. Child learns how to do things (basic problem solving) and that doing things is desirable.	Provide opportunities for exploring new places or activities. Allow play to include activities involving water, clay (for modeling), or finger paint.
School-age child	Latent stage: Child's personality development appears to be nonactive or dormant.	Help children have positive experiences with learning so their self-esteem continues to grow and they can prepare for the conflicts of adolescence.	Developmental task is to form a sense of industry versus inferiority. Child learns how to do things well.	Provide opportunities such as allowing child to assemble and complete a short project so that child feels rewarded for accomplishment.
Adolescent	Genital stage: Adolescent develops sexual maturity and learns to establish satisfactory relationships with the opposite sex.	Provide appropriate opportunities for the child to relate with opposite sex; allow child to verbalize feelings about new relationships.	Developmental task is to form a sense of identity versus role confusion. Adolescents learn who they are and what kind of person they will be by adjusting to a new body image, seeking emancipation from parents, choosing a vocation, and determining a value system.	Provide opportunities for an adolescent to discuss feelings about events important to him or her. Offer support and praise for decision making.

Adapted from Erikson, E. H. (1993). *Childhood and society.* New York: W. W. Norton; and Freud, S. (1962). *Three essays on the theory of sexuality.* New York: Hearst Corporation, with permission.

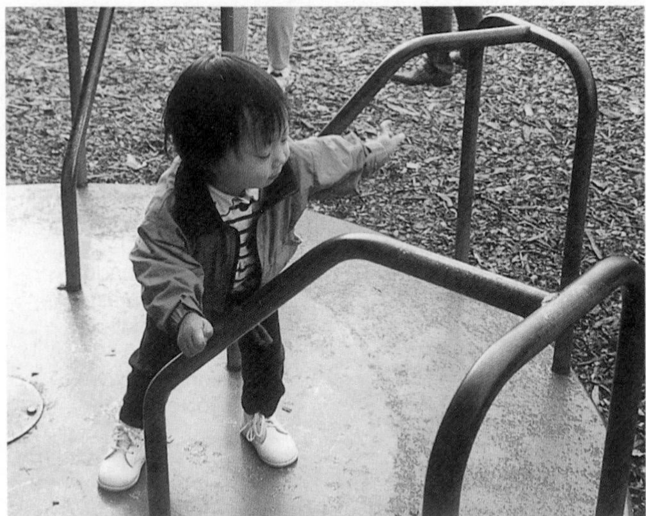

FIGURE 28.4 A toddler enjoys active, independent exploration as part of building a sense of autonomy.

The Toddler

Erikson defines the developmental task of the toddler age as learning **autonomy versus shame or doubt.** Autonomy (self-government or independence) builds on children's new motor and mental abilities. Children take pride in new accomplishments and want to do everything independently, whether it is pulling the wrapper off a piece of candy, selecting a vitamin tablet out of the bottle, flushing the toilet, or replying, "No!" If parents recognize toddlers need to do what they are capable of doing, at their own pace and in their own time, then children develop a sense of being able to control their muscles and impulses during this time. When caregivers are impatient and do everything for them, this enforces a sense of shame and doubt. If children are never allowed to do things they want to do, they will eventually doubt their ability to do them; they will stop trying and cannot do them. If children leave this stage with less autonomy than shame or doubt, they can be disabled in their attempts to achieve independence and may lack confidence in their abilities to achieve well into adolescence and adulthood (Fig. 28.4).

The Preschooler

The developmental task of the preschool period is learning **initiative versus guilt.** Learning initiative is learning how to do things. Children can initiate motor activities of various sorts on their own and no longer merely respond to or imitate the actions of other children or of their parents. The same is true for language and fantasy activities.

Whether children leave this stage with a sense of initiative outweighing a sense of guilt depends largely on how parents respond to self-initiated activities. When children are given much freedom and opportunity to initiate motor play such as running, bike riding, sliding, and wrestling or are exposed to such play materials as finger paints, sand, water, and modeling clay, their sense of initiative is reinforced. Initiative is also encouraged when parents answer a child's questions (intellectual initiative) and do not inhibit fantasy or play activity. If children are made to feel their motor activity is bad (perhaps in a small apartment or a hospital), their questions are a nuisance, or their play is silly and stupid, they may develop a sense of guilt over self-initiated activities that will persist in later life. Those who do not develop initiative may later have limited brainstorming and problem-solving skills; they wait for clues or guidance from others before acting.

What if... John's father does not allow his preschool twins to play freely because he demands an orderly household? They begin to show signs of poor initiative. How would you counsel this parent?

The School-Age Child

Erikson viewed the developmental task of the school-age period as developing **industry versus inferiority,** or accomplishment rather than inferiority. During the preschool period, children learned initiative—how to do something. During school age, children learn how to do things *well.* A school-age child, while doing a project will ask, "Am I doing a good job? Am I doing this right?" When they are encouraged in their efforts to do practical tasks or make practical things and are praised and rewarded for the finished results, their sense of industry grows (Fig. 28.5). Parents who see their children's efforts at making and doing things as merely "busy work" or who do not show appreciation for their children's efforts may cause them to develop a sense of inferiority rather than pride and accomplishment.

During the elementary school years, a child's world grows to include the school and community environment, and success or failure in those settings can have a lasting impact. Children with an intelligence quotient of 80 or 90 (slightly below normal), for example, may have a particularly traumatic school experience, even when their sense of industry is rewarded and encouraged at home. Their learning style may be so different from the average child's they have difficulty competing with children of average ability; this causes repeated failures in their efforts to learn, reinforcing their sense of inferiority. On the other hand, children whose sense of industry has not been supported at home may have it revital-

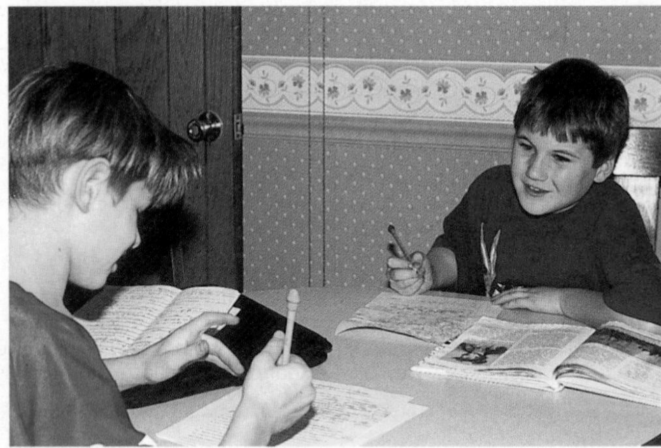

FIGURE 28.5 School-age children develop a sense of industry by working on projects that result in a feeling of accomplishment.

ized at school through the efforts of a committed teacher. A nurse during a hospitalization could also fulfill this role.

The Adolescent

Erikson believed the new interpersonal dimension that emerges during adolescence is a sense of **identity versus role confusion.** To achieve this, adolescents must bring together everything they have learned about themselves as a son or daughter, an athlete, a friend, a fast-food cook, a student, a garage band musician, and so on, and integrate these different images into a whole that makes sense. If adolescents cannot do so, they are left with role confusion; that is, they are left unsure of what kind of person they are and are uncertain what they can do or what kind of person they can become. Some adolescents seek a negative identity: being identified as a drug abuser or runaway may be preferable to having no identity at all. Body piercing and tattooing can help establish identity as they are outward expressions of who adolescents think they are (Box 28.4).

The Young Adult

The developmental crisis of the young adult is achieving a sense of **intimacy versus isolation.** Intimacy is the ability to relate well with other people, not only with members of the opposite sex but also with one's own sex to form long-lasting friendships.

A sense of intimacy grows out of earlier developmental tasks, because people need a strong sense of identity before they can reach out fully and offer deep friendship or love. Because there is always the risk of being rejected or hurt when offering love or friendship, individuals cannot offer it if they do not have confidence they can cope with rejection or if they did not develop a sense of trust as an infant. Parents without a sense of intimacy may have more difficulty than others accepting a pregnancy and beginning to love a newborn child.

The Middle-Aged Adult

The developmental task of middle age is to establish a sense of **generativity versus stagnation.** People extend their concern from just themselves and their families to the community and the world. They may become politically active, work to solve environmental problems, or participate in far-reaching community or world-based decisions.

People with a sense of generativity are self-confident and better able to juggle their various lives (mother, soccer coach, church member, teacher, political party chairperson, gourmet cook). People without this sense become stagnated or self-absorbed. Those who have devoted themselves to only one role are more likely to find themselves at the end of middle age with a narrow perspective and lack of ability to cope with change. Women without a sense of generativity may have more difficulty than others accepting a late-in-life pregnancy and a new role of childbearing and childrearing.

The Older Adult

Older adults play a role in childrearing today because many of them give childcare to young children while parents work. The developmental task of older adults is **integrity versus despair.** Older adults with integrity feel good about the life choices they have made; those with a feeling of despair wish life could begin over again so that things could turn out differently. A sense of integrity is helpful in a grandparent who provides childcare, as it helps children develop a sense of trust and learn initiative (Bernal & Anuncibay, 2008).

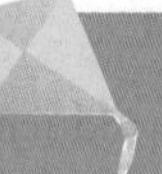

BOX 28.4 * Focus on Evidence-Based Practice

Is body piercing or tattooing increasing in incidence in adolescents?

Body piercing or tattooing can be a means of establishing identify in adolescents. To establish whether the incidence of students with either a body piercing or tattoo is increasing, researchers asked 454 undergraduate college students in 2001 and 661 students in 2006 at an eastern U.S. university if they presently had a piercing or tattoo. In the year 2001 group, 60% of females and 42% of males had a body piercing; 26% of females and 22% of males had a tattoo. In the 2006 group, 62% of females and 36% of males had a body piercing; 21% of females and 23% of males had a tattoo. Researchers did not count pierced earlobes in females in the results but they did count ear cartilage as piercing (accounting for the substantially higher incidence in females). Overall, both body piercing (51% and 49%) and tattooing (24% and 22%) stayed roughly the same during these time periods. The medical complications reported for piercing (17% and 19%) also remained the same but was a cause for concern as almost one-fifth of students reported having a complication, most frequently an infection, at the piercing site.

Based on the above study, what symptoms would you want adolescents to inspect for following a body piercing to be certain they aren't developing a complication?

Source: Mayers, L. B., & Chiffriller, S. H. (2008). Body art (body piercing and tattooing) among undergraduate university students: "then and now". *Journal of Adolescent Health, 42*(2), 201–203.

Criticism of Erikson's Theory

Erikson's main contribution to human development was the creation of stages so that development can be broken down into separate phases for study. A criticism of his theory is that life does not occur in easily divided stages, and trying to divide it that way can create superficial divisions.

✔ Checkpoint Question 28.2

John, 6 years old, is a school-age child. What must he learn, according to Erikson, to complete the developmental task of this period?

a. How to be creative.
b. How to think abstractly.
c. How to trust others.
d. How to do things well.

Piaget's Theory of Cognitive Development

Jean Piaget (1896–1980), a Swiss psychologist, introduced concepts of **cognitive development** or the way children learn and think that have roots similar to those of both Freud and Erikson and yet separate from each (Wadsworth, 2003). Piaget defined four stages of cognitive development; within each stage are finer units or **schemas.** Each period is an advance over the previous one. To progress from one period to the next, children reorganize their thinking processes to bring them closer to adult thinking. These stages of cognitive development are summarized in Table 28.6.

The Infant

Piaget referred to the infant stage as the **sensorimotor stage.** Sensorimotor intelligence is practical intelligence, because words and symbols for thinking and problem solving are not yet available at this early age. At the beginning of infancy, babies relate to the world through their senses, using only reflex behavior. As infants progress through this stage (which includes the schemas of primary and secondary circular reactions and coordination of secondary reactions, as defined in Table 28.6), they learn the basic concept that people are entities separate from objects. Piaget used the term "primary" to refer to activities related to a child's own body and the term "circulatory reaction" to show that repetition of behavior occurs (infants accidentally bring their thumb to their mouth, enjoy the sensation of sucking, and so repeat it).

The term "secondary" refers to activities that are separate from a child's body. An example of secondary schema learning is when a baby hits a mobile, notices that this makes it move, and so hits it again. During this secondary schema, infants also learn that objects in the environment—bottle, blocks, bed, or even a parent—are permanent and continue to exist even though they are out of sight or changed in some way. For example:

- Infants will search for a block hidden by a blanket, knowing the block still exists.
- Infants can recognize that a parent remains the same person whether dressed in a robe and slippers or pants and a T-shirt.
- Infants play peek-a-boo because they realize the person playing with them exists behind his or her hands.
- Infants learn they are a separate entity from objects. They learn where their body stops and their bed, playthings, or parent begins.

A great deal of the mouthing and handling of objects by infants and the delight of watching a caregiver appear is part of primary and secondary schemas and discovering **permanence.** The world begins to make sense and the developmental task of achieving trust falls into place when the concept of permanence has been learned (infants know their parents exist and will return to them). Gaining a concept of permanence also contributes to "eighth-month anxiety," a stage in which infants continue to cry for their parents because they know their parents still exist even when out of sight.

During the final phase of the infant year (coordination of secondary reactions), infants begin to demonstrate goal-directed behavior. After noticing that hitting a mobile makes it move, infants then reach for and hit a music box nearby, in this way actively seeking new experiences. It is important for infants to have stimulating objects around for exploring in this way so that experimenting and learning can proceed.

The Toddler

The toddler period is one of transition as children complete the final stages of the sensorimotor period (defined in Table 28.6 as tertiary circular reaction and invention of new means) and begin to develop some cognitive skills of the preoperative period, such as symbolic thought and egocentric thinking. In the tertiary circular reaction schema, children use trial and error to discover new characteristics of objects and events. A toddler sitting in a high chair who keeps dropping objects over the edge of the tray is exploring both permanence and the different actions of toys. During the schema of "invention of new means," children become able to think through actions or mentally project the solution to a problem. If given a box, a toddler will investigate how the top of the box can be removed; if given a second box, even one that varies in shape, the child can foresee how the top can be removed. Toddlers following a ball that has rolled under a coffee table no longer have to follow the ball's path to retrieve it but can project where it will have rolled and walk around the coffee table to find it again.

During the period of *preoperational thought*, children relearn on a conceptual level some of the lessons they mastered as infants at the sensorimotor level, before having language. Now, children are able to use symbols to represent objects. They may have difficulty viewing one object as being different from another, however. On a walk through a department store decorated with teddy bears, for example, children are not sure whether they are seeing a succession of bears or if the same bear keeps reappearing as if it is following them, asking to be taken home.

Toddlers draw conclusions only from obvious facts they see: Daddy is shaving; therefore he must be going to work, because he went to work after he shaved yesterday. This type of faulty reasoning (prelogical reasoning) can lead children to wrong conclusions and faulty judgment.

How children think has many implications for nursing. If you made John's bed yesterday and then he went to surgery, he may cry at the sight of you approaching with clean sheets today, thinking he will have to go to surgery again.

The Preschooler

Piaget saw preschool children as moving on to a substage of preoperational thought termed *intuitive thought.* During this time, children tend to look at an object and see only one of its characteristics (referred to as **centering).** For example, they see that a banana is yellow but do not notice it is also long. Centering is noticeable when children are learning about medicine (they observe it tastes bitter but cannot understand it is also good for them).

Centering contributes to the preschooler's lack of **conservation** (the ability to discern truth, even though physical properties change) or **reversibility** (ability to retrace steps). For example, if preschoolers see water being poured from

TABLE 28.6 ✻ Piaget's Stages of Cognitive Development

Stage of Development	Age Span	Nursing Implications
Sensorimotor		
Neonatal reflex	1 mo	Stimuli are assimilated into beginning mental images. Behavior entirely reflexive.
Primary circular reaction	1–4 mo	Hand–mouth and ear–eye coordination develop. Infant spends much time looking at objects and separating self from them. Beginning intention of behavior is present (the infant brings thumb to mouth for a purpose: to suck it). Enjoyable activity for this period: a rattle or tape of parent's voice.
Secondary circular reaction	4–8 mo	Infant learns to initiate, recognize, and repeat pleasurable experiences from environment. Memory traces are present; infant anticipates familiar events (a parent coming near him will pick him up). Good toy for this period: mirror; good game: peek-a-boo.
Coordination of secondary reactions	8–12 mo	Infant can plan activities to attain specific goals. Perceives that others can cause activity and that activities of own body are separate from activity of objects. Can search for and retrieve toy that disappears from view. Recognizes shapes and sizes of familiar objects. Because of increased sense of separateness, infant experiences separation anxiety when primary caregiver leaves. Good toy for this period: nesting toys (i.e., colored boxes).
Tertiary circular reaction	12–18 mo	Child is able to experiment to discover new properties of objects and events. Capable of space perception and time perception as well as permanence. Objects outside self are understood as causes of actions. Good game for this period: throw and retrieve.
Invention of new means through mental combinations	18–24 mo	Transitional phase to the preoperational thought period. Uses memory and imitation to act. Can solve basic problems, foresee maneuvers that will succeed or fail. Good toys for this period: those with several uses, such as blocks, colored plastic rings.
Preoperational thought	2–7 yr	Thought becomes more symbolic; can arrive at answers mentally instead of through physical attempt. Comprehends simple abstractions but thinking is basically concrete and literal. Child is egocentric (unable to see the viewpoint of another). Displays static thinking (inability to remember what they started to talk about so that at the end of a sentence children are talking about another topic). Concept of time is now, and concept of distance is only as far as they can see. Centering or focusing on a single aspect of an object causes distorted reasoning. No awareness of reversibility (for every action there is an opposite action) is present. Unable to state cause–effect relationships, categories, or abstractions. Good toy for this period: items that require imagination, such as modeling clay.
Concrete operational thought	7–12 yr	Concrete operations includes systematic reasoning. Uses memory to learn broad concepts (fruit) and subgroups of concepts (apples, oranges). Classifications involve sorting objects according to attributes such as color; seriation, in which objects are ordered according to increasing or decreasing measures such as weight; multiplication, in which objects are simultaneously classified and seriated using weight. Child is aware of reversibility, an opposite operation or continuation of reasoning back to a starting point (follows a route through a maze and then reverses steps). Understands conservation, sees constancy despite transformation (mass or quantity remains the same even if it changes shape or position). Good activity for this period: collecting and classifying natural objects such as native plants, sea shells, etc. Expose child to other viewpoints by asking questions such as, "How do you think you'd feel if you were a nurse and had to tell a boy to stay in bed?"
Formal operational thought	12 yr	Can solve hypothetical problems with scientific reasoning; understands causality and can deal with the past, present, and future. Adult or mature thought. Good activity for this period: "talk time" to sort through attitudes and opinions.

From Piaget, J. (1961). *The growth of logical thinking from childhood to adolescence.* New York: Basic Books, with permission.

one glass into another glass that is taller and thinner than the first one, they will notice only one changing characteristic. They might say that there is now more water in the second glass (because the level has risen), or there is less water (because the second glass is narrower), even when told that no water has been added or removed. When the water is poured back into the first glass, they still will not understand that the amount of water is unchanged. This immature perception leads children, as it did during the toddler period, to make faulty conclusions. It takes more years of development for children to learn that when thought processes such as knowing that the amount of water did not change and perceptions conflict, thought processes are more trustworthy.

Preschool thinking is also influenced by **role fantasy,** or how children would like something to turn out. Children use **assimilation** (taking in information and changing it to fit their existing ideas) as a part of this. For example, because a child wants to go outside and play, he says the outside is calling him to come and play. Children believe their wishes are as real as facts and dreams are as real as daytime happenings during this stage. They perceive animals and even inanimate objects as being capable of thought and feeling (they say a dog took their doll because the dog was feeling sad; they say a footstool meant to trip them). This is often called "magical thinking." Later, children learn **accommodation** (they change their ideas to fit reality rather than the reverse).

Egocentrism, or perceiving that one's thoughts and needs are better or more important than those of others, is also strong during this period. Preschoolers cannot believe that not everyone knows facts they know; if asked, "What is your name?" they may reply, "Don't you know my name?" As a part of this, children define objects mainly in relation to themselves, so that a spoon is "what I eat with," not just a curved metal object.

The School-Age Child

Piaget viewed school age as a period during which *concrete operational thought* begins as school-age children can discover concrete solutions to everyday problems and recognize cause-and-effect relationships. A child who understands water does not change in amount just because it is poured from one glass to another has grasped the concept of conservation. Conservation of numbers is learned as early as age 7 years, conservation of quantity at age 7 or 8 years, conservation of weight at age 9 years, and conservation of volume at age 11 years. Reasoning during school age tends to be inductive, proceeding from specific to general: school-age children tend to reason that a toy they are holding is broken, the toy is made of plastic, so all plastic toys break easily.

The Adolescent

Piaget saw adolescence as the time when cognition achieves its final form, that of formal operational thought. When this stage is reached, adolescents are capable of thinking in terms of possibility—what could be **(abstract thought)**—rather than being limited to thinking about what already is (concrete thought). This makes it possible for adolescents to use scientific reasoning or also understand deductive reasoning, or reasoning that proceeds from the general to the specific (plastic toys break easily, the toy they are holding is plastic; it will break easily).

Criticism of Piaget's Theory

Piaget has been criticized because he used only a small sample of subjects (his own children) to develop his theory. Because children today begin activities to learn reading much earlier than they did at the time the theory was devised, the age groups and "norms" may no longer be accurate. Learning computer skills at an early age may be changing both the rate and type of children's cognitive development.

Kohlberg's Theory of Moral Development

Lawrence Kohlberg (1927–1987), a psychologist, studied the reasoning ability of boys and, based on Piaget's development stages, developed a theory on the way children gain knowledge of right and wrong or moral reasoning. These stages, as described by Kohlberg (1984), are summarized in Table 28.7.

Recognizing where a child is at according to these stages can help identify how children may feel about an illness such as whether children think it is fair that they are ill. Recognizing moral reasoning also helps determine whether children can be depended on to carry out self-care activities such as administering their own medicine or whether children have internalized standards of conduct so they do not "cheat" when away from external control. Moral stages closely approximate cognitive stages of development, because children must be able to think abstractly (be able to conceptualize an idea without a concrete picture) before being able to understand how rules apply even when no one is there to enforce them.

The Infant

The infant period is a *prereligious stage.* Infants have little concept of any motivating force beyond that of their parents. Infants learn that when they do certain actions, parents give affection and approval; for other actions, parents scold and label the behavior "bad." To support this stage of development, it is important for caregivers to praise infants for doing what they have been asked to do. Caregivers should also know the average infant is trying hard to please; if an infant falls short of doing this, it is probably because of immature development rather than any effort to displease.

The development of trust is important in moral development because infants who develop a sound sense of trust can better develop a spiritual orientation in future years or be bound by a moral conscience (they can trust in a spiritual being as well as humans around them).

The Toddler

Toddlers begin to formulate a sense of right and wrong, but their reason for doing right is centered most strongly in "mother or father says so" rather than in any spiritual or societal motivation. Kohlberg referred to this as a "punishment obedience orientation" (a child is good because a parent says a child must be good, not because it is "right" to be good).

TABLE 28.7 ✻ Kohlberg's Stages of Moral Development

Age (Year)	Stage	Description	Nursing Implications
Preconventional (Level I)			
2–3	1	Punishment/obedience orientation ("heteronymous morality"). Child does right because a parent tells him or her to and to avoid punishment.	Child needs help to determine what are right actions. Give clear instructions to avoid confusion.
4–7	2	Individualism. Instrumental purpose and exchange. Carries out actions to satisfy own needs rather than society's. Will do something for another if that person does something for the child.	Child is unable to recognize that like situations require like actions. Unable to take responsibility for self-care, because meeting own needs interferes with this.
Conventional (Level II)			
7–10	3	Orientation to interpersonal relations of mutuality. Child follows rules because of a need to be a "good" person in own eyes and eyes of others.	Child enjoys helping others because this is "nice" behavior. Allow child to help with bed making and other like activities. Praise for desired behavior such as sharing.
10–12	4	Maintenance of social order, fixed rules, and authority. Child finds following rules satisfying. Follows rules of authority figures as well as parents in an effort to keep the "system" working.	Child often asks what are the rules and is something "right." May have difficulty modifying a procedure because one method may not be "right." Follows self-care measures only if someone is there to enforce them.
Postconventional (Level III)			
Older than 12	5	Social contract, utilitarian law-making perspectives. Follows standards of society for the good of all people.	Adolescents can be responsible for self-care because they view this as a standard of adult behavior.
	6	Universal ethical principle orientation. Follows internalized standards of conduct.	Many adults do not reach this level of moral development.

From Kohlberg, L. (1984). *The psychology of moral development.* New York: Harper & Row, with permission.

Toddlers may not obey requests from people other than their parents because they do not view their authority as being at the same level as their parents' authority. This means that while providing nursing care, it might be necessary to ask a parent to reinforce instructions to be certain a toddler will follow them.

The Preschooler

Preschoolers tend to do good out of self-interest rather than out of true intent to do good or because of a strong spiritual motivation. When asked why it is wrong to steal from a neighbor, for example, a preschooler will answer, "Because my mother won't like me any more." Because of egocentrism, a preschooler may do things for others only in return for things done for him or her. This means it may be necessary to remind children of actions taken on their behalf or trade off actions such as, "Lie still now for me while I change your dressing and I'll read you a story when I'm through."

Children at this age also imitate what they see, so if they see less-than-perfect role models, they may copy those wrong actions, assuming those actions are correct. Preschoolers have great difficulty knowing what rules apply to new situations because they cannot judge whether a previously learned principle of right or wrong can be applied to this new situation (does not recognize that stealing money in a hospital setting is the same as stealing it at home).

The School-Age Child

School-age children enter a stage of moral development termed *conventional development,* a level at which many adults continue to function. Young school-age children adhere to a phase of development termed the "nice girl, nice boy" stage. Children engage in actions that are "nice" or "fair" rather than necessarily right. Sharing, for example, is "nice." Taking turns is "fair." Stealing is not. Young school-age children may lie about their actions to disguise that they have been involved in an action that is not "nice." When asked why it is wrong to steal from a neighbor, the school-age child most often answers, "Because it's not nice or fair."

Later in the school-age period, as children learn about community resources, they become aware that community laws are enforced by crossing guards or police. They may have difficulty following self-care measures reliably when out of a nurse's or parent's sight during this time because they feel it is necessary to obey rules only when the rules can be clearly enforced. At this point, they might answer the question about stealing from a neighbor with, "You shouldn't steal because the police will put you in jail."

The Adolescent

As adolescents become capable of abstract thought, they become capable of internalizing standards of conduct (they do what they think is right regardless of whether anyone is watching). This is termed *postconventional development* and is the mature form of moral reasoning. In this stage, if asked why it is wrong to steal from a neighbor, adolescents answer, "Because it deprives my neighbors of possessions they have earned." Adolescents can carry out self-care measures even when someone else is not present when they enter this stage because they can understand not only the importance of the measures to themselves but also the principle that certain things should be done simply because they are right to do. Many adolescents do not enter this phase of development, however, and as adults they continue at a school-age level, doing right things only when obvious authority or set rules are present.

Criticism of Kohlberg's Theory

Kohlberg's theory is frequently challenged as being male-oriented because his original research was conducted entirely with boys. Carol Gilligan (1993), a sociologist, has suggested that girls may not score well on Kohlberg's scale because, being more concerned with relationships than boys, they make moral decisions based on individual circumstances, a different criterion for decision making.

USING GROWTH AND DEVELOPMENT IN PRACTICE

An assessment of children's growth and development should be included in all children's nursing care plans as whether they are growing and developing within usual parameters is a significant mark of wellness (see Focus on Nursing Care Planning Box 28.5).

✓ Checkpoint Question 28.3

Suppose John, 6 years old, tells you his broken leg wants to get better. What type of thinking is he using?

a. Magical thinking.
b. Deductive reasoning.
c. Concrete operational thinking.
d. Sensorial thought.

BOX 28.5 ✻ Focus on Nursing Care Planning

A Multidisciplinary Care Map for a Child With a Developmental Concern

John Olson is a 6-year-old boy you see in an emergency department because he has a broken leg from a bicycle accident. His parents tell you although John has lived with them for 3 years, they find him cold and unloving. They ask you what they can do to change this.

Family Assessment ✻ Family lives in a three-bedroom house in suburbs. Father works as a plumber; mother has a part-time job as a substitute grade-school teacher.

Client Assessment ✻ At 4 months of age, John was taken away from his mother because she was not caring for him adequately. He was then moved back and forth among 12 different foster homes until he was finally adopted at age 3½. His adoptive parents have 3-year-old twins of their own.

Nursing Diagnosis ✻ Interrupted family processes related to inability of child to meet parents' developmental expectations

Outcome Criteria ✻ Child demonstrates greater participation in family activities and improved response to parents' attempts to bond with him by 3 months' time.

Team Member Responsible	Assessment	Intervention	Rationale	Expected Outcome
Activities of Daily Living				
Nurse	Assess if family has thought through impact of bicycle accident on daily activities.	Suggest some obvious accommodations needed for cast care: no tub bathing, difficulty with stairs, no bike riding.	If a family is already under stress, an accident can compound the problem.	Family members state that accidents are not anyone's "fault"; are prepared to make adjustments needed.

		Consultations		
Nurse/ physician	Assess if parents feel that psychological counseling would be appropriate for child.	Assist parents with gaining a consultation if they feel they would welcome this.	Consultation with a skilled professional can offer parents information on specific actions to take.	Parents state whether they feel situation merits more skilled help at this time.
		Procedures/Medications		
Physician/ nurse	Assess what emergency actions are necessary for fractured tibia.	Apply cast; give instructions for cast care. Keep pain or discomfort to a minimum.	Definite measures to prevent pain are important in promoting a sense of trust.	Client states he understands cast care; states that emergency department experience was an adventure, not an ordeal.
		Nutrition		
Nurse	Employ a 24-hour recall dietary history to assess for usual calcium and vitamin D intake.	Suggest additional sources of calcium or vitamin D if needed.	Calcium is important for good bone healing and absorbed best in the presence of vitamin D.	Client states he understands calcium will help healing and is willing to ingest more as needed.
		Patient/Family Education		
Nurse	Assess what parents understand about the development of trust in early life.	Suggest ways to initiate a sense of trust by demonstrating dependability and a warm, loving relationship.	A sense of trust can be reinstated at a later developmental stage if it has been lost.	Parents state they are willing to begin more active steps toward improving relationship with son.
		Psychosocial/Spiritual/Emotional Needs		
Nurse	Assess what type of child parents expected to adopt.	Suggest measures that could bring parents and child closer together such as a "game night," always eating meals together, quiet "talk times" before bed.	Identifying differences between expectations and reality can help people understand dissatisfactions.	Client and parents state they are willing to begin active program of shared activities.
		Discharge Planning		
Nurse	Assess if client or parents have any further needs they would like to discuss.	Discuss with client and parents adjustments client will have to make to attend school with a cast in place.	Small needs not met can grow into major needs before a return appointment and interfere further with a sense of trust.	Client and parents state they understand adjustments that need to be made and will work them out together.

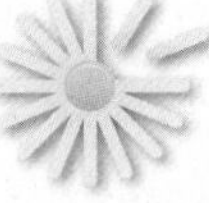

Key Points for Review

- Knowledge of growth and development is important in health promotion and illness prevention because it lays the basis for assessment and anticipatory guidance.
- Genetic factors that influence growth and development are gender, ethnicity, intelligence, and health.
- Environmental influences include quality of nutrition, socioeconomic level, parent–child relationship, ordinal position in the family, and environmental health.
- To meet growth and development milestones, children need to follow basic guidelines for a healthy diet, such as eating a variety of foods; maintaining ideal weight; avoiding extreme levels of saturated fat and cholesterol; eating foods with adequate starch and fiber; and avoiding too much sugar, the same as adults.
- Temperament is a child's characteristic manner of thinking, behaving, or reacting. Helping parents understand the effect of temperament is a nursing role.
- Common theories of development are Freud's psychoanalytic theory and Erikson's theory of psychosocial development. Both of these theories describe specific tasks children must complete at each stage of development to become a well-adapted adult.
- Piaget's theory of cognitive development describes ways that children learn. Kohlberg advanced a theory of moral development, or how children use moral reasoning to solve problems they face.
- Although growth and development occur in known patterns, their rate varies from child to child. Caution parents not to be concerned because two siblings are very different as long as they both fit within usual parameters.

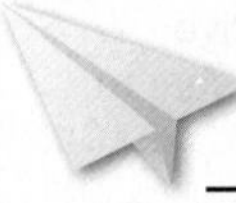

CRITICAL THINKING EXERCISES

1. John is the 6-year-old boy you met at the beginning of the chapter. He had lived in many foster homes before he was adopted. His parents state that they find him cold and unloving. What developmental task was John unable to complete because of these frequent moves at such a young age? What actions could his new parents take to try to strengthen this developmental task at this point?
2. John's mother describes her 3-year-old twins as "totally different" from each other. One is shy and quiet and agreeable; the other is aggressive and persistent. What characteristic is she describing? Which child does she probably view as easier to care for? What anticipatory guidance could you give her to help her better understand these differences in her children?
3. Children who are hospitalized for long periods may fall behind in development. What specific measures could you take to promote developmental growth and encourage a sense of autonomy if John were a hospitalized 2-year-old? To promote a sense of industry if he were hospitalized at age 10 years?
4. Examine the National Health Goals related to growth and development of children. Most government-sponsored funds for nursing research are allotted based on these goals. What would be a possible research topic to explore pertinent to these goals that would be applicable to John's family and also advance evidence-based practice?

CRITICAL THINKING SCENARIO

Open the accompanying CD-ROM or visit http://thePoint.lww.com and read the Patient Scenario included for this chapter, then answer the questions to further sharpen your skills and grow more familiar with NCLEX style questions related to principles of growth and development. Confirm your answers are correct by reading the rationales.

REFERENCES

Barnes-Powell, L. L. (2007). Infants of diabetic mothers: the effects of hyperglycemia on the fetus and neonate. *Neonatal Network: The Journal of Neonatal Nursing, 26*(5), 283–290.

Bernal, J. G., & Anuncibay, R. (2008). Intergenerational grandparent/grandchild relations: the socioeducational role of grandparents. *Educational Gerontology, 34*(1), 67–88.

Carey, W. B., & McDevitt, S. C. (1978). Revision of the infant temperament questionnaire. *Pediatrics, 61*(4), 735–739.

Carey, W. B., & McDevitt, S. C. (1994). *Prevention and early intervention: Individual differences as risk factors for the mental health of children.* New York: Brunner/Mazel.

Chess, S., & Thomas, A. (1995). *Temperament in clinical practice.* New York: Guilford Publications.

Coles, R. (2001). *The Erik H. Erikson reader.* New York: W.W. Norton.

Coren, E., & Barlow, J. (2009). Individual and group-based parenting programmes for improving psychosocial outcomes for teenage parents and their children. *Cochrane Database of Systematic Reviews, 2009*(1), (CD002964).

Cox, S. R. (2008). Staying healthy on a vegetarian diet during pregnancy. *Journal of Midwifery and Women's Health, 53*(1), 91–92.

Demicheli, V., et al. (2009). Vaccines for measles, mumps and rubella in children. *Cochrane Database of Systematic Reviews, 2009*(1), (CD004407).

Dooley, M., & Stewart, J. (2007). Family income, parenting styles and child behavioural-emotional outcomes. *Health Economics, 16*(2), 145–162.

Edmundson, M. (2007). *The death of Sigmund Freud: the legacy of his last days.* New York: Bloomsbury.

Erikson, E. H. (1993). *Childhood & society. New York:* W. W. Norton.

Fisler, J. S., & Warden, C. H. (2007). The current and future search for obesity genes. *American Journal of Clinical Nutrition, 85*(1), 1–2.

Fitzgerald, H. E., & Das Eiden, R. (2007). Paternal alcoholism, family functioning, and infant mental health. *Zero to Three, 27*(4), 11–18.

Foley, M. (2007). School-age temperament: implications for school nurses. *Journal for Specialists in Pediatric Nursing, 12*(2), 128–131.

Freud, S. (1962). *Three essays on the theory of sexuality.* New York: Hearst Corporation.

Gilligan, C. (1993). *In a different voice: Psychological theory and women's development.* Cambridge, MA: Harvard University Press.

Goldson, E., & Reynolds, A. (2008). Child development and behavior. In W. W. Hay, et al. (Eds.). *Current pediatric diagnosis and treatment* (18th ed.). Columbus, OH: McGraw-Hill.

Green, M., & Solnit, A. (1964). Reactions to the threatened loss of a child: A vulnerable child syndrome. *Pediatrics, 34*(8), 58–62.

Hale, R. (2007). Infant nutrition and the benefits of breastfeeding. *British Journal of Midwifery, 15*(6), 368–371.

Horowitz, F. D. (1994). John B. Watson's legacy: learning and environment. In D. Ross, et al. (Eds.). *A century of developmental psychology.* Washington, DC: American Psychological Association.

Hussain, A., et al. (2007). Prevention of type 2 diabetes: a review. *Diabetes Research and Clinical Practice, 76*(3), 317–326.

Kline, A. M. (2008). Pediatric obesity in acute and critical care. *AACN Advanced Critical Care, 19*(1), 38–46.

Knitzer, J. (2008). Giving infants and toddlers a head start: getting policies in sync with knowledge. *Infants and Young Children, 21*(1), 18–29.

Kohlberg, L. (1984). *The psychology of moral development.* New York: Harper & Row.

Mayers, L. B., & Chiffriller, S. H. (2008). Body art (body piercing and tattooing) among undergraduate university students: "then and now". *Journal of Adolescent Health, 42*(2), 201–203.

McCann, J. C., & Ames, B. N. (2007). An overview of evidence for a causal relation between iron deficiency during development and deficits in cognitive or behavioral function. *American Journal of Clinical Nutrition, 85*(4), 931–945.

Motz, M., Leslie, M., & DeMarchi, G. (2007). Breaking the cycle: using a relational approach to address the impact of maternal substance use on regulation and attachment in children. *Zero to Three, 27*(4), 19–25.

Ondrak, K. S., & Morgan, D. W. (2007). Physical activity, calcium intake and bone health in children and adolescents. *Sports Medicine, 37*(7), 587–600.

O'Shea, T. M., et al. (2007). Follow-up care for infants with chronic lung disease: a randomized comparison of community- and center-based models. *Pediatrics, 119*(4), e947–e957.

Piaget, J. (1961). *The growth of logical thinking from childhood to adolescence.* New York: Basic Books.

Rolfes, S. R., Pinna, K., & Whitney, E. N. (2009). *Understanding normal and clinical nutrition.* New York: Wadsworth/Cengage Learning.

Shulruf, B., et al. (2007). Designing multidisciplinary longitudinal studies of human development: analyzing past research to inform methodology. *Evaluation and the Health Professions, 30*(3), 207–228.

Thomas, K. A., & Uran, A. (2007). How the NICU environment sounds to a preterm infant. *MCN: The American Journal of Maternal/Child Nursing, 32*(4), 250–253.

Ulrich, B. (2007). Nature and nurture in the development of children with a disability, I: dynamic systems approach to organisms' inherent plasticity that underlies options for therapeutic intervention. *Developmental Medicine and Child Neurology, 49*(Suppl 110), 5–6.

U.S. Department of Agriculture (USDA). (2005). *Dietary guidelines for Americans.* Washington, DC: Author.

Vartanian, L. R., Schwartz, M. B., & Brownell, K. D. (2007). Effects of soft drink consumption on nutrition and health: a systematic review and meta-analysis. *American Journal of Public Health, 97*(4), 667–675.

Wadsworth, B. J. (2003). *Piaget's theory of cognitive and affective development: foundations of constructivism* (5th ed.). New York: Longman.

SUGGESTED READINGS

Acolet, D. (2008). Quality of neonatal care and outcome. *Archives of Disease in Childhood Fetal and Neonatal Edition, 93*(1), F69–F73.

Caughy, M. O., Hayslett-McCall, K. L., & O'Campo, P. J. (2007). No neighborhood is an island: incorporating distal neighborhood effects into multilevel studies of child developmental competence. *Health and Place, 13*(4), 788–798.

Chumlea, C. (2007). Which growth charts are the best for children today? *Nutrition Today, 42*(4), 148–150.

Darbyshire, P. (2007). 'Childhood': are reports of its death greatly exaggerated? *Journal of Child Health Care, 11*(2), 85–97.

Kristjansson, E. A., et al. (2009). School feeding for improving the physical and psychosocial health of disadvantaged students. *Cochrane Database of Systematic Reviews, 2009*(1), (CD004676).

Sullivan, M. C., & Msall, M. E. (2007). Functional performance of preterm children at age 4. *Journal of Pediatric Nursing: Nursing Care of Children and Families, 22*(4), 297–309.

Talen, M. R., et al. (2007). Well-child check-up revised: an efficient protocol for assessing children's social-emotional development. *Families, Systems and Health, 25*(1), 23–35.

Tedder, J., & Register, N. (2007). The "HUG": an innovative approach to pediatric nursing care... (help, understanding, and guidance for young families). *MCN: The American Journal of Maternal/Child Nursing, 32*(4), 210–214.

Wagner, S. (2007). Knowledge of normal development key in diagnosis. *Patient Education Management, 14*(8), 89–90.

Ward, T. M., Rankin, S., & Lee, K. A. (2007). Caring for children with sleep problems. *Journal of Pediatric Nursing: Nursing Care of Children and Families, 22*(4), 283–296.

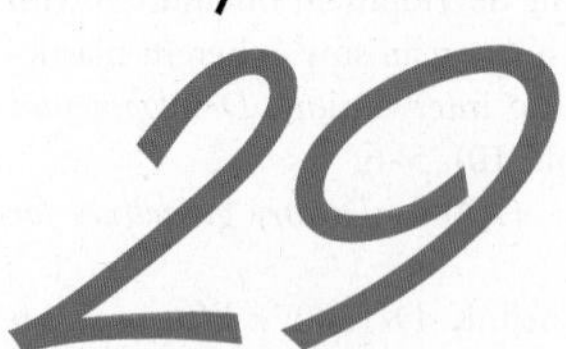

Chapter 29 Nursing Care of a Family With an Infant

KEY TERMS

- baby-bottle syndrome
- binocular vision
- deciduous teeth
- eighth-month anxiety
- extrusion reflex
- hand regard
- natal teeth
- neck-righting reflex
- neonatal teeth
- object permanence
- pincer grasp
- seborrhea
- social smile
- thumb opposition

OBJECTIVES

After mastering the contents of this chapter, you should be able to:

1. Describe normal infant growth and development and associated parental concerns.
2. Identify National Health Goals related to infant growth and development that nurses can help the nation achieve.
3. Use critical thinking to analyze methods of care for an infant to be certain care is family centered.
4. Assess an infant for normal growth and development milestones.
5. Formulate nursing diagnoses related to infant growth and development and associated parental concerns.
6. Identify expected outcomes to promote optimal infant growth and development needs.
7. Plan nursing care to meet an infant's growth and development needs such as teaching parents to childproof their home.
8. Implement nursing care related to normal growth and development of an infant such as encouraging eye/hand coordination.
9. Evaluate expected outcomes for achievement and effectiveness of care.
10. Identify areas related to nursing care of an infant that could benefit from additional nursing research or application of evidence-based practice.
11. Integrate knowledge of infant growth and development with nursing process to achieve quality maternal and child health nursing care.

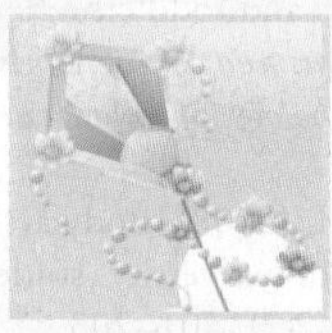

You meet Ms. Simpson, 19, at a pediatric clinic when she brings in her 2-month-old son, Bryan. She looks tired. She tells you she is exhausted because her baby is "awake all night, crying constantly." She stopped breastfeeding and changed him to formula to see if that would help. It didn't. She tells you his bowel movements are normal. When you weigh Bryan, you find he has gained weight well. When you talk to him, he demonstrates a social smile. Previous chapters described the newborn and the capabilities with which children are born. This chapter adds information about the dramatic changes, both physical and psychosocial, that occur during the first year. Such information can build a base for care and health teaching for the age group.

What condition common to early infancy might Ms. Simpson be describing? Is this normal infant behavior? What factors might be playing a role? What suggestions could you make to help her enjoy caring for Bryan more?

Traditionally, infancy is designated as the period of time from 1 month to 1 year of age. In these important months, an infant undergoes such rapid development that parents sometimes believe their baby looks different and demonstrates new abilities every day. During this time, an infant triples birth weight and increases length by 50%. Infant's reflexes develop and senses sharpen and, with the process of attachment to primary caregivers, they form a first social relationship. Because of the growth and learning potential that occurs, this first year is a crucial one. Without proper nutrition, a baby will not grow and physically thrive, and without proper stimulation and nurturing care by consistent caregivers, an infant may not develop a healthy interest in life or a feeling of security essential for future development.

As a result, infant health promotion is the subject of much concern. National Health Goals addressing this important developmental stage are highlighted in Box 29.1.

Although infant health care visits are scheduled less frequently than formerly, a standard schedule is for 2-week, 2-month, 4-month, 6-month, and 12-month visits (American Academy of Pediatrics [AAP], 2009). These visits are as important for the parents as they are for an infant because they provide an opportunity for parents to ask questions about their child's growth pattern and developmental progress. They also provide opportunities for health care providers to assess for potential problems. Anticipatory guidance offered at these visits can help parents prepare for the rapid changes that mark the first year of life. When appropriate, encouraging parents to join clubs or networking groups helps to increase their knowledge base and confidence level as well.

Table 29.1 details the usual procedures for infant health maintenance visits. The vaccines administered during the first year are discussed in Chapter 34 and also listed in Appendix J.

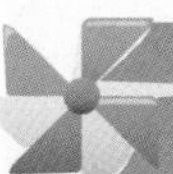

BOX 29.1 * Focus on National Health Goals

A number of National Health Goals focus on promotion of health during the infant year. These are:

- Increase the proportion of mothers who breastfeed until 1 year of age from a baseline of 16% to 25%.
- Reduce the incidence of early childhood caries such as those caused by baby-bottle syndrome from a baseline of 18% to 11%. Special target population: parents and caregivers with less than high school educations.
- Reduce the rate of fetal and infant deaths from a baseline of 7.5 per 1000 to 4.5 per 1000.
- Increase the rate of use of child automobile restraints in children 4 years and under from a baseline of 92% to 100%.
- Increase the percentage of healthy full-term infants who are put down to sleep on their backs from a baseline of 35% to 70%.
- Increase to at least 90% the proportion of infants who receive all recommended immunizations for an infant at appropriate intervals (http://www.nih.gov).

Nurses can help the nation achieve these goals by educating parents about the importance of not putting an infant to bed with a bottle of milk or juice, the use of infant car seats, and continuing breastfeeding for a full year. A number of areas related to these topics that could benefit from additional nursing research include effective ways mothers can comfort an infant in a car seat without removing the infant from the seat; characteristics of programs that are successful in promoting breastfeeding; and effective ways to teach about immunizations so that parents secure those recommended for infants.

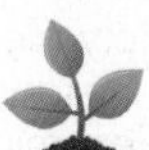

Nursing Process Overview

For Healthy Development of an Infant

Assessment

Nursing assessment of an infant begins with an interview with the primary caregiver. Important areas to discuss include nutrition, growth patterns, and development. An infant's height, weight, and head circumference are important indicators of growth, so they should be measured and plotted on standard growth charts (Brayden, Daley, & Brown, 2008). These charts represent average growth and can determine if the baby's growth remains within the same relative percentile at each checkup.

Physical assessment of an infant must be done quickly yet thoroughly because a baby can tire or become hungry, making it difficult to judge overall behavior and temperament. The primary caregiver should be present to make a child feel comfortable. Using a calm approach helps the infant remain calm as well.

Nursing Diagnosis

Much of your assessment of an infant and family will focus on basic needs such as sleep, nutrition, and activity and the parents' adjustment to their new role. Examples of nursing diagnoses are:

- Ineffective breastfeeding related to maternal fatigue
- Disturbed sleep pattern (maternal) related to baby's need to nurse every 2 hours
- Deficient knowledge related to normal infant growth and development
- Imbalanced nutrition, less than body requirements, related to infant's difficulty sucking
- Health-seeking behaviors related to adjusting to parenthood
- Delayed growth and development related to lack of stimulating environment
- Risk for impaired parenting related to long hospitalization of infant
- Readiness for enhanced family coping related to increased financial support
- Social isolation (maternal) related to lack of adequate social support
- Ineffective role performance related to new responsibilities within the family

Outcome Identification and Planning

Outcomes established for infant care need to be realistic based on the family's new circumstances. Parents of infants,

TABLE 29.1 ✻ Health Maintenance Schedule, Infant Period

Area of Focus	Methods	Frequency
Assessment		
Developmental milestones	History, observation	Every visit
	Denver Developmental Screening Test (DDST II)	At 3 months and 1 year
Growth milestones	Height, weight, head circumference plotted on standard growth chart; physical examination	Every visit
Nutritional adequacy	History, observation	Every visit
Parent-child relationship	History, observation	Every visit
Sleep positioning counseling	Discussion of placing infants on back to sleep	Every visit up to 9 months
Injury and violence counseling	Discussion of safety measures to take with infants	Every visit
Vision and hearing screening	Observation and history	Every visit
Dental health	History, physical examination	Every visit after teeth erupt
Anemia	Hematocrit, hemoglobin	9- or 12-month visit
Lead screening	Finger stick	9- or 12-month visit
Tuberculosis screening	PPD test	12-month visit
Immunizations		
Diphtheria, pertussis, tetanus (DPT) vaccine	Review of history and health record; teaching caregiver about any risks and side effects; administering immunization in accordance with health care agency policies	2-, 4-, and 6-month visits
Haemophilus influenzae type B (HiB) vaccine		2-, 4-, 6-, and 12-month visits
Hepatitis A vaccine		12-month visit
Hepatitis B vaccine		Birth, 2-month, and 12-month visits
Inactivated poliomyelitis vaccine		2-, 4-, and 6-month visits
Influenza vaccine		Yearly at 6-month or more visit.
Pneumococcal vaccine		2-, 4-, 6-, and 12-month visits
Rotovirus vaccine		2-, 4-, and 6-month visit
Varicella vaccine		12-month visit

Source: American Academy of Pediatrics (AAP). (2009). *Recommendations for preventive pediatric health care.* Washington, DC: Author.

especially first-time parents, must do a lot of adjusting, and this takes time. Try to suggest activities that can be easily incorporated into the family's lifestyle. If your assessment data indicate that a child needs more exposure to language and you know both parents work during the day, for example, you might suggest the parents ask their child's caretaker to talk to their infant more. Encourage parents to spend additional time each evening reading or reciting nursery rhymes to their baby. The combined interventions should increase the baby's language skills. Helpful Web sites about growth and development to recommend are the BabyCenter (http://www. Babycenter.com) and Dr. Greene (http://www.DrGreene.com). Helpful Web sites to alert parents about safety are the American Association of Poison Control Centers (http://www.aapcc. org) and the AAP (http://www.aap.org). For questions about car seats, parents can consult the U.S. Department of Transportation National Highway Traffic Safety Administration (http://www.nhtsa.dot.gov). The national 800 telephone number for a poison control center is 1-800-222-1222.

Implementation

One of the most important interventions of the infant period is teaching new parents about how to care for their infant and keep the infant safe. Whenever possible, this information should be anticipatory so parents can prepare for ways to care for and protect their infant as the infant grows.

Outcome Evaluation

Evaluate expected outcomes at each visit to detect changes in parents' understanding of caring for their infant. Help parents understand all aspects of infant care, not just a single element.

Examples of expected outcomes include:

- Mother states she feels fatigued but able to cope with sleep disturbance from night waking.
- Parents state five actions they are taking daily to encourage bonding.
- Father states both he and spouse are adjusting to new roles as parents.
- Parents verbalize appropriate techniques they use to stimulate infant.
- Infant demonstrates age-appropriate growth and development.
- Infant exhibits weight, height, and head and chest circumference within acceptable norms.

GROWTH AND DEVELOPMENT OF AN INFANT

WATCH & LEARN

Infants grow rapidly both in size and in their ability to perform tasks. Although development follows set patterns, some of it is dependent on cultural factors. One difference is in the way mothers carry their infants. Many mothers tend to carry infants in their arms, while other women carry their infant in a shoulder sling or on their hip or in a forward-facing harness, positions that allow a woman to continue to work or walk while holding an infant close.

The amount of infant bathing that is done is also inconsistent across cultures. In the United States, most infants are bathed daily. In colder climates or countries where clean water is not readily available, infant bathing is more limited. The use of diapers varies also. In hot climate countries, infants are often not diapered. Being aware of these cultural differences leads to better understanding of the reasons for an individual woman's particular method of childrearing. Box 29.2 shows the typical appearance of a well infant.

Physical Growth

The physiologic changes that occur in the infant year reflect both the increasing maturity and growth of body organs. The following sections will discuss the changes that are typically seen in the first year of life.

Weight

As a rule, most infants double their birth weight by 6 months of age and triple it by 1 year. During the first 6 months, infants typically average a weight gain of 2 lb per month. During the second 6 months, weight gain is approximately 1 lb per month. The average 1-year-old boy weighs 10 kg (22 lb); the average girl weighs 9.5 kg (21 lb). An infant's weight, however, is relevant only when plotted on a standard growth chart and compared to that child's own growth curve (see Appendix E).

Height

An infant increases in height during the first year by 50%, or grows from the average birth length of 20 inches to about 30 inches (50.8 to 76.2 cm). Height, like weight, is best assessed if it is plotted on a standard growth chart. Infant growth is most apparent in the trunk during the early months. During the second half of the first year, it becomes more apparent as lengthening of the legs. At the end of the first year, the child's legs may still appear disproportionately short and bowed. For accuracy, measure infants lying supine on a measuring board (see Nursing Procedure 34.8, Chapter 34).

Head Circumference

By the end of the first year, the brain has already reached two thirds of its adult size. Head circumference increases rapidly during the infant period to reflect that rapid brain growth.

Some infants' heads appear asymmetric until the second half of the first year. This may occur from always being placed in one sleeping position, causing the skull bones to flatten on that side. Suggest to parents that they place the infant on the back to sleep and prone when playing to prevent this. This early head distortion gradually corrects itself as the

Box 29.2 Assessment
Assessing the Average Infant

Follow across midline at 3 months
Social smile at 2 months; first tooth erupts at 6 months
Respiratory rate slows to 20–30 bpm by end of year
Heart rate slows to 100–120 bpm by end of first year
Pincer grasp at 10 months
Abdomen protuberant
Liver remains immature
Triples weight by 1 year
Legs may appear short and bowed
Grows in height by 50% (20 to 30 inches)

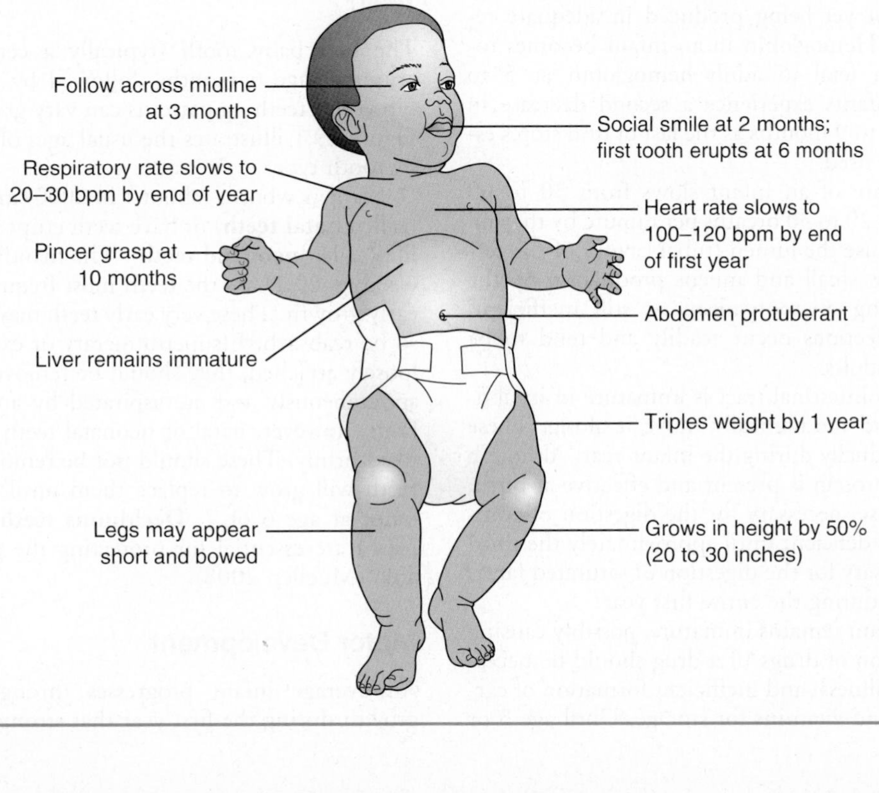

child sleeps less and spends more time with the head in an erect position. Persistence of asymmetry may suggest an infant is not receiving enough stimulation or is spending the majority of time lying in bed.

Body Proportion

Body proportion changes during the first year from that of a newborn to a more typical infant appearance. The mandible becomes more prominent as bone grows. By the end of the infant period, the lower jaw is prominent and remains that way throughout life.

The circumference of the chest is generally less than that of the head at birth by about 2 cm. It is even with the head circumference in some infants as early as 6 months and in most by 12 months. The abdomen remains protuberant until the child has been walking well for some time, generally well into the toddler period. Cervical, thoracic, and lumbar vertebral curves develop as infants hold up their head, sit, and walk.

Lengthening of the lower extremities during the last 6 months of infancy readies the child for walking and often changes the appearance from "baby-like" to "toddler-like."

Body Systems

In the cardiovascular system, heart rate slows from 120 to 160 beats per minute to 100 to 120 beats per minute by the end of the first year. The heart continues to occupy a little over half the width of the chest. Pulse rate may begin to slow with inhalation (sinus arrhythmia), but this does not become marked until preschool age. That the heart is becoming more efficient is shown by a decreasing pulse rate and a slightly elevated blood pressure (from an average of 80/40 to 100/60 mm Hg).

Infants are prone to develop a physiologic anemia at 2 to 3 months of age. This occurs because the life of a red cell is 4 months so the cells the child had at birth are disintegrating, but new cells are not yet being produced in adequate replacement numbers. Hemoglobin in an infant becomes totally converted from fetal to adult hemoglobin at 5 to 6 months of age. Infants experience a second decrease in serum iron levels at 6 to 9 months as the last of iron stores established in utero are used.

The respiratory rate of an infant slows from 30 to 60 breaths per minute to 20 to 30 breaths per minute by the end of the first year. Because the lumen (tubal cavity) of the respiratory tract remains small and mucus production by the tract to clear invading microorganisms is still inefficient, upper respiratory infections occur readily and tend to be more severe than in adults.

At birth, the gastrointestinal tract is immature in its ability to digest food and mechanically move it along. These functions mature gradually during the infant year. Although the ability to digest protein is present and effective at birth, the amount of amylase, necessary for the digestion of complex carbohydrates, is deficient until approximately the third month. Lipase, necessary for the digestion of saturated fat, is decreased in amount during the entire first year.

The liver of an infant remains immature, possibly causing inadequate conjugation of drugs (if a drug should be necessary for treatment of illness) and inefficient formation of carbohydrate, protein, and vitamins for storage. Until age 3 or 4 months, an **extrusion reflex** (food placed on an infant's tongue is thrust forward and out of the mouth) prevents some infants from eating effectively. Infants can drink from a cup almost as newborns as long as a parent controls the fluid flow. An infant can independently drink from a cup by age 8 or 10 months.

The kidneys remain immature and not as efficient at eliminating body wastes as in an adult. The infant is also unable to concentrate urine as much as an adult, which causes them to be more prone to dehydration. The endocrine system remains particularly immature in response to pituitary stimulation, such as adrenocorticotropic hormone, or insulin production from the pancreas. Without these hormones functioning effectively, an infant may not be able to respond to stress effectively.

An infant's immune system becomes functional by at least 2 months of age; an infant can actively produce both IgG and IgM antibodies by 1 year. The levels of other immunoglobulins (IgA, IgE, and IgD) are not plentiful until preschool age, the reason infants continue to need protection from infection.

The ability to adjust to cold is mature by age 6 months. By this age, an infant can shiver in response to cold (which increases muscle activity and provides warmth) and has developed additional adipose tissue to serve as insulation. The amount of brown fat, which protected the newborn from cold, decreases during the first year.

Although the fluid in body compartments shifts to some extent, extracellular fluid accounts for approximately 35% of an infant's body weight, with intracellular fluid accounting for approximately 40% by the end of the first year, in contrast to adult proportions of 20% and 40%, respectively. This proportional difference increases an infant's susceptibility to dehydration from illnesses such as diarrhea, because loss of extracellular fluid could result in loss of over a third of an infant's body fluid.

Teeth

The first baby tooth (typically a central incisor) usually erupts at age 6 months, followed by a new one monthly. However, teething patterns can vary greatly among children. Figure 29.1 illustrates the usual ages of baby tooth eruption by tooth type.

Some newborns (about 1 in 2000) may be born with teeth (called **natal teeth**) or have teeth erupt in the first 4 weeks of life (called **neonatal teeth**). The mandibular central incisors (see Fig. 29.1) are the teeth most frequently involved in this early growth. These very early teeth may be membranous and so be reabsorbed (supernumerary or extra teeth). If they are loosely attached, they should be removed before they loosen spontaneously and are aspirated by an infant. In most infants, however, natal or neonatal teeth are deciduous or are fixed firmly. These should not be removed because no other teeth will grow to replace them until the permanent teeth erupt at age 6 or 7. **Deciduous teeth** (temporary or baby teeth) are essential for protecting the growth of the dental arch (Mueller, 2008).

Motor Development

An average infant progresses through systematic motor growth during the first year that strongly reflects the princi-

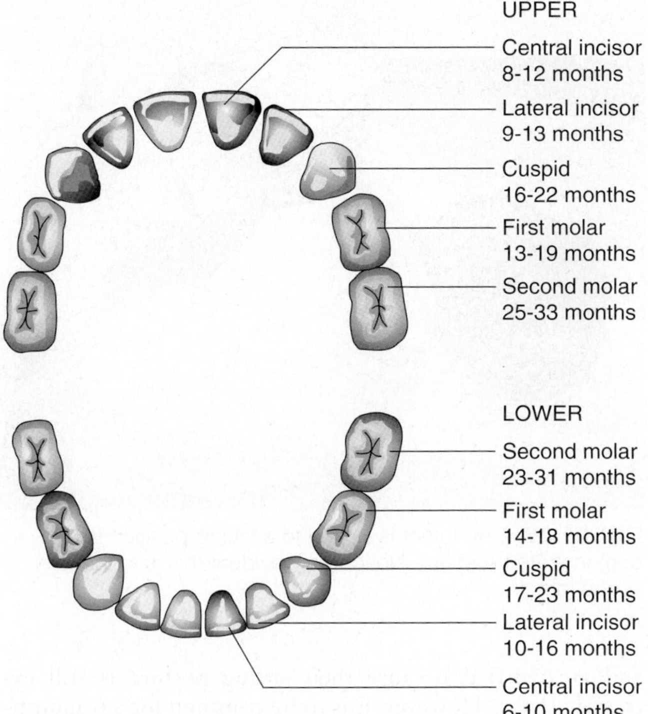

FIGURE 29.1 Eruption pattern of deciduous teeth.

ples of cephalocaudal and gross to fine motor development. Control proceeds from head to trunk to lower extremities in a progressive, predictable sequence. Different infants show individual variations in accomplishing different tasks; the ages given here are averages.

To assess motor development, both *gross motor development* (ability to accomplish large body movements) and *fine motor development*, which is measured by observing or testing *prehensile ability* (ability to coordinate hand movements), should be evaluated.

Gross Motor Development

To assess gross motor development, an infant is observed in four positions: ventral suspension, prone, sitting, and standing.

Ventral Suspension Position. *Ventral suspension* refers to an infant's appearance when held in midair on a horizontal plane, supported by a hand under the abdomen (Fig. 29.2A). In this position, the newborn allows the head to hang down with little effort at control. A 1-month-old child lifts the head momentarily, then drops it again. Two-month-old children hold their heads in the same plane as the rest of their body, a major advance in muscle control. A 3-month-old child lifts and maintains the head well above the plane of the rest of the body in ventral suspension.

A *Landau reflex* develops at 3 months. When held in ventral suspension, an infant's head, legs, and spine extend. When the head is depressed, the hips, knees, and elbows flex. This reflex continues to be present in most infants during the second 6 months of life, but then it becomes increasingly difficult to demonstrate. A child with motor weakness, cerebral palsy, or other neuromuscular defect will not be able to demonstrate the reflex.

At 6 to 9 months, an infant also demonstrates a *parachute reaction* from a ventral suspension position. When infants are suddenly lowered toward an examining table from ventral suspension, the arms extend as if to protect themselves from falling. In children with hemiplegia, the response is noticeable only on the unaffected side. Children with cerebral palsy do not demonstrate this response because they flex their extremities too tightly.

Prone Position. When lying on their stomach, newborns can turn their heads to move them out of a position where breathing is impaired, but they cannot hold them raised (see Fig. 29.2B). By 1 month of age, infants lift their heads and turn them easily to the side. They still tend to keep their knees tucked under the abdomen as they did as a newborn. Two-month-old infants can raise their heads and maintain the position, but they cannot raise their chests high enough to look around yet. Their head is still held facing downward.

A 3-month-old child lifts the head and shoulders well off the table and looks around when prone. The pelvis is flat on the table, no longer elevated. Some children can turn from a prone to a side-lying position at this age.

Four-month-old children lift their chests off the bed and look around actively, turning their heads from side to side. They can turn from front to back. The first time, this tends to occur as an extension of lifting the chest combined with a

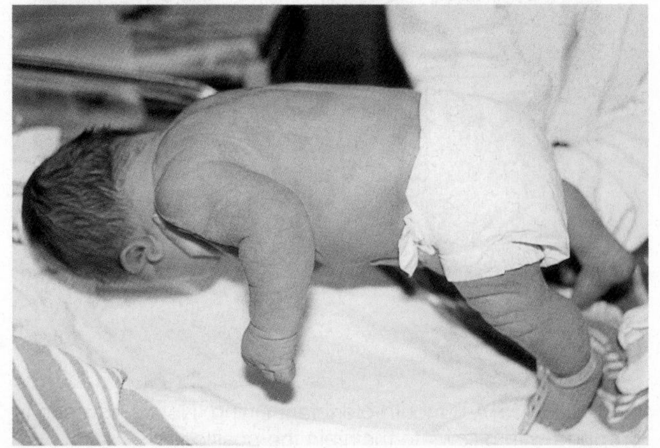
A

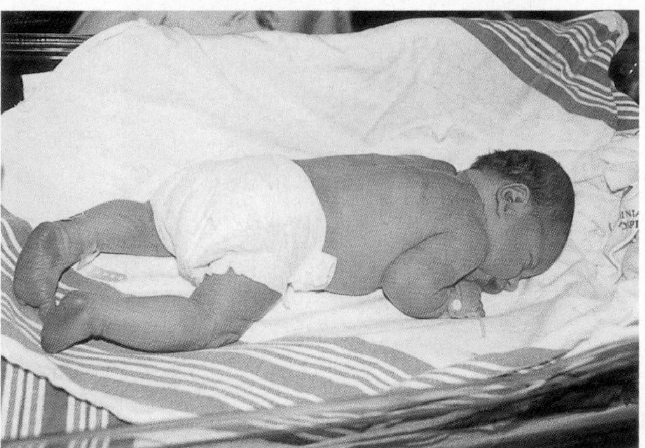
B

FIGURE 29.2 (**A**) Ventral suspension position. (**B**) Prone position.

neck-righting reflex, which begins at this age. When an infant turns the head to the side, the shoulders, trunk, and pelvis turn in that direction, too. This reflex causes babies to lose their balance and roll sideways when lifting the head up. The baby is frightened by the sudden feeling of rolling free and probably cries. After this happens a few more times, however, a baby begins to delight in this new accomplishment. Most babies turn front to back first and then, 1 month later, back to front. When taking a health history, ask which way a child turned first. Those with spasticity may turn first back to front. This is not necessarily an indication of spasticity, however, because some healthy babies turn back to front first also.

Five-month-old children rest weight on their forearms when prone. They can turn completely over, front to back and back to front. At 6 months, infants rest their weight on their hands with extended arms. They can raise their chests and the upper part of their abdomens off the table.

By 9 months, a child can creep from the prone position. Creeping is a new skill, advanced from hitching (in which infants slide along the floor) that they may have been doing. Creeping means the child has the abdomen off the floor and moves one hand and one leg and then the other hand and leg, using the knees on the floor to locomote (Fig. 29.3).

Sitting Position. When placed on the back and then pulled to a sitting position, a 1-month-old child has gross head lag as in the first days of life (Fig. 29.4). In a sitting position, the back appears rounded and an infant demonstrates only momentary head control. Two-month-olds can hold their head fairly steady when sitting up, although it does tend to bob forward. An infant at this age still has head lag when pulled to a sitting position.

A 3-month-old child has only slight head lag when pulled to a sitting position. A 4-month-old child reaches an important milestone by no longer demonstrating head lag when pulled to a sitting position.

A 5-month-old infant can be seen to straighten the back when held or propped in a sitting position. By 6 months, children sit momentarily without support. They anticipate being picked up and reach up with their hands from this position. Some parents expect a child this age to sit securely and are worried because their sitting posture is still extremely shaky. However, it is more common for a 6-month-old child to have only a limited ability to sit independently (Fig. 29.5). Six-month-old children often sit with their legs spread and their arms stiffened between them, hands on the floor, as a prop. Infants are capable of movement by hitching or sliding backward from this position. Alert parents an infant this young is capable of moving from one spot to another in this way, so they are prepared for this and can prevent accidents.

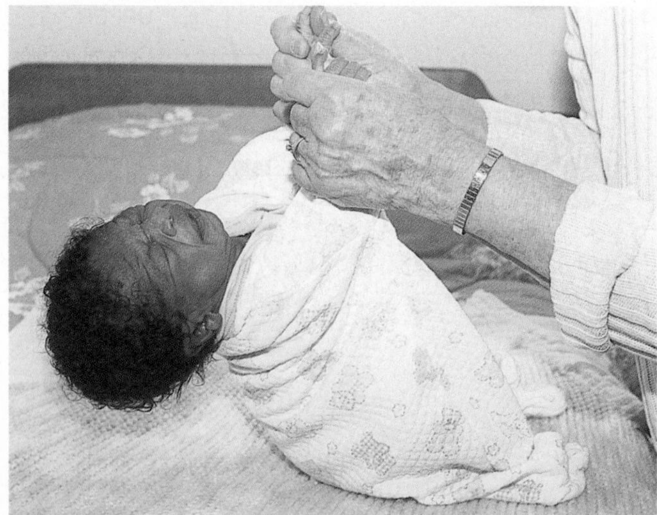

FIGURE 29.4 An infant is pulled to a sitting position to demonstrate head lag. Notice how evident this is in the very young infant.

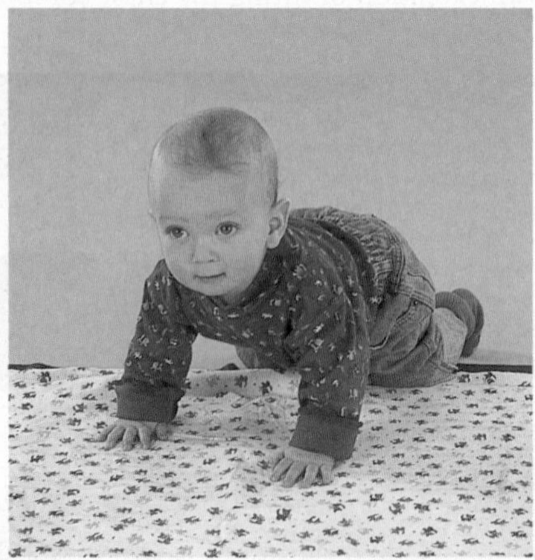

FIGURE 29.3 Creeping. The older infant moves forward, carrying his torso above and parallel to the floor.

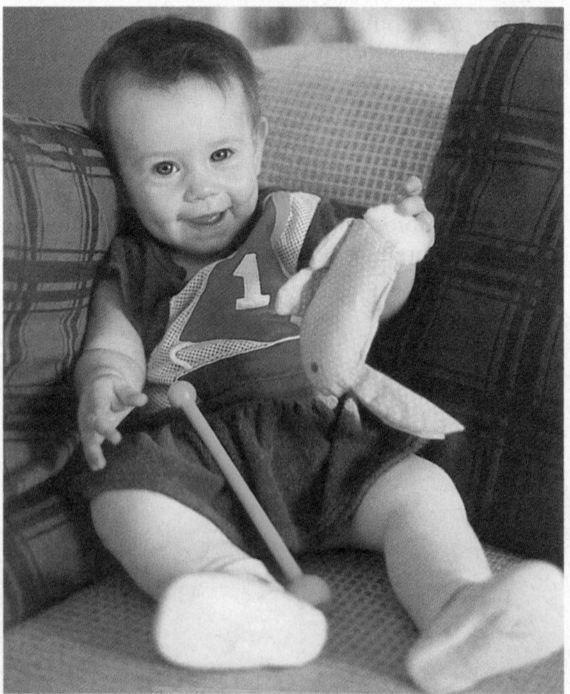

FIGURE 29.5 A 6-month-old infant sitting. Notice how she is propped with pillows to maintain the position.

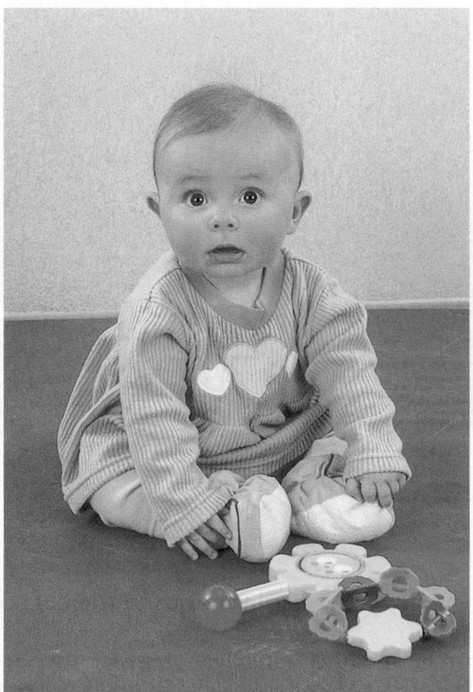
FIGURE 29.6 At 8 months an infant sits independently.

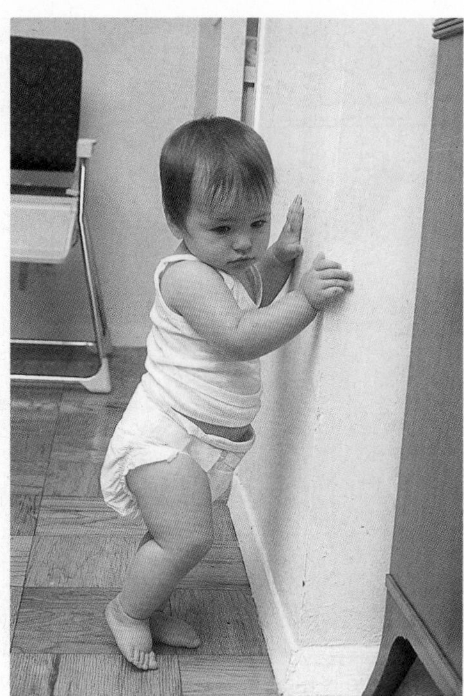
FIGURE 29.7 An 11-month-old child cruising along the walls. Further childproofing of the house will be necessary to keep her safe. (From Photo Researchers, Inc.)

A 7-month-old child sits alone, but only when the hands are held forward for balance. An 8-month-old child can sit securely without any additional support (Fig. 29.6). This is a major milestone in development that should always be considered in assessment. Children with delayed cognitive or motor development may not accomplish this step at this time.

At 9 months, infants sit so steadily they can lean forward and regain their balance. They may still lose their balance if they lean sideways, a skill not achieved for another month.

Standing Position. A newborn stepping reflex can still be demonstrated at 1 month of age. In a standing position, an infant's knees and hips flex rather than support more than momentary weight. Two-month-old children, when held in a standing position, hold their head up with the same show of support as in a sitting position. At 3 months, infants begin to try to support part of their weight.

At 4 months, infants begin to be able to support their weight on their legs. They are successful at doing this because the stepping reflex has faded.

A 5-month-old child continues the ability to sustain a portion of weight. The tonic neck reflex should be extinguished, and the Moro reflex is fading. By 6 months, infants support nearly their full weight when in a standing position. A 7-month-old child bounces with enjoyment in a standing position.

Nine-month-old children can stand holding onto a coffee table if they are placed in that position. Some 9-month-old children can pull up to that position. Ten-month-old children can pull themselves to a standing position by holding onto the side of a playpen or a low table, but they cannot let themselves down again as yet.

At around 11 months, a child learns to "cruise" or move about the crib or room by holding onto objects such as the crib rails, chairs, walls, and low tables (Fig. 29.7). At 12 months, children stand alone at least momentarily. Some parents expect children to walk at this time and are disappointed to see they are merely standing. A child has until about 22 months of age to walk and still be within the normal limit, however (Fig. 29.8).

✔ Checkpoint Question 29.1

Bryan is 2 months old. At what age would you expect him to sit securely?

a. 2.5 months.
b. 6 months.
c. 8 months.
d. 12 months.

Fine Motor Development

One-month-old infants still have a strong grasp reflex, and they hold their hands in fists so tightly it is difficult to extend the fingers. As the grasp reflex begins to fade, a 2-month-old child will hold an object for a few minutes before dropping it. The hands are held open, not closed in fists.

At 3 months, infants reach for attractive objects in front of them. Their grasp is unpracticed, however, so they usually miss them. Assure parents this is part of normal development. Otherwise, they may think their child is nearsighted or farsighted or has poor coordination.

By 4 months, infants bring their hands together and pull at their clothes. They will shake a rattle placed in their hand. **Thumb opposition** (ability to bring the thumb and fingers

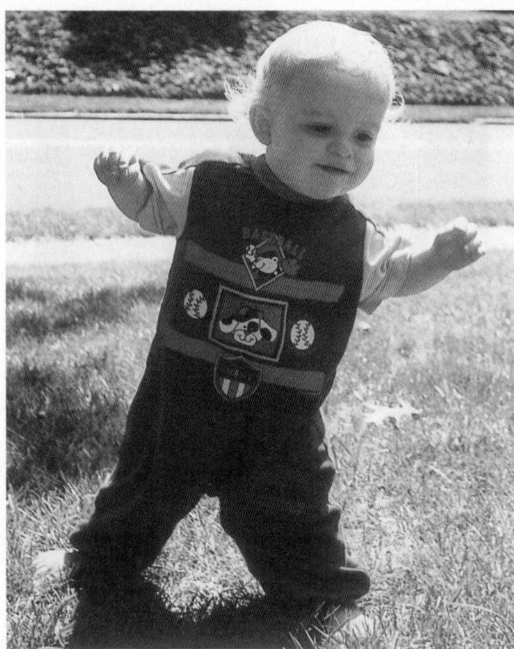

FIGURE 29.8 There is a wide variation in the age at which children take a first step, typically ranging from 8 to 15 months. Here a child has mastered walking by 1 year.

together) is beginning, but the motion is a scooping or raking one, not a picking-up one, and is not very accurate. An infant is limited to handling large objects (Fig. 29.9). Palmar and plantar grasp reflexes have disappeared.

Five-month-old children can accept objects that are handed to them by grasping with the whole hand. They can reach and pick up objects without the object being offered and often play with their toes as objects. Fisting that persists beyond 5 months suggests a delay in motor development. Unilateral fisting suggests hemiparesis or paralysis on that side.

By 6 months, grasping has advanced to a point where a child can hold objects in both hands. Infants at this age will drop one toy when a second one is offered for the same hand. They can hold a spoon and start to feed themselves (with much spilling). Moro, palmar grasp, and the tonic neck reflex have completely faded. A Moro reflex that persists beyond this point should arouse suspicion of neurologic disease.

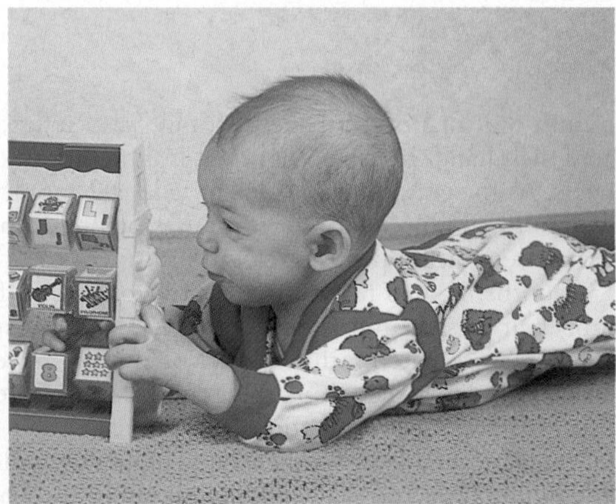

FIGURE 29.9 By age 4 months, an infant is able to manipulate large objects.

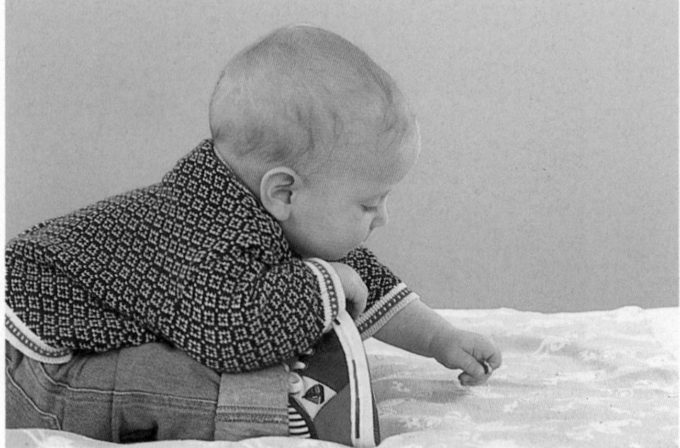

FIGURE 29.10 An infant almost ready to demonstrate a pincer grasp.

Seven-month-old children can transfer toys from one hand to the other. They hold a first object when a second one is offered. By 8 months, random reaching and ineffective grasping have disappeared as a result of advanced eye–hand coordination.

A major milestone of 10 months is the ability to bring the thumb and first finger together in a **pincer grasp** (Fig. 29.10). This enables children to pick up small objects such as crumbs or pieces of cereal from a highchair tray. They use one finger to point to objects. They offer toys to people but then cannot release them.

At 12 months, infants can draw a semistraight line with a crayon. They enjoy putting objects such as small blocks in containers and taking them out again. They can hold a cup and spoon to feed themselves fairly well (if they have been allowed to practice) and can take off socks and push their hands into sleeves (again, if they have been allowed to practice). They can offer toys and release them.

What if... Bryan learns to pick up very small articles such as marbles by 10 months? How would being able to do this affect an infant's safety?

Developmental Milestones

In addition to the gross and fine motor skills developing at this time, language and play behavior also reach major milestones. Motor and cognitive development and play throughout this year are summarized in Table 29.2.

Language Development

A child begins to make small, cooing (dovelike) sounds by the end of the first month. A 2-month-old child differentiates a cry. For example, caregivers can distinguish a cry that means "hungry" from one that means "wet" or from one that means "lonely." This is an important milestone in development for an infant and also in marking how far a parent has progressed in the task of learning the infant's cues. A first-time parent has more difficulty making the distinction in crying than one who

TABLE 29.2 ✻ Summary of Infant Growth and Development

Month	Motor Development	Fine Motor Development	Socialization and Language	Play
0–1	Largely reflex	Keeps hands fisted; able to follow object to midline		Enjoys watching face of primary caregiver, listening to soothing sounds
2	Holds head up when prone	Has social smile	Makes cooing sounds; differentiates cry	Enjoys bright-colored mobiles
3	Holds head and chest up when prone	Follows object past midline	Laughs out loud	Spends time looking at hands or uses them as toy during the month (hand regard)
4	Grasp, stepping, tonic neck reflexes are fading			Needs space to turn
5	Turns front to back; no longer has head lag when pulled upright; bears partial weight on feet when held upright			Handles rattles well
6	Turns both ways; Moro reflex fading	Uses palmar grasp	May say vowel sounds (*oh-oh*)	Enjoys bathtub toys, rubber ring for teething
7	Reaches out in anticipation of being picked up; first tooth (central incisor) erupts; sits unsteadily (still needs support)	Transfers objects hand to hand	Shows beginning fear of strangers	Likes objects that are good size for transferring
8	Sits securely without support		Has peak fear of strangers (ability to tell known from unknown people)	Enjoys manipulation, rattles and toys of different textures
9	Creeps or crawls (abdomen off floor)		Says first word (*da-da*)	Needs space for creeping
10	Pulls self to standing	Uses pincer grasp (thumb and finger) to pick up small objects		Plays games like patty-cake and peek-a-boo
11	"Cruises" (walks with support)			"Cruises"
12	Stands alone; some infants take first step	Holds cup and spoon well; helps to dress (pushes arm into sleeve)	Says two words plus *ma-ma* and *da-da*	Likes toys that fit inside each other (pots and pans); nursery rhymes; will like pull toys as soon as walking

has experienced this before. An infant's ability to make throaty, gurgling, or cooing sounds also increases at this time.

In response to a nodding, smiling face or a friendly tone of voice, a 3-month-old child will squeal with pleasure. This is an important step in development because it makes a baby even more fun to be with. Parents spend increased time with infants at this age, not just to care for them but because they enjoy their company.

By 4 months, infants are very "talkative," cooing, babbling, and gurgling when spoken to. They definitely laugh out loud. By 5 months, an infant says some simple vowel sounds (for example, "goo-goo" and "gah-gah"). At 6 months, infants learn the art of imitating. They may imitate a parent's cough, for example, or say "Oh!" as a way of attracting attention.

The amount of talking infants do increases at 7 months. They can imitate vowel sounds well (for example, "oh-oh," "ah-ah," and "oo-oo"). By 9 months, an infant usually speaks a first word: "da-da" or "ba-ba." Occasionally a mother may need reassurance that "da-da" for daddy is an easier syllable to pronounce than "ma-ma" for mommy. German mothers report the first word their babies say is "here," as that is "da" in German. By 10 months, an infant masters another word such as "bye-bye" or "no." By 12 months, infants can generally say two words besides "ma-ma" and "da-da"; they use those two words with meaning.

Play

Parents often ask what toys their infant would enjoy. Because 1-month-olds can fix their eyes on an object, they are interested in watching a mobile over their crib or playpen. Mobiles are best if they are black and white or brightly colored and light enough in weight so they move when someone walks by. They should face down toward the infant, not toward an adult standing beside the crib. Musical mobiles provide extra stimulation. One-month-old children also spend a great deal of time watching their parent's face, appearing to enjoy this activity so much a face may become their favorite "toy." Help parents understand they are not spoiling infants by sitting and holding them for long periods of time in their early months. Parents will enjoy recalling such calm moments later, when they are stacking blocks, winding up toys, or playing table games with their growing child.

Hearing is a second sense that is a source of pleasure for children in early infancy. Even newborns "listen" to the sound of a music box or a musical rattle. They stir and seem apprehensive at the sound of a raucous rattle.

Two-month-old infants will hold light, small rattles for a short period of time but then drop them. They are very attuned to mobiles or cradle gyms strung across their crib. They continue to spend a great deal of time just watching the people around them.

Three-month-old children can handle small blocks or small rattles. Four-month-old children need a playpen or a sheet spread on the floor so they have an opportunity to exercise their new skill of rolling over. Rolling over is so intriguing it may serve as a "toy" for the entire month.

Five-month-old infants are ready for a variety of objects to handle, such as plastic rings, blocks, squeeze toys, clothespins, rattles, and plastic keys. All these should be small enough an infant can lift them with one hand, yet big enough the baby cannot possibly swallow them.

A 6-month-old child can sit steadily enough to be ready for bathtub toys such as rubber ducks or plastic boats. Because they are starting to teethe, infants enjoy a teething ring to chew on at this time.

Because 7-month-old children can transfer toys, they are interested in items such as blocks, rattles, or plastic keys that are small enough to be used for this. As their mobility increases, they begin to be more interested in brightly colored balls or toys that previously rolled out of reach.

Eight-month-old children are sensitive to differences in texture. They enjoy having toys that have different feels to them, such as velvet, fur, fuzzy, smooth, or rough items.

The 9-month-old infant needs the experience of creeping. This means time out of a crib or playpen so there is room to maneuver. Many 9-month-olds begin to enjoy toys that go inside one another, such as a nest of blocks or rings of assorted sizes that fit on a center post. Some are more interested in pots and pans that stack rather than toys.

By 10 months, infants are ready for peek-a-boo and will spend a long time playing the game with their hands or with a cloth over their head that they can reach and remove. They can clap and are also ready to play patty-cake. These games have a positive value, just as laughing out loud did for the 3-month-old child. They make a baby feel like an active part of the household. A family feeling begins to grow as the baby can participate in active games.

At 11 months, children have learned to cruise or walk along low tables by holding on. They often find this so absorbing they spend little time doing anything else during the month.

Twelve-month-old infants enjoy putting things in and taking things out of containers. They like little boxes that fit inside one another or dropping small blocks into a cardboard box. As soon as they can walk, they will be interested in pull toys. A lot of time may be spent listening to someone saying nursery rhymes or listening to music.

✔ Checkpoint Question 29.2

How many words does a typical 12-month-old infant use?

a. Two, plus "ma-ma" and "da-da."
b. About 12 words.
c. Twenty or more words.
d. About 50 words.

Development of Senses

Like other facets of development, maturation of the senses proceeds step by step during the infant year.

Vision

One-month-old infants regard an object in the midline of their vision (something directly in front of themselves) as soon as it is brought in as close as about 18 inches (46 cm) away. They follow it a short distance, but not across the midline as yet. They study or regard a human face with a fixed stare. Two-month-old infants focus well (from about age 6 weeks) and follow objects with the eyes (although still not past the midline). Ability to follow and focus this way is a major milestone in development, indicating an infant has achieved **binocular vision**, or the ability to fuse two images into one (Fig. 29.11). Teach parents to make a point of initiating eye-to-eye contact with newborns right from the beginning as a method of stimulating vision as well as promoting socialization.

Three-month-old infants can follow an object across their midline. They typically hold their hands in front of their face and study their fingers for long periods of time (**hand**

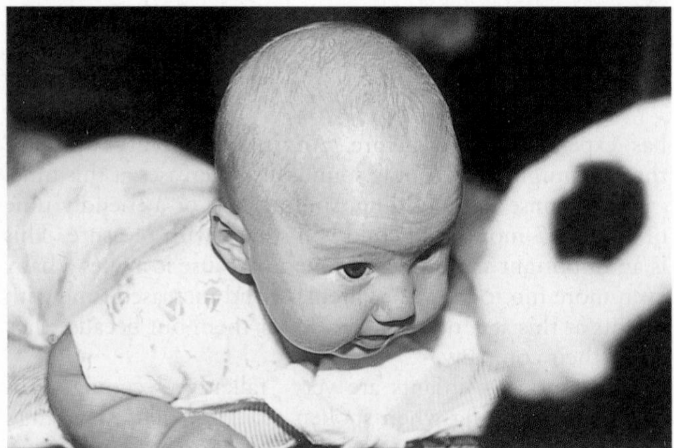

FIGURE 29.11 A 2-month-old infant focuses steadily and lifts her head up while prone. Note her interest in the stuffed bear.

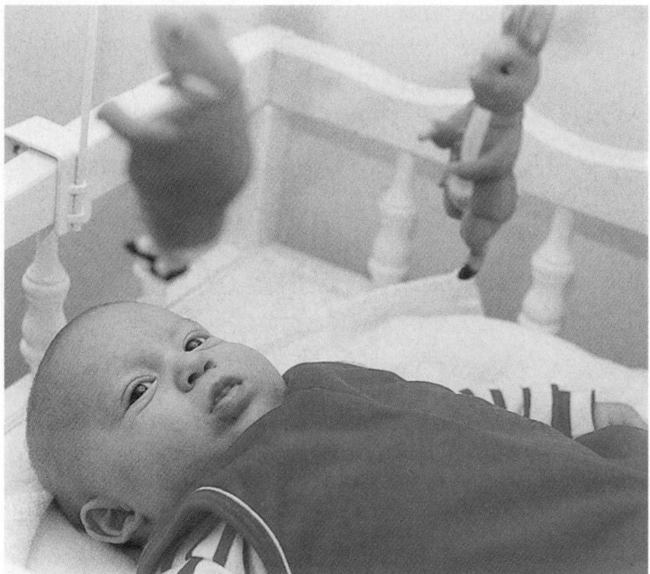

FIGURE 29.12 A 2-month-old infant enjoys watching a simple mobile.

regard). Blind children also demonstrate this phenomenon, however, so it may not be so much a test of vision as of cognitive or exploratory development. Up until 6 months of age, infants may experience difficulty in establishing eye coordination. After 3 months, however, an infant whose eyes still "cross" should be examined by a physician.

Four-month-old infants recognize familiar objects, such as a frequently seen bottle, rattle, or toy animal. They follow their parents' movements with their eyes eagerly. At 6 months, infants are capable of organized depth perception. This increases the accuracy of their reach for objects as they begin to perceive distances accurately.

Seven-month-old children pat their image in a mirror. Their depth perception has matured to the extent they can perform such tasks as transferring toys from hand to hand. By 10 months, an infant looks under a towel or around a corner for a concealed object (beginning of object permanence).

Most parents are aware that infants enjoy mobiles and also a crib mirror (Fig. 29.12). Occasionally they supply so many of these they can overdo the amount of visual stimulation, overwhelming their infant with too many patterns and objects dangling above the crib. Ask parents to consider how all these trappings must appear from an infant's view.

In a hospital environment, assess that an infant is receiving visual stimulation. Add or reduce objects as appropriate. If a child's movement is restricted in any way, move the position of the mobile from time to time. Photographs of family members brought from home or pictures drawn by older brothers or sisters can be posted near an infant's crib. Ask the parents if there are any items from home an infant would normally see during the course of the day while being fed, changed, or bathed. It may be possible to bring those items into the hospital for visual stimulation.

Hearing

Hearing is demonstrated by the 1-month-old child who quiets momentarily at a distinctive sound such as a bell or a squeaky rubber toy. Hearing awareness becomes so acute by 2 months of age that infants will stop an activity at the sound of spoken words. Many 3-month-old infants turn their heads to attempt to locate a sound. At 4 months of age, when infants hear a distinctive sound they turn and look in that direction.

By 5 months of age, infants demonstrate they can localize sounds downward and to the side, by turning their head and looking down. Six-month-olds have progressed to being able to locate sounds made above them. By 10 months, infants can recognize their name and listen acutely when spoken to. By 12 months, infants can easily locate sound in any direction and turn toward it. A vocabulary of two words plus "ma-ma" and "da-da" also demonstrates an infant can hear.

Infants appear to enjoy soft, musical sounds or soft, cooing voices; they are startled by harsh, raucous rattles or loud bangs. Urge parents to choose for an infant's first toys ones that make these types of welcoming sounds. Tape recordings of maternal heart sounds can be soothing to very young infants. For the hospitalized infant, an audiotape of family voices might be a soothing reminder of their presence. Encourage parents to read to their child daily from the beginning of life through the early school-age years, not only because the sound of the parent's voice is comforting but also because this increases language development dramatically (Box 29.3).

Touch

An infant needs to be touched to experience skin-to-skin contact. Clothes should feel comfortable and soft rather than

BOX 29.3 * Focus on Communication

You listen while Bryan's mother dresses her son after a clinic visit.

Less Effective Communication

Ms. Simpson: Don't move. And take your thumb out of your mouth. I have to put on your sweater. All right. Let's go.

Mrs. Ortello is also the mother of a 2-month-old child. You listen to her as she dresses her son as well.

More Effective Communication

Mrs. Ortello: Are you ready to go? It's time to get dressed. Next, we'll pick up Daddy. Then we're going shopping. Remember shopping? That's when you ride in the red car seat while I buy things. I hope you have my shopping gene because we do a lot of shopping. This is your yellow sweater Aunt Mary gave you. Remember her? The funny lady who said you were cute except you have no hair? Okay. We're ready. As soon as I put on my coat, we'll go.

These two women's approaches to talking to their children differ because the second mother seems to understand and appreciate that infants enjoy the sound of a parent's voice. In the first scenario, the mother is only giving instructions. Which infant might you anticipate will develop the largest vocabulary? Which one will be more aware of the names of colors sooner? Nurses can assist parents with more effective communication techniques such as this.

rough; diapers should be dry rather than wet. Teach parents to handle infants with assurance and gentleness. Remind parents that right now their child is a baby; there will be time enough later on to become a strong man or woman.

Because premature infants need to be kept warm while being held, parents are often advised to cuddle an infant next to their bare chest ("skin-to-skin contact"). This is also effective with term infants as a way of promoting close physical contact (Moore, Anderson, & Bergman, 2009).

Taste

Infants demonstrate that they have an acute sense of taste by turning away from or spitting out a taste they do not enjoy. Urge parents to make mealtime a time for fostering trust as well as supplying nutrition by being certain feedings are done at an infant's pace and the amount offered fits the child's needs and not the parent's idea of how much should be eaten.

Smell

Infants can smell accurately within 1 or 2 hours after birth. They respond to an irritating smell by drawing back from it. They appear to enjoy pleasant odors and learn early in life to identify the familiar smell of breast milk. Teach parents to be alert to substances that cause sneezing when sprayed into the air, such as room deodorizers or cleaning compounds, and to keep irritating odors out of the child's environment.

Emotional Development

Socialization, or learning how to interact with others, is an extensive phenomenon. One-month-old infants show they can differentiate between faces and other objects by studying a face or the picture of a face longer than other objects. They quiet best and eat best for the person who has been their primary caregiver.

When an interested person nods and smiles at a 6-week-old infant, the infant smiles in return. This is a **social smile** and is a definite response to the interaction, not the faint, quick "smile" that younger infants, even newborns, demonstrate. It is a major milestone for assessing several areas, most notably vision, motor control, and intelligence. Cognitively challenged children or children with spasticity may not demonstrate a social smile until much later.

By 3 months, infants demonstrate increased social awareness by readily smiling at the sight of a parent's face (Fig. 29.13). Three-month-old infants laugh out loud at the sight of a funny face.

By 4 months, when a person who has been playing with and entertaining an infant leaves, an infant is likely to cry to show how enjoyable is this type of interaction. Infants at this age recognize their primary caregiver and prefer that person's presence to others. By 5 months, infants may show displeasure when an object is taken away from them. This is a step beyond showing displeasure when a person leaves.

By 6 months, infants are increasingly aware of the difference between people who regularly care for them and strangers. They may begin to draw back from unfamiliar people. Seven-month-old infants begin to show obvious fear of strangers. They may cry when taken from their parent, attempt to cling to the parent, and reach out to be taken back. Parents may view this as a bad trait or a regression in socialization. Help them appreciate it is actually a big step forward, because it shows their infant can differentiate between persons and recognizes the difference between persons to trust and others.

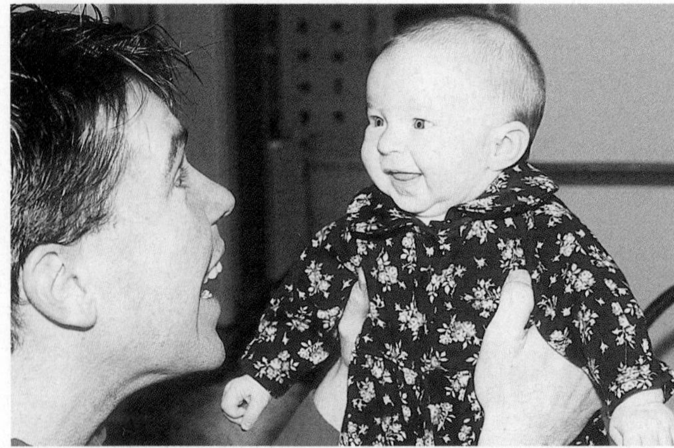

FIGURE 29.13 A 3-month-old smiles delightedly at her father's happy face. This indicates increased social awareness.

Fear of strangers reaches its height during the eighth month, so much so this phenomenon is often termed **eighth-month anxiety**, or stranger anxiety (Goldson & Reynolds, 2008). An infant at the height of this phase will not go willingly from a parent's arms to a nurse's. Taking a few minutes to talk to the child and parent first is time well spent.

Nine-month-old infants are very aware of changes in tone of voice. They will cry when scolded, not because they understand what is being said but because they sense their parent's displeasure.

By 12 months, most children have overcome their fear of strangers and are alert and responsive again when approached. They like to play interactive nursery rhymes and rhythm games and "dance" with others. They like being at the table for meals and joining in family activities.

Cognitive Development

In the first month of life, an infant mainly uses simple reflex activity. There is little evidence that infants at this age see themselves as separate from their environment. However, this does not mean they cannot respond actively or interact with people. They tend to enjoy people and faces more than they do objects.

Primary Circular Reaction

By the third month of life, a child enters a cognitive stage identified by Piaget (1966) as *primary circular reaction.* During this time, an infant explores objects by grasping them with the hands or by mouthing them (Fig. 29.14). Infants appear to be unaware of what actions they can cause or what actions occur independently. For example, if an infant's hand should accidentally strike a mobile across the crib, an infant appears to enjoy watching the brightly colored birds move in front of him, but makes no attempt to

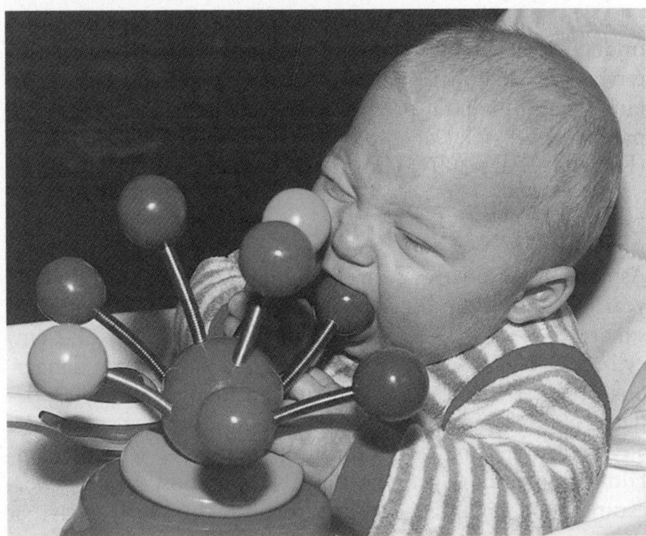

FIGURE 29.14 Infants explore the world by mouthing objects or fingering them. This also helps them separate self from environment.

hit the mobile again because he does not realize his hand caused the movement.

Secondary Circular Reaction

At about 6 months of age (cognitive development has wide variation), infants pass into a stage Piaget (1966) called *secondary circular reaction.* During this time, infants can grasp the idea their actions can initiate pleasurable sensations. Now when infants reach for a mobile above the crib, hit it, and watch it move, they realize it was their hand that initiated the motion, and so hit it again.

Infants are still unaware of the permanence of objects by the end of this stage. For example, if an object is hidden from vision (a baby drops it from her hand or it is hidden by a blanket), an infant will not search for it: gone is gone. If any part of the object is exposed, the infant can visualize the whole object and will reach to obtain it.

Coordination of Secondary Schema

Infants of 10 months discover **object permanence**, or become aware an object out of sight still exists. Infants are ready for peek-a-boo once they have gained the concept of permanence. They know their parent still exists even when hiding behind a hand or blanket and wait excitedly for the parent to reappear. If a baby drops a piece of breakfast cereal or a spoon from a highchair tray, although it is out of sight, an infant knows it still exists and will reach for it. Piaget (1966) called this stage of cognitive development *coordination of secondary schema.*

As infants reach 1 year of age, they are capable of reproducing interesting events (they deliberately hit a mobile once; it moves; they hit it again) and producing new events. They drop objects from a highchair or playpen and watch where they fall or roll. This is a frustrating activity for caregivers because it involves a great deal of reaching and picking up. It is an important activity for infants, however, because it confirms their awareness of the permanence of objects and how they are able to control events in their world.

✓ Checkpoint Question 29.3

Which action would show that an infant has developed object permanence?

a. He looks for a Cheerio that falls off his highchair tray.
b. He cries when he is either hungry or lonely.
c. He prefers a large yellow ball to a small red one.
d. He smiles when the mobile on his crib jingles.

HEALTH PROMOTION OF AN INFANT AND FAMILY

The nursing role with infants is wide-ranging because infants are so dependent on their caregivers for safety, learning, and emotional development.

Promoting Achievement of Developmental Task: Trust Versus Mistrust

Erikson (1993) proposed that the developmental task of the infant period is to form a sense of trust. When an infant is hungry, a parent feeds and makes the infant comfortable again. When an infant is wet, a parent changes a diaper and the infant is dry again. When an infant is cold, a parent holds the baby closely. By this process, infants learn to trust that when they have a need or are in distress, a person will come and meet that need.

A synonym for trust in this connotation is love. By the way infants are handled, fed, talked to, and held, they learn to love and recognize they are loved. Infants who have numerous caregivers, who may be fed one day on a rigid schedule and the next only when they are hungry, who sometimes are treated roughly and sometimes gently, can have difficulty learning to trust. If infants cannot trust, they cannot enjoy deeply satisfying interactions with others and can have difficulty trusting themselves or experiencing high self-esteem. They may have difficulty establishing close relationships as adults.

It is important for infants to establish the ability to love, or trust, early in life this way because development is sequential. If a first developmental step is inadequate, this inadequacy can pervade all future steps. In reference to trust, the end result could be an adult unable to instill a sense of trust in a child, perpetuating the inadequacy from generation to generation.

How do parents (or a nurse) encourage a sense of trust in an infant? Trust arises primarily from a sense of confidence that one can predict what is coming next. This does not mean parents should set up a rigid schedule of care for a child. It does imply establishing some schedule—for example, breakfast, bath, playtime, nap, lunch, walk outside, quiet playtime, dinner, story, and bedtime. This gentle rhythm of care gives infants a sense of being able to predict what is going to happen and gives life some consistency. Infants thrive on routine such as the same story read over and over again at bedtime, or the same spoon every day for lunch. Infancy is not too early for children to learn family traditions such as decorating for a holiday that will help them feel secure in the world as they grow. Some parents have difficulty accepting routine as important to a child. They may be so

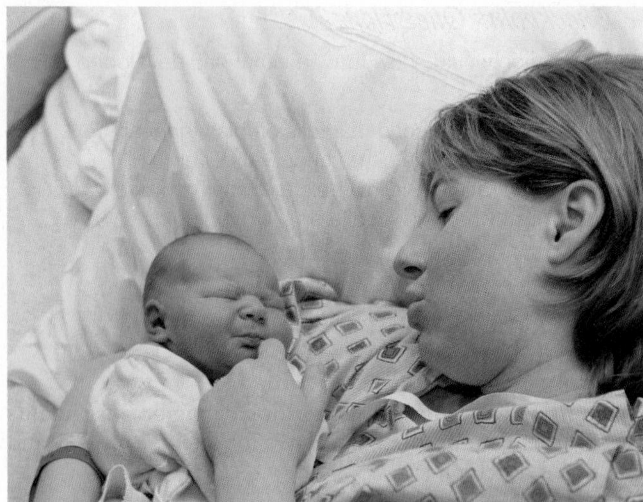

FIGURE 29.15 An infant's sense of trust develops through warm interpersonal relationships. Here a mother and baby share a "together" moment.

tired of their own work treadmill they want to raise their children as free spirits. Do not discourage this philosophy; however, you might suggest a few modifications to instill some order into infants' lives.

As important to an infant as the rhythm of care is that the care be given largely by one person (Fig. 29.15). This person can be the mother, father, grandparent, a conscientious babysitter, a foster parent, or anyone who can give consistent care. For infants ill at birth who are hospitalized for months, this person is often a primary nurse or case manager. You may have to encourage parents not to feel self-conscious talking to a baby who does not talk back. Pointing out the importance of such interactions and role-modeling them while caring for children help parents use this type of stimulation as they care for their baby's physical needs.

Women who work outside their home during the first year of a baby's life (at least 90% of women today) should try to arrange for one person to care for their child while they are away from home or choose a day care center that will provide a consistent caregiver. Urge them to discuss their methods of child care with alternative caregivers to prevent disrupting an infant's routine. When a child is admitted to a hospital, document and use this information.

Parents should make sure the caretaker they choose will actively interact with their child to provide a sense of trust. Passively caring for infants—not talking to them or touching or stroking them while feeding or changing them—amounts to not being with them. An increasing number of parents are installing video cameras to make sure a caretaker is actively interacting with their baby to instill a sense of trust in their child. Nursing actions designed to help an ill infant develop a sense of trust are detailed in Table 29.3.

Promoting Infant Safety

Accidents are a leading cause of death in children from 1 month through 24 years of age. They are second only to acute infections as a cause of acute morbidity and physician visits (National Vital Statistics System [NVSS], 2009).

Most accidents in infancy occur because parents either underestimate or overestimate a child's ability. Nursing interventions that help parents become sensitive to their infant's developmental progress not only help establish sound parent–child relationships but also guard infant safety (Forsythe et al., 2007) (Box 29.4).

Aspiration Prevention

Aspiration is a potential threat to infants throughout the first year. Round, cylindrical objects are more dangerous than square or flexible objects in this regard. A 1-inch (3.2-cm) cylinder, such as a carrot or hot dog, is particularly dangerous because it can totally obstruct an infant's airway. A deflated balloon can be sucked into the mouth, obstructing the airway in the same way. Educate parents who feed their infant formula not to prop bottles. By doing this, they are overestimating their infant's ability to push the bottle away, sit up, turn the head to the side, cough, and clear the airway if milk should flow too rapidly into the mouth and an infant begins to aspirate.

Other instances of aspiration occur because parents underestimate their infant's ability to grasp and place objects in their mouth. Even a newborn can wiggle to a new position to reach an attractive object such as a teddy bear with small button eyes. Newborns' grasp and sucking reflexes automatically cause them to grasp and pull the object into their mouth. Caution parents to be certain nothing comes within an infant's reach that would not be safe to put into the mouth. Using clothing without decorative buttons, and checking toys and rattles to ensure they have no small parts that could snap off or fall out, are good steps for parents to follow. A test of whether a toy could be dangerous if an infant puts it inside the mouth is whether it fits inside a toilet paper roll. If it does, it is small enough to be aspirated. When solid foods are introduced, encourage parents to offer small pieces of hot dogs or grapes, not large chunks for this reason. Children under about 5 years should not be offered popcorn or peanuts because of this danger of aspiration.

As infants become more adept at handling toys, parents need to reassess toys for loose pieces or parts. If parents are going to offer an infant a pacifier, they should use one that has a one-piece construction with a flange large enough to keep it from completely entering the child's mouth (Fig. 29.16).

Fall Prevention

Falls are a second major cause of infant accidents. As a preventive measure, no infant, beginning with a newborn, should be left unattended on a raised surface. Normal wiggling can bring a baby to the edge of a bed, couch, or table top, resulting in a fall.

Teach parents to be prepared for their infant to roll over by 2 months of age. From that time on, they must be especially vigilant not to leave the baby unattended on a changing table or counter. If the child sleeps in a crib, the mattress should be lowered to its bottom position so the height of the side rails increases; rails should be 2⅜ inches apart, narrow enough so children cannot put their head between them. Two months is about the maximum length of time infants can safely sleep in a bassinet; they need the protection of a crib and high siderails before they turn over.

TABLE 29.3 ✻ Ways for Nurses to Help an Ill Infant Develop a Sense of Trust

Area of Care	Nursing Actions
Nutrition	Encourage mothers to breastfeed if possible; provide privacy and support as necessary. Hold the infant no matter what feeding method is used (gavage, total parenteral, oral, enteral). If this is not possible, hold infants for a time after or between feedings so they receive holding equal to what they would ordinarily receive. If infant feeding is not oral, provide a pacifier (medical condition considered) five or six times daily for sucking pleasure. Hold and comfort after an episode of vomiting, even if not noticeably disturbing to an infant.
Dressing change	Use nonallergenic tape to avoid irritation while applied and pain when removed. Use a minimum of tape so the least amount has to be pulled free from sensitive skin (consider using stockinette, rolled gauze, or Kling gauze to hold a bandage in place rather than tape). To prevent chilling, be certain irrigation solutions are warm. Minimize exposure of the child during dressing changes to conserve warmth. Restrain only those body parts necessary for security. Talk to the infant. Hearing an explanation of what you are doing is comforting, not for the meaning of the words but for the nonthreatening tone of your voice.
Medicine administration	Flavor oral medicine to disguise disagreeable taste (being careful not to increase the amount to beyond what the child will take readily). Offer a drink of flavorful fluid afterward to counter medicinal taste. Never administer medicine in an infant's formula to prevent changing the formula's taste. Comfort the infant after injections or intravenous insertion by holding and rocking, or give immediately to a parent for this. Check intravenous sites frequently (every 30 min) for swelling to prevent infiltration and pain. Hold and play with infants despite tubing and restraints.
Rest	Encourage parents to sit and hold infants; infants sleep in a parent's arms as soundly as they do in bed. Rock infants to sleep if this is comforting. If contagion is not a problem, bring cribs to the nursing desk where infants can see you until they fall asleep. Always wake infants gently, because it is frightening (for anyone) to be awakened by a stranger. If bed rest is necessary, check for irritated elbows, heels, and knees from the infant's skin rubbing against sheets; protect with long sleeves or pants.
Hygiene	Check the temperature of bath water for comfort and to prevent chilling. Change diapers frequently to reduce discomfort from irritation. To avoid caries and prevent pain, begin tooth-brushing with first tooth.
Pain	Hold and comfort an infant in pain. Do not ask parents to hold a child during a painful procedure; it is difficult for them to see their child in pain. Allow them to comfort the child afterward. Reduce painful procedures to a minimum; combine blood drawing so only one puncture is necessary for many tests, etc.
Stimulation	Talk to infants while you care for them so they come to know you. Remember that infants focus longest on a human face. Provide a crib mirror or a mobile, because visual stimulation is satisfying to an infant. If no mobile is available, create one from a wire coat hanger, string, or strips of adhesive tape and objects that will suspend easily and are light enough to move from motion of the crib or an air current (colored paper, cotton balls, colored tongue blades). For safety, hang the mobile high enough for the infant to see but not reach. During the second half of the first year, remember that infants need to try to crawl. Put a pad or sheet on the floor and encourage infants to come to you or to explore on their own while you stand by to offer reassurance (this is almost impossible to accomplish in a crib).

All of these safety precautions apply to the hospital environment as well as to the home. Be sure crib sides are raised and secure before anyone walks away from the crib, even for just a moment. Also ensure that the space between the mattress and headboard is small enough an infant's head could not become trapped. Make sure cords from nursing call bells or safety pins are out of an infant's reach.

Car Safety

Teaching car safety for infants (as well as for the whole family) is a vital preventive health measure. The use of car seats for newborns is discussed in Chapter 18. Car seats should continue to be used without interruption through the preschool age, or until the child reaches 40 to 60 lb. If parents are firm about keeping infants in car seats even when they get fussy or impatient, children will eventually become more comfortable in seats than outside them. Infants up to 20 lb and 1 year old should be placed in rear-facing seats in the back seat because an inflating front-seat airbag could suffocate an infant (AAP, 2009).

Safety with Siblings

As infants become more fun to play with at about 3 months, older brothers and sisters grow more interested in interacting

BOX 29.4 ✻ Focus on Family Teaching

Accident Prevention Measures for Infants

Q. Bryan's mother is worried about keeping him safe. She asks, "How can I prevent accidents at this age?"

A. Here are some tips to help prevent specific types of accidents:

Potential Accident	Prevention Measures
General	Know the whereabouts of infants at all times. Be aware that the frequency of accidents is increased when parents are under stress. Take special precautions at these times. Choose babysitters carefully and explain and enforce all precautions when sitters are in charge.
Aspiration	Be certain any object that an infant can grasp and bring to the mouth is either safe to eat or too big to fit in the mouth. Do not feed an infant foods such as popcorn or peanuts, because these are easily aspirated. Store baby products such as powder out of infant's reach; powder is high risk for aspiration. Inspect toys and pacifiers for small parts that could be aspirated if broken off; do not make homemade pacifiers.
Falls	Never leave an infant on an unprotected surface, such as a bed or couch, even if the child is in an infant seat. Place a gate at the top and bottom of stairways; do not allow an infant to walk with a sharp object in the hands or mouth (it could pierce the throat in a fall). Raise crib rails and make sure they are locked before walking away from crib. Do not leave a child unattended in a highchair; avoid using an infant walker.
Motor vehicle	Never transport unless an infant is buckled into an infant car seat in the back seat of the car. Be aware of the proper technique for placing an infant in a car seat. Do not be distracted by an infant while driving. Do not leave an infant unattended in a parked car (can become dehydrated from excess heat, move gear shift, or be abducted).
Suffocation	Allow no plastic bags within infant's reach. Do not use pillows in a crib. Store unused appliances such as refrigerators or stoves with the doors removed. Buy a crib that is approved for safety (spacing of rails is not over 2⅜ in [6 cm] apart). Remove constricting clothing such as a bib from neck at bedtime.
Drowning	Do not leave infants alone in a bathtub or unsupervised near water (even buckets of cleaning water).
Animal bites	Do not allow an infant to approach a strange dog; supervise play with family pets.
Poisoning	Never present medication as a candy. Buy medications in containers with safety caps; put away immediately after use. Never take medication in front of infants. Place all medication and poisons in locked cabinets or overhead shelves. Never leave medication in a pocket or handbag. Use no lead-based paint in any area of the home. Hang plants or set on high surfaces. Post telephone number of the poison control center by the telephone.
Burns	Test warmth of formula and food before feeding (use extra precaution with microwave warming). Do not smoke or drink hot liquids while holding or caring for infant. Buy flame-retardant clothing for infants. Use a sunscreen on a child over 6 months when out in direct or indirect sunlight; limit the child's sun exposure to less than 30 min at a time. Turn handles of pans toward back of stove. Use a cool-mist, not a hot-mist, vaporizer; remain in room to monitor so child cannot reach vaporizer. Keep a screen in front of a fireplace or heater. Monitor infants carefully near candles. Do not leave infants unsupervised near hot-water faucets. Do not allow infants to blow out matches (don't teach children that fire is fun). Keep electric wires and cords out of reach; cover electrical outlets with safety plugs.

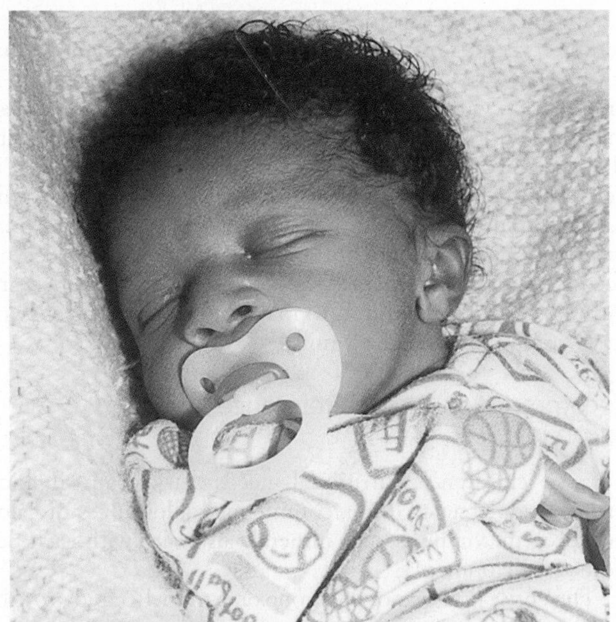

FIGURE 29.16 Many infants enjoy sucking on a pacifier to help them fall asleep. This may also help prevent sudden infant death syndrome.

with them. You may need to remind parents that children under 5 years of age, as a group, are not responsible enough or knowledgeable enough about infants to be left unattended with them. They might introduce an unsafe toy or engage in play that is too rough for an infant. Some preschoolers may be so jealous of a new baby they will physically harm an infant if left alone.

Bathing and Swimming Safety

As babies begin to develop good back support, many parents begin to bathe them in an adult tub. Caution parents never to leave an infant unattended in a tub, even when propped up out of the water or sitting in a bath ring or bath seat. Normal wiggling can easily cause a baby to slip down under the water. This applies to a hospital setting as well.

Many communities offer infant swim programs for babies as young as 6 months. If their child is enrolled in one of these programs, parents may become overconfident about their infant's ability to operate safely in water. Because children can dog-paddle momentarily in a swimming pool does not mean they can sustain that position for any length of time in a bathtub or pool. Being able to swim momentarily may also cause children to lose their instinctive fear of water and so be in more danger when around water than children who are still naturally more cautious. Such programs may also cause hypothermia and spread microorganisms because infants this age are not yet toilet-trained. Exposure to chlorinated water can damage lung epithelium that may be a precursor to childhood asthma (Bernard et al., 2007).

Childproofing

When infants begin teething at 5 to 6 months, they chew on any object within reach to lessen gum-line pain. Remind parents to check for possible sources of lead paint, such as painted cribs, playpen rails, or windowsills (Keefe, 2007). Paints safe for baby furniture should be marked "Safe for use on surfaces that might be chewed by children." If an infant is going to be allowed to play on the floor, parents should move furniture in front of electrical fixtures or buy protective caps for outlets. Infants are especially fascinated by the holes and will probe them with (often wet) fingers. Parents may need to install safety gates at the top and bottom of stairways as other safety measures.

Urge parents to move all potentially poisonous substances from bottom cupboards and store them well out of their infant's reach. Infants of any age should not be left unattended in carriages, highchairs, grocery shopping carts, or strollers. Baby walkers are extremely dangerous because infants can maneuver them near stairways and fall the length of the stairs.

When infants begin creeping, remind parents to recheck bottom cupboards and stairways for safety. When the child begins to walk, higher areas, such as coffee tables, need to be cleared of dangerous items. In a hospital setting, assess low counter areas for dangerous objects. Do not leave possibly dangerous supplies in an infant's room.

By 10 months, achievement of a pincer grasp makes infants able to pick up very small objects. Remind parents to check play areas or areas such as table tops for pins or other sharp objects that could be swallowed. Some of an infant's toys are now also 10 months old and need to be checked to be certain they are still intact and safe.

Children who can walk may venture into the street or a swimming pool if not carefully supervised (Fig. 29.17). Although they seem very independent and able to take care of themselves, their judgment about what is dangerous is immature. In a hospital setting, a 12-month-old child can

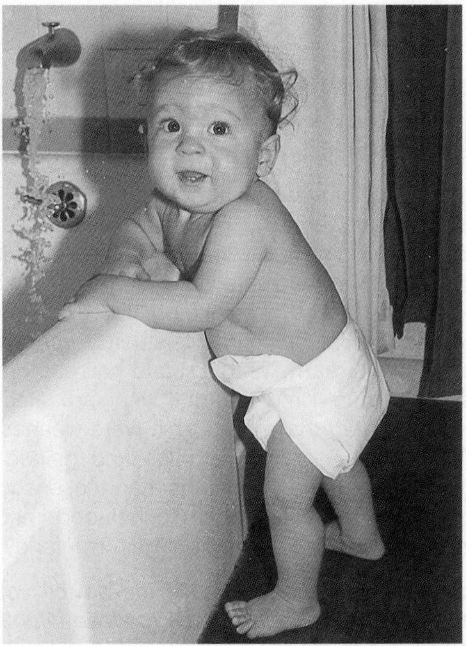

FIGURE 29.17 Once walking begins, the extended range of activities brings an infant in contact with potentially dangerous places or objects unless the house is childproofed. The bathroom is an important place to begin.

wander onto an elevator, out of the hospital, or into a laboratory area, or fall down a flight of stairs if not supervised (Forsythe et al., 2007).

✔ Checkpoint Question 29.4

You review infant safety with Bryan's mother. What are two of the most common types of accidents in infants?

a. Drowning and homicide.
b. Poisoning and burns.
c. Falls and auto accidents.
d. Aspiration and falls.

Promoting Nutritional Health of an Infant

The first choice for feeding an infant during the first 12 months of life is breast milk (see Chapter 19). All the necessary nutrients, vitamins, minerals, and water are provided by human milk for the first 6 months of life, with exception of vitamin K (1 mg intramuscularly is administered at birth); vitamin D (200 IU of oral vitamin D drops is administered daily beginning during the first 2 months of life if there is limited sunlight exposure); vitamin B_{12} if the mother is a strict vegetarian and takes no B_{12} supplement; and fluoride, but only if this is not included in the water supply (Thilo & Rosenberg, 2008). If a woman was iron deficient during pregnancy or has a low iron intake, supplemental iron may be indicated. How long mothers continue to breastfeed is an individual choice, although it is recommended through the entire first year (American College of Obstetricians and Gynecologists [ACOG], 2007). Early weaning from breastfeeding can lead to an increased incidence of obesity (Box 29.5). Prolonged breastfeeding into the preschool period can limit nutrients and might impair a child's growth.

BOX 29.5 ✻ Focus on Evidence-Based Practice

Does the timing of weaning affect infant weight?

Interested in answering this question, researchers assessed the feeding practices of 1-year-old infants through semistructured interviews with their mothers. They also had weights taken at birth, 8 weeks, 7 months, and 14 months. Half of the infants studied were weaned before 4 months (early weaning) and half of them were weaned later than 4 months (late weaning). Results of the study revealed that infants who were weaned early were heavier at 7 and 14 months and gained more weight between 8 and 14 months than those who were weaned later. The researchers concluded that early weaning is related to rapid weight gain in infancy.

Would the above study influence the advice you give parents on when is the ideal time to wean infants from breast or bottle to a cup?

Source: Sloan, S., et al. Early weaning is related to weight and rate of weight gain in infancy. *Child: Care, Health and Development, 34*(1), 59–64.

For infants whose mothers choose not to breastfeed, a commercial iron-fortified formula will supply adequate nutrition (Lawson, 2007) (see Appendix B). Supplementation is unnecessary with iron-fortified commercial formula unless the water supply does not contain fluoride. Infants who are changed to cow's milk before 1 year of age (a practice that is not recommended because the protein in cow's milk is difficult for an infant to digest, possibly leading to such intestinal irritation that slight but continuous gastrointestinal bleeding occurs, resulting in anemia) should receive a supplementary form of vitamin C and iron to make up for the deficiency of these components in cow's milk.

Recommended Dietary Reference Intakes for an Infant

Because children's nutritional needs vary from infancy through adolescence, the recommended allowances of calories, protein, vitamins, and minerals also vary with each period of development.

The entire first year of life is one of extremely rapid growth, so a high-protein, high-calorie intake is necessary. Both commercial formulas and breast milk contain 20 calories/oz. Calorie allowances can be gradually reduced during the first year from a level of 120 per kilogram of body weight at birth to approximately 100 per kilogram of body weight at the end of the first year to prevent babies from becoming overweight.

Although heredity plays a role, a baby who is overweight during the first year of life is more likely to become an obese adult than one whose weight is within normal limits as, once formed, fat cells (adipocytes) remain for life. Breastfed infants gain less weight than those who are formula fed. Delaying the introduction of solid food until 4 to 6 months and avoiding sweet drinks for infants can help avoid obesity in formula fed infants (Thilo & Rosenberg, 2008).

Introduction of Solid Food

From a nutritional standpoint, a normal full-term infant can thrive on breast milk or a commercial iron-fortified formula without the addition of any solid food until 4 to 6 months (Gomella & Haist, 2007). Delaying solid food until this time helps prevent overwhelming an infant's kidneys with a heavy solute load that can occur when protein is ingested. Although difficult to document, it also may delay the development of food allergies in susceptible infants and be another way to help prevent future obesity (Sass, 2007).

Most parents are eager to begin feeding their infant solid food, hoping this will help their child sleep through the night. Some parents do begin solid food before 6 months without apparent ill effects, possibly because much of the food is not processed by the gastrointestinal tract, passing through undigested because of the immaturity of the digestive system and decreased amylase and lipase secretion.

Generally speaking, infants are physiologically ready for solid food when they are nursing vigorously every 3 to 4 hours and do not seem satisfied or taking more than 32 oz (960 mL) of formula a day and do not seem satisfied. Infants are not ready to digest complex starches until amylase is present in saliva at approximately 2 to 3 months. Biting movements begin at approximately 3 months. Chewing movements do not begin until 7 to 9 months. Therefore, foods that require chewing should not be given until this age (Box 29.6).

BOX 29.6 ✻ Focus on Family Teaching

Tips to Help Introduce Solid Foods to Infants

Q. Bryan's mother has already started feeding him solid food. She asks, "When and how should I have begun solid foods?"

A. Infants typically are ready for solid food at 4 to 6 months of age. Use these guidelines to help when you start feeding your infant solid foods:

- Introduce one food at a time, waiting 5 to 7 days between new items.
- Introduce the food before formula or breastfeeding when an infant is hungry.
- Introduce small amounts of a new food (1 or 2 tsp) at a time.
- Respect infant food preferences; a child cannot be expected to like all new tastes equally well.
- Use only minimal to no salt and sugar on solid foods to minimize the number of additives.
- Remember that the extrusion reflex is present for the first 4 to 6 months of life, so any food placed on an infant's tongue will be pushed forward.
- To prevent aspiration, *do not* place food in bottles with formula.
- Introduce foods with a positive, "You'll like this" attitude.

Loss of Extrusion Reflex

When anything is placed on the anterior third of a newborn's tongue, it is automatically extruded or thrust out of the mouth by the tongue (extrusion reflex; Fig. 29.18). This is a life-saving reflex because it prevents infants from swallowing or aspirating foreign objects that touch the mouth. Infants extrude food when a spoonful of it is placed on the tongue in the same way. The reflex fades at 3 to 4 months. Until this time, it may be difficult to get an infant to eat solid food.

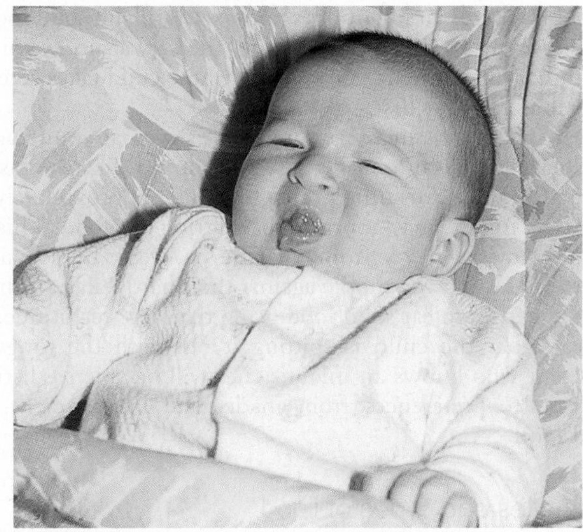

FIGURE 29.18 A 3-month-old baby demonstrates an extrusion reflex. Caution parents not to interpret this action as a food dislike but recognize it as the reflex action that it is.

Techniques for Feeding Solid Food

Table 29.4 shows the usual times and patterns for introducing solid food. Teach parents to offer new foods one at a time and allow a child to eat that item for about 1 week before introducing another new food. This system helps parents to detect possible food allergy. For example, if they start egg yolk on Monday and by Tuesday evening the child is breathing noisily or has a rash, they could suspect the child is allergic to eggs. If two new foods had been started on Monday, it would be hard to know which one was suspect. Introducing foods one at a time also helps to establish a sense of trust in infants, because it minimizes the number of new experiences in any one day.

It is best for the first solid food feeding if an infant is held in the parent's arms as if for bottle-feeding or breastfeeding. This reduces the newness of the experience and minimizes the amount of stress associated with it. Some infants accept new experiences of this type readily, whereas other infants

TABLE 29.4 ✻ Suggested Schedule for Introduction of Solid Foods

Age (mo)	Food to Introduce*	Rationale
5–6	Iron-fortified infant cereal mixed with breast milk, orange juice, or formula	Aids in preventing iron-deficiency anemia; the least allergenic type of food; an easily digested food
7	Vegetables	Good source of vitamin A; adds new texture and flavors to diet
8	Fruit	Best source of vitamin C, good source of vitamin A; adds new texture and flavors to diet
9	Meat	Good source of protein, iron, and B vitamins
10	Egg yolk	Good source of iron

*Wheat, tomatoes, oranges, fish, and egg whites should be omitted if there are allergies in the family, because these foods are most likely to cause allergies.

resist heartily. If an infant does not take readily to solid food, advise parents to wait a few days and then try again. Remind them that this is not a contest to see whose child takes cereal, vegetables, or fruit first.

Babies have distinct taste preferences even at young ages and may spit out a food because they do not like the taste. Even after the extrusion reflex has faded (at approximately 4 months), infants may appear to be spitting out food. This is because infants drink from a bottle or breast by pressing their tongue and the nipple against their hard palate. When an infant tries to eat solid food using the same technique, it appears that the child is spitting it out with the tongue. A parent who knows an infant's cues will be able to distinguish taste preferences from inadequate management of solid food.

Quantities and Types of Food

Infants take different quantities of food according to their preferences and needs. A newborn's stomach can hold approximately 2 tablespoons (30 mL). By 1 year, a stomach can hold no more than about 1 cup (240 mL). For this reason, when they begin eating solid food, infants rarely take more than 2 tablespoons (30 mL) at a time.

Cereal. The first food generally given to infants is infant cereal fortified with B vitamins and iron. These are precooked, fine dry powders to which expressed breast milk or infant formula is added. Initially, cereal should be mixed with enough fluid to make the mixture fairly liquid. As an infant adjusts to eating food from a spoon, parents can gradually thicken it. Adding sugar to cereal is unnecessary. Extra sugar in the diet can lead to diarrhea in young infants and beginning caries in older infants.

Fortified cereal costs no more than unfortified cereal, so remind parents to buy the fortified product. The first cereal introduced is usually rice cereal, because fewer children are allergic to rice products than to wheat and corn products. Usually, it is offered twice a day, morning and evening. Once the child has taken rice cereal for 1 week, parents can try another kind.

Some parents mix cereal with an infant's formula and give it to the child from a bottle. Caution parents to avoid this practice because (a) it is necessary to cut a larger hole in the bottle nipple for the cereal and milk mixture to flow freely, and there is a danger an infant may aspirate if the hole cut is too big; (b) there is a real danger of aspiration if the parent then uses that nipple for formula without cereal added; and (c) it denies the child the opportunity of learning to eat from a spoon and experiencing different food tastes and textures.

Infant cereal is so rich in iron parents should continue feeding it at least through the first year. Ideally, children should eat infant cereal until age 3 or 4 years, as few popularly advertised products can match the nutrients of fortified infant cereal.

Vegetables and Fruit. Because their iron content is generally higher than that of fruits, vegetables are usually the second food added to the diet (at 5–7 months of age). Parents who have a blender, strainer, or grinder can prepare their own. They simply cook a vegetable and then blend or strain it so it does not have to be chewed. Caution parents not to add butter or salt to the preparation, because infants have difficulty digesting fats until almost the end of the first year, and the added salt is unnecessary. Additional sugar is also unnecessary. By filling ice-cube trays with the blended vegetables, parents can make a 1-week supply and defrost a cube at a time. An ice cube is approximately 1 oz, or one-fourth the size of a jar of baby food.

If parents use commercial baby food, they should feed it from a dish rather than directly from the jar. This is because if the spoon carries salivary enzymes from an infant's mouth to the food, the enzymes will quickly liquefy what remains in the jar. Also, there is danger of transferring bacteria (principally streptococci) from an infant's mouth to the jar. Then, if the parent keeps the jar for another feeding in the next 24 hours, bacteria will multiply rapidly because the contents serve as a culture medium. Baby food jars should be refrigerated once they are opened, and manufacturers recommend they be used no longer than 48 hours after they were first opened.

When vegetables are added to the diet, they are usually offered at lunch. Remind parents to offer both green and yellow vegetables. Help them to remember that their own dislike of a particular vegetable does not mean their child will feel the same way about it. If they do convey distaste for a food, their child will pick up on the feeling and will not like the vegetable either.

Fruit is usually offered 1 month after beginning vegetables (at 6–8 months). It can be given in addition to cereal for breakfast and dinner. Raw mashed banana is easy to prepare with just a fork; peaches are easily prepared in a blender. As with vegetables, parents should offer a selection so an infant is exposed to different tastes and textures.

Meat and Eggs. Meat is usually introduced at 9 months. Parents can grind a portion of the meat they have prepared for their own meal so it is tender, or they can use commercially prepared products. If they use commercial baby meat, urge them to use the plain meat products, not vegetable and meat dinners, because these contain mostly vegetables. Chicken has the advantage of being low in cholesterol, but this is not a priority with infants. Beef and pork have more iron than chicken, so encourage parents to offer these more frequently than chicken. When meat is added to an infant's diet, it is usually added as part of the evening meal in place of cereal.

Egg yolks are offered by 10 months of age. Egg yolks contain the bulk of the iron content of eggs; the white contains the bulk of protein. Egg yolk alone should be given at first, because the protein of the egg white can lead to allergy or can be difficult for an infant to digest. Eggs may be prepared by hard-boiling (then adding a little formula or breast milk to the mashed yolk to make it more liquid) or purchased as commercial baby food. Soft-boiling or poaching is not usually recommended, because salmonella, the chief offending microorganism that may be in eggs, may not be killed by these methods. Also, thorough cooking makes protein easier to digest.

Table Food. With the introduction of solid food, encourage parents to establish a three-meal-a-day pattern, if that is the family's lifestyle, and to have the infant join the family at the table. Generally, encourage parents to use homemade foods rather than relying on commercially prepared junior foods, although commercial foods are now prepared without excessive additives and are convenient for parents who have little preparation time. Mashed potatoes or peas and cut-up meatloaf are examples of table foods that infants older than 6 months of age like to eat and busy parents can prepare quickly. If hot dogs are offered, caution parents to cut them into small bite-size portions; otherwise, they can be aspirated. As infants begin teething, they enjoy dried bread, teething biscuits, or zwieback.

Some infants are too distracted by the activity at a family table to eat well. Parents may find these children eat more if they are fed first and then allowed to have a small amount to "feed themselves" or a cracker to chew on while just sitting at the table and being with the family.

Remind parents that highchairs are one of the most dangerous pieces of baby equipment they own. Urge them always to fasten the restraint and never leave an infant unattended in a highchair, because even a 6-month-old can squirm out of a chair with little effort. Nurses must also keep this in mind when feeding infants in a hospital setting.

Establishment of Healthy Eating Patterns

Some parents may need to be reminded that although rules for infant feeding are designed to promote healthy nutrition, they should individualize their approach according to the cues their child is giving them for readiness.

A child who adapts to change poorly may have difficulty accepting the first solid food, for example, and may have difficulty with each new food. Parents may need support to remember a child is not conducting this struggle out of a desire for conflict but because this is a characteristic of temperament. Giving food to others is interpreted by many as giving love, so refusing food is equated with refusing love. Help parents understand this is not what is happening. Refusing a teaspoonful of carrots is refusing a teaspoonful of carrots, nothing more.

Most infants, however, eat hungrily so feeding problems tend to be reported more frequently as a second-year or toddler problem than as an infant concern. If an infant does refuse to eat, ask the parents what foods they are offering. Have them list exactly the types and amounts of foods the child ate the day before (a 24-hour dietary recall history). It may be apparent from this that enough is being eaten in a day's time and that the parents' expectations are unrealistic for the child's size and age.

If intake is inadequate and the child is, indeed, a fussy eater, ask about the parents' methods of feeding. For example, ask if they are offering a bottle first and then infant food. Infants generally accept the new experience of eating from a spoon better when they are hungry, not when their stomach is full. On the other hand, some babies, particularly those with an intense temperament, may be so hungry at mealtime they cannot tolerate the frustration of spoon-feeding until some of their hunger is relieved. They may need to drink 2 or 3 oz of formula or nurse at the breast for a few minutes before they will eat a spoonful of food.

An infant who is fatigued or overstimulated may not eat well. Providing a quiet environment away from older brothers or sisters before mealtime may solve this problem.

Encourage parents not to force infants to eat if they do not seem hungry. Healthy, happy infants will be hungry at mealtime and will eat. Those who refuse a meal may be tired, distracted, or perhaps ill. Forcing only leads to regurgitation or, if they are ill, vomiting. It also can result in feeding problems or a situation in which infants refuse to eat altogether. Infants who are eating and not thriving or not eating and therefore not thriving should be examined to determine if a cause such as a metabolic disorder or failure to thrive exists (see Chapters 48 and 55).

Weaning

Infants are capable of approximating their lips to a cup so they can drink effectively from one at about 9 months of age. The sucking reflex begins to diminish in intensity between ages 6 and 9 months, which makes this the time to consider weaning.

To wean from formula or breast milk, the mother chooses one feeding a day and then begins offering fluid by the new method at that feeding. She should choose a time of day that is not an infant's fussy period; other than that, the time is immaterial. After 3 days to 1 week, when an infant has become acclimated to the one change, the mother changes a second feeding. Should an illness such as an upper respiratory infection occur or should the child have teething discomfort, there will be setbacks, so no set number of weeks should be prescribed to complete weaning. Infants usually need more fluid during hot weather than cold weather because of increased perspiration. This may make it more difficult to begin weaning during the summer.

Self-Feeding

At approximately 6 months of age, infants become interested in handling a spoon and beginning to feed themselves. Their coordination, unfortunately, has not developed enough for them to use a spoon without a great deal of spilling, so they are much more adept at feeding themselves with their fingers (Fig. 29.19). Parents concerned with neatness can spread newspapers, a plastic tablecloth, or a towel on the floor around a highchair to catch most of the dropped food, and then let the child practice. When an infant becomes fatigued or frustrated at attempts of self-feeding, a parent can then quietly help without

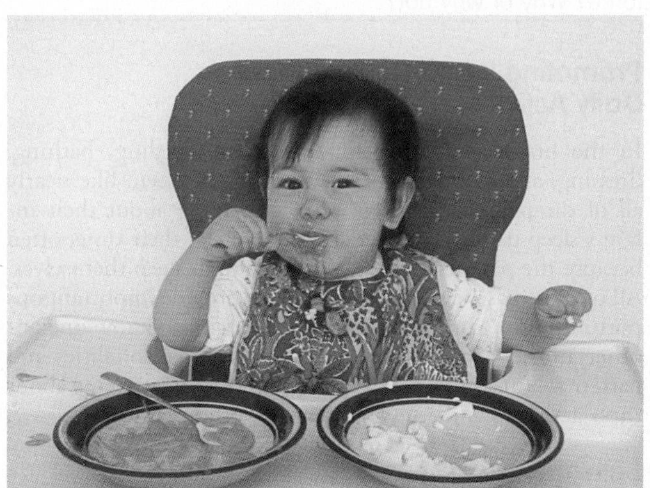

FIGURE 29.19 Self-feeding is not always a neat process for an infant.

making an issue of it. Parents who insist on continuing to spoon-feed past the time infants want to feed themselves can cause infants to balk at eating. Often, a compromise is helpful. If a parent gives the infant a spoon, the child can poke at a cereal dish with it while the parent continues to offer bites from a second spoon. In this way, a child is "in charge" of the feeding yet receptive to taking food from the parent.

When infants no longer attempt to feed themselves at a meal but merely begin to play with their food by squeezing it through their fingers or dabbing it in their hair, it is time to end the meal. This behavior indicates that they have had enough.

Adequate Intake With a Vegetarian Diet

An infant eating a vegetarian diet should continue to be breastfed or ingest an iron-fortified, balanced, commercial formula for the entire first year. If a milk allergy is present, a soy-based formula can be used. When solid foods are added at 6 months, an assortment of foods should be provided, including vegetables such as avocados, potatoes, and broccoli; fruits such as apples, prunes (high in iron), and bananas; infant cereal; tofu; wheat germ; legumes; brewer's yeast; and synthetic vitamin D. Feeding fortified cereal throughout the first year will ensure that iron stores are built. If the diet is to include dairy products, these can be added toward the end of the first year as usual (Conti, 2008).

Because vegetarian diets are high in fiber, infants who eat them may have more frequent and looser-than-normal bowel movements. Teach parents to change diapers frequently to avoid skin irritation. Using less fibrous, more concentrated forms of protein, such as tofu and powdered nuts rather than cereal mixtures, can minimize this problem.

A sound vegetarian diet can be easily designed for the older infant who prefers finger foods, because many vegetables, fruits, and grains such as pieces of oranges, peaches, tomatoes, and crackers and protein or Quom for protein are easily eaten this way (Theobald, 2007).

What if... Bryan's grandmother tells you she believes children should always finish everything on their plate, so as not to waste food? Is always cleaning a plate a good or bad habit for parents to enforce? Why or why not?

Promoting Infant Development in Daily Activities

In the first year, caring for an infant—feeding, bathing, dressing, and so forth—occupies what may seem like nearly all of the parents' waking hours. Worrying about their infant's sleep patterns may take up the rest of their time, often because the parents are not getting enough sleep themselves. All of these basic care-related activities provide important opportunities for caregivers and infants to get to know one another and to become used to each other's personalities and patterns. Nurses can play a key role in teaching parents about these activities and stressing their importance.

Bathing

Except in very hot weather, an infant does not need a bath every day. If a parent is tired and would not enjoy bath time or if some days are just too rushed, a complete bath can be omitted, with only an infant's face, hands, and diaper area washed. Some infants do need their head and scalp washed frequently (every day or every other day) to prevent **seborrhea,** a scaly scalp condition often called cradle cap (Smoker, 2007). If seborrhea lesions do develop, they adhere to the scalp in yellow, crusty patches. The skin beneath them may be slightly erythematous. The patches can be softened by oiling the scalp with mineral oil or petroleum jelly and leaving it on overnight. The crusts can then be removed by shampooing the hair the next morning. A soft toothbrush or fine-toothed comb can be used to help remove crusts.

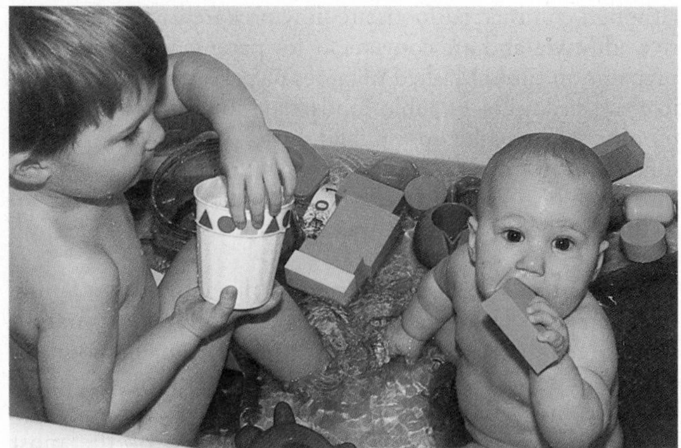

FIGURE 29.20 An 8-month-old enjoys bath time with his big brother. Parents should always watch carefully while infants and toddlers are in the tub.

Bath time should be fun for an infant and can serve many functions other than just the obvious one of cleanliness (Fig. 29.20). Especially during the second half of the first year, an infant enjoys poking at soap bubbles on the surface of the water or playing with bath toys. Bath time also helps an infant learn different textures and sensations and provides an opportunity to exercise and kick, as well as a good opportunity for a parent to touch and communicate with the child. Teach parents *not* to leave infants alone in tubs as they could easily slip under the water.

Diaper-Area Care

The most effective means of promoting good diaper-area hygiene is to change diapers frequently, about every 2 to 4 hours. However, it is rarely good practice to interrupt the child's sleep to change diapers. If an infant develops a rash from sleeping in wet diapers, air drying or sleeping without a diaper may be a solution.

At each diaper change, the parents should wash the skin with clear water or with a commercial alcohol-free diaper wipe (and perfume-free if an infant has sensitive skin), then pat or allow to air dry. Routinely using an ointment such as Desitin or A&D ointment to keep urine and feces away from an infant's skin is good prophylaxis. Parents do not need to use baby powder. If they choose to, advise them to sprinkle the powder on their hands first, and then apply it to an infant's skin. Caution them not to shake the powder on an infant, to reduce the possibility of aspiration. They should place the container out of the infant's reach afterward, or an infant could easily spill it into his mouth and aspirate it.

Care of Teeth

It is well accepted that exposing developing teeth to fluoride is one of the most effective ways to promote healthy tooth formation and prevent tooth decay. The most important time for children to receive fluoride is between 6 months and 12 years of age. A water level of 0.6 ppm fluoride is recommended because this is the level that protects tooth enamel yet does not lead to staining of teeth. In communities where the water supply does not provide enough fluoride, the use of an oral fluoride supplement beginning at 6 months or the use of fluoride toothpaste or rinses after tooth eruption is recommended (Armfield & Spencer, 2007).

Teach parents to ask about the presence of fluoride in the drinking water in their community and help them to determine what, if any, supplementation is necessary. Breastfed infants do not receive a great deal of fluoride from breast milk, so it may be recommended they be given fluoride drops once a day. Teach parents to begin "brushing" even before teeth erupt by rubbing a soft washcloth over the gum pads. This eliminates plaque and reduces the presence of bacteria, creating a clean environment for the arrival of the first teeth. Once teeth erupt, all surfaces should be brushed with a soft brush or washcloth once or twice a day. Children lack the coordination to brush effectively until they are school-age, so parents must be responsible for this activity well past infancy. Toothpaste is not necessary for an infant, because it is the scrubbing that removes the plaque.

The initial dental checkup should be made by 1 year of age; checkups should continue at 6-month intervals until adulthood.

Dressing

Clothing for infants should be easy to launder and simply constructed, so dressing and undressing are not a struggle. Infants enjoy kicking and making gross body movements, so their clothing should not be binding. When they begin to creep, they need long pants to protect their knees. Until they begin to walk, they need only soft-soled shoes or merely socks or booties to keep their feet warm. Even when they begin walking, the soles of their shoes need only be firm enough to protect their feet against rough surfaces. Extremely hard soles and high ankle sides are unnecessary.

Sleep

Sleep needs and habits vary greatly among infants, but most require 10 to 12 hours of sleep at night and one or several naps during the day. Parents are usually advised to let a baby sleep in a separate space rather than in their bed so the parents do not awaken at every toss and squeak. Doing so allows infants to learn to quiet themselves and go back to sleep should they awaken briefly. This may help prevent sleep problems such as night waking in the future. Other parents prefer to have infants sleep with them in a family bed, as they believe this practice promotes a feeling of security (Baddock et al., 2007). Bed sharing also promotes breastfeeding but also has the danger of accidental suffocation. Caution parents not to place pillows in an infant's bed to avoid suffocation. Always place infants on their back to sleep because this position markedly reduces the incidence of sudden infant death syndrome (SIDS). Use of a pacifier while an infant sleeps may further reduce this risk (Damato, 2007). See Chapter 26 for a further discussion of SIDS.

Exercise

Infants benefit from outings in a carriage or stroller because sunlight provides a natural source of vitamin D. In hot weather, caution parents to protect an infant from sunburn by exposing the child to the sun for only very short periods, beginning with 3 to 5 minutes the first day, a little more the next day, and so on up to 15 to 20 minutes at a time. The sun is most intense between 10 AM and 3 PM, so early mornings and late afternoons are the best times for infants to be outside. These short time spans are necessary because the use of sunscreen is not recommended in children until they are at least 6 months old (Lim, 2008).

Toward the end of the first year, infants need space to crawl and then to walk, such as in an enclosed outdoor play space. In addition to providing fresh air, going for leisurely walks while pointing out the sights of the world—trees, birds, dogs, houses, neighbors—helps children develop language.

Parents can judge how much outdoor clothing to put on an infant by how much they need themselves. If an adult needs a winter coat, an infant will need a snowsuit; sweaters may be adequate for both; if an adult needs no outer clothing, an infant probably does not either.

It is not necessary to enroll infants in formal exercise programs for them to secure adequate exercise. Such programs may put unusual strain on muscles and tendons. Infants using infant walkers must be closely supervised, because they can be injured if they maneuver the walker too near a stairway and fall.

Promoting Healthy Family Functioning

A primary task of parents during the infant year is to learn to interpret infants' cues to decipher their needs. It is helpful if they can learn early on to perceive an infant as a separate individual with unique needs. This becomes an easier task by 2 months, when infants can indicate by their particular cry whether they are feeling cold, hungry, wet, or lonely. Parents spend a great deal of time with their infant in these first months, which gives them the opportunity to learn and recognize nonverbal cues and to become aware of their baby's needs.

Parental Concerns and Problems Related to Normal Infant Development

Some of the difficulties parents are apt to have in evaluating the health of infants are shown in Table 29.5. New parents may need reassurance and answers to questions about child-care procedures or health during an infant period because they have not yet learned their child's cues. However, the need for reassurance may be just as great in experienced parents. The unique characteristics of each child require some adjustment from parents.

Teething

Most infants have little difficulty with teething, but some appear very distressed. Generally, the gums are sore and tender

TABLE 29.5 ✻ Common Difficulties Parents Experience in Evaluating the Health of Infants

Difficulty	Suggestions for Improving Assessment
Evaluating pain	Infants manifest pain by fussiness. They can reveal arm and leg pain by immobility of the body part; ear pain by brushing or tugging at the ear; stomach pain by pulling up the legs against the abdomen.
Evaluating degree of reduced activity	Lack of interest in smiling or interaction is an important observation. Increased sleeping or lying supine with legs nonflexed (frog-legged) as if exhausted is important.
Evaluating infant temperature	All parents should learn how to take an axillary or tympanic temperature so they can report a specific degree of fever rather than a subjective finding, such as "feels hot."
Evaluating amount of vomiting or diarrhea	Knowing the number of times vomiting and/or diarrhea has occurred is important. Estimating amount in comparisons with what the child has eaten is helpful as well as estimating an amount (a cupful, etc.). Knowing whether diapers are "soaked" or "stained" with stools is important in estimating amount. Caution parents that vomiting and diarrhea are always serious in infants.

before a new tooth breaks the surface. As soon as the tooth is through, the tenderness passes.

Because of this pain, infants can be resistant to chewing for a day or two and be slightly cranky, possibly because they are a little hungry from not eating as much as usual. High fever, seizures, vomiting or diarrhea, and earache are never normal signs of teething. An infant with any of these symptoms has an underlying infection or disease process requiring further evaluation.

Many over-the-counter medicines are sold for teething pain. As a rule, their use should be discouraged if they contain benzocaine, a topical anesthetic, because if applied too far back in the throat, this could interfere with the gag reflex. Acetaminophen (Tylenol), 10 to 15 mg/kg every 4 hours, up to four times a day, may be used for teething discomfort but parents should check with their infant's health care provider before giving any over-the-counter drug this way. Teething rings that can be placed in the refrigerator provide soothing coolness against the tender gums. An infant who is teething will place almost any object in the mouth, so parents must screen articles within the baby's reach to be certain they are edible or safe to chew.

Thumb-sucking

Sucking is a surprisingly strong need: prenatal ultrasounds even demonstrate fetal thumb-sucking in utero. Many infants begin to suck a thumb or finger at about 3 months of age and continue the habit through the first few years of life. The sucking reflex peaks at 6 to 9 months, whereas thumb-sucking peaks at about 18 months.

Parents can be assured that thumb-sucking is normal and does not deform the jaw line as long as it stops by school age. It does not cause "baby talk" or any of the other symptoms commonly attributed to it. The best approach is to be certain an infant has adequate sucking pleasure and then to ignore thumb-sucking. Making an issue of it rarely causes a child to stop; if anything, it usually intensifies and prolongs it.

Use of Pacifiers

Whether to use pacifiers is a question parents must settle for themselves, depending on how they feel about them and their infant's needs. Infants rarely have such a need for sucking they must have a pacifier in their mouth constantly. Discussing a few pros and cons with the parents clarifies the subject. Use of a pacifier at bedtime may reduce the risk of SIDS as, with a pacifier, a baby rouses periodically from sleep to suck and so does not continue for an extended time in deep phases of sleep.

An infant who completes a feeding and still seems restless and discontent, who actively searches for something to put into the mouth, or who sucks on hands and clothes may need a pacifier. Babies who have colic crave sucking and enjoy pacifiers because their abdomen hurts, and they interpret this as a hunger sensation. If a child is formula fed, parents should check nipples to be certain the holes are small and the rubber is sturdy, so that an infant can suck hard enough to derive pleasure. If the nipples are satisfactory, parents could offer a pacifier after feeding for more sucking. Freudian theory proposes that a child whose sucking needs are met in infancy will not crave as much oral stimulation later in life and is less likely to become a pencil chewer, cigarette smoker, or nail biter or develop pica, the eating of nonfood substances (Nurcombe, 2008).

A major drawback of pacifiers is the problem of cleanliness. If used at times other than bedtime, they tend to fall on the floor or sidewalk and are then put back into an infant's mouth. If not well constructed, they may come apart and be aspirated. Hanging a pacifier on a string around an infant's neck could cause strangulation.

Parents should attempt to wean a child from a pacifier any time after 3 months of age and certainly during the time the sucking reflex is fading at 6 to 9 months unless used at night for sleeping, as the AAP recommends using pacifiers at bedtime as a possible way to reduce the incidence of SIDS (Damato, 2007). Weaning after this age is difficult because a pacifier becomes a comfort mechanism, like a warm blanket or fuzzy toy to which a child may cling.

Head Banging

Some infants rhythmically bang their heads against the bars of a crib for a period of time before falling asleep. This is distressing behavior for parents. Besides fearing that children will hurt themselves, some parents may have heard that blind children or those with mental illness do this and worry that their child is ill in some way.

Head banging in this limited fashion—beginning during the second half of the first year of life and continuing through to the preschool period, associated with naptime or bedtime, and lasting under 15 minutes—can be considered normal. Children use this measure to relax and fall asleep. Investigating stress factors operating in the house may be helpful. If some of them can be relieved such as parents' overestimation of the child's development, marital discord, illness in another family member, the head banging may decrease, or it may have already become such a strong habit that it will persist for months or even years.

Advise parents to pad the rails of cribs so infants cannot hurt themselves, and reassure them this is a normal mechanism for relief of tension in children of this age. No therapy should be necessary. Excessive head banging done to the exclusion of normal development or activity, or head banging past the preschool period, suggests a pathologic basis, and such children then need a referral for counseling and further evaluation.

Sleep Problems

Sleep problems develop in early infancy because of colic or because an otherwise healthy infant takes longer than usual to adjust to sleeping through the night. Breastfed babies tend to wake more often than those who are formula fed because breast milk is more easily digested, so infants become hungry sooner. In late infancy, the problem of waking at night and remaining awake for an hour or more becomes common. Although an infant may be content and not cry during this time, parents are reluctant to sleep while the child is awake, so they may become extremely fatigued. This is an increasing concern because more and more families today consist of two wage-earning parents; there is no time for parents to nap during the day to make up for sleep lost at night. Suggestions for eliminating or at least coping with night waking are (a) delay bedtime by 1 hour; (b) shorten an afternoon sleep period; (c) do not respond immediately to infants at night so they can have time to fall back to sleep on their own; and (d) provide soft toys or music to allow infants to play quietly alone during this wakeful time. Reassuring parents that infants take varying lengths of time to adjust to night sleeping is helpful in assuring them their child is normal. Suggesting parents use the time they are awake at night to do such things as solve a problem at work, watch the late show, or plan a shopping list may help them view the situation as a constructive time rather than a problem.

Constipation

Breastfed infants are rarely constipated because their stools tend to be loose. Constipation may occur in formula-fed infants if their diet is deficient in fluid. This can be corrected simply with the addition of more fluid.

Some parents misinterpret the normal pushing movements of a newborn to be constipation. When infants defecate, their faces do turn red, and they grimace and grunt. As long as stools are not hard and contain no evidence of fresh blood (as might occur with a rectal fissure), this is normal infant behavior.

If constipation persists beyond 5 or 6 months of age, encourage parents to check with the infant's health care provider about measures to relieve this. Adding foods with bulk, such as fruits or vegetables, and increasing fluid intake generally relieves the problem. Apple juice (3 or 4 oz) or prune juice (0.5 to 1 oz daily) may be given as a temporary measure.

All infants with a history of constipation for more than 1 week should be examined for an anal fissure or tight anal sphincter. Softening stools and thereby relieving the pain of defecation often solves the problem and helps the fissure to heal. If an unusually tight anal sphincter exists, parents will be given instructions to manually dilate the sphincter two or three times daily until it dilates sufficiently. One of the first symptoms of Hirschsprung's disease (aganglionic megacolon, or lack of nerve innervation to a portion of the colon) is constipation. If no stool is present in the rectum of a constipated infant on rectal examination, this disease is suggested (Sondheimer, 2008). A careful history must then be taken to assess for other symptoms of Hirschsprung's disease: ribbon-like stools, bouts of diarrhea, and a distended abdomen (see Chapter 45).

Chronic constipation also may occur in children with congenital hypothyroidism (decreased functioning of the thyroid gland). Therefore, an infant with constipation also should be carefully observed for characteristic signs of hypothyroidism, such as lethargy, protruding tongue, and failure to meet developmental milestones (see Chapter 48). Infants with either Hirschsprung's disease or hypothyroidism need therapy to correct the disorder.

Loose Stools

Many new parents are unfamiliar with the consistency or color of normal newborn stools, so they mistakenly report normal stooling as diarrhea. Stools of breastfed infants are generally softer than those of formula-fed infants. If a mother takes a laxative while breastfeeding, an infant's stools may be very loose. An infant who is formula fed can have loose stools if the formula is not diluted properly.

Occasionally, loose stools may begin with the introduction of solid food, such as fruit. Malabsorption syndrome (celiac disease), or an inability to digest fat, may manifest themselves first by loose stools and a distended abdomen and deficiency of fat-soluble vitamins (see Chapter 45).

When talking to a parent about loose stools, ask about the duration of the loose stools, the number of stools per day, their color and consistency, and whether there is any mucus or blood in them. Is there associated fever, cramping, or vomiting? Does an infant continue to eat well? Appear well? Seem to be thriving? Is an infant wetting at least six diapers daily?

Infants with associated signs and symptoms such as fever, cramping, vomiting, loss of appetite, a decrease in voiding, and weight loss should be examined by their health care provider because this suggests an infectious process. Dehydration occurs rapidly in a small infant who is not eating and is losing body fluid through loose stools.

Colic

Colic is paroxysmal abdominal pain that generally occurs in infants under 3 months of age and is marked by loud, intense crying (Bolte, 2007). An infant cries loudly and pulls the legs up against the abdomen. The infant's face becomes red and flushed, the fists clench, and the abdomen becomes tense. If offered a bottle, the infant will suck vigorously for a few minutes as if starved, then stop as another wave of intestinal pain occurs.

The cause of colic is unclear. It may occur in susceptible infants from overfeeding or from swallowing too much air while drinking. Formula-fed babies are more likely to have colic than breastfed babies, possibly because they swallow more air while drinking or because formula is harder to digest.

Although infants continue to thrive despite colic, the condition should not be dismissed as unimportant. It is a distressing and frightening problem for parents not only because an infant appears to be in acute pain, but also the distress persists for hours, usually into the middle of the night, so no one in the family gets adequate rest. This is a difficult beginning to a parent–child relationship, which needs to be strong and binding for the parents to enjoy parenting and for an infant to thrive in their care (see Focus on Nursing Care Planning Box 29.7).

Take a thorough history of an infant with signs of colic because intestinal obstruction or infection may mimic an at-

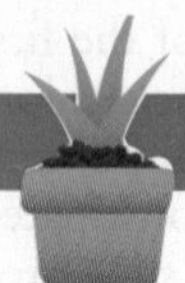

BOX 29.7 ✻ Focus on Nursing Care Planning

A Multidisciplinary Care Map for an Infant With Colic

You meet Ms. Simpson, 19, at a pediatric clinic when she brings in her 2-month-old son, Bryan. She looks tired. She tells you that she is exhausted because her baby is "awake all night, crying constantly." She stopped breastfeeding and changed him to formula to see if that would help. It didn't. She tells you his bowel movements are normal. When you weigh Bryan, you find he has gained weight well. When you talk to him, he demonstrates a social smile.

Family Assessment ✻ Infant lives with single parent and her family (grandfather, grandmother, 26-year-old uncle, and 22-year-old aunt). Grandmother cares for infant while mother works as an exotic dancer from 12 noon to 6 PM.

Client Assessment ✻ Well-proportioned 2-month-old boy. Height and weight at 50th percentile on growth chart. Bottle feeding with intake of approximately 4 oz of commercial formula every 4 hours. Experiencing 2 or 3 soft yellow bowel movements daily. The mother reports, "He's been crying every night lately from about 6 PM till 9 PM. His face gets red, and he pulls his legs up against his belly. I give him a bottle, he sucks for a few minutes like he's starving, and then stops, pulls up his legs, and starts to cry. He's good for my mother in the afternoon; cries from six to nine at night for me. I'm at the end of my rope." Physical examination within normal limits. Diagnosis of colic is made.

Nursing Diagnosis ✻ Compromised family coping related to difficulty managing infant crying episodes

Outcome Criteria ✻ Parent expresses increased confidence in caring for infant and increased feeling of control over situation within 1 week; infant sleeps for at least some of 6 PM to 9 PM period.

Team Member Responsible	Assessment	Intervention	Rationale	Expected Outcome
		Activities of Daily Living		
Nurse	Assess what infant's total day is like to try and identify why crying seems confined to evenings.	Make suggestions as needed to see that different caregivers use consistency in care.	Infants with several daily caretakers can have difficulty adjusting to changing feeding techniques.	Parent details a day history for infant.
		Consultations		
Nurse	Determine which nurse practitioner is available for consultation.	Contact nurse practitioner to do physical exam to ensure infant is healthy.	A physical exam will differentiate symptoms of colic from another more serious problem.	Nurse practitioner completes physical exam and makes recommendations.
		Procedures/Medications		
Nurse	Assess what steps parent has taken to try and relieve symptoms.	Suggest the use of a pacifier, sitting infant upright, feeding in quiet environment, riding in car, etc.	Sucking on a pacifier may increase peristalsis and promote passage of gas. An upright position may prevent distention.	Parent states she is willing to try new measures such as a pacifier.

		Nutrition		
Nurse	Assess how parent prepares formula; what technique she uses for bottle feeding and burping infant.	Review methods for formula preparation, bottle holding, and burping as needed; be certain other family members are consistent.	Proper techniques can minimize the amount of air swallowed and possible subsequent development of intestinal gas.	Parent describes formula preparation and infant feeding methods. Confirms other family members are consistent.
		Patient/Family Education		
Nurse	Assess what parent knows about colic, including its incidence, usual timing, symptoms, etc.	Educate parent about common characteristics of colic, including duration, timing, and intensity of crying.	Education promotes better understanding of the problem, alleviating some of the stress and anxiety associated with it.	Parent states she understands symptoms of colic and how common it is in newborns.
		Psychosocial/Spiritual/Emotional Needs		
Nurse/nurse practitioner	Assess what parent thinks is the cause of her infant crying so much in the evening.	Reassure parent she is not the cause of the child's discomfort. It's a coincidence she is giving care at the time colic occurs.	A parent can feel guilty if she is unable to soothe child. Reassurance the problem is not her fault can aid in objective problem solving.	Parent states she understands the problem is not a personal one.
Nurse	Assess parent's level of stress about constant crying.	Caution parent that crying in infants produces frustration in adults. Help parent plan respite time if possible to give relief.	Acknowledging their frustration helps to validate their feelings. A plan of action provides opportunities to regain some control over the situation. Time away can help relieve feelings of frustration and tension.	Parent states she is frustrated but also ready to work on solving problem.
		Discharge Planning		
Nurse	Urge the parent to call for further suggestions if further help is needed. Explain colic generally resolves by 3 months of age.	Advise parent to contact clinic if measures are ineffective by 1 week.	Medication to reduce colic symptoms may be prescribed if nonpharmacologic measures are not effective.	Parent agrees to call in 1 week if crying has not improved.

tack of colic and be misinterpreted by the casual interviewer. Ask parents about the duration of the problem and its frequency (it usually lasts up to 3 hours a day and occurs at least 3 days every week). Ask what happens just before the attack (Colic usually occurs at a time removed from a feeding), and ask the parent to describe the attack itself and associated symptoms. Document the number and type of bowel movements the infant has, because bowel movements are not abnormal with colic. Constipation; narrow, ribbonlike stools; and the presence of blood or mucus in the stool all suggest other problems. A family medical history is important to obtain because allergy to milk may simulate colic.

Determine the baby's feeding pattern (breastfed or bottle fed). If bottle fed, ask about the type of formula and how it is prepared. Ask parents if they are holding the baby upright so air bubbles can rise and whether they burp the infant adequately after feeding. For a breastfed baby, a change in maternal diet such as avoiding "gassy" foods like cabbage might be helpful to reduce or limit colicky periods. It may be helpful to recommend that both breast- and formula-fed infants receive small, frequent feedings to prevent distention and discomfort. Offering a pacifier may be comforting.

Some parents try placing a hot water bottle on their infant's stomach for comfort, but this should be discouraged. A basic rule for any abdominal discomfort is to avoid heat in case appendicitis is developing. This is highly unlikely in so young an infant, but parents will remember they once used heat and may use it again when the child is older. Hot water bottles and heating pads also might burn the delicate skin of infants.

Changing formula bottles to the type with disposable bags that collapse as the baby sucks may help minimize the amount of air swallowed. Taking infants for car rides is often reported as being helpful in soothing colicky babies. Some music boxes simulate the sound of a heartbeat, which also may be helpful. Antiflatulent agents such as simethicone have not been shown to be helpful but may be tried (Srinivasan & Middleton, 2008).

It is important to think of colic as a family problem or else a vicious circle may begin. An infant cries and the parents become tense and unsure. An infant senses the tension and develops more colic. Help parents plan relief time from infant care to relieve their stress level and prevent this cycle.

In most infants, colic disappears almost magically at 3 months of age, probably because it becomes easier to digest food and an infant maintains a more upright position by this time, which allows less gas to form.

Spitting Up

Almost all infants spit up, although formula-fed babies appear to do it more than breastfed babies. Parents who did not handle their infant much in the health care facility where their child was born may discover spitting up only after they take the baby home. They may interpret this as vomiting or think an infant is developing an infection. Ask them to describe carefully what they mean by "spitting up." How long has the baby been doing it? How frequently? What is the appearance of the spit-up milk? Almost all milk that is spit up smells at least faintly sour, but it should not contain blood or bile.

A baby who spits up a mouthful of milk (rolling down the chin) two or three times a day (or sometimes after every meal) is experiencing normal, early-infancy spitting up. Associated signs such as diarrhea, abdominal cramps, fever, cough, cold, or loss of activity suggest illness. If an infant is spitting up so forcefully that milk is projected 3 or 4 feet away, it may be beginning pyloric stenosis (an abnormally tight valve between the stomach and duodenum), which requires surgical intervention. If the spitting up is a large amount with each feeding, parents may be describing gastroesophageal reflux, in which a lax cardiac sphincter from the stomach into the esophagus allows regurgitation of gastric contents into the esophagus. This also requires medical attention (see Chapter 45).

Burping a baby thoroughly after a feeding often limits spitting up. Parents may try sitting an infant in an infant chair for half an hour after feeding. Changing formulas generally is of little value. Reassure parents that spitting up decreases in amount as the baby becomes better at coordinating swallowing and digestive processes (the cardiac sphincter matures). In the meantime, a bib can protect the baby's clothing and the parent. After a few months, the child will naturally stay in an upright position longer, and gravity will help to correct the problem.

Diaper Dermatitis

Some infants have such sensitive skin that diaper dermatitis (diaper rash) is a problem from the first few days of life. It occurs for several reasons.

When parents do not change a child's diaper frequently, feces is left in contact with skin, and irritation may result in the perianal area. Urine that is left in diapers too long breaks down into ammonia, a chemical that is extremely irritating to infant skin. Ammonia dermatitis of this type is generally a problem in the second half of the first year of life, when an infant is producing a larger quantity of urine than before. For some infants, however, it is a problem from the first week.

Frequent diaper changing, applying A&D or Desitin ointment, and exposing the diaper area to air may relieve the problem. Some infants may have to sleep without diapers at night to control the problem.

Whenever the entire diaper area is erythematous and irritated so that the outline of the diaper on the skin can be identified, one must suspect an allergy to the material in the diaper or to laundry products if a commercially washed or home-washed diaper is being used. Changing the brand or type of diaper or washing solution usually alleviates this problem.

If a diaper area is covered with lesions that are bright red, with or without oozing, last longer than 3 days, and appear as red pinpoint lesions, suspect a fungal (monilial or candidiasis) infection. This is discussed in Chapter 43.

Miliaria

Miliaria, or prickly heat rash, occurs most often in warm weather or when babies are overdressed or sleep in overheated rooms. Clusters of pinpoint, reddened papules with occasional vesicles and pustules surrounded by erythema usually appear on the neck first and may spread upward to around the ears and onto the face or down onto the trunk.

Bathing an infant twice a day during hot weather, particularly if a small amount of baking soda is added to the bath water, may improve the rash. Eliminating sweating by reducing the amount of clothing on an infant or lowering the room temperature should bring almost immediate improvement and prevent further eruptions.

Infant Caries (Baby-Bottle Syndrome)

Putting an infant to bed with a bottle of formula, breast milk, orange juice, or glucose water can result in aspiration. It also can lead to decay of all the upper teeth and the lower posterior teeth (Fig. 29.21) (Yost & Li, 2008). Decay occurs

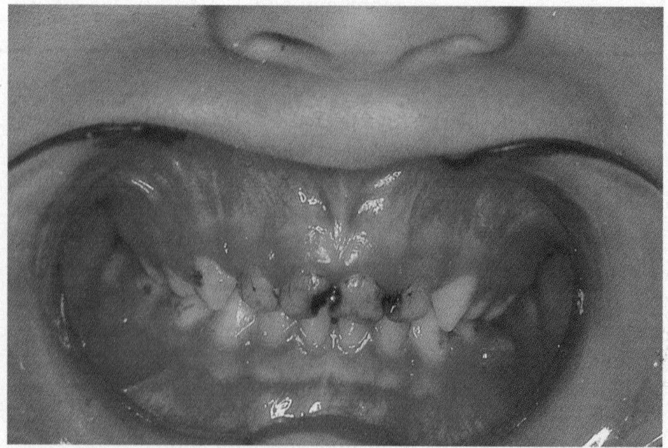

FIGURE 29.21 Baby-bottle syndrome. Notice the extensive decay in the upper teeth. (From K. L. Boyd, DDS/Custom Medical Stock Photograph.)

because while an infant sleeps, liquid from the propped bottle continuously soaks the upper front teeth and lower back teeth (the lower front teeth are protected by the tongue). The problem, called **baby-bottle syndrome**, occurs because the carbohydrate in solutions such as formula or glucose water ferments to organic acids that demineralize the tooth enamel until it decays.

To prevent this problem, advise parents never to put their baby to bed with a bottle. If parents insist a bottle is necessary to allow a baby to fall asleep, encourage them to fill it with water and use a nipple with a smaller hole to prevent the baby from receiving a large amount of fluid. If the baby refuses to drink anything but milk, the parents might dilute the milk with water more and more each night until the bottle is down to water only.

Obesity in Infants

Obesity in infants is defined as a weight greater than the 90th to 95th percentile on a standardized height/weight chart. Obesity occurs when there is an increase in the number of fat cells because of excessive calorie intake. Preventing obesity in infants is important because the extra fat cells formed at this time are likely to remain throughout childhood and even into adulthood. If a child becomes obese because of overingestion of milk, iron-deficiency anemia may also be present because of the low iron content of both breast and commercial milk. Once infant obesity begins, it is difficult to reverse, so prevention is the key (Farrow & Blissett, 2008).

Overfeeding in infancy often occurs because parents were taught to eat everything on their plate, and they continue to instill this concept in their children. This occurs most often with formula-fed infants whose parents urge them to empty their bottle or finish a cereal serving. It can occur any time parents automatically feed an infant when the child cries, rather than investigating what the cry might really mean. As a general rule, an infant should take no more than 32 oz of formula daily. When solid food is introduced, a bottle of water can be substituted for formula at one feeding. Nonfat milk should not be given because it contains so little fat that essential fatty acid requirements may not be sufficient to ensure cell growth.

Another way to help prevent obesity is to add a source of fiber, such as whole-grain cereal and raw fruit, to an infant's diet. These prolong the stomach-emptying time, so they can help reduce food intake. Caution parents about giving obese infants foods with high amounts of refined sugars, such as pudding, cake, cookies, and candy. Encourage parents to learn more about balanced nutrition and to provide this for their entire family.

Concerns of the Family With a Cognitively or Physically Challenged or Chronically Ill Infant

An infant born with a cognitive or physical challenge or an illness is usually hospitalized immediately after birth for diagnosis and treatment. This can result in delayed bonding because the newborn is separated from the parents during this time. Encourage parents to visit an intensive care nursery regularly to help form a strong parent–child attachment. If parents cannot visit, urge them to call the hospital as frequently as they can to inquire about their child. In addition, nurses can supply digital photographs of an infant for parents to take home.

Many of the developmental events of the infant year (social smile, laughing out loud, reaching for an object, uttering the first word, sitting, talking) are activities that encourage parent–child interaction because they make an infant fun to be with and naturally make a parent want to spend more time with the child. Children who are cognitively challenged may not reach these milestones. Children who are physically challenged may be unable to achieve them as well if they cannot reach up and pat their mother's face or hold out arms to be picked up by a father. If children cannot interact with parents in these ways, parents may find themselves equally unable to interact with their children. If infants leave the hospital with a cast or other equipment such as a ventilator for care, parents may be so concerned with these items that they cannot initiate normal singing and playing activities with their children.

To encourage a good parent–child relationship, point out the positive things an infant can do. Perhaps the child's facial expression says, "Pick me up," even though he does not reach up with his hands; perhaps his eyes follow his mother's actions even though he cannot yet call to her.

Helping parents to interact more fully with their infants helps to build a sense of trust in an infant. Without a sense of trust, children have difficulty expressing themselves to others; they may not believe they are lovable or people would want to interact with them. Physically challenged individuals, no matter what their ages, need people around them to give them help at whatever point they cannot meet their own needs. It is unfortunate when physically challenged children cannot reach out for help because they do not have a sense of trust.

Infants who are cognitively or physically challenged or chronically ill experience the same health and growth problems as other infants. Parents may be reluctant to bring up these concerns at health care visits because they believe such problems pale in comparison to the primary illness or condition. When taking the health histories of children with chronic or longstanding medical problems, ask parents about secondary concerns. "What about everyday things? Any problems there?" Treat these concerns seriously, so parents can feel confident about bringing them to your attention at future health care visits. Also mention they are part of normal infant development so parents can begin to view their child apart from the primary illness.

Teething pain, discomfort from diaper rash, and colic are all potential problems in infancy and may occur even more frequently in babies with other illnesses. For instance, parents may not want to "bother" an ill infant with physical care as often as they would a well child. Before homes were well-heated, bathing an ill infant could cause extensive chilling, and many people still believe bathing is not appropriate for ill children. Colic may occur because parents are reluctant to tire ill infants by burping them after a feeding. Parents' attention may be so focused on the primary health problem rather than on everyday concerns, such as diaper care, that diaper dermatitis occurs. The bowel movements of physically disabled or chronically ill children may be looser than normal because of a liquid diet or medicine. Their urine may be more concentrated because of reduced intake. These conditions may also lead to diaper rash. Offering anticipatory guidance to parents can go a long way toward helping them avoid this special concern of infancy.

Nutrition and the Cognitively or Physically Challenged Infant

Nutrition is often a concern for infants who are born physically challenged or are ill at birth. Infants who have fevers because of illness have increased metabolic needs and require more calories than normal. To compound the problem, ill children may become too fatigued to take adequate feedings. If any degree of neurologic involvement exists, sucking and swallowing reflexes may not be coordinated. With gastrointestinal involvement, feeding may be impossible.

To ensure adequate calorie and protein intake, infants may need to be maintained on nasogastric tube or gastrostomy feedings, or total parenteral nutrition. These methods limit the amount of sucking that is possible. Because sucking provides pleasure as well as satisfying thirst, this is a major loss. Provide an infant with nonnutritive sucking experiences if possible to fill this need.

Infants who are ill for a long time may not eat solid foods eagerly once they are introduced because they are not hungry enough to be interested in a new eating method. Help parents to experiment with different foods to find a taste that does appeal to ill children, or teach them to limit foods to only those the child appears to like most from all five food groups to ensure the infant receives adequate nutrition.

✔ Checkpoint Question 29.5

Bryan's mother is concerned about him developing baby-bottle syndrome. What would be her best action to prevent this?

a. Use plastic rather than glass bottles.
b. Boil formula to reduce the curd.
c. Do not put Bryan to bed with a bottle.
d. Check the expiration date on formula.

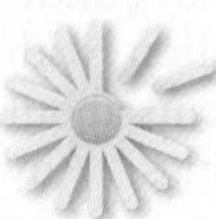

Key Points for Review

- The infant period is from 1 month to 12 months. Children typically double their birth weight at 4 to 6 months and triple it at 1 year.
- Infants develop their first tooth at about 6 months; by 12 months, they have six to eight teeth.
- Important gross motor milestones during the infant year are lifting the chest off a bed at 2 months, sitting at 6 to 8 months, creeping at 9 months, "cruising" at 10 to 11 months, and walking at 12 months.
- Important fine motor accomplishments are the ability to pass an object from one hand to the other (7 months) and a pincer grasp (10 months).
- Important milestones of language development during the first year are differentiating a cry (2 months), making simple vowel sounds (5 to 6 months), and saying two words besides "ma-ma" and "da-da" (12 months). The more infants are spoken to, the easier it is for them to acquire language.
- Providing infants with proper toys for play helps development. All infant toys need to be checked to be certain they are too large to be aspirated.
- Important milestones of vision development are the ability to follow a moving object past the midline (3 months) and ability to focus securely without eyes crossing (3 months).
- According to Erikson, the developmental task of the infant year is the development of a sense of trust versus mistrust.
- Safety is important. Infants must be protected from falls and aspiration of small objects. A skill an infant cannot accomplish one day, such as crawling, may be accomplished the next.
- Solid food is generally introduced into an infant's diet at 4 to 6 months of age. Before infants can eat solid food, they must lose their extrusion reflex.
- Common concerns related to infant development include teething, thumb-sucking, use of pacifiers, sleep problems, constipation, colic, diaper dermatitis, baby-bottle syndrome (decayed teeth from sucking on a bottle of formula while they sleep), and obesity. Nurses play a key role in teaching parents about these problems and measures to deal with them.
- Remember that parent–infant attachment is critical to mental health. Urge parents to continue to give as much care as possible to sick infants to maintain this important relationship.

CRITICAL THINKING EXERCISES

1. Bryan, the 2-month-old boy you met at the beginning of the chapter, was diagnosed with colic. What are common suggestions you could make to his parents to help reduce his discomfort and crying?
2. Bryan's mother wants to "childproof" her house. What questions would you ask to assess whether the infant's house is safe for him?
3. Bryan's father tells you that he has difficulty feeding Bryan solid food because Bryan "spits out" everything he tries to get him to eat. How could you help this father parent better?
4. Examine the National Health Goals related to growth and development of the infant. Most government-sponsored funds for nursing research are allotted based on these goals. What would be a possible research topic to explore pertinent to these goals that would be applicable to Bryan's family and also advance evidence-based practice?

CRITICAL THINKING SCENARIO

Open the accompanying CD-ROM or visit http://thePoint.lww.com and read the Patient Scenario included for this chapter, then answer the questions to further sharpen your skills and grow more familiar with NCLEX style questions related to nursing care of the family with an infant. Confirm your answers are correct by reading the rationales.

REFERENCES

American Academy of Pediatrics (AAP) Committee on Practice and Ambulatory Medicine. (2009). *Recommendations for preventive pediatric health care.* Washington, DC: Author.

American Academy of Pediatrics (AAP). (2009). Car safety seats: a guide for families. http://www.aap.org/family/carseatguide.htm.

American College of Obstetricians and Gynecologists (ACOG). (2007). Special report from ACOG: breastfeeding: maternal and infant aspects. *ACOG Clinical Review, 12*(1), 1S–16S.

Armfield, J. M., & Spencer, A. J. (2007). Community effectiveness of fissure sealants and the effect of fluoridated water consumption. *Community Dental Health, 24*(1), 4–11.

Baddock, S. A., et al. (2007). Sleep arrangements and behavior of bed-sharing families in the home setting. *Pediatrics, 119*(1), e200–e207.

Bernard, A., et al. (2007). Infant swimming practice, pulmonary epithelium integrity, and the risk of allergic and respiratory diseases later in childhood. *Pediatrics, 119*(6), 1095–1103.

Bolte, R. (2007). The crying child: potential causes. What are they trying to tell us? *Contemporary Pediatrics, 24*(5), 74–81.

Brayden, R. M., Daley, M. F., & Brown, J. M. (2008). Ambulatory and community pediatrics. In W. W. Hay, et al. (Eds.). *Current pediatric diagnosis and treatment* (18th ed.). Columbus, OH: McGraw-Hill.

Conti, T. D. (2008). Breastfeeding and infant nutrition. In J. E. South-Paul, S. C. Matheny, & E. L. Lewis (Eds.). *Current diagnosis and treatment in family medicine* (2nd ed.). Columbus, OH: McGraw-Hill.

Damato, E. G. (2007). Safe sleep: can pacifiers reduce SIDS risk? *Nursing for Women's Health, 11*(1), 72–76.

Erikson, E. (1993). *Childhood and society* (3rd ed.). New York: W. W. Norton.

Farrow, C. V., & Blissett, J. (2008). Controlling feeding practices: cause or consequence of early child weight? *Pediatrics, 121*(1), e164–e169.

Forsythe, P. L., et al. (2007). Infant safety at home. *Advances in Neonatal Care, 7*(2), 78–79.

Goldson, E., & Reynolds, A. (2008). Child development and behavior. In W. W. Hay, et al. (Eds.). *Current pediatric diagnosis and treatment* (18th ed.). Columbus, OH: McGraw-Hill.

Gomella, L. G., & Haist, S. A. (Eds.). (2007). *Clinician's pocket reference* (11th ed.). Columbus, OH: McGraw-Hill.

Keefe, S. (2007). Heavy burden. *Advance for Nurses, 9*(23), 31.

Lawson, M. (2007). Contemporary aspects of infant feeding. *Paediatric Nursing, 19*(2), 39–45.

Lim, H. W. (2008). Photoprotection and sun protective agents. In K. Wolff, et al. (Eds.). *Fitzpatrick's dermatology in general medicine* (7th ed.). Columbus, OH: McGraw-Hill.

Moore, E. R., Anderson, G. C., & Bergman, N. (2009). Early skin-to-skin contact for mothers and their healthy newborn infants. *Cochrane Database of Systematic Reviews, 2009*(1), (CD003519).

Mueller, W. A. (2008). Oral medicine and dentistry. In W. W. Hay, et al. (Eds.). *Current pediatric diagnosis and treatment* (18th ed.). Columbus, OH: McGraw-Hill.

National Vital Statistics System (NVSS). (2008). *Health of Americans.* Hyattsville, MD: Author.

Nurcombe, B. (2008). Developmental disorders of attachment, feeding, elimination and sleeping. In M. H. Ebert, et al. (Eds.). *Current diagnosis and treatment: psychiatry* (2nd ed.). Columbus, OH: McGraw-Hill.

Piaget, J. (1966). *The origins of intelligence in children.* New York: International University Press.

Sass, P. (2006). Evidence in nutrition. Does early introduction of solid food (before 4 months of age) lead to an increased risk of adult obesity? *Evidence-Based Practice, 9*(7), 9–11.

Sloan, S., et al. Early weaning is related to weight and rate of weight gain in infancy. *Child: Care, Health and Development, 34*(1), 59–64.

Smoker, A. L. (2007). On top of cradle cap. *Journal of Family Health Care, 17*(4), 134–136.

Sondheimer, J. M. (2008). Gastrointestinal tract. In W. W. Hay, et al. (Eds.). *Current pediatric diagnosis and treatment* (18th ed.). Columbus, OH: McGraw-Hill.

Srinivasan, S., & Middleton, D. B. (2008). Well child care. In J. E. South-Paul, S. C. Matheny, & E. L. Lewis (Eds.). *Current diagnosis and treatment in family medicine.* (2nd ed.). Columbus, OH: McGraw-Hill.

Theobald, H. (2007). Childhood nutrition. *Journal of Community Nursing, 21*(2), 25–28.

Thilo, E. H., & Rosenberg, A. A. (2008). The newborn. In W. W. Hay, et al. (Eds.). *Current pediatric diagnosis and treatment* (18th ed.). Columbus, OH: McGraw-Hill.

Yost, J., & Li, Y. (2008). Promoting oral health from birth through childhood: prevention of early childhood caries. *MCN: The American Journal of Maternal/Child Nursing, 33*(1), 17–25.

SUGGESTED READINGS

Blanchard, D. S., & Vermilya, H. L. (2007). Bedsharing: toward a more holistic approach in research and practice. *Holistic Nursing Practice, 21*(1), 19–25.

Chumlea. C. (2007). Which growth charts are the best for children today? *Nutrition Today, 42*(4), 148–150.

Darbyshire, P. (2007). 'Childhood': are reports of its death greatly exaggerated? *Journal of Child Health Care, 11*(2), 85–97.

Eronen, R., Pincombe, J., & Calabretto, H. (2007). Support for stressed parents of young infants. *Neonatal, Paediatric and Child Health Nursing, 10*(2), 20–27.

Kramer, M. S., & Kakuma, R. (2009). Optimal duration of exclusive breastfeeding. *Cochrane Database of Systematic Reviews, 2009*(1), (CD003517).

Limbo, R., & Pridham, K. (2007). Mothers' understanding of their infants in the context of an internal working model of caregiving. *Advances in Nursing Science, 30*(2), 139–150.

Morin, K. H. (2008). Oral health: getting off to a good start. *MCN: The American Journal of Maternal/Child Nursing, 33*(1), 58.

Wagner, S. (2007). Knowledge of normal development key in diagnosis. *Patient Education Management, 14*(8), 89–90.

Ward, T. M., Rankin, S., & Lee, K. A. (2007). Caring for children with sleep problems. *Journal of Pediatric Nursing: Nursing Care of Children and Families, 22*(4), 283–296.

Underdown, A., et al. (2009). Massage intervention for promoting mental and physical health in infants aged under six months. *Cochrane Database of Systematic Reviews, 2009*(1), (CD005038).

Chapter 30 Nursing Care of a Family With a Toddler

KEY TERMS

- assimilation
- autonomy
- deferred imitation
- discipline
- lordosis
- parallel play
- preoperational thought
- punishment
- tertiary circular reaction stage

OBJECTIVES

After mastering the contents of this chapter, you should be able to:

1. Describe normal growth and development of a toddler as well as common parental concerns.
2. Identify National Health Goals related to the toddler age group that nurses can help the nation achieve.
3. Use critical thinking to analyze methods of care for toddlers to be certain care is family centered.
4. Assess a toddler for normal growth and development milestones.
5. Formulate nursing diagnoses related to toddler growth and development or parental concerns regarding growth and development.
6. Identify expected outcomes for nursing care of a toddler.
7. Plan nursing care to meet a toddler's growth and development needs, such as anticipatory guidance to prevent problems such as sleep disturbances.
8. Implement nursing care to promote normal growth and development of a toddler, such as discussing toddler developmental milestones with parents.
9. Evaluate expected outcomes for achievement and effectiveness of care.
10. Identify areas related to care of a toddler that could benefit from additional nursing research or application of evidence-based practice.
11. Integrate knowledge of toddler growth and development with nursing process to achieve quality maternal and child health nursing care.

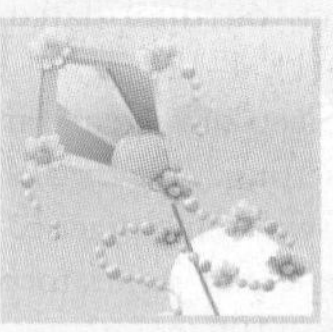

Jason is a 2½-year-old boy you see at a pediatric clinic. His mother tells you he has changed completely in the past 6 months from an easy-to-care-for baby into a "monster" who refuses to do anything she asks. The only word he says anymore is "no." He has a temper tantrum every night at dinner over some type of food. She tells you this has changed parenting from "fun" to "a real chore."

The previous chapter discussed the growth and development of infants and abilities infants develop in the first year. This chapter adds information about the dramatic changes, both physical and psychosocial, that occur during the toddler years. These changes form the basis for care and health teaching for this age group.

What advice could you give Jason's mother to help her regain a positive view of parenting?

During the toddler period, the age span from 1 to 3 years, enormous changes take place in a child and, consequently, in a family. During this period, children accomplish a wide array of developmental tasks and change from largely immobile and preverbal infants who are dependent on caregivers for the fulfillment of most needs to walking, talking young children with a growing sense of **autonomy** (independence). To match this growth, parents must also change during this period. If a parent enjoyed being the parent to an infant because time could be spent rocking or singing to the child, they may not enjoy being the parent of a toddler as now their task is to support their child's growing independence with patience and sensitivity and to learn methods for handling the child's frustrations that arise from the quest for autonomy. Because healthy children and families are constantly being challenged by the process of normal development, parents often have questions about how to guide their children in different situations and how to cope with special needs and concerns relevant to this age. National Health Goals related to the toddler age group are shown in Box 30.1.

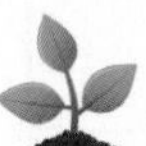

Nursing Process Overview

For Healthy Development of a Toddler

Assessment

Whether a child is seen for a routine checkup or has come to a health care center because of a specific health concern, assessment begins with taking a careful health history. Asking parents about a toddler's ability to carry out activities of daily living offers assessment information not only on the child's developmental progress but also important clues about the child–parent relationship.

Careful observation is another crucial element of nursing assessment of a toddler. This is because parents may become so emotionally involved in a health concern they may not describe it with complete objectivity. On the other hand, parents see their children daily and so are the best source of information and opinion on when a child seems to be acting "out of sorts" or "different" (a typical sign a child may not be feeling well).

Nursing Diagnosis

Nursing diagnoses related to normal growth and development of toddlers usually focus on the parents' eagerness to learn more about the parameters of normal growth and development or issues of safety or care. Examples are:

- Health-seeking behaviors related to normal toddler development
- Deficient knowledge related to best method of toilet training
- Risk for injury related to impulsiveness of toddler
- Interrupted family process related to need for close supervision of 2-year-old
- Readiness for enhanced family coping related to parents' ability to adjust to new needs of child
- Readiness for enhanced parenting related to increased awareness for poison prevention
- Disturbed sleep pattern related to lack of bedtime routine

Outcome Identification and Planning

To help parents resolve a concern during the toddler period, focus largely on family education and anticipatory guidance. Urge them to establish realistic goals and outcomes so they can meet the rapidly changing needs of their toddler and learn to cope with typical toddler behaviors. Otherwise, parents can expect too much of a toddler and grow frustrated instead of enjoying being a parent of a child this age. Helpful Web sites about growth and development to recommend are the BabyCenter (http://www.Babycenter.com) and Dr. Greene (http://www.Dr Greene.com). Helpful Web sites to alert parents about safety are the American Association of Poison Control Centers (http://www.aapcc.org) and the American Academy of Pediatrics (http://www.aap.org). For questions about car seats, parents can consult the U.S. Department of Transportation National Highway Traffic Safety Administration (http://www.nhtsa.dot.gov). The national 800 telephone number for a poison control center is 1-800-222-1222.

Implementation

When teaching about typical toddler behavior, teach parents a good rule is to think of a toddler as a visitor from a foreign land who wants to participate in everything the family is doing but does not know the customs or the language. They need to help their toddler learn these the same as they would that stranger.

Also teach parents not only how to approach a current problem but also how to learn adequate methods for resolving similar situations that are sure to arise in the future. If parents do not learn methods that can be applied throughout their child's growing years, they may win bat-

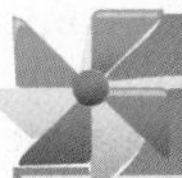

BOX 30.1 * Focus on National Health Goals

Several National Health Goals relate specifically to safety during the toddler years. These are:

- Increase the rate of use of child automotive restraints in children 4 years and younger to 100% from a baseline of 92%.
- Eliminate elevated blood lead levels in children or improve from a baseline level of 4.4% of children 1 to 16 years of age to 0%.
- Reduce the proportion of children 2 to 4 years of age who have dental caries in their primary or permanent teeth from a baseline of 18% to 11%.
- Reduce the rate of deaths caused by poisonings, from a baseline of 6.8 per 100,000 to 1.5 per 100,000 (http://www.nih.gov).

Nurses can help the nation achieve these goals by continuing to educate parents about the importance of using car seats and childproofing their homes against poisoning. Areas that could benefit from additional nursing research are methods parents can use to keep their toddlers entertained while in automobiles and specific home situations in which poisoning is apt to occur.

tles but lose wars. For instance, parents may find that promising children a treat when they are in the middle of a temper tantrum will stop the tantrum, but it will not prevent other tantrums from occurring in the future (and, in fact, may encourage them). Health visits provide opportunities to help parents learn healthy coping techniques. In addition, demonstrating good communication skills with toddlers can serve as a model for healthy communication behavior with them.

Outcome Evaluation

Expected outcomes must be evaluated frequently during the toddler period because children change so much and learn so many new skills during this time that their abilities and associated parental concerns can change from day to day. Examples of expected outcomes are:

- Parents state child maintains a consistent bedtime routine within the next 2 weeks.
- Parents state they have childproofed their home by putting a lock on kitchen cupboard by next clinic visit.
- Grandmother states she has modified usual activities to conserve strength to care for toddler granddaughter by 1 week's time.

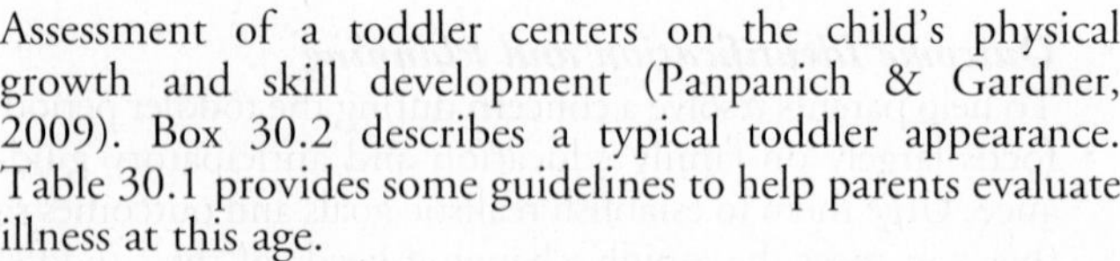

GROWTH AND DEVELOPMENT OF A TODDLER

Assessment of a toddler centers on the child's physical growth and skill development (Panpanich & Gardner, 2009). Box 30.2 describes a typical toddler appearance. Table 30.1 provides some guidelines to help parents evaluate illness at this age.

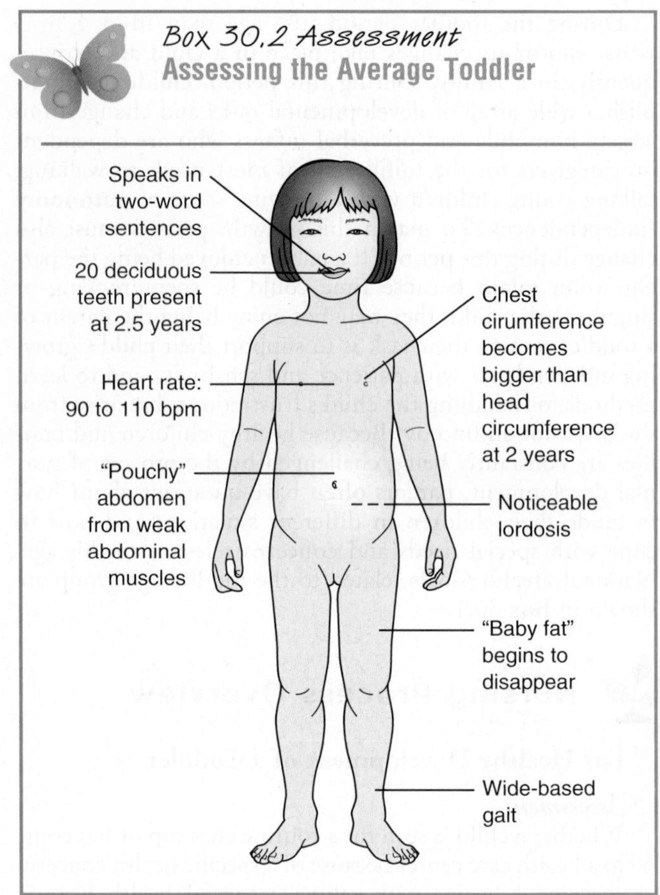

Physical Growth

While toddlers are making great strides developmentally, their physical growth begins to slow.

Weight, Height, and Head Circumference

Plot weight and height on a standard growth chart at each health care visit (see Appendix E) to determine if progress is normal for that particular child. A child gains only about 5 to 6 lb (2.5 kg) and 5 in (12 cm) a year during the toddler period, much less than the rate of infant growth. As subcutaneous tissue, or baby fat, begins to disappear toward the end of the second year, the child changes from a plump baby into a leaner, more muscular little girl or boy. A toddler's appetite decreases accordingly, yet adequate intake of all nutrients is still essential to meet energy needs (Rolfes, Pinna, & Whitney, 2009).

Head circumference increases only about 2 cm during the second year compared to about 12 cm during the first year. Head circumference equals chest circumference at 6 months to 1 year of age. By 2 years, chest circumference has grown greater than that of the head.

Body Contour

Toddlers tend to have a prominent abdomen because although they are walking well, their abdominal muscles are not yet strong enough to support abdominal contents as well as they will later (Fig. 30.1A). They also have a forward curve of the spine at the sacral area **(lordosis).** As they become more experienced at walking, this will correct itself naturally. Many toddlers, in addition, waddle or walk with a wide stance (see Fig. 30.1B). This stance seems to increase the lordotic curve, but it keeps them on their feet.

Body Systems

Body systems continue to mature during this time:

- Respirations slow slightly but continue to be mainly abdominal.
- The heart rate slows from 110 to 90 beats per minute; blood pressure increases to about 99/64 mm Hg.
- The brain develops to about 90% of its adult size.
- In the respiratory system, the lumens of vessels enlarge progressively so the threat of lower respiratory infection becomes less.
- Stomach secretions become more acid; therefore, gastrointestinal infections also become less common.
- Stomach capacity increases to the point a child can eat three meals a day.
- Control of the urinary and anal sphincters becomes possible with complete myelination of the spinal cord so toilet training is possible.
- IgG and IgM antibody production becomes mature at 2 years of age. The passive immunity obtained during intrauterine life is no longer operative.

TABLE 30.1 ✻ Parental Difficulties in Evaluating Illness in a Toddler

Problem	Guidelines for Parents
Evaluating seriousness of illness	Toddlers typically answer "No" to almost all questions. A question such as "Does your arm hurt?" may bring a "No" response even if the arm does hurt. Observing children for indications of illness (holding an arm stiffly, rubbing abdomen, crying when they void) is more helpful. Many toddlers do not know the words to describe a feeling of nausea or a sore throat. They reveal these symptoms by not eating. If the child is normally a light eater, as many are, it is difficult for a parent to appreciate these signs.
Differentiating tiredness from illness	Toddlers tend to whine or sleep when they are either tired or ill. Reviewing the child's day and activity often helps to evaluate what is happening. If the child is not tired (it is not nap or bedtime), or there is not a break in usual routine, crying and whining or temper tantrums suggest illness.
Evaluating nutritional intake	Toddlers are normally fussy eaters compared to infants. Evaluating children regarding whether they are active and growing is better than assessing any one day's food intake. Check weekly intake history.
Age-specific diseases to be aware of	The toddler period is an important age to assess speech development; children should be further evaluated if they cannot use simple sentences composed of a noun and verb ("me go") by 2 years of age. As children begin to walk, they should be observed for abnormal gait. Osteomyelitis (bone infection) occurs with a high frequency in toddlers; symptoms of limping, swollen joints, or arm or leg pain should be regarded as serious until ruled otherwise. Toddlers contract 10–12 mild upper respiratory infections a year. Otitis media (middle ear infection) may occur as a complication of these. The child with an upper respiratory infection who suddenly develops a high fever and pulls or manipulates ears should be seen by a physician. Children who attend day care programs have a high incidence of hepatitis A, *Giardia*, and *Shigella* infections. Teach parents to report jaundice or diarrhea promptly to a health care provider to detect these infections.

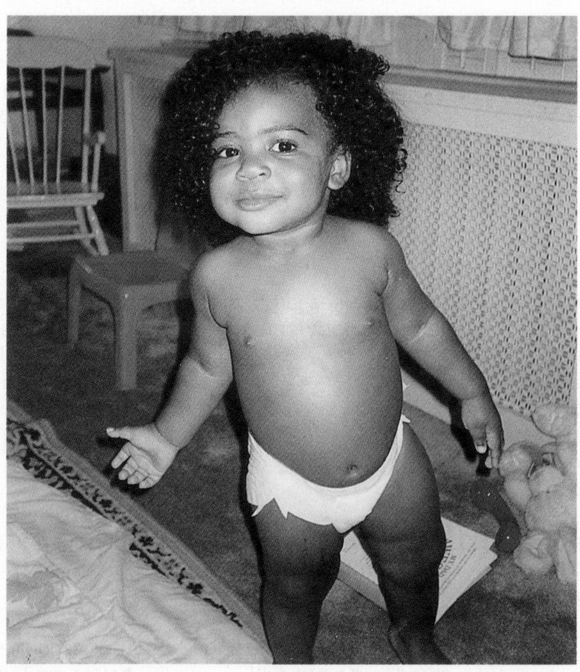
A

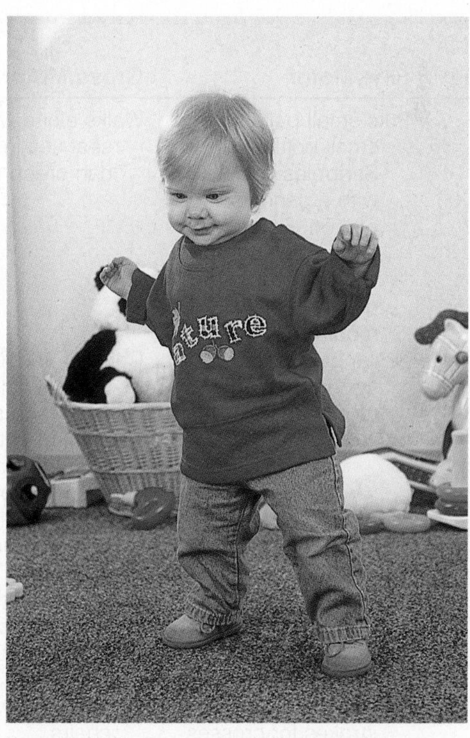
B

FIGURE 30.1 Physical characteristics of toddlers. (**A**) Toddlers typically have a prominent abdomen. (**B**) Toddlers typically walk with an unsteady gait for better stability.

Teeth

Eight new teeth (the canines and the first molars) erupt during the second year. All 20 deciduous teeth are generally present by 2.5 to 3 years of age (Gonsalves, 2008).

Developmental Milestones

The developmental milestones of the toddler years are less numerous but no less dramatic than those of the infant year, because this is a period of slow and steady, not sudden, growth. Toddler development is influenced to some extent by the amount of social contact and the number of opportunities children have to explore and experience new degrees of independence. It is strongly influenced by individual readiness for a new skill. Table 30.2 highlights growth and development milestones of gross and fine motor, language, and play development of the toddler years.

Language Development

Toddlerhood is a critical time for language development, although even this varies among children, because to master language, children need practice time. A child who is 2 years old and does not talk in two-word, noun–verb simple sentences needs a careful assessment to determine the cause. This is beyond a point of normal development. Parents are often worried that lack of language means their child has autism (Johnson, 2008). A delay in language can represent only a temporary setback in development, however.

A word that is used frequently by toddlers and that is a manifestation of their developing autonomy is "no." Toddlers may use the word to mean they are refusing a task, or they do not understand it, or they may only be practicing a sound that they have noticed has potent effects on those around them.

To learn other words, children need exposure to conversation and need to be read to often. Language develops most quickly if parents respect what toddlers have to say so children grasp the use and purpose of language.

Urge parents to encourage language development by naming objects as they play with their child ("ball," "block," "music box," "doll") or when they give their toddler something ("Here is your drink of water," "Let's put on these pajamas," and so on). This helps children grasp the fact that words are not meaningless sounds; they apply to people and objects and have uses. Always answering a child's questions is another good way to do this. Be sure answers for toddlers are simple and brief because they have such a short attention span.

Some toddlers do not develop language readily because they are not called on to use it. When they point at an object, someone hands it to them; when they climb into their highchair, someone places a meal in front of them. In other families, an older child may speak for a younger one. To assess whether parents are encouraging language development, ask them what happens when the child wants something. Do they provide opportunities for the child to ask for things before they supply them? Children should not be made to name an object before they can have it (because their vocabulary is so limited, the objects they could have would be

TABLE 30.2 ✻ Milestones of Toddler Growth and Development

Age (Months)	Fine Motor	Gross Motor	Language	Play
15	Puts small pellets into small bottles. Scribbles voluntarily with a pencil or crayon. Holds a spoon well but may still turn it upside down on the way to mouth	Walks alone well; can seat self in chair; can creep upstairs	4–6 words	Can stack 2 blocks; enjoys being read to; drops toys for adult to recover (exploring sense of permanence)
18	No longer rotates a spoon to bring it to mouth	Can run and jump in place. Can walk up and down stairs holding onto a person's hand or railing. Typically places both feet on one step before advancing.	7–20 words, uses jargoning; names 1 body part	Imitates household chores, dusting, etc.; begins parallel play (playing beside not with another child)
24	Can open doors by turning doorknobs, unscrew lids	Walks up stairs alone still using both feet on same step at same time	50 words, 2-word sentences (noun-pronoun and verb), such as "Daddy go," "me come"	Parallel play evident
30	Makes simple lines or strokes for crosses with a pencil	Can jump down from chairs	Verbal language increasing steadily. Knows full name; can name one color and holds up fingers to show age	Spends time playing house, imitating parents' actions; play is "rough-housing" or active

restricted to 10 or fewer), but parents can reinforce language by rewording a question; for example, "You want the ball?" Reading aloud strengthens vocabulary in the same way. Reading the exact words in a book is not as important to toddlers as pointing to the pictures that accompany them. For example, Jane threw the ball ("See Jane throwing the ball?") or the dog ran away with the ball ("Look, that dog took that ball!").

Children who are very active may use fewer words than children who are less active. Active children are too busy doing things to describe what they are doing or too busy obtaining objects to need to ask for many things. Such children probably have a large unexpressed vocabulary, however, or understand more words (comprehensive vocabulary) than can be expressed (expressive vocabulary).

Because children learn language from imitating what they hear, they will speak like those around them. If they are spoken to in baby talk, their enunciation of words can be poor; if they hear examples of bad grammar, they will not use good grammar. Remind parents that pronouns are difficult for children to use correctly; many children are 3½ or 4 years of age before they can separate the different uses of "I," "me," "him," and "her." Bilingual children interchange words from both languages.

✔ Checkpoint Question 30.1

What type of sentence should Jason, a 2-year-old, have mastered?

a. "Red ripe tomatoes."
b. "Daddy come."
c. "Old MacDonald."
d. "Please, please."

Emotional Development

Children change a great deal in their ability to understand the world and how they relate to people during the toddler years.

Autonomy. The developmental task of the toddler years according to Erikson (1993) is the development of a *sense of autonomy versus shame or doubt.* Children who have learned to trust themselves and others during the infant year are better prepared to do this than those who cannot trust themselves or others.

To develop a sense of autonomy is to develop a sense of independence. A healthy level of autonomy is achieved when parents are able to encourage independence while still maintaining consistently sound rules for safety. Children who are constantly told not to try things because they will hurt themselves may be left with a stronger sense of doubt than confidence at the end of the toddler period. Children who are made to feel it is wrong to be independent may leave the toddler period with a stronger sense of shame than autonomy.

Infants appear to have difficulty differentiating between their bodies and those of others; they think of their bodies as extensions of their parents or their primary caregivers. When infants approach toddlerhood, they begin to make the differentiation. As they recognize they are separate individuals, they also realize they do not always have to do what others want them to do. From this realization comes the reputation toddlers have for being negativistic, obstinate, and difficult to manage.

This reputation is little deserved, however, and exists largely because parents misinterpret children's cues. For example, children's refusal to accept help putting on shoes may be seen by a parent as disobedience, whereas children may view this as insisting on performing a task they can do independently—a positive expression of autonomy.

Socialization. Once toddlers are walking well, they become resistant to sitting in laps and being cuddled. This is not lack of a desire for socialization but a function of being independent. At 15 months, children are still enthusiastic about interacting with people, providing those people are willing to follow them where they want to go. By 18 months, toddlers imitate the things they see a parent doing, such as "study" or "sweep," so they seek out parents to observe and initiate interactions. By 2 or more years, children become aware of gender differences and may point to other children and identify them as "boy" or "girl."

Play Behavior. All during the toddler period, children play beside children next to them, not with them. This side-by-side play (called **parallel play**) is not unfriendly but is a normal developmental sequence that occurs during the toddler period (Fig. 30.2). Caution parents that if two toddlers are going to play together, they must provide duplicate toys or an argument over one toy is likely to occur (Goldson & Reynolds, 2008). Toddlers who have an aggressive personality probably have the most difficulty adapting to play groups (Box 30.3).

The toys toddlers enjoy most are those they can play with by themselves and that require action. Trucks they can make go, squeaky frogs they can squeeze, waddling ducks they can pull, rocking horses they can ride, pegs they can pound, blocks they can stack, and a toy telephone they can talk into are all favorites. These are all toys children can control, giving them a sense of power in manipulation, an expression of autonomy (Fig. 30.3).

Some parents are not prepared for this change in play habits in their child. They wonder why a child who used to

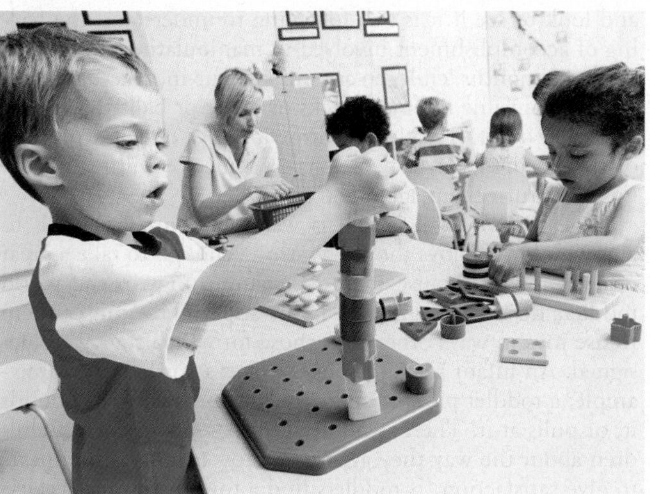

FIGURE 30.2 Parallel play. The toddler usually plays alongside another child rather than cooperatively.

BOX 30.3 * Focus on Evidence-Based Practice

Do aggressive preschool children have lower cognitive ability than nonaggressive children?

To explore the association between cognitive ability and temperament, researchers evaluated 31 children who had previously been rated as aggressive on the Aggressive Behavior Scale of the Achenbach Child Behavior Checklist. Their cognitive ability and temperament were then assessed using the Differential Ability Scale and the Carey Temperament Behavioral Styles Questionnaire respectively. Analysis showed that three different groups of children emerged. The first group (41.9% of the sample) demonstrated low adaptability, low persistence, high activity, negative mood, and low rhythmicity, along with borderline-deficient cognitive scores. The second group (38.7%) demonstrated low adaptability, low persistence, high activity, and negative mood, along with average cognitive scores. The third group (19.4%) demonstrated essentially midrange temperament characteristics and average cognitive scores. All three groups shared the temperamental tendency of a high threshold of response. The researchers concluded that children with varying temperaments and cognitive ability manifest aggressive tendencies. Knowing that they demonstrate a high level of response could help parents to accept this aspect of temperament and possibly avoid situations where it might be most intense.

Based on this study, would it be surprising to find a child with average cognitive scores demonstrating aggressive behavior at preschool?

Source: Sakimura, J. N., et al. (2008). Cognitive and temperament clusters in 3- to 5-year-old children with aggressive behavior. *Journal of School Health, 78*(1), 38–45.

play quietly in her crib is now more interested in banging trucks together. However, they need only watch a toddler tug a pull toy, stop to see if it is following, walk again, and stop and look to see if it is still following to understand the feeling of accomplishment involved in manipulating toys.

At 15 months, children are still in a put-in, take-out stage, so they continue to enjoy stacks of boxes or balls that fit inside each other. They enjoy throwing toys out of a playpen or from a highchair tray as long as someone will pick them up and return them again and again.

The 18-month-old child is walking securely enough to enjoy pull toys. Toys should be strong enough to take a great deal of abuse, because there are many things in the world toddlers do not recognize or know about. This causes them to use toys in ways other than those for which they were designed. An infant sits and softly strokes a stuffed cat, for example; a toddler picks it up by the tail and swings it, pounds it, or pulls at it. There is no need for parents to correct children about the way they are using a toy as long as it appears to give satisfaction. If toddlers find a toy frustrating because they are holding or using it incorrectly, showing them the right way will ease frustration.

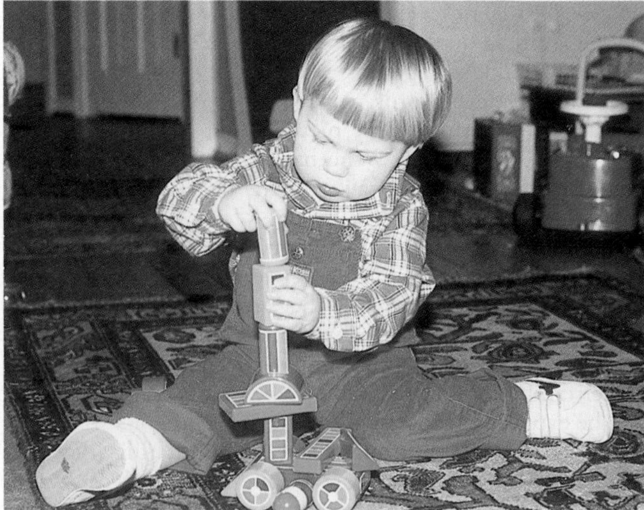

FIGURE 30.3 Toddlers enjoy toys that they can manipulate.

By age 2, when toddlers begin to spend time imitating adult actions in their play such as wrapping a doll and putting it to bed, "setting the table," or "driving the car," they begin to use fewer toys than before. The act of imitating has become their play. By the end of the toddler period, both boys and girls begin to like rough-housing and spend at least part of every day in this very active, stimulating type of play (Fig. 30.4). Encouraging parents to schedule this type of play outdoors, where vases or other prized possessions cannot be broken, makes it more acceptable. A child who feels a need for active play is unable to sit down and eat, fall asleep, or play quiet games so may be described as "trouble." It is good to explore with parents the amount of outside or rough-housing time they allow a child each day. A trip in a stroller is not the same kind of activity as walking and running. Stroller walks are good because they provide fresh air and sunshine, but toddlers also need opportunities to engage in strenuous activity. Because of this rough activity, most toddlers have at least one black-and-blue mark on their legs at all times from tripping over their feet while trying to run too fast or jumping or bumping into a chair or doorway.

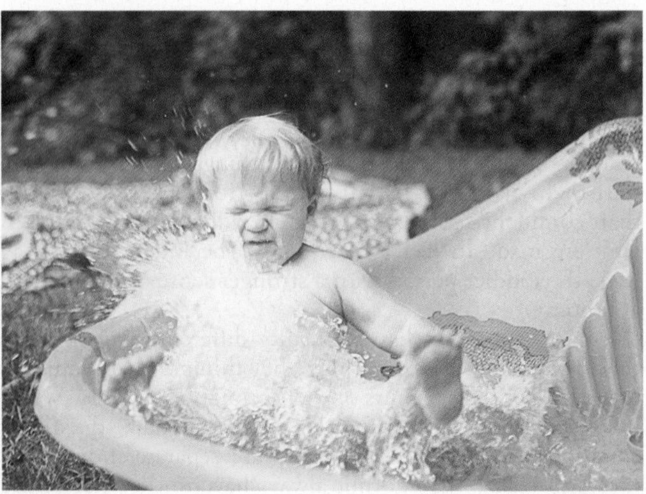

FIGURE 30.4 Toddlers usually enjoy rough and tumble play.

TABLE 30.3 ✻ Cognitive and Psychosocial Development of a Toddler

Age in Months	Stage	Task
Cognitive		
12–18	Sensorimotor 5	Child experiments by trial and error methods
18–24	Sensorimotor 6	Can pretend and use deferred imitation; object permanence is complete
24	Preoperational thought	Able to use assimilation or change situation to fit thoughts
Psychosocial		
24–36	Autonomy vs. shame or guilt	Learn independence and the beginning of problem solving

From Piaget, J. (1969). *The theory of stages in cognitive development.* New York: McGraw-Hill; and Erikson, E. H. (1993). *Childhood and society.* New York: W. W. Norton; with permission.

Cognitive Development

A toddler enters the fifth and sixth stages of Piaget's sensorimotor thought (Table 30.3). Piaget referred to stage 5 (between 12 and 18 months) as a **tertiary circular reaction stage**, describing a toddler in this stage as "a little scientist" because of the child's interest in trying to discover new ways to handle objects or new results that different actions can achieve (Piaget, 1969). For instance, by trial and error, toddlers discover that cats do not like baths and that cookies on the center of a table can be reached by crawling up onto the table or pulling on the tablecloth. Obviously, this type of scientific investigation can lead to errors or injury. Toddlers have also advanced beyond what they could do as infants in terms of dropping objects and watching where they roll. As infants, to retrieve an article that rolled under a chair, they would crawl under the chair along the same path the object took. Many children at 15 months are able to follow a different path (walk in back of the chair) to obtain the object. This results from increased awareness that the object is permanent and, even if it follows a different direction from the one the child must take, it will be there to retrieve.

By stage 6 (between 18 and 24 months), toddlers are able to try out various actions mentally rather than having to actually perform them—the beginning of problem solving or symbolic thought. Children at this stage are also able to remember an action and imitate it later **(deferred imitation);** they can do such things as pretend to drive a car or put a baby to sleep because they have not seen this just previously but at a past time. Object permanence becomes complete.

At the end of the toddler period, children enter a second major period of cognitive development: **preoperational thought.** During this period, children deal much more constructively with symbols than they did while still in the sensorimotor period of cognition. They begin to use a process termed **assimilation.** Because they are not able to change their thoughts to fit a situation, they learn to change the situation (or how they perceive it) to fit their thoughts. This ability is what causes toddlers to use toys in the "wrong" way. For example, if they are given a toy hammer, instead of pounding with it, they might shake it to see if it rattles, using the toy in a way they had previously played (they have changed the toy's use to fit thoughts, or used assimilation).

HEALTH PROMOTION FOR A TODDLER AND FAMILY

Toddlers tend to develop many upper respiratory and ear infections but otherwise come to health care facilities most often for health maintenance visits (recommended at 15, 18, and 24 months) and the immunizations important at these times. These visits allow you to focus on health promotion and provide an opportunity for early detection of any growth and development delays. Table 30.4 lists specific areas to assess during these visits.

Routine health maintenance visits also provide opportunities to support parents through the normal crises of the toddler period. Ways to encourage parents to promote healthy development of independence in their toddler include listening carefully to their concerns, asking questions to help separate the objective circumstances surrounding a problem from the parents' possible emotional biases, and providing guidelines on how to handle specific problems.

Promoting Toddler Safety

Accidents are the major cause of death in children of all ages. Accidental ingestions (poisoning) are the type of accident that occurs most frequently in toddlers (Dart & Rumack, 2008). Although poisoning can involve medicine such as acetaminophen, it most often occurs from ingestion of cleaning products. Aspiration or ingestion of small objects such as watch or hearing aid batteries, pencil erasers, or crayons is also a major danger for children of this age (Dutta & Barzin, 2008). Urge parents to childproof their home by putting all poisonous products, drugs, and small objects out of reach by the time their infant is crawling, and certainly by the time their infant is walking (Myers, Li, & Shaheen, 2007).

Other accidents that occur frequently in toddlers include motor vehicle accidents, burns, falls, drowning, and

TABLE 30.4 ✻ Health Maintenance Schedule, Toddler Period

Area of Focus	Methods	Frequency
Developmental milestones	History, observation	Every visit
	Formal Denver Developmental Screening Test (DDST II)	18th-month visit
Growth milestones	Height, weight plotted on standard growth chart; physical examination	Every visit
Nutrition	History, observation; height/weight information	Every visit
Parent–child relationship	History, observation	Every visit
Behavior problems	History, observation	Every visit
Vision and hearing defects	History, observation	Every visit
Dental health	History, physical examination; first dental appointment	Every visit; first at 12 months
Anemia	Hematocrit/hemoglobin	24th-month visit
Lead screening	Whole blood lead level	Depending on risk level; 24th-month visit
Tuberculosis	PPD test	Depending on prevalence in community
Urinalysis	Clean-catch urine	24th-month visit
Immunizations		
Diphtheria, tetanus, and pertussis (DPT) vaccine	Check history and past records; inform caregiver about any risks and side effects.	15th- or 18th-month visit (4th)
Haemophilus influenzae type B (HiB) vaccine	Administer immunization in accordance with health care agency policies	12th- or 15th-month visit (4th)
Hepatitis A vaccine		12th- & 18th-month visit (1st & 2nd)
Hepatitis B vaccine		15th- or 18th-month visit (3rd)
Influenza vaccine		Yearly
Measles, mumps, and rubella (MMR) vaccine		12th- or 15th-month visit (1st)
Pneumococcal vaccine		12th- or 15th-month visit (4th)
Varicella vaccine		12th- or 15th-month visit (1st)
Anticipatory Guidance		
Toddler care	Active listening and health teaching	Every visit
Expected growth and developmental milestones before next visit	Health teaching	Every visit
Poison and accident prevention	Educate parents about toddler safety, such as using car seats and bicycle helmets, locking up poisons, and such precautions as removing drawstrings from hooded clothing to prevent strangulation.	Every visit
	Provide telephone number and location of nearest poison control center.	
Problem Solving		
Any problems expressed by caregiver during course of the visit	Active listening and health teaching regarding temper tantrums, toilet training, negativity	Every visit

Source: American Academy of Pediatrics. (2009). *Recommendations for preventive pediatric health care.* Washington, DC: Author.

playground injuries. These occur because toddlers' motor ability jumps ahead of their judgment. To prevent serious injury, a toddler must be supervised at all times. Toddlers can walk surely and swiftly enough so that if they are left outside to play, they can very quickly travel a block away. Because they have no judgment concerning moving cars, they walk across streets with no regard for oncoming cars. Because they cannot swim well, parents need to check whether backyard pools are securely fenced (Thompson & Rivara, 2009). Until children weigh 40 to 60 lb, they need a toddler-size car seat for safety in automobiles (Fig. 30.5). They should be placed in the back seat if the car has a passenger seat airbag (American Academy of Pediatrics [AAP], 2009). They need to wear a helmet as soon as they begin riding a tricycle.

Some 15-month-old children can climb over the side rails of their cribs and enjoy exploring the house early in the morning before anyone else is awake. Parents might have to move their child to a regular bed with a side rail as early as this time to keep the child from falling when climbing out of

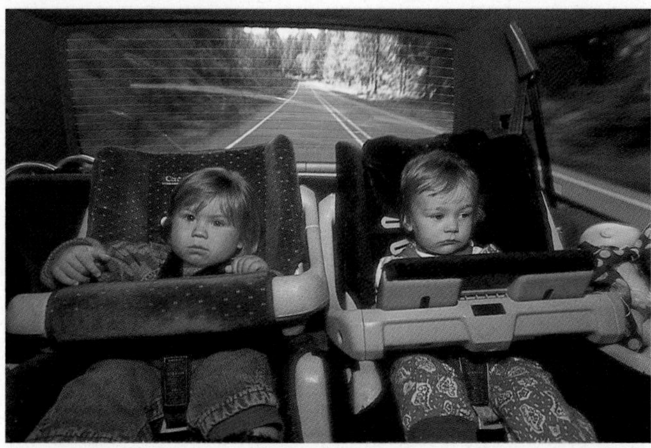

FIGURE 30.5 Toddlers should use a car seat for safety while riding in an automobile. (From David J. Sams/Stock Boston.)

a crib. A safety gate on the door of the room is another way to keep a toddler contained and safe.

As the child reaches 2 years of age and begins to imitate housework or repairing a car, parents must be sure the child does not use real cleaning compounds or sharp tools. Box 30.4 summarizes accident prevention measures to encourage parents to take with their toddler.

Lead Screening

The Centers for Disease Control and Prevention (CDC) has set as a goal the elimination of elevated blood lead levels in children (CDC, 2008). All children between the ages of 6 months and 6 years who live in communities with buildings built before 1950 should be tested periodically for the presence of too much lead in their body (lead poisoning). Elevated lead levels are caused by eating, chewing, or sucking on objects (such as windowsills, paint chips, or furniture) that are covered with lead-based paint. Although federal law has prohibited the use of lead in the manufacture of interior and exterior paints since the mid-1970s, many older houses still contain lead paint (Brown, 2008). Additional sources of lead poisoning can include:

- Soil around the exterior of the house and potentially contaminated food grown there
- Dust or fumes created by home renovation
- Pottery made with lead glazes
- Jewelry made from lead or lead alloys
- Colored print in newspapers
- Old water pipes
- Lead-based gasoline—children who live in high-traffic areas are at high risk for contamination by lead fumes
- Lead dust brought home on the clothing of parents who work with lead products such as batteries
- Toys or cribs that were painted with lead-based paint
- Sources in other countries (pertains to immigrant children)

Because lead is toxic to body tissue, ingestion of it leads to serious damage in the brain and nervous system, kidneys, and red blood cells. Levels as low as 10 μg/dL can cause learning and behavioral problems (Keefe, 2007). High levels may result in seizures, cognitive challenges, coma, and even death.

Beginning symptoms of lead poisoning include irritability, headache, fatigue, and abdominal pain (Chen et al., 2007). Often, however, there are no symptoms before damage occurs, which is why blood screening is essential. The AAP Committee on Practice and Ambulatory Medicine (2009) recommends screening for all children between the ages of 9 and 12 months at least once and again at 24 months of age. A small amount of blood taken by a finger prick is analyzed. A positive result (over 10 μg/dL) must be confirmed by further testing. Therapy for lead poisoning is discussed in Chapter 52.

Promoting Nutritional Health of a Toddler

Because growth slows abruptly after the first year of life, a toddler's appetite is smaller than an infant's. Children who ate hungrily 2 months earlier now sit and play with their food. If feeding problems begin at this time, it is often because parents are unaware their toddler's appetite has decreased so food consumption will be less. Because the actual amount of food eaten daily varies from one child to another, teach parents to place a small amount of food on a plate and allow their child to eat it and ask for more rather than serve a large portion the child cannot finish. One tablespoonful of each food served is a good start. Also, cleaning a plate gives a child a feeling of independent functioning, whereas leaving food uneaten may suggest that parents expected something more. It is important to educate parents while the child is still an infant that this decline in food intake will occur so they will not be concerned when it happens.

Allowing self-feeding is a major way to strengthen independence in a toddler. Offering finger foods and allowing a choice between two types of food helps promote independence while exposing children to varied foods (Williamson, 2007). Nutritious finger foods that toddlers enjoy include pieces of chicken, slices of banana, pieces of cheese, and crackers. Most toddlers insist on feeding themselves and generally will resist eating if a parent insists on feeding them. An individual child may react to repeated attempts at being fed by refusing to eat at all. Many toddlers prefer to eat the same type of food over and over because of the sense of security this offers.

Toddlers usually do not like food that is "mixed up" such as casseroles (except maybe spaghetti); they often prefer that different foods do not touch one another on their plate. Frequently they eat all of one item before going on to another. They often prefer brightly colored foods to bland colors.

Toddler Nutrition

Parents may become frustrated when trying to provide adequate nutrition for their toddler because of a toddler's varying and unpredictable appetite and food preferences. Although a toddler's daily food consumption may vary greatly, energy needs are generally met when sufficient food is supplied in a positive environment. Sedentary children ages 1 to 3 years should consume 1000 kcal daily; active children in this age group may need up to 1400 kcal daily (U.S. Department of Agriculture [USDA], 2005). Calories are best supplied by a variety of foods spaced into three meals a day (Krebs & Primak, 2008). Protein and carbohydrate needs are often those most easily met during the toddler period; diets high in sugar should be avoided. Fats should generally not be restricted for children under 2 years old; however, children

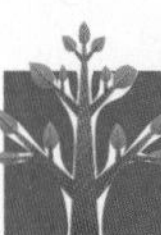

BOX 30.4 * Focus on Family Teaching

Common Safety Measures to Prevent Accidents During the Toddler Years

Q. Ms. Matthis tells you, "My toddler is constantly on the go. How can I keep him safe?"

A. Accident prevention must be ongoing while your child is a toddler. Try the following precautions:

Potential Accident	Prevention Measure
Motor vehicles	Maintain child in car seat; do not be distracted from safe driving by a child in a car.
	Do not allow child to play outside unsupervised. Do not allow child to operate electronic garage doors.
	Supervise toddler who is too young to be left alone on a tricycle.
	Teach safety with pedaling toys (look before crossing driveways; do not cross streets) but do not expect that toddler will obey these rules at all times (in other words, stay close by).
Falls	Keep house windows closed or keep secure screens in place.
	Place gates at top and bottom of stairs. Supervise at playgrounds.
	Do not allow child to walk with sharp object in hand or mouth.
	Raise crib rails and check to make sure they are locked before walking away from crib.
Aspiration	Examine toys for small parts that could be aspirated; remove toys that appear dangerous.
	Do not feed toddler popcorn, peanuts, etc.; urge children not to eat while running. Do not leave toddler alone with a balloon.
Drowning	Do not leave toddler alone in a bathtub or near water (including buckets of cleaning water and washing machines).
Animal bites	Do not allow toddler to approach strange dogs.
	Supervise child's play with family pets.
Poisoning	Never present medication as candy. Buy medications with childproof caps; put away immediately after use.
	Never take medication in front of child.
	Place all medication and poisons in locked cabinets or overhead shelves where child cannot reach them.
	Never leave medication in parents' purse or pocket, where child can reach it.
	Always store food or substances in their original containers.
	Know the names of house plants and find out if they are poisonous. (Call regional poison control center for information.)
	Hang plants or set them on high surfaces beyond toddler's grasp.
	Be certain that small batteries or magnets are out of reach.
	Post telephone number of nearest poison control center by the telephone.
	Inspect toys to be certain they are free of lead-based paint.
Burns	Buy flame-retardant clothing.
	Cook on the back burners of stove if possible and turn handles of pots toward back of stove to prevent toddler from reaching up and pulling them down.
	Use cool-mist vaporizer rather than steam vaporizer or remain in room when vaporizer is operating so child is not tempted to play with it.
	Keep screen in front of fireplace or heater.
	Monitor toddlers carefully when they are near lit candles.
	Do not leave toddlers unsupervised near hot-water faucets.
	Check temperature setting for hot-water heater and turn down thermostat if it is over 125° F.
	Do not leave coffee/tea pots on a table where child can reach them.
	Never drink hot beverages when a child is sitting on your lap or playing within reach.
	Do not allow toddlers to blow out matches (teach that fire is not fun); store matches out of reach.
	Keep electric wires and cords out of toddler's reach; cover electrical outlets with safety plugs.
General	Know whereabouts of toddlers at all times. Toddlers can climb onto chairs, stools, etc., they could not manage before; can turn door knobs and go places they could not go before.
	Be aware that the frequency of accidents increases when the family is under stress and therefore less attentive to children. Special precautions must be taken at these times.
	Be aware some children are more active, curious, and impulsive and therefore more vulnerable to accidents than others.

over 2 years old should have a total fat intake between 30% and 35% of calories, with most fat coming from sources of polyunsaturated and monounsaturated fatty acids, such as fish, nuts, and vegetable oils—the same as for adults. *Trans*–fatty acids should be kept to a minimum. Adequate calcium and phosphorus intake is important for bone mineralization. Milk should be whole milk until age 2 years, after which 2% milk can be introduced (Rolfes, Pinna, & Whitney, 2009).

Promoting Adequate Intake With a Vegetarian Diet

Vegetarian diets are adequate for toddlers if parents are well informed about needed vitamins and minerals (Theobald,

2007). A vegetarian diet can be easily designed for a toddler who prefers finger foods, because many vegetables, fruits, and grains such as pieces of oranges, peaches, raisins, chickpeas, tomatoes, and crackers are easily eaten this way. The use of fortified soy milk prevents fluid, protein, B_{12}, and calcium deficiencies. Tofu or Quom should be part of every meal to supply protein.

Promoting Toddler Development in Daily Activities

A toddler's new independence and developing abilities in self-care, such as dressing, eating, and, to a limited extent, hygiene, present special challenges for parents. Learning how to promote autonomy yet maintain a safe, healthful environment should be a major goal for the family.

Dressing

By the end of the toddler period, most children can put on their own socks, underpants, and undershirt (Fig. 30.6). Some may also be able to pull on slacks, pullover shirts (the sleeves of a shirt often confuse a toddler), or simple dresses. Parents may be reluctant to encourage toddlers to dress themselves as it is often easier and quicker to put their clothes on for them because a toddler who is dressed by parents will (usually) be wearing clothes in the correct way. When toddlers dress themselves, they invariably put shoes on the wrong feet and shirt and pants on backward. Encourage parents to give up perfection for the benefit of the child's developing sense of autonomy. If children end up with underpants or shirt on backward, in most instances it does not make that much difference, and toddlers are not likely to feel independent and confident if their attempts at dressing are criticized. If parents feel they must change the child's clothes, they should begin with a positive statement, such as "You did a good job," before making the switch.

During a health assessment, ask parents if their child can put on any clothing. Parents who allow this name those items the child can manage. Parents who do not allow self-dressing will probably describe the daily battle they have about dressing: "She puts up such a fuss, I don't think she will ever do it on her own." These parents may need help to understand the situation: the child may be resisting because she wants to dress herself. Do not judge how much independent exploration parents encourage by what they do in a physician's office or pediatric clinic. In these settings, they may dress a child quickly to show the child the examination is over, or they may simply be in a hurry to get home.

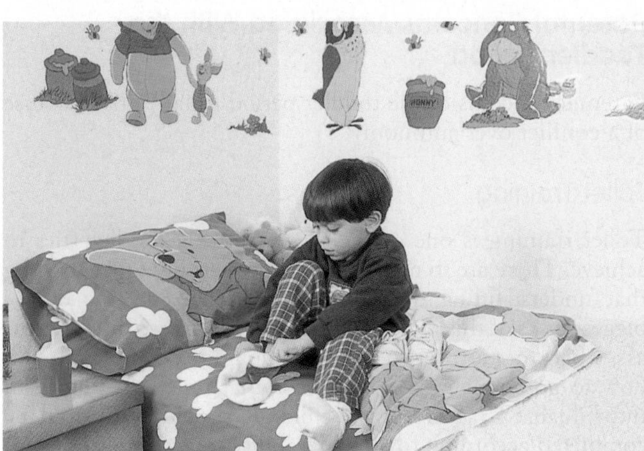

FIGURE 30.6 Getting dressed by himself is a fun morning activity for this older toddler.

As soon as children are up on their feet and walking, they need shoe soles that are firm enough to provide protection from rough surfaces. However, toddlers do not need extremely firm or ankle-high shoes. Because a toddler's arches are still developing, it is better for their arches to provide foot support rather than having it provided by shoes. Sneakers are an ideal toddler shoe because the soles are hard enough for rough surfaces and arch support is limited.

Sleep

The amount of sleep children need gradually decreases as they grow older (Goldson & Reynolds, 2008). They may begin the toddler period napping twice a day and sleeping 12 hours each night, and end it with one nap a day and only 8 hours' sleep at night. Parents who are not aware that the need for sleep declines at this time may view a child's disinterest in sleeping as a problem. A parent's insistence that a child get more sleep may lead to sleeping problems or refusal to sleep at all. If a child cannot fall asleep at night, maybe it is time to omit or shorten an afternoon nap. If a child is so short-tempered at dinnertime that eating is impossible, perhaps the child needs two naps a day. Some toddlers begin having night terrors or wake crying from a bad dream so they receive little sleep as they are reluctant to fall back asleep (Petit et al., 2007).

Usually, toddlers naturally fall asleep when they are tired. They may begin to resist naps, however, as well as nighttime sleep when they become aware for the first time that activities go on while they sleep, so they do not want to miss anything. Caution parents that when they say, "We'll do this after naptime," they wait until then to do it. Otherwise, a child may be reluctant to nap the next day for fear of missing another activity. Also, parents must be sure older siblings do not point out to a toddler all the exciting things a toddler missed while napping.

Other toddlers resist naptime as part of their developing negativism. Parents might minimize this by including a nap as part of lunchtime routine, not as a separate activity: the child always goes from the table directly to bed. The parent can state simply, "It's naptime now," and then give a secondary choice: "Do you want to sleep with your teddy bear or your rag doll?" Toward the end of the toddler period, when children are ready to omit their afternoon naps, they may still be agreeable to a "shoes-off" or quiet-play period until they begin to attend school full time.

As with any other activity of this period, a toddler loves a bedtime routine: bath, pajamas, a story, brushing teeth, being tucked into bed, having a drink of water, choosing a toy to sleep with, and turning out the lights. Parents must be careful, however, not to let a child maneuver them into such a long procedure that sleep is delayed considerably past the time initially set. Although toddlers need to be independent, they also need a feeling of security. Just as adults like to know there are guardrails along steep mountain roads, toddlers, especially when they are tired, like to see parents as firm, consistent people who can be counted on to be reliable over and over (Ward, Rankin, & Lee, 2007).

Many toddlers are ready to be moved out of a crib into a youth bed or regular bed with protective side rails or a chair strategically placed beside it by the end of the toddler period. Moving children to a more grown-up bed is usually preferable to forcing them to sleep in a crib if they no longer feel they should be there. Either children will not fall asleep in the crib or they will scale the side rail and perhaps fall.

Remind parents to stress that sleeping in a regular bed does not give children the right to get in and out of bed as they choose. Some toddlers do well if they are allowed to sleep in a regular bed and a folding gate is placed across the door to their room. This arrangement gives them a feeling of independence but still keeps them safe. When first moved to a bed without side rails, many children are found sleeping on the floor of the room in the morning. There is no harm in this unless it is cold or drafty. Dressing the child in warm pajamas or putting a blanket on the floor might be solutions to help parents accept this.

Bathing

The time for a toddler's bath should depend on the parents' and the child's wishes and schedule. Some parents prefer to bathe a toddler before the evening meal because it has a quieting effect and prepares a child for eating; others prefer to give it at bedtime because it has a relaxing effect and helps a child sleep. The time, however, is not as important as the attempt to establish a sense of routine, a sense that life has order. Learning to be independent is sometimes frightening, and there is security in knowing certain events are predictable.

Toddlers usually enjoy bath time, and parents should make an effort to make it fun by providing a toy, such as a rubber duck, boat, or plastic fish. Bath time is usually so enjoyable for toddlers that parents can use it as a recreational activity or something to do on a rainy day when they can find nothing else to interest their child. Remind parents that although toddlers can sit well in a bathtub, it is still not safe to leave them alone unsupervised. They might slip and get their head under water or reach and turn on the hot-water faucet and scald themselves (Ring, 2007).

Care of Teeth

Toddlers often need between-meal snacks. Encourage parents to offer fruit (bananas, pieces of apple, orange slices) or protein foods (cheese or pieces of chicken) rather than high-carbohydrate items for snacks such as cookies not only for the nutrition involved but also because protein snacks help prevent caries more than sugar snacks by limiting exposure of the child's teeth to carbohydrate. Calcium (found in large amounts in milk, cheese, and yogurt) is especially important to the development of strong teeth and are good for snacks. In addition, children should continue to drink fluoridated water, if it is available, so that all new teeth form with cavity-resistant enamel (Armfield & Spencer, 2007).

For tooth care, toddlers need to have a toothbrush they recognize as their own. Toward the end of the toddler period, they can begin to do the brushing themselves under supervision (almost all children need some supervision until about age 8). Remind parents it is better for a child to brush thoroughly once a day, probably at bedtime, than to do it poorly many times a day. After brushing, parents can use dental floss to clean between the child's teeth and remove plaque.

Urge parents to schedule a first visit to a dentist skilled in pediatric dental care at about 12 months of age for assessment of dentition (Mueller, 2008). Parents can prepare their child for this first and subsequent visits by reading a story about a dentist visit, maintaining a positive attitude about the visit, avoiding the use of frightening words like "drill" or "shot," and answering their child's questions honestly without going into too much detail. Because children rarely have cavities this early, the visit is usually painless and sets a positive stage for future dental supervision visits.

Promoting Healthy Family Functioning

Because learning self-reliance is the primary goal of a child during the toddler period, some parents who enjoyed caring for their child as an infant may find it difficult to have their authority challenged by a toddler. Help parents to understand their responses to these attempts at independence are crucial to the healthy development of their child. Although the child still needs firm limits to feel secure, a child must be given some room to make independent decisions in areas that the parents feel they do not need to control. An outside person, such as a nurse, can provide an important perspective on this issue.

If parents punish children excessively at each move toward independence, children will not fight them indefinitely. Instead, they will begin to feel guilty for wanting to do things independently. Adults without a sense of autonomy feel this way about independent thought. They may follow orders well, but when the job calls for a new program or function, they cannot reach into unknown areas without a great deal of consultation and help.

You may need to caution some parents not to begin to function at the same level as their toddler. An easy reaction to a toddler's refusal to allow a parent to help is, "You won't let me help you with this, so I won't do anything for you." This is a defense mechanism that prevents parents from feeling rejected. Teach parents that refusing to accept help is not refusing to accept love. Refusing to let mother put on a shoe is an instance of refusing to let mother put on a shoe, nothing more.

At bedtime, naptime, or anytime they are tired, toddlers may become much more like their old selves, wanting to sit on a parent's lap and be rocked or picked up and carried. This does not signal babyish behavior or regression in a toddler; it is a natural state between infant and preschool ages.

Parental Concerns Associated With the Toddler Period

Parental concerns of the toddler period usually arise because of a conflict over autonomy.

Toilet Training

Toilet training is one of the biggest tasks a toddler tries to achieve. There are so many theories concerning toilet training that understanding the procedure can become one of the biggest tasks of this period for parents. Most first-time parents ask when to start, when training should be completed, and how to go about it. The answer is that toilet training is an individualized task for each child. It should begin and be completed according to a child's ability to accomplish it, not according to a set schedule. In the United States, toilet training is usually introduced during the toddler period. Like so many other aspects of childrearing, though, the time when parents begin these activities is culturally determined. In other countries, toilet training may be started as soon as a child can sit, at about 6 months. Although praise is used in the United States as a common means of encouraging toddlers to learn new tasks, other cultures believe praise will bring a child harm by attracting evil spirits; strategies of shame or strict discipline are used instead. Being aware that childrearing practices are not consistent across the world is a help in understanding why parents approach childrearing problems differently and why childrearing advice must be individualized.

Before children can begin toilet training, they must have reached three important developmental levels, one physiologic and the other two cognitive:

- They must have control of rectal and urethral sphincters, usually achieved at the time they walk well.
- They must have a cognitive understanding of what it means to hold urine and stools until they can release them at a certain place and time.
- They must have a desire to delay immediate gratification for a more socially accepted action.

Because physiologic development is cephalocaudal, the rectal and urethral sphincters are not mature enough for control in most children until at least the end of the first year, when tracts of the spinal cord are myelinated to the anal level. A good way for a parent to know that a child's development has reached this point is to wait until the child can walk well independently.

Toilet training need not start this early, however, because cognitively and socially, many children do not understand what is being asked of them until they are 2 or even 3 years old. The markers of readiness are subtle, but as a rule children are ready for toilet training when they begin to be uncomfortable in wet diapers. They demonstrate this by pulling or tugging at soiled diapers; they may bring a parent a clean diaper after they have soiled so they can be changed (Fig. 30.7).

Teach parents not to underestimate the difficulty of the task they are expecting their child to achieve. Infants live by a pleasure principle: they want what they want when they want it. Before they can complete toilet training, they must be able to give up an immediate pleasure—relieving themselves whenever they have the urge—to gain other pleasure later on—improved physical comfort and another step in growing up. For specific tips on how to potty train a toddler, see Box 30.5.

Some toddlers smear or play with feces, often at about the same time that toilet training is started. This occurs because they have become aware of body excretions but have no adult values toward them; stools seem little different from the modeling clay they play with. This activity can be minimized by providing toddlers with play substances of similar texture and by changing diapers immediately after defecation. Teach parents to accept this behavior for what it is: enjoyment of the body and of the self, and the discovery of a new substance. After a child is fully toilet trained, this activity rarely persists.

Ritualistic Behavior

Although toddlers spend a great deal of time every day investigating new ways to do things and doing things they have never done before, they also enjoy ritualistic patterns. They will use only "their" spoon at mealtime, only "their" washcloth at bath time. They will not go outside unless mother or father locates their favorite cap.

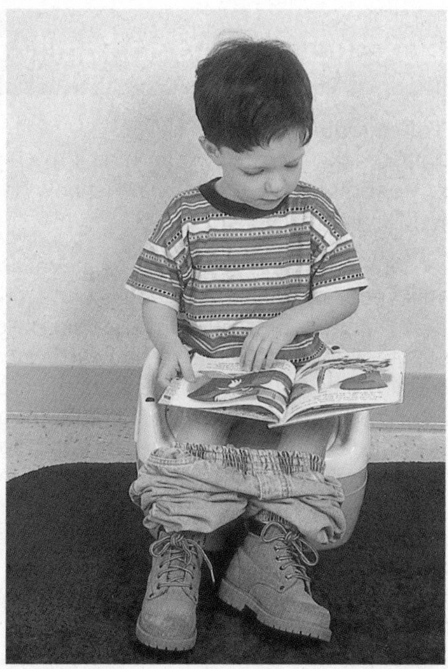

FIGURE 30.7 Toddlers are interested in toilet training as an expression of autonomy.

The child who seems to need an excessive number of objects to cling to or an excessive number of routines, however, may be trying to say, "I need more guidelines, more rules. Don't let me be quite so independent."

What if... Jason's mother tells you he is toilet-trained, but in the hospital he refuses to use a toilet? What would you do?

Negativism

As part of establishing their identities as separate individuals, toddlers typically go through a period of extreme negativism. They do not want to do anything a parent wants them to do. Their reply to every request is a very definite "no."

It is easy for parents to believe their authority is being questioned when this happens and to worry children are becoming so disrespectful they will have difficulty getting along in the world. They can be baffled by the extreme change from happy, cooperative infants who lived to please them to irritating, uncooperative toddlers. They may need some help to realize this is not only a normal phenomenon of toddlerhood but also a positive stage in development. This change indicates that toddlers have learned they are separate individuals with separate needs. It is important that toddlers do this if they are to grow up to be persons who are independent and able to take care of their own needs and desires.

Parents who went away from home for the first time to college or camp might remember they behaved similarly. They may recall they rarely slept or ate sensibly; they tried, in effect, to break every rule their parents used to enforce on them. Most regained their equilibrium in time to find a midpoint between irresponsible independence and common sense.

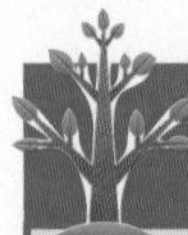

BOX 30.5 * Focus on Family Teaching

How to Toilet Train a Toddler

Q. Ms. Matthis asks you, "How can I tell if my 2-year-old is ready for potty training? And if he is, how do I start?"

A. Try the following suggestions:

1. Children are physically ready for toilet training when they walk securely. Plan 1 or 2 weeks of psychological "readiness" activities, which will help your child realize the task of toilet training is a step toward growing up. If your child feels toilet training is something only toddlers do, he may react with extreme negativism. Readiness activities may include showing your child that other family members use the toilet; making it clear that bigger people customarily leave urine and feces in the toilet, without suggesting that these materials are dirty or distasteful; and introducing training pants and showing your child that bigger people wear underpants too.
2. Check that training pants pull down readily and that slacks are free of complicated buttons or grippers; otherwise, your child will have accidents because he cannot undress quickly enough.
3. Purchase either a potty chair that sits on the floor or an infant seat that is placed on the regular toilet. The potty chair is low and potentially less frightening to a child, but it must be emptied and cleaned after each use. If you choose an infant seat, place a footstool in front of the toilet so your child has some support for his feet.
4. Put your child on the potty chair or toilet at regular intervals (e.g., when the child wakes up in the morning, after breakfast, during midmorning, before lunch, after lunch).
5. Praise your child if he does urinate or defecate. Remind him to wash his hands.
6. Be careful not to flush the toilet while the child is sitting on it. Two-year-old children are unable to realize they will not be flushed away and may become frightened. Encourage your child to flush the toilet independently after you have helped him get redressed.
7. Do not allow a child to remain on a potty chair for much longer than 10 minutes (less than that if he is resistant). Also, do not allow your child to use the chair to eat or as a play table, so he does not become confused regarding its purpose.
8. If your child is not ready or does not successfully use the potty on a day-to-day basis, have him return to diapers for a short period. Be careful not to make him feel as if this represents failure. Be careful not to equate "good" with being dry and "bad" with being wet. Continue with readiness activities. Reintroduce training pants and attempt toilet training again when your child seems more ready.
9. When boys have mastered defecation, it is time to include urination. Boys enjoy standing to urinate and aiming at objects in a toilet bowl, such as several pieces of breakfast cereal.
10. Some toddlers have difficulty remaining dry at night until they are 3 to 4 years old. Do not pressure your child to accomplish nighttime dryness, but assume that he is doing the best he can do. Put him into training pants for the night by explaining (not punitively) that it is hard to keep dry while he sleeps. After your child has been dry during the night for about 1 month, he has probably mastered nighttime dryness.
11. Do not wake your child during the night and carry him to the bathroom to void. This system may keep him dry during the night, but it does not help him stay dry for long periods. It may even prolong nighttime wetness, because it conditions him to void every 4 hours or so instead of retaining urine for 12 hours while he sleeps.

If parents can recall such circumstances, it helps them to understand this behavior in their toddler is not specific to the age but to the first feeling of independence. They can also remember they meant no vindictiveness by their behavior, so they can realize their child means none. This understanding can help to put the child's "no" into a better light.

Once it runs its course, extreme negativism passes. In the meantime, the more parents try to make children obey them, the more children are likely to resist. Some long-term parent–child interaction problems begin during this period because parents insist on being obeyed totally or are inconsistent in their approach.

A toddler's "no" can best be eliminated by limiting the number of questions asked of the child. A father does not really mean, for example, "Are you ready for dinner?" He means, "Come to the table. It's dinnertime." A mother asks, "Will you come take a bath now?" She means, "It's time for your bath." Making a statement instead of asking a question can avoid a great many negative responses.

A toddler needs experience in making choices, however. To provide the opportunity to do this, a parent could give a secondary choice. "No" is not allowed for the major task, so the parent states, "It's bath time now" but then says, "Do you want to take your duck or your toy boat into the tub with you?" Other examples are, "It's lunchtime. Do you want to use a big or little plate?" or "It's time to go shopping. Do you want to wear your jacket or your sweater?" Although this solution is simple, it is one that parents may not arrive at by themselves because finding a solution is always more difficult for a person in the middle of a problem than for an objective observer. Once they are helped to practice this approach, however, parents usually find it helpful in smoothing out the friction caused by the negativism of the toddler period (Box 30.6).

Discipline

Some parents ask during the last part of the infant year or the early toddler period when they should start to discipline their child or when toddlers are old enough to be punished. Remind parents that "discipline" and "punishment" are not interchangeable terms. **Discipline** means setting rules or

BOX 30.6 ✻ Focus on Communication

Ms. Matthis has brought her 2-year-old son, Jason, to the clinic for a health maintenance visit. Jason is rambunctious and uncooperative. Ms. Matthis is obviously frustrated.

Less Effective Communication

Nurse: Come on, Jason, sit quietly so I can hear your heartbeat.
Jason: No!
Ms. Matthis: Jason, listen to the nurse.
Jason: No!
Nurse: If you promise to sit still, I'll let you play with the stethoscope.
Jason: Okay.
Jason plays with the stethoscope.
Ms. Matthis: Jason, now it's time to give the stethoscope back to the nurse.
Jason: No.
Nurse: There are other children waiting to see me. I really must listen to your heart now.
Ms. Matthis takes the stethoscope from Jason. Jason starts crying.
Ms. Matthis: Jason, if you stop crying and sit still, I'll take you for ice cream on our way home.
Jason: (whimpering a bit) Okay.
Ms. Matthis: Sometimes he can be so difficult.
Nurse: Oh, those terrible twos!

More Effective Communication

Nurse: Jason, I need to listen to your heart so you must be very quiet. Would you rather sit quietly on the chair or the table?
Jason: The table.
Nurse: All right, Jason, jump up.
Jason climbs onto the table and starts to fidget.
Ms. Matthis: Jason, sit still for the nurse.
Jason: No!
Nurse: If you'd like, you can play with the stethoscope for a few seconds. Do you want to listen to your mom's heart or my heart?
Jason: Mom's.
Nurse: Great, now we will both be very quiet so you can hear.
Jason listens to his mother's heart.
Nurse: Good, now it's my turn.
Jason: Okay. (Jason hands back the stethoscope.)
Ms. Matthis: How did you get him to listen so well? At home he never listens. It can be so frustrating.
Nurse: Yes, this can be a frustrating period. By giving Jason choices, you can help him feel more in control without having to directly challenge your authority.

Toddlerhood can be a challenging and frustrating time for parents. You can teach parents effective communication skills to help toddlers assert their independence, while allowing parents to maintain discipline. It is important to show parents that offering choices rather than bribes is a far more effective and long-lasting method of modifying a toddler's behavior. In the first scenario, the nurse and mother both bribe Jason. Jason finally does what they want, but the situation is still frustrating, and his behavior change will not likely be long-lasting. In the second scenario, the nurse demonstrates how to better communicate by offering choices. The situation is much more enjoyable for everyone.

road signs so children know what is expected of them. **Punishment** is a consequence that results from a breakdown in discipline, from the child's disregard of the rules that were learned.

Parents should begin to instill some sense of discipline early in life because part of it involves setting safety limits and protecting others or property: for example, a child must stay away from the fireplace or heater; she must not go into the street; she must not hit other children. Enforcing limits, however, arises out of the day-to-day interaction with the child, out of the rhythm of child care, not out of a set procedure such as, "Today, I'm going to teach discipline." Two general rules to follow are (a) parents need to be consistent and (b) rules are learned best if correct behavior is praised rather than wrong behavior punished.

"Timeout" is a technique to help children learn that actions have consequences. To use "timeout" effectively, parents first need to be certain their child understands the rule they are trying to enforce: for instance, "If you hit your brother, you'll have timeout." Parents should give one warning. If the child repeats the behavior, parents select an area that is nonstimulating, such as a corner of a room or a hallway. The child is directed to go immediately to the "timeout" space. The child then sits there for a specified period of time. If the child cries or shows any other disruptive behavior, the timeout period does not begin until there is quiet. When the specified time period has passed, the child can return to the family. A guide regarding how long children should remain in their "timeout" chair is 1 minute per year of age. Using a timer that rings when time is up lets children know when they can return to the family.

Separation Anxiety

As discussed in Chapter 29, fear of being separated from parents begins at about 6 months of age and persists throughout the preschool period. This universal fear of this age group is known as *separation anxiety*. For this reason, toddlers have difficulty accepting being separated from their primary caregiver to spend the day at a day care center or if they or their primary caregiver is hospitalized. Chapter 36 discusses nursing responsibility for care of toddlers in the hospital as well as the reactions of toddlers to the separation caused by hospitalization and the methods used to minimize these reactions.

Parents may ask what they can do about this problem. They believe they have a right to leave their child in a babysitter's or center's care, but how can they tolerate the crying at the door? Most toddlers react best to separation if a regular babysitter is employed or the day care center is one with consistent caregivers. Many are more comfortable if they are cared for in their own home. It helps if they have fair warning that they will have a babysitter. For example, they could be told, "Mommy is fixing dinner early because Mommy and Daddy are going to visit some friends tonight. Marsha is going to come and babysit for you. She'll put you to bed. When you wake up in the morning, Mommy and Daddy will be here again."

No matter how well prepared toddlers are, they may cry when the babysitter actually appears or may greet the babysitter warmly only to cry when the parents reach for their coats. It helps if parents say goodbye firmly, repeat the explanation they will be there when the child wakes in the morning, and then leave. Prolonged goodbyes only lead to more crying. Sneaking out prevents crying and may ease the parents' guilt, but it can strengthen fear of abandonment so should be discouraged. This applies to hospital visits as well.

✔ Checkpoint Question 30.2

Jason answers every request of his mother by saying, "No!" How would you suggest she minimize this?

a. Tell Jason she does not want him to say "No" anymore.
b. Answer all Jason's questions by saying, "No!"
c. Reduce the number of questions she asks Jason.
d. Explain he is not using good communication skills.

Temper Tantrums

Almost every toddler has a temper tantrum at one time or another. The child may kick, scream, stamp feet, shout "No, no, no," lie on the floor, flail arms and legs, and bang the head against the floor. Children may even hold their breath until they become cyanotic. If breath holding, the child develops a distended chest (a halt after inspiration), often air-filled cheeks, and increasing distress as the child's body registers oxygen want. This is harmless breath holding; ignoring it will make it ineffective and the child will give it up. True breath holding is a neurologic problem in which children, under stress, appear to "forget" to breathe in or halt breathing after expiration, usually at the peak of anger. They become so short of breath that they slump to the floor. Breath holding can be mistaken for seizures because of the fall to the floor (see Chapter 49). Guidelines that are helpful in differentiating simple breath holding from neurologic disorders are shown in Table 30.5.

Temper tantrums occur as a natural consequence of toddlers' development (Taylor, 2007). They occur because toddlers are independent enough to know what they want, but they do not have the vocabulary or the wisdom to express their feelings in a more socially acceptable way. For example, temper tantrums occur most often when children are tired, just before naptime or bedtime, or during a long shopping trip or visit. Tantrums may be a response to an unrealistic request by a parent: asking children to comb their hair before they are coordinated enough to do so, asking them to pick up toys before they have a feeling of family responsibility, or asking them to share before they can understand what that means. Also, tantrums may occur if parents are saying "no" too frequently in regard to such things as touching the coffee table, getting dirty, using a spoon, or running and jumping so that children feel constantly thwarted. A tantrum may be a response to difficulty making choices or decisions or to pressure from activities such as toilet training. Such children need to express feelings in some way and do so with temper tantrums. These episodes are taxing for the parents; they are also energy-consuming for children.

Box 30.7 offers suggestions for managing temper tantrums. Probably the best approach is for parents to tell a child simply that they disapprove of the tantrum and then ignore it. They might say, "I'll be in the bedroom. When you're done kicking, you come into the bedroom, too." Children who are left alone in a room this way will usually not continue a tantrum but will stop after 1 or 2 minutes and rejoin their parents. Parents should then accept the child warmly and proceed as if the tantrum had not occurred. This same approach works well for nurses caring for hospitalized toddlers.

Nursing Diagnoses and Related Interventions

Nursing Diagnosis: Risk for compromised family coping related to toddler behavior

Outcome Evaluation: Family states temper tantrums now occur less than two times daily.

Helping parents correct problems early may limit the number of tantrums they must deal with; it will not prevent them, however, because parents cannot anticipate all the circumstances that will cause this reaction. In fact, parents should not feel they must prevent all of them; they are, after all, parents, not mind readers (see Focus on Nursing Care Planning Box 30.8). As the child matures, increases in vocabulary, and is capable of better responses to stress situations, tantrums begin to fade by themselves.

TABLE 30.5 ✱ Differentiating Temper Tantrums, Breath Holding, and Seizures

Assessment	Temper Tantrums	Breath Holding	Seizures
Provocation	Usually provoked—parent can state a reason for it (she asked toddler to come to dinner, toddler wanted to finish an activity)	Usually provoked; child very angry; child breathes out and forgets to breathe in	Not provoked
Appearance of cyanosis	Child holds breath, becomes cyanotic, then slumps to floor	Child breathes out, becomes cyanotic, then slumps to floor	Child slumps to floor first, then becomes cyanotic

BOX 30.7 ✻ Focus on Family Teaching

Managing Toddler's Temper Tantrums

Q. Suppose Jason's mother tells you, "I've had it with temper tantrums. I can't stand to watch another one."

A. Here are suggestions to prevent them:

Try to determine the reason for the behavior:

- Do tantrums always occur just before bedtime? If so, you might schedule an earlier bedtime or an afternoon nap.
- Do tantrums occur every time you go shopping? If so, perhaps it would help to schedule two shorter trips each week rather than one long one.
- Do tantrums occur whenever you ask the child to do something? If so, is the child being asked to perform tasks not age-appropriate?
- Do tantrums occur in response to not being able to make a decision? If so, you may have to limit the number of choices you are asking of the child.

Next, be certain it seems like a tantrum, not something more:

- Is there a possibility you are mistaking seizure activity for temper tantrums?
- Could you be confusing neurologic breath holding with a temper tantrum?

Lastly, think through what you do when the child has a tantrum:

- Do you give either material or emotional bribes (e.g., "Come and get a cookie," or "Stop and I'll give you a kiss")? This method is rarely effective because by acceding to the child's wishes, you are encouraging your child to have more tantrums because they are so successful.
- Do you punish the child? Toddlers have a right to express opinions; they just need to be guided to learn a more controlled and mature way of doing that.
- Do you demonstrate adult behavior in managing temper tantrums? For example, if the child shouts or kicks, do you respond, "I can shout as loud as you. I can kick as hard as you"? Instead of showing the child a better way to express feelings, this reinforces the way the child is responding.

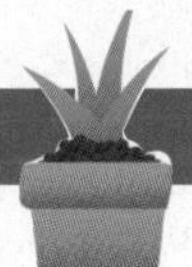

BOX 30.8 ✻ Focus on Nursing Care Planning

A Multidisciplinary Care Map for a Toddler With Temper Tantrums

Jason is a 2½-year-old boy you see at a pediatric clinic. His mother tells you he has changed completely in the past 6 months from an easy-to-care-for baby into a "monster" who refuses to do anything she asks. The only word he says anymore is "no." He has a temper tantrum every night at dinner over some type of food. She tells you this has changed parenting from "fun" to "a real chore."

Family Assessment ✻ Child lives with two parents in three-bedroom home. Father is a ferry boat captain; works 6 days a week. Mother works as a secretary at local university. Finances are "Good. We've worked hard to get where we are."

Client Assessment ✻ Well-nourished 2-year-old boy. Physical findings within normal limits. Mother reports the child is having temper tantrums "at least 20 times a day. He throws himself on the floor and pounds his head and fists." Mother unable to describe any precipitating factors for the tantrums. She states, "He seems to have them just when I start to do something. I could be playing with him one minute, and then I get up to do something, like answer the phone or start dinner, and he starts." Mother reports picking up the child immediately because she fears he will hurt himself. "I just don't know what to do anymore."

Nursing Diagnosis ✻ Health-seeking behaviors related to measures for dealing with and reducing the number of temper tantrums.

Outcome Criteria ✻ Mother describes measures to manage tantrums; reports tantrums have decreased to fewer than 4 a day by end of 1 week.

Team Member Responsible	Assessment	Intervention	Rationale	Expected Outcome
		Activities of Daily Living		
Nurse	Ask mother to describe a typical day and to document when tantrums occur and situations that seem to provoke them.	Make suggestions to eliminate periods of stress as revealed by assessment.	Temper tantrums can increase with stress and inability of child to feel independent.	Mother reviews a typical day and identifies times when tantrums are most apt to occur.

(continued)

BOX 30.8 ✻ Focus on Nursing Care Planning (continued)

Consultations				
Physician	Assess if child has possible neurologic symptoms.	Refer child for full neurologic workup if physical exam suggests the need.	Temper tantrums can be confused with seizures if a careful history is not taken.	Mother agrees to further neurologic testing if suggested.
Procedures/Medications				
Nurse/nurse practitioner	Assess what measures mother thinks would prevent temper tantrums best.	Work with the mother to develop actions (e.g., ignoring the tantrum, telling child she disapproves of behavior). Encourage mother not to pick up child unless there is actual danger of injury.	Temper tantrums are a way of expressing frustration. Rewarding the behavior prevents the child from learning more mature methods of coping with frustration.	Mother voices agreement to try suggested solutions and to telephone clinic in 5 days if there is no improvement.
Nutrition				
Nurse practitioner	Assess if child appears well nourished; assess usual dietary pattern.	As eating is a time when tantrums occur, review with mother if her actions are different at this time than others.	Eating is an area in which children can express independence.	Mother lists foods that allow child independent eating, which she will try to serve, to keep meals tantrum-free.
Patient/Family Education				
Nurse	Assess mother's knowledge of toddler behavior and temper tantrums.	Review normal toddler growth and development, explaining some temper tantrums during this period are natural occurrences.	Information about normal toddler growth and development provides a foundation for further teaching and instruction.	Mother states she understands that tantrums occur because of toddler's limited capabilities to express emotion.
Nurse	Assess why mother is so fearful child will hurt himself during a tantrum.	Inform the mother children rarely hurt themselves during tantrums.	Increased knowledge about the minimal risk of injury during tantrums should help to alleviate the mother's anxiety.	Mother states she has increased understanding about the danger of tantrums.
Psychosocial/Spiritual/Emotional Needs				
Nurse/nurse practitioner	Assess what mother feels would be most helpful to relieve her degree of stress and frustration.	Suggest she arrange for "time out" breaks for herself by having husband or friend relieve her.	Short periods away from the child can allow her to regroup her thinking.	Mother describes a plan by which she can receive more help with child care from friend, as husband is home only 1 day a week.
Discharge Planning				
Nurse/nurse practitioner	Review with mother the plan for added support and interventions.	Instruct the mother to keep a diary of the child's behavior and measures used during the next week. Set up an appointment for a telephone conference with the mother next week to review the diary and discuss the child's behavior.	Keeping a diary and reviewing it over the telephone aids in evaluating the child's behavior and the effectiveness of the methods used. Follow-up telephone call also provides an additional opportunity for feedback, teaching, and support.	Mother states she will follow suggestions for managing tantrums; will keep telephone and clinic appointments for follow-up care.

What if... Jason, whom you are caring for in the hospital, has a temper tantrum in the middle of a busy hallway? Would you ignore it or move him to a quieter place?

Concerns of the Family With a Physically Challenged or Chronically Ill Toddler

It may be difficult for children with handicaps or disabilities to achieve a sense of autonomy or independence because they may never be totally independent. It is important for these children to develop as strong a sense of autonomy as possible, though, so they see themselves as independent and can work to become increasingly self-sufficient as they grow older. It takes courage for an adult to do such things as move a wheelchair through a busy airport or a concert crowd. Nursing actions designed to help the challenged or chronically ill child develop a sense of autonomy are outlined in Table 30.6. Most important are actions that allow toddlers to do as much for themselves as possible. If toddlers have physical limitations, for example, they may be unable to explore freely or may not have the physical ability to pound and manipulate toys as the average toddler does. They do have the ability to work at a project while they sit in a chair at a table.

A toddler with a long-term illness or who is physically challenged can be expected to exhibit normal toddler behaviors, such as temper tantrums, and to have normal outlooks, such as negativism. Parents whose child is uncoordinated or has a neurologic disease may mistake temper tantrums for seizure activity. Investigate such activity carefully, and explain to parents the difference between the two. Parents may also mistake particular toddlers' insistence on having their own way as a manifestation of illness. Remind these parents the behavior is more often an indication of age and development rather than of illness so they can respond appropriately.

Toilet training is difficult for a child who is hospitalized at periodic intervals, as success usually requires a consistent caregiver; in addition, hospitalization can result in regressive behaviors. If a chronically ill child has difficulty with ambulation, soiling accidents may occur beyond the usual age because of inability to reach a bathroom easily.

Children who survive a long-term illness are sometimes referred to as medically fragile or vulnerable children (Green & Solnit, 1964). Some parents tend to protect and shelter such a child, and you may have to remind them even though

TABLE 30.6 * Nursing Interventions to Help a Physically Challenged or Chronically Ill Child Develop a Sense of Autonomy

Area	Nursing Action
Nutrition	A special diet may limit typical finger foods. Use imagination to offer other foods not usually eaten this way as finger foods. Allow child to help pour liquid diet for a tube feeding. Toddlers are frightened by vomiting because they have no control over it. Check for possibility of nausea; toddlers have no way to express this other than by not eating.
Dressing changes	A child can hold pieces of tape or put tape in place to maintain sense of control. The child can remove an old bandage if it is not contaminated. Allow children to view their incisions and watch dressing changes; explaining each step of a procedure as you perform it helps a child maintain control. Restrain only those body parts necessary during a procedure to allow a child a sense of control. Remove all supplies after a procedure, or the child may "redo" the dressing.
Medication	Allow children no choice regarding whether a medicine will be taken. Do allow a child to choose a "chaser," such as milk or juice, after oral medicine. Do not ask a toddler to indicate a choice of site for an injection or intravenous insertion; this is too advanced a decision for a toddler to handle.
Rest	Locate or create a ritual for bedtime (put child into bed, tuck him in, say, "Goodnight, Bobby." Tuck in bear. Say, "Goodnight, Bear"). Allow a choice of toy or cover but not a choice of bedtime or naptime hour.
Hygiene	Allow a child a choice of bathtub toy or clothing. Allow a child to wash face and hands to gain control of the situation. Allow the child to put toothpaste on a brush, but you should brush or "touch up" teeth afterward to ensure that all plaque has been removed.
Pain	Encourage a child to express pain ("Say 'ouch' when I pull off the tape"). Help channel a child's self-expression to what is acceptable (e.g., the child may shout but may not kick).
Stimulation	Provide a toddler with a toy that can be manipulated, such as boxes that fit inside one another and can be taken out again, trucks that can be pushed, and pegs that can be pounded. In a health care setting, items can usually be found that fit together (boxes from central supply or plastic vials from the pharmacy). Another action toy: buy a non-latex balloon and tie it to the crib side to be used as a punching bag; another one tied to the foot of the crib can serve as a leg exerciser.
Elimination	A child who is toilet trained needs to be encouraged to use a potty chair or toilet during an illness. Help children with ureter or bowel stomas to help with changing bags so they are as independent in bowel function as possible.

chronically ill, a toddler will demand independence and has the right to explore. A child who uses a lower-extremity prosthesis, for example, might prefer to crawl somewhere rather than wait for help to put the prosthesis in place. Although this degree of independence is good, parents may have to limit how it is expressed so the child will learn how to use the prosthesis (for example, they could make a rule the child must use the prosthesis to walk but can choose whether to use a spoon when eating).

Nutrition and the Physically Challenged or Chronically Ill Toddler

Toddlers need experience feeding themselves if at all possible. Help parents accept the accidents that occur with self-feeding, particularly if the child has difficulty with coordination; suggest finger foods if possible.

If on a special diet, children may not be allowed to eat finger foods; if they are tube fed, they receive no experience with finger foods at all. For these toddlers, parents should try to provide other, comparable experiences in independence, such as letting them choose what toy to take to bed.

✔ Checkpoint Question 30.3

Jason's mother uses "timeout" for punishment. What is a good rule for this?

a. The child should sit still for as many minutes as his age.
b. The child should sit still for as many minutes as he misbehaved.
c. Timeout activities can include quiet play or reading books.
d. Children are not ready for timeout until school age.

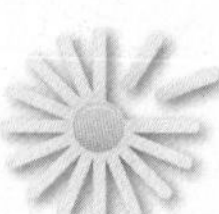

Key Points for Review

- Erikson's developmental task for the toddler period is to form a sense of autonomy or independence versus shame or doubt.
- Toddlers make great strides forward in development, but their physical growth slows.
- A critical milestone of toddler development is being able to form two-word sentences (a noun and a verb) by 2 years of age.
- Toddlers are capable of preoperational thought or are able to deal much more constructively with symbols than they could while infants.
- Important aspects of care are promoting toddler safety, including screening for lead poisoning; promoting toddler development, such as promoting daily activities; and healthy family functioning.
- Toddler appetites decrease from those of the infant, so children eat proportionally less than they did as infants.
- Common concerns of parents during the toddler period are toilet training, ritualistic behavior, negativism, temper tantrums, discipline, and separation anxiety.
- Promoting autonomy in the child who is physically challenged or chronically ill calls for creative planning, because there may be many tasks that must be done for the child to be certain they are done safely.

CRITICAL THINKING EXERCISES

1. Jason is the toddler you met at the beginning of the chapter. His mother tells you he refuses to do anything she tells him to do. What are three questions you would want to ask his mother to help her explore the problem?
2. Jason's father tells you Jason eats "almost nothing." What is the best way to evaluate if a child's intake is adequate? Why does the intake of toddlers decrease from what it was during the infant year?
3. Because his parents both work, Jason is cared for in the morning by his grandmother, a child care teacher in the afternoon, and his parents in the evening. What suggestions could you offer to make toilet training easier with multiple caregivers?
4. Examine the National Health Goals related to growth and development of the toddler. Most government-sponsored funds for nursing research are allotted based on these goals. What would be a possible research topic to explore pertinent to these goals that would be applicable to Jason's family and also advance evidence-based practice?

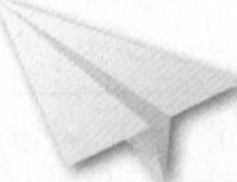

CRITICAL THINKING SCENARIO

Open the accompanying CD-ROM and read the Patient Scenario included for this chapter, then answer the questions to further sharpen your skills and grow more familiar with NCLEX types of questions related to toddler growth and development. Confirm your answers are correct by reading the rationales.

REFERENCES

American Academy of Pediatrics (AAP) Committee on Practice and Ambulatory Medicine. (2009). *Recommendations for preventive pediatric health care.* Washington, DC: Author.

American Academy of Pediatrics. (2009). Car safety seats: a guide for families. Retrieved from http://www.aap.org/family/carseatguide.htm.

Armfield, J. M., & Spencer, A. J. (2007). Community effectiveness of fissure sealants and the effect of fluoridated water consumption. *Community Dental Health, 24*(1), 4–11.

Brown, M.J. (2008). Childhood lead poisoning prevention: getting the job done by 2010. *Journal of Environmental Health, 70*(6), 56–57.

Centers for Disease Control and Prevention (CDC). (2008). *Lead poisoning prevention program.* Atlanta, GA: Author.

Chen, A., et al. (2007). Lead exposure, IQ, and behavior in urban 5- to 7-year-olds: does lead affect behavior only by lowering IQ? *Pediatrics, 119*(3), e650–658.

Dart, R. C., & Rumack, B. H. (2008). Poisoning. In W. W. Hay, et al. (Eds.). *Current pediatric diagnosis and treatment* (18th ed.). Columbus, OH: McGraw-Hill.

Dutta, S., & Barzin, A. (2008). Multiple magnet ingestion as a source of severe gastrointestinal complications requiring surgical intervention. *Archives of Pediatrics and Adolescent Medicine, 162*(2), 123–125.

Erikson, E. H. (1993). *Childhood and society.* New York: W. W. Norton.

Goldson, E., & Reynolds, A. (2008). Child development and behavior. In W. W. Hay, et al. (Eds.). *Current pediatric diagnosis and treatment* (18th ed.). Columbus, OH: McGraw-Hill.

Gonsalves, W. (2008). Oral health. In J. E. South-Paul, S. C. Matheny, & E. L. Lewis (Eds.). *Current diagnosis and treatment in family medicine.* (2nd ed.). Columbus, OH: McGraw-Hill.

Green, M., & Solnit, A. (1964). Reactions to the threatened loss of a child: a vulnerable child syndrome. *Pediatrics, 34*(1), 58–64.

Johnson, C. P. (2008). Recognition of autism before age 2 years. *Pediatrics in Review, 29*(3), 86–96.

Keefe, S. (2007). Heavy burden. *Advance for Nurses, 4*(23), 31.

Krebs, N. F., & Primak, L. E. (2008). Normal childhood nutrition and its disorders. In W. W. Hay, et al. (Eds.). *Current pediatric diagnosis and treatment* (18th ed.). Columbus, OH: McGraw-Hill.

Mueller, W. A. (2008). Oral medicine and dentistry. In W. W. Hay, et al. (Eds.). *Current pediatric diagnosis and treatment* (18th ed.). Columbus, OH: McGraw-Hill.

Myers, R. P., Li, B., & Shaheen, A. A. M. (2007). Emergency department visits for acetaminophen overdose: a Canadian population-based epidemiologic study (1997–2002). *CJEM: Canadian Journal of Emergency Medical Care, 9*(4), 267–274.

Panpanich, R., & Garner, P. (2009). Growth monitoring in children. *Cochrane Database of Systematic Reviews, 2009*(1), (CD001443).

Petit, D., et al. (2007). Dyssomnias and parasomnias in early childhood. *Pediatrics, 119*(5), e1016–e1025.

Piaget, J. (1969). *The theory of stages in cognitive development.* New York: McGraw-Hill.

Ring, L. M. (2007). Kids and hot liquids—a burning reality. *Journal of Pediatric Health Care, 21*(3), 192–194.

Rolfes, S. R., Pinna, K., & Whitney, E. N. (2009). *Understanding normal and clinical nutrition.* New York: Wadsworth/Cengage Learning.

Sakimura, J. N., et al. (2008). Cognitive and temperament clusters in 3- to 5-year-old children with aggressive behavior. *Journal of School Health, 78*(1), 38–45.

Taylor, T. (2007). Managing unwanted behaviour in pre-school children. *Community Practitioner, 80*(4), 30–35.

Theobald, H. (2007). Childhood nutrition. *Journal of Community Nursing, 21*(2), 25–28.

Thompson, D. C., & Rivara, F. P. (2009). Pool fencing for preventing drowning in children. *Cochrane Database of Systematic Reviews, 2009*(1), (CD001047).

U.S. Department of Agriculture (USDA). (2005). *Nutrition and your health: dietary guidelines for Americans.* Hyattsville, MD: Author.

Ward, T. M., Rankin, S., & Lee, K. A. (2007). Caring for children with sleep problems. *Journal of Pediatric Nursing: Nursing Care of Children and Families, 22*(4), 283–296.

Williamson, C. (2007). Nutrition for toddlers: practical advice to give parents. *The Journal of Family Health Care, 17*(1), 19–22.

SUGGESTED READINGS

Darbyshire, P. (2007). 'Childhood': are reports of its death greatly exaggerated? *Journal of Child Health Care, 11*(2), 85–97.

Dooley, M., & Stewart, J. (2007). Family income, parenting styles and child behavioural-emotional outcomes. *Health Economics, 16*(2), 145–162.

Lewis, C. W., et al. (2007). Preventive dental care for children in the United States: a national perspective. *Pediatrics, 119*(3), e544–e553.

Morin, K. H. (2007). Toddlers: start off on the right foot. *MCN: The American Journal of Maternal/Child Nursing, 32*(2), 122.

Needham, L., et al. (2007). Supporting healthy eating among preschoolers: challenges for child care staff. *Canadian Journal of Dietetic Practice and Research, 68*(2), 107–110.

Talen, M. R., et al. (2007). Well-child check-up revised: an efficient protocol for assessing children's social-emotional development. *Families, Systems and Health, 25*(1), 23–35.

Wagner, S. (2007). Knowledge of normal development key in diagnosis. *Patient Education Management, 14*(8), 89–90.

Yost, J., & Li, Y. (2008). Promoting oral health from birth through childhood: prevention of early childhood caries. *MCN: American Journal of Maternal Child Nursing, 33*(1), 17–23.

Zierold, K. M., Havlena, J., & Anderson, H. (2007). Exposure to lead and length of time needed to make homes lead-safe for young children. *American Journal of Public Health, 97*(2), 267–270.

Zoritch, B., Roberts, I., & Oakley, A. (2009). Day care for pre-school children. *Cochrane Database of Systematic Reviews, 2009*(1), (CD000564).

Chapter 31 Nursing Care of a Family With a Preschool Child

KEY TERMS

- broken fluency
- bruxism
- conservation
- ectomorphic body type
- Electra complex
- endomorphic body type
- genu valgus
- intuitional thought
- Oedipus complex
- secondary stuttering

OBJECTIVES

After mastering the contents of this chapter, you should be able to:

1. Describe normal growth and development as well as common parental concerns of the preschool period.
2. Identify National Health Goals related to the preschool period that nurses can help the nation achieve.
3. Use critical thinking to analyze methods of care for preschoolers to be certain care is family centered.
4. Assess a preschooler for normal growth and developmental milestones.
5. Formulate nursing diagnoses related to preschool growth and development and common parental concerns.
6. Identify expected outcomes for nursing care of a preschooler.
7. Plan nursing care to meet a preschooler's growth and development needs, such as planning age-appropriate play activities.
8. Implement nursing care related to normal growth and development of a preschooler, such as preparing a preschooler for an invasive procedure.
9. Evaluate expected outcomes for achievement and effectiveness of care.
10. Identify areas related to care of the preschool-age child that could benefit from additional nursing research or application of evidence-based practice.
11. Integrate knowledge of preschool growth and development with nursing process to achieve quality maternal and child health nursing care.

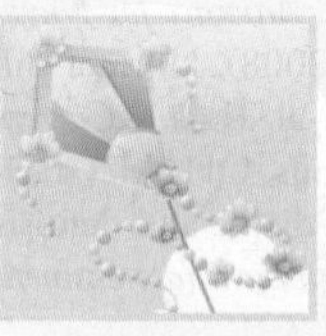

Cathy Edwards is a 3-year-old girl. Her father cares for her because her mother is hospitalized as a result of preterm labor for a second pregnancy. Her father tells you he is concerned because Cathy talks constantly with an imaginary friend named Emma. She makes up stories about events that cannot possibly be true. When corrected, Cathy stutters so badly no one can understand her.

The previous chapter described toddler growth and development and the abilities children develop during that period. This chapter adds information about the changes, both physical and psychosocial, that occur during the preschool years. Such information builds a base for care and health teaching for the age group.

Is Cathy's father describing typical preschool behavior, or does Cathy need a referral to a child guidance counselor?

The preschool period traditionally includes ages 3 to 6 years. Although physical growth slows considerably during this period, personality and cognitive growth continue at a rapid rate. This is also an important period of growth for parents. They may be unsure about how much independence and responsibility for self-care they should allow their preschooler. Most children of this age want to do things for themselves—choose their own clothing and dress by themselves, feed themselves completely, wash their own hair, and so forth. As a result, parents of a preschooler may find their child dressed in one red sock and one green sock, going to preschool with unwashed ears, or trying to eat soup with a fork. They need reassurance that this behavior is typical as it is the way that children adjust to new experiences. Parents may also need some guidance in separating those tasks a preschooler can accomplish independently from those that still require some adult supervision so they can set sensible limits. Setting limits this way protects children from harming themselves or others while participating in all the interesting experiences available to them (Thompson & Rivera, 2009). Box 31.1 lists National Health Goals related to the period.

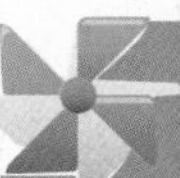

BOX 31.1 * Focus on National Health Goals

A number of National Health Goals are designed to target the preschool population:

- Increase the number of states with laws requiring helmets for bicycle riders under 15 years of age from a baseline of 10 states to 50 states.
- Reduce infectious diarrhea by at least 25% among children in licensed child care centers.
- Reduce acute middle ear infections among children age 4 and younger from a baseline of 344.7 health care visits per 1000 children to 294 visits per 1000 children.
- Increase the rate of use of child auto restraints among children age 4 and younger from a baseline of 92% to 100%.
- Reduce the proportion of children 2 to 4 years of age who have dental caries in their primary or permanent teeth from a baseline of 18% to 11%.
- Reduce the rate of deaths caused by poisoning from a baseline of 6.8 per 100,000 to 1.5 per 100,000 (http://www.nih.gov).

Nurses can help the nation achieve these goals by serving as consultants at day care and preschool settings to be certain that protection from the spread of infectious diseases in these settings is provided and by urging parents to protect against poisoning and to fit their children with helmets before beginning bicycle riding.

A number of questions could benefit from additional nursing research, such as: What practices seem most effective in reducing the spread of infection in day care or preschool settings? What are the barriers to parents buying helmets for this age child? What proportion of parents know the signs and symptoms of common illnesses their child might contract in a child care or preschool setting?

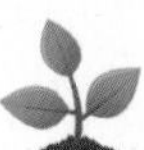

Nursing Process Overview

For Healthy Development of the Preschooler

Assessment

Regular assessment of a preschooler includes obtaining a health history and performing both a physical and developmental evaluation. Preschoolers speak very little during a health assessment; they may even revert to baby talk or babyish actions such as thumb-sucking if they find a health visit stressful. A history that details their usual performance level is therefore very important for accurate evaluation.

Assess a child's weight and height according to standard growth charts (see Appendix E). Keep in mind these charts are based on average weights and heights of white American children, so those for children from other ethnic or cultural backgrounds may not completely agree with these norms. Also assess a child for general appearance. Does the child appear alert? Happy? Active? Healthy? Ask whether a child can play actively without becoming exhausted. Assess the teeth for presence of cavities. Evaluate for a symmetrical gait. As preschoolers develop frequent upper respiratory infections (the average preschooler may have 6 to 12 a year), assess for these as well.

Nursing Diagnosis

Nursing diagnoses for preschoolers typically concern health promotion. Examples are:

- Health-seeking behaviors related to developmental expectations
- Readiness for enhanced parenting related to parent's pride in child

Other nursing diagnoses include:

- Risk for injury related to increased independence outside the home
- Delayed growth and development related to frequent illness
- Risk for poisoning related to maturational age of child
- Parental anxiety related to lack of understanding of childhood development
- Imbalanced nutrition related to child's many food dislikes

Outcome Identification and Planning

For many parents, preschool is a difficult time because a child is at an in-between stage: no longer an infant, although not yet ready for formal school. Planning and establishing expected outcomes for care of the preschooler often begin with establishing a schedule for discussing normal preschool development with the parents (this should be done at all health maintenance visits). Planning for accident prevention such as how to cross streets safely becomes increasingly important as children begin to enjoy experiences away from home. It is important to plan opportunities for adventurous activities or messy play. When asking parents to incorporate adventurous activities or messy material into a preschooler's play, you may be asking them to do something they do not personally enjoy. Most parents do initiate these activities with their child if they believe they are important, but some are able to do this better than others. Allowing children choices may also be difficult for parents because they want to protect them from making errors. Helpful Web sites about growth and development to recommend are the BabyCenter (http://www.Babycenter.com) and Dr. Greene (http://www.DrGreene.com). Helpful Web sites to alert parents about safety are the American Association of Poison Control Centers (http://www.aapcc.org) and the American Academy of Pediatrics (http://www.aap.org). For questions about car seats, parents can consult the U.S. Department of Transportation National Highway Traffic Safety Administration (http://www.nhtsa.dot.gov). The national 800 telephone number for a poison control center is 1-800-222-1222.

Implementation

Preschool children imitate moods as well as actions. An important nursing intervention, then, is role playing a mood or attitude you would like a child to learn. To project an attitude that health assessment is an enjoyable activity, you might suggest preschoolers participate by listening to their heart or coloring the table paper. Accident prevention is also best taught by role modeling (a parent always crosses streets at the corner and does not start the car until seatbelts are in place).

Outcome Evaluation

Evaluation of expected outcomes needs to be continuous and frequent. Because growth during this period is more cognitive and emotional than physical, parents may report little growth. Evaluating specific areas helps them to see that progress has occurred. Examples of expected outcomes might be:

- Child states importance of holding parent's hand while crossing streets.
- Parent states realistic expectations of 3-year-old's motor ability by next visit.
- Mother reports she has prepared 4-year-old for new baby by next visit.

GROWTH AND DEVELOPMENT OF A PRESCHOOLER

Assessment of preschoolers needs to include physical, cognitive, and developmental growth (Box 31.2).

Physical Growth

A definite change in body contour occurs during the preschool years. The wide-legged gait, prominent lordosis, and protuberant abdomen of the toddler change to slimmer, taller, and much more childlike proportions. Contour changes are so definite that future body type—**ectomorphic** (slim) or **endomorphic** (large)—becomes apparent. Handedness begins to be obvious. A major step forward is a child's ability to learn extended language, which is achieved not only by motor but also by cognitive development. Children of this age who are exposed to more than one language or who live in a bilingual family have a unique opportunity to master two languages with relative ease because of this increased cognitive ability.

Box 31.2 Assessment

Assessing the Average Preschooler

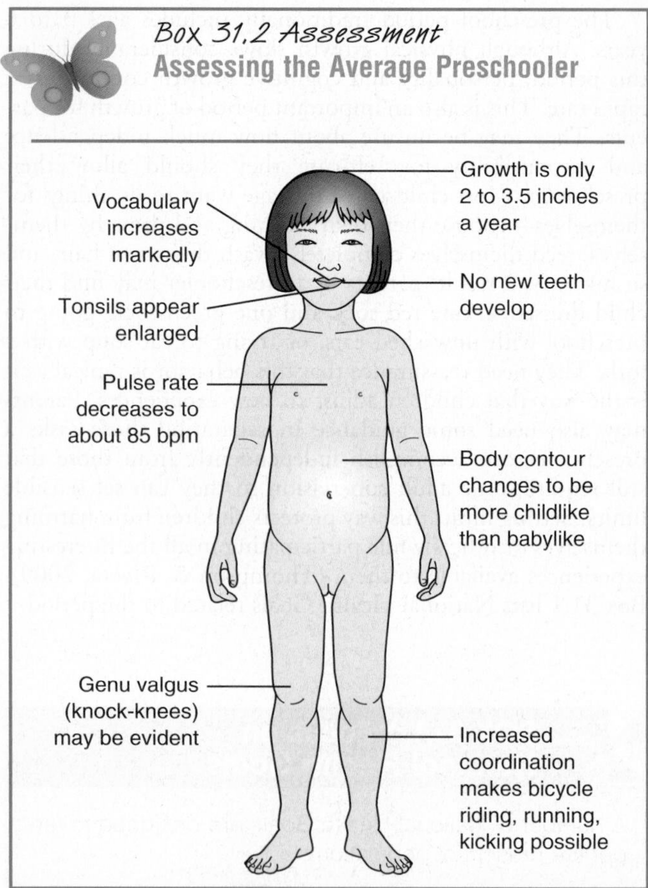

Lymphatic tissue begins to increase in size, particularly the tonsils, and levels of IgG and IgA antibodies increase. These changes tend to make preschool illnesses more localized (an upper respiratory infection remains localized to the nose with little systemic fever).

Physiologic splitting of heart sounds may be present for the first time on auscultation; innocent heart murmurs may also be heard for the first time. This type of murmur occurs because of the changing size of the heart in reference to the thorax as the anteroposterior and transverse diameters of the chest reach adult proportions. Pulse rate decreases to about 85 beats per minute; blood pressure holds at about 100/60 mm Hg.

The bladder is easily palpable above the symphysis pubis; voiding is frequent enough (9 or 10 times a day) that play must be interrupted, and accidents may occur if a child becomes absorbed in an activity.

A child who earlier in life had an indeterminate longitudinal arch in the foot generally demonstrates a well-formed arch now. Muscles are noticeably stronger and make activities such as gymnastics possible. Many children at the beginning of the period exhibit **genu valgus** (knock-knees); this disappears with increased skeletal growth at the end of the preschool period.

Weight, Height, and Head Circumference

Weight gain is slight during the preschool years: the average child gains only about 4.5 lb (2 kg) a year. Appetite remains as it was during the toddler years, which is considerably less than some parents would like or expect. Parents may bring a preschooler to a health care facility because they fear their child is losing weight. When the child's weight is plotted on a growth chart, however, it is evident the child is gaining weight; what parents are noticing is the age-appropriate change in body shape from rounded to slim.

Height gain is also minimal during this period: only 2 to 3.5 in (6 to 8 cm) a year on average (see Appendix E). Head circumference is not routinely measured at physical assessments on children over 2 years of age.

Teeth

Children generally have all 20 of their deciduous teeth by 3 years of age. Preserving these teeth is important as they hold the position for the permanent teeth as the child's jaw grows larger (Mueller, 2008).

Developmental Milestones

Each year during the preschool period marks a major step forward in gross motor, fine motor, and language development. Play activities change focus as the preschooler learns new skills and understands more about the world (Fig. 31.1). Table 31.1 summarizes the major milestones of the period.

Language Development

A 3-year-old child has a vocabulary of about 900 words. These are used to ask questions constantly, up to 400 a day, mostly "how" and "why" questions, such as "Why is snow cold? How do worms hear? What does your tongue do?" A child needs simple answers to such questions so curiosity, vocabulary building, and questioning are encouraged, and also because the depth of a child's understanding is often deceptive. For example, if a parent tells a child shoes should go on with the buckles on the outside, a child may seem to understand but may return in a few minutes to ask, "Why do I have to go outside to put on my shoes?" Words that sound alike but mean different things such as whether and weather can be truly confounding to children of this age.

Four- and 5-year-old children continue to ask many questions. They enjoy participating in mealtime conversation and can describe something from their day in great detail. Preschoolers imitate language exactly, so if they hear less-than-perfect language, this is the language pattern they adopt. They may imitate and use "bathroom language" if not corrected because of the attention from adults this generates.

Preschoolers are egocentric, so they define objects in relation to themselves (a key is not a metal object but "what I use

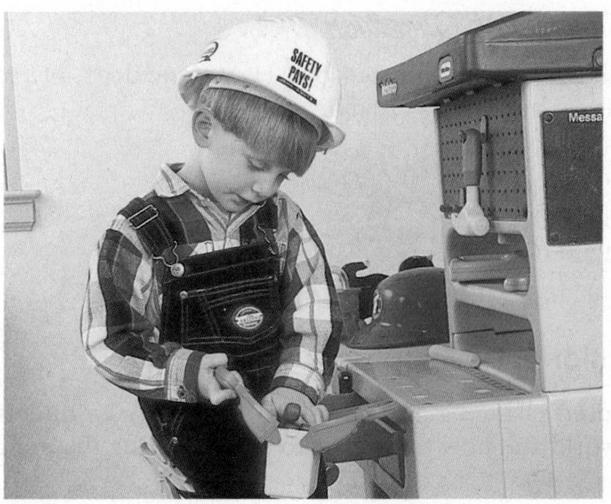

FIGURE 31.1 Preschoolers like to imitate the roles of adults, as they learn about the world around them.

to open a door," and a car is not a means of transportation but "what Mom uses to take me to school").

Whether children are allowed to ask questions is culturally determined and can make a difference in how much vocabulary a child uses. In a society in which children are expected to be seen and not heard, a preschool child may not have the same expressive vocabulary as a child who has been encouraged to ask questions. Recognition that differences among cultures can affect levels of development means that assessment must be individualized and meaningful in terms of the cultural milieu.

Play

Preschoolers do not need many toys. Their imaginations are keener than they will be at any other time in their lives, so they enjoy games that use imitation such as pretending to be teachers, cowboys, firefighters, and store clerks. They imitate exactly what they see parents doing: eating meals, mowing the lawn, cleaning the house, arguing, and so forth, so parents' actions directly influence their behavior (Dooley & Stewart, 2007). Many preschoolers have imaginary friends as a normal part of having an active imagination (Goldson & Reynolds, 2008). These often exist until children formally begin school.

Four- and 5-year-olds divide their time between roughhousing and imitative play. Five-year-olds are interested in group games or songs they have learned in kindergarten or preschool.

TABLE 31.1 ✻ Summary of Preschool Growth and Development

Age (yr)	Fine Motor	Gross Motor	Language	Play
3	Undresses self; stacks tower of blocks; draws a cross	Runs; alternates feet on stairs; rides tricycle; stands on one foot	Vocabulary of 900 words	Able to take turns; very imaginative
4	Can do simple buttons	Constantly in motion; jumps; skips	Vocabulary of 1500 words	Pretending is major activity
5	Draws a 6-part man; can lace shoes	Throws overhand	Vocabulary of 2100 words	Likes games with numbers or letters

✔ *Checkpoint Question 31.1*

Cathy asks constant questions. How many does a typical 3-year-old ask in a day's time?

a. Less than 50.
b. 100–200.
c. 300–400.
d. 1200 or more.

Emotional Development

Children change a great deal in their ability to understand the world and how they relate to people during the preschool years.

Developmental Task: Initiative Versus Guilt

The developmental task of the preschool years, according to Erikson, is to form a sense of initiative versus guilt (Erikson, 1993).

A child with a well-developed sense of initiative has discovered that learning new things is fun.

If children are criticized or punished for attempts at initiative, they develop a sense of guilt for wanting to try new activities or have new experiences. Those who leave the preschool period with guilt may carry it with them into new situations, such as starting elementary school. They may even have difficulty later in life making decisions about everything from changing jobs to choosing an apartment, because they cannot envision they are capable of solving associated problems.

To gain a sense of initiative, preschoolers need exposure to a wide variety of experiences and play materials so they can learn as much about the world as possible. They are ready to reach outside their homes for new experiences, such as a trip to the zoo or an amusement park (Fig. 31.2). They are interested in seeing new places, and so enjoy going with the family on vacation. These types of experiences lead to increased vocabulary; for instance, at the zoo, preschoolers not only learn words such as *giraffe*, *elephant*, and *bear*, but they also learn to transfer them from abstract concepts to the animals they name.

Urge parents to provide play materials that encourage creative play, such as finger paints, soapy water to splash or blow into bubbles, mud to make into pies, sand to build castles, and modeling clay or homemade dough to mold into figures or make into pretend cookies. These are messy activities, and many parents cannot let a child indulge in them more than once a week, but any experience with free-form play is helpful.

Preschoolers tend to have such active imaginations that they need little guidance in this type of play. They smear both hands into clay or finger paint and create instinctively. Urge parents to support this kind of play but not try to make models. If a parent draws a tree with finger paint, for example, and says, "Now you draw one," a child may decide it is no fun to finger paint because he knows his tree will not look as good as his parent's. As he is not ready for competition, he will drop out of the activity rather than have his drawing shown up as inferior.

Preschoolers may make nothing recognizable out of clay or finger paint, preferring simply to handle the medium. As long as they enjoy the feel of the material, they do not need to make anything. Pressure to make things is not fun and can discourage their interest in learning.

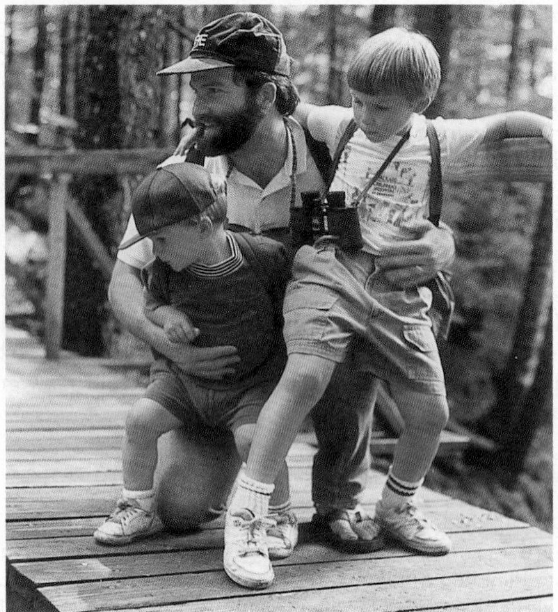

FIGURE 31.2 Preschoolers like exposure to new events and places. Here a 3-year-old is eager to explore the woods during a hike with the family.

Imitation. Preschoolers need free rein to imitate the roles of the people around them. Again, role playing should be fun and does not have to be accurate. If a boy is pretending to be a police officer and is busy putting out fires, or a firefighter and is stopping playmates from speeding, the fact he is freely imitating a role is more important than getting the role absolutely correct. If a parent is concerned a child should separate these two roles accurately, it is usually best not to stop the play to do so. Rather, the next time they are driving past the fire station, the parent could explain this is where firefighters work, and they put out fires, or the police station is where police officers work, and they make sure that people drive safely.

Children generally imitate those activities best that they see their parents performing at home. A young girl will set the table for breakfast, eat with her "husband," help clean off the table, and leave for work. A young boy might cook, pretend to feed a doll, and put the doll to bed as he has seen his father do with a younger sibling. In addition to learning what activities adults carry out at home, preschoolers should also be introduced to their parents' work environments. Such visits not only provide a visual context for the parent's job but also let a child learn such words as photocopier, cash register, assembly line, legal brief, or fax machine.

Today, as many as 90% of mothers of childbearing age work outside the home at least part time. Remind a mother to introduce her preschooler to her "other" self—lawyer, secretary, or telephone repair person—in the same way a child is exposed to the father's outside work side.

Fantasy. Toddlers cannot differentiate between fantasy and reality; they believe cartoon characters or children in books are real. Preschoolers begin to make this differentiation. They may become so engrossed in a fantasy role, however, they become afraid they have lost their own identity or have become "stuck" in their fantasies. Such intense involvement in play is part of "magical thinking," or believing thoughts and wishes can come true.

Parents sometimes strengthen this feeling without realizing it: they (and you) need to be careful in this regard. A preschooler, for example, may be pretending she is a white rabbit. Her mother walks into the room, is aware of the game, and decides to participate. She says, "That's strange, I don't see Cindy anywhere. All I see is a white rabbit." Then she leaves the room. Cindy can be frightened she has actually become a white rabbit. A better response for the mother would be to support the imitation—this is age-appropriate behavior and a good way of exploring roles—while helping a child maintain the difference between pretend and real. She might say, "What a nice white rabbit you're pretending to be," both supporting the fantasy and yet reassuring a child she is still herself.

In a health care setting, it is particularly important that you let children know they are still recognizable. When examining the ears of a girl who tells you she is a rabbit, comment her ears are all better again, rather than play to the make-believe with remarks about long, furry rabbit ears.

Oedipus and Electra Complexes

Although the development of Oedipus and Electra complexes may have been overstated by Freud because of gender bias, many children do appear to manifest such behavior (Luborsky & Barrett, 2007). An **Oedipus complex** refers to the strong emotional attachment a preschool boy demonstrates toward his mother; an **Electra complex** is the attachment of a preschool girl to her father. Each child competes with the same-sex parent for the love and attention of the other parent. Parents who are not prepared for this behavior may feel hurt or rejected. For example, a daughter prefers to sit beside her father at the table or in the car; she asks her father to tuck her in at night. She is "Daddy's girl." The mother may feel left out of the family interaction when this happens. On the other hand, a boy will ask his mother for the same favors. He wants to sit beside her, to have her read to him, and to tuck him in for the night, and the father may feel left out.

Parents can be reassured that this phenomenon of competition and romance in preschoolers is normal. Parents may need help in handling feelings of jealousy and anger, however, particularly if a child is vocal in expressing feelings toward a parent. It is difficult for a mother to reply calmly to a 3-year-old daughter who is shouting at her, "I hate you! I only love Daddy!" By understanding the motivation behind such a statement, the parent may be able to calmly react by stating, "Well, I don't like to be shouted at, but I still love you."

Gender Roles

Preschoolers need exposure to an adult of the opposite gender so they can become familiar with opposite gender roles. Encourage single parents to plan opportunities for their children to spend some time with adults other than themselves, such as a grandparent, a friend, or a relative of the opposite sex, for this exposure. A preschool teacher may serve as this person. Because most preschool teachers are women, a mother may have to look elsewhere to find an adult male role model. If a child is hospitalized during the preschool period, a male nurse could fill this role.

Children's gender-typical actions are strengthened by parents, strangers, preschool teachers, other family members, and other children. Many parents do not want their child to grow up as they did, with a fixed role as a result of gender stereotyping. Help them understand they reinforce such attitudes by their actions as well as by their words. For example, a father may tell his son it is important for both boys and girls to do housework, but if the father never does dishes, he is teaching his son that managing a household is not a man's job.

Socialization

Because 3-year-olds are capable of sharing, they play with other children their age much more agreeably than do toddlers, which is why the preschool period is a sensitive and critical time for socialization. Children who are exposed to other playmates have an easier time learning to relate to people than those raised in an environment where they never see other children of the same age (Fig. 31.3).

Although 4-year-olds continue to enjoy play groups, they may become involved in arguments more than they did at age 3, especially as they become more certain of their role in the group. This development, like so many others, may make parents worry a child is regressing. However, it is really forward movement, involving some testing and identification of their group role.

Five-year-olds begin to develop "best" friendships, perhaps on the basis of who they walk to school with or who lives closest to them. The elementary rule that an odd number of children will have difficulty playing well together pertains to children at this age: two or four will play, but three or five will quarrel.

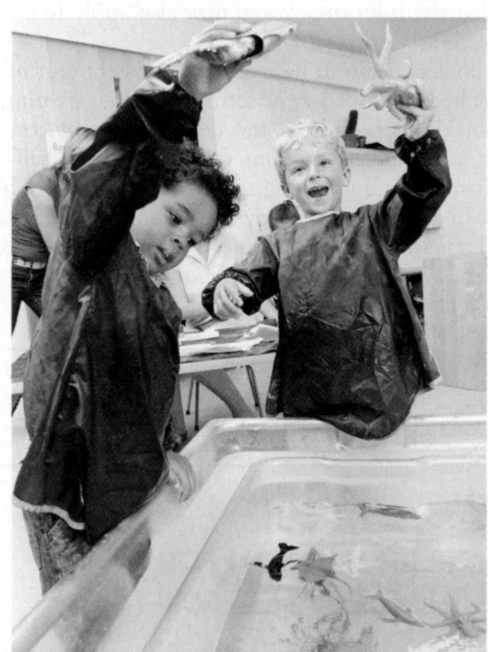

FIGURE 31.3 The preschool child begins to develop friendships.

Cognitive Development

At age 3 years, cognitive development according to Piaget is still preoperational (Piaget, 1969). Although children during this period do enter a second phase called **intuitional thought**, they lack the insight to view themselves as others see them or put themselves in another's place (termed *centering*). Because preschoolers cannot make this kind of mental substitution, they feel they are always right. This causes them to argue with the forcefulness that comes from believing they are 100% correct. This is an important point to remember when explaining procedures to preschoolers. They cannot see your side of the situation; they cannot hurry because you must have something done by 10:00 o'clock; they cannot hold still just because you want them to.

Also, preschoolers are not yet aware of the property of **conservation.** This means that if they have two balls of clay of equal size, but one is squashed flatter and wider than the other, preschoolers will insist the flatter one is bigger (because it is wider) or that the intact one is bigger (because it is taller). They cannot see that only the form, not the amount, has changed. This inability to appreciate conservation has implications for nursing care. Preschoolers are not able to comprehend that a procedure done two separate ways is the same procedure. Therefore, if the nurse before you told a child to turn on his right side and then his left side while his bed was made, you may have to allow him to turn those same ways.

Moral and Spiritual Development

Children of preschool age determine right from wrong based on their parents' rules. They have little understanding of the rationale for these rules or even whether the rules are consistent. If asked the question, "Why is it wrong to hit other children?" the average preschooler answers, "Because my mother says it's wrong." When pressed further, the preschooler justifies that conviction with, "It just is, that's all." Because preschoolers depend on their parents to supply rules for them, when faced with a new situation they have difficulty seeing that the rules they know may also apply to a new situation such as a hospital.

Preschoolers begin to have an elemental concept of God if they have been provided some form of religious training. Belief in an outside force aids in the development of conscience; however, preschoolers tend to do good out of self-interest rather than because of strong spiritual motivation (Kohlberg, 1984). Children this age enjoy the security of religious holidays and religious rituals such as prayer and grace before meals because these rituals offer them the same reassurance and security as a familiar nursery rhyme read over and over.

What if... Cathy, 3 years old, understands the rule "Don't steal from stores"? Would she also understand "Don't steal from a hospital"?

HEALTH PROMOTION FOR A PRESCHOOLER AND FAMILY

Preschoolers are old enough to begin to take responsibility for their own actions. The preschooler's safety, nutritional health, daily activities, and family functioning are all affected by this increased responsibility.

Promoting Preschooler Safety

As preschoolers broaden their horizons, safety issues increase. By age 4, children may project an attitude of independence and the ability to take care of their own needs. Part of this is pseudo-independence; they still need supervision to be certain they do not injure themselves or other children while roughhousing and to ensure they do not stray too far from home. Their interest in learning adult roles may lead them into exploring the blades of a lawn mower or an electric saw or a neighbor's pool (Thompson & Rivara, 2009). It is not too early to think about gun safety or being sure that any gun in their home is locked away (DuRant, 2007). They must be reminded repeatedly not to walk in back of or in front of automobiles. Otherwise, a preschooler's thought "I want to play with Mary across the street" can be so quick and so intense a child will run into the middle of the street before remembering the rules "Watch out for cars" and "Don't cross the street."

Because preschoolers imitate adult roles so well, they may imitate taking medicine if they see family members doing so (Box 31.3). A good rule for parents is never to take medicine

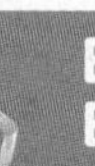

BOX 31.3 * Focus on Evidence-Based Practice

Does medicine given for upper respiratory infections pose a major threat for poisoning in preschoolers?

Preschool children usually develop a number of upper respiratory infections a year as this is a time when they are first exposed to other children through preschool or Head Start programs. That makes this the time when children are first introduced to pleasant tasting cough and cold medicines. To investigate whether adverse drug events including poisoning related to common cough and cold medications frequently occur in preschool children, researchers surveyed the emergency departments of 63 U.S. hospitals for a year. During the survey year, 158,520 patients 18 years or younger were treated in emergency departments for unanticipated or adverse drug events. Almost half (49.4%) of these visits occurred in preschool children between 1 and 4 years of age. Unintentional overdose (poisoning) was the most common reason that children were seen (44.9%), followed by allergic reactions (35%) and adverse effects (12.6%). Antimicrobial agents, analgesic medications, and respiratory medications accounted for almost half of adverse drug events (25.2%, 13.7%, and 10.6%, respectively). Fortunately, fewer than 1 in 10 patients (9.5%) required hospitalization or extended observation following these events.

Based on the above, what advice would you want to give parents about using cough or cold medications with preschool children?

Source: Cohen, A. L., et al. (2008). National surveillance of emergency department visits for outpatient adverse drug events in children and adolescents. *Journal of Pediatrics, 152*(3), 416–421.

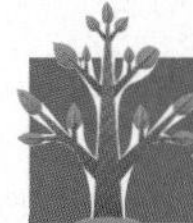

BOX 31.4 * Focus on Family Teaching

Common Safety Measures to Prevent Accidents During the Preschool Years

Q. Cathy's father says to you, "My preschooler is so active! How can I keep her safe?"

A. All of the safety measures that apply to toddlers also apply to preschoolers. In addition, try these tips:

Possible Accident	Prevention Measure
Motor vehicles	Teach safety with tricycle (look before crossing driveways; do not cross streets). Teach child to always hold hands with a grownup before crossing a street. Teach parking lot safety (hold hands with grownup; do not run behind cars that are backing up). Children should wear helmets when riding bicycles.
Falls	Supervise preschooler at playgrounds. Remove drawstrings from hooded clothing. Help child to judge safe distances for jumping or safe heights for climbing.
Drowning	Teach beginning swimming.
Animal bites	Do not allow child to approach strange dogs. Supervise child's play with family pets.
Poisoning	Never present medication as a candy. Never take medication in front of a child. Never store food or substances in containers other than their own. Post telephone number of local poison control center by the telephone. Teach child that medication is a serious substance and not for play.
Burns	Store matches in closed containers. Do not allow preschooler to help light birthday candles, fireplaces, etc. (fire is not fun or a "treat").
Community safety	Teach preschooler that not all people are friends ("Do not talk to strangers or take candy from strangers"). Define a stranger as someone a child does not know, not someone odd-looking. Teach child to say "no" to people whose touching the child does not enjoy, including family members. (When a child is sexually abused, the offender is usually a family member or close family friend.)
General	Know whereabouts of preschooler at all times. Be aware that frequency of accidents is increased when parents are under stress. Special precautions must be taken at these times. Some children are more active, curious, and impulsive and therefore more vulnerable to accidents than others.

in front of children. Additional safety points for the preschool period are summarized in Box 31.4.

Keeping Children Safe, Strong, and Free

The preschool years are not too early a time to educate children about the potential threat of harm from strangers or even how to address bullying behavior from people (children or adults) they meet at preschool or at play. This includes:

- Warning a child never to talk with or accept a ride from a stranger
- Teaching a child how to call for help in an emergency (yelling or running to a designated neighbor's house if outside, or dialing 911 if near a telephone)
- Describing what police officers look like and explaining that police officers can help in an emergency situation
- Explaining that if children or adults ask them to keep secrets about anything that has made them uncomfortable, they should tell their parents or another trusted adult, even if they have promised to keep the secret
- Explaining that bullying behavior from other children is not to be tolerated and should be reported so they can receive help managing it

It is often difficult for parents to impart this type of information to preschoolers because they cannot imagine their child will ever be in situations in which the information will be needed, nor do they want to terrify their child about the world. However, if the information is presented in a calm yet serious manner, children can begin to use it to build safe habits that will help them later when they are old enough to walk home from school alone or play with their friends, unsupervised, at a public playground.

Motor Vehicle and Bicycle Safety

With more and more cars being equipped with front-seat air bags, make certain parents safely buckle preschoolers into car seats in the back seat (American Academy of Pediatrics [AAP], 2009). Parents should stress the important role of seat belts in preventing injury in accidents and should make it a rule that the car does not move until seatbelts are fastened. Many preschoolers outgrow their first car seats during this period (when they reach 40 lb) and need to graduate to a booster-type seat. Remind parents to check the position of the shoulder harness so it does not go across a child's face or throat.

Preschool is also the right age to promote bicycle safety (Pardi, 2007). Head injuries are a major cause of death and injury to preschoolers, and bicycle accidents are among the major causes of such injuries. Some parents may have already purchased a helmet for their child when the child was a toddler and riding in a bicycle seat. Once children begin riding independently, however, they definitely need a safety helmet approved for children their age and size. Encourage parents who ride bicycles to demonstrate safe riding habits by wearing helmets as well. Seeing a parent routinely wearing a helmet may well be the most compelling reason for a preschooler to wear one.

What if... Cathy tells you she knows not to leave preschool with anyone who is strange? Is that the same as knowing not to leave with a stranger?

Promoting Nutritional Health of the Preschooler

Like the toddler period, the preschool years are not a time of fast growth, so preschool children are not likely to have ravenous appetites. Offering small servings of food is still a good idea, so a child is not overwhelmed by the amount on a plate and is allowed the successful feeling of cleaning a plate and asking for more. Parents need to check that children are not snacking so frequently that they miss out on planned meals to be certain children receive a complete range of nutrients (Gable, Chang, & Krull, 2007).

Most children are hungry after preschool and enjoy a snack when they arrive home. Because sugary foods can dull a child's appetite for dinner and it is not too soon to begin measures to prevent childhood obesity, urge parents to offer foods such as fruit, cheese, or milk rather than cookies and a soft drink (Rolfes, Pinna, & Whitney, 2009).

Teach parents to make mealtime a happy and enjoyable part of the day for everyone. Some preschool children learn to eat as quickly as possible (and perhaps incompletely) to escape from the table before something unpleasant happens, such as an argument they can sense is brewing. Initiative, or learning how to do things, can be strengthened by allowing a child to prepare simple foods, such as making a sandwich or spreading jelly on toast.

Recommended Dietary Reference Intakes

As with all age groups, foods selected for preschoolers should be based on food pyramid groups, making sure to offer a variety. Preschoolers may not eat a great deal of meat because it can be hard to chew. Many parents ask whether their preschooler needs to take supplementary vitamins because they eat so little. As long as a child is eating foods from all pyramid food groups and meets the criteria for a healthy child such as being alert and active, with height and weight within normal averages, additional vitamins are probably unnecessary.

If parents do give vitamins, remind them a child will undoubtedly view a vitamin as candy rather than medicine because of the attractive shapes and colors of preschool vitamins, so they must be stored out of reach. Caution parents not to give more vitamins than the recommended daily amount, because poisoning from high doses of fat-soluble vitamins or iron can result.

Promoting Nutritional Health With a Vegetarian Diet

A vegetarian diet is usually colorful and therefore appeals to preschoolers. Many vegetables, fruits, and grains are also good snack foods and so are convenient for a child who eats frequently during the day.

If vegetarian diets are deficient in any aspects, they usually lack calcium, vitamin B_{12}, and vitamin D. Check to see a child is ingesting a variety of calcium sources (green leafy vegetables, milk products) as this is so important for bone growth. Vitamin D is found in fortified cereals and milk. Vitamin B_{12} is found almost exclusively in animal products, so a child may need a supplemental source of this (Rolfes, Pinna, & Whitney, 2009).

Promoting Development of the Preschooler in Daily Activities

The preschooler has often mastered the basic skills needed for most self-care activities, including feeding, dressing, washing (with supervision), and brushing teeth (again, with supervision).

Dressing

Many 3-year-olds and most 4-year-olds can dress themselves except for difficult buttons, although there may be a conflict over what a child will wear. Preschoolers prefer bright colors or prints and so may select items that do not match. As with other preschool activities, however, children need the experience of choosing their own clothes. One way for parents to solve the problem of mismatching is to fold together matching shirts and pants so a child sees them as a set rather than individual pieces. If children insist on wearing mismatched clothes, parents should make no apologies for their appearance. A simple statement such as "Mark chose his own clothes today" explains the situation. Anyone who understands preschoolers appreciates that the experience children gain in being able to select their own clothing is worth more than a perfect appearance by adult standards.

Sleep

Many toddlers, going through a typical negative phase, resist taking naps no matter how tired they are. Preschoolers, on the other hand, are more aware of their needs; when they are tired, they often curl up on a couch or soft chair and fall asleep. Many, particularly those who attend afternoon child care or preschool, give up afternoon naps. If they nap at a preschool, they may have some difficulty going to sleep at the usual bedtime established at home.

Children in this age group, however, may refuse to go to sleep because of fear of the dark. Night waking from nightmares or night terrors reaches its peak (Hiscock et al., 2007). This means preschoolers may need a night light, although they did not need one before. A helpful suggestion for parents is to screen out frightening stories or television watching just prior to bedtime and continue familiar bedtime routines.

Exercise

The preschool period is an active phase, so children receive a great deal of exercise. Rough-housing is a good way of getting rid of tension and should be allowed as long as it does not become destructive. In addition, preschoolers love time-honored games such as ring-around-the-rosy, London Bridge, or other more structured games they were not ready for as toddlers. Promoting this type of active game and reducing television watching can help children develop motor skills as well as be a step toward preventing childhood obesity (Kline, 2008).

Hygiene

Preschoolers can wash and dry their hands adequately if the faucet is regulated for them so they do not scald themselves with hot water. Also, when possible, parents should turn down the temperature of the water heater in their home to under 120° F to help prevent scalds. Preschoolers do not clean their fingernails very well, so these often need "touching up" by a parent or older sibling. The child may also need the assistance of a parent or older sibling to clean the ears during bath time. Hair washing can be a problem, as well. Preschoolers are too heavy for a parent to hold over the sink to rinse their hair, and children may have difficulty keeping the eyes closed well enough or long enough to keep soap out because they insist on opening them to see whether the parent is finished. Hanging a mobile over the tub so they have a reason to look up for rinsing and using a nonirritating shampoo are good suggestions. Although preschoolers may sit well in bathtubs, they should still not be left unsupervised at bath time. Caution parents about not using bubble bath with preschoolers as some girls develop vulvar irritation (and perhaps bladder infections) from exposure to such products.

Care of Teeth

If independent toothbrushing was not started as a daily practice during the infant or toddler years, it should be started during the preschool years. A child should continue to drink fluoridated water or receive a prescribed oral fluoride supplement if fluoride is not provided in the water supply (Armfield & Spencer, 2007).

One good toothbrushing period a day is often more effective than more frequent half-hearted brushings. Although many preschoolers do well brushing their own teeth, parents must check that all tooth surfaces are cleaned. They should floss the teeth, because this is a skill beyond a preschooler's motor ability.

Toothbrushing is generally well accepted by preschoolers because it imitates adults. Electric or battery-operated toothbrushes are favorites because of the adult responsibility involved in handling them. Children must be supervised when using an electric toothbrush, however, and must be taught not to use it or any other electrical appliance near a basin of water.

Encouraging children to eat apples, carrots, celery, chicken, or cheese for snacks rather than candy or sweets is yet another way to attempt to prevent tooth decay. If a child is allowed to chew gum, it should be the sugar-free variety.

Children should have made a first visit to a dentist by 2½ years of age for evaluation of tooth formation. Because this visit usually shows no cavities, this should have been a pain-free experience, so a child should not fear the dentist, and the idea that dentists like to help rather than hurt should have been implanted. If parents did not take a child for this visit previously, it should be done during the preschool period. Deciduous teeth must be preserved to protect the dental arch. If teeth have to be pulled as a result of disease, the permanent teeth can drift out of position or the jaw may not grow enough to accommodate them.

Night Grinding. **Bruxism**, or grinding the teeth at night (usually during sleep), is a habit of many young children (Goddard, 2008). Teeth grinding may be a way of "letting go," similar to body rocking, that children do for a short time each night to release tension and allow themselves to fall asleep. Children who grind their teeth extensively may have greater-than-average anxiety. Children with cerebral palsy may do it because of the spasticity of jaw muscles. If the grinding is extensive, the crowns of the teeth can become abraded. The condition can advance to such an extent that tooth nerves become exposed. If the problem seems to stem from anxiety, identifying and relieving the source of anxiety is essential for treatment. If some damage is evident, refer the family to a pedodontist so the teeth can be evaluated, repaired (capped), and conserved.

Promoting Healthy Family Functioning

Some parents who enjoyed maintaining a rhythm of care for an infant and allowed for ritualistic behavior of a toddler may have difficulty being the parents of a preschooler because more flexibility and creativity are required. Others come into their own as the parents of a preschooler; they delight in encouraging imaginative games and play.

A major parental role during this time is to encourage vocabulary development. One way to do this is to read aloud to a child; another is to answer questions so a child sees language as an organized system of communication. Answering a preschooler's questions can be difficult because the questions are frequently philosophical; for example, "Why is grass green?" A child may listen to an explanation of chlorophyll but then repeat the question, regardless of the clarity of the explanation, because the parent underestimated the extent of the question: a child did not want to know what makes grass green, but why, philosophically, it is not red or blue or yellow. The obvious answer to that is, "I don't know." Parents who are confident can give this answer without feeling threatened. Parents who are less sure of themselves may feel extremely uncomfortable when they realize they do not know the answers to a 4-year-old's questions (Box 31.5).

Discipline

Preschoolers have definite opinions on things such as what they want to eat, where they want to go, and what they want to wear. This may bring them into opposition with parents. A major parental responsibility when this happens is to guide a child through these struggles without discouraging the child's right to have an opinion. "Timeout" is a good technique to correct behavior for parents throughout the preschool years (see Chapter 30). This technique allows parents to discipline without using physical punishment and allows a child to learn a new way of behavior without extreme stress.

Parental Concerns Associated With the Preschool Period

A number of common health problems and fears usually arise during the preschool years.

Common Health Problems of the Preschooler

The mortality of children during the preschool years is low and becoming lower every year as more infectious diseases

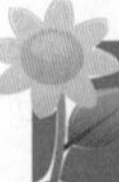

BOX 31.5 * Focus on Communication

Cathy's father brings her for a well-child visit. You overhear him talking to his daughter in the waiting room.

Less Effective Communication

Cathy: Why do we have to wait so long?
Mr. Edwards: It's how things work here.
Cathy: Why?
Mr. Edwards: I have no idea.
Cathy: Why is that girl here? Is she sick?
Mr. Edwards: I have no idea.
Cathy: When are we going home?
Mr. Edwards: I have no idea.
Cathy: What's that girl's name?
Mr. Edwards: I have no idea.

More Effective Communication

Cathy: Why do we have to wait so long?
Mr. Edwards: It's how things work here.
Cathy: Why?
Mr. Edwards: People have to take turns. We're waiting for our turn.
Cathy: Why is that girl here? Is she sick?
Mr. Edwards: She might be. Some children are here because they're sick and some are just in for a check-up like you.
Cathy: When are we going home?
Mr. Edwards: As soon as the nurse practitioner checks you over.
Cathy: What's that girl's name?
Mr. Edwards: I don't know. Do you want to ask her?

Preschoolers ask 300 to 400 questions a day as they explore their world. In the first scenario, the father tries to discourage questions by offering almost no answers. In the second scenario, when he tries to answer a child's questions, he is not only supplying information but is also helping a child build vocabulary. Because preschoolers ask so many questions, you may have to encourage parents to continue to answer questions this way. Otherwise, discouraging questions can become the method of interaction.

are preventable. This results in the major cause of death being automobile accidents, followed by poisoning and falls (Centers for Disease Control and Prevention [CDC], 2008).

The number of minor illnesses, such as colds, ear infections, and flu symptoms, is also high. Children who live in homes in which parents smoke have a higher incidence of ear (otitis media) and respiratory infections than others (Kaul & Stevens-Simon, 2008). Children who attend child care or preschool programs also have an increased incidence of gastrointestinal disturbances (such as vomiting and diarrhea) from the exposure to other children (Butterton & Calderwood, 2008).

Many parents find it extremely difficult to cope with the parade of constant minor infections that occur, causing stress between parent and child, an almost monthly battle of "Stay indoors until you feel better," conflict. Children may demonstrate frequent whining or clinging behavior because they do not feel completely well. Such constant illness can cause parents to perceive a child as sickly or not able to cope with everyday life. Whereas parents encouraged independence before, they may now begin to overprotect (to shelter to too great a degree). Give reassurance that frequent minor illnesses are common in preschoolers. As parents become more experienced in handling these conditions, their perception of whether an illness is a problem will change.

Table 31.2 shows the usual health maintenance schedule for preschoolers. Table 31.3 lists common problems parents may have in evaluating a preschooler's illness.

Common Fears of the Preschooler

Because preschoolers' imagination is so active, this can lead to a number of fears. Fears of the dark, mutilation, and separation or abandonment are all very real to a preschooler. These can rise in incidence when combined with the stress of an illness or hospitalization (Anderzen-Carlsson et al., 2007). Although most of these fears can be handled by comforting from parents, in some children, fears are so intensified that they need therapy such as desensitization to the fear (Gordon et al., 2007).

Fear of the Dark. The tendency to fear the dark is an example of a fear heightened by a child's vivid imagination: a stuffed toy by daylight becomes a threatening monster at night. Children awaken screaming because of nightmares. They may be reluctant to go to bed or to go back to sleep by themselves.

If parents are prepared for this fear and understand it is a phase of growth, they are better able to cope with it. It is generally helpful if they monitor the stimuli their children are exposed to, especially around bedtime. This includes television, adult discussions, and frightening stories. Parents are sometimes reluctant to leave a child's light on at night because they do not want to cater to the fear. Burning a dim night light, however, can solve the problem and costs only pennies. Children who awake terrified and screaming need reassurance they are safe, that whatever was chasing them was a dream and is not in their room. They may require an understanding adult to sit on their bed until they can fall back to sleep again (Fig. 31.4). Most preschoolers do not remember in the morning that they had such a dream; they remember for a lifetime they received comfort when they needed it.

If parents take sensible precautions against fear of the dark or nightmares and a child continues to have this kind of disturbance every night, it may be a reaction to undue stress. In these instances, the source of the stress needs to be investigated. Giving sleep medication to counteract the sleep disturbance does not help solve the basic problem, so this is rarely recommended. Fear of the dark can become intensified in a hospital setting and requires careful planning to relieve.

Fear of Mutilation. Fear of mutilation is also significant during the preschool age, as revealed by the intense reaction of a preschooler to even a simple injury such as falling and scraping a knee or having a needle inserted for an immunization. A child cries afterward not only from the pain but also from the intrusiveness of the injury or procedure. Part of this fear

TABLE 31.2 ✻ Health Maintenance Schedule, Preschool Period

Area of Focus	Methods	Frequency
Assessment		
Developmental milestones	History, observation	Every visit
	Formal Denver Developmental Screening Test (DDST II)	Before start of school
Growth milestones	Height, weight plotted on standard growth chart; physical examination	Every visit
Hypertension	Blood pressure	Every visit
Nutrition	History, observation; height/weight information	Every visit
Parent–child relationship	History, observation	Every visit
Behavior problems	History, observation	Every visit
Vision and hearing defects	History, observation	Every visit
	Formal Preschool E and audiometer testing	Before start of school
Dental health	History, physical examination	Every visit
Tuberculosis	PPD test (if there are high-risk factors)	Before start of school
Immunizations		
Diphtheria, pertussis, and tetanus vaccine (DTaP)	Check history and past records; inform caregiver about any risks and side effects; administer immunization in accordance with health care agency policies	Before start of school (4–6 years)
Hepatitis A vaccine		If not previously immunized
Influenza vaccine		Yearly
Measles, mumps, and rubella (MMR) vaccine		Before start of school (4–6 years)
Pneumococcal polysaccharide vaccine (PVV)		If underlying medical conditions
Poliomyelitis (inactivated) vaccine		Before start of school (4–6 years)
Varicella vaccine		4–6 years (2nd)
Anticipatory Guidance		
Preschool care	Active listening and health teaching	Every visit
Expected growth and developmental milestones before next visit	Active listening and health teaching	Every visit
Accident prevention	Counseling about street and personal safety	Every visit
Any problems expressed by caregiver during course of the visit	Active listening and health teaching regarding preschool illnesses and need for imaginative play	Every visit

Source: American Academy of Pediatrics. (2009). *Recommendations for preventive pediatric health care.* Washington, DC: Author.

arises because preschoolers do not know which body parts are essential and which ones—like an inch of scraped skin—can be easily replaced. Boys develop a fear of castration because developmentally they are more in tune with their body parts and are starting to identify with the same-sex parent as they go through the Oedipal phase. Preschoolers can worry that if some blood is taken out of their bodies, all of their blood will leak out. They often lift a bandage to peek at an incision or cut to see if their body is still intact underneath. They dislike procedures such as needlesticks, rectal temperature assessment, otoscopic examination, or having a nasogastric tube passed into their stomach. They need good explanations of the limits of health care procedures such as a tympanic thermometer does not hurt or a finger prick heals quickly or distraction techniques in order to feel safe (Windich-Biermeier et al., 2007).

Fear of Separation or Abandonment. Fear of separation continues to be a major concern for preschoolers. For some children, it intensifies because their keen imagination allows them to believe they have been deserted when they are safe. Their sense of time is still so distorted they cannot be comforted by assurances such as, "Mommy will pick you up from preschool at noon." Their sense of distance is also limited, so making a statement such as "I work only a block away" is not reassuring. Relating time and space to something a child knows, such as meals, television shows, or a friend's house, is most effective. For example, stating, "Mommy will pick you up from preschool after you have had your snack" or showing a child the work site might be more comforting.

Caution parents to be sensitive to such fears when they talk about missing children or if they have their preschooler's fingerprints taken for identification. Children whose chief

TABLE 31.3 ✻ Parental Difficulties Evaluating Illness in a Preschool Child

Difficulty	Helpful Suggestions for Parents
Evaluating seriousness of illness or condition	Preschoolers are eager to please and tend to answer all questions such as, "Does your stomach hurt?" with a yes. Observing the child for signs of illness—refusing to eat, holding an arm stiffly, having to go to the bathroom frequently—is often more productive as an evaluation technique.
Evaluating bowel and bladder problems	Preschoolers are independent in toilet habits for the first time, so parents do not have diaper contents to evaluate. Frequent trips to the bathroom, rubbing the abdomen, and holding genitals are the usual signs of bowel or bladder dysfunction.
Evaluating nutritional intake	Preschoolers begin to eat away from home at friends' houses or at child care, or to stay overnight with grandparents, so parents do not observe daily food intake as accurately as before. Observing whether a child is growing and active is better than monitoring any one day's food intake.
Evaluating bedwetting	Many preschoolers continue to have occasional enuresis at night until school age. If other signs are present—pain, low-grade fever, listlessness—a child should have a urine culture, as persistent bedwetting can indicate a low-grade urinary tract infection.
Evaluating activity vs. hyperactivity	Many lay magazines have articles on hyperactivity in children. Parents often wonder whether their active child is truly hyperactive. As a rule of thumb, if a child can sit through a meal (when he is hungry), watch a half-hour television show (that is his favorite), or sit still while his favorite story is read to him, he is not hyperactive.
Age-specific diseases to be aware of	Preschool age is a time for vision and hearing assessment. For the first time, a child is able to be tested by a standard chart or by audiometry. Urinary tract infections tend to occur with a high frequency in preschool-age girls. Language assessment should be done if a child is not able to make wants known by complete, articulated sentences by age 3 (exceptions are transposing *w* for *r* and broken fluency: "I want-want-want to go").

fear is that they will be abandoned or kidnapped might not hear that fingerprints are being taken to keep them safe, only that someone might take them away from their parents.

A hospital admission or going to a new school often brings a child's fear of separation to the forefront. Help parents thoroughly prepare preschoolers for these experiences so they can survive them in sound mental health (Chapter 36).

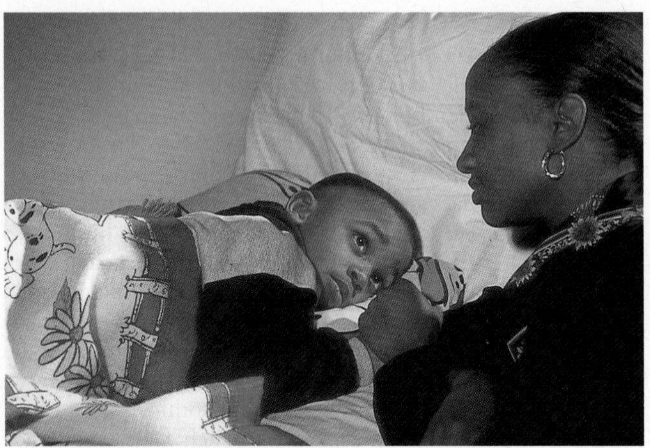

FIGURE 31.4 Having mom close by after a bad dream is a comfort to the preschooler.

Behavior Variations

A combination of a keen imagination and immature reasoning results in common behavior variations in preschoolers.

Telling Tall Tales. Stretching stories to make them seem more interesting is a phenomenon frequently encountered in this age group. After a trip to the zoo, for example, if you ask a child of this age, "What happened today?" a child perceives you want something exciting to have happened, so might answer, "A bear jumped out of his cage and ate up the boy next to me." This is not lying, but merely supplying an expected answer. Caution parents not to encourage this kind of storytelling, but instead help the child separate fact from fiction by saying, "That's a good story, but now tell me what really happened." This conveys the idea a child has not told the truth, yet does not squash imagination or initiative.

Imaginary Friends. Many preschoolers have an imaginary friend who plays with them (Goldson & Reynolds, 2008). They tell a parent to "wait for Eric" or "set a place at the table for Lucy." Although imaginary friends are a normal, creative part of the preschool years and can be invented by children who are surrounded by real playmates as well as by those who have few friends, parents may find them disconcerting. If so, ask parents to make certain their child has exposure to real playmates. As long as imaginary playmates do not take center stage in children's lives or prevent them from socializing with other children, they should not pose a problem and often leave as quickly as they come. In the meantime, they can encourage language development and may provide an outlet for a child to express innermost feelings or serve as a handy scapegoat for behavior about which a child has some conflict.

Parents can help their preschooler separate fact from fantasy about their imaginary friend by saying, "I know Eric isn't real, but if you want to pretend, I'll set a place for him." This response helps a child understand what is real and what is fantasy without restricting a child's imagination or creativity.

Difficulty Sharing. Sharing is a concept that first comes to be understood around the age of 3 years. Before this, children engage in parallel play (two children need two toys and two spaces to play, because they cannot pass one toy back and forth or play together). Around 3 years of age, children begin to understand that some things are theirs, some belong to others, and some can belong to both. For the first time, they can stand in line to wait for a drink, take turns using a shovel at a sandbox, and share a box of crayons. Sharing does not come easily, however; children who are ill or under stress have even greater difficulty with it than usual. Assure parents that sharing is a difficult concept to grasp and that, as with most skills, preschoolers need practice to understand and learn it.

Parents need to accompany experiences with sharing with experiences in learning property rights: "This is my private drawer and no one touches what is in it but me." "That is your dresser top, and no one touches the things on it but you." "A shovel is ours and can be used by everyone playing in the sand pile." Defining limits and exposing children to these three categories (*mine, yours, ours*) helps them determine which objects belong to which category.

Regression. Some preschoolers, generally in relation to stress, revert to behavior they previously outgrew, such as thumb-sucking, negativism, loss of bladder control, and inability to separate from their parents. Although the stress that causes this may take many forms, it is usually the result of such things as a new baby in the family, a new school experience, seeing frightening and graphic television news, stress in the home from financial or other problems, marital difficulties, or separation caused by hospitalization.

Help parents understand that regression in these circumstances is normal, and a child's thumb-sucking is little different from the parents' reaction to stress (smoking many cigarettes, nail biting, overeating), to make it easier for them to accept and understand. Obviously, removing the stress is the best way to help a child discontinue this behavior. The stresses mentioned, however, are not easily removed. New babies cannot be returned, irreparable marriages cannot be patched together, frightening news happens every day, and hospitalizations do occur.

Techniques for minimizing the stress of hospitalization for preschoolers are discussed in Chapter 36. Children's reactions to severe and prolonged stress are discussed in Chapter 54. Children undergoing less severe stress can be assured that although situations are changing, the important aspect of their life—someone still loves them and will continue to take care of them—is not. Thumb-sucking or other manifestations of stress are best ignored; calling them to a child's attention merely causes more stress, because it makes children aware they are not pleasing parents, in addition to experiencing the primary stress.

Sibling Rivalry. Jealousy of a brother or sister may first become evident during the preschool period (Taylor, 2007). This occurs partly because this is the first time that children have enough vocabulary to express how they feel (know a name to call) and partly because preschoolers are more aware of family roles and how responsibilities at home are divided. For many children, this is also the time when a new brother or sister is born.

A firstborn child is rarely allowed the privileges of a second child. The parents were untried, unsure of how far they should let a child venture or what level of responsibility a child could accept when the child was younger, or the firstborn serves as the "trial run" for all children who come after. This phenomenon can lead to sibling rivalry, because children as young as preschool can sense that a younger sibling is being allowed behavior that was not tolerated in them. They are little appeased by the explanation, "Your brother is just a baby."

To help preschoolers feel secure and promote self-esteem, supplying them with a private drawer or box for their things that parents or other children do not touch can be helpful. This can help defend their possessions against younger children who do not appreciate their property rights.

Preparing for a New Sibling

Introduction of a new sibling is such a major happening that parents need to take special steps to be certain their preschooler will be prepared. There is no rule as to when this preparation should begin, but it should be before the time the child begins to feel the difference the new baby will make. This is perhaps when the mother first begins to look pregnant. It is certainly before parents begin to make physical preparations for the new child. It is always less frightening for a child of any age to understand why things are happening, no matter how distasteful they may be, rather than hear people whispering or having parents obviously evading the issue. The unknown is always more fearful than a definite event that can be faced and conquered.

Help parents not to underestimate the significance of a bed to a preschool child. It is security, consistency, and "home." If their preschooler is sleeping in the crib that is to be used for the new baby, it is usually best if the preschooler is moved to a bed about 3 months in advance of the birth. The parents might explain, "It's time to sleep in a new bed now because you're a big boy." The fact that he is growing up is a better reason for such a move than because a new brother or sister wants the old bed. The latter is a direct route to sibling rivalry and jealousy.

If children are to start preschool or child care, they should do so either before the new baby is born or 2 or 3 months afterward, if possible. That way, children can perceive starting school as a result of maturity and not of being pushed out of the house by the new child.

If the mother will be hospitalized for the birth, she should be certain her child is prepared for this separation in advance. As the mother is likely to go to the hospital during the night, it is unrealistic to expect a child in the morning to be happy about the arrival of a new sibling when he realizes the new baby has taken away his mother. Some communities offer preparation for birth classes for preschoolers, the same as for parents, or include children in adult preparation courses to help them master this new experience.

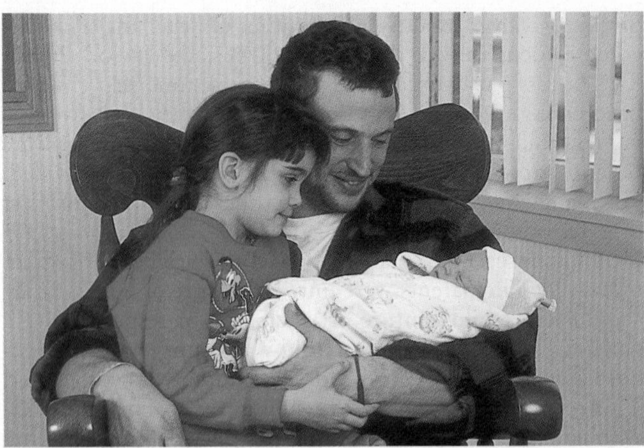

FIGURE 31.5 A preschooler greets a new baby sister. She feels special as dad explains how important it is to be a big sister.

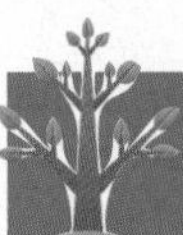

BOX 31.6 * Focus on Family Teaching

Suggestions to Help Minimize Sibling Rivalry

Q. Cathy's father says to you, "Cathy's acting jealous of her new sister and she's not even born yet. How can I reduce sibling jealousy?"

A. This isn't a simple problem, but the following suggestions might help:

- After returning home from the hospital, devote attention to your preschooler and spend some special time together after the baby has gone to bed.
- When friends and family visit, encourage them to spend time with the preschooler as well as the baby. If they bring gifts for the baby, it is often wise for them to bring a small present for the preschooler as well.
- So that your preschooler does not come to expect gifts (promoting sibling rivalry), teach her to help open the baby's gifts. Explain to her that it is the baby's birthday and on her birthday she will receive gifts, too.
- Do not ask your preschooler a question such as, "Do you like your new sister?" It is better to express feelings of empathy such as, "New babies cry a lot. It's hard to get used to that, isn't it?"
- Provide special time for your preschooler during each day, so that when you say, "Mother and Daddy love you just the same," it seems real. This might be a quiet time for talking or reading.
- While feeding the baby, read or tell a story to your preschooler. Some children enjoy feeding a doll while a parent feeds the baby or giving a doll a bath while the baby has one.

Encourage women to maintain contact with their preschooler during the short time they are hospitalized for the new birth. Some preschoolers may react very coldly to their mothers, turning their head away and refusing to come to them after even a few days' separation when they return home. This is a reaction not to the new baby but to the separation, the same phenomenon that may occur when a child returns home after being hospitalized (see Chapter 36). Allowing the child to visit in the hospital can help relieve this type of separation anxiety.

Ask pregnant women or couples what kind of preparation such as this they are making for older children; ask the mother of a new baby how everything is working out. Most parents find the problem of jealousy is bigger than they anticipated and welcome a few suggestions about how to provide more time for their preschooler during the day and which activities a preschooler would especially enjoy (Fig. 31.5; Box 31.6).

✔ Checkpoint Question 31.2

Cathy will need to change to a new bed because her baby sister will need Cathy's old crib. What measure would you suggest that her parents take to help decrease sibling rivalry between Cathy and her new sister?

a. Ask her to get her crib ready for the new baby.
b. Tell her she will have to share with the baby.
c. Move her to the new bed before the baby arrives.
d. Explain that sisters grow up to become best friends.

Sex Education

Children during the preschool age become acutely aware of the difference between boys and girls, possibly because it is a normal progression in development and possibly because this may be the first time in their lives they are exposed to the genitalia of the opposite sex as they watch while a new brother or sister has diapers changed, they see other children using the bathroom at a preschool, or they see a parent nude.

Preschoolers' questions about genital organs are simple and fact-finding; for example, "Why does James look like that?" or "How does Jasmine pee?" Explanations should be just as simple: "Boys look different from girls. The different part is called a penis." It is important for parents not to convey that these body parts are never to be talked about to leave an open line of communication for sexual questions. Occasionally, girls attempt to void standing up as they have seen boys doing; boys may try sitting down to void as they try to use this new body knowledge.

It is common for preschoolers to engage in masturbation while watching television or being read to or before they fall asleep at night. The frequency of this may increase under stress, as does thumb-sucking. If observing a child doing this bothers parents, suggest they explain that certain things are done in some places but not in others. Children can relate to this kind of direction without feeling inhibited, just as they can accept the fact that they use a bathroom in private or eat only at the table. Calling unnecessary attention to the act can increase anxiety and cause increased, not decreased, activity.

An important part of sex education for preschoolers is teaching them to avoid sexual abuse, such as not allowing anyone to touch their body unless they agree it is all right (see Chapter 32, Box 32.5). Because children have been taught this, remember to ask permission before giving nursing care that involves touching.

Because this may be the time a new brother or sister comes into the family, it is also the most likely time for questions such as, "Where do babies come from?" Because a child

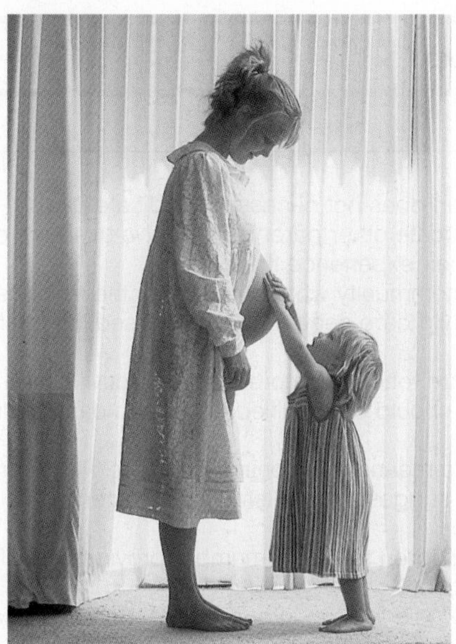

FIGURE 31.6 Preschool children are interested in learning where babies grow and have beginning sexual awareness. (From Taeke Henstra/Science Source/Photo Researchers, Inc.)

is asking a simple fact-finding question, parents usually find a simple, factual answer to this type of question is best: "Babies grow in a special place in a mother's body called a uterus." Saying "uterus" rather than "tummy" prevents children from envisioning babies and food all mixed together in their mother's stomach (Fig. 31.6).

It is so natural for preschoolers to ask about where babies come from that those who do not ask are exceptions. Preschoolers who do not ask may be reticent because they sense from a preliminary exploratory question that the subject is closed. A parent could introduce the subject by visiting a new baby in the neighborhood with the child or pointing out a neighbor who is pregnant. The birth of kittens or puppies can also offer the chance to introduce the subject. If a new brother or sister will be born at a birthing center or at home, many parents allow preschoolers to watch the birth. Encourage parents to prepare children well for this experience, or else the sight of their mother in pain and the wonder of birth can become an overwhelming and negative experience rather than a positive one for them.

Preschool children generally do not ask how babies get inside mothers to start growing or how babies get out at the end of the process. Should they ask, a suitable explanation might be, "When a woman and a man love each other and decide they want a baby, the man plants a seed inside the woman. The man's seed and the woman's seed grow together in the special place inside the mother into a new baby." Some parents prefer to say, "God plants a seed." This answer may leave preschool boys feeling cheated that men have such a little role in this wondrous process. Perhaps a compromise statement is, "God helps the man plant a seed." If preschoolers ask how the baby gets out, an answer might be, "The woman goes to the hospital and the doctor or nurse helps the baby get out from the vagina."

Many new books for children explain where babies come from, including descriptions of sexual relations and orgasm. These are helpful for parents to read to a child to increase understanding.

Choosing a Preschool or Child Care Center

A school or child care experience is helpful for preschoolers, as peer exposure appears to have a positive effect on social development (Zoritch, Roberts, & Oakley, 2009). Children who have learned to be comfortable in a preschool group approach school comfortably and ready to learn; children who have played only infrequently in groups during the preschool age are forced into this new situation in kindergarten or first grade. They can be so busy adjusting to this new concept they are left behind in learning new skills. The terms "child care center," and "preschool," are often used interchangeably, so parents cannot depend on the name of a school to define its structure. Traditionally, the main purpose of a child care center is to provide child care while parents work or are otherwise occupied. A preschool is dedicated to stimulating children's sense of creativity and initiative and introducing them to new experiences and social contacts they would not ordinarily receive at home. Head Start programs and many modern child care centers fulfill both functions (Olsen & DeBoise, 2007).

If there are other 3- or 4-year-old children in a neighborhood with whom a child has almost daily contact, and if a parent can supervise organized play dates and projects (providing peer interaction, in which working together is the key), a preschool program may not be necessary. On the other hand, if all the neighborhood children are either older or younger or there is only one other child available to play with during the day, a preschool experience will probably be beneficial. Parents with large families point out that their child gets ample exposure to groups, that every meal is a "group session." This is not a peer group, however. Older siblings give in to the 3- or 4-year-old child, and younger siblings are not capable of peer competition. This situation does not offer the same experience as does preschool.

Be sure parents investigate preschools or child care centers carefully before they enroll their child to be certain their child will be safe there and have an enjoyable experience. Guidelines to aid parents in this assessment are shown in Table 31.4.

To continue to evaluate their child's school experience, urge parents to make a habit of asking children what happened at school, what they learned, and the names of any new friends. For the remainder of the growing years, school will have important effects on their child's development. By taking an active role in education, parents influence what and how their child learns.

Child care centers are often blamed for the spread of infectious disease among the 5-and-under population because bringing together children from so many different homes to one setting each day does increase the risk of spreading contagious disease. Preschoolers in day care settings may develop frequent upper respiratory infections or gastrointestinal illnesses. Outbreaks of cytomegalovirus and human parvovirus (fifth disease) make working in such centers a particular hazard to pregnant women as these are potentially teratogenic. To prevent the spread of infection, children need to wash their hands frequently and cover their mouths when coughing. Child care centers where infants as well as older children are enrolled need to take special precautions against hepatitis A or parasitic infections, as these can be spread by caregivers' not washing their hands or the changing table after changing diapers. Hepatitis may be subclinical in the preschooler,

TABLE 31.4 ✻ Questions to Use in Evaluating Child Care Centers

Question	Finding
Management	
How long has the center been in operation?	Length of operation does not necessarily indicate quality, but it allows you to locate other parents who have used the center to ask about their experience there.
Is the center licensed, registered, approved, or inspected by the appropriate agency?	Ask in your local community what agency has the responsibility for licensing child care centers. If not licensed, its quality is suspect.
What are the qualifications of staff members?	If staff members are teachers, more learning activities will be provided; staff should be qualified to perform cardiopulmonary resuscitation.
Is there a fast turnover rate of staff?	A fast turnover rate means little continuity of care will be provided (and probably suggests dissatisfaction with center administration).
What is the child–staff ratio?	A ratio of 3 or 4 children to 1 staff member provides time for quality interaction.
What is the center's policy on parental visits?	Parents should be able to drop in at any time. Be wary of facilities that restrict parental visiting in any way.
Physical Environment	
Is there adequate space in the center?	There should be opportunities for rough-and-tumble and imaginative play and naptime as well as table activities.
Does the space appear safe?	Stairways should be fenced. No paint should be peeling.
Can children get in and out of the building easily?	A first-floor plan is safest. Fire exits should be well marked. An evacuation plan should be practiced.
Is there a safe play area for children outside?	Find out how often children are taken outside: once or twice a day, or only occasionally for "outings"?
Is there a quiet place for naps?	Ask if a child can nap if tired or has to wait until a set naptime.
Can the bathroom be reached easily?	Both potty chairs and small toilet seats should be available.
If food is provided, does it meet preschool recommendations?	Food should be "preschool friendly."
Is there adequate refrigeration?	Food poisoning is a concern without refrigeration.
Staff Philosophy	
Are the workers warm and affectionate toward the children?	Watch how they greet children. They should ask questions and listen to answers.
Do caretakers spend more of their time performing janitorial tasks (cleaning) and reprimanding children, or can they devote their time to the children?	It is best if cleaning staff is separate from care staff.
Is each child assigned to a particular caregiver on a continuing basis?	Ask staff to describe their care pattern; if this is not planned, little continuity of care results.
Are the children provided stimulating toys and equipment?	Imaginative items, such as a puppet theater, finger paint, and water play, should be included.
How do the staff discipline children? Do they yell or treat the children roughly?	The method should reflect the parents' philosophy. Staff should be able to talk to children calmly without raising their voices in anger.
Is there a planned curriculum?	There should be specific individualized goals the staff hopes to accomplish.
Can the child pursue an individual interest?	Play or learning activities should be individualized.
Health Care Protocols	
How does the center care for an ill child?	There should be access to a nurse. Staff should be able to evaluate for illness. They should know actions to take in an emergency.
What precautions does the staff take to prevent spread of infection?	Counter where diapers are changed should be wiped with a disinfectant; tissues and handwashing facilities should be present.
Does the center follow good sanitary practices?	Be sure the center requires waterproof disposable diapers to minimize contamination of the environment and other children, and separates diaper-changing areas from other activities, especially anything related to food handling. Observe adult caregivers changing diapers. Do they wash hands after each change?

Under what conditions are children not allowed to attend the center?	A center should have a very specific policy on what illness symptoms require a child to be kept home—and they should enforce this policy strictly. For instance, a runny nose may be acceptable, but a fever is not; children with chickenpox should be kept at home until the scabs are healed over. Talk to parents whose children have been at the center long enough to have experienced some illnesses, and find out what the family did and how the center responded.
Children's Behavior	
Do the children appear happy and relaxed?	Observe for at least one morning.
Do they rush to greet any new visitors?	This could be a sign of boredom with their center's activities and a strong need for adult attention.

but other members of the preschooler's family can develop overt symptoms as the illness spreads through the family (Friedman, 2009).

Preparing a Child for School

At the end of the preschool period, children begin a formal school experience as they enter kindergarten. Parents may wonder whether their child is old enough for this, especially if a child's birthday is in the late summer or early fall. If this is so, urge parents to discuss their concern with school officials to determine whether their child should be registered for kindergarten or delayed for a year. As school involves a great deal of children's time and influences their future greatly, it is important for parents to take time to prepare preschoolers not only physically by being certain their immunizations are up to date but emotionally as well.

Essential to this preparation is the parents' attitude. If school is always discussed as something to look forward to, as an adventure that will be satisfying and rewarding, a child comes to view it as a positive experience. If school is presented as a punishment ("Wait until you get into first grade—your teacher will make you sit up and behave"), there can be little delight in anticipating it.

If a child was not attending preschool, some parents may have to change their child's daily routine a few months in advance of beginning school to accustom a child to waking earlier or going to bed earlier. School has so many new components that it is wise to try to eliminate as many distractions like this as possible.

If a child is to ride a bus to school, a parent might take a child on a municipal bus as an introduction to this form of transportation. If a child is to walk, a trial walk is in order. In either instance, safety should be stressed: "Don't walk behind the bus because the driver can't see you" and "Wait for the crossing guard to help you cross the street."

If a child will be required to take a lunch to school, a parent can introduce this new experience by preparing a bagged lunch at home some noon. If a child is to purchase lunch at school, the parent can play "cafeteria" at home by serving a meal buffet-style and letting a child practice walking from one dish to another to select food.

Some kindergartens suggest children know how to tie their shoes, name basic colors, and print their name before they begin. Parents should familiarize themselves with any such suggestions from the school, but the wisdom of requiring these skills can be questioned. Identifying colors should be established by this age, but some children are not coordinated enough at 4½ years to tie their shoes or print. A better contribution for parents to make toward their children's achievement in school is to instill in their children the concept that learning is fun and a certain child may not always be able to do all the things other children can do, but trying to do individual best is what is important. Trying to make children complete fine motor tasks for which they are not developmentally prepared does not instill that concept.

For children to do well in a formal school setting, they must be able to follow instructions and sit at a table and chair for a short work period. When some parents examine their child's day, they are surprised to realize how few instructions they give their child in a day. They put on the child's coat, pick up the child's toys, and lead the child to the table for dinner. Similarly, they never encourage their child to spend any time in a chair, which is something the child will have to do for at least short periods in school. Coloring at a table rather than on the floor will introduce this situation without any problem.

Finally, going to school is a form of separation and a new experience if a child has not attended child care or preschool, so parents must make preparations for this. It might be good to arrange to have a child stay with another caregiver for part of a day. Staying at school can then be compared with that event.

These are minimum preparations parents can complete to ready their child for school. Caution both parents and children that no matter how hard they try, not everything can be anticipated; school will bring some new happenings that can not be predicted. If a child has been led to believe that learning is fun and new experiences are enjoyable (creating a strong sense of initiative), these unpredictable instances can be accepted as fun. The concept that new experiences are enjoyable will prepare a child not only for a first day at school but for thousands of profitable days and experiences ahead (see Focus on Nursing Care Planning Box 31.7).

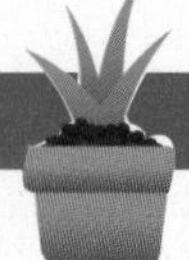

BOX 31.7 ✻ Focus on Nursing Care Planning

A Multidisciplinary Care Map for a Preschooler With Fears

Cathy Edwards is a 3-year-old girl. Her father cares for her because her mother is hospitalized with preterm labor for a second pregnancy. Her father tells you he is concerned because Cathy talks constantly with an imaginary friend named Emma. She makes up stories about events that cannot possibly be true. When corrected, Cathy stutters so badly no one can understand her. At a well-child visit, her father says he is concerned about his daughter's crying at day care.

Family Assessment ✻ Family lives in rented apartment in inner city. Mother is hospitalized with complications of second pregnancy. Father works as city police detective. Mother is stay-at-home mom.

Client Assessment ✻ 3-year-old girl within normal limits for height, weight, and development. Child currently enrolled in all-day preschool program while mother is hospitalized. Father picks child up after his work. Father arrived late to pick child up from preschool last week. She states, "He forgot me." Child refuses to return to preschool. Cries, sticks finger in mouth to make herself vomit, and complains that her stomach hurts when he tries to drop her off now.

Nursing Diagnosis ✻ Fear related to separation and abandonment during preschool period

Outcome Criteria ✻ Child verbalizes fear. Father demonstrates measures to minimize child's fears; reports by 2 weeks that crying episodes at school have decreased.

Team Member Responsible	Assessment	Intervention	Rationale	Expected Outcome
		Activities of Daily Living		
Nurse	Ask father to detail a 24-hour day in family to gain clear picture of child's role and capabilities.	Father describes differences in family life since wife has been hospitalized, strain it causes on Cathy.	People are unable to solve a problem until the extent of the problem is clear.	Father details a typical day and may express his wish to continue the preschool experience
		Consultations		
Nurse	Assess if father feels referral to child guidance service is necessary to help reduce fear.	Encourage the father to talk with the preschool staff about the problem and common methods to decrease a child's fear.	Discussion with care providers can help reinforce the measures used by the father, providing consistency and thereby helping to minimize a child's fears.	Father states he will consult with preschool staff to help solve problem.
		Procedures/Medications		
Nurse	Assess what father knows about measures to reduce fear in preschoolers.	Instruct the father in measures to help reduce child's fear, such as reinforcing the time he will return. Will call if he's running late. Post memo to self to pick her up.	Reassurance helps to reduce a child's fear of abandonment.	Father describes steps he will take to be certain he will not be late again at preschool for pick up.
		Nutrition		
Nurse	Assess if child uses threat of vomiting at any other time.	Stress effect of eating disorders is potentially dangerous.	Frequent vomiting in young children can lead to fluid and electrolyte imbalances.	Father states whether he has ever seen pseudovomiting before.

Patient/Family Education				
Nurse/nurse practitioner	Assess father's knowledge of typical preschool fears such as abandonment, fear of the dark.	Review with the father the typical fears experienced by the preschooler, including those of separation and abandonment.	Knowledge of normal growth and development helps to reduce the father's anxiety about the behavior and possible causes.	Father acknowledges he deals with adults in his business; expresses desire to learn more about preschool period.
Psychosocial/Spiritual/Emotional Needs				
Nurse	Explore with child why she is so fearful her father will not return for her.	Encourage the father to set up a special time for himself and his daughter in the evening or on weekends, so they have a consistent close time.	Special time for a father and daughter enhances the parent–child relationship. Consistently adhering to this time helps to foster a sense of trust and security and show he is dependable.	Father states he will plan for a special time each week, even if it is difficult to arrange because of wife's hospitalization and his irregular work schedule.
Discharge Planning				
Nurse	Assess if father would find a follow-up telephone call helpful.	Arrange for a follow-up telephone call (if desired) in one week.	Follow-up provides additional support and means for evaluating the effectiveness of the methods used.	Father states he is receptive to follow-up care.

Broken Fluency

Developing language is such a complicated process that children from 2 to 6 years of age typically have some speech difficulty. A child may begin to repeat words or syllables, saying, "I-I-I want a n-n-new spoon-spoon-spoon." This is called **broken fluency** (repetition and prolongation of sounds, syllables, and words). It is often referred to as **secondary stuttering** because the child began to speak without this problem and then, during the preschool years, developed it. Unlike the adult who stutters, children are unaware that they are not being fluent unless it is called to their attention. It is a part of normal development and, if accepted as such, will pass. It is associated with rapid speech patterns that may also be present in the parents (Savelkoul et al., 2007). A parent who knows a persistent stutterer or who was a persistent stutterer as a child may react to this normal broken fluency of the preschooler in a more emotional way than the problem deserves. If a child becomes conscious of a disrupted speech pattern, it is less likely the problem will correct itself. It is resolved most quickly if parents follow a few simple rules, listed in Box 31.8.

"Bathroom Language"

Many preschoolers imitate the vocabularies of their parents or older children in the family so well during this time that they incorporate swear words into their vocabularies. Parents may have to be reminded that children do not necessarily understand what the words mean; they have simply heard them, just as they have heard hundreds of other words and have decided to use them. Correction should be unemotional; for example, "That's not a word I like to hear you say. When you're angry, why don't you say 'fudge' (or whatever)?" The correcting is no different from that involved when a child uses poor grammar. If parents become emotional, a child realizes the value of such words and may continue using them for the attention they create.

Concerns of the Family With a Physically Challenged or Chronically Ill Preschooler

Learning how to do things when you have physical limitations can be frustrating. Being unable to understand how to do things because of physical or mental limitations can be even more so. To learn problem solving, however, is part of developing a sense of initiative. A preschooler with a disability such as cerebral palsy has a greater need for problem-solving skills than the average child, because even simple procedures such as eating or getting dressed can be difficult if a physical challenge limits the options.

Physically challenged or chronically ill preschoolers should attend a preschool program if at all possible because of the socialization benefits. Many of the learning activities that preschoolers enjoy, such as playing with paint, clay, or soap bubbles, are messy. If a child must remain in bed,

BOX 31.8 * Focus on Family Teaching

Suggestions to Reduce Stuttering in the Preschool Child

Q. Mr. Edwards says to you, "My 3-year-old daughter stutters. What can I do to stop this?"

A. What sounds like stuttering in a preschooler is often broken fluency. Helpful tips to improve fluency are:

- Do not discuss in a child's presence the difficulty she is having with speech. Do not label her a "stutterer." This makes her conscious of her speech patterns and compounds the problem. If you have to think about every word you say, it is difficult not to have trouble speaking.
- Listen with patience to what a child is saying. Do not interrupt or fill in a word for her. Do not tell her to speak more slowly or to start over. These actions make a child conscious of her speech, and her broken fluency increases.
- Talk to her in a calm, simple way. It is difficult for a child to keep up with adult speech. If adults talk slowly to her, she sees no need to rush and so speaks more clearly.
- Protect space for her to talk if there are other children in the family. Rushing to say something before a second child interrupts is the same as rushing to conform to adult speech.
- Do not force a child to speak if she does not want to. Do not ask her to recite or sing for strangers.
- Do not reward her for fluent speech or punish her for nonfluent speech. Broken fluency is a developmental stage in language formation, not an indication of regression or a chronic speech pattern.

parents may be reluctant to offer these types of experiences. A large tray of dry oatmeal or other breakfast cereal with sand shovels or cars and trucks is a good substitute activity for such a child. Although not necessarily neat, these substances (which are available even in a hospital setting) can be swept away easily at the finish of play. Table 31.5 lists nursing actions that can aid a chronically challenged child to solve problems and develop a sense of initiative.

Nutrition and the Physically Challenged or Chronically Ill Preschooler

Experiences with eating help to reinforce a sense of initiative in preschoolers. Chronically ill preschoolers who are limited in the foods they can eat (perhaps they have to maintain a diet of soft foods) or in their ability to help with food preparation may miss this reinforcement. If their appetite is diminished because of illness to the point where they take little or nothing orally, it is still important they continue to join the family at meals. In most households, this is a time for socialization, and preschoolers are ripe for the learning that goes with this type of daily interaction. Encourage parents to include the ill child in family meals and other social occasions whenever possible.

✓ Checkpoint Question 31.3

Cathy's parents want to know how to react to her when she begins to masturbate while watching television. What would you suggest?

a. They give her "timeout" when this begins.
b. They refuse to allow her to watch television.
c. They remind her some activities are private.
d. They schedule a health check-up for vaginal disease.

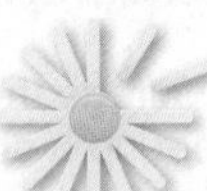

Key Points for Review

- Although preschoolers grow only slightly and gain just a little weight, they seem much taller than when they were toddlers because their contour changes to more childlike proportions.
- Erikson's developmental task for the preschool period is to gain a sense of initiative or learn how to do things. Play materials ideal for this age group are those that stimulate creativity, such as modeling clay or colored markers.
- Promoting childhood safety is a major role because preschoolers' active imaginations can lead them into dangerous situations.
- Appetite is not large in this age group because this is not a rapid growth time. Preschoolers can be interested in helping with food preparation.
- Common parental concerns during the preschool period are broken fluency, imaginary friends, difficulty sharing, and sibling rivalry.
- Preschool is often the time when a new sibling is born. Good preparation for this is necessary to prevent intense sibling rivalry.
- Preschoolers have a number of universal fears, including fear of the dark, mutilation, and abandonment. All care provided for this age group should include active measures to reduce these fears as much as possible.
- Preschoolers are still operating at a cognitive level that prevents them from understanding conservation (objects have not changed substance although they have changed appearance). This means they need an explanation, for example, of how they will be the same person postoperatively as they were preoperatively.
- Preschoolers are self-centered (egocentric). This makes it difficult for them to share and view someone else's side of a problem. They need good explanations of how a procedure will benefit them before they can agree to it.
- Many preschoolers begin preschool programs or child care. Late in the preschool period, they may be enrolled in kindergarten. Parents often appreciate guidance on how to prepare their children for these new experiences.
- Preschoolers who are physically challenged or who have chronic illnesses may have difficulty achieving a sense of initiative, because they may be limited in their ability to participate in activities that stimulate initiative. They may need special playtimes set aside for stimulation and learning.

TABLE 31.5 ✻ Nursing Actions That Encourage a Sense of Initiative in a Physically Challenged or Chronically Ill Preschooler

Consideration	Nursing Actions
Nutrition	Serving toast or sandwiches cut into animal shapes with cookie cutters, cereal in the form of alphabet characters, or food arranged on a plate to make a face appeals to the imagination and may make a preschooler more interested in food. Respect child's food preferences.
Dressing change	Allow preschooler to measure and cut tape or draw a face on it. Allow child to see incision site. Explain steps of dressing change as you work to reduce unknowns and areas of fear. Provide extra bandages to put on a doll so child can see that bandages themselves are not to be feared.
Medicine	Allow child to choose a chaser such as juice or milk after oral medicine. Choosing site for injection or intravenous line is too advanced for the preschooler; do not suggest such choices.
Rest	Provide a light in the room or bring child's bed into hallway so fear of the dark is reduced and child can deal with only reality problems. Identify sounds the preschooler might hear in the hospital, such as an air conditioner turning on.
Hygiene	Allow child to choose bathtub toys, clothing. Allow child to wash own hands and face. Allow child to splash in water as a play activity as well as for cleanliness.
Pain	Encourage preschooler to express pain. Allow child to handle syringe or suction catheter, and give "shots" or suction to a doll to alleviate anger or fear. Encourage child to ask for analgesic if necessary.
Stimulation	Guessing games encourage a sense of initiative. Draw a dog or a house and ask child to close his or her eyes while you add one more detail to the drawing, such as an ear or a chimney; ask child to identify new item. Reverse the game and ask child what you erased from the drawing, or allow child to do own drawing. Provide manipulative toys, such as finger paint, soapy water, clay, or dry cereal to use as sand. Allow preschooler to accompany you to other departments as a way of teaching more about the hospital. Use "Simon Says" games not only for socialization but also to urge treatments, such as deep-breathing exercises. Encourage use of playroom for socialization. Encourage child to interact with family by drawing pictures for siblings or using the telephone to call home.

CRITICAL THINKING EXERCISES

1. Cathy is the 3-year-old girl you met at the beginning of the chapter. Cathy's father is concerned because Cathy tells exaggerated stories about events at her preschool. How would you recommend her father handle this?
2. Because her family is moving, Cathy will be starting a new preschool next week. What suggestions could you make to her father about choosing a safe setting? How should he prepare Cathy for this experience?
3. Cathy's parents tell you she keeps the entire family awake at night because she is so afraid of the dark. What suggestions could you make to help relieve this problem?
4. Examine the National Health Goals related to growth and development of the preschooler. Most government-sponsored funds for nursing research are allotted based on these goals. What would be a possible research topic to explore pertinent to these goals that would be applicable to Cathy's family and also advance evidence-based practice?

CRITICAL THINKING SCENARIO

Open the accompanying CD-ROM or visit http://thePoint.lww.com and read the Patient Scenario included for this chapter, then answer the questions to further sharpen your skills and grow more familiar with NCLEX style questions related to preschool growth and development. Confirm your answers are correct by reading the rationales.

REFERENCES

American Academy of Pediatrics (AAP) Committee on Practice and Ambulatory Medicine. (2009). *Recommendations for preventive pediatric health care.* Washington, DC: Author.

American Academy of Pediatrics. (2009). Car safety seats: a guide for families. Retrieved from http://www.aap.org/family/carseatguide.htm

Anderzen-Carlsson, A., et al. (2007). Children's fear as experienced by the parents of children with cancer. *Journal of Pediatric Nursing, 22*(3), 233–244.

Armfield, J. M., & Spencer, A. J. (2007). Community effectiveness of fissure sealants and the effect of fluoridated water consumption. *Community Dental Health, 24*(1), 4–11.

Butterton, J. R., & Calderwood, S. B. (2008). Acute infectious diarrheal diseases and bacterial food poisoning. In Fauci, A. S., et al (Eds.). *Harrison's principles of internal medicine* (17th ed.). New York: McGraw-Hill.

Centers for Disease Control and Prevention (CDC). (2008). *Injuries Among Children and Adolescents.* Atlanta, GA: Author.

Cohen, A. L., et al. (2008). National surveillance of emergency department visits for outpatient adverse drug events in children and adolescents. *Journal of Pediatrics, 152*(3), 416–421.

Dooley, M., & Stewart, J. (2007). Family income, parenting styles and child behavioural-emotional outcomes. *Health Economics, 16*(2), 145–162.

DuRant, R. H. (2007). Firearm ownership and storage patterns among families with children who receive well-child care in pediatric offices. *Pediatrics, 119*(6), e1271–e1279.

Erikson, E. H. (1993). *Childhood and society.* New York: W. W. Norton.

Friedman, L. S. (2009). Hepatology. In McPhee, S. J., & Papadakis, M. A. (Eds.). *Current Medical Diagnosis and Treatment.* Columbus, OH: McGraw-Hill.

Gable, S., Chang, Y., & Krull, J. L. (2007). Television watching and frequency of family meals are predictive of overweight onset and persistence in a national sample of school-aged children. *Journal of the American Dietetic Association, 107*(1), 53–61.

Goddard, G. (2008). Temporomandibular disorders. In A. K. Lalwani (Ed.). *Current diagnosis and treatment in otolaryngology* (2nd ed.). Columbus, OH: McGraw-Hill.

Goldson, E., & Reynolds, A. (2008). Child development and behavior. In W. W. Hay, et al. (Eds.). *Current pediatric diagnosis and treatment* (18th ed.). Columbus, OH: McGraw-Hill.

Gordon, J., et al. (2007). Treatment of children's nighttime fears: the need for a modern randomised controlled trial. *Clinical Psychology Review, 27*(1), 98–113.

Hiscock, H., et al. (2007). Adverse associations of sleep problems in Australian preschoolers: national population study. *Pediatrics, 119*(1), 86–93.

Kaul, P., & Stevens-Simon, C. (2008). Substance abuse. In W. W. Hay, et al. (Eds.). *Current pediatric diagnosis and treatment* (18th ed.). Columbus, OH: McGraw-Hill.

Kline, A. M. (2008). Pediatric obesity in acute and critical care. *AACN: Advanced Critical Care, 19*(1), 38–46.

Kohlberg, L. (1984). *The psychology of moral development.* New York: Harper & Row.

Luborsky, L., & Barrett, M. S. (2007).The history and empirical status of key psychoanalytic concepts. *Annual Review of Clinical Psychology, 2007*(2), 1–19.

Mueller, W. A. (2008). Oral medicine and dentistry. In W. W. Hay, et al. (Eds.). *Current pediatric diagnosis and treatment* (18th ed.). Columbus, OH: McGraw-Hill.

Olsen, L., & DeBoise, T. (2007). Enhancing school readiness: the Early Head Start model. *Children and Schools, 29*(1), 47–50.

Pardi, L. A., et al. (2007). Issues in pediatrics. The effect of bicycle helmet legislation on pediatric injury. *Journal of Trauma Nursing, 14*(2), 84–87.

Piaget, J. (1969). *The theory of stages in cognitive development.* New York: McGraw-Hill.

Rolfes, S. R., Pinna, K., & Whitney, E. N. (2009). *Understanding normal and clinical nutrition.* New York: Wadsworth/Cengage Learning.

Savelkoul, E. M., et al. (2007). Coordinated interpersonal timing in the conversations of children who stutter and their mothers and fathers. *Journal of Fluency Disorders, 32* (1), 1–32.

Taylor, T. (2007). Managing unwanted behaviour in pre-school children. *Community Practitioner, 80*(4), 30–35.

Thompson, D. C., & Rivara, F. P. (2009). Pool fencing for preventing drowning in children. *Cochrane Database of Systematic Reviews, 2009*(1), (CD001047).

Windich-Biermeier, A., et al. (2007). Effects of distraction on pain, fear, and distress during venous port access and venipuncture in children and adolescents with cancer. *Journal of Pediatric Oncology Nursing,24*(1), 8–19.

Zoritch, B., Roberts, I., & Oakley, A. (2009). Day care for pre-school children. *Cochrane Database of Systematic Reviews, 2009*(1), (CD000564).

SUGGESTED READINGS

Chumlea, C. (2007). Which growth charts are the best for children today? *Nutrition Today, 42*(4), 148–150.

Darbyshire, P. (2007). 'Childhood': are reports of its death greatly exaggerated? *Journal of Child Health Care, 11*(2), 85–97.

Jellinek, M. S. (2008). Caring for the psychosocial needs of children: from advocacy to structural change. *Ambulatory Pediatrics, 8*(1), 8–10.

Klig, J. E. (2007). Violence and children: a view from the emergency department. *Current Opinion in Pediatrics, 19*(3), 245–246.

Kochanska, G., Aksan, N., & Joy, M. E. (2007). Children's fearfulness as a moderator of parenting in early socialization: two longitudinal studies. *Developmental Psychology, 43*(1), 222–237.

Lewis, C. W., et al. (2007). Preventive dental care for children in the United States: a national perspective. *Pediatrics, 119*(3), e544–e553.

Needham, L., et al. (2007). Supporting healthy eating among preschoolers: challenges for child care staff. *Canadian Journal of Dietetic Practice and Research, 68*(2), 107–110.

Powell, C., et al. (2009). Screening for amblyopia in childhood. *Cochrane Database of Systematic Reviews, 2009*(1), (CD005020).

Sullivan, M. C., & Msall, M. E. (2007). Functional performance of preterm children at age 4. *Journal of Pediatric Nursing: Nursing Care of Children and Families, 22*(4), 297–309.

Talen, M. R., et al. (2007). Well-child check-up revised: an efficient protocol for assessing children's social-emotional development. *Families, Systems and Health, 25*(1), 23–35.

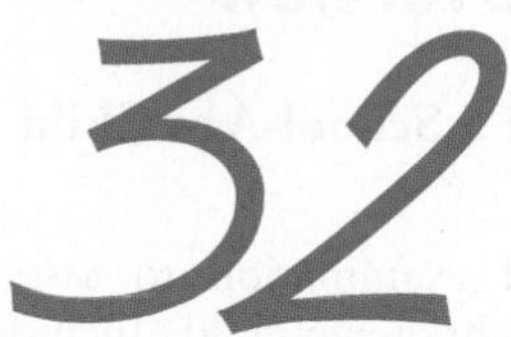

Chapter 32 Nursing Care of a Family With a School-Age Child

KEY TERMS

- accommodation
- caries
- class inclusion
- conservation
- decentering
- inclusion
- latchkey children
- malocclusion
- nocturnal emissions

OBJECTIVES

After mastering the contents of this chapter, you should be able to:

1. Describe the normal growth and development pattern and common parental concerns of the school-age period.
2. Identify National Health Goals related to school-age children that nurses can help the nation achieve.
3. Use critical thinking to analyze ways in which the care of school-age children can be more family centered.
4. Assess a school-age child for normal growth and development milestones.
5. Formulate nursing diagnoses that speak to both school-age children and their families.
6. Identify expected outcomes for nursing care of a school-ager.
7. Plan anticipatory guidance to prevent problems of growth and development in a school-age child such as teaching about normal puberty.
8. Implement nursing care to help achieve normal growth and development of a school-age child, such as counseling parents about helping their child adjust to a new school.
9. Evaluate expected outcomes for achievement and effectiveness of care.
10. Identify areas related to care of school-age children that could benefit from additional nursing research or application of evidence-based practice.
11. Integrate knowledge of school-age growth and development with nursing process to achieve quality maternal and child health nursing care.

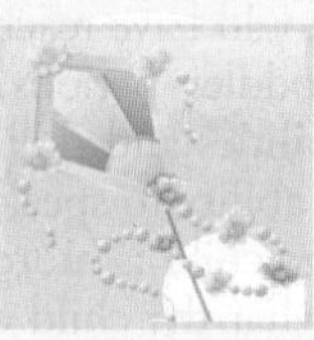

Shelly Lewis is a 12-year-old girl who recently started middle school. Her mother tells you that although Shelly, who is overweight, says she likes school, she has developed a lot of nervous habits such as nail biting since school started. Her mother asks if this is normal.

The previous chapter discussed the preschooler and the abilities children develop in those years. This chapter adds information about the dramatic changes, both physical and psychosocial, that occur during the school-age years. Such information builds a base for care and health teaching for this age group.

How would you advise Shelly's mother?

The term "school age" commonly refers to children between the ages of 6 and 12. Although these years represent a time of slow physical growth, cognitive growth and development continue to proceed at rapid rates. Because of this, there are many differences among children from one year to the next. For example, 7- and 10-year-old children have very different needs and outlooks, as do 11- and 12-year-old children. Because of these big differences, always assess children as individuals to understand the particular developmental needs of each child based on what developmental status has been achieved, not on what stage you think the child should have reached (AAP, 2009).

Unlike the infant or toddler periods, whose progress is marked by obvious new abilities and skills such as the ability to sit up or roll over or the ability to speak a full sentence, the development of a school-age child is more subtle and may be marked by mood swings; what the child enjoys on one occasion may not be acceptable on the next. For instance, a child may ask his parents for a guitar and lessons, but then after the family invests in these, he may quickly lose interest in music and prefer soccer. Children of school age may also be more influenced by the attitudes of their friends than previously. They may choose not to do something that was previously enjoyable because no friends are interested in the activity. Parents who make too much of these likes and dislikes may find themselves engaged in unnecessary conflicts with their child. The school-age period is usually the first time children begin to make truly independent judgments. As parents may not be prepared for this, this may also create conflicts with parents. Box 32.1 lists National Health Goals related to the school-age period.

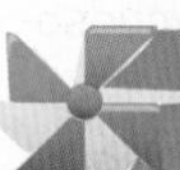

BOX 32.1 * Focus on National Health Goals

A number of National Health Goals address the health of the school-age population:

- Increase the proportion of public and private schools that require daily physical education for all students from a baseline of 17% to a target of 25%.
- Reduce the rate of deaths caused by motor vehicle accidents to no more than 9.2 per 100,000 children from a baseline of 15.6 per 100,000.
- Reduce the proportion of children who have dental caries (in permanent or primary teeth) to no more than 11% from a baseline of 18%.
- Increase children's rate of safety belt use in automobiles from a baseline of 69% to 92%.
- Increase the number of states that require helmet use by bicyclists from 10 to 50 states (http://www.nih.gov).

Nurses can help the nation achieve these goals by urging children to begin and maintain a consistent exercise program, brush teeth and go for dental checkups regularly, and follow safety rules both in and around automobiles. Additional nursing research that would be helpful includes these questions: What is the ideal exercise program that is interesting enough to children that it will hold their attention for a long span of time? What are effective ways to teach street safety to children in the early school years? What strategies are most effective in helping school-age children brush teeth daily?

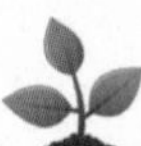

Nursing Process Overview

For Healthy Development of a School-Age Child

Assessment

Use both history and physical examination to assess growth and development of a school-age child. Include questions about school activities and progress. School-age children are interested and able to contribute to their own health history; to allow for this, it is useful to interview children 10 years or older at least in part without their parents present. During the physical examination, show your respect for children's adult-level modesty by furnishing a cover gown.

Parents of school-age children often mention behavioral issues or conflicts during yearly health visits. Some parents feel they are losing contact with their children during these years. This can cause them to misinterpret a normal change in behavior, especially if they are not prepared for what to expect from their child. Other parents may consider children who behave differently from their siblings as "abnormal" when children are just expressing their own personality.

When problems are discussed in the health care setting, take the history from the parent but also allow the child to express the problem. It may be necessary to obtain the opinion of school personnel (with the parents' permission) regarding the problem or even just determine whether school personnel feel a problem exists. In some instances, a counselor's opinion may be necessary. If the problem is related to a medical condition, its effect on the family should also be assessed, because the illness of a child affects the functioning of the entire family.

Nursing Diagnosis

Common nursing diagnoses pertinent to growth and development during the school-age period are:

- Health-seeking behaviors related to normal school-age growth and development
- Readiness for enhanced parenting related to improved family living conditions
- Anxiety related to slow growth pattern of child
- Risk for injury related to deficient parental knowledge about safety precautions for a school-age child
- Imbalanced nutrition, more than body requirements, related to frequent consumption of snack foods
- Delayed growth and development related to speech, motor, psychosocial, or cognitive concerns

Outcome Identification and Planning

When identifying expected outcomes and planning care, keep in mind that school-age children tend to enjoy small or short-term projects rather than long, involved ones. A child with diabetes, for example, in her early school years may gain a feeling of achievement by learning to assess her own serum glucose level, but she may have difficulty continuing glucose assessment on a regular basis.

Behavior problems need to be well defined before outcomes are identified and interventions planned. Often, it is enough for parents to accept the problem as one consistent with normal growth and development. A helpful Web site to recommend to parents to learn more about school-age growth and development is the American Academy of Pediatrics (http://www.aap.org). For questions about car seats, parents can consult the U.S. Department of Transportation National Highway Traffic Safety Administration (http://www.nhtsa.dot.gov).

Implementation

School-age children are interested in learning about adult roles, so this means they will watch you to see your attitude as well as your actions in a given situation. When giving care, keep in mind children this age feel more comfortable if they know the "hows" and "whys" of actions. They may not cooperate with a procedure until they are given a satisfactory explanation of why it must be done.

Outcome Evaluation

Yearly health visits covering both physical and psychosocial development are important at this age. It may be useful for parents to look back on problems identified at the last visit and discuss if and how they were resolved. Often, some problems and conflicts fade away without anyone really noticing. As some problems recede, however, others may emerge. At times, the same concerns of parents and the child may appear to be unresolved at each visit. Make sure no underlying problem exists that prevents resolution. Examples of expected outcomes are:

- Parent states he allows child to make own decisions about how to spend allowance.
- Child lists books she and her parents have read together in past 2 weeks.
- Child states he understands his growth is normal, even though he is the shortest boy in his eighth-grade class.
- Child does not sustain injury from sports activities during the summer recess.

GROWTH AND DEVELOPMENT OF A SCHOOL-AGE CHILD

Growth and development for a school-age child occur slowly, and over a relatively long time span so children grow and develop extensively during this period.

Physical Growth

School-age children's annual average weight gain is approximately 3 to 5 lb (1.3 to 2.2 kg); the increase in height is 1 to 2 in (2.5 to 5 cm). Children who did not lose the lordosis and knock-kneed appearance of toddlers during the preschool period lose these now. Posture becomes more erect (Goldson & Reynolds, 2008).

By 10 years of age, brain growth is complete, so fine motor coordination becomes refined. As the eye globe reaches its final shape at about this same time, an adult vision level is achieved. If the eruption of permanent teeth and growth of the jaw do not correlate with final head growth, **malocclusion** (a deviation from the normal) with teeth malalignment may be present.

The immunoglobulins IgG and IgA reach adult levels, and lymphatic tissue continues to grow up until about age 9. Because the lymphatic system grows so rapidly, this results in an abundance of tonsillar and adenoid tissue in the early school years, which is often mistaken for disease during respiratory illness as the tonsils seem so enlarged in the back of the throat. Enlarged tonsils may also result in temporary conduction deafness from eustachian tube obstruction until this tissue recedes normally.

The appendix is also lined with lymphatic tissue, so swelling of this tissue in the narrow tube can lead to trapped fecal material and inflammation (appendicitis) in the early school-age child. Frontal sinuses develop at about 6 years, so sinus headache becomes a possibility (before then, headache in children is rarely caused by a sinus infection).

The left ventricle of the heart enlarges to be strong enough to pump blood to the growing body. Innocent heart murmurs may become apparent because of the extra blood crossing heart valves. The pulse rate decreases to 70 to 80 beats per minute; blood pressure rises to about 112/60 mm Hg. Maturation of the respiratory system leads to increased oxygen–carbon dioxide exchange, which increases exertion ability and stamina. Scoliosis may become apparent for the first time in late childhood. All school-age children over age 8 should be screened for this at all health appraisals (see Chapter 51).

Sexual Maturation

At a set point in brain maturity, the hypothalamus transmits an enzyme to the anterior pituitary gland to begin production of gonadotropic hormones, which activate changes in testes and ovaries and produce puberty. Hormone changes that occur with puberty are discussed in Chapter 5. Table 32.1 describes the usual order for secondary sex characteristics to develop.

Timing of the onset of puberty varies widely, between 10 and 14 years of age. The length of time it takes to pass through puberty until sexual maturity is complete also varies. Sexual maturation in girls usually occurs between 12 and 18 years; in boys, between 14 and 20 years. Puberty is occurring increasingly earlier, however, and, in a class of 10-year-old sixth graders, it is not unusual to discover that more than half of the girls are already menstruating. This means that for sex education to be effective, parents must introduce this material when their children are in grade school, not in middle school or high school.

Sexual and Physical Concerns. The changes in physical appearance that come with puberty can lead to concerns for both children and their parents. School age is a time for parents to discuss with children the physical changes that will occur and the sexual responsibility these changes dictate. This is also a time to reinforce previous teaching with children that their body is their own, to be used only in the way they choose. Specific measures for children to help prevent sexual abuse are discussed later in this chapter. School nurses can play a major role in this type of education as well.

In both sexes, puberty brings changes in the sebaceous glands. Under the influence of androgen, glands become more active, setting the stage for acne (see Chapter 33). Vasomotor instability commonly leads to blushing; perspiration also increases (Kaplan & Love-Osborne, 2008).

Concerns of Girls. Prepubertal girls are usually taller, by about 2 in (5 cm) or more, than preadolescent boys because their typical growth spurt begins earlier. In a culture in which

TABLE 32.1 ✻ Chronologic Development of Secondary Sex Characteristics

Age (yr)	Boys	Girls
9–11	Prepubertal weight gain occurs.	Breasts: elevation of papilla with breast bud formation; areolar diameter enlarges.
11–12	Sparse growth of straight, downy, slightly pigmented hair at base of penis. Scrotum becoming textured; growth of penis and testes begins. Sebaceous gland secretion increases. Perspiration increases.	Straight hair along the labia. Vaginal epithelium becomes cornified. pH of vaginal secretions acid; slight mucous vaginal discharge present. Sebaceous gland secretion increases. Perspiration increases. Dramatic growth spurt.
12–13	Pubic hair present across pubis. Penis lengthens. Dramatic linear growth spurt. Breast enlargement occurs.	Pubic hair grows darker; spreads over entire pubis. Breasts enlarge, still no protrusion of nipples. Axillary hair present. Menarche occurs.

boys are expected to be taller than girls, this can cause concern. Sometimes a girl notices the change in her pelvic contour when she tries on a skirt or dress from the year before and realizes her hips are becoming broader. She may misinterpret this finding as a gain in weight and attempt a crash diet. She can be reassured that broad bone structure of the hips is part of an adult female profile.

Girls are usually conscious of breast development, and whether they are overdeveloped or underdeveloped. Also, breast development is not always symmetrical, so it is not unusual for a girl to have breasts of slightly different sizes. After the condition has been checked during a physical examination, she can be reassured that this development is normal. Supernumerary (additional) nipples may darken or increase in size at puberty. Be sure girls understand that a supernumerary nipple is affected by the hormones in her body in the same way as other breast tissue, so she understands these changes are normal.

Early preparation for menstruation is important for future childbearing and for the girl's concept of herself as a woman (Box 32.2). In addition to an explanation of the reason for menstrual flow, girls need an explanation of good hygiene and reassurance they can bathe, shower, and swim during their periods. They can use either sanitary napkins or tampons; if they choose tampons, they must take precautions to avoid toxic shock syndrome (see Chapter 47).

BOX 32.2 ✻ Focus on Communication

Shelly is a 12-year-old girl who comes to the nurse's office at her school.

Less Effective Communication

Nurse: Hello, Shelly. What can I do for you?
Shelly: I'm having cramps.
Nurse: Are you having your period?
Shelly: No. I haven't started them yet.
Nurse: Describe your cramps to me.
Shelly: Both my sisters started their periods when they were 10.
Nurse: Are you sick to your stomach?
Shelly: I'm the only girl in my gym class who doesn't have her period yet.
Nurse: Let's talk about the cramps. What do you think is causing those?
Shelly: They're not really bad. I'll go back to class.

More Effective Communication

Nurse: Hello, Shelly. What can I do for you?
Shelly: I'm having cramps.
Nurse: Are you having your period?
Shelly: No. I haven't started them yet.
Nurse: Describe your cramps to me.
Shelly: Both my sisters started their periods when they were 10.
Nurse: Are you sick to your stomach?
Shelly: I'm the only girl in my gym class who doesn't have her period yet.
Nurse: You sound as if you're more worried about that than what you came in for.
Shelly: I need to know if I'm all right.
Nurse: Let's talk about that.

In the past, when topics such as menstruation were discussed only in whispers and neither television nor magazines advertised sanitary pads or medicine for menstrual discomfort, most 12-year-old children had little idea about what to expect at puberty. Today, with this information readily available to the public, it is easy to forget that preadolescents, because they may not read magazines or watch adult television shows, still may not know much about what to expect at puberty. Be aware that almost all prepubescent girls are concerned about puberty changes. Through effective communication and listening, you can help them talk about their problems and concerns.

The average age at which menarche (the first menstrual period) occurs is 12.4 years (McDowell, Brody, & Hughes, 2007). Most girls have some menstrual irregularity during the first year or two after menarche. This occurs primarily because a girl's cycles are anovulatory at first. With maturity and the onset of ovulation, cycles become more regular. A preadolescent who is experiencing consistent irregularities in her period should be assessed for malnourishment and obesity as possible influences. Emotions can also cause irregularity. If irregularity continues beyond the first year, a careful history of the girl's school, social, nutrition, level of exercise, and home adjustment should be taken. Dysmenorrhea, or painful menstruation, is discussed in Chapter 47.

Girls also need to know that vaginal secretions will begin to be present. If this is not explained, a girl may fear needlessly that she has contracted an infection. Explain that any secretions that cause vulvar irritation should be evaluated at a health care facility, because this does suggest infection.

Concerns of Boys. Boys who are not prepared for the physical changes of puberty are as equally concerned about them as are girls. Just as girls are keenly aware of breast development, boys are aware of increasing genital size. If they do not know testicular development precedes penis growth, they can worry that their growth will be inadequate. Boys should also be informed that hypertrophy of breast tissue (gynecomastia) can occur in prepuberty (most often in stocky or obese boys), and that this is a transitory phenomenon and, although it may cause self-conscious reactions, it will fade as soon as the male hormones become more mature and active.

Some boys also become concerned because, although they have pubic hair, they cannot yet grow a beard or do not have chest hair—outward, easily recognized signs of maturity. You can assure them that pubic hair normally appears first and that chest and facial hair may not grow until several years later.

As seminal fluid is produced, boys begin to notice ejaculation during sleep, termed **nocturnal emissions.** Preadolescent boys may believe an old myth that loss of seminal fluid is debilitating; also, boys may have heard the term "premature ejaculation" and worry this is a forewarning of a problem in years to come. Both are fallacies.

Teeth

Deciduous teeth are lost and permanent teeth erupt during the school-age period (Fig. 32.1). The average child gains 28 teeth between 6 and 12 years of age: the central and lateral incisors; first, second, and third cuspids; and first and second molars (Fig. 32.2).

Developmental Milestones

As with all ages, you can measure school-age children's progress by whether they meet typical developmental milestones.

Gross Motor Development

School-age development is summarized in Table 32.2. At the beginning of the school-age period (age 6), children endlessly jump, tumble, skip, and hop. They have enough coordination to walk a straight line. Many can ride a bicycle. They can skip rope with practice. A 7-year-old appears quiet compared

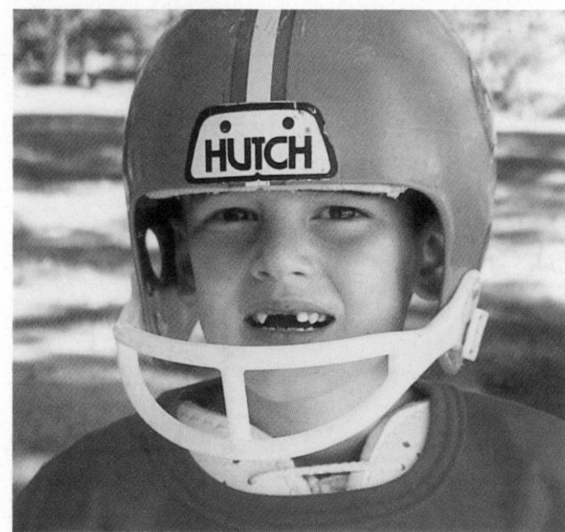

FIGURE 32.1 Early-school-age children typically have a missing upper incisor as deciduous teeth are replaced by permanent teeth.

with a rough-and-tumble 6-year-old. Gender differences usually begin to manifest in play: there are "girl games," such as dressing dolls, and "boy games," such as pretending to be pirates.

The movements of 8-year-olds are more graceful than those of younger children, although as their arms and legs grow, they may stumble on furniture or spill milk and food. They ride a bicycle well and enjoy sports such as gymnastics, soccer, and hockey.

Nine-year-olds are on the go constantly, as if they always have a deadline to meet. They have enough eye–hand coordination to enjoy baseball, basketball, and volleyball. By 10 years of age, they are more interested in perfecting their athletic skills than they were previously.

At age 11, many children feel awkward because of their growth spurt and drop out of sports activities rather than look ungainly in their attempts. They may channel their energy into constant motion instead: constantly drumming fingers and tapping pencils or feet. This fall in sports participation may bother parents who see sports as the key to popularity or self-esteem.

Twelve-year-olds plunge into activities with intensity and concentration. They often enjoy participating in sports events for charities such as walk-a-thons. They may be refreshingly cooperative around the house, able to handle a great deal of responsibility, and complete given tasks.

Fine Motor Development

Six-year-olds can easily tie their shoelaces. They can cut and paste well and draw a person with good detail. They can print, although they may routinely reverse letters. Seven-year-olds concentrate on fine motor skills even more than they did the year before. This has been called the "eraser year" because children are never quite content with what they have done. They set too high a standard for themselves and then have difficulty performing at that level.

By 8 years of age, children's eyes are developed enough so they can read regular-size type. This can make reading a greater pleasure and school more enjoyable (Fig. 32.3).

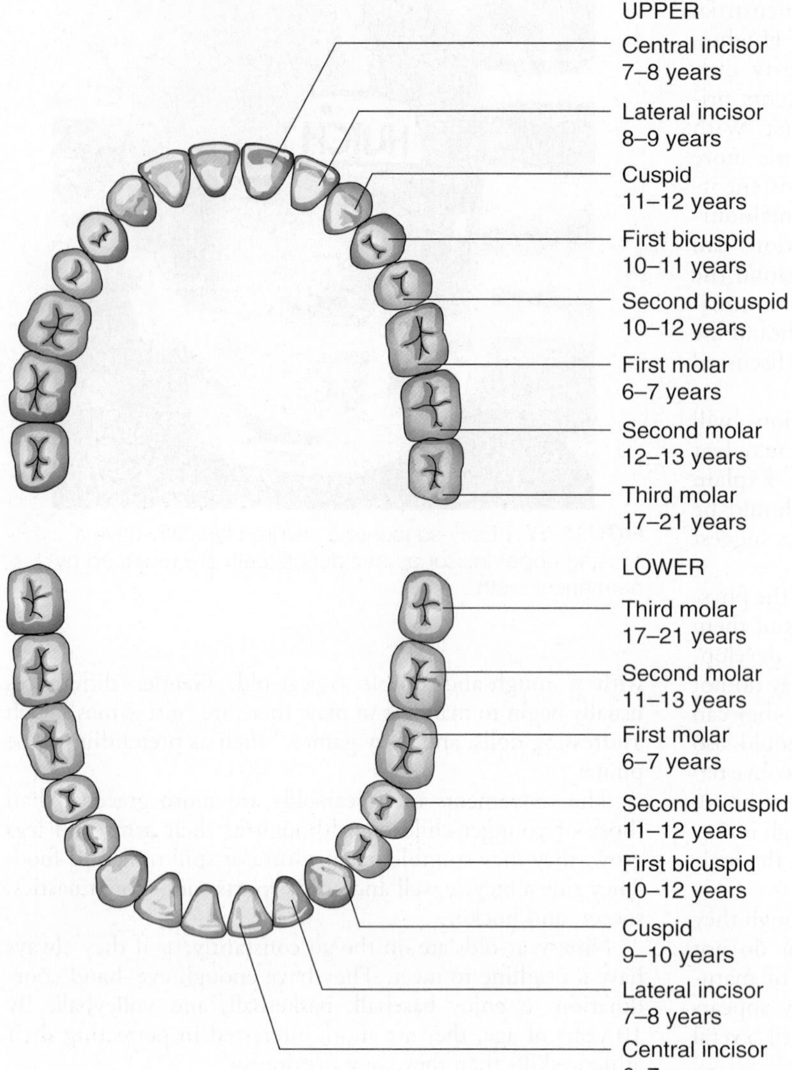

FIGURE 32.2 Eruption pattern of permanent teeth.

Eight-year-olds learn to write script rather than print. They enjoy showing off this new skill in cards, letters, or projects. By age 9, their writing begins to look mature and less awkward.

Older school-age children begin to evaluate their teachers' ability and may perform at varying levels, depending on each teacher's expectations. The middle school curriculum involves more challenging science and mathematics courses than previously and includes good literature. This may be a child's first exposure to reading as a fulfilling and worthwhile experience rather than just as an assignment and may be the time a child is "turned on" to reading.

Play

Play continues to be rough at age 6; however, when children discover reading as an enjoyable activity that opens doors to other worlds, they can begin to spend quiet time with books. Many children spend hours playing increasingly challenging video games, an activity that can either foster a healthy sense of competition or create isolation from others.

By 7 years of age, children require more props for play than when they were younger, which indicates the start of a decline in imaginative play; this may continue unless a child receives adequate encouragement to use imagination. Children also begin to develop an interest in collecting items such as baseball cards, dolls, rocks, or marbles. The type of item may not be as important as the quantity. By age 8, collections may become increasingly structured as children develop skills for sorting and cataloging.

Competitive behaviors can develop and cause children to change the rules in the middle of a game to keep from losing. At about 10 years of age, children become very interested in rules and fairness in competitive play situations (Fig. 32.4). Children also begin discovering the Internet and how other children out there are waiting to talk to them in chat rooms. Not yet wise enough to recognize the dangers talking to strangers can create, this is an activity parents need to supervise. Music and artistic expression also become important during this time. During preteen years, listening to music and learning popular dances take the place of earlier simple games. Both boys and girls seem to feel they are on the verge of something great and anxiously wait to turn 13 and be a teenager.

TABLE 32.2 ✲ Summary of School-Age Development

Age (yr)	Physical Development	Psychosocial and Cognitive Development
6	A year of constant motion; skipping is a new skill; first molars erupt.	First-grade teacher becomes authority figure; adjustment to all-day school may be difficult and lead to nervous manifestations of fingernail biting, etc. Defines words by their use: a key is to unlock a door, not a metal object.
7	Central incisors erupt; difference between sexes becomes apparent in play (video games vs. dolls); spends time in quiet play.	A quiet year; striving for perfection leads to this year being called an eraser year. Conservation (water poured from tall container to a wide, flat one is the same amount of water) is learned; can tell time; can make simple change.
8	Coordination definitely improved; playing with gang becomes important; eyes become fully developed.	"Best friends" develop; whispering and giggling begin; can write as well as print; understands concepts of past, present, and future.
9	All activities done with gang.	Gang age; a 9-year-old club is formed to spite someone, has secret codes, is all boy or all girl; gangs disband and reform quickly.
10	Coordination improves.	Ready for camp away from home; collecting age; likes rules; ready for competitive games.
11	Active, but awkward and ungainly.	Insecure with members of opposite sex; repeats off-color jokes.
12	Coordination improves.	A sense of humor is present; is social and cooperative.

Language Development

Six-year-olds talk in full sentences, using language easily and with meaning. They no longer sound as though talking is an experiment but appear to have incorporated language permanently. They still define objects by their use: a key is to unlock a door; a fork is to eat with.

Most 7-year-olds can tell the time in hours, but they may have trouble with concepts such as "half past" and "quarter to," especially with the prevalence of digital clocks and watches. They know the months of the year and can name the months in which holidays fall. They can add and subtract and make simple change (if they have had experience), so they can go to the store and make simple purchases. Much of children's talk is concerned with these concepts as they practice them and show them off for family or friends.

As children discover "dirty" jokes at about age 9, they like to tell them to friends or try to understand those told by adults. They use swear words to express anger or just to show other children they are growing up. They may have a short period of intense fascination with "bathroom language," as they did during preschool years. As before, if they want to discourage this, parents should make it clear they find such language unacceptable and refrain from using it themselves in their child's presence.

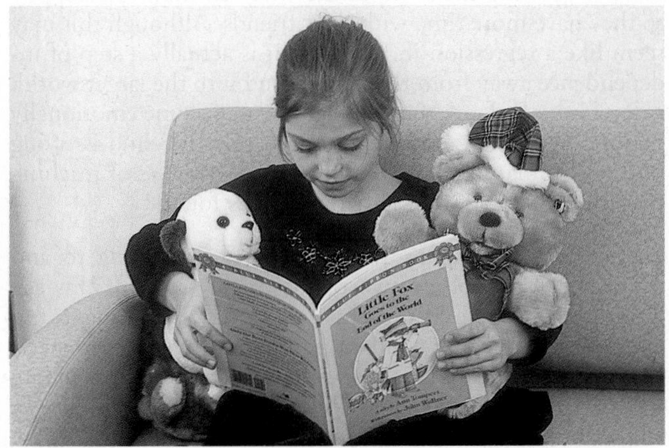

FIGURE 32.3 One of the biggest discoveries of childhood is that reading and writing are fun. Both are activities that can help a child pass the hours of illness.

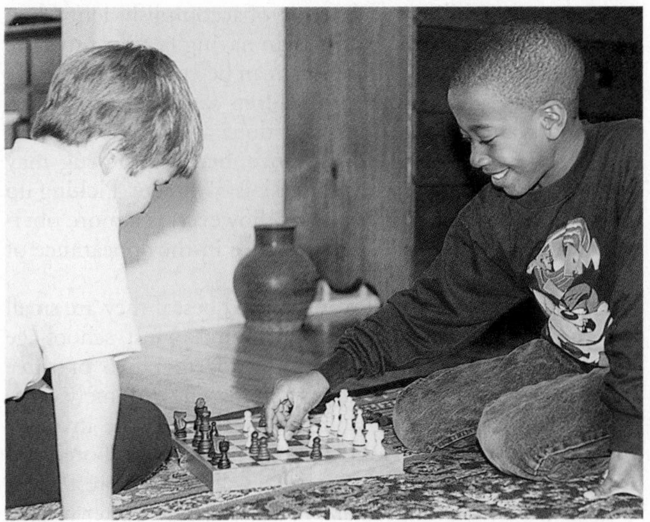

FIGURE 32.4 By 10 years of age, children are ready for competition. These two children enjoy a game of chess.

By 12 years of age, a sense of humor is apparent. Twelve-year-olds can carry on an adult conversation, although stories are limited because of their lack of experience.

Emotional Development

Ideally, children enter the school-age period with the ability to trust others and with a sense of respect for their own worth. They can accomplish small tasks independently because they have gained a sense of autonomy. They should have practiced or mimicked adult roles and had the opportunity to explore at preschool or other social environments. They should have learned to share, to have discovered that learning is fun and an adventure, and have learned that doing things is more important and more rewarding than watching things being done (a sense of initiative).

Developmental Task: Industry Versus Inferiority

During the early school years, children attempt to master yet another developmental step: learning a sense of industry or accomplishment (Erikson, 1993). If gaining a sense of initiative can be defined as learning how to do things, then gaining a sense of industry is learning how to do things well.

If children are prevented from achieving a sense of industry or do not receive rewards for accomplishment, they can develop a feeling of inferiority or become convinced they cannot do things they actually can do. These children will have difficulty tackling new situations later in life (new job, new school, new responsibility) because they cannot envision how they could be successful in handling them. This can result in frustration in school or work activities.

The questions a preschool child asks reflect curiosity, such as "how," "why," and "what." During the early school years, children concentrate their questions on the "how" of tasks: "Is this the right way to do this?" "Am I making this right?" "Is this good?" Often school-age children will comment, "I can't do anything right" because their craft project does not look perfect or falls short of expectations. School-age children need reassurance they are doing things correctly and this reassurance is best if it comes frequently rather than infrequently after long waits.

The best type of book for school-age children has many short chapters; children feel a sense of accomplishment when they finish each chapter, rather than having to wait until the end of the book. Small chores that can be completed quickly also give this type of reward. Children can survey their finished work and see that they have done a good job. A child may dislike vacuuming, for instance, because the rug may not look very different when the task is complete. Picking up the scattered contents of a toy box, however, is a more obvious task that clearly makes a difference in the appearance of the room.

Hobbies and projects also are enjoyed best if they are small and can be finished within a short time. Most school-age children, for example, prefer putting together two or three fairly simple model-car kits to assembling one extremely complicated kit. The three kits offer three rewards; the involved one delays the reward so long the child may become bored and never complete it. With adolescence will come more respect for quality. Children will realize if they want the better model, they will have to spend the extra energy and attention—quality products involve quality work (Fig. 32.5).

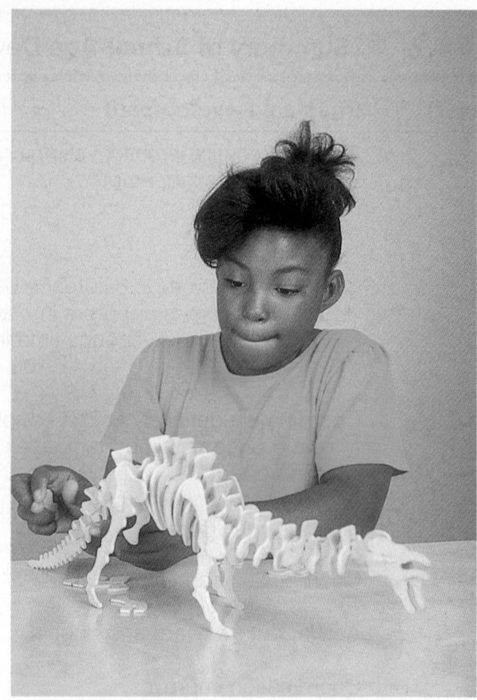

FIGURE 32.5 Assembling this simple model in a short time helps a school-age child gain a sense of industry. (© Stephen Frisch/Stock Boston.)

Home as a Setting to Learn Industry. Parents of a school-age child need to take a step forward in development along with their child. For the first time, they realize their child looks to other role models than themselves. Parents who enjoyed fostering imagination in a preschooler may feel frustrated when a school-age child begins to conform to rules and insists on the "right way" to do things. They may feel they have failed to encourage the child's creativity, but conformity is vital to children at this age. It is how they learn more about their world's rules.

Eight- or 9-year-olds begin to spend more and more time with their peers and less time with their family. They forget to do household chores they once enjoyed, such as setting the table or mowing the lawn, or they may do the work sloppily so they have more time with their friends. Although this may seem like a regression in behavior, it is actually a step of independence away from the parents and into the larger world, a developmental task that will help them become emotionally mature. This is an example of a new role the child is trying out, one of many that will be tried in the process of reaching maturity, when an eventual "right-fit" is found.

School as a Setting to Learn Industry. Adjusting to and achieving in school are two of the major tasks for this age group. Ideally, a child's teacher will think of learning as fun and will encourage a child to plunge into new experiences. Unfortunately, parents must monitor teachers and school activities to make sure their children are being led this way while not being pushed too hard.

Schools are increasingly assuming responsibility for education about sex, safety, avoidance of substances of abuse, and preparation for family living. These discussions are generally superficial, however, and if the classes are large, they may raise more questions than they answer. Although learning these skills with peers helps children learn other people's opinions in these areas, such classes should not replace parental teaching. If given adequate encouragement and preparation by health care providers, most parents are eager to maintain such responsibility.

Structured Activities. Girl Scouts, Boy Scouts, Campfire Girls, and 4-H clubs are respected school-age activities. If the local chapters are well run by leaders who understand children's needs, they can provide hours of constructive activity and strengthen a sense of industry. Merit badge systems are geared to the needs of school-age children, offering small but frequent rewards. As with school activities, parents should determine the worth of each organization for their individual child.

Urge parents to evaluate competitive sports programs as well. Before children can compete successfully, they must be able to lose a game without feeling devastated—in other words, to be able to say, "I lost because I played badly," not "I lost because I am a bad person." Children do not usually develop sufficient ego strength to do this until they are about 10 years old.

Another problem to consider with organized contact sports is the possibility of athletic injuries. Encourage parents to consider their child's maturity and the risk of injury (see Chapter 51) before they decide whether team competition is right for their child.

Problem Solving. An important part of developing a sense of industry is learning how to solve problems. Parents and teachers can help children develop this skill by encouraging practice. When a child asks, "Is this the right way to do this?" a parent can encourage problem solving by saying, "Let's talk about possible ways of doing it" rather than offering a quick solution.

The world depends on machinery, so mishaps and breakdowns (and therefore sudden changes) do occur. A child who can create an indoor playhouse with a card table and blanket when it is too wet or cold to use an outdoor playhouse will be able, as an adult, to problem solve another solution to a data distribution problem when a computer malfunctions. This attitude of optimism rather than pessimism toward problem solving produces adults who rarely say, "It can't be done." Just as important, it leaves these adults with confidence and a sense of pride, feeling good about themselves because they have control of their environment and abilities.

Learning to Live With Others. School-age children are sometimes so interested in tasks and in accomplishing physical projects that they forget they must work with people to achieve these goals. A good time to urge children to learn compassion and thoughtfulness toward others is during the early school years, when children are first exposed to large groups of other youngsters. Writing thank-you letters and shoveling an older neighbor's sidewalk are examples of activities that can help children develop empathy toward others.

Learning to give a present without receiving one in return or doing a favor without expecting a reward is also a part of this process, and this can be taught by example. Children should see their parents doing such things with an attitude not of "What will I get?" but "What can I contribute?"

Children may show empathy toward others as early as 20 months, but cognitively they cannot relate others' experiences to their own until about 6 years of age. Therefore, it is usually ineffective to lecture a child by saying, "That was cruel to call Mary names." The child may feel she had every right to do so. A better technique is to ask children to put themselves in Mary's place for a minute and imagine how they would feel if they were Mary. A school-age child will generally be able to do this and understand why name-calling hurts and makes children feel rejected. Following this, a simple statement such as, "It doesn't feel good to be called names, does it?" may suffice.

Socialization

Six-year-old children play in groups, but when they are tired or under added stress, they prefer one-to-one contact. In a first-grade classroom, students compete actively for a few minutes of special time with their teacher. At the end of a day, they enjoy time spent individually with parents. You may have to remind parents this is not babyish behavior but that of a typical 6-year-old.

Seven-year-olds are increasingly aware of family roles and responsibility. Promises must be kept, because 7-year-olds view them as definite, firm commitments. These children tattle because they have a strong sense of justice. This tattling may dissolve play groups quickly.

Eight-year-olds actively seek the company of other children. Most 8-year-old girls have a close girlfriend; boys have a close boyfriend. Girls begin to whisper among themselves as they share secrets with close friends, annoying both parents and teachers.

Nine-year-olds take the values of their peer group very seriously. They are much more interested in how other children dress than in what their parents want them to wear. This is typically the gang age because children form clubs, usually "spite clubs." This means if there are four girls on the block, three form a club and exclude the fourth. The reason for exclusion is often unclear; it might be that the fourth child has a chronic disease, that she has more or less money than the others, that she was at the dentist's the day the club was formed, or simply that the club cannot exist unless there is someone to exclude. Such clubs typically have a secret password and secret meeting place. Membership is generally all girls or all boys. If an excluded child does not react badly to being shut out, the club will probably disband after a few days because its purpose is lost. The next day, the excluded member may meet with two others and snub a different child. Parents have to be careful not to intervene with this type of play, because loyalties shift quickly: the child they defend today may be the excluded one tomorrow.

Because they are so ready for social interaction, 9-year-olds are ready for activities away from home, such as a week at camp. They can take care of their own needs and are mature enough to be separated from their parents for this length of time. Going to camp before this age usually results in homesickness and can be a negative introduction to being away from home.

Although 10-year-olds enjoy groups, they also enjoy privacy. They like having their own bedroom or at least their own dresser, where they can store a collection and know it is free from parents' or siblings' eyes. One of the best gifts for a 10-year-old is a box that locks.

Girls become increasingly interested in boys and vice versa by 11 years of age. Favorite activities are mixed-sex rather than single-sex ones. Children of this age are particularly insecure, however, and girls tend to dance with girls while boys talk together in corners. Better socialization patterns need not be rushed. Just as infants crawl before they walk, so 11-year-olds must attempt many awkward and uncomfortable social experiences before they become comfortable forming relationships with the opposite sex.

Twelve-year-olds feel more comfortable in social situations than they did the year before. Boys experience erections on small provocation so may feel uncomfortable being pushed into boy–girl situations until they know how to control their bodies better. As some children develop faster than others, every group has some members who are almost adolescent and some who are still children, making social interests sometimes difficult.

✔ Checkpoint Question 32.1

Shelly has belonged to a series of clubs for 9-year-olds. A usual characteristic of clubs for this age child is:

a. The club has formal rules and regulations.
b. It is designed to help shy children socialize.
c. It is designed to spite or exclude another child.
d. Clubs include both boys and girls.

Cognitive Development

The period from 5 to 7 years of age is a transitional stage where children undergo a shift from the preoperational thought they used as preschoolers to concrete operational thought or the ability to reason through any problem they can actually visualize (Piaget, 1969) (Fig. 32.6).

Children can use concrete operational thought because they learn several new concepts, such as:

- **Decentering,** the ability to project oneself into other people's situations and see the world from their viewpoint rather than focusing only on their own view.

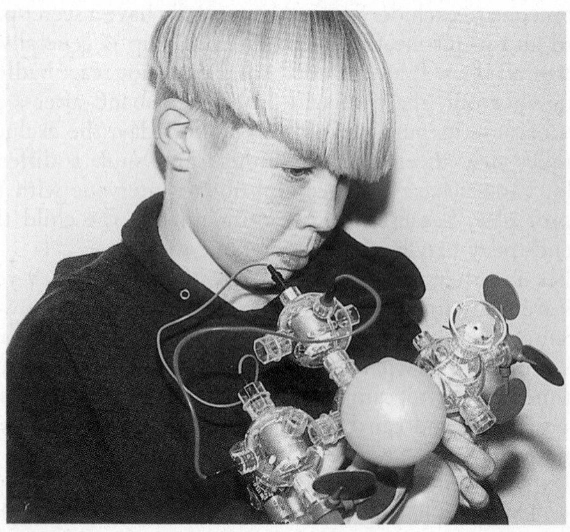

FIGURE 32.6 School-age children learn concrete operational thought or concentrate on phenomena they can actually see occurring.

- **Accommodation,** the ability to adapt thought processes to fit what is perceived such as understanding that there can be more than one reason for other people's actions. A preschooler might expect to see the same nurse in the morning who was there the evening before; a school-age child can understand that different nurses work different shifts.
- **Conservation,** the ability to appreciate that a change in shape does not necessarily mean a change in size. If you pour 30 mL of cough medicine from a thin glass into a wide one, the preschooler will say that one glass holds more than the other; a school-age child will say both glasses hold an equal amount.
- **Class inclusion,** the ability to understand that objects can belong to more than one classification. A preschooler can categorize items in only one way, for example, such as stones and shells are found at the beach; a school-age child can categorize them in many ways such as stones and shells are both found at the beach but are made of different materials, are different in sizes, etc.

These cognitive developments lead to some of the typical changes and characteristics of the school-age period. Decentering enables a school-age child to feel compassion for others, which was not possible in younger years. Because understanding conservation is possible, a school-age child is not fooled by perceptions as often as before; because of this, sibling arguments over food (your piece of pie is bigger than mine, his glass of cola is bigger than mine) decrease during the school-age years. The ability to classify objects leads to the collecting activities of the school-age period. Class inclusion is also necessary for learning mathematics and reading, systems that categorize numbers and words.

What if... ? You make a child's hospital bed one day and then give him an injection. What if the next day the child starts to cry while you're making the bed? The lack of what cognitive process led him to believe your action would be the same the second day?

Moral and Spiritual Development

School-age children begin to mature in terms of moral development as they enter a stage of *preconventional reasoning*, sometimes as early as 5 years of age (Kohlberg, 1984). During this stage, if asked, "Why is it wrong to steal from your neighbor?" school-age children will answer, "The police say it's wrong," or "Because if you do, you'll go to jail." They concentrate on "niceness" or "fairness" and cannot see yet that stealing hurts their neighbor, the highest level of moral reasoning.

School-age children begin to learn about the rituals and meaning behind their religious practices, so the distinction between right and wrong becomes more important to them than it was when they were preschoolers. Parent role modeling is also important. Remember that school-age children are rule-oriented; when they pray, they may expect their God to follow rules also (if you are good and pray for something, you should receive it). This makes children of this age confused if a prayer is not immediately answered. Because they are still limited in their ability to understand others' views, they may interpret something as being right because it is good for them, not because it is right for humanity as a whole.

What if... Shelly understands stealing from a neighbor is wrong? Will she also understand that stealing from a large department store or taking things from a health clinic is wrong?

HEALTH PROMOTION FOR A SCHOOL-AGE CHILD AND FAMILY

Because of still limited judgment, school children need guidelines in reference to safety, nutrition, and daily care. These are always excellent topics for discussion at health care visits (Box 32.3).

Promoting School-Age Safety

School-age children are ready for time on their own without direct adult supervision. Many children as young as 8 or 9 stay by themselves after school (see the section on latchkey children later in this chapter). Children are generally ready for this type of experience if they can reliably follow instructions (don't use the fireplace; don't open the door) and can occupy themselves for an hour's time. Be certain school-age children know to use seatbelts in cars and bicycle safety around cars (AAP, 2009). As with adults, accidents tend to occur when children are under stress. Box 32.4 lists common measures helpful in preventing accidents in this age group.

School age is not too early for parents to look at the effect of carrying heavy backpacks on children's posture. A backpack that weighs more than 10% of the child's body weight is enough to cause a child to have to lean forward chronically to bear the weight. This can lead to chronic back pain (Shilt & Barnett, 2007).

Sexual abuse is an unfortunate and all-too-common hazard for children. Teaching points to help children avoid sexual abuse are summarized in Box 32.5 (see also Chapter 55).

BOX 32.3 * Focus on Evidence-Based Practice

Does family structure make a difference in how much health care children receive?

Single-father families have increased in recent years to now represent 6% of American families with children. Families headed by single fathers are less likely to be poor, are more likely to be employed, and are better off overall economically than families with single mothers but they are worse off economically, measured both by poverty status and labor force participation, than married couples with children. To investigate whether single-father parents are as conscientious in obtaining health care for children, researchers studied a total of 62,193 children. Three percent of sample children lived in single-father families and 22% of sample children lived in single-mother families. Single-father families had significantly better health care coverage than single-mother families as health insurance is associated with employment and single fathers held more full-time jobs than single mothers in this survey. Despite the difference in insurance coverage, 86% of children in single-mother and 87% of two-parent families had had a health provider visit in the past year while children in single-father households had a rate of 80 percent. Children living in single-father households had lower overall rates of well-child care (57% compared with 69% for children in single-mother households and 67% for children in two-parent households) and a lower likelihood of having a usual source of care (87% compared with 91% for children in single-mother households and 95% for children in two-parent households).

Would the above study influence how closely you assessed a child for up-to-date immunizations?

Source: Leininger, L. J., & Ziol-Guest, K. M. (2008). Reexamining the effects of family structure on children's access to care: the single-father family. *Health Services Research, 43*(1.1), 117–133.

Promoting Nutritional Health of a School-Age Child

Most school-age children have good appetites, although any meal is influenced by the day's activity. If children have had a full day of activities, they may come to the dinner table ready to eat anything. If a day was filled with frustration—a child received a poor mark in school, had an argument with a friend, or has a big game to think about—the child may pick and poke at food. This is no different from the way adults feel at times, so should be respected.

Establishing Healthy Eating Patterns

School-age children need breakfast to provide enough energy to get them through active mornings at school. They eat best if parents get up in the morning and eat some themselves. Children react badly to the instruction, "Do as I say, not as I do."

If children take a packed lunch to school, urge parents to allow them some say in the meal, because packed lunches become tedious for everyone after a while. Whether they take lunch or buy it at school, school-age children should know some elementary facts of nutrition so they do not trade a sandwich for cake or choose only desserts from the cafeteria. Ideally, children should receive guidance from school personnel, but this often is impossible in a busy lunchroom. Health care personnel, therefore, should play an active role in nutrition education at health maintenance visits.

Many children qualify for a free or reduced-price school lunch and breakfast (Kristjansson et al., 2009). A government-regulated school lunch (type A) provides milk (8 oz), protein (2 oz), one starch serving, vegetable (¾ cup), and fruit (¾ cup). Serving sizes vary according to age to provide one third of a child's nutrition requirements for a day (Fig. 32.7). Check that children are actually eating school lunches, not trading items they do not want, so they receive the full benefit of the program.

Most children are hungry after school and enjoy a snack when they arrive home. Because sugary foods may dull a child's appetite for dinner, urge parents to make the snack nutritious: fruit, cheese, or milk, rather than cookies and a soft drink.

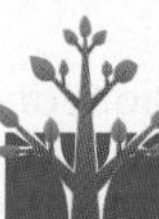

BOX 32.4 * Focus on Family Teaching

Common Safety Measures to Prevent Accidents During the School Years

Q. Shelly's mother tells you, "My school-ager is constantly on the go. How can I keep her free from accidents when I'm not always with her?"

A. Putting preventive steps in place is the key.

Accident	Preventive Measure
Motor vehicle accidents	Insist children use seat belts in a car; role model their use.
	Teach street-crossing safety; stress that streets are no place for rough-housing, pushing, or shoving.
	Teach bicycle safety, including advice not to take "passengers" on a bicycle and to use a helmet.
	Teach parking lot and school bus safety (do not walk in back of parked cars, wait for crossing guard, etc.).
Community	Avoid unsafe areas, such as train yards, grain silos, back alleys.
	Do not go with strangers (parents can establish a code word with child; child does not leave school with anyone who does not know the word).
	Children should say "no" to anyone who touches them if they do not wish it, including family members (most sexual abuse is by a family member, not a stranger).
	For late school-age, teach rules of safer sex (use of condoms; inspecting partner, etc.).
Burns	Teach safety with candles, matches, campfires—fire is not fun.
	Teach safety with beginning cooking skills (remember to include microwave oven safety, such as closing firmly before turning on oven; not using metal containers).
	Teach safety with sun exposure—use sun block.
	Do not climb electric poles.
Falls	Teach that rough-housing on fences, climbing on roofs, etc., is hazardous.
	Teach skateboard, scooter, and skating safety.
Sports injuries	Teach that wearing appropriate equipment for sports (face masks for hockey; mouthpiece and cup for football; helmet for bicycle riding, skateboarding, or in-line skating; batting helmets for baseball) is not babyish but smart.
	Stress not to play to a point of exhaustion or in a sport beyond physical capability (no pitching baseball or toe ballet for an early grade-school child).
	Use trampolines only with adult supervision to avoid serious neck injury.
Drowning	Teach how to swim; dares and rough-housing when diving or swimming are not appropriate. Do not swim beyond limits of capabilities.
Drugs	Help your child avoid all recreational drugs and take prescription medicine only as directed. Avoid tobacco and alcohol.
Firearms	Teach safe firearm use. Keep firearms in locked cabinets with bullets separate from gun.
General	School-age children should keep adults informed regarding where they are and what they are doing.
	Be aware that the frequency of accidents increases when parents are under stress and therefore less attentive. Special precautions must be taken at these times.
	Some children are more active, curious, and impulsive and therefore more vulnerable to accidents than others.

Early school age is not too young to put in place preventive measures against cardiovascular changes later in life. Limiting salty foods, for example, can help prevent hypertension (He, Marrero, & Macgregor, 2008). Excessive saturated fat can lead to the formation of artery plaques and cardiovascular disease.

Teach parents to make every attempt to make mealtime a happy and enjoyable part of the day for everyone. Some school-age children learn to eat as quickly as possible (and so incompletely) to escape from the table before something unpleasant happens, such as an argument they can sense is brewing.

Fostering Industry

As a part of fostering industry, school-age children usually enjoy helping to plan meals. They can prepare foods such as instant pudding, Jell-O, salads, scrambled eggs, and sandwiches. They may eat meals they have planned or prepared more willingly than ones that are just set in front of them.

Most parents would like children to develop better table manners. Because they are in a hurry to finish eating, school-age children tend to gulp their food. Many meals are interrupted by spilled milk. As children become teenagers and are more aware of the impression they make on others, manners often improve dramatically. It is often comforting for parents to know that children typically display better table manners in other people's homes than in their own.

Recommended Dietary Reference Intakes

Although parents may have less to say about what a school-age child eats, it is important that the increasing energy requirements that come with this age (often in spurts) are met daily with foods of high nutritional value.

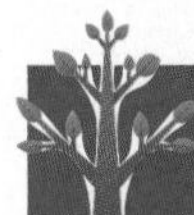

BOX 32.5 * Focus on Family Teaching

Teaching Points to Help Children Avoid Sexual Abuse

Q. Shelly's mother wants to protect her daughter from sexual abuse. She asks you, "What are good rules to teach children without scaring them?"

A. A number of common rules are:

1. Your body is your property and you can decide who looks at it or touches it.
2. Secrets are fun things to keep. If a person asks you not to tell about something that was done to you that you did not like, it is not a secret. It is all right to tell about it.
3. Do not go anywhere with a stranger (a stranger is someone you do not know, not someone "strange"). Do not be fooled by people asking you to give them directions or to go with them because your mother is sick or hurt or they have lost a pet.
4. Being touched by someone you like is a good feeling. You do not have to allow anyone to touch you in a way you do not like. Do not allow yourself to be left alone with a person you are uncomfortable with because that person touches you in a way you do not like.
5. A "private part" is the part of you a bathing suit touches. If anyone asks you to show them a private part or touches a private part, tell them to stop, and tell someone else.
6. If the person you tell does not believe you, keep telling people until someone does believe you.

During the late school years, the recommended dietary intakes for children begin to be separated into categories for girls and boys because boys require more calories and other nutrients at this time. Because school-age children typically dislike vegetables, their intake may be deficient in fiber. Both girls and boys require more iron in prepuberty than they did between the ages of 7 and 10. Adequate calcium and fluoride intake remains important to ensure good teeth and bone growth.

Promoting Nutritional Health With a Vegetarian Diet

School-age children who are raised in vegetarian homes need to learn aspects of vegetarian nutrition if they are going to eat in a school cafeteria. Unfortunately, many school lunch programs offer mainly milk and meat or cheese foods, such as sloppy Joe sandwiches, macaroni and cheese, or pizza. This forces children who are vegetarians to carry packed lunches. Vegetarian packed lunches can be varied with foods such as cucumber, tomato, or peanut butter sandwiches on whole-grain bread; hot soups; salads; vegetable sticks; and fruit. When eating at a friend's house, children need to learn to notify the host that they eat a special diet or know how to choose correctly from foods they are served.

A potential problem to assess with vegetarian school-age children is whether they are obtaining enough protein and calcium to be prepared for the rapid growth spurt of puberty. Foods high in calcium are green, leafy vegetables such as spinach and turnip greens, prunes, nuts, enriched bread, and cereals. Soybeans, legumes, nuts, grains, and immature seeds like green beans, lima beans, and corn are relatively high in protein. As with any individual on a vegetarian diet, children may need a vitamin B_{12} supplement. Encourage outside activities for sun exposure to increase vitamin D. Iron may need to be supplemented, especially in girls with heavy menstrual flows (Rolfes, Pinna, & Whitney, 2009).

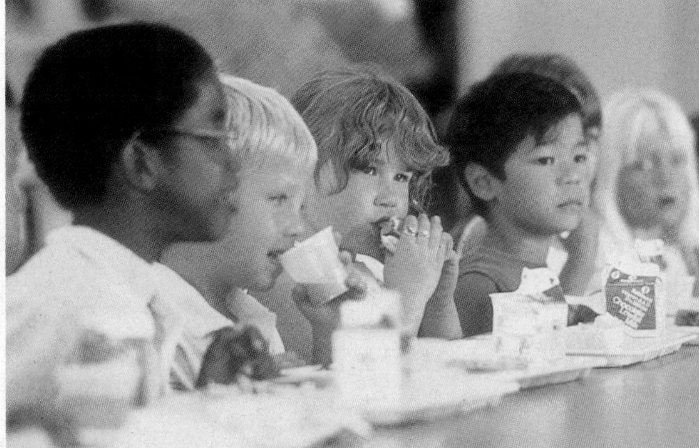

FIGURE 32.7 School lunch programs provide nutritious meals to help school-age children meet nutrition requirements.

Promoting Development of a School-Age Child in Daily Activities

With life centered on school activities and friends, a school-age child still needs parental guidance for most daily activities, because the habits and lifestyle patterns gained during this period will form the basis for the patterns of living later in life. Figure 32.8 shows a day in the life of a family with school-age children. Along with nutritional needs, areas of concern for a school-age child and family include dressing, sleep needs, exercise, hygiene, and dental care.

Dress

Although school-age children can fully dress themselves, they are not good at taking care of their clothes until later in the school-age years. This is the right age, however (if not started already), to teach children the importance of caring for their own belongings. School-age children have definite opinions about clothing styles, often based on the likes of their friends or a popular sports or rock star rather than the preferences of their parents. Help parents be aware that a child who wears different clothing than others may become the object of exclusion from a school club or group. In schools with a gang culture, children may not be able to wear a certain color or style lest they be mistaken for a gang member. Many schools have begun requiring school uniforms to avoid this problem.

Sleep

Sleep needs vary among individual children. Younger school-age children typically require 10 to 12 hours of sleep each night, and older ones require about 8 to 10 hours. Most 6-year-olds are too old for naps but do require a quiet time after school to get them through the remainder of the day. Nighttime terrors may continue during the early school years

7:00 AM: The family sits down to a healthy breakfast. Claudia helps Laura with the butter.

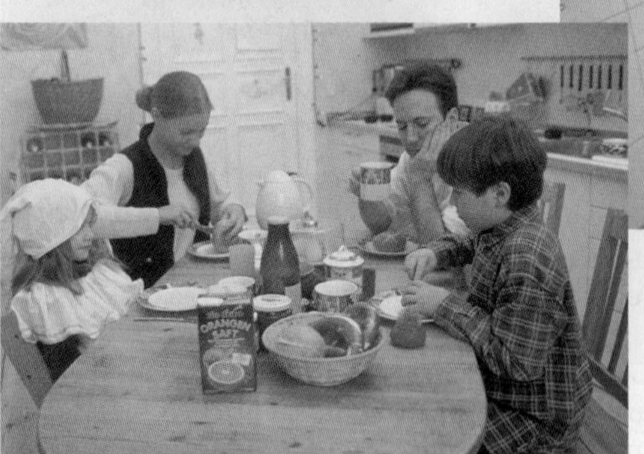

7:30 AM: John walks Marc to school, emphasizing safety when crossing the street.

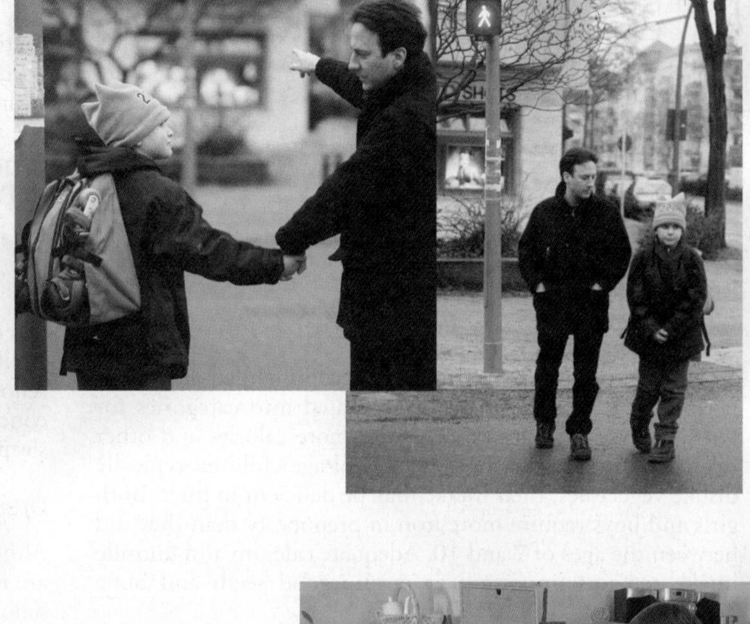

10:00 AM: Claudia and Laura bake a cake for the night's dessert. Four-year-old Laura enjoys practicing adult roles.

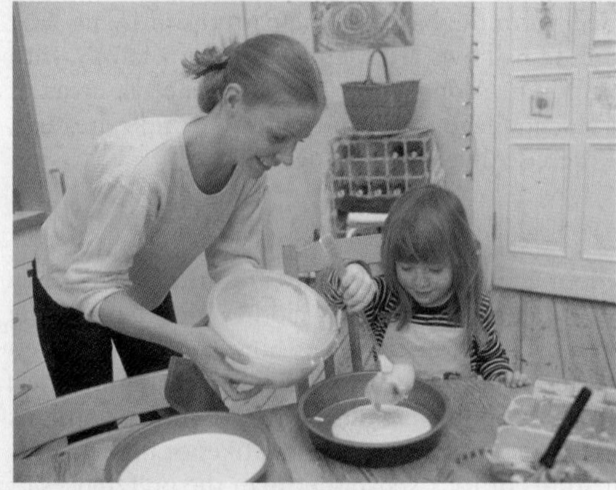

3:00 PM: Marc and Laura play together after Marc gets home from school. Their cooperative play is punctuated by an occasional argument.

FIGURE 32.8 A day in the life of a family with young children.

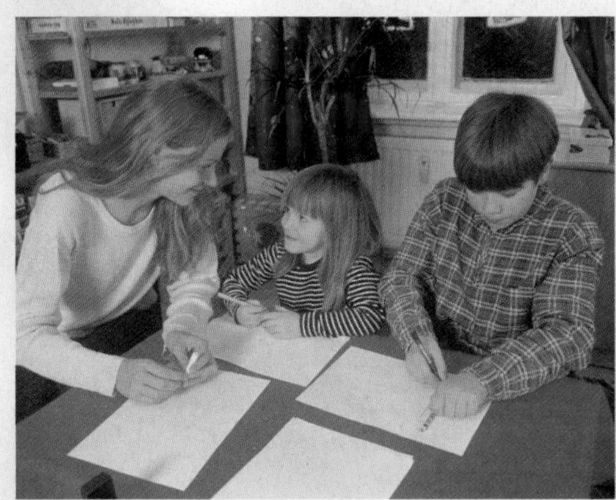

4:00 PM: Claudia helps Marc with his homework. Laura likes to draw alongside her big brother.

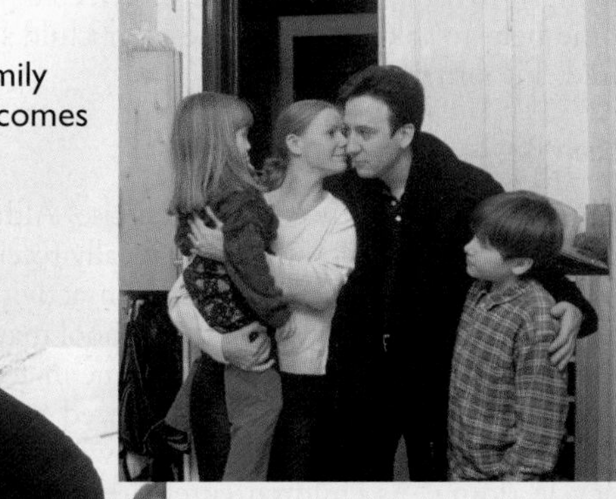

5:00 PM: The family greets John as he comes home from work.

5:30 PM: John and Marc go rollerblading before dinner. John makes sure Marc's protective gear is in place.

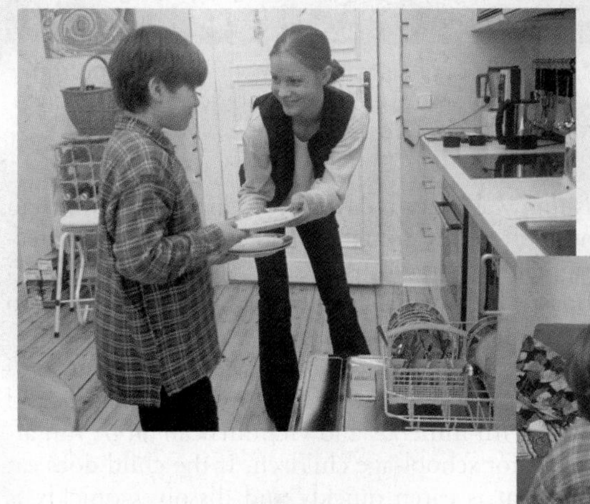

7:00 PM: After dinner, Marc helps with the dishes; then the family spends time together playing a game.

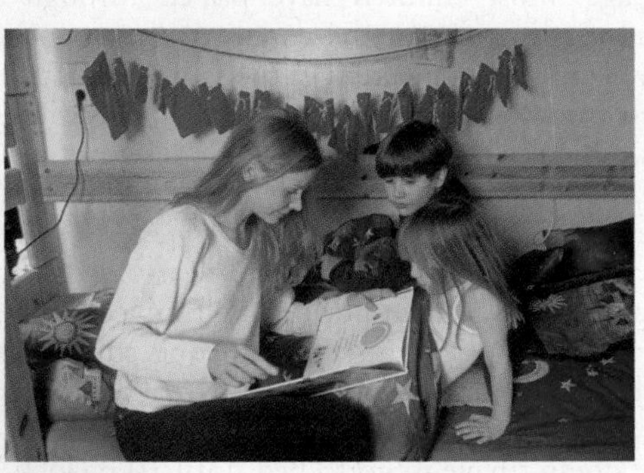

8:30 PM: Time to get ready for bed! Claudia helps the kids clean up and brush their teeth. And there's always time to read them a story.

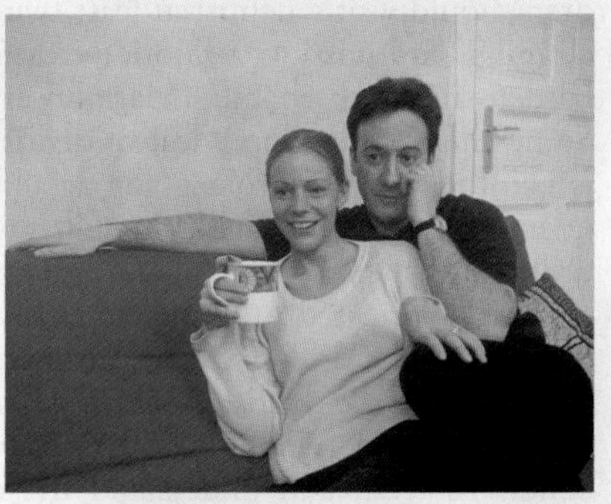

9:00 PM: John and Claudia relax together at the end of the day.

FIGURE 32.8 *(continued)*

and may actually increase during the first-grade year as a child reacts to the stress of beginning school.

During early school years, many children enjoy a quiet talk or a reading time at bedtime. At about age 9, when friends become more important, children generally are ready to give up pre-bedtime talks with parents in preference to calling or text messaging a friend. Some parents react strongly to this change and feel rejected. They may need some help to take at face value their child's statement, "I'm tired. I'd rather go to sleep."

Exercise

School-age children need daily exercise. Although they go to school all day, they do not automatically receive much exercise because school is basically a sit-down activity. Children who are bussed or driven by a parent to school may therefore return home without having spent much time in active exercise.

Exercise need not involve organized sports. It can come from neighborhood games, walking with parents or a dog, or bicycle riding. As children enter preadolescence, those with poor coordination may become reluctant to exercise. Urge them to participate in some daily exercise, or else obesity, or osteoporosis later in life, can result.

Hygiene

Children of 6 or 7 years of age still need help in regulating bath water temperature and in cleaning their ears and fingernails. By age 8, children are generally capable of bathing themselves but may not do it well because they are too busy to take the time or because they do not find bathing as important as do their parents.

Both boys and girls become interested in showering as they approach their teens. This can be encouraged as perspiration increases with puberty, along with sebaceous gland activity. When girls begin to menstruate, they may be afraid to take baths or wash their hair during their period if they have heard this is not safe. They need information on the importance and safety of good hygiene during their menses. Boys who are uncircumcised may develop inflammation under the foreskin from increased secretions if they do not wash regularly.

Care of Teeth

With proper dental care, the average child today can expect to grow up cavity free. To ensure this happening, school-age children should visit a dentist at least twice yearly for a checkup, cleaning, and possibly a fluoride treatment to strengthen and harden the tooth enamel (Marinho et al., 2009) (Fig. 32.9). Some children develop a fear of dentists and, if a dentist visit is painful, want to avoid going at all. The advantage of frequent visits is that if cavities are filled when they are small, the drilling required is minimal and little pain is involved. If cavities are not treated promptly in this way but are allowed to grow large, the drilling hurts, causing these children to refuse to go back to the dentist. More large cavities then grow, and a vicious circle develops. Pedodontists specialize in caring for children's teeth and understand the developmental level of their patients. Children who tend to develop caries (cavities) might be encouraged to visit a pedodontist if one is available and affordable.

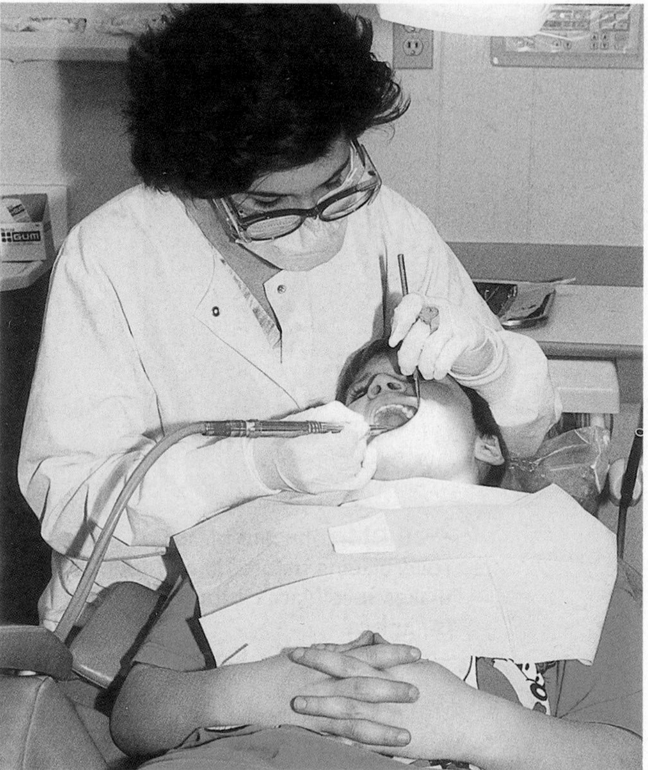

FIGURE 32.9 Dental caries are the number one health problem in school-age children. Teach children good dental health and encourage them to visit a dentist twice a year.

School-age children have to be reminded to brush their teeth daily. If brushing becomes an area of conflict for the family, brushing well once a day may be more effective than brushing more often but doing an inadequate job. For effective brushing, a child should use a soft toothbrush, fluoride-based toothpaste, and dental floss to clean between teeth to help remove plaque.

Snacks are best limited to high-protein foods such as chicken and cheese rather than candy. Fruits, vegetables, and cereals fortified with minerals and vitamins can all be fun afterschool snacks for school-age children. If the child does eat candy, a type that is eaten quickly and dissolves quickly is better than slowly dissolving or sticky candy, which stays in contact with the teeth longer.

Promoting Healthy Family Functioning

At 6 years of age, most children have passed through a preschool phase of attraction for the parent of the opposite sex and identify again with the parent of the same sex (Freud, 1962). Children from single-parent homes, or those with a parent who has difficulty being a good role model, may need help in finding a suitable adult to serve as this important person in their life.

To their parents' annoyance, many 6-year-olds often quote their teacher as the final authority on all subjects. This may be the first time the parents see someone surpassing them in their child's eyes, and accepting the situation can be painful. Children also cite their friends as guides for behavior: "Mary Jane doesn't have to go to bed until 10 o'clock," or "Carlos' mother lets him go to the movies every Saturday." Parents may require help to realize these remarks are a normal consequence of being exposed to other adults and children. A simple statement such as, "There are all kinds of ways to do things, but in our house, the rule is this," shows no criticism of Carlos' or Mary Jane's family, yet conveys a special "our house" feeling and offers security to a child.

Parents often must be reminded that even the simplest tasks of everyday life require repeated practice before they can be accomplished well. The way parents correct children as they learn these tasks can influence children's opinions of themselves and their ability to continue learning. "Putting all the silverware in a pile is one way of putting it away; another way would be to divide spoons, forks, and knives separately" is always preferable to "What a silly way to put away silverware!" Comments such as, "Can't you do anything right?" or "Why don't you ever do what I say?" should always be avoided because children will rise only to the level expected of them. Children who are constantly told they are stupid, thoughtless, bad, or ill-behaved may begin to act that way to conform to their parents' expectations.

If parents have difficulty telling what a child's completed project is supposed to be, the time-honored "Tell me about it" is preferable to "What is it?" It is good for parents to find a redeeming characteristic in a project, no matter how shakily put together it is: "I like the bright color you painted it" or "That must have been fun to make." Displaying and using children's gifts are part of having school-age children in a family. A finger painting hung on the refrigerator door will enhance, not detract from, the most elegant home. The best-dressed woman looks even more radiant wearing her child's necklace made of macaroni on a string. Both examples are gestures of love, which goes well with everything.

In talking to parents of school-age children, good questions to ask to estimate the degree of interaction that occurs in the home and whether parents are strengthening a child's sense of accomplishment are:

- How do you correct John when he does something wrong?
- Do you display his school projects?
- Does he have chores that are his to accomplish?

Common Health Problems of the School-Age Period

Children in their early school years have one of the lowest rates of death and serious illness of any age group. The two leading causes of death are accidents and cancer. Minor illnesses are largely because of dental caries, gastrointestinal disturbances, and upper respiratory infections.

Table 32.3 shows the usual health maintenance pattern for a school-age child (AAP, 2009). Table 32.4 lists problems that parents may have in evaluating illness in school-age children. Many communities are establishing school-based community health care clinics to improve the health care available for school-age children.

Dental Caries

Caries (cavities) are progressive, destructive lesions or decalcification of the tooth enamel and dentin. When the pH of the tooth surface drops to 5.6 or below (which happens after children eat readily fermented carbohydrates, such as table sugar), acid microorganisms (acidogenic lactobacilli and aciduric streptococci) found in dental plaque attack the organic cementing medium of teeth and destroy it. Plaque tends to accumulate in deep grooves of the teeth and contact areas between teeth, making these areas most susceptible to dental decay. The enamel on primary teeth is thinner than that on permanent teeth, so they are even more susceptible to destruction than permanent teeth. The distance from the enamel to the pulp is shorter, too, so invasion of the tooth nerve can occur quickly. Neglected caries result in poor chewing and therefore poor digestion, abscess and pain, and sometimes osteomyelitis (bone infection).

As stated earlier, dental caries are largely preventable with proper brushing and use of fluoridated water or fluoride application. When caries do occur, it is important they be treated quickly and the child's dental hygiene practices be evaluated and improved if necessary. Most important, children must believe they have a stake in the health or disease of their teeth so they willingly undertake the self-care measures necessary to ensure healthy teeth, with parental support rather than parental command.

Malocclusion

The upper jaw in children matures rapidly in early childhood along with skull growth; the lower jaw forms more slowly, forcing teeth to make a prolonged series of changes until they reach their final adult alignment and position. Good tooth occlusion, in which the upper teeth overlap the lower teeth by a small amount and teeth are evenly spaced and in good alignment, is necessary for optimal formation of teeth, health of the supporting tissue, optimal speech development, and what most people view as a pleasant physical appearance. *Malocclusion* (a deviation from the normal) may be congenital and related to conditions such as cleft palate, a small lower jaw, or familial traits tending toward malocclusion. The condition can result from constant mouth breathing or abnormal tongue position (tongue thrusting). Thumb-sucking appears to have little role in malocclusion as long as this does not persist past the time of eruption of the permanent front teeth (6 to 7 years). The loss of teeth because of extraction or accident may lead to malocclusion if not properly treated to maintain alignment.

Malocclusion may be either crossbite (sideways) or anterior or posterior. Children with a malocclusion should be evaluated by an orthodontist to see if orthodontic braces or other therapy is necessary. The time to begin correction varies with the extent of the malocclusion and the jaw size. Braces are expensive and painful when they are first applied and at periodic visits when they are tightened to maintain pressure for further straightening. Some children develop mild, shallow ulcerations (canker sores) on the buccal membrane from friction of metal wires. Rubbing the offending wire with dental wax dulls the surface and gives relief. Oral acetaminophen or an agent such as Ora-Jel (an over-the-counter drug) rubbed on the ulceration also gives relief. Children who wear braces need to have their teeth assessed frequently to see they are brushing properly around the braces (a Water Pik is often recommended for thorough cleaning) and that they are using dental floss to remove plaque from around wires (Harrison, O'Brien, & Worthington, 2009).

After removal of braces, many children must wear retainers to maintain the correction the braces achieved. Although braces are wired into place, retainers are not. Wearing a retainer can prove troublesome for a child as it

TABLE 32.3 ✻ Health Maintenance Schedule, School-Age Period

Area of Focus	Methods	Frequency
Assessment		
Developmental milestones	History, observation	Every visit
Growth milestones	Height, weight plotted on standard growth chart; physical examination	Every visit
Hypertension	Blood pressure	Every visit
Nutrition	History, observation; height/weight information	Every visit
Parent–child relationship	History, observation	Every visit
Behavior or school problems	History, observation	Every visit
Vision and hearing disorders	History, observation	Every visit
	Formal Snellen or Titmus testing	At 7–8 and 10–12 years
	Audiometer testing	At 6 and 10–12 years
Dental health	History, physical examination	Every visit
Scoliosis	Physical examination	Yearly after age 8 years
Thyroid	Physical examination, history	Every visit after age 10 years
Tuberculosis	PPD skin test	Depending on prevalence of tuberculosis in community
Bacteriuria	Clean-catch urine	At 6–7 years
Anemia	Hematocrit/hemoglobin	At 11–12 years
Immunizations		
Diphtheria and tetanus (Tdap) vaccine	Check history and past records; inform caregiver about any risks and side-effects; administer immunization in accordance with health care agency policies.	11–12 years
Hepatitis A vaccine		If not previously administered
Hepatitis B vaccine		If not administered in infancy or three injections were not completed
Human papillomavirus vaccine (HPV or Gardasil) in girls		11 or 12 years; 2nd injection 2 months later; 3rd injection 6 months after 1st dose
Influenza vaccine		Yearly
Meningococcal vaccine		11–12 years
Pneumococcal vaccine		To children at high risk
Varicella vaccine		At any age after 1 year if not previously immunized or at 11–12 years if lacking reliable history of chickenpox
Anticipatory Guidance		
School-age care	Active listening and health teaching	Every visit
Expected growth and developmental milestones before next visit	Active listening and health teaching	Every visit
Accident prevention	Counseling about street and personal safety	Every visit
Problem Solving		
Any problems expressed by caregiver during course of the visit	Active listening and health teaching regarding cigarette smoking, drug abuse, sex education, school adjustment	Every visit

Source: American Academy of Pediatrics Committee on Practice and Ambulatory Medicine. (2009). *Recommendations for preventive pediatric health care.* Washington, DC: Author.

must be removed when eating such as in the school cafeteria or in a restaurant. Show appropriate sympathy and help children problem-solve if they are bothered by the appearance of braces or wearing a retainer. For instance, if removing the retainer in front of friends is embarrassing for a child, perhaps it could be removed in the bathroom before going to the cafeteria each day. Braces and retainers, once thought of as implements to be made fun of, have become such a common feature of life for schoolchildren today that most children who wear them find comfort in not being the only one to suffer this indignity and, once used to their own appliances, experience little reluctance in letting their classmates see them. Some even view them as a mark of pride or badge of courage.

TABLE 32.4 ✻ Parental Difficulties Evaluating Illness in the School-Age Child

Difficulty	Helpful Suggestions for Parents
Evaluating seriousness of illness	For the first time, a school-age child may view illness as a way to avoid unpleasant activities (school, a coach who asks too much, household chores). Evaluating whether the child has symptoms when he is asked to do something he likes to do often reveals the difference between exaggeration and an ill child (too sick to eat spinach, not too sick to eat ice cream; too sick to go to school, not too sick to go ice skating). If the child uses symptoms of illness as a means of avoiding situations, parents must evaluate what it is that the child wants so badly to avoid and see if some change should be made in expectations.
Evaluating nutritional intake	Many school-age children eat lunch at school; they may spend weekends away from home and weeks away at camp. As with all ages, noting whether they are growing and active is better than monitoring any one day's food intake.
Evaluating puberty changes	There is a wide variation in the time that secondary sex characteristics occur (9–17 years for girls; 10–18 years for boys). Children should be examined if and when they or their parents are concerned that pubertal changes are delayed.
Age-specific diseases to be aware of	School age is a time to evaluate vision; children normally develop vision changes as maturity of the eye globe increases. Squinting, rubbing eyes, or poor marks in school may be signs of poor vision. Streptococcal sore throats occur frequently in early-school-age children. Those with sore throats should be examined by a health care provider to prevent complications, such as glomerulonephritis or rheumatic fever, from developing. Girls, in particular, must be evaluated for scoliosis (curvature of the spine). Parents detect this by noticing that the girl's skirts hang unevenly or bra straps are uneven. Parents may need to be cautioned that vomiting or headache in the morning that passes fairly quickly (at about the same time the school bus leaves) may be a symptom of school phobia, but physical examination is in order because these are also symptoms of other conditions. Absence seizures, a neurologic condition that typically arises in school-age years, can be confused with behavior problems if observation is not thorough (see Chap. 49). Attention-deficit/hyperactivity disorder (ADHD) (see Chap. 54) can also lead to behavior or inattention disorders.

✔ Checkpoint Question 32.2

If Shelly eats candy, what is the best type in terms of preventing caries?

a. Saltwater taffy
b. A chocolate bar
c. Chewy caramels
d. Hard candy

Concerns and Problems of the School-Age Period

One of the most important disorders of the school-age period is attention-deficit/hyperactivity disorder (ADHD) because it interferes so dramatically with school progress (see Chapter 54). Other problems concern language, fears, and responsibility.

Nursing Diagnoses and Related Interventions

✻

Nursing Diagnosis: Parental anxiety related to behavior of school-age child

Outcome Evaluation: Parent states undesired behavior has decreased in frequency; parent feels less stress about child's health or future.

Problems Associated With Language Development

The common speech problem of the preschool years is broken fluency; the most common problem of a school-age child is articulation. The child has difficulty pronouncing *s, z, th, l, r,* and *w* or substitutes *w* for *r* ("westroom" instead of "restroom") or *r* for *l* ("radies' room" instead of "ladies' room"). This is most noticeable during the first and second grades; it usually disappears by the third grade. Unless it persists, speech therapy for this normal developmental stage is not necessary.

Common Fears and Anxieties of a School-Age Child

School-age children are old enough to experience adult reactions to problems at home or school.

Anxiety Related to Beginning School. Adjusting to grade school is a big task for 6-year-olds. Even if they attended preschool, grade school is different: the rules are firmer, and

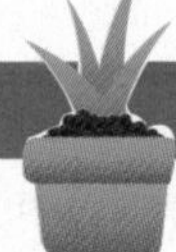

BOX 32.6 ✻ Focus on Nursing Care Planning

A Multidisciplinary Care Map for a School-Age Child Starting Middle School

Shelly Lewis is a 12-year-old girl who recently started middle school. Her mother tells you that although Shelly, who is overweight, says she likes school, she has developed a lot of nervous habits such as nail biting since school started.

Family Assessment ✻ Child lives with mother, stepfather, and 3 younger stepsisters in 4-bedroom home. Family owns a boarding kennel for dogs; both parents work full time at business. Mother describes finances as "Okay. It's hard with a big family."

Client Assessment ✻ Child has been "chubby" since preschool. States she likes to read rather than play sports. Has just started middle school (seventh grade). Observed to be restless in chair during conversation with mother about the new school. Mother states, "Her sisters have no trouble with change; she always does. Don't you think if she lost weight she'd fit in better?"

Nursing Diagnosis ✻ Anxiety related to beginning a new school.

Outcome Criteria ✻ Child states she feels more comfortable with new school setting; nail biting has decreased in intensity; agrees to begin weight-reduction program.

Team Member Responsible	Assessment	Intervention	Rationale	Expected Outcome
		Activities of Daily Living		
Nurse	Assess what activities client enjoys.	Review with client advantage of participating in activities that involve more exercise than reading. Suggest listening to taped books while walking with a friend.	Effective weight reduction calls for increased exercise. Taped books still supply reading enjoyment.	Child states she will try some active activity for at least 20 minutes each day.
		Consultations		
Nurse	Assess if child would like to be referred to a weight-reduction class at health center.	Suggest different options available such as weight-loss group or commercial weight-reduction program.	Children respond well to group activities. Other group members supply friendship as well as increase motivation.	Child states whether she would like to join a weight-reduction group.
		Procedures/Medications		
Nurse	Ask child to try to identify if she feels something is upsetting about the new school; if so, what is that thing?	Help child "walk through" a day at school and discuss how small changes could affect her fitting into school.	Talking with the child allows her to share feelings and concerns openly and safely, possibly increasing the child's awareness of them and their impact on her.	Child describes a typical day and points she would like to see changed.
		Nutrition		
Nurse/nutritionist	Assess child's intake by 24-hour recall history.	Review with child changes that would reduce calories yet maintain her lifestyle.	Twelve-year-old children are old enough to take responsibility for what and when they eat.	Client reviews her dietary intake; makes at least three suggestions on things she will attempt to change.

Patient/Family Education				
Nurse	Assess if family members appreciate the stress a new school setting can create.	Review with mother and child ways to reduce stress when encountering new situations, such as equating them with something already known.	It is easy for parents to view 12-year-olds as able to handle new situations better than they can because of pseudo-maturity.	Mother states she may have been taking the change in school too lightly; needs to offer more support.
Psychosocial/Spiritual/Emotional Needs				
Nurse/nurse practitioner	Assess family functioning with child's mother.	Stress that all children are individuals and what works for stepsisters may not work for client.	Being constantly compared to siblings can create feelings of low self-esteem, which can lead to difficulty solving problems.	Mother states she will try to reduce comparisons to stepsisters, to help reduce stress at home.
Discharge Planning				
Nurse	Assess if child or mother thinks an early follow-up appointment would be helpful.	Arrange for a follow-up clinic appointment within 1 month with the mother and daughter if desired.	It is difficult for a family to make internal changes if they are too emotionally involved to be objective.	Mother and child express their preferences based on their future plans.

the elective feeling ("If I don't like it, I can quit") is gone. School is for keeps until age 16 or longer, a time span too long for a young child to even imagine. Whereas preschool learning was carried out through fun activities, part of every day in grade school involves obvious work (see Focus on Nursing Care Planning Box 32.6).

Because school is an adjustment, a health assessment of all school-age children should include an inquiry about progress in school. You can obtain information by asking a parent, "How is Susan doing in school?" followed by a second question, "How does her teacher say she is doing?" If there is a discrepancy between the answers, the situation bears study. The answer to the first question reveals the parent's attitude toward the child's progress. The answer to the second may indicate a child who is having trouble adjusting to a structured school environment. Some parents have to alter their expectations of how much their child should be achieving to conform to their child's actual ability. This can be difficult.

One of the biggest tasks of the first year of school is learning to read. It is best if parents have prepared children for this by reading to them since infancy, pointing to the words and pictures as they go along. This helps children realize sentences flow from left to right and the words, not the pictures, tell the story. Box 32.7 offers some useful hints to help parents encourage reading in their young school-age child.

Many first-graders are capable of mature action at school but appear less mature when they return home. Their pseudo-sophistication of the day is gone. They may bite their nails, suck their thumb, or talk baby talk. Some develop tics (irregular movements of isolated muscle groups), such as wrinkling the forehead, shrugging the shoulders, twisting the mouth, coughing, clearing the throat, or frequently blinking

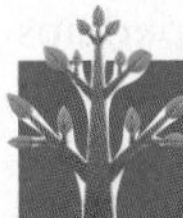

BOX 32.7 * Focus on Family Teaching

Tips to Help Make Reading More Enjoyable for a Child

Q. Shelly's grandmother says to you, "I want my grandchild to enjoy reading more. How can I encourage this?"

A. Integrating reading into a total lifestyle is the best approach.

- Read yourself to set an example, so your child associates learning to read with adult activity. If you spend most of your free time watching television, your child will think reading is mainly for children and assume that it is not important.
- Make reading more fun by encouraging your child to make practical use of reading. Ask her to read recipes while you cook or to read road signs during a car trip.
- Play a treasure hunt game in which you hide a small object, such as a favorite toy, then write simple clues on slips of paper—"Look under a lamp," then, under the lamp, "Look in a book," and so on until your child has been led to the hidden object. Such games help your child see reading as an important means of obtaining information. Your child can develop writing skills by playing the same game for you to follow.
- Suggest to relatives that a gift certificate from a bookstore would be a good present. Let your child browse the store to select the book.
- Talk about books the child has read—what was good, what was bad, or what the child learned.
- Read a book together as a pre-bedtime family activity.

or rolling the eyes. Such movements may occasionally be confused with seizure activity. Tics, however, disappear during sleep and occur mainly when the child is subjected to stress or anxiety. Scolding, nagging, threatening, or punishing does not stop either tics or nail biting; it invariably makes these problems worse. Methods such as using bad-flavored nail polish and restraining the child's hands to prevent nail biting are also ineffective.

These behaviors stop when the underlying stress is discovered and alleviated. Urge parents to spend some time with a child after school or in the evening so the child continues to feel secure in the family and does not feel pushed out by being sent to school. If such behavior manifestations persist despite attempts to eliminate their cause, the family might benefit from formal counseling.

School Refusal or Phobia. School refusal is fear of attending school. It is a type of "social phobia" similar to agoraphobia (fear of going outside the home). Children who resist attending school this way may develop physical signs of illness, such as vomiting, diarrhea, headache, or abdominal pain on school days (Tyrrell, 2007). This lasts until after the school bus has left or the child is allowed to stay home for the day.

A particular child may be reacting to a situation such as a harsh teacher, having to shower in gym class, or facing a class bully every day. In these instances, the child's fear may be well grounded. Counseling may help the child manage the situation better. If not, parents can attempt to have the child transferred to another classroom or perhaps excused from a disliked situation such as showering to stop the school resistance.

School refusal may occur from fear of separation from parents. The child may be overly dependent on the parents or may be reluctant to leave home because of worry that younger siblings will usurp the parents' affection. The anxiety of separation may also result because the parent is overprotective of the child or is the one having the most difficulty separating.

Because the problem of school refusal is usually only partly the child's, the entire family generally requires counseling to resolve the issue. As a rule, once it has been established the child is free of any illness and the resistance stems from separation anxiety or phobia, the child should be made to attend school. Reinforcement by parents to go to school this way helps to prevent problems such as school failure, peer ridicule, or a pattern of avoiding difficulties. Some children may benefit from a gradual program of school involvement, such as walking to school but not going in for one day, then going to school but staying for only 1 hour the next day, then staying for half a day, and so on, until the child can stay all day every day. Give support to parents so they can treat the child's illness symptoms matter-of-factly (a great deal of reassurance that these symptoms are not major will be necessary) so they can take the child firmly to the bus or to the classroom.

Managing school refusal requires coordination among the school, school nurse, and health care provider who diagnoses the problem. A nurse is the ideal person to coordinate such efforts and to help parents allow the child some independence not only in going to school but in other activities. A few children have such difficulty they require psychiatric therapy to resolve their difficulties with school.

Home Schooling

Because of religious or personal preference or because of disillusionment with the school system, a growing number of children are home schooled today (Gaither, 2008). It is important to identify these children at a health care visit because with their less extensive experience with peers than other children, they may not be as comfortable with peer interaction. As their main contact has been with parents at home, their vocabulary may be advanced or can suggest they are older than their real age. They may be experts at computer searching but know less than other children about health prevention measures as they have not had contact with school nurses or health courses. When discussing home schooling with parents, assess if children do have peer experiences, perhaps through participation in community sports teams. Ask if they receive exposure to other cultures or families so they can better adjust to people different from themselves at college or a first work position.

Latchkey Children

Latchkey children are schoolchildren who are without adult supervision for part of each weekday. The term alludes to the fact they generally carry a key so they can let themselves into their home after school.

Latchkey children have become a prominent concern because in as many as 90% of families today in the United States, both parents work at least part-time outside the home. Few parents have work hours so flexible they can always be at home when a child leaves for or returns from school. Extended family members who once watched children after school are often working as well or may no longer be close at hand; many communities are no longer close-knit enough to have neighbors who can be depended on to help out with informal child care.

A major concern of children staying alone is that they will develop an increased tendency toward accidents, delinquent behavior, alcohol or beginning drug abuse, or decreased school performance from lack of adult supervision. For children who feel safe in their community, however, a short period of independence every day may actually be beneficial; it encourages problem solving in self-care.

Suggestions for parents whose children must spend time alone before or after school are given in Box 32.8. Many communities offer special afterschool programs so children do not have to be home alone. Nurses are in a position to educate parents about such services so their children can feel both safe and stimulated creatively during this time. Boy Scouts and Campfire Girls are examples of organizations that offer programs to help children adjust to being home alone. Many communities are organizing hotline numbers a child who is alone can call if a problem arises. At health visits, assess whether parents and a child appear to have a problem with or are uncomfortable about afterschool arrangements. For a child who is extremely fearful or impulsive or who finds problem solving difficult, time alone after school may not be appropriate. Determine the individual circumstances, and recommend changes when appropriate.

Sex Education

It is important that school-age children be educated about pubertal changes and responsible sexual practices so they are

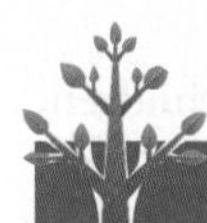

BOX 32.8 ✻ Focus on Family Teaching

Tips for Latchkey Children and Parents

Q. Shelly stays by herself after school for a half-hour. Her father asks you, "What are good tips for being sure it's safe to let her do this?"

A. Think of several areas:

Safety Teaching for Children

- Always lock doors and never show keys to others or indicate that you stay home alone.
- When answering the telephone, say a parent is busy, not absent from home.
- Have a plan in event you lose your key (stay with a neighbor, etc.).
- Do not go into the house if the door is open or a window is broken.
- Learn fire safety (practice a fire drill from all rooms of the house).
- Check in with parents by telephone when you first arrive home from school.
- Identify a caller before opening the door. Agree on a secret code word; you should not open the door or go with a person unless the person knows the word.
- Learn how to change light bulbs safely if it will be dark before parents return home. If appropriate, learn how to change fuses or reset circuit-breaker switches.
- Learn how to report a fire and telephone police (practice this with your parents).

Safety Responsibilities for Parents

- Prepare a safety kit and keep it filled; include a flashlight in case of a power failure so children do not need to light candles.
- Plan afterschool snacks that do not require cooking to prevent burns.
- Keep firearms locked, with the key in a place unknown to child.
- Keep a list of emergency telephone numbers (including parents' work numbers) by the telephone.
- Arrange with a neighbor who is usually home during the late afternoon for child to stay with in an emergency.
- If an older child will be watching a younger one, be certain both children understand the rules laid down and the degree of responsibility expected.
- Be certain child understands that rules that apply during other times (never swim alone; do not play by the railroad tracks) also apply during independent time.

Parental Actions to Prevent Loneliness

- Be certain to make additional time available after work so children can describe their day.
- Each morning help children plan an activity for that day so they have something purposeful to look forward to during time alone.
- Allow special privileges such as listening to music that other members of the family do not like as well; allow extra television hours during this time.
- Consider a pet. Even a caged animal, such as a hamster or a bird, offers companionship in a quiet house.
- Call children if there will be a delay in arriving home; unexpected time alone is very frightening.
- Leave messages on the refrigerator or in the bathroom that just say hi.
- Leave a tape- or video-recorded message for children to play (make sure it is not full of tasks to do, but is a welcoming message).
- Encourage children to read; fictional characters serve as friends as well as help to pass time.
- Urge children to network with other latchkey children regarding how they use time effectively; talking on the telephone or e-mailing another child reduces loneliness for both.

Parental Actions to Increase Socialization

- Help children plan afterschool activities such as joining a science club for one afternoon a week.
- Explore sports programs at school or in the community, as these often are held after school.
- Explore child care programs at the school the child attends, a public library, or a church or synagogue.
- Network with other parents or ask for flex time so child supervision can be alternated after school.
- Be sure children have opportunities to socialize with friends on weekends or on days when either parent is home.

Parental Actions to Increase Self-Esteem

- Praise children for the ability to take care of themselves for short time intervals (rather than scold that there are cracker crumbs on the carpet).
- Walk with children through the empty house and together identify sounds (the click of the furnace turning on, the refrigerator starting to defrost, etc.), so they can determine the cause of sounds when home alone and not be frightened.
- Help children to view quiet time as beneficial time in which they can do some things more efficiently than at noisy times such as homework.
- Do not allow child to use the latchkey role to provoke parental guilt. Allow children to have some say in family spending so they can see how their time alone (which allows both parents to work) contributes to family unity and progress.

well prepared for these. Also, preteens should have adults to whom they can turn for answers to questions about sex. Ideally, these should be their parents, but because sex is an emotionally charged topic, some parents may be extremely uncomfortable discussing it with their children. As a result, health care personnel often become resource persons.

Sex education should be incorporated into health education throughout the school years in a manner that is appropriate to age and development. Topics to teach and discuss in a sex education course for both preadolescent boys and girls include:

- Reproductive organ function
- Secondary sexual characteristics, so children will know what is going on in their bodies
- Physiology of reproduction, so they understand what menstruation is and why it occurs
- Male sexual functioning, including why the production of increased amounts of seminal fluid leads to nocturnal emissions
- Explanation of the physiology of pregnancy and the possibility that comes with sexual maturity for unplanned or unwanted pregnancies
- Social and moral implications of sexual maturity
- Birth control measures and the principles of safer sex if appropriate to the cultural setting (see Chapters 5 and 6)

A sex education course that includes films and discussions is helpful but never answers all of a preteen's questions (most youngsters would rather avoid asking a question than risk appearing ignorant in front of their peers in such a setting). Handing children booklets or showing films with the words, "If you have any questions after you've read (or watched) this, come and ask me" is equally ineffective because it implies they should have no questions. Urge parents or other health educators to watch films or read booklets with children to show they are truly available to answer questions.

Stealing

During early school age, most children go through a period during which they steal loose change from their mother's purse or father's dresser. This usually happens at around 7 years of age, when children first learn how to make change and also discover the importance of money. Stealing occurs because, although a child is gaining an appreciation for money, this appreciation is not yet balanced by strong moral principles.

Parents should explore the reason for the stealing:

- Do other children on the block receive an allowance and so have money for small items?
- Did their child make a bet that must be paid?
- Is a child buying a bully's friendship by purchasing gum or candy for that child?
- Does a child need more security and view money as security?

As a rule, early childhood stealing is best handled without a great deal of emotion. A parent should tell the child the money is missing. The importance of property rights should be reviewed: mother's and father's money is theirs; the child's money is the child's; they are not interchangeable. Youngsters who continue to steal past 9 years of age may require counseling because they should have progressed beyond this normal developmental step by this age.

Some shoplifting occurs with early school-age children, but the major problem with this arises during preadolescence. Some of this happens for the same reason that past generations tipped over outhouses or untied the preacher's horse and buggy: it is a public act of rebellion against authority, a "coming of age" ritual. It usually occurs because of peer pressure such as when children believe they must have a certain type of clothing to belong to the "in" crowd. It can also be an initiation ritual for gang membership.

Shoplifting must be taken seriously by parents because it is a punishable crime, not a prank. Just as money missing from a purse should not be ignored, shoplifting should be confronted immediately to prevent children who succeed once from taking something even bigger the second time. Children should be asked how they came to possess the article and should not be allowed to use it. Children should then be denied access to stores until they demonstrate more responsibility. A child who shoplifts more than once may need counseling; it reflects more than simple confusion about property rights.

As an overall principle, parents should set good examples if they expect their child to be honest. If one parent takes money from the other without permission, neither should be surprised to find their child attempting to do the same. If a parent changes price tags or unwraps items and eats them without paying for them in the supermarket, a parent cannot expect a child to do otherwise.

Violence or Terrorism

Children basically view their world as safe, so it is a shock when violence such as a school shooting or reports of terrorists enter their lives (Gaffney, 2008). Common recommendations for parents to help children feel safe are:

- Assure children they are safe; the violence is isolated to another part of the world and they are out of danger.
- Assure children their parents are actively involved in keeping them safe.
- Observe for signs of stress such as sleep disturbances, fatigue, lack of pleasure in activities, or signs of beginning substance abuse.
- Not allow children or adolescents to view footage of traumatic events over and over, as this decreases their ability to feel safe.
- Watch news programs with children so they can explain that the situation portrayed is not near them and that their child is safe.
- Explain there are bad people in the world, and bad people do bad things, but help children appreciate not all people in a particular group or who look a particular way are bad. Lashing out at people who resemble them only causes more harm.
- Prepare a family disaster plan, including such things as bottled water, blankets, toiletries, pet supplies, appropriate clothing, flashlights, and information such as what immunizations their children have had (particularly tetanus) and, if a child is ill, a history of medical needs or care so that in an emergency, these items are ready.
- Designate a "rally point" where the family will meet if ever separated by a disaster or evacuation.

Some parents may be reluctant to talk to their children about a disaster plan for the family, believing that these preparations will frighten children unnecessarily, but such preparations should have the major effect of increasing a feeling of safety, not decreasing it. Fear of the unknown is always more intense than fear of something tangible.

Bullying

A frequent reason school-age children cite for feeling so unhappy that they turn guns on classmates is that they were ridiculed or bullied to the point they could no longer take such abuse (Fitzpatrick, Dulin, & Piko, 2007). Why do some children become bullies and some become victims? Traits commonly associated with school-age bullies are:

- Advanced physical size and strength for their age
- Aggressive temperament (both male and female)
- Parents who are indifferent
- Parents who are permissive with an aggressive child
- Parents who typically resort to physical punishment
- Presence of a child who is a "natural victim" (underweight, small, anxious, insecure, cautious, or sensitive, with low self-esteem)

Suggestions for school personnel to deal with bullies are:

- Supervise recreation periods closely.
- Intervene immediately to stop bullying.
- Insist that if such behavior does not stop, both school and parents will become involved.
- Therapy may be needed to correct bullying behavior if it is ingrained.

Advise parents to discuss bullying with their school-age child and tell them how it should be reported, so that adults can intervene. School bullying has long-term effects on mental health from the view of both the bully and the victim (Sourander et al., 2007).

Recreational Drug Use

Once considered a college or high school problem, illegal drugs such as marijuana are now available to children as early as elementary school and certainly by the time they reach the seventh and eighth grades (Reboussin, Hubbard, & Ialongo, 2007). Cocaine and amphetamines are also becoming increasingly easy for children to obtain. Because alcohol is available in so many homes and often can be purchased in small stores without proof of age, this is yet another commonly abused drug of this age group (Wright, 2007).

The use of hard drugs and alcohol and ways to encourage children to avoid their use are discussed in Chapter 33. Inhalants that are easily available to school-age children, and so may be abused by them, are airplane glue (toluene) and aerosolized cooking oil (Ding et al., 2007). Children do not become physically addicted to glue but do become psychologically dependent on it. To achieve the desired effect, they drop quantities of the glue into a paper bag, then sniff the fumes and experience a feeling of exhilaration or giddiness. This may seem a harmless procedure, but in high concentrations glue fumes can cause extensive liver damage or pulmonary edema that can be fatal. Inhalants such as cooking spray or computer keyboard cleaner give this same effect. Because these products contain Freon, they can cause severe respiratory and cardiac irregularity.

Parents should suspect glue sniffing or some other form of recreational drug use if their child regularly appears irritable, inattentive, or drowsy. School health personnel should be aware of the increase in this practice among students and look for warning signs as substance abuse in middle school children may be associated with suicide attempts (Dunn et al., 2008).

Abuse of steroids to improve muscle mass can be found in children as young as sixth grade, particularly those interested in weight-lifting. Counsel children against this because abuse of steroids leads to cardiovascular irregularities, uncontrollable aggressiveness, and possible cancer in later life (Vertalino et al., 2007).

Cigarette smoking also begins in school-age children. With the sure knowledge that cigarette smoking plays a large part in the development of lung cancer and other serious respiratory illnesses, many parents assume their children will know not to start. Smoking is considered by children to be an adult activity, however, so adopting the habit can be considered a giant step on the road to adulthood. Although the amount of cigarette advertising targeting young people as consumers has decreased, school-age children should be taught to recognize advertising manipulation aimed at them. Caution children against experimenting with smokeless tobacco as well as this can lead to mouth and throat cancer. Children may try this after seeing professional athletes using it.

To discourage use of tobacco by school-age children, health care professionals and parents need to be role models of excellent health behaviors in hopes children will follow their good examples.

Children of Alcoholic Parents

As many as one in five children live with an alcoholic parent (Hussong et al., 2007). Such children are at greater risk for having emotional problems than are others because of the frequent disruption in their lives. Alcoholism may have a genetic cause, so children of alcoholics may be more likely to become alcoholics. They also can learn poor coping behavior. Immediate problems that can occur with children of alcoholics are:

- A feeling of guilt that they are the cause of the parent's drinking
- Constant worry that the alcoholic parent will become sick or die, leaving the child; at the same time, fear of violence from the alcoholic parent and a wish the parent would leave
- A feeling of shame that prevents the child from inviting friends home or asking for help
- Decreased ability to trust adults because the parent has been unreliable so many times
- Concern because the alcoholic parent's behavior is so erratic that no regular schedule of bedtime and meals exists
- Anger at the alcoholic parent for drinking and at the nonalcoholic parent for not doing more to correct things
- Helplessness to change the situation

Such fears may be revealed by failing marks in school, withdrawal from friends or social activities, and delinquent behavior such as stealing. With adolescence may come depression, suicidal thoughts, or abuse of drugs or alcohol. School nurses are in an excellent position to identify such children, monitor their school progress, and refer them to organizations such as Al-Anon or Alateen (http://www.al-anon-alateen.org) for support.

Nursing Diagnoses and Related Interventions

*

Nursing Diagnosis: Altered family dynamics related to lack of motivation to reduce weight

Outcome Evaluation: Child states reasonable weight loss and exercise goals; discusses feelings about being overweight and reactions from schoolmates; expresses positive feelings about self-worth.

Motivating preteens to lose weight can be difficult because they often have little regard for what will happen to them in the future. They are not upset when told obese people do not live as long as slimmer persons and have more heart attacks, because this will happen far in the future. They do, however, have a great respect for adults who are sympathetic to their problems. They are also aware slim children are usually the most popular, and they wish they could look that way. They follow better dietary regimens, therefore, if they are asked to do so by a respected adult, such as a nurse, or if they fear being left out of social interactions

Obesity

As many as 50% of school-age children are obese by body mass index guidelines for ideal weight. Some of these children have been overweight since infancy; their prepubertal natural weight gain makes them obese. Children with an endomorphic build (a natural tendency to accumulate body fat) are more likely to be obese at any time of life than those with a mesomorphic (normal) or ectomorphic (slender) build. Many families rely on fast-food meals several times a week, and such foods tend to be high in calories and fat and can lead to obesity. Soft drink machines in grade schools add to the problem (LaRowe, Moeller, & Adams, 2007). Children of obese parents are also inclined to obesity; perhaps genetic influences have some bearing. If parents ingest a diet full of excessive calories, the child is encouraged to eat similarly; this makes environmental factors also play a role.

Obese children begin to develop many of the same health problems as obese adults, such as hypertension, type 2 diabetes, and an elevated total cholesterol level, with possible atherosclerosis. They also may be ridiculed for their size and be unable to participate on sports teams. This is strong evidence for the need for active measures to help preteens regulate their weight.

Those who become so obese that friends leave them out of activities or who cannot play sports because they tire so quickly may develop such a poor self-image that they have little motivation for self-improvement. A weight-reduction program for school-age children that emphasizes long-term lifestyle changes is best. It should contain features such as:

- Intake of about 1200 calories (no more than 30% as fat), with lifestyle changes such as a structured family meal, eliminating eating or snacking in front of the television, decreased portion sizes, and elimination of sugar-rich drinks
- An active exercise program, including such things as monitoring and limiting time spent in physical inactivity (watching television, playing computer and video games, surfing the Internet, and talking on the telephone)
- A counseling program to discuss aspects such as self-image and motivation to reduce weight (Haines & Neumark-Sztainer, 2007).

Total caloric intake cannot be reduced too drastically because children need calories to form new body tissue for continued growth. If carbohydrate intake is restricted too greatly, protein is broken down for body energy and a negative nitrogen balance is produced. Caution children not to try faddish high-protein diets (as most adults should not), because such diets do not supply enough carbohydrates and may produce a heavy renal solute load (the breakdown product of proteins) for the kidneys. It helps if children aim to lose 5 lb over a short time rather than 50 lb over a year. This short-term goal coincides better with the task of developing industry.

Surgical techniques such as stomach banding are obviously extreme measures and inappropriate for children. Obese children might request one, however, in an attempt to avoid the not insignificant difficulty of long-term weight loss.

Overweight school-age children often do well if a dieters' club is formed. They are not too young to participate in formal weight-control organizations. Having tangible support from other group members helps them follow tedious and monotonous nutrition patterns. Behavior modification can also be useful in teaching children how to eat in a healthier manner.

As a way of increasing daily activity, preadolescents do well with formal exercise classes because they enjoy the support from other children. In addition, encourage them to increase informal exercise, such as walking to and from school. Encourage coaches of childhood sports to accept obese children as part of a team, not because the child will necessarily benefit the team, but because the exercise will benefit the child. Exercise burns up calories, and if children's daylight hours are filled with activities and friends, they have less time to eat.

Lifestyle change is the ultimate goal for the entire family, because obesity is usually a family problem. Rather than preparing special meals for just the obese child, the entire family probably needs to eat in a healthier manner. Because preadolescents do not generally prepare their own food, the person in the home who prepares meals requires as much information on the planned weight loss as the child. The old concepts that used to hold ("A clean plate is good; how can you leave food when people in other countries are starving?") may have to be changed so children and other family members reduce their intake appropriately. The importance of exercise should also be reflected in the home. Family members should not only encourage the obese child to exercise but also should partake in some form of daily activity themselves.

There is some danger in pointing out to preadolescents that they are terribly overweight because some children become so obsessed with losing weight that they become bulimic or anorexic (Honey & Halsle, 2007) (see Chapter 54). Stressing that children "become healthier" or "improve stamina" may be better advice than talking about dieting.

Concerns of the Physically Challenged or Chronically Ill School-Age Child

One of the biggest problems facing school-age children with long-term illness or physical challenge is time lost from school. This threatens not only academic achievement but also children's relationships with peers. It may make a child the "odd person out" with respect to making friends or joining gangs. Whether children are confined to the home or hospitalized, helping them to keep in contact with friends by telephone, e-mail, or letters can help foster the socialization that is important for continued development. Encourage parents (or school friends) to obtain schoolwork and help these children with their homework so they can progress with learning at a usual pace and continue to build self-esteem.

Most children with physical or cognitive challenges attend regular schools and classes (**inclusion**) because federal law (PL 99-457) stipulates all children must receive equal education in the least restrictive situation possible. Placement in classrooms is determined by a committee in each school system. You may need to advocate for a child with such a committee to demonstrate, for example, that although children use wheelchairs or need continuous oxygen, they can participate in regular classroom settings; or that a particular child would benefit from a period each day with a special resource teacher. It may be necessary to meet with a school nurse, teacher, or the child's classmates (with the parents' permission) to increase their understanding and acceptance of a child's illness.

Urge parents of children with physical or cognitive challenges to assign them household chores just like other children their age and to allow them to participate in activities, such as Girl or Boy Scouts, in which accomplishment is encouraged. It is important for such children to develop a sense of industry or accomplishment so they can persevere in measures that will help them to be as independent as possible (Fig. 32.10).

When you are caring for a school-age child who is chronically ill or physically challenged, choose short-term activities that can be completed independently, as with all school-age children. Conversely, be careful not to insult a child with tasks that are obviously not age-appropriate. Table 32.5 describes some nursing actions to help foster a sense of industry in children who are physically challenged or chronically ill.

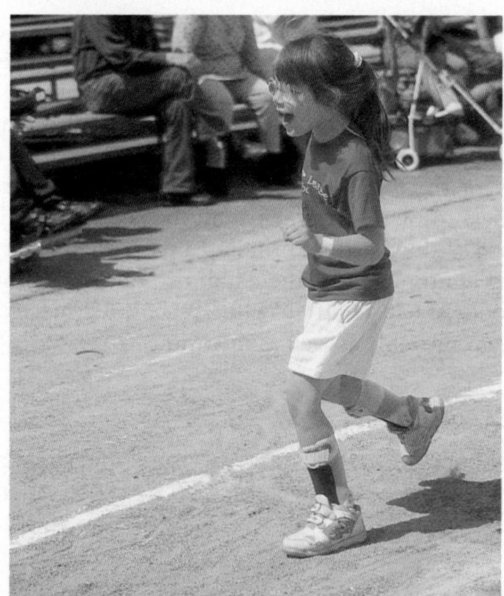

FIGURE 32.10 A school-age child who is physically challenged is elated at a finish line. This accomplishment can go far toward her developing a sense of industry. (© Jose Carillo/Stock Boston.)

Nutrition and the Challenged School-Age Child

Food preparation and dishwashing are times for socializing in most households. A school-age child who cannot be involved in these activities because of a physical challenge needs extra time during the day to make up for these lost socializing experiences, such as a specific hour set aside for talking or sharing a project that can be accomplished in one sitting.

TABLE 32.5 ✻ Nursing Actions That Encourage a Sense of Industry in a Physically Challenged or Chronically Ill School-Age Child

Category	Actions
Nutrition	Allow choices of food and respect food preferences. Provide small food servings that child can finish, encouraging sense of accomplishment.
Dressing	Allow child to make out requisitions for supplies. Ask for suggestions regarding how bulky the child wants dressing, where to apply tape.
Medicine	Teach child name and action of medicine. Encourage child to keep track of medication times by clock or record. Child may feel more in control of injections or intravenous insertions if allowed to choose the site from among options offered. Allow child to choose oral medicine form (capsules or liquid) if possible.
Rest	Establish clear rules for rest periods (reading or watching television is all right; playing a game is not, etc.).
Hygiene	Respect modesty of school-age child at an adult level. Allow as much choice as possible such as own clothing, timing of self-care.
Pain	Encourage child to express and rate pain. Encourage child to use distraction techniques, such as counting backward from 100 or imagery, during episodes of pain. Explain source and cause of pain to give child sense of mastery.
Stimulation	Encourage school work. Encourage activity that ends in a product (putting together a picture puzzle rather than listening to a CD). Encourage paper-and-pencil games, such as connect the dots, tic tac toe. Card games provide social interaction and also encourage simple addition skills (make a deck from paper if one is not available). Do not suggest competitive games for children less than age 10 years. Encourage using playroom for socialization. Encourage child to keep in contact with school friends by telephoning or text messaging.

When eating in cafeterias or at a friend's home, children who must eat special diets are usually tempted to select the same food as everyone else rather than limit what they choose. They may decline invitations rather than admit to requiring a special diet or needing help with eating. Ask at health care visits if any of these problems are present. Help children with special diets to plan ways they could be comfortable in social food-based settings such as bringing a party snack that is easily eaten and appropriate for the child, or politely declining particular foods. Help children who are hospitalized to select a diet that is enjoyable as well as nutritious.

✔ Checkpoint Question 32.3

School-agers can begin drug abuse. What is a common household product frequently abused by school-agers?

a. Grated orange peel
b. Laundry bleach
c. Aerosol cooking oil
d. Shredded cabbage

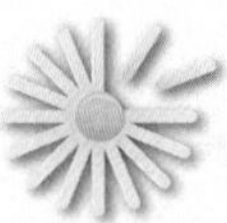

Key Points for Review

- School-age children mature slowly but steadily. Their average annual weight gain is 3 to 5 lb; their increase in height is 1 to 2 inches.
- At about age 10, children begin to develop secondary sex characteristics. Preparation for this helps them accept these changes positively.
- Deciduous teeth are lost and permanent teeth erupt during the school-age period.
- Erikson's developmental task for the school-age period is to gain a sense of industry, or how to do things well.
- Common health problems during the school-age period include minor respiratory and gastrointestinal infections as well as dental caries and malocclusion.
- Common parental concerns during this period are language development, fears and anxieties, and behavior problems such as stealing and using recreational drugs.
- As many as 90% of parents of school-age children are dual-earner families. This means many school-age children return home before their parents. Counseling families on ways to turn this independent time alone into a positive experience is a nursing responsibility.
- Children in a concrete stage of operational thought are limited to understanding concepts they can actually see. When health teaching, use concrete examples (actually let them hold a syringe, do not just talk about it) to increase their understanding.
- School-age children thrive on rules. It is confusing for them when rules are changed (medicine will now be taken four rather than three times a day) unless they have a clear explanation of why the change is occurring.
- School-age children are looking for good adult role models; it is hard for them to feel confidence in an adult who is not honest with them or who fails to live up to their expectations by not following through on promises.
- School-age children with a family tendency toward obesity may become overweight. Helping the family learn a healthier lifestyle is important.

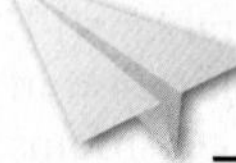

CRITICAL THINKING EXERCISES

1. Shelly is the 12-year-old you met at the beginning of the chapter. Her mother told you that she has developed many nervous habits since she started middle school. She asks you if this is normal. How would you answer? What suggestions would you make to her mother regarding this?
2. Shelly has become obese in the last year. School-age children develop obesity because of excessive nutritional intake, lack of exercise, and inheritance or family factors. What are suggestions you could make to help prevent Shelly from gaining more weight? What is a possible consequence of telling school-age children they are overweight?
3. Shelly's best friend is a 12-year-old boy who is confined to a wheelchair because of muscular dystrophy. Why might developing a sense of industry be particularly difficult for him? What suggestions could you make to encourage this?
4. Examine the National Health Goals related to school-age children. Most government-sponsored funds for nursing research are allotted based on these goals. What would be a possible research topic to explore pertinent to these goals that would be applicable to the Lewis family and also advance evidence-based practice?

CRITICAL THINKING SCENARIO

Open the accompanying CD-ROM or visit http://thePoint.lww.com and read the Patient Scenario included for this chapter, then answer the questions to further sharpen your skills and grow more familiar with NCLEX style questions related to school-age growth and development. Confirm your answers are correct by reading the rationales.

REFERENCES

American Academy of Pediatrics (AAP). (2009). Car safety seats: a guide for families. Retrieved from http://www.aap.org/family/carseatguide.htm.

American Academy of Pediatrics Committee on Practice and Ambulatory Medicine. (2009). *Recommendations for preventive pediatric health care.* Washington, DC: Author.

Ding, K., et al. (2007). Inhalant use among Indiana school children. *American Journal of Health Behavior, 31*(1), 24–34.

Dunn, M. S., et al. (2008). Substance use behavior and suicide indicators among rural middle school students. *Journal of School Health, 78*(1), 26–31.

Erikson, E. H. (1993). *Childhood and society.* New York: W. W. Norton.

Fitzpatrick, K. M., Dulin, A. J., & Piko, B. F. (2007). Not just pushing and shoving: school bullying among African American adolescents. *Journal of School Health, 77*(1), 16–22.

Freud, S. (1962). *Three essays on the theory of sexuality.* New York: Hearst Corporation.

Gaffney, D. A. (2008). Families, schools, and disaster: the mental health consequences of catastrophic events. *Family and Community Health, 31*(1), 44–53.

Gaither, M. (2008). Why homeschooling happened. *Educational Horizons, 86*(4), 226–237.

Goldson, E., & Reynolds, A. (2008). Child development and behavior. In W. W. Hay, et al. (Eds.). *Current pediatric diagnosis and treatment* (18th ed.). Columbus, OH: McGraw-Hill.

Haines, J., & Neumark-Sztainer, D. (2007). Addressing weight-related issues in an elementary school: what do students, parents, and school staff recommend? *Eating Disorders, 15*(1), 5–21.

Harrison, J. E., O'Brien, K. D., & Worthington, H.V. (2009). Orthodontic treatment for prominent upper front teeth in children. *Cochrane Database of Systematic Reviews, 2009*(1), (CD003452).

He, F. J., Marrero, N. M., & Macgregor, G. A. (2008). Salt and blood pressure in children and adolescents. *Journal of Human Hypertension, 22*(1), 4–11.

Honey, A., & Halse, C. (2007). Looking after well siblings of adolescent girls with anorexia: an important parental role. *Child: Care, Health and Development, 33*(1), 52–58.

Hussong, A. M., et al. (2007). Externalizing symptoms among children of alcoholic parents: entry points for an antisocial pathway to alcoholism. *Journal of Abnormal Psychology, 116*(3), 529–542.

Kaplan, D. W., & Love-Osborne, K. (2008). Adolescence. In W. W. Hay, et al. (Eds.). *Current pediatric diagnosis and treatment* (18th ed.). Columbus, OH: McGraw-Hill.

Kohlberg, L. (1984). *The psychology of moral development.* New York: Harper & Row.

Kristjansson, E. A., et al. (2009). School feeding for improving the physical and psychosocial health of disadvantaged elementary school children. *Cochrane Database of Systematic Reviews, 2009*(1), (CD004676).

LaRowe, T. L., Moeller, S. M., & Adams, A. K. (2007). Beverage patterns, diet quality, and body mass index of US preschool and school-aged children. *Journal of the American Dietetic Association, 107*(7), 1124–1133.

Leininger, L. J., & Ziol-Guest, K. M. (2008). Reexamining the effects of family structure on children's access to care: the single-father family. *Health Services Research, 43*(1.1), 117–133.

Marinho, V. C. C., et al. (2009). Topical fluoride (toothpastes, mouthrinses, gels or varnishes) for preventing dental caries in children and adolescents. *Cochrane Database of Systematic Reviews, 2009*(1), (CD002782).

McDowell, M. A., Brody, D. J., & Hughes, J. P. (2007). Has age at menarche changed? Results from the National Health and Nutrition Examination Survey. *Journal of Adolescent Health, 40*(3), 227–231.

Piaget, J. (1969). *The theory of stages in cognitive development.* New York: McGraw-Hill.

Reboussin, B. A., Hubbard, S., & Ialongo, N. S. (2007). Marijuana use patterns among African-American middle-school students: a longitudinal latent class regression analysis. *Drug and Alcohol Dependence, 90*(1), 12–24.

Rolfes, S. R., Pinna, K., & Whitney, E. N. (2009). *Understanding normal and clinical nutrition.* New York: Wadsworth/Cengage Learning.

Shilt, J. S., & Barnett, T. M. (2007). Evaluating and managing back pain in children. *Journal of Musculoskeletal Medicine, 24*(2), 73–76.

Sourander, A., et al. (2007). What is the early adulthood outcome of boys who bully or are bullied in childhood? *Pediatrics, 120*(2), 397–404.

Tyrrell, M. (2007). School phobia. *Journal of School Nursing, 21*(3), 147–151.

Wright, L. S. (2007). A norm changing approach to drug prevention. *Journal of Drug Education, 37*(2), 191–215.

Vertalino, M., et al. (2007). Participation in weight-related sports is associated with higher use of unhealthful weight-control behaviors and steroid use. *Journal of the American Dietetic Association, 107*(3), 434–440.

SUGGESTED READINGS

Bell, M. L., et al. (2007). Can first and second grade students benefit from an alcohol use prevention program? *Journal of Child and Adolescent Substance Abuse, 16*(3), 89–107.

Champion, K. M., & Clay, D. L. (2007). Individual differences in responses to provocation and frequent victimization by peers. *Child Psychiatry and Human Development, 37*(3), 205–220.

Hoagwood, K. E., et al. (2007). Empirically based school interventions targeted at academic and mental health functioning. *Journal of Emotional and Behavioral Disorders, 15*(2), 66–92.

Khattab, N., & Jones, C. P. (2007). Growing up girl: preparing for change through group work. *Journal for Specialists in Group Work, 32*(1), 41–50.

Kearney, C. A., & Bensaheb, A. (2007). School absenteeism and school refusal behavior: a review and suggestions for school-based health professionals. *Journal of School Health, 76*(1), 3–7.

Lilja, J., Giota, J., & Hamilton, D. (2007). How cultural factors influence school-based substance use prevention programs. *Substance Use and Misuse, 42*(2-3), 485–494.

Logue, J. N. (2008). Violent death in American schools in the 21st century: reflections following the 2006 Amish school shootings. *Journal of School Health, 78*(1), 58–61.

Murphy, M., & Polivka, B. (2007). Parental perceptions of the schools' role in addressing childhood obesity. *Journal of School Nursing, 23*(1), 40–46.

Powell, C., Wedner, S., & Hatt, S. (2009). Vision screening for correctable visual acuity deficits in school-age children and adolescents. *Cochrane Database of Systematic Reviews, 2009*(1), (CD005023).

Russell-Mayhew, S., Arthur, N., & Ewashen, C. (2007). Targeting students, teachers and parents in a wellness-based prevention program in schools. *Eating Disorders, 15*(2), 159–181.

Chapter 33 Nursing Care of a Family With an Adolescent

KEY TERMS

- adolescence
- comedones
- formal operational thought
- glycogen loading
- identity
- puberty
- role confusion
- stalking
- substance abuse

OBJECTIVES

After mastering the contents of this chapter, you should be able to:

1. Describe normal growth and development and common parental concerns of the adolescent period.
2. Identify National Health Goals related to adolescents that nurses could help the nation achieve.
3. Use critical thinking to analyze ways in which care of an adolescent could be more family centered.
4. Assess an adolescent for normal growth and development milestones.
5. Formulate nursing diagnoses for the family of an adolescent.
6. Identify expected outcomes for nursing care of an adolescent.
7. Plan nursing care related to growth and development concerns of an adolescent, such as planning health teaching necessary to accept pubertal changes.
8. Implement nursing care related to growth and development or special needs of an adolescent, such as organizing a discussion group on ways to prevent drug abuse.
9. Evaluate expected outcomes for achievement and effectiveness of care.
10. Identify areas related to care of adolescents that could benefit from additional nursing research or application of evidence-based practice.
11. Integrate knowledge of adolescent growth and development with nursing process to achieve quality maternal and child health nursing care.

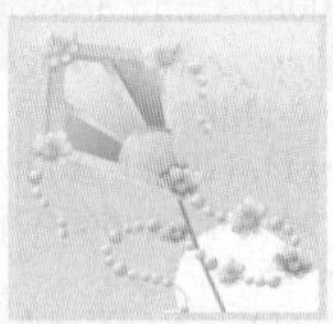

Raul is a 15-year-old teenager you see at an adolescent clinic. His chief concern is a head cold. He has numerous acne lesions on his forehead and cheeks. His parents tell you Raul seemed depressed for a long time after his girlfriend broke up with him but now seems happy again. They are pleased to see him maturing so much that he recently gave away his collection of baseball cards to a young neighbor. You mention to Raul that a decongestant would probably make him feel better. He asks you how many pills it would take to kill someone, then jokes he was kidding. The physician in the clinic prescribes a decongestant and suggests Raul return in 6 months.

The previous chapter discussed school-age children and the capabilities children develop during that time period. This chapter adds information about the changes, both physical and psychosocial, that occur during adolescence. Such information builds a base for care and health teaching for this age group.

Did Raul have some needs that were not met by his clinic visit?

Adolescence is generally defined as the period between 13 and 18 or 20 years, a time that serves as a transition between childhood and young adulthood. It can be divided into an early period (13 to 14 years), a middle period (15 to 16 years), and a late period (17 to 20 years). During all periods, adolescence is defined not so much by chronologic age as by physiologic, psychological, and sociologic changes. The drastic change in physical appearance and the change in expectations of others (especially parents) that occur during the period can lead to both emotional and physical health problems.

Adolescents invariably feel a sense of pressure throughout this period because they are mature in some respects but still young in others. For example, an adolescent's sexual interests are awakening, yet personal or parental pressures discourage sexual exploration. An adolescent may not feel mature enough to live away from home yet parents and teachers are urging the adolescent to apply for an out-of-town college. This duality causes a major dilemma for an adolescent, leading to many of the growth and developmental concerns of the age (Lovato et al., 2009).

There is such a strong adolescent subculture today parents may feel from the minute their child enters the teenage years that they will have difficulty guiding their child or understanding teenage values, as though entering this period locks their adolescent into a shell or pulls down a curtain between child and parents. This can become a self-fulfilling prophecy, whereby the parents actually cause the communication breakdown. At other times, communication problems can begin when a teenager refuses to respect parents' opinions or stops asking for them. Many of the problems adolescents bring to health care personnel arise from this communication impasse, no matter how it started. They also often come to health care facilities with many misconceptions, seeking adult help and guidance. National Health Goals related to adolescence are shown in Box 33.1.

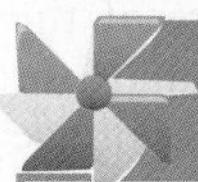

BOX 33.1 ✻ Focus on National Health Goals

Health teaching in the adolescent years is important, because healthy habits begun at this time can influence health over a lifetime. For this reason, a number of National Health Goals relate to adolescent health:

- Reduce the number of adolescents who are overweight or obese to a prevalence of no more than 5% from a baseline of 11%.
- Reduce tobacco use by adolescents to a rate of 16% from a baseline of 35%.
- Reduce the rate of smokeless tobacco use by adolescents to no more than 1% from a baseline of 8%.
- Reduce the rate of deaths caused by alcohol-related motor vehicle accidents among people ages 15 to 24 to no more than 9.2% from a baseline of 13.5%.
- Reduce the rate of suicide attempts by adolescents to no more than 1% from a baseline of 2.6%.
- Increase to 35% the proportion of adolescents who exercise at least 30 minutes a day, 5 days a week, from a baseline of 27% (http://www.nih.gov).

Nurses can help the nation achieve these goals by educating adolescents against the use of cigarettes, smokeless tobacco, alcohol, drug abuse, and acts of violence and by acting as support people for adolescents during times of crisis to help prevent suicide. Areas that could benefit from additional nursing research are identifying effective programs that reduce the use of smokeless tobacco or cigarette smoking, documenting the best actions for nurses to take in emergency rooms when adolescents are admitted after suicide attempts, and constructing rapid surveys to identify adolescents who are abusing drugs.

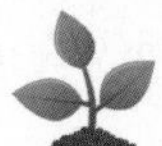

Nursing Process Overview

For Healthy Development of an Adolescent

Assessment

Parents rarely bring adolescents for routine health maintenance visits the way they did when their children were younger, and adolescents generally do not come to health care facilities on their own unless they are ill. Unless adolescents need a physical examination for athletic clearance, therefore, they are often not seen for health assessments. When adolescents are accompanied by their parents at health visits, it is best to obtain a health history separately from parents to promote independence and responsibility for self-care. When performing physical examinations on adolescents, be aware they may be very self-conscious. They also need health assurance and appreciate comments such as "Your hair has a nice, healthy feel," or "This is an accessory nipple. Have you ever wondered about it?" so they can learn more about their rapidly changing bodies.

Nursing Diagnosis

Nursing diagnoses for adolescents cover a wide range. Frequently used diagnoses related to adolescents and their families are:

- Health-seeking behaviors related to normal growth and development
- Low self-esteem related to facial acne
- Anxiety related to concerns about normal growth and development
- Risk for injury related to peer pressure to use alcohol and drugs
- Readiness for enhanced parenting related to increased knowledge of teenage years

Outcome Identification and Planning

When planning care with adolescents, respect the fact they have a strong desire to exert independence or do things their own way. This means they are not likely to adhere to a plan of care that disrupts their lifestyle or makes them appear different from others their age. Including them in planning is essential so the plan will be agreeable and accepted. Establishing a contract such as asking an adolescent to agree to take medication daily may be the most effective means to reach a mutual understanding.

Adolescents are very present oriented, so a program that provides immediate results, such as increased respiratory function, will usually be carried out well. In contrast, a regimen oriented toward the future, with long-term goals such as preventing hypertension, may not be as successful. This does not mean it is not important to teach adolescents about the necessity of reducing future health risks—by eating well, *not* smoking, and generally taking care of their bodies—but that information will be best accepted if geared as much as possible to specific, short-term benefits to their health.

Teaching by peers is another effective way to motivate teens. Organizing peer support groups this way can be a major contribution of school nurses. Helpful Web sites for teenage referral are Mothers Against School Hazing (http://www.mashinc.org) and Mothers Against Drunk Driving (http://www.madd.org). Other organizations that address some of the concerns of adolescence are the American Association of Suicidology (http://www.suicidology.org), Partnership for a Drug-Free America (http://www.drugfreeamerica.org), Al-Anon/Alateen (http://www.alateen.com), Planned Parenthood Federation of America, Inc. (http://www.plannedparenthood.org), and Sexual Information and Education Council of the United States (SIECUS) (http://www.siecus.org).

Implementation

Adolescents do poorly with tasks that someone tells them they *must* do. If they help to plan tasks, however, they can typically carry them out successfully. Adolescents have little patience with adults who do not demonstrate the behavior they are being asked to achieve; a parent or nurse who smokes and asks an adolescent not to smoke, for example, will probably not be successful. For best results, evaluate how an intervention appears from an adolescent's standpoint before beginning teaching.

Outcome Evaluation

Evaluation of expected outcomes should include not only whether desired outcomes have been achieved but whether adolescents are pleased with their success. Individuals will have difficulty accomplishing desired goals as adults unless they have high self-esteem that includes feeling secure in their new body image.

Examples of outcome criteria that might be established are:

- Client states she is able to feel good about herself even though she is the shortest girl in her class.
- Client states he has not consumed alcohol in 2 weeks.
- Parents state they feel more confident about their ability to parent an adolescent.
- Client states she feels high self-esteem despite persistent facial acne.

GROWTH AND DEVELOPMENT OF AN ADOLESCENT

Adolescents grow both rapidly and mature dramatically during this period. In the United States, as in most developed countries, adolescence covers a long time span. In developing countries, in contrast, adolescence tends to be much shorter because children must take full-time jobs early in life to help support their families. Socioeconomic factors definitely influence the length of adolescence across all cultures. Recognizing that adolescents may have differing responsibilities and life experiences based on cultural expectations can be useful when making an assessment. In a family in which an adolescent is expected to begin working full-time or to marry at an early age, you may need to include factors such as occupational hazards or the effects of job, family, and financial stress on an adolescent. Readiness for early childbearing may also be important.

Physical Growth

The major milestones of development in the adolescent period are the onset of puberty at 9 to 12 years of age, and the cessation of body growth at 16 to 20 years. Between these milestones, physiologic growth and development of adult coordination occur. At first, the gain in physical growth is mostly in weight, leading to the stocky, slightly obese appearance of prepubescence; later comes the thin, gangly appearance of late adolescence.

Most girls are 1 to 2 in (2.4 to 5 cm) taller than boys coming into adolescence but generally stop growing within 3 years from menarche. Those girls who started menstruating at 10 years of age, therefore, may reach their adult height by age 13.

Boys grow about 4 to 12 in (10 to 30 cm) in height and gain about 15 to 65 lb (7 to 30 kg) during adolescence. Girls grow 2 to 8 in (5 to 20 cm) in height and gain 15 to 55 lb (7 to 25 kg). Growth stops with closure of the epiphyseal lines of long bones. This occurs at about 16 or 17 years of age in females and about 18 to 20 years of age in males.

The increase in body size does not occur in all organ systems at the same rate. For example, adolescents' skeletal system grows faster than muscles, and muscle mass increases more rapidly than heart size. These differences in growth rates make adolescents appear long-legged and awkward during a rapid growth spurt because their extremities elongate first, followed by trunk growth. Both sexes may lack coordination during these times. A 13-year-old child, for example, typically reaches to pick up a glass of milk at the dinner table and spills it, having reached beyond it because an arm is longer than the child realized.

Because the heart and lungs increase in size more slowly than the rest of the body, blood flow and oxygen availability are reduced. This means adolescents may have insufficient energy and become fatigued trying to finish the various activities that interest them. Pulse rate and respiratory rate decrease slightly (to 70 beats per minute and 20 breaths per minute, respectively), and blood pressure increases slightly (to 120/70 mm Hg), reaching adult levels by late adolescence. With adulthood, blood pressure becomes slightly higher in males than females because more force is necessary to distribute blood to the larger male body mass.

All during adolescence, androgen stimulates sebaceous glands to extreme activity, sometimes resulting in acne, a common adolescent skin problem. Apocrine sweat glands (glands present in the axillae and genital area) form shortly after puberty. Apocrine sweat glands produce a strong odor in response to emotional stimulation. Therefore, adolescents begin to notice they must shower or bathe more frequently than when they were younger in order to be free of body odor.

Teeth

Adolescents gain their second molars at about 13 years of age and their third molars (wisdom teeth) between 18 and 21 years of age. Third molars may erupt as early as 14 to 15 years of age. The jaw reaches adult size only toward the end of adolescence, however. As a result, adolescents whose third molars erupt before the lengthening of the jaw is complete may experience pain and may need these molars extracted because they do not fit their jawline (Mettes et al., 2009).

Puberty

Puberty is the time at which an individual first becomes capable of sexual reproduction. A girl has entered puberty when she begins to menstruate; a boy enters puberty when he begins to produce spermatozoa. These events usually occur between ages 11 and 14 years. The age of first menstruation in girls is gradually decreasing from a mean of 13 years to 12.4 years, probably related to more weight gain in girls (Lee et al., 2007; McDowell, Brody, & Hughes, 2007). Puberty creates many questions for early teenagers about what is normal and what is not (Cousineau et al., 2007).

Secondary Sex Changes

Secondary sex characteristics such as body hair configuration and breast growth are those characteristics which distinguish the sexes from each other but play no direct part in reproduction. The secondary sex characteristics that began in the late school-age period (see Chapter 32) continue to develop during adolescence. Typical stages of sexual maturation are shown in Table 33.1.

Sexual maturity in males and females is classified according to Tanner stages, named after the original researcher on sexual maturity (Tanner, 1962). Tanner stages of female sexual development are shown in Figure 33.1; stages of male genital growth are shown in Figure 33.2.

✔ Checkpoint Question 33.1

Raul is concerned about developing body odor. What body glands are responsible for this?

a. Adipose glands
b. Apocrine glands
c. Sebaceous glands
d. Dermal pod glands

Developmental Milestones

The same assessment categories of younger children continue to apply to adolescents.

Play or Recreation

Thirteen-year-old children change from school-age activities of active games to more adult forms of recreation such as listening to music, chatting on computers, or following a sports team's wins and losses. Team (or school) loyalty is intense, and following a coach's instructions becomes mandatory. This attitude is similar to the loyalty 6-year-old children show toward their first-grade teacher.

Young adolescents who do not have the physical ability to compete successfully in sports do their best to avoid these activities. Urge parents to encourage youngsters to play sports for their own health and well-being and the companionship involved, however, even though they do not excel. If adolescents thought they would be successful at a sport but then are not, they need a sympathetic person to listen to the frustration they feel and to be encouraged to try other activities in which they can excel, such as science, music, or art. Overuse injuries from athletics occur in early adolescence until adolescents learn more about their limits and begin to respect the advice of adults on being well prepared and trained for sports participation.

TABLE 33.1 ✲ Sexual Maturation in Adolescents

Age (yr)	Males	Females
13–15	Growth spurt continuing; pubic hair abundant and curly; testes, scrotum, and penis enlarging further; axillary hair present; facial hair fine and downy; voice changes happening with annoying frequency	Pubic hair thick and curly, triangular in distribution, breast areola and papilla form secondary mound; menstruation is ovulatory, making pregnancy possible
15–16	Genitalia adult; pubic hair abundant and curly; scrotum dark and heavily rugated; facial and body hair present; sperm production mature	Pubic hair curly and abundant (adult); may extend onto medial aspect of thighs; breast tissue adult and nipples protrude; areolas no longer project as separate ridges from breasts; may have some degree of facial acne
16–17	Pubic hair curly and abundant (adult), may scrotum, and penis adult in size; may have some degree of facial acne; gynecomastia (enlarged breast tissue), if present, fades	End of skeletal growth extend along medial aspect of thighs; testes,
17–18	End of skeletal growth	

Source: Tanner, J. M. (1962). *Growth at adolescence* (2nd ed.). Oxford: Blackwell.

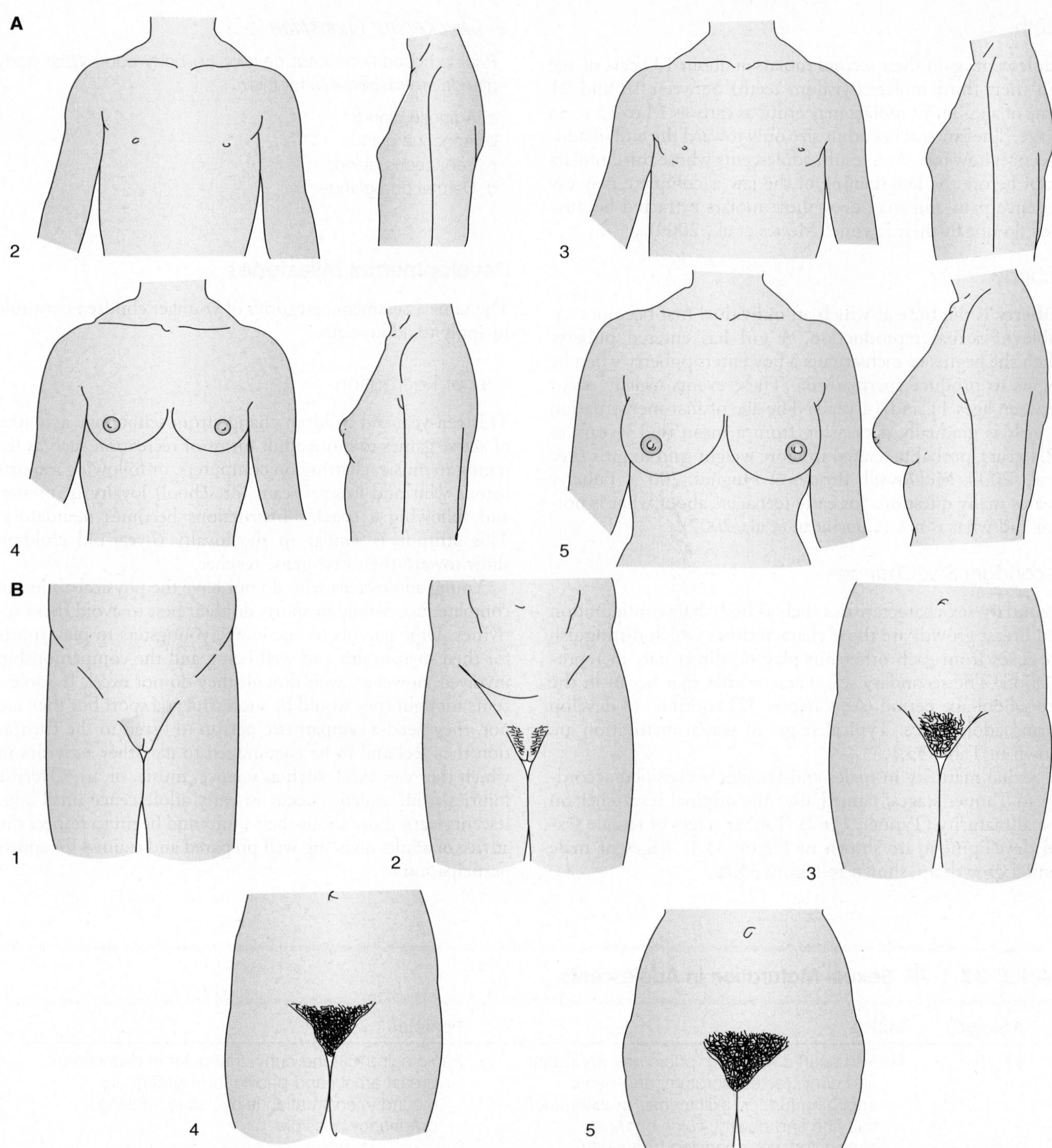

FIGURE 33.1 (**A**) Female breast development. *Sex maturity rating 1* (not shown), prepubertal; elevation of papilla only. *Sex maturity rating 2:* breast buds appear; areola is slightly widened and projects as small mound. *Sex maturity rating 3:* enlargement of the entire breast with no protrusion of the papilla or the nipple. *Sex maturity rating 4:* enlargement of the breast and projection of areola and papilla as a secondary mound. *Sex maturity rating 5:* adult configuration of the breast with protrusion of the nipple; areola no longer projects separately from remainder of breast. (**B**) Female pubic hair development. *Sex maturity rating 1:* prepubertal; no pubic hair. *Sex maturity rating 2:* straight hair extends along the labia and, between rating 2 and 3, begins on the pubis. *Sex maturity rating 3:* Pubic hair increased in quantity, darker, and present in the typical female triangle but in smaller quantity. *Sex maturity rating 4:* pubic hair more dense, curled, and adult in distribution but less abundant. *Sex maturity rating 5:* abundant, adult-type pattern; hair may extend onto the medial part of the thighs. (Adapted from Tanner, J. M. [1962]. *Growth at adolescence* [2nd ed.]. Oxford: Blackwell.)

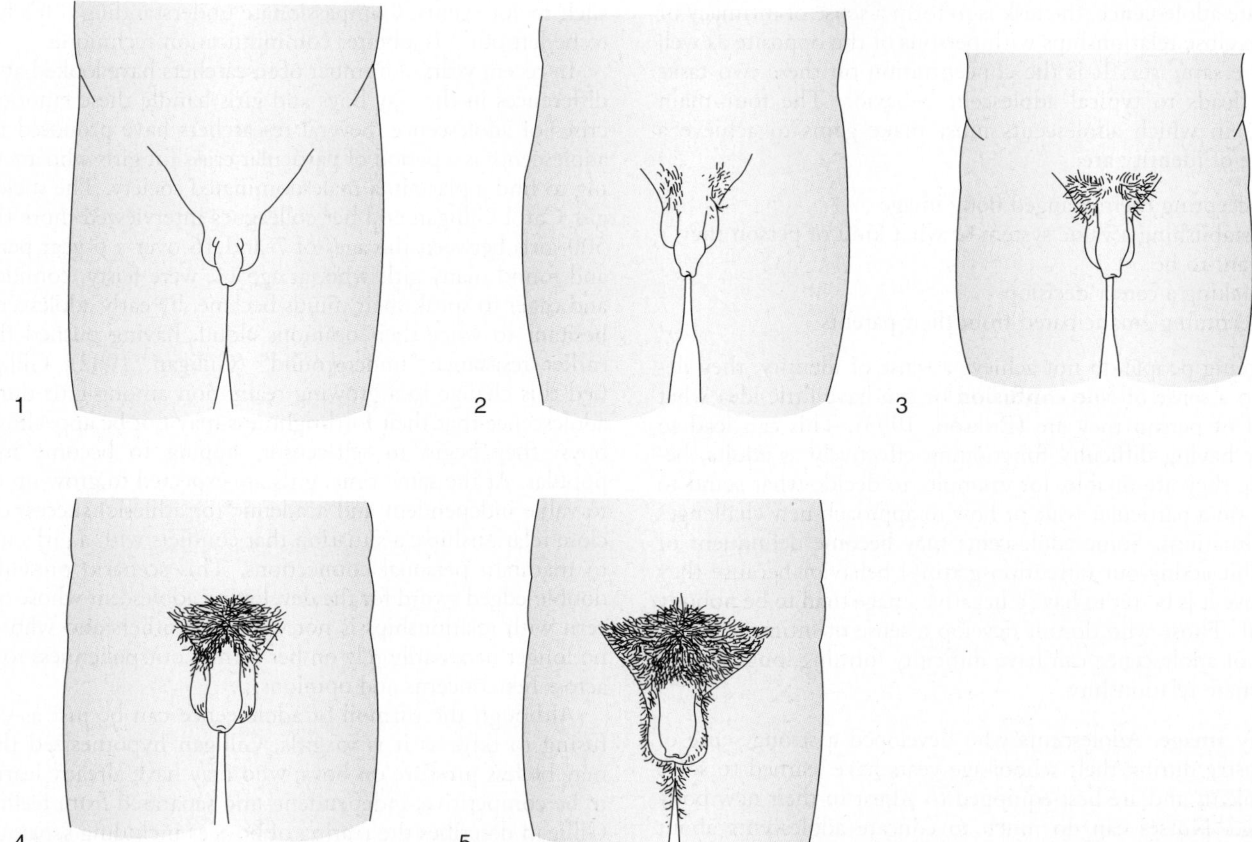

FIGURE 33.2 Male genital and pubic hair development. Ratings for pubic hair and for genital development can differ in a typical boy at any given time, since pubic hair and genitalia do not necessarily develop at the same rate. *Sex maturity rating 1:* prepubertal; no pubic hair; genitalia unchanged from early childhood. *Sex maturity rating 2;* light, downy hair develops laterally and later becomes dark; penis and testes may be slightly larger; scrotum becoming more textured. *Sex maturity rating 3:* pubic hair has extended across the pubis, testes and scrotum are further enlarged; penis is larger, especially in length. *Sex maturity rating 4:* more abundant pubic hair with curling; genitalia resemble those of an adult; glans has become larger and broader, scrotum is darker. *Sex maturity rating 5:* adult quantity and pattern of pubic hair, with hair present along inner borders of thighs; testes and scrotum are adult in size. (Adapted from Tanner, J. M. [1962]. *Growth at adolescence* [2nd ed.]. Oxford: Blackwell.)

Most adolescents spend a great deal of time just talking with peers as social interaction. Some parents disapprove of the number of hours spent in this activity, afraid their children are wasting important time, or at least exchanging a great deal of trivial conversation. For an adolescent, however, talking is no more a waste of time than was imaginative play as a preschooler. It is a major way to learn about the world.

Fifteen-year-old children may spend a great deal of time in their room or, if they do not have a room of their own, in a quiet corner of the home away from traffic and conversation areas. If they cannot find privacy somewhere in the house, they tend to spend time elsewhere.

Beginning at age 16, most adolescents want part-time jobs to earn money. Such jobs can teach young people how to work with others, accept responsibility, and spend money wisely.

When families were larger, each older child had responsibility for a younger sibling and baby care was a natural activity. With small nuclear families, many adolescents have never had the responsibility of caring for anyone younger than themselves. For their own sake and that of the children they will care for, adolescents who plan to babysit should learn some basic rules of child care and safety. Many schools or Red Cross organizations offer courses in babysitting just for the teenager.

Many adolescents engage in charitable endeavors during middle to late adolescence. They learn they are strong and capable enough not only to take care of themselves but also to help less fortunate people in their community. Adolescents do well organizing and supervising swimming or gym programs for physically challenged children, cooking and delivering food to older shut-ins, or raising money to purchase equipment for a hospital. High school clubs may be organized to send money to children overseas. These activities fulfill an adolescent's need for satisfying interaction with others and are indications of maturity and willingness to accept adult roles.

Emotional Development

Developmental Task: Identity Versus Role Confusion

According to Erikson (1993), the developmental task in early and mid-adolescence is to form a sense of **identity** or decide who they are and what kind of person they will be.

In late adolescence, the task is to form a sense of intimacy or form close relationships with persons of the opposite as well as the same sex. It is the concentration on these two tasks that leads to typical adolescent behavior. The four main areas in which adolescents must make gains to achieve a sense of identity are:

1. Accepting their changed body image
2. Establishing a value system or what kind of person they want to be
3. Making a career decision
4. Becoming emancipated from their parents

If young people do not achieve a sense of identity, they develop a sense of **role confusion** or can have little idea what kind of person they are (Erikson, 1993). This can lead to their having difficulty functioning effectively as adults, because they are unable, for example, to decide what stand to take on a particular issue or how to approach new challenges or situations. Some adolescents may become delinquent or exhibit acting-out (attention-getting) behavior because they believe it is better to have a negative image than to be nobody at all. Those who do not develop a sense of intimacy at the end of adolescence can have difficulty forming long-term or intimate relationships.

Body Image. Adolescents who developed a strong sense of industry during their school-age years have learned to solve problems and are best equipped to adjust to their new body image. Nurses can do much to educate adolescents about their bodies and help them to accept the changes that mark maturity. Some adolescents, for example, are disappointed with their final height; they had hoped to be 6 ft tall and are only 5 ft 6 in tall. In other instances, they have seen themselves as "ugly ducklings" and dreamed they would emerge as beautiful swans. They are depressed to find, at the end of adolescence, they still look much like ducks.

Adolescents are usually their own worst critics, never pleased with any aspect of their bodies. Those with low self-esteem may need parental or health care provider support to understand that a person's worth is based on more than physical appearance. They may need help to realize the characteristics that make someone creative, compassionate, and fun to be with are the qualities on which lasting relationships are built.

Self-Esteem. Like body image, self-esteem may undergo major changes during the adolescent years and can be challenged by *all* the changes that occur during adolescence, including:

- Changes in one's body and physiologic functioning
- Changes in feelings and emotional focus
- Changes in social relationships (including relationships with both family and friends)
- Changes in family and school expectations

All of these factors can have an effect on adolescents' feelings about themselves, sometimes resulting in crisis.

Help parents understand how important it is for adolescents to have immediate successes such as making the high school basketball team or having a date for the senior prom. Parental comments, such as "When you're older, these things won't be so important," are not likely to erase the hurt that comes from being 16 years old and not being included in such major events. Compassionate understanding ("It's hard to be left out") is a better communication technique.

In recent years, a number of researchers have looked at the differences in the way boys and girls handle these emotional crises of adolescence. Several researchers have proposed that adolescence is a period of particular crisis for girls who are trying to find a place in a male-dominated society. The sociologist Carol Gilligan and her colleagues interviewed more than 500 girls between the ages of 7 and 16 over a 5-year period and found many girls who, at age 11, were feisty, confident, and eager to speak their minds became, by early adolescence, hesitant to voice their opinions aloud, having pushed their earlier resistance "underground" (Gilligan, 1982). Gilligan tied this change to a growing realization among girls during adolescence that their forthrightness may not be appealing to boys; they begin to self-censor, hoping to become more popular. At the same time, girls are expected to grow up and to value independent and academic (or athletic) success over close relationships, a situation that conflicts with a girl's need to maintain personal connections. This scenario presents a double-edged sword for the developing adolescent whose concern with relationships is not valued by others and who can no longer necessarily rely on her former outspokenness to get across her concerns and opinions.

Although the turmoil of adolescence can be just as confusing to boys as it is to girls, Gilligan hypothesized there may be less pressure on boys, who may have already learned to be competitive, independent, and separated from feelings. Gilligan describes the rearing of boys as including separation from emotions and feelings at an earlier age, whereas girls are encouraged to maintain their concern for people throughout their childhood. This makes girls at risk for more conflicting feelings throughout adolescence.

Parents can help adolescent girls deal with these conflicts by encouraging them to maintain their honesty and forthrightness. According to Gilligan, however, this option puts adolescents at risk for criticism from other adults. The cost of going underground, by repressing one's views and feelings, may, however, be higher. Long-term psychological problems, notably eating disorders, which by some statistics are said to affect as many as one in five women in the United States, may be one unfortunate result of such repression.

Value System. Adolescents develop values through talking to peers. They also need an attentive adult ear, someone who will listen to their fears, hopes, dreams, and the pressure they feel to be somebody, the pressure of wanting to do something and yet not knowing what or how.

In early adolescence, girls tend to band together with girls and boys with boys. They dress identically with other members of their group: jeans and sweatshirts, special jackets, or whatever the fashion may be. On the surface, this makes adolescents appear to be losing their identities rather than finding them (Fig. 33.3). Adolescents who are different for any reason such as overweight or from a different socioeconomic, racial, or cultural background often are excluded from groups in the same way they were from clubs as 9-year-olds. This behavior may seem immature, but, like banding together, it is a necessary way for adolescents to establish a sense of identity. They know they are like the rest of the group because they dress, talk, and think the same way and go to the same places. They know they are not like the excluded member. Knowing who they are *not* is one step in discovering who

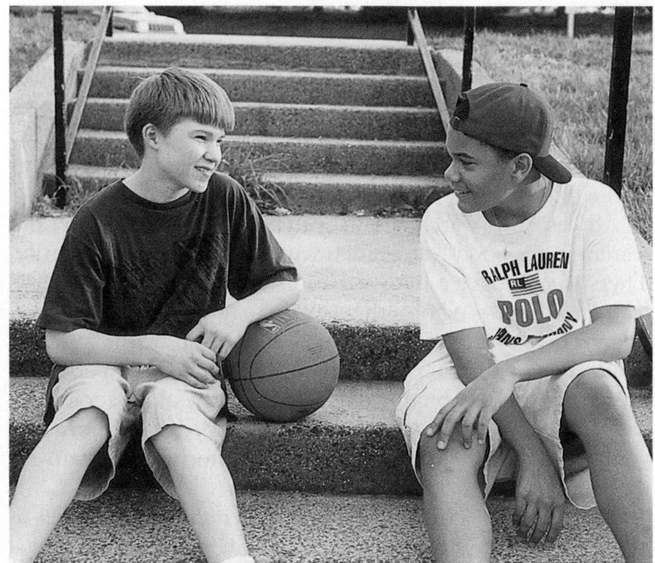

FIGURE 33.3 Adolescents have a need to interact with peers to learn more about themselves and others.

they are. Helping adolescents to appreciate that it is not fair to exclude others on the basis of superficial characteristics helps them move more quickly through this stage.

Some parents may be concerned about an early adolescent's lack of interest in the opposite sex. Occasionally, they worry about an intensely close girl–girl or boy–boy relationship. You can assure parents that adolescents must feel secure and pleased with their own sex before they can relate comfortably to the opposite sex.

Career Decisions. Part of the feeling of knowing what kind of person you are is knowing what kind of occupation will be a fit. Because of the thousands of opportunities available today, making a career decision becomes more and more difficult.

Many adolescents are encouraged to wait until they have been in college for 2 years before choosing a major. This delay may be an advantage because of the wide range of available options. It delays settling on a concrete goal until about 20 years of age, however, and therefore puts off a choice that strengthens an adolescent's sense of identity. Some school-age children do poorly in school during preadolescence but, as adolescents, show increased interest in learning as they select a job field and come to see education as relevant to their future.

Emancipation From Parents. Emancipation from parents can become a major issue during the middle and late adolescent years for two reasons. Some parents may not yet be ready for their child to be totally independent, and some adolescents may not yet be sure they want to be on their own. They may fight bitterly for a right—for example, to stay out until midnight or later on a weekend—then never use the privilege once they have gained it. Winning the battle was more important than exercising the newly won right.

In some instances, the closer the tie adolescents feel with their parents, the more severe can be their struggle. Because they love and feel loved, severing bonds is difficult. As long as parents are reasonable in their restrictions, the amount of noise being made may be proof the ties are strong and separation or emancipation is not easy.

Encourage parents to give adolescents more freedom such as allowing them to buy their own clothes, use their own judgment about allotting time for studying, choose their friends, join clubs, or choose afterschool activities; at the same time, help parents continue to place some restrictions on adolescent behavior ("You must drive the car safely or you can't use it," "You must continue to take responsibility for household chores," "We must know where you go after school"). These are not unreasonable rules and actually help adolescents accept the responsibility that must come with independence.

Help parents also make emancipation a gradual reeling-out process. Some parents err on one side or the other, either by neglecting to let out the line at all until adolescents, feeling trapped, have no other choice but to break free and swim away; or letting it all out at once, leaving adolescents to flounder because they cannot yet swim effectively on their own.

In some instances, friction and misunderstandings arise because parents had such traumatic experiences as adolescents themselves that they fear seeing their children reach this stage. Their own experiences may cause them to react so strongly that they are unable to discuss anything with their children. This makes adolescents feel they have offended their parents in some way. They do not understand that the parental attitudes are based not on anything they may have done, but on old, unresolved conflicts being brought to the surface. In other instances, parents may view adolescent growth as threatening. Seeing their adolescent grow up may make them feel old or, if a marriage is not strong, fear that once their child becomes independent their marriage may dissolve. They may strive to keep their child immature (producing conflict) in an effort to keep these thoughts from entering the corners of their minds.

Both parents and adolescents may need help to understand that emancipation does not mean severance but a change in a relationship. People who are independent of one another can have even better relationships than those who are dependent on one another. This step is actually no different from the one children accomplished when they grew from infants to toddlers, when they changed from wanting to be held and rocked to wanting to run. If parents can think of it in this light, they will gain a better perspective and may realize they will not lose their children because they become adults. There are ex-wives and ex-husbands. There are no ex-children.

By the time children are 18 years of age, they have survived leaving high school. They are in college or have found a beginning job and have begun to manage their own lives, perhaps even their own apartment. They are like swimmers who have discovered the water is not as cold as they thought it would be.

Many 18-year-olds so enjoy their new independence they find it difficult to understand why adulthood is thought to be challenging. A little more maturity will help them realize that initial success as an independent young adult does not necessarily guarantee additional success, that beginning adult life may be far easier than continuing it in the years ahead.

Sense of Intimacy. Once adolescents have achieved a sense of identity in early or mid-adolescence, they are ready to work on a second developmental task, that of achieving a sense of intimacy (Erikson, 1993). The ability to form intimate relationships is strongly correlated with the sense of trust, the first developmental task in infancy. Infants who are unable to form a sense of trust may be unable to relate to others on a deep enough level to form lasting and close relationships as adults. Conversely, adults unable to gain a sense of intimacy may be unable to foster a sense of trust in an infant.

Some adolescents require help from parents or other adults to differentiate between sound relationships and those that are based only on sexual attraction. Never do adolescents need an adult to listen to them more than when they are struggling with the heart-rending feelings of young love or wondering whether a particular love relationship is temporary or lasting. It helps to put this into perspective if parents or health care personnel who counsel adolescents remember that first love is such an intense emotion, it physically hurts.

Some parents may not be able simply to listen without interjecting their own opinions, because they worry that love between adolescents will lead to a sexual relationship. Parents should feel an obligation to inform their children of their feelings about early sexual relationships. They also should be realistically aware some adolescents will not follow their advice. Rates of teenage pregnancy and sexually transmitted diseases, including human immunodeficiency virus (HIV) infection, are high and still rising. If parents suspect their adolescent is sexually active, counsel them to be sure their child is knowledgeable about safer sex practices (see Chapter 5, Box 5.4, for guidelines regarding safer sex; see Chapter 22 for a discussion of adolescent pregnancy).

Some adolescents may believe that intense sexual yearnings or peer pressure can be alleviated only by a sexual act. They can be reassured they are pleasant people to be with because of the many fine qualities they possess and that sexual intercourse can be delayed until two persons have come to know these qualities in each other and have made a mutual commitment based on a deeper level than simply physical passion.

Intimacy involves this deeper level of relationships or developing a sense of compassion or concern for people of both sexes. It means being able to discern when words will hurt, when a companion is unhappy and needs encouragement, or when a friend is floundering and needs support.

In our busy modern society in which adolescents can engage in such a variety of activities, they may need help learning how to project themselves into another person's situation and to ask themselves how the world looks from that position. This ability, *empathy,* is feeling for another or a developed sense of intimacy in its finest form.

Socialization

Early teenagers may feel more self-doubt than self-confidence. They want to look grown up, but they still look like children. The voices of most boys have not yet dependably deepened; this makes them unable to trust their voices to carry the serious tone they wish to convey. Most girls' bodies have not yet fully developed; they may look at themselves in a mirror and compare their profiles with those of models in popular magazines and feel inadequate.

Both male and female 13-year-olds tend to be loud and boisterous, particularly when peers of the opposite sex whose attention they would like to attract are nearby. They are impulsive and very much like 2-year-old children in that they want what they want immediately, not when it is convenient for others.

Many 13-year-olds fall "in love." At this age, however, they may spend more time longing for someone than they do instituting an in-depth and rewarding relationship. They have too little experience with life, too limited a frame of reference yet to know how to offer a deep commitment to another or accept one from that person.

Fourteen-year-olds are often quieter and more introspective than they were the year before. They are becoming used to their changing bodies, have more confidence in themselves, and feel more self-esteem.

Adolescents watch adults carefully during this period, searching for good role models with whom they can identify. They usually have a hero—a film star, writer, scientist, doctor, or athlete—whom they want to grow up to be like. Fourteen-year-olds often form a friendship with an older adolescent of the same sex, trying to imitate that person in everything from thoughts to clothing. If the older adolescent has dropped out of school or plays a particular sport, the younger person may express a wish to drop out or train for that sport, too.

Idolization of famous people or older adolescents fades as adolescents become more interested in forming reciprocal friendships. Attachments to older adolescents are often severed abruptly and painfully as older teenagers make it clear they are more interested in being with people their own age. Rejection by an older member of a pair this way forces the younger member to turn to own-age friends and ends the intense hero worship so typical of early adolescence.

Most 15-year-olds fall in love five or six times a year. However, many of these relationships are based on attraction because of physical appearance, not because of inner qualities or characteristics that are necessarily compatible with their own. Because infatuation is fleeting, it can lead to extremely intense but brief attachments that fade once the two young people discover they really have little in common. Falling in love this often, however, does not mean their feelings are any less strong or they feel any less pain when the relationship ends (Fig. 33.4).

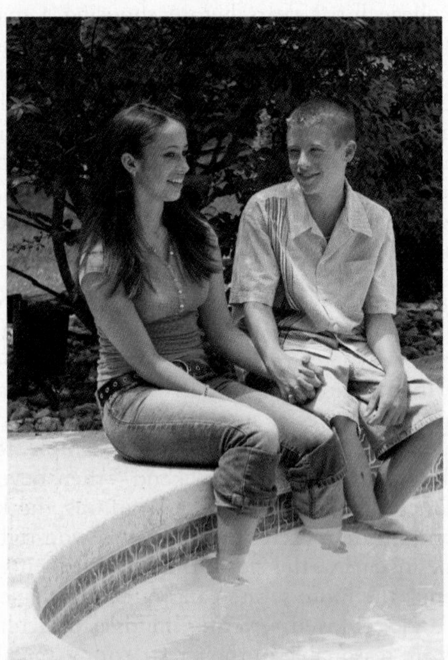

FIGURE 33.4 Although love can be fleeting, adolescents feel intensely for another.

By age 16, boys are becoming sexually mature (although they continue to grow taller until about 18 years of age). Both sexes are better able to trust their bodies than they were the year before. By age 17, they tend to be quieter and thoughtful about interactions. They have left behind the childish behaviors they used in early adolescence—shoving and punching—to get the attention of the opposite sex.

Cognitive Development

The final stage of cognitive development, the stage of **formal operational thought,** begins at age 12 or 13 years and grows in depth over the adolescent years (Piaget, 1969). This step involves the ability to think in abstract terms and use the scientific method to arrive at conclusions. The problems that adolescents are asked to solve in school depend on this type of thought such as a boy rowing upstream at 5 miles per hour against a current of 2 miles per hour will go how far in 1 hour? Problem solving in any situation depends on the ability to think abstractly and logically.

With the ability to use scientific reasoning, adolescents can plan their future. They can create a hypothesis (What if I go to college? What if I don't go to college?) and think through the probable consequences. Thinking abstractly is what allows adolescents to project themselves into the minds of others and imagine how others view them or their actions (display compassion).

Moral and Spiritual Development

Because adolescents enlarge their thought processes to include formal reasoning, they are able to respond to the question, "Why is it wrong to steal from your neighbor's house?" with "It would hurt my neighbor by requiring him to spend money to replace what I stole," rather than with the immature response of the school-age child, "The police will punish me." Some adolescents, however, may have difficulty envisioning a department store or a large corporation as capable of suffering economic loss from stealing, a concept that can contribute to the frequent practice of petty shoplifting at this age.

Almost all adolescents question the existence of God and any religious practices they have been taught (Kohlberg, 1984). This questioning is a natural part of forming a sense of identity and establishing a value system at a time in life when they draw away from their families.

✔ Checkpoint Question 33.2

Raul is entering the final stage of cognitive development. This stage is termed:

a. Formal operational thought.
b. Cognitive attainment.
c. Concrete operational thought.
d. Scientific formulating.

HEALTH PROMOTION FOR AN ADOLESCENT AND FAMILY

Because of still limited judgment, adolescents still need guidelines in reference to safety, nutrition, and daily care. These are always excellent topics for discussion at health care visits.

Promoting Adolescent Safety

Accidents, most commonly those involving motor vehicles, are the leading cause of death among adolescents. Although teenagers are at the peak of physical and sensorimotor functioning, their need to rebel against authority or to gain attention leads them to take foolish chances while driving, such as speeding or driving while intoxicated.

In the interest of an adolescent's safety and that of others, parents need to have the courage to insist on emotional maturity rather than age as the qualification for obtaining a driver's license. Because there is a worry that driver education classes lead to more teenage drivers on the road and there is little proof that they actually reduce traffic accidents, many schools no longer offer these courses (Roberts, 2009). Encourage adolescents to seek out a community-sponsored course not only to learn the techniques of safe driving but also to learn a sense of responsibility toward others. Some adolescents dismiss seat belts as childish, and they need convincing that it is only sensible to use every safety precaution available when in a motor vehicle.

Equally dangerous for adolescents are motorcycles, motorbikes, and motor scooters, which are appealing because of their low cost and convenience in parking. Both drivers and riders should wear safety helmets to prevent head injury; long pants to prevent leg burns from exhaust pipes; and full body covering to prevent abrasions in case of an accident. Advise adolescents who choose these forms of transportation to be as familiar with safety rules as automobile drivers. They need to wait to drive motorcycles or scooters until they are emotionally mature enough to use sound driving judgment.

Drowning is another chief accident of adolescence, even though it is largely preventable. Teaching all children to swim is not the only preventive measure, because some drownings occur when good swimmers go beyond their capabilities on dares or in hopes of impressing friends. Teaching water safety, such as not swimming alone or when tired, is as important as teaching the mechanics of swimming.

Other common causes of death in adolescents are homicide and suicide, related to the easy accessibility of guns to teenagers. Gang violence and the desire to protect themselves from this can add to this problem. Accidental gunshot injuries increase in early adolescence, often for the same reason that drowning increases: youngsters want to impress friends. Some teenagers play gunshot Russian roulette to prove to friends they are courageous. It is important that both water and firearm safety be taught creatively to adolescents by encouraging problem solving rather than by lecturing, because they tend to rebel against such lectures or claim that they have heard it all before.

Athletic injuries tend to increase in number during adolescence because of the vigorous level of competition that occurs in organized sports. These are often overuse injuries because of poor conditioning. Types of athletic injuries are discussed in Chapter 51. Health teaching measures to prevent accidents and athletic injuries are summarized in Box 33.2.

Promoting Nutritional Health for an Adolescent

Adolescents are experiencing so much growth they may always feel hungry (Fig. 33.5). If adolescents' eating habits are unsupervised, they tend to eat faddish or quick snack foods rather than more nutritionally sound ones because of both

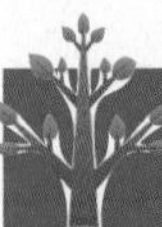

BOX 33.2 * Focus on Family Teaching

Measures to Prevent Accidents in Adolescents

Q. Raul's mother tells you, "My son doesn't always use mature judgment. How can I keep him safe from accidents?"

A. Teach the following points:

Accident	Health Teaching Measure
Motor vehicle	Use a seat belt whether as a driver or passenger. Do not drink alcohol while driving, and refuse to ride with anyone who has been drinking. Wear helmet and long trousers as driver or passenger on a motorcycle. Accepting dares has no place in safe driving. Take a driver education course to learn safe driving habits for both two-wheel and four-wheel vehicles.
Firearms	Always consider all guns loaded and potentially lethal. Learn safe gun handling before attempting to clean a gun or hunt.
Drowning	Learn how to swim. Follow safe water rules, such as never swimming alone, no diving into shallow end of swimming pools, no hyperventilating before swimming under water, no swimming beyond own limit. Taking dares has no place in water safety.
Sports	Use protective equipment, such as face masks for hockey, pads for football. Do not attempt participation beyond physical limits. Careful preparation for sports through training is essential to safety. Recognize and set own limit for sports participation.

hunger and peer pressure. Some adolescents turn away from the five pyramid food groups to eat great quantities of sweets, soft drinks, or empty-calorie snacks so they are left poorly nourished despite their large intake. One form of adolescent rebellion is to refuse to eat foods that parents stress are good for them. Parents who stock their kitchens with more nutritious foods, always keep plenty of milk and healthy snacks such as fruit and vegetables on hand, and are willing to meet their adolescents halfway in terms of food preferences such as serving pizza once a week can be more certain their child is eating nutritious foods during the day. Giving an adolescent some responsibility for food planning or meals such as making dinner every Wednesday night can teach some important lessons about nutrition without conflict.

Adolescents who are slightly obese because of prepubertal changes may begin low-calorie or starvation diets to lose excess weight. Some develop eating disorders such as bulimia or anorexia nervosa (see Chapter 54). A weight-loss diet may be appropriate during adolescence, but it must be supervised to ensure that an adolescent consumes sufficient calories and

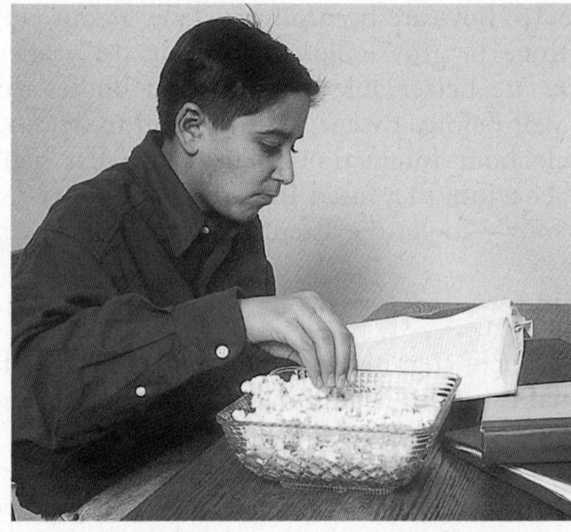

FIGURE 33.5 Adolescents experience rapid physical growth, so typically, they are always hungry. (© Billy Barnes/Stock Boston.)

nutrients for growth. For example, many adolescents omit breads and cereals entirely to lose weight rather than just reducing the amounts they consume. Diets such as these may be deficient in thiamine and riboflavin.

Recommended Dietary Reference Intakes

An adolescent needs an increased number of calories to support the rapid body growth that occurs. As shown in Appendix E, males grow more than females during this period. One of the most important things adolescents can learn is that just filling their stomachs will not provide adequate nutrition. Foods that supply the necessary carbohydrates, vitamins, protein, and minerals are essential.

The nutrients that are most apt to be deficient in both male and female adolescent diets are iron, calcium, and zinc. Large amounts of iron are necessary to meet expanding blood volume requirements. Females require a high iron intake not only because of increasing blood volume but also because iron begins to be lost with menstruation. Girls with a heavy menstrual flow (menorrhagia) may need to take an additional iron supplement to prevent iron-deficiency anemia (Selby, 2007) (see Chapter 44). Increased calcium plus physical exercise is necessary for rapid skeletal growth as well as to "stockpile" calcium to prevent osteoporosis later in life (Ondrak & Morgan, 2007). Zinc is necessary for sexual maturation and final body growth. Good sources of iron are meat and green vegetables; calcium is abundant in milk and milk products; meat and milk are also high in zinc.

Promoting Nutritional Health With a Varied Diet

Vegetarian Diets. Because vegetables generally contain fewer calories than meat, adolescents need to consume large amounts of them to achieve an adequate caloric intake with a vegetarian diet. Textured vegetable protein such as tofu or Quom can be added to meals to increase the amount of protein supplied and to help meet adolescent growth needs (Theobald, 2007). Some adolescents may find it difficult to follow a vegetarian diet because it makes them different from their peers and limits the foods they can eat at parties or at school, such as pizza, meat tortillas, or hot dogs. Whether to continue to follow this type of diet is a decision an adolescent must make as part of achieving a sense of identity. Well-balanced vegetarian diets can supply enough energy for an active athlete (Rolfes, Pinna, & Whitney, 2009). Be certain all adolescent vegetarians are following a diet and not eating only fruits and vegetables as a method to lose weight.

Glycogen Loading. Athletes need more carbohydrate or energy than do people who do not engage in strenuous activity, and the source of carbohydrate that best sustains athletes comes from the breakdown of glycogen because this supplies a slow steady release of glucose. **Glycogen loading** is a procedure used to ensure there is adequate glycogen to sustain energy through an athletic event. Several days before a sports event, athletes lower their carbohydrate intake and exercise heavily to deplete muscle glycogen stores. They then switch to a diet high in carbohydrate. With the renewed carbohydrate intake, muscle glycogen is stored at approximately twice the usual level, ready to supply twice the glucose for sustained energy. The effects of frequent glycogen loading are unknown, however, so the practice is not recommended for adolescents. As a rule, the goals of nutrition that are best for everyone, such as eating a well-balanced diet, are also the best rules for athletes, rather than diets that interfere with carbohydrate, fluid, or fat intake (Griffin, 2007).

Promoting Development of an Adolescent in Daily Activities

Maintaining adequate nutrition to support rapid adolescent growth is essential to continued healthy development, as discussed earlier. Adequate sleep, hygiene, and exercise are also important and should become an adolescent's responsibility rather than the parents'. Parents can, however, encourage adolescents to engage in healthy patterns of living—primarily through role modeling.

Dress and Hygiene

Adolescents are capable of total self-care and, because of their body awareness, may even be overly conscientious about personal hygiene and appearance. They often wash their hair every day but then grow dissatisfied because their hair has lost so much natural oil it is dull and stringy. Both sexes try many types of shampoo, deodorant, breath fresheners, and toothpaste. They may take seriously (without admitting it) the content of ads showing toothpastes or deodorants can help win an attractive person or gain instant success. Remember this when caring for hospitalized adolescents. Providing time for self-care, such as shampooing hair, is important to include in an adolescent's nursing care plan.

Adolescents are acutely aware of what their peers are wearing. When adolescents cannot trust or are disappointed in their bodies, it is very reassuring to be dressed exactly like everyone else. When they first begin to work, many adolescents spend their first paychecks entirely on clothing. This seems inappropriate to many parents; they want their child to learn to spend money on more lasting items or to show an interest in saving. Adolescents may have to mature fully, however, before they discover their real person shows through their clothing.

Remembering how important clothing is for adolescents also helps you plan care for them during a hospitalization. Most teenagers seem to improve markedly when allowed to wear their own clothing rather than a hospital gown.

Care of Teeth

Adolescents are generally very conscientious about toothbrushing because of a fear of developing bad breath. They should continue to use a fluoride paste rather than a brand advertised as providing white teeth. They should continue to drink fluoridated water to ensure firm enamel growth (Armfield & Spencer, 2007). They tend to snack a great deal, so their teeth are always exposed to bacterial erosion, and so some may develop cavities for the first time during this period. Teens with braces must be extremely conscientious about toothbrushing to prevent plaque buildup on hidden tooth surfaces.

Sleep

Although it is widely believed that everyone needs 8 hours of sleep a night, some need more and others can adjust to considerably less. Because protein synthesis occurs most readily during sleep and adolescents are building so many new cells, adolescents may need proportionately more sleep than any other age group. In addition, because this is a stress period similar to first grade, adolescents may sleep restlessly as their mind reworks the day's tensions; even long periods of sleep, therefore, may not leave them feeling refreshed (Brand et al., 2007).

Many adolescents attempt to get by with too little sleep, because they are constantly busy and because staying up late is a symbol of the adult status they long for. Frequent lack of sleep can lead to chronic fatigue or depression, however. This is why adolescents, admitted to a hospital for even a minor illness, may sleep as if exhausted as they make up for a chronic lack of sleep.

Exercise

Just as with younger children, adolescents need exercise every day both to maintain muscle tone and to provide an outlet for tension. Unlike younger children, although they are constantly on the go, adolescents often receive little real exercise. They ride a bus to school, sit for classes, sit at a mall after school and talk to friends, sit and watch a basketball game in the evening. They have put in a full day from 7 in the morning until 11 at night, yet they have had little exercise compared with the amount they used to get when they came home from school and played tag or hide-and-seek for several hours before dinner. Because of this, adolescents who have had an injury and must learn an activity such as crutch walking need to do muscle-strengthening exercises at first, just as adults must.

Adolescents who are involved in structured athletic activities do receive daily exercise. If they have not participated in competitive sports before, however, they may need advice on increasing exercise gradually so they do not overdo and consequently develop muscle sprains or other overuse injuries.

Promoting Healthy Family Functioning

Early adolescents may have many disagreements with parents that stem partly from wanting more independence and partly from being so disappointed in their bodies. It is frustrating for children to be told by parents they are too old to behave in a certain manner when they still do not feel or look older. At other times, just when they begin to accept their maturing appearance, parents tell them they are too young to do something. It may be helpful to counsel parents to appreciate that although it is not easy to live with a teenager, it is equally difficult to be the teenager.

When a child reaches about age 15, parent–child friction tends to peak. By this age, adolescents have discovered from careful observation that most adults are far from perfect. Teachers they previously thought of as all-knowing are revealed to have very human shortcomings: they are not able to answer every question asked; some may make it clear they do not have the time or interest for questions. Even a favorite coach may be discovered to be imperfect. School marks may slump as a reflection of this "fallen angel" syndrome.

Adolescents find even more fault in their parents and wonder how they can exist with their outdated ideas. They have trouble respecting parents who are so obviously imperfect. These adolescents may follow health advice poorly because they view health care personnel in the same light.

By the time they are 16 years old, adolescents generally become more willing to listen and to talk about problems. As a result, they may learn that adults are not as inadequate as they previously thought. Their parents, for example, may not be exactly the kind of persons these adolescents might wish they were, but, generally, 16-year-old children can understand adults are only human. This changed perception does not mean an adolescent of 16 is calm and quiet, free of parent–child discord. Adolescents may comprehend how hard it was for parents to get where they are, but they may not understand, for example, why they themselves are not allowed to stay out beyond midnight on weekends.

Seventeen-year-old adolescents who have stayed in school are usually high school seniors; for most of them, this year is likely to be stormy. Looking ahead to leaving a school system with which they have been involved since they were very young may give some 17-year-old adolescents a feeling of losing security. Even if going away to college or beginning a full-time job seems exciting, it can also be an unwelcome change from the people and routines they feel so comfortable with to new contacts and new regulations that appear strange and even hostile.

The ambivalence that such feelings create makes 17-year-olds difficult to understand. They like to see parents perpetuating family traditions: a vacation in an old familiar place, the house decorated for a holiday in the same way, or the traditional birthday meal. Parents should appreciate that clinging to security this way is not the step backward it may seem. Instead, this behavior may be the preliminary working through to a time of separation that will be a major milestone in growing up.

Unfortunately, to prove they are old enough to leave high school and to enter into a more mature college or work world, adolescents this age may begin to experiment with drugs or alcohol, interpreting their use as the mark of being an adult.

Common Health Problems of an Adolescent

A health maintenance schedule for the adolescent period and the assessments to be included at visits are shown in Table 33.2.

Hypertension

Hypertension is present if blood pressure is above the 95th percentile, or 127/81 mm Hg for 16-year-old girls and 131/81 for 16-year-old boys for two consecutive readings in different settings (see Appendix G). Adolescents who are obese, who are African American, who eat a diet high in salt, or who have a family history of hypertension are those most susceptible to developing this disease. Prevention and management of hypertension are discussed in Chapter 41. All children over 3 years of age should have their blood pressure taken routinely at health assessments to detect this (AAP, 2009). This is particularly true for adolescents as new medication plus education in risk factors makes treatment at this age successful (Seikaly, 2007).

Poor Posture

Many adolescents demonstrate poor posture, a tendency to round shoulders, and a shambling, slouchy walk. This is due in part to the imbalance of growth that arises from the skeletal system growing a little more rapidly than the muscles attached to it. Poor posture particularly seems to develop in adolescents who reach adult height before their peers. They slouch to appear no taller than anyone around them. Girls, especially, may slouch so as not to appear taller than boys in the belief that boys only like girls shorter than themselves. Girls may also slouch to diminish the appearance of their breast size if they are developing more rapidly than their friends. This also can occur from carrying backpacks that are too heavy (Moore, White, & Moore, 2007).

Urge children of both sexes to use good posture during these rapid-growth years. Tall adolescents of both sexes are generally picked out by basketball or track coaches and so may have the incentive, if properly guided, to maintain good posture. Assess posture at all adolescent health appraisals to detect the difference between simple poor posture and the beginning of scoliosis (lateral curvature of the spine; see Chapters 34 and 51).

Body Piercing and Tattoos

Body piercing and tattoos are a strong mark of adolescence (Armstrong, 2007). Both sexes have ears, lips, chins, navels, and breasts pierced and filled with studs, or tattoos applied to arms, legs, or their central body. These acts have become a way for adolescents to make a statement that they are different from their parents. Be certain they know the symptoms of infection at a piercing or tattoo site (redness, warmness, drainage, swelling, mild pain) and to report these to a health care provider if they occur as serious staphylococcal or streptococcal infections can occur at piercing sites. Caution adolescents that sharing needles for piercing or tattooing carries the same risk as sharing needles for intravenous drug use.

Fatigue

So many adolescents comment they feel fatigued to some degree that this can be considered normal for the age group. Because fatigue may be a beginning symptom of disease, however, it is important it be investigated as a legitimate concern and not underestimated. Assess an adolescent's diet, sleep patterns, and activity schedules, because all can contribute greatly to fatigue. Note when the fatigue began. A short period of extreme tiredness is more likely to suggest disease than a long, ill-defined report of always feeling tired.

If an adolescent's sleep and diet appear to be adequate, the activity schedule is reasonable (in an attempt to be popular, some adolescents take on a schedule that would exhaust three

TABLE 33.2 ✻ Health Maintenance Schedule, Adolescent Period

Area of Focus	Methods	Frequency
Assessment		
Developmental milestones	History, observation	Every visit
Growth milestones	Height, weight plotted on standard growth chart; physical examination	Every visit
Hypertension	Blood pressure	Every visit
Nutrition	History, observation; height/weight information	Every visit
Hypercholesterolemia	Total cholesterol and triglycerides	During adolescence for children with family members with the disorder
Parent–child relationship	History, observation	Every visit
Behavior or school problems	History, observation	Every visit
Vision and hearing disorders	History, observation	Every visit
	Formal Snellen or Titmus testing	At 15 and 18 years
	Audiometer testing	At 15 and 18 years
Dental health	History, physical examination	Every visit
Scoliosis	Physical examination	Every visit to 16 years
Thyroid disease	Physical examination, history	Every visit
Tuberculosis	PPD test	Depending on prevalence of tuberculosis in community
Bacteriuria	Dipstick	Annually if sexually active
Anemia	Hematocrit or hemoglobin	Annually for menstruating females
Cervical or vaginal cancer	Pap test, pelvic examination	Every 1 to 3 years for sexually active females
Sexually transmitted diseases	History, observation	Every visit if sexually active
Immunizations		
Hepatitis A vaccine	Check history and past records; inform caregiver about any risks and side effects; administer vaccine in accordance with health care agency policies	If not previously immunized
Hepatitis B vaccine		If not previously immunized
Human papillomavirus vaccine (HPV; Gardasil)		Females if not previously vaccinated
Influenza vaccine		Yearly
Measles, mumps, and rubella vaccine		If not previously vaccinated; not to pregnant adolescents.
Meningococcal vaccine		If not previously vaccinated
Pneumococcal vaccine		To high-risk groups if not previously vaccinated
Tetanus and diphtheria vaccine (Tdap)		If 5 years since last booster
Varicella vaccine		If not previously vaccinated
Anticipatory Guidance		
Adolescent care including violence and nutrition counseling	Active listening and health teaching	Every visit
Expected growth and developmental milestones before next visit	Active listening and health teaching	Every visit
Injury prevention	Counseling about street and personal safety	Every visit
Problem Solving		
Any problems expressed by caregiver or adolescent during visit	Active listening and health teaching regarding cigarette smoking, drug abuse, school adjustment	Every visit

Source: American Academy of Pediatrics. (2009). *Recommendations for preventive pediatric health care*. Washington, DC: Author.

people), and physical assessment suggests no illness, then the fatigue may be of emotional origin. It can be a means of avoiding school, avoiding conflict with parents (when children appear ill, parents are more sympathetic), or avoiding social situations. Those who are understimulated by school may develop fatigue as a sign of boredom.

Blood tests may be indicated to rule out anemia and the infection that is so common in adolescents—infectious mononucleosis (see Chapter 43). Chronic fatigue syndrome may need to also be ruled out (Knoop et al., 2008). If it is determined that teenagers do not have these conditions, they can be assured they are healthy and offered guidance to solve the problem with better diet, more sleep, fewer activities, and development of better problem-solving techniques to relieve tensions.

Menstrual Irregularities

Menstrual irregularities can be a major health concern of adolescent girls as they learn to adjust to their individual body cycles. Chapter 47 discusses these problems in detail.

Acne

Acne is a self-limiting inflammatory disease that involves the sebaceous glands that empty into hair shafts (the pilosebaceous unit). It is the most common skin disorder of adolescence, occurring in as many as 80% to 95% of adolescents (Knox, 2008). It occurs slightly more frequently in boys than in girls. The peak age for the lesions to occur in girls is 14 to 17 years; for boys, 16 to 19 years. Although not proved, genetic factors may play a part in their development. Cigarette smoking may also increase the number of inflammatory lesions.

Before the rapid increase in androgen secretion occurs with puberty, the sebaceous glands that enter into hair follicles are small and relatively inactive, so acne is nonexistent. Changes associated with puberty cause acne to develop:

- As androgen levels rise in both sexes, sebaceous glands become active.
- Abnormal keratinization (cell growth) of the lining of the ducts occurs; this overgrowth obstructs the ducts.
- The output of sebum increases. Sebum is largely composed of lipids, mainly triglycerides.
- If all of the material formed cannot be eliminated to the skin surface because of the narrow gland ducts, the glands enlarge, and trapped sebum causes whiteheads, or closed **comedones.**
- As trapped sebum darkens from accumulation of melanin and oxidation of the fatty acid component on exposure to air, blackheads, or open comedones, form.
- Bacteria (generally, *Propionibacterium acnes*) lodge and thrive in the retained secretions, forming papules.
- Leakage of free fatty acid causes a dermal inflammatory reaction.
- If glands rupture, sebum is extruded into adjacent skin, which produces reddened inflammatory cysts.

Acne is categorized as mild (comedones are present), moderate (papules and pustules are also present), or severe (cysts are present). The most common locations of acne lesions are the face, neck, back, upper arms, and chest (Fig. 33.6). Flare-ups are associated with emotional stress, menstrual periods, or the use of greasy hair creams or makeup that can further plug gland ducts. Lesions are less noticeable in summer months, probably because of increased exposure to the sun, which increases epidermic peeling, or the reduction in stress as a result of being out of school.

Assessment. Always ask adolescents at health assessments if they are troubled with acne and to what extent it interferes with their self-image as this can be a major cause of stress in adolescents (Reich et al., 2007). Inspect for facial, chest, and back lesions on physical examination.

Therapeutic Management. The goal of therapy for acne is threefold: (a) decrease sebum formation, (b) prevent comedones, and (c) control bacterial proliferation.

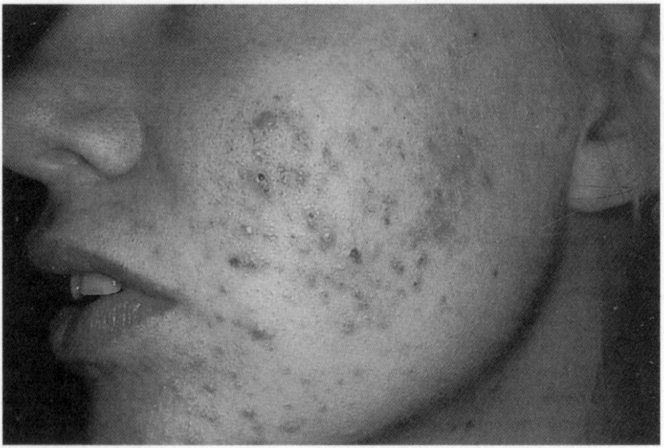

FIGURE 33.6 Facial acne in an adolescent.

External Medication. Medications that are applied externally peel away the superficial skin layer to prevent sebum plugs from forming and are sufficient if only comedones are present. The most frequently used over-the-counter medications contain benzoyl peroxide. A common prescription medication is tretinoin (Retin-A cream). This reduces keratin formation and plugging of ducts. Caution adolescents using a vitamin A cream to avoid prolonged sun exposure or to use a sunblock of SPF 15 or higher, because the preparation makes their skin more susceptible than usual to ultraviolet rays. Caution adolescents also that, for the first week or two of therapy, peeling or oxidizing may make the complexion actually appear worse rather than better. Topical antibiotic creams such as erythromycin and clindamycin may be prescribed to reduce the bacterial level on skin, but usually only after oxidizing agents have not succeeded; these creams may sensitize adolescents unnecessarily to antibiotics (Karch, 2009).

Systemic Medication. Isotretinoin (Accutane), a form of vitamin A, is an extremely effective oral drug for reducing sebum production and abnormal keratinization of gland ducts; it is prescribed for cystic acne (Box 33.3).

In pustular and cystic acne, systemic (oral) antibiotics are also helpful. Tetracycline (500 mg twice daily the first week, then tapered to 250 mg daily for maintenance) is effective against the anaerobic bacteria that break down sebum to form irritating acids. Improvement is not generally seen for 2 weeks, so you may need to support adolescents to continue to take the medication during the waiting period. Without noticeable improvement, adolescents have a tendency to continue taking the higher dose or even increase the dose, hoping to initiate a faster effect. Tetracycline is not prescribed for children under age 12, because it can cause permanent staining of teeth and possibly interfere with growth of long bones. Likewise, tetracycline should not be given to females who may be pregnant, because it causes faulty bone growth in a fetus (Karch, 2009). Because tetracycline may interfere with oral contraceptives, adolescent girls should use another method of birth control while taking the antibiotic.

Food impairs the absorption of tetracycline so the drug should be taken on an empty stomach (2 hours before or after eating). Adolescents must be certain of the date of expiration of the drug; outdated tetracycline breaks down into an

BOX 33.3 ✻ Focus on Pharmacology

Isotretinoin (Accutane)

Classification Isotretinoin is a vitamin A metabolite.
Action: Reduces sebum secretion
Pregnancy Risk Category: X
Dosage: 0.5–2 mg/kg PO per day for 15 to 20 weeks
Possible adverse effects: Nausea, vomiting, dry skin, pruritus, fatigue, headache, epistaxis, dry nose, dry mouth, eye irritation, elevated sedimentation rate, hypertriglyceridemia, proteinuria, hematuria (Karch, 2009)

Nursing Implications

- Drug may be associated with an increased risk of suicide.
- Drug is highly teratogenic (destructive to fetal growth). Girls should have a pregnancy test before treatment and before prescription renewal to be certain they are not pregnant. Suggest girls use a form of birth control to prevent pregnancy while on the drug and for 1 month afterward.
- Serum levels of both triglycerides and cholesterol and liver function studies should be obtained, both baseline and monitoring, because both triglycerides and cholesterol serum are raised by the drug.
- Drug is extremely drying to skin; caution adolescents to discontinue all other acne medications during therapy to reduce this effect.
- Caution adolescents to continue to avoid sunlight or use a sunblock. If eyes become too dry, patient may need to discontinue the use of contact lenses.
- Advise adolescents to take drug with meals, to avoid gastric irritation.
- Adolescents with severe headache or visual disturbances should report these symptoms, and the medication should be discontinued.
- Advise adolescents not to donate blood while taking the drug, because of potential damage to the fetus of a recipient.

extremely toxic composition. Females taking systemic antibiotics for long periods of time become susceptible to developing candidal vaginitis and need to be instructed about the symptoms of this: a white, pruritic vaginal discharge. Alternative antibiotics prescribed are erythromycin, minocycline, or clindamycin. Although these drugs avoid the complications of tetracycline, they may not produce the same effective results.

Other Treatment Methods. If inflammatory reactions from acne are extreme, a corticosteroid such as prednisone or a nonsteroidal anti-inflammatory drug (NSAID) may be prescribed. Steroids must be used with caution in growing adolescents, because they can lead to stunted growth. Cortisone may be injected directly into cystic lesions to reduce inflammation. This type of injection may reduce keloid formation, which is why it is usually reserved for adolescents who are prone to this permanent form of scarring.

Estrogen, alone or in combination with progesterone, suppresses sebaceous gland activity and is therefore useful therapy in some girls. However, isotretinoin is more often prescribed instead of estrogen for two reasons: (a) high estrogen levels tend to close epiphyseal centers of long bones, causing bone growth to stop; and (b) long-term therapy does have potential side effects, including embolism and thrombophlebitis and possibly breast and uterine cancer.

Some degree of scarring may result from acne lesions. Laser therapy is a follow-up possibility to reduce the effect of scarring.

Nursing Diagnoses and Related Interventions

✻

Nursing Diagnosis: Risk for low self-esteem related to development of acne during adolescence and lack of knowledge regarding treatment possibilities

Outcome Evaluation: Adolescent verbalizes positive aspects of self; states acne does not affect self-image; or, if client admits to feelings of negative self-esteem, is able to discuss feelings and concerns about condition; describes ways to prevent or reduce acne outbreaks and states realistic short- and long-term goals of treatment.

It is important to respect how devastating acne can be to an adolescent. The actual extent of the condition often is not as important as an adolescent's feelings about it. With a face constantly covered by red marks, it is extremely difficult for adolescents to feel good about themselves (see Focus on Nursing Care Planning Box 33.4).

When carrying out interventions, remember that acne is a potentially destructive disease; if left untreated, it can cause irreparable physical and emotional scarring. Therefore, advise parents and adolescents to seek medical treatment rather than self-medicate if the condition is severe. At the same time, overconcern may lead to undue self-consciousness that affects performance in school and establishment of social relationships. Common health teaching measures for the prevention and treatment of acne are summarized in Box 33.5.

Obesity

Most overweight adolescents have obese parents, suggesting that both inheritance and environment play a part in the development of adolescent obesity. It can be difficult for adolescents to learn to like themselves (achieve a sense of identity) if they do not like their reflection in a mirror. It is equally difficult if they are always excluded from groups because of their weight. This has led to the suicide rate for obese adolescents being higher than for non-obese adolescents (Whetstone, Morrissey, & Cummings, 2007). Some adolescents may be unaware their food intake is excessive, because they have been told they need excess nutrients for healthy adolescent growth and everyone in their family eats large portions. They may state that their friends are

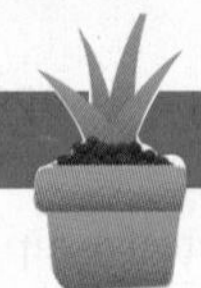

BOX 33.4 ✻ Focus on Nursing Care Planning

A Multidisciplinary Care Map for an Adolescent With Acne

Raul is a 15-year-old boy you see at an adolescent clinic. His chief concern is a head cold. He has numerous acne lesions on his forehead and cheeks. His parents tell you Raul seemed depressed for a long time after his girlfriend broke up with him but now seems happy again. They are pleased to see him maturing so much that he recently gave away his collection of baseball cards to a young neighbor. You mention to Raul that a decongestant would probably make him feel better. He asks you how many pills it would take to kill someone, then jokes he was kidding.

Family Assessment ✻ Client lives with two parents and two younger siblings. Father manages a funeral parlor; mother works as a beautician for funeral parlor. Client describes finances as "all right, if you think burying people is a good way to earn money."

Client Assessment ✻ 15-year-old male with history of acne for the last 6 months. Reports washing his face approximately 5 or 6 times a day with abrasive soap and covering lesions with cocoa butter cream twice a day. He states, "Look at my skin. It's horrible! I don't eat chocolate. But no matter how much I wash it, my skin is getting worse instead of better. I dread going to school, and forget about getting my picture taken. My mom says to just wait it out." Physical examination reveals scattered pustules and comedones on forehead and face, very prominent on nose and both cheeks. Two lesions on right cheek with large erythematous base and tender to touch. Remainder of physical examination unremarkable.

Nursing Diagnosis ✻ Knowledge deficit related to cause and treatment for acne

Outcome Criteria ✻ Adolescent states causes of acne; identifies measures for prevention and treatment; demonstrates appropriate skin care measures.

Team Member Responsible	Assessment	Intervention	Rationale	Expected Outcome
		Activities of Daily Living		
Nurse/nurse practitioner	Assess adolescent's understanding of acne and its causes.	Instruct adolescent in measures to prevent and control acne, including twice-daily washing with mild soap and water; avoidance of picking or squeezing lesions; and avoidance of greasy or oily skin preparations.	Daily washing removes irritating fatty acids; excessive washing can rupture glands and exacerbate acne. Picking or squeezing lesions ruptures glands and spreads sebum. Greasy or oily skin preparations can plug gland ducts, increasing comedone formation.	Client states intent to follow recommendations to decrease acne symptoms.
		Consultations		
Physician	Evaluate if client requires a psychiatric referral for depression.	Arrange for consultation if assessment suggests client may be contemplating suicide.	Client shows typical signs of pre-suicide behavior.	Psychiatric case worker meets with client at end of clinic visit and makes recommendations.
		Procedures/Medications		
Nurse/nurse practitioner	Assess what measures client has been using to self-treat acne.	Discuss treatment options available.	Discussion provides the adolescent with information about the numerous treatment options available for acne.	Client describes full range of therapies he has been using for self-treatment.
Physician	Determine if a topical or oral medication will be best to treat acne.	Prescribe medications to reduce acne symptoms. Caution results will not be immediate.	Vitamin A preparations and antibiotics are both effective in reducing inflammation of acne.	Client states he will follow medication regimen although results will not occur instantaneously.

Nutrition				
Nurse/ nutritionist	Assess client's understanding of the effect of nutrition on acne.	Counsel client to follow a well-balanced diet.	No particular food is associated with development of acne, despite old beliefs.	Client states he understands food intake is not the major cause of acne.
Patient/Family Education				
Nurse	Assess family's communication level, overall coping techniques, and abilities.	Discuss how better communication can aid in helping adolescent cope with life changes.	Parents seem unaware they are discussing a child potentially at serious risk.	Parents discuss family communication pattern; make suggestions for better patterns.
Psychosocial/Spiritual/Emotional Needs				
Nurse	Assess how acne affects client's self esteem.	Review and reinforce with adolescent positive attributes about self.	Positive attributes provide a foundation for rebuilding self-esteem.	Client states he knows others value his friendship above his appearance.
Discharge Planning				
Nurse	Review if any additional teaching is necessary regarding acne, self-esteem, or pre-suicide behavior.	Clarify any misconceptions about acne. Review and reinforce positive attributes about self.	Misconceptions can negatively affect self-esteem. Positive attributes provide a foundation for rebuilding self-esteem.	Client agrees he will telephone if sadness increases.
Nurse/nurse practitioner	Assess if client can safely return home.	Give client hotline telephone number; instruct to use as needed.	Knowing a support source is available can be as valuable as actually contacting the source.	Client assures staff that he has the hotline number available and will call if necessary.

overweight but their own weight seems all right, even though they are considerably overweight. Health teaching with these adolescents needs to begin with a discussion of "normal" weight. If they do not begin this as adolescents, they will become obese adults.

A reducing diet of fewer than 1400 to 1600 calories per day can rarely be tolerated by adolescents. Such a diet would not provide sufficient protein and could be deficient in vitamins. If adolescents eat a diet that is too low in protein for any length of time, they can develop a faulty nitrogen balance, which can lead to seriously impaired growth. They generally can adhere to a diet closer to 1800 calories per day.

Nursing Diagnoses and Related Interventions

Nursing Diagnosis: Ineffective individual coping by overeating related to stresses of adolescent period that has led to obesity

Outcome Evaluation: Adolescent identifies stressful situations in life that lead to overeating; describes ways to avoid those situations or methods that would help coping with them.

Adolescents who are overweight because of stress need support until their pleasure in eating diminishes and their satisfaction with themselves as a "new" person or their friends' satisfaction with them can sustain them. They may need to visit a health care facility once or twice a week for encouragement and praise for their efforts. National weight-control organizations are good if other adolescents also attend the meetings. They are ineffective if all the other members are adults because adolescents generally cannot relate to adult problems. It is important that adolescent self-esteem is maintained or an adolescent may switch to binge eating or such severe dieting that the opposite—extreme weight loss—occurs.

In addition to reducing calories consumed, encourage activities that use up calories, such as swimming or participation in gym classes and other school activities (Stephens, 2008).

Adolescents could perhaps walk to school rather than ride, or walk the dog for three blocks rather than one. These activities are generally preferable to formal exercises, such as situps and push-ups, which can be viewed as punishment.

BOX 33.5 ✻ Focus on Family Teaching

Guidelines for the Prevention and Treatment of Acne

Q. Raul says to you, "I've had acne for the last 3 months. How can I make this go away?"

A. Most adolescents have some acne. Try the following suggestions:

1. Do not pick or squeeze acne lesions, which ruptures glands and spreads sebum into the skin, increasing symptoms. The times you are most likely to do this are during periods of stress, such as when you are taking a test. When you find your hand on your face, distract yourself with some other motion, such as interlocking your fingers.
2. Makeup, greasy hair preparations, or tight sweatbands can plug ducts of glands and increase comedone formation. Avoid these, if possible. Using medicated makeup both covers and helps lesions heal.
3. Topical acne preparations work by unplugging glands. You must use them consistently to make them effective. Plan enough time in the morning before school and a time in the evening to apply these. Post a chart by your bathroom mirror to remind yourself.
4. Washing daily to remove irritating fatty acids is helpful. Excessive washing is not necessary to prevent lesion formation. In fact, excessive washing can actually harm healing by rupturing glands.
5. Oral medications work by reducing sebum secretions or preventing bacterial invasion. These work only if you take them conscientiously. Make a chart to post in your bathroom or kitchen to remind yourself to take these, also. Remember that tetracycline must be taken on an empty stomach or it is not effective.
6. If you are taking oral vitamin A (Accutane), do not take another source of vitamin A in a tablet. Accutane is very harmful to fetal growth. Girls taking Accutane should take measures to prevent pregnancy while taking the drug and for 1 month afterward. If a girl does become pregnant while taking the drug, she should stop taking it immediately and notify her physician.
7. Both topical and oral vitamin A make your skin very sensitive to sunlight. Avoid long exposures to sunlight, or you will sunburn readily.
8. No acne medication works immediately. While you are waiting for lesions to heal, keep yourself occupied with a new activity (join a school club, try dancing lessons). When your skin is clear once more, these experiences will help make you an interesting person as well as one with clear skin.
9. Although diet does not influence the development of acne lesions, you should eat a healthy, well-balanced diet for good general health.

Adolescents who use overeating as their main reaction to stress may require psychological counseling rather than diet counseling if they are to develop a more mature emotional response. Behavior modification is sometimes successful with adolescents as a means of helping them lose weight, but it is rarely recommended for obesity alone. If the obesity is causing serious body image problems, lowered self-esteem, and depression, behavior modification might be suggested (see Chapter 35).

General measures to help adolescents decrease overeating include:

- Making a detailed log of the amount they eat, the time, and the circumstances (including how they felt while they were eating), and then changing those circumstances
- Always eating in one place (the kitchen table) instead of while walking home from school or watching television
- Slowing the process of eating by counting mouthfuls and putting the fork down beside the plate between bites, and being served food on small plates so helpings look larger

These measures may be of little use, however, unless they are combined with a suitable diet and adequate exercise. Despite all these interventions, weight reduction may not always be effective with adolescents. For some, a more realistic goal might be to prevent additional weight gain until they reach adulthood.

Concerns Regarding Sexuality and Sexual Activity

Because of increasing exposure to and acceptance of premarital sexual relations in society, more adolescents than ever before engage in high-risk sexual behaviors exposing them to sexually transmitted infections or conception (Fergus, Zimmerman, & Caldwell, 2007). Because of this, as part of routine health assessment of adolescents and preadolescents, ask if they are sexually active or are concerned about sexual risk behaviors (Hornor, 2007).

Adolescents are usually interested in discussing sexuality concerns with a health care provider because they are concerned they are exposing themselves to HIV infection or other sexually transmitted diseases and to pregnancy. At the same time, it is a difficult topic for them to discuss. Some adolescents may feel trapped into engaging in sex even though they are unwilling, because they perceive it as a way of having friends. For adolescents who want to have intercourse, the primary reasons given are sexual curiosity (50% of boys; 24% of girls) and affection for their partner (25% of boys; 48% of girls). For adolescents who agree to have intercourse but do not really want to, the primary reasons given are peer pressure (about 30%), curiosity (50% of boys; 25% of girls), and affection for their partner (> 33%) (Nusbaum & Katsufrakis, 2008).

Counseling can help adolescents improve their perspective and learn how to say no. In contrast, some adolescents would like to be sexually active but are not because they believe myths: early sexual relations will drain their strength and make them poor athletes; having sex too early in life will stretch the vagina and make sexual relations later on unenjoyable. Unless these falsehoods are explored through discussion, adolescents who believe them may never be comfortable with sexual relationships.

Adolescence is also the time when teenagers deal with the realization they are gay or lesbian. Although this orientation is something they have been aware of for years, actually facing it and accepting it is another step—and for many families, a difficult one (Benson et al., 2007). Offer support to adolescents who are having difficulty telling their parents about their perceived sexual orientation. To their surprise, they often discover their parents already know what they are going to say before it is voiced.

Sometimes adolescents use a mild cold or a mild acne condition as a reason to come to a health care facility, where they hope that someone will stumble onto their real concern about sexual activity. After asking adolescents at health maintenance visits if they are sexually active, ask if they have any questions or problems they want to discuss with you about this. Ask if they are interested in learning more about contraception. Be certain they are practicing safer sex measures (see Chapter 5, Box 5.4). Overall guidelines on counseling an adolescent with respect to sexual activity are summarized in Box 33.6.

Be certain to provide information on date rape and rape prevention as well when discussing sexual behaviors, because adolescents are in a high-risk age group for date rape (Yamawaki, 2007) (Box 33.7; see also Chapter 55).

BOX 33.6 * Focus on Family Teaching

Health Teaching Guidelines for Adolescents Regarding Sexuality

Q. Raul asks you, "How does a guy know when he's ready for sex?"

A. Here are a few common guidelines:

1. It is your choice whether to participate in sexual relations. Do not be influenced by friends who may be exaggerating stories to impress you or who ask you for involvement you do not want. When you say no, be firm and clear about your wishes.
2. Pregnancy can occur with *any* sexual encounter unless you use some prevention to avoid it. Be direct with a sexual partner in discussing abstinence or birth control measures.
3. Sexual relations neither add to nor detract from your physical strength or general wellness.
4. The mark of an adult sexual relationship is that the activity is pleasurable to both partners. If sexual partners are not interested in your enjoyment as well as their own, you should reconsider the relationship.
5. There is no "normal" mode of sexual expression. Any activity that is pleasurable to both partners is normal.
6. Learn about safer sex techniques. Practice them (see Box 5.4, Chapter 5).

Caution adolescents about the dangers of flunitrazepam (Rohypnol), the "date-rape drug," a colorless, odorless, and flavorless benzodiazepine drug that, if dropped into a drink, can remain undetected but cause drowsiness, impaired motor skills, and amnesia (Karch, 2009). Adolescents who are seen for sexual assault who appear intoxicated or have amnesia for the event should be suspected of unknowingly ingesting flunitrazepam. In these instances, a urine specimen analysis will reveal the drug's metabolites. If a clinic does not have the ability to do this type of test, the manufacturer of the drug (Hoffmann-LaRoche Inc.) will assess for the presence of the drug.

Stalking

Stalking refers to repetitive, intrusive, and unwanted actions directed at an individual to gain the individual's attention or evoke fear. The usual stalker is a male who stalks a female who has rejected him. Stalkers instill fear into their victims by constant and threatening pursuit. In some instances, the stalker can resort to attacking a victim and even murder if further rejected.

Stalking behavior begins as early as adolescence; either males or females can become stalkers or victims (Dietz & Martin, 2007). It is difficult to prevent stalking because no one can evaluate when they begin a relationship that it will end so badly. Stalking may take place as mainly Internet correspondence (cyberstalking), but sending unwanted e-mails or instant messages is still stalking. Measures to help avoid being stalked are the same as those for avoiding rape, such as advising adolescents not to put themselves in positions where they will be vulnerable to being alone with a stalker, and report stalking to law enforcement officers so they can obtain a restraining order to prevent the stalker from coming near them any longer.

Concerns Regarding Hazing

Hazing refers to demeaning or humiliating rituals that prospective members have to undergo to join sororities, fraternities, adolescent gangs, or sports teams (MASH, 2008). Most rituals are secret and in the past were accepted as "rites of passage." In recent years, hazing has become so extreme that the practice has moved out of the "just fun" category into activities that can cause physical and certainly psychological harm. Rituals may be as subtle as being called names, forced to wear ridiculous clothing, or engage in crude or lewd skits. Unfortunately, they also can be played to an extreme where adolescents are punched or kicked, asked to pretend to perform a sexual act towards another, sodomized, left out in the cold so long, frostbite develops, or forced to drink alcohol until they vomit or pass out or even die from alcohol intoxication. Many of the rituals found in this last category constitute criminal acts which will hold up in court if the evidence is available (Sodl et al., 2008). Initiation for street gangs can require prospective members to steal or destroy property or even kill. Parents need to be aware of what clubs or organizations their adolescent is attempting to join and what the requirements for membership will be. Health care providers can help adolescents make sound decisions about what type of hazing their organization advocates by asking teenagers about the subject at health assessments.

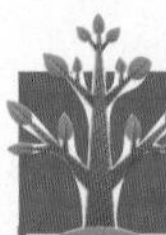

BOX 33.7 * Focus on Family Teaching

Health Teaching Guidelines for the Prevention of Rape in Adolescents

Q. Raul's sister asks you, "Are there rules for how to avoid rape?"

A. Several suggestions are:

Home

1. Do not advertise that you stay alone while a parent works or is on vacation.
2. Ask for identification from meter readers or repairmen before admitting them into the home.
3. Insist on adequate lighting for hallways in an apartment building or around your own home.
4. Have your house key in your hand when you approach your door; do not stand fumbling for it by the doorway.
5. Keep your doors and windows locked when you are alone at home.

Car

1. Avoid isolated parking places; park near a building or in a lot with a parking attendant.
2. Lock your car when waiting in it and after parking it.
3. Look in the back seat before unlocking and entering your car.
4. Have your car key ready when you approach your car; do not stand fumbling for it.

Work or School

1. Do not enter an elevator with a stranger.
2. Lock the outside door, and do not admit people you do not know when working alone at night.
3. Ask for security protection to walk out to your car after hours.
4. When going to and from school or work after dark, walk in the street rather than next to shrubs or dark buildings.

Dates

1. Be clear with your date that when you say no, you mean no.
2. Limit alcohol use, because it can lead to risk-taking behavior.
3. Make it clear that you consider date rape the same as any rape and you will press charges.
4. Rohypnol is a sedative, known as a "date rape" drug. Do not date any individual who brags that he knows how to obtain it or use it.

Personal Actions

1. Do not wear chains around your neck that could be used to strangle you.
2. Learn self-defense; scratch the attacker to obtain skin and blood specimens under fingernails.
3. Be aware that an attacker could take any weapon away and use it on you; use caution carrying a weapon or Mace.
4. Fight or struggle cautiously to prevent harm to you beyond the rape itself. Actions such as kicking or gouging eyes may not be effective and may cause more violence.
5. If an attack occurs, observe the attacker's appearance as carefully as possible. Note identifying characteristics, such as a birthmark, scar, tattoo, words, or manner of speech, to be able to identify the individual later.
6. Press charges in court to make rape a crime of extreme magnitude and as an opportunity to fight back.
7. Work to provide rape prevention information and a united front against rape in your community.

Concerns Regarding Substance Abuse

Substance abuse refers to the use of chemicals to improve a mental state or induce euphoria. This is so common among adolescents that as many as 50% of high school seniors report having experimented with some form of drug (CDC, 2008a). Drug use occurs in adolescence from a desire to expand consciousness or to feel more confident and mature; it also can be a response to peer pressure or a form of adolescent rebellion (Box 33.8). This type of rebellion is more emotionally charged than acts such as staying out late or wearing clothing other than those approved by parents, because it is not only harmful but also illegal. Usual stages of substance abuse are shown in Table 33.3.

Types of Abused Substances

Drugs that adolescents abuse are those they can obtain on limited budgets and through limited contacts.

Prescription and Over-the-Counter Drugs. Adolescents may begin drug experimentation by taking sedatives, pain medication, or cough syrup containing dextromethorphan, abbreviated DXM, prescribed for another family member or a pet. A small amount of DXM causes lightheadedness. In larger doses, it can resort in distortions of color and sound, visual hallucinations, or "out-of-body" experiences. This is called "pharming"; unaware of usual dosages, adolescents who use drugs this way can easily overdose (Levine et al., 2007). Methylphenidate (Ritalin) is a drug frequently prescribed for attention-deficit/hyperactivity disorder. When oral Ritalin tablets are crushed and injected intravenously, they offer a feeling of giddiness and extreme well-being. Unfortunately, because they do not completely dissolve, the resultant small particles remaining in the bloodstream can result in pulmonary embolus or emphysema. Ketamine is an anesthetic used in veterinary medicine that is also frequently abused. Every house has a number of inhalants, such as a spray-type oil for cooking or gas, butane, or lighter fluid, that can also be abused by adolescents. Screening for abuse of

BOX 33.8 ✻ Focus on Evidence-Based Practice

Do adolescents who are religiously active engage in more or less substance abuse?

It is usually assumed that adolescents who attend their religious center at least once weekly abuse substances less than others. To establish whether this is true, researchers surveyed a large number (33,007) of adolescents in grades 9 through 12 as to their religious attendance and substance abuse. The results of this survey showed tobacco, marijuana, and alcohol were used regularly by 11% to 13% of all students. There were marked differences in alcohol, marijuana, and cigarette use, however, among adolescents who never, occasionally, or regularly participated in religious activity. Weekly religious attendance was consistently associated with less substance use whereas occasional religious participation sometimes was associated with greater use compared to those students who had no religious activity.

Based on the above study, would you ask an adolescent who you know attends church at least monthly if he abuses any substance such as alcohol and marijuana or could you safely assume that he would not be abusing these substances?

Source: Steinman, K. J., Ferketich, A. K., & Sahr, T. (2008). The dose-response relationship of adolescent religious activity and substance use: variation across demographic groups. *Health Education and Behavior, 35*(1), 22–43.

inhalants or readiness to abuse such substances is important, as inhalants can lead to cardiac failure even on a first-time use (Williams & Storck, 2007).

Tobacco. Although it is well documented that cigarette smoking leads to increased cardiovascular and respiratory illnesses by middle age, every day approximately 4000 American youth aged 12 to 17 years try their first cigarette. About 23% of high school students report current cigarette use and 14% report current cigar use. Eight percent of high school students and 18% of white male high school students report current smokeless tobacco use (CDC, 2008b). Adolescents usually begin smoking because the habit conveys a stamp of maturity; smoking may be viewed as especially desirable by those who are having difficulty demonstrating maturity in other areas. One of the strongest determinants of whether adolescents will begin smoking is whether their friends smoke. Although at one time proportionately more males than females smoked, adolescent girls now are the population most likely to begin smoking. As cigar smoking becomes more popular with adults, it also is becoming more popular with adolescents.

It is well documented that adolescents are influenced to begin smoking by advertising (Lovato et al., 2009). Most school systems have extensive programs as early as grade school to caution children against cigarette smoking and advertising. Unfortunately, the ultimate danger of illness or death in middle age is not a strong threat to young persons who are interested only in the present.

More effective, therefore, might be campaigns that point out cigarette smoking causes foul-smelling hair, clothes, and breath and this detracts from physical appearance. Helping adolescents find other methods to demonstrate their maturity, such as allowing them opportunities for increased decision making, and emphasizing that being able *not* to smoke is a sign of true maturity, may also be effective.

Adolescents can be urged to quit cigarette smoking through enrolling in a formal cigarette withdrawal program. Nicotine gum and nicotine patches have both been successfully used with adolescents.

Remember that adolescents are very reluctant to follow instructions that are given from a "do as I say, not as I do" standpoint. Nurses who smoke, therefore, can have extreme difficulty launching an effective campaign against the habit with adolescents.

TABLE 33.3 ✻ Stages of Substance Abuse

Stage	Name	Characteristics
0	Preabuse	Curious about drugs, need for peer acceptance; anger or boredom
1	Experimentation	Learning the high; little behavior change except lying; commonly used drugs: tobacco, alcohol, and marijuana; use is confined to social situations on weekends in the company of others, with others supplying the drugs.
2	Early regular use	Adolescent actively seeks the drug-induced mood swing; drugs are no longer just on social occasion but to relieve everyday stress. Use is frequent and may be solitary, regularly on weekends and occasionally on weekdays. Adolescents have their own supply. Drugs used include stimulants, sedatives, and inhalants. Behavior changes include change in dress, friends, deteriorating school performance, mood swings, lying, and stealing.
3	Late regular use	Dependent on substance of abuse; deteriorating behavior, fighting, lying, stealing, prostitution; often depressed, suicidal ideation, self-destructive or risk-taking behaviors
4	End stage	Substance use to avoid dysphoria; withdrawal; continued deterioration of behavior and mental state

Source: Muramoto, M. L., & Leshan, L. (1993). Adolescent substance abuse. *Primary Care, 20*(3), 141–144.

Stopping smoking is especially difficult during periods of stress or inactivity. Trying to introduce such an action during exam week, for example, is not good planning. During an illness is also a bad time, unless not feeling well has reduced the urge to smoke. A return visit for follow-up and health maintenance care might be a better time to introduce the topic.

Another source of nicotine that school-age children and adolescents may abuse is "smokeless tobacco," or chewing tobacco (Percy, 2008). Many baseball players use this form of tobacco, and adolescents who admire them may be particularly drawn to this tobacco source. Although chewing tobacco does not have the potential dangers of smoking tobacco in relation to lung disease, it can cause gingival recession and lip and mouth cancer and can be just as habit-forming as cigarettes.

Alcohol. As many as 90% of high school seniors report having used alcohol. As many as 25% of high school students report having engaged in episodic heavy or binge drinking. At least 10% of high school students report driving a car or other vehicle when they had been drinking alcohol. Twenty-nine percent of students report having ridden in a car or other vehicle driven by someone who had been drinking alcohol (CDC, 2008a). Although its use is correlated with motor vehicle accidents, homicide, and suicide in adolescents, alcohol has never carried the stigma of other drugs. Some parents are actually relieved when they realize their child's strange behavior on returning home from a party is caused by drunkenness and not illegal drugs. Alcohol use cannot be taken lightly, however, because it is linked to diseases such as cirrhosis, cognitive challenge, and destructive behaviors such as addiction, depression, and vulnerability to date rape.

Environment has a definite role in the use of alcohol, but heredity may play a part in whether an adolescent becomes addicted. Remind parents they have a responsibility to set good examples for adolescents in the use of alcohol or not drink indiscriminantly.

Most adolescents will admit they use alcohol if asked two specific questions: (a) Do you think you have a drinking problem? and (b) When was your last drink? Adolescents who answer yes to the first and "within the last 24 hours" to the second are candidates for further assessment.

Athletes tend to drink more than nonathletes probably due to their greater exposure to social situations (Wetherill & Fromme, 2007). Once adolescents face the fact that they have become alcohol dependent, an organization such as Alcoholics Anonymous can be invaluable to help them stop drinking. Encourage the remainder of their family to join Al-Anon, the organization for families of alcoholics, so both children and families can restructure their lives to find satisfaction without the use of this drug.

Many adolescents are not primary alcohol abusers but are the children of alcoholic parents. Make an effort to identify this group of children as well, not only to prevent them from becoming users of alcohol but also to help them build self-esteem and coping abilities for the difficulties they face living in a possibly disorganized household.

Performance-Enhancing Drug Abuse. Anabolic steroids are derivatives of the natural hormone testosterone. Common names are stanozolol, an oral compound, and testosterone propionate, an injectable form. Adolescents take steroids (obtained illegally) to enhance lean body mass and muscular development and so improve their athletic ability or appearance (Van den Berg et al., 2007). Anabolic steroids also have the side effects of euphoria and lessened fatigue, which make them doubly appealing (Vertalino et al., 2007).

To obtain maximum effects, teenagers may be taking up to 30 times the therapeutic dose. This can lead to adverse effects, such as early closure of the epiphyseal line of long bones, acne, elevated triglyceride levels, hypertension, aggressiveness, possibly psychosis, abnormal liver function, and, perhaps, liver cancer.

Students using anabolic steroids need to be identified so they can be cautioned that the use of such drugs is illegal in sports competition as well as being detrimental to their health. There is also concern that the use of such drugs serves as a gateway to additional drug use (Wagner & Anthony, 2007). If needles are shared, this can lead to hepatitis B or HIV infection. Human growth hormone has the ability to increase muscle strength and stamina and is more difficult to detect so is also becoming a commonly abused substance in athletes (Gibney, Healy, & Sonksen, 2007).

Marijuana. Marijuana (widely known as *pot* or *grass*) is derived from the leaves and stems of the Indian hemp plant, *Cannabis sativa.* It is generally rolled into cigarettes ("joints" or "reefers") and smoked, although it can be mixed with food or sniffed. Scraping the resin from the flowering leaves produces a much stronger substance called hashish. *Sinsemilla* is a seedless form that is even more potent.

Breakdown products of marijuana are not readily eliminated from the body but remain in the fatty cells of the brain. This residue results in synaptic gaps that can delay electrical brain waves and memory storage, especially for short-term memory. Physical and psychological effects of all forms of marijuana are euphoria and a sense of well-being, temporary impairment of coordination or motor activities, altered sensory perceptions, rapid mood swings, altered self-image, decreased attention span, and loss of memory for recent events (up to 1 hour time). Withdrawal symptoms include irritability, drowsiness, and cravings for high-carbohydrate snacks (Mendelson & Mello, 2008).

Long-term side effects can include disorders such as sinusitis, bronchitis, emphysema, and perhaps lung cancer (these can develop after only 1 year of use compared with 20 years of use for cigarette smoking), and lack of sperm formation or testicular cancer in males (Daling et al., 2009).

Despite its known dangers, marijuana is the most common illicit substance, next to alcohol, used by adolescents. Help adolescents realize that marijuana is more than an amusing leisure activity or a way to relieve stress so they can put its use into long-term perspective. Because it is used medically to relieve nausea and vomiting, adolescents may view it as harmless.

Amphetamines. The amphetamines are a group of drugs sometimes used in the treatment of hyperactivity and narcolepsy, among other central nervous system disorders. They are easily manufactured in "meth labs" in people's homes and so are readily available to adolescents. Amphetamines are called *uppers* or *speed* because they give the user a false sense of well-being, alertness, or self-esteem (Degenhardt et al., 2007). A newer, stronger form that produces intense symptoms is known as *ice.* Some of the side effects that can occur are aggressive or demanding behavior, paranoia, and extreme restlessness. Chronic methamphetamine abuse results in severe blackened, crumbling teeth. Because amphetamines suppress the appetite, adolescents may lose weight or eat only sporadically while taking them. Their use without a prescription is illegal.

Cocaine. Cocaine is one of the most popular drugs of abuse for young adults and its use may begin in adolescents. The drug may be sniffed into the nose (snorted), smoked, or injected intravenously. Occasionally it is combined with heroin and injected (termed a speedball). Common street names for cocaine are *snow* and *white lady,* because of its fine, white powder. A stronger form, called *crack,* is manufactured by heating cocaine powder with baking soda and water. This preparation process is dangerous in itself because it involves using volatile solvents that can ignite or explode. The resulting drug, often called *freebase* or *rock,* is so strong it can cause immediate cardiac and respiratory arrhythmias (Murphy & Benowitz, 2007).

It is difficult to document how many adolescents use cocaine, but estimates range from 3% to 9%. Cocaine that is either inhaled or smoked is absorbed through the mucous membrane into the bloodstream. After absorption, blood levels rise rapidly for the first 20 minutes, peak at 60 minutes, and then decline over the next 3 hours. Although a toxic dose of cocaine is usually considered to be 600 to 700 mg, toxicity has been reported with doses as low as 20 mg (a single line).

Cocaine produces the physical effects of increased pulse and respiration rates, increased temperature, increased blood pressure, and decreased appetite. Psychological effects produced are euphoria, excitement and restlessness, increased sociability, and possible hallucinations.

Toxic symptoms include seizures, tachyarrhythmias, tachypnea, hypertension, increased deep tendon reflexes, decreased response to stimuli, nausea and vomiting, abdominal pain, headaches, and chills and fever. It is a major cause of cardiovascular arrest in young adults (Kaul & Stevens-Simon, 2008).

Cocaine is rarely ingested orally, but occasionally adolescents swallow it when trying to hide a supply from parents or school personnel. Gastric acid destroys the action of cocaine, so it is potentially harmless when swallowed in this way. Cocaine has been swallowed in plastic pouches with the idea this will allow it to pass harmlessly through the gastrointestinal tract and also allow it to be recovered later in stool. If peristaltic action in the intestine causes the bag to break, this amount of cocaine is absorbed into the bloodstream at toxic levels. This can lead to sudden cardiac and respiratory arrest.

Teach adolescents that although cocaine sniffing may be fascinating and offer temporary pleasure and relief from stress, it also causes psychological dependency and is potentially extremely dangerous because of its cardiac and respiratory effects. Chronic inhalation of cocaine can cause ulceration in the mucous membrane of the nose, and injection of the substance exposes an adolescent to the risk of HIV/acquired immunodeficiency syndrome (AIDS), hepatitis, and other diseases contracted through contaminated equipment. Cocaine taken during pregnancy can cause separation of the placenta with potential fetal and maternal death.

Hallucinogens. Examples of hallucinogenic drugs used by adolescents are lysergic acid diethylamide (LSD), dimethyltryptamine (DMT), 2,5-dimethoxy-4-methamphetamine (STP), phencyclidine hydrochloride (PCP), and methaqualone (Quaalude). The use of LSD has increased in popularity substantially since the 1960s when it first became available, because it is a drug that can be manufactured by an informed adolescent in a "kitchen lab."

All of these drugs cause bizarre mind reactions such as distortion in vision, smell, or hearing. Adolescents report seeing colors more vividly than they have ever seen before, hearing sounds so clear they cause physical pain, and perceiving themselves as being totally impervious to harm.

The effect of such drugs can be extremely pleasurable (described as a "good trip") or extremely terrifying (a "bad trip"). Recurrences or flashbacks of drug-induced experiences may, unfortunately, recur at unpredictable times and in unexpected places. Such flashbacks are not only disconcerting but can be dangerous, especially if they occur while a person is driving a motor vehicle. They can be so frightening that some users believe they are becoming mentally deranged.

It is illegal to produce, sell, or possess hallucinogens in the United States. A hallucinogen related to mescaline, methylenedioxymethamphetamine (MDMA, or known as *ecstasy*), was previously used by some psychotherapists to make patients more receptive to therapy. It has been added to Schedule I of the Controlled Substances Act because it was found to cause brain damage. Chronic use destroys the serotonin system of the brain so it is associated with progressive decline of immediate and delayed memory and with alterations in mood (Medina & Shear, 2007).

Opiates. Opiates are drugs such as heroin, meperidine (Demerol), and morphine. At one time, these were not typically used by adolescents because they are expensive, but they now are gaining popularity among teens.

Opiates can be extremely dangerous because of their tendency to decrease respiratory rate. Addiction to opiates can cause such a physiologic craving that adolescents, like adults, will steal, defraud, turn to prostitution, or resort to whatever method is available to secure enough money to buy a day's supply. In addition to the direct danger of opiates, adolescents who use them risk the danger of contracting HIV/AIDS and hepatitis B infection if they share contaminated needles. "Snorting" heroin can lead to acute cerebral vascular accident and death.

Methadone or LAAM (Levomethadyl acetate) programs may be prescribed to help adolescents wean themselves from opiates (Maremmani et al., 2007). The users report to a center every day and receive an oral dose of methadone, which fulfills the same physiologic need as heroin. Although methadone is a narcotic itself, because adolescents do not have to pay for it, they no longer have to steal or prostitute themselves to obtain it. It allows them to continue in school or hold a job and become productive citizens. Caution them that a methadone overdose can occur the same as with any narcotic. After a time, LAAM is gradually substituted. The advantage of LAAM over methadone is that its effect lasts longer—72 rather than 24 hours—so less frequent administration is necessary. If a methadone program is not available, teenagers may be treated with buprenorphine (Levy et al., 2007).

Assessment of Substance Abuse

If adolescents trust health care personnel, they will generally admit they have engaged in drug experimentation (Box 33.9). Some common findings on the health history that suggest an adolescent is abusing some substance are:

- Failure to complete assignments in school
- Demonstration of poor reasoning ability
- Decreased school attendance
- Frequent mood swings
- Deteriorating physical appearance
- Recent change in peer group
- Expressed negative perceptions of parents

These are not necessarily diagnostic findings, however, because they can also be part of an adolescent's search for identity. Substance abuse can be strongly suspected in an adolescent who is hospitalized for hepatitis B or who is HIV positive, as well as one who appears overly anxious to leave a health care facility or who receives no benefit from usual analgesic agents. General physical symptoms that indicate drug abuse are summarized in Table 33.4.

Nursing Diagnoses and Related Interventions

Nursing Diagnosis: Risk for injury related to the use of alcohol or illegal chemical substances

Outcome Evaluation: Adolescent states he is not experimenting with drugs; can describe a way to respond to peers who encourage such use; shows no evidence of drug use such as lethargy, confusion, positive urine drug screen, or parental suspicion.

In addition to any physical damage that substance abuse may cause, one of the greatest dangers of early drug experimentation is it affects an adolescent's ability to solve problems, with a consequent delay in maturity. Adolescents may cling to peers to shield drug use and stay away from adults they are afraid might detect it, removing themselves from exposure to adult role models. It is important to help adolescents plan ways they can feel satisfaction in life without substance use, such as how to feel secure enough to interact with others without relying on cocaine or marijuana, or how to accomplish activities to increase self-esteem so alcohol is not needed.

When establishing expected outcomes with adolescents who are chemically dependent, remember it is difficult for them to appreciate how much they depend on a drug until they try to stop using it. A goal of not using a drug for 24 hours at a time may be the only one possible at first.

Try to caution adolescents against substance abuse in the same manner you would caution about the unwise use of motor vehicles or swimming beyond personal limits. Scare stories (soft drugs automatically lead to hard drugs, marijuana destroys your brain, drug addicts are sex perverts) cloud the issue and make adolescents dismiss all advice given them about drugs as worthless.

To maintain a realistic approach to the problem, health care personnel and parents should counsel (not lecture) that substance abuse is both illegal and harmful but also remember how difficult it is for adolescents to say no to peer pressure. Important teaching points to prevent substance abuse are summarized in Box 33.10.

Therapeutic communities or 24-hour facilities in which adolescents can live while they recover from chemical dependency may be necessary for some adolescents. The aim of all these programs is to increase adolescents' sense of self-esteem, improve problem-solving ability, realign them with society's values, and increase their self-awareness so they can function effectively without the aid of substances of abuse. Unfortunately, campaigns against substance abuse for adolescents have not been very successful, so the problem continues. Adolescents who are no longer chemically dependent should be evaluated by a history and physical examination at all health care visits because, if the circumstances that initially caused them to become chemically dependent recur, they may return to a dependency pattern. A continuing relationship with health care personnel not only allows time for this evaluation but also provides concrete role models of nonchemical, productive behavior.

BOX 33.9 * Focus on Communication

You talk to Raul, 15, in an adolescent clinic.

Less Effective Communication

Nurse: Here's a pamphlet about adolescents and drug use. I hope you haven't been using any.
Raul: No problem.
Nurse: Drugs can be really harmful. It takes an absolutely stupid person to use them.
Raul: No problem.
Nurse: Have you been doing any?
Raul: No problem.

More Effective Communication

Nurse: Here's a pamphlet about adolescents and drug use. I hope you haven't been using any.
Raul: No problem.
Nurse: Sometimes it's difficult for children to talk to parents or other adults about such things.
Raul: No problem.
Nurse: Have you been doing any?
Raul: No problem.

Raul answered with the same response in both conversations. Do you think he meant the same thing in both conversations? Was the nurse wise to announce that only stupid people use drugs and then ask if Raul was using any?

Concerns Regarding Depression and Attempted Suicide

Suicide is deliberate self-injury with the intent to end one's life. Successful suicide occurs more frequently in males than in

TABLE 33.4 ✲ Symptoms to Help Identify Drug Abusers

Drugs Used	Symptoms of Use	Dangers
Glue	Violence, drunken appearance, dreamy or blank expression Glue smears on clothing or fingers; tubes of glue, paper bags in possession	Lung, brain, or liver damage; death through suffocation or choking; anemia
Heroin, morphine, codeine	Stupor, drowsiness, needle marks on body, watery eyes, loss of appetite, bloodstains on shirt sleeve, runny nose Needle or hypodermic syringe, cotton, tourniquet string, burnt bottle caps or spoons, glassine envelopes in possession	Death from overdose; addiction; liver and other infections due to unsterile needles
Cough medicine containing codeine and opium	Drunken appearance, lack of coordination, confusion, excessive itching Empty bottle of cough medicine in possession	Addiction
Marijuana	Sleepiness, wandering mind, enlarged pupils, lack of coordination Strong odor of burnt leaves, small seeds in pocket lining, cigarette paper, discolored fingers	Psychological dependence; possibly testicular cancer
Hallucinogens (LSD, DMT, PCP)	Severe hallucinations, feelings of detachment, incoherent speech, cold hands and feet, laughing and crying, vomiting Possession of cube sugar with discoloration in center, strong body odor	Suicidal tendencies, unpredictable behavior; chronic exposure may have neurologic effects
Stimulants (methamphetamine, cocaine)	Aggressive behavior, giggling, silliness, rapid speech, confused thinking, no appetite, extreme fatigue, black caries, dry mouth, shakiness, insomnia. Pills or capsules of varying colors in possession; absence of nasal hair; possession of a glass pipe	Death from overdose; hallucinations; psychosis
Depressants (barbiturates, alcohol)	Drowsiness, stupor, dullness, slurred speech, drunken appearance, vomiting Pills or capsules of varying colors in possession; odor of alcohol on breath	Death or unconsciousness from overdose; addiction; seizures from withdrawal
Steroids	Aggressive behavior; increase in muscle strength and mass	Violent actions; possibly tumor growth

females, although more females apparently attempt suicide than males (about 8:1). Adolescent suicides are attempted most often in the spring or the fall, reflecting school stress at these times of year, and between 3 PM and midnight, reflecting depression that increases with the dark. Suicide is so common in adolescents that it ranks third as a cause of death in the 15- to 19-year-old group (CDC, 2008a). This statistic may actually be underestimated, because some well-meaning coroners or physicians may report these deaths as accidents to spare the family additional pain.

Some automobile or hiking accidents may be attempts at self-destruction; in addition, some homicides may be caused by deliberately provoking another person in the hope of being killed. Incest, abuse, increased chemical dependency, marital instability in the family, and poor problem-solving ability are reasons that may lead an adolescent to decide that death may be easier than coping with overwhelming problems. A wish to "get even" over some hurt or drug and alcohol use may contribute to suicide by further impairing judgment (Kaplan & Love-Osborne, 2008).

Some degree of depression is present in most adolescents, because they are not only losing their parents at this time as they grow apart from them, but they are also losing their carefree childhood. If school failure or loss of a friend or losing a competition is superimposed on an existing depression, the pressure may be great enough to cause some adolescents to attempt suicide. Some other reasons for attempting suicide include anger with others and manipulation (psychological blackmail) as a way of having one's needs met. Loss of a parent, loss of a girlfriend or boyfriend, loss of a community, and loss of self-esteem are all significant and can trigger a suicide. Because some adolescents may be unable to believe that a parent was at fault in the case of divorce or that the death of a parent could not have been prevented, they may believe, instead, they somehow caused the parent to leave or to die. The loss of a girlfriend or boyfriend is particularly significant because it involves two types of loss: friendship and self-esteem. Rejection from a peer group, sports team, or school club may cause a similar loss of self-esteem.

Assessment

Adolescents need to have thorough physical examinations at health maintenance visits to assure them they are in good physical health. Assess for signs of depression such as anorexia, insomnia, excessive fatigue, or weight loss. In younger adolescents, depression may be manifested by behavior problems such as disobedience, temper tantrums,

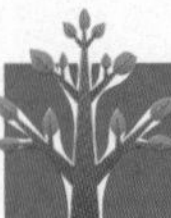

BOX 33.10 * Focus on Family Teaching

Health Teaching Guidelines for the Prevention of Substance Abuse in Adolescents

Q. Raul, at 15, is very aware drugs are readily accessible in his neighborhood. He asks you, "What are guidelines to help avoid substance abuse?"

A. Below are some common suggestions:

1. All chemicals are harmful to the body, at least to some extent (alcohol, for example, causes liver disease).
2. Relying on drugs to give you courage to solve problems (or help to forget you have problems) prevents you from learning to handle life situations and maturing.
3. The bottom line of drug abuse is that you have the final say: you are the only one who can stop chemical dependency from happening.
4. Whether a drug is inhaled, swallowed, or injected, it still is absorbed and enters your body.
5. Despite their social acceptability, alcohol and nicotine are drugs. A month of daily use of either can make you addicted.

truancy, and running away from home. Self-destructive behavior or accident proneness may be noted. Difficulties in school; acting out with chemicals, alcohol, or sexual promiscuity; or trouble with legal authorities may be further clues. Occasionally, depressed adolescents find it so hard to be alone they seek constant activity as a means of escape. In contrast, others may withdraw from contact with other persons and become completely isolated. Either behavior can be detected through assessment of activity and interaction levels.

Adolescents who attempt suicide fall into no one category, although many tend to be loners or to have difficulty expressing their feelings to others and, therefore, do not receive emotional support from friends. Others are "perfect" students. The stress of trying to achieve continually at this level, however, is the trigger that provokes suicide. Gay and lesbian youths appear to have higher levels of suicide than others, reflecting the level of stress they may be experiencing. Assess for these lifestyles as well.

If another member of a family or a close friend committed suicide, the chance that an adolescent will do so is greater than usual, as adolescents then see suicide as a method of coping and use it. The anniversary of a family member's suicide is an especially vulnerable time as wishing to join the dead family member may appear attractive. When one adolescent in a high school commits suicide, there is a good chance another will take similar action soon afterward. Adolescent suicide rates may actually reach epidemic proportions after a popular student's suicide. Students who have Internet contacts may arrange a group suicide as a method of making a statement or gaining support.

Because suicide usually reflects a problem in family interaction, family assessment is helpful. A thorough family history may reveal conflict with one or both parents. A frequent comment heard is, "They'll be sorry when I'm dead." School friends may often be aware an adolescent is contemplating suicide before the parents. Caution parents not to discount reports from their child's friends who tell them they are concerned about their child. Close to the chosen time of suicide, some adolescents may demonstrate characteristic behaviors that show they are making preparations to end their life. Teach family and friends these typical danger signs (Box 33.11).

After a suicide attempt, ask enough questions on a health history so you know whether an adolescent made a detailed suicide plan. For example, a young person who took four aspirins and left the empty aspirin container conspicuously on the kitchen counter just before his mother was due to arrive home from work is more likely to be only crying for help; one who took 100 aspirins and hid the container under the bed just after his mother left for 8 hours of work is much more apt to be making a serious attempt. You may be the first person in a health care facility to realize that an adolescent talking about suicide is not "just talking" (it is a fallacy that people who talk about suicide do not attempt it) but has a definite, well-thought-out plan to accomplish it. An adolescent who has been admitted to a hospital unit after a

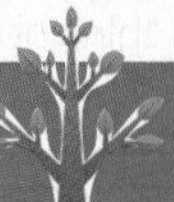

BOX 33.11 * Focus on Family Teaching

Suicide Warning Signs

Q. Raul's father says to you, "Our neighbor's son recently committed suicide. What are warning signs of this to look for in our son?"

A. The following are commonly seen clues:

- Giving away prized possessions
- Organ donation questions, such as "How do you leave your body to a medical school?"
- Sudden, unexplained elevation of mood. Mood elevation may indicate that the individual has reached a decision about the suicide and feels relief.
- Accident proneness, carelessness, and death wishes
- A statement such as, "This is the last time you will see me."
- Decrease in verbal communication
- Withdrawal from peer activities or previously enjoyed events
- Previous attempt (80% of all completed suicides have been preceded by a failed attempt)
- Preference for art, music, and literature with themes of death
- Recent increase in interpersonal conflict with significant others
- Running away from home
- Recent experience of a friend or famous person committing suicide
- Inquiring about the hereafter
- Asking for information (supposedly for a friend) about suicide prevention and intervention
- Almost any sustained deviation from the normal pattern of behavior

serious suicide attempt may formulate a new plan that will be successful the next time unless some action is taken and the adolescent's life can be changed in some way.

Nursing Diagnoses and Related Interventions

Nursing Diagnosis: Risk for violence, self-directed, related to symptoms of depression or expressed desire to hurt oneself

Outcome Evaluation: Client expresses feelings of depression to health care providers or other adults; states she will contact support person should the desire to commit suicide become overwhelming.

Crisis intervention for adolescents who are contemplating suicide includes trying to alleviate their pain and depression and counseling them in an effort to help them change their perspective on the value of life. Be aware that establishing expected outcomes with adolescents who are contemplating suicide or who have made an attempt will be difficult because they are often too depressed to come up with an alternative solution to their problems (their goal is to kill themselves, not solve problems).

Try to find out the things in the child's life that are still viewed as important; build a plan that will help view life as worth living enough to work through problems. Show them no one can change everything, but everyone can make one or two changes that can make a difference. After these small changes are made, a domino effect can be created to change more and more of one's circumstances.

Because adolescents resort to suicide as a method of solving problems, helping them in this area is a prime intervention strategy. Asking "what would happen if" questions such as "Suppose you did fail a course; what would happen?" "Are there ways you can reverse the finality of the problem perhaps by talking to a teacher about make-up assignments, asking a friend for help in reviewing material, or buying a review book to help in studying?" Do not count on everyone in an adolescent's life being willing to help. A high school teacher may feel that to be asked to do outside tutoring is an imposition so for you to advise adolescents to seek this kind of help will only add to their depression. You may have to make these contacts yourself (with an adolescent's permission) because, generally, persons who are depressed have difficulty initiating this type of action because they do not believe anyone cares enough about them to help.

A general measure is to help adolescents speak honestly about thoughts of suicide and the problems that have led them to think that death is a solution. Most problems begin to seem manageable if they can be put into words in this way. It is important not to underestimate adolescents' determination to end their life, however. In most instances, an adolescent at this point needs referral to a consultant well versed in suicide prevention to improve self-image and offer alternative solutions to problems.

For an adolescent's safety, a period of observation in a hospital setting is desirable after a suicide attempt to prevent the adolescent from inflicting personal injury again and to allow assessment in a neutral setting, away from the stress that precipitated the attempt. This can take place in an adolescent service rather than a psychiatric service.

Antidepressant medicine alone, a therapy used with depressed adults, may be of little value in treating depressed adolescents. Tricyclic antidepressants generally are ineffective and may cause serious adverse effects. Evidence for the effectiveness of selective serotonin reuptake inhibitors is limited. All antidepressants have a black box warning because some antidepressants have been associated with elevating the mood of depressed children enough to allow them to formulate a plan and commit suicide after taking them (Bhatia & Bhatia, 2007). Fluoxetine is an example of a drug approved for the treatment of depression in children 8 to 17 years of age.

Continuing evaluation by both history taking and physical examination is necessary, because the young person who has attempted suicide may attempt it again if support people and better problem-solving ability are not available at another time.

What if... Raul seems unusually happy at a clinic visit, when usually he is sad? Would you worry that this change in mood is a warning sign that he might be contemplating suicide?

Concerns Regarding Runaways

A *runaway* is commonly defined as a child between the ages of 10 and 17 years who has been absent from home at least overnight without permission of a parent or guardian. The frequency of running away for adolescents may be as high as one in eight. Fortunately, most do not go far or stay away long (less than 1 week) (Milburn et al., 2007); about 1 in 20 adolescent runaways stays away as long as 1 year; some never return home. Runaway adolescents are most likely to be from low- or high-income families. Unemployment, alcoholism, sexual abuse, attempted suicide, and poverty are frequent characteristics (Chen et al., 2007). They are slightly more likely to be male than female. Events they encounter may be so traumatic they develop a posttraumatic syndrome (Thompson et al., 2007).

Assessment

Running away is usually preceded by an argument with parents that is often the last straw after a number of long-term disagreements. Other reasons may be personal concerns such as loneliness, pregnancy, and problems with friends, school, or the police. Incest can also be a precipitating cause, as can other parental abuse. A school history often reveals frequent truancy, failing grades, possible drug use, and runaway behavior by friends. It is a sad fact that some adolescents are "throwaways" or cannot remain at home because they have been rejected by their families.

Common health reasons for which runaway adolescents are seen at health care facilities are sexually transmitted diseases, including HIV/AIDS, rape, pregnancy, substance abuse, hepatitis, and vaginitis. They also have a high incidence of suicide attempts. When caring for adolescents with these concerns, be certain to secure a thorough history so the fact they are no longer living at home will not be missed. Be sure to be nonjudgmental in questioning. Revealing you are shocked by a report an adolescent has been sleeping on a park bench for 2 months, has been robbed, or steals to obtain money could prevent you from learning even greater concerns, such as having a sexually transmitted disease, being pregnant, or using drugs. Ask if the adolescent wants to return home. Even though being homeless is high stress, and many adolescent runaways want to take the first step back toward their parents, they may not know how to begin the process.

Nursing Diagnoses and Related Interventions

Nursing Diagnosis: Ineffective individual coping related to stress of adolescent period and inadequate family resources

Outcome Evaluation: Adolescent states stress level at home is manageable; is able to describe how he can use family and community resources to help solve problems and aid in a crisis.

Adolescents may run away because they cannot solve a problem in any other way; therefore, setting goals with them may be difficult. A short-term goal to stay home through a holiday rather than a long-term one of finishing high school may be all you can achieve.

Because adolescent runaways lack references for jobs and do not necessarily qualify for public assistance programs, they generally have no secure source of income. This can cause both males and females to resort to prostitution to support themselves, or they may resort to stealing. Police consider them to be juvenile delinquents and are required to return them to their homes if discovered. If they leave home again, they may be sentenced to an institution for care; unfortunately, these facilities are often crowded and may not have the means to meet adolescent needs other than food and clothing.

Try to imagine yourself in adolescent runaways' circumstances to determine whether your health instructions are sensible for their lifestyle. Giving them instructions to eat a high-protein diet or iron-rich foods, for example, may be ludicrous. If they do not have a source of running water, soaking a lesion or changing a dressing may be difficult. They may have no way to pay for health care, making it impossible to obtain a prescription medication, so giving them a sample of a drug is often more practical. If they do not have a means of transportation, they may be unable to return to the health care facility for frequent follow-up visits. Try to meet as many of the runaway's needs as possible, therefore, at one visit. Remember that many runaways have associated school failure so may be poor readers; discuss the information with them when giving them a pamphlet.

Be certain runaway adolescents are familiar with the national Youth Crisis Hotline, which they can call day or night when they want to return home. The telephone number is 1-800-448-4663 (1-800-HIT HOME). Remember also that they are runaways because, for some reason, their home was intolerable. Although they agree to return home, they may not remain there unless circumstances have been or can be changed.

Nursing Diagnosis: Impaired parenting related to inability of family to adjust to adolescent needs

Outcome Evaluation: Parents list definite changes they have made in family life to better accommodate an adolescent, such as providing increased privacy or using "contracting" with adolescent.

In some instances, it is impossible for a family to reestablish itself after a child has run away because the family is dysfunctional (incest or abuse has occurred). In other instances, family life can be modified to welcome the runaway adolescent back home.

So that parents and an adolescent can learn to communicate better, it is helpful to urge them to establish ground rules for communication (shouting or threats are not allowed; no subject is too difficult to be discussed calmly; no emotion or feeling is to be called "foolish"). Once ground rules are laid, parents and the adolescent should meet to discuss how difficult it is to be an adolescent and how equally difficult it is to be the parent of an adolescent; in the past, they became so engaged in arguing that they did not appreciate the other side of the controversy.

Helping parents and adolescents establish a contract for behavior can be effective (for the right to have her own private room, an adolescent cannot do drugs; for the right to stay overnight at a friend's house on Friday, she must eat with the family all other nights, for example). Contracting is effective with adolescents, but it does carry the responsibility for parents to be certain they are abiding by their half of the contract (not invading the private room) and of being prepared to enforce the contract. Some families benefit by calling on a mediator (a relative, a close friend, a minister or rabbi) to listen to both sides of an issue and make a ruling.

What if... After a fair trial of trying to make adjustments, an adolescent's parents are still unable to maintain a functional home life for him? What other arrangements would you suggest to them to arrange for safe care of their adolescent?

Unique Concerns of the Family With a Physically Challenged or Chronically Ill Adolescent

Achieving a sense of identity may be difficult for adolescents who have a chronic illness or other challenge. It is vital, however, for such individuals to learn to look past their particular condition to their real selves. For example, a 16-year-old girl in a wheelchair must learn to perceive herself as a teenager who is normal intellectually, is a good conversationalist, has a good sense of humor, enjoys watching football, and only incidentally uses a wheelchair to ambulate.

TABLE 33.5 ✻ Nursing Actions That Encourage a Sense of Identity in the Physically Challenged or Chronically Ill Adolescent

Category	Actions
Nutrition	If adolescent is on special diet, discuss role of food preferences with dietitian (hot dogs, pizza, etc.). Respect food preferences.
Dressing change	Allow adolescent to order supplies. Ask for suggestions as to final appearance of dressing. If soaks are included, have adolescent time the treatment. Allow adolescent to choose time for dressing change.
Medicine	Offering the adolescent a choice of site for injection or intravenous insertion encourages a sense of control. Teach name, action, and possible side effects of medicine.
Rest	Contract with adolescent for time and length of rest periods.
Hygiene	Respect modesty of the adolescent as being at adult level. Contract with adolescent for extent of self-care (will give own bath and make bed, not medicate self).
Pain	Encourage adolescent to express pain; teach distraction technique for sharp pain, such as deep breathing, counting backward from 100. Encourage adolescent to ask for analgesics as needed.
Stimulation	Provide tapes of favorite music with earphones. Provide a radio for adolescent to listen to talk show to foster active involvement. Encourage school work, crossword puzzles (you may need to help adolescents divide school assignments so they do not become overly fatigued and frustrated). Provide cards for games to increase socialization (make or have the adolescent make a card deck from pieces of paper if one is not available). Encourage adolescents to network with one another. Encourage adolescents to keep in contact with friends through telephoning, e-mail, or writing notes.

Some of the biggest problems of chronically ill adolescents are likely to be difficulties in being as independent as they would like to be, achieving in school, and establishing intimate relationships. Those who cannot learn to drive when their friends are learning to do so, who are not invited to dances and parties because of a disability, or who are too hesitant to ask someone to go with them, may feel acute losses of self-esteem. Moreover, the loss of many hours of school because of illness or frequent hospitalization may result in the inability to pursue a desired career, at least without a delay. Adolescence may be the first time these children realize that certain occupations or opportunities, such as a military career, may be closed to them. As they prepare to leave the security of a familiar school system, it may be the first time they examine just how they will be able to function on their own. Some may come to realize they will never be able to do so with complete independence.

Chronic hospitalization or the realization they will never be free of symptoms can cause depression in adolescents, placing them at high risk for substance abuse or suicide. Helping these adolescents realize that even completely well people must compromise life decisions for other reasons such as lack of money, lack of ability or qualifications, or extra personal responsibilities helps them feel they are not so different from others. This type of guidance can be time consuming, but sometimes the fact that an adult is willing to make this time commitment with them is enough to give these adolescents the self-esteem they need to alter aspirations and plans and find a future role consistent with their capabilities. Nursing actions that encourage a sense of identity in an adolescent with a long-term illness or who is physically challenged are summarized in Table 33.5.

Nutrition and the Chronically Ill Adolescent

Adolescents who are not fully mobile must be aware of their total calorie intake, or as growth needs decline at the end of adolescence they can become obese. They should also be knowledgeable about good nutrition, so they can participate in meal planning, an action that helps them feel a sense of control over this area of their life. Assess how often they have a chance to eat at fast-food restaurants; although this is not a source of excellent nutrition, eating there occasionally provides an important social experience and a chance to be like their peers.

✔ Checkpoint Question 33.3

Raul admits he has experimented with cocaine. A typical change in facial appearance that occurs with cocaine use is:

a. Frown lines in the forehead.
b. Thin, fissured lips.
c. Loss of eyebrow hair.
d. Absent nasal hair.

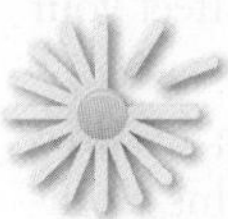

Key Points for Review

- The major milestones of development in the adolescent period are the onset of puberty and the cessation of body growth. Between these milestones, physical growth is rapid, although the development of adult coordination and thought processes is slow.

- The development of secondary sex characteristics is completed during adolescence. These are rated according to Tanner stages.
- The developmental task of an adolescent according to Erikson is to establish independence from parents by gaining a sense of identity versus role confusion. Adolescents, therefore, usually respond best to health care personnel who respect their attempts at independence and allow them as many choices as possible in care.
- Adolescents reach a point of cognitive development termed *formal operational thought.* With this gained, they are able to think in abstract terms and use the scientific method to arrive at conclusions.
- Adolescents need to consume adequate calories and especially protein, iron, calcium, and zinc to meet their increased growth needs.
- To appear older than they are, some adolescents present an assured, "I know that" attitude. To be effective, health teaching may have to be introduced with "I know you know this, so I'll just review it" approach that allows an adolescent to maintain a mature front, while gaining additional information.
- Being an adolescent is difficult in today's world. Be aware that, to reduce stress, some adolescents begin to use substances of abuse. Asking about an adolescent's drug experiences, if any, during a health assessment is not intruding on privacy; it is conducting safe health interviewing.
- Promoting adolescent safety is an important nursing role. Motor vehicle accidents, homicide, drowning, and suicide are leading causes of death in this age group.
- Common health problems in an adolescent are sometimes minor and include poor posture, fatigue, or acne; they can also be serious, such as beginning hypertension, substance abuse, and scoliosis. Identifying these problems and referring an adolescent for help are important nursing actions.

CRITICAL THINKING EXERCISES

1. Raul is the 15-year-old teenager you met at the beginning of the chapter. His parents tell you he was depressed after the loss of a girlfriend but now is suddenly happy. He has been collecting baseball cards since he was 8. Recently, he gave his collection away to a neighborhood boy because "I won't need them where I'm going." Why might you be concerned about him? What additional questions might you ask him? If you learned he is about to leave to be an exchange student in England, how would this affect your assessment of the situation?
2. Suppose Raul tells you during history taking he does not smoke, but you smell cigarette smoke on his clothing. Although he says he does not use drugs, a number of blue-and-white capsules fall out of his shirt pocket when he unbuttons his shirt. What questions would you ask to determine if he is smoking cigarettes or using drugs? Describe your next action if he does admit he is not only heavily into drugs but does not intend to stop using them.
3. A shy, quiet, 14-year-old girl you care for in a hospital setting tells you she is concerned because she has not menstruated yet. This is making her feel "left out" at school. How would you counsel her? What if she were 16 and had the same concern?
4. Examine the National Health Goals related to growth and development of adolescents. Most government-sponsored funds for nursing research are allotted based on these goals. What would be a possible research topic to explore pertinent to these goals that would be applicable to Raul's family and also advance evidence-based practice?

CRITICAL THINKING SCENARIO

Open the accompanying CD-ROM or visit http://thePoint.lww.com and read the Patient Scenario included for this chapter, then answer the questions to further sharpen your skills and grow more familiar with NCLEX style questions related to adolescent growth and development. Confirm your answers are correct by reading the rationales.

REFERENCES

American Academy of Pediatrics (AAP). (2009). *Recommendations for preventive pediatric health care.* Washington, DC: Author.

Armfield, J. M., & Spencer, A. J. (2007). Community effectiveness of fissure sealants and the effect of fluoridated water consumption. *Community Dental Health, 24*(1), 4–11.

Armstrong, M. L. (2007). A brief overview of body art: regulation and standardization are needed as the popularity of tattooing and body piercing increases. *American Journal of Nursing, 107*(4), 56–57.

Benson, P. A., et al. (2007). Access to health care issues among gay, lesbian, and bisexual adolescents: examination of the Project Q Survey. *Journal of Adolescent Health, 40*(2), S7–S8.

Bhatia, S. K., & Bhatia, S. C. (2007). Childhood and adolescent depression. *American Family Physician, 75*(1), 73–84.

Brand, S., et al. (2007). Romantic love, hypomania, and sleep patterns in adolescents. *Journal of Adolescent Health, 41*(1), 69–76.

Centers for Disease Control and Prevention (CDC). (2008a). *Alcohol and drug use.* Atlanta, GA: Author.

Centers for Disease Control and Prevention (CDC). (2008b). *Tobacco use and the health of young people.* Atlanta, GA: Author.

Chen, X., et al. (2007). Onset of conduct disorder, use of delinquent subsistence strategies, and street victimization among homeless and runaway adolescents in the midwest. *Journal of Interpersonal Violence, 22*(9), 1156–1183.

Cousineau, T. M., et al. (2007). Improving young adolescents' puberty knowledge: a randomized controlled trial. *Journal of Adolescent Health, 40*(2), S7–S8.

Daling, J. R., Doody, D. R., Sun, X., et al. (2009). Association of marijuana use and the incidence of testicular germ cell tumors. *Cancer Early View* [Epub 2/9/09].

Dietz, N. A., & Martin, P. Y. (2007). Women who are stalked: questioning the fear standard. *Violence Against Women, 13*(7), 750–776.

Degenhardt, L., et al. (2007). The predictors and consequences of adolescent amphetamine use. *Addiction, 102*(7), 1076–1084.

Erikson, E. H. (1993). *Childhood and society.* New York: W. W. Norton.

Fergus, S., Zimmerman, M. A., & Caldwell, C. H. (2007). Growth trajectories of sexual risk behavior in adolescence and young adulthood. *American Journal of Public Health, 97*(6), 1096–1101.

Gibney, J., Healy, M. L., & Sonksen, P. H. (2007). The growth hormone/insulin-like growth factor-I axis in exercise and sport. *Endocrine Reviews, 28*(6), 603–624.

Gilligan, C., et al. (1982). *In a different voice: psychological theory and women's development.* Cambridge, MA: Harvard University Press.

Griffin, J. (2007). Nutrition for the serious young athlete—the educational approach. *SportEX Dynamics, 1*(12), 7–9.

Hornor, G. (2007). Genitourinary assessment: an integral part of a complete physical examination. *Journal of Pediatric Health Care, 21*(3), 162–170.

Kaplan, D. W., & Love-Osborne, K. (2008). Adolescence. In W. W. Hay, et al. (Eds.). *Current pediatric diagnosis and treatment* (18th ed.). Columbus, OH: McGraw-Hill.

Karch, A. M. (2009). *Lippincott's nursing drug guide.* Philadelphia: Lippincott Williams & Wilkins.

Kaul, P., & Stevens-Simon, C. (2008). Substance abuse. In W. W. Hay, et al. (Eds.). *Current pediatric diagnosis and treatment* (18th ed.). Columbus, OH: McGraw-Hill.

Knox, M. A. (2008). Skin diseases in infants and children. In J. E. South-Paul, S. C. Matheny, & E. L. Lewis. (Eds.). *Current diagnosis and treatment in family medicine* (2nd ed.). Columbus, OH: McGraw-Hill.

Knoop, H., et al. (2008). Efficacy of cognitive behavioral therapy for adolescents with chronic fatigue syndrome: long-term follow-up of a randomized, controlled trial. *Pediatrics, 121*(3), e619–e625.

Kohlberg, L. (1984). *The psychology of moral development.* New York: Harper & Row.

Lee, J. M., et al. (2007). Weight status in young girls and the onset of puberty. *Pediatrics, 119*(3), e624–e630.

Levy, S., et al. (2007). Buprenorphine replacement therapy for adolescents with opioid dependence: early experience from a children's hospital-based outpatient treatment program. *Journal of Adolescent Health, 40*(5), 477–482.

Levine, D. A. (2007). 'Pharming': the abuse of prescription and over-the-counter drugs in teens. *Current Opinion in Pediatrics, 19*(3), 270–274.

Lovato, C., et al. (2009). Impact of tobacco advertising and promotion on increasing adolescent smoking behaviours. *Cochrane Database of Systematic Reviews, 2009*(1), (CD003439).

Maremmani, I., et al. (2007). Alcohol and cocaine use and abuse among opioid addicts engaged in a methadone maintenance treatment program. *Journal of Addictive Diseases, 26*(1), 61–70.

McDowell, M. A., Brody, D. J., & Hughes, J. P. (2007). Has age at menarche changed? Results from the National Health and Nutrition Examination Survey (NHANES) 1999–2004. *Journal of Adolescent Health, 40*(3), 227–231.

Medina, K. L., & Shear, P. K. (2007). Anxiety, depression, and behavioral symptoms of executive dysfunction in ecstasy users: contributors of polydrug use. *Drug and Alcohol Dependence, 87*(2–3), 303–311.

Mettes, T. G., et al. (2009). Interventions for treating asymptomatic impacted wisdom teeth in adolescents and adults. *Cochrane Database of Systematic Reviews, 2009*(1), (CD003879).

Mendelson, J. H., & Mello, N. K. (2008). Cocaine and other commonly abused drugs. In Fauci, A. S., et al. (Eds.). *Harrison's principles of internal medicine* (17th ed.). Columbus, OH: McGraw-Hill.

Milburn, N. G., et al. (2007). Newly homeless youth typically return home. *Journal of Adolescent Health, 40* (6), 574–576.

Moore, M. J., White, G. L., & Moore, D. L. (2007). Association of relative backpack weight with reported pain, pain sites, medical utilization, and lost school time in children and adolescents. *Journal of School Health, 77*(5), 232–239.

Mothers Against School Hazing (MASH). (2008). Available at http://www.mashinc.org.

Muramoto, M. L., & Leshan, L (1993). Adolescent substance abuse. *Primary Care, 20*(3), 141–144.

Murphy, N. G., & Benowitz, N. L. (2007). Cocaine. In K. R. Olson (Ed.). *Poisoning and drug overdose* (5th ed.). Columbus, OH: McGraw-Hill.

Nusbaum, M. R. H., & Katsufrakis, P. J. (2008). Adolescent sexuality. In J. E. South-Paul, S. C. Matheny, & E. L. Lewis. (Eds.). *Current diagnosis and treatment in family medicine* (2nd ed.). Columbus, OH: McGraw-Hill.

Ondrak, K. S., & Morgan, D. W. (2007). Physical activity, calcium intake and bone health in children and adolescents. *Sports Medicine, 37*(7), 587–600.

Percy, M. S. (2008). Oral health of adolescents—it's more than dental caries. *MCN: American Journal of Maternal Child Nursing, 33*(1), 26–31.

Piaget, J. (1969). *The theory of stages in cognitive development.* New York: McGraw-Hill.

Reich, A., et al. (2007). Acne vulgaris: what teenagers think about it. *Dermatology Nursing, 19*(1), 49–54.

Roberts, I. (2009). School-based driver education for the prevention of traffic crashes. *Cochrane Database of Systematic Reviews, 2009*(1), (CD003201).

Rolfes, S. R., Pinna, K., & Whitney, E. N. (2009). *Understanding normal and clinical nutrition.* New York: Wadsworth/Cengage Learning.

Seikaly, M.G. (2007). Hypertension in children: an update on treatment strategies. *Current Opinion in Pediatrics, 19*(2), 170–177.

Selby, M. (2007). Menstrual problems: from menarche to menopause. *Practice Nurse, 33*(5), 33–36.

Sodl, J. F., et al. (2008). Traumatic myositis ossificans as a result of college fraternity hazing. *Clinical Orthopaedics & Related Research, 466*(1), 225–230.

Steinman, K. J., Ferketich, A. K., & Sahr, T. (2008). The dose-response relationship of adolescent religious activity and substance use: variation across demographic groups. *Health Education & Behavior, 35*(1), 22–43.

Stephens, M. B. (2008). Physical activity in adolescents. In J. E. South-Paul, S. C. Matheny, & E. L. Lewis. (Eds.). *Current diagnosis and treatment in family medicine* (2nd ed.). Columbus, OH: McGraw-Hill.

Tanner, J. M. (1962). *Growth at adolescence* (2nd ed.). Oxford: Blackwell.

Theobald, H. (2007). Childhood nutrition. *Journal of Community Nursing, 21*(2), 25–28.

Thompson, S. J., et al. (2007). Predictors of posttraumatic stress symptoms among runaway youth utilizing two service sectors. *Journal of Traumatic Stress, 20*(4), 553–563.

Van den Berg, P., et al. (2007). Steroid use among adolescents: longitudinal findings from Project EAT. *Pediatrics, 119*(3), 476–486.

Vertalino, M., et al. (2007). Participation in weight-related sports is associated with higher use of unhealthful weight-control behaviors and steroid use. *Journal of the American Dietetic Association, 107*(3), 434–440.

Wagner, F. A., & Anthony, J. C. (2007). Male-female differences in the risk of progression from first use to dependence upon cannabis, cocaine, and alcohol. *Drug and Alcohol Dependence, 86*(2–3), 191–198.

Whetstone, L. M., Morrissey, S. L., & Cummings, D. M. (2007). Children at risk: the association between perceived weight status and suicidal thoughts and attempts in middle school youth. *Journal of School Health, 77*(2), 59–66.

Williams, J. F., & Storck, M. (2007). Inhalant abuse. *Pediatrics, 119*(5), 1009–1017.

Wetherill, R. R., & Fromme, K. (2007). Alcohol use, sexual activity, and perceived risk in high school athletes and non-athletes. *Journal of Adolescent Health, 41*(3), 294–301.

Yamawaki, N. (2007). Rape perception and the function of ambivalent sexism and gender-role traditionality. *Journal of Interpersonal Violence, 22*(4), 406–423.

SUGGESTED READINGS

Agrawal, A., et al. (2007). Correlates of cannabis initiation in a longitudinal sample of young women: the importance of peer influences. *Preventive Medicine, 45*(1), 31–34.

Costello, E. J., et al. (2007). Pubertal maturation and the development of alcohol use and abuse. *Drug and Alcohol Dependence, 88*(Suppl 1), S50–S59.

Deardorff, J., et al. (2007). Puberty and gender interact to predict social anxiety symptoms in early adolescence. *Journal of Adolescent Health, 41*(1), 102–104.

Ding, C., & Parks, S. (2007). Fast food and body weight among adolescents. *International Electronic Journal of Health Education, 10*(3), 65–77.

Gosselt, J. F., et al. (2007). Mystery shopping and alcohol sales: do supermarkets and liquor stores sell alcohol to underage customers? *Journal of Adolescent Health, 41*(3), 302–308.

Hempstead, K. (2007). The geography of self-injury: spatial patterns in attempted and completed suicide. *Social Science & Medicine, 62*(12), 3186–3196.

Kinsman, S. B., et al. (2007). How do young drivers view peer passengers? *Journal of Adolescent Health, 40*(2), S53–S54.

Papathanasiou, I., & Lahana, E. (2007). Adolescence, sexuality and sexual education. *Health Science Journal, 1*(1), 1–8.

Rauscher, K. J., & Myers, D. J. (2008). Socioeconomic disparities in the prevalence of work-related injuries among adolescents in the United States. *Journal of Adolescent Health, 42*(1), 50–57.

Thomas, R., & Perera, R. (2009). School-based programmes for preventing smoking. *Cochrane Database of Systematic Reviews, 2009*(1), (CD001293)

Chapter 34 Child Health Assessment

KEY TERMS

- antitoxins
- audiogram
- auscultation
- bruit
- chief concern
- conjunctivitis
- deep tendon reflexes
- diaphragmatic excursion
- epispadias
- esotropia
- exotropia
- gamma globulin
- geographic tongue
- hordeolum
- hydrocele
- hypospadias
- inspection
- intelligence
- intercostal spaces
- kwashiorkor
- palpation
- percussion
- physiologic splitting
- point of maximum impulse
- ptosis
- retractions
- review of systems
- sinus arrhythmia
- strabismus
- temperament
- toxoid
- turgor
- varicocele

OBJECTIVES

After mastering the contents of this chapter, you should be able to:

1. State the purposes of health assessment in children of all ages.
2. Identify National Health Goals related to health assessment of children nurses can help the nation achieve.
3. Use critical thinking to analyze ways health assessment skills can be incorporated into nursing care procedures to maintain family centered care.
4. Assess a child and family by health interview, physical examination, and development screening.
5. Formulate nursing diagnoses based on health assessment findings.
6. Identify expected outcomes based on health assessment findings.
7. Plan nursing care based on health assessment findings such as informing parents of health deviations.
8. Implement nursing care such as conducting an age-appropriate health interview or physical examination by modifying techniques based on the child's age.
9. Evaluate expected outcomes for achievement and effectiveness of care.
10. Identify areas related to health assessment of children that could benefit from additional nursing research or application of evidence-based practice.
11. Integrate nursing process with knowledge of health assessment to achieve quality maternal and child health nursing care.

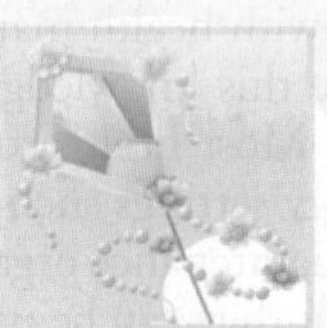

Keoto Wiser is a 13-year-old you meet in an ambulatory clinic. Her father has brought both her and her 2-year-old sister, Candy, for health assessments before Keoto begins seventh grade. Her father is worried Keoto does not see well because she always sits close to the television set. Keoto's mother did not want to bring her for a preschool assessment because she is worried that if glasses are prescribed, her daughter will not be able to play on a school soccer team.

Previous chapters described the normal growth and development of children. This chapter adds information about techniques for assessing the health of children, including history taking, physical examination, related screening procedures for hearing, vision, and development, and immunizations. This information builds a base for care and health teaching for differing age groups throughout childhood.

What questions would you want to ask Keoto? What screening tests for vision would be best for this 13-year-old child? What could you do to help her adjust to wearing glasses, if they are prescribed?

Nursing assessment is not only the first step in the nursing process but also the fundamental means by which health care personnel establish and maintain contact with children and their families. Child health assessment is especially important as an opportunity to provide families with information about health promotion, signs of health and illness, and expected developmental progress in their children. This anticipatory guidance can have a long-lasting positive impact on the health of children and their families.

Effective assessment for the maternal–child population first requires you to be familiar with health maintenance standards and usual findings, because this knowledge is essential to the ability to recognize illness. Most health screening procedures are performed in ambulatory settings such as pediatric clinics, physicians' offices, health maintenance organizations, community clinics, and schools, but they can be used to evaluate children in all settings (Sleeper, Ariza, & Binns, 2009).

Sometimes it is necessary to complete just a partial history or a partial physical examination, such as when a child is referred for vision examination. This chapter, however, covers all aspects of physical examination so that, when necessary, a complete examination can be performed. Assessment procedures specific to particular illnesses are discussed in later chapters with the illness they detect.

Findings and techniques in children differ depending on racial and ethnic characteristics. Whether people establish eye contact with an interviewer, for example, is a characteristic that is culturally determined. Assessing for cyanosis, as another example, is more difficult in dark-skinned than in fair-skinned children (mucous membrane is the best place to detect this). Because height and weight charts are standardized on middle-class white children, measurements of children who do not fit this description may not plot well on these charts. In Vietnam, touching the head of a child during physical assessment is thought to be harmful because the head is considered to be the seat of the soul.

Recognizing that people hold differing cultural expectations and characteristics such as these can help in establishing rapport with children and their families and help make health assessment more meaningful.

Some cultures are much more aware of the role of communicable disease in childhood illnesses than others and so advocate for all children to be immunized against these disorders. Even if awareness about the danger of disease spread exists, however, it does not mean all people in a community are conscientious about having their children immunized. Other factors such as cost and convenience and ethical beliefs are also important.

Some religious groups, such as the Amish, do not encourage immunizations. In these communities, the prevalence of illnesses such as measles can rise to high numbers. Being aware that immunization rates are not consistent from place to place aids in understanding the importance of planning health education and health surveillance based on individual community needs. Box 34.1 lists National Health Goals related to health assessment in children.

BOX 34.1 ✻ Focus on National Health Goals

A number of National Health Goals relate directly to health assessment of children. These are:

- Increase the proportion of territories and states that have service systems for children with special health care needs from a baseline of 15% to a target of 100%.
- Increase the proportion of children and youth, 17 years of age and younger, who have a specific source of ongoing care from a baseline of 93% to a target of 97%.
- Achieve and maintain effective vaccination coverage levels for universally recommended vaccines among young children from baselines of 84% (DTaP); 87% (hepatitis B); 91% (polio); 43% (varicella); and 92% (MMR) to an overall target level of 90% (http://www.nih.gov).

Nurses can help the nation achieve these goals by participating actively in health assessment and conscientiously screening for and administering vaccines. Nursing research that might add more information in this area would include techniques that can be used to orient preschoolers quickly to a health care setting, effective techniques for eliciting health interview information from adolescents, and methods to help parents better record or remember what immunizations their children have received.

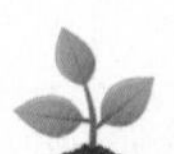

Nursing Process Overview

For Health Assessment of the Child and Family

Assessment

Health assessment of children can be a positive, educational experience for a child and family if time is taken to listen carefully to the family's concerns and responses to questions. Never rush either an interview or a physical examination. Be sure children have time to familiarize themselves with the environment and equipment that will be used.

Obtaining health histories and performing physical examinations can be done independently or as part of a total preventive health care program for a child. The recommendations for standard preventive pediatric health care for the United States are shown in Table 34.1.

Nursing Diagnosis

Health assessment provides the data used to identify potential problems and serves as the basis for the establishment of nursing diagnoses. Be certain not to overlook diagnoses that accentuate the healthy functioning of a child and family, even when diagnoses that address specific problems have been identified. These wellness diagnoses are crucial components of the entire assessment picture and often provide an avenue for addressing identified problems. For instance, the nursing diagnosis of "Impaired social interaction related to lack of self-esteem secondary to disability" would be appropriate for a 4-year-old child who ambulates by wheelchair who, according to the parents, feels uncomfortable around other children.

If the parents have difficulty adapting to their child's disability but are eager to accept advice from health care experts on how to provide the most stimulating environment for their child, the diagnosis "Readiness for enhanced family coping" would also be appropriate. Using both these diagnoses allows the development of a plan of care that takes the best advantage of this family's strengths.

Outcome Identification and Planning

Health promotion and illness prevention are vital parts of outcome identification following health assessment. Helping parents plan for their child's next developmental stage or keeping them aware of important safety measures and other ways to keep children well are also important. Remind them about immunizations needed in the future and be certain they know when to schedule the next health visit. A current immunization schedule is always available at the Centers for Disease Control and Prevention (CDC) Web site (http://www.CDC.gov). Growth charts for children are available at both the CDC (http://www.CDC.gov/growthcharts) and the World Health Organization (http://www.WHO.int/childgrowth) Web sites.

Implementation

Health interviewing and physical examination both require a great deal of skill, skill that can be perfected only through practice. To perfect skills and judgment with children of different ages, take advantage of every opportunity to practice interviewing and physical examination techniques.

Outcome Evaluation

Health assessment of children is an ongoing process that does not end when the first database is obtained. Data must be added at all future interactions so the database remains current and meaningful. Examples suggesting that expected outcomes have been achieved would include:

- Parents state after health examination that they are satisfied with child's motor development.
- Child states after Snellen test that she is aware her vision needs correction.
- Parents state they will continue to assess child's growth by weighing child weekly.

HEALTH HISTORY: ESTABLISHING A DATABASE

The assessment of a young child begins with an interview of the child's parents. An adolescent or preadolescent may choose to be interviewed without the parents present, although many preadolescents and adolescents still prefer to have a parent with them for support.

The purpose of a health interview is to gather information that will direct physical or laboratory examinations to complete a thorough health evaluation. An extensive interview elicits facts such as parental problems in childrearing or detection of future health problems. It lays a foundation for health education and health promotion. Important principles of child health interviewing include the interview setting, the types of questions asked, and the type of information collected.

Interview Setting

An interview is best conducted in a private room with all parties seated comfortably; if not seated, a health care provider appears rushed and cannot interact at eye level. During the interview, call the parents by their names. This lets them know their input and opinions about how their child is developing are valued. A question such as, "Does Candy speak in sentences yet, Mr. Wiser?" is far more personal and a better form than, "Does your baby sit up yet?" As children grow, they are able to answer questions directly.

Types of Questions Asked

The phrasing of questions varies depending on the type of answer desired. Closed-ended and open-ended questions are two types of effective questions; compound, expansive, and leading questions, on the other hand, are three types of questions to avoid.

Closed-Ended Question

This simplest form of question asks directly for a fact: "Does Candy walk yet?" "Did you take Candy's temperature?" This is an effective type of question if a particular point is being sought. It is limited in scope, however, because the response usually will be only a yes or no, with no further elaboration.

Open-Ended Question

An open-ended question allows a parent to elaborate. In contrast to a closed-ended question like "Did you take Candy's temperature?" the question "What did you do for Candy?" is open-ended. The parent answers with a listing of all the things he did: took Candy's temperature, had her lie on the couch, gave her extra fluid, and so on. It is important to ask open-ended questions with school-age children and adolescents so they are encouraged to describe a problem fully.

Compound Question

Compound questions are confusing and should be avoided because the information they elicit is often inaccurate and must be followed by a clarifying question. An example is, "Did Candy have nausea and vomiting?" The parent answers yes, but it still is not known whether Candy had vomiting and nausea, just vomiting, or just nausea.

Expansive Question

This is an open-ended question gone wrong because it is too vague to answer. "What can you tell me about Candy?" leaves a parent wondering where to start. "How has Candy been since her last visit?" limits the question and makes it answerable.

Leading Question

A leading question supplies its own answer so also should be avoided. "Candy has had all her immunizations, hasn't she?" implies that Candy should have had them and perhaps the parent is a poor caregiver if he answers that question any way

(text continues on page 953)

TABLE 34.1 ✻ Recommendations for Preventive Pediatric Health Care

Each child and family is unique; therefore, these **Recommendations for Preventive Pediatric Health Care** are designed for the care of children who are receiving competent parenting, have no manifestations of any important health problems, and are growing and developing in satisfactory fashion. **Additional visits may become necessary** if circumstances suggest variations from normal.

Developmental, psychosocial, and chronic disease issues for children and adolescents may require frequent counseling and treatment visits separate from preventive care visits.

These guidelines represent a consensus by the American Academy of Pediatrics (AAP) and Bright Futures. The AAP continues to emphasize the great importance of **continuity of care** in comprehensive health supervision and the need to avoid **fragmentation of care.**

The recommendations in this statement do not indicate an exclusive course of treatment or standard of medical care. Variations, taking into account individual circumstances, may be appropriate.

	INFANCY								EARLY CHILDHOOD						
Age[a]	**Prenatal[b]**	**Newborn[c]**	**3–5[d]**	**By 1 mo**	**2 mo**	**4 mo**	**6 mo**	**9 mo**	**12 mo**	**15 mo**	**18 mo**	**24 mo**	**30 mo**	**3 y**	**4 y**
HISTORY															
Initial/interval	•	•	•	•	•	•	•	•	•	•	•	•	•	•	•
MEASUREMENTS															
Length/height and weight		•	•	•	•	•	•	•	•	•	•	•	•	•	•
Head circumference		•	•	•	•	•	•	•	•	•	•	•			
Weight for length		•	•	•	•	•	•	•	•	•	•				
Body mass index												•	•	•	•
Blood pressure[e]		★	★	★	★	★	★	★	★	★	★	★	★	•	•
SENSORY SCREENING															
Vision		★	★	★	★	★	★	★	★	★	★	★	★	•[f]	•
Hearing		•[g]	★	★	★	★	★	★	★	★	★	★	★	★	•
DEVELOPMENTAL/ BEHAVIORAL ASSESSMENT															
Developmental screening[h]								•			•		•		
Autism screening[i]											•	•			
Developmental surveillance[h]		•	•	•	•	•	•		•	•		•		•	•
Psychosocial/behavioral assessment		•	•	•	•	•	•	•	•	•	•	•	•	•	•
Alcohol and drug use assessment															
PHYSICAL EXAMINATION[j]		•	•	•	•	•	•	•	•	•	•	•	•	•	•
PROCEDURES[k]															
Newborn metabolic/ hemoglobin screening[l]		←	•	→	→										
Immunization[m]		•	•	•	•	•	•	•	•	•	•	•	•	•	•
Hematocrit or hemoglobin[n]						★			•		★	★		★	★
Lead screening[o]							★	★	•or★[p]		★	•or★[p]		★	★
Tuberculin test[q]				★			★		★		★	★		★	★
Dyslipidemia screening[r]												★			★
STI screening[s]															
Cervical dysplasia screening[t]															
ORAL HEALTH[u]							★	★	•or★[u]		•or★[u]	•or★[u]	•or★[u]	•[v]	
ANTICIPATORY GUIDANCE[w]	•	•	•	•	•	•	•	•	•	•	•	•	•	•	•

	MIDDLE CHILDHOOD						ADOLESCENCE										
Age[a]	5 y	6 y	7 y	8 y	9 y	10 y	11 y	12 y	13 y	14 y	15 y	16 y	17 y	18 y	19 y	20 y	21 y
HISTORY																	
Initial/interval	•	•	•	•	•	•	•	•	•	•	•	•	•	•	•	•	•
MEASUREMENTS																	
Length/height and weight	•	•	•	•	•	•	•	•	•	•	•	•		•	•	•	•
Head circumference																	
Weight for length																	
Body mass index	•	•	•	•	•	•	•	•	•	•	•	•	•	•	•	•	•
Blood pressure[e]	•	•	•	•	•	•	•	•	•	•	•	•	•	•	•	•	•
SENSORY SCREENING																	
Vision	•	•	★	•	★	•	★	•	★	★	•	★	★	•	★	★	★
Hearing	•	•	★	•	★	•	★	★	★	★	★	★	★	★	★	★	★
DEVELOPMENTAL/ BEHAVIORAL ASSESSMENT																	
Developmental screening[h]																	
Autism screening[i]																	
Developmental surveillance[h]	•	•	•	•	•	•	•	•	•	•	•	•	•	•	•	•	•
Psychosocial/behavioral assessment	•	•	•	•	•	•	•	•	•	•	•	•	•	•	•	•	•
Alcohol and drug use assessment							★	★	★	★	★	★	★	★	★	★	★
PHYSICAL EXAMINATION[j]	•	•	•	•	•	•	•	•	•	•	•	•	•	•	•	•	•
PROCEDURES[k]																	
Newborn metabolic/ hemoglobin screening[l]																	
Immunization[m]	•	•	•	•	•	•	•	•	•	•	•	•	•	•	•	•	•
Hematocrit or hemoglobin[n]	★	★	★	★	★	★	★	★	★	★	★	★	★	★	★	★	★
Lead screening[o]	★	★															
Tuberculin test[q]	★	★	★	★	★	★	★	★	★	★	★	★	★	★	★	★	★
Dyslipidemia screening[r]		★		★		★	★	★	★	★	★	★	★	←	—	•	→
STI screening[s]							★	★	★	★	★	★	★	★	★	★	★
Cervical dysplasia screening[t]							★	★	★	★	★	★	★	★	★	★	★
ORAL HEALTH[u]		•[v]															
ANTICIPATORY GUIDANCE[w]	•	•	•	•	•	•	•	•	•	•	•	•	•	•	•	•	•

• = to be performed ★ = risk assessment to be performed, with appropriate action to follow, if positive ← • → = range during which a service may be provided, with the symbol indicating the preferred age

[a] If a child comes under care for the first time at any point on the schedule, or if any items are not accomplished at the suggested age, the schedule should be brought up to date at the earliest possible time.

[b] A prenatal visit is recommended for parents who are at high risk, for first-time parents, and for those who request a conference. The prenatal visit should include anticipatory guidance, pertinent medical history, and a discussion of benefits of breastfeeding and planned method of feeding per AAP statement "The Prenatal Visit" (2001) [URL: http://aappolicy.aappublications.org/cgi/content/full/pediatrics;107/6/1456].

[c] Every infant should have a newborn evaluation after birth, breastfeeding encouraged, and instruction and support offered.

[d] Every infant should have an evaluation within 3 to 5 days of birth and within 48 to 72 hours after discharge from the hospital, to include evaluation for feeding and jaundice. Breastfeeding infants should receive formal breastfeeding evaluation, encouragement, and instruction as recommended in AAP statement "Breastfeeding and the Use of Human Milk" (2005) [URL: http://aappolicy.aappublications.org/cgi/content/full/pediatrics;115/2/496]. For newborns discharged in less than 48 hours after delivery, the infant must be examined within 48 hours of discharge per AAP statement "Hospital Stay for Healthy Term Newborns" (2004) [URL: http://aappolicy.aappublications.org/cgi/ content/full/ pediatrics;113/5/1434].

[e] Blood pressure measurement in infants and children with specific risk conditions should be performed at visits before age 3 years.

[f] If the patient is uncooperative, rescreen within 6 months per AAP statement "Eye Examination and Vision Screening in Infants, Children, and Young Adults" (1996) [URL: http://aappolicy.aappublications.org/ cgi/reprint/ pediatrics;98/1/153.pdf].

(continued)

TABLE 34.1 * Recommendations for Preventive Pediatric Health Care (continued)

[g] All newborns should be screened per AAP statement "Year 2000 Position Statement: Principles and Guidelines for Early Hearing Detection and Intervention Programs" (2000) [URL: http://aappolicy.aappublications.org/cgi/content/full/pediatrics;106/4/798]. Joint Committee on Infant Hearing. Year 2007 position statement: principles and guidelines for early hearing detection and intervention programs. *Pediatrics.* 2007;120:898–921.

[h] AAP Council on Children With Disabilities, AAP Section on Developmental Behavioral Pediatrics, AAP Bright Futures Steering Committee, AAP Medical Home Initiatives for Children With Special Needs Project Advisory Committee. Identifying infants and young children with developmental disorders in the medical home: an algorithm for developmental surveillance and screening. *Pediatrics.* 2006;118:405–420 [URL: http://aappolicy.aappublications.org/cgi/content/full/pediatrics;118/1/405].

[i] Gupta VB, Hyman SL, Johnson CP, et al. Identifying children with autism early? *Pediatrics.* 2007;119:152–153 [URL: http://pediatrics.aappublications.org/cgi/content/full/119/1/152].

[j] At each visit, age-appropriate physical examination is essential, with infant totally unclothed, older child undressed and suitably draped.

[k] These may be modified, depending on entry point into schedule and individual need.

[l] Newborn metabolic and hemoglobinopathy screening should be done according to state law. Results should be reviewed at visits and appropriate retesting or referral done as needed.

[m] Schedules per the Committee on Infectious Diseases, published annually in the January issue of *Pediatrics.* Every visit should be an opportunity to update and complete a child's immunizations.

[n] See AAP *Pediatric Nutrition Handbook,* 5th Edition (2003) for a discussion of universal and selective screening options. See also Recommendations to prevent and control iron deficiency in the United States. *MMWR Recomm Rep.* 1998;47(RR-3):1–36.

[o] For children at risk of lead exposure, consult the AAP statement "Lead Exposure in Children: Prevention, Detection, and Management" (2005) [URL: http://aappolicy.aappublications.org/cgi/content/full/pediatrics;116/4/1036]. Additionally, screening should be done in accordance with state law where applicable.

[p] Perform risk assessments or screens as appropriate, based on universal screening requirements for patients with Medicaid or high prevalence areas.

[q] Tuberculosis testing per recommendations of the Committee on Infectious Diseases, published in the current edition of *Red Book: Report of the Committee on Infectious Diseases.* Testing should be done on recognition of high-risk factors.

[r] "Third Report of the National Cholesterol Education Program (NCEP) Expert Panel on Detection, Evaluation, and Treatment of High Blood Cholesterol in Adults (Adult Treatment Panel III) Final Report" (2002) [URL: http://circ.ahajournals.org/cgi/content/full/106/25/3143] and "The Expert Committee Recommendations on the Assessment, Prevention, and Treatment of Child and Adolescent Overweight and Obesity." Supplement to *Pediatrics.* In press.

[s] All sexually active patients should be screened for sexually transmitted infections (STIs).

[t] All sexually active girls should have screening for cervical dysplasia as part of a pelvic examination beginning within 3 years of onset of sexual activity or age 21 (whichever comes first).

[u] Referral to dental home, if available. Otherwise, administer oral health risk assessment. If the primary water source is deficient in fluoride, consider oral fluoride supplementation.

[v] At the visits for 3 years and 6 years of age, it should be determined whether the patient has a dental home. If the patient does not have a dental home, a referral should be made to one. If the primary water source is deficient in fluoride, consider oral fluoride supplementation.

[w] Refer to the specific guidance by age as listed in Bright Futures Guidelines. (Hagan JF, Shaw JS, Duncan PM, eds. *Bright Futures: Guidelines for Health Supervision of Infants, Children, and Adolescents.* 3rd ed. Elk Grove Village, IL: American Academy of Pediatrics; 2008.)

but yes. The penalty for such an exchange could be a child left vulnerable to disease.

Categories of a Health Interview

Data gathering for an initial health assessment can be divided into nine categories, which are all discussed later and in sequence. At return visits, the categories used generally include only introduction and explanation, chief concern, health and family profile, interval history, and day history.

While conducting a health interview, be certain to make a transition statement before shifting from one section of an interview to another. Without a transition, a parent can be left wondering what is the importance of the next question, possibly misinterpreting its significance. For instance, if a parent has been providing information on the family's hospital insurance policy and, without a transition statement, is asked whether the child has been vomiting, a parent may think the interviewer believes the child needs hospitalization when that is not the intent at all. A statement such as, "Before we talk about Candy's current symptoms, let me ask you some general questions about your family as a whole," is an example of a good transition statement.

Introduction and Explanation

As a matter of courtesy, parents and a child should be told to whom they are talking and what topics they will be discussing. "Hello, Ms. Wiser, I'm Janet Dickson, a nurse here in the One-Day Surgery Department. I'd like to talk to you about Candy" is an example of a suitable introduction. Because some families have never had the benefit of in-depth health care, it is also helpful to include a statement about the subjects that will be discussed during the interview. For example, "So that I can get a picture of Candy's overall health, I'd like to ask you questions about why you've brought her here today, your pregnancy with her, concerns you've had in the past, and questions about your typical day with Candy," would be appropriate. Hearing that, parents begin to concentrate on those areas because they realize health care providers in this setting are interested not just in Candy's health this particular day but in her total health.

Demographic Data

To begin collecting demographic data, obtain a child's name, address, gender, and the name of the person who will be providing information. To provide culturally competent care and make provisions for special needs, a child's culture, ethnicity, place of birth, religious or spiritual practices, and primary and secondary language should also be identified. Ask if the child has a Social Security number.

Be certain to identify the child's primary caregiver. If the parents are divorced or deceased, it is especially important to identify who has custody of the child and who has the right to sign a consent for health care.

Chief Concern

After gathering demographic data, begin data collection with the reason the parents have brought the child to the health care agency: the **chief concern.** This is what parents are most anxious to discuss, so it is important they get this immediate concern off their mind early in the interview. An effective way to elicit this information is to ask an open-ended question such as, "Why did you bring Candy to the clinic today, Ms. Wiser?" Such an opening allows the parent freedom to answer in a number of areas of concern: physical, emotional, nutritional, and developmental. If asked, "How is Candy feeling today?" or "Is Candy ill?" a parent is left to think about only physical aspects and may not voice the biggest concern: Candy's teething difficulty or frequent temper tantrums. For more details on eliciting information about children's chief concern, see Box 34.2. Record a Chief Concern in the child's record exactly as it is stated ("He has constant headaches," not, "Headache") as the parent's description often reveals not only information about a disease condition but also the depth of the parent's concern about the symptom (Geller, 2007).

History of Chief Concern

Once a parent has voiced a chief concern, ask him or her to describe at least six aspects of the problem, including duration, intensity, frequency, description, associated symptoms, and actions taken.

In discussing *duration,* determine when children were last well to determine when they became ill. For example, on Saturday morning, Candy began having long crying periods. On Monday night, she developed a fever. On Tuesday afternoon, her mother brought her into the clinic for a checkup. The parent states Candy vomited three times Monday morning and thinks this was caused by teething. Unless the parent is asked when Candy was last well, she may pinpoint Monday as the beginning of the illness (the vomiting) when actually it was Saturday (the crying).

In this example, the *intensity* of the illness refers to the kind of vomiting the child is having. Is it drooling, spitting up, or actual vomiting? *Frequency* refers to how often the vomiting occurs throughout the duration of the illness. The *description* is the amount (a cupful? a mouthful?) and color (whether it contains blood, bile, or mucus). *Associated symptoms* might include fever, abdominal pain, difficulty eating, or signs of respiratory illness. A good question to use to obtain this information is, "Is Candy ill in any other way?"

Knowing the parent's *actions* can be important for a number of reasons. First, it helps to know whether anything a parent has been doing such as offering a great deal of fluid to replace that vomited and by doing so causing more vomiting or using a home remedy or alternative therapy that actually induces vomiting could have made the illness worse. The parent's actions also reveal what the parent has previously tried but found ineffective. Telling a parent to give a child 2 tablets of acetaminophen (Tylenol) every 4 hours for fever if the parent has already done that and the fever has not improved would be unproductive. This information also reveals the parent's response to caring for an ill child. A parent who says, "I tucked her into bed and gave her a little tea to drink" is different from one who replies, "Nothing. I fall apart when my child is ill." If the child is going to return home under the parents' care, the second set of parents in the example need more instructions and support before they leave the health care setting than the first parent.

Obtaining information about the chief concern also puts the parent's observations in proper perspective. In the previous example, the parent is probably not describing

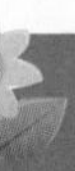

BOX 34.2 * Focus on Communication

You see Keoto at another time at an ambulatory clinic because she has frequency and burning on urination. Her mother accompanies her for the visit.

Less Effective Communication

Nurse: Hello, Keoto. What's the reason you've come into the clinic today?
Mrs. Wiser: It hurts when she urinates.
Nurse: How long ago did that start, Keoto?
Mrs. Wiser: She started complaining about it yesterday.
Nurse: Has she had any blood in her urine?
Mrs. Wiser: She hasn't said anything about that. The important thing is the pain.
Nurse: Okay. I'm sure we need a urine specimen for culture. Let's get that to get started here.

More Effective Communication

Nurse: Hello, Keoto. What's the reason you've come into the clinic today?
Mrs. Wiser: It hurts when she urinates.
Nurse: Let's let Keoto answer for herself, Mrs. Wiser. Tell me what you think is the problem, Keoto.
Keoto: It hurts when I go to the bathroom.
Nurse: How long ago did that start, Keoto?
Mrs. Wiser: She started complaining about it yesterday.
Nurse: Keoto, when do *you* think it started?
Keoto: About an hour after I came in from my date last night.
Nurse: Have you had any blood in your urine?
Mrs. Wiser: She hasn't said anything about that.
Nurse: Keoto, have you noticed your urine is red or dark brown?
Keoto: I had bright blood last night.
Nurse: Let me take you down to the lavatory and explain about a urine specimen. While we're there, I'd like to ask you some more questions about last night.

At about 10 years of age, children are able to supply much of a health history by themselves. As children become teenagers, it is increasingly important for them to do this because they may not have shared a total history with a parent. In the above scenario, for example, when the child is asked directly for information, she supplied more than when her history was given by the mother. Some urinary tract infections occur in girls after their first sexual relations. It would be important to ask Keoto if she is sexually active (what her date last night included), not only to document the probable cause of the urinary tract infection but also to be certain she is knowledgeable about pregnancy prevention and safer sex practices.

teething difficulty (teething does not cause vomiting); more likely, the child has a viral gastroenteritis. Unless the problem is investigated, it is easy to accept the parent's statement at face value as a teething problem without appreciating its full significance.

During this phase of the interview, it is also important to gather information about related or other health concerns. After the chief concern is documented, ask another open-ended question to elicit additional information: "Is there anything else that worries you about Candy?" Now the parent might want to talk about Candy's temper tantrums. Unless asked about a second problem, a parent can go home with the first problem cared for but the second one still not addressed. When the parent arrives home and Candy begins stomping her feet in the car, unwilling to go into the house, the parent will feel that the health care Candy received was less than adequate because she did not receive help with this concern.

Do not assume parents will always reveal their most important concern in the initial minute of an interview: discussing certain symptoms such as constipation can be embarrassing for parents (Bisanz, 2007). It also can be frightening to put a fear a child has a serious illness into words. As long as a concern hangs as a nebulous thought in the mind, it is easy to tell oneself it may not be true. Only when a parent voices the thought ("Do you think Candy is retarded?" "Do you think this is leukemia?" "Could this be inherited?") does the fear become real. Before parents dare to speak openly this way, they must trust health care providers not to treat their statement lightly. For this reason, it is helpful to repeat the question about a second concern once more at the very end of the interview.

Health and Family Profile

Before pursuing the past history or development of a child, document the circumstances in which the child lives. A good introduction to a health and family profile is a sentence such as, "Before we talk about any past illnesses or happenings with Candy, let me ask you some questions about her health and your family as a whole."

Important information concerning a child's current health status includes:

- Who is the child's primary health care provider?
- How often is the child seen for routine health examinations?
- Are the child's immunizations up to date?
- What is the child's general state of health? How does it compare to the child's health 1 and 5 years ago (if appropriate)?
- Does the child have any known allergies?
- Does the child have a chronic illness or disability?
- Is the child taking any prescription medications? Over-the-counter medications? Home or folk remedies, such as herbal remedies?
- Is the child undergoing any treatments?

Important information concerning the family includes:

- Is the parent married, single, or divorced?
- Is the family nuclear or extended?
- How many children are in the family?
- What are the family's current living arrangements?
- What are the parents' occupations? (This helps establish the family's socioeconomic level, and time available for child care.)
- If both parents work, how do they manage child care?

Obtaining a health and family profile is sometimes delayed by medical interviewers until the end of the interview, when, theoretically, a parent or child is more comfortable and will answer these personal questions more readily. However, by following a nursing model and obtaining the information earlier in the interview, the health care practitioner can better assess the child and evaluate data.

Day History

The child's current skills, sleep patterns, hygiene practices, eating habits, and interactions with the family can all be elicited by asking a parent to describe a typical day. Day histories are fun to obtain because most parents are eager to describe their day with their child and information gained this way is surprisingly rich and pertinent, much more so than if parents are just asked how their child sleeps, eats, or plays.

Begin by asking, "Was yesterday a fairly typical day for Candy?" (The parent says yes, it was.) "Describe for me everything Candy did yesterday, beginning with when she first woke up." Some parents offer this information in great detail; with others, it is necessary to backtrack for particular details: "What did she eat for breakfast? Does she use a fork and spoon? Does she sit in a high chair or on your lap?"

Play. Play, the work of children, reveals a great deal about the child's development and overall well-being. Important questions to ask about play include:

- Is Candy kept in a playpen or given room to run?
- What is Candy's favorite toy?
- Does she play active, chasing games or engage in quiet, pretending types of activities?
- Do you (the parent) spend time reading to the child?
- Do you (the parent) play with the child or let the child play alone? (This allows for an estimation of the quality of interaction during the day.)

Sleep. Every child needs adequate rest for healthy growth and development. Poor sleep patterns can often reveal a psychosocial or physical health problem. Important questions regarding sleep include:

- When the child sleeps, how long does she sleep?
- Is falling asleep a problem?
- Where does she sleep? Does she have night terrors?
- Does she sleepwalk?
- Does she wet her bed (depending on whether the child is toilet-trained)?

Hygiene. Good hygiene practices promote healthy teeth, gums, and skin, prevent infections, and improve self-esteem. Poor hygiene may reflect neglect, depression, drug abuse, or poor living conditions. Important questions regarding hygiene include:

- How much self-care does the child do?
- Does the child take baths or showers?
- Does the child brush her teeth? How often? Does she floss regularly? (Responses depend on the age of the child.)
- Does the child wash her hands before snacks and meals?
- Has there been a recent change in hygiene practices?

Nutrition. Nutritional assessment is an important portion of a health assessment because it influences health so strongly (Rolfes, Pinna, & Whitney, 2009). Characteristics of a nutritionally healthy child that can be revealed by assessment are summarized in Table 34.2. Food and nutrient intake risk factors are summarized in Box 34.3.

TABLE 34.2 ✻ Physical Signs of Adequate Nutrition

Assessment	Finding
Overall impression	Alert, with good energy level; positive mood
Hair	Shiny, strong, with good body
Eyes	Good eyesight, particularly at night; conjunctiva moist and pink
Mouth	No cavities in teeth; no swollen or inflamed gingivae; no cracks or fissures at corners of mouth; mucous membrane moist and pink; tongue smooth and nontender
Neck	Normal contour of thyroid gland
Skin	Smooth; normal color and turgor; no ecchymotic or petechial areas present
Extremities	Normal muscle mass and circumference; normal strength and mobility; no edema present; no tender joints; normal reflexes; legs not bowed
Gastrointestinal	No diarrhea or constipation present
Finger and toenails	Smooth, pink; not cracked or broken
Height and weight	Within normal limits on growth chart
Blood pressure	Normal for age

Taking a history of a child's food intake can help determine whether there are any foods missing in a typical meal plan or whether any quantities seem inadequate or excessive. Be certain to assess not only the quantity of food eaten but the quality as well; for example, for the infant, cereal should be iron fortified.

Food intake is best obtained by asking a parent to describe a typical day (24-hour recall), listing what the child ate for each meal and between meals as well. With an older child, the 24-hour recall can be a joint parent–child venture. Providing this history can be difficult when the child consumes some meals at home and others at day care or school. It may be necessary to ask for a weekend history to get a complete picture.

When assessing the adolescent, take a 24-hour recall nutritional history without a parent present, if possible. In front of a parent, adolescents may add nutritional foods to a food intake history or leave out foods they have eaten, such as milkshakes, potato chips, or pizza, to avoid a lecture later; on the other hand, they may leave out healthy items or add less desirable ones because they may enjoy the obvious parental disapproval, indicative of their rebellion against adult authority.

BOX 34.3 ✻ Food and Nutrient Intake Risk Factors

History or evidence of any of the following may pose a potential nutritional risk:

- Intake less or greater than standard for age, calories, protein, or activity
- Intake less or greater than standard for nutrients such as vitamins and minerals
- Unusual food habits, such as pica, faddism, and meal skipping
- Inappropriate use of supplements (vitamins, minerals, fortified food products)
- A physician's order for NPO or a clear liquid diet for more than 3 days without enteral or parenteral nutrition
- Inadequate transitional feeding, enteral support, or parenteral support
- Minimal or no intake from a major food group
- Fluid intake less than output
- Eating or feeding disorders such as bulimia
- Food allergies
- Restricted diet

After taking a history of a child's food intake, determine whether the child is receiving foods that comply with the recommendations of the food guide pyramid (see Appendix K). If whole food groups are absent or grossly inadequate, follow-up evaluation should include a food frequency record as a double-check to see if the 24-hour recall was truly representative of a usual day. Remember that children do not have to eat food from all groups at every meal, as long as they eat from them every day. If parents think in terms of days rather than meals, it allows them to exert less pressure on a child to eat at each meal.

Be sure to consider the role of food preferences and cultural, lifestyle, and financial variations when assessing food intake. The number of meals eaten at home versus outside the home, the form and content of traditional meals cooked at home, and the pattern of meals should all be considered. Any religious dietary restrictions should also be obtained. Do not appear critical of a child's diet. If you convey dismay at erratic eating habits, parents or older children (especially adolescents) may begin to fabricate a food history to make it seem more acceptable.

Past Health History

For a past health history, ask whether a child has ever had any serious illnesses. Parents do not generally think of childhood diseases such as measles, chickenpox, and mumps as serious illnesses; inquire about these separately. Also inquire about the child's immunization history and whether the immunizations are up to date for the child's age. (See the discussion of immunizations later in this chapter.) Has a child had any accidents (unintentional injuries)? Any surgery? Parents may not think of a tonsillectomy as surgery because there were no stitches; ask about that separately. Did a child ever ingest anything that was inedible or harmful? Has a child been hospitalized for any reason? How many times has a child been seen in an emergency department? These last questions provide information about the degree of adult supervision, and possibly clues to abuse (Riley, 2007).

Information about the outcome of past illnesses is as important to obtain as information about the illnesses themselves. If the child had otitis media (middle ear infection) at age 2 years and received an antibiotic and recovered without complications, the parent has every reason to be confident that the child will get better from a present illness also; the parent has confidence in health care personnel. If the child had an allergic reaction to the antibiotic or was left with a hearing difficulty from the previous illness, parents may distrust the care being given to their child now; they may not follow instructions well, thinking nothing works anyway. Or the parents may need extra support to follow instructions. This is important information for planning care.

When parents report a past health concern or illness, be sure to ask for details of the illness. This can help to minimize inaccurate data and ensure that the present and future care of the child is appropriate. For example, parents might believe their child is allergic to an antibiotic because while the child was taking the drug he developed diarrhea. There is a strong possibility the diarrhea was associated with the reason for taking the antibiotic, not with the drug itself. In this example, you would want to ask about specific symptoms and record what the parent says about allergies so the person who prescribes medication for the child can decide whether a true allergy exists.

The health of children is affected by their mother's health during pregnancy. For children under age 5 years, therefore, a pregnancy history is usually obtained.

Pregnancy History. For a pregnancy history, document which pregnancy this was for the mother. Were there complications in any past pregnancies? Abortions or miscarriages? Stillbirths? Children born prematurely? A history of the pregnancy of the child being assessed can begin with a question such as, "How was your pregnancy with Candy?" This allows the mother to answer in both physical and emotional areas. After exploring details mentioned by the mother, ask about specific events that are known to occur with pregnancy that may have had an effect on a fetus, such as:

- Did the mother have any complications such as bleeding, falls, swelling of hands and feet, high blood pressure, or unusual weight gain?
- Did she take any medication?
- Were any radiographs taken?
- Did she smoke cigarettes, drink alcohol, or use recreational drugs?
- Did the pregnancy end early or late?

Because life contingencies such as loss of finances or illness in the family during a pregnancy may affect a parent's ability to form a bond with a child, the emotional experiences of a woman during pregnancy are also important to obtain. Ask if the parents planned the pregnancy. A question such as, "A lot of pregnancies come as a sort of surprise. Is that how it was with Candy?" or "Some unmarried women want to have children and some don't. How was it with you?" lets parents know you will nonjudgmentally accept any answer they give.

Next, review labor and birth. Questions to ask include:

- How long was labor? Was it what you expected it to be?
- Were there any complications? Was the birth vaginal or cesarean?
- Was anesthesia used for birth?
- Was the baby born vertex (head-first) or breech?

Ask about the health of the child at birth as well. Questions to ask include:

- Did the baby cry right away?
- Did the infant room in or need care in a special nursery?
- Did the infant need special procedures or equipment at birth?
- Was there cyanosis or jaundice?
- Was the infant discharged from the birth setting with the mother?
- How did the parents feel about having a boy or girl?
- How did it feel for them to be new parents?

Family Health History

Because some diseases are inherited or familial, it is important to know which ones occur in a family. Ask if any family member has heart disease (childhood or adult type), kidney disease, a congenital anomaly, seizures, diabetes (type 1 or 2), tuberculosis, a sexually transmitted infection, or allergies or is cognitively challenged.

Review of Systems

The last step in a health interview is a summary of body symptoms or a **review of systems.** Again, make certain to introduce this part of the history with a transition statement; otherwise, parents may think that the local problem (vomiting) they were describing suggests other problems. For example, a statement, such as, "I'd like to ask about different parts of Candy's body, from her head down to her toes, just to be certain I don't miss anything" provides a transition.

Although the important items to be covered in a review of systems differ according to the age of the child, a basic list is shown in Box 34.4.

A review of systems covers a lot of ground, but it generally takes no more than 5 minutes. However, do not rush through the questions so quickly that a parent does not have time to answer or begins to believe this part of the interview is only an unimportant exercise ("Has Candy ever had nausea/vomiting/diarrhea/painful joints/broken bones?") All the questions are important. If a child has any of the symptoms described, an entirely new area needs to be explored.

BOX 34.4 ✻ Review of Systems

The following questions provide a guide when completing a review of systems:

Neuropsychiatric symptoms: Has the child ever had seizures? Head injury? Attention problems? Depression? Aggressive behavior? Has the parent ever had such difficulty rousing the child that the parent believed the child was unconscious? Have there been any problems with suspected substance abuse?

Eyes: Has the child had difficulty with eyes not focusing? Eye infection? Does the parent have any reason to believe that the child does not see well? Does the child wear eyeglasses? Contacts?

Ears: Ear infections? Drainage from the ears? Ear aches? Tubes in ears? Any infection from piercing? Reason to believe the child does not hear well?

Nose: Frequent drainage or cold symptoms? Difficulty breathing? Nosebleeds?

Mouth: Difficulty with teeth or teething? Mouth infections? Has the child seen a dentist (if older than age 2 years)? Does the child chew tobacco?

Throat: Throat infections? Difficulty swallowing?

Neck: Masses or swelling? Stiffness? Does the child hold the head and neck straight? (Torticollis or wry neck will make the child hold the head crookedly; children with poor vision also may cock their heads to the side to try to see better.)

Chest: Is breast development in girls appropriate for age? For adolescent girls over 14 years and Tanner stage V, ask about yearly breast examination.

Lungs: Breathing problems? Infections? Pneumonia? Asthma? Does the child smoke any substance?

Heart: Has a physician ever said there was difficulty? What exactly was said?

GI system: Has there been an eating problem? Frequent nausea? Vomiting? (Ask separately from nausea; children with pyloric stenosis [obstruction of the pyloric opening of the stomach] have vomiting but no nausea; children with a brain tumor may also have vomiting but no nausea; pregnant teenagers may have nausea but not vomiting.) Diarrhea? Any constipation? Is the child toilet-trained? Any difficulty with this?

Genitourinary system: Pain or burning on urination? Blood in urine? Does the child have a good urine stream? If a girl is age 10 years or older, has she started menstruation? Any problems with menstruation? If an adolescent male, has he begun testicular self-examination? If an adolescent, is the child sexually active? Using contraception? Want more information on contraception? Ever had an STI? (To protect privacy, it is essential to ask the adolescent, not the parents, questions regarding sexuality.)

Extremities: Painful or swollen joints? Broken bones? Muscle sprains? Is the parent pleased with the child's coordination?

Skin: Rashes? Lesions such as warts?

Immunizations: What immunizations has the child received to date?

Conclusion

A health history should close with one last open-ended question: "Is there anything more about Candy we should know?" or "Is there anything I didn't mention you want to ask about?" A parent may have been reluctant to bring up something earlier. Asking this final question gives a parent a final opportunity to do this.

✔ Checkpoint Question 34.1

You take a health history on Keoto from her father. What question should you ask at the end of every interview?

a. Do you have a ride so you can get home?
b. Is there anything else you'd like to discuss?
c. Am I a good interviewer? I'm trying hard.
d. Do you have another child who also needs care?

PHYSICAL ASSESSMENT

Mastery of physical examination technique is essential to incorporating physical assessment data into the assessment step of the nursing process, so physical assessment, along with health interviewing, is one of the most frequently practiced skills of a nurse. The scope and extent of pediatric physical assessment vary, like health interviewing, depending on the circumstances of each health visit. Sometimes only a single segment is required to obtain the information needed. For example, if a child has a gastrointestinal disorder, assessment might be only a brief, multisystem examination concentrating on the gastrointestinal system such as mouth, abdomen, and rectum and fluid status (condition of skin turgor, lips, and mucous membranes). At a first health care encounter, however, children usually receive a complete physical examination.

Purpose and Techniques

The actual process of physical examination involves four separate techniques (see also Box 34.5):

Inspection is used to determine whether there is redness or swelling or any break in the skin.
Palpation yields information on warmth and edema.
Percussion helps determine the consistency of tissue beneath the surface.
Auscultation reveals the presence of sound.

These techniques are usually carried out in the above order in each area of the body except the abdomen (auscultation should follow inspection and precede palpation of the abdomen, because handling the abdomen may obliterate bowel sounds). Findings from performing these techniques strengthen or validate history findings and help determine whether a problem requires immediate action (Askin, 2007).

Use physical examination to complement the questions asked when a parent describes some symptom a child is experiencing. If parents say they think their child has pain, for example, ask about the duration, intensity, frequency, associated symptoms, and any action or activity that precipitates the pain. Then examine the area for signs of inflammation and palpate for tenderness.

Effective use of physical assessment skills takes practice. Palpating an abdomen, for example, is a simple procedure; recognizing abdominal pathology through palpation is a more complicated skill. It is difficult to distinguish between normal liver tissue and a distended liver, for example, until both these conditions have been felt many times.

BOX 34.5 ✻ Techniques of Physical Examination

Inspection: Examining a child or adolescent initially with your eyes or nose, being alert to visual indications or odors that may point to a health problem.

Palpation: Examining by touch and can be either light or deep touch. Use light palpation before deep palpation so the child or adolescent does not tense muscles and make light palpation difficult. The tips of your fingers are most sensitive to texture, vibration, consistency, and contour; the back of your hand is most sensitive to warmth. *If a child has a sensitive or painful body part, palpate that area last.* Otherwise, the child may be unwilling to allow you to touch other parts for fear of additional pain.

Percussion: The assessment of a body structure by determining the sound you hear in response to striking the part with an examining finger and then interpreting the sound. Dense body areas such as bone have a dull, flat sound; those filled with air, such as lungs, are resonant. If an organ is stretched (a distended bladder), it has a hyperresonant or low and hollow sound. An organ stretched to an even greater point of distention has a tympanic or extremely hollow, ringing sound.

Auscultation: Listening to sounds that are either discernible to the ear (wheezing or heavy breathing) or, as in most cases, made louder by means of a stethoscope. Always listen for four qualities of sound: duration, frequency, intensity (loudness), and pitch (high or low).

Equipment, Setting, and Approach

When performing a complete physical assessment, you will need the following equipment: a thermometer, a stethoscope, a tongue depressor, an ophthalmoscope, an otoscope, a sphygmomanometer, a tape measure, a tuning fork, a reflex (percussion) hammer, rubber gloves, and perhaps a client drape or gown. Nurses who work in community settings or clients' homes must be sure to carry any equipment that may be needed with them.

Be certain the temperature in an examining room is comfortable, and provide privacy. Change paper table covers between children to avoid possible spread of illness.

During a complete physical examination, every part of the child's body should be exposed for inspection. To protect against chilling and to provide for modesty, expose body parts individually and only for the amount of time necessary for the examination. As examining body parts such as the mouth or an open lesion exposes your hands to body fluids, as part of infection control precautions, wear gloves as appropriate during an examination.

People have the right not to have another person touch their body unless they permit them to do so. It is essential, therefore, to inform children it is necessary to touch them for a physical examination, and tell them what is happening at each step during the examination so they know when they will be touched such as saying, "Next I want to look at your throat." If some action will cause discomfort, such as deep palpation of the abdomen, offer fair warning: "You'll feel pressure for a minute." Such explanations are also psychologically reassuring because they prevent surprises.

Assume that adolescents will cooperate in placing themselves in whatever position is required to inspect body parts unless they are short of breath or in some other way unable to cooperate. Small children may not cooperate as readily and may need to be restrained during an examination of body parts such as the nose, throat, and ears. Proper restraint enables an examiner to see well and also to ensure that the instrument used will not accidentally injure a child. As a rule, do not ask parents to restrain during any procedure in which a child will feel threatened or feel pain; parents are best used as protectors and comforters. Some procedures, such as ear examination, do require a strong restraining hand, and this can be frightening to children. Urge parents to do this with a positive approach such as, "I'll help you keep your head still."

Variations for Age and Developmental Stage

Techniques of physical examination should be tailored to the age and developmental stage of the individual being assessed (Table 34.3). Expected findings also depend on the child's age and developmental stage.

TABLE 34.3 ✻ Techniques of Physical Examination Based on Child's Age

Age	Techniques
Newborn	Undress only the body part being examined or use a radiant heat warmer to conserve heat (be certain all body parts are exposed during examination). Examine heart and respiratory systems first before the newborn cries, then follow head-to-toe procedure, performing all manipulative procedures such as throat and eyes last. Examine newborn with parents present, using this assessment time to teach them about normal appearance and development.
Infant	As with newborns, begin examination with heart and respiratory assessment, then follow head-to-toe procedure, performing all manipulative procedures such as throat and ears last. Begin examination while parent holds infant in arms or lap to calm the child. Talk to the infant as you proceed; infants calm to sound of your voice or the feeling tone that you radiate as much as they do to what you actually say. A positive tone ("This is like a game") therefore often brings better cooperation than a strict, businesslike approach. Infants older than 3 mo like to handle tongue blades. They can be distracted by brightly colored toys while you listen to their heart or lungs. They cooperate best if a parent holds them for major portion of examination. Offering a bottle of water or pacifier may be necessary during heart assessment.
Toddler	Allow toddler to handle equipment; include games, such as blowing out otoscope light, to relax child. Ask parent to remove clothing or allow child to do it independently. Use head-to-toe procedure; leave uncomfortable procedures such as throat and ear examination for last.
Preschooler	Use games such as "Simon Says" to ease child's fright. Ask child to undress; do not remove underpants. Keep in mind that preschoolers are extremely threatened by intrusive procedures. Thus, they are frightened of examining instruments. Allow them to handle instruments before use. Assure them that instruments do not hurt. Children up to school age often need to be restrained for ear and throat examination because they grow fearful about procedures performed on a part of the body they cannot see (ears) or about a throat examination that may be uncomfortable.
School-age child	Ask whether child wants parent present or not. Proceed with head-to-toe assessment; leave genitalia for last. Allow child to undress except for underpants; supply gown. Explain equipment and reasons for procedures. Teach whys and hows of procedures.
Adolescent	Ask if the adolescent wants parent present or not. Teach adolescent about good health care during examination. Comment on body parts as you examine them: "Your heart sounds good," "Ears look fine." Sometimes adolescents are so concerned with a part of their body (a supernumerary nipple, for example) that they are unable to voice this concern. A comment such as, "This is a supernumerary (extra) nipple. Does it ever worry you that you have that?" may help the adolescent to talk about what has indeed been a concern for years. Use head-to-toe procedure; leave genitalia for last. Include health teaching on testicular self-examination.

Newborn

All newborns receive a physical examination immediately after birth and again after the first 24 hours of life. When examining newborns, remember that maintaining body temperature is one of the newborn's most difficult tasks (McCall et al., 2009). Cover body areas that are not being directly examined. Take axillary or tympanic temperatures to prevent rupture of rectal mucosa. Assess the heart rate apically because peripheral pulses may be too faint to be counted accurately. Be certain to take femoral pulses in newborns to rule out coarctation of the aorta. Include newborn reflexes, head circumference, and an assessment of gestational age (see Chapter 18) as routine parts of the examination.

Infant

Infants are usually examined most effectively if a parent holds them during most of the examination. Use an "isn't this fun?" or "this is a game" approach. As a rule, assess heart and lung function first; do intrusive procedures such as ear and throat assessment last so an infant does not cry and complicate the remainder of the examination. Blood pressure is still not taken routinely. Include assessment of newborn reflexes until 6 months of age; continue to take the heart rate apically and the temperature in the axilla or by tympanic membrane. Measure head circumference for a full year.

Toward the end of the first year, children become fearful of strangers. Taking an extra minute to become well acquainted with an infant at the beginning of an examination can help to counteract this problem.

Toddler and Preschooler

Both toddlers and preschoolers may be afraid of examining equipment. To alleviate their fears, let them handle items such as stethoscopes, otoscopes, and blood pressure cuffs before the examination (Fig. 34.1). Leave intrusive procedures such as assessment of the genitalia, ears, and throat until last. Give generous praise for cooperation (anything short of hysterical screaming or kicking is good cooperation for intrusive procedures in this age group). Box 34.6 describes ways parents can prepare children of this age for assessment.

Begin to include blood pressure as part of routine assessment at 3 years of age; taking an oral temperature by an electronic thermometer, rather than a tympanic temperature, can also begin at this age. Before beginning an examination, establish a good rapport with the child's parents, because children this age sense parental trust or suspicion.

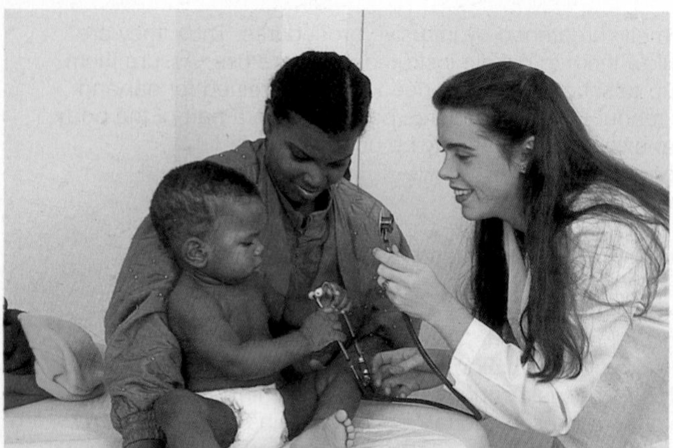

FIGURE 34.1 Children need the opportunity to play with examining equipment so they become more familiar with it and less frightened by it.

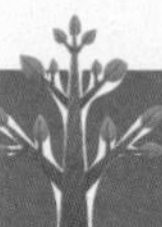

BOX 34.6 * Focus on Family Teaching

Suggestions for Preparing a Child for a Health Assessment

Q. Candy's father asks you, "How can I best prepare my 2-year-old for a preschool health exam?"

A. Here are some suggestions to help prepare a child for a health assessment:

- Promote the attitude that a health visit will be a positive experience.
- Bring a comfort item from home (favorite doll or toy).
- Never threaten the child that if she is not good, a doctor or nurse will punish her.
- Review with your daughter what she can expect during an assessment (a health care provider will ask some questions of her parent; she or he will then look at the child's head, hands, etc.).
- If she has been taught not to let strangers touch her body (as she should have been taught), reassure her that it is all right for the health care provider to examine her.
- Dress your daughter in clothing that is easy to remove and replace so you can dress her quickly after an examination. This is a way of assuring her that the examination is over.

School-Age Child and Adolescent

Some children of this age may still be unaware of what a physical examination includes and whether it will cause discomfort. Offer good explanations so they are not frightened by the unknown. Provide older children with a choice about having a parent with them during the examination. Some may enjoy having a parent with them; others may resent their presence. Adolescents are often worried about some normal physical finding such as a mole or supernumerary (extra) nipple. Make a habit of commenting on such findings—"This is a mole on your hand; that's normal"—as a means of both reassurance and health teaching. Be certain to assess height and weight as more children are obese than ever before. It is increasingly important to take blood pressure beginning in early school age also because as more children are overweight today, more have elevated blood pressure (Chiolero et al., 2007). Obesity in school-age children and adolescents is also associated with the development of type 2 diabetes mellitus and future cardiovascular disorders. There is also an association between overweight and suicide in children (Whetstone, Morrissey, & Cummings, 2007).

School-age children and adolescents are particularly modest. Respect this by careful use of gowns or drapes. Teach testicular self-examination for boys beginning at about age 13. The American Cancer Society (ACS) recommends that women should be taught to perform monthly breast self-examinations when they reach 20 years of age (ACS, 2008).

✔ Checkpoint Question 34.2

Keoto's sister is 2 years old. At what age should you include blood pressure as a routine procedure?

a. 1 year.
b. 2 years.
c. 3 years.
d. 6 years.

Components of Physical Examination

Presented here are the components of a routine or general physical assessment. Physical examination may be done in any order, but traditionally the order proceeds from head to toe, examining each body part thoroughly before moving on to the next. With infants and young children, however, it is easiest to begin with the heart and lungs; this is because if the infant cries, findings in these areas become difficult to assess over the sound of crying.

If abnormalities are discovered during an examination, further assessment will be necessary. A complete neurologic examination, for example, is not routine and so is not included here (see Chapter 49 for details on a neurologic examination). It is important to recognize what a "general" physical examination of this nature entails so you can interpret the extent of assessment a child has received when the parent states, "He had a routine physical."

Vital Sign Assessment

Vital signs refer to temperature, pulse, respiration, blood pressure, and whether the child has pain (the state of vital bodily functions including heart and lung function, metabolic rate, and comfort level). Temperature is an important assessment in children because it can reveal subtle infection that has not as yet become obvious by other signs (Sur & Bukont, 2007). Because of the important information they provide, measurements of these signs are recorded not only with complete physical examinations but in many other instances of care. Techniques of these measurements and the nursing responsibilities that accompany them are discussed in Chapter 37. Remember that blood pressure in children can be elevated if they are anxious in a medical setting the same as happens to adults (Howell et al., 2007).

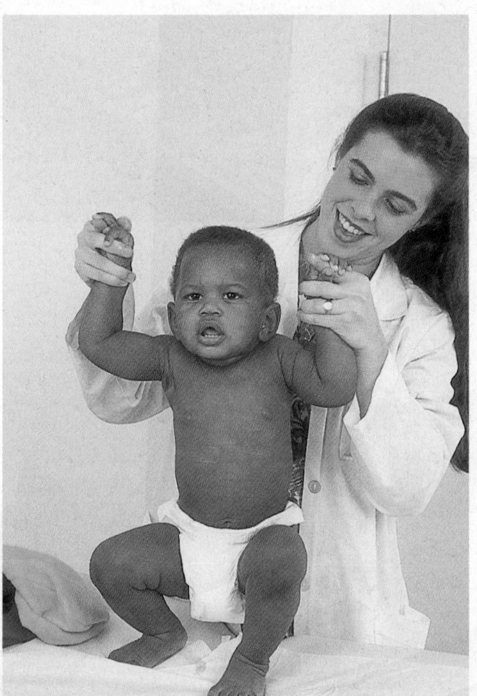

FIGURE 34.2 General appearance assessment reveals that this child is well proportioned and active.

General Appearance

Physical examination begins with inspection of general appearance to form an overall impression of a child's health and well-being and to pinpoint specific body areas that will need detailed assessment (Fig. 34.2 and Box 34.7). Assess such areas as:

- Does the child appear well or ill overall?
- Is the child's height and weight proportional?

Box 34.7 Assessment
Assessing the Child Overview

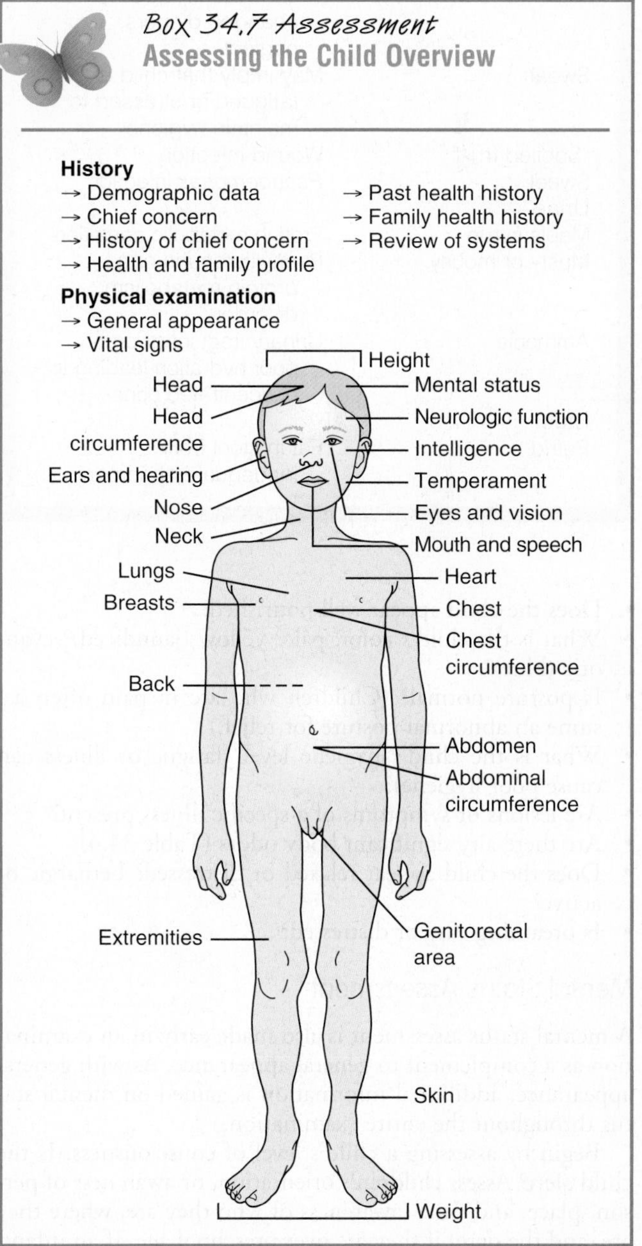

TABLE 34.4 ✻ Significant Body Odors

Source of Odor	Possible Cause
Breath	
Alcohol	Possible recent ingestion (important if coma or neurologic symptoms are present as cause of abnormal functioning)
Camphor	Mothball ingestion
Halitosis (bad breath)	Poor dental hygiene, lung infection; foreign body in respiratory tract
Burnt rope	Marijuana use
Sweet	Acidosis (seen in a child in diabetic coma)
Body	
Stale urine	Incontinence; poor kidney functioning leading to uremia; infrequently changed diapers; neglect
Sweat	May imply that child is too fatigued or stressed to maintain hygiene
"Spoiled fruit"	Wound infection
Sweet	*Pseudomonas* infection
Urine	
Maple syrup	Protein metabolic condition
Musty or mousy	Phenylketonuria or a protein metabolism disorder
Ammonia	Urinary tract infection or poor hydration leading to concentrated urine
Stool	
Putrid	Fat in stool from inadequate absorption

- Does the child appear well nourished?
- What is the child's color: pale? yellow (jaundiced)? cyanotic (blue)?
- Is posture normal? (Children who are in pain often assume an abnormal posture for relief.)
- What is the child's hygiene level (fatigue or illness can cause poor hygiene)?
- Are lesions or symptoms of a specific illness present?
- Are there any significant body odors (Table 34.4)?
- Does the child appear relaxed or distressed? Lethargic or active?
- Is breathing easy or distressed?

Mental Status Assessment

A mental status assessment is also made early in an examination as a complement to general appearance. As with general appearance, additional information is gained on mental status throughout the entire examination.

Begin by assessing a child's level of consciousness: Is the child alert? Assess children's orientation, or awareness of person, place, and time (awareness of who they are, where they are, and the date) if they are over preschool age. If an infant, does the child "attune" or look aware of surroundings? Assess the appropriateness of behavior and mood: for example, is a child hostile, frightened, or relaxed? At some point in the examination of children above preschool age, ask questions that test recent memory (what they ate for breakfast) and distant memory (who was their first-grade teacher).

Body Measurements

Body measurements are important determinants of health in children because with chronic illness the body expends so many nutrients combating the destructive process of the disease that normal height and weight cannot be maintained. Conversely, overweight (obesity) can lead to illnesses such as heart and lung disease later in life. Obesity has become such a health problem that it is considered an epidemic in many parts of the United States (Singhal, Schwenk, & Kumar, 2007).

Weight and Height. In children, both height and weight are good determinants of health and normal nutrition. Until they can stand well, infants are weighed laying or sitting on an infant scale. Because diapers can be heavy in proportion to total body weight, weigh infants nude. Always keep a protective hand over an infant on an infant scale (hovering but not touching), as infants squirm readily and there is danger of them falling. Always cover scales with scale paper before weighing to prevent spread of infection from one child to another (Fig. 34.3).

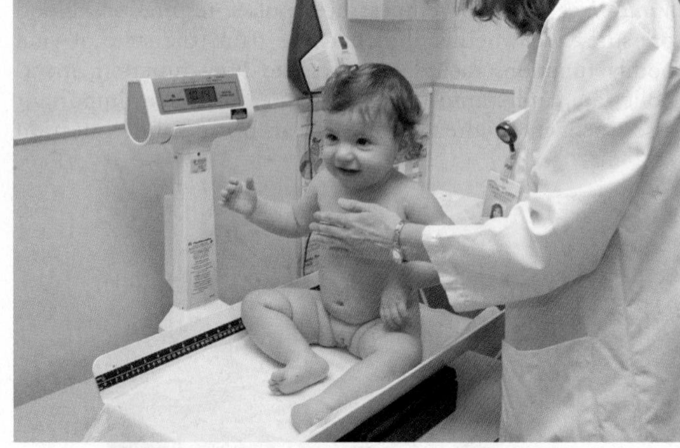

A

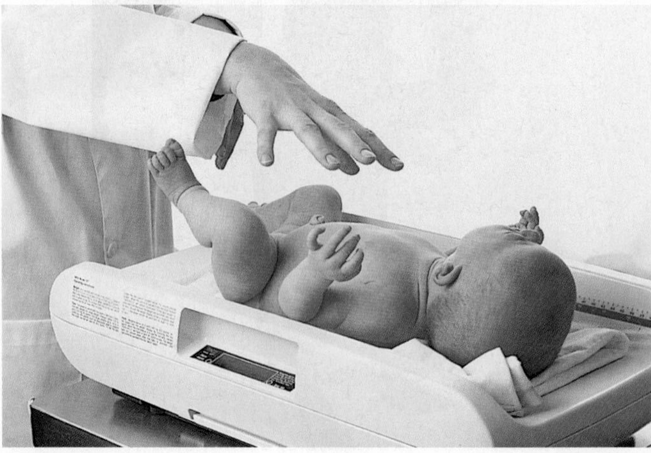

B

FIGURE 34.3 A nurse or caregiver should remain nearby while weighing the infant or toddler.

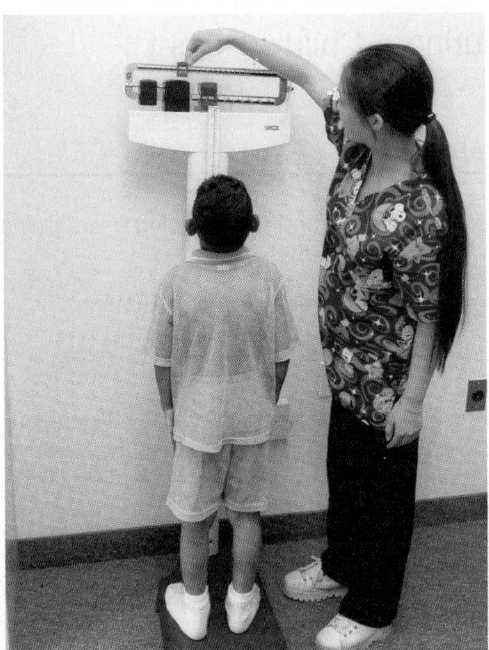

FIGURE 34.4 Children who can stand independently can be weighed on a regular standing balance scale.

Children older than age 2 years are weighed on standing scales, in street clothes (no shoes), or, if in a hospital, in a gown or pajamas (see Fig. 34.4). If children are going to have serial weights (weighed every day), be sure they wear the same clothing every time they are weighed so any discrepancy in weight is truly a difference in body weight and not a weight change as the result of more or less clothing. Take the weight at the same time each day (preferably before breakfast) on the same scale for greatest accuracy.

Most children and their parents want to know their weight. To convert from kilograms to pounds, multiply the kilogram amount by 2.2 (50 kg × 2.2 = 110 lb).

For accurate measurement of height for infants and older children, see Box 34.8. Plot height measurements for children on a standard graph, the same as for weight. Height and weight should follow the same percentiles. Remember that height/weight charts have been standardized for middle-class white American children, so there will be variations among children from different cultural backgrounds. The important thing to look for is consistency of measurements over time (always at the same percentile).

To assess whether weight is average for height, compare the child's weight with a standardized height/weight graph (Appendix E). In the standardized scale for children, all weights between the 10th and 90th percentiles are considered normal (statistically, a range of weights that includes two standard deviations from the mean or the 50th percentile). All children with weight below the 25th or above the 75th percentiles need close examination as they are moving close to the end points of the usual weight continuum (Chumlea, 2007).

As important as the fact that children's weight falls between the 10th and 90th percentile on growth charts is that over time the weight follows one of the percentile curves—in other words, children are not at the 80th percentile the first time they are weighed and a month later at the 40th percentile. Although both readings are within the normal range, they reflect a weight loss that would need investigation. Gaining weight in the same way could be equally serious. A child is defined as "failing to thrive" if height or weight drops below the third percentile on a standardized growth chart (Black et al., 2007). Any height or weight in this category definitely needs to be reported so its cause can be investigated.

U.S. growth charts were compiled by the CDC in the 1960s when almost all infants were formula fed, not breastfed, so breastfed infants tend to score lower on these charts (often at the 25th percentile) than might be expected. The World Health Organization has published growth charts that better reflect the weight of breastfed infants. It can be helpful to plot infant weight on these alternative growth charts to reassure parents their breastfed infant is thriving (Chumlea, 2007).

Another method to determine whether a child's weight is consistent with height is to compute the body mass index (BMI). Table 34.5 describes the formula used to calculate BMI and the implications of the values obtained (see also Appendix E).

What if... Keoto, 13 years old, weighs 93 lb? Would you be concerned? What if 6 months earlier she had weighed 110 lb and a year earlier she had weighed 105 lb?

Head Circumference. Head circumference is measured at birth and routinely on physical assessment until 1 year of age (some health care agencies measure it routinely until 2 years of age). Head growth occurs because the brain is growing, so head circumference reflects brain growth and potential neurologic function. The measurement is made by placing a tape measure around an infant's head just above the eyebrows and around the most prominent portion of the back of the head, the occipital prominence (Fig. 34.5). Babies generally push any object away from their head, so it may be difficult to carry out this otherwise simple procedure. Plot measurements on a standardized graph (see Appendix E). Head circumference should correlate with the child's length; that is, if length is in the 40th percentile, head circumference also should be. If measurements of head circumference plot at different percentiles over time, this should be reported because it implies that brain or skull growth is in some way abnormal and needs investigation.

Chest and Abdominal Circumference. Measurements of chest and abdominal circumference are not done routinely, but only when specific pathology warrants. Chest circumference is measured at the nipple line, abdominal circumference at the level of the umbilicus.

Skin

Skin is assessed in conjunction with the examination of each body region. Assess temperature, color, dryness, texture, **turgor** (amount of fluid in body tissue; Fig. 34.6), and presence of any lesions that might reveal a communicable illness of childhood.

Table 34.6 summarizes various findings that may be detected. Be certain to examine a child's total skin surface at some time during an examination. As necessary, remove and replace adhesive bandages and other dressings that could hide important findings. Be certain there is adequate lighting, especially when assessing dark-skinned children.

Box 34.8 Nursing Procedure ✻ Measuring a Child's Height

Purpose: To assess for optimal growth.

Procedure	Principle
Infant	
Until they can stand securely (at approximately age 2 years), the most accurate method for obtaining a length measurement for infants is the recumbent measuring board (Figure A).	
1. Align the infant's head snugly against the top bar of the frame and ask an assistant to secure it there. Parents can help you restrain infants for height measurements because it is a painless procedure.	**1.** Provides a starting point for measurement.
2. Straighten the infant's body.	**2.** Straightens knees to ensure accuracy. Knees are difficult to straighten in infants because they always keep them flexed.
3. Hold the infant's feet in a vertical position. Bring the foot board up snugly against the bottom of the foot.	**3.** Completes measurement.
4. If an examining table is used, mark the spots at the top of the child's head and bottom of feet and then measure between the marks.	**4.** Provides for an alternative approach.
5. Plot height measurement on a standard graph.	**5.** Allows for interpretation of findings.

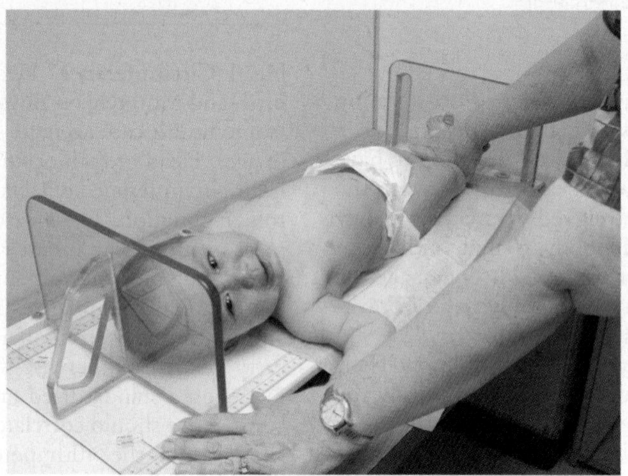

A

Procedure	Principle
Older Child	
For older children, a stadiometer is the most accurate method for measurement (Figure B).	
1. Have the child remove shoes.	**1.** Promotes accuracy.
2. Have the child stand straight with head held level.	**2.** Puts the child in the proper position for accurate measurement.
3. Align the measuring bar of a standing scale with the top of the head.	**3.** Determines the measurement.
4. If stadiometer is not available, place a flat object such as a clipboard on the child's head in a horizontal position and read the height at the point at which the object touches a measuring tape on the back of the scale or a flat wall surface.	**4.** Provides for an alternative approach.
5. Plot height measurement on a standard graph.	**5.** Allows for interpretation of findings.

Box 34.8 Nursing Procedure ✻ Measuring a Child's Height

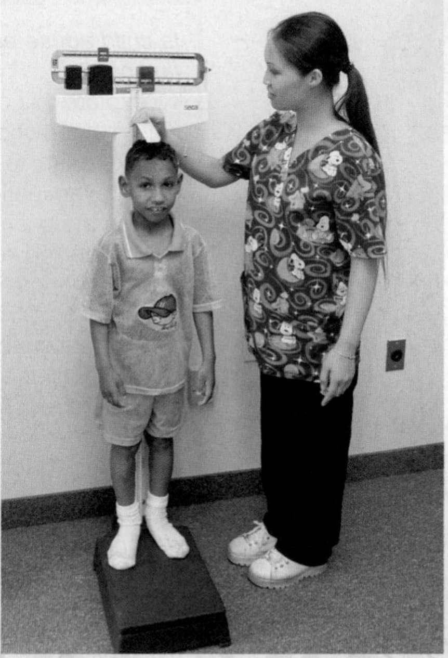

B

Newborn and Infant. Newborns may appear ruddy because their layer of subcutaneous fat is thin and the intense redness of their blood circulation is visible. Erythema toxicum (newborn rash) or birthmarks (hemangiomas, mongolian spots, or nevi) may be present (see Chapter 18). After the first few days of life, a diaper rash may be present.

Toddler, Preschooler, and School-Age Child. Many children this age have minor lesions from mosquito bites or from flea bites if they own a pet. They also typically have a number of ecchymotic spots on their lower extremities from bumping into objects during active play. Ecchymotic spots on upper extremities are less common and may suggest a blood coagulation problem. In evaluating ecchymotic spots on children of all ages, though, consider the possibility of child abuse (Newton & Vandeven, 2007) (Box 34.9). Lesions, scratch marks, or excessive dryness can reveal atopic dermatitis, a common childhood disorder (Findlay, 2007).

Adolescent. At least a few acne lesions on the face or back are usually present in the adolescent. Lesions or rashes caused by allergies to cosmetics also may be seen. If a child has a tattoo or body piercing, assess the site for inflammation to be certain an infection is not beginning.

TABLE 34.5 ✻ Body Mass Index Calculation

To calculate the body mass index (BMI), divide the child's weight in kilograms by the square of the child's height in meters:

BMI (kg/m^2)	Implication
<18.5	Underweight
18.5–24.9	Normal
25.0–29.9	Overweight
>30	Obese

Head

To examine a child's head, slide a hand over the skull, assessing for irregular configurations or tenderness. Most children have a prominent occipital outgrowth; do not mistake

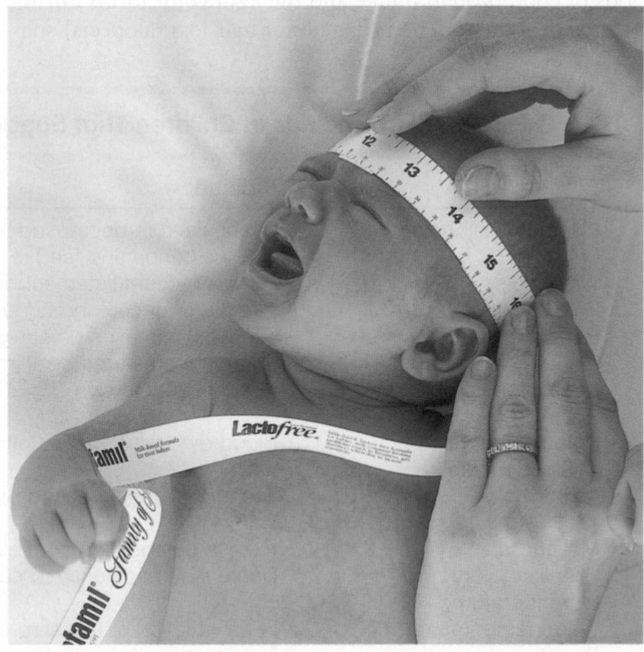

FIGURE 34.5 Measuring head circumference. The measuring tape passes just above the eyebrows and around the prominent posterior aspect of the head.

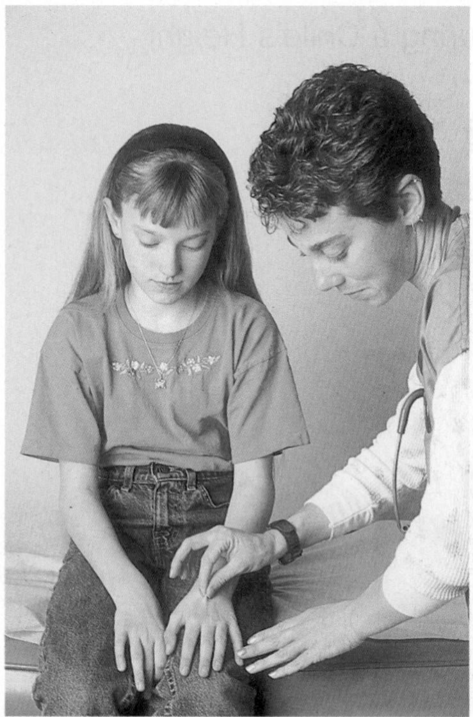

FIGURE 34.6 Assessing skin turgor. If the ridge of tissue does not immediately return to place, this suggests that the child is poorly hydrated.

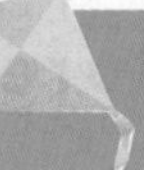

BOX 34.9 * Focus on Evidence-Based Practice

Is child abuse easy to detect from physical examination findings?

To explore this question, researchers asked 22 pediatricians, all of whom had substantial academic and clinical expertise, to evaluate and rate whether findings from child examinations indicated physical abuse. Even though the scenarios were taken from children who had been referred for abuse investigation, results showed that scenarios were rarely rated as "definite abuse" (likelihood ≥95%). Seven of 156 scenarios were rated as "no reasonable concern for abuse" (≤15% chance). Because of the wide variability in responses, the researchers recommend that health care agencies use a peer-review or multidisciplinary team approach when assessing for child abuse.

Based on the above, would you ask a colleague for a second opinion if you suspect physical abuse in a child following a physical examination?

Source: Lindberg, D. M., Lindsell, C. J., & Shapiro, R. A. (2008). Variability in expert assessments of child physical abuse likelihood. *Pediatrics, 121*(4), e945–e953.

this natural head contour for an abnormality. Assess the texture and cleanliness of hair. Children who are well nourished usually have hair of good texture; poorly nourished children tend to have dry, brittle, or limp hair. If hair is exceptionally oily, it may suggest a lack of adequate hygiene, possibly from fatigue because of an unidentified illness. If a serious protein deficiency such as **kwashiorkor** is present, the hair becomes striped with dark and light color; dark hair forms during periods of good protein intake and the light color forms during periods of protein deficit. Patches of hair loss (alopecia) suggest a fungal infection (tinea capitis), child abuse, or a possible drug reaction (chemotherapy will cause total hair loss, not patches).

Newborn and Infant. In a newborn, the head usually shows molding (an elongated shape because of pressure against the cervix before birth). A caput succedaneum or cephalhematoma from the pressure of birth may be present (see Chapter 18). Skull suture lines may be palpable. In both newborns and infants, sit the child upright and palpate the

TABLE 34.6 * Skin Findings in Children That Suggest Illness

Finding	Indication
Central bluish color	Cyanosis from decreased respiratory function or cyanotic heart disease. Acrocyanosis (blue hands and feet) is normal in newborn for first 48 hours.
White color	Edema (accumulated subcutaneous fluid is stretching the skin)
Pale color	Anemia or decreased circulation to a body part
Reddened area	Local inflammation or increased systemic temperature
Linear abrasion	Scratch marks from local irritation from an insect bite, or allergic reaction
Ecchymoses (black and blue marks)	Recent injury to skin
Petechiae (pinpoint blood marks)	Blood dyscrasia (poor clotting ability)
Yellow color	Jaundice from increased bilirubin in subcutaneous tissue; carotenemia (excess carotene in skin)
Moistness	Excess perspiration from elevated temperature
Localized cold temperature	Decreased circulation to particular body part
Warm temperature	Local irritation or elevated systemic temperature
Poor turgor	Dehydration
Rash	Infectious childhood illness, excessive heat, allergy

skull for the presence of fontanelles (the places where the skull bones fuse). The anterior fontanelle is at the junction of the two parietal bones and the two fused frontal bones. It is diamond shaped and measures 2 to 3 cm (0.8 to 1.2 in) in width and 3 to 4 cm (1.2 to 1.6 in) in length. The posterior fontanelle is at the junction of the parietal bones and the occipital bone. It is triangular and measures approximately 1 cm (0.5 in) in length (see Fig. 15.2).

With the infant sitting, fontanelles should be felt as soft spots but should not appear indented (a sign of dehydration) or bulging (a sign of increased intracranial pressure). When an infant cries, cerebral pressure increases so with crying, the fontanelles may feel tense, and sometimes even the fluctuation of a pulse can be observed. The anterior fontanelle normally closes at 12 to 18 months and the posterior fontanelle by the end of 2 months. They should not be palpable after these times. The closing of fontanelles too early or too late can indicate decreased or increased brain or ventricle growth from excessive cerebral spinal fluid.

A scalp problem commonly encountered in infants is seborrhea (scaling, greasy-appearing, salmon-colored patches), or "cradle cap." Increasing the frequency of hair washing to once a day and applying baby oil to the scalp typically reduces this problem.

Toddler, Preschooler, and School-Age Child. Examine the hair of children who attend school or day care carefully for small white-yellow, sand-sized particles attached to hair strands—the eggs (nits) of pediculi (head lice). Pediculi spread easily in school-age children because of the sharing of combs and towels in school. Nits cling and cannot be readily removed from hair by running fingers the length of the hair (Sciscione & Krause-Parello, 2007). The child may have recent scratch marks on the scalp or state that the scalp feels itchy.

Also examine the scalp carefully for round circular areas (perhaps weeping in the center, crusting and scaling on the edges) that would suggest tinea capitis (ringworm, a fungal infection). Like pediculi, fungal infections can spread readily among school-age children; a prescription medication is necessary to best cure both conditions (see Chapter 43).

Adolescent. Adolescents may streak their hair with dye or arrange it in a way that requires gel, hair extensions, or use of a curling iron. Inspect to see that their scalp and hair are healthy underneath the styling.

Eyes

Observe eyes for symmetry and signs of redness (erythema), frequent blinking, crusting, squinting, or rubbing as these are signs of **conjunctivitis,** an infection of the thin conjunctiva that covers the eye globe (Patel et al., 2007). Observe lids and lashes for redness or abnormalities as well to detect a **hordeolum** or stye (an infection of the gland that lubricates an eyelash). Both conditions require an antibiotic for therapy (see Chapter 50).

Assess the location of eyes in relation to the nose (not unusually wide or narrow spaced) and the relationship of the globe to the socket (neither sunken nor protruding from the socket [exophthalmos]). Abnormalities in these areas occur in chromosomal or metabolic illnesses such as hyperthyroidism. Inspect the sclera of the eye for spots of hemorrhage (called subconjunctival hemorrhage) or yellowing. African American children often have a slight yellowing of the sclera and small black spots on the sclera; do not mistake these for abnormal findings. Assess that no sclera shows above the pupil (if it does, this is termed a sunset sign, an indication of increased intracranial pressure).

Palpate each eye globe with the eyelid closed to assess for tenseness, a finding suggesting glaucoma (rare in children). Determine whether the eyelids completely close (edema or neurologic illnesses may make eyelids too short to do this) when the child shuts the eyes. Also determine whether the lids retract far enough so they do not obscure vision when the child opens the eyes. When a lid obscures vision, a condition termed **ptosis,** it generally denotes neurologic involvement. Differences in Western and Eastern eye creases are shown in Figure 34.7.

Examine the inner lining of the lower eyelid (the conjunctiva) by pulling the lid down slightly with a fingertip. Here, the mucous membrane should appear pink and moist. In children with anemia, it often appears pale; with allergy or infection, it may appear unusually red and irritated. Do not initiate a blink reflex by touching the cornea with a wisp of cotton, as can be done in adults; this is momentarily painful and frightening to children.

In addition, observe whether the eyes appear to be in good alignment. **Strabismus** refers to eyes that are not evenly aligned. If an eye is always turning in, the condition is **esotropia;** if it always turns out, **exotropia.** Two screening procedures for straight eye alignment include a Hirschberg's test and a cover test. During a Hirschberg's test, the light of

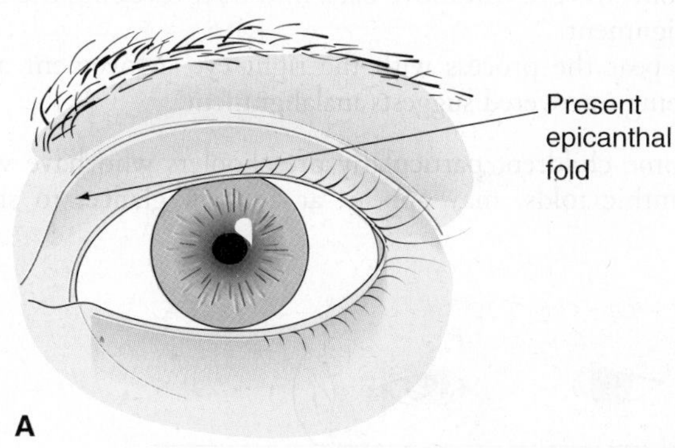

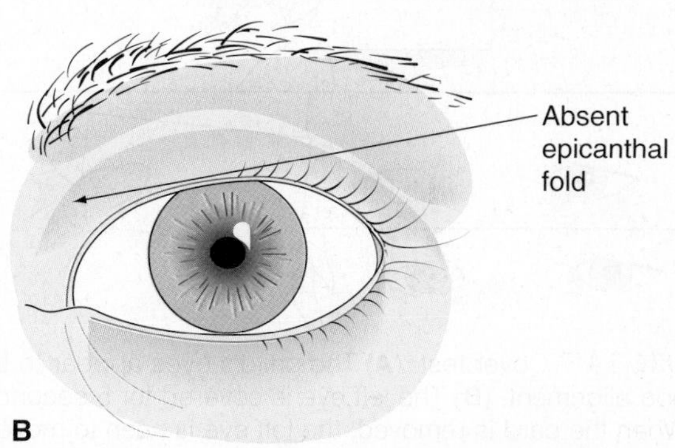

FIGURE 34.7 Differences in eye formation. (**A**) Western. (**B**) Eastern. The extra inner fold of tissue is an epicanthal fold.

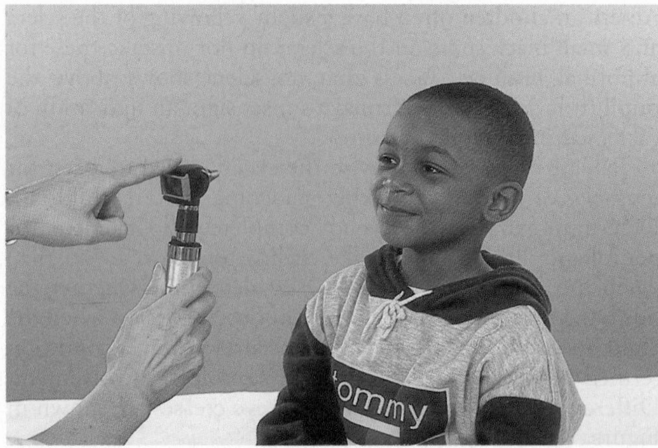

FIGURE 34.8 Testing good eye alignment by Hirschberg's test. The child is asked to look directly at the light of the otoscope. The light reflex on the pupils of both eyes will be equal if the eyes are in straight alignment.

an otoscope should reflect evenly off both pupils if they are in equal alignment (Fig. 34.8).

To perform a cover test (Fig. 34.9),

- Have children look at an attractive object approximately 4 ft in front of them.
- Hold a 3 × 5-inch card over the left eye for a count of 5. If any degree of strabismus is present, the eye will wander to its misaligned position while covered.
- Remove the card and observe the eye for movement.
- As the child again fixes vision on the specified object in front, the eye will move back into line, revealing the misalignment.
- Repeat the process with the right eye. Movement after being uncovered suggests malalignment.

Some children, particularly preschoolers who have wide epicanthic folds, may appear, at a quick glance, to show

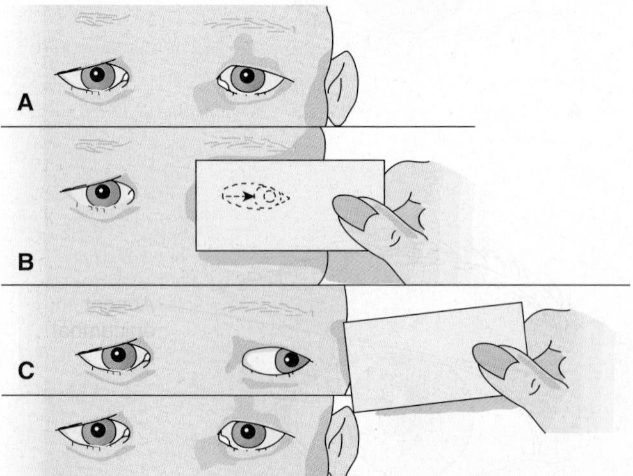

FIGURE 34.9 Cover test. (**A**) The child's eyes appear to be in good alignment. (**B**) The left eye is covered for 5 seconds. (**C**) When the card is removed, the left eye is seen to move perceptibly back to good alignment. This movement indicates that it "drifted" into a deviant position while covered, that is, that an exophoria (misalignment) is present.

misalignment. A cover test is helpful in these children. There will be no eye movement after removal of the card because there is no misalignment present, only the temporary appearance of misalignment. Reasons for true misalignment are discussed in Chapter 50.

Test the eyes for their ability to focus in all fields of vision also:

- Ask the child to follow a moving light (or catch the attention of an infant with a moving light) while holding the child's chin stationary.
- Move the light out to the side, then up, then down.
- Cross to the opposite side and move it up and down.
- Bring the light back to the midline and observe whether the child's eyes converge (follow the light to the nose) as the light moves in toward the nose. Infants under age 3 months cannot follow past the midline; the eyes of children under school age do not converge well.

Observe if the pupil constricts (reduces in size) in response to a light, an indication the third cranial nerve is intact. It is best to approach the child's eye from the forehead so the light suddenly appears on the pupil rather than advancing it toward the child slowly. This makes the pupil constrict more dramatically. This should occur in response to a light shining directly on a pupil (direct constriction); when one pupil constricts, constriction will also occur in the opposite eye (consensual constriction). Record that pupils are equal in size and react to light as "PERL" (pupils equivalent, react to light). If the pupil converges (moves to follow a light in toward the nose), this is charted as "PEARL" or "PERLA" (pupils equal, react to light, accommodate).

For a final step, shine a flashlight or ophthalmoscope light into the pupil. A red reflex or the red pupil that occurs with a flash photograph should appear. This is evidence that the retina is intact and the lens and cornea are clear (no tumor, cataract, scarring, or infection is present).

Newborn and Infant. Newborns often have a small, bright-red spot on the sclera (a subconjunctival hemorrhage) because the pressure of birth has ruptured a small conjunctival blood vessel. This is normal and will fade in 7 to 10 days as the blood is absorbed.

Infants can easily be tested for a red reflex, but until they are about 3 months, they cannot follow an object or light across the midline or follow a light into all six positions of gaze. Even a newborn, however, can follow a bright light to the midline. Assessing for a red reflex is important in newborns because a congenital cataract can lead to loss of central vision if not discovered early.

Toddler and Preschooler. Most young children are reluctant to let someone look into their eyes. Explaining what will happen during an eye examination is effective in reducing the child's anxiety about this part of the assessment.

School-Age Child and Adolescent. Many older children wear contact lenses (a red reflex is visible with a contact lens in place); some may be nervous about having their eyes examined because they know they should be wearing prescribed eyeglasses but are not wearing them because they do not like their appearance. Observe carefully for pupillary appearance and ability to constrict in adolescents to rule out drug abuse. Many adolescent girls are anemic and so have pale conjunctiva.

Nose

Observe the nose for flaring of the nostrils (a sign of need for oxygen). Using an otoscope light, observe the mucous membrane of the nose for color (it should be pink; pale suggests allergies, redness suggests infection). Note and describe any discharge. Document the septum is in the midline (displaced septa such as those that occur after facial injuries can interfere with respiration and make nasal intubation in emergencies difficult). Gently press one nostril closed and ask the child to inhale; repeat on the opposite side to ensure that both sides of the nose are patent, that is, no choanal atresia or membrane obstructing the posterior nares exists. Sinuses do not fully develop until about 6 years. For children 6 or older, palpate the areas over the frontal and maxillary sinuses for tenderness, a symptom of sinus infection. Assess the sense of smell in school-age children and adolescents by asking them to identify a familiar odor such as chocolate or an orange.

Newborn and Infant. Infants are obligate nose breathers. They cannot coordinate mouth breathing, so they become disturbed when the nose is temporarily blocked to check for patency; do this only momentarily to avoid discomfort. Most newborns have milia (small white papules) on the surface of the nose.

Older Children. Many children, preschool age and older, have upper respiratory infections that cause reddened nasal mucous membranes and a purulent discharge. In contrast, allergies cause a clear discharge and pale mucous membranes. Children who have dry mucosa because of dry air (which leads to cracking and nosebleed) may be reluctant to allow inspection of their nose. Adolescents who sniff cocaine lose nasal hair and may have excoriations or abscesses in the mucous membrane. If the child has a nose piercing, inspect the site for redness or drainage.

Ears

Observe ears for proper alignment. In the average child, a line drawn from the inner canthus of the eye to the outer canthus and then to the ear will touch the top of the pinna of the ear (Fig. 34.10). Ears set lower than this are associated with chromosomal disorders such as trisomy 13. Observe the opening to the ear canal for any discharge. Touch the pinna and watch for evidence of pain (a sign of external canal infections). Observe the area immediately in front of the ear for a dermal sinus or a skin tag (a finding that is usually innocent but may be associated with kidney abnormalities). Observe the ear lobes for redness or drainage from infected piercing sites.

To examine the ear canal:

- Straighten the ear canal by pulling the pinna gently down and back in the child under 2 years of age and up and back in the older child.
- Select an otoscope tip. Otoscope tip sizes vary; use the smallest size possible that still gives adequate visibility.
- With the ear canal held straight, insert an otoscope tip into the external canal.
- Rest the instrument on a hand, not on the child's head (Fig. 34.11). In this position, the otoscope will move with a child, avoiding the danger that the plastic tip will scratch the canal if a child should move suddenly.
- Inspect the sides of the ear canal and then locate landmarks on the surface of the tympanic membrane.

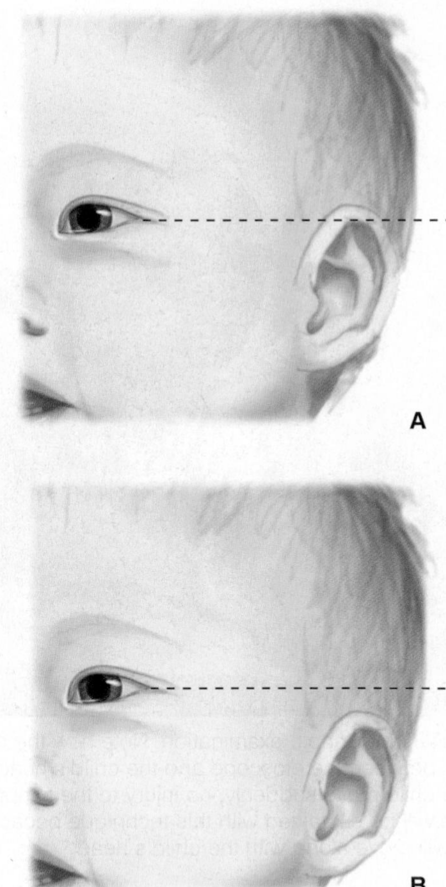

FIGURE 34.10 Normal ear alignment. When a line is drawn from the inner canthus through the outer canthus to the ear, the top of the ear pinna should meet the line (**A**). Abnormal ear alignment (**B**) is associated with certain chromosomal abnormalities.

The outline of the malleus of the inner ear through the translucent membrane is a key landmark to visualize (Fig. 34.12). The color of the membrane is pinkish gray; if the tension of the membrane is normal, a cone of light (the light reflex) should be present in one of the lower corners (at either the 5 o'clock or 7 o'clock position).

Although many children have wax (cerumen) in their ear canals, appearing as a dark-brown, glistening substance, viewing the tympanic membrane past the wax is almost always possible.

If an ear infection is present, the tympanic membrane appears reddened and often bulges forward so the malleus is no longer discernible and the cone of light is absent (Legros et al., 2008). If there is fluid in the middle ear, it may be possible to see bubbles of air through the membrane. With chronic middle ear disease (serous otitis media), the tympanic membrane may be retracted, the malleus is extremely prominent, and the cone of light is again missing. If the membrane has been torn from trauma or rupture, the jagged edge and opening to the middle ear are discernible. Inspect

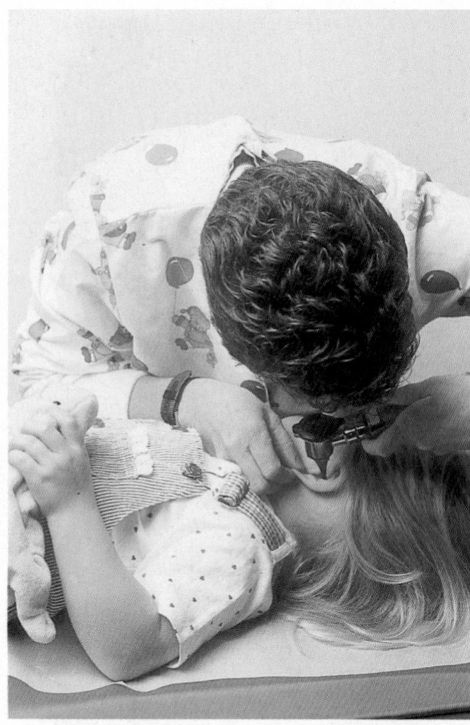

FIGURE 34.11 Otoscopic examination. Note how the nurse's hand rests between the otoscope and the child's head. Should the child move suddenly, no injury to the tympanic membrane will be sustained with this technique because the otoscope will move along with the child's head.

also for any ulcerated areas that could be a cholesteatoma or an ingrowing tumor (see Chapter 50).

Although not a routine procedure, the mobility of the eardrum can be tested by injecting a column of air into the ear canal against the drum by a pneumatic attachment on an otoscope that looks like the bulb of a blood pressure cuff (Fig. 34.13). A normal drum is freely mobile and can be seen to move with pressure on the bulb; one with fluid behind it has decreased mobility. Before introducing air, warn the child that this "tickles."

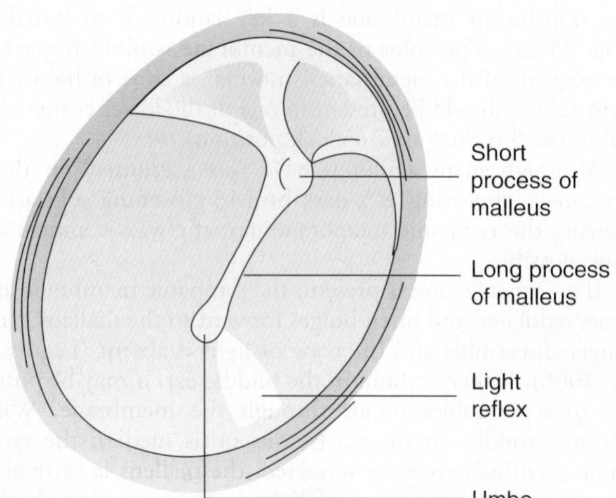

FIGURE 34.12 A tympanic membrane as viewed with an otoscope.

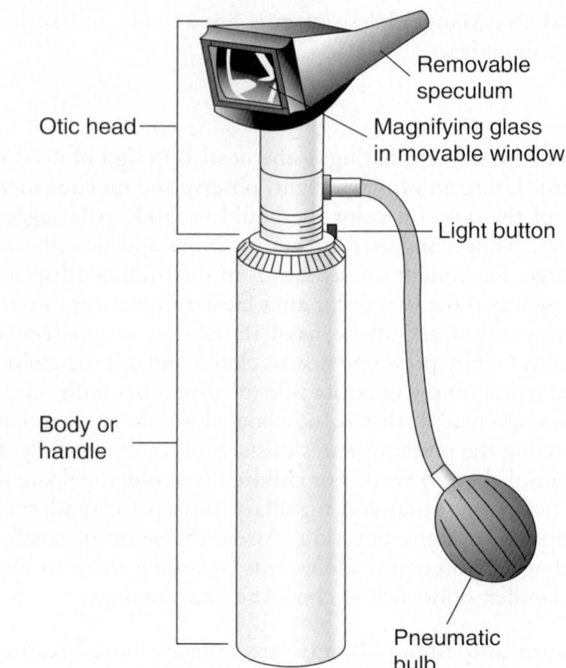

FIGURE 34.13 Otoscope with pneumatic attachment.

Finally, appraise hearing. Appraisal can be done grossly in older children by assessing their response to questions. Distract an infant with a toy; then make a sound behind the infant's back, out of peripheral vision, and watch for the response. Hearing infants will show some noticeable reaction, although they have difficulty looking directly toward or locating the sound until about 4 months of age.

Newborn and Infant. Many newborns still have amniotic fluid or vernix caseosa in their ear canal, so inspecting the ear canal is ineffective. Be certain to assess for ear level and normal pinna contour. Assess gross hearing ability—for example, by watching the infant startle to a sudden sound or quiet to the calming effect of quiet talking.

Older Children. Middle ear infection (otitis media) is a common childhood illness. This causes the ear to be painful when examined. An external ear infection (often called swimmer's ear) causes any movement of the pinna to be painful. For these reasons and because children are told many times never to put anything into their ears, they usually resist ear examinations. Explaining what is happening helps to allay any fears. Beginning with preschool age, children may have myringotomy tubes (small circular plastic tubes placed into the tympanic membrane) to relieve chronic fluid collected in the middle ear. Inspect that the area surrounding the tube is not inflamed and the tube is not merely lying in the external canal and no longer inserted into the membrane (see Chapter 50).

Mouth

Assess the external appearance of the lips, looking for symmetry and color. Ask a child to smile and frown to evaluate the mobility of facial muscles. Count the number of teeth present

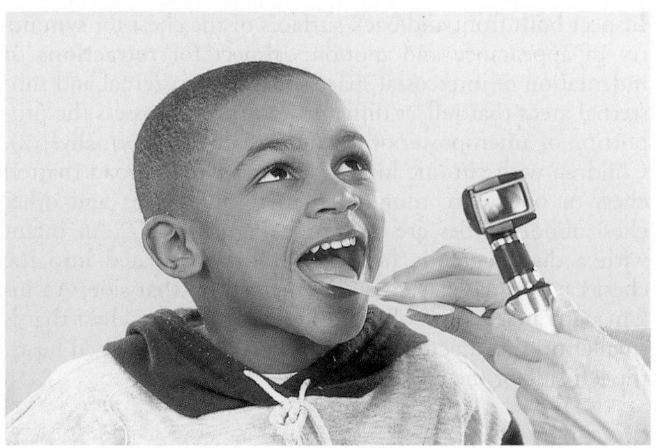

FIGURE 34.14 Inspecting the pharynx in a schoolager.

and assess their condition (number missing or cavities present). Inspect the gum line (gingivae) for redness, tenderness, and edema, symptoms of periodontal disease. Inspect the buccal membrane and palate for color (pink) and the presence of any lesions. Ask a child to stick out the tongue and assess for midline position and no fasciculations (trembling). Inspect the area under the tongue for lesions in school-age children and adolescents who smoke or chew tobacco because this is the most common first site for oral cancer.

A child's tongue is normally smooth and moist. With dehydration present, it often appears roughened and dry. **Geographic tongue** is a term for the rough-appearing tongue surface that often accompanies general symptoms of illness such as fever; it may also occur normally. If a child has a pierced tongue, inspect for redness at the site. Assess that the object is secure so there is little chance of aspiration or that it is not striking tooth enamel and wearing this away.

Inspect the uvula to be certain it is in the midline. Use a tongue blade to press down and forward on the back of the tongue (Fig. 34.14). The epiglottis can usually be observed with the tongue depressed. Observe for abnormal enlargement, palatine redness, or drainage of tonsils. Although tonsillar tissue differs greatly in size, it should not be reddened or have pus in the crypts (indentations). After initiating the gag reflex in infants to view the back of their throat, always turn their head to the side so they do not choke on any saliva that accumulated in the mouth during the throat examination. Infants are less able to manage this than are adults.

Do not depress the tongue of any child who is suspected to have epiglottitis or whose glottis is inflamed. Symptoms of this condition are a sore throat, drooling, fever, difficulty with respiration, dysphagia, and a barking cough. If a swollen, inflamed epiglottis rises with the pressure of a tongue blade, it can obstruct the respiratory tract so completely the child is immediately unable to breathe.

Newborn and Infant. Many newborns have considerable mucus in their mouths because they are less able to handle swallowing because of immature muscle coordination. If a newborn has teeth, evaluate them for stability; if loose, they may need to be removed to prevent aspiration. Assess for white patches that do not scrape away from the buccal membrane or tongue (thrush), a common but abnormal finding in infants that needs antifungal therapy (see Chapter 43).

Older Children. Tonsillar tissue in children reaches its maximum growth at early school age, making many preschool children appear to be "all tonsils." As long as the tissue does not appear reddened or tender, it can be assumed to be normal for the age. Many children have irregular, pale-pink, elevated projections on the posterior pharynx as a normal finding. A stream of mucopurulent discharge in the posterior pharynx is not unusual if an upper respiratory infection and a "post-nasal" flow of secretions are present. For a child with orthodontic appliances such as braces, assess carefully for pinpoint ulcers to be certain the wires are not causing undue discomfort or infection. Cavities appear as dark-brown areas on the tooth enamel. Many school-age children or adolescents have at least one present and need a dental care referral.

✔ Checkpoint Question 34.3

You typically gag children to inspect the back of their throat. When is it important *not* to elicit a gag reflex?

a. When children are under 5 years of age.
b. When a child has symptoms of epiglottitis.
c. When a boy has a possible inguinal hernia.
d. When a girl has a geographic tongue.

Neck

Assess the neck for symmetry (the trachea should be in the midline; any deviation suggests lung pathology). Observe the outline of the thyroid gland (barely noticeable before puberty because it is obscured by the sternocleidomastoid muscle) on the anterior neck. Palpate the area in front of the ear (location of the parotid gland) and smooth a hand over the location of lymph nodes at the sides of the neck and under the chin to palpate for swelling. Figure 34.15 shows the location of lymph node chains of the head and neck. Because children have so many upper respiratory infections, a few nodes that are freely movable, about the size of peas, termed "shotty" nodes because they simulate the feel of buckshot under the skin, are often present. Commonly, preauricular and postauricular nodes are palpable after ear infections, and postoccipital nodes are palpable after a scalp infection. Submental nodes generally denote a tooth abscess. Palpable submaxillary, anterior, and posterior cervical nodes follow throat infections.

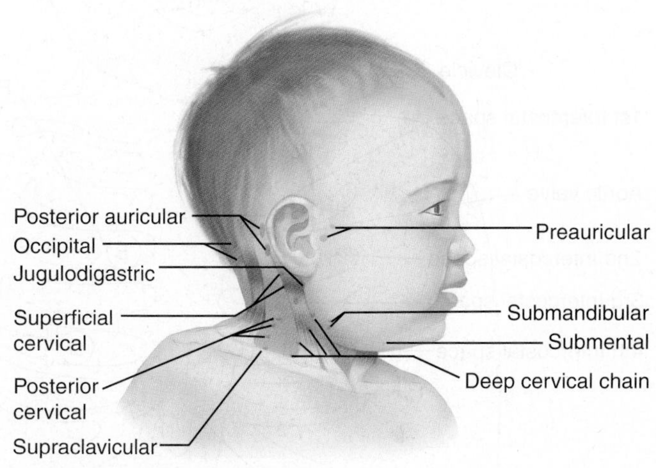

FIGURE 34.15 Location of lymph nodes.

Ask the child to move the head (or move it for the child) through flexion (touch chin to chest) and extension (raise chin as high as possible), and turn it right and left (rotation) to see that a child does this easily. Pain on forward flexion is an important sign of neurologic (meningeal) irritation.

Newborn and Infant. With infants, always assess the ability to control the head by laying the infant supine and pulling the child to a sitting position. Babies younger than 4 months of age will let their heads lag backward as they are pulled up this way; they right their heads only as they reach a sitting position. After 4 months, infants should bring their head up with them (no head lag) if their neuromuscular coordination is adequate for their age. This simple but important test yields information about overall neuromuscular control as well as neck strength.

Adolescent. In adolescents, palpate the thyroid gland for symmetry and possible nodes. To do this, press on the right side of the gland, causing it to be more prominent on the left side. Then palpate the left half to discern any irregularities (areas of hardness). Repeat on the right side. A finding of a thyroid node needs to be investigated. It may be only an innocent transient cyst, or it may be the first indication of thyroid malignancy. Many adolescents have some increase in the size of the thyroid at puberty; this hypertrophy should not be accompanied by any nodes.

Chest

For ease in specifying the location of chest pathology, the chest is divided into sections by imaginary lines drawn through the mid-clavicle, mid-mammary, and midsternum points on the front; the mid-axilla on the side; and the mid-scapula on the back. Pathology is described in terms of these lines such as "abnormal lung sound heard at left mid-axillary line". Other helpful means of locating pathology is by the suprasternal notch, the ribs, and the spaces between them **(intercostal spaces).** Intercostal spaces are numbered according to the ribs immediately above them (Fig. 34.16). Inspect both front and back surfaces of the chest for symmetry of appearance and motion. Inspect for **retractions** or indentation of intercostal spaces or the suprasternal and substernal areas that reflect difficult respirations. Assess the proportion of anteroposterior to lateral diameter (normally 1:2). Children with chronic lung disease develop a broad (barrel) chest or one more rounded than normal. This and other chest abnormalities are shown in Figure 34.17. An infant with a diaphragmatic hernia (intestine herniated into the chest cavity) may have a chest enlarged on that side. An infant with atelectasis (collapsed lung) may have a chest that is smaller on the affected side. If a child has an enlarged heart, the left side of the chest may appear larger.

Breasts

The degree of breast assessment depends on the child's age and development. As part of a normal breast assessment, inspect and palpate the breasts of all children to detect any abnormalities.

Newborn. Both male and female newborns may have breast edema from the influence of maternal hormones. A few drops of clear fluid may even be present from the nipples. This is normal and will fade in a few days time. Document if a supernumerary nipple is present for baseline data.

School-Age Child and Adolescent. Perform a breast examination on all girls past puberty. If a girl younger than 8 years is beginning breast development, precocious puberty (see Chapter 48) should be suspected. Many preadolescent boys develop hypertrophy of breast tissue because of increased hormonal influences (gynecomastia); they are generally concerned and need reassurance this is normal for their age and will fade as soon as androgen becomes their dominant hormone. Adolescent girls may be concerned their breast tissue is inadequate or that breast growth is uneven. They can be assured that not all women have completely symmetric breasts.

Inspection of breast tissue is easiest if a child sits on the examining table, arms at the sides, with both breasts exposed.

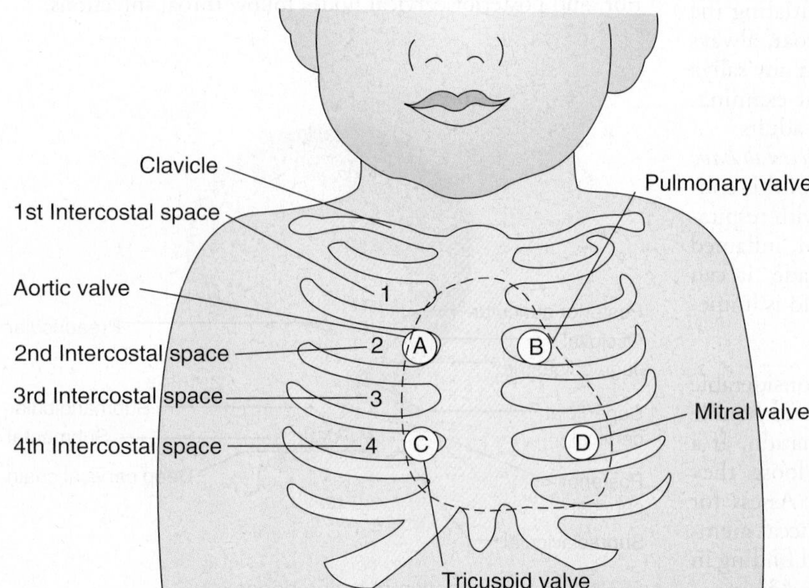

FIGURE 34.16 Intercostal (between rib) spaces are numbered according to the ribs immediately above them. The points (**A, B, C,** and **D**) to which the sounds of the heart valves radiate or where the sounds can be heard best are the listening posts of the heart.

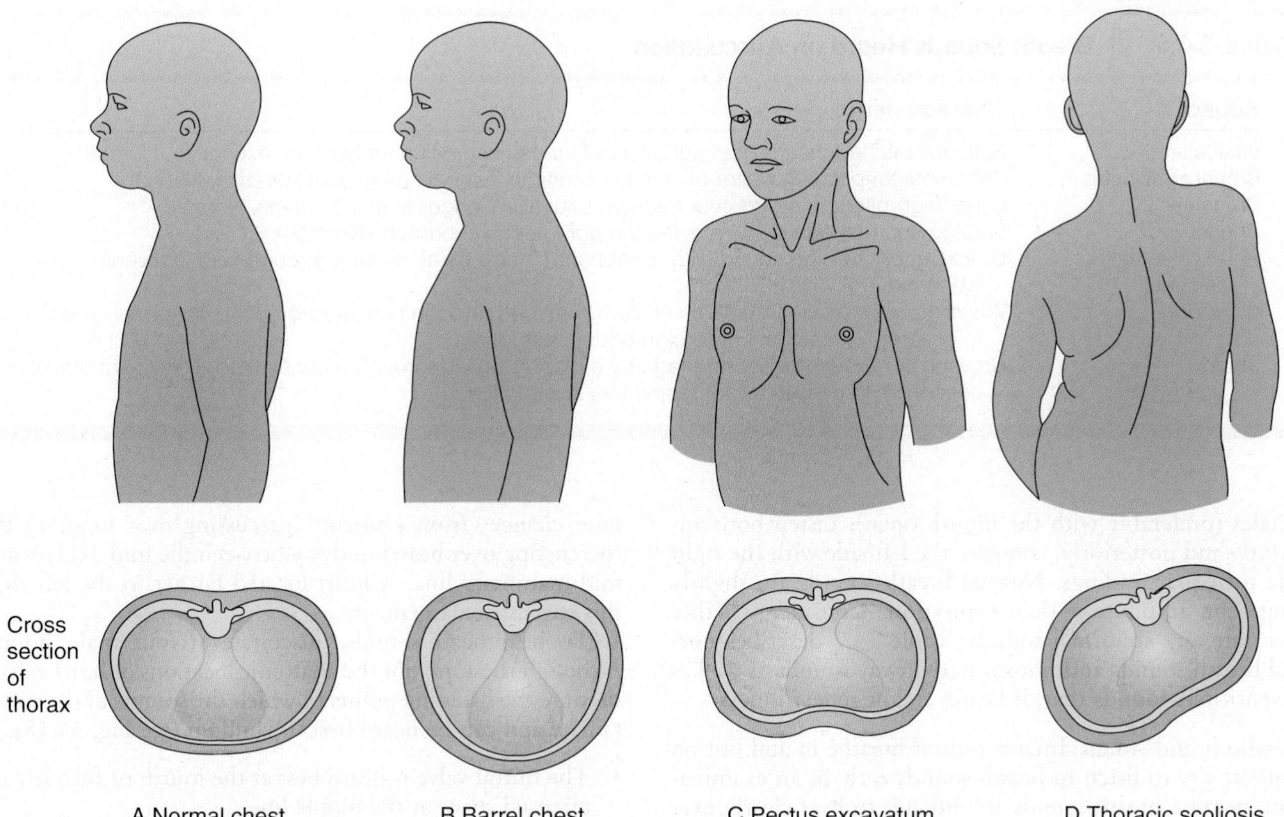

FIGURE 34.17 Chest contours that can be assessed by inspection. (**A**) Normal chest. (**B**) Barrel chest. (**C**) Funnel chest (pectus excavatum). (**D**) Thoracic kyphoscoliosis.

Inspect for symmetry. As mentioned, it is normal and not unusual for a girl to have breasts of slightly unequal size.

Inspect breasts for edema, erythema, wrinkling, retraction, or dimpling of the skin; all suggest that a tumor is growing in deeper layers of the tissue. Erythema occurs from inflammation because of abnormal, rapidly growing tissue; edema results from the blockage of lymph channels because of tumor pressure. Breast edema makes the skin appear not only swollen but also pitted (an orange-peel effect). Note any nipple discharge or "pulled" nipple placement as another way to detect edema.

With the girl's arms at her sides to take pressure off breast tissue, palpate well into each axilla (because breast tissue extends that far), and also palpate to assess axillary lymph nodes. Normally, no nodes should be felt. Ask the girl to lie down; place a folded towel under her near shoulder. Palpate the near breast with her lying down with her arm raised and placed under her head because this spreads out breast tissue; begin at the nipple and palpate outward in a circular motion. The lower edge of each breast feels hard; do not mistake this or rib prominences underneath for a tumor.

Lungs

Various findings reveal respiratory distress in children. Assess the rate of respirations and whether respirations are easy and relaxed or if accessory muscles are necessary for effective ventilation. Palpate over lung areas for vibrations that suggest air is having difficulty moving through air passages (Aylott, 2007).

On the anterior chest, lung tissue extends from above the clavicles to the sixth or eighth rib. On the posterior chest, lung tissue is as low as the 10th to 12th thoracic vertebrae. The right lung has three lobes; the left, only two. Attempt to evaluate all five lobes during lung assessment because lung disease can be specific for a lobe or involve the entire lung.

Following palpation, percuss over lung tissue. Normal lung is resonant in older children; in infants and younger children it is hyperresonant because of the thinness of the chest wall. Overexpanded lungs sound hyperresonant in older children; and lungs filled with fluid sound dull in older children and less resonant in younger children. The lower anterior lobe of the right lung will sound dull because the liver covers it on the anterior surface below the fourth or fifth intercostal space. The space over the heart will also percuss as dull.

Diaphragmatic excursion (the distance the diaphragm descends with inhalation) is an estimation of lung volume. To establish this:

- Ask the child to take in a deep breath and hold it.
- Percuss downward to locate the bottom of the lungs (the percussion note changes from resonant to flat at that point).
- Ask the child to expire fully and momentarily hold that position.
- Percuss upward to locate the expired or empty lung position (the percussion note changes from flat to resonant).

The difference between these two points is the diaphragmatic excursion. Children who have overexpanded lungs from obstructive disease will have little diaphragmatic excursion in relation to others.

Ausculate breath sounds by listening with the diaphragm of a stethoscope over each lung lobe while a child inhales and

TABLE 34.7 ✻ Breath Sounds Heard on Auscultation

Sound	Characteristics
Vesicular	Soft, low-pitched, heard over periphery of lungs, inspiration longer than expiration. Normal.
Bronchovesicular	Soft, medium-pitched, heard over major bronchi; inspiration equals expiration. Normal.
Bronchial	Loud, high-pitched, heard over trachea; expiration longer than inspiration. Normal.
Rhonchi	Snoring sound made by air moving through mucus in bronchi. Normal.
Rales (also called crackles)	Crackling or crinkling sound (like cellophane) made by air moving through fluid in alveoli. Abnormal.
Wheezing	Whistling on expiration made by air being pushed through narrowed bronchi. Abnormal; seen in children with asthma or foreign body obstruction.
Stridor	Crowing or rooster-like sound made by air being pulled through a constricted larynx. Abnormal; seen in children with upper respiratory obstruction.

exhales (preferably with the mouth open). Listen both anteriorly and posteriorly; compare the left side with the right side for equal findings. Normal breath sounds are slightly longer on inspiration than expiration. Consider whether there are any abnormal sounds. Table 34.7 describes normal breath sounds and transmitted airway sounds as well as adventitious sounds that, if heard, might reflect illness.

Newborn and Infant. Infants cannot breathe in and out on request. Try to listen to breath sounds early in an examination, because breath sounds are difficult to hear clearly over the sound of crying.

Heart and Heart Sounds

Heart assessment begins with asking children if they have ever had heart pain (Galioto, 2007). Visual inspection to see if there is a point on the chest where the heartbeat can be observed follows this. This point represents the location of the left ventricle or the point where the apical heartbeat can be heard best. In children younger than 7 years, this point is generally lateral to the nipple line and at the fourth intercostal space. In children older than 4 years, it is at the nipple line or just medial to it and at the fifth intercostal space. This point is termed the **point of maximum impulse (PMI)** and is observable in approximately 50% of children.

Percuss the left side of the chest to discern the left side of the heart. Percussing in from the axilla, the sound will become dull as the heart is identified. Normally, the percussion note changes from resonant (percussing over lung) to flat (percussing over heart) midway between the mid-axillary and mid-mammary line. A heart located farther to the left than this suggests enlargement.

To hear heart sounds, auscultate at four main points. Although these are not the anatomic locations of heart valves, they are the listening points to which the sounds of the valves radiate and can be heard best in children (see Fig. 34.18).

- The mitral valve is heard best at the fourth or fifth left intercostal space at the nipple line.
- The tricuspid valve is heard best near the base of the sternum (fourth or fifth right intercostal space).
- The pulmonary valve is heard best at the second left intercostal space.
- The aortic valve is heard best at the second right intercostal space.

Table 34.8 describes normal and abnormal heart sounds that may be heard on auscultation. Abnormal sounds are heard best if the diaphragm of the stethoscope is used first, followed by the bell of the stethoscope.

To understand heart sounds, recall heart physiology. The first sound heard (S_1) is that of the mitral and tricuspid valves closing and the ventricles contracting (described as a "lub" sound). The second sound (described as a "dub"; S_2) is made by the closure of the aortic and pulmonary valves and atrial contraction. The first sound is generally longer and lower-pitched than the second sound. It is louder than

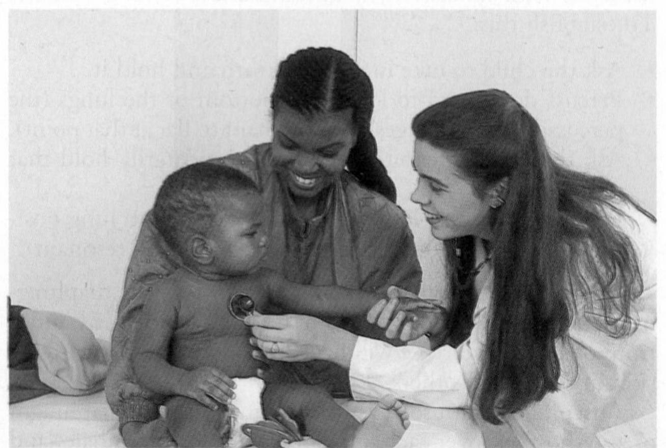

FIGURE 34.18 Auscultating heart sounds.

TABLE 34.8 ✻ Heart Sounds Heard on Auscultation

Sound	Cause
S_1 (first heart sound)	Closure of tricuspid and mitral valves with beginning of ventricular contraction (systole)
S_2 (second heart sound)	Closure of pulmonary and aortic valves with beginning of atrial contraction (diastole)
S_3 (third heart sound)	Rapid ventricular filling
S_4 (fourth heart sound)	Abnormal filling of ventricles

TABLE 34.9 ✻ Description of Accessory Heart Sounds

Assessment	Information to be Gathered
Location	At which listening post is the sound most distinct?
Quality	Can sound be described as blowing, rubbing, rasping, musical?
Intensity	*Murmurs* are graded according to the following criteria: Grade 6: So loud it can be heard with stethoscope not touching the chest wall; has a thrill (palpable vibration). Grade 5: Very loud but must touch stethoscope to chest to hear; has a thrill. Grade 4: Loud; may or may not have a thrill. Grade 3: Moderately loud; no thrill. Grade 2: Quiet but easily discernible. Grade 1: Very quiet; difficult to hear.
Timing	When in relation to S_1 and S_2 did you hear it? A sound superimposed between S_1 and S_2 is a *systolic murmur*, one between S_2 and the next S_1 is a *diastolic murmur*. Innocent murmurs (functional, denoting no pathology) are usually systolic, although there are exceptions to this; pathologic murmurs are more likely to be diastolic.
Pitch	Can the sound be described as high- or low-pitched?
Radiation and thrills	Is there an accompanying thrill? Does sound radiate so it can be heard at another location, such as back of chest?

the second sound over the heart ventricles; otherwise, it is slightly quieter.

Note the rhythm of the heart sounds. This should be regular. **Sinus arrhythmia** is a phenomenon that most school-age and adolescent children demonstrate. With sinus arrhythmia, a marked heart rate increase occurs as a child inspires and a marked decrease in heart rate is noted as the child expires. This is a normal finding. Ask the child to take and hold a breath, and the rhythm of the heart remains the same.

With inspiration and the normal resulting increase of pressure in the lungs, the pulmonary valve tends to close slightly later than the aortic valve. This is termed **physiologic splitting** and is heard as "lub d-dub." As long as this is associated with inspiration, it is a normal finding. Fixed splitting implies there is always difficulty with the pulmonary valve closing and suggests pathology.

At times, a distinct third heart sound (S_3) may be heard because of rapid filling of the ventricles. Although this is not necessarily a serious finding, further investigation is warranted. The presence of a fourth heart sound (S_4) generally signifies heart pathology because this sound (a gallop rhythm) is caused by abnormal filling of the ventricles.

Listen to the heart in all areas; assess rate and compare this to the child's age to determine if it is a normal rate. A heart murmur is caused by the sound of blood flowing with difficulty or in an abnormal pathway within the heart (sounds like a swishing sound) and can be either innocent (functional) or pathogenic (organic). If a heart is pumping with abnormal force, there may be a palpable vibration termed a thrill on the chest wall. Palpate the precordium (area over the heart) for evidence of this (feels like a cat purring) or a heave (a definite outward chest movement), which also denotes a struggling heart. On hearing or palpating any accessory heart sounds or movements, try to describe them with reference to Table 34.9.

All unusual heart sounds need further identification and investigation of their cause. The skills of listening to and identifying normal and abnormal heart sounds require considerable practice. Determining the cause of an abnormal heart sound requires a cardiac specialist. Determining that an abnormal sound exists, however, and securing proper referral is an important nursing role.

Newborn, Infant, and Toddler. Listen to heart sounds in young children early in an examination, before a child begins to cry, because it is almost impossible to evaluate heart sounds over the sound of crying. Allowing a parent to hold a child while listening to the heart helps reduce fear.

School-Age Child and Adolescent. Listen carefully for sounds of murmurs in children of school age and older. Be particularly conscientious with student athletes; it seems paradoxical that they could have heart disease, but, if present, it can be fatal to them during athletic events (Drezner et al., 2007). Refer them to a physician for further evaluation if any abnormalities are detected. Parents are always frightened by an unusual heart sound, but unless the child has other symptoms, they can be assured that most murmurs are innocent (functional) and caused only by the normal flow of blood across valves.

✔ Checkpoint Question 34.4

Keoto has a sinus arrhythmia. This refers to:

a. A widely spaced rib cage
b. Faint, barely audible heart sounds
c. Increased heart rate on inspiration
d. An abnormal heart rate in a child

Abdomen

The abdomen is divided anatomically into four quadrants. The quadrants and the organs that lie within them are shown in Fig. 34.19. To assess an abdomen, first inspect the surface for symmetry and contour. It will be slightly protuberant in infants and scaphoid in older children. Note any skin lesions or scars.

Auscultate the abdomen for bowel sounds before palpating, because palpating may alter bowel movement (peristalsis) and therefore disturb bowel sounds. Bowel sounds can normally be heard in all quadrants of the abdomen. They are high "pinging" sounds that occur normally at intervals of approximately 5 to 10 seconds. Since these sounds are high-pitched sounds, they may be heard best with the bell of a stethoscope. If the bowel is distended, the sounds occur more frequently; if the

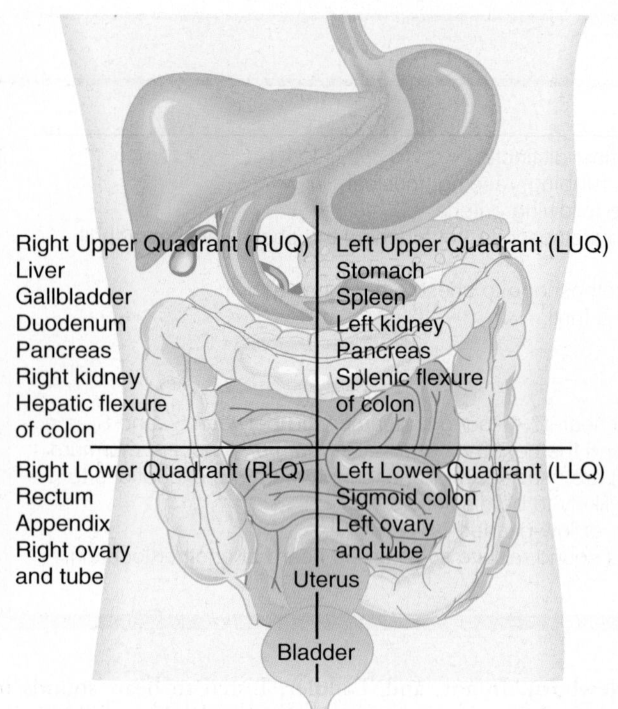

FIGURE 34.19 Quadrants of the abdomen and underlying structures.

bowel is blocked so that there is no movement of contents, the sounds will be absent below the obstruction. Listen for 3 to 5 minutes before concluding that no bowel sounds are present to be certain they are not just widely spaced.

Listen along the middle of the abdomen over the aorta for irregular sounds. A **bruit** is a swishing or blowing sound that occurs if there is an outpouching of the aorta (an aneurysm), a condition that can be congenital, although it usually occurs with aging.

Palpate the abdomen in a systematic manner to include all four quadrants. First palpate lightly, then deeply. Ascertain whether any area is tender by watching the child's face while palpating; observe for guarding or the child tensing the abdominal muscles to keep you from pressing deeply at that point. If a child indicates any portion of the abdomen is tender, begin assessment at the farthest point and work toward the tender area. If no tenderness is present, the order of palpation is unimportant as long as it is thorough. Note any hard areas or masses. If a tender area is detected, attempt to elicit rebound tenderness to determine its cause. To do this, press in on the abdomen, then lift your hand suddenly. This causes internal organs to vibrate. Although all children do not show this sign, the occurrence of more pain with the vibration than with the original pressure is one of the standard diagnostic criteria for appendicitis (Becker, Kharbanda, & Bachur, 2007).

By palpating from the right lower quadrant to the right upper quadrant, the hand will bump against the lower edge of the liver 1 to 2 cm below the right ribs. On the left side, the lower edge of the spleen may be discernible in the same way. A liver or spleen larger than this is suggestive of disease. Palpate the umbilicus to try to identify the presence of an umbilical hernia. A fascial ring at the umbilicus of more than 2 cm in diameter in an infant denotes a ring of fascia larger than will normally close spontaneously; when this is present, the child will generally need surgery to prevent an umbilical hernia. Liver, spleen, and bladder size can all be documented further by percussion.

Newborn and Infant. Kidneys may be located by deep abdominal palpation in newborns and infants. The right kidney is slightly lower than the left and so is easier to locate. The optimal time to palpate the kidney of a newborn is during the first few hours of life, before the bowel begins to fill with air and obscures palpation. To palpate the kidneys:

- Place a hand under an infant's back just below the 12th rib.
- Press upward.
- Place the other hand on that side of the abdomen just below the umbilicus.
- Press deeply.
- Locate the kidney, which can be felt as a firm mass approximately the size of a walnut between the hands.

Preschooler and School-Age Child. Children's abdomens at this age are often "ticklish," and children may tense or guard their abdominal muscles when touched, making it difficult to palpate. Distract a child by asking a question about home or school, or let a child place a hand under the examiner's to help relax (Fig. 34.20).

Genitorectal Area

In both sexes, the rectum should be inspected for any protruding hemorrhoidal tissue (rare in children) or fissures. Fissures may signify chronic constipation, intra-abdominal pressure, or sexual abuse.

Female Genitalia. Inspection of external female genitalia and assessment of femoral nodes are included in every complete health assessment (Hornor, 2007). An external examination consists of inspecting for Tanner stage of hair growth and configuration (an inverted triangle) and inspection of external genitalia (clitoris, labia majora, and labia minora) for normal contours. Look for signs of discharge or irritation. A vaginal discharge that suggests infection or a fourchette tear in a young child may be an indication of sexual abuse, in an adolescent of rape (Lewin, 2007). A pelvic examination is usually scheduled at the time the girl becomes sexually active or at age 18 (American Academy of Pediatrics [AAP], 2009). The technique for an internal pelvic examination is discussed in Chapter 11.

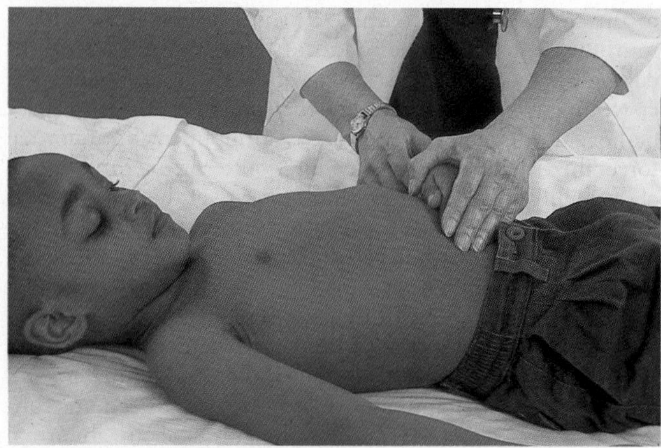

FIGURE 34.20 Decrease ticklishness during abdominal palpation by placing the child's hand under yours.

Male Genitalia. Inspection of male genitalia consists of observing:

- The distribution and Tanner stage of hair, which has a diamond shape
- The penis, for lesions that might suggest a sexually transmitted infection
- Appearance and placement of the urethral opening, which should be slitlike and centered at the penis tip. Children with repeated urinary tract infections develop scarring of the meatal opening, making it small and round (Hornor, 2007).
- The ability to retract the foreskin, if a boy is uncircumcised. Phimosis exists when the foreskin of a child older than 6 to 12 months is too tight to retract.

Hypospadias is a term for a urethral opening located on the inferior or ventral (under) surface of the penis; **epispadias** denotes a urethral opening on the superior or dorsal (upper) surface. Both these conditions need to be identified. If more than a slight deviation is present, repair is usually initiated before school age because such a urethral placement may interfere with self-image if not corrected. With adulthood, it can interfere with fertility.

Inspect the scrotum for size and the presence of testes. In most boys, the left testicle is slightly lower than the right, so the scrotum does not appear truly symmetric. Palpate to check that both testes are present by placing one hand over the top of the scrotum at the inguinal ring and then palpating the testis on that side (see Chapter 18, Fig. 18.17). This hand position prevents the testis from slipping up into the inguinal ring and appearing to be absent on palpation. Any swelling or mass in the scrotum needs to be identified. The most likely cause of such a condition is a **hydrocele,** or a fluid-filled sac, but it could represent a serious finding such as testicular cancer in adolescents. Hydroceles can be transilluminated: when a flashlight is held in back of the scrotum, the fluid-filled cyst glows. A **varicocele** (enlarged vein of the epididymis) may be palpated. These are not important findings in young boys, but they could possibly interfere with fertility in later life.

Assess the urethral meatus for any discharge that could reveal a sexually transmitted infection such as gonorrhea or any lesions that would suggest herpes 2 infection or syphilis (see Chapter 47). Beginning at puberty, teach boys to do testicular palpation every month. The technique for this is shown in Box 34.10.

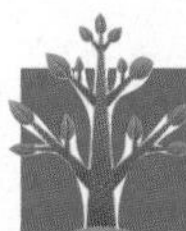

BOX 34.10 ✻ Focus on Family Teaching

Testicular Self-Examination

Q. Keoto's father asks you, "What is the best technique for testicular self-examination?"

A. Starting in the adolescent years, all males need to perform testicular self-examination. Follow these guidelines:

- Select a certain day each month (first day, last day, and so forth) to perform the examination.
- Perform the examination in or immediately after a shower, because that is when scrotal skin is most relaxed.
- Gently roll each testicle between your thumb and fingers, feeling for any hard lumps or nodules, change in consistency, or difference in size.
- If you notice any of these changes, call your doctor.
- Also feel for the epididymis, found at the rear of the testes. It should feel like a strong cord.
- Remember that for most males, one testicle is slightly larger than the other and hangs a little lower in the scrotal sac.

Inguinal Hernia

To assess for the presence of an inguinal hernia in an infant, simply observe the groin area for any bulging (especially while the infant is crying). In a school-age child or adolescent, with the child standing, place a fingertip against the inguinal ring in the groin area and ask the child to cough. If the tendency for a hernia is present, coughing tightens the abdominal muscles and forces the abdominal contents to bulge against the finger. Palpate femoral nodes (located in the groin and on the inner surface of the upper thigh) for any swelling, which suggests infection.

Extremities

Observe the upper extremities for good color and warmth. Inspect the fingernails for color, contour, and shape. Normally, nails are pink, smooth, and convex. They should feel hard to the touch and not so brittle that they break readily. Signs of bitten fingernails in the school-age child may reflect a high level of stress. Darker-skinned children's nails are more deeply pigmented. A blue or purple tinge denotes cyanosis; a yellow tinge is jaundice. Children who have decreased respiratory function or heart disease develop clubbed fingers (Fig. 34.21); children with endocarditis often have characteristic linear hemorrhages under the nails. Iron-deficiency anemia may cause extremely concave surfaces (spoon-shaped). Press against a fingernail, release the pressure, and time the refilling interval (should be under 5 seconds). Count the fingers and check for webbing between fingers. Examine that fingerprints are present. Distinctive dermatoglyphics are present on fingertips from the third month of intrauterine life; these are unique to every person and show patterns of circular grooves. Abnormal fingerprints may occur with chromosomal anomalies. Check for normal palmar creases. Children with chromosomal abnormalities

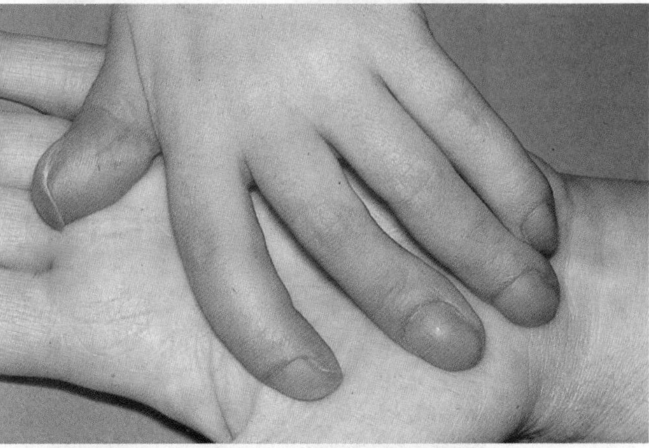

FIGURE 34.21 Clubbed fingers are a sign of cyanosis from heart or respiratory disease. (From NMSB/Custom Medical Stock Photograph.)

may have only one central palm crease (a simian line) on each hand rather than the normal three (see Chapter 7). Check the wrist, elbow, and shoulder joints for movement and normal range of motion; palpate joints for swelling or warmth. Palpate to be certain no lymph nodes are present in the antecubital space; palpate to check the radial pulse is present.

Inspect the lower extremities for color and warmth. Count the toes and check for webbing between toes. Check the ankle, knee, and hip joints for normal range of motion. Check for developmental hip dysplasia in infants by attempting to abduct the hip fully (see Chapter 27, Box 27.9). Palpate to ensure no enlarged lymph nodes are present in the groin or popliteal areas and that femoral pulses are present and equal bilaterally. Ask the older child to walk, and observe for ease of gait, limping, or any foot displacement such as toeing in or out. Toddlers typically walk with a wide-based gait; they walk best if allowed to walk toward their parent (a safe action) rather than away. Many adolescents are self-conscious and slouch or amble rather than presenting their true, natural gait. Children who limp need further evaluation. A limp can be the result of something as simple as a blister on the foot from wearing new shoes but can also be a sign of a serious hip or bone condition (Paton, 2007).

Back

Inspect the back for symmetry and the spinal column for any deviation. Inspect the base of the spine for a dermal sinus (a pinpoint opening) or for a tuft of hair or a hemangioma that might reveal a spina bifida occulta (a defect of the bony structure of the canal). Inspect also for any dimpling that might denote a dermal cyst (pilonidal cyst). This is an innocent finding unless it becomes infected or connects to deeper tissue layers. Assess for tenderness along the spinal column by palpating each vertebra as chronic lower back pain can be present as early as school age (Shilt & Barnett, 2007).

Routine assessment of the school-age child beginning at 12 years and through adolescence should include a scoliosis (sideways curvature of the spine) screening (Sponseller, 2007). Box 34.11 details the steps to follow for a scoliosis screen. (See Chapter 51 for more details on scoliosis.)

Box 34.11 Nursing Procedure ✻ Scoliosis Screening

Purpose To assess for scoliosis (sideways curvature of the spine).

Procedure	Principle
1. Have the child remove clothing, except for undergarments. Ask the child to stand up straight, with feet together and arms at sides. Observe the child from a posterior view.	1. Promotes optimal view of back.
2. Inspect for unequal shoulder or hip level, prominence of one scapula, or a curved spinal column (See Fig.).	2. Denotes signs of spinal curvature.

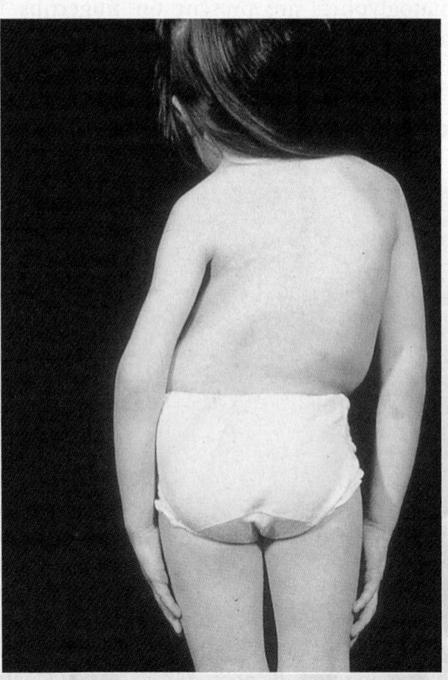

Box 34.11 Nursing Procedure ✻ Scoliosis Screening

Procedure	Principle
Ask yourself the following questions: • Is one shoulder higher than the other? • Is one shoulder blade more prominent than the other? • Does one hip seem higher or more prominent than the other? • Does the child seem to lean to one side? • Does the spinal column appear curved?	
3. Compare the level of the elbows in relation to the iliac crests. Be sure the arms are hanging down at the sides. Ask yourself the following questions: • Is the distance between one arm and body greater than on the other side? • Are the elbows uneven? • Do the elbows fall at the level of the crest or closer to the crest on one side? (Normally the elbows fall above the iliac crest.)	**3.** Helps to determine uneven posture because it will affect level of elbows.
4. Ask the child to bend over and touch toes while you continue to observe the back. Ask yourself the following questions: • Is there a hump in the back? • Does the spinal column appear to curve? • Is one shoulder blade more prominent than the other?	**4.** Provides evidence of spinal rotation. As the child bends, the rotation of the spine accompanying scoliosis becomes more prominent.
5. Refer the child to a physician for further examination if the answer to any of the above questions is yes.	**5.** Provides for proper referral.
6. Educate the child to inform parents or health care providers if signs of scoliosis begin to develop, such as a skirt hanging unevenly, or bra straps that need to be adjusted.	**6.** Encourages health promotion.

Neurologic Function

A full neurologic examination takes at least 20 minutes to complete, so it is not included in a routine physical examination. It is important, however, to assess for **deep tendon reflexes** (such as triceps, biceps, patellar, and Achilles reflexes) to test for motor and sensory function and balance and coordination. Techniques for eliciting deep tendon reflexes are shown in Figure 34.22. Grade reflexes according to the scale in Table 34.10. The biceps reflex tests the fifth and sixth cervical nerves; the triceps reflex tests the seventh and eighth cervical; the patellar reflex tests the second, third, and fourth lumbar; and the Achilles reflex tests the first and second sacral. Test the sole of the foot for a Babinski reflex (see Fig. 18.8). Fanning of the toes will occur in an infant younger than 3 months; a downward reflex of the toes will occur beyond 3 months. (Some normal infants demonstrate a flaring Babinski response until they are 2; in the absence of other neurologic findings, this is not significant.)

Test for superficial reflexes: abdominal reflexes in both sexes, cremasteric reflex in boys. An abdominal reflex is elicited by lightly stroking each quadrant of the abdomen. Normally, the umbilicus moves perceptibly toward the stroke. Presence of the reflex indicates integrity of the 10th thoracic nerve and the first lumbar nerve of the spinal cord. A cremasteric reflex is elicited by stroking the medial aspect of the thigh in boys. The testes move perceptibly upward. The presence of this reflex indicates integrity of the first and second lumbar nerves.

Motor and Sensory Function

Test general facial nerve function by asking a child to make a face. The child's ability to grasp with the hands and push against a surface with the feet establishes general motor ability. Recall whether gait was adequate when the child was observed walking to assess for balance and coordination.

To test sensory function, ask children to close their eyes and identify the location where they are touched at six points (at least) on different body parts.

ASSESSING VISION, HEARING, AND SPEECH

Assessing vision, hearing, and speech is an important part of physical assessment because these are important to the development of age-appropriate skills.

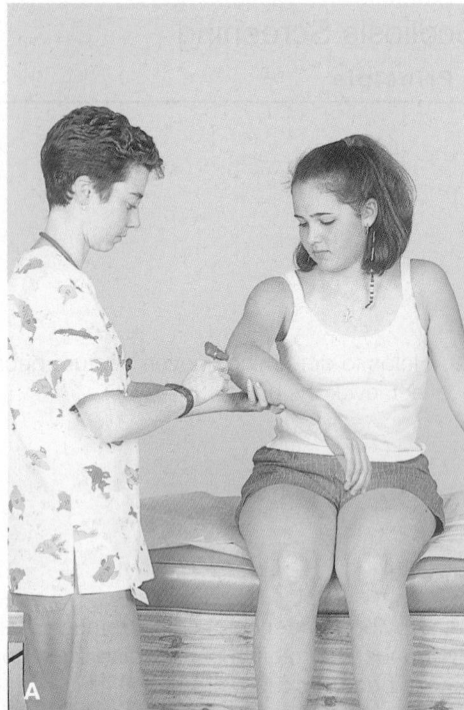

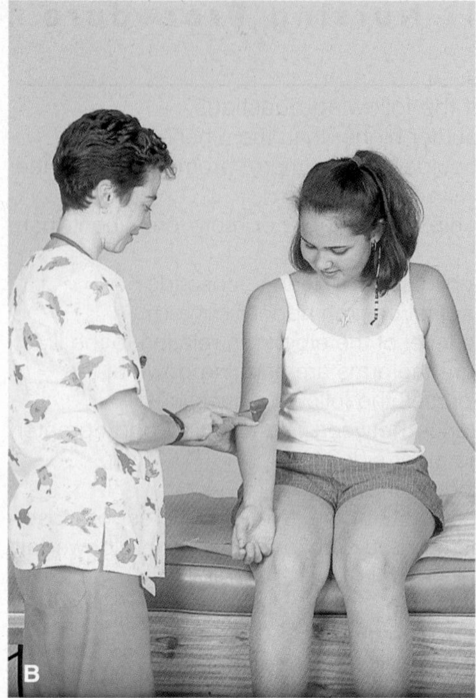

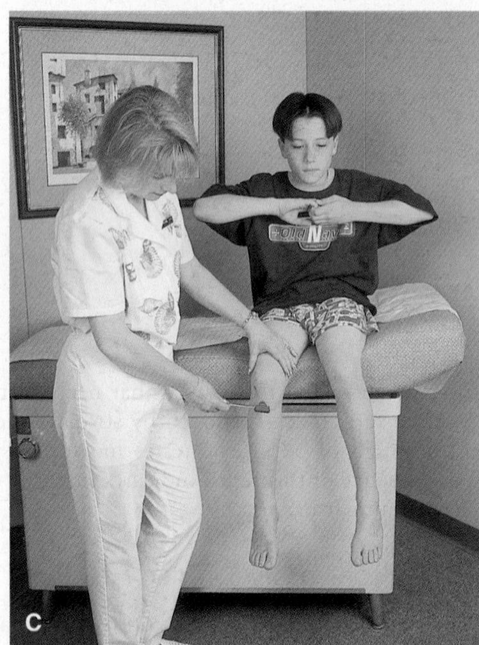

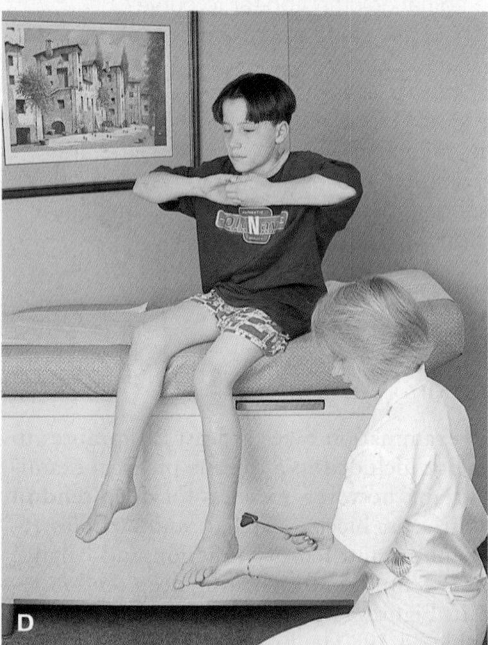

FIGURE 34.22 Deep tendon reflexes. (**A**) Triceps reflex. The triceps tendon is struck. The forearm will move perceptibly if the reflex is elicited. (**B**) Biceps reflex. The examiner's thumb is placed over the biceps tendon. The reflex hammer actually strikes the examiner's thumb. The examiner will feel the child's forearm move when the reflex is elicited. (**C**) Patellar reflex. (**D**) Achilles reflex. In both **C** and **D**, the child grasps his hands together and pulls as a means of distracting him away from what the nurse is testing. This helps to decrease muscle tension, facilitate the reflex arc, and elicit more accurate results.

TABLE 34.10 ✻ Grading of Deep Tendon Reflexes

Grade	Interpretation
4+	Hyperactive; extremely marked reaction; abnormal
3+	Stronger than average but within normal range
2+	Average response
1+	Less than average response but within normal range
0	No response; abnormal

Vision Assessment

Assessing vision is an important part of physical assessment because good vision is so important to childhood development. The extent of testing depends on the age of the child.

Any child with congenital anomalies, low birth weight, or fetal alcohol syndrome is at risk for eye abnormalities, as is a child who received oxygen at birth. During an assessment, if you notice an unreported injury or infection or signs of neglected vision, make a special note. Because the average parent is careful of a child's eyes, these findings may be indicative of child neglect.

Vision Screening

Routine vision screening is usually begun at 3 years of age. Common vision screening indicators and techniques for children of different ages are summarized in Table 34.11. Parents can provide important clues to possible problems: listen carefully any time a parent expresses concern about or questions a child's ability to see well.

Newborn and Infant. Newborns should be able to focus on a moving object such as a finger and follow it to the midline.

TABLE 34.11 ✻ Common Vision Screening Indicators and Procedures

Age	Common Test
Newborn	General appearance*
	Ability to follow moving object to midline; focus steadily on an object at 10–12 in
Infant and toddler	General appearance*
	Ability to follow light past midline
3 yr–school age	General appearance*
	Random dot E for stereopsis (depth perception)
	Allen cards or preschool E chart for visual acuity
	Ishihara's plates for color awareness
School age–adolescent	General appearance*
	Snellen's test for visual acuity

* Note redness, blinking, squinting, or crusting.

Infants see black and white objects better than they do colored objects. They seem to see objects that are closest to them (a distance of about 19 cm [8 to 10 in]) best. Ask the parents if an infant's eyes follow them as they move around the room. Does an infant who is older than 6 weeks return their smile? Do the parents have any reason to think their child has difficulty seeing?

Toddler and Preschooler. Ask the parents of older infants, toddlers, or preschoolers if their children do any of the following:

- Rub their eyes, blink frequently, squint, or frown
- Cover one eye to look at objects
- Tilt the head to see things better
- Stumble over objects in their path
- Hold books and toys extremely close or extremely far away to look at them

Asking whether children sit close to a television set is meaningless because almost all children do that if allowed.

School-Age Child and Adolescent. Ask the parents if their child does any of the following:

- Reports frequent headaches
- Does poorly with classwork
- Avoids sports that require long-distance vision, such as baseball or softball
- Avoids watching movies
- Skips over words when reading aloud
- Reports blurriness or double vision
- Has reddened conjunctivae or drainage from the eyes
- Blinks at bright light

Techniques of Vision Testing

Vision is tested by asking a child to read an eye chart. All children need good orientation to such testing so they can appreciate this is not a test in the usual sense of the word; otherwise, they may be unusually anxious or try to pass it by cheating. Vision testing needs to be started in the preschool period so children with amblyopia (lazy eye; see Chapter 50), a potentially serious vision disorder, can be identified while the condition is still correctable (Wallace et al., 2007). In addition to usual testing, a Polaroid or digital photograph of a child can be used to help identify strabismus (uneven gaze).

Snellen Chart. As soon as children can identify letters of the alphabet (early school age), their vision can be tested at a health checkup by using a Snellen eye chart. This chart is standardized, so set procedures must be followed when using it to test vision (Box 34.12).

Preschool E Chart. Between 3 years of age and the age they can read the alphabet, children can have their vision tested by using an LEA chart that uses symbols such as squares and circles instead of letters, or a preschool E chart (Fig. 34.23). These charts are also helpful in testing children who are cognitively challenged or those who do not speak fluent English. To test using a preschool E chart, the procedure is similar to that of the standard Snellen chart:

1. The child stands 20 ft from the chart and then should read first with the right eye, then with the left, then both eyes, as with standard testing. Young children do

Box 34.12 Nursing Procedure ✻ Snellen Eye Chart Assessment

Purpose To assess vision.

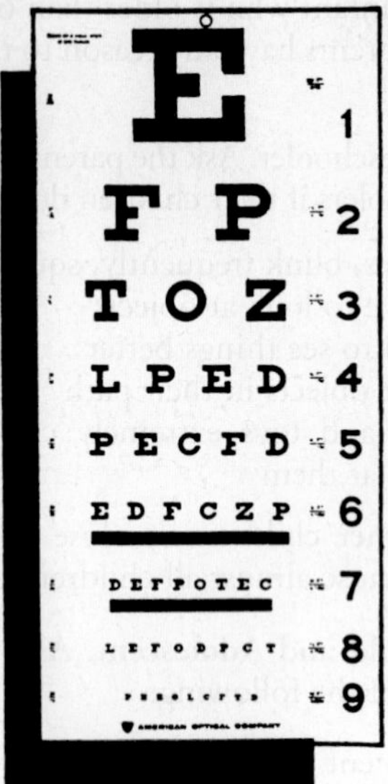

Procedure	Principle
1. Hang the chart so the 20-ft line is at the child's eye level.	1. The child who has to look up or down must look farther than the child who is looking straight across at the chart. A possible solution to avoid moving the chart is to have smaller children stand and taller children sit. To accommodate children in wheelchairs, the chart needs to be lowered (or else have all children sit for the test).
2. Provide a good light for the chart and place it so there is no glare. A light intensity of 20 foot-candles is recommended.	2. Appropriate lighting provides for optimal test conditions.
3. Measure a distance of 20 ft from the chart. Mark the floor at this point with a piece of masking tape or other similar mark. For younger children, it is helpful to cut out paper footprints and paste them to the floor with the heels of the footprints touching the 20-ft line. If the child sits in a chair, the back legs of the chair should touch the 20-ft line.	3. Twenty feet is the optimal distance from the chart for testing.
4. Provide an individual 3 × 5-in card (to cover the eye not being tested) for each child who is examined.	4. Covering the other eye allows for one eye to be tested at a time.
5. If the child wears glasses, screen while he or she is wearing the glasses. If a child has forgotten to bring glasses, defer the screening until the child can bring the glasses. Do not screen the child first without glasses and then with them, because this forces the child to strain to read the chart.	5. Testing with corrective lenses screens for corrected eyesight. After squinting, a child may have difficulty readjusting to reading with glasses, and this makes the prescription appear too weak or too strong.
6. To begin testing, tell the child to stand with his or her shoes on the footprints (heels against the line); keep both eyes open; and cover the left eye with the occluding card. Be certain the child does not press the card against the eye (instead, the edge of the card should rest across the child's nose).	6. Covering the eye not being tested provides optimal test conditions. Pressure will cause blurred vision when the child removes the card to test that eye.

Box 34.12 Nursing Procedure ✻ Snellen Eye Chart Assessment

Procedure	Principle
7. Begin at the 40-ft line of the chart and, using a pointer or pencil, point to each symbol on the line from left to right (the order in which children are taught to read). If the child reads a majority of symbols in a line, he or she sees the line satisfactorily.	**7.** Starting at the 40-ft line is the standardized testing procedure.
8. If the child "passes" the 40-ft line, have the child read the 30- and 20-ft lines or the last line the child can read. Record the last line read. If the child fails to read the 40-ft line satisfactorily, then begin at the top of the chart and move downward to identify the last line the child can read. Record this reading. Because the 200-ft, 100-ft, and 70-ft lines have so few symbols, the child must read all the symbols on them to have read satisfactorily.	**8.** Moving to the 30-ft line or less reflects use of standardized testing procedure.
9. Visual acuity is always stated as a fraction. The top number is the distance in feet the child stands from the chart (always 20). The bottom of the fraction represents the last line the child read correctly. The adult with good (average) vision can read the 20-ft line from 20 ft away and thus is said to have 20/20 vision.	**9.** Using a fraction for visual acuity is the standardized reporting procedure.
10. It is important to test the eyes separately, then together. For example, Tony reads all the symbols on the 40-ft line with his right eye; he misses three out of four on the 30-ft line. His visual acuity for his right eye is 20 (the distance from the chart) over 40 (the last line he read correctly). With his left eye, Tony reads the 40-ft, 30-ft, and 20-ft lines correctly. His vision in that eye is 20/20. With both eyes, Tony reads the 40-ft, 30-ft, and 20-ft lines correctly. His visual acuity for both eyes is 20/20.	**10.** If only this last reading were taken, the right eye weakness (a symptom of amblyopia or "lazy eye") would be missed.
11. Observe children for straining or squinting as they read the chart.	**11.** By squinting and changing the shape of the eyeball, children can improve their vision and will score higher. Children will appear to see better than they actually do in everyday situations.

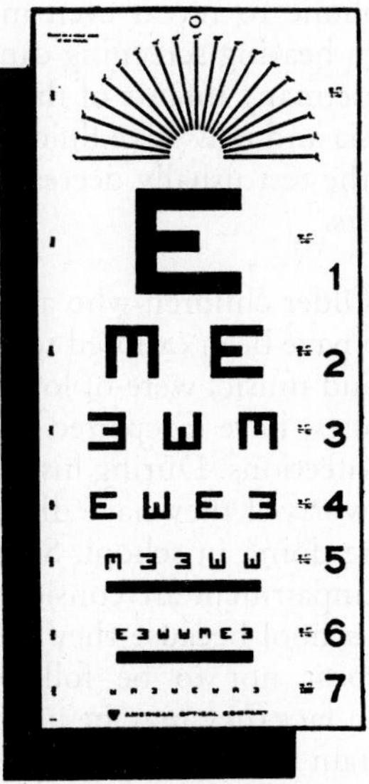

FIGURE 34.23 Astigmatic and preschool E chart. (From the American Optical Corporation, with permission.)

not understand the importance of not pressing an occluder card against their eye or of not peeking, so a second person is often needed to hold the card for children of this age. Using a pair of plastic eyeglasses with one side patched is another way to solve this problem.

2. It is helpful to compare the E with a table with three legs and ask the child which way the legs of the table point. By 3 years, children are familiar with tables, but Es are strange symbols. Tell the child to point with the entire arm and hand in the direction the legs point so you do not confuse the hand motion.
3. Begin at the 40-ft line, as with the standard Snellen chart, and work downward until the child passes all lines or cannot read the majority of symbols on a line.

Allen Cards. Preschool children may also be tested with Allen cards, which consist of pictures of common objects such as a horse and rider, car, house, and birthday cake. These are shown to the child at a 15-ft distance, and the child is asked to identify the pictures (proof the child sees them). Be certain children have time to examine the cards before the test so they know the names of the objects.

STYCAR Cards. For this test, the child is given cards with nine letters: H, C, O, L, U, T, X, V, and A. The child holds up the card that matches the one pointed to on a chart.

Titmus Vision Tester. Another useful method for testing the vision of children is the Titmus Vision Tester. This is the same instrument used by many motor vehicle licensing offices. As the child looks into the eyepieces of the machine, alphabet letters or preschool Es are projected onto a well-lighted screen for the child to identify. Closed vision testers such as the Titmus have an advantage over wall charts in that a child is less easily distracted during testing. Also, because children cannot see the vision chart beforehand, they cannot memorize the letters while waiting to be tested.

Color Vision Discrimination Testing. The inability to discern colors is a sex-linked recessive characteristic that tends to occur in males rather than in females, although females carry the gene for the disorder. All male children should be screened once for the disorder during their early school years.

To test a child for color awareness, ask the child to identify the colored stripes at the top of a Snellen eye chart or show the child a series of colored diagrams (Ishihara's plates). With the latter, a person with color vision can see hidden figures such as butterflies, but people with red-green or yellow-blue color vision deficits cannot. Detecting color vision deficit in children is important because many educational materials and some occupations depend on the ability to identify color. Even such a simple childhood pleasure as riding a bicycle safely on city streets depends on being able to distinguish colors, such as red from green on a traffic light.

Vision Referrals

Screen children twice before referring them to a physician for corrective eye care, as some children do not perform well on eye tests because they are easily distracted or do not know their alphabet as well as they pretend to know it. For example, they may say they do not see a letter when they really mean they do not know or remember its name. Testing twice helps eliminate or identify this type of misleading result.

After a second screening, the following children generally require a vision referral:

- Preschool children (3 to 5 years of age) who have 20/50 vision in one or both eyes
- Children 6 years of age or older who have 20/40 vision or worse in one or both eyes
- Any child with a two-line difference between the eyes, which might be the beginning of amblyopia
- Any child who states or shows symptoms of visual disturbance

Hearing Assessment

A thorough health assessment should also include an evaluation of hearing, including both history and observation, because good hearing is necessary for the development of age-appropriate skills. Parents and grandparents are usually attuned to hearing difficulty in children and may be suspicious of it in advance of its official detection. When taking an auditory history, be certain to ask the accompanying adult or parent an overall question such as, "Do you have any reason to believe your child doesn't hear as well as other children?"

Auditory Screening

Routine screening for adequate hearing levels is usually begun at 3 years of age. Testing requires knowledge of the technique, use of an audiometer, and a quiet, undistracted setting.

Newborn and Infant. In most hospitals, all newborns are routinely screened for hearing. Certain infants are high risk for hearing deficits so definitely should be screened. This includes infants with:

- History of childhood hearing impairment in the family
- Perinatal infection, such as cytomegalovirus, rubella, herpes, toxoplasmosis, or syphilis
- Anatomic malformations involving the head or neck
- Birth weight less than 1500 g
- Hyperbilirubinemia at a level exceeding indication for exchange transfusion
- Bacterial meningitis, especially when caused by *Haemophilus influenzae*
- Severe birth asphyxia: infants with an Apgar score of 0 to 3, those who failed to breathe spontaneously within 10 minutes of birth, or those with hypotonia persisting to 2 hours of age
- Newborns who received an antibiotic

A newborn's hearing is usually assessed through simple response testing—observing whether an infant stirs or responds to a sound delivered to the child with a commercial device (Young & Tattersall, 2007). It can also be done by brainstem auditory-evoked response (BAER) testing. For this method, an earphone is placed on the infant and an electrode is attached to the scalp. When sound is transmitted to the child's ear through the earphone, the electrical potential created as the sound is processed by the brainstem is read by the scalp electrode, processed by a microcomputer, and plotted on a graph. This type of testing may be used at any age and is successful even in children who are comatose or anesthetized. Smaller units using transient evoked otoacoustic emissions (TEOAEs) are also available. With these, a click stimulus delivered to a normal ear produces an echo from the cochlea. This can be detected by a miniature microphone to reveal even minor hearing loss. Although newborn hearing screening can lead to false-positive results because many infants of this age are still sleepy from birth analgesia and may have fluid- or vernix-filled ear canals, repeating the test usually decreases the incidence of false-positive results.

Older Children. Older children who are at risk for hearing loss are those who have been exposed to loud noises such as an explosion or loud music, were of low birth weight, have congenital anomalies, have a repaired cleft palate, or have had repeated ear infections. During history taking, ask children if they ever worry if they have difficulty hearing. Ask them how they are doing in school. Some children with a minimal hearing impairment are considered to have behavioral problems in school because they do not follow directions well or appear not to be following the teacher's discussion when in fact they may be unable to hear what is being said. Be certain not to confuse difficulty hearing with shyness or recalcitrance in answering. Children with an ear infection (otitis media) or allergies should be tested after the fluids in their ears clear because their hearing may be temporarily affected by these conditions. Cerumen in the ear canal is not documented to substantially decrease hearing.

Principles of Audiometric Assessment

Frequency. Sound is the result of vibration; frequency is the number of vibrations a sound creates per second. When frequency is increased, the pitch of the sound increases. For audiometric testing, frequency is measured in Hertz units. Normal speech sounds fall into a narrow range, 500 to 2000 Hz, so to function adequately and speak effectively, a child must be able to hear in this range. Children are tested for a wider frequency range than this, from 500 to 6000 Hz, on a routine screening assessment.

Loudness. Decibels are an expression of the intensity of loudness of a sound (or vigor of the vibrations). A decibel level of 0 dB is the softest sound that can be heard. Normal conversation is approximately 50 to 60 dB. The sound level at which inner ear damage can occur is about 90 dB. Sound levels of 140 dB are so intense they actually cause pain. Screening audiometry is done at 25 dB.

Hearing Loss. Table 34.12 lists levels of hearing loss. The inability of a child to hear sounds softer than 30 dB indicates a child will have some difficulty hearing normal instructions and questions. If a child cannot hear sounds softer than 50 dB, the child misses most normal conversation and will have difficulty achieving in a regular classroom environment. Hearing loss at this level is so severe that the child will also be speech-challenged because normal speech sounds cannot be heard.

If children can hear all frequencies at the 25-dB level, they have passed an audiometric screening check. If a child fails to hear two or more frequencies at 25 dB, in either or both ears, the child has failed a screening audiometry test and should be referred to a physician or an otologist. An **audiogram** is a record of audiometric testing. Figure 34.24 shows an audiogram of a child with normal hearing in the right ear (the child heard all frequencies at the 20-dB level) but an inability to hear sounds softer than 45 dB in the left ear at frequencies of 1000, 2000, and 4000 Hz.

Acoustic Impedance Testing

Acoustic impedance testing is based on the principle that sound entering the ear canal meets resistance at the tympanic membrane. If the middle ear is functioning normally, there will be a symmetric pattern of resistance on a tympanogram printout. If the middle ear is functioning abnormally, the level of resistance will be greater or less than normal, so the pattern will be abnormal.

Acoustic impedance testing is performed by audiologists. For the assessment, the ear to be tested is plugged with a rubber disc. Sound is then administered to the ear through the center of the disc. The resistance met at the eardrum is registered and recorded as a graph. Tympanograms are inaccurate in children younger than 7 months because the tympanic membrane is too compliant under that age to register normal impedance.

Conduction Loss Testing

Both the Rinne and the Weber tests are helpful assessments that can be used to help determine the cause of hearing loss in older children (Box 34.13).

Speech Assessment

Speech problems are directly related to hearing problems: infants who do not hear will make preliminary babbling sounds but then will not develop intelligible speech because they cannot hear and repeat sounds. Speech difficulties may also be related to:

- Motor development such as when the child cannot control tongue and facial muscles well enough to form proper words
- Cognitive development such as when the cognitively challenged child cannot grasp the concept of speech or word use until later than normal, or possibly not at all
- Cultural influences such as when the parents speak two languages, making it difficult for a child to accurately learn and articulate either language or when parents spoke "baby talk" for so long the child mimicked that instead of pronouncing words clearly

Speech screening begins by asking children a few simple questions to determine their language pattern. Also ask parents

TABLE 34.12 ✻ Levels of Hearing Loss

Hearing Loss (DB Level)	Hearing Level Present
Slight (<30)	Inability to hear whispered words or faint speech No speech challenge present Possible lack of awareness of hearing difficulty Achievement in school and home is attained by leaning forward, speaking loudly
Mild (30–50)	Beginning speech challenge possibly present Difficulty hearing if not facing speaker; some difficulty with normal conversation
Moderate (55–70)	Speech challenge present, possibly requiring speech therapy Difficulty with normal conversation
Severe (70–90)	Difficulty with any but nearby loud voice Vowels easier to hear than consonants Speech therapy required for clear speech. Possible ability to still hear loud sounds such as jets or whistle of train.
Profound (>90)	Almost no sound heard

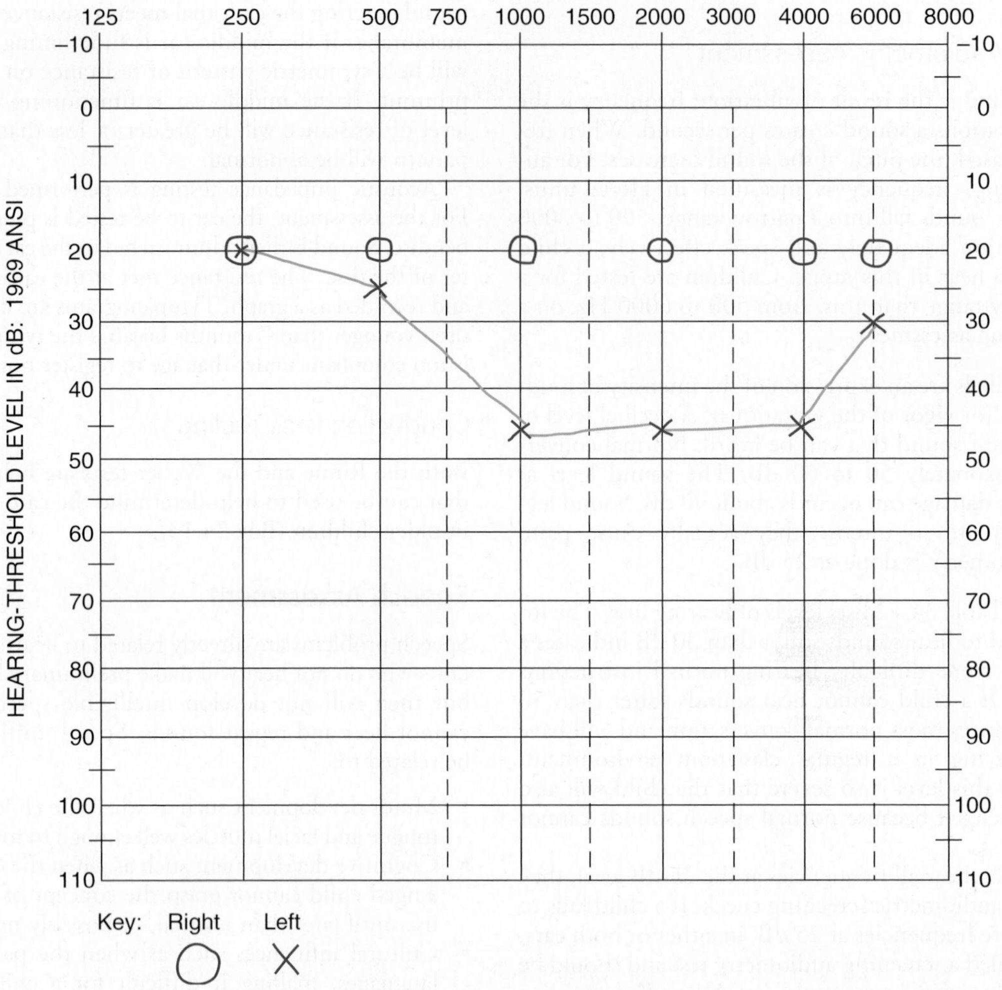

FIGURE 34.24 An audiogram done as a screening procedure. Notice that hearing is normal in the right ear (all frequencies are heard at the 20-dB level). In the left ear there is hearing loss (the frequencies 1000, 2000, and 4000 Hz are heard only at the 45-dB level). (Courtesy of Dr. H. Schill, Speech Pathology and Audiology Department, Boston University.)

if they have noticed any difficulties with their child's pronunciation or comprehension. Standardized tests, such as the Denver Articulation Screening Examination (DASE), may also be administered.

Denver Articulation Screening Examination

The DASE is designed to detect significant developmental delays and normal variations in the acquisition of speech sounds. Because it is a standardized test, its directions must be followed carefully. The test is useful only with English-speaking children.

Administration. Before the test, explain that the child will need to repeat some words she hears. Give enough examples so she will understand what she is to do: "When I say 'boat,' then you say 'boat.'" When you are certain the child understands the directions, say each of the 22 words shown on the DASE form (Fig. 34.25A). Convey the impression that there is no right or wrong answer. Give the child approval for responding and following directions correctly, no matter how inaccurately the child repeats the word.

Scoring. The DASE is designed for use with children between ages 2.5 and 6 years. In scoring, consider the child's age to be the closest previous age shown on the percentile rank chart (see Fig. 34.25B). Score the child's pronunciation of the underlined sounds or blends in each word on the test form. A perfect raw score is 30 correctly articulated sounds. Match this raw score on the percentile rank chart with the column representing the child's age. The number at which the raw score line and the age column meet is the percentile rank of the child (how the child compares with other children of that age). Percentiles shown above the heavy line are abnormal; those below the line are normal—for example, a 3-year-old who says only 12 sounds correctly ranks in the

BOX 34.13 ✻ Rinne and Weber Tests

Rinne and Weber tests are assessments for air and bone conduction.

Rinne Test
Strike a 500-Hz tuning fork and hold the stem of it against the child's mastoid bone. Ask the child to say when the tuning fork's ringing sound can no longer be heard. When the child says it is no longer audible, move the fork forward so it is at the auditory meatus (Figure A). Because air conduction is normally better than bone conduction, the child should hear it when it is held in front of the meatus, although it can no longer be heard when it was held against the bone. If the child does not hear it when it is brought forward, then the child's air conduction is probably reduced.

Weber Test
Strike a 500-Hz tuning fork and hold the stem of it against the top of the child's head (Figure B). The child with normal hearing in both ears will hear the sound equally well with both ears. If the child has an air conduction loss in one ear, the child will hear the sound better in that ear than in the good ear. The test must be used in conjunction with other evaluation tools because if the sound is intensified in one ear, it may mean that there is no hearing perception (there is nerve loss) in the opposite ear.

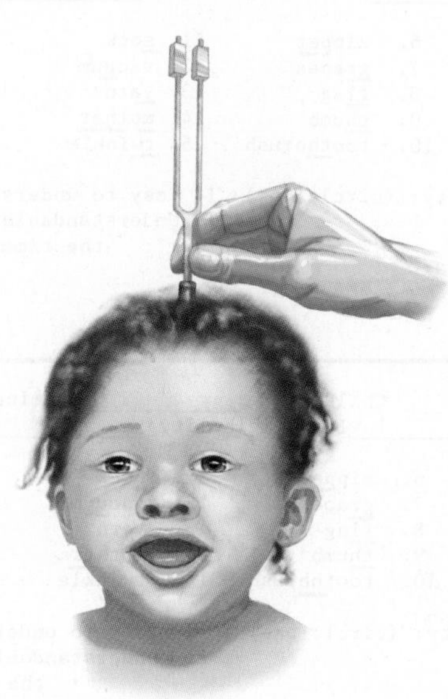

B

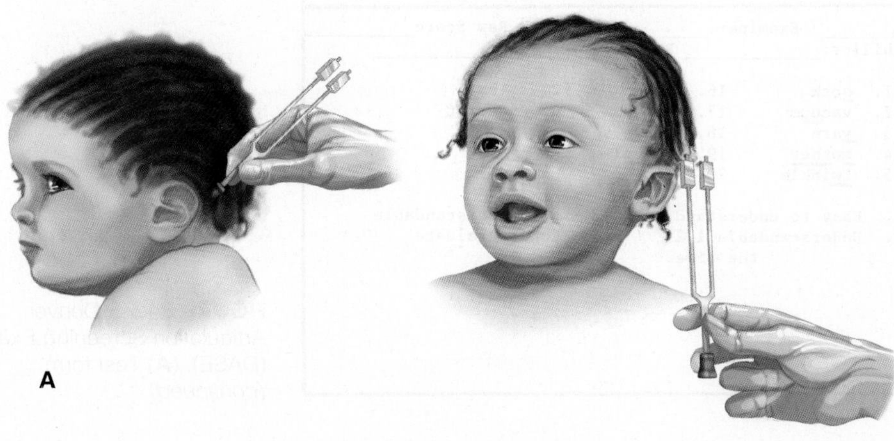

A

DENVER ARTICULATION SCREENING EXAM
for children 2 1/2 to 6 years of age

Instructions: Have child repeat each word after you. Circle the underlined sounds that he pronounces correctly. Total correct sounds is the Raw Score. Use charts on reverse side to score results.

NAME

HOSP. NO.

ADDRESS

Date: ________ Child's Age: ________ Examiner: ________ Raw Score: ________
Percentile: ________ Intelligibility: ________ Result: ________

1. table 6. zipper 11. sock 16. wagon 21. leaf
2. shirt 7. grapes 12. vacuum 17. gum 22. carrot
3. door 8. flag 13. yarn 18. house
4. trunk 9. thumb 14. mother 19. pencil
5. jumping 10. toothbrush 15. twinkle 20. fish

Intelligibility: (circle one) 1. Easy to understand 2. Understandable 1/2 the time. 3. Not understandable 4. Can't evaluate

Comments:

Date: ________ Child's Age: ________ Examiner: ________ Raw Score ________
Percentile: ________ Intelligibility: ________ Result: ________

1. table 6. zipper 11. sock 16. wagon 21. leaf
2. shirt 7. grapes 12. vacuum 17. gum 22. carrot
3. door 8. flag 13. yarn 18. house
4. trunk 9. thumb 14. mother 19. pencil
5. jumping 10. toothbrush 15. twinkle 20. fish

Intelligibility: (circle one) 1. Easy to understand 2. Understandable 1/2 the time. 3. Not understandable 4. Can't evaluate

Comments:

Date: ________ Child's Age: ________ Examiner: ________ Raw Score ________
Percentile: ________ Intelligibility: ________ Result: ________

1. table 6. zipper 11. sock 16. wagon 21. leaf
2. shirt 7. grapes 12. vacuum 17. gum 22. carrot
3. door 8. flag 13. yarn 18. house
4. trunk 9. thumb 14. mother 19. pencil
5. jumping 10. toothbrush 15. twinkle 20. fish

Intelligibility: (circle one) 1. Easy to understand 2. Understandable 1/2 the time. 3. Not understandable 4. Can't evaluate

Comments:

A

FIGURE 34.25 Denver Articulation Screening Exam (DASE). (**A**) Test form. *(continued)*

To score DASE words: Note Raw Score for child's performance. Match raw score line (extreme left of chart) with column representing child's age (to the closest previous age group). Where raw score line and age column meet number in that square denotes percentile rank of child's performance when compared to other children that age. Percentiles above heavy line are ABNORMAL percentiles, below heavy line are NORMAL.

PERCENTILE RANK

Raw Score	2.5 yr.	3.0	3.5	4.0	4.5	5.0	5.5	6 years
2	1							
3	2							
4	5							
5	9							
6	16							
7	23							
8	31	2						
9	37	4	1					
10	42	6	2					
11	48	7	4					
12	54	9	6	1	1			
13	58	12	9	2	3	1	1	
14	62	17	11	5	4	2	2	
15	68	23	15	9	5	3	2	
16	75	31	19	12	5	4	3	
17	79	38	25	15	6	6	4	
18	83	46	31	19	8	7	4	
19	86	51	38	24	10	9	5	1
20	89	58	45	30	12	11	7	3
21	92	65	52	36	15	15	9	4
22	94	72	58	43	18	19	12	5
23	96	77	63	50	22	24	15	7
24	97	82	70	58	29	29	20	15
25	99	87	78	66	36	34	26	17
26	99	91	84	75	46	43	34	24
27		94	89	82	57	54	44	34
28		96	94	88	70	68	59	47
29		98	98	94	84	84	77	68
30		100	100	100	100	100	100	100

To Score intelligibility:

	NORMAL	ABNORMAL
2 1/2 years	Understandable 1/2 the time, or, "easy"	Not Understandable
3 years and older	Easy to understand	Understandable 1/2 time Not understandable

Test Result: 1. NORMAL on Dase and Intelligibility = NORMAL

2. ABNORMAL on Dase and/or Intelligibility = ABNORMAL

* If abnormal on initial screening rescreen within 2 weeks. If abnormal again child should be referred for complete speech evaluation.

B

FIGURE 34.25 *(continued)* **(B)** Percentile rank form. (Reprinted by permission. Copyright 1971 by Amelia F. Drumwright, University of Colorado Medical Center, Denver, CO.)

9th percentile (abnormal ranking), and a 3-year-old who says 20 sounds correctly ranks in the 58th percentile (normal ranking).

In addition to determining the percentile ranking, rate the child's spontaneous speech in terms of intelligibility as 1, easy to understand; 2, understandable half the time; 3, not understandable; or 4, cannot evaluate (maybe the child did not speak in sentences or phrases during your contact with the child). Score intelligibility according to the chart in Figure 34.25B. For a final score, rate the child's total test result (normal or abnormal on the DASE or intelligibility).

Children who score abnormally on this screening test should be retested in 2 weeks. If they still score abnormally, they should be referred for complete speech evaluation.

ASSESSING DEVELOPMENTAL MILESTONES

It would be ideal if children demonstrated all the developmental skills of which they are capable every time they are asked to demonstrate them. Rarely, however, do they accomplish this. Infants become hungry, sleepy, or upset during testing. Older children may become shy. A portion of developmental information on almost all health assessments, therefore, must be elicited by history taking. All previous developmental milestones must be obtained this way.

Developmental History

Many parents keep careful records of their first child's development, a less careful record of their second, a scanty record of the third, and so on. The best information, therefore, generally depends on parents' memories.

Parents may not be able to recall the month during which a skill was first demonstrated. It is often helpful to ask them to try to remember in terms of holidays or seasons. For example, they may not know at which month their infant first used a pincer grasp (grasped cleanly with index finger and thumb) but do recall the way the child pinched the ear of the family dog at a summer picnic.

If parents seem to have no recall at all of developmental milestones that are important for the child's present evaluation, suggest they ask other family members or look through family photographs to jog their memories and then call with as much information as they can gather.

In addition to getting the parents' description of the skills a child has mastered, it is helpful to watch children perform skills and rate them according to standard criteria.

Denver II Developmental Screening Test

The Denver II Developmental Screening Test (see Appendix H) is the most widely used tool to assess childhood development (Frankenburg, 1994). The test can detect delays during infancy and the preschool years. Four main categories of development are rated:

1. Personal–social
2. Fine motor-adaptive
3. Language
4. Gross motor skills

Administration

The Denver II ideally should be completed when a child is approximately 3 or 4 months of age, again at about 10 months, and again at 3 years. It is a supplement to the developmental evaluation by history that should be a part of every well-child assessment.

The materials to administer the test must be purchased as a kit. They include a skein of red wool, a box of raisins, a small bottle, a bell, a rattle with a narrow handle, a tennis ball, ten 1-inch brightly colored blocks, a small plastic doll, a toy baby bottle, a plastic cup, and a pencil.

Although administration of the Denver II is not difficult, it should not be attempted except by health care providers trained specifically in its procedures and interpretation. This precaution is necessary to ensure the validity of its developmental norms. Periodic retraining and proficiency testing are recommended to sustain a high degree of accuracy in administration.

A parent should be cautioned before administration that this is not a test of intelligence but of the child's level of development. The child's inability to perform a task that most children of the same age can accomplish indicates a delay in that area. Further evaluation is then needed to determine the reason for this delay.

Scoring

The child is scored P (passed), F (failed), R (refused), or N.O. (no opportunity) on each item according to guidelines in the instruction manual. Each item is represented on the test form (see Appendix H) by a bar showing the ages by which 25%, 50%, 75%, and 90% of children normally have mastered that item. The left end of the bar is the 25% mark; the tick mark at the top of the bar, 50%; the left end of the colored (gray) area, 75%; and the right end of the bar, 90%. Looking at the form, notice, for example, the item "plays pat-a-cake" in the area of personal-social development. With this item, 25% of children show the trait at 7 months, 50% between 9 and 10 months, 75% between 10 and 11 months, and 90% by ages 11 to 12 months. Interpretation of performance is detailed in the manual.

Prescreening Test

A Denver Prescreening Developmental Questionnaire (R-PDQII) is available in addition to the Denver II. The PDQII is designed to identify children who require further testing with a full Denver II. It is a questionnaire completed by the parents addressing 10 developmental items. A child who scores 8 out of 10 or fewer should be retested in approximately 2 weeks. If the initial score is under 6 or the retest score is 8 or below, the child should have a full Denver II. Encouraging parents to complete a questionnaire this way can detect developmental delays that otherwise might be missed in a busy office or clinic (Hix-Small et al., 2007).

Cognitive Development

Children must learn many important concepts or ideas such as near, far, here, there, number sequences, how to judge time intervals, how to reason and solve problems, and how to judge weight before they can function effectively in the world.

This type of learning—gaining concepts—is cognitive learning and is measured by intelligence tests. **Intelligence** can be defined as the ability to think abstractly, to adjust to new situations, and to profit from experience. Almost everyone has had their intelligence quotient (IQ) rated at some point in a school career. Although intelligence tests are not part of routine health appraisals, it is helpful to be familiar with those that are used for childhood measurements because these findings are helpful in predicting children's school success.

The IQ is the ratio of mental age as measured by an intelligence test to chronologic age. The formula for IQ is (mental age/chronologic age) multiplied by 100. A child aged 9 years old (chronologic age) who passes all the items on an intelligence test that an average 9-year-old child passes would be (9 [mental age]/9 [chronologic age]) × 100 = 100 (child's IQ). If a child passes no more items than the average 5-year-old child would, the IQ would be (5 [mental age]/9 [chronologic age]) × 100 = 55. If a child passed all the items that a 12-year-old child normally passes, the IQ would be (12 [mental age]/9 [chronologic age]) × 100 = 133.

Intelligence scores are not always accurate because children may score poorly because of test anxiety. Cultural bias and past experience can also affect how children score. Therefore, labeling children by IQ and classifying them into divisions based on IQ is often unfair and must be done with considerable thought and study.

It is difficult to test very young children with any degree of accuracy because they lack the ability to complete tasks in the areas used for scoring intelligence tests: comprehension, imagination, reasoning, memory, and vocabulary. The most common tests used with infants include the Cattell Infant Intelligence Scale, the Bayley Mental Scale, and the Gesell

Developmental Schedule. These tests rely heavily on perceptual and motor skills as rating devices.

The two most frequently used tests for older children are the Wechsler Intelligence Scale for Children and the Stanford-Binet test. All schoolchildren take one of these tests during the primary school grades. The results are made available to child health care teams if they can demonstrate to school officials that such information is necessary for total health care or planning. If the information is unavailable, the child can be referred to a psychologist or a psychological testing clinic for assessment.

Goodenough-Harris Drawing Test

A child's drawing can reveal information on developmental or emotional problems. A Goodenough-Harris Drawing Test is a quick intelligence measurement that can be administered without special training (Goodenough, 1926). Give a child between 3 and 10 years of age a pencil and paper and tell the child to draw a person. Urge the child to draw it carefully and to take enough time to do it well.

The child receives 1 point for each of the items in the drawing listed in Box 34.14. For each 4 points scored, 1 year is added to a base age of 3 years to calculate the child's mental age. The image shown in Box 34.14 was drawn by a 4½-year-old child: it was given 8 points. The child's IQ level is therefore (5.0/4.5) times 100 = 111.

Scores on the test are reasonably reliable, correlating well with a Stanford-Binet test, although results may not be as reliable with children who are mentally ill. A child who scores significantly lower than chronologic age (after allowing for

BOX 34.14 ❋ Goodenough-Harris Drawing Test

Score one point for each characteristic listed below that is present on drawing. For every four points, 1 year is added to a base mental age of 3 years.

1. Head present
2. Legs present
3. Arms present

4a. Trunk present
  b. Length of trunk greater than breadth
  c. Shoulders indicated

5a. Both arms and legs attached to trunk
  b. Legs attached to trunk; arms attached to trunk at correct point

6a. Neck present
  b. Neck outline continuous with head, trunk, or both

7a. Eyes present
  b. Nose present
  c. Mouth present
  d. Nose and mouth in two dimensions, two lips shown
  e. Nostrils indicated

8a. Hair shown
  b. Hair nontransparent, over more than circumference

9a. Clothing present
  b. Two articles of clothing nontransparent
  c. No transparencies, both sleeves and trousers shown
  d. Four or more articles of clothing defnitely indicated
  e. Costume complete, without incongruities

10a. Fingers shown
  b. Correct number of fingers shown
  c. Fingers in two dimensions, length greater than breadth, angle less than 180°
  d. Opposition of thumb shown
  e. Hand shown distinct from fingers or arms

11a. Arm joint shown, either elbow, shoulder, or both
  b. Leg joint shown, either knee, hip, or both

12a. Head in proportion
  b. Arms in proportion
  c. Legs in proportion
  d. Feet in proportion
  e. Both arms and legs in two dimensions

13. Heel shown

14a. Firm lines without overlapping at junctions
  b. Firm lines with correct joining
  c. Head outline more than circle
  d. Trunk outline more than circle
  e. Outline of arms and legs without narrowing at point of junction with body
  f. Features symmetric, correct position

15a. Ears present
  b. Ears in correct position and proportion

16a. Eye detail: brow and lashes shown
  b. Eye detail: pupil shown
  c. Eye detail: proportion correct
  d. Eye detail: glance directed to front in profile drawing

17a. Both chin and forehead present
  b. Projection of chin shown

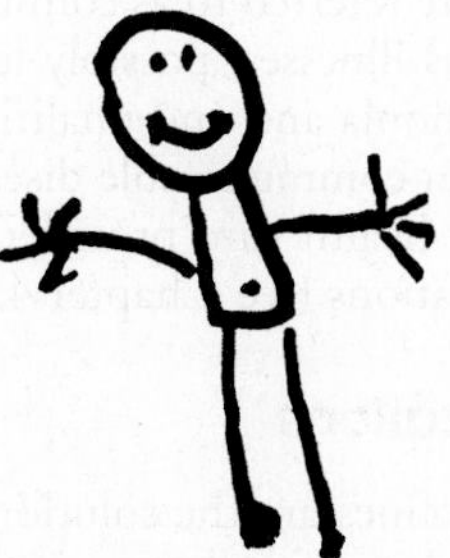

An 8-point drawing

From Goodenough, F.L. (1926). *Measurement of intelligence by drawings.* New York: World Book Company, with permission.

fatigue, illness, strange surroundings, nervousness, physical ability to use a pencil, and previous practice using a pencil and paper) should be referred for more refined testing.

Temperament

Temperament refers to a child's innate behavioral characteristics, such as activity level, rhythmicity, tendency to approach or withdraw, and adaptability to situations (see Chapter 28). A child with an "easy" temperament is generally adaptable and easy to care for; a child with a "difficult" temperament, in contrast, will almost automatically create childrearing concerns. Helping parents assess their children's temperament helps them, in turn, recognize their children's uniqueness and so anticipate and ideally prevent personality conflicts as a child grows older and expresses identified reactions to situations. If a behavior or parent–child interaction problem is already present, a nursing assessment can be useful to determine whether temperament is a factor in the problem and to assist parents with constructive solutions (Thomas & Chess, 1977).

IMMUNIZATION STATUS

One of the most important health assessment and promotion measures for children is to establish that their immunization status is up to date (AAP, 2009; Tables 34.13 and 34.14). Routine immunization schedules call for children to receive immunity against a number of dangerous infections, including measles, mumps, rubella, diphtheria, tetanus, pertussis, hepatitis B, poliomyelitis, pneumococcal pneumonia, *H. influenzae* meningitis, varicella (chickenpox), and rotavirus. New influenza vaccines are developed yearly to help ward off influenza viruses. Human papillomavirus vaccination (HPV) is recommended for prepubertal girls. Research continues on the development of vaccines to combat other diseases, including HIV infection and West Nile virus.

Teach parents about the need for children to be immunized and the need to be able to describe the record of immunizations their child has received. If gaps occur in a child's immunizations, remind the child's primary care provider about this lack in protection and prepare to administer the necessary vaccines.

Help parents understand that although diseases such as measles and mumps are referred to as common childhood illnesses, they are serious illnesses, possibly leading to complications such as pneumonia and encephalitis. When children develop these common communicable diseases, they need to be seen by a primary health care provider to minimize the risk for these complications (see Chapter 43).

Types of Immunizations

Immunizations or vaccines are the solutions used to immunize children to provide artificially acquired active or passive immunity. Box 34.15 reviews characteristics of active and passive immunity.

Vaccines are prepared in a number of forms. Attenuated vaccines are made from live organisms that have been reduced in virulence to a point where they will not cause active disease but will ensure a good antibody response. Because they are strong and effective solutions, a single dose usually provides a good degree of active immunity.

Because some bacteria, such as diphtheria, cause disease by producing a toxin, the vaccine against such a disease, a **toxoid,** is actually an extract of the toxin with reduced virulence. The antibodies produced against toxin-producing bacteria are **antitoxins.** The solution given for passive immunity against diphtheria is an antitoxin.

Gamma globulin is serum obtained from the pooled blood of many people. Because it combines the serum of many people, it probably has antibody protection against measles, rubella, poliomyelitis, varicella, and hepatitis B, among many other infectious diseases. When administered, it offers artificially acquired passive immunity.

Immune serums are serums available against specific diseases such as diphtheria, tetanus, the pit viper snake, black widow spider, and respiratory syncytial virus. Like general immune globulin, these provide passive immunity.

Available Vaccines

The AAP and CDC issue specific recommendations for childhood immunization (see Table 34.13 and Appendix J).

Diphtheria, Tetanus, Pertussis (DTaP) Vaccines

Diphtheria, tetanus toxoid, and acellular pertussis (whooping cough) vaccines are supplied in a single vial as DTaP and given in one intramuscular injection. It is recommended that children receive a primary series of four immunizations with the vaccine (2, 4, 6, and 15 to 18 months). A booster is then given between 4 and 6 years, or before entry into school. In the past, no further pertussis vaccine was administered after this point. Now, because of whooping cough outbreaks in the teenage or young adult population, a combined injection of diphtheria, tetanus toxoid, and acellular pertussis (Tdap vaccine) is recommended at 11 to 12 years. Teenagers who did not receive the 11/12-year booster or received only diphtheria/tetanus injection at that time are encouraged to receive one dose of Tdap 5 years after the last Td/DTaP dose. It is recommended that adults continue with tetanus prophylaxis every 10 years throughout life to keep tetanus immunization current.

In the past, a great deal of controversy arose about the safety of the diphtheria-tetanus-pertussis vaccine, most of it directed at the pertussis component. Severe reactions, such as high fever, persistent crying, and even seizures, were reported. For this reason, the former DTP vaccine has been modified to DTaP or contains a less reactive pertussis component. Side effects can still include drowsiness, fretfulness, low-grade fever, and redness and pain at the injection site.

Some parents, after hearing about reactions to the former vaccine, may refuse immunizations for their children. This is their right, but children who are not immunized against pertussis (unless there is a medical or moral contraindication) may be refused admittance to preschool or beginning school programs. Parents should be informed of this when they refuse to sign consent for immunization.

Pertussis vaccination is contraindicated in children who have a progressive or unstable neurologic disorder or who have had a severe allergic reaction to pertussis in a previous DTaP vaccination. If pertussis immunization is contraindicated, the Td, or diphtheria-tetanus vaccine, is substituted.

TABLE 34.13 ✻ Recommended Immunization Schedule for Persons Aged 0 Through 6 Years—United States • 2009 (For those who fall behind or start late, see the catch-up schedule)

Vaccine ▼ Age ►	Birth	1 month	2 months	4 months	6 months	12 months	15 months	18 months	19–23 months	2–3 years	4–6 years
Hepatitis B[1]	HepB	HepB		see footnote 1		HepB					
Rotavirus[2]			RV	RV	*RV*[2]						
Diphtheria, Tetanus, Pertussis[3]			DTaP	DTaP	DTaP	see footnote 3	DTaP				DTaP
Haemophilus influenzae type b[4]			Hib	Hib	*Hib*[4]	Hib					
Pneumococcal[5]			PCV	PCV	PCV	PCV				PPSV	
Inactivated Poliovirus			IPV	IPV		IPV					IPV
Influenza[6]								Influenza (Yearly)			
Measles, Mumps, Rubella[7]						MMR			see footnote 7		MMR
Varicella[8]						Varicella			see footnote 8		Varicella
Hepatitis A[9]							HepA (2 doses)			HepA Series	
Meningococcal[10]										MCV	

Legend: Range of recommended ages; Certain high-risk groups

This schedule indicates the recommended ages for routine administration of currently licensed vaccines, as of December 1, 2008, for children aged 0 through 6 years. Any dose not administered at the recommended age should be administered at a subsequent visit, when indicated and feasible. Licensed combination vaccines may be used whenever any component of the combination is indicated and other components are not contraindicated and if approved by the Food and Drug Administration for that dose of the series. Providers should consult the relevant Advisory Committee on Immunization Practices statement for detailed recommendations, including high-risk conditions: http://www.cdc.gov/vaccines/pubs/acip-list.htm. Clinically significant adverse events that follow immunization should be reported to the Vaccine Adverse Event Reporting System (VAERS). Guidance about how to obtain and complete a VAERS form is available at http://www.vaers.hhs.gov or by telephone, 800-822-7967.

1. Hepatitis B vaccine (HepB). ***(Minimum age: birth)***

At birth:
- Administer monovalent HepB to all newborns before hospital discharge.
- If mother is hepatitis B surface antigen (HBsAg)-positive, administer HepB and 0.5 mL of hepatitis B immune globulin (HBIG) within 12 hours of birth.
- If mother's HBsAg status is unknown, administer HepB within 12 hours of birth. Determine mother's HBsAg status as soon as possible and, if HBsAg-positive, administer HBIG (no later than age 1 week).

After the birth dose:
- The HepB series should be completed with either monovalent HepB or a combination vaccine containing HepB. The second dose should be administered at age 1 or 2 months. The final dose should be administered no earlier than age 24 weeks.
- Infants born to HBsAg-positive mothers should be tested for HBsAg and antibody to HBsAg (anti-HBs) after completion of at least 3 doses of the HepB series, at age 9 through 18 months (generally at the next well-child visit).

4-month dose:
- Administration of 4 doses of HepB to infants is permissible when combination vaccines containing HepB are administered after the birth dose.

2. Rotavirus vaccine (RV). ***(Minimum age: 6 weeks)***
- Administer the first dose at age 6 through 14 weeks (maximum age: 14 weeks 6 days). Vaccination should not be initiated for infants aged 15 weeks or older (i.e., 15 weeks 0 days or older).
- Administer the final dose in the series by age 8 months 0 days.
- If Rotarix® is administered at ages 2 and 4 months, a dose at 6 months is not indicated.

3. Diphtheria and tetanus toxoids and acellular pertussis vaccine (DTaP). ***(Minimum age: 6 weeks)***
- The fourth dose may be administered as early as age 12 months, provided at least 6 months have elapsed since the third dose.
- Administer the final dose in the series at age 4 through 6 years.

4. *Haemophilus influenzae* type b conjugate vaccine (Hib). ***(Minimum age: 6 weeks)***
- If PRP-OMP (PedvaxHIB® or Comvax® [HepB-Hib]) is administered at ages 2 and 4 months, a dose at age 6 months is not indicated.
- TriHiBit® (DTaP/Hib) should not be used for doses at ages 2, 4, or 6 months but can be used as the final dose in children aged 12 months or older.

5. Pneumococcal vaccine. ***(Minimum age: 6 weeks for pneumococcal conjugate vaccine [PCV]; 2 years for pneumococcal polysaccharide vaccine [PPSV])***
- PCV is recommended for all children aged younger than 5 years. Administer 1 dose of PCV to all healthy children aged 24 through 59 months who are not completely vaccinated for their age.
- Administer PPSV to children aged 2 years or older with certain underlying medical conditions (see *MMWR* 2000;49[No. RR-9]), including a cochlear implant.

6. Influenza vaccine. ***(Minimum age: 6 months for trivalent inactivated influenza vaccine [TIV]; 2 years for live, attenuated influenza vaccine [LAIV])***
- Administer annually to children aged 6 months through 18 years.
- For healthy nonpregnant persons (i.e., those who do not have underlying medical conditions that predispose them to influenza complications) aged 2 through 49 years, either LAIV or TIV may be used.
- Children receiving TIV should receive 0.25 mL if aged 6 through 35 months or 0.5 mL if aged 3 years or older.
- Administer 2 doses (separated by at least 4 weeks) to children aged younger than 9 years who are receiving influenza vaccine for the first time or who were vaccinated for the first time during the previous influenza season but only received 1 dose.

7. Measles, mumps, and rubella vaccine (MMR). ***(Minimum age: 12 months)***
- Administer the second dose at age 4 through 6 years. However, the second dose may be administered before age 4, provided at least 28 days have elapsed since the first dose.

8. Varicella vaccine. ***(Minimum age: 12 months)***
- Administer the second dose at age 4 through 6 years. However, the second dose may be administered before age 4, provided at least 3 months have elapsed since the first dose.
- For children aged 12 months through 12 years the minimum interval between doses is 3 months. However, if the second dose was administered at least 28 days after the first dose, it can be accepted as valid.

9. Hepatitis A vaccine (HepA). ***(Minimum age: 12 months)***
- Administer to all children aged 1 year (i.e., aged 12 through 23 months). Administer 2 doses at least 6 months apart.
- Children not fully vaccinated by age 2 years can be vaccinated at subsequent visits.
- HepA also is recommended for children older than 1 year who live in areas where vaccination programs target older children or who are at increased risk of infection. See *MMWR* 2006;55(No. RR-7).

10. Meningococcal vaccine. ***(Minimum age: 2 years for meningococcal conjugate vaccine [MCV] and for meningococcal polysaccharide vaccine [MPSV])***
- Administer MCV to children aged 2 through 10 years with terminal complement component deficiency, anatomic or functional asplenia, and certain other high-risk groups. See *MMWR* 2005;54(No. RR-7).
- Persons who received MPSV 3 or more years previously and who remain at increased risk for meningococcal disease should be revaccinated with MCV.

The Recommended Immunization Schedules for Persons Aged 0 Through 18 Years are approved by the Advisory Committee on Immunization Practices (www.cdc.gov/vaccines/recs/acip), the American Academy of Pediatrics (http://www.aap.org), and the American Academy of Family Physicians (http://www.aafp.org).

DEPARTMENT OF HEALTH AND HUMAN SERVICES • CENTERS FOR DISEASE CONTROL AND PREVENTION

TABLE 34.14 ✻ Recommended Immunization Schedule for Persons Aged 7 Through 18 Years—United States • 2009 (For those who fall behind or start late, see the schedule below and the catch-up schedule)

Vaccine ▼ Age ►	7–10 years	11–12 years	13–18 years
Tetanus, Diphtheria, Pertussis[1]	*see footnote 1*	Tdap	Tdap
Human Papillomavirus[2]	*see footnote 2*	HPV (3 doses)	HPV Series
Meningococcal[3]	MCV	MCV	MCV
Influenza[4]		Influenza (Yearly)	
Pneumococcal[5]		PPSV	
Hepatitis A[6]		HepA Series	
Hepatitis B[7]		HepB Series	
Inactivated Poliovirus[8]		IPV Series	
Measles, Mumps, Rubella[9]		MMR Series	
Varicella[10]		Varicella Series	

Range of recommended ages

Catch-up immunization

Certain high-risk groups

This schedule indicates the recommended ages for routine administration of currently licensed vaccines, as of December 1, 2008, for children aged 7 through 18 years. Any dose not administered at the recommended age should be administered at a subsequent visit, when indicated and feasible. Licensed combination vaccines may be used whenever any component of the combination is indicated and other components are not contraindicated and if approved by the Food and Drug Administration for that dose of the series. Providers should consult the relevant Advisory Committee on Immunization Practices statement for detailed recommendations, including high risk conditions: http://www.cdc.gov/vaccines/pubs/acip-list.htm. Clinically significant adverse events that follow immunization should be reported to the Vaccine Adverse Event Reporting System (VAERS). Guidance about how to obtain and complete a VAERS form is available at http://www.vaers.hhs.gov or by telephone, 800-822-7967.

1. **Tetanus and diphtheria toxoids and acellular pertussis vaccine (Tdap).** ***(Minimum age: 10 years for BOOSTRIX® and 11 years for ADACEL®)***
   - Administer at age 11 or 12 years for those who have completed the recommended childhood DTP/DTaP vaccination series and have not received a tetanus and diphtheria toxoid (Td) booster dose.
   - Persons aged 13 through 18 years who have not received Tdap should receive a dose.
   - A 5-year interval from the last Td dose is encouraged when Tdap is used as a booster dose; however, a shorter interval may be used if pertussis immunity is needed.
2. **Human papillomavirus vaccine (HPV).** ***(Minimum age: 9 years)***
   - Administer the first dose to females at age 11 or 12 years.
   - Administer the second dose 2 months after the first dose and the third dose 6 months after the first dose (at least 24 weeks after the first dose).
   - Administer the series to females at age 13 through 18 years if not previously vaccinated.
3. **Meningococcal conjugate vaccine (MCV).**
   - Administer at age 11 or 12 years, or at age 13 through 18 years if not previously vaccinated.
   - Administer to previously unvaccinated college freshmen living in a dormitory.
   - MCV is recommended for children aged 2 through 10 years with terminal complement component deficiency, anatomic or functional asplenia, and certain other groups at high risk. See *MMWR* 2005;54(No. RR-7).
   - Persons who received MPSV 5 or more years previously and remain at increased risk for meningococcal disease should be revaccinated with MCV.
4. **Influenza vaccine.**
   - Administer annually to children aged 6 months through 18 years.
   - For healthy nonpregnant persons (i.e., those who do not have underlying medical conditions that predispose them to influenza complications) aged 2 through 49 years, either LAIV or TIV may be used.
   - Administer 2 doses (separated by at least 4 weeks) to children aged younger than 9 years who are receiving influenza vaccine for the first time or who were vaccinated for the first time during the previous influenza season but only received 1 dose.
5. **Pneumococcal polysaccharide vaccine (PPSV).**
   - Administer to children with certain underlying medical conditions (see *MMWR* 1997;46[No. RR-8]), including a cochlear implant. A single revaccination should be administered to children with functional or anatomic asplenia or other immunocompromising condition after 5 years.
6. **Hepatitis A vaccine (HepA).**
   - Administer 2 doses at least 6 months apart.
   - HepA is recommended for children older than 1 year who live in areas where vaccination programs target older children or who are at increased risk of infection. See *MMWR* 2006;55(No. RR-7).
7. **Hepatitis B vaccine (HepB).**
   - Administer the 3-dose series to those not previously vaccinated.
   - A 2-dose series (separated by at least 4 months) of adult formulation Recombivax HB® is licensed for children aged 11 through 15 years.
8. **Inactivated poliovirus vaccine (IPV).**
   - For children who received an all-IPV or all-oral poliovirus (OPV) series, a fourth dose is not necessary if the third dose was administered at age 4 years or older.
   - If both OPV and IPV were administered as part of a series, a total of 4 doses should be administered, regardless of the child's current age.
9. **Measles, mumps, and rubella vaccine (MMR).**
   - If not previously vaccinated, administer 2 doses or the second dose for those who have received only 1 dose, with at least 28 days between doses.
10. **Varicella vaccine.**
    - For persons aged 7 through 18 years without evidence of immunity (see *MMWR* 2007;56[No. RR-4]), administer 2 doses if not previously vaccinated or the second dose if they have received only 1 dose.
    - For persons aged 7 through 12 years, the minimum interval between doses is 3 months. However, if the second dose was administered at least 28 days after the first dose, it can be accepted as valid.
    - For persons aged 13 years and older, the minimum interval between doses is 28 days.

The Recommended Immunization Schedules for Persons Aged 0 Through 18 Years are approved by the Advisory Committee on Immunization Practices (www.cdc.gov/vaccines/recs/acip), the American Academy of Pediatrics (http://www.aap.org), and the American Academy of Family Physicians (http://www.aafp.org).

DEPARTMENT OF HEALTH AND HUMAN SERVICES • CENTERS FOR DISEASE CONTROL AND PREVENTION

BOX 34.15 ✻ Active Versus Passive Immunity

Immunity, the ability to combat a particular antigen, may be either active or passive.

Active Immunity. When a child produces antibodies after the natural invasion of a pathogen (the child has measles, for example), the child is said to have *naturally acquired active immunity.* Active antibodies (or the child's ability to produce antibodies rapidly should the specific antigen [measles] invade again) last a lifetime. When pathogens are artificially injected into the child by immunization, the child receives *artificially acquired active immunity.* If the specific antigen should enter again, antibodies are produced against the pathogen that are just as lasting as those produced in naturally acquired active immunity.

Passive Immunity. IgG antibodies that a woman possesses either through immunization or through having had a disease are transferred across the placenta to a fetus in utero. Because the fetus does not make these antibodies but merely receives them, this is termed *naturally acquired passive immunity.* Passive immunity lasts only months. Some antibodies transferred across the placenta may have slightly longer lifetimes than this. For example, measles antibodies have been isolated up to age 1 year, and that is why measles immunization must be delayed until age 15 months (AAP, 2009).

When children are exposed to a disease against which they have no antibodies, antibodies made synthetically or obtained from animal serum may be injected into the child to give rapid immunity (*artificially acquired passive immunity*). Like naturally acquired passive antibodies, these last only approximately 6 weeks. A child who is susceptible to tetanus, for example, would receive tetanus antibodies after a stab wound.

Polio Vaccines

Inactivated polio vaccine (IPV) contains all three strains of poliovirus and is the type preferred for routine immunization. IPV is administered in a primary series of three doses and given along with DTaP at 2, 4, and 6 to 18 months of age. A fourth booster dose is given between the ages of 4 and 6 years, before school entry (AAP, 2009).

Measles, Mumps, Rubella (MMR) Vaccines

Measles-mumps-rubella vaccine is furnished in one injection and routinely administered between 12 and 15 months. A second dose of MMR is generally given between the ages of 4 to 6 years or, if the child did not receive the 4- to 6-year dose, at 11 to 12 years. Although MMR may be given as early as 12 months, it is usually recommended that the vaccine not be administered to children younger than 15 months because children receive a great deal of passive immunity to measles from their mothers across the placenta. Until this passive immunity has faded, the injected vaccine will be neutralized by passive antibodies and no immunity will result. For the same reason, children who have recently received immune globulin or other blood products that contain antibodies should not receive MMR vaccination for about 3 months because the passively acquired antibodies could interfere with the child's immune response to the vaccine.

Side effects of the vaccine include transient rash and a fever, which may begin 5 to 12 days after vaccination and last several days. Adverse reactions include joint pain, low-grade fever, rash, and lymphadenopathy 5 to 12 days after vaccination.

Children should be skin-tested for tuberculosis before measles vaccine administration because measles virus can cause tuberculosis to become systemic. Tuberculosis skin tests also may show false-negative reactions if given shortly after measles immunization (a child who has active tuberculosis would be wrongly identified as not having it).

Formerly, there was a concern that the administration of the MMR vaccine was associated with the development of autism in children, as symptoms of autism often begin to be apparent during the second year or close to the time of MMR vaccine administration. Further research has shown there to be no causal relationship between the vaccine and autism, dispelling this fear (Clifton, 2007). Parents may ask about this, however, and refuse to have their child immunized against MMR for this reason.

Hepatitis B Vaccine

The vaccine for hepatitis B virus (HBV) is recommended for all infants in the United States as Hepatitis B is associated with liver cancer later in life. Three doses are required. Those born to hepatitis B surface antigen (HBsAg)-negative mothers should receive the first dose in the newborn period before hospital discharge, a second dose 1 month after the first dose, and a third dose 2 months later but not before 6 months of age. Those born to HBsAg-positive mothers should receive hepatitis B immune globulin within 12 hours of birth plus HBV. A second dose of HBV is recommended at 1 to 2 months, and a third dose at 6 months. If the mother's HBsAg status is unknown, infants should receive the vaccine within 12 hours of birth, the second dose at 1 month of age, and the third dose at 6 months of age. Children who did not receive the vaccine at birth may begin a two-injection or three-injection series, depending on the vaccine used at any well-child visit. In addition, HBV immunization is recommended for populations at increased risk for contracting hepatitis B infection, including (but not limited to) health care workers with significant exposure to blood, clients receiving hemodialysis, those with hemophilia and others receiving clotting factor concentrates, illicit injectable drug users, and sexually active individuals with multiple sexual partners.

Hepatitis A Vaccine

Two doses of hepatitis A vaccine, administered 6 months apart, are recommended for all children between 1 and 2 years of age. Children who did not receive this as toddlers can be vaccinated against hepatitis A at any time.

Rotavirus Vaccine

Rotaviruses are responsible for the majority of severe gastrointestinal disease in infants so immunization against these viruses is important in preventing outbreaks of diarrhea in infants, particularly those who attend a day care setting. The vaccine is given at 2, 4 and 6 months. No doses should be given after children are older than 32 weeks.

H. influenzae Type B Vaccines

H. influenzae type b conjugate vaccine (Hib) protects against *H. influenzae* bacteria, a major cause of meningitis in children. You may need to explain the difference between *H. influenzae* (a bacteria) and influenza virus, so that parents do not think that a "flu shot" protects against this. Several formulations of this vaccine are available, and three of them are currently licensed for use in infancy. Depending on the individual vaccine, they are administered in a two-dose (at age 2 and 4 months) or a three-dose regimen (at 2, 4, and 6 months, with an additional booster at 12 months). Local reactions include tenderness at the injection site. Systemic reactions such as crying and fever may occur (AAP, 2009).

Varicella Vaccine

Varicella (chickenpox) vaccine was a difficult vaccine to develop because of the complex structure of the herpes-zoster virus. It is an important vaccine because once a generation of children has been successfully immunized, it should mark the end of epidemic childhood diseases. Infants may receive varicella vaccine at any visit after their first birthday (usually scheduled at 12 to 18 months) and again at 4 to 6 years. Those who did not receive the vaccine as infants and who lack a reliable history of chickenpox should be immunized during adolescence with two doses of vaccine, administered at least 1 month apart.

Pneumococcal Pneumonia Vaccine

The pneumococcal vaccine is recommended for all children between 2 and 23 months. The vaccine is administered at 2, 4, 6, and 12 months and provides protection for 6 to 10 years (AAP, 2009). It is especially recommended for children (and adults) who would be prone to a pneumococcal infection (those with pulmonary or cardiac disease, those without a spleen, those who are immunosuppressed).

Human Papillomavirus Vaccine

The human papillomavirus (HPV) is associated with the development of cervical cancer in women. To help prevent HPV, it is recommended that all girls receive three injections of this vaccine beginning at 11 to 12 years of age. The second dose should be administered 2 months after the first and the third dose 6 months after the first dose. Those who did not receive the vaccine in early adolescence can receive it at any time, respecting the proper monthly intervals for administration. Some teenagers who have taken abstinence pledges not to have sexual relations until they are married may voice that they do not need the vaccine. Counseling them about the safety of prophylaxis may be necessary.

Meningococcal Vaccine

Children who have immunologic deficiencies or have had their spleen removed because of trauma or therapy for a blood dyscrasia are prone to develop meningitis caused by meningococcal bacteria. Children in these high-risk groups are, therefore, advised to receive a meningococcal vaccine between 2 and 10 years of age. As meningitis occurs frequently on college campuses, previously unvaccinated college freshmen living in dormitories should also receive the vaccine.

Lyme Disease Vaccine

Lyme disease is a serious and debilitating infection caused by *Borrelia burgdorferi* and transmitted by the bite of a deer tick. A vaccine to guard against it is available for high-risk populations such as workers who maintain power lines and hunters. Although the initial trials are favorable, it has not yet been approved for children under 15 years of age (AAP, 2009).

Influenza Vaccine

Influenza is caused by A, B, or C retroviruses, which mutate so easily it has been impossible to design a vaccine that is effective for longer than 1 year. All children, infants through adolescents, particularly those who have chronic pulmonary or cardiovascular disorders or are immunosuppressed, should receive a yearly injection of the vaccine. As the vaccine can be supplied as a nasal spray, receiving the vaccine is painless (AAP, 2009).

Anthrax and Smallpox Vaccines

Anthrax is a potentially fatal disease caused by a gram-positive spore-forming anthracis bacillus spread by farm animal feces. It is extremely rare, but parents may ask about a vaccine for it because of the threat of biologic warfare associated with terrorism. A vaccine is available for people in high-risk occupations, such as hunters, taxidermists, or veterinarians, but it is not recommended for children yet.

Smallpox is an extremely infectious disease caused by the smallpox virus and transmitted by direct or indirect contact. Smallpox vaccination has not been required in the United States for over 30 years because the disease is theoretically extinct across the world. As with anthrax, parents may ask about vaccination for it because it is a disease associated with biologic warfare and terrorism. Both a vaccine (active artificial immunity) and passive artificial immunity are available, should a child be exposed to the virus. In some high-risk communities, health care providers are asked to be immunized to be certain that they will not contract the virus in a terrorist attack (Wiser, Balicer, & Cohen, 2007).

Administration of Immunizations

Assess well children at health maintenance visits and assess the immunization status of ill children at clinic or hospital admission to identify those who need their immunizations updated. Children who are seriously ill should not receive immunizations, but a slight upper respiratory tract infection (a stuffy nose with no fever) is not a contraindication. So many infants and preschoolers have common cold symptoms (the average toddler has 10 to 12 colds a year) that if children were not immunized at health maintenance visits when they have slight cold symptoms, many would never receive basic immunizations. Table 34.13 shows current recommended childhood immunizations, Table 34.14 displays recommended adolescent recommendations, and Table 34.15 displays immunizations for children who did not receive primary immunizations

TABLE 34.15 ✻ **Catch-up Immunization Schedule for Persons Aged 4 Months Through 18 Years Who Start Late or Who Are More Than 1 Month Behind—United States • 2009**

The table below provides catch-up schedules and minimum intervals between doses for children whose vaccinations have been delayed. A vaccine series does not need to be restarted, regardless of the time that has elapsed between doses. Use the section appropriate for the child's age.

CATCH-UP SCHEDULE FOR PERSONS AGED 4 MONTHS THROUGH 6 YEARS					
	Minimum Age for Dose 1	Minimum Interval Between Doses			
VACCINE		Dose 1 to Dose 2	Dose 2 to Dose 3	Dose 3 to Dose 4	Dose 4 to Dose 5
Hepatitis B[1]	**Birth**	**4 weeks**	**8 weeks** (and at least 16 weeks after first dose)		
Rotavirus[2]	**6 wks**	**4 weeks**	**4 weeks**[2]		
Diphtheria, Tetanus, Pertussis[3]	**6 wks**	**4 weeks**	**4 weeks**	**6 months**	**6 months**[3]
***Haemophilus influenzae* type b**[4]	**6 wks**	**4 weeks** if first dose administered at younger than age 12 months **8 weeks (as final dose)** if first dose administered at at age 12–14 months **No further doses needed** if first dose administered at age 15 months or older	**4 weeks**[4] if current age is younger than 12 months **8 weeks (as final dose)**[4] if current age is 12 months or older and second dose administered at younger than age 15 months **No further doses needed** if previous dose administered at age 15 months or older	**8 weeks (as final dose)** This dose only necessary for children aged 12 months through 59 months who received 3 doses before age 12 months	
Pneumococcal[5]	**6 wks**	**4 weeks** if first dose administered at younger than age 12 months **8 weeks (as final dose for healthy children)** if first dose administered at age 12 months or older or current age 24 through 59 months **No further doses needed** for healthy children if first dose administered at age 24 months or older	**4 weeks** if current age is younger than 12 months **8 weeks (as final dose for healthy children)** if current age is 12 months or older **No further doses needed** for healthy children if previous dose administered at age 24 months or older	**8 weeks (as final dose)** This dose only necessary for children aged 12 months through 9 months who received 3 doses before age 12 months or for high-risk children who received 3 doses at any age	

1. **Hepatitis B vaccine (HepB).**
   - Administer the 3-dose series to those not previously vaccinated.
   - A 2-dose series (separated by at least 4 months) of adult formulation Recombivax HB® is licensed for children aged 11 through 15 years.
2. **Rotavirus vaccine (RV).**
   - The maximum age for the first dose is 14 weeks 6 days. Vaccination should not be initiated for infants aged 15 weeks or older (i.e., 15 weeks 0 days or older).
   - Administer the final dose in the series by age 8 months 0 days.
   - If Rotarix® was administered for the first and second doses, a third dose is not indicated.
3. **Diphtheria and tetanus toxoids and acellular pertussis vaccine (DTaP).**
   - The fifth dose is not necessary if the fourth dose was administered at age 4 years or older.
4. ***Haemophilus influenzae* type b conjugate vaccine (Hib).**
   - Hib vaccine is not generally recommended for persons aged 5 years or older. No efficacy data are available on which to base a recommendation concerning use of Hib vaccine for older children and adults. However, studies suggest good immunogenicity in persons who have sickle cell disease, leukemia, or HIV infection, or who have had a splenectomy; administering 1 dose of Hib vaccine to these persons is not contraindicated.
   - If the first 2 doses were PRP-OMP (PedvaxHIB® or Comvax®), and administered at age 11 months or younger, the third (and final) dose should be administered at age 12 through 15 months and at least 8 weeks after the second dose.
   - If the first dose was administered at age 7 through 11 months, administer 2 doses separated by 4 weeks and a final dose at age 12 through 15 months.
5. **Pneumococcal vaccine.**
   - Administer 1 dose of pneumococcal conjugate vaccine (PCV) to all healthy children aged 24 through 59 months who have not received at least 1 dose of PCV on or after age 12 months.

(continued)

TABLE 34.15 ✻ Catch-up Immunization Schedule for Persons Aged 4 Months Through 18 Years Who Start Late or Who Are More Than 1 Month Behind—United States • 2009 (continued)

VACCINE	Minimum Age for Dose 1	Minimum Interval Between Doses: Dose 1 to Dose 2	Dose 2 to Dose 3	Dose 3 to Dose 4	Dose 4 to Dose 5
CATCH-UP SCHEDULE FOR PERSONS AGED 4 MONTHS THROUGH 6 YEARS					
Inactivated Poliovirus[6]	**6 wks**	**4 weeks**	**4 weeks**	**4 weeks**[6]	
Measles, Mumps, Rubella[7]	**12 mos**	**4 weeks**			
Varicella[8]	**12 mos**	**3 months**			
Hepatitis A[9]	**12 mos**	**6 months**			
CATCH-UP SCHEDULE FOR PERSONS AGED 7 THROUGH 18 YEARS					
Tetanus, Diphtheria/ Tetanus, Diphtheria, Pertussis[10]	**7 yrs**[10]	**4 weeks**	**4 weeks** if first dose administered at younger than age 12 months **6 months** if first dose administered at age 12 months or older	**6 months** if first dose administered at younger than age 12 months	
Human Papillomavirus[11]	**9 yrs**	**Routine dosing intervals are recommended**[11]			
Hepatitis A[9]	**12 mos**	**6 months**			
Hepatitis B[1]	**Birth**	**4 weeks**	**8 weeks** (and at least 16 weeks after first dose)		
Inactivated Poliovirus[6]	**6 wks**	**4 weeks**	**4 weeks**	**4 weeks**[6]	
Measles, Mumps, Rubella[7]	**12 mos**	**4 weeks**			
Varicella[8]	**12 mos**	**3 months** if the person is younger than age 13 years **4 weeks** if the person is aged 13 years or older			

- For children aged 24 through 59 months with underlying medical conditions, administer 1 dose of PCV if 3 doses were received previously or administer 2 doses of PCV at least 8 weeks apart if fewer than 3 doses were received previously.
- Administer pneumococcal polysaccharide vaccine (PPSV) to children aged 2 years or older with certain underlying medical conditions (see *MMWR* 2000;49[No. RR-9]), including a cochlear implant, at least 8 weeks after the last dose of PCV.

6. **Inactivated poliovirus vaccine (IPV).**
   - For children who received an all-IPV or all-oral poliovirus (OPV) series, a fourth dose is not necessary if the third dose was administered at age 4 years or older.
   - If both OPV and IPV were administered as part of a series, a total of 4 doses should be administered, regardless of the child's current age.
7. **Measles, mumps, and rubella vaccine (MMR).**
   - Administer the second dose at age 4 through 6 years. However, the second dose may be administered before age 4, provided at least 28 days have elapsed since the first dose.
   - If not previously vaccinated, administer 2 doses with at least 28 days between doses.
8. **Varicella vaccine.**
   - Administer the second dose at age 4 through 6 years. However, the second dose may be administered before age 4, provided at least 3 months have elapsed since the first dose.
   - For persons aged 12 months through 12 years, the minimum interval between doses is 3 months. However, if the second dose was administered at least 28 days after the first dose, it can be accepted as valid.
   - For persons aged 13 years and older, the minimum interval between doses is 28 days.
9. **Hepatitis A vaccine (HepA).**
   - HepA is recommended for children older than 1 year who live in areas where vaccination programs target older children or who are at increased risk of infection. See *MMWR* 2006;55(No. RR-7).
10. **Tetanus and diphtheria toxoids vaccine (Td) and tetanus and diphtheria toxoids and acellular pertussis vaccine (Tdap).**
    - Doses of DTaP are counted as part of the Td/Tdap series
    - Tdap should be substituted for a single dose of Td in the catch-up series or as a booster for children aged 10 through 18 years; use Td for other doses.
11. **Human papillomavirus vaccine (HPV).**
    - Administer the series to females at age 13 through 18 years if not previously vaccinated.
    - Use recommended routine dosing intervals for series catch-up (i.e., the second and third doses should be administered at 2 and 6 months after the first dose). However, the minimum interval between the first and second doses is 4 weeks. The minimum interval between the second and third doses is 12 weeks, and the third dose should be given at least 24 weeks after the first dose.

Information about reporting reactions after immunization is available online at **http://www.vaers.hhs.gov** or by telephone, **800-822-7967**. Suspected cases of vaccine-preventable diseases should be reported to the state or local health department. Additional information, including precautions and contraindications for immunization, is available from the National Center for Immunization and Respiratory Diseases at **http://www.cdc.gov/vaccines** or telephone, **800-CDC-INFO (800-232-4636).**

DEPARTMENT OF HEALTH AND HUMAN SERVICES • CENTERS FOR DISEASE CONTROL AND PREVENTION

or are behind in a vaccination schedule (a catch-up schedule). Because these schedules change yearly based on the introduction of new vaccines or new potential health threats, consult the AAP web site (http://www.aap.org) for up-to-date information before immunizing a specific child.

Because children with chronic illnesses may be hospitalized when an injection is due, such children often fall behind schedule. Children who miss the scheduled time for an immunization should not have the series started over but simply continued where they left off.

Primary care providers may choose to alter the sequence of immunization schedules if specific infections are prevalent at the time. For example, measles vaccine might be given on a first health maintenance visit (providing a child is older than 12 months) if an epidemic were currently under way in the community.

Children who are immunosuppressed, receiving corticosteroids, or receiving chemotherapy or radiation therapy should not receive live virus vaccines. The live-attenuated viruses such as measles, rubella, oral polio (OPV), and mumps must not be given to girls who are pregnant because these vaccines could cross the placenta, causing actual disease in the fetus. Before traveling internationally, parents should consult their local public health service to see what additional vaccines are required for overseas travel.

When preparing to administer an immunization, be sure to follow the manufacturer's recommendations for storage and handling of vaccines such as whether to expose to light or whether to refrigerate. Failure to follow these precautions may significantly reduce the potency and effectiveness of vaccines.

Although measles, mumps, and rubella vaccines are prepared from chick embryo cultures, egg sensitivities are not likely to occur because egg albumin and yolk components of the egg are absent from the culture. Children with egg allergy should have their allergist's permission for immunization, however, to rule out the possibility of a hypersensitivity reaction.

What if... Keoto's father tells you they have moved so often he does not know what immunizations she has had, but he knows she has never received a full series of anything. What would you do? Should Keoto have everything repeated?

Providing Teaching about Immunizations

A major reason parents do not bring children for routine immunizations is they do not know what is required or have misconceptions about immunity. Fully inform parents and, when old enough, children about what immunizations are needed in childhood. When vaccines are given, be certain parents know what is being given and what side effects may be expected. Because children may develop a low-grade fever after any immunization, counsel parents they may need to give acetaminophen (Tylenol) or children's ibuprofen for a fever of greater than 101° F (38.4° C).

Unfavorable reactions are most likely to occur within a few hours or days of administration. With live attenuated virus vaccines, viruses can multiply, so reactions may occur up to 30 days later. With rubella vaccine, a reaction (serum sickness) may occur up to 60 days later. Ask parents to report any untoward symptoms of immunization such as these.

When giving a vaccine, record the date, type of vaccine, vaccine manufacturer, lot number, and name and address of the vaccine provider so that if a vaccine reaction should occur, the instance can be investigated. Make a copy of the child's immunization record and urge parents to keep such records at home as well. They will need this information to admit their child to school and to feel safe in the event of an epidemic of a particular disease. They will need to know their child's record of tetanus immunization if the child should receive a puncture wound so that the correct therapy can be given for this.

CONCLUDING A HEALTH ASSESSMENT

At every health maintenance visit, inform parents and the child (or ask the child's physician to inform them, depending on agency policy) of any available results of screening procedures performed. After learning the results, some parents may require counseling to assist them with health or behavior concerns (see Focus on Nursing Care Planning Box 34.16).

Ask parents if they have any other remaining questions. If the health assessment revealed some health concerns and follow-up procedures are planned, be certain parents understand the reason for the upcoming tests. Suggest to parents that follow-up telephone calls are welcome after they return home from a health assessment so additional questions can be answered. Provide parents with the best hours to call so someone will be available to answer questions for them.

✓ Checkpoint Question 34.5

Keoto's father wants to be sure Keoto's immunizations are up to date. When is the immunization for varicella usually given?

a. At 12 to 18 months of age.
b. At 2 and 4 months of age.
c. At 16 years of age.
d. It is not recommended for children.

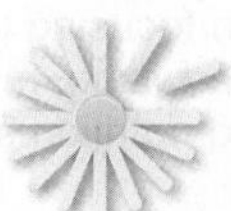

Key Points for Review

- Health assessment always causes some degree of apprehension for both parents and children because of worry some illness will be detected. Giving reassurance of wellness during examinations helps to alleviate this worry.
- A health history is an important part of a health assessment. The purpose is to gather information that will supplement physical or laboratory examinations to provide a more thorough health evaluation.
- The parts of a complete health history are introduction, chief concern, present health, family profile, history of past illnesses, day history, family health history, and review of systems.
- Physical examination involves four techniques: inspection, palpation, percussion, and auscultation. Techniques and approaches must be varied according to the child's age.
- Be certain to use examining instruments safely such as supporting an otoscope base so that if a child moves, the otoscope moves with the child. Be certain young children

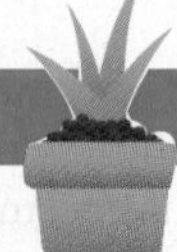

BOX 34.16 ✻ Focus on Nursing Care Planning

A Multidisciplinary Care Map for a Child in Need of a Presports Health Assessment

Keoto Wiser is a 13-year-old you meet in an ambulatory clinic. Her father has brought her for health assessment before Keoto begins seventh grade.

Family Assessment ✻ Child lives with two parents and 2-year-old sister, Candy. Father works as a paramedic for the fire department; mother is a notary public employed by a bank. Father rates finances as "good."

Child Assessment ✻ Keoto was born with a lung cyst that was removed by surgery at 6 months of age. Her father is concerned her lessened lung size may make her ineligible for competitive sports participation. Asking if carbohydrate loading would give her enough energy to make up for any decreased lung function. Is also concerned she needs eyeglasses, as she always sits close to the television set.

Nursing Diagnosis ✻ Anxiety related to ability to participate in school sports program

Outcome Criteria ✻ Client participates in school sports program to the degree based on physical findings.

Team Member Responsible	Assessment	Intervention	Rationale	Expected Outcome
		Activities of Daily Living		
Nurse	Assess child's development by taking a 24-hour day history.	Discuss with parent and child any areas that cause concern.	Parents can "get behind" in expectations of child, as preteenage children are growing and developing rapidly.	Parent or child gives day history; discusses any areas they see as problematic.
		Consultations		
Physician	Determine which school physician determines eligibility for sports teams.	Consult with school physician to determine eligibility for sports.	Schools may have restrictions on children who do not have both pairs of duplicate organs like lungs.	Qualifications for sports participation are outlined for parents and child.
		Procedures/Medications		
Nurse practitioner	Obtain health history, particularly in regard to stamina, nutrition, and past ability to participate in structured activities.	Perform complete physical examination focusing on heart, lung, muscle, and nutrition status.	Physical examination can reveal additional findings regarding lung capacity and stamina.	Physical examination determines child's overall health.
Nurse	Assess whether child is familiar with Snellen vision testing.	Test child's eyesight using a Snellen eye chart.	A Snellen eye chart is a standardized test for vision appraisal.	Child completes eye exam. Mother agrees to any recommendations.
		Nutrition		
Nurse/ nutritionist	Assess what parent and child know about carbohydrate loading.	Counsel regarding disadvantages of carbohydrate loading and sports participation for children.	Children and parents who are well informed can make informed choices on the benefit of nutrition practices.	Parent and child state they understand carbohydrate loading is not recommended for children.
		Patient/Family Education		
Nurse	Assess past health history and recommended immunizations.	Review with parent and child the child's current immunization status and any immunizations needed.	Parents are often unfamiliar with required immunizations so need to be reminded of recommended schedules.	Parent and child agree to any immunization necessary before child returns to school.

		Psychosocial/Spiritual/Emotional Needs		
Nurse	Assess what will be child's reaction if she cannot participate in school sports program.	If child is unable to participate in school sports, review with child other options: join a club; petition school sports committee.	Planning ahead can help child adjust to less-than-desired results from health assessment.	Child lists alternate ways to participate with other children at school, if sports are not an option, or describes sensible plan for petitioning for exception to rules.
		Discharge Planning		
Nurse	Assess if parent or child has had questions answered by health assessment.	Answer remaining questions; schedule a return visit as needed.	If questions remain unanswered at a health assessment, needs are not fully met.	Parent and child state they have no further questions; describe plans for next action.

are not left unsupervised on an examining table so they do not fall.

- The components of a physical examination are vital sign assessment; general appearance; mental status assessment; body measurements; and assessment of head, eyes, nose, ears, mouth, neck, chest, breasts, lungs, heart, abdomen, rectogenital area, extremities, back, and neurologic function.
- Adolescent boys should be taught testicular self-examination at the time of a health appraisal. The American Cancer Society recommends that women should be taught to perform monthly breast self-examinations when they reach 20 years of age.
- Vision assessment consists of asking children to read a standardized chart such as a Snellen or Preschool E Chart, cover testing, or color discrimination assessment.
- Hearing assessment consists of such assessments as audiometric testing and a Rinne and Weber test.
- Development is an important part of total assessment. The Denver II Developmental Screening Test and the Denver Articulation Screening Examination are specific development tests.
- The Goodenough-Harris Drawing Test correlates well with IQ and is an easy test to administer to children between the ages of 3 and 10 years to assess intelligence.
- Temperament refers to a child's innate behavioral characteristics, such as activity level, rhythmicity, and tendency to approach or withdraw and adapt to situations. Assessing this can help parents better understand behavior in their child.
- Assessment of immunization status is included as part of health assessment. Childhood immunizations are a major safeguard for children against common illnesses.

CRITICAL THINKING EXERCISES

1. Keoto is the 13-year-old girl you met at the beginning of the chapter. Her father has brought her to your ambulatory clinic for a middle school checkup because he is worried she needs glasses (she always sits close to the television set). Her mother was reluctant to bring her because she does not want her to be prescribed glasses. What questions on history would be important to ask the father or Keoto? What type of eye chart would you use with Keoto to assess her vision?
2. Keoto's 2-year-old sister, Candy, is very resistant to being examined. What techniques would you use to help this toddler adjust better to a physical examination?
3. Children should be completely undressed for physical examinations and all body surfaces inspected. What would be your response if Candy's father said he did not want to undress his child? What if he did not want to remove a Band-Aid from Candy's back?
4. Examine the National Health Goals related to health assessment of children. Most government-sponsored funds for nursing research are allotted based on these goals. What would be a possible research topic to explore pertinent to these goals that would be applicable to Keoto's family and also advance evidence-based practice?

CRITICAL THINKING SCENARIO

Open the accompanying CD-ROM or visit http://thePoint.lww.com and read the Patient Scenario included for this chapter, then answer the questions to further sharpen your skills and grow more familiar with NCLEX style questions related to child health assessment. Confirm your answers are correct by reading the rationales.

REFERENCES

American Academy of Pediatrics (AAP) Committee on Practice and Ambulatory Medicine. (2009). *Recommendations for preventive pediatric health care.* Washington, DC: Author.

American Cancer Society (ACS). (2008). *Breast self-examination.* Atlanta, GA: Author.

Askin, D. F. (2007). Physical assessment of the newborn: inspection through palpation. *Nursing for Women's Health, 11*(3), 304–315.

Aylott, M. (2007). Observing the sick child: respiratory palpation. *Paediatric Nursing, 19*(1), 38–45.

Becker, T., Kharbanda, A., & Bachur, R. (2007). Atypical clinical features of pediatric appendicitis. *Academic Emergency Medicine, 14*(2), 124–129.

Bisanz, A. (2007). Chronic constipation. *American Journal of Nursing, 107*(4), 72–78.

Black, M. M., et al. (2007). Early intervention and recovery among children with failure to thrive: follow-up at age 8. *Pediatrics, 120*(1), 59–69.

Chiolero, A., et al. (2007). Has blood pressure increased in children in response to the obesity epidemic? *Pediatrics, 119*(3), 544–553.

Chumlea, C. (2007). Which growth charts are the best for children today? *Nutrition Today, 42*(4), 148–150.

Clifton, J. C. (2007). Mercury exposure and public health. *Pediatric Clinics of North America, 54*(2), 237–269.

Drezner, J. A., et al. (2007). Inter-Association Task Force recommendations on emergency preparedness and management of sudden cardiac arrest in high school and college athletic programs: a consensus statement. *Journal of Athletic Training, 42*(1), 143–158.

Findlay, J. (2007). Treating atopic dermatitis. *Contemporary Pediatrics, 24*(6), S4–S12.

Frankenburg, W. K. (1994). Preventing developmental delays: is developmental screening sufficient? *Pediatrics, 93*(4), 586–589.

Galioto, F. M, Jr. (2007). Child chest pain: a course of action. *Contemporary Pediatrics, 24*(5), 47–48.

Geller, K. H. (2007). Advice of counsel. Quote parents in pediatric patient history. *RN, 70*(8), 23.

Goodenough, F. L. (1926). *Measurement of intelligence by drawings.* New York: World Book Company.

Hix-Small, H., et al. (2007). Impact of implementing developmental screening at 12 and 24 months in a pediatric practice. *Pediatrics, 120*(2), 381–389.

Hornor, G. (2007). Genitourinary assessment: an integral part of a complete physical examination. *Journal of Pediatric Health Care, 21*(3), 162–170.

Howell, C. C., et al. (2007). The relationships among anxiety, anger, and blood pressure in children. *Applied Nursing Research, 20*(1), 17–23.

Legros, J. M., et al. (2008). Clinical qualitative evaluation of the diagnosis of acute otitis media in general practice. *International Journal of Pediatric Otorhinolaryngology, 72*(1), 23–30.

Lewin, L. C. (2007). Sexually transmitted infections in preadolescent children. *Journal of Pediatric Health Care, 21*(3), 153–161.

Lindberg, D. M., Lindsell, C. J., & Shapiro, R. A. (2008). Variability in expert assessments of child physical abuse likelihood. *Pediatrics, 121*(4), e945–e953.

McCall, E. M., et al. (2009). Interventions to prevent hypothermia at birth in preterm and/or low birthweight babies. *Cochrane Database of Systematic Reviews, 2009*(1), (CD004210).

Newton, A. W., & Vandeven, A. M. (2007). Update on child maltreatment. *Current Opinion in Pediatrics, 19*(2), 223–229.

Patel, P. B., et al. (2007). Clinical features of bacterial conjunctivitis in children. *Academic Emergency Medicine, 14*(1), 1–5.

Paton, E. A. (2007). Evaluating the child with a limp. *Advanced Emergency Nursing Journal, 29*(1), 68–72.

Riley, J. (2007). Do you know how to recognize child abuse? *Nursing Made Incredibly Easy! 5*(2), 54–63.

Rolfes, S. R., Pinna, K., & Whitney, E. N. (2009). *Understanding normal and clinical nutrition.* New York: Wadsworth/Cengage Learning.

Sciscione, P., & Krause-Parello, C. A. (2007). No-nit policies in schools: time for change. *Journal of School Nursing, 23*(1), 13–20.

Shilt, J. S., & Barnett, T. M. (2007). Evaluating and managing back pain in children. *Journal of Musculoskeletal Medicine, 24*(2), 73–76.

Singhal, V., Schwenk, W. F., & Kumar, S. (2007). Evaluation and management of childhood and adolescent obesity. *Mayo Clinic Proceedings, 82*(10), 1258–1264.

Sleeper, E. J., Ariza, A. J., & Binns, H. J. (2009). Do hospitalized pediatric patients have weight and blood pressure concerns identified? *Journal of Pediatrics, 154*(2), 213–217.

Sponseller, P. D. (2007). Scoliosis. In F. J. Frassica, P. D. Sponseller, & J. H. Wilckens (Eds.). *5-minute orthopaedic consult.* Philadelphia, PA: Lippincott Williams & Wilkins.

Sur, D. K., & Bukont, E. L. (2007). Evaluating fever of unidentifiable source in young children. *American Family Physician, 75*(12), 1805–1811.

Thomas, A., & Chess, S. (1977). *Temperament and development.* New York: Brunner/Mazel.

Wallace, D. K., et al. (2007). Treatment of bilateral refractive amblyopia in children three to less than 10 years of age. *American Journal of Ophthalmology, 144*(4), 487–496.

Whetstone, L. M., Morrissey, S. L., & Cummings, D. M. (2007). Children at risk: the association between perceived weight status and suicidal thoughts and attempts in middle school youth. *Journal of School Health, 77*(2), 59–66.

Wiser, I., Balicer, R. D., & Cohen, D. (2007). An update on smallpox vaccine candidates and their role in bioterrorism related vaccination strategies. *Vaccine, 25*(6), 976–984.

Young, A., & Tattersall, H. (2007). Universal newborn hearing screening and early identification of deafness: parents' responses to knowing early and their expectations of child communication development. *Journal of Deaf Studies and Deaf Education, 12*(2), 209–220.

SUGGESTED READINGS

Bolte, R. (2007). The crying child: evaluation and management. What are they trying to tell you? *Contemporary Pediatrics, 24*(6), 90–95.

Eppich, W. J., & Zonfrillo, M. R. (2007). Emergency department evaluation and management of blunt abdominal trauma in children. *Current Opinion in Pediatrics, 19*(3), 265–269.

Jennissen, C. (2007). Evaluating fever in neonates and infants. *Emergency Medicine, 39*(6), 41–48.

Jurbergs, N., et al. (2008). Adaptive style and differences in parent and child report of health-related quality of life in children with cancer. *Psycho-Oncology, 17*(1), 83–90.

McCaskey, M. S. (2007). Pediatric assessment: the little differences. *Home Healthcare Nurse, 25*(1), 20–24.

Phillips, S., et al. (2007). Ideal body weight in children. *Nutrition in Clinical Practice, 22*(2), 240–245.

Podoll, A., et al. (2007). Inaccuracy in pediatric outpatient blood pressure measurement. *Pediatrics, 119*(3), e538–e543.

Powell, C., Wedner, S., & Hatt, S. (2009). Vision screening for correctable visual acuity deficits in school-age children and adolescents. *Cochrane Database of Systematic Reviews, 2009*(1), (CD005023).

Surkan, P. J., et al. (2008). Maternal depressive symptoms, parenting self-efficacy, and child growth. *American Journal of Public Health, 98*(1), 125–132.

Sutton, D., et al. (2008). Preventing or accelerating emergency care for children with complex healthcare needs. *Archives of Disease in Childhood, 93*(1), 17–22.

Chapter 35 Communication and Teaching With Children and Families

KEY TERMS

- affective learning
- behavior therapy
- clarifying
- cognitive learning
- communication
- demonstration
- empathy
- feedback
- focusing
- nontherapeutic communication
- paraphrasing
- perception checking
- positive reinforcement
- psychomotor learning
- redemonstration
- reflecting
- teaching plan
- therapeutic communication

OBJECTIVES

After mastering the contents of this chapter, you should be able to:

1. Describe principles of effective communication and teaching and learning as they relate to health teaching with children.
2. Identify National Health Goals related to communication and teaching with children that nurses could help the nation achieve.
3. Use critical thinking to analyze ways therapeutic communication and health teaching can be further incorporated into the nursing care of children and families to make it more family centered.
4. Assess children for their ability to communicate and readiness to learn.
5. State nursing diagnoses related to communication and health teaching with children.
6. Identify expected outcomes for a specific child based on the child's age, developmental maturity, emotional needs, and communication or learning style.
7. Plan nursing care based on the use of communication and health teaching priorities.
8. Implement health teaching such as devising a puppet show using principles of effective communication and teaching–learning.
9. Evaluate expected outcomes for achievement and effectiveness of care.
10. Identify areas of care related to effective communication or health teaching of children that could benefit from additional nursing research or application of evidence-based practice.
11. Integrate knowledge of effective communication and teaching–learning with the nursing process to achieve quality maternal and child health nursing care.

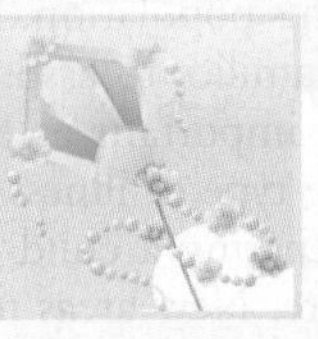

You meet two patients of very different ages in an outpatient clinic. Wolf Whitefeather is a 3-year-old boy with chronic asthma who is scheduled for repair of syndactyly (webbed fingers) next week. One of his favorite activities is coloring. His mother tells you she is concerned Wolf will be hard to entertain after surgery because the large pressure bandage he will have afterward will prevent him from coloring with that hand. "I don't even want to begin to talk to him about surgery," she tells you.

What would be a good strategy for teaching about this type of surgery to a 3-year-old child?

Barry Sandoz is a 15-year-old with a recurring peptic ulcer. His mother tells you health teaching with Barry will be ineffective because he never listens to a thing adults say.

Would you try to teach Barry more about his condition? How would your communications with these children vary because of their age difference?

Previous chapters discussed normal growth and development and how children's understanding increases with age. This chapter adds information about techniques for effective communication and health teaching with children. This type of information is what builds successful bases for disease prevention and health promotion for an age group.

Communication and health teaching are independent nursing actions that accompany all nursing care. They are probably the most frequently used interventions for nurses working with childbearing and childrearing families because health promotion is such a priority for this population. Education is a prime method for empowering families to assume responsibility for their own health. It is as important as any intervention for families experiencing some type of illness or injury; it is especially important when preparing a child for surgery or some other health care procedure. New areas that require teaching are constantly arising as the health care environment continues to grow more technical.

Learning to communicate is one of the most important skills that children learn (Barlow & Parsons, 2009). Communication with children can be either formal or informal. Health teaching may be offered to an individual or to a group of children with similar learning needs. It can also be both formal, such as teaching a group of preschoolers about hospitalization, or informal, such as assuring a parent a child is getting enough nutrition, even though the child snacks rather than sits down to regular meals. The same principles of effective teaching and learning apply no matter which technique is used or whether it is offered to an individual or to a group. National Health Goals related to health teaching and children are shown in Box 35.1.

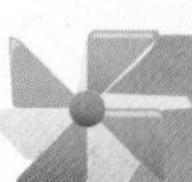

BOX 35.1 ✻ Focus on National Health Goals

Several National Health Goals address good communication or health teaching, because it is such an important mechanism of preventive health care. These goals include:

- Increase the proportion of middle, junior high, and senior high schools that provide school health education to prevent unintentional injuries, violence, suicide, tobacco use and addiction, alcohol and other drug use, unintended pregnancy, HIV infection, AIDS, and other STIs, unhealthy dietary patterns, inadequate physical activity, and environmental health problems from a baseline of 28% to 70%.
- Increase the proportion of the nation's elementary, middle, junior high, and senior high schools that have a nurse-to-student ratio of at least 1:750 from a baseline of 28% to 50%.
- Increase the proportion of local health departments that have established culturally appropriate and linguistically competent community health-promotion and disease-prevention programs, from a baseline of 35% to 50% (http://www.nih.gov).

Nurses can help the nation achieve these goals by consulting with schools and health care organizations to develop health teaching programs and by teaching such programs. Areas that could benefit from nursing research include ways in which busy health care providers can better incorporate health teaching into care; what special techniques are needed to be certain that underserved populations are addressed; and whether material with immediate application requires different teaching techniques than material necessary for long-term care.

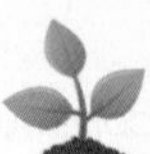

Nursing Process Overview

For Health Teaching With Children

Assessment

Communication and health teaching are best accomplished when they are placed within the context of the nursing process. Learner needs and characteristics, teacher characteristics, available support people, and level of content are all factors that affect learning or whether communication will be received. Assessing these allows nursing diagnoses that clearly state the specific health needs to be formulated.

Nursing Diagnosis

Common examples of nursing diagnoses related to communication or health teaching are:

- Impaired verbal communication related to use of Russian as primary language
- Deficient knowledge related to importance of taking medicine daily
- Health-seeking behaviors related to ways to improve the child's nutritional intake
- Impaired verbal communication related to placement of endotracheal tube
- Anxiety related to perceived amount of material needed to be learned for home care of child

Outcome Identification and Planning

After formulation of a nursing diagnosis, an individualized plan for communication or teaching should be constructed. A plan should detail not only what is to be communicated or learned but also methods regarding how this will be accomplished and evaluated. The most effective way to ensure that expected outcomes are achieved is to ask a child or family to join in planning. Be certain outcomes are concrete and measurable (not "Child will discuss general aspects of his disease," but "Child will list three steps to help prevent disease reoccurrence"). Helpful tips for health education can be found at the American Association for Health Education Web site (http://www.aahperd.org/AAHE).

Implementation

The step of implementation involves the actual communication or teaching carried out. Teaching children is not always easy and requires practice and knowledge of each child's particular developmental level and needs.

Outcome Evaluation

As a final step of communication or teaching, what was communicated or learned must be evaluated. A new plan may need to be developed and teaching continued if communication or learning was less than optimal. Examples of outcome criteria are:

- Child demonstrates good technique in self-injection of insulin.
- Child demonstrates anger by language rather than punching wall.
- Child lists five foods to include in a high-protein diet.
- Family demonstrates improved family communication techniques by next clinic visit.
- Parents demonstrate effective cardiopulmonary resuscitation technique at home visit.

COMMUNICATION

Communication is the exchange of ideas between two or more persons. It can be verbal, using words, or nonverbal, using actions such as touch or eye contact or even a remote system such as mail or e-mail. It is an important process in the care of children because it can make or break an effective relationship. As a process, communication can be divided into two major categories: nontherapeutic (casual, everyday conversation) and therapeutic (helpful and constructive interchanges).

Nontherapeutic Communication

Nontherapeutic communication is identified by its lack of structure or planning—that is, it lacks deliberate purpose other than socializing. Dinner conversation is an example of nontherapeutic communication.

Therapeutic Communication

Therapeutic communication is an interaction between two people that is planned (you deliberately intend to determine the true way a child feels), has structure (you use specific wording techniques that will encourage the response you expect to elicit), and is helpful and constructive (at the end of the exchange you will know more about the child than you did at the beginning, and the child, ideally, also knows more about a particular problem or concern).

In some instances, there is no cure for a child you care for—no surgery, no medication, no pain relief. If you practice therapeutic communication, however, you still have something to offer this child: support by your words or nonverbal communication such as touch. This is often the most valued, most appreciated, and most helpful aspect of all the care you offer (Fig. 35.1).

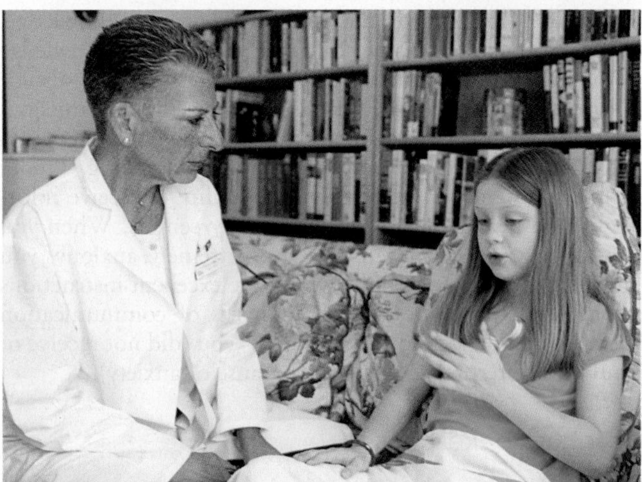

FIGURE 35.1 Sitting at the child's level and allowing the child time for self-expression are steps that improve therapeutic communication.

Components of Good Communication

Cultural differences between a teacher and a learner can complicate techniques of health teaching and evaluation of its effectiveness. Even when language is not a barrier, the way children show that they are listening or comprehending may vary from culture to culture. Looking directly at a speaker, for example, is considered disrespectful in some Asian countries. The "OK" sign traditional in the United States can be interpreted as vulgar, not positive, in Spain. In South Africa or some Middle Eastern countries, a "thumbs up" sign is insulting. In India, the way people move their head to express "yes" and "no" can be opposite to those used in the United States.

Being aware of these cultural differences is important when planning health teaching for diverse cultural groups so that neither teaching nor reactions to teaching are misinterpreted. Communication can be broken down and diagrammed according to its essential components: the encoder, the code, the decoder, and response or feedback.

The Encoder

The encoder is the person who originates a message. Such a person desires to share a thought or feeling with someone else. The person molds this thought into a form suitable for transferring to another person (a code). Communication can be ineffective if a person omits cognitive processing or speaks without thinking, chooses the wrong words for the message, or accompanies the spoken words with a facial expression, tone of voice, or gesture inappropriate for the message.

The Code

The code is the message that is conveyed, as well as the medium or system used to convey it. Although this usually involves a simple spoken system, messages can also be conveyed by such methods as a painting, poem, novel, Morse code, Braille, computer, television, CD, radio, audio or videotape, DVD, camcorder, movie projector, telephone, or text messaging. Communication can be ineffective because a person chooses the wrong medium for a message such as delivering a lecture with many technical words when a drawing with carefully labeled parts would have made the message much clearer, or e-mailing when confronting a person directly would have been more effective.

The Decoder

The receiver (decoder) of the message is the person who not only receives it (hears it, reads it, views it) but interprets or decodes its meaning (cognitive processing). Messages are interpreted in light of the receiver's previous knowledge. They may be misinterpreted if a receiver's store of knowledge is too different from that of the sender. Messages may also be misinterpreted if the receiver misses part of the transmission, such as the wink accompanying the spoken words that would have let the receiver know the sender was joking. Under stress, children tend to narrow their ability to receive information to a small area of concern (they center). When you are dealing with children who are extremely anxious, you may find, therefore, although you gave excellent instructions (both sender and message components of communication were adequate), a child did not "hear" you (did not receive or could not interpret the message because of anxiety).

Feedback or Response

Feedback is the reply the decoder returns to the sender to acknowledge the message has been received and interpreted. This could be a spoken statement, a nod of the head, a facial grimace, a return e-mail, or the sudden slamming of a telephone receiver. With feedback, the roles of sender and receiver become reversed and another communication cycle is begun. Communication can be ineffective if children do not offer feedback (the message was either not received or understood) or offer feedback before the message is fully interpreted (acting before thinking). When you are caring for children with sensory challenges such as vision or hearing problems, you may need to change your usual feedback mechanisms in order to be understood, because a nod of the head or quiet response may not be received.

The Development of Language

Development of language involves not only physically being able to form and voice words but also comprehension of what they mean and how they are used (Marshall, Goldbart, and Phillips, 2007) (Box 35.2). One of the first responses an infant makes at birth is to communicate. A first cry is important because it signals the infant is breathing well. It also announces to the parents the birth is real and stimulates the beginning of parent–child interaction. Early in life, when infants cry, they kick their legs and thrash their arms or react with their whole body. Some new parents comment that their newborns have bad tempers because the infant seems so angry. They are actually commenting on the way newborns respond with their total body to stimuli. Infants discontinue gesturing wildly with every need as soon as they learn the more refined communication system of language.

By age 2, children have mastered language well enough to be able to put together two-word sentences (a noun and a verb). By preschool age, they not only have a vocabulary of about 900 words but also can code them into simple jokes or stories (Goldson & Reynolds, 2008).

School-age children enlarge their ability to communicate from oral exchanges to use of e-mail or the telephone. They can write poetry and, by the end of the period, show an adult sense of humor by the jokes they create. Adolescents progress to a new phase in which they originate new words for objects or feelings ("cool" and "whatever" as responses). This form of communication helps them separate their world from adults and keeps their adolescent culture separate.

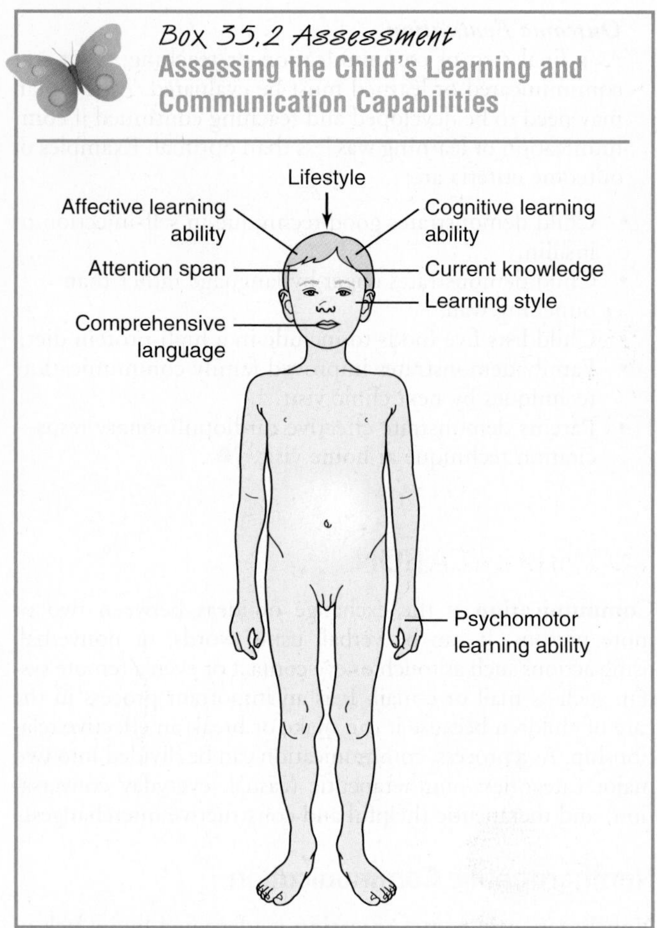

Levels of Communication

Not every conversation you engage in has the same depth level, nor should it. Throughout a day, a person may use as many as five levels, from clichés to peak communication.

First-Level: Cliché Conversation

Cliché conversation is pleasant chatting or comments such as, "Have a nice day" between people who do not intend their relationship to extend beyond a superficial level. It is important when meeting a child for the first time that you introduce yourself not only with your name but also your position and function ("I'm a student nurse who is going to take care of you"; "I'm a nurse who will be visiting you in your home"). This information leads the family to move the conversation from the cliché level to a more meaningful one.

Second Level: Fact Reporting

Fact reporting is simply stating facts about oneself ("I'm 12; I'm in sixth grade"). Fact reporting is necessary for you to understand children, but it does not tell you anything about their feelings or needs. Children can move from this level to a higher level of communication only when they feel they can trust you with more information.

Third Level: Shared Personal Ideas and Judgments

When children know you well, they are able to share ideas such as, "I always wanted to be an astronaut" and judgments ("This is too hard for me; I need to learn a different way"). This level of communication exposes them to loss of self-esteem if their views are not respected. It is the level that is the beginning of therapeutic interactions.

Fourth Level: Shared Feelings

It is difficult to share feelings until you truly trust one another, because feelings are tenuous, fragile concepts, easily destroyed and crushed by inept or uncaring comments. Listen carefully for an expression of feeling from children such as, "I hate always being sick." These admissions are telling you much more than how a child experiences the world; they represent trust in you and the depth of the relationship the child has established with you.

Fifth Level: Peak Communication

The fifth level of communication is a sense of oneness, or being able to know what the other person is experiencing without it actually being voiced. It sometimes occurs spontaneously in high-intensity situations but generally arises out of long-term relationships. For example, you notice that a parent sits soundlessly beside her daughter's bedside for hours at a time. When she leaves, the daughter says, "She makes me feel so much better when she's here." It would be easy to view this mother as nonsupportive (she says almost nothing during the time she's there), but by using fifth-level communication, she has given her daughter more comfort than other visitors who talk the entire time they visit.

Nonverbal Communication

Nonverbal communication involves a variety of factors that are important as accomplishments to effective communication. Nonverbal communication can be especially important in areas such as intensive care units when a child may be unable to speak because of endotracheal tubes and ventilators. Nonverbal communication can be expressed in a variety of ways.

Distance

Although it is affected by cultural and personal variables, the distance at which you position yourself from the person you are talking to can indicate your feelings or the type of conversation you want to have. People generally consider the space directly surrounding them (up to 18 inches) as *intimate* space, to be crossed only by people who know them well or with whom they are comfortable having close body contact. Sometimes you will notice in a heated discussion that one person moves aggressively into this space and the other automatically steps back to protect it. People in elevators usually separate themselves from others by this much space if the car is not full.

Whenever you touch a child, you violate this space, so always ask permission to touch ("Okay if I change your bandage now?"), or with small children, announce what you are going to do ("It's time to change your bandage now"). If children agree to let you enter this space, it means they see you as safe, protective, and helpful.

The space between 18 inches to 4 feet is sensed by most people as *personal* space. This is the distance people usually stand apart from each other for casual conversation. It is a comfortable hand-shaking distance. When you stand by the side of a crib or bed or sit next to a person at home, you are within this space. It is a concerned, I-care-about-you distance but does not invade intimate space.

The distance between 4 feet and 12 feet is *social* space, the distance used to conduct business or teach a class. Conversation spoken at this distance is readily heard by others. Do not use social space to ask a personal question. If you ask a child, "How are you feeling?" as you pass in a hallway, for example, the child will probably answer, "Fine, thank you," a programmed reply almost everyone is taught in early childhood. In contrast, if you ask that same question from a personal or intimate distance, providing privacy, the answer might be, "I'm scared I'm never going home again."

Although it is carried out miles apart, most people perceive speaking on the telephone or using the mail or e-mail as either social or personal space. The tone of voice or the words used help to differentiate which area they consider it to be. A message such as, "Have I got news for you!" suggests social space. "Can you keep a secret?" brings it into intimate space.

Distance beyond 12 feet is *public* space. To communicate from this distance, you need to shout; privacy is not respected at all. Waving to a friend in a hallway or across a parking lot is an example of public space communication.

Genuineness

Genuineness is a quality of projecting sincerity or being yourself. Children will have difficulty trusting you and therefore will be unable to move to a deep relationship with you if you change your behavior from one day to the next such as from maximum patience to short-tempered, because they have to spend energy every day testing to see who you are that day. The way to achieve a feeling of genuineness is not to try to be what you are not as the insecurity that comes from pretending can manifest itself as negative feelings such as aggressiveness or a bored attitude.

Warmth

Warmth is an innate quality, and some people manifest it more spontaneously than others. Basic ways in which warmth is demonstrated are direct eye contact, use of a gentle tone of voice, listening attentively, approaching a child within a comfortable space of 1 to 4 feet (closer may be threatening; farther away may be distancing), and using touch appropriately. Warmth is a quality that you display best when you know another person well. Any action that helps you to know a person better (taking a health history, talking about school or family or how a child feels about the present situation) not only lets you plan care but also allows you to become increasingly comfortable with the child and deepen the warmth of your relationship.

Empathy

Empathy is the ability to put yourself in another person's place and experience a feeling the same as that person is experiencing. People who are capable of empathy are the best support people because they can anticipate a child's reactions or fears. At first, it seems empathy would require you to have experienced all the situations that children experience. This is not necessarily true, however, because you understand the common emotion of all situations in other ways. If you have hoped for something very strongly and then not attained it, loved someone and not had that emotion returned, lost someone or something that was so important to you that you felt actual pain, you can feel empathy for children who have received a disappointing diagnosis or who are unhappy for other reasons you have never experienced. Feeling empathy is emotionally draining because, when you assume another person's emotions, you experience them at the same depth as that person. Nurses who are capable of empathy need to surround themselves with good support people so they have refueling resources when they need them.

Gestures

Children vary a great deal in the gestures they use to accompany their spoken words. Although this is culturally influenced, it is also an individual trait. Be careful not to assess emotion only by a child's gestures; some children wave their arms wildly describing an everyday occurrence; others would use that degree of expression only when in extreme distress. Be aware also that your own gestures are always being read by children. A statement that you approve of something is contradicted by placing your arms across your chest in a disapproving, stern manner. Saying that broccoli is good to eat because it contains antioxidants but then making a sour face makes your healthy eating message ineffective.

Body Posture and Gait

Children who feel good about themselves usually assume an upright body posture and walk rapidly and surely; those who are depressed or insecure tend to slouch and move more slowly and timidly; those who are threatened tend to either draw back or act aggressively. Children who are in agreement with you usually maintain eye contact with you as you speak to them. Very depressed or insecure children do not do that (they feel too inferior), nor do children who are very angry. Children from some cultures may not meet your gaze because it is not culturally appropriate.

Facial expression is an important accompanying gesture. Clenched teeth, frowns, and smiles are easily interpreted by everyone. The degree of pain a child is experiencing may be more evident by facial expression than words.

General Appearance

Children who have good self-esteem tend to maintain good body hygiene and care about their appearance. Those who are depressed may not feel the effort involved in grooming is worthwhile. Personal hygiene varies, however, and it is difficult to assess on your first contact with a child. What you see as ill-kempt may be neat and trim for that particular child; what you think of as well groomed may be comparatively sloppy for that child.

Be aware that your impression of how children dress registers very strongly on your subconscious. Do not let an unconscious dislike for a mode of dress of some child (body piercing or a turban) cause you to draw back. Preparing to give nursing care is not the same kind of activity as evaluating whether you wish to invite someone to dinner.

Touch

Touch is the most intimate and meaningful of nonverbal techniques. When words are inadequate, touch rarely is. Learn to use touch such as clapping a child's shoulder or squeezing a hand to accompany reassuring words or in place of words as a strong support signal (I'm here; I understand; it's all right to be afraid). On the other hand, be aware that some children enjoy being touched more than others. Because of individual preferences or cultural variations, some children do not like you to use this nonverbal signal with them. Assess individually for the appropriateness of using touch.

Use of Humor

Some people have a natural knack for finding humor in any situation; others do not instinctively have this quality and must cultivate it. Those who can laugh at their own mistakes are usually enjoyable people to have around, because their laughter at themselves suggests that, when you make a mistake, they will be able to accept it the same way (or at least not be angry about it).

Be careful of the use of humor with children because they are school-age before they appreciate most adult jokes. If they are fatigued or ill, they may be looking for a firm support person to be with them more than one who is amusing. You can often measure a child's progress by noting the first time after a procedure the child responds to you with a humorous statement. Remember, though, that laughter and joking can also be signs of increasing anxiety. Evaluate the use of humor to be certain a child really finds a situation amusing.

Use of Drawings

A useful nonverbal technique to learn how children feel about a frightening experience is to ask them to draw a picture of what happened or a picture of themselves. A child hospitalized for heart surgery, for example, might draw her heart prominently. She's revealing that she realizes she cannot survive if something happens to such an important body part.

A child's use of color may be a clue regarding mood (happy children tend to use bright colors; depressed children use black or dark colors). A child with good self-esteem usually fills the full page with a drawing; one with less self-esteem crowds a drawing into a corner. These observations are quite variable, however; a child may have had only a black crayon with which to color or may be saving the rest of the paper for a second drawing.

Use of Music

The type of music to which children prefer to listen to often also conveys their mood. The better they feel about themselves, the more likely they are to choose lively music; if they are sad, they often choose a quieter, more comforting type.

Children enjoy repetition, however, and so may play the same music over and over, independent of their mood.

Techniques To Encourage Therapeutic Communication

Several techniques are effective in deepening communication patterns and relationships. These techniques can be learned if they are not a spontaneous part of your present communication pattern (Box 35.3).

Attentive Listening

No one likes to talk to someone who does not appear to be listening or responding. Good listening, therefore, like speaking, is not passive but active. Be aware that your posture reveals to a great extent whether you are listening (sitting, not standing, to convey that you are not on the run; leaning forward, not backward; stooping to meet a child's level). Nodding, maintaining eye contact, and stopping all other activities are strong indicators you are attuned to what is being said. Making it clear that you are concentrating on what another is saying by such a motion as nodding indicates you value what the other person is saying. Children who feel valued are much more likely to confide feelings and concerns than those who sense you consider them not important.

In some instances, it is necessary to repeat a part of what a child said, interject an appropriate "uh-huh" or "m-m-m," or make a direct statement ("I'm listening. Go on") to indicate you are listening. Be certain that when you are listening to the 20th child on any given day, you do not exhibit "end-of-the day" behavior. To be therapeutic, you have to give everyone's concerns the same alert attention.

BOX 35.3 ✻ Focus on Family Teaching

Listening to Children

Q. Barry's mother says to you, "My son always tells me I don't listen to him. How can I be a better listener?"

A. Try the following tips:

1. Stop talking. You cannot listen if you are talking.
2. Look and act interested. Do not read or write while he talks. Listen to understand rather than to reply.
3. Remove distractions. Do not doodle, tap, or shuffle papers. Would it be quieter if you turned off the television?
4. Empathize. Try to put yourself in your child's place so you can see his point of view.
5. Be patient. Allow plenty of time. Do not interrupt. Do not edge toward the door or walk away.
6. Hold your temper. An angry person gets the wrong meaning from words.
7. Hold argument or criticism, which puts children on the defensive. They may stop talking or get angry.
8. Ask questions. This is proof that you have been listening.
9. Stop talking. This is the first and last suggestion, because all others depend on it.

Open-Ended Questions

A pointed or direct question used in discussing asks for a specific task; it implies all you are interested in hearing about is that one fact. An example of a direct question is, "Do you take Tylenol when you have a headache?" An open-ended question is not limited to a simple answer but invites a wide variety of responses because it is so comprehensive such as, "Tell me what you do when you have a headache." A child might answer this question by not only describing the amount of analgesic she takes but also putting a cold towel on her forehead, staying home from school, and closing her eyes to stop the pain. Three or four times more information has been elicited.

Open-ended questions are not effective if the topic is difficult for a child to describe (a preschooler has difficulty responding even yes or no; a paragraph of material would be impossible) or if the child is naturally shy or defensive about the subject (he knows he has not been doing the things you told him to do and would rather not admit it).

Most communication is a combination of direct and open-ended questions. Listen carefully the next time you ask someone to explain something to see if you make use of mostly direct (information-limiting) questions or open-ended (information-expanding) ones.

Reflecting

Reflecting is another technique, like attentive listening, that is so simple that its importance is easy to discount. **Reflecting** is restating the last word or phrase a child has said when there is a pause in the communication. A child says, "I'm worried," and then stops. You repeat the last word. "Worried?" The child, assured you are listening and interested, will generally enlarge on the first statement: "I'm worried I won't make the football team this year." Older school-age children may not respond well to reflection; they may interpret it as imitating them, not seeking information.

Clarifying

Clarifying consists of repeating statements others have made so both of you can be certain you understood them. This is particularly helpful if a child has been describing a set of symptoms or series of actions. You would clarify such a statement by saying, "Let me see if I understand this. You said you always get the pain first in your stomach. Then it spreads to your chest." If you are not quoting correctly, the child will interrupt and restate the problem: "No, the chest pain comes first."

Paraphrasing

Paraphrasing is restating what children have said not only to assure them you have heard correctly (as in clarifying) but also to help them explain what they have been trying to say in other words. In clarifying, you repeat a child's exact words; in paraphrasing, you retain the meaning of the words but repeat them in a clearer or more condensed form. The child says, for example, "I don't talk about my problems with my parents." A paraphrasing statement might be, "You're telling me you and your parents haven't discussed home care. Is that right?" When paraphrasing, ask for confirmation that your interpretation is correct; otherwise, you may find yourself putting words in children's mouths.

When the topic is embarrassing or emotionally charged (an adolescent discussing sexual orientation), the child might use such vague terms that the explanation becomes difficult to follow. Paraphrasing using basic terms would let him know not only that you understand him but that, if he can describe the problem better with such words than with medical terminology, it is acceptable to you.

Perception Checking

Perception checking documents a feeling or emotion reported to you. This makes it a step deeper than paraphrasing. In paraphrasing, you document a statement or fact; in perception checking, you document a feeling or emotion. The child says, "I'm not at all worried about surgery. I know a lot of kids have the same thing done every day. I mean, what could happen?" You say, "You're telling me you're not worried, but the number of times you've said it makes me wonder if you really are worried. Are you?"

Always ask for validation that your perception is correct so you do not make false assumptions. Perception checking is helpful because, as a rule, children are not ready to deal with emotions until they can admit they are experiencing them. When you bring an emotion out on the table this way, it allows them to confront it and deal with it for the first time. They may lose their reluctance to admit other worries because you have implied that worrying is acceptable.

Focusing

Focusing helps children to center on a subject you suspect is causing them anxiety because they comment about it indirectly or else completely avoid it. It is done by repeating something they said ("You mentioned you feel tired all the time") or by mentioning the avoided topic ("You haven't said a word about how you feel about this surgery. Is that a problem?"). Once a subject is brought up for discussion, most children respond to it. As long as it can be avoided, however, they do not have to face the problem and begin to solve it.

Supportive Statements

Supportive statements let children know you accept their behavior or at least appreciate they have dealt well with unfortunate circumstances. For example, an adolescent says, "My girlfriend dumped me while I've been here in the hospital." Such a statement deserves a supportive reply such as, "That must not feel good." The adolescent will take this response to mean you want to discuss the topic and, encouraged by your empathy, may elaborate on it as it still affects him.

Silence

If you ask a question and a child does not respond immediately, it is natural to ask another question or perhaps change the subject, assuming the child is not interested in the topic. This is a social custom that allows you not to put someone into the awkward position of having to discuss a sensitive topic. Silence, however, is an effective therapeutic technique. If you ask an emotion-laden question ("Are you worried?") and the child does not answer immediately, allow a period of silence to pass. Because you do not hurry to fill in the silence, the child is likely to respond by hurrying an answer (to fill in the silence); when this happens, the answer is usually spontaneous and often open and uninhibited. In other instances, a child may answer the question deliberately and cautiously and, because you have provided a period of time to answer, offer additional information.

Do not overdo silence, however, either by the number of times you use it or the length of time you allow it to extend. In this era of constant noise, many individuals are extremely uncomfortable with silence. Too much silence can indicate to a child you are not interested enough to maintain the conversation.

Process Recording

Process recording is a method to examine how effective you are at therapeutic communication. After your next interaction with a child, take a few minutes and write down in the left column of a sheet of paper a statement the child made to you. In the middle column, write what you thought on hearing the statement. In a third column, write your response. Try to record both statements and responses verbatim or as close to the actual words used as possible. The average person can accurately recall about 3 minutes of communication this way.

Next, examine your responses to each statement: Did I encourage the child to tell me more by my response, or did I block communication? Were my responses supportive or critical or trite? Did I use open-ended questions or closed, direct ones? Did I check perceptions or did I just assume that I understood correctly what was told to me? See Box 35.4 for an example of a process recording with an adolescent.

✔ Checkpoint Question 35.1

Barry tells you he hates school. Which response would be the best example of paraphrasing?

a. "Tell me again what you said."
b. "School?"
c. "You're telling me you're unhappy with school?"
d. "Hate is a strong emotion for a teenager to feel."

Factors That Can Interfere With Effective Communication

Because so much of nursing care is influenced by verbal communication, it is important to avoid miscalculations in communication and to recognize common situations in which meanings can easily be distorted.

Age and Developmental Level

Age and developmental levels are important to communication ability because they influence vocabulary and reading ability so greatly (Oakhill & Petrides, 2007). A 3-year-old child may not have the vocabulary to explain the way her knee feels (she has heard the word "ache" but only in connection with headache; she does not know that knees can ache as well). Early school-age children have difficulty describing the blurring they experience as they focus on a blackboard with less-than-perfect eyesight, because this is the way they have always seen. The ability to describe inner feelings such as anger, sadness, and fear comes only with adolescence.

BOX 35.4 ✻ A Process Recording

The following is a record of an interaction between a nursing student and Barry Sandoz, a 15-year-old boy who is hospitalized. Barry has been diagnosed as having a peptic ulcer.

What Client Said and Did	What I Thought and Felt	What I Said and Did
	I felt anxious meeting a new patient, although I thought he'd be friendly because he was so close to my age.	I walked into his room and said, "Good morning."
He was sitting up in bed holding his hands on his abdomen. He said, "Get me something for this pain," without even looking at me.	I felt attacked. As if he thought I should have done something sooner, but I had just arrived.	I asked, "What kind of pain are you having?"
He said, "I need a student nurse like a hole in the head. Isn't there anyone else around?"	Now, I really felt attacked.	I said, "I can get you something for pain. I just need to know what kind of pain you have."
He said, "Hydrochloric acid is carving a hole into my stomach. Is that enough explanation for you to get me something?"	I felt angry that he insisted on putting me down so.	I said, "It certainly is. And I appreciate that if I had pain like that I would not want to answer questions either." I left to find my instructor and get him something for pain. I returned in 15 minutes and said, "I have an injection for you."
He asked, "Did you have to take so long to do that?"	I was getting really angry.	I said nothing. I just checked his ID band and gave him the injection.
He asked, "Now could you get me my purple pill?"	I was angry at his demanding tone and threatened because I didn't even know what he meant by his "purple pill."	I said, "I'll have to check your medication sheet."
He said, "Any chance you could do that in a hurry?"	Even more angry.	I said, "Are you always so demanding?"
He turned on his side so his back was to me, clenched his teeth, and pushed his hands into his abdomen again.	I realized that my criticism was unfair because he was in pain. But it was too late to take it back.	I said, "I'm sorry. I know you're uncomfortable."
He shouted, "I am not uncomfortable! I am having my stomach ripped out! Could you help me out in any decent way with that?"	I realized I was in over my head. I thought I'd limit any further interaction so he couldn't make me angry again.	I said nothing. I just left to check on whether he could have any other medicine. I returned (quickly as I could) with Prilosec (his purple pill).
He asked, "Do you know if Dr. M. is still in surgery?"	Threatened again; I didn't even know how to find that out.	I said, "I can find out for you."
He said, "Hand me that book on the chair over there, before you go, will you?"	Trying to concentrate on not being angry at his demanding tone, yet I had medicine I had to give safely.	I said, "Let me see your ID band again first."
He turned his wrist over so I couldn't read his ID.	I thought: I am tired of him demanding things and getting the book was not as important as what I was doing.	I said nothing.
He said, "If I don't get to that book today, I might as well cash it in."	Getting angry again, but also "hearing" what he had said for the first time.	I said, "Cash it in?"
He said, "Don't you think I ought to? I can't go back to school with pain like this. Wouldn't dying be better than failing out?"		I was surprised how one quick response on my part had brought out so much emotion. I also knew I was in over my head again (but in a nice way).

(continued)

BOX 35.4 ✻ A Process Recording (continued)

Evaluation

My overall interaction with Barry would have been better if I hadn't been caught so off guard in the beginning by assuming that he was going to be someone who had a lot in common with me (student–student, close age group). His initial response to me seemed so much more intense because I had stereotyped him that way.

My responses to him were adequate up to the point that I became angry. I should have answered his comment, "Do you always take so long to do something?" with a supportive one such as, "I know it's hard to be in pain." (I heard a nurse answer that question for a client with, "Believe it or not, sometimes I take longer," and all of us laughed. I think the client felt good about being able to appreciate something funny, but I'm glad I didn't try humor here. Silence was inadequate but at least not irritating.)

If I had been more sensitive to what Barry was saying (and less angry), I would have noticed that after I gave the injection he became nicer to me (asking if I could get him his Prilosec, not just demanding it). I was too angry to notice his change in behavior though, so I cut off his preliminary attempt to interact with me by criticizing him ("Are you always so demanding?") My supportive statement ("I'm sorry; I know you're uncomfortable") was ineffective after the criticism.

In the final interaction, I was so concerned with my own needs (get my work done) that I completely missed what he said about why the book was important to him. Fortunately, at the last minute, I got my mind off my problem and onto his and was able to produce a therapeutic response for him. He shouldn't have had to describe something with the impact of driving a truck over me before he caught my attention, though. Better listening (and thinking while I'm listening) would make me hear better and be more helpful sooner in this type of interaction.

Intellectual Level

Intellectual level, like age, affects vocabulary and ability both to encode and decode messages. It influences the number of languages a child speaks, reading ability, and the depth of explanation a child is capable of understanding.

Physical Factors

Physical factors such as speech impairments and hearing or vision challenges interfere with the transmission and reception of messages. When children are distracted by such sensations as fatigue or pain, they also may have a reduced ability to transmit or receive messages correctly.

Technical Terminology

Adults have heard common medical words and so usually have little difficulty understanding an explanation of one. Children, in contrast, have not heard many medical words. Listen to the explanations you give them to be certain you would have understood your explanation at their age.

Showing Disapproval

Parents and children do not come for health care to be criticized; they come to learn more about how to stay well or recover from illness. If you criticize them, they may not reveal any further information to you because they do not want you to react in the same way you did to their preliminary statements.

Suppose an adolescent says, "I never drink milk. That's for babies." Knowing milk is an important source of calcium, you respond, "That's not healthy. You should drink at least two glasses a day." This discourages the adolescent from telling you any more about her eating habits (she does not eat much protein either, but you will miss this information because she will not expose herself to your criticism again).

Be aware that nonverbal disapproval (frowning, sighing) can be just as conversation stopping as spoken disapproval. On the other hand, this does not mean you should show approval of wrong actions. Merely listen to them with no action or comment and make a mental note. At the end of your interaction, introduce the change in behavior you'd like to see ("Let's plan some ways you can include more calcium with your meals without drinking milk").

Not Showing Approval When Warranted

Every student has had the experience of completing a difficult assignment and receiving only criticism from a teacher—no comment that, aside from the part that was not satisfactory, the rest of the assignment was done well. This happens because the instructor assumed the student would do a good job; no reward was given for meeting minimum criteria. From the other side of the desk, however, it would have been satisfying—and offered motivation to continue to do well—to have heard the words "good job."

When discussing health care problems with children, it is easy to forget that what you accept as standard behavior may take a great deal of effort for an ill child to accomplish (coughing and deep breathing after surgery seems simple but is actually very difficult to do because it is so painful). Giving children praise for what they do well encourages them to tell you more about themselves and to try other things. If a topic is difficult for them to talk about, saying that you realize it is a sensitive topic helps them continue to discuss it.

Being Defensive

In the same way that children who request health care do not enjoy being criticized, neither does the average health care provider. If a child makes a critical remark, therefore, it is easy to respond with a defensive or protective comment rather than a therapeutic one. An adolescent might say, "We have to wait so long here; this is a really dumb clinic." It is easy to reply, "Don't say that. This is a good clinic." This type of response implies that any complaint is out of line. Try to respond instead with a supportive comment such as, "I know it makes a long day for you." No health care agency is so good that there is nothing to criticize.

Cliché Advice

Cliché advice (advice given from a formula, not individualized to the situation) is meaningless because it is too general to be helpful. Statements such as, "Rome wasn't built in a day" and "You have to walk before you can run" are examples of this kind of advice. Children consider their problem unique and resent being given advice that could apply to everyone.

Topping Up

"Topping up" is minimizing a child's views by telling a better story. A child tells you, for example, he has a headache; you say, "You should feel the one I have." A child says she has a problem; you say, "You want to know what problems really are? Come and work here." This implies to children their problems are inconsequential, at least in respect to yours. They will not be likely to tell you any more about themselves after such responses.

Communication Situations That Require Special Skills

Some communication situations require special skills in addition to the usual therapeutic communication techniques to promote understanding.

The Shy Child

The amount of verbal communication children use varies culturally and individually. Some children talk excessively when they are nervous; those who are shy may stop talking completely. Children who are comfortable with verbal communication reach out to secure the help they need from others by talking; shy individuals are more likely to have their needs go unrecognized. It is difficult to assess how shy children feel when they are reluctant to communicate about such things as whether they are psychologically ready for surgery or if they understand the long-term effect a disease is going to have. If they do not give you much verbal feedback, the tendency is to believe they do not have a concern. That leaves them without support people when they most need them.

Fortunately, in most instances, once children realize they know and can trust you, shyness fades. A therapeutic response, therefore, would be not to leave them alone but to maintain an active relationship despite the lack of feedback. This does not necessarily involve talking to children but may involve checking on them frequently, remaining in the room while a physician completes an examination, helping with the adhesive strip after a technician obtains a blood sample, or sitting with them for a few minutes while a medication takes effect.

The Angry Child

It is difficult to work with angry children because you feel yourself being pulled into their anger. The typical response at hearing an angry outburst is to imitate it (a child is radiating anger as tight-lipped silence, so you say nothing as well; a child shouts at you, and you shout back). This is not therapeutic, however. Make a point of not allowing yourself to be drawn into children's anger, while at the same time acknowledging it is all right to be angry (I understand that you're angry but please don't shout"). Help them to focus their anger if at all possible so they can better understand it and begin to deal with it.

To encourage focusing, ask children to detail why they are angry. An adolescent who feels angry at the entire health care delivery system is highly frustrated because he cannot begin to handle the whole bureaucracy; establishing that what he is really angry about is one nurse's action, for example, builds a base for resolving the problem. If a child uses silence as a method of maintaining anger, suggesting possible reasons for the anger may be helpful ("I know Dr. Smith was just talking to you. Are you angry about something she said?" or, "I know you were asking about crutch walking before. Does it have something to do with that?"). Once the subject is out in the open, few children can resist describing the extent of or reason for their anger. Be aware, too, that when you ask someone to explain why they are angry, you ask for the emotion and the distress that go with it to be expressed as well. Even if you are the object of the anger, you are committed to listening to the child's views.

Helping children focus anger this way moves them toward a constructive solution (focusing anger at the physical therapy department because that is where the offense occurred seems justified, but calling you names, not eating dinner, or shouting at a parent does not). If necessary, censor the way the anger is expressed, not the right to be angry. Keep anger from affecting you by reacting to the explanation, not the tone or force of it. Keep any response on your part a tone gentler and quieter than that used toward you.

The Demanding Child

Nursing has few equals in job satisfaction (provided salary and other working conditions are adequate) because the majority of people you care for are grateful for everything you do for them. It can be upsetting, therefore, to discover a particular child who is not grateful for or even satisfied with anything you do. This type of child is also easy to back away from or avoid.

Demanding behavior generally stems from insecurity or fear (so afraid that something will happen to them while you are out of the room they constantly find more for you to do to keep you in the room, or so afraid of unplanned events that they structure things so that nothing unexpected can happen). Give more of yourself, not less, to counteract this response. When you have proven you are dependably there for them, children do not feel so insecure, and the need to be demanding usually fades. Withdrawing may increase the child's insecurity and the demanding behavior. Ask instead, "Is there anything else I can do for you?" not, "Haven't I already done enough?"

The Sexually Aggressive Adolescent

Sexually aggressive behavior stems from the same cause as every other aggressive and demanding behavior: insecurity. It can be manifested as telling unwelcome jokes or inappropriate physical touching. This may be pronounced in adolescents who worry that illness or surgery will interfere with sexual function. Adolescents with this degree of insecurity may benefit from counseling to help them channel coping responses into more socially acceptable behaviors. Be sure they have factual information regarding the extent or effect of their illness. Set limits, as necessary, to make giving care acceptable to you. Always censor the action, not the adolescent. Be aware that sexually aggressive behavior occurs in both males and females.

The Child Who Is Not Proficient in English

It is not unusual in any nursing care setting to encounter children who have a different primary language from yours; in other instances, a child's speech may be limited or difficult to understand because of an accent, dialect, or speech impairment; some children may speak your language but their use of words is so different from yours that the words have different meanings (Uccelli & Paez, 2007).

Most children who speak another language have a support person who can serve as an interpreter. Anticipate the instructions you will need to give the child (cough, deep breathe, save urine, and so forth) and ask the interpreter to write them out in the child's language for times the interpreter may not be present. Post them conspicuously in the room or the child's care plan so everyone giving care can be familiar with them.

Most health care facilities have a list of people who serve as translators as needed; many times, you can contact such a person by telephone to ask for a specific word you want to know. If you have to give instructions and no translator is present, do not be self-conscious about using hand gestures or drawing a picture to express the action you want (a child lying in bed), an arrow pointing to a chair, and a child sitting in a chair for, "I'm going to help you get out of bed." Allow children ample paper to draw pictures to show what they want to tell you. Supply pictures for preschool children so they can select the one they want.

Everyone has a tendency to shout at children who speak a different language as if loudness will increase understanding. Try to avoid doing this. When using an interpreter, be certain to speak slowly and use common words that can be translated literally. "I need to stick Mary's arm for blood" could be interpreted literally to mean putting a stick in the child's arm.

The Unconscious Child

Hearing is the last sense lost with unconsciousness and the first sense regained with consciousness. This means you always need to be aware that children who do not respond to you may be able to hear and interpret anything you say. Never say anything to unconscious children or within their hearing, therefore, that you would not say if they were fully alert. Continue to use nonverbal communication such as touch to help convey your message.

The Hearing-Challenged Child

It is difficult for hearing challenged children to enunciate words clearly because they are not aware that the voice sound they are forming is not clear (Toe, Beattie, & Barr, 2007). When communicating with hearing-challenged children, check whether they use a hearing aid; if so, be certain it is turned on. Face them when you speak so they can follow your lip movements. Use hand gestures as necessary to convey your message, or write out instructions. If you have difficulty understanding what they are trying to say, ask them to write it down if they are old enough. Use common sense about how loud to raise your voice to facilitate communication. As a rule, at the point that privacy is lost, it is time to resort to written words or sign language. Children who use sign language to communicate have a right to have an interpreter present to facilitate communication, the same as children who do not use English as their primary language.

The Vision-Challenged Child

When speaking to a child who is challenged visually, be careful not to rely on nonverbal communication techniques such as hand gestures, as these cannot be seen. A statement such as, "Take a piece of gauze about this long" is meaningless. Never touch children who cannot see you without speaking to them first so you do not startle them.

HEALTH TEACHING IN A CHANGING HEALTH CARE ENVIRONMENT

In the past, when children were admitted to hospitals well in advance of surgery and remained in the hospital after surgery or therapy until they were almost totally well, there was a wide window of time for health teaching. Today, when surgery is often a 1-day experience, the window for teaching has greatly narrowed (Cabana et al., 2008). This means nurses must use more creative approaches to achieve the same health education results. Discharge instructions may require both verbal and written approaches (Johnson, Sandford, & Tyndall, 2009).

Children's sophistication about learning techniques has also changed. Children today are exposed to such a diet of clever animation on television or in movies that a simple lecture on good nutrition can seem dull and uninteresting. Children who are adept at arcade or computer games where dexterity is the requirement may no longer find handling a syringe or a feeding tube a challenging feat. Before beginning, assess each child to find out what the child expects to learn, identify individual learning style, and determine what teaching techniques would suit the child best.

The Teacher–Learner Relationship

Effective teaching and learning depend a great deal on the teacher–learner relationship, because, as a teacher, you can only influence an individual to learn; you cannot force learning. Before teaching can be considered effective, learning has to have occurred in a way in which change in behavior is measurable. Conversely, before learning occurs, teaching must have occurred in some form. For example, a parent teaching a child about the need to brush teeth daily must not only elicit the child's statement that daily brushing is important but also see that the child is, in fact, brushing her teeth every day. If the topic is abstract, such as helping a child change a concept about a chronic illness, change can still be measured (the child not only talks about the illness but also begins to take actions to prevent complications). Common principles of teaching are summarized in Table 35.1. Principles of effective learning are summarized in Table 35.2.

TABLE 35.1 ✻ Principles of Teaching

Principle	Rationale
Know the subject.	To effectively teach children, you must be able not only to present material but also to answer questions about it. Children's questions can be as probing as an adult's and they can often be more frequent, because children are used to asking questions of a teacher or a parent.
Know the audience.	Children vary a great deal in cognitive development depending on their age group. To teach preschoolers about health, you might choose to teach how to brush teeth using puppets as a teaching aid. The same clever puppet and toothbrushing presentation likely would not be well received among adolescents.
Know yourself.	Analyze which teaching techniques (lecture, role playing, small group discussion, audiovisual aids) fit your teaching style. Using techniques that are comfortable allows teaching to be most effective.
Assess individual learning styles.	Most children respond well to visual images (seeing a demonstration or drawing) to complement learning. Assessing individual learning styles helps to meet each child's best way of learning.
Define expected outcomes.	Expected outcomes serve as guidelines to help you select from all you know about a subject that part which is most pertinent to an individual child. They should be realistic, measurable, and mutually established. Instruction on how to walk using crutches for an early school-age child would include how to carry school books while using crutches; for an adolescent, instruction might include how to board a city bus so he or she could get to and from a part-time job.
Provide an environment conducive for learning.	Children are easily distracted from learning because of so many new experiences in their world. Divide material into segments to keep teaching sessions short; avoid competing factors such as television or mealtime.
Be consistent.	Nothing is more confusing to a person learning something for the first time than to be told two different ways to do it. Choose one method that should work best for a child and then consistently stress that method. After a child has learned the one method, then suggest alternative methods if the child is interested.
Be honest.	Abstract concepts such as "little white lies" cannot be understood by children younger than adolescents.
Recognize that actions teach as much as or sometimes more than verbal statements.	Children watch facial expressions and nonverbal gestures as much as they listen. Be certain that a nonverbal statement is not contradicting a verbal one.
Teach from the simple to the complex.	Fundamentals must be grasped before extensive learning can proceed. Many children have little idea of body anatomy. Often you need to begin with the basics; when these are mastered, you can proceed to teach about a disease condition.
Teach principles.	Teaching children the principle behind why they are doing something gives them reason to do it. It expands learning in that it allows children to modify and change to an alternative method as long as the principle is fulfilled.
Emphasize what the child should do; mention, but do not emphasize what the child should not do.	Teaching from a positive standpoint makes learning more enjoyable. Because health care information should last a lifetime, thinking of it in a positive way makes it applicable to lifetime use. However, children need to know both the do's and don'ts regarding health issues.
Include evaluation as a final step.	The only way to determine the effectiveness of teaching is to test or evaluate if learning has occurred. Structure the time and method of evaluation when first establishing a teaching plan.

An equal partnership encourages learning more readily than a relationship in which a teacher maintains ultimate control and authority. A teacher–learner relationship based on mutual sharing empowers and motivates an individual to learn. To foster mutual sharing in the learning process, first negotiate with the learner to establish learning needs and goals. Allow this negotiation to continue throughout the entire learning process as needs and goals change. Next, focus on the whole person by considering the learner's cognitive and developmental abilities, values, beliefs, feelings, experiences, and learning style. Finally, the teacher–learner relationship should be interactive. The teacher and learner should both actively participate in the process and modify the teaching plan as they learn from one another.

Types of Learning

There are several different types of learning. Learning the mathematical formula necessary to change pounds to kilograms, for example, is different from learning how to fill a

TABLE 35.2 ✻ Principles of Learning

Principle	Rationale
Learning occurs best when children are ready to learn.	Interferences with learning may be physical (e.g., pain or hunger) or psychological (e.g., fear or anxiety). The first time children are told that they must inject insulin daily, for example, they may be too anxious to learn about it.
Learning occurs most quickly if children can see how the new information will benefit them.	Sixteen-year-old children learn how to drive a car quickly because they grasp readily that being able to drive will immediately enlarge their world. Children are not ready to learn insulin injections until they can see an advantage of giving them. Make a habit of including the benefit of learning in the introduction of learning.
Learning occurs best if rewards, not penalties, are offered.	Notice the amount of shoulder patting and back slapping that high school coaches engage in (rewarding by praise). Giving positive reinforcement immediately like this makes it more effective than if such reinforcement is delayed. If you must criticize the way a task was done, first compliment children on some aspect they did well and then explain the part that needs improvement. This increases self-esteem and allows children to feel good enough about themselves so that they can accept the criticism. Never be reluctant to praise in public; always criticize in private.
Children learn best by actively participating in learning.	Active participation requires involvement in learning. Ask questions to involve participation; allow children to touch and handle equipment to increase participation.
Learning occurs best in a non-stressful and accepting environment.	No one wants to take a chance redemonstrating a procedure or asking a question if they believe that actions or opinions will not be respected. People do learn from "top sergeants," but the learning experience has so many unpleasant memories attached to it that they may not retain the learning. Health teaching is too important to be presented in a way that will lead to its being quickly discarded.
Children learn best those things that hold a particular interest for them.	Everyone is more interested in some things than in others. A child with diabetes mellitus who enjoys dancing might be most interested in learning regulation of insulin for exercise; an adolescent anxious to leave for college might be most interested in selecting a diabetic diet from a cafeteria.
Learning ability plateaus.	Children learn to the point of saturation; learning and interest in learning halt at that point and do not continue until the material learned is thoroughly digested and understood. Wait until information is processed, and, at that point, the child will be interested once more.

syringe. Learning to be kind to a brother with a chronic illness is yet another type. Before you begin teaching, for best results, analyze the type of learning you want to see take place. This helps in setting goals and designing teaching strategies.

Cognitive Learning

Cognitive learning involves a change in the individual's level of understanding or knowledge. Learning the principle behind why a particular medicine must be injected into a muscle, as opposed to subcutaneous tissue, is cognitive learning. Cognitive learning requires adequate development, intelligence, and attention span. It can be gained through exposure to any teaching technique but is usually learned through lecture, reading, and audiovisual aids. Techniques for teaching when cognitive learning is the goal must be based on the learner's cognitive ability (Barlow & Parsons, 2009). During the school-age years, learning capability is concrete (children have difficulty picturing body parts functioning unless they actually see them doing this); during the adolescent years, it becomes possible to learn abstract concepts, and children at that point can accept that liver enzymes are released with liver damage even though they never see that occur (Piaget, 1969).

Psychomotor Learning

Psychomotor learning requires a change in a person's ability to perform a skill. Learning to hold a syringe, fill the syringe with medicine, and inject it into a muscle is an example of psychomotor learning. Acquiring psychomotor skills depends on muscle and neurologic coordination. It is mastered best through demonstration and redemonstration.

Affective Learning

Affective learning involves a change in a person's attitude and is the most difficult area in which to bring about change. To teach a child the reason for and the skill of giving a self-injection, for example, may be easy; teaching the child to *like* giving a self-injection may never be possible. The best goal accomplished could be that the child will *value* the procedure because it will prevent him from developing hyperglycemia. Affective learning is gained best though role modeling, role playing, or shared-experience discussion.

Influence of Age and Stage on Ability to Learn

Learning ability varies a great deal depending on a child's stage of development and the past experiences the child has had in the specific area of learning (Heard, 2008).

The Infant

Infants learn by exploring the environment with their senses (psychomotor learning). They learn best from a primary caregiver because that is whom infants most want to please. Few health care points are actually taught at this age. Any that are taught must be presented not as a structured activity but as a game or an amusing or attractive activity. You could teach an infant to exercise a leg by showing how to kick a balloon tied to a crib rail or rolling a ball and encouraging the infant to move and creep after it, for example.

The Toddler

Toddlers are developing a sense of autonomy that is, learning to be independent (Erikson, 1993). Trying to teach toddlers a new activity such as eating a new food or brushing their teeth may be met with a sharp "No!" as children this age enjoy exerting their new independence. This retort does not mean the activity is unappealing to a child, however, only that the child is aware he does not have to do everything he is told to do. Toddlers also sometimes resist a change in routine because they need rituals to feel secure. If an activity will allow children to increase a level of independent functioning, they will usually learn it rapidly. Teaching activities such as exercise or deep breathing by having children imitate the action is an effective teaching method because it presents the activity as a game (so there is nothing to be resisted). Parents can be instrumental in maintaining a new skill their child has learned by incorporating it into a daily routine or a ritual.

The Preschooler

Preschool children are interested in learning, because developing a sense of initiative is the main developmental task of the period. Provided that instructions are geared to their small vocabularies, they "soak up" new methods of doing things. Because they are so imaginative and uninhibited, they have few reservations about the "right" way to do things. They will experiment with trial-and-error methods. They will both watch eagerly and freely redemonstrate a skill. They ask many questions about equipment and procedures. Keep explanations short and words simple; a preschooler's attention span rarely exceeds 5 minutes.

In terms of cognitive development, preschool children "center" or can learn only one characteristic of an object. This can limit their ability to learn all aspects of care or more than one method of doing something on any one day (Piaget, 1969).

Preschoolers tend to be frightened of intrusive procedures such as rectal temperature taking, bladder catheterization, or nasopharyngeal suction. They typically remove adhesive bandages minutes after application to check on the condition of their skin underneath (that it has not disappeared); they worry that any blood removed may be the last they have. Teaching this type of procedure or explaining to children why it is necessary calls for clear explanations and praise for learning. Use dolls or puppets to help children visualize details whenever possible, because pointing to a place on a puppet's body is not as intrusive as pointing to the child's own body (Fig. 35.2).

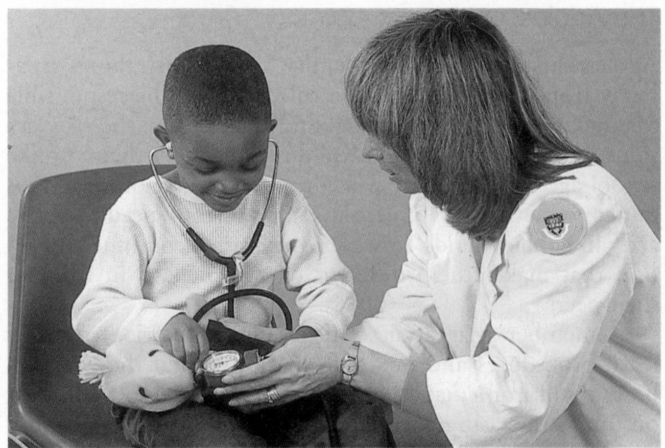

FIGURE 35.2 Teaching with dolls or toys can help to make an intrusive procedure seem less frightening for a preschooler.

Parents are often most aware of the technique that will be best to motivate their preschooler. Often, this begins with reading or telling a story about the problem (Ono et al., 2008).

The School-Age Child

School-age children enjoy short projects that offer an immediate reward. Therefore, they learn best if a procedure is broken down into different stages and presented as separate short procedures rather than one long one. They enjoy games, so playing "Simon Says" may be an effective way to have school-age children learn deep breathing, for example.

School-age children are used to learning things and accept learning a new procedure or new information as just another experience in a busy day. The "staying power" of school-age children is notoriously short, however; the ability to continue to perform at the level taught tends to decrease sharply if learning is not reinforced. Be certain, therefore, that a backup person in the home knows the health care information as well as the child so that person can reinforce it or carry out a procedure if necessary.

Toward the end of the school-age period, children become interested in doing only those things their friends are also doing. Children may interpret as unreasonable, therefore, a request to do something after school (come home and take a medication) that is different from what all their friends are doing such as stopping at the playground or mall. Modify a teaching plan as necessary to help children fit what they must learn into a school and social schedule. Otherwise, the teaching may be very short-lived.

As part of moral development, school-age children thrive on rules or the "right way" to do things (Kohlberg, 1984). This means if two or more people are going to be involved in teaching, they must be consistent in their approach. It is frustrating for school-age children to be shown two ways or not have a "right way" to do something.

Parents who have been supervising their child's school learning through checking homework easily assume a role in supervising health learning also. Parents who have not been monitoring learning previously may need support to fulfill this role.

The Adolescent

Adolescents, struggling for identity, like to learn things separately from their parents. As a rule, they can be responsible for their own self-care; if they understand how the new actions they have been taught will directly benefit them, unlike school-age children, they will continue to carry those actions out conscientiously. Adolescents have a strong need to be exactly like their friends, however; they rarely continue any action that makes them different or conspicuous in front of their peers.

Remember that adolescents are present-oriented; they learn procedures and new information best if they can see how it will immediately benefit them. They also focus best on things they can do rather than on things they cannot do. They learn poorly if the only benefit of new information presented to them is something that will affect them at some future date. Rotating insulin injection sites, for example, prevents "pockmark" formations (*lipoatrophy*) in the skin when the person reaches approximately 30 years of age. Given this information, adolescents tend not to rotate injection sites because the benefit is not relevant to them at the moment. An explanation such as, "Rotating injection sites will ensure insulin absorption and allow you to play basketball this semester" (an equally true statement) is a better adolescent motivator.

For the first time, adolescents are able to think abstractly or use scientific reasoning. This means they can create hypotheses ("what if" questions) and think through what will be the consequences of an action (Piaget, 1969). This allows them to understand the principle of what they are being taught and reinforces the reason for the learning. Parents may find they are not as effective with teaching their child as they were when the child was younger. They may need to "step aside" and let you introduce the subject until the phase of adolescent rebellion passes.

✔ Checkpoint Question 35.2

You want Barry to increase his cognitive understanding of his condition. Which statement from him would best show he has increased cognitive knowledge?

a. "I feel so much better now about the care I need."
b. "I understand I have to take two types of medicine."
c. "I've finally learned how to swallow big capsules."
d. "I hate having to take medicine but I will take it."

DEVELOPING AND IMPLEMENTING A TEACHING PLAN

A **teaching plan** is a design of the content to be taught and the teaching–learning techniques to be used. The first step in developing a teaching plan consists of assessing a child's current level of knowledge, ability, and motivation to learn new knowledge.

Areas of Assessment

Important areas for assessment include a child's current level of understanding; cognitive, physical, psychosocial aspects; and how the new knowledge will meld with the child's and family's lifestyle.

Language Level

Assessing language development includes assessing both the child's spoken vocabulary (how well the child speaks) and comprehensive vocabulary (how many words the child understands). Most children have a comprehensive vocabulary well above their speaking one or can understand about three times the words they actually use. Assess also "family vocabulary" or specific words the family uses. Be aware that if English is not a child's primary language, comprehensive vocabulary may not be greater than spoken vocabulary in English. Additional pictures, drawings, or diagrams may be necessary to convey meaning (Timler, Vogler-Elias, & McGill, 2007).

Child's Current Knowledge

Assessing how much a child currently knows about the health area in question helps to establish the needs and goals for the teaching plan. Current knowledge is in part developmentally based and in part experience based. Parents can tell you if a young child has had experience with the subject area. Some school-age children have had excellent anatomy and health classes as part of their science curriculum and are well aware of body organs. Children who are home schooled may have researched the subject as an independent project. Children who have lived with a family member with an illness may already know what home care problems occur with that particular illness; on the other hand, what they know about the illness may be accompanied by so many misconceptions that they need a great deal of teaching to prevent being hampered by half-truths or unnecessary restraints. A helpful method of assessment, which promotes mutual sharing in the learning process, is asking children to list what they know about the health area on one side of a piece of paper and what they want to know more about on the opposite side. To reveal this type of information, young children can be asked to draw pictures of themselves, of someone with their illness, or of a good thing to do to keep well.

Child's Intellectual Capability

In many instances, intellectual capability can be inferred from developmental milestones such as a child spoke in two-word sentences at 2 years or from educational level such as attending the age-appropriate class in school. However, most children regress at least slightly with illness; what one would normally expect from a 10-year-old, therefore, may be impossible for an *ill* 10-year-old. Children with chronic illnesses may not have met developmental milestones because of their lack of experiences, not because they do not have the cognitive ability to learn.

Child's Physical/Cognitive Capabilities

If a procedure that requires a certain level of psychomotor skill, such as medicine injection, will be necessary for care, assess a child's physical ability to perform the procedure (Hughes, 2007). If you omit this step, the procedure will be frustrating because you will be asking a child to perform a skill above capability. Assess vision and hearing ability and right- or left-hand dominance as well; these are important considerations for determining not only whether a child can accomplish procedures but also how the material will be presented.

Child's Psychological or Emotional Capabilities

To learn best, children need some motivation to learn or at least appreciate how their life will be improved through learning this new skill. It may be difficult for young children to grasp how the new skill will make them feel better. Some children are too ill or too exhausted or have too much pain to be ready for learning until these factors can be alleviated. With early hospital discharge, a great deal of health education may have to be delayed until a particular child has returned home and feels better.

Children, like adults, may have difficulty learning about an aspect of their care if they find it distasteful. A child who uses food as comfort, for example, may have trouble learning about a restrictive diet because it conflicts with the way the child views food. Children with urinary or bowel disorders may have difficulty learning about these body parts if they view them as "dirty" or distasteful. School-age and adolescent children may have difficulty discussing and asking questions about a reproductive tract illness not only because they lack knowledge of the subject but also because they sense sexual functioning is not an "open" topic in their family.

Children with low self-esteem are less capable of learning self-care than others because they do not feel as capable as others. For some children, it may be necessary to plan ways to increase self-esteem first before planning active teaching.

Child's Sociocultural Values

Different cultures have different values related to good health. If a child from a family that values sports develops an illness that impairs the ability to run, for example, the family might consider the disability overwhelming. If the family believes that being able to write and read well are the keys to succeeding in life, the same leg impairment might be viewed as merely a minor complication. Study each family individually to determine which aspect of health will be most important to emphasize when teaching (Box 35.5).

An important aspect of culture is whether children are raised in an environment where they are urged to be active participants in learning (allowed a lot of "hands-on" experimentation) or whether they are encouraged to be "watchers." Male/female roles also are culturally determined. This means a girl from a female-passive culture might not be enthusiastic about learning a self-care procedure because self-care is not expected of her. How long children are expected to be children (carefree, no responsibility) also varies culture to culture. In a family where children are expected to be out working and contributing to the family income by age 15, a child might have a very different attitude toward learning a self-care activity than the same-age child in a family where children are expected to remain noncontributing family members until after college (at least 21 years of age).

Child's Attention Span

The attention span of children and the capability to comprehend concepts and perform psychomotor skills differ a great deal depending on individuality and age. In general, the younger the child, the shorter is the attention span (under school age, 5 minutes of attention is all that can be expected). This means you must use more "attention-getting" teaching to hold attention in younger children. Think about the clever puppet shows or animation children are exposed to today.

BOX 35.5 * Focus on Communication

Wolf Whitefeather is the 3-year-old boy scheduled for a syndactyly (webbed fingers) repair next week. You speak with him through a puppet at a clinic visit to assess his understanding of the surgery.

Less Effective Communication

Nurse: Hello. Could you tell me what the little boy named Wolf is going to have done in surgery?
Wolf: His fingers got sick when he was born.
Nurse: When is he having them fixed?
Wolf: The day after we go to church.
Nurse: Will it hurt?
Wolf: No. His fingers are going to sleep.
Nurse: Will he have a big bandage afterward?
Wolf: So big he can't see how his fingers got cut.
Nurse: Okay. Thank you for talking to me. I'll see you Monday.

More Effective Communication

Nurse: Hello. Could you tell me what the little boy named Wolf is going to have done in surgery?
Wolf: His fingers got sick when he was born.
Nurse: When is he having them fixed?
Wolf: The day after we go to church.
Nurse: Will it hurt?
Wolf: No. His fingers are going to sleep.
Nurse: Will he have a big bandage afterward?
Wolf: So big he can't see how his fingers got cut.
Nurse: What does that mean? Cut?
Wolf: Cut so they're not there anymore.
Nurse: Why do you think that's going to happen?
Wolf: I think he's been bad.

The two scenarios above are good examples of what asking children about what they expect to happen in surgery can reveal. When asked what he means by "cut," it becomes obvious that Wolf needs additional teaching, probably using a drawing to illustrate what will be done. After surgery, when his fingers are covered by a pressure dressing so he cannot see them, he will need additional reassurance that his fingers are still intact underneath the gauze.

Teaching that is not accompanied by these same attention-holding techniques needs to be very short to be effective.

Child's Lifestyle

Lifestyle refers to the common pattern of a child's life. For example, a child who attends school daily and returns home every day at 3 PM has a fairly consistent lifestyle. A busy adolescent who works part-time, participates in several clubs after school, and socializes on weekends may have a varied pattern of activity every day.

Knowing family patterns helps to plan the timing of such activities as medication administration or exercise or meal times. If both parents work during the day and do not return home until 6 PM, medication may have to be administered after this time; exercises may have to be supervised in the evening, not the morning. A family that goes camping every weekend will need to plan ways to carry out a health routine at remote camp sites.

Child's Learning Style

Some children learn well from oral descriptions. Others have to see a statement in print before they can fully comprehend it. Still others are so visually oriented that they need to see a picture or a diagram before they can grasp the explanation. These different learning styles vary from child to child; few children are aware of their own learning style, so they cannot explain what it is. After caring for them for a time, it becomes easier to detect the way children learn best. Tailor a teaching plan to a learning style for the most effective learning situation.

Formulating the Plan

Formulating a teaching plan begins with establishing expected outcomes and techniques of teaching. It may need to include communication strategies for parents as well as children.

Identifying Personal Strengths and Limitations

When formulating a teaching plan, be honest about your capabilities. If you feel uncomfortable teaching a child about surgery with clever puppets dressed in scrub suits, it might be better to avoid this approach; in the wrong hands, such a method can sound so flat or complicated a child is left feeling more frightened by the presentation than comforted. Attempting to use a teaching method that is uncomfortable can cause children to interpret your insecurity as evidence there is something wrong with them, not with the method.

Some health teaching involves giving instructions in areas of care that may be personally embarrassing such as instructing a member of the opposite sex how to obtain a clean-catch urine specimen, for example. Proceeding blindly may not result in effective teaching, because the child may be so embarrassed by your discomfort that concentrating on instructions becomes difficult. In doing this type of teaching, nothing serves you as well (as in any client contact) as honesty. Admit to children that you are not used to giving this type of instruction. This approach will probably evoke a response from children that they are not used to having anyone talk about it either. Once you have found common ground (this is not the most comfortable discussion for either of you), there is a basis for effective health teaching. Honesty also allows a child to know that your discomfort is not from lack of knowledge on the subject (the child can trust what is being said) and also not the child's fault (the subject, not the child, is the disturbing factor).

Preparing Expected Outcomes

Planning outcomes is most effective when they are planned collaboratively with a child and family. They should reflect the type of learning desired: cognitive, psychomotor, or affective. They should help to establish both content and time guidelines based on both the child's cognitive ability to learn and the time frame it will take to learn. It is unnecessary (and often overwhelming) for a child to learn everything about an illness in the first day or week after a diagnosis. Likewise, information on how to stay well does not need to be presented in one setting. In many instances, it is effective to teach only part of the information needed; another nurse in another setting such as an ambulatory clinic or in the child's home can teach the remainder. For best results, state outcomes as behavioral objectives or as the activity the child is expected to demonstrate when the child has learned the new knowledge—not "Tim understands the importance of deep-breathing exercises daily" but "Tim does deep-breathing exercises daily."

Identifying Teaching Formats

Teaching techniques vary with the content to be covered, teacher–learner characteristics, and the environment for teaching.

Formal Versus Informal Teaching. Both formal and informal teaching formats are used in health education. Careful assessment is necessary to determine which format would be the best technique for a given situation. An example of formal teaching would be conducting a class on healthy eating as part of a health education course. An example of informal teaching would be explaining to a child who refuses to eat that he needs to at least drink something because his body needs more fluids to get better. Sometimes informal teaching occurs so spontaneously that it is easy to be unaware of it. It may occur, for example, in response to a question such as, "How long will I have to take this medicine?" If you answer, "For 2 weeks," that is just answering a question. If you answer, "For 2 weeks because. . .," that is teaching.

Be careful not to equate informal teaching with disorganized, or unnecessary, teaching. It is just as important as formal teaching; it is just communicated in a less structured way. Informal teaching requires that teaching and learning principles that include knowing the subject, recognizing individual learning styles, providing an effective environment, limiting time span, and so forth are followed, just as with more formal teaching. Table 35.3 lists suggestions for incorporating informal teaching into care.

Group Versus Individual Teaching. Although most health teaching is done on an individual basis, teaching groups of children is common in some situations. Individual instruction more directly addresses a child's unique needs; group teaching can meet individual needs while adding depth to learning as children discuss information within the group. For many children, hearing that they are not the only person with their problem is comforting. Hearing another child discuss how to solve a problem may be more meaningful than hearing the same information from an adult. Peer learning in this way, therefore, not only improves knowledge but may also improve attitude and motivation to learn.

Consider the following important guidelines when group teaching:

1. Assess for common interests and goals so that the information will appeal to as many in the group as possible.
2. Be certain that all members of the group can see and hear all others.
3. Encourage all members of the group to participate in discussions by calling on them if necessary.
4. Limit any one person from dominating the group by a statement such as, "That's a good point, Reneé. Has anyone else had a similar experience?"

TABLE 35.3 ✻ Ways to Incorporate Informal Teaching Into Care

Activity	Type of Teaching
Medication administration	Children as young as early school age should know the type and action and any expected side effects of all medication they are taking. Present medicine not by saying, "Here is your pill" but "Here is your [name of medication], medicine to help your temperature come back to normal. After you take this, you might feel yourself start to sweat. That means it's working."
Vital sign measurement	When taking vital signs such as blood pressure, temperature, and pulse, tell children what normal levels are: "Your blood pressure is 100/70. That's normal." If the child is in a high-risk category for hypertension, add some prevention measures to teaching.
Any procedure	Always tell children the purpose and principle of procedures, not "You need to drink a lot of fluid," but "You need to drink a lot of fluid because . . ."
Dressing changes	Dressing changes provide an opportunity to teach the danger of introducing infection into an open wound. The parents or child may not change this dressing, but they will apply bandages to small cuts in the future and so will benefit from teaching.
Mealtime	Provide information about nutrition: "I know you're not hungry enough to eat the entire sandwich, but could you try the meat? Meat is high in protein and that's important for healing."
Hygiene	Emphasize the necessity of good perineal hygiene to decrease the possibility of urinary tract infection.
Physical assessment	Explain aspects of testicular self-examination and describe "normal" findings as both education and reassurance.
Positioning	Teach the hazards of immobility and how change of position and ambulation increase circulation and respiratory function.
Sleep	Teach that sleep is a healing therapy and should not be considered a waste of time.
Bowel elimination	Teach children that elimination patterns vary; occasional variations in their elimination patterns are normal.

5. Avoid competition in the group. No one is always right; no one is always wrong.
6. Ask group members to evaluate the experience afterward to be certain it met the group's needs.

Home Versus Institutional Teaching. Health teaching is just as important in the home as it is in a health care agency, school, or community setting. Teaching in the health care agency usually focuses on immediate acute care concerns. Teaching in the school may focus on topics such as basic health promotion and hygiene, reproductive and sex education, and drug prevention. Teaching in the home may focus on medication regimens, dressing changes, or measures to prevent complications of a particular illness. It may also involve helping a child and parents adapt a procedure to the home setting, such as accommodating a wheelchair at home. Be certain parents have obtained the supplies they will need to learn and perform the procedure in the home.

Teaching in the home offers the advantage of being able to assess a child's environment, interactions with other family members, and overall family functioning. This may yield data that prove useful for further planning and implementation of care. It may also provide an opportunity to include other family members—siblings, grandparents, and so forth—in the teaching plan, which could strengthen the impact of teaching and ensure that all family members understand the procedures in the same way.

Always include evaluation as a step of teaching in all settings so you can feel confident that learning has occurred.

What if... Barry, who is overweight, needs to begin a lower-calorie nutrition pattern as well as a lower-cholesterol one? Who would you need to teach? Barry? His mother who prepares his food? Or his father, who does the family grocery shopping?

Determining Teaching Strategies

Because children's knowledge base, capabilities, learning styles, and attention spans vary, teaching strategies are most effective when they are intermixed and when they are selected in response to the individual situation and child to be taught. The more interactive the method, the more appealing it might be to a particular child.

Lecture. Lecture (or directly explaining information) is the most efficient and time-saving method of offering information to both individual children and groups. A lecture, however, does not allow for much participation, and it is effective only in short, well-structured periods. It is rarely effective for children who are not yet school age.

Demonstration. Demonstration is actually performing a procedure such as a dressing change or instillation of eye drops so the child can see clearly how the procedure should be done. Do not demonstrate a procedure unless you have all the necessary equipment to do it. If you stop in the middle of a demonstration to say, "Be sure to use a sterile syringe, not what I'm using," the poor technique demonstrated may be the lesson learned, not the good technique. The purpose of demonstration is to show how the procedure actually is done; having to imagine steps is little different than reading about it. School-age children, because of their stage of cognitive development (concrete operations), learn best by demonstration (Fig. 35.3).

Redemonstration. To determine whether a child has truly grasped a demonstration, ask the child to perform a **redemonstration,** or exact imitation of the procedure. Redemonstration is best if it immediately follows demonstration. Praise the effort to redemonstrate even if the redemonstration is not of the quality desired. No one likes to be put on the spot, and children may be unwilling to expose themselves again by a second demonstration if criticized. Be aware that there are many different ways to do almost everything. Children do not have to follow your motions exactly, as long as their technique accomplishes the same goal. An effective way to correct a wrong action is to say, "That's one way of doing that; most children, however, find it easier to. . . ." This type of criticism is nonthreatening because it acknowledges the child's effort in a positive way before offering a correction.

Discussion. Discussion is a shared learning experience in which children ask questions about particular concerns and these are answered based on their individual circumstances, or children are asked questions about some problem, such as how they anticipate managing some aspect of care, and together the problem is solved. At the beginning of health education, children tend to ask few questions because they do not know enough about an illness or health issue to anticipate concerns. As their knowledge increases, so does their ability to project and modify information to fit their own lifestyle. Remember that children tend to think in the present: a problem that will arise once tomorrow is usually more important to a child than one that can be predicted to arise repeatedly in years to come. Because it recognizes and respects their opinions, school-agers and adolescents enjoy discussion.

Role Modeling. Role modeling is demonstrating a certain attitude or behavior you want a child to learn. Be certain when health teaching not only to present facts but also to radiate a positive attitude. Showing frustration at getting a bubble out of medicine in a syringe demonstrates, for example, that giving injections is frustrating; showing a bored attitude toward nutrition instructions implies that nutrition information is boring. The child picks up the role modeling cues as readily as the spoken message. Role modeling is an important technique used to teach new parents newborn care; as they watch a nurse hold, comfort, and talk to their newborn, they quickly learn to model these behaviors.

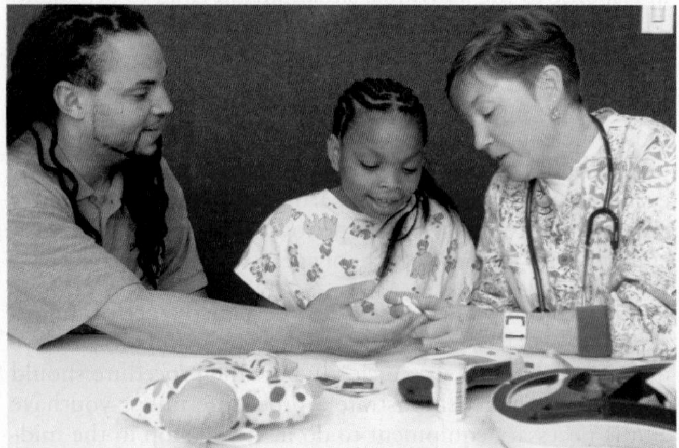

FIGURE 35.3 A school-age child watches a demonstration of insulin injections.

Behavior Therapy. Typically, learning occurs best with **positive reinforcement** (a child tries to understand a new procedure, is praised for the effort, and tries even harder). **Behavior therapy,** also called *behavior modification,* is a term used for a system aimed at *erasing* some form of behavior that interferes with healthy functioning. It was originally designed to help people who are cognitively challenged erase socially unacceptable behavior such as poking their fingers in their eyes. Currently it has many uses, including concerns such as controlling disruptive classroom behavior. The basic premise of behavior modification is that a child is rewarded for healthful behavior, whereas unhealthful behavior is ignored or unrewarded. For example, a cognitively challenged child may have a socially unacceptable habit of constantly rocking back and forth. The child is not scolded or criticized for rocking, but the action is ignored. On the other hand, preferred behavior (sitting for 5 minutes without rocking) is praised. As another example, a child might be ignored for being a picky eater, then praised for the few bites he does eat well. Children respond best to behavior modification if, in addition to praise, they receive a tangible reward such as a star on a chart or an extra privilege of some sort for good behavior.

A behavior modification program must be discussed with the child before it is begun, because no behavior can be modified, just as no new behavior can be learned, until a child truly wants a change to occur. It might be necessary to ask older children to sign a learning contract to be certain that both teacher and learner agree on the method to be used. Many older children are able to use self-rewards to reinforce a behavior modification program such as rewarding themselves by playing a video game or going to a movie after an afternoon of efficient studying or an hour of doing breathing exercises.

Behavior modification is a technique that must be used with common sense and concern so that children are not being manipulated more than they are being helped to achieve a more healthful lifestyle. It is a legitimate device to use in helping a child with attention deficit/hyperactivity disorder sit still long enough to eat a meal or learn in school. It can be helpful in encouraging children to do as much self-care as possible or discourage disorders such as obsessive compulsive behavior (O'Kearney, Anstey, & von Sanden, 2009).

Trying to modify beliefs or values by behavior modification is unethical and is one reason why behavior modification is often criticized as a learning technique. However, some behavior changes also require a change in values to be effective and long term. For example, a child's behavior of talking back to parents can be extinguished by ignoring or not responding to the behavior and praising polite communication. This method teaches the child to value improved communication and parental approval in order to meet his or her needs.

Selecting Teaching Tools

Teaching tools are the mechanical devices used to present content. They vary based on content, teacher–learner characteristics, and environment.

Visual Aids. "A picture is worth a thousand words" is not an idle quotation but a realistic one. Because small children know little about their bodies or where body organs are located, using visual aids such as drawings or photographs of anatomy can be very helpful. Figure 35.4 shows abdominal contents as an example of such a drawing. You could use such an illustration to show a preschooler how food moves through the body. Figure 35.5 is an example of a good tool to use while naming body parts. Pointing to a figure drawing and saying, "This is the part of your tummy the doctor will fix," is less threatening than actually pointing to the child's abdomen. Clarifying body parts this way is important because young children may have no clear understanding of where a body part such as a hand ends and an arm begins.

Do not be afraid to draw a picture of a heart, a kidney, a bladder, or any other organ to make a point about anatomic structure. Children are more interested in understanding procedures or the reason for a health maintenance measure than criticizing your artwork (they likely do not know anatomy well enough to be able to tell if a drawing is distorted).

Pamphlets. Pamphlets are helpful teaching aids with school-age children and adolescents because they usually contain brief, easy to read, easily understood information and are often cleverly illustrated with cartoon characters to make them enjoyable. Be certain to read any pamphlet before offering it to a child to be certain the information included in it is accurate. Medical advances are made so quickly that a 1-year-old pamphlet may contain a gross inaccuracy in the light of subsequent knowledge.

If a pamphlet contains some statements that are inaccurate or that do not apply to a child, do not simply cross out the information that would be contradictory before offering it (most children deliberately read what they have been told not to read); take the time to explain why it does not apply. Also, do not be misled into believing that because children are given clever pamphlets, they will necessarily read them and learn from them. Sit with a school-age child and read the pamphlet together; talk with an adolescent about the pamphlet's contents later to ensure it has been read.

Learning Games. For memorizing certain kinds of information, such as what foods are high or low in potassium or sodium, flash cards are a helpful learning tool. Many children enjoy playing trivia-type board games. Instead of the usual

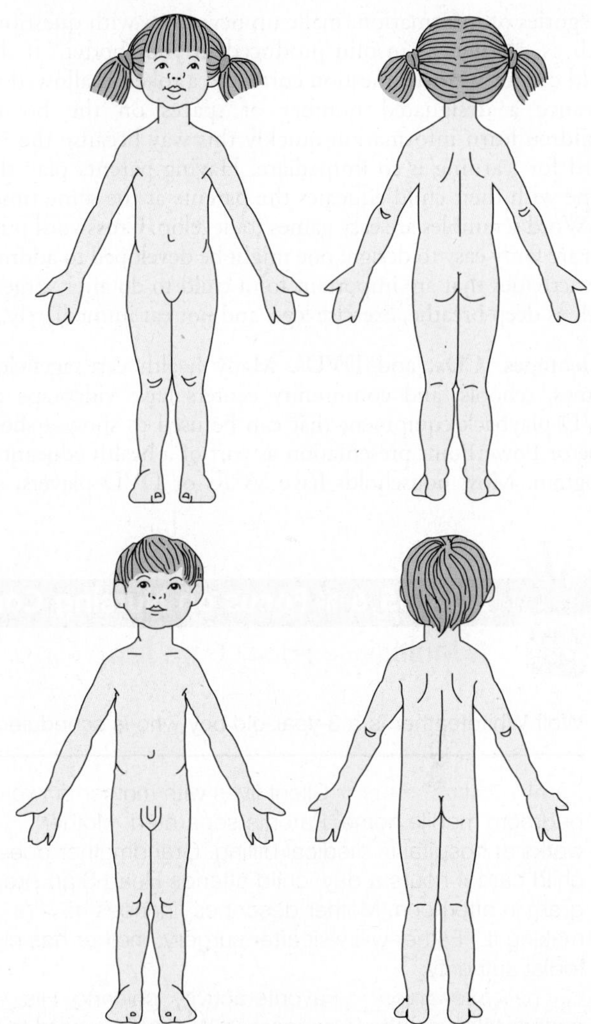

FIGURE 35.5 Simple line drawings such as these can be used to explain to a child exactly what part of his or her body will be "fixed" in surgery. For many children, having this pointed out on a drawing seems much less intrusive than having it pointed to on their own body.

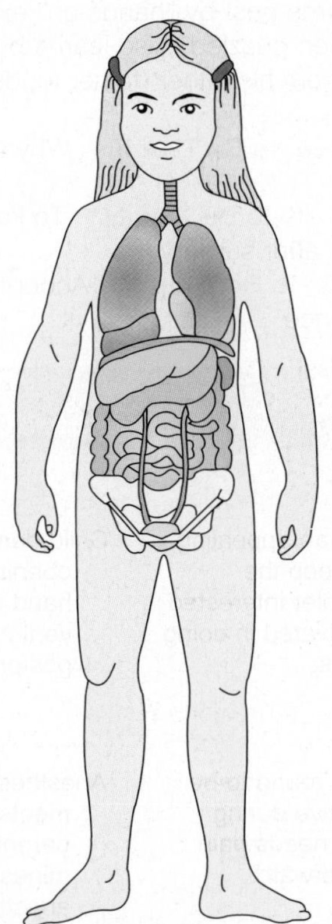

FIGURE 35.4 Anatomic drawings are helpful to illustrate basic health education topics as well as health care procedures.

categories of information, make up new cards with questions such as, "Where is insulin produced in your body?" If the child can answer the question correctly, a token is allowed to advance a designated number of spaces on the board. Children learn information quickly this way because the reward for learning is so immediate. Having parents play the game with their child educates the parents at the same time.

Word scrambles are easy games to develop. Crossword puzzles are fairly easy to design; one might be developed to address the activities that are important for a child to do after surgery such as deep breathe, exercise legs, and not eat immediately.

Videotapes, CDs, and DVDs. Many health care agencies, homes, schools, and community centers have videotape or DVD playback equipment that can be used to show a short tape or PowerPoint presentation as part of a health education program. Most households have VCRs or DVD players, so tapes or disks can be sent home for families to view. Viewing such programs can give children a sense of power in that the program seems to be talking directly to them. It can also be used over and over to refresh children's knowledge of the steps they need to take to remain well (Yoon & Godwin, 2007). As with pamphlets, view the material first before showing it; be certain to check that the vocabulary used is appropriate for an individual child or family (Bauman et al., 2007).

Puppets and Dolls. Many children are shy about talking to strangers; this shyness, in addition to their concern about what will happen to them, may make it difficult for them to discuss or explain what they know about their health, illness, or intended surgery. However, they may be able to open up to an uncritical puppet or doll (see Focus on Nursing Care Planning Box 35.6). Preschool children are particularly receptive to puppets and dolls because, with their imagination

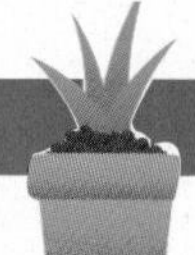

BOX 35.6 * Focus on Nursing Care Planning

A Multidisciplinary Care Map for a Preschooler Having Surgery

Wolf Whitefeather is a 3-year-old boy who is scheduled for repair of syndactyly (webbed fingers) next week.

Family Assessment * Client lives with mother in two-bedroom mobile home. Parents separated. Mother works at hospital in medical billing. Grandmother does child care 4 hours a day; child attends Head Start program in afternoon. Mother describes finances as "I'm making it." Father will visit after surgery; mother has custodial authority.

Client Assessment * Favorite activity: coloring. His mother tells you she is concerned Wolf will be hard to entertain after surgery because the large pressure bandage he will have afterward will prevent him from coloring with that hand. "I don't even want to begin to talk to him about surgery," she tells you. When nervous or frightened, child has a habit of biting his hand; he has done this constantly since admission.

Nursing Diagnosis * Deficient knowledge related to what to expect in surgery

Outcome Criteria * Child describes expected outcomes of surgery. Demonstrates a minimum of nervous behaviors such as biting hand, can play "Simon Says" for hand exercises postsurgery, and describes how pain will be relieved by "special button" (patient-controlled analgesia).

Teaching Points * Child is shy with strangers; mother states that he learns best by "hands-on" experiences; "cocks head" when puzzled. Also learns better from his mother than from his father (father tends to be authoritarian).

Cognitive Learning to Be Taught * Why surgery is necessary

Psychomotor Skills to Be Taught * To keep hand in elevated position after surgery

Affective Aspects to Be Taught * Accepts surgery as a growth experience

Team Member Responsible	Assessment	Intervention	Rationale	Expected Outcome
Activities of Daily Living				
Nurse	Assess what child and parent understand about care necessary postoperatively.	Introduce postoperative hand exercises child will need to do by playing "Simon Says."	Games are an appealing way to keep the preschooler interested and motivated in doing exercises.	Child demonstrates opening and closing hand to help prevent contractions postprocedure.
Consultations				
Surgeon	Assess which anesthesiologist or nurse anesthetist is available for consult.	Request anesthesia/analgesia consult.	Child is too young to be cooperative during surgery; needs pain relief afterward.	Anesthesia service meets with child and parent and determines best form of anesthesia and pain management.

		Procedures/Medications		
Nurse practitioner/ resident physician	Assess health history.	Complete physical exam.	Health assessment helps ensure readiness for surgery.	Child cooperates with history and exam.
Nurse	Assess Wolf's and parent's knowledge of surgery and postoperative procedures.	Introduce dressing and show how child's hand will be suspended postoperatively by letting Wolf dress and suspend puppet's hand.	Therapeutic play provides an excellent medium for teaching and learning with toddlers and preschoolers.	Child demonstrates he understands how hand will be positioned by showing position with puppet.
		Nutrition		
Nurse	Assess if child and parent know child will be NPO for general anesthesia for surgery.	Teach parent importance of NPO preoperatively and immediately postoperatively.	Maintaining NPO status helps prevent aspiration with anesthesia.	Child and parent state they understand necessity for NPO status and will adhere to requirement.
		Patient/Family Education		
Nurse	Assess child's cognitive level and ability to learn.	Using puppets, teach that child's hand must be washed with antiseptic wash solution before surgery.	Reducing skin bacteria prior to surgery can help prevent osteomyelitis.	Child cooperates with preprocedure washes.
Nurse	Reassess who is child's main support person.	Ask mother, as support person, to reinforce preparation.	Wolf learns best from mother; reinforcement from her could help Wolf go into the operation viewing it as a growth experience.	Mother reinforces necessity for surgery and accompanying pre- and postoperative procedures.
		Psychosocial/Spiritual/Emotional Needs		
Nurse/pain management team member	Assess what past experiences, if any, child has had with pain.	Teach that child will have pain after surgery but that it can be relieved by a "special button" on his intravenous line.	Preparing a child for postoperative procedures and explaining how pain will be relieved before surgery (when the child still feels well) can help reduce the amount of learning the child needs to accomplish after surgery, when he doesn't feel well.	Child and parent state they know there will be pain and understand method to be used for control.
		Discharge Planning		
Nurse	Assess if child and parent feel equipped to change bandages, carry out hand exercises at home.	Review with parent a schedule of care based on Head Start and grandmother involvement.	Helping a parent walk through how postprocedure activities can be managed helps ensure adherence.	Mother states that she has a plan for how to consistently arrange care given by three caregivers.
Nurse/ physician	Assess when return visit is needed and is convenient for parent.	Schedule return visit for postsurgery evaluation.	Follow-up care is necessary to evaluate success of surgery.	Parents states she understands importance of follow-up visit and will keep appointment.

at its peak, they believe the puppet or doll is actually talking to them (Wright et al., 2007).

Teaching preschool children about what to expect from a hospital experience is often taught by using a series of puppets to represent different hospital personnel such as a surgeon, a nurse, and a nurse's assistant. Children can practice giving the doll "shots" or submitting it to the procedures they will experience (see Chapter 36 for a discussion of therapeutic play).

Mass Media. Television and radio are examples of effective mass media that teach many children topics about self-help or self-care. Consulting on the topics to present or helping develop the material used in these types of health messages can be an important role for nurses. Messages originated for these media must be attention-getting and brief to compete with the programs and commercial messages that precede or follow them.

Computers. Many children learn to solve problems using computers as early as preschool age and are exposed to computers at home, child care, or school. Using a computer application to answer questions about an illness is effective because this type of activity can be both entertaining and informative (Gielen et al., 2007). Caution children that not all information posted on the web is reliable and participating in chat rooms can lead to exposure to Internet predators.

Health Fairs. Health fairs are displays presenting health-related information to large numbers of people. They are effective with children if they encourage active participation through interactive displays or computer games.

Preparing Teaching Supplies

To avoid having to reorganize equipment or instructions each time a procedure is taught, put together a basket or box containing all the information and equipment needed to teach a particular task. This helps ensure that teaching is organized and is economical in that everyone on a hospital unit is not opening new equipment for demonstrations. It also helps to ensure that everyone is teaching the same information. Nothing is more confusing to anyone learning a new skill than to be taught two different principles for doing it or two different techniques.

Implementing the Plan

Health teaching can begin immediately and flow easily if goals have been developed well and strategies for teaching have been designed carefully.

Resource People

Many health care agencies, including home care agencies, have specific people who are available for health teaching about specific subjects such as diabetes, stomal care, or respiratory exercises or drug prevention. Using such people is helpful because they know all the "tricks of the trade" for teaching that particular subject.

Some children do not learn as well from such designated teachers, however, because they see them only infrequently, where they see a primary nurse daily. Some parents react badly to the thought that it takes an expert to tell them about the care needed (if care is so complicated, how can they possibly learn it?). They also find it inconvenient to be told that their questions cannot be answered until the following day when the designated teacher is available to answer them. Be sure that if a designated teacher does teach a subject, you coordinate your teaching with that person. Make a point of introducing the person to a child so the child does not view the person as a suspicious stranger.

Parent Education

With very young children, parents as well as children need teaching. It is good practice with all children to be certain that at least one adult in the household has the necessary information or can perform the required skill as well as the child. Let the child choose this person as the individual who everyone assumes is a child's chief support person may not be the person the child perceives as the most reliable choice and, therefore, not the one the child wants as a health care backup. This person, when identified, needs as much information as the child does about why the health measure is important.

What if... Wolf, 3 years old, refuses to tell you whether he has pain because you are a "stranger" and he doesn't talk to strangers? What would you do?

Evaluating the Effectiveness of Teaching

Evaluation, or assessing whether teaching has been effective, is the final step in teaching. Evaluation occurs not only after the teaching plan has been implemented but throughout the entire learning process. This ongoing evaluation helps both teacher and learner modify the teaching plan to better meet changing needs.

There is some advantage in asking children questions before and after teaching to prove that teaching was effective and the child has safely learned a new health care measure. Demonstration of a change of behavior or attitude, however, is the real proof that learning has occurred.

HEALTH TEACHING FOR A SURGICAL EXPERIENCE

Teaching to prepare a child for surgery is an example of teaching that requires planning for several stages of learning. The child and the child's parents often feel anxious about surgery because this is always a potentially frightening experience, so teaching must first address this anxiety. Such preparation differs according to the type of surgery being performed, but certain activities apply to all surgery and all children. Psychological preparation of both child and parents is aimed at reducing a child's fears about the procedure and consists primarily of providing health teaching and opportunities for therapeutic play. Physical preparation includes providing for restrictions on food and fluid intake before surgery, preparing the incision site on the child's skin, and arranging for transportation of the child to surgery. Because many children's surgical procedures are done on an ambulatory basis, preparation must also include informing parents about the details of the preparation techniques, the surgery, the postoperative period, and the steps they must take toward preparation. Do not downplay a family's fears, but allow the child and family opportunities to express their concerns as part of the teaching–learning process.

Assessing Current Level of Knowledge

On admission to an inpatient surgical or an ambulatory unit, discuss with parents the preparation they have made for this experience and what specifically they have told a child about what will happen. It is good to ask also whether a child's concerns about the experience seem more or less than the parents had anticipated. Is the child emotionally prepared? Ask if there has been an unpleasant surgery or hospitalization in the family that a child might have heard discussed. Has the child seen anything recently on a medical show on television that might have been upsetting?

Emotional Preparation

Preparing a child emotionally for surgery requires minimizing fears common to all children such as fear of separation, fear of mutilation, or fear of death. This can be accomplished by telling a child about the procedure and describing any specific equipment and techniques that will be used, such as anesthesia, eye bandages, nasogastric tubes, sutures, or special aftercare. Be certain all preparation is appropriate to the child's age. More children who need surgery receive a general anesthetic rather than a local or regional anesthetic, as might be used with adults, because this minimizes their fears of intrusive or mutilating procedures, and because children who are not yet adolescent are not mature enough to cooperate adequately during surgery if they are not fully anesthetized.

It is best to prepare a child for surgery or hospitalization in stages because it is difficult for a child to absorb everything at once. However, contact before surgery may be limited to only one office or clinic visit, so time constraints can force information to be more compacted.

Be certain to discuss preparations for surgery such as coming for blood work and not eating the morning of surgery. If the child will have general anesthesia, it is important to emphasize that anesthetized sleep is "special" sleep. Otherwise, toddlers or preschoolers may be reluctant to fall asleep after surgery for fear people will come and do strange things to them. Do not say a child will be "put to sleep." Dogs and cats who are "put to sleep" are not seen again. To help prepare a young child for surgery, a doll could be used: its abdomen washed, an injection given to make it sleepy, and a hospital gown put on. It could be carried to a cart made from a cardboard box. After saying goodbye to its parents, the doll could be wheeled to surgery by a puppet nurse.

The surgery procedure should be discussed but minimized. "After you're asleep, the doctor will fix your tummy. You won't feel anything because of the special sleep. When you wake up, you'll be in a room called a recovery room where you'll stay until you're wide awake." Be honest concerning pain: "Your tummy will feel sore afterward, but I'll give you something to make it feel better" is a fair statement.

It is important to alert children that nurses and doctors in surgery wear surgical masks. Assure toddlers and preschoolers that the persons behind the masks are doctors and nurses, some of whom the child has probably already met, not superheros or bandits.

It is good to mention recovery rooms in preparation, because this is often an area parents neglect to mention. In fact, parents may not be aware that, in some institutions, they will not be allowed in the recovery room and may have promised the child, "As soon as you wake up, I'll be there." Clarify the parents' misconceptions about recovery rooms, and reiterate that the child will get to see his parents back in his own room once he is fully awake. This both makes the parents' preparation correct and saves the child from feeling deceived.

Explain postsurgery items, such as the use of oxygen, monitors, bedpans, bandages, or intravenous equipment. Furnishing a doll with such equipment is especially helpful in preparing younger children (Fig. 35.6). This prevents preschoolers from feeling overwhelmed by being taken to an intensive care unit and shown actual monitors and respirators. After surgery, be certain to evaluate whether a child's preparation was adequate, both to document that the experience was as trauma free as it could be and to evaluate your expertise in teaching children (Li, Lopez, & Lee, 2007).

Physical Preparation

Most children will be placed on nothing by mouth (NPO) status for surgery. The length of the time a child will remain NPO depends on the child's age. Adolescents and school-age children may be restricted from taking food or fluid from midnight until the time of surgery the following morning; however, if infants younger than 6 months were held NPO for as long a time as this, they would be taken to surgery in dehydration. Therefore, infants younger than 6 months may be kept NPO for as little as 4 hours. At the end of the 4 hours, as the infant becomes hungry, the infant will begin to cry and fuss for fluid. Parents need an explanation that infants who vomit during surgery because of recent feedings may aspirate; therefore, even though an infant is becoming hungry, it is important that fluid not be ingested. Although a hungry child will usually not suck on one for long, a pacifier can be offered.

Preparation of surgical sites varies. In most instances, shaving of the area and final cleansing are done in a holding room adjacent to the operating room after the child is anesthetized. A povidone–iodine wash may be ordered before

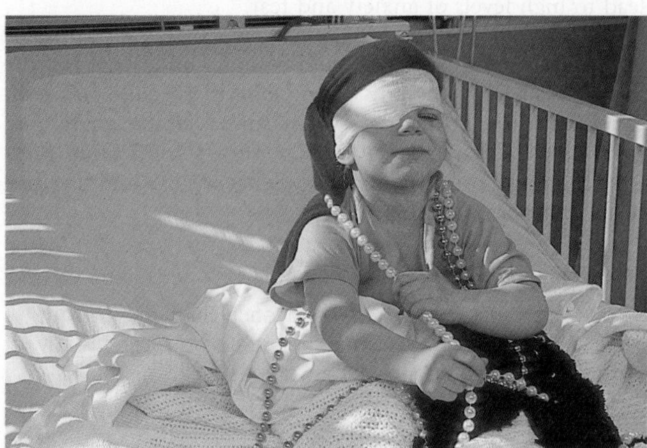

FIGURE 35.6 Pretending to be a pirate helps this young child prepare for having to wear an eye patch after surgery.

transport to the operating room for some types of surgery. Washing a particular body part in this manner can be interpreted as an intrusive procedure by a preschooler. Give a great deal of assurance that the solution being used will not sting but is only cleaning.

Implementing the Plan

Check children's identification bands to ensure they are legible and secure before the child is transported to surgery. If not, replace or secure them before surgery. Immediately before transport, remove barrettes and bobby pins from a child's hair and check the mouth for loose teeth (particularly in children aged 6, 7, and 8 years, who are losing their central and lateral incisors) or for dental appliances. It is rare to find a child with full dentures but not uncommon to find a post or screw-in tooth that may have to be removed before surgery or a retainer used to maintain orthodontic correction after brace removal. Teeth braces do not need to be removed. Make certain the anesthesiologist knows about any loose teeth before an airway for surgery is inserted (a loose tooth could be knocked totally free and aspirated during the procedure).

For some children, having to give up their own pajamas or their bedroom slippers or outside shoes to change to a hospital gown is a terrifying moment. Giving up underpants is a step that many preschool and early school-age children cannot tolerate. For this reason, many children are allowed to wear their own pajamas or clothes until they are under an anesthetic.

In ambulatory settings, children may walk to surgery. If they will ride in a cart, this should have been introduced during preparation. Be sure to fasten a restraining strap for safety (presented with, "Here's your seat belt; it's just like going in a car."). Preschoolers may enjoy taking a favorite toy or blanket to surgery with them. Ideally, they should be allowed to keep this with them until they are under an anesthetic. Parents should be allowed to accompany children to the operating suite. Some parents can accompany a child into an anesthesiologist's induction room; for others, this is inappropriate or too anxiety-producing. A nurse whom the child knows should accompany the child to the operating room and remain there until the child is under the anesthetic, if possible. Even if a child has been well prepared for the surgical experience and the change in personnel on arrival to the surgical suite, saying goodbye to parents at the door of the surgical suite and the actual sight of strange personnel can lead to high levels of anxiety and fear.

Although it may not be cost-effective to have a staff nurse wait with a child until the child is under an anesthetic, the nurse's wait will probably not be long if the child has been called for surgery when the surgical suite is almost ready. The psychological benefit of a familiar nurse's comforting presence can make the difference between a positive and negative hospital experience (Box 35.7).

✔Checkpoint Question 35.3

You want to use a board game to teach Barry more about his hypercholesterolemia. At what age are children first ready for competition and so enjoy board games?

a. 3 years.
b. 6 years.
c. 10 years.
d. 14 years.

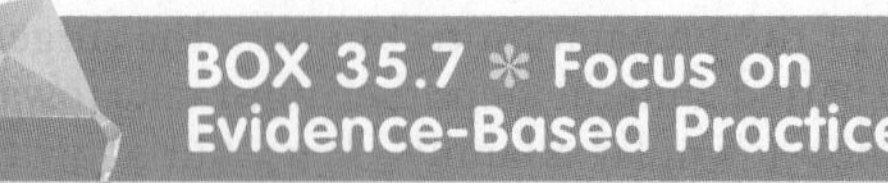

BOX 35.7 ✻ Focus on Evidence-Based Practice

What type of information do the parents of children with head injuries want from health care providers?

To answer this question, nurse researchers mailed a questionnaire asking, "What questions did you have when your child injured his/her head?" to parents of children who were seen in a hospital emergency department for head injury. The mean age of the 24 girls and 33 boys was 5.2 years (with a range from 1 month to 15 years), with 36 (63%) of the children having been less than 5 years old at the time of their injury. The head injuries were caused by falls (76%), bicycle accidents (8%), trauma to the head (8%), or sporting accidents (8%). Despite differences in the severity of the child's head injury and requirement for hospitalization, all the families expressed the same informational needs and the need for emotional support. The concerns that parents voiced were categorized into four divisions: (1) Information about the head injury by responses such as, "Is there a brain injury?" "Is there bleeding into the brain?" (2) Need for information on everyday living by such responses as, "Are there any restrictions?" "What should we be aware of?" (3) Need for reassurance by responses such as, "Is there any risk for delayed development?" or "Will she/he recover?" and (4) Need to share the emotional burden by responses such as, "Should we have come to the hospital by ambulance?" or "Should we have come to the hospital sooner?"

Based on this study, would it be important to include emotional support for children as a part of information they need following an injury?

Source: Falk, A. C., von Wendt, L., & Klang, B. (2008). Informational needs in families after their child's mild head injury. *Patient Education and Counseling, 70*(2), 251–255.

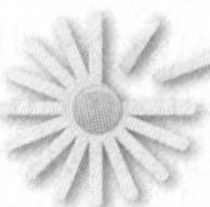

Key Points for Review

- Communication is the exchange of ideas between two or more persons. It can be verbal or nonverbal.
- Therapeutic communication is a planned interaction, has structure, and is constructive. Nontherapeutic communication lacks deliberate purpose other than socializing.
- Successful communication requires an encoder, a code, a decoder, and feedback or response.
- Levels of communication are (a) cliché, (b) fact reporting, (c) shared ideas, (d) shared feelings, and (e) a sense of knowing what another wants without it needing to be voiced.
- Typical methods of nonverbal communication are using distance, gestures, body posture and gait, touch, use of drawings, and empathy.
- Techniques that encourage therapeutic communication are attentive listening, open-ended questions, reflecting, clarifying, paraphrasing, perception checking, focusing, supportive statements, and silence.

- Some situations require special communication techniques such as interacting with demanding or shy children, children who are visually or hearing challenged, or children who are not proficient in English.
- Establishing a teacher–learner relationship based on mutual input and setting expected outcomes are effective ways to meet the unique needs and goals of a child and family.
- There are three types of learning: cognitive, psychomotor, and affective. For something to be learned well, all of these areas may need to be involved.
- To individualize a teaching program for a child, assess the child's attention span, cognitive or intellectual capability, lifestyle, and learning style and your own teaching strengths and limitations.
- In many instances, there is a great deal of material a child must learn about an illness. If possible, divide material into lessons that must be taught immediately and lessons that can be taught at spaced return health visits.
- The format and strategies of teaching used with children vary depending on a child's age and developmental level. Various types to consider are formal versus informal, single or group teaching, lecture, discussion, and role playing.
- Behavior modification is a special technique aimed at erasing some form of behavior that interferes with good health.
- Children are learning many other things besides health information every day. This may make the retention of information not as great as you would like. You may need to schedule frequent reviews and updates to keep information current.

CRITICAL THINKING EXERCISES

1. Wolf Whitefeather is the preschooler you met at the beginning of the chapter. He will be having surgery in a week for bilateral syndactyly (webbed fingers). His mother asks you how to prepare him for this. What suggestions would you make? The child will be left with a noticeable scar and some lack of function after surgery, so he cannot be reassured that everything will be all right. How will this affect your teaching?
2. Barry Sandoz's family has hypercholesterolemia. It is recommended that Barry begin a low-cholesterol diet. He says, "Don't tell me anything about foods I can't eat. I've heard it all." You say, "Heard it all?" He says, "Don't repeat what I said. That really bugs me." You know he needs to learn more about foods to eat so he can eat safely in the school cafeteria. What would you do?
3. Wolf has to learn how to use a peak flowmeter at least once daily to monitor asthma symptoms. How would you teach this skill to so young a child? Suppose his mother says there is no reason to teach him how to read the meter because she will do it for him. Would your teaching plan be different?
4. Examine the National Health Goals related to communication and teaching with children. Most government-sponsored funds for nursing research are allotted based on these goals. What would be a possible research topic to explore pertinent to these goals that would be applicable to the Whitefeather family and also advance evidence-based practice?

CRITICAL THINKING SCENARIO

Open the accompanying CD-ROM or visit http://thePoint.lww.com and read the Patient Scenario included for this chapter, then answer the questions to further sharpen your skills and grow more familiar with NCLEX style questions related to communication and children. Confirm your answers by reading the rationales.

REFERENCES

Barlow, J., & Parsons, J. (2009). Group-based parent-training programmes for improving emotional and behavioural adjustment in 0–3 year old children. *Cochrane Database of Systematic Reviews, 2009*(1), (CD003680).

Bauman, M. E., et al. (2007). Developing educational materials to facilitate adherence: pediatric thrombosis as a case illustration. *Journal of Pediatric Health Care, 21*(3), 198–206.

Cabana, M. D., et al. (2008). Selective provision of asthma self-management tools to families. *Pediatrics, 121*(4), e900–e905.

Erikson, E. H. (1993). *Childhood and society.* New York: W. W. Norton.

Falk, A. C., von Wendt, L., & Klang, B. (2008). Informational needs in families after their child's mild head injury. *Patient Education and Counseling, 70*(2), 251–255.

Gielen, A. C., et al. (2007). Using a computer kiosk to promote child safety: results of a randomized, controlled trial in an urban pediatric emergency department. *Pediatrics, 120*(2), 330–339.

Goldson, E., & Reynolds, A. (2008). Child development and behavior. In W. W. Hay, et al. (Eds.). *Current pediatric diagnosis and treatment* (18th ed.). Columbus, OH: McGraw-Hill.

Heard, L. (2008). Taking care of the little things: preparation of the pediatric endoscopy patient. *Gastroenterology Nursing, 31*(2), 108–112.

Hughes, L. J. (2007). Creating a farm and food learning box curriculum for preschool-aged children and their families. *Journal of Nutrition Education and Behavior, 39*(3), 171–172.

Johnson, A., Sandford, J., & Tyndall, J. (2009).Written and verbal information versus verbal information only for patients being discharged from acute hospital settings to home. *Cochrane Database of Systematic Reviews, 2009*(1), (CD003716).

Kohlberg, L. (1984). *The psychology of moral development.* New York: Harper & Row.

Li, H. C. W., Lopez, V., & Lee, T. L. I. (2007). Effects of preoperative therapeutic play on outcomes of school-age children undergoing day surgery. *Research in Nursing and Health, 30*(3), 320–332.

Marshall, J., Goldbart, J., & Phillips, J. (2007). Parents' and speech and language therapists' explanatory models of language development, language delay and intervention. *International Journal of Language and Communication Disorders, 42*(5), 533–555.

Oakhill, J. V., & Petrides, A. (2007). Sex differences in the effects of interest on boys' and girls' reading comprehension. *British Journal of Psychology, 98*(Part 2), 223–235.

O'Kearney, R. T., Anstey, K. J., & von Sanden, C. (2009). Behavioural and cognitive behavioural therapy for obsessive compulsive disorder in children and adolescents. *Cochrane Database of Systematic Reviews, 2009*(1), (CD004856).

Ono, S., et al. (2008). Preparation of a picture book to support parents and autonomy in preschool children facing day surgery. *Pediatric Nursing, 34*(1), 82–88.

Piaget, J. (1969). *The origins of intelligence in children.* New York: International Universities Press.

Timler, G. R., Vogler-Elias, D., & McGill, K. F. (2007). Strategies for promoting generalization of social communication skills in preschoolers and school-aged children. *Topics in Language Disorders, 27*(2), 167–181.

Toe, D., Beattie, R., & Barr, M. (2007). The development of pragmatic skills in children who are severely and profoundly deaf. *Deafness and Education International, 9*(2), 101–117.

Uccelli, P., & Paez, M. M. (2007). Narrative and vocabulary development of bilingual children from kindergarten to first grade: developmental changes and associations among English and Spanish skills. *Language, Speech, and Hearing Services in Schools, 38*(3), 225–236.

Wright, N. D., et al. (2007). The school yard kids: a puppet show to promote a healthful lifestyle. *Journal of Nutrition Education and Behavior, 39*(5), 290–291.

Yoon, S. L., & Godwin, A. (2007). Enhancing self-management in children with sickle cell disease through playing a CD-ROM educational game: a pilot study. *Pediatric Nursing, 33*(1), 60–63.

SUGGESTED READINGS

Bell, M. L., et al. (2007). Can first and second grade students benefit from an alcohol use prevention program? *Journal of Child and Adolescent Substance Abuse, 16*(3), 89–107.

Brown, S. L., Teufel, J. A., & Birch, D. A. (2007). Early adolescents perceptions of health and health literacy. *Journal of School Health, 77*(1), 7–15.

Chiang, H., & Lin, Y. (2008). Expressive communication of children with autism. *Journal of Autism and Developmental Disorders, 38*(3), 538–545.

Gritz, E. R., et al. (2007). Effects of a preschool staff intervention on children's sun protection: outcomes of Sun Protection Is Fun! *Health Education and Behavior, 34*(4), 562–577.

Hammer, C. S., Lawrence, F. R., & Miccio, A. W. (2007). Bilingual children's language abilities and early reading outcomes in Head Start and kindergarten. *Language, Speech, and Hearing Services in Schools, 38*(3), 237–248.

Hay, I., et al. (2007). Language delays, reading delays, and learning difficulties: interactive elements requiring multidimensional programming. *Journal of Learning Disabilities, 40*(5), 400–409.

James, A., Soler, A., & Weatherall, R. (2009). Cognitive behavioural therapy for anxiety disorders in children and adolescents. *Cochrane Database of Systematic Reviews, 2009*(1), (CD004690).

Welsh, C. (2007). Harry Potter and the underage drinkers: can we use this to talk to teens about alcohol? *Journal of Child and Adolescent Substance Abuse, 16*(4), 119–126.

Wolf, F. M., et al. (2008). Educational interventions for asthma in children. *Cochrane Database of Systematic Reviews, 2009*(1), (CD000326).

Wu, Y., & Newfield, S. A. (2007). Comparing data collected by computerized and written surveys for adolescence health research. *Journal of School Health, 77*(1), 23–28.

Unit 6

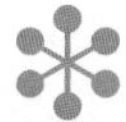

The Nursing Role in Supporting the Health of Ill Children and Their Families

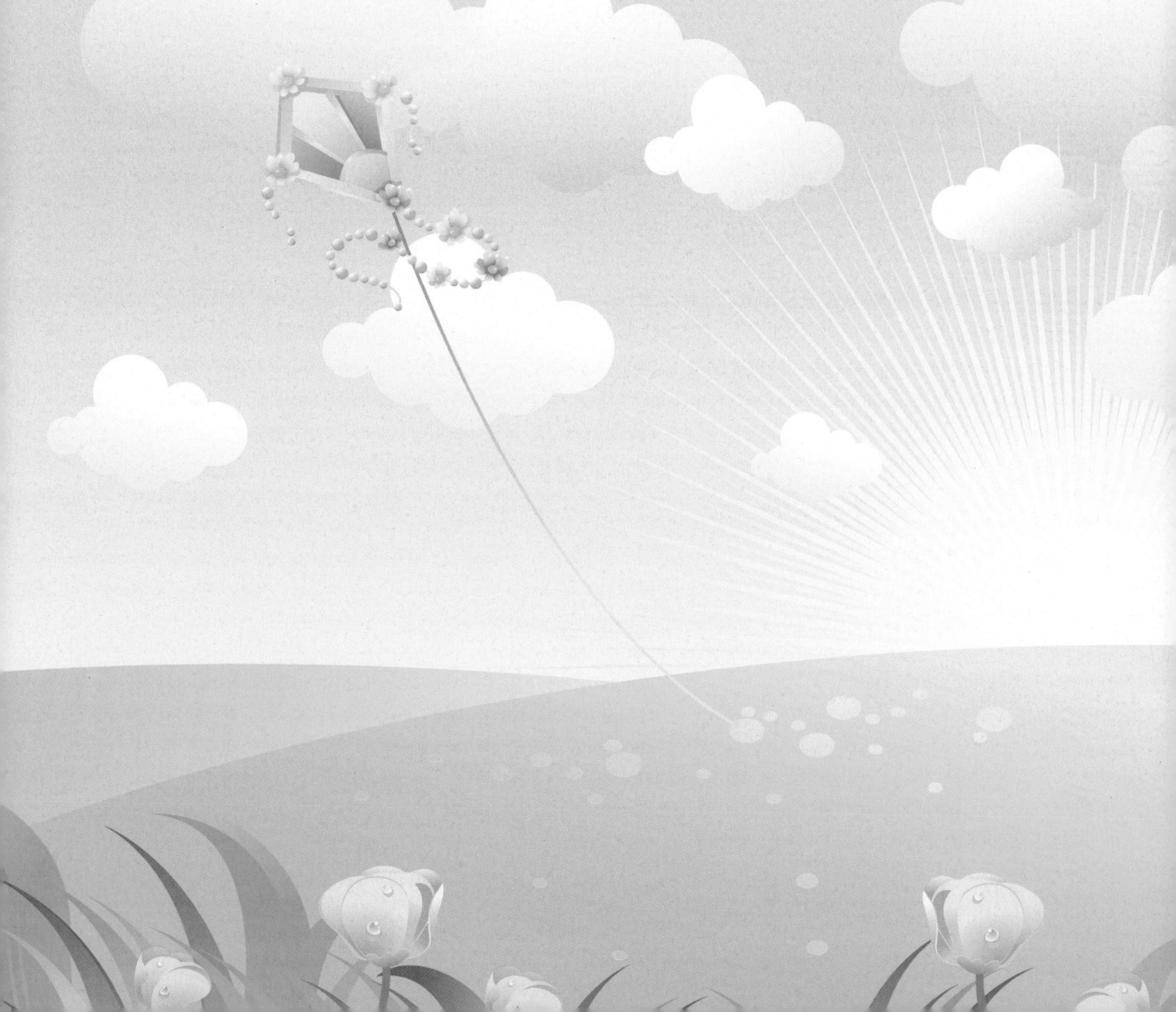

Chapter 36 Nursing Care of a Family With an Ill Child

KEY TERMS

- calorie counting
- case management nursing
- non–rapid eye movement (NREM) sleep
- play therapy
- primary nursing
- rapid eye movement (REM) sleep
- sensory deprivation
- sensory overload
- sleep deprivation
- therapeutic play

OBJECTIVES

After mastering the contents of this chapter, you should be able to:

1. Describe illness and illness experiences as they must appear to children.
2. Identify National Health Goals related to care of ill children nurses can help the nation achieve.
3. Use critical thinking to analyze ways in which illness care can be made more family centered and less traumatic for children.
4. Assess the impact of an illness, especially one requiring a hospital stay, on a child.
5. Formulate nursing diagnoses related to the stress of illness in children.
6. Establish expected outcomes for an ill child.
7. Plan nursing care to reduce the stress of illness, such as helping parents plan for ambulatory care or hospitalization.
8. Implement measures such as orientation, education, and therapeutic play to reduce the stress of illness.
9. Evaluate expected outcomes for achievement and effectiveness of care.
10. Identify areas related to illness in children that could benefit from additional nursing research or application of evidence-based practice.
11. Integrate knowledge about a child's response to illness with the nursing process to achieve quality maternal and child health nursing care.

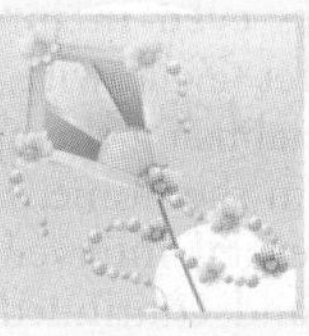

Becky is a 7-year-old who burned her foot in a campfire accident. She is going to be admitted to the hospital for 1-day surgery to have the wound debrided. Becky's parents tell you that Becky "hasn't been herself" since the injury. She has reverted to temper tantrums and sulking, more like a 3-year-old than one of early school age. Even though she has been told eating meat is important because it provides protein for healing, she refuses to eat anything but Jell-O or soup. In the admission suite of the hospital, she picked up a doll and twisted its leg off. "How can we get our old daughter back again?" her mother asks you.

Previous chapters described the normal growth and development of children and their special needs at each stage of development. This chapter adds information about the additional needs of children when they become ill. Such information builds a base for nursing care and health teaching.

Becky is obviously showing some effects of her accident. What type of additional explanation might be helpful to her? What advice would you give her mother to help her better prepare Becky for the upcoming debridement procedure?

Illnesses that require the attention of health care professionals are outside the usual occurrences of childhood, so most children typically have little knowledge about them. Helping a child and family prepare for or adjust to such an experience is a fundamental nursing role. This role goes well beyond just providing information on what to expect throughout an illness. It involves providing emotional support as well.

Nurses need to provide orientation programs before hospital admissions and advocate for more open parental visiting and overnight stay policies even in intensive care areas if these are not already in effect (Zelkowitz, 2009). In addition, nurses can help families establish a therapeutic environment for the care of an ill child in the home. For individual families, nurses can perform several interventions that promote comfort, safety, security, and continued growth and development. Therapeutic play is one of the more powerful tools available to a nurse working toward this objective. National Health Goals related to children and illness are shown in Box 36.1.

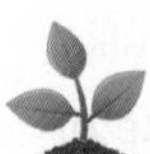

Nursing Process Overview

For an Ill Child

Assessment

Assessment for an ill child begins with an interview of the child and parents to identify ways they think the illness will change their lives. This could include a wide range of situations such as increased expenses, changes in schedules to visit or stay with a hospitalized child, the need for one parent to take a leave from work to care for an ill child at home, the need to schedule frequent ambulatory visits, consultation to handle body image changes, and the need to arrange for child care for other children. Because these needs change as the course of an illness changes, assessment must be ongoing.

Nursing Diagnosis

Nursing diagnoses vary greatly depending on the extent of a child's illness, the care needed, and the age of a child. Those often used with families of children seen in ambulatory and in-hospital settings include:

- Health-seeking behaviors related to lack of knowledge regarding illness
- Anxiety related to pending hospital admission
- Risk for social isolation related to hospitalization
- Fear related to being away from home for first time
- Activity intolerance realted to fatigue from illness
- Potential for injury related to high-tech therapy equipment

Outcome Identification and Planning

Planning for the care of an ill child requires consideration of all aspects of the child's and family's life: financial, social, and personal. When children become ill, many of their needs, such as those for nutrition, play, and family support, change. If a child will need long-term care or hospitalization, the entire family may find their priorities changing. Unless these changing needs are examined, recognized, and met, a child may achieve physical wellness again but not mental or emotional health. A family may be left severely disadvantaged. Identifying additional needs in this way and putting in place necessary services or interventions is an important nursing role. An organization that offers helpful information on hospitalization of children is the National Association of Child Care Professionals (http://www.naccp.org).

Implementation

Five hazards that may occur with children with all illnesses are (a) experiencing harm or injury, such as physical discomfort, pain, mutilation, and death; (b) being separated from routines, parents, peers, and respected adults; (c) facing the unknown (new and strange sights and sounds and happenings); (d) facing uncertain limits (unclear definition of acceptable and expected behavior); and (e) experiencing a loss of control (loss of competence or loss of the ability to make decisions).

Being aware of these potential problems is important to guard against those that are preventable and to reduce a child's anxiety associated with those that cannot be prevented (such as facing new sights and sounds). Discussing these hazards with older children is important so that implementations to reduce their impact can be tailored to each child. Reading to a child, role playing, and puppetry are all useful techniques for reducing the number of new experiences and easing the impact on the child. Be certain that the techniques you use are appropriate not only for a child's age but also for the child's individual learning style and level of illness. Be certain that children participate in making any decision that is age appropriate for them.

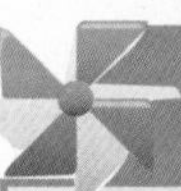

BOX 36.1 * Focus on National Health Goals

Illness and hospitalization can be major stressors for children. Two National Health Goals speak directly to this:

- Increase the number of states and the District of Columbia that have implemented statewide pediatric protocols for online medical direction.
- Increase the number of states and the District of Columbia that have implemented guidelines for prehospital and hospital pediatric care (http://www.nih.gov).

Helping with assessment of children's stress level and reducing the stress of hospitalization or health care are ways that nurses can help the nation achieve these goals. Areas where additional nursing research or evidence-based practice could aid understanding are: What measures do parents need to make them feel most comfortable in a hospital setting? What are the deterrents to therapeutic play on hospital units, and how could these be removed? And are there additional contributions nurses could make to shorten hospital stays for children?

Outcome Evaluation

Evaluation of expected outcomes for ill children should include specific measures such as whether discomfort was kept to a minimum during the experience. Indicators to evaluate outcomes that are long term should include whether children were able to return to usual behaviors after the experience. The following are examples that suggest achievement of outcomes regarding a hospital experience:

- Parents state their level of anxiety regarding hospitalization of their infant is now at a tolerable level.
- Parents have effectively changed work schedules to be able to stay with their child in the hospital.
- Social isolation of toddler is minimized through case manager nursing assignment.

THE MEANING OF ILLNESS TO CHILDREN

The response of children to illness depends on their cognitive ability, past experiences, and level of knowledge. From early school age, children generally know quite a bit about the workings of their major body parts. As general guidelines, early grade-school children are usually able to name the function of the heart, lungs, and stomach. They may not be able to do that for the bowel, kidneys, or bladder; this reflects the difficulty some parents have in discussing these body parts with their children.

Younger children may think the cause of illness is magical (no one knows where it comes from) or that it occurs as a consequence of breaking a rule such as walking in the rain or eating candy after school. With this perspective, they may also think that getting well again is possible only if they follow another set of rules, such as staying in bed and taking medicine. By fourth grade, children are generally aware of the role that germs play in illness but may be fooled by thinking that all illness is caused by germs. Because of this, they may see a passive role for themselves in getting well, because illness comes from outside influences. At about eighth grade, children are able to voice an understanding that illness can occur from several causes, such as being susceptible to chickenpox because they did not get the vaccine or they carelessly caused an accident. Once they understand this, they can take an active role in getting better. These concepts parallel cognitive development (see Chapter 28).

Knowing how children of each age view illness affects the planning of nursing care, influencing how explanations should be worded. For example, saying that you are going to "stick" a child for blood work could be interpreted by young children as meaning you are actually going to put a stick in their arm. Saying a child will receive a dye for a test could be interpreted as meaning the child will "die" during the procedure. Children who think illness comes as punishment for breaking rules can interpret nursing procedures such as giving an injection as punishment. They can be confused about explanations of procedures because some words sound alike or have double meanings ("drawing" as in making a picture versus drawing blood). Because of these distorted perceptions, explanations of procedures do not always relieve children's stress.

Differences in Responses of Children and Adults to Illness

Keeping in mind that children are not just small adults is important when evaluating how children react to illness, perceive an illness, or react to health care (Fig. 36.1). Their body images, as evidenced in their drawings, are different from those of adults. They can have difficulty telling which body parts are indispensable and which are not (this is why it is wise to talk to preschool and early school-age children about "fixing" body parts, such as tonsils, rather than "taking them out").

Inability to Communicate

Very young children do not have the vocabulary to describe symptoms. Headache is an example of a symptom that children younger than 5 years have a great deal of difficulty describing. Dizziness and nausea can be equally bewildering because children this age do not know the words to express these phenomena.

By the time they reach school age, most children can describe symptoms with accuracy. They may intensify their concerns, however, if they believe someone expects symptoms to be more serious. They may minimize symptoms if they are afraid illness will interfere with an activity.

Because of this, evaluate a child's symptoms as much by observation as by a child's report. A crying, whining preschooler who is "just not herself" probably has a symptom she cannot describe. A school-age child who guards her abdomen (keeps abdominal muscles rigid) is in pain just as clearly as a child who verbalizes a source of discomfort. This makes keen, astute observations necessary to ascertain the extent of a child's illness at any given time.

Inability to Monitor Own Care and Manage Fear

Adults who are ill often ask about medications prescribed for them or procedures they are scheduled to undergo. For example, if a hospitalized man knows he is to receive a diuretic three times a day and by 10 AM has not been given it, he usually reminds someone of the oversight. School-age and younger children cannot monitor their own care this way because they may not know which medicine or procedures they

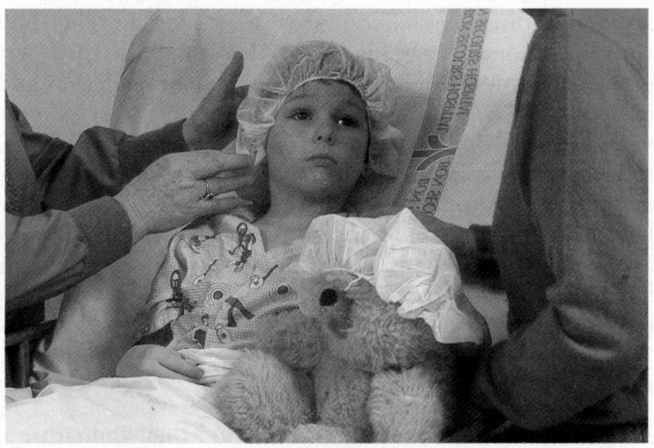

FIGURE 36.1 Illness is potentially traumatic because of the unknown and pain and discomfort that may be involved. Children need extra attention and reassurance to calm their fears.

are to receive. If they do know, they may be confused about time. In addition, children have fears that adults do not experience. The infant, for example, fears separation above all else; the toddler and preschooler fear such things as separation, the dark, the unknown, intrusive procedures, and mutilation of body parts. The school-age child and adolescent are concerned about the loss of body parts, loss of life, and loss of friends. Adults have fears also, but most have learned to cope with them. Children in a strange environment (such as a hospital) require proportionally more support and active intervention to cope with their stress and fears or hospitalization can result in a posttraumatic stress disorder (PTSD) (Pao, Ballard, & Rosenstein, 2007).

Nutritional Needs

In addition to psychological differences, there are major physiologic differences in the way illness affects children compared with adults. This is because children have different physiologic needs and respond to imbalances in different ways.

Children need more nutrients (calories, protein, minerals, and vitamins) per pound of body weight than adults, for example, because their basic metabolic rate is faster, and they must take in not only enough to maintain body tissues but also enough to allow for growth. The infant requires 120 kcal per kilogram of body weight per day; the adult requires only 30 to 35. An ill child who must limit food intake because of nausea or vomiting, therefore, may require hospitalization, even though this might be unnecessary for an adult under the same circumstances.

Fluid and Electrolyte Balance

In the adult, extracellular water (that in plasma and outside body cells) represents approximately 23% of total body water; in a newborn, extracellular water is closer to 40%. This means that an infant does not have as much water stored in the cells as an adult does and so is more likely to lose a devastating amount of body water with diarrhea or vomiting. Because of this, there is no such thing as "only diarrhea" or "simple diarrhea" in a child younger than 1 year. The full implications of both vomiting and diarrhea are discussed in Chapter 45.

Systemic Response to Illness

Because their bodies are immature, young children tend to respond to disease systemically rather than locally. The child with pneumonia, for example, may be brought to an emergency department not because of a cough (although the child has one) but because of accompanying systemic symptoms such as fever, vomiting, and diarrhea. Nausea and vomiting, in fact, occur so frequently in children with any type of illness these symptoms do not have the diagnostic value they have in adults. Systemic reactions of these kinds can delay diagnosis and therapy and cause increased fluid and nutrient loss, circumstances that compound an initial illness and can result in hospitalization.

Age-Specific Diseases

Because of their growth requirement and their immaturity, children are susceptible to some diseases that do not affect adults. For example, because infants are growing, a lack of vitamin D will cause rickets or abnormal bone growth, but this same lack does not cause these condition in adults. Most adults have achieved immunity to common infectious diseases; children, however, are susceptible to childhood diseases such as measles, mumps, and chickenpox. Children younger than 5 years who have a high temperature may respond with generalized seizures (febrile seizures), a phenomenon that rarely occurs after this age (Pavlidou, 2008). When children do not receive adequate iron, those younger than 1 year of age are subject to iron-deficiency anemia because fetal red blood cells are destroyed after birth and are replaced by mature red blood cells only very slowly.

✔ Checkpoint Question 36.1

Young children are more at risk for dehydration with vomiting than are adults. This is because:

a. They have a smaller stomach and intestines than do adults.
b. They have proportionally more extracellular water than do adults.
c. Children metabolize fluid more slowly than do most adults.
d. They maintain more fluid inside body cells than do adults.

CARE OF THE ILL CHILD AND FAMILY IN THE HOSPITAL

The parents of children admitted to intensive care or neonatal intensive care units (ICUs and NICUs) can be predicted to experience a high degree of stress during their child's hospitalization both because of the severity of their child's illness and the high-tech pediatric ICU or NICU setting (Koh et al., 2007). They can experience a second round of stress when their child is transferred from an NICU or pediatric ICU (PICU) to a regular hospital unit (Rowe & Jones, 2008). Based on this theory that hospitalization creates a high degree of stress for children, only those children who cannot be managed successfully on an ambulatory basis are now admitted to the hospital. This was not always true. For example, in the past, most children with head injuries automatically stayed overnight for observation. Currently, unless a child is unconscious or shows other signs of neurologic injury, the child is sent home to be observed by parents for signs of increased intracranial pressure. This policy requires that time be spent to teach parents skills such as how to take a pulse or evaluate consciousness. Teaching them requires patience because parents under stress can have difficulty comprehending instructions. However, because psychological trauma and excessive health care costs are prevented by allowing a child to return home, it is important teaching. Children who are seen in the emergency departments for acute gastritis and vomiting were also once automatically admitted to the hospital so they could receive intravenous fluid. Today, they are given an oral hydrating solution or probiotics so they no longer need to be admitted (Marcos & DuPont, 2007).

As yet another example, many pediatric surgery procedures such as tonsillectomy or herniorrhaphy can be done on an ambulatory or outpatient basis. This prevents the major problem of separation anxiety, but it does not necessarily reduce parents' or children's anxiety about the procedure. Some parents actually feel less confident and more anxious with ambulatory procedures than they did with in-hospital admissions because they sense their responsibility for preparation and follow-up care will be significantly greater (Heard, 2008). They often comment that modern care is not as good as when children were admitted, and that this change is a result of cost containment by insurance companies. Although it is true that short hospital stays reduce cost, it is helpful to inform parents that ambulatory or outpatient procedures are as safe as those performed with hospital admissions, and that ambulatory procedures can be helpful in preventing the detrimental effects of separation.

The Effect of Hospital Separation and Children

Decreasing Separation Anxiety

It is difficult to explain the meaning that a primary caregiver has for a child, but the intensity of the relationship can be demonstrated. As early as 4 months of age, the infant registers disapproval if a primary caregiver walks away. As early as 5 months of age, an infant registers anxiety when strangers are present or when a person other than the usual caregiver gives care. Infants fix their eyes on the stranger, become restless, perhaps thrash arms or legs, and begin to cry. This activity peaks at approximately 8 months of age, so it is commonly called "8-month anxiety." It is a developmental milestone that shows an infant is able to distinguish a primary caregiver from other persons. It also means the child has reached a vulnerable stage in emotional development and will react poorly to separation or to the threat of it (Smith, Hefley, & Anand, 2007).

Toddlers and preschoolers can be as affected by separation as infants. In many instances, they express their feelings better, louder, and longer than infants. Although many toddlers and preschoolers attend day care and have had prior experiences with separation, others may have had only limited experiences. Being hospitalized may be the first time they are away from parents in a strange setting or away from home overnight. If this is so, many preschoolers may wonder whether they will ever live with their parents again. Problems of separation are especially intense in younger children because they do not understand time. Statements such as, "Mom will visit again tomorrow" or "Dad will be here by 6 o'clock" are meaningless to children younger than 5 years because they do not know what either "tomorrow" or "6 o'clock" means.

School-age children and adolescents react better than younger children to the separation imposed by hospitalization because they have experiences they can use for comparison. They have been to school for whole days; perhaps they have stayed with a grandparent or a friend overnight; they may have been to camp. This can make hospitalization a time for developing self-esteem and confidence in their ability to be independent. Even in light of this, ill school-age children and adolescents may still feel anxious about being separated from their parents. They appreciate their parents' presence and need reassurance that their parents support and love them.

Remember that parents may have an equally difficult time being separated from children. You may need to spend time with them assuring them that their child will receive good care at all times, even if they are absent.

To appreciate why preventing separation is so important, it is helpful to review the research that provided the foundation for this method of care. Spitz (1945) was one of the first researchers who documented the effects of separation on children. He observed children in a penal nursery and in a foundling home who were separated from their mothers for both short and long periods. From this observation, he was able to document how poorly children responded to separation from their parents. Bowlby conducted additional studies after World War II (Bowlby, 1966). Building on Spitz's and Bowlby's work, Robertson (1958) studied the effect of hospitalization on children and supplied labels for separation effects (Table 36.1). Although defined over 50 years ago, these findings are still applicable to children today.

Effects of hospitalization can be so severe that they can be compared to posttraumatic stress disorder, the development of characteristic symptoms following exposure to an extremely traumatic situation (Mulvihill, 2007). Children who develop this condition demonstrate persistent symptoms of anxiety such as difficulty falling asleep, irritability, outbursts of anger, difficulty concentrating or completing tasks, or stomachaches and headaches. They re-experience the traumatic event through dreams or flashbacks.

Reducing the ill effects of separation and hospitalization to the extent possible should be a high priority for health care providers. Nurses play a major role in this on both direct care and management levels. Unfortunately, despite the best preparation by parents or nurses, not all of these effects of hospitalization can be prevented.

✔ Checkpoint Question 36.2

Suppose Becky shows signs of separation anxiety. The first stage of separation anxiety is marked by:

a. Loud, demanding crying.
b. Silent, sullen protest.
c. Quiet introspective thought.
d. Inability to respond verbally.

TABLE 36.1 ✻ Stages of Separation Anxiety

Stage	Manifestations
Protest	The child cries loudly and demandingly; rejects any attempts to be comforted by nurse or substitute primary caregivers.
Despair	The child becomes less active and cries monotonously or wails in a state of mourning; may turn away from parent's approach; often lies on abdomen, facial expression flat; may lose weight and develop insomnia; loses developmental skills; prone to minor ailments such as upper respiratory infections; IQ will measure lower than previous measurement.
Denial	The child is silent, face expressionless; represses feelings for absent caregiver to protect self; deterioration in developmental milestones is apparent; may respond quickly but superficially to all caregivers; may have difficulty forming close relationships later in life.

Be certain that parents have the necessary factual information themselves so that they can provide accurate and appropriate explanations to school-age children. If they do not know the answer to a question, caution them that the best response is simply, "I don't know" rather than a guess. This prevents a child from feeling betrayed when the real answer is different.

Many community hospitals sponsor hospital orientation programs for children's groups or school groups during which hospitalization is discussed. These programs are beneficial because they lay a foundation for all children about what to expect in a hospitalization; then, if they must be admitted on an emergency basis, they may not be so frightened. Programs are offered by nurses at the hospital or on visits to children's groups or schools (Fig. 36.2). Box 36.4 provides guidelines for setting up hospital tours or discussions for early school-age children.

At approximately 9 years of age, when children first begin to understand the full meaning of death, parents need to be especially careful to explain that an anesthetic causes a "special sleep," not that a child is "put to sleep." Animals that are "put to sleep" are not seen again. Talking to another child who has undergone the same experience and come through it intact is yet another helpful way to introduce children and adolescents to hospitalization. Although parents cannot usually supply such a person in advance, on admission to the hospital, a visit to a recovering patient is often possible and is a constructive way to give reassurance.

If hospitalization is to be more than 1 week long, a parent must think about the means to continue the child's schooling. Advise parents to ask their physician at what point their child will be able to do homework. Many school systems provide tutors; children's hospitals often have their own teachers from the local school system to carry out this service.

What if... Becky's mother brought pots and pans to the hospital as Becky's favorite play items? Would you suggest she bring an actual toy?

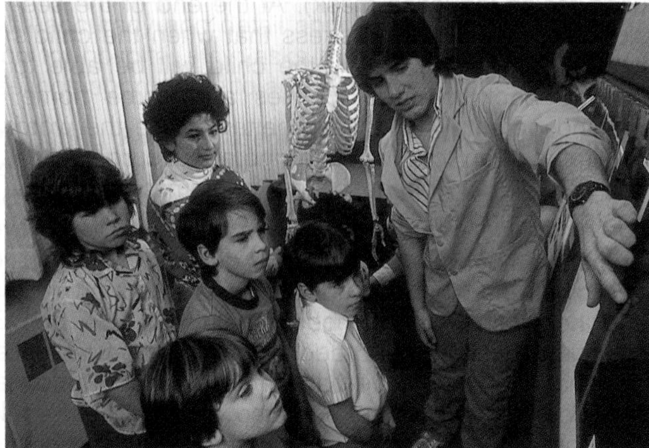

FIGURE 36.2 Children learn what to expect from hospitalization during a prehospital program.

Box 36.4 Guidelines for Conducting Hospital Tours With Early School-Age Children

1. Keep groups small (about 10 children per group) so individual reactions to the presentations can be assessed.
2. Allow or encourage parents to join the tour so their anxiety about the hospital can also be relieved.
3. Conduct the tour for only 20 to 30 minutes to meet the short attention span of children.
4. Use an indirect method to present various aspects of a hospital, such as puppets, films, or a slide show, to decrease anxiety.
5. Present the features of a hospital in a nonthreatening environment, such as the hospital playroom. Avoid the emergency department, ICUs, or operating rooms while touring, because these are anxiety-producing areas for children. Talk about these areas by using slides or photographs instead.
6. Present explanations about hospitalization in concrete terms and at the child's level of understanding. Include only what the child will see, hear, and feel.
7. Avoid dwelling on unpleasant and threatening events or intrusive procedures, such as blood drawing or anesthesia, that may create anxiety.
8. Allow children opportunities to ask questions.
9. Allow children opportunities to play with dolls and hospital equipment, to both decrease anxiety and satisfy curiosity.

Preparing a Child With a Different Cultural Background. Perhaps the most important aspect to consider when preparing a child from a different culture for hospitalization is to identify what traditions or practices will be in opposition to health care facility practices. Ask enough questions and practice good listening skills to gain information about the particular needs of a child and family. When cultural differences do exist, be prepared to act as a liaison between the family and the health care team. If a different language is interfering with communication, a translator may be necessary in this preparation phase. Provide the opportunity for parents to voice their fears and ask questions at the time of hospitalization or treatment. When families speak a different language or are unfamiliar with hospital routine, allow more time and more opportunities for discussion and communication so these are not slighted.

Preparing a Physically Challenged or Chronically Ill Child. Physically challenged or chronically ill children frequently come to ambulatory health care settings for care; they often are admitted to the hospital for care, possibly remaining in the hospital for an extended time with continuing care at home. Think through ways in which a new hospitalization or visit will be like past ones and other ways in which it will be different to determine how best to prepare the child. Help children to maintain contact with their families and school friends during a long hospitalization by encouraging telephone calls, e-mails, text messaging, letters, and visits.

Admitting an Ill Child and Family

Whether an ambulatory or inpatient hospital unit admission, children and parents need to be admitted as a single entity to encourage parents to feel they are true partners in care. A child coming to a hospital for an elective admission generally arrives at a reception area, where significant facts are obtained, such as name, age, address, and hospital insurance coverage. The child and parents are then brought to the hospital unit. Remember that first impressions count. If parents are left standing at a counter while nurses chat, they can easily feel that no one appreciates their concern and that possibly their child will not receive optimal care. Some days are busier than others and it is true that at certain times on a children's unit all nurses are busy finishing treatments for other children before they can take the time to admit a new child (Box 36.5). Even so, one nurse should take the time to meet and greet the parents and child and find a comfortable place for the family to wait until someone is available. When introducing yourself to children, stoop down so that your face is level with the child's face (Fig. 36.3). Call the child by name or ask for a nickname. Calling all children "honey" or "pumpkin" can cause children to worry they have been confused with another child.

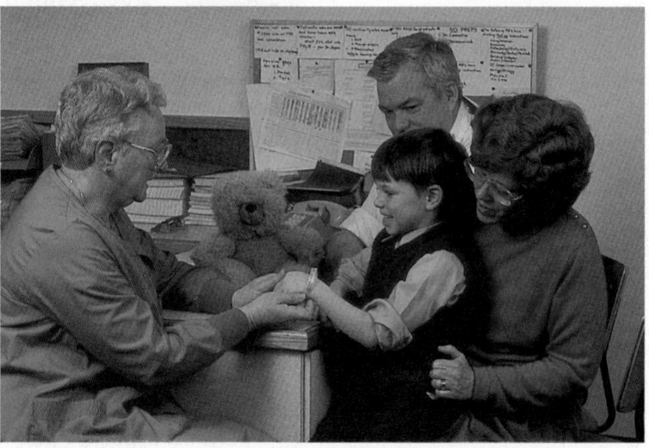

FIGURE 36.3 A child is admitted to a hospital unit. Notice how the nurse greets the child at the child's own level.

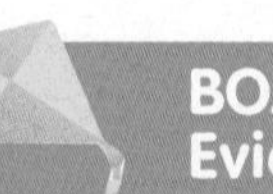

BOX 36.5 * Focus on Evidence-Based Practice

Is the length of children's hospital stay influenced by how full or empty the hospital is on the day of admission?

If a hospital is crowded, it is assumed that children who are newly admitted may be discharged earlier than usual in order to reduce the hospital's patient census. To discover if this is true, researchers analyzed the length of hospital stays for children aged 1 to 17 years. Results of the study showed that for children who were admitted with nonrespiratory disease, patient census had no effect. For children admitted with respiratory diseases, when admission-day occupancy rate was 60% to 100% children had an increase in their average length of stay over children admitted when occupancy rate was below this. Also, increased admission-day occupancy was associated with longer lengths of stay for less complicated respiratory admissions but not for children who were admitted with the most serious conditions. The researchers concluded that medical professionals, during times of increased workload, first focus their attention on more acutely ill children with a complicated course and thus delay treatment of children who have less complicated courses. This extends those children's hospitalization.

Based on the above, for which child would it be more important to advocate for to be certain a hospital stay is not longer than average? A child with pneumonia who is seriously ill or one admitted for diagnostic tests for a possible allergy?

Source: Lorch, S. A., et al. (2008). Impact of admission-day crowding on the length of stay of pediatric hospitalizations. *Pediatrics, 121*(4), e718–e730.

On admission to a health care facility, all children should have an armband attached giving their name and hospital chart number. Because their hands are not much larger than their wrists and their feet are not much larger than their ankles, neonates (infants younger than 1 month of age) often need two bands in place as an extra safeguard. If a band falls off, secure it back onto the child: never tape it to the crib or bedside stand, as this is not adequate protection: if an infant is placed in the wrong crib by mistake, the infant could be given a medicine that is lethal before the mistake is realized.

Assessment on Admission

Assess each child's level of preparation for a hospitalization on admission to the facility (Box 36.6). Be aware of not only what the child describes orally but also what facial expressions or nervous manifestations may be indicating.

Interview parents on hospital admission for a nursing history to obtain the information needed to plan nursing care (Chapter 34 describes a full child database interview history). Many hospitals have information checklists for parents to bring with them. Obtaining information in this way is highly efficient, but it may not be as satisfying to worried parents as hearing a nurse taking a few minutes to ask questions personally or specifically review the completed form. Typical information that is necessary to obtain about a child is shown in Table 36.2. This is then included in the child's plan of care as a vital step of assessment (see Focus on Nursing Care Planning Box 36.7).

Make a note of any medication or food allergy on the child's plan of care and, if pertinent, post this information by the child's bed because unlike an adult, a child cannot call these things to the attention of health care personnel when food or medication is offered.

Take and record the child's temperature, pulse, and respirations. Measure height and weight to determine overall

Box 36.6 Assessment
Assessing a Child for Effects of Illness

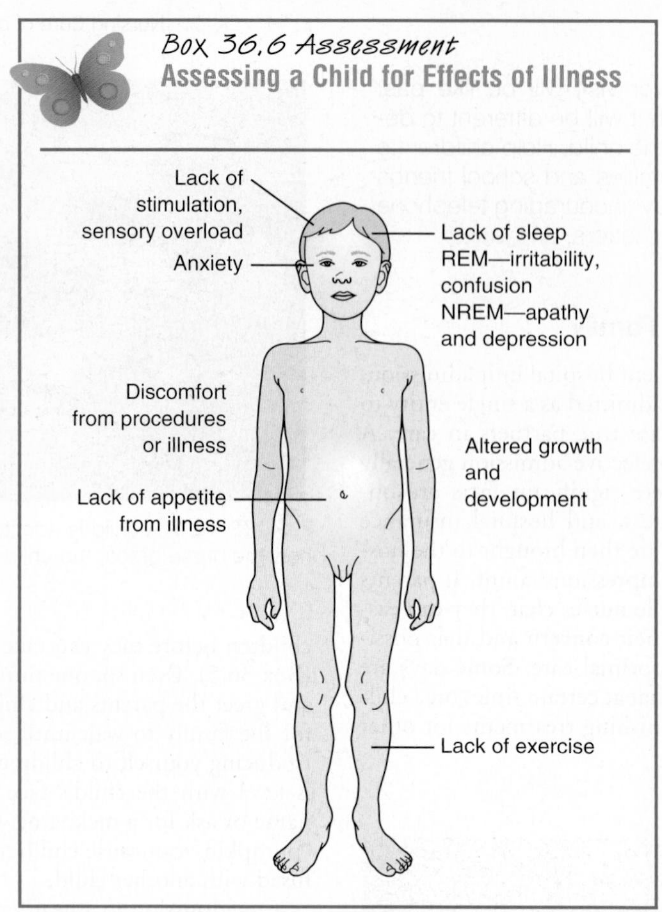

TABLE 36.2 ✻ Information Necessary for the Child's Plan of Care on Admission

Area of Information	Specific Knowledge
Chief concern	Determine what the parents' understanding is of why the child is being admitted. (This view may differ widely from the physician's view regarding the reason the child is being admitted.) What has the child been told about the reason for hospitalization?
Family profile	Obtain child's name and birthday. Who lives at home (include pets)? Ask about parents' occupation and education levels. Who is the child's primary caregiver? Have there been any disruptive happenings lately in the child's life, such as a move or a divorce, that would make the child particularly insecure at this time? Will a parent be staying with the child? If parents are separated or divorced, what will arrangements be? Who has legal authority to sign medical permission?
Past experience with illness or separation	Ask about previous hospital experiences and how the child feels about them. Has there been a recent hospitalization for anyone in the family that resulted in a bad outcome? Has the child been away from the parents before? Overnight at a grandparent's? Summer camp? What is the child's past experience with taking medicine? Has the child swallowed pills before? Does the child have any known allergies to food or medications? (Document these by asking for exact symptoms and happenings.)
Daily routines	Ask about the child's regular bedtime and sleep times. Does the child nap? Does the child have a bedtime ritual? What type of bed does the child sleep in? Does the child sleep with a favorite toy or blanket? What is bath time routine? Does the child need help brushing teeth or combing hair or is this done independently? What words does the child use for voiding and defecating? Is the child completely toilet trained? If a preschooler, is the child accustomed to using a potty chair or toilet? Does the child have enuresis (bedwetting)? What is the child's usual meal plan? Are there foods the child does not eat? What is the child's favorite toy? Did the child pack it for the hospital? What are the child's favorite games and hobbies or interests? Are there television programs the parents especially like the child to see or not see?
Developmental survey	Ascertain the child's developmental level. Does child feed self? Use a spoon, cup, bottle? Dress self? If school age, what grade in school?
Special information	Obtain any special information about the child that would make him or her more comfortable in the hospital.

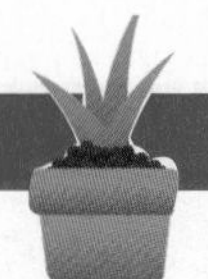

BOX 36.7 ✻ Focus on Nursing Care Planning

A Multidisciplinary Care Map for a Child Having 1-Day Surgery

Becky is a 7-year-old who burned her foot in a campfire accident. She is going to be admitted to the hospital for 1-day surgery to have the wound debrided.

Family Assessment ✻ Child lives with parents and two older brothers (10 and 14 years) in a three-bedroom suburban home. Father works as sound technician at a recording studio; mother was a grade-school teacher, now is stay-at-home mom; home schools all three children. Father rates finances as, "All right. We have everything we need."

Client Assessment ✻ Client burned left foot on a campfire while on a family weekend camping trip. Was playing hide and seek with brothers and ran into fire. Treated at local hospital for third-degree burn; transferred to burn center for follow-up care. Becky's parents tell you that Becky "hasn't been herself" since the injury. She has reverted to temper tantrums and sulking, more like a 3-year-old than one of early school age. Even though she has been told eating meat is important because it provides protein for healing, she refuses to eat anything but Jell-O or soup. In the admission suite of the hospital, she picked up a doll and twisted its leg off. "What can I do with her?" her mother asks you. "How can we get our old daughter back again?"

Nursing Diagnosis ✻ Anxiety related to hospital admission and burn debridement

Outcome Criteria ✻ Child accurately describes what debridement will entail; cooperates with procedures with age-appropriate responses. Describes measures she will need to take after returning home to aid burn healing.

Team Member Responsible	Assessment	Intervention	Rationale	Expected Outcome
		Activities of Daily Living		
Nurse	Assess the degree of self-care child usually carries out.	Allow child maximum inclusion in procedures.	Ability to carry out self-care helps "normalize" hospital procedures.	Child participates in self-care to extent possible with post-procedure bandage.
		Consultations		
Nurse	Consult with Child Life service on what type of therapeutic play would be most beneficial.	Conduct therapeutic play with child before and after debridement procedure.	Therapeutic play can be helpful to children to relieve their anxiety about a hurtful procedure.	Child participates in therapeutic play; demonstrates less anxious behaviors following debridement.
		Procedures/Medications		
Nurse	Assess what is child's greatest concern about debridement procedure.	Prepare child for surgery, stressing anesthesia will be used to relieve pain during procedure; analgesia will be available after procedure.	A clear understanding of what is to happen helps to relieve anxiety; knowing pain relief is available is invaluable to well-being.	Child and parent state they understand what procedure will entail; child cooperates in age-appropriate ways.
		Nutrition		
Nurse/ nutritionist	Assess what are child's favorite foods.	Suggest ways mother could incorporate protein into soup (meat soups) to increase protein in child's diet.	Jell-O is a protein source; adding meat to what child eats will provide protein yet respect child's choice of food.	Mother details ways she can increase child's protein intake without opposing child's food preferences.

(continued)

BOX 36.7 ✻ Focus on Nursing Care Planning (continued)

Patient/Family Education				
Nurse/nurse practitioner	Assess what child and parent understand about debridement procedure.	Educate family about procedure and pre- and postoperative care.	Well-prepared child and family can better cooperate with care to make experience a positive one for child.	Child and parents ask questions about procedure; state they understand what it will entail.
Psychosocial/Spiritual/Emotional Needs				
Nurse/nurse practitioner	Take history about burn accident.	Review with mother what she believes has caused the change in child's attitude. Does she think child or parent feels guilt about accident?	Children can believe they are being punished by procedures if they believe an accident was their fault; guilt can also influence parent's relationship with child.	Child and parent state they both should have been more diligent to avoid accident, but accidents happen even in the best circumstances.
Discharge Planning				
Nurse	Assess what will be a typical day for child after return home.	Plan with parent what measures child will need to carry out to keep bandage clean, exercise foot, return to home schooling.	Prospective planning can help avoid problems in home care.	Child and parent review a typical day and decide on actions that will promote healing.
Nurse/physician	Assess when follow-up visit will be necessary.	Schedule follow-up visit as determined by surgeon.	A follow-up visit will help ensure burn is healing without further complications.	Child and parent state they understand importance of follow-up visit and will keep appointment.

growth and to allow for determination of surface area, the measurement on which medication dosage is calculated. Whether blood pressure needs to be taken depends on the age (usually in children over 3 years of age) and condition of the child. Obtain a specimen for urinalysis as another routine procedure. Be sure to explain all equipment used and allow the child to touch and handle it as much as possible to help reduce anxiety.

Inspect for gross motor ability when weighing a child and measuring height. Listen for language ability (although children in strange situations may say nothing). Perform a physical examination (see Chapter 34) to gain the information necessary for nursing diagnosis and planning.

The way children deal with hospitalization is based on the same factors that determine how they deal with any crisis: perception of the event, whether support people are available, and effectiveness of past coping experiences or skills. After assessment, analyze whether a child's coping ability seems to be enough to balance the hazards of inpatient or ambulatory care hospitalization.

Nursing Diagnoses and Related Interventions

✻

Nursing Diagnosis: Parental and child anxiety related to the need for child's hospitalization

Outcome Evaluation: Parents and child state accurately the reason for child's hospital admission and therapy child will receive; state that although worried, they feel confident they can manage their anxiety.

To help reduce family anxiety regarding hospitalization, be certain a family is oriented to a hospital stay by discussing the need for hospitalization and what they can expect when the hospitalization is first suggested to them in an ambulatory care setting. When children are admitted for emergency care, this type of orientation must be completed immediately, as soon as their physical needs are met. Whether children are admitted for an ambulatory care admission or are being hospitalized for a potentially longer stay, be certain that the parents and the child are oriented to the unit, the personnel who will be caring for them, and any pertinent routines they will need to follow.

On admission, both parents and child need at least basic information. If the child's diagnosis is uncertain, what steps are being taken to confirm it? It helps if these steps are named specifically: for instance, blood work, x-ray studies, observation, recording of vital signs, or calling in a consultant. What is the tentative plan for the child? Complete bedrest or infection control procedures until the results of blood work or cultures are back? Special diet? Special procedures? If the primary care provider has written no orders as yet, be honest: "The specific plan of care isn't written yet. I'll let you know as soon as I'm sure what it will be." Although this answer does not provide a family with information, it does tell them you appreciate how difficult and bewildering it can be when a child is admitted to a health care facility.

For an emergency admission, parents may have little understanding of their child's condition or the treatment plan. Conversely, someone might have taken a great deal of time to explain what was happening while the child was being cared for in the emergency department or brought to the unit. To determine the parents' knowledge level, ask them if they have any questions about their child's condition or the course of treatment they want to discuss with the inpatient facility's health care team.

If parents must leave rather than remain with a child, be certain they see the child's room before they go. This is important to convince children that parents will know where they can find them when they return. If there are other children in the room, introduce a new child to them. Let children wear their own clothes if possible rather than change into hospital gowns.

Promoting a Positive Hospital Stay

Promoting a positive hospital stay is important to the health of both children and their families. Several nursing actions are important to make the difference between a successful and an unsuccessful hospital experience.

Minimizing Length of Hospital Stay

Hospitalization should be limited to the shortest time possible. Be certain that diagnostic procedures are scheduled for a child's, not the hospital's, convenience so that no child stays in a hospital longer than is necessary. Pressure from concerned nurses who insist on having a voice in policies can make a big difference in a department's willingness to cooperate with scheduling.

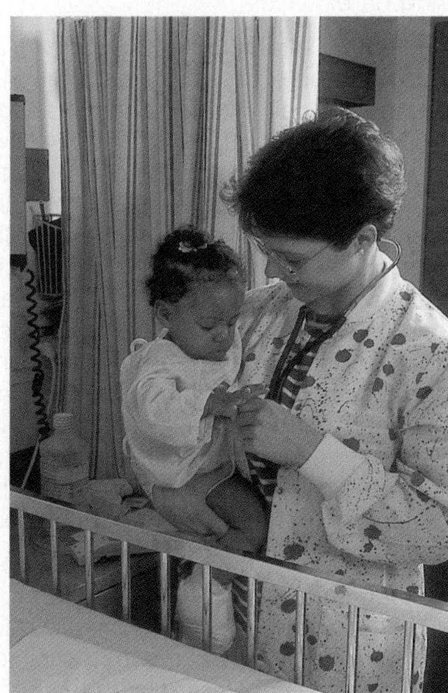

FIGURE 36.4 Hospitalized children should have one nurse who is "theirs" to minimize the effect of separation from parents (primary care nursing). (From Susan Leavines/Photo Researchers, Inc.)

Providing Continuity of Care

To ensure that children are exposed to as few substitute care people as possible and to maintain the consistency and quality of care, nursing assignments are best if one nurse gives as much care to the same child as possible (either **primary nursing** or **case management nursing;** Fig. 36.4). These staffing patterns allow the same nurse to admit the child, take the nursing history, establish nursing diagnoses, set goals for care in cooperation with the parents and the child, and evaluate progress toward achieving goals. It allows children to have one main nurse to call their own. It allows parents to establish meaningful contact with hospital staff and maintains continuity of care, planning, and implementation.

Nursing Diagnoses and Related Interventions

Nursing Diagnosis: Anxiety of child related to separation during hospitalization

Outcome Evaluation: Child actively relates to hospital personnel and hospital routine in ways appropriate to child's age and stage of development; manifests a minimum of nervous symptoms.

Promoting Open Parent Visiting. When possible, children younger than 5 years should have their primary caregiver room-in with them when they are in a hospital (Fig. 36.5). Children younger than 10 to 12 years continue to enjoy the feeling of security this provides. This policy is expensive for a hospital because a bed or cot must be provided for this person as well as for the child, and despite the presence of this person, no reduction in nursing staff is possible. In many instances, because so much parental education is

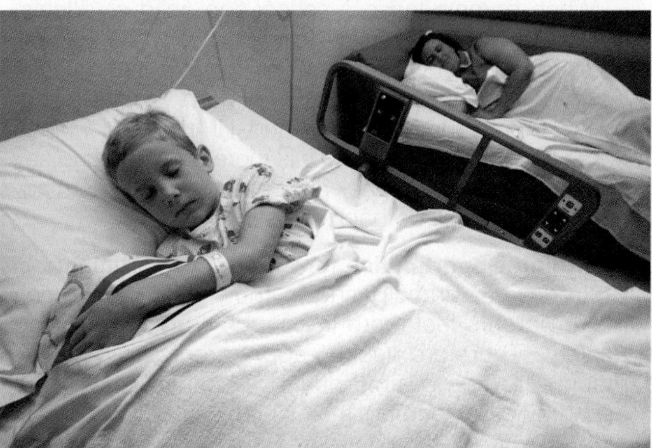

FIGURE 36.5 Rooming-in helps alleviate separation anxiety for both the child and the caregiver.

needed, requirements for health care personnel actually increase. However, such policies greatly reduce symptoms of separation anxiety.

Not all parents can stay in the hospital continuously. Mothers and fathers who cannot stay may need help in smoothing the transition of their coming or going. For example, when a toddler first sees his parents after being separated, his reaction might be to ignore them (a sign of despair). This is a defense mechanism: "I won't show them I love them until they show me they love me; that way I won't be hurt again." The parents' reaction to being treated this way may be anger. If this makes the parents go and play with a child in the next bed—a "well, be that way then" reaction—the toddler's worst fears are fulfilled: his parents do not love him anymore. However, if you urge the parents to speak to the child for a few minutes or try to interest the child in a toy, a child will generally reach out to be comforted and act relieved the parents are there.

Parents often need help in saying goodbye when it is time to leave a child to go eat a meal or go home for the night (if the parent is not sleeping in). Assure parents that although someone will not be in their child's room every minute while they are gone, the child will be well cared for. When the parents of an infant are leaving, go into the room a few minutes before they leave and hold or play with the infant. Help a parent to say once, "I have to go now," and then go. Prolonged departures only delay the process and do not reduce the amount of crying that may occur. After parents leave, infants may cry until they fall asleep from exhaustion. Hold and rock them, letting them know that they are safe.

If the parents of a toddler or preschooler have to leave, urge them first to give a warning they will soon have to go: "I have to leave now to fix dinner." When the time to go has come, parents should say firmly that it is time to go and then explain the time they will return. Time for a preschooler is best measured in terms of events rather than clock hours. "I'll be back after you've eaten supper," "after you wake up tomorrow," or "after nap time" gives the child a concrete event by which to measure time. Like infants, toddlers need someone with them when their parents leave; they like to be held or played with so they know they are not alone.

When parents leave a school-age child or adolescent, urge them to provide definite times when they will return and to leave suggestions for activities a child could do to occupy the time ("Why don't you finish your book? Start your homework and I'll check it when I come back"). Remind them it is more comforting to say specifically, "I will be back around 9 tomorrow morning" rather than, "I will be back sometime tomorrow."

Providing Opportunities for Parents to Participate in Child's Care. Participating in their child's care can make parents feel more in control, thereby reducing anxiety. Therefore, encourage parents to give as much care as possible during a hospital stay, such as bathing or feeding their child, giving oral medicine, helping with procedures such as warm soaks, or checking their child is awake from anesthesia. Most parents are eager to help and do these things spontaneously. Be certain they receive proper instruction on the tasks they will be able to do. Be sure parents who change diapers or feed children know whether the number of diaper changes or the amount of food intake should be recorded; ask them to report when they do these things or write them down on a flow sheet attached to the child's door or crib. Do not have them restrain childen for a procedure that will be painful.

Occasionally parents may be reluctant to give care for fear of being judged inadequate. You can assure them they are the persons from whom their child would most like to receive care. Parents may point out that they are paying for nursing care and so want a nurse to give care. This type of parent will usually soften if approached professionally and assured that nurses are willing to help but for the best interests of the child, the parent is the better caregiver.

Children may be apprehensive about undergoing a procedure without a parent present. There is rarely any reason a parent cannot accompany a child into a treatment room to help with undressing, measuring weight and height, and taking a temperature or accompanying a child to another department for a procedure such as an ultrasound or blood work. Most importantly, the mother or father can comfort the child in these strange surroundings.

Although helping with procedures can strengthen the parent–child relationship, remind parents their most important role is being parents. Sitting and rocking or reading to their child and just being there will be their best role to minimize the adverse effects of hospitalization. When a child is to have surgery, it may be especially difficult for parents to separate from their child so the child can leave for the operating room. Helping them do this is an important part of preoperative nursing care.

Supporting Sibling Visitations. Children in a family are under considerable stress while a sibling is hospitalized because their world changes so much (Gursky, 2007). Sibling visitation refers to allowing the brothers and sisters of hospitalized children to visit the ill child in the hospital. Allowing this alleviates loneliness on both sides and helps prevent other children at home from imagining the ill child is sicker than is true. It helps the ill child continue to feel part of the family. Siblings who visit need to be free of communicable disease. Nurses may need to help parents divide their time between the ill child and siblings during a visit (short, frequent visits may be better for young children than long ones). Before a visit, ensure that the ill child's room is safe for younger children's visits by such things as receiving poisonous substances or electric wires within reach.

Minimizing Negative Effects of Procedures. Ill children often undergo numerous diagnostic and therapeutic procedures that have the potential to cause pain, fear, and anxiety. Details related to specific procedures are discussed in Chapter 37. General guidelines to make any procedure less painful or frightening are discussed in the following sections.

Nursing Diagnoses and Related Interventions

Nursing Diagnosis: Fear or anxiety related to diagnostic or therapeutic procedures

Outcome Evaluation: Child voices satisfaction with comfort measures; describes self-participation in a procedure.

Reducing or Eliminating Pain. Some pain and discomfort are unavoidable in association with health care. Limit this whenever possible, however, by such measures as advocating for the use of intermittent infusion devices such as heparin locks (see Chapter 37) to eliminate multiple punctures for intravenous medication or blood sampling, administering ample analgesia, including alternative therapy techniques such as distraction or imagery, providing traditional comforts such as a change of clothing or position, reading to a child, and planning a special project. Children do not always express discomfort as freely as adults; therefore, closer assessment may be necessary to reveal how they feel. Because pain increases with anxiety, reducing a child's anxiety with good preparation and encouraging a sense of control can also help to eliminate discomfort (see Chapter 39). Distraction by such a method as music may also be effective (Caprilli et al., 2007).

Maintaining the Child's Bed as a Safe Area. To assure children that their bed is an area that is safe, all painful procedures should be done in a treatment room, away from the child's bed. Be sure this rule is not broken, because only one painful experience at the bedside can be enough to significantly increase a child's anxiety. This rule should include finger punctures for blood work; although done quickly, these can cause as much pain and stress as venipunctures. In addition, dressing changes, although not necessarily painful, can cause worry and so should be done in a treatment room, not at a child's bedside as well.

Helping Children to Maintain Control. Events are always more frightening if they appear to be beyond our control. Explaining to children what will happen such as what they will feel or what they will see and helping them to make choices whenever possible limits this type of fear because these actions offer a sense of control (Fig. 36.6). In almost any procedure, there is some choice a child can make (use a straw to drink or not, decide what size of tape to use on a bandage, or walk one way in the hall or the other). Letting a child participate in signing a consent form can be an additional way to help the child feel a sense of control.

Providing Adequate Play Facilities

Play is the medium through which children learn. To continue development during hospitalization, children need to be able to play as normally as possible, no matter how long their stay. Children's hospital units should be equipped with

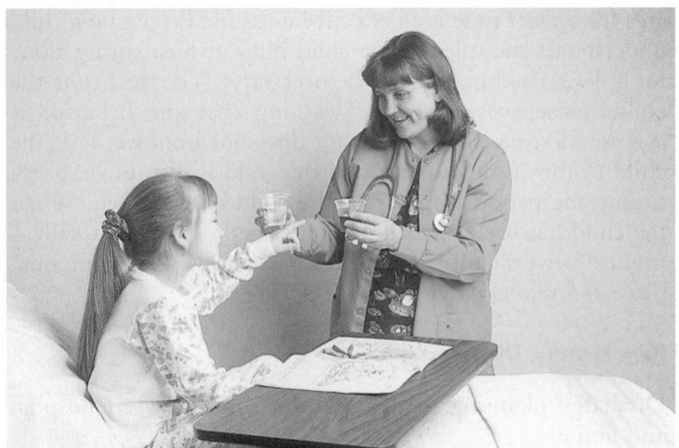

FIGURE 36.6 Include children in procedures whenever possible to offer them a feeling of control. Here a nurse gives a child a choice of fluids to drink with her medication.

a playroom or play space in which children can feel secure and in which they know they will not be hurt. No medical procedures, not even painless ones, should be performed in this area. Children who are on bedrest need toys or crafts supplied for them in addition.

Because hospitalization is a traumatic experience, children need the opportunity to express their feelings through therapeutic play before painful procedures (Li, Lopez, & Lee, 2007). The uses of play and guidelines for providing therapeutic play are discussed later in this chapter.

Setting Limits on Behavior

Setting limits on behavior can help promote a positive hospital stay because it can help to provide a sense of security and safety for a child. Average children are motivated to follow instructions and demonstrate good behavior during a hospital stay because they want to get well again and return home as soon as possible. Occasional children who misbehave in a hospital setting usually do so because they lack a clear understanding of what is expected of them or are making a strong statement that their personal needs have not been recognized and met.

A child who needs frequent reminders to stop running in the hallway, for example, is probably bored with staying in a room. Providing more activities (playing a game with the child) or allowing more structured exercise (letting the child accompany a nursing aide to take a blood specimen to a laboratory) can prevent further unsafe activity.

Children who refuse to cooperate for procedures generally do so out of fear of the unknown rather than deliberate misbehavior. The better prepared a child is for such a procedure, therefore, the better a child is apt to accept it. For potentially painful procedures such as a bone marrow aspiration, lumbar puncture, blood sampling, or cast removal, any behavior short of hysterical screaming can be considered "good" behavior. If limit setting is necessary, such as with a child who hits or bites other children, confer with the child's parents about the need for limit setting and what measures they would suggest. Gain their cooperation and approval so that what you do is consistent with their care (Pao, Ballard, & Rosenstein, 2007). Using "time out" periods or removing the child to a nonstimulating area for a short time is an effective measure. Be certain a child understands the rules (if the child bites or hits, sitting alone for a designated period will be necessary). The next time the child misbehaves, give one warning that the behavior is against the rules; if the behavior does not improve, take the child to the "time out" spot. If the child is disruptive, begin timing the period from when the child quiets down. When the child has been quiet for the specified duration (usually 1 minute per year of age), the child can leave the "time out" place and rejoin activities.

Discharge Planning

Discharge planning is an important link between hospital and home.

Nursing Diagnoses and Related Interventions

Nursing Diagnosis: Parental health-seeking behaviors related to care for child at home after hospital discharge

Outcome Evaluation: Parents state accurately the care their child will need at home; describe and demonstrate any procedures they will need to perform with child.

Many children, particularly those having surgery, are hospitalized for only a few hours; as soon as they are able to take and retain fluid and have voided once, they are discharged. This represents such a short time that preparation for discharge must start even before they are admitted to the hospital (Melnyk et al., 2007).

If a child has been admitted on an inpatient basis, preparation for discharge should begin on the day of admission. If some procedures will need to be continued at home, allow parents to perform them in the hospital at least once so that they can become comfortable with the necessary technique and discover any problems while help is still available. Urge parents to think through problems they might have with a procedure at home. Suppose a parent will be doing warm sterile soaks for an open lesion at home. How will the parent sterilize water? Where can the parent buy dressings? Can the parent afford them? What can be used to keep the soaks warm for 20 minutes? What suggestions would be helpful to give the parent for keeping the child quiet and content for 20 minutes, so that the child does not move a great deal and knock off the dressing? These are real problems that must be worked out before a parent can perform the procedure at home. Do not leave this kind of instruction until the last day, because then there will not be time left to solve such problems (Wolf et al., 2009).

Discharge planners can be indispensable in helping ready parents for home care. In a general hospital setting, however, if a discharge planner is unfamiliar with specific procedures (or children), such a person may not be as helpful on a practical level as anticipated. Some parents require follow-up help in their homes that will be provided by a community or home health care nurse. Do not leave the full responsibility for teaching to these home care nurses either. Teach the parents what they must do on the first day they are at home before further help arrives. Be certain they know the person to contact if plans do not work out as anticipated and that they have a definite return appointment for follow-up care.

Many preschool children manifest behavior problems such as thumb-sucking, bed wetting, temper tantrums, and nightmares after returning home from a hospital stay; school-age children may manifest these behaviors to a lesser extent. You can assure parents these behaviors are part of a child's normal response to hospitalization. These behaviors do not happen because the child has been "spoiled" by the hospital staff or by the parents during the illness but because the experience was too intense for the child to handle easily, even with all the precautions taken to prevent stress. As children realize they are safely back home and the experience is over, these behavior reactions become less frequent and eventually disappear.

NURSING RESPONSIBILITIES FOR CARE OF AN ILL CHILD AND FAMILY

Nursing responsibilities will vary, naturally, with the type, extent, and seriousness of a child's illness, age, care setting, and individual circumstances. Several responsibilities, however, such as promotion of normal growth and development, sleep, stimulation, and play, cross all ages and phases of care. Chapter 37 discusses specific responsibilities related to diagnostic tests or interventions. Chapter 39 discusses the important role of promoting comfort in an ill child.

Promoting Growth and Development of an Ill Child

It is easy for children to fall behind in growth and development because of an illness unless health care providers monitor for this.

Nursing Diagnoses and Related Interventions

Nursing Diagnosis: Risk for delayed growth and development related to effects of illness

Outcome Evaluation: Child demonstrates only limited signs of regression to previous stage; is able to continue doing the activities most recently accomplished.

Illness represents a crisis event. In a crisis state, children, like adults, are susceptible to change or growth with only the slightest intervention. Without intervention, they are likely to be overwhelmed.

Promoting Growth and Development of an Ill Infant. To promote optimal growth and development, try to change an infant's normal routine as little as possible. Sameness provides security to a child and encourages the development of trust. When admitting an infant to a hospital, ask parents what type of bed the child usually sleeps in. A child who is used to sleeping in a bassinet may feel loose and insecure in a large crib. You would need to swaddle such a child in a receiving blanket in a large crib to offer the same close, bound feeling of a smaller sleeping area.

Also, attempt to change the infant's diet as little as possible. Unless a child is diagnosed with failure to thrive or is obviously underweight, illness is not an ideal period in which to introduce new foods or formula. Unless their physical condition warrants a change, infants who breastfeed should continue to do so for as many feedings as possible. Expressed breast milk can be given by bottle to the child when the mother is not available. Overall, because infants cannot begin to understand the strange feelings accompanying illness, they need increased swaddling and comforting. As their condition improves, they need to be provided with stimulation and play opportunities.

Promoting Growth and Development of an Ill Toddler or Preschooler. Because illness can limit autonomy and prevent children from learning how to do new things, try to find opportunities to promote both autonomy in toddlers and initiative in preschoolers. Urge parents to encourage children to make choices about their care whenever possible. For example, coloring in a medication schedule is the kind of task that helps to encourage initiative in a preschooler.

If admitted to the hospital, toddlers and preschoolers who are not used to sleeping in cribs may resent being put in a crib unless the reason is explained to them ("All our beds here have side rails"). Watch toddlers closely to be certain they do not climb over crib rails to get out of bed. A child who does try may be safer in a bed than a crib.

As with infants, illness is a poor time to change the eating habits of toddlers and preschoolers. Because children of this age insist on self-feeding, they generally do poorly eating in bed and often do better sitting at low tables. Many child-care units in hospitals organize tables for toddlers and preschoolers to eat together. Some children do well at these tables, but others are too distracted by the activity and the noise and may need a separate low table by their bed to eat well. All children may eat better when their parents are present.

Illness is also a poor time to begin toilet training, even if it is appropriate to the child's age. If the parents have already begun toilet training, continue it with as normal a routine as possible.

Promoting Growth and Development of an Ill School-Age Child. School-age children need to continue to work on a sense of industry while ill. This means learning more about how and why things are done. Explain about specific procedures and involve them as much as possible in planning their care to help foster a sense of industry.

Remember that children who are ill are not at their best and so may not act as mature as usual. This means a 7-year-old whose parents describe him as very mature may seem to function at the level of a 5-year-old. Children of any age should not be held to their chronologic age when they are ill. In a hospital, school-age children enjoy sharing a room with another child close in age so they can play games together. School-age children do well with competition when they are healthy but often do poorly with competition when they are ill. They may revert to playing types of games they would normally dismiss as too young for them.

School-age children and adolescents should continue schooling if they are ill for a long time, provided their condition will allow it. Because it is age appropriate, ill children do well with school activities or working with a tutor. It is such a normal, everyday activity that it provides security in an otherwise insecure situation. It also reassures them that they are expected to get better and to return to school when this is over.

During the times a child will not be attending school, working on projects such as needlecraft, helping plan family menus, writing for brochures about the place the family plans to visit on vacation next year, or viewing videotapes on science or nature are activities that not only help pass the time but also encourage learning. School-age children also are developing moral responsibility and may find comfort in spiritual practices. Ways to assist with spiritual needs are shown in Table 36.3.

Encourage school-age children to carry out self-care and, if cared for at home, to contribute to household routines, such as helping with dishes or picking up after themselves, as much as they are able. This not only takes some burden off caregivers but also makes a child feel like an intrinsic part of the family.

Promoting Growth and Development of an Ill Adolescent. An adolescent who is struggling to develop a sense of identity may find it very difficult to be ill because the limitations imposed by an illness can make the development of a sense of identity difficult. Help adolescents to continue to participate in activities they did before becoming ill, if possible, to help them feel their world is not totally changing. Encourage them to maintain self-care activities and good hygiene practices to help preserve self-esteem.

Illness can be difficult for adolescents also because peer relationships are so important to them. They may miss acting in a school play, playing on a sports team, or competing for a scholarship. A girlfriend or boyfriend may fall in love with someone else while an adolescent is hospitalized. This makes them feel excluded and hurt. For these reasons, it is important for them to have visitors from their peer group, just as much as infants need visits from parents. Using a cell phone to text message is an easy way to contact friends and maintain relationships with individuals who are important to them.

Adolescents appreciate being hospitalized in a special adolescent unit or at least in a room free of childish decor. Adolescent hospital units should be organized with the same considerations for visiting parents as other children's units; anxiety and pain of separation are not limited to the under-13 set. Urge parents to stay overnight if they and the adolescent wish. Although adolescents enjoy having parents stay overnight because it is reassuring to know they

✔ Checkpoint Question 36.3

You want to encourage Becky to drink a lot of water. Which action would do this best?

a. Scold her for not cooperating to make herself well again.
b. Offer her small glasses of fluid so she can drink these frequently.
c. Offer her large glasses of fluid so she does not have to drink so often.
d. Alert her if she does not drink fluid, she will have to receive an IV.

PROMOTING SAFETY FOR AN ILL CHILD

A prime consideration of nursing interventions is to keep children safe during illness care.

Nursing Diagnoses and Related Interventions

Nursing Diagnosis: Risk for injury related to procedures or therapy necessary for care

Outcome Evaluation: Child remains free of injuries and accidents, such as a fall from bed or injury from medical equipment.

Promoting safety for children is a responsibility for all health care providers. Care of an ill or physically challenged child at home includes assessing the safety of the house and providing family teaching. It also includes making provisions for emergencies. For example, a family may need to install a counter-level telephone or purchase a cell phone so a child in a wheelchair can call for emergency help. They might need to make a plan for how to evacuate an ill child from the home in an emergency such as a fire.

Safety on a children's unit or clinic is the responsibility of everyone, from the administrator of the institution to part-time health care personnel. Important steps to follow to make a child health care environment a safer place are:

- Always be sure of the location of all children in your care.
- Ensure that doors or gates are provided near stairways or elevators.
- Ensure that back doors of health care facilities have working alarms to prevent children from going out and strangers from coming in.
- Be sure windows are covered by screens or guards so children cannot climb up on sills and fall out.
- Check that the side rails of beds and cribs are in good repair and raised appropriately.
- Always raise bedside rails after a child has received preoperative or sedative medication.
- Test a crib rail after it is raised to ensure the lock has caught so the rail will remain raised.
- Push bedside tables or stands away from cribs so a child cannot climb over the railing and use the stand as a step down.
- Be certain crib caps are provided for small children to prevent them from climbing out of bed.
- Fasten the seat belt restraint for infants in highchairs. Never leave an infant in a highchair (at home or in a hospital) without someone close enough to reach the child as infants can easily squirm out of a highchair restraint.
- Ensure that electrical cords or appliances such as hair dryers are not used in bathrooms, where they could come in contact with water.
- Be careful of the placement of television/call cords or Venetian blind cords so they cannot lead to strangulation.
- Never leave children younger than 5 years alone in a bathtub; they could turn on the hot water and scald themselves or slip under the water and drown.
- Never leave equipment or items that would be harmful to eat within the reach of children.
- Adhere to all fire precaution measures.
- Closely follow standard infection precautions to prevent the spread of infections.

Promoting Fire Safety. Fire precautions both in the home and in the hospital are essential in preserving the safety of ill or disabled children. Adults can usually take responsibility for removing themselves from a burning structure, but children depend on care providers. Ensure that there is a plan of action in case of a fire and that everyone in the home, in the clinic, or on a hospital unit knows it. To be certain a home is safe, having a smoke detector on each floor is a wise precaution. A downstairs bedroom is not only safest in case of a fire but also allows a child more self-care ability. Fire departments supply free decals for the bedroom windows of children or those who are physically challenged so they can be easily located in a fire. Encourage parents to contact their local fire department for this safety measure.

Electrical equipment such as respiratory and cardiac monitors, radiant heat warmers, special-care equipment, and electrical heating pads are often used in the care of children. Do not use equipment with frayed cords or equipment that is not properly grounded. Plugs should be three-pronged for extra safety; do not overload circuits with additional plugs. Electrical outlets should have safety caps to cover them when they are not in use so toddlers cannot poke objects into them and electrocute themselves.

Adhering to Standard Infection Precautions. In every health care setting, closely follow standard infection precautions to protect ill children, family, and staff from infections. Because of a compromised immune system, ill children may be more susceptible to repeat or secondary infections than usual, especially drug resistant strains of bacteria such as methicillin-resistant *Staphylococcus aureus* (MRSA), that can spread easily if not everyone is conscientious about precautions (Raymond et al., 2007). Proper handwashing technique, disposal of tissues and waste materials, and efforts to minimize exposure of other ill children or adults are all effective methods to decrease the risk of infection. For more details on infection control, see Chapter 43.

PROMOTING ADEQUATE SLEEP FOR AN ILL CHILD

Ill children need adequate rest and sleep so their body tissues can effectively use nutrients for repair and normal growth can continue (Meltzer et al., 2007). Children may not sleep well when they are ill because of discomfort, pain, administration of medications, or intensified symptoms of chronic sleep problems. They may not sleep well in a hospital because it is a strange setting; they may have to undergo so many procedures that they also do not nap or rest as much during the day as usual. Children who are recovering from trauma such as injuries from a car accident or burns may be unable to sleep because of nightmares about the accident. These nightmares can cause them to suffer sleep deprivation in the same way as a child who is frequently awakened for procedures during the night. Encourage parents to stay with these children for support and comfort. Remember, though, that parents who sleep in hospital rooms do not obtain adequate sleep either (Lee et al., 2007). Although their presence is healthy for children, it can lower the parent's ability to handle stress or interpret happenings.

Sleep Patterns

Sleep is influenced by anxiety level, state of health, habit, medication, and environment at the time of sleep. Stages of sleep are summarized in Table 36.5. Figure 36.8A shows a pattern of normal sleep. As a sleep cycle begins, children first enter **non–rapid eye movement (NREM) sleep.** This type of sleep occurs in up to 80% of total sleep time. As children fall deeper and deeper asleep, they pass from stage I to stages II, III, and IV of NREM sleep over a period of 20 to 30 minutes. **Rapid eye movement (REM) sleep** follows. In infants, most of sleep time is REM sleep, whereas young adults have the least amount of this type of sleep. The sleep pattern of a child who is awakened frequently during the night for procedures would resemble that shown in Figure 36.8B.

The purpose of NREM sleep, the first phase of sleep, is rest and restoration of the body; this stage keeps body cells functioning and healthy. During the periods of stage III and IV NREM sleep, the secretion of growth hormone (somatotropic hormone) from the pituitary is at its highest level. Growth hormone is necessary for protein synthesis and growth of new cells and for repair and maintenance of all cells. Corticosteroids and adrenaline from the adrenal gland, which are instrumental in the catabolism or breakdown of cells, are at their lowest levels. This balance of hormones produces the ideal combination for protein synthesis and cell growth and repair.

The purpose of REM sleep is less clear. The rapid eye movements may serve to coordinate binocular vision. Dreams that occur during this time apparently serve as a release of tension or help to integrate new knowledge and experience with old in the brain's memory system. Vital signs may fall during NREM sleep. During REM sleep, vital signs rise to near-normal levels. These periods of REM sleep interspersed with NREM sleep, therefore, may be a fail-safe measure to prevent vital signs from falling too low during sleep.

TABLE 36.5 ✻ Stages of Sleep in Children

Stage	Description	Nursing Implications
NREM		
I	A feeling of drifting or falling. Often described as twilight sleep. Temperature and heart rate decrease slightly; EEG waves show peaked, frequent waves (alpha waves).	A child can be roused easily from this early sleep by the slightest noise or even the silent presence of another person in the room. Reduce noise level in room to promote sleep.
II	Sleep deepens. Temperature and heart rate decrease slightly more.	It is more difficult to wake a child from sleep when this point has been reached.
III	Sleep deepens still further. An EEG tracing reveals mixed spindle and delta (slow) waves. Temperature and heart rate decrease further. This period lasts about 10 min.	It is very difficult to wake a child from stage III sleep. Use patience to wake a child fully to offer medicine.
IV	Approximately 20 to 30 min after beginning to fall asleep, a child enters stage IV sleep. Respirations are slow and deep, temperature and heart rate slow even more, and blood pressure decreases; EEG shows delta (slow, steady) waves. Children remain at a stage IV sleep level for approximately 30 min, then progress back through stages III and II until they then pass into a phase of REM sleep.	Children may be confused and unable to orient themselves readily if awakened from stage IV sleep. Use patience until a child is fully awake, particularly if asking a question.
REM	Eyes move in rapid, involuntary motions. Respirations are irregular; body turnings, movements, and penile erections may occur. Lasts 10 to 30 min and then a new sleep cycle with NREM sleep begins.	Dreaming occurs during REM sleep. Although children appear to be close to waking because of the active eye movements, they are really very soundly asleep. Children may wake afraid and crying, disturbed by a frightening dream.

there—or encourage the child to join the rest of the family for activities by resting on the couch in the living room, a lounge chair in the backyard, or sitting in the kitchen. This principle applies to hospitalized children as well. To interact more easily, a toddler may rest in a parent's lap rather than in a bed.

Providing Stimulation for Children on Transmission-Based Precautions. Children who are placed on transmission-based precautions because of the possibility of contagious illness may experience severe sensory deprivation if everyone who enters the room must wear a gown and mask or if the number of visitors must be kept to a minimum. If gloves are part of precautions, a child can experience a significant loss of skin-to-skin contact as well. Transmission-based precautions are discussed in Chapter 43. Careful planning must be done to ensure that a child who is isolated this way is not psychologically isolated and that every possible measure is carried out to maintain sensory, social, physical, and cognitive stimulation. For example, try to visit with a child at a time in addition to those times in which you must perform procedures so you can simply talk; place the bed so the child can see out of the room; encourage the child to telephone or text message friends; make posters for the walls so they're no longer bare; or encourage interactive play such as electronic games. For ideas on providing stimulation to children in specific age groups, refer to Chapters 29 to 33.

Sensory Overload

Sensory overload, in contrast to deprivation, occurs when children receive more stimulation than they can tolerate or process. Children with sensory overload react similarly to those with sensory deprivation or feel confused, unable to make decisions, and feel severely fatigued. Sometimes it is difficult to determine the cause of these symptoms (whether they are caused by sensory deprivation or overload) unless assessed carefully.

The lights in ICUs, for example, are never turned out. Although children may find this comforting, it can also result in excessive stimulation. In addition to constant light, there is excessive sound such as the whir of machines, buzzing of ventilators, ringing of alarms, or mix of voices in consultation. Most ICUs have no windows because the wall space is used for monitoring equipment; therefore, night and day are not easily distinguished. It is easy for a child to become confused about time and place in such a setting. For children who are cared for at home in a family room where people talk constantly, the television is always on, and activity never ceases, sensory overload may also occur. An important nursing role is reducing sensory stimulation attributed to overload. Orient children to the time of day by making frequent references to it or by providing calendars and clocks. If necessary, provide eye covers or ear plugs to reduce stimulation.

PROMOTING PLAY FOR AN ILL CHILD 

Play, often described as "the work of children," is an invaluable component of child health care. Providing a space and opportunity for play can help children feel more comfortable and allow for an important release of energy for children who are confined to a room or bed. Play also may be used to help assess children's level of knowledge and feelings about their condition so that more individualized nursing care can be planned. Depending on a child's age, play can also be a useful tool in health teaching (see Chapter 35).

Defining play is not a simple task because play activities vary greatly from child to child and among different age, cultural, and socioeconomic groups. A common definition is that play is any voluntary activity engaged in for the purpose of enjoyment. If a child views an activity as enjoyment, therefore, no matter what it is and whether it would be fun or not for an adult, it is play.

Play is clearly the means by which children develop increasing cognitive, psychomotor, and social capabilities. Touching a soft rabbit, passing colored blocks from one hand to the other, pounding with a plastic hammer, feeding a doll, and playing board games are all ways in which children are exposed to and learn about different textures and colors, experience the feeling of possessing and owning, and learn about competition, winning, and losing. A soft toy tells a child more clearly than can be described that this is what the word "soft" means. Colored blocks reveal how parts can join to make a whole, how things stacked too high will fall (there are limits one cannot go beyond), and practice makes perfect. As children talk with playmates during play, they develop both language and social skills. The repetitive acts involved in most games encourage the development of musculoskeletal skills. Play is not something children do when they have nothing else to do then; it is something children *have* to do. During illness, it provides a feeling of security because it is an activity that has continuity with everyday life.

The manner in which children play differs as they mature. Types of play and the age groups in which these types are seen most frequently are shown in Box 36.8.

Assessing Child Health Through Play

Children who are acutely ill do not play or play very little because they do not have the strength, the attention span, or the interest in activities required for play. They continue, however, to enjoy being read to, and they find comfort in holding a favorite toy even if they do not actively manipulate it. Once children are over the acute phase of an illness, interest in play returns. Whether a child is spontaneously playing, then, is a good index of health. The toys children use at play are a good indication of their growth and development level and emotional state.

The average parent knows a child's play preferences and current favorite game or toy. Asking for this information at a health interview helps to assess a child's developmental level and whether it is age-appropriate. It also helps to assess the quality of parenting (if parents view play as important or are familiar with the child's activities).

Providing Play in Ambulatory Settings

Children in ambulatory departments are under a great deal of stress. They sit in a waiting room and glance fearfully at the door that leads to the examining room. They hear children crying beyond the door and wait in terror for what lies in store for them when it is their turn.

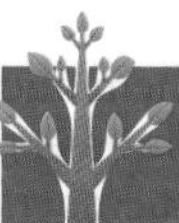

BOX 36.8 * Focus on Family Teaching

Understanding Different Play Types

Q. Becky's mother tells you, "When Becky was younger, she didn't like toys as much as the boxes they came in. What's normal for children and play?"

A. Children play differently at different ages. Examples of typical play patterns include:

Type of Play/Age	Description	Example
Observation/Infant	Child watches particular play intently, although not actively engaged in it.	Watching a mobile
Parallel/Toddler	Two children play side by side but seldom attempt to interact with each other.	Playing separately with similar push toy
Associative/Preschooler	Children play together in a similar activity; there is little organization of responsibilities	Engaging in typical backyard play
Cooperative/School-age	Children play with an organized structure or compete for desired goal or outcome.	Playing organized games with rules

Most parents know that when their child is coming to a hospital to be admitted, they should pack the child's favorite toy. Often they do not think of an ambulatory visit as a sufficiently threatening circumstance to warrant bringing a favorite toy, however, so the child has nothing to play with. Having a parent sit beside them is so comforting they may ignore or hesitate moving 4 feet away to get the toys furnished by the health care facility unless they are urged to do so.

It is best if ambulatory departments are stocked with toys that can be played with quickly and by single children. There should be a low table and chairs so a parent can come to a table and play with a child. Examining rooms should have toys also—they may be used to distract a child while a procedure such as an ear examination is performed, and because the wait in an examining room may be as long as the wait in a waiting room. Well siblings who accompany a parent and sick child to the facility can play with toys to distract them as well so that a parent can concentrate on the ailing child. Some hospitals furnish computer games for older children for this reason. Examples of ways that play can be used in an ambulatory care setting are shown in Table 36.6.

TABLE 36.6 * Ways to Incorporate Play Into Ambulatory Nursing Care

Nursing Care	Play Activity
Aid with physical assessment	Distract child's attention with puppet during respiratory and cardiac assessment. Play "Simon Says" to encourage child to take deep breaths for respiratory assessment. Allow child to listen to own heart with stethoscope. Play "Follow the Leader" to assess gait. Draw a face on the tongue blade used to assess throat. Show child how to "blow out" the otoscope light. Draw child's outline on the table examining paper and give it to the child to take home to color.
Health teaching	Use puppets as teacher. Create word scrambles or crossword puzzles.

Providing Play in the Hospital

Ideally, all hospital units in which children are cared for should have a play space big enough for most of the children on the unit to come to. There should be enough space to accommodate children who are not fully ambulatory, such as those with casts or in wheelchairs (Fig. 36.10). Tables for board games and play materials such as crayons and paints should be available. Children can release a great deal of anger or tension by splashing water, squeezing or pouring sand, or smearing finger paint.

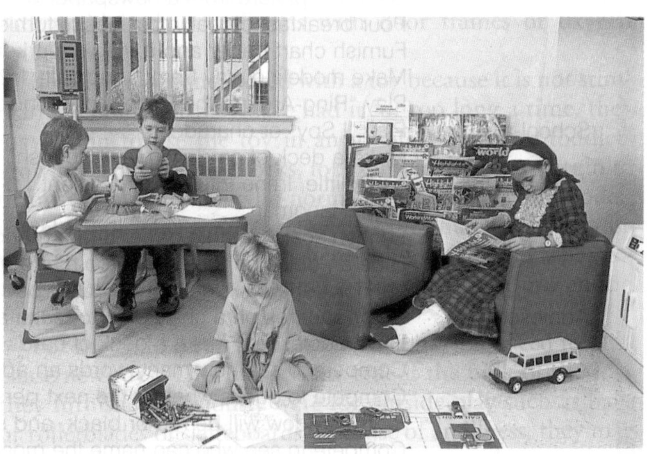

FIGURE 36.10 Children enjoying themselves in a hospital playroom, which is spacious and well equipped with age-appropriate toys and activities.

Child Support Programs

Child support programs are incorporated into all major children's hospitals and are an integral feature of child health care (Wilmot, 2007). As part of a child support program, a specialist offers children the opportunity to re-enact and thereby master the anxiety associated with illness. Through therapeutic play, child specialists provide programs that prepare children for hospitalization and, once hospitalized, prepare children for surgery or for procedures that could be painful. They consult with parents about good toys to choose for home care. These specialists help children air their frustration about painful or intrusive procedures, prevent social isolation of children by means of an active recreation program, and ensure that the total health care environment is conducive to children's well-being.

Such a program not only aids in promoting children's mental health but also leads to more cooperative responses of children to treatments or procedures. It is complementary to play programs initiated by nurses.

✔ Checkpoint Question 36.4

You worry about Becky aspirating a toy you give her. Which of the following items is most apt to be aspirated?

a. Pages in a coloring book.
b. Clothing from a baby doll.
c. Pieces of colored chalk.
d. Blocks 2 inches square.

Therapeutic Play

Anything almost automatically becomes less threatening when a person can talk about it. Many children cannot talk about what is happening to them during illness, however, because of fear or because their vocabulary is so limited they cannot describe their feelings.

Because play is the language of children, children who have difficulty voicing their thoughts in words can often speak clearly through play. **Play therapy** is a psychoanalytic technique used by psychiatrists to help children understand their feelings and thoughts and motivations better. In play therapy, the therapist attempts to interpret the child's verbal and nonverbal cues. Interpreting nonverbal cues and helping the child understand them this way requires the skill of a psychiatric nurse-clinician or others with specialized training. **Therapeutic play** is a play technique that can be used by nurses to better understand children's feelings and thoughts (William, Lopez, & Lee, 2007). For therapeutic play, only the child's verbal cues are used as responses.

Therapeutic play can be divided into three types:

1. Energy release
2. Dramatic play
3. Creative play

Energy Release

Children release energy by pounding, hitting, running, punching, or shouting. Furnishing children with materials that allow them to do these things helps them release anxiety as well. Toddlers pound pegs with a plastic hammer or pretend to cut wood with a toy saw. Other examples include giving modeling clay to a preschooler (an anxious child often pounds it flat; a relaxed child, however, will build it into shapes) or tying a balloon to an overbed trapeze for a school-age child or adolescent to punch.

Dramatic Play

Dramatic play is acting out an anxiety-producing situation. It is most effective with preschool children because they are at the peak of imagination. During illness, the situations about which children need to express feelings are illness related, and therefore the equipment needed for therapeutic play is common health care equipment: dolls, doll beds, play stethoscopes, intravenous equipment, syringes, masks, and gowns. Puppets of doctors, nurses, mothers, fathers, and children help young children express their feelings. Anatomically correct dolls are used to help children describe their feelings about sexual abuse.

It is good to have a play session with a child near the beginning of an illness to see whether the child communicates any fears about this experience through play. This initial session also serves as a way of preparing the child for events that will occur during the illness (Fig. 36.11). Repeat a play session after any painful or traumatic procedure such as surgery so that the child can express new feelings. A list of procedures that fall into this category is shown in Table 36.9. If such play sessions reveal fears, a child should be scheduled for other play sessions, perhaps once daily.

Furnish children with a wide range of equipment and then let them choose those items with which they wish to play. Children invariably choose a piece of equipment that has been used with them. They poke at a doll with a syringe or enjoy giving it a "shot." They wrap the doll in bandages or put tubes into its mouth or stomach, acting out things that were done to them or that they saw done to other children on a nursing unit or at a clinic visit they fear will be done to them. Allow play to be nondirective (let children proceed at their own pace, choosing freely what equipment to play with and what they want to do with equipment). As a child works through an experience this way, the experience becomes less fearful and the child gains increased control over it.

Observe for children who may be using equipment in an unusual way, such as hitting dolls with stethoscopes or poking them in the eye with a thermometer (suggesting they are

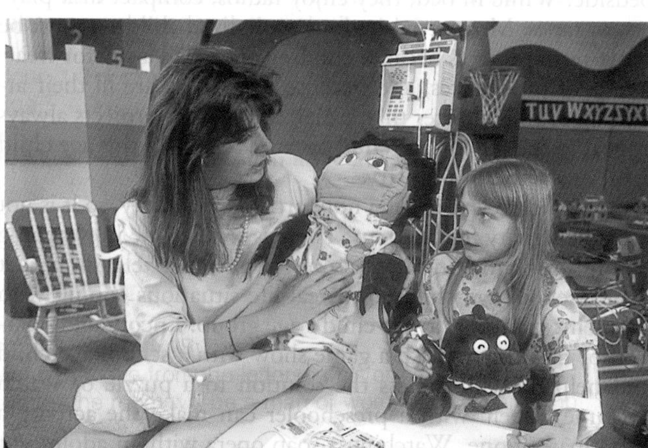

FIGURE 36.11 Therapeutic play allows children the opportunity to voice their fears of illness and procedures. (From Daemmrich/Stock Boston.)

TABLE 36.9 ✻ Therapeutic Play Techniques for Children After Procedures

Procedure	Play Activity (Provide a doll and. . .)
Radiograph	Table and box labeled "x-ray machine"; children sometimes worry that x-rays have injured them, just as laser rays in science fiction shows do.
Blood drawing	Syringe, alcohol wipes, tourniquet, or finger lancets; remember that finger sticks are as frightening for children as are needles.
Clean-catch urine	Alcohol wipes and a collection cup; children are often more embarrassed by urine collection than adults realize.
Intravenous therapy	Intravenous tubing, as well as restraints and armboard; some children are as angry about being restrained as having the needle inserted.
Endoscopy such as bronchoscopy, cystoscopy	Catheters or a penlight to simulate a scope
Scans	Intravenous fluid and tubing, because scans usually require the intravenous injection of isotopes
Bone marrow	Alcohol wipes, syringe
EEG, EKG	Electrode leads that attach to a box; children might be afraid of these procedures because of their fear of electricity.
Surgery	An anesthesia mask and a blunt kitchen knife; watch and listen for where the child cuts and how the experience is described.
Dental examination	Suction catheter, a penlight to simulate a drill, and a 4 × 4 piece of plastic to simulate a dental dam; some children are angered by the use of plastic in their mouth.
Dressing changes	Gauze and adhesive tape
Cast application or removal	Provide plaster to soak and apply; simulate a cast cutter with an electric razor or hair dryer.
Nasogastric tube insertion, enema, catheterization	Appropriate tubes
Temperature assessment	Thermometer

confused about the purpose of such equipment). Such behavior can alert you to the importance of explaining the purpose of equipment to children. Listen to what children say as they play. A comment such as, "I'm giving shots to all the bad dolls" suggests the child thinks injections are punishment. It would be important to stress the next time the child needs an injection that medicine is to make the child feel well again. A comment such as, "This doll is going to surgery, so you won't have her anymore" could suggest the child thinks she will not return from surgery (she may have heard a family member describe someone who died after surgery and is asking for reassurance that such a thing is not going to happen to her). Do not be surprised about the force with which children insert nasogastric tubes into dolls. In part, this reflects how they perceive these procedures, but it also represents energy or anxiety release, in the way that pounding or hitting releases anger.

To better understand how a child feels, repeat what the child says verbally: "You're giving the bad dolls shots?" or ask the child to tell you more about the activity: "Do you think that's the only kind of children who get shots—bad children?" Do not rush to reassure ("Don't worry, that isn't going to happen to you"). Quick reassurance tells children they should not ask any more questions or that the topic is not open for discussion.

Sometimes even children who seem well prepared may be taken by surprise during a procedure. For example, 7-year-old Tanya, seen in an ambulatory setting for a diagnostic workup after a urinary tract infection, showed little interest in dolls and syringes and tubing in the playroom. She had been prepared by her mother for the experience and seemed to understand what would happen during her x-ray procedure. After returning from the x-ray room, where she had a voiding cystourethrogram, however, she was obviously upset. Her nurse brought her a rag doll, a doctor and a nurse figure, a play x-ray machine, and some tubing that could simulate a urinary catheter and encouraged Tanya to play with them. Tanya picked up the girl doll and put her under the x-ray machine. She imitated the doctor doll shouting, "Pee in front of everybody!" Tanya's mother had not realized that she would have to void during a cystourethrogram and so had not prepared her for that. Tanya felt betrayed by not being really prepared for this embarrassing situation. Her play brought her emotion out in the open, where it could be talked about and handled. When Tanya was scheduled the next day for ureteral reflux surgery, her nurse was alerted to make the preparation absolutely thorough.

Children older than 9 or 10 years find playing with dolls too childish to be of benefit. They enjoy handling syringes, however, and being able to see and handle such equipment as nasogastric tubes in advance of their being placed. Active handling helps to eliminate fear because it identifies exactly what the child has to face; it meets their concrete-level learning needs.

Creative Play

Some children are too angry to be able to act out their feelings through dramatic play. However, they may be able to draw a picture that expresses their emotions or conveys the extent of their knowledge. To encourage this, give a child a

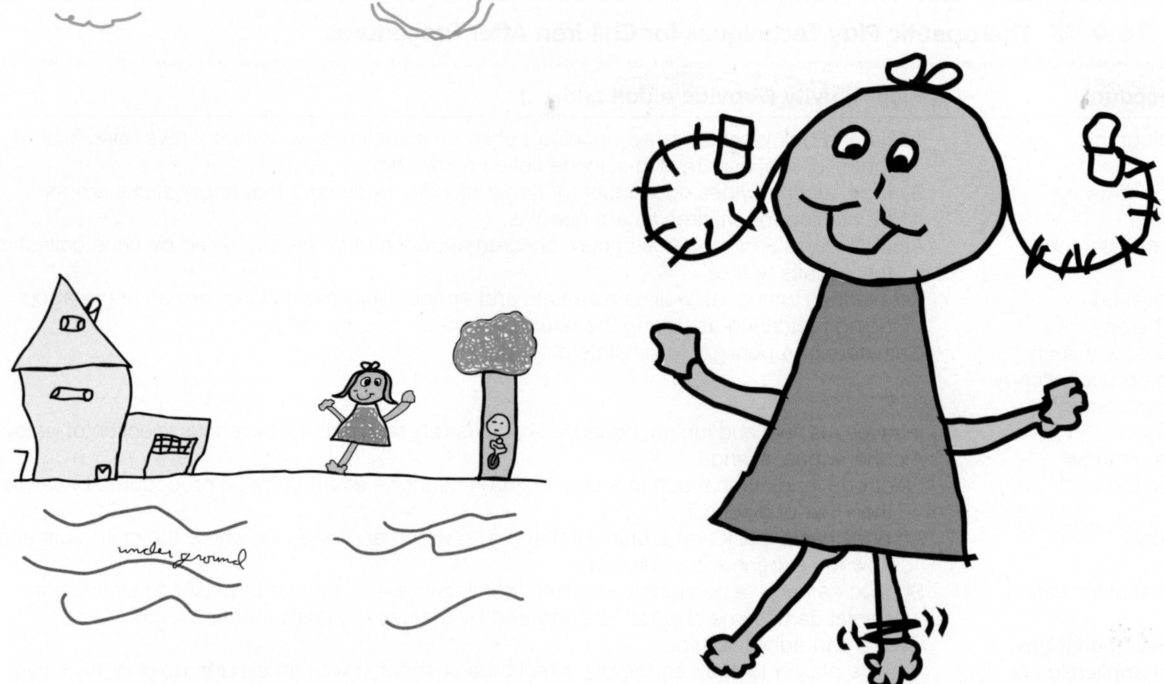

FIGURE 36.12 (**A**) Children who are concerned about body parts may draw pictures with that part missing or exaggerated. Note the missing left leg here. (**B**) After reassurance that her leg will be all right, the girl who did the drawing in *A* now draws a girl with two legs.

blank paper and crayons or markers. If a child seems reluctant to draw something spontaneously, suggest a topic: "Why don't you draw a picture of yourself?"

Some children are so concerned with particular parts of their bodies that when asked to draw pictures of themselves, they draw only the body part about which they are worried. Such children generally are saying they need to talk about that part of the body, to be given reassurance that it is going to be all right. Figure 36.12A shows a picture drawn by Becky when she was admitted to the hospital for 1-day surgery for debridement of a campfire burn on her left foot. She stated on admission she was being admitted to have the burn on her foot "cleaned out." This sounds like a child who understands what debridement involves. Note, however, that the figure she drew has no left leg. One has to wonder whether she was concerned she was going to surgery to have more than debridement. After the word "debridement" was explained to her, she drew the picture in Figure 36.12B. The child in the drawing now has a left and a right leg, the left leg covered by a bandage. Through a drawing, this child was able to say something she could not express without this help.

Many ill children draw pictures that reflect punitive images: a boy or girl tied to a bed or shut behind bars, or doctors and nurses frowning at them, obviously unhappy with them. Such children may need assurance that they are not being punished; they need to stay in bed or are being cared for by doctors and nurses to be made well (Fig. 36.13). Other children draw pictures that are symbolic of death: airplanes crashing, boats sinking, buildings on fire, children in graveyards. They need assurance that they will not die.

Other concerns such as fear of abandonment and loss of independence may also be manifested in drawings. For example, preschoolers may draw a child in one corner of a picture and an adult in a far corner. They may comment that the parent cannot find the child because she's gone to the hospital. They need to be reassured their parents know where

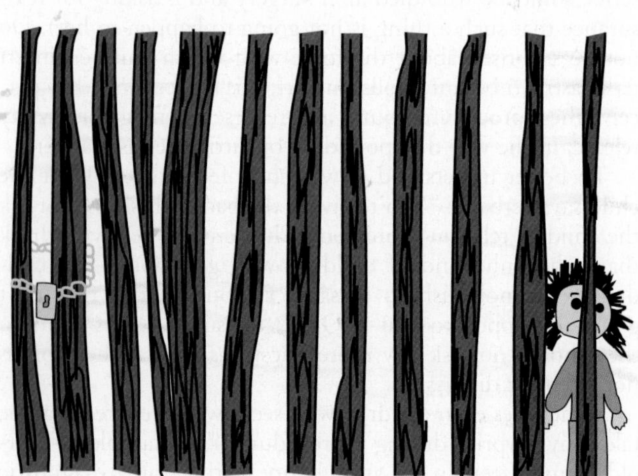

FIGURE 36.13 A picture drawn by a hospitalized child. Note the prison-like appearance of the crib. (Courtesy of Rita Crever.)

Fosdal, M. B., & Wojner-Alexandrov, A. W. (2007). Events of hospitalization among children with sickle cell disease. *Journal of Pediatric Nursing: Nursing Care of Children and Families, 22*(4), 342–346.

Knutsson, S., et al. (2008). Children's experiences of visiting a seriously ill/injured relative on an adult intensive care unit. *Journal of Advanced Nursing, 61*(2), 154–162.

Mayer, M. L., Skinner, A. C., & Freed, G. L. (2009). Interspecialty differences in the care of children with chronic or serious acute conditions: review of the literature. *Journal of Pediatrics, 154*(2), 164–168.

Norton, S. P., et al. (2007). Effect of a clinical pathway on the hospitalisation rates of children with asthma: a prospective study. *Archives of Disease in Childhood, 92* (1), 60–66.

Scott, J. T., et al. (2009). Interventions for improving communication with children and adolescents about their cancer. *Cochrane Database of Systematic Reviews, 2009*(1), (CD002969).

Spilkin, A., & Ballantyne, A. (2007). Behavior in children with a chronic illness. *Families, Systems and Health, 25*(1), 68–84.

Yang, J., et al. (2007). Patient and hospital characteristics associated with length of stay and hospital charges for pediatric sports-related injury hospitalizations in the United States, 2000–2003. *Pediatrics, 119*(4), e813–e820.

Zerr, D. M., et al. (2008). Hospital-based influenza vaccination of children: an opportunity to prevent subsequent hospitalization. *Pediatrics, 121*(2), 345–348.

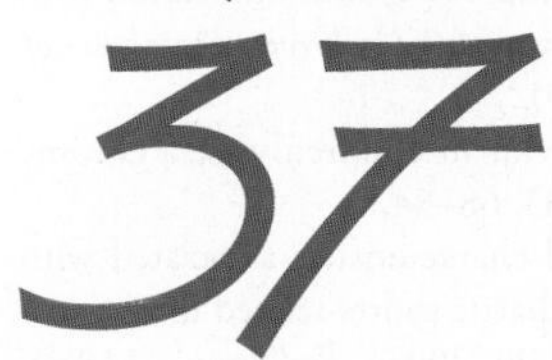

Chapter 37 Nursing Care of a Family When a Child Needs Diagnostic or Therapeutic Modalities

KEY TERMS

- aspiration studies
- barium contrast studies
- bronchoscopy
- clean-catch urine specimen
- colonoscopy
- computed tomography (CT)
- electrical impulse studies
- endoscopy
- gavage feedings
- magnetic resonance imaging (MRI)
- positron emission tomography (PET)
- radiopharmaceuticals
- single-photon emission computed tomography (SPECT)
- total parenteral nutrition (TPN)
- ultrasound

OBJECTIVES

After mastering the contents of this chapter, you should be able to:

1. Describe common nursing interventions used in the health care of children to aid diagnosis and therapy.
2. Identify National Health Goals related to diagnostic and therapeutic procedures for children that nurses could help the nation achieve.
3. Use critical thinking to analyze ways diagnostic and therapeutic procedures can be modified to be more family centered.
4. Assess children regarding developmental stage and knowledge level before beginning diagnostic or therapeutic procedures.
5. Formulate nursing diagnoses related to common diagnostic or therapeutic procedures used with children.
6. Identify expected outcomes for a child who needs a diagnostic or therapeutic procedure.
7. Plan nursing interventions to aid in diagnosis or therapy for children.
8. Implement nursing interventions relevant to diagnostic or therapeutic procedures such as preparing a child for magnetic resonance imaging.
9. Evaluate expected outcomes for achievement and effectiveness of care.
10. Identify areas related to nursing procedures with children that could benefit from additional nursing research or application of evidence-based practice.
11. Integrate knowledge of common diagnostic and therapeutic procedures with nursing process to achieve quality maternal and child health nursing care.

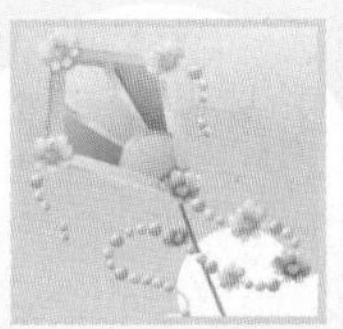

T.J. Balliff is a preschooler who is scheduled to have a magnetic resonance imaging (MRI) study because of a head injury. "How can I agree to this?" his mother asks you. "He's afraid of the dark. How can I allow him to be wheeled into a long dark machine that way?"

Previous chapters described the growth and development of well children. This chapter adds information about how to care for children who are having diagnostic or therapeutic procedures. This is important information because it builds a base for both care and health teaching.

How would you explain MRI to T.J.to make the procedure more acceptable to him?

Illness can be particularly stressful if many diagnostic and therapeutic procedures are necessary for care. In today's health care climate, there is less time for teaching and preparation than once available, so good planning and follow-through become essential when these are scheduled. Chapter 36 described measures to make an illness experience a more positive one. Health teaching, discussed in Chapter 35, is also a cornerstone in this process. Everything that nurses do with and for ill children can have a major influence on children's progress toward health as well as on children's and families' perception of professional health care and the ability to carry out healthful practices in the future (Shah & Ohlsson, 2009).

Many nursing actions offer an opportunity to accomplish several goals. Supporting a child and family during a diagnostic procedure, for instance, not only can aid in efficient diagnosis but also may help establish a trusting relationship between the family and health care providers that will make all future interactions more successful. This chapter describes the most common diagnostic and therapeutic techniques used in the care of ill children, including modifications needed to make these procedures safe and reduce associated stress, depending on the child's age and condition. National Health Goals that address this area of child health practice are shown in Box 37.1.

BOX 37.1 ✻ Focus on National Health Goals

A key component of minimizing the stress of hospitalization and procedures for children, and thereby maximizing safety, is to limit the length of time children spend in the hospital. Several National Health Goals address reducing the length of time that children spend in hospitals. One example is:

- Reduce hospitalization rates for three ambulatory care–sensitive conditions—pediatric asthma, uncontrolled diabetes, and immunization-preventable pneumonia and influenza—from baseline levels of 23 per 10,000, 7.2 per 10,000, and 10.6 per 10,000 hospital admissions to target levels of 17.3 per 10,000, 5.4 per 10,000, and 8.0 per 10,000 hospital admissions.

A major role of health care providers is to keep children free from disease so that they undergo a minimal number of procedures. A National Health Goal also addresses this:

- Increase the proportion of persons appropriately counseled about health behaviors (http://www.nih.gov).

Nurses can help the nation achieve these goals by providing health counseling to aid in preventing children from becoming ill and subsequently requiring hospitalization.

Areas related to these goals that could benefit from additional nursing research and application of evidence-based practice include determining what teaching techniques are most effective in keeping children well; what methods are efficient at ensuring that children's hospitalizations are as short as possible; and what techniques or supplies are most satisfactory to children when procedures are performed.

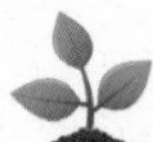

Nursing Process Overview

For a Child Who Needs Diagnostic or Therapeutic Procedures

Assessment

Before performing procedures such as assisting with a diagnostic test or collecting laboratory specimens, first carefully evaluate a child's age and developmental stage, as well as any special needs a child may have. Even the most common and painless procedures create a certain amount of stress for children and parents. During complex diagnostic procedures, this stress level is almost certain to increase even further. Unfamiliar doctors and nurses, high-tech supplies and equipment, and strange surroundings all add up to a frightening experience for most adults; imagine how frightening they can seem to children.

Assess a child's level of anxiety associated with unfamiliar equipment, circumstances, and surroundings as well as the child's knowledge concerning a technique before initiating a therapeutic procedure or beginning health teaching. Respecting a child's past experience with similar procedures can lay a foundation for knowledge and cooperation.

Nursing Diagnosis

Common nursing diagnoses related to diagnostic and therapeutic procedures are as varied as the procedures themselves. Some examples are:

- Fear related to new and strange surroundings of the procedure room
- Pain related to lumbar puncture
- Deficient knowledge related to technique for 24-hour urine collection
- Deficient diversionary activity related to hospitalization and lengthy procedures
- Imbalanced nutrition, less than body requirements, related to need for food restriction preprocedure and postprocedure
- Risk for injury related to need for intrusive procedures

Outcome Identification and Planning

As every procedure can result in even more stress than that caused by the primary illness, an important nursing goal is to cause the least degree of anxiety possible while completing interventions. To achieve this goal, plan specific ways to prepare children in advance, such as the best way to explain a procedure to a particular child. Also ensure the child is not overwhelmed by the number of diagnostic or therapeutic procedures performed in any one day. With small children, it may make more sense to stagger ambulatory diagnostic tests over several days to preserve a child's coping ability. Conversely, some older children (and parents) do better if they can complete all necessary tests in 1 day, so they do not have to anticipate more testing over a long period. Use nursing judgment and data from periodic assessments to help primary care providers determine the type of schedule that is in the child's and family's best interest. A helpful Web site to recommend for parents to help them prepare children for procedures is http://www.kidshealth.org.

Implementation

Whether assisting with a procedure or performing a therapeutic intervention, it is necessary to function in several roles at the same time: performing (or assisting with) the procedure, providing active support to the child and parents, and observing and then documenting the child's reactions. Providing support is a major role, and there are many ways to do this, such as holding a child's hand or placing a hand on the parent's shoulder. Playing a distracting game with an older child can also be helpful. Important observations to be made include signs of discomfort, changes in vital signs, or other signals of distress such as pallor or dizziness. Maintain a flow sheet of observations during a procedure. After a procedure the child's reaction, and specimens obtained can then be documented accurately and efficiently in the child's record.

As a final follow-through step, think of therapeutic play techniques to introduce that would be helpful in relieving stress caused by the procedure.

Outcome Evaluation

Evaluating expected outcomes related to diagnostic and therapeutic procedures not only helps in determining the effect of the procedure on a child but also aids in future planning, should other procedures be required. Recording that a particular child who did not appear nervous during a procedure later admitted to being "more scared than I've ever been before," for example, can help another nurse provide reassurance to this child, even when the child is masking emotions the next time. Examples suggesting achievement of expected outcomes are:

- Child says she is able to cope with second bone marrow aspiration.
- Child lists steps to take to collect 24-hour urine at home.
- Child participates in 1 hour of active exercise daily.
- Child eats a minimum of 1000 calories per day.
- Child experiences minimal loss of blood (less than 10 mL) during diagnostic procedure.
- Parent outlines plan to use alternative therapies to reduce the child's anxiety.

NURSING RESPONSIBILITIES WITH DIAGNOSTIC AND THERAPEUTIC TECHNIQUES

The most efficient way to reduce children's stress from hospitalization is to reduce the number of hospitalizations necessary. When hospitalization does become necessary, reducing the stress of the experience through being certain that procedures are carried out in the least stressful way possible is necessary. Responsibilities when assisting with procedures performed on children include:

- Helping obtain informed consent as needed
- Explaining the procedure to the child and the parents to be certain both are well informed
- Scheduling the procedure
- Preparing the child physically and psychologically
- Obtaining necessary equipment for the procedure
- Accompanying a child to a treatment room or hospital department where the procedure will be performed
- Providing support during the procedure using the least amount of restraint possible
- Ensuring adherence to standard infection precautions
- Assessing a child's response to the procedure
- Providing care to a child and specimens obtained once the procedure is completed
- Overseeing or cooperating with other health care disciplines to ensure the safety and efficacy of all procedures

Obtaining Informed Consent

Consent to perform a procedure must be obtained if a procedure carries any risk that would not be present if it were not performed. For a parent to sign a consent form, the parent must be knowledgeable about the content of the procedure and the risks of having or not having it performed. Although obtaining consent is the physician's responsibility, assuring that it is obtained is a nursing responsibility. Acting as an advocate for a family if they do not understand the consent form, the procedure, or the risks of the procedure is an important nursing role. Be certain the rights of emancipated minors are respected and that, in single-parent families, the custodial parent is the one who is asked to give the permission.

Explaining Procedures

To be able to explain procedures clearly and answer questions about them appropriately, try to observe as many procedures as you can. Asking children after any procedure what sensations they experienced can help children work through possibly frightening situations (often called "debriefing") and also increase your knowledge of common procedures (Wennstrom, Hallberg, & Bergh, 2008) (Box 37.2).

As a general guide, a child needs a detailed description of the procedure, such as, "I'll clean your finger. You will feel a small pinprick," as well as an explanation of:

- Why the procedure is being performed—for example, "The doctor needs to look at your blood to see why you're so sick."
- Where the procedure will be done—for instance, the radiography department or a treatment room
- Any unusual sensations to be expected during the procedure, such as, "Alcohol for cleaning your skin will feel cold."
- Any pain involved: "The needle will sting, although I'll put some cream on first to dull the feeling."
- Any strange equipment used, such as an x-ray machine
- The approximate length of time the procedure will take
- Any special care after the procedure—for example, "You will need to lie quietly for 15 minutes afterward."

Be certain to use age-appropriate language when explaining procedures. Also be careful not to use words that might be confusing during an explanation, such as "transducer" or "electrode," without defining them. Try to associate the procedure with something with which a child is already familiar and comfortable such as describing an x-ray machine as "a big camera." Try not to use the word "test" in explanations because school-age children associate the word "test" with a pass/fail situation. This can make them unduly worried after a procedure about whether they have "passed" it.

BOX 37.2 * Focus on Evidence-Based Practice

Does "debriefing" help children adjust to surgical procedures?

Fear of separation, unfamiliar routines, anesthetic/operation expectations/experiences, and pain and needles are all potential sources of fear or worry in children. To see if perioperative discussions would help relieve stress, researchers selected 15 boys and 5 girls (aged 6–9 years) scheduled for elective day surgery. They collected data on the children's response to surgery by a tape-recorded preoperative interview, participant observations, and asking children to make a preoperative and postoperative drawing. Results of the study showed that the main problem children revealed was feeling forced into an unpredictable and distressful situation. Preoperatively, they did not know what to expect and did not like "breaking away from their daily routine." A common reaction was "trying to gain control" over the situation. During the perioperative period, the categories "losing control" and "cooperating despite fear and pain" were reported. Postoperatively, the categories "breathing a sigh of relief" and "regaining normality in life" emerged.

Based on the above, would it be important to talk to children about a surgical experience afterward or would it be less stressful if the subject wasn't brought up again?

Source: Wennstrom, B., Hallberg, L. R., & Bergh, I. (2008). Use of perioperative dialogues with children undergoing day surgery. *Journal of Advanced Nursing, 62*(1), 96–106.

If you are unfamiliar with what a procedure entails, do not guess as nothing is more confusing to children or parents than being told two different versions of something. Most technical personnel will take the time to describe important information a child should know about a study or procedure to you so you can relay this to the child. Having a well-informed patient makes the technician's job easier. Be certain parents receive an explanation of the procedure as well as the child. A child has difficulty relaxing if parents are still anxious because they do not understand what is going to happen. Encourage parents to stay with a child during most procedures, because they can be extremely helpful in reducing a procedure's threatening aspects (Pruitt et al., 2008).

Scheduling

Most diagnostic procedures are scheduled on an ambulatory basis. Try to arrange for a child to have time for meals and some free play time between procedures. If food or fluid must be restricted for procedures, monitor the child's degree of discomfort and physiologic needs related to this; advocate as necessary for a time lapse between examinations or improved coordination in scheduling to decrease the time spent without food or fluid. Most of the time, small sips of water or ice chips are acceptable, depending on the procedure.

Preparing a Child and Family Physically and Psychologically

Physical preparation varies depending on what procedure is to be performed. In many instances, preparing a child for an examination such as a barium enema involves another procedure such as a saline enema, so physical preparation becomes education for the actual examination. In all instances, explain both the preparative and actual procedures. Appropriate explanations aid in reducing anxiety and fear.

For many procedures, especially those that may be painful such as a bronchoscopy (see section on Direct Visualization Procedures), children may be administered nitrous oxide (Farrell et al., 2008). Conscious sedation may also be used (Hertzog & Havidich, 2007). Conscious sedation refers to a depressed level of consciousness induced by the intravenous administration of a sedative such as midazolam in combination with a narcotic such as morphine sulfate and perhaps a hypnotic such as propofol. About 60 minutes before the procedure, children may be given oral chloral hydrate to relieve both apprehension and make them feel sleepy.

While under conscious sedation, children are able to maintain their ability to breathe independently and also respond appropriately to verbal commands such as to lift their head. They feel minimal pain, however, because of the analgesic administered. Conscious sedation is used in both ambulatory and inpatient settings. Before conscious sedation is begun, emergency equipment, including respiratory and pharmacologic measures, must be readily available. The child's level of consciousness and ability to respond, heart rate, respiratory rate, blood pressure, and oxygen saturation are monitored during the procedure. Using conscious sedation is very effective to allow children to accept a potentially painful procedure emotionally and physically. If this is used, be certain a child is prepared both for the diagnostic procedure and for the use of conscious sedation.

Accompanying the Child

If a procedure will be done at a different site from the primary care clinic or hospital unit with which a child is comfortable, ideally a nurse whom the child knows should accompany the child as well as a parent to the other department and remain with the child for the procedure, or at least until the child has met a primary person who will be responsible for the procedure. Having a parent accompany a child is of additional invaluable help. Older children do well with being accompanied by only a nursing assistant as long as they have been introduced in advance to the new person who will give them care.

Before leaving the child's patient care unit or clinic, have the child void for comfort unless this is contraindicated. Check for any medication or specific assessment procedures such as a blood pressure recording that should be given or done before leaving the unit for another department, in case the child is away from the primary unit for an extended time. If a child is an inpatient, check also that the identification band is securely in place and readily visible despite any intravenous equipment. If there will be a considerable wait in another department, ask children if they would like to bring along an activity such as a game or book. Hallways can be cool. Provide adequate blankets for comfort, especially for infants. Always use cart straps and side rails for safety.

Providing Support

Children do well with diagnostic and evaluative procedures as long as they have adequate support from a concerned provider or parent. Try to provide this both verbally (explain what is going to happen; assure the child everything is going well) and nonverbally (a hand on the arm or a nearby presence).

Modifying Procedures According to a Child's Age and Developmental Stage

A child's age and potential understanding of procedures must be considered when planning the number and order of tests and the way they are performed.

The Infant

The number of painful or uncomfortable procedures done on infants should be kept to an absolute minimum to avoid interfering with an infant's developing sense of trust. Parents should be allowed to accompany their infant to hospital departments and remain during procedures to offer support. Some parents may ask to hold their child during a procedure that causes pain, but do not ask parents to restrain the child during such a procedure. Their role should be a supportive and comforting one, not a policing one.

Infants become dehydrated quickly so the time they can remain NPO for procedures must be limited. You may need to advocate for time for breastfeeding before and after procedures for both an infant's and mother's comfort. If a procedure continues longer than 3 to 4 hours, provide the mother a room in which to use a breast pump, if needed.

Infants need to be picked up and comforted after procedures (a child of any age likes a hug or honest compliment for cooperation). It is important that obtaining blood specimens (which can deplete an infant's small blood stores) and x-rays (which are possibly harmful to immature bone marrow) are also kept to a minimum in infants. Help parents understand why these procedures are being limited so they do not think their infant's care is being compromised by so few diagnostic procedures.

The Toddler and Preschooler

Toddlers and preschoolers resist any diagnostic testing that involves any degree of discomfort or pain or that is unfamiliar to them. Give children of this age short explanations of what to expect, close to the time of the procedure, so that little time can be spent worrying about it. Try to associate any new equipment with things which they are already familiar.

The School-Age Child and Adolescent

School-age children are interested in the theory and reason for procedures. Often they can be persuaded to cooperate for a procedure by being promised a look at their radiograph or a point-of-care meter readout afterward. Be careful to ensure that viewing the results is actually possible before promising this to children; otherwise, it can be difficult to obtain any further cooperation. Adolescents may project an air of maturity or sophistication beyond their years to remain in control of themselves in the face of frightening procedures. Do not be misled into thinking a child this age would not appreciate an explanation or a comforting hand on a shoulder during a procedure.

What if... A 14-year-old adolescent who is scheduled for a series of diagnostic tests, says, "I'm not a kid, you know," and refuses to listen when you start to explain a procedure? Later, he acts angry because he has been "tricked" into having the procedure. How could you give explanations to him without offending him? What do you think is the basis for his actions?

Promoting Safety During Procedures

Safety is an important component of all patient care. Children's immaturity, which makes them unable to form mature judgments, leaves them vulnerable to harm unless their caretakers give special consideration to promoting safety during procedures.

Nursing Diagnoses and Related Interventions

Nursing Diagnosis: Risk for injury related to diagnostic procedures

Outcome Evaluation: Child remains free of injury from diagnostic equipment.

As a basic safety measure, before giving any food or performing any procedure, read the name on a child's identification armband. If an armband must be removed because it interferes with an intravenous infusion site, cut it away but immediately anchor it to another extremity with adhesive tape. Ask the admissions department to provide a new armband as soon as possible. Do not leave the old one off while waiting for a replacement band; this leaves the child susceptible to the danger of mistaken identity during the waiting period.

Because of their natural curiosity, children tend to fuss with equipment to see what will happen if they turn a knob or spin a dial. This means they need close monitoring while procedures are performed to ensure they do not touch any buttons or in other ways accidentally harm themselves. After a procedure, be sure to remove all equipment from a room. Children may pick up scissors or forceps left at bedsides and injure an eye; syringes and needles can cause puncture injuries. They may drink antiseptics such as alcohol or povidone-iodine left at bedsides and poison themselves. Young children can choke on small objects such as needle covers.

Use of Restraints

The purpose of a restraint is to keep a child safe during a procedure. Always use the least amount of restraint necessary and apply with care, because if improperly applied, restraints can cause extreme stress and possibly more harm than help (Brenner, 2007). Children can have difficulty distinguishing between restraint and punishment, so restraint should never be used more often or for any longer a time than necessary. Be certain parents receive an explanation of why their child

has a restraint in place—for example, because of a particular danger of this procedure, it is safer for their child.

If restraints are in place, check them every 15 minutes to be certain they are not occluding circulation; remove them temporarily every hour so the body part can be exercised (provided the exercise does not dislodge a device or interfere with a treatment). No part of a child's body other than that which is necessary should be restrained. When infants have scalp vein infusions in place, such as for injection of a radioactive isotope for a nuclear medicine scan, for example, their arms may need to be immobilized so that they do not touch the infusion site. Their trunk may need to be immobilized so they do not turn. Their lower extremities may not have to be restrained, however, so they can still actively kick and exercise. When a nurse or a parent is with a child, in most instances, all restraints can be removed.

Various types of restraints are described in Table 37.1 and shown in Figure 37.1.

Providing Care After Procedures

After a procedure, assess how well a child reacted to the procedure by both observation and history. Allowing children to explain what happened helps them retrace the procedure in their mind so they can conquer their fear of it. Fill in gaps in information as necessary to improve a child's perception of

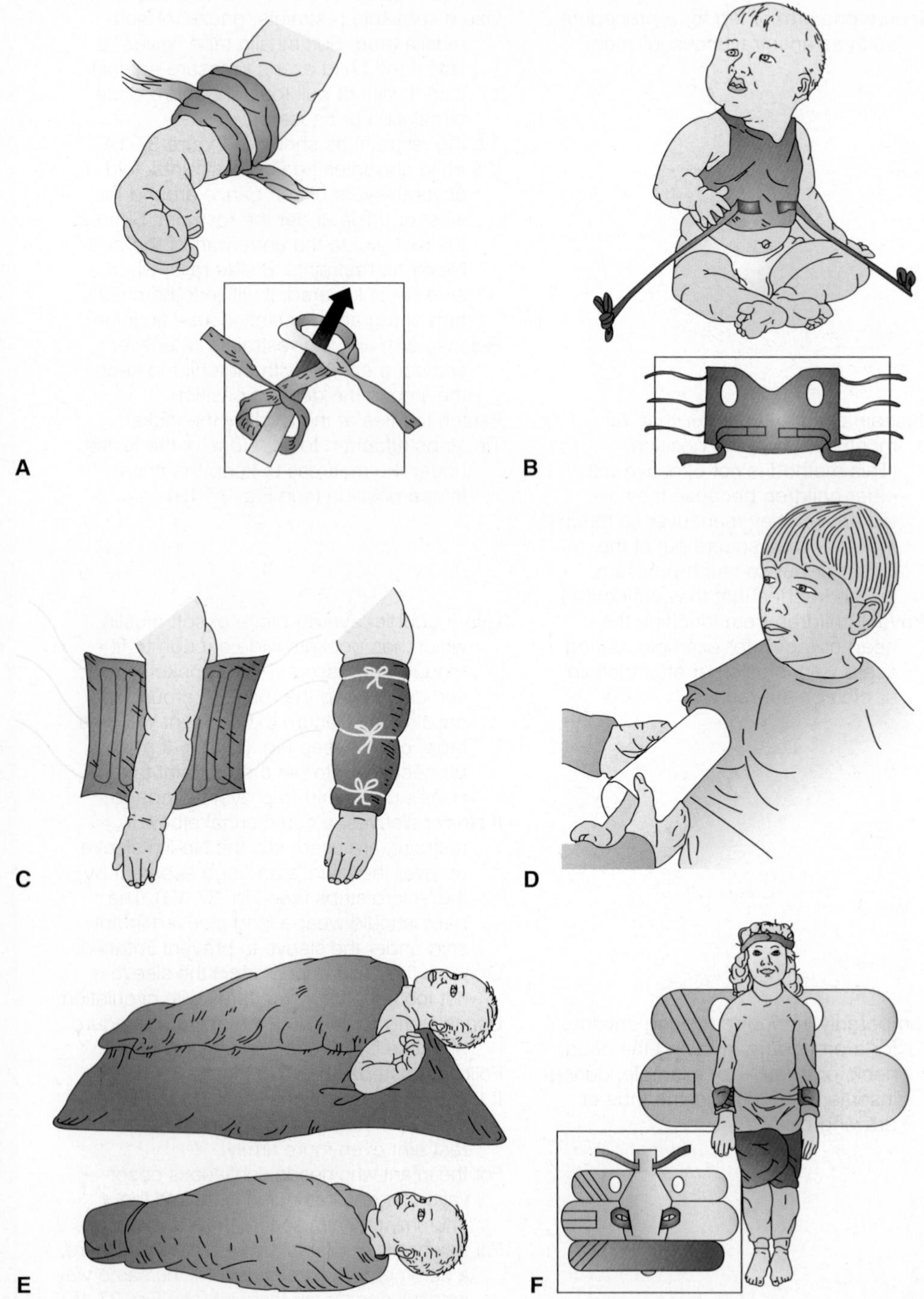

FIGURE 37.1 (**A**) Clove hitch restraint. (**B**) Jacket restraint. (**C**) Elbow restraint. (**D**) No-No sleeve or commercial elbow restraint. (**E**) Mummy restraint. (**F**) Papoose board.

TABLE 37.1 ❋ Safety Restraints

Type of Restraint	Purpose	Method
Wheelchairs and carts	Promote safety while transporting children to and from a procedure. Remind children to stay in a wheelchair while being transported. Prevent children from rolling off a cart while being transported.	For a wheelchair, use a vest restraint. Attach straps to the frame of the wheelchair with enough slack so the child has some mobility. For a cart, fasten a restraining belt and raise the side rails. Even with restraints in place, never leave a child unattended in hallways outside departments in a wheelchair or on a cart. Not only is this unsafe because the child may attempt to get down from the cart or wheelchair, but the anxiety of waiting in a strange department for a procedure is too acute for him or her to handle.
Clove-hitch restraints	Secure one arm or leg for a procedure, such as an intravenous infusion.	Use disposable restraints, gauze, or soft muslin tape. Soft muslin tape "gives" a little if the child exerts pressure against it so it will not pull too tight and reduce circulation or cause pain. Tie the restraint as shown in Figure 37-1A. If a child struggles against restraints, fold several layers of soft gauze around the wrist or ankle under the restraint. Secure the restraint to the underpart of the bed. Never tie restraints to side rails: when a side rail is lowered, it will jerk the child's arm or leg and possibly cause an injury. Release arm and leg restraints whenever someone can be with the child to keep the limb in the desired position.
Jacket restraints	Restrain children younger than 6 months in a supine position. (This method is not effective with older children because they are too active: they maneuver so much that they may squirm out of the jacket or put so much pressure on the trachea that they suffocate.)	Fasten the ties at the back of the jacket. Tie strips attached to the sides of the jacket under the mattress to keep the child in one position (see Fig. 37-1B).
Elbow restraints	Prevent children from touching the head or face—for example, during scalp vein infusion or after cleft lip or cleft palate repair.	Use a double-layered piece of soft muslin, which has pockets wide enough to fit tongue depressors. Place pockets vertically. Wrap the restraint around the child's arm. Secure the restraint with ties, tape, or pins (see Fig. 37-1C). It may be necessary to pin the restraint to the child's undershirt to prevent slippage. If No-No sleeves, a commercial elbow restraint, are used, slip the No-No sleeve up over the infant's arm and secure it by the Velcro strips (see Fig. 37-1D). The baby should wear a long-sleeved infant shirt under the sleeve to prevent irritation. Observe the child to be certain the sleeve is not too tight that it interferes with circulation.
Mummy restraints	Temporarily immobilize young children for a procedure involving the head, neck, or throat—for example, during insertion of a nasogastric tube or drawing blood.	Use this only for the duration of the procedure because it is a total body restraint. Follow the steps shown in Figure 37-1E. If the child is exceptionally strong, a few safety pins can be used to hold the restraint even more firmly. For the infant who needs continuous observation for respiratory function, fold the mummy restraint so the chest is exposed. For newborns or infants, use a "Papoose Board," a commercial restraint used in the same way as a full or mummy restraint (see Fig. 37-1F).

Activity:	Description:	Score:
Activity	Able to move four extremities	2
	Able to move two extremities	1
	Able to move no extremities	0
Respiration	Regular, able to deep breathe/cough	2
	Dyspnea, limited and obstructed breathing	1
	Apneic	0
Circulation	BP within 20 mm Hg of preprocedure	2
	BP within 20–25 mm Hg of preprocedure	1
	BP 25 mm Hg above preprocedure level	0
Level of consciousness	Awake, alert	5
	Drowsy, but easily aroused	4
	Stupor, aroused by vigorous stimuli	2
	Responds to pain only	1
	No response to pain	0
Skin color	Pink, warm, dry	2
	Pale, dusky, blotchy, clammy	1
	Cyanotic, diaphoretic, cold	0
Ambulation	Ambulates with minimum help	5
	Ambulates with minimum support	4
	Unable to ambulate	2

FIGURE 37.2 Post-Anesthesia Recovery Score. A passing score is at least 10 with a level of consciousness score no lower than 4. (From Tolia, V., et al. [2000]. Sedation for pediatric endoscopic procedures. *Journal of Pediatric Gastroenterology and Nutrition, 30*[5], 477–485.)

the procedure. Providing therapeutic play is another measure to reduce anxiety (see Chapter 36).

Be certain tissue samples obtained after a procedure such as bone marrow aspiration are sent to the proper department for analysis as soon as possible. Guard against specimens being dropped or improperly labeled; children do not have extra body fluids such as blood to sacrifice for additional specimen collection.

If conscious sedation was used, be sure children are awake before they are discharged home or return to an inpatient hospital unit. Using a postanesthesia score sheet (Fig. 37.2) is an effective method to rate recovery from anesthesia.

Children can be discharged as soon as 30 minutes after conscious sedation if they are awake and oriented, the airway is patent and respiratory status is stable (no retraction, stridor, or wheezing), oxygen saturation is 95% or greater in room air, and blood pressure, heart rate, and respiratory rates are appropriate for age, and the child is reasonably free of pain.

Parents often have questions about what care their child will need after they return home. Tips for parents following conscious sedation are highlighted in Box 37.3.

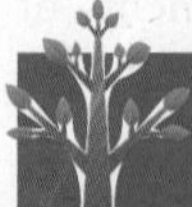

BOX 37.3 ✻ Focus on Family Teaching

Care After Conscious Sedation

Q. T.J.'s mother asks you, "My son received conscious sedation for his MRI. What special care will he need when he comes home?"

A. Here are some tips to help you when you get your son home:

- Keep in mind that most children sleep after leaving the ambulatory care facility or hospital. Some are sleepy for the remainder of the day.
- Do not allow the child to walk alone for at least 4 hours. The child may suddenly feel dizzy and fall without warning.
- Wait until getting home to give the child something to eat or drink, to avoid car sickness. Conscious sedation may cause children to feel nauseated more easily than usual.
- For the first 12 hours after the child wakes, do not ask him to do any activity that requires alertness, coordination, or balance, such as riding a bicycle, swimming, or doing homework. The sedative can affect the child's coordination and balance.
- Remember that the child may forget things readily for the rest of the day. This forgetfulness should go away after a night's sleep.
- Keep in mind that a sedative may cause children to behave in unexpected ways, such as losing self-control or becoming very emotional. By the next day, the child's behavior should return to normal.
- Give infants clear liquids (water, apple juice, tea) after getting home. Wait approximately 30 minutes to make sure the child does not choke or vomit. Then milk, formula, or other foods may be given.
- Do not allow children to drink until they can hold a cup without help, to make sure they are awake enough to keep from choking. Wait approximately 30 minutes. If there is no vomiting or choking, the child can be given food.
- Call your primary care provider if the child has pain or recurrent vomiting, or if any of the effects above last for more than 12 hours.

✔ **Checkpoint Question 37.1**

You are going to restrain T.J. to obtain a blood sample from his hand. What type of restraint would be best?

a. Ask his mother to hold him tightly on her lap.
b. Apply a jacket restraint to confine his body.
c. Ask a fellow nurse to hold his hand firmly.
d. Use a mummy restraint so he can't be hurt.

MEASURING VITAL SIGNS

Vital signs for children consist of temperature, pulse, respiratory rate, blood pressure, and pain assessment. All of these need to be recorded both conscientiously and with knowledge of the child's underlying condition so they can be analyzed meaningfully. Be especially alert that assessing any of these measures is not enough; if they are abnormal or if a child has pain, a measure to relieve the problem needs to be initiated (Schiavenato, 2008). Appendix G shows the average pulse rates, respiration rates, and blood pressures for children of different ages, as these differ according to the size and age of the child. Pain assessment is discussed in Chapter 39.

Temperature

Normal temperature values in children are the same as in adults: axillary, 97.6° F (36.5° C); oral or tympanic, 98.6° F (37.0° C); and rectal, 99.6° F (37.6° C). Thermometers that assess tympanic membrane temperature are ideal for assessment in children because they register within 2 seconds and therefore cause less fear in a child because a child has to be restrained for only a few seconds (Fig. 37.3A). Tympanic membrane temperatures may not be effective in newborns because of the vernix still present in their ears.

Newborns should not have their temperature taken rectally because of the danger of damaging their rectal mucosa with a thermometer; it should be taken by the axillary route instead (see Fig. 37.3B). Because preschoolers generally fear intrusive procedures, consider taking axillary or tympanic temperatures in children until 4 or 5 years of age.

For a tympanic temperature recording, insert the tip of the tympanic thermometer gently into the child's ear canal. Straighten the ear canal by pulling down on the earlobe in a child younger than age 2 and pulling up on the pinna of the child older than age 2. This directs the sensor beam toward the center of the tympanic membrane and not the sides of the canal. Tympanic membrane temperature is not affected by the presence of earwax, so it gives consistently accurate results. By 4 years of age, children are usually old enough to close their mouth sufficiently for oral temperature recording by an electronic thermometer.

For an axillary recording, place the tip of an electronic thermometer in the axilla and hold the child's arm down to the side to keep the thermometer firmly in place until it registers. For the rare occasions when a rectal temperature must be taken, insert a thermometer only to the length of the bulb (½ inch) in infants and not over 1 inch in older children, and hold it in place for 5 minutes.

Pulse Rate

As children grow older, the heart rate slows and the range of normal values narrows. If possible, measure a child's pulse rate at rest. An apical pulse (listening at the heart apex through a stethoscope) is taken in children younger than 1 year because their radial (wrist) pulse is too faint to be palpated accurately. In an infant, the point of maximum intensity, or the point on the chest wall where the heartbeat can be heard most distinctly, is just above and outside the left nipple (just lateral to the midclavicular line at the third or fourth intercostal space). This point gradually becomes more medial and slightly lower up to 7 years of age. By 7 years, it is at the fourth or fifth interspace at the midclavicular line. For greatest accuracy, count the pulse rate for 1 full minute.

Respiratory Rate

Respirations also should be measured before an infant is disturbed because the respiratory rate increases with crying. Take this while a child is sitting in a parent's lap or lying quietly in a crib before lowering the side rail if possible. Infants tend to breathe with their abdominal muscles; therefore, it is as accurate to take respirations by counting movements of the abdomen as it is to count chest movements. Again, for greatest accuracy, count respirations for 1 full minute.

Blood Pressure

Blood pressure is included in the routine physical assessment of all children older than 3 years of age. Offer a good expla-

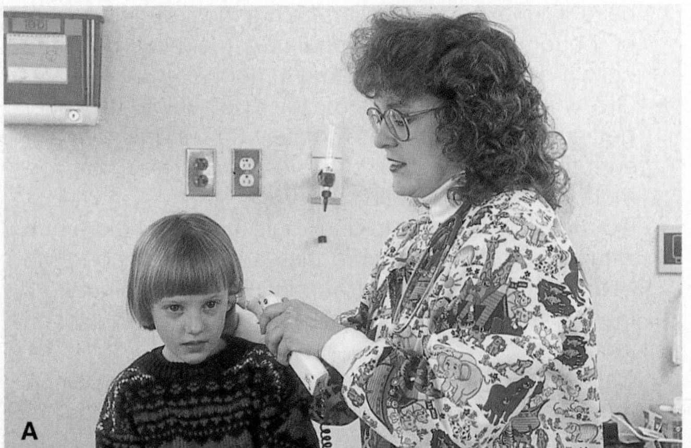
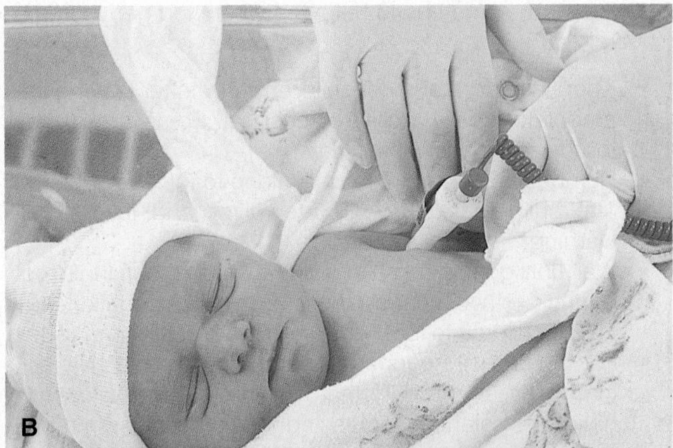

FIGURE 37.3 Temperature taking. (**A**) Tympanic membrane temperature. (**B**) Axillary temperature.

nation of the procedure, especially to young children, because wrapping their arm and applying pressure can be frightening if they are not prepared for it.

Systolic pressure in children is read as the manometer pressure is dropping, at the moment that sound first appears. The point at which the sound disappears is considered the diastolic pressure. Blood pressure is difficult to measure in infants because of mechanical problems. The cuff used should be no more than two-thirds and not less than one-half the length of their upper arm; a wider cuff (larger bladder size) gives a lower reading and a narrower cuff gives a higher reading (Fig. 37.4). Doppler ultrasound blood pressure recording is especially effective with infants. This technique bounces high-frequency sound waves off body parts; the rate and pitch at which they return depends on the density of the body part that is struck. If a Doppler lead is placed over an artery, either the movement of the blood (pulse wave) or its tension (blood pressure) can be registered on a digital readout or monitor print. Doppler examinations can be adapted to broadcast the sound of the pulse waves for auscultatory assessment.

Electronic blood pressure recording is most helpful when a continuous assessment is necessary, but it can be used for a single recording. Watching the digital readout numbers is interesting for preschoolers. Electronic pressure readings are typically 5 mm Hg higher for diastolic and 10 mm Hg higher for systolic blood pressure compared with auscultatory techniques (Brayden, Daley, & Brown, 2008). Direct measurement (intra-arterial monitoring by an indwelling catheter into the radial or femoral artery) is used with children who are critically ill. This technique is reviewed in Chapter 41.

Lower extremity blood pressure can be obtained by wrapping the cuff over the thigh and palpating or auscultating the popliteal pulse (posterior knee). In infants younger than 1 year, the thigh and arm blood pressure should be equal. In children older than 1 year, the systolic pressure in the thigh tends to be 10 to 40 mm Hg higher, while diastolic pressure remains the same. If the thigh blood pressure reading is lower than that in the arm, suspect that coarctation of the aorta or an interference with circulation to the lower extremities may be causing this.

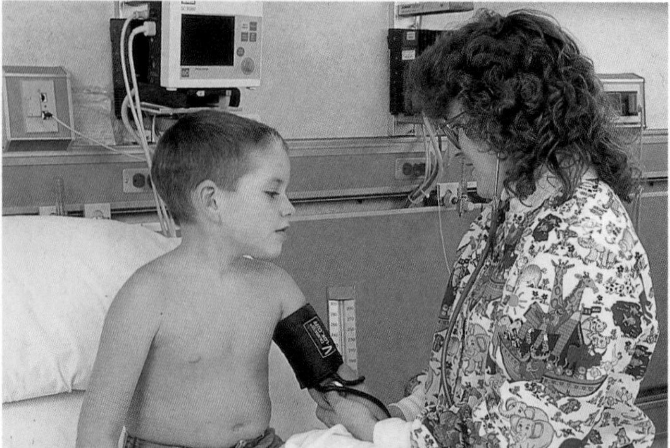

FIGURE 37.4 Measurement of blood pressure is essential during routine health assessments and before diagnostic or therapeutic procedures. Here a nurse assesses a child's blood pressure in preparation for a procedure.

When assessing blood pressure, be certain to pay attention to the pulse pressure—the difference between systolic and diastolic readings. Both unusually wide (more than 50 mm Hg) or narrow (less than 10 mm Hg) ranges may suggest congenital heart disease. An abnormally narrow pulse pressure, for instance, is a sign of aortic stenosis. An abnormally low diastolic pressure (causing a wide pulse pressure) occurs with patent ductus arteriosus.

REDUCING ELEVATED TEMPERATURE IN CHILDREN

Fever is such a common symptom in children that reducing temperature or giving a parent instructions on how to reduce a child's temperature at home is a common intervention with children.

Nursing Diagnoses and Related Interventions

Nursing Diagnosis: Risk for hyperthermia related to illness affecting temperature regulation, medications, or surgery

Outcome Evaluation: Child's temperature returns to 98.6° F (37° C) orally within 2 hours.

Because the temperature-regulating mechanism in children is immature, fever tends to be more marked in children than in adults and may even be out of proportion to the seriousness or extent of their disease. An increased temperature occurs because a child's temperature-regulating point (set point) has been elevated. The child's temperature cannot be reduced until the set point returns (or is returned) to normal.

Tylenol and Motrin are excellent antipyretics, so they are the drugs most often prescribed to reduce fever in children (Boxes 37.4 and 37.5).

BOX 37.4 * Focus on Pharmacology

Acetaminophen (Tylenol)

Action: Used for moderate temperature elevation or pain; does not have anti-inflammatory properties (Karch, 2009)

Pregnancy risk category: B

Dosage: Oral: 10–15 mg/kg every 4–6 hours as needed; may repeat 4 or 5 times per day; do not exceed 5 doses in 24 hours

Possible adverse effects: Elevated liver enzymes, jaundice, rash

Nursing Implications

- Caution parents that drug can cause severe liver toxicity with overdose.
- Educate parents not to administer a larger dose or more frequently than prescribed.
- Encourage parents to increase the child's fluid intake to aid in reducing fever.

BOX 37.5 ✻ Focus on Pharmacology

Ibuprofen (Advil, Pediaprofen)

Action: Used to reduce inflammation, fever, and mild to moderate pain

Pregnancy risk category: B; D if used in last trimester

Dosage: (for fever or pain) 5–10 mg/kg every 6–8 hours; do not exceed 40 mg in 24 hours

Possible adverse effects: Gastric upset, headache, dizziness, nausea, occult blood loss, prolonged bleeding, peptic ulceration

Nursing Implications

- Use with caution in children with gastrointestinal irritation.
- Drug can cause renal failure if child becomes dehydrated; encourage fluid intake.
- Administer with food or drink to minimize gastrointestinal irritation.

Parents often do not give an adequate dose of an antipyretic such as acetaminophen because they are afraid their child will have a bad reaction to it. This results in the high fever continuing. Encourage them to give a full dose of the antipyretic every 4 hours, up to five doses a day, until their child's temperature is reduced. Teach parents that fever is actually a body protection measure, and unless it is exceptionally high (more than 106° F [41.1° C]), it does no specific harm. In fact, there is some evidence that fever may be of value in helping to combat infection, because it aids in destroying microorganisms (Edwards et al., 2007). For this reason, caution parents that fever itself is not harmful so they don't give too high a dose of an antipyretic or a severe overdose where liver or kidney toxicity can occur (Karch, 2009). An antipyretic is generally ordered for any child whose oral or tympanic temperature is more than 101° F (38.4° C) or whose rectal temperature is more than 102° F (39.0° C). Caution parents not to give acetylsalicylic acid (aspirin) to children with fever because aspirin is associated with Reye's syndrome, a severe neurologic disorder (see Chapter 49).

In addition to antipyretic administration, parents should dress children with fever in lightweight clothing, such as summer pajamas. Remove all clothing but the diaper from an infant. Many parents dress febrile children warmly in flannel nightgowns to keep them from "getting a chill." This actually increases the child's temperature and does not prevent the shaking, trembling reaction that comes with high fever. Placing a cool cloth (not ice) on a child's forehead can feel comforting. Although sponging children to lower temperature may be effective in a small group of children, it is no longer recommended for children as a whole, because it can lead to extreme chilling and shock to an immature nervous system and has little advantage over the use of oral antipyretics (Meremikwu & Oyo-Ita, 2009).

Caution parents that common antipyretics for children's fever taste like candy. Be sure they know to lock antipyretics away or children can help themselves to more "candy" when a parent's back is turned.

COMMON DIAGNOSTIC PROCEDURES

Diagnostic and therapeutic procedures used with children vary depending on a child's condition and age but are similar to those used with adults. Blood, urine, and stool studies are commonly ordered. Respiratory illnesses require special procedures; these are discussed in Chapter 40 with respiratory disorders. Biopsies (surgical procedures to remove tissue for examination) are discussed in Chapter 53. Stress testing for cardiovascular pathology is discussed in Chapter 41.

Electrical Impulse Studies

Electrical impulse studies are those that include electrical conduction. Children need special preparation for studies such as electrocardiograms (ECGs; Fig. 37.5) or electroencephalograms (EEGs) because they have been warned not to play with electric wires and so may worry about being burned or electrocuted. They can be reassured that the electricity passes from their body to the machine, not the other way around; except for electromyelograms (study of the conduction paths of the spinal cord), children can be assured that these tests are painless. Electrodes are attached to the body by paste, which is easily removable. If possible, give the child a portion of the test strip afterward as a souvenir.

X-Ray Studies

A variety of x-ray studies are used to inspect internal body tissues. These range from simple x-rays to the more complicated computed tomography (CT) scan or dye contrast study.

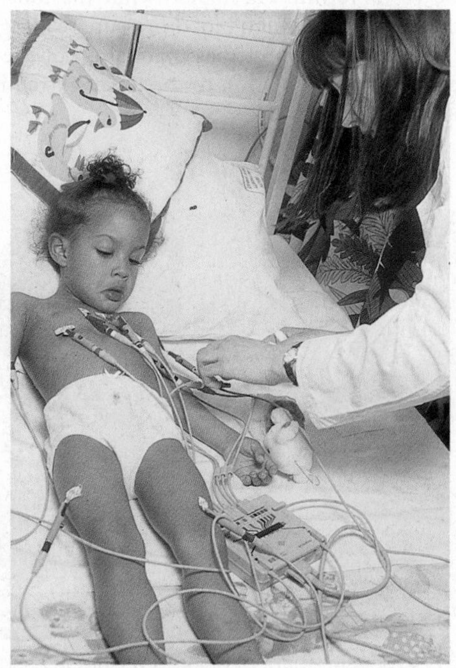

FIGURE 37.5 Administering an ECG. Children can be assured this is a painless procedure. (From John Watney/Photo Researchers, Inc.)

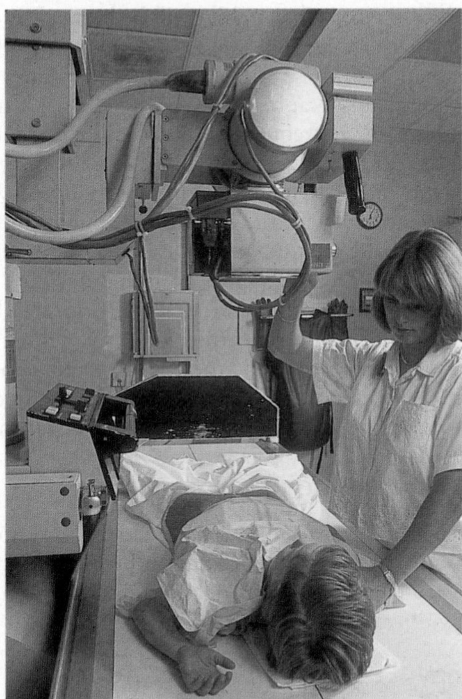

FIGURE 37.6 Positioning of a child for an x-ray. (© Bachmann/Stock Boston.)

Flat-Plate Radiographs

Radiographs are used both to diagnose illness and check the placement of apparatus such as gastrointestinal feeding tubes. As a rule, children accept radiographs well because an x-ray machine can be compared with a camera, an instrument with which they are familiar (Fig. 37.6). Caution children that although you or a parent may be able to accompany them to the x-ray department, you will not be allowed to stay in the room while the picture is actually taken. If it is necessary for you to remain in the room to restrain a child, do not do this without lead apron and lead glove protection. Such protection is also necessary for portable radiographs taken at a child's or infant's bedside.

Dye Contrast Studies

To visualize a body cavity, some type of radiopaque dye may be swallowed or injected into the cavity and then examined on radiography. **Barium contrast studies,** for example, are used to observe the outline of the gastrointestinal tract. Barium may be swallowed to outline the upper gastrointestinal tract or instilled by enema to outline the lower portion. Caution a child that barium, even if flavored, does not taste terribly good. In studies such as an intravenous pyelogram (IVP), dye is injected intravenously; as it circulates to the kidneys, a radiograph is taken. Because iodine is incorporated in most radiopaque material, be sure to check whether a child is allergic to iodine before the procedure. When the dye is injected, the child may feel a hot flush, a sensation that can be frightening if the child is unprepared for this. Try not to use the word "dye" while describing the procedure to prevent young children from worrying they will be dyed like an Easter egg or will "die." Say "medicine" instead.

Children easily grow bored during this type of procedure because of the time involved waiting for the dye to reach the specific organ to be studied. Have the child take along an activity to make the time pass faster. If children are not allowed to eat for the duration of a long procedure, be certain that they receive supervision or else, not realizing the importance of this, they may decide to snack. Ensure that parents understand that children do not "radiate" x-rays or radioactivity after the procedure, so they will not be afraid to hold a child closely for comfort.

Computed Tomography

Computed tomography (CT) is an x-ray procedure in which many views of an organ or body part are obtained to represent what the organ would look like if it were cut into thin slices. As with any radiograph, dense structures appear white and less dense structures appear gray to black on the films.

The procedure may require injection of an iodine-based contrast medium. If a radioisotope is added, the study is referred to as **positron emission tomography (PET)** or **single-photon emission computed tomography (SPECT).**

Because a CT scan involves so many films, it is a lengthy procedure. The machinery is complex, large, and potentially frightening (Fig. 37.7A). Children must lie still during the long procedure to avoid creating shadows on the film. To help them lie still for an extended period, they may be given a sedative such as chloral hydrate before the procedure to make them sleepy. Conscious sedation also may be used. You

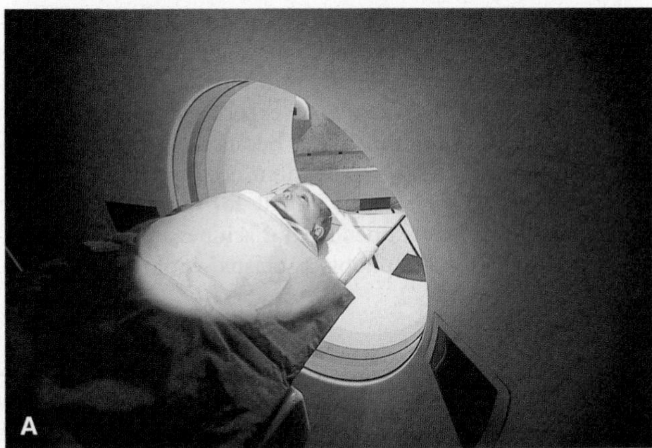

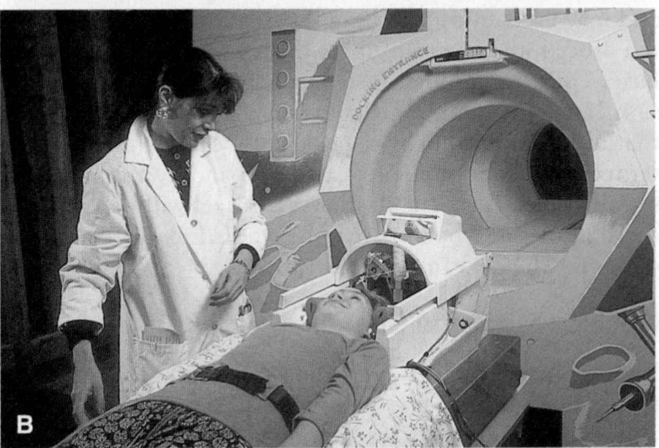

FIGURE 37.7 Some procedures are potentially frightening because of the size of the machinery used. (**A**) A CT scanner. (From Alexander Tsiara/Photo Researchers, Inc.) (**B**) An MRI scanner. (From Richard Nowitz/Photo Researchers, Inc.)

can assure parents that although the radiation exposure from CT scans occurs over a long period, such low doses are used that the actual exposure is comparable to a regular x-ray. Repeated CT scans, however, can carry a threat of excessive radiation exposure (Rice et al., 2007).

Magnetic Resonance Imaging

Magnetic resonance imaging (MRI) combines a magnetic field, radiofrequency, and computer technology to produce diagnostic images to aid in the diagnosis of disorders such as the cause of renal or brain pathology (Akpinar, Koroglu, & Ptak, 2007). The child lies on a moving pallet that is pushed into the core of the machine—the magnet (see Fig. 37.7B). When the magnetic field surrounding the child is turned on, it causes tissue atoms to line up in a parallel fashion. As radio waves are turned on and off, the atoms change position. This change is sensed and converted into a visual display on a computer screen.

The procedure has an advantage over radiography in that it has no apparent ill effects, it can reveal astonishingly clear structural defects in soft tissue, and if a contrast medium is required, it is not iodine based, so the danger of a reaction is minimal. Because metal may deflect the magnetic waves, children with a metal prosthesis or metal dental braces may be poor candidates for the procedure. Hairpins and eye makeup (which often has a metallic base), watches, or other jewelry or medals should be removed. Be certain a child's hospital gown does not have a metal snap at the neckline.

When the radio waves are turned on and off during the procedure, a booming noise occurs. Prepare children for this sound (often compared with the sound of drums) as well as the feeling of claustrophobia they may experience (see Focus on Nursing Care Planning Box 37.6). Because the procedure may take up to 45 minutes, some children need a sedative or conscious sedation so they can lie quietly for the duration of the procedure. Newer, more open MRI machines are able to alleviate the feeling of claustrophobia associated with the procedure.

Ultrasound

Ultrasound is a painless procedure in which images of internal tissue and organs, such as the appendix, are produced by the use of sound waves (Gracey & McClure, 2007). Because it is noninvasive, children accept ultrasound easily and may even enjoy watching the oscilloscope screen during the procedure. The transducer that is used on the body surface to pick up internal images can be compared to a television camera (Fig. 37.8). Be certain that parents understand that ultrasound is not an x-ray and appears to have no long-term effects, so it can be repeated over and over for serial determinations. Alert a child that a clear gel will be applied to the skin over the body part to be studied to aid sound conduction. The gel can feel cold and sticky.

Nuclear Medicine Studies

Radiopharmaceuticals are radioactive-combined substances that, when given orally or by injection, flow to designated body organs. When a scintillation machine (a form of Geiger counter) is passed over the organ where the radiopharmaceutical has collected, the pattern of the collected material outlines the organ; the pattern can be produced as a screen image or a photograph.

Parents may worry that a child will be harmed by such exposure to a radioactive substance. You can assure them the dose of radiation in these studies is no greater than that used for a diagnostic radiograph, so this is not a danger. Tagged iodine (iodine-131) is frequently the medium used for such studies. A danger of iodine is that it will go immediately to the thyroid gland rather than the organ to be studied when injected intravenously, with the result that enough concentrated radioactivity could accumulate to destroy the thyroid gland. For this reason, a blocking agent such as potassium perchlorate that prevents thyroid gland accumulation may be given prior to the test. This prevents the radioactive substance from concentrating in the thyroid, thereby protecting the gland. Always check whether a blocking agent is required before transporting a child to the nuclear medicine department.

Direct Visualization Procedures

Direct visualization procedures involve the observation of an internal body cavity by way of a thin tube inserted through a body surface opening. Types of direct visualization include endoscopy, bronchoscopy, and colonoscopy.

Endoscopy

Endoscopy involves an endoscope passed through the mouth to examine the gastrointestinal tract. It has become a common method of diagnosis for gastrointestinal disorders in children. When first developed, endoscopes were straight, stiff, metal instruments, so their use was limited. Currently, endoscopes are fiberoptic (using a flexible, easily maneuvered, brightly lit tube), so these examinations have become more common and certainly not as uncomfortable as before.

The procedure is often frightening, however, as manipulation is necessary. A child can easily understand an explanation of the procedure (the physician will extend the child's head and pass a tube down into the child's stomach for direct observation), but the child is uncomfortable at the thought of someone doing it. Children are placed on nothing by mouth (NPO) status for about 4 hours before the procedure. They may need a sedative or conscious sedation so they can lie quietly for the time needed. Good support during the procedure is also important. Ask whether a child can have a digital photograph taken during the procedure to keep as a souvenir. Endoscopy is also used as an emergency measure to remove objects such as quarters or safety pins swallowed by children.

After an endoscopy study, edema may occur from the pressure of the scope on the esophagus and pharynx. This means that the child requires close observation afterward to be certain edema is not interfering with a vital function such as respiration or causing discomfort. After the procedure, it is important to check that the child's gag reflex has returned before offering any fluid to drink. Observe closely the first time the child drinks after the procedure to ensure that the gag reflex is intact despite throat edema from the procedure or the effect of a local pharyngeal anesthetic that may have been sprayed into the throat before the procedure.

Bronchoscopy

Bronchoscopy is the direct visualization of the larynx, trachea, and bronchi through a lit, flexible, fiberoptic tube (a

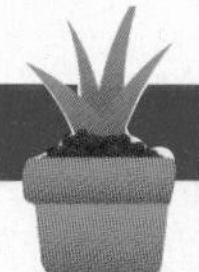

BOX 37.6 ✻ Focus on Nursing Care Planning

A Multidisciplinary Care Map for a Child in Need of Diagnostic Tests

T.J. Balliff is a preschooler who is scheduled to have a magnetic resonance imaging (MRI) study for a possible head injury.

Family Assessment ✻ Child lives with single-parent mother in two-bedroom loft in refurbished inner-city warehouse. Mother is a commercial artist. Rates finances as "healthy."

Client Assessment ✻ Child was playing at community playground with nanny. Was pushed off top of slide by another child. Fell approximately 6 feet onto head. Brought to ER by mother. Neck brace applied. T = 100.6 tympanic; P = 90; BP = 100/65. Crying from pain in neck and upper back. "How can I agree to an MRI?" his mother asks you. "He's afraid of the dark. How can I allow him to be wheeled into a long dark machine?"

Nursing Diagnosis ✻ Anxiety (child and parent) related to necessary diagnostic procedure

Outcome Criteria ✻ Mother listens to explanation of advantages of MRI for diagnosis of head, neck, or spine injury. Voices agreement to allow procedure. Helps prepare child for anxiety-filled experience.

Team Member Responsible	Assessment	Intervention	Rationale	Expected Outcome
		Activities of Daily Living		
Nurse	Assess by history if child has change of behavior from usual.	Review with parent that traumatic events can affect all body systems.	Head injury, if severe, can affect vital signs and thinking.	Parents states she feels child is reacting normally except for neck pain.
		Consultations		
Physician	Complete physical and neurologic exam. Assess if further neurologic consultation will be necessary.	Consult as necessary with neurologist about child's condition and continued care based on MRI findings.	A 6-foot fall could cause considerable intracranial swelling depending on whether child broke fall or not.	Neurologist on call completes necessary consult and any needed additional procedures.
		Procedures/Medications		
Nurse	Assess what medicine child is usually given for pain.	Administer acetaminophen per physician order to child.	Relieving pain is a prime responsibility with injured children.	Child swallows oral analgesic without complications.
Pain management nurse	Assess if child has past allergies or reactions to any medication.	Prepare child and administer conscious sedation.	Conscious sedation will allow child to sleep during an otherwise frightening procedure.	Child and mother consent to conscious sedation. Sedation is used during procedure without complication.
Nurse	Assess which MRI technician is available for procedure.	Meet with MRI technician to review child's fear of the dark.	Reducing children's fears often requires a multidisciplinary approach.	MRI technician takes active measures to try to reduce fear during procedure.
		Nutrition		
Nurse	Assess last time child ate or drank.	Keep child NPO prior to procedure.	Conscious sedation can cause aspiration in children with full stomachs.	Child remains NPO until postprocedure.

(continued)

BOX 37.6 ✻ Focus on Nursing Care Planning (continued)

Patient/Family Education				
Nurse/nurse practitioner	Assess parent's understanding of the need and technique of MRI.	Fill in gaps of knowledge for parent about procedure.	A well-informed parent is able to make well-informed decisions about care.	Mother states she understands why procedure is needed. Signs procedure consent.
Psychosocial/Spiritual/Emotional Needs				
Nurse/pain management nurse	Assess if child is mature enough to understand increasing increments.	Ask child to rate his pain by a FACES pain scale.	As pain is a subjective symptom, self-rating best reveals its nature.	Child uses pain scale to establish a baseline preprocedure and again postprocedure.
Nurse	Assess if child is still frightened from bullying episode at playground.	Review with child that bad things happen to good people.	Discussion of an accident can help to relieve guilt and increase self-esteem.	Child discusses what happened; states accident was not his fault.
Discharge Planning				
Nurse/physician	Assess if parent understands importance of assessing child's temperature and pulse every 4 hours after return home.	Review with parent technique for temperature and pulse assessment.	An increasing temperature and decreasing pulse rate can indicate increased intracranial pressure.	Parent confirms she will be able to take vital signs accurately; will notify ER if vital signs vary from norms given her.

bronchofiberscope). The procedure is used with children who have aspirated a foreign object such as a peanut or to take culture and biopsy specimens (Righini et al., 2007). Before the procedure, the child may be given atropine by injection to reduce bronchial secretions and to encourage bronchial relaxation. Typically, the throat is sprayed with a local pharyngeal anesthetic to numb the area. Because the procedure can be frightening and this makes it difficult for a child to cooperate, a sedative or conscious sedation usually is administered. Any manipulation of the airway has the potential to cause increased bronchial secretions and edema, leading to narrowing of the airway. Therefore, closely observe the child's respiratory function and airway for at least 4 hours after the procedure. An ice bag applied to the neck often helps reduce the possibility of edema and relieve throat discomfort. Assess for the presence of a gag reflex before offering any oral fluids to the child after the procedure. Observe children carefully the first time they drink after the procedure to be certain their gag reflex is intact and they do not choke.

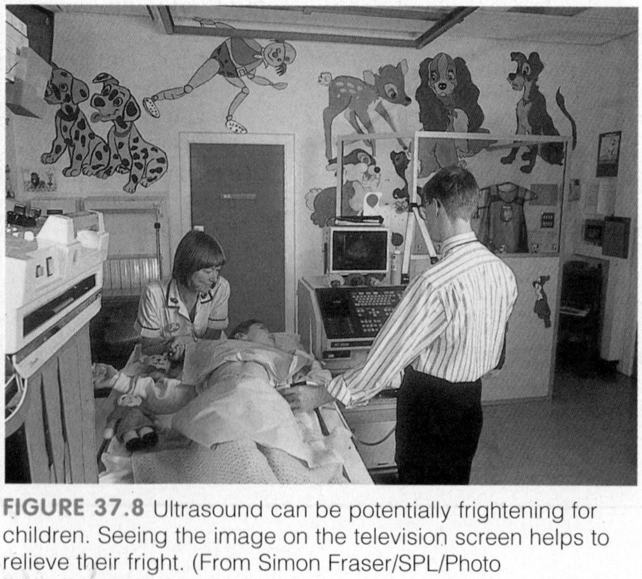

FIGURE 37.8 Ultrasound can be potentially frightening for children. Seeing the image on the television screen helps to relieve their fright. (From Simon Fraser/SPL/Photo Researchers, Inc.)

Colonoscopy

Colonoscopy is endoscopic examination of the large intestine with a flexible fiberscope inserted through the anus and advanced as far as the ileocecal valve. Air is then infused to expand the bowel walls. The technique allows the colon walls to be visualized; if abnormalities are found, photographs can be taken for analysis. It is used to diagnose inflammatory bowel disease or obtain biopsies if a malignancy is suspected (de Ridder et al., 2007).

Before the procedure, children are given a clear liquid diet for about 24 hours. Then they are given an isotonic saline laxative that causes fluid diarrhea so their bowel is clean for the procedure. It can be difficult for younger children to drink as much of the laxative solution as is needed to clear their bowel completely of stool. Playing games such as "Simon Says" can be helpful to gain their cooperation. If the laxative cannot be taken, a saline enema may be necessary. Conscious sedation is used during the procedure to reduce discomfort.

Box 37.8 Nursing Procedure ✻ Technique for fingertip or heel capillary puncture

Purpose: To obtain a blood sample from a peripheral capillary.

Procedure	Principle
1. Wash your hands; identify child; explain procedure to child.	**1.** Prevents spread of microorganisms from you to child. Confirms you are performing procedure on the right child. Promotes safety and well-being.
2. Assess status of puncture site.	**2.** Site must be warm and free of lesions.
3. Analyze appropriateness of procedure; adjust plan to individual circumstances.	**3.** Nursing care is always individualized based on professional judgment of client need.
4. Plan and give health teaching and preparation information as necessary.	**4.** Health teaching and preparation is an independent nursing action always included in care.
5. Assemble necessary equipment: gloves, alcohol swab, lancet, collecting capillary blood tube, dry compress or cotton ball, adhesive bandage.	**5.** Organization and preparation help conserve energy and maximize efficiency.
6. Assess the temperature of the selected site. Fingertips and heels must be warm. Warm by holding finger or heel in your hand for a moment or two. Warming heels or fingers by immersing them in warm water or covering with a warm compress is not advised.	**6.** Although warmth helps to dilate vessels and allows blood to flow more freely, warm water methods increase the flow of blood so much that values become comparable with arterial, not venous, values.
7. Select the exact puncture site: sides of tip of finger; right or left of medial artery of heel (see figure below). Allow child to choose finger if appropriate.	**7.** Using the child's nondominant hand avoids the child from having to use the tender finger on dominant hand afterward. Allowing choices adds to child's feelings of control and self-esteem.

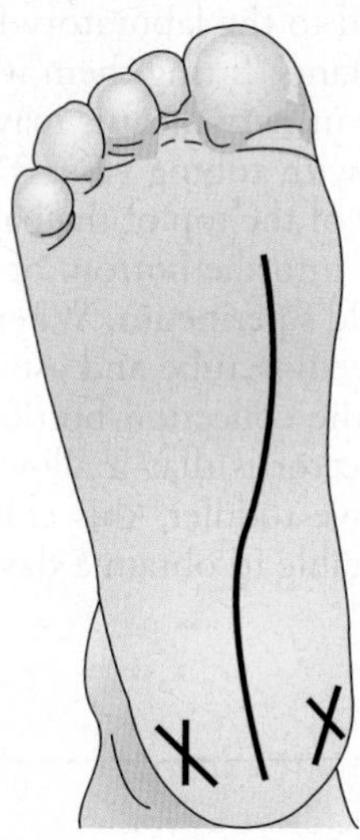

Procedure	Principle
8. Apply gloves. Swab site with alcohol and allow to dry. Puncture with a quick thrusting movement; wipe away first drop of blood with dry cotton ball.	**8.** Allowing the alcohol to dry prevents burning from the puncture. Wiping away first drop prevents contamination or dilution of the specimen.
9. Hold heel or finger lower than proximal extremity; touch capillary tube to blood drop and tip to encourage flow. Do not squeeze tissue around site.	**9.** Capillary action will quickly fill the collecting tube; squeezing causes tissue injury.
10. After filling required number of blood tubes, apply dry compress to site; apply adhesive bandage.	**10.** Applying dry compress to site halts bleeding.
11. Label specimen appropriately and send to proper laboratory for analysis.	**11.** Labeling and prompt transport ensure continuity of care.
12. Evaluate effectiveness, efficiency, cost, safety, and comfort aspects of procedure; record procedure and child's reaction.	**12.** Evaluation determines effectiveness of care. Documentation provides evidence of nursing care and the child's status.

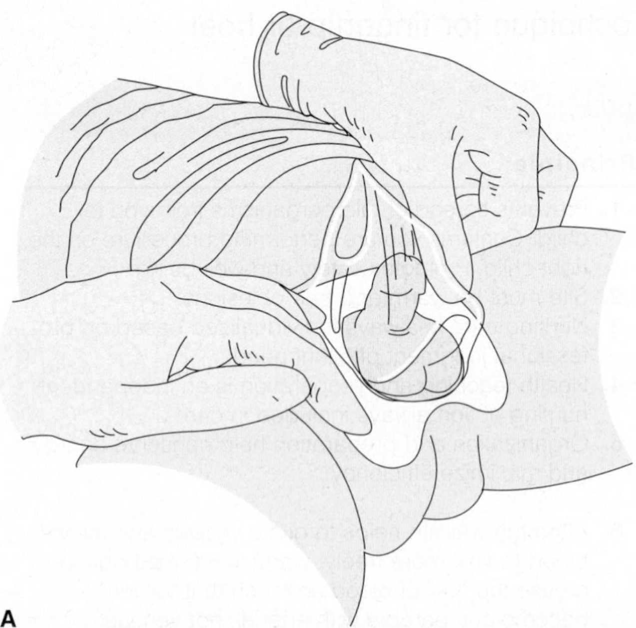

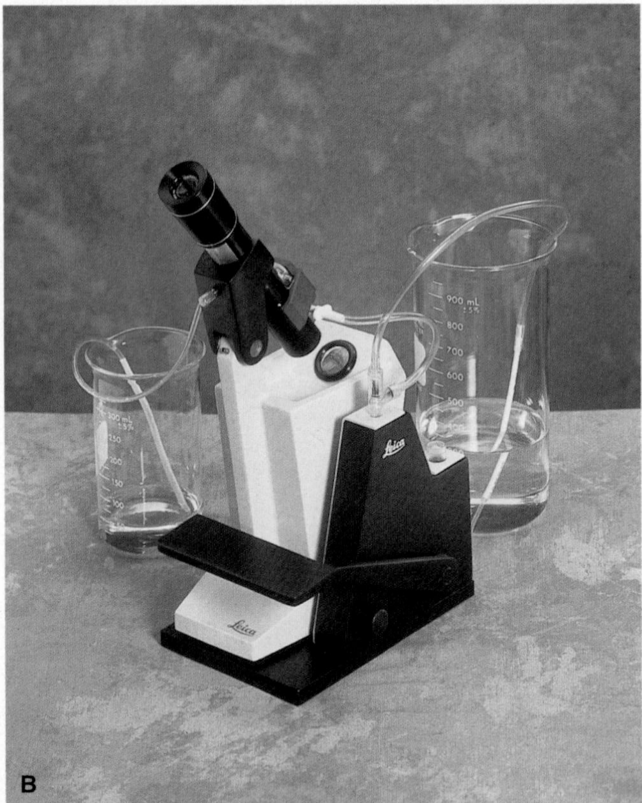

FIGURE 37.10 (**A**) Urine collector for infants. The trick to making the collector adhere is to be certain the child's skin is dry. (**B**) Testing specific gravity of urine with a refractometer. The advantage of this is that only one drop of urine is required.

is known. If the urine collection was started early in the morning and this first specimen was counted as part of the collection, the urine collected during the next 24 hours would include urine that had been forming all night, resulting in an approximately 32-hour collection period that would distort the analysis.

Record the start of the collection period as the time of the discarded urine. Save all urine voided for the next 24 hours and place it in one collection bottle. Have the child void (or watch for an infant to void) at the end of the 24-hour period and add the final specimen to the collection bottle. Record the time of the collection as being from the time of the discarded urine to the final specimen added to the collection.

For an infant, use a 24-hour rather than a single specimen urine collector. These types of collectors will adhere for this length of time only if a child's perineum is thoroughly dry at the time of application. Apply tincture of benzoin or a commercial product to toughen the perineal skin and make the skin somewhat tacky. Doing so helps to ensure the collector firmly adheres to the skin and also eases removal of the collector. After the collector is applied, place an infant in a semi-Fowler's position, if possible, to encourage urine to flow freely into the collector. Make certain the tubing from the collector is pinned out of the infant's reach or the infant may pull the collector free. It may be necessary to place a diaper on the infant to keep the apparatus out of sight. Provide activities; make sure the parents understand that they can pick up infants and hold them during this time, as long as they take care not to kink or pull the tubing.

To keep the bacterial count to a minimum, 24-hour collections are generally kept on ice or poured into a container that is then refrigerated during the 24-hour period until they can be transported to the laboratory for analysis.

With active infants, fitting them with a colostomy bag applied to cover the urinary meatus may be more effective than using a collector with tubing (Fig. 37.11). Puncture a small hole in the corner of the top of the bag. Insert a small feeding tube through this into the bottom of the bag and then apply the bag to the child's perineum. When the child voids, attach a syringe to the feeding tube and aspirate the urine. Transfer the specimen to the collection bottle. The advantage of this type of urine collector is that it allows a child to be ambulatory. For the active toddler, this collector may be the only type that is acceptable to obtain a day-long specimen.

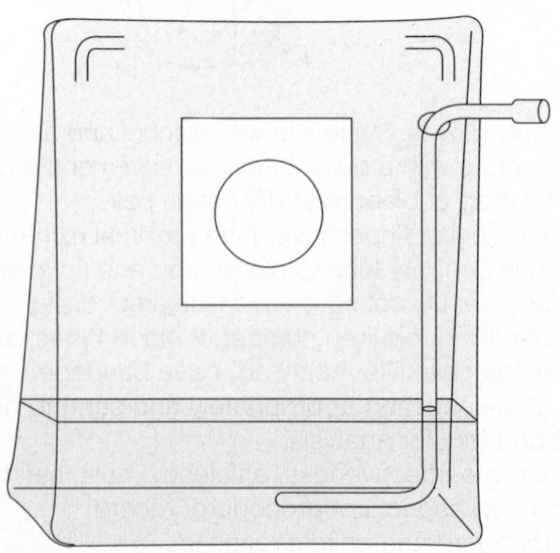

FIGURE 37.11 A 24-hour urine collector made from a colostomy bag. When the infant voids the bag fills with urine, which can be aspirated from the bag by the inserted feeding tube.

Clean-Catch Specimens

A **clean-catch urine specimen** is ordered when a urine culture for bacteria is desired. The objective of the specimen is to obtain urine that is uncontaminated by external organisms that would increase the organism count of the urine. Specimens used for protein or blood analysis may be ordered as clean-catch specimens also because this careful cleaning also reduces the possibility that vaginal or foreskin secretions, which contain protein or blood, would be added to the specimen. This type of specimen requires that the urinary meatus and the surrounding structures be cleaned before voiding.

The technique for obtaining a clean-catch urine specimen from an older child is the same as that for an adult (see Nursing Procedure 11.6). Some modifications are necessary for the young child or infant, as it is not always possible to obtain a midstream urine specimen from young children. To collect a specimen from a young child, ask the child to void into a sterile emesis basin or sterile container attached to a toilet or potty seat after you have washed the perineum or penis. Then dip a sterile container into the urine stream to obtain the specimen. If the child voids only a small amount, send that in the sterile container, marked "not midstream." To collect a specimen from an infant, wash the genitalia and apply a sterile urine collector. If the infant does not void within 2 hours, remove the collecting bag and recleanse the perineum or penis because some microorganisms will have collected after this period of time. After the area is recleansed, then reapply a new sterile bag. Again, mark specimens as "not midstream" or "obtained by a collector" for laboratory purposes.

Clean-catch urine specimens have a major advantage over bladder catheterized specimens: they are not intrusive, so they carry no risk of introducing a bladder infection. If clean-catch specimens are obtained with care, they practically eliminate the need for catheterization. A clean-catch specimen with a bacterial colony count of more than 100,000 per milliliter is considered a positive specimen, or evidence that a urinary tract infection exists.

It is almost impossible for young girls to wash their perineum thoroughly because they cannot see it well, so they usually need assistance. Young boys also must be assisted to wash until they have enough coordination to do it themselves. Be aware that this is embarrassing for children. Ask a parent to confirm for a child that the procedure is all right, because they have been told not to let adults touch this part of their body.

To be certain that school-age children and adolescents understand the procedure, have them repeat the instructions given to them; then send them to a nearby bathroom to carry out the procedure by themselves.

Suprapubic Aspiration

Suprapubic aspiration is the withdrawal of urine by insertion of a sterile needle into the bladder through the anterior wall of the abdomen. The technique is used to obtain urine for culture in infants who cannot void on command (Thilo & Rosenberg, 2008). It is usually done by physicians, although nurse practitioners or nurses in specialty units may perform it. The steps for suprapubic aspiration are:

1. The anterior abdominal wall is cleaned with an antiseptic.
2. The urinary meatus is blocked by gloved finger pressure, confining urine in the bladder.

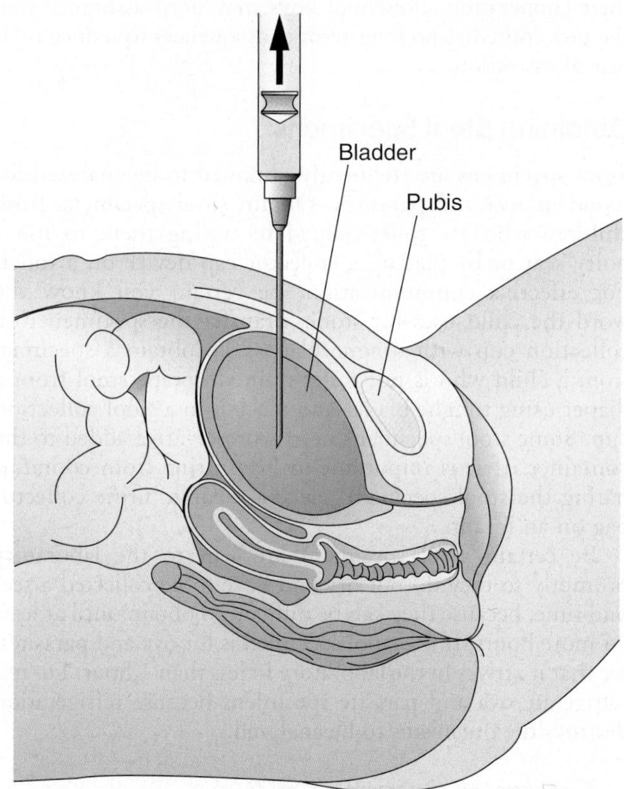

FIGURE 37.12 A suprapubic bladder aspiration. The full bladder is easily accessible by an abdominal puncture.

3. A needle is inserted just above the pubis into the bladder.
4. Urine is aspirated through the needle into a sterile syringe and the syringe and needle are withdrawn.

Although suprapubic aspiration for urine appears complicated, it is not. The bladder is the most anterior of abdominal organs and, when distended with urine, is easily accessible just under the abdominal wall (Fig. 37.12). Because the needle can cause a bladder spasm, however, it can produce sharp discomfort. Parents may not have heard of this procedure and may wonder why their child had urine drawn by needle and syringe instead of by catheter. The method is used because theoretically the risk of bladder infection from needle insertion is less than that from catheter insertion.

Catheterization

Bladder catheterization is accomplished most easily in children up to school age if a small (No. 5 or No. 8) feeding tube is used instead of a urinary catheter. This thin tube passes readily through the meatus of even an infant. Before beginning catheterization, be certain to observe the perineum of girls to locate the urinary meatus; it is not as readily observable in infants and young children as it is in adult women. Cleanse the perineum or penis well before inserting the tube to reduce the risk of infection.

Catheterization is an invasive procedure, so children must be prepared in advance. Caution children that the catheter will sting for an instant as it is inserted and they will have to lie still until the urine specimen is obtained. They need both support to submit to the procedure and praise afterward for their cooperation. Preschool boys may need assurance that the procedure has no long-term consequences to reduce their fear of castration.

Obtaining Stool Specimens

Stool specimens are frequently obtained to be analyzed for blood or ova and parasites. Obtain stool specimens from children who are toilet-trained by asking them to use a potty seat or by placing a collector cap device on a toilet. For effective communication, be certain you know the word the child uses for stool. Transfer the specimen to a collection cup with tongue blades. To obtain a specimen from a child who is not toilet-trained, scrape stool from a diaper using tongue blades and place it in a stool collection cup. Some stool specimens need a preservative added to the container. If it is important to keep urine from contaminating the stool specimen, place a separate urine collector bag on an infant.

Be certain stool specimens are sent to the laboratory promptly so they do not dry and have to be collected a second time, because they can be difficult to obtain until at least 24 more hours. If the stool specimen is for ova and parasites, see that it arrives in the laboratory in less than 1 hour. Do not refrigerate ova and parasite specimens because refrigeration destroys the organisms to be analyzed.

✔ Checkpoint Question 37.2

T.J. will have a 24-hour urine specimen collected. You would time this from:

a. The time of the discard specimen.
b. The first urine voided in the morning.
c. A set time, such as 8 AM.
d. The first voiding after the discard urine.

HOT AND COLD THERAPY

Children who sustain muscle sprains or undergo procedures such as bronchoscopy or tonsillectomy may have cold applications prescribed to prevent inflammation and edema (Fig. 37.13). If inflammation or edema is already present, application of heat may be prescribed to help it resolve. It is important to implement measures to prevent both burns and boredom in the child during treatments. Guidelines for hot and cold applications are shown in Box 37.9.

BOX 37.9 ✻ Focus on Family Teaching

Guidelines for Hot and Cold Applications With Children

Q. T.J.'s mother tells you, "I need to apply cold compresses to my child's head to reduce swelling. How do I do this?"

A. When applying any type of hot or cold therapy such as cold or warm compresses, use the following guidelines:

- Apply neither heat nor cold for longer than 20 minutes unless prescribed otherwise, because after this time, the vasoconstriction caused by cold and the vasodilatation caused by heat is reversed.
- When using electrical sources of heat with toddlers and preschoolers, never make a game of plugging in and pulling out the apparatus that makes the light come on or a dial glow. Otherwise, the child may play with it after you leave.
- Supply a special activity for a child to enjoy while a hot or cold application is in place (playing a board game or reading a story to the child), so that the procedure is not viewed as a chore but as a pleasant time to look forward to.
- Put tape on the gauge of an electric appliance at the point where you want it, so that you will be able to tell if the child changes the setting.
- To be certain that solutions or heat sources are not too hot, always test them with your inner wrist or the dorsal surface of your hand before applying them to the child.
- Do not apply ice packs or ice directly to the skin. Cover the pack or ice with a towel or other cover to prevent frostbite and cell damage from cold.
- Be cautious using heat or cold applications with a child who is receiving an analgesic, because the child's perception of heat or cold may be reduced, and the site could easily be burned.

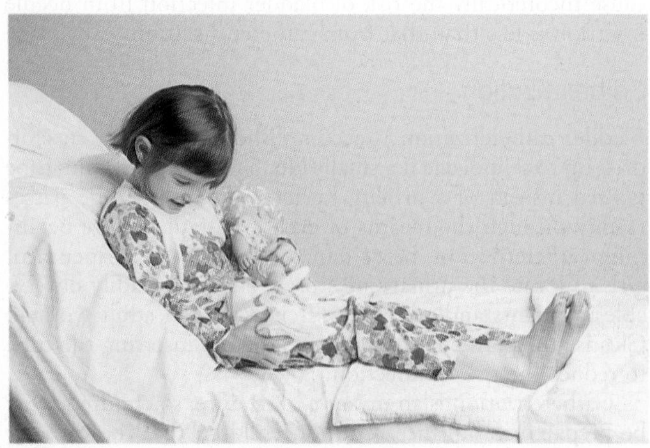

FIGURE 37.13 A rubber glove used as an ice pack. A face drawn on it helps to make it seem friendlier. Wrap gloves in washcloths to help avoid latex allergy.

NUTRITIONAL CARE

Because almost all illnesses affect children's nutritional and fluid balance, assessment of these areas sheds a great deal of light on a child's general health. Nutritional assessment begins by asking a child or parent for a 24-hour recall of all the foods eaten during that time, followed by more specific measures such as intake and output measurements. Common therapies for nutritional deficiencies include enteral feeding, gastrostomy, and total parenteral nutrition (TPN).

Nursing Diagnoses and Related Interventions

Nursing Diagnosis: Risk for imbalanced nutrition, less than body requirements, related to chronic illness

Outcome Evaluation: Skin turgor is good; no signs of dehydration are present; child gains a minimum of 1 pound weekly as evidence that nutritional needs are being met.

Measuring Fluid Intake and Output

Fluid is an essential element of nutrition because of the water supplied and because it can also be a source of calories and vitamins. To document fluid balance, some children may have fluid intake and output measured and recorded. This is especially true for children with vomiting, diarrhea, burns, hemorrhage, dehydration, cardiac and kidney disease, draining wounds, gastrointestinal suction, edema, and diuretic or intravenous therapy.

Fluid Intake

Estimating the intake of infants who are formula fed is simply a matter of estimating the kind and amount of fluids that were swallowed. Intake in breastfed infants is merely recorded as "breastfed." If it is necessary to estimate the amount more closely than this, an infant can be weighed before and after a feeding. The difference in weight (in grams) is the number of milliliters of breast milk ingested. This measurement is not very accurate, however, because if the child voided or had a bowel movement, weight is affected by these losses.

With preschool children, be certain to record fluids ingested during snacks as well as meals, because children this age usually have many during the day. At approximately 10 years of age, children can be depended on to record their own intake as long as they have a list of how many milliliters are contained in each glass or cup they use (an average cup is 150 mL; a glass, 180 mL). Remind them that soup, flavored frozen ice such as Popsicles, and sherbet are liquids and should be counted.

Fluid Output

Diapers can be readily used as a method of measuring urine output. Weigh a diaper before it is placed on an infant and record this weight conspicuously (mark it on the front of the plastic covering with a ballpoint pen). Reweigh the diaper after it is wet and subtract the difference to determine the amount of urine present. This difference will be in grams. Because 1 g = 1 mL, the amount can be recorded in milliliters. In infants who have liquid stools, it is difficult to separate stool from urine because these blend together in a diaper. Separate urine from stool by applying a urine collector; check it frequently for filling.

Girls often void along with bowel movements when they use a toilet, which means that a urine specimen is easily lost. To separate urine from bowel movements, teach older children to void first before trying to move their bowels.

Enteral Feedings

Enteral feedings, also called nasogastric tube feedings, are a common means of supplying adequate nutrition to an infant who is unable to suck or tires too easily when sucking, or to an older child who cannot eat. Enteral feedings have the advantage over parenteral nutrition because they preserve the stomach mucosa and also decrease the risk of intravenous infection. In infants, such feedings are traditionally called **gavage feedings** (Box 37.10 and Table 37.2).

Whether enteral catheters should be passed through the nares or the mouth is controversial. Orogastric insertion allows for easier breathing because the nose is not blocked. Because newborns are nose breathers, it seems reasonable that passing a catheter through the mouth in this size infant will lead to less distress than passing it through the nose. Orogastric insertion can also decrease the possibility of striking the vagal nerve and causing bradycardia. If the tube is to be left in place, however, it may be passed through a nostril. For the older child, insertion through a nostril is more comfortable.

Tube placement can be confirmed by x-ray; then at each feeding, measuring the length of the tubing is a method to make certain it has not moved. Children are generally offered bolus or intermittent feedings rather than continuous infusions to more closely mimic a normal feeding pattern. The formula used should be at room temperature to prevent chilling. Before a feeding, elevate the child's upper trunk 30 to 40 degrees so the fluid will remain in the stomach and not flow upward into the esophagus, possibly causing aspiration. Do this by holding an infant in the lap or placing the infant in an infant seat. For an older child, use pillows or elevate the head of the bed. If ordered, use a syringe to aspirate the tube for any stomach residual (this is important if there is a question regarding whether an infant is absorbing the quantity of fluid being given and also confirms tube placement is in the stomach). After noting the amount, replace this fluid so the child does not lose the electrolytes it contains. To administer the feeding, attach a syringe to the tube and allow the specified amount to flow by gravity only (to prevent reflux and possible aspiration).

After the feeding, flush the tube with a specified amount of clear water to clear it of the feeding solution. Keep the child's head elevated for at least 1 hour after a feeding to help prevent esophageal reflux.

Children with long-term neurologic disabilities may have enteral tubes left in place for continuous feedings administered by an enteric feeding pump. Give mouth care at least twice a day to children who are receiving nasogastric tube feedings; otherwise, their mouths become dry and ulcers can form.

Gastrostomy Tube Feedings

Children may have gastrostomy tubes inserted for feeding. Such feedings may be necessary for children who cannot swallow or have an esophageal stricture (Ramelli et al., 2007). With the use of regional anesthesia, the tube is inserted through a puncture wound in the abdominal wall into the stomach (Fig. 37.14). The tube used in children is usually actually an indwelling urinary catheter (Foley catheter) rather than a true gastrostomy tube. This is because a Foley catheter can be removed easily and changed should it become plugged. In addition, the balloon used to secure the tube is small enough so it does not obscure and fill the small stomach space.

Box 37.10 Nursing Procedure ✻ Initiating an Enteral Feeding for an Infant

Purpose: To supply nutrition by an enteral tube..

Procedure	Principle
1. Loosely swaddle the infant using a mummy restraint.	**1.** Mummy restraints effectively contain arms and legs without causing any unwarranted pressure on the infant.
2. Measure the space from the bridge of the infant's nose to the earlobe to a point halfway between the xiphoid process and the umbilicus using a no. 8 or no. 10 feeding tube. If the infant is older than 1 year of age, measure from the bridge of the nose to the earlobe to the xiphoid process.	**2.** Measuring the tube ensures that it will be long enough to enter the stomach. If a tube is passed too far, it will curl and end up in the esophagus; if not passed far enough, it will also be in the esophagus. Both situations could lead to aspiration of the feeding.

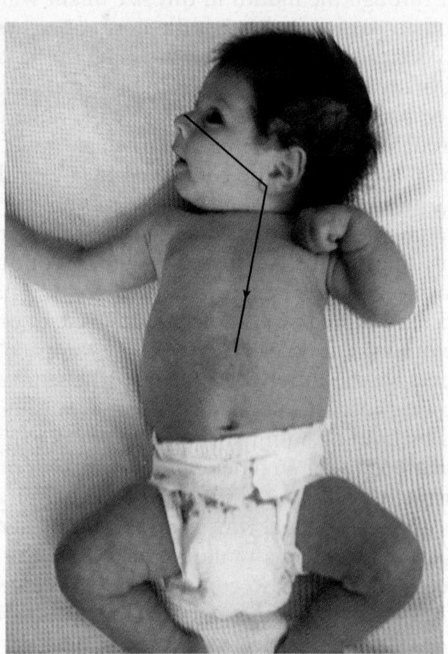

Procedure	Principle
3. Mark the tube at the measured point with a small clamp or piece of tape. Lubricate the tip of the catheter with water.	**3.** Lubrication helps the tube pass through the esophagus without trauma. An oil lubricant is never used because although the tube is going to be passed into the stomach, occasionally it can accidentally pass into the trachea. Oil left in the trachea could lead to lipoid pneumonia, a complication an infant already burdened with a disease may not be able to tolerate.
4. Pass the catheter with gentle pressure to the point of the clamp or tape. If the catheter is inadvertently passed into the trachea rather than the esophagus, the infant usually will cough and become dyspneic. If this happens, withdraw and replace the catheter.	**4.** Using gentle pressure helps to ensure comfort and safety.
5. Assess the catheter for position (confirm that it is not in the trachea) before administering a feeding (see Table 37.2).	**5.** Assessing for proper placement helps to ensure that the feeding will enter the stomach, not the infant's respiratory tract.
6. Aspirate stomach contents to assess amount. If the amount aspirated is small (a few milliliters), merely replace it at the beginning of the feeding. If large (large is determined by comparing it to the physician's order), replace it through the tubing, and reduce the amount of the feeding by that amount.	**6.** Assessing stomach content amount aids in determining if the previous feeding was absorbed. Replacing stomach secretions rather than discarding them helps prevent electrolyte loss.

Box 37.10 Nursing Procedure ✻ Initiating an Enteral Feeding for an Infant

Procedure	Principle
7. After being certain that the catheter is in the stomach, attach a syringe or special feeding funnel to the tube. Elevate the infant's head and chest slightly to encourage fluid to flow downward into the stomach.	**7.** Elevating the infant's upper body allows the feeding to flow by gravity.
8. Add the specific kind and amount of feeding prescribed to the syringe or funnel and allow it to flow by gravity into the infant's stomach. Don't elevate the syringe end of the tube more than 12 inches above the infant's abdomen (see figure below).	**8.** Excessive elevation can cause the feeding to flow too quickly, filling the esophagus and increasing the risk for aspiration. Hurrying feedings by using the plunger of the syringe or a bulb attachment for more pressure also can lead to aspiration.
9. Offer a pacifier (nonnutrient sucking) during the feeding if the infant appears to enjoy this.	**9.** Nonnutrient sucking can help satisfy the infant's normal need to suck, which would otherwise go unsatisfied with gavage feedings.
10. When the feeding has passed through the tube, reclamp the tube securely and gently and rapidly withdraw it.	**10.** Clamping the tube before it is withdrawn is important to prevent any milk remaining in the tube from flowing out as the tube is removed and thereby reduce the risk of aspiration.

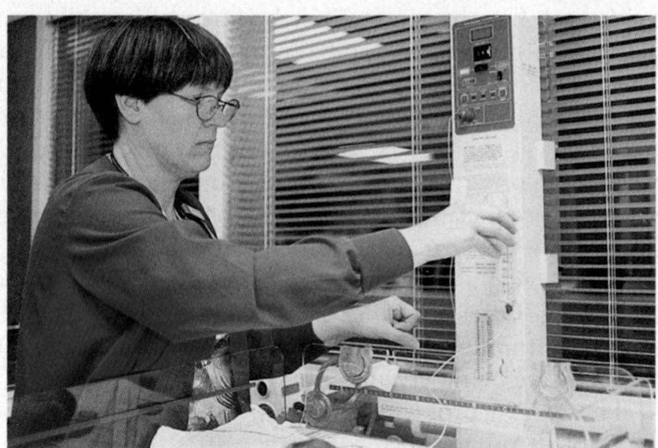

Procedure	Principle
11. If the tube is to remain in place, flush it with 1 to 5 mL of clear water and cap it.	**11.** Flushing a tube helps prevent clogging and plugging of the tube with the feeding solution. Capping a tube helps to prevent air and bacteria from entering.
12. If the tube is to be left in place, tape it below the nose and to the cheek. Do not tape it to the forehead.	**12.** Taping a tube to the forehead can put pressure on the anterior naris, leading to ulceration.
13. Bubble the baby after an enteral feeding as you would after a bottle or breast feeding. If a parent is present, encourage him or her to do this.	**13.** Bubbling helps in preventing air accumulation and regurgitation of feeding. Encouraging parental participation aids in promoting close contact, which is essential to the baby's development.
14. Unswaddle and place the infant on the right side with the head slightly elevated or hold and rock the infant in this position.	**14.** Placing on the right side helps the feeding solution enter the pyloric valve, promoting stomach emptying.
15. Assess that the infant appears comfortable. If a parent observed the procedure, answer any questions or concerns.	**15.** Assessing the infant after the feeding aids in outcome evaluation. Helping parents feel comfortable with alternative feeding methods can help increase their self-esteem and promote bonding with the infant.

TABLE 37.2 ✻ Methods to Determine Proper Gavage Tube Placement

Method	Considerations
If an x-ray is obtained to document correct tube placement, measure the length of the tube evident at that time. Remeasure the length of tube before a feeding to document that the tube has not pulled out or advanced further.	This system has inherent problems as it requires an x-ray and does not verify that the tube is actually in the stomach but can be used if it is health care policy.
Attach syringe to the tube and aspirate stomach contents. Test for pH (below 7 is acid).	In most instances, stomach contents aspirated this way are returned to the stomach before the feeding; in small infants, the amount of stomach contents is subtracted from the prescribed amount of feeding; because stomach contents are highly acid, discarding them at each feeding can lead to alkalosis.
Inject 5 mL air into the gavage tube and listen over the stomach with a stethoscope to the sound of injected air.	The injected air is heard as a whistling or growling sound; do not use an adult-size stethoscope on small infants to listen for it; the diaphragm of the stethoscope will be partially over lung, and where one is hearing the air injection is unknown.

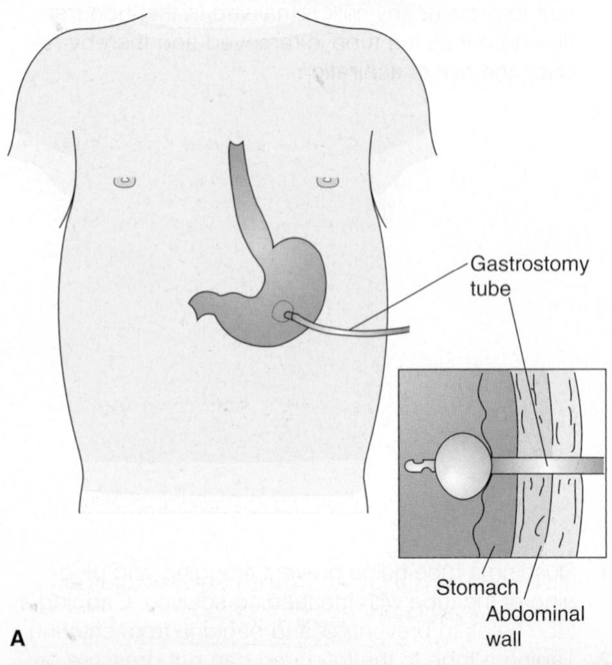

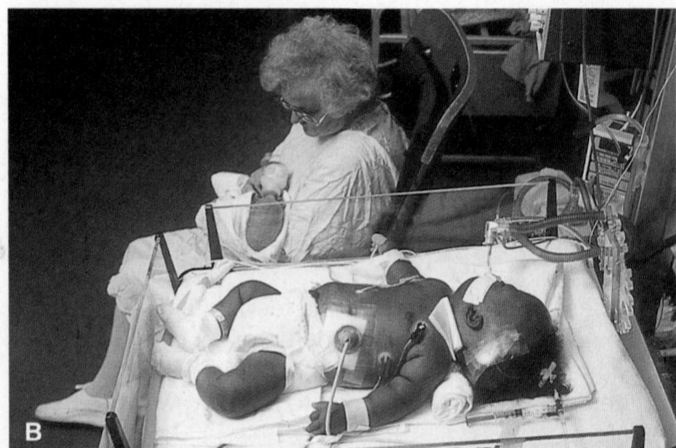

FIGURE 37.14 Children who are ill often need supplemental feeding by nasogastric or gastrostomy tube feedings. (**A**) Internal placement of a gastrostomy tube. (**B**) An infant with a gastrostomy tube in place. (From W. McIntyre/Photo Researchers, Inc.)

As with nasogastric feedings, gastrostomy feedings should be at room temperature to prevent chilling. Be certain to aspirate for stomach secretions before the feeding and allow the formula to flow by gravity, not be forced. If a child has had esophageal surgery, suspend the unclamped tube in an elevated position after the feeding. Leaving the tube unclamped and elevated this way ensures that if the child should vomit, vomitus will be evacuated from the stomach by the tube rather than past new sutures in the esophagus. If a tube is left elevated and unclamped, cover it with a clean piece of porous gauze to prevent bacteria from entering it.

Infants who are fed by gastrostomy tube miss the pleasure of sucking. Offer a pacifier to suck on during the procedure unless contraindicated. Talk or sing to the child as if the feeding were being given orally.

The biggest problem with gastrostomy tubes is that they may not fit snugly, so formula or gastric secretions can leak around the tube onto the abdominal skin. Gastric secretions are irritating because of their high hydrochloric acid content. To protect infant skin, consult a wound, ostomy, continence nurse specialist (WOCN) for wound care. Often commercially available skin protectants can be placed around the tube to protect the skin. One method of helping to provide a snug fit for the tube is to place a soft nipple used with premature infants (enlarge the nipple opening slightly) over the catheter (nipple tip up) so the base of the nipple fits against the skin protectant. Tape the tube to the nipple at the tip, which brings the balloon of the tube up against the stomach wall and prevents leakage. Tape the nipple to the skin and skin protectant securely using nonadhesive tape. Clean the skin around the nipple daily with a product such as half-strength hydrogen peroxide; change the skin protectant as directed by the manufacturer's instructions. At the time of the change, expose the skin to air for approximately 1 hour.

A major complication associated with the use of a gastrostomy tube is that it can move into the duodenum through the pyloric sphincter and cause obstruction. Observe and report any vomiting, abdominal distention, or brown or green tube drainage (duodenal secretions that would suggest the tube has moved). Testing residual aspiration fluid to see that it is acid is a guarantee that the tube is in the stomach (stomach secretions are acid; duodenal secretions are alkaline). Putting a mark on the tube with an indelible pen just above the nipple lets you check that the tube has not migrated into the stomach but is remaining securely in place.

Tubes are replaced approximately every 6 weeks. To replace a tube, deflate the catheter balloon by withdrawing the water in it and then gently pull the tube free. Insert a clean catheter into the stomach opening approximately 1 inch beyond the balloon; inflate the balloon with 2 to 4 mL water. Attach a nipple and tape in place.

Most children receiving gastrostomy feedings will have the tube in place for an extended time. Teach the child's parents how to feed the child by this method, how to remove and to replace a tube, and the danger signs to watch for such as vomiting, abdominal discomfort, or skin excoriation. Help parents to view this as an alternative way of feeding rather than a totally different one. Be certain they are comfortable with the procedure before the child is discharged from the hospital, so they can effectively feed the child by this method. Reinforce with them the understanding that it does not hurt their child to have the tube replaced or to have pressure put against the tube, so that they need not worry about holding their child snugly. Many children on long-term gastrostomy feedings have gastrostomy buttons implanted for easier stomach access (Fig. 37.15). For feeding, a catheter is inserted through the device; the catheter is removed following the feeding. With a gastrostomy button in place, only a small access device is visible, not a large bulky tube.

Percutaneous endoscopic gastrostomy (PEG) tubes are feeding tubes that are passed using endoscopy through the esophagus into the stomach and then pulled through a stab wound to the outside of the abdominal wall. The tube is then held in place by an external restraining disc. Although tubes may be passed so formula is introduced into the jejunum by this same method, such tubes bypass normal stomach digestion rather than support it so they may not be appropriate for all children (McDermott, Tomkins, & Lazonby, 2007). The overall use of such tubes is limited because a small child's esophagus may not be wide enough to insert the tube by this route.

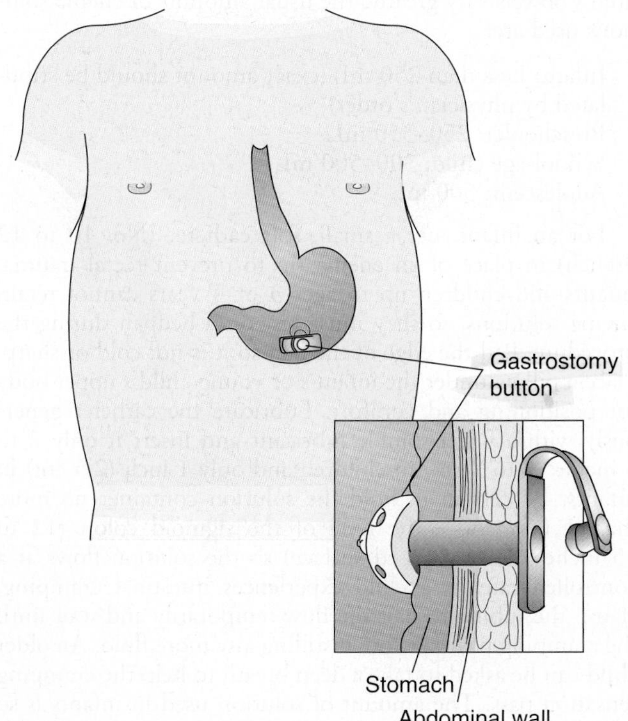

FIGURE 37.15 Placement of a gastrostomy button.

What if... A parent whose child has a gastrostomy tube in place tells you she's going to take the child to a restaurant so the child learns about "eating out." Would you agree with her that this is a good idea?

Total Parenteral Nutrition

Total parenteral nutrition (TPN) has become one of the most important therapies for children who have gastrointestinal illnesses that prevent proper absorption of basic caloric or fluid requirements or respiratory illnesses that make infants too exhausted to suck.

Nursing Diagnoses and Related Interventions

Nursing Diagnosis: Imbalanced nutrition, less than body requirements, related to malabsorption of nutrients

Outcome Evaluation: Skin turgor is good; no signs of dehydration are present; child loses no weight during therapy; intestinal cramps and distention lessen.

Traditional intravenous therapy contains fluid, electrolytes, and sugars but not protein and fat, which are essential for the maintenance and growth of body tissues. With TPN, all of a child's nutritional needs can be met by a concentrated hypertonic solution of intravenous therapy containing glucose, vitamins, electrolytes, trace minerals, and protein. An intralipid solution (emulsified fat able to be administered intravenously) given once or twice per week supplies needed fatty acids. Children with chronic diarrhea or vomiting, inflammatory bowel disease, bowel obstruction, anorexia, or extreme immaturity are examples of children who benefit greatly from TPN.

TPN solutions may be administered via a central intravenous access site or via a peripherally inserted central venous catheter (PICC). If a central access site is chosen, a catheter is inserted through the right external jugular vein into the superior vena cava or directly into the subclavian vein under strict aseptic conditions (see Chapter 38). The catheter is secured at the site of insertion with sutures and covered with a sterile dressing to help reduce bacterial contamination. A major vein of this type is chosen to avoid inflammation reactions and resulting venous thrombosis from the high-caloric and high-osmotic fluid that will be infused (Ainsworth, Clerihew, & McGuire, 2009).

TPN solution is prepared in a pharmacy under sterile conditions according to prescription. A Millipore filter, which removes small particles in the solution that might cause an embolus to form, is inserted into the tubing. The solution should be administered by means of a constant infusion pump so the rate can be governed. As a general rule, if the rate should fall behind, do not increase it the next hour to make up the amount of fluid, or serious cardiovascular overload could result because of the concentrated fluid being administered.

Infection is a major danger of TPN because the solution is a perfect medium for the growth of bacteria or *Candida* organisms. The dressing over the insertion site and the intravenous tubing are changed every 1 to 2 days to avoid infection; the tubing should not be used for obtaining blood or for adding medications (unless a double-barreled tube is used), because either process has the potential to introduce infection. Sterile technique is required in changing bottles of solution so that the tubing is not contaminated. Some health care facilities require nurses to wear both masks and gloves while doing this to avoid airborne and direct contamination. Fewer restrictions are necessary for home care. The insertion site should be inspected at the time of the dressing change for indications of local infection, such as redness, tenderness, or discharge as infection at the insertion site can lead to a serious sepsis or thrombosis (Marra et al., 2007).

A second major problem that can occur with TPN is dehydration. A TPN solution contains approximately twice the amount of glucose normally administered in an intravenous solution to ensure that the amino acids in the solution will be used for protein synthesis, not for energy. Dehydration may occur as the kidneys recognize the amount of glucose in the bloodstream as excessive and start to reduce it by excreting it (the same phenomenon that leads to high urine output in persons with diabetes mellitus). When TPN is begun, test urine for glucose and for specific gravity with each voiding. If two or more consecutive samples indicate a 3+ or 4+ glucose level, either the rate of the infusion or the amount of glucose in the solution may need to be decreased, or insulin my need to be added to the solution, to counteract the excess glucose. Generally, decreasing the concentration of glucose and then gradually increasing it again allows the child's body to adjust to the glucose overload.

After the first few days of TPN, a rebound effect (the child's body produces increased insulin) may cause hypoglycemia. A urine sample that suddenly is negative for glucose after several serial specimens have been highly positive is therefore not necessarily an encouraging sign; rather, it may be a warning that the child's glucose level has become dangerously low. TPN solution should never be discontinued abruptly but gradually tapered, or a glucose rebound effect could also occur. If a TPN catheter should be accidentally pulled out by a child, the child must be immediately assessed for hemorrhage from the insertion site and closely observed in the next few hours for signs of hypoglycemia such as lethargy, incoordination, fidgeting, or seizures. Parents need to be alerted to these concerns for safe home care.

Remember that to a child, eating is more than a means of receiving nourishment; it is also a means of receiving comfort and love. Even though children are able to voice the reason they must have TPN and appear to understand that they are receiving all the needed nutrients by infusion, they still may miss eating food and the natural social interaction that comes with it. While in a hospital, they may be upset by the smell of food from a hospital unit kitchen or by the fact that playmates have to leave to eat a meal. Finding an activity for a child receiving TPN while other children eat such as helping to check supplies on the emergency cart or stamping laboratory slips may be helpful to supply the interaction a child misses. Ask whether a child can be allowed chewing gum or occasional hard candy for chewing and taste sensations. Tooth brushing twice a day helps to keep oral mucous membranes healthy because the child is not chewing. An infant enjoys sucking pleasure from a pacifier.

Many children on long-term TPN are cared for by parents at home. Careful coordination with the home care agency is necessary to ensure that parents are familiar with the system and know how to obtain TPN fluid so the child's care continues safely. Make sure parents arrange for special time each day with the child to make up for the time normally spent interacting at meals.

ASSISTANCE WITH ELIMINATION

Two aspects of intestinal elimination that require special care are administration of enemas and ostomy care.

Administering Enemas

Enemas are rarely used with children unless they are therapy for Hirschsprung's disease or a part of preparation for surgery or an x-ray study. If an enema is necessary, offer a careful explanation of what the child can expect. As the sizes of children's bowels vary greatly, the usual amounts of enema solutions used are:

- Infant: Less than 250 mL (exact amount should be stipulated by physician's order)
- Preschooler: 250–350 mL
- School-age child: 300–500 mL
- Adolescent: 500 mL

For an infant, use a small, soft catheter (No. 10 to 12 French) in place of an enema tip to prevent rectal trauma. Infants and children up to ages 3 or 4 years cannot retain enema solutions, so they must rest on a bedpan during the procedure. Pad the edge of the pan so it is not cold or sharp. Place a pillow under the infant's or young child's upper body for positioning and comfort. Lubricate the catheter generously with a water-soluble lubricant and insert it only 2 to 3 inches (5 to 7 cm) in children and only 1 inch (2.5 cm) in infants. Be certain to hold the solution container no more than 1 foot above the level of the sigmoid colon (12 to 15 inches above the bed surface) so the solution flows at a controlled rate. If a child experiences intestinal cramping, clamp the tubing to halt the flow temporarily and wait until the cramping passes before instilling any more fluid. An older child can be asked to take a deep breath to help the cramping sensation pass. The amount of solution used in infants is so small that this is not usually a problem. If the enema solution

- Children enjoy adults who are secure in their actions. Practice as necessary the steps of a procedure before you begin so you can demonstrate confidence and skill.
- Once you have announced that a procedure needs to be done, proceed to do it; waiting for something to happen is often as stressful as actually having it done.
- Involve children in procedures, as this gives them a sense of control. Allow a child to examine electrodes or apply gel for electrode contact before a procedure. Give children a portion of an ECG strip as a badge of courage after the procedure, or let children apply their own adhesive bandage.
- Praise children for cooperation even if none was visibly obvious. For painful procedures, any behavior short of hysterical screaming counts as cooperation.
- Following the use of conscious sedation, observe children carefully until they are fully awake. Check for the return of the child's gag reflex before offering any fluids to minimize the risk of aspiration.
- Help make feeding by a route such as a gastrostomy tube as close to normal as possible by talking to the child to simulate mealtime conversation and socialization.

CRITICAL THINKING EXERCISES

1. T.J. is the 4-year-old you met at the beginning of the chapter who is frightened of dark places. He is scheduled to have an MRI of his head, which means he will be wheeled into a huge, dark, noisy, hollow tube. How would you prepare him for this?
2. T.J. is also scheduled for a CT scan with dye injected. His mother asks you to assure her that her son will not have a reaction to the dye. How will you answer her?
3. T.J.'s new brother had bowel surgery at birth and now has a temporary colostomy. His grandmother cares for him two mornings a week while his mother attends school. The grandmother tells you that she cannot imagine how she can care for an infant with a colostomy. What could you do to try to make her feel more comfortable with the baby's care? Will his care really be much different from that for other newborns?
4. Examine the National Health Goals related to health care of children. Most government-sponsored funds for nursing research are allotted based on these goals. What would be a possible research topic to explore pertinent to these goals that would be applicable to the Balliff family and also advance evidence-based practice?

CRITICAL THINKING SCENARIO

Open the accompanying CD-ROM or visit http://thePoint.lww.com and read the Patient Scenario included for this chapter, then answer the questions to further sharpen your skills and grow more familiar with NCLEX style questions related to diagnostic procedures or therapy in children. Confirm your answers are correct by reading the rationales.

REFERENCES

Ainsworth, S. B., Clerihew, L., & McGuire, W. (2009). Percutaneous central venous catheters versus peripheral cannulae for delivery of parenteral nutrition in neonates. *Cochrane Database of Systematic Reviews, 2009*(1), (CD004219).

Akpinar, E., Koroglu, M., & Ptak, T. (2007). Diffusion tensor MR imaging in pediatric head trauma. *Journal of Computer Assisted Tomography, 31*(5), 657–661.

Brayden, R. M., Daley, M. F., & Brown, J. M. (2008). Ambulatory and community pediatrics. In W. W. Hay, et al. (Eds.). *Current Pediatric Diagnosis and Treatment* (18th ed.). Columbus, OH: McGraw-Hill.

Brenner, M. (2007). Child restraint in the acute setting of pediatric nursing: an extraordinarily stressful event. *Issues in Comprehensive Pediatric Nursing, 30*(1–2), 29–37.

de Ridder, L., et al. (2007). Rectal bleeding in children: endoscopic evaluation revisited. *European Journal of Gastroenterology and Hepatology, 19*(4), 317–320.

Edwards, H., et al. (2007). Improving paediatric nurses' knowledge and attitudes in childhood fever management. *Journal of Advanced Nursing, 57*(3), 257–269.

Ekenze, S. O., Agugua-Obianyo, N. E. N., & Amah, C. C. (2007). Colostomy for large bowel anomalies in children: a case controlled study. *International Journal of Surgery, 5*(4), 273–277.

Farrell, M. K., et al. (2008). Creation of a registered nurse-administered nitrous oxide sedation program for radiology and beyond. *Pediatric Nursing, 34*(1), 29–36.

Gracey, D., & McClure, M. J. (2007). The impact of ultrasound in suspected acute appendicitis. *Clinical Radiology, 62*(6), 573–578.

Hertzog, J. H., & Havidich, J. E. (2007). Non-anesthesiologist-provided pediatric procedural sedation: an update. *Current Opinion in Anesthesiology, 20*(4), 365–372.

Karch, A. M. (2009). *Lippincott's nursing drug guide.* Philadelphia: Lippincott Williams & Wilkins.

Marra, A. R., et al. (2007). Epidemiology of bloodstream infections in patients receiving long-term total parenteral nutrition. *Journal of Clinical Gastroenterology, 41*(1), 19–28.

McDermott, A., Tomkins, N., & Lazonby, G. (2007). Nasojejunal tube placement in paediatric intensive care. *Paediatric Nursing, 19*(2), 26–28.

Meremikwu, M., & Oyo-Ita, A. (2009). Physical methods for treating fever in children. *Cochrane Database of Systematic Reviews, 2009*(1), (CD004264).

Pruitt, L. M., et al. (2008). Parental presence during pediatric invasive procedures. *Journal of Pediatric Health Care, 22*(2), 120–127.

Ramelli, G. P., et al. (2007). Gastrostomy placement in paediatric patients with neuromuscular disorders: indications and outcome. *Developmental Medicine & Child Neurology, 49*(5), 367–371.

Rice, H. E., et al. (2007). Review of radiation risks from computed tomography: essentials for the pediatric surgeon. *Journal of Pediatric Surgery, 42*(4), 603–607.

Righini, C. A., et al. (2007). What is the diagnostic value of flexible bronchoscopy in the initial investigation of children with suspected foreign body aspiration? *International Journal of Pediatric Otorhinolaryngology, 71*(9), 1383–1390.

Schiavenato, M. (2008). Facial expression and pain assessment in the pediatric patient: the primal face of pain. *Journal for Specialists in Pediatric Nursing, 13*(2), 89–97.

Shah, V., & Ohlsson, A. (2009). Venipuncture versus heel lance for blood sampling in term neonates. *Cochrane Database of Systematic Reviews, 2009*(1), (CD001452).

Thilo, E. H., & Rosenberg, A. A. (2008). The newborn infant. In W. W. Hay, et al. (Eds.). *Current Pediatric Diagnosis and Treatment* (18th ed.). Columbus, OH: McGraw-Hill.

Wennstrom, B., Hallberg, L. R., & Bergh, I. (2008). Use of perioperative dialogues with children undergoing day surgery. *Journal of Advanced Nursing, 62*(1), 96–106.

Windich-Biermeier, A., et al. (2007). Effects of distraction on pain, fear, and distress during venous port access and venipuncture in children and adolescents with cancer. *Journal of Pediatric Oncology Nursing, 24*(1), 8–19.

SUGGESTED READINGS

Berkowitz, C. D. (2007). Approach to the febrile infant: a changing paradigm. *Family Practice Recertification, 29*(3), 41–47.

Folk, L. A. (2007). Foundations in newborn care. Guide to capillary heelstick blood sampling in infants. *Advances in Neonatal Care, 7*(4), 171–178.

Fralick, S. L. (2007). A restraint utilization project. *Nursing Administration Quarterly, 31*(3), 219–225.

Mulvihill, D. (2007). Nursing care of children after a traumatic incident. *Issues in Comprehensive Pediatric Nursing, 30*(1–2), 15–28.

Pao, M., Ballard, E. D., & Rosenstein, D. L. (2007). Growing up in the hospital. *Journal of the American Medical Association, 297*(24), 2752–2755.

Plant, K. M., & Sanders, M. R. (2007). Predictors of care-giver stress in families of preschool-aged children with developmental disabilities. *Journal of Intellectual Disability Research, 51*(Part 2), 109–124.

Rogers, J., & Saunders, C. (2008). Urine collection in infants and children. *Nursing Times, 104*(5), 40–42.

Root, N. (2007). Creating a safe environment for pediatric ED patients. *Journal of Emergency Nursing, 33*(3), 286–289.

Scott, J. T., et al. (2009). Interventions for improving communication with children and adolescents about their cancer. *Cochrane Database of Systematic Reviews, 2009*(1), (CD002969).

Smith, A. B., Hefley, G. C., & Anand, K. J. (2007). Parent bed spaces in the PICU: effect on parental stress. *Pediatric Nursing, 33*(3), 215–221.

Chapter 38 Nursing Care of a Family When a Child Needs Medication Administration or Intravenous Therapy

KEY TERMS

- absorption
- distribution
- excretion
- intermittent infusion devices
- intracath
- metabolism
- pharmacokinetics
- vascular access port

OBJECTIVES

After mastering the contents of this chapter, you should be able to:

1. Describe common methods of medication and intravenous therapy used in the health care of children.
2. Identify National Health Goals related to medication or intravenous therapy that nurses could help the nation achieve.
3. Use critical thinking to analyze ways that medicine or intravenous therapy can be modified to be more family centered.
4. Assess the developmental stage and knowledge level of children and adolescents before beginning medication or intravenous therapy.
5. Formulate nursing diagnoses related to medication or intravenous therapy with children.
6. Identify expected outcomes for children receiving medication or intravenous therapy.
7. Plan nursing interventions to aid in making medicine and intravenous therapy maximally effective.
8. Implement nursing interventions concerned with medication and intravenous therapy and children, such as introducing patient-controlled analgesia.
9. Evaluate expected outcomes for achievement and effectiveness of care.
10. Identify areas related to medication or intravenous therapy with children that could benefit from additional nursing research or application of evidence-based practice.
11. Integrate knowledge of medication and intravenous therapy with nursing process to achieve quality maternal and child health nursing care.

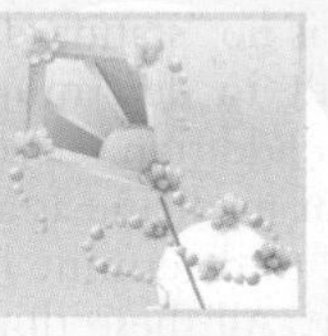

Terry, an 8-year-old with Down syndrome, is brought to the emergency department by her parents because she has pain in her ankle. She is diagnosed with osteomyelitis, a bone infection. When you give her a tablet of acetaminophen (Tylenol) for pain, she spits it out. She does the same when you repeat with a second tablet. Her mother tells you Terry can't swallow pills. Her father tells you, "You'll have to give her medicine intravenously." Previous chapters described the difficulty children may have adjusting to illness and also diagnostic and therapeutic procedures that are frequently used with children. This chapter adds information about techniques for administering medication and intravenous (IV) therapy to children. As therapy for almost all illnesses today involves some form of medicine or IV administration, this information is pertinent to the care of almost all children.

What technique would you use to help Terry learn to swallow pills? How would you gain her cooperation?

Most adults have little difficulty understanding that taking medicine will be important to relieve whatever symptoms they are experiencing from an illness. Because children do not necessarily have this same level of understanding, they may resist taking medicine unless its importance is thoroughly explained to them and the medication is given to them by a method that best meets their preference. Many children do not have enough coordination to swallow tablets or pills until they are 6 or 7 years of age. This can make taking oral medication difficult unless it is furnished in a liquid or melt-away form. Almost all children fear intrusive procedures. This can make them resist accepting medication given by a rectal, nasal, intramuscular (IM), or intravenous (IV) route. Because children range in size from as small as 1 pound (0.5 kg) if premature to over 200 (90.9 kg) pounds by late adolescence, there is no "standard" dose of medicine. This can make it difficult to determine the correct dose (Hartling et al., 2009). In addition, children have difficulty reporting adverse effects of medicine as accurately as adults. This can make it difficult to determine if side effects or adverse effects are occurring. All these things make medicine administration for children one of the most challenging interventions in nursing. National Health Goals that address this area of child health practice are shown in Box 38.1.

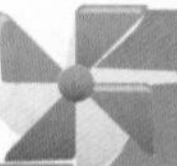

BOX 38.1 * Focus on National Health Goals

When administering medicine to children or teaching children and parents how to take medicine, remember that medicines can be as dangerous in overdoses as they are helpful in the correct doses. They can be ineffective if the doses are inadequate or missed. Poisoning and drug abuse are addressed by the following national health goals:

- Reduce the incidence of childhood poisonings, from a baseline of 348 per 100,000 population to a target of 292 per 100,000 population.
- Increase the proportion of adolescents not using alcohol or any illicit drug during the past month from a baseline of 79% to a target of 89%.
- Reduce the rate of steroid use among adolescents in the past year from a baseline of 1.5% to 0.4% (http://www.nih.gov).

Nurses can help the nation achieve these goals by educating parents about safe drug storage (locked in elevated cabinets) and teaching children and parents about effective nonpharmacologic ways to relieve stress or anxiety to help reduce drug dependence.

Areas related to these goals that could benefit from additional nursing research to strengthen evidence-based practice would include studies on the most effective ways to teach parents about safe drug storage, the phenomenon that drug poisoning increases when families are under stress, and effective ways to impart information to adolescents about the seriousness of drug abuse and its possible consequences.

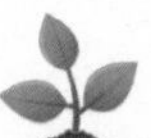

Nursing Process Overview

For a Child Needing Medication/Intravenous Therapy

Assessment

Because children vary so greatly in size and individual need, medication administration to children begins by assessing the child's height and weight so a correct dose of medicine or amount of IV fluid can be calculated based on the child's surface area. Also crucial to assessment is the child's developmental age. This is important because it will reveal if a child can swallow oral medicine or can use such self-medication methods as patient-controlled analgesia; in addition, it will1 help you determine which site would be best for an IM or IV injection. Also assess the child's chronological age and cognitive level to aid in planning the level of explanation that will be needed. Include an assessment of the child's past experience with taking medicine to help predict what a present response to medicine administration might be. Last, inquire about the family's cultural beliefs and attitudes toward medications, including use of herbal or folk remedies.

People's attitude about the worth or wisdom of medicine is not consistent across cultures. Not all families, therefore, can be expected to accept medicine administration as enthusiastically as others; some families believe an herb or home remedy would be preferable. Because of this, a family may accept a prescription but then not fill it or administer the medicine. In addition to prescribed medicine, some families give herbal remedies that can duplicate or counteract a medicine's effect. Keep in mind, too, that medicine is expensive and difficult for many families without health insurance to afford.

As part of health histories, always ask if a child commonly takes any type of herbal or home remedy or if the child has been given anything specific for the present illness. When you give parents a prescription, ask them if they think they will have any difficulty with obtaining or giving it, assessing for the medicine's effect, or returning for a follow-up appointment to evaluate the medicine's effect. Such questions allow parents to say they have questions about the medicine or are uncertain whether they should give it because of a cultural belief.

Following medicine administration, careful observation must continue to determine if the medication is having its desired effect and if any unwanted or adverse effects are occurring.

Nursing Diagnosis

Common nursing diagnoses related to medicine administration vary widely. Some examples are:

- Disturbed sleep pattern related to q4h (every 4 hours) timing of medication administration
- Deficient knowledge related to action and side effects of medicine
- Fear related to IV administration of medicine
- Discomfort related to rash as side effect of medicine
- Health-seeking behaviors by parent related to desire to learn more about different types of medicine available for child's illness

Outcome Identification and Planning
Planning for medicine administration for children involves the same safe rules of administration as those for adults. Extra consideration is necessary at each step, however, because determining the right form and route of medicine such as liquid or capsule, oral or IM, varies so widely. Establishing that a dose is accurate for that size child can involve recalculating the dose using a nomogram that shows body surface area. The schedule for administration must be not only one that is effective for the drug's action but also one that will not interfere with school activities, eating, or sleep.

Explain to children the effects that can be expected from any medicine. Be certain to give this explanation at an age-appropriate level, and be sure it is consistent with any prior explanation that a parent or other health care provider has given. The American Academy of Pediatrics Web site (http://www.aap.org/) offers information on general medicine administration and tips on how to read medicine labels and is a useful site to recommend to parents. The RN Voice site (http://www.ManageIVpain.com) offers helpful tips on how to reduce insertion pain.

Implementation
Medicine and IV interventions with children include both administering medicine to ill children and teaching parents and children how to continue to take the medicine when at home or at school. As long as a child is uncomfortable or has definite disease symptoms, parents tend to give medicine conscientiously. However, when symptoms fade, a child returns to school, or the family returns to its busy everyday schedule, it is easy for parents to forget to give medicine. This can leave children open to a recurrence of the condition or symptoms, such as pain or recurrent infection, because the organisms causing the illness were only suppressed, not killed. Helping parents fill out administration schedules to post in a readily visible location, such as on the refrigerator or a bathroom mirror, can be as important an act as explaining the drug's action to help ensure all doses of medicine will be given.

Outcome Evaluation
Expected outcomes associated with medication administration should ensure that a child received the medicine as prescribed and that the medicine had the desired effect. Specific examples suggesting outcome achievement are:

- Child states she understands she must continue to take thyroid hormone for a lifetime.
- Parents list the adverse effects of the drug and state the telephone number they will call if adverse symptoms occur.
- Adolescent describes an administration program that includes four doses daily but allows time for sports activities after school.
- Child contracts to allow IV therapy if it is inserted into nondominant hand.

MEDICATION ADMINISTRATION

Medications in children are given by a variety of routes: orally, intranasally, transdermally, topically, rectally, and via injection (subcutaneous, IM, IV, intraosseous, or epidural) or by inhalation. Epidural administration is described in Chapter 16. Inhalation techniques are discussed in Chapter 40.

To administer drugs safely, it is important to have a good understanding of **pharmacokinetics** (the way drugs are absorbed, distributed throughout the body, metabolized, inactivated, and excreted).

Pharmacokinetics in Children

The four basic processes of absorption, distribution, metabolism, and excretion determine the intensity and duration of a drug's action. The immaturity of body systems in children (and especially in newborns) plays a major role in drug action throughout each of these processes (Stavroudis, Miller, & Lehmann, 2008).

Absorption

Drug **absorption** (transfer of the drug from its point of entry in the body into the bloodstream) is influenced by the route of administration as well as by the concentration and acidity of the drug. Some routes of administration in children are limited and so are rarely used. For example, children younger than school age usually cannot hold tablets under their tongue for sublingual administration; they tend to swallow them instead. The small muscle size of young children limits sites for IM injection. Infants pull off transdermal patches because they do not understand that this is a drug. Gastrointestinal absorption may be so immature at birth that oral absorption in newborns can be reduced. Vomiting and diarrhea, frequent symptoms of childhood illnesses, also interfere with absorption because a drug would not remain in the gastrointestinal tract long enough to be absorbed.

Distribution

Distribution refers to the movement of the drug through the bloodstream to a specific site of action. Many drugs are distributed bound to serum albumin (manufactured by the liver). This binding action limits the amount of free drug in the circulation, thereby providing protection against toxic levels of a drug. As free drug is used, the bound drug is released to maintain a therapeutic level. Newborns with immature liver function may not have enough serum albumin to transport drugs readily. This is particularly true if elevated bilirubin levels are present, because bilirubin is also carried by serum albumin. Bound to serum albumin this way, bilirubin is harmless. In free form, however, it can leave the bloodstream and enter other body tissues. If it enters the brain cells, it destroys their ability to function (kernicterus). If a newborn who has a high level of bilirubin from destruction of fetal hemoglobin receives a drug such as sulfonamide that competes for albumin binding sites, a large quantity of bilirubin may be left unbound and the infant may develop kernicterus or not receive benefit for the sulfonamide because it can not be carried to the infection site. In addition, newborns have sluggish peripheral circulation, so distribution in children this young may not be effective. Any child with cardiovascular disease also may have limited distribution of drugs because of poor circulation.

Metabolism

Metabolism involves the conversion of the drug into an active form (biotransformation) or an inactive form (inactivation). Because a child's basic metabolic rate is faster than that of an adult, certain drugs are metabolized more rapidly in children. This means the drug must be administered more frequently to a child to maintain effective drug levels than it would be in adults. Some drugs, such as the salicylates and chloramphenicol, are metabolized directly by liver enzymes. Because liver enzymes are not fully developed in newborns, these drugs cannot be metabolized and so will reach toxic levels rapidly. Older children with liver disease who have impaired liver enzymes also have a decreased ability to inactivate or transform drugs.

Excretion

The **excretion** (elimination of raw drug or drug metabolites, a process that largely prevents properly administered drugs from becoming toxic) of drugs is potentially limited until about 12 months of age, when kidney function becomes mature. If a child has kidney disease, excretion potential is limited at any age. A few drugs such as digitoxin are excreted in bile. In the newborn with sluggish bile formation, excretion of these drugs is questionable. Monitoring intake and output is important in children receiving drugs to be certain that urine excretion or an outlet for drug metabolites is adequate.

What if... Terry's mother tells you her child's school has a "no drug" policy, so the school nurse will not be able to give Terry even a prescription drug in school? How would you advise her?

Adverse Drug Effects in Children

Children respond to drugs in much the same way as adults, but they may experience unique or exaggerated side effects because of immature liver function or rapid metabolism during periods of rapid growth. The newborn may suffer adverse effects from drugs taken by the mother prenatally or from drugs taken by a breastfeeding mother.

Safe Storage of Drugs

Because young children do not appreciate that overdoses of medicine can be serious and even fatal, they may help themselves to additional medicine and poison themselves (Dart & Rumack, 2008).

Adolescents can deliberately take extra doses of drugs such as steroids or pain medicine, hoping for an added effect. Oxycodone (OxyContin), for example, is an analgesic that may be prescribed for adolescents (Baker & Jenkins, 2008); it is also frequently abused by them. Ritalin (methylphenidate), administered to children with attention-deficit/hyperactivity disorder, is a second prescription drug that is also frequently abused (Szobot & Bukstein, 2008).

As with adults, always be certain medicine is stored in a safe place. A toddler walking past a medicine cart, for example, could easily explore it and remove a handful of pills. For the same reason, never leave medicine on a bedside table for children to take later if they are playing a game or taking a shower; a nearby toddler could take the medicine first.

When teaching parents about administering medicine at home, stress that they also need to keep drugs in a safe place. In most homes, this is in a locked medicine cabinet or drawer above the height their child could reach. Remind parents that most childhood poisonings occur when a family is under stress because, during these times, the family may forget usual procedures. Reinforce the need to take special precautions to lock away medications at these times. Be certain to teach parents they should never take medicine in front of children (children can imitate this action with the parent's medication when the parents are out of sight). Another caution is not to pour or prepare medicine in the dark. Because almost all medicine bottles dispensed from local pharmacies look and feel the same, it is easy to pour the wrong liquid, extract the wrong pills, or read the bottle instructions incorrectly without adequate light.

Safe Administration of Drugs

Administering drugs safely to children requires that you first determine that you are giving the right drug to the right child, in the right dosage and by the right route, at the right time. You also need to ensure that the parents or child have the right information about the medicine.

Right Medicine

Most medication errors are made in situations where the number of medications being given is high and speed in administration is crucial. Intensive care units and emergency departments, therefore, are the highest areas at risk for medication errors (Root, 2007). A prescriber may write an order using a generic or a trade name. As the number of medicines available grows, so does the possibility that two drugs have similar names. That makes the step in medicine administration—identifying you have the correct drug—even more important than ever.

Right Child

Children cannot be depended on to give their correct names. Anxious to please, a preschooler will answer the question, "Are you Johnny Jones?" with "yes." He may also agree with any other name you propose. School-age children who want to avoid taking a medicine may deny they are the person whose name you called. To prevent these types of errors, never ask children their names for identification. Instead, read their identification arm bands and compare them with the medication sheet or medical record. In ambulatory care settings or homes, ask a parent to confirm the child's identity.

Right Dosage

The correct dosage of most drugs for children is based on body surface area using a nomogram (Fig. 38.1). To calculate surface area using such a chart, find the child's height in the left column (40 cm, for example); next, find the child's weight in the right column (20 kg). Hold a ruler or straightedge to connect the two points. The mark at which the ruler crosses the center column is the child's body surface area (0.38 m^2 in the example). Before administering any medication to a child, confirm that the dose ordered is correct for the child's weight or this body surface area. Take and record height and weight measurements at health visits or on hospi-

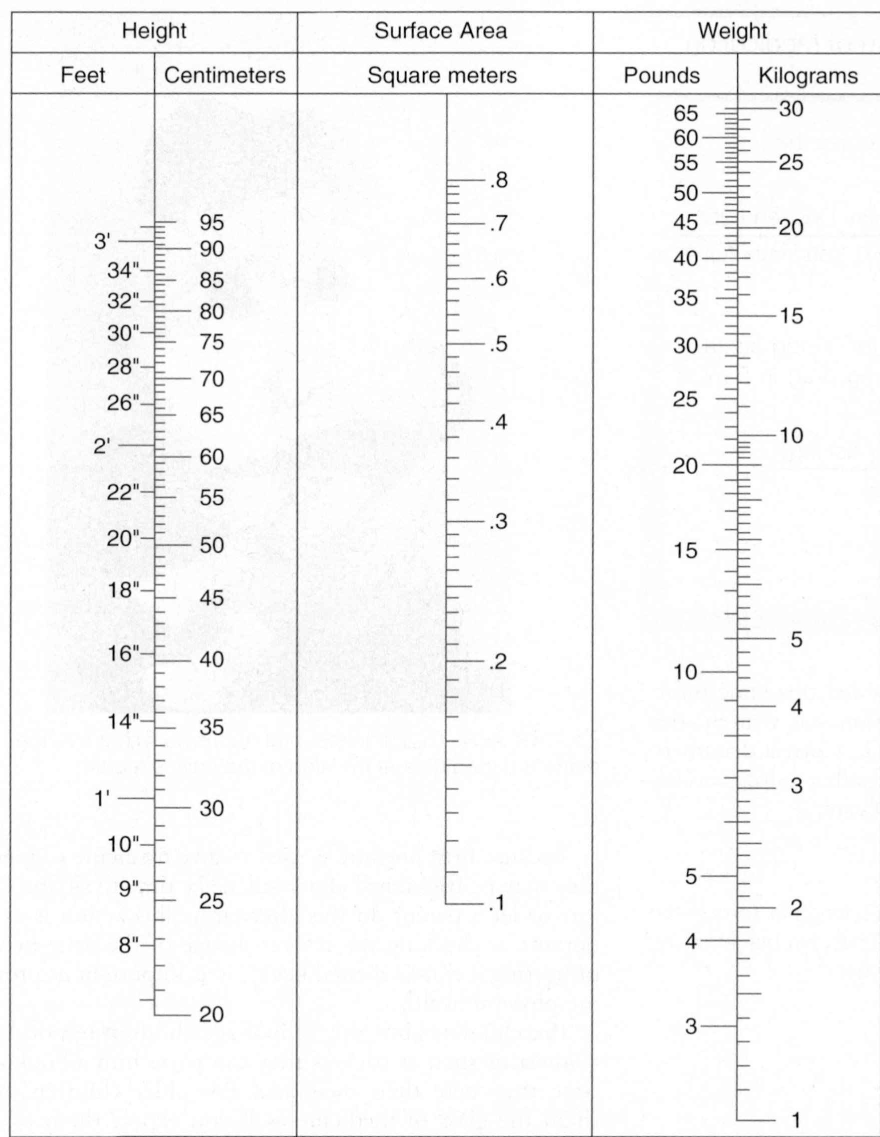

FIGURE 38.1 A nomogram to estimate body surface area. To use such a chart, draw a line from the child's height to the child's weight. The point at which it crosses the middle line is the child's surface area.

tal admission (or as frequently as daily during an admission) to obtain this information for dose calculation.

Many hospitals use color coding to help identify a correct drug dose. Every pediatric unit or clinic should have a drug reference, such as the *Physicians' Desk Reference*, to help determine safe drug doses. However, there are always exceptions to a rule. For example, a child with a gunshot wound may receive more than the usual dose of antibiotics because the risk of infection is so high. A 3-year-old weighing only as much as a 1-year-old would receive a dose of an antibiotic consistent with that given to a 1-year-old (not the child's actual age) because of small body size. Because of such exceptions, an ordered dose that does not conform to the standard dose may still be correct; however, recheck the dose for accuracy with the prescriber before it is administered. Preventing medication errors in children is everyone's responsibility.

Although most medication on hospital units is supplied in unit doses, nurses may still need to calculate fractional dosages (Box 38.2). By verifying drug dosages, nurses serve as a child's first line of defense against dosage error. When talking to parents about giving medicine, stress that if a medicine comes supplied with a dropper or dosing cap, they should use that to measure the amount of medicine (Sobhani et al., 2008).

Right Route and Time

Possible routes of administration for medicine in children are discussed below. Each of these methods requires special techniques, as most children do not enjoy taking medicine and need strong support during administration.

Right Information and Documentation

Because so many medications are advertised directly today on television or in magazines, many parents are already aware of drug names and the action of individual drugs. However, because they have been given only snatches of information (or listened to or read only that much), they also may have misconceptions about a particular drug. Be certain when giving medicine to a child or handing a prescription to a parent that you explain the drug's purpose and action, when and how it should be taken, and any side or adverse effects the parent should be aware of. People under stress do not "hear" well, so

BOX 38.2 ✻ Fractional Calculation of Medication Dosages

To calculate a fractional drug dose use the formula:

$$\frac{\text{Strength Desired (D)}}{\text{Strength You Have (H)}} \quad \frac{\text{Quantity Desired (QD)}}{\text{Quantity You Have (QH)}}$$

= Answer

For example, you have an order for 90 mg acetaminophen. It is supplied as 125 mg drug in 5 mL liquid. Using the formula:

$$\frac{\text{90 mg (D)}}{\text{125 mg (H)}} \times \frac{\text{QD (what you are asking)}}{\text{5 mL (QH)}} = ?$$

125 QD = 450(5 × 90)

450 divided by 125 = 3.6 mL

although the prescriber may have reviewed this same information with them when the prescription was written, this may be the first time they actually hear it. Correct documentation assures other health care providers that a drug was administered and allows for continuity of care.

✔ Checkpoint Question 38.1

You are going to give acetaminophen (Tylenol) to Terry in the emergency department. She has no ID band in place as yet. What would be the best way to identify her?

a. Ask her what is her name.
b. Tell her you need to know her name.
c. Ask a parent to identify her for you.
d. Ask to see her school bus pass I.D.

Oral Administration

Children younger than 9 years often have difficulty swallowing tablets. For children younger than 3 years of age, it is virtually impossible. Most oral medication for young children, therefore, is furnished in liquid form, chewables, or meltaways (Sammons & Conroy, 2008).

In infants, oral medication can be given with a medicine dropper or a unit dose syringe (without a needle). Gently restrain the child's arms and head by holding the child against your body with the head raised. Never give medicine with the child lying completely flat; otherwise, a child could choke and aspirate. A crying child is already opening the mouth for you; otherwise, gently open the mouth by pressing on the child's chin. Press the bulb of the medicine dropper or use the plunger of the syringe so that the fluid flows slowly into the side of the child's mouth. Be certain that the end of the syringe or dropper rests at the side of the infant's mouth to help prevent aspiration (Fig. 38.2). An infant also may be given fluid from a small glass or spoon. Allow the fluid to flow a little at a time so that the child has time to swallow between small sips. As oral solutions are pleasantly flavored, most infants resist the first drop but then suck the remainder of the medicine into their mouth.

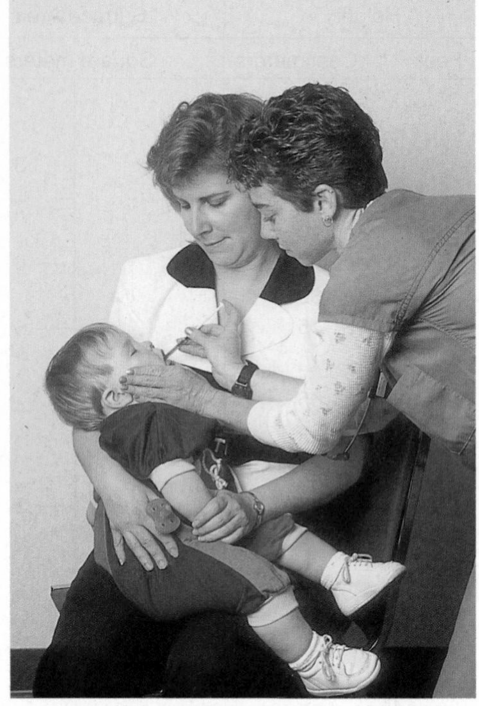

FIGURE 38.2 To administer oral medicine with a syringe, place the medicine at the side of the child's mouth.

Because firm pressure is used to give medicine to infants, they may be frightened afterward. Take time to sit and comfort or let a parent do this afterward. This action is as important as checking the correct dosage of the drug because protecting a child's mental health is as important as protecting physical health.

Preschoolers and early school-age children respond well to rewards such as stickers they can paste into a book each time they take their medicine. For older children, hand them the glass of medicine as if you expect them to take it. Offer a "chaser" if necessary and not contraindicated (Box 38.3). If a child has difficulty swallowing tablets, they can be crushed and added to a teaspoonful of applesauce or a flavored syrup. If pills are not to be chewed (capsules or enteric-coated tablets), be certain a child knows not to chew them. Some children are old enough to swallow tablets but have never done it before. You can use small bits of ice for practice; they melt rapidly and do not stick in the back of the throat or esophagus. Have the child put the ice on the back of the tongue, tip the head slightly to the side, take a sip of water, and swallow the water. Praise the child for learning this new skill. Do not use candy for practice; you do not want to suggest that medicine is the same as candy.

Another useful technique to help a child swallow pills is to push them into a teaspoonful of ice cream or pudding. Children tend not to chew this type of food; rather, they swallow it along with the pill. If using this technique, push the pill into the ice cream or pudding in front of the child. The intent is not to hide the pill, but to help the child learn to swallow medicine.

Box 38.4 gives additional guidelines for administering oral medication to children or teaching parents how to give medicine at home.

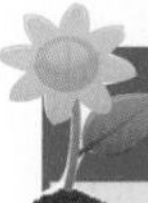

BOX 38.3 * Focus on Communication

You want to give acetaminophen (Tylenol) to Terry, 8 years old, to help relieve her pain.

Less Effective Communication

Nurse: I have your medicine, Terry. Swallow these for me?
Terry: No. My ankle is too sore.
Nurse: If you don't swallow them, I'll put them into a shot and give it that way. And that will really hurt.
Terry: I'd rather get a shot, my ankle is so sore.
Nurse: Well, I can't do that. Tylenol doesn't come that way.
Terry: Then I'm not going to take it.

More Effective Communication

Nurse: I have your medicine, Terry. Swallow these for me.
Terry: No. My ankle is too sore.
Nurse: That's why I want you to swallow the pill. It'll take away the hurt.
Terry: I'd rather get a shot, my ankle is so sore.
Nurse: This type of medicine has to be swallowed. Do you want orange juice or soda pop to drink after it?
Terry: Soda pop.
Nurse: Okay. Take a big swallow and it'll be gone.

The nurse in the first scenario makes some important medication administration errors: first, he *asks* the child if she will swallow the tablets rather than *telling* her to swallow them; second, he threatens the child; even worse, he threatens with a measure he cannot enforce (acetaminophen does not come in an injectable form). When the child refuses the request and contradicts his threat, he is left powerless. A better approach is shown in the second scenario: here, the nurse explains the advantage of taking the medicine and conveys that he expects the child to be cooperative. Allowing a secondary choice, such as a choice of beverage, offers children a sense of control but does not allow them to say no to the primary request.

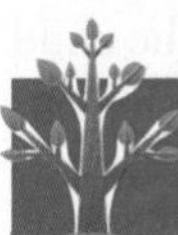

BOX 38.4 * Focus on Family Teaching

Guidelines for Administering Oral Medication

Q. Terry's mother tells you, "All my children fight me anytime they need to be given medicine. How can I get them to take medicine without a battle?"

A. Use the following guidelines to help make this task a bit easier:

- Do not say, "*Can* you drink this for me?" If an adult seems unsure whether children can do a task, children can develop grave doubts themselves.
- Do not say, "*Will* you drink this for me?" This leaves a child the opportunity to say no and creates the awkward position of having to admit that the child really does not have a choice in the matter; the child *must* take the medicine.
- State firmly, "It's time for you to drink your medicine now." Give the child a secondary choice that allows a sense of control: "It is time to drink your medicine now; do you want milk or water to swallow after it?" is a suitable choice, assuming both milk and water are compatible with the medication.
- Never refer to medicine as candy. If they think it is candy, children may help themselves to fatal amounts of medicine when everyone's back is turned.
- Do not bribe children to take medicine. Bribing may work for one dose, but when a second dose is due, the child will ask for a bigger bribe; for a third dose, an even bigger one. At some point (generally reached quickly), it is impossible to supply such large bribes and therefore it is impossible to enforce the rules.
- Do not threaten. Statements such as, "Take this quickly or I'll ask the doctor to make it into a shot" cannot be followed through. The child calls the bluff (many medicines do not come in a form that can be injected intramuscularly), and once more the child is in control. A statement such as, "Take this or I'll call your doctor" is unfair (the physician has been made the villain) and ultimately undermines your authority (it is obvious that you must not have much power, or you would not need help).
- Do not lie about the taste of medicine. Children expect honesty from adults. If in doubt about the taste, taste it (with the obvious exception of drugs such as digitoxin). Most children's medicines are artificially flavored with raspberry, orange, or cherry syrup, so they do not taste bad.
- If a medicine tastes bitter, mix it with a spoonful of strained applesauce or a teaspoonful of flavored syrup. Do not mix medicine with a full jar of baby food, because the child will then have to eat the entire jar of food to get all of the medicine. As a rule, encourage children to take medicine straight, then follow it with a pleasant-tasting drink to take away any bitter taste.
- If a medicine is supplied in tablet form, crush or dissolve it in water and mix it with syrup or applesauce for a better taste if appropriate. Be certain before removing the particles from a capsule that the medicine will work properly when not in capsule form: some are encapsulated to keep them from dissolving in the stomach and to bring them into the intestine, where they have their therapeutic effect. The same precaution must be followed when giving enteric-coated tablets.
- Never leave medicine by a child's bed for the child to take "in a minute" or "after your shower." The child may become involved with another activity "in a minute" and will not take it, or a smaller child could find the medicine appealing and swallow it.

What if . . . Terry's father tells you Terry is such a "picky eater" that she rarely eats a full meal? When should he give a medicine that should be taken with a meal?

Intranasal Administration

More medications are supplied as nose drops or spray every year (Holsti et al., 2007). These are advantageous in that a nasal spray is easy for a parent to administer. Having someone drop medicine into the nose can be very uncomfortable, though. Tell the child you understand this, but that the medicine is important because it will help the child get better. Explain what you are going to do: "I'm going to place two drops of medicine into your nose. Then I want you to sniff for me [demonstrate]. Then I'll put two drops into the other side of your nose and I want you to sniff again."

Turn the child onto the back. A school-age child could extend the head over the side of the bed so that it is lower than the trunk. Preschoolers generally are too frightened by this strange position and do better with a pillow under their shoulders so that their head extends over the pillow and rests downward. An infant may need to be restrained in a mummy restraint for nose drop administration (see Chapter 37 for a discussion of appropriate restraints).

Instill the appropriate number of drops into one nostril. Turn the child's head to the side—to the left after the left nostril, to the right after the right nostril—so that the medicine stays in the nose longer. If the child is a preschooler or older, ask him or her to further "sniff" the medicine. Have the child remain in the head-flat position for at least 1 minute to let the medicine come in contact with the mucous membrane of the nose. If a child gets up immediately, the medicine will flow out and will be less effective.

Give children high praise even if they did not cooperate well. Praise tells children you understand how hard it was to stay still.

Children over about age 6 can use nasal sprays competently after they have been introduced to the technique. Acknowledge that spraying a liquid into the nose is uncomfortable because it tickles or causes a sneezing sensation. Have the child sit or stand upright, hold the spray bottle upright with the tip just inside one side of the nose, and gently squeeze the spray bottle. In most instances, a child should then tip the head to the side (the right side for the right nostril, the left side for the left nostril) or sniff, depending on the bottle instructions, for best absorption. The administration is then repeated for the second nostril. Stress that although this form of medication administration seems simple and "fun," drugs are well absorbed across the nasal mucosa so this route is an effective means of drug administration and can be a route for important and even life-sustaining drugs. Spray bottles should be individually prescribed for children and not used by any other child to prevent the spread of disease organisms. As influenza vaccine is now supplied in this form, in the near future, children will be more and more familiar with this route of medicine administration and, hopefully, less resistant to the method (Carpenter et al., 2007).

Ophthalmic Administration

Eye medications, in particular antibiotics to treat eye infections, are most often administered by being dropped into the conjunctival sac of the eye (Renouf, 2007). This type of administration, like nose drops, is frightening for children because they have been warned many times never to put anything into their eyes. Also, children know that getting something in the eye, such as dust, which has probably happened at some point, can be painful. As a result, infants and preschoolers generally must be restrained in a mummy restraint for eye drop administration. Always explain what you are going to do and that the medicine will not hurt (assuming that is true). Place the child on the back. Open the eyes of infants and preschoolers by gently but firmly pressing on the lower lid with the thumb and on the upper lid with the index finger. A school-age child or adolescent will open eyes cooperatively, but you may need to rest a hand on the eyelid to keep the eye open long enough for the drug to be administered (Fig. 38.3). Be sure that your fingernails are cut short to avoid scratching the child's cornea.

Instill the correct number of drops into the conjunctiva of the lower lid. Allow the eyelid to close. Avoid placing the drops directly on the cornea, because that can be painful. To prevent the conjunctiva from drying, do not hold the eyelids apart any longer than necessary. After the child has blinked two or three times, allow the child to get up. Praise the child for cooperation even if cooperation was not evident; the child accomplished a major feat by allowing you to touch and invade an eye this way.

To instill an ophthalmic ointment, apply a fine line of the ointment along the inside rim of the conjunctival sac, working from the inner to the outer eye canthus. If the eye is pus-filled, applying medication under pressure toward the midline can force pus across to the other eye or down the lacrimal duct, so applying the medicine from the medial aspect to the outer one may prevent transferring infected mucus from one eye to the other. Eye medicine should be individually prescribed and not used by other children, because if the tip of the dropper or tube touches the conjunctival sac it is contaminated with body fluid.

Otic Administration

Otic administration refers to administering medicine, primarily drops, into the ear canal. Like other forms of medicine, this is difficult for children to accept because they have been told many times not to put anything into their ears.

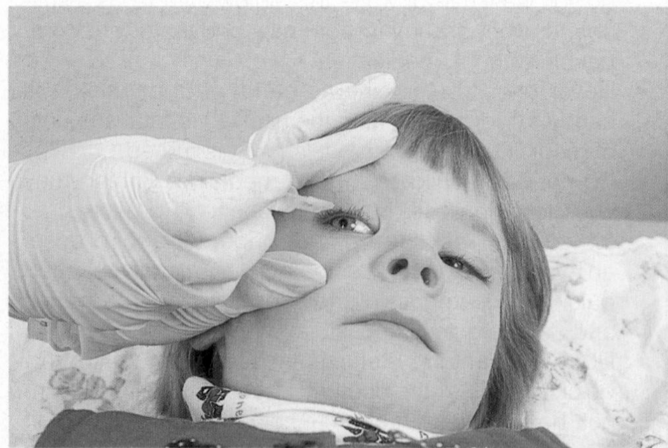

FIGURE 38.3 Administering eye drops.

Also, because ear drops are generally administered for earache, which is sharp, excruciating pain, a child may worry that having medicine put into the ear will make the pain even worse. In addition, a child cannot watch what is happening (always frightening), and the odd sensation of drops of fluid running into an ear can cause a tickling, uncomfortable sensation. Assuming that you have been honest with the child up to this point, remind the child, "Remember how I told you the injection would hurt a little? Well, if this would hurt, I'd tell you now, too. But this doesn't hurt." Remind the child that ear drops can feel funny, however, as if someone were tickling the ear. Ear drops must always be used at room temperature or warmed slightly. Cold fluid, such as medication taken from a refrigerator, does cause pain and may also cause severe vertigo as it touches the tympanic membrane.

Place the child on the back, in a mummy restraint if necessary. Turn the head to one side (Fig. 38.4). The slant of the ear canal in children is shown in Chapter 50. If the child is younger than 2 years, straighten the external ear canal by pulling the pinna down and back. If the child is older than 2 years, pull the pinna of the ear up and back. Instill the specified number of drops into the ear canal. Hold the child's head in the sideways position for at least 1 minute to ensure that the medication fills the entire ear canal. Praise the child for cooperation after the procedure.

Rectal Administration

A good route for administering medication to children who are unconscious is by rectal insertion, because this avoids the danger of aspiration and allows a drug to be absorbed across the mucous membrane of the intestine (Kleiber, 2008). Rectal administration may be used to give a drug such as Tylenol to uncooperative young children or those who are vomiting. Most children, however, rate this as the least desirable method for receiving medication so it is not a major route of administration.

Some medications are given by rectal suppository; a few are given by retention enema. Because the child cannot see what is happening with rectal administration, a child can be easily frightened by this procedure. Show the child the medication so that the child can be certain it is not an injection. Having been honest with the child up to this point will be helpful again: "If it were anything else, I would tell you so."

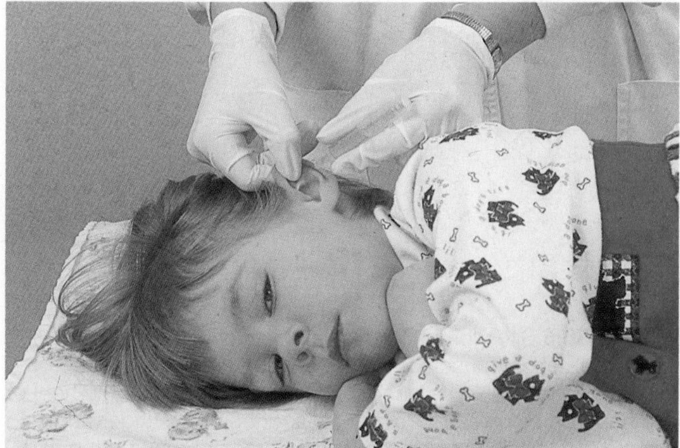

FIGURE 38.4 Administering ear drops. For the child over 2 years old, the pinna of the ear is pulled up and back.

Many suppositories are supplied already lubricated. If not, add a drop of water-based lubricant such as K-Y Jelly to the tip. Use a glove and insert the suppository gently but quickly beyond the rectal sphincters (approximately ½ inch or as far as the first knuckle of the little finger for infants, and approximately 1 inch or as far as the first knuckle of the index finger for older children). Withdraw your finger and press the child's buttocks together firmly for a count of approximately 10, or until the child's urge to evacuate the suppository passes.

If the medication is to be administered by a retention enema to a young child, use usual enema technique, but with as small an amount of fluid as possible so the child can retain it. Press the child's buttocks firmly together for approximately 15 seconds after administering the enema or a child will expel the solution almost immediately and the medicine will be lost. Using a distraction technique, such as asking the child to count backward or saying the alphabet backward, can also help a defecation reflex to pass. Remember that invasive procedures are particularly threatening to the preschooler. Give lavish praise for cooperation.

Transdermal/Topical Administration

Children who have skin irritation or need medicine to relieve itching or dryness may have topical creams or lotions prescribed. Most children accept this type of application well because the medicine brings almost immediate relief. Children as young as toddlers can help apply this type of medicine with your supervision. Be certain they wash their hands afterward so they do not lick any extra off their fingers and inadvertently take it orally.

Several children's medicines are available by transdermal patch, because absorption of drugs through the skin can be yet another effective and pain-free route for administration. Be certain that the child's skin is dry and intact at the site where the patch will be applied. Apply patches over the trunk or a major muscle, not on distal extremities, for best absorption. Assess the skin under the patch every time a patch is changed to be certain the site is not becoming irritated. Change the site every time a new patch is applied to decrease the possibility of irritation to the skin.

Young children tend to remove transdermal patches the same as they do Band-Aids because of normal curiosity about what is underneath. Putting clothes on the young child immediately so the patch is out of sight is helpful. Be certain patches applied to children wearing diapers are not placed where a leaking diaper could wet the patch and irritate the skin or dilute the medicine.

Intramuscular and Subcutaneous Administration

IM injections are rarely prescribed for children because many children do not have sufficient muscle mass for easy deposition of medication, and they are often painful. For IM injections in infants, the mandatory site for administration is the vastus lateralis muscle of the anterior thigh (Fig. 38.5). Use the lateral aspect rather than the medial portion, where an injection would cause more pain. Using the gluteal muscle in

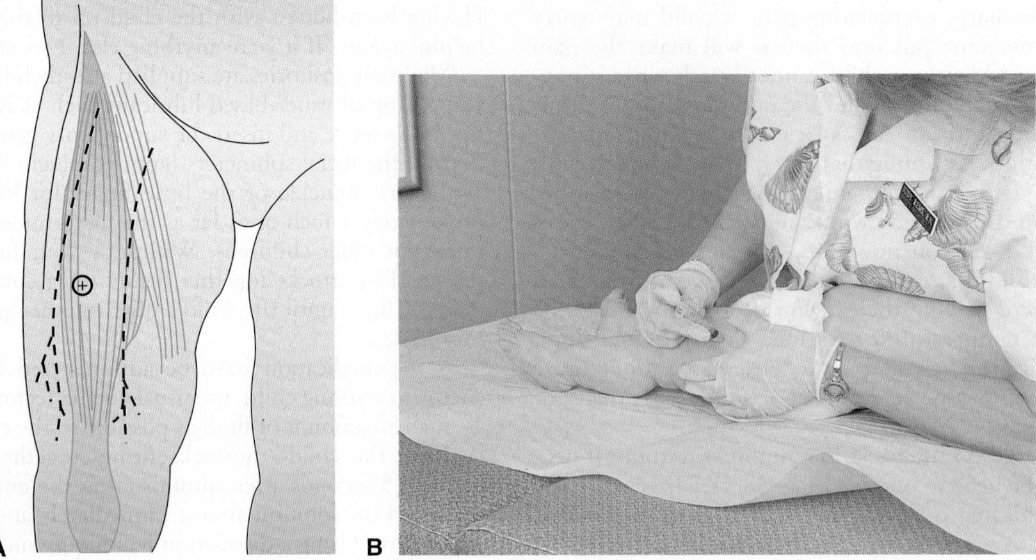

FIGURE 38.5 (**A**) For infants under walking age, use the vastus lateralis muscle for intramuscular injections. (**B**) Technique for administering an intramuscular injection to an infant. Note the way the nurse uses her body to restrain and stabilize the infant.

children younger than 1 year is extremely hazardous as this muscle does not develop until a child walks. This means that the sciatic nerve occupies a larger portion of the area than later on and could be permanently damaged by gluteal injections. Figure 38.5 shows an effective restraining technique for giving injections to infants. In older children, as in adults, the deltoid muscle (see Fig. 38.6A) or a ventrogluteal site (see Fig. 38.6B) should be used.

Never give injections to children who are sleeping in the hope they will not wake up and notice what is happening. They will wake up and will be terrified at being attacked. Instead, always give a short explanation of what you are about to do. Be honest about the pain involved; try to describe it accurately so that the child knows it has limits (a small amount of pain for a short time) with an explanation such as, "I have some medicine for you. I'm going to put it into your leg. It will sting for a second just like a pinprick. Then it will be over." To reduce pain further, ask for a prescription for an analgesic cream to be applied an hour before the injection (see Chapter 39). Most children react well to injections if you acknowledge that even with an anesthetic cream, injections can still hurt.

When giving injections, once you have described the drug's purpose and what you are going to do, do not delay giving the injection further by trying to distract the child or make a case it will not be bad. The suspense the child can feel while waiting can be worse than the actual injection. Give the injection quickly, but always use good technique. Remember to aspirate (if indicated). Quickness counts, but safety is your priority. Massage the area briefly after the injection to help ensure absorption of the medication, but remember that the rubbing may be painful and may be experienced as intrusive.

Statements such as "Don't cry" are not therapeutic. When children feel pain, they should be allowed to cry. As a way of giving children a better sense of control, you can tell them to say "ouch" or yell or scream when the needle is inserted. Most children appreciate being given approval to vent their feelings this way.

If necessary, ask for help in restraining a child when giving an injection to ensure safe administration. School-age children, however, may be proud they are able to lie still; being re-

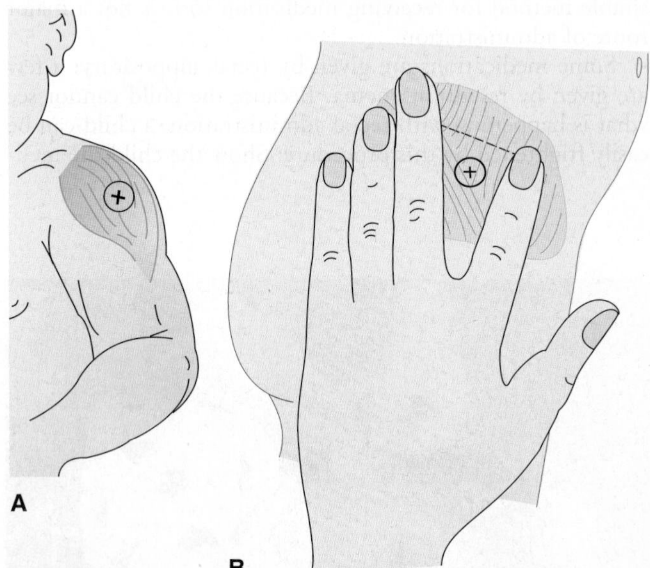

FIGURE 38.6 Sites for intramuscular injection. (**A**) In older children, the deltoid muscle is an acceptable site. (**B**) A ventrogluteal site may also be used in older children. Place the heel of the hand on the greater trochanter and the index finger angled toward the child's anterosuperior iliac crest, spreading the middle finger along the crest posteriorly. The triangle formed by the space between the index and middle fingers is the correct site.

strained would shame them. Hold and comfort a young child after all painful procedures, or let a parent do this.

Record the site of an IM injection as well as the medication injected, so that sites can be rotated for better absorption.

Continuous Subcutaneous Pump Infusion

Continuous subcutaneous pump infusion is administration of a medication by the constant infusion of a medication into the subcutaneous tissue using a medication pump (Khan & Younger, 2007). Continuous pump infusions supply a constant level of medicine to sustain consistent blood levels. The disadvantage is that a child must be careful to protect the pump from damage.

With an infusion pump, the drug is instilled into the subcutaneous tissue by the constant forward movement of a plunger of a medicine-filled syringe. The site chosen is usually the abdomen, as this both protects the pump and allows it to be out of sight. Insulin (see Chapter 48) and heparin are two drugs often prescribed for use with infusion pumps. Based on the success of this infusion technique for long-term drug administration, the system likely will be even more frequently used in the future.

The syringe is filled with medicine, and a small tube with the needle attached at the distal end is attached to the hub of the syringe. The syringe is then clamped to the pump, and the skin site is cleaned with alcohol and the needle inserted at a 45-degree angle (usual subcutaneous insertion technique). As soon as the needle is taped in place, the pump is turned on (see Fig. 20.5).

The insertion site should be changed every 1 to 2 days to reduce the possibility of infection. The pump should be removed to shower (the syringe, tubing, and needle can be left taped in place). For swimming or tub bathing, the entire pump, syringe, tubing, and needle should be removed. In children who are not toilet-trained, it is important to keep the pump and insertion site away from an area that could be soiled with urine or stool.

Older children, like adults, can be worried at first that the pump will fail to operate, so they check it often to be certain the syringe is emptying. With small children, cover the pump with clothing to prevent them from touching or trying to manipulate the syringe.

✔ Checkpoint Question 38.2

Suppose Terry needs to have ear drops. What is the best technique for giving these?

a. Have her place them herself to give a sense of control.
b. Refrigerate the drug first so it numbs the ear canal.
c. Pull the pinna of her ear down to straighten the canal.
d. Keep her head turned to the side to help retain the drops.

INTRAVENOUS THERAPY

In the past, IV therapy was used extensively as a rapid means of hydrating children who had become dehydrated because of diarrhea. Today, oral rehydration therapy is most often used in this way (Hartling et al., 2009). IV therapy is a fast and effective means of administering medicine to ill infants or children, however, so it still has a common place in care. It can be used to maintain fluid and electrolyte balance, to produce therapeutic levels of drugs in the body quickly, and to provide rehydration and nutritional support (Ford, 2008). Blood or blood product replacement is another common therapy (see Chapter 44). IV fluid may be infused into a peripheral vein, a central venous access device, or a peripherally inserted central venous catheter. The amount, type, and rate of IV fluids for children are prescribed carefully to prevent fluid overload.

Determining Fluid and Caloric Needs of the Child

IV fluid administered to children and infants must be isotonic (exerts the same osmotic pressure as their bloodstream) to prevent destruction of red blood cells or water intoxication. Using isotonic fluid prevents a pressure gradient that would lead to fluid shifting into the interstitial tissue (as would happen if the IV fluid were hypotonic) or fluid shifting from interstitial tissue into the bloodstream (as would happen if the IV fluid were hypertonic). Lactated Ringer's and 0.9% normal saline are two isotonic IV fluids commonly used in children. Normal saline 0.45% is a hypotonic solution that may be used with children who are dehydrated to restore blood volume quickly. Dextrose 10% in 0.9% sodium chloride is an example of a hypertonic solution that might be used to cause fluid to shift into the bloodstream to relieve cerebral edema for a child with a head injury. A typical fluid used for maintenance is 5% dextrose in 0.2% normal saline.

It is important to understand the principles of IV therapy, including the fluid and caloric needs of the child (which differ significantly from those of the adult) so you can act as a second level of protection against overhydration or underhydration.

Table 38.1 shows a method of calculating fluid requirements for children. Fluids administered using this table should contain 5% dextrose and 25 mEq sodium and 20 mEq potassium per liter so nutrients for energy and electrolytes are also replaced. Common IV solutions and oral rehydration formulas used with infants (rehydalyte and pedialyte) contain these proportions. According to Table 38.1, a child weighing 45 kg would need 2000 mL of a maintenance solution containing 5% dextrose, 25 mEq sodium, and 20 mEq potassium per liter. A flow rate would be calculated for this amount (2000 mL fluid in 24 hours = 83 mL/hr).

TABLE 38.1 ✻ A Method to Calculate Fluid Requirement

Body Weight	Fluid Requirement per 24 Hours
Up to 10 kg	100 mL/kg
11–20 kg	1000 mL + 50 mL/kg for each additional kg over 10 kg
More than 20 kg	1500 mL + 20 mL/kg for each additional kg over 20 kg

Box 38.5 Nursing Procedure ✻ Initiating a Scalp Vein Infusion

Purpose: To provide a route for intravenous therapy.

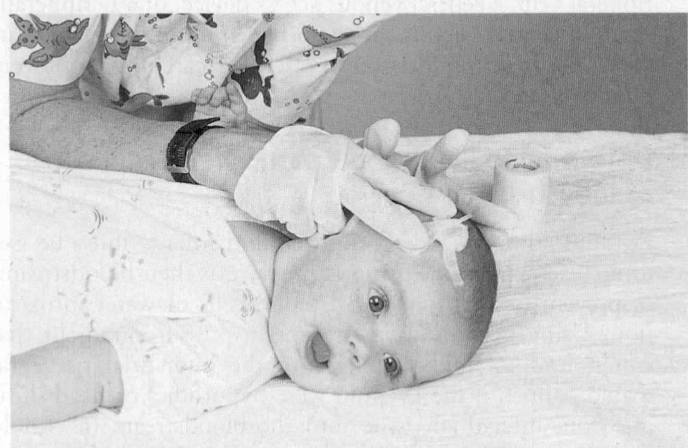

© Lesha Photography

Procedure	Principle
1. Adequately restrain the infant, using a mummy restraint.	**1.** Restraining the infant promotes safety. Mummy restraints are useful because it is physically exhausting to try to hold the infant's arms and legs still.
2. Press the child's head to the side and hold it firmly in that position, one hand on the occiput, the other securing the front of the head. Be certain that the hand resting over the child's face does not obstruct the child's breathing.	**2.** This positions the child without interfering with respirations.
3. Lather the site over the temporal bone with a cleaning solution.	**3.** The cleaning solution reduces the possibility of infection.
4. Carefully shave the hair. Assure parents that the hair will grow in quickly after the procedure. Ask parents if they want to save the clippings of hair if it is their child's first haircut.	**4.** Hair removal allows a clear view of the insertion site and possibly reduces the risk of infection.
5. Apply EMLA cream to the chosen site. After 60 minutes, place a rubber band around the infant's head at the level of the forehead.	**5.** A tourniquet is needed to dilate scalp veins. EMLA cream decreases discomfort but takes time to anesthetize the site.
6. Reswaddle the infant. Wash the shaved area with an antiseptic solution.	**6.** Washing the scalp further reduces the possibility of infection.
7. Insert a special small scalp vein needle or polytetrafluoroethylene (Teflon) catheter. Scalp vein needles have protruding plastic "wings" (often referred to as butterflies) on the sides to allow easy manipulation.	**7.** Use of an appropriate insertion device establishes a fluid route.
8. Continue to hold the infant firmly until the needle is securely taped in place, and until satisfied that the infusion is running well.	**8.** Securing the infant and device ensures an effective insertion site.
9. Cover the infusion needle with a piece of gauze (a plastic protector taped onto the site provides additional protection).	**9.** Covering the site keeps the infant from brushing the needle out of place when he or she turns the head.
10. If necessary, pin the shirt sleeves to the sides of the diaper or use a trunk or jacket restraint for an infant who is old enough to turn over.	**10.** Pinning the shirt keeps the infant from brushing at the site. Using restraints prevents the infant from turning over.
11. Spend some time comforting the child, talking and smiling at him or her, and lightly touching and stroking. Many infants enjoy sucking a pacifier after painful procedures; being held and rocked is the best comfort.	**11.** The infant may be frightened by the pinprick of the needle insertion, as well as by having been held so firmly for a length of time.

Obtaining Venous Access

The needle size for IV therapy varies depending on the solution and the rate at which it will be administered. Commonly used needle sizes include 22 gauge, 24 gauge, and 25 gauge (in newborns). "Butterfly" needles are metal needles with a flange of plastic added on both sides of the needle hub to give the person starting the infusion a wider surface to grasp, thereby making it easier to guide needle placement. Butterflies are also termed "scalp vein needles" because they were originally designed for use in infant scalp veins. A length of narrow tubing leads from the needle to the fluid administration tubing. This tubing must be flushed with IV solution before the needle is inserted to avoid an air embolus.

Sites frequently used for IV insertion in young children or infants include the veins on the dorsal surface of the hand or on the flexor surface of the wrist. Leg and foot veins also may be used. Another site is a scalp vein over the temporal area. An infusion placed in a scalp vein can be frightening to parents because it seems a much more serious procedure than an infusion administered into a hand. Explain to parents that scalp vein infusion is an effective method of administering fluid or medicine to infants and ultimately might cause the least discomfort for their child because needles there do not infiltrate readily (Box 38.5).

Preschoolers and older children often express a preference regarding where they want an infusion inserted. Offer a choice, if possible, or suggest the nondominant hand. Act as the child's advocate and see that wishes are respected.

Children who have IV infusions for long periods may require the placement of an **intracath** (a slim, pliable catheter threaded into a vein). The advantage of this type of device is that it cannot be dislodged as easily as a normally inserted IV needle, allowing a child to move about more freely.

For all children (including adolescents), IV infusions are usually secured in place with at least a small armboard. Although children may say they will be careful not to move their arms, without an armboard it is easy to move unintentionally to turn off the television set or reach for something that fell off the bed and accidentally dislodge the needle. Tape a board to the arm of an older child with the words, "This is just to remind you to keep your arm still"—an explanation more acceptable than if children think you doubt their ability to hold their hands still.

Determining Rate and Amount of Fluid Administration

Because children's hearts and circulatory systems are smaller than those of adults, IV fluid must be infused at a slower rate. If administered at an adult rate, the child's cardiovascular system could quickly become overloaded. Automatic rate-flow infusion pumps are useful when giving potent medications, and they should be mandatory for small children because they regulate the flow accurately to a few drops per minute (Fig. 38.7). Overloading of IV fluid in infants and children can also be prevented by use of fluid chambers, devices that allow only 50 to 100 mL of fluid into the drip chamber at a time. With these in place, even if the pump fails, only the amount of fluid in the drip chamber will be allowed to enter the child's circulation, not the entire contents of the bag suspended above the child's head.

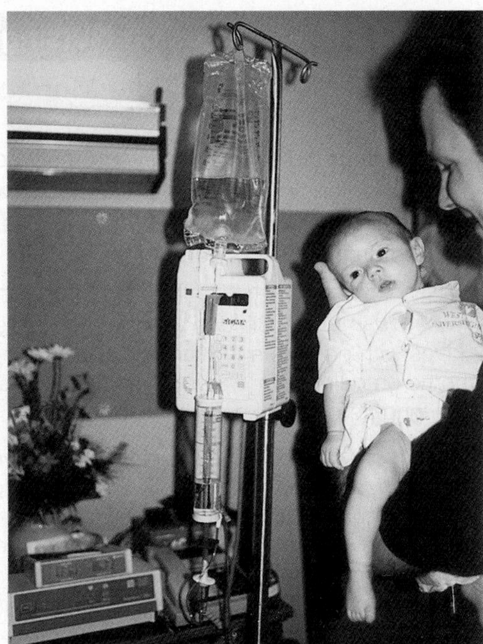

FIGURE 38.7 An infusion pump and calibrated infusion chamber are safety features used with children's intravenous infusions.

A third fluid safety measure is the use of a minidropper, a device that reduces the size of the drop in the control chamber to 60 drops per mL (usually there are 10 to 15 drops per mL). With a normal dropper in place, an infusion regulated to administer 30 mL/hr drops at a rate of 7 or 8 drops per minute, so it is difficult to regulate. With a minidropper in place, the drops are smaller: the same infusion (still providing the same amount of fluid per hour) drops at 30 drops per minute. This flow is easier to regulate and provides more accurate IV administration.

Keep a careful record of both the rate and amount of IV fluid administered to guard against fluid overload. At least once an hour, record the type and amount of fluid; the rate of flow (including the number of drops per minute); and, for a cross-check, the amount of fluid remaining in the bag. Signs of fluid overload are those of congestive heart failure: increased pulse rate and blood pressure. As the heart becomes overwhelmed by excessive fluid, blood pressure falls and signs of edema develop. Watch for changes in vital signs such as these when children are receiving IV fluids. In addition, assess the specific gravity of urine at least every 4 hours to detect extremely dilute urine (specific gravity under 1.003) as this suggests the child is excreting a large quantity of fluid in an effort to reduce overloaded circulating volume.

It is difficult for children to lie still and wait for an IV infusion to finish (see Focus on Nursing Care Planning Box 38.6). Provide them with activities and allow them out of bed as much as possible. Infants and preschoolers may need to have their other arm restrained to keep them from playing with an infusion needle. Be sure parents understand the importance of the IV therapy and help guard the infusion site as well. Infants who receive total fluids by IV infusion generally enjoy sucking on a pacifier to fulfill their oral needs.

Parents and children often have numerous questions about IV therapy; Box 38.8 supplies appropriate answers.

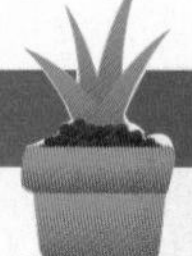

BOX 38.6 ✻ Focus on Nursing Care Planning

A Multidisciplinary Care Map for a Child Receiving Medication

Terry is an 8-year-old with Down syndrome whom you see in the emergency room. She is diagnosed with osteomyelitis, a bone infection. When you give her a tablet of acetaminophen (Tylenol) for pain, she spits it out. She does the same when you repeat with a second tablet. Her mother tells you Terry cannot swallow pills. Her father tells you, "You'll have to give her medicine intravenously."

Family Assessment ✻ Child is youngest of four siblings. Lives with parents and other siblings in five-bedroom home on dairy farm. Parents rate finances as, "Fine, as long as people keep drinking milk."

Client Assessment ✻ Child diagnosed with Down syndrome at birth; IQ approximately 60. Lacerated right foot on farm equipment by fall from hay loft 2 weeks ago. Laceration cleaned and bandaged by mother; not seen by health care provider. Today, wound has not healed; is open and erythematous; foot swollen; pain radiates up leg from foot. X-ray reveals abscess in bone (osteomyelitis). Child is so frightened by injections that she screams at the sight of any kind of needle. Child placed on bedrest and prescribed intravenous antibiotic and Demerol.

Nursing Diagnosis ✻ Pain related to disease process (infection) in foot

Outcome Evaluation ✻ Child rates pain on pain scale as 2 or below. Cooperates with IV medication therapy to supply antibiotic and pain relief.

Team Member Responsible	Assessment	Intervention	Rationale	Expected Outcome
		Activities of Daily Living		
Nurse	Assess what self-care measures child can complete by herself while on bedrest.	Explain resting foot and maintaining IV therapy are crucial measures.	Rest and antibiotic therapy will best cure condition and relieve pain.	Child, nurse, and parent agree on plan of care for activities of daily living.
		Consultations		
Nurse/physician	Assess if pain management team advice will be necessary.	Meet with pain consultant to discuss problem: child is in pain but needs to remain still for IV therapy.	Sustained antibiotic therapy is necessary to treat bone infection; consultation can help avoid infiltration.	Pain management consultant meets with child and parent as appropriate; agrees on pain management plan.
		Procedures/Medications		
Nurse	Assess if child has a preference for IV therapy site.	Begin IV therapy in nondominant hand if possible per M.D. order.	Allowing a child as much freedom as possible helps to prevent a feeling of entrapment.	Child helps to identify insertion site; cooperates to the best of ability with IV insertion.
Nurse	Ask child to rate pain by FACES pain scale.	Explain to child and parents how IV will supply pain medication; begin IV infusion.	IV Demerol will effectively control child's pain.	Child agrees to use of IV for pain relief. Rates pain level hourly.
		Nutrition		
Nurse	Assess if child has had past experience with eating in bed.	Discuss with child and parent the importance of continuing nutrition while on bedrest. Suggest taking pain medication bolus before meals.	Hospitalization can be a major stress to children. Pain can interfere with nutrition.	Child discusses intent not to let hospitalization or pain interfere with nutrition.

Patient/Family Education				
Nurse	Assess if child has had experience with IV therapy in the past.	Review importance and plan for IV therapy with child and parents.	Knowledgeable patients and parents can aid in the success of therapy.	Child and parents state they understand why antibiotic and analgesia is needed and why administration method is required.
Psychosocial/Spiritual/Emotional Needs				
Nurse	Explore (if known) why child is so afraid of needles.	Discuss advantages of IV therapy, which will minimize injections yet supply antibiotic.	Fear of needles is common in children; advocating for IV therapy can help relieve this fear.	Child states she understands IV therapy will involve a needle but needle will be inserted only once.
Discharge Planning				
Nurse	Assess if parents have questions about child's care at home.	Explain the importance of continuing oral antibiotic, adequate oral pain relief.	Continuing antibiotic administration will be necessary to combat deep-seated infection.	Parents state they understand importance of continuing medicine administration. Keep follow-up visit for evaluation.

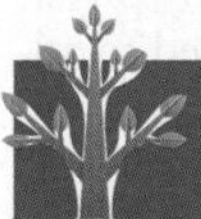

BOX 38.7 * Focus on Family Teaching

General Considerations for Intravenous Therapy

Q. Terry's mother asks you a lot of questions about intravenous therapy, such as "Why can't Terry just drink fluid?"

A. Parents and children often want to know more about IV therapy. Some of the typical questions parents ask are:

- Will the insertion hurt? (Yes, but only as the needle is inserted; after that the infusion will be pain-free.)
- How long will the infusion be necessary? (The duration differs depending on the medicine and fluid prescription and can vary depending on the effect of the medicine or fluid.)
- Isn't there another way to administer the same medicine? (Usually, no. IV administration allows medicine to reach the bloodstream immediately and so is the method of choice when immediate effect is important; also, some medications can only be given intravenously.)
- What can the child do during the infusion? (Any activity that will not interfere with the infusion. If a child will have medicine administration daily, help the child plan a special activity such as play a board game, listen to special music, or watch a favorite TV program, an activity reserved for only that time. This changes the IV infusion from a dreaded activity to a "can't wait for" activity.)
- Will it hurt when the needle is removed? (No, although taking off the tape that holds the needle in place may cause some discomfort.)

Intravenous Medication Administration

Medications may be added to an IV line as a small, one-time administration (bolus) or by piggyback for longer infusions. As with any medication administration, identify the child before adding medicine to an IV line. Also ensure that the drug to be injected is compatible with the IV fluid being infused.

To administer medicine by a bolus technique, clamp the IV tubing above the medicine port in the IV line; clean the port with alcohol; insert the needle of the syringe filled with the prescribed medicine into the port; and inject the medicine slowly and gently based on the manufacturer's instructions. Once the medication has been given, remove the syringe and needle and reopen the IV line immediately to allow the IV solution to flush the medicine into the child.

For a piggyback infusion of medicine, medication is provided by the pharmacy and prepared and diluted in small fluid-filled plastic bags. To begin a piggyback infusion, hang the piggyback bag, clean the medicine port on the IV line, and insert the piggyback system into the port. Lower the level of the main infusion bag and adjust the flow rate to that desired to allow the piggyback system to operate. As soon as the piggyback bag has emptied, elevate the maintenance bag of fluid again and make sure the IV line is flowing well and at the proper rate.

Children accept piggyback administrations of fluid well because it seems no different from receiving maintenance IV fluid. Older children can take an active role in alerting health care providers that the total medication amount has infused and it is time to return to maintenance fluid.

Analgesics are commonly administered to older children by patient-controlled analgesia machines (D'Arcy, 2008). Because these machines are set with lockout time intervals, they are safe to use with children as young as early school age (see Chapter 39). Although, when programmed, such pumps help protect against medication errors, they are not foolproof (Box 38.8).

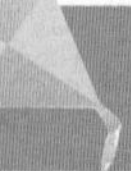

BOX 38.8 * Focus on Evidence-Based Practice

Does use of patient-controlled analgesia help reduce medication errors?

One of the advantages of patient-controlled analgesia is that the system can reduce medication errors, because if the pump is programmed correctly, no further thought toward medication administration seems necessary. To see if PCA administration does reduce errors, researchers analyzed medication errors from a national reporting service over a 5-year period. Of all the orders reported only 1% were related to PCA pumps. Of that 1% of errors, over one third (38%) involved an improper dosage or quantity, while 17.4% involved an omission and 17.3% an unauthorized or wrong drug. Overwhelmingly, human factors were the main cause of PCA errors. Equipment issues (19.5%) and similar drug names and product packaging (11.6%) were also implicated. Distractions (37.8%) and inexperienced staff (26.3%) were the leading contributing factors.

Based on the above study, do you need to check that a PCA pump that was programmed by another nurse is programmed correctly or should you just assume that the child is protected from a medication error because of the pump?

Source: Hicks, R. W., et al. (2008). Medication errors involving patient-controlled analgesia. *AJHP: American Journal of Health-System Pharmacy, 65*(5), 429–440.

Using Intermittent Infusion Devices

Intermittent infusion devices, still sometimes called heparin locks, are devices that maintain open venous access for medicine administration while allowing children to be free of IV tubing so that they can be out of bed and more active (Fig. 38.8). The veins of the back of the hand are generally chosen as the IV site. Scalp vein tubing is used and capped at the end with a specially designed rubber stopper or a commercial trap. The tubing is filled with a dilute solution of heparin or normal saline through the rubber stopper and flushed again with solution every 2 to 8 hours (depending on hospital policy) to keep it patent. IV medication can be added to the site as needed. The tubing and stopper must be firmly secured to the wrist and an armboard taped in place to remind a child to protect the site from trauma.

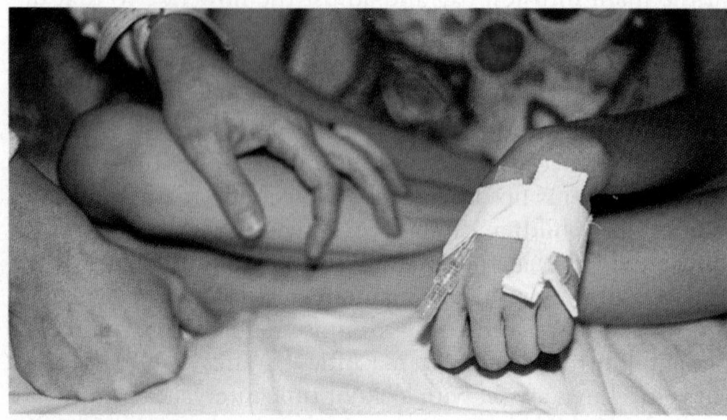

FIGURE 38.8 An intermittent infusion device in place. Advocating for this type of apparatus minimizes pain.

Children who are hospitalized or receiving home care for a long time and who need only IV medication, not additional fluid, are good candidates for such devices. Intermittent infusion devices also can be used if frequent venous blood samples are required. If blood is drawn from the already inserted tubing, the child is pricked only once (when the device is originally placed) no matter how many samples are drawn. Similar devices may be inserted into arteries when arterial blood is required—for example, for the child who is having blood gases monitored frequently.

Using Central Venous Access Catheters and Devices

Venous access for long-term IV therapy can be obtained using a catheter inserted into the vena cava just outside the right atrium; the catheter exits the chest just under the clavicle (Fig. 38.9). Typical catheters used in this way include Broviac, Hickman, and Groshong catheters. Such catheters have a wrinkle-resistant fabric (Dacron) cuff that adheres to the subcutaneous tissue and helps to seal the catheter in place and keep out infection. These catheters are inserted by physicians or nurses who are specially prepared and are used to administer bolus or continuous infusions of medications and fluid (Jardine, Inglis, & Davies, 2009). Care of the catheters (depending on agency policy) consists of daily or weekly changes of dressings over the exit site and periodic irrigation with heparin or saline to ensure patency.

Such catheters are advantageous because discomfort from further skin punctures is avoided. One disadvantage is that the catheter could become snagged on something and accidentally be pulled out. If this happens, it is an emergency situation because the child could lose an appreciable amount of blood from the point of entrance into a vein as major as the vena cava. Unless there is a waterproof dressing covering the insertion site, children with central venous catheters in place are usually not allowed to swim or take showers, to avoid infection.

Vascular access ports (VAPs; infusion ports that can be implanted) are small plastic devices that are implanted under the skin, usually on the anterior chest just under the clavicle, for long-term fluid or medication administration via bolus or continuous administration (see Fig. 38.9D). A small catheter threads from the port internally into a central vein. Common brands include Port-A-Cath, Infus-A-Port, and Groshong Venous Port. After skin cleansing, blood samples can be removed or medication can be injected by a puncture through the chest skin into the port. Although this device requires a skin puncture (causes pain), it may be well accepted by children because it is not as visible as a central venous catheter, no dressing is required, and it allows a full range of activities, such as showering and swimming. Be certain when accessing these ports to use only the needle supplied by the manufacturer, because a regular needle tends to "core" or remove a small circle of the membrane over the port and destroy the integrity of the device. Use EMLA cream to decrease discomfort as necessary.

2. Suppose Terry needs to have an intraosseous infusion. How would you explain what this is to her parents?
3. Suppose Terry's mother tells you that she does not believe in introducing any "foreign" substance into her child's body, so she does not intend to give her the antibiotic for her infected foot. Would there be a way to change her mind? How would you counsel her?
4. Examine the National Health Goals related to medicine administration in children. Most government-sponsored funds for nursing research are allotted based on these goals. What would be a possible research topic to explore pertinent to these goals that would be applicable to Terry's family and also advance evidence-based practice?

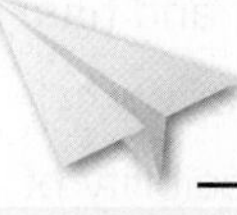

CRITICAL THINKING SCENARIO

Open the accompanying CD-ROM or visit http://thePoint.lww.com and read the Patient Scenario included for this chapter, then answer the questions to further sharpen your skills and grow more familiar with NCLEX style questions related to medication or intravenous therapy in children. Confirm your answers are correct by reading the rationales.

REFERENCES

Baker, D. D., & Jenkins, A. J. (2008). A comparison of methadone, oxycodone, and hydrocodone related deaths in Northeast Ohio. *Journal of Analytical Toxicology, 32*(2), 165–171.

Carpenter, L. R., et al. (2007). Mass distribution of free, intranasally administered influenza vaccine in a public school system. *Pediatrics, 120*(1), e172–e178.

D'Arcy, Y. (2008). Keep your patient safe during PCA. *Nursing, 38*(1), 50–56.

Dart, R. C., & Rumack, B. H. (2008). Poisoning. In W. W. Hay, et al. (Eds.). *Current pediatric diagnosis and treatment* (18th ed.). Columbus, OH: McGraw-Hill.

de Caen, A. (2007). Venous access in the critically ill child: when the peripheral intravenous fails! *Pediatric Emergency Care, 23*(6), 422–426.

Ford, D. M. (2008). Fluid, electrolyte and acid-base disorders and therapy. In W. W. Hay, et al. (Eds.). *Current pediatric diagnosis and treatment* (18th ed.). Columbus, OH: McGraw-Hill.

Hartling, L., et al. (2009). Oral versus intravenous rehydration for treating dehydration due to gastroenteritis in children. *Cochrane Database of Systematic Reviews, 2009*(1), (CD004390).

Hicks, R. W., et al. (2008). Medication errors involving patient-controlled analgesia. *AJHP: American Journal of Health-System Pharmacy, 65*(5), 429–440.

Holsti, M., et al. (2007). Prehospital intranasal midazolam for the treatment of pediatric seizures. *Pediatric Emergency Care, 23*(3), 148–153.

Jardine, L. A., Inglis, G. D. T., & Davies, M. W. (2009). Prophylactic systemic antibiotics to reduce morbidity and mortality in neonates with central venous catheters. *Cochrane Database of Systematic Reviews, 2009*(1), (CD006179).

Khan, M., & Younger, G. (2007). Promoting safe administration of subcutaneous infusions. *Nursing Standard, 21*(31), 50–56.

Kleiber, C. (2008). Acetaminophen dosing for neonates, infants, and children. *JSPN: Journal for Specialists in Pediatric Nursing, 13*(1), 48–49.

Linck, D. A., Donze, A., & Hamvas, A. (2007). Neonatal peripherally inserted central catheter team: evolution and outcomes of a bedside-nurse-designed program. *Advances in Neonatal Care, 7*(1), 22–29.

Renouf, P. (2007). Immediate or delayed prescribing of antibiotics reduced duration of symptoms in acute infective conjunctivitis. *Evidence-Based Nursing, 10*(1), 10.

Root, N. (2007). Creating a safe environment for pediatric ED patients. *Journal of Emergency Nursing, 33*(3), 286–289.

Sammons, H., & Conroy, S. (2008). How do we ensure safe prescribing for children? *Archives of Disease in Childhood, 93*(2), 98–99.

Sobhani, P., et al. (2008). Accuracy of oral liquid measuring devices: comparison of dosing cup and oral dosing syringe. *Annals of Pharmacotherapy, 42*(1), 46–52.

Szobot, C. M., & Bukstein, O. (2008). Attention deficit hyperactivity disorder and substance use disorders. *Child & Adolescent Psychiatric Clinics of North America, 17*(2), 309–323.

Stavroudis, T. A., Miller, M. R., & Lehmann, C. U. (2008). Medication errors in neonates. *Clinics in Perinatology, 35*(1), 141–161.

SUGGESTED READINGS

Berry, K. A. (2008). Rx to improve medication safety. *Behavioral Healthcare, 28*(2), 36–38.

Bridge, L. (2007). Reducing the risk of wrong route errors. *Paediatric Nursing, 19*(6), 33–35.

Cescon, D. W., & Etchells, E. (2008). Barcoded medication administration: a last line of defense. *JAMA: Journal of the American Medical Association, 299*(18), 2200–2202.

Cohen, M. R. (2008). Medication errors. *Nursing, 38*(1), 12.

Holliday, M. A., Ray, P. E., & Friedman, A. L. (2007). Fluid therapy for children: facts, fashions and questions. *Archives of Disease in Childhood, 92*(6), 546–550.

Ludeman, K. (2007). Choosing the right vascular access device. *Nursing, 37*(9), 38–41.

Rinke, M. L., et al. (2008). Patient safety rounds in a pediatric tertiary care center. *Joint Commission Journal on Quality and Patient Safety, 34*(1), 5–12.

Simpson, K. R. (2008). Perinatal patient safety. Medication safety with heparin. *MCN: The American Journal of Maternal/Child Nursing, 3*(2), 135.

Stokes, T., et al. (2009). Self-management education for children with epilepsy. *Cochrane Database of Systematic Reviews, 2009*(1), (CD004724).

Zandieh, S. O., et al. (2008). Risk factors in preventable adverse drug events in pediatric outpatients. *Journal of Pediatrics, 152*(2), 225–231.

Chapter 39 Pain Management in Children

KEY TERMS

- acute pain
- conscious sedation
- chronic pain
- cutaneous pain
- distraction
- epidural analgesia
- gate control theory
- nociceptors
- pain
- pain threshold
- pain tolerance
- patient-controlled analgesia
- referred pain
- somatic pain
- substitution of meaning
- thought stopping
- transcutaneous electrical nerve stimulation
- visceral pain

OBJECTIVES

After mastering the contents of this chapter, you should be able to:

1. Describe the major methods and techniques of pain management for children.
2. Identify National Health Goals related to pain management in children that nurses can help the nation achieve.
3. Use critical thinking to analyze ways nursing care for a child in pain could be more family centered.
4. Assess a child regarding whether pain management is needed or adequate.
5. Formulate nursing diagnoses for a child in pain.
6. Identify expected outcomes for a child in pain.
7. Plan nursing care for a child in pain.
8. Implement nursing care related to a child in pain such as suggesting an alternative therapy.
9. Evaluate outcomes for achievement and effectiveness of care of a child in pain.
10. Identify areas related to care of children in pain that could benefit from additional nursing research or application of evidence-based practice.
11. Integrate knowledge of pain in children with nursing process to achieve quality maternal and child health nursing care.

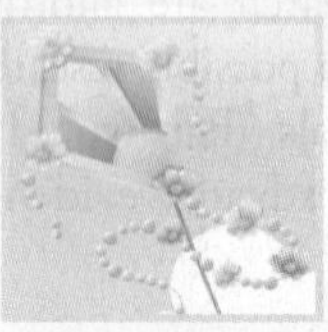

Robin Harvey is a 3-year-old girl who was admitted to your hospital unit and has just returned from a bone marrow aspiration to rule out the possibility of leukemia. Robin received intravenous morphine sulfate during the procedure. Her mother asks you if Robin could have some more. "I know she's not having pain yet," her mother tells you, "but I want her to have something before the pain comes back."

Previous chapters described the growth and development of children and general care of ill children. This chapter adds information about care of children when they need pain management. Such information builds a base for care and health teaching in a crucial area.

Is this mother's assessment or Robin's assessment of her pain apt to be most accurate? Would anticipating pain in this way be the best intervention for Robin?

Pain is a difficult concept to define because it is experienced uniquely. It is important to remember that it is subjective (experienced by the person), not objective (able to be determined by observation). McCaffery's classic description of pain (Pasero & McCaffery, 2004) is the one most useful with children: "The sensation of pain is whatever the person experiencing it says it is, and it exists whenever the person says it does."

For children, pain is not only a hurting sensation, but it can also be a confusing one because a child did not anticipate the pain, does not have words to explain how it feels, and cannot always understand its cause. In addition, preschoolers and younger children lack an understanding of time, which makes it difficult to explain when the pain will go away. Children may feel frustrated or angry because no one can prevent their hurt or give them relief. Because children may have difficulty describing pain in a manner adults can understand, it is difficult to assess the extent of their discomfort. Because pain is an individualized sensation, it may be experienced and expressed differently by different children. In some families, for example, pain may be expressed very openly and freely. In others, children are expected to be stoic about pain. Because the expression of pain is culturally determined this way, two children who have the same degree of pain may express it very differently (Eccleston et al., 2009).

Additionally, children's perception of the situation influences their response to the situation, independent of the intensity of the pain. This means that children experiencing procedures that are less intrusive but who are feeling maximum anxiety may describe the degree of pain felt as more intense than they otherwise might, because of the accompanying anxiety.

Both helping children describe the type and extent of pain they are feeling and performing active interventions to relieve pain are important nursing roles. Assessing for pain is so important that pain can be considered the "fifth vital sign."

National Health Goals do not address pain relief in children directly, but they do address the reduction of accidental injury, which is a major source of pain in children. These goals are shown in Box 39.1.

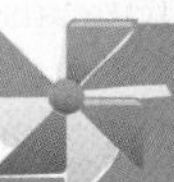

BOX 39.1 ✻ Focus on National Health Goals

Although National Health Goals do not speak directly to alleviating pain in children, many of the goals speak to reducing unintentional accidents, which are a major source of pain in children. Some of these objectives are:

- Increase the rate of use for automobile safety belts and infant safety seats to 100% for children under age 4 from a baseline of 92%.
- Increase the rate of helmet use to at least 79% of motorcyclists from a baseline of 67%.
- Increase the number of states with laws requiring bicycle helmets for riders under the age of 15 from a baseline of 10 states to all states.
- Increase the presence of functional smoke detectors to 100% of all inhabited residential dwellings from a baseline of 88%.
- Reduce the rate of hospital emergency department visits for nonfatal dog bite injuries to 114 per 100,000 of the population from a baseline of 151 per 100,000 (http://www.nih.gov).

Nurses can be help the nation to reduce pain among children by teaching about the importance of using safety belts and bicycle helmets. As primary care providers, they can lead the effort to be certain that children and parents receive counseling on safety precautions. Additional nursing research that is needed in the area of pain relief concerns identifying the best way for children to rate pain and the nonpharmacologic measures that work best with different age groups.

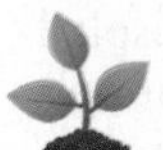

Nursing Process Overview

For a Child in Pain

Assessment

Children, like adults, experience pain differently depending on the type and cause of the pain, their temperament, their previous experience with pain, and their expectation of relief. Infants and young children cannot verbalize what they are feeling so have the most trouble communicating how they feel.

Beginning with preschool age, children can indicate where they feel pain and can learn to express the degree of pain through a system such as comparing it to a number of poker chips or drawings of faces. Older school-age children and adolescents can be asked to rate their pain on a scale of 1 to 10. Be aware that children may be reluctant to admit pain because they are trying to be brave. Some may be reluctant to say they have pain because they are afraid they will receive a "shot" to relieve it, and that will cause more pain. As a rule, including assessment of pain level along with vital sign measurement is an efficient way to ensure that pain is assessed. Be alert that this is only the first step in pain management, though. If children have pain, they need some intervention as a second step to relieve it. Let children know that admitting to having pain is necessary for them to obtain adequate relief.

Parents often are unclear what role they should assume in pain management. Frequently parents believe nurses and doctors are the experts and so will automatically treat their child's pain. Nurses, on the other hand, may assume that parents will speak up if their child is in pain. How pain will be assessed, the parents' role, and what is available for pain relief should be discussed clearly and openly so these misunderstandings do not occur. Be certain that you also reassess pain to be certain that interventions such as administration of an analgesic or distraction or improved positioning were effective.

Nursing Diagnosis

Nursing diagnoses for children with pain focus not only on the pain but also on the stress, fear, or anxiety that pain produces. Examples of nursing diagnoses are:

- Pain related to frequent invasive procedures
- Fear related to anticipation of painful procedures

- Disturbed sleep pattern related to chronic pain
- Anxiety related to planned dressing changes that cause pain

Outcome Identification and Planning

The mark of efficient pain control is to anticipate when pain will occur and plan interventions to prevent it rather than let it occur and then relieve it. Three common reasons why nurses may not provide adequate pain relief to children are a belief that infants and young children do not experience pain, a fear that children will become addicted to pain relief medications, and a fear of causing respiratory depression from analgesics. Infants and young children do experience pain, and there is no confirmation that children receiving narcotics during a short hospital stay will become addicted to pain medication or that opiates cause greater respiratory depression in children than in adults. Although the use of opiates can lead to dependency, this is very different from addiction and can be addressed with a weaning regimen if needed. The American Academy of Pediatrics' pain management suggestions are available at http://www.aap.org/.

Implementation

Implementation for pain relief includes choosing the specific method of pain relief best for each child. All persons involved in a child's care need to be aware of the signs and symptoms an individual child uses to express pain and specific ways that will help the child manage pain. If children are reluctant to admit they have pain because of the fear of receiving an injection, advocate for an oral form of analgesia or an intermittent intravenous (IV) infusion device or patient-controlled analgesia (PCA) as appropriate options. Many parents are unsure about the safety of using strong analgesics for pain relief so often give less than the prescribed dose. Therefore, educating parents about the need for pain relief, proper doses, and taking actions to involve them in the assessment and evaluation process are essential. Planning and assisting with complementary therapies is yet another area to consider.

Outcome Evaluation

Evaluation of expected outcomes is a key aspect of managing pain because no one pain relief measure is effective for everyone. After a child is given an analgesic, look for nonverbal clues, assess vital signs, and listen to the child's statements about pain to determine whether a drug was effective. Based on these findings, it may become clear that the technique of pain management being used may need to be modified or increased. A new technique may need to be added to the regimen so a child receives maximum pain relief.

Possible examples indicating achievement of expected outcomes are:

- Child states pain is now at a tolerable level.
- Adolescent says she has managed her fear through imagery.
- Child rates pain as no greater than 2 on a 1-to-10 scale.
- Child describes ways he will help reduce pain when it returns.
- Child resumes age-appropriate behaviors following analgesia administration.

PHYSIOLOGY OF PAIN

As in adults, pain in children occurs for one of four reasons: reduced oxygen in tissues from impaired circulation, pressure on tissue, external injury, or overstretching of body cavities with fluid or air. The stimuli causing pain are not always visible or measurable. In addition, anxiety can lead to increased pain regardless of the physical stimuli.

Pain conduction consists of four major steps: transduction (sensing the pain sensation), transmission (routing the pain sensation to the spinal cord), perception (the brain interprets the sensation as pain), and modulation (steps taken to relive pain).

Transduction begins in the peripheral nerves when a mechanical, thermal, or chemical stimulus activates **nociceptors,** a specialized group of sensory receptors. Several neurotransmitters (e.g., substance P) are also stimulated and involved in conducting pain. Sharp pain impulses are conducted by both A-alpha and A-beta fibers (large fibers that are myelinated and conduct the response at a rapid rate). Light pressure and vibration are conducted by A-delta fibers, fibers that are smaller and conduct at a slower rate. C fibers are smaller yet and conduct at an even slower rate.

Pain impulses join central nervous system (CNS) fibers in the dorsal horn of the spinal cord. Here the impulses are projected upward to the brain, where they will be perceived as pain.

- **Acute pain** is sharp pain. It generally occurs abruptly after an injury. Paper cuts are examples of lacerations that cause acute pain.
- **Chronic pain** is pain that lasts for a prolonged period (often defined as 6 months). Acute pain usually causes extreme distress and anxiety; chronic pain can lead to depression and less ability to achieve (Eccleston et al., 2009).
- **Cutaneous pain** is pain that arises from superficial structures such as the skin and mucous membrane. A paper cut is an example.
- **Somatic pain** is pain that originates from deep body structures such as muscles or blood vessels. The pain of a sprained ankle is somatic pain.
- **Visceral pain** involves sensations that arise from internal organs such as the intestines. The pain of appendicitis is visceral pain.
- **Referred pain** is pain that is perceived at a site distant from its point of origin. Right lower lobe pneumonia, for example, is often first thought to be abdominal pain because the pain of this is referred to the abdomen.

A child's **pain threshold** refers to the point at which the child first feels pain. This varies greatly from person to person and is probably most influenced by heredity. All people also have a point above which they are not willing to bear any additional pain. This is a person's **pain tolerance.** Pain tolerance levels are probably most affected by cultural influences.

When pain is felt the pituitary and hypothalamus glands attempt to modify pain by releasing *endorphins* or polypeptide compounds that simulate opiates in their ability to produce analgesia and a sense of well-being. Children also modify pain by physical actions such as shifting position or rubbing the body part.

Several theories have been proposed to explain the transmission of pain and how pain can best be managed. Of these, the gate control theory is the best known.

Gate Control Theory of Pain

The **gate control theory** of pain (Melzack & Wall, 1965) attempts to explain how pain impulses travel from a site of injury to the brain, where the impulse is actually registered as pain. This theory envisions gating mechanisms in the substantia gelatinosa of the dorsal horn of the spinal cord that, when activated, can halt an impulse at that level of the cord. This prevents the pain impulse from being received at the brain level and interpreted as pain. Gating mechanisms can be stimulated by three techniques: cutaneous stimulation, distraction, and anxiety reduction.

Cutaneous stimulation has an effect because when the peripheral nerves next to an injury site are stimulated, the ability of the A-delta or C-fiber nerves at the injury site to transmit pain impulses appears to decrease. Rubbing an injured part such as a stubbed toe and applying heat or cold to the site are effective maneuvers to suppress pain because they activate these nearby fibers. This technique is especially effective with children because the rubbing is not only comforting from a physical standpoint but also conveys psychological warmth.

Distraction allows the cells of the brainstem that register an impulse as pain to be preoccupied with other stimuli so a pain impulse cannot register. Having a child focus on an action or a thought is a common form of distraction. Telling a child to say "ouch" while an injection is administered is the simplest use of this technique.

Pain impulses are perceived more quickly by the brain if anxiety is also present. Therefore, attempts to reduce a child's anxiety as much as possible can help reduce the feeling of pain. Teaching a school-age child about what to expect with a procedure is the kind of technique that does this. As well as knowing when something is going to happen, children also should know when nothing is going to happen. Being told that a clinic visit will not involve painful procedures allows a child to relax and feel less anxiety.

The effectiveness of gate control theory techniques varies with a child's age, ability to cooperate, degree of pain, and time allowed for learning and applying the techniques. Because memory may influence the sensation of pain (expecting to have pain produces anxiety, which increases pain), these techniques are best taught to children before they begin to have pain. In all instances, children should know to use them just before or at the moment they first feel the pain. If they wait until pain is intense, the pain may be so distracting they cannot concentrate on using a technique. Children who were able to use a distraction technique in the past but can no longer do so need to be evaluated for what is changing. Is it their ability to cope with the pain, or is the pain increasing in intensity? Contrary to common belief, familiarity with diagnostic or therapeutic procedures does not necessarily lessen either the fear or the pain experienced.

ASSESSING TYPE AND DEGREE OF PAIN

Pain assessment is difficult with children, not only because children have difficulty describing pain but also because some children will suffer with pain rather than report it, unaware that someone could make it go away. Other children may distract themselves by methods such as concentrating on play. Some children may sleep, not from comfort but from the exhaustion caused by pain. Cultural differences also influence how pain is expressed (Box 39.2). All of these things can make using only subjective measures, such as observation, to assess pain misleading.

Pain assessment in children is also difficult because techniques vary widely from assessment of a nonverbal infant to an older adolescent. Keep in mind a child's developmental level as well as chronological age when assessing for pain.

Box 39.2 Assessment
Assessing a Child With Pain

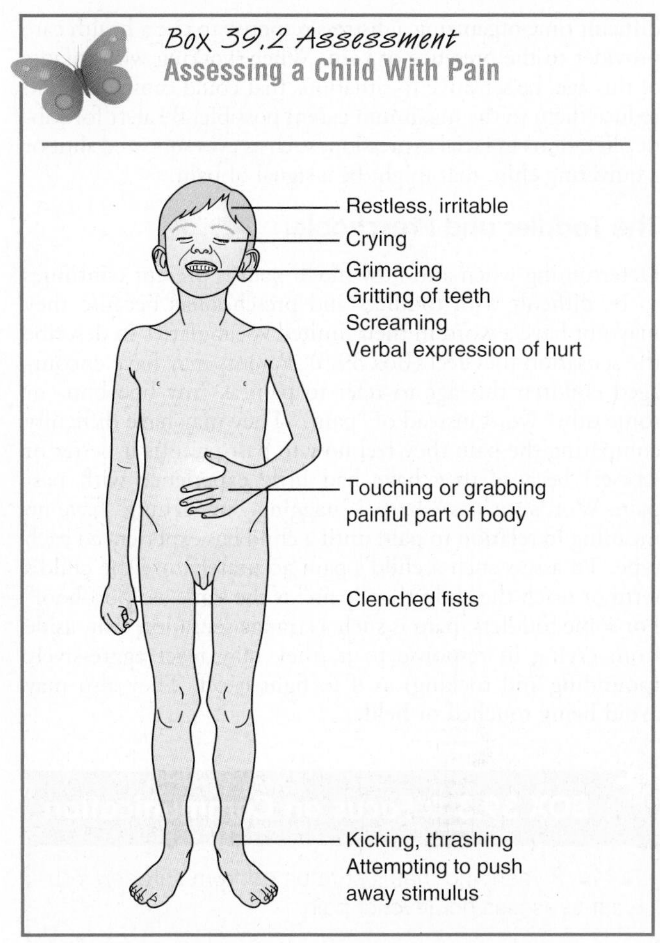

The Infant

In the past, it was believed that infants do not feel pain because of incomplete myelinization of peripheral nerves. This is no longer believed to be true, because myelinization is not necessary for pain perception.

A second argument against needing to provide pain relief to infants was that they have no memory. It can be shown, however, that physiologic changes occur with pain even in premature infants, so even with a lack of memory, it is clear pain is experienced. In all ages, pain has been shown to have the potential for serious physical harm. Because they are preverbal, observing for cues such as diffuse body movement; tears; a high-pitched, sharp, harsh cry; stiff posture; lack of play; and fisting are all cues to reveal discomfort (American Academy of Pediatrics [AAP], 2007). Even newborns instinctively guard a body part by holding an extremity still or tensing the abdomen. Perhaps the chief mark of pain in infants is that when pain is present, they cannot be comforted completely. Preterm neonates may have a particularly difficult time organizing a distress response to cue a health care provider to the presence of pain. When working with infants of this age, be sensitive to situations that could cause pain and reduce them to the maximum extent possible. Be alert for subtle alterations in facial expression, such as eyes squeezed shut or a quivering chin, that might be a signal of pain.

The Toddler and Preschooler

Determining when and how much pain is present continues to be difficult with toddlers and preschoolers because they may not have a word in their limited vocabularies to describe the sensation they feel (Box 39.3). Parents may have encouraged children this age to refer to pain as "my boo-boo" or some other word instead of "pain." They may have difficulty comparing the pain they feel now to past pain (is it better or worse?) because they have had little experience with past pain. Words such as "sharp," "nagging," or "aching" have no meaning in relation to pain until a child has experienced each type. To assess such a child's pain accurately, use the child's term or teach the child that "pain" is the same as "boo-boo." For some toddlers, pain is such a strange sensation that, aside from crying in response to it, they may react aggressively (pounding and rocking) as if to fight it off. They also may avoid being touched or held.

BOX 39.3 * Focus on Communication

Robin, 3 years old, has just returned from surgery. You want to assess her level of pain.

Less Effective Communication

Nurse: Robin? How are you feeling?
Mrs. Harvey: I don't think she hurts yet.
Nurse: I'm going to show you some faces, Robin. Just point to the one that looks the way you feel. If you point to a sad one, I'll get you a shot to take away your pain.
Robin: (Points to the first face—the "no pain" face.)
Nurse: No pain? Good. That's probably because your anesthetic is still working.

More Effective Communication

Nurse: Robin? How are you feeling?
Mrs. Harvey: I don't think she hurts yet.
Nurse: Robin? Remember the faces we looked at this morning before surgery? I want you to use them to tell me how you feel. This one means "no hurt." This one means "the most hurt you could have." Point to the one that shows how much hurt you have.
Robin: (Points to the middle face—the "hurts even more" face.)

It is important when using pain rating scales to introduce them to children before surgery or before they have pain from procedures, so that both the pain and the rating tool are not new to the child all at once. It is important also to give the correct instructions for standardized assessment tools, or the results will not be accurate. Mentioning a "shot for pain" can cause children not to report pain because they imagine the injection will cause even more pain, rather than relieve it.

Preschool children can describe they have pain but continue to have difficulty describing its intensity. They begin to use comforting mechanisms, such as gritting teeth, pressing a hand against a forehead, pulling on their ear, holding their throat, rubbing an arm, or grimacing, to control or express pain. Some preschoolers do not think to mention they have pain because they believe it is something to be expected or, because of their egocentric thinking, they assume adults are already aware of their pain. They may think pain is punishment for some act, so this is what they deserve. It is sometimes difficult to comfort children this age during painful procedures because they do not yet have a perception of time. Soothing statements such as, "It's only for a minute" are not comforting to the preschooler who does not know how long that is.

For all young children who cannot fully verbalize their pain state, carefully examine their behavior. In addition to behaviors already discussed, young children may regress or become very withdrawn when in pain. Ask yourself, "What would this child normally be doing (for example, playing, eating, sleeping)?" Deviations from usual behavior may, in the absence of any other verbal description, be signs a child is in pain. Input from parents on how their child usually behaves can be valuable in evaluation. Keep in mind that any procedure or condition that would normally cause pain in an adult will cause pain in a child. In a nonverbal child, a trial dose of analgesia may be used. You can then evaluate behavior changes after the dose is given. Children who resume their usual behavior after analgesia were probably in pain before the analgesia took effect.

The School-Age Child and Adolescent

Children who think concretely (preadolescents) can have difficulty envisioning that a word like "sharp" applies both to knives and to the feeling in their abdomen. Because of this, they continue to have difficulty describing pain. They may also assume that you, as an authority figure, already know they have pain (Schiavenato, 2008).

Some children of school age will regress with pain such as baby-talk or lying in a fetal position. Children this age can understand that if pain will last only an instant, such as with an injection, it can be controlled through nonpharmacologic activities such as distraction techniques.

Children may be in middle school before they can understand how to use a numerical pain rating scale or that the scale intensifies from left to right. Doing some preassessment work with them, such as giving them 10 different-sized triangles and asking them to arrange them from smallest to largest, is a good way to evaluate if they understand incremental measurements. The child who can arrange triangles this way understands the concept of least to most. Once children have grasped this concept, they can describe pain intensity in a very measurable way. A scale of 1 to 5 can be used in younger children if 1 to 10 seems overwhelming. Yet another technique is to turn the scale vertically so it measures bottom (little pain) to top (a lot of pain).

Adolescents commonly use adult mechanisms for controlling pain. Some are even more stoic in the face of pain than adults, trying to avoid stereotypes of "crybaby" or "chicken." This tendency makes assessment for body motions that could indicate pain, such as clenched hands, clenched teeth, rapid breathing, and guarding of body parts, not as helpful as it may be in adults.

PAIN ASSESSMENT

Common fallacies about pain in children are shown in Table 39.1. The techniques to assess pain must vary depending on the age of the child and the type and extent of pain. Although monitoring for physiologic findings such as a change in pulse or blood pressure may give some indication that a child is under stress, these are not the most dependable indicators of pain. Because pain is a subjective finding, once children can speak, asking them to tell you about their pain (self-reporting on a pain rating scale) is the most accurate method for assessment.

A variety of pain rating scales have been devised for use with children. None has been proven to be consistently better than the others, mainly because both children and the type of pain they can be experiencing vary so much. As a rule, pick a well-documented effective scale and use that consistently for a child rather than asking a child to adapt to different assessment techniques. Be sure to follow the specific instructions for that scale.

Pain Experience Inventory

The Pain Experience Inventory is a tool consisting of eight questions for children and eight questions for the child's parents. It is designed to elicit the terms a child uses to denote pain and what actions a child thinks will best alleviate the pain. Such a form can be used when a child is admitted to an acute care facility or on an initial home care visit (Box 39.4). If possible, it should be used before the child has pain.

CRIES Neonatal Postoperative Pain Measurement Scale

The CRIES inventory is a 10-point scale on which five physiologic and behavioral variables frequently associated with neonatal pain can be assessed and rated (Krechel & Bildner, 1995):

- Amount and type of crying
- Need for oxygen administration
- Increased vital signs
- Facial expression
- Sleeplessness

Each area is scored from 0 to 2, and then a total score is obtained (Table 39.2). On the scale, infants with a score of 4 or more are most likely to be in pain and need interventions to reduce discomfort. The scale cannot be used with infants

BOX 39.4 ✻ Pain Experience Inventory

Questions for Child

Tell me what pain is.
Tell me about the hurt you have had before.
What do you do when you hurt?
Do you tell others when you hurt?
What do you want others to do for you when you hurt?
What do you not want others to do for you when you hurt?
What helps the most to take away your hurt?
Is there anything special that you would like me to know about you when you hurt? (If yes, have child describe.)

Questions for Parents

Describe any pain your child has had before.
How does your child usually react to pain?
Does your child tell you or others when pain is experienced?
How do you know when your child is in pain?
What do you do for your child when your child is hurting?
What does your child do to help relieve pain?
Which of these actions work best to decrease or take away your child's pain?
Is there anything special that you would like me to know about your child and pain? (If yes, have parents describe.) (Hester & Barcus, 1986.)

TABLE 39.1 ✻ Common Fallacies About Pain in Children

Fallacy	Fact
Nurses can accurately estimate children's pain from physical appearance or activity.	Nurses commonly underestimate children's pain when they do not rely on children's self-reports.
Young children, particularly newborns, do not feel pain.	Newborns and children do feel pain.
A child who resumes usual activity or sleeps cannot be in pain.	Some children distract themselves with play or music while in pain. They may sleep from exhaustion from the pain.
Because of the possible adverse effects, narcotic. analgesics are too dangerous for young children.	Narcotics can be used safely with children, including low-birth-weight infants.
Experiencing pain will not harm an infant or young child.	Newborns with pain can become cyanotic and bradycardic; no one knows the psychological stress of pain at this age.
If children deny they are feeling pain, you should believe them.	Children may deny pain to avoid a procedure, such as an injection, which they view as more painful. They may be afraid, fearing that they are being punished, or believe others know how they feel.

TABLE 39.2 ✱ CRIES Neonatal Postoperative Pain Measurement Scale

	Infant's Score		
Assessment	*0*	*1*	*2*
Crying	No	High-pitched	Inconsolable
Oxygen required for saturation above 95%	No	>30%	>30%
Increased vital signs	Heart rate and blood pressure within 10% of preoperative values	Heart rate or blood pressure 11–20% higher than preoperative value	Heart rate or blood pressure 21% or more above preoperative value
Expression	None	Grimace	Grimace/grunt
Sleepless	No	Waking at frequent intervals	Constantly awake
Total infant score			

Source: Krechel, S. W., & Bildner, J. (1995). CRIES: A new neonatal postoperative pain management score. *Pediatric Anesthesia, 5*(1), 53.

who are intubated or paralyzed for ventilatory assistance because they would have no score for cry, and because their faces are obscured, it is difficult to rate them for facial expression.

The COMFORT Behavior Scale

The COMFORT behavior scale is a pain rating scale devised by nurses to rate pain in very young infants (van Dijk et al., 2005). On the first part of the scale, six different categories (alertness, calmness/agitation, crying, physical movement, muscle tone, and facial expression) are rated from 1 to 5. Six is the lowest score (no pain), and 30 is the highest (a great deal of pain). In addition to rating physical parameters, the infant is then observed for 2 minutes and the evaluation of the baby's pain is documented on an analogue (1-to-10) visual scale.

FLACC Pain Assessment Tool

The FLACC Pain Assessment Tool (Merkel et al., 1997) is a scale by which health care providers can rate a child's pain when a child cannot give input, such as during circumcision (Brady-Fryer, Wiebe, & Lander, 2009). It incorporates five types of behaviors that can be used to rate pain: facial expression, leg movement, activity, cry, and consolability. Data indicate the scale is reliable and valid. Because a child does not provide active input, an older child may experience a loss of the self-control that can come from active participation by using this scale.

Poker Chip Tool

The Poker Chip Tool (Hester & Barcus, 1986) uses four red poker chips placed in a horizontal line in front of the child. The technique can be used with children as young as 4 years of age, provided the child can count or has some concept of numbers. To use the tool, tell the child, "These are pieces of hurt." Beginning at the chip nearest the child's left hand and ending at the one nearest the child's right hand, point to the chips and say, "This is a little bit of hurt, this is a little more hurt, this is more hurt, and this [the fourth chip] is the most hurt you could ever have." Then ask the child, "How many pieces of hurt do you have right now?" Children without pain will reply they don't hurt; others will point to one of the poker chips. To gain more understanding of how much pain the child is feeling, clarify the child's answer by a follow-up question such as, "Oh, you have a little hurt? Tell me about the hurt." This is an effective tool for young children because the poker chips are concrete items and children are concrete thinkers (Fig. 39.1).

FACES Pain Rating Scale

This scale consists of six cartoon-like faces ranging from smiling to tearful (Fig. 39.2). Explain to the child that each face from left to right corresponds to a person who has no hurt up to a lot of hurt (Wong & Baker, 1996). Use the words under each face to describe the amount of pain the face represents. Next, ask the child to choose the face that best describes the child's pain and record the number under the face the child chooses. Children as young as 3 years can effectively use this scale. The scale appeals to health care providers because it is cute; however, because it is not as concrete a measure as the

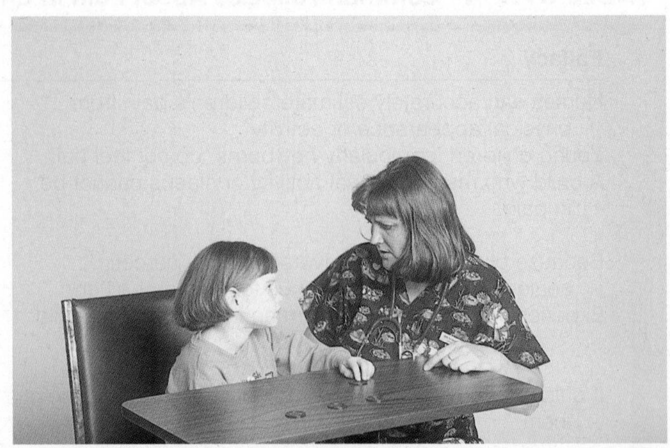

FIGURE 39.1 Use a pain rating tool to assess children's pain. Here, a child points to the poker chip indicating the degree of pain she is experiencing.

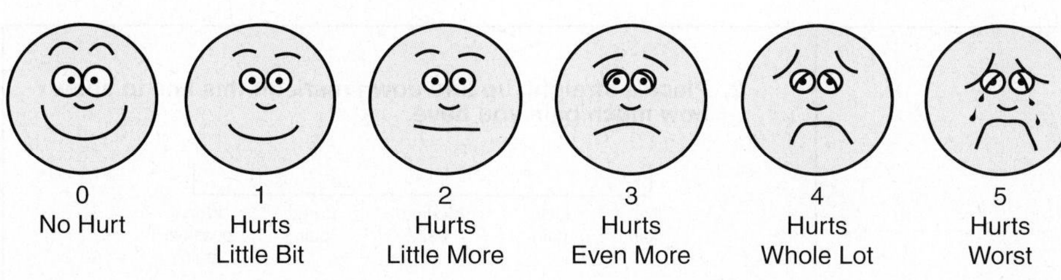

FIGURE 39.2 The FACES pain rating scale. (From *Whaley and Wong's essentials of pediatric nursing* [5th ed., p. 1216] [1997]. Copyright by Mosby–Year Book, Inc. Reprinted by permission.)

Poker Chip Tool, it, therefore, may not be as effective with all children.

Oucher Pain Rating Scale

The Oucher (Beyer, Denyes, & Villarruel, 1992) scale consists of six photographs of children's faces representing "no hurt" to "biggest hurt you could ever have." Also included is a vertical scale with numbers from 0 to 100. To use the photograph portion, point to each photograph and explain what each photo represents. Ask the child to point to the photo that best represents the child's degree of hurt.

To use the numbered scale portion, point to each section of the scale and explain 0 means "no hurt"; 1 to 29 means "a little hurt"; 30 to 69 means "middle hurt"; 70 to 99 means "big hurt"; and 100 means "the biggest hurt you could ever have." Ask the child to point to the section of the scale that represents the present level of hurt. Children as young as 3 can use the tool by pointing to the photograph that best describes their level of pain. If the child can count to 100 by ones and understands the concept of increasing value, the numbered scale can be used. The Oucher scale has white, African American, and Hispanic American photograph versions. Allow children to select the version they want to use or present the version that most closely matches the cultural characteristics of the child.

Numerical or Visual Analog Scale

A numerical or visual analog scale (Fig. 39.3) uses a line with end points marked "0 = no pain" on the left and "10 = worst pain" on the right. Divisions along the line are marked in units from 1 to 9. Explain to children that the left end of the line (the 0) means a person feels no pain. At the other end is a 10, which means a person feels the worst pain possible. The numbers 1 to 9 in the middle are for "a little pain" to "a lot of pain." Ask children to choose a number that best describes their pain. As soon as they can count and have a concept of numbers, children can use a numerical scale. Be certain to show school-age children the scale; do not just say score your pain from 0 to 10. Until children reach late adolescence, they use concrete thought processes so need the help of seeing the line to rate their pain accurately.

Adolescent Pediatric Pain Tool

The Adolescent Pediatric Pain Tool (APPT) combines a visual activity and a numerical scale (Savedra et al., 1992). On one half of the form (Fig. 39.4) is an outline figure showing the anterior and posterior view of a child. To use the tool, tell a child to color in the figure drawing where pain is felt. In addition, on the right side of the form, tell the child to rate present pain in reference to "no pain," "little pain," "medium pain," "large pain," and "worst possible pain." For a third activity, tell children to point to or circle as many words as possible on the form that describe their pain (words such as horrible, pounding, cutting, and stinging). The scale is suggested for use in children 8 through 17 years. As many children below this level need so much help reading and interpreting the multitude of words that describe pain it makes the form impractical below this age. This is a useful tool for involving parents to talk with their child about pain. Reading the words together helps children examine the type, location, and level of pain they are experiencing. It also helps parents to better understand what their child is experiencing.

Logs and Diaries

Having children keep logs or diaries in which they note when pain occurs and then rate the pain each time it occurs is useful for assessing children with chronic but intermittent pain. Examining such a diary can not only reveal when pain occurs but also provide direction for pain management. For example, if the diary shows the child always awakens with pain in the morning, the child may need a longer-acting analgesic to take at bedtime; if pain is worse during weekends spent at a

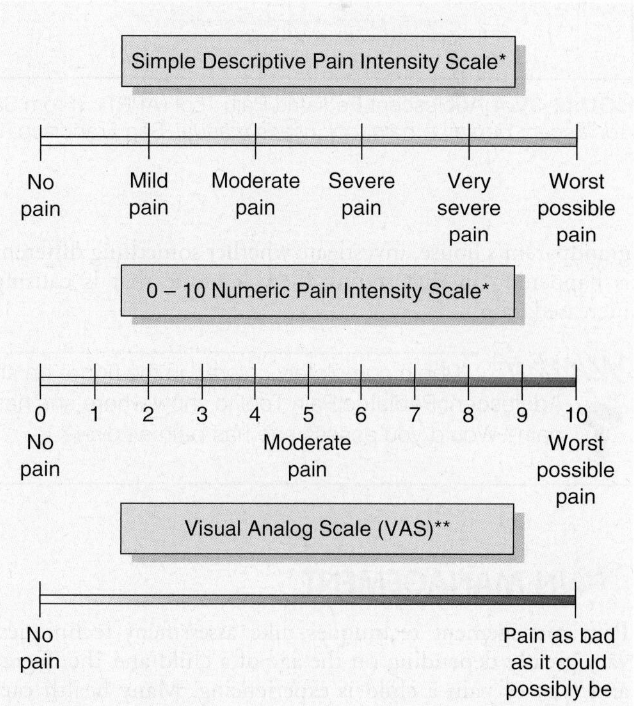

FIGURE 39.3 Numerical and visual analog scales.

CODE __________

DATE __________

Adolescent and Pediatric Pain Tool (APPT)

1. INSTRUCTIONS

Color in the areas on these drawings to show where you have pain. Make the marks as big or as small as the place where the pain is.

Right Left Left Right

2. Place a straight, up and down mark on this line to show how much pain you have.

No pain — Little pain — Medium pain — Large pain — Worst possible pain

3. Point to or circle as many of these words that describe your pain

1
annoying
bad
horrible
miserable
terrible
uncomfortable
2
aching
hurting
like an ache
like a hurt
sore
3
beating
hitting
pounding
punching
throbbing
4
biting
cutting
like a pin
like a sharp knife
pin like
sharp
stabbing

5
blistering
burning
hot
6
cramping
crushing
like a pinch
pinching
pressure
7
itching
like a scratch
like a sting
scratching
stinging
8
shocking
shooting
splitting
9
numb
stiff
swollen
tight

10
awful
deadly
dying
killing
11
crying
frightening
screaming
terrifying
12
dizzy
sickening
suffocating
13
never goes away
uncontrollable
14
always
comes and goes
comes on all of a sudden
constant
continuous
forever

15
off and on
once in a while
sneaks up
sometimes
steady

If you like you may add other words:

____

____

____

For office use only

BSA: ______
IS: ______

#S (2-9)	____/37=	____ %
#A (10-12)	____/11=	____ %
#E (1,13)	____/8=	____ %
#T (14,15)	____/11=	____ %
Total	____/67=	____ %

FIGURE 39.4 Adolescent Pediatric Pain Tool (APPT). (From Savedra, M. C., Tesler, M. D., Holzemer, W. L., et al. [1992]. *Adolescent pediatric pain tool: user's manual.* San Francisco: University of California–San Francisco.)

grandparent's house, investigate whether something different is happening in that setting than at home that is causing increased pain.

What if... Robin completely colored in the figure on an Adolescent Pediatric Pain Tool to show where she has pain? Would you assess she has pain all over?

PAIN MANAGEMENT

Pain management techniques, like assessment techniques, vary greatly depending on the age of a child and the degree and type of pain a child is experiencing. Many health care agencies employ nurses specially prepared in pain management to serve on an interdisciplinary team of health care providers, including physicians, anesthesiologists, patient advocates, and wound therapy nurses, to plan individual pain management programs for children (Box 39.5).

Children with chronic pain or pain not relieved with standard approaches may benefit from a referral to a pain management specialist or team. Relief of frequent pain episodes or prolonged pain may require intense, consistent assessment and intervention, which is difficult to achieve in an acute care setting or during infrequent office visits. Whatever assessment tools or methods of pain relief are used, staff should become familiar and comfortable with their use. It is important that pain be assessed in an organized and consistent manner so relief and interventions do not vary based on the health care provider.

In the past, children frequently were not prescribed potent analgesics because of the fear that the drugs commonly used, such as morphine, would decrease their respiratory rate to an unsafe level. Children who had adequate analgesia prescribed may not have received it because a nurse was overly concerned about causing respiratory distress. Today, it is recognized that if the dosage of an opiate such as morphine is based on the child's size, there is no more danger of respiratory depression in children than in adults. Therefore, after checking that the correct dosage has been

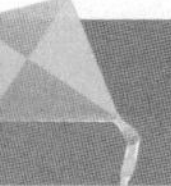

BOX 39.5 * Focus on Evidence-Based Practice

Can nurses be instrumental in teaching other health care providers about pain management?

Pain management programs work best if all health care providers are aware of both assessment and management aspects of the program. To see if pain management on a hospital unit could be improved, researchers asked five senior house officers to take a 1-hour education program on pain management provided by the hospital play specialist. Following care by the newly educated house officers, nurses reported on the clinicians' adherence to best practice, and 21 children who had undergone painful procedures were interviewed with their parents to assess their levels of pain, distress, satisfaction, and coping style. Results of the study showed that house officers had increased their knowledge of how to work with children undergoing painful procedures. The main changes in knowledge were involving nurses and the play specialist, preparing the equipment out of sight of the child, and using distraction techniques. Parents and children reported low levels of distress during painful procedures and high levels of satisfaction with procedures and listed several coping strategies such as distraction that helped the child, and the parent, to cope during the procedure.

Based on the above study, would you try to change the attitude of health care providers toward pain management or rate that as too difficult to attempt?

Source: Lawes, C., et al. (2008). Impact of an education programme for staff working with children undergoing painful procedures. *Paediatric Nursing, 20*(2), 33–37.

prescribed, opiates can be given with confidence to decrease pain without untoward effects. To give nurses more leeway in pain management, it is helpful if a range is given for a dose, rather than a set number so the dose can be adjusted based on the degree of pain (Pasero, Manworren, & McCaffery, 2007).

A good rule for determining whether children need pain relief for a procedure is to remember that if the procedure would cause pain in an adult, it will also cause pain in a child. Often a combination of nonpharmacologic and pharmacologic methods is most effective for pain relief (see Focus on Nursing Care Planning Box 39.6). Many health care professionals such as laboratory technicians, physicians, and x-ray or endoscopic assistants are called on to perform procedures with a child that could cause pain. Health care is a collaborative enterprise. Assist these individuals to schedule procedures at times when a child can be administered optimal pain relief. Help them institute nonpharmacologic measures of pain management such as distraction (Gatlin & Schulmeister, 2007).

General measures to alleviate pain that are helpful to parents as well as health care providers are summarized in Box 39.7. These guidelines are based primarily on the gate control theory.

NONPHARMACOLOGIC PAIN MANAGEMENT

Nonpharmacologic pain relief measures can be used independently or as complements to pharmacologic pain relief. They fit under the umbrella of alternative and complementary therapies.

Distraction

Distraction techniques aim at shifting a child's focus from pain to another activity or interest (Fig. 39.5). Blowing soap bubbles, for example, could be used during an injection to accomplish this. If oral glucose is offered to infants during painful procedures, the pain they experience appears to be significantly less (Hatfield et al., 2008). It is hypothesized that drinking glucose not only serves as a distraction technique but also activates endorphins and produces a central analgesic effect (Stevens, Yamada, & Ohlsson, 2009). Breastfeeding may also be used in this way but is not advised to avoid the infant making an association between breastfeeding and pain. When helping parents teach a distraction technique such as blowing soap bubbles to their child, be certain they do not interpret "distraction" as just talking to the child or suggesting a video game to divert attention. Although these are distractions, simple distraction like this can allow pain to break through.

Substitution of Meaning or Imagery

Substitution of meaning or guided imagery is a distraction technique to help a child place another meaning (a nonpainful one) on a painful procedure (Russell & Smart, 2007). Children are often more adept at imagery than adults because their imagination is less inhibited. Success with this technique requires practice, so it has limited application in an acute care setting. This technique works well with quick, simple procedures such as venipunctures or chronic pain. A venipuncture, for example, could be viewed as a silver rocket probing the moon to transport specimens back to earth or a submarine diving under the water to escape torpedoes just in time. Be certain a child thinks of a specific image. Help the child elaborate on the image to make it more concrete each time it is used so the child's mind stays on the image (what color is the rocket ship? Are there stripes on the sides? What does the pilot look like?).

Thought Stopping

Thought stopping is a technique in which children are taught to stop anxious thoughts by substituting a positive or relaxing thought. As with imagery, this technique requires a great deal of practice before it is used in a painful situation. Anticipatory anxiety is a negative force because it increases the pain experience during a procedure and makes the time before it full of anxiety as well. For this technique, help children to think of a set of positive things about the approaching feared procedure. For a bone marrow aspiration, for example, this might include, "It doesn't take long; the doctor and nurse who do it are helping me; it's important to help me get better." Whenever children start to think about the impending procedure, they should stop whatever they are doing and recite the list of positive thoughts to themselves if

BOX 39.6 ✻ Focus on Nursing Care Planning

A Multidisciplinary Care Map for a Child Requiring Pain Management

Robin Harvey, a 3-year-old girl admitted to your hospital unit, has just returned from a bone marrow aspiration to rule out the possibility of leukemia. Robin received IV morphine sulfate during the procedure. Unfortunately, the bone marrow obtained for analysis is not adequate, so a repeat procedure is scheduled for 3 hours from now.

Family Assessment ✻ Child is only daughter of two parents. Father works as a welder in a local steel mill; mother works part time at a local convenience store. Family rates finances, "Doing good."

Client Assessment ✻ A 3-year-old girl with a history of frequent nosebleeds, petechiae, and bruising admitted for diagnostic testing. First experience with hospitalization. Screams at the sight of a syringe and needle. Both parents at bedside talking with child. Child upset and crying, "Don't let them hurt me!"

Nursing Diagnoses ✻ Anxiety related to fear of the unknown and anticipation of painful procedure

Outcome Criteria ✻ Child identifies pain as no higher than 1 with Oucher Pain Rating Scale; exhibits few to no nonverbal indicators of pain; exhibits age-appropriate coping behaviors, including one nonpharmacologic pain relief technique.

Team Member Responsible	Assessment	Intervention	Rationale	Expected Outcome
		Activities of Daily Living		
Nurse	Assess if IV morphine provided adequate pain relief for last procedure.	Review with parents the necessity for the repeat procedure and possible methods to help child with pain.	Being prepared for coming procedure can reduce anxiety in both parents and child.	Parents state they understand why repeat procedure must be done; are satisfied with pain relief measures to be used.
Nurse	Assess vital signs and child's present pain rating.	Engage the child in quiet activities for the first hour post-procedure.	The child is at risk for bleeding from the puncture site. Quiet activities reduce the risk for bleeding and also provide distraction.	Vital signs remain stable; pain rating is not over 1 on child rating scale. Child colors quietly.
		Consultations		
Nurse/physician	Assess if pain management team member is available for consultation.	Consult with pain management team member for best pain relief for frightened preschool child.	Well-planned pain relief can best meet the needs of an anxious child.	Pain management team member meets with parents and child; determines best method of pain relief.
		Procedures/Medications		
Nurse	Assess if bone aspiration site is free of inflammation.	Apply anesthetic cream to aspiration site and cover with an occlusive dressing 1 hour before scheduled procedure per MD order.	An anesthetic cream anesthetizes skin. An occlusive dressing enhances absorption and tissue penetration.	Child cooperates with application procedure. Occlusive dressing remains in place preprocedure.
Nurse	Assess reddened or blanched skin at site of anesthetic cream just prior to procedure.	Just prior to the procedure, remove the occlusive dressing and wipe away the EMLA cream.	Removal prior to the procedure is necessary to cleanse skin. Reddened or blanched skin indicates that the drug has been effective.	Child cooperates with removal of occlusive dressing and anesthetic cream. Skin appears as if anesthetic effect has been achieved.

Nurse	Assess if child or parents have preference for where IV line should be inserted.	IV analgesia or conscious sedation is administered by IV route.	A bone marrow aspiration is painful, so a route for pain relief is necessary. Allowing choice of IV site offers a sense of control.	IV line is safely inserted; child chooses site that will best allow her to color quietly following the procedure.
		Nutrition		
Nurse	Assess when child last ate.	Keep NPO for 30 minutes preprocedure.	Heavy analgesia can lead to aspiration if stomach is full.	Parents state they understand temporary restriction for fluid.
		Patient/Family Education		
Nurse	Assess what child and parents believe was most traumatic aspect of previous bone marrow aspiration.	Review with child feeling of pressure with needle insertion.	Anticipatory knowledge of events and feelings helps to prepare the child and aids in coping.	Child and parents state they feel prepared for new procedure.
Nurse	Assess if pain assessment tool was used with child during prior procedure.	Introduce the child to Oucher Pain Rating Scale.	Introducing the child to the tool prior to the onset of pain minimizes anxiety associated with a new experience and increases the tool's usefulness and accuracy in determining the child's pain level.	Child rates her pain preprocedure as 0 to 10 to demonstrate she understands how to use scale. Sets a baseline for comparison.
Nurse	Assess the child's understanding about the reason for the bone marrow aspiration.	Review procedure with child and parents.	Assessment and review reveal information about the child, her knowledge base, and possible clues to her anxiety, providing a foundation on which to build future strategies and teaching.	Child and parents voice accurate understanding of the procedure of bone marrow aspiration and importance for diagnosis.
		Psychosocial/Spiritual/Emotional Needs		
Nurse	Assess if child has had experience with therapeutic play.	Provide opportunities for therapeutic play with a doll and syringe before and after procedure.	Therapeutic play helps the child express her feelings about painful procedures and possibly reduces anxiety.	Child plays with doll and syringe under nurse supervision. Does not demonstrate behavior suggestive of extreme anxiety or fright.
		Discharge Planning		
Nurse	Assess if child is free of pain postprocedure; if parents received adequate information on outcome of procedure.	Ask child to rate pain on Oucher scale; ask parents if they have received procedure report and understand results.	Postprocedure evaluation helps to meet further needs of child and parents and improve skills of health care providers.	Child rates pain as 1 or below on pain rating scale. Parents state they have results of procedure and understand the next step needed for diagnosis and treatment.

BOX 39.7 * Focus on Family Teaching

Pain Management With Children

Q. Mrs. Harvey asks you, "How can I be sure I can keep my daughter free from pain after she returns home from the hospital?"

A. Here are some ways to offer pain relief in addition to just giving medicine:

- Let the child know it is important to you to try to take the pain away, and you will work with her to relieve it. Use a positive approach: "This medicine will take away your pain," not "Take this and let's hope it works."
- Administer pain medication before pain becomes intense to help prevent pain rather than just relieve it. If a child is in the hospital, inform the staff if a particular approach works or does not work.
- Never just give an analgesic. Make the child comfortable in ways such as straightening the sheets or offering a backrub.
- Ask your child about measures she thinks will be helpful, such as an additional pillow, the television turned on, a favorite toy nearby.
- Help your child talk about and describe the pain she is experiencing. This can help make it more concrete and not as psychologically frightening.
- Relieve anxiety about other phases of life, if possible. Relaxation reduces muscle strain and tension that add to pain.
- Offer emotional support to your child. Pain never seems as bad when a support person is present. Reassuring your child that she is loved and that you will be there for her can be very comforting.
- Try not to use such statements as, "Be a big girl" or "Stop crying" when a child is in pain from a procedure such as an injection. Say instead, "It's all right to cry. I know it hurts," to avoid shaming a child who cannot stop crying.

others are present or out loud if they are alone or only important support people are present. Children can then return to a usual activity. Every time the anxious thoughts appear, however, a child should stop and recite the list.

Thought stopping is an effective technique because it allows children to feel in control of their thoughts, which is different from merely saying, "Don't think about it." This technique does not suppress thoughts; rather, it changes them into positive ones. The secret for success is for the child to use the technique every time the disturbing, anxious thought appears even if, at first, such thoughts crowd in as frequently as every few minutes.

Hypnosis

Hypnosis is not a common pain management technique with children but can be very effective when a child is properly trained in the technique (Robertson, 2007). For best results, a child needs to train with a therapist before anticipated pain, so at the time of the pain, the child can produce a trance-like state to avoid sensing pain (Shakibaei et al., 2008).

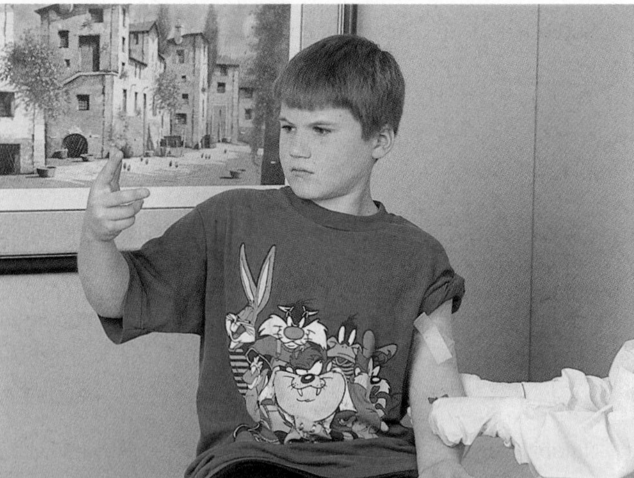

FIGURE 39.5 A child using distraction as a pain management technique.

Aromatherapy and Essential Oils

Aromatherapy is based on the principle that the sense of smell plays a significant role in overall health. When an essential oil is inhaled, its molecules are transported via the olfactory system to the limbic system in the brain. The brain responds to particular aromas with emotional responses. When applied externally, the oils are absorbed by the skin and then carried throughout the body. Essential oils may be able to penetrate cell walls and transport nutrients or oxygen to the inside of cells. Jasmine and lavender are oils thought to be responsible for relieving pain. When a drop of lavender oil is placed on the skin, a child should be able to taste it within 15 seconds.

Magnet Therapy

Magnet therapy is based on the belief that magnets can control or shift body energy lines to restore health or relieve pain. Magnets can be applied as jewelry or sewn into clothing or shoes. Although many people find relief from magnet therapy, the relief may be more of a placebo effect than an actual change in pain level (Pope & McNally, 2007). Copper also is believed to have pain-relieving ability and is often incorporated into rings and bracelets for this reason.

Music Therapy

Music therapy is the use of music for calming or improving well-being and can be effective even for premature infants. It can help to relieve pain both because it can be relaxing and is a distraction (Windich-Biermeir et al., 2007). Children may "blast" music not because they enjoy hearing it that loud but because they are feeling great pain and need that level of distraction to feel free of pain.

Yoga and Meditation

Yoga, a term derived from the Sanskrit word for union, involves a series of exercises that were originally designed to bring people who practice it closer to God. It offers a significant variety of proven health benefits, such as increasing the efficiency of the heart, slowing the respiratory rate, improving fitness, lowering blood pressure, promoting relaxation, reducing stress, and allaying anxiety. Exercises consist of deep-breathing exercises, body postures to stretch and strengthen muscles, and meditation to focus the mind and relax the body. Yoga may be helpful in reducing pain through its ability to relax the body and possibly through the release of endorphins (Galantino, Galbavy, & Quinn, 2008).

Acupuncture

Acupuncture involves the insertion of needles into critical positions (meridian lines) in the body to achieve pain relief (Vas et al., 2007). Although acupuncture is almost painless, children can be very afraid of it at first because of the sight of the needles. This level of stress can make it an unattractive option for pain management for children. Children who consent to having it done, however, particularly those with chronic pain, report that the overall process is pleasant and the method offers good pain relief.

Crystal or Gemstone Therapy

Some people believe that gemstones or crystals have healing powers, which are magnified when they are positioned around the body. If these are being used, be careful when changing bedding or rearranging equipment in a child's room that you do not tip them over. A child may feel they may lose their pain-relieving powers if placed in a different position (Vantol, 2008).

Herbal Therapies

Parents may believe that specific herbs are helpful in relieving pain for their child and in general improving their child's health. Some examples include chamomile tea (inflammation reduction), garlic (anti-inflammatory, anticancer), ginger (nausea or vomiting reduction), goldenrod (urinary tract inflammation reduction), or peppermint (abdominal pain relief) (DerMarderosian & Beutler, 2007). Always ask when taking health histories if a child is being given any herbs, both to be informed about common herbs and to be certain that what the child is receiving will complement, not interfere with, the effects of a pain medication.

Biofeedback

Biofeedback is based on the belief that people can regulate internal events such as heart rate and pain response (Tsai et al., 2007). A biofeedback apparatus is used to measure muscle tone or the child's ability to relax. Biofeedback can be effective with adolescents but is less effective with school-age and younger children because they tend to resist the biofeedback information or cannot concentrate for long enough for training to be effective. Children who want to use biofeedback need to attend several sessions to condition themselves to regulate their pain response.

Therapeutic Touch and Massage

Therapeutic touch is the use of touch to provide comfort and relieve pain (Dowd et al., 2007). It is based on the concept that the body contains energy fields. When these are plentiful, they lead to health, but when they are in lesser supply, ill health results. Proponents believe it is possible to redirect energy fields to increase the release of endorphins. Therapeutic touch may also be effective as it serves as a form of distraction.

Transcutaneous Electrical Nerve Stimulation

Transcutaneous electrical nerve stimulation (TENS) involves applying small electrodes to the dermatomes that supply the body portion where pain is experienced (Poole, 2007). When children sense pain, they push a button on a control box, which then delivers a small electrical current to the skin. The principle underlying this technique is the same as rubbing an injured part: the current interferes with the transmission of the pain impulse across small nerve fibers.

TENS can be used to manage either acute or chronic pain. Some children (and parents) dislike TENS therapy because they are afraid or nervous about the electric current. Assure them the current is a very mild one and will not harm their child. TENS is not recommended if the child is incontinent or has a wound that is likely to cause the electrodes to get wet.

Heat or Cold Application

Cold reduces pain by constricting capillaries and therefore reducing vessel permeability and edema and pressure at an injured site. After the first 24 hours of an injury, applying heat may be more helpful because this dilates capillaries, increases blood flow to the area, and again helps reduce edema.

✔ Checkpoint Question 39.1

You teach Robin imaging to help reduce pain. Why does a technique such as imagery work well for children?

a. Children's pain is not as acute as is adults' pain.
b. Intravenous pain relief is not effective in children.
c. Children's imaginations are at their peak.
d. Children's muscles are less tense than adults' muscles.

PHARMACOLOGIC PAIN RELIEF

Pharmacologic pain relief refers to the administration of a wide variety of analgesic medications (D'Arcy, 2007). Many children need analgesic agents in addition to nonpharmacologic techniques for pain relief, especially for acute pain. Medications can be applied topically or given orally, intramuscularly, intravenously, or by epidural injection. As a rule, intramuscularly administered analgesia should be avoided in children because children dislike injections. Be certain children understand it is acceptable to ask for medication for pain; they may not know they can unless this is stressed by health care providers.

Topical Anesthetic Cream

To reduce the pain of procedures such as venipuncture, lumbar puncture, and bone marrow aspiration, a local anesthetic cream or a solution of lidocaine and epinephrine can be used (Subramanian et al., 2008).

BOX 39.8 * Focus on Pharmacology

EMLA Cream

Classification: EMLA (an eutectic mixture of local anesthetics) is a topical analgesic cream containing lidocaine and prilocaine.

Action: Acts to anesthetize skin before potentially painful procedures (Karch, 2009).

Pregnancy risk category: B

Dosage: Dollop of cream to intended skin site for at least 1 hour before procedure (2–3 hours before deeper procedures such as lumbar puncture or bone marrow aspiration)

Possible adverse effects: Hypersensitivity

Nursing Implications

- Explain to the child that the cream will help prevent pain during a procedure.
- Apply a dollop of cream to the intended site and cover with a transparent occlusive dressing at least 1 hour before the procedure. Do not spread cream or rub it in.
- If the cream is to be applied at home, instruct the parents how to apply the cream and the occlusive dressing. Suggest that the parents use plastic wrap, such as Saran Wrap, for the occlusive dressing.
- Instruct the child not to touch the dressing while it is in place. If necessary, cover the occlusive dressing with an opaque material to prevent the child from touching or playing with the dressing.
- Just before the procedure, remove the dressing and then wipe the skin to remove cream.
- Observe the skin. Look for reddened or blanched skin, which indicates that the drug has penetrated the skin.
- Do not use the drug for a child with a known history of sensitivity or allergy to local anesthetics such as lidocaine.
- The drug is not approved for use in infants younger than 1 month.

The cream is applied to the skin, and the site is then covered with an occlusive dressing or plastic wrap. To be most effective, it must be applied at least 1 hour before an expected procedure (Box 39.8). Parents can apply anesthetic cream at home before bringing a child to a clinic visit for a procedure such as bone marrow aspiration (Fig. 39.6). Caution them not to allow their child to remove the dressing and eat the cream (it could anesthetize the gag reflex). It also is potentially dangerous if rubbed into the eyes. Anesthetic creams have changed procedures such as obtaining blood from painful ones to painless ones. They also can be used effectively for pain relief with circumcision (Taddio, Ohlsson, & Ohlsson, 2009). A disadvantage of EMLA cream is that it must be applied at least 1 hour before the procedure; however, it can be applied up to 3 hours before a procedure and still be effective. A newer compound, ELA-MAX (LMX), containing only lidocaine, takes effect in 30 minutes or less

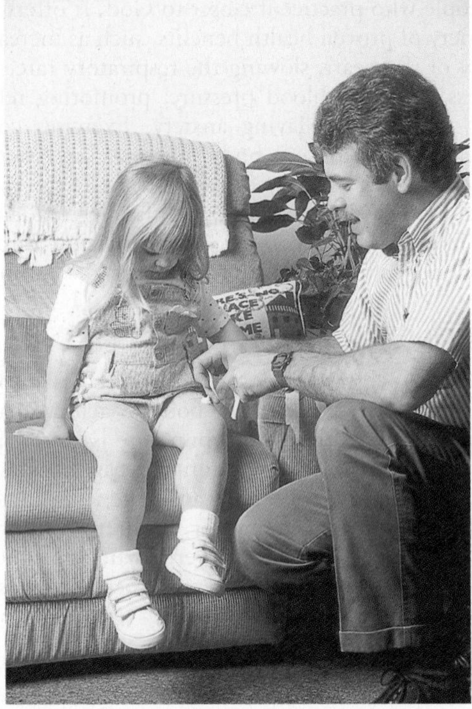

FIGURE 39.6 A father applies an anesthetic cream at home prior to a painful procedure.

(Subramanian et al., 2008). It can be purchased without a prescription.

What if... Robin is scheduled to have blood drawn at 10 AM and, to prepare her for this, you apply an anesthetic cream that takes an hour to be effective at 9 AM, but then the technician who will take the blood arrives early? Would you ask the technician to wait, or explain to Robin the cream is not going to work?

Oral Analgesia

Oral analgesia is advantageous because it is cost-effective and relatively easy to administer. Many analgesics can be prepared as elixirs or suppositories for children unable to swallow pills. Analgesia can be adequately achieved if dosing is correct.

Over-the-counter analgesics, such as acetaminophen (Tylenol), are flavored to make them taste good. Caution parents that even though such drugs taste sweet, they should never refer to medicine as "candy." Reinforce with them the need for proper storage (locked or out of the child's reach). Otherwise, children may help themselves to more when the parent leaves the room. Toxicity from too-frequent or overly large doses of acetaminophen can lead to severe liver damage in children (Karch, 2009).

Nonsteroidal anti-inflammatory drugs (NSAIDs) are excellent for reducing the pain that accompanies inflammation in injuries such as sprained ankles or rheumatic conditions. Examples of NSAIDs include ibuprofen and naproxen. Long-term administration of any NSAID can lead to severe gastric irritation and may be associated with heart attacks, so it should not be used longer than prescribed. Help parents giving any analgesia around the clock for several days to make out a medication sheet to hang on their refrigerator door. This reminds them when the next dose is due and alerts them not to give the drug doses too close together.

Children should not receive acetylsalicylic acid (aspirin) for routine pain relief, especially in the presence of flulike symptoms, because there is an association between aspirin administration and the development of Reye syndrome (see Chapter 49).

For managing severe or acute pain, such as postoperative pain or the pain of a sickle-cell crisis, opioids, such as morphine, codeine, and hydromorphone (Dilaudid), are the usual drugs of choice. Codeine may be given in combination with acetaminophen. Because this class of drugs is also referred to as narcotics, parents may be reluctant to give their children these medications, concerned their child will become addicted. Acknowledge their concern but reassure them the risk for addiction during short-term use is remote. Reinforce that the main concern is supplying adequate pain relief for their child.

Intramuscular Injection

Opiates are available as intramuscular injections. Analgesia for children is rarely given by this route, however, as injections are associated with pain on administration and also produce great fear in children. It is also associated with several risks, including uneven absorption, unpredictable onset of action, and nerve and tissue damage. Other routes should be used whenever possible.

Intravenous Administration

IV administration of analgesia, the most rapid-acting route, is the method of choice in emergency situations, in the child with acute pain, and in a child requiring frequent doses of analgesia but in whom the gastrointestinal tract cannot be used. Common opioids given by this route include morphine, fentanyl, and hydromorphone (Dilaudid). Hydromorphone is 8 to 10 times stronger than morphine but very similar to morphine in action. Fentanyl has a shorter duration of action than morphine. Side effects of pruritus and vasodilatation are less. These features make it an ideal drug to use for short, painful procedures, such as debriding a burn or inserting a chest tube to relieve a pneumothorax.

These analgesics can be given by bolus injection or by continuous infusion. If doses will be given periodically by an IV line, advocate for the use of an intermittent infusion device to avoid repeated venipunctures with each dose or the need for a confining IV line to be in place.

If a child's pain is frequent or constant, continuous IV administration may be necessary to reduce the level of pain. As the child becomes able to take medications by mouth, oral forms of analgesics are then administered. When switching from IV to oral medications, it is important to use equianalgesic doses. As-needed (PRN) dosing should be avoided because it leads to inconsistent administration.

All opioids have the potential to decrease respiratory rate, although this is not a worry with accurate dosing. Other side effects include nausea, pruritus, vasodilatation, cough suppression, and constipation. If toxicity with opioids should occur, naloxone (Narcan) can be administered to counteract the effects.

✔ Checkpoint Question 39.2

Robin was given analgesia intravenously. Why is the intramuscular route infrequently used to administer analgesia to children?

a. The average child has a tremendous fear of injections.
b. IM doses must be larger in children than in adults.
c. IM medications must be administered cold or chilled.
d. IM solutions are readily confused with IV solutions.

Patient-Controlled Analgesia

Patient-controlled analgesia (PCA) is a form of IV administration that allows a child to self-administer boluses of medication, usually opioids, with a medication pump (see also Chapter 16). Children as young as 5 or 6 years may be able to assess when they need a bolus of medicine and press the button on the pump to deliver the new dose through an established IV line. Parents or a nurse can administer a new dose to children younger than this. Morphine is a common analgesic used for PCA administration (Cho, Ha, & Rhee, 2007). The pump is set with a lock-out time so that after each dose the pump will not release further medication even if the button is pushed again; because of this, children cannot overmedicate themselves. If pain is constant, a continuous infusion should be used so that pain relief continues even while the child sleeps. The pump can still be programmed for bolus dosing to cover episodes of increased pain.

Conscious Sedation

Conscious sedation refers to a state of depressed consciousness usually obtained through IV analgesia therapy (Hertzog & Havidish, 2007). The technique allows a child to be both pain-free and sedated for a procedure. Unlike with the use of general anesthesia, protective reflexes are left intact and a child can respond to instructions during the procedure. The technique is used for procedures such as extensive wound care; bone marrow aspiration, which is potentially very painful; magnetic resonance imaging, which may require a child to lie still for a long period of time; and endoscopy, which is both potentially frightening and requires a child to lie still for a period of time. In many health care settings, conscious sedation is administered and monitored by nurses specially prepared in the technique (Fig. 39.7). Drugs used for conscious sedation can be something as common as chloral hydrate or as involved as a sedative-hypnotic-analgesic combination that relieves both anxiety and pain and depresses the child's memory of the event.

Intranasal Administration

Intranasal administration is becoming an attractive way to dispense medicine for children. Influenza vaccine, for example, is now available in an intranasal form (Carpenter et al., 2007). Midazolam (Versed) is a short-acting adjuvant sedative that can be administered intranasally by nasal drops or nasal spray before surgery or procedures such as nuclear medicine scanning (Karch, 2009). Because it has a very short duration of action, it may require repeat administration. Because midazolam has no analgesic action, analgesia, such as with morphine, should also be used if the procedure will be painful.

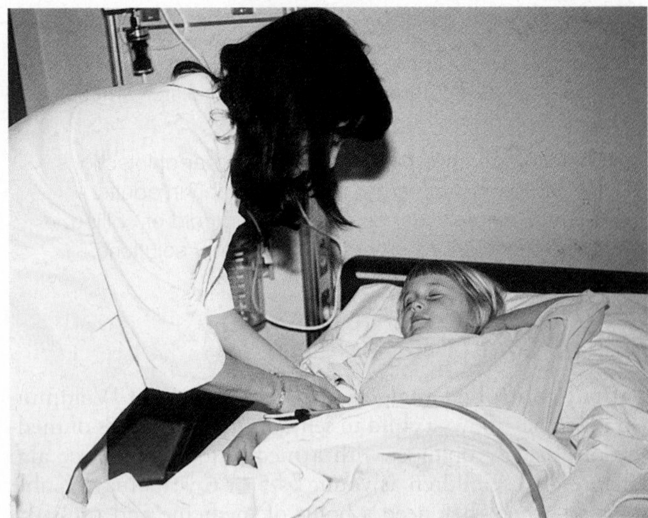

FIGURE 39.7 A nurse monitors the vital signs of a child who has received conscious sedation.

Local Anesthesia Injection

Local anesthetics stop pain transmission by blocking nerve conduction of the impulse at the site of pain. Children receive local anesthetic injections, such as lidocaine, before procedures such as bone marrow aspiration and peritoneal dialysis. For many children, the sight of the anesthetic needle is so frightening that they cannot listen to the assurance that the momentary needlestick will actually prevent further pain. The use of an anesthetic cream before the injection relieves the needlestick pain and allows the anesthetic to numb the deeper tissues.

Epidural Analgesia

Epidural analgesia, injection of an analgesic agent into the epidural space just outside the spinal canal, can be used to provide analgesia to the lower body for 12 to 24 hours. An opioid, often combined with a long-acting anesthetic, is instilled continuously or administered intermittently. Opiate receptors in the spinal cord are affected directly, providing analgesia. Epidural anesthesia is commonly used for childbirth (see Chapter 16). Children who have orthopedic or chest surgery, for example, may have an epidural catheter inserted in the operating room and continue to receive analgesia by this method to relieve postsurgical pain (Schoen, 2007). This is a very effective route of analgesia in the postoperative child in the first few days.

Some parents may be reluctant to allow this type of analgesia because they equate it with spinal anesthesia, which can be followed by severe headaches. You can assure them that an epidural needle does not enter the cerebrospinal fluid, so spinal headaches are rare.

ONGOING PAIN RELIEF

Be certain children who begin a pain management program in a health care setting are provided with support and follow-up pain management to the extent necessary when they return home. Early discharge and the increased use of outpatient surgery necessitate adequate pain management in the home setting. Otherwise, lack of pain relief at home can be overwhelming.

Either oral or IV analgesia may be needed in a home setting. Be certain parents have instructions on dosing, administration, frequency, expected outcomes, and expected level of relief. Provide them with the name and telephone number of a health care professional whom they can call if they have questions about pain management.

✔ Checkpoint Question 39.3

Suppose Robin is scheduled for conscious sedation to have her repeat bone marrow aspiration. Which would be the best explanation to prepare her for this?

a. "You'll be given a special medicine to put you to sleep for surgery."
b. "I'll give you some medicine, but you'll still be awake and feel pain."
c. "Conscious sedation is an analgesic, not anesthetic, method of pain relief."
d. "I'll give you medicine so you're very sleepy but can still talk to me."

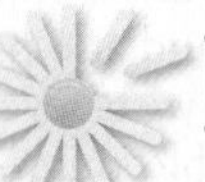

Key Points for Review

- Many children and infants are undermedicated for pain relief because of common misperceptions by health care personnel, such as that infants do not feel or remember pain.
- Inviting parents and the child, if preschool age or older, to participate in assessment and pain management is an important aspect of pain therapy.
- Pain in children is best assessed by means of a standardized self-report tool such as the Poker Chip or FACES tool. Without self-report forms, both nurses and parents may underestimate children's pain.
- Many children benefit from a combination of nonpharmacologic and pharmacologic methods of pain management.
- Many nonpharmacologic pain relief measures such as imagery, distraction, and TENS are based on the gate control theory of pain management.
- Few analgesics are administered intramuscularly to children. Instead, IV administration is the method of choice for the child with acute pain. Patient-controlled analgesia, commonly used to administer morphine, can be used effectively with children.
- Conscious sedation is useful for potentially frightening procedures. Protective reflexes are left intact, and the child can respond to instructions during the procedure.

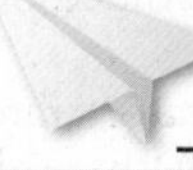

CRITICAL THINKING EXERCISES

1. Robin is the 3-year-old girl you met at the beginning of the chapter. She was given IV morphine in surgery 1 hour ago for a bone marrow aspiration. Her mother asks

you now if Robin can have some more, not because her pain has returned, but because the mother wants it given before any pain comes back. Is this mother's assessment or Robin's assessment of her pain apt to be most accurate? Would anticipating pain in this way be the best intervention for Robin?

2. Robin is prescribed an intravascular antibiotic twice daily. She always screams the second she sees the syringe even though the addition of the medicine to her IV line should cause minimal pain. What type of pain management should be used? How should the child's anxiety be addressed?
3. A fellow nurse tells you that she does not use self-report tools with children; she feels they take the place of her nursing judgment. You like to use rating scales. How would you justify your view? What are the pros and cons of pain assessment tools?
4. Examine the National Health Goals related to pain assessment and management in children. Most government-sponsored funds for nursing research are allotted based on these goals. What would be a possible research topic to explore pertinent to these goals that would be applicable to Robin's family and also advance evidence-based practice?

CRITICAL THINKING SCENARIO

Open the accompanying CD-ROM or visit http://thePoint.lww.com and read the Patient Scenario included for this chapter, then answer the questions to further sharpen your skills and grow more familiar with NCLEX style questions related to pain management in children. Confirm your answers are correct by reading the rationales.

REFERENCES

American Academy of Pediatrics (AAP), Committee on Fetus and Newborn. (2007). Prevention and management of pain in the neonate: an update. *Pediatrics, 18*(5), 2231–2241.

Beyer, J. E., Denyes, M. J., & Villarruel, A. M. (1992). The creation, validation, and continuing development of the Oucher: a measure of pain intensity in children. *Journal of Pediatric Nursing, 7*(5), 335–346.

Brady-Fryer, B., Wiebe, N., & Lander, J. A. (2009). Pain relief for neonatal circumcision. *Cochrane Database of Systematic Reviews, 2009*(1), (CD004217).

Carpenter, L. R., et al. (2007). Mass distribution of free, intranasally administered influenza vaccine in a public school system. *Pediatrics, 120*(1), e172–e178.

Cho, N. S., Ha, J. H., & Rhee, Y. G. (2007). Patient-controlled analgesia after arthroscopic rotator cuff repair: subacromial catheter versus intravenous injection. *American Journal of Sports Medicine, 35*(1), 75–79.

D'Arcy, Y. (2007). Controlling pain. New pain management options: delivery systems and techniques. *Nursing,* 37(2), 26–27.

DerMarderosian, A., & Beutler, J. A. (2007). *The review of natural products.* St. Louis, MO: Wolters Kluwer Health.

Dowd, T., et al. (2007). Comparison of a healing touch, coaching, and a combined intervention on comfort and stress in younger college students. *Holistic Nursing Practice, 21*(4), 194–202.

Eccleston, C., et al. (2009). Psychological therapies for the management of chronic and recurrent pain in children and adolescents. *Cochrane Database of Systematic Reviews, 2009*(1), (CD003968).

Galantino, M. L., Galbavy, R., & Quinn, L. (2008). Therapeutic effects of yoga for children: A systematic review of the literature. *Pediatric Physical Therapy, 20*(1), 66–80.

Gatlin, C. G., & Schulmeister, L. (2007).When medication is not enough: Nonpharmacologic management of pain. *Clinical Journal of Oncology Nursing, 11*(5), 699–704.

Hatfield, L. A., et al. (2008). Analgesic properties of oral sucrose during routine immunizations at 2 and 4 months of age. *Pediatrics, 121*(2), e327–e334.

Hertzog, J. H., & Havidich, J. E. (2007). Non-anesthesiologist-provided pediatric procedural sedation: an update. *Current Opinion in Anesthesiology, 20*(4), 365–372.

Hester, N. O., & Barcus, C. S. (1986). Assessment and management of pain in children. *Pediatrics: Nursing Update, 1*(14), 2–6.

Karch, A. M. (2009). *Lippincott's nursing drug guide.* Philadelphia: Lippincott Williams & Wilkins.

Krechel, S. W., & Bildner, J. (1995). CRIES: A new neonatal postoperative pain measurement score. *Paediatric Anesthesia, 5*(1), 53–57.

Lawes, C., et al. (2008). Impact of an education programme for staff working with children undergoing painful procedures. *Pediatric Nursing, 20*(2), 33–37.

Melzack, R., & Wall, P. (1965). Pain mechanisms: A new theory. *Science, 150*(4), 971–976.

Merkel, S. I., et al. (1997). The FLACC: a behavioral scale for scoring postoperative pain in young children. *Pediatric Nursing, 23*(3), 293–298.

Pasero, C., Manworren, R. C. B., & McCaffery, M. (2007). Pain control: IV opioid range orders for acute pain management. *American Journal of Nursing, 107*(2), 52–60.

Pasero, C., & McCaffery, M. (2004). Comfort-function goals: A way to establish accountability for pain relief. *American Journal of Nursing, 104*(9), 77–81.

Poole, D. (2007). Use of TENS in pain management, part one: how TENS works. *Nursing Times, 103*(7), 28–29.

Pope, K. W., & McNally, R. J. (2007). Nonspecific placebo effects explain the therapeutic benefit of magnets. *Scientific Review of Alternative Medicine, 6*(1), 13–16.

Robertson, J. (2007). Review: distraction, hypnosis, and combined cognitive-behavioural interventions reduce needle related pain and distress in children and adolescents. *Evidence-Based Nursing, 10*(3), 75.

Russell, C., & Smart, S. (2007). Guided imagery and distraction therapy in paediatric hospice care. *Paediatric Nursing, 19*(2), 24–25.

Savedra, M. C., Tesler, M. D., Holzemer, W. L., et al. (1992). *Adolescent pediatric pain tool: user's manual.* San Francisco: University of California–San Francisco.

Schoen, D. C. (2007). Pain in the orthopaedic patient. *Orthopaedic Nursing, 26*(2), 140–144.

Schiavenato, M. (2008). Facial expression and pain assessment in the pediatric patient: The primal face of pain. *Journal for Specialists in Pediatric Nursing, 13*(2), 89–97.

Shakibaei, F., et al. (2008). Hypnotherapy in management of pain and reexperiencing of trauma in burn patients. *International Journal of Clinical and Experimental Hypnosis, 56*(2), 185–197.

Stevens, B., Yamada, J., & Ohlsson, A. (2009). Sucrose for analgesia in newborn infants undergoing painful procedures. *Cochrane Database of Systematic Reviews, 2009*(1), (CD001069).

Subramanian, A., et al. (2008). *Drug facts and comparisons.* St. Louis: Wolters Kluwer Health.

Taddio, A., Ohlsson, K., & Ohlsson, A. (2009). Lidocaine-prilocaine cream for analgesia during circumcision in newborn boys. *Cochrane Database of Systematic Reviews, 2009*(1), (CD000496).

Tsai, P., et al. (2007). Effects of electromyography biofeedback—assisted relaxation on pain in patients with advanced cancer in a palliative care unit. *Cancer Nursing, 30*(5), 347–353.

van Dijk M., et al. (2005). The COMFORT Behavior Scale: A tool for assessing pain and sedation in infants. *American Journal of Nursing, 105*(1), 33–36.

Vantol, L. (2008). Case study: the power of crystal therapy. *Positive Health, 147*(5), 40–41.

Vas, J., et al. (2007). Effectiveness of acupuncture and related techniques in treating non-oncological pain in primary healthcare: An audit. *Acupuncture in Medicine, 25*(1–2), 41–46.

Windich-Biermeier, A., et al. (2007). Effects of distraction on pain, fear, and distress during venous port access and venipuncture in children and adolescents with cancer. *Journal of Pediatric Oncology Nursing, 24*(1), 8–19.

Wong, D., & Baker, C. (1996). *Reference manual for the Wong-Baker FACES pain rating scale.* Duarte, CA: CHNMC.

SUGGESTED READINGS

Bellieni, C. V., & Buonocore, G. (2008). Neonatal pain treatment: ethical to be effective. *Journal of Perinatology, 28*(2), 87–88.

Bhargava, R., & Young, K. D. (2007). Procedural pain management patterns in academic pediatric emergency departments. *Academic Emergency Medicine, 14*(5), 479–482.

Cadden, K. A. (2007). Better pain management. *Nursing Management, 38*(8), 30–35.

Jeffs, D. A. (2007). A pilot study of distraction for adolescents during allergy testing. *Journal for Specialists in Pediatric Nursing, 12*(3), 170–185.

Kwekkeboom, K. L., et al. (2008). Oncology nurses' use of nondrug pain interventions in practice. *Journal of Pain & Symptom Management, 35*(1), 83–94.

Manworren, R. C. B. (2007). Ask the expert. It's time to relieve children's pain. *Journal for Specialists in Pediatric Nursing, 12*(3), 196–198.

Matharu, L., & Ashley, P. F. (2009). Sedation of anxious children undergoing dental treatment. *Cochrane Database of Systematic Reviews, 2009*(1), (CD003877).

Reschreiter, H., & Lawson, A. D. (2007). Pain management in the intensive care unit. *Care of the Critically Ill, 23*(1), 15–20.

Rieman, M. T., & Gordon, M. (2007). Pain management competency evidenced by a survey of pediatric nurses' knowledge and attitudes. *Pediatric Nursing, 33*(4), 307–314.

Twycross, A. (2007). What is the impact of theoretical knowledge on children's nurses' post-operative pain management practices? An exploratory study. *Nurse Education Today, 27*(7), 697–707.

Unit 7

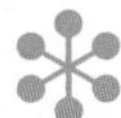

The Nursing Role in Restoring and Maintaining the Health of Children and Families With Physiologic Disorders

Chapter 40 Nursing Care of a Family When a Child Has a Respiratory Disorder

KEY TERMS

- adventitious sounds
- anoxia
- arterial blood gases
- aspiration
- atelectasis
- clubbing
- cyanosis
- expiration
- hypoxemia
- hypoxia
- inspiration
- paroxysmal coughing
- percussion
- pneumothorax
- rales
- retraction
- steatorrhea
- stridor
- tachypnea
- tracheostomy
- tracheotomy
- vibration
- wheezing

OBJECTIVES

After mastering the contents of this chapter, you should be able to:

1. Describe common respiratory disorders in children.
2. Identify National Health Goals related to children with respiratory disorders that nurses could help the nation achieve.
3. Use critical thinking to analyze ways nursing care for a child with a respiratory disorder could be more family centered.
4. Assess a child with a respiratory disorder.
5. Formulate nursing diagnoses related to respiratory disorders in children.
6. Identify expected outcomes that address the priority needs of a child with a respiratory disorder.
7. Plan nursing care for a child with a respiratory disorder.
8. Implement nursing care for a child with a respiratory disorder such as administering oxygen to a child.
9. Evaluate expected outcomes for achievement and effectiveness of care.
10. Identify areas related to care of children with respiratory disorders that could benefit from additional nursing research or application of evidence-based practice.
11. Integrate knowledge of respiratory disorders in children with nursing process to achieve quality maternal and child health nursing care.

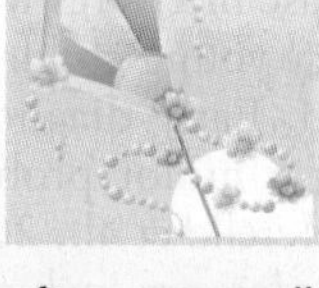

Michael is a 4-year-old who is brought to the emergency department by paramedics after responding to an emergency call by his grandmother at his home. He has a sharp, barking cough, is crying loudly, and is obviously short of breath. "He can't breathe!" his grandmother shouts at you. "I gave him some chocolate. Is he allergic to that?" his grandmother asks. Michael is diagnosed as having laryngotracheobronchitis (croup) and admitted to an ambulatory care unit.

Previous chapters described the growth and development of well children. This chapter adds information about the dramatic changes, both physical and psychosocial, that occur when children develop respiratory disorders.

What emergency care does Michael need? What about Michael's action would lead you to believe his airway is not yet completely obstructed?

Respiratory disorders are among the most common causes of illness and hospitalization in children. Overall, respiratory dysfunction in children tends to be more serious than in adults because the lumens of a child's respiratory tract are smaller and therefore more likely to become obstructed. Because respiratory disorders range from minor illnesses such as a simple upper respiratory tract infection to life-threatening lower respiratory tract diseases, such as pneumonia, and because the level of acuity can change quickly, respiratory disorders are often difficult for parents to evaluate. Both a child and parents need a great deal of nursing support when disease interferes with the function of breathing, because even very young children can panic when breathing becomes labored. Early diagnosis and treatment are essential in preventing a minor problem from turning into a more serious one (Merelle et al., 2009).

Because respiratory disorders are such a common cause of childhood illness and hospitalization, National Health Goals have been established for children with respiratory illnesses (Box 40.1).

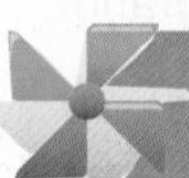

BOX 40.1 * Focus on National Health Goals

Several National Health Goals focus on respiratory illness in children:

- Reduce the rate of asthma deaths in children aged 5 to 14 years from a baseline of 3.3 per million to a target level of 0.9 per million.
- Reduce the rate of hospital emergency department visits for children with asthma younger than 5 years from a baseline of 150 per 10,000 to 80 per 10,000.
- Reduce the rate of cigarette use by adolescents from a baseline of 35% to a target of 16%; cigar use from 18% to 8%, oral tobacco use from 8% to 1%, and bidis use from 4% to 2%.
- Reduce the incidence of invasive pneumococcal infections in children younger than 5 years from a baseline of 76 per 100,000 to a target of 46 per 100,000.
- Reduce the incidence of tuberculosis from a baseline of 6.8 per 100,000 cases yearly to a target level of 1.0 per 100,000 (http://www.nih.gov).

Nurses can help the nation achieve these goals by teaching children to avoid beginning cigarette smoking, including the use of bidis (chocolate-flavored tobacco products), teaching children ways to help avoid respiratory infections such as good handwashing, and reminding parents to come for child health maintenance visits so that children can receive pneumococcal immunization or screening for tuberculosis, as appropriate.

Additional nursing research is needed about the accuracy of parents in self-reading and interpreting tuberculosis screening tests and information required by new parents to better manage respiratory illness in infants and young children.

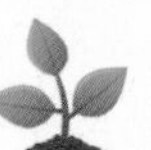

Nursing Process Overview

For a Child With a Respiratory Disorder

Assessment

Respiratory illness can begin as early as moments after birth if a newborn has difficulty initiating a first breath or establishing regular respirations. Rating a newborn using an Apgar score can help to quickly identify a newborn who may be experiencing respiratory difficulty at this early stage.

As a nurse in an emergent care or health maintenance organization, you are often the first health care provider to talk to a parent about a child's respiratory illness. It is important to establish both the onset and duration of the problem so that its seriousness can be rapidly determined. An episode of sudden coughing is suggestive of an acute respiratory disorder. Infants who cannot finish a bottle feeding because of exhaustion or rapid breathing or children who cannot run with other children because they do not have enough breath should be suspected of having a chronic respiratory disorder.

A child admitted to the hospital with a respiratory disorder is usually in an acute stage of the illness. A child's condition may worsen rapidly in the first few hours until a prescribed medication, such as an antibiotic or bronchodilator, begins to take effect. Nursing assessment that a child is developing tachypnea or retractions may be the first indication of a child's worsening condition.

Nursing Diagnosis

Nursing diagnoses established for children with respiratory disorders focus both on the alteration in mechanisms of breathing and on the emotional distress such problems can create. "Ineffective airway clearance" is a common diagnostic category used in this area. The problem may be related to any one of a variety of factors, such as ineffective cough, fatigue, weakness, viscous secretions, pain, aspiration (inhalation of a foreign object into the airway), or lack of knowledge about the importance of coughing.

The diagnostic categories "Impaired gas exchange" and "Ineffective breathing pattern" also may be used, although because a nurse does not generally prescribe definitive treatment for these problems (except when caused by hyperventilation), it may be more appropriate for a nursing diagnosis to focus on the effects of impaired gas exchange or ineffective breathing on daily activities and psychosocial health. Examples of nursing diagnoses are:

- Activity intolerance related to insufficient oxygenation
- Fatigue related to impaired gas exchange
- Fear related to inability to breathe without effort
- Impaired social interaction related to difficulty in keeping up with physical activities of peers
- Deficient knowledge related to need for continued treatment

Outcome Identification and Planning

If a child is experiencing an acute respiratory problem, the expected outcomes and plan of care will focus on supporting the child and family through prescribed therapy and keeping parents informed about their child's health status and response to treatment. Often the treatment period for respiratory illness is prolonged, so parents of children with chronic conditions need to learn how to continue therapy at home. Helping parents to plan programs of exercise and teaching chest physiotherapy and the actions of prescribed medications are important nursing activities. Parents also need to understand that their approach to these programs must change as their child grows older. With an infant, they simply need to perform the prescribed procedures. A game might be a good way to get a toddler or preschooler to breathe deeply ("Simon says, cough. Simon says, take five deep breaths"). Parents need to plan exercise programs for school-age children and adolescents around their school day. Otherwise, children may have difficulty carrying out the program or carry it out only sporadically. If parents include other family members, such as older siblings (within reason) or grandparents, in a respiratory therapy program, this can help to diffuse the burden of care and also to unite the family in working toward a common goal. Helpful Web sites for parents to consult about respiratory illnesses are http://www.kidshealth.org and http://www.everydayhealth.com. Some organizations to recommend as support to parents of the child with a respiratory disorder include American Lung Association (http://www.lungusa.org), National Asthma Education and Prevention Program (http://www.nhlbi.nih.gov), National Easter Seal Society (http://www.easterseals.com), and Cystic Fibrosis Foundation (http://www.cff.org).

Implementation

Collaborative nursing interventions in the care of a child with respiratory dysfunction include suctioning to remove respiratory secretions, administering oxygen, and providing humidification and expectorant therapy to help maintain clear airways. Some of the most important nursing interventions in this area are independent nursing functions: placing a child in an upright position to help the child cough more effectively; providing an interesting game to teach a child the importance of strengthening chest muscles; supporting a child and family through the anxiety created when a child is not breathing normally; and teaching parents of a child with chronic respiratory dysfunction the basics of percussion or chest physiotherapy techniques. All of these interventions require sound nursing judgment and skill to carry out or teach effectively.

Outcome Evaluation

An acute respiratory illness such as pneumonia is extremely frightening for parents as well as the child. After the child has recovered, talk with the parents to determine whether they have come to terms with their fear and can treat the child as a well child again. Otherwise, overprotection of a child by the parents may result in a well but dependent child. This pattern is one that nursing evaluation can help to prevent.

Expected outcomes for a child with chronic respiratory disease will change as a child grows and develops. No matter what the specific concerns are, however, evaluation should always include examination of how well a child individually and the family as a whole have adapted to managing the limitations imposed by the disorder while maintaining a lifestyle that fosters growth and development for all family members.

Examples of expected outcomes that would indicate achievement of goals are:

- Infant, at 3 months, maintains respiratory rate of at least 30 breaths per minute.
- Child describes a reduced program of school activities he will maintain to reduce fatigue.
- Child's PO_2 is maintained at 80 to 100 mm Hg in room air.
- Child lists steps she will take if breathing becomes impaired while at school.
- Parents demonstrate correct techniques for performing respiratory therapy at home.

ANATOMY AND PHYSIOLOGY OF THE RESPIRATORY SYSTEM

The respiratory system can be separated into two divisions: the upper respiratory tract, composed of the nose, paranasal sinuses, pharynx, larynx, and epiglottis; and the lower tract, composed of the bronchi, bronchioles, and alveoli. Through **inspiration** (breathing in), the respiratory system delivers warmed and moistened air to the alveoli, transports oxygen across the alveolar membrane to hemoglobin-laden red blood cells, and allows carbon dioxide to diffuse from red blood cells back into the alveoli. Through **expiration** (breathing out), carbon dioxide–filled air is discharged to the outside. Levels of oxygen and carbon dioxide in the lungs, blood, and body cells are shown in Figure 40.1.

The respiratory center is located in the medulla of the brain. Peripheral receptors located in the aortic arch and carotid arteries sense diminished PO_2 levels and respond by increasing the respiratory rate. Central respiratory receptors in the medulla sense increased PCO_2 levels along with body acidity, temperature, and blood pressure as another stimulus to respiration. Depth of respiration is influenced by proprioceptors located in the lung periphery that register lung fullness. An inhibitory center in the pons halts inspiratory impulses before the lungs become overextended. Often children with chronic lung disease such as cystic fibrosis have adapted so well to a chronically high PCO_2 level that central receptor sites no longer register this as abnormal. In these instances, the main stimulus for respiration is a low oxygen level. In such children, administering high levels of oxygen can be dangerous because it alleviates oxygen want or their main respiratory stimulus.

Respiratory Tract Differences in Children

Embryologic development of the respiratory tract is discussed in Chapter 9. Because the respiratory tract continues to mature during childhood, children have several important differences in respiratory anatomy and physiology than adults. The ethmoidal and maxillary sinuses are present at birth; the frontal sinuses (the sinuses most frequently involved in sinus infection) and the sphenoidal sinuses do not develop until 6 to 8 years of age. Due to rapid growth of lymphoid tissue, tonsillar tissue is normally enlarged in early school-age children.

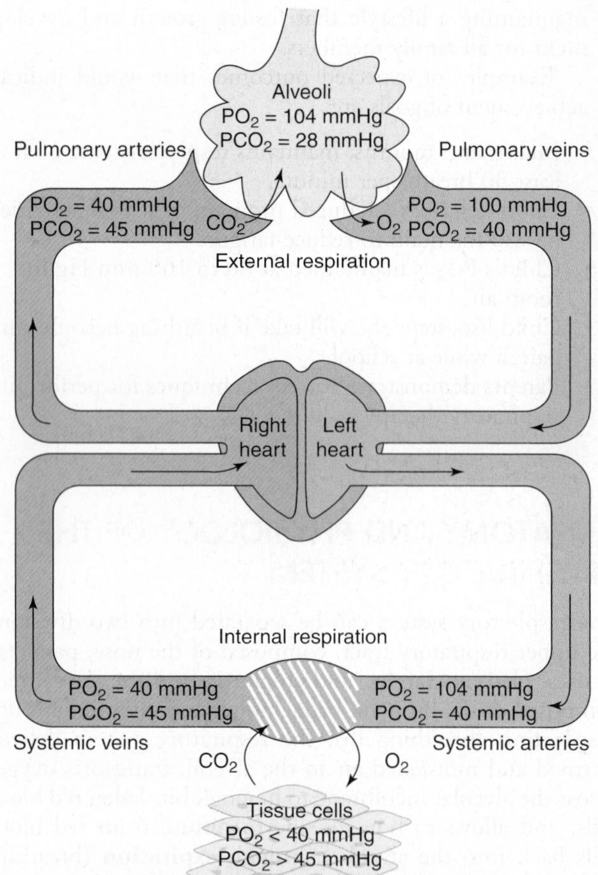

FIGURE 40.1 Partial pressure of gas (mm Hg) as measured in peripheral and systemic circulation. Because of the differences in partial pressure of the gases in the different areas, O_2 moves from alveoli to pulmonary capillaries (i.e., the gas moves from the area of greater concentration to one of a lesser concentration). When it reaches the tissue capillaries, O_2 partial pressure in cells is less, so O_2 goes into the tissues and CO_2 moves out.

Respiratory mucus functions as a cleaning agent by moving invading organisms or other particles out of the lungs. However, newborns produce little respiratory mucus, which makes them more susceptible to respiratory infection than older children. Excessive production of mucus in children up to 2 years of age can actually lead to obstruction because the bronchial lumens are so small in children of this age.

After 2 years of age, the right bronchus is noticeably shorter, wider, and more vertical than the left. This is the reason that inhaled foreign bodies most often lodge in the right bronchus. Infants' chest muscles are not fully developed, so they use their abdominal muscles to assist in inhalation. The change to thoracic breathing begins at 2 to 3 years of age and is complete at 7 years. Because accessory muscles are used more in children than in adults, weakness of these muscles from disease may more easily result in respiratory failure in children than in adults.

In infants, the walls of the airways have less cartilage than in older children and adults and so are not as strong and more likely to collapse after expiration. An advantage of immature development is that a lessened amount of smooth muscle in the airway means an infant does not develop bronchospasm as readily as an older child or adult. Therefore, **wheezing** (the sound of air being pushed through constricted bronchioles) may not be a prominent finding in infants even when the lumen of the airway is severely compromised.

ASSESSING RESPIRATORY ILLNESS IN CHILDREN

Assessment of respiratory illness in children includes an interview, physical examination, and laboratory testing. If the child is in acute distress, the interview and health history may cover only the most important details: when the child first became ill and what symptoms are present. It is important, however, to get as accurate a picture as possible, because the problem could be the result of a variety of circumstances (Box 40.2).

Symptoms of **hypoxemia** (deficient oxygenation of the blood), for example, are often insidious. Peripheral vasoconstriction (a mechanism to save the available oxygen for central life-sustaining body organs) leads to a pale appearance. Tachypnea and tachycardia (efforts to oxygenate cells better) can lead to anxiety and confusion (caused by limited cerebral

Box 40.2 Assessment
Assessing a Child for Signs and Symptoms of Respiratory Dysfunction

History

Chief concern: Cough, rapid respirations, noisy breathing, rhinitis, reddened sore throat, lethargy, cyanosis, difficulty sucking, fever.

Past medical history: Poor weight gain, difficulty with respirations at birth, prematurity.

Family history: History of family member with asthma; other family members with respiratory infection.

Physical examination

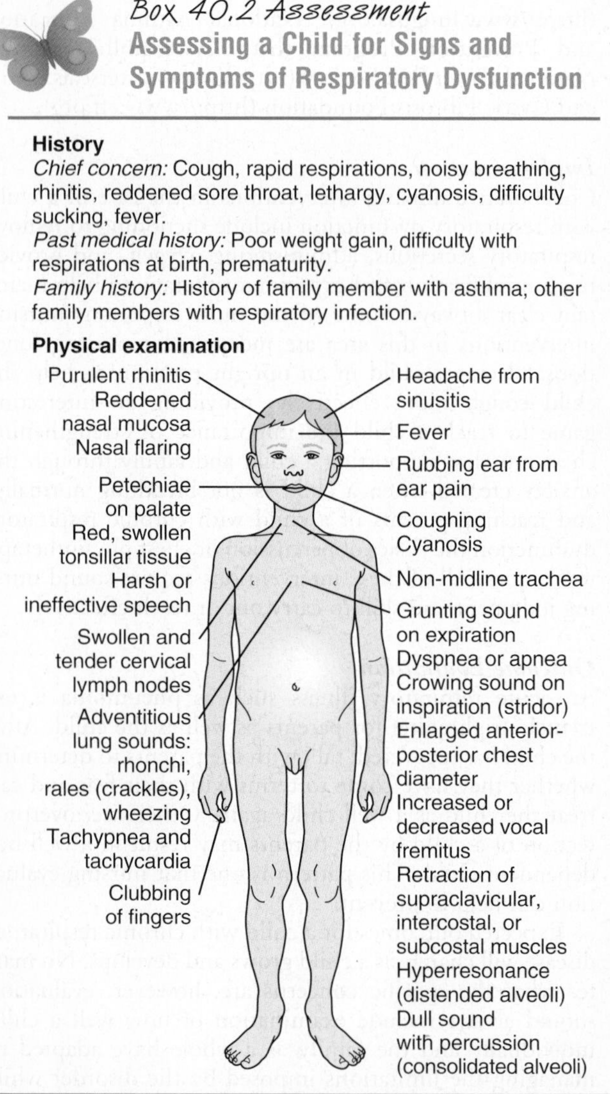

perfusion). A poor feeding pattern may be one of the first signs noted in the infant because an infant cannot suck and breathe rapidly at the same time. Cardiac arrhythmia may occur because of inadequate cardiac tissue perfusion. Always ask about home remedies that may have been used in an attempt to increase breathing space or effort.

Physical Assessment

Physical assessment of a child with a respiratory disorder includes observation of symptoms such as cough, cyanosis, or pallor, as well as evaluation of respirations and breath sounds (Hueston, 2008). Breath sounds are best heard if an infant or child is not crying. Spending time comforting a child to prevent crying is time well spent.

Cough

A cough reflex is initiated by stimulation of the nerves of the respiratory tract mucosa by the presence of dust, chemicals, mucus, or inflammation. The sound of coughing is caused by rapid expiratory air movement past the glottis. Coughing is a useful procedure to clear excess mucus or foreign bodies from the respiratory tract. It only becomes harmful and needs suppression when there is no mucus or debris to be expelled and the amount of coughing becomes exhausting. This might occur with respiratory tract inflammation. **Paroxysmal coughing** refers to a series of expiratory coughs after a deep inspiration. Commonly, this occurs in children with pertussis (whooping cough) or those who have aspirated a foreign body or a liquid they attempted to drink.

Although helpful in removing mucus, coughing increases chest pressure and so may decrease venous return to the heart. This lowers cardiac output and can lead to fainting (syncope). Paroxysmal coughing may increase the pressure in the central venous circulation to such an extent that bleeding into the central nervous system (CNS) can result. Because young children often vomit after a series of coughs, they may be suspected initially of having a gastric disturbance even though their main illness is respiratory.

Rate and Depth of Respirations

Tachypnea (an increased respiratory rate) often is the first indicator of airway obstruction in young children. When assessing respiratory rate, particularly in infants, try to count respiratory rate before waking them, because crying distorts respiratory rate. Assess also the depth and quality of respiration, as these also reveal **anoxia** or lack of oxygen in body cells.

Retractions

When children must inspire more forcefully than normally to inflate their lungs because of an airway obstruction or stiff, noncompliant lungs (as in newborns with pulmonary dysplasia), intrapleural pressure is decreased to the point that the nonrigid parts of the chest (the intercostal spaces) draw inward, creating **retractions** (Fig. 40.2). Retractions occur more commonly in newborns and infants than in older children because the intercostal tissues are weaker and less developed in younger children. Retraction of upper chest muscles (supraclavicular or suprasternal) suggests upper airway obstruction; retraction of intercostal or subcostal muscles suggests lower airway obstruction.

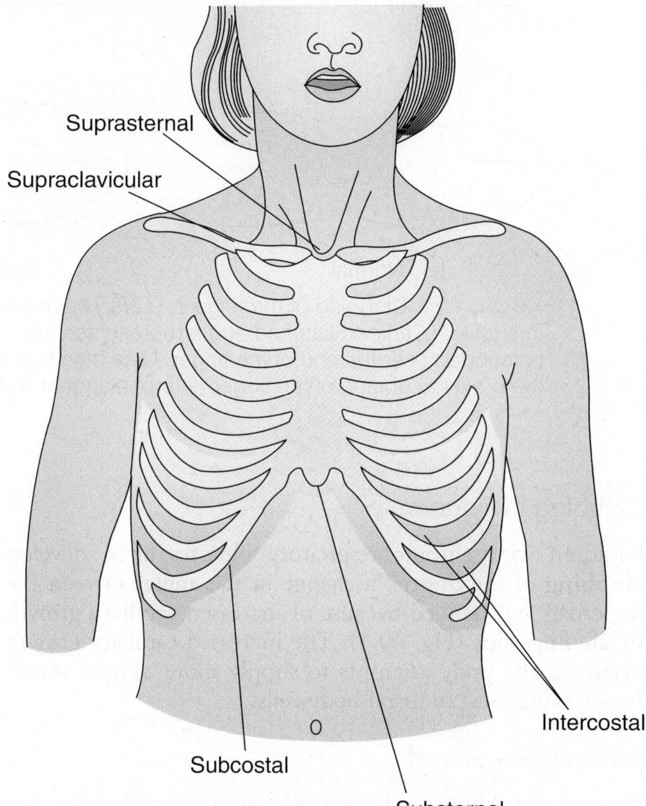

FIGURE 40.2 Sites of respiratory retraction.

Restlessness

When children or infants have decreased oxygen in body cells **(hypoxia),** they become anxious and restless. Be careful not to interpret the excessive movements of infants with respiratory distress as a sign that they are improving; anxious, restless stirring may be their only way of signaling that their respiratory obstruction is becoming acute; it may be one of the first signs of airway obstruction.

Cyanosis

Cyanosis (a blue tinge to the skin) indicates hypoxia. It becomes apparent when the PO_2 is under 40 mm Hg or the level of unoxygenated hemoglobin increases to over 3 g/100 mL (because incompletely oxygenated red blood cells in the circulation are what give blood a dark color). If children have a low red blood cell count, cyanosis may not be apparent because there are not enough red blood cells to give the arterial blood its blue tinge. This occurs at hemoglobin levels below 5 g/100 mL. The degree of cyanosis present, therefore, is not always an accurate indication of the degree of airway difficulty. When children have accompanying peripheral vasoconstriction caused by shock, cyanosis of the extremities also may or may not be apparent.

As the PO_2 drops and cyanosis results, children increase their respiratory effort in an attempt to supply more oxygen to their tissues. When they do this, the difference in pressure between the intralumen of a not yet fully developed trachea and the surrounding tissue becomes so great that the trachea may collapse, compounding the obstruction problem.

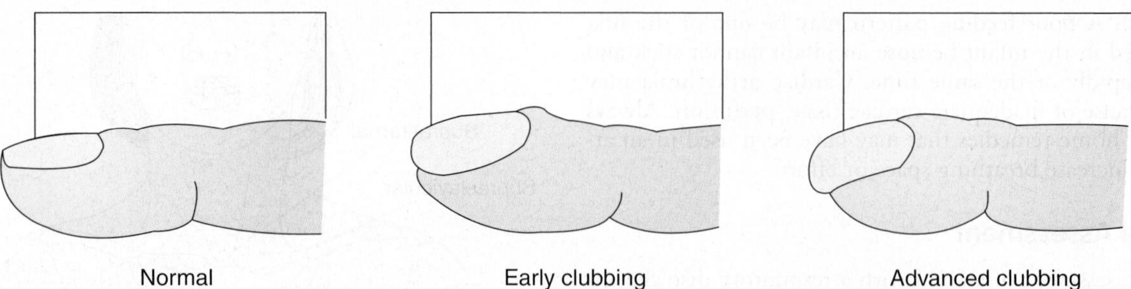

FIGURE 40.3 Clubbing of the fingers. (*Left*) The angle between the nail and digit is normally about 20 degrees in a child. (*Center*) Flattened angle represents early stage of clubbing. (*Right*) In advanced clubbing, the nail is rounded over the end of the finger. Note also that the distal phalanx is bulbous and of greater depth than the proximal portion of the finger (interphalangeal depth).

Clubbing of Fingers

Children with chronic respiratory illnesses often develop **clubbing** of the fingers, a change in the angle between the fingernail and nailbed because of increased capillary growth in the fingertips (Fig. 40.3). The increased capillary growth occurs as the body attempts to supply more oxygen routes (more capillaries) to distal body cells.

Adventitious Sounds

Normal breath sounds are reviewed in Chapter 34. **Adventitious sounds** (extra or abnormal breathing sounds) are caused by pathologic conditions and can be heard on lung assessment in children with respiratory disorders. Normally, on chest auscultation, the inspiratory sound is softer and longer than the expiratory sound. This is referred to as *vesicular breathing*. If you listen over the trachea, this pattern in terms of the length of inspiration and expiration is reversed. This is *bronchial or tubular breathing*. If you hear bronchial breath sounds in the periphery of the lungs, where normally you would expect to hear a vesicular pattern, it indicates that gas exchange in peripheral alveoli is so compromised (as in pneumonia) that you are listening to transmitted tracheal sounds.

Accessory sounds of respiration result from the vibrations produced as air is forced past obstructions such as mucus. If the obstruction is in the nose or pharynx, the noise produced is a snoring sound (*rhonchi*). If the obstruction is at the base of the tongue or in the larynx, you will hear a harsh, strident sound on inspiration. This is laryngeal *stridor*. It is often most marked when a child is in a supine position and less marked when a child sits upright. If an obstruction is in the lower trachea or bronchioles, it is most noticeable on expiration. An expiratory whistle sound (*wheezing*) occurs. If alveoli become fluid-filled, fine crackling sounds **(rales)** are heard. Diminished or absent breath sounds occur when the alveoli are so fluid-filled that little or no air can enter them.

Chest Diameters

With chronic obstructive lung disease, children may be unable to exhale completely, allowing air to be chronically trapped in lung alveoli (hyperinflation). This produces an elongated anteroposterior diameter of the chest, sometimes termed a "pigeon breast." There is an accompanying tympanic or hyperresonant (loud and hollow) sound heard on percussion (see later discussion on chest physiotherapy) over lung spaces.

Laboratory Tests

Several laboratory tests can be used to confirm or rule out the presence of a respiratory disorder and to help identify the cause and severity of the problem. These include analysis of arterial blood gases, nasopharyngeal culture, and sputum analysis.

Blood Gas Analysis

Blood gas analysis is an invasive method for determining the effectiveness of ventilation and acid–base status. The normal values of **arterial blood gases (ABGs)**—the amount of oxygen and carbon dioxide in the blood—are shown in Table 40.1.

Blood gas analysis provides important information about oxygenation of the blood, as values may indicate not only whether the arterial partial pressure of oxygen (PO_2) is adequate but also whether the oxygen saturation of hemoglobin is adequate. The oxygen saturation level will fall if adequate oxygen cannot reach the bloodstream because of respiratory distress or if the hemoglobin is defective and cannot carry a full complement of oxygen (as with sickle cell anemia or thalassemia major). If a child has a severe anemia, the saturation level may be adequate (95% to 100%), but body cells may still not be receiving enough oxygen because of the limited number of red blood cells carrying oxygen. With increased PCO_2 or decreased PO_2, a low pH, or decreased temperature, the ability of hemoglobin to accept oxygen diminishes so, again, cells may become hypoxic.

PCO_2 measures the efficiency of ventilation. In children who are hypoventilating (breathing very shallowly), PCO_2 will be increased because they cannot blow off CO_2; in children who are hyperventilating (breathing deeply), PCO_2 will be decreased because children are blowing off too much. When children cannot evacuate accumulated CO_2 because of an obstruction or hypoventilation, the partial pressure of CO_2 in the arterial blood rises and the concentration of carbonic acid (formed when carbon dioxide dissolves in H_2O in plasma) also rises. This leads to acidosis (a decrease in serum pH or an increase in acidity).

The body can compensate for developing acidity for a long time by gradually increasing the amount of bicarbonate in the bloodstream by decreasing the amount of bicarbonate excreted by the kidneys. When respiratory distress is relieved (by removal of an obstruction or by assisted ventilation), the amount of bicarbonate present in the bloodstream may ex-

TABLE 40.1 ✻ Arterial Blood Gas Values

Measure	Definition	Normal Value	Clinical Significance
Po_2	Partial pressure of oxygen in arterial blood	80–100 mm Hg	Decreased if child cannot inspire adequately
Pco_2	Partial pressure of carbon dioxide in arterial blood	35–45 mm Hg	Increased if child cannot expire adequately
O_2 saturation	The percentage of hemoglobin carrying oxygen	95%–100%	Decreased if O_2 cannot reach red blood cells, if unoxygenated cells are being mixed with oxygenated ones, or if hemoglobin is defective
pH	The hydrogen ion concentration of blood	7.35–7.45	Decreased if CO_2 is being retained as carbonic acid in blood
HCO_3	The bicarbonate concentration in blood	22–26 mEq/L	Increased in respiratory alkalosis; decreased in respiratory acidosis
Base excess	Bicarbonate available for buffering	−2.5 or +2.5 mEq/L	(+) = alkaline excess (−) = alkaline deficit

ceed the amount of acid produced at that point, and the child's condition may change from acidosis to alkalosis. With alkalosis, the respiratory rate decreases as the child tries to conserve CO_2. As a result, periods of apnea may occur. Children require close observation during this time, including frequent blood gas and electrolyte determinations to ensure prompt treatment to detect and reverse these changes. Respiratory alkalosis and respiratory acidosis are compared in Table 40.2. Box 40.3 shows steps for evaluating ABGs.

To analyze blood gases, arterial blood rather than venous blood must be used (arterial blood will reflect how well the lungs are oxygenating the blood, whereas venous blood will reflect only the oxygenation of the particular extremity from which the blood was drawn). In the young infant, the temporal artery may be used as a site for blood gasses; in newborns, an umbilical artery catheter can be used. In older children, the radial artery is the site of choice because of the collateral circulation present at the wrist. (If clotting should occur in the radial artery, the hand would still be well nourished by collateral circulation; see the Allen test in Box 40.4.)

For an ABG assessment, a specimen is withdrawn into a heparinized syringe (to prevent clotting). After any arterial puncture, always firmly compress the site. Otherwise, blood from the punctured vessel can seep into subcutaneous tissue, possibly causing a large hematoma and obscuring the site for further assessment. If frequent specimen collections are required, an arterial catheter, inserted either peripherally or centrally, may be used. Doing so allows frequent specimen collections without the trauma of additional punctures. Be sure to apply dressings over the area where an arterial catheter exits the skin to help prevent a young child from fussing or playing with the site. Soft restraints, such as an elbow or hand restraint, may be needed to keep a child from dislodging the catheter.

TABLE 40.2 ✻ Comparison of Respiratory Alkalosis and Respiratory Acidosis

Acid–Base Condition	Cause	Findings
Respiratory alkalosis	Hyperventilation	Rapid, deep breathing Confusion, unconsciousness Elevated plasma pH (above 7.45) Elevated urine pH (above 7) Decreased Pco_2 (below 40 mm Hg) Plasma bicarbonate –Initially normal –Compensated: below 20 mEq/L Base excess: 0 or a negative reading such as −4
Respiratory acidosis	Hypoventilation trapping carbon dioxide in alveoli	Shallow breathing; inability to expire freely Confusion, disorientation Decreased plasma pH (below 7.35) Decreased urine pH (below 6) Elevated Pco_2 (over 40 mm Hg) Plasma bicarbonate –Initially normal or elevated –Compensated: above 25 mEq/L Base excess: 0 or a positive reading such as +4

BOX 40.3 ✻ Quick Assessment of Arterial Blood Gases

Use a systematic format to assess ABGs quickly:

1. Evaluate the pH: Normally, pH falls between 7.35 and 7.45. A pH below 7.35 denotes acidemia; one above 7.45 reflects alkalemia. If the patient has more than one acid–base imbalance at work, the pH identifies the process in control.
2. Evaluate PCO_2: The partial pressure of arterial CO_2 (PCO_2) normally ranges between 35 and 45 mm Hg. A PCO_2 greater than 45 mm Hg indicates ventilatory failure and respiratory acidosis from CO_2 accumulation. A PCO_2 less than 35 mm Hg indicates alveolar hyperventilation and respiratory alkalosis.
3. Evaluate HCO_3: A bicarbonate (HCO_3^-) less than 22 mEq/L or a base excess (BE) less than −2 mEq/L denotes metabolic acidosis. A bicarbonate level greater than 26 mEq/L or a BE greater than 2 mEq/L reflects metabolic alkalosis. If the two measurements conflict, the BE is the better indicator of metabolic status.
4. Determine which is the primary and which is the compensating disorder: Often, two acid–base imbalances coincide; one is primary, the other is the body's attempt to return the pH to normal. When both the PCO_2 and the HCO_3^- are abnormal, one denotes the primary acid–base disorder and the other denotes the compensating disorder.
   a. To decide which is which, check the pH. *Only a process of acidosis can make the pH acidic; only a process of alkalosis can make the pH alkaline.* For example, if steps 2 and 3 indicate that the patient has respiratory acidosis and metabolic alkalosis and the pH is 7.25, the primary disorder must be respiratory acidosis. The remaining disorder is compensating for the primary problem.
   b. When pH rises (becomes alkalotic), PCO_2 decreases in amount (will be below 35 mm Hg). When pH decreases (becomes acidotic), PCO_2 increases (will be above 45 mm Hg). When an opposite problem exists this way (pH increased; PCO_2 decreased), the problem is respiratory in origin.
   c. pH and HCO_3 normally move in the same direction (when pH is elevated, HCO_3 is elevated). When these two measurements correspond this way (pH decreased, HCO_3 decreased), then the cause of the problem is metabolic in origin.
   d. Three states of compensation are possible: *noncompensation,* reflected in an alteration of only PCO_2 or HCO_3^-; *partial compensation,* in which both PCO_2 and HCO_3^- are abnormal and, because compensation is incomplete, the pH is also abnormal; and *complete compensation,* in which both PCO_2 and HCO_3^- are abnormal but, because compensation is complete, the pH is normal. To identify the primary disorder when compensation is complete, consider a pH between 7.35 and 7.40 indicative of primary acidosis and a pH between 7.40 and 7.45 indicative of primary alkalosis.
5. Evaluate oxygenation: Normally PO_2 remains between 80 and 100 mm Hg. A PO_2 between 60 and 80 mm Hg reflects mild hypoxemia; between 40 and 60 mm Hg, moderate hypoxemia; and below 40 mm Hg, severe hypoxemia.
6. Interpret the findings: Your final analysis should include the degree of compensation, the primary disorder, and the oxygenation status; for example, "partially compensated respiratory acidosis with moderate hypoxemia."

BOX 40.4 ✻ Allen Test

Before obtaining an ABG from the radial artery, it is important to establish that a child has collateral circulation to the hand. Otherwise, the needle puncture may block the artery and block blood flow to the hand.

To prove that there is collateral circulation, compress both the radial and ulnar arteries on the inner side of the wrist and elevate the hand until color disappears. Release the pressure over the ulnar artery and observe for a color change in the hand. If the hand does not pinken (proof the blood has flowed into the hand), the radial artery on that wrist should not be used for catheter insertion.

In small infants, when it is impossible to obtain arterial blood directly, heel or finger punctures may be used. If the heel or finger is warmed for about 20 minutes with a warm compress before the procedure, local blood flow increases so much that the blood gas levels of the capillaries approach those of arteries.

Be certain to note the use of oxygen, if any, and its liter flow on laboratory slips for ABG assessments. Also note the site where the specimen was obtained. While being transported to the laboratory, ABG specimens should be kept on ice to ensure accurate results (CO_2 levels decline in room air).

The oxygen saturation of hemoglobin can also be obtained noninvasively using pulse oximetry and transcutaneous oxygen monitoring.

Pulse Oximetry. Pulse oximetry is a noninvasive technique for measuring oxygen saturation. For the measurement, a sensor and a photodetector are placed around a vascular bed, most often a finger in a child or a foot in an infant (Fig. 40.4). Infrared light is directed through the finger from the sensor to

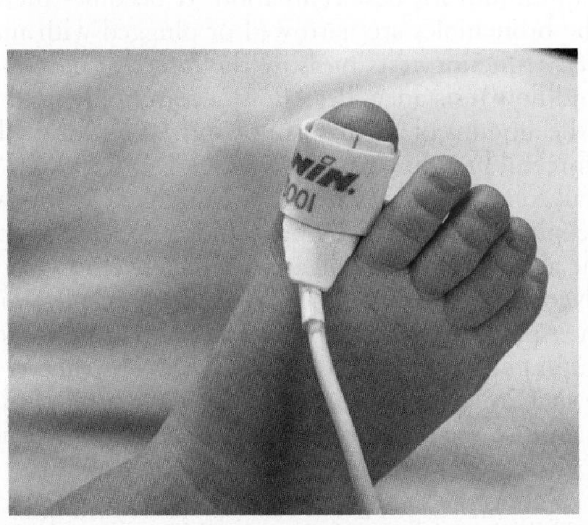

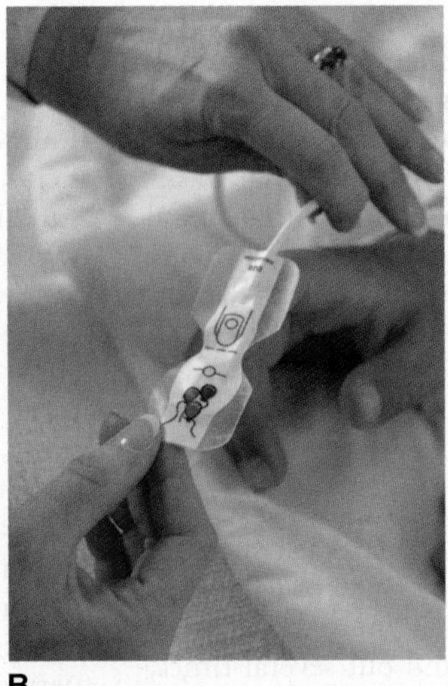

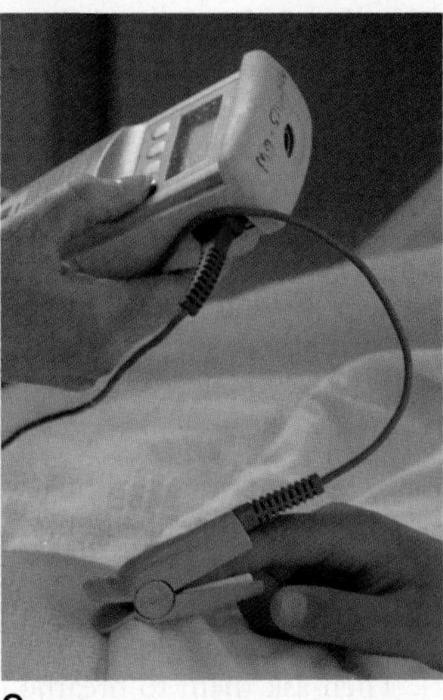

FIGURE 40.4 Types of pulse oximetry probes include (**A**) infant continuous; (**B**) finger continuous; and (**C**) finger intermittent. (From *Maternity and Pediatric Nursing.* Philadelphia: Lippincott Williams & Wilkins.)

the photodetector. Because hemoglobin absorbs light waves differently when it is bound to oxygen than when it is not, the oximeter can detect the degree of oxygen saturation (SaO_2) in the hemoglobin.

Oxygen saturation is closely aligned with PO_2 (Fig. 40.5). When SaO_2 is 95%, the PO_2 is within the normal range of 80 to 100 mm Hg. When SaO_2 has fallen to 90%, the PO_2 is 60 mm Hg. An easy rule to remember concerning the relationship between SaO_2 and PO_2 is the 60 to 30, 90 to 60 rule: when SaO_2 is 60, PO_2 is 30; when SaO_2 is 90, PO_2 is 60. Any SaO_2 reading under 90, therefore, is a cause for concern.

One advantage of pulse oximetry is that it is noninvasive. A second advantage is that the continuous monitoring provided by a pulse oximeter allows you to modify your care appropriately. If an oxygen level should begin to fall while you are handling an infant, for example, you could immediately stop care until the infant's PO_2 again returns to normal. A

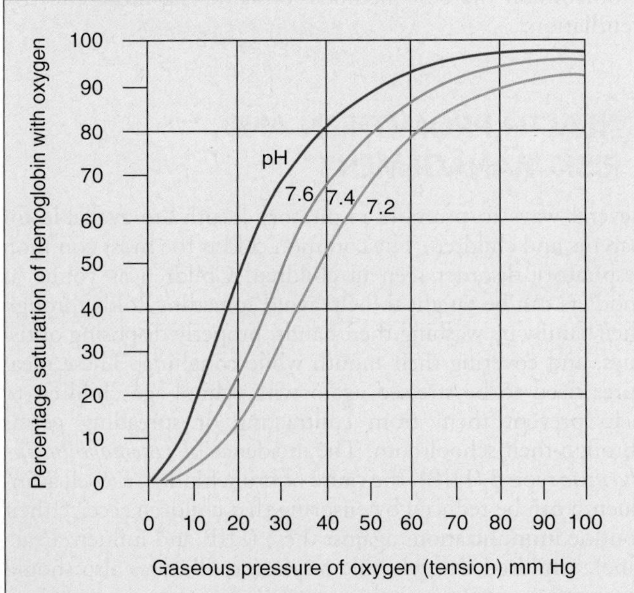

FIGURE 40.5 Oxyhemoglobin dissociation curve.

disadvantage is that the sensor is small and must be checked frequently to see that it remains in place. Excess light in a room can distort the reading. Therefore, the sensor may need to be covered with a blanket in a neonatal intensive care unit or brightly lit nursery for readings to be accurate. Young children also tend to remove the sensors just as they frequently remove adhesive bandages from their fingers.

Transcutaneous Oxygen Monitoring. Transcutaneous monitoring is another means of continuous, noninvasive measurement of oxygen saturation. For this determination, electrodes heated to 44° C are attached to an infant's chest. The heat causes vasodilation underneath the skin and brings the peripheral arterial blood to the surface to be read for oxygen content. This is converted to mm Hg for a monitor readout. The oxygen saturation level read by this method correlates with intra-arterial PO_2, the same as with pulse oximetry. Transcutaneous monitoring has a disadvantage compared with pulse oximetry because the probe position needs to be changed about every 3 to 4 hours to prevent a burn to the skin, and sensor recalibration is necessary with each position change.

Nasopharyngeal Culture

When done efficiently, nasopharyngeal cultures cause little discomfort and reveal a great deal of information about the microorganisms causing a disease. However, most children are terribly frightened by having something placed in their noses or throats and so may resist accordingly. Firm, calm support during the procedure while you touch a moistened swab to the mucus membrane of the nose or throat is essential. Nose and throat cultures can reveal only the organisms present in the upper respiratory tract. As a result, they may not show organisms causing a lower respiratory tract infection. A throat culture will miss pathogenic organisms if the culture tip is not touched to the infected aspect of the pharynx.

Respiratory Syncytial Virus Nasal Washings

Nasal washings are obtained to diagnose an infection by the respiratory syncytial virus (RSV). For this, a child is placed in the supine position, and 1 to 2 mL sterile normal saline is dropped with a sterile needleless syringe into one nostril. The nose is then aspirated using a small, sterile bulb syringe. The secretions removed are placed in a sterile container to be sent to the laboratory for analysis. Nasal washings are even more uncomfortable for children than nasal swabbing because of the saline that is instilled. Provide comfort to a child afterward and assure the child the specimen collection is over.

Sputum Analysis

Because they cannot raise sputum with a cough, sputum collection is rarely feasible in children younger than school age. Older children, however, are able to cough and raise sputum. Teach them exactly what you want (a specimen of what they are coughing up, not just clearing from the back of their throat). Then ask them to breathe in and out several times, cough deeply and spit mucus they have raised into a sterile specimen jar.

Diagnostic Procedures

In addition to cultures, several other diagnostic procedures are used to identify respiratory disorders in children. Many of these procedures are also used with adults, with modifications to account for the physical and developmental differences of children. Bronchoscopy (visualization of the bronchi through a bronchoscope) is discussed in Chapter 37.

Chest Radiography

Chest x-ray films will show areas of infiltration or consolidation in the lungs; if a foreign body is opaque, an x-ray study will show its location. Chest x-ray films are more difficult to obtain in infants than in older children, because infants cannot take a breath and hold it when instructed. It is therefore difficult to picture the lungs at their most expanded position. Computed tomography (CT) scans may be ordered for children with chronic lung disease because this technique can best mark disease progress.

Bronchography

On a chest radiography, the air-filled larynx, trachea, and major bronchi are revealed as dark spaces. Any obstruction or distortion in the organs is apparent. For further definition of structures, a radiopaque solution may be introduced into the respiratory tract by an ultrasonic nebulizer or by a catheter inserted into the trachea before the x-ray study is performed. Children may require conscious sedation for this because nebulization or having a catheter passed into the airway can be frightening. Afterward, children may have increased mucus production from bronchial irritation by the procedure. Observe them carefully after such a procedure for possible respiratory obstruction from accumulating mucus.

Pulmonary Function Studies

The process of ventilation, or the work of breathing, involves three main forces: (a) an inertial force that must be overcome to change the speed and direction of air when the lungs change from exhalation to inhalation; (b) an elastic force to help the lungs expand with inhalation; and (c) the flow resistance force or resistance to the movement of air through the bronchial tree that must be overcome. Flow resistance must be at a minimum for best ventilation. It becomes increased when the bronchioles are narrowed or plugged with mucus. Pulmonary function tests measure the forces of inertia, elasticity, and flow resistance. Peak flow, a commonly used measure, is the amount of air that can be moved out of the lungs with a forceful breath.

The alveoli of the lungs are never completely empty at the end of expiration because the bronchioles collapse, trapping air in the alveoli before alveoli are completely empty. In contrast, alveoli are never completely filled on inspiration because their potential for expansion exceeds that necessary for good respiratory function. Children with obstructive lung diseases such as asthma or bronchiolitis have some difficulty moving air into the lungs, but they have even more difficulty moving air out of the lungs. Even if they do expire the same amount of air as the average child, they expire it over a longer period. Children with restrictive ventilatory disorders, such as neuromuscular disorders, have equal difficulty with inspiration and expiration.

Several lung capacity studies can be done to determine the degree of obstruction or restricted ventilation ability. For these studies, the child breathes into a spirometer, a device that records the force of air exchange.

Children younger than 4 years of age are usually unable to participate in pulmonary function tests because these tests require their cooperation. All children need good preparation and teaching for these tests because they must breathe forcefully through the mouth into a mouthpiece on cue. Some tests require the nose be closed by a clamp or clip or an assistant's hand while the child blows out. This can be a frightening feeling for children with respiratory disease. They may need some trial runs to assure themselves that they can breathe with the clamp in place. Without good orientation to the equipment, they may become so anxious about their performance that they develop tachypnea or fail to inhale or exhale at their full capacity, so the test results are skewed.

Common pulmonary function tests are outlined in Table 40.3. The results of pulmonary function studies help determine the nature and extent of a child's respiratory problem and the best methods for achieving more effective ventilation.

HEALTH PROMOTION AND RISK MANAGEMENT

Several ways to promote respiratory health are available for parents and children. The common cold is the most common respiratory disorder seen in children. Children as young as toddlers can be taught to help avoid spreading colds through their family by washing their hands, properly disposing of tissues, and covering their mouth while coughing. These measures need to be stressed again with school-age children to help prevent them from contracting or spreading germs through their schoolroom. The incidence of *Haemophilus influenzae* type B (HIB), the cause of bronchiolitis, as well as influenza can be reduced by ensuring that children receive their routine immunizations against these (HIB and influenza vaccine). Children with chronic respiratory illnesses also should receive the pneumococcal vaccine. Reducing respiratory irritation by reducing secondary smoke can help prevent upper

Box 40.5 Nursing Procedure ✻ Chest Physiotherapy

Purpose: To encourage the loosening and raising of mucus from the respiratory tract through the use of postural gravity drainage and percussion (clapping) and vibrating techniques.

Procedure	Principle
1. Wash your hands; identify child; explain procedure to child.	**1.** Handwashing prevents spread of microorganisms. Identifying the child ensures that you are performing the procedure on the right child. Explaining the procedure beforehand promotes child's understanding and adherence and helps to minimize anxiety.
2. Assess child as to status; analyze appropriateness of procedure; modify plan as necessary.	**2.** Chest physiotherapy is physically exhausting; can increase intracranial pressure when head is lowered in dependent position. Wait 1 h after meals to avoid inducing vomiting with coughing.
3. Assemble supplies: pillow or slant board, disposable tissues (sputum cup if specimen for culture is desired); percussion device (if infant); nebulizer with correct fluid and medicine if prescribed.	**3.** Organizing care increases efficiency and helps prevent tiring child. Nebulization before postural drainage may be prescribed to promote bronchodilation, dilute mucus, and aid mobility of secretions.
4. Select a drainage position (see Fig. 40.8). Position child appropriately but comfortably. Auscultate and percuss lung area for baseline determinations.	**4.** Positions aid in the gravity drainage of secretions.
5. Use percussion and clapping technique (see figure) for 1–2 min and vibrate during 4 or 5 exhalations the section of chest indicated for the position. Observe child closely for respiratory distress. 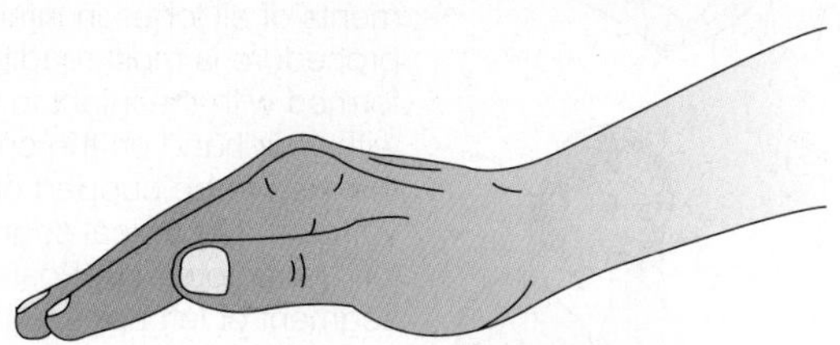	**5.** Percussion and vibration loosen bronchial mucus and allow it to be coughed from the respiratory tract. As mucus moves, it may plug a bronchus; observe for cyanosis, tachypnea, dyspnea, and violent coughing as signs of this.
6. Ask child to deep breathe and cough to raise secretions. Auscultate lung section to ascertain clearing of secretions.	**6.** Coughing also helps move secretions.
7. Reposition; percuss and vibrate the chest areas in additional drainage positions as prescribed. Continue to observe for signs of respiratory distress. Provide rest as necessary between positions.	**7.** Position changes allow for loosening and drainage in other lung segments. Child may grow tired after repeated percussion/vibration.
8. At finish of prescribed positions, return child to bed. Provide mouthwash if desired (and age-appropriate); discard used tissues.	**8.** Coughed sputum may taste unpleasant. Use standard infection precautions to avoid touching soiled tissues.
9. Evaluate effectiveness, cost, comfort, and safety of procedure. Plan health teaching as necessary, such as benefits of procedure.	**9.** Evaluation allows for determining effectiveness of the procedure and need for modifications for future treatments. Health teaching is an independent nursing action always included in nursing care.
10. Record procedure, description of sputum raised, and child's reaction to procedure. If sputum specimen is obtained, send to laboratory for analysis.	**10.** Documentation provides evidence of nursing care, child's status, and effectiveness of interventions.

demonstrate the proper technique by taking a deep breath, blowing it out, taking a second deep breath, blowing that out, taking a third deep breath, and then coughing. The irritation of mucus in the major airway by the third breath makes a cough happen almost spontaneously.

Formerly, CPT was done in hospital settings by respiratory therapists. However, in today's health care climate of managed care, nurses are now often the health care provider who perform CPT and teach it to parents. One or both parents may need to learn the technique before their child is discharged so that it can be continued conscientiously at home. The technique is used most frequently with children with bronchiolitis or cystic fibrosis (van der Schans, Prasad, & Main, 2009).

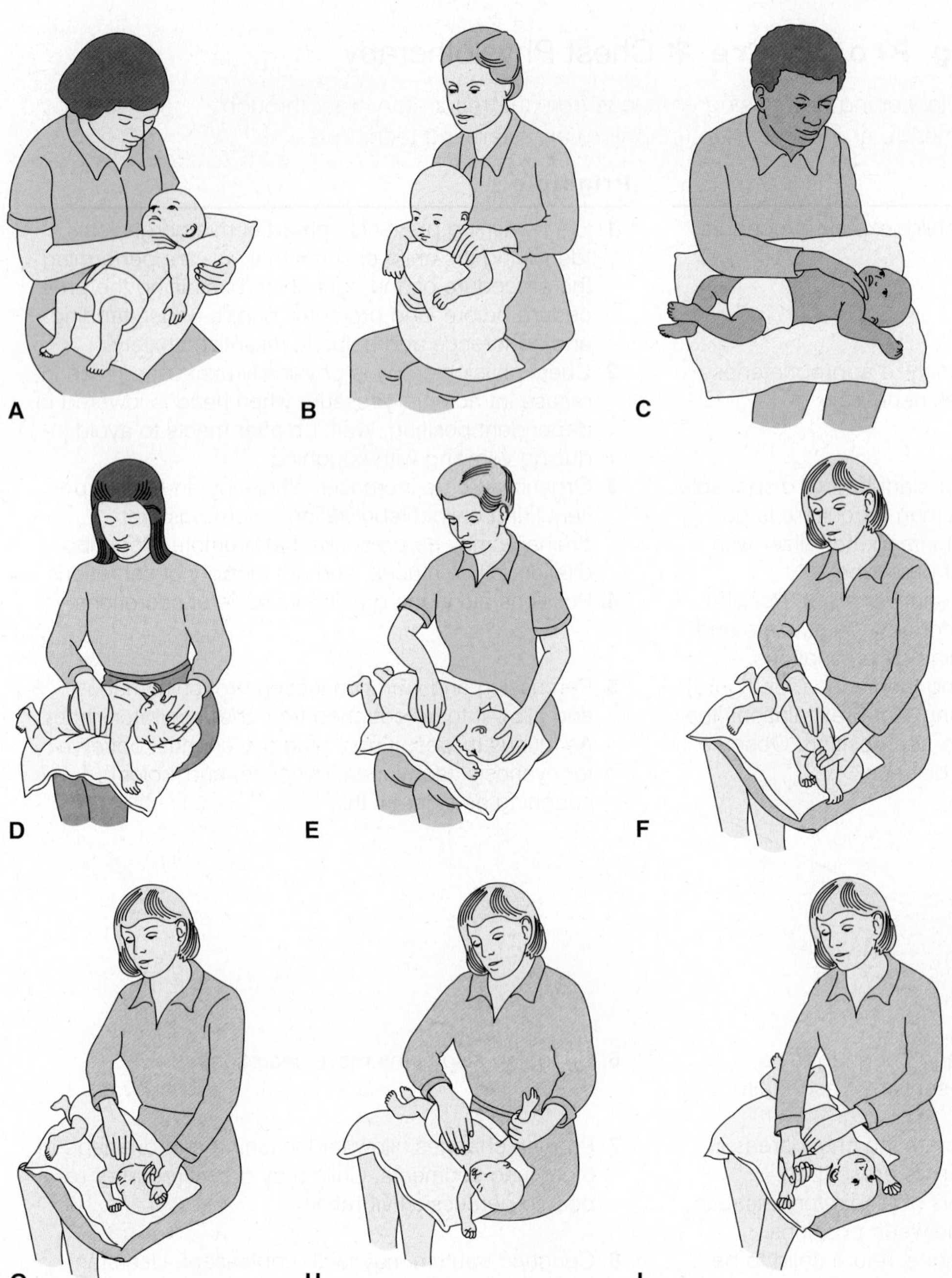

FIGURE 40.8 Positions for bronchial drainage for major segments of all lobes in infants. This procedure is most readily performed with the infant in your lap, with your hand on the chest over the area to be cupped or vibrated. (**A**) Apical segment of left upper lobe. (**B**) Posterior segment of left upper lobe. (**C**) Anterior segment of left upper lobe. (**D**) Superior segment of right lower lobe. (**E**) Posterior basal segment of right lower lobe. (**F**) Lateral basal segment of right lower lobe. (**G**) Anterior basal segment of right lower lobe. (**H**) Medial and lateral segments of right middle lobe. (**I**) Lingular segments (superior and inferior) of left upper lobe.

What if... Michael needs to cough to raise bronchial mucus. What if he refuses to? How can you get him to cough?

Therapy to Improve Oxygenation

Improving oxygenation almost automatically relieves breathing distress.

Oxygen Administration

Oxygen administration elevates the arterial oxygen saturation level by supplying more oxygen to red blood cells through the respiratory tract. Oxygen may be delivered to infants by flooding an incubator or by using a plastic hood, mask, or cannula. Plastic oxygen hoods are tight-fitting enclosures that can keep oxygen concentration at nearly 100% (Fig. 40.10). Always check that a hood fits snugly over the infant's head, making sure it does not rub against the infant's neck, chin, or shoulders. Be sure the gas does not blow directly into the infant's face.

Although a nasal catheter or nasal prongs can be used for infants, they are usually reserved for older children. These provide a concentration of approximately 50% with an oxygen flow of 4 L/min. Most children do not like nasal prongs or catheters because they are intrusive. Assess their nostrils carefully when using these as the pressure of prongs can cause areas of necrosis, particularly on the nasal septum.

A snug-fitting oxygen mask is a method for supplying nearly 100% oxygen and is the method frequently used in

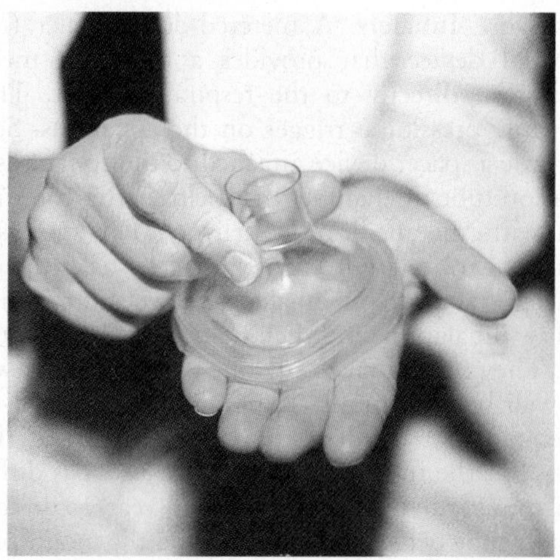

FIGURE 40.9 Alternative percussion device. To assist with percussing an infant or small child, a nipple or mask such as that from a manual resuscitation bag may be used.

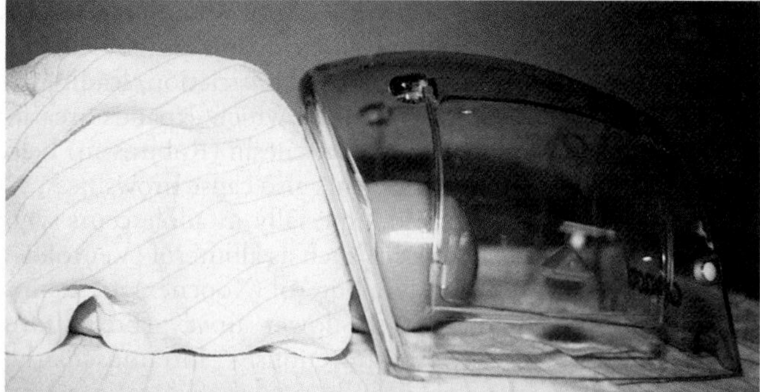

FIGURE 40.10 Oxygen hood for an infant.

emergencies (Fig. 40.11). Masks, like prongs or catheters, are often not well tolerated by children because they tend to slip and obstruct their view. If necessary, let them hold a mask rather than strapping it in place to allow them more control.

Regardless of the delivery method used, oxygen must be administered warmed and moistened. Without proper humidification, oxygen dries mucous membranes and thickens secretions, compounding breathing difficulty. Oxygen, like any other drug, requires careful administration and follow-up assessment. If concentrations are too low, oxygen is not therapeutic; in concentrations greater than those desired, it can be toxic. If newborns are subjected to oxygen concentrations over 100 mm Hg for an extended time, retinopathy of prematurity can occur (see Chapter 26). In any child, administering oxygen concentrations of 70% to 80% for an extended period may lead to a thickening of the lung alveoli and a loss of lung pliancy (oxygen toxicity or bronchopulmonary dysplasia). For these reasons, oxygen should not be given in high concentrations for long periods unless adequate facilities for blood gas analysis are available (Marino, 2007).

When caring for a child with any form of oxygen equipment, follow good safety rules. Because oxygen supports combustion, keep open flames away from oxygen and minimize the risks of sparks. Since oxygen is humidified, oxygen equipment is a good source of microbial contaminants. Change equipment according to your agency's policy, but at least once a week to keep bacterial counts within safe limits. Monitor and record a child's oxygen saturation level via pulse oximetry or transcutaneous pulse oximetry as indicated. Obtain ABG measurements with any change in condition or oxygen flow or as otherwise ordered.

Pharmacologic Therapy

Children notice difficulty with exchange of air when their airways become obstructed because of unusual mucus production, bronchoconstriction, or inflammation. Several drugs may be used in children to reverse these processes. Nasal sprays such as normal saline can be administered to

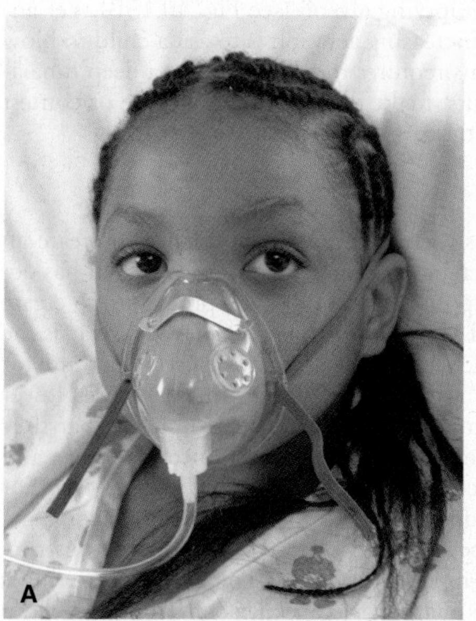

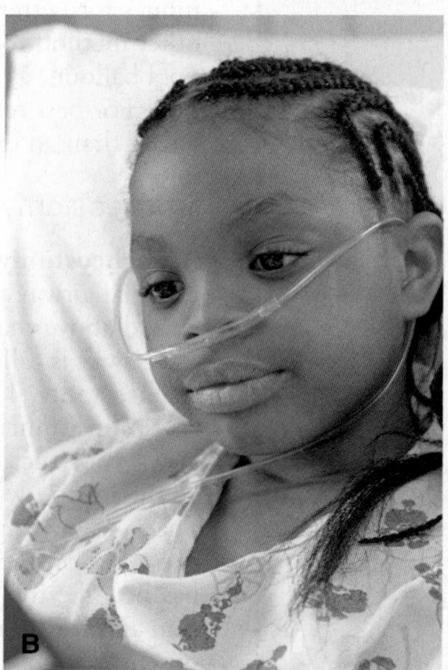

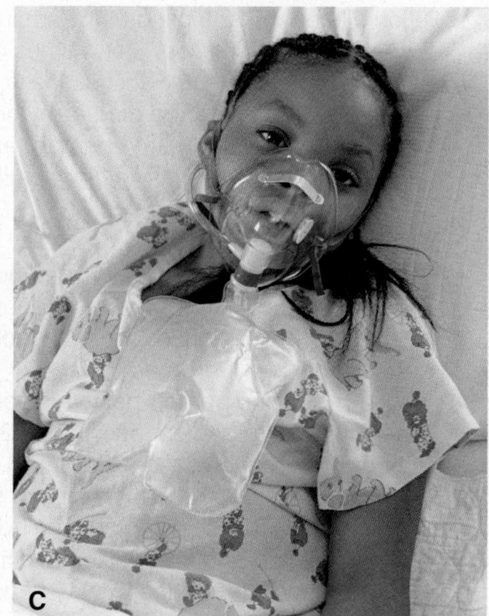

FIGURE 40.11 Types of oxygen administration include (**A**) simple oxygen mask, (**B**) nasal cannula, and (**C**) a nonrebreather mask. (From *Maternity and Pediatric Nursing*. Philadelphia: Lippincott Williams & Wilkins.)

moisten and loosen nasal secretions. Antihistamines given by this route can reduce mucus production and thereby enlarge the airway. Decongestants cause vasoconstriction, leading to shrinkage of the mucous membranes, which expands breathing space. Expectorants such as guaifenesin (Robitussin) help to raise mucus. Most of these agents also cause drowsiness, so their doses must be regulated, especially in adolescents who will be driving. Bronchodilators such as albuterol (Ventolin), terbutaline (Brethine), and levalbuterol (Xopenex) are examples of drugs used to open the lower airway (Box 40.6). Antibiotics may be given intravenously, intramuscularly, orally, or inhaled through nebulization to reduce infection and limit purulent mucus and inflammation. Corticosteroids taken either orally or by inhalation enlarge the airway by reducing further inflammation (Deglin & Vallerand, 2008). Caution parents not to give cough and cold medications to children under 2 years of age unless specifically prescribed by their health care provider (DHHS, 2008).

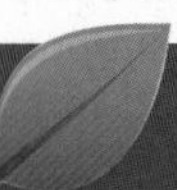

BOX 40.6 * Focus on Pharmacology

Albuterol Sulfate (Proventil, Ventolin)

Classification: Albuterol is a beta-2–adrenergic agonist.

Action: Acts selectively to cause bronchodilation and vasodilation for relief of bronchospasm (Karch, 2009).

Pregnancy risk category: C

Oral Dosage:

- Children older than 14 years—2 or 4 mg, 3 or 4 times daily; not to exceed 32 mg/day
- Children ages 6 to 14 years—2 mg, 3 or 4 times daily, not to exceed 24 mg/day
- Children ages 2 to 6 years—0.1 mg/kg, 3 times daily, not to exceed 2 mg/day; gradually increasing to 0.2 mg/kg, 3 times daily, not to exceed 4 mg/day

Inhaled Dosage: Children 12 years of age and older—2 puffs every 4 to 6 hours: 2.5 mg (0.5 mL of 0.5% solution diluted with 2.5 mL of 0.9% sodium chloride) OR 3 mL of 0.083% solution, 3 or 4 times daily

Possible adverse effects: Restlessness, apprehension, anxiety, fear, nausea, cardiac arrhythmias, paradoxical airway resistance with repeated, excessive use of inhalation preparations, sweating, pallor, and flushing

Nursing Implications

- Instruct parents and child in method to administer drug. Teach child and parents about use and care of nebulized solution or metered-dose inhaler and spacer devices, if ordered.
- Caution child and parents not to exceed the number of ordered puffs, to prevent possible tolerance to drug.
- If more than one inhalation is ordered, advise child to wait 1 to 2 minutes before taking the second puff.
- If the child is also receiving an inhaled corticosteroid, advise the child and parents to have the child use the albuterol first to open the airways and then wait approximately 5 minutes before using the corticosteroid, to maximize its effectiveness.

Metered-Dose Inhalers. A metered-dose inhaler (MDI) is a hand-held device that provides a route for medication administration directly to the respiratory tract. The child inhales while pressing a trigger on the apparatus. Some devices include a spacer device attached to the apparatus, a plastic extension tube or chamber that helps better coordinate inhalation with the medication delivery. For successful use, children need to follow five general rules: shake the canister, exhale deeply, activate the inhaler as they begin to inhale, take a long slow inhalation, and then hold their breath for 5 to 10 seconds. They should take only one puff at a time, with a 1-minute wait between puffs (Karch, 2009). Metered-dose inhalers require that children trigger the inhaler at the same time they breathe in (Fig. 40.12A). Because it is difficult for children younger than approximately 12 years to do this, placing a spacer tube between the inhaler and the mouthpiece better coordinates inhaling and trigger release (Fig. 40.12B).

Incentive Spirometry

Incentive spirometers are devices that encourage children to inhale deeply to aerate the lungs fully or move mucus. Although manufactured in different configurations, a common type consists of a hollow plastic tube containing a brightly colored ball or dome-shaped disk that will rise in the tube when a child inhales through the attached mouthpiece and tubing. The deeper the inhalation, the higher the ball rises in the tube.

Children need instruction on how to use this type of device, because their first impression is that they should blow out against the mouthpiece rather than inhale (Fig. 40.13A). Incentive spirometry is effective with children because the device and procedure resemble a game more than an actual treatment.

Breathing Techniques

Some children need exercises prescribed to help them better inflate alveoli or more fully empty alveoli. Blowing a piece of cotton or a plastic ball across a table, blowing through a straw, or blowing out with the lips pursed are effective techniques for better emptying alveoli (see Fig. 40.13B). Yet another method for increasing aeration is to ask a child to blow up a balloon, as this requires the child to take a deep inhalation. For best results, make these activities a game or contest rather than an exercise.

Tracheostomy

A **tracheostomy** is an opening into the trachea to create an artificial airway to relieve respiratory obstruction that has occurred above that point (Yu, 2008). The procedure to create the airway is called a **tracheotomy;** the resultant airway is the tracheostomy. Tracheostomies also may be used as a route for suctioning mucus when accumulating mucus causes lower airway obstruction. A danger of tracheostomies is that they eliminate the warming and filtering action of the nose and pharynx, making children more susceptible to infection. For these reasons, endotracheal intubation, not tracheostomy, has become the method of choice to relieve airway obstruction and for short-term oxygenation. The exception to this is obstruction in the pharynx, because it is often impossible to pass an endotracheal tube beyond obstruction at this point. Tracheostomies are also still used for long-term home care.

Emergency Intubation. Few medical emergencies are as frightening to a child or parents as an acute obstruction of a child's upper airway requiring a tracheotomy or endotracheal intubation. The child suddenly becomes limp and breathless, with color changing quickly to systemic cyanosis. Tracheotomies are done more easily on a treatment room table than on a bed or crib, so it is generally best to carry a child immediately to a treatment room for the procedure. If a child cannot be moved quickly, however, because of accessory equipment, do not lose time in transport. For tracheotomy, the cricoid cartilage of the trachea is swabbed with an antiseptic; if readily available, a local anesthetic may be injected into the cartilage ring. (This is not necessary in the unconscious child.) An incision is made just under the ring of cartilage and a tracheostomy tube with its obturator in place is inserted into the opening (Fig. 40.14A). When the obturator is removed, the child can breathe through the hollow tracheostomy tube (see Fig. 40.14B). Have suction equipment available for immediate use to clear any blood caused by the incision (this is minimal) and any obstructing mucus from the trachea.

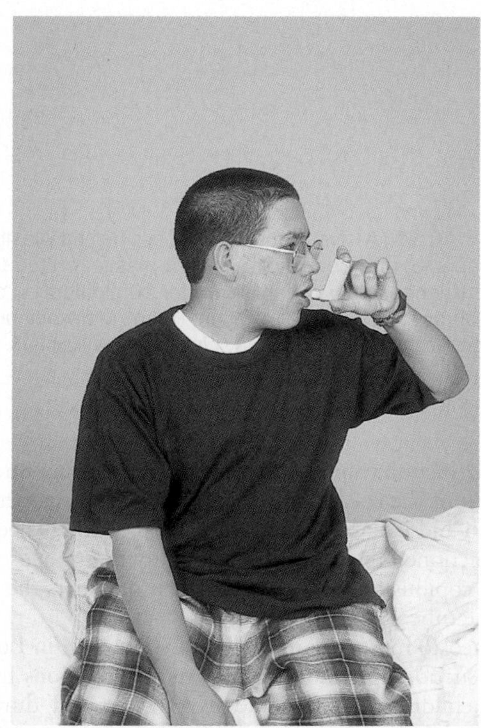

A

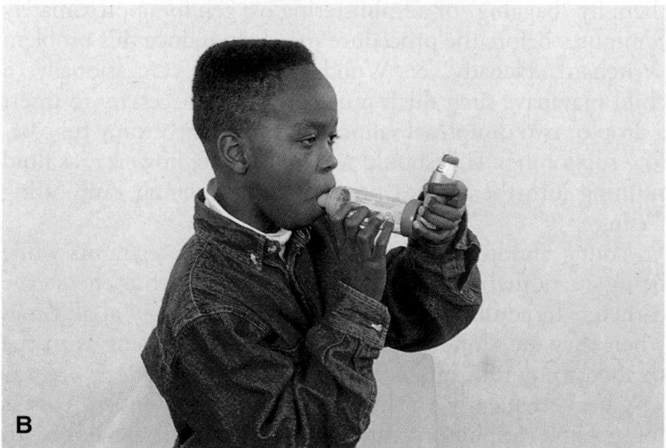

B

FIGURE 40.12 (**A**) Many children use a metered-dose inhaler to administer a bronchodilator to themselves. Be certain children respect such medicine as medicine so they use sensible precautions. (**B**) Younger children need a "spacer" with inhalers so they do not need to correlate administration with inhalation.

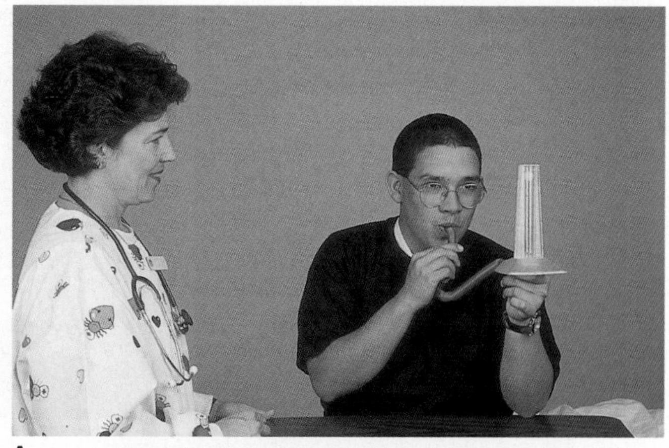

A

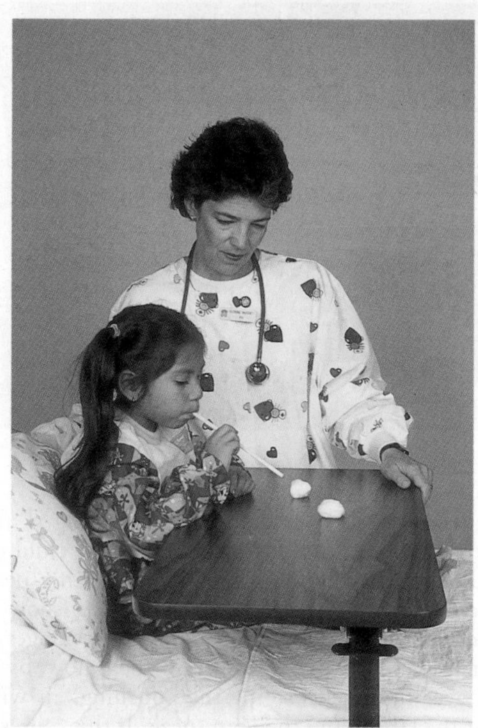

B

FIGURE 40.13 (**A**) Incentive spirometry is an appealing method to encourage children to aerate their lungs. (**B**) Encouraging children to take a deep breath and try to blow a cotton ball across the table is also an entertaining way to help them fully expand their lungs.

The color change in children after tracheostomy is usually dramatic. They inhale deeply several times through the tube, and color returns to normal. A few sutures may be necessary at the tube insertion site to halt bleeding or to reduce the size of the incision so the tube fits snugly.

As children begin to breathe normally and, if unconscious, regain consciousness, they often thrash and push at people around them, both from oxygen deficit and from fright. They call for a parent but can make no sound, adding

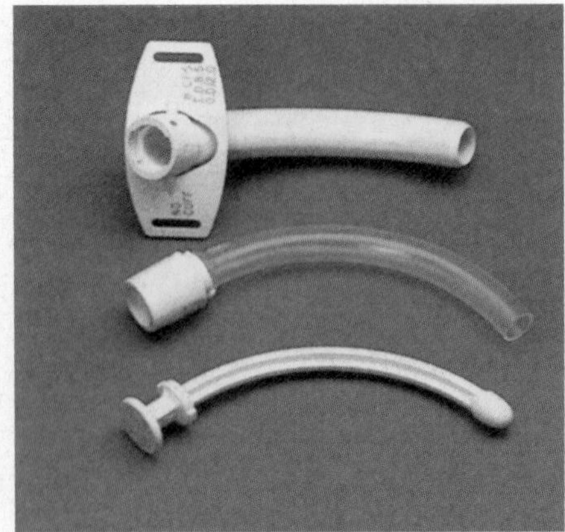
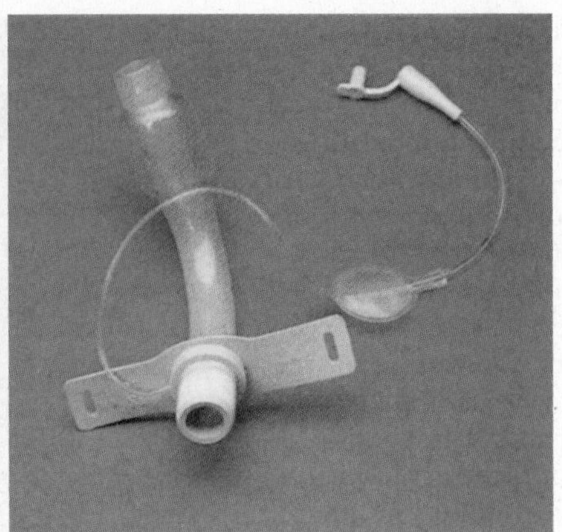
A

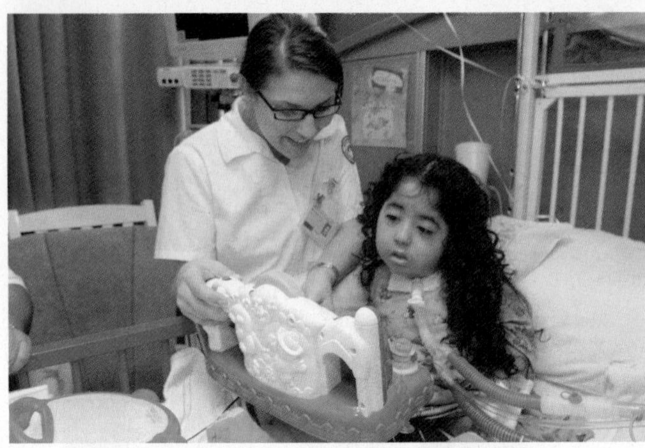
B

FIGURE 40.14 (**A**) Tracheostomy tubes: (*left*) a plastic tube, inner cannula, and obturator; (*right*) a plastic, cuffed tube. (**B**) The tracheostomy collar allows for humidification of inspired air or supplemental oxygen. (From *Maternity and Pediatric Nursing*. Philadelphia: Lippincott Williams & Wilkins.)

to their fright. Assure children that everything is all right, even though they cannot speak. A school-age child can understand a simple explanation such as, "You can't speak right now because of the tube in your throat." As soon as children's respirations are even and they are no longer experiencing acute respiratory distress, show them how, by placing a finger over the tracheostomy tube opening, air will again flow past the larynx and they can speak. If this causes a child to become short of breath, supply a paper and pencil or chalkboard for communication.

Be certain parents understand why the tube is in place and how important it is that it remain patent. Assure them that it is a temporary measure to provide oxygen (provided this is true). If they were not present in the room for the procedure, encourage them to visit the child as soon as possible to assure themselves their child is again all right. Children have difficulty relaxing enough to accept this strange new way of breathing until their parents can relax and accept it also. Some children hyperventilate, not because of respiratory difficulty, but because of this fear.

Suctioning Technique. Most tracheostomy tubes used with children today are plastic. They do not include an inner cannula that would require removal and regular cleaning. Most children, however, do require frequent suctioning (perhaps as often as every 15 minutes) to keep their airway free of mucus. Use sterile technique to prevent introducing microorganisms, and suction gently yet thoroughly. Ineffective suctioning does not remove obstructive mucus and because of irritation can actually cause more mucus to form. Be certain you know how deeply to suction. Some children need to be suctioned only the length of the tracheostomy tube so that the catheter does not touch and irritate the tracheal mucosa. Others need to be deeply suctioned to reduce the possibility that mucus will become so copious or so thickened that it obstructs the trachea below the tube.

Tracheostomy suctioning technique is shown in Box 40.7. Because suctioning removes air as well as secretions from the trachea, children may become oxygen-deprived during the procedure. Although not evidence-based, preoxygenating them by "bagging" or administering oxygen for approximately 5 minutes before the procedure may help reduce this problem (Pritchard, Flenady, & Woodgate, 2009). Occasionally, a child may have such thick mucus that it is necessary to insert a drop or two of normal saline into the tracheostomy tube before suctioning. This should not be routine, however, as fluid running into the trachea produces a frightening, suffocating feeling.

Young children may need to wear elbow restraints while being suctioned to keep their hands away from the sterile catheter. In addition, restraints may be necessary at all times when they are alone to prevent them from fussing with the tracheostomy tube and accidentally removing it.

Check frequently on children with tracheostomies to assess for possible respiratory difficulty. Spend time playing with them or just sitting and rocking them so they can think of you in ways other than as the person who comes to suction them. If parents cannot stay with the child, assure them that you check on their child more frequently than what is necessary for suctioning alone, so they can feel confident if the child should

Box 40.7 Nursing Procedure ✻ Tracheostomy Suction

Purpose: To remove mucus from the trachea.

Procedure	Principle
1. Wash hands; identify child; explain procedure to child.	**1.** Handwashing minimizes the risk for spread of microorganisms; identifying the child ensures that you are performing the procedure on the right child; explaining the procedure helps to encourage cooperation and minimize anxiety.
2. Assess child, especially breath sounds; analyze appropriateness of procedure. Plan ways to modify care based on individual circumstances.	**2.** Assessment prior to procedure provides a baseline for future evaluation. Modifications enhance individualization of nursing care based on client need.
3. Assemble supplies: suction source and tubing, sterile suction catheter (#12 or 14F) or sterile suction kit, sterile gloves, bottle of sterile normal saline, sterile medicine dropper or syringe, manual resuscitator. Plan method to keep child from touching sterile catheter (placing a restraint, distraction, or asking assistance from another nurse).	**3.** Organizing supplies will increase efficiency of procedure.
4. Open the bottle of sterile normal saline and suction catheter or kit. Pour a small amount of saline solution into disposable container included in kit. Prepare syringe or dropper with small amount of sterile normal saline; put on sterile gloves.	**4.** Sterile technique is important to prevent introducing microorganisms.
5. Hold suction catheter with one gloved hand, suction tubing with other gloved hand, and attach tubing to sterile catheter; dip tip of catheter into normal saline and suction a small amount through catheter.	**5.** Proper handling of equipment using sterile technique reduces the risk of contamination because once a sterile glove touches suction tubing, it is no longer sterile. Using sterile normal saline to suction through the catheter and tubing ensures patency.
6. If necessary, instruct assistant to hyperoxygenate child with manual resuscitator.	**6.** Hyperoxygenation prevents child from developing hypoxia during suctioning.

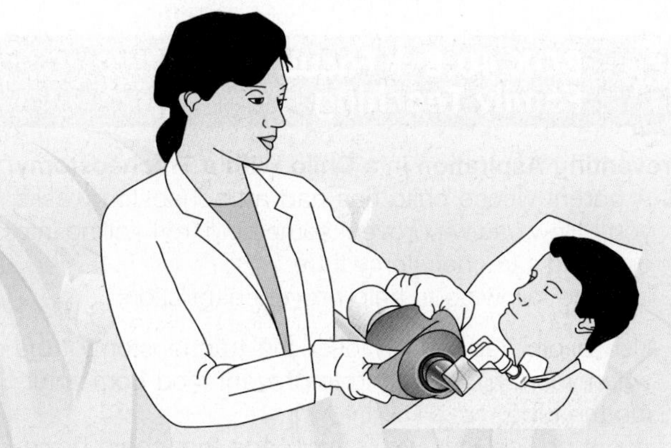

(continued)

Box 40.7 Nursing Procedure * Tracheostomy Suction (continued)

Procedure	Principle
7. Hold your breath; introduce sterile catheter into tracheostomy tube to desired length. Apply suction for 5 to 10 sec and gently withdraw, rotating gently.	**7.** Holding your breath helps you not to suction longer than is comfortable. Applying suction only on withdrawal allows the catheter to pass freely without irritating the trachea and prevents oversuctioning. Prolonged suctioning longer than 10 sec can cause hypoxia.
8. Rinse catheter by dipping tip in normal saline and applying suction.	**8.** Rinsing catheter ensures that it remains patent.
9. Repeat procedure until airway sounds clear. Be careful not to suction longer than necessary.	**9.** Suctioning is fatiguing to children. Extended suctioning can lead to airway irritation and further mucus production.
10. Assess effectiveness and efficiency of procedure; plan teaching such as importance of procedure to parents; document procedure.	**10.** Comparing initial baseline assessments with post-procedure status provides information about effectiveness of the procedure. Teaching is an important independent nursing care activity for the child and parents.
11. Comfort child; remain with child for support. Provide opportunities for therapeutic play.	**11.** Suctioning is frightening; offering support and comfort after all such procedures helps to decrease fears and anxieties.

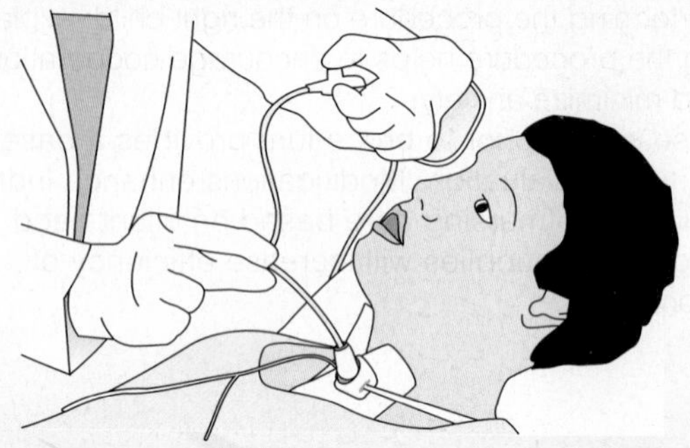

have another episode of acute obstruction, someone will be nearby. If the tracheostomy tube is to be left in place after discharge from the hospital, be certain parents have enough experience with changing tubes if that will be necessary or suctioning so they can safely care for their child at home.

Tracheostomy tubes are held in place by cloth ties that fasten at the back of the child's neck. Change ties when they become soiled or loose, and check them frequently to be certain they remain tied. Children may fuss with and untie such things, whereas adults will not. Assess that the ties fit snugly but allow for one finger to be inserted underneath them so they do not rub and cause pain. For preschoolers or younger children, it is a good idea to cover the tracheostomy opening with a gauze square tied to the child's neck like a bib while they eat. This prevents crumbs or spilled liquids from entering the tracheostomy opening. Do not give children small toys that could fit into the lumen of the tube and cause obstruction (Box 40.8).

Each child is considered individually regarding when it is time to remove a tracheostomy tube. Tubes are generally sealed off partially by adhesive tape or a commercial occlusion device for a day or two before removal; then they are completely occluded (but not removed) for another day. This provides a weaning period where suctioning is still possible if it is needed. Occasionally, children cough so forcefully that they dislodge a tracheostomy tube. You might be with a child when this occurs, or you might walk into the room and find the tube lying beside the child on the bedclothes. As long as the child is

BOX 40.8 * Focus on Family Teaching

Preventing Aspiration in a Child With a Tracheostomy

Q. A parent whose child has had a tracheostomy asks you, "How can we prevent something from falling into our child's tracheostomy tube"?

A. Use the following to help prevent aspiration:

- Use a bib tied loosely over the tracheostomy tube when your child is eating to prevent food from entering the tube.
- Avoid buying toys with small parts that could be removed and dropped into the tube.
- Inspect stuffed toys to be certain they are intact and do not shed (fur or stuffing could enter the tube).
- Supervise play with other children to be certain they do not place anything in the tube.
- Stay with your child in the bathtub, to be certain water does not splash into the tube.
- Keep use of sprays such as perfume or room fresheners to a minimum, because they can be irritating to the trachea.
- Avoid cold air, because it can cause tracheal spasm (cover the child's throat with a loose fleece scarf when out in cold weather).

not in distress, this is not an emergency. Because the incision site usually does not close completely to occlude the tracheal opening when a tube is dislodged, the child still has a patent airway. Always keep a new tube and inserter (obturator) at the bedside in case replacement is necessary. Slide the obturator into the tube and gently replace it in the tracheal opening. Remove the obturator and secure the new tube in place. If you do this quickly yet calmly, the average child is not alarmed and so will not protest. If, however, a child senses your excitement or if you indicate that something is terribly wrong, a child may begin to cry and turn away, making it difficult to replace the tube without assistance.

Endotracheal Intubation

Endotracheal intubation (nasal or oral intubation) is the preferred means of bypassing upper airway obstruction and allowing free entry of air to the trachea. There is little difference in efficiency between oral and nasal methods (Spence & Barr, 2009). However, since intubation tubes cause edema and local irritation, they cannot be left in place as a permanent solution. As with tracheostomies, children cannot speak while intubated. Supply those old enough to write with a pencil and paper for effective communication. Preschoolers can point to pictures to indicate what they need. Providing simple drawings or photos (a drink, a straw, a blanket, the television turned on, a urinal) to make needs known is helpful. Endotracheal tubes are held in place by being taped to the face. Make sure tubes are carefully secured, because children can easily dislodge them. As much as possible, limit the number of tape changes to protect the skin on the child's cheeks.

A capnometer is a device that measures the amount of CO_2 in inhaled or exhaled breaths. It uses infrared technology and is attached to the distal end of the endotracheal tube. By measuring the percentage of CO_2 in expired air, the arterial CO_2 (PCO_2) can be estimated. Used in this way, a capnometer can reduce the number of arterial punctures needed for ABG analysis.

Assisted Ventilation

When it is not possible to improve oxygen saturation to sufficient levels by the methods described above, assisted ventilation may be necessary (Carpenter et al., 2008). Positive-pressure machines deliver moistened or nebulized air or oxygen to the lungs under enough pressure and with appropriate timing to produce artificial, periodic inflation of alveoli; they rely on the elastic recoil of the lungs to empty the alveoli.

Depending on the type of ventilator, the inspiration–expiration cycle is determined by a timed interval, a volume limit, or a pressure limit, depending on the child's condition. Ventilators can supply high tidal volumes at a low frequency rate or low tidal volumes at rates as high as 200 to 300 breaths per minute. Hyperinflation of lungs can occur with high-frequency ventilation because there is not enough time for expiration to occur. For this reason, some high-frequency ventilators are set so air is sucked out of the lungs rather than depending on the normal elastic recoil of the lungs. Some commonly used terms associated with ventilator therapy are shown in Table 40.4.

Children who need respiratory assistance are frightened. A great many fight ventilators or refuse to lie quietly and let the ventilator breathe for them. Pancuronium (Pavulon) may be administered intravenously to a point of abolishing spontaneous respiratory action to overcome resistance and allow mechanical ventilation to be accomplished at lower pressures because without normal respiratory action, there is no normal muscle resistance to overcome (Box 40.9). Clearly, children who receive pancuronium have no spontaneous respiratory function and need critical observation and frequent ABG analysis because they depend totally on caregivers at that point.

Mechanical ventilation for a prolonged period requires that children either have a tracheotomy performed or have an endotracheal tube passed (Fig. 40.15). A cuffed tube is used with ventilators so the seal at the trachea is airtight. Infants need a nasogastric tube inserted to prevent stomach distention from air entering the esophagus. Providing adequate nutrition may be difficult for children on ventilators. Enteric (nasogastric) feedings or total parenteral nutrition solves this problem. Providing a balance of rest, stimulation, and assurance for the child is a challenge for nursing personnel and parents.

Once children become accustomed to assisted ventilation, it can be difficult to discontinue a device, even when there is no longer a clinical indication for it. This is most pronounced

TABLE 40.4 ✻ Terms Commonly Used With Ventilator Therapy

Term	Definition	Clinical Application
IMV	Intermittent mandatory ventilation	Number of mandatory breaths the ventilator will deliver each hour. A child may breathe most of the time without assistance, but a set (mandatory) number of breaths per minute is delivered to ensure adequate lung expansion and oxygenation.
PEEP	Positive end-expiratory pressure	Pressure delivered to lungs at the end of each expiration to keep alveoli from collapsing on expiration and to ensure adequate oxygenation
Sigh	A deep inhalation delivered by the ventilator	Method used to fully inflate the lungs several times each minute
CPAP	Continuous positive airway pressure	A constant pressure exerted on the alveoli to keep them from collapsing on expiration
FIO_2	Concentration of oxygen the child is receiving (inspiring)	A child on oxygen therapy will have an FIO_2 from 22% to 100%

BOX 40.9 * Focus on Pharmacology

Pancuronium Bromide (Pavulon)

Classification: Pancuronium bromide is a neuromuscular blocking agent.

Action: Relaxes skeletal muscles during assisted mechanical ventilation or endotracheal intubation (Karch, 2009).

Pregnancy risk category: C

Dosage: 0.03–0.04 mg/kg intravenously initially, then 0.03–0.1 mg/kg intravenously, repeated every 30 to 60 minutes as needed.

Possible adverse effects: Prolonged dose-related apnea; tachycardia, excessive salivation, and sweating.

Nursing Implications

- Keep in mind that the child's respiratory muscles do not function after administration; maintain assisted ventilation.
- Know that the drug's action peaks in approximately 2 to 3 minutes and lasts approximately 1 hour (longer in children with poor renal perfusion).
- Remember that the drug does not alter state of consciousness. Anticipate the need for sedation or analgesia for procedures.
- Keep equipment for emergency resuscitation (Ambu bag) at bedside in case of a power or mechanical ventilator failure.
- Be sure to explain all events and procedures to the child; even though the respiratory muscles may be paralyzed, the child can still hear. Also encourage the parents to talk to the child when they visit.
- Be prepared to reverse the effects of the drug by administering atropine and neostigmine methylsulfate (Prostigmin).
- Monitor all physiologic parameters, including vital signs, heart rate, and blood pressure. Obtain electrolyte levels as ordered, because electrolyte imbalances can potentiate neuromuscular effects.

in adolescents, who are aware of the role of oxygen and proper ventilation for life function. You may need to provide several trial periods free of the ventilator with someone remaining close by so they can be assured that if they do have difficulty breathing, someone is standing by to help. Many children are too afraid to fall asleep on the first night off a ventilator unless someone is with them and has assured them they will be there through the night.

Lung Transplantation

Lung transplantation is a possibility for children with a chronic respiratory illness such as cystic fibrosis (Visner & Goldfarb, 2007). The transplant may involve a single lung, or it can be done in conjunction with heart transplantation if chronic respiratory disease has caused ventricular hypertrophy of the heart. The donor lung can be from a live donor or a cadaver.

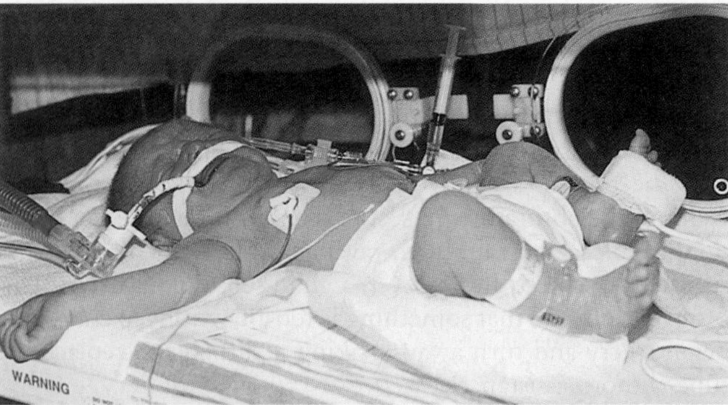

FIGURE 40.15 An infant with an endotracheal tube receiving assisted ventilation.

As with any organ transplantation, children need continued immunosuppression therapy with drugs such as cyclosporine or azathioprine (Imuran) following a lung transplant to decrease cell-mediated immunity. Although this level of immunosuppression is the key to successful transplantation, it also makes posttransplant children susceptible to fungal, bacterial, and viral lung infections. In addition, families experience a tremendous psychosocial toll as they wait to see whether the new transplant will be rejected. Children may need to have chest physiotherapy or use a portable spirometry device daily to help mobilize secretions resulting from loss of nerve innervation or a reaction to accumulating mucus in the transplanted lung.

DISORDERS OF THE UPPER RESPIRATORY TRACT

The upper respiratory tract warms, humidifies, and filters the air that enters the body (Fig. 40.16). As such, the structures of the upper respiratory tract constantly come into contact with a barrage of foreign organisms, including pathogens, that can lead to airway irritation and illness. Congenital malformations of respiratory structures also cause some upper respiratory tract disorders.

Upper respiratory illnesses occur universally, making them a concern of parents the world over. Home remedies for such illnesses vary greatly, however. Hanging garlic around a child's neck is a frequent therapy in Mediterranean countries. "Cupping" or applying pressure to the back to "draw out" an infection (which leaves red circular ecchymotic marks on the child's back) may be used in Asian cultures. Although the therapeutic value of these remedies may not be proved, it is important to the nurse–patient and nurse–family relationships to respect family traditions.

Choanal Atresia

Choanal atresia is congenital obstruction of the posterior nares by an obstructing membrane or bony growth, preventing a newborn from drawing air through the nose and down into the nasopharynx (Kelley et al., 2008). It may be either unilateral or bilateral.

Newborns up to approximately 3 months of age are naturally nose-breathers. Infants with choanal atresia, therefore,

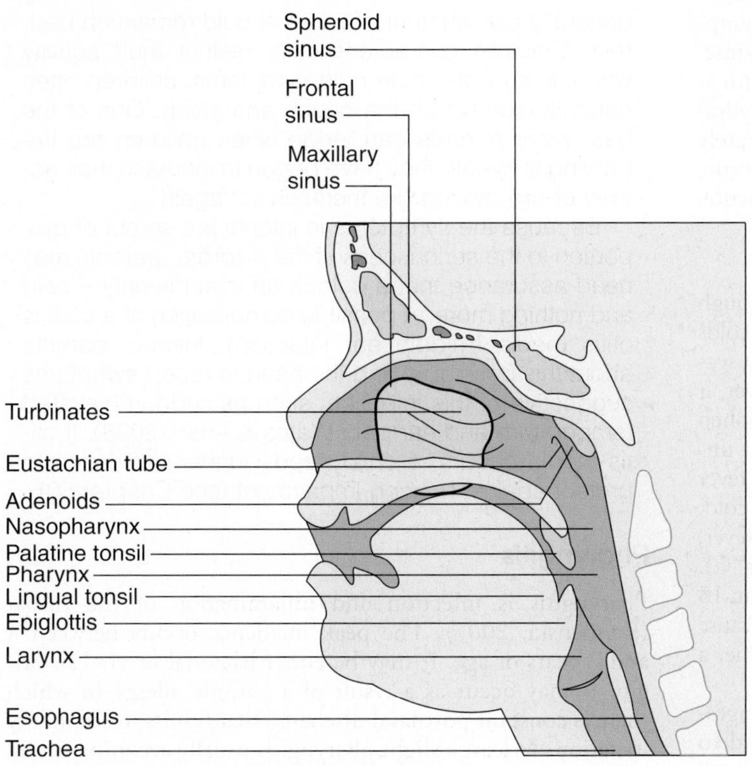

FIGURE 40.16 Structures of the upper respiratory tract.

develop signs of respiratory distress at birth or immediately after they quiet for the first time and attempt to breathe through their nose. Passing a soft no. 8 or 10 French catheter through the posterior nares to the stomach is a part of birthing room procedure in many health care facilities. If such a catheter will not pass bilaterally, the diagnosis of choanal atresia is confirmed immediately at birth.

Choanal atresia can also be assessed by holding the newborn's mouth closed, then gently compressing first one nostril, then the other. If atresia is present, infants will struggle as they experience air hunger when their mouth is closed. Their color improves when they open their mouth to cry. Atresia is also suggested if infants struggle and become cyanotic at feedings because they cannot suck and breathe through the mouth simultaneously.

The treatment for choanal atresia is either local piercing of the obstructing membrane or surgical removal of the bony growth. Because infants with choanal atresia have such difficulty with feeding, they may receive intravenous fluid to maintain their glucose and fluid level until surgery can be performed. Some infants may need an oral airway inserted so they can continue to breathe through their mouths. Following surgery, children have no further difficulty or symptoms.

✔ Checkpoint Question 40.1

Suppose Michael was born with choanal atresia. What would be the best way to assess if this is present?

a. Observe if a newborn can breathe while lying on his stomach.
b. Close the infant's mouth to see if he can breathe through his nose.
c. Assess if the infant's palatine tonsils are blocking his airway.
d. Listen for the sound of either stridor or wheezing on inhalation.

Acute Nasopharyngitis (Common Cold)

The common cold is the most frequent infectious disease in children—in fact, toddlers have an average of 10 to 12 colds a year. School-age children and adolescents have as many as four or five yearly. The incubation period is typically 2 to 3 days. Most occur in the fall and winter (Kelley et al., 2008).

They are caused by one of several viruses, most predominantly by rhinovirus, coxsackievirus, RSV, adenovirus, and parainfluenza and influenza viruses. Children are exposed to colds at school or while playing with other children. If they are in ill health from some other cause, or if their immune system is compromised, they are more susceptible than others to the cold viruses. Although difficult to prove, stress factors also appear to play a role in the development of common colds in children.

Assessment

Symptoms begin with nasal congestion, a watery rhinitis, and a low-grade fever. The mucous membrane of the nose becomes edematous and inflamed, constricting airway space and causing difficulty breathing. Posterior rhinitis, plus local irritation, leads to pharyngitis (sore throat). Upper airway secretions that drain into the trachea lead to a cough. Cervical lymph nodes may be swollen and palpable. The process lasts about a week and then symptoms fade. In some children, a thick, purulent nasal discharge occurs because bacteria such as streptococci invade the irritated nasal mucous membrane and cause a secondary purulent infection.

Infants can be critically ill yet not develop a fever because their temperature-regulating system is still immature. With the common cold, they often develop a fever elevated out of proportion to the symptoms, possibly as high as 102° to 104°

F (38.8° to 40° C). Infants also may develop secondary symptoms, such as vomiting and diarrhea, as a general response. Because they cannot suck and breathe through their mouth at the same time, they refuse feedings. This can lead to dehydration. Older children rarely develop as high a fever, rarely above 102° F (38.8° C). Because older children can breathe through their mouth, nasal congestion does not seem as acute.

Therapeutic Management

There is no specific treatment for a common cold. Although many parents ask to have antibiotics prescribed, because colds are caused by a virus, antibiotics are not effective unless a secondary bacterial invasion has occurred. If a child has a fever, it can be controlled by an antipyretic such as acetaminophen (Tylenol) or children's ibuprofen (Motrin). Help parents understand that these drugs are effective only in controlling fever symptoms; they do not reduce congestion or "cure" the cold. Therefore, they should not be given unless the child has a fever, generally defined as an oral temperature over 101° F (38.4° C). You may need to remind parents that children younger than 18 years should not be given acetylsalicylic acid (aspirin) because this is associated with the development of Reye syndrome, a potentially fatal neurologic disorder (see Chapter 49).

If infants have difficulty nursing because of nasal congestion, saline nose drops or nasal spray may be prescribed to liquefy nasal secretions and help them drain. Removing nasal mucus via a bulb syringe before feedings also allows infants to breathe more freely and be able to suck more efficiently. Caution parents that if they use a bulb syringe, they must compress the bulb first, then insert it into the child's nostril. If they insert the bulb syringe first, then depress the bulb, they will actually push secretions further back into the nose, causing increased obstruction.

There is little proof that oral decongestants relieve congestion to an appreciable degree with the common cold. Cough suppressants are not necessary either as coughing raises secretions, preventing pooling of secretions and the danger of consequent lower respiratory infection. Guaifenesin is an example of a drug that loosens secretions but does not suppress a cough so is safe to use. Parents may use a cool mist vaporizer to help loosen nasal secretions if they wish. The efficiency of home vaporizers is questionable, however, and safe use of a vaporizer, including proper cleaning, must be stressed or it can serve as a reservoir for microorganisms.

Nursing Diagnoses and Related Interventions

*

Nursing Diagnosis: Parental health-seeking behaviors related to management of child's upper respiratory symptoms

Outcome Evaluation: Parents state intention to use cool mist vaporizer to loosen secretions, to encourage oral fluid, to administer an antipyretic to reduce fever, and to avoid cough medicine.

Care of the child with a cold is primarily supportive until the infection runs its course. Because they may have a loss of appetite, children may prefer simple liquids to solid food for the first few days of the illness. Parents generally ask whether children should remain on bedrest. Children characteristically restrict their activity when ill, so with acute cold symptoms, children often naturally curl up on the couch and sleep. One of the best ways parents can judge when children are improving is to note they have begun to increase their activity or are "acting like themselves" again.

Because the symptoms in infants are so out of proportion to the seriousness of the disorder, parents may need assurance that a cold in an infant is only a cold and nothing more. A possible complication of a cold is otitis media (middle ear infection). Instruct parents about this possibility and the need to report symptoms suggestive of this infection, such as sudden elevated temperature and ear pain (Yates & Anari, 2008). If otitis media occurs, a child needs further evaluation to protect against hearing impairment (see Chapter 50).

Pharyngitis

Pharyngitis is infection and inflammation of the throat (Kamienski, 2007). The peak incidence occurs between 4 and 7 years of age. It may be either bacterial or viral in origin. It may occur as a result of a chronic allergy in which there is constant postnasal discharge that results in secondary irritation. At least a slight pharyngitis usually accompanies all common upper respiratory infections.

Viral Pharyngitis

The causative agent of pharyngitis is usually an adenovirus (Levin & Weinberg, 2008). The symptoms are generally mild: a sore throat, fever, and general malaise. On physical assessment, regional lymph nodes may be noticeably enlarged. Erythema will be present in the back of the pharynx and the palatine arch. Laboratory studies will indicate an increased white blood cell count.

If the inflammation is mild, children rarely need more than an oral analgesic such as acetaminophen or ibuprofen for comfort. Warm heat applied to the external neck area using a warm towel or heating pad also can be soothing. By school age, children are capable of gargling with a solution such as warm water to help reduce the pain. Before this age, children tend to swallow the solution unless the procedure is well explained and demonstrated to them.

Because children's throats feel so sore, they often prefer liquids to solid food. Infants, especially, must be observed closely until the inflammation and tenderness diminish to be certain that they take in sufficient fluid to prevent dehydration.

Streptococcal Pharyngitis

Group A beta-hemolytic streptococcus is the organism most frequently involved in bacterial pharyngitis in children. All streptococcal infections must be taken seriously because they can lead to cardiac and kidney damage from the accompanying autoimmune process (Ogle & Anderson, 2008).

Assessment. Streptococcal infections are generally more severe than viral infections. The fact that symptoms are mild, however, does not rule out streptococcal infection. With a streptococcal pharyngitis, the back of the throat and palatine tonsils are usually markedly erythematous (bright red); the tonsils are enlarged and there may be a white exudate in the tonsillar crypts. Petechiae may be present on the palate. A child typically appears ill with a high fever, an extremely sore throat, difficulty swallowing, and overall lethargy. Temperature is usually elevated to as high as 104° F (40° C). The child often has a headache. Swollen abdominal lymph nodes may cause abdominal pain. A throat culture, often completed as a quick office procedure, confirms the presence of the *Streptococcus* bacteria.

Therapeutic Management. Treatment consists of a full 10-day course of an oral antibiotic such as penicillin G or clindamycin. Cephalosporins or broad-spectrum macrolides such as erythromycin may be prescribed if resistant organisms are known to be in the community. Help parents understand the importance of completing the full prescribed days of therapy. The recommended treatment days are necessary to ensure the streptococci are eradicated completely. If they are not, the child may develop a hypersensitivity or autoimmune reaction to group A streptococci that can result in rheumatic fever (although the chance of rheumatic fever occurring is probably as low as 1%) or glomerulonephritis.

Symptoms of acute glomerulonephritis (blood and protein in urine) appear in 1 to 2 weeks after the pharyngitis. For this reason, 2 weeks after treatment, children may be asked to return to the health care facility with a urine specimen to be examined for protein so that developing acute glomerulonephritis can be detected (Steer, Danchin, & Carapetis, 2007).

To ensure that a child receives the full antibiotic course, help parents make a reminder sheet to place on a cabinet or refrigerator door. In addition, instruct them about measures for rest, relief of throat pain, and maintaining hydration, the same actions as for a common cold. Because it is impossible for parents to discriminate between a pharyngitis caused by a virus (and needing no therapy other than comfort measures) and a streptococcal pharyngitis (needing definite therapy to prevent life-threatening illnesses), a child with pharyngitis always should be examined by health care personnel.

✔ Checkpoint Question 40.2

Suppose Michael is diagnosed as having a streptococcal pharyngitis. The chief danger of such an infection is:

a. Lymph nodes will swell and obstruct the airway.
b. Infection may spread and cause a tooth abscess.
c. A small number of children develop kidney disease.
d. Four of five children will develop lung abscesses.

Retropharyngeal Abscess

In infants, the lymph nodes that drain the nasopharynx are located just behind the posterior pharynx wall. These nodes may become infected following an acute nasopharyngitis or pharyngitis. Since these nodes disappear by preschool age, the problem is usually limited to young infants (Page, Bauer, & Lieu, 2008).

Assessment. Typically, infants have an upper respiratory tract infection or sore throat for a few days. Suddenly, they refuse to eat. They develop a high fever and may drool because they cannot swallow saliva past the obstruction in the back of their throat. They "snore" with respirations as the pharynx becomes further occluded. To allow themselves more breathing space, they may hyperextend the head, a very unusual position for infants.

Physical assessment reveals enlargement of the regional lymph nodes. The mass in the posterior pharynx may not be visible if it is below the point of vision. An ultrasound or x-ray study using a swallowed contrast medium will reveal the bulging tissue in the pharynx. Laboratory studies will reveal leukocytosis.

Therapeutic Management. Because the most common cause of retropharyngeal abscess is group A beta-hemolytic streptococcus, benzathine penicillin G or penicillin V is effective. As a result of their poor swallowing, infants' mouths may need to be suctioned to remove secretions. Be careful not to touch the suction catheter to the posterior pharynx because this might rupture the abscess, possibly leading to aspiration of the abscess contents (producing respiratory obstruction or a pneumonia caused by the aspirated purulent material). Blood vessels invade some retropharyngeal abscesses, so rupture of the structure also could lead to profuse bleeding (dangerous to the child both because of the loss of blood from major arteries such as the carotid artery and because the blood could be aspirated).

Place infants in a side-lying position to allow difficult-to-swallow mouth secretions to drain forward. Limit oral intake to fluids. A hard food such as a toast crust (a food often recommended for teething) could rupture the abscess with its hard edges.

Although some postpharyngeal abscesses resolve on their own, some need to be incised by a surgeon to promote drainage. This is done with the child in a Trendelenburg position so that drainage from the abscess can be suctioned away to prevent aspiration. After surgery, maintain the child in a Trendelenburg or a side position as prescribed to encourage further drainage and prevent aspiration. Monitor vital signs closely. Observe any drainage from infants' mouths to detect fresh bleeding. Frequent swallowing is also a sign of postpharyngeal bleeding. Increased respiratory rate suggests airway obstruction.

Oral fluid is introduced as soon as an infant's swallowing and gag reflexes are intact after surgery. Although the throat is undoubtedly still sore, most infants suck eagerly and need supplemental intravenous fluid administration following surgery for only a short time.

On admission to the hospital, parents may have been thoroughly frightened by the extent of the child's symptoms (gurgling or snoring sound, high temperature, dyspnea). Allow parents to give care while in the hospital to help them allay their fears and regain confidence in their ability to care for the child again.

Tonsillitis

"Tonsillitis" refers to infection and inflammation of the palatine tonsils. "Adenitis" refers to infection and inflammation of the adenoid (pharyngeal) tonsils.

Tonsillar tissue is lymphoid tissue that filters pathogenic organisms from the head and neck area. The palatine tonsils are located on both sides of the pharynx; the adenoids are in the nasopharynx. Tubal tonsils are located at the entrance to the eustachian tubes. Lingual tonsils are located at the base of the tongue. All of the tonsils, referred to collectively as Waldeyer's ring, are easily infected because of the bacteria that pass through or are screened through them with lymph.

Assessment

Infection of the palatine tonsils presents with all of the symptoms of a severe pharyngitis. Children drool because their throat is too sore for them to swallow saliva. They may describe swallowing as so painful it feels as if they are swallowing bits of metal or glass. In addition, they usually have a high fever and are lethargic. Tonsillar tissue appears bright red and may be so enlarged the two areas of palatine tonsillar tissue meet in the midline. Pus can be detected on or expelled from the crypts of the tonsils (Millar et al., 2007).

In addition to fever, lethargy, pharyngeal pain, and edema, the symptoms of adenoidal tissue infection also include a nasal quality of speech, mouth breathing, difficulty hearing, and perhaps halitosis or sleep apnea. The mouth breathing, change in speech, and apnea result from the postpharyngeal obstruction by the enlarged tissue. The difficulty with hearing occurs because of eustachian tube obstruction. Long-term obstruction this way can further cause serous and acute otitis media.

Tonsillitis occurs most commonly in school-age children. The responsible organism is identified by a throat culture. In children younger than 3 years of age, the cause is often viral. In school-age children, the organism is generally a group A beta-hemolytic streptococcus (Steer, Danchin, & Carapetis, 2007).

Therapeutic Management

Therapy for bacterial tonsillitis includes an antipyretic for fever, an analgesic for pain, and a full 10-day course of an antibiotic such as penicillin or amoxicillin. If the cause is viral, no therapy other than comfort or fever reduction strategies is necessary. Although the pain of the infection will subside a day or two after the antibiotic administration is begun, remind parents that children need the full 10-day course of antibiotic to eradicate streptococci completely from the back of the throat. After a tonsillar infection, tonsillar tissue may remain hypertrophied, or it may atrophy and appear smaller than it did previously.

Tonsillectomy. Tonsillectomy is removal of the palatine tonsils. *Adenoidectomy* is removal of the pharyngeal tonsils. In the past, tonsillectomy was a common procedure following an episode of tonsillitis, but today it is not recommended unless all other measures to prevent frequent infections prove ineffective. Tonsillar tissue is removed by ligating the tonsil or by laser surgery. Because sutures are not placed, the chance for hemorrhage after this type of surgery is higher than after surgery involving a closed incision. The danger of aspiration of blood at the time of surgery and the danger of a general anesthetic compound the risk.

Chronic tonsillitis is about the only reason for removal of palatine tonsils. Adenoids may be removed if they are so hypertrophied they cause obstruction or sleep apnea. At one time, adenoids and palatine tonsils were always removed together; today, depending on the symptoms and the extent of hypertrophy and infection, children may have a tonsillectomy, an adenoidectomy, or both.

Tonsillectomy or adenoidectomy is never done while the organs are infected, because an operation at such a time might spread pathogenic organisms into the bloodstream, causing septicemia. Parents often ask why an operation to remove tonsils must be delayed until the child is well again. They think that as long as the tonsils are sore, they should be immediately removed. Help them understand why it is safer to schedule surgery for a later date. Most parents report an improvement in their child's general health and performance after tonsillectomy surgery, as this ends the chronic infections.

Nursing Diagnoses and Related Interventions

Nursing Diagnosis: Risk for fluid volume deficit related to blood loss from surgery

Outcome Evaluation: Child's pulse and blood pressure remain normal for age; there is absence of extensive bleeding; intake and output are within acceptable parameters.

Tonsillectomies are done as ambulatory or 1-day surgery following completion of a complete history and physical examination and laboratory tests, including bleeding and clotting times, complete blood count, and urinalysis. Teach parents to use common sense in their child's care during the week before hospital admission so that the child does not have a cold or recurrent tonsillitis at the time planned for surgery. An important aspect of immediate assessment on the day of surgery is to observe for loose teeth; if present, they could be dislodged during surgery and aspirated. If loose teeth are present, mark this on the front of the child's chart and report it to the anesthesiologist.

After surgery, observe vital signs carefully to make certain the child is not bleeding from the denuded surgical area. Place the child on the side or abdomen with a pillow under the chest so that the head is lower than the chest. This allows blood and unswallowed saliva to drain from the child's mouth rather than back to the pharynx, where it might be aspirated (Fig. 40.17).

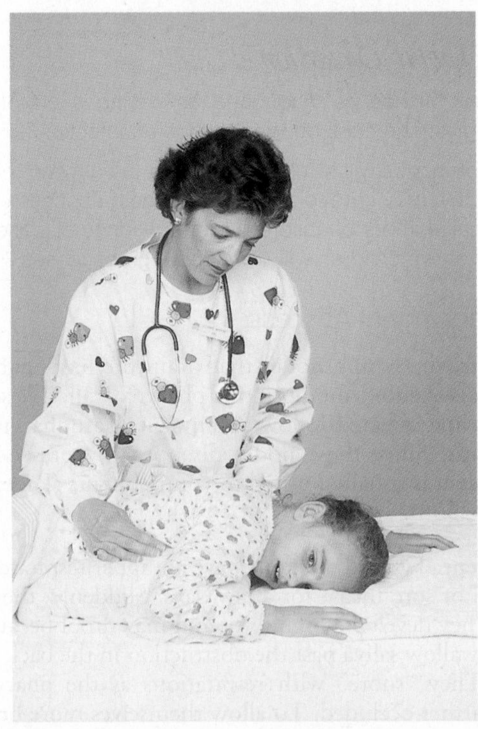

FIGURE 40.17 Positioning a child after tonsillectomy. The pillow under the chest helps secretions flow out of the mouth.

If hemorrhage occurs after tonsillectomy, it can be acute and intense. Because children will swallow any blood that is oozing from the surgical site, a child can be bleeding heavily and yet little blood is apparent. To detect bleeding, assess for subtle signs of hemorrhage, such as an increasing pulse or respiratory rate, frequent swallowing, throat clearing, or a feeling of anxiety. A child's first line of defense against hemorrhage is a nurse who recognizes these subtle signs of bleeding before the bleeding becomes so intense that signs of shock occur.

If you find that the surgical site is bleeding, elevate the child's head to reduce vascular pressure on the operative site. Use a good light to inspect the posterior throat. Have a dental mirror available so the surgeon can thoroughly inspect the bleeding area. If the surgical area is bleeding heavily, the child may need to be returned to surgery for a suture or two to halt bleeding.

The most dangerous periods for a child after a tonsillectomy are the first 24 hours, when the clots covering the denuded surgical area are forming, and days 5 to 7, when the clots begin to lyse or dissolve. If new granulation tissue is not yet present when the clots dissolve, hemorrhage from the denuded surface can occur.

If children have no complications from surgery, are able to swallow fluids, and have voided, they are discharged later the same day of surgery. Parents need careful instructions concerning the danger signs to watch for during the first day home (frequent swallowing, clearing the throat, increasing restlessness). They are usually advised to restrict their child's activity (no gymnastics, swimming) until after the seventh day, when firm healing should have taken place. The child needs a return appointment to a health care facility approximately 2 weeks after surgery for follow-up assessment to make sure the surgical area has healed without complication.

Nursing Diagnosis: Pain related to surgical procedure

Outcome Evaluation: Child states level of pain is tolerable.

Tonsillectomy is an uncomfortable and painful procedure for children. Be sure they receive good preparation for the procedure and for the sensations they will experience afterward. Although tonsils are removed, it is better to talk about tonsils being "fixed" rather than taken out; children may be extremely frightened to know that a body part will be removed, however small it is.

Children's throats are extremely sore following a tonsillectomy. Liquid analgesics are better tolerated than pills or tablets because they are easier to swallow. Rectal administration is a possibility for very young children. Occasionally, a child may require intravenous pain relief.

Most children are thirsty immediately after surgery, and drinking is helpful because swallowing fluid causes active pharyngeal movement, increasing the blood supply to the area and reducing edema and pain. Children commonly are promised by well-meaning people they can have all the ice cream they want after a tonsillectomy. However, because milk products form tenacious secretions that are difficult to swallow, ice cream is not a food of choice. Offer instead frequent sips of clear liquid, Popsicles, or ice chips. Avoid acid juices because these sting the denuded tissue. Carbonated beverages also can irritate the area unless they stand for a time to become "flat." Avoid red fluid such as Kool-Aid, which if vomited can be mistaken for swallowed blood.

Children can then gradually advance after 24 to 48 hours to a diet of soft foods such as gelatin, mashed potatoes, soups, and cooked fruits. They should continue to eat only soft foods for the first week (no toast crusts or other foods that could cause pharyngeal irritation if not chewed well). Be certain parents know whom they should call (clinic, hospital, or pediatrician) if they have a question or concern about their child's condition or care. Caution parents that some children develop a mild earache after tonsillectomy for the first week, probably caused by shifting pressure on the eustachian tube.

✔ Checkpoint Question 40.3

Suppose Michael's 4-year-old roommate spits up dark-red blood following her tonsillectomy. Your best action in relation to this would be:

a. Suction the back of her throat.
b. Encourage her to cough vigorously.
c. Perform a subdiaphragmatic thrust.
d. Continue to observe her for bleeding.

Epistaxis

Epistaxis (nosebleed) is extremely common in children and usually occurs from trauma, such as picking at the nose, from falling, or from being hit on the nose by another child (Burton & Doree, 2009). In homes that lack humidification, the hot dry environment causes children's mucous membranes to dry, feel uncomfortable, and be susceptible to cracking and bleeding. In all children, epistaxis tends to occur during respiratory illnesses. It also may occur after strenuous exercise, and it is associated with several systemic diseases, such as rheumatic fever, scarlet fever, measles, or varicella infection (chickenpox). It can occur with nasal polyps, sinusitis, or allergic rhinitis. Some families show a familial predisposition.

Nosebleeds are always frightening because of the visible bleeding and a choking sensation if blood should run down the back of the nasopharynx. The fear is generally out of proportion to the seriousness of the bleeding.

Keep children with nosebleeds in an upright position with their head tilted slightly forward to minimize the amount of blood pressure in nasal vessels and to keep blood moving forward, not back into the nasopharynx. Apply pressure to the sides of the nose with your fingers (Fig. 40.18). Make every effort to quiet the child and to help stop crying, because crying increases pressure in the blood vessels of the head and prolongs bleeding. If these simple measures do not control the bleeding, epinephrine (1:1000) may be applied to the bleeding site to constrict blood vessels. A nasal pack may be necessary to provide continued pressure.

Every child has an occasional nosebleed. Chronic nasal bleeding, however, should be investigated to rule out a systemic disease or blood disorder.

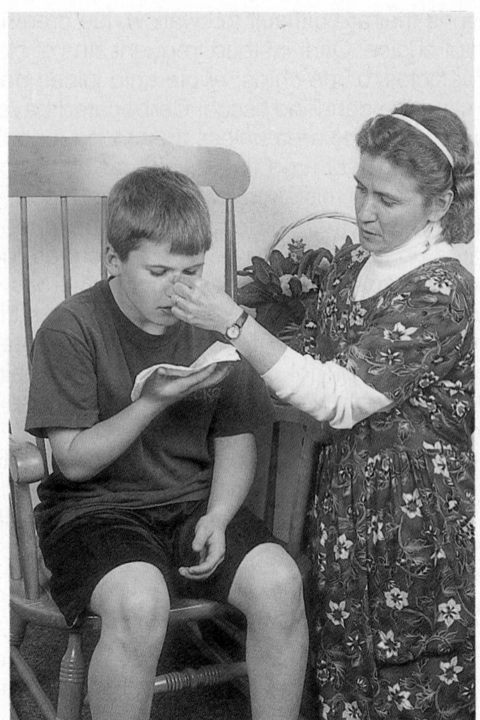

FIGURE 40.18 Emergency therapy for a nosebleed is to sit the child up and apply pressure to the sides of the nose.

Sinusitis

Sinusitis is infection and inflammation of the sinus cavities. It is rare in children younger than 6 years of age because the frontal sinuses do not develop fully until age 6. It can occur as a primary infection or a secondary one in older children when streptococcal, staphylococcal, or *H. influenzae* organisms spread from the nasal cavity (Revai et al., 2007). Children develop a fever, a purulent nasal discharge, headache, and tenderness over the affected sinus. A nose and throat culture will identify the infectious organism.

Treatment for acute sinusitis consists of an antipyretic for fever, an analgesic for pain, and an antibiotic for the specific organism involved. Oxymetazoline hydrochloride (Afrin), supplied as nose drops or a nasal spray, shrinks the edematous mucous membranes and allows infected material to drain from the sinuses and relieve pain. To avoid a rebound effect, this type of nasal spray should be used for only 3 days at a time; otherwise, it actually causes more nasal congestion than was present originally. Warm compresses to the sinus area may also encourage drainage and relieve pain. Some children need acetaminophen (Tylenol) for pain.

Sinusitis is considered by many adults to be a minor illness. It needs to be treated, however, because it can have serious complications if the infection spreads from the sinuses to invade the facial bone (osteomyelitis) or the middle ear (otitis media). Chronic sinusitis can also interfere with school and social interactions because of the constant pain.

Laryngitis

Laryngitis is inflammation of the larynx. It results in brassy, hoarse voice sounds or inability to make audible voice sounds. It may occur as a complication of pharyngitis or from excessive use of the voice, as in shouting or loud cheering. Laryngitis is as annoying for children as it is for adults. Sips of fluid (either warm or cold, whichever feels best) offer relief from the annoying tickling sensation often present. The most effective measure, however, is for the child to rest the voice for at least 24 hours, until inflammation subsides. For infants with laryngitis, attempt to meet their needs before they have to cry for things. Simply caution older children not to speak. Provide them with a paper and pencil or chalkboard for communication.

Congenital Laryngomalacia/Tracheomalacia

Congenital laryngomalacia means that an infant's laryngeal structure is weaker than normal and collapses more than usual on inspiration (Richter et al., 2008). This produces laryngeal **stridor** (a high-pitched crowing sound on inspiration) present from birth, possibly intensified when the infant is in a supine position or when sucking.

Assessment

The infant's sternum and intercostal spaces may retract on inspiration because of the increased effort needed to pull air into the trachea past the collapsed cartilage rings. Many infants with this condition must stop sucking frequently during a feeding to maintain adequate ventilation and to rest from their respiratory effort, which is exhausting.

Therapeutic Management

Most children with congenital laryngomalacia need no routine therapy other than to have parents feed them slowly, providing rest periods as needed. The condition improves as infants mature and cartilage in the larynx becomes stronger at about 1 year of age. When parents wake at night and listen in a quiet house to the sound of stridor, it seems unbearably loud. This makes it difficult for them to believe it is safe for them to care for the infant at home.

Many parents sleep at night with the child's crib next to their bed or with one hand resting on the infant's chest so they can be assured during the night the child is continuing to breathe. At health care visits, assess whether the parents are receiving enough sleep and are not becoming too exhausted to be able to continue their daily activities. Showing them a weight chart that demonstrates their child is growing and thriving despite this problem can be reassuring.

Be certain parents know the importance of bringing the child for early care if signs of an upper respiratory tract infection develop. If not, laryngeal collapse will be even more intense during these times, and complete obstruction of the trachea could occur. If stridor becomes more intense, advise parents to have the infant seen by their primary care provider, because generally this indicates beginning obstruction and probably the beginning of an upper respiratory tract infection. As parents become more accustomed to the sound their infant makes while breathing, they will become astute reporters of change in their infant's condition; listen to them carefully when they report a change to prevent overlooking this important information.

Croup (Laryngotracheobronchitis)

Croup (inflammation of the larynx, trachea, and major bronchi) is one of the most frightening diseases of early childhood for both parents and children. In children between 6 months and 3 years of age, the cause of croup is usually a viral infection such as parainfluenza virus. In previous years, the most common cause was *H. influenzae.* However, since immunization against this organism has been included in a routine immunization series, the incidence of croup from this cause has declined by 90% (Kerby et al., 2008).

Assessment

With croup, children typically have only a mild upper respiratory tract infection at bedtime. Temperature is normal or only mildly elevated. During the night, they develop a barking cough (croupy cough), inspiratory stridor, and marked retractions. They wake in extreme respiratory distress. The larynx, trachea, and major bronchi are all inflamed. These severe symptoms typically last several hours and then, except for a rattling cough, subside by morning. Symptoms may recur the following night. Cyanosis is rarely present, but the danger of glottal obstruction from the laryngeal inflammation and hypoxemia is very real. Pulse oximetry and transcutaneous SaO_2 monitors are helpful measures to document whether hypoxemia is occurring.

Therapeutic Management

One emergency method of relieving croup symptoms is for a parent to run the shower or hot water tap in a bathroom until the room fills with steam, then keep the child in this warm, moist environment. If this does not relieve symptoms, parents should bring the child to an emergency department for further evaluation and care. When a child is seen at an emergency room, cool moist air with a corticosteroid such as dexamethasone, or racemic epinephrine, given by nebulizer, reduces inflammation and produces effective bronchodilation to open the airway. Intravenous therapy may be prescribed to keep the child well hydrated. Maintain accurate intake and output records and test urine specific gravity to ensure that hydration is adequate.

Nursing Diagnoses and Related Interventions

Nursing Diagnosis: Ineffective airway clearance related to edema and constriction of airway

Outcome Evaluation: Respiratory rate is below 22 breaths per minute; no cyanosis is present; PO_2 is 80 to 100 mm Hg; SaO_2 is over 95%.

Attach a sensor for pulse oximetry monitoring and remain constantly with a child with croup, not only to observe closely for increasing respiratory distress but also to reduce the child's anxiety. Take vital signs as often as every 15 minutes, because extreme restlessness and thrashing, increased stridor, increased heart and respiratory rates, and cyanosis are symptoms of oxygen deprivation. In some children, it is difficult to distinguish between fright from the newness of the experience (and their sense of their parents' fright) and the anxiety that comes from oxygen deprivation. Keep a continuous record of vital signs and activity as a way to demonstrate increasing respiratory rate and restlessness. ABGs may be obtained to assess for sufficient oxygenation if pulse oximetry is not being used. A tracheostomy or endotracheal intubation along with oxygen therapy may be necessary if symptoms do not diminish. (It is difficult to intubate children with croup because of the severe respiratory tract edema.)

Laryngospasm with total occlusion of the airway can occur when a child's gag reflex is elicited or when the child is crying. Therefore, do not elicit a gag reflex in any child with a croupy, barking cough, and provide comfort to prevent crying.

Croup is a frightening disease for parents because their child is suddenly ill with severe symptoms. When the severe symptoms disappear by morning, parents may feel foolish they rushed to a hospital with the child in the middle of the night. Assure them that their initial judgment was correct. When they brought the child in, the child was seriously ill. Parents may be reluctant to see their child discharged in the morning until they are convinced that their child is now well enough to go home (see Focus on Nursing Care Planning Box 40.10).

What if... Michael, who had loud stridor when he was admitted, suddenly has no stridor present? Would you be relieved (his condition must be improving) or worried (his airway may be so blocked that not enough air is entering to make the sound of stridor)? How should you respond?

Epiglottitis

Epiglottitis is inflammation of the epiglottis (the flap of tissue that covers the opening to the larynx to keep out food and fluid during swallowing). Although it is rare, inflammation of the epiglottis is an emergency because the swollen epiglottis cannot rise and allow the airway to open. It occurs most frequently in children from 2 to about 7 years of age (Ogle & Anderson, 2008).

Epiglottitis can be either bacterial or viral in origin. *H. influenzae* type B has been replaced as the most common bacterial cause of the disorder by pneumococci, streptococci, or staphylococci. Echovirus and RSV also can cause the disorder.

Assessment

Symptoms begin as those of a mild upper respiratory tract infection. After 1 or 2 days, as inflammation spreads to the epiglottis, the child suddenly develops severe inspiratory stridor, a high fever, hoarseness, and a very sore throat. Children may have such difficulty swallowing that they drool saliva. They may protrude their tongue to increase free movement in the pharynx.

If a child's gag reflex is stimulated with a tongue blade, the swollen and inflamed epiglottis can be seen to rise in the back of the throat as a cherry-red structure. It can be so edematous, however, that the gagging procedure causes complete obstruction of the glottis and shuts off the ability of the child to inhale. Therefore, in children with symptoms of epiglottitis (dysphagia, inspiratory stridor, cough, fever, and hoarseness), *never attempt to visualize the epiglottis directly with a tongue blade or obtain a throat culture* unless a means of providing an

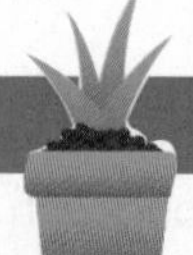

BOX 40.10 ✻ Focus on Nursing Care Planning

A Multidisciplinary Care Map for a Child With Laryngotracheobronchitis (Croup)

Michael is a 4-year-old who is brought to the emergency department by paramedics who responded to an emergency call by his grandmother at his home. He has a sharp, barking cough, is crying loudly, and is obviously short of breath. His grandmother shouts at you. "I gave him some chocolate. Is he allergic to that?" Michael is diagnosed as having laryngotracheobronchitis (croup) and admitted to an ambulatory care unit.

Family Assessment ✻ Child lives with two parents in four-bedroom suburban home. Father works as a bartender at local restaurant; mother works part-time as a beautician. Parents are out of town on vacation. Were notified of child's condition and gave oral permission for therapy by telephone to W. Burton, M.D. (witnessed by C. Finacca, R.N.); will fax consent and signatures from vacation hotel.

Client Assessment ✻ Child was born with choanal atresia. Is allergic to seafood, especially shrimp (develops hives and shortness of breath). Age-acceptable parameters for height and weight. Has had a "slight head cold" for last 2 days; woke from nap this afternoon gasping for breath. Has audible stridor. Tympanic temperature 102.2° F (39.0° C); pulse 146; respirations 40. Nasal flaring and intercostal retractions noted. Sharp, frequent, nonproductive cough.

Nursing Diagnosis ✻ Fear related to inability to breathe without effort, heightened by absence of parents.

Outcome Criteria ✻ Respiratory rate, oxygen saturation, and arterial blood gas levels are within age-acceptable parameters without the use of supplemental oxygen. No stridor is present on auscultation. Child states he can breathe more easily; is aware parents are concerned although absent.

Team Member Responsible	Assessment	Intervention	Rationale	Expected Outcome
		Activities of Daily Living		
Nurse	Assess if child is able to complete any self-care despite fatigue and shortness of breath.	Place the child in a semi-Fowler's to high Fowler's position. Reposition the child frequently.	An upright position facilitates breathing and promotes optimal lung expansion by lowering diaphragm. Frequent repositioning prevents pooling and stasis of secretions.	Child cooperates with procedures to extent possible, given degree of fatigue and fear.
		Consultations		
Nurse practitioner	Assess if anesthesiologist is available.	Consult with anesthesiologist about the possibility that intubation or tracheostomy may be necessary.	If tracheolaryngeal edema occludes airway, intubation or tracheostomy can be life-saving.	Anesthesiology team examines child; prepares equipment for emergency intubation if necessary.
		Procedures/Medications		
Nurse	Assess temperature by tympanic thermometer.	Administer acetaminophen liquid orally as prescribed.	Oral temperature would be inaccurate because of rapid respirations.	Child's temperature decreases one degree per hour until it reaches 98.6° F.
Nurse	Assess if child has experience with vital sign procedures or breath sound assessment.	Assess pulse, respirations, and lung sounds every 15 minutes.	An increasing pulse or respiratory rate or increased stridor can signal decreasing oxygenation.	Child agrees to allow chest leads to be applied to monitor heart rate. Pulse and respiratory rate do not increase any further.

Nurse	Assess if child has ever received medicine by nebulizer or humidifier.	Administer racemic epinephrine by nebulizer every 3 hours as prescribed. Keep room infused with cold humidification.	Epinephrine causes bronchodilation, widening lumen of airway. Cold moisture helps reduce inflammation and moisten mucus.	Child cooperates with nebulizer therapy to extent possible, given fear. Respiratory rate and stridor decrease following treatment.
Nurse	Assess which method of oxygen administration (face mask or nasal prongs) would be most acceptable to child.	Administer humidified oxygen at prescribed rate. Obtain arterial blood gases (ABGs) as ordered and monitor oxygen saturation levels via pulse oximetry.	Humidified oxygen improves ventilation without drying the mucous membranes, to reduce hypoxemia. ABGs and pulse oximetry provide objective evidence of the child's oxygenation.	Child chooses method for oxygen administration; cooperates with oxygen administration; Po_2 and Sao_2 improve to adequate levels.
		Nutrition		
Nurse	Assess what is child's favorite fluid to drink.	Offer the child sips of fluid frequently. Maintain intravenous fluid as prescribed.	Dehydration can occur from rapid respirations. Adequate hydration can help keep mucus moist.	Child drinks 80% of fluid offered; IV is maintained at correct rate.
		Patient/Family Education		
Nurse	Assess grandparent's knowledge of child's condition.	Review that croup is a viral infection, not an allergic disorder.	Understanding why a disease occurs can help grandparent to cooperate with therapy.	Grandparent states that she understands the cause of croup, its usual course, and its prognosis.
		Psychosocial/Spiritual/Emotional Needs		
Nurse/nurse practitioner	Assess if child has had prior experiences with hospitalization. Ask child to state if he feels afraid or anxious of procedures.	Use play to encourage child to cough, deep breathe, and drink fluid. Involve the grandparent in these activities.	Games and play are effective methods for encouraging fluid intake in a child. Involving the grandparent promotes participation in child's care.	Child states he understands the nebulizer, oxygen mask, etc. are to help him breathe, not punishment for eating candy.
		Discharge Planning		
Nurse	Assess if grandparent is comfortable with taking child home.	Review child's condition and careful watching grandparent will need to continue.	Croup is a frightening illness. Grandparent needs good preparation to continue care at home.	Grandparent states she is prepared to take child home; will telephone if child's symptoms return.
Nurse	Assess if grandparent knows action to take if child should develop croup again.	Review how to flood bathroom with warm moist steam.	Warm steam can help reduce airway inflammation.	Grandparent states she is prepared to initiate home therapy if a second incidence of croup should occur. Knows to call 911 if child's condition does not improve.

artificial airway, such as tracheostomy or endotracheal intubation, is readily available. This is especially important for the nurse who functions in an expanded role and performs physical assessments and routinely elicits gag reflexes.

When epiglottitis is present, laboratory studies will show leukocytosis (20,000 to 30,000 mm^3), with the proportion of neutrophils increased. A blood culture to evaluate for septicemia and ABGs to evaluate respiratory sufficiency may be ordered. However, because excessive crying can precipitate entrapment of the epiglottis and obstruction, such tests may be delayed in preference to a lateral neck x-ray film or ultrasound, which will show the enlarged epiglottis. Do not allow a child with possible epiglottitis to go to these departments accompanied only by parents or a nursing aide, in case obstruction occurs in the radiograph or ultrasound room.

Therapeutic Management

Children need moist air to reduce the epiglottal inflammation. If cyanosis is present, they need oxygen. An antibiotic, such as a third-generation cephalosporin such as cefotaxime, may be prescribed until a throat culture indicates a specific antibiotic drug. Because they cannot swallow, children need intravenous fluid therapy to maintain hydration. They may need a prophylactic tracheostomy or endotracheal intubation to prevent total airway obstruction, although it is often difficult to intubate children with epiglottitis because the tube cannot be passed beyond the edematous epiglottis. After antibiotic therapy begins, the epiglottal inflammation recedes rapidly. By 12 to 24 hours, it has reduced enough that the airway may be removed. Antibiotic administration will continue for a full 7 to 10 days. Siblings of the ill child may be prescribed prophylactic antibiotic therapy to prevent them from developing the same symptoms.

Initially, the symptoms of epiglottitis are not unlike those of croup. As a result, parents may not realize the extent of the occlusion in their child, especially if the child has had croup on other occasions. They may question why a prophylactic tracheostomy was necessary this time when it was not used when the child had croup. Explain to them the difference between the two diseases (Table 40.5).

Some infants with epiglottitis die because obstruction occurs before a tracheotomy can be accomplished. If this should happen, parents can be assured they could not realize the seriousness of their child's symptoms. This may make them overcautious, bringing other children to health care settings repeatedly for symptoms that are obviously not serious. It will take time for them to regain confidence in themselves as parents and in their ability to judge a child's health.

✔ Checkpoint Question 40.4

Michael has a barking cough, sore throat, and high fever. You want to see if his throat looks sore. Your best procedure to do this would be:

a. Gag him with a tongue blade to inspect his tonsils.
b. Ask him to press down on his tongue with a finger.
c. Elicit a gag reflex using only one gloved finger.
d. Inspect his throat visually only.

Aspiration

Aspiration (inhalation of a foreign object into the airway) occurs most frequently in infants and toddlers. When a child aspirates a foreign object such as a coin or a peanut, the immediate reaction is choking and hard, forceful coughing. Usually, this dislodges the object. However, if the airway becomes so obstructed that coughing is impossible (no sound with cough), or if there are signs of increased respiratory difficulty accompanied by stridor, some intervention is essential. A series of subdiaphragmatic abdominal thrusts are recommended for children, the same as for adults. This recommendation does not extend to infants, however, because of the great risk of rupturing the liver (American Heart Association, 2008).

For this maneuver, stand behind the child and place a fist just under the child's diaphragm (a point immediately below the anterior rib cage). Embrace the child, grip your fist with your other hand, and pull back and up with a rapid thrust. The pressure created by this action of pushing up on the diaphragm forces the aspirated material out of the trachea (Fig. 40.19).

TABLE 40.5 ✻ Comparison of Laryngotracheobronchitis (Croup) and Epiglottitis

Assessment	Laryngotracheobronchitis	Epiglottitis
Causative organism	Usually viral	Usually pneumococci or streptococci
Usual age of child	6 mo–3 years	3–6 years
Seasonal occurrence	Late fall and winter	None
Onset pattern	Preceded by upper respiratory infection; cough becomes worse at night	Preceded by upper respiratory infection; suddenly very ill
Presence of fever	Low grade	Elevated to about 103° F
Appearance	Retractions and stridor; prolonged inspiratory phase of respirations; not very ill-appearing	Drooling; very ill-appearing; neck hyperextended to breathe. (Do not attempt to view enlarged epiglottis, or immediate airway obstruction can occur.)
Cough	Sharp, barking	Muffled cough
Radiographic findings	Lateral neck radiograph showing subglottal narrowing	Lateral neck radiograph showing enlarged epiglottis
Possible complications	Asphyxia because of subglottic obstruction	Asphyxia because of supraglottic obstruction

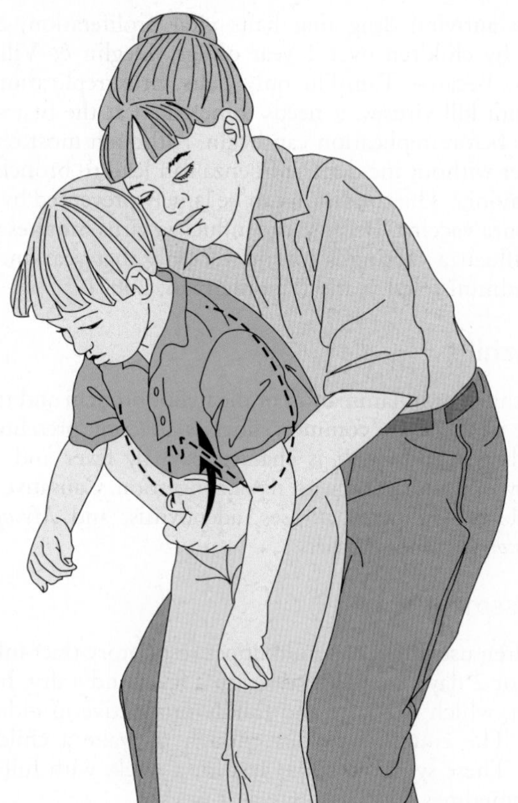

FIGURE 40.19 Subdiaphragmatic abdominal thrust on a school-age child.

If a child is lying on his or her back at the time of the aspiration, stand at the head of the bed or table, place your hands in the same position as described above, and exert the same inward and upward thrust. A subdiaphragmatic abdominal maneuver may cause a child to vomit as well as expel an aspirated object. Turn the child's head to the side to prevent aspiration of vomitus.

For infants, use back thrusts to dislodge an aspirated object. Turn the infant prone over your arm and administer up to five quick back blows forcefully between the infant's shoulder blades, using the heel of the hand (Fig. 40.20A). If the object is not expelled, turn the infant while carefully supporting the head and neck and hold the infant in a supine position draped over your thigh. Be sure to keep the infant's head lower than his or her chest. Provide up to five quick downward thrusts in the lower third of the sternum (Fig. 40.20B; American Heart Association, 2008). This is generally enough to dislodge the foreign object. However, if this does not occur, rescue breathing may then be attempted.

Bronchial Obstruction

The right main bronchus is straighter and has a larger lumen than the left bronchus in children older than 2 years of age. For this reason, an aspirated foreign object that is not large enough to obstruct the trachea may lodge in the right bronchus, obstructing a portion or all of the right lung. The alveoli distal to the obstruction will collapse as the air remaining in them becomes absorbed (atelectasis), or hyperinflation and pneumothorax may occur if the foreign body serves as a ball valve, allowing air to enter but not leave the alveoli (see later discussion on disorders of the lower respiratory tract).

Assessment

After aspirating a small foreign body, the child generally coughs violently and may become dyspneic. If the article is not expelled, hemoptysis, fever, purulent sputum, and leukocytosis will generally result as infection develops. Localized wheezing (a high whistling sound on expiration made by air passing through the narrowed lumen) may occur. Because this is localized, it is different from the generalized wheezing of a child with asthma.

A chest radiograph will reveal the presence of a radiopaque object. Objects most frequently aspirated include bones, popcorn, nuts, and coins. As a rule, nuts or popcorn should not be given to children younger than school age. These objects are coated with oil, and as they swell with moisture in the respiratory tract, they cause not only obstruction but also lipid pneumonia, a persistent and difficult-to-treat type of pneumonia. Foreign bodies that are inhaled this deeply are rarely coughed

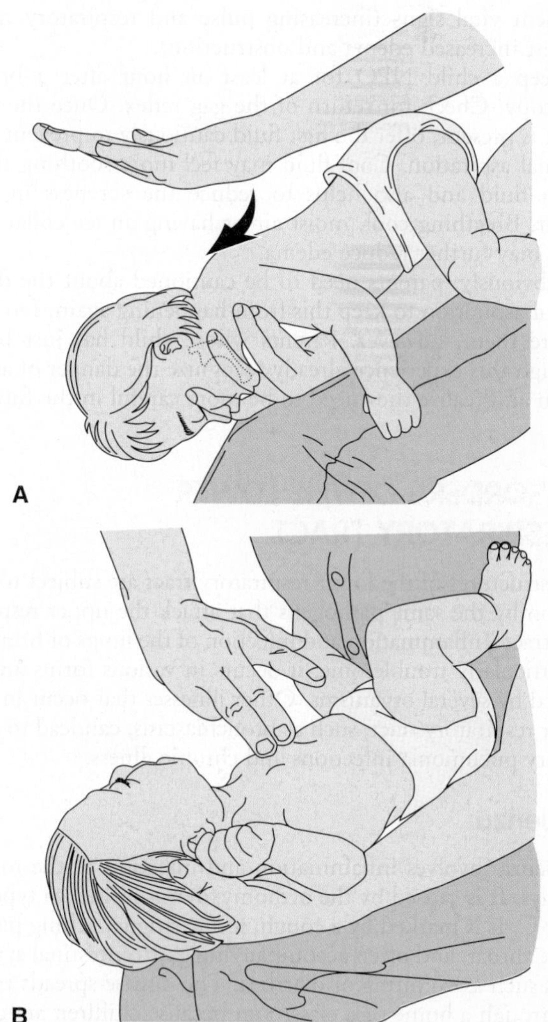

FIGURE 40.20 Back blows (**A**) and chest thrusts (**B**) to relieve complete foreign body airway obstruction in an infant. (From American Heart Association. [2008]. *Resuscitation in the newborn.* Dallas, TX: Author.)

up spontaneously, despite the severe coughing that ensues. Because objects such as plastic and nuts cannot be visualized well on x-ray film, an x-ray study may be inconclusive.

Therapeutic Management

Children who are seen in emergency departments after aspirating a foreign body are in distress from pain and are choking and coughing. Their parents are frightened by the degree of distress. Parents may feel bad about having offered the child (or allowed the child to reach) a food such as a peanut. Children need quick orientation to the treatment environment, as they move from the emergency department to radiography and then possibly to surgery or a treatment room. If possible, allow the parents to go with them. Throughout, be vigilant in observing the child for coughing up the foreign body or developing increasing respiratory distress.

A bronchoscopy may be necessary to remove the foreign body (Rosbe, 2008). Children are often given conscious sedation for a bronchoscopy (for details of a bronchoscopy procedure and conscious sedation, see Chapter 37). After bronchoscopy, assess the child closely for signs of bronchial edema and airway obstruction that occurs from mucus accumulation because of the bronchus manipulation. Obtain frequent vital signs (increasing pulse and respiratory rates suggest increased edema and obstruction).

Keep a child NPO for at least an hour after a bronchoscopy. Check for return of the gag reflex. Once the gag reflex is present, offer the first fluid cautiously to prevent additional aspiration. Cool fluid may feel more soothing than warm fluid and also helps to reduce the soreness in the throat. Breathing cool, moist air or having an ice collar applied may further reduce edema.

Obviously, parents need to be cautioned about the dangers of aspiration to keep this from happening again. Do not lecture them, however. Parents whose child has just been through this experience already recognize the danger of aspiration and realize they need to be more careful in the future.

DISORDERS OF THE LOWER RESPIRATORY TRACT

The structures of the lower respiratory tract are subject to infection by the same pathogens that attack the upper respiratory tract. Inflammation and infection of the lungs or bronchi is particularly troublesome: it occurs in various forms and is caused by several organisms. Other illnesses that occur in the lower respiratory tract, such as bronchiastasis, can lead to secondary pneumonia infections and chronic illness.

Influenza

Influenza involves inflammation and infection of the major airways. It is caused by the orthomyxovirus influenza type A, B, or C. It is marked by a cough, fever, fatigue, aching pains, a sore throat, and often accompanying gastrointestinal symptoms such as vomiting or diarrhea. The disease spreads readily through a home or a classroom because children are contagious on the day before symptoms appear and for about the next 5 days.

Children usually need an antipyretic such as acetaminophen (Tylenol) to control fever. Oseltamivir (TamiFlu), a new antiviral drug that halts viral proliferation, can be taken by children over 1 year of age (Deglin & Villerand, 2008). Because TamiFlu only halts virus replication, and does not kill viruses, it needs to be taken at the first sign of illness before replication can begin. Although most children recover without incident, influenza can lead to bronchitis or pneumonia. The condition can be largely prevented by yearly influenza vaccine. Because the influenza virus mutates yearly, the influenza vaccine is specific for only that year and must be readministered yearly (Zimmerman, 2007).

Bronchitis

Bronchitis, or inflammation of the major bronchi and trachea, is one of the more common illnesses affecting preschool and school-age children. It is characterized by fever and cough, usually in conjunction with nasal congestion. Causative agents include the influenza viruses, adenovirus, and *Mycoplasma pneumoniae*, among others.

Assessment

Children usually have a mild upper respiratory tract infection for 1 or 2 days; they then develop a fever and a dry, hacking cough, which is hoarse and mildly productive in older children. The cough is serious enough to wake a child from sleep. These symptoms may last for a week, with full recovery sometimes taking as long as 2 weeks.

On auscultation, rhonchi and coarse crackles (the sound of rales) can be heard. A chest radiograph will reveal diffuse alveolar hyperinflation and some markings at the hilus of the lung.

Therapeutic Management

Therapy is aimed at relieving respiratory symptoms, reducing fever, and maintaining adequate hydration. An antibiotic is prescribed for bacterial infections. If mucus is viscid, an expectorant may be necessary to help the child raise sputum. It is important that children with bronchitis cough to raise accumulating sputum. Cough syrups to suppress coughing, therefore, are rarely indicated.

Bronchiolitis

Bronchiolitis is inflammation of the fine bronchioles and small bronchi. It is the most common lower respiratory illness in children younger than 2 years, peaking in incidence at 6 months of age. The infection occurs most often in the winter and spring. Many children who develop asthma later in life have numerous instances of bronchiolitis during their first year of life. Viruses, such as adenovirus, parainfluenza virus, and RSV, in particular, appear to be the pathogens most responsible for this illness (Quintero & Gershan, 2007).

Assessment

Typically, infants have 1 or 2 days of an upper respiratory tract infection, then suddenly begin to demonstrate nasal flaring, intercostal and subcostal retractions on inspiration, and an increased respiratory rate. They may have a mild fever, leukocytosis, and an increased erythrocyte sedimentation rate, indicating the amount of bronchial inflammation present. Both accumulating mucus and inflammation block the small bronchioles, so air can no longer enter or leave alveoli freely. Most infants develop alveolar hyperinflation because air enters more easily than it leaves inflamed, narrowed bronchioles. This increases the expiratory phase of respiration and can create wheezing. After initial hyperinflation, areas of atelectasis in alveoli may occur as the air that cannot be expired is absorbed. Tachycardia and cyanosis develop from hypoxia. Infants soon become exhausted from rapid respirations. A chest radiograph may show pulmonary infiltrates caused by a secondary infection or collapse of alveoli (atelectasis). Pulse oximetry shows low oxygen saturation. A throat culture will identify the offending organism.

Therapeutic Management

For children with less severe symptoms, antipyretics, adequate hydration, and maintaining a watchful eye for progression to more serious illness is all that is necessary. Hospitalization is warranted for children in severe distress such as when an infant is tachypneic, has marked retractions, seems listless, or has a history of poor fluid intake.

Antibiotics are not commonly used in the treatment of bronchiolitis, because bacteria are rarely a causative factor (Spurling et al., 2009). Children with chronic pulmonary disease may receive anti-RSV immunoglobulin if RSV (respiratory syncytial virus) was identified as the causative agent.

If symptoms are severe, children need humidified oxygen to counteract hypoxemia and adequate hydration to keep respiratory membranes moist. Nebulized bronchodilators, epinephrine, and anti-inflammatory medications such as nebulized budesonide (a glucocorticoid steroid) may be used, although there is little evidence they make a major difference in reducing symptoms. Some children need ventilatory assistance to achieve adequate ventilation. All infants with bronchiolitis need to be carefully observed because if RSV is the cause, apnea may occur. In some infants, extracorporeal membrane oxygenation (the same as that used for heart surgery) is necessary to maintain adequate oxygenation.

Feeding is often a problem because infants tire easily and therefore cannot finish a feeding. Intravenous fluids may be given for the first 1 or 2 days of illness to eliminate the need for oral feeding.

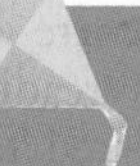

BOX 40.11 ✻ Focus on Evidence-Based Practice

How do you know when it is safe to discharge an infant with bronchiolitis from the emergency room?

During 2004 and 2006, researchers studied the outcome of 1456 infants under 2 years of age seen in 30 U.S. emergency departments with a diagnosis of bronchiolitis. Of these children, 57%, or 837, were discharged home. Factors that predicted a safe discharge to home (the child's condition improved on home care) were infant was over 2 months of age, there was no history of intubation, respiratory rate was specific for age (under 45 breaths per minute for 0–1.9 months, under 43 breaths per minute for 2–5 months, and under 40 breaths per minute for 6–23.9 months), there were no or only mild retractions, initial oxygen saturation was at or greater than 94%, few albuterol or epinephrine treatments were needed in the first hour, and the infant took in an adequate oral intake.

Based on the above research, suppose a parent of an infant, diagnosed with bronchiolitis, who is 1 month of age, has a respiratory rate of 55, moderate retractions, and an oxygen saturation level of 94.5% tells you she cannot wait in the emergency department any longer. Would you advise her that it is safe to leave and take her infant home?

Source: Mansbach, J. M. (2008). Prospective multicenter study of bronchiolitis: predicting safe discharges from the emergency department. *Pediatrics, 121*(4), 680–688.

Nursing Diagnoses and Related Interventions

✻

Nursing Diagnosis: Parental anxiety related to respiratory distress in child

Outcome Evaluation: Parents state that their anxiety level is tolerable as signs and symptoms of disease decrease.

Be certain that parents receive a good explanation of their child's condition. Most parents are aware of bronchi but are unfamiliar with the word *bronchiole*. This leaves them unsure how a simple cold has become so severe. They wonder whether they should have sought medical attention sooner. This may cause them to lose confidence in themselves as parents. Assure them that bronchiolitis begins as only a cold and that it was impossible to know that this cold would take a more serious turn but their child is now safe for discharge (Box 40.11).

The acute phase of bronchiolitis lasts 2 or 3 days. After this time, the child's condition improves rapidly. Although mortality from bronchiolitis is less than 1%, it is a serious disorder of infancy; without treatment, a larger number of infants certainly would die. Some children develop an increased incidence of airway hyperreactivity that may persist for years and be manifested later as asthma (Boguniewicz, 2008).

Respiratory Syncytial Virus Bronchiolitis

RSV is a pathogenic RNA virus that is the most common cause of bronchiolitis in young children. Symptoms begin as a mild upper respiratory infection that quickly extends to include the bronchioles. The infant becomes lethargic and possibly cyanotic. Dehydration occurs as the child becomes too fatigued to suck. Respiratory distress with nasal flaring, retractions, grunting, rales, rhonchi, and expiratory wheezing noted on auscultation occur. All infants with an RSV infection must be monitored closely because the virus tends to cause apnea or periodic halting of respirations. The diagnosis is confirmed by throat or nasal culture.

Therapy is supportive (supplemental oxygen and hydration therapy), although life-threatening apnea may require ventilatory support with mechanical ventilation. Ribavirin, an antiviral agent, is effective against RSV, but ribavirin aerosol treatment is controversial as the drug is teratogenic and could be harmful to pregnant caregivers (Ventre & Randolph, 2009). Because RSV infection spreads readily from one child to the next, infants should be isolated for care. Nursing care should be organized so nurses do not care for other infants than those infected with RSV.

The disease peaks in severity between 48 to 72 hours. Recurrent apneic episodes are rare, so home monitoring for apneic episodes is usually not necessary. Two products are available for the prevention of RSV infection: RSV immune globulin intravenous (RSV-IGIV), made from RSV antibody–positive donor serum, and Palivizumab, a humanized monoclonal antibody produced by recombinant DNA technology. These may be given prophylactically to premature infants during the winter months (Kerby et al., 2008).

Asthma

Asthma, an immediate hypersensitivity (type I) response, is the most common chronic illness in children, accounting for a large number of days of absenteeism from school and many hospital admissions each year. It tends to occur initially before 5 years of age, although in these early years it may be diagnosed as frequent occurrences of bronchiolitis rather than asthma (Table 40.6). The condition may be intermittent, with symptom-free periods, or chronic, with continuous symptoms.

Asthma tends to occur in children with atopy or those who tend to be hypersensitive to allergens. Mast cells release histamine and leukotrienes that result in diffuse obstructive and restrictive airway disease because of a triad of inflammation, bronchoconstriction, and increased mucus production. Most children with asthma can be shown to have sensitization to inhalant antigens such as pollens, molds, or house dust. Food also may be involved. Severe bronchoconstriction can also occur because of exposure to cold air or irritating odors, such as turpentine or smog, as well as inhalation of a known allergen. Air pollutants such as cigarette smoke may lower the threshold for hypersensitivity reactions and worsen the condition. Although there may be a seasonal factor responsible for a particular child's symptoms, most children have multiple sensitivities and are affected all year long. Aspirin can be a trigger, so caution adolescents with asthma that if they begin to take aspirin as an adult, it may initiate an attack.

Mechanism of Disease

Asthma primarily affects the small airways and involves three separate processes: bronchospasm, inflammation of bronchial mucosa, and increased bronchial secretions (mucus). All three processes act to reduce the size of the airway lumen, leading to acute respiratory distress. Bronchial constriction occurs because of stimulation of the parasympathetic nervous system (cholinergic mediated system), which initiates smooth muscle constriction. Inflammation and mucus production occur because of mast cell activation to release leukotrienes, histamine, and prostaglandins. Once viewed as a long-term, poorly controlled disorder, newer therapy makes this a reversible or manageable disorder (Boguniewicz, 2008).

Assessment

The word *asthma* is derived from the Greek word for "panting," a description of the child's distress. Typically, after exposure to an allergen or trigger, an episode begins with a dry cough, often at night as bronchoconstriction begins. Because bronchioles are normally larger in lumen on inspiration than expiration even with bronchoconstriction, children may inhale normally or have little difficulty. They develop increasing difficulty exhaling, however, as it becomes more and more difficult to force air through the narrowed lumen of the inflamed bronchioles filled with mucus. This causes the typical dyspnea and wheezing (the sound caused by air being pushed forcibly past obstructed bronchioles) typically associated with the disorder. Wheezing is heard primarily on expiration. However, when severe, it may be heard on inspiration as well. Hearing it on inspiration means a child is having extreme breathing difficulty. If a child coughs up mucus, it is generally copious and may contain white casts bearing the shape of the bronchi from which it was dislodged.

History. Assessment should include a thorough history of the development of a child's symptoms—for example, what the child was doing at the time of the attack, and what actions were taken by the parents or child to decrease or arrest the symptoms. When an acute attack has passed, ask the parent or child to describe the home environment, including any pets, the child's bedroom, outdoor play space, classroom environment, and type of heating in the house, to see whether more environmental control could reduce future occurrences.

Physical Assessment. A physical assessment includes examining for the specific symptoms of asthma. In many children, the initial wheezing is so loud it can be heard without a stethoscope. In others, it is evident only by auscultation. Asthma affects all lobes of the lungs, so although the wheezing may be more prominent in one lobe than in another, it is generally audible in all lung fields. Audible wheezing in only one lobe suggests that only one bronchus is plugged, which suggests that a foreign body such as a peanut is more likely responsible than asthma. Cyanosis may be present. The eosinophil count is elevated.

Bronchospasm leads to CO_2 trapping and retention; therefore, arterial oxygen saturation monitored by a pulse oximeter will begin to decrease because of the child's inability to fully aerate the lungs. The child becomes frightened because of an acute feeling of suffocation. A peak flow meter shows decreased ability to exhale (Fig. 40.21).

Air-filled lungs are hyperresonant to percussion or they make a louder, hollower noise on percussion than usual. With normal respiration, the inspiration phase of breathing is longer than the expiration phase. During an asthma attack, however, a child must work so hard to exhale that the expiration phase becomes longer than the inspiration phase. Time the two phases to demonstrate this. Also observe for retractions (the chest wall is drawn inward with breaths) because children have to use intercostal accessory muscles to achieve full breaths.

As constriction becomes acute, the sound of wheezing may decrease because so little air can leave the alveoli. Hypoxemia and possibly cyanosis will become severe. When blood gases show an increased P_{CO_2} level and the sound of wheezing suddenly stops, respiratory failure is imminent.

During attacks, children with asthma are generally more comfortable in a sitting or standing position rather than lying down. If seated in a chair, they lean forward and raise their shoulders to give themselves more breathing space. Do not urge children to "lie down and relax," as this can cause severe anxiety and increased difficulty in breathing. Children who

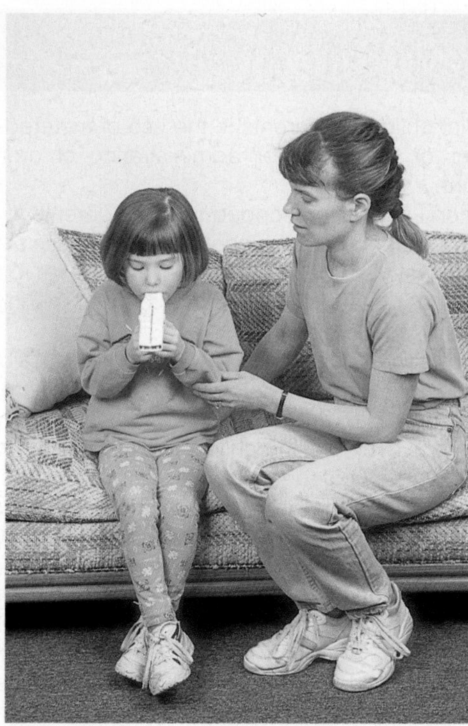

FIGURE 40.21 Here a child with asthma practices using a peak flow meter to track her peak expiratory flow readings on a daily basis.

do agree to lie down are either at the end of an attack and beginning to feel less threatened by the dyspnea or are so exhausted by the paroxysms of coughing they no longer have the strength to sit upright.

Over time, as children have many bouts of asthma, they develop a shield-like or barrel-shaped chest from constant overinflation of air in alveoli. Clubbing of the fingers (from the growth of excess capillaries initiated when oxygen deprivation is sensed in distal parts) may be noticeable. If children are treated for a long period with high doses of steroids, they may fall behind in growth.

Pulmonary Function Studies

Good pulmonary function depends on good ventilation (both drawing adequate air into the lungs and expelling it again), adequate transfer of gases across the alveolar capillary membranes, and adequate volume and distribution of pulmonary capillary blood flow to transport oxygen to body cells. In children with asthma, the vital capacity (air that they are able to exhale) may be low or the capacity may be normal, but, because of narrowed bronchioles as a result of bronchospasm, the expiratory rate will be abnormally long (more than 10 seconds, rather than the normal 2 or 3 seconds). If a child has bronchial plugging, the vital capacity will be low because of air absorption behind blocked bronchi. A gross measure of vital capacity is to ask a child to blow out a match. A child with an average vital capacity should be able to do this when the match is held at 6 inches. Children with asthma may not have the expiratory pressure to do this.

Peak Expiratory Flow Rate Monitoring. Children with asthma often use a home peak flow meter daily to measure gross changes in peak expiratory flow over time and help in planning an appropriate therapeutic regimen (Fig. 40.21). Children with asthma should be able to tell you their usual reading and personal best score.

To use a peak flow meter, a child places the indicator on the apparatus at the bottom of the numbered scale, and takes a deep breath. A child then places the meter in the mouth and blows out as hard and fast as possible. The child then repeats this two more times and records the highest number achieved as the peak flow meter result. During a 2-week period when a child feels well, this should be done daily. The highest number achieved during this time is recorded as the child's personal best.

Children are assigned "zones" to rate their expiratory compliance:

- Green zone (80% to 100% of their personal best) means no asthma symptoms are present, and they should take their routine medications.
- Yellow zone (50% to 80% of personal best) signals caution. An episode of asthma may be beginning.
- Red zone (below 50% of personal best) indicates an asthma episode is beginning. Children should immediately take their prescribed medication such as an inhaled beta-2–agonist, then repeat the peak flow assessment. If the second reading is not in the green zone, their parents should alert their primary care provider of the impending asthma attack.

Therapeutic Management

Therapy for children with asthma involves planning for the three goals of all allergic disorders: avoidance of the allergen by environmental control; skin testing and hyposensitization to identified allergens; and relief of symptoms by pharmacologic agents. Parents need good instructions to be able to continue to address all three concerns over an extended period of time (McMullen et al., 2007).

Cough suppressants are contraindicated with asthma because, as a rule, as long as children can continue to cough up mucus, they are not in serious danger. When they stop coughing up mucus, thick plugs form that then may lead to pneumonia, atelectasis, and further acidosis.

A child with mild but persistent asthma usually is prescribed an inhaled anti-inflammatory corticosteroid such as fluticasone (Flovent) daily. Children who have moderate persistent symptoms usually are prescribed a long-acting bronchodilator at bedtime in addition to the inhaled anti-inflammatory daily corticosteroid. Children who have severe persistent asthma symptoms take a high dose of both an oral corticosteroid and an inhaled corticosteroid daily as well as a long-acting bronchodilator at bedtime. In addition, children may be prescribed a short-acting beta-2–agonist bronchodilator, such as albuterol or terbutaline, to use if an attack should begin (see Box 40.6). Cromolyn sodium is a mast cell stabilizer given by a nebulizer or metered-dose inhaler (see Figures 40.6 and 40.12A,B). This can prevent bronchoconstriction and thereby prevent the symptoms of asthma (Box 40.12). Cromolyn sodium is not effective once symptoms have begun.

Another group of drugs used in the treatment of asthma are leukotriene receptor antagonists such as montelukast (Singulair) (Scow, Luttermoser, & Dickerson, 2007). These drugs are used for prophylaxis and chronic treatment of

BOX 40.12 * Focus on Pharmacology

Cromolyn Sodium (Intal)

Classification: Cromolyn sodium is a mast cell inhibitor.

Action: Inhibits the release of histamine, slow-releasing substance of anaphylaxis, and leukotriene, thereby decreasing the overall allergic response. In asthma, it is used prophylactically to prevent severe bronchospasms (Karch, 2009).

Pregnancy risk category: B

Dosage: Initially, 20 mg inhaled (via spinhaler inhalant or as nebulized solution) 4 times daily at regular intervals; one ampule orally 4 times daily 1/2 hour before meals and at bedtime (ampule is not recommended for use in children under the age of 5 years)

Possible adverse effects: Dizziness, headache, nausea, dry and irritated throat, cough, nasal congestion, epistaxis, sneezing

Nursing Implications

- Instruct parents and child that this drug is not effective in an acute attack.
- Caution child and parents to take the drug exactly as prescribed and to continue other agents, such as bronchodilators.
- Instruct child and parents in the use of metered-dose inhaler or nebulizer for administration of cromolyn sodium.
- If the oral form is prescribed, instruct parents to open the ampule and pour the contents into a glass of water and to wait for the medication to dissolve. Caution parents not to substitute the oral form for the inhalant form and vice versa.
- Instruct parents and child to watch for a possible recurrence of asthma symptoms if dosage is decreased.
- Know that this drug is only given once the acute episode is over and the child's airway is clear, to prevent a further episode.
- Caution child and parents not to exceed the number of ordered puffs via inhaler, to prevent possible tolerance to drug.
- If more than one inhalation is ordered, advise child to wait 1 to 2 minutes before taking the second puff.
- If the child is also receiving an inhaled bronchodilator, advise the child and parents to have the child use the bronchodilator first to open the airways and then wait approximately 5 minutes before using the cromolyn sodium, to maximize its effectiveness.

asthma in children over 6 years of age. They are not effective in an acute attack.

If children are to receive medication by nebulizer or inhaler, be certain they know how to use these properly. It is easy for children to take this type of medication lightly (the belief it is "not really medicine" because it is not swallowed). As a result, overdose from constant use of nebulizers or metered-dose inhalers can occur.

Dehydration occurs rapidly in children during an asthma attack because they have decreased oral intake (children stop drinking because they are coughing, or coughing makes them vomit and parents stop offering fluid) as well as increased insensible loss that occurs from tachypnea. Dehydration may contribute to increased mucus plugging and further airway obstruction. Encourage children to continue to drink fluids (ask about favorite beverages and offer small sips of them). Avoid milk or milk products because they cause thick mucus and difficulty swallowing. In an emergency setting, an intravenous line is established to supply continuous fluid therapy and also provide a route for emergency drug administration.

Nursing Diagnoses and Related Interventions

*

Nursing Diagnosis: Fear related to sudden onset of asthma attack

Outcome Evaluation: Parents and child express confidence in their ability to prevent attacks and effectively manage any that occur.

Asthma is a frightening disease. At the time it is diagnosed, parents may have already gone through a long period of wondering why their child was always tired and had episodes of difficulty with breathing. After diagnosis, parents may be afraid to allow a child to sleep overnight away from them or leave the child alone with a babysitter. Help parents find a middle ground: to allow a child enough freedom for growth and development while still being certain the child is safe. Taking steps to slow breathing, better emptying alveoli through pursed-lip breathing, and administering medications to prevent symptoms are key measures for children to learn. Many children have long periods without attacks. When a new one occurs after a long absence, it is almost as frightening as the original attack because everything seems so new again.

Nursing Diagnosis: Health-seeking behaviors related to prevention of and treatment for asthma attacks

Outcome Evaluation: Parents and child accurately state triggers that cause an attack; child correctly demonstrates breathing exercises, use of inhaler, and peak expiratory flow meter.

Children need to learn how to avoid possible triggers through environmental control. If foods are a trigger, children need to learn to be responsible for their own diets so they can avoid these foods. Children as young as 6 years can learn what foods they cannot eat and can take responsibility for telling a friend's parent or a schoolteacher that they must not eat certain foods. They must learn to use a metered-dose inhaler or nebulizer if prescribed. At the same time, they must not become inhaler-dependent or use the inhaler constantly, afraid to go anywhere without it. This will invariably result in their using the inhaler much more often than is necessary.

To prevent children with asthma from losing chest mobility and to decrease their tendency to develop a barrel chest, they can be taught several breathing or mobility exercises to do daily at home. Such exercises are aimed at increasing expiratory function (diaphragmatic or side expansion breathing). Recommended activities include bending side to side, bending forward and touching the left foot with the right hand, and swinging the arms rhythmically in front of the body like a windmill (jumping jacks). These exercises can be incorporated into a bedtime or after-school routine. (Parents [and nurses] who do mobility exercises with children find the exercises are helpful to them as well, as they help tighten the abdominal muscles.) Using an incentive spirometer daily is another method for children to use to exercise the lungs and keep chest muscles supple.

The prognosis in children who develop asthma is good if they adhere to their treatment regimen. Children do not outgrow asthma, although most of them may become symptom-free as adults, probably because the lumens of major airways enlarge with adulthood.

Do not convey to parents the impression that asthma is a disease that will be simply outgrown, however. Although asthma may not always last into adulthood, parents need to maintain careful environmental control, conscientious administration of medication, and hyposensitization, if indicated, to keep the child free of symptoms during childhood.

Status Asthmaticus

Under ordinary circumstances, an asthma attack responds readily to the aerosol administration of a bronchodilator such as albuterol, terbutaline, levalbuterol (Xopenex), or salmeterol (Serevent). When children fail to respond and an attack continues, they are in *status asthmaticus*. This is an extreme emergency because, if the attack cannot be relieved, a child may die of heart failure caused by the combination of exhaustion, atelectasis, and respiratory acidosis from bronchial plugging.

Assessment

A child with status asthmaticus is in acute respiratory distress. Both heart rate and respiratory rate are elevated. Both oxygen saturation and PO_2 are low; PCO_2 is elevated because the bronchi are so constricted the child cannot exhale, resulting in CO_2 accumulation. The rising PCO_2 rapidly leads to acidosis. In contrast to the loud wheezing initially heard in an asthma attack, children with status asthmaticus may have so little air able to pass in or out of their lungs that breath sounds are limited. Pulse oximetry will reveal the low oxygen saturation level.

Status asthmaticus is often initiated by a respiratory infection, which acts as the triggering mechanism for the prolonged attack. If this occurs, obtain cultures from coughed sputum, and be prepared to administer a broad-spectrum antibiotic until the culture results are available. Be certain the sputum obtained for culture was coughed from deep in the respiratory tract and not just from the back of the child's throat.

Therapeutic Management

By definition, a child in status asthmaticus has failed to respond to first-line therapy (Mannix & Bachur, 2007). Continuous nebulization with an inhaled beta-2-agonist and intravenous corticosteroids may be necessary to reduce symptoms. Oxygen is given by face mask or nasal prongs to maintain the PO_2 at more than 90 mm Hg. These methods supply good oxygen concentrations and yet leave the child's face unobscured for easy observation. To prevent drying of pulmonary secretions, always give oxygen with humidification. It is best administered at a concentration of 30% to 40%, not 100%. If concentrations greater than 40% are needed, a Venturi mask that allows for rebreathing may be used. Some children in severe status asthmaticus have such a carbon dioxide buildup (because they cannot exhale properly) that they develop carbon dioxide narcosis with no stimulation for inhalation. The child's respiratory stimulus, therefore, is hypoxia, or lack of oxygen. If 100% oxygen were administered, the oxygen lack would disappear, and respirations would cease. The idea "if a little is good, a lot is better" does not apply here. After it has been ascertained that the child is not in acidosis (from blood gas and pH studies), oxygen levels may be increased, but for initial therapy, unless prescribed otherwise, keep the level at 40%.

During the acute stage of status asthmaticus, children need increased fluid to combat dehydration and keep airway secretions moist. Drinking tends to aggravate coughing, so an intravenous infusion such as 5% glucose in 0.45 saline is usually prescribed to supply fluid. If a child can drink, do not offer cold fluids because these tend to aggravate bronchospasm.

Monitor intake and output; measure the specific gravity of urine. Under stress, antidiuretic hormone is released, so fluid retention and overhydration may occur.

An increasing PCO_2 is a danger sign because it indicates the degree of hypoventilation. In severe attacks, endotracheal intubation and mechanical ventilation may be necessary to maintain effective respirations (Carpenter et al., 2008).

Bronchiectasis

Bronchiectasis is chronic dilatation and plugging of the bronchi. It may follow pneumonia, aspiration of a foreign body, pertussis, or asthma.

Children develop a chronic cough with mucopurulent sputum (Kerby et al., 2008). Young infants may have accompanying wheezing or stridor. If a large area of lung is involved, children may have cyanosis. As the disease becomes chronic, children develop symptoms of chronic lung disease, such as clubbing of the fingers and easy fatigability. Their physical growth may become restricted. Their chest may become enlarged from overinflation of alveoli caused by the air trapped behind inflamed bronchi.

Inhaled mucolytic agents or bronchodilators and chest physiotherapy may be necessary to raise the tenacious sputum. An antibiotic will be necessary if infection is present. The cause of the bronchiectasis such as an aspirated seed or nut must be identified and relieved before the chronic process can be relieved. In rare instances, surgery to remove the affected lung portion may be necessary.

Pneumonia

Pneumonia (infection and inflammation of alveoli) occurs at a rate of 2 to 4 children in 100. It may be of bacterial origin (pneumococcal, streptococcal, staphylococcal, or chlamydial) or viral in origin, such as RSV. Aspiration of

products are a common cause of childhood poisonings and result in hydrocarbon pneumonia.

Assessment. Children who swallow a hydrocarbon-based product usually exhibit gastrointestinal symptoms such as nausea and vomiting. Next, they become drowsy and develop a cough from inhalation as vapors from the stomach rise and are inhaled. As bronchial edema occurs from irritation and inflammation, respirations become increased and dyspneic.

Physical assessment shows an increased percussion sound caused by the presence of air trapped in the alveoli beyond the point of inflammation. Rales may be heard as air passes through collecting mucus. Because air cannot reach and inflate the alveoli fully, breath sounds may be diminished.

Therapeutic Management. Irritation from fumes of hydrocarbon ingestion may occur when children initially swallow the fluid. If they are given an emetic to induce vomiting, it can cause them to aspirate vomitus or cause additional irritation. Parents should telephone a poison control center to ask for advice if their child has swallowed any poison, rather than induce vomiting to prevent this secondary complication. In the emergency room, gastric lavage may be done by health care personnel with great care to remove the substance from the stomach and help prevent inhalation.

The child is usually admitted to a hospital observation unit for a short time. Obtain vital signs and observe the child's general appearance carefully for evidence of increased respiratory tract obstruction or increasing drowsiness or other symptoms of CNS involvement from CNS intoxication. Cool, moist air administered by a nebulizer with supplemental oxygen may be prescribed to decrease lung inflammation. If febrile, a child needs an antipyretic. Frequent changes of position will prevent pooling of secretions, which could lead to a secondary infection. Chest physiotherapy will help to move secretions and reduce areas of stasis.

The initial inflammation reaction from hydrocarbon aspiration may lead to such occlusion that emphysema (pocketing of air in alveoli) occurs, causing rupture of the alveoli into the pleural space, with consequent pneumothorax and atelectasis.

Often, children who swallow a household cleaner or other substance are aware they should not have been handling substances kept under the sink. As a result, they cannot help but interpret the hospitalization, blood drawing, and other uncomfortable procedures as punishments for their action. They may benefit from therapeutic play with puppets or dolls that will help alleviate their guilt and anger at being "punished" so severely.

Hydrocarbon pneumonia is slow to resolve, so the child will be ill for some time. After the illness, reinforce with parents the need to keep poisons in a safe place. Offer a listening ear so they can explain they were unaware of the extreme danger of these everyday household products.

Atelectasis

Atelectasis is the collapse of lung alveoli. It may occur in children as a primary or secondary condition. It must be considered as a possibility in all children with respiratory distress.

Primary Atelectasis

Primary atelectasis occurs in newborns who do not breathe with enough respiratory strength at birth to inflate lung tissue or whose alveoli are so immature or so lacking in surfactant that alveoli cannot expand. This is seen most commonly in immature infants or in infants with CNS damage. It may occur if infants have mucus or meconium plugs in the trachea.

When atelectasis occurs, the newborn's respirations become irregular, with nasal flaring and apnea. After a few minutes, a respiratory grunt and cyanosis may occur. The sound of a respiratory grunt is caused by the newborn's glottis closing on expiration. At first, this is a helpful action because it increases pressure in the respiratory tract, keeps alveoli from collapsing, and allows for better alveoli exchange surfaces. This action is also tiring, however, and as the infant tires, hypoxemia will increase, and the infant will become hypotonic and flaccid. The Apgar score will invariably be low.

As infants cry or are administered oxygen, more alveoli become aerated and cyanosis may decrease. The cause of the atelectasis must be established, however, so that therapy directed to the specific cause can be initiated.

Secondary Atelectasis

Secondary atelectasis occurs in children when they have a respiratory tract obstruction that prevents air from entering a portion of the alveoli. As the residual air in the alveoli is absorbed, the alveoli collapse. The causes of obstruction in children include mucus plugs that may occur with chronic respiratory disease or aspiration of foreign objects. In some children, atelectasis occurs because of pressure on lung tissue from outside forces, such as compression from a diaphragmatic hernia, scoliosis, or enlarged thoracic lymph nodes (Fig. 40.22).

The signs of secondary atelectasis depend on the degree of collapse. Asymmetry of the chest may be noticed. Breath sounds on the affected side are decreased. If the process is extensive, tachypnea and cyanosis will be present. A chest radiograph will show the collapsed alveoli (a "whiteout").

Children with atelectasis are prone to secondary infection because mucus, which provides a good medium for bacteria, becomes stagnant without air exchange.

Therapeutic Management. Atelectasis caused by inspiration of a foreign object will not be relieved until the object is removed by bronchoscopy. Atelectasis caused by a mucus plug will resolve when the plug resolves or is moved or expectorated. Children may need oxygen and assisted ventilation to maintain adequate respiratory function until this time (Groeben et al., 2008).

Make certain the chest of a child with atelectasis is kept free from pressure so that lung expansion is as full as possible (to allow as much breathing space as possible). If restraints are being used to keep an infant positioned, make certain that body restraints are not crossing the chest area and interfering with chest expansion. Check clothing to be certain it is loose and nonbinding. Make certain the child's arms are not positioned across the chest, where their weight could interfere with deep inspiration.

A semi-Fowler's position generally allows for the best lung expansion because it lowers abdominal contents and increases chest space. Increase the humidity of the child's environment to prevent further bronchial plugging; suction and chest physiotherapy may be necessary to keep the respiratory tract clear and free of mucus. Observe closely for increased respirations or cyanosis, as these indicate failing oxygenation.

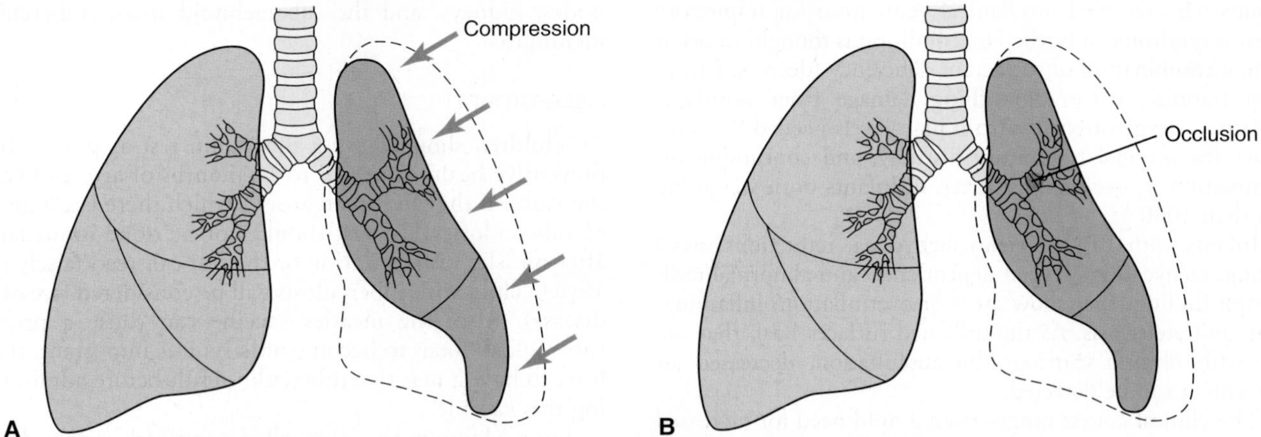

FIGURE 40.22 (A) Atelectasis caused by compression of lung tissue. (B) Atelectasis caused by obstruction.

Pneumothorax

Pneumothorax is the presence of atmospheric air in the pleural space; its presence causes the alveoli to collapse (atelectasis) (Fig. 40.23). Pneumothorax in children usually occurs when air seeps from ruptured alveoli and collects in the pleural cavity. It also can occur when external puncture wounds allow air to enter the chest (Chauvin, Chen, & Anthony, 2007).

Pneumothorax occurs in approximately 1% of newborns, probably because of rupture of the alveoli from the extreme intrathoracic pressure needed to initiate a first inspiration. The infant develops tachypnea, grunting respirations, flaring of the nares, and cyanosis. Auscultation reveals absent or decreased breath sounds on the affected side. Percussion may not be revealing, despite the hollow air space; as so much air is present, this may be hyperresonant. A more revealing sign may be the shift of the apical pulse (mediastinal shift) away from the site of the pneumothorax and the resulting atelectasis. A chest film will show the darkened area of the air-filled pleural space.

A child with a pneumothorax needs oxygen therapy to relieve respiratory distress. A thoracotomy catheter or needle may be placed in the pleural space and atmospheric air aspirated or low-pressure suction with water-seal drainage applied to remove accumulated air. In most children with pneumothorax, symptoms are relieved within 24 hours after suction is begun. The use of water-seal drainage with children is discussed in Chapter 41.

If the air in the pleural space is from a puncture wound such as a stab wound, cover the chest wound immediately with an impervious material, such as petrolatum gauze, to prevent further air from entering and help decrease the possibility of atelectasis. In an emergency, an impervious object can be your gloved hand.

Pneumothorax is always a potentially serious respiratory problem. The extent of the symptoms and the outcome will depend on the cause of entry of air into the pleural space and whether it can be removed.

Bronchopulmonary Dysplasia

Bronchopulmonary dysplasia (BPD) is chronic pulmonary involvement that occurs in 10% to 40% of infants who are treated for acute respiratory distress in the first days of life (Yost & Soll, 2009). The condition most often occurs in

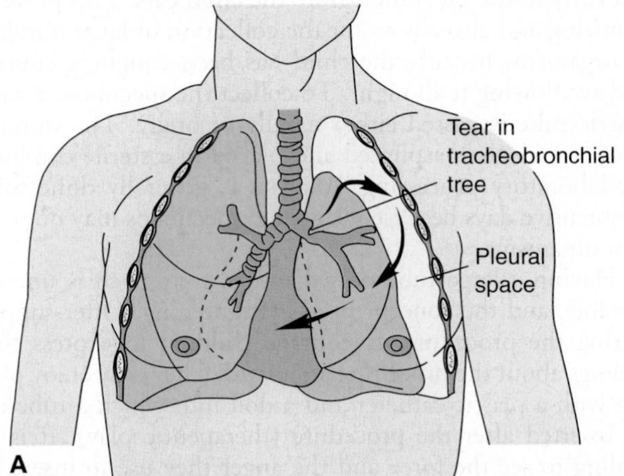

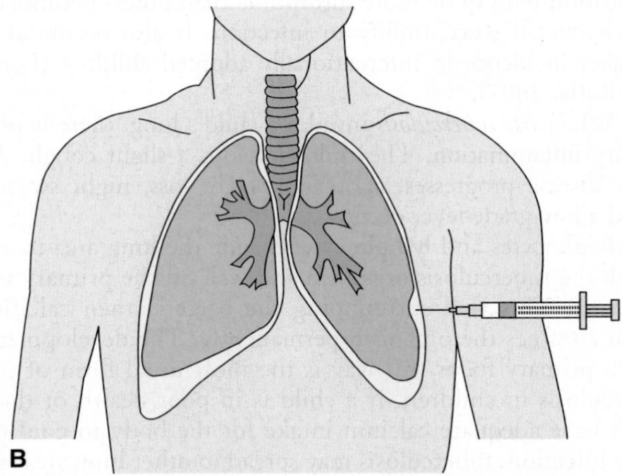

FIGURE 40.23 (A) Pneumothorax. A tear in the tracheobronchial tree has caused air to move into the pleural space; the lung collapses and the mediastinum shifts to the unaffected side. (B) Aspiration of air from the pleural space allows lung to re-expand after a pneumothorax.

infants who received mechanical ventilation for respiratory distress syndrome at birth. The condition is thought to occur from a combination of surfactant deficiency (decreased from lung trauma), barotrauma (lung damage from ventilator pressure), oxygen toxicity (from high levels needed to counteract the original respiratory distress), and continuing inflammation. It occurs most often in infants born weighting less than 1000 g.

Infants with BPD develop tachypnea, retractions, nasal flaring, tachycardia, oxygen dependence, and abnormal radiograph findings that show areas of overinflation, inflammation, and atelectasis. As the inflamed surfaces heal, they are left with fibrotic scarring. On auscultation, decreased air movement can be detected.

The clinical course ranges from a mild need for increased oxygen requirements that will gradually resolve over a few months to severe disease requiring chronic tracheostomy and mechanical ventilation for as long as the first 2 years of life. A respiratory infection greatly compromises the infant's ability to breathe.

Administration of a corticosteroid to reduce inflammation and a bronchodilator by nebulizer greatly improves respiratory function. Infants need to be monitored carefully for nutrition and fluid intake, especially if ventilator dependent. Because of the long hospitalization involved, parents need support to continue to visit and care for the child as what seemed to be a miracle at birth (their very small newborn survived) becomes years of specialized and expensive health care.

Tuberculosis

Tuberculosis is a highly contagious pulmonary disease. The causative agent is *Mycobacterium tuberculosis* (tubercle bacillus). The mode of transmission is inhalation of infected droplets. The incubation period is 2 to 10 weeks (Starke, 2007).

Children generally contract this disease from someone in the immediate family. When any member of a family contracts tuberculosis, all family members must be tested (a Mantoux skin test) to screen for the disease. In some children, the contact is not known, and the disease is first detected when symptoms appear. Children who are homeless or severely impoverished or who have chronic illness or malnutrition tend to be more susceptible than others because of their overall susceptibility to infection. It also occurs at a higher incidence in internationally adopted children (Long & Boffa, 2007).

When *M. tuberculosis* invades a child's lung, there is primary inflammation. The child develops a slight cough. As the disease progresses, anorexia, weight loss, night sweats, and a low-grade fever occur.

Leukocytes and lymphocytes invade the lung area to attack the tuberculosis organism and wall off the primary infection. This wall surrounding the bacteria then calcifies and confines the organism permanently. The development of a primary focus this way is the most usual form of tuberculosis in children. If a child is in poor health or does not have adequate calcium intake for the body to confine the infection, tuberculosis may spread to other lung areas or to other parts of the body (miliary tuberculosis). Common body sites that may be affected are bones and joints, lymph nodes, kidneys, and the subarachnoid space (tuberculous meningitis).

Assessment

All children should have a tuberculin test as part of basic preventive health care at 9 to 12 months of age, and yearly thereafter if they live in an area in which there is a high risk of tuberculosis. The test should not be done immediately after measles immunization or the test can read falsely negative (a child with tuberculosis will be considered free of the disease). Also, the measles vaccine can cause a primary tuberculosis focus to become miliary; it is important, therefore, to have a negative tuberculin result before administering this vaccine.

For a Mantoux test, also called a purified protein derivative (PPD) test, 5 units of protein derivative vaccine is injected intradermally, usually on the left lower arm. A health care professional inspects the area in 72 hours and notes the reaction. A positive reaction (the formation of 5 to 15 mm of reddened induration) indicates the child has been exposed to tuberculosis or has developed antibodies to the foreign products of the tuberculosis organism. Children with positive reactions need follow-up with a chest radiograph to ascertain the importance of the reaction; that is, whether a current infection exists. Skin testing should not be done on children who are known to have had tuberculosis. Such a child will have such an intense reaction that the skin at the site of the test may slough and necrose.

In the early course of tuberculosis, because the initial focus of the tuberculosis is so small, it may not be evident on a chest radiograph. As local inflammation occurs, however, cloudiness in the inflamed area will be noticeable on the film, as will calcification as it occurs.

To confirm a diagnosis of active disease, sputum may be analyzed. Make certain children understand that you want them to expectorate mucus raised from the lungs, not just from the back of the throat. Have a child demonstrate a deep cough to you so you can be sure you are both talking about the same thing. Infants and children younger than 5 years do not raise sputum but swallow it. In young children, therefore, gastric lavage may be necessary to obtain the sputum specimen (because tuberculosis bacteria are acid-fast, they are not destroyed by gastric secretions). Schedule this test early in the morning before the child eats. This prevents vomiting and also allows for the collection of large numbers of organisms because the child has been coughing sputum and swallowing it all night. To collect the specimen, a nasogastric tube is passed either nasally or orally. The stomach contents are then aspirated and placed in a sterile container for laboratory processing. Analysis is generally done for 3 consecutive days because individual specimens may not contain organisms.

Having a large tube passed into the stomach is uncomfortable, and the concept itself is frightening. Offer support during the procedure. Encourage children to express their feelings about the procedure afterward. They may enjoy playing with a plastic catheter and a doll into which a tube can be inserted after the procedure (therapeutic play). It is revealing to see the force and the anger they use to insert the tube into the doll. This helps you to understand how they envision the procedure.

Children who have primary tuberculosis are not infectious because they have a minimal pulmonary lesion and little or no cough. They need not be isolated. As soon as drug therapy has been started, they can return to regular activities, including school.

Before drug therapy was available, a diagnosis of tuberculosis meant a hospital stay of approximately a year. Parents who believe that tuberculosis is still treated this way will need assurance that it is all right for their child to return home and attend regular school as soon as their child begins taking medication.

Therapeutic Management

Several medications are effective against tuberculosis. Isoniazid (INH) is the drug of choice. INH may produce peripheral neurologic symptoms if pyridoxine (vitamin B_6) is not administered concurrently. Rifampin is a secondary drug often used in combination with INH. Para-aminosalicylic acid (PAS) is bacteriostatic to *M. tuberculosis* and for a long time served as the mainstay of therapy. However, PAS administration may lead to such gastrointestinal disturbances in children that it is not used as much as in the past. If it is prescribed, it should be administered after meals, never on an empty stomach.

Ethambutol is used with older children. It must be used with caution with infants because one side effect is optic neuritis; the inability to do adequate eye examinations in children under school age to discover this side effect can make ethambutol unsafe for long-term use.

In addition to drug therapy, children should ingest a diet high in protein, calcium, and pyridoxine, especially if INH is being used as they help supply nutrients necessary to wall off organisms in lung tissue.

Because tuberculosis therapy can last up to 18 months, a major concern during treatment is that the tuberculosis organism will become resistant to commonly used drugs. Children should have periodic chest radiographs for the rest of their life to make certain their disease does not become active again later in life. A woman who had tuberculosis as a child should tell her primary care provider about this when she becomes pregnant; lung changes that occur in pregnancy as a result of the pressure of the growing uterus against the lungs can break down calcifications and reactivate tuberculosis. Children who develop another chronic disease that interferes with appetite, and therefore with calcium intake, also have a high risk of reactivation of calcium-contained tuberculosis.

Because children will be taking medicine for a long time, they need periodic health care visits to evaluate the extent of drug adherence. Assess that they receive regular childhood immunizations so they do not contract a second disease until they have fully recovered from tuberculosis. It is most important to prevent pertussis (whooping cough) because the paroxysmal cough caused by this illness could easily reactivate tuberculosis lesions.

The Bacille Calmette-Guérin (BCG) vaccine is available against tuberculosis, but it is not used routinely in the United States. A skin test will be strongly positive after effective BCG vaccination. For this reason, most people advocate placing children on prophylactic INH when there is known tuberculosis in the home rather than vaccinating them against tuberculosis. With this method, as long as a repeat PPD test remains negative, you know that they are disease-free. After BCG vaccine is administered, the value of skin testing would be lost.

Cystic Fibrosis

Children with cystic fibrosis (CF) have a generalized dysfunction of the exocrine glands (Gardner, 2007). Mucus secretions of the body, particularly in the pancreas and the lungs, are so tenacious that they have difficulty flowing through gland ducts. There is also a marked electrolyte change in the secretions of the sweat glands (chloride concentration of sweat is two to five times above normal). The cause of the disorder is an abnormality of the long arm of chromosome 7. This results in the inability to transport small molecules across cell membranes; this leads to dehydration of epithelial cells in the airway and pancreas and dried secretions.

The disorder is inherited as an autosomal recessive trait. It occurs in approximately 1 in 2500 live births. It occurs most commonly in Caucasian children and rarely in black or Asian children. Although the disease can be fatal in early life, as many as 50% of children now live to be more than 30 years of age. With the availability of lung transplants, full life expectancy is possible. Because the gene that causes the disorder can be isolated, chorionic villi sampling or amniocentesis can be done early in pregnancy to detect fetuses who have the disease. All newborns can be screened at birth by a simple heel puncture blood sample for the disorder (Merelle et al., 2009). In the future, it is expected that gene therapy will be available to reverse the effect of the involved gene.

Boys with CF may not be able to reproduce because they have persistent plugging and blocking of the vas deferens from tenacious seminal fluid. Girls may have such thick cervical secretions that sperm penetration is limited. Artificial insemination or in vitro fertilization can be accomplished if they desire to become pregnant.

Pancreas Involvement

The acinar cells of the pancreas normally produce lipase, trypsin, and amylase, enzymes that flow into the duodenum to digest fat, protein, and carbohydrate. With CF, these enzyme secretions become so thickened that they plug the ducts; eventually, there is such back-pressure on the acinar cells that they become atrophied and then are no longer capable of producing the enzymes. The islets of Langerhans and insulin production are little influenced by this process until late in the disease because they have endocrine (ductless) activity.

Without pancreatic enzymes in the duodenum, children cannot digest fat, protein, and some sugars. The child's stools become large, bulky, and greasy **(steatorrhea).**The intestinal flora increases because of the undigested food; this, when combined with the fat in the stool, gives the stool an extremely foul odor, often compared to that of a cat's stool. The bulk of feces in the intestine leads to a protuberant abdomen. Because children are benefiting from only about 50% of the food they ingest, they show signs of malnutrition—emaciated extremities and loose, flabby folds of skin on their buttocks. The fat-soluble vitamins, particularly A, D, and E, cannot be absorbed because fat is not absorbed, so children develop symptoms of low levels of these vitamins. These four symptoms—malnutrition, protuberant abdomen, steatorrhea, and fat-soluble vitamin deficiencies—are the same four symptoms that are part of celiac disease (malabsorption syndrome), so they are referred to as a celiac syndrome (see Chapter 45).

Meconium in a newborn is normally thick and tenacious. In approximately 10% of children with CF, it may be so thick, because pancreatic enzymes are lacking, that it obstructs the intestine (meconium ileus). The newborn develops abdominal distention with no passage of stool. Meconium ileus should be suspected in any infant who does not pass a stool by 24 hours of life (Jawaheer et al., 2007). Rectal prolapse from straining to evacuate hard stool is another common finding in infants with CF.

Lung Involvement

Thickened mucus pools in bronchioles. Pockets of infection then begin in these secretions. The organisms most frequently cultured are *Staphylococcus aureus, Pseudomonas aeruginosa,* and *H. influenzae.* Secondary emphysema (overinflated alveoli) occurs because air cannot be pushed past the thick mucus on expiration, when all bronchi are narrower than they are on inspiration. Bronchiectasis and pneumonia occur. Respiratory acidosis may develop because obstruction interferes with the ability to exhale carbon dioxide. Atelectasis occurs as a result of absorption of air from alveoli behind blocked bronchioles. The child's fingers become clubbed because of the inadequate peripheral tissue perfusion. The anterior-posterior diameter of the chest becomes enlarged.

Sweat Gland Involvement

Although the sweat glands themselves do not appear to be changed in structure, the electrolyte composition of perspiration is changed. The level of chloride to sodium is increased two to five times above normal. Some parents report they knew their newborn had the disease before they had laboratory tests done because when they kissed their child, they could taste such strong salt in the perspiration.

Assessment. If CF is not diagnosed by a screening blood sample at birth, it can be diagnosed by documenting the chromosomal abnormality, or by the history and the combination of the abnormal concentration of chloride in sweat, the absence of pancreatic enzymes in the duodenum, the presence of immunoreactive trypsinogen in the blood, and pulmonary involvement.

CF may be suspected in a newborn when a newborn loses the normal amount of weight at birth (5% to 10% of birth weight), but then, because the infant cannot make use of the fat in milk, does not gain it back at the usual time of 7 to 10 days and perhaps not until 4 to 6 weeks of age. Nurses often weigh newborn babies and infants at well child health visits so may be the first to detect this lack of weight gain. Nurses may also be the first health care provider to suspect CF because meconium is so tenacious an infant is unable to pass stool (meconium ileus). Chromosome analysis or analysis of serum immunoreactive trypsin (IRT) in the stool, which is elevated because obstruction in the pancreas occurs as early as during fetal life, confirms the diagnosis.

Children who are not diagnosed at birth may be seen in a health care setting at about 1 month of age because of a feeding problem. Using only about 50% of their intake because of their poor digestive function, they are always hungry. This causes them to eat so ravenously they tend to swallow air. This leads to colic or abdominal distention and vomiting. The appearance of typical CF stools (large and greasy) is an important finding because children with simple colic do not show these changes in stool consistency.

Respiratory infections develop at 4 to 6 months of age. Even at this early stage of the disease, wheezing and rhonchi may be heard on chest auscultation.

By the time a child with CF is a preschooler, a cough is a prominent finding. On percussion, the chest is hyperresonant, reflecting the emphysema present. Rales and rhonchi are heard. Clubbing of the fingers may already be apparent. It is rare for a child to go undiagnosed beyond this time because the symptoms of the illness have become so persistent and evident.

Sweat Testing. Sweat testing is a time-honored method for detecting the abnormal concentrations in sweat in children with CF. Sweat is collected by placing a filter paper on the skin and analyzed for sodium chloride content. With chromosomal determination available, sweat tests are no longer necessary, but parents may ask about the procedure if they hear about it from friends. A normal concentration of chloride in sweat is 20 mEq/L. A level of more than 60 mEq/L chloride in children is diagnostic of CF.

Duodenal Analysis. Analysis of duodenal secretions for detection of pancreatic enzymes reveals the extent of the pancreatic involvement. This is done by passing a nasogastric tube into the duodenum and then aspirating secretions for analysis. This test may take a considerable amount of time because the tube is allowed to pass through the pylorus and into the duodenum by natural peristaltic action. You can tell that a tube has passed from the stomach into the duodenum by aspirating secretions from the tube and testing them for pH. Stomach secretions are acid (pH less than 7.0); duodenal secretions are alkaline (pH more than 7.0). The initial insertion of the tube typically is frightening to children because they may choke and gag as it passes the pharynx. Children, however, are generally surprised that once the initial insertion is done, the tube is not uncomfortable. They need a great deal of support during the procedure, however, because it is so unusual for them and initially so uncomfortable. Duodenal analysis may also be done by endoscopy; for this, children usually receive conscious sedation (Lee et al., 2008).

The secretions removed from the duodenum are sent to the laboratory for analysis of trypsin content, the easiest pancreatic enzyme to assay. Keep the secretions cold during transport. They should be analyzed immediately for accurate results.

Stool Analysis. Stool may be collected and analyzed for fat content and lack of trypsin, although description of the large greasy appearance may be all that is necessary.

Pulmonary Testing. A chest radiograph generally confirms the extent of the pulmonary involvement (pockets of emphysema and perhaps beginning pneumonia infiltration are present). Pulmonary function tests may be done to determine if atelectasis and emphysema are present.

Therapeutic Management. Therapy for children with CF consists of measures to reduce the involvement of the pancreas, lungs, and sweat glands. Because so many organs are involved, care works best if it is a collaborative process (Rideout, 2007).

Nursing Diagnoses and Related Interventions

Nursing Diagnosis: Imbalanced nutrition, less than body requirements, related to inability to digest fat

Outcome Evaluation: Child's height and weight follow percentile growth curves; quantity of stool decreases; signs and symptoms of vitamin deficiency are absent.

Children with CF are placed on a high-calorie, high-protein, moderate-fat diet. Water-miscible forms of vitamins A, D, and E are supplemented. Medium-chain triglycerides are used with the diet because these are more readily digested than other oils. During the hot months of the year, extra salt may be added to food to replace that lost though perspiration.

Generally, infants with CF cannot be totally breast-fed because there is not enough protein in breast milk for them (they need large amounts because they cannot make use of all the protein they ingest). Breastfeeding with supplementary formula is required. Some of these children, unfortunately, are initially diagnosed as having a milk allergy and are treated by being placed on a soybean formula. This does not contain enough protein either, and their malnutrition increases greatly while they are taking this formula. A high-protein formula, such as Probana, is generally recommended as a supplement.

Because children with CF have a ravenous appetite, they eat well. Before each meal or snack, they need to take a synthetic pancreatic enzyme, pancreatic lipase (Cotazym or Pancrease), to replace the enzyme they cannot produce (Box 40.14). These synthetic enzymes are supplied in large capsules that must be opened for young children because they cannot swallow such a big capsule; infants, in particular, may not have enough gastric acids to dissolve the capsule. The powder from the capsule is then added to a small amount (no more than a teaspoonful) of food. It should not be added to hot food, or a large portion of enzyme activity can be destroyed. Also, it must not be added to the infant's bottle of formula, because the infant may not drink the entire bottle and therefore will not receive the total benefit of the enzyme. When children are taking a synthetic source of pancreatic enzyme this way, the size of stools and the accompanying foul odor decreases. Children begin to gain weight. In adolescence, children may have a great deal of difficulty eating enough to maintain weight, even with enzyme therapy, because their growth spurt requires so many additional calories.

If children with CF become overheated, they begin to lose excessive sodium and chloride through perspiration and become dehydrated. Caution parents to keep their house temperature at 72° F or below and to offer water frequently. They also need to supervise outside play to guard against overexertion or heat exposure.

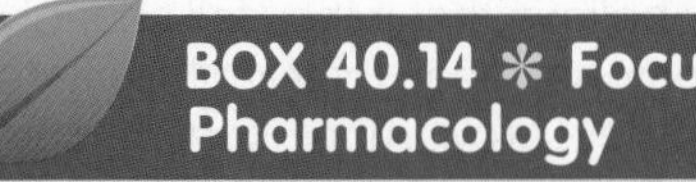

BOX 40.14 * Focus on Pharmacology

Pancrelipase (Cotazym)

Classification: Pancrelipase is an enzyme replacement.

Action: Used to aid digestion in children with cystic fibrosis (Karch, 2009).

Pregnancy risk category: C

Dosage:

- Children 6 months to 1 year of age: 2000 U orally per meal
- Children 1 to 6 years of age: 4000 to 8000 U orally with each meal and 4000 U with snacks
- Children 7 to 12 years of age: 4000 to 12,000 U orally with each meal and with snacks

Possible adverse effects: Nausea, abdominal cramps, diarrhea, hypersensitivity

Nursing Implications

- Administer the drug before or with meals and snacks. Instruct parents and child to do the same.
- Caution child and parents to avoid inhaling powder or spilling it on the hands, because it may irritate the skin or mucous membranes.
- Do not crush or let the child chew the enteric form of the drug.
- Instruct the child and parents about possible adverse effects and encourage them to contact their health care provider should any become severe.

Nursing Diagnosis: Ineffective airway clearance related to inability to clear mucus from the respiratory tract

Outcome Evaluation: Child's temperature is below 100.4° F (38.0° C); Po_2 is 80 to 90 mm Hg; Pco_2 is less than 40 mm Hg.

Unfortunately, the pulmonary effects of CF progress despite supplementation with pancreatic enzyme; infection from plugged airways is always a possibility. Therefore, it is important to try to keep bronchial secretions as moist and freely flowing as possible so they can drain from the bronchial tree. This is done by frequent nebulization or aerosol therapy followed by chest physiotherapy.

Be certain to observe children with CF frequently because their condition can change rapidly. If a portion of a lung becomes obstructed from a plug of mucus, a child can quickly experience respiratory difficulty. The right side of the heart tends to enlarge in children with chronic respiratory disease because the congestion in the lungs increases pressure in the pulmonary artery and the right ventricle. After a period of stress or exercise, children may begin to show signs of cardiac failure because their already enlarged heart cannot compensate any further.

Humidified Oxygen. Oxygen is supplied to children by mask, prongs, ventilators, or nebulizers. Mist can be supplied by an ultrasonic compressor and delivered through a nebulizer mask, which makes the droplet size so small the mist reaches the smallest bronchial spaces.

Aerosol Therapy. Three or four times a day, children may be given aerosol therapy by means of a nebulizer to provide antibiotics or bronchodilators. Antibiotics are specifically determined by culture. A mucolytic, such as acetylcysteine (Mucomyst), can be added to the mist to aid in diluting and liquefying secretions. Children's coughs will become loose and productive after using aerosol therapy. Provide a box of tissues so a child can cough up these loose secretions. Observe children to ensure that they can cough and keep the airway clear. Never give cough syrups to suppress a cough, because getting secretions out is essential for air exchange and to prevent infection. Likewise, question an order for codeine as an analgesic, because codeine suppresses the cough reflex.

Chest Physiotherapy. Because the bronchial secretions with CF are so tenacious, even with liquefaction by mist or aerosol therapy, children may be unable to raise them. To aid drainage of secretions, children need chest physiotherapy frequently, approximately three or four times a day.

Activity. Children with CF need to maintain their usual activities as much as possible. When in bed, they need frequent position changes so that, at various times of the day, all lobes of their lungs will be encouraged to drain by being in a superior position. Be certain they sit up part of each day to drain the upper lobes. This change in position also helps to prevent skin breakdown over bony prominences.

Respiratory Hygiene. The sputum that a child coughs up may have a disagreeable taste or odor. Offer frequent mouth care, toothbrushing, and a good-tasting mouthwash to make the child's mouth feel fresh.

Nursing Diagnosis: Risk for impaired skin integrity related to acid stools

Outcome Evaluation: Child's skin does not exhibit areas of erythema or ulceration; rectal prolapse is not present.

Until children are regulated on pancreatic enzymes, their stool is particularly irritating because of its high fat content. Children who are not toilet-trained need to have their diapers changed immediately after they wet or pass stool so that they do not develop skin irritation and breakdown in the diaper area.

After a bowel movement, check the rectum for rectal prolapse. Because of weak musculature of the rectal area, this is a common complication. A prolapse of rectal mucosa appears as a bright-red mass protruding from the anal sphincter. This mucosa must be replaced promptly before its blood supply is compromised. Place the child on the slant board used for chest physiotherapy with the head lower than the buttocks; then, with a lubricated, gloved hand, gently replace the prolapsed rectal mass. Afterward, compress the buttocks together to maintain gentle pressure on the anus for a few minutes. This is much less of a problem in children who are receiving pancreatic enzymes than in those who are not, because the incidence of rectal prolapse decreases with better nutrition.

Nursing Diagnosis: Risk for compromised family coping related to chronic illness in a child

Outcome Evaluation: Family members state they have adequate resources to cope with current circumstances.

The parents of children with CF are asked to assume a great deal of responsibility for care of their child. Begin discharge planning when a child is first admitted to a hospital in terms of what changes need to be made to accommodate the child at home and to familiarize parents with the necessary care measures. For example, many children with this disorder sleep with oxygen by cannula at night when they are at home. Parents need to be taught the functions of oxygen and how to regulate the flow. This type of learning is most effective if a little is taught every day (for example, "Could you turn the oxygen on for me, Mrs. Smith? I'm ready to tuck Brian in to sleep" rather than a sit-down, let-me-tell-you-how-oxygen-works lecture given close to the day of discharge). Teach parents how to do chest physiotherapy the same way.

The family will have to think through how the care of this child will affect their home life. They are going to be spending a great deal of time caring for the child, so they will need to balance work, care of the child, and care of the rest of the family. Many parents become fatigued after the first week of having the child at home; they may believe that if they fall soundly asleep at night, they may not hear their child call to them if in distress. As they grow more confident in their ability to evaluate their child's condition before bedtime, their apprehension will lessen, but real confidence may not come for months, even years. This may always be a problem for some parents.

Be sure that parents have the telephone number of the health care provider they should call if they feel overwhelmed. Encourage parents to join a support group, so that there are other people available who understand and to whom they can voice their concerns. At these times, one of the most important needs they have is to verbalize to someone what it feels like to be the parent of a child with CF, including feelings of guilt they may be experiencing because the disease is inherited.

Adequate Rest and Comfort. Any child who has compromised lung function has a degree of dyspnea that leads to exhaustion. To counteract this, provide periods of rest during the day, but do not group too many activities or procedures together all at once, as this could exhaust a child. Plan a rest period before meals so that a child is not too tired to eat. Also plan for a long rest period before chest physiotherapy so that a child will be able to tolerate it better. Achieving a balance between allowing periods of rest and yet not doing all procedures at once is not an easy task.

Growth and Development. Children need to be exposed to as many normal life experiences as possible. This may be difficult because it is important not to tire the child out or expose the child to crowds of people (possibly increasing the risk for infection). Assist parents with planning age-appropriate activities with the child.

Children should attend regular school if at all possible so they are provided with socialization experiences with other children. If this is not possible, a home tutor can be arranged for them. Urge children to participate to the extent they can in physical fitness activities in school or with friends. Use a reminder sheet as necessary so they can remember to take pancreatic enzymes with them if they are going to be eating lunch in the school cafeteria or outside the home.

Continuing Care. Ensure that children with CF receive periodic health assessments and routine childhood immunizations. It is not unusual for children with a chronic disease to fall behind in routine checkups and immunizations if they are hospitalized at the times these are routinely done. It is particularly important that children with CF receive the pertussis and measles vaccines, because these two infections cause severe respiratory complications. Children also should receive influenza, meningococcal, and pneumococcal vaccines.

As children with CF reach adolescence, they are candidates for lung transplants. Some of these are done as lower lobe transplants from a living donor. People who donate a single lobe in this manner report that they feel little loss of lung capacity afterward. A lung transplant is advantageous for children with CF because the new lung does not possess the defective gene that caused mucus to be so thick. Life span can greatly improve.

✔ Checkpoint Question 40.5

Children with cystic fibrosis take the pancreatic enzyme pancrelipase before each meal. You would prepare this by:

a. Opening the capsule and adding it to warm tea.
b. Adding it to at least 8 ounces of milk to drink.
c. Sprinkling it on a small amount of applesauce.
d. Teaching the child how to swallow large capsules.

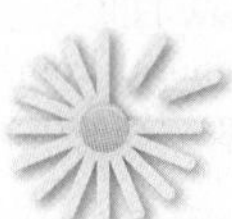

Key Points for Review

- Respiratory tract disorders tend to occur more frequently in children than adults, because the lumens of children's bronchi are narrow and obstruction and infection can occur more easily.
- Infants with respiratory illness need extremely close observation because they cannot describe oxygen deprivation. Young children do not comprehend the fact that oxygen supports combustion. Observe them more frequently than adults to be certain that no flames, such as birthday candles, are brought within 10 feet of an oxygen source.
- Acute nasopharyngitis (common cold) is the most common infectious disease in children. There is no specific therapy for a common cold other than comfort measures.
- Tonsillitis is infection and inflammation of the palatine tonsils. Adenitis is infection and inflammation of the adenoid tonsils. Children with recurring infections may have their tonsils surgically removed.
- Laryngotracheobronchitis (croup) is inflammation of the larynx, trachea, and major bronchi. Epiglottitis is inflammation of the epiglottis. Both of these conditions can cause severe impairment of the airway. Children with epiglottitis should never be assessed for a gag reflex with a tongue blade because the elevated epiglottis can completely occlude the airway.
- Bronchitis is inflammation of the major bronchi and trachea. Bronchiolitis is inflammation of the fine bronchioles. Both conditions are caused by bacterial or viral invasion.
- Respiratory syncytial virus infection is an infection that accounts for the majority of lower respiratory infections in young children. Infants with RSV infections must be observed closely because they are prone to apnea.
- Pneumonia may occur from a variety of organisms (viral, pneumococcal, chlamydial, mycoplasmal, lipid, and hydrocarbon). Except for viral pneumonia, children need specific antibiotics, depending on the organism present.
- Asthma, a type I hypersensitivity reaction, is a diffuse and obstructive airway disease with wheezing as the most common symptom. Newer drugs such as leukotriene receptor antagonists and careful environmental control have aided in the management of this disorder.
- Tuberculosis is a lung infection that is growing in incidence, with some strains becoming very resistant to the usual therapy. The entire family needs drug therapy if one member develops a primary lesion.
- Cystic fibrosis is a disease in which there is generalized dysfunction of the exocrine glands. This results in malabsorption and tenacious pulmonary secretions, leading to infection and pneumonia. Lung transplantation can be used to replace the diseased lung tissue and increase the child's life span.

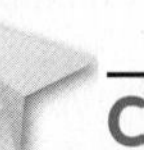

CRITICAL THINKING EXERCISES

1. Michael is the 4-year-old you met at the beginning of the chapter. His grandmother brought him to the emergency room because his respirations were rapid and he had a sharp, barking cough. He is diagnosed as having laryngotracheobronchitis (croup). He was crying loudly. What about Michael's actions would lead you to believe his airway is not yet extremely constricted? Would you encourage him to lie down and rest? What emergency care does Michael need?
2. One of Michael's observation unit roommates has a permanent tracheostomy tube in place from pulmonary dysplasia as an infant. Her parents are going to enroll her in kindergarten starting next month. What

precautions would you want to review with her parents to keep this experience safe?

3. When the 4-year-old in the ambulatory bed next to Michael returns from tonsillectomy surgery, what observations would be most important to make? Why is the 7th day after tonsillectomy surgery a particularly important day for close observation?
5. Examine the National Health Goals related to respiratory disorders in children. Most government-sponsored funds for nursing research are allotted based on these goals. What would be a possible research topic to explore pertinent to these goals that would be applicable to Michael's family and also advance evidence-based practice?

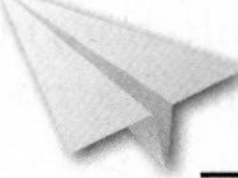

CRITICAL THINKING SCENARIO

Open the accompanying CD-ROM or visit http://thePoint.lww.com and read the Patient Scenario included for this chapter, then answer the questions to further sharpen your skills and grow more familiar with NCLEX style questions related to respiratory disorders in children. Confirm your answers are correct by reading the rationales.

REFERENCES

American Heart Association. (2008). *Pediatric advanced life support.* Dallas, TX: Author.

Awasthi, S., et al. (2008). Does 3-day course of oral amoxicillin benefit children of non-severe pneumonia with wheeze? *PLoS ONE, 3*(4), e1991.

Boguniewicz, M. (2008). Allergic disorders. In W. W. Hay, et al. (Eds.). *Current pediatric diagnosis and treatment* (18th ed.). Columbus, OH: McGraw-Hill.

Burton, M. J., & Doree, C. J. (2009). Interventions for recurrent idiopathic epistaxis (nosebleeds) in children. *Cochrane Database of Systematic Reviews, 2009*(1), (CD004461).

Carpenter, T. C., et al. (2008). Critical care. In W. W. Hay, et al. (Eds.). *Current pediatric diagnosis and treatment* (18th ed.). Columbus, OH: McGraw-Hill.

Chauvin, N. A., Chen, M. Y., & Anthony, E. Y. (2007). Air in all the wrong places. *Contemporary Pediatrics, 24*(2), 32–36.

Deglin, J. H., & Vallerand, A. H. (2008). *Davis's drug guide for nurses* (10th ed.). Philadelphia: F.A. Davis.

Department of Health and Human Services. (2008). *Recommendations regarding use of over-the-counter cough and cold products.* Washington, DC: Author.

Gardner, J. (2007).What you need to know about cystic fibrosis. *Nursing, 37*(7), 52–55.

Groeben, H., et al. (2008). Different mechanisms of atelectasis formation require different treatment strategies. *Experimental Lung Research, 34*(3), 115–124.

Hueston, W. J. (2008). Respiratory problems. In J. E. South-Paul, S. C. Matheny, & E. L. Lewis. (Eds.). *Current diagnosis and treatment in family medicine* (2nd ed.). Columbus, OH: McGraw-Hill.

Jawaheer, J., et al. (2008). Primary resection and anastomosis for complicated meconium ileus: a safe procedure? *Pediatric Surgery International, 23*(11), 1091–1093.

Kamienski, M. (2007). Emergency. When sore throat gets serious: three different cases, three very different causes. *American Journal of Nursing, 107*(10), 35–38.

Karch, A. M. (2009). *Lippincott's nursing drug guide.* Philadelphia: Lippincott Williams & Wilkins.

Kelley, P. E., et al. (2008). Ear, nose and throat. In W. W. Hay, et al. (Eds.). *Current pediatric diagnosis and treatment* (18th ed.). Columbus, OH: McGraw-Hill.

Kerby, G. S., et al. (2008). Respiratory tract and mediastinum. In W. W. Hay, et al. (Eds.). *Current pediatric diagnosis and treatment* (18th ed.). Columbus, OH: McGraw-Hill.

Lee, K. K., et al. (2008). Modifications in endoscopic practice for pediatric patients. *Gastrointestinal Endoscopy, 67*(1), 1–9.

Levin, M. J., & Weinberg, A. (2008). Infections: viral and rickettsial. In W. W. Hay, et al. (Eds.). *Current pediatric diagnosis and treatment* (18th ed.). Columbus, OH: McGraw-Hill.

Long, R., & Boffa, J. (2007). Why internationally adopted children should be screened for tuberculosis. *CMAJ: Canadian Medical Association Journal, 177*(2), 172–173.

Mannix, R., & Bachur, R. (2007). Status asthmaticus in children. *Current Opinion in Pediatrics, 19*(3), 281–287.

Mansbach, J. M. (2008). Prospective multicenter study of bronchiolitis: Predicting safe discharges from the emergency department. *Pediatrics, 121*(4), 680–688.

Marino, P. L. (2007). *The ICU book.* Philadelphia: Lippincott Williams & Wilkins.

McMullen, A., et al. (2007). Asthma care of children in clinical practice: do parents report receiving appropriate education? *Pediatric Nursing, 33*(1), 37–44.

Merelle, M. E., et al. (2009). Newborn screening for cystic fibrosis. *Cochrane Database of Systematic Reviews, 2009*(1), (CD001402).

Millar, K.R., et al. (2007). Suspected peritonsillar abscess in children. *Pediatric Emergency Care, 23*(7), 431–438.

Ogle, J. W., & Anderson, M. S. (2008). Infections: bacterial and spirochetal. In W. W. Hay, et al. (Eds.). *Current pediatric diagnosis and treatment* (18th ed.). Columbus, OH: McGraw-Hill.

Page, N. C., Bauer, E. M., & Lieu, J. E. (2008). Clinical features and treatment of retropharyngeal abscess in children. *Otolaryngology-Head and Neck Surgery, 138*(3), 300–306.

Pritchard, M., Flenady, V., & Woodgate, P. (2009). Preoxygenation for tracheal suctioning in intubated, ventilated newborn infants. *Cochrane Database of Systematic Reviews, 2009*(1), (CD000427).

Quintero, D. R., & Gershan, W. M. (2007). Diagnosis and treatment of infants with bronchiolitis. *Journal of Clinical Outcomes Management, 14*(4), 205–210.

Raab, E. L. (2007). The resuscitation and care of the newborn at risk. In A. H. Decherney & L. Nathan (Eds.). *Current diagnosis and treatment in obstetrics and gynecology* (10th ed.). Columbus, OH: McGraw-Hill.

Revai, K., et al. (2007). Incidence of acute otitis media and sinusitis complicating upper respiratory tract infection: the effect of age. *Pediatrics, 119*(6), e1408–e412.

Richter, G. T., et al. (2008). Late-onset laryngomalacia: a variant of disease. *Archives of Otolaryngology-Head & Neck Surgery, 134*(1), 75–80.

Rideout, K. (2007). Evaluation of a PNP care coordinator model for hospitalized children, adolescents, and young adults with cystic fibrosis. *Pediatric Nursing, 33*(1), 29–36.

Rosbe, K.W. (2008). Foreign bodies. In A. K. Lalwani (Ed.). *Current diagnosis and treatment in otolaryngology—head and neck surgery* (2nd ed.). Columbus, OH: McGraw-Hill.

Ryan, T., Brewer, M., & Small, L. (2008). Over-the-counter cough and cold medication use in young children. *Pediatric Nursing, 34*(2), 174–180.

Scow, D. T., Luttermoser, G. K., & Dickerson, K. S. (2007). Leukotriene inhibitors in the treatment of allergy and asthma. *American Family Physician, 75*(1), 65–70.

Spence, K., & Barr, P. (2009). Nasal versus oral intubation for mechanical ventilation of newborn infants. *Cochrane Database of Systematic Reviews, 2009*(1), (CD000948).

Spurling, G. K. P., et al. (2009). Antibiotics for bronchiolitis in children. *Cochrane Database of Systematic Reviews, 2009*(1), (CD005189).

Starke, J. R. (2007). New concepts in childhood tuberculosis. *Current Opinion in Pediatrics, 19*(3), 306–313.

Steer, A. C., Danchin, M. H., & Carapetis, J. R. (2007). Group A streptococcal infections in children. *Journal of Paediatrics & Child Health, 43*(4), 203–213.

Subramanian, A., et al. (2008). *Drug facts and comparisons.* St. Louis: Wolters Kluwer Health.

van der Schans, C., Prasad, A., & Main, E. (2009). Chest physiotherapy compared to no chest physiotherapy for cystic fibrosis. *Cochrane Database of Systematic Reviews, 2009*(1), (CD001401).

Ventre, K., & Randolph, A. G. (2009). Ribavirin for respiratory syncytial virus infection of the lower respiratory tract in infants and young children. *Cochrane Database of Systematic Reviews, 2009*(1), (CD000181).

Visner, G. A., & Goldfarb, S. B. (2007). Posttransplant monitoring of pediatric lung transplant recipients. *Current Opinion in Pediatrics, 19*(3), 321–326.

Yates, P. D., & Anari, S. (2008). Otitis media. In A. K. Lalwani (Ed.). *Current diagnosis and treatment in otolaryngology—head and neck surgery* (2nd ed.). Columbus, OH: McGraw-Hill.

Yost, C. C., & Soll, R. F. (2009). Early versus delayed selective surfactant treatment for neonatal respiratory distress syndrome. *Cochrane Database of Systematic Reviews, 2009*(1), (CD001456).

Yu, K. C.Y . (2008). Airway management and tracheotomy. In A. K. Lalwani (Ed.). *Current diagnosis and treatment in otolaryngology—head and neck surgery* (2nd ed.). Columbus, OH: McGraw-Hill.

Zimmerman, R. K. (2007). Influenza. In F. J. Domino. (Ed.). *The 5-minute clinical consult.* Philadelphia: Lippincott Williams & Wilkins.

SUGGESTED READINGS

Aly, H. (2007). Is there a strategy for preventing bronchopulmonary dysplasia? Absence of evidence is not evidence of absence. *Pediatrics, 119*(4), 818–820.

Asensio, O., et al. (2009). Home intravenous antibiotics for cystic fibrosis. *Cochrane Database of Systematic Reviews, 2009*(1), (CD001917).

Baum, S. G., & Carey, J. (2007). Preventing and treating influenza. *Infections in Medicine, 24*(1), 13–17.

Burton, M. J., Towler, B., & Glasziou, P. (2009). Tonsillectomy versus non-surgical treatment for chronic/recurrent acute tonsillitis. *Cochrane Database of Systematic Reviews, 2009*(1), (CD001802).

Collins, J. D. (2007). A young child with a history of foreign body aspiration. *Family Practice Recertification, 29*(3), 12–15.

Karr, C., et al. (2007). Effects of subchronic and chronic exposure to ambient air pollutants on infant bronchiolitis. *American Journal of Epidemiology, 165*(5), 553–560.

Moore, M., & Little, P. (2009). Humidified air inhalation for treating croup. *Cochrane Database of Systematic Reviews, 2009*(1), (CD002870).

Murphy, M. F., et al. (2008). The young airway: Prehospital assessment and management of pediatric respiratory distress. *JEMS: Journal of Emergency Medical Services, 33*(6), 58–60.

Verhulst, S. L., et al. (2007). Sleep-disordered breathing in overweight and obese children and adolescents: Prevalence, characteristics and the role of fat distribution. *Archives of Disease in Childhood, 92*(3), 205–208.

Willis, K. C. (2007). Bronchiolitis: Advanced practice focus in the emergency department. *Journal of Emergency Nursing, 33*(4), 346–351.

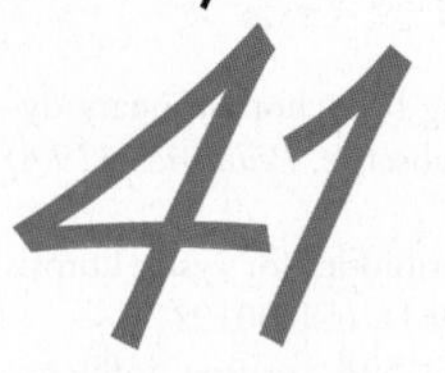

Chapter 41 Nursing Care of a Family When a Child Has a Cardiovascular Disorder

KEY TERMS

- acyanotic heart disease
- afterload
- balloon angioplasty
- cardiac catheterization
- congestive heart failure
- contractility
- cyanosis
- cyanotic heart disease
- diastole
- innocent heart murmur
- left-to-right shunt
- organic heart murmur
- polycythemia
- postcardiac surgery syndrome
- postperfusion syndrome
- preload
- right-to-left shunt
- systole
- vasculitis

OBJECTIVES

After mastering the contents of this chapter, you should be able to:

1. Describe the common cardiovascular disorders of childhood.
2. Identify National Health Goals related to children with cardiovascular disorders that nurses could help the nation achieve.
3. Use critical thinking to analyze ways that nursing care of children with cardiovascular disorders could be more family centered.
4. Assess a child with a cardiovascular dysfunction.
5. Formulate nursing diagnoses for a child with a cardiovascular disorder.
6. Identify appropriate outcomes based on the priority needs of a child with a cardiovascular disorder.
7. Plan nursing care for a child with a cardiovascular disorder.
8. Implement nursing care for a child with a cardiovascular disorder such as teaching about the importance of taking prescribed medication.
9. Evaluate expected outcomes for achievement and effectiveness of care.
10. Identify areas related to the care of children with cardiovascular disorders that could benefit from additional nursing research or application of evidence-based practice.
11. Integrate knowledge of cardiovascular disorders with nursing process to achieve quality maternal and child health nursing care.

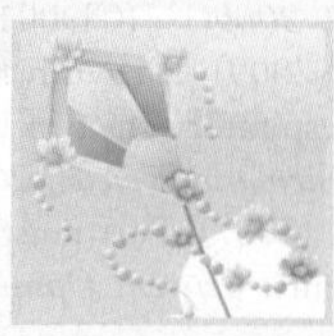

Megan is a newborn who was born with tetralogy of Fallot. By 1 hour of age, she developed rapid respirations, tachycardia, and cyanosis. An echocardiogram revealed the typical four structural defects of the syndrome. Megan's parents will be taking her home for a month to await cardiac surgery. They tell you their doctor instructed them to "watch her carefully" during that time. "What does that mean?" they ask you. Will they be able to take her outside in a stroller? Should she sleep in their bedroom? Exactly what should they watch for?

Previous chapters described the growth and development of well children. This chapter adds information about the child who is ill with a cardiovascular disorder and the stress that such a serious diagnosis places on families. Such information builds a base for care and health teaching for children with these disorders.

What advice would you give Megan's parents?

The cardiovascular system, the body system on which all other systems depend, consists of the heart, which acts as a pump; the blood, which provides the fluid and cells for transport of oxygen and nutrients; and the blood vessels, which provide the means and routes for transport throughout the body. The regular pumping of the heart propels oxygen and needed nutrients through the bloodstream to cells and allows waste products to be removed from cells and transported to the lungs or kidneys for excretion. The cardiovascular system also transports regulatory materials such as hormones, enzymes, and antibodies to the body systems. It can adapt to changing body needs by adjusting the rate and force of heart pumping, modifying the size of the blood vessels, and altering the volume and composition of the blood (Bashore & Granger, 2009).

Most cardiovascular disorders in children occur as a result of a congenital anomaly; either the heart developed inadequately in utero, or the heart cannot adapt to extrauterine life for some reason. Open-heart surgery often is the only treatment that will correct the primary congenital problem. Children also may experience acquired cardiovascular disorders, such as rheumatic fever or Kawasaki disease. All these disorders can lead to inadequate heart function.

Cardiovascular disorders are frightening for both children and parents, as even small children realize the importance of their hearts in sustaining life, and they recognize the seriousness of any illness that undermines the heart's activity. For the families of children with a cardiovascular disorder, understanding the functioning of the heart and circulation is an important first step toward coping with the illness. Cardiac disorders are a major focus of health promotion and disease prevention measures in both adults and children. National Health Goals related to cardiovascular illness and children are shown in Box 41.1.

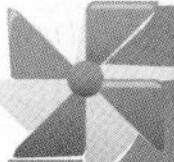

BOX 41.1 * Focus on National Health Goals

Cardiovascular illness is a major health problem in adults. However, the illness and its effects can be prevented or at least minimized by instituting measures early in childhood. A number of National Health Goals address ways that children should modify nutrition or exercise to achieve better cardiovascular health:

- Increase the proportion of adolescents who engage in vigorous physical activity that promotes cardiorespiratory fitness 3 or more days per week for 20 or more minutes per occasion from a baseline of 65% to at least 85%.
- Increase the proportion of persons aged 2 years and older who consume less than 10% of calories from saturated fat from a baseline of 36% to a target level of 75%.
- Reduce the proportion of children and adolescents who are overweight or obese from a baseline of 11% to a target level of 5% (http://www.nih.gov).

Nurses can help the nation achieve these goals by educating parents and children about the importance of reducing obesity and planning exercise and nutrition programs for sound cardiovascular health. It is equally important for nurses to caution parents not to start their children on reduced-fat diets until they are 2 years old, to allow for myelination of nerve cells.

Nursing research is needed to determine what weight loss programs are the most effective for children, what reduced-fat foods make the best finger foods for preschoolers, what snacks schools could provide in snack machines that would have a reduced fat content and would also be eaten by children, and what are effective ways to increase physical activity in adolescents who do not participate in any type of organized sport or exercise program.

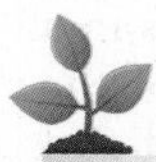

Nursing Process Overview

For Care of a Child With a Cardiovascular Disorder

Assessment

Assessment of a child with a cardiovascular disorder includes both careful history taking and physical examination, because many of the signs and symptoms of heart disease in children are subtle. A variety of diagnostic studies such as echocardiography or electrocardiography or cardiac catheterization may be used to confirm the diagnosis and prepare a child for surgery. Teaching about these tests and providing psychological support to children and their families are two major responsibilities of nurses throughout the assessment process.

Remember that hypertension, hypercholesterolemia, and congenital heart disorders occur at higher incidences in some families than others because these disorders tend to be familial. Hypertension, for example, occurs at a higher rate in African Americans than in other groups. Nurses have a responsibility to educate adolescents about the importance of maintaining a sensible weight and sodium intake and reducing saturated fat and cholesterol intake, in an attempt to minimize these familial disorders. Be knowledgeable about cultural preferences in foods when planning preventive health care.

Nursing Diagnosis

Nursing diagnoses associated with heart disease in children usually speak to the effect of poor circulation on body tissues or the effect a serious disorder can create on the child or parents. Examples are:

- Decreased cardiac output related to congenital structural disorder
- Ineffective tissue perfusion related to inadequate cardiac output
- Deficient knowledge related to care of the child pre- and postoperatively
- Fear related to lack of knowledge about child's illness
- Interrupted family processes related to stresses of the diagnosis and care responsibilities
- Ineffective coping related to lack of adequate support people
- Impaired parenting related to inability to bond with critically ill newborn

If the concerns in the latter three diagnoses are not identified when a child is ill, they may continue long after a child is treated and returns home.

If a child will be undergoing surgery or cardiac catheterization, nursing diagnoses will focus on the psychological needs of the child and family for preparation and postprocedure care in addition to physical concerns after the procedure such as hypothermia related to cooling during surgery; powerlessness related to conscious sedation during cardiac catheterization.

Outcome Identification and Planning

Nursing planning is essential to help parents and children understand heart anatomy. A sound knowledge base will help them understand the need for diagnostic testing. Additional teaching is necessary to prepare parents and children for procedures or surgery and recovery at home. Teaching parents to conscientiously administer cardiac medications is another area where planning plays an important role. Part of this planning includes establishing appropriate outcomes to help a child and parents adjust to a serious diagnosis, now and in the future, such as coping with their present fears and caring for the child at home. Parents may wish to contact the American Heart Association (www.americanheart.org) for educational materials and family support groups in their area.

Implementation

Nursing interventions in the care of children with a cardiovascular disorder include teaching, providing an opportunity for children and their families to express fears about a child's illness and treatment plan, providing physiologic and psychological support such as comfort measures after surgery, and caring for a child in cardiac failure. An equally important role is teaching prevention of heart disease. Measures such as promoting nonsmoking and exercise, maintaining appropriate weight, and eating a low-fat diet are discussed in Chapter 32.

Outcome Evaluation

Outcome evaluation should be both short and long term for the child and family. It is important for families to receive adequate immediate support during procedures and treatment. If long-term care is necessary, evaluating the family's ability to think of their child not in terms of illness but in terms of wellness is also key. Provide opportunities for parents to express their concerns about their child at follow-up visits to help address any misconceptions about their child's future.

Examples suggesting achievement of outcomes are:

- Child's heart rate remains within accepted parameters for age.
- Child demonstrates age-appropriate coping skills related to diagnosis and possible surgery.
- Parents demonstrate competence with procedures required for care of their child.
- Parents exhibit positive coping skills related to their child's diagnosis and required care to foster optimal growth and development in their child.
- Parents verbalize positive aspects about their child.

THE CARDIOVASCULAR SYSTEM

Embryologic development of the heart is described in Chapter 9. Cardiac adaptations at birth are described in Chapter 18. After these adaptations, the heart can be thought of as consisting of two pumps: the right side pumps blood to the lungs, where it is oxygenated before returning to the left side of the heart; the left side pumps the oxygenated blood to the peripheral tissues through systemic arteries. After supplying nutrients and collecting wastes, the blood returns through the veins to the right side of the heart, where the cycle begins again. Contraction of the chambers is termed **systole**; relaxation is termed **diastole**. Normal heart anatomy is shown in Figure 41.1.

Most heart disease in children occurs because embryonic structures necessary for fetal life did not close at birth or the heart originally formed inappropriately. For example, a septal defect between the right and left sides of the heart may remain open. Because pressure and volume on the left side of the heart are greater than on the right side, blood will flow through the connecting opening left to right, or from the area of stronger heart action to the area of weaker heart action, compromising right-sided function.

Cardiac output (CO) is the volume of blood pumped by the ventricles each minute. It is calculated by multiplying stroke volume (the volume of blood a ventricle ejects during systole) by the heart rate (beats per minute). CO is affected by three main factors: preload, contractility, and afterload. **Preload** is the volume of blood in the ventricles at the end of diastole (the point just before contraction). **Afterload** refers to the resistance against which the ventricles must pump. **Contractility,** the ability of the ventricles to stretch, refers to the force of contraction generated by the myocardial muscle. The Frank-Starling law predicts that the stroke volume can be increased by increasing the stretch of the fibers. Excessive stretch, however, results in a decrease in cardiac output as the heart tires. Much of the therapy of heart disease is aimed at reducing preload and afterload and increasing contractility to promote better cardiac output.

ASSESSMENT OF HEART DISORDERS IN CHILDREN

The assessment of heart disease in children begins with a thorough history and a physical assessment. More specific diagnostic studies, such as electrocardiography or echocardiography, are ordered as indicated. Because all children with heart disorders have an increased risk of poor tissue perfusion, which may affect growth and development, developmental testing also is incorporated into the assessment.

History

Some congenital heart disorders, such as atrial septal defects, may have a polygenic inheritance pattern. Because the heart arises from the same embryonic origin as the kidney, heart disorders often occur in conjunction with renal disease. Heart disorders also occur as an anomaly in chromosomal disorders such as Down syndrome (Marian, Brugada, & Roberts, 2008).

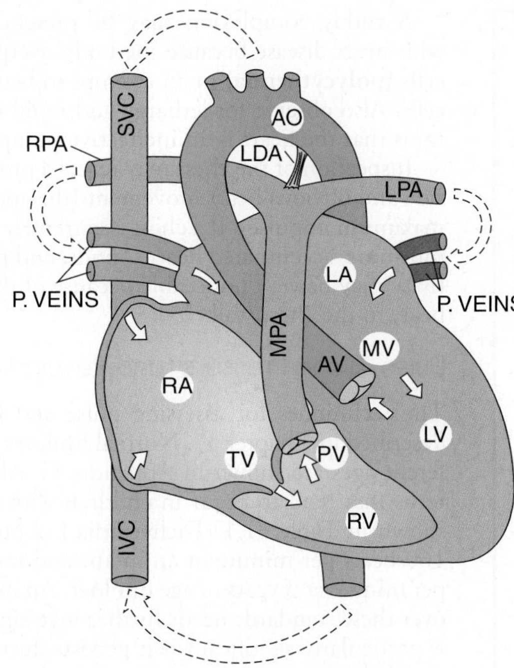

AO–Aorta
AV–Aortic valve
IVC–Inferior vena cava
LA–Left atrium
LPA–Left pulmonary artery
LV–Left ventricle
MPA–Main pulmonary artery
MV–Mitral valve
LDA–Ligamentum ductus arteriosus
PV–Pulmonary valve
P. Vein–Pulmonary vein
RA–Right atrium
RPA–Right pulmonary artery
RV–Right ventricle
SVC–Superior vena cava
TV–Tricuspid valve

FIGURE 41.1 Anatomy of the normal heart.

As a result of technological advances in prenatal health care, such as prenatal ultrasound, which can show poor heart action or a enlarged heart, heart disease may be recognized as early as fetal life. However, even with these advances, heart disease may not be detected before birth. In the newborn period, because the newborn heart rate is so rapid that extra sounds of abnormal circulation may not be heard, heart disease still may not be detected. Because of relatively high pulmonary resistance, defects of the septum may not be readily apparent until about 2 weeks after birth. Infants with heart disease generally have tachycardia and tachypnea. The infant who is breathing rapidly has to stop sucking on a bottle or breast frequently to breathe. The infant who is easily fatigued because of ineffective heart action has to stop sucking to rest before finishing a feeding. Heart disease may be first discovered, therefore, when an infant is brought to a primary care setting at 1 or 2 weeks of age because the child is so fatigued the child is unable to suck long enough to obtain adequate calories or fluid.

A history should include a thorough pregnancy history to try to determine whether an intrauterine insult could have led to poor fetal formation. Cardiac anomalies can occur as a result of intrauterine infections such as toxoplasmosis, cytomegalovirus, or rubella. Also ask whether the mother took any medication during pregnancy, whether nutrition was adequate, or whether she was exposed to any radiation, because these may also contribute to congenital heart disorders.

A mark of older children with heart disease is that they become easily fatigued. When obtaining the history, ask how much activity it takes before a child becomes tired: an hour of strenuous play? A short walk? Be sure parents are not confusing sedentary activities (the child who prefers to sit and read) with activities that are the result of fatigue such as coming home from school and falling asleep day after day.

Ask about a child's usual position when resting. Some infants with congenital heart disease prefer a knee–chest position, whereas older children often voluntarily squat. These positions are unusual in children but trap blood in the lower extremities because of the sharp bend at the knee and hip, allowing the child to oxygenate the blood remaining in the upper body more fully and easily. Also ask about frequency of infections, because children with heart disease have a higher incidence of lower respiratory tract infections than do other children, probably due to less than usual pulmonary circulation. Children with left-to-right shunts tend to perspire excessively because of sympathetic nerve stimulation. Ask if there is an indication of this. Urine is produced only when cardiac function is adequate to perfuse the kidneys. Ask if an infant is wetting diapers or if an older child is voiding normally to discover this. Edema from retained fluid is a late sign of heart disease in children. If it does occur, periorbital edema generally occurs first. **Cyanosis** (a blue tinge to the skin) may occur if a shunt allows deoxygenated blood to enter the arterial system. Such infants generally fail to thrive and are below usual height and weight on a standard growth chart. Children with coarctation of the aorta, discussed below, who have high blood pressure in the head and upper extremities, have a history of nosebleeds and headaches. Because of corresponding low blood pressure in the lower extremities, such children may have pain in the legs on running (reported as "growing pains").

Physical Assessment

Physical assessment of a child with a suspected heart disorder begins with measuring height and weight and comparing these findings against standard growth charts. A thorough physical examination should then be done, with particular emphasis on certain body parts or systems (Box 41.2).

Because a major part of the physical assessment will include inspection, palpation, and auscultation of the chest for heart function, it is best if a child is relaxed and not crying. Provide age-appropriate toys that can distract a child readily.

Box 41.2 Assessment
Assessing a Child With a Cardiovascular Disorder

History
Chief concern: Fatigue, cyanosis, frequent upper respiratory infections, feeding difficulty, poor weight gain, growth failure.
Past medical history: Infection during pregnancy, difficulty with resuscitation at birth.
Family history: Other members with heart disorders.

Physical examination
Decreased height and weight
Easily fatigued

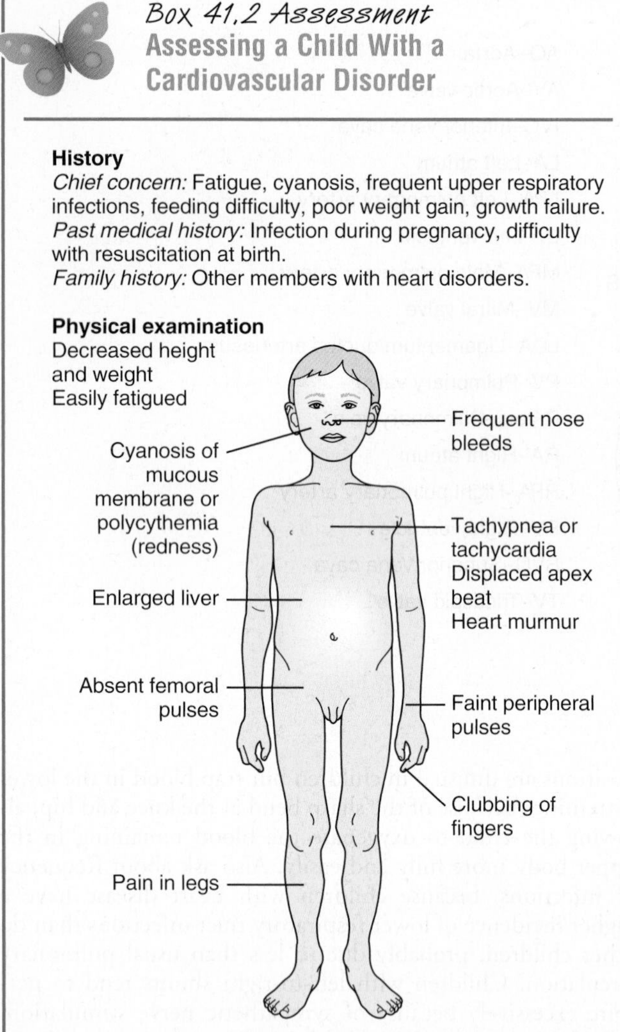

A bottle of formula or breast milk (or asking the mother to breastfeed) can help comfort an infant. Play with both children and infants if possible before an examination so they are acquainted and are not afraid of you.

General Appearance

Inspect toes and fingers (particularly the thumbs) for clubbing and color. Assess capillary refill time by applying slight pressure on a fingernail and quickly releasing. The nailbed will blanch white and then quickly return to pink in a child with good circulation and oxygenation. In a child with poor tissue perfusion, the pink color returns slowly (more than 5 seconds).

The mucous membranes of the mouth are the most likely place for cyanosis to be visible, so always assess the buccal membrane and lips for a blue color. Any time hemoglobin is reduced below 4 to 6 g per 100 mL, cyanosis may not be evident because the severe anemia masks it. Cyanosis persisting for over 20 minutes after birth (except for acrocyanosis) suggests serious cardiopulmonary dysfunction. If the cyanosis increases with crying, cardiac dysfunction is suggested, as this implies the infant cannot meet the increased circulatory demands of extrauterine life. If the cyanosis decreases with crying, pulmonary dysfunction is suggested because crying deepens respirations and aerates more lung tissue.

A ruddy complexion may be present in some children with heart disease because the body overproduces red blood cells **(polycythemia)** in an attempt to better oxygenate body cells. Also observe for lethargy and rapid respirations, symptoms that the heart is an ineffective pump.

Inspection of the chest may reveal a prominence of the left side and obvious heart movement (the apex beat, or point of maximum impulse). If a chest is extremely flat, loud innocent murmurs, accentuated heart sounds, and palpable cardiac activity may be very noticeable because of the proximity of the heart to the chest wall.

Pulse, Blood Pressure, and Respirations

The techniques for assessing pulse and blood pressure are described in Chapter 37. Normal findings for children of different ages are shown in Appendix G. Abnormal pulse patterns that tend to occur in children with heart disorders are shown in Table 41.1. Tachycardia is a pulse rate more than 160 beats per minute in an infant and more than 100 beats per minute at 3 years of age or older. An increase in pulse rate over these standards needs further investigation. Tachycardia is particularly significant if it persists during sleep, when the possibility of excitement and activity is removed.

Murmurs of no significance are termed functional, insignificant, or innocent murmurs. In discussing such murmurs with parents, the term **innocent heart murmur** is best to use because it most clearly describes that the sound heard is not important or is nothing to worry about. Such murmurs probably reflect a normal variation of vibration in the heart or pulmonary artery.

Although innocent murmurs are of no consequence, parents need to be told when their child has one because this finding will undoubtedly be discovered again at a future health assessment. Activities need not be restricted when a child has an innocent murmur and the child requires no more frequent health appraisals than other children. Innocent murmurs do not turn into serious murmurs so parents should not view them as a prelude to heart disease. Innocent murmurs may become more pronounced during

TABLE 41.1 ✻ Abnormal Pulse Patterns

Pulse Pattern	Description
Water hammer	Very forceful and bounding pulse (Corrigan's pulse); capillary pulsations possibly apparent even in the fingernails; suggestive of cardiac insufficiency, as in patent ductus arteriosus
Pulsus alternans	A pulse of one strong beat and one weak beat; suggestive of myocardial weakness
Dicrotic	A double radial pulse for every apical beat; symptomatic of aortic stenosis
Thready	Weak and usually rapid pulse; suggestive of ineffective heart action

TABLE 41.2 ✻ Comparison of Innocent and Organic Murmurs

Characteristic	Innocent	Organic
Timing	Systolic	Systolic or diastolic
Duration	Short	Longer
Quality	Soft, musical	Harsh, blowing
Intensity	Soft	Loud
Position in which heard	Usually supine position	Heard in all positions
Affected by exercise	Yes	No

febrile illness, anxiety, or pregnancy. This is why they may be audible for the first time at a hospital admission or at a sick-child visit. At future health assessments, parents may need to be reassured again that a murmur is innocent.

If a murmur occurs as the result of heart disease or a congenital defect, it is an **organic heart murmur.** The characteristics of innocent and organic murmurs are compared in Table 41.2.

To help differentiate innocent from organic murmurs, describe any murmur that you hear according to:

- Its position in the cardiac cycle, that is, early systolic, midsystolic, late diastolic, etc.
- Duration (how long the sound lasts)
- Quality (blowing, rasping, rumbling)
- Pitch (high- or low-sounding noise)
- Intensity (loudness)
- Location (where it is heard best or the point of maximum intensity)
- Presence of a thrill (a palpable purring sensation)
- The response of the murmur to exercise or change of position.

The intensity, or loudness, of the murmur is graded according to standard criteria shown in Table 34.9, Chapter 34.

Diagnostic Tests

The diagnostic studies performed on a child with suspected heart disease vary with the specific lesion suspected.

Electrocardiogram

An *electrocardiogram* (ECG) is a written record of the electrical voltages generated by the contracting heart. It provides information about heart rate, rhythm, state of the myocardium, presence or absence of hypertrophy (thickening of the heart walls), ischemia or necrosis due to inadequate cardiac circulation, and abnormalities of conduction. It also can provide information about the presence or effect of various drugs and electrolyte imbalances (Morelli, Biancaniello, & Chandran, 2007).

On an ECG waveform tracing, an upward pattern indicates a positive voltage, whereas a downward pattern indicates a negative voltage. The heartbeat is initiated by the sinoatrial (SA) node in the right atrial wall near the entrance of the superior vena cava. From the SA node, the electrical impulse spreads over the atria, reaching the atrioventricular (AV) node in the lower right atrium. From there, it spreads through the AV bundle (bundle of His) and the Purkinje fibers to the walls and septum of the ventricles. At the point that the ventricles have filled, the electrical flow has reached a peak, causing the ventricles to contract.

A normal ECG consists of an atrial wave (the P wave, denoting atrial contraction), a brief hesitation before the AV node is activated, then the prominent peak as the ventricles contract (the QRS spike), another brief hesitation, and then a large slow wave caused by ventricular recovery (the T wave) and often an incompletely understood additional slow wave (the U wave; Fig. 41.2). A longer-than-normal P wave suggests that the atria are hypertrophied and it is taking longer than usual for the electrical conduction to spread over the atria. A lengthened P-R interval suggests that there is difficulty in coordination between the SA and AV nodes (first-degree heart block). A heightened R wave indicates that ventricular hypertrophy is present. An R wave that is decreased in height means that the ventricles cannot contract fully, as happens if they are surrounded by fluid (pericarditis).

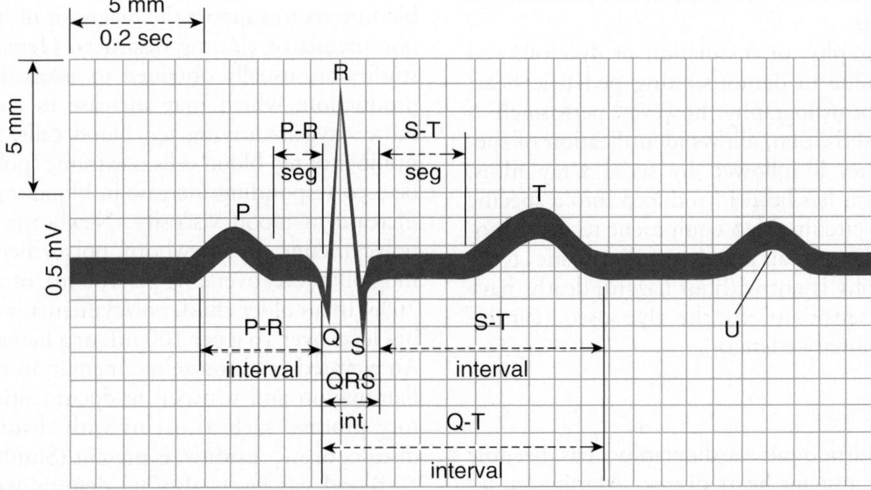

FIGURE 41.2 A normal ECG configuration.

Elongation of the T wave occurs in hyperkalemia; depression of the T wave is associated with anoxia; depression of the ST segment is associated with abnormal calcium levels.

✓ Checkpoint Question 41.1

Megan has a heart murmur from tetralogy of Fallot, a congenital heart disorder. This type of murmur is termed:

a. Innocent
b. Functional
c. Organic
d. Symmetrical

Radiography

X-ray examination can furnish an accurate picture of the heart size and the contour and size of the heart chambers. It can reveal fluid collecting in the lungs or pulmonary artery from cardiac failure. It also can be used to confirm the placement of pacemaker leads. In a posteroanterior view (in children over 1 year of age), if the cardiac width is more than half the chest width, it indicates that the heart is unusually enlarged. In infants, because of the more horizontal position of the heart, this ratio must be increased to more than half.

In addition to a chest radiograph, an upper gastrointestinal (UGI) series may be done. This is because the esophagus is located so close to cardiac chambers that when it is visualized with barium, it can help define cardiovascular structures. Even with this technique, interpretation of atrial or ventricular hypertrophy in infants and children by radiography is difficult. X-ray findings are therefore usually complemented by ECG, a more sensitive and accurate measure of ventricular enlargement.

Fluoroscopy, a form of x-ray, provides a permanent motion-picture record of the size and configuration of the heart and great vessels, lungs, thoracic cage, and diaphragm. Because prolonged observation is necessary to record this information, special precautions must be taken to protect a child and health care personnel from radiation during an assessment.

In radioangiocardiography, a radioactive substance such as technetium is injected intravenously into the bloodstream. As the substance circulates through the heart, it may be traced and recorded on videotape. The procedure involves a low dose of radiation and may be used to demonstrate, in particular, septal shunts.

Generalized angiography, or instillation of dye followed by x-rays, has little value in demonstrating pediatric heart defects. Selective angiocardiography, however, performed as part of a cardiac catheterization, allows identification of specific heart abnormalities if followed by serial x-ray films. After a contrast medium has been introduced into a specific heart chamber, closed-circuit video equipment records fluoroscopy pictures. Although an excellent diagnostic technique, angiocardiography is not without hazard: deaths have been reported from sensitivity to the dye used, cardiac arrhythmias, and pulmonary edema.

Echocardiography

Echocardiography, or ultrasound cardiography, has become the primary diagnostic test for heart disease (Marijon et al., 2007). High-frequency sound waves, directed toward the heart, are used to locate and study the movement and dimensions of cardiac structures, such as the size of chambers, thickness of walls, relationship of major vessels to chambers, and the thickness, motion, and pressure gradients of valves. This technique is referred to as M-mode, a single beam that reveals chamber contractility; two-dimensional, a technique used to reveal chamber and vessel size; and Doppler technique, which reveals the velocity of blood flow. Remind parents that echocardiography does not use x-rays so it can be repeated at frequent intervals without exposing children to the possible risk of radiation. It may be done using a transesophageal probe to better reveal heart chambers (Lim et al., 2007). Fetal echocardiography can reveal heart anomalies as early as 18 weeks into a pregnancy. This can alert staff to be prepared with immediate resuscitation or other needed equipment at the baby's birth (DeMaria & Blanchard, 2008).

Phonocardiography and Magnetic Resonance Imaging

A *phonocardiogram* is a diagram of heart sounds translated into electrical energy by a microphone placed on the child's chest and then recorded as a diagrammatic representation of heart sounds. The technique can measure the timing of heart sounds that occur too quickly or at too high or too low a sound frequency for the human ear to detect by direct auscultation. Magnetic resonance imaging (MRI) may also be used to evaluate heart structure or size or blood flow (Laifer-Narin et al., 2007).

Exercise Testing

Exercise tests using treadmill walking to demonstrate that the pulmonary circulation can increase to meet the increased respiratory demands of exercise may be performed with children, although these tests are not used as extensively with children as they are with adults. With children who have heart defects that obstruct the flow of blood to the lungs (such as pulmonary stenosis), accommodation to exercise is not possible, and such a test can cause extreme exertional dyspnea. Such tests are difficult to perform successfully with young children because they require the child's cooperation.

Laboratory Tests

Children with heart disease usually undergo a number of blood tests to support the diagnosis of heart disease or to rule out anemia or clotting disorders. Hematocrit or hemoglobin studies are usually obtained to assess the rate of erythrocyte production, which may increase in an attempt to produce more oxygen-carrying red blood cells. If the increase in the number of red blood cells is extreme (polycythemia), there will be a corresponding increase in blood volume and possibly an increase in blood viscosity. Newborns are normally slightly polycythemic. In a newborn, polycythemia is defined as a hemoglobin level over 25 g per 100 mL or a hematocrit level over 70%. In an older child, polycythemia is defined as a hemoglobin level over 16 g per 100 mL or a hematocrit level over 55%. An elevated erythrocyte sedimentation rate (ESR) denotes inflammation and is useful in documenting that an inflammatory process, such as occurs with rheumatic fever, Kawasaki disease, or myocarditis, is present (Smith, 2008).

Blood gas levels also are determined. To test for this, a child is given 100% oxygen for about 15 minutes. If the child still has a Po_2 less than 150 mm Hg after this time, a shunt directing deoxygenated blood into oxygenated blood can be suspected. Oxygen saturation levels also are assessed; children with a deoxygenated to oxygenated shunt will have a lower-than-normal oxygen saturation level in arterial blood. Normally, arterial blood oxygen saturation is 95% to 100%; oxygen saturation is usually less than 92% when venous arterial shunts are present.

Before cardiac catheterization or surgery, blood clotting must be assessed. Expect prothrombin and partial thromboplastin times and platelet count studies to be completed before the procedure. Some children with polycythemia from heart disease have an associated reduced platelet count (thrombocytopenia). Because platelet formation is necessary for blood coagulation, the platelet count must be corrected before cardiac surgery.

In children with heart failure, a serum sodium level may be obtained to ensure that an increased sodium level is not causing edema. All children receiving diuretics should have serum potassium levels determined periodically because diuretics tend to deplete the body of potassium. Low serum potassium levels potentiate or increase the effect of cardiac glycosides, such as digoxin. For this reason, serum potassium levels are also usually obtained in children receiving these medications.

HEALTH PROMOTION AND RISK MANAGEMENT

Cardiac disease prevention in adults has received extensive attention in health literature. Because the risk factors that lead to adult heart disease, such as obesity, high cholesterol serum levels, and lack of consistent exercise, involve health habits that begin in childhood, prevention of cardiac disease has shifted from an adult to a child focus. Early interventions to reduce risk factors in early life should have a major impact on reducing the incidence of heart disease in the next generation.

Risk Management for Congenital Heart Disease

The cause of congenital heart disease often cannot be documented, although it is associated with familial patterns of inheritance and possibly triggers such as infection during pregnancy. All women of childbearing age should be immunized against rubella (German measles) and varicella (chickenpox) because these viruses are known to cause heart damage in a fetus if the mother contracts them during pregnancy. Because some types of congenital heart disorders have a familial incidence, parents who have a family member born with a heart defect need to alert their primary care provider so that other children can be carefully screened prenatally and at birth for a similar disorder.

Risk Management for Acquired Heart Disease

Acquired heart diseases in children that have identified risk factors include rheumatic fever, hypertension, and hyperlipidemia. Rheumatic fever is an autoimmune response that follows a group A beta-hemolytic streptococcal infection. Ensuring that all parents know that children with streptococcal infections from otitis media, streptococcal pharyngitis, and impetigo should receive adequate antibiotic therapy is essential for disease prevention (Chakko & Bisno, 2008).

Although hypertension (elevated blood pressure) occurs mainly because of a genetic predisposition, a high intake of sodium (such as table salt), lack of exercise, and obesity increase the chances that a susceptible child will develop the disorder by late childhood (Sondheimer, Yetman, & Miyamoto, 2008). If infants are never introduced to high-sodium foods, perhaps by the time they are selecting their own meals they will continue to eat a low-sodium diet, helping to prevent the development of hypertension in later life. For this reason, baby food manufacturers have stopped adding salt and monosodium glutamate to infant food. Urging school-age children and adolescents to reduce their intake of canned soups, cheese, lunch meats, and hot dogs, all foods with high sodium content, can reduce salt intake in these age groups. School nurses can play an important role in this effort by monitoring the foods served daily in school cafeterias and advocating for more nutritious menus. Beginning when a child is 3 years of age, blood pressure should be included as part of routine assessment to detect hypertension as early as possible (AAP, 2009).

Although the tendency toward hyperlipidemia is inherited as an autosomal dominant trait, a diet high in saturated fat has been implicated in the development of the syndrome. It is important that fat intake not be restricted in infants because they need fat and the calories it provides for brain growth. School-age children and adolescents, however, should reduce their fat intake to 30% of total calories (the same recommendation as for adults). The use of vegetable oils in place of saturated fat should begin when children begin solid food. Children from high-risk families (a family member has had an early myocardial infarction or hyperlipidemia) should be regularly screened for elevated cholesterol and triglyceride levels beginning at about 3 years of age. Children with low-density lipoprotein (LDL) levels greater than 130 mg/dL on two successive tests should receive nutritional counseling and instruction about a regular exercise program to enhance their health (Sondheimer, Yetman, & Miyamoto, 2008).

NURSING CARE OF THE CHILD WITH A CARDIAC DISORDER

Most parents have many questions about how to care for a child with heart disease. Encourage them to learn as much as possible about their child's disorder. Encourage them to handle and feed their newborn in the hospital so they can feel secure in caring for the infant at home. Be certain parents recognize that not all children with heart disease have the same disease or need the same degree of restriction. If this is not made clear to parents, they may unnecessarily limit their child's activity, assuming that because another child was told not to do some activity, their child should not do it either.

Nursing Diagnoses and Related Interventions

*

Nursing Diagnosis: Parental health-seeking behaviors related to desire to be informed about child's disorder

Outcome Evaluation: Parents accurately state the nature of their child's illness and unique needs of the child; can name primary care providers who will follow child's progress; state they will telephone or e-mail if they have any questions.

Provide Information About Care. Parents generally ask whether it is safe to let a baby with heart disease cry. If the infant has a cardiac disorder such as tetralogy of Fallot in which hypercyanotic episodes tend to develop, the baby should not be allowed to cry for long periods of time (no baby should). However, crying for a few minutes while a parent warms formula or fully awakens at night will, as a rule, not harm the baby.

Another common question is, "Does our child need special nutrition?" As with all newborns, breastfeeding is the preferred method of feeding, and the average infant with heart disease can be successful at this. Salt is rarely restricted during early life because infants need sodium to regulate water balance. Because anemia stresses the heart, infants are generally given an iron supplement, either with formula or separately, to prevent iron deficiency anemia during the first year. They may be prescribed supplemental vitamins with formula or when breastfeeding is stopped. Because some infants with congenital heart disease tire readily, frequent small feedings during the day may be necessary. If a child is an extremely poor eater, a high-calorie formula or enteral or gastrostomy feedings may be necessary to supply enough calories for growth.

"How much activity can we allow the baby?" This answer depends on the type and extent of the heart disorder. As a rule, infants or young children naturally limit their own activity. Parents may need guidance, however, in setting sensible limits. Roughhousing with infants, such as tossing them up in the air and watching them squeal and laugh, or playing games such as chasing a ball, may not be advisable. Encourage parents to observe their infant carefully to recognize the first signs of respiratory distress and the point at which a child's activity is beginning to exceed tolerance. Caution parents to observe a child carefully and thoughtfully as new activities are introduced and new interests are gained, so that the child's activity is limited to what the heart can accommodate.

"What do we do if our child becomes ill?" Although children with congenital heart disorders are usually seen by a cardiologist for health supervision, it is important that they are also seen by health care personnel for routine care who can ensure they are receiving normal childhood immunizations and health guidance. As a rule, infants with heart disorders need prompt treatment for minor illnesses. The fever that accompanies a cold, for instance, can increase the metabolic rate of a child who has a severe congenital heart disorder to beyond the point at which the child's heart can compensate. Dehydration must be avoided in children with polycythemia or the polycythemia may become so severe that clotting or thrombophlebitis may result. It is also important that infections be treated vigorously to avoid infectious endocarditis.

Children with congenital heart disorders or rheumatic fever need prophylactic antibiotic therapy before they have oral surgery (tooth extractions or tonsils removed). This is because the streptococcal organisms generally present in the mouth can lead to infectious endocarditis if the organisms enter the bloodstream during surgery (Sykes & Farrington, 2007). It is a good rule for parents of children with structural heart defects to ask that their children be given prophylactic antibiotics before they visit the dentist at all, because they cannot always anticipate what procedures the dentist will do at any one visit. Oral penicillin is the preferred prophylactic antibiotic; erythromycin can be used for a child sensitive to penicillin. Some parents need reassurance that their child will not become immune to penicillin if it is taken this way over long periods. Children with congenital heart disorders should receive routine immunizations and influenza vaccines and should be considered for pneumonia vaccine.

Review Steps for Follow-Up Care and Emergencies. Before parents leave the hospital with a newborn who has a congenital heart disorder, be certain they have the name and number of the person to call if they have a question about their infant's health (their primary care provider and an emergency telephone number as a back-up). Review with them the steps to take if their child should become cyanotic, such as placing the child in a knee–chest position. Be certain they have an appointment for a first health assessment. This helps to reassure them that the responsibility of caring for this child will not be theirs alone but will be shared by concerned health care personnel. In many instances, parents are first-time parents. If they are unsure whether their child is in distress or ill, urge them to err on the side of caution by telephoning or bringing the child to their primary care setting. Everyone who cares for infants or children with heart disease appreciates the responsibility parents feel and the difficulty they can have in making health judgments about their child.

Most parents feel relieved to know they can have home follow-up after a hospitalization. In addition to providing opportunities for child and family assessment, home visits allow parents to discuss the frightening responsibility they feel and to obtain a second opinion about their child's health. Teach cardiopulmonary resuscitation (CPR) and how to activate the community's emergency medical system (EMS) before they leave the hospital. It may be reassuring for the parents to visit their closest EMS station so they know the staff is acquainted with their child should an emergency call be necessary.

The Child Having Cardiac Catheterization

Cardiac catheterization, a procedure in which a small radiopaque catheter is passed through a major vein in the arm, leg, or neck into the heart to secure blood samples or inject dye, helps to evaluate cardiac function (Sondheimer, Yetman, & Miyamoto, 2008). Diagnostic cardiac catheterization is used to help diagnose specific heart disorders in anticipation of surgery. Interventional cardiac catheterization is used to correct an abnormality, such as dilating a narrowed valve by the use of a balloon catheter or other device. With both types, the pressure of blood flow in all heart chambers and total cardiac output can be evaluated. Blood specimens can be obtained to determine oxygen saturation levels, or a contrast dye can be injected for angiography. Electrodes can be introduced to record electrical activity and diagnose arrhythmias.

This procedure is usually completed as ambulatory or 1-day surgery using conscious sedation. Children must have a recent chest radiograph, ECG, and electrolyte levels, and blood must be typed and cross-matched before the procedure. Take and record pedal pulses for a baseline assessment. Also measure and record height and weight. This information is used to determine catheter size and the amount of sedation to be administered. Because the vessel site chosen for catheterization must not be infected at the time of catheterization (or obscured by a hematoma), do not draw blood specimens from the projected catheterization entry site before the procedure (generally a femoral vein). Children scheduled for the procedure are usually kept NPO for 2 to 4 hours beforehand to reduce the danger of vomiting and aspiration during the procedure.

In the cardiac catheterization room, ECG and pulse oximetry leads are attached. The site for catheter insertion is locally anesthetized with EMLA cream or intradermal lidocaine, and a catheter is threaded through a large-bore needle into a blood vessel. The specific vessel used differs according to the technique being planned. In neonates, an umbilical artery can be catheterized. For right-side heart catheterization, a right femoral vein or a vein in the antecubital fossa usually is used. Left-side heart catheterization can be performed using either a venous or an arterial approach. If done by the arterial route, a catheter is inserted into either the femoral or brachial artery. If a venous route is used, the catheter is inserted into the right femoral vein. Under fluoroscopy, the catheter is advanced to the right atrium and then through the foramen ovale. Once the catheter is in a selected heart chamber, radiopaque dye can be injected to outline the heart configuration (Fig. 41.3).

Cardiac catheterization has a mortality rate of under 0.1% when done as an elective procedure and approximately 2% to 5% when performed in a severely distressed child (Kern & King, 2008). Arrhythmias may occur while the catheter is being passed through the heart chambers or when contrast dye is being injected. Such arrhythmias generally are transitory or stop abruptly with withdrawal of the catheter. Inadvertent perforation of the heart may occur during passage of the catheter. Other complications include bleeding from the insertion site (secondary to heparin introduced into the catheter to reduce the possibility of clot formation) and thrombophlebitis (from platelet aggregation due to irritation by the catheter, a foreign body). Because cardiac catheterization may be necessary so that the cardiac surgeon can visualize and plan a cardiac repair, the key to making cardiac surgery safe, the benefit of the procedure outweighs these risks.

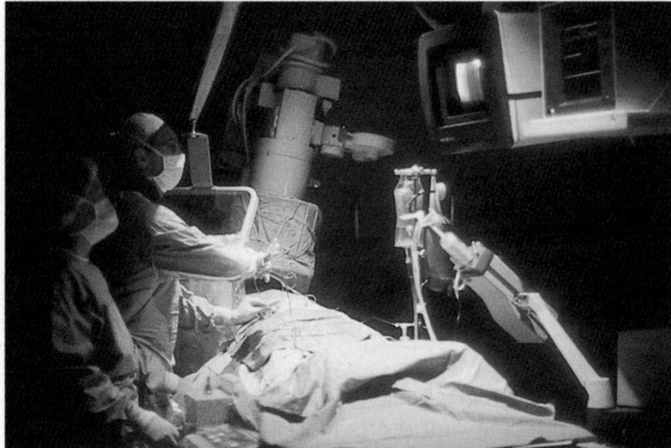

FIGURE 41.3 A child undergoing a cardiac catheterization. (© Hough/Custom Medical Stock Photograph.)

Nursing Diagnosis and Related Interventions: Preprocedure Phase

Nursing Diagnosis: Anxiety related to lack of knowledge about cardiac catheterization procedure

Outcome Evaluation: Parents and child state goal of procedure and reasons for preparation and aftercare measures; state that anxiety is less after teaching.

Because most cardiac catheterizations are done with children under conscious sedation, children may need more information about what is going to happen during this procedure than they will need for cardiac surgery, when they will be fully anesthetized. Provide explanations about the procedure for the child with the parents present, if possible. This allows parents to help reinforce the information. After this explanation, provide parents with a more detailed explanation of the procedure and allow time to ask any questions they do not want to ask in the child's presence.

Parents often need a review of heart anatomy. Although the cardiologist may have already done this, many parents appreciate reinforcement and a review of this information. Show them the pathway the catheter will take during the procedure.

Be aware that consenting to a cardiac catheterization experience brings with it the realization that cardiac surgery may be necessary. As a result, parents may be so concerned with what the procedure may reveal that they cannot listen well to preprocedure explanations. Allow them to accompany their child to the catheterization room and, if possible and appropriate, to remain there for support during the procedure if they choose.

Review with children what they will see in the catheterization room. Small children can become overwhelmed by seeing the actual equipment. Therefore, try building a facsimile room out of small cardboard boxes (representing the x-ray machine, the fluoroscopy screen, the ECG machine, and so forth). A puppet or small doll can serve as the patient in the miniature room. Dress the puppets in surgery suits and masks like those worn by cardiac catheterization personnel and act out what the child can expect to happen. Older children prefer a tour of the cardiac catheterization area and the opportunity to meet the personnel.

If children have never seen ECG leads or restraints before, let them touch and feel the equipment. Caution them the total procedure may be as long as 3 to 4 hours and that they will need to lie still during this time. Help them master imagery or another stress-reduction technique to help reduce apprehension.

Do not underestimate what children know about their heart's purpose and function; even preschoolers know their heart is vital to their body. Reassure them that the doctors are only taking a look at their heart during this procedure, not cutting it or removing any part of it.

Teach children of all ages that when the catheter is inserted, it will not hurt. Caution them, however, that they may feel a momentary speeding up of their heart, a feeling that is uncomfortable. When dye is inserted, they may feel a stinging sensation. Do not use the word "dye," which young children may misinterpret as "die." Instead, say "medicine." Caution them that the lights will be turned off after the medicine is injected so a doctor can watch the medicine on a television screen (fluoroscopy) as it passes through the heart. Let children know that after the procedure, a pressure dressing will be placed over the catheter insertion site to reduce the risk of bleeding. They will need to keep that extremity flat and unbent to prevent the dressing from loosening.

Nursing Diagnoses and Related Interventions: Postprocedure Phase

Nursing Diagnosis: Risk for ineffective cardiopulmonary and peripheral tissue perfusion related to cardiac catheterization

Outcome Evaluation: Child's vital signs remain within established parameters; absence of arrhythmia; absence of bleeding or hematoma formation at catheter insertion site; pedal pulse is present distal to catheter insertion site.

When a child returns from the procedure, assess the pressure dressing over the catheter insertion site to be certain the dressing is snug and intact and no bleeding is present. Instruct the child not to bend the hip (if the femoral site was used) or the elbow (if the brachial site was used) to keep the pressure dressing secure and to prevent hematoma formation. This is particularly important when an artery was used for catheterization; a loose dressing on an artery will cause a large blood loss in a very short time. Palpate pulses and assess color, temperature, and circulation (blanch the toe or fingernail and watch to see that it turns pink again readily) distal to the insertion site to ensure that blood flow in the extremity is unobstructed. If there is bleeding at the insertion site, apply firm, continuous pressure and notify the physician who performed the procedure immediately.

Children often appreciate being asked to describe their experience afterward. Saying out loud how frightened they were—by the x-ray machine being pushed in over them or by the thought of a tube going all the way into their heart—helps alleviate their fear and allows better acceptance of the procedure. Praise them for their cooperation during a very stressful experience. Introduce therapeutic play if needed.

Keep the child flat in bed for 2 to 3 hours until the child is completely awake from conscious sedation. This helps to prevent not only oozing at the insertion site but also postural hypotension, which may occur when a child rises suddenly after lying flat while under sedation for such a long period. In the immediate postcatheterization period, a child's blood pressure may be 10% to 15% lower than the precatheterization level because of the hypotensive effect of the radiopaque dye.

Cardiac arrhythmias and bradycardia may occur from the mechanical action of the catheter having touched the conduction nodes of the heart. Assess pulse, blood pressure, and respirations at frequent intervals (about every 15 minutes) for the first several hours to help detect if this has occurred. Monitor the pulse for a full minute to aid in recognizing abnormalities. Be alert for signs of arrhythmias. Small children cannot describe the odd feeling that accompanies an arrhythmia. Older children might describe it as their heart "fluttering" or "skipping beats." Therefore, be alert for signs of increasing anxiety in children after a catheterization; this may be a child's way of reporting these feelings.

Infants may need intravenous (IV) fluid during the procedure and for several hours afterward to prevent dehydration, which could result from being NPO for a long period of time. If an infant is polycythemic, IV fluid helps minimize the risk of vessel thrombi. Regulate IV fluid carefully to prevent heart failure from fluid overload.

Assess temperature immediately after the procedure to determine a baseline. Some children have a transient elevation in temperature already due to physiologic dehydration as a result of having been NPO or as a reaction to the dye. Others have slightly subnormal temperature readings from lying in a cool procedure room for a lengthy period. This below-normal body temperature quickly compromises respiratory and heart action because, to raise body temperature, infants must increase their metabolic rate. This requires rapid breathing and increased heart action, which can lead to exhaustion. Infants may need to be placed under radiant heat warmers to help regain and maintain normal body temperature and also to allow accurate temperature determinations.

The adverse effects of cardiac catheterization may be episodes of apnea, sternal retractions, or dyspnea. If oxygen was administered during the catheterization procedure, it may be continued for a period of time after the procedure to reduce the stress of respirations. Like arrhythmias, dyspnea, bradycardia, and blood pressure anomalies may be transient, but all should be reported so they can be evaluated.

Nursing Diagnosis: Risk for infection related to presence of cardiac catheterization incision site

Outcome Evaluation: The child's temperature remains less than 100.4° F (38.0° C) axillary; the catheter insertion site appears free of erythema or drainage.

If the dressing for a cardiac catheterization is over the femoral artery or vein, keep it clean of stool and urine. Waterproofing the dressing with plastic may be necessary. Also check the insertion site for signs of infection, because any opening in the skin is a portal of entry for bacteria. Alert parents to observe the catheter insertion site daily for redness. Most parents are advised to monitor their child's temperature daily for about 3 days and to omit tub baths and strenuous exercise for their child for 2 to 3 days to aid healing.

✔ Checkpoint Question 41.2

Megan is scheduled for a cardiac catheterization. Why might a child develop cardiac arrhythmias after this procedure?

a. The dye inserted can create inflamed heart chambers.
b. The many radiographs taken lead to a weakened heart muscle.
c. The catheter can irritate nerves in the heart septum.
d. Latex allergy can cause symptoms of unusual heart rate.

The Child Scheduled for Cardiac Surgery

There are many different types of congenital heart disorders, and many different procedures are available to correct them. Open-heart or intra-catheter surgery, however, remains the chief cure for congenital heart disease (Fulton & Freed, 2008). Open-heart surgery is made possible by the use of cardiopulmonary bypass or extracorporeal membrane oxygenation (ECMO). With this, the venous return to the heart is diverted from the right atrium or inferior and superior vena cava to a heart–lung machine, where it is artificially oxygenated. It is returned to the body's arterial system by way of the aorta, bypassing the heart. The heart, practically bloodless, now can be opened and operated on. Blood returns to the coronary and pulmonary capillary beds under pressure from the aorta so that even though blood bypasses the heart, it still receives an adequate blood supply for self-maintenance during the bypass procedure (Fynn-Thompson & Almond, 2007). Very ill infants may be maintained on ECMO using the same technique after surgery.

During surgery, hypothermia (reducing the child's body temperature to 68° to 79° F [20° to 26° C]) is used to reduce the child's metabolic needs and slow the heart rate. If extreme hypothermia is used (59° to 68° F [15° to 20° C]), usually in an infant, the body temperature drops so low that the heart stops beating and the surgeon can work in a quiet and bloodless field. Measuring temperature to be certain the infant is rewarmed is a major responsibility afterward.

Preoperative Care

Before surgery, obtain vital signs (blood pressure, temperature, pulse, and respirations) to establish baselines. Count pulse and respiratory rates for a full minute for accuracy. Some children may need baseline pulse determinations done at several pulse points or blood pressures taken in both upper and lower extremities. Before obtaining a blood pressure, have a child rest for about 15 minutes and take the recording with the child lying down so it closely mimics what the child's position will be following surgery. Also record height and weight, because these parameters are necessary for the estimation of blood volume for the heart–lung machine and for medication dosages. Weighing also is helpful in estimating blood loss or edema after surgery. In children receiving digoxin, it is usually withheld 24 hours before surgery because cardiac surgery may cause arrhythmias in the presence of cardiac glycosides.

The immediate surgical preparation of children varies from one institution to another but usually includes preparing the skin incision site. The skin over the surgical incision area is scrubbed with an antiseptic solution to ensure as clean a surgical field as possible. Most children and parents are startled to learn that cardiac surgery may be performed through the sternal bone or the back, not over the left side of the chest, and may question the area being prepared for the incision. An enema also may be given to keep children from straining to pass stool in the immediate postoperative period and placing additional strain on the newly operated heart.

Nursing Diagnoses and Related Interventions: Preoperative Phase

Nursing Diagnosis: Deficient knowledge related to cardiac surgery and its outcome

Outcome Evaluation: Parents and child accurately state the reason for surgery and expected outcome.

Bringing a child to the hospital for cardiac surgery is a large responsibility for parents. They want their child to be made well, but they are also aware there is a definite risk from this surgery. They may have been protecting and guarding their child for months or years, and they feel no less protective the morning of surgery. For this reason, parents of children being readied for cardiac surgery may watch preoperative procedures more carefully than usual. Review with them what they already know about the surgery to correct any misconceptions and inform them what laboratory tests will be scheduled. Prepare them for the amount of equipment that will surround their child after surgery, such as cardiac monitors, oxygen and IV equipment, chest tubes, and a ventilator. Parents usually appreciate visiting the intensive care unit (ICU) where their child will be cared for after surgery. Be certain they have an opportunity to meet the ICU staff, especially if those nurses are not the same ones who are caring for the child preoperatively.

Prepare Child for Surgery and Postoperative Care. It is best if a child is prepared for surgery with the parents present. This allows parents the opportunity to reinforce your teaching and shows children that their parents approve and feel secure with these surgery plans. Parents will then need additional time to discuss the surgical procedure with you and ask questions they might not have wished to ask in the presence of their child.

Children can be very frightened about cardiac surgery (Fig. 41.4). Remember when caring for them preoperatively (or any time) not to make careless remarks so children can maintain confidence in health care personnel. For example, statements such as, "These syringes never work right" (when all you mean

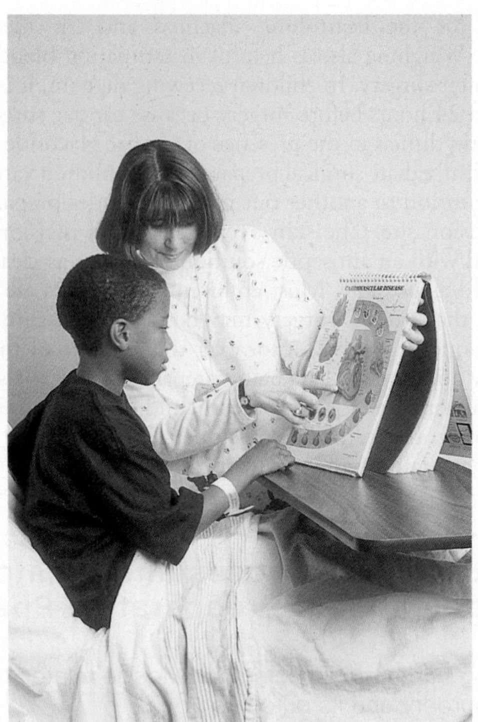

FIGURE 41.4 Orientation for cardiac surgery includes time for talking and learning more about the heart. (© Lesha Photography.)

is you prefer another brand) or "Amy [an ICU nurse] is a real clown" (when you mean she is not only a competent nurse but has a good sense of humor besides) could be interpreted by anxious parents or children to mean a child is in less-than-competent hands. Because many children having cardiac surgery have had previous cardiac catheterizations, talking to them about their previous hospitalization experiences is helpful. Talking will reveal the things they fear the most this time. Any misconceptions they have about past experiences can then be discussed and clarified.

Both parents and children may have questions about the difference between cardiac catheterization and cardiac surgery. One important difference is that children are sedated but awake for the former but anesthetized for the latter. For some children, knowing they will be fully asleep is more reassuring; for others, it is more frightening. When they were awake, they knew that they were all right; asleep, how can they know? Encourage them to express these feelings so they can receive reassurance that anesthetized sleep is a special sleep from which they will have no difficulty waking. Meeting the anesthesiologist and receiving reassurance directly from the person who will be watching over them while they are asleep is often helpful.

As with cardiac catheterization, it may help to make models of the equipment that will surround the child postoperatively. Parents and older children can be taken to the ICU where they will return after surgery and be shown the actual equipment and setting.

After surgery, a child will need to cough and deep-breathe and use incentive spirometry to help the lungs expand. Introduce these exercises preoperatively to let a child know what will be expected. Familiarize children with chest tubes. Caution both children and parents that chest tubes must stay in place until it is time for them to be removed. If children want to turn over with tubes in place, they need to ask for help to prevent the tubes from being dislodged. Caution parents that a chest-tube drainage reservoir must remain below the level of the child's chest and must not be raised for any reason. If children are not familiar with ECG leads, introduce these as part of preoperative preparation. Comparing these tubes or leads to being "hooked up" like an astronaut is often appealing to children. In addition, introduce children to the form of oxygen therapy they will receive after surgery (mask, cannula, or ventilator) to avoid surprises. Orienting children to oxygen equipment is discussed in Chapter 40.

Postoperative Care

After surgery and before leaving the operating room, an x-ray film is taken and the child is weighed. Future estimates of lung expansion and weight, to reveal whether edema is accumulating from poor heart function, will be checked against these two measurements.

Nursing Diagnoses and Related Interventions: Postoperative Phase

Nursing Diagnosis: Risk for ineffective cardiopulmonary tissue perfusion related to cardiac surgery

Outcome Evaluation: Vital signs are within normal limits; central venous pressure (CVP) or pulmonary artery wedge pressure is within established parameters.

Taking accurate vital signs, as often as every 15 minutes, is essential in the immediate postoperative period following cardiac surgery. Continuous cardiac monitoring and assisted ventilation with endotracheal intubation also are usually necessary. Blood pressure will probably be monitored directly by means of an intra-arterial catheter or indirectly with an automated blood pressure recording device. Hemodynamic monitoring by way of a pulmonary artery or central venous catheter will reveal information on chamber pressures and oxygen saturation (Fig. 41.5).

Adequate voiding after surgery indicates that the kidneys are receiving an adequate blood flow or the heart is working effectively. An indwelling urinary (Foley) catheter is usually inserted at the time of surgery so urine output can be carefully recorded postoperatively (it should be 1 mL/kg/hr). Be certain to mark the amount of urine drainage present when children first return from surgery so that lack of or diminished urinary output will not be missed or misinterpreted. Individual samples may be tested for specific gravity and pH. A specific gravity below 1.010 implies that the kidneys are not concentrating urine well, perhaps because of the stress of surgery. The pH should remain slightly acid; however, extreme acidity may indicate respiratory acidosis from poor pulmonary perfusion.

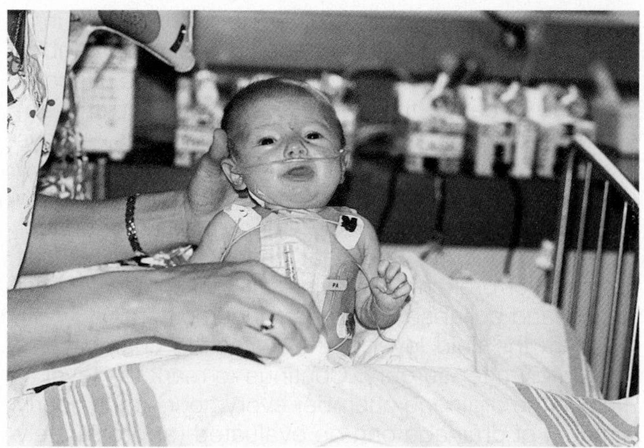

FIGURE 41.5 Because children after cardiac surgery typically have a myriad of wires and tubes attached to monitors, pumps, and equipment, parents need to be prepared for how their child will look. As the child's condition improves, use of the equipment is discontinued. Here, an infant is 2 days post-cardiac surgery. Note his level of alertness and the use of only a few monitoring devices and equipment. (© Caroline Brown, RNC, MS, DEd.)

Carefully record all IV fluid administered to the child after surgery. Fluid overload can pose a severe threat to the heart during the immediate postoperative period. Use an infusion control device to regulate the amount and rate of infusion.

Laboratory tests such as arterial blood gases (Po_2 and Pco_2), hemoglobin, hematocrit, clotting time, and electrolytes (particularly sodium and potassium) will be monitored closely to assess cardiac and pulmonary function postoperatively. Oxygen saturation levels may be monitored by pulse oximetry or transcutaneous oxygen monitoring. A drug such as dopamine may be administered to improve cardiac output.

Central Venous Pressure Monitoring. CVP may be recorded by inserting a catheter into a brachial, jugular, or subclavian vein, and ultimately into the right atrium (Fig. 41.6). CVP is an excellent way to evaluate a child's fluid volume status. CVP will rise with heart failure, indicating that the heart cannot handle the blood arriving at the atria.

Pulmonary Artery Pressure Monitoring. To assess pressure in the left side of the heart parallel to CVP measurement, a multilumen pulmonary artery catheter, such as a Swan-Ganz catheter, can be threaded through the venous circulation through the right side of the heart and into the pulmonary artery. The pressure, registered there as a waveform on a cardiac monitor, reflects both the resistance of the lungs to the passage of blood (pulmonary artery resistance) and the ability of the left side of the heart to handle the circulating fluid volume. Such catheters must be kept from clotting with frequent irrigations or with a constant infusion system. When withdrawing blood specimen samples from the catheter, make sure no air is allowed to enter, because this would immediately flow into the left side of the heart and possibly to a cerebral artery as an embolus.

Nursing Diagnosis: Impaired gas exchange related to unexpanded lung space and collection of lung excretions.

Outcome Evaluation: Child's respiratory rate remains within age-appropriate parameters; absence of rales or other adventitious breath sounds; chest tubes function normally.

Measures to Prevent Pooling of Secretions in Lungs. Suction as necessary while a child is receiving ventilatory assistance to prevent pooling of secretions in the respiratory tract. As soon as the endotracheal

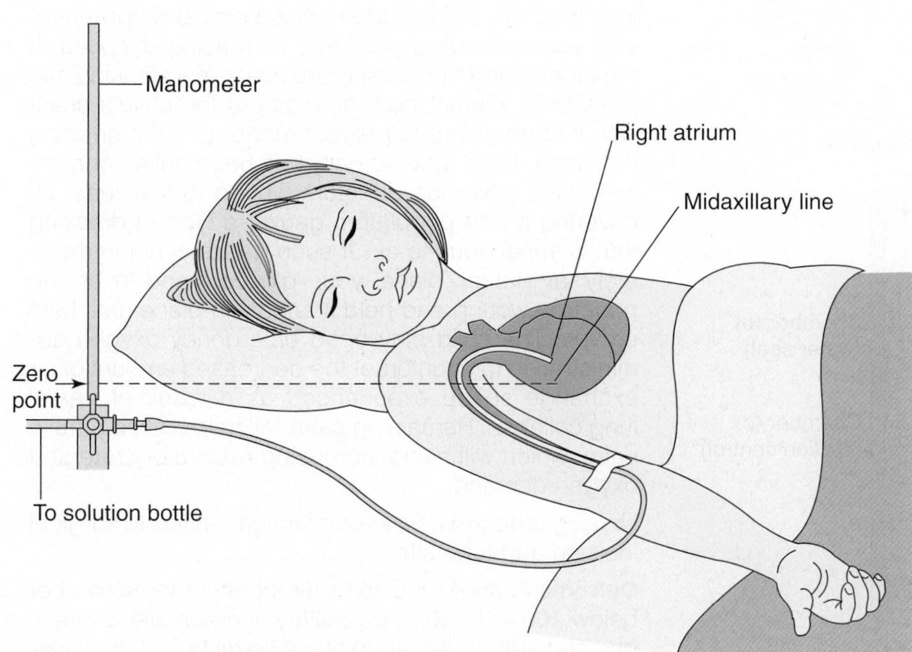

FIGURE 41.6 A CVP catheter may be inserted after cardiac surgery to monitor fluid volume. The zero point on the scale is at the level of the right atrium.

tube and ventilator are removed, encourage the child to cough and deep-breathe or use an incentive spirometer at hourly intervals to help mobilize secretions. Although children may have practiced such procedures preoperatively, they may have difficulty carrying them out now because, unless continuous epidural anesthesia is used for pain relief, coughing or deep-breathing can be very painful. To minimize pain, administer the prescribed analgesia or alert the child to use the patient-controlled analgesia (PCA) pump 10 to 15 minutes before it is time to deep-breathe. For optimal effectiveness, demonstrating coughing again, sometimes deep-breathing with the child, may be necessary. Chest physiotherapy with percussion and vibration may be prescribed to keep lung secretions mobile. Be certain parents understand that games such as blowing cotton balls or blowing up a balloon are not really games but important exercises to help achieve lung expansion. Otherwise, they may interpret these exercises as too tiring for the child and discourage them.

Most children have two thoracotomy chest tubes inserted following surgery. The upper tube drains air to aid lung re-expansion and the lower one drains fluid to encourage lung expansion and decrease the possibility of infection. These tubes are connected to a water-seal drainage apparatus (a Pleur-Evac; Fig. 41.7).

Pleur-Evacs consist of three chambers: one to collect drainage, one to furnish a water seal, and one that can be attached to suction. A thoracotomy tube connects to the first drainage compartment. Because of the water seal, atmospheric air cannot enter the tube and flow back into the pleural space. Note how much drainage is occurring and if the level of fluid fluctuates (proof that the apparatus is airtight). On the third or fourth postoperative day, the fluctuation will cease, indicating that the lungs are fully expanded. Then it is time for the tubes to be removed.

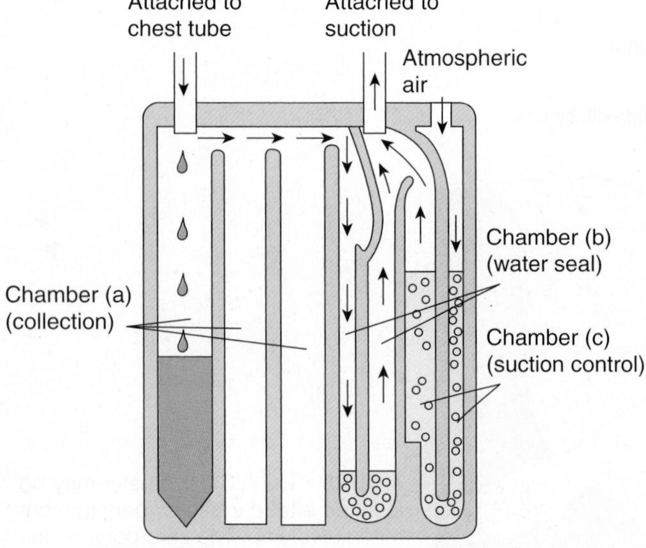

FIGURE 41.7 Pleur-Evac system for chest tube drainage.

Maintain children with chest tubes in place in a semi-Fowler's position because thoracotomy tubes drain best in this position; often there is less dyspnea as well, because the chest is elevated and the abdominal contents do not press on the lungs. Always keep thoracotomy chest tube drainage systems below the level of the child's chest so that fluid does not flow back into the pleural space. Check that tube connections are secure and that the Pleur-Evac is not cracked or broken. Otherwise, air can enter the chest cavity and collapse the lungs (pneumothorax).

Mark the fluid level in the collecting chamber immediately after surgery. Continue to mark the level of fluid in the drainage chamber every hour so the hourly amount of drainage can be evaluated (approximately 5 mL/kg/hr is typical). Also note the color and the presence of any clots in the drainage. Drainage fluid may be blood-tinged but should not contain fresh blood. If it does, this suggests active bleeding.

A chest radiograph taken on the third or fourth postoperative day will confirm that full lung expansion has returned. The tubes are then removed by a physician or nurse practitioner while an impervious dressing is simultaneously applied to the puncture wound. Provide emotional support during thoracotomy tube removal. Children know these tubes are important for their well-being. Aside from worrying about the momentary pain of removal, they may believe that something bad will happen after the tubes are removed. Do not change any dressings over former thoracotomy tube sites, because lifting them to change them could allow air to enter.

Occasionally, despite being cautioned not to, children may turn so suddenly after surgery that they pull a thoracotomy tube out accidentally. This creates an emergency situation because air rushing into the child's chest can cause a pneumothorax with sudden dyspnea, tachycardia, cyanosis, and perhaps sharp chest pain. If a tube is only loosened or air is leaking slowly through a connection, the symptoms may be less dramatic but include restlessness and apprehension accompanying gradually increasing dyspnea. If the air entering the chest is the result of air leaking into the tubing, clamp the tube close to the child's chest with a large clamp to prevent further air from entering the chest. If the tube actually has been pulled out, immediately close the puncture wound to the chest by covering it with petrolatum gauze, a type of dressing that is impervious to air. If such gauze is not immediately available, place your gloved hand over the puncture wound and hold it snugly in place until help arrives. The child may need emergency oxygen administration to counteract the decreased amount of air exchange space experienced as a result of partial lung collapse. Remaining calm will help a child remain calm, which will avoid increasing respiratory rate and oxygen demand.

Nursing Diagnosis: Risk for infection related to surgical incision and tube sites

Outcome Evaluation: Child's temperature remains at or below 100.4° F (38.0° C) axillary; incision site is clean, dry, and without evidence of erythema or foul drainage.

Some children are begun on a prophylactic course of a broad-spectrum antibiotic before surgery. If so, this will be continued for 24 to 48 hours postoperatively. Frequently monitor temperature postoperatively to assess for infection. Frequently assess the dressing over the surgical incision and the points of insertion of the thoracotomy tubes for drainage and erythema. Use strict aseptic technique when changing the incisional dressing to avoid introducing pathogens.

Nursing Diagnosis: Hypothermia related to cooling during surgery

Outcome Evaluation: Child's temperature is above 96.8° F (36.0° C) axillary. Capillary refill is less than 5 seconds.

If hypothermia was induced for surgery, the child's temperature will be low postoperatively and a hyperthermia blanket, warm blankets, or radiant heat may be necessary to elevate the temperature to normal. Alternatively, a child's temperature may be above normal because of an inflammatory response to hypothermia. Unless infection is developing, these temperature readings will gradually return to normal in a few days.

Nursing Diagnosis: Risk for excess or deficient fluid volume related to fluid shifts accompanying cardiac surgery

Outcome Evaluation: Child maintains weight; skin turgor is good; central venous pressure or pulmonary artery pressure is within established parameters.

Children tend to develop hypervolemia after cardiac surgery because of increased production of aldosterone by the adrenal glands and an increase in antidiuretic hormone secretion by the pituitary gland in response to stress. Also, if cardiopulmonary bypass was used, some fluid may have been shifted from the intravascular system to the interstitial spaces during surgery. After surgery, this fluid returns by osmosis to the vessels, causing hypervolemia. On the other hand, an individual child may have experienced excessive bleeding because of the heparin used during surgery and may subsequently develop hypovolemia.

Monitor central venous or pulmonary artery pressure to evaluate a child's hemodynamic status. Monitor IV fluid administration carefully to prevent fluid overload. Typically, oral fluid intake is withheld for at least the first 24 hours after surgery. Once bowel sounds have returned, oral fluids can be introduced gradually.

Nursing Diagnosis: Parental anxiety related to lack of knowledge of postoperative routine and exercises

Outcome Evaluation: Family members accurately state plans for child's postoperative recovery; relate less anxiety after teaching and support.

Most children recover quickly from heart surgery. Passive range-of-motion exercises may be prescribed the day of surgery. By 24 hours, children are out of bed and ambulating. Encourage parents to do whatever they want to do for their child's care during this period. It is difficult for them to accept the fact the surgery is over and their child is now a well child (or will be at the end of the recovery period).

Offering the child sips of water or helping the child with bathing (under supervision) helps parents see that their child is returning to usual activities and doing well. Be certain that in the midst of the postoperative excitement, the child receives adequate rest the first postoperative days. You may need to monitor and regulate visits by staff and outside visitors to make sure a child is undisturbed for sustained rest periods. Urge parents to read to children or play music for them as a way to provide quiet rest periods. Caution parents not to pick up an infant under the arms, because this pulls on the chest incision. Show them how to lift an infant by placing their hands under the shoulders and buttocks instead.

Once the immediate postoperative period has passed, the child will be moved from the ICU to a routine patient unit. This may be a difficult move for both the child and the parents because they have developed confidence in the ICU staff and are reluctant to entrust the child to new personnel (even if the patient unit is the one to which the child was initially admitted before surgery). It helps the transition if the regular nursing staff visits the child daily in the ICU. Generally, place children returning from the ICU in a room near the nursing station, and place the bed so it can be easily seen from the hallway. Although you are not providing the constant attendance that the child received in the ICU, you can show that you are very observant and aware of individual needs. Stopping to look in every time you pass the room reassures the family that you are always close by. Allow parents an opportunity to voice their concern over the change in personnel and surroundings. Accepting this change can help prepare them for the day of hospital discharge, when they will be observing and caring for their child on their own.

At hospital discharge, parents need clear explanations of the activities in which the child will and will not be able to participate. Be sure they have an appointment for a checkup for the child and the telephone number they should call if they have any questions regarding their child's care. The protectiveness they felt for the child before surgery does not diminish instantly, even though surgery has been completed. They may find themselves saying, "Don't run" for months after the child has been allowed full activity. They may appreciate a listening ear for their concerns, which may include feeling they are not as important to their child as they were when the child was ill. Emphasize that well children also need continued parental supervision and guidance (Box 41.3).

Complications of Cardiac Surgery

A number of complications can arise after cardiac surgery because of the use of cardiopulmonary bypass and the extent of the surgery (Box 41.4). The first of these is hemorrhage, because heparin is used to prevent blood coagulation during the cardiopulmonary bypass. Although protamine sulfate (the antidote for heparin) is administered IV immediately after surgery, some heparin is still present in the

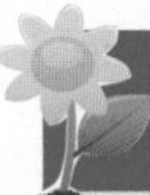

BOX 41.3 * Focus on Communication

Megan is a 3-month-old infant who is being discharged after cardiac surgery. You stop at her hospital room to give discharge instructions to her mother.

Less Effective Communication

Nurse: Good morning, Mrs. Carver. Let me review a few instructions with you.

Mrs. Carver: The most important thing you can tell me is how to keep a baby on bedrest.

Nurse: Most infants are so exhausted from surgery, they automatically reduce their activity, so that's not a problem. You can let her return to her usual activities at as near normal a level as possible.

Mrs. Carver: She likes to kick a mobile. It'll be hard to keep her from doing that.

Nurse: Her appetite should be back to normal in a few days. Check back with the clinic if it doesn't improve.

Mrs. Carver: I don't understand how she'll eat well if she has to be in bed all the time.

Nurse: Megan will need to continue to take digoxin until she returns for her checkup in 1 week. Do you have any questions about the dose?

Mrs. Carver: No. It'll be hard to get her to cooperate, though, when she's unhappy about having to stay in bed all the time.

Nurse: You'll need to check the incision daily and report any redness or increasing pain.

Mrs. Carver: I can do that. The thing I'll have trouble with is keeping her on bedrest.

Nurse: Infants generally limit their own activity, so that shouldn't be a problem. Wait here, now, until I call transportation to take you downstairs.

More Effective Communication

Nurse: Good morning, Mrs. Carver. Let me review a few instructions with you.

Mrs. Carver: The most important thing you can tell me is how to keep a baby on bedrest.

Nurse: Most infants are so exhausted from surgery, they automatically reduce their activity, so that's not a problem. You can let her return to her usual activities at as near normal a level as possible.

Mrs. Carver: She likes to kick a mobile in bed. It'll be hard to keep her from doing that.

Nurse: You'll need to check the incision daily and report any redness or increasing pain.

Mrs. Carver: I can do that. The thing I'll have trouble with is keeping her on bedrest.

Nurse: You've mentioned bedrest several times. Megan doesn't have to stay on bedrest. Let's talk about what activities she can do.

Because cardiac surgery is such serious surgery, most parents assume that it will take their child a very long time to recover from it. In the above scenarios, the mother has overestimated the time it will take her child to return to normal activities. Only when really listening to what the mother is saying, rather than just continuing to review discharge instructions, does the nurse recognize that the mother has not heard the first instruction—let the child return to activities at as near normal a level as possible.

child's system. Monitor the coagulation time and vital signs and observe thoracotomy tube drainage to identify early signs of bleeding.

Shock, another possible complication, is revealed by hypotension, oliguria, acidosis, and cyanosis. It may result from hypovolemia or cardiac tamponade (bleeding into the heart muscle or pericardium, interfering with the heart's ability to contract forcibly), or it may be a reaction to prolonged extracorporeal perfusion. It is treated according to individual needs, including plasma volume expanders, continued mechanical ventilation, and perhaps a return to surgery to stop the bleeding. Heart block or arrhythmias may occur as the result of edema or trauma compromising the effectiveness of the bundle of His. An artificial pacemaker may be inserted to correct these problems. If the child had congestive heart disease before surgery, this may persist for a week or more after surgery. If it occurs as a new entity, it suggests that the surgery has caused a stricture to circulation at some point, causing either the right or left side of the heart to become overwhelmed. Measures for treating postoperative congestive heart failure are the same as those in children who have this syndrome from any cause. Neurologic symptoms, also a possible complication, may occur if the child experienced hypoxia during surgery.

A **postcardiac surgery syndrome** may develop at the end of the first postoperative week. This is a febrile illness with pericarditis and pleurisy (fluid collecting in the pleural space) that appears to be a benign inflammatory response to the surgical procedure. Anti-inflammatory therapy and bedrest reduce the symptoms. The symptoms may recur months after surgery.

Postperfusion syndrome may occur 3 to 12 weeks after surgery. The child develops a fever, an enlarged spleen, general malaise, and a maculopapular rash. Increased liver size also may be present. The white blood count reveals a leukocytosis, with lymphocytes as the predominant cell type. Such a reaction is usually caused by a cytomegalovirus infection contracted from the donor blood used in the cardiopulmonary bypass machine. The illness runs a short course, with no permanent effect.

✔ Checkpoint Question 41.3

Megan will be scheduled for open-heart surgery. What type of fluid imbalance is apt to occur after cardiac surgery?

a. Hypervolemia from aldosterone production.
b. Hypercalcemia from calcium release from bones.
c. Hypernatremia from excess sodium retention.
d. Hypokalemia from excess urine diuresis.

BOX 41.4 * Focus on Evidence-Based Practice

Do parents rate their child's quality of life as improved following cardiac surgery?

Because children's physical abilities improve following cardiac surgery, it is usually assumed that both children and parents will be happier afterward. To investigate whether parents reported that as being true, researchers asked the parents of 110 children (mean age, 10.4 years) to rate their children's health-related quality of life on a questionnaire. The mean age of the children's surgery was 2.3 years, and the mean duration of cardiopulmonary bypass was 95 minutes. Circulatory arrest had been performed in 9% of the children. Parents reported that most dimensions of quality of life including autonomy and motor, social, emotional, and cognitive functioning were impaired. Factors such as the duration of cardiopulmonary bypass, the length of hospitalization, the need for current cardiac medication, and adverse family relationships all had negative impacts on the parent's ratings of their child's quality of life.

Based on the above study, would you promise parents that their child will be "perfect" following cardiac surgery?

Source: Landolt, M. A., Valsangiacomo Buechel, E. R., & Latal, B. (2008). Health-related quality of life in children and adolescents after open-heart surgery. *Journal of Pediatrics, 152*(3), 349–355.

The Child with an Artificial Valve Replacement

A number of congenital heart anomalies, such as aortic stenosis, and diseases, such as rheumatic fever or Kawasaki disease, can require artificial heart valve replacement. Valve replacement is technically more complicated in children than adults because children's hearts are smaller. Because children have a longer life expectancy than adults, valve durability also is a prime consideration. In addition, the advantage of the long-term anticoagulation therapy necessary to prevent clots from forming at the valve site must be weighed against the problem of extensive bleeding from normal childhood accidents.

Artificial valves were first obtained from pigs (porcine) or cows (bovine), but synthetic material (prosthetic) or human donors (homografts) are most often used today because synthetic materials or a child's own tissue provide the best long-term replacement. After surgery to place an artificial valve, a child is given either anticoagulation or antiplatelet therapy to prevent thrombi from forming at the valve implantation site. The drugs prescribed most commonly for anticoagulation therapy are heparin or warfarin sodium (Coumadin). Antiplatelet therapy also may be used, most often acetylsalicylic acid (aspirin) and dipyridamole (Persantine). Aspirin decreases platelet aggregation; dipyridamole decreases platelet adhesiveness. The dosage for these drugs must be periodically monitored by blood analysis to ensure they remain adequate as the child grows.

If a child should develop a bacterial infection with an artificial valve in place, organisms tend to cluster and colonize at the valve site. For this reason, a child generally is prescribed prophylactic antibiotic therapy to prevent this from becoming endocarditis. Additional therapy with amoxicillin will be prescribed if a child is scheduled for dental work or any other invasive procedure (Sykes & Farrington, 2007).

Adolescent girls need counseling about avoiding pregnancy until they become adults because the artificial valve may be unable to accommodate the increased blood volume associated with pregnancy and support the adolescent's growth as well. In addition, because warfarin is teratogenic, any girl contemplating pregnancy needs to be changed to a heparin regimen before conception. Girls with artificial valves in place should not use an estrogen-based birth control pill, because this can increase blood coagulation and possibly lead to thrombi. They also should not use an intrauterine device (IUD) because IUDs have been associated with an increased rate of pelvic inflammatory disease, which could spread to the valve site.

Hemolytic anemia may occur as a complication of artificial valve replacement. The extreme turbulence of blood through the prosthetic valve apparently results in breakage of red blood cells. Blood replacement may be necessary if the hemolytic process persists.

The Child Undergoing Cardiac Transplantation

Children who have a hypoplastic left ventricle or extensive cardiomyopathy from any cause are candidates for heart transplantation (Schroeder et al., 2008). Children are usually maintained on extracorporeal membrane oxygenation (ECMO) or a trial ventricular assist device while waiting for surgery (Fynn-Thompson & Almond, 2007).

Children who will be having heart transplants may be at home or in the hospital when their family is notified that a donor heart is available. After removal from the donor, the transplant heart is perfused with a balanced electrolyte solution and chilled immediately. It can be maintained this way for 2 to 3 hours using cardiopulmonary bypass technique before being transplanted. For the procedure, the aorta of the child who will be receiving the heart is cross-clamped, and the original heart is removed except for the upper portion of the right atrium, which contains the SA node. Once the new heart is transplanted and the major cardiac vessels are reattached, intrathoracic hemodynamic monitoring lines and ventricle pacing wires are implanted. Transplanted hearts beat normally except for autonomic nervous system control. This means the transplanted heart varies its rate in response to the amount of blood arriving at it and the response to catecholamines rather than by nervous system control. An ECG will show two P waves (one from the residual original heart and one from the donor heart) because both SA nodes are intact.

Postoperative care is similar to that for any child undergoing cardiac surgery. The child has the same potential problems: decreased cardiac output, impaired gas exchange, risk for infection, imbalanced nutrition, and ineffective family coping. Children are prone to arrhythmias because of possible injury to the SA node during transport or transplant.

Although a long-term consequence of cardiac transplantation is severe atherosclerosis, apparently as a result of inflammation, rejection of the transplant is the number one cause of death in cardiac transplant patients (Law, 2007). An antithymocyte antibody preparation and drugs such as cyclosporine A, prednisone, and azathioprine are commonly used for immunosuppression in an attempt to reduce the risk of rejection. However, rejection still can occur in hyperacute, acute, or chronic forms. Hyperacute rejection occurs immediately and is manifested by coronary thrombosis. Acute rejection occurs in about 7 days and is manifested by low-grade fever, tachycardia, edema, and ECG changes. Cardiac catheterization is usually performed a week after transplant to obtain a biopsy sample from the heart muscle to evaluate for signs of acute rejection (tissue necrosis will have started to occur). Long-term or chronic rejection may begin as early as 6 months. At any point that rejection is beginning, additional antithymocyte globulin (ATG) or monoclonal antibodies to CD3T-lymphocytes (OKT-3) may be infused to help stop the process.

Once past the rejection period, most children adjust well to cardiac transplant. They can participate in normal growth and development activities after the procedure. Depending on the specific protocol, they return to the transplant center about once yearly for a repeat cardiac catheterization and evaluation of progress.

The Child with a Pacemaker

A child whose heart has ineffective SA node function or has difficulty in transmitting impulses from the SA node to the ventricles may have an artificial pacemaker inserted to control the heartbeat by stimulating the ventricles electronically (Karpawich, 2007). The pacing system consists of two components: a pulse generator that contains the battery and programmed instructions, and wire leads that connect to the heart. Most leads placed in children are an epicardial type and are attached to the epicardium (the outside wall of the heart) by suture. The generator is placed under the skin in the subxiphoid or mid- or lower abdomen. Heart disorders that will need pacing can be detected during intrauterine life by fetal monitoring. In these children, pacemakers can be implanted as soon as they are born.

Commonly, the type of pacemaker and its functions are denoted by either a three- or five-letter code. With the three-letter system, the first letter identifies the chamber paced, the second the chamber sensed, and the third the pacemaker's response to the intrinsic activity of the heart. If a fourth letter is used, it denotes whether rate modulation is possible; a fifth letter denotes whether antitachyarrhythmia function, such as the ability to produce a shock to defibrillate, is possible (Vijayaraman & Ellenbogen, 2008). For example, a pacemaker that is set to pace the ***v***entricle, sense the ***v***entricle, and be ***i***nhibited (cannot modify the rate and does not respond as long as the heart initiates a normal beat) is a VVI pacemaker.

Teach the parents of the child with a pacemaker how to take the child's pulse accurately. They will need to do this daily at home and report any alterations in the pulse rate to their primary care provider until it is certain that the paced rate is appropriate. They also may need to telephone the health care center periodically and transmit a recording of the child's heart action to the center by means of a telephone attachment to ensure that the paced rate remains accurate.

Some parents stay awake at night worrying that the pacemaker batteries will suddenly stop operating and their child will die. Because of this fear, they may be afraid to take vacations or allow the child to go away to camp. How long a pacemaker battery lasts depends on the percentage of time pacing is needed (continuous or intermittent), the battery energy output in amplitude (the amount of battery voltage needed to create each pacing impulse), and the pulse width (the length of time the impulse is being delivered). With usual pacemaker parameters, such as an intermittent pattern, low amplitude, and narrow pulse width, a battery can last 12 to 15 years. In all instances, parents can be reassured that pacemaker batteries lose power slowly, not abruptly. They will have ample time to recognize weakening batteries through signs in their child such as dizziness, fatigue, fainting, or a slow pulse rate and arrange to have the pacemaker replaced before the child's heart would fail.

Occasionally, pacemaker leads in the right ventricle of infants lie in such close proximity to the diaphragm that they stimulate the diaphragm to contract with each ventricular contraction. This causes constant hiccupping. If this occurs, the leads may need a position adjustment. Another problem with infants is that there is not room to implant the generator deeply, so it can trigger airport security systems.

Help parents learn to evaluate whether toys are safe. As a rule, magnets should be avoided. Toys that emit an electrical current can interfere with a pacemaker's operation and so are not recommended. Also question the use of MRI (which involves the use of magnets) or electrocautery (which involves the use of electricity) with these children. Children should not participate in contact sports such as football that could injure the pacemaker. Sports such as gymnastics and basketball that involve a high degree of shoulder action could dislodge pacemaker leads.

CONGENITAL HEART DISORDERS

About 8% of term newborns are born with a congenital cardiovascular abnormality (Fulton & Freed, 2008). This rate is even higher in preterm infants. Overall, these disorders affect equal numbers of male and female infants, but specific defects show a tendency toward sex differences. Patent ductus arteriosus and atrial septal defect, for example, are found more commonly in girls. Conditions such as valvular aortic stenosis, coarctation of the aorta, tetralogy of Fallot, and transposition of the great vessels occur more often in boys.

The usual cause of congenital heart disorders is failure of a heart structure to progress beyond an early stage of embryonic development. Maternal rubella is an example of an infection known to lead to disorders such as patent ductus arteriosus, pulmonary or aortic stenosis, atrial or ventricular septal defects, or pulmonary stenosis. Atrial and ventricular septal defects can also be familial. If a parent has an aortic stenosis, atrial septal defect, ventricular septal defect, or pulmonic stenosis, the incidence of this occurring also in the child is about 10% to 15% (Fulton & Freed, 2008).

Classification

Formerly, congenital heart disorders were classified based on the physical sign of cyanosis, or these disorders were classified as either cyanotic or acyanotic disorders.

Acyanotic heart disease involves heart or circulatory anomalies that involve either a stricture to the flow of blood or a shunt that moves blood from the arterial to the venous system (oxygenated to unoxygenated blood, or **left-to-right shunts**). These disorders cause the heart to function as an ineffective pump and make the child prone to heart failure. **Cyanotic heart disease** occurs when blood is shunted from the venous to the arterial system as a result of abnormal communication between the two systems (deoxygenated blood to oxygenated blood, or **right-to-left shunts**). Although helpful, this classification system led to difficulties because children with acyanotic heart disease can develop cyanosis, and children with cyanotic disease may not exhibit cyanosis until they are seriously ill.

To solve this problem, a second classification system has been established that addresses the hemodynamic and blood flow patterns of the disorders rather than their effect, allowing a more uniform and predictable set of signs and symptoms. As identified by this system, the four classifications identify disorders with:

- Increased pulmonary blood flow
- Obstruction to blood flow leaving the heart
- Mixed blood flow (oxygenated and deoxygenated blood mixing in the heart or great vessels)
- Decreased pulmonary blood flow

Disorders With Increased Pulmonary Blood Flow

Congenital heart disorders associated with increased pulmonary blood flow involve blood flow from the left side of the heart, which is under greater pressure, to the right side of the heart, which is under less pressure, through some abnormal opening or connection between the two systems or the great arteries. Disorders of this type include ventricular septal defect (VSD), atrial septal defect (ASD), atrioventricular canal (AVC) defect, and patent ductus arteriosus (PDA).

Ventricular Septal Defect

VSD, the most common type of congenital cardiac disorder seen, accounts for about 30% of all instances of congenital heart disease, or about 2 in every 1000 live births (Fulton & Freed, 2008). With this defect, an opening is present in the septum between the two ventricles. Because pressure in the left ventricle is greater than that in the right ventricle, blood shunts from left to right across the septum (an acyanotic disorder). This impairs the effort of the heart because blood that should go into the aorta and out to the body is shunted back into the pulmonary circulation, resulting in right ventricular hypertrophy and increased pressure in the pulmonary artery (Fig. 41.8).

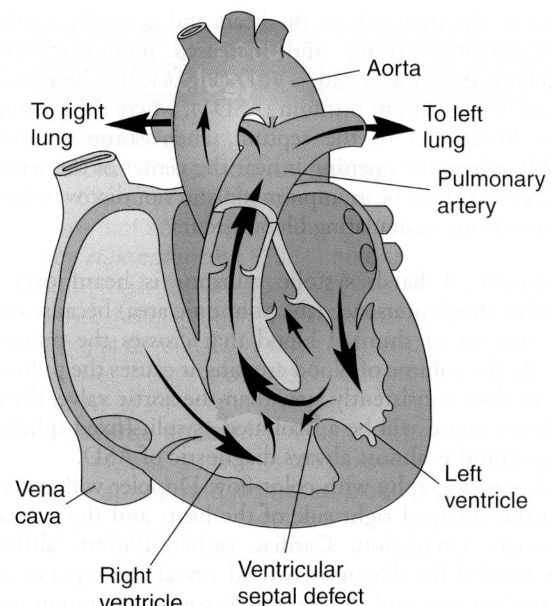

FIGURE 41.8 A ventricular septal defect.

Assessment. A VSD may not be evident at birth. With incomplete opening of the alveoli, there is still high pulmonary artery resistance, so little blood is shunted through the defect. At about 4 to 8 weeks of age, as shunting begins, the infant demonstrates easy fatigue, and a loud, harsh pansystolic murmur becomes evident along the left sternal border at the third or fourth interspace. This typical murmur is generally widely transmitted. A thrill (vibration) also may be palpable. The diagnosis of VSD is based on examination by echocardiography with color flow Doppler or MRI, which reveals right ventricular hypertrophy and possibly pulmonary artery dilatation from the increased blood flow. An ECG will also reveal right ventricular hypertrophy.

Therapeutic Management. Up to 85% of VSDs are so small they close spontaneously (Sondheimer, Yetman, & Miyamoto, 2008). Those that are moderate in size may be closed during cardiac catheterization. Larger ones (over 3 mm) require open-heart surgery. This is usually scheduled before 2 years of age to prevent pulmonary artery hypertension. Closure is important because if the defect is left open, cardiac failure from the artery hypertension can result. The heart can become infected (endocarditis) because of the recirculating blood flow.

Surgery requires the use of extracorporeal circulation and a quiet heart. In surgery, after cardiopulmonary bypass, the edges of the septal opening are approximated and sutured. If the defect is exceptionally large, a Silastic or Dacron patch can be sutured into place to occlude the space. With time, septal tissue will grow across the synthetic patch and knit it firmly into place. Postoperatively, be alert for arrhythmias because edema in the septum can interfere with ventricular conduction. Children may receive prophylactic antibiotics to prevent bacterial endocarditis for 6 months afterward. If there are no complications, children can expect to participate in normal activities after the repair.

Atrial Septal Defect

An ASD is an abnormal communication between the two atria, allowing blood to shift from the left to the right atrium (an acyanotic defect). It is more common in girls than boys (Fulton & Freed, 2008). Blood flow is from left to right (oxygenated to deoxygenated) because of the stronger contraction of the left side of the heart. This causes an increase in the

Disorders With Obstruction to Blood Flow

A number of congenital anomalies cause the blood flow leaving the heart to be obstructed because a vessel or a valve is narrower than usual. Pressure from blood flow increases prior to the narrowing and decreases after the narrowing. These are problematic defects in that they prohibit enough blood from reaching its intended site, the lungs or the rest of the body; they threaten to overwhelm the heart because of back-pressure. Obstructive defects of this category include pulmonary stenosis, aortic stenosis, and coarctation of the aorta.

Pulmonary Stenosis

Pulmonary stenosis is narrowing of the pulmonary valve or the pulmonary artery just distal to the valve (Fig. 41.12). It accounts for about 10% of congenital heart anomalies (Fulton & Freed, 2008). Inability of the right ventricle to evacuate blood by way of the pulmonary artery because of the obstruction leads to right ventricular hypertrophy.

Assessment. Infants with pulmonary artery stenosis may be asymptomatic or have signs of mild (right-sided) heart failure. If the narrowing is severe, cyanosis may be present from inability of adequate blood to reach the lungs for oxygenation or right-to-left shunting across the foramen ovale because of the increased right-sided heart pressure. A typical systolic ejection murmur, grade IV or V crescendo–decrescendo in quality, can be heard, usually loudest at the upper left sternal border. It may radiate to the suprasternal notch. A thrill may be present in the upper left sternal area or at the suprasternal notch. The second heart sound may be widely split because of late closure of the pulmonary valve. An ECG or echocardiography will reveal right ventricular hypertrophy. Cardiac catheterization is rarely necessary for diagnosis but is used for interventional enlargement of the stenosed valve.

Therapeutic Management. Management of the defect depends on the severity of the stenosis and the child's age. **Balloon angioplasty** by way of cardiac catheterization is the procedure of choice. With this procedure, a catheter with an uninflated balloon at its tip is inserted and passed through the heart into the stenosed valve. As the balloon is inflated, it breaks valve adhesions and relieves the stenosis. Following the procedure, although children may always have a residual heart murmur, they can expect a normal life span.

Aortic Stenosis

Stenosis, or stricture, of the aortic valve prevents blood from passing freely from the left ventricle of the heart into the aorta. Because the heart cannot force blood through the strictured valve, increased pressure and hypertrophy of the left ventricle occur (Fig. 41.13). If the left ventricular pressure becomes acute, pressure in the left atrium also increases, resulting in back-pressure in pulmonary veins and possibly pulmonary edema. Aortic stenosis accounts for about 7% of congenital cardiac abnormalities (Fulton & Freed, 2008).

Assessment. Most children with aortic stenosis are asymptomatic, but physical assessment generally reveals a typical murmur, a rough systolic sound heard loudest in the second right interspace (the aortic space). The murmur may be transmitted to the right shoulder, clavicle, and up the vessels of the neck; it may also be transmitted to the heart's apex. A thrill may be present, particularly at the suprasternal notch. If severe, decreased cardiac output evidenced by faint pulses, hypotension, tachycardia, and inability to suck for long periods may be present. When the child is active, chest pain similar to angina occurs, because the coronary arteries receive inadequate blood. Sudden death can occur when the amount of oxygen needed by the heart muscle on exertion far exceeds what is available.

ECG or echocardiography will reveal left ventricular hypertrophy. Cardiac catheterization is rarely necessary unless interventional therapy by this route is planned.

Therapeutic Management. Stabilization with a beta-blocker or a calcium channel blocker may be necessary to reduce cardiac

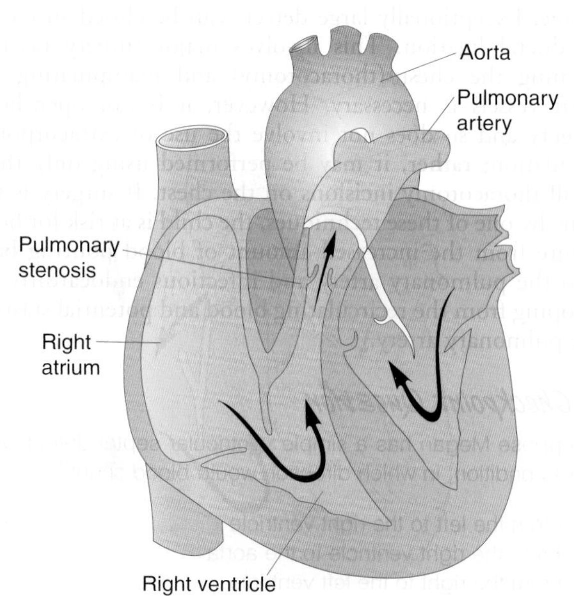

FIGURE 41.12 Pulmonary stenosis.

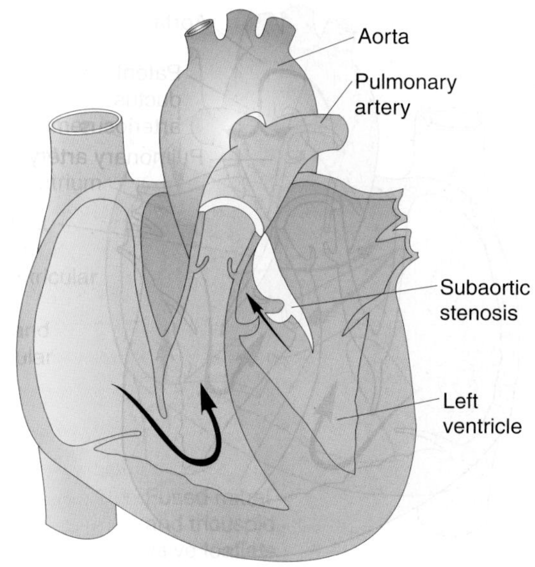

FIGURE 41.13 Aortic stenosis.

hypertrophy before the defect is corrected. Balloon valvuloplasty is the surgical treatment of choice. Surgery that involves dividing the stenotic valve or dilating an accompanying constrictive aortic ring can be used for severe defects. Such a repair may lead to aortic valve insufficiency in later life, at which time further surgery may be needed. Some children will need artificial valve replacement for correction. If a prosthetic valve is used, children generally continue to receive anticoagulation or antiplatelet therapy and antibiotic prophylaxis against endocarditis. In addition, children need exercise testing before participating in competitive sports if an artificial valve is in place.

Coarctation of the Aorta

Coarctation of the aorta, a narrowing of the lumen of the aorta due to a constricting band (Fig. 41.14), accounts for about 6% of instances of congenital heart disease (Keller, Wessels, & Markwald, 2008). It occurs more frequently in boys than in girls and is the leading cause of congestive heart failure in the first few months of life. There are two locations in which this commonly occurs. In the first, termed "preductal," the constriction occurs between the subclavian artery and the ductus arteriosus. In the second, postductal, the constriction is distal to the ductus arteriosus.

Because it is difficult for blood to pass through the narrowed lumen of the aorta, blood pressure increases proximal to the coarctation and decreases distal to it. This results in increased blood pressure in the heart and upper portions of the body as pressure in the subclavian artery increases. Elevated upper-body blood pressure produces headache and vertigo. Because a child under 3 years of age has difficulty describing these sensations, exceptional irritability may be the main clue that these symptoms are present. Epistaxis (nosebleed) and cerebrovascular accident, an event not generally associated with children, can occur from this dangerously elevated blood pressure.

Assessment. If the coarctation is slight, absence of palpable femoral pulses may be the only symptom. For this reason, always include evaluation of femoral pulses in all initial newborn assessments and admission inspections to newborn nurseries. Children who have an obstruction proximal to the left subclavian artery may have absent brachial pulses as well. As children with coarctation of the aorta grow older, they may experience leg pain on exertion because of the diminished blood supply to their lower extremities. Because collateral circulation is necessary to allow blood to flow around the constriction, collateral arteries enlarge and may be seen on the ribs as obvious nodules as the child grows older.

The diagnosis of coarctation of the aorta may be made on the basis of the history and physical assessment. On examination, the blood pressure in the arms will be at least 20 mm Hg higher than in the legs, a reversal of the normal pattern. Echocardiography, ECG, MRI, or x-ray examination of older children will reveal left-sided heart enlargement from back-pressure and also notching of the ribs from the enlarged collateral vessels. Occasionally, a murmur is present, but this is variable in position, intensity, and character. The most frequent type is a soft or moderately loud systolic murmur, especially prominent at the base of the heart and transmitted to the left interscapular area. The absence of a murmur, however, does not rule out coarctation of the aorta.

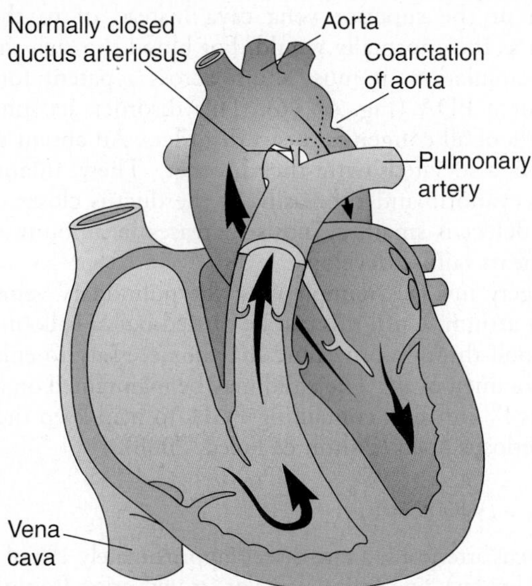

FIGURE 41.14 Coarctation of the aorta.

Therapeutic Management. Management of coarctation of the aorta is by interventional angiography (a balloon catheter) or surgery. With surgery, the narrowed portion of the aorta is removed and the new ends of the aorta are anastomosed. A graft of transplanted subclavian artery may be necessary if the narrowed section is so extensive that an anastomosis cannot be accomplished readily.

Many infants with coarctation of the aorta require therapy with digoxin and diuretics in the time before surgery can be performed. This drug therapy aims to reduce the severity of the congestive heart failure from hypertension.

Planning a time for correction of the condition is important. It would be ideal if children could achieve the greater part of their adult height before surgical correction, as this might prevent a strain on the incision line as they grow. At the same time, in terms of self-image, correction is best done before children begin to think of themselves as chronically ill or before they develop a complication, such as chronic hypertension. Girls must have the defect repaired before childbearing age, or the extra blood volume during pregnancy can cause heart failure. Surgical repair is usually scheduled, therefore, by 2 years of age. If the surgery is successful, the child can expect to live a normal life. After surgery, abdominal vessels receive more blood than they did previously. This may result in abdominal pain or generalized abdominal discomfort, but this is a short-term problem. Some children continue to have elevated upper body hypertension after the repair. They need continued treatment with antihypertensive agents. Some children require repeat balloon angioplasty at adolescence to re-enlarge the aortic lumen and help reduce this upper body hypertension.

Disorders With Mixed Blood Flow

Mixed disorders are cardiac anomalies that involve mixing of blood from the pulmonary and systemic circulation in the heart chambers. This mixing results in a relative deoxygenation of systemic blood flow, although cyanosis is not always visible. Mixed defects include transposition of the great arteries, total anomalous pulmonary venous return, truncus arteriosus, and hypoplastic left heart syndrome.

Transposition of the Great Arteries

In transposition of the great arteries, the aorta arises from the right ventricle instead of the left, and the pulmonary artery arises from the left ventricle instead of the right. Blood enters the heart from the vena cava to the right atrium, then flows to the right ventricle, and goes out into the aorta to the body completely deoxygenated; it returns again by the vena cava. A secondary source of blood enters the heart from the pulmonary veins, goes to the left atrium, left ventricle, and out the pulmonary artery to the lungs to be oxygenated, and returns to the left atrium, a second closed circulatory system (Fig. 41.15). This severe a defect is incompatible with life. In most instances, atrial and ventricular septal defects occur in connection with this transposition, making the entire heart one mixed circulatory system. It tends to occur in large newborns (9 to 10 lb) and occurs more often in boys than in girls. This disorder accounts for about 5% of congenital heart anomalies (Fulton & Freed, 2008).

Assessment. Infants with this defect are usually cyanotic from birth. There may be no murmur, or there may be various murmurs, depending on the shunting of blood through atrial or ventricular defects or through the ductus arteriosus, which usually remains open. Echocardiography generally reveals an enlarged heart. An ECG may or may not reveal heart changes. Cardiac catheterization will reveal the low oxygen saturation resulting from the mixing of blood in the heart chambers.

Therapeutic Management. If no septal defect exists or if the defect is too small to allow enough mixing of blood to sustain life, PGE_1, a prostaglandin, will be administered to keep the ductus arteriosus patent. A balloon atrial septal pull-through operation to enlarge the septal openings may also need to be done in the infant's first few days. With this procedure, done by cardiac catheterization, a deflated balloon catheter is passed

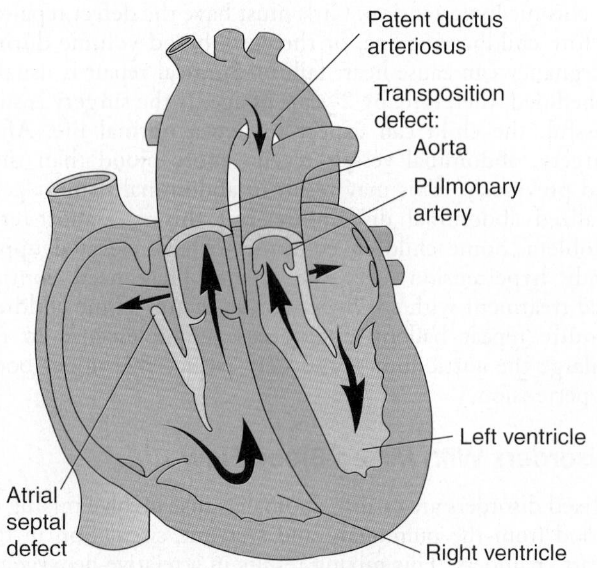

FIGURE 41.15 Transposition of the great vessels.

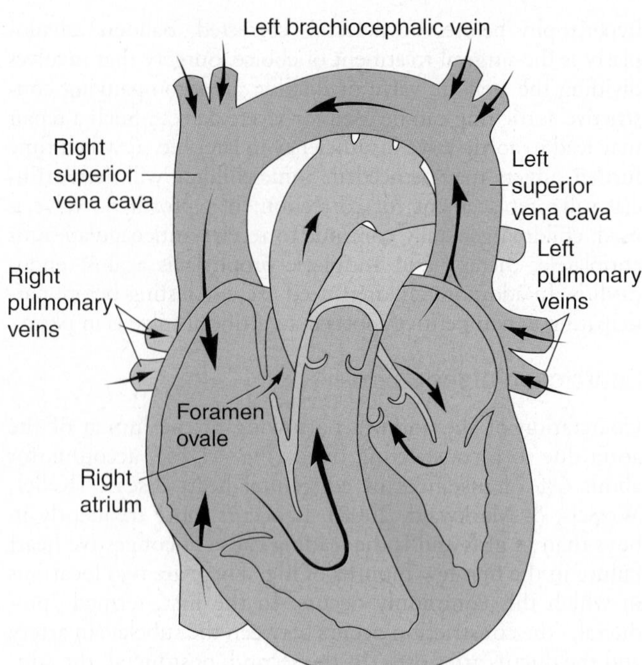

FIGURE 41.16 Total anomalous pulmonary venous return.

from the right atrium through the foramen ovale into the left atrium. The balloon is then inflated, and the catheter is drawn back into the right atrium. This enlarges the opening of the foramen ovale and creates an artificial ASD.

Surgical correction of transposition of the great vessels, done at 1 week to 3 months of age, involves an arterial switch procedure in which the major vessels are switched in position (DeBord, Cherry, & Hickey, 2007). The child will be transported to a major center for the surgery and care as soon as a disorder of this magnitude is diagnosed. The survival rate following surgery is as high as 95%.

Total Anomalous Pulmonary Venous Return

In this disorder, the pulmonary veins return to the right atrium or the superior vena cava instead of to the left atrium as they normally would. For blood to reach the systemic circulation, it must shunt across a patent foramen ovale or a PDA (Fig. 41.16). This disorder accounts for only 2% of all congenital heart disorders. An absent spleen is often associated with the disorder. These infants are mildly cyanotic and tire easily. If the ductus closes or the septal defect is small, cyanosis increases in amount; right-sided heart failure develops.

Surgery involves reimplanting the pulmonary veins into the left atrium. Until this can be carried out, a balloon atrial septal pull-through procedure may be necessary to enlarge a small foramen ovale. The child may be maintained on a continuous IV infusion containing PGE_1 to help keep the ductus arteriosus open (Fulton & Freed, 2008).

Truncus Arteriosus

In truncus arteriosus, a rare defect (approximately 1% of initial cardiac lesions), one major artery or "trunk" arises from the left and right ventricles in place of separate aorta and pulmonary

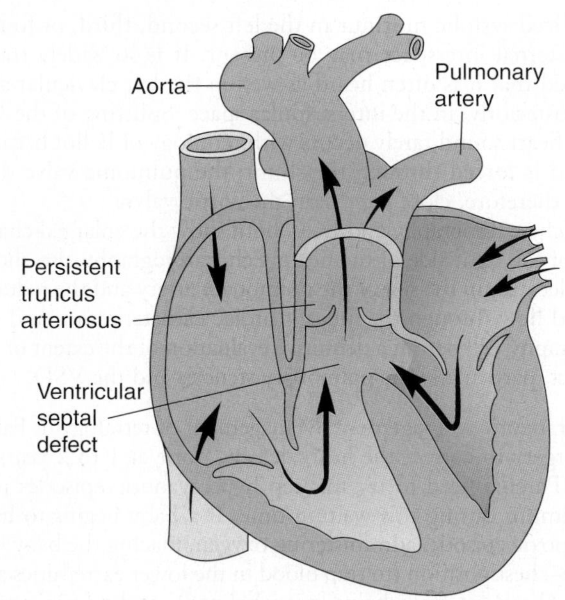

FIGURE 41.17 Truncus arteriosus.

artery vessels (Fig. 41.17). There is usually an accompanying VSD. The child is cyanotic and may have a typical VSD murmur. Repair involves restructuring the common trunk to create separate vessels. Some children need a second surgical procedure by school age as the graft inserted to separate the aorta and pulmonary artery is outgrown.

Hypoplastic Left Heart Syndrome

In hypoplastic left heart syndrome, a rare disorder accounting for only 1% to 3% of congenital heart disease, the left ventricle is nonfunctional. There may be accompanying mitral or aortic valve atresia. The nonfunctioning left ventricle lacks adequate strength to pump blood into the systemic circulation. This causes the right ventricle to hypertrophy as it tries to maintain the entire heart action (Alsoufi et al., 2007). The disorder may be detected by ultrasound prenatally (Rasiah et al., 2008). At birth, mild to moderate cyanosis develops as deoxygenated blood is shunted across the foramen ovale because of the greater pressure on the right. Echocardiography effectively diagnoses this condition. Prostaglandin therapy to maintain a PDA will be initiated to increase blood supply to the aorta. Inhaled nitrogen combined with oxygen may be prescribed to decrease Po_2; this increases pulmonary resistance and allows the right heart to shift more blood into the left heart and aorta. Surgery has limited success in this syndrome, although a great deal of research is being done in this area and a two- or three-stage procedure (restructuring of the heart; a Norwood procedure) is possible. Heart transplantation is the ultimate answer for prolonging the child's life, but the number of donor hearts available for newborns is limited (Tjang et al., 2007).

Disorders With Decreased Pulmonary Blood Flow

As the category implies, disorders with decreased pulmonary blood flow involve some type of obstruction to blood flow in the pulmonary artery. Because of the obstruction, pressure increases in the right side of the heart. If an ASD or VSD also is present, deoxygenated blood shunts from right to left. This results in deoxygenated blood invading the systemic circulation. Common disorders include tricuspid atresia and tetralogy of Fallot.

Tricuspid Atresia

Tricuspid atresia is an extremely serious disorder because the tricuspid valve is completely closed, allowing no blood to flow from the right atrium to the right ventricle (Bartlett et al., 2007). Instead, blood crosses through the patent foramen ovale into the left atrium, bypassing the lungs and the step of oxygenation. It reaches the lungs for oxygenation by being shunted back through a PDA (Fig. 41.18). As long as the foramen ovale and ductus arteriosus remain open, the child can obtain adequate oxygenation. At the point they close, however, the infant will develop extreme cyanosis, tachycardia, and dyspnea. An IV infusion of PGE_1 is begun to ensure that the ductus remains open. Surgery consists of the construction of a vena cava-to-pulmonary artery shunt, which deflects more blood to the lungs, or a Fontan procedure (sometimes termed a Glenn Shunt baffle), which restructures the right side of the heart.

Tetralogy of Fallot

Tetralogy of Fallot, one of the first types of congenital heart disease described, occurs in about 10% of children with congenital cardiac disease (Dambro, 2008). It is called a tetralogy because four anomalies are present: pulmonary stenosis, VSD (usually large), dextroposition (overriding) of the aorta, and hypertrophy of the right ventricle. Because of the pulmonary stenosis, pressure builds up in the right side of the heart. Blood then shunts from this area of increased pressure into the left ventricle and the overriding aorta. The extra effort involved to force blood through the stenosed pulmonary artery causes the fourth deformity, hypertrophy of the right ventricle (Fig. 41.19). A number of children with this disorder show a

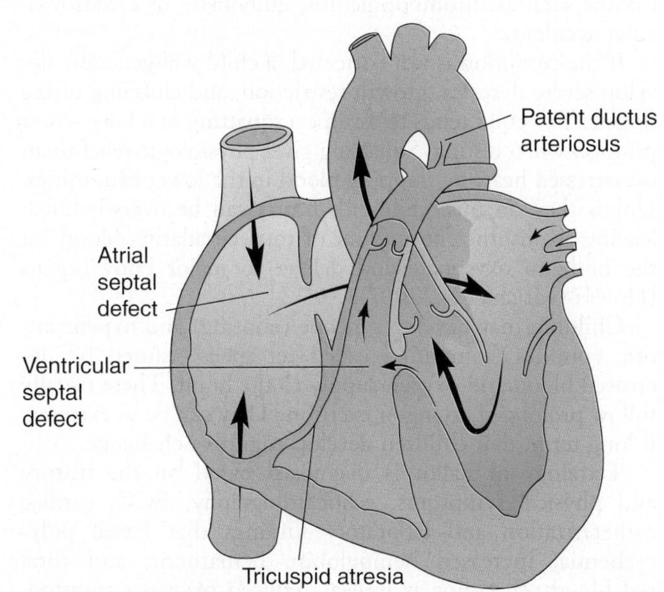

FIGURE 41.18 Tricuspid atresia.

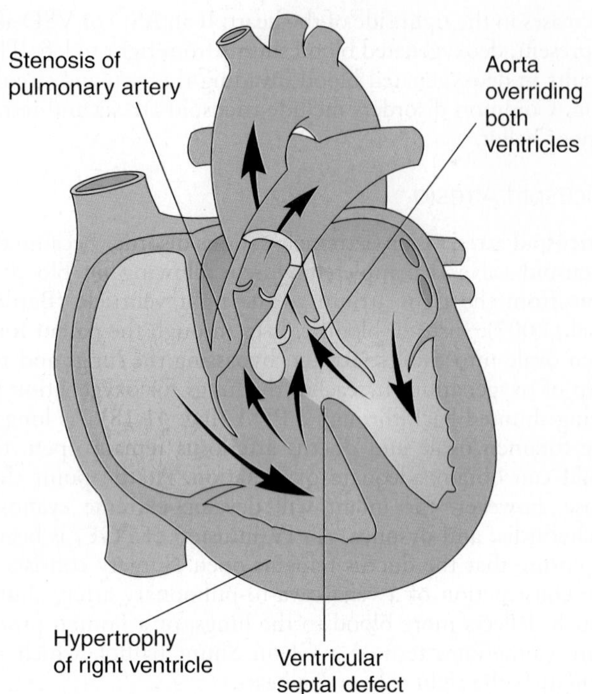

FIGURE 41.19 Tetralogy of Fallot.

deletion abnormality of chromosome 22 (22q11.2), or the disorder can result from a documented chromosome disorder.

Assessment. Although this is an extremely serious form of heart disease, newborns may not exhibit a high degree of cyanosis immediately after birth. As they become more active, however, their skin acquires a bluish tint as cyanosis begins. Polycythemia (an increase in the number of red blood cells) occurs as the body attempts to provide enough red blood cells to supply oxygen to all body parts. This is an additional potential danger because the increased concentration of red blood cells causes the blood to become thick (increased viscosity), and clots in blood vessels may occur, with complications such as thrombophlebitis, embolism, or cerebrovascular accident.

If the condition is not corrected, a child will generally develop severe dyspnea, growth restriction, and clubbing of the fingers. The child tends to assume a squatting or a knee–chest position when resting. Squatting gives physiologic relief to an overstressed heart by trapping blood in the lower extremities. Unless they do this, children's hearts can be overwhelmed, leaving an insufficient amount of total circulating blood for the body to oxygenate and deliver to major body organs (Hovels-Gurich et al., 2007).

Children may develop syncope (fainting) and hypercyanotic episodes (sometimes called tet spells) caused by decreased blood and oxygen supply to the brain. These usually follow prolonged crying or exertion. They can be so extreme, if long term, that children develop cognitive challenge.

Tetralogy of Fallot is diagnosed based on the history and physical symptoms, echocardiography, ECG, cardiac catheterization and laboratory findings that reveal polycythemia, increased hemoglobin, hematocrit, and total red blood cell count as well as reduced oxygen saturation. A loud, harsh, widely transmitted murmur or a soft, scratchy, localized systolic murmur in the left second, third, or fourth parasternal interspace may be present. It is so widely transmitted that it is often heard as well in the left clavicular area or posteriorly, in the interscapular space. Splitting of the second heart sound rarely occurs with tetralogy of Fallot because blood is forced through the shunt; the pulmonic valve does not, therefore, close later than the aortic valve.

Echocardiography and ECG both show the enlarged chamber of the right side of the heart. Echocardiography also shows the decrease in the size of the pulmonary artery and the reduced blood flow through the lungs. Cardiac catheterization and angiography will permit a definitive evaluation of the extent of the defect, particularly the pulmonary stenosis and the VSD.

Therapeutic Management. Management of tetralogy of Fallot is surgery to correct the heart defects, done at 1 to 2 years of age. Parents need to try to keep hypercyanotic episodes to a minimum during this waiting time. If a baby begins to have a hypoxic episode, administering oxygen, placing the baby in a knee–chest position (to trap blood in the lower extremities and keep the heart from being overwhelmed), and administering morphine sulfate generally reduces symptoms. If not, propranolol (Inderal, a beta-blocker) may be given orally to aid pulmonary artery dilation. A temporary or palliative surgical repair, called the Blalock-Taussig procedure, can create a shunt between the aorta and the pulmonary artery (creating a ductus arteriosus). This will allow blood to leave the aorta and enter the pulmonary artery, oxygenate in the lungs, and return to the left side of the heart, the aorta, and the body. Because the subclavian artery is used in a Blalock-Taussig procedure, a child will not have a palpable pulse in the right arm after this procedure. For this reason, blood pressure and venipunctures should be avoided in the affected arm.

A full repair that relieves the pulmonary stenosis, VSD, and overriding aorta will then be scheduled (a Brock procedure). Postoperatively, observe for arrhythmias, which may result from any ventricular septal repair, edema, and conduction interference.

What if... You noticed Megan, who has tetralogy of Fallot, always draws her knees up tightly against her chest? Would this be a concern for you? Why or why not?

ACQUIRED HEART DISEASE

The most commonly acquired heart disease in children is congestive heart failure (CHF), or a condition where the heart is overwhelmed and unable to effectively pump blood forward.

Congestive Heart Failure

Congestive heart failure (CHF) usually occurs as a result of a congenital heart disorder or a disease such as rheumatic fever, Kawasaki disease, or infectious endocarditis. This occurs when the myocardium of the heart cannot pump and circulate enough blood to supply oxygen and nutrients to body cells (Fenton & Burch, 2007). Blood pools in the heart (excessive preload) or in the pulmonary or venous systems. This may result from a congenital disorder that lessens the effectiveness of the heart's pumping action, or it may occur after cardiac surgery or rheumatic fever, when the myocardium is weakened. Severe anemia, hypocalcemia, and myocarditis may contribute to the heart's inability to function effectively. CHF is most apt to occur in children under 1 year of age (Fulton & Freed, 2008).

The heart can compensate in several ways to move blood forward and attempt to increase cardiac output. The muscle fibers can lengthen, causing the ventricles to enlarge in an attempt to handle more blood with each heart stroke (ventricular hypertrophy). The heart can also increase the number of beats per minute. As long as these mechanisms allow for adequate cardiac output, the signs of heart failure are not apparent. However, the heart's capacity for compensation is limited, particularly in infants, an age group in which hypertrophy is restricted. Eventually, in children of all ages, the heart can no longer compensate and becomes overwhelmed by the amount of blood present, which cannot be pushed forward effectively.

Sympathetic nervous system stimulation causes the frequently seen symptoms of excessive sweating and pallor. As blood flow to the kidneys decreases, the glomerular filtration rate slows, resulting in stimulation of the renin-angiotensin system, which causes fluid and sodium retention. Aldosterone secretion by the adrenal glands further promotes sodium retention in an attempt to increase blood flow to the kidneys. Antidiuretic hormone secretion by the pituitary is also increased to help retain fluid. This additional fluid results in dependent edema.

Assessment

One of the first signs of CHF is tachycardia as the heart attempts to beat faster to move blood forward more effectively; this is quickly followed by tachypnea or rapid breathing. When a child has primary right heart failure, increased venous pressure and hepatomegaly (enlarged liver) occur from back-pressure in the portal circulation. The child may feel irritable and restless from the abdominal pain caused by the liver distention. Lower extremity edema, usually a primary sign in adults, is often a late sign of heart failure in children (Box 41.6).

With left-sided heart failure, back-pressure causes blood to accumulate in the pulmonary system. Dyspnea is usually the dominant symptom, especially when a child lies flat (this is orthopnea or difficulty breathing except in an upright position; it occurs due to increased pulmonary congestion). A child may have rales and may produce bloody sputum on coughing (from lung capillaries broken under increased pulmonary blood pressure). A child may appear cyanotic from interference with gas exchange in the alveoli, which begin to fill with fluid (pulmonary edema). Left-sided heart failure can ultimately lead to right-sided heart failure as extensive pressure in the pulmonary system prevents blood from leaving the right ventricle.

In an infant, heart failure is often difficult to detect because it presents with very subtle signs. The infant becomes breathless from rapid respirations, tires easily, and has difficulty feeding because of the exhaustion and dyspnea present. Often an infant becomes diaphoretic from the effort of feeding. If edema is present, it is generalized rather than dependent and often is first noticed as periorbital edema. An abrupt gain in weight may be the most obvious indication that extra fluid is accumulating. On physical examination, an infant will have an enlarged liver (a liver palpable more than

Box 41.6 Assessment
Assessing a Child With Heart Failure

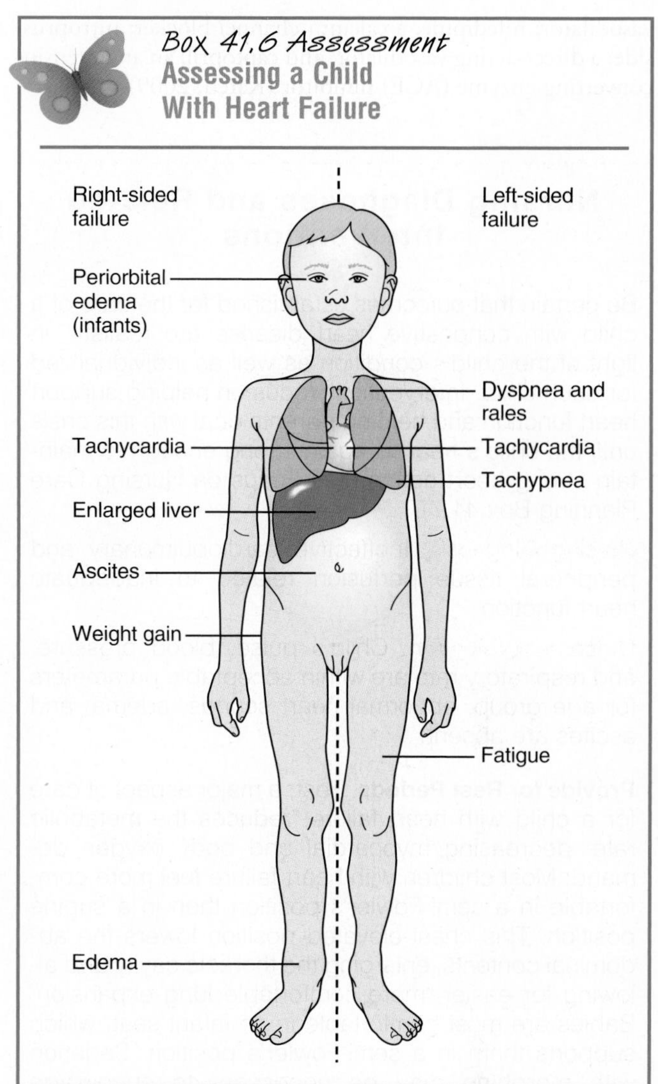

2 cm below the right costal margin) and may have ascites or fluid in the peritoneal space.

The apical heartbeat is displaced laterally and downward. As a rule, if the width of the heart is more than half the width of the chest (in a child over 1 year of age), the heart is enlarged. In addition, a galloping heart rhythm or an accentuated third heart sound may be heard because of the sudden distention of the ventricle during the rapid filling phase. Heart failure may be confirmed by echocardiography, which reveals the enlarged heart. Ventricular hypertrophy can be confirmed by ECG.

Therapeutic Management

Therapy for heart failure consists of reducing the workload of the heart by measures such as evacuating the accumulated fluid (reduces preload) with diuretics, slowing the heart rate and strengthening cardiac function (increases contractility) by administering an inotropic (heart-strengthening) drug, and reducing afterload with a vasodilator.

Commonly used diuretics include furosemide (Lasix) and spironolactone (Aldactone). The most common drug used to increase contractility and slow tachycardia is digoxin. Drugs that decrease afterload include hydralazine, an arterial vasodilator; nifedipine, a calcium channel blocker; nitroprusside, a direct-acting vasodilator; and captopril, an angiotensin-converting enzyme (ACE) inhibitor (Karch, 2009).

Nursing Diagnoses and Related Interventions

Be certain that outcomes established for the care of a child with congestive heart disease are realistic in light of the child's condition as well as individualized for each child. Interventions focus on helping support heart function and helping parents deal with this crisis until the child's heart is again strong enough to maintain strong heart action (see Focus on Nursing Care Planning Box 41.7).

Nursing Diagnosis: Ineffective cardiopulmonary and peripheral tissue perfusion related to inadequate heart function

Outcome Evaluation: Child's pulse, blood pressure, and respiratory rate are within acceptable parameters for age group; abnormal heart sounds, edema, and ascites are absent.

Provide for Rest Periods. Rest, a major aspect of care for a child with heart failure, reduces the metabolic rate, decreasing myocardial and body oxygen demand. Most children with heart failure feel more comfortable in a semi-Fowler's position than in a supine position. This chest-elevated position lowers the abdominal contents, enlarging the thoracic cavity and allowing for easier, more comfortable lung expansion. Babies are most comfortable in an infant seat, which supports them in a semi-Fowler's position. Sedation with morphine may be necessary to encourage bedrest in some children. Most children with heart failure, however, automatically limit their activity, so the need for sedation must be considered on an individual basis.

Organize nursing care to allow periods of sustained rest. At the same time, do not attempt to perform too many procedures at once or you will exhaust the child. Be certain that both you and the child's parents understand how much rest the child is to have each day. The term "complete bedrest" is often loosely used and has different meanings to different people. Does it mean a child may eat by herself, or must she be fed? Does it mean bathroom privileges or not? Playtime or not? Unless children are exceptionally exhausted, most children need to be entertained or played with to remain on bedrest. Activities such as watching television, being read to, or listening to music can quiet a child and promote better rest than if the child is expected to rest quietly without any diversion.

Provide Oxygen as Necessary. If a child has dyspnea, hypoxemia, or cyanosis, supplemental oxygen by way of hood, mask, or nasal prongs is usually necessary.

Remember that oxygen is considered to be a drug so must be prescribed according to amount or oxygen parameters except when associated with resuscitation, and oxygen saturation should be monitored with pulse oximetry. Assess the nostrils of the child receiving oxygen with nasal prongs every 4 hours to prevent pressure and subsequent irritation and breakdown of the interior nostrils (this is a major problem in newborns). For a child with heart failure, it is a strain to be submitted to strange, frightening equipment. Orient a child to oxygen equipment before it is brought to the bedside. Children generally experience such relief from dyspnea when they are receiving oxygen that their apprehension quickly disappears.

Administer Drugs as Prescribed to Improve Heart Action. Digoxin, a cardiac glycoside made from digitalis, acts directly on the heart to increase the contractility of the myocardium (and the force of contraction). It also slows the ventricular response in atrial arrhythmias. Digoxin is a potent drug, so doses must be prepared with extreme accuracy. For safest administration, digoxin should be prescribed with the dose designated in both milligrams and milliliters. When this is done, the milligram dose can be checked against the milliliter dose to be certain the decimal point of the milligram dose has not been inadvertently misplaced (0.03 mg, not 0.3 mg, for example). Digoxin may also be ordered in micrograms or μg (0.02 mg = 20 μg). Digoxin preparations are typically administered IV first in a large dose (the digitalizing dose). Six to 8 hours later, one fourth of the initial dose is given; another one fourth is given again in 6 to 8 more hours. An ECG and serum digoxin level are generally obtained before the second or third dose of digoxin to assess the adequacy of the dose. Following this, maintenance doses are given once daily. For children under 10 years of age, the dosage could be divided into two doses given at 12-hour intervals.

Before administering a dose of digoxin, to be certain that the child's heart rate is not abnormally low, always obtain a child's apical pulse. As a rule, the pulse rate should be above 100 beats per minute in infants and above 70 beats per minute in older children. When effective, digoxin improves the strength of the heart's contraction. Diuresis begins and relieves any edema present. Changes in the ECG (a lengthening of the P-R interval or a depression of the S-T segment) confirm that digitalization has taken place.

The "window" between effective digitalization and digoxin toxicity is very narrow. Monitor serum digoxin levels closely as prescribed. Symptoms of toxicity include anorexia, nausea and vomiting, dizziness, diarrhea, headache, and arrhythmia.

Many children are discharged on long-term administration of digoxin (Lanoxin). If parents will be administering the drug after their child's discharge from the hospital, be certain they understand the drug's correct dose and frequency of administration. Help them choose a specific time for administration to which they can adhere faithfully. Make out a reminder sheet to

BOX 41.7 ✻ Focus on Nursing Care Planning

A Multidisciplinary Care Map for an Infant With Congestive Heart Failure

Megan is a newborn who was born with tetralogy of Fallot. By 1 hour of age, she developed rapid respirations, tachycardia, and cyanosis. An echocardiogram revealed the typical four structural defects of the syndrome. An hour later, Megan is in heart failure.

Family Assessment ✻ Child's parents were divorced 1 month ago; dual custody of infant granted. Child will spend weekdays with mother, weekends with father. Father is a city bus driver; mother is a paralegal. Father to pay child support; with child support, mother rates finances as "workable."

Client Criteria ✻ One-hour-old infant girl who appears pale to cyanotic, tachycardic, and dyspneic. Child born by vaginal birth; Apgars 9 and 6. Afebrile; pulse 150 bpm; respirations 36. Oxygen saturation via pulse oximetry 90 mm Hg. Apical heart rate displaced down and laterally. S3 heart sound noted. Lungs with harsh rhonchi and rales on auscultation. Generalized edema with hepatomegaly.

Nursing Diagnosis ✻ Ineffective cardiopulmonary tissue perfusion related to impaired cardiac function and increased cardiac workload

Outcome Evaluation ✻ Child's vital signs are within age-acceptable parameters; skin color pink and warm; dyspnea seems lessened. Absence of S3 heart sound; oxygen saturation more than 95 mm Hg. Lungs clear to auscultation.

Team Member Responsible	Assessment	Intervention	Rationale	Expected Outcome
		Activities of Daily Living		
Nurse	Assess vital signs as prescribed. Auscultate heart and lung sounds. Monitor arterial blood gas values and oxygen saturation levels via pulse oximetry.	Place infant in infant seat to elevate head and chest 30° to 60°.	Elevating the head and chest relieves pressure on the diaphragm, enhancing lung expansion and heart function.	Child's vital signs remain within prescribed parameters. O_2 saturation is at 95%. Po_2 is 80–100 mm Hg.
Nurse	Assess actions that appear to allow the infant to be most comfortable.	Remove any constricting clothing from child's chest. Limit procedures to those that are necessary to provide adequate rest periods.	Constricting clothing interferes with chest expansion. Activity increases metabolic and myocardial oxygen demands, further impairing cardiopulmonary tissue perfusion.	Infant appears to rest comfortably in infant seat.
		Consultations		
Physician	Determine whether additional consultation will be necessary.	Consult with cardiac specialist on call as necessary.	Infants with congestive heart failure have few resources to use to compensate for failing heart action.	Cardiac specialist consults as necessary to better stabilize infant's condition.
		Procedures/Medications		
Nurse	Assess apical pulse before administering digoxin. Obtain serum digoxin levels as ordered.	Administer digoxin as prescribed.	Digoxin improves myocardial contractility.	Infant receives digoxin based on adequate heart rate and serum level.
Nurse	Obtain baseline weight. Assess electrolytes for hypokalemia before administering diuretics.	Monitor weight daily at same time. Administer diuretics, such as furosemide, as ordered.	Weight is an indicator of fluid balance. Diuretics reduce edema and diminish afterload. Potassium can be removed with urine.	Infant receives diuretics as prescribed, based on weight and potassium status.

(continued)

BOX 41.7 ✻ Focus on Nursing Care Planning (continued)

Nurse/ respiratory therapist	Assess O_2 saturation with continuous pulse oximetry.	Administer oxygen by infant hood.	Oxygen enhances tissue perfusion; Infant hoods provide oxygen without obscuring infant's face.	Infant's O_2 saturation remains at 95% or above.
		Nutrition		
Nurse	Assess child's intake and output for adequacy.	Feed 1 oz commercial formula q4h as prescribed. Allow to rest halfway through feeding.	Eating requires energy expenditure, which could compromise heart function and interfere with nutrition.	Infant takes in prescribed formula without evidence of undue tiredness.
Nurse	Determine when mother will be present in hospital.	Urge mother to feed infant at least once daily.	Feeding can promote mother–child interaction.	Mother visits and feeds at least one feeding daily. States she is comfortable feeding ill infant.
		Patient/Family Education		
Nurse	Assess parents' understanding of child's condition.	Educate parents as needed about congenital heart disease and congestive heart failure.	Parents need an understanding of child's illness to respect need for rest and medications.	Parents both state that they understand child's condition; necessary because both will be caregivers.
		Psychosocial/Spiritual/Emotional Needs		
Nurse/nurse practitioner	Assess whether parents feel they have enough emotional support to care for an ill infant at home.	Discuss necessity for vigilance and keeping infant free of infection.	Respiratory infection could quickly worsen child's condition.	Parents state that they understand the strain caring for an ill infant can cause. Have made arrangements for continuous care.
		Discharge Planning		
Nurse	Assess whether parents have any further questions about child's condition or needs.	Review care necessary for infant. Give parents written instructions.	Parents will be taking responsibility for a potentially ill infant.	Parents state that they feel confident in their ability to care for infant prior to corrective surgery.
Nurse	Assess whether parents are familiar with CPR technique for infants.	Teach parents infant CPR technique using CPR mannequin.	Well-prepared parents can be the child's first line of defense.	Parents correctly demonstrate infant CPR technique on CPR mannequin.
Nurse	Assess whether parents will be able to return infant in 1 week for follow-up visit.	Schedule appointment for 1-week follow-up visit.	Weekly evaluation will help ascertain that child's condition remains stable until corrective surgery.	Parents state that they understand importance of follow-up visit and will keep appointment.

help them remember to give the drug. Additional instructions for home administration of digoxin are shown in Box 41.8.

Diuretics such as furosemide (Lasix) may be administered to decrease pulmonary edema, which will reduce afterload. This choice appears to be more effective than restricting salt and fluid in young children. Daily weights are a good way to gauge the diuretic's effectiveness. Be certain children are weighed at the same time, with the same scale, in the same clothing (or nude) every day so measurements are as accurate as possible and any weight loss can be noted easily. As large quantities of fluid can be lost through diuretics, so can potassium, which could lead to hypokalemia

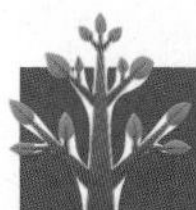

BOX 41.8 * Focus on Family Teaching

Giving Digoxin Safely at Home

Q. Megan's mother says to you, "The doctor has prescribed our daughter digoxin to take at home. Are there any special things we should do?"

A. Use the guidelines below to ensure safe digoxin administration at home:

- Always assess an apical pulse before administration; do not administer the drug if your child's heart rate is below 100 beats per minute (or as specifically instructed as she grows older).
- Always use the same measuring device (spoon or dropper) each time, so the dose given remains consistent.
- Do not change the amount or timing of the dose without specific instructions from your primary care provider.
- If you omit a single dose, give the next dose on time as prescribed.
- If you omit more than one dose, telephone your primary care provider for further instructions.
- Give digoxin 1 hour before or 2 hours after feeding, to avoid a dose being lost if the child spits up.
- If a dose is vomited, do not repeat the dose. Give the next dose at the scheduled time. If the child vomits the next dose, call your primary care provider.
- Notify your primary care provider if the child vomits more than once each day, because vomiting is a sign of digoxin overdose (toxicity).
- Notify your primary care provider if administration of the medicine or the timing of the dose is difficult for your lifestyle.

(low serum potassium levels). For these reasons, monitor urine output and serum electrolyte levels, including the potassium level. Normal urine output is 1 to 2 mL/kg/hr. If hypokalemia occurs, the risk for digoxin toxicity increases. Hydrochlorothiazide (HCTZ) is a typical diuretic used for long-term therapy. Because HCTZ, a thiazide diuretic, also promotes potassium excretion, a diet high in potassium and perhaps oral potassium supplementation may be prescribed to maintain potassium levels. Liquid potassium is irritating to the gastrointestinal tract and should be given mixed with fruit juice.

Nursing Diagnosis: Risk for imbalanced nutrition, less than body requirements, related to fatigue

Outcome Evaluation: Child maintains percentile curve on growth chart; skin turgor is good.

Maintaining proper nutrition may be a problem for children with heart failure because they tire easily. Eating six to eight small meals daily is often less tiring than eating three large meals. Smaller meals also prevent the child's stomach from pressing upward on the diaphragm and compromising an enlarged heart. Sucking is hard work, so infants may need to drink smaller amounts frequently to maintain adequate fluid intake or receive a higher-calorie formula to allow for adequate calories without added fluid volume. Using soft "preemie" nipples may be helpful because they make sucking easier. If an infant is breastfed, the mother may need to consult a lactation consultant to coordinate a program of frequent feedings.

Nursing Diagnosis: Fear related to child's ill appearance and possible disease outcome

Outcome Evaluation: Parents and child openly discuss fears and concerns, actively question, and express confidence in treatment plan and health care team.

By school age, children with heart failure are usually aware of the seriousness of their condition. They learn this from the frequent procedures and visits to cardiologists and from the exhaustion they feel because their heart is not working well. They may lie stiffly in bed, afraid to move, afraid to burden their already overtaxed heart with even simple activities such as turning pages in a book. Offer reassurance that although their heart is a little behind in its action, the oxygen and medication they are receiving are helping. Reassure them that people are checking on them frequently and observing them closely in between as well as during procedures. Give them time to talk and use play to express their fears.

Parents of a child with heart failure need the same reassurance (provided, of course, the statements are true). They are as frightened by what the physician has told them as by their child's obviously ill appearance. It is often helpful to point out subtle signs of improvement in their child that they may not notice on their own, such as a slower heart rate or slower, less distressed respirations.

If the child will be cared for at home, review CPR technique to be certain parents know what to do in an emergency. Be certain they have a follow-up appointment scheduled and a telephone number they can call if they have any concerns about their child's condition.

Persistent Pulmonary Hypertension

Persistent pulmonary hypertension (PPH) results when the pulmonary vascular resistance present at birth because of unopened alveoli fails to fall to normal. The disorder occurs most often in full-term infants who have experienced perinatal asphyxia from conditions such as postterm birth (Hernandez-Diaz et al., 2007). PPH occurs because hypoxia and acidosis from respiratory difficulty cause vasoconstriction of the pulmonary artery. The infant develops tachypnea. Pulse oximetry shows a low Po_2 from inability of blood to perfuse the lungs because of the pulmonary artery constriction. The resulting hypoxia and acidosis cause even greater vasoconstriction of the pulmonary artery. An echocardiogram slows right-to-left shunting across the patent ductus or foramen ovale.

Treatment consists of supportive therapy such as oxygen, high-frequency oscillatory ventilation, IV glucose to provide calories, antibiotics to combat infection, medications to reduce pulmonary resistance, and other drugs, such as low-dose dopamine, to elevate systemic blood pressure. Sildenafil citrate has promising effects for vasodilation and reduced resistance

(Leibovitch, Matok, & Paret, 2007). Sodium bicarbonate may be necessary to relieve acidosis and to help reverse pulmonary vasoconstriction. Inhaled nitric oxide may be administered to promote pulmonary vasodilatation (Tanaka et al., 2007). Infants who do not respond to these usual measures may require ECMO to allow the lungs to rest until adequate pulmonary vasodilatation and the return of alveoli perfusion can be achieved.

PPH is a serious threat to newborns, both because of the original insult from respiratory distress that produced the syndrome and the prolonged therapy course. Because of this, a newborn may be left with neurologic challenge from severe hypoxia and inadequate brain cell oxygen perfusion.

Rheumatic Fever

Rheumatic fever is an autoimmune disease that occurs as a reaction to a group A beta-hemolytic streptococcal infection (Bashore & Granger, 2009). Inflammation from the immune response leads to fibrin deposits on the endocardium and valves, in particular the mitral valve, as well as in the major body joints. The disease often follows an attack of pharyngitis, tonsillitis, scarlet fever, "strep throat," or impetigo, because the organism common to these infections is a group A beta-hemolytic streptococcus. In 95% of children with acute rheumatic fever, an elevation of one or more antistreptococcal antibodies, an indication of a recent streptococcal infection, can be documented. Although the incidence of rheumatic fever has declined greatly in recent years, the disease has not been eradicated, and in some inner cities and developing countries, the incidence is rising (Carapetis, 2007). It occurs most often in children 6 to 15 years of age, with a peak incidence at 8 years. It is seen most often in poor, crowded urban areas. Because children do not develop immunity to streptococcal infections, streptococcal infections recur; rheumatic fever also recurs.

The symptoms of the original streptococcal infection subside in a few days with or without antimicrobial therapy. Children appear well again. After 1 to 3 weeks, however, if the child was not treated with an appropriate antibiotic for the original infection, the onset of rheumatic fever symptoms can begin. Because nurses are the primary people who advise parents when to seek health care and how to adhere to medicine administration, nurses have contributed greatly to the decline of this disorder.

Assessment

The signs and symptoms of rheumatic fever are divided into major and minor symptoms according to the Jones criteria (Box 41.9). Of these, the heart involvement is the most serious. The child usually has a systolic murmur from mitral insufficiency and prolonged P-R and Q-T intervals on the ECG that reflect inflammation and slowing of impulse conduction. Sydenham's chorea (sudden involuntary movement of the limbs) is a striking symptom (Weiner & Normandin, 2007). This loss of voluntary muscle control due to inflammation of basal ganglia occurs most often in children between 7 and 14 years of age (rarely after age 20). It occurs more frequently in girls than boys. Dysfunctional speech from chorea may be demonstrated by asking the child to count rapidly. Children with chorea begin with clear speech, but then suddenly the sounds become garbled or they cannot speak for several seconds. If asked to protrude the tongue, children cannot keep from making undulating, jerky movements. If asked to extend their arms in front of them, they soon hyperextend their wrists and fingers. Hand grasp may be weak or may consist of spasmodic contractions and relaxation. If asked to smile, the facial expression may change rapidly from a "Cheshire cat" grin to a flat, expressionless affect or grimace. Erythema marginatum, a macular rash found predominantly on the trunk, subcutaneous nodules or painless lumps on tendon sheaths by the joints, and tender swollen large joints (polyarthritis) are additional manifestations. Important laboratory findings include the presence of an antibody antistreptococcal titer (ASO) and an increased ESR and C-reactive protein levels (Smith, 2008).

Therapeutic Management

The full course of rheumatic fever is 6 to 8 weeks. Children are maintained on bedrest only during the acute phase of illness or until congestive heart disease is not present, the ESR decreases, and the C-reactive protein level and pulse rate return to normal. Because pulse rate is a valuable sign of improvement, monitoring vital signs is essential during the acute phase. Obtaining an apical pulse for a full minute is preferred. It may be ordered when the child is asleep as well

Box 41.9 Assessment
Assessing a Child With Rheumatic Fever

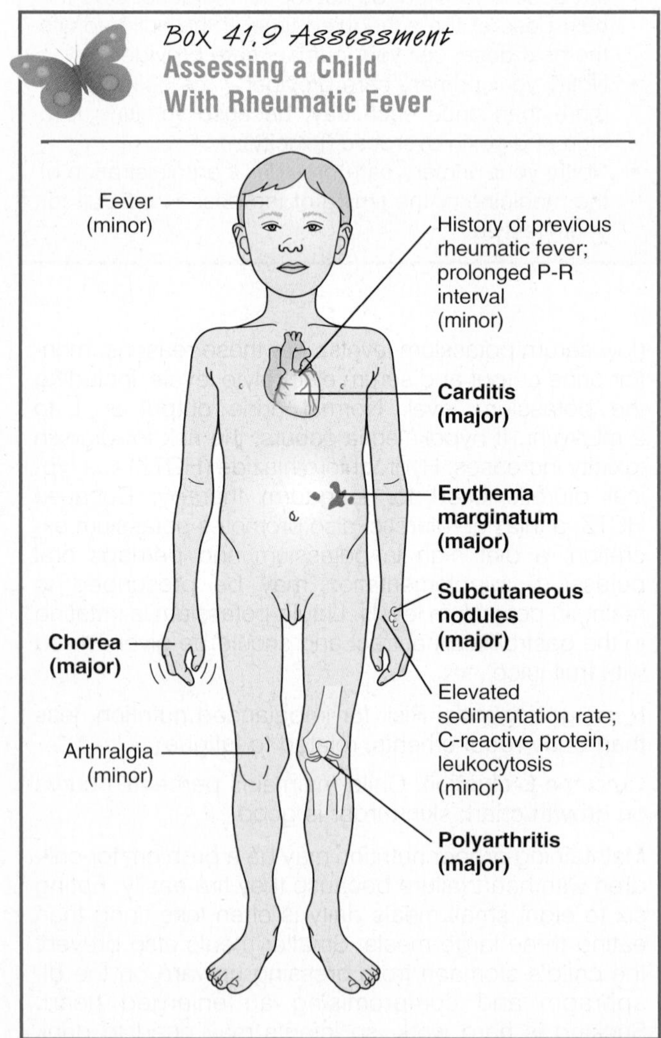

as when the child is awake to measure the effect of activity on the pulse rate.

A course of penicillin therapy or a single intramuscular injection of benzathine penicillin is used to eliminate group A beta-hemolytic streptococci completely from the child's body. Oral ibuprofen is prescribed to reduce inflammation and joint pain. Corticosteroids may be prescribed to reduce inflammation in children who are not responding to ibuprofen therapy alone. Possible side effects of corticosteroid therapy include hirsutism, a round moon face (Cushing's syndrome), and an increased susceptibility to infection.

Phenobarbital and diazepam are both effective in reducing the purposeless movements of chorea. If heart failure is present, measures to reduce heart failure such as digoxin and diuretics will be prescribed.

The prognosis for the child with rheumatic fever depends on the extent of myocardial involvement. Valve destruction from formation of Aschoff's bodies (fibrin deposits) may result in permanent valve dysfunction, especially of the mitral valve. With severe myocarditis the heart dilates, but when it cannot maintain this compensation, it eventually fails to contract effectively. Children may be left with mitral valve insufficiency, which is especially hazardous for girls, because this may lead to heart failure during pregnancy. Some children need mitral valve replacement to restore heart function. Usually, there are no residual effects from joint or chorea involvement.

Nursing Diagnoses and Related Interventions

Nursing Diagnosis: Risk for nonadherence to drug therapy related to knowledge deficit about importance of long-term therapy

Outcome Evaluation: Child takes oral penicillin daily; absence of symptoms of throat infection; vital signs are within age-acceptable parameters.

Therapy for Initial Attack. A child who has had rheumatic fever is at great risk for a recurrence (Sondheimer, Yetman, & Miyamoto, 2008). To eliminate the bacteria from the upper respiratory tract, either amoxicillin or penicillin is prescribed. To be effective, a drug level must be maintained for 10 to 14 days. Erythromycin is used in children sensitive to penicillin; it, too, must be continued for at least 10 days. One intramuscular injection of a long-acting penicillin, such as benzathine penicillin (Bicillin), can be used with children if there is a question whether the parent will give, or the child will take, the full course of oral penicillin. Be sure to repeat prescription instructions for parents in ambulatory settings so they understand how often and how much of a drug is to be given and the need to give the drug for the full 10 to 14 days. Usually a child's symptoms will fade before then, and if the parents are not cautioned about the importance of the drug, they may give the drug for only 2 or 3 days and then discontinue it.

Prevent Recurrent Attacks. Children who have had rheumatic fever must be prevented from contracting the disease again to prevent valve damage from occurring a second time. To do this, they must take prophylactic antibiotic therapy for at least 5 years after the initial attack, or until they are 18 years of age. If some valve involvement is present, many physicians advocate maintaining the child on penicillin indefinitely. Penicillin may be prescribed as monthly injections of benzathine penicillin G or daily oral doses of aqueous penicillin (penicillin V).

Additional prophylactic measures should be instituted when dental or tonsillar surgery is planned, because most children have streptococci in their throats (Sykes & Farrington, 2007). With an open incision in the mouth, the risk of streptococcal invasion of the bloodstream increases.

Nursing Diagnosis: Situational low self-esteem related to chorea movements secondary to rheumatic fever

Outcome Evaluation: Child expresses frustration with inability to control movements; continues to feed and dress self with help as needed.

Children may have difficulty feeding themselves because of chorea. They may also be emotionally unstable and cry easily. Emphasize the transitory nature of the chorea; stress that it is frustrating to have to be fed and to be unable to use your hands meaningfully, but that this lack of coordination will pass without permanent effects. Provide toys and games that do not require fine coordination, because it may be frustrating to try to do something such as move checkers or chessmen on a board (a typical low-activity game). Children with chorea who are on bedrest may need to have the bedrails padded so they do not injure themselves from thrashing movements.

Kawasaki Disease

Kawasaki disease (mucocutaneous lymph node syndrome) is a febrile, multisystem disorder that occurs almost exclusively in children before the age of puberty. It has replaced rheumatic fever as the most likely cause of acquired heart disease in children. The peak incidence is in boys under 4 years of age. The incidence is higher in late winter and spring. **Vasculitis** (inflammation of blood vessels) is the principal (and life-threatening) finding because it can lead to formation of aneurysm and myocardial infarction (Rowley & Shulman, 2007).

The cause of Kawasaki disease is unknown, but it apparently develops in genetically predisposed individuals after exposure to an as-yet-unidentified infectious agent. After the infection (perhaps an upper respiratory infection), altered immune function occurs. An increase in antibody production creates circulating immune (antibody–antigen) complexes that bind to the vascular endothelium and cause inflammation. The inflammation of blood vessels leads to aneurysms, platelet accumulation, and the formation of thrombi or obstruction in the heart and blood vessels.

Assessment

Kawasaki disease begins with an acute phase (stage I) of high fever (102° to 104° F [39.0° to 40.0° C]) that does not respond to antipyretics (Box 41.10). The child acts lethargic or irritable and may have reddened and swollen hands and feet.

Box 41.10 Assessment
Assessing a Child With Kawasaki Disease

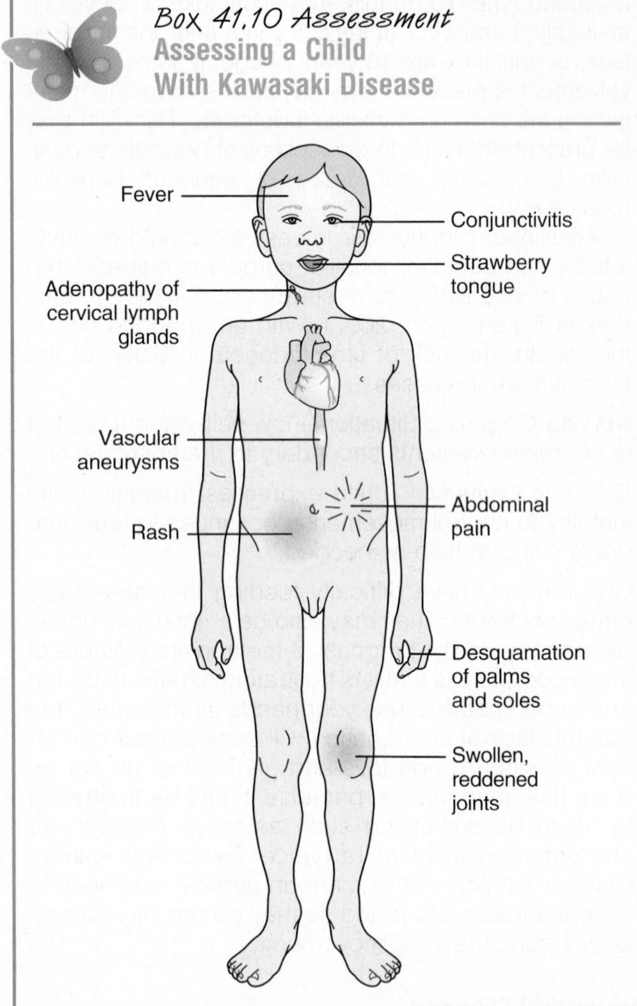

Soon the bulbar mucous membranes of the eyes become inflamed (conjunctivitis) and the child develops a "strawberry" tongue and red, cracked lips. A variety of rashes occur, often confined to the diaper area. Cervical lymph nodes become enlarged. As internal lymph nodes swell, children may develop abdominal pain, anorexia, and diarrhea. Joints may swell and redden, simulating an arthritic process. White blood cell count and the ESR are both elevated.

About 10 days after the onset, a subacute phase begins. The skin desquamates, particularly on the palms and soles. The platelet count rises; this increases the possibility of clotting, which could result in necrosis of distant body cells, particularly the fingertips, if they no longer receive adequate blood. Aneurysms may form in coronary arteries, compromising heart activity. Sudden death from accumulating thrombi or rupture of an aneurysm may occur, making this the most dangerous phase.

The convalescent phase (stage II) begins at about the 25th day and lasts until 40 days. Stage III lasts from 40 days until the ESR returns to normal. To be diagnosed with Kawasaki disease, a child must manifest fever and four of the typical symptoms shown in Box 41.11, plus echocardiographic confirmation of artery disease. Children are followed by sequential echocardiograms to monitor for development of aneurysms.

BOX 41.11 ✻ Criteria for Diagnosis of Kawasaki Disease

1. Fever of 5 or more days' duration
2. Bilateral congestion of ocular conjunctivae
3. Changes of the mucous membrane of the upper respiratory tract, such as reddened pharynx; red, dry, fissured lips; or protuberance of tongue papillae ("strawberry" tongue)
4. Changes of the peripheral extremities, such as peripheral edema, peripheral erythema, desquamation of palms and soles
5. Rash, primarily truncal and polymorphous
6. Cervical lymph node swelling

Therapeutic Management

The administration of acetylsalicylic acid (aspirin) or ibuprofen decreases inflammation and blocks platelet aggregation. Abciximab is a platelet receptor inhibitor specific for Kawasaki disease (Karch, 2009). IV immune globulin (IVIG) can also be administered to reduce the immune response (Oates-Whitehead et al., 2009). Caution parents that children should not receive routine immunizations while taking IVIG or the immunization will be ineffective. Steroids, which may increase aneurysm formation, are contraindicated. If the child is left with coronary artery disease from stenosis of the coronary arteries, coronary artery bypass surgery may be necessary in the future.

Nursing Diagnoses and Related Interventions ✻

Nursing Diagnosis: Risk for ineffective peripheral tissue perfusion related to inflammation of blood vessels

Outcome Evaluation: Child's pulse, blood pressure, and respiratory rate are within age-established parameters; capillary filling time is less than 5 seconds.

Observe for signs of heart failure such as tachycardia, dyspnea, rales, and edema. Inspect the extremities for color and palpate for warmth and capillary filling in toes and fingers to evaluate peripheral tissue perfusion. If a child is developing myocarditis, be alert for chest pain, arrhythmias, and ECG changes. All these are findings that need to be reported and documented.

Nursing Diagnosis: Pain related to swelling of lymph nodes and inflammation of joints

Outcome Evaluation: Child states level of pain is tolerable; rates it below 2 on a standard scale.

A child with Kawasaki disease is uncomfortable from the joint involvement, edema, pruritic rash, abdominal discomfort, and the frequent blood sampling necessary to monitor the platelet count. The high fever can lead to dry, cracked lips. Ibuprofen, administered for its anti-inflammatory action, helps reduce both the pain and itchiness (which is a low level of pain). Provide additional comfort measures such as rocking and holding. Protect edematous areas from pressure; make certain clothing is not constricting and irritating areas of rash. Applying lip balm protects lips from drying and cracking.

Because the fever remains high, offer extra fluid to help maintain hydration and reduce mouth tenderness. Keep the child free of heavy blankets or clothing and prevent overexertion. Monitor IV fluid to prevent fluid overload.

Children with Kawasaki disease lose their appetite and generally eat poorly because of the systemic illness, mouth soreness from cracks and fissures, and abdominal pressure from swollen lymph nodes. Carefully monitor and record the child's intake and output. Encourage the child to continue brushing his or her teeth (use a soft toothbrush or a padded tongue blade), even though the oral mucous membrane is tender. Soft, nonirritating foods such as gelatin (Jell-O) may be better tolerated than foods that require chewing and acidic fluids, such as orange juice, that might sting. Observe for signs of gastrointestinal obstruction, such as vomiting.

Most children with Kawasaki disease recover fully, but a few will need cardiac bypass surgery to treat aneurysms that developed in the coronary arteries.

What if... A child with Kawasaki disease has ibuprofen ordered every 4 hours but tells you she no longer has pain or fever? Should you continue to give it?

Endocarditis

Endocarditis is inflammation and infection of the endocardium or valves of the heart (Tulathimutte, 2008). It may occur in a child without heart disease but more commonly occurs as a complication of congenital heart disease such as tetralogy of Fallot, VSD, or coarctation of the aorta. The infection is generally caused by streptococci of the viridans type, although staphylococcal or fungal organisms may be at fault. The streptococcal infection tends to invade the body during oral surgery, such as with dental extractions. It also can enter from a urinary tract infection or a skin infection, such as impetigo. As the disease progresses, vegetation composed of bacteria, fibrin, and blood appears on the endocardium of the valves and heart chambers. This tends to occur more commonly on the left side of the heart, although if a heart defect is present the erosion begins at the site of the defect. Over a period of time, the invading process destroys the endocardial lining of the heart, underlying muscle and valves (Sondheimer, Yetman, & Miyamoto, 2008).

Assessment

The onset of the illness is insidious. Children often appear pale, with anorexia and weight loss. Arthralgia (pain in joints), malaise, chills, or periods of sweating, especially at night, occur. As the vegetative process begins to erode the heart's valves, significant murmurs become audible. Signs of heart failure appear. Petechiae of the conjunctiva or oral mucosa or hemorrhages of the fingernails or toenails (that simulate a splinter inserted under the nail) may be present. The child may notice left upper quadrant abdominal pain from infarction of the spleen; on physical assessment, the spleen may be enlarged. Laboratory studies may reveal proteinuria or hematuria; a normochromic, normocytic anemia may also be present. There may be leukocytosis and an increased ESR. An echocardiogram shows vegetative growths on the heart valves. The diagnosis is confirmed by a blood culture that reveals the presence of the invading organism.

Therapeutic Management

All children with congenital heart disease and those who have had rheumatic fever should have prophylactic administration of an antibiotic before ear, nose, throat, tonsil, or mouth surgery (and before childbirth) to prevent infectious endocarditis. If it does occur despite these preventive measures, therapy is directed toward the underlying infection and also includes supportive measures to reduce heart failure. Because the invading organism is generally a streptococcus, a penicillinase-resistant penicillin such as nafcillin (Unipen) is prescribed and given IV through a central venous access device. Giving the drug into a large vessel allows quick dilution and distribution. Children need long-term follow-up care to be certain the invading organism is eliminated and the disease process has halted. Prognosis is good unless an embolus from the vegetations on the valves causes a complication such as renal occlusion or cerebrovascular accident.

Arrhythmias

Children have fewer cardiac arrhythmias than do adults, but the number of these is increasing as more and more children survive cardiac surgery for congenital heart disease but are left with a cardiac arrhythmia due to septal trauma (Prystowsky & Foge, 2008). Better means of monitoring cardiac rhythm patterns through the use of Holter monitors has also made detection of cardiac arrhythmia easier. Remember that most children show a normal sinus arrhythmia or a slowing of the heart rate during inspiration (increased lung size slows lung perfusion, putting enough back-pressure on the heart to slow the heartbeat), with the normal rate resuming on expiration.

Ventricular tachycardia and atrial fibrillation are syndromes that occur because of multiple or abnormal initiation of the heartbeat and can occur following surgery for congenital heart disease. These can cause episodes of syncope, palpitations, and exercise intolerance. If bradycardia occurs, it can be treated with a drug such as atropine to counteract vagal stimulation; digoxin is commonly used for decreasing and strengthening the heart rate if needed. A few children may require pacemakers implanted to maintain a steady heart rhythm.

Cryo- or radioablation are nonsurgical transvenous catheter techniques that can permanently disrupt an abnormal arrhythmia focus (Tuzcu, 2007).

Hypertension

Although primary hypertension may occur in children, hypertension in children usually occurs as a secondary manifestation of another disease such as a kidney disorder. It has a higher incidence among black children than other ethnic groups and occurs in about 1% of schoolchildren and adolescents. As obesity in children is increasing, the incidence of hypertension in children is also increasing.

It is difficult to define hypertension in children because normal blood pressure varies with the age of the child. A systolic pressure reading above the 95th percentile for a given age may be used as a practical criterion (AAP, 2009).

Assessment

Beginning at 3 years of age, blood pressure should be included as a part of routine health assessment. Normal blood pressure and the technique of blood pressure recording in children are discussed in Chapter 34. To ensure accuracy, be sure a child is relaxed, after at least 1 or 2 minutes of rest, before taking a blood pressure. When children are discovered on routine physical assessment to have hypertension, the reading should be repeated at a successive visit to confirm that the abnormal reading was not a reaction to the stress of the examination or some other emotional event of that day. Only when the blood pressure is still elevated on a third occasion is hypertension diagnosed.

When a child has hypertension, a number of additional studies are performed to discover underlying disease conditions. The most common diseases associated with hypertension in children are renal and cardiac diseases such as coarctation of the aorta, Cushing's syndrome, primary hyperaldosteronism, adrenogenital syndrome, pheochromocytoma (a tumor of the adrenal gland), and brain tumor. If blood pressure is elevated, record a blood pressure in both lower extremities and upper extremities to help rule out coarctation of the aorta (which results in low pressure in the lower extremities). Obtain a urine specimen for analysis of microalbuminuria, a finding that accompanies hypertension. If red blood cells are present in urine, this suggests glomerulonephritis, a kidney disease that increases blood pressure. Children with suspected hypertension should have a funduscopic examination of their eyes to determine the presence of papilledema or spasm, or hemorrhage of the retinal arteries from the consistently elevated blood pressure. If papilledema is present, children need immediate care to prevent optic nerve damage. Further studies to rule out adrenal or renal disease may be ordered if these preliminary assessment procedures do not reveal a cause for the hypertension (Armstrong, 2007).

Therapeutic Management

Therapy for hypertension depends on the underlying primary disease. Although the underlying disease conditions that lead to hypertension are serious disorders, they are also ones that can respond to therapy. Therefore, hypertension must not be dismissed lightly.

If essential hypertension (elevated blood pressure for no identifiable reason) is present and a child is obese, a child is placed on a reducing diet and urged to increase the level of exercise to reduce weight. Salt intake is rarely limited, but it may be if salt intake has been excessive; girls are advised not to use oral contraceptives, which elevate blood pressure. Unfortunately, because mild hypertension produces few symptoms, often children do not adhere to nutritional suggestions or suggested exercise programs well. For these children, a single medication such as an angiotensin-converting enzyme (ACE) inhibitor such as captopril [Capoten] may be prescribed. A diuretic such as furosemide (Lasix) or vasodilators such as hydralazine (Apresoline) may also be added.

Children with hypertension need continued counseling at health care visits. Educate them and their parents about the long-term effects of hypertension (increased risk of heart and blood vessel disease). Only if children understand these long-term consequences can they see the benefits of taking medication today.

Dyslipidemia

Dyslipidemia (increased lipids in blood serum) can involve cholesterol or triglycerides. Risk factors include familial hypercholesterolemia, a dominantly inherited disease occurring in 5% to 25% of children; obesity; a sedentary lifestyle; and a high-fat diet (Pignone & McPhee, 2009). For this reason, all children of parents with premature coronary artery disease (disease before the age of 55) or a family history of hypercholesterolemia (parents with blood cholesterol levels above 200 mg/dL or low-density lipoprotein [LDL] levels above 130 mg/dL) should be screened for total serum cholesterol, because there is an association between high total cholesterol and LDL and the incidence of coronary artery disease. This is particularly important if the child smokes, is obese, or has a sedentary lifestyle.

Acceptable levels of total cholesterol and LDL in children are less than 170 mg/dL and less than 110 mg/dL, respectively. Levels are borderline if they are 170 to 199 mg/dL and 110 to 129 mg/dL. They are high if over 200 mg/dL and 130 mg/dL (AAP, 2009).

If the total triglyceride, cholesterol, or LDL level is found to be elevated, the child's diet should be regulated in an attempt to lower these levels. Exercise also should be increased. Adolescents may be placed on the American Heart Association's step 1 diet (total fat no more than 30% of calories; cholesterol less than 300 mg/day) to attempt to bring them into adulthood with sound nutritional habits. Children rarely are placed on low-fat diets because they need calories for growth. Use of low-fat diets in infants under 2 years of age is even less common because fat is needed for myelinization of nerves.

If the child becomes an adolescent and the diet has not been effective, one of the many cholesterol-reducing agents such as cholestyramine (Questran) may be prescribed. These agents reduce the cholesterol level by binding bile acids and decreasing their reabsorption. Side effects of these drugs include large, bulky stools and possible gastrointestinal discomfort. If this therapy is ineffective, an HMG-CoA inhibitor such as atorvastatin (Lipitor) may be prescribed.

Because hypercholesterolemia has no symptoms, it is difficult to motivate children to continue a special diet and take medication unless the entire family changes to a lower fat diet (Poustie & Rutherford, 2009). They need continued counseling at health care visits so they understand the damage that excess lipids can cause.

Cardiomyopathy

The term "cardiomyopathy" refers to a structural or functional abnormality of the ventricular myocardium that occurs following an infection such as adenovirus, cytomegalovirus, or

HIV/AIDS infection and results in severe dilation of the left or both ventricles (Colam et al., 2007). This impairs systolic function and leads to heart failure. Idiopathic dilated cardiomyopathy (IDC) is a rare form that presents before 2 years of age, usually after a viral respiratory or gastrointestinal illness. Hypertrophic cardiomyopathy (HCM) is a relatively common autosomal dominant disease that occurs at an incidence of about 1 in 500 young adults (Marian, Brugada, & Roberts, 2008).

In the older child, symptoms appear gradually. Physical examination reveals an ill-appearing child with severe respiratory distress. Peripheral pulses are weak and blood pressure is decreased. Pulsus alternans (beat-to-beat variation) is a common finding. The liver is enlarged from backflow pressure. A chest radiograph, echocardiogram, and ECG all reveal the enlarged heart.

Therapy is directed at controlling the heart failure by bedrest, fluid restriction, and pharmacologic agents to decrease the cardiac load, improve myocardial contractility, and decrease afterload. Immune globulin may help reverse the process. If a child fails to respond to medical therapy, the prognosis is poor unless the child is eligible for cardiac transplantation.

CARDIOPULMONARY ARREST

Children with heart disease are at high risk for cardiopulmonary arrest, although this may occur in any child for reasons such as airway obstruction, trauma, anaphylactic reaction, central nervous system depression, drowning, or electrocution. Management of cardiopulmonary arrest may vary according to the cause of the arrest and the age of the patient, but the basic considerations are the same.

Many health care facilities and public buildings provide automated external defibrillators (AEDs) for use in cardiac resuscitation. Nurses who respond to emergencies need to familiarize themselves with this equipment as well as CPR technique (AHA, 2008).

Assessment

Respiratory failure is the most frequent cause of cardiac arrest because anoxia in the heart muscle quickly leads to cardiac arrest. When cardiac arrest occurs, no audible heart sounds or pulses can be obtained. No blood pressure can be recorded (do not waste time trying to obtain one). If a cardiac monitor was attached before the arrest, it will show no ECG complex. This is a helpful assessment if available, but again do not waste time attaching monitor leads if they are not already in place. The outcome for the child in arrest will depend to a great extent on the speed with which resuscitation is begun, so it is better to err on the side of unnecessary resuscitation rather than delayed resuscitation. The steps for resuscitation can be remembered as "ABCs" (*airway, breathing, and circulation*).

Airway

The first step in resuscitation is to shake the child and call the child's name to verify that a child is not just sound asleep. If a child does not respond to this action, call for help. Turn the child onto the back and open the mouth. Tip the child's head backward slightly to a neutral position or place a rolled towel or other fairly firm object under the neck to hyperextend the head slightly (a "sniffing" position). Do not overextend the neck, however, or you will occlude, not clear, the airway (AHA, 2008).

Breathing

Emergency equipment such as an Ambu-bag should be readily available in all health care settings so that mouth-to-mouth resuscitation is not necessary. If no breathing bag is available, use a protective one-way valve mask for mouth-to-mouth resuscitation to protect yourself from body secretions.

For small infants, place the bag mask over the infant's mouth and nose, creating a seal. For larger infants and children, make a bag-to-mouth seal, pinching the child's nose tightly with the thumb and forefingers. Provide two slow breaths (1 to 1.5 seconds per breath). It may be necessary to adjust the head-tilt chin position to obtain optimal airway patency, although this should not be done if neck or spine trauma is suspected (AHA, 2008).

If oxygen is available, attach it to the resuscitation bag, running at a rate of about 4 L/min. However, do not wait for oxygen if it is not available. Room air's oxygen content is about 21%, so additional oxygen is helpful but not necessary for resuscitation.

Observe the child's chest with each breath you administer to see if it rises. If it does not, the airway is obstructed and air cannot reach the lungs; you need to alert the EMS system for help. Perform back blows and chest thrusts for an infant or subdiaphragmatic abdominal thrusts for an older child to help relieve the obstruction (see Chapter 40). Continued breaths should be given at the rate of normal respirations (20/min) in both infants and older children. When respiratory arrest has occurred and mechanical ventilation is anticipated, the child can be intubated to provide an open airway, as discussed in Chapter 40.

Circulation

After the two initial ventilations, feel for a carotid pulse (in an infant, the brachial pulse) or assess for other signs of circulation, such as adequate color (Fig. 41.20). It is better to use the carotid than a peripheral pulse as an indicator of cardiac function in older children, because with shock, the peripheral pulses may be absent while the heart is still beating. The carotid pulse is also the easiest to assess from your position near the child's head. In an infant, however, the neck may be too chubby for you to easily palpate a carotid pulse, so the brachial pulse is easiest to assess.

If you feel no pulse, begin chest compressions. In a newborn, enough pressure will be generated by two fingers pressed on the midsternum about a fingerbreadth below the nipple line to a depth of ½ to 1 inch (Fig. 41.21). Midsternal compression is used with newborns and infants to prevent excessive pressure on the ribs and the possibility of breaking either a rib or the xiphoid process (which then might puncture the heart or liver). In the older child, you need to apply the heel of your palm over the sternum (measure one or two fingerbreadths up from the sternal-costal notch and place the palm there) and compress 1 to 1½ inches (Fig. 41.22). Compress the chest at a rate of 100 beats per minute in both infants and older children (AHA, 2008).

Breathing and cardiac compression must be carried out concurrently but not exactly at the same time. If there are two

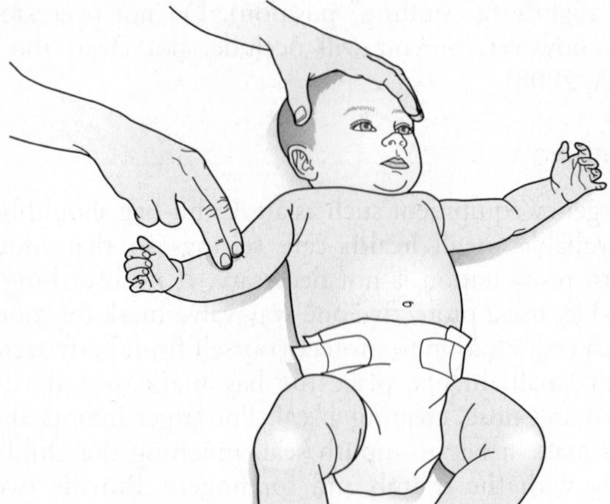

FIGURE 41.20 Assessing a brachial pulse in an infant.

people available for resuscitation, one can administer breaths to the child while the other compresses the chest. If you are by yourself, you must do both. For infants, administer two breaths, then compress the chest 30 times; administer another two breaths, then compress the chest 30 more times, and so forth. This 2:30 ratio of ventilations to compressions is necessary to effectively ventilate and circulate blood for this size child. For older children, use a 2:15 ratio as with adults. A 2:15 ratio reduces the number of times compressions must be interrupted for breaths. Be certain that you release the pressure on the chest between compressions; this allows the heart to fill more readily. Do not lift your fingers or hands off the chest, however, because doing so requires time spent to properly reposition them. Also make sure to maintain a patent airway by using the head-tilt chin lift using the hand not performing the compressions. If the resuscitation attempt is successful, the

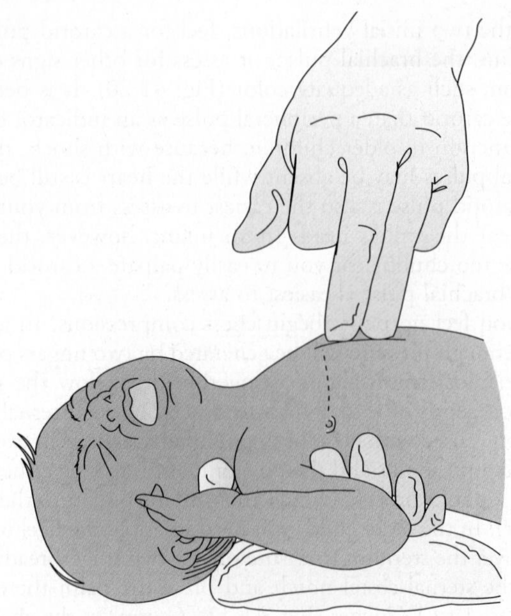

FIGURE 41.21 With cardiac resuscitation in a newborn or infant, chest compression is best done by pressing two fingers on the midsternum. Notice the slight extension of the infant's head to maintain a patent airway.

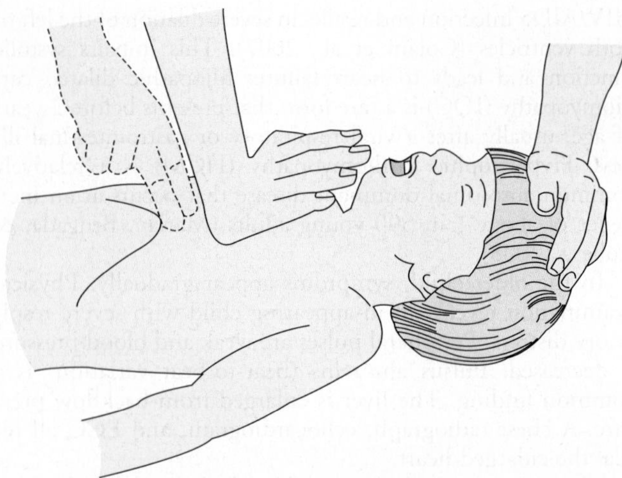

FIGURE 41.22 Locating hand position for cardiac compression in an older child.

child's color will improve (especially the oral mucous membrane, which is readily visible) and the carotid pulse will become palpable.

These three techniques (clearing the airway, ventilating the lungs, and circulating blood by cardiac compression) will provide adequate oxygenation to major body organs for several minutes until additional personnel arrive who can then initiate further resuscitation measures. The outcome of these secondary measures depends on how well and promptly the initial measures were performed.

Secondary Measures

IV access for drug administration must be accomplished as a fourth step. If it is not possible after several attempts to locate an accessible vein, an intraosseous catheter can be inserted (see Chapter 38). Drugs administered through an intraosseous route reach the circulation as rapidly as IV administration because of the rich blood supply in bone. Drugs such as epinephrine, lidocaine, and atropine also may be given by an endotracheal tube. An endotracheal dose is calculated by multiplying the IV dose by 2 or 3. The drug is then diluted with normal saline, administered by a catheter inserted deeply into the tube, and followed by an additional 1 or 2 mL of normal saline and several positive-pressure breaths to move the drug into the lungs.

Common drugs helpful in resuscitation procedures that should be available on a pediatric emergency resuscitation cart include:

- *Atropine:* Reduces bronchial secretions, keeping the airway clear during resuscitation attempts. It also reduces vagus nerve effects, relieving bradycardia.
- *Calcium chloride:* Increases heart contractility. A contraindication to its use is the presence of digitalis toxicity.
- *Epinephrine:* Strengthens or initiates cardiac contractions; increases heart rate and blood pressure; bronchodilates
- *Adenosine:* Relieves arrhythmias
- *Lidocaine:* Counteracts ventricular arrhythmias
- *Amiodarone (Cordarone):* An antidysrhythmic
- *Bretylium tosylate:* Like lidocaine, counteracts ventricular arrhythmias

- *Dopamine:* Increases cardiac output. It acts on alpha-receptors to cause vasoconstriction.
- *Dobutamine:* Acts as a direct-acting beta-agonist that increases contractility and heart rate

Psychological Support

A cardiopulmonary arrest is an acute emergency, and everyone who arrives at the scene should know what course of action to take. Even after heart action has been initiated, ventricular fibrillation may occur, requiring defibrillation. As soon as children begin to respond to resuscitation, be aware that they begin to hear. Children are obviously frightened by the number of people and all the equipment surrounding them, such as cardiac monitor leads, IV tubing, and possibly an endotracheal tube. A child may have vivid memories of frightening body sensations just before going into cardiac arrest. A child may regain consciousness, therefore, struggling and fighting. Assure the child that everyone is there to help. It is extremely frightening for parents to see their child suddenly cease breathing. Although it is comforting to see emergency personnel arrive promptly and efficiently, parents are frightened to realize their child is ill enough to need such skilled personnel. Assist, inform, and comfort parents, therefore, as well as the child.

Provide specific information on the child's condition as soon as it is available, and update the parents often. Allow them to see their child as soon as possible after the resuscitation attempt is complete so they can assure themselves their child is breathing and has heart function once again. Be certain they know that follow-up procedures such as ECG monitoring or blood-gas measurements are being scheduled to prevent another emergency. In contrast, offer support to help them begin grieving if the child does not survive.

✓ Checkpoint Question 41.5

You need to teach CPR to Megan's parents before hospital discharge. What is the ratio of ventilation to compressions used for resuscitating an infant (one person rescue)?

a. 2:30
b. 1:10
c. 2:15
d. 3:15

Key Points for Review

- Cardiovascular disorders in children may be either structural, such as congenital heart disease, or acquired, such as Kawasaki disease, rheumatic fever, or cardiomyopathy. Assessment of children with heart disease includes history and physical examination. Echocardiogram, magnetic resonance imaging, and cardiac catheterization are procedures used frequently for diagnosis.
- Children with cardiac disease may fall behind in development because they do not have the energy to play usual childhood games. Help parents to think of games that are intellectually or developmentally stimulating without being physically exhausting.
- Limiting saturated fat intake and following a consistent exercise program are important strategies for children to prevent heart disease in later life.
- A number of therapies are available for children with cardiac disease. For example, children born with a septal defect undergo open-heart surgical repairs; those with hypoplastic left heart syndrome may undergo cardiac transplant. Children born with ineffective sinoatrial node function may have pacemakers implanted to improve heart function.
- The families of children undergoing cardiac surgery need a great deal of support from health care personnel so they can cope well enough with this major event to provide effective support to their child.
- Postcardiac surgery syndrome and postperfusion syndrome are two complications that may occur after cardiac surgery. They are related to the extracorporeal circulation used during the procedure.
- Congenital heart disorders are classified as those associated with increased pulmonary blood flow, decreased pulmonary blood flow, obstruction to blood flow, and mixed blood flow.
- Common signs of heart failure seen in children include tachycardia, tachypnea, enlarged liver, dyspnea, and cyanosis. Signs tend to be subtle in infants and may be manifested chiefly by difficulty in feeding from exhaustion and dyspnea.
- Rheumatic fever is an autoimmune disease that occurs after a group A beta-hemolytic streptococcal infection. Common signs and symptoms include fever, chorea, arthralgia, polyarthritis, erythema marginatum, subcutaneous nodules, and an elevated ESR. Taking prophylactic penicillin after the illness until age 18 helps prevent further recurrence and cardiac involvement. Some children with congenital heart disease may also need this same protective routine.
- Kawasaki disease results from altered immune function. An inflammation of blood vessels leads to platelet aggregation and formation of thrombi and aneurysms.
- Infectious endocarditis is an infection of the endocardium of the heart. It may be a complication of congenital heart disease.
- Hypertension in children usually occurs as a result of a secondary disorder. A diet that is moderate in cholesterol content along with regular exercise and maintenance of weight proportional to height can help prevent this condition.
- Children with heart disease are at high risk for cardiopulmonary arrest. Nurses and parents need to know how to perform CPR to be prepared for this emergency.

CRITICAL THINKING EXERCISES

1. Megan is the newborn with tetralogy of Fallot whom you met at the beginning of the chapter. Her parents are taking her home for a month while they wait for cardiac surgery to be scheduled. They asked you what "watch her

carefully" means and how much exercise they should allow her. What advice would you give them about how to care for Megan?

2. Megan is admitted to the hospital with beginning heart failure. Her most important need is to have sustained periods of rest. How would you schedule your nursing care to avoid tiring her? What advice would you give to her parents at hospital discharge about home care?
3. Megan will need to take prophylactic penicillin until she is an adolescent. She will be living with her mother during the week and visiting her father on weekends. What steps would you take to ensure adherence over this long period?
4. Examine the National Health Goals related to heart disease in children. Most government-sponsored funds for nursing research are allotted based on these goals. What would be a possible research topic to explore pertinent to these goals that would be applicable to Megan's family and also advance evidence-based practice?

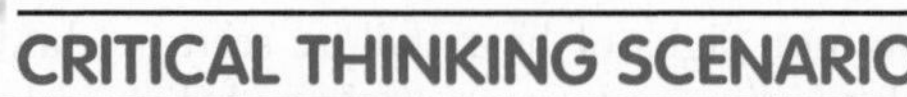

CRITICAL THINKING SCENARIO

Open the accompanying CD-ROM or visit http://thePoint.lww.com and read the Patient Scenario included for this chapter, then answer the questions to further sharpen your skills and grow more familiar with NCLEX style questions related to cardiovascular disorders in children. Confirm your answers are correct by reading the rationales.

REFERENCES

Alsoufi, B., et al. (2007). New developments in the treatment of hypoplastic left heart syndrome. *Pediatrics, 119*(1), 109–117.

American Academy of Pediatrics (AAP), Committee on Practice and Ambulatory Medicine. (2009). *Recommendations for preventive pediatric health care.* Washington, DC: Author.

American Heart Association. (2008). *Pediatric advanced life support.* Dallas, TX: Author.

Armstrong, C. (2007). Practice guidelines. Cardiovascular risk reduction in children. *American Family Physician, 75*(12), 1873–1876.

Bartlett, H. L., et al. (2007). Early outcomes of tricuspid valve replacement in young children. *Circulation, 115*(3), 319–325.

Bashore, T. M., & Granger, C. B. (2009). Cardiology. In S. J. McPhee & M. A. Papadakis (Eds.). *Current medical diagnosis and treatment.* Columbus, OH: McGraw-Hill.

Carapetis, J. R. (2007). Rheumatic heart disease in developing countries. *New England Journal of Medicine, 357*(5), 439–441.

Chakko, S., & Bisno, A. L. (2008). Acute rheumatic fever. In V. Fuster, et al. (Eds.). *Hurst's the heart* (12th ed.). Columbus, OH: McGraw-Hill.

Colam, S. D., et al. (2007). Epidemiology and cause-specific outcome of hypertrophic cardiomyopathy in children: findings from the pediatric cardiomyopathy registry. *Circulation, 115*(6), 773–781.

Dambro, M. R. (2008). Tetralogy of Fallot. In F. J. Domino. (Ed.). *The 5-minute clinical consult.* Philadelphia: Lippincott Williams & Wilkins.

DeBord, S., Cherry, C., & Hickey, C. (2007). The arterial switch procedure for transposition of the great arteries. *AORN Journal, 86*(2), 211–226.

DeMaria, A. N., & Blanchard, D. G. (2008). The echocardiogram. In V. Fuster, et al. (Eds.). *Hurst's the heart* (12th ed.). Columbus, OH: McGraw-Hill.

Fenton, M., & Burch, M. (2007). Understanding chronic heart failure. *Archives of Disease in Childhood, 92*(9), 812–816.

Fulton, D. R., & Freed, M. D. (2008). The pathology, pathophysiology, recognition, and treatment of congenital heart disease. In V. Fuster, et al. (Eds.). *Hurst's the heart* (12th ed.). Columbus, OH: McGraw-Hill.

Fynn-Thompson, F., & Almond, C. (2007). Pediatric ventricular assist devices. *Cardiology, 28*(2), 149–155.

Hernandez-Diaz, S., et al. (2007). Risk factors for persistent pulmonary hypertension of the newborn. *Pediatrics, 120*(2), e272–e282.

Hovels-Gurich, H. H., et al. (2007). Long-term behavior and quality of life after corrective cardiac surgery in infancy for tetralogy of Fallot or ventricular septal defect. *Pediatric Cardiology, 28*(5), 346–354.

Karch, A. M. (2009). *Lippincott's nursing drug guide.* Philadelphia: Lippincott Williams & Wilkins.

Karpawich, P. P. (2007). Pediatric cardiac resynchronization pacing therapy. *Current Opinion in Cardiology, 22*(2), 72–76.

Keller, B. B., Wessels, A., & Markwald, R. R. (2008). Molecular development of the heart and vasculature. In V. Fuster, et al. (Eds.). *Hurst's the heart* (12th ed.). Columbus, OH: McGraw-Hill.

Kern, M. J., & King, S. B. (2008). Cardiac catheterization, cardiac angiography, and coronary blood flow and pressure measurements. In V. Fuster, et al. (Eds.). *Hurst's the heart* (12th ed.). Columbus, OH: McGraw-Hill.

Laifer-Narin, S., et al. (2007). Fetal magnetic resonance imaging: A review. *Current Opinion in Obstetrics & Gynecology, 19*(2), 151–156.

Landolt, M. A., Valsangiacomo Buechel, E. R., & Latal, B. (2008). Health-related quality of life in children and adolescents after open-heart surgery. *Journal of Pediatrics, 152*(3), 349–355.

Law, Y. M. (2007). Pathophysiology and diagnosis of allograft rejection in pediatric heart transplantation. *Current Opinion in Cardiology, 22*(2), 66–71.

Leibovitch, L., Matok, I., & Paret, G. (2007). Therapeutic applications of sildenafil citrate in the management of paediatric pulmonary hypertension. *Drugs, 67*(1), 57–73.

Lim, D. S., et al. (2007). Transesophageal echocardiographic guidance for surgical repair of aortic insufficiency in congenital heart disease. *Journal of the American Society of Echocardiography, 20*(9), 1080–1085.

Lim, D. S., & Matherne, G. P. (2007). Percutaneous device closure of atrial septal defect in a premature infant with rapid improvement in pulmonary status. *Pediatrics, 119*(2), 398–400.

Marian, A. J., Brugada, R., & Roberts R. (2008). Cardiovascular diseases due to genetic abnormalities. In V. Fuster, et al. (Eds.). *Hurst's the heart* (12th ed.). Columbus, OH: McGraw-Hill.

Marijon, E., et al. (2007). Prevalence of rheumatic heart disease detected by echocardiographic screening. *New England Journal of Medicine, 357*(5), 470–476.

Morelli, P., Biancaniello, T., & Chandran, L. (2007). The essentials of pediatric ECGs. *Contemporary Pediatrics, 24*(9), 49–53.

Oates-Whitehead, R. M., et al. (2009). Intravenous immunoglobulin for the treatment of Kawasaki disease in children. *Cochrane Database of Systematic Reviews, 2009*(1), (CD004000).

Pignone, M., & McPhee, S. J. (2009). Disease prevention and health promotion. In S. J. McPhee & M. A. Papadakis (Eds.). *Current medical diagnosis and treatment.* Columbus, OH: McGraw-Hill.

Poustie, V. J., & Rutherford, P. (2009). Dietary treatment for familial hypercholesterolaemia. *Cochrane Database of Systematic Reviews, 2009*(1), (CD001918).

Prystowsky, E. N., & Foge, R.I. (2008). Approach to the patient with cardiac arrhythmias. In V. Fuster, et al. (Eds.). *Hurst's the heart* (12th ed.). Columbus, OH: McGraw-Hill

Rasiah, S. V., et al. (2008). Antenatal perspective of hypoplastic left heart syndrome: 5 Years on. *Archives of Disease in Childhood Fetal and Neonatal Edition, 93*(3), F192–F197.

Rowley, A. H., & Shulman, S. T. (2007). New developments in the search for the etiologic agent of Kawasaki disease. *Current Opinion in Pediatrics, 19*(1), 71–74.

Schroeder, J. S., et al. (2008). Surgical treatment of heart failure, cardiac transplantation, and mechanical ventricular support. In V. Fuster, et al. (Eds.). *Hurst's the heart* (12th ed.). Columbus, OH: McGraw-Hill.

Smith, H. G. (2008). Rheumatic fever. In F. J. Domino. (Ed.). *The 5-minute clinical consult.* Philadelphia: Lippincott Williams & Wilkins.

Sondheimer, H. M., Yetman, A. T., & Miyamoto, S. D. (2008). Cardiovascular diseases. In W. W. Hay, et al. (Eds.). *Current pediatric diagnosis and treatment* (18th ed.). Columbus, OH: McGraw-Hill.

Sykes, R. B., & Farrington, E. (2007). Prophylaxis for bacterial endocarditis prior to dental procedures in children. *Journal of Pediatric Health Care, 21*(4), 256–260.

Tanaka, Y., et al. (2007). Inhaled nitric oxide therapy decreases the risk of cerebral palsy in preterm infants with persistent pulmonary hypertension of the newborn. *Pediatrics, 119*(6), 1159–1164.

Thilo, E. H., & Rosenberg, A. A. (2008). The newborn. In W. W. Hay, et al. (Eds.). *Current pediatric diagnosis and treatment* (18th ed.). Columbus, OH: McGraw-Hill.

Tjang, Y. S., et al. (2007). Heart transplantation in children: clinical outcomes in a single center. *Annals of Thoracic Surgery, 84*(5), 1640–1644.

Tulathimutte, N. (2008). Infective endocarditis. In F. J. Domino. (Ed.). *The 5-minute clinical consult.* Philadelphia: Lippincott Williams & Wilkins.

Tuzcu, V. (2007). Cryoablation of accessory pathways in children. *Pacing and Clinical Electrophysiology, 30*(9), 1129–1135.

Vijayaraman, P., & Ellenbogen, K. A. (2008). Bradyarrhythmias and pacemakers. In V. Fuster, et al. (Eds.). *Hurst's the heart* (12th ed.). Columbus, OH: McGraw-Hill.

Weiner, S. G., & Normandin, P. A. (2007). Sydenham chorea: a case report and review of the literature. *Pediatric Emergency Care, 23*(1), 20–24.

SUGGESTED READINGS

Baumer, J. H., et al. (2009). Salicylate for the treatment of Kawasaki disease in children. *Cochrane Database of Systematic Reviews, 2009*(1), (CD004175).

Brosig, C. L., et al. (2007). Psychosocial outcomes for preschool children and families after surgery for complex congenital heart disease. *Pediatric Cardiology, 28*(4), 255–262.

Canter, C. E., et al. (2007). Indications for heart transplantation in pediatric heart disease. *Circulation, 115*(5), 658–676.

Carberry, K. E., et al. (2007). Mechanical circulatory support for the pediatric patient. *Critical Care Nursing Quarterly, 30*(2), 121–142.

Haney, E. M., et al. (2007). Screening and treatment for lipid disorders in children and adolescents: systematic evidence review for the US Preventive Services Task Force. *Pediatrics, 120*(1), e189–e214.

Lane, J. R., & Ben-Shachar, G. (2007). Myocardial infarction in healthy adolescents. *Pediatrics, 120*(4), e938–e943.

McGrath, J. M. (2007). Early detection and immediate management of congenital heart disease is important to long-term outcomes. *Journal of Perinatal and Neonatal Nursing, 20*(4), 285–286.

O'Brien, P. (2007). The role of the nurse practitioner in congenital heart surgery. *Pediatric Cardiology, 28*(2), 88–95.

O'Connor, M., McDaniel, N., & Brady, W. J. (2008). The pediatric electrocardiogram, part II: dysrhythmias. *American Journal of Emergency Medicine, 26*(3), 348–358.

Valdez, R., et al. (2007). Is family history a useful tool for detecting children at risk for diabetes and cardiovascular diseases? *Pediatrics, 120*(2), S78–S86.

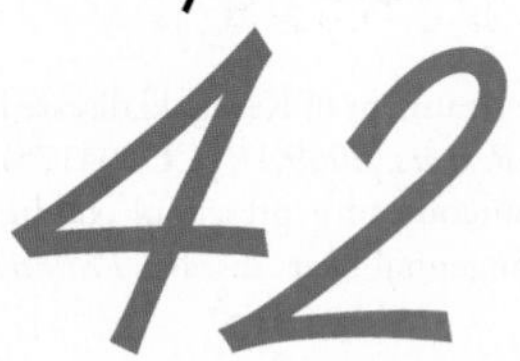

Chapter 42 Nursing Care of a Family When a Child Has an Immune Disorder

KEY TERMS

- allergen
- anaphylaxis
- antigen
- autoimmunity
- cell-mediated immunity
- chemotaxis
- complement
- cytotoxic response
- delayed hypersensitivity
- environmental control
- humoral immunity
- hypersensitivity response
- hyposensitization
- immune response
- immunity
- immunogen
- immunoglobulins
- lymphokines
- lysis
- macrophage
- phagocytosis
- tolerance

OBJECTIVES

After mastering the contents of this chapter, you should be able to:

1. Describe the immune process as it relates to childhood illnesses.
2. Identify National Health Goals related to immune disorders in children that nurses could help the nation achieve.
3. Use critical thinking to analyze ways that nursing care for a child with an immune disorder can be more family centered.
4. Assess a child with a disorder of the immune system.
5. Formulate nursing diagnoses for a child with a disorder of the immune system.
6. Establish outcomes for a child with a disorder of the immune system.
7. Plan nursing care pertinent to a child with an immune system disorder.
8. Implement nursing care for a child with an immune disorder such as teaching about environmental control.
9. Evaluate expected outcomes for achievement and effectiveness of care.
10. Identify areas related to care of a child with an immune disorder that could benefit from additional nursing research or application of evidence-based practice.
11. Integrate knowledge of immune disorders and the nursing process to achieve quality maternal and child health nursing care.

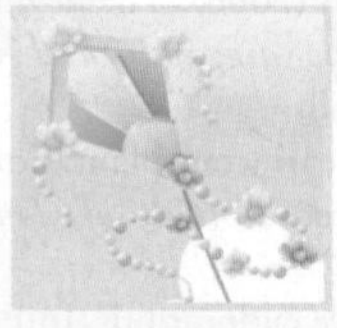

Dexter Goodenough is a 6-year-old boy you meet in an ambulatory setting. He had atopic dermatitis (infantile eczema) as an infant. Today, his eyes look reddened and are watering; his nose is draining a clear discharge. His mother tells you he is constantly listless and other children make fun of him because of his appearance. His grades are "terrible" because the minute he gets to school, his symptoms begin. Dexter is diagnosed as having atopic rhinitis (hay fever). "Thank heavens," his mother exclaims. "I thought when I heard he had an immune system disease he had AIDS. What a relief to know it's only an allergy."

Previous chapters described normal growth and development of children. This chapter adds information about the dramatic changes, both physical and psychosocial, that can occur when a child is born with or develops a disorder of the immune system.

In light of the effect this condition is having on Dexter's life, is this "only" an allergy? What additional information would you want his mother to know about his condition? Knowing his problem is worse at school, what environmental control measures would you want to suggest for Dexter?

The immune system consists of a complex network of cells interacting to protect the body against invasion by foreign substances. The study of the immune system has grown immensely over the past several years, and almost every day brings new findings. More diseases are being attributed at least in part to malfunctioning of the immune system, all of which makes an understanding of how the immune system works in health and disease essential for safe nursing care.

Disorders of the immune system include deficiencies of immune substances and function that affect the body's ability to ward off infection (immunodeficiency disorders); abnormal and excessive immune response to foreign substances (hypersensitivity disorders, or allergies); and abnormal and excessive immune response to self (autoimmune disorders). Immune disorders are a focus of much research and study because they may hold the key to understanding why major illnesses such as HIV/AIDS and possibly cancer occur. Immunodeficiencies and examples of allergic disorders are described in this chapter. Autoimmune disorders, which include a wide range of illnesses, often affect a particular body system. These are addressed in the chapters that discuss the affected system (rheumatoid arthritis, which affects the joints, for example, is discussed in Chapter 51). National Health Goals related to immune disorders and children are shown in Box 42.1.

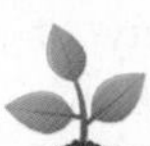

Nursing Process Overview

For a Child With an Immune Disorder

Assessment

The immune system provides protection for the body from invading organisms or antigens. A deficiency of *immunocompetent* cells (cells capable of resisting these types of foreign invaders) or alteration in their function can limit this protection. Assessment focuses on analysis of blood components, particularly the white blood cells, to determine exactly what components are altered, missing, or not functioning properly. When the immune system reacts excessively or inappropriately to the invasion of certain antigens, a thorough history and analysis of presenting symptoms is usually the best way to identify the problem and develop appropriate interventions.

Nursing Diagnosis

Several nursing diagnoses associated with immune dysfunction are:

- Risk for infection related to altered immune response
- Impaired skin integrity related to inadequate lymphocyte protection
- Activity intolerance related to chronic illness

Nursing diagnoses for children experiencing allergic responses focus on their particular allergic symptoms. Examples of these are:

- Situational low self-esteem related to effects of contact dermatitis
- Ineffective breathing pattern related to bronchospasm of anaphylaxis
- Anxiety related to continued allergic response
- Powerlessness related to difficulty determining cause of allergy
- Risk for delayed growth and development related to chronicity of HIV/AIDS

Outcome Identification and Planning

Outcome identification and planning for a child with an immune disorder focus both on present and future concerns.

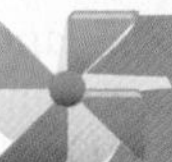

BOX 42.1 * Focus on National Health Goals

Allergies affect at least 25% of the population so efforts to reduce them are reflected in several National Health Goals:

- Reduce indoor allergen levels such as dust mites from a baseline of 46.2% to 37% of homes.
- Increase or maintain the number of territories or states that monitor diseases that can be caused by exposure to environmental hazards from a baseline of 6 to 25.

Of the immunologic disorders, human immunodeficiency virus (HIV) infection is the most serious, not only because it is still ultimately fatal but also because its spread has been so difficult to contain. National Health Goals that address HIV/AIDS are:

- Increase the proportion of adolescents who abstain from sexual intercourse or use condoms if sexually active from a baseline of 72% to at least 83%.
- Reduce occupational needlestick injuries among health care workers from a baseline of 600,000 per year to 420,000 per year, a 30% improvement.
- Reduce AIDS among adolescents and adults from a baseline of 19.5 new cases per 100,000 of the population to a target level of 1.0 per 100,000.
- Reduce the incidence of new cases of perinatally acquired HIV infection from 82 to 75 yearly.
- Increase the proportion of middle, junior high, and senior high schools that provide education on HIV and AIDS from a baseline of 65% to a target level of 90% (http://www.nih.gov).

Nurses can help the nation achieve these goals by initiating educational programs for children that include teaching children and adolescents about the way HIV is transmitted (sexual relations and unclean intravenous needles) and protective measures they can take to avoid contracting the disease (using safer sex practices and not using intravenous drugs).

Nursing research that could add helpful information to the area includes research that attempts to answer questions such as: How can school nurses best help children with food allergies select a nutritious meal from a cafeteria menu? How can parents of school-age children be persuaded that safer sex practices should be part of usual school-age health awareness curricula? What methods work best to educate adolescents about the danger of unprotected sex?

Relief of immediate symptoms is the first priority. This is followed by planning for long-term care and prevention of future attacks. Looking into organizations that could supply information for parents or children could be key. Informational and support organizations that can be helpful are Eczema Association for Science and Education (http://www.nationaleczema.org), The Asthma and Allergy Foundation of America (http://www.aafa.org/), and the Elizabeth Glaser Pediatric AIDS Foundation (http://www.pedaids.org).

Implementation

A major nursing intervention in the care of children with immune disorders is client and family teaching. The family of a child with an immunodeficiency may need help in identifying ways to keep the child from contracting life-threatening infections while at the same time providing enough stimulation and social contact to promote normal growth and development. A similar teaching goal must be established for a child with a chronic allergic disorder. Parents need to learn ways to help their child avoid triggers or situations that provoke allergy, but they must not keep the child so isolated or fearful that the child misses out on important experiences.

Outcome Evaluation

Outcome evaluation with immune disorders must be ongoing because new triggers for allergies can arise at any time. New therapies for HIV/AIDS are constantly being suggested. Because the field of immunology is continually evolving, theories about immune diseases and associated treatments may change from visit to visit. Be certain parents are kept abreast of developments in the field, especially those that will affect their ability to provide an environment that is safest for their child.

Examples of outcomes suggesting achievement of goals include:

- Child voices high self-esteem even if contact dermatitis rash has not completely faded.
- Child's respiratory rate is maintained at 20 breaths per minute with minimal wheezing.
- Child and parents state they can cope with their present level of anxiety.
- Child lists three actions she takes daily to help feel a greater sense of control.
- Child demonstrates achievement of developmental milestones within age-acceptable parameters despite chronic illness.

THE IMMUNE SYSTEM

The immune system functions to protect the body from invasion by foreign substances by several mechanisms. First, body surfaces such as the skin, cilia, and mucous membranes act as physical protective barriers. When an invading pathogen does get through this barrier, the process of **phagocytosis** (destruction of invaders) begins. **Macrophages** (mature white blood cells) engulf, ingest, and neutralize the pathogen. At the same time, an inflammatory response creates vascular and cellular changes that help to rid the body of dead tissue and the inactivated antigens. The immune system maintains cells ready to attack this way whenever necessary, directing the efforts of macrophages and supplementing the inflammatory response as necessary. It also singles out specific antigens for interactions (antibody–antigen reactions). This immune response not only furnishes immediate protection but also creates a template for how to destroy that particular antigen again in the future.

Immune Response

The **immune response** is the body's action plan devised to combat invading organisms or substances by leukocyte and antibody activity. An **antigen** is any foreign substance (molecule) capable of stimulating an immune response. Most antigens are proteins, but other large molecules such as polysaccharides may also function as antigens. Penicillin, although not antigenic by itself, may become antigenic when it combines with a higher-weight molecule, usually a protein (a process called *hapten formation*; this explains why penicillin reactions occur). If an antigen is one that can be readily destroyed by an immune response, and **immunity** (the ability to destroy like antigens) results, the antigen may be referred to as a simple **immunogen.** If, during the immune response, mediating substances are released that cause tissue injury and allergic symptoms, the antigen is termed an **allergen.** Allergens may enter the body through a variety of routes. They may be ingested (foods such as eggs or wheat), inhaled (pollen, dust, or mold spores), injected (drugs), or absorbed across the skin or mucous membranes (poison ivy).

Immune System Organs and Cells

The organs of the immune system consist of the lymph nodes, bone marrow, thymus, spleen, and tonsils. Bone marrow produces two types of lymphocytes, *B lymphocytes* and *T lymphocytes*. After being produced, lymphocytes travel throughout the lymphoid system and are stored in the lymph nodes and spleen. Both T and B lymphocytes recognize invading organisms and provide for attack of specific antigens (Fig. 42.1).

B Lymphocytes

Originating in the bone marrow (the reason for their name), the B lymphocytes develop into *plasma cells* and *memory cells* when exposed to antigens. Plasma cells secrete large quantities of immunoglobulins or antibodies, which bind to and destroy specific antigens (termed *humoral immunity*). When an antibody is formed in response to a particular antigen this way, it is specific to that antigen. An antibody against the pertussis antigen, for instance, will not have any effect on the tetanus antigen. Memory cells are responsible for retaining the formula or ability to produce specific **immunoglobulins.** Immunoglobulins are classified as IgG, IgA, IgM, IgD, and IgE. Those involved in immunity are IgG, IgA, and IgM. IgM reaches adult levels at approximately 1 year of age, IgG at 4 years, and IgA at adolescence. IgE is primarily responsible for allergic or hypersensitivity responses. It is present at proportions capable of extreme response early in infancy. The functions of the immunoglobulins are summarized in Table 42.1.

T Lymphocytes

T lymphocytes account for 70% to 80% of blood lymphocytes and are responsible for *cell-mediated immunity*. They

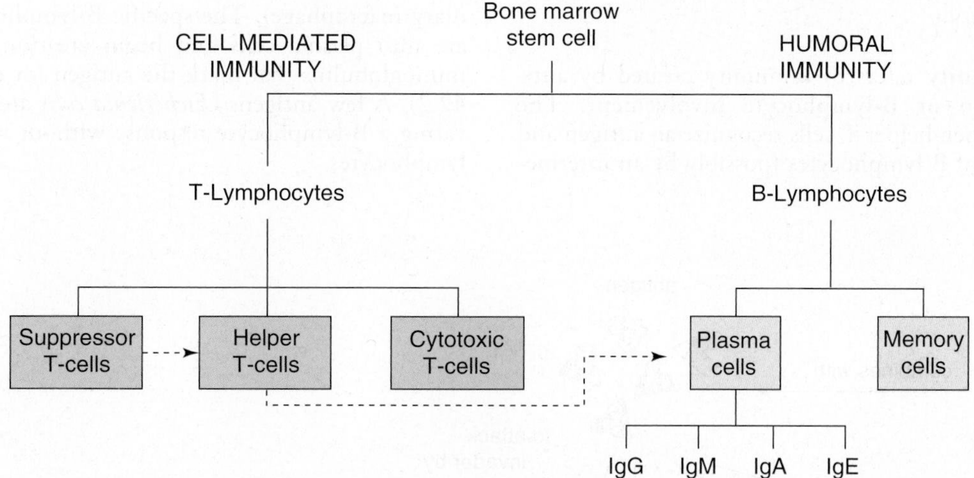

FIGURE 42.1 Lymphocyte production. From the bone marrow stem cell, T and B lymphocytes are formed. T-lymphocyte action leads to cell-mediated immunity. B-lymphocyte action results in humoral immunity.

are produced by the bone marrow but mature under the influence of the thymus gland (hence their name). When mature, T lymphocytes leave the thymus to enter specific body regions (thymus-dependent zones), mostly in the lymph nodes and spleen; there, they react specifically to viruses, fungi, and parasites but have an effect on all antigens. T cells can be differentiated into three subtypes.

The first type, *cytotoxic (killer) T cells*, are T lymphocytes that have the specific feature of binding to the surface of antigens and directly destroying the cell membrane and therefore the cell (phagocytes). As a part of this process, cytotoxic cells secrete **lymphokines;** lymphokines contain or prevent migration of antigens and call other lymphocytes into the area. Interferon is an example of a lymphokine important in preventing viral spread and helping to call leukocytes into the area (the property of **chemotaxis**).

The second type, *helper T cells* (CD4 cells), stimulate B lymphocytes to divide and mature into plasma cells and begin secreting immunoglobulins. The IgA antibody response, especially, depends on stimulation by helper T cells. Helper T cells can be identified in blood because of specific markers on their surface. Analysis of these (CD4 counts) is an important assessment of the competency of the immune system (Kishiyama & Adelman, 2009).

The third type, *suppressor T cells*, are T cells that reduce the production of immunoglobulins against a specific antigen and prevent their overproduction.

Types of Immunity

The action of B and T lymphocytes leads to two different types of immunity: humoral and cell-mediated immunity.

TABLE 42.1 ✻ Location and Function of Immunoglobulins

Immunoglobulin	Description
IgM	Effective in agglutinating antigen as well as lysing cell walls; discovered early in the course of an infection in the bloodstream
IgG	Most frequently occurring antibody in plasma; during secondary response, it is the major immunoglobulin to be synthesized; it freely diffuses into extravascular spaces to contact antigens; in prenatal life, it diffuses across the placenta to supply passive immune protection to the fetus and until the infant can effectively produce immunoglobulins; it has the major responsibility for neutralizing bacterial toxins and in activating phagocytosis (destruction of bacteria)
IgA	Found in external body secretions such as saliva, sweat, tears, mucus, bile, and colostrum; provides defense against pathogens on exposed surfaces, especially those of the gastrointestinal tract and respiratory tract, apparently by preventing adherence of pathogens to mucosal cells
IgD	Found in plasma; may be the receptor that binds antigens to lymphocyte surfaces
IgE	Involved in immediate hypersensitivity reactions; exists bound to mast cells on tissue surfaces; when contacted by an antigen, cellular granules are released; associated with allergy and parasitic infections

Humoral Immunity

Humoral immunity refers to immunity created by antibody production or B-lymphocyte involvement. The process begins when helper T cells recognize an antigen and cause activation of B lymphocytes (possibly by an intermediary macrophage). The specific B lymphocytes differentiate into plasma cells and begin creation of specific immunoglobulins that mark the antigen for destruction (Fig. 42.2). A few antigens (*Escherichia coli*) are capable of activating a B-lymphocyte response without recognition by T lymphocytes.

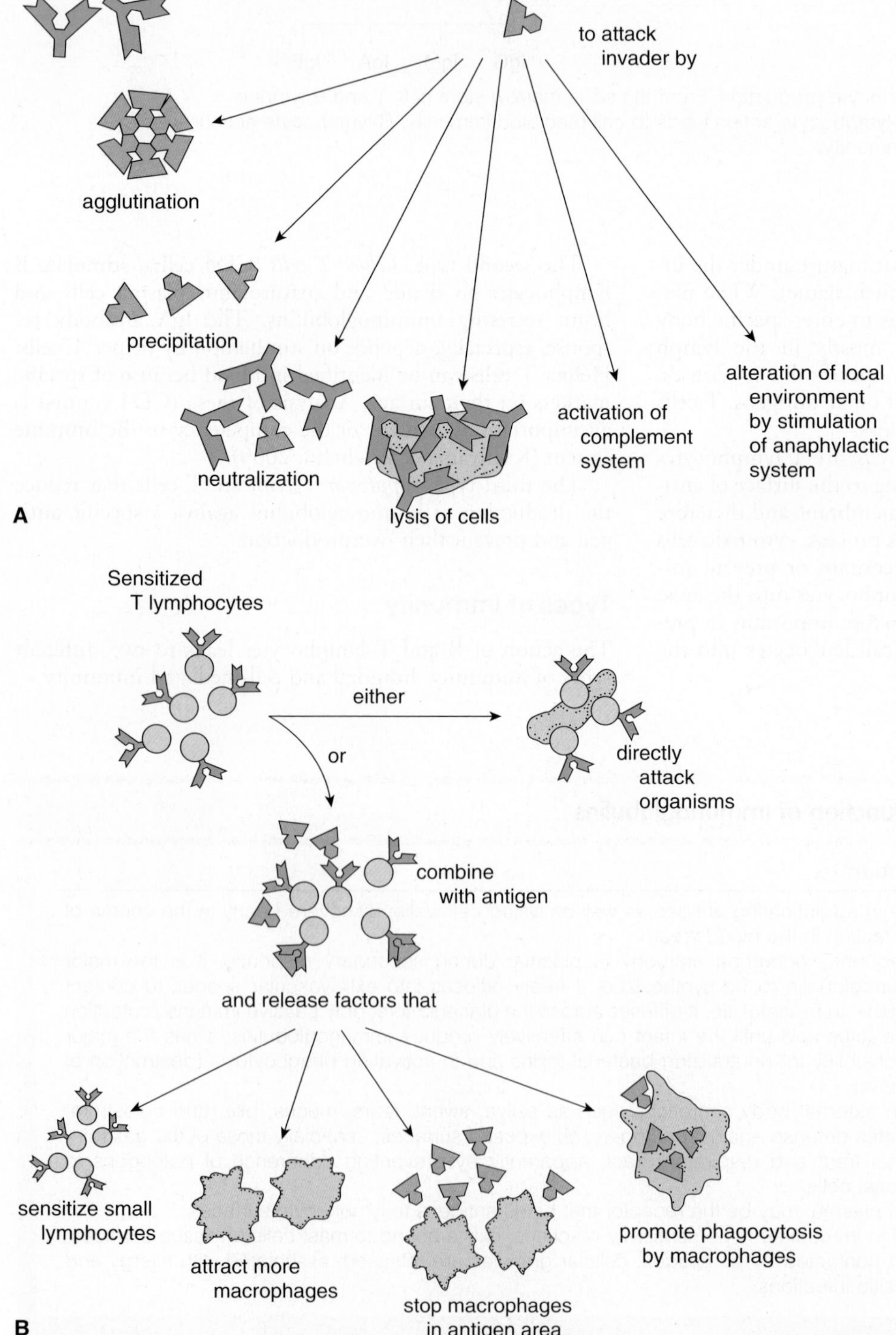

FIGURE 42.2 Mechanism of immunity response. (**A**) Humoral immunity. (**B**) Cell-mediated immunity.

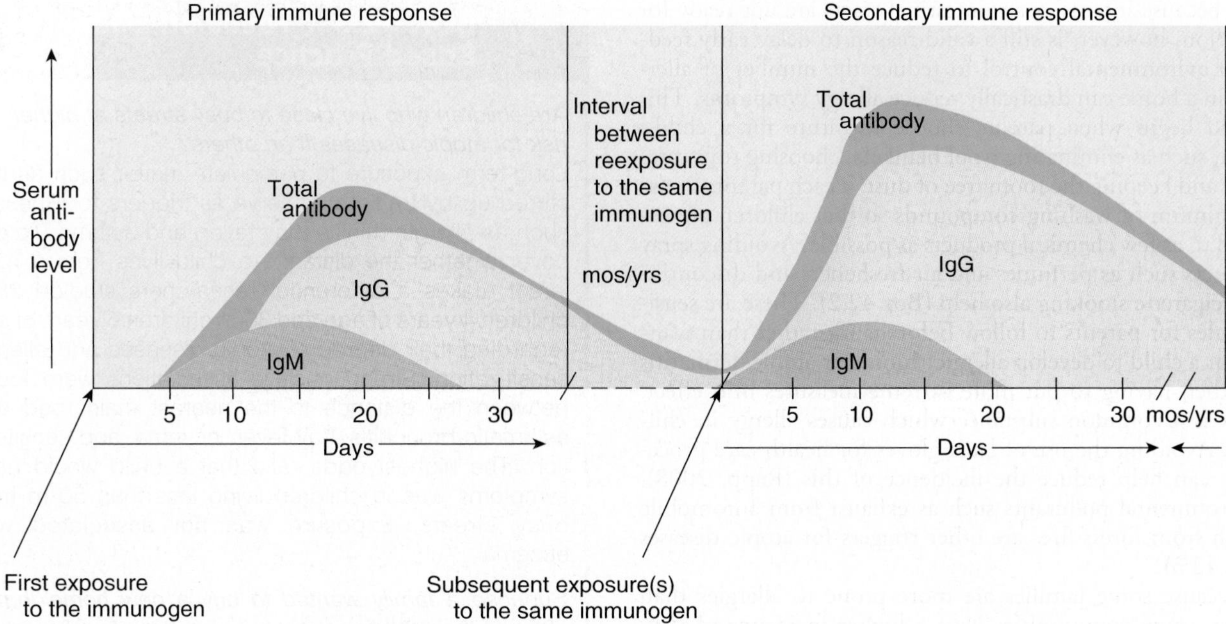

FIGURE 42.3 Primary and secondary humoral responses. IgM is the first immunoglobulin to appear in the serum.

Primary Response. The first time a specific antigen enters the body and is identified by T lymphocytes, B-cell differentiation and growth begin. Within 6 days, IgM antibodies specific to the antigen can be measured in the bloodstream. The production of IgM antibodies peaks at 14 days and then declines until, within a few weeks, few are any longer present. At approximately day 10, IgG production begins and remains high for several weeks (Fig. 42.3).

Secondary Response. When a specific antigen enters the body a second or additional time, antibody production begins immediately because of memory cells. The main type of immunoglobulin produced in a secondary response is IgG (see Fig. 42.3).

Complement Activation. **Complement** is composed of 20 different proteins that are normally nonfunctional molecules; however, when activated by antigen–antibody contact, these molecules begin a cascade response that leads to increased vascular permeability, smooth muscle contraction, chemotaxis ("calling" leukocytes into the area), phagocytosis, and **lysis** (killing) of the foreign antigen. The affected area feels warm and looks reddened and swollen, indicating an inflammatory reaction. Although an inflammatory reaction causes some local injury to tissue around the antigen, it is helpful overall because it produces an environment harmful to the antigen. Complement reactions that persist beyond the usual time for resolution (2 to 3 days) may be responsible for many of the autoimmune disorders.

Cell-Mediated Immunity

Cell-mediated immunity is the type of immune response caused by T-lymphocyte activity. Cytotoxic T cells attack and directly destroy invading antigens through the release of chemical compounds on the antigen membrane, injection of a toxin directly into the antigen, or secretion of lymphokines. A wheal-and-flare response occurs because of accumulation of lymphocytes around small blood vessels, resulting in minor destruction of blood vessels (see Fig. 42.2). This response is termed **delayed hypersensitivity** if the T-lymphocyte activity occurs solely without an accompanying humoral response. It is this response that causes transplant rejection.

Autoimmunity

Autoimmunity results from an inability to distinguish self from nonself, causing the immune system to carry out immune responses against normal cells and tissue. Autoimmune responses may be organ-specific or limited to one organ, as happens with attachment to the thyroid gland in Hashimoto's disease (see Chapter 48), or generalized and systemic (not organ-specific), as in rheumatoid arthritis and systemic lupus erythematosus (see Chapter 20). There is currently much research oriented toward the study of autoimmune responses and their possible implications in a wide variety of disorders, such as multiple sclerosis. Autoimmune disorders occur at a greater rate in some families than in others and in girls and women more than boys and men.

HEALTH PROMOTION AND RISK MANAGEMENT

As many as 15% to 30% of children today have some form of allergy or involvement of the immune system (Boguniewicz, 2008). Preventing allergies, therefore, could have a major impact on the health of children. Early prevention can begin with encouraging women to breastfeed so that infants are not exposed to cow milk protein. Delaying the introduction of solid food until 6 months of age, once thought to reduce the development of allergies, may not be as beneficial as once thought (Filipiak et al., 2007). Delaying solid food because infants' gastrointestinal tracts are not ready for digestion, however, is still a valid reason to delay early feeding. Environmental control to reduce the number of allergens in a home can drastically reduce allergy symptoms. This should begin when parents choose furniture for a child's room, such as eliminating wool blankets, choosing toys carefully, and keeping the room free of dust. Teach parents to use a minimum of washing compounds so that children are exposed to as few chemical products as possible. Avoiding spray products such as perfumes and air fresheners and discontinuing cigarette smoking also help (Box 42.2). These are sensible rules for parents to follow beforehand, rather than waiting for a child to develop allergic rhinitis or atopic dermatitis and then having to put more extreme measures into effect. Latex is a common substance which causes allergy in children. Avoiding the use of latex gloves for health care procedures can help reduce the incidence of this (Rapp, 2008). Environmental pollutants such as exhaust from automobile or ash from forest fires are other triggers for atopic diseases (Box 42.3).

Because some families are more prone to allergies than others, some communities have a higher incidence of children with allergies than others. As a result, these communities may have more services and specialists to treat these children, a situation that develops a "community culture" of allergy acceptance and treatment. Children typically may leave school early for immunotherapy. School cafeterias commonly offer allergy-free foods. In other communities where fewer children have allergies, a child with an allergy is viewed as unique or not typical, so may need additional support.

Allergies are a type of disorder that typically causes chronic rather than acute symptoms. For this reason, children who develop allergies often need to be encouraged to be vigilant in taking their medicine. For the same reason, once parents begin a child on an immunotherapy program, they may need to be encouraged to continue it. It helps if children and their parents understand how allergic reactions lead to symptoms and how important it is for them to play a role in their own therapy.

Although it is probably impossible to keep children with atopic allergies free of reactions and manifestations of allergies, parents who know of familial allergy patterns can take some preventive steps in this direction. If parents are going to prepare allergy-free foods, be sure they consider the child's likes and dislikes and think through the child's weekly intake to ensure the child receives all essential nutrients. If a child eats at school or has a meal prepared every day at a child care center, remind parents to make sure the center, babysitter, or school dietitian is aware of the child's allergies. If a child is allergic to wheat products and cannot eat bread for sandwiches, preparing a bag lunch for school may be a difficult daily problem that only good planning can eliminate.

If a child's allergies involve pollen sensitivities, planning vacations at a time when the pollen count is lowest may make the vacation more pleasant for the family. If desensitization against a specific pollen is necessary, assist parents in planning to start desensitization so it will be effective by the time the pollen count of the offending allergen rises.

Health promotion is also important to prevent HIV/AIDS. Teaching children safer sex practices is an important part of this. All health care providers can help prevent the spread of HIV/AIDS by using standard infection precautions. The parents of children with immune deficiencies may need to be reminded periodically to take measures to keep their children free of disease, such as keeping immunizations updated and seeking help immediately for infections.

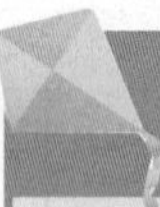

BOX 42.3 * Focus on Evidence-Based Practice

Are children who live close to busy streets at higher risk for atopic diseases than others?

Long-term exposure to particulate matter such as that stirred up by traffic may serve as triggers for illnesses such as allergic rhinitis (hay fever) and asthma. To discover whether the distance a child lives from a busy street makes a difference, researchers studied 2860 children 4 years of age and 3061 children 6 years of age regarding their degree of atopic diseases and allergic sensitization. Strong positive associations were found between the distance to the nearest main road and asthmatic bronchitis, hay fever, eczema, and sensitization. The highest odds ratio that a child would have symptoms was in children living less than 50 m from busy streets. Exposure was not associated with eczema.

Suppose a family wanted to buy a new home that is close to their child's school but also close to a busy traffic area? Based on the above, would you advise the family to do so?

Source: Morgenstern, V., et al. (2008). Atopic diseases, allergic sensitization, and exposure to traffic-related air pollution in children. *American Journal of Respiratory and Critical Care Medicine, 177*(12), 1331–1337.

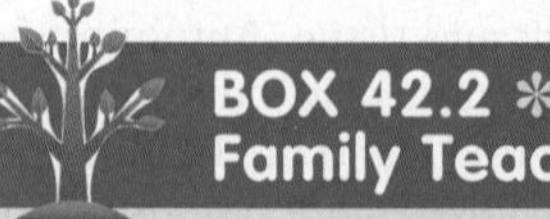

BOX 42.2 * Focus on Family Teaching

Avoiding Secondary Smoke

Q. Dexter's mother says to you, "Neither my husband nor I smoke, but some of our relatives and friends do. How can we keep our child from being exposed to secondary smoke?"

A. Use the following guidelines to help avoid secondary smoke:

- Declare your home a smoke-free zone.
- If family members smoke, ask them to smoke outside.
- If at a restaurant, ask to sit in a no-smoking area, or visit only smoke-free restaurants.
- If staying at a hotel, ask for a nonsmoking room.
- Do not be reluctant to ask people around your child at a social gathering to stop smoking.
- As smoke adheres to people's clothing, suggest a person who smokes not hold a young baby.
- Encourage your friends or family members who smoke to take quit-smoking courses (for their own benefit as well as yours).

IMMUNODEFICIENCY DISORDERS

When any one portion of the immune system is not functioning adequately, an immunodeficiency results. The immunodeficiency disorder may be primary (congenital) or acquired (secondary to viral invasion or exposure to a toxic substance). Only a part or the entire system may fail in its goal of protecting the body from invading organisms.

Primary (Congenital) Immunodeficiency

Children with primary congenital immunodeficiencies are born without an essential immune substance or function or with inadequate amounts of immune substances. Usually these deficiencies become apparent relatively early in life. However, it may take a few months for B-lymphocyte deficiencies to produce symptoms, because a newborn is born with enough maternal IgG (which crossed the placenta during pregnancy) to supply protection for approximately the first 6 months of life.

B-Lymphocyte Deficiencies

B-lymphocyte deficiencies create abnormally low levels of immunoglobulins either selectively (as in an IgA deficiency) or totally, which is referred to as hypogammaglobulinemia or agammaglobulinemia (Liu, Stewart, & Johnston, 2008).

Hypogammaglobulinemia. Although hypogammaglobulinemia can occur as a result of chemotherapy or critical illness, it most often presents as an inherited X-linked recessive defect in the maturation of B lymphocytes that results in abnormally low levels of all immunoglobulins (Estrella, Foley, & Cunningham-Rundles, 2007). At approximately 6 months of age, when passively transferred maternal antibodies fade, male infants begin to develop frequent bacterial respiratory, digestive, or throat infections. Autoimmune diseases such as rheumatoid arthritis and systemic lupus erythematosus may occur in later life. The cellular or T-lymphocyte response remains adequate, allowing the child to resist viral, fungal, and parasitic infections.

This deficiency is treated with monthly intravenous immune globulin (IVIG) injections to supply immunoglobulins. Bone marrow transplantation may be successful in restoring immune competency. Parents and children, as they grow older, need to be taught the importance of recognizing infection early. Also help them set up a schedule for IVIG injections so these are not forgotten.

Common Variable Immunoglobulin Deficiencies. The most common disorder in this group is deficiency of IgA in surface secretions. The overall level of B lymphocytes is normal, but IgA production is reduced or absent, perhaps because of an increase of IgA suppressor cells or a defect in T-helper cells important for IgA synthesis. Without IgA, infections of surfaces exposed to the external environment and normally protected by mucus become common. Sinusitis, upper respiratory tract illness, and inflammatory bowel disease are apt to occur. There are associated atopic diseases (allergies) because without IgA on the surface mucosa, many more antigens than usual can enter the body, permitting more antigens to interact with IgE and produce allergic symptoms. Chronic irritation because of these large numbers of antigens predisposes exposed tissue to malignant transformation, so malignancy of the respiratory, gastrointestinal, and lymphoid systems occurs more readily. There is an increased risk that an antibody will cross-react with a self-antigen to cause autoimmune illness, so diseases such as systemic lupus erythematosus and rheumatoid arthritis also occur at increased rates. IgA deficiency can occur as a secondary type because of treatment with phenytoin (an anticonvulsant) and penicillamine (a copper chelating agent). IVIG contains little IgA, so therapy with IVIG does not greatly reduce symptoms. Because prevention, not treatment, is the key, parents need to be conscientious about preventing infections and perhaps administering prophylactic antibiotics to prevent respiratory infections (Liu, Stewart, & Johnston, 2008).

T-Lymphocyte Deficiencies

T-lymphocyte immunodeficiencies involve inadequate numbers or inadequate functioning of one or more types of T lymphocytes; this affects cell-mediated immunity and also, because of helper T-lymphocyte function, possibly humoral immunity as well. DiGeorge anomaly (which includes failure of the thymus to develop) and chronic mucocutaneous candidiasis are two disorders caused by T-lymphocyte deficiency or malfunction. DiGeorge syndrome is a defect of chromosome 22 or 22q11.2 (Van Aken et al., 2007).

Combined T- and B-Lymphocyte Deficiency

Severe combined immunodeficiency syndrome (SCIDS) is the most frequently seen disorder characterized by an absence or reduction of both humoral and cell-mediated immunity. SCIDS occurs as either an X-linked or autosomal recessive disorder (Liu, Stewart, & Johnston, 2008). It is caused by a developmental abnormality (sometimes but not always related to the absence of a particular enzyme), which prevents the formation of T lymphocytes (a stem cell abnormality). This, in turn, prevents the maturation of both T and B lymphocytes. Children cannot respond directly to antigen invasion and no antibodies are produced. Bone marrow (stem cell) transplantation has proven to be an effective treatment for this disorder (Waruiru et al., 2007).

Secondary (Acquired) Immunodeficiency

Secondary immunodeficiency, or loss of immune system response, can occur from factors such as severe systemic infection, cancer, renal disease, radiation therapy, severe stress, malnutrition, immunosuppressive therapy, and aging. There can be complete or partial loss of both B- and T-lymphocyte response.

Stress appears to alter the immune response by stimulating the release of corticosteroids from the adrenal gland. This suppresses the inflammatory response by inhibiting macrophage action. Immunosuppressive drugs, such as prednisone, can also suppress the inflammatory response. Radiation or chemotherapy can act to limit or destroy rapidly growing cells. Because both T and B lymphocytes are rapidly growing and dividing cells, they are killed by these drugs or radiation. Extreme infection is yet another cause for a decreased immune response because the body's continued ability to combat infection becomes exhausted.

Malnutrition can decrease immunity because rapidly growing cells need protein for synthesis; renal disease with protein loss will also deplete the amount of protein available for new lymphocyte production.

HIV Infection and AIDS

AIDS is the end stage of acquired immunodeficiency caused by infection with the RNA human immunodeficiency retrovirus HIV (McFarland, 2008). The virus has at least two divisions, HIV-1 and HIV-2, with a variety of further subtypes. The virus acts by attacking the lymphoreticular system, in particular CD4-bearing helper T lymphocytes.

The virus enters, substitutes its own RNA and DNA for the cell's DNA, and replicates in these lymphocytes, destroying them in the process.

There is no defense against the virus, so it remains in the body for life. Infection results in loss of CD4 lymphocytes and the ability to initiate an effective B-lymphocyte response. A CD4 cell count in the laboratory determines how many cells are still present and functioning. Because B-lymphocyte or humoral immune function, which initiates the production of antibodies, is affected, antibody formation will be decreased (hypogammaglobulinemia). When monocytes and macrophages become affected as well, the person with HIV infection cannot resist normal infection. When this CD4 count falls below 500 cells/mm^3 or the viral load rises above 5000 copies/mL, it is difficult for infected individuals to resist opportunistic infections such as fungal infections. The final result is that both the immune response and the ability to screen and remove malignant cells from the body are lost.

Transmission. HIV infection is spread by exposure to blood and other body secretions through sexual contact, sharing of contaminated needles for injection, transfusion of contaminated blood or blood products, perinatally from mother to fetus or newborn, and through breastfeeding. A few children have acquired the infection because of sexual abuse. Health care providers must maintain vigilance to guard against needle punctures, as these injuries are a source of blood transfer.

Pediatric AIDS accounts for only 1% to 2% of the total instances of AIDS (CDC, 2008a). Although it is decreasing in incidence, transmission of HIV from mother to child by placental spread is still the most common reason for childhood HIV infection in the United States. This transmission can occur during pregnancy, at birth, and possibly during breastfeeding. Transmission by this route has declined to less than 3% since HIV-positive women have been identified during pregnancy and prescribed antiviral therapy (Suksomboon, Poolsup, & Ket-Aim, 2007).

In the past, many children with hemophilia, because they receive so many blood product transfusions during childhood, received HIV-contaminated blood and were infected. This source of transmission now almost never occurs. The increasing rate of sexual activity and the rapidly rising incidence of sexually transmitted infections among adolescents make this group, next to newborn infants who received the virus from their mother, the most vulnerable to growing rates of HIV infection (McFarland, 2008). HIV is not transmitted by animals or through usual casual contact, such as shaking hands or kissing, or in households, day care centers, or schools.

Assessment. HIV has a long incubation period of about 10 years in adults. The disorder appears to progress more rapidly in children and infants who receive the virus through placental transmission if they do not receive treatment. These individuals are usually HIV positive by 6 months and develop clinical signs by 1 to 3 years of age. Children who receive the virus from another source usually convert to HIV positivity by 2 to 6 weeks, or at least by 6 months after exposure. During this preconversion time, a child may display preliminary symptoms such as poor resistance to infection, fever, swollen lymph nodes, respiratory tract infections, and thrush.

All infants born to infected mothers test positive for antibodies to the virus at birth because of passive antibody transmission. This persists for about 18 months. The disease is diagnosed, therefore, by recovery of the HIV antigen in children under this age and antibodies to the virus in children over this age. Tests to detect the antigen are termed PCR (polymerase chain reaction) tests; those for the antibody are termed ELISA (enzyme-linked immunosorbent assay) and Western blot confirmation. CD4 counts are used to document the disease status and predict disease progression. Normal counts vary according to age because the lymphocyte count normally varies by age. Table 42.2 shows the use of Centers for Disease Control and Prevention (CDC) guidelines and CD4 counts to determine disease progress. Severe suppression indicates a condition serious enough to cause life-threatening infections (CDC, 2008a).

The CDC classification of HIV infection in children has three categories:

- Category A, *Mildly Symptomatic*: two or more symptoms such as enlarged lymph nodes, liver, or spleen, or recurrent or persistent upper respiratory infections, sinusitis, or otitis media
- Category B, *Moderately Symptomatic*: more serious illnesses such as oropharyngeal candidiasis, bacterial meningitis, pneumonia, or sepsis, cardiomyopathy, cytomegalovirus infection, hepatitis, herpes simplex virus (HSV), bronchitis, pneumonitis, or esophagitis, herpes zoster (shingles), lymphoid interstitial pneumonia (LIP), pulmonary lymphoid hyperplasia complex, or toxoplasmosis

TABLE 42.2 ✻ CD4 Cell Counts Related to Progress of HIV/AIDS in Children

	Age of Child		
	Under 12 Months	*1–5 Years*	*6–12 Years*
No evidence of suppression	1500 cells/μL	1000 cells/μL	500 cells/μL
Evidence of moderate suppression	750–1499 cells/μL	500–999 cells/μL	200–499 cells/μL
Severe suppression	750 cells/μL	500 cells/μL	200 cells/μL

Source: Centers for Disease Control and Prevention. (2008a). *HIV/AIDS recommendations.* Washington, DC: Author.

- Category C, *Severely Symptomatic (AIDS),* serious bacterial infections such as septicemia, pneumonia, meningitis, bone or joint infection, or abscess of an internal organ or body cavity; candidiasis (esophageal or pulmonary), encephalopathy, herpes simplex lasting over 1 month, histoplasmosis, lymphoma, tuberculosis, Mycobacterium or *Pneumocystis carinii* pneumonia.

In addition to these symptoms, children may develop a malignant neoplasm, most noticeably Kaposi's sarcoma or non-Hodgkin's lymphoma (Engels et al., 2008).

Therapeutic Management. Because of the success of zidovudine administration during the pregnancy of HIV-positive women, many fewer infants are born with HIV infection today (Suksomboon, Poolsup, & Ket-Aim, 2007). Those who are born with a perinatal infection, once thought to have a short life expectancy, now have an opportunity for long-term survival. To accomplish this, therapy involves a complex regimen of nutritional supplements to prevent weight loss, vaccines to prevent infections, and highly active antiretroviral therapy (HAART) as well as antibacterial agents to combat the HIV virus and opportunistic infections (Casado et al., 2007).

BOX 42.4 ✻ Focus on Pharmacology

Zidovudine (ZDV)

Classification: Zidovudine is a thymidine analog.

Action: Zidovudine inhibits the replication of some retroviruses, including HIV (Karch, 2009).

Pregnancy risk category: C

Dosage: 2 mg/kg every 6 hours to infants born to HIV-positive mothers, starting within 12 hours of birth to 6 wk of age. 180 mg/m^2 (720 mg/m^2/dose) orally or intravenously every 6 hours to children ages 3 mo to 12 y (dosage not to exceed 200 mg every 6 hours).

Possible adverse effects: Nausea, loss of appetite, change in taste, paresthesia, headache, fever, agranulocytopenia, and rash

Nursing Implications

- When administering the drug intravenously, infuse the drug over 60 min to avoid too rapid an infusion.
- Administer the drug around the clock for maximum effectiveness.
- Monitor blood studies frequently for changes.
- Advise child to eat frequent small meals to counteract change in taste and loss of appetite.
- If the child experiences paresthesias, institute safety precautions and instruct the child and parents in measures to prevent injury related to loss of feeling.
- Caution child and parents that ZDV does not reduce the risk of HIV transmission, except placentally. Reinforce the importance of hygiene and infection control measures.

Nursing Diagnoses and Related Interventions

✻

Nursing Diagnosis: Risk for infection related to decreased immune function

Outcome Evaluation: Child's temperature is within normal parameters; no cough or skin lesions are present.

Children with HIV infection and their families must maintain strict personal hygiene by measures such as frequent handwashing and avoid close contact between the child and anyone who has a respiratory infection to try to prevent the child from contracting dangerous opportunistic infections. It is important to assess the oral cavity of children with AIDS for herpes and thrush lesions (Gennaro, Naidoo, & Berthold, 2008). When infections do occur, antiviral and antifungal treatment should be prompt and aggressive.

Combating the infection requires specific antiretroviral medications to prevent progressive deterioration of the immune system and to provide prophylactic measures against opportunistic infections. Three classes of drugs are the mainstay of therapy: nucleoside reverse transcriptase inhibitors (NRTIs), nonnucleoside reverse transcriptase inhibitors (NNRTIs), and protease inhibitors. NRTIs are designed to block production of viral DNA, limiting the ability of the virus to infect cells; zidovudine is an example (Box 42.4). NNRTIs also inhibit the DNA synthesis of viruses but act at different sites on the viral enzyme; nevirapine and efavirenz are examples. Protease inhibitors stop the ability of the virus to produce protease, limiting metastasis; amprenavir, nelfinavir, atazanavir, and ritonavir are examples of protease inhibitors used in children (Chadwick et al., 2008). Children are prescribed a regimen involving multiple drugs, such as one protease inhibitor plus two NRTIs.

In addition, many children are given prophylactic therapy for *P. carinii* pneumonia (trimethoprim/sulfamethoxazole [TMP-SMZ]) beginning at 6 months of age. Children with HIV infection are more susceptible to tuberculosis than other children, so they also must be safeguarded against contracting this. If a child develops tuberculosis, a combination of antituberculosis drugs, such as isoniazid or rifampin, is used. Preventing tuberculosis is becoming more difficult because strains of tuberculosis have become resistant to the usual drugs (Wells et al., 2007).

Children with HIV infection should receive routine immunizations with the killed virus vaccines, including the new pneumococcal vaccine, according to the usual schedule. Symptomatic children should not receive the varicella vaccine, and those with low CD4 counts should not receive MMR. If a child is exposed to varicella, intravenous varicella zoster immune globulin (VZIG) is prescribed in an attempt to prevent this disease. Yearly influenza vaccinations should begin at 6 months of age (CDC, 2008b).

Nursing Diagnosis: Risk for compromised family coping related to diagnosis of HIV infection in child

Outcome Evaluation: Parents state ability to continue providing child's physical care; identify outside resources for help with care and decision making.

The diagnosis of HIV infection in an infant or child can prove devastating for a family. When the infection is transmitted maternally, this diagnosis may be the first indication of the existence of HIV infection in the mother; as such, this signals tremendous stress for the whole family. If the child contracted HIV infection from a contaminated blood transfusion or organ donation (rare with current protocols for donor screening), the family can feel so betrayed and angry that they are unwilling to cooperate with health care providers who, in their minds, are responsible for their child's illness. When it occurs in an adolescent, parents may blame themselves for not supervising the child's activities more closely or providing better safer sex information. In any instance, the family's coping skills are sure to be compromised. Siblings may feel left out of the family circle because of the many health care appointments needed for the ill child. They may fear contracting the infection themselves. One of the first nursing priorities in the care of such a family should be to help the family re-establish their previous level of functioning so they can turn their attention to their child's emotional and physical care needs and to their own needs as well.

Physical care requirements for the child with HIV infection may be extensive, depending on the child's symptoms and disease progression. No matter what the child's physical needs, however, love and emotional support are essential to the child's well-being and psychological health. Parents or caregivers need extensive support, education, and anticipatory guidance from nurses and other members of the health care team. Encourage parents to seek medical care for their child at the first sign of illness or infection to prevent unnecessary hospitalization and pain.

A Pregnant Woman With HIV Infection

One fourth of the nearly one million people in the United States infected with this virus are female. The infection has become the leading cause of death in women 25 to 44 years of age. One percent to 2% of every 1000 women giving birth are HIV positive. When the disorder is discovered during pregnancy, pregnancy does not appear to accelerate the progression of the disease.

Risk factors for contracting an HIV infection in women include:

- Multiple sexual partners of the individual or sexual partner
- Bisexual partners
- Intravenous drug use by the individual or sexual partner

Assessment. Unlike other sexually transmitted infections, HIV infection rarely begins with reproductive tract irritation. Instead, early symptoms are more subtle and often difficult to differentiate from those of other diseases or even from the symptoms of early pregnancy (e.g., fatigue, anemia, diarrhea, and weight loss).

Without therapy, HIV infection may progress through the following stages:

- The initial invasion of the virus, which may be accompanied by mild, flulike symptoms
- Seroconversion, in which a woman converts from having no HIV antibodies in her blood serum (HIV serum negative) to having antibodies against HIV (HIV serum positive). Seroconversion happens 6 weeks to 1 year after exposure.
- An asymptomatic period during which a woman appears to be disease-free except for symptoms such as weight loss and fatigue (a wasting syndrome), although the virus can be replicating during this time. The length of this period varies but averages 3 to 11 years.
- A symptomatic period during which a woman develops opportunistic infections and possibly malignancies (e.g., toxoplasmosis, oral and vaginal candidiasis, gastrointestinal illness, herpes simplex, *P. carinii* pneumonia [PCP], *Candida* esophagitis, Kaposi sarcoma, and HIV-associated dementia). At this point, the CD4 count is usually below 200 cells/mm^3.

Although women are not as yet routinely screened for this infection during pregnancy (as a rule, no screening program is initiated for any disease until there is a cure for the disease), women who practice high-risk sexual behaviors should be asked if they want to be screened. A woman with HIV infection may also have contracted other STIs such as syphilis, gonorrhea, chlamydia, and hepatitis B, and so should be screened for these as well. Because HIV-positive women are at higher risk for developing toxoplasmosis and cytomegalovirus infections, the health history should include questions about cat ownership, ingestion of raw meat, and recent mild, flulike symptoms (see Chapter 12). Ordinarily, toxoplasmosis presents with few symptoms. However, in the HIV-positive woman, it may invade the cerebrospinal fluid and cause extreme neurologic involvement. Tuberculosis also occurs at a higher rate in HIV-positive people than in others and may worsen during pregnancy, so a test for tuberculosis should also be included.

If a woman is found to be HIV positive (has developed antibodies from having been exposed to the virus) through an ELISA antibody reaction or a Western blot analysis, the issues of safer sex practices, testing of sexual contacts, continuation or termination of the pregnancy, and treatment during pregnancy need to be addressed. HIV infection is associated with low birth weight and preterm birth. About 20% to 50% of infants born to untreated HIV-positive women will contract the virus and develop AIDS in the first year of life. However, if zidovudine (ZVD) is administered to the woman beginning with the 14th week of pregnancy and the newborn receives antiviral therapy beginning with birth, the risk of developing AIDS falls below 10% (Zanchetta et al., 2008).

Therapeutic Management. Women who are identified as HIV positive are usually advised not to become pregnant until more is learned about how to prevent transmission to a fetus. Often, however, the existence of HIV is discovered only after pregnancy is already present. Progression of the disease is assessed by frequent CD4 cell counts and viral load levels during the coming months.

A goal of therapy is to maintain the CD4 cell count at greater than 500 cells/mm^3 by administering (in addition to oral ZVD) one or more protease inhibitors, such as ritonavir (Norvir) or indinavir (Crixivan), in conjunction with a nucleoside reverse transcriptase inhibitor (NRTI) drug.

If *P. carinii* pneumonia develops, a woman is treated with trimethoprim with sulfamethoxazole (Bactrim), a combination drug not without consequences, as trimethoprim may be teratogenic in early pregnancy; sulfamethoxazole (Gantanol) may lead to increased bilirubin levels in the newborn if administered late in pregnancy. Pentamidine (Pentam), the drug of choice for PCP in nonpregnant women, is yet another option.

Kaposi's sarcoma, a rare malignancy that tends to occur with AIDS, is normally treated with chemotherapy. Chemotherapy is contraindicated during early pregnancy because of the potential for fetal injury but can be used later in pregnancy to halt these malignant growths.

Thrombocytopenia (lowered platelet count) may be present as a part of the disease pathology or as a response to zidovudine therapy. This may make a woman a poor candidate for an epidural injection for anesthesia during labor or for episiotomy. She may need a platelet transfusion close to birth to restore coagulation ability. To reduce the risk of mother-to-newborn transmission, women are offered the option of cesarean birth.

Follow-up testing of newborns being treated with zidovudine for the first 6 weeks is important. If the child has two negative HIV cultures at 4 months of age, HIV infection can be reasonably excluded.

Nursing Diagnoses and Related Interventions

Nursing Diagnosis: Risk for infection (opportunistic) related to dysfunction of the immune system secondary to invasion of HIV

Outcome Evaluation: CD4 counts remain above 500/mm^3; viral load less than 5000 copies/mL; no symptoms of lung, vaginal, esophageal, or central nervous system infections are present.

Pregnant women who have CD4 counts below 200/mm^3 may be prescribed drugs to help prevent opportunistic infections. Such drugs include acyclovir (Zovirax) for herpes simplex, clotrimazole troches (Mycelex) for oral thrush, pyrimethamine (Daraprim) and sulfadiazine for toxoplasmosis, and trimethoprim with sulfamethoxazole (Bactrim) for PCP. They may be immunized against pneumonia, influenza, and hepatitis B.

During pregnancy and at birth, active interventions are necessary to reduce the possibility of fetal exposure to maternal blood, often the mode of transmission to the fetus. Amniocentesis, for example, presents a risk for exposure to maternal blood and therefore is avoided if at all possible for diagnosing fetal maturity. During labor, internal fetal monitors, scalp blood sampling, forceps, and vacuum extraction are avoided to prevent the creation of a source of bleeding (that is, an open lesion on the fetal scalp). Episiotomy also is avoided to limit this as a possible blood source. Although the risk may be lower than previously believed, breast milk can transmit HIV and as breastfeeding also increases the incidence of mastitis in an immunosuppressed woman, women are advised not to breastfeed (Chasela et al., 2008). Breastfeeding could also be exhausting for a debilitated woman.

Women who are HIV positive need to be aware that they can still spread this illness to others through unprotected sexual relations or unintentional contamination by blood, even though they are being treated with antibiotics or zidovudine. Nurses can help reduce this risk by providing patient education about the mode of HIV transmission and safer sex practices.

Health care providers must use standard infection precautions (see Chapter 43) to protect against the spread of HIV. This includes the use of gloves when there is a possibility of contact with body secretions; cover gowns if clothing will be exposed to secretions; and goggles at birth, when there may be splashing of amniotic fluid. Gloves should be worn when handling the newborn until all maternal blood has been removed by a first bath. No blood sampling or injections should be completed on the neonate until after a first bath and the removal of maternal blood.

Caring for a woman who is HIV positive during pregnancy and childbirth calls for great sensitivity to respect a woman as a patient with a possibly fatal disease while at the same time encouraging her to continue with prenatal care. Because research into the cause and treatment of this disease is ongoing, recommendations constantly change. Nurses need to remain current on recommendations for therapy or prevention.

✓Checkpoint Question 42.1

When Dexter's mother learned he had an immunologic disease, she was concerned that he had developed acquired immunodeficiency syndrome (HIV infection or AIDS). What is the transmission method by which most children acquire HIV infection?

a. Blood transfusion.
b. Shared bath towels.
c. Placental transfer.
d. Sneezing and coughing.

ALLERGY

Allergic diseases occur as a result of an abnormal antigen–antibody response. Allergic symptoms can be chronic and minor, such as those that occur with seasonal rhinitis, or acute and severe, as in an anaphylactic reaction. They can disrupt a child's life and development and the life of the family. When the cause of an allergic response is difficult to pinpoint, the child and parents often become frustrated. Even when the child has a known allergy, symptoms can vary from minor to acute without warning, ultimately disrupting family functioning (Box 42.5).

Hypersensitivity

The underlying cause of all allergic disorders appears to be an excessive antigen–antibody response when the invading organism is an allergen rather than a simple immunogen. This is termed a type I response or a **hypersensitivity response** when it happens immediately. It can also occur as a type II, III, or IV response (Table 42.3). Types I, II, and III are mediated by antibodies (humoral response), whereas type IV is mediated by the T lymphocytes (cell-mediated response).

Type I: Anaphylaxis

With a type I allergic response, IgE receptor sites attached to the surface of mast cells bind to IgE antibodies responding to

Box 42.5 Assessment
Assessing a Child With an Immune Disorder

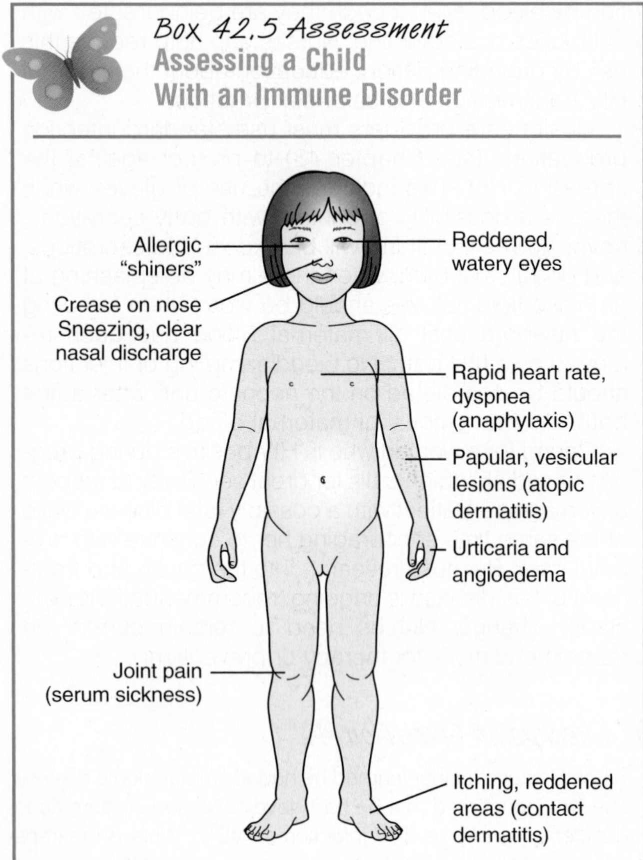

the presence of an antigen. Mast cells are specialized cells found lining blood vessels and in connective tissue, the mucous membranes, and skin. The IgE immunoglobulin triggers mast cells to release intracellular granules. These contain histamine, leukotrienes, a slow-reacting substance of anaphylaxis (SRS-A), and chemotactic substances (substances to draw leukocytes into the area). Histamine and leukotrienes cause peripheral vasodilation and permeability of blood vessels. This leads to vascular congestion and edema. SRS-A causes extreme bronchial constriction and reduced vasodilation and permeability. **Anaphylaxis** is an acute reaction characterized by extreme vasodilation that leads to circulatory shock and extreme bronchoconstriction that decreases the airway lumens (Lane & Bolte, 2007).

Type II: Cytotoxic Response

In a **cytotoxic response,** cells are detected as foreign and immunoglobulins directly attack and destroy them without harming surrounding tissue. Foreign red blood cells that are introduced to an Rh-negative woman by an Rh-positive fetus are destroyed by this process (see Chapter 26). Tumor cells may be destroyed by this process. Why this immune response fails when malignant cells begin to proliferate is not understood. Current research is attempting to devise ways to activate the natural immune response as a method of destroying malignant cells. Care of the child with a malignancy (neoplasm) is discussed in Chapter 53.

Type III: Immune Complex

A type III response is an IgG- or IgE-mediated antigen–antibody complex reaction that involves complement and initiates the inflammatory response. Complement reactions that persist beyond the usual inhibition may serve as the basis for many of the autoimmune illnesses, such as glomerulonephritis and systemic lupus erythematosus (see Chapter 46). Serum sickness also occurs as a result of a type III response.

Type IV: Cell-Mediated Hypersensitivity

In a delayed hypersensitivity response, T lymphocytes react with antigens and release lymphokines to call macrophages into the area. An inflammatory response occurs that helps to destroy the foreign tissue. A Mantoux or purified protein derivative (PPD) tuberculin test is an example of this. Redness and induration of the site do not begin initially but only after approximately 12 hours from the injection. The reaction peaks in 24 to 72 hours (a delayed response).

Contact dermatitis is another example of a delayed hypersensitivity response. Certain substances, such as cosmetics,

TABLE 42.3 Classification of Hypersensitivity Reactions

Type	Involved Cell	Mechanism	Effect
I Anaphylaxis	IgE	IgE attached to surface of mast cell triggers release of intracellular granules from mast cells on contact with antigens	Allergies, asthma, atopic dermatitis, anaphylaxis
II Cytotoxic	IgG or IgM	Antigen–antibody reaction leading to antigen destruction; complement is activated	Hemolytic anemia, transfusion reaction, erythroblastosis fetalis
III Immune complex disease	IgG or IgE	Antigen–antibody complexes precipitate; complement is activated, leading to inflammatory response	Rheumatoid arthritis, systemic lupus erythematosus
IV Delayed	T lymphocyte	T cells combine with antigen to induce inflammatory reactions by direct cell involvement or release of lymphokines	Contact dermatitis, transplant graft reaction

household products, or cured leather, alter the protein of skin cells so that they become an antigen, or the foreign substance combines with the protein (hapten formation) to become an antigenic protein. Lymphocytes and macrophages infiltrate the area and attempt to destroy the offending protein. Redness and vesicles occur, and pruritus may be intense.

Assessment of Allergy in Children

History

Taking a health history of a child with an allergy can be time-consuming because many factors must be considered. A family history is important because there are familial tendencies with allergic diseases. Obtaining the exact symptoms of the allergy is important to help identify the allergen: rhinitis, for example, is probably because of an airborne antigen; urticaria (swelling and itching) is often caused by ingested antigens; and contact dermatitis (often a rash) must be from something that contacts the skin in that area. The time of the year that the allergy occurs also may give a clue to its cause. If the child's allergy exists all year, the antigen must be one that is present all year (house dust mites, pet dander, or a common food). If it occurs in the spring, it may be because of a tree pollen; in summer, a grass pollen; if it occurs just in August, ragweed is a prime suspect.

Children with allergic rhinitis (hay fever) develop common symptoms such as a horizontal crease across the nose (called a Dennie's line) from their habit of constantly wiping away nasal secretions. They also may develop dark patches under their eyes from back-pressure from nasal congestion.

Many symptoms of allergy are vague, described as "colds all winter," "itching," or "runny nose." Listen carefully: even though no one symptom is acute, together such symptoms can interfere with a child's comfort, school experience, and long-term health. Having the parents and the child keep a chart of when symptoms are worse and better often helps identify a specific allergen. Children with allergic rhinitis (hay fever), for example, have more symptoms on a windy day and fewer after a rainstorm (the rain washes pollen out of the air). Children are often poor reporters of when they have symptoms because they cannot remember clearly whether they had the same rhinitis and watery eye symptoms last summer as they do this summer. A record that details when symptoms start—for example, on arising, or only after the child reaches school—also can help identify an allergen.

Laboratory Testing

Few laboratory tests are helpful in establishing a diagnosis of allergy. A determination of IgE serum antibodies can be made. Most children with an allergy have an increased eosinophil count. Five percent or more of eosinophils on a differential count, or an eosinophil count of 250 or more cells per cubic millimeter, is significant. Another main cause of an increased eosinophil count is invasion by ova or parasites. This is why a stool specimen for ova and parasites is generally collected to rule out these problems as the cause of the increased eosinophil count. A radioallergosorbent test (RAST) may be ordered. This is an indirect radioimmunoassay in which the child's serum IgE is allowed to react with specific allergens impregnated in laboratory disks (Schafer et al., 2007).

Skin Testing

Skin testing is done to detect the presence of IgE in the skin, or to isolate an antigen (allergen) to which the IgE is responding or to which a child is sensitive. When an allergen is introduced into the child's skin and the child is sensitive to that allergen, a wheal or flare response appears at the site of the test. This is because of the release of histamine, which leads to local vasodilation. Because this reaction appears quickly, the test should be read in 20 minutes. Systemic or aerosol administration of an antihistamine will inhibit the flare response, so the child should not receive these drugs for 8 hours before skin testing. Corticosteroid therapy does not affect immediate skin reactivity and so may be continued during skin testing.

Skin testing may be done by applying a patch or using a scratch or an intracutaneous injection technique. Patch testing has become the method of choice because it is painless and more efficient. For the child with rare allergies not typically provided by commercial patches, scratch or intracutaneous testing still may be necessary. Scratch testing is done by placing a drop of allergen solution on the skin, then scratching through the drop of liquid with a sterile needle. A relatively concentrated extract of allergen must be used for scratch testing because little allergen enters the child's skin.

Intracutaneous injections are done by injecting a small amount of a solution of allergen below the epidermis of the skin. This is usually done on the forearm so that if a sensitivity reaction does occur, a tourniquet can be applied proximal to the test site to prevent further absorption of the antigen. If the categories to be tested are extensive, the back can be used. Solutions used for intracutaneous injections are more dilute than those used for scratch testing (1:500 dilution compared with 1:5 for scratch testing). This means that the allergen extracts are not interchangeable from a group prepared for scratch testing to a group prepared for intracutaneous injections (or vice versa).

Because intracutaneous injections are given just below the epidermal layer of skin, they are almost painless. This is the same phenomenon as passing a needle or pin under the top layer of skin of a fingertip, a trick every school-age child does at least once to the horror of friends. The child needs a great deal of support for this type of skin testing, however, because it looks as if it will be painful, and the sight of a needle is frightening.

After all forms of skin testing, if the child is allergic to the test solution, a wheal and erythema (redness) will occur at the test site (Fig. 42.4). The size of the reaction is measured and graded as 1+ to 4+ or as slight, moderate, or marked. The allergens chosen for skin testing depend on the child's symptoms. Few children need more than 30 test media tried. This is because most allergies are worse at certain times of the year, and only the allergens prevalent at that time of year need to be evaluated.

Have a syringe filled with 1 mL epinephrine (Adrenalin) 1:1000 on hand to counteract an unexpected anaphylactic reaction from skin testing. Epinephrine is given subcutaneously in doses of 0.01 mg/kg, up to 0.5 mg. Children should stay in the health care setting for at least 30 minutes after skin testing so they are there when such a reaction is most apt to occur.

Skin testing with food extracts is largely ineffective. Food allergies are best identified by eliminating a suspected

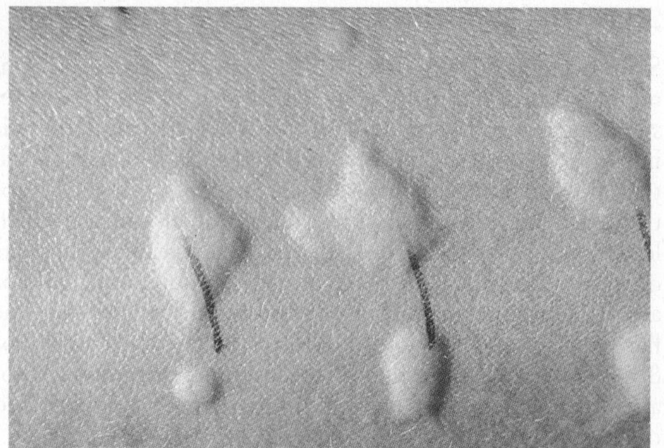

FIGURE 42.4 Allergy skin testing. Note the positive reactions. (© SPL/Custom Medical Stock Photograph.)

food from the diet and observing whether there is an improvement in symptoms. After a time of improvement, the food is reintroduced. If it is one to which the child is allergic, symptoms will return with its reintroduction (termed "rechallenging").

Therapeutic Management

No matter what the symptoms of a child's allergy, there are three goals for therapy: reduce the child's exposure to the allergen, hyposensitize the child to produce a state of increased clinical **tolerance** (a state of not responding) to the allergen, and modify the child's response to the allergen with a pharmacologic agent.

Reducing the child's exposure to the allergen is possible when the offending allergen is a drug, food, or irritant. Reducing exposure is much more difficult when the child is found to be allergic to allergens such as molds, dust, feathers, or other substances found almost everywhere.

Environmental Control

Environmental control means removal of as many common allergens as possible from a child's environment. Common measures of environmental control are shown in Table 42.4 and Box 42.6. Some parents carry out instructions to reduce potential allergens in their house without difficulty, but for others the process seems too involved to undertake. Help parents understand that environmental control can make a great deal of difference in their child's

TABLE 42.4 ✻ Common Measures for Environmental Control of Allergens

Area of Concern	Measures	Rationale
Child's bedroom	Encase mattress and pillow in sturdy plastic.	Reduces dust and dust mites
	Cover the zipper of plastic pillow and mattress case with adhesive tape.	Keeps dust confined
	Use blankets or quilts made of or stuffed with smooth, synthetic material; avoid wool.	Minimizes dust; wool is a good dust collector or may be an allergen itself
	Take down any ornamental items, such as a bed canopy.	Prevents dust collection
	Remove stuffed chairs and replace with wooden ones.	Removes dust collectors
	Remove venetian blinds and curtains that need to be dry-cleaned; replace with easily laundered types.	Removes dust collectors
	Remove stuffed toys unless filled with synthetic material.	Removes dust collectors and possible sources of allergens
	Remove aquariums and plants.	Removes mold spores
	Clean closet so it contains only currently used items.	Eliminates dust collectors
	Remove any fur or woolen items from child's wardrobe.	Removes possible allergens
Living room	Remove all carpets. If a rug is necessary, replace an animal hair pad with a foam rubber one.	Avoids containers for dust collection
	Provide a wooden chair for sitting.	Provides space free from allergens
	Vacuum frequently.	Minimizes dust collection
	Use linoleum or plastic laminate surface on carpet if child sits on the floor.	Provides space free from allergens
	Discourage child from lying on rug.	Reduces exposure to allergens
Bathroom	Use nonscented toilet paper, soaps, cleaners.	Minimizes exposure to potential irritants
School room	Have child sit away from blackboard, caged animals, or fish tanks.	Minimizes exposure to chalk, mold spores, and animal dander, which are allergens
	Keep locker free of collectibles	Reduces dust collection
General	Purchase a dehumidifier; add compounds to paint to decrease mold spores.	Reduces mold spores
	Use HEPA filters on furnaces, vacuums.	Filters air of possible allergens
	Do not keep a pet.	Reduces exposure to animal dander
	Dust daily with a moist cloth.	Controls dust better than dry dusting

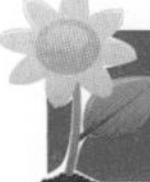

BOX 42.6 * Focus on Communication

The Goodenough family has been instructed on environmental control measures because Dexter has severe allergic rhinitis. Despite this, Dexter's symptoms have not improved. You meet with his parents to confirm they are carrying out these measures.

Less Effective Communication

Nurse: Have you made the changes around your house that we discussed to reduce dust?

Mrs. Goodenough: As many as we can.

Nurse: What about Dexter's bedroom? Do you have the mattress covered? Any frilly curtains down? Any stuffed animals taken out?

Mrs. Goodenough: I've done everything I can.

Nurse: In the living room, it's important he has a protected floor space, also that he doesn't sit in overstuffed chairs.

Mrs. Goodenough: I've done everything I can.

Nurse: Okay, you sound in good shape. It's puzzling, though, why, in the face of all you've done, Dexter's symptoms haven't improved.

More Effective Communication

Nurse: Have you made the changes around your house that we discussed to reduce dust?

Mrs. Goodenough: As many as we can.

Nurse: What about Dexter's bedroom? Do you have the mattress covered? Any frilly curtains down? Any stuffed animals taken out?

Mrs. Goodenough: I've done everything I can.

Nurse: It's puzzling why Dexter's symptoms haven't improved. Why don't you tell me exactly what steps you've taken?

Mrs. Goodenough: I covered the mattress. I had to leave the curtains up, though, because they match the rug. I took out a lot of the toys, but I had to leave the stuffed bears because they match the wallpaper.

Nurse: Let's review again what environmental control means and the effect it can have on reducing Dexter's symptoms.

By taking the parent's statement that she has done "everything possible" to mean she has done everything that needs to be done, the nurse makes an incorrect assumption. Following up by asking the parents to be more specific reveals better information.

symptoms. If environmental control is effective with a child, this is preferable to hyposensitization, which involves many visits to the doctor and many injections.

Hyposensitization

Hyposensitization, or immunotherapy, is done when the child's allergy symptoms cannot be controlled by avoidance of an allergen or conventional drug therapy. Because it is expensive and may not be successful, it is usually considered only after environmental control has been tried.

Hyposensitization works by increasing the plasma concentration of IgG antibodies. IgG acts to prevent or block IgE antibodies from coming in contact with the allergen. After specific allergens have been recognized with skin testing, small amounts of the allergy extract (dilute enough to be clinically subreactive) are injected into the child subcutaneously at 3- to 5-day intervals. The dose of antigen is increased in strength each time until a peak concentration is reached. The peak dose corresponds to the greatest strength that does not give clinical symptoms after injection. Following this, the child's allergy symptoms should be greatly reduced or absent. The child then needs periodic injections every 3 to 4 weeks to maintain hyposensitization to the allergen. If a child is going to have an anaphylactic reaction to an injected allergen, it generally occurs within 30 minutes after the injection. Therefore, always have children wait in the health care setting for 30 minutes after injection before going home.

Immunotherapy is generally continued for 2 to 3 years because the longer it is used, the longer the period of relief from symptoms after it is stopped. Be certain that parents know at the beginning of therapy that this therapy will not "cure" their child. It will make the child symptom-free or will decrease symptoms for a length of time, however, and it may prevent a mild atopic disorder such as hay fever (allergic rhinitis) from turning into a severe atopic disorder such as asthma (see Chapter 40). Be certain children have adequate preparation for the procedure. Help them understand the importance of returning for additional injections.

A newer technique of immunotherapy is the sublingual administration of chosen allergen solutions. SLIT (sublingual immunotherapy) is administered for an equal length of time as injection therapy, but SLIT has the advantage of being painless while producing equal results.

Pharmacologic Therapy

Several pharmacologic preparations can be used to reduce the symptoms of childhood allergies. Like hyposensitization procedures, these drugs do not change the sensitivity to allergens; they only relieve the symptoms.

Antihistamines block histamine release and as a result control itching, sneezing, and rhinorrhea. Diphenhydramine hydrochloride (Benadryl) is the prototype of this drug class (Box 42.7). It is effective but causes severe drowsiness. Second- and third-generation antihistamines, such as cetirizine (Zyrtec) and loratadine (Claritin), cause less drowsiness and provide a longer effect.

Decongestants, such as pseudoephedrine (Sudafed), decrease nasal edema and can help enlarge breathing space. Intranasal corticosteroids reduce inflammation, producing an effect similar to decongestants. Intranasal cromolyn sodium can be used prophylactically to prevent symptoms.

COMMON IMMUNE REACTIONS

Anaphylactic Shock

Anaphylactic shock is an immediate, life-threatening, type I hypersensitivity reaction that occurs after exposure to an

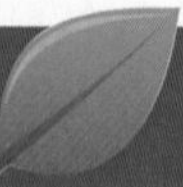

BOX 42.7 * Focus on Pharmacology

Diphenhydramine Hydrochloride (Benadryl)

Classification: Diphenhydramine is a first-generation antihistamine.

Action: Blocks the effects of histamine at H_1 receptor sites, resulting in relief of symptoms associated with histamine release disorders such as allergic rhinitis (Karch, 2009).

Pregnancy risk category: B

Dosage: 12.5 to 25 mg three times to four times daily or 5 mg/kg/day or 150 mg/m^2/day orally (in children weighing over 10 kg [20 lb]) up to a maximum dose of 300 mg/day

Possible adverse effects: Drowsiness, dizziness, sedation, epigastric distress, dry mouth, thickening of bronchial secretions, hypotension

Nursing Implications

- Administer drug with food if gastrointestinal upset occurs.
- Use a humidifier to keep nasal mucosa moist.
- Be alert for drowsiness, which may interfere with school or sports performance; notify the health care provider for possible change in dosage or drug.
- Encourage the child to suck on sugarless lozenges to combat dry mouth.
- Notify health care provider if child develops a lower respiratory tract disorder. Antihistamines should not be used when secretions need to be kept moist to enhance expectoration.
- Do not use this drug if the child has glucose-6-phosphate dehydrogenase deficiency. Severe hemolysis may occur.

allergen in a previously sensitized child. Within minutes of antigen invasion (being stung by an insect or receiving an injection of a drug to which a child has been sensitized), symptoms begin (Boguniewicz, 2008).

Assessment

Initially, a child may become nauseated, with vomiting and diarrhea, because of the sudden increase in gastrointestinal secretions produced by the stimulation of histamine. This is followed by urticaria and angioedema. Bronchospasm can become so severe the child becomes dyspneic and hypoxemic. Continued bronchospasm leads to hypoxia. As blood vessels dilate, the blood pressure and pulse rate fall. Seizures and death may follow as soon as 10 minutes after the allergen was introduced into the child's body.

It is sometimes difficult to distinguish anaphylactic shock from fainting (syncope). Children, as a rule, however, do not faint after an injection or a bee sting. Syncope rarely occurs if a person is lying down, so if the reaction occurred while the child was lying on the treatment table, it is most likely that the reaction is anaphylactic. With syncope, although the child falls and is momentarily unconscious, the pulse and blood pressure remain normal. The child appears pale and may have intense perspiration, but can be roused readily after breathing amyl nitrite (smelling salts). The child with an anaphylactic reaction cannot be roused this way.

Therapeutic Management

Preventing and recognizing anaphylaxis are as important as knowing how to respond when it occurs. Before giving drugs that are known to have a high incidence of anaphylactic reactions such as penicillin, aspirin, or antitoxin serums, be certain to ask parents if their child has ever had a reaction to the drug before. If in doubt, withhold the drug until its safety can be confirmed. Check the child's chart to be certain that no prior reactions are noted. People who have hypersensitivity reactions to any injectable substance should wear a bracelet or necklace identifying the drug to which they are allergic. Some children object to this safety measure because they do not want to look conspicuous, but assure them this is important. Generally, children who have hypersensitivity reactions to insect stings are advised to undergo hyposensitization therapy because they cannot totally avoid insects.

Epinephrine is the drug of choice to treat anaphylaxis (Box 42.8) (Pongracic & Kim, 2007). Additional emergency interventions for anaphylactic shock are summarized in

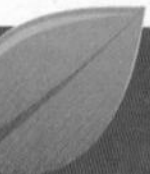

BOX 42.8 * Focus on Pharmacology

Epinephrine Hydrochloride (Adrenalin)

Classification: Epinephrine is a sympathomimetic drug.

Action: Acts on both alpha- and beta-receptor sites of sympathetic receptor cells to cause increased blood pressure and heart rate. It also relaxes the smooth muscles of the bronchi. It is used to counteract the symptoms of anaphylaxis (Karch, 2009).

Pregnancy risk category: C

Dosage: 0.01 mg/kg or 0.3 mL/m^2 of a 1:1000 solution subcutaneously every 20 min or more often if needed for 4 hours, not to exceed 0.5 mL (0.5 mg) in a single dose (for children and infants); 0.005 mL/kg (0.025 mg/kg) subcutaneously of a 1:200 suspension (in infants and children 1 mo to 1 y)

Possible adverse effects: Anxiety, restlessness, headache, nausea, arrhythmias, hypertension, palpitations, pallor

Nursing Implications

- Be sure to calculate the drug dosage and check the solution strength carefully; solution is available in different concentrations, and epinephrine is a very potent drug.
- Obtain blood pressure, pulse, and respirations and auscultate breath sounds before and immediately after administration. Assess the child for signs indicating resolution of anaphylaxis.
- Rotate injection sites to prevent necrosis.
- Have a rapidly acting alpha-adrenergic blocking agent or vasodilator readily available in case of hypertensive reaction; have a beta-adrenergic blocking agent readily available in case of arrhythmias.
- Protect the drug from light and heat. Use only solutions that are clear and colorless.

BOX 42.9 ✻ Emergency Measures for Anaphylactic Shock

Anaphylaxis is an emergency, and fast action is necessary.

- Position the child with head even with the body to counteract hypotension.
- Administer aqueous epinephrine (Adrenalin) 1:1000 subcutaneously at a dosage of 0.01 mg per kilogram of body weight up to 0.5 mg. This relieves laryngeal edema and severe bronchospasm.
- Administer nebulized bronchodilators such as albuterol to halt wheezing.
- If hypoxia is present, administer oxygen by mask or nasal cannula.
- Notify the cardiac arrest team because both respiratory and cardiac arrest may occur.
- Anticipate use of diphenhydramine (Benadryl) IM or IV as a secondary medication, particularly if urticaria (itching and swelling) is present.
- Anticipate the need for an IV fluid line as a route for a vasopressor such as dopamine and fluid to help restore blood pressure.
- If the child is experiencing seizures, prepare to administer phenobarbital or diazepam.
- Be prepared to administer corticosteroids as second-line drugs. Corticosteroids do not act immediately but reduce inflammation, which is necessary. IV methylprednisolone is a typical drug given.
- Keep the child and family members calm; anxiety adds to bronchospasm and decreases breathing ability.

Box 42.9. If anaphylaxis follows an injection or an insect sting, give the epinephrine in the opposite arm. Place a tourniquet on the extremity of the allergenic injection or sting proximal to the injection site to prevent further absorption of the allergen. Release the tourniquet every 15 minutes for a few seconds to avoid totally compromising blood flow.

If a sensitized child receives an injection or is stung by an insect while at home, parents must know the proper procedure to follow so they can give their child immediate help. In place of a tourniquet, they can apply ice to the injection or sting site to slow absorption. If a child has been prescribed an antihistamine, they should give that. Then the parents should notify their emergency response system (911) that their child is having a severe reaction. Caution them not to attempt to give an oral medication if the child is comatose. Parents may purchase an emergency kit (Ana-Kit), an insect sting treatment kit that contains measured doses of epinephrine (often in a device called an EpiPen, which injects the epinephrine; Box 42.10) and an antihistamine. Parents and children need practice to inject EpiPens correctly or they can accidentally puncture their thumb. If that happens, the vasoconstriction action of the epinephrine could disrupt circulation in their thumb (Mehr, Robinson, & Tang, 2007).

Evaluation of the child after an anaphylactic reaction involves not only a physical examination but also evaluation to help the child avoid such a serious reaction from occurring again. This involves health teaching about the substance that caused the reaction and related substances that could have the same effect.

✓ Checkpoint Question 42.2

Any child can have an anaphylactic reaction to a food or drug. What is the drug of choice you would want to have available to treat anaphylactic reactions?

a. Prednisone.
b. Epinephrine.
c. Penicillin.
d. Ibuprofen.

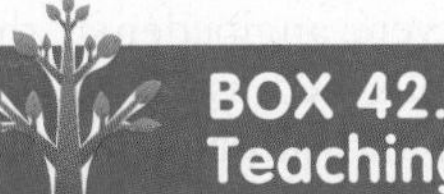

BOX 42.10 ✻ Focus on Family Teaching

Guidelines for Using an EpiPen

Q. Dexter's father says to you, "If my child is stung by a bee, I'm supposed to inject epinephrine. How do I do that?"

A. It is important you think about this in advance, because at the moment your child is stung, it will be an emergency situation.

- Purchase an EpiPen, a commercial syringe with a designated dose of epinephrine for use in emergencies.
- If necessary, purchase additional EpiPens so you have one at home, provide one for your child's school, and maybe keep one in your car to avoid having to remember to carry a single one with you.
- Store EpiPens at room temperature; don't refrigerate.
- Inspect the color of the solution in the EpiPen once a month; replace it if it is cloudy or discolored.
- If your child is stung, remove the gray safety cap from the device and wipe the outer fleshy portion of your child's thigh with an alcohol wipe.
- Place the EpiPen against the thigh until the device activates, injecting the solution into your child's thigh. If necessary, you can place the device on top of your child's clothing. The needle is long enough to pass through the clothing and into your child's skin.
- Be careful before injecting that you are holding the EpiPen with the needle toward your child. If not, you will accidentally inject your own thumb (a serious circumstance, as the dose of epinephrine could seriously injure your thumb).
- Keep in mind that the EpiPen is designed so that not all the solution in the pen will be ejected. Do not try to give the remainder of the solution.
- Remember that epinephrine will control symptoms for about 20 minutes. After administering the dose, therefore, call 911 for transportation assistance or transport your child to an emergency facility for further care.

Urticaria and Angioedema

Urticaria, or hives, refers to flat wheals surrounded by erythema arising from the chorion layer of skin; they are intensely pruritic (often described as a burning sensation). Elevations may occur so close together they tend to coalesce (blend together). Urticaria occurs from a type I or immediate hypersensitivity reaction created by the release of histamine from an antibody–antigen reaction, similar to but of lesser intensity than anaphylaxis. In chronic urticaria, no causative allergen may be found. There is dilatation of capillaries and venules with increased permeability.

Angioedema is edema of the skin and subcutaneous tissue. This occurs most frequently on the eyelids, hands, feet, genitalia, and lips—areas where skin is loosely bound by subcutaneous tissue. Angioedema can be distinguished from other edemas because it is not dependent, is generally asymmetrically distributed, and usually occurs with urticaria. One type is inherited as an autosomal disorder on chromosome 11 (Chawla & Riederer, 2007). With severe angioedema, the larynx may be involved. This is serious because laryngeal edema may lead to airway obstruction and subsequently asphyxiation and death.

The allergens that most frequently cause urticaria and angioedema include drugs, foods, and insect stings. Exposure to hot or cold can also cause these reactions. The cause of the reaction should be identified so it can be avoided in the future. Although hot and cold exposure is a rare cause, children with this form must be identified because if they swim in cold water, the sudden release of histamine could cause dizziness so severe that they could drown. Therapy for urticaria or angioedema is subcutaneous epinephrine or an oral antihistamine.

Serum Sickness

Serum sickness is a type III hypersensitivity response of the body to a foreign serum antigen or drug (Segal, 2007). Examples of foreign sera given to children include tetanus antitoxin, diphtheria antitoxin, and rabies antiserum. These are obtained from horse serum. Children may also experience a serum sickness reaction to a drug such as penicillin, but this is rare.

Assessment

Symptoms of serum sickness begin 7 to 12 days after the serum injection. If the child has received the same type of foreign serum previously, symptoms may occur as early as 1 to 5 days. Children notice itching, edema, and erythema at the injection site. There is generalized urticaria (hives) with or without angioedema (generalized edema). Erythematous maculopapular rashes, erythema multiforme (a generalized macular eruption with dark red papules), or purpura (hemorrhage into the skin) may result.

There may be fever and arthralgia (joint pain). Swollen lymph nodes may be present, especially of the regional nodes near the site of the injection. The child may have weight gain, nausea, vomiting, and abdominal pain. In more extreme instances, the child's nervous system may be involved and optic neuritis, stupor, and coma may occur. If edema is severe, laryngeal edema will become the paramount symptom that needs treatment.

Therapeutic Management

Serum sickness lasts days or weeks. In its usual form (symptoms of urticaria, edema, arthralgia, or pruritus), the treatment is only symptomatic because the condition will improve by itself with time. However, an antihistamine such as diphenhydramine (Benadryl) or epinephrine may be helpful in relieving symptoms. A nonsteroidal anti-inflammatory drug (NSAID) such as ibuprofen (Motrin) or a corticosteroid may be necessary to relieve the fever and joint pain.

Like anaphylactic reactions, serum sickness reactions are frightening to a child and parents. Parents need an explanation of why the reaction occurred (their child has a low threshold of sensitization to this particular substance), that it was not anyone's fault, and that it did not occur from administration of the wrong compound (assuming that proper precautions to ascertain sensitivity to the solution were taken before the incident). Because serum sickness mimics so many other disorders, parents need reassurance that it is not arthritis (the arthralgia may make them think it is) and that their child will not have long-term effects from it.

The child should not receive the foreign serum or drug that was responsible for this primary occurrence of serum sickness again. Otherwise, if administered again, the manifestation of the reaction may be anaphylaxis. Children should wear a bracelet or necklace stating the solutions to which they are hypersensitive. Children should have their immunizations (and records) kept current so there is never a need to give sera such as tetanus or diphtheria antitoxins.

ATOPIC DISORDERS

Individuals with atopy are prone to all allergic responses. Three disorders occur most frequently: hay fever (allergic rhinitis), eczema (atopic dermatitis), and asthma (discussed in Chapter 40). Although these diseases show a familial tendency, different family members may have different symptoms. In one family, for example, the father may have allergic rhinitis, one child may have asthma, and another may have atopic dermatitis.

The gene responsible for an immune response is located near the human leukocyte antigen that is responsible for graft rejection. In certain children, a tendency for sensitivity to antigens or abnormality of this gene is apparently inherited. These children have a higher-than-normal production of IgE antibody that makes them more responsive to allergens than other people. However, there is also a strong environmental component to these diseases. Children whose parents smoke have a greater incidence of atopic disorders compared with children of parents who do not smoke (Goodwin, 2007).

Allergic Rhinitis

Allergic rhinitis is caused by a type I or immediate hypersensitivity immune response. It occurs in 10% to 40% of children (Al Sayyad et al., 2009).

Assessment

Common symptoms of allergic rhinitis include sneezing, nasal engorgement, and a profuse watery nasal discharge. The mucous membrane of the nose is generally paler than normal. It may be edematous, adding to nasal congestion.

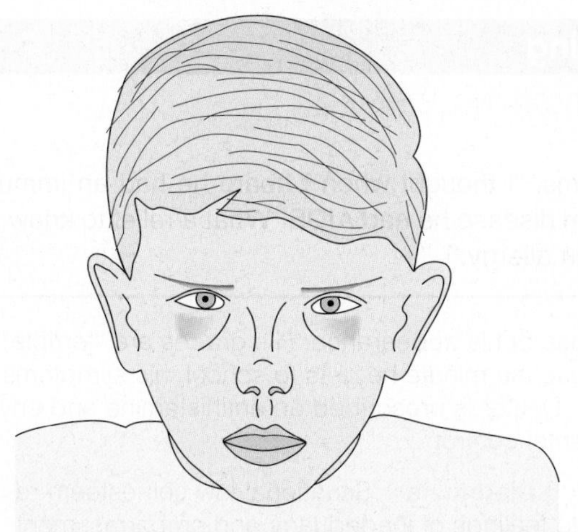

FIGURE 42.5 Back-pressure to the blood circulation around the eye orbit from allergic rhinitis may lead to dark areas under the eyes (allergic shiners). The frequent rubbing of the nose in an upward direction can lead to a peculiar horizontal crease (Dennie's line).

The eyes tend to water. The conjunctivae may be pruritic, often with a distinctive pebbly appearance. Children constantly rub their noses in an upward motion, termed an allergic salute. Over a long period, rubbing the nose this way leads to a horizontal crease across the tip of the nose, called an allergic crease. Because of congestion in the nose, there tends to be back-pressure to the blood circulation around the eye orbit, which leads to blackened areas under the eyes, termed allergic shiners (Fig. 42.5).

Children older than 6 years (when frontal sinuses develop) may report a full frontal headache. This becomes more marked with adolescence. Some children feel exhausted and lethargic and cannot function well in school. Recurrent otitis media may occur because of the swollen pharyngeal tissue (eustachian tubes are blocked to the middle ear). A smear of the nasal discharge will reveal an increased eosinophil count (more than 10% of the white cell count). RAST analysis may reveal the offending allergens.

The allergens that cause allergic rhinitis are generally pollens or molds rather than foods or drugs. Many of these children are brought to a health care setting during peak pollen months because parents think they have a "summer cold." However, with an upper respiratory infection, the mucous membrane of the nose is more apt to be reddened than pale, and the secretions draining from the nose are apt to be thick white or yellow rather than the thin, watery secretions of allergic rhinitis. Children with an upper respiratory infection often have a fever; children with allergic rhinitis do not. With an upper respiratory infection, a sore throat and cervical adenopathy may be present, but these are rare with allergic rhinitis.

Therapeutic Management

Allergic rhinitis is managed by avoidance of allergens, use of pharmacologic agents (antihistamines, leukotriene inhibitors, or corticosteroids), or immunotherapy. Parents usually ask how sick children should be before they need to see an allergist about skin testing and definite treatment (an expensive, time-consuming, and potentially painful procedure). Individual circumstances dictate the direction of treatment. As a rule, a child whose symptoms are increasing in intensity, who has associated lower respiratory tract involvement, or whose condition interferes with activities in which the child wants to participate needs definitive testing and treatment. Others can be managed by environmental control and medications to reduce symptoms.

Intranasal corticosteroids or antihistamines are effective in reducing symptoms in most children. Caution children and parents that antihistamines tend to cause sleepiness. Assess whether this will interfere with schoolwork or if an adolescent, if it could interfere with driving an automobile. Be certain that parents understand that if nasal antihistamine sprays are given for more than 3 days, a rebound effect may occur (the nasal mucosa becomes more edematous rather than less edematous).

Avoidance of allergens may be ineffective with allergic rhinitis because a child has a sensitivity to many different pollens or grasses. If children always show symptoms at one particular time of the year, parents may be able to carry out environmental control for that period of the year. Some children with allergic rhinitis are more comfortable in air-conditioned buildings; others have strong symptoms in the presence of air conditioning, probably accounting for the high incidence of headaches that occur at school (Aamodt et al., 2007).

Allergic rhinitis is often considered a minor illness by parents, something that children will outgrow. However, for children who have the condition, it may not be a minor illness and it may keep them from interacting with other children during certain months because they dread going outside and initiating symptoms. Help parents understand the importance of avoiding allergens and the need for conscientious administration of intranasal corticosteroids or antihistamines to minimize symptoms (see Focus on Nursing Care Planning Box 42.11).

Perennial Allergic Rhinitis

Allergic rhinitis becomes perennial (year-round) when the allergen is one that is capable of affecting the child year-round, such as house dust mites or pet hair. Although the child's symptoms may not result in the obvious distress associated with seasonal allergic rhinitis, the child needs treatment just as much because the symptoms occur constantly. Because the agent that causes perennial allergic rhinitis is often house dust, environmental control plays a big role in the control of the disorder. Serous otitis media may be a long-term consequence of perennial allergic rhinitis (see Chapter 50).

Atopic Dermatitis (Infantile Eczema)

Atopic dermatitis is primarily a disease of infants, beginning as early as the second month of life and possibly lasting until the child is 2 to 3 years old. It may be related to food allergy because it tends to occur more often in formula-fed infants than in breastfed infants and is more common if infants are fed solid food before 6 months. Sweating, heat, tight clothing, and contact irritants such as soap increase the pruritus. Symptoms may be more annoying in the winter, when additional irritating clothing is present, with marked improvement in the summer.

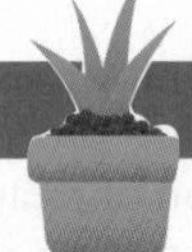

BOX 42.11 ✻ Focus on Nursing Care Planning

A Multidisciplinary Care Map for a Child With Allergic Rhinitis

Dexter Goodenough is a 6-year-old boy you meet in an ambulatory setting. Dexter is diagnosed as having allergic rhinitis (hay fever). "Thank heavens," his mother exclaims. "I thought when I heard he had an immune system disease he had AIDS. What a relief to know it's only an allergy."

Family Assessment ✻ Child lives with his mother and his stepfather in a beach-front cottage. Also in the family is a brother, 8 years; a stepbrother, 16 years; and a paternal grandmother. His stepfather owns a jewelry store. His mother is a stay-at-home mom. Finances are rated as "not a problem."

Client Assessment ✻ Child's eyes are reddened and watery; his nose drains a clear discharge. His mother tells you he frequently has a headache and is constantly listless, and other children make fun of him because of his appearance. His grades are "terrible" because the minute he gets to school, his symptoms begin. Dexter is prescribed an antihistamine and environmental control.

Nursing Diagnosis ✻ Situational low self-esteem related to feelings of inadequacy and embarrassment

Outcome Criteria ✻ Client states he is able to function in school in spite of allergy symptoms and discomfort; is taking active measures to avoid allergens.

Team Member Responsible	Assessment	Intervention	Rationale	Expected Outcome
		Activities of Daily Living		
Nurse	Assess what Dexter's classroom is like to identify potential allergens, as child's symptoms are most intense when he is at school.	Discuss potential source of allergens with mother; ask her to meet with teacher to see if modifications could be made.	Environmental control can reduce the number of allergens causing symptoms.	Child describes classroom. Mother visits classroom as necessary to suggest changes.
		Consultations		
Physician	Assess if child's symptoms could be reduced with hyposensitization.	Consult with allergist about possibility of hyposensitization.	Hyposensitization can greatly reduce allergy symptoms if specific allergens can be identified.	Parent and child agree to hyposensitization if prescribed.
		Procedures/Medications		
Nurse	Assess if child has had experience with taking medicine before.	Help mother set up a medicine chart that will help with antihistamine adherence.	Allergy medicine is most effective when it is taken conscientiously.	Parent states she will be conscientious about antihistamine administration.
		Nutrition		
Nurse	Assess if there are any foods child or mother feel contribute to allergy symptoms.	If foods are identified, review with mother list of foods to avoid.	Respiratory allergens are more likely involved in allergic rhinitis, but foods should be ruled out.	Mother and child describe any foods that cause discomfort for child and measures to avoid them.

Patient/Family Education				
Nurse	Assess environmental aspects at home that could be causing child's symptoms.	Discuss environmental control with parents.	Reducing allergens in the home can also aid in reducing child's symptoms.	Parents agree to any modifications necessary in their home.
Nurse	Assess if the child is exposed to secondary smoke in home.	Educate family on the damage that secondary smoke can cause.	Secondary smoke is a potent allergen and also may contribute to lung and heart disease.	Parents agree to make home smoke-free.
Psychosocial/Spiritual/Emotional Needs				
Nurse	Assess the extent of ridicule child undergoes at school.	Discuss coping measures with child. Urge mother to report bullying to school authorities.	Psychological health is as important as physical health.	Child describes experiences at school. States he is no longer bullied.
Discharge Planning				
Nurse	Assess if parent has other questions about child's allergies.	Schedule a follow-up visit for reevaluation of new medication.	Allergy control can involve a range of medicine, so it can be confusing for children or parents.	Mother states she understands the importance of follow-up visit and will keep appointment.

Assessment

With infantile atopic dermatitis, capillary permeability increases, causing a loss of serous fluid out into the tissues. Children develop papular and vesicular skin eruptions with surrounding erythema. The vesicles rupture and exude yellow, sticky secretions that form crusts on the skin as they dry. Because the lesions are extremely pruritic, the child scratches and further irritates the lesions, causing linear excoriations. Secondary infections of open lesions may then occur. As the infected lesions heal, the skin becomes depigmented and lichenified (shiny), and dry, flaky scales form. If secondary infection occurs, local lymph nodes will be swollen. The child may have a low-grade fever. An increased eosinophil count reveals that the condition is allergy-based.

The common sites for lesions include the scalp and forehead, the cheeks, neck, behind the ears, and the extensor surfaces of the extremities (Fig. 42.6). The palms of the hands and the soles of the feet are uninvolved. Because the lesions are uncomfortable, children with infantile atopic dermatitis may be overly fussy and irritable. They may not eat well because of this generalized discomfort.

Although infantile atopic dermatitis is generally diagnosed while taking the family history (considering other allergic individuals in the family) and noticing the characteristic lesions and their patterns, it is sometimes difficult to distinguish from seborrheic dermatitis (cradle cap; see Chapter 29). The findings in seborrheic dermatitis and infantile atopic dermatitis are compared in Table 42.5. Seborrheic dermatitis is a benign condition of infants, requiring little treatment other than frequent shampooing of the hair and soaking the lesions in mineral oil and combing them away (Smoker, 2007). A child with infantile atopic dermatitis, on the other hand, will not respond to these measures but must be referred for additional treatment. Also, children with infantile atopic dermatitis should have a repeat test for phenylketonuria (PKU) done because children with PKU often have atopic dermatitis (Itin & Goldsmith, 2008).

Skin testing is ineffective because the allergen causing infantile atopic dermatitis is often a food allergen. However, it may also be caused by pollens, dust, or mold spores. For this reason, skin testing may be attempted to isolate a causative allergen.

Therapeutic Management

The treatment of atopic dermatitis is aimed at reducing the amount of allergen exposure, if such allergens can be identified. The most likely foods to which infants are allergic are

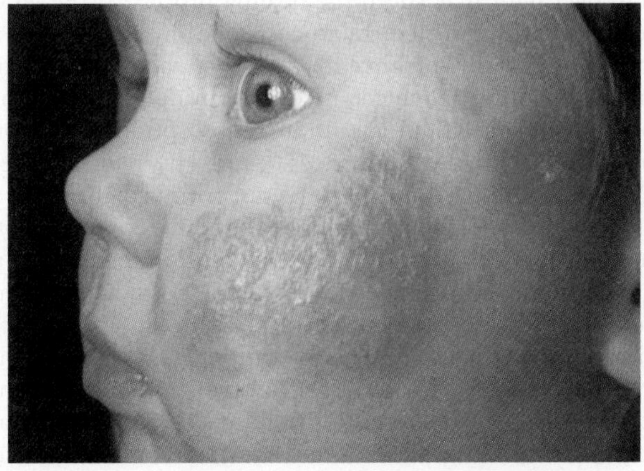

FIGURE 42.6 Infant with atopic dermatitis. (From Sauer, G. C., & Hall, J. C. [1996]. *Manual of skin diseases* [7th ed.]. Philadelphia: Lippincott-Raven Publishers.)

TABLE 42.5 ✻ Comparison of Seborrheic Dermatitis and Atopic Dermatitis

Finding	Seborrheic Dermatitis	Atopic Dermatitis
Age at onset	0–6 months	2–6 months
Length of disease	Rarely 1 year	2–3 years
Mood of child	Happy; parents happy	Irritable; parents tired
Location of lesions	Scalp, behind ears, near umbilicus	Cheeks, extensor surfaces, some flexor surfaces
Types of lesions	Salmon-colored erythematous lesions with greasy scales	Papulovesicular erythematous lesions with weeping and crusting
Itching	No	Severe
Depigmentation	No	Yes
Lichenification	No	Yes
White dermographism	No	Yes
Eosinophilia	No nasal mucus or blood eosinophilia	Nasal mucus or blood eosinophilia
IgE serum levels	Low	High

milk, eggs, wheat, chocolate, fish, tomatoes, and peanuts. The use of elimination diets to identify food allergens is discussed later in this chapter. A second major consideration in treatment is aimed at reducing pruritus so children do not irritate lesions and cause secondary infections by scratching. Hydrating the skin by bathing or applying wet dressings (wet with tap water or Burow's solution) for 15 to 20 minutes, followed by application of a hydrating emollient such as petroleum jelly (Vaseline) or even vegetable shortening (Crisco), is helpful. Do not allow infants to become chilled if a large portion of the body is to be covered with wet dressings. A stockinette dressing with holes cut out for the eyes, nose, and mouth pulled over the head will hold wet dressings in place on the face and neck. To prevent corneal irritation, be careful that such dressings do not come in contact with the eyes.

Some infants need an antihistamine to reduce itching. Topical steroids such as 1% hydrocortisone cream do a great deal to relieve the discomfort and appearance of lesions by reducing the inflammation and pruritus. If the lesions are dry, a corticosteroid ointment is most effective; if moist, a lotion may be most effective. Applying the cream or lotion and then covering the area with an occlusive dressing such as plastic wrap overnight may speed the healing process. If the lesions are secondarily infected, hydrocortisone mixed with an antibiotic (generally neomycin) and a suitable base is prescribed. Caution parents not to discontinue application of cortisone cream abruptly. Although absorption with topical application is limited, some does occur. This reduces adrenal gland functioning. If the cream is discontinued abruptly, the infant's adrenal response (ability to produce epinephrine) in an emergency might be limited. Also caution the parents not to overuse the cortisone cream. More is not better and may increase the risk of systemic absorption. Because of the complications that steroid creams can create, the new immunomodulators tacrolimus (Protopic) and pimecrolimus (Elidel) may be prescribed for children over 2 years of age. Because these drugs have been associated with the development of skin cancer, they are FDA approved but with a "Black Box" warning that they should be prescribed at the lowest possible dose (Patel, Greer, & Skinner, 2007).

Nursing Diagnoses and Related Interventions

✻

Nursing Diagnosis: Risk for impaired parenting related to feelings of inadequacy secondary to infant's chronic atopic dermatitis

Outcome Evaluation: Parents express confidence in their ability to follow recommended therapy; express positive aspects of infant; hold infant close and smile and talk to infant.

Parents of children with infantile atopic dermatitis need a great deal of support through the course of the disease because infants can be irritable from the constant pruritus. No matter how hard parents try, they cannot seem to make their child happy. Parents need a listening ear so they can vent these concerns and maintain their self-esteem as parents. Support groups also can help meet this need.

Nursing Diagnosis: Impaired skin integrity related to infantile atopic dermatitis

Outcome Evaluation: Infant does not scratch lesions; parents state infant is less irritable and easier to care for. Lesions show signs of healing.

When lesions begin to heal, a skin emollient and moisturizer, such as Eucerin, or baths with a substance to lubricate the skin, such as Alpha-Keri, are prescribed to prevent excessive skin dryness. The infant should soak in the bath with the lubricant for approximately 15 minutes, then be patted, not rubbed, dry so the lesions are not aggravated. Caution parents not to use soap, because it can be drying.

Suggest that parents trim their infant's fingernails short or cover hands with cotton socks to prevent scratching. Exposure to the herpes virus can cause a generalized reaction. Caution parents to screen babysitters or alert child care personnel with active herpes lesions not to care for their infants while atopic dermatitis is active.

In most infants, the lesions of infantile atopic dermatitis clear by the time a child is 3 years old. Unless secondary infection with scarring results, the skin surface will not be marked. Many of these children go on to develop other allergies, however, as they grow older. In the preschool years, the child's parents may report that the child has "one cold after another" (allergic rhinitis). By early school years, the child may show signs of asthma.

Atopic Dermatitis in the Older Child

Atopic dermatitis in the older child may occur at any age, but frequently it occurs at puberty or late adolescence (Horii et al., 2007). Atopic dermatitis that occurs at these later ages is prominent on the flexor surface of the extremities and on the dorsal surfaces of the wrists and ankles. It often occurs in the eyebrows; if the child scratches the lesions, the child may be left with scant eyebrows. Depigmentation or hyperpigmentation is usually present, and lichenification is marked. The fingernails often have a glossy sheen from the buffing action of constant rubbing and scratching. In some children, an itch–scratch cycle in response to stress may lead to an exacerbation of symptoms. For example, children begin to feel pressured in school or upset because they are left out of the neighborhood group of children. Children rub their skin, a nervous, comforting mannerism, and the rubbing or scratching leads to irritation of lesions. Then the lesions itch, and the child scratches vigorously because of discomfort. The more a child scratches, the worse the lesions become; the more lesions there are, the more the child scratches, and so on.

Therapeutic Management

Atopic dermatitis is a difficult disease for older children. Because they can see that the scratching leads to depigmentation or lichenification, they know they should stop scratching to keep the disorder under control. The itching is so intense, however, that they wake at night scratching and cannot stop. Adolescents are acutely aware of their appearance, so this is an especially difficult illness for them. Suggest they not use soap or use only a prescription soap to prevent skin drying. They should avoid swimming in chlorinated pools. Encourage other summer sports if possible. If children are required to swim in school, encourage them to shower well afterward to remove chlorine from the skin and apply a skin emollient and moisturizer such as Eucerin after swimming. After a period of activity in which sweating occurs, suggest that the child take a shower to remove perspiration, which is irritating to skin. Avoiding tight clothing at the flexor portions of the extremities may also help. Caution children not to use medication intended for acne cover-up on atopic dermatitis lesions because these medications are designed to dry the skin and will increase itching.

Medical treatment is basically the same as for the infant with atopic dermatitis: keeping the skin hydrated and identifying allergens and any psychological problems that are initiating an itch–scratch cycle. Application of hydrocortisone cream can make a big difference in helping lesions improve. Phototherapy with ultraviolet light may be prescribed.

Evaluation for the older child with atopic dermatitis should include evaluating how well the lesions are healing and also how well the child is adjusting to school and family. A child who enters adulthood with poor self-esteem because of a chronic allergic disorder during childhood could have difficulty achieving a high level of adult wellness.

What if... Dexter's atopic dermatitis is worse every December and every June at the end of school semesters? What might you suspect as the cause of an itch–scratch cycle at this time?

DRUG AND FOOD ALLERGIES

Drug Allergies

One of the hazards of giving any medication is the risk that a child may experience a reaction to it or exhibit allergic symptoms. Because reactions to drugs differ, it is important to be familiar with the symptoms of an allergic reaction, a toxic reaction, or a known side effect to a drug.

A *toxic reaction* is one that occurs when a child has received too much of a drug. *Side effects* of drugs are those that are known to occur in addition to a therapeutic effect. When an *allergic effect* occurs, unpredictable symptoms occur. The drug itself may not be an allergen, but when the drug combines with body protein, it becomes an allergen. This is why allergic responses occur not with the initial administration of a drug but only after the protein interaction (hapten formation or sensitivity) has occurred. When drugs are applied to skin or mucous membrane, the chance of a drug allergy is highest. With the exception of acetylsalicylic acid (aspirin), allergy occurs rarely to orally administered drugs. Children with atopic diseases appear to be most prone to allergic drug reactions, although anyone can have such a reaction.

Reactions to drugs differ, but skin manifestations seen frequently include urticaria, angioedema, allergic contact dermatitis, pruritus, and purpura. Respiratory symptoms include wheezing or rhinitis. Thrombocytopenia and hemolytic anemia may develop. Anaphylactic shock and serum sickness may occur. Children with a known drug allergy should wear a medical identification bracelet stating the drug to which they are sensitive.

Drugs that are frequently involved in allergic reactions are parenteral penicillin and vaccines. In most instances, discontinuing the drug or never again administering the vaccine is the only therapy needed. If urticaria or serum sickness occurs, an antihistamine (such as diphenhydramine hydrochloride [Benadryl]) is needed to relieve the symptoms. If anaphylaxis results, the treatment would be the same as for any anaphylaxis.

Food Allergies

Food allergies manifest themselves differently from one child to another, but urticaria, angioedema, pruritus, stomach pain, colic, cramps, diarrhea, respiratory symptoms, and atopic dermatitis are common symptoms (Roberts, 2007).

A symptom such as urticaria begins to manifest itself only minutes after an offending food is eaten. Other symptoms may be delayed, making the offending food difficult to recognize. Whole protein is probably the cause of immediate reactions; delayed reactions are probably the result of sensitivity to some protein breakdown product.

Skin testing is unreliable with food allergies because it is done with whole protein extracts. Delayed reactions, therefore, will not be detected this way. The most common foods that cause immediate allergy symptoms include egg white, fish and other seafood, berries, and nuts. Delayed food reactions are commonly caused by cereals (wheat and corn), milk, chocolate, pork, legumes, white potatoes, beef, food additives and colorings, and oranges. If children are allergic to milk, caution them that they are probably allergic to milk products as well. Children who are allergic to eggs often cannot eat any foods that contain egg, such as pudding or baked goods. As some vaccines have an egg ingredient, children with an egg hypersensitivity should not routinely receive these vaccines (Allen, Campbell, & Kemp, 2007).

Assessment

Young children cannot describe why they do not enjoy eating because they do not know the word for "headache," "stomachache," or "itchiness," but they tend to avoid foods that affect them. This gives them a reputation of being "fussy eaters." This is not diagnostic of food allergies, however, because children may refuse to eat foods as a form of toddler rebellion or may be reported as fussy eaters because parents are expecting them to eat more than their small size requires.

Encouraging a child or parents to keep a food diary or a record of everything a child eats each day often is the best way to spot offending foods. They should note the presence of symptoms, if any. A food that is found on lists when symptoms were few, but not on days when the child is in distress, is not an offending food. A food that appears only on "bad days," however, can be strongly suspected as an allergen.

An elimination diet is another method that can be used to detect food allergens. For this, parents feed the child only foods that rarely cause allergy, such as rice, lamb, carrots, peas, and sweet potatoes, for about 7 days. Then they add, one by one, at 2- to 3-day intervals, foods that are suspected of causing allergy. When a food is introduced this way, the child must be encouraged to eat a lot of it that day. If symptoms occur, the food is then eliminated from the child's meals on a permanent basis. If no symptoms occur, the child can continue to eat the food.

Therapeutic Management

The treatment of food allergy is to permanently eliminate offending foods from the child's diet. This is relatively easy to do if there are only a few offending foods, but it becomes difficult when the foods are great in number or, like milk, wheat, or eggs, are found in many products. Parents must become careful shoppers, reading labels carefully to be certain the foods they are buying do not contain products to which their child is sensitive. Help school-age children learn to choose foods they can safely eat at the school cafeteria or at summer camp.

Milk Hypersensitivity

The true incidence of milk hypersensitivity is probably not as high as the number of diagnoses made. Allergy to milk is typified by failure to gain weight, diarrhea, perhaps vomiting, and abdominal pain. Because these symptoms may also occur in a gastroenteritis infection, an infant may be misdiagnosed with an infection. Some infants with colic (characterized by abdominal pain, no change in stools, and no failure to gain weight) or those with lactase deficiency (they cannot ingest the lactose in milk) may also be incorrectly diagnosed as having a milk allergy. If milk allergy is suspected, children are given a casein hydrolysate or soybean formula (Sondheimer, 2008). When this is done, symptoms are usually dramatically relieved.

Caution parents to read food labels carefully to be certain that frozen foods or hot dogs do not contain milk as milk can be used as a filler in these products. As milk is a major source of vitamin D and calcium, children who have to avoid all milk may need a vitamin and calcium supplement. To establish whether the problem is truly a milk allergy, milk should be reintroduced at a later date. If the problem is a true milk allergy, signs will recur.

Peanut Hypersensitivity

A growing number of children are identified yearly as being so allergic to peanuts that even smelling peanut butter in a cafeteria or another child's lunch can provoke acute wheezing or anaphylaxis (Banerjee et al., 2007). School nurses need to be very aware of this danger and may need to advocate for "peanut-free" lunch rooms. Desensitization to peanuts can minimize children's responses.

STINGING INSECT HYPERSENSITIVITY

Children may have severe hypersensitivity reactions to stings from bees, wasps, hornets, or yellow jackets. Although a serum sickness reaction may occur, the usual reaction to these stings is an immediate type I hypersensitivity reaction (anaphylaxis). They can receive so many stings from "killer bees" the reaction is fatal. The peak season for insect stings is summer, and more boys than girls have allergic reactions to insect stings (Bledsoe, 2007).

Assessment

The first time a child is stung, the total reaction is probably only local edema at the site. The second time, generalized urticaria, pruritus, and edema may develop. The third time, symptoms may progress to wheezing and dyspnea. The next time, the reaction could be so severe that shock and death result. The progression of symptoms may be slower than this (involving 10 to 12 stings) if the stings occur far apart; if the stings are received close together (1 or 2 days apart, or even 3 weeks apart), the progression to fatal symptoms may occur as early as the second or third exposure.

The time interval between the fatal sting and death is extremely short, approximately 10 minutes. For this reason, these children must be identified and given medication to combat shock immediately (there is no time to transport them for emergency care).

Therapeutic Management

The best way to protect children with allergies to stinging insects is to begin hyposensitization against insect stings after the first reaction. An extract of wasp, yellow jacket, hornet, and honeybee venom accomplishes this.

The child who has not been hyposensitized must be treated immediately after the sting. This can be done by subcutaneous injection of epinephrine, which will give rapid relief (EpiPens are available for self-injection; see Box 42.10). If children are going on a hiking or camping expedition away from parents, caution parents that children need to learn to administer this to themselves, or be certain that a responsible adult accompanying them will be able to do it. Someone at school should be given the responsibility of administering this if a child is stung during recess or an outside gym period. If a school nurse is in attendance, this certainly is the nurse's responsibility. In schools where there is no full-time nurse, another person must be designated and taught how to give the injection. If the child has antihistamine medication in addition to epinephrine, this should be taken also. Ice applied to the site minimizes the amount of venom absorbed. The child should then be transported to the nearest hospital in case additional epinephrine is needed (the initial injection will be effective for only approximately 20 minutes).

Teach children who are allergic to stinging insects not to use scented preparations such as hair spray, deodorants, lotions, or perfume because these attract bees and wasps. They should not go outside barefoot because bees are often found in ground clover. They should not be assigned household chores such as mowing the lawn or weeding the garden, actions that might stir up bees. Because insects tend to cluster around garbage containers, taking out the trash is also an inappropriate chore for these children. Caution a child to have a fast-acting insecticide handy when out of doors to use on flying insects. Encourage a child to refrain from drinking from open soda cans at picnics and outside activities; bees and wasps are drawn to the sugar in the soda, and the child may be unaware that an insect has entered the open can.

✔ Checkpoint Question 42.3

Dexter is atopic or prone to allergies. In the hospital he has no toys. What would be a poor choice of a toy to make for him?

a. A paper deck of cards.
b. A cloth beanbag.
c. A latex glove balloon.
d. A tongue-blade puppet.

CONTACT DERMATITIS

Contact dermatitis is an example of a delayed or type IV hypersensitivity response; it is a reaction to skin contact with an allergen (a substance irritating to the child only with prior sensitization). The first reaction is generally erythema, followed by intensely pruritic papules and then vesicles. The allergen causing the irritation is often suggested by the part of the child's body that is affected. For example, dermatitis from a diaper-washing compound appears in the diaper area. Allergy to cosmetics appears on the face. Oozing at the site of pierced ears suggests an allergy to the nickel used in earring posts. Poison ivy appears on the hands and arms where the child brushed against the plant (Fig. 42.7). Many children, especially those who have had many surgical procedures such as children with spina bifida as well as health care providers, are developing reactions to latex gloves (Cremer et al., 2007). Footwear, because of the chemicals used to tan leather, is also a frequent offender.

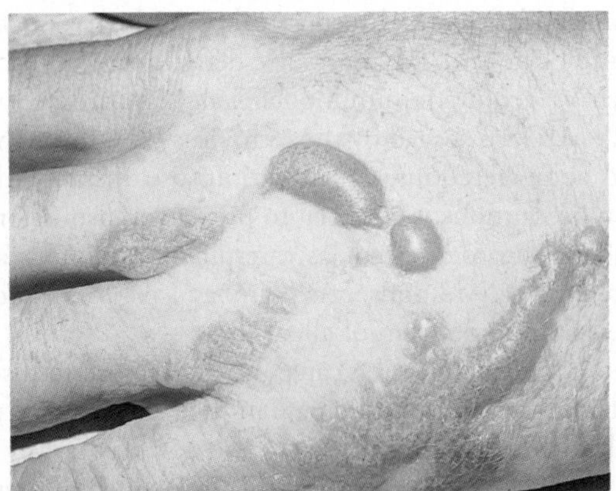

FIGURE 42.7 Poison ivy on a child's hand. (© Beckman/Custom Medical Stock Photograph.)

Assessment

Patch testing may be used to identify contact dermatitis allergens. A child should not be taking a corticosteroid at the time of patch testing because these drugs reduce delayed hypersensitivity reactions. However, a child may continue to take antihistamines or sympathomimetic drugs because these do not interfere with delayed reactions. After 48 hours, the patches used for testing are removed and the reactions are graded 1+ to 4+, the same as in regular skin testing.

Therapeutic Management

Treatment for contact dermatitis consists of removing the identified allergen from the child's environment. In children, this is generally not difficult to do. In adults, because allergens may be job-related, this is much more difficult.

Dressings moistened with water, saline, or Burow's solution relieve itching. Calamine or Caladryl lotion are also generally effective. Hydrocortisone lotions or creams reduce itching and also promote healing. Baths with baking soda or oatmeal in the water may be helpful if a large area of the body is involved. Some children need a sedative to relieve their discomfort during the period of intense pruritus.

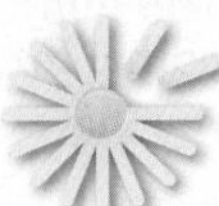

What if... Dexter, who is allergic to leather, develops an erythematous, pruritic area on his right buttock? What would be a likely object causing the irritation?

Key Points for Review

- An antigen is a foreign substance capable of stimulating an immune response. The immune system protects the body from invasion by foreign substances.
- Humoral immunity refers to immunity created by antibody production. B lymphocytes are involved in this type of reaction. Cell-mediated immunity refers to T-lymphocyte involvement.
- Autoimmunity results from an inability to distinguish self from nonself, causing the immune system to carry out immune responses against normal cells.

- Immunodeficiency disorders can be primary, such as B-lymphocyte and T-lymphocyte deficiencies, or secondary, such as acquired immunodeficiency syndrome (AIDS). HIV/AIDS is spread by the retrovirus HIV through blood and body secretions. Conscientious use of standard infection precautions is essential to prevent transmission.
- Allergic disorders occur as a result of an abnormal antigen–antibody response. As many as 15% to 30% of children have some form of allergy.
- Immune disorders, as a category, are long-term disorders, and children must participate in their own care to remain well such as avoiding allergens and conscientiously taking an antihistamine to remain well. Involving children from the start helps them play an active role in their own care.
- Anaphylactic shock is an acute type I hypersensitivity reaction characterized by extreme vasodilation and bronchoconstriction. If action is not taken immediately, the reaction can be fatal. Subcutaneous epinephrine is the drug of choice to reduce symptoms.
- Atopic disorders include allergic rhinitis (hay fever), atopic dermatitis, and asthma.
- Environmental control refers to ways to reduce the number of allergens to which children are exposed. Hyposensitization is a method to increase the plasma concentration of IgG antibodies to prevent or block IgE antibody formation and allergic symptoms.
- Promoting breastfeeding may be a prime intervention to help prevent food allergies in allergy-prone families.

CRITICAL THINKING EXERCISES

1. Dexter, the 6-year-old boy you met at the beginning of the chapter, was diagnosed as having allergic rhinitis. His symptoms begin when he arrives at school. Knowing this problem is worse at school, what environmental control measures would you suggest for Dexter?
2. When Dexter had atopic dermatitis (infantile eczema) as an infant, almost his entire face was covered with weeping, crusting lesions. His forehead was lined with scratch marks. His mother was exhausted because Dexter never slept because of the constant itching. What suggestions could you have made to his mother to make him more comfortable? What would you have suggested she do for herself?
3. Dexter's mother was concerned he might have AIDS. What would you want to explain to Dexter's mother about how the HIV virus is spread?
4. Examine the National Health Goals related to immune disorders and children. Most government-sponsored funds for nursing research are allotted based on these goals. What would be a possible research topic to explore pertinent to these goals that would be applicable to Dexter's family and also advance evidence-based practice?

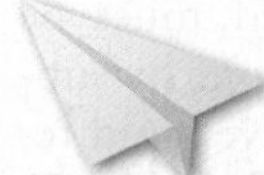

CRITICAL THINKING SCENARIO

Open the accompanying CD-ROM or visit http://thePoint.lww.com and read the Patient Scenario included for this chapter, then answer the questions to further sharpen your skills and grow more familiar with NCLEX style questions related to immune system disorders in children. Confirm your answers are correct by reading the rationales.

REFERENCES

Aamodt, A. H., et al. (2007). Is headache related to asthma, hay fever, and chronic bronchitis? *Headache, 47*(2), 204–212.

Allen, C. W., Campbell, D. E., & Kemp, A. S. (2007). Egg allergy: are all childhood food allergies the same? *Journal of Paediatrics and Child Health, 43*(4), 214–218.

Al Sayyad, J. J., et al. (2009). Topical nasal steroids for intermittent and persistent allergic rhinitis in children. *Cochrane Database of Systematic Reviews, 2009*(1), (CD003163).

Banerjee, D. K., et al. (2007). Peanut-free guidelines reduce school lunch peanut contents. *Archives of Disease in Childhood, 92*(11), 980–982.

Bledsoe, B. E. (2007). Attacking insects. Unwelcome visitors: is EMS ready for fire ants and killer bees. *Emergency Medical Services, 36*(8), 68–72.

Boguniewicz, M. (2008). Allergic disorders. In W. W. Hay, et al. (Eds.). *Current pediatric diagnosis and treatment* (18th ed.). Columbus, OH: McGraw-Hill.

Casado, C., et al. (2007). Coinfection and superinfection in patients with long-term, nonprogressive HIV-1 disease. *Journal of Infectious Diseases, 196*(6), 895–899.

Centers for Disease Control and Prevention (2008a). *HIV/AIDS recommendations.* Washington, DC: Author.

Centers for Disease Control and Prevention. (2008b). *Recommended immunization schedule for ages 0-6 years.* Washington, DC: Author.

Chadwick, E. G., et al. (2008). Pharmacokinetics, safety and efficacy of lopinavir/ritonavir in infants less than 6 months of age: 24 week results. *AIDS, 22*(2), 249–255.

Chasela, C., et al. (2008). Risk factors for late postnatal transmission of human immunodeficiency virus type 1 in sub-Saharan Africa. *Pediatric Infectious Disease Journal, 27*(3), 251–256.

Chawla, S., & Riederer, M. (2007). Angioedema. *Clinical Pediatrics, 46*(8), 748–751.

Cremer, R., et al. (2007). Natural rubber latex sensitisation and allergy in patients with spina bifida, urogenital disorders and oesophageal atresia compared with a normal paediatric population. *European Journal of Pediatric Surgery, 17*(3), 194–198.

Engels, E. A., et al. (2008). Cancer risk in people infected with human immunodeficiency virus in the United States. *International Journal of Cancer, 123*(1), 187–194.

Estrella, L., Foley, M. E., & Cunningham-Rundles, C. (2007). X-linked agammaglobulinemia in a 10-year-old child: a case study. *Journal of the American Academy of Nurse Practitioners, 19*(4), 205–211.

Filipiak, B., et al. (2007). Solid food introduction in relation to eczema: results from a four-year prospective birth cohort study. *Journal of Pediatrics, 151*(4), 352–358.

Gennaro, S., Naidoo, S., & Berthold, P. (2008). Oral health & HIV/AIDS. *MCN, American Journal of Maternal Child Nursing, 33*(1), 50–57.

Goodwin, R. D. (2007). Environmental tobacco smoke and the epidemic of asthma in children: the role of cigarette use. *Annals of Allergy, Asthma, & Immunology, 98*(5), 447–454.

Horii, K. A., et al. (2007). Atopic dermatitis in children in the United States, 1997-2004: visit trends, patient and provider characteristics, and prescribing patterns. *Pediatrics, 120*(3), e527–e534.

Itin, P. H., & Goldsmith, L. A. (2008). Cutaneous changes in errors of amino acid metabolism. In K. Wolff, et al. (Eds.). *Fitzpatrick's dermatology in general medicine* (7th ed.). Columbus, OH: McGraw-Hill.

Karch, A. M. (2009). *Lippincott's nursing drug guide.* Philadelphia: Lippincott Williams & Wilkins.

Kishiyama, J. L., & Adelman, D. C. (2009). Basic immunology. In S. J. McPhee & M. A. Papadakis (Eds.). *Current medical diagnosis and treatment.* Columbus, OH: McGraw-Hill.

Lane, R. D., & Bolte, R. G. (2007). Pediatric anaphylaxis. *Pediatric Emergency Care, 23*(1), 49–60.

Liu, A. H., Stewart, L. J., & Johnston, R. (2008). Immunodeficiency. In W. W. Hay, et al. (Eds.). *Current pediatric diagnosis and treatment* (18th ed.). Columbus, OH: McGraw-Hill.

McFarland, E. J. (2008). Human immunodeficiency virus infection. In W. W. Hay, et al. (Eds.). *Current pediatric diagnosis and treatment* (18th ed.). Columbus, OH: McGraw-Hill.

Mehr, S., Robinson, M., & Tang, M. (2007). Doctor—How do I use my EpiPen? *Pediatric Allergy & Immunology, 18*(5), 448–452.

Morgenstern, V., et al. (2008). Atopic diseases, allergic sensitization, and exposure to traffic-related air pollution in children. *American Journal of Respiratory and Critical Care Medicine, 177*(12), 1331–1337.

Patel, T. S., Greer, S. C., & Skinner, R. B. (2007). Cancer concerns with topical immunomodulators in atopic dermatitis: overview of data and recommendations to clinicians. *American Journal of Clinical Dermatology, 8*(4), 189–194.

Pongracic, J. A., & Kim, J. S. (2007). Update on epinephrine for the treatment of anaphylaxis. *Current Opinion in Pediatrics, 19*(1), 94–98.

Rapp, S. M. (2008). Hospitals adopt latex-safe practices for patient, health care worker safety. *Orthopedics Today, 28*(5), 83.

Roberts, G. (2007). Anaphylaxis to foods. *Pediatric Allergy and Immunology, 18*(6), 543–548.

Schafer, J. A., et al. (2007). Penicillin allergy skin testing: what do we do now? *Pharmacotherapy, 27*(4), 542–545.

Segal, A. R., et al. (2007). Cutaneous reactions to drugs in children. *Pediatrics, 120*(4), e1082–e1096.

Smoker, A. L. (2007). On top of cradle cap. *Journal of Family Health Care, 17*(4), 134–136.

Sondheimer, J. M. (2008). Gastrointestinal tract. In W. W. Hay, et al. (Eds.). *Current pediatric diagnosis and treatment* (18th ed.). Columbus, OH: McGraw-Hill.

Suksomboon, N., Poolsup, N., & Ket-Aim, S. (2007). Systematic review of the efficacy of antiretroviral therapies for reducing the risk of mother-to-child transmission of HIV infection. *Journal of Clinical Pharmacy & Therapeutics, 32*(3), 293–311.

Van Aken, K., et al. (2007). Motor development in school-aged children with 22q11 deletion (velocardiofacial/DiGeorge syndrome). *Developmental Medicine and Child Neurology, 49*(3), 210–213.

Waruiru, C., et al. (2007). Outcome of hematopoietic stem cell transplantation in severe combined immune deficiency with central nervous system viral infection. *Pediatric Infectious Disease Journal, 26*(2), 129–133.

Wells, C. D., et al. (2007). HIV infection and multidrug-resistant tuberculosis: the perfect storm. *Journal of Infectious Diseases, 196*(Suppl 1), S86–S107.

Zanchetta, M., et al. (2008). Early therapy in HIV-1-infected children: Effect on HIV-1 dynamics and HIV-1-specific immune response. *Antiviral Therapy, 13*(1), 47–55.

SUGGESTED READINGS

Butz, A. M., et al. (2007). Shared decision making in school age children with asthma. *Pediatric Nursing, 33*(2), 111–118.

Chen, C. M., et al. (2007). Longitudinal study on cat allergen exposure and the development of allergy in young children. *Journal of Allergy and Clinical Immunology, 119*(5), 1148–1155.

Dowdee, A., & Ossege, J. (2007). Assessment of childhood allergy for the primary care practitioner. *Journal of the American Academy of Nurse Practitioners, 19*(2), 53–62.

Ersser, S. J., et al. (2009). Psychological and educational interventions for atopic eczema in children. *Cochrane Database of Systematic Reviews, 2009*(1), (CD004054).

Fortunato, J. E., & Scheimann, A. O. (2008). Protein-energy malnutrition and feeding refusal secondary to food allergies. *Clinical Pediatrics, 47*(5), 496–499.

Gillespie, C. A., et al. (2007). "Living with risk": mothering a child with food-induced anaphylaxis. *Journal of Pediatric Nursing: Nursing Care of Children and Families, 22*(1), 30–42.

Hayden, M. L., & Womack, C. R. (2007). Caring for patients with allergic rhinitis. *Journal of the American Academy of Nurse Practitioners, 19*(6), 290–298.

Krouse, H. J. (2007). Diagnostic testing for inhalant allergies. *Society of Otorhinolaryngology Nurses: Head and Neck Nursing, 25*(2), 9–14.

Palmer, C. M., & Lyon, V. B. (2008). Stepwise approach to topical therapy for atopic dermatitis. *Clinical Pediatrics, 47*(5), 423–434.

Usmani, N., & Wilkinson, S. M. (2007). Allergic skin disease: investigation of both immediate- and delayed-type hypersensitivity is essential. *Clinical and Experimental Allergy, 37*(10), 1541–1546.

Chapter 43

Nursing Care of a Family When a Child Has an Infectious Disorder

KEY TERMS

- catarrhal stage
- chain of infection
- convalescent period
- enanthem
- exanthem
- exotoxin
- fomites
- incubation period
- interferon
- Koplik's spots
- means of transmission
- portal of entry
- portal of exit
- prodromal period
- reservoir
- septicemia
- susceptible host

OBJECTIVES

After mastering the contents of this chapter, you should be able to:

1. Describe the causes and course of common infectious disorders of childhood.
2. Identify National Health Goals related to infectious disorders in children that nurses could help the nation achieve.
3. Use critical thinking to analyze ways that care of a child with an infectious disorder could be more family centered.
4. Assess a child with an infectious disorder.
5. Formulate nursing diagnoses for a child with an infectious disorder.
6. Establish outcomes for the care of a child with an infectious disorder.
7. Plan nursing care for a child with an infectious disorder.
8. Implement nursing care specific to the child with an infectious disorder, such as helping alleviate the pruritus of a rash.
9. Evaluate expected outcomes for achievement and effectiveness of care.
10. Identify areas of nursing care related to children with infectious diseases that could benefit from additional nursing research or application of evidence-based practice.
11. Integrate knowledge of infectious diseases and nursing process to achieve quality maternal and child health nursing care.

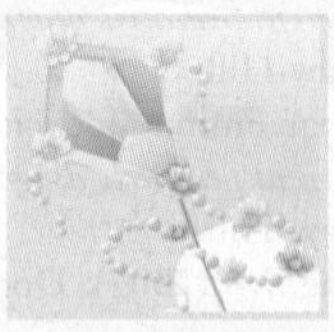

Marty Ireland, a 10-year-old boy, was admitted to the hospital for appendicitis. The morning after surgery, his throat was painful and his arms were covered by a very itchy, red, macular rash. Marty was diagnosed as having scarlet fever. "How could this have happened?" his mother asks you. "He's not a bad kid. How could two bad things happen to him at once?"

Previous chapters described the growth and development of well children. This chapter adds information about the dramatic changes, both physical and psychosocial, that can occur when children contract an infectious disorder. This is important information to protect child health because many of these disorders spread easily to other children.

What advice would you give Marty's mother? Is it likely that Marty contracted this new disease while he was in the hospital, or before he was admitted? What is a measure you would recommend to help reduce the itching?

Despite the number of preventive measures available, infectious diseases remain a leading cause of morbidity in children. Nurses play a key role in educating parents and the public about common childhood infectious disorders and appropriate preventive steps. They must be able to identify the symptoms of common infectious diseases of childhood, because nurses are often the first to see evidence of infection. For example, a school nurse is asked to be an expert on screening children for potentially communicable infections such as impetigo or tinea capitis (ringworm). In health care settings, nurses often perform triage, identifying children who must be seen immediately, those who can wait to be seen, and those who should not stay in a waiting room with other children because they may have an infectious disorder. Occasionally, children admitted to an inpatient unit develop diarrhea soon after admission. It is vital that a nurse quickly recognize that this could be contagious so other children in the hospital, especially those who are immunosuppressed, can be protected (Chambers, 2009).

Several National Health Goals, shown in Box 43.1, are related to the prevention of infectious disorders in children.

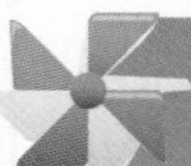

BOX 43.1 * Focus on National Health Goals

Several National Health Goals address ways to prevent and reduce the incidence of infectious disease in children. Examples of these are:

- Reduce the annual incidence of Lyme disease from a baseline of 17.4 per 100,000 to a target of 9.7 per 100,000 population.
- Reduce the rate of hospital-acquired central line–associated bloodstream infections among people in intensive care units from 5.3 per 1000 days stay to 4.8 per 1000 days stay.
- Reduce the rate of hospital-acquired central line–associated bloodstream infections among infants weighing 1000 grams or less at birth in intensive care from 12.2 per 1000 days stay to 11 per 1000 days stay.
- Achieve and maintain the rate of effective vaccination coverage levels for universally recommended vaccines among young children, such as varicella vaccine, from a baseline of 43% to a target level of 90% (http://www.nih.gov).

Nurses can help the nation achieve these goals by educating parents about the importance of immunizations and ways to avoid infections such as Lyme disease. They can also help prevent the spread of infection in hospital units by adhering scrupulously to infection control precautions.

Nursing research that could increase understanding in this area includes studies aimed at answering questions such as the following: What precautions can summer camps or camp sites take to discourage children from petting wild animals to prevent contracting rabies or being exposed to ticks? What information do parents need to convince them to obtain full immunizations for children? What types of orientation do new staff nurses need to help them learn or better follow infection prevention techniques?

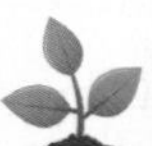

Nursing Process Overview

For a Child With an Infectious Disorder

Assessment

Many infectious diseases begin subtly. Parents report symptoms such as, "he doesn't act like himself" or "she's so listless." In many syndromes, children are infectious during this time. Following the prodomal period, an **exanthem** (rash) can develop. Rashes can be difficult to identify, so it is important to obtain as full a description and history of a rash as possible.

Nursing Diagnosis

Common nursing diagnoses used with children directly related to the infectious process are:

- Pain related to pruritus from skin lesions
- Impaired skin integrity related to rash, pruritus, and scratching
- Risk for infection related to presence of infective organism in sibling
- Altered body temperature, fever, related to systemic infection
- Fluid volume deficit related to insensible fluid loss from increased body temperature

Additional diagnoses when children must be separated from others to prevent infection transmission might include:

- Social isolation related to precautions required to prevent infection transmission
- Deficient diversional activity related to activity restriction and precautions to prevent disease transmission

Outcome Identification and Planning

When establishing outcomes for care of children with infectious disorders, include those that help parents deal with the current infection and also prevent another infection such as teaching about necessary infection control precautions and immunizations. Parents often ask about communicability to their other children and to the infected child's playmates or schoolmates, so these issues need to be addressed. Planning care for a child who requires restrictions to prevent disease transmission requires thoughtful consideration to prevent boredom. Two organizations helpful for referral are the National Foundation for Infectious Diseases (http://www.nfid.org) and the Centers for Disease Control (http://www.cdc.gov).

Implementation

Nursing responsibilities when caring for a child with an infectious disorder depend on the setting in which the child is seen. Often, a child will not be brought into a clinic if the disease can be easily identified over the telephone. Counseling parents about techniques to relieve the irritation of rashes and other symptoms of infectious illness can then be given over the telephone as well. Administering antibiotics and being alert for potential adverse effects are other major nursing responsibilities.

Outcome Evaluation

Evaluation of outcomes for the child with an infectious disease should determine not only whether the child is returning to wellness but also whether the child and family have learned more about ways to prevent infectious diseases. If one member of the family is receiving steroid therapy or has an immune system dysfunction, prevention of transmission takes on even greater importance.

Examples of expected outcomes that would indicate achievement of goals are:

- Child states pain from pruritus and skin lesions is at a tolerable level.
- Sibling remains free of signs and symptoms of infectious disorder.
- Parent names activities he has planned to provide diversional activities.

THE INFECTIOUS PROCESS

A *pathogen* is any organism that causes disease. Pathogens can be classified into five types of microorganisms: viruses, bacteria, rickettsiae, helminths, and fungi. The properties of these organisms are discussed in conjunction with the common diseases that they cause.

Stages of Infectious Disease

Infectious diseases follow certain stages during which the communicability (ability to be spread to others) or severity of the illness can be predicted (Fig. 43.1).

- The **incubation period** is the time between the invasion of an organism and the onset of symptoms of infection. During this time, microorganisms grow and multiply. The incubation period varies depending on the pathogen. A common interval is 7 to 10 days, but it can be longer. The incubation period for tetanus, for example, is 2 to 21 days.
- A **prodromal period** is a time between the beginning of nonspecific symptoms and disease-specific ones. Nonspecific symptoms include lethargy, low-grade fever, fatigue, and malaise. Children are infectious (capable of spreading the microorganisms to others) during this time, but because their symptoms are so vague they do not generally take any precautions against spreading disease. Therefore, during a prodromal period, infectious diseases spread readily through communities to any susceptible individuals. Prodromal stages are generally short, ranging from hours to a few days.
- *Illness* is the stage during which specific symptoms are evident. Most illnesses have local symptoms related to the body organ affected and also systemic symptoms that affect the entire body, such as fever, increased white blood cell count, or headache. Many childhood infections have an accompanying rash on the skin (exanthem) or mucous membrane **(enanthem)** (Box 43.2).
- The **convalescent period** is the interval between when symptoms first begin to fade and the child returns to full wellness. Because fatigue is often an accompanying symptom of infection, the convalescent period, or the time until full energy is restored, is often longer than anticipated.

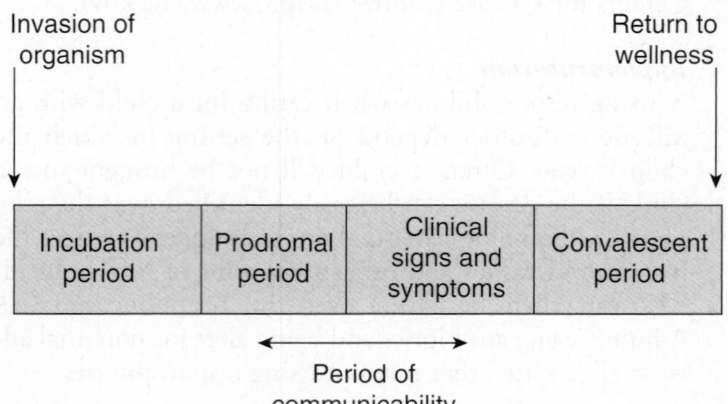

FIGURE 43.1 Time frame for infectious diseases. Period of communicability is the time during which the disease can be transmitted to other people.

Box 43.2 Assessment
Assessing a Child With Common Signs and Symptoms of Infectious Disorders

History

Chief concern: Does child have a fever, general malaise, vomiting, or diarrhea? Was child recently exposed to someone with an infection?

Past medical history: Are child's immunizations current?

Physical examination

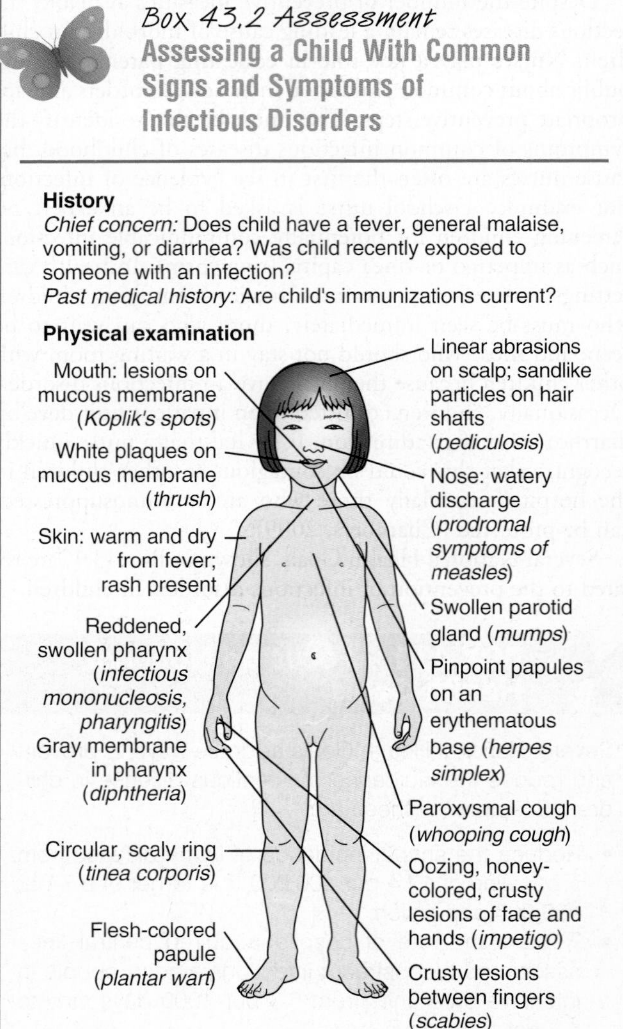

Chain of Infection

Chain of infection is the method by which organisms are spread and enter a new individual to cause disease. An important method of preventing infection is to break the chain of infection. Nurses are instrumental in teaching parents how to prevent the spread of infection in homes and how to carry out safe practices so infection does not spread in health care facilities.

Reservoir

The **reservoir** is the container or place in which organisms grow and reproduce. The source of a human pathogen could be another human with the disease, a human carrying the disease, soil, or an animal or insect. Immunizations are helpful in limiting organisms' use of children as reservoirs for growth.

Portal of Exit

The **portal of exit** is the method by which organisms leave an infected child's body to be spread to others. This could be by upper respiratory excretions, feces, vomitus, saliva, urine, vaginal secretions, blood, or lesion secretions (Table 43.1). To break a chain of infection at this point, follow good aseptic technique and prescribed transmission-based precautions such as wearing a gown, gloves, or mask as appropriate. Teach parents good handwashing technique after the use of a bathroom or after handling diapers. Be sure to supply an adequate number of disposable tissues so droplet or airborne spread from coughing or sneezing can be limited.

Means of Transmission

The **means of transmission** is the way that infection is spread. This can be by direct or indirect contact. **Fomites** are inanimate objects such as soil, food, water, bedding, towels, combs, or drinking glasses that lead to indirect spread. Insects, rats, or other vermin (vectors) also cause indirect spread.

Head lice (tinea capitis) can be spread by a fomite such as a comb if it is passed from one child to another. Insects carry and spread rickettsial diseases. Soil always contains some anaerobic organisms (those that grow without oxygen), such as tetanus bacilli. When a child receives a puncture wound, such as from stepping on a rusty nail, some dirt may be left in the closed wound, and tetanus bacilli contained in the soil can begin to multiply in the closed area. Staphylococcal gastrointestinal disorders can be spread by improperly refrigerated food.

Direct contact implies body-to-body touching. Sexually transmitted infections (STIs) and skin disorders are spread this way. The most common means of indirect contact is the spread of mouth and nose secretions (droplet infection) through talking, sneezing, coughing, breathing, and kissing. Some droplets containing pathogenic organisms are spread immediately to another individual in this way. Some droplets fall to the ground, where the organisms dry and then are spread by dust. If small, the organisms become suspended in the air (airborne transmission) and can move with the wind to infect people at a distance. Common respiratory tract infections, for example, are spread by indirect contact.

To break a chain of infection at this point, use transmission-based precautions as appropriate and wash hands before, between, and after client care. Teach parents and children good handwashing technique and other measures as necessary.

Portal of Entry

The **portal of entry** or the opening through which a pathogen can enter a child's body can be by inhalation, ingestion, or breaks in the skin such as bites, abrasions, and burns. To break a chain of infection at this point, teach children to wash their hands after sneezing or coughing and before eating and after using the bathroom. Teach girls to wipe their perineum from front to back after defecating or voiding to prevent organisms from spreading from the rectum to the urethra. Teach parents to wash cuts and abrasions before bandaging them.

Susceptible Host

For infection to occur, a child must be susceptible to the infection **(susceptible host).** Certain characteristics make some individuals more prone to infection than others:

- Age—infection occurs most readily in the very young and the very old

TABLE 43.1 ✻ Methods by Which Infections Spread

Portal of Exit	Means of Transmission	Portal of Entry	Prevention Measures
Blood	Arthropod vectors Blood sampling Transfusion	Injection into the bloodstream	Decreasing vector incidence Careful handling of blood sampling equipment Screening of transfused blood for organisms such as human immunodeficiency virus (HIV) or hepatitis B
Respiratory secretions	Airborne droplets Fomites	Respiratory tract	Wearing mask Droplet precautions Airborne precautions Handwashing
Feces	Water, food Fomites Vectors such as flies	Gastrointestinal tract	Handwashing before eating, after using bathroom, or handling diapers
Exudate from lesions	Direct contact Contact with soiled dressings	Skin, mucous membranes	Contact precautions Self-screening for sexual contacts Gloves

TABLE 43.2 ✻ Types and Functions of White Blood Cells (Leukocytes)

Type	Percentage of Total Count	Origin	Function
Granular Forms			
Neutrophils	60 at birth 33 at 2 years 60 thereafter	Bone marrow	Active in acute bacterial infections
Eosinophils	1–4	Bone marrow	Increased in parasitic infection
Basophils	0.0–0.5	Bone marrow	Increased with inflammation
Nongranular Forms			
Lymphocytes	30 at birth 50 at 2 years 30 thereafter	Bone marrow Divides into B cells and T cells	Direct reaction with antigens (T lymphocytes—centered in thymus gland); antibody production by B lymphocytes against antigens
Monocytes	5–10	Bone marrow	Backup for neutrophils in acute infection; macrophages are mature form

- Gender—girls, for example, have more urinary tract infections than boys
- Virulence—some organisms are stronger than others or cause disease more readily
- Body defenses present—physical, chemical, and immune responses all protect against foreign invaders. Children with immunosuppression are more susceptible than others.

Immune Response to Organisms

When a foreign organism (antigen) is identified, it can be destroyed by the phagocytic (cell-engulfing) action of white blood cells or by activation of the body's immune system. Phagocytes are unique white blood cells that are capable of cell destruction. The cells chiefly responsible for this function are neutrophils. Monocytes serve as backup cells for phagocytosis. The action of all white blood cells is summarized in Table 43.2.

The action of phagocytes on organisms produces pus (remnants of the organisms, phagocytes, and destroyed tissue). Children and parents alike may need a review of the purpose of pus because they think its presence indicates that an infection is becoming worse. More likely, it indicates that phagocytosis is occurring and the infection is resolving.

If bacteria escape the action of the phagocytes, they enter the blood and lymph systems and are then transported to other body locations, activating the immune system. Pathogenic organisms in the bloodstream create **septicemia,** which is always a serious development because it means the organism is being spread systemically.

With activation of the immune system, B lymphocytes (humoral immunity) and T lymphocytes (cell-mediated immunity) are produced. B lymphocytes form antibodies specific to offending antigens that either actively destroy cells or activate *complement,* a special body protein that is capable of lysing cells (see Chapter 42).

T lymphocytes (thymus-dependent) can destroy antigens by direct contact or release of lymphokines. An example of a lymphokine is **interferon,** a substance that prevents cells from being host to more than one virus at a time. This is why it is rare to see a child with two viral diseases at the same time, although it is not impossible to see a child with both a viral and a bacterial disease (perhaps scarlet fever and a common cold) at the same time. This is also why two virus vaccines are not given to a child at the same time unless they are specially designed to be given together (such as measles, mumps, and rubella). (See Chapter 42 for a more detailed discussion of the immune response and Chapter 34 for a discussion of immunizations.)

HEALTH PROMOTION AND RISK MANAGEMENT

Preventing infectious diseases is important because these disorders are responsible for a high percentage of hospital admissions in children (Box 43.3). Prevention begins with being certain all children are in general good health. Adequate nutrition is important to provide protein and vitamins to supply adequate white blood cells so that both phagocytic and antibody-producing B lymphocytes are available to destroy invading organisms.

A second important step is to be certain all parents are aware of the need for their children to be immunized. Nurses need to ensure that immunizations are offered to children at well-child and many illness health care visits.

It is important that parents also understand that although diseases such as scarlet fever, chickenpox (varicella), and mumps (infectious parotitis) are referred to as "common" childhood illnesses, they have the potential to be serious illnesses, leading to complications such as pneumonia and encephalitis. When children develop these common communicable diseases, they need to be seen by a primary health care provider to minimize the risk for these complications.

The responsibility expected of parents and children to help prevent the spread of communicable diseases differs from country to country and varies among cultures. In the United States, both federal and state governments have taken an active role in preventing the spread of infectious disease by requiring children to have immunizations against the most common illnesses. Parents are expected to obtain such immunizations for children by school age. Schools and school nurses, as the school system's front-line health officers, take an active role in enforcing these regulations. Community

BOX 43.3 ✻ Focus on Evidence-Based Practice

Is infectious disease still a major reason for hospitalization in infants?

Because children receive so many immunizations today, many parents are surprised to learn their child has an infectious disease. The are shocked when they are told their child needs to be hospitalized as a part of therapy. To discover what is the rate of hospitalization for infectious diseases today in infants, researchers analyzed the reason for hospital admission of infants in the United States for a full year. Results of this analysis revealed that 42.8% of all hospitalizations for infants were for infectious diseases. This averages about 1 hospitalization for every 14 infants in the United States. The rates of hospitalization were highest for boys and nonwhite infants and averaged 3 days in length. The most commonly seen diagnoses among the infant infectious disease hospitalizations were lower respiratory tract infections (59.0%), kidney, urinary tract, and bladder infections (7.6%), upper respiratory tract infections (6.5%), and septicemia (6.5%). The median cost of an infectious disease hospitalization was $2235, with total annual hospital costs of approximately $690 million, among infants in the United States.

Based on the above study, would you assure the parents of an infant diagnosed with an infectious disease that the child can be cared for safely at home?

Source: Yorita, K. L., et al. (2008). Infectious disease hospitalizations among infants in the United States. *Pediatrics, 121*(2), 244–252.

health nurses are also instrumental in administering immunizations and counseling families on how to prevent the spread of disease in their home. Nurses can also make certain that parents are aware of the latest studies available on the safety of vaccines so they do not associate common vaccines with the development of autism, for example.

War-torn countries have a great deal of difficulty maintaining this same level of disease prevention. Remember when caring for children newly arrived from another country that the child may not have the same level of immunization as usually seen. This opens an important area of health teaching, as the parents may not be aware of the importance of immunizations, which ones are required, or what community services are available to supply them.

Preventing the Spread of Infections

Nosocomial or health care-associated infections (HAI) are infections that are contracted while in a hospital or other health care setting. They represent a major threat to hospitalized children. The overall rate of nosocomial, or hospital-acquired, infection in children ranges from 0% in low-risk settings to 23% in high-risk settings such as intensive care units. Children younger than 2 years, children with a nutritional deficit, those who are immunosuppressed, those who have indwelling vascular lines or catheters, those receiving multiple antibiotic therapy, or those who remain in the hospital for longer than 72 hours are at highest risk for contracting such an infection. Nurses provide a line of defense against such infections by adhering to strict aseptic technique, such as frequent and thorough handwashing, and by following protective transmission-based precautions when indicated (Mark, Harless, & Berman, 2007). Nurses and other health care providers must also take precautions to protect themselves from acquiring communicable diseases, including HIV and hepatitis, by adhering to standard infection precautions recommended by the Centers for Disease Control and Prevention (CDC, 2008a). Box 43.4 and Appendix I summarize standard infection precautions and transmission-based infection control precautions (CDC, 2008b).

CARING FOR THE CHILD WITH AN INFECTIOUS DISEASE

As almost all childhood infectious diseases include a fever or rash, nursing care must address identification and relief of these symptoms.

Nursing Diagnoses and Related Interventions

✻

Nursing Diagnosis: Pain related to pruritus from skin lesions

Outcome Evaluation: Child states he is more comfortable; reports less itching; is not seen scratching rash; no signs of excessive scratching or bleeding are present.

Providing comfort for the pruritus of skin lesions is important for many childhood infections. No matter what agent is causing the disease, a rash tends to be extremely itchy and uncomfortable. Fortunately, several simple remedies are available for reducing discomfort. Because pruritus is a minimal form of pain, an analgesic, such as acetaminophen (Tylenol), may be helpful. An antihistamine, such as diphenhydramine hydrochloride (Benadryl), is extremely helpful. Calamine lotion is a nonprescription lotion that is cooling and soothing and often helps to relieve itching. Colloidal baths, such as baking soda or oatmeal (approximately 1 cup to 3 inches of bath water), are soothing for some children. Warn parents to take precautions to prevent clogging the drain if oatmeal is used. Caution parents to use only lukewarm water, not hot, because heat usually increases the sensation of itching. Bathing serves two purposes: it can be not only soothing but also distracting. A child, especially a preschooler, may splash for 15 to 20 minutes in a bathtub without noticing the discomfort of a rash.

Some parents bundle up children with rashes, believing that the extra clothing brings out the rash, and that if a rash does not come out, it will go in and affect a child's heart or brain. In reality, bundling up only serves to make a rash more uncomfortable and probably increases any accompanying fever. Instead,

BOX 43.4 ✻ Standard and Transmission-Based Precautions for Infection Control

To reduce the risk of disease transmission in the health care setting:

1. Wash hands immediately with soap and water before and after examining patients and after any contact with blood, body fluids, and contaminated items—whether or not you wear gloves. Use of a plain, nonantimicrobial soap is recommended.
2. Wear clean, nonsterile gloves anytime contact with blood, body fluids, mucous membrane, or broken skin is likely. Change gloves between tasks or procedures on the same patient. Before going to another patient, remove gloves promptly and wash hands immediately and then put on new gloves.
3. Wear a mask, protective eyewear, and gown during any patient care activity when splashes or sprays of body fluids are likely. Remove the soiled gown as soon as possible and wash hands.
4. Handle needles and other sharp instruments safely. Do not recap needles. Make sure contaminated nondisposable equipment is not reused with another patient until it has been cleaned, disinfected, and sterilized properly. Dispose of nonreusable needles, syringes, and other sharp patient care instruments in puncture-resistant containers.
5. Routinely clean and disinfect frequently touched surfaces including beds, bedrails, examination tables, and bedside tables.
6. Do not touch linens soiled with blood or body fluids with bare hands. Use plastic bags to transport soiled linen.
7. Place a patient whose blood or body fluids are likely to contaminate surfaces or other patients in an isolation room or area.
8. Minimize the use of invasive procedures to avoid the potential for injury and accidental exposure. Use oral rather than injectable medications whenever possible.
9. When a specific diagnosis is made, find out how the disease is transmitted. Use precautions according to the transmission risk.

Airborne Precautions

Airborne precautions reduce the risk of small-particle organisms being transmitted through the air. Microorganisms carried by this route can be carried widely. If airborne transmission is possible:

1. Place the patient in an isolation room that is not air-conditioned or where air is not circulated to the rest of the health care facility. Make sure the room has a door that can be closed.
2. Wear a HEPA or other biosafety mask when working with the patient and in the patient's room.
3. Limit movement of the patient from the room to other areas. Place a surgical mask on the patient who must be moved.

Droplet Precautions

Droplet precautions reduce the risk of pathogens being spread through large-particle droplet contact by acts such as coughing, sneezing, and talking or through procedures such as suctioning or bronchoscopy. Large droplets do not remain suspended in the air for long periods and generally travel only short distances, so close proximity is required for spread of disease. If droplet transmission is possible:

1. Place the patient in an isolation room.
2. Wear a HEPA or other biosafety mask when working with the patient.
3. Limit movement of the patient from the room to other areas. If the patient must be moved, place a surgical mask on the patient.

Contact Precautions

Contact precautions reduce the risk of transmission of pathogens by direct contact such as skin-to-skin contact (shaking hands) or indirect contact through an intermediate object such as a comb or soiled dressing. If contact transmission is possible:

1. Place the patient in an isolation room and limit access.
2. Wear gloves during contact with patient and with infectious body fluids or contaminated items. Reinforce handwashing throughout the health facility.
3. Wear two layers of protective clothing.
4. Limit movement of the patient from the isolation room to other areas.
5. Avoid sharing equipment between patients. Designate equipment for each patient, if supplies allow. If sharing equipment is unavoidable, clean and disinfect it before use with the next patient.

Source: Centers for Disease Control and Prevention. (2008b). *Recommendations for isolation precautions in hospitals.* Washington, DC: Author.

dress a child in light cotton clothing. Remove wool blankets from the bed. Cut the child's fingernails short so scratching will not open up lesions, causing secondary infection. Placing cotton gloves on the child, especially at night, may help. Comfort measures of this type for relieving the discomfort of rashes are summarized in Box 43.5.

None of these measures is foolproof. Some may provide great relief to some children and little or none to others. Regardless of whether they offer direct relief, they do give a parent a constructive and comforting activity to carry out, providing parents with an opportunity to soothe their children and themselves.

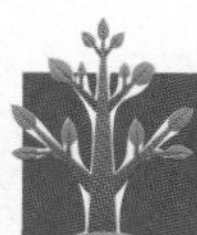

BOX 43.5 * Focus on Family Teaching

Relieving the Itchiness of a Rash

Q. Marty's mother says to you, "Our son is miserable because his rash is so itchy. What can we do to help him?"

A. Itching is a very uncomfortable sensation. Use the following to help relieve the itch of a rash:

- Dress your child in light cotton clothing so overheating and perspiration do not occur. Perspiration can make itching worse.
- Avoid wool clothing, because it can irritate skin and increase itching.
- Offer adequate fluid to maintain good hydration, because dry skin increases discomfort.
- Keep your child's fingernails short, to avoid injury to the skin from scratching.
- Teach your child to press on an itchy area rather than scratching to relieve discomfort; cold cloths applied to an area can also be helpful.
- Administer an analgesic, such as acetaminophen, as needed for comfort.
- Adding a few teaspoonfuls of baking soda to bath water can be soothing. Use lukewarm rather than hot water.
- Keep in mind that some children need an antihistamine such as diphenhydramine (Benadryl) to reduce itching. Ask your primary care provider about using it.

Most infectious diseases also involve fever. Measures to combat fever in children are discussed in Chapter 37.

Nursing Diagnosis: Social isolation related to required activity restriction associated with precautions to prevent disease transmission

Outcome Evaluation: Child states reasons for restrictions; expresses interest in activities proposed by nurses or parents.

A child who is restricted from others because of infection control precautions can begin to feel lonely and depressed unless stimulation and social needs are met.

Children easily associate isolation and restriction with being punished. In a hospital setting, make as few trips as possible in and out of the room to limit the possibility of pathogen spread; on the other hand, do not make care visits seem hurried. If there is a procedure scheduled at 9:00 AM and another at 9:30 AM, stay in the room rather than leave to return again, if possible. Use the time to read a story to the child, play a card game, or talk about how strange and lonely it feels to be separated from other people.

When a child is hospitalized and requires transmission-based infection control precautions, parents must follow these precautions just as all hospital personnel do when they visit. Some parents feel so self-conscious about having to gown and wash they may stay away rather than visit. Making them feel comfortable with these procedures is a nursing responsibility. Remember that when children are admitted to a hospital, parents may not hear everything that is said to them during admission because of their anxiety. If the gowning technique was explained on admission, therefore, do not expect parents to remember the next day what was said. Explain the technique as many times as necessary.

Parents may be reluctant to give children who require transmission-based precautions their favorite toy, thinking that the hospital will insist on destroying it after the precautions are discontinued. Few pathogens exist that are not destroyed by exposure to sunlight, however, and few articles are available that cannot be further gas-sterilized to ensure that pathogens have been removed, so there is no reason to restrict toys. Check the rooms of children requiring transmission-based precautions for favorite toys, therefore, the same as in all rooms. Never leave children in a room before checking that they have a toy to play with or an activity that will keep them busy for the length of time they will be alone. See Chapter 36 for a discussion of interventions that can be used to promote adequate stimulation for a child requiring transmission-based precautions.

VIRAL INFECTIONS

Viruses are the smallest infectious agents known, so small they cannot be seen through an ordinary microscope. They are actually not true cells because they contain either ribonucleic acid (RNA) or deoxyribonucleic acid (DNA), but not both. Because they are incomplete, viruses increase in number by replication inside bacteria, plant, animal, or human cells using the biochemical products of living cells to function. Although a body cell may not be outwardly altered by a virus invasion, it could fail to function or die because of lysis of internal components or rupture. Symptoms usually do not become apparent until many cells have been interrupted in this way, so the incubation period of viral infections can be long. Some viruses are capable of invading only specific cells. The Epstein-Barr virus, for example, invades only B lymphocytes, HIV viruses invade CD4 T lymphocytes, and influenza viruses affect specific receptor sites in tracheal cells.

Viral Exanthems

The majority of childhood exanthems (rashes) are caused by viruses, and each of these diseases has specific symptoms, characteristic lesions, and a specific distribution or pattern to the rash that allows it to be identified (Figs. 43.2 and 43.3).

Exanthem Subitum (Roseola Infantum)

- Causative agent: Human herpesvirus 6 (HHV-6)
- Incubation period: Approximately 10 days
- Period of communicability: During febrile period
- Mode of transmission: Unknown
- Immunity: Contracting the disease offers lasting natural immunity; no artificial immunity is available.

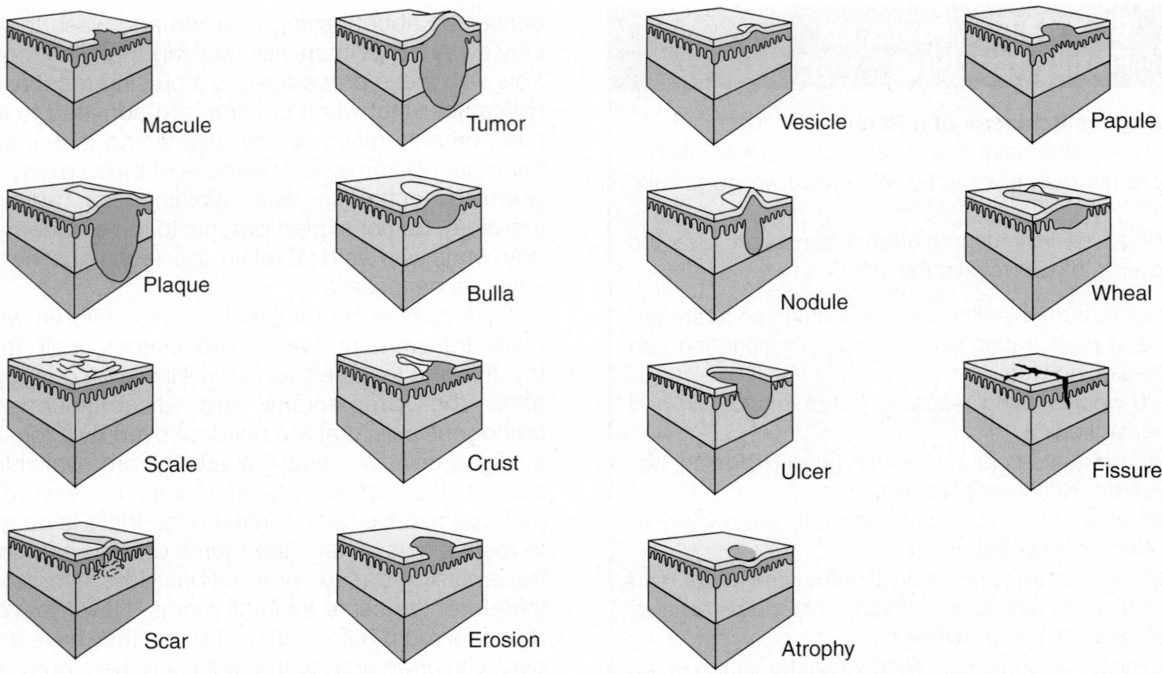

FIGURE 43.2 Primary and secondary skin lesions and their characteristics.

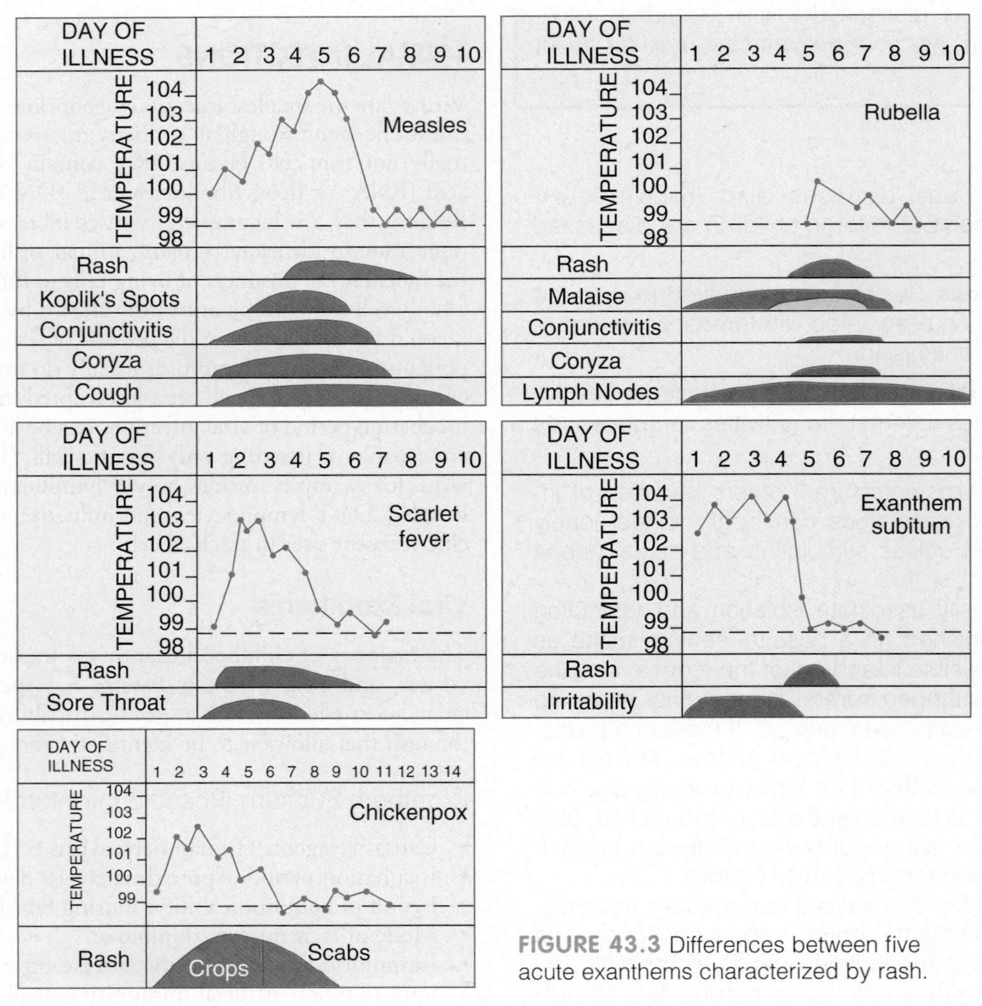

FIGURE 43.3 Differences between five acute exanthems characterized by rash.

Assessment. Roseola is a disease with symptoms that appear to be more severe than is warranted. It generally occurs in children between 6 months to 3 years, mainly in the spring and fall, although it can occur any time of the year. The first symptom is a high fever (104° to 105° F [40.0° to 40.6° C]). Infants may be irritable and anorexic but rarely appear as ill as this high a fever suggests. They usually remain playful and alert. The pharynx may be slightly inflamed. The occipital, cervical, and postauricular lymph nodes may be enlarged. The white blood count is usually decreased, with the proportion of lymphocytes increased.

After 3 or 4 days, the fever falls abruptly and a distinctive rash appears (see Fig. 43.3). The lesions are discrete, rose-pink macules approximately 2 to 3 mm in size. They fade on pressure and occur most prominently on the trunk. The rash resembles that of rubella or measles, but it is darker, and children have no accompanying coryza (upper respiratory symptoms), conjunctivitis, or cough. Because it occurs mainly on the child's trunk, parents may report it as a heat rash. The rash lasts 1 to 2 days. The diagnosis of roseola is based on the physical signs and symptoms. The hallmark of roseola is the appearance of a rash immediately after the sharp decline in fever (Dyer, 2007).

Therapeutic Management. Treatment focuses on measures to reduce the discomfort of the rash and fever. The fever will respond to acetaminophen (Tylenol) or ibuprofen (Motrin), but after 4 hours it is apt to rise again to the high level. The most frequent complication of roseola is a febrile seizure with the onset of the disease because the temperature rises so rapidly. Management of this type of seizure is discussed in Chapter 49.

There are no long-term effects of roseola. If an infant develops this exanthem in the hospital, follow standard infection precautions.

Rubella (German Measles)

- Causative agent: Rubella virus
- Incubation period: 14 to 21 days
- Period of communicability: 7 days before to approximately 5 days after the rash appears
- Mode of transmission: Direct and indirect contact with droplets
- Immunity: Contracting the disease offers lasting natural immunity; a high rubella titer reveals infection has occurred.
- Active artificial immunity: Attenuated live virus vaccine
- Passive artificial immunity: Immune serum globulin is considered for pregnant women.

Assessment. Rubella is a disease rarely seen today, but when it does occur, it affects older school-age and adolescent children; it occurs most commonly during the spring. The symptoms begin with a 1- to 5-day prodromal period, during which children or adolescents have a low-grade fever, headache, malaise, anorexia, mild conjunctivitis, possibly a sore throat, a mild cough, and swollen lymph nodes such as those in the suboccipital, postauricular, and cervical chains (Levin & Weinberg, 2008).

After the 1 to 5 days of prodromal signs, a discrete pink-red maculopapular rash (see Fig. 43.3) begins on the face, then spreads downward to the trunk and extremities. On the third day, the rash disappears. There is generally no desquamation (peeling); if present, it is primarily fine flaking of the skin.

Fever with rubella is not marked, although arthritis (joint pain) with effusion into the joints occurs in some children on the second or third day, lasting as long as 5 to 10 days.

Therapeutic Management. Children need comfort measures for the rash and an antipyretic such as acetaminophen (Tylenol) or ibuprofen (Motrin) for fever or joint pain. If a child develops rubella while in the hospital, follow droplet precautions for 7 days after the onset of the rash in addition to standard infection precautions.

If rubella occurs during pregnancy, it can cause extensive congenital malformation in the fetus (see Chapter 12). Because of this, it can never be considered a simple disease. It is important that girls be immunized against it before they reach child-bearing age (Thilo & Rosenberg, 2008).

Measles (Rubeola)

- Causative agent: Measles virus
- Incubation period: 10 to 12 days
- Period of communicability: Fifth day of incubation period through the first few days of rash
- Mode of transmission: Direct or indirect contact with droplets
- Immunity: Contracting the disease offers lasting natural immunity.
- Active artificial immunity: Attenuated live measles vaccine
- Passive artificial immunity: Immune serum globulin

Assessment. Measles is sometimes called brown or black, regular, or 7-day measles to differentiate it from rubella (German, or 3-day, measles). Like rubella, because of high vaccination rates, it is rarely seen today except for periodic outbreaks that occur in newly underimmunized immigrant populations or an underimmunized college-age population (Muller et al., 2007). The incidence of the disease is highest in the winter and spring.

The disease has a 10- to 11-day prodromal period, during which lymphoid tissue, particularly postauricular, cervical, and occipital lymph nodes, becomes enlarged. Children develop a high fever (103° to 104° F [39.5° to 40.0° C]) and malaise. By the second day of the prodromal period, coryza (rhinitis and a sore throat), conjunctivitis with photophobia (sensitivity to light), and a cough develop. **Koplik's spots** (small, irregular, bright-red spots with a blue-white center point) appear on the buccal membrane. Unfortunately, the coryza of measles is indistinguishable from that of a common cold (nasal congestion, a mucopurulent discharge, and a deep brassy, bronchial cough) when it begins. As a result, many children with measles are diagnosed as having a simple upper respiratory infection at this point.

Koplik's spots distinguish the disease because none of the other exanthems has this finding. They appear first on the buccal membrane opposite the molars and then extend to cover the entire buccal surface (Fig. 43.4). The raised base of the spots may coalesce so that the blue-white centers stand out as grains of salt on the erythematous membrane.

By the fourth day of fever, the rash appears. A deep-red maculopapular eruption begins at the hairline of the forehead, behind the ears, and at the back of the neck and then

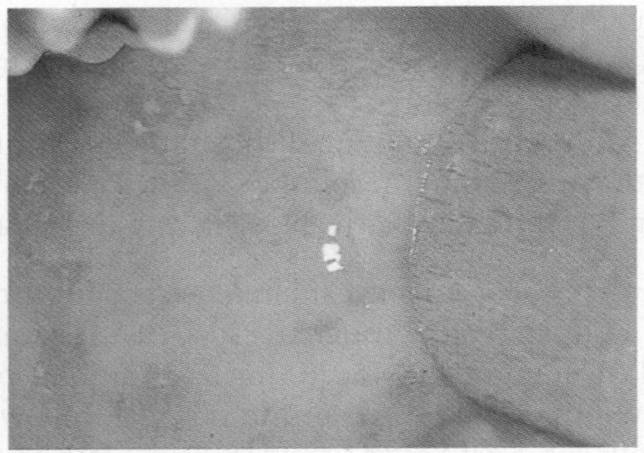

FIGURE 43.4 Koplik's spots on the oral mucous membrane. (SPL/Custom Medical Stock Photograph.)

spreads to the face, the neck, upper extremities, trunk, and finally the lower extremities (Fig. 43.5). After several days, the rash typically turns from red to brown. While the rash is red, it fades on pressure; when it is brown, it does not fade. This differentiates it from the rash of scarlet fever, which always fades on pressure. After 5 to 6 days, the rash completely fades. There is a fine desquamation after this. However, the skin of the hands and feet does not desquamate, a feature again differentiating it from scarlet fever.

Children with measles appear very ill because their cough is loud and frequent, the coryza is acute, the fever is high, and the rash is pruritic. Fortunately, on the third or fourth day of rash, when the temperature begins to fall, the other symptoms clear quickly and children feel better. Fever that lasts beyond the third or fourth day of rash or coughing that continues generally suggests that a complication of measles, such as pneumonia, has occurred.

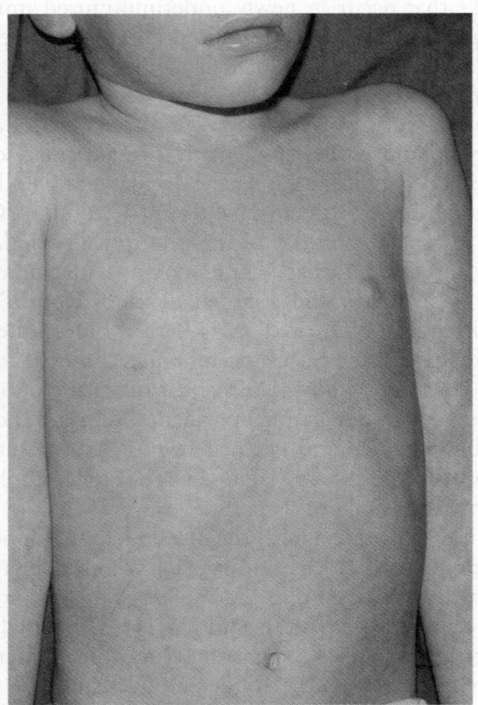

FIGURE 43.5 The typical rash of measles on a child's upper body. (© NMSB/Custom Medical Stock Photograph.)

Therapeutic Management. Children with measles need comfort measures for the rash and an antipyretic for the fever. The coryza, which does not respond to decongestants, fortunately lasts only a few days. The skin below the nose may become excoriated from the constant nasal drainage. Applying a lubricating jelly or an emollient (A&D ointment) to the area may help prevent excoriation. A child may need a cough suppressant to control the cough; otherwise, the throat can become painful from frequent irritation. Because children with measles have photophobia, it is painful for them to look at bright lights, so it may be painful for them to watch television. They are often more comfortable with the shades or curtains drawn or wearing dark glasses, so these measures should be instituted. Children need to be seen by a health care provider because the complications of measles include otitis media (middle ear infection), pneumonia, airway obstruction, and acute encephalitis (Levin & Weinberg, 2008). If a child is hospitalized, follow airborne precautions for the duration of the illness in addition to standard infection precautions.

Chickenpox (Varicella)

- Causative agent: Varicella-zoster virus
- Incubation period: 10 to 21 days
- Period of communicability: 1 day before the rash to 5 to 6 days after its appearance, when all the vesicles have crusted
- Mode of transmission: Highly contagious; spread by direct or indirect contact of saliva or vesicles
- Immunity: Contracting the disease offers lasting natural immunity to chickenpox; because the same virus causes herpes zoster, it may be reactivated at a later time as herpes zoster (shingles).
- Active artificial immunity: Attenuated live virus vaccine
- Passive artificial immunity: There is little passive placental immunity to chickenpox. Children who are immunosuppressed, such as those with leukemia or HIV/AIDS, or those who are being treated with corticosteroids are given varicella-zoster immune globulin (VZIG). This may prevent or modify chickenpox if given within 72 hours of exposure.

Assessment. Chickenpox is another common childhood infection that is decreasing in incidence because of required immunization. The people most prone to it are those who have not been immunized, such as older children and college students. The disease is marked by a low-grade fever, malaise, and, in 24 hours, the appearance of a rash (see Fig. 43.3). The lesion begins as a macula, then progresses rapidly within 6 to 8 hours to a papule, then a vesicle that first becomes umbilicated and then forms a crust. Each lesion is approximately 2 to 3 mm in diameter and is surrounded by an erythematous area. When the first crop of lesions appears, the child's temperature may rise markedly to 104° or 105° F (40.0° or 40.6° C).

Most of the chickenpox lesions are found on the trunk, although the face, scalp, palate, and neck also may be involved. They appear in approximately three separate series or crops, with each new lesion moving through progressive stages (Fig. 43.6). At one time, all four stages of lesions (macule, papule, vesicle, and crust) are present.

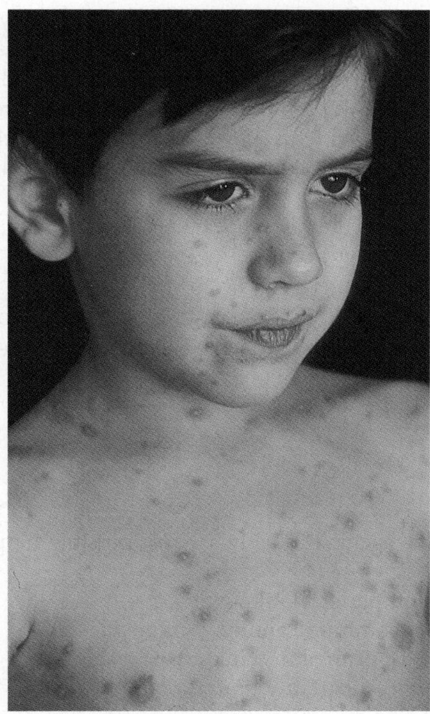

FIGURE 43.6 An older school-age boy with varicella. (© Martin/Custom Medical Stock Photograph.)

Therapeutic Management. If the scabs from crusting are allowed to fall off naturally and lesions do not become secondarily infected, no scarring results. Scabs removed prematurely may leave a white, round, slightly indented scar at the site. For this reason, it is important that children not scratch and remove scabs, but because the rash of chickenpox is extremely pruritic, preventing scratching becomes a difficult problem for parents. A prescribed antihistamine usually helps to reduce the itchiness to a bearable level, and an antipyretic will counteract the high fever. Acyclovir may be prescribed to reduce the number of lesions and shorten the course of the illness (Koo & Shandera, 2009). The development of Reye syndrome has been associated with aspirin use during varicella and influenza virus illnesses (see Chapter 49), so caution parents to avoid aspirin and to use acetaminophen or ibuprofen to control fever instead.

If the child is hospitalized, follow airborne and contact precautions until all lesions are crusted, in addition to standard infection precautions. Children may return to school as soon as all the lesions are crusted (the crusts are not infectious). Complications include secondary infections of the lesions, pneumonia, and encephalitis.

Herpes Zoster

Herpes zoster is caused by the varicella-zoster virus, the same virus that causes chickenpox (Weinberg, 2007). Apparently, the first time the virus invades, children have symptoms of chickenpox. With a second invasion, herpes zoster symptoms appear due to reactivation of a latent virus. Herpes zoster tends to occur in older children or young adults, although it can occur at any age.

The first manifestations are pruritus and cutaneous vesicular lesions on erythematous bases that follow the distributions of the lumbar and thoracic nerves (usually on the trunk, face, or upper back) and cause deep nagging pain (Fig. 43.7).

Treatment for herpes zoster includes measures to reduce pruritus and analgesia for pain. Acyclovir, which inhibits viral DNA synthesis, may be effective in limiting the disease. VZIG may minimize symptoms.

Smallpox (Variola)

- Causative agent: Smallpox virus
- Incubation period: 7 to 17 days
- Period of communicability: From onset of rash until all crusts have been shed
- Mode of transmission: Direct or indirect contact
- Immunity: Lasting natural immunity after contracting the disease
- Active artificial immunity: No longer recommended
- Passive artificial immunity: Vaccinia immune globulin (VIG)

Smallpox is a disease that has been extinct in the world since 1995. However, health care providers need to be able to recognize symptoms of it because viruses, colonies of which are stored in various laboratories throughout the world, could be used as an agent of biologic terrorism.

The disease has a 3- to 4-day prodromal period of chills, fever, headache, and vomiting. A child appears extremely ill and exhausted. On day 3 or 4, a rash and high fever appear. The lesions, most prominent on the distal extremities and face, begin as macules, then progress to papules, vesicles, and pustules, eventually crusting over a 10- to 14-day period.

Although the lesions of smallpox resemble those of chickenpox, they can be differentiated by the appearance of the pustular stage (not seen with chickenpox) and the fact that they arise as one crop of lesions and all progress at the same rate (chickenpox occurs in stages). The crusts of chickenpox are not contagious; the crusts of smallpox are (Berger, 2009).

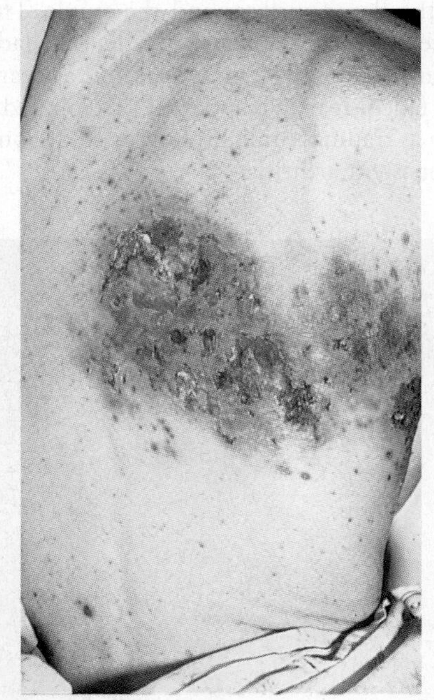

FIGURE 43.7 Herpes zoster on a child's back. (© Dr. P. Marazzi/SPL/Science Source/Photo Researchers.)

Smallpox is a serious illness: its mortality rate is as high as 50% and it can be spread readily from one infected person to another. Children are treated with VIG to suppress symptoms and an antibiotic to prevent secondary infection of lesions. They may need oxygen or other measures to support respiratory function and measures such as a cardiac glycoside to support cardiac function.

✔ Checkpoint Question 43.1

If a smallpox epidemic should occur, it will be important to be able to distinguish chickenpox (varicella) from smallpox. What are the stages of chickenpox lesions?

a. Macular, papular, vesicular, and crusting.
b. Macular, crusting, and extensive peeling.
c. Papular, vesicular, and pruritic crusting.
d. Maculopapular lesions with fine flaking.

Erythema Infectiosum ("Fifth Disease")

- Causative agent: Parvovirus B19
- Incubation period: 6 to 14 days
- Period of communicability: Uncertain
- Mode of transmission: Droplet
- Immunity: None

Assessment. Erythema infectiosum (the fifth important childhood exanthem) occurs most often in children 2 to 12 years of age. The first phase of the infection includes fever, headache, and malaise. A week later, a rash, which erupts in three stages, appears. The rash is intensely red and appears first on the face. The lesions are maculopapular and coalesce on the cheeks to form a "slapped face" appearance (Fig. 43.8). The facial lesions fade in 1 to 120 days (Servey, Reamy, & Hodge, 2007).

A day after the facial lesions appear, a rash appears on the extensor surfaces of the extremities. One day later, the rash appears on the flexor surfaces and the trunk. These lesions last for 1 week or more. When they fade, they fade from the center outward, giving the lesions a lacelike appearance. After the rash has faded, it may reappear if precipitated by skin irritation such as trauma, sunlight, hot, or cold. Some children develop a persistent arthritis.

Therapeutic Management. Treatment is typically supportive, with antipyretics and analgesics. Children also may need additional comfort measures for the rash (see Box 43.5). There are no known complications of fifth disease for a child; it is teratogenic in a fetus, however, so children with this disorder should avoid contact with pregnant women. Use droplet precautions in a hospital. Children can return to school as soon as the rash appears because they are no longer infectious after this point.

What if... Marty's parents tell you their doctor is ruling out fifth disease? What are the other four diseases that gave this disease its name?

Pityriasis Rosea

- Causative agent: Probably a virus, possibly herpesvirus 6 or 7
- Incubation period: Unknown
- Period of communicability: Unknown
- Mode of transmission: Unknown
- Immunity: Apparently none

Pityriasis rosea occurs in school-age and older children. Children may have a short, mild prodromal period of fever and sore throat. A herald patch, an erythematous round lesion with a scaly border, usually appearing on the trunk, is the first obvious lesion (Fig. 43.9). Approximately 1 week after the appearance of the herald patch, a generalized rash of papules, vesicles, or urticaria appears. This is generally also confined to the trunk. The rash follows skin lines, giving it the unique configuration of a Christmas tree (Morelli & Burch, 2008).

The rash lasts 6 to 8 weeks. It is pruritic and, because it lasts so long, is particularly worrisome to children and parents. Because the lesions, particularly the herald patch, are scaly at the edges, they are often confused with tinea corporis (ringworm). Treatment is limited to oral antihistamines and other comfort measures for rash.

Pityriasis rosea appears to have no sequelae or complications; in fact, it is difficult to demonstrate in what manner it is infectious. It is a baffling rash of childhood but needs to be differentiated from serious (severe) exanthems.

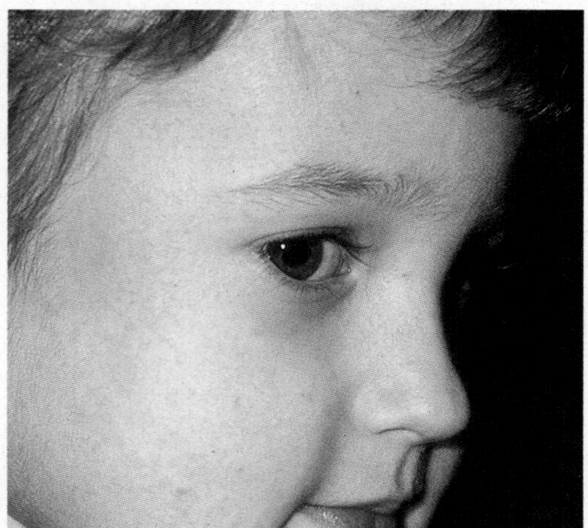

FIGURE 43.8 The rash of fifth disease. (© Dr. P. Marazzi/SPL/Science Source/Photo Researchers.)

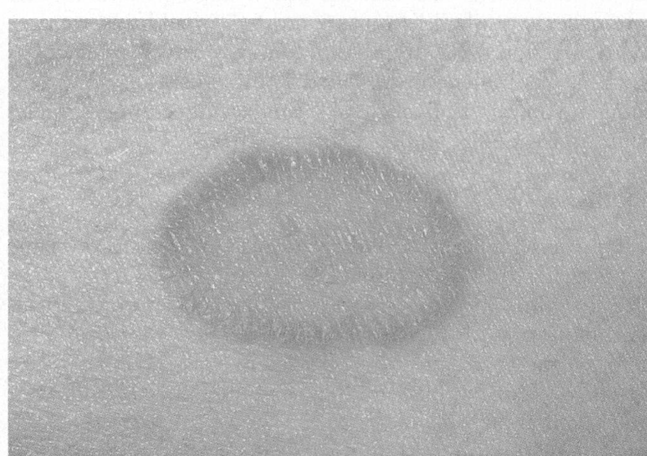

FIGURE 43.9 The "herald patch" of pityriasis rosea. (Dr. H. C. Robinson/SPL/Science Source/Photo Researchers.)

Enteroviruses

There are three main types of enteroviruses: echoviruses (33 subdivisions), coxsackievirus A (24 subdivisions) and coxsackievirus B (6 types), and polioviruses (3 subdivisions).

Echovirus Infections

The echoviruses are responsible for several childhood diseases, including aseptic meningitis, diarrhea, acute respiratory illness, and maculopapular rashes. Such infections are usually benign and self-limiting. Treatment involves supportive measures. If a child is hospitalized, follow contact precautions for the duration of the illness, in addition to standard infection precautions.

Coxsackievirus Infections

The coxsackievirus groups are responsible, like the echovirus groups, for a variety of diseases. One of the most frequently found diseases of children caused by coxsackievirus A is herpangina. With herpangina, children have an abrupt elevation of temperature, up to 104° or 105° F (40.0° or 40.6° C) for 1 to 4 days. Anorexia, difficulty swallowing, sore throat, and vomiting may be present. Children may have headache and abdominal pain. Small lesions, generally discrete grayish vesicles, pinpoint in size, appear on the tonsillar fauces, soft palate, and uvula (Koo & Shandera, 2009). Lesions may be present elsewhere in the mouth or throat as well. The lesions gradually change to shallow ulcers surrounded by a red areola. They disappear within a few days after the temperature returns to normal. There are generally no complications.

Children need to be maintained on soft or liquid foods while their mouth and throat are sore. They may need an antipyretic for fever. If a child is hospitalized, follow contact precautions for the duration of the illness, in addition to standard infection precautions.

Poliovirus Infections: Poliomyelitis (Infantile Paralysis)

- Causative agent: Poliovirus
- Incubation period: 7 to 14 days
- Period of communicability: Greatest shortly before and after onset of symptoms, when virus is present in the throat and feces (1 to 6 weeks)
- Mode of transmission: Direct and indirect contact
- Immunity: Contracting the disease causes active immunity against the one strain of virus causing the illness.
- Active artificial immunity: Inactivated polio virus vaccine (IPV)
- Passive artificial immunity: None

Polio is Greek for "gray," the color of the spinal cord after it atrophies from the effect of the poliomyelitis virus. No longer seen in the United States thanks to effective vaccination programs, poliomyelitis may be caused by any of the three strains of poliovirus, the rationale for immunizing children with the trivalent (three-strain) vaccine. Poliomyelitis still does occur in other parts of the world, and in war-torn or developing nations such as India and parts of Africa, the incidence is still high.

Assessment. The poliovirus enters the child's gastrointestinal tract, where it multiplies and produces symptoms such as fever, headache, nausea, vomiting, or abdominal pain. Moderate pain of the neck, back, and legs soon develops. The cerebrospinal fluid shows increased protein and lymphocytes.

These initial symptoms are followed by intense pain and tremors of the extremities and then paralysis, occurring either immediately or over a period of 1 to 7 days as the virus invades the central nervous system. Kernig's sign, a test for meningeal irritation, is positive (see Chapter 49). Children demonstrate a tripod sign—when sitting on the floor or on an examining table, they cannot sit without placing both the arms and hands behind them to brace themselves. Their deep tendon reflexes are hyperactive at first and then diminish as the central nervous system is fully invaded. Laryngeal paralysis makes swallowing or talking difficult, and respiratory paralysis can halt respiration (National Immunization Program, 2008).

Therapeutic Management. Treatment for poliomyelitis is bedrest with analgesia and moist hot packs to relieve pain. If the respiratory muscles are involved, long-term ventilation is necessary. Survivors tend to develop progressive muscle atrophy (postpoliomyelitis muscular atrophy syndrome) or severe arthritis in late adulthood, further reducing their ability to be self-sufficient (Sheth & Keenan, 2007).

Viral Infections of the Integumentary System

Viral infections of the skin include the herpes infections and warts (verrucae).

Herpesvirus Infections

Herpesviruses are responsible for several infections in children.

- Causative agent: Herpes simplex or herpes type 1 or type 2 virus
- Incubation period: 2 to 12 days
- Period of communicability: Greatest early in the course of the infection
- Mode of transmission: Direct contact
- Immunity: Immunity to a primary herpes response is gained after one incident. There is no immunity to recurrent herpes infections because the virus lies dormant in the body until it is activated by stress, sun exposure, fever, other illness, or menstruation.

About 30% of children in the United States are or have been infected by the herpes virus (Lauri, 2007). When children are first invaded by a herpesvirus, they have no antibodies against the virus, so a primary form of the disease such as herpetic gingivostomatitis occurs. The virus remains latent in the neurons of local sensory ganglia, or children become permanent carriers of the herpes simplex virus.

Acute Herpetic Gingivostomatitis. Acute herpetic gingivostomatitis is the most common form of herpes simplex invasion in young children (Berger, 2009). It is an example of the primary, not the recurrent, response. It occurs in children aged 1 to 4 years. Children have a high fever (104° to 105° F [40.0° to 40.6° C]), are restless, and have anorexia and a sore mouth. Their gumline is swollen and reddened and bleeds easily. White plaques or shallow ulcers with red areolae appear on the buccal mucosa, tongue, and palate and perhaps on the tonsillar fauces. The anterior cervical lymph nodes are enlarged and tender. The disease runs its course in 5 to 7 days.

Children need an antipyretic to reduce fever. They also need soft, acid-free foods that they can eat with minimal irritation or abrasion. Popsicles are soothing against inflamed mucous membranes. Oral acyclovir helps with healing. Use contact precautions with hospitalized children.

Children with gingivostomatitis appear very ill. The disease can become very serious, especially in infants, if their mouths become so sore that they cannot swallow readily and they become malnourished and dehydrated.

Herpes Simplex (Herpes Labialis). Herpes simplex infection, popularly known as a cold sore or fever blister, represents the recurrent form of a type 1 herpesvirus invasion that has remained dormant in the ganglia of the trigeminal or fifth cranial nerve. Herpes simplex typically appears as clusters of painful, grouped vesicles surrounded by an erythematous base on the lips or skin surrounding the mouth. After 2 or 3 days, vesicles crust, then gradually dry. Keeping lesions dry helps them to fade sooner, but keeping them lubricated with an ointment reduces pain. Topical or oral acyclovir reduces pain and increases healing. Children feel conspicuous about the appearance of herpes simplex lesions. They may need counseling to assure them that the lesions are not as obvious to others as they seem to them (Berger, 2009).

Acute Herpetic Vulvovaginitis (Genital Herpes). Genital herpes is caused by the herpesvirus type 2, which remains dormant in the ganglia of the sacral nerves. Because this form is spread primarily by sexual contact, it is discussed in Chapter 47 with other STIs. The occurrence of this in a young child suggests child sexual abuse (Reading & Rannan-Eliya, 2007).

Warts (Verrucae)

Warts, one of the most common dermatologic diseases in children, are caused by the papillomavirus. The virus has an incubation period of 1 to 6 months. The mode of transmission is unknown, but it is probably by direct contact (Androphy & Lowy, 2008).

Warts are flesh-colored, dirty-appearing papules. They generally occur on the dorsal surface of the hands, although they may occur anywhere. Plantar warts appear on the soles of the feet and are painful when children walk. They may be differentiated from calluses in that they obliterate skin lines as they grow, whereas calluses do not.

Warts on the hands or the face are generally removed if they are cosmetically unattractive to children. Plantar warts may have to be removed because of the discomfort they cause. Parents can use over-the-counter wart-removing preparations, such as Compound W, to dissolve them. Application of 40% salicylic acid may be prescribed to remove plantar warts. Carbon dioxide snow, liquid nitrogen, electrodesiccation, and curettage are also effective for removal, but these methods are painful and rarely necessary.

Children need reassurance that people do not catch warts from frogs or toads and even if left without any treatment, warts will eventually fade by themselves after about 24 months. Anogenital warts need special consideration as they can be a mark of sexual abuse (Reading & Rannan-Eliya, 2007).

Viruses Causing Central Nervous System Diseases

Viruses are responsible for causing several central nervous system disorders such as rabies, encephalitis, and meningitis. Encephalitis and meningitis are discussed in Chapter 49.

Rabies

- Causative agent: Rabies virus
- Incubation period: 2 to 6 weeks, possibly as long as 12 months
- Period of communicability: 3 to 5 days before the onset of symptoms through the course of the disease
- Mode of transmission: The bite of rabid animals; rarely through saliva from infected animals being transferred to open lesions on a child's skin
- Immunity: Contracting the disease apparently offers active immunity, but few people have ever survived the illness to verify this.
- Active artificial immunity: Human diploid cell rabies vaccine
- Passive artificial immunity: Rabies immune globulin (RIG)

Any warm-blooded animal can contract rabies. Wild animals, such as skunks, squirrels, raccoons, and bats, constitute the most important sources of infection from rabies in the United States. However, children receive more bites and, therefore, more treatments for rabies from bites of dogs or cats. Bites of rodents are seldom found to be rabid. Bites from other children are not rabid, although therapy is required because such bites usually contain streptococci. In the animal infected with rabies, the virus can be cultured from the central nervous system, saliva, urine, lymph, and blood. When a child is bitten by an infected animal, the virus migrates from the bite area to the child's central nervous system. Cranial nerve and spinal cord nuclei become acutely damaged. Negri bodies (cytoplasmic inclusion bodies) can be isolated from nerve cells for diagnosis (Fishbein, 2008).

Assessment. The diagnosis of rabies is established largely from the history of an animal bite and the clinical symptoms. After the long incubation period of the virus, children begin to show prodromal signs of malaise, fever, anorexia, nausea, sore throat, drowsiness, irritability, and restlessness. They may notice numbness or hyperesthesia at the area of the bite and along the course of the involved nerves. The white blood cell count will show slight leukocytosis. The cerebrospinal fluid is usually normal, with perhaps only a slight elevation in protein and cells. As the symptoms increase, there is high fever, anxiety, and hyperexcitability. Involuntary twitching movements and generalized seizures may occur. When children try to drink, there are violent contractions of the muscles of the mouth. They may drool saliva rather than swallow it because swallowing is extremely painful. These two phenomena give the disease its popular name, hydrophobia ("water-fear") (Shandera & Corrales-Medina, 2009).

As symptoms progress, children become comatose, with possible total body paralysis. Peripheral vascular collapse and death follow quickly in only 5 or 6 days. Postmortem examination will reveal the diagnostic Negri bodies in brain cells.

Therapeutic Management. Once the disease process begins, rabies is almost invariably fatal. The key is preventing the active process. All children who receive an animal bite should be seen by a primary care provider to evaluate the circumstances surrounding the bite and to decide whether to begin rabies prevention measures. The decision to treat must be made immediately if treatment is to be effective.

Taking a history of the incident to determine the type of animal is of primary importance. Most children are sure they know the type of animal if it was a dog; they may be unsure if it was a wild animal. Do not lead children into naming an animal just to please. If asked, "Was it a skunk? A raccoon? A squirrel?" children may choose an animal name because they think that is the answer expected. Instead, ask children to describe the animal; from that description, establish the kind of animal that bit the child. It helps in rural health facilities to have a picture book of animals handy so that preschoolers, in particular, can identify the animal that bit them. A rabid animal usually does not act normally. It runs blindly, often staggering; it may dribble saliva rather than swallow it. It is easy to assess whether a household pet is acting this way. It is sometimes difficult to assess the actions of a wild animal because the fear it experiences at being trapped or cornered may make it run about frantically.

An unprovoked attack is highly suggestive that the animal is rabid, rather than if the bite happens during a provoked attack. Let children know that they will not be punished if they were provoking an animal so they feel free to say so. Statements such as "I was only hugging him" or "I was just feeding him" may sound innocent but may have constituted a provoked attack to the animal.

The kind of wound that a child receives also is instrumental in deciding whether to begin treatment. A bite mark is much more serious than a scratch from an animal's claws. The immunization status of the animal should be checked if available. Whether rabies exists in the community at the time of the attack will also influence the decision. An animal that has been properly immunized against rabies will rarely transmit the virus. If there have been no other reported instances in domestic animals, the chance that this dog bite is serious in terms of rabies is lower than if dogs with rabies have been reported in the area.

Inspect the wound carefully to see whether it was caused by teeth marks or scratch marks. Wash the wound well with an antiseptic. If puncture wounds are present, the wound must not be sutured and closed, because tetanus (organisms that are anaerobic and grow in deep, closed wounds, where oxygen does not reach) can develop in the wound. The animal that caused the bite should be located if possible and then confined for 5 to 10 days. If it develops any signs of rabies during this period, it will be destroyed and the brain examined for evidence of rabies. Domestic animals are not destroyed unless they show signs of rabies; if people are unaware of this, they may resist surrendering an animal for observation.

If the animal is found to be rabid, children receive both rabies vaccine and antirabies serum (RIG). This applies also if the animal escapes and its condition is unknown (it is assumed to be rabid). A portion of the RIG dose is injected into the wound site and the remainder is given intramuscularly. Antirabies vaccine is given immediately and then again on days 3, 7, 14, and 28 (Fishbein, 2008).

It may seem contradictory to give an active immunization serum (administering antigen to children) when they have received an animal bite (which administers antigen to them). This is done because the rabies virus has a long incubation period before antibody production is stimulated; administering RIG provides antibodies against the rabies virus immediately. Administering rabies vaccine allows the child to begin additional antibody formation so that by the time the rabies virus from the bite begins to have an effect (2 to 6 weeks after the bite), the child has developed sufficient antibodies to combat it and prevent the illness.

West Nile Virus Disease

Although the West Nile virus may be transmitted by contaminated blood products, it is usually spread by the bite of a mosquito after the mosquito has bitten, and acquired the infection from, a natural host such as an infected bird (CDC, 2007).

Fortunately, most children who contract the disease remain asymptomatic. A small number develop flulike symptoms such as fever, fatigue, and malaise. A few develop encephalitis, with symptoms such as mental confusion, lethargy, photophobia, headache, muscle weakness, and coma, leading to death. West Nile virus disease is diagnosed when antibodies to the virus are recovered from blood serum. There is no specific therapy for the disorder, except for supportive measures to maintain function.

Parents can help prevent the spread of West Nile disease in several important ways:

- Urge children to wear long sleeves and pants to avoid mosquito bites.
- Have children apply insect repellent with DEET if hiking near swampy areas where mosquitoes may breed.
- Urge children to avoid outside activities between dusk and dawn, when mosquitoes are most likely to bite.
- Empty potential stagnant water sources, such as bird baths, to prevent mosquitoes from breeding close to the house.

Other Viral Infections

Mumps (Epidemic Parotitis)

- Causative agent: Mumps virus
- Incubation period: 14 to 21 days
- Period of communicability: Shortly before and after onset of parotitis
- Mode of transmission: Direct or indirect contact
- Immunity: Contracting the disease gives lasting natural immunity.
- Active artificial immunity: Attenuated live mumps vaccine
- Passive artificial immunity: Mumps immune globulin

Assessment. Mumps is now a rare disease in the United States due to successful immunization programs. It is most likely to be seen in adolescents who have not been immunized. If the disease occurs, it begins with fever, headache, anorexia, and malaise. Within 24 hours, an "earache" occurs. When the child points to the site of the pain, however, the child points, not to the ear, but to the jawline just in front of the ear lobe. Chewing movements aggravate the pain. By the next day, the parotid gland (located just in

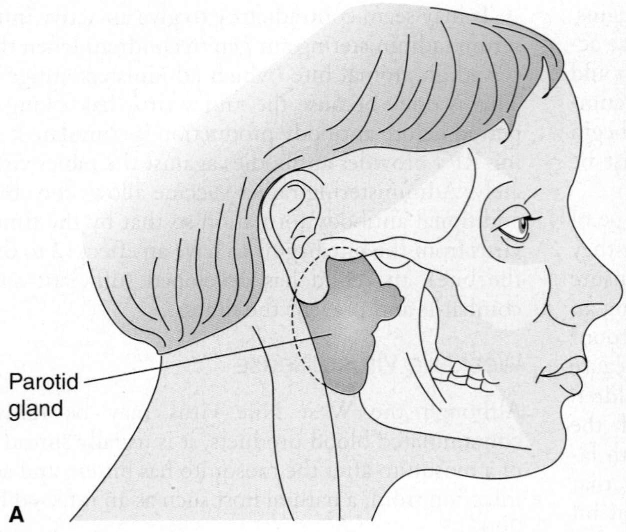

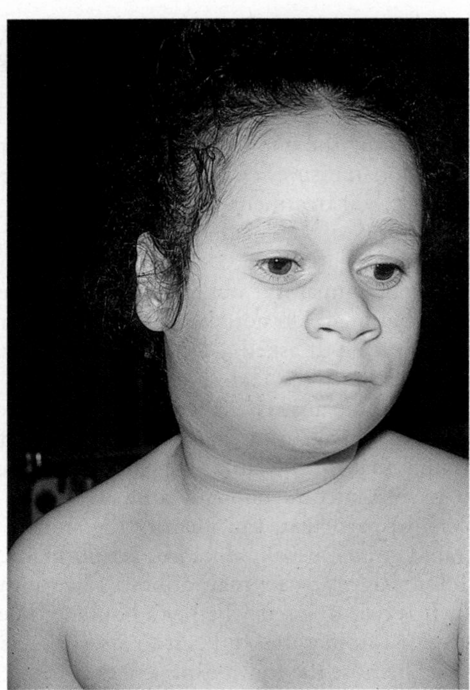

FIGURE 43.10 Infectious parotitis. (**A**) The parotid gland is located just in front of the ear. (**B**) A boy with parotitis (mumps). (© Morris Huberland/Science Source/Photo Researchers.)

front of the earlobe) is swollen and tender. As the parotid gland swells, it displaces the ear upward and backward. Boys also may develop testicular pain and swelling (orchitis).

It is often difficult to differentiate mumps from submaxillary adenitis (swelling of lymph nodes). The best method of differentiation is to place a hand along the child's jaw line. If the major amount of swelling is above the hand, it is probably mumps. If the largest amount of swelling is below the hand line, it is probably adenitis (Fig. 43.10).

Therapeutic Management. Because chewing movements are so painful, children may need soft or liquid foods until the major portion of the swelling recedes (about 6 days). It is also more difficult for them to swallow sour foods than sweet ones. They may need an analgesic for pain and an antipyretic for fever. If a child is hospitalized, follow droplet precautions in addition to standard infection precautions. Children are still infectious for at least 5 days after symptoms appear so shouldn't return to school until this time (Levin & Weinberg, 2008).

One attack of mumps gives lasting immunity. Some parents worry that because their child has swelling only on one side, the child will develop mumps on the opposite side in the future. If a child does appear to have mumps twice, the diagnosis was probably confused with cervical adenitis one of the two times.

Mumps is a potentially serious illness because several serious complications can occur. If mumps orchitis develops, it is generally unilateral. A single testis swells rapidly and is painful and tender. When the fever declines, testicular swelling also decreases, although the tenderness may exist for weeks. Atrophy of the testis may result leading to a low sperm count. The chance that mumps orchitis will lead to complete sterility is exaggerated, however (Butel, 2007).

The complication of meningoencephalitis occurs in a few children. Severe permanent hearing impairment is a rare complication that may occur because of neuritis of the auditory nerve.

✔ Checkpoint Question 43.2

Which is the best description of mumps (infectious parotitis)?

a. Cervical lymph nodes become swollen.
b. Swelling behind the child's ear occurs.
c. Swelling above the jaw line occurs.
d. The adenoid tonsils are red and swollen.

Infectious Mononucleosis

- Causative agent: Epstein-Barr virus
- Incubation period: Unknown; probably 2 to 8 weeks
- Period of communicability: Unknown; probably only during acute illness
- Mode of transmission: Direct and indirect contact
- Immunity: One episode apparently gives lasting immunity. No vaccination is available.

Infectious mononucleosis is also known as glandular fever or, because it was first discovered as a disease that is transferred readily from one person to another by kissing, the *kissing disease*. It occurs most commonly in adolescents and young adults, although it may occur in any age child (Butel, 2007).

Assessment. The beginning symptoms include chills, fever, headache, anorexia, and malaise. Children develop enlarged lymph nodes and a severe sore throat. The fever is generally high (103° F [39.5° C]) and lasts approximately 6 days.

The cervical lymph nodes, most markedly affected, feel firm and tender. The tonsils feel painful and are enlarged and erythematous. A thick, white membrane may cover the ton-

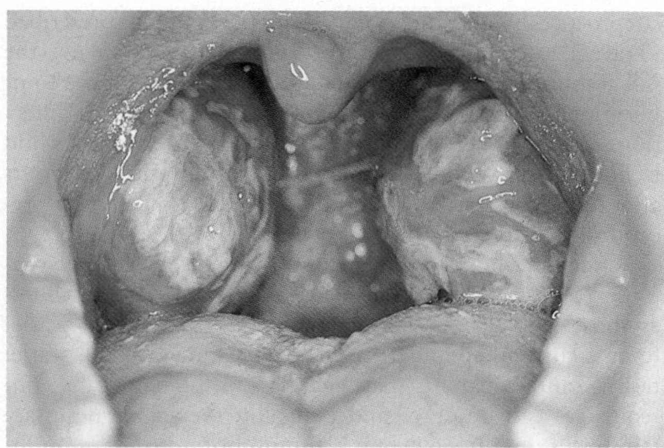

FIGURE 43.11 Appearance of the tonsils in a child with infectious mononucleosis. Note the degree of erythema, enlargement, and purulent covering. (© Dr. P. Marazzi/SPL/Science Source/Photo Researchers.)

sils and often petechiae appear on the palate (Fig. 43.11). If the mesenteric lymph nodes enlarge, children may experience abdominal pain so sharp it simulates appendicitis. The spleen enlarges, placing the child at risk for spontaneous rupture. Hepatitis, a maculopapular eruption similar to the rash of rubella, pneumonitis, and central nervous system involvement such as encephalitis, meningitis, or polyneuritis may occur.

Lymphocytosis, or lymphocytes representing more than 50% of the total white blood cell count, occurs. Of these lymphocytes, a significant number (more than 20%) are atypical; they are larger-than-normal, mature lymphocytes, and their nuclei are somewhat less dense. A serologic test, known as the heterophil antibody test, is based on the fact that the antibody produced in infectious mononucleosis will agglutinate sheep red blood cells. A technique known as the Monospot test has also been developed, using horse red blood cells. This test can be performed in minutes. A positive test, along with the increased number of atypical lymphocytes apparent on a blood slide, confirms the diagnosis of infectious mononucleosis. Epstein-Barr virus antibodies can be recovered from blood serum for a final diagnosis.

Therapeutic Management. Children with infectious mononucleosis need bedrest during the acute stage of the illness (7 to 10 days) because with the splenomegaly there is a danger of spleen rupture with any trauma to that area. If a child is hospitalized, follow standard infection precautions. Be careful in helping children with this disease turn in bed so that no pressure is placed over the splenic area. If palpating the spleen, do so gently to avoid inadvertent rupture.

Teach children and parents the importance of maintaining a good fluid intake despite the sore throat. Cool, nonacidic fluids are often tolerated best.

Neurologic complications such as meningitis or encephalitis may occur. Children may notice weakness and general fatigue for up to 6 weeks after the illness. Caution them to avoid contact sports as long as their spleen is enlarged. Because infectious mononucleosis occurs primarily in young adults, it may interrupt school or career plans. Help these young adults to voice their frustration with this illness. Offer support to help them through this unexpected interruption in their life.

✔ *Checkpoint Question 43.3*

For a child with infectious mononucleosis, why must abdominal palpation be performed gently?

a. Regional lymph nodes are painful.
b. The enlarged spleen can rupture.
c. Red cells pocket just under the skin.
d. Petechiae form easily from bruising.

Hantavirus Pulmonary Syndrome Infection

The hantavirus is a member of the arbovirus group. The virus infects small rodents and perhaps cats who have eaten mice. In the Far East, the virus produces an illness marked by extreme purpura from thrombocytopenia and severe gastrointestinal symptoms. In 1993, an outbreak of severe illness from a previously undiscovered hantavirus occurred in the United States. Outbreaks continue to occur sporadically. Major symptoms are fever, muscle aches, thrombocytopenia, gastrointestinal symptoms, and hypotension. Death can occur from rapid progressive pulmonary edema.

Supportive care is necessary, as antiviral medications do not seem to be effective (Koo & Shandera, 2009). Caution families not to touch dead mice and to have mice exterminated from their homes to avoid the possibility of contracting this disease.

BACTERIAL INFECTIONS

Bacteria reproduce by fission, in which one cell enlarges and duplicates itself, then divides into two equal parts. They are usually single-celled organisms occurring in three main shapes: spheres (cocci), rods (bacilli), and spirals (spirochetes). Bacteria are independent, living organisms. They have a nucleus, cytoplasm, and a cell wall, and they contain both DNA and RNA.

Bacteria are most commonly observed under a microscope after being fixed to a slide by heating followed by staining. Bacteria that stain violet are gram-positive organisms; those that stain red are gram-negative organisms. Those that cannot be decolorized with acid after being stained are acid-fast. As some bacteria grow, they produce **exotoxins,** or poisons. If this happens, disease symptoms arise not from the bacteria itself but from the effect of these toxins on the body. Tetanus, botulism, and diphtheria are diseases caused by the systemic spread of toxins produced by bacteria.

Some bacteria are capable of producing enzymes as they grow. Hemolytic streptococci, for example, produce streptokinase, which enables the bacteria to pass through blood clots. Penicillinase, an enzyme produced by certain bacteria, can destroy penicillin. Many first-generation penicillins are therefore ineffective against such organisms.

Streptococcal Diseases

Streptococci, gram-positive organisms, are found normally in the respiratory, alimentary, and female genital tracts. Most severe diseases in children result from infection with

Streptococcus pyogenes (beta-hemolytic streptococci, group A). Beta-hemolytic, group B streptococcal infection can be contracted from vaginal secretions at birth (see Chapter 26) and so tends to occur in newborns. Streptococcal pharyngeal infection is discussed in Chapter 40 with other throat infections. Rheumatic fever and glomerulonephritis, conditions that may result as an autoimmune response to streptococci, are discussed in Chapters 41 and 46, respectively.

Scarlet Fever

- Causative agent: Beta-hemolytic streptococci, group A
- Incubation period: 2 to 5 days
- Period of communicability: Greatest during acute phase of respiratory illness; 1 to 7 days
- Mode of transmission: Direct contact and large droplets
- Immunity: One episode of disease gives lasting immunity to scarlet fever toxin. No vaccination is available.

Assessment. Scarlet fever occurs most commonly in the 6- to 12-year-old age group, although it may be seen in preschoolers. The incidence is highest in temperate climates, and the disease occurs usually in late winter or early spring.

The symptoms of scarlet fever begin abruptly and are those of a streptococcal pharyngitis: fever, sore throat, perhaps headache, chills, and malaise. As the beta-hemolytic, group A streptococcus grows in the child's body, it produces several toxins; erythrogenic toxin is the one responsible for the rash of scarlet fever. The rash appears 12 to 48 hours after the onset of the pharyngeal symptoms (see Fig. 43.3). The fever is high (103° to 104° F [39.5° to 40.0° C]) on the first day of throat symptoms and again on the day the rash appears, and then gradually returns to normal. The pulse rate may be increased out of proportion to the fever.

The rash of scarlet fever is both enanthematous and exanthematous (on both mucous membrane and skin). The tonsils are inflamed and enlarged and usually covered with white exudate. The uvula and pharynx are beefy red. The palate is usually covered with erythematous punctiform (pinpoint) lesions and perhaps scattered petechiae. The tongue, during the first 2 days of the illness, is white and appears furry. By day 3, papillae enlarge and protrude through the white coat, giving the tongue a "white strawberry" appearance. By day 4 or 5, the white coat disappears and the prominent papillae of the tongue give it a "red strawberry" appearance. A "strawberry tongue" is distinctive for scarlet fever and helps to differentiate the disease from other rashes. A throat culture reveals streptococci.

The skin rash is typically red, pinpoint lesions that blanch on pressure and feel as rough as sandpaper. Lesions are densest on the trunk and in skin folds. Few lesions appear on the face. The area around the mouth tends to be abnormally pale (circumoral pallor). There are areas of hyperpigmentation in skin folds at the joints (Pastia's sign). The rash persists for approximately 1 week. It desquamates, with large areas of skin peeling off in fine flakes.

Therapeutic Management. Children with scarlet fever usually appear ill. They need a soft or liquid diet for a few days until their throat soreness has diminished. They may need an analgesic and antipyretic, such as acetaminophen (Tylenol) or children's ibuprofen (Motrin) for pain and fever. The rash of scarlet fever tends to be pruritic, so comfort measures are necessary. Because the underlying cause of the illness is a streptococcal infection, a course of penicillin is prescribed (Travers & Mousdicas, 2008). Caution parents to give the full amount prescribed for the full course to prevent the complications of beta-hemolytic, group A streptococcal infections (acute glomerulonephritis or rheumatic fever). If a child is hospitalized, follow droplet precautions until 24 hours after therapy is started, in addition to standard infection precautions (see Box 43.4).

Children who receive penicillin may not develop the typical extreme rash and do not have as severe a systemic illness as those who do not receive penicillin. As a result, scarlet fever is currently popularly termed scarlatina (a small, scarlet rash). Caution parents that regardless of the name, the consequences can be grave and penicillin therapy is necessary (see Focus on Nursing Care Planning Box 43.6).

✔ Checkpoint Question 43.4

Marty has developed scarlet fever. What is the mark of scarlet fever lesions?

a. They appear on skin and mucous membranes.
b. The crusts that form are mildly contagious.
c. The lesions weep a clear, sticky fluid.
d. Lesions are dark brown to black.

Impetigo

- Causative agent: Beta-hemolytic streptococcus, group A (nonbullous); *Staphylococcus aureus* (bullous)
- Incubation period: 2 to 5 days
- Period of communicability: From outbreak of lesions until lesions are healed
- Mode of transmission: Direct contact with lesions
- Immunity: None

Impetigo is only mildly infectious because it seems to be transmitted only by direct contact (Cole & Gazewood, 2007). It is not uncommon to see several children in a family with identical lesions, however. Parents may be upset at being told their child has impetigo because at one time the lesions (dirty and crusty-appearing) were associated with poverty and poor hygiene.

Assessment. Impetigo is a superficial infection of the skin. It begins as a single papulovesicular lesion surrounded by localized erythema. As more vesicles appear, they become purulent, ooze, and form honey-colored crusts (Fig. 43.12). They are found most commonly on the face and extremities. They are often seen as secondary infections of insect bites or in children who have body piercings. If there are several lesions, children may have local swollen lymph nodes.

Therapeutic Management. Treatment is oral administration of penicillin or erythromycin or the application of mupirocin (Bactroban) ointment for 7 to 10 days (Box 43.7). The lesions heal most quickly if a parent or the child washes the crusts daily with soap and water.

Although rare, complications of rheumatic fever or acute glomerulonephritis may occur after impetigo, as they may after other streptococcal infections. If a child develops impetigo while in the hospital, follow contact precautions until 24 hours after initiation of therapy.

(text continues on page 1279)

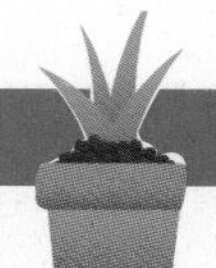

BOX 43.6 ✻ Focus on Nursing Care Planning

A Multidisciplinary Care Map for a Hospitalized Child With Scarlet Fever

Marty, a 10-year-old boy, was admitted to the hospital for appendicitis. The morning after surgery, his throat was painful and his arms were covered by a very itchy, red, macular rash. Marty was diagnosed as having scarlet fever. "How could this have happened?" his mother asks you. "He's not a bad kid. How could two bad things happen to him at once?"

Family Assessment ✻ Child has two siblings: a 6-year-old brother and a 10-day-old newborn. Parents are migrant crop workers. Move yearly from Florida to Connecticut to follow crops. Mother rates finances as: "We have no money."

Client Assessment ✻ Macular, pinpoint erythematous rash on abdomen, groin folds, and chest. Lesions blanch with pressure. Groin fold areas hyperpigmented. Child scratching lesions constantly. Uvula and pharynx beefy red. Tonsils inflamed and enlarged with white exudate. Temperature 103° F (39.5° C). Pinpoint lesions with two or three scattered petechiae noted on palate. Tongue white and furry. Throat culture positive for streptococcus. Other physical examination findings within normal limits for postoperative course. Child upset and crying. "I wish my Mom was here to stay with me. I'm all by myself. I can't even go to the playroom." Mother usually visits once a day in the late afternoon.

Nursing Diagnosis ✻ Social isolation related to required restrictions associated with infection control precautions

Outcome Evaluation ✻ Child states reason for restrictions; identifies time when restrictions will be lifted; expresses interest in activities proposed.

Team Member Responsible	Assessment	Intervention	Rationale	Expected Outcome
		Activities of Daily Living		
Nurse	Assess what child understands about how communicable diseases are spread.	Explain the reasons for restrictions and infection control precautions. Institute droplet precautions.	Child may associate precautions and restrictions with feelings of being punished. Droplet precautions help reduce the spread of the disease.	Child states he understands reason for isolation. Cooperates to maintain infection precautions.
Nurse	Assess what play activity would provide stimulation.	Visit the child frequently, at least every hour, and provide him with opportunities for therapeutic play.	Frequent visits help to decrease feelings of being alone. Therapeutic play helps the child deal with resentment about condition.	Child states that although he wants to go to playroom, he has found an enjoyable activity to occupy his time in his hospital room.
		Consultations		
Physician	Determine whether hospital infection control committee is aware of contagious illness in a postoperative patient.	Consult with infection control members on the possibility surgical personnel may have been exposed to scarlet fever.	Scarlet fever is contagious for 2 to 7 days prior to outbreak of rash.	Infection control committee members state they are aware of possible spread of illness to health care personnel and institute needed precautions, such as prescribed penicillin for exposed health care personnel.

(continued)

BOX 43.6 ✻ Focus on Nursing Care Planning (continued)

		Procedures/Medications		
Nurse	Determine whether child has ever had a reaction to penicillin.	Begin antibiotic therapy (penicillin V) as prescribed.	Penicillin is effective for group A beta-hemolytic streptococcus, the causative organism of scarlet fever.	Child's parents are contacted and report child has not had a previous reaction to penicillin. Child cooperates to take oral penicillin as prescribed.
Nurse	Ask child to rate pain of sore throat and itchiness of rash on scales of 1 to 10.	Administer analgesia and antihistamine prescribed. Caution child antihistamine may make him feel sleepy.	An antihistamine such as Benadryl can greatly reduce the pruritus of a rash.	Child states the itchiness of rash and pain of sore throat have decreased to tolerable levels.
		Nutrition		
Nurse/ nutritionist	Assess what fluid child would find most appealing to drink.	Provide frequent oral fluids. When soft diet is begun (child is postop appendicitis), provide soft foods.	Adequate fluid intake is important to prevent skin dryness, which increases discomfort. A soft or liquid diet is less irritating to the child's sore throat.	Child identifies favorite fluid to drink. States he is able to eat soft foods even with painful throat.
		Patient/Family Education		
Nurse/ physician	Determine whether other members of family will need prophylactic antibiotic.	Explain the purpose of prophylactic penicillin for susceptible family members.	As family members were near child during prodromal period, they are susceptible to also contract the disease.	Parent identifies susceptible family members; states she will be able to fill prescription for susceptible family members and supervise them to ensure they take prescribed antibiotic.
		Psychosocial/Spiritual/Emotional Needs		
Nurse	Assess whether child and parent understand the cause of scarlet fever.	Discuss the spread of infectious diseases is not related to "good or bad."	Mother voiced she was concerned because two diseases happened to her child at the same time.	Mother and child state they understand diseases are caused by infectious organisms, not moral status.
		Discharge Planning		
Nurse	Assess if parent is aware child's rash will be itchy for about a week.	Discuss possible measures parent can take to reduce pruritus (loose clothing, cool compresses) and measures to reduce pain of sore throat (analgesic).	If children scratch pruritic lesions, they can cause secondary infection. Sore throats interfere with comfort and ability to eat well.	Parent states she understands common measures to reduce pruritus and will begin them.

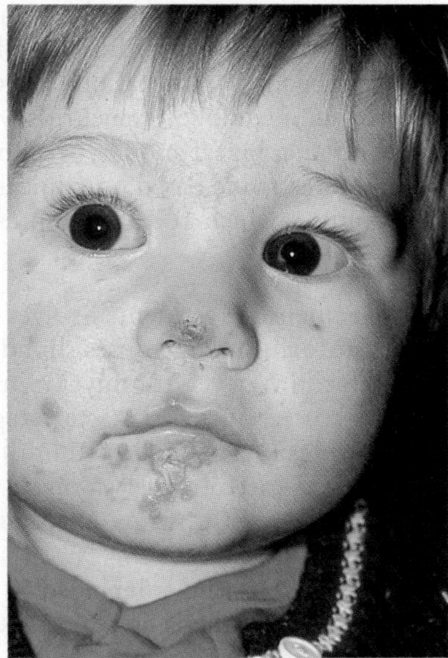

FIGURE 43.12 Impetigo in a toddler. Note the honey-colored crust appearance of some of the lesions. (© Dr. P. Marazzi/SPL/Science Source/Photo Researchers.)

Cat-Scratch Disease

- Causative agent: *Bartonella henselae* bacteria
- Incubation period: 3 to 10 days
- Period of communicability: Unknown
- Mode of transmission: Bite or scratch from a cat or kitten
- Immunity: One episode of disease gives lasting immunity; no passive artificial immunity

Cat-scratch disease occurs most commonly in preschool children because children at that age play roughly with cats or pick them up against their will and so receive scratches. At the time the child contracts the disease, the cat does not appear ill.

The first symptom for the child is a single skin papule or pustule that lasts 1 to 3 weeks. Approximately 2 weeks after the scratch, a single but severe local swollen lymph node also develops. The node most markedly involved is of the head, neck, or axilla. The node enlargement generally lasts 2 to 3 months. In some children, there is node suppuration (a node breaks open to the skin and drains sterile pus) (Fisher, 2007).

Some children have a low-grade fever and malaise. Occasionally, central nervous system involvement, such as encephalitis or meningitis, occurs. A positive reaction to a skin test of cat-scratch disease antigen is present. This, along with the history of a cat scratch and the aspiration of sterile pus from the enlarged lymph node, is diagnostic. Treatment is symptomatic, although an antibiotic may be prescribed to help shorten the course of the disease. Children may need an analgesic to relieve pain from the swollen lymph node. Aspiration of the involved node may be necessary to relieve pain.

Parents may ask if the cat should be destroyed. Because an attack of cat-scratch disease gives lifetime immunity and fewer than 10% of children scratched by the same cat contract cat-scratch disease, there is no need to destroy the cat for an act it may have seen as defending its safety.

BOX 43.7 * Focus on Pharmacology

Mupirocin (Bactroban)

Classification: Mupirocin is a topical antibiotic.

Action: Mupirocin is used to treat impetigo caused by *Staphylococcus aureus* and *Streptococcus pyogenes.*

Pregnancy risk category: B

Dosage: Small amount applied three times a day to the affected areas for 10 days

Possible adverse effects: Erythema, dry skin, pruritus, burning, stinging (Karch, 2009)

Nursing Implications

- Advise parents to wash the lesions with soap and water and pat dry before applying ointment, to soften crusts for better absorption.
- Caution parents that causative organisms are infectious by direct contact. Instruct them to wash their own hands before and after applying the ointment.
- Urge parents to continue to use the ointment to ensure eradication of the causative germs. The lesions may begin to improve before 10 days have elapsed.
- Instruct the parents to use caution when applying the ointment around the eyes. Ointment is irritating to the eyes.
- Teach the parents about the signs and symptoms of secondary fungal infection that may occur and instruct them to notify a health care provider should any occur.

Staphylococcal Infections

Staphylococcal organisms are gram-positive. Colonies of staphylococci are normally found on the skin, so they are generally the organisms involved in skin infections (pyodermas). Because the organisms grow rapidly in cream foods that are not well refrigerated, such as potato salad or cream pies, they are often the organisms involved in summer food poisoning episodes. Because food poisoning produces gastrointestinal symptoms, these infections are discussed in Chapter 45.

Furunculosis (Boils)

A furuncle is a staphylococcal infection of a hair follicle. A yellow pustule forms at the site. There is localized redness, pain, and edema of the surrounding skin. Moist heat for 20 minutes applied to the lesion can help relieve pain. Urge children not to rupture these lesions but rather to allow them to run their self-limiting course so the infection is not spread to surrounding tissue and does not become a cellulitis.

Cellulitis

Cellulitis is a staphylococcal inflammation of the deeper layers of skin. It occurs generally on the extremities or face, or surrounding wounds. The skin feels warm and is edematous and reddened. Cellulitis is treated with a systemic antibiotic. Warm soaks relieve pain and inflammation.

Methicillin-Resistant *Staphylococcus Aureus*

Methicillin-resistant *Staphylococcus aureus* (MRSA) is a strain of staphylococcus that causes skin infections and has become resistant to common broad-spectrum antibiotics. When an infection occurs in a health care setting, it is referred to as health care–associated MRSA or HA-MRSA. If it occurs in a community setting, it is CA-MRSA. Children with weakened immune systems are at most risk of contracting the infection.

An infection usually begins as a boil. It can spread to become a painful abscess or invade deeper body structures such as joints and heart valves. Children who are identified as having MRSA are isolated to help prevent spread of the bacteria to others. Vancomycin is the drug of choice for treatment of hospital based lesions because the bacteria are still susceptible to its design. Trimethoprim-sulfamethoxazole is commonly used with community infections. Use strict standard infection precaution measures when caring for a child with an MRSA infection. Teach children that the best way to prevent staphylococcal infections of the skin is good handwashing and reporting skin wounds to a health care provider before an open wound can become infected (Pallin et al., 2008).

Scalded Skin Disease

Scalded skin disease (Ritter's disease) is a staphylococcal infection seen primarily in newborns. Children develop rough-textured skin and general erythema. Large bullae (vesicles), filled with clear fluid, form. The epidermis separates in large sheets, leaving a red, glistening, scalded-looking surface. Children need intensive intravenous antibiotic therapy to survive this extreme infection (Painter, Trevillion, & Snape, 2007).

Other Bacterial Infections

Diphtheria

- Causative agent: *Corynebacterium diphtheriae* (Klebs-Löffler bacillus)
- Incubation period: 2 to 6 days
- Period of communicability: Rarely more than 2 weeks to 4 weeks in untreated persons; 1 to 2 days in children treated with antibiotics
- Mode of transmission: Direct or indirect contact
- Immunity: Contracting the disease gives lasting natural immunity.
- Active artificial immunity: Diphtheria toxin given as part of DTaP vaccine
- Passive artificial immunity: Diphtheria antitoxin

Assessment. Although diphtheria is an illness that should be extinct because of available immunization, it still occurs in isolated outbreaks. When diphtheria bacilli invade and grow in the nasopharynx of children, they produce an exotoxin (a potent protein poison) that causes massive cell necrosis and inflammation. The necrosing material lends itself well to the growth of the bacilli, so the bacilli reproduce rapidly. The inflammation and necrosing cells form a characteristic gray membrane on the nasopharynx. This may extend up into the nose and down into the major bronchi, causing a purulent nasal discharge and a brassy cough. The toxin is absorbed from the membrane surface and spread systemically by the bloodstream to affect major organs, such as the heart and nervous system. If untreated, myocarditis with heart failure and conduction disturbances may occur. Central nervous system involvement can include severe neuritis with paralysis of the diaphragm and pharyngeal and laryngeal muscles. The diagnosis of diphtheria is made based on clinical appearance and on a throat culture, which reveals the presence of the bacilli (Chambers, 2009).

Therapeutic Management. Treatment involves intravenous administration of antitoxin in large doses. In addition, children are given penicillin or erythromycin intravenously. Complete bedrest is crucial during the acute stage of the illness. Droplet precautions must be followed until cultures are negative. Children need careful observation at all times to prevent airway obstruction. If obstruction occurs, endotracheal intubation may be necessary.

Because the diphtheria vaccine is included in routine immunizations for infants, diphtheria is almost extinct in the United States. However, isolated instances do occur, and when they do, prompt recognition and treatment are necessary.

Whooping Cough (Pertussis)

- Causative agent: *Bordetella pertussis*
- Incubation period: 5 to 21 days
- Mode of transmission: Direct or indirect contact
- Period of communicability: Greatest in catarrhal (respiratory illness) stage
- Immunity: Contracting the disease offers lasting natural immunity.
- Active artificial immunity: Pertussis vaccine given as part of DTaP vaccine
- Passive artificial immunity: Pertussis immune serum globulin

Pertussis is a serious disease of childhood. Like diphtheria, pertussis has become quite rare because of required immunizations, but it still occurs sporadically and is actually making a comeback in some locales and in adolescents (Judelsohn & Koslap-Petraco, 2007). Those most susceptible are children who have not been immunized because a previous vaccine had possible side effects that led parents to refuse immunization.

Assessment. Pertussis manifests itself in three stages: catarrhal, paroxysmal, and convalescent. The **catarrhal stage** begins with upper respiratory symptoms such as coryza, sneezing, lacrimation, cough, and a low-grade fever. Children are irritable and listless. In some children, a mild cough is the only symptom during this stage. It lasts from 1 to 2 weeks (Knox, 2008).

The paroxysmal stage lasts 4 to 6 weeks. During this time, the cough changes from a mild one to a paroxysmal one, involving 5 to 10 short, rapid coughs, followed by a rapid inspiration, which causes the "whoop," or high-pitched crowing sound, of whooping cough. Children are in obvious distress while coughing. They may become cyanotic or red-faced, and their nose may drain thick, tenacious mucus. They often vomit after a paroxysm of coughing, and they are exhausted afterward from the effort. Attacks of coughing tend to be more severe at night.

During the convalescent stage, there is a gradual cessation of the coughing and vomiting. The cough may be present for some time, but as single, not paroxysmal, coughs. During the next year, if children develop an upper respiratory infection, they may again have a return of the paroxysmal coughing with vomiting.

Pertussis is diagnosed by its striking symptoms, although in children younger than 6 months of age, the "whoop" of the cough may be absent, making it more difficult to diagnose. The *B. pertussis* bacillus may be cultured from nasopharyngeal secretions during the catarrhal and paroxysmal stages. The white cell count, particularly the lymphocyte count, increases with whooping cough: it may be as high as 20,000 to 30,000/mm^3 at the end of the catarrhal stage (normal is 5000 to 10,000/mm^3).

Therapeutic Management. Children with pertussis are maintained on bedrest until the paroxysms of coughing subside. They need to be secluded from environmental factors, such as cigarette smoke, dust, and strenuous activity, that initiate coughing episodes. Nutrition may be a problem if the child is constantly coughing and vomiting. As a rule, frequent small meals are vomited less than larger meals. Infants with pertussis may be admitted to a health care facility for observation because they may have such tenacious secretions with coughing episodes that they need airway suction. Place an intercom in the infant's room so personnel can listen for paroxysms of coughing.

A full 10-day course of erythromycin or azithromycin may be prescribed as these drugs have the potential to shorten the period of communicability and may shorten the duration of symptoms. Droplet precautions are used until 5 days after a child starts effective therapy. Complications of pertussis include pneumonia, atelectasis, or emphysema from plugged bronchioles. Seizures from asphyxia as a result of severe paroxysms of coughing may occur. Epistaxis, subconjunctival and subarachnoid bleeding from the force of coughing, may occur. If sufficient fluid intake cannot be maintained, alkalosis and dehydration from persistent vomiting can occur.

Prevention. Little passive immunity is transferred to the newborn, so children in their early months are particularly susceptible to this disease. This is why pertussis vaccine is one of the first immunizations scheduled. Infants who have not yet been immunized or are immunocompromised and are exposed may be given pertussis immune serum globulin to protect them from contracting the disease (Wood et al., 2008).

What if... An adolescent with pertussis vomits after an episode of coughing? Should you urge him to try to eat again immediately, or do you think he would be too nauseated to do so?

Anthrax

- Causative agent: *Bacillus anthracis,* a bacteria
- Incubation period: 1 to 7 days (inhalational), 1 to 12 days (cutaneous), 1 to 7 days (gastrointestinal)
- Mode of transmission: Originally contracted from contact with cow or sheep feces; not transmissible from person to person
- Immunity: Unstudied
- Active artificial immunity: A vaccine is available for people in high-risk occupations, such as veterinarians, but it is not recommended for children.
- Passive artificial immunity: Not available

Anthrax is an acute infectious disease that is contracted from exposure to the bacteria or its spores (Bravata et al., 2007). Such bacteria live in the feces of infected cows or sheep. As the organism grows inside the human body, a toxin is produced that is the actual source of the symptoms. Children, like adults, may be affected by all three clinical forms: cutaneous, inhalational, or gastrointestinal.

Inhalational anthrax begins with a brief prodromal period of flulike symptoms, followed shortly by dyspnea, severe systemic shock, and marked evidence of mediastinal widening and pleural effusion on radiography. The mortality for this form is over 90%. Because it can be fatal and spread through coughing, inhalational anthrax has been proposed as bacteria that could be used in bioterrorism (Place et al., 2007).

Cutaneous anthrax is characterized by a skin lesion that begins as a papule, then passes through a vesicle stage to a painless depressed black eschar. Fever, malaise, and headache and regional swollen lymph nodes may accompany the skin lesion. The mortality of cutaneous anthrax is as low as 1% with antibiotic therapy.

Gastrointestinal anthrax is contracted by eating undercooked meat infected with the organism. The child develops severe abdominal pain, fever, bloody diarrhea, and septicemia. Mortality is about 25%.

If a child is exposed to anthrax, prophylaxis with ciprofloxacin (Cipro) for those over 18 years and doxycycline for younger patients should be started. Drug therapy is continued for 60 days because of the potential persistence of spores.

Tetanus (Lockjaw)

- Causative agent: *Clostridium tetani*
- Incubation period: 3 days to 3 weeks
- Period of communicability: None
- Mode of transmission: Direct or indirect contamination of a closed wound
- Immunity: Development of the disease gives lasting natural immunity.
- Active artificial immunity: Tetanus toxoid contained in DTaP vaccine
- Passive artificial immunity: Tetanus immune globulin

Tetanus, a highly fatal disease if untreated, is caused by an anaerobic, spore-forming bacillus. The bacillus, found in soil and the excretions of animals, enters the body through a wound. If the wound is deep, such as a puncture wound, where the distal end of the wound is shut off from an oxygen source, the tetanus bacilli begin to reproduce. The organism may also enter through a burn site, which crusts, creating an anaerobic environment. As the bacilli grow, they produce exotoxins that cause the disease symptoms by affecting the motor nuclei of the central nervous system (Ogle & Anderson, 2008).

The entrance site of the bacillus does not appear infected (no pus or reddened area is present unless a secondary infection also exists). After the incubation period, the exotoxins have developed to such an extent, however, that they are capable of disrupting the nervous system. In the United States most children are vaccinated against tetanus; in developing countries it continues to have a high incidence, caused by infection of an entry point such as the umbilical cord at birth (Roper, Vandelaer, & Gasse, 2007).

Assessment. The first symptoms that are noticeable are stiffness of the neck and jaw (lockjaw). Within 24 to 48 hours, muscular rigidity of the trunk and extremities develops. The back becomes arched (opisthotonos), the abdominal muscles are stiff and boardlike, and the face assumes an unusual appearance, with wrinkling of the forehead and distortion of the corners of the mouth (a "sardonic grin" sign). Any stimulation, such as a sudden noise, a bright light, or a touch, causes painful, paroxysmal spasms. The sensorium is clear throughout the course of the disease, so the child is aware of the pain associated with muscle spasms. As these spasms begin to include laryngospasm, respiratory obstruction, and a collection of secretions in the respiratory tract, death by asphyxiation may occur.

Fever is an ominous sign accompanying tetanus. Children who survive the disease rarely have more than a low-grade fever.

Therapeutic Management. A child needs to be cared for in a quiet, stimulation-free room. If the wound has necrotic tissue, it may be débrided to ensure that no secondary infections arise. Enteral or total parenteral nutrition may be necessary to prevent aspiration from laryngeal spasm. Tetanus immune globulin (human) is administered to supply passive antitoxins to combat the growing organisms.

Parenteral penicillin G or erythromycin is administered to reduce the number of growing forms of the bacillus. Sedation and a muscle relaxant may be necessary to reduce the severity and pain of the muscle spasms. A child may need to be intubated and mechanical ventilation begun to maintain respiratory function.

Prevention. Tetanus is a serious disease, but it can be prevented through active immunization and suitable booster immunization. Children routinely receive tetanus immunization as part of routine DTaP immunization and a booster dose at school age; thereafter they should receive a booster dose every 10 years. At the time of a wound, the wound site should be cleaned well with soap and water and a suitable antiseptic. If the wound is deep, such as a knife stab, a nail puncture, or a dog bite, it should not be sutured but should be left open to heal by secondary intention. This reduces the possibility of an anaerobic pocket forming in the wound. If the child received basic immunization against tetanus and it has been fewer than 10 years since the last injection, no booster or antitoxin management is needed at the time of the wound.

If a child's immunization record cannot be obtained, or if it has been more than 10 years since the child received a booster injection or an initial injection for tetanus, a child will probably be treated with a booster injection and tetanus immune globulin. A booster injection provides tetanus antigen to the child. If the child received initial immunization for this disease, the booster will cause the body to "remember" how to make tetanus antibodies, and the body will begin to produce them rapidly. By the time the invading tetanus organisms from the wound have passed their long incubation period (3 days to 3 weeks), the child will have antibodies in the system prepared to eradicate the organisms. If the initial immunizations were incomplete or are unknown, in addition to tetanus antigen the child will also receive the passive antibodies included in tetanus immune globulin (Ogle & Anderson, 2008).

Lyme Disease

- Causative agent: *Borrelia burgdorferi,* a spirochete
- Incubation period: 3 to 30 days
- Period of communicability: Not communicable from one person to another
- Mode of transmission: Deer tick
- Active artificial immunity: Lyme disease vaccine

Lyme disease is caused by a spirochete, *Borrelia burgdorferi,* that is transmitted by a tick often carried on deer (Philip & Jacobs, 2009). The disease is the most frequently reported vector-borne infection in the United States, occurring most often in the summer and early fall. Almost immediately after the tick bite, an erythematous papule is noticeable at the site, which spreads over the next 3 to 30 days (the incubation period) to become a large, round ring with a raised swollen border (erythema chronicum migrans; Fig. 43.13). This is followed by systemic involvement that leads to cardiac, musculoskeletal, and neurologic symptoms. Cardiac involvement may be so severe that it includes heart block from atrioventricular conduction abnormalities. Neurologic symptoms commonly include stiff neck, headache, and cranial nerve palsy. Musculoskeletal symptoms occur in 50% of children and include painful swollen arthritic joints, particularly the knee.

Amoxicillin or penicillin V is administered at the time of the bite to young children. Doxycycline is given to those older than 8 years of age. A vaccine for the disease has been approved for use in adults who live or work in high-risk areas but not yet for children.

Parents should be cautioned to inspect the skin of children who have been playing in wooded areas for tick bites to help identify the disorder before debilitating symptoms occur. Other suggestions for avoiding Lyme disease are shown in Box 43.8.

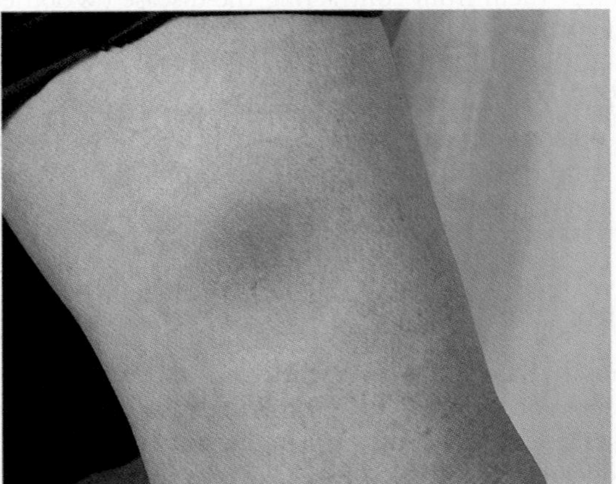

FIGURE 43.13 The rash of Lyme disease. (© Larry Mulvehill/Science Source/Photo Researchers.)

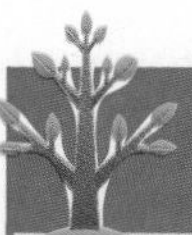

BOX 43.8 * Focus on Family Teaching

Tips for Avoiding Exposure to Lyme Disease

Q. Marty's father tells you, "My children love to play in the woods, but I'm so afraid that they'll get Lyme disease. What can I do to protect them?"

A. Here are some suggestions for you and your children to help reduce the risk for exposure to Lyme disease:

- Wear protective clothing when hiking or playing in wooded areas: long sleeves, high necklines, long slacks. Tuck bottom of slacks into socks or boots.
- Wear light-colored clothing, so any tick present on clothing can be readily observed.
- Inspect skin for ticks thoroughly after hiking or playing in wooded areas. Remove any ticks found with tweezers.
- Report any area of inflammation that might be a tick bite to a health care provider for early diagnosis.
- Ask your primary care provider about the availability of Lyme disease vaccine. Currently, it is administered only to adults with high-risk occupations, but it is anticipated that the vaccine will soon be available for children living in high-risk areas.

OTHER INFECTIOUS PATHOGENS

Rickettsial Diseases

Rickettsiae are organisms that resemble viruses both in size and in their inability to reproduce except inside the cells of a host organism. They reproduce by fission, however, as bacteria do; like bacteria, they are complete organisms containing both RNA and DNA. They multiply inside ticks, lice, mites, or fleas (arthropods) without causing disease. They are transmitted to humans through the bite or feces of the infected arthropod. An exception is Q fever, which is spread by droplet infection. All rickettsial diseases include fever, and almost all include a rash caused by rickettsial multiplication in the endothelial cells of small blood vessels. Rickettsiae invasion triggers an immune response.

Rocky Mountain Spotted Fever

- Causative agent: *Rickettsia rickettsii*
- Incubation period: 3 to 12 days
- Period of communicability: Not communicable from one person to another
- Mode of transmission: Wood, dog, or rabbit tick
- Active artificial immunity: Rocky Mountain spotted fever vaccine

Rocky Mountain spotted fever is the second most common rickettsial disease seen in the United States. It is most prevalent in the western United States and is transmitted by a tick (Buckingham et al., 2007). It is seen most often during the spring and early summer, when ticks are most commonly seen. A reddened area develops at the site of the tick bite. In 2 to 8 days, a typical rash, persistent headache, fever (as high as 104° F [40° C]), and mental confusion begin. The rash is distinctive, beginning with reddened macules, then changing to petechiae. It begins on the wrists and ankles, then spreads up the arms and legs onto the trunk. Unlike most rashes, it can cover the palms and soles (Fig. 43.14).

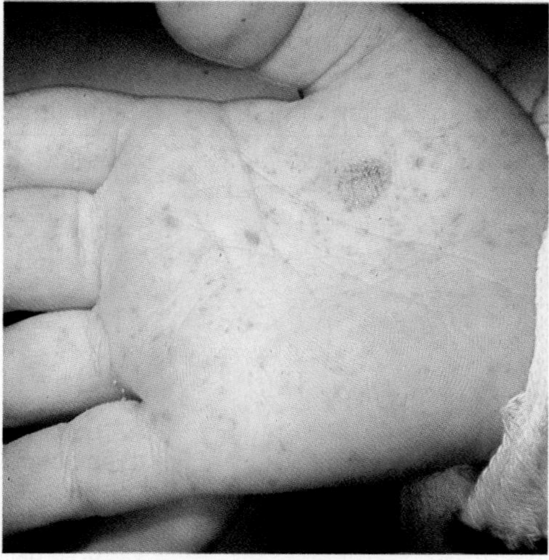

FIGURE 43.14 Typical rash of Rocky Mountain spotted fever. (Courtesy of Stuart Starr, MD, The Children's Hospital of Philadelphia.)

In untreated children, symptoms worsen to include central nervous system involvement (stiff neck and seizures) and cardiac and pulmonary symptoms such as heart failure and pneumonia. Nitrogen loss in the urine becomes extreme. An accompanying hyponatremia may also be present.

Therapy is with tetracycline or erythromycin for 7 to 10 days. Caution parents to administer the drug for the full course of therapy to ensure disease eradication and prevent the risk of complications. Rocky Mountain spotted fever was a serious childhood illness before antibiotic therapy was available, and it still has the potential to be serious if the symptoms are not reported when they first occur.

Murine Typhus

Murine typhus is seen almost exclusively in the southern United States. It is transmitted by mites and fleas that live on rats. Its symptoms are almost identical to those of Rocky Mountain spotted fever. It responds to tetracycline or a third-generation antibiotic such as ciprofloxacin (Cipro).

Chlamydial Infections

Chlamydiae are gram-negative nonmotile organisms similar to rickettsiae. Chlamydial pneumonia or vaginitis may occur in children (see Chapters 40 and 47). Psittacosis is a chlamydial infection commonly found in children.

Psittacosis

Psittacosis, caused by *Chlamydia psittaci,* is a disease transmitted to children by birds, such as parakeets, lovebirds, parrots, chickens, turkeys, and pigeons (Ogle & Anderson, 2008). The bird has no apparent symptoms of illness. Children develop symptoms of an upper respiratory infection, possibly accompanied by a low-grade fever, a dry cough, weakness, and anorexia out of proportion to the fever. An enlarged spleen may also be present. Children may

TABLE 43.3 ✻ Common Parasitic Infections

Infection	Organism	Symptoms	Treatment
Pediculosis capitis	Head lice	Small, white flecks on hair shaft (nits or eggs of lice) Extreme pruritus	Wash hair with shampoo such as lindane (Kwell). Comb nits from hair with fine-toothed comb. Wash bed sheets, recently worn clothes. Vacuum pillows, mattresses, or other items unable to be washed. Teach children not to exchange combs, hair barrettes, or other personal items.
Pediculosis	Pubic lice	Same as for head lice except on pubic hair	Same as head lice
Scabies	Female mite (*Acarus scabiei*)	Black burrow filled with mite feces 1–2 inches long, usually between fingers and toes, on palms, or in axilla or groin	Caution adolescent that groin infestations might be spread by physical intimacy. Wash area with lindane (Kwell) lotion or permethrin (Elimite).

develop patchy bronchopneumonia. The course of the disease is as long as 3 to 4 weeks. Treatment is with erythromycin for young children and tetracycline for children over the age of 8 years.

Parasitic Infections

Parasites are organisms that live on and obtain their food supply from other organisms. Frequently seen parasites in children include head lice and scabies (Table 43.3). Parents are often embarrassed when they learn that their child has lice. Reassure them that this infestation can happen to any child (Box 43.9).

BOX 43.9 ✻ Focus on Communication

When Marty's 6-year-old brother Joshua visits him, you notice he has scratch marks on his neck and forehead. His hair shafts are covered by sandlike particles. You suspect he has pediculosis capitis or head lice.

Less Effective Communication

Nurse: Mrs. Ireland, I'm wondering if you've noticed these sandlike particles in your son's hair.

Mrs. Ireland: Well, you know boys. They don't always wash well.

Nurse: I'm concerned they may be the eggs of head lice.

Mrs. Ireland: We're not that poor. Don't insult us.

Nurse: I didn't mean to. Like you said, it's probably something else.

More Effective Communication

Nurse: Mrs. Ireland, I'm wondering if you've noticed these sandlike particles in your son's hair.

Mrs. Ireland: Well, you know boys. They don't always wash well.

Nurse: I'm concerned they may be the eggs of head lice.

Mrs. Ireland: We're not that poor. Don't insult us.

Nurse: Let's talk about head lice, and how easy it is for anyone to get them.

The above scenario is an example of what can happen if people believe one of the myths that circulate related to communicable diseases. Head lice can be spread easily in locker rooms or classrooms, so any child can contract them.

Helminthic Infections

Helminths are pathogenic or parasitic worms. They may be roundworms (nematodes), flukes (trematodes), or tapeworms (cestodes). Most helminths begin life when the eggs or larvae are eliminated in the feces or urine of humans. They are then transmitted to the oral cavity by contaminated foods or hands. Because children tend to be careless about washing their hands before eating or tend to suck their thumbs, they are prone to these infections (Wilson & Caumes, 2008).

Roundworms (Ascariasis)

The roundworm parasite lives in the intestinal tract. Eggs are excreted in the feces. Children typically ingest the eggs when they eat food with hands that are improperly washed. Larvae, which hatch from the ingested eggs, penetrate the intestinal wall and enter the circulation. From there, they may migrate to any body tissue. Children have a loss of appetite and perhaps nausea and vomiting. Intestinal obstruction may occur from a mass of roundworms in the intestinal tract. Ascariasis can be prevented by the sanitary disposal of feces to prevent contamination of the soil. A single dose of an anthelmintic such as pyrantel pamoate (Antiminth) controls the infection.

Hookworms

Hookworm eggs, like roundworm eggs, are found in human feces. They enter children's bodies through the skin and then migrate to the intestinal tract, where they attach themselves onto the intestinal villi. They suck blood from the intestinal wall to sustain themselves. If a great number of hookworms are present, severe anemia may result. Treatment is with anthelmintics to destroy the worms. Children may also need therapy for the anemia.

Pinworms

Pinworms are small, white, threadlike worms that live in the cecum. At night, the female pinworm migrates down the intestinal tract and out the anus to deposit eggs on the skin in the anal and perianal region. The movement of the worms causes the anal area to itch, and the child awakens at night crying and scratching. Some of the eggs are then carried from the child's fingernails to the mouth. They hatch in the child's intestinal tract, and the cycle is repeated (Weinberg & Levin, 2008).

The worms are large enough that they can be seen if children's buttocks are separated when they are sleeping. Pressing a piece of cellophane tape against the anus and then looking at it under a microscope will generally reveal pinworm eggs.

Treatment is with a single dose of mebendazole (Vermox) or pyrantel pamoate (Antiminth). Both drugs destroy pinworms. All family members are treated for pinworm infestation because the worms are easily transmitted from person to person. Underclothing, bedding, towels, and nightclothes should be washed before reuse. Teach children to avoid nail-biting and to wash their hands before food preparation or eating to avoid transfer of pinworm eggs to the gastrointestinal tract.

Protozoan Infections

Protozoa are unicellular organisms. They absorb fluid through the cell membrane and can move from place to place by pseudopod, flagella, or cilia action. They are most pathogenic in the gastrointestinal, genitourinary, and circulatory systems. Some protozoa reproduce by simple binary fission; other forms have complex life cycles. Protozoa have the ability to form cysts or surround themselves with a membrane; this makes them resistant to destruction.

Giardiasis

Giardia lamblia is a protozoan infection that is responsible for epidemic outbreaks of diarrhea, particularly in travelers to Europe and in day care centers in the United States (Yoder et al., 2007).

Transmission occurs when the child ingests the cysts of the organism on unclean hands. In the intestine, the cysts develop into the mature form of the organism, causing symptoms such as diarrhea, weight loss, abdominal cramps, and nausea.

Diagnosis is made by history and recognition of the mature form of the organism in the stool or on duodenal aspiration. Therapy is with metronidazole (Flagyl) for 7 days (Escobedo & Cimerman, 2007).

Fungal Infections

Fungi are larger than bacteria; some are unicellular (yeasts), but generally they are multicellular (molds). Fungal infections are most often divided into groups according to the body tissue they infect. Deep mycoses invade internal organs. Transmission is by the inhalation of spores. Subcutaneous mycoses invade skin, subcutaneous tissue, and bone. Infections usually occur from introduction of the fungi into a wound. Superficial mycoses invade only the hair, skin, or nails.

Superficial Fungal Infections

Four superficial fungal infections are seen frequently in children: tinea cruris, pedis, capitis, and corporis.

Tinea Cruris. Tinea cruris (jock itch) occurs on the inner aspects of the thighs and scrotum. It is pruritic. Local application of clotrimazole (Lotrimin) or econazole (Spectazole) liquid or powder destroys the infection (Karch, 2009).

Tinea Pedis. Tinea pedis (athlete's foot) produces skin lesions between the toes and on the plantar surface of the foot. Pruritic, pinpoint vesicles and fissuring, especially between the toes, may occur. It is treated with liquid preparations of an antifungal agent such as clotrimazole (Lotrimin).

Tinea Capitis. Tinea capitis (ringworm) is a fungal infection that begins as an infection of a single hair follicle but spreads rapidly in a circular pattern to produce a lesion usually approximately 1 inch in diameter. The hairs involved in the lesion generally break off. The circle becomes filled with dirty-appearing scales. Some strains of tinea capitis may be detected because they glow green under a Wood's light. Newer strains of the organism do not do this, so the test is losing its accuracy.

Treatment is with griseofulvin given orally. Adolescents should be cautioned not to use alcohol while taking this drug; this may cause tachycardia. Safety during pregnancy is not established. Children need to avoid strong sunlight during therapy because photosensitivity may occur.

Tinea capitis is not as contagious as was once assumed. Children need not be kept home from school, although they should be cautioned not to exchange towels or combs or other potential fomites. The course of the disease may be long; it may be 3 months before all lesions have faded (Ali, Graham, & Forgie, 2007).

Tinea Corporis. Tinea corporis is fungal infection of the epidermal layer of the skin. It presents as a scaly ring of inflammation with a clear area in the center anywhere on the body (Fig. 43.15). Treatment is with a topical antifungal agent such as clotrimazole (Lotrimin).

Candidiasis

Candida albicans is the fungus responsible for candidal (monilial) infections. Candidal organisms grow in the vagina of many adult women and adolescents (candidal vaginitis) (see Chapter 47). Newborns born vaginally may develop an infection of the mucous membrane of the mouth (thrush or oral candidal infection). Thrush is characterized by white plaques on an erythematous base on the buccal membrane and the surface of the tongue. It resembles a milk curd left from a recent milk feeding. Thrush plaques do not scrape away, however, whereas milk curds do. The mouth is painful, and the child does not eat well due to the inflammation and local pain.

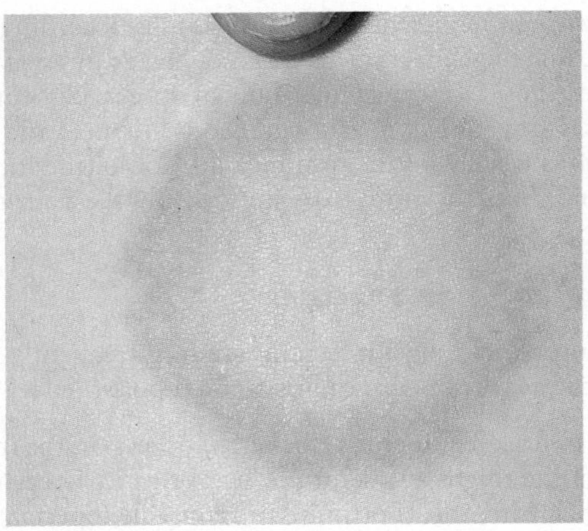

FIGURE 43.15 Ringworm. The fungus spreads rapidly, producing a circular, ringlike lesion. (© SPL/Science Source/Photo Researchers.)

C. albicans can also cause a severe, bright red, sharply circumscribed diaper-area rash (Fig. 43.16). Satellite lesions are usually also present. The rash is marked by its intense color, and it does not improve with the usual diaper rash measures, such as Desitin ointment, frequent changing of diapers, or exposure to air.

Nystatin is an example of an effective antifungal drug (Karch, 2009). For oral thrush, it is generally administered by mouth approximately four times a day. It should be dropped into the mouth after feedings so it will remain in contact with the lesions rather than being washed away immediately by a feeding. For diaper rash, a nystatin ointment is prescribed.

Candidiasis can become a generalized infection, especially in a newborn. It can spread easily through a newborn nursery (Mohan, Eddama, & Weisman, 2009). There is a tendency to think of thrush as a common, almost expected disease of infants. It needs treatment, however, to prevent it from becoming more serious or systemic or epidemic.

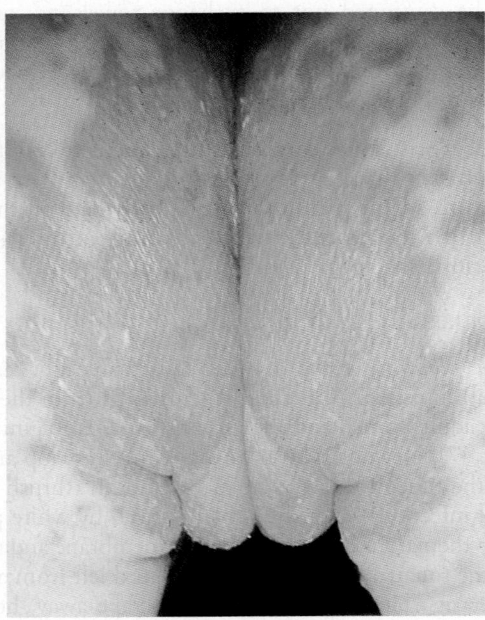

FIGURE 43.16 Monilial diaper rash. Note the intense red color of the rash. (© Custom Medical Stock Photograph.)

✓ Checkpoint Question 43.5

Marty had a pinworm infection last year. A typical symptom of this infection to assess for would be:

a. Nausea and vomiting.
b. Anal itching on awakening.
c. Loose, bloody stools.
d. Mild jaundice and itching.

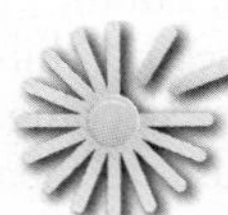

Key Points for Review

- The incubation period of an infectious disease is the time between the invasion of an organism and the onset of symptoms. The prodromal period is the time between the beginning of nonspecific symptoms and specific symptoms. Children are infectious during the prodromal period. Illness is the stage during which specific symptoms are evident. The convalescent period is the interval between the time symptoms begin to fade and the time the child returns to full wellness.
- The chain of infection depends on the presence of a reservoir, a portal of exit, a means of transmission, a portal of entry, and a susceptible host. To reduce the spread of infection, use standard infection precautions. Transmission-based precautions—airborne, droplet, and contact—also may be necessary.
- Common viral infections of childhood include exanthem subitum (roseola), rubella (German measles), measles (rubeola), chickenpox (varicella), herpes zoster, erythema infectiosum (fifth disease), pityriasis rosea, mumps (epidemic parotitis), infectious mononucleosis, and cat-scratch disease. Other important viral infections include poliomyelitis (now almost extinct), herpesvirus infections, verrucae (warts), rabies, and West Nile virus disease.
- Streptococcal diseases include scarlet fever and impetigo. Staphylococcal infections include furunculosis (boils), cellulitis, and scalded skin disease. Outbreaks of diphtheria, whooping cough (pertussis), and tetanus (lockjaw) still occur.
- Important tick-borne diseases are Rocky Mountain spotted fever and Lyme disease. Parasitic infections are pediculosis capitis (head lice), pediculosis pubis, and scabies. Helminthic infections are roundworms, hookworms, and pinworms. Fungal infections are tinea capitis and tinea corporis (ringworm).
- Teaching parents and children about infection control measures and the need for keeping immunizations up to date is essential to reduce the risk of infectious disorders in children.

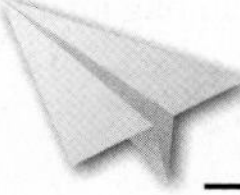

CRITICAL THINKING EXERCISES

1. Marty Ireland is the 10-year-old boy you met at the beginning of the chapter. He was diagnosed as having scarlet fever the morning after surgery for appendicitis. Is it likely that Marty contracted this infection while he was hospitalized, or is it more likely that the contact occurred before hospitalization? What is the typical pattern of scarlet fever lesions? What would you recommend to his parents to help reduce the itchiness of the rash?
2. Suppose Marty's mother tells you one disease she is not worried about is Lyme disease, as her children never eat limes. How would you respond to her?
3. Suppose Marty's mother tells you she doesn't intend to have her newborn immunized because she feels the risk of developing a complication from vaccine administration is higher than letting her child contract simple childhood illnesses. How would you counsel her?
4. Examine the National Health Goals related to infectious diseases in children. Most government-sponsored funds for nursing research are allotted based on these goals. What would be a possible research topic to explore pertinent to these goals that would be applicable to the Ireland family and also advance evidence-based practice?

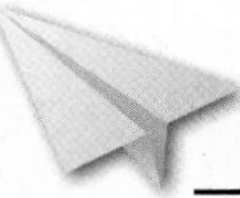

CRITICAL THINKING SCENARIO

Open the accompanying CD-ROM or visit http://thePoint.lww.com and read the Patient Scenario included for this chapter, then answer the questions to further sharpen your skills and grow more familiar with NCLEX style questions related to infectious disorders in children. Confirm your answers are correct by reading the rationales.

REFERENCES

Ali, S., Graham, T. A., & Forgie, S. E. (2007). The assessment and management of tinea capitis in children. *Pediatric Emergency Care, 23*(9), 662–665.

Androphy, E. J., & Lowy, D. R. (2008). Warts. In K. Wolff, et al. (Eds.). *Fitzpatrick's Dermatology in general medicine* (7th ed.). Columbus, OH: McGraw-Hill.

Berger, T. G. (2009). Dermatology. In S. J. McPhee & M. A. Papadakis (Eds.). *Current medical diagnosis and treatment.* Columbus, OH: McGraw-Hill.

Bravata, D. M., et al. (2007). Inhalational, gastrointestinal, and cutaneous anthrax in children: a systematic review of cases: 1900 to 2005. *Archives of Pediatrics and Adolescent Medicine, 161*(9), 896–905.

Buckingham, S. C., et al. (2007). Clinical and laboratory features, hospital course, and outcome of Rocky Mountain spotted fever in children. *Journal of Pediatrics, 150*(2), 180–184.

Butel, J. S. (2007). Paramyxoviruses and rubella virus. In G. F. Brooks, et al. (Eds.). *Jawetz, Melnick, and Adelberg's Medical Microbiology* (24th ed.). Columbus, OH: McGraw-Hill.

Centers for Disease Control and Prevention. (2007). West Nile virus update—United States, January 1–November 13, 2007. *MMWR Morbidity and Mortality Weekly Report, 56*(45), 1191–1192.

Centers for Disease Control and Prevention. (2008a). *HIV/AIDS recommendations.* Washington, DC: Author.

Centers for Disease Control and Prevention. (2008b). *Recommendations for isolation precautions in hospitals.* Washington, DC: Author.

Chambers, H. F. (2009). Infectious diseases: bacterial and chlamydial. In S. J. McPhee & M. A. Papadakis (Eds.). *Current medical diagnosis and treatment.* Columbus, OH: McGraw-Hill.

Cole, C., & Gazewood, J. (2007). Diagnosis and treatment of impetigo. *American Family Physician, 75*(6), 859–864.

Dyer, J. A. (2007). Childhood viral exanthems. *Pediatric Annals, 36*(1), 21–29.

Escobedo, A. A., & Cimerman, S. (2007). Giardiasis: a pharmacotherapy review. *Expert Opinion on Pharmacotherapy, 8*(12), 1885–1902.

Fishbein, D. B. (2008). Rabies. In F. J. Domino. (Ed.). *The 5-minute clinical consult.* Philadelphia: Lippincott Williams & Wilkins.

Fisher, W. (2007). Images in emergency medicine. *Bartonella henselae* lymphadenitis. *Annals of Emergency Medicine, 50*(1), 90–97.

Judelsohn, R. G., & Koslap-Petraco, M. B. (2007). Public health perspectives on the rising incidence of pertussis. *Public Health Nursing, 24*(5), 421–428.

Karch, A. M. (2009). *Lippincott's nursing drug guide.* Philadelphia: Lippincott Williams & Wilkins.

Knox, M. A. (2008). Common infections in children. In J. E. South-Paul, S. C. Matheny, & E. L. Lewis. (Eds.). *Current diagnosis and treatment in family medicine* (2nd ed.). Columbus, OH: McGraw-Hill.

Koo, H., & Shandera, W. X. (2009). Infectious diseases: viral and rickettsial. In S. J. McPhee & M. A. Papadakis (Eds.). *Current medical diagnosis and treatment.* Columbus, OH: McGraw-Hill.

Lauri, E. (2007). Seroprevalence of herpes simplex virus type 1 in children in the United States. *Journal of Pediatrics, 151*(4), 374–377.

Levin, M. J., & Weinberg, A. (2008). Infections: viral and rickettsial. In W. W. Hay, et al. (Eds.). *Current pediatric diagnosis and treatment* (18th ed.). Columbus, OH: McGraw-Hill.

Mark, B. A., Harless, D. W., & Berman, W. F. (2007). Nurse staffing and adverse events in hospitalized children. *Policy, Politics, & Nursing Practice, 8*(2), 83–92.

Mohan, P., Eddama, O., & Weisman, L. E. (2009). Patient isolation measures for infants with Candida colonization or infection for preventing or reducing transmission of Candida in neonatal units. *Cochrane Database of Systematic Reviews, 2009*(1), (CD006068).

Morelli, J. G., & Burch, J. M. (2008). Skin. In W. W. Hay, et al. (Eds.). *Current pediatric diagnosis and treatment* (18th ed.). Columbus, OH: McGraw-Hill.

Muller, C. P., et al. (2007). Reducing global disease burden of measles and rubella. *Vaccine, 25*(1), 1–9.

National Immunization Program. (2008). *Epidemiology and prevention of vaccine-preventable diseases* (3rd ed.). Atlanta, GA: CDC.

Ogle, J. W., & Anderson, M. S. (2008). Infections: bacterial and spirochetal. In W. W. Hay, et al. (Eds.). *Current pediatric diagnosis and treatment* (18th ed.). Columbus, OH: McGraw-Hill.

Painter, D., Trevillion, N., & Snape, T. (2007). Staphylococcal scalded skin syndrome. *Emergency Nurse, 14*(10), 20–21.

Pallin, D. J., et al. (2008). Increased US emergency department visits for skin and soft tissue infections, and changes in antibiotic choices, during the emergence of community-associated methicillin-resistant *Staphylococcus aureus. Annals of Emergency Medicine, 51*(3), 291–298.

Place, R. C., et al. (2007). Bioterrorism-related inhalational anthrax: Can extrapolated adult guidelines be applied to a pediatric population? *Biosecurity and Bioterrorism, 5*(1), 35–42.

Philip, S. S., & Jacobs, R. A. (2009). Infectious diseases: spirochetal. In S. J. McPhee & M. A. Papadakis (Eds.). *Current medical diagnosis and treatment.* Columbus, OH: McGraw-Hill.

Reading, R., & Rannan-Eliya, Y. (2007). Evidence for sexual transmission of genital herpes in children. *Archives of Disease in Childhood, 92*(7), 608–613.

Roper, M. H., Vandelaer, J. H., & Gasse, F. L. (2007). Maternal and neonatal tetanus. *Lancet, 370* (9603), 1947–1959.

Servey, J. T., Reamy, B. V., & Hodge, J. (2007). Clinical presentations of parvovirus B19 infection. *American Family Physician, 75*(3), 373–376.

Shandera, W. X., & Corrales-Medina, V. F. (2009). Viral and rickettsial infections. In S. J. McPhee & M. A. Papadakis (Eds.). *Current medical diagnosis and treatment.* Columbus, OH: McGraw-Hill.

Sheth, N. P., & Keenan, M. A. (2007). Orthopedic surgery considerations in post-polio syndrome. *American Journal of Orthopedics, 36*(7), 348–353.

Thilo, E. H., & Rosenberg, A. A. (2008). The newborn infant. In W. W. Hay, et al. (Eds.). *Current pediatric diagnosis and treatment* (18th ed.). Columbus, OH: McGraw-Hill.

Travers, J. B., & Mousdicas, N. (2008). Gram-positive infections associated with toxin production. In K. Wolff, et al. (Eds.). *Fitzpatrick's dermatology in general medicine* (7th ed.). Columbus, OH: McGraw-Hill.

Weinberg, J. M. (2007). Herpes zoster: epidemiology, natural history, and common complications. *Journal of the American Academy of Dermatology, 57*(6 Suppl), S130–S135.

Weinberg, A., & Levin, M. J. (2008). Infections: parasitic and mycotic. In W. W. Hay, et al. (Eds.). *Current pediatric diagnosis and treatment* (18th ed.). Columbus, OH: McGraw-Hill.

Wilson, M. E., & Caumes, E. (2008). Helminthic infections. In K. Wolff, et al. (Eds.). *Fitzpatrick's dermatology in general medicine* (7th ed.). Columbus, OH: McGraw-Hill.

Wood, N., et al. (2008). Pertussis in infants: Preventing deaths and hospitalisations in the very young. *Journal of Paediatrics and Child Health, 44*(4), 161–165.

Yoder, J. S., et al. (2007). Giardiasis surveillance—United States, 2003-2005. *Morbidity and Mortality Weekly Report, 56*(7), 11–18.

Yorita, K. L., et al. (2008). Infectious disease hospitalizations among infants in the United States. *Pediatrics, 121*(2), 244–252.

SUGGESTED READINGS

Aber, C., Alvarez, C. E., & Schachner, L. A. (2007). Fever and rash in a child: when to worry? *Pediatric Annals, 36*(1), 30–38.

Douglas, R. M., et al. (2009). Vitamin C for preventing and treating the common cold. *Cochrane Database of Systematic Reviews, 2009*(1), (CD000980).

Gordon, R. A., Kaestner, R., & Korenman, S. (2007). The effects of maternal employment on child injuries and infectious disease. *Demography, 44*(2), 307–333.

Hilton, S., Hunt, K., & Petticrew, M. (2007). Gaps in parental understandings and experiences of vaccine-preventable diseases: a qualitative study. *Child: Care, Health and Development, 33*(2), 170–179.

Hviid, A., & Melbye, M. (2007). The impact of birth weight on infectious disease hospitalization in childhood. *American Journal of Epidemiology, 165*(7), 756–761.

Popovich, D., & McAlhany, A. (2007). Accurately diagnosing commonly misdiagnosed circular rashes. *Pediatric Nursing, 33*(4), 315–320.

Putukian, M., et al. (2008). Mononucleosis and athletic participation: an evidence-based subject review. *Clinical Journal of Sport Medicine, 18*(4), 309–315.

Senior, K. (2008). Climate change and infectious disease: a dangerous liaison? *The Lancet Infectious Diseases, 8*(2), 92–93.

Sethuraman, U., & Kamat, D. (2007). Management of child with fever after international travel. *Clinical Pediatrics, 46*(3), 222–227.

Vessey, J. A., et al. (2007). Comparing hand washing to hand sanitizers in reducing elementary school students' absenteeism. *Pediatric Nursing, 33*(4), 368–372.

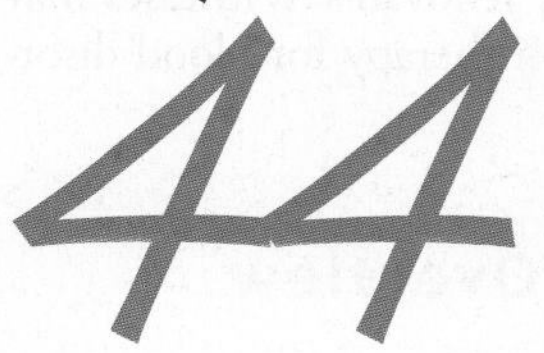

Chapter 44 Nursing Care of a Family When a Child Has a Hematologic Disorder

KEY TERMS

- agranulocytes
- allogeneic transplantation
- autologous transplantation
- blood dyscrasias
- erythroblasts
- erythrocytes
- erythropoietin
- granulocytes
- hemochromatosis
- hemolysis
- hemosiderosis
- hypodermoclysis
- leukocytes
- leukopenia
- megakaryocytes
- normoblasts
- pancytopenia
- petechiae
- plethora
- poikilocytic
- priapism
- purpura
- reticulocytes
- synergeneic transplantation
- thrombocytes
- thrombocytopenia

OBJECTIVES

After mastering the contents of this chapter, you should be able to:

1. Describe the major hematologic disorders of childhood.
2. Identify National Health Goals related to children with hematologic disorders that nurses could help the nation achieve.
3. Use critical thinking to analyze ways that nursing care for a child with a hematologic disorder could be more family centered.
4. Assess a child with a hematologic disorder.
5. Formulate nursing diagnoses for a child with a hematologic disorder such as sickle-cell anemia.
6. Identify expected outcomes for a child with a hematologic disorder.
7. Plan nursing care for a child with a hematologic disorder.
8. Implement nursing care related to a child with a hematologic disorder, such as reducing the possibility of infection.
9. Evaluate expected outcomes for achievement and effectiveness of care.
10. Identify areas related to care of children with hematologic disorders that could benefit from additional nursing research or application of evidence-based practice.
11. Integrate knowledge of hematologic disorders in children with nursing process to achieve quality maternal and child health nursing care.

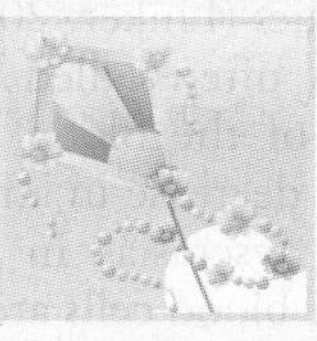

Lana is a 4-year-old girl diagnosed with thalassemia major. She has a prominent mandible and wide-spaced upper front teeth from overgrowth of bone marrow centers. Her skin is bronze from the number of transfusions (64) she has received in her short lifetime. Joey, a 7-year-old with sickle-cell anemia, is seen at the same clinic. His growth is only in the 5th percentile, and he's had two vaso-occlusive crises in the past year. "Why did this happen?" Lana's mother asks you. "Why were our two families so unlucky? What could we do to help our children have better lives?" Previous chapters described the growth and development of well children. This chapter adds information about the dramatic changes, both physical and psychosocial, that occur when children have a hematologic disorder.

What additional health teaching does Lana's mother need to help her better understand these hematologic diseases?

The blood and blood-forming tissues that make up the hematologic system play a vital role in body metabolism: transporting oxygen and nutrients to body cells, removing carbon dioxide from cells, and initiating blood coagulation when vessels are injured. As a result, any alteration in the substance or function of blood or its components can have immediate and life-threatening effects on the functioning of all body systems. For instance, an alteration in the process of coagulation can result in death from acute and uncontrollable blood loss. Inadequate red cell formation results in decreased oxygenation in tissues (Linker, 2009).

Hematologic disorders, often called **blood dyscrasias,** occur when components of the blood are formed incorrectly or either increase or decrease in amount beyond normal ranges. Most blood dyscrasias in children originate in the bone marrow, where blood cells are formed. National Health Goals related to blood disorders are shown in Box 44.1.

Blood dyscrasias do not occur at equal rates in all countries, because many of these disorders are inherited. Sickle-cell anemia, for example, occurs mainly in African Americans; thalassemia occurs in children from Mediterranean countries. Iron-deficiency anemia, an example of a noninherited disorder, tends to occur in children from lower socioeconomic areas of many countries, because iron-rich foods often are expensive. Being aware of the differences in the incidence of blood dyscrasias this way can be helpful in planning care and providing health care services for children and communities. Treatment for blood disorders can be culturally influenced as well. For example, families who are Jehovah's Witnesses may refuse blood transfusions, a common therapy for blood disorders, on religious grounds.

BOX 44.1 ✻ Focus on National Health Goals

National Health Goals have been set to address both iron-deficiency anemia and sickle-cell anemia, two common blood disorders in children:

- Reduce the incidence of iron deficiency among children aged 1 to 2 years to less than 5% and among women of childbearing age to less than 7% from baselines of 9% and 11%.
- Reduce hospitalization for sickle-cell disease yearly among children aged 9 years and under from a baseline of 41.3 hospitalizations per 100,000 children to 33 per 100,000 (http://www.nih.gov).

Nurses can help the nation achieve these goals by educating parents about the importance of women taking an iron supplement during pregnancy and adding iron-rich cereal to their infants' diets. They could help reduce hospital admissions by being certain that parents are well informed about their child's sickle-cell disease and precautions they can take to help avoid disease crises. Nursing research questions that could add important information for prevention for iron-deficiency anemia include: what are ways of increasing adherence among pregnant women that would help ensure that all women take an iron supplement during pregnancy and do infants maintain higher iron levels when cereal is eaten with milk or orange juice?

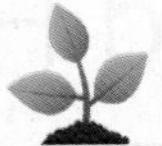

Nursing Process Overview

For a Child With a Hematologic Disorder

Assessment

Many of the symptoms of hematologic disorders begin insidiously, with symptoms such as pallor, lethargy, and bruising. These are such minor symptoms that parents may not bring their child to a health care facility for some time. They are surprised to learn when they do that such subtle symptoms can signify the presence of a serious illness.

Many hematologic disorders are inherited. When a child is diagnosed with one, parents may feel guilty or blame themselves or their partner for their child's disease. It may be difficult for parents to support a child during an illness when they need intensive support themselves because they feel the illness is their fault. Be certain both parents and children receive the support and comfort that they need.

Asking at routine checkups about a child's dietary intake often reveals iron-deficiency anemia. Many infants with this problem have been drinking too much milk and not eating enough iron-containing foods. This makes them iron-deficient, but aside from paleness and irritability, they appear plump and "healthy." Their parents do not suspect their baby's appearance masks a nutritional deficiency.

Nursing Diagnosis

Nursing diagnoses commonly used with children who have hematologic disorders are:

- Deficient knowledge related to the cause of child's illness
- Imbalanced nutrition, less than body requirements, related to parental lack of knowledge of need for iron-rich foods
- Anxiety related to frequent blood-sampling procedures
- Pain related to tissue ischemia
- Compromised family coping related to long-term care needs of child with a chronic hematologic disorder

Outcome Identification and Planning

When helping parents plan outcomes, be certain that the outcomes are realistic for both the child and family. It may not be possible to reduce the number of blood-sampling procedures, for example, but a child can be helped, with distraction techniques, to deal with the pain and anxiety the procedures produce.

Children with hematologic disorders often are prescribed long-term medication such as a corticosteroid. When a child appears very ill, parents are usually very conscientious about giving such medicine. When a child has a disorder with few symptoms, however, like a blood dyscrasia, it is easy for parents to forget to give the medication. In addition, a child may refuse to take the medication for a long time because it tastes bad or upsets the stomach. Planning includes helping parents devise ways to disguise the taste or remember to give the medication over the long term.

Nutritional planning is another area that needs consideration. Parents of children with iron-deficiency anemia, for example, may need to modify meal plans not only for the child but also for the entire family; this is not necessarily easy to do, because iron-rich foods are expensive. If children are "fussy eaters," parents may need a great deal of support to insist that children eat foods containing iron rather than giving them what they want to eat. If a child will be restricted in activity for long periods because the immune system is compromised as a part of the illness, planning must include ways to keep the child engaged with friends to promote development. Parents may need help investigating possible resources for education and support to do this.

Because of the chronicity of some of the hematologic disorders, parents and children often need the support of outside agencies. Some organizations helpful for referral are the Aplastic Anemia Foundation of America (http://www.aplastic.org), Sickle-cell Disease Association of America (http://www.sicklecelldisease.org), American Society of Pediatric Hematology and Oncology (http://www.aspho.org), and National Hemophilia Foundation (http://www.hemophilia.org).

Implementation

Nursing interventions for children with hematologic disorders include helping to obtain specimens for testing and assisting with blood or hematopoietic stem cell transfusions. Remember that a finger puncture for blood is often as painful as a venipuncture (and more painful afterward because the fingertip is irritated every time the child attempts to use it). Suggesting that blood be drawn by means of an intermittent device may reduce the number of times a child is subjected to venipuncture. Applying an anesthetic cream (mixtures of lidocaine and prilocaine) before finger punctures or venipunctures also helps to reduce pain and improve cooperation with these procedures. Even so, children may need some therapeutic playtime with a syringe and a doll to express their anger about constant invasion by needles.

Outcome Evaluation

Evaluation focuses on whether short-term outcomes such as moderation of pain or elimination of anxiety in a child undergoing diagnosis or treatment were achieved and progress is being made toward the achievement of long-term outcomes such as improving the ability of the family to manage the stress of raising a child with a chronic illness or deal with frequently occurring health crises.

Examples of expected outcomes that suggest goals were achieved are:

- Parents correctly state the most frequent causes of iron-deficiency anemia.
- Child states she feels better able to cope with blood-sampling procedures through the use of imagery.
- Parents describe realistic plans to ensure adherence to long-term medication administration.
- Parents voice they understand importance of preventing dehydration in school-age child with sickle-cell anemia.

ANATOMY AND PHYSIOLOGY OF THE HEMATOPOIETIC SYSTEM

Blood components originate in the bone marrow, circulate through blood vessels, and ultimately are destroyed by the spleen.

Blood Formation and Components

The formation of blood cells begins in the fetal yolk sac as early as week 2 of intrauterine life. By month 2 of intrauterine life, the liver and spleen begin forming blood components. At approximately month 4, the bone marrow becomes and remains the active center for the origination of blood cells. As in extrauterine life, the spleen serves as the organ for the destruction of blood cells once their normal life span has passed.

The total volume of blood in the body is roughly proportional to body weight: 85 mL/kg at birth, 75 mL/kg at 6 months of age, and 70 mL/kg after the first year. The *blood plasma* (the liquid portion containing proteins, hormones, enzymes, and electrolytes) is in equilibrium with the fluid of the interstitial tissue spaces. Although it is important in diseases causing vomiting and diarrhea (when this fluid may become depleted, leading to dehydration), plasma is not a major site of hematologic disease. The formed elements—the erythrocytes (red blood cells), leukocytes (white blood cells), and thrombocytes (platelets)—are the portions most affected by hematologic disorders in children.

Erythrocytes (Red Blood Cells)

Erythrocytes (red blood cells [RBCs]) function chiefly to transport oxygen to and carry carbon dioxide away from body cells. RBCs are formed under the stimulation of **erythropoietin,** a hormone produced by the kidneys that is stimulated whenever a child has tissue hypoxia. Children with kidney disease often have a low number of RBCs because erythropoietin secretion is inadequate in diseased kidneys. *Polycythemia*, or an overproduction of RBCs, can occur in children who experience prolonged systemic hypoxia because of erythropoietin overproduction.

RBCs form first as **erythroblasts** (large, nucleated cells), then mature through **normoblast** and **reticulocyte** stages to mature, nonnucleated erythrocytes. Approximately 1% of RBCs are in the reticulocyte stage at all times. An elevated reticulocyte count indicates that rapid production of new RBCs is occurring. This is seen in children with iron-deficiency anemia once iron therapy is begun and the body is again able to produce RBCs. The absence of a nucleus in the mature red blood cell allows for increased space for oxygen transport, but it also limits the life of cells because metabolic processes are limited. At the end of their life span (about 120 days), erythrocytes are destroyed through phagocytosis by reticuloendothelial cells, found in the highest proportion in the spleen.

In infants, the long bones of the body are filled with red marrow actively producing RBCs. In early childhood, yellow marrow begins to replace this in long bones, so blood element production is then carried out mainly in the ribs, scapulae, vertebrae, and skull bones. The yellow marrow remaining in the extremities can be activated if necessary to produce additional blood products.

At birth, an infant has approximately 5 million RBCs per cubic millimeter of blood. This concentration diminishes rapidly in the first months, reaching a low of approximately 4.1 million per cubic millimeter at 3 to 4 months of age. The number then slowly increases until adolescence, when the adult value of approximately 4.9 million per cubic millimeter is reached.

Hemoglobin. The component of RBCs that allows them to carry out the transport of oxygen is *hemoglobin*, a complex protein. Hemoglobin is composed of globin, a protein (like all proteins) dependent on nitrogen metabolism for its formation, and heme, an iron-containing pigment. Deficiency of either iron stores or nitrogen, therefore, will interfere with the synthesis of hemoglobin. It is the heme portion that combines with oxygen and carbon dioxide for transport.

The hemoglobin in erythrocytes during fetal life is different from that formed after birth. Fetal hemoglobin has a special affinity for oxygen, so it can absorb oxygen at the low oxygen tension that exists in utero. It is composed of two alpha and two gamma polypeptide chains. At birth, 40% to 70% of the infant's hemoglobin is fetal hemoglobin (hemoglobin F). This is gradually replaced by adult hemoglobin (hemoglobin A) during the first 6 months of life. Hemoglobin A is composed of two alpha and two beta chains. For this reason, diseases such as sickle-cell anemia or the thalassemias, which are disorders of the beta chains, do not become apparent clinically until this hemoglobin change has occurred (at approximately 6 months of age). However, because some hemoglobin A is present even in early intrauterine life, they can be diagnosed prenatally by hemoglobin analysis or electrophoresis.

The hemoglobin amount in blood varies according to the number of RBCs present and the average amount of hemoglobin each cell contains. Hemoglobin levels are highest at birth (13.7 to 20.1 g/100 mL); they reach a low at approximately 3 months of age (9.5 to 14.5 g/100 mL), and then gradually rise again until adult values are reached at puberty (11 to 16 g/100 mL).

Bilirubin. After a RBC reaches its life span of approximately 120 days, it disintegrates and its protein component is preserved by specialized cells in the liver and spleen (reticuloendothelial cells) for further use. Iron is released for reuse by the bone marrow to construct new RBCs. As the heme portion is degraded, it is converted into protoporphyrin. Protoporphyrin is then further broken down into indirect bilirubin. Indirect bilirubin is fat soluble and cannot be excreted by the kidneys in this state. It is therefore converted by the liver enzyme glucuronyl transferase into *direct bilirubin*, which is water soluble. This is then excreted in bile.

In the newborn, generally liver function is so immature that the conversion from indirect to direct bilirubin cannot be made. Because of this, bilirubin remains in the indirect form. When the level of indirect bilirubin in the blood rises to more than 7 mg/100 mL, it permeates outside the circulatory system, and the infant shows signs of yellowing or jaundice. If excessive **hemolysis** (destruction) of RBCs occurs from other than natural causes, a child will also show signs of jaundice.

Leukocytes (White Blood Cells)

Leukocytes (white blood cells [WBCs]) are nucleated cells. They are few in number compared with RBCs, with approximately 1 WBC to every 500 RBCs. Their primary function is defense against antigen invasion. There are two main forms of WBCs: **granulocytes** (those with granules in the cell cytoplasm) and **agranulocytes** (those without granules in the cell cytoplasm). Granulocytes (often referred to as polymorphonuclear forms) are further differentiated as neutrophils, basophils, and eosinophils. The agranulocytic leukocytes are further differentiated as lymphocytes and monocytes.

A typical total white cell count is 5000 to 10,000 cells per cubic millimeter of blood. The WBC count in newborns is approximately 20,000 per cubic millimeter, a high level caused by the trauma of birth. In the newborn, granulocytes are the most common WBCs. By 14 to 30 days of life, the total WBC count falls to approximately 12,000 per cubic millimeter, and lymphocytes become the dominant type. By 4 years of age, the WBC count reaches an adult level (5000 to 10,000 cells/mm^3), and granulocytes are again the dominant type. Leukocytes are produced in response to need. Their life span varies from approximately 6 hours to unknown intervals.

Thrombocytes (Platelets)

When blood is centrifuged in a test tube, plasma rises to the top as a clear yellow fluid; red cells sink to the bottom as a dark-red paste. Between these two layers a thin white strip (often termed a buffy coat) forms that consists of the WBCs and thrombocytes. **Thrombocytes** are round, nonnucleated bodies formed by the bone marrow. Their function is capillary hemostasis and primary coagulation. The normal range is 150,000 to 300,000 per cubic millimeter after the first year. Immature thrombocytes are termed **megakaryocytes.** If large numbers of these are present in serum, it indicates that rapid production of platelets is occurring.

Blood Coagulation

Effective blood coagulation depends on a complex series of events including a combination of blood and tissue factors released from the plasma (the intrinsic pathway) and from injured tissue (the extrinsic pathway). The plasma-released factors are factors VIII, IX, and XII. Factors released from injured tissues are a tissue factor (an incomplete thromboplastin or factor III), plus factors VII and X. Together, these pathways form factor V. The names for coagulation factors are given in Box 44.2.

BOX 44.2 ✻ Blood Coagulation Factors

I	Fibrinogen
II	Prothrombin
III	Thromboplastin
IV	Calcium
V	Labile factor (platelet phospholipids)
VII	Stable factor
VIII	Antihemophilic factor
IX	Christmas factor; antihemophilic factor B; plasma thromboplastin component
X	Stuart factor
XI	Plasma thromboplastin antecedent (antihemophilic factor C)
XII	Hageman factor
XIII	Fibrin stabilizing factor

Numbers refer to the order in which factors were discovered, not to the order of action in coagulation.

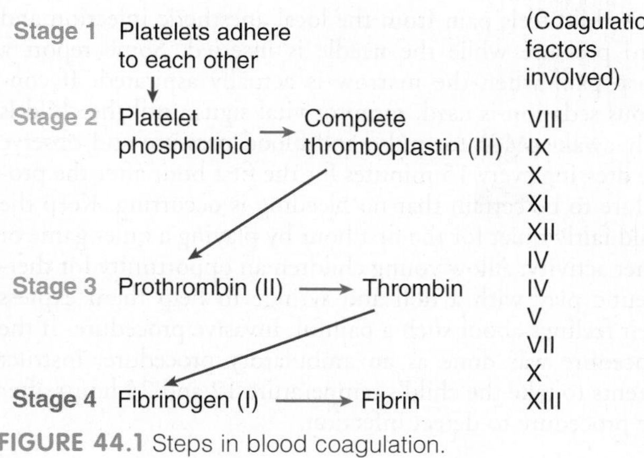

FIGURE 44.1 Steps in blood coagulation.

When a vessel is injured, vasoconstriction occurs in the area proximal to the injury, narrowing the vessel lumen and reducing the amount of blood to the injured area. Platelets begin to adhere to the damaged vessel site and to one another, forming a platelet plug. This is the first stage of clotting (Fig. 44.1).

In the second stage, factors from either the intrinsic or the extrinsic system combine with platelet phospholipid to form complete thromboplastin.

In the third stage, thromboplastin converts prothrombin (factor II) to thrombin if ionized calcium is present. The production of prothrombin and factors VII, IX, and X depends on the presence of vitamin K. This stage will be incomplete if levels of any of factors VIII through XII, vitamin K, or calcium are deficient.

In the fourth stage, thrombin converts fibrinogen (factor I) to fibrin. Fibrin strands form a mesh incorporating RBCs, WBCs, and platelets to form a permanent protective seal at the site of injury. Factor XIII (fibrin stabilizing factor) acts to make the fibrin clot insoluble and permanent.

To prevent too much coagulation after the seal is complete, plasminogen is then converted to plasmin (a fibrinolysin) near the injury to halt the clotting sequence. Blood coagulation problems will result if any step or factor in the process is inadequate. Common tests for blood coagulation are described in Table 44.1.

TABLE 44.1 ✻ Tests for Blood Coagulation

Test	Definition	Normal Value
Prothrombin time (PT)	Measures action of prothrombin after complete thromboplastin is added to the blood in a test tube; reveals deficiencies in prothrombin, factors V, VII, and X. International Normalized Ratio (INR) is a comparative rating of PT ratios that allows for more sensitive analysis.	11–13 seconds (PT) 2.0–3.0 (INR)
Partial thromboplastin time (PTT)	Measures activity of thromboplastin after incomplete thromboplastin is added to blood in a test tube; reveals deficiencies in thromboplastin, factors VIII–XII	30–45 seconds
Bleeding time	Measures the time required for bleeding at a stab wound on the earlobe to cease; reveals deficiencies in platelet formation and vasoconstrictive ability	3–10 minutes
Clot retraction	Measures platelet function; interval from placement of blood in a tube to the point clot shrinks and expels serum	Retraction at side of test tube in 1 hour; complete in 24 hours
Tourniquet	Measures capillary fragility and platelet function; response of tissue to application of tourniquet to forearm for 5–10 minutes	0–2 petechiae per 2-cm area
Prothrombin consumption time	Evaluates thromboplastin function; child's blood is allowed to clot and PT is then done on the serum; if clot formation used a great deal of prothrombin (as it should), serum prothrombin time will be brief; prolongation denotes defects in thromboplastin function	Approximately 20 seconds
Thromboplastin generation time	Tests basic ability to form thromboplastin; difficult test to do; ordered rarely to distinguish factor VIII from factor IX defects	12 seconds or less
Plasma fibrinogen	Measures stage 4 clotting process; level of fibrinogen in blood	200–400 mg/100 mL plasma
Venous clotting time (Lee-White)	Measures factor defects in stages 2 and 4; time it takes venous blood to clot in a test tube	9–12 minutes

ASSESSMENT OF AND THERAPEUTIC TECHNIQUES FOR HEMATOLOGIC DISORDERS

Assessment of children with hematologic disorders begins with a history to identify inherited disorders. For specific diagnosis, children generally require several diagnostic procedures such as blood cell or bone marrow analysis.

Bone Marrow Aspiration and Biopsy

Bone marrow aspiration provides samples of bone marrow so that the type and quantity of cells can be determined (Beattie, 2007). In children, the aspiration sites used are the iliac crests or spines (rather than the sternum, which is commonly used in adults; Fig. 44.2) because these sites have larger marrow compartments during childhood. Also, performing the test at these sites is usually less frightening for children. In neonates, the anterior tibia can be used.

For a bone marrow aspiration, a child lies prone on a treatment table. Use of a hard table rather than a bed is advantageous because pressure is needed to insert the needle through the surface of the bone into the marrow compartment. Conscious sedation may be used to help reduce the child's fear. Topical anesthesia helps reduce pain.

The area of the aspiration is cleaned with an antiseptic solution and draped. The overlying skin is infiltrated with a local anesthetic. After a few minutes, a large-bore needle and stylus is introduced through the overlying tissue into the bone. This involves considerable pressure. When the marrow cavity is reached, the stylus is removed, a syringe is attached to the needle, and bone marrow is aspirated (appears as thick blood in the syringe). The syringe is then removed, and marrow is expelled onto a slide and allowed to dry. After being sprayed with a preservative, it is taken to the laboratory for analysis. The aspiration needle is removed, and pressure is applied to the puncture site to prevent bleeding. After another few minutes, a pressure dressing is applied.

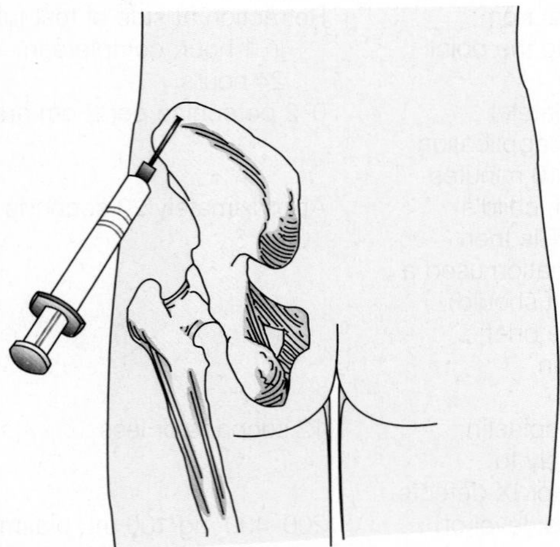

FIGURE 44.2 A common site used for bone marrow aspiration in children is the iliac crest. In neonates, the anterior tibia may be used.

A child feels pain from the local anesthetic injection and hard pressure while the needle is inserted. Some report a sharp pain when the marrow is actually aspirated. If conscious sedation is used, monitor vital signs until the child is fully awake. Monitor pulse and blood pressure and observe the dressing every 15 minutes for the first hour after the procedure to be certain that no bleeding is occurring. Keep the child fairly quiet for the first hour by playing a quiet game or other activity. Allow young children an opportunity for therapeutic play with a doll and syringe to help them express their feelings about such a painful, invasive procedure. If the procedure was done as an ambulatory procedure, instruct parents to take the child's temperature 12 and 24 hours after the procedure to detect infection.

Blood Transfusion

Transfusions of blood or its products are used in the treatment of many disorders, including the anemias and primary immunodeficiency disorders (see Chapter 42). A variety of forms of blood are available, including whole blood, packed RBCs, washed RBCs (as much "foreign" matter is removed as possible to reduce the possibility of blood reaction), plasma, plasma factors, platelets, WBCs, and albumin. No matter what is the blood product, it is important that it has been carefully matched with the child's blood type. Blood must be infused accompanied with a solution as nearly isotonic as possible (normal saline). If blood is given with a hypertonic solution, fluid will be drawn out of the RBCs, causing them to shrink; if infused with a hypotonic solution, fluid will be drawn into the cells, and they will burst. In both instances, they will be destroyed.

Packed RBCs is the most common form of transfusion used with children because they help minimize the risk of fluid overload. The usual amount of blood transfused to children is 15 mL/kg body weight. The commonly accepted rate for transfusions in a child is 10 mL/kg/hr unless the child has hypovolemic shock and volume equilibrium needs to be established. An infusion of packed RBCs at a proportion of 15 mL/kg can be expected to raise the hematocrit level 5 points. A transfusion of platelets will elevate the platelet count by approximately 10,000 cells. Platelets last only approximately 10 days, however, so transfusions of these must be repeated every 10 days.

Even if given slowly, a blood transfusion is always a strain on a child's circulation beyond that of a regular intravenous infusion, because the circulatory system must accommodate a thick, difficult-to-mobilize fluid.

Before any transfusion, ensure that a signed consent form is obtained to respect sociocultural or religious beliefs. Also obtain vital signs to establish a baseline. Monitor vital signs about every 15 minutes during the first hour and approximately every half hour for the remainder of the transfusion. Give the infusion slowly for the first 15 minutes; then increase the rate to 10 mL/kg/hr if no reaction occurs. Common symptoms of blood transfusion reactions are shown in Table 44.2.

Provide an enjoyable activity for children during transfusions. Without this, a child can become bored and could attempt to increase the infusion rate to speed up the process.

TABLE 44.2 ✻ Common Symptoms of Blood Transfusion Reactions

Symptoms	Cause	Time of Occurrence	Nursing Interventions
Headache, chills, back pain, dyspnea, hypotension, hemoglobinuria (blood in urine)	Anaphylactic reaction to incompatible blood; agglutination of red blood cells occurs; kidney tubules may become blocked, resulting in kidney failure	Immediately after start of transfusion	Discontinue transfusion. Maintain normal saline infusion for accessible intravenous line. Administer oxygen as necessary. Anticipate physician order for diuretic to increase renal tubule flow and reduce tubule plugging and/or heparin to reduce intravascular coagulation.
Pruritus, urticaria (hives), wheezing	Allergy to protein components of transfusion	Within first hour after start of transfusion	Discontinue transfusion temporarily. Give oxygen as needed. Anticipate physician order for antihistamine to reduce symptoms.
Increased temperature	Possible contaminant in transfused blood	Approximately 1 hour after start of transfusion	Discontinue transfusion. Obtain blood culture to rule out bacterial invasion as ordered.
Increased pulse, dyspnea	Circulatory overload	During course of transfusion	Discontinue transfusion. Give oxygen as needed. Provide supportive care for pulmonary edema and congestive heart failure. Anticipate physician order for diuretic to increase excretion of fluid.
Muscle cramping, twitching of extremities, convulsion	Acid-citrate-dextrose anticoagulant in transfusion is combining with serum calcium and causing hypocalcemia	During course of transfusion	Discontinue transfusion. Anticipate physician order for calcium gluconate intravenously to restore calcium level.
Fever, jaundice, lethargy, tenderness over liver	Hepatitis from contaminated transfusion	Weeks or months after transfusion	Obtain transfusion history of any child with hepatitis symptoms. Refer for care of hepatitis.
Bronze-colored skin	Hemosiderosis or deposition of iron from transfusion in skin	After repeated transfusions	Support self-esteem with altered body image. Administer iron-chelating agent (deferoxamine) as ordered to help reduce level of accumulating iron.

Hematopoietic Stem Cell Transplantation

Stem cell transplantation is the intravenous infusion of hematopoietic stem cells from bone marrow obtained by marrow aspiration or from peripheral or umbilical cord blood drawn from a donor to reestablish marrow function in a child with defective or nonfunctioning bone marrow. Donors are compatible when their human leukocyte antigen (HLA) system matches that of the recipient.

Hematopoietic stem cell transplantation has become a relatively common procedure for children with blood disorders such as acquired aplastic anemia, sickle-cell anemia, thalassemia, and leukemia and some forms of immune dysfunction diseases. Although a stressful procedure to undertake, it offers children the opportunity for a complete reversal of symptoms (Nuss & Wilson, 2007). There is no guarantee that the graft will be accepted by the recipient, or that improvement will occur. However, with good tissue compatibility in the absence of infection, this can be effective in most children.

Hematopoietic stem cells can be recovered from circulating peripheral blood after the stimulation of stem cell production by a cytokine or stem cell colony-stimulating factor. Stem cell transplants are most successful when recipients have not already received multiple blood transfusions that have sensitized them to blood products. Success also depends on the HLA compatibility of donated stem cells to the child's blood. An identical twin is the ideal donor; a parent or sibling may be next best, although compatibility is not guaranteed. Siblings have about a 25% chance of being HLA compatible.

Stem cell transplants are allogeneic, synergeneic, or autologous. **Allogeneic transplantation** involves the transfer of stem cells from an immune-compatible (histocompatible) donor, usually a sibling, although a national registry allows compatible volunteer donors to be located. **Synergeneic transplantation** involves a donor and recipient who are genetically identical (are identical twins). **Autologous transplantation** involves use of the child's own stem cells. The source of most autologous transfusions is cord blood that was banked at the child's birth (Tse, Bunting, & Laughlin, 2008). If this is not available, stem cells are aspirated from the bone marrow or obtained from circulating blood, treated to remove abnormal cells, and then reinfused.

Parents who are found to be incompatible donors may feel guilty and frustrated they can not do more for their child. If the most compatible person for transplant is a young sibling, health care personnel and parents alike may have some reservations about submitting the young child to bone marrow aspiration (Weiner et al., 2007).

To prevent a child from rejecting newly transplanted donor stem cells by the T lymphocytes, a drug such as cyclophosphamide (Cytoxan) will be administered intravenously to the child before the procedure to suppress marrow and T-lymphocyte production. This may cause nausea and vomiting. Total body irradiation to destroy the child's marrow also may be done. This is a difficult time for the child because even with antiemetic therapy, total body irradiation causes extreme nausea, vomiting, and diarrhea.

To obtain hematopoietic stem cells from peripheral blood, donors receive 5 days of a colony-stimulating factor to promote the release of stem cells into the peripheral blood. Blood is then collected by a plasmapheresis technique. If umbilical cord blood is used, it is drained from the placenta immediately after birth. It is then cryopreserved in a cord blood bank and infused into the recipient by usual blood infusion technique.

If the marrow will be taken directly from a donor, on the day of the procedure, the donor is admitted to the hospital for a 1-day stay and receives epidural anesthesia or conscious sedation, as multiple bone marrow aspirations from the posterior iliac crests are necessary for retrieval. The marrow is strained to remove fat and bone particles and any other unwanted cells. An anticoagulant is added to prevent clotting. It is then infused intravenously into the recipient's bloodstream.

Because an infused hematopoietic stem cell solution is fairly thick, the infusion takes 60 to 90 minutes. Do not use a filter that is normally used for the infusion of blood products, because this would filter out marrow tissue. Monitor the child's cardiac rate and rhythm during the infusion to detect circulatory overload or pulmonary emboli from unfiltered particles.

Fever and chills are common reactions to a hematopoietic stem cell transplant infusion. Acetaminophen (Tylenol), diazepam (Valium), or diphenhydramine hydrochloride (Benadryl) may be prescribed to reduce this reaction.

After the infusion, take the child's temperature at 1 hour and then every 4 hours to detect infection that could occur because the child's WBCs are nonfunctional from radiation or immunosuppression. Reinforce strict handwashing and limit the child's diet to cooked foods to reduce exposure to bacteria.

Almost immediately after the infusion, stem cells begin to migrate from the child's bloodstream into the marrow. If engraftment occurs (the transplant is accepted), new RBCs can be detected in the peripheral blood in approximately 3 weeks. WBCs and platelet cells may not return to normal for up to 1 year after a transplant; weight gain may also be delayed (Box 44.3).

At first, the WBC count must be measured daily; bone marrow aspirations or venous blood samples are scheduled at regular intervals to assess the growth of the new marrow.

What if... Lana's 12-year-old sister donates hematopoietic stem cells to Lana, but the transplant does not "take"? How would you explain to the donor child that she did not fail?

BOX 44.3 * Focus on Evidence-Based Practice

Do children continue to grow following hematopoietic stem cell transplantation?

To analyze the growth patterns of children following hematopoietic stem cell transplantation, researchers secured anthropometric measurements on 35 children who received a transplant in a tertiary children's hospital prior to their transplant and again at 2 and 4 months afterward. The results of the study showed that although height showed an increase, weight, skinfold triceps, and mid-arm circumference showed a decrease over the 4-month measurement period. Almost all children experienced gastrointestinal symptoms such as constipation, diarrhea, nausea, vomiting, change in taste, dry mouth, and loss of appetite that could have interfered with nutrition and be a cause of the delayed growth.

Based on the above study, would you be surprised if a child gained no weight in the 3 months since a hematopoietic stem cell transplant? Would it be important to assess gastrointestinal symptoms in all posttransplant children?

Source: Rodgers, C., et al. (2008). Growth patterns and gastrointestinal symptoms in pediatric patients after hematopoietic stem cell transplantation. *Oncology Nursing Forum, 35*(3), 443–448.

Nursing Diagnoses and Related Interventions

Nursing Diagnosis: Anxiety related to lack of knowledge about procedure and expected outcome of hematopoietic stem cell transplant

Outcome Evaluation: Parents state the reason for the transplant; state they are agreeable to the procedure even though they know the transplant may not be successful, depending on immunologic factors that are not totally known to science.

Hematopoietic stem cell transplantation is an emotional experience not only for the child but also for the parents and the marrow donor. Be certain that both the child who receives the transplant and the donor understand they are not responsible for the outcome of the transplant. Its success does not depend on their behavior or what kind of person they are but on immunologic factors over which they have no control. Be certain donors know that if bone marrow aspiration was done, the donor sites will feel tender afterward. Conscious sedation will leave them feeling exhausted for several days. Donors who have undergone bone marrow aspiration generally are asked to return to their primary care provider in 24 to 48 hours to be certain the aspiration sites are not infected (no local swelling, redness, intense pain, or fever).

Nursing Diagnosis: Risk for delayed growth and development related to extended restrictions and infection control precautions in hospital or at home

Outcome Evaluation: Parents express satisfaction with child's ongoing development. Objective tests of developmental stage show child within age-appropriate ranges.

Children may be restricted from interacting with other children to prevent them from contracting an infection following stem cell transplantation until the WBC count returns to a safe range. Because of this restriction, be certain they are not isolated from health care providers. Visit the room frequently; provide sterilized play materials as appropriate. Most children grow tired of a restricted diet and may crave fresh fruits and vegetables. Thick-skinned fruits such as bananas and oranges can be given soon after the procedure, but unwashed foods are avoided as they could carry bacteria.

Be certain children are well prepared for all procedures. Allow them to make as many choices as they can about their care to help them preserve a sense of control over their life. Children who receive a transplant need periods of therapeutic play incorporated into their care so they can begin to express their anger and frustration at the number of intravenous therapies or follow-up bone marrow aspirations they require. Measures to help children cope with pain, such as imagery, can help a child accept one more painful procedure. Encourage parents to spend time with their child during long periods of hospitalization for additional support.

Provisions for completing schoolwork need to be made as soon as a child has a return of RBCs in the peripheral blood (approximately 3 weeks). On the day of discharge, parents may be surprised that the child's blood replacement is not complete and that they will need to continue infection control measures and restrictions at home. Help them locate a support group in their community if possible. Be certain they feel free to call the transplant center after discharge if they have any problems. Once the danger of infection has passed and the restrictions can be discontinued, some parents may still be reluctant to allow their child outside, fearing that the child may still be susceptible to infection. Frequent follow-up for the next year not only is necessary to ensure that a child is free of infection but assesses whether the parents allow their child to pursue age-appropriate activities.

If children are prepared adequately for these painful or restrictive procedures and supported throughout, they should have no long-term consequences. Not all hematopoietic stem cell transplants are successful, however, and some children will die of the original disease that necessitated the transplant. A risk is that some children develop an infection despite all precautions and die of sepsis in the weeks immediately after the transplant.

Graft-Versus-Host Disease

Graft-versus-host disease (GVHD) is a potentially lethal immunologic response of donor T cells against the tissue of the bone marrow recipient (Saria & Gosselin-Acomb, 2007). The symptoms range from mild to severe and include a rash and general malaise beginning 7 to 14 days after the transplant. Latent virus infections may become active. Severe symptoms include high fever and diarrhea and liver and spleen enlargement as cells are destroyed.

Because there is no known cure for GVHD, prevention is essential. Careful tissue typing; intravenous administration of an immunosuppressant such as methotrexate, a corticosteroid, or cyclosporine before transplant; and irradiation of blood products (which helps to inactivate mature T lymphocytes) before stem cell infusion all can help reduce the incidence of this complication. Drugs such as methotrexate and cyclosporine kill all rapidly growing cells, including WBCs and T lymphocytes, so administration of these drugs after transplantation cannot be continued because they would also slow the growth of the host's new stem cells. Depletion of mature T lymphocytes from donor bone marrow before it is infused into the child offers good results, as does the administration of corticosteroids or antithymocyte globulin (ATG), an immune serum, to children after the transplant (Grosskreutz et al., 2007).

✔ Checkpoint Question 44.1

Lana, who has thalassemia major, is scheduled for a bone marrow transplant. Which is the best instruction for her regarding this?

a. She must not move while the bone marrow is infused into her.
b. She will not be allowed to eat raw fruit following the transplant.
c. Her hip bones will feel tender from the marrow transplantation.
d. She will not need any further bone marrow aspirations after this.

Splenectomy

One of the purposes of the spleen is to remove damaged or aged blood cells. This poses a problem with diseases such as sickle-cell anemia and the thalassemias because the spleen recognizes the typical cells of these diseases as damaged and destroys them. This causes children with these disorders to have a continuous anemia, with hemoglobin levels as low as 5 to 9 g/mL. In some children, therefore, removal of the spleen (splenectomy) will not cure the basic defect of the blood cells but will limit the degree of anemia (Owusu-Ofori & Hirst, 2009). Splenectomy formerly required a large abdominal incision but today it can be performed by laparoscopy.

A second function of the spleen is to strain the plasma for invading microorganisms so that phagocytes and lymphocytes can destroy them. This causes children who have had their spleen removed to be very susceptible to pneumococcal infections because this bacteria is no longer removed systematically from the body (Riddington & Owusu-Ofori, 2009). After surgery, oral penicillin is given as a prophylactic antibiotic for a year or two to guard against infection. The child should receive pneumococcal and meningococcal vaccines as well as routine immunizations, including influenza vaccine. Teach parents about signs of infection (cough, fever, general malaise), and encourage them to report any such signs immediately.

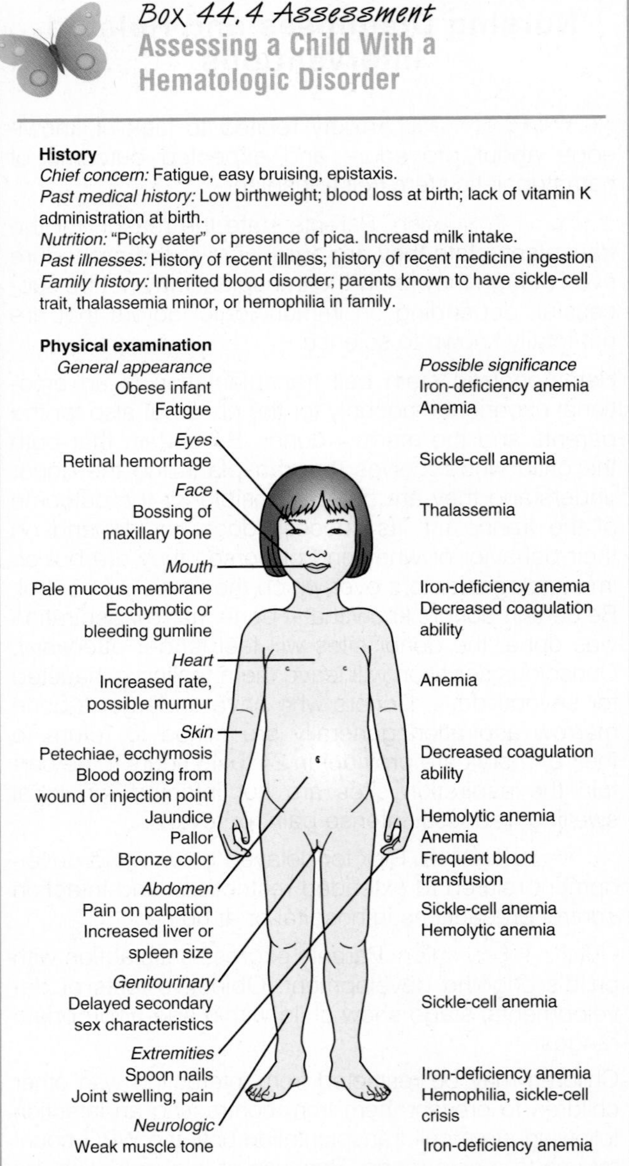

Box 44.4 Assessment
Assessing a Child With a Hematologic Disorder

History

Chief concern: Fatigue, easy bruising, epistaxis.
Past medical history: Low birthweight; blood loss at birth; lack of vitamin K administration at birth.
Nutrition: "Picky eater" or presence of pica. Increasd milk intake.
Past illnesses: History of recent illness; history of recent medicine ingestion
Family history: Inherited blood disorder; parents known to have sickle-cell trait, thalassemia minor, or hemophilia in family.

Physical examination

Physical examination	Possible significance
General appearance	
Obese infant	Iron-deficiency anemia
Fatigue	Anemia
Eyes	
Retinal hemorrhage	Sickle-cell anemia
Face	
Bossing of maxillary bone	Thalassemia
Mouth	
Pale mucous membrane	Iron-deficiency anemia
Ecchymotic or bleeding gumline	Decreased coagulation ability
Heart	
Increased rate, possible murmur	Anemia
Skin	
Petechiae, ecchymosis Blood oozing from wound or injection point	Decreased coagulation ability
Jaundice	Hemolytic anemia
Pallor	Anemia
Bronze color	Frequent blood transfusion
Abdomen	
Pain on palpation	Sickle-cell anemia
Increased liver or spleen size	Hemolytic anemia
Genitourinary	
Delayed secondary sex characteristics	Sickle-cell anemia
Extremities	
Spoon nails	Iron-deficiency anemia
Joint swelling, pain	Hemophilia, sickle-cell crisis
Neurologic	
Weak muscle tone	Iron-deficiency anemia

HEALTH PROMOTION AND RISK MANAGEMENT

Hematologic disorders cover a wide range of diseases and produce multiple symptoms in children (Box 44.4). Many disorders such as sickle-cell anemia and hemophilia are inherited. Health promotion and disease prevention, therefore, begins with ensuring that families have access to genetic counseling so they can be aware of the incidence of a disorder in their family and the potential for the disease to develop in their child.

The most frequently occurring anemia in children, iron-deficiency anemia, is preventable. This condition could be virtually eliminated if all infants were breastfed and those infants who are formula-fed were fed iron-fortified formula for the full first year. Also, when cereal is introduced, iron-fortified types should be used. The disorder occurs again with a high incidence in adolescents because adolescent diets tend to be low in meat and green vegetables, the chief dietary sources of iron. Adolescents who begin vegetarian diets become especially prone to developing the disorder. Counseling parents of young children to maintain well-child health care visits and urging adolescents to ingest iron-rich foods could have a major impact on decreasing the incidence of the disorder.

Aplastic anemia, or the inability to form blood elements, can be acquired if a child is exposed to a toxic drug or chemical. Educating parents about the importance of keeping poisons out of the reach of children could help decrease the incidence of this disorder.

Nurses can also help make the therapy for these disorders much less painful and distressing than it was in the past. All hematologic disorders require obtaining blood specimens for diagnosis and continued testing for follow-up. Many therapies include blood product transfusion. The use of EMLA cream or topical lidocaine can greatly reduce the pain of venipuncture. Helping a child to use a distraction technique such as imagery can reduce apprehension or fear associated with the procedures or treatments.

DISORDERS OF THE RED BLOOD CELLS

Most RBC disorders fall into the category of the anemias, or a reduction in the number or function of erythrocytes. Polycythemia, or an increase in the number of RBCs, can also occur and may be as dangerous to a child as a reduction in RBC production.

Anemia occurs when the rate of RBC production falls below that of cell destruction, or when there is a loss of RBCs, causing their number and the hemoglobin level to fall below the normal value for a child's age. Anemias are classified according to the changes seen in RBC numbers or configuration, or according to the source of the problem.

Although any reduction in the amount of circulating hemoglobin lessens the oxygen-carrying capacity, clinical symptoms are not apparent until the hemoglobin level reaches 7 to 8 g/100 mL. Average values for hemoglobin and RBC number are shown in Appendix F.

Normochromic, Normocytic Anemias

Normochromic, normocytic anemias are marked by impaired production of erythrocytes by the bone marrow, or by abnormal or uncompensated loss of circulating RBCs, as with acute hemorrhage. The RBCs are normal in both color and size, but there are simply too few of them.

Acute Blood-Loss Anemia

Blood loss sufficient to cause anemia might occur from trauma such as an automobile accident with internal bleeding; from acute nephritis in which blood is lost in the urine; or in the newborn from disorders such as placenta previa, premature separation of the placenta, maternal–fetal or twin-to-twin transfusion, or trauma to the cord or placenta, as might occur with cesarean birth. It can also occur from intestinal parasites such as tapeworm (Barnett et al., 2007).

Children are in shock from acute blood loss and appear pale. As the heart attempts to push the reduced amount of blood through the body more rapidly, tachycardia will occur. Loss of RBCs needed for oxygen transport causes body cells to register an oxygen deficit, and children begin to breathe rapidly. Newborns may have gasping respirations, sternal retractions, and cyanosis. They will not respond to oxygen therapy because they lack RBCs to transport and use the oxygen. Such infants become listless and inactive.

This type of acute blood-loss anemia generally is transitory because the sudden reduction in available oxygen stimulates the release of erythropoietin from the kidney and a regeneration response in the bone marrow. The reticulocyte count becomes elevated, evidence the bone marrow is trying to increase production of erythrocytes to meet the sudden shortage.

Treatment involves control of bleeding by addressing its underlying cause. The child or infant should be placed in a supine position to provide as much circulation as possible to brain cells. Keep the child warm with blankets; place an infant in an incubator or under a radiant heat warmer. Blood transfusion may be necessary to provide an immediate increase in the number of erythrocytes. Until blood is available for transfusion, a blood expander such as plasma or intravenous fluid such as normal saline or Ringer's lactate may be given to expand blood volume and improve blood pressure.

Anemia of Acute Infection

Acute infection or inflammation, especially in infants, may lead to increased destruction or decreased production of erythrocytes. Common conditions include osteomyelitis, ulcerative colitis, and kidney infection. Management involves treatment of the underlying condition. When this is reversed, the blood values will return to normal.

Anemia of Renal Disease

Either acute or chronic renal disease can cause loss of function in kidney cells, and this causes an accompanying decrease in erythropoietin production. This decreases the stimulation for RBC production in the bone marrow, and a resultant normocytic, normochromic anemia occurs. Administration of recombinant human erythropoietin can increase RBC production and correct the anemia, but not the renal disease (Tse, Bunting, & Laughlin, 2008).

Anemia of Neoplastic Disease

Malignant growths such as leukemia or lymphosarcoma (common neoplasms of childhood) result in normochromic, normocytic anemias because invasion of bone marrow by proliferating neoplastic cells impairs RBC production. There may be accompanying blood loss if platelet formation also has decreased. The treatment of such an anemia involves measures designed to achieve remission of the neoplastic process and transfusion to increase the erythrocyte count.

Hypersplenism

Under normal conditions, blood is filtered rapidly through the spleen. If the spleen is enlarged and functioning abnormally, blood cells pass through more slowly, with more cells being destroyed in the process. This increased destruction of RBCs can cause anemia and may lead to pancytopenia (deficiency of all cell elements of blood). Virtually any underlying splenic condition can cause this syndrome.

Therapeutic management consists of treating the underlying splenic disorder, including possible splenectomy. Although the spleen's role in the body's defense mechanisms against infection is not well documented, the organ appears to be relatively important in early infancy. Its function decreases as a child grows older, and it may serve no immune function at all in adulthood. If the spleen is removed, there is no decrease in general immunity or in gamma globulin or antibody formation. With the removal of the spleen's filtering function, however, there seems to be an increased susceptibility to meningitis or pneumonia due to pneumococci. For this reason, a splenectomy may be delayed until after 2 years of age, when the risk of meningitis decreases. Such children should receive immunization against influenza, pneumococci, and *H. influenzae* in addition to prophylactic penicillin for 2 years after the splenectomy.

Aplastic Anemias

Aplastic anemias result from depression of hematopoietic activity in the bone marrow. The formation and development of WBCs, platelets, and RBCs can all be affected.

Congenital aplastic anemia (Fanconi syndrome) is inherited as an autosomal recessive trait. A child is born with several congenital anomalies, such as skeletal and renal abnormalities, hypogenitalism, and short stature. Between 4 and 12 years of age, a child begins to manifest symptoms of **pancytopenia,** or reduction of all blood cell components (Linker, 2009).

Acquired aplastic anemia is a decrease in bone marrow production that can occur if a child is exposed excessively to radiation, drugs, or chemicals known to cause bone marrow damage. Drugs that may cause this include chloramphenicol, sulfonamides, arsenic (contained in rat poison, sometimes eaten by children), hydantoin, benzene, or quinine. Exposure to insecticides also may cause severe bone marrow dysfunction. Chemotherapeutic drugs temporarily reduce bone marrow production. A serious infection such as meningococcal pneumonia might cause autoimmunologic suppression of the bone marrow.

Assessment. When symptoms begin, a child appears pale, fatigues easily, and has anorexia. These symptoms reflect the lower RBC count (anemia) and tissue hypoxia. Because of reduced platelet formation **(thrombocytopenia),** the child bruises easily or has **petechiae** (pinpoint, macular, purplish-red spots caused by intradermal or submucous hemorrhage). A child may have excessive nosebleeds or gastrointestinal bleeding. As a result of a decrease in WBCs **(leukopenia),** a child may contract an increased number of infections and respond poorly to antibiotic therapy. Observe closely for signs of cardiac decompensation such as tachycardia, tachypnea, shortness of breath, or cyanosis from the long-term increased workload on the heart. Ask about any exposure to drugs or chemicals or recent infection. Bone marrow samples will show a reduced number of blood elements; blood-forming spaces become infiltrated by fatty tissue.

Therapeutic Management. The ultimate therapy for both congenital and acquired aplastic anemia is hemopoietic stem cell transplantation (Gluckman et al., 2007). If a donor cannot be located, the disease is managed by procedures to suppress T-lymphocyte–dependent autoimmune responses with antithymocyte globulin (ATG) or cyclosporine or transfusion of new blood elements (Ambruso, Hays, & Goldenberg, 2008). ATG, given intravenously, must always be administered cautiously because of the high risk for anaphylaxis. Packed RBCs and platelet transfusions are generally necessary to maintain adequate blood elements. Prophylactic platelet transfusions may be given (Ferrara et al., 2007). An RBC-stimulating factor (erythropoietin) may be helpful. Colony-stimulating factors may also improve bone marrow function. Some children show improvement with a course of an oral corticosteroid (prednisone). Testosterone to stimulate RBC growth may be tried.

For children who receive a hematopoietic stem cell transplant, chances of complete recovery are good. For others, the course is uncertain. A decreased platelet count may persist for years after other blood elements have returned to normal. Bleeding, therefore, especially petechiae or purpura, may be a long-term problem. Any drug or chemical suspected of causing the bone marrow dysfunction must be discontinued at once and the child must never be exposed to that substance again. Children with aplastic anemia are apt to be irritable because of their fatigue and recurring symptoms. Their parents may feel responsible for causing the illness if it originated from exposure to a chemical such as an insecticide. Many parents will have less confidence in health care personnel if the illness followed treatment with a drug such as chloramphenicol. They wonder how they can trust in a drug to cure the illness if they believe that one drug caused the illness. How can they trust that their child will not be harmed further?

When discussing with parents the outcome of this disease, be conservatively optimistic. It may be easier for parents to deal with this problem if they face only one day or one blood test at a time rather than trying to predict the outcomes of all the blood tests to come. They need to feel they can discuss their frustration and bitterness about continual abnormal results with health care personnel. Establishing good communication with these parents does much to establish their trust in everyone caring for their child.

Nursing Diagnoses and Related Interventions

Nursing Diagnosis: Risk for infection related to dramatic decrease in number of WBCs

Outcome Evaluation: Child's temperature remains below 100° F (38.0° C) axillary; symptoms of infection such as cough, vomiting, or diarrhea are absent.

Exposure to other children must be limited as long as WBC production is inadequate to prevent infection. Remind parents of the signs and symptoms of infection and advise them to come for treatment promptly if their child shows any of these signs. In the absence of granulocytes, however, antibiotic therapy may be ineffective, and severe septicemia can result. WBCs (granulocytes) may be transfused to counteract a severe infection.

Nursing Diagnosis: Risk for disturbed body image related to changed appearance occurring as medication side effect

Outcome Evaluation: Child views self as a worthwhile person; does not appear to be excessively shy or reluctant to interact with peers.

Children who receive corticosteroids such as prednisone to suppress the immune response almost always experience some of the drug's side effects, such as a cushingoid appearance, hirsutism, hypertension, and marked weight gain. Long-term therapy with testosterone can result in masculinizing effects, such as growth of facial and body hair, the development of acne, and deepening of the voice. Be sure both children and their parents know that these effects are related to the medication and that they will remain for an extended period but will fade when the medication is withdrawn.

Adolescents may have an especially difficult time accepting weight gain and increased acne. They need a chance to express their feelings about their changed appearance. Reinforce and emphasize positive attributes.

Nursing Diagnosis: Risk for injury related to ineffective blood clotting mechanisms secondary to inadequate platelet formation

Outcome Evaluation: Child exhibits no ecchymotic skin areas, gingival bleeding, or epistaxis; stools are negative for occult blood.

Inadequate platelet formation interferes with blood coagulation, placing a child at risk for bleeding (Box 44.5).

Hypoplastic Anemias

Hypoplastic anemias also result from depression of hematopoietic activity in bone marrow; they can be either congenital or acquired. Unlike aplastic anemias, in which WBCs, RBCs, and platelets are affected, in hypoplastic anemias only RBCs are affected.

Congenital hypoplastic anemia (Blackfan-Diamond syndrome) is a rare disorder that shows symptoms as early as

BOX 44.5 ✻ Techniques for Reducing Bleeding With Thrombocytopenia

Some techniques for reducing bleeding due to inadequate platelet formation include:

- Limit the number of blood-drawing procedures; combine samples whenever possible.
- Use a blood pressure cuff instead of a tourniquet to reduce the number of petechiae.
- Apply pressure to any puncture site for a full 5 minutes before applying a bandage.
- Minimize use of adhesive tape to the skin (pulling for removal may tear the skin and cause petechiae).
- Pad side and crib rails to prevent bruising.
- Protect intravenous sites to avoid numerous reinsertions.
- Administer medication orally or by intravenous infusion when appropriate to minimize the number of injection sites.
- Assess that the child is offered foods that can be chewed without irritation (avoid toast crusts, for example).
- Urge the child to use a soft toothbrush.
- Check toys for sharp corners, which may cause scratches. Urge the child to be careful with paper, because paper cuts can bleed out of proportion to their size.
- Assess the need for routine blood pressure determinations. Tight cuffs could lead to petechiae.
- Distract the child from rough play; suggest stimulating but quiet activities to minimize risk of injury.
- Keep a record of blood drawn; do not draw extra amounts "just in case" so children do not become more anemic.

the first 6 to 8 months of life. It affects both sexes and is apparently caused by an inherent defect in RBC formation. No changes in the leukocytes or platelets occur. An acquired form is caused by infection with parvovirus, the infectious agent of fifth disease (Servey, Reamy, & Hodge, 2007).

The onset of hypoplastic anemia is insidious, and at first it may be difficult to differentiate from iron-deficiency anemia. In iron-deficiency anemia, blood cells appear hypochromic and microcytic; in hypoplastic anemia, they are normochromic and normocytic but few in number.

With acquired hypoplastic anemia, the reduction of RBCs is transient, so no therapy is necessary. Children with the congenital form show increased erythropoiesis with corticosteroid therapy. Long-term transfusions of packed RBCs are needed to raise erythrocyte levels. As a result of the necessary number of transfusions, **hemosiderosis** (deposition of iron in body tissue) can occur. Therefore, an iron chelation program such as subcutaneous infusion **(hypodermoclysis)** of deferoxamine (Desferal) may be started concurrently with transfusions. Deferoxamine binds with iron and aids its excretion from the body in urine; it is given 5 or 6 days a week over an 8-hour period. This is one of the few times that an infusion is given subcutaneously. Parents can do this at home after careful instruction, often while their child is asleep at night. The parent must assess that voiding is present and specific gravity is normal (1.003 to 1.030) before drug administration.

For such an infusion, an area beside the scapula or on the thigh is cleaned with alcohol; a short 25-gauge needle is inserted at a low angle into only the subcutaneous tissue. The medication is then allowed to infuse slowly. Periodic slit-lamp eye examinations should be scheduled to check for cataract formation, a possible adverse effect of deferoxamine.

Congenital hypoplastic anemia is a chronic condition. However, approximately one fourth of affected children will undergo spontaneous permanent remission before age 13 years. If not, they are candidates for hematopoietic stem cell transplantation. Both the child and the parents need support from health care personnel to help them accept the many procedures and tests required.

✔ Checkpoint Question 44.2

Lana has received iron chelation therapy in the past. Iron chelation therapy is:

a. A procedure to remove excess iron from the child's body.
b. A procedure to help iron move effectively into hemoglobin.
c. A therapy to increase the iron level in bone and muscle cells.
d. A therapy to convert iron into calcium to increase heart action.

Hypochromic Anemias

When hemoglobin synthesis is inadequate, the erythrocytes appear pale (hypochromia). Hypochromia is generally accompanied by a reduction in the diameter of cells (RBCs are also microcytic).

Iron-Deficiency Anemia

Although the incidence of iron-deficiency anemia is decreasing in the United States due to improved infant nutrition, it is still the most common anemia of infancy and childhood, occurring when the intake of dietary iron is inadequate. Most iron in the body is incorporated in hemoglobin, but an additional amount is stored in the bone marrow to be available for hemoglobin production. Inadequate dietary iron prevents proper hemoglobin formation. With iron-deficiency anemia, RBCs are both small in size (hypocytic) and pale (hypochromic) due to the stunted hemoglobin.

Children are at high risk for iron-deficiency anemia because they need more daily iron in proportion to their body weight to maintain an adequate iron level than do adults. This results in a necessary daily intake of 6 to 15 mg of iron. Iron-deficiency anemia occurs most often between ages 9 months and 3 years; its frequency rises again in adolescence, when iron requirements increase for girls who are menstruating. It also is found in overweight teenagers if they ingest most of their calories from high-carbohydrate, not iron-rich, foods (Brotanek et al., 2007).

Causes in Infants. Several causes lead to iron-deficiency anemia. When an infant's diet lacks sufficient iron, the infant usually has enough in reserve to last for the first 6 months. After that, if the infant's diet continues to be iron deficient, there will be difficulty forming adequate RBCs. Infants of low birth weight have fewer iron stores than those born at term because iron stores are laid down near the end of gestation. Because low-birth-weight infants also grow rapidly and their need for RBCs expands accordingly, they tend to develop iron-deficiency anemia before 5 to 6 months. As a preventive measure, they may be given an iron supplement beginning at about 2 months of age.

Women with iron deficiency during pregnancy tend to give birth to iron-deficient babies because the babies do not receive iron stores. Low hemoglobin levels from iron-deficiency anemia lead to diffusion of plasma proteins such as albumin and gamma globulin out of the bloodstream by osmosis. The loss of transferrin, a plasma protein responsible for binding iron to protein to facilitate its transportation to bone marrow after absorption from the gastrointestinal tract, further depletes this system of iron transport.

Infants born with structural defects of the gastrointestinal system, such as gastroesophageal reflux (chalasia—an immature valve between the esophagus and stomach, resulting in regurgitation) or pyloric stenosis (narrowing between the stomach and duodenum, resulting in vomiting), are particularly prone to iron-deficiency anemia. Although their diet is adequate, they cannot make use of the iron because it is never adequately digested. Infants with chronic diarrhea are also prone to this form of anemia due to inadequate absorption. Some infants develop minimal gastrointestinal bleeding if fed cow's milk; this is why breast milk or commercial formula is recommended for the full first year.

Iron-deficiency anemia can be prevented in formula-fed infants by giving them iron-fortified formula. If an infant is breastfed, iron-fortified cereal should be introduced when solid foods are introduced in the first year. Fortunately, these cost no more than nonfortified foods. Occasionally, an infant becomes constipated while ingesting iron-rich formula, but this is the exception rather than the rule.

Causes in Older Children. In children older than 2 years, chronic blood loss is the most frequent cause of iron-deficiency anemia. This is caused by gastrointestinal tract lesions such as polyps, ulcerative colitis, Crohn's disease, protein-induced enteropathies, parasitic infestation, or frequent epistaxis.

Adolescent girls can become iron deficient because of frequent attempts to diet and overconsumption of snack foods low in iron. Without sufficient iron, their body cannot compensate for the iron lost with menstrual flow.

Assessment. Common symptoms of iron-deficiency anemia are shown in Box 44.6. Children with iron-deficiency anemia appear pale. Because the pallor develops slowly, however, parents may not realize how extensive it is. They may describe their child as "fair-skinned" even though the child's pallor is so extreme the skin is transparent. In dark-skinned infants, pale mucous membranes may be the most significant finding.

Infants may show poor muscle tone and reduced activity. They are generally irritable from fatigue. Their heart may be enlarged, and there may be a soft systolic precordial murmur as the heart increases its action, attempting to supply body cells with more oxygen. The spleen may be slightly enlarged. Fingernails become typically spoon-shaped or depressed in contour.

A 24-hour dietary history generally reveals an abnormally high milk intake. As a rule, infants should not ingest more than 32 oz of milk a day. Infants with iron-deficiency anemia may be drinking up to 50 oz a day. One quart of milk provides only approximately 0.5 mg of iron. In contrast, 1 tablespoon of iron-fortified baby cereal supplies 2.5 to 5.0 mg of iron.

Box 44.6 Assessment

Assessing a Child With Iron-Deficiency Anemia

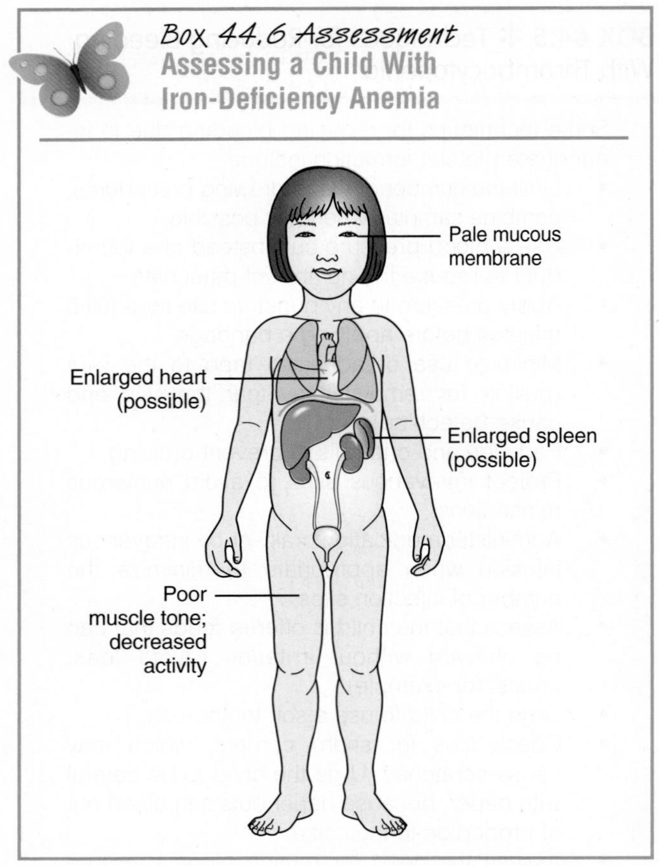

As iron-deficiency anemia develops, laboratory studies will reveal a decreased hemoglobin level (a hemoglobin level less than 11 g/100 mL of blood) and reduced hematocrit level (below 33%). The RBCs are microcytic and hypochromic and possibly **poikilocytic** (irregular in shape). The mean corpuscular volume is low. The mean corpuscular hemoglobin may be reduced. Serum iron levels are normally 70 μg/100 mL; with iron-deficiency anemia the level is often as low as 30 μg/100 mL, with an increased iron-binding capacity (more than 350 μg/100 mL). The level of serum ferritin reflects the extent of iron stores so is less than 10 μg/100 mL (normal is 35 μg/mL). Without iron, heme precursors cannot be used, so free erythrocyte protoporphyrins increase to more than 10 μg/g from a normal of 1.9 μg/g.

Monoamine oxidase (MAO) is an enzyme important for central nervous system maturation. Iron is incorporated into MAO, so without iron this necessary enzyme is absent and central nervous system maturation may be affected.

There may be an association in school-age children between iron-deficiency anemia and poor school achievement, probably related to chronic fatigue. Iron-deficiency anemia is also associated with pica (the eating of inedible substances such as dirt and paper). Eating ice cubes is common in adolescents. Until the anemia is corrected, parents need to supervise the child's environment to keep inedible materials out of his or her reach.

BOX 44.7 ✻ Focus on Pharmacology

Ferrous Sulfate (Feosol)

Classification: Ferrous sulfate is an iron salt.

Action: Supplies iron for red cell production. It elevates the serum iron concentration and then is converted to hemoglobin or trapped in the reticuloendothelial cells for storage and eventual conversion to a usable form of iron (Karch, 2009).

Pregnancy risk category: A

Dosage: For severe iron-deficiency anemia: 4 to 6 mg/kg/day, in three divided doses. For mild iron-deficiency anemia: 3 mg/kg/day in two divided doses.

Possible adverse effects: Gastrointestinal upset, anorexia, nausea, vomiting, constipation, dark stools, stained teeth (liquid preparations)

Nursing Implications

- Instruct parents to administer the drug on an empty stomach with water to enhance absorption. If this causes gastrointestinal irritation, administer it after meals. Avoid giving it with milk, eggs, coffee, or tea.
- If the liquid preparation is ordered, advise parents to mix it with water or juice to mask the taste and prevent staining of teeth. Encourage the parents to have the child drink the medication through a straw to avoid staining of the teeth.
- Keep in mind that iron is absorbed best in the presence of vitamin C. Suggest parents give the iron with a citrus juice such as orange juice to help absorption. Some children may be prescribed vitamin C to take concurrently to increase absorption.
- Inform child and parents that iron may turn stools black.
- Encourage parents to include high-fiber foods in the child's diet to minimize the risk of constipation.
- Reinforce the need for thorough brushing of teeth to prevent staining.
- Remind parents about the need for follow-up blood studies to evaluate the effectiveness of the drug.

Therapeutic Management. Therapy for iron-deficiency anemia focuses on treatment of the underlying cause. Sources of gastrointestinal bleeding must be ruled out. The diet must be rich in iron and should contain extra vitamin C, as this enhances iron absorption. An iron compound such as ferrous sulfate for 4 to 6 weeks is the drug of choice to improve RBC formation and replace iron stores (Domellof, 2007) (Box 44.7).

Nursing Diagnoses and Related Interventions

✻

Nursing Diagnosis: Imbalanced nutrition, less than body requirements, related to inadequate ingestion of iron

Outcome Evaluation: Parents report child's dietary intake includes iron-rich foods; parents administer ferrous sulfate as prescribed; serum iron levels increase to normal by 6 months.

When planning care for an infant with iron-deficiency anemia, it is helpful to minimize the child's activities to prevent fatigue, particularly at mealtime, as a fatigued child is more reluctant to eat any food, let alone eat iron-rich foods.

Counsel parents on measures to improve their infant's nutrition, such as adding iron-rich foods while decreasing formula or breast milk intake. If the child is not fond of meat, suggest parents substitute cheese, eggs, green vegetables, or fortified cereal. Because iron-rich foods are often expensive, remind parents that these items are important and that they should not substitute less expensive, high-carbohydrate foods. Before iron therapy is started, help parents create reminder sheets so they can manage to give the supplement over a long period of time. Alert parents to possible side effects, such as stomach irritation, constipation, and that liquid iron preparations can stain teeth if not taken through a straw. Iron is absorbed best with an accompanying acid medium so ascorbic acid may also be prescribed (or the parent be advised to give the iron medication with orange juice) to increase absorption. To avoid constipation, the child may need additional fiber like that supplied by green leafy vegetables. If oral iron is not tolerated or if there is a doubt the child will take it, an iron-dextran injection (Imferon) can be given intramuscularly. Imferon stains the skin and is extremely irritating unless it is given by deep Z-track intramuscular injection.

Of all age groups, adolescents tend to do the least well with taking medicine consistently. Help them plan a daily time for taking their iron supplement with a medication reminder chart. At first, they may reject this as childish, but assure them that everyone needs these charts. Review with them the iron-rich foods they will need to eat daily. An iron supplement is effective only if taken with iron-rich foods.

After 7 days of iron therapy, a reticulocyte count is usually obtained. If elevated, this means the child is now receiving adequate iron and the rapid proliferation of new erythrocytes is correcting the anemia. Iron medication must be taken for at least 4 to 6 weeks after the RBC count is normal to rebuild iron levels in the blood. In some children, maintenance therapy may continue for as long as a year.

Chronic Infection Anemia

Acute infection interferes with RBC production, producing a normochromic, normocytic anemia. When infections are chronic, anemia of a hypochromic, microcytic type occurs. This is probably caused by impaired iron metabolism as well as impaired RBC production.

The degree of anemia is rarely as severe as that occurring with iron deficiency. Administration of iron has little effect until the infection is controlled (Adamson & Longo, 2008).

Macrocytic (Megaloblastic) Anemias

A macrocytic anemia is one in which the RBCs are abnormally large (Primack & Mahaniah, 2008). These cells are actually immature erythrocytes or megaloblasts (nucleated immature red cells). For this reason, these anemias are often referred to as megaloblastic anemias. Because these anemias are caused by nutritional deficiencies, they occur less frequently in the United States than in developing countries.

Anemia of Folic Acid Deficiency

A deficiency of folic acid combined with vitamin C deficiency produces an anemia in which the erythrocytes are abnormally large. There is often accompanying neutropenia and thrombocytopenia. Mean corpuscular volume and mean corpuscular hemoglobin are increased, whereas mean corpuscular hemoglobin concentration is normal. Bone marrow will contain megaloblasts, indicating inhibition of the production of erythrocytes at an early stage. Megaloblastic arrest, or inability of RBCs to mature past an early stage, may occur in the first year of life from the continued use of infant food containing too little folic acid or from an infant drinking goat's milk, which tends to be deficient in folic acid. Treatment is daily oral administration of folic acid. Response to treatment is dramatic.

Pernicious Anemia (Vitamin B_{12} Deficiency)

Vitamin B_{12} is necessary for maturation of RBCs. Pernicious anemia results from deficiency or inability to use the vitamin (Waterbury, 2007). In children, the cause is more often lack of ingestion of vitamin B_{12}. The vitamin is found primarily in foods of animal origin, including both cow's milk and breast milk. Adolescents may be deficient in vitamin B_{12} if they are ingesting a long-term, poorly formulated vegetarian diet.

For absorption of vitamin B_{12} from the intestine, an intrinsic factor must be present in the gastric mucosa. In adults, lack of the intrinsic factor is the most frequent cause of the disorder. If a child has an intrinsic factor deficiency, symptoms can occur as early as the first 2 years of life (once the intrauterine stores of vitamin B_{12} have been exhausted). The child appears pale, anorexic, and irritable, with chronic diarrhea. The tongue appears smooth and beefy red due to papillary atrophy. In children, neuropathologic findings such as ataxia, hyporeflexia, paresthesia, and a positive Babinski reflex are less noticeable than in adults.

Laboratory findings reveal low serum levels of vitamin B_{12}. The rate and efficiency of absorption of vitamin B_{12} can be tested by the ingestion of the radioactively tagged vitamin. The dose absorbed in the presence and absence of a dose of intrinsic factor can be measured.

If the anemia is caused by a B_{12}-deficient diet, temporary injections of B_{12} will reverse the symptoms. If the anemia is caused by lack of the intrinsic factor, lifelong monthly intramuscular injections of B_{12} may be necessary. Parents and the child need to understand that lifelong therapy will be necessary.

Hemolytic Anemias

Hemolytic anemias are those in which the number of erythrocytes decreases due to increased destruction of erythrocytes. This may be caused by fundamental abnormalities of erythrocyte structure or by extracellular destruction forces.

Congenital Spherocytosis

Congenital spherocytosis is a hemolytic anemia that is inherited as an autosomal dominant trait. It occurs most frequently in the white Northern European population (Adamson & Longo, 2008). RBCs are small and defective, apparently due to abnormalities of the protein of the cell membrane that make them unusually permeable to sodium. The life span of erythrocytes is diminished.

The disease may be noticed shortly after birth, although symptoms may appear at any age. The hemolysis of RBCs appears to occur in the spleen, apparently from excessive absorption of sodium into the cell. The abnormal cell swells, ruptures, and is destroyed. Chronic jaundice and splenomegaly develop. The mean corpuscular hemoglobin concentration is increased because the cells are small. Gallstones may be present in the older school-age child and adolescent because of the continuous hemolysis, bilirubin release, and incorporation of bilirubin into gallstones.

Infections may precipitate a crisis or cause bone marrow failure. During such a period, the anemia increases rapidly as the hemolysis continues. Blood transfusion will be necessary to maintain a sufficient number of circulating erythrocytes until the crisis passes.

The diagnosis of the disease is based on family history, the obvious hemolysis, and the presence of the abnormal spherocytes. The treatment is generally splenectomy at approximately 5 to 6 years. This measure will increase the number of RBCs present but will not alter their abnormal structure.

Glucose-6-Phosphate Dehydrogenase Deficiency

The enzyme glucose-6-phosphate dehydrogenase (G6PD) is necessary for maintenance of RBC life. Lack of the enzyme results in premature destruction of RBCs. The disease is transmitted as a sex-linked recessive trait. It occurs most frequently in children of African American, Asian, Sephardic Jewish, and Mediterranean descent. Approximately 10% of African American males have the disorder (Waterbury, 2007). Because the disease is sex-linked, males of high-risk groups should be screened in infancy.

G6PD occurs in two identifiable forms. Children with congenital nonspherocytic hemolytic anemia have hemolysis, jaundice, and splenomegaly and may have aplastic crises. Other children have a drug-induced form in which the blood pattern is normal until the child is exposed to fava beans or drugs such as antipyretics, sulfonamides, antimalarials, and naphthaquinolones (the most common drug in these groups is acetylsalicylic acid [aspirin]). Approximately 2 days after ingestion of such an oxidant drug, the child begins to show evidence of hemolysis.

A blood smear will show *Heinz bodies* (oddly shaped particles in RBCs). The degree of RBC destruction depends on the drug and the extent of exposure to it. The child may have accompanying fever and back pain. Occasionally a newborn is seen with marked hemolysis because the mother ingested an initiating drug during pregnancy.

G6PD deficiency may be diagnosed by a rapid enzyme screening test or electrophoretic analysis of RBCs. Drug-induced hemolysis usually is self-limiting, and blood transfusions are rarely necessary. Both parents and children should be told of the abnormality in the child's metabolism so they can avoid common drugs such as acetylsalicylic acid.

Sickle-Cell Anemia

Sickle-cell anemia is the presence of abnormally shaped (elongated) RBCs. It is an autosomal recessive inherited disorder on the beta chain of hemoglobin; the amino acid valine takes the place of the normally appearing glutamic acid. The erythrocytes become characteristically elongated and crescent-shaped (sickled) when they are submitted to low oxygen tension (less than 60% to 70%), a low blood pH (acidosis), or increased blood viscosity, such as occurs with dehydration or hypoxia. When RBCs sickle, they can not move freely through vessels. Stasis and further sickling occur (a *sickle-cell crisis*). Blood flow halts and tissue distal to the blockage becomes ischemic, resulting in acute pain and cell destruction (Linker, 2009).

Because fetal hemoglobin contains a gamma, not a beta, chain, the disease usually will not result in clinical symptoms until a child's hemoglobin changes from the fetal to the adult form at approximately 6 months. However, the disease can be diagnosed prenatally by chorionic villi sampling or from cord blood during amniocentesis. If these were not done, it can be identified at birth by neonatal screening (Lees, Davies, & Dezateux, 2009). The abnormal form of hemoglobin in this disorder is designated hemoglobin S. A child with sickle-cell disease is said to have hemoglobin SS (homozygous involvement).

Sickle-cell disease occurs in about 1 of every 400 African American infants in the United States. Sickle-cell trait occurs in approximately 1 in 12 (Ambruso, Hayes, & Goldenberg, 2008).

Both parents of the child with the disease will have both normal adult and hemoglobin S or be carriers (heterozygous) of the *sickle-cell trait* (have hemoglobin AS). In people with the trait, approximately 25% to 50% of hemoglobin produced is abnormal. They produce enough normal hemoglobin to compensate for the hemoglobin that is sickled and therefore show no symptoms. A child with the disease (homozygous) produces no normal hemoglobin and so shows characteristic symptoms of sickle-cell anemia. A very few children have combinations of hemoglobin S and hemoglobin C or E, leading to mild anemia (Creary, Williamson, & Kulkarni, 2007).

Sickle-Cell Crisis. *Sickle-cell crisis* is the term used to denote a sudden, severe onset of sickling. Symptoms of crisis occur from pooling of many new sickled cells in vessels and consequent tissue hypoxia beyond the blockage (a *vaso-occlusive crisis*). A sickle-cell crisis can occur when a child has an illness causing dehydration or a respiratory infection that results in lowered oxygen exchange and a lowered arterial oxygen level, or after extremely strenuous exercise (enough to lead to tissue hypoxia). Sometimes no obvious cause of a crisis can be found (Box 44.8). Symptoms are sudden, severe, and painful (see Focus on Nursing Care Planning Box 44.9). Laboratory reports reveal a hemoglobin level of only 6 to 8 g/100 mL. A peripheral blood smear demonstrates sickled cells. The WBC count is often elevated to 12,000 to 20,000/mm^3. Bilirubin and reticulocyte levels are increased.

Further complications that may occur are aseptic necrosis of the head of the femur or humerus with increased joint pain or a cerebrovascular accident that occurs from a blocked artery, causing loss of motor function, coma, seizures, or even death (Owusu-Ofori & Hirst, 2009). If there is renal involvement, hematuria or flank pain may be present.

Box 44.8 Assessment
Assessing a Child With Sickle-Cell Crisis

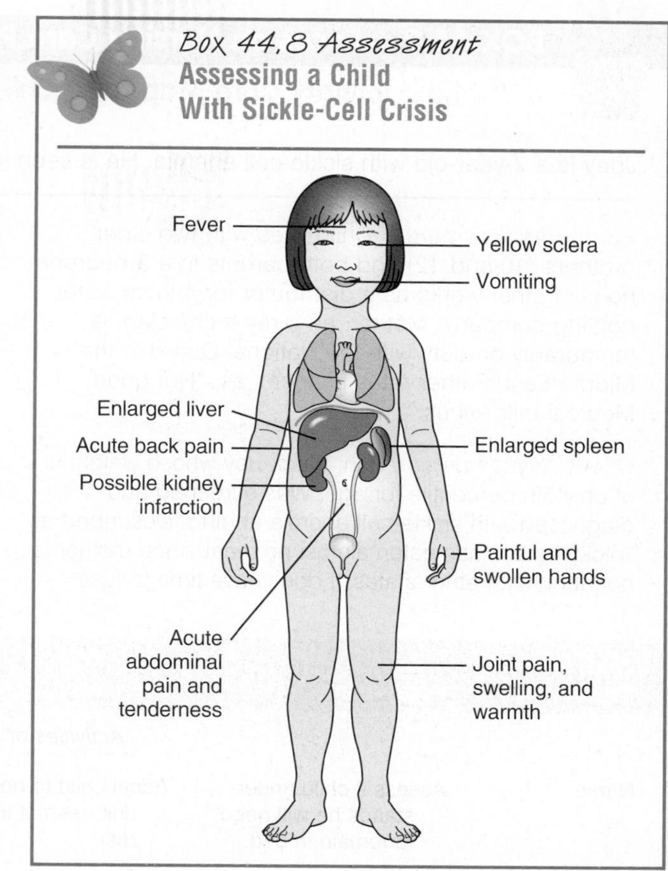

Additional types of crisis may occur.

- A *sequestration crisis* may occur when there is splenic sequestration of RBCs or severe anemia occurs due to pooling and increased destruction of sickled cells in the liver and spleen). This leads to shock from hypovolemia. The spleen is enlarged and tender.
- A *hyperhemolytic crisis* can occur when there is increased destruction of RBCs. A *megaloblastic crisis* may occur if the child has folic acid or vitamin B deficiency (new RBCs cannot be fully formed due to lack of these ingredients).
- An *aplastic crisis* is manifested by severe anemia due to a sudden decrease in RBC production. This form usually occurs with infection.

Assessment for Sickle-Cell Anemia. Hemoglobin electrophoresis is used to diagnose sickle-cell anemia at birth from the few red cells that have already converted to their adult form. At approximately 6 months of age, children with sickle-cell disease begin to show initial signs of fever and anemia. Stasis of blood and infarction may occur in any body part, leading to local pain. Some infants have swelling of the hands and feet (a hand–foot syndrome) probably caused by aseptic infarction of the bones of the hands and feet. Children with sickle-cell anemia tend to have a slight build and characteristically long arms and legs. They may have a protruding abdomen because of an enlarged spleen and liver. In adolescence, the spleen size may decrease from

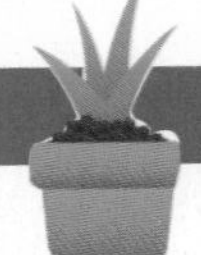

BOX 44.9 * Focus on Nursing Care Planning

A Multidisciplinary Care Map for a Child With Sickle-Cell Anemia

Joey is a 7-year-old with sickle-cell anemia. He is seen in the emergency room for a vaso-occlusive crisis.

Family Assessment * Child lives with two older brothers (10 and 12) and both parents in a 3-bedroom home. Father works as a distributor for a local water bottling company. Mother, an x-ray technician, is temporarily on duty with the National Guard in the Middle East. Father rates finances as, "Not good. Medical bills kill us."

Client Assessment * Thin, black boy whose weight is at only 5th percentile for age. Was screened and diagnosed with sickle-cell anemia at birth. Described as "picky eater"; has eaten almost no meat since mother is not at home. Father states "I don't have time to fuss" over meals. Has a history of two former vaso-occlusive crises. Missed last regularly scheduled health assessment 2 weeks ago, as father had difficulty taking off from work for visit. Was playing "tag" with older brothers on local beach this afternoon. Sclera was jaundiced and child was crying from pain by time father returned from work. Hemoglobin 6 g/100 mL; hematocrit 31%.

Nursing Diagnosis * Altered tissue perfusion related to vaso-occlusive crisis

Outcome Criteria * Oxygen saturation level is maintained at 95% or higher; pain decreases to tolerable level; symptoms of hemolytic crisis decrease.

Team Member Responsible	Assessment	Intervention	Rationale	Expected Outcome
		Activities of Daily Living		
Nurse	Assess if child understands he will need to remain in bed.	Admit child to hospital unit; restrict to bed rest.	Bedrest reduces the need for oxygen in body cells.	Child complies with bedrest; plays non-action games with parent or health care personnel.
		Consultations		
Nurse practitioner/ physician	Assess if hematology service is needed for consult.	Meet with hematology service as needed for emergency and long-range consult.	Repeated vaso-occlusive crises suggest family needs better management strategies.	Hematology service meets with physician/nurse practitioner and parent and child as indicated.
		Procedures/Medications		
Nurse/nurse practitioner	Assess degree of child's pain by use of FACES pain scale.	Administer prescribed narcotic as required.	Vaso-occlusive crises can cause sharp pain that requires strong analgesia.	Child rates pain as no higher than 2 following analgesia administration.
Nurse	Assess O_2 saturation level by pulse oximetry.	Administer oxygen by face mask to keep O_2 saturation above 95% or as prescribed.	O_2 saturation decreases as sickled cells are unable to carry a full complement of oxygen.	Child cooperates with pulse oximetry and oxygen administration. SO_2 remains above 95%.
Nurse	Determine whether child has been taking folic acid at home.	Administer folic acid as prescribed.	Folic acid is necessary to build new red cells to replace those that have been hemolyzed.	Child takes folic acid cooperatively.
		Nutrition		
Nurse	Assess child's intake and output.	Begin IV therapy as prescribed.	IV therapy helps restore hydration and reduce sickle-cell clotting.	Child names best hand to start infusion; cooperates with arm board restriction.

Nurse/ nutritionist	Assess child's usual dietary intake by 24-hour dietary recall history.	Demonstrate child's reduced weight to parent using height/weight chart. Plan ways to increase calorie intake.	Even "picky eaters" need to take in enough food daily to meet growth and maintenance needs.	Parent states he will try harder to serve foods child likes; child voices intent to eat at least one meat helping daily.
		Patient/Family Education		
Nurse	Assess family members' understanding of the causes of sickle-cell vaso-occlusive crises.	Review with family members the importance of child avoiding dehydration and oxygen deficiency.	Dehydration leads to clumping of sickled cells, cutting off circulation in distant body parts.	Family members state they are aware they must be as responsible as child for avoiding sickling circumstances.
		Psychosocial/Spiritual/Emotional Needs		
Nurse	Assess the stress level of the family in light of absent mother and child with chronic illness.	Review with family ways to maintain a tight family unit (game night, common activities) to maintain family until mother returns.	When families miss a support person, they need to rally together to devise other support methods.	Father states he will try harder to meet children's needs although worrying about wife's safety is a major concern.
		Discharge Planning		
Nurse	Determine whether parent has any questions about care of a child with sickle-cell anemia.	Schedule a follow-up visit in 3 days for evaluation.	Care of a chronically ill child can be a major strain on a family. Follow-up visits help share responsibility for care.	Father states he understands importance of follow-up visit and will keep appointment with child.

repeated infarction and atrophy. An atropic spleen leaves a child more susceptible to infection than normal because the spleen can no longer filter bacteria. Pneumococcal meningitis and salmonella-induced osteomyelitis become frequent illnesses; prophylactic antibiotics and pneumococcal vaccine may be prescribed to prevent these infections (Davies et al., 2009).

An acute chest syndrome with symptoms of pulmonary infiltrates with chest pain, fever, tachypnea, wheezing, or cough that leads to pneumonia may also occur. Acute chest syndrome develops because, when areas of the lung become inflamed and hypoxic, sickle cells adhere to the activated endothelium and then fail to be reoxygenated (Adamson & Longo, 2008). Blood transfusion is used to increase the oxygen-carrying capacity of blood, and broad-spectrum antibiotics are given to resolve the pneumonia.

Another common complication occurs when the liver becomes enlarged from stasis of blood flow. Eventually, cirrhosis (fibrotic degeneration) will occur from infarcts and tissue scarring. The kidneys may have subsequent scarring also, so kidney function may be decreased. The sclerae are generally icteric (yellowed) from release of bilirubin from destruction of the sickled cells; small retinal occlusions may lead to decreased vision. Regular eye examinations are necessary in children with sickle-cell disease to detect this. Cell clusters in the blood vessels of the penis may cause **priapism,** or persistent, painful erection (Chinegwundoh & Anie, 2009).

Therapeutic Management. The child in sickle-cell crisis has three primary needs: pain relief and adequate hydration and oxygenation to prevent further sickling and halt the crisis.

Acetaminophen (Tylenol) may be adequate pain relief for some children; for others, a narcotic analgesic such as intravenous morphine may be needed. Once children are pain free, they are able to relax, reducing the metabolic demand for oxygen and helping to end the sickling. Hydration is generally accomplished with intensive intravenous fluid replacement therapy. Tissue hypoxia leads to acidosis. The acidosis must be corrected by electrolyte replacement. Some kidney infarction may have occurred, so do not administer potassium intravenously until kidney function has been determined (the child is voiding). Otherwise, excessive potassium levels may occur, possibly leading to cardiac arrhythmias. If infection appears to be the precipitator for a sickling crisis, blood and urine cultures, a chest radiograph, and a complete blood count will be taken and the infection will be treated by antibiotics. Blood transfusion (usually packed RBCs) may be necessary to maintain the hemoglobin above 12 g/dL (termed hypertransfusion).

Hydroxyurea, an antineoplastic agent that has the potential to increase the production of hemoglobin F (fetal hemoglobin), can be used in children with sickle-cell disease to increase their overall hemoglobin level (Jones, Davies, & Olujohungbe, 2009). The drug, given orally, can cause anorexia. Therefore, monitor the child's nutrition intake during this drug therapy. If none of the above measures appears to be effective, children may be given an exchange transfusion to remove most of the sickled cells and replace them with normal cells. Exchange transfusion (see Chapter 26) must be done with small amounts of blood at each exchange. Otherwise, the pressure changes can cause such irregularities in blood volume that heart failure results. Hematopoietic stem cell transplantation is possible for the child who does not respond to usual therapies.

✓ Checkpoint Question 44.3

Joey, who has sickle-cell anemia, has had two vaso-occlusive crises in the past year. A vaso-occlusive crisis occurs because:

a. An enlarged spleen causes blood to pool there.
b. Dehydration leads to thrombosed sickle cells.
c. Hemorrhage reduces a child's total blood volume.
d. Decreased platelet number leads to poor coagulation.

Nursing Diagnoses and Related Interventions

Nursing Diagnosis: Ineffective tissue perfusion related to generalized infarcts due to sickling

Outcome Evaluation: Child's respiratory rate is 16 to 20/min; cyanosis is absent; arterial blood gases within acceptable parameters including P_{CO_2} = 40 mm Hg; P_{O_2} = 80 to 90 mm Hg; oxygen saturation of 95%; urine output greater than 1 mL/kg/hr.

Oxygen may be administered by nasal cannula or mask if arterial blood gases reveal a low P_{O_2} level. Oxygen may not reach every distal body part effectively, however, if blood flowing to the part is obstructed by the sickled cells. When hemoglobin S is below 40%, there generally is adequate blood flow to body cells. High concentrations of oxygen are not used because hypoxia is a stimulant to erythrocyte production—production badly needed to replace damaged cells. Monitor the flow rate carefully and use pulse oximetry to evaluate oxygen saturation levels for changes. Encourage bed rest to relieve the pain and reduce oxygen expenditure (Box 44.10).

It is important to maintain accurate intake and output records and to test urine for specific gravity and hematuria to detect the extent or presence of kidney damage from infarcts.

Nursing Diagnosis: Ineffective health maintenance related to lack of knowledge regarding long-term needs of child with sickle-cell anemia

Outcome Evaluation: Parent accurately describes disease process and identifies special precautions necessary to prevent sickle-cell crisis.

In many children, episodes of sickling grow less severe as a child reaches adolescence. Such children will have a normal life expectancy but still experience the stresses of chronic illness. Other children experience such devastating episodes in early childhood that the disease becomes fatal at an early age. Parents need support to supervise children carefully day by day when they are aware that, due to the intense episodes, the child may die despite the precautions.

Between crises, care focuses on preventing recurring crises. Although the hemoglobin level of children may remain as low as 6 to 9 g/100 mL, children adjust well to this chronic state. Children who receive frequent blood transfusions should not be given supplementary iron or iron-fortified formula or vitamins or they may receive too much iron; high levels of excess iron are deposited in body tissues **(hemochromatosis)** to a point of staining body tissue or being incorporated into body tissue with fibrotic scarring (hemosiderosis). Oral folic

BOX 44.10 ✻ Focus on Communication

Joey, who has sickle-cell disease, is seen in the emergency department with a new vaso-occlusive crisis. His right knee is discolored by a large brush burn. He's crying from pain.

Less Effective Communication

Nurse: Hello, Mr. Harrow. I need to ask some questions to see if anything triggered this new crisis.
Mr. Harrow: He better not have been doing something he's not allowed to do.
Nurse: His knee looks like he fell. Were you running, Joey? So you got dehydrated?
Mr. Harrow: He better not say he was doing that!
Nurse: Joey, how did you hurt your knee?
Joey: I don't know.
Nurse: Okay. Let's get you better and not worry about what started this.

More Effective Communication

Nurse: Hello, Mr. Harrow. I need to ask some questions to see if anything triggered this new crisis.
Mr. Harrow: He better not have been doing something he's not allowed to do.
Nurse: His knee looks like he fell. Were you running, Joey? So you got dehydrated?
Mr. Harrow: He better not say he was doing that!
Nurse: Mr. Harrow, I need to get an accurate history of what happened. I'd like Joey to tell us how he thinks the accident happened. Then later on, we can talk about what are good rules for him to be following.

Children with blood disorders have to follow a great many rules to avoid clotting or bleeding episodes, such as not playing contact sports or playing too hard in the sun. Because these forbidden activities are appealing, children occasionally break the rules. In an emergency room, it is important that children and parents both recognize that the priority at the moment is obtaining an accurate history. Until they realize this, they may be so concerned with the broken rule that they are unable to move beyond that to secure adequate therapy.

acid may be prescribed to help rebuild hemolyzed RBCs.

Children with sickle-cell anemia need to be followed at regular health care visits. They must receive childhood immunizations so they are not vulnerable to common childhood infections such as measles or pertussis. They are also candidates for meningococcal, pneumococcal, and influenza vaccines to prevent infection. They may be prescribed oral penicillin as prophylaxis for the first 5 years. Puberty may be delayed, and both parents and children may need counseling to accept this. Once puberty changes do occur, they are adequate, just later than usual. Parents and children with sickle-cell disease also need support and positive reinforcement to enhance the child's self-esteem and to learn how to deal with problems that occur as a result of this chronic hematologic disorder (Box 44.11).

Caution parents to bring their child to a health care facility at the first indication of infection. Some parents are reluctant to do this, afraid that they will be labeled overprotective. Assure them that health care personnel are knowledgeable about sickle-cell anemia, and they know that a child with even a minor infection could become very ill.

Parents must make decisions regarding children's activity levels. Children should attend regular school and should be allowed to participate in all school activities except contact sports (such as football), which could result in rupture of an enlarged spleen or liver. Long-distance running is also inadvisable because it can lead to dehydration. During the summer, parents need to offer the child frequent drinks to prevent dehydration, especially on long hikes and at the beach. Caution parents against taking the child on board an unpressurized aircraft in which the oxygen concentration may fall during flight.

Some children who have had kidney infarcts and lessened ability to concentrate urine have chronic nocturnal enuresis (bedwetting).

Children with sickle-cell disease are at high risk if they need surgery. The hours of being held on nothing-by-mouth status, as well as being unable to eat afterward, may lead to dehydration. Anesthesia may cause a transient hypoxia leading to sickling. Parents must be cautioned that even for such a simple operation as tooth extraction, therefore, they must alert health care personnel about their child's condition.

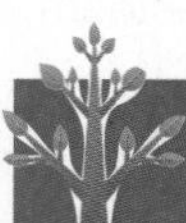

BOX 44.11 * Focus on Family Teaching

School Safety Precautions for Children with Sickle-Cell Disease

Q. Joey's father says to you, "My son has sickle-cell disease. What can I do to help keep him safe at school?"

A. Use these guidelines to help ensure your son's safety at school:

- Be certain your child either takes fluid with him or buys adequate fluid for lunch. Children with sickle-cell anemia need to maintain a high fluid intake to prevent their blood from becoming thick.
- Provide additional fluid in the summer, when dehydration is more apt to happen. Anticipate ways to provide fluid during long hikes or school trips; time spent on a hot beach may need to be limited.
- Learn about sources high in folic acid, such as vegetables and fruit, and be certain these foods are included in your son's diet every day.
- Encourage the boy to get adequate sleep at night as a general measure to prevent illness.
- With the exception of contact sports (to avoid damage to an enlarged spleen) and long-distance running (to prevent dehydration), encourage your son to participate in normal school activities.
- Know that bedwetting may occur as part of the illness. Encourage your son to take baths in the morning if this occurs so his clothes don't smell of urine.
- Maintain routine health care such as immunizations to prevent common childhood illnesses such as measles and mumps, which cause fever and dehydration.
- Call your primary health care provider at the first sign of illness, such as an upper respiratory infection, so therapy can be begun immediately.

What if... Joey's parent tells you he restricts Joey, who has sickle-cell anemia, from drinking any fluid after 4 PM to prevent bedwetting? Is this a good solution to bedwetting for this child? How would you counsel this parent?

Thalassemias

The thalassemias are autosomal recessive anemias associated with abnormalities of the beta chain of adult hemoglobin (HgbA). Although these anemias occur most frequently in the Mediterranean population, they also occur in children of African and Asian heritage (Waterbury, 2007).

Thalassemia Minor (Heterozygous Beta-Thalassemia)

Children with thalassemia minor, a mild form of this anemia, produce both defective beta hemoglobin and normal hemoglobin. Because there is some normal production, the RBC count will be normal, but the hemoglobin concentration will be decreased 2 to 3 g/100 mL below normal levels. The blood cells are moderately hypochromic and microcytic because of the poor hemoglobin formation.

Children may have no symptoms other than pallor. They require no treatment, and life expectancy is normal. They should not receive a routine iron supplement because their inability to incorporate it well into hemoglobin may cause them to accumulate too much iron. The condition represents the heterozygous form of the disorder or can be compared with children having the sickle-cell trait.

Thalassemia Major (Homozygous Beta-Thalassemia)

Thalassemia major is also called Cooley's anemia or Mediterranean anemia. Because thalassemia is a beta chain

TABLE 44.3 ✻ Effects of Thalassemia Major

Body Organ or System	Effect of Abnormal Cell Production
Bone marrow	Overstimulation of bone marrow leads to increased facial-mandibular growth
Skin	Bronze-colored from hemosiderosis and jaundice
Spleen	Splenomegaly
Liver and gallbladder	Cirrhosis and cholelithiasis
Pancreas	Destruction of islet cells and diabetes mellitus
Heart	Failure from circulatory overload

hemoglobin defect, symptoms do not become apparent until a child's fetal hemoglobin has largely been replaced by adult hemoglobin during the second half of the first year of life. Effects of thalassemia major on body systems are summarized in Table 44.3. Unable to produce normal beta hemoglobin, the child shows symptoms of anemia: pallor, irritability, and anorexia (Muncie, 2008).

RBCs are hypochromic (pale) and microcytic (small). Fragmented poikilocytes and basophilic stippling (unevenness of hemoglobin concentration) are present. The hemoglobin level is less than 5 g/100 mL. The serum iron level is high because iron is not being incorporated into hemoglobin; iron saturation is 100%.

Assessment. To maintain a functional level of hemoglobin, the bone marrow hypertrophies in an attempt to produce more RBCs. This may cause bone pain; the ineffective attempt often leads to the formation of target cells or large macrocytes that are short-lived and nonfunctional. As bone marrow becomes hyperactive, this results in a characteristic change in the shape of the skull (parietal and frontal bossing) and protrusion of the upper teeth, with marked malocclusion. The base of the nose may be broad and flattened; the eyes may be slanted with an epicanthal fold, as in Down syndrome. A radiograph of bone shows marked osteoporotic (of lessened density) tissue, possibly resulting in fractures. The child may have hepatosplenomegaly due to excessive iron deposits and fibrotic scarring in the liver and the spleen's increased attempts to destroy defective RBCs. Abdominal pressure from the enlarged spleen may cause anorexia and vomiting. Epistaxis is common, as is diabetes mellitus due to pancreatic hemosiderosis (deposition of iron) and cardiac dilatation with an accompanying murmur. Arrhythmias and heart failure are frequent causes of death.

Therapeutic Management. Digitalis, diuretics, and a low-sodium diet may be prescribed to prevent heart failure, which could result from the decompensation that accompanies anemia, and from myocardial fibrosis caused by invasion of iron (hemosiderosis). Transfusion of packed RBCs every 2 to 4 weeks (hypertransfusion therapy) will maintain hemoglobin between 10 and 12 g/100 mL. With this level of hemoglobin, erythropoiesis is suppressed and cosmetic facial alterations, osteoporosis, and cardiac dilatation are minimized. Hypertransfusion therapy also reduces the possibility that splenectomy will be necessary. Frequent blood transfusions, unfortunately, increase the risk of blood-borne disease, such as hepatitis B, and hemosiderosis. Children may receive an oral iron-chelating agent to remove this excessive store of iron, such as deferasirox (Stumpf, 2007). Others receive deferoxamine given subcutaneously over 6 to 8 hours as they sleep at night (Karch, 2009).

Splenectomy may become necessary to reduce discomfort and also to reduce the rate of RBC hemolysis and the number of transfusions needed. Bone marrow stem cell transplantation can offer a cure. With treatment, the overall prognosis of thalassemia is improving but still grave. Most children with the disease die of cardiac failure during adolescence or as young adults if they do not receive a hematopoietic stem cell transplant (Muncie, 2008).

Nursing Diagnoses and Related Interventions

Nursing Diagnosis: Risk for situational low self-esteem related to changed physical appearance

Outcome Evaluation: Child states he can accept altered appearance and interacts with peers.

Children with thalassemia major may have delayed growth and sexual maturation. They usually develop a marked change in facial appearance because of the overgrowth of marrow-producing centers of the facial bones. This can be demoralizing because these changes will be permanent. In addition, the child who receives frequent blood transfusions may develop such hemosiderosis that skin color appears bronze.

Children should be allowed as much activity as possible and should attend regular school, if possible, to maintain a nearly normal childhood. Discussions about other children's reactions to their changing facial appearance can be helpful.

Autoimmune Acquired Hemolytic Anemia

Occasionally, autoimmune antibodies (abnormal antibodies of the IgG class) attach themselves to RBCs, destroying them or causing hemolysis. This may occur at any age, and its origin is generally idiopathic, although the disorder may be associated with malignancy, viral infections, or collagen diseases such as rheumatoid arthritis or systemic lupus erythematosus. A child may recently have had an upper respiratory infection, measles, or varicella virus infection (chickenpox). Such hemolysis may occur after the administration of drugs such as quinine, phenacetin, sulfonamides, or penicillin.

The exact cause is unknown but appears to involve a change in the RBCs themselves, making them act as antigens, or a change in antibody production, making antibodies destructive to other substances.

Assessment. The onset is insidious. Children have a low-grade fever, anorexia, lethargy, pallor, and icterus from release of indirect bilirubin from the hemolyzed cells. Both urine and stools appear dark because the excess bilirubin is being excreted. In some children, the illness begins abruptly with high fever, hemoglobinuria, marked jaundice, and pallor. The liver and spleen may be enlarged.

Laboratory findings reveal that the RBCs are extremely small and round (spherocytosis), resembling hereditary spherocytosis. The reticulocyte count is increased as the body attempts to form replacement RBCs. A direct Coombs' test result is positive, indicating the presence of antibodies attached to red cells. Hemoglobin levels may fall as low as 6 g/100 mL.

Therapeutic Management. In some children, the disease process runs a limited course and no treatment is necessary. In others, a single blood transfusion may correct the disturbance. For these children, it is difficult to cross-match blood for transfusion because the red cell antibody tends to clump or agglutinate all blood tested. If cross-matching is impossible, the child may be given type O Rh-negative blood. Observe the child carefully during any transfusion for signs of transfusion reaction.

If anemia is persistent, corticosteroid therapy (oral prednisone) to reduce the immune response is generally effective, increasing the RBC count and hemoglobin concentration in a short period. For some children, stronger immunosuppressive agents such as cyclophosphamide (Cytoxan) or azathioprine (Imuran) are necessary to reduce antibody formation. If these are ineffective, splenectomy may be necessary.

Often it is difficult for parents to understand the process causing their child's condition. How could a child's body turn on itself? How long will this last? What will stop it from happening again? There are no answers to these questions. Provide the parents and child with support as they wait for this unexplainable process to run its course and for their child to be well again.

✔ Checkpoint Question 44.4

Autoimmune acquired hemolytic anemia can occur in any child. The usual cause of this disorder is:

a. Allergy to the protein found in fish.
b. A mutant gene similar to sickle cell.
c. An elevated eosinophil cell count.
d. Antibody production against red cells.

Polycythemia

Polycythemia is an increase in the number of RBCs (Zull, 2007). The condition results from increased erythropoiesis, which occurs as a compensatory response to insufficient oxygenation of the blood in order to help supply more oxygen to body cells. Chronic pulmonary disease and congenital heart disease are the usual causes of polycythemia in childhood. Also, it may occur from the lower oxygen level maintained during intrauterine life in newborns or with twin transfusion at birth (one twin receives excess blood while a second twin is anemic).

Plethora (marked reddened appearance of the skin) occurs because of the increase in total RBC volume. Erythrocytes are usually macrocytic (large) and the hemoglobin content is high. This means that the mean corpuscular hemoglobin will be elevated; the mean corpuscular hemoglobin concentration, however, will be normal, indicating that, although many in number, each erythrocyte is normally saturated with hemoglobin. The RBC count may be as high as 7 million/mm^3. Hemoglobin levels may be as high as 23 g/100 mL.

Treatment of polycythemia involves treatment of the underlying cause. Because of the high blood viscosity from so many crowded blood cells, cerebrovascular accident or emboli may occur. The risk increases particularly if the child becomes dehydrated, such as with fever or during surgery. Exchange transfusion or phlebotomy to reduce the RBC count may be necessary.

DISORDERS OF THE WHITE BLOOD CELLS

Most disorders characterized by a decrease or increase in the number of WBCs or specific WBC components occur in response to another disease (often infection or an allergic reaction) in the body (Table 44.4). Laboratory values of WBCs, therefore, provide one of the first objective indicators of infectious disease, often aiding in specific diagnoses. These diseases are discussed in Chapter 43. Leukemia, overproduction of WBCs, is discussed with other malignant conditions in Chapter 53.

DISORDERS OF BLOOD COAGULATION

Platelets are necessary for blood coagulation, so disorders that limit the number of platelets limit the effectiveness of this process. A normal platelet level is 150,000/mm^3. Thrombocytopenia (decreased platelet count) is defined as a platelet count of less than 40,000/mm^3. Thrombocytopenia often leads to purpura, or blood seeping from vessels into the skin. In one rare disorder, children are born with thrombocytopenia and are also missing the radius bone in the forearm (TAR [thrombocytopenia/absent radius] syndrome).

Purpuras

Purpura refers to a hemorrhagic rash or small hemorrhages in the superficial layer of skin. Two main types of purpura occur in children: idiopathic thrombocytopenia purpura and Henoch-Schönlein syndrome.

Idiopathic Thrombocytopenic Purpura

Idiopathic thrombocytopenic purpura (ITP) is the result of a decrease in the number of circulating platelets in the presence of adequate megakaryocytes (precursors to platelets). The cause is unknown, but it is thought to result from an increased rate of platelet destruction due to an antiplatelet antibody that destroys platelets making this an autoimmune illness (Schmidt & Aldeen, 2007).

In most instances, ITP occurs approximately 2 weeks after a viral infection such as rubella, rubeola, varicella, or an upper respiratory tract infection. Congenital ITP may occur in the newborn of a woman who has had ITP during pregnancy. An antiplatelet factor apparently crosses the placenta and causes platelet destruction in the newborn in the same way that Rh incompatibility or hemolytic disease of the newborn develops (see Chapter 26). However, in ITP, the platelets, not the RBCs, are sensitized.

TABLE 44.4 ✻ Disorders of White Blood Cells

Disorder	Description	Causes/Treatment
Neutropenia	Reduced number of white blood cells	Transient phenomenon with nonpyrogenic infections such as viral disease Response to therapy with some drugs, such as 6-mercaptopurine or nitrogen mustard Possible side effect from drugs such as phenytoin sodium (Dilantin), chloramphenicol, or chlorpromazine Treatments: Possibly white blood cell transfusion; prophylactic antibiotics
Neutrophilia	Increased number of circulating white blood cells, primarily neutrophils (total number of cells increases and the proportion of mature neutrophils changes, with an increase in immature cells)	Usually in response to infection or inflammation (see Chapter 43) Treatment: antibiotic therapy to eliminate infectious organisms
Leukemia	Uncontrolled proliferation of white blood cells	Neoplastic disorder (see Chapter 53)
Eosinophilia	Increased number of eosinophils	Associated with many allergic disorders, such as atopic dermatitis, and with parasitic invasion (see Chapters 42 and 43)
Lymphocytosis	Increased number of lymphocytes	Normally occurs in the preschool period, when there is a marked predominance of lymphocytes in relation to neutrophils Abnormally elevated in childhood illnesses such as pertussis, infectious mononucleosis, and lymphocytic leukemia Treatment: Therapy for the underlying condition

Assessment. Manifestations often begin abruptly, first evidenced as miniature petechiae or as large areas of asymmetric ecchymosis most prominent over the legs, although they may occur anywhere on the body (Fig. 44.3). Epistaxis or bleeding into joints may be present.

Laboratory studies reveal marked thrombocytopenia. The platelet count may be as low as $20{,}000/mm^3$. Bone marrow examination reveals a normal number of megakaryocytes.

Therapeutic Management. Oral prednisone to reduce the immune response and intravenous immunoglobulin (IVIG) or, in Rh-positive children, anti-D immunoglobulin to supply anti-ITP antibodies are used to treat ITP (Giulino, Bussel, & Neufeld, 2007). Platelet transfusion will temporarily increase the platelet count, but because the life span of platelets is relatively short, a platelet transfusion has only limited effect. Children with central nervous system bleeding may require a splenectomy although this is rarely necessary.

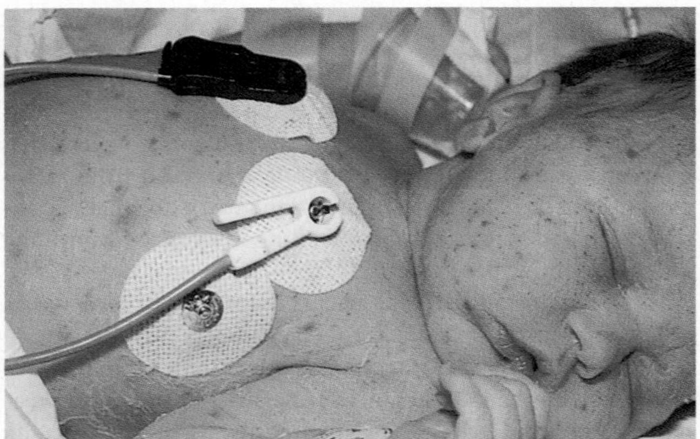

FIGURE 44.3 An infant with ITP. Notice the tiny petechiae and larger ecchymotic areas. (From Zitelli, B. J., & Davis, H. W. [1997]. *Atlas of pediatric physical diagnosis* [3rd ed.]. St. Louis: Mosby–Year Book, Inc.)

If the child experiences joint pain from bleeding, acetaminophen (Tylenol) rather than salicylates or ibuprofen is prescribed for pain. Both salicylates and ibuprofen increase the chance for bleeding as they prevent the aggregation of platelets at wound sites.

In most children, ITP runs a limited, 1- to 3-month course. A few children develop chronic ITP. A course of immunosuppressive drugs may be attempted if the chronic state persists.

All children need to be vaccinated against the viral diseases of childhood so that diseases such as rubella, rubeola, and varicella are eradicated and can no longer lead to this defective coagulation process.

Nursing Diagnoses and Related Interventions

Nursing Diagnosis: Health-seeking behaviors related to injury-prevention measures

Outcome Evaluation: Parents state precautions they will take to reduce possibility of bleeding; repeat correct dose and timing of medication therapy; child's skin is free of ecchymotic areas; platelet count rises to normal values.

The techniques for reducing bleeding described earlier in the chapter such as padding surfaces where the child plays (see Box 44.5) can be used to reduce the possibility of bleeding for the child with ITP. Parents cannot eliminate the possibility of a serious bleeding injury, however, until the platelet count returns to normal. The chief danger to the child from ITP, aside from the psychological stress of a perplexing illness, is intracranial hemorrhage. Although this is rare, be alert for signs such as persistent headache, nuchal rigidity, and lethargy.

Nursing Diagnosis: Risk for compromised family coping related to diagnosis of child's illness

Outcome Evaluation: Parents state they understand the nature of their child's illness and have identified ways to carry out daily activities despite the illness.

Because symptoms such as the easy bruising of ITP mimics the beginning ones of leukemia, parents may be extremely frightened when symptoms first occur. You can assure them after the diagnosis is made that this bruising is not leukemia. If the ITP follows a long course (2 or 3 months), reassure them that this process will not later become leukemia. A child may have so many bruises that the parents are initially suspected of child abuse. This can cause them to become very defensive and angry at health care personnel. Allow them time to express their anger and regain confidence in their health care team.

It is always bewildering for parents to be told that no one knows exactly what is causing their child's illness. To feel comfortable that health care personnel can manage their child's care without knowing the exact cause, they need careful explanations of all procedures.

Henoch-Schönlein Syndrome

Henoch-Schönlein purpura (also called anaphylactoid purpura) is caused by increased vessel permeability. Although no definite allergic correlation can be identified, it is generally considered to be a hypersensitivity reaction to an invading allergen. It occurs most frequently in children between 2 and 8 years of age, and more frequently in boys than girls (Hellmann & Imboden, 2009). Usually, there is a history of a mild infection before the outbreak of symptoms. The syndrome presents (because of the purpura) as a possible platelet disorder until a differential diagnosis is made.

Assessment. The purpural rash occurs typically on the buttocks, posterior thighs, and extensor surface of the arms and legs (Fig. 44.4). The tips of the ears may be involved. The rash begins as a crop of urticarial lesions that change to pink maculopapules. These become hemorrhagic (bright red) and then fade, leaving brown macular spots that remain for several weeks. The child's joints are tender and swollen. The child may have gastrointestinal symptoms such as abdominal pain, vomiting, or blood in stools. Gross or microscopic hematuria may be present from kidney involvement. A biopsy shows granulocytes in the walls of small arterioles.

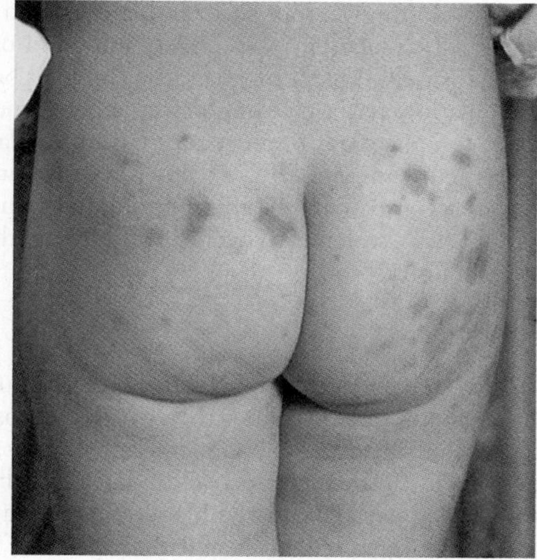

FIGURE 44.4 The distinctive purpural rash of Henoch-Schönlein syndrome appearing on the buttocks of a young child. (From Zitelli, B. J., & Davis, H. W. [1997]. *Atlas of pediatric physical diagnosis* [3rd ed.]. St. Louis: Mosby–Year Book, Inc.)

Laboratory studies show a normal platelet count. Sedimentation rate, WBC count, and eosinophil count are elevated.

Therapeutic Management. Treatment involves oral corticosteroid therapy (prednisone) and mild analgesics for a short period. Nose and throat cultures rule out continuing bacterial involvement. Urine should be assessed for protein and glucose to detect kidney involvement. Typically the disease runs a course of 4 to 6 weeks. A few children develop chronic nephritis as a complication (Butani & Morgenstern, 2007).

Disseminated Intravascular Coagulation

Disseminated intravascular coagulation (DIC) is an acquired disorder of blood clotting that results from excessive trauma or some similar underlying stimulus (Bowman, 2007). Normal blood clotting is a balance between the hemostatic (clotting) system and the fibrinolytic (dissolving) system of the bloodstream. After a blood vessel injury, local vasoconstriction rapidly prevents additional blood loss at the site. With the tear in the vessel wall, the underlying collagen is exposed. This causes platelets to swell and become adherent and irregular in shape. They release adenosine diphosphate, which attracts additional platelets and binds them together (platelet aggregation). This phenomenon results in a platelet plug to seal the vessel. The plug is strengthened by fibrin threads that form as a result of an intrinsic and extrinsic coagulation process into a firm, fixed structure. To prevent too much clotting from occurring, plasmin or fibrinolysin, a proteolytic enzyme formed from plasminogen, digests fibrin threads and causes lysis of the clot along with consumption of blood clotting factors. As plasmin, fibrinogen, and fibrin are lysed, fibrin degradation products are formed. These products prevent the laying down of further fibrin and platelet aggregation.

With DIC, an imbalance occurs between clotting activity and fibrinolysis. Extreme clotting due to endothelial damage begins at one point in the circulatory system, depleting the availability of clotting factors such as platelets and fibrin from the general circulation. A secondary initiation of fibrinolysis begins as well. A paradox exists: the child has both increased coagulation and a bleeding defect at the same time. Many of the complications of pregnancy (abruptio placentae or death of a fetus) initiate DIC, so this is a common complication seen accompanying bleeding during pregnancy (see Chapter 21). DIC also tends to occur in children with acute infections or trauma.

Assessment

A child begins to have uncontrolled bleeding from puncture sites from injections or intravenous therapy. Ecchymoses and petechiae form on the skin. The toes and fingers may appear pale, cyanotic, or mottled and feel cold because small blood vessels are so filled with coagulated blood that circulation to the extremities is impaired. If coagulation is acute, neurologic or renal symptoms may occur from occlusion of vessels supplying the brain and kidneys. Observe all children with a serious illness carefully for signs of increased bleeding such as petechiae or oozing from blood-sampling sites to help identify that this is happening.

With DIC, laboratory tests usually reveal:

- Thrombocytopenia (level depends on the rate at which bone marrow can replace platelets)
- Large platelets on blood smear, possibly fragmented (from passing through meshes of collecting fibrin)
- Prolonged prothrombin and partial thromboplastin times
- Markedly low serum fibrinogen levels (less than 100 mg/100 mL)
- Elevated fibrin split products

Therapeutic Management

To halt the process of DIC, the underlying insult that began the phenomenon must be halted. Intravenous heparin administration helps to interfere with the marked coagulation. Although blood transfusion may be necessary to correct blood loss, it may be delayed until after heparin has been administered so that the new blood factors are not also consumed by the coagulation process. Fresh-frozen plasma, platelets, or fibrinogen may be administered.

With adequate therapy, the results of blood coagulation studies will return to normal. If renal or brain cells were damaged from occluded capillaries, permanent injury to these areas can result.

Nursing Diagnoses and Related Interventions

Nursing Diagnosis: Deficient knowledge about blood clotting disorder related to its paradoxical nature

Outcome Evaluation: Client or parents accurately state nature of illness and proposed therapy; state signs and symptoms of disease; verbalize understanding of treatments.

Parents may be bewildered by the paradoxical problems of bleeding on the one hand and clotting on the other. If they understand the action of heparin—to discourage blood coagulation—their child's need and the medication seem directly contradictory. Be certain that both children and parents are given a full explanation. The child has an increased risk of hemorrhage because part of the coagulation system has used up coagulation factors; heparin is acting to stop this coagulation. This explanation will help parents understand what is happening and foster trust and confidence in caregivers.

Hemophilias

Hemophilia is an inherited disorder of blood coagulation. There are numerous hemophilia types, each involving deficiency of a different blood coagulation factor.

Hemophilia A (Factor VIII Deficiency)

The classic form of hemophilia is caused by deficiency of the coagulation component factor VIII, the antihemophilic factor. It is transmitted as a sex-linked recessive trait. In the United States, the incidence is approximately 1 in 10,000 white males. The female carrier may have slightly lowered but sufficient levels of the factor VIII component so that she does not manifest a bleeding disorder. Males with the disease also have varying levels of factor VIII, and their bleeding tendency varies accordingly, from mild to severe (Ambruso, Hays, & Goldenberg, 2008).

Factor VIII is an intrinsic factor of coagulation, so the intrinsic system for manufacturing thromboplastin is incomplete. The child's coagulation ability is not absent because the extrinsic or tissue system remains intact. Because of this system, the child's blood will eventually coagulate after an injury.

Assessment. Hemophilia often is recognized first in the infant who bleeds excessively after circumcision. If the disease has not shown itself for several generations in a family, the parents may be unaware of its existence. For this reason, all infants need careful and thoughtful observation after circumcision.

Because infants do not receive many injuries, children's bleeding tendencies may not become apparent until they become active (crawling, climbing, or walking).

Suddenly the lower extremities (where the child bumps things) become heavily bruised. There is soft tissue bleeding and painful hemorrhage into the joints, which become swollen and warm. The child holds the injured joint stiffly. Repeated bleeding into a joint causes damage to the synovial membrane (hemarthrosis), possibly resulting in severe loss of joint mobility.

Severe bleeding may also occur into the gastrointestinal tract, peritoneal cavity, or central nervous system. Interestingly, nosebleeds are common but are not as severe as with the platelet deficiency syndromes. The child must be identified as having hemophilia before surgery is performed for any reason; otherwise, fatal bleeding could occur.

With hemophilia, the platelet count and prothrombin time are normal. The whole blood clotting time is markedly prolonged or normal, depending on the level of factor VIII present. A thromboplastin generation test is abnormal. Partial thromboplastin time (PTT) is the test that best reveals the low levels of factor VIII.

Therapeutic Management. With even minor abrasions, bleeding must be controlled by the administration of factor VIII. This may be supplied by fresh whole blood or by fresh or frozen plasma, but it is best supplied by a concentrate of factor VIII. One bag of concentrate per 5 kg body weight is usually sufficient. This provides protection for approximately 12 hours; another transfusion may be necessary after that time. Powdered forms of factor VIII that can be stored at home and reconstituted as needed are available. In some children, administration of desmopressin (DDAVP), which stimulates the release of factor VIII, may be helpful. Prophylactic administration, although expensive, may best reduce bleeding episodes.

In a few children, antibodies (termed inhibitors) to factor VIII develop, rendering the factor ineffective. If this happens, epsilon-aminocaproic acid, a fibrinolytic enzyme that helps to stabilize clot formation and promote wound healing, can be self-administered every 6 hours if needed. Children with inhibitors to factor VIII can also be given a factor IX concentrate (Proplex or Konyne). This concentrate enters the coagulation cascade after factor VIII and halts bleeding.

Nursing Diagnoses and Related Interventions

Nursing Diagnosis: Parental health-seeking behaviors related to strategies for protecting child from injury

Outcome Evaluation: Child's skin is free of ecchymotic areas; frequent epistaxis is absent; blood pressure is within age-appropriate parameters; swelling or warmth at joints is absent.

Parents need information about how to prevent bleeding episodes and also how to respond when one occurs. Prevention of injury is the most important intervention with these children. Help parents to set appropriate limits. An active infant may need to have crib sides padded; all toys need to be inspected for sharp edges or parts.

Parents (and the child as soon as approximately 10 years of age) can be taught to administer a replacement factor intravenously to prevent bleeding immediately after an injury. Although the child needs to be assessed by a health care provider, this action, combined with immobilization of the injured extremity and an ice pack applied locally, almost always eliminates the need for hospital admission. Pressure should be applied to a laceration to halt bleeding directly. "Butterfly bandages" are used in place of suturing for lacerations whenever possible, because sutures make additional puncture sites that could bleed.

Nursing Diagnosis: Pain related to joint infiltration by blood

Outcome Evaluation: Child states that pain is at a tolerable level.

The child with hemophiliac bleeding experiences discomfort because of the bleeding into joints and may be frightened because his parents are so frightened. Immobilization of the affected joint helps to decrease bleeding and also helps provide relief. Be certain that immobilized joints are in good alignment. As soon as the acute bleeding episode has halted (approximately 48 hours), perform passive range of motion as ordered to maintain function. Acetaminophen (Tylenol) rather than ibuprofen is ordered as an analgesic because ibuprofen may prolong bleeding. As soon as effective levels of factor VIII have been provided, the pain in the bleeding joint is generally relieved, despite the continued heat or swelling.

Nursing Diagnosis: Risk for interrupted family processes related to fears regarding child's prognosis and long-term nature of illness

Outcome Evaluation: Family members voice their fear regarding illness; state that they can cope despite stress level; demonstrate positive coping responses.

Parents of children with hemophilia are frightened during a time of acute bleeding, not just because of what is currently happening but also because they may have seen other family members or even a previous child die of the disease. Be certain to give them a chance to talk about how the bleeding began ("I should have noticed that toy had a sharp edge," "He fell from his bike. I should have watched him more closely"). It is extremely important for parents to allow the child to lead a normal life. Remind them that it is impossible to prevent all injuries. Assist them with measures that offer them a sense of control over the situation. As children reach school age, they must learn to monitor their own activities to prevent bleeding episodes.

von Willebrand's Disease

von Willebrand's disease, an inherited autosomal dominant disorder affecting both sexes, is often referred to as angiohemophilia. Along with a factor VIII defect, there is also an inability of the platelets to aggregate. In addition, the blood vessels cannot constrict to aid in coagulation. Bleeding time is prolonged, with most hemorrhages occurring from mucous membrane sites.

Epistaxis is a major problem, because all children tend to rub or pick at their nose as a nervous mechanism. In girls, menstrual flow is unusually heavy and may cause embarrassment from stained clothing. Childbirth is obviously a risk for women with von Willebrand's disease (James & Jamison, 2007). Bleeding is controlled with factor VIII replenishment as with hemophilia, or by administration of DDAVP, which stimulates factor VIII release.

Christmas Disease (Hemophilia B, Factor IX Deficiency)

Christmas disease, caused by factor IX deficiency, is transmitted as a sex-linked recessive trait. Only approximately 15% of people with hemophilia have this form. Treatment is with a concentrate of factor IX, available for home administration (Linker, 2009).

Hemophilia C (Factor XI deficiency)

Hemophilia C or plasma thromboplastin antecedent deficiency, caused by factor XI deficiency, is transmitted as an autosomal recessive trait occurring in both sexes. The symptoms are generally mild compared with those in children with factor VIII or factor IX deficiencies. Bleeding episodes are treated with administration of DDAVP or transfusion of fresh blood or plasma (Ambruso, Hays, & Goldenberg, 2008).

✔ Checkpoint Question 44.5

Disseminated intravascular coagulation can occur in any child with a critical illness. The drug of choice you would expect to administer for this condition is:

a. Erythropoietin, to stimulate new red cells.
b. Methotrexate, to decrease red cell number.
c. Heparin, to halt abnormal coagulation.
d. Prednisone, to decrease the immune reaction.

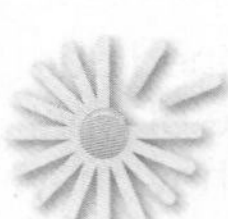

Key Points for Review

- Hematopoietic stem cell transplantation is the main therapy for numerous blood dyscrasias. Transplantation can be allogeneic (from a histocompatible donor) or autologous (using the child's own marrow or umbilical cord blood) or synergeneic (the donor and recipient are identical twins).
- Splenectomy, another possible treatment, may increase a child's susceptibility to pneumococcal infections. Assess whether a child has received pneumococcal vaccine after a splenectomy.
- Disorders of the red blood cells that commonly occur in children include acute blood-loss anemia and anemia of acute infection. Aplastic and hypoplastic anemias occur from depression of hematopoietic activity in bone marrow. These anemias can be congenital or acquired.
- A major hypochromic anemia that develops in children is iron-deficiency anemia. Children invariably fatigue easily because they cannot oxygenate body cells well. Their care must include measures to keep them from tiring; oxygen administration may be necessary.
- Macrocytic anemias occur from folic acid deficiency and pernicious anemia (vitamin B_{12} deficiency).
- Hemolytic anemias include congenital spherocytosis, glucose-6-dehydrogenase deficiency, sickle-cell anemia, thalassemia, and autoimmune acquired hemolytic anemia. Sickle-cell anemia occurs most often in African American children.
- Disorders of white blood cells that occur include neutropenia (reduced number of white blood cells) and neutrophilia (increased number). Neutropenia makes children susceptible to infection.
- Disorders of blood coagulation include the purpuras (idiopathic thrombocytopenic purpura and Henoch-Schönlein syndrome), disseminated intravascular coagulation, and the hemophilias.
- Children with blood coagulation disorders must carefully guard against injury. This includes monitoring types of toys and activities. It may include padding a crib or side rail.
- Disorders of the blood tend to be long-term illnesses. Education of the parents and child is important to promote adaptation to the condition and enhance long-term medication therapy.

CRITICAL THINKING EXERCISES

1. Lana is the 4-year-old girl diagnosed with thalassemia major whom you met at the beginning of the chapter. She has a prominent mandible and wide-spaced upper front teeth from overgrowth of bone marrow centers. Her skin is bronze from the number of transfusions (64) she has received in her short lifetime. "Why is my daughter starting to look different?" Lana's mother asks you. What additional health teaching does Lana's mother need to help her better understand her daughter's disease? How would you explain why skin color changes have happened to her daughter?
2. Joey, a 7-year-old with sickle-cell anemia, is seen at the same clinic as Lana. His growth is only in the fifth percentile, and he has had two vaso-occlusive crises in the past year. Every summer for the past 2 years, while he has been home from school on summer vacation, he has had an acute episode of his illness. What assessments would you want to make of his family before this summer? What precautions would you want to discuss with them?
3. Justin is a 5-year-old boy with hemophilia who wants to join a preschool soccer program. How would you counsel his family regarding this plan?
4. Examine the National Health Goals related to hematologic disorders in children. Most government-sponsored funds for nursing research are allotted based on these goals. What would be a possible research topic to explore pertinent to these goals that would be applicable to Lana's family and also advance evidence-based practice?

CRITICAL THINKING SCENARIO

Open the accompanying CD-ROM or visit http://thePoint.lww.com and read the Patient Scenario included for this chapter, then answer the questions to further sharpen your skills and grow more familiar with NCLEX style questions related to hematologic disorders in children. Confirm your answers are correct by reading the rationales.

REFERENCES

Adamson, J. W., & Longo, D. L. (2008). Anemia and polycythemia. In A. S. Fauci (Ed.). *Harrison's principles of internal medicine* (17th ed.). Columbus, OH: McGraw-Hill.

Ambruso, D. R., Hays, T., & Goldenberg, N. (2008). Hematologic disorders. In W. W. Hay, et al. (Eds.). *Current pediatric diagnosis and treatment* (18th ed.). Columbus, OH: McGraw-Hill.

Barnett, K., et al. (2007). Tapeworm infestation: a cause of iron deficiency anemia shown by capsule endoscopy. *Gastrointestinal Endoscopy, 66*(3), 625–627.

Beattie, S. (2007). Hands-on help: bone marrow aspiration and biopsy. *RN, 70*(2), 41–43.

Bowman, S. H. (2007). Disseminated intravascular coagulation. In J. Schaider, et al. (Eds.). *Rosen & Barkin's 5-minute emergency medicine consult.* Philadelphia: Lippincott Williams & Wilkins.

Brotanek, J. M., et al. (2007). Iron deficiency in early childhood in the United States: risk factors and racial/ethnic disparities. *Pediatrics, 120*(3), 568–575.

Butani, L., & Morgenstern, B. Z. (2007). Long-term outcome in children after Henoch-Schonlein purpura nephritis. *Clinical Pediatrics, 46*(6), 505–511.

Chinegwundoh, F. I., & Anie, K. A. (2009). Treatments for priapism in boys and men with sickle-cell disease. *Cochrane Database of Systematic Reviews, 2009*(1), (CD004198).

Creary, M., Williamson, D., & Kulkarni, R. (2007). Sickle-cell disease: current activities, public health implications, and future directions. *Journal of Women's Health, 16*(5), 575–582.

Davies, E. G., et al. (2009). Pneumococcal vaccines for sickle-cell disease. *Cochrane Database of Systematic Reviews, 2009*(1), (CD003885).

Domellof, M. (2007). Iron requirements, absorption and metabolism in infancy and childhood. *Current Opinion in Clinical Nutrition and Metabolic Care, 10*(3), 329–335.

Ferrara, M., et al. (2007). Prophylactic platelet transfusion in children with thrombocytopenic disorders: a retrospective review. *Hematology, 12*(4), 297–299.

Giulino, L. B., Bussel, J.B., & Neufeld, E. J. (2007). Treatment with rituximab in benign and malignant hematologic disorders in children. *Journal of Pediatrics, 150*(4), 338–344.

Gluckman, E., et al. (2007). Results of unrelated cord blood transplant in Fanconi anemia patients: risk factor analysis for engraftment and survival. *Biology of Blood and Marrow Transplantation, 13*(9), 1073–1082.

Grosskreutz, C., et al. (2007). Graft versus host disease after stem cell allotransplantation with low-dose total body irradiation, fludarabine, and antithymocyte globulin. *Transplantation, 84*(5), 598–604.

Hellmann, D. B., & Imboden, J. B. (2009). Musculoskeletal disorders. In S. J. McPhee & M. A. Papadakis (Eds.). *Current medical diagnosis and treatment.* Columbus, OH: McGraw-Hill.

James, A. H., & Jamison, M. G. (2007). Bleeding events and other complications during pregnancy and childbirth in women with von Willebrand disease. *Journal of Thrombosis and Haemostasis, 5*(6), 1165–1169.

Jones, A. P., Davies, S. C., & Olujohungbe, A. (2009). Hydroxyurea for sickle-cell disease. *Cochrane Database of Systematic Reviews, 2009*(1), (CD002202).

Karch, A. M. (2009). *Lippincott's nursing drug guide.* Philadelphia: Lippincott Williams & Wilkins.

Lees, C., Davies, S. C., & Dezateux, C. (2009). Neonatal screening for sickle-cell disease. *Cochrane Database of Systematic Reviews, 2009*(1), (CD001913).

Linker, C. A. (2009). Hematology. In S. J. McPhee & M. A. Papadakis (Eds.). *Current medical diagnosis and treatment.* Columbus, OH: McGraw-Hill.

Muncie, H. L. (2008). Thalassemia. In F. J. Domino (Ed.). *The 5-minute clinical consult.* Philadelphia: Lippincott Williams & Wilkins.

Nuss, S. L., & Wilson, M. E. (2007). Health-related quality of life following hematopoietic stem cell transplant during childhood. *Journal of Pediatric Oncology Nursing, 24*(2), 106–115.

Owusu-Ofori, S., & Hirst, C. (2009). Splenectomy versus conservative management for acute sequestration crises in people with sickle-cell disease. *Cochrane Database of Systematic Reviews, 2009*(1), (CD003425).

Primack, B. A., & Mahaniah, K. J. (2008). Anemia. In J. E. South-Paul, S. C. Matheny, & E. L. Lewis (Eds.). *Current diagnosis and treatment in family medicine* (2nd ed.). Columbus, OH: McGraw-Hill.

Riddington, C., & Owusu-Ofori, S. (2009). Prophylactic antibiotics for preventing pneumococcal infection in children with sickle-cell disease. *Cochrane Database of Systematic Reviews, 2009*(1), (CD003427).

Rodgers, C., et al. (2008). Growth patterns and gastrointestinal symptoms in pediatric patients after hematopoietic stem cell transplantation. *Oncology Nursing Forum, 35*(3), 443–448.

Saria, M. G., & Gosselin-Acomb, T. K. (2007). Hematopoietic stem cell transplantation: implications for critical care nurses. *Clinical Journal of Oncology Nursing, 11*(1), 53–63.

Servey, J. T., Reamy, B. V., & Hodge, J. (2007). Clinical presentations of parvovirus B19 infection. *American Family Physician, 75*(3), 373–376.

Schmidt, M., & Aldeen, A. (2007). Idiopathic thrombocytopenic purpura. In J. Schaider, et al. (Eds.). *Rosen & Barkin's 5-minute emergency medicine consult.* Philadelphia: Lippincott Williams & Wilkins.

Stumpf, J. L. (2007). Deferasirox. *AJHP: American Journal of Health-System Pharmacy, 64*(6), 606–616.

Tse, W., Bunting, K. D., & Laughlin, M. J. (2008). New insights into cord blood stem cell transplantation. *Current Opinion in Hematology, 15*(4), 279–284.

Waterbury, L. (2007). Anemia. In N. H. Fiebach, et al. (Eds.). *Principles of ambulatory medicine* (7th ed.). Philadelphia: Lippincott Williams & Wilkins.

Wiener, L. S., et al. (2007). Hematopoietic stem cell donation in children: a review of the sibling donor experience. *Journal of Psychosocial Oncology, 25*(1), 45–66.

Zull, D. N. (2007). Polycythemia. In J. Schaider, et al. (Eds.). *Rosen & Barkin's 5-minute emergency medicine consult.* Philadelphia: Lippincott Williams & Wilkins.

SUGGESTED READINGS

Anie, K. A., & Massaglia, P. (2009). Psychological therapies for thalassaemia. *Cochrane Database of Systematic Reviews, 2009*(1), (CD002890).

Bartle, C. (2007). Developing a service for children with iron deficiency anaemia. *Nursing Standard, 21*(19), 44–49.

Gray, A., et al. (2007). Safe transfusion of blood and blood components . . . art and science. *Nursing Standard, 21*(51), 40–47.

Justice, H. M., & Mason, J. D. (2007). Recognizing acquired thrombocytopenic coagulopathies. *Emergency Medicine, 39*(7), 7–12.

Kyles, D. (2007). Is your patient having a transfusion reaction? *Nursing 2007, 37*(4), 1–4.

Mahat, G., Scoloveno, M. A., & Donnelly, C. B. (2007). Written educational materials for families of chronically ill children. *Journal of the American Academy of Nurse Practitioners, 19*(9), 471–476.

Mattson, M. R. (2007). Graft-versus-host disease: review and nursing implications. *Clinical Journal of Oncology Nursing, 11*(3), 325–328.

Peirano, P. D., et al. (2007). Iron deficiency anemia in infancy is associated with altered temporal organization of sleep states in childhood. *Pediatric Research, 62*(6), 715–719.

Rees, D. C. (2007). Neonatal sickle-cell disease and thalassaemia. *Infant, 3*(1), 31–35.

Saulsbury, F. T. (2007). Clinical update: Henoch-Schonlein purpura. *Lancet, 369*(9566), 976–978.

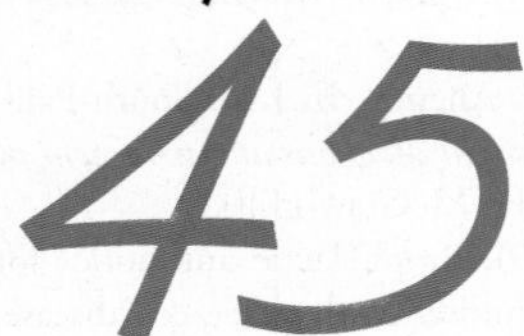

Chapter 45 Nursing Care of a Family When a Child Has a Gastrointestinal Disorder

KEY TERMS

- beriberi
- celiac disease
- dehydration
- gastroesophageal reflux
- hiatal hernia
- inguinal hernia
- insensible loss
- intussusception
- irritable bowel syndrome
- keratomalacia
- kwashiorkor
- liver transplantation
- McBurney's point
- Meckel's diverticulum
- necrotizing enterocolitis
- nutritional marasmus
- overhydration
- pellagra
- rickets
- scurvy
- steatorrhea
- volvulus
- xerophthalmia

OBJECTIVES

After mastering the contents of this chapter, you should be able to:

1. Describe common gastrointestinal disorders seen in children.
2. Identify National Health Goals related to gastrointestinal disorders and children that nurses could help the nation achieve.
3. Analyze ways that nursing care of a child with a gastrointestinal disorder could be more family centered.
4. Assess a child with a gastrointestinal disorder.
5. Formulate nursing diagnoses for a child with a gastrointestinal disorder.
6. Develop expected outcomes for a child with a gastrointestinal disorder.
7. Plan nursing care for a child with a gastrointestinal disorder.
8. Implement nursing care for a child with a gastrointestinal disorder, such as preparing the child for surgery.
9. Evaluate expected outcomes for achievement and effectiveness of care.
10. Identify areas of care related to gastrointestinal disorders and children that could benefit from additional nursing research or application of evidence-based practice.
11. Integrate knowledge of gastrointestinal disorders with nursing process to achieve quality maternal and child health nursing care.

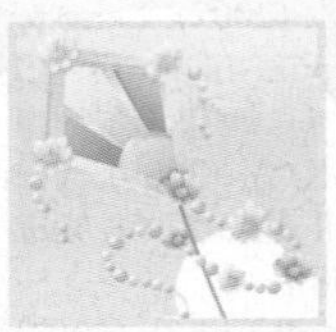

Barry Abraham is a 2-year-old boy diagnosed with celiac disease whom you see at a birthday party. His abdomen is protuberant, yet his arms and legs seem thin and wasted. He refuses to eat a piece of birthday cake even though his mother sits beside him insisting on it. "See the problem I have with him?" she asks you. "He eats nothing. When he does, he gets diarrhea."

Previous chapters described the growth and development of well children and the nursing care for children with disorders of other systems. This chapter adds information about the dramatic changes, both physical and psychosocial, that can occur when children develop gastrointestinal disorders. Such information builds a base for care and health teaching for children with these disorders.

Does Barry's mother understand her son's disease? Is she choosing wise food selections for him?

The gastrointestinal (GI) system involves a long body tract and numerous organs. Because it is so long and diverse, a multitude of possible disorders can occur along it, including both congenital disorders and acquired illnesses. Because the GI system is responsible for taking in and processing nutrients for all parts of the body, any problem with the system can quickly affect other body systems and, if not adequately treated, can affect overall health, growth, and development.

Health education is extremely important for children with GI disorders and their families because it can be difficult to appreciate the seriousness of GI illness. Often, parents are surprised to find that what they thought was a simple "stomach flu" has caused serious electrolyte imbalances and possibly a life-threatening state for their child. Some GI disorders require both parents and child to learn new nutritional patterns. When children are young, the parents need education concerning this topic. As children grow older, counseling to help them maintain self-esteem and learn nutritional requirements so they can become independent become important.

Food poisoning and hepatitis are examples of GI illnesses that are so pervasive that national health goals have been set to limit their incidence (see Box 45.1).

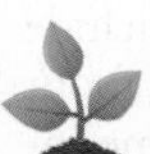

Nursing Process Overview

For a Child With a Gastrointestinal Disorder

Assessment

Children with GI disorders quickly become dehydrated, especially if vomiting or diarrhea is a symptom. This means they need to be assessed for signs of fluid loss, such as poor skin turgor, dry mucous membranes, or lack of tearing. When talking to parents about a child's symptoms, ask exactly what they mean when they say "spitting up" or "a little vomiting." Also ask how many times a child has voided or how many diapers have been wet in the past 24 hours, and whether this is less than usual. Compare the child's current weight with past weight measurements, if available. Unless the child is an adolescent who has been actively dieting, there is never a normal reason for weight loss in children.

Ask parents to describe what they mean by diarrhea as some parents mistakenly confuse normal newborn or infant stools with diarrhea. As a rule, all children with diarrhea, especially small children, need to be seen by a health care provider because fluid and electrolyte changes occur rapidly in children because of the greater percentage of fluid held extracellularly rather than intracellularly.

For many children, a GI tract disorder is diagnosed largely by presenting symptoms such as those just described. In other instances, x-ray studies with a contrast medium (barium) or an endoscopic examination may be needed to confirm the presence of an anomaly. Ultrasound or magnetic resonance imaging (MRI) also may be helpful. Another important assessment area is laboratory testing for electrolyte balance through serum analysis or fluid concentration through urinalysis.

Nursing Diagnosis

Nursing diagnoses relevant to children with GI disorders invariably center on imbalanced nutrition, because most GI diseases alter the kind and amount of nutrients ingested or absorbed into the body in some way. However,

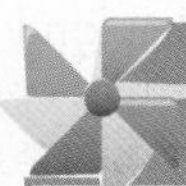

BOX 45.1 ✻ Focus on National Health Goals

Nutrition deficiencies, unsafe food preparation, and hepatitis are three areas that could be reduced in incidence if people knew more about them and took active interventions to reduce their occurrence or spread. National Health Goals addressing these include:

- Reduce infections caused by key food-borne pathogens such as *Salmonella* infection from 13.6 per 100,000 to 6.8 per 100,000, *Listeria* infection from 0.47 per 100,000 to 0.24 per 100,000, and *E. coli* infection from 22 per 100,000 to 11 per 100,000.
- Increase the proportion of persons 2 years of age and older who meet the daily recommendation of calcium from 45% to 74%.
- Reduce the incidence of chronic hepatitis B viral infections in infants and young children (perinatal infections) from a baseline of 1682 instances per year to a target level of 400 instances per year.
- Reduce the rate of hepatitis B infections in adolescents 19 to 24 years of age from 24 per 100,000 population to 2.4 per 100,000 population.
- Reduce the incidence of hepatitis C from a baseline of 2.4 new cases per 100,000 population to 1 new case per 100,000 population.
- Reduce the rate of hepatitis A infection from a baseline of 11.3 per 100,000 to 4.5 per 100,000 (http://www.nih.gov).

Nurses can help the nation achieve these goals by counseling parents about safe food preparation and the need for children to ingest adequate calcium for sound bone growth, by serving as consultants to day care providers to reduce the spread of stool contamination in these settings, and by actively administering hepatitis A and B vaccines to infants and adolescents to eradicate these forms of the illness in another generation. Nursing research in several areas could be helpful: What is the best media to use to educate parents about safe food preparation? Does the brand of diapers used by children in day care influence the spread of infectious stool? How many infants are not being brought for follow-up care and so do not receive all three immunizations against hepatitis B? Do most parents appreciate the devastating outcome that can result from hepatitis?

GI disorders also take an emotional toll on the ill child and family. Feeding is one of the primary ways mothers bond with their newborns, so bonding can be seriously threatened when a newborn develops a GI disorder, especially when hospitalization is required. The process of eating and the types of food eaten are also integral components of family life and culture, so any disruption caused by illness can place a strain on the entire family. Examples of nursing diagnoses are:

- Impaired parenting related to interference with establishing parent–infant bond
- Interrupted family processes related to chronic illness in child
- Risk for deficient fluid volume related to chronic diarrhea
- Imbalanced nutrition, less than body requirements, related to malabsorption of necessary nutrients
- Situational low self-esteem related to feelings of being different resulting from special dietary restrictions

Outcome Identification and Planning

Planning care for a child with a GI disorder often includes nutritional planning with the child and parents. Be certain when helping to plan a new nutritional pattern that the person who actually prepares or supervises the child's nutrition is included. In many instances, some of the foods that a child eats may be prepared by a babysitter, day care center staff, the child's other parent, or a grandparent. Many children eat breakfast and lunch at school cafeterias. That means it may be necessary to contact school staff to ask them to make meal exceptions for a child or to supervise a choice of foods (or to see that a child eats only the packaged lunch brought to school, not extra items the child trades for with friends).

Some parents are unfamiliar with basic food categories and the importance of providing food from the food pyramid in children's diets. When a special diet is requested, they may have little understanding of which foods have high or low fiber content, or which foods are "bland" or "clear." Many parents have difficulty keeping children restricted to "nothing by mouth" (NPO) for tests or to rest the GI tract as they have been told that dehydration happens quickly in infants (which it does). They need support to follow the necessary restrictions when those restrictions are so opposed to basic parenting, which involves giving food.

If feedings will be given by nasogastric or gastrostomy tube, parents need enough practice time to be comfortable with the equipment and the technique before they are given the responsibility of doing it alone at home. If a child is going to gag or become distressed when a new tube is passed, parents need to have this happen where there are calm, supportive people nearby, not when they are by themselves at home.

Anticipate the need for additional support for the family and child with a chronic GI disorder. Agencies that might be helpful for referral are the Celiac Disease Foundation (http://www.celiac.org), Crohn's and Colitis Foundation of America (http://www.ccfa.org), International Foundation for Functional Gastrointestinal Disorders (http://www.iffgd.org), and North American Society for Pediatric Gastroenterology, Hepatology and Nutrition (http://www.naspgn.org).

Implementation

Never underestimate the difficulty family members may experience adapting to alternative nutrition methods such as total parenteral nutrition or enteric or gastrostomy feedings, or caring for a child with a colostomy. Parents need a great deal of support to adapt their busy life to these alternative methods of feeding or care.

GI disorders that occur at birth are discussed in Chapter 27. Insertion of a nasogastric tube, enteral and parenteral nutrition, and administration of an enema are discussed in Chapter 37. Be certain to give clear, simple explanations, and praise both parents and child after they demonstrate these procedures. Children can easily interpret enemas as punishment because of the extreme intrusiveness. Provide therapeutic play before and after these procedures to reduce children's anxiety.

Outcome Evaluation

Recording children's height and weight is a primary method to evaluate nutritional outcomes. Even if a diet is limited in a special way, if it is adequate, children should gain weight and maintain growth.

Because children will ultimately be responsible for their own nutrition, expected outcomes should include making certain that children gradually learn more about their specific nutritional measures so they can become increasingly responsible for their own intake. Often, only when they are at this stage can their parents feel secure enough to let them stay overnight with a friend, visit a relative in a distant city, go to summer camp—activities that become important to children as they reach school age.

The saying "people are what they eat" has some relevance. Children who require special nutritional plans need to be evaluated for self-esteem at periodic health visits. Do children think of themselves as inferior to or different from others because of food restrictions? What kind of positive experiences can be offered to such children, or what can parents do to provide children with experiences that would improve self-esteem?

Some examples of expected outcomes are:

- Child lists examples of bland foods to select for lunch from school cafeteria menu.
- Parent states steps she will take to seek medical care if child has a second episode of severe diarrhea.
- Family members state they have adjusted to care of a child with celiac disease.

ANATOMY AND PHYSIOLOGY OF THE GASTROINTESTINAL SYSTEM

Embryonic development of the GI tract is discussed in Chapter 9. Digestion begins in the mouth, where food is broken down into small particles and mixed with saliva from the sublingual, submandibular, and parotid glands. Both gagging and swallowing reflexes are present even in newborns to prevent aspiration with swallowing. Digestion continues in the stomach and small intestine, the same as in adults.

The esophagus pierces the diaphragm to serve as a passageway to the stomach (Fig. 45.1). Occasionally, an infant is born with a portion of the bowel or stomach protruding

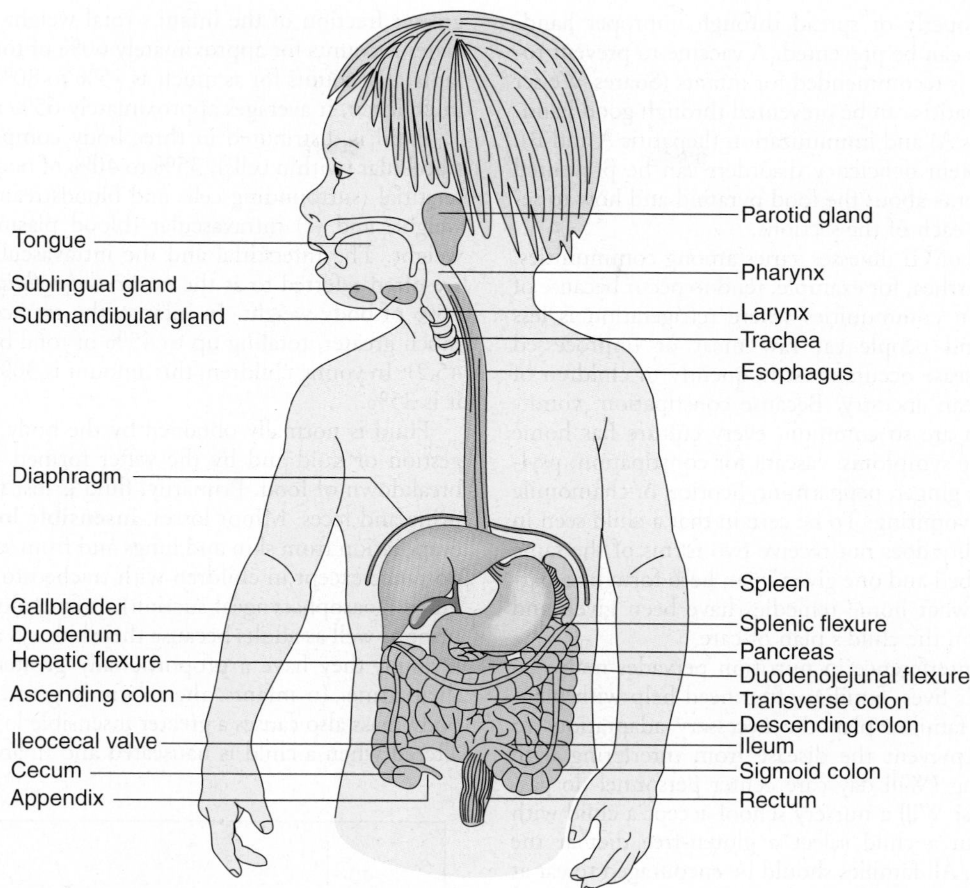

FIGURE 45.1 The gastrointestinal tract.

through the diaphragm's esophageal opening (hiatal or diaphragmatic hernia). At the junction of the esophagus and the stomach is the gastroesophageal (cardiac) sphincter. In some newborns, this sphincter is so lax that fluid regurgitates into the esophagus (gastroesophageal reflux). At the distal end of the stomach is the pyloric sphincter. In some infants, this valve is narrowed (stenosed), preventing food from flowing out of the stomach freely (pyloric stenosis). Originally, it was believed that the stomach was sterile because the action of hydrochloric acid could easily kill invading organisms and limit infections. However, since the discovery that a bacterium, *Helicobacter pylori,* is the cause of peptic ulcer disease, it is obvious that organisms can and do survive in the stomach. Vomiting and diarrhea are symptoms that arise because of stomach or intestinal infections (McQuaid, 2009).

The small intestine is divided into three sections: duodenum, jejunum, and ileum. The large intestine is divided into the cecum, ascending colon, transverse colon, descending colon, sigmoid colon, and rectum. The appendix, which frequently becomes diseased in children, is attached to the cecum.

DIAGNOSTIC AND THERAPEUTIC TECHNIQUES

Several typical procedures are used in the diagnosis and therapy of GI disorders. Common diagnostic procedures include fiberoptic endoscopy, colonoscopy, and barium enema. Children need good preparation for these procedures because they are potentially frightening. If children receive conscious sedation for a procedure, they need preparation for this as well as the actual procedure.

Therapy may include alternative methods of feeding such as enteral (nasogastric or gastrostomy tube feedings) or nutrition sources such as total parenteral nutrition and intravenous (IV) therapy to rest the GI tract. A colostomy or ileostomy may be created to further rest the GI tract. As these are used for other disorders as well, these procedures, their meaning, their impact on children, and nursing responsibilities are discussed in Chapters 37 and 38.

HEALTH PROMOTION AND RISK MANAGEMENT

Health promotion related to GI disorders focuses on a wide area because the causes of these disorders cover a wide range. Some disorders, such as appendicitis, cannot be prevented because they occur for unpredictable causes. Some, such as celiac disease (sensitivity or abnormal immunologic response to protein), involve genetic aspects that cannot be changed. Some, such as Crohn's disease and ulcerative colitis, are associated with an autoimmune response. Other conditions, such as vomiting and diarrhea, are often caused by foods that were refrigerated improperly or spread through improper handwashing and thus can be prevented. A vaccine to prevent rotavirus infections is recommended for infants (Soares-Weiser et al., 2009). Hepatitis can be prevented through good handwashing (hepatitis A) and immunization (hepatitis A and B). Vitamin and protein deficiency disorders can be prevented by educating parents about the food pyramid and how to select foods that fit each of the sections.

The incidence of GI illnesses varies among communities. Vomiting and diarrhea, for example, tend to occur because of food poisoning in communities where refrigeration is less than optimal, and people eat raw meat or unprocessed cheese. Celiac disease occurs most frequently in children of Northern European ancestry. Because constipation, vomiting, and diarrhea are so common, every culture has home remedies for these symptoms: cascara for constipation; psyllium for diarrhea; ginger, peppermint, licorice, or chamomile tea for nausea or vomiting. To be certain that a child seen in a health care facility does not receive two forms of the same drug (one prescribed and one given in an herb form by a parent), always ask what home remedies have been given and document these on the child's plan of care.

Because any interference in nutrition pervades many aspects of children's lives, families often need help with planning care. Help families plan the necessary adaptations to their lifestyle to prevent the disease from interfering with family functioning (Will day care center personnel do gastrostomy feedings? Will a nursery school accept a child with a colostomy? Can a child select a gluten-free diet at the school cafeteria?). All families should be encouraged to eat at least one meal a day together so they can have time to share experiences and "touch base" with each other. For the family with a child who has a feeding problem such as a gastrostomy feeding or total parenteral nutrition, this can be difficult. Urge such families to bring the child to the table for a social time even if the child cannot eat with the family. If watching family members eat while the child cannot is too difficult, urge the family to provide a "together" time in some other way so they do not miss out on this valuable family activity.

Some GI disorders in children, such as aganglionic megacolon, are diagnosed late because parents think the child's refusal to eat is just the sign of being a "picky eater" or a manifestation of 2-year-old autonomy. Educating parents about normal nutrition and how to distinguish things such as vomiting from illness from normal "spitting up" or severe diarrhea from a simple GI upset helps parents bring their children for care at the earliest possible time. Early intervention prevents the child from becoming dehydrated and seriously ill.

FLUID, ELECTROLYTE, AND ACID–BASE IMBALANCES

The GI system plays a major role in maintaining fluid, electrolyte, and acid–base balance. It is the main route by which substances are taken into the body and can be a major source of loss if vomiting or diarrhea occurs (Holliday, Ray, & Friedman, 2007).

Fluid Balance

Retaining fluid is of greater importance in the body chemistry of infants than that of adults because fluid constitutes a greater fraction of the infant's total weight. In adults, body water accounts for approximately 60% of total weight. In infants, it accounts for as much as 75% to 80% of total weight; in children, it averages approximately 65% to 70%.

Fluid is distributed in three body compartments: (a) intracellular (within cells), 35% to 40% of body weight; (b) interstitial (surrounding cells and bloodstream), 20% of body weight; and (c) intravascular (blood plasma), 5% of body weight. The interstitial and the intravascular fluid together are often referred to as the *extracellular fluid* (ECF), totaling 25% of body weight. In infants, the extracellular portion is much greater, totaling up to 45% of total body weight (Fig. 45.2). In young children, this amount is 30%; in adolescents, it is 25%.

Fluid is normally obtained by the body through oral ingestion of fluid and by the water formed in the metabolic breakdown of food. Primarily, fluid is lost from the body in urine and feces. Minor losses, **insensible losses,** occur from evaporation from skin and lungs and from saliva (of little importance except in children with tracheostomies or those requiring nasopharyngeal suction). Infants do not concentrate urine as well as adults because their kidneys are immature. As a result, they have a proportionally greater loss of fluid in their urine. In infants, the relatively greater surface area to body mass also causes a greater insensible loss. Fluid intake is altered when a child is nauseated and unable to ingest fluid

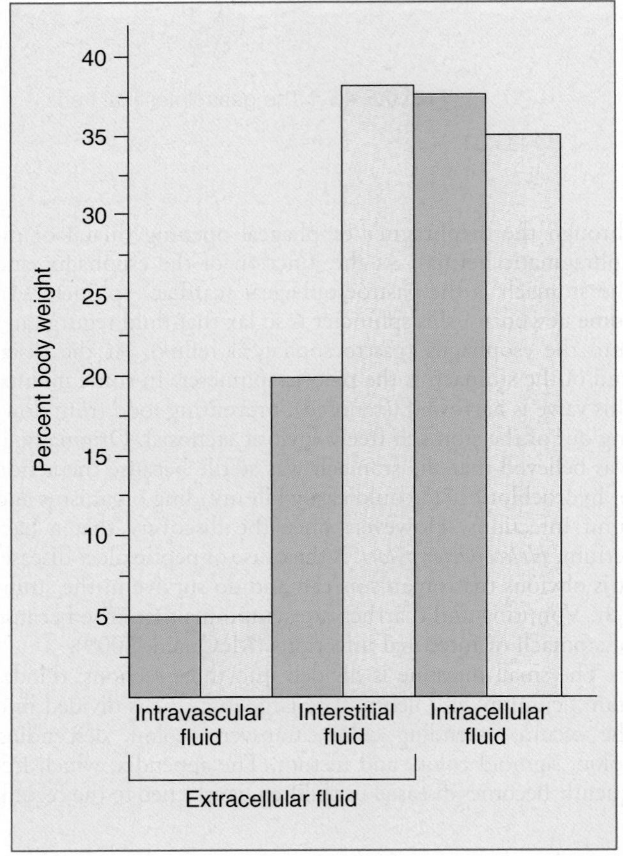

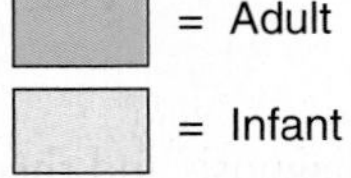

FIGURE 45.2 Distribution of fluid in body compartments.

TABLE 45.1 ✻ A Method to Calculate Fluid Requirement

Body Weight	Fluid Requirement per 24 h
Up to 10 kg	100 ml/kg
11–20 kg	1000 ml + 50 ml/kg for each additional kg over 10 kg
More than 20 kg	1500 ml + 20 ml/kg for each additional kg over 20 kg

or is vomiting and losing fluid ingested. When diarrhea occurs, or when a child becomes diaphoretic because of fever, the fluid output can be markedly increased. **Dehydration** occurs when there is an excessive loss of body water (Scherb, Stevens, & Busman, 2007).

In an adult's weighing 70 kg, the extracellular fluid volume is approximately 14,000 mL. Each day, the well adult's ingests approximately 2000 mL of fluid and excretes approximately 2000 mL as urine. This means that approximately 14% of the adult's total ECF (2000 mL of 14,000 mL) is exchanged each day. In contrast to this, 7-kg infants have an ECF volume of only 1750 mL. They ingest approximately 700 mL daily and excrete approximately 700 mL daily. Therefore, they exchange approximately 40% of their volume daily. As a result of this increased exchange rate, infants' fluid balance may be more critically affected when they are ill. Adults, when they do not eat for a day because of a GI upset, and whose kidneys continue to excrete at the normal rate, will have 14% less fluid in the extracellular space by the end of the day. Infants who do not eat for a day (providing kidney function remains constant) will be 40% short of ECF by the end of the day. This is obviously a more important loss of fluid than the same loss would be in an adult; therefore, dehydration is always a more serious problem in infants than in older children and adults. Requirements of fluid for infants and children are shown in Table 45.1.

Fluid Imbalances

Under most circumstances, water and salt are lost in proportion to each other (*isotonic dehydration*). Occasionally, water is lost out of proportion to salt or water depletion or *hypertonic dehydration* occurs. Occasionally, electrolytes are lost out of proportion to water (*hypotonic dehydration*). Each of these abnormal states produces specific symptoms.

Isotonic Dehydration

When a child's body loses more water than it absorbs (as with diarrhea) or absorbs less fluid than it excretes (as with nausea and vomiting), the first result will be a decrease in the volume of blood plasma. The body compensates for this rapidly by shifting interstitial fluid into the blood vessels. The composition of fluid in these two spaces is similar, so the replacement by this fluid does not change plasma composition. However, this replacement phenomenon can proceed only until the interstitial fluid reserve is depleted—a danger point for a child because it is difficult for the body to replace interstitial fluid from the intracellular fluid (the fluids in these two compartments have different electrolyte contents). If an infant continues to lose fluid after this point, the volume of the plasma will continue to fall rapidly, resulting ultimately in cardiovascular collapse. Typical signs and symptoms of isotonic dehydration are summarized in Table 45.2.

Hypertonic Dehydration

Water is apt to be lost in a greater proportion than electrolytes when fluid intake decreases in conjunction with a fluid loss increase, as might occur in a child with nausea (preventing fluid intake) and fever (increased fluid loss through perspiration); profuse diarrhea, where there is a greater loss of fluid than salt; or renal disease associated with polyuria such as nephrosis with diuresis. In these instances, fluid loss is out of proportion to the loss of electrolytes, and, with such an increased loss of fluid, electrolytes concentrate in the blood. Fluid shifts from the interstitial and intracellular spaces into the bloodstream (from areas of less osmotic pressure to areas of greater pressure). Dehydration occurs in the interstitial and intracellular compartments. The red blood cell count and hematocrit will be elevated because the blood is more concentrated than usual. Levels of electrolytes such as sodium, chloride, and bicarbonate will also likely be increased. Additional signs and symptoms are summarized in Table 45.2.

Hypotonic Dehydration

With hypotonic dehydration, there is a disproportionately high loss of electrolytes relative to fluid lost. The plasma concentration of sodium and chloride will be low. This could result from excessive loss of electrolytes by vomiting or from low intake of salt associated with extreme losses through diuresis. It also occurs when there is extreme loss of electrolytes in diseases such as adrenocortical insufficiency or diabetic acidosis. When low levels of electrolytes occur, the osmotic pressure in

TABLE 45.2 ✻ Signs and Symptoms of Dehydration

	Isotonic	Hypotonic	Hypertonic
Thirst	Mild	Moderate	Extreme
Skin turgor	Poor	Very poor	Moderate
Skin consistency	Dry	Clammy	Moderate
Skin temperature	Cool	Cool	Warm
Urine output	Decreased	Decreased	Decreased
Activity	Irritable	Lethargic	Very lethargic
Serum sodium level	Normal	Reduced	Increased

extracellular spaces decreases. The kidneys begin to excrete more fluid to decrease ECF volume and bring the proportion of electrolytes and fluid back into line. This may lead to a secondary extracellular dehydration (see Table 45.2).

Overhydration

Overhydration may be as serious as dehydration. It generally occurs in children who are receiving IV fluid. The excess fluid in these instances is usually extracellular. The condition is serious because the ECF overload can lead to cardiovascular overload and cardiac failure.

When large quantities of salt-poor fluid (hypotonic solutions) such as tapwater are ingested or are given by enema, the body transfers water from the extracellular space into the intracellular space to restore normal osmotic relationships. This transfer results in intracellular edema manifested by headache, nausea, vomiting, dimness and blurring of vision, cramps, muscle twitching, and seizures. A situation in which intracellular edema may occur is when tap water enemas are given to a child with aganglionic disease of the intestine.

Acid–Base Imbalance

The GI system often is involved with two severe acid–base imbalances: metabolic acidosis and metabolic alkalosis. These imbalances occur with severe diarrhea or vomiting.

When dealing with acid–base balance, a key component is pH. The abbreviation "pH" refers to two French words that mean the "power of hydrogen." pH denotes whether a solution is acid or alkaline, determined by the proportion of hydrogen (H^+) ions in relation to hydroxide (OH^-) ions—the two substances that disassociate when water is broken down into its basic components ($H_2O = H^+$ and OH^-). A solution is acid (pH below 7.0) if it contains proportionately more H^+ ions than OH^- ions. It is alkaline (pH above 7.0) if the proportion of OH^- ions exceeds that of H^+ ions.

Whether body serum is becoming acidotic is determined by analyzing a sample of arterial blood for blood gases. The pH of blood is normally slightly alkaline, ranging from 7.35 to 7.45. PCO_2 (the amount of dissolved carbon dioxide in arterial blood) is normally 35 to 45 mm Hg. The level of bicarbonate (HCO_3) in arterial blood is normally 22 to 26 mEq/L.

Metabolic Acidosis

Metabolic acidosis may result from diarrhea. When diarrhea occurs, a great deal of sodium is lost with stool. This excessive loss of Na^+, in turn, causes the body to conserve H^+ ions in an attempt to keep the total number of positive and negative ions in serum balanced. As a result, a child becomes acidotic as the number of H^+ ions in the blood increases proportionately over the number of OH^- ions present. With metabolic acidosis, arterial blood gas analysis will reveal a decreased pH (under 7.35) and a low HCO_3 value (near or below 22 mEq/L). The lower the HCO_3 value is, presumably the more Na^+ ions that have been lost or the more extensive the diarrhea has been.

To correct this problem (a pH too low is incompatible with life), the body uses both its kidney and respiratory buffering systems. The respiratory buffering system attempts to correct the imbalance quickly. H^+ ions combine with HCO_3^- ions to form carbonic acid. This, in turn, is broken down into CO_2 and water, which is then eliminated by the lungs during expiration. This process works immediately, and, as it continues for a time, the bicarbonate level in the serum falls lower and lower as the body uses up its bicarbonate store.

In the kidneys, H^+ ions are excreted directly or combine with other substances, such as phosphate and ammonia, to form a weak acid, which is excreted. Unfortunately, this process is slow, taking up to 24 hours.

The child breathes rapidly (hyperpnea) to "blow off" CO_2 to prevent it from combining with H_2O and reforming HCO_3. Urine becomes more acid as ammonia formation in the urine is increased.

Metabolic Alkalosis

With vomiting, a great deal of hydrochloric acid is lost. When Cl^- ions are lost this way, the body has to decrease the number of H^+ ions present so the number of positive and negative charges remains balanced. This causes the child to become alkalotic as the number of H^+ ions becomes proportionately lower than the number of OH^- ions present. To further reduce the number of H^+ ions, the lungs conserve CO_2 and water by slowing respirations (hypopnea). The excessive CO_2 retained by this maneuver dissolves in the blood as carbonic acid and then is converted into excessive H^+ and HCO_3^-. With metabolic alkalosis, therefore, the serum HCO_3 invariably will be high. The higher the value, presumably the more Cl^- ions have been lost or the more extensive the vomiting has been.

The child will breathe slowly and shallowly; pH will be elevated (near or above 7.45), and HCO_3 level will be near or above 28 mEq/L.

When alkalosis occurs from vomiting, a secondary electrolyte problem often occurs. As the kidneys begin to help conserve H^+ ions, K^+ ions are exchanged for H^+ ions—that is, K^+ ions are excreted in order to retain H^+ ions. As a result of this loss of K^+ into the urine, low K^+ levels (hypokalemia) invariably accompany metabolic alkalosis.

✓ Checkpoint Question 45.1

Barry has frequent bouts of vomiting. What secondary electrolyte problem often occurs when metabolic alkalosis results from vomiting?

a. Acidosis.
b. Hyponatremia.
c. Hypokalemia.
d. Hyperchlorosis.

COMMON GASTROINTESTINAL SYMPTOMS OF ILLNESS IN CHILDREN

Vomiting and diarrhea in children commonly occur as symptoms of disease of the GI tract as well as symptoms of disease in other body systems (Box 45.2). Pneumonia or otitis media, for example, may present first with vomiting or diarrhea. The danger is that either can lead to a disturbance in hydration, electrolyte, or acid–base balance. In many infants, these secondary disturbances can be more threatening to the child than the primary disease.

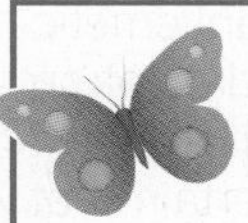

Box 45.2 Assessment
Assessing a Child With Altered GI Function

History
Chief concern: Vomiting, diarrhea, constipation, abdominal pain, abdominal distention, weight below normal standard, lethargy, paleness.
Past medical history: History of past vomiting or diarrhea or abdominal pain; hydramnios in pregnancy.
Family history: Relatives have a similar disorder; high stress level because of home or school environment.

Physical examination

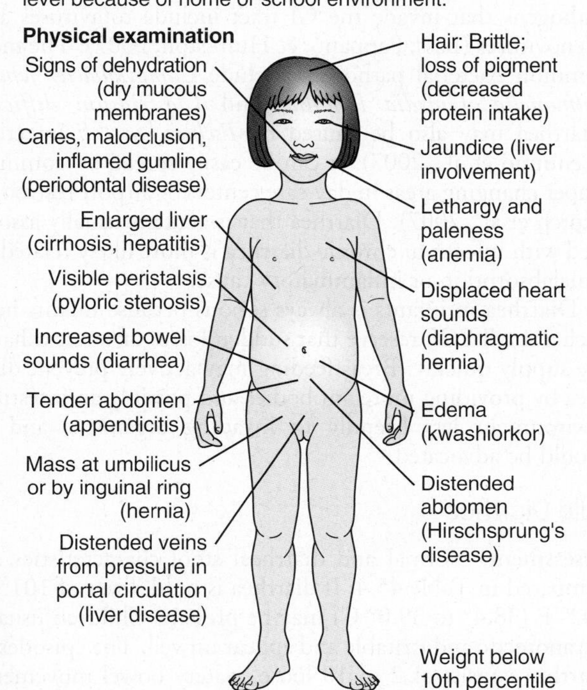

Vomiting

Many children with vomiting are suffering from a mild gastroenteritis (infection) caused by a viral or bacterial organism. The adolescent who is pregnant may also experience vomiting. Some children develop persistent or cyclic vomiting (Fitzpatrick et al., 2007). In all forms, vomiting is always potentially serious because a metabolic alkalosis and dehydration may result.

Assessment

In describing symptoms of vomiting, be certain to differentiate between the various terms that are used (Table 45.3). It is important that vomiting be described correctly this way because different conditions are marked by different forms of vomiting, and a correct description of the child's actions can aid greatly in diagnosis.

Therapeutic Management

The treatment for vomiting is to withhold food from the stomach for a time as if there is nothing in the stomach, vomiting cannot occur. Most parents treat vomiting in the opposite way. Every time a child vomits, they attempt to feed the child again. The child vomits again and they feed again, and so on. This prolongs the vomiting and intensifies the potential for electrolyte imbalance.

Nursing Diagnoses and Related Interventions

Nursing Diagnosis: Risk for deficient fluid volume related to vomiting

Outcome Evaluation: Skin turgor remains good; specific gravity of urine is 1.003 to 1.030; urine output is more than 1 mL/kg/hr; episodes of vomiting decrease in frequency and amount.

TABLE 45.3 ✻ Differentiation Between Regurgitation and Vomiting

Characteristic	Regurgitation	Vomiting
Timing	Occurs with feeding	Timing unrelated to feeding
Forcefulness	Runs out of mouth with *little force*	Forceful; often projected 1 ft away from the infant; *projectile vomiting*—projected as much as 4 ft (most often related to increased intracranial pressure in newborns; in infants age 4–6 wk, possibly because of pyloric stenosis)
Description	Smells barely sour; only slightly curdled	Extremely sour smelling, appearing curdled, yellow, green, clear or watery, or black; perhaps fresh blood or old blood staining from swallowed maternal blood (in newborns)
Distress	Nonpainful; child does not appear to be in distress and may even smile as if sensation is enjoyable	Possible crying just before vomiting as if abdominal pain is present, and after vomiting as if the force of action is frightening
Duration	Occurs once per feeding	Continuing until stomach is empty; followed by dry retching
Amount	1–2 tsp	Full stomach contents

To decrease vomiting, withhold food and fluid for a time (nothing by mouth [NPO]), depending on the age of the child. On the average, a period of 3 to 6 hours is usually sufficient. In the older child, after this period of fasting, offer a few ice chips, then water in small amounts—approximately 1 tbsp every 15 minutes, four times; then 2 tbsp every half-hour, four times. Popsicles can be substituted for water. If this is retained, children can be given small sips of clear liquids, such as tea, ginger ale, or a rehydration fluid such as Pedialyte. The World Health Organization provides a home recipe for fluid rehydration of 2 tablespoons of sugar (or honey) with ¼ teaspoon of table salt and ¼ teaspoon of baking soda dissolved in 1 liter (1 qt) of water.

Children may become hungry and want whole glasses of fluid, but keeping the quantity to small sips prevents vomiting. Once the child is able to retain sips of clear liquids, the child can be offered portions of broth, clear soup, and skim milk in addition to clear liquids. Dry crackers or toast will help assuage hunger. By the second day, children can take a soft diet; by the third day, they should be back to their regular diet.

For the infant, introduce fluid after a fasting period of approximately 3 hours in the same slow manner: 1 tbsp every 15 minutes for 2 hours, then 1 oz every 2 hours for the next 12 to 18 hours. Glucose water or a commercial hydration solution such as Pedialyte may be given as fluid during this time to help the infant maintain electrolyte balance. Infants progress, as do older children, gradually to clear liquids or breast milk, then a soft diet, then a regular diet. If vomiting is prolonged, infants may need IV therapy or an antiemetic to restore hydration (Leung et al., 2007).

Teach parents the importance of following these routines of gradually increasing fluid at intervals. Assure them that if children receive a small amount of fluid and do not vomit it, they will ultimately receive more fluid than if they take a large amount but, because of gastroenteritis, vomit that amount. Parents are capable of understanding that stomach secretions are lost along with vomitus each time, and the preservation of these stomach secretions is important to keep their child well. Antiemetic medicine is rarely necessary for children because acute gastroenteritis is a self-limiting condition and vomiting may actually be helpful if it rids the child's body of toxic substances. If vomiting is severe, however, an antiemetic such as promethazine (Phenergan) or Ondansetron (Zofran) may be prescribed. Always ask parents if they have used an herbal remedy, to be certain that any medication prescribed will be safe with the alternative treatment.

Diarrhea

Diarrhea caused by a virus is the major cause of infant gastroenteritis in developing countries. The most common viral pathogens that invade the GI tract include rotaviruses and adenoviruses (Bass, Pappano, & Humiston, 2007). The most common bacterial pathogens include *Campylobacter jejuni, Salmonella, Giardia lamblia,* and *Clostridium difficile.* Diarrhea may also be caused by *Escherichia coli* infection (Cennimo et al., 2007). It can be easily spread by common diaper changing areas in day care centers or airport restrooms (Kotch et al., 2007). Diarrhea that is acute is usually associated with infection; chronic diarrhea is more likely related to a malabsorption or inflammatory cause.

Diarrhea in infants is always serious because infants have such a small ECF reserve that sudden losses of water exhaust the supply quickly. Breastfeeding may actively prevent diarrhea by providing more antibodies and possibly an intestinal environment less friendly to invading organisms and so should be advocated.

Mild Diarrhea

Assessment. Normal and diarrheal stool characteristics are compared in Table 45.4. If diarrhea is mild, fever of 101° to 102° F (38.4° to 39.0° C) may be present. Children usually are anorectic and irritable and appear unwell. The episodes of diarrhea consist of 2 to 10 loose, watery bowel movements per day.

The mucous membrane of the mouth appears dry and the skin feels warm although skin turgor will not yet be decreased. The pulse will be rapid and out of proportion to the low-grade fever. Urine output is usually normal.

Therapeutic Management. At this stage, diarrhea is not yet serious, and children can be cared for at home. As with vomiting, treatment for diarrhea must involve resting the GI tract, but this is necessary for only a short time. At the end of approximately 1 hour, parents can begin to offer an oral rehydration solution such as Pedialyte in small amounts on a

TABLE 45.4 ✻ Differentiation Between Infant Normal Stool and Diarrheal Stool

Characteristic	Infant Normal Stool	Diarrheal Stool
Frequency	1–3 daily	Unlimited number
Color	Yellow	Green
Effort of expulsion	Some pushing effort	Effortless; may be explosive
pH	More than 7.0 (alkaline)	Less than 7.0 (acidic)
Odor	Odorless	Sweet or foul smelling
Occult blood	Negative	Positive; blood may be overt
Reducing substances	Negative	Positive

regimen similar to that for vomiting (Freedman, 2007). For breastfed infants, breastfeeding should continue. Again, it may be difficult for parents to restrict fluid for a short time if they think they should overfeed children to make up for the fluid loss. Children also need measures to reduce the elevated temperature. In developing countries, where children may be zinc deficient, zinc may be administered. Probiotics (dietary supplements containing potentially beneficial bacteria or yeasts) to change the bacterial flora of the intestine may be administered (Walter & Isolauri, 2007).

Caution parents to contact their health care provider rather than use over-the-counter drugs such as loperamide (Imodium) or kaolin and pectin (Kaopectate) to halt diarrhea because, as a rule, these are too strong for young children (Karch, 2009). Also caution parents to wash their hands after changing diapers to prevent the spread of infection to themselves and to notify their health care provider if fever, pain, or diarrhea worsens.

Infants may develop a lactase deficiency after diarrhea that leads to lactose intolerance. With lactose intolerance, a child cannot take formula or breast milk or new diarrhea will begin. Such an infant will need to be introduced to a lactose-free formula initially before being returned to the usual formula or to breast milk.

Severe Diarrhea

Assessment. Severe diarrhea may result from progressive mild diarrhea, or it may begin in a severe form. Infants with severe diarrhea are obviously ill. Rectal temperature is often as high as 103° to 104° F (39.5° to 40.0° C). Both pulse and respirations are weak and rapid. The skin is pale and cool. Infants may appear apprehensive, listless, and lethargic. They have obvious signs of dehydration such as a depressed fontanelle, sunken eyes, and poor skin turgor. The episodes of diarrhea usually consist of a bowel movement every few minutes. The stool is liquid green, perhaps mixed with mucus and blood, and it may be passed with explosive force. Urine output will be scanty and concentrated. Laboratory findings will show elevated hematocrit, hemoglobin, and serum protein levels because of the dehydration. Electrolyte determinations will indicate a metabolic acidosis (Sondheimer, 2008).

It is difficult to measure the amount of fluid a child has lost, but an estimate can be derived from the loss in body weight, if known. For example, if a child weighed 10.4 kg yesterday at a health maintenance visit and today weighs 8.9 kg, the child has lost more than 10% of body weight. Mild dehydration occurs with a loss of 2.5% to 5% of body weight. In contrast, severe diarrhea quickly causes a 5% to 15% loss. Any infant who has lost 10% or more of body weight requires immediate treatment.

Therapeutic Management. Treatment focuses on regulating electrolyte and fluid balance by oral or IV rehydration therapy, initiating rest for the GI tract, and discovering the organism responsible for the diarrhea.

All children with severe diarrhea or diarrhea that persists longer than 24 hours should have a stool culture taken so definite antibiotic therapy can be prescribed. Stool cultures may be taken from the rectum or from stool in a diaper or a bedpan. Blood specimens need to be drawn for a hemoglobin level (an estimation of hydration as well as anemia); white blood cell and differential counts (to attempt to establish whether infection is present); and determinations of P_{CO_2}, Cl^-, Na^+, K^+, and pH (to establish electrolyte needs). If a child can drink, the most effective way to replace fluid is by offering oral rehydration therapy. For a child who will not drink, an IV solution such as normal saline or 5% glucose in normal saline is begun. The solution will provide replacement of fluid, sodium, and calories. Although infants usually have a potassium depletion, potassium cannot be given until it is established that they are not in renal failure. Giving potassium IV when the body has no outlet for excessive potassium can lead to excessively high potassium levels and heart block. *Before this initial IV fluid is changed to a potassium solution, therefore, be certain that the infant or child has voided—proof that the kidneys are functioning.*

Fluid must be given to replace the deficit that has occurred, for maintenance therapy, and to replace the continuing loss until the diarrhea improves. If infants have lost less than 5% of total body weight, their fluid deficit is approximately 50 mL/kg of body weight. If infants have lost 10% of body weight, they need approximately 100 mL/kg of body weight to replace their fluid deficit. If the weight loss suggests a 12% to 15% loss of body fluid, they require 125 mL/kg of body weight to replace the fluid lost. This fluid will be given rapidly in the first 3 to 6 hours, and then it will be slowed to a maintenance rate. Once infants void, a potassium additive can be ordered to restore serum potassium.

Nursing Diagnoses and Related Interventions

Nursing Diagnosis: Deficient fluid volume related to loss of fluid through diarrhea

Outcome Evaluation: Skin turgor remains good; specific gravity of urine is 1.003 to 1.030; urine output is more than 1 mL/kg/hr; bowel movements are formed and fewer than four per day. Stool tests negative for reducing substances and blood pH is more than 7.

Promote Hydration and Comfort. During the time infants are NPO, wet infants' lips with a moisturizing cream or jelly such as Vaseline if they appear to be dry. Offer them a pacifier to suck if this seems to comfort them. (They want to suck because they are very thirsty, and, if they have intestinal cramping with the diarrhea, they interpret this as hunger.)

As the infant's condition improves, oral intake can be increased, changing to a soft then a regular diet. Some children become lactose intolerant after diarrhea and will need a lactose-free formula for rehydration (Misra et al., 2007).

If the child with severe diarrhea also has a fever, measures to reduce the fever will be necessary (see Chapter 37). Do not obtain rectal temperatures to assess fever, because stimulating the anal sphincter could initiate more diarrhea. Assess perianal skin for irritation from liquid stools, and keep the skin clean and dry.

Record Fluid Intake and Output. Much of the nursing care of children with diarrhea focuses on careful recording of fluid intake and output. Because children have dehydration when first seen, oral rehydration or IV therapy serves as their lifeline. Be sure to maintain proper functioning of an IV infusion and site if this is used. An arm board may be necessary to prevent catheter dislodgment or interference with the infusion. Soft restraints applied to the affected and unaffected extremities may be necessary to prevent a child from pulling, playing with, or poking at the tubing or site. If soft restraints are used, be sure to release them every hour and passively exercise the child's extremities. Give parents an explanation of why the IV infusion is important so they will understand the need for the soft restraints.

In children who are not toilet trained, apply a disposable urine collection bag to help separate urine from feces. This makes it obvious that the child is voiding, confirming kidney function. Confirmation of adequate kidney function is necessary for IV K^+ replacement therapy, if ordered.

Separating urine from stools also helps to judge the appearance of stools or their water content. For each stool passed, record its color, consistency, odor, size, and the presence of any blood or mucus. Weigh soiled diapers to reveal the number of grams of stool in the diaper (1 g = 1 mL fluid). Testing the stool for acidity and for reducing substances (sugars) indicates how quickly the stool has passed through the irritated tract. A stool positive for sugar indicates that little absorption occurred, because sugar is normally absorbed rapidly from ingested food. Acid stool (pH less than 7.0) shows the presence of unabsorbed sugar also (a process occurs similar to the process that causes acid to invade tooth enamel in the presence of glucose on teeth). Diarrheal stools are green from lack of time for bile to be modified in the intestine. As diarrhea improves and stool remains in the intestine for a longer period, the stool deepens in color and the acid and sugar contents fade. Testing stools for occult blood shows the extent of bowel irritation that is occurring from the acid stool. As the diarrhea improves and the irritation to the bowel lessens, the finding of occult blood disappears.

Nursing Diagnosis: Risk for impaired skin integrity related to presence of diarrheal stool on skin

Outcome Evaluation: Skin in diaper area is not erythematous or ulcerated.

Because diarrheal stool is extremely irritating to the skin, change diapers immediately after infants pass any stool. Wash the skin of the diaper area well after each stool, and cover it with an ointment such as Vaseline or A&D to protect it from further irritation. If the child is older, caution the child to wipe away stool thoroughly.

If infants already have skin excoriation from the number of stools they have had at home, an ointment such as Desitin may help soothe the irritated skin. Exposing infants' buttocks to air is generally helpful in healing irritation. Assure older children that loss of stool by diarrhea is not "shameful" or "babyish" but to be expected because they are ill.

Nursing Diagnosis: Anxiety related to traumatic experience

Outcome Evaluation: Child interacts with parents in age-appropriate way; can be comforted after painful procedures.

All children with diarrhea are assumed to have an infectious form of gastroenteritis and therefore need contact and standard infection precautions. Children usually are uncomfortable from the diarrhea, exhausted, and confused with these new body sensations. They need the security of someone to stay with them. When a child with severe diarrhea is admitted to the hospital, many emergency procedures must be performed, such as collecting specimens, reducing temperature, and beginning rehydration. During all of these procedures, try to remember how all of this must seem to the child in the bed. Be sure to take time during initial procedures to touch and soothe children and talk to them; once the initial admission procedures are done, sit by the bed and hold a child or gently stroke a child's head. Teach parents how to adhere to standard infection precautions and follow contact precautions if necessary. Encourage them to give any care possible. Children need this support to counteract the strange world into which they have suddenly been plunged.

What if... Barry's mother tells you her doctor has told her to "force fluids" for Barry whenever he has diarrhea? She asks how much she should force the child to drink. How would you answer her?

Bacterial Infectious Diseases That Cause Diarrhea and Vomiting

Several common microorganisms are responsible for diarrhea in children.

Salmonella

- Causative agent: One of the *Salmonella* bacteria
- Incubation period: 6 to 72 hours for intraluminal type; 7 to 14 days for extraluminal type
- Period of communicability: As long as organisms are being excreted (may be as long as 3 months)
- Mode of transmission: Ingestion of contaminated food, especially chicken and raw eggs

Salmonella is the most common type of food poisoning in the United States and a major cause of diarrhea in children. The diagnosis of the infection can be made from stool culture. Children develop diarrhea, abdominal pain, vomiting, high temperature, and headache. They are listless and drowsy. The diarrhea is severe and may contain blood and mucus (Chambers, 2009). *Salmonella* infection may remain in the bowel as an intraluminal disease. When it does, it is treated, like severe diarrhea, with fluid and electrolyte replacement. Antibiotics are rarely prescribed as they may actually prolong the length of the infection (Sirinavin & Garner, 2009). If the infection becomes systemic (extraluminal disease), it is treated with the addition of an antibiotic such as ampicillin or a third-generation cephalosporin (Ogle & Anderson, 2008).

Complications such as meningitis, bronchitis, and osteomyelitis may occur. Because the source of *Salmonella* generally is infected food (contaminated chicken and eggs are common sources), caution parents to wash utensils used to prepare raw chicken such as cutting boards well and to cook eggs thoroughly. Although rare, *Salmonella* also may be transmitted to children by infected turtles (Box 45.3).

Listeriosis

- Causative agent: *Listeria monocytogenes*
- Incubation period: Variable, ranging from 1 day to more than 3 weeks

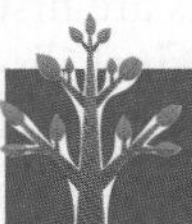

BOX 45.3 ✻ Focus on Family Teaching

Preventing *Salmonella*- or *Listeria*-Caused Gastroenteritis

Q. Barry's mother says to you, "Our son had severe diarrhea from food poisoning. How can we make sure he doesn't get that again?"

A. Anyone can get food poisoning. However, it can be prevented by using the following measures:

- Wash your hands well before preparing any foods, but especially chicken and eggs.
- Remember that chicken may become contaminated with *Salmonella* at the factory where it was prepared. Wash your hands well after handling raw chicken to prevent the spread of infection to other foods being prepared.
- Clean cutting boards or food preparation surfaces with hot, soapy water and dry thoroughly after use to prevent them from becoming reservoirs of infection.
- Make a habit of preparing chicken last, after other foods are prepared.
- Cook eggs well (do not use raw eggs in milkshakes; cook soft-boiled or poached eggs at least 3 min).
- Refrigerate chicken and eggs after preparation.
- Wash hands well after playing with or feeding a pet turtle or changing the turtle's water.
- Wash raw vegetables thoroughly before eating.
- Avoid soft cheeses such as feta, Brie, Camembert, blue-veined, and Mexican queso fresco cheese. Hard cheeses; processed cheeses, including sliced cheese, cream cheese, cheese spreads, and cottage cheese; and yogurt need not be avoided.
- Cook leftover foods or ready-to-eat foods such as hot dogs until steaming hot before eating.
- Avoid foods from delicatessen counters such as prepared salads, meats, and cheeses or heat/reheat these foods until steaming before eating.
- Avoid refrigerated pates and other meat spreads or heat/reheat these foods before eating; canned or shelf-stable pate and meat spreads need not be avoided.
- Avoid raw or unpasteurized milk, including goat's milk, or milk products or foods that contain unpasteurized milk or milk products.

- Mode of transmission: Ingestion of unpasteurized milk or cheeses or vegetables grown in contaminated soil

Listeriosis is a serious infection caused by eating food contaminated with the gram-positive bacterium *Listeria monocytogenes*. The cause of the infection may be difficult to locate as the incubation period can last for almost a month. After this time, however, a child develops fever, muscle aches, nausea, and diarrhea. If infection spreads to the nervous system, symptoms such as headache, stiff neck, confusion, loss of balance, or convulsions can occur. The infection is particularly important to avoid during pregnancy as infections during pregnancy can lead to miscarriage or stillbirth, prematurity, or infection of the newborn. The bacteria is found in soil and water. Vegetables can become contaminated by being grown in contaminated soil. The most frequent source, however, is unpasteurized (raw) milk or foods made from unpasteurized milk such as soft cheese. Therapy is intravenous ampicillin and an aminoglycoside such as gentamicin. If a child is hospitalized, standard infection precautions should be instituted. Measures to avoid the infection are shown in Box 45.3.

Shigellosis (Dysentery)

- Causative agent: Organisms of the genus *Shigella*
- Incubation period: 1 to 7 days
- Period of communicability: Approximately 1 to 4 weeks
- Mode of transmission: Contaminated food, water, or milk products

Shigella organisms, like the *Salmonella* group, cause extremely severe diarrhea that contains blood and mucus. As the organism becomes more resistant, ampicillin or trimethoprim–sulfamethoxazole, typical drugs used for therapy in the past, are being replaced by cephalosporins. The child needs intense fluid and electrolyte replacement. *Shigella* infection can be prevented by safe food handling and cautioning families to drink only from safe water sources (Ogle & Anderson, 2008).

Staphylococcal Food Poisoning

- Causative agent: Staphylococcal enterotoxin produced by some strains of *Staphylococcus aureus*
- Incubation period: 1 to 7 hours
- Period of communicability: Carriers may contaminate food as long as they harbor the organism
- Mode of transmission: Ingestion of contaminated food

With staphylococcal food poisoning, a child has severe vomiting and diarrhea, abdominal cramping, excessive salivation, and nausea within 2 to 6 hours of eating (Ogle & Anderson, 2008). Organisms are most often spread through creamed foods such as potato salad. It is often difficult to culture the causative organism from the contaminated food because although the staphylococci may have been destroyed by cooking, the enterotoxin that actually causes the disorder will not have been destroyed. The child needs intensive supportive therapy with fluid and electrolyte replacement and perhaps administration of a drug effective against *Staphylococcus,* such as cefotaxime. Food poisoning from this source can be prevented by proper refrigeration of food.

✔ Checkpoint Question 45.2

Barry's mother tells you she often makes milkshakes with raw eggs. What infectious organism is easily spread this way?

a. Pneumococcus.
b. *Salmonella.*
c. Streptococcus A.
d. *H. pylori.*

COMMON DISORDERS OF THE STOMACH AND DUODENUM

Disorders of the upper GI tract in children tend to involve inadequate valve function or infection.

Gastroesophageal Reflux

Gastrointestinal reflux or the regurgitation of stomach secretions into the esophagus through the gastroesophageal (cardiac) valve occurs mainly in infants and adolescents.

Gastroesophageal Reflux in Infants

Gastroesophageal reflux in infants occurs from a neuromuscular disturbance in which the gastroesophageal (cardiac) sphincter and the lower portion of the esophagus spasm and allow easy regurgitation of gastric contents into the esophagus. It usually starts within 1 week after birth and may be associated with a hiatal hernia (see later discussion). Children with cerebral palsy or other neurologic involvement are at particular risk. The regurgitation occurs almost immediately after feeding or when the infant is laid down after a feeding. If the amount of the reflux is large or constant, an infant does not retain sufficient calories and will fail to thrive. In addition, aspiration pneumonia or esophageal stricture from the constant reflux of hydrochloric acid into the esophagus can occur (Sondheimer & Sundaram, 2008).

Assessment. The diagnosis is suggested by the history. Vomiting appears effortless and is not projectile; it begins much earlier in life than the vomiting associated with pyloric stenosis. The child may be irritable and may experience periods of apnea. Inserting a probe or catheter through the nose into the distal esophagus and determining the pH from secretions can show whether gastric secretions are entering the esophagus (if the pH is less than 7.0, then acid is present). Esophageal manometry is used to measure the strength of the esophageal sphincter. Fiberoptic endoscopy or esophagography (barium swallow) will further show the involved sphincter and the reflux of stomach contents into the esophagus, especially if the infant's head is tilted downward.

Therapeutic Management. The traditional treatment of GI reflux is to feed infants a formula thickened with rice cereal (1 tbsp of cereal per 1 oz of formula or breast milk) while holding them in an upright position and then keeping them upright in an infant chair for 1 hour after feeding so gravity can help prevent reflux (Craig et al., 2009). An H_2 receptor antagonist such as ranitidine (Zantac) or a proton pump inhibitor such as omeprazole (Prilosec) may be prescribed daily to reduce the possibility of the stomach acid contents irritating the esophagus.

Gastroesophageal reflux is usually a self-limiting condition. As the esophageal sphincter matures and the child begins to eat solid food and is maintained in a more upright position, the problem disappears. If not, botulinum toxin may be injected into the lower esophageal sphincter to temporarily relieve symptoms of obstruction. If medical therapy this way is ineffective, a laparoscopic or surgical myotomy procedure (narrowing of the esophageal sphincter) may be performed. After this procedure, the child will temporarily have a nasogastric tube in place that is attached to intermittent low suction. It is usually irrigated with normal saline every 2 hours to ensure patency. Assess nasogastric tube drainage and any vomitus for coffee-colored drainage (although this is normal for the first 24 hours) that would indicate bleeding from the surgical site. When infants are first fed after surgery, they may display signs of abdominal discomfort and distention because food can no longer reflux into the esophagus as readily as it could before surgery. As their stomach adjusts to this, symptoms fade. Before this happens, however, the distention may be so extreme that it leads to bradycardia and dyspnea. Be alert for the development of these important signs and symptoms.

Nursing Diagnoses and Related Interventions

Nursing Diagnosis: Risk for imbalanced nutrition, less than body requirements, related to regurgitation of food with esophageal reflux

Outcome Evaluation: Skin fold returns to place quickly when turgor is assessed; specific gravity of urine is 1.003 to 1.030; intake is 50 cal/lb/24 hr.

Teach parents the importance of monitoring intake, output (urination), and weight. Also reinforce the need to keep the infant upright, such as in an infant seat, after a feeding. Be certain parents understand how much cereal to mix with formula or breast milk. Encourage parents to feed the infant during the short time that the infant remains in the hospital after surgery so that they can regain their confidence as parents.

Gastrointestinal Reflux in Adolescents

Gastroesophageal reflux disease (GERD) affects about 20% of adults; symptoms frequently begin in adolescence. Irritation to the esophagus occurs when stomach contents, including hydrochloric acid, reflux through the lower esophageal sphincter and irritate the esophageal lining. Reflux occurs because of an incompetent sphincter especially when the adolescent lies supine or when intra-abdominal pressure is increased by a full stomach, lifting or bending, or tight clothing. It is potentially dangerous because it can lead to erosion of the esophagus with perforation or stricture of the esophagus. It may be associated with the development of esophageal cancer in later life (Zagaria, 2008).

The typical symptom is heartburn that occurs 30–60 minutes after a meal. Diagnosis is based on history (typical symptoms of heartburn) and, if symptoms are severe, endoscopy to reveal the irritated esophagus (esophagitis). The goal of treatment is to provide symptomatic relief and to heal any esophagitis identified.

Adolescents should avoid lying down until 3 hours after a meal and should sleep at night with their upper body elevated on a foam wedge. They should avoid acidic foods such as tomato products, citrus fruits, or spicy foods. Avoiding foods that delay gastric emptying such as fatty foods, chocolate, or alcohol and eating smaller portions may also be helpful. Weight loss, avoiding bending after meals, and removing tight belts are also recommended steps.

Antacids relieve pain immediately by decreasing the concentration of the stomach acid and are sold over the counter. H_2-receptor antagonists such as cimetidine (Pepcid) or ranitidine (Zantac) are also available over the counter and can be taken before meals to prevent heartburn symptoms. Proton pump inhibitors such as omeprazole (Prilosec) or rabeprazole (Aciphex), drugs that halt the release of stomach acids, are prescription drugs that offer the best long-term relief. Adolescents generally take these for 6 to 8 months until esophageal healing is complete.

As adults, esophageal reflux may return. Some adults require surgery in later life to relieve esophageal strictures or recurring ulcers from returning irritation.

Pyloric Stenosis

The pyloric sphincter is the opening between the lower portion of the stomach and the beginning portion of the intestine, the duodenum. If hypertrophy or hyperplasia of the muscle surrounding the sphincter occurs, it is difficult for the stomach to empty, a condition called *pyloric stenosis* (Fig. 45.3). With this condition, at 4 to 6 weeks of age, infants begin to vomit almost immediately after each feeding. The vomiting grows increasingly forceful until it is projectile, possibly projecting as much as 3 to 4 feet. The incidence is high, approximately 1:150 in males and 1:750 in females. It tends to occur most frequently in first-born white male infants. The exact cause is unknown, but multifactorial inheritance is the likely cause. It occurs less frequently in breastfed infants than in formula-fed infants. Formula-fed infants typically begin having symptoms at approximately 4 weeks of age. Breastfed infants begin having symptoms at 6 weeks because the curd of breast milk is smaller than that of cow's milk, and it passes through a hypertrophied muscle more easily. For unknown reasons, an increased incidence is seen in infants who receive a macrolide antibiotic such as erythromycin (Maheshwai, 2007).

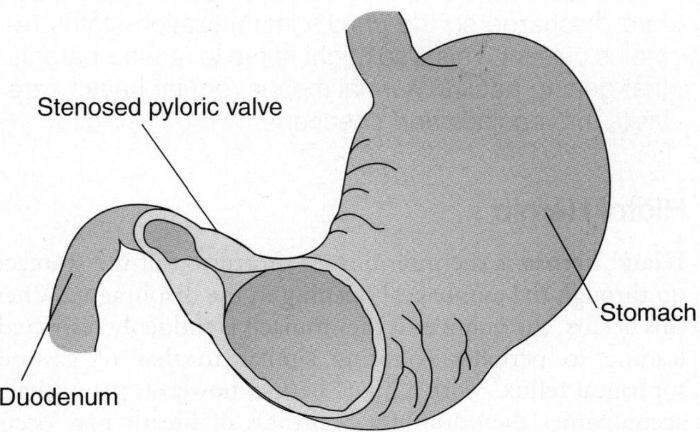

FIGURE 45.3 Pyloric stenosis. Fluid is unable to pass easily through the stenosed and hypertrophied pyloric valve.

Vomitus usually smells sour because it has reached the stomach and has been in contact with stomach enzymes. There is never bile in the vomiting of pyloric stenosis because the feeding does not reach the duodenum to become mixed with bile. Infants are usually hungry immediately after vomiting because they are not nauseated. Although it is difficult to assess whether nausea is present in infants, signs such as a disinterest in eating, excessive drooling, or chewing on the tongue may suggest this.

Assessment

The diagnosis of pyloric stenosis is made primarily from the history. Whenever parents say that their baby is vomiting or spitting up, be certain to get a full description:

- What is the duration? *Begins at 6 weeks of age*
- What is the intensity? *Projectile vomiting*
- What is the frequency? *Immediately after eating*
- What is the description of the vomitus? *Sour but contains no bile*
- Is the infant ill in any other way? *No.*

Many infants have signs of dehydration from the vomiting when they are first seen. Lack of tears (many infants younger than age 6 weeks do not tear), dry mucous membrane of the mouth, sunken fontanelles, fever, decreased urine output, poor skin turgor, and weight loss are common signs seen. Alkalosis also may be present because of the excessive loss of Cl^- ions from stomach fluid, along with accompanying hypochloremia, hypokalemia, and starvation. Hypopnea (slowed respirations) occurs as the body attempts to compensate for the alkalosis. This will cause the HCO_3 content of plasma generally to be above 30 mEq/L (normal is 22 to 28 mEq/L). Tetany may occur with alkalosis because the increased HCO_3^- ions may combine with Ca^{2+} ions, trying to effect homeostasis and thereby lowering the level of ionized calcium. Low serum calcium levels lead to tetany.

A definitive diagnosis is made by watching the infant drink. Before the child drinks, attempt to palpate the right upper quadrant of the abdomen for a pyloric mass. If one is present, it feels round and firm, approximately the size of an olive. As the infant drinks, observe for gastric peristaltic waves passing from left to right across the abdomen. The olive-size lump becomes more prominent. The infant vomits with projectile emesis. If the diagnosis is still in doubt, an ultrasound will show the hypertrophied sphincter (Oldham & Aiken, 2007). Endoscopy also may be used for diagnosis by directly visualizing the hypertrophied sphincter.

Therapeutic Management

Treatment is surgical or laparoscopic correction (a pyloromyotomy), performed before electrolyte imbalance from the vomiting or hypoglycemia from the lack of food occurs. Before surgery, if electrolyte imbalance, dehydration, and starvation have already occurred, these must be corrected by administration of IV fluid, usually isotonic saline or 5% glucose in saline. Oral feedings are withheld to prevent further electrolyte depletion. An infant who is receiving only IV fluid generally needs a pacifier to meet nonnutritive sucking needs and be comfortable. If tetany is present, verified by a low calcium level on blood analysis, IV calcium also must be administered. The infant usually needs additional potassium, but as a rule this can not be administered until it is determined that the child's kidneys are functioning (the child is voiding). Otherwise, the potassium buildup could cause cardiac arrhythmias.

For surgical correction, the muscle of the pylorus is split down to the mucosa, allowing for a larger lumen. Although the procedure sounds simple, it is technically difficult to perform, and there is a high risk for infection afterward because the abdominal incision is near the diaper area.

The prognosis for infants with pyloric stenosis is excellent if the condition is discovered before an electrolyte imbalance occurs.

Nursing Diagnoses and Related Interventions

Nursing Diagnosis: Risk for deficient fluid volume related to inability to retain food

Outcome Evaluation: Skin turgor remains good; specific gravity of urine is 1.003 to 1.030; vomiting episodes have ceased; weight is within acceptable age-appropriate parameters.

Preoperative Care. Preoperative management consists of fluid and electrolyte replacement based on laboratory determinations. A baseline weight is essential for establishing the extent of dehydration. Note carefully the frequency of urination, the specific gravity of the urine, and the number of stools passed to help assess dehydration and starvation. Parents may be impatient with preoperative management because it may take 24 hours or more to restore a severe fluid imbalance. They need an explanation that infants cannot go to surgery with an electrolyte imbalance; these hours before surgery are as important to the welfare of their child as the operation itself.

Postoperative Care. Infants will return from surgery or laparoscopy with an IV line in place. The postoperative feeding regimen differs from one surgeon to another but usually involves frequent feedings of small amounts of fluid. Approximately 4 to 6 hours after surgery, infants are started on a small amount of an oral rehydrating solution by bottle. If no vomiting occurs, the amount is increased or half-strength formula or breastfeeding is begun. Finally, by 24 to 48 hours, infants are taking their full formula diet or being fully breastfed. They are usually discharged from the hospital at the end of 48 hours.

Postoperatively, it is important that infants be given no more than the amount of fluid ordered at a time so the surgical repair site is not overwhelmed. Infants need to ingest these small amounts because a small quantity of fluid passing through the sphincter in the immediate postoperative days helps to keep adhesions of the sphincter from forming. As the amount taken orally increases, the IV fluid will be decreased and then discontinued. Infants should be bubbled well after a feeding so there is no pressure from air in the stomach. Lay them on their side after feeding so that if vomiting does occur, there is little chance of aspiration. Laying them on their right side may aid the flow of fluid through the pyloric valve by gravity. Continue to monitor daily weights to confirm that the child is receiving adequate intake. Usually no vomiting occurs postoperatively, but if it does occur, report it immediately. The feeding regimen may need to be adjusted accordingly, and the infant may require a longer hospital stay. Some infants have a short-term diarrhea (dumping syndrome) after surgery because of rapid functioning of the pyloric sphincter, but this tends to resolve without additional therapy.

Nursing Diagnosis: Risk for infection at site of surgical incision related to danger of contamination from feces because of proximity of incision to diaper area

Outcome Evaluation: Infant's temperature is below 98.6° F (37.0° C) axillary; incision is clean, dry, and intact without erythema or drainage.

The surgical incision for pyloric stenosis may be covered with collodion, a solution similar to clear nail polish, or a similar commercial compound to help keep urine and feces from touching it. Keep diapers folded low to prevent the incision from being contaminated, and change diapers frequently. If the incision should be exposed to feces, wash the collodion well with soap and water.

Nursing Diagnosis: Risk for impaired parenting related to infant's feeding difficulty and illness

Outcome Evaluation: Parents hold and feed infant; express positive characteristics about infant.

Encourage the parents to "room in" with their child so they can grow comfortable and confident in caring for the child again. When the child first began vomiting so forcefully, parents may have felt they were doing something wrong and so may have lost confidence in themselves as parents. Explain to them that the vomiting was caused by a physical problem and not by anything they did.

Hospitalization often occurs near the infant's second month, when the child would normally receive diphtheria-tetanus-pertussis, rotavirus, pneumococcal, oral poliomyelitis, and *Haemophilus influenzae* immunizations. Ask if they could be administered before discharge so the child's immunization status remains current. This also might serve to remind parents that getting back to normal means regular health care visits for vaccines and checkups.

Hiatal Hernia

Hiatal hernia is the intermittent protrusion of the stomach up through the esophageal opening in the diaphragm. When this occurs, the volume of the stomach is suddenly restricted, leading to periodic vomiting similar to that of gastroesophageal reflux. With a hiatal hernia, however, pain usually accompanies the vomiting. Shortness of breath may occur from compression of the lung space by the stomach (Skandalakis, 2007).

Hiatal hernia is diagnosed by history and an ultrasound or barium swallow. Keeping a baby in an upright position helps prevent the condition from recurring. Medication to reduce acid secretions may also be helpful. If the condition has not corrected itself by the time the infant is 6 months old, even with maintaining an upright position most of the day, laparoscopic surgery may be performed to reduce the stomach's ability to protrude through the diaphragm.

Peptic Ulcer Disease

A *peptic ulcer* is a shallow excavation formed in the mucosal wall of the stomach, the pylorus, or the duodenum. In infants, ulcers tend to be gastric; in adolescents, they are usually duodenal. Such ulcers occur in a primary form caused by infection of *H. pylori* bacteria and a secondary form that follows severe stress such as burns or chronic ingestion of medications such as acetylsalicylic acid or prednisone (Lebwohl, 2007).

Peptic ulcer disease occurs in only 1% to 2% of children. It occurs more frequently in males than in females. In addition to infection from *H. pylori,* associated factors in adolescents may include a genetic tendency and use of nonsteroidal anti-inflammatory drugs (NSAIDs), alcohol, caffeine, and cigarettes (Barba, Fitzgerald, & Wood, 2007).

The small ulceration of the gastric or duodenal lining leads to pain, blood in the stool, and vomiting (with blood). If left uncorrected, peptic ulcer disease can lead to bowel or stomach perforation with acute hemorrhage or pyloric obstruction (Hua et al., 2007). A chronic ulcer condition may lead to anemia from the constant, gradual blood loss.

Assessment

An ulcer occurring in a neonate usually presents with hematemesis (blood in vomitus) or melena (blood in the stool). Such ulcers are usually superficial and heal rapidly, although they can lead to rupture, with symptoms of respiratory distress, abdominal distention, vomiting, and, if extensive, cardiovascular collapse. If an ulcer occurs in a toddler, the first symptoms are usually anorexia or vomiting. Bleeding follows in several weeks. If an ulcer begins when children are of preschool or early school age, pain may be the presenting symptom. The child may report pain as mild, severe, colicky, or continuous. It is often poorly localized, although it may be in the epigastric area as in adults. If the pain occurs in the right lower quadrant, it can be confused with appendicitis.

In older, school-age children and adolescents, symptoms are generally those of the adult: a gnawing or aching pain in the epigastric area before meals that is relieved by eating. Vomiting (because of spasm and edema of the pylorus) occurs in a small number of children. On abdominal palpation, epigastric tenderness is noted.

Fiberoptic endoscopy is the most reliable diagnostic test to confirm the diagnosis of peptic ulcer disease; it allows for visual inspection and cultures for *H. pylori*. Because childhood ulcers are shallow, they may not show up well on radiography. In many children, little increase in gastric activity can be demonstrated by gastric analysis. Children with this condition must have blood tests done periodically to be monitored for blood loss anemia.

Therapeutic Management

Children with peptic ulcer disease are treated with a combination of medications to reduce the bacteria count and suppress gastric acidity. Adolescents are prescribed an antibiotic such as amoxicillin or clarithromycin (Biaxin) and a proton pump inhibitor such as omeprazole (Prilosec). Bismuth subsalicylate (Pepto-Bismol) is soothing and mildly antibiotic and so may be prescribed concurrently. Younger children are prescribed cimetidine (Tagamet) because safe levels of omeprazole have yet to be established for this age group. With current therapy, only a few children experience the potential complications of perforation, blood loss anemia, and intestinal obstruction, although some school-age children and adolescents will have recurring symptoms as they grow older. Most important to prevent an ulcer reoccurring seems to be evacuation of *H. pylori* from the child's stomach or intestine (Bose et al., 2007).

Nursing Diagnoses and Related Interventions

Having peptic ulcer disease can be difficult for children because it is painful, and remembering to take medicine daily may be a problem.

Nursing Diagnosis: Pain related to ulceration in intestinal tract

Outcome Evaluation: Child exhibits verbal and nonverbal signs of decreased pain; the infant appears comfortable without excessive crying.

Children with peptic ulcer disease should be able to eat a normal diet, avoiding heavily spiced food such as pizza or sausage if such food causes discomfort. Work with them to devise a schedule so they can remember to take their medications.

Be certain that the outcomes planned are realistic. It may not be possible to relieve symptoms of peptic ulcer immediately. However, children can be helped immediately to understand why the pain occurs and what they can do to help relieve it.

✓ Checkpoint Question 45.3

Barry's older sister had pyloric stenosis as an infant. Vomiting with pyloric stenosis typically occurs:

a. Immediately after feeding.
b. An hour after feeding.
c. On arising in the morning.
d. When the infant cries.

HEPATIC DISORDERS

Hepatic disorders include both acquired disorders, such as hepatitis or cirrhosis, and congenital disorders, such as obstruction or atresia of the biliary duct.

Liver Function

The liver lies immediately under the diaphragm on the right side. In infants, 1 or 2 cm of liver is readily and normally palpable. The organ is essential for the normal metabolism of carbohydrates, proteins, and fats. It plays a role in the maintenance of normal blood sugar level by changing glucose to glycogen and storing it until needed by body cells. It then reverses the process and changes glycogen back to glucose and releases it into the blood when cells need it (Jonas & Perez-Atayde, 2007).

The liver assists in the catabolism of fatty acids and protein and serves as a temporary storage space for both fat and protein. The liver, by the means of the enzyme glucuronosyltransferase, converts indirect (or unconjugated) bilirubin into direct (or conjugated) bilirubin so it can be excreted in bile and eliminated from the body. This is an important function in the newborn, and jaundice can result if the level of glucuronosyltransferase is low because of immaturity.

The liver manufactures bile, a secretion necessary for the digestion of fat; fibrinogen and prothrombin, substances essential for blood clotting; heparin, a substance necessary to keep blood from clotting in intact vessels; and blood proteins. It produces large amounts of body heat. It destroys red blood cells and detoxifies many harmful absorbed substances, such as drugs. Because the liver, a life-sustaining organ, performs all of these functions, any disorder involving the liver is always serious. Several common liver function tests are used to diagnose the nature of liver pathology (Table 45.5).

Hepatitis

Hepatitis (inflammation and infection of the liver) is caused by invasion by hepatitis A, B, C, D, or E virus (Tan & Lok, 2007).

Hepatitis A

- Causative agent: A picornavirus, hepatitis A virus (HAV)
- Incubation period: 25 days on average
- Period of communicability: Highest during 2 weeks preceding onset of symptoms
- Mode of transmission: In children, ingestion of fecally contaminated water or shellfish; day care center spread from contaminated changing tables
- Immunity: Natural; one episode induces immunity for the specific type of virus
- Active artificial immunity: HAV vaccine (recommended for all children 12 to 23 months of age and workers in day care centers) (AAP, 2009)
- Passive artificial immunity: Immune globulin

Hepatitis B

- Causative agent: A hepadnavirus; hepatitis B virus (HBV)
- Incubation period: 120 days on average
- Period of communicability: Later part of incubation period and during the acute stage
- Mode of transmission: Transfusion of contaminated blood and plasma or semen; inoculation by a contaminated syringe or needle through IV drug use; may be spread to fetus if mother has infection in third trimester of pregnancy
- Immunity: Natural; one episode induces immunity for the specific type of virus
- Active artificial immunity: Vaccine for the HBV virus recommended for routine immunization beginning at birth and also to all health care providers (AAP, 2009)

TABLE 45.5 ✻ Liver Function Tests

Test	Description
Serum bilirubin	Indirect bilirubin found in large quantities in bloodstream indicates that the child is not converting it to direct bilirubin; hence, liver cell function may be impaired; the normal value of total bilirubin in serum is 1.5 mg per 100 mL; if large amounts of direct bilirubin are found in serum, it implies obstruction of the bile duct, preventing the excretion of the converted substance.
Stool and urine bilirubin	If bile pigments can be obtained from stool (excreted as urobilinogen in stool and urine), it is evidence that bile is being manufactured and excreted from the liver; without the presence of bile pigment, stool appears light in color (clay colored). Even trace amounts of bilirubin in urine are abnormal, possibly indicating liver dysfunction.
Alkaline phosphatase	Alkaline phosphatase is an enzyme produced by the liver and bone and excreted in the bile; with bile duct obstruction, increased levels of alkaline phosphatase will be in the blood.
Prothrombin time	This test is associated with blood coagulation. In chronic liver disease, the level of prothrombin produced by the liver may fall so severely that the prothrombin time is increased; there is little change in prothrombin time in mild or short-term liver disease.
Aspartate transaminase (AST; serum glutamic-oxaloacetic transaminase [SGOT])	AST (SGOT) is an enzyme found in the heart and liver; when there is acute cellular destruction in either organ, the enzyme is released into the bloodstream from the damaged cells; the blood levels are increased by 8 hours after injury; the level reaches a peak in 24 or 36 hours and then falls to normal in 4 to 6 days.
Alanine transaminase (ALT; serum glutamate pyruvate transaminase [SGPT])	ALT (SGPT) is an enzyme found mostly in the liver; it rises for the same reasons as AST (SGOT) but is not as sensitive an indicator of liver damage.
Lactic dehydrogenase (LDH)	LDH is another enzyme found in the heart and liver; it is a relatively insensitive indicator of liver destruction, however; infectious mononucleosis is the one disease in which increased levels of LDH are seen frequently.
Serum albumin	Albumin, a serum protein, is chiefly synthesized in the liver; most acute or chronic liver disease will cause decreased serum albumin.

- Passive artificial immunity: Specific hepatitis B immune serum globulin

Hepatitis C, D, and E

Although hepatitis A and B are the viruses that most frequently cause hepatitis, hepatitis C, D, and E viruses may also be involved. Hepatitis C (HCV) is a single-strand RNA virus. Transmission, as with HBV, is primarily by blood or blood products, IV drug use, or sexual contact. The virus produces mild symptoms of disease, but there is a high incidence of chronic infection with the virus.

Hepatitis D (HDV) or the delta form is similar to HBV in transmission, although it apparently requires a coexisting HBV infection to be activated. Disease symptoms are mild, but there is a high incidence of fulminant hepatitis after the initial infection.

The E form of hepatitis is enterically transmitted similarly to hepatitis A (fecally contaminated water). Disease symptoms from the E virus are usually mild, except in pregnant women, in whom they tend to be severe (Patra et al., 2007).

Assessment. No matter which virus is involved, hepatitis is a generalized body infection with specific intense liver effects. Type A occurs in children of all ages and accounts for approximately 30% of instances. Hepatitis B tends to occur in newborns from placental-fetal transfer and in adolescents after intimate contact or the use of contaminated syringes for drug injection.

Clinically, it is impossible to differentiate the type of hepatitis from the signs that are present. All hepatitis viruses cause liver cell destruction, leading to increased serum aspartate amino transaminase (AST), alanine aminotransaminase (ALT), and alkaline phosphatase levels. Albumin synthesis decreases, and bile formation and excretion are impaired. The type of virus causing the disease can be determined by the recognition of a specific antibody against the virus (anti-HAV IgM, anti-HBV IgM, and so forth).

Children notice headache, fever, and anorexia. Symptoms with hepatitis A are generally mild. Jaundice occurs as liver function slows. This lasts for approximately a week, and then symptoms fade with full recovery. Symptoms of hepatitis B are more marked. Children report generalized aching, right upper quadrant pain, and headache. They may have a low-grade fever. They feel ill; they are irritable and fretful from pruritus (itching). After 3 to 7 days of such symptoms, the color of the urine becomes darker (brown) because of the excretion of bilirubin. In another 2 days, the sclerae of the eyes become jaundiced; soon a child has generalized jaundice. With the generalized jaundice, there is little excretion of bilirubin into the stool, so the stools become white or gray. This icteric (jaundiced) phase lasts for a few days to 2 weeks. Some children have an anicteric form of infection, in which they develop the beginning symptoms but then never develop the jaundice. They are as infectious, however, as children with overt jaundice.

Laboratory studies will show elevations of the liver enzymes AST (SGOT) and serum alanine transaminase (ALT; serum glutamate pyruvate transaminase [SGPT]). Levels of bilirubin are increased in the urine. Bile pigments in the stool are decreased. Serum bilirubin levels are increased.

Therapeutic Management. All health care providers should receive prophylaxis against hepatitis with the hepatitis vaccine. Infants should also receive routine immunization against HBV. All women should be screened during pregnancy for hepatitis B surface antigen (HBsAg). Infants born to hepatitis-positive mothers receive both HBIG and active immunization at birth to prevent them from contracting the disease (Lee et al., 2009). Hepatitis A vaccine is available for health care providers and included in routine immunization programs for infants beginning at one year of age (AAP, 2009).

Strict handwashing and infection control precautions are mandatory when caring for children with hepatitis. Feces must be disposed of carefully because the type A virus can be cultured from feces. Syringes and needles must be disposed of with caution because the type B virus can be transmitted by blood. Contacts should receive immune globulin (hepatitis A) or hepatitis B immune globulin (HBIG) as appropriate.

The treatment for hepatitis A is increased rest and maintenance of a good caloric intake. A low-fat diet, once recommended, is not required and, in any event, is difficult to enforce. Children are generally hungrier at breakfast than later in the day, so encourage them to eat a healthy breakfast. Children can be cared for at home. They should not return to school or a day care center until 2 weeks after the onset of symptoms.

Lamivudine (Epivir), an antiviral agent, may be effective in reducing viral replication with hepatitis B. Interferon also may be prescribed. Of those with type B, 90% will recover completely, but 10% will develop chronic hepatitis and become hepatitis carriers. Hepatitis B is always potentially serious because newborns who contract the disease at birth have an increased risk for liver carcinoma later in life (Perrillo & Jacobson, 2007). As hepatitis B is a sexually transmitted disease, preadolescent children with the infection need to be screened for the possibility of sexual abuse (Lewin, 2007).

Nursing Diagnoses and Related Interventions

Nursing Diagnosis: Pain related to pruritus of jaundice and liver inflammation

Outcome Evaluation: Child states level of itching is tolerable; no scratch marks on skin; reports right upper quadrant pain is minimal.

Pruritus from jaundice results in extreme discomfort for some children (Cies & Giamalis, 2007). Being certain that a child is not overheated and not perspiring reduces the itching. A cool bath is often comforting. Skin moisturizers such as Eucerin or an antihistamine may be prescribed. Cholestyramine (Questran) is a bile acid sequestrant, which binds bile in the GI tract to prevent its reabsorption so helps prevent pruritus. Teaching a child distraction techniques such as putting pressure on a pruritic area or trying imagery to lessen the urge to scratch can also be helpful.

Chronic Hepatitis

Hepatitis is considered chronic when it persists for longer than 6 months. This is most often the result of hepatitis B,

palpated, but, once an examiner's hand is withdrawn, the child experiences acute pain caused by the shifting of the abdominal contents. This is diagnostic for appendicitis, but it should be done with children only when necessary because it does cause acute pain. Caution children that the maneuver may cause pain. On auscultation, bowel sounds will be reduced: only one or two are heard in the same length of time that 30 are normally heard. Absence of bowel sounds on auscultation suggests peritonitis or an appendix that has already ruptured.

Laboratory findings usually indicate leukocytosis (white blood cell count between 10,000 and 18,000/mm^3), which is actually low for the extent of the infection that may be present. Ketone levels in the urine are inordinately elevated as a symptom of starvation from poor intestinal absorption.

An ultrasound reveals the swollen appendix. It can also be confirmed by a CT scan. Pain in the right lower quadrant may also occur as a manifestation of right lower lobe pneumonia. Therefore, children may have a chest x-ray taken to rule this out as the source of pain. Because, in the past, assessment of appendicitis depended on being able to detect abdominal pain, both parents and health care providers may be reluctant to administer analgesia to children with abdominal pain. Because ultrasound can successfully reveal appendicitis, however, analgesia to make the child comfortable can be given (Bromberg & Goldman, 2007).

Therapeutic Management

Therapy for appendicitis is surgical removal of the appendix by laparoscopy before it ruptures (Sauerland, Lefering, & Neugebauer, 2009). Achieving surgery before rupture occurs is easier in older children, who are more capable of relating the progression of symptoms. It is more difficult in young children, whose history is not as accurate, who do not have the words to describe their symptoms, or who will not relax their abdominal muscles enough to allow for manual examination. Also, the wall of the appendix is thinner and perforates more readily in young children.

Nursing Diagnoses and Related Interventions

Priorities for nursing care must be established quickly because this is an emergency, and the child must be prepared immediately for surgery (see Focus on Nursing Care Planning Box 45.4).

Nursing Diagnosis: Pain related to inflamed appendix

Outcome Evaluation: Child states that level of pain is tolerable.

Once a diagnosis is made by ultrasound, a child needs an analgesic for pain. Cathartics and heat to the abdomen are contraindicated, because these increase the possibility of rupture of the appendix. The abdomen will be shaved and washed with an antiseptic solution immediately before surgery. If you are assisting with the procedure, be gentle because the abdomen is tender, and compression could cause the appendix to rupture. Use lukewarm, not hot water, because heat can increase the possibility of appendix rupture by increasing edema in the appendix. Urge the child to find the best position of comfort, and assure both parents and the child that surgery is being scheduled as soon as possible.

Nursing Diagnosis: Fear related to emergency nature of disorder and immediate surgery

Outcome Evaluation: Parents and child state that they understand what interventions are necessary and cooperate as necessary.

Admission for appendicitis often occurs rapidly. A parent telephones a primary care provider, who recommends the child be seen in an emergency room. Surgery is scheduled as soon as it can be arranged. A mere 30 minutes may pass from the time of the first phone call until the child is wheeled into surgery. During this time, the parent and child both need to be told exactly what is happening ("I'm going to take some blood; I'm putting your name tag on your arm") and who the people are who are caring for them ("This is Dr. Brown, the anesthesiologist. I'm Ms. Henry, a registered nurse."). Parents do not think clearly in this type of emergency, and their reactions to situations may not be their usual ones. Explain that the procedures being done for the child such as blood studies or a short wait while an operating room is prepared are necessary for safe surgery and that the danger of the appendix rupturing is not as acute a danger as they may have believed under these controlled circumstances.

Remember that these children have had no preparation for hospitalization. The axiom "What they don't know won't hurt them" is not true. Lack of knowledge can make appendicitis a harrowing experience for parents as well as children. Praise them for the things they did well, such as recognizing the child was ill and bringing the child immediately for care, to help offer a sense of control.

Nursing Diagnosis: Risk for deficient fluid volume related to NPO status

Outcome Evaluation: Child's skin fold returns to place quickly when turgor is assessed; pulse and blood pressure are within normal age limits; weight is maintained.

Preoperatively, obtain a urine sample for urinalysis and blood for a complete blood count. IV fluid therapy may be initiated to hydrate a child who has been vomiting a great deal. Postoperatively, children may have a nasogastric tube in place; they will be maintained on IV fluids until they can take adequate oral feedings (approximately 24 hours). With unruptured appendicitis, the postoperative course is uneventful; children are up a few hours after surgery and are discharged within several days. They generally return to school in another week.

Ruptured Appendix

If a child's appendix has already ruptured when the child is seen in the emergency department, the potential for peritonitis increases greatly. Children generally appear severely ill.

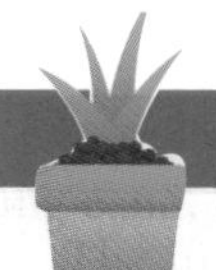

BOX 45.4 ✻ Focus on Nursing Care Planning

A Multidisciplinary Care Map for a Child With Appendicitis

Barry's parents bring his older sister, 10-year-old Leann, to the emergency department because of nausea, vomiting, and abdominal pain since yesterday. Father states, "We thought it was just an upset stomach, but it isn't getting any better, and the pain is much worse now."

Family Assessment ✻ Child lives with 2 younger siblings and both parents on a rural horse farm. Father works as a newspaper printer in town; mother cares for horses and stable. Mother reports finances as, "Good. We're enjoying this time of life."

Client Assessment ✻ Well-nourished, 10-year-old female with a history of no major medical problems. Temperature 101.2° F; pulse 100; respirations 24. Mother reports that yesterday the child stated she was not feeling well. "She wasn't eating, and she had pains in her stomach. Last night, the pain got worse and she started vomiting." Pain now localized in right lower quadrant. Legs drawn up against abdomen. Bowel sounds sluggish. Rebound tenderness present. White blood cell count of 17,000/mm^3. Ultrasound confirms appendicitis. Child is scheduled for emergency appendectomy.

Nursing Diagnosis ✻ Pain related to presence of appendicitis

Outcome Criteria ✻ Child states pain is not above a 2 on 1–10 pain scale.

Team Member Responsible	Assessment	Intervention	Rationale	Expected Outcome
		Activities of Daily Living		
Nurse	Assess what is child's most comfortable position.	Do not palpate child's abdomen.	Palpating could rupture inflamed appendix.	Child states she knows not to put pressure on abdomen.
		Consultations		
Physician	Assess what anesthetist is available for emergency surgery.	Consult with anesthetist about emergency surgery.	Emergency surgery has added risks because of lack of preparation.	Anesthesiology service consults and readies for surgery.
		Procedures/Medications		
Nurse	Assess if child has ever had surgery before.	Wash abdomen and shave from nipple line to groin.	Removing abdominal hair helps prevent infection.	Abdominal preparation is completed prior to surgery.
Nurse	Assess if child's armband is in place.	Complete preoperative checklist.	Safety precautions are important to prevent misidentification during surgery.	Child's armband is in place; preoperative checklist completed and signed.
		Nutrition		
Nurse	Assess when was the last time child ate or drank. Assess skin turgor.	Keep child NPO while awaiting surgery.	Eating could evoke vomiting with aspiration during surgery.	Child cooperates to remain NPO until surgery.
Nurse	Assess if child has had prior experience with IV fluid administration.	Begin IV fluid as prescribed.	IV fluid can help prevent dehydration from previous vomiting while NPO.	Child states she understands why IV is prescribed; protects infusion site from trauma.

(continued)

BOX 45.6 ✻ Focus on Pharmacology

Sulfasalazine (Azulfidine)

Classification: Sulfasalazine is a combination anti-inflammatory agent and antibiotic.

Action: Reduces the inflammation of ulcerative colitis and Crohn's disease (Karch, 2009).

Pregnancy risk category: C (D at term)

Dosage: Varied, based on severity of illness, 20 to 75 mg/kg/day. Initially, 40 to 60 mg/kg/24 hr orally in four to six divided doses in children older than age 2 years. Maintenance therapy usually 20 to 30 mg/kg/day in four equally divided doses.

Possible adverse effects: Sensitivity to sunlight; dizziness; drowsiness, nausea, abdominal pains, crystalluria, and hematuria

Nursing Implications

- Caution the parents and child that the drug may turn urine orange-red and soft contact lenses yellow.
- Advise children to take with or just after meals to avoid GI irritation.
- Ensure adequate fluid intake to avoid crystallization of sulfa component in urine.
- Anticipate prescription for folic acid concurrently. Drug decreases folic acid absorption.
- Instruct the child and parents about the need to use sunscreens and protective clothing while outside.

Beattie, 2007). A child can remain home during this period as long as parents have thorough education about the child's nutritional needs (see Chapter 37).

When food is reintroduced after the resting period, a high-protein, high-carbohydrate, high-vitamin diet is prescribed to replace nutrients. Children may eat cautiously at first to avoid reintroducing diarrhea so assess intake and output. A combination of an anti-inflammatory drug such as prednisone (a corticosteroid), sulfasalazine (Azulfidine; a sulfonamide and salicylic acid), azathioprine (Imuran; an immunosuppressive agent), or monoclonal antibodies (infliximab) generally bring about a great improvement in symptoms (Box 45.6). For ulcerative colitis, cyclosporine may be used. If medical therapy is ineffective, bowel resection to remove a portion of the bowel (colectomy) followed by an ileoanal pull-through may be necessary. In some children, such a large portion of the bowel may be removed that a colostomy or a continent ileostomy needs to be constructed (for continent ileostomy, an internal reservoir is created using a section of bowel and emptied by insertion of a catheter; Fig. 45.9).

Bowel surgery is a serious step. Because it reduces the possibility of the child's developing intestinal cancer in association with ulcerative colitis, it may be necessary in children whose disease is running a long-term, debilitating course that does not improve (Ba'ath et al., 2007). Children who recover from inflammatory bowel disease should have a colonoscopy yearly for the rest of their lives.

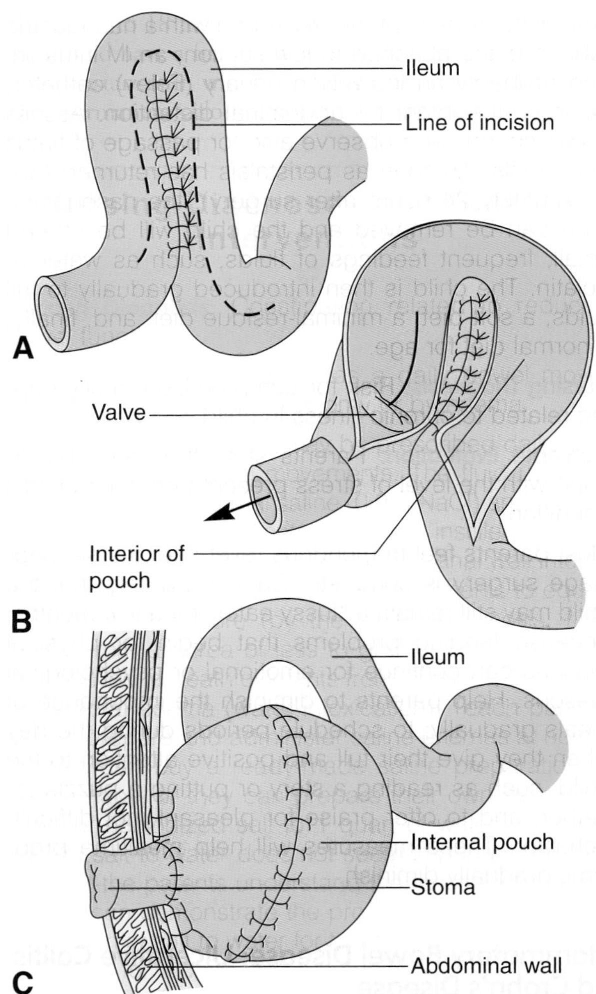

FIGURE 45.9 A continent ileostomy. (**A**) Segment of bowel is anastomosed. (**B**) Pouch for stool collection is formed. (**C**) Liquid stool is contained in pouch until drained by catheter.

Nursing Diagnoses and Related Interventions

Nursing Diagnosis: Imbalanced nutrition related to poor absorption because of disease process

Outcome Evaluation: Child's weight follows a percentile growth curve; urine specific gravity is 1.003 to 1.030. Child states that alternative feeding method is tolerable.

Nutrition is a priority concern for children with both Crohn's disease and ulcerative colitis because malnutrition can occur from the combination of poor intestinal absorption and chronic diarrhea. Unless active steps are taken to supplement nutrition, children with inflammatory bowel disease can be left both short in stature and light in weight. Anorexia with protein, vitamin, fat, and mineral deficiencies all may occur.

When nutrition is supplied by enteral or total parenteral nutrition solutions, allowing the enteral infusion to flow during the night and removing the tube during the day can make feedings more tolerable. Remember that food provides social experiences as well as nutrition. Help parents provide opportunities for usual mealtime stimulation in other ways.

Nursing Diagnosis: Risk for ineffective coping related to chronic illness

Outcome Evaluation: Child expresses feelings, states that she understands the disease and therapy, and suggests ways to minimize stress.

Caution children about the possible side effects, such as excessive weight gain, a round facial appearance, and facial acne, that may occur if corticosteroid therapy, such as prednisone, is used so they are not surprised by this. Assess blood pressure, intake and output, weight, and sleep patterns for any child taking steroids. Caution children that sulfasalazine (Azulfidine) turns urine an orange-yellow so they do not mistake this color change as bleeding.

Provide time to listen so children have someone outside their family to talk to about their symptoms and family or stress problems (Box 45.7). The disorder follows a chronic course and can involve embarrassing episodes of diarrhea or acute abdominal pain.

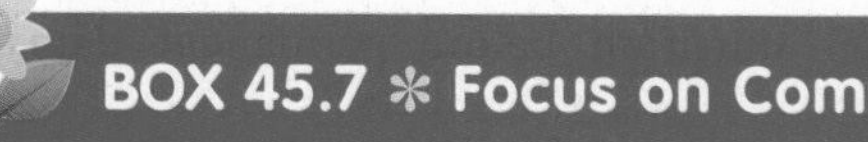

BOX 45.7 * Focus on Communication

Barry's older sister Addie has Crohn's disease. Her doctor has told her parents she won't need surgery but will need long-term therapy. You see Mrs. Abraham filling out forms by Addie's bedside.

Less Effective Communication

Nurse: Mrs. Abraham, can I help you with anything?

Mrs. Abraham: No. With Addie well again in a short time, I'm going to start back to college. I'm filling out the forms.

Nurse: Do you mean Addie doesn't need parenteral nutrition?

Mrs. Abraham: She doesn't need anything. Not even surgery.

Nurse: That's wonderful. She's very lucky.

More Effective Communication

Nurse: Mrs. Abraham, can I help you with anything?

Mrs. Abraham: No. With Addie well again in a short time, I'm going to start back to college. I'm filling out the forms.

Nurse: Do you mean Addie doesn't need parenteral nutrition?

Mrs. Abraham: She doesn't need anything. Not even surgery.

Nurse: Let's review exactly what the doctor has told you.

People under stress often do not hear instructions well. When this happens, they may need them repeated several times before they truly comprehend what was said. An easy solution when you are aware that a parent has not heard potentially bad news is to ignore the loss of information, as in the first scenario above. A better solution is to explore with the parents what they did hear and help them receive more accurate information.

Irritable Bowel Syndrome (Chronic Nonspecific Diarrhea)

Irritable bowel syndrome involves intermittent episodes of loose and normal stools or recurrent abdominal pain. It appears slightly more often in girls than in boys. It is most often seen in infants 6 to 36 months of age. Most children outgrow the symptoms by 3 years of age. The cause is unknown, but it is associated with low fat intake (without fat slowing absorption, stool passes rapidly through the bowel). Excessive fluid intake also may play a role.

The symptoms are usually vague. The episodes of diarrhea may occur several times a week or as frequently as twice a day. There seems to be no relationship to meals.

Children are encouraged to eat a regular diet. Psyllium bulk agents will almost always reduce the frequency of symptoms. Probiotics or foods supplemented with lactic acid-producing bacteria may improve symptoms (Walter & Isolauri, 2007).

Chronic Recurrent Abdominal Pain

Some children develop episodes of recurring abdominal pain. Although such episodes can occur for reasons such as lactose intolerance or muscle strain from sports activities, in most instances the cause is unknown (Sondheimer, 2008). Children who experience this are commonly 6 or 7 years of age or in prepuberty (11 to 12 years of age). The pain is not accompanied by a change in bowel habits. There is no association with meals. Episodes of pain can last for only a few minutes or for hours. The intensity of the pain is mild or "annoying" rather than severe. It is generally poorly localized, although children may point to the umbilicus as the primary site. On physical examination, there is no abdominal tenderness, distention, guarding, or muscle spasm.

Symptoms of stress such as sleep disturbances, fears, or eating problems may be present. A family history may indicate problems in the family such as marital discord, financial problems, or physical illness in parents or siblings.

Although the cause of the pain cannot be identified, the pain is real. For some children, just having the opportunity to talk to an understanding person about the problem is all that is necessary to stop the attacks of pain. Other families need counseling regarding the underlying problem, such as allowing children to express their anger, reducing excessive demands on them, or giving them more attention by spending more time with them. The family may need to be referred to a family service agency for counseling (Huertas-Ceballos et al., 2009).

DISORDERS CAUSED BY FOOD, VITAMIN, AND MINERAL DEFICIENCIES

There are many underfed and malnourished children in every part of the world. Although extreme diseases of food or vitamin deprivation are rare in the United States, they do exist. Such children need early identification so they can receive better nutrition before permanent damage occurs.

The average child does not develop a deficient intake of essential nutrients because, even if the child is occasionally a fussy eater, over the space of a week, a child does ingest foods containing the necessary nutrients. Carefully assess any child who has an interference in nutrition such as a GI illness or a child is receiving enteric feedings or total parenteral nutrition to make sure that nutrient deficiencies do not exist. Assess abused or neglected children closely for nutritional deficiencies, because they may not have been given adequate food.

Kwashiorkor

Kwashiorkor, a disease caused by protein deficiency, occurs most frequently in children ages 1 to 3 years, because this age group requires a high protein intake. It is a disease found almost exclusively in developing countries in Africa, Asia, and Latin America, although it does occur in the United States (Baron, 2009). It tends to occur after weaning, when children change from breast milk to a diet consisting mainly of carbohydrates. Growth failure is a major symptom. Because edema is also a symptom, however, children may not appear light in weight until the edema is relieved. There is a severe wasting of muscles, but, again, this is masked by the edema.

Edema results from hypoproteinemia, which causes a shift of body fluid from the intravascular compartments to the interstitial space, causing ascites (Fig. 45.10). This is the same phenomenon that causes extensive edema in children with nephrosis. The edema tends to be dependent, so it is first noted in the lower extremities. Children are generally irritable and uninterested in their surroundings. They fall behind other children of the same age in motor development.

If the child had a period of good protein intake, then poor protein intake, then good intake again, hair shafts develop a striped appearance of brown, then white, and so on—a "zebra sign." Children also have diarrhea, iron-deficiency anemia, and enlarged livers.

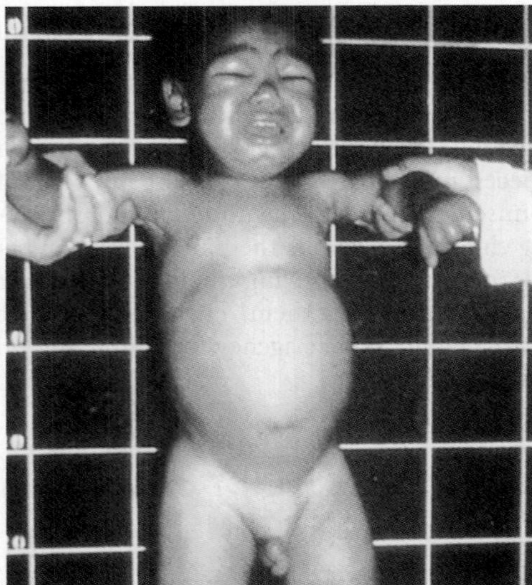

FIGURE 45.10 A child with kwashiorkor. Here the extensive generalized edema masks the severe muscle wasting. Notice the severe abdominal distention from ascites.

Without treatment, kwashiorkor is fatal. For therapy, a diet rich in protein is essential. Even so, there is evidence to suggest that protein malnutrition early in life, even if corrected later, may result in failure of children to reach their full potential of intellectual and psychological development.

Nutritional Marasmus

Nutritional marasmus is caused by a deficiency of all food groups, basically a form of starvation. Although it is seen most commonly in developing countries where food supplies are short, it can be seen in grossly neglected children or those with failure to thrive in the United States (see Chapter 55). These children are most commonly younger than 1 year of age. They have many of the same symptoms as children with kwashiorkor, including growth failure, muscle wasting, irritability, iron-deficiency anemia, and diarrhea. Whereas children with kwashiorkor are anorectic, children with nutritional marasmus are invariably hungry (starving) and will suck at any object offered them, such as a finger or their clothing. Treatment is a diet rich in all nutrients.

Vitamin and Mineral Deficiencies

Both vitamin and mineral deficiencies occur at a low rate in children of the United States because so many foods are enriched (restoration of ingredients removed by processing) or fortified (additional vitamins and minerals not normally present have been added). Milk, for example, is fortified with vitamins D and A. Orange juice is fortified with calcium. White bread is enriched with B vitamins. Vitamin deficiency diseases are summarized in Table 45.7.

Iodine Deficiency

Because iodine is not supplemented in food except as iodized salt, a diet deficient in iodine may lead to either hypothyroidism or overgrowth (*goiter*) of the thyroid gland as the gland struggles to produce thyroxine in the face of deficient iodine. Goiter tends to occur most commonly in girls at puberty and during pregnancy. It is potentially dangerous as an enlarged thyroid gland may lead to difficulty breathing. In the United States, areas where goiter is endemic are mainly the states bordering Canada, especially the Great Lakes area, and the states between the Rocky Mountains and the Appalachians (Rolfes, Pinna, & Whitney, 2009).

Supplemental iodine or synthetic thyroxine (Synthroid) is needed to correct the deficiency. Children must also be maintained on a diet adequate in iodine, found most abundantly in seafood (Rolfes, Pinna, & Whitney, 2009).

✔ Checkpoint Question 45.5

Kwashiorkor is a disorder common in developing countries. This disorder occurs because of lack of which nutrient?

a. Water-soluble vitamins.
b. Fats and triglycerides.
c. Quality protein.
d. Vitamin K.

TABLE 45.7 * Vitamin Deficiency Disorders

Vitamin	Cause of Deficiency	Signs and Symptoms
Vitamin A	Lack of yellow vegetables in diet	Tender tongue; cracks at corners of mouth Night blindness **Xerophthalmia** (dry and lusterless conjunctivae) **Keratomalacia** (necrosis of the cornea with perforation, loss of ocular fluid, and blindness)
Vitamin B_1	Most common in children who eat polished rice as dietary staple, because B_1 is contained in hull of rice	**Beriberi** (tingling and numbness of extremities; heart palpitations; exhaustion) Diarrhea and vomiting Aphonia (cry without sound) Anesthesia of feet
Niacin	Common in children who eat corn as dietary staple, because corn is low in niacin	**Pellagra** (dermatitis; resembles a sunburn) Diarrhea Mental confusion (dementia)
Vitamin C	Lack of fresh fruits in diet	**Scurvy** (muscle tenderness; petechiae) Poor muscle tone; delayed tooth formation
Vitamin D	Lack of sunlight	**Rickets** (poor bone formation) Craniotabes (softening of the skull) Swelling at joints, particularly of wrists and cartilage of ribs Bowed legs Tetany (muscle spasms)

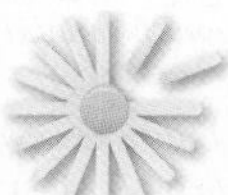

Key Points for Review

- Children with gastrointestinal disorders need to join the family for mealtime if possible. Even if they cannot eat the same foods as other family members, they benefit from the social interaction.
- Some gastrointestinal disorders lead to long-term therapies such as colostomy or gastrostomy feedings. Because these disorders interfere with common body functions such as eating and elimination, they are difficult for children to accept without the support of concerned health care providers.
- Children lose proportionately more fluid with vomiting and diarrhea than adults, so they need rapid assessment and interventions to avoid dehydration.
- Fluid, electrolyte, and acid–base imbalances tend to occur rapidly with vomiting and diarrhea. Vomiting leads to alkalosis. Diarrhea leads to acidosis.
- Gastrointestinal disorders almost always interfere with nutrition to some degree. This is a greater problem in children than adults because children need to ingest adequate nutrients and fluid daily for growth as well as body maintenance.
- Gastroesophageal reflux is a neuromuscular disturbance in which the cardiac sphincter is lax, allowing for easy regurgitation of gastric contents into the esophagus. It is treated by feeding a thickened formula and keeping an infant upright after feedings.
- Pyloric stenosis is hypertrophy of the valve between the stomach and duodenum. It impedes the passage of feedings, leading to vomiting.
- Peptic ulcer disease may occur in children of all ages. The disorder causes a shallow excavation to form in the mucosal wall of the stomach. It is treated, like adult ulcers, with antibiotics and agents to suppress gastric acidity.
- Forms of hepatitis seen in children include hepatitis A and C (caused usually by eating contaminated shellfish) and hepatitis B, D, and E (caused by contaminated blood or placental transfer).
- Congenital obstruction of the bile ducts occurs from failure of the bile duct to recanalize in utero. This can lead to fibrotic scarring of the liver (cirrhosis). Most of these children need a liver transplant to restore liver function.
- Intussusception is the invagination of one portion of the intestine into another. Volvulus is twisting of intestine. Both may lead to bowel obstruction.
- Necrotizing enterocolitis is the development of necrotic patches on the intestine. It occurs almost exclusively in immature infants.
- Appendicitis is inflammation of the appendix. It is always an emergency and is the most common reason for abdominal surgery in children. Laparoscopy is done to remove the appendix, ideally before it ruptures.
- Celiac disease (gluten-induced enteropathy) is a change in the ability of the intestinal villi to absorb. It is a dominantly inherited illness.
- Both inguinal and hiatal hernia can occur in children. These are surgically corrected when recognized.
- Hirschsprung's disease (aganglionic megacolon) is absence of ganglionic innervation in a section of the lower bowel. Therapy may involve a temporary colostomy followed by surgery in 6 to 12 months to remove the affected bowel portion.

- Inflammatory bowel disease can occur as either ulcerative colitis or Crohn's disease. Therapy is long-term. If medical therapy is unsuccessful, portions of the bowel may be surgically removed. Ulcerative colitis is associated with the development of colon cancer later in life.
- Kwashiorkor (protein deficiency), nutritional marasmus (starvation), vitamins A and D (rickets), B_1 (beriberi), and C (scurvy) deficiencies, or iodine deficiencies occur in children when they are not provided or cannot absorb adequate nutrients. Although more common in developing countries, they can occur in a child in any community.

CRITICAL THINKING EXERCISES

1. Barry is the 2-year-old boy you met at the beginning of the chapter. He was diagnosed with celiac disease. When you met him, his mother was insisting that he eat a piece of birthday cake. What health education does his mother need to help her choose a better diet for her son? What would have been a better food, probably available at a birthday party, that he could have eaten?
2. Suppose Barry is seen in a hospital emergency department with severe diarrhea. What emergency interventions does he need to prevent an electrolyte or fluid imbalance? What measures could you take to reduce his fear of the strange hospital environment?
3. Barry's older sister, who has Crohn's disease, is being cared for at home with total parenteral nutrition. How can you help her keep pace with her friends at school? How can you help her maintain a sense of high self-esteem in light of her many hospitalizations and home care?
4. Examine the National Health Goals related to gastrointestinal disorders in children. Most government-sponsored funds for nursing research are allotted based on these goals. What would be a possible research topic to explore pertinent to these goals that would be applicable to the Abraham family and also advance evidence-based practice?

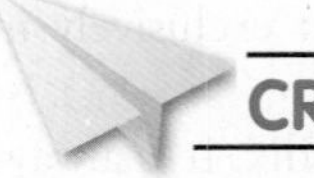

CRITICAL THINKING SCENARIO

Open the accompanying CD-ROM or visit http://thePoint.lww.com and read the Patient Scenario included for this chapter, then answer the questions to further sharpen your skills and grow more familiar with NCLEX style questions related to gastrointestinal disorders in children. Confirm your answers are correct by reading the rationales.

REFERENCES

Al Faleh, K., & Bassler, D. (2009). Probiotics for prevention of necrotizing enterocolitis in preterm infants. *Cochrane Database of Systematic Reviews, 2009*(1), (CD005496).

American Academy of Pediatrics (AAP), Committee on Practice and Ambulatory Medicine. (2009). *Recommendations for preventive pediatric health care.* Washington, DC: Author.

Applegate, K. E. (2008). Intussusception in children: imaging choices. *Seminars in Roentgenology, 43*(1), 15–21.

Ba'ath, M. E., et al. (2007). Surgical management of inflammatory bowel disease. *Archives of Disease in Childhood, 92*(4), 312–316.

Barba, K., Fitzgerald, P., & Wood, S. (2007). Managing peptic ulcer disease. *Nursing 2007, 37*(7), 56–57.

Baron, R. B. (2009). Nutritional requirements and disorders. In S. J. McPhee & M. A. Papadakis (Eds.). *Current medical diagnosis and treatment.* Columbus, OH: McGraw-Hill.

Barter, C., & Dunne, L. (2008). Abdominal pain. In J. E. South-Paul, S. C. Matheny, & E. L. Lewis. (Eds.). *Current diagnosis and treatment in family medicine* (2nd ed.). Columbus, OH: McGraw-Hill.

Bass, E. S., Pappano, D. A., & Humiston, S. G. (2007). Rotavirus. *Pediatrics in Review, 28*(5), 183–191.

Bose, A. C., et al. (2007). *Helicobacter pylori* eradication prevents recurrence after simple closure of perforated duodenal ulcer. *Journal of Gastroenterology and Hepatology, 22*(3), 345–348.

Brandt, M. L. (2008). Pediatric hernias. *Surgical Clinics of North America, 88*(1), 27–43.

Bromberg, R., & Goldman, R. D. (2007). Pediatric pearls: current practice. Does analgesia mask diagnosis of appendicitis among children? *Canadian Family Physician, 53*(1), 39–41.

Bueno, J., et al. (2007). Liver transplantation in childhood with more than 10 years of follow-up: analysis of a single-center experience. *Transplantation Proceedings, 39*(7), 2288–2289.

Carter, B. M. (2007). Treatment outcomes of necrotizing enterocolitis for preterm infants. *JOGNN: Journal of Obstetric, Gynecologic, and Neonatal Nursing, 36*(4), 377–385.

Cennimo, D. J., et al. (2007). Enteroaggregative *Escherichia coli*: a review of trends, diagnosis, and treatment. *Infections in Medicine, 24*(3), 100–110.

Chambers, H. F. (2009). Infectious diseases: bacterial and chlamydial. In S. J. McPhee & M. A. Papadakis (Eds.). *Current medical diagnosis and treatment.* Columbus, OH: McGraw-Hill.

Cies, J. J., & Giamalis, J. N. (2007). Treatment of cholestatic pruritus in children. *AJHP: American Journal of Health-System Pharmacy, 64*(11), 1157–1161.

Cochran, J. B., & Losek, J. D. (2007). Acute liver failure in children. *Pediatric Emergency Care, 23*(2), 129–135.

Craig, W. R., et al. (2009). Metoclopramide, thickened feedings, and positioning for gastro-oesophageal reflux in children under two years. *Cochrane Database of Systematic Reviews, 2009*(1), (CD003502).

Dasgupta, R., & Langer, J. C. (2008). Evaluation and management of persistent problems after surgery for Hirschsprung disease in a child. *Journal of Pediatric Gastroenterology and Nutrition, 46*(1), 13–19.

Della Rocca, J. (2007). Minimizing the perils of appendicitis. *Nursing 2007, 37*(1), 1–3.

Ebell, M. H. (2008). Diagnosis of appendicitis: part II. Laboratory and imaging tests. *American Family Physician, 77*(8), 1153–1155.

Fitzpatrick, E., et al. (2007). Outcome for children with cyclical vomiting syndrome. *Archives of Disease in Childhood, 92*(11), 1001–1004.

Freedman, S. B. (2007). Acute infectious pediatric gastroenteritis: beyond oral rehydration therapy. *Expert Opinion on Pharmacotherapy, 8*(11), 1651–1665.

Friedman, L. S. (2009). Hepatology. In S. J. McPhee & M. A. Papadakis (Eds.). *Current medical diagnosis and treatment.* Columbus, OH: McGraw-Hill.

Goldin, A. B., et al. (2007). Aminoglycoside-based triple-antibiotic therapy versus monotherapy for children with ruptured appendicitis. *Pediatrics, 119*(5), 905–911.

Grave, G. D., et al. (2007). New therapies and preventive approaches for necrotizing enterocolitis: report of a research planning workshop. *Pediatric Research, 62*(4), 510–514.

Hartman, E. E., et al. (2007). Explaining change in quality of life of children and adolescents with anorectal malformations or Hirschsprung disease. *Pediatrics, 119*(2), e374–e383.

Holliday, M. A., Ray, P. E., & Friedman, A. L. (2007). Fluid therapy for children: Facts, fashions and questions. *Archives of Disease in Childhood, 92*(6), 546–550.

Hua, M. C., et al. (2007). Perforated peptic ulcer in children: a 20-year experience. *Journal of Pediatric Gastroenterology and Nutrition, 45*(1), 71–74.

Huertas-Ceballos, A., et al. (2009). Psychosocial interventions for recurrent abdominal pain (RAP) and irritable bowel syndrome (IBS) in childhood. *Cochrane Database of Systematic Reviews, 2009*(1), (CD003014).

Ingoe, R., & Lange, P. (2007). Ladd's procedure for correction of intestinal malrotation with volvulus in children. *Association of Operating Room Nurses: AORN Journal, 85*(2), 300–312.

Jonas, M. M., & Perez-Atayde, A. R. (2007). Liver disease in infancy and childhood. In E. R. Schiff, M. F. Sorrell, & W. C. Maddrey. (Eds.). *Schiff's diseases of the liver* (10th ed.). Philadelphia: Lippincott Williams & Wilkins.

Kaiser, A. D., Applegate, K. E., & Ladd, A. P. (2007). Current success in the treatment of intussusception in children. *Surgery, 142*(4), 469–475.

Kamath, B. M. (2008). Neonatal cholestasis. In M. W. Schwartz (Ed.). *The 5-minute pediatric consult* (5th ed.). Philadelphia: Lippincott Williams & Wilkins.

Karch, A. M. (2009). *Lippincott's nursing drug guide.* Philadelphia: Lippincott Williams & Wilkins.

Kotch, J. B., et al. (2007). Hand-washing and diapering equipment reduces disease among children in out-of-home child care centers. *Pediatrics, 120*(1), e29–e36.

Lebwohl, J. M. (2007). Peptic ulcer. In J. Schaider, et al. (Eds.). *Rosen & Barkin's 5-minute emergency medicine consult.* Philadelphia: Lippincott Williams & Wilkins.

Lee, C., et al. (2009). Hepatitis B immunisation for newborn infants of hepatitis B surface antigen-positive mothers. *Cochrane Database of Systematic Reviews, 2009*(1), (CD004790).

Leung, A. K., & Robson, W. L. (2007). Acute gastroenteritis in children: role of anti-emetic medication for gastroenteritis-related vomiting. *Paediatric Drugs, 9*(3), 175–184.

Lewin, L. C. (2007). Sexually transmitted infections in preadolescent children. *Journal of Pediatric Health Care, 21*(3), 153–161.

Maheshwai, N. (2007). Are young infants treated with erythromycin at risk for developing hypertrophic pyloric stenosis? *Archives of Disease in Childhood, 92*(3), 271–273.

McQuaid, K. R. (2009). Gastroenterology In S. J. McPhee & M. A. Papadakis (Eds.). *Current medical diagnosis and treatment.* Columbus, OH: McGraw-Hill.

Merchant, A. (2007). Inflammatory bowel disease in children: an overview for pediatric healthcare providers. *Gastroenterology Nursing, 30*(4), 278–284.

Misra, S., et al. (2007). A prospective study of rotavirus diarrhea in children under 1 year of age. *Clinical Pediatrics, 46*(8), 683–688.

Nandish, S., Weston, M. J., & Wolstenhulme, S. (2007). Perforated Meckel's diverticulum: a cause for haemoperitoneum. *Ultrasound, 15*(2), 93–95.

Niramis, R., et al. (2008). Quality of life of patients with Hirschsprung's disease at 5-20 years post pull-through operations. *European Journal of Pediatric Surgery, 18*(1), 38–43.

Ogle, J. W., & Anderson, M. S. (2008). Infections: Bacterial and spirochetal. In W. W. Hay, et al. (Eds.). *Current pediatric diagnosis and treatment* (18th ed.). Columbus, OH: McGraw-Hill.

Oldham, K. T., & Aiken, J. J. (2007). Congenital pyloric stenosis and duodenal obstruction. In J. E. Fischer (Ed.). *Mastery of surgery.* Philadelphia: Lippincott Williams & Wilkins.

Patra, S., et al. (2007). Maternal and fetal outcomes in pregnant women with acute hepatitis E virus infection. *Annals of Internal Medicine, 147*(1), 28–33.

Perrillo, R. P., & Jacobson, I. M. (2007). Halting the natural history of hepatitis B viral infection: a paradigm shift. *Seminars in Liver Disease, 27*(Suppl 1), 3–8.

Philichi, L. (2008). When the going gets tough: pediatric constipation and encopresis. *Gastroenterology Nursing, 31*(2), 121–130.

Reading, R. (2007). Clinical review: chronic constipation in children. *Child: Care, Health and Development, 33*(3), 350–351.

Rolfes, S. R., Pinna, K., & Whitney, E. N. (2009). *Understanding normal and clinical nutrition.* New York: Wadsworth/Cengage Learning.

Sauerland, S., Lefering, R., & Neugebauer, E. A. M. (2009). Laparoscopic versus open surgery for suspected appendicitis. *Cochrane Database of Systematic Reviews, 2009*(1), (CD001546).

Scherb, C. A., Stevens, M. S., & Busman, C. (2007). Outcomes related to dehydration in the pediatric population. *Journal of Pediatric Nursing, 22*(5), 376–382.

Sirinavin, S., & Garner, P. (2009). Antibiotics for treating salmonella gut infections. *Cochrane Database of Systematic Reviews, 2009*(1), (CD001167).

Skandalakis, P. N. (2007). Surgical anatomy of the diaphragm. In J. E. Fischer (Ed.). *Mastery of surgery.* Philadelphia: Lippincott Williams & Wilkins.

Soares-Weiser, K., et al. (2009). Rotavirus vaccine for preventing diarrhoea. *Cochrane Database of Systematic Reviews, 2009*(1), (CD002848).

Sondheimer, J. M. & Sundaram, S. (2008). Gastrointestinal tract. In W. W. Hay, et al. (Eds.). *Current pediatric diagnosis and treatment* (18th ed.). Columbus, OH: McGraw-Hill.

Tan, J., & Lok, A. S. F. (2007). Update on viral hepatitis. *Current Opinion in Gastroenterology, 23*(3), 263–267.

Treem, W. R. (2007). Beyond five years: long-term follow-up in pediatric liver transplantation. *Current Gastroenterology Reports, 9*(3), 230–236.

Tully, A. (2008). Pediatric celiac disease. *Gastroenterology Nursing, 31*(2), 132–142.

Walter, A., & Isolauri, E. (2007). Understanding the use of probiotics in pediatric populations. *Contemporary Pediatrics, 24*(5), 1–6.

Wiskin, A. E., Wootton, S. A., & Beattie, R. M. (2007). Nutrition issues in pediatric Crohn's disease. *Nutrition in Clinical Practice, 22*(2), 214–222.

Zagaria, M. A. E. (2008). Pediatric GER & GERD: overview of management. *The American Journal for Nurse Practitioners, 12*(1), 36–42.

SUGGESTED READINGS

Ainsworth, S. B., Clerihew, L., & McGuire, W. (2009). Percutaneous central venous catheters versus peripheral cannulae for delivery of parenteral nutrition in neonates. *Cochrane Database of Systematic Reviews,* (3), (CD004219).

Brown-Guttovz, H. (2007). Action stat. Intussusception. *Nursing 2007, 37*(2), 80.

Ceballos, C. (2008). Growth and early onset inflammatory bowel disease. *Gastroenterology Nursing, 31*(2), 101–106.

Ekenze, S. O., Agugua-Obianyo, N. E., & Amah, C. C. (2007). Colostomy for large bowel anomalies in children: a case controlled study. *International Journal of Surgery, 5*(4), 273–277.

Gibson, L., Saeed, S. A., & Turner-Henson, A. (2007). Pediatric management problems. Stomach pain. *Pediatric Nursing, 33*(2), 136–137.

Lee, C. K., & Jonas, M. M. (2007). Pediatric hepatobiliary disease. *Current Opinion in Gastroenterology, 23*(3), 306–309.

Murphy, M. S. (2008). Management of bloody diarrhoea in children in primary care. *BMJ: British Medical Journal, 336*(7651), 1010–1015.

Peterson, K. D. (2008). Inflammatory bowel disease: impact on early teenage years. *Gastroenterology Nursing, 31*(3), 235–236.

Simpson, T., Ivey, J., & Vincent, J. L. (2008). Pediatric management problems. Neonate with gastrointestinal issues. *Pediatric Nursing, 34*(1), 60–61.

Tobias, N., et al. (2008). Management principles of organic causes of childhood constipation. *Journal of Pediatric Health Care, 22*(1), 12–23.

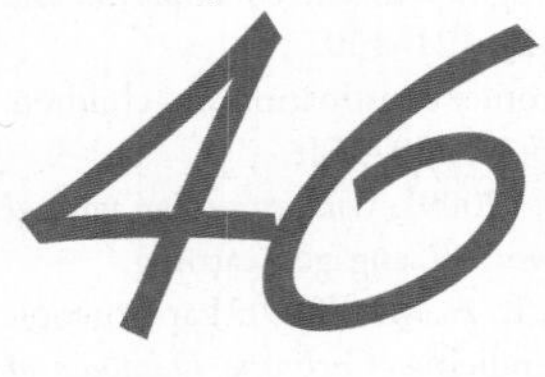

Chapter 46 Nursing Care of a Family When a Child Has a Renal or Urinary Tract Disorder

KEY TERMS

- Alport's syndrome
- azotemia
- Bowman's capsule
- dialysis
- enuresis
- epispadias
- exstrophy of the bladder
- glomerular filtration rate
- glomerulonephritis
- hydronephrosis
- hypospadias
- nephrosis
- patent urachus
- polycystic kidney
- postural proteinuria
- prune belly syndrome
- vesicoureteral reflux

OBJECTIVES

After mastering the contents of this chapter, you should be able to:

1. Describe common renal and urinary disorders that occur in children.
2. Identify National Health Goals related to renal or urinary tract disorders in children that nurses can help the nation achieve.
3. Analyze methods for making nursing care of the child with a renal or urinary disorder more family centered.
4. Assess a child for a renal or urinary tract disorder.
5. Formulate nursing diagnoses related to renal or urinary disorders in children.
6. Establish expected outcomes for a child with a renal or urinary disorder.
7. Plan nursing care related to urinary or renal disorders in children.
8. Implement nursing care for a child with a renal or urinary disorder such as preparing a child for peritoneal dialysis.
9. Evaluate expected outcomes for achievement and effectiveness of care.
10. Identify areas related to care of the child with a renal or urinary disorder that would benefit from additional nursing research or application of evidence-based practice.
11. Integrate knowledge of renal and urinary tract disorders with the nursing process to achieve quality maternal and child health nursing care.

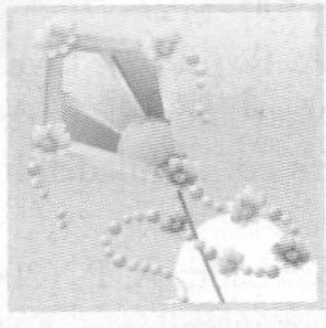

Carol Hendricks is a 4-year-old girl admitted to the hospital with nephrotic syndrome. She has marked ascites and edema. "I kept asking everyone why she was gaining so much weight when she doesn't eat anything," her grandmother tells you. "My daughter said this happened because she drank part of a beer I left on the coffee table. Do you think that's what caused it? What if she needs a kidney transplant? Will I be allowed to give a kidney to her?" Previous chapters described the growth and development of well children and the nursing care of children with disorders of other systems. This chapter adds information about the dramatic changes, both physical and psychosocial, that occur when children develop urinary tract or renal disorders. This information builds a base for assessment, care, and health teaching.

How would you answer Carol's grandmother? What information does she need to better understand her grandchild's condition?

Normally, the urinary system maintains the proper balance of fluid (water) and electrolytes in the blood. When disease occurs, such as with structural abnormalities or kidney malfunction, children may be left with excessive amounts of fluid in the body or with an imbalance of electrolytes essential to their body's functioning. Disorders involving the kidneys and urinary tract often are long term. Urinary tract disorders can ultimately (if not originally) affect the kidneys, resulting in kidney dysfunction, with potentially fatal consequences (Watnick & Morrison, 2009).

Unfortunately, because symptoms may be vague, or because a child or parents do not realize the seriousness of urinary disease or are embarrassed to discuss it, children may not be evaluated at the first sign of illness. Health education to increase the awareness of the symptoms of urinary tract and kidney disorders is an important area of family health teaching. National Health Goals related to renal or urinary tract disorders and children are shown in Box 46.1.

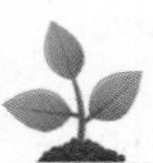

Nursing Process Overview

For Care of a Child With a Renal or Urinary Tract Disorder

Assessment

Because the symptoms of many urinary tract and renal disorders such as mild abdominal pain, slowly increasing edema, or low-grade fever are subtle, parents may not bring their child for evaluation as early in the disease as they might if symptoms were more definite. School nurses can play an important role in recognizing the seriousness of minor symptoms and making proper referrals for care.

The ease with which parents and children can discuss illnesses of the kidneys or urinary tract is culturally influenced. As a general rule, because elimination functions are typically regarded as private, this is not a body system that people discuss as comfortably as they do illnesses of other body systems. The more that modesty is stressed in a culture, the more difficult it may be for people to ask questions about this system's disorders. By being aware that this is a difficult area for parents to discuss, health care personnel can better observe whether added health education is needed when caring for a child with one of these disorders.

A hallmark of kidney or bladder infection is pain. If children have had bladder surgery, they also may experience pain on urination or pain from bladder spasms. Be sure to assess the degree of any pain, including its location and intensity, before administering an analgesic or antispasmodic. Urine specimens also provide valuable assessment information. Techniques for obtaining urine samples such as clean-catch, catheterization, 24-hour collections, suprapubic aspiration, and urinalysis are described in Chapter 37.

Nursing Diagnosis

Nursing diagnoses used with children with urinary tract or renal disorders are related to the symptoms these disorders cause. Some examples are:

- Pain related to bladder irritation from urinary tract infection
- Excess fluid volume related to decreased kidney function and fluid accumulation
- Fear related to as yet unknown outcome of kidney transplantation
- Imbalanced nutrition, less than body requirements, related to effects of dietary restrictions
- Social isolation related to immunosuppressant therapy
- Risk for injury related to body's inability to excrete waste products properly

Because the entire family becomes involved in long-term renal disease, other appropriate nursing diagnoses might include:

- Interrupted family processes related to the effects and stresses of child's chronic illness
- Compromised family coping related to the chronic nature of child's illness

Outcome Identification and Planning

Be certain that outcomes established for care are relevant to a child's age and condition. Because renal disease may become chronic, expected outcomes may need to be modified frequently to meet changing needs.

Planning for a child with a urinary tract or renal disorder often involves helping parents remember to give medicine. A child with nephrotic syndrome or a renal transplant, for example, may take three or four different types of medicine every day at home. Be certain parents understand

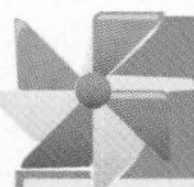

BOX 46.1 * Focus on National Health Goals

Renal disease can lead to long-term illness, so preventing it is important to improving the health of the nation. The following National Health Goals address this concern:

- Reduce the rate of new cases of end-stage renal disease from a baseline of 300 per 1 million population to a target rate of 221 per 1 million population.
- Increase the proportion of patients with treated chronic kidney failure who receive a transplant within 3 years of end-stage renal disease (ESRD) from a baseline of 23.1 per 1000 to 30.5 per 1000 (http://www.nih.gov).

Nurses can help the nation achieve these goals by educating parents to give antibiotics conscientiously for streptococcal throat infections and being active advocates for organ transplant procedures.

Areas that would benefit from nursing research include: determining parents' or children's ability to accurately self-assess for proteinuria after streptococcal infections, identifying the specific needs of children on ambulatory peritoneal dialysis, designing ways to make low-potassium diets more appealing to children with end-stage renal disease, or designing ways that organ donation can be presented to make it more appealing to potential donors.

the types of medicine prescribed and the expected action of each. If school-age children cannot take medicine in school, they need a schedule that allows them to take medicine before they leave home in the morning or after they return in the afternoon. If a child's school allows medication to be given during school hours, an order from the prescriber and the reason for the medication is usually required.

If a child has severe renal impairment, parents may be asked to make decisions regarding kidney removal and transplantation. Provide them with ample time for discussion. If a kidney donor is sought among relatives, the parents must help decide whether the person whose tissue matches the child's really wants to donate a kidney or is being pressured to do so. Helping parents to schedule times for hemodialysis or peritoneal dialysis or to supervise continuous cycling peritoneal dialysis (CCPD), to care for their other children, and to provide a life apart from their child requires nursing planning. Referrals to support organizations such as the following may be helpful: National Kidney Foundation (http://www.kidney.org) and Kidney Dialysis Foundation (http://www.kdf.org.sg/).

Implementation

Parents may or may not understand the function of the urinary system because it is not a system that receives much discussion. For example, they may confuse the words "ureter" and "urethra." A nurse can play a major role as a resource person, explaining anatomy and the tests and procedures and why they are being done.

Many children with kidney disease take a corticosteroid for immunosuppression and so develop a typical cushingoid appearance. They may have edema or ascites, which makes them appear obese. A child may be teased or criticized by classmates because of this "different" appearance. Contacting the school nurse or making the reason for the child's appearance known to the child's teacher may be necessary to help minimize this. Frequent contact and discussion with the child's siblings are also important to help them understand the reason for so many tests and health care visits and why their sibling is receiving so much attention. Discussion also helps open up channels of communication with all members of the family.

If kidney damage is extensive and the child's kidneys fail or a transplant is rejected, nursing care needs to be refocused on helping the family to face the possibility of the child's death. Nursing interventions can begin to prepare the child, parents, and family for this event (see Chapter 56).

Outcome Evaluation

Children with urinary or renal disease often need follow-up care after their acute illness. Because they are followed by a specialty renal group or clinic, parents may assume that routine health maintenance care is being given as well. Check to see that children are receiving routine childhood immunizations (remember that children taking steroid or other immunosuppressive therapy should not receive live virus immunizations) and that parents have their questions about day-to-day childrearing concerns answered.

Children returning to health care agencies for re-evaluation usually need as much preparation for procedures as those having them for the first time. Memory blurs events and sometimes confuses children. For example, they may recall that a particular test involved an injection when it did not, making them worry needlessly unless their memories are refreshed. Parents wait anxiously for the results of re-evaluation studies. Ensure they are given test results as soon as a comprehensive opinion of the child's progress is available. Be sure that all involved are aware of how anxious a particular parent is to hear the results of the re-evaluation.

Examples suggesting achievement of outcomes are:

- Child reports pain is at a tolerable level and decreasing in intensity after treatment.
- Family members state they are able to cope with long-term illness in child.
- Child states the purpose of a low-sodium diet and lists the ingredients of a low-sodium meal.
- Child states she can accept the need for kidney transplantation.
- Child states the precautions he must follow to reduce possibility of infection while on immunosuppressive therapy.
- Child remains free of any signs and symptoms of complications related to accumulated waste products.

ANATOMY AND PHYSIOLOGY OF THE KIDNEYS

Embryonic development of the urinary tract is discussed in Chapter 9. Figure 46.1 identifies the structures of the tract. Kidneys are located slightly lower in relation to the ribs than in adults. They also do not have as much perinephric fat to pad them. This makes them more susceptible to trauma.

Nephron

A *nephron,* the functioning unit of the kidney, consists of a glomerulus (a filtrating unit) and a complex set of tubules with accompanying blood supply (Fig. 46.2). Enclosed by a

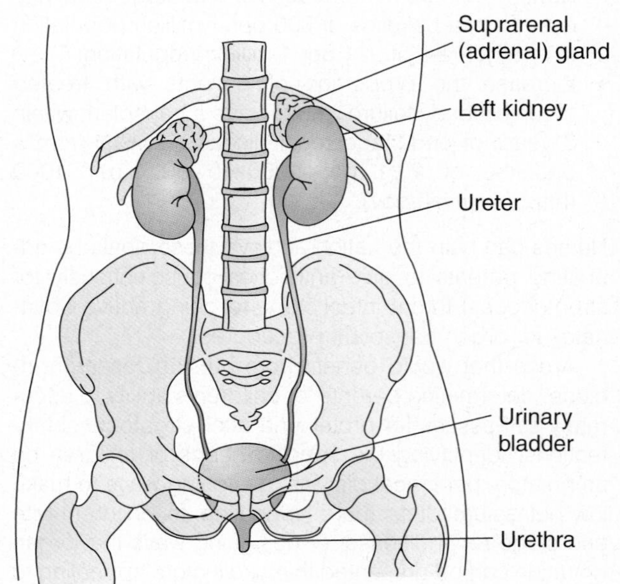

FIGURE 46.1 The urinary system.

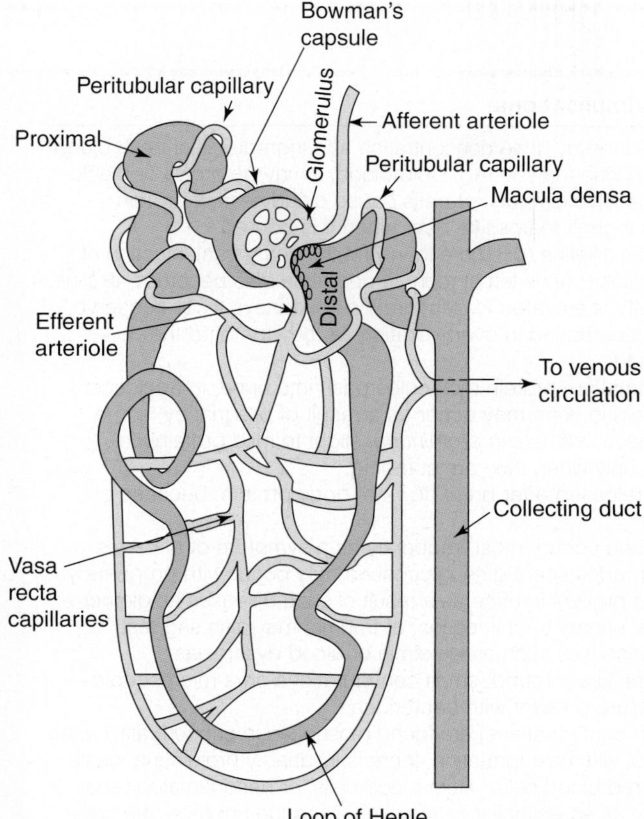

FIGURE 46.2 Basic structure of a nephron with its accompanying blood vessels.

TABLE 46.1 ✻ Functions of the Nephron

Site	Activity
Glomerulus	Secretion of water and all solutes except protein from blood
Proximal convoluted tubule	Reabsorption of 80% of glomerular filtrated water, all of glucose, amino acids, vitamins, and proteins; most of sodium, chloride, and ascorbic acid; secretion of creatinine
Descending and ascending loop of Henle	Reabsorption of additional water; fluid becomes neutral in reaction; specific gravity 1.010; additional reabsorption of sodium and chloride
Distal convoluted tubule	Reabsorption of water, sodium, chloride, phosphate, and sulfate as needed; secretion of potassium, H^+ ions, and ammonia (secretion of $NH4^+$ and H^+ ions conserves base because H^+ ions are substituted for sodium ions; sodium is reabsorbed as sodium bicarbonate)

double-walled chamber called a **Bowman's capsule,** the *glomerulus* is a capillary tuft supplied by a large afferent (ingoing) and a small efferent (outgoing) arteriole. It is invaginated within a tubule with a proximal and distal portion. In the glomerulus, water and solutes are filtered from the blood. This passage of water and solutes from the blood into the glomeruli is effective only as long as the blood pressure in glomerular arteries exceeds that in the tubule. The smaller efferent arteriole normally causes back-pressure in the glomerular arterioles, increasing the existing pressure and allowing filtration to occur readily. If blood pressure in these arterioles should fall below the tubular pressure or the tubular pressure should rise above that of the arterioles, little or no filtration will occur. For this reason, renal function must be assessed carefully in children who are hemorrhaging or are in shock with lowered blood pressure for any reason.

The solution that filtered into the tubule from afferent arterioles passes through the proximal portion, the loop of Henle, and then the distal portion. Beginning with the loop of Henle, water and electrolytes diffuse back into blood capillaries, reducing the volume of the filtrate by approximately 90%.

The glomerular filtrate enters the proximal tubule at a rate of approximately 120 mL/min. So much water is reabsorbed that the final end product (urine) left in the tubule is excreted at a rate of only approximately 1 mL/min. The proximal portion of the tubules reabsorbs most of the water, glucose, sodium chloride, phosphate (PO_4^-), sulfate (SO_4^-), and some bicarbonate (HCO_3) ions. This is a passive process, not particularly affected by body needs. In contrast, the distal portion of the tubule responds selectively to body needs. If necessary, Na^+ and HCO_3^- ions and additional water can be reabsorbed. The functions of nephron structures are summarized in Table 46.1.

Urine

The amount of urine excreted in a 24-hour period depends on fluid intake, kidney health, and age. Approximate urine output from different age groups is shown in Table 46.2. A significant decrease in urine production is *oliguria;* absence of urine production is *anuria.*

When renal disease occurs and glomerular or tubular function becomes impaired, nonprotein nitrogenous substances such as creatinine, urea, ammonia, and purine bodies are retained in the blood rather than being excreted. Urea is

TABLE 46.2 ✻ Child's Average Urine Output in 24 Hours

Age	Amount of Urine (mL)
6 mo–2 yr	540–600
2–5 yr	500–780
5–8 yr	600–1200
8–14 yr	1000–1500
Over 14 yr	1500

TABLE 46.3 ✻ Characteristics of Urine

Assessment	Normal Finding	Description/Implications
Color	Pale yellow	Color is influenced by urine concentration and ingredients; if fresh blood is present, urine may be red; if old blood, it may be brown or black.
Appearance	Clear	Bacteria, excessive crystals, or cells cause cloudiness; if protein content is high, it foams like beer when it is poured.
pH	4.6–8.0	Urine becomes alkaline (pH more than 7) with urinary tract infection or severe alkalosis; urine left at room temperature also becomes alkaline.
Specific gravity	1.003–1.030	Specific gravity is elevated in dehydration as kidneys try to conserve fluid, and decreased in overhydration as they try to rid the body of fluid.
Protein	0	Due to inflammation, protein molecules pass into urine; in adolescent girls, protein in urine may occur as a result of pregnancy; some children have *orthostatic proteinuria,* slight to mild proteinuria occurring only when they are standing.
Ketones	0	Ketones are released after breakdown of body protein, because of starvation.
Glucose	0	Glucose in urine occurs most frequently as a symptom of diabetes mellitus; in adolescent girls, glucosuria may occur with pregnancy.
Red blood cells	Less than 1 per high-power field Negative on dipstick	Blood may be present in urine as a result of such diseases as glomerulonephritis, urinary tract infection, or trauma; may also suggest systemic diseases such as leukemia or blood dyscrasias.
White blood cells	Less than 5 per high-power field	White blood cells are round, small configurations on a microscopic slide; they are present with bacteriuria.
Casts	0	Casts (protein configurations) are found most often in concentrated urine specimens; with cast formation, there is invariably proteinuria; casts comprise red blood cells, white blood cells, or desquamated renal epithelium; as an epithelial cast moves along the nephron, the cells begin to disintegrate, leaving a coarse granular cast; some disintegrate still further to become fine granular casts. The last stage of the process is a configuration in the shape of the tubule, termed a *waxy cast* (translucent and may be shiny and reflect light). The stage of the cast is important in indicating the flow of urine through the kidney. Hyaline casts are formations of protein appearing dull and reflecting light poorly; fatty casts are casts caused by the degeneration of tubular epithelial cells and are found in children with nephrosis. Red blood cells, white blood cells, and fatty casts are evidence of disease; other casts suggest urine stasis and probably proteinuria.
Crystals	Possibly present or not	Crystal formation is possibly indication of urine pH; uric acid, cystine, and calcium oxalate crystals are examples of crystals found in acid urine; phosphate crystals tend to be present in alkaline urine. Infection (particularly *Proteus* infection) is the most usual cause of alkaline urine. Sulfur crystals may be present if the child is receiving a sulfa drug (such as sulfamethoxazole [Gantanol]).

formed from the breakdown of amino acids by the liver. The amount of urea in urine is an indirect indication of kidney and liver function.

Creatinine is a product released during muscle cell metabolism. The amount excreted in urine normally remains constant, regardless of the amount of protein in the diet or body processes. When it is less in amount, therefore, it means that kidneys are not functioning as well as usual. When kidney function is impaired, not only is creatinine level reduced, but also some constituents that normally are retained such as albumin, glucose, blood, bile pigments, and casts will be allowed to enter the urine. Bile pigments that stain urine a green/yellow/brown color appear in the urine when the child has elevated levels of indirect or direct bilirubin in the blood plasma (hemolysis of red blood cells or jaundice will cause this). Casts are formed when there is an abnormal condition that causes the kidney tubule to become lined with protein formed from red and white blood cells, epithelial cells, or fatty cells that harden into the shape of the tubule. After urine washes the casts out, they can be detected by microscopic examination of urine. As protein deposits in this way only when fluid is slow-moving, their presence suggests slow filtration. Normal constituents of urine are shown in Table 46.3.

ASSESSMENT OF RENAL AND URINARY TRACT DYSFUNCTION

Assessment of urinary or renal tract disorders is based on the history, physical examination, and laboratory/diagnostic tests (Box 46.2).

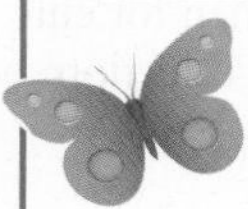

Box 46.2 Assessment
Assessing a Child for Renal and Urinary Tract Dysfunction

History
Chief concern: Child reports burning or cries on urination; bloody or "dark" urine, frequency of urination; abdominal pain, flank pain, enuresis. Parents report increase in size of abdomen, periorbital edema, poor appetite, frequent thirst, weight gain, strong odor to urine; diaper rash in infants. A school-age child may be described as a behavior problem because he or she frequently asks to use the bathroom.
Family history: History of renal disease, such as polycystic kidney, enuresis; hypertension.
Pregnancy history: Exposure to nephrotoxic drugs (antibiotics) during pregnancy. Oligohydramnios at birth.
Past illness history: Child recently had a throat or skin infection.

Physical assessment
General appearance
Fatigue, paleness
Growth restriction
Low-grade temperature

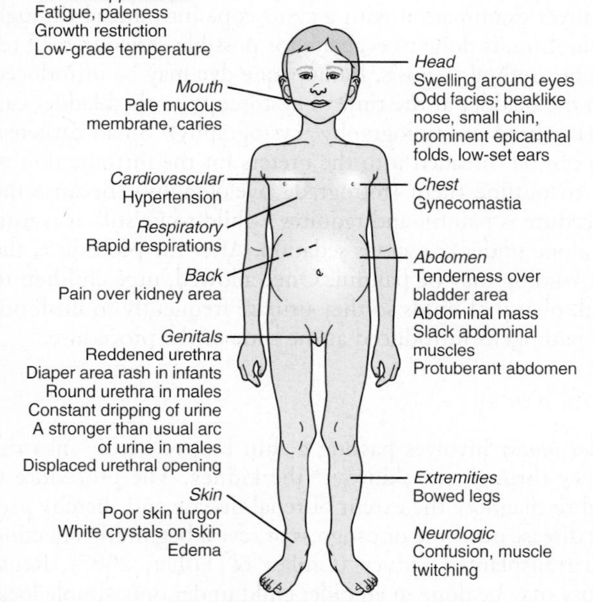

Laboratory/Diagnostic Tests

A variety of diagnostic tests may be performed, either in an ambulatory department or on an inpatient basis, to document renal or urinary tract disease.

Urinalysis

One of the most revealing tests of kidney function is also one of the simplest: urinalysis. For best results, specimens collected should be fresh because urine that stands at room temperature for any length of time changes composition. Devices used to collect urine specimens and the method for obtaining urine specimens from diapers are described in Chapter 37. A chemical reagent strip can be used to detect glucose, protein, and occult blood and to measure pH. Specific gravity is best determined by use of a refractometer (requires only a single drop [see Chapter 37]).

Creatinine Clearance Rate

Glomerular filtration rate is the rate at which substances are filtered from the blood to the urine. It is measured by the amount of creatinine (the breakdown product of creatine from muscle contraction) excreted in 24 hours as determined by a 24-hour urine sample. A venous blood sample is taken during the 24-hour period and compared with the urine findings (if urine creatinine is decreased, this will be increased). A normal creatinine clearance rate is 100 mL/min. A normal urine creatinine level is 0.7 to 1.5 mg/100 mL; creatinine in blood serum rarely exceeds 1 mg/dL (Watnick & Morrison, 2009).

Radioisotope Scanning

The administration of radioisotopes (a technetium scan) is a second way to assess glomeruli filtration ability. Radioactively tagged substances are given intravenously (IV); the rate at which these substances can be observed flowing through the kidney and excreted in urine is then determined. The level of radioisotopes used in these studies is small, and urinating removes the substance from the body immediately afterward. Children do not remain radioactive, so parents should not be afraid to stay near them or to hold them after such a study.

Urine Culture

A urinary tract infection (UTI), the presence of bacteria in urine, is diagnosed by a urine culture. Because bladder catheterization can introduce bacteria into the bladder and also is painful and intrusive, most urine specimens in children are obtained by a clean-catch procedure or sterile suprapubic aspiration (see Chapter 37). Several instant-read commercial kits for culturing urine are available for use in ambulatory settings.

Blood Studies

A blood urea nitrogen (BUN) test measures the level of urea in blood and is used to assess glomerular function, or how well the kidneys can clear this from the bloodstream. However, this level may not increase until approximately 50% of glomeruli are destroyed, because the remaining glomeruli can increase in size and function to accommodate urine production. A normal value is 5 to 20 mg/100 mL.

Ultrasonography and Magnetic Resonance Imaging

An *ultrasound* or *magnetic resonance imaging* (MRI) can detect differing sizes of kidneys or ureters and can differentiate between solid or cystic kidney masses. They do not involve x-rays and so may be repeated at frequent intervals for follow-up without danger of radiation exposure (Riccabona, 2007).

X-Ray Studies

A plain flat-plate abdominal x-ray film can provide information about the size and contour of the kidneys. This radiograph may be referred to as a *KUB* (*k*idney, *u*reters, and *b*ladder). A small kidney shown this way is generally a hypoplastic or an underdeveloped organ. A large kidney may indicate hydronephrosis or a polycystic kidney.

Computed Tomography

Computed tomography (CT) scans of the kidneys are used to show the size and density of kidney structures and adequacy of urine flow. Conscious sedation may be given before a CT scan because a child must lie still for an extended time during the procedure, and the size of a CT scanner and the fact that it surrounds the child may be frightening. Be sure to prepare the child for this. A contrast medium may be injected before the procedure to better outline urine flow. If this medium is iodine based, be certain to ask about allergy to iodine before the study. Because a support person is not allowed to remain in the room during the procedure, thoroughly prepare children so they can comfortably remain still for the procedure.

Intravenous Pyelogram. An *intravenous pyelogram* (IVP) is an x-ray study of the upper urinary tract. It used to be a mainstay of diagnosis for kidney disorders but now is used less frequently because ultrasounds, MRIs, or CT scans reveal so much information. For an IVP, a radiopaque dye is injected into a peripheral vein, circulates through the bloodstream, and is almost immediately identified as a foreign substance by the kidney and filtered out into the urine by the glomeruli. X-ray films taken at frequent intervals show the outline of collecting systems in the kidney and of the ureters as the radiopaque dye passes through them.

In preparing children for an IVP, tell them that they will receive an injection. Say "medicine," not "dye" (or compare coloring kidneys to coloring with crayons or coloring Easter eggs), because the child may mistake "dye" for "die." Be sure children know that, after this injection, they must lie still in whatever position they are placed until all films are taken. This may be difficult for young children because x-ray tables are hard and cold and the x-ray camera overhead can be frightening. When explaining the test, compare the x-ray machine to a camera. Caution children that they may experience flushing of the face, warmth, and a salty taste in their mouth after the injection of medicine. Because the dye used is iodine based, ask the parents if the child has a known allergy to iodine. This is rarely known in children because they may have had no previous studies of this kind.

Voiding Cystourethrogram. A *voiding cystourethrogram* (VCUG), a study of the lower urinary tract, reveals the structure of the urethra and bladder and the presence of reflux into the ureters (Gomella & Haist, 2007). After bladder catheterization, a radiopaque dye is injected into the bladder, and the catheter is then removed. The child is asked to void into a bedpan while serial x-ray films are taken. Although the catheterization is unpleasant, being asked to void while they are observed on an x-ray table may be the most stressful part of the procedure for most children because they have been taught that voiding is a private act. Be sure that children are told in advance that they will be asked to do this. Caution a child that a first voiding this way after catheterization may be painful. A few children have difficulty voiding a second time later in the day because they worry that the second voiding will also sting. Pouring warm water over the perineal area while sitting on a toilet or sitting in a bathtub of warm water and voiding into the water may help relieve pain. Most children, once they void this second time and realize that it is not painful, usually have no further difficulty.

A VCUG should not be done if a child has an active UTI because there is danger that the radiopaque material injected into the bladder could spread, carrying bacteria from the infection into the ureters and kidneys. Report any symptoms of UTI such as frequency, pain on voiding, or low back pain to the radiologic physician. A clean-catch urine specimen for culture may be ordered before the VCUG to rule out infection.

✔ Checkpoint Question 46.1

Carol had a voiding cystourethrogram last year to help diagnose a urinary tract infection. Why is a voiding cystourethrogram a difficult test for preschool children?

a. Reading the instructions for the test is difficult.
b. Lying in an MRI machine is dark and scary.
c. They feel uncomfortable voiding in public.
d. The dye capsules may be too large to swallow.

Cystoscopy

Cystoscopy, examination of the bladder and ureter openings by direct examination with a cystoscope introduced through the urethra, is done to evaluate for possible vesicoureteral reflux or urethral stenosis. Radiopaque dye may be introduced into the bladder at the time of cystoscopy so the bladder can be visualized on radiography (cystography). Small catheters also can be threaded into the ureters for the introduction of dye to outline them (retrograde pyelography). Because the procedure is painful and requires a child to lie still, it is usually done under conscious sedation. After the procedure, the first voiding may be painful. Once allowed, urge children to drink plenty of fluids so they urinate frequently to flush out any pathogens introduced at the time of the procedure.

Renal Biopsy

Renal biopsy involves passing a thin biopsy needle into the kidney through the skin over the kidney. The procedure is used to diagnose the extent of renal disease and thereby predict disease outcome or progress or reveal beginning rejection of a transplanted kidney (Croker & Tisher, 2007). Renal biopsy may be done in an older child under only simple local anesthesia, but conscious sedation may be necessary for a younger child who cannot cooperate easily. The kidney is located first by ultrasound to accurately locate the place of the biopsy. The child lies prone with a sandbag under the abdomen for firmness. If the procedure is done under a local anesthetic, prepare children for the feel of a pinprick as the local anesthetic is injected; after this, they should not feel any further pain. What they will feel is pressure as the biopsy needle is inserted. Caution children that they need to lie still while the biopsy specimen is taken (if the child moved suddenly, the needle might puncture a renal artery or vein or tear vital glomeruli). Be certain children have support people to accompany them for this procedure so that they have someone to hold their hand or comfort them when they feel the pressure of the needle.

After the biopsy, press a sterile gauze square against the biopsy site for approximately 15 minutes to halt bleeding, and then apply a pressure dressing. Caution parents that a large dressing will be used and that the size of this dressing does not reflect the size of the specimen taken (the amount of tissue removed is no more than the lumen of the needle used, or approximately the size of a pencil lead).

If the procedure was done on an ambulatory basis, children can be discharged 2 to 4 hours after the procedure if vital signs are stable and they have voided. Measure vital signs and observe the biopsy site every 15 minutes for at least the first hour. Do not lift the dressing to assess bleeding, because doing so destroys the protective function of the pressure dressing. Encourage children to drink a considerable amount of fluid (a glass every hour while awake) during the first 24 hours to keep urine flowing freely and prevent blood from clotting in the kidney tubules and blocking urine flow. Play games with the child, if necessary, to encourage a high fluid intake (the child must take a drink each time before a turn at a game; play "Simon Says" and have Simon frequently say, "Drink").

The first voiding after renal biopsy is invariably blood-tinged. Advise parents to keep children on restricted activity for 24 hours or until no more hematuria is present. Instruct parents how to keep serial urine samples, comparing each specimen with the previous one, to detect whether hematuria is becoming more or less marked. When urine no longer appears bloody, they can test it for occult blood to confirm that bleeding has stopped. A hematocrit may be ordered 24 hours after the procedure to ensure that no bleeding is continuing.

What if... Carol's grandmother telephones you after a kidney biopsy and says Carol is voiding black urine? Is there a possibility this is blood? What questions would you ask to elicit additional information? What recommendations would you make to the grandmother?

THERAPEUTIC MEASURES FOR THE MANAGEMENT OF RENAL DISEASE

As kidney function is necessary for life, if it deteriorates, some method to replace function must be instituted.

Peritoneal Dialysis

Dialysis is the separation and removal of solutes from body fluid by diffusion through a semipermeable membrane. *Peritoneal dialysis* uses the membrane of the peritoneal cavity to do this. Hemodialysis uses an outside synthetic membrane to do this. Unlike hemodialysis, peritoneal dialysis does not require elaborate equipment or expense, but it does take more time.

Peritoneal dialysis may be used as a temporary measure for children who experience sudden renal failure caused by trauma or shock. It is used for fairly long periods with children with chronic renal disease both in the hospital or at home to allow them to live until a kidney transplantation can be arranged (Coe & Lail, 2007). It is usually begun when the serum creatinine level reaches 10 mg/100 mL. Other indications are congestive heart failure, BUN of more than 100 mg/100 mL, hyperkalemia (potassium level of more than 6 mEq/L), and uremic encephalopathy (confusion or coma). CCPD allows the procedure to be done at home because less rigorous monitoring of the procedure is necessary.

Method for Performing Peritoneal Dialysis

Before peritoneal dialysis begins, a child's weight and vital signs are obtained to provide baseline information. Ask the child to void to reduce bladder size so that the bladder occupies as little anterior space as possible. If a child cannot void, catheterization may be necessary. Following this, the child's abdomen is cleaned just below the umbilicus with an antiseptic solution and covered with a sterile drape; a local anesthetic is injected into the abdominal wall, and a large-bore needle is inserted into the peritoneal cavity. If ascites fluid is present, a quantity of this fluid is removed and then a warmed hypertonic glucose solution (approximately 50 to 100 mL/kg of body weight) or a commercial dialysis solution is infused by gravity flow into the peritoneal cavity. This distends the abdominal wall and allows safe insertion of a peritoneal catheter, which is sutured in place and covered with a sterile dressing (Fig. 46.3). This catheter will remain in place for the duration of dialysis.

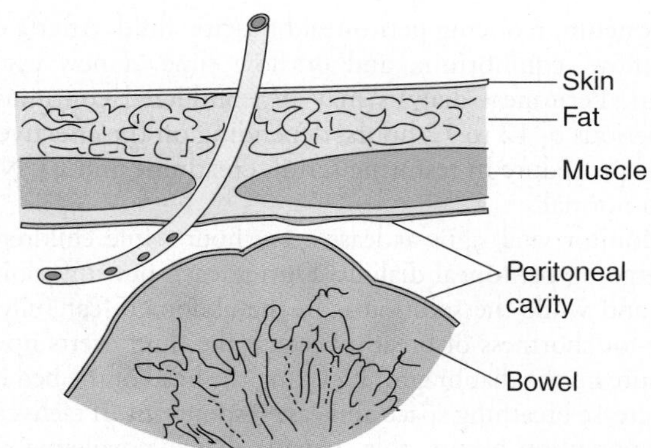

FIGURE 46.3 Insertion site for peritoneal dialysis catheter.

As for any procedure, children need to be well prepared for peritoneal dialysis but if the procedure is presented in a matter-of-fact way, children usually accept it with no more apprehension than IV therapy. Both procedures involve a needle penetration. You can assure children that they will feel the initial prick of the needle that administers the local anesthetic but will feel only pressure after that as the peritoneal needle or catheter is inserted. The procedure is intrusive, however, and frightening. Provide opportunities for therapeutic play such as letting the child handle a cloth doll, a dialysis tube, IV tubing, a doll's bed, or syringes and needles.

With the dialysis tube in place, a prescribed amount of dialysis solution is then infused into the peritoneal cavity by gravity drainage. This takes approximately 10 minutes and is recorded as inflow time. Be certain that the infusion fluid is warmed to room temperature to prevent the child from becoming chilled; warming the solution to near body temperature also appears to improve diffusion efficiency. It can be warmed in a basin of warm water or with the use of commercial warm packs at the child's bedside. Heparin is generally added at least to the first infusion to keep any initial bleeding from the abdominal puncture from plugging the tube.

Infused fluid is allowed to remain in the child's peritoneal cavity for 15 to 60 minutes (called the *equilibrium* or *dwell time*). Because the infused solution is hypertonic, fluid from extracellular spaces diffuses across the semipermeable peritoneal membrane to dilute the hypertonic solution (the law of osmosis). Urea and electrolytes diffuse with this fluid. After this designated equilibrium time, drain the fluid from the peritoneal catheter into a collecting bottle (this takes approximately 10 minutes and is recorded as outflow time). More fluid generally drains from the peritoneal cavity than was infused, because excessive fluid has diffused across the peritoneum, reducing peritoneal or ascitic fluid. After a cycle of inflow, equilibrium, and outflow time, a new cycle is begun. Peritoneal dialysis may be conducted continuously for periods of 12 to 72 hours, depending on the effectiveness of the procedure in restoring serum creatinine and BUN levels to normal.

Monitor vital signs at least every hour while children are undergoing peritoneal dialysis. During each new infusion period and while the solution is in the abdomen, carefully observe for shortness of breath, because the fluid exerts upward pressure on the diaphragm. Elevating the head of the bed helps to increase breathing space and ease respirations. If tachycardia or hypotension occurs, this suggests that hypovolemia is occurring. An increasing temperature (after 24 hours) may indicate peritoneal infection, a serious complication (Auron et al., 2007). Frequent blood studies are necessary during periods of peritoneal dialysis to determine electrolyte concentrations. If electrolyte imbalances occur, electrolytes may be added to the infusion solution or administered IV.

The longer the peritoneal catheter remains in place, the greater the risk of peritoneal infection at the catheter insertion site. Assess the insertion site daily for signs of infection, such as redness or drainage. Obtain temperature about every 4 hours. Ask children to report any abdominal pain or diarrhea. Assess for abdominal guarding or tenderness once daily by palpating the abdomen; a rigid abdomen suggest peritonitis or infection. Follow the agency's policy for cleaning and covering the end of the peritoneal catheter if there are periods when dialysis is halted (Fig. 46.4).

Once cycles of dialysis begin, children often grow bored lying in bed waiting for this procedure to be finished. They need planned interaction for these times—perhaps a toy or game that is allowed only during the procedure, so that it remains special. Children generally do not feel hungry while having peritoneal dialysis, because the bulk of peritoneal fluid causes pressure on the stomach and makes them feel uncomfortably full. They do well on a liquid diet or small frequent feedings during this time. So that children can feel that they have a sense of control over what is happening, let them help with the procedure by doing such things as recording the amount of solution infused and drained, and allowing them to select liquids they like for meals.

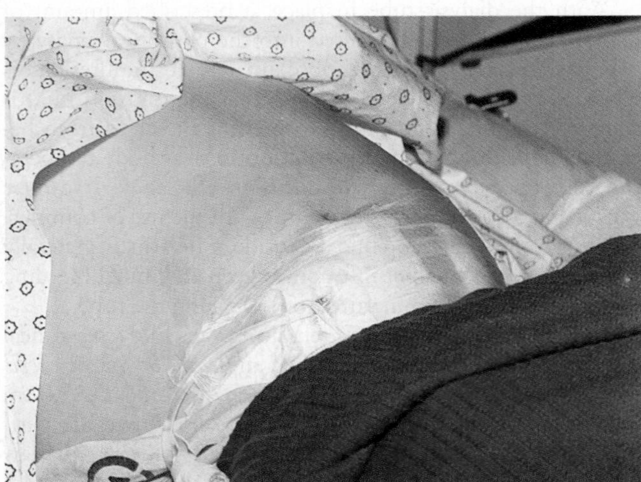

FIGURE 46.4 Peritoneal catheter inserted into a child's abdomen. A secure dressing surrounds the insertion site to prevent infection. (Courtesy of Karen M. Polise, MSN, RN, Division of Nephrology, The Children's Hospital of Philadelphia.)

Peritoneal dialysis is a simple yet important concept. Help parents understand its importance so they can demonstrate a positive attitude toward it. The parents' acceptance of the procedure helps the child accept it as well.

Continuous Cycling Peritoneal Dialysis

CCPD allows a child to go to school or participate in other activities while receiving dialysis. With CCPD, a permanent dialysis catheter is inserted and sutured into place at the abdomen. Each day, the child or parent attaches a bag of dialysis fluid and tubing to this and infuses a prescribed dialysis solution by gravity drainage; the bag and tubing are then rolled into a compact square under the child's clothes. The infused solution remains in the child for 4 to 6 hours during the day (8 hours at night); the dialysate bag is then lowered and the solution drains from the peritoneal cavity into it. The bag and fluid are then discarded and a new bag of dialysate solution is attached and raised, and new solution is infused.

CCPD requires careful monitoring and attention by the child or family. They must keep accurate records of infusions. Children can participate in gym programs but should not participate in contact sports or swimming. Teach parents to think ahead for holidays or family trips so they do not run short of supplies.

Because CCPD is continuous, electrolytes in the bloodstream are maintained at more constant levels than when intermittent dialysis is used although because a great deal of potassium is removed, children may become hypokalemic (Factor, 2007). CCPD also allows greater freedom because children can return home and go back to school. There are disadvantages, however. Infection can occur because of the long-term placement of the catheter. Dehydration or hypernatremia may occur because of excess fluid removal. Because the tube remains in place at all times and the peritoneal solution constantly distends the abdomen, the child appears obese and clothing is difficult to fit, the child is frequently reminded of the illness and may have difficulty accepting this change in body image. Possible complications of CCPD are summarized in Table 46.4.

Hemodialysis

Hemodialysis removes body wastes by using an external membrane as the diffusion surface. For hemodialysis, a catheter is inserted into an artery and blood is removed from the child and circulated through a dialysis coil. Urea and electrolytes in the blood diffuse into the surrounding fluid bath as the blood passes through the coil (Ahmad et al., 2007). After diffusion is complete, the blood is returned to the child's venous circulation (Fig. 46.5).

Hemodialysis can be done as a continuous process, but it is so effective that 3 hours of hemodialysis accomplishes as much as 12 hours of peritoneal dialysis. Children who have renal failure or whose kidneys have been removed while they await a kidney transplant can be maintained almost indefinitely by hemodialysis sessions two or three times a week or by continuous ultrafiltration or continuous arteriovenous hemofiltration (Schon et al., 2007). It can be used in infants as well as older children (Sousa et al., 2008).

TABLE 46.4 ✻ Possible Complications of Continuous Ambulatory Peritoneal Dialysis

Assessment	Problem	Interventions
Redness or pain or swelling at tube insertion site	Infection	Take culture at site; administer antibiotics as prescribed; continue site care as ordered; notify physician.
Abdominal pain, increased temperature, nausea and vomiting, cloudy return in drainage solution	Peritonitis	Notify physician; administer antibiotics as prescribed; auscultate for bowel sounds.
Cramps as fluid is infused	Irritation of peritoneal cavity	Infuse solutions more slowly; warm temperature of solution to body temperature.
Difficulty with infusion or drainage of fluid	Kinked or clotted tubing; malpositioned catheter	Assess tubing for kinking; change position of child; ask child to cough to increase abdominal pressure; add prescribed amount of heparin to dialysate bag (prevents clotting).
Weight increase; moist cough, shortness of breath	Fluid overload	Decrease sodium and fluid oral intake; assess blood pressure and weight; use 4.25% exchange solution until weight is again decreased.
Weight loss, hypotension, poor skin turgor, tachycardia	Fluid loss	Increase fluid and sodium intake; assess blood pressure and weight; do not use 4.25% solution.
Blood-tinged dialysis return	Ruptured blood vessel	Assess pulse and blood pressure; observe for further bleeding in drainage; flush catheter with prescribed amount of heparin to keep clots from forming.

To establish a site for initial blood removal, children may have a double-lumen central catheter inserted into a central vein, such as the subclavian or internal jugular vein.

A permanent technique is subcutaneous anastomosis of a vein and artery, creating an arteriovenous fistula (usually the brachial artery and brachiocephalic vein; Fig. 46.6A) or internal anastomosis of the artery and vein using a subcutaneous graft (see Fig. 46.6B). The possibility of infection is reduced with internal anastomosis, although, unfortunately, two venipunctures, one from a low point in the shunt to remove blood and one high in the shunt to return it, are necessary for dialysis (use lidocaine or EMLA cream to reduce pain). The ability to feel a thrill (vibration) or hear a bruit over the fistula or graft site is proof that it is open.

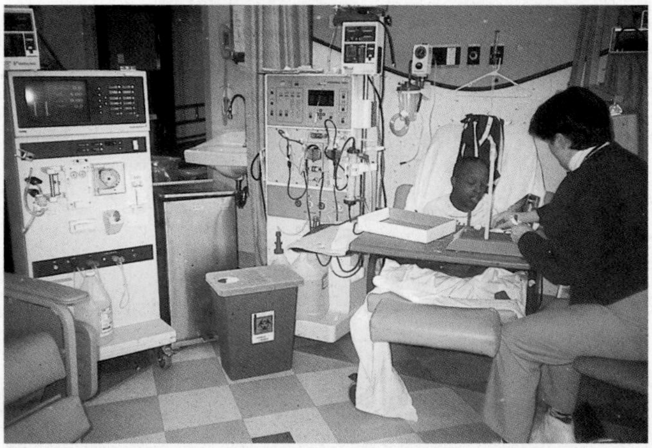

The risks of hemodialysis include infection introduced with venipuncture (severe because the infection automatically is septicemia) and clotting of the access site, which can lead to emboli. During hemodialysis, children may begin to show signs of confusion, vomiting, visual blurring, or hallucinations from a *dialysis disequilibrium syndrome.* This occurs because the hemodialysis is removing urea from the blood at too rapid a rate—faster than urea can be shifted from the brain to the blood. This causes fluid to shift into the brain, resulting in cerebral edema. The procedure must be temporarily halted to allow equalization to return. Muscle cramping may occur from sodium depletion. A "first use" syndrome or symptoms such as dizziness or muscle cramping may occur from a reaction to the fibers in the dialysis machine coil.

Children grow bored during hemodialysis as they do during peritoneal dialysis. They need entertainment so the procedure remains acceptable. Help parents provide stimulating activities such as a play board, a ball to throw, or rings to stack for the infant. Parents may envision the infant as so ill that lying still without an activity would be best. Children need stimulation and play to avoid missing normal developmental milestones, however, even during a long therapy such as dialysis.

When children's kidneys are removed prior to transplantation so they must remain on a continuous program of hemodialysis, they may come to resent a machine as "owning" or "controlling" them. They become aware that they cannot exist apart from it. Allowing them to plan special activities to

FIGURE 46.5 An adolescent receiving hemodialysis. A catheter from the child is connected to the hemodialysis equipment (in the background). Blood flows from the child through the catheter to the hemodialysis equipment for waste removal and is then returned to the child's venous circulation. (Courtesy of Karen M. Polise, MSN, RN, Division of Nephrology, The Children's Hospital of Philadelphia.)

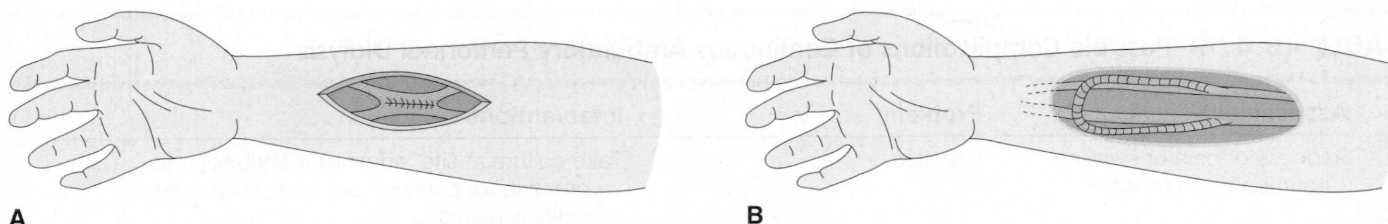

FIGURE 46.6 (**A**) An internal arteriovenous fistula. (**B**) An internal arteriovenous graft.

do during hemodialysis time can help to give them a feeling of control.

HEALTH PROMOTION AND RISK MANAGEMENT

Several important interventions can help prevent urinary and renal disease in children. The first intervention is to educate parents and caregivers about wiping from front to back when changing diapers of female infants. The second intervention is to prevent urinary tract infection in girls by beginning education about perineal hygiene measures from the time they are first toilet-trained. Remind parents of simple ways to prevent UTI, such as not allowing children to bathe with bubble bath. Teach parents to recognize the normal appearance of urine (clear and yellow) so that they can recognize abnormalities, such as red, black, or cloudy urine and the signs and symptoms of UTI, such as urgency, frequency, and pain.

Educating parents about the importance of giving the full course of antibiotics prescribed for UTI can help prevent reinfection. Also important is educating parents about the importance of giving the full course of antibiotics after a streptococcal infection to prevent acute glomerulonephritis.

STRUCTURAL ABNORMALITIES OF THE URINARY TRACT

Because the urinary tract is a system of hollow tubes, congenital disorders can rise from faulty recanalization in intrauterine life.

Patent Urachus

When the bladder first forms in utero, it is joined to the umbilicus by a narrow tube, the *urachus.* When this fails to close properly during embryologic development, a fistula is left between the bladder and umbilicus **(patent urachus).** This occurs more commonly in males than in females. Nurses are frequently the ones to discover this condition as they notice clear fluid draining from the base of the umbilical cord while changing a newborn's diaper. If you test the fluid with Nitrazine paper for pH, its acid content will identify it as urine. An ultrasound will confirm the patent connection.

A few patent urachus abnormalities heal spontaneously, but most require surgical correction to prevent pathogens from entering the fistula site and causing persistent bladder infection. This can be done in the immediate neonatal period using only a small subumbilical incision (Ashley, 2007).

Exstrophy of the Bladder

Exstrophy of the bladder is a midline closure defect that occurs during the embryonic period of gestation (first 8 weeks). As a result, the bladder lies open and exposed on the abdomen. It occurs more frequently in males than females at a ratio of 2:1 (Atala, 2007).

Assessment

Exstrophy is often revealed by fetal ultrasound as there is no anterior wall of the bladder and no anterior skin covering on the lower anterior abdomen (Fig. 46.7A). The bladder appears bright red and continually drains urine from the open

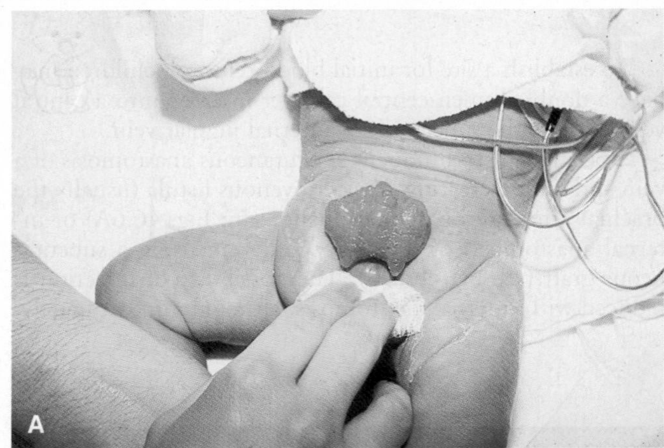

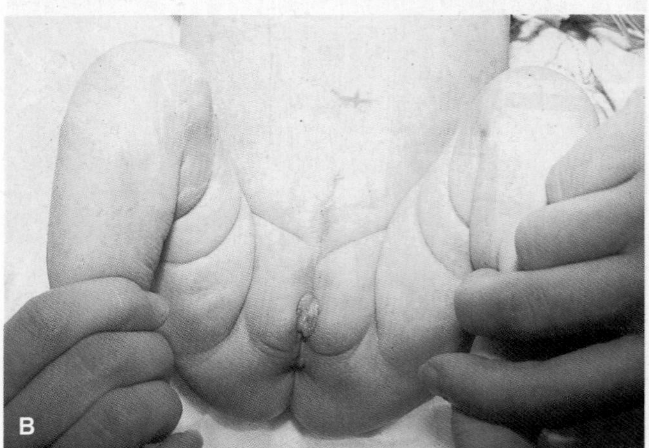

FIGURE 46.7 Bladder exstrophy. (**A**) Prior to surgical reconstruction. Note the bright-red color of the bladder. (**B**) Following surgical reconstruction. (Courtesy of Karen M. Polise, MSN, RN, Division of Nephrology, The Children's Hospital of Philadelphia.)

surface. In males, the penis is often unformed or malformed. In females, the urethra may also be abnormally formed. Pelvic bone defects, particularly nonclosure of the pubic arch, and urethral defects such as epispadias—opening of the urinary meatus on the dorsal or superior surface of the penis—may be present. The skin around the bladder quickly becomes excoriated because of constant exposure to acid urine. Untreated bladder exstrophy leads to kidney infection from ascending organisms. When children with this disorder begin to walk, they may demonstrate a "waddling" gait from the effect of the nonfused pubic arch.

Therapeutic Management

The treatment of bladder exstrophy begins with surgical closure of the bladder and, if necessary, the anterior abdominal wall and construction of a urethra (Gearhart, Baird, & Nelson, 2007; see Fig. 46.7B).

Preoperative Interventions. To minimize the possibility of infection in the bladder while the infant is waiting for initial surgery, keep the exposed bladder covered by a sterile plastic bowel bag. This prevents the bladder surface from adhering to bedclothes or diapers and the mucosal surface from being injured. To prevent the skin of the abdomen from excoriation due to the constant irritation of urine, protect it with a substance such as A&D ointment, Karaya Gum, or Maalox. Consult a wound, ostomy, continence nurse for the best approach. To reduce pressure and prevent further separation of the symphysis, the orthopedic physician may ask that the infant's legs be flexed, brought together, and wrapped in Ace bandages to hold them in that position. If this is done, do not separate the infant's legs to apply diapers; just place them under the child instead. Be certain to change diapers promptly after defecation so feces are not brought forward to the open bladder. Position the infant on the back, the same as for all infants, so urine drains freely. Sponge bathe rather than tub bathe the infant to prevent water from entering the ureters and becoming a source of infection.

Parents often need support to view their child as normal in all other ways but the unusual bladder formation. In some instances, the bladder repair will not be done immediately, so parents will need instructions on how to care for the child at home while waiting for surgery.

Postoperative Interventions. Surgery may be completed either as a one-step or two-step procedure. In the first step, the bladder tissue is reconstructed; in the second, a urethra is created. After bladder construction, the surgical incision over the bladder area must be kept free of infection. Position the infant on the back or in an infant chair to prevent feces from coming forward and contaminating the incision line. A suprapubic or indwelling urethral catheter for urine drainage will be in place to allow the newly constructed bladder to rest. Immediately after surgery, urine draining from the catheter may be blood-stained, but this should clear after the first few hours. Children may notice sharp painful bladder contractions for the first few days after surgery. Analgesics and antispasmodics may be needed to keep the child comfortable. To prevent the nonfused pubic bone from separating and putting stress on the suture line, at the time of surgery, the child may be fitted with an external fixation device after an osteotomy to hold the pubic bones in approximation until they fuse (4 to 6 weeks).

After the second-stage urethra repair, children can be expected to experience some stress incontinence (loss of urine on physical exertion) from the constructed urethra. When they are older, Kegel exercises can help strengthen the perineal muscles.

Surgical repair may be limited if inadequate bladder tissue is present. For this reason, in some instances, the bladder is surgically removed and a ureterocecal implantation (ureters directed into the small intestine) or a *continent urinary reservoir* (an artificial bladder) is constructed (Fig. 46.8).

To construct a continent urinary reservoir, a small segment of the intestine, usually the cecum, is separated from the intestinal tract. The intestinal tract is then anastomosed so that a normal gastrointestinal (GI) tract is maintained. The separated segment is attached to the internal abdominal wall using the appendix to create an artificial urethra. The ureters are anastomosed to this segment.

Urine drains from the kidneys into the ureters, and then into the collecting bowel segment. The parent or child catheterizes the abdominal urethra three or four times daily to empty urine. The procedure is theoretically simple, but it is technically difficult to accomplish. Parents need a good review of anatomy to aid their understanding of the procedure. As the child reaches school age and begins school activities, such as showering, that exposes the condition to others, adjusting to a continent urinary reservoir can be difficult. Ensure that the child has a plan for follow-up care during the school years and in adolescence so the function of the reservoir and also the child's adjustment can continue to be assessed.

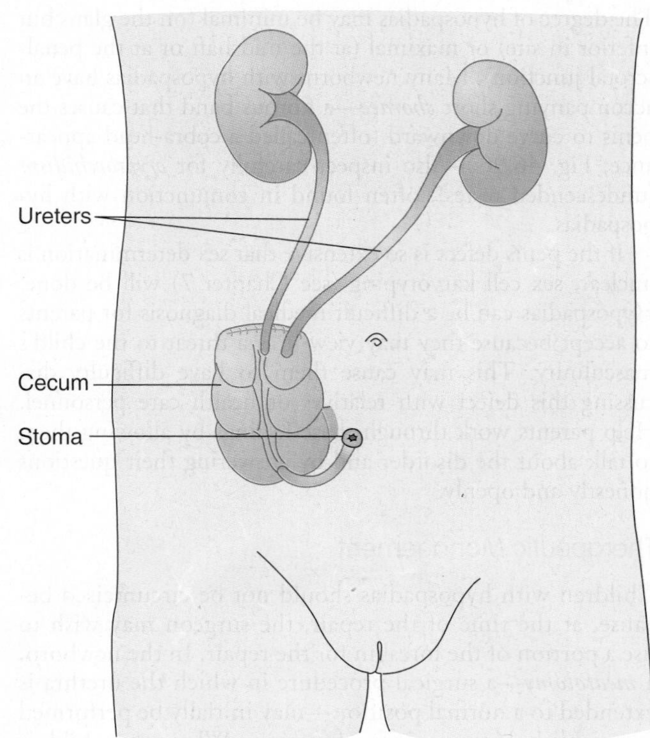

FIGURE 46.8 A continent urine reservoir. A portion of intestine is isolated; the attached ureters drain into it. The appendix creates an abdominal stoma for catheterization.

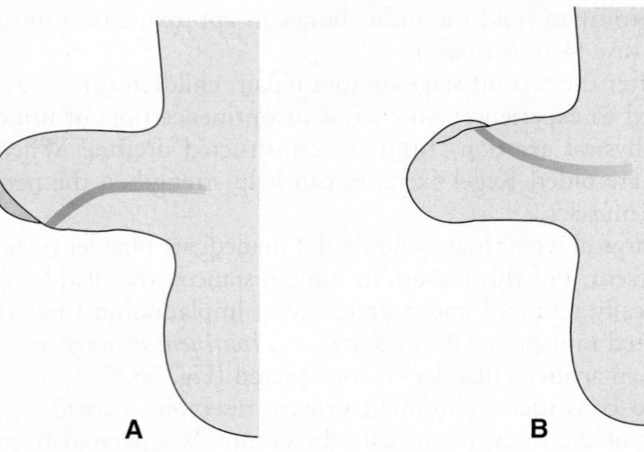

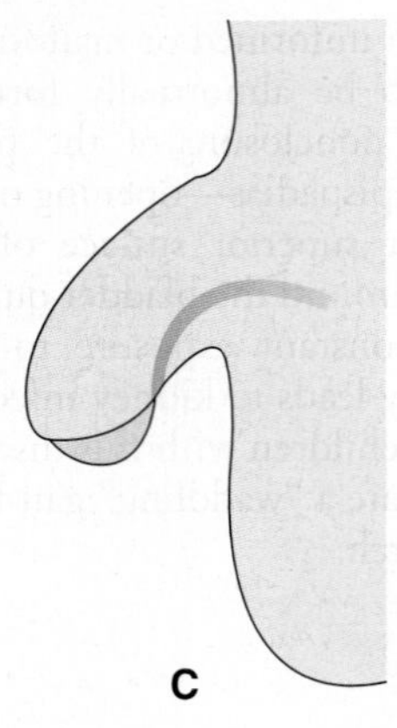

FIGURE 46.9 Urethral defects. (**A**) Hypospadias. (**B**) Epispadias. (**C**) Hypospadias with chordee.

Hypospadias

Hypospadias is a urethral defect in which the urethral opening is not at the end of the penis but on the ventral (lower) aspect of the penis (Fig. 46.9A). The meatus may be near the glans, midway back, or at the base of the penis (Hutton & Babu, 2007). This anomaly is fairly common, occurring in approximately 1 in 300 male newborns. It tends to be familial or may occur from a multifactorial genetic focus. **Epispadias** is a similar defect in which the opening is on the dorsal surface of the penis (Fig. 46.9B); this is corrected the same way.

Assessment

Be certain to inspect all male newborns at birth for hypospadias or epispadias as part of the routine physical examination. The degree of hypospadias may be minimal (on the glans but inferior in site) or maximal (at the midshaft or at the penal-scrotal junction). Many newborns with hypospadias have an accompanying short *chordee*—a fibrous band that causes the penis to curve downward (often called a cobra-head appearance; Fig. 46.9C). Also inspect carefully for *cryptorchidism* (undescended testes), often found in conjunction with hypospadias.

If the penis defect is so extensive that sex determination is unclear, sex cell karyotyping (see Chapter 7) will be done. Hypospadias can be a difficult medical diagnosis for parents to accept because they may view it as a threat to the child's masculinity. This may cause them to have difficulty discussing this defect with relatives or health care personnel. Help parents work through these feelings by allowing them to talk about the disorder and by answering their questions honestly and openly.

Therapeutic Management

Children with hypospadias should not be circumcised because, at the time of the repair, the surgeon may wish to use a portion of the foreskin for the repair. In the newborn, a *meatotomy*—a surgical procedure in which the urethra is extended to a normal position—may initially be performed to establish better urinary function. When the child is older (age 12 to 18 months), adherent chordee may be released. If the repair will be extensive, all surgery may be delayed until the child is 3 to 4 years of age. To encourage penis growth and make the procedure easier, the child may have testosterone cream applied to the penis or receive daily injections of testosterone. It is important that hypospadias be corrected before school age so the child looks and feels like other children (Dodson et al., 2007). If left uncorrected, in later years, a meatal opening at an inferior penile site may interfere with fertility, because it does not allow sperm to be deposited close to the female cervix during coitus. Repair must be made before this time to prevent subfertility.

After surgical repair, a urethral urinary drainage catheter will be inserted to allow urine output without putting tension against the urethral sutures. The child may notice painful bladder spasms as long as the catheter is in place (3 to 7 days). An analgesic such as acetaminophen (Tylenol) and an antispasmodic medication such as oxybutynin (Ditropan) may be prescribed for pain relief.

After hypospadias repair, children can be expected to have usual urinary and reproductive function unless accompanying anomalies of the penis were present.

✔Checkpoint Question 46.2

The appearance of a child with hypospadias is:

a. The urethra opens on the underside of the penis.
b. The bladder opens on the surface of the abdomen.
c. Urine drains into the rectum and is excreted with stool.
d. The child is unable to void, as there is no urethral meatus.

INFECTIONS OF THE URINARY SYSTEM AND RELATED DISORDERS

As the urinary system drains to the outside of the body, infection can easily spread to the bladder or kidneys.

Urinary Tract Infection

UTI occurs more often in females than in males at a rate of about 8% to 2% (Lum, 2008). Pathogens appear to enter the urinary tract most often as an ascending infection from the perineum. Most urinary pathogens are gram-negative rods. *E. coli* is a frequent offender. UTIs also are a common cause of nosocomial or health care–acquired infections in children with urinary catheters.

UTIs tend to occur more often in girls than in boys because the urethra is shorter in girls and because it is located close to the vagina (allowing the spread of vulvovaginitis) and close to the anus, from which *E. coli* spread. Changing diapers frequently can help reduce the risk for infection in infants. Girls should be taught early (when they are toilet-trained) to wipe themselves from front to back after voiding and defecating to avoid contaminating the urethra. There is a suggested correlation between the use of products such as bubble bath, feminine hygiene sprays, and hot tubs and UTI in girls so use of these should be discouraged or minimized (Schilling McCann et al., 2007). Infection also often occurs after sexual intercourse. Teach both adolescent males and females to void after sexual intercourse. Additional measures to prevent UTIs are summarized in Box 46.3.

UTIs need vigorous treatment in childhood so they do not spread to involve the kidneys (pyelonephritis). Girls who have more than three UTIs or boys with their first UTI should be referred to a urologist to determine whether they have a congenital anomaly such as urethral stenosis or bladder–ureter reflux that causes recurrent urinary stasis. A secondary problem is more likely in boys with a UTI.

BOX 46.3 ✻ Focus on Family Teaching

Preventing Urinary Tract Infection (UTI) in Females

Q. Carol's grandmother tells you, "Carol had a urinary tract infection last year. How can we prevent that from happening again?"

A. Here are some important tips to help prevent UTI:

- Encourage your granddaughter to drink periodically during the day, especially in warm weather or during exercise, to keep urine flowing freely and prevent stasis of urine in ureters.
- Urge her to urinate at least every 4 hours to prevent stasis of urine in the bladder.
- Teach her not to bathe with bubble bath; this can cause vulvar and urethral irritation.
- Help your granddaughter learn to wipe from front to back after moving her bowels or urinating, to prevent moving rectal contamination forward to the urethra.
- Have your granddaughter wear cotton, not synthetic, underwear to decrease perineal irritation.
- Instruct your granddaughter to wash her vulva daily to lower the bacterial count on the perineum.
- When your granddaughter begins menstruating, encourage her to change sanitary pads at least every 4 hours to reduce the possible growth of bacteria near the urethra.
- If symptoms of UTI should occur (pain on urination, frequency, blood in urine), call your primary health care provider. If an antibiotic is prescribed, make sure that your granddaughter takes it for the full prescribed course, so all bacteria are completely eradicated. Otherwise, after a short time, bacteria will proliferate, and the infection will recur.
- When your granddaughter becomes sexually active, teach her to urinate immediately after intercourse to remove any bacteria forced into the urethra by pressure.

Assessment

Although it may be possible to locate a UTI precisely as urethritis, cystitis, ureteritis, or pyelonephritis, the signs and symptoms in young children often are not clear-cut. When the exact location or extent of the infection is unknown, it is referred to simply as a UTI. The typical symptoms that occur in older children or in adults—pain on urination, frequency, burning, and hematuria—may not be present. If the infection is confined to the bladder (cystitis), the child may have a low-grade fever, mild abdominal pain, and enuresis (bedwetting). If the infection is a pyelonephritis, the symptoms generally are more acute, with high fever, abdominal or flank pain, vomiting, and malaise. Any child with a fever and no demonstrable cause on physical examination should be evaluated for UTI (Wan, Liu, & Chen, 2007).

Urine for culture can be collected by a clean-catch technique, suprapubic aspiration, or catheterization, so that bacteria from the vulva or foreskin do not contaminate the sample and give a false reading. Suprapubic aspiration is generally limited to infants because the sight of the syringe is so frightening to older children; plus, the procedure can introduce infection. The use of catheterization, also frightening and a potential source of infection, is limited in children of all ages.

Urine obtained from suprapubic aspiration is generally sterile, so any growth from this source is significant. A clean-catch urine specimen is said to be positive for bacteriuria if the bacterial colony count is more than 100,000/mL. A count of less than 10,000/mL is considered a negative culture. Counts between 10,000 and 100,000/mL are repeated. Usually, the urine also is positive for proteinuria (because of the presence of bacteria). Microscopic examination may indicate the presence of red blood cells (hematuria) because of mucosal irritation. The presence of red or white blood cells and bacteria tends to make urine more alkaline, so the pH will be elevated (greater than 7).

Therapeutic Management

The medical treatment for UTI is the oral administration of an antibiotic specific to the causative organism that is cultured (Lum, 2008).

In addition to the antibiotic, a child needs to drink a large quantity of fluid to "flush" the infection out of the urinary tract. Cranberry juice is often recommended as being highly effective in acidifying urine and making it more resistant to bacterial growth. In actual practice, there is little proof of its effectiveness, so offer any fluid the child drinks readily. If the child experiences moderate to severe pain on urination that interferes with the ability to void, suggest that the child sit in a bathtub of warm water and void into the water. A mild analgesic, such as acetaminophen (Tylenol), may help reduce pain enough to allow voiding.

With a UTI, treatment with antibiotics must be continued for the full prescription or the infection will return. Create a reminder sheet for parents to post in a readily visible location, such as on the refrigerator door, to help ensure adherence. A repeat clean-catch urine sample is usually obtained at 72 hours to assess the effectiveness of the antibiotic treatment.

After antibiotic therapy is stopped, it is helpful if parents obtain another clean catch urine specimen to be tested to prove that bacteria are not still present. After recurrent UTIs, children may be prescribed a prophylactic antibiotic for 6 months. At periodic health checkups for the next few years, a child should void a clean-catch specimen for culture or microscopic analysis.

"Honeymoon" Cystitis

Honeymoon cystitis refers to lower UTI seen in young women shortly after they initiate a first sexual relationship. Such infections occur in connection with the local irritation and inflammation caused by initial coitus.

Like most UTIs, these respond quickly to antibiotic therapy. Voiding as soon as possible after coitus may help to flush pathogenic organisms from the urethra and prevent such infections. When cystitis is seen in adolescent girls, it should alert health care providers to the possibility that a girl may be sexually active. In addition to needing counseling about personal hygiene measures to prevent UTI, the girl may need information on sexually transmitted infections, reproductive planning, and her responsibility for her maturing body. Recurrent UTIs in a school-age or preschool girl may suggest sexual abuse.

Vesicoureteral Reflux

Normally, urine flows from the ureters into the bladder, with almost no flow re-entering the ureters from the bladder. This is because the ureters enter the bladder obliquely, and a bladder skin flap or "valve" obscures the end of the ureter, preventing backflow. **Vesicoureteral reflux** refers to retrograde flow of urine from the bladder into the ureters (Watnick & Morrison, 2009). This reflux occurs because the valve that guards the entrance from the bladder to the ureter is defective, either from birth or because of scarring from repeated UTIs, bladder pressure that is stronger than usual, or ureters that are implanted at abnormal sites or angles. This backflow of urine happens at micturition (voiding) when the bladder contracts (Fig. 46.10).

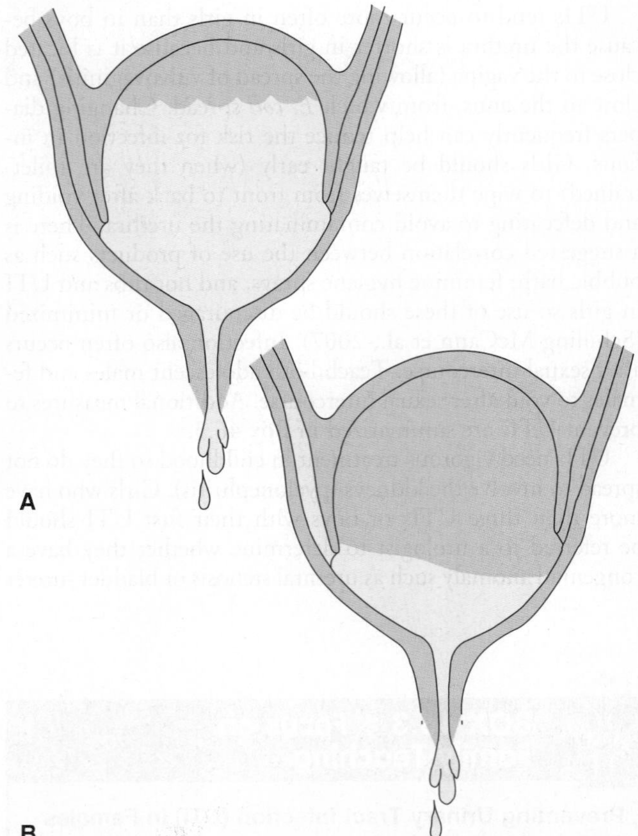

FIGURE 46.10 Vesicoureteral reflux. (**A**) Normal voiding pattern. (**B**) Reflux into ureters with voiding.

Reflux leads to bladder infection because urine is retained in the ureters after voiding, and stasis of any fluid is subject to infection. It also appears that the capacity for normal bladder tissue to lyse bacteria becomes reduced due to the large residual urine volume that is always present. In addition, reflux is a potentially serious condition because it can lead to back-pressure on the kidneys, possibly leading to nephron destruction and, subsequently, hydronephrosis or dilatation of the renal pelvis. As it is prone to appear in families, it is most likely a heterogeneous disorder (Kelly et al., 2007).

Assessment

A child with reflux is usually first seen by health care personnel because of a history of repeated UTI. A voiding cystourethrogram, CT scan, cystoscopy, or cystography with contrast material will show the ureteral reflux. Based on diagnostic studies, reflux is graded from I to V by degree of reflux, with V being the most serious.

Therapeutic Management

The majority of instances of vesicoureteral reflux resolve with maturity without a need for surgery. Until this normal growth occurs, however, the condition must be rigorously treated to decrease the possibility of glomerular scarring from infection or back-pressure. Teaching double voiding (having the child void, then in a few minutes attempt to void again) may help to empty the bladder and prevent recurrent infection from urinary stasis. Some girls need to remain on prophylactic antibiotics to prevent bladder infection. Long-term maintenance with antibiotics may be as effective as surgery in reducing renal scarring from recurrent urinary tract infection in lower grades of reflux (Hensle, Grogg, & Eaddy, 2007).

If continuous antibiotic therapy does not prevent recurrent UTIs, reflux can be corrected by cystoscopy. Under general anesthesia or conscious sedation, a cystoscope is passed, and an agent such as Deflux (dextranomer–hyaluronic acid) is injected to stabilize the ureter valves (Sutherland et al., 2007). Laparoscopic surgery to correct the placement of ureters may be scheduled to reinsert the ureters at a more oblique angle, creating the usual valve effect.

After surgery, a suprapubic catheter remains in place to keep the bladder empty and prevent pressure against the surgical area. Two ureteral catheters (stents), threaded into the ureters to drain urine directly from the kidney pelvis, also exit at the suprapubic tube site. Tubes are attached as a closed drainage system to collecting bags. Sterile gauze dressings and antibiotic cream are placed around the tube insertion sites.

In preparing children for this type of surgery, be certain to prepare them for the number of tubes that will be inserted. Explain that even with the tubes in place, the child will be allowed to walk and move about soon after the operation (and should do this). Be sure that the child and parents understand the importance of keeping the urine collection bags below the level of the child's bladder to prevent urine from flowing back into the bladder. Caution them not to raise the bags above the child's bladder level when helping the child out of bed.

Observe the catheter drainage tubes closely, every hour for the first 24 hours and then at least every 4 hours. Note the color and the amount of drainage (urine), and carefully measure and record it. Initially, drainage will be bloody, but this should clear in 1 or 2 days. Assess drainage for clots (should not be over pinpoint in size). The stents should drain an equal amount, to ensure that kidney production is equal on both sides. Urine will drain primarily from the stents for approximately the first 3 days after surgery; thereafter, drainage will flow around the stents and will be mainly from the suprapubic tube.

Be sure that the ends of the catheters do not become contaminated, because then infection can spread to the surgical area or the kidneys. An antiseptic solution may be ordered placed in the drainage bags to limit the growth of bacteria in the collecting urine. Be certain any amount added is subtracted from the output amount. As soon as urine drainage from the stent catheters has decreased and blood has cleared, the stent catheters will be removed. To show that urine is clearing of blood, obtain serial urine specimens each time collecting bags are emptied and label it with the time of removal. Comparing the color of these samples will show that urine is clearing of blood. School-age children can help label the containers, which can help to add to their sense of accomplishment and control over the situation. Many children become frightened when they learn the stent catheters will be removed. Assure them that this will not be painful and can be done at an ambulatory visit without anesthesia.

Incisional pain and painful bladder spasms may occur for the first 3 days after surgery, so antispasmodics may be prescribed to reduce bladder spasm. Also, not touching or not moving the suprapubic tube helps to reduce spasms because this limits bladder irritation. The suprapubic tube is removed between 4 and 7 days after surgery (again, a nearly painless procedure). There may be slight urine leakage from the puncture site of the tube for 1 or 2 days after removal of the tube. Keep a sterile dressing in place to absorb the leaking urine. Remind the child and parents to avoid tub baths until the suprapubic tube site has closed completely.

A few children continue to have bladder reflux after ureter reimplantation. All children need follow-up care such as repeated urine cultures or perhaps an IVP or ultrasound at a later date to establish that surgery was effective in halting the reflux.

Hydronephrosis

Hydronephrosis is enlargement of the pelvis of the kidney with urine as a result of back-pressure in the ureter (Watnick & Morrison, 2009). The back-pressure is generally caused by obstruction, either of the ureter or of the point where the ureter joins the bladder, as with vesicoureteral reflux. Although this may occur at any age, it occurs most often in the first 6 months of life. If it occurs during intrauterine life, it will be revealed by fetal ultrasound (Hubert & Palmer, 2007).

Children with hydronephrosis are usually asymptomatic. They may have repeated UTIs from urinary stasis (difficult to detect in a child this age except as general irritability or crying on voiding). Elevated blood pressure caused by increasing tubular pressure (which activates the renin-angiotensin system) may be detected on a routine health assessment, although blood pressure is not taken routinely in a child of this age. With severe back-pressure, the infant experiences flank or abdominal pain. Abdominal palpation may reveal an abdominal mass (the dilated kidney pelvis). An IVP or ultrasound will show the enlarged pelvis and the point of obstruction.

Hydronephrosis is a serious disorder because, if the pressure in the pelvis becomes too acute, back-pressure on the kidney will interfere with tubular function or destroy the nephrons. The treatment is surgical correction of the obstruction before glomerular or tubular destruction occurs.

DISORDERS AFFECTING NORMAL URINARY ELIMINATION

Interferences with urine elimination can arise from innocent conditions such as enuresis or extremely serious disorders such as kidney agenesis.

Enuresis

Enuresis is involuntary passage of urine past the age when a child should be expected to have attained bladder control (Weaver & Dobson, 2007). Because this is expected at age 2 to 3 years of age for daytime and age 4 years for nighttime, enuresis is said to occur at approximately 5 to 7 years. Enuresis may be nocturnal (occurs only at night), diurnal (occurs during the day), or both. It is primary if bladder training was never achieved, acquired or secondary if control was established but has now been lost.

Most enuresis is nocturnal; daytime enuresis occurs only rarely, except during naptime. Functional nocturnal enuresis (that with no known cause) occurs in approximately 8% to 12% of children age 8 years or younger. It is found more frequently in boys than in girls. It also tends to be familial (if it is present in a child, one of the parents probably experienced it, too).

Assessment

Children with enuresis who are older than 5 years of age need an evaluation to determine whether there is an organic cause for the disorder. During the history, ask how parents have tried to correct the problem; identify whether it is primarily a problem for the child or the parents (treatment will be most effective if the child wants the situation corrected). Assess whether there are stresses in the family, such as parents who expect more mature behavior of a child than the child can handle such as the introduction of a new brother or sister, an uncomfortable school situation such as being assigned to a "shouting" teacher, or marital discord.

If they wet only on nights when they are exceptionally tired or troubled, a functional rather than an organic cause is suggested. If children wet only when they are engrossed in an interesting activity, they may simply need more reminders to empty their bladder. If children have symptoms other than bedwetting, such as abdominal pain, burning, or frequency, UTI is suggested. It is a common practice for many parents to get children out of bed every night and take them to the bathroom. At any point parents stop this practice, children may begin bedwetting because they have been conditioned to empty their bladder at that time of night.

Some children with enuresis have abnormal electroencephalographic patterns. Other children with the same abnormal patterns do not have enuresis, however, so this by itself is not a sufficiently specific finding to be helpful. In others, bedwetting seems to occur as children pass from a period of rapid eye movement sleep pattern to a type IV level, or it is primarily a sleep disorder. It may be associated with small bladder capacity (which would explain why the condition is familial).

Although usually not necessary to aid diagnosis, an IVP, VCUG, or ultrasound may be done to rule out organic disease. A clean-catch urine specimen should be collected to rule out bacteriuria. Specific gravity is assessed to rule out a defect in urine concentration. Protein and glucose levels are evaluated to determine evidence of kidney disease.

Therapeutic Management

The treatment of enuresis may be complex because the cause is generally unknown. If stress factors have been identified, an attempt should be made to correct these. Some stress factors, such as birth of a new sibling, cannot be changed, but frank discussion with children regarding what causes the stress and attempts to help children cope better with their daytime activities may improve enuresis (Box 46.4).

In many children, it helps to limit fluids after dinner. Urge parents to exercise common sense in this area. Remind them that a child may not be able to go every night without a drink from dinner until breakfast. Caution parents of children with sickle-cell anemia not to restrict fluid this way because increased sickling of cells occurs with dehydration.

BOX 46.4 ✻ Focus on Evidence-Based Practice

Does bedwetting (nocturnal enuresis) affect the quality of life of families?

For this study, 28 women who reported that their child had nocturnal enuresis and 38 women whose child had no urinary symptoms were asked to fill in three separate questionnaires: one on general health, one on risk of depression, and one on risk of anxiety. Results of the inventories showed that the mothers of children with nocturnal enuresis had significantly lower quality-of-life scores related to bodily pain and emotional well-being than did mothers whose child was symptom-free. They also scored significantly higher on a depression scale.

Suppose a parent tells you that her child has nocturnal enuresis but she knows it is only a stage of growth so she is not worried. Based on the above study, would you ask any further questions?

Source: Egemen, A., et al. (2008). An evaluation of quality of life of mothers of children with enuresis nocturna. *Pediatric Nephrology, 23*(1), 93–98.

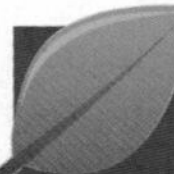

BOX 46.5 ✻ Focus on Pharmacology

Desmopressin acetate (DDAVP)

Classification: A synthetic form of human antidiuretic hormone

Action: Promotes resorption of water in the renal tubule or decreases bladder filling; drug of choice for enuresis (Karch, 2009)

Pregnancy Risk Category: B

Dosage: In children 6 years of age and older, 20 μg (0.2 mL) intranasally at bedtime, possibly increasing the dose up to 40 μg if necessary; or 0.2 mg orally at bedtime, titrated up to 0.6 mg to obtain the desired response

Possible Adverse Effects: Transient headache, nausea, flushing, mild abdominal cramps, fluid retention

Nursing Implications

- Instruct parents and child that child should restrict fluid after dinnertime in addition to taking medication.
- If given intranasally, advise parents to refrigerate the solution.
- Teach parents and child the proper method for intranasal administration.
- Caution child and parents that nasal administration is less effective if the child develops a cold with draining rhinitis.

Alarm bells that ring when children wet at night are effective in some children. This type of system does not actually stop bedwetting. The alarm wakes the child, the child stops voiding, and then gets up and uses the bathroom. Over time, this type of conditioning may be effective, but once the urine alarm is removed, children may relapse. Bladder-stretching exercises—drinking a large quantity of water and then refraining from voiding as long as possible—to increase the functional size of the bladder can be helpful in some children. A bladder that can hold 300 to 350 mL of fluid will generally be large enough to contain urine during a night's sleep.

If these measures are not effective, synthetic antidiuretic hormone (ADH; desmopressin [DDAVP]) administered intranasally or orally is the drug of choice to reduce urinary output and enuresis (Glazener, Evans, & Peto, 2009; Box 46.5).

Enuresis is not a minor problem for either parents or for the child. As a general measure, children who wet their beds need to take baths in the morning rather than at bedtime to minimize urine odor and avoid teasing. Parents may find planning a vacation with hotel stays difficult. They may resent the daily linen washing. Children may exclude themselves from activities such as slumber parties or camping trips with friends to avoid embarrassment.

Enuresis may occur in hospitalized children because of the stress of their new surroundings. Preschool children may experience it because they are uncomfortable using strange bathrooms or do not understand which bathroom is theirs to use. As a rule, place as little stress or importance on enuresis as possible during an illness, and encourage parents to do the same.

Postural (Orthostatic) Proteinuria

A few children will spill albumin into the urine when they stand upright for an extended period (**postural proteinuria,** also called postural albuminuria). The amount of spilling decreases when they rest in a supine position. Children with this condition have no apparent damage to glomeruli; the phenomenon is apparently attributable to the effect of gravity on glomerular function.

To determine whether postural proteinuria exists, urine is collected after the child has been recumbent during the night (a first-voided specimen) and then again after the child has been up and active for several hours. Make certain when collecting these urine specimens to record the child's activity accurately. If the child stood by the crib rail crying for a parent or was held in a nurse's lap for most of the night, the urine may show protein in the morning specimen because it is not truly a "resting specimen." Likewise, for the specimen to be collected after the child has been active, make certain that the child is up and active, not lying in a supine position reading a book for most of the time. Play a game if necessary, such as follow the leader, so the child is active.

Postural proteinuria needs no therapy. However, be sure to document the condition because some of these children develop some form of kidney disorder later in life.

Kidney Agenesis

Agenesis means lack of growth (literally, lack of a beginning) or that no organ formed in utero. Absence of kidneys in a newborn is suggested when the volume of amniotic fluid on ultrasound or at birth is less than normal (oligohydramnios). This occurs because urine normally adds to the volume of amniotic fluid in utero. The infant with kidney agenesis often has *Potter's syndrome* or accompanying misshapen, low-set ears and hypoplastic (stiff, inflexible) lungs from the lack of amniotic fluid in utero. Without kidneys, the fetus cannot void urine. Bilateral absence of kidneys this way is obviously incompatible with life unless a renal transplantation can be accomplished, but the associated condition of nonfunctioning lungs makes a successful transplantation highly unlikely.

Polycystic Kidney

Polycystic kidney means that large, fluid-filled cysts have formed in place of normal kidney tissue. The most frequent type of polycystic kidney seen in children is inherited as an autosomal recessive trait. A more rare form is inherited as an autosomal dominant trait (Boyer et al., 2007). With either type, there is abnormal development of the collecting tubules. The kidneys are large and feel soft and spongy. If the disorder is bilateral, an infant will not pass urine. The mother will have had oligohydramnios during pregnancy. Children often have a typical appearance (*hypertelorism*—wide-spaced eyes, epicanthal folds, flattened nose; or *micrognathia*—small jaw), the findings of Potter's syndrome. Either *transillumination* or *ultrasound* will show the fluid-filled cysts.

If the condition is unilateral, urine production will be decreased (oliguria), not absent. Because kidneys are difficult to locate in newborns, a unilateral polycystic kidney may be missed until later in life, when, with increased kidney growth, an abdominal mass can be palpated. The cystic growth offers such resistance to blood circulation that systemic hypertension often results by school age.

In many children, the liver is filled with identical cysts. This is most evident later in life when increased difficulty with portal circulation occurs (blood cannot perfuse the cystic liver structures either).

The treatment for polycystic formation is surgical removal of a kidney if only one is cystic. If both kidneys are cystic, treatment is renal transplantation (difficult in the young child, because few infant kidneys are available for transplantation and because of the technical challenge presented by such small blood vessels).

Because this kidney disease is inherited, parents, and children at adolescence, need genetic counseling to inform them that future children may also have this problem.

Renal Hypoplasia

Hypoplasia means reduced growth. Hypoplastic kidneys contain fewer lobes than normal kidneys and are small and underdeveloped. The child with hypoplastic kidneys, in addition to having poor kidney function, may develop hypertension from stenosis of the renal arteries. If hypoplasia is bilateral, the child may need a kidney transplant in later life to maintain kidney function and prevent extreme hypertension.

Prune Belly Syndrome

Prune belly syndrome is severe urinary tract dilation that develops as early as intrauterine life from an unknown cause. Occurring mainly in boys, the severe dilation causes backpressure and destruction of kidneys. The infant is born with oligohydramnios and pulmonary dysplasia because of the lack of amniotic fluid in utero (Woods & Brandon, 2007).

The condition is marked by the presence of three symptoms: deficiency of usual abdominal muscle tone, bilateral undescended testes, and the dilated faulty development of the bladder and upper urinary tract. The infant's abdomen appears wrinkled (like a prune) because of the poorly developed abdominal muscles (Fig. 46.11). Without surgical remodeling, the infant will develop repeated UTIs, leading eventually to end-stage renal disease. Teach parents to protect their child's abdomen from trauma such as can happen from lap belts or baby walkers because their child lacks abdominal support. Some children need kidney transplants as

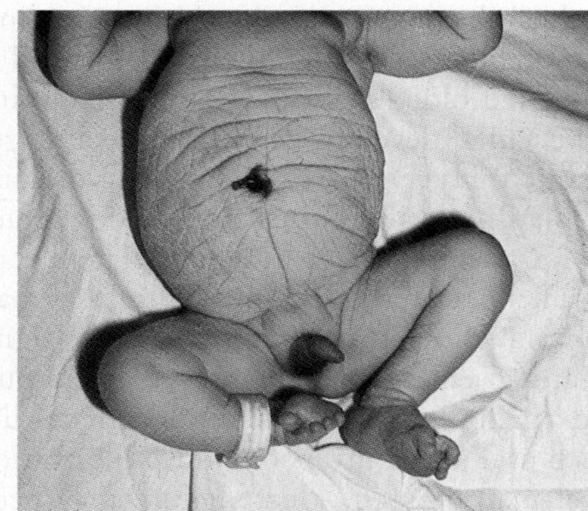

FIGURE 46.11 Prune belly syndrome. (Courtesy of Karen M. Polise, MSN, RN, Division of Nephrology, The Children's Hospital of Philadelphia.)

they reach school age because of destruction of glomeruli from back-pressure (Kamel et al., 2007).

Acute Poststreptococcal Glomerulonephritis

Glomerulonephritis, inflammation of the glomeruli of the kidney, may occur as a separate entity but usually occurs as an immune complex disease after infection with nephritogenic streptococci (most commonly subtypes of group A beta-hemolytic streptococci). Tissue damage occurs from a complement fixation reaction in the glomeruli (*complement* is a cascade of proteins activated by antigen–antibody reactions and actually plugs or obstructs glomeruli). IgG antibodies against streptococci may be detected in the bloodstream of children with acute glomerulonephritis, proof that the illness follows a streptococcal infection (Sinha et al., 2007).

Intravascular coagulation occurs in the minute renal vessels. Ischemic damage leads to scarring and decreased glomerular function. This results in a reduction in the glomerular filtration rate, leading to an accumulation of sodium and water in the bloodstream. Inflammation of the glomeruli increases permeability, allowing protein molecules to escape into the filtrate.

Assessment

Acute glomerulonephritis is most common in children between the ages of 5 and 10 years, the age group most susceptible to streptococcal infections. Boys appear to develop the disease more often than girls; it occurs more often during the winter and spring, as do pharyngeal streptococcal infections. The child typically has a history of a recent respiratory infection (within 7 to 14 days) or impetigo (within 3 weeks). All children who have had a "strep" throat, tonsillitis, otitis media, or impetigo caused by streptococcal infection, ideally, should have a urinalysis 2 weeks after the infection to evaluate that glomerulonephritis is not occurring. Many children do not receive this follow-up step, however, because of lack of health insurance coverage or compliance.

Acute glomerulonephritis is characterized by a sudden onset of hematuria and proteinuria. The protein content both of individual urine specimens and of total 24-hour urine volume is measured. Testing a single specimen will show 1+ to 4+ protein; a 24-hour urine specimen may contain as much as 1 g protein (normally, urine contains none).

The hematuria associated with acute glomerulonephritis is usually so gross that the child's urine appears tea-colored, reddish-brown, or smoky. Urinary sediment will contain white blood cells, epithelial cells, and hyaline, granular, and red blood cell casts. After these initial urine changes, the child develops oliguria. Specific gravity of urine is elevated. Hypertension from hypervolemia occurs. The child may have abdominal pain, a low-grade fever, edema, anorexia, vomiting, or headache. There may be cardiac involvement related to the difficulty in managing the excessive plasma fluid. Such children show signs of orthopnea, cardiac enlargement, enlarged liver, pulmonary edema, and a galloping heart rhythm. Electrocardiographic changes such as T-wave inversion and prolongation of the P-R interval may be seen. Heart failure may occur from circulatory overload.

Blood analysis will indicate a lowered blood protein level (hypoalbuminemia) caused by the massive proteinuria. Low serum complement will be present, and, as the blood volume expands, a mild anemia also will occur. As in all inflammatory diseases, the erythrocyte sedimentation rate will increase. Because the glomeruli cannot filter properly, concentrations of urea, nonprotein nitrogen (BUN), and creatinine in blood will increase. The antistreptolysin O (anti–DNase B) titer or antibody formation against streptococci is generally elevated.

If blood pressure reaches 160/100 mm Hg as part of the acute process, encephalopathy may occur, with symptoms of headache, irritability, seizures, vomiting, coma or lethargy, and perhaps transitory paralysis. This extreme elevation in blood pressure is probably related to the expanded circulatory volume. The cerebral symptoms are caused by *cerebral ischemia* (vasoconstriction of cerebral vessels to reduce cranial pressure).

Therapeutic Management

The course of acute glomerulonephritis is 1 to 2 weeks. During this time, there is little therapy specific for the disorder. Antibiotics usually are ineffective because the disease is caused not by an active infection but by an antigen–antibody inflammatory response to a past infection. Diuretics are of little value because obstructed glomeruli bases cannot be made to function; a course of ethacrynic acid or furosemide (Lasix) may be tried. If heart failure occurs, specific measures such as placing the child in a semi-Fowler's position, digitalization, and oxygen administration may be necessary. If diastolic blood pressure rises to more than 90 mm Hg, antihypertensive therapy with a calcium channel blocker may be necessary. Phosphate binders, such as aluminum hydroxide to reduce phosphate absorption in the GI tract, or a potassium-removing resin agent, such as sodium polystyrene sulfonate (Kayexalate), may be necessary in children who have rising phosphate and potassium levels.

Bedrest is unnecessary, although children should be encouraged to participate in quiet play activities. They can attend school and engage in normal activities after 1 or 2 weeks, but competitive activity is limited until kidney function has returned to normal to avoid overstressing the kidneys.

Diet is controversial. Although limiting protein intake reduces the amount of protein lost in urine, many children who are losing large quantities of protein need high-protein diets to supplement this loss. Salt restriction may be needed to reduce severe edema. Most children do well on a normal diet for their age, however, with normal salt and protein content. Weighing the child every day and calculating intake and output are important assessments in following the course of the disease.

In most children, acute glomerulonephritis runs a limited, benign course. After most symptoms fade, proteinuria and impaired clearance of urea and creatinine may remain for as long as 2 months, however. Caution parents that the results of a urine protein test may remain abnormal for up to a year; caution them that, if their child has this test as a routine screening procedure at a health checkup, they should not worry that this finding means reinfection or the beginning of further disease.

A few children will not completely recover from acute glomerulonephritis but will develop chronic nephritis. These children appear to suffer destruction from the initial inflammation that results in chronic renal insufficiency.

Nursing Diagnoses and Related Interventions

Nursing Diagnosis: Situational low self-esteem, related to feelings of responsibility for onset of serious illness

Outcome Evaluation: Child (parent) admits guilt about inadequate treatment of initial infection; discusses plans and ways to maintain health; participates in care.

Glomerulonephritis is a frightening disease for both children and their parents. Children may be frightened by the initial hematuria. They may be upset at the appearance of periorbital edema, which makes their reflection in the mirror so strange to them. Children as young as early school age are aware that kidneys are necessary for life, and this means they recognize the seriousness of kidney disease.

If children were prescribed penicillin for pharyngitis 2 weeks before the development of the nephritis but refused to take it, they may believe that they caused this disease. The parents may feel guilty because they did not insist the child take the medicine. They worry that their child will develop chronic glomerulonephritis or die during the acute phase of this attack. These parents and children need to talk about their feelings openly. Provide frequent reports of subtle positive changes in a child's condition such as "His blood pressure is staying down by itself now; he does not need medicine for that anymore." "He weighs 2 pounds less today than 4 days ago; that generally means his kidneys are beginning to function more efficiently again."

Be certain that parents know the date and place of a return visit for follow-up care. Because this is a perplexing disease, be sure they have a telephone number to call if they have questions about their child's care or condition.

The most frequent type of acute glomerulonephritis can be avoided by the prevention or effective early treatment of group A beta-hemolytic streptococcal infections. Acute glomerulonephritis tends not to recur with subsequent streptococcal infections, so prophylactic penicillin to prevent further streptococcal infections is unnecessary.

IGA Glomerulonephritis

Acute glomerulonephritis may occur when there is no evidence of a prior infection (Watnick & Morrison, 2009). In these children, immunoglobin A is elevated. The gross hematuria resolves within a few days and is not apt to produce serious sequelae. Because of the benign course of the illness, no therapy is indicated except for careful observation for more serious signs such as severe proteinuria, hypertension, or renal insufficiency. If these symptoms occur, corticosteroids will halt the disease process. Omega-3 fatty acids present in fish oils may be prescribed but their use is not well established.

✔ Checkpoint Question 46.3

What is typically the first symptom of acute glomerulonephritis?

a. Low blood pressure from excessive aldosterone
b. "Old blood" in urine from kidney bleeding
c. Dependent edema from protein accumulation
d. Pain on urination from urethra inflammation

Chronic Glomerulonephritis

Although chronic glomerulonephritis occasionally follows acute glomerulonephritis or nephrotic syndrome, it also occurs as a primary disease (or after acute glomerulonephritis that was clinically so mild it was undiagnosed). The child is found to have proteinuria at a routine checkup. Further investigation may indicate hypertension and the presence of red cell or white cell casts and occult blood in urine. The specific gravity of the child's urine is below normal (below 1.003). Blood studies may indicate an increased BUN or creatinine level. A renal biopsy will show permanent destruction of glomeruli membranes.

Chronic glomerulonephritis may result in either diffuse or local nephron damage. The remaining functioning nephrons increase their glomerular filtration rate to compensate for those that are damaged. At some point in this chronic disease destruction process, however, compensatory mechanisms fail, and renal insufficiency or failure will result. **Alport's syndrome** that also includes hearing loss and ocular changes is a progressive chronic glomerulonephritis inherited as a X-linked or autosomal recessive disorder (Shaw et al., 2007).

During the illness, if the child has acute symptoms of edema, hematuria, hypertension, or oliguria, bedrest may be necessary. If children have only a chronic manifestation, such as proteinuria, and if they feel well, they can maintain normal activity, including attending school. Children should not engage in competitive activities such as contact sports, however, because of the risk of kidney injury.

Therapy is nonspecific and directed at symptom relief rather than the disease process itself, because the cause of the disease is unknown. Therapy with antihypertensive drugs such as hydralazine (Apresoline) or with diuretics to increase urine output such as ethacrynic acid (Edecrin) may be necessary. Corticosteroid therapy may reduce or halt the progress of the disorder by reducing inflammation. Children have difficulty accepting long-term corticosteroid therapy because of the side effects, in particular a typical "moon face" and extra body hair (Cushing's syndrome). Talk with them about these body changes and assure them that these changes will reverse when the drug is discontinued.

Children receiving corticosteroids are at an increased risk for infection because of the immunosuppressive activity of these drugs. They need to be shielded from other children and health care personnel with infection. Parents need to learn to take their child's temperature and recognize and report the earliest signs of infection.

Generally, the prognosis for children with chronic glomerulonephritis is poor. Although the illness may run a long-term course, eventually it leads to renal insufficiency and renal failure. Children may be maintained for long periods by peritoneal dialysis or hemodialysis. Kidney transplantation is a possibility.

Because children as young as early school age are aware of the importance of kidney function to life, most children with chronic renal disease are aware of the likely outcome of their disease. Most children are adolescents or young adults before the disease runs its ultimate course. They indicate that they appreciate having health care personnel face this outcome with them honestly if kidney transplantation cannot be performed to prolong their life.

Nephrotic Syndrome (Nephrosis)

Nephrosis, altered glomerular permeability due to fusion of the glomeruli membrane surfaces, causes abnormal loss of protein in urine. Immunologic mechanisms are involved in instigating the process. The cause may be hypersensitivity to an antigen–antibody reaction or an autoimmune process. A T-lymphocyte dysfunction may be responsible. The highest incidence is at 3 years of age, and it occurs more often in boys than in girls (Lum, 2008).

Nephrotic syndrome in children occurs in three forms: (a) congenital, which occurs as an autosomal recessive disorder; (b) secondary, as a progression of glomerulonephritis or in connection with systemic diseases such as sickle cell anemia or systemic lupus erythematosus (SLE); or (c) idiopathic (primary). The congenital form is rare; in children, the idiopathic form is most common (Tkaczyk et al., 2008).

Nephrosis can be further classified according to the amount of membrane destruction. Minimal change nephrotic syndrome (MCNS) is the type most often seen in children (80%). As the name implies, with this type, little scarring of glomeruli occurs. Children with this degree of scarring respond well to therapy. Other types are focal glomerulosclerosis (FGS) and membranoproliferative glomerulonephritis (MPGN). Both of these types involve scarring of glomeruli, and these children will have a poorer response to therapy (Lu et al., 2007).

The four characteristic symptoms of nephrotic syndrome are proteinuria, edema, hypoalbuminemia (low serum albumin level), and hyperlipidemia (increased blood lipid level). Proteinuria occurs because increased glomerular permeability leads to protein loss in the urine and, subsequently, hypoalbuminemia. With a low level of protein in the bloodstream, osmotic pressure causes fluid to shift from the bloodstream into interstitial tissue, causing edema. As the blood volume decreases, the kidneys begin to conserve sodium and water, adding to the potential for edema. The hyperlipidemia occurs because the liver increases production of lipoproteins to try to compensate for protein loss. Lipids are too large to be lost in urine, so they rise to high levels in the blood serum. Some children have such high lipid levels that, when blood is drawn and placed into a test tube, a circle of white fat forms on the top of it. Figure 46.12 illustrates the process that leads to these common symptoms.

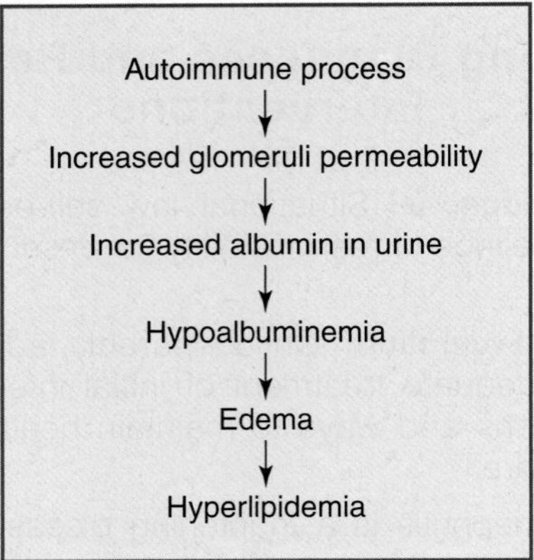

FIGURE 46.12 The process that results in the signs and symptoms of nephrotic syndrome.

Assessment

Symptoms usually begin insidiously. Children develop edema around the eyes (periorbital edema), most noticeable when they wake in the morning from a head-dependent position. Parents may notice that clothing no longer fits a child around the waist, because edematous fluid is beginning to collect in the abdominal cavity (ascites). It is easy to dismiss these first symptoms as those of an upper respiratory tract infection and the normal "paunchy" belly of a toddler or preschooler. As edema progresses, the child's skin becomes pale, stretched, and taut. In boys, scrotal edema becomes extremely marked. Ascites may become so extensive that the resultant pressure on the stomach leads to anorexia or vomiting. Children may have diarrhea caused by intestinal edema and poor absorption by the edematous membrane. Because of poor nutrition, growth may stop. The child may become malnourished but yet appear deceptively obese because of the extensive edema (Fig. 46.13). When the ascites becomes even more extensive, children may have difficulty breathing as the abdominal fluid presses against the diaphragm, decreasing lung expansion. Parents report that children are irritable and fussy, probably from the feeling of abdominal fullness and generalized edema. An increased risk for clotting can occur from the decreased intravascular fluid volume.

Laboratory studies will reveal marked proteinuria. A single test will show a 1+ to 4+ protein; a 24-hour total urine test will show up to 15 g protein (normally urine contains no protein). The protein loss with nephrotic syndrome is almost entirely albumin, differentiating it from the proteinuria of glomerulonephritis, in which protein loss tends to be non-

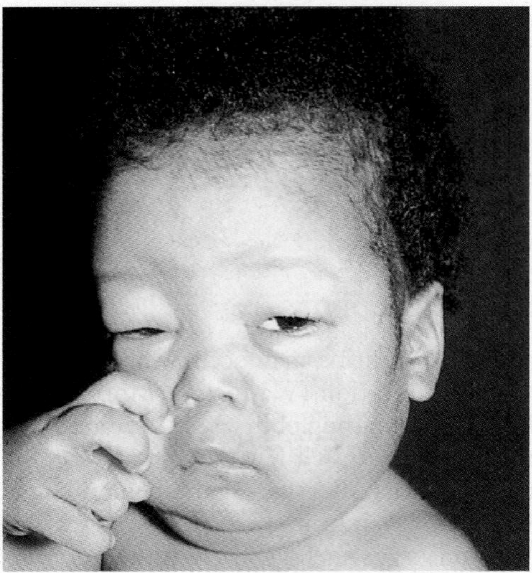

FIGURE 46.13 A 2-year-old with nephrotic syndrome. Note the extensive edema of the face and hand. (From B. J. Zitelli & H. W. Davis [1997]. *Atlas of pediatric physical diagnosis* [3rd ed.]. St. Louis: Mosby–Year Book, Inc.)

TABLE 46.5 ✻ Comparison of Features of Acute Glomerulonephritis and Nephrotic Syndrome

Factor	Acute Glomerulonephritis	Nephrotic Syndrome
Cause	Immune reaction to group A beta-hemolytic streptococcal infection	Idiopathic; possibly a hypersensitivity reaction
Onset	Abrupt	Insidious
Hematuria	Profuse	Rare
Edema	Mild	Extreme
Hypertension	Marked	Mild
Hyperlipidemia	Rare or mild	Marked
Peak age frequency	5–10 yr	2–3 yr
Interventions	Limited activity; antihypertensives as needed; symptomatic therapy for congestive heart failure	Corticosteroid administration; cyclophosphamide administration; possibly a diuretic and potassium supplement
Diet	Normal for age	High-protein, low-sodium diet
Prevention	Prevention or thorough treatment of group A beta-hemolytic streptococcal infections	None known

specific. Some children with nephrotic syndrome exhibit hematuria at the onset, but it is minimal in contrast to that seen with acute glomerulonephritis. The erythrocyte sedimentation rate (demonstrating the inflammation of the glomeruli membrane) is elevated. Features of acute glomerulonephritis and nephrotic syndrome are compared in Table 46.5. A renal biopsy may be done to determine whether there is scarring of the glomerular membrane and document the type of nephrotic syndrome present.

Therapeutic Management

Therapy for a child with nephrotic syndrome is directed toward reducing the proteinuria and subsequently the edema with a course of corticosteroids, such as IV methylprednisolone or oral prednisone, and keeping the child free of infection while the immune system is suppressed. An initial dose of prednisone is given until diuresis without protein loss is accomplished; the dosage is then reduced for maintenance and continued for as long as 1 to 2 months.

Instruct parents to test the first urine specimen of the day for protein with a chemical reagent strip and keep an accurate chart showing the pattern of protein loss. Approximately once a week, they are usually asked to collect a 24-hour urine specimen so total protein loss can be measured.

After the initial 4 weeks, prednisone is generally given every other day rather than every day. Prednisone has the potential to halt growth and to suppress adrenal gland secretion. However, growth is apparently not delayed when the drug is given on alternate days and there is less alteration of adrenal steroid production (Karch, 2009). Parents may need to be assured that alternate-day therapy is best to keep them from changing the schedule to every day or giving twice the calculated dose by adding extra tablets on alternate days. To help parents remember to give medication on alternate days, have them choose either even or odd calendar days as the day of administration. Help them design a reminder chart. Prednisone tastes bitter, so parents may welcome suggestions regarding how to disguise the taste, such as by mixing it with applesauce.

Be certain both the parents and the child are aware that prednisone causes a cushingoid appearance or a "moon face," extra fat at the base of the neck, and increased body hair. Urge parents to plan ahead when getting pharmacy refills so that the prednisone therapy is not stopped abruptly because they ran out of medication; an abrupt stop can lead to adrenal insufficiency.

Diuretics are not commonly used to reduce the edema because they tend to decrease blood volume, which is already decreased. This could lead to acute renal failure. Children who respond poorly to prednisone alone, however, may need diuretic therapy with a drug such as furosemide (Lasix). When children are taking furosemide for extended periods, there is always a danger that too much potassium will be excreted, causing hypokalemia. Children on long-term diuretic therapy usually need frequent blood studies to determine that electrolyte levels, especially potassium, are adequate. They may need supplemental potassium and should eat foods high in potassium. IV albumin may be administered to temporarily correct hypoalbuminemia. As the serum albumin level rises, fluid shifts from subcutaneous spaces into the bloodstream. Children are then administered a rapidly acting diuretic to remove the extra fluid. It is important that the diuretic be administered after the albumin infusion or the child could develop a fluid overload and, subsequently, heart failure.

Some children are prednisone resistant or do not respond to corticosteroid therapy. A course of cyclophosphamide (Cytoxan), cyclosporine (Sandimmune), or mycophenolate mofetil (CellCept), stronger immunosuppressant agents, may be effective in reducing symptoms or preventing further relapses of the disease in these children (Pena et al., 2007). It is important to ensure adequate fluid intake with these drugs to prevent bladder irritation and bleeding. Cyclophosphamide is also used in chemotherapy for malignancy (see Chapter 53). Be certain that parents are not misled into believing that their child has cancer because their child is receiving a chemotherapeutic drug.

The prognosis for children with nephrotic syndrome varies. Almost all children with MCNS respond initially to steroid therapy. Although they may have a relapse, they will then remain free of the disease. Those with FGS and MPGN types will have relapses at frequent or infrequent intervals over the next several years. Children who have frequent relapses have a relatively poorer chance of ever being free of the disorder. Many develop renal failure later. Kidney transplantation may be necessary to sustain life. All children and families need emotional support while the disease runs a long-term course.

✔ Checkpoint Question 46.4

What is an important nursing intervention for children with nephrotic syndrome?

a. Caution them not to eat salt, as salt irritates the bladder.
b. Encourage them to walk a mile daily for exercise.
c. Teach them to test their urine for proteinuria.
d. Teach them to take their temperature daily.

Nursing Diagnoses and Related Interventions

Nursing Diagnosis: Imbalanced nutrition, less than body requirements, related to poor appetite, restricted diet, and protein loss

Outcome Evaluation: Child follows normal growth curve on standard growth chart.

For children with nephrosis, a good protein intake is necessary to offset protein loss. A good potassium intake through consumption of fruits and fruit juices, particularly bananas, is necessary to maintain sufficient serum potassium levels, especially if the child is receiving a potassium-losing diuretic (Table 46.6). This may be difficult for children, however, because they have poor appetites. During acute phases of the disease, fluid or sodium may be temporarily restricted. If this is so, most children are happiest with many small glasses of fluid spaced throughout the day, rather than several large drinks. It helps to make a chart showing the amount of fluid a child is allowed each day. As fluid is given, color in a portion of the chart corresponding to the amount given. This allows the child to tell from the uncolored portion how much more fluid is allowed that day. This is easier for toddlers and preschoolers (the age group usually affected by this disease) to understand rather than talking in terms of milliliters or even glassfuls.

TABLE 46.6 ✻ Foods High in Potassium

Food Group	Examples
Fruits	Bananas, peaches, prunes, raisins, oranges, and orange juice
Vegetables	Carrots, celery, lima beans, potatoes, collards, dandelion greens, spinach
Meat	Nuts, peanuts, red meat
Dairy products	Milk, whole or skim; low-sodium milk
Miscellaneous	Salt substitutes, chocolate and cocoa, bran

Parents need to weigh children daily to detect fluid accumulation (use the same scale with the child in the same clothing at the same time of day), and they also must measure intake and output accurately. If the child is hospitalized, taking pulse rate and blood pressure every 4 hours will help detect hypovolemia from excessive fluid shifts to interstitial tissue.

Nursing Diagnosis: Risk for impaired skin integrity related to edema

Outcome Evaluation: Child's skin is intact without erythema.

The edematous skin of children with nephrotic syndrome tends to break down easily, so they need frequent position changes while in bed. Check clothing to make certain that the elastic band at the waist of pajamas or other constricting parts is not tight. Soft gauze placed between skin surfaces, especially around the scrotum, tends to prevent skin irritation and breakdown. Edematous tissue does not heal well, so breaks in the skin easily become secondarily infected. The child who is not toilet-trained needs frequent diaper changes and thorough cleaning at each change to prevent skin breakdown in the diaper area.

Generally, children are more comfortable if they sleep with their head elevated in a semi-Fowler's position rather than a supine or prone position because this reduces periorbital edema. If children sleep in a head-flat position, edema can be so severe by morning that their eyes are swollen completely shut; their tongues are also swollen, so they cannot speak. At home, parents can provide a semi-Fowler's position by placing extra pillows on the child's bed or slipping a cardboard box under the head of the mattress to raise the end of the mattress.

Because medications are poorly absorbed from edematous skin areas, intramuscular (IM) injections should be kept to a minimum. Medication should be administered orally if possible (see Focus on Nursing Care Planning, Box 46.6).

Nursing Diagnosis: Knowledge deficit related to chronic illness

Outcome Evaluation: Parents describe course and nature of nephrosis and their role in care of child at home.

Parents often need support to manage children with a chronic illness at home. They need clear instructions about their responsibilities, including keeping their child free of infection, perhaps by limiting exposure to friends, and giving prednisone or oral diuretics and a potassium supplement. Review medication instructions with parents and have them repeat the instructions. Make certain they understand where and when they are to return for a follow-up visit and make certain they have a telephone number to call if they have questions or concerns about their child's care or health.

What if... You need to give an IM injection to Carol, who has extensive dependent edema from nephrotic syndrome? Would it be best to give it in a thigh or deltoid muscle, and why?

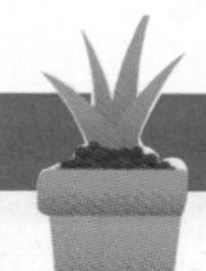

BOX 46.6 ✻ Focus on Nursing Care Planning

A Multidisciplinary Care Map for a Child With Nephrotic Syndrome

Carol is a 4-year-old girl admitted to the hospital with nephrotic syndrome. She has marked ascites and edema. "I kept asking everyone how she could be gaining so much weight, yet she doesn't eat anything," her grandmother tells you. "My daughter said this happened because Carol drank part of a beer I left on the coffee table. I didn't give her the beer; she just picked it up and drank it. Do you think that's what caused this?"

Family Assessment ✻ Child lives with grandparents in a trailer park while mother is incarcerated on a drug charge. Grandparents are both retired. Grandfather rates finances as, "Okay. I saved some money and we both get Social Security."

Client Assessment ✻ Child began "gaining weight" and becoming irritable a week ago. Yesterday, her face appeared "very puffy." Appetite has declined sharply in last 2 weeks. States she's "always full." Marked dependent edema (4+ over tibia) present. Urine tested and found to be 4+ for protein.

Nursing Diagnosis ✻ Excess fluid volume related to decreased kidney function and fluid accumulation

Outcome Criteria ✻ Child's edema decreases; urine proteinuria is less than 2+.

Team Member Responsible	Assessment	Intervention	Rationale	Expected Outcome
		Activities of Daily Living		
Nurse	Assess whether child is able to carry out routine activities with ascites or edema.	Review with grandparents advantage of allowing child to continue usual activities.	Child's mobility may interfere with physical tasks; other children may make fun of her appearance at nursery school.	Child and grandparents state that child can continue with usual activities.
		Consultations		
Physician	Assess whether grandparents have legal guardianship for child and can give permission for health care.	Contact renal service and suggest child be admitted to service for evaluation.	Nephrotic syndrome is a chronic disorder that requires conscientious, specialized health supervision.	Grandparents state they have or will obtain legal guardianship; renal service personnel meet with child and grandparents for consultation.
		Procedures/Medications		
Nurse	Assess if child has experience with oral medication.	Administer oral prednisone as prescribed.	Prednisone, a corticosteroid, reduces immune response and proteinuria.	Child accepts oral prednisone and helps make out reminder sheet.
Nurse	Assess if grandparents have experience with dipstick urine testing and 24-hour urine collection.	Observe grandparents' technique for dipstick urine testing and urine collection and recording results.	Testing for protein in urine will reveal extent of protein loss.	Grandparents state they feel able to test and collect urine conscientiously and record results in diary.
		Nutrition		
Nurse/ nutritionist	Assess child's typical food intake for last 24 hours.	Suggest grandmother monitor child's intake to be certain it includes all food groups daily.	Ascites crowds stomach, so it can give a feeling of fullness and cause undernutrition.	Child describes yesterday's intake; grandmother voices intent to supervise child's intake to be certain it is nutritious.

(continued)

BOX 46.6 * Focus on Nursing Care Planning (continued)

Patient/Family Education				
Nurse	Assess grandparents' knowledge about kidney function and kidney disease.	Teach grandparents about kidney function and disease process as needed.	Understanding disease process can help grandparents to better carry out therapy.	Grandparents state they understand why edema has occurred and describe action of medicine to reverse this.
Psychosocial/Spiritual/Emotional Needs				
Nurse	Assess whether grandparents are having childrearing concerns.	Review natural inquisitiveness of preschool children, which can lead them into unsafe areas.	Grandparent states she didn't supervise child well so child drank beer off coffee table.	Grandparent states that although caring for a preschooler is difficult, she feels adequate to give care.
Discharge Planning				
Nurse	Assess if grandparents have transportation to return for follow-up appointment.	Schedule return appointment for 1 week at kidney clinic.	As nephrotic syndrome is a long-term disorder, child will need continued follow-up for years to come.	Grandparents state they are aware of long-term nature of disorder and will keep follow-up appointments.

Henoch-Schönlein Syndrome Nephritis

Henoch-Schönlein purpura is discussed in Chapter 44. Approximately one quarter of the children who develop this type of purpura develop renal disease as a secondary complication. The renal involvement becomes apparent within a few days after the manifestations of purpuric symptoms. Children may show only urinary abnormalities such as proteinuria or may have a rapidly progressing glomerulonephritis. Fortunately, most children recover completely. Only a few develop chronic symptoms, but in those who do, long-term kidney disease can develop (Ambruso, Hays, & Goldenberg, 2008).

Systemic Lupus Erythematosus

SLE is an autoimmune disease in which autoantibodies and antigens cause deposits of complement in the kidney glomerulus (see Chapter 20). Because of this, some children with SLE develop symptoms of acute or chronic glomerulonephritis, the ultimate cause of death in many adults with SLE (Hellmann & Imboden, 2009). Therapy with corticosteroids or cytotoxic agents may be effective. If kidney transplantation is required, the same damage rarely occurs in the transplanted kidney.

Hemolytic-Uremic Syndrome

With hemolytic-uremic syndrome, the lining of glomerular arterioles becomes inflamed, swollen, and occluded with particles of platelets and fibrin. The child's red blood cells and platelets are damaged as they flow through the partially occluded blood vessels. As the damaged cells reach the spleen, they are destroyed by the spleen and removed from circulation. This leads to hemolytic anemia.

Ninety percent of children who develop this syndrome have recently experienced an *E. coli* GI infection. The most likely source of the *E. coli* is undercooked hamburger, because *E. coli* is found in the intestine of beef cattle. It occurs more frequently in infants who have their initial *E. coli* infection treated with an antibiotic than those who are not treated (Raffaelli et al., 2007).

Assessment

The syndrome occurs most often during the summer and in children 6 months to 4 years of age. Children usually develop only a transient diarrhea, although this can progress to severe fluid loss and bowel wall necrosis. Fever may be so elevated that the child experiences stupor and hallucinations. Oliguria accompanied by proteinuria, hematuria, and urinary casts in urine follows. The oliguria will lead to increased serum creatinine, BUN, and extensive edema. Children appear pale from anemia; easy bruising or petechiae may be present from *thrombocytopenia* (reduced platelet level). Laboratory studies will show fibrin split products in the serum as the fibrin deposits in glomerular vessels are degraded. Thrombocytopenia is present because platelets are damaged by the irregular blood vessels. An increased reticulocyte count indicates that red blood cells are rapidly being replaced.

Therapeutic Management

The child needs supportive therapy to maintain kidney and heart function. The extreme oliguria can be treated with peritoneal dialysis; anemia can be corrected by careful transfusion of packed red cells. Peritoneal dialysis can be extremely frightening to parents and the child because it involves penetration of the child's abdomen. Be certain they understand that the actual dialysis procedure is not painful and they can hold the child during infusion.

Ensure that parents understand the importance of follow-up care and have an appointment for this. Help them begin to view the child as well again so they do not continue to shelter the child unnecessarily but allow for normal growth and development.

Despite the extent of the illness, most infants with hemolytic-uremic syndrome recover completely. Some children, however, die of the acute illness or continue to have chronic renal involvement.

Acute Renal Failure

Renal failure occurs in either an acute or chronic form. The acute form most often occurs because of a sudden body insult, such as severe dehydration. The chronic form results from extensive kidney disease, such as hemolytic-uremic syndrome or glomerulonephritis (Reddy & Murra, 2009).

Other causes of acute renal failure include prolonged anesthesia, hemorrhage, shock, severe diarrhea, or sudden traumatic injury. It also can occur in children who are placed on cardiopulmonary bypass while undergoing heart surgery, who receive common antibiotics (aminoglycosides, penicillin, cephalosporins, and sulfonamides), who swallow a poison such as arsenic (found in rat poison), or who are exposed to industrial wastes such as mercury. All of these conditions appear to lead to renal ischemia, which ultimately leads to acute renal failure.

Assessment

One of the first symptoms noted with acute renal failure is *oliguria,* a urine output of less than 1 mL/kg of the child's body weight/hour. An indwelling urinary catheter may be inserted to rule out the possibility that urinary retention in the bladder rather than kidney dysfunction is causing the severe oliguria.

Azotemia (accumulation of nitrogen waste in the bloodstream) will occur because of the oliguria. *Uremia* (extra accumulation of nitrogen wastes in the blood, with additional toxic symptoms such as cerebral irritation) also may occur. The BUN rises progressively as renal insufficiency continues and the breakdown products of protein cannot be excreted. A BUN level greater than 80 to 100 mg/100 mL is toxic and needs correction, usually by dialysis. Urine creatinine is another measure that can be used as an indicator of function, because it is normally excreted at a uniform rate. A rate of less than 10 mg/100 mL indicates severe renal failure. As the kidneys become unable to dilute or concentrate urine, the specific gravity of urine often becomes "fixed" at 1.010.

Hyperkalemia (elevated potassium level) may occur if potassium cannot be excreted. Hyperkalemia is manifested by a weak, irregular pulse, abdominal cramps, lowered blood pressure, and muscle weakness. Acidosis will follow shortly with acute renal failure from the inability of H^+ ions to be excreted. As total output decreases, phosphorus levels will rise in the bloodstream. A high serum phosphorus level leads to a low calcium serum level (recall that phosphorus and calcium have an inverse proportional relationship). Severe hypocalcemia can lead to muscle twitching and seizures (*tetany*); chronic hypocalcemia can lead to withdrawal of calcium from bones (*osteodystrophy*).

An IVP or radioactive uptake scan may be ordered to substantiate the lack of kidney function. Parents and children need support for this type of study, because the results may be disappointing and so different from what they hoped they would be.

Therapeutic Management

Because acute renal failure is a reaction to body stress caused by acute disease or insult, attempts to treat it focus on supporting the child's body systems while correcting the underlying condition. If the child is dehydrated (as with diarrhea or hemorrhage), IV fluid is needed to replace plasma volume. Administer such fluid slowly enough to avoid heart failure; extra fluid cannot be removed by the kidneys because they are not functioning. The fluid should not contain potassium until it is established that kidney function is adequate; buildup of potassium may otherwise cause heart block. Potassium levels greater than 6 mEq/L are corrected by the IV administration of calcium gluconate (as the glucose moves into cells, it carries potassium with it), by the oral administration of a cation exchange resin such as Kayexalate, or by dialysis. Administering sodium bicarbonate may cause a shift of potassium from the bloodstream into cells, temporarily reducing the circulating potassium level. Administration of a combination of IV glucose and insulin may also be effective (insulin helps glucose move into cells).

A diuretic such as furosemide (Lasix) may be ordered in an attempt to increase urine production. Diet should be low in protein, potassium, and sodium and high in carbohydrate to supply enough calories for metabolism yet limit urea production and control serum potassium levels. Fluid intake may be limited to prevent heart failure due to accumulating fluid that cannot be excreted. Weigh children daily (same scale, same clothing, same time of day) and maintain accurate intake and output recordings to evaluate fluid status. If children are so ill that they cannot eat, total parenteral nutrition may be necessary. Regulate amounts carefully to prevent fluid overload (see Chapter 37 for administration techniques).

When recovery from acute renal failure begins, children generally have a degree of diuresis as the extra fluid accumulated by the body is cleared. The increase in urine must be noted, because children may need additional fluid intake at this point to prevent hypovolemia, which could lead once more to renal failure. Parents usually remain anxious for an extended period after an episode of acute renal failure because they fear that the restoration of kidney function is only temporary. Reassure them that urine output is remaining at a normal level. This helps them to relax and interact effectively with their child.

Chronic Renal Failure

Chronic renal failure results from developmental abnormalities, when acute failure becomes long term, or when chronic kidney disease has caused extensive nephron destruction (Lum, 2008). The nephrons that are not destroyed by long-term disease appear to function normally; they simply are inadequate in number to sustain kidney function. Glomeruli can adjust so that kidney functions continue normally until 50% of nephrons are destroyed. After this point, kidney function diminishes by degrees until the child develops end-stage kidney disease, where the kidneys cannot maintain normal function.

Assessment

With loss of nephron function, kidneys cannot concentrate urine. This results in polyuria, possibly manifested as enuresis.

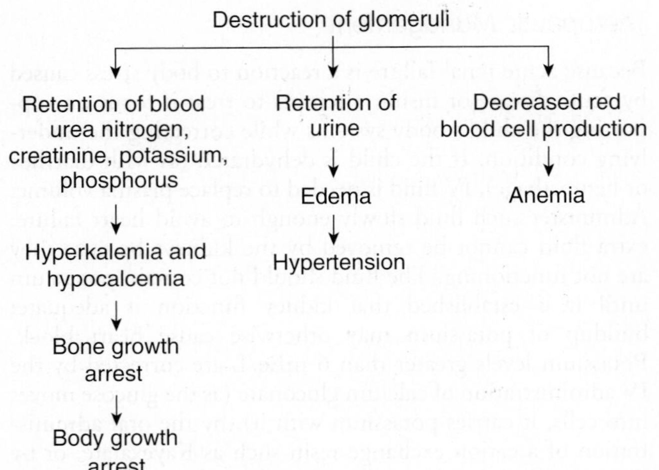

FIGURE 46.14 Pathology of chronic renal failure.

The few functioning nephrons present cannot reabsorb enough sodium to maintain a functioning level of body fluid, so dehydration occurs. As additional nephrons are lost, oliguria and anuria occur. Inability to excrete H^+ ions leads to acidosis. Hypocalcemia and hyperphosphatemia occur from the kidney's inability to excrete phosphate. Osteodystrophy occurs as calcium is withdrawn from bones to compensate. Kidneys are responsible for synthesizing vitamin D to its active form. With poor kidney function, vitamin D cannot be used. Without this, calcium cannot be absorbed from the GI tract and deposited in bones. Bones become so calcium depleted that growth halts and the bones lose strength (renal rickets).

Erythropoietin, formed by the kidneys, stimulates red cell production. With decreased erythropoietin production, anemia develops. Pruritus may be present from skin irritation due to excretion of nitrogenous wastes in sweat from high levels of BUN and serum creatinine. These changes are summarized in Fig. 46.14.

Therapeutic Management

Children with chronic renal failure are generally placed on a low-protein, low-phosphorus, low-potassium diet to prevent rapid urea and phosphate buildup. Children may take aluminum hydroxide gel with meals to bind phosphorus in the intestines and prevent absorption. Milk usually is not given because it is high in sodium, potassium, and phosphate—electrolytes children may have difficulty clearing. Meat is restricted and even beans are high enough in protein to be eliminated from the diet. This can be difficult for parents and children to understand because they are taught that meats are high in protein but vegetables are not. Letting children have some choice about what foods they eat each day helps to promote adjustment to this restricted diet. Whoever prepares meals needs good instructions on selecting low-protein foods. Low-electrolyte, low-protein formulas are commercially available for infants with renal failure.

Total daily fluid intake may need to be restricted, although restriction should be as minimal as possible or it can present an area of tremendous conflict between the child and parents. Many children need sodium intake restricted, and others need a normal sodium intake (but no excessively salty foods such as lunch meats, potato chips, or pretzels). Other children may actually need additional salt because, due to poor tubular reabsorption, they dump sodium in urine. Low-sodium formulas such as Lonalac are recommended for children with heart failure who need a low-sodium intake. Use them cautiously in children with renal insufficiency, because their high potassium content can lead to toxic potassium blood levels. Diuretics may be ordered to help children regulate sodium and fluid levels and prevent edema.

As renal failure becomes prolonged, a child may need supplemental calcium to prevent muscle cramping, rickets, tetany, or seizures. As hypertension becomes more and more acute from the accumulating blood volume, a daily antihypertensive drug may be prescribed. A blood transfusion may be needed to correct anemia, but it must be given cautiously so volume overload does not occur. Recombinant human erythropoietin may be prescribed to stimulate red blood cell formation. Effective excretion of urea can be accomplished by dialysis or by replacing the nonfunctioning kidneys with kidney transplantation. Growth hormone may increase height in some children who have fallen behind in stature (Vimalachandra et al., 2009).

Nursing Diagnoses and Related Interventions

Nursing Diagnosis: Risk for interrupted family processes related to chronically ill family member

Outcome Evaluation: Family members express feelings about illness to each other and to health care providers; participate in care of ill member.

Children with renal failure grow poorly because of the alteration in calcium metabolism. It is easy for them to become depressed because of chronic fatigue and an unappetizing diet. If children are taking corticosteroids or other immunosuppressive drugs because of glomerulonephritis, they may be angry or disheartened about their change in appearance. Help them stay as active as possible by doing age-appropriate activities.

Caring for a child with chronic renal disease is not only time-consuming but also financially and socially devastating for parents. Parents caring for such children at home need opportunities at periodic health assessments to voice their frustrations, fears, and anxieties. They need time to do those things important to them as individuals, whether taking a weekend trip or attending an evening show or program. Ask parents at clinic or follow-up visits, "Do you ever get out of the house or have the opportunity to do anything for yourself?" "What can we do for *you*?" Help of this kind ultimately improves children's care, because it improves the lives and mental attitudes of those around them.

KIDNEY TRANSPLANTATION

The ultimate possibility for prolonging the life of children with renal failure is kidney transplantation. With complete renal failure, children who have extensive hypertension may have their damaged kidneys removed and may be placed on hemodialysis or CCPD to await kidney transplantation. Kidney removal this way is an important step for parents and the child. Although parents realize that their child's kidneys are no longer functioning, this step removes all hope that a miracle might happen and make them function once more. Parents may ask whether it is possible to leave one of the child's kidneys, because only one kidney will be transplanted (this is not recommended, because the hypertension would continue). Parents need a thorough explanation of why hypertension is destructive, that is, it could lead to cerebrovascular accident or coronary artery disease. They must understand that renal biopsy shows that, short of a miracle, their child's kidneys will not function again, so that removal of them is not a loss but only recognition of a loss.

Preoperative Care

Kidney transplantation is most effective (the kidney is less likely to be rejected) if the kidney is taken from a living twin, parent, or sibling (Lim, 2007). In these instances, the success rate is as high as 90% (Chan et al., 2007). Rejection occurs at a higher incidence if a kidney comes from a cadaver or recently deceased child. Most people consider that children should be of legal age to give consent to supply a kidney for transplantation, so few children have a sibling who is eligible to donate a kidney. Tissue studies done to determine the best donor (matched for human leukocyte antigens [HLA]) may show that the person in a family most willing to donate a kidney is not the best person in terms of tissue compatibility. This can cause bitterness and hopelessness in the family, compounding an already stressed family life. Many children anticipate that the characteristics of the donor will be transmitted to them by the kidney, so they are reluctant to accept the kidney of a family member with a character trait they do not like (perhaps a bad temper). They need to be assured that transplanted organs do not carry this type of problem with them. Adult-sized kidneys may be transplanted into children, although if the child weighs less than 10 kg, a kidney this large may lead to hypertension, excessive diuresis, and abdominal complications because of the lack of space. Transplanted kidneys are placed in the abdomen, not the usual kidney space.

People who cannot donate a kidney include those with multiple bilateral small renal arteries, bilateral renal disease, renal infection, advanced medical illness, severe obesity, or hypertension. Although kidney removal can be done by laparoscopy, donors must understand that removal of a kidney involves major surgery. Tests that kidney donors can expect to have preoperatively include HLA typing, electrolyte blood analysis, complete blood count, bleeding time, urinalysis and urine culture, 24-hour urine sample for protein, a renal arteriogram, and IV pyelography. They will have urine samples collected after surgery to assess that their remaining kidney is capable of maintaining full function and they are still in good health.

Before surgery, children who are to receive a transplant may be dialyzed to clear their body of excessive potassium and fluid. If the donated kidney will be from a relative, there is adequate time for thorough preoperative preparation. If the donor kidney is from a cadaver, the announcement of surgery will be sudden and time for preoperative instruction and procedures may be limited.

Children who receive pretransplantation blood transfusions have an improved chance of transplant success (Suthanthiran, Hartono, & Strom, 2007). Most children, therefore, receive at least five blood transfusions while awaiting surgery. The mechanisms by which this operates are unclear, but transfusion-induced production of antibodies or immune complexes appears to mediate graft survival.

Human Leukocyte Antigen Typing

HLAs are a group of antigens found on the surfaces of all cells with a nucleus, including blood components such as leukocytes and platelets. The name is derived from the fact that they were first identified on white blood cells. Such antigens are inherited from both parents and are specific for each individual. They denote tissue type or determine which tissue the immune system identifies as foreign tissue. They are carried on the short arm of chromosome 6 in each cell.

Such antigens also serve as the basis for paternity typing. They may cause reactions to blood product transfusions and bone marrow and organ transplants. When two people have like HLA antigens, they are said to be *histocompatible.* Identical twins have complete histocompatibility and family members have partial histocompatibility; any two people can have histocompatibility at least on one antigen site.

Children who are awaiting kidney transplantation are tissue typed, and this information is circulated to major medical centers. When a kidney is available for transplantation, the child's tissue type is compared with the donor kidney. For tissue typing, lymphocytes from both a donor and recipient are grown together in a culture medium and then examined for like characteristics. With new immune suppressive drugs, however, even unmatched donor kidneys have a chance to successfully graft.

Postoperative Care

After renal transplantation, children are cared for in an environment that is as sterile as possible. They are placed on immunosuppressive therapy such as cyclosporine, azathioprine [Imuran], and methylprednisolone [Solu-Medrol]) to reduce the possibility of kidney rejection. Antilymphocyte globulin and antithymocyte globulin may be added to aid immunosuppression.

Although some transplanted kidneys begin to function immediately, hemodialysis may be continued until the implanted kidney can fully function after the insult of transplantation. Be prepared to help a child and parents through a "honeymoon" period after the transplantation.

Help children understand that acceptance or rejection of a kidney depends on a multitude of factors—the condition of renal veins and arteries, the transplanted kidney, or antigen–antibody formation—but none of these factors is related to whether the child is good or bad or deserves or does not deserve to have the transplantation work (Box 46.7).

Children with end-stage renal disease usually fail to grow despite treatment. Although the rate of growth is improved after kidney transplantation, they will probably never reach full height. Part of this growth restriction is related to the need for corticosteroid maintenance therapy to continue immunosuppression.

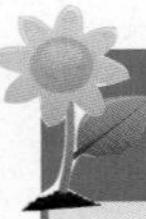

BOX 46.7 * Focus on Communication

Carol's grandmother tells you Carol has "changed completely" since she became ill.

Less Effective Communication

Nurse: Mrs. Hendricks, in what way has Carol changed?

Mrs. Hendricks: She used to whine all the time, and constantly ask for things. Now she entertains herself. It's like heaven.

Nurse: That sounds wonderful. Let's review her medicine routine to be sure that's going well.

Mrs. Hendricks: That's another thing she does perfectly: never fusses a bit about anything she has to take.

More Effective Communication

Nurse: Mrs. Hendricks, in what way has Carol changed?

Mrs. Hendricks: She used to whine all the time, and constantly ask for things. Now she entertains herself. It's like heaven.

Nurse: Do you think she's acting a little too perfect?

Mrs. Hendricks: Well, it does seem a bit strange for her.

Nurse: Do you think she could be worrying that if she misbehaves, her medicine won't work?

Mrs. Hendricks: I never thought of that. I would feel better if she started to act like her old self.

What the grandmother above is describing is a "honeymoon" period that children may pass through after being told their kidneys are important for life. Parents often need help seeing this for what it is so they can begin to reassure children that behaving perfectly will not influence the outcome of their illness and that, because they loved them as they were, they will continue to love them regardless.

Transplant Rejection

Acute transplant rejection, if it occurs, usually develops within the first 3 months after transplantation. Children begin to develop fever, proteinuria, oliguria, weight gain, hypertension, and tenderness over the kidney. Serum creatinine and BUN levels will rise. Increasing the dose of immunosuppressants may be effective in relieving this type of rejection.

Rejection may also be *chronic,* in which the transplanted kidney gradually loses function after the first 6 months. Hypertension and anemia result. A biopsy will show vascular changes such as narrowing of arterial lumens and interstitial changes such as fibrosis and tubular atrophy. This type of rejection is difficult to halt, although it may be such a slow, steady process that it is 2 or 3 years before the kidney fails. If a kidney is rejected, it is removed and a child is returned to a program of hemodialysis. Because one kidney was rejected does not mean that a second transplant will be rejected also. Unfortunately, however, the number of kidneys available for transplantation is limited, so kidney rejection becomes an ominous sign for the child's long-term survival.

Malignant disease is more common in transplantation recipients than in the normal population, probably because of the long-term immunosuppression (Villeneuve et al., 2007). The original disease for which the child underwent transplantation may recur in the transplanted kidney. This is most apt to occur in glomerulonephritis. During adolescence, typically an age of poor adherence to medication regimens, kidney recipients need to be followed closely to be certain they are taking their immunosuppressive therapy. Parents cannot help but overprotect the child; they worry that a rough-housing session with a sibling or playing a game such as baseball may injure the transplanted kidney. The child may be afraid to engage in any activity for the same reason unless you help a family fully adjust to this major life change.

✔ Checkpoint Question 46.5

How would you best explain kidney transplantation to a child?

a. A new kidney will be placed in your abdomen.
b. The new kidney will be placed in your bladder.
c. You must never eat eggs after a kidney transplant.
d. Your urine will be brown for the rest of your life.

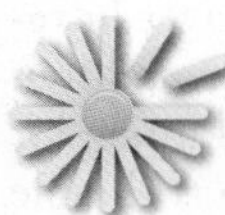

Key Points for Review

- Many urinary tract disorders, such as polycystic kidneys, urethral obstruction, and bladder exstrophy, are evident on a fetal ultrasound. Early identification this way allows therapy to begin in utero or immediately at birth.
- Many urinary tract disorders, such as polycystic kidneys or chronic renal failure, are long-term conditions requiring years of therapy. Be certain that parents are well informed about their child's condition so they can continue to participate in planning their child's care.
- Congenital structural abnormalities of the urinary tract include patent urachus, exstrophy of the bladder, hypospadias, and epispadias. Surgical correction is required for all of these.
- Urinary tract infection tends to occur more often in girls than boys. "Honeymoon cystitis" refers to a urinary tract infection occurring with first-time sexual intercourse.
- Vesicoureteral reflux is the backflow of urine into ureters with voiding. It occurs because the valve that guards the entrance to the ureters is lax or misplaced. Surgical correction may be necessary to prevent repeated urinary tract infection.
- Kidney dysfunction can occur for structural reasons such as kidney agenesis, polycystic kidney, and renal hypoplasia.
- Acute poststreptococcal glomerulonephritis is inflammation of the glomeruli after a streptococcal infection. It is characterized by an acute episode of hematuria and proteinuria.
- Nephrotic syndrome is an immunologic process that results in altered glomerular permeability.
- Diminished kidney function leads to both fluid and electrolyte imbalances. Creative techniques are necessary to encourage children to continue to ingest a restricted-protein diet.

- Renal failure can be acute or chronic. Peritoneal dialysis or hemodialysis may be used to remove body wastes until kidney function can be restored.
- Kidney transplantation may be an option for some children with kidney disorders. This is extensive surgery and requires the child to remain on immunosuppressive therapy to counteract transplant rejection.

CRITICAL THINKING EXERCISES

1. Carol is the preschooler with nephrotic syndrome whom you met at the beginning of the chapter. Her grandmother asked you whether a sip of beer could have caused Carol's kidney disease. What would you tell her is the cause of nephrosis? What discharge instructions can you anticipate you will need to review with Carol's grandmother?

2. Carol's grandmother is afraid Carol will need a kidney transplant. Carol tells you she hopes she has been good enough to deserve being chosen for a transplant. What would you want to teach this family about the transplantation selection process?

3. Suppose Carol receives continuous ambulatory peritoneal dialysis and wants to go to her church camp this summer. Her grandmother asks you whether this would be a good experience for her. What factors would you want to know about the camp? About Carol? About her procedure?

4. Examine the National Health Goals related to renal disorders and children. Most government-sponsored funds for nursing research are allotted based on these goals. What would be a possible research topic to explore pertinent to these goals that would be applicable to Carol's family and also advance evidence-based practice?

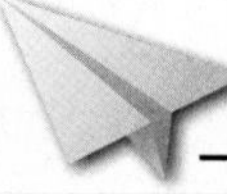

CRITICAL THINKING SCENARIO

Open the accompanying CD-ROM or visit http://thePoint.lww.com and read the Patient Scenario included for this chapter, then answer the questions to further sharpen your skills and grow more familiar with NCLEX style questions related to renal or urinary tract disorders in children. Confirm your answers are correct by reading the rationales.

REFERENCES

Ahmad, S., et al. (2007). Hemodialysis apparatus. In J. T. Daugirdas, P. G. Blake, & T. S. Ing (Eds.). *Handbook of dialysis*. Philadelphia: Lippincott Williams & Wilkins.

Ambruso, D. R., Hays, T., & Goldenberg, N. (2008). Hematologic disorders. In W. W. Hay, et al. (Eds.). *Current pediatric diagnosis and treatment* (18th ed.). Columbus, OH: McGraw-Hill.

Ashley, R. A., (2007). Urachal anomalies: a longitudinal study of urachal remnants in children and adults. *Journal of Urology, 178*(4.2), 1615–1618.

Atala, A. (2007). Congenital urologic anomalies. In R. W. Schrier (Ed.). *Diseases of the kidney and urinary tract*. Philadelphia: Lippincott Williams & Wilkins.

Auron, A., et al. (2007). Prevention of peritonitis in children receiving peritoneal dialysis. *Pediatric Nephrology, 22*(4), 578–585.

Boyer, O., et al. (2007). Prognosis of autosomal dominant polycystic kidney disease diagnosed in utero or at birth. *Pediatric Nephrology, 22*(3), 380–388.

Chan, L., et al. (2007). Outcomes and complications of renal transplantation. In R. W. Schrier (Ed.). *Diseases of the kidney and urinary tract*. Philadelphia: Lippincott Williams & Wilkins.

Coe, K., & Lail, C. (2007). Peritoneal dialysis in the neonatal intensive care unit: management of acute renal failure after a severe subgaleal hemorrhage. *Advances in Neonatal Care, 7*(4), 179–186.

Croker, B. P., & Tisher, C. C. (2007). Indications for and interpretation of the renal biopsy. In R. W. Schrier (Ed.). *Diseases of the kidney and urinary tract*. Philadelphia: Lippincott Williams & Wilkins.

Dodson, J. L., et al. (2007). Outcomes of delayed hypospadias repair: implications for decision making. *Journal of Urology, 178*(1), 278–281.

Egemen, A., et al. (2008). An evaluation of quality of life of mothers of children with enuresis nocturna. *Pediatric Nephrology, 23*(1), 93–98.

Factor, K. F. (2007). Potassium management in pediatric peritoneal dialysis patients: can a diet with increased potassium maintain a normal serum potassium without a potassium supplement? *Advances in Peritoneal Dialysis, 23*(2), 167–169.

Gearhart, J. P., Baird, A., & Nelson, C. P. (2007). Results of bladder neck reconstruction after newborn complete primary repair of exstrophy. *Journal of Urology, 178*(4.2), 1619–1622.

Glazener, C. M. A., Evans, J. H. C., & Peto, R. E. (2009). Drugs for nocturnal enuresis in children (other than desmopressin and tricyclics). *Cochrane Database of Systematic Reviews, 2009*(1), (CD002238).

Gomella, L. G., & Haist, S. A. (2007). *Clinician's pocket reference* (11th ed.). Columbus, OH: McGraw-Hill.

Hellmann, D. B., & Imboden, J. B. (2009). Musculoskeletal disorders. In S. J. McPhee & M. A. Papadakis (Eds.). *Current medical diagnosis and treatment*. Columbus, OH: McGraw-Hill.

Hensle, T. W., Grogg, A. L., & Eaddy, M. (2007). Pediatric vesicoureteral reflux: treatment patterns and outcomes. *Nature Clinical Practice Urology, 4*(9), 462–463.

Hubert, K. C., & Palmer, J. S. (2007). Current diagnosis and management of fetal genitourinary abnormalities. *Urologic Clinics of North America, 34*(1), 89–101.

Hutton, K. A., & Babu, R. (2007). Normal anatomy of the external urethral meatus in boys: implications for hypospadias repair. *BJU International: British Journal of Urology, 100*(1), 161–163.

Kamel, M. H., et al. (2007). Deceased-donor kidney transplantation in prune belly syndrome. *Urology, 69*(4), 666–669.

Karch, A. M. (2009). *Lippincott's nursing drug guide*. Philadelphia: Lippincott Williams & Wilkins.

Kelly, H., et al. (2007). A genome-wide scan for genes involved in primary vesicoureteric reflux. *Journal of Medical Genetics, 44*(11), 710–717.

Lim, W. H., et al. (2007). Parental donors in live-donor kidney transplantation associated with increased rejection rates and reduced glomerular filtration rates. *Transplantation, 84*(8), 972–980.

Lu, D. F., et al. (2007). A descriptive study of individuals with membranoproliferative glomerulonephritis. *Nephrology Nursing Journal: Journal of the American Nephrology Nurses' Association, 34*(3), 295–302.

Lum, G. M. (2008). The kidney and urinary tract. In W. W. Hay, et al. (Eds.). *Current pediatric diagnosis and treatment* (18th ed.). Columbus, OH: McGraw-Hill.

Pena, A., et al. (2007). Steroid-resistant nephrotic syndrome: long-term evolution after sequential therapy. *Pediatric Nephrology, 22*(11), 1875–1880.

Raffaelli, R. M ., et al. (2007). Child care-associated outbreak of *Escherichia coli* O157:H7 and hemolytic uremic syndrome. *Pediatric Infectious Disease Journal, 26*(10), 951–953.

Reddy, B., & Murra, P. (2009). Acute renal failure. In S. J. McPhee & M. A. Papadakis (Eds.). *Current medical diagnosis and treatment.* Columbus, OH: McGraw-Hill.

Riccabona, M. (2007). Paediatric magnetic resonance urography: just fancy images or a new important diagnostic tool? *Current Opinion in Urology, 17*(1), 48–55.

Schilling McCann, J. A., et al. (Eds.). (2007). *Professional guide to signs and symptoms.* Philadelphia: Lippincott Williams & Wilkins.

Schon, D., et al. (2007). Increasing the use of arteriovenous fistula in hemodialysis: economic benefits and economic barriers. *CJASN: Clinical Journal of The American Society of Nephrology, 2*(2), 268–276.

Shaw, E. A., et al. (2007). Characterization of the peripheral retinopathy in X-linked and autosomal recessive Alport syndrome. *Nephrology Dialysis Transplantation, 22*(1), 104–108.

Sinha, R., et al. (2007). Acute rheumatic fever with concomitant poststreptococcal glomerulonephritis. *American Journal of Kidney Diseases, 50*(1), A33–A35.

Sousa, C. N., et al. (2008). Haemodialysis for children under the age of two years. *Journal of Renal Care, 34*(1), 9–13.

Suthanthiran, M., Hartono, C., & Strom, T. B. (2007). Immunobiology and immunopharmacology of renal allograft rejection. In R. W. Schrier (Ed.). *Diseases of the kidney and urinary tract.* Philadelphia: Lippincott Williams & Wilkins.

Sutherland, R. W., et al. (2007). Endoscopic treatment of VUR: who, when, and how? *Contemporary Urology, 19*(8), 28–30.

Tkaczyk, M., et al. (2008). Markers of endothelial dysfunction in children with idiopathic nephrotic syndrome. *American Journal of Nephrology, 28*(2), 197–202.

Villeneuve, P. J., et al. (2007). Cancer incidence among Canadian kidney transplant recipients. *American Journal of Transplantation, 7*(4), 941–948.

Vimalachandra, D. et al. (2009). Growth hormone for children with chronic kidney disease. *Cochrane Database of Systematic Reviews, 2009*(1), (CD003264).

Wan, K. S., Liu, C. K., & Chen, L. H. (2007). Primary urinary tract infection in infants: prophylaxis for uncomplicated pyelonephritis. *Nephrology, 12*(2), 178–181.

Watnick, S., & Morrison, G. (2009). Nephrology. In S. J. McPhee & M. A. Papadakis (Eds.). *Current medical diagnosis and treatment.* Columbus, OH: McGraw-Hill.

Weaver, A., & Dobson, P. (2007). Nocturnal enuresis in children. *Journal of Family Health Care, 17*(5), 159–161.

Woods, A. G., & Brandon, D. H. (2007). Prune belly syndrome. A focused physical assessment. *Advances in Neonatal Care, 7*(3), 132–143.

SUGGESTED READINGS

Chaturvedi, S., & Jones, C. (2009). Protein restriction for children with chronic renal failure. *Cochrane Database of Systematic Reviews, 2009*(1), (CD006863).

Hodson, E. M., Willis, N. S., & Craig, J. C. (2009). Antibiotics for acute pyelonephritis in children. *Cochrane Database of Systematic Reviews, 2009*(1), (CD003772).

Maizels, M., & Saldano, D. D. (2007). Childhood bed-wetting. *Contemporary Urology, 19*(7), 18–23.

Marks, S. D. (2007). How have the past 5 years of research changed clinical practice in paediatric nephrology? *Archives of Disease in Childhood, 92*(4), 357–361.

Murphy, F. (2007). The role of the nurse post-renal transplantation. *British Journal of Nursing, 16*(11), 667–675.

Prelog, M., et al. (2007). Acute nosocomial urinary tract infection in children. *Infection Control and Hospital Epidemiology, 28*(8), 1019–1023.

Warady, B. A., & Chadha, V. (2007). Chronic kidney disease in children: the global perspective. *Pediatric Nephrology, 22*(12), 1999–2009.

Watkins, J. (2007). Urinary tract infections in children. *Practice Nursing, 18*(10), 516.

Williams, G. J., et al. (2009). Long-term antibiotics for preventing recurrent urinary tract infection in children. *Cochrane Database of Systematic Reviews, 2009*(1), (CD001534).

Zioni, N. (2007). Improving the nutritional condition of infants and young children undergoing hemodialysis. *EDTNA/ERCA Journal of The European Dialysis and Transplant Nurses Association/European Renal Care Association, 33*(1), 11–16.

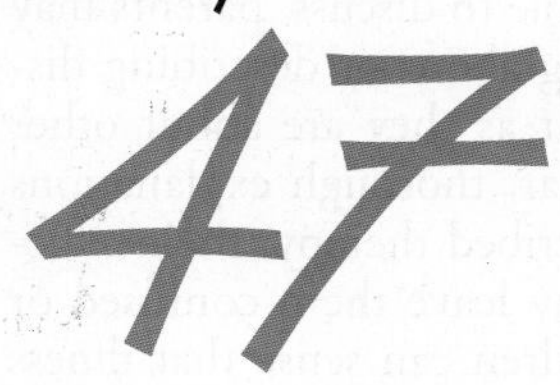

Chapter 47 Nursing Care of a Family When a Child Has a Reproductive Disorder

KEY TERMS

- amenorrhea
- anovulatory
- cryptorchidism
- dysmenorrhea
- endometriosis
- fibrocystic breast disease
- gynecomastia
- hermaphrodite
- hydrocele
- menorrhagia
- metrorrhagia
- mittelschmerz
- orchiectomy
- orchiopexy
- pelvic inflammatory disease (PID)
- premenstrual dysphoric disorder
- pseudohermaphrodite
- sexually transmitted infection (STI)
- toxic shock syndrome
- varicocele
- vulvovaginitis

OBJECTIVES

After mastering the contents of this chapter, you should be able to:

1. Describe common reproductive disorders in children.
2. Identify National Health Goals related to reproductive disorders that nurses can help the nation achieve.
3. Analyze ways that nursing care for a child with a reproductive disorder can be more family centered.
4. Assess a child with a reproductive disorder.
5. Formulate nursing diagnoses for a child with a reproductive disorder.
6. Develop expected outcomes for a child with a reproductive disorder.
7. Plan nursing care related to reproductive disorders in children.
8. Implement nursing care for a child with a reproductive disorder, such as teaching about normal menstruation.
9. Evaluate expected outcomes for achievement and effectiveness of care.
10. Identify areas related to the care of children with reproductive disorders that could benefit from additional nursing research or application of evidence-based practice.
11. Integrate knowledge of reproductive disorders in children with the nursing process to achieve quality maternal and child health nursing care.

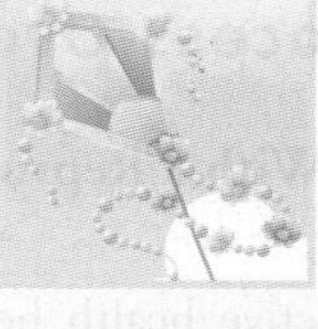

Navi is a 15-year-old girl you meet in a pediatric clinic. She has been diagnosed with gonorrhea because of a purulent vaginal discharge and burning on urination. When you ask her if she is sexually active, she says no; she thinks she contracted the infection from sharing a towel in a locker room. As she leaves the clinic, you hear her tell the receptionist, "I'm glad I got this early in life. Now I won't have to worry about getting it again."

Previous chapters described the growth and development of well children and illnesses that occur in other body systems. This chapter adds information about the dramatic changes, both physical and psychosocial, that occur when children develop reproductive disorders. Such information forms the basis for care and health teaching in this area.

What kind of health education does Navi need?

Reproductive disorders in children range from mild infections to serious anatomic malformations. All of these disorders require prompt and careful treatment so that children can reach adulthood in good reproductive health, with unaltered fertility, and with a positive sense of sexuality. Reproductive infections may suggest child abuse, so children with these also need careful assessment to rule out this possibility (see Chapter 55). National Health Goals related to reproductive disorders in children are highlighted in Box 47.1.

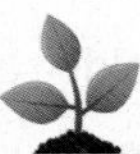

Nursing Process Overview

For Care of a Child With a Reproductive Disorder

Assessment

Assessment of reproductive health begins with the first physical examination at birth and continues at health assessments throughout childhood and adolescence. As this is a sensitive area for many people to discuss, parents may not be as comfortable inquiring about or describing disorders of the reproductive tract as they are about other disorders. Unless they have clear, thorough explanations of the disease process and prescribed therapy, their reluctance to pursue the subject may leave them confused or misinformed. Even young children can sense that illness affecting the genitalia or their reproductive tract is viewed by some adults as different from other diseases so may not ask as many questions as they do about other diseases.

Nursing Diagnosis

Nursing diagnoses formulated for reproductive illnesses in children focus not only on the result of the disease symptoms but on the anxiety this type of disorder can cause. Examples of nursing diagnoses are:

- Risk for infection transmission related to lack of knowledge of safer sex practices
- Pain related to symptoms of vaginal infection
- Disturbed body image related to fibrocystic breast disease
- Anxiety related to absence or irregularity of menstrual periods in adolescent
- Fear related to surgery on genital organs

Outcome Identification and Planning

Assessment of a child's knowledge about the reproductive system and ways that illness can affect reproductive and sexual functioning forms the foundation for developing appropriate outcomes. Educating the child about reproductive health may be one of the first areas to plan. When establishing expected outcomes with adolescents, work with them to establish a plan that will correlate with their schedules. Adolescents need to be involved in the decision making process.

Organizations helpful for referral for adolescents include the National Women's Health Network (http://www.womenshealthnetwork.org) and the National Adolescent Health Information Center (http://nahic.ucsf.edu).

Implementation

Interventions for children with reproductive disorders should always include education about reproductive functioning and measures for maintaining reproductive and sexual health and preventing illness. Health education regarding the importance of testicular self-examination for adolescent males should be stressed at health care visits (see Chapter 34). Guidelines for teaching about menstrual health and safer sex (covered in Chapter 5) are also important.

Essential nursing interventions also include supporting parents and children through difficult decisions and frightening procedures and providing close observation and empathic counseling after surgery. For example, surgery for undescended testes is a procedure that can be traumatic for a child, especially if it is performed during a developmental stage in which a boy views such surgery as castrating (a psychological reason in addition to a physical reason why it is done early in life). As all children with any reproductive disorder reach puberty, they need honest explanations about any effect such a condition will have on

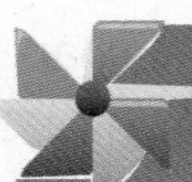

BOX 47.1 * Focus on National Health Goals

Because sexually transmitted infections (STIs) not only cause short-term distress as a result of painful lesions but also can have long-term implications for fertility and future childbearing, several National Health Goals specifically address them. These goals are:

- Reduce the proportion of adolescents with *Chlamydia trachomatis* infections from baselines of 12% (females) and 15% (males) to a target of 3%.
- Reduce the annual incidence of new cases of gonorrhea in adolescent females from a baseline of 279 cases per 100,000 people to no more than 42 cases per 100,000 people.
- Reduce the incidence of primary and secondary syphilis from a baseline of 3.2 per 100,000 people to no more than 0.2 case per 100,000 people.
- Reduce the incidence of congenital syphilis from a baseline of 28 per 100,000 live births to 1 per 100,000 live births.
- Reduce the incidence of genital herpes from a baseline of 17% to no more than 14%.
- Reduce the proportion of females with human papillomavirus infection (no target set as yet).
- Reduce the incidence of pelvic inflammatory disease among women aged 15 through 44 years from a baseline of 8% to no more than 5% (http://www.nih.gov).

Nurses can help the nation achieve these goals by educating adolescents about effective ways to prevent STIs and how to recognize the signs and symptoms of these illnesses. Areas that could benefit from additional nursing research and evidence-based practice in this area include the most effective ways to teach adolescents about safer sex practices, the reasons adolescents continue to believe that they cannot contract infectious diseases, and strategies that would make it easier for parents to discuss this topic with adolescents.

interpersonal relationships, sexual functioning, or childbearing.

Outcome Evaluation

The responses of children to reproductive dysfunction vary both with the severity of the illness and with the specific age and fears of the child. It is safe to assume, however, that children who have experienced such an illness are at risk for a loss of self-esteem or confusion about their body image. Therefore, outcome evaluation should include long-term evaluation of the child's coping abilities and self-image. If a child contracts a sexually transmitted infection (STI), evaluation should also address the child's knowledge about avoiding STIs in the future and willingness to seek help should an infection recur.

The following are examples suggesting achievement of outcomes:

- Adolescent states that discomfort from vaginal infection is tolerable after beginning medication.
- Adolescent states she is able to view self as competent despite fibrocystic breast disease.
- Child states that she is able to wait 6 months without worrying about not yet having a menstrual period.
- Child states that he feels less fearful about impending surgery after talking with his health care provider.

ASSESSING REPRODUCTIVE DISORDERS IN CHILDREN

Reproductive disorders in children may be congenital or acquired so assessment for these must be ongoing throughout childhood (Box 47.2) (Fitzgerald, 2009).

As with other parts of a health interview, questions regarding reproductive health and illness are generally addressed to the parents until the child is able to answer history questions reliably and independently. Once a girl has reached adolescence, a gynecologic history (Box 47.3) should be included in the health assessment. To preserve their privacy, adolescents of both genders may prefer not to be accompanied by a parent during a physical examination for reproductive dysfunction.

Some adolescents visit health care facilities on their own. They may be worried that they have contracted an STI. They may suspect that they have become pregnant or want to receive some form of contraception. Before they can admit their chief concern, however, they may "test" a health care provider by eliciting a reaction to a minor problem. Be aware that an adolescent who consults a health care provider with a seemingly minor concern may be misinterpreting symptoms and be truly worried that a minor symptom is serious; on the other hand, the adolescent actually may be seeking help for another problem. Asking the adolescent, "Is there anything else that worries you? Is there any other way we can help you today?" may help you elicit the adolescent's primary concern (Box 47.4).

A pelvic examination is unnecessary for girls who have not yet reached adolescence. However, if vaginal walls need to be inspected (because of an inflammation or infection or the suspicion of sexual abuse), an otoscope and ear tip can be used in place of a speculum. Cotton-tipped applicators can be used to take culture specimens without causing discomfort.

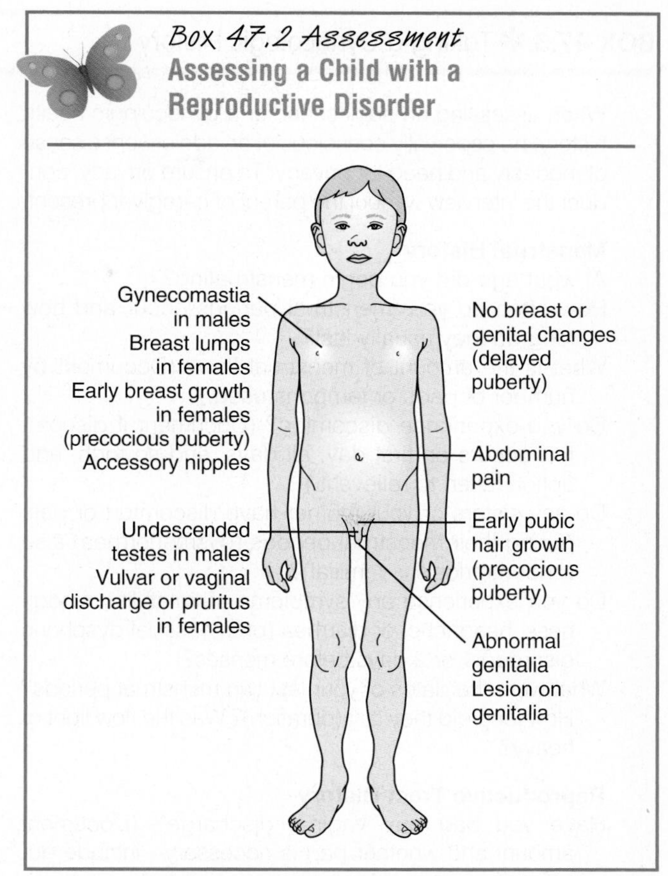

For the adolescent girl, the pelvic examination becomes part of routine health care around the age of 18 to 20 years if the teen is not sexually active and is not having problems. Because the first pelvic examination can be stressful for some teens, spend time with the girl before the procedure to teach her about what is being assessed. A three-dimensional model of internal organs and some representative instruments may be more useful when describing the examination than a verbal description of anatomy. A small speculum should be used for examining young girls. For their comfort, warm the speculum first. Let the girl look at and handle a speculum before it is used.

Remaining beside an adolescent as a support person helps to reduce the stress the teen may be experiencing. To protect her self-esteem, be sure a girl meets the person who will examine her before she is placed in a lithotomy position. Different cultures have different attitudes toward reproductive disorders. Adolescents in Middle Eastern countries, for example, are extremely modest, and so they are extremely uncomfortable having pelvic examinations done for reproductive disorders. Girls from these countries may be more comfortable if the examiner is a woman.

A young adolescent may be uncomfortable in a lithotomy position and can be examined in a dorsal recumbent position instead (see Chapter 11 for information on assisting with a pelvic examination). Allow an adolescent to choose whether she wants a parent to remain in the room with her.

BOX 47.3 ✻ Taking a Gynecologic History

When assessing an adolescent for a gynecologic health history, be especially conscious of an adolescent's sense of modesty and need for privacy. To ensure privacy, conduct the interview without the parent or caregiver present.

Menstrual History

At what age did you begin menstruating?

How often do your menstrual periods occur and how long do they usually last?

What is the amount of menstrual flow? (Document by number of pads or tampons used.)

Do you experience discomfort? (Document if discomfort occurs on first day, all days, and so forth, and action taken to relieve it.)

Do any sisters or your mother have discomfort or pain during their menstrual periods (dysmenorrhea) also (endometriosis is familial)?

Do you experience any symptoms of irritability, moodiness, headache, or diarrhea (premenstrual dysphoric disorder) 1 or 2 days before menses?

What were the dates of your last two menstrual periods? How long did they last (duration)? Was the flow light or heavy?

Reproductive Tract History

Have you had any vaginal discharge? (Document amount and whether pad is necessary—include duration, frequency, description, associated symptoms, actions taken.)

Is there vaginal itching (pruritus)?

Is there any vaginal odor?

Have you had reproductive tract surgery? Have you ever been pregnant? Have you ever had an abortion or miscarriage?

Sexual History

Have you had a sexually transmitted infection such as herpes, gonorrhea, or syphilis?

Are you currently sexually active? What is the gender of your partner?

Do you experience any discomfort during sexual activity (dyspareunia) or any spotting afterward (postcoital spotting)?

Do you have any concerns such as being worried about frequency, position, partner's satisfaction with coitus? Do you experience orgasm?

Contraception History

Do you use any type of birth control? If so, what contraceptive do you use? (Document length of time used, satisfaction, any problems.)

Have you used any other type in the past?

Breast Health

Have you ever noticed any abnormality such as a lump, discharge, or pain in your breasts?

Have you ever had breast surgery?

Have you breastfed a child?

Do you have a yearly breast examination by a health care provider?

BOX 47.4 ✻ Focus on Communication

Navi, age 15 years, is seen at your pediatric clinic. She has mild upper respiratory tract symptoms.

Less Effective Communication

Nurse: Navi? Doctor Jensen doesn't believe you need anything for your cold. Just drink a little extra fluid and take it easy for a couple days.

Navi: Don't I need a prescription? Some penicillin or something?

Nurse: No. Colds are caused by viruses. Penicillin isn't necessary.

Navi: I want to be sure I get over this. I'd really like an antibiotic of some kind.

Nurse: One really isn't necessary.

Navi: I have a bad cough. I don't think I mentioned that.

Nurse: Doctor Jensen listened to your chest. You don't have anything serious there.

Navi: My stomach doesn't feel very good either. Can't I have something?

Nurse: Sorry. Goodbye now.

More Effective Communication

Nurse: Navi? Doctor Jensen doesn't believe you need anything for your cold. Just drink a little extra fluid and take it easy for a couple days.

Navi: Don't I need a prescription? Some penicillin or something?

Nurse: No. Colds are caused by viruses. Penicillin isn't necessary.

Navi: I want to be sure I get over this. I'd really like an antibiotic of some kind.

Nurse: One really isn't necessary.

Navi: I have a bad cough. I don't think I mentioned that.

Nurse: Doctor Jensen listened to your chest. You don't have anything serious there.

Navi: My stomach doesn't feel very good either. Can't I have something?

Nurse: It seems that you have more symptoms than you mentioned. Are you worried about something other than cold symptoms?

Navi: Well, I have this rash and . . .

Nurse: And . . . ? Go on . . .

Navi: And I'm scared I might have a sex disease.

Adolescents can have difficulty discussing reproductive tract symptoms. If they have too much difficulty, they can try to obtain an antibiotic by describing respiratory or abdominal symptoms. Being alert to this possibility helps you to recognize a "growing" history of this type.

HEALTH PROMOTION AND RISK MANAGEMENT

Newborns need a thorough examination at birth to rule out congenital reproductive disorders so these can be diagnosed and management can begin. All children need education about sexually healthy decisions and caring for their bodies. Adolescents may state they are not interested in this information because they are certain that they are choosing abstinence. It is still important to provide the education in regards to making sexually healthy decisions and reward positive choices to staying healthy.

DISORDERS CAUSED BY ALTERED REPRODUCTIVE DEVELOPMENT

Genetic sex or *biologic gender* (sex chromosomes XX or XY) is determined at conception. However, development of the reproductive system, including external genitalia, occurs over two distinct periods. Reproductive organs and genitalia begin to differentiate in utero by the 8th week, with growth and refinement occurring over the next several months. This period constitutes the first phase of reproductive development. The second phase occurs with specific endocrine changes that are triggered during puberty; this is a period of maturation of primary and secondary sexual characteristics.

Ambiguous genitalia, which is a rare condition with various causes that occurs during fetal development, and precocious puberty or delayed puberty, which are second phase disorders, are examples of altered reproductive development. (For a discussion of genetic disorders, see Chapter 7.)

Ambiguous Genitalia

Ambiguous genitalia refers to genitalia that are not clearly defined in a newborn (Gollu et al., 2007). Understanding how reproductive organs develop in utero is important to the understanding of why ambiguous genitalia occur. Although external sexual characteristics generally follow from the presence of the XX or XY chromosomes, under certain circumstances it is possible for structures usually considered "male" or "female" to develop in individuals of either chromosomal gender. Usually, a diagnosis of ambiguous genitalia means that external sexual organs in the child did not follow the normal course of development, so that, at birth, they are so incompletely or abnormally formed that it is impossible to clearly determine the child's gender by simple observation. For instance, a male infant with *hypospadias* (urethral opening on the underside of the penis) and cryptorchidism (undescended testes) may appear more female than male on first inspection (see Chapter 46 for a discussion of hypospadias). A chromosomal female (XX) fetus may become "masculinized" with exposure to androgen in utero; in such children, the clitoris may be so enlarged that it appears more like a penis, the labia may be partially fused and difficult to tell from a male perineum, or the urethra may be displaced so far forward that it is located on the clitoris. When this occurs, the newborn will appear to be a boy on initial inspection. Likewise, under certain conditions, a chromosomal male (XY) may become "feminized," with a lack of fusion of the labioscrotal folds and an incompletely formed penis.

The most common cause of in vitro virilization of females is *congenital adrenocortical syndrome.* The adrenal gland produces androgen instead of adequate cortisone, causing the clitoris to become the size of a typical newborn male's penis (see Chapter 48).

If testosterone was produced in utero but development of the müllerian duct (female) was not suppressed, a child may be intersexed (formerly termed **hermaphrodite**), with both ovaries and testes and either male or female external genitalia. Children with ambiguous genitalia are often termed pseudointersexed or **pseudohermaphrodites** because, as infants, they have some external features of both sexes, although only either ovaries or testes (or neither) are present.

Assessment

If there is any question about a child's gender, karyotyping helps to establish whether the child is genetically male or female (see Chapter 7). This involves drawing a specimen of blood, allowing the white blood cells to reach a division stage, and then examining them. *Laparoscopy* (introduction of a narrow laparoscope into the abdominal cavity through a half-inch incision under the umbilicus) or possibly exploratory surgery may be necessary to determine if ovaries or undescended testes are present. Intravenous pyelography or ultrasound can be used to establish whether a male has a complete urinary tract.

Therapeutic Management

Once the child's true chromosomal gender has been documented, the extent of necessary reconstructive surgery is determined in consultation with the parents. This may involve correction of a hypospadias or cryptorchidism, removal of labial adhesions, or surgical removal of an enlarged clitoris. If removal of an enlarged clitoris is involved, the parents must consider what the absence of this organ will mean to the girl in terms of later sexual enjoyment. Parents may be well advised to delay this type of surgery until the girl can decide for herself whether she wants it done (Verkauskas et al., 2007). If a vagina will be constructed, surgery for this is usually delayed until adolescence when growth is complete.

If an infant is chromosomally male but does not have an adequate penis, a decision to raise the child as a female might be made, although construction of an artificial penis is more likely. Nonfunctioning ovaries or testes are generally removed to prevent malignancy later in life.

Nursing Diagnoses and Related Interventions

When identifying expected outcomes, be aware that parents under stress may have difficulty making long-range plans. The birth of a child with a perplexing defect produces a particularly high level of stress, hampering parents' ability to think clearly and calmly about their situation.

Nursing Diagnosis: Anxiety related to ambiguous gender of child at birth

Outcome Evaluation: Parents voice willingness to support treatment plan, including additional necessary tests, and state they are prepared to make decisions with guidance from health care team.

If the gender of a child is unclear, the parents should be told this immediately. If told first that their child is a boy, only to be told 24 hours later that "he" is really a girl, parents can have difficulty accepting this drastic change. During this period when the baby's gender is yet to be determined, avoid calling the baby "it." Rather, say "the baby" or "your child." Explain how sexual organs form in utero and that every child has the potential to be externally female or male.

To promote bonding, help parents understand that their child is otherwise perfect (assuming this is true). As the child grows, additional counseling may be needed to provide education about the congenital defect.

Precocious Puberty

Although development of breasts or pubic hair before age 8 years or menses before age 9 years may be just early maturation, such development has traditionally been considered precocious sexual development (Cesario & Hughes, 2007). Often, such development is limited to breast tissue or pubic hair growth but can proceed to complete secondary sex characteristics, spermatogenesis, or menstrual function. Precocious puberty occurs more often in girls than in boys (Carel & Leger, 2008).

This condition is caused by the early production of gonadotropins by the pituitary gland; gonadotropins stimulate the ovaries or testes to produce sex hormones. Such stimulation can occur because of a pituitary tumor, cyst, or traumatic injury to the third ventricle next to the pituitary gland. It also can occur because of estrogen-secreting cysts or tumors of the ovary or testosterone-secreting cysts of the testes. In rare instances, it occurs because of an estrogen- or testosterone-secreting adrenal tumor. In girls, ingestion of a mother's oral contraceptive pills can initiate menarche-like changes. Overstimulation by the enzyme aromatase which converts androgens into estrogens by a process called aromatization may be yet anther cause.

In children affected by precocious puberty, a tumor must be ruled out. If no physical cause, such as a tumor, is detected, the phenomenon appears to occur only because the *gonadostat* of the hypothalamus (the trigger that begins the development of secondary sex characteristics) was turned on several years too early. It is categorized as either central precocious puberty (gonadotropin-releasing hormone [GnRH]–dependent), in which gonadotrophic hormones are elevated, or as peripheral precocious puberty (Gn-RH–independent), which is basically elevation of sexual steroids produced by the gonads or adrenals.

Assessment

With precocious puberty, children have increased breast and genital development and accelerated skeletal maturation. Girls have menstrual bleeding with little pubic or axillary hair because of still low androgen secretion. Boys have obvious genital growth. The diagnosis of early puberty is confirmed by serum analysis for estrogen or androgen; these will be at adult levels.

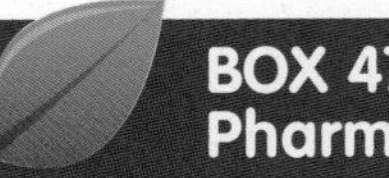

BOX 47.5 ✻ Focus on Pharmacology

Leuprolide acetate (Lupron)

Classification: Leuprolide is a hormonal agent, specifically a luteinizing hormone-releasing hormone (LH-RH) agonist.

Action: Occupies pituitary gonadotropin-releasing hormone (GnRH) receptors, preventing GnRH from functioning (Karch, 2009).

Pregnancy Risk Category: X

Dosage: Daily subcutaneous (SQ) or monthly intramuscular (IM) injection

Possible Adverse Effects: Nausea, vomiting, anorexia, hot flashes, headache, pain at injection site

Nursing Implications

- Administer only with the syringes supplied with the drug.
- Vary injection sites to decrease local irritation.
- Monitor injection sites for bruising and rash.
- Instruct parents in method for proper administration.
- If monthly doses are prescribed, assist parents with preparing a realistic schedule for administration. Encourage the use of a calendar for accurate timing.

Therapeutic Management

A synthetic analog to GnRH is available as leuprolide acetate (Lupron) (Box 47.5). Administration of this analog desensitizes GnRH receptors, making stimulation by GnRH ineffective and halts sexual maturation at the point to which it has advanced (Nebesio & Eugster, 2007). The preparation is administered subcutaneously every day. After it is discontinued at age 12 or 13 years, puberty progresses normally. Therapy may also include use of aromatase inhibitors, which are able to block the enzyme aromatase and therefore decrease signs of estrogen effects (Shulman et al., 2008).

Nursing Diagnoses and Related Interventions

Nursing Diagnosis: Disturbed body image related to precocious puberty

Outcome Evaluation: Child voices an understanding of what is happening and does not evidence excessive shyness or reluctance to interact with peers.

Children who develop precociously may have difficulty interacting with peers because they appear so different from other members of their age group. Parents may worry about children becoming sexually active, particularly about girls becoming pregnant. Both parents and children need reassurance that, after reaching the age of normal puberty, the child will maintain normal growth and development.

Parents must also understand that the child is fully fertile and able to inseminate or conceive when early puberty occurs. Oral contraceptives are not advisable for girls this young, because the increased load of estrogen hastens the closing of epiphyseal lines of long bones too early, possibly stunting the child's growth permanently.

Parents may need to be reminded that, although their child appears to be much older, the changes are only in sexual characteristics. Household tasks, responsibility, and expectations must be geared to the child's chronologic age, not to outward appearance.

Delayed Puberty

Secondary sex characteristics normally are present by age 14 years in girls and 15 years in boys. Delayed puberty, as the name implies, is the failure of pubertal changes to occur at the usual age. The family history of many children reveals a family tendency for late maturation. If so, the child needs a thorough physical examination to disclose whether some secondary sex characteristics are present or whether endocrine stimulation is beginning.

If girls have not begun to menstruate by age 17 years and pathology has been ruled out, menstrual cycles can be initiated by administering estrogen. Many girls worry considerably about delayed menstruation, but, once reassured that development is merely delayed, they are usually willing to wait for menarche to occur on its own. Similarly, boys who are distressed by their lack of development may receive testosterone supplements to stimulate pubic hair and genital growth.

✔ Checkpoint Question 47.1

Suppose a school-age girl develops precocious puberty. What advice would you give her parents?

a. Excess estrogen causes children to be intersexed or hermaphrodites.
b. Although her sexual appearance is advanced, the girl cannot conceive.
c. Treat the child appropriately for her chronologic, not appearance, age.
d. To not allow the child to eat processed meats, which contain hormones.

REPRODUCTIVE DISORDERS IN MALES

Common reproductive disorders in males include structural alterations in the penis or testes such as phimosis and cryptorchidism, inflammation such as balanoposthitis, and, in adolescents, testicular cancer.

Balanitis (Balanoposthitis)

Balanoposthitis is inflammation of the glans and prepuce of the penis. It is usually caused by poor hygiene and may accompany a urethritis or a regional dermatitis.

Assessment

The prepuce and glans become red and swollen; a purulent discharge may be present. The boy may have difficulty voiding because of crusting at the meatal opening and because acidic urine touching the denuded surface of the glans causes pain (Hsieh, Chang, & Chang, 2007).

Therapeutic Management

Medical treatment involves local application of heat; this can be carried out with warm wet soaks or warm baths. A local antibiotic ointment may be prescribed. If *phimosis* (a tight foreskin) appears to be contributing to the condition, circumcision may be advocated after the inflammation subsides to prevent the condition from recurring.

Although balanoposthitis is painful, a boy may tolerate the discomfort for several days because he is too embarrassed to discuss the problem. He may think it was caused by masturbation (which can contribute to the irritation) or by sexual activity and may be reluctant to seek help for fear of being criticized. He can be reassured that the problem is local and will have no long-range effect. Any discharge should be cultured to rule out an STI such as gonorrhea. On the other hand, in developing countries where balanitis can become chronic because of lack of bathing or shower facilities, it may be associated with the development of penile cancer (Bunker, 2008).

Phimosis and Paraphimosis

Phimosis is the inability to retract the foreskin from the glans of the penis. The foreskin is tight at birth and may even be held fast by adhesions so cannot be retracted in newborns. After a few months, the adhesions dissolve and the foreskin becomes retractable; if it does not, the infant has phimosis. If a foreskin is extremely tight it can interfere with voiding. Balanoposthitis may develop because the foreskin cannot be retracted for cleaning. Circumcision of newborns (discussed in Chapter 18) is no longer routinely advised but is used to relieve phimosis (Johnson et al., 2007). Paraphimosis is the inability to replace the prepuce over the glans once it has been retracted. This is an emergency situation to address before circulation to the glans is impaired (Yigiter, Arda, & Hicsonmez, 2008).

Cryptorchidism

Cryptorchidism is failure of one or both testes to descend from the abdominal cavity into the scrotum (Kollin et al., 2007). Normally, the testes descend into the scrotal sac during months 7 to 9 of intrauterine life. They may descend any time up to 6 months after birth; they rarely descend after that time.

The cause of undescended testes is unclear. It may be associated with caffeine intake during pregnancy (Mongraw-Chaffin et al., 2008). Fibrous bands at the inguinal ring or inadequate length of spermatic vessels may prevent descent. Testes apparently descend because of stimulation by testosterone; hence, it is possible that a lower than normal level of testosterone production prevents descent. About 17% of premature infants and 3% to 4% of full-term infants are born with undescended testes.

Assessment

Early detection of undescended testes is important, because the warmth of the abdominal cavity may inhibit development of the testes, ultimately affecting spermatogenesis. After puberty, sperm production deteriorates rapidly in undescended testes, and the testes may even undergo a malignant change (Walsh et al., 2007). Anchoring the testes in the scrotal sac may not prevent malignancy, but it will allow the boy to perform preventive measures such as testicular self-examination.

It is more common for the right testis to remain undescended than the left one. In approximately 20% of all boys, both testes remain undescended. Some boys may be diagnosed with undescended testes when, in fact, the testes have retracted and have made the palpation assessment difficult.

If the child is supine or the examining room is chilly, the scrotal sac may appear to be empty. Excessive palpation or stroking of the inner thigh may also stimulate the cremasteric reflex and cause retraction. In these instances, testes descend when the child is standing or after a warm bath.

An undescended testis may be at the inguinal ring (true undescended testis) or ectopic (still in the abdomen). Laparoscopy is effective in identifying undescended testes. Because testes arise from the same germ tissue as the kidneys, the kidney function of a child with ectopic testes is usually evaluated. If undescended testes and other factors such as ambiguous genitals pose questions about the child's gender, a *karyotype* may be done to determine true gender.

Therapeutic Management

Because the testes sometimes descend spontaneously during the first year of life, treatment is usually delayed for 6 to 12 months. Boys may be given chorionic gonadotropin hormone for about 5 days to stimulate testicular descent, but this therapy is successful only in approximately 25% of infants (Fitzgerald, 2009).

If necessary, surgery **(orchiopexy)** by laparoscopy by 1 year of age corrects the condition.

Nursing Diagnoses and Related Interventions

If an orchiopexy is scheduled, the focus is on parent and child teaching, preoperative preparation, and postoperative care.

Nursing Diagnosis: Deficient knowledge related to parents' and child's inexperience with surgical procedure and postoperative treatment plan

Outcome Evaluation: Parents (and child, if old enough) accurately describe what will be accomplished by surgery.

Boys who are old enough to understand need good preparation for this type of surgery. Use an anatomically correct picture to point out the exact site at which surgery will be performed. Reassure the boy that the penis itself will not be cut. The child may not voice a fear of mutilation, but you can assume that it exists, especially in preschool children.

During surgery, internal sutures may be inserted to hold the testis in place. Although the child may be discharged from the hospital on the same day, his activity will be limited until approximately the second day after surgery, to ensure that the internal suture line remains intact.

Nursing Diagnosis: Disturbed body image related to change in physical appearance

Outcome Evaluation: Child (if verbal) states that he views self as a whole person and interacts with peers without excessive shyness or hesitancy.

Postoperative evaluation should reveal that the suture line is healing well and that both testes can be palpated in the scrotum. It should also address the boy's feelings about the surgery and the changes in his body. He may need an opportunity to express his fears about mutilation or castration by playing with puppets or dolls after surgery. Even after a repair, boys who had bilateral cryptorchidism may be less fertile as adults. When boys reach puberty, teach them testicular self-examination to assess any early symptoms of malignancy, such as nodules or abnormal growth (see Chapter 34).

Hydrocele

When a testis descends into the scrotum in utero, it is preceded by a fold of tissue, the *processus vaginalis.* Occasionally, fluid collects in this fold. If this occurs, **hydrocele** (the fluid) can be revealed by prenatal ultrasound. At birth, the collection of fluid makes the scrotum of the newborn appear enlarged (Bouhadiba, Godbole, & Marven, 2007). On *transillumination* (the shining of a light through the scrotal sac), the area is illuminated by the water and shines or glows. Ultrasound also can reveal this fluid collection. If the hydrocele is uncomplicated, the fluid will gradually be reabsorbed and no treatment is necessary. The child's parents can be assured that the hydrocele is only excess fluid and that the scrotal enlargement is not caused by an abnormal testis, tumor, or hernia.

A hydrocele may form later in life due to *inguinal hernia* (abdominal contents extruding into the scrotum through the inguinal ring, with accompanying fluid). If this happens, the hernia must be repaired for the hydrocele to be reabsorbed (see Chapter 45). Injection of a drug to decrease fluid production (*sclerotherapy*) may also be effective.

Varicocele

A **varicocele** is abnormal dilation of the veins of the spermatic cord (Fig. 47.1). It is important to identify varicoceles in adolescents because although it may not cause a difference, the increased heat and congestion in the testicles could be a cause of subfertility (Zampieri et al., 2007). No treatment is necessary unless fertility becomes a concern, at which time the varicocele can be surgically removed. The adolescent may report some local tenderness and edema for a few days after surgery. Edema can be minimized by applying ice for the first few hours postoperatively.

Testicular Torsion

Testicular torsion (twisting of the spermatic cord) is a surgical emergency. Although it can be present in newborns, it occurs most frequently during early adolescence (Brown-Guttovz, 2007). Less than normal testicular support apparently allows the spermatic cord to twist. Testicular torsion

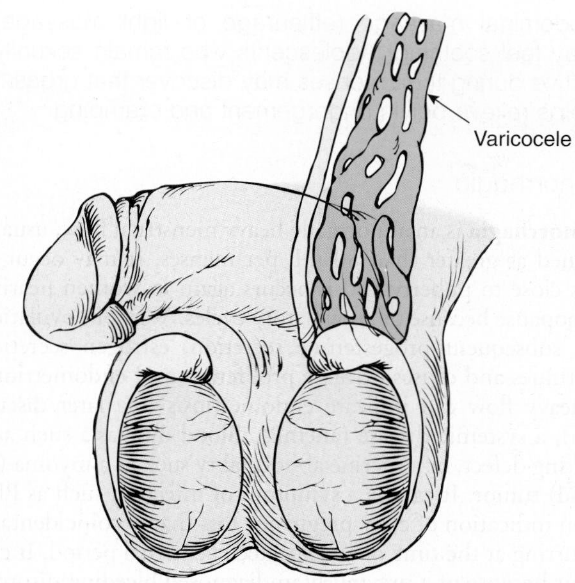

FIGURE 47.1 A varicocele. Identifying varicocele in adolescent males is important because the condition may be associated with subfertility.

usually results from a sports activity. The boy experiences severe scrotal pain and perhaps nausea and vomiting from the severity of the pain. The testis feels tender to palpation, and edema begins to develop. If the condition is not recognized promptly (within 4 hours), irreversible change in the testis can occur from lack of circulation to the organ. Boys need to be educated about the phenomenon so that they report symptoms promptly. The torsion can be reduced manually under ultrasound guidance (Park et al., 2007). Laparoscopic surgery, however, is usually necessary to reduce the torsion and re-establish circulation.

Testicular Cancer

Testicular cancer is rare (only 1% of all malignancies). It usually occurs between ages 15 and 35 years, often in association with cryptorchidism (Walsh, 2007). Symptoms include painless testicular enlargement and a feeling of heaviness in the scrotum. The disease metastasizes rapidly, leading to abdominal and back pain due to retroperitoneal node extension, weight loss, and general weakness. Human chorionic gonadotropin (hCG) and alpha-fetoprotein (AFP), tumor markers, can be detected in blood serum. **Gynecomastia** (enlargement of the breasts) may arise because of hCG produced by the tumor.

Therapy for testicular malignancy is **orchiectomy** (removal of the testis) followed by radiation or chemotherapy (Einhorn et al., 2007). After surgical removal, a gel-filled prosthesis can be inserted to provide a symmetric appearance to the scrotum. Subfertility in the opposite testis results after radiation therapy. For some patients, "sperm banking," or preserving frozen sperm before the procedure, may be presented as an option for future family planning.

Teaching males to perform testicular self-examination for early cancer detection is important to help them detect symptoms at an early point (see Chapter 34).

REPRODUCTIVE DISORDERS IN FEMALES

The most frequent reproductive disorders in females involve vaginal or menstrual irregularities. Other disorders are caused by structural alterations of the reproductive organs such as imperforate hymen, by pelvic inflammatory disease (PID), or infections caused by STIs.

Menstrual Disorders

Because menstruation is an ongoing process throughout half of a woman's life, it affects her self-image significantly. An irregularity such as painful cycles can exert a major influence on daily activities.

Menstrual disorders fall into two categories: (a) menstruation that is painful or uncomfortable and (b) infrequent or too-frequent cycles.

Mittelschmerz

Some women experience abdominal pain during ovulation from the release of accompanying prostaglandins. Pain may also be caused by a drop or two of follicular fluid or blood that spills into the abdominal cavity. This pain, called **mittelschmerz,** can range from a few sharp cramps to several hours of discomfort. It is typically felt on one side of the abdomen (near an ovary) and may be accompanied by scant vaginal spotting.

An advantage of mittelschmerz is that it clearly marks ovulation. If pain is felt in the right lower quadrant, it can be differentiated from appendicitis by the lack of associated symptoms such as nausea, vomiting, fever, abdominal guarding, and rebound tenderness as well as by its occurrence in the menstrual cycle. Usually mittelschmerz is of limited discomfort. It can be relieved by a mild analgesic such as acetaminophen.

Dysmenorrhea

Dysmenorrhea is painful menstruation. For generations, it was thought to be mainly psychological, needing no treatment other than reassurance that it was a normal phenomenon and something women should endure. Today, it is known that the pain is caused by the release of prostaglandins in response to tissue destruction during the ischemic phase of the menstrual cycle (Harel, 2007). Prostaglandin release causes smooth muscle contraction and pain in the uterus.

Dysmenorrhea can also be a preliminary symptom of an underlying illness such as PID, uterine myomas (tumors), or endometriosis (abnormal formation of endometrial tissue).

Assessment. During the first year or two of menstruation, dysmenorrhea rarely occurs, because early menstrual cycles are usually **anovulatory** (without ovulation). As ovulation begins, typical menstrual discomfort also begins. Dysmenorrhea can be categorized as mild (no interference with normal activities), moderate (some interference), or severe (interference with the majority of everyday activities). As many as 80% of adolescents have some discomfort with menstruation; in approximately 10%, the discomfort seriously interferes with daily living (Rapkin & Howe, 2007).

Dysmenorrhea is *primary* if it occurs in the absence of organic disease; it is *secondary* if it occurs as a result of organic disease. Symptoms may begin with a "bloated" feeling and light cramping 24 hours before menstrual flow. Pain is mainly noticed, however, when the flow begins. Colicky (sharp) pain is superimposed on a dull, nagging pain across the lower abdomen. Accompanying this is an "aching, pulling" sensation of the vulva and inner thighs. Some adolescents have mild diarrhea with the abdominal cramping. Mild breast tenderness, abdominal distention, nausea and vomiting, headache, and facial flushing may also be present.

Therapeutic Management. Painful symptoms can usually be controlled by an analgesic such as acetylsalicylic acid (aspirin) or ibuprofen (Advil, Motrin). Acetylsalicylic acid (aspirin) works well as an analgesic for dysmenorrhea because it is a mild prostaglandin inhibitor. Although adolescents are usually advised not to take aspirin because of its link to Reye's syndrome, girls may take it safely at the beginning of a menstrual period as long as they do not have additional flulike symptoms. Ibuprofen is a stronger prostaglandin inhibitor and relieves more severe menstrual pain. Naproxen sodium (Aleve) is also effective. Be certain that girls know not to take these drugs on an empty stomach, because they can be extremely irritating to gastric mucosa. Low-dose oral contraceptives to prevent ovulation may also be effective if pregnancy is not desired. One disadvantage of this therapy is the possible adverse effects of long-term estrogen administration. Adolescents may choose to be prescribed long-acting oral contraceptives so that they have menstrual periods only every 3 months (Pavone & Burke, 2007). Several alternative therapies such as imagery and transcutaneous electrical nerve stimulation (TENS) are also effective to relieve menstrual pain (Proctor et al., 2009)

Nursing Diagnoses and Related Interventions

Nursing Diagnosis: Pain related to dysmenorrhea

Outcome Evaluation: Client states that she has some control over pain through nonpharmacologic or pharmacologic methods.

Several nonpharmacologic solutions such as yoga and exercise may help relieve dysmenorrhea (Hall, 2009). Decreasing sodium intake for a few days before an expected menstrual flow, by omitting salty foods such as potato chips, pretzels, ham, and other luncheon meats and by not adding salt to foods, may help reduce "bloated" feelings. Abdominal breathing (breathing in and out slowly, allowing the abdominal wall to rise with each inhalation) may also be helpful. Applying heat to the abdomen with a heating pad or taking a hot shower or tub bath may relax muscle tension and relieve pain. Acupressure, although short lived, might also be of help (Jun et al., 2007). Caution young girls not to apply heat to their abdomen for abdominal pain until their menstrual flow begins; if the pain results from an inflamed appendix, heat can cause rupture of the appendix and life-threatening peritonitis. Resting may help to relieve vulvar pain; abdominal massage (effleurage or light massage) may feel soothing. Adolescents who remain sexually active during their menses may discover that orgasm helps relieve pelvic engorgement and cramping.

Menorrhagia

Menorrhagia is an abnormally heavy menstrual flow, usually defined as greater than 80 mL per menses. It may occur in girls close to puberty and it occurs again in women nearing menopause because of anovulatory cycles. Without ovulation and subsequent progesterone secretion, estrogen secretion continues and causes extreme proliferation of endometrium. A heavy flow can indicate endometriosis (see later discussion), a systemic disease (anemia), blood dyscrasia such as a clotting defect, or a uterine abnormality such as a myoma (fibroid) tumor. It can be a symptom of infection such as PID or an indication of early pregnancy loss that is coincidentally occurring at the time of an expected menstrual period. It can occur because of a previously undiagnosed bleeding disorder such as von Willebrand disease (Aydinok, Egemen, & Balkan, 2007). It can occur from breakthrough bleeding from an oral contraceptive (Grover, 2007). There is often an unusual amount of flow in girls using intrauterine devices (IUDs). With oral contraceptives, the flow is often light; for this reason, it may seem alarmingly heavy once pills are discontinued, when this is just a return of the adolescent's normal flow.

Assessment and Therapy. It is difficult to determine when a menstrual flow is abnormally heavy, but one method is to ask the girl how long it takes her to saturate a sanitary napkin or tampon. A sanitary napkin or tampon holds approximately 25 mL of fluid. If a pad or tampon is saturated in less than 1 hour, the flow is considered heavier than usual.

Determining the cause of menorrhagia is important, because it can lead to anemia from excessive iron loss. If anemia occurs, iron supplements may be necessary to achieve sufficient hemoglobin formation. The adolescent who is losing excessive blood because of anovulatory cycles may be prescribed progesterone during the luteal phase to prevent proliferative growth during this phase of the cycle; if the ability to conceive is unimportant, adolescents may be prescribed a low-dose oral contraceptive or GnRH inhibitor to decrease the flow.

Metrorrhagia

Metrorrhagia is bleeding between menstrual periods (Gray & Emans, 2007). This is normal in some adolescents who have spotting at the time of ovulation ("mittelstaining"). It may also occur in teenagers taking oral contraceptives (breakthrough bleeding) during the first 3 or 4 months of use. Additionally, vaginal irritation from infection can cause midcycle spotting. Spotting may also represent a temporarily low level of progesterone production and endometrial sloughing (dysfunctional uterine bleeding or a luteal phase defect), although this condition most often occurs near the end of the reproductive years.

If metrorrhagia occurs for more than one menstrual cycle in a teenager who is not taking oral contraceptives, she should be referred to her primary care provider for examination, because abnormal vaginal bleeding can be an early sign of uterine carcinoma or ovarian cysts.

Endometriosis

Endometriosis is the abnormal growth of extrauterine endometrial cells, often in the cul-de-sac of the peritoneal cavity or on the uterine ligaments or ovaries. This abnormal tissue results from excessive endometrial production and a reflux of blood and tissue through the fallopian tubes during a menstrual flow. As many as 25% of women in the United States have endometriosis, and as many as 50% of adolescents seen for dysmenorrhea have endometriosis (Yates & Vlahos, 2007).

The condition tends to occur most often in white nulliparous women, but there is also a familial tendency. Daughters of women with endometriosis may develop symptoms of dysmenorrhea early in life. They may want to consider having children before overgrowth of the endometrium becomes so extensive that it interferes with conception.

The excessive production of endometrial tissue may be related to a deficient immunologic response. In many women, it appears to be related to excess estrogen production or a failed luteal menstrual phase. Many women with endometriosis do not ovulate or ovulate irregularly. Therefore, endometriosis is discovered at a higher than usual rate among women undergoing subfertility testing (Vercellini et al., 2007).

In these women, estrogen secretion continues through the cycle rather than becoming secondary to progesterone late in the cycle, as happens with normal ovulation. The resulting proliferation of tissue forces the blood back into the fallopian tubes.

Endometriosis causes dysmenorrhea when the abnormal tissue responds to estrogen and progesterone stimulation by swelling and then sloughing its layers in the same manner as the uterine lining. This causes inflammation of surrounding tissue in the abdominal cavity and an even greater release of prostaglandins. Abnormal tissue in the pelvic cul-de-sac can cause *dyspareunia* (painful coitus) because it puts pressure on the posterior vagina. Subfertility may result if the fallopian tubes become immobilized and blocked by tissue implants or adhesions, preventing peristaltic motion and transport of ova (see Chapter 8).

Assessment. Pelvic examination may show that the uterus is displaced by tender, fixed, palpable nodules. Nodules in the cul-de-sac or on an ovary also may be palpable. If the endometriosis is minimal, the girl will not experience related symptoms. If the condition is moderate or extensive, she may experience extreme dysmenorrhea or dyspareunia.

Therapeutic Management. Treatment for endometriosis can be medical or surgical, depending on the extent of the condition. Estrogen/progesterone-based oral contraceptives may stimulate implant regression as the tissue sloughs under the influence of the progesterone. Danazol (Danocrine), a synthetic androgen, can be prescribed to help shrink the abnormal tissue. Administration of a GnRH agonist, such as leuprolide acetate (Lupron), can reduce hormone stimulation and cause the same effect (see Box 47.5). Laparotomy with excision by laser surgery is the most effective measure, but, because this is a highly invasive procedure, a course of conservative medical treatment may be tried first.

Amenorrhea

Amenorrhea, or absence of a menstrual flow, strongly suggests pregnancy but is by no means definitive, because it can also result from tension, anxiety, fatigue, chronic illness, extreme dieting, or strenuous exercise. Amenorrhea as a sign of pregnancy is discussed in Chapter 10. Competitive swimmers, long-distance runners (50 to 75 miles weekly), and ballet dancers notice that intensive training causes their periods to become scant and irregular. This appears to be associated with their low ratio of body fat to body muscle, which leads to excessive secretion of prolactin. An elevation in prolactin causes a decrease in GnRH from the hypothalamus, followed by declines in follicle-stimulating hormone (FSH), follicular development, and estrogen secretion. Menstrual cycles usually return to normal within 3 months after discontinuation of strenuous training and conditioning.

Adolescents who wish to maintain a normal cycle while training for a sports event may take bromocriptine (Parlodel), which can reduce high prolactin levels by acting on the hypothalamus and initiating menstruation each month. Many adolescents, however, view the absence of menstrual periods as a benefit during sports training. If a menstrual flow is delayed and pregnancy is suspected, bromocriptine should be discontinued, because it is potentially teratogenic.

Amenorrhea also occurs among females who diet excessively, partially as a natural defense mechanism to limit ovulation and as a means of conserving body fluid. Adolescents with *anorexia nervosa* or *bulimia* (eating disorders described in Chapter 54) often develop amenorrhea after approximately 3 months of excessive dieting or binging and dieting; as in athletes, this is caused by an increase in prolactin.

Premenstrual Dysphoric Disorder

Premenstrual dysphoric disorder (PDD) is a condition that occurs in the luteal phase of the menstrual cycle and is relieved by the onset of menses. It has both behavioral and physiologic symptoms. Because of the variety of possible symptoms, as many as 30% of women experience some degree of PDD; at least 3% experience a cluster of symptoms that include anxiety, fatigue, abdominal bloating, headache, appetite disturbance, irritability, and depression. For about 3% of women, these symptoms are so extreme that they are incapacitating (Stotland, 2007).

The cause of PDD is unproved but, contrary to previous beliefs, it must be due to more than a drop in progesterone just before menses. A syndrome similar to PDD can occur in women after tubal ligation; a decrease in the blood supply to the ovary apparently results in decreased luteal function. In some women, a vitamin B–complex deficiency may lead to estrogen excess, causing an abnormal ratio of estrogen to progesterone; other related causes may be poor renal clearance leading to water retention, or hypoglycemia leading to a surge of epinephrine and low calcium levels and interference with serotonin synthesis.

Symptoms of PDD vary from cycle to cycle and throughout life. Therapy is aimed at correcting specific symptoms (Yonkers, O'Brien, & Eriksson, 2008).

Adolescents who think they have PDD should keep a diary of when symptoms occur. If they are aware of recurring patterns that indicate PDD, they will be better able to recognize the cause. They should be certain their diet is high in vitamins and calcium and low in salt. Agents that suppress ovarian function, such as oral contraceptives or the GnRH agonist leuprolide, may be prescribed. If depression is a major symptom, an antidepressant such as buspirone

(BuSpar) can be helpful. Paroxetine (Paxil) is a selective serotonin reuptake inhibitor that is specifically designed for PDD therapy in adults. Antidepressants are prescribed with caution in adolescents, however, because they may be responsible for an increase in suicidal behavior (Kaplan & Love-Osborne, 2007).

Additional Reproductive Disorders in Females

Female Circumcision

Female circumcision is incision and removal of the clitoris (Elnashar & Abdelhady, 2007). There is no medical reason or advantage of the procedure but it is regarded as a coming of age ritual in some cultures. Although not a custom practiced in the United States, adolescents or women who have had this done in another country may be seen in gynecology settings. They may have difficulty with childbirth because of vulvar scarring and contraction.

Imperforate Hymen

The *hymen* is the membranous ring of tissue that partly obstructs the vaginal opening. An *imperforate hymen* totally occludes the vagina, preventing the escape of vaginal secretions and menstrual blood (Dane et al., 2007).

Before menarche, the child with an imperforate hymen usually has no symptoms. With onset of menstruation, the menstrual flow is obstructed. It builds up in the vagina, causing increased pressure in the vagina and uterus and eventually abdominal pain. Palpation of the abdomen reveals a lower abdominal mass. On vaginal examination, an intact, bulging hymen is evident.

The treatment is surgical incision or removal of the hymenal tissue. The girl may have local pain after the incision, which can be relieved by a mild analgesic and warm baths.

Careful explanation of this condition will help the girl understand that it will not interfere with sexual relations or future childbearing. Because most girls of early menstrual age have scant knowledge of anatomy, pictures of the reproductive tract help to explain that this is a local and minor problem.

Toxic Shock Syndrome

Toxic shock syndrome (TSS) is an infection that usually is caused by toxin-producing strains of *Staphylococcus aureus* organisms. Although organisms can enter the body by other means, they typically enter through vaginal walls that have been damaged by the insertion of tampons at the time of a menstrual period (Kansal et al., 2007).

Assessment. The symptoms of TSS are described in Box 47.6. Some women have mild diarrhea as a normal accompaniment to dysmenorrhea, but any female who develops fever with diarrhea and vomiting during a menstrual period should suspect TSS.

Therapeutic Management. Women or adolescents with suspected TSS need a careful vaginal examination and removal of any tampon particles, as well as cervical and vaginal cultures for *S. aureus.* Iodine douches may reduce the number of organisms present vaginally. *S. aureus* is usually resistant to penicillin but not to penicillinase-resistant antibiotics such as the cephalosporins, oxacillins, or clindamycins, so these are prescribed. Intravenous fluid therapy to restore circulating fluid volume and increase blood pressure, or vasopressors such as dopamine (Intropin), may be necessary to increase the blood pressure. Osmotic therapy to shift fluid back into the intravascular circulation may be necessary to prevent renal and cardiac failure. Recovery occurs in 7 to 10 days; fatigue and weakness may remain for months afterward.

The rate of TSS recurrence is 28% to 64%, usually within 2 months after the first attack. Recurrence probably happens because the organism is not completely eliminated from the body. Therefore, be certain that girls complete their entire antibiotic prescription. Be sure to educate girls about menstrual hygiene (Box 47.7). All girls should use the lowest-absorbency tampon appropriate for their individual flow. Girls who develop TSS should avoid tampon use in the future.

BOX 47.6 ✻ Symptoms of Toxic Shock Syndrome*

- Temperature greater than 102° F (38.9° C)
- Vomiting and diarrhea
- A macular (sunburn-like) rash that desquamates on palms and soles 1 to 2 weeks after illness
- Severe hypotension (systolic pressure less than 90 mm Hg)
- Shock, leading to poor organ perfusion
- Impaired renal function with elevated blood urea nitrogen or creatinine at least twice the upper limit of normal
- Severe muscle pain or creatine phosphokinase at least twice the upper limit of normal
- Hyperemia of mucous membrane
- Impaired liver function with increased total bilirubin and increased serum glutamate oxaloacetate transaminase (aspartate aminotransferase) at twice the upper limit of normal
- Decreased platelet count
- Central nervous system symptoms of disorientation, confusion, severe headache

*Three symptoms must be present for diagnosis.

Vulvovaginitis

In **vulvovaginitis,** inflammation of the vulva or vagina is accompanied by pain, odor, pruritus, and a vaginal discharge (Hansen et al., 2007). Vaginal bleeding may be present. This condition may occur in a girl of any age, but it tends to be more frequent as girls reach puberty. The change to adult pH and the presence of vaginal secretions make the vagina more receptive to infections. Box 47.8 discusses common measures to relieve discomfort.

Preschool and School-Age Children. Vaginal discharge may occur before menarche, but bleeding is rarely seen at this age. If bleeding is present, its cause must be determined. Cystitis can cause urethral bleeding; scratching due to rectal pruritus can lead to rectal bleeding. The cause of true vaginal bleeding in this early age group is usually either irritation caused by an inserted foreign object in the vagina, infestation of

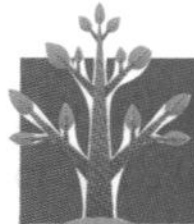

BOX 47.7 ✻ Focus on Family Teaching

Preventing Toxic Shock Syndrome

Q. Navi says to you, "I've heard so much about a disease called toxic shock syndrome. What is it and how can I make sure that I don't get it?"

A. Although toxic shock syndrome can occur for other reasons, it most often occurs during a menstrual flow when tampons are used. The following are measures to help prevent the syndrome:

- Use only tampons made of natural materials such as cotton, not synthetics such as cellulose or polyester, and avoid high-absorbency tampons.
- Change tampons at least every 4 hours during use.
- Alternate use of tampons with use of sanitary pads.
- Avoid handling the portion of the tampon that will be inserted vaginally.
- Do not use tampons near the end of a menstrual flow, when excessive vaginal dryness can result from scant flow.
- Do not insert more than one tampon at a time, to avoid abrasions and to keep the vaginal walls from becoming too dry.
- Avoid deodorant tampons, deodorant sanitary pads, and feminine hygiene sprays; these products can irritate the vulvar–vaginal lining.
- If fever, vomiting, or diarrhea occurs during a menstrual period, discontinue tampon use and immediately consult a health care provider, because these are symptoms of TSS.
- Anyone who has had one episode of TSS is well advised not to use tampons again, or at least not until two vaginal cultures for *Staphylococcus aureus*, the bacteria usually responsible for TSS, are negative.

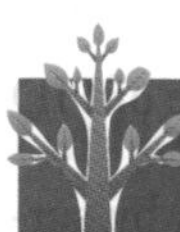

BOX 47.8 ✻ Focus on Family Teaching

Tips for Relieving the Pain of Vulvitis

Q. Navi says to you, "I have a vaginal discharge. The itching is awful. Is there anything I can do to relieve it?"

A. Here are some tips that might help:

- Wash the area twice a day with mild, nonperfumed soap and water, and pat dry. This removes secretions and decreases irritation. Wash and dry from front to back, to prevent spreading rectal contamination forward.
- Take sitz baths or apply warm, moist compresses three times a day to soothe the area and keep it free of irritating drainage.
- After drying the cleansed area, apply cornstarch for comfort and to absorb residual moisture.
- Avoid bubble baths and feminine hygiene sprays, because the ingredients may cause additional local irritation or contribute to urinary tract infections.
- Take acetaminophen (Tylenol) every 4 hours. Acetaminophen is an analgesic that relieves pain and reduces itching, a mild pain sensation.
- Avoid scratching, which may increase abrasions and introduce a secondary infection. Instead, apply a cold compress to relieve the itching sensation.
- Wear cotton underwear, which allows air to circulate and moisture to evaporate, rather than nylon or silk, which prevents air circulation and retains moisture.
- Sleep without underwear.
- Use an anesthetic spray or hydrocortisone cream only as prescribed.
- Carefully follow instructions from your health care provider about caring for a vaginal infection; only after the infection subsides will the vulvitis clear.

pinworms, or *vaginitis* (vaginal inflammation or infection). Sexual abuse must be investigated as a cause of any bleeding, tenderness, or infection (see Chapter 55). Precocious puberty must also be ruled out.

Treatment for pinworm is discussed in Chapter 43. If there is a foreign body in the vagina, it obviously should be removed. Vaginal examination is necessary, first to locate the object and then to confirm that it has been fully removed. This may be difficult for girls to accept, because vaginal manipulation and stretching can be painful. Use of a small speculum helps reduce the pain. A local antibiotic ointment or warm bath may be ordered to reduce accompanying infection and inflammation afterward. Sometimes, daily bubble baths cause vulvar irritation. This can be quickly remedied by discontinuing the bubble baths; irritation from such compounds can lead not only to local discomfort but to urinary tract infection as well (Schilling McCann et al., 2007).

A few preschool or school-age children develop a vaginitis due to *Streptococcus* or to *Escherichia coli* introduced from the anus by improper perineal care after voiding or bowel movements. A tight hymen then traps the microorganisms in the vagina and leads to infection. The girl needs to be reminded to wipe from front to back after voiding or bowel movements.

Adolescents. As a girl enters puberty, she may notice a slight vaginal discharge caused by increased vaginal secretions. She can be reassured that this is normal. To keep from developing vulvar irritation, caution girls to wear cotton underpants rather than nylon (so that moisture is absorbed better) and to dry the vulva thoroughly after bathing or swimming.

Some girls develop vulvar irritation after using personal hygiene sprays or douches. These products are unnecessary so should be discontinued. Good hygiene can be achieved by daily washing and frequent changing of tampons or sanitary pads during menstruation. This will prevent chafing or stasis of menstrual blood and help prevent irritation and excessive odor.

Pelvic Inflammatory Disease

Pelvic inflammatory disease (PID) is infection of the pelvic organs: the uterus, fallopian tubes, ovaries, and their supporting structures. The infection can extend to cause pelvic peritonitis. Although sexual transmission accounts for approximately 75% of all instances of PID (gonorrheal and chlamydial organisms are frequently responsible), infections from other causes such as *E. coli* or *Streptococcus* are beginning to occur more frequently and may be as severe.

other strenuous activity. This discomfort can be relieved with a simple analgesic, such as acetaminophen (Tylenol), or warm compresses, avoidance of trauma, and firm bra support. The formation of fibrocystic lesions may be increased in some women with the use of methylxanthines found in caffeine, theophylline, and theobromine. Avoiding foods such as coffee, cola drinks, tea, chocolate, some toffee candy, and medications such as aspirin compound or Excedrin that contain caffeine reduces pain. Discontinuing smoking can also decrease the occurrence of fibrocystic lesions. Decreased sodium intake or short-term use of a mild diuretic just before menses can reduce fluid retention.

If these measures do not decrease the fibrocystic symptoms, cysts may be aspirated under a local anesthetic by injection of a thin sterile needle attached to a small syringe. This procedure not only reduces the size of the cyst but also provides fluid for biopsy (Chaiwun & Thorner, 2007).

Danazol (Danocrine), a synthetic androgen, may help reduce the symptoms by suppressing estrogen formation in the ovaries (Giuliano, 2009). In addition to being physically distressed, women with fibrocystic breasts may worry that each lump could be malignant. They can be reassured that the disease itself does not lead to breast carcinoma. Breast carcinoma does occur in women with fibrocystic breast disease, however, and it may even metastasize before a woman seeks health consultation, if she assumes that all her breast lesions are benign. Therefore, in addition to a yearly breast examination, women need an annual breast ultrasound, which involves no x-ray exposure and can efficiently locate fluid-filled cysts.

Fibroadenoma

Fibroadenomas are tumors that consist of both fibrotic and glandular components and occur in response to estrogen stimulation. The tumors may increase in size during adolescence, during pregnancy and lactation, or when a woman takes an estrogen source such as an oral contraceptive (Chang & McGrath, 2007).

Unlike fibrocystic lesions, fibroadenomas are round and well delineated, feeling firmer and more rubbery than fluid-filled cysts. Occasionally, they calcify and feel extremely hard. They are typically painless and freely movable and tend not to cause skin retraction. Like fibrocystic lesions, they do not become malignant.

Such tumors can be surgically excised so that a woman no longer has to worry about them. Because the incision is small, it leaves little scarring at the site.

✓ Checkpoint Question 47.2

Navi, 15, asks if she is too young to have breast augmentation. What advice would you give her?

a. She will not be able to breastfeed after augmentation.
b. Breast implants cause a high degree of fibrocystic disease.
c. Breast growth may not be fully complete at age 15.
d. Implants increase the risk of breast cancer and so are dangerous.

Mastitis

Mastitis is inflammation or infection of the breast (Betzold, 2007). As this usually occurs as a complication of breastfeeding, it is discussed in Chapter 25.

SEXUALLY TRANSMITTED INFECTIONS

Sexually transmitted infections (STIs) are diseases that are spread through sexual contact with an infected partner. They range in severity from easily treated infections, such as trichomoniasis, to human immunodeficiency virus (HIV) infection, which, despite advances in therapy, is life-threatening. If these diseases are discovered in young children, the possibility of sexual abuse has to be considered (Reading & Rannan-Eliya, 2007). STIs may be spread among women having sex with women or men having sex with men (Evans et al., 2007). Male circumcision does not appear to reduce the spread (Box 47.9).

Abstinence or condom use provides the best protection against STIs. Additional measures are voiding immediately after coitus, washing the genitals well with soap and water, and choosing sexual partners who are at low risk for infection (avoiding persons who are intravenous drug users or those with multiple sexual partners). Educating adolescents about safer sex practices, including the need for condom use (see Chapter 5) and the importance of health screening for these disorders, is an important nursing responsibility. STIs are becoming more difficult to treat because the causative organisms are becoming more and more resistant to antibiotics. Always reinforce the fact that little immunity develops from STIs, so such diseases can be contracted repeatedly. In most instances, an infected partner should also be treated or the disease can recur from cross-infection. Treatment of most STIs begins with determining the causative organism so that the appropriate antimicrobial or antifungal agent can be prescribed.

BOX 47.9 ✻ Focus on Evidence-Based Practice

Does male circumcision help prevent sexually transmitted infections?

It is often theorized that male circumcision might help reduce the possibility of contracting or transmitting sexually transmitted infections. To discover if this is true, researchers enrolled a cohort of children born in 1972–1973 and asked them about their sexual experiences at 21, 26, and 32 years of age. Of the 499 men studied, 201 (40.3%) had been circumcised. The circumcised and uncircumcised groups differed little in socioeconomic characteristics and sexual behavior. Overall, up to age 32 years, the incidence rates for all STIs were not statistically significantly different—23.4 and 24.4 per 1000 person-years for the uncircumcised and circumcised men, respectively.

Based on the above, if an adolescent asks you if circumcision would reduce his risk for gonorrhea, how would you advise him?

Source: Dickson, N. P., et al. (2008). Circumcision and risk of sexually transmitted infections in a birth cohort. *Journal of Pediatrics, 152*(3), 383–387.

Pregnancy and Sexually Transmitted Infections

Several STIs such as syphilis are known to be teratogenic. All of them are suspected of being a causative factor of preterm birth. Chapter 26 discusses care for the newborn affected by these diseases.

Candidiasis

Candidiasis is a vaginal infection spread by the fungus *Candida,* an organism that thrives on glycogen. Candidiasis is so common that as many as 90% of women will have it sometime in their life. As many as 40% of sexually active females have asymptomatic candidal vaginal infections; this rate rises even higher during pregnancy, when high estrogen levels lead to glycogen levels that produce a favorable environment for fungal growth. Because oral contraceptives produce a pseudopregnancy state, women using oral contraceptives also have frequent vaginal candidal infections. When a woman is being treated with an antibiotic (which destroys normal vaginal flora and lets fungal organisms grow more readily), she is also particularly susceptible to this infection. Incidence is also strongly associated with immune suppression and diabetes mellitus, because hyperglycemia provides a glucose-rich environment for candidal growth (Tanner & Alexander, 2007).

Assessment

Because of the scant mucus production in the period before menses, symptoms may be most acute at this time. An adolescent will notice vulvar and vaginal reddening, burning and itching, and even bleeding from hairline fissures. The vagina sometimes shows white "patches" on the walls. The patches are adherent and cannot be scraped away without bleeding. A thick, cream cheese–like discharge can usually be observed at the vaginal introitus. There may be pain on coitus or on tampon insertion. Candidal infections may also be present at other body sites, such as the oral cavity or a moist area such as the umbilicus. In immunosuppressed individuals, it can become systemic (Blyth, Palasanthiran, & O'Brien, 2007).

Candidal infections are diagnosed by removing a sample of the discharge from the vaginal wall and placing it on a glass slide; three or four drops of a 20% potassium hydroxide (KOH) solution are then added, and the mixture is protected by a coverslip. Under a microscope, typical fungal hyphae indicate the presence of *Candida* organisms (Table 47.1). An at-home test kit (Vagasil Screening Kit) is available that gives results instantly. A woman inserts a pH wand into her vagina and in a few seconds compares the color of the swab to a pH color chart. If the reading is above 5.0, it suggests that she may have a bacterial infection and should see a doctor. A normal pH level of 4.5 plus itching and/or burning, unusual discharge, or a yeasty odor suggests a yeast infection and it would be all right for her to use an over-the-counter treatment.

Therapeutic Management

Therapy for candidal infections includes vaginal suppositories or cream applications of antifungal preparations such as miconazole (Monistat) or clotrimazole (Lotrimin), once a day for 3 to 7 days. Oral fluconazole (Diflucan) can be ad-

TABLE 47.1 ✻ Common Vulvovaginal Infections

Causative Agent	Symptoms	Common Therapy
Candida	Vulvar reddening and pruritus; thick, white, cheeselike vaginal discharge	Nystatin or miconazole (Monistat) suppositories or fluconazole (Diflucan) orally; bathing with dilute sodium bicarbonate solution may relieve pruritus
Trichomonas	Thin, irritating, frothy, gray-green discharge; strong, putrid odor; itching	Metronidazole (Flagyl) orally; douching with weak vinegar solution to reduce pruritus
Herpesvirus type II	Painful pinpoint vesicles on an erythematous base with a watery vaginal discharge possible; voiding may be irritating and painful	Bathing with dilute sodium bicarbonate solution, applying lubricating jelly to lesions or an oral analgesic such as aspirin may be necessary for pain relief; topically applied acyclovir (Zovirax) helps heal lesions
Gardnerella	Edema and reddening of vulva, milky gray discharge, fishlike odor	Metronidazole (Flagyl) or clindamycin
Chlamydia trachomatis	Watery, gray-white vaginal discharge, vulvar itching	Tetracycline or doxycycline; erythromycin during pregnancy
Neisseria gonorrhoeae	Possibly symptomless; may have profuse yellow-green vaginal discharge	Ceftriaxone and doxycycline; oral amoxicillin
Enterobius vermicularis (pinworm)	Rectal pruritus, especially on rising in the morning	Oral administration of an anthelmintic, such as mebendazole (Vermox)
Treponema pallidum (syphilis)	Painless ulcer on vulva or vagina	Benzathine penicillin, administered intramuscularly
Streptococcus	Vaginitis, vulvar itching; edema and reddening of vulva	Antibiotic (e.g., amoxicillin)
Foreign body	Vaginal discharge; odor	Removal of foreign body during pelvic examination

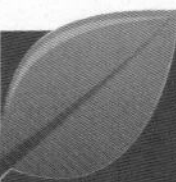

BOX 47.10 * Focus on Pharmacology

Fluconazole (Diflucan)
Classification: Antifungal agent
Action: Increases fungal cell wall permeability, thereby exerting fungicidal or fungostatic action (Karch, 2009)
Pregnancy Risk Category: C
Dosage: 150 mg orally as a single dose
Possible Adverse Effects: Nausea, vomiting; diarrhea, abdominal pain, headache

Nursing Implications

- Instruct the adolescent that this drug is given as a one-time single dose.
- Teach the adolescent about safer sex measures and hygiene practices to help prevent reinfection after therapy.
- Urge the adolescent to watch for signs and symptoms of possible reinfection and report them to the primary care provider.

ministered as a one-time oral dose (Box 47.10). Antifungal creams are purchased over-the-counter. Teach women to insert these or antifungal suppositories at bedtime so the drug does not drain from the vagina immediately afterward. During the day, a girl may want to wear a sanitary pad to avoid staining from vaginal discharge. Treatment should not be interrupted until it is complete, even during a menstrual period. Because miconazole and clotrimazole are available without prescription, be certain that adolescents know how to differentiate a candidal infection from other infections or to consult a health care provider for assistance and treatment if they are not sure.

If a girl has frequent candidal infections, her urine should be tested for glucose to rule out diabetes mellitus. If she is using an oral contraceptive, she might be counseled to use another contraceptive method. If an adolescent is sexually active, treatment of the male partner may be necessary to break a reinfection cycle.

Pregnancy and Candidiasis. Candidiasis occurs more frequently during pregnancy than usual because of the increased estrogen level present during pregnancy, which causes the vaginal pH to be less acidic. It occurs frequently in pregnant women with gestational diabetes and in women with HIV infection. Women with repeated infections should have their urine tested for glucose to determine whether gestational diabetes is present.

Both miconazole (Monistat) for 7 days or a single dose of oral fluconazole (Diflucan) are approved for use during pregnancy. Treating the infection during pregnancy is important not only because the profuse vaginal discharge and pruritus can be uncomfortable but if the infection is still present in the vagina at the time of childbirth, it may cause a candidal infection, or thrush, in the newborn (see Chapter 43). Caution pregnant women to call their primary health care provider before using an over-the-counter product to double-check the product is safe to use during pregnancy and so that her primary care provider can know that a vaginal infection is occurring because, although it is not well established, antifungal use during the first trimester of pregnancy is possibly associated with hypoplastic heart disease in newborns (Carter et al., 2008).

What if... Navi tells you she feels safe from contracting an STI because she knows she is up to date with her immunizations? How would you counsel her?

Trichomoniasis

Trichomonas vaginalis is a single-cell protozoan that is spread by coitus and affects between 3% and 13% of adult men and women in the United States (Sutton et al., 2007). The incubation period is 4 to 20 days.

Assessment

With a trichomonal infection, females notice vaginal irritation and a frothy white or grayish-green vaginal discharge. The frothiness of the discharge is an important typical finding. The upper vagina is reddened and may have pinpoint petechiae. Extreme vulvar itching is present. By contrast, males with the same infection rarely report any symptoms.

The infection is diagnosed by microscopic examination of a sample of the vaginal discharge after it is combined with lactated Ringer's or normal saline solution. Trichomonads typically appear as rounded, mobile structures. Be aware that *Trichomonas* infections cause such inflammatory changes in the cervix or vagina that a Pap test taken during this time may be misinterpreted as showing abnormal tissue.

Therapeutic Management

Oral metronidazole (Flagyl) eradicates trichomonal infections. Treatment with Flagyl and use of condoms by sexual partners help prevent recurrence of *Trichomonas* in both parties. Because the drug interacts with alcohol to cause acute nausea and vomiting, advise women not to drink alcoholic beverages during the course of treatment.

Pregnancy and Trichomoniasis. Trichomoniasis infections are associated with preterm labor, premature rupture of membranes, and postcesarean infection (Hay & Czeizel, 2007). The drug of choice is single-dose oral metronidazole. Metronidazole was once thought to be teratogenic but is now considered to be safe in either early or late pregnancy (Karch, 2009).

Bacterial Vaginosis

Bacterial vaginosis is the invasion of an organism such as *Gardnerella vaginalis.* This organism thrives in the vagina, a body area with a reduced oxygen level. When the infection is present vaginal discharge appears milk-white to gray and has a fishlike odor. Pruritus can be intense. Microscopic examination of the discharge in normal saline solution shows gram-negative rods adhering to vaginal epithelial cells, which are termed *clue cells* (Burke & Rogers, 2007).

The treatment is oral or vaginal metronidazole for 7 days; the woman's sexual partners should also be treated to prevent recurrence of the infection.

Pregnancy and Bacterial Vaginosis

The treatment during pregnancy is oral metronidazole or clindamycin for 7 days. Untreated *G. vaginalis* infections are associated with amniotic fluid infections and, perhaps, preterm labor as well as premature rupture of the membranes (Soper, 2007).

Chlamydia trachomatis Infection

Chlamydia trachomatis infections have become the most common bacterial cause of STI in the United States (Wendel & Zenilman, 2007). Symptoms include a heavy, grayish-white discharge and vulvar itching. The incubation period is 1 to 5 weeks. Diagnosis is made by culture of the organism. Therapy is oral doxycycline or tetracycline for 7 days or azithromycin in a single dose. Because it has become so common, most public health departments require that cases now be reported. Long-term effects of chlamydial infections are PID, possibly leading to subfertility. Because there is a strong association between gonorrhea and *Chlamydia*, if a chlamydial infection is documented, women are usually tested for gonorrhea as well. Home tests are available for both *Chlamydia* and gonorrhea. Encouraging women to use these could increase the number of infections treated yearly (Cook et al., 2007).

Pregnancy and *Chlamydia*

Screening for *Chlamydia* via a vaginal culture is usually done during a woman's first prenatal visit. If a woman has multiple sexual partners, screening may be repeated again in the third trimester. Doxycycline (Vibramycin), the therapy for nonpregnant women, is contraindicated during pregnancy because of possible fetal long-bone deformities; azithromycin (Zithromax) or amoxicillin (Amoxil) is used instead (Tanner & Alexander, 2007). A woman's partner also should be treated to prevent her from becoming reinfected. As with nonpregnant women, because there is a strong association between gonorrhea and *Chlamydia*, if a chlamydial infection is documented, women are usually tested for gonorrhea as well.

Chlamydial infections must be treated during pregnancy because they are associated with premature rupture of the membranes, preterm labor, and endometritis in the postpartum period. An infant who is born while a chlamydial infection is present can suffer conjunctivitis or pneumonia after birth (Hahn & Giunta, 2007) (see Chapters 50 and 40).

Human Papillomavirus

The human papillomavirus (HPV) causes fibrous tissue overgrowth (sometime called genital warts) on the external vulva, vagina, or cervix (condyloma acuminatum). At first, lesions appear as discrete papillary structures; they then spread, enlarge, and coalesce to form large, cauliflower-like lesions. The infection may be present in as many as 10% to 30% of women and is most common in women who have multiple sexual partners (Howley & Lowy, 2007). Therapy for such lesions is aimed at dissolving the lesions and also ending any secondary infection present. Small growths may be removed by applying podophyllin (Podofin). Large lesions may be removed by laser therapy, cryocautery, or knife excision. With cryocautery, edema at the site is evident immediately; lesions become gangrenous, and sloughing occurs in 7 days. Healing will be complete in 4 to 6 weeks with only slight depigmentation at the site. Sitz baths and a lidocaine cream may be soothing during the healing period. Children (both male and female) with HPV infections should be further investigated for sexual abuse (Reading & Rannan-Eliya, 2007). HPV infections are serious because they are associated with the development of cervical cancer later in life (Soper, 2007). Women who have had one episode of infection should be conscientious about having yearly Pap tests for the rest of their lives. The vaccine, Gardasil, is recommended to be routinely administered to early teenage girls in three doses. A second dose is 2 months after the first dose and the third dose is 6 months after the first dose. Immunizing young teenage girls against HPV infection should reduce not only the incidence of HPV infections in the future but the rate of cervical cancer as well (Deglin & Villarand, 2009).

Pregnancy and Human Papillomavirus Infection

HPV lesions tend to increase in size during pregnancy because of the high vascular flow in the pelvic area. They may become secondarily ulcerated and infected; when this occurs, a foul vulvar odor may develop.

Podophyllum is contraindicated during pregnancy because of possible toxic effects on the fetus. Trichloroacetic acid (TCA) or bichloroacetic acid (BCA) applied to the lesions weekly may be effective and can be used during pregnancy. Women who do not find the lesions bothersome may choose to leave them in place during pregnancy and have them removed during the postpartum period.

The presence of vulvar lesions appears to have no effect on the fetus during pregnancy, but if they are present at the time of birth and so large that they obstruct the birth canal, a cesarean birth may be scheduled.

Herpes Genitalis (Herpes Simplex Type 2)

Genital herpes is caused by *herpesvirus hominis* type 2 (also called herpes simplex virus type 2, or HSV-2). This is one of four similar herpesviruses: cytomegalovirus, Epstein-Barr, varicella-zoster, and herpes types 1 and 2. Genital herpes occurs in epidemic proportions in the United States, and its incidence appears to be growing yearly (Wendel & Zenilman, 2007). Unlike most other STIs, although the virus can be contained, there is no known cure. The disease involves a lifelong process, therefore, and, although it is not a precursor to cervical cancer, women with cervical cancer tend to have more antibodies against herpes genitalis than others or probably have been exposed to the virus more than others. The virus is spread by skin-to-skin contact, entering through a break in the skin or mucous membrane. In the newborn, the virus can be systemic or even fatal (see Chapter 26).

Assessment

Herpes is diagnosed by culture of the lesion secretion from its location on the vulva, vagina, cervix, or penis or by isolation of HSV antibodies in serum. The incubation period is 3 to 14 days. On first contact, extensive primary lesions originate as a group of pinpoint vesicles on an erythematous base. Within a few days, the vesicles ulcerate and become moist, painful, draining, open lesions. An adolescent may have accompanying flulike symptoms with increased temperature;

vaginal lesions may cause a profuse discharge. Pain is intense on contact with clothing or acidic urine.

After the primary stage that lasts approximately 1 week, lesions heal but the virus lingers in a latent form, affecting the sensory nerve ganglia. The condition will flare up and become an active infection during illness, just prior to menstruation, fever, overexposure to sunlight, or stress. A secondary response usually produces only local lesions rather than systemic symptoms.

Therapeutic Management

Acyclovir (Zovirax) is an example of an antiviral that controls the virus by interfering with deoxyribonucleic acid reproduction and decreasing symptoms (Watkins, 2008). The drug is available as a topical ointment. If applying this to a client, be certain to protect yourself with a finger cot or glove so that you do not contract the virus or absorb the drug. Sitz baths three times a day may be helpful to reduce discomfort. An emollient (A&D Ointment) can also reduce discomfort, but its moisture tends to prolong the active period of the lesions. Topical imiquimod (Aldara) or Foscarnet (Foscavir) may be prescribed for resistant lesions.

Condoms (male or female) help prevent the spread of herpes among sexual partners. Valacyclovir (Valtrex) may be prescribed as a preventive measure to help limit the disease spread. Because of the possible association with cervical cancer, any female with genital herpes should have yearly Pap tests for the rest of her life.

People with herpes may have difficulty establishing sexual relationships for fear of infecting a partner. Because herpes is communicated only by direct contact, infected people need to inform their partners when they have any active lesions and avoid sexual contact or use a condom to decrease the danger of spreading the virus.

Pregnancy and Herpes Simplex Virus Type 2 Infection. If a woman contracts a herpes type 2 infection during pregnancy, herpes can be transmitted across the placenta to cause congenital infection in the newborn. If a woman has primary or secondary active lesions in the vagina or on the vulva at the time of birth, herpes infection can be transmitted to the newborn at birth. When infection in the newborn occurs, congenital herpes, a severe systemic infection that is often fatal, can result (see Chapter 26). To help avoid transmission, women with active lesions are scheduled for cesarean birth. If no lesions are present, a vaginal birth is preferable (Tanner & Alexander, 2007).

Diagnosis of the disorder is made by the appearance of the lesions and on the results of a Pap smear and an enzyme-linked immunosorbent assay (ELISA). The drug of choice for the treatment of herpes infection is the same as for nonpregnant women (acyclovir [Zovirax] or valacyclovir [Valtrex]) (Karch, 2009). Women can reduce the pain of the lesions by taking sitz baths or applying warm, moist tea bags to the area.

Hepatitis B and Hepatitis C

Both hepatitis B and hepatitis C can be spread by semen as well as blood and therefore are considered STIs. These are discussed in Chapter 45, with other forms of hepatitis. Because hepatitis B can be spread by sexual intercourse, adolescents who did not receive immunization against this as an infant need immunization against this updated.

Gonorrhea

Gonorrhea is transmitted by *Neisseria gonorrhoeae,* a gram-positive diplococcus that thrives on columnar transitional epithelium of the mucous membrane. Symptoms begin after a 2- to 7-day incubation period. In males, they include *urethritis* (pain on urination and frequency of urination) and a urethral discharge. Without treatment, the infection may spread to the testes, scarring the tubules and causing permanent sterility. Untreated, the infection is easily spread among sexual partners. It often occurs concurrently with chlamydial infection (Wendel & Zenilman, 2007).

Although symptoms of gonorrhea in females are not as visible, there may be a slight yellowish vaginal discharge. Bartholin's glands may become inflamed and painful. If left untreated, the infection may spread to pelvic organs, most notably the fallopian tubes (PID). Tubal scarring can result in permanent sterility. In both males and females, untreated gonorrhea can lead to arthritis or heart disease from systemic involvement.

Assessment

A urine culture for the gonococcal bacillus, in addition to vaginal and urethral cultures, should be obtained from all children with vulvovaginitis or a urethral discharge. In males, a first voiding may reveal gonococci if a midstream urine specimen is inconclusive.

Therapeutic Management

Although gonorrhea has traditionally been treated with amoxicillin and probenecid, the incidence of penicillinase-producing strains has made this traditional therapy ineffective. Therefore, oral cefixime (Suprax) or intramuscular ceftriaxone (Rocephin) plus oral doxycycline (Vibramycin) for 7 days is the current recommended therapy. This treatment regimen is effective for both gonorrhea and *Chlamydia.* Sexual partners should receive the same treatment.

Approximately 24 hours after treatment, gonorrhea is no longer infectious. Approximately 7 days after treatment, a client should return for a follow-up culture to verify that the disease has been completely eradicated (few adolescents take this precaution). Adolescents are usually assessed for syphilis along with the gonorrheal culture, although the dose of ceftriaxone and doxycycline is also effective treatment for syphilis. Most states require that gonorrhea be reported to the health department; adolescents are asked to name sexual contacts.

Nursing Diagnoses and Related Interventions

Nursing Diagnosis: Anxiety related to having contracted a reportable STI

Outcome Evaluation: Adolescent voices confidence in ability to cope with this problem and demonstrates understanding of the illness, the treatment regimen, and future prevention options.

People who seek treatment for an STI need to believe that they can trust health care personnel and reveal information without fear of criticism. Assure the adolescent of absolute confidentiality in naming sexual contacts. Without being told who put them at risk, these people can then be notified by a health department investigator that they have been exposed to a particular STI. This vital information helps prevent further spread of the disease.

Reassure people that the treatment is not prolonged and as simple as taking medication. This is an insidious disease, and, even though no symptoms are apparent, it can have disastrous long-term effects if left untreated (see Focus on Nursing Care Planning Box 47.11).

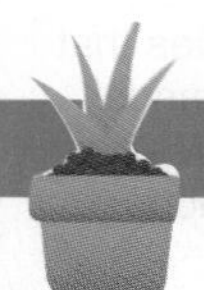

BOX 47.11 ✻ Focus on Nursing Care Planning

A Multidisciplinary Care Map for an Adolescent With Gonorrhea

Navi is a 15-year-old female high school student you meet at a pediatric clinic. She describes intense vulvar irritation from a yellowish vaginal discharge.

Family Assessment ✻ Navi lives with mother in studio apartment in inner city. Mother works at home as a freelance journalist. Mother describes finances as "good."

Client Assessment ✻ Well-proportioned female; sexual maturity Tanner stage 3. Has not had first menstrual period as yet. Sexually active for approximately 1 year with same partner. "He doesn't use a condom anymore because he's only dating me."

Vulva reddened and excoriated. Yellow-green discharge noted at vaginal introitus. Reddened areas noted on vaginal walls. One dose of intramuscular (IM) ceftriaxone (Rocephin), plus oral doxycycline (Vibramycin) for 7 days, is prescribed. She asks, "How did I get this? From my boyfriend? Does he need to be treated too?"

Nursing Diagnosis ✻ Deficient knowledge related to cause and treatment of sexually transmitted infection (STI).

Outcome Evaluation ✻ Adolescent states that she understands cause of STI; reports boyfriend has an appointment within 48 hours for evaluation.

Team Member Responsible	Assessment	Intervention	Rationale	Expected Outcome
		Activities of Daily Living		
Nurse	Assess whether adolescent understands importance of washing hands well after using bathroom and avoiding sexual intercourse during treatment.	Discuss how disease can be spread to other body parts by unclean hands.	Gonorrhea is particularly hazardous, because it can cause eye infections with corneal scarring.	Adolescent states that she will take precautions to wash hands well; she will avoid sexual intercourse until repeat culture.
		Consultations		
Nurse	Confer with STI counselor.	Meet with STI counselor regarding procedure for STI contacts.	Gonorrhea is a reportable disease.	STI counselor assumes responsibility for securing STI contacts.
		Procedures/Medications		
Nurse	Assess whether adolescent has experience with taking medicine. Assess if a reminder sheet would be helpful.	Administer ceftriaxone (Rocephin) IM; give instructions for oral doxycycline (Vibramycin) for 7 days as prescribed.	The antibiotics chosen for gonorrhea treatment are also effective against *Chlamydia*, which is frequently associated with gonorrhea.	Adolescent accepts IM injection; states she understands importance of taking oral antibiotic for full 7 days.
Nurse	Assess whether adolescent has access to a bathtub at home.	Recommend the use of sitz baths before and after school.	Sitz baths are soothing and help keep the area free of irritating discharge.	Adolescent states she will use home bathtub for sitz baths twice daily.

(continued)

BOX 47.11 * Focus on Nursing Care Planning (continued)

Nutrition				
Not applicable	NA	NA	NA	NA
Patient/Family Education				
Nurse	Assess whether adolescent is aware that STIs are spread through sexual intercourse.	Teach adolescent about the cause, means of spread, and treatment for gonorrhea.	Adolescent must be aware of STIs to prevent them in the future.	Adolescent states that she understands STIs are spread by sexual relations.
Psychosocial/Spiritual/Emotional Needs				
Nurse	Assess intensity of adolescent's pruritus or pain from vulvitis on a scale of 1 to 10.	Discuss the use of acetaminophen or ibuprofen for pain and pruritus as prescribed.	Acetaminophen and ibuprofen are effective analgesics for mild pain and itching.	Adolescent describes correct dosage of analgesics and states intention to use them.
STI counselor	Assess whether adolescent has had sexual contacts other than current boyfriend.	Ask adolescent to name any additional sexual contacts.	Sexual contacts need to be notified so they also can receive treatment.	Adolescent names any other sexual contacts; possibility of rape or abuse is ruled out.
Discharge Planning				
Nurse	Assess whether adolescent understands that she must ask boyfriend to use a condom for sexual relations.	Discuss the possibility that, because he contracted an STI, his relationship with her may not be monogamous. Explain that nonmonogamous relations make condom use even more important, not less important.	STI was spread to her by a sexual contact.	Adolescent states she will be more conscientious about insisting boyfriend use a condom.
Nurse	Assess whether child or parent has any questions about disease or therapy.	Schedule child for a return appointment in 1 week for reculture.	A repeat culture will reveal whether antibiotic therapy has been effective.	Child and parent state that they understand the importance of a repeat culture and will keep return appointment.

Pregnancy and Gonorrhea. Gonorrhea is associated with spontaneous miscarriage, preterm birth, and endometritis in the postpartum period. Pregnant women cannot be administered doxycycline because it has the potential to be teratogenic. Instead, they are prescribed amoxicillin or azithromycin. It is important that gonorrhea be identified and treated during pregnancy because if the infection is present at the time of birth, it can cause a severe eye infection that can lead to blindness in the newborn (ophthalmia neonatorum; see Chapter 26) (Heidary & Kazlas, 2008).

Syphilis

Syphilis is a systemic disease caused by the spirochete *Treponema pallidum.* It is transmitted by sexual contact with a person who has an active spirochete-containing lesion (Tanner & Alexander, 2007). Like gonorrhea and *Chlamydia*, it must be reported to public health departments.

After an incubation period of 10 to 90 days, a typical lesion appears, usually on the genitalia (penis or labia) or on the mouth, lips, or rectal area from oral–genital or genital–anal contact. The lesion (termed a *chancre*) is a deep ulcer and is usually painless despite its size. Swollen lymph nodes may be present but these are unlikely to be noticed by the affected person. A lesion in the vagina may not be detected. Without treatment, a chancre lasts approximately 6 weeks and then fades.

Approximately 2 to 4 weeks after the chancre disappears, a generalized, macular, copper-colored rash appears. Unlike many other rashes, it affects the soles and the palms. A serologic test for syphilis yields a positive result at this time. There may be secondary symptoms of generalized illness, such as low-grade fever. With or without treatment, this stage of syphilis also fades.

The next stage is a latency period that may last from only a few years to several decades. The only indication of the disease is the serologic test, which continues to yield a positive result.

The final stage of syphilis is a destructive neurologic disease that involves major body organs such as the heart and the nervous system. Typical symptoms are blindness; paralysis; severe, crippling neurologic deformities; mental confusion; slurred speech; and lack of coordination. This third stage must be identified before the disease becomes fatal.

Assessment

Syphilis is diagnosed by recognition of the various symptoms of the three stages and by serologic serum tests, usually the Venereal Disease Research Laboratory test (VDRL), the automated reagin test (ART), the rapid plasma reagin test (RPR), or the fluorescent treponemal antibody–absorption test (FTA-ABS).

Therapeutic Management

Benzathine penicillin G, given intramuscularly in two sites, is effective therapy. For the adolescent who is sensitive to penicillin, either oral erythromycin or tetracycline can be given for 10 to 15 days. Sexual partners are treated in the same way as the person with the active infection. Therapy effectively arrests the disease at whatever stage it has reached. After therapy, adolescents may experience a sudden episode of hypotension, fever, tachycardia, and muscle aches. This is called a Jarisch-Herxheimer reaction and is caused by the sudden destruction of spirochetes. The reaction lasts about 24 hours and then fades (Wendel & Zenilman, 2007). Because syphilis can be treated so easily, one would think it would be easy to eradicate. In reality, however, because the primary chancre is painless, many people are either unaware of it or choose to ignore it, thereby transmitting the disease to unsuspecting partners. Adolescents, in particular, need accurate information about syphilis to become aware of the symptoms and safer sex practices. They should believe that they can report the disease to health care personnel and can name sexual contacts without fear of being criticized (Leung-Chen, 2008).

Pregnancy and Syphilis. Early in pregnancy (before week 18), the placenta appears to provide some protection against syphilis. After this time, however, the spirochete crosses the placenta freely and may be responsible for spontaneous miscarriage, preterm labor, stillbirth, or congenital anomalies in the newborn (see Chapter 12). All pregnant women are screened for syphilis at a first prenatal visit with a VDRL, ART, or FTA-ABS antibody reaction test. Those who have multiple sexual partners are tested again at about week 36 of pregnancy. In some institutions, women are screened again at the beginning of labor and newborns are screened for congenital syphilis by a cord blood sample. One injection of benzathine penicillin G is the drug of choice for the treatment of syphilis during pregnancy the same as for those who are not pregnant.

If a woman does contract syphilis during pregnancy and it is untreated, a congenital form of the disease can occur in the newborn as the spirochete crosses the placenta readily in the last four months of pregnancy. Severely infected infants will be stillborn; others, less infected, are born with congenital anomalies. Moist lesions of the infant (the cord and nasal secretions) are generally infectious.

Unlike adults, the infant does not develop a chancre but about a week after birth, will develop a typical copper-colored rash, most prominent over the face, soles of feet, and palms of hands. Bullous lesions on the palms and soles may also develop. The infant's nose may show a severe rhinitis (snuffles). Radiography of the long bones reveal changes of epiphyseal lines at about 1 to 3 months of age. By 5 to 6 months, these bone changes may no longer be visible and so may be missed.

When the child's permanent teeth erupt at 5 or 6 years of age, they may be pegged or notched (Hutchinson's teeth). This is most noticeable in the upper central incisors. All teeth tend to be of poor quality and decay easily. If the disease remains untreated, interstitial keratitis, an inflammatory reaction of the cornea that can result in scarring and blindness, may develop when the child is school age. As the disease progresses further, it may become tertiary or lead to severe neurologic symptoms.

Infants born to a woman with a positive VDRL are given a course of penicillin at birth. FTA-ABS is a sensitive, specific test for IgM antibodies against syphilis and may be helpful for diagnosis in the newborn.

Group B Streptococcal Infection

Although streptococcus B infection is a less publicized disease than STIs such as herpes type 2 or gonorrhea, it may actually occur at a higher incidence than those diseases. It produces few symptoms. For a pregnant adolescent, however, consequences can be urinary tract infection (UTI), intra-amniotic infection, perhaps preterm birth, and postpartum endometritis.

Pregnant women are screened for streptococcus B at 35 to 38 weeks of pregnancy. This screening is important, because approximately 40% to 70% of neonates whose mothers have an active infection at the time of birth will become infected from placental transfer or from direct contact with the organisms. Infected neonates may develop severe pneumonia, sepsis, respiratory distress syndrome, or meningitis (Heath & Schuchat, 2007). These effects on the neonate are discussed in Chapter 26.

A broad-spectrum penicillin such as ampicillin is the treatment of choice. Women who experience rupture of membranes at less than 37 weeks of pregnancy and so have not yet been screened may be treated with intravenous ampicillin to reduce the risk of spreading the infection to the newborn.

Human Immunodeficiency Virus (HIV)

HIV is carried by semen as well as other body fluids, so infection with this virus is considered an STI. Invasion of the virus is discussed with other immune disorders in Chapter 42.

✓Checkpoint Question 47.3

Candidal vaginal infections can occur as an opportunistic infection when adolescents are prescribed antibiotics. What are the typical symptoms of a candidal vaginal infection?

a. Yellow pinpoint vaginal lesions.
b. Pruritic reddened vaginal walls.
c. White, cheeselike vaginal discharge.
d. Vaginal atrophy with final scarring.

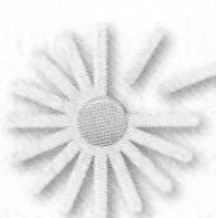

Key Points for Review

- Children who are born with a reproductive tract disorder frequently adjust well when young. They may need counseling at puberty or when they become aware of the impact of their disorder on sexual functioning or their ability to reproduce.
- The cause of ambiguous genitalia is unknown but may be related to the level of testosterone produced in utero. The true gender of children is established by a karyotype of chromosomes.
- The development of breast or pubic hair before age 8 years or menses before age 9 years is considered precocious sexual development. Children may be treated with a synthetic analog of gonadotropin-releasing hormone to reduce development. Without effective support, such children are at high risk for disturbed body image.
- Delayed puberty is the failure to develop secondary sex characteristics by the age of 17 years. Girls may be administered estrogen to promote development; boys may be administered testosterone.
- Balanoposthitis (inflammation of the glans and prepuce of the penis) and phimosis (constricted foreskin) occur in boys. Phimosis can be treated with circumcision.
- Cryptorchidism is failure of one or both testes to descend during intrauterine life. The condition is surgically corrected to prevent subfertility and to detect testicular cancer later in life.
- Testicular cancer is rare but tends to occur in young men. Boys need to be taught testicular self-examination for early detection.
- Dysmenorrhea, or painful menstruation, occurs frequently in adolescent girls. Therapy is the use of a prostaglandin inhibitor such as ibuprofen.
- Untreated endometriosis (the abnormal growth of extrauterine endometrial tissue) can lead to subfertility later in life. Therapy is administration of a synthetic androgen or gonadotropin-releasing hormone receptor inhibitor or surgery to reduce the size of the abnormal tissue.
- Vulvovaginitis (inflammation of the vulva and vagina) and pelvic inflammatory disease are infections that can occur in adolescents. Therapy to prevent fallopian tube scarring and subfertility later in life is essential. Girls need to be taught, in addition, ways to avoid toxic shock syndrome.
- Conditions such as fibrocystic breast disease can occur in adolescents. Reducing intake of caffeine and sodium can minimize symptoms.
- Sexually transmitted infections (STIs) such as candidiasis, trichomoniasis, *C. trachomatis* infection, genital warts, herpes genitalis, gonorrhea, and syphilis are increasing in incidence in the adolescent population. An important health-teaching area for adolescents is the need to follow safer sex practices.
- STIs such as candidiasis, trichomoniasis, *Chlamydia*, syphilis, herpes type 2, gonorrhea, papilloma, and HIV may occur during pregnancy. These illnesses need to be treated promptly. Women need to use safer sex practices to help prevent these diseases.
- When teaching about STIs, it is important to stress that they do not confer immunity and therefore can be contracted more than once. If an STI occurs in a young child, the potential for child abuse should be investigated.

CRITICAL THINKING EXERCISES

1. Navi is the 15-year-old girl you met at the beginning of the chapter, who was diagnosed as having gonorrhea. She says she is glad she contracted the disease early in life, because now she will never get it again. She also states that she is not sexually active. What health teaching does Navi need to be better informed about her disease? What other follow-up is needed?
2. Navi has almost no breast development and also has not menstruated yet. She asks you if it is time to worry. How would you counsel her?
3. Ryan, the boy whom Navi dates, was born with undescended testes. He had surgery for this condition when he was 2 years old. He is concerned now that he is at high risk for testicular cancer. How would you counsel him?
4. Examine the National Health Goals related to reproductive disorders in children. Most government-sponsored funds for nursing research are allotted based on these goals. What would be a possible research topic to explore pertinent to these goals that would be applicable to Navi's family and also advance evidence-based practice?

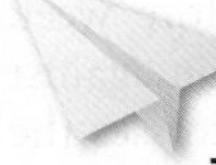

CRITICAL THINKING SCENARIO

Open the accompanying CD-ROM or visit http://thePoint.lww.com and read the Patient Scenario included for this chapter, then answer the questions to

further sharpen your skills and grow more familiar with NCLEX style questions related to reproductive disorders in children. Confirm your answers are correct by reading the rationales.

REFERENCES

Aydinok, Y., Egemen, A., & Balkan, C. (2007). Menorrhagia due to abnormalities of the platelet function: evaluation of two young patients. *Pediatrics International, 49*(1), 106–108.

Betzold, C. M. (2007). An update on the recognition and management of lactational breast inflammation. *Journal of Midwifery and Women's Health, 52*(6), 595–605.

Blyth, C. C., Palasanthiran, P., & O'Brien, T. A. (2007). Antifungal therapy in children with invasive fungal infections: a systematic review. *Pediatrics, 119*(4), 772–784.

Bouhadiba, N., Godbole, P., & Marven, S. (2007). Laparoscopic excision of abdominoscrotal hydrocele. *Journal of Laparoendoscopic and Advanced Surgical Techniques, 17*(5), 701–703.

Brown-Guttovz, H. (2007). Testicular torsion. *Nursing 2007,* 37(10), 72.

Bunker, C. B. (2008). Diseases and disorders of the male genitalia. In K. Wolff, et al. (Eds.). *Fitzpatrick's dermatology in general medicine* (7th ed.). Columbus, OH: McGraw-Hill.

Burke, A. E., & Rogers, L. C. (2007). Nonmalignant vulvovaginal disorders, pelvic inflammatory disease, and chronic pelvic pain. In N. H. Fiebach, et al. (Eds.). *Principles of ambulatory medicine* (7th ed.). Philadelphia: Lippincott Williams & Wilkins.

Carel, J. C., & Leger, J. (2008). Clinical practice. Precocious puberty. *New England Journal of Medicine, 358*(22), 2366–2377.

Carter, T. C., et al. (2008). Antifungal drugs and the risk of selected birth defects. *American Journal of Obstetrics and Gynecology, 198*(2), 191–197.

Cesario, S. K., & Hughes, L. A. (2007). Precocious puberty: a comprehensive review of literature. *JOGNN: Journal of Obstetric, Gynecologic, and Neonatal Nursing, 36*(3), 263–274.

Chaiwun, B., & Thorner, P. (2007). Fine needle aspiration for evaluation of breast masses. *Current Opinion in Obstetrics and Gynecology, 19*(1), 48–55.

Chang, D. S., & McGrath, M. H. (2007). Management of benign tumors of the adolescent breast. *Plastic and Reconstructive Surgery, 120*(1), 13e–19e.

Cook, R. L., et al. (2007). Home screening for sexually transmitted diseases in high-risk young women: randomized controlled trial. *Sexually Transmitted Infections, 83*(4), 286–291.

Dane, C., et al. (2007). Imperforate hymen—a rare cause of abdominal pain: two cases and review of the literature. *Journal of Pediatric and Adolescent Gynecology, 20*(4), 245–247.

Deglin, J. H., & Vallerand, A. H. (2009). *Davis's drug guide for nurses* (11th ed.). Philadelphia: F. A. Davis Company.

Diamantopoulos, S., & Bao, Y. (2007). Gynecomastia and premature thelarche: A guide for practitioners. *Pediatrics in Review, 28*(9), e57–e68.

Dickson, N. P., et al. (2008). Circumcision and risk of sexually transmitted infections in a birth cohort. *Journal of Pediatrics, 152*(3), 383–387.

Einhorn, L. H., et al. (2007). High-dose chemotherapy and stem-cell rescue for metastatic germ-cell tumors. *New England Journal of Medicine, 357*(4), 340–348.

Elnashar, A., & Abdelhady, R. (2007). The impact of female genital cutting on health of newly married women. *International Journal of Gynaecology and Obstetrics, 97*(3), 238–244.

Evans, A. L., et al. (2007). Prevalence of bacterial vaginosis in lesbians and heterosexual women in a community setting. *Sexually Transmitted Infections, 83*(6), 470–475.

Fitzgerald, P. A. (2009). Endocrine disorders. In S. J. McPhee & M. A. Papadakis (Eds.). *Current medical diagnosis and treatment.* Columbus, OH: McGraw-Hill.

Giuliano, A. E. (2009). Breast disorders. In S. J. McPhee & M. A. Papadakis (Eds.). *Current medical diagnosis and treatment.* Columbus, OH: McGraw-Hill.

Gollu, G., et al. (2007). Ambiguous genitalia: an overview of 17 years' experience. *Journal of Pediatric Surgery, 42*(5), 840–844.

Gray, S. H., & Emans, S. J. (2007). Abnormal vaginal bleeding in adolescents. *Pediatrics in Review, 28*(5), 175–182.

Grover, S. (2007). Bleeding disorders and heavy menses in adolescents. *Current Opinion in Obstetrics and Gynecology, 19*(5), 415–419.

Grube, B. J., & Giuliano, A. E. (2007). Benign breast disease. In J. S. Berek (Ed.). *Berek & Novak's obstetrics & gynecology.* Philadelphia: Lippincott Williams & Wilkins.

Hahn, B., & Giunta, Y. P. (2007). Images in emergency medicine. *Chlamydia* conjunctivitis. *Annals of Emergency Medicine, 49*(6), 823–831.

Hall, J. E. (2009). Menstrual disorders and pelvic pain. In A. S. Fauci, (Ed.). *Harrison's principles of internal medicine* (17th ed.). Columbus, OH: McGraw-Hill.

Hansen, M. T., et al. (2007). *Streptococcus pyogenes* pharyngeal colonization resulting in recurrent, prepubertal vulvovaginitis. *Journal of Pediatric and Adolescent Gynecology, 20*(5), 315–317.

Harel, Z. (2007). Dysmenorrhea in adolescents and young adults: etiology and management. *Journal of Pediatric and Adolescent Gynecology, 19*(6), 363–371.

Hay, P., & Czeizel, A. E. (2007). Asymptomatic trichomonas and candida colonization and pregnancy outcome. *Best Practice and Research in Clinical Obstetrics and Gynaecology, 21*(3), 403–409.

Heath, P. T., & Schuchat, A. (2007). Perinatal group B streptococcal disease. *Best Practice and Research in Clinical Obstetrics and Gynaecology, 21*(3), 411–424.

Heidary, G., & Kazlas, M. (2008). Pediatric ophthalmology. In D. Pavan-Langston (Ed.). *Manual of ocular diagnosis and therapy.* Philadelphia: Lippincott Williams & Wilkins.

Howley, P. M., & Lowy, D. R. (2007). Papillomaviruses. In D. M. Knipe & P. M. Howley (Eds.). *Fields virology.* Philadelphia: Lippincott Williams & Wilkins.

Hsieh, T. F., Chang, C. H., & Chang, S. S. (2007). Foreskin development before adolescence in 2149 schoolboys. *International Journal of Urology, 13*(7), 968–970.

Johnson, T. R., et al. (2007). Why and how a Department of Obstetrics and Gynecology stopped doing routine newborn male circumcision. *Obstetrics and Gynecology, 109*(3), 750–752.

Jun, E. M., et al. (2007). Effects of acupressure on dysmenorrhea and skin temperature changes in college students: A non-randomized controlled trial. *International Journal of Nursing Studies, 44*(6), 973–981.

Kansal, R., et al. (2007). Structural and functional properties of antibodies to the superantigen TSST-1 and their relationship to menstrual toxic shock syndrome. *Journal of Clinical Immunology, 27*(3), 327–338.

Kaplan, D. W., & Love-Osborne, K. (2007). Adolescence. In W. W. Hay, et al. (Eds.). *Current pediatric diagnosis and treatment* (18th ed.). Columbus, OH: McGraw-Hill.

Karch, A. M. (2009). *Lippincott's nursing drug guide.* Philadelphia: Lippincott Williams & Wilkins.

Kast, R. E. (2007). Some fibrocystic breast change may be caused by sexually transmitted *H. pylori* during oral nipple contact: supporting literature and case report of resolution after gut *H. pylori* eradication treatment. *Medical Hypotheses, 68*(5), 1041–1046.

Kollin, C., et al. (2007). Surgical treatment of unilaterally undescended testes: testicular growth after randomization to orchiopexy at age 9 months or 3 years. *Journal of Urology, 178*(4.2), 1589–1593.

Leung-Chen, P. (2008). Syphilis makes another comeback: nurses can help in containing transmission, above all through education. *American Journal of Nursing, 108*(2), 28–31.

Majeski, J. (2007). Shoulder restraint injury of the female breast. *International Surgery, 92*(2), 99–102.

Mongraw-Chaffin, M. L., et al. (2008). Maternal smoking, alcohol consumption, and caffeine consumption during pregnancy in relation to a son's risk of persistent cryptorchidism. *American Journal of Epidemiology, 167*(3), 257–261.

Nebesio, T. D., & Eugster, E. A. (2007). Current concepts in normal and abnormal puberty. *Current Problems in Pediatric and Adolescent Health Care, 37*(2), 50–72.

Oztas, M. O., & Gurer, M. A. (2007). Dermoscopic features of accessory nipples. *International Journal of Dermatology, 46*(10), 1067–1068.

Park, S. J., et al. (2007). Manual reduction of torsion of an intrascrotal appendage under ultrasonographic monitoring. *Journal of Ultrasound in Medicine, 26*(3), 293–299.

Pavone, M. E., & Burke, A. (2007). Fertility control: contraception, sterilization and abortion. In K. B. Fortner, et al. (Eds). *The Johns Hopkins manual of gynecology and obstetrics.* Philadelphia: Lippincott Williams & Wilkins.

Proctor, M. L., et al. (2009). Transcutaneous electrical nerve stimulation and acupuncture for primary dysmenorrhoea. *Cochrane Database of Systematic Reviews, 2009*(1), (CD002123).

Rapkin, A. J., & Howe, C. N. (2007). Pelvic pain and dysmenorrhea. In J. S. Berek, (Ed.). *Berek & Novak's obstetrics and gynecology.* Philadelphia: Lippincott Williams & Wilkins.

Reading, R., & Rannan-Eliya, Y. (2007). Evidence for sexual transmission of genital herpes in children. *Archives of Disease in Childhood, 92*(7), 608–613.

Schilling McCann, J. A., et al. (Eds.). (2007). *Professional guide to signs and symptoms.* Philadelphia: Lippincott Williams & Wilkins.

Shulman, D. I., et al. (2008). Use of aromatase inhibitors in children and adolescents with disorders of growth and adolescent development. *Pediatrics, 121*(4), e975–e983.

Sigurdson, L., et al. (2007). Symptoms and related severity experienced by women with breast hypertrophy. *Plastic and Reconstructive Surgery, 119*(2), 481–486.

Soper, D. E. (2007). Genitourinary infections and sexually transmitted diseases. In J. S. Berek, (Ed.). *Berek & Novak's obstetrics and gynecology.* Philadelphia: Lippincott Williams & Wilkins.

Stotland, N. L. (2007). Common psychiatric problems. In J. S. Berek, (Ed.). *Berek & Novak's obstetrics and gynecology.* Philadelphia: Lippincott Williams & Wilkins.

Sutton, M., et al. (2007). The prevalence of *Trichomonas vaginalis* infection among reproductive-age women in the United States, 2001-2004. *Clinical Infectious Diseases, 45*(10), 1319–1326.

Tanner, E., & Alexander, C. J. (2007). Infections of the genital tract. In K. B. Fortner, et al. (Eds.). *The Johns Hopkins manual of gynecology and obstetrics.* Philadelphia: Lippincott Williams & Wilkins.

Vercellini, P., et al. (2007). Association between endometriosis stage, lesion type, patient characteristics and severity of pelvic pain symptoms: a multivariate analysis of over 1000 patients. *Human Reproduction, 22*(1), 266–271.

Verkauskas, G., et al. (2007). The long-term followup of 33 cases of true hermaphroditism: a 40-year experience with conservative gonadal surgery. *Journal of Urology, 177*(2), 726–731.

Walsh, T. J., et al. (2007). Prepubertal orchiopexy for cryptorchidism may be associated with lower risk of testicular cancer. *Journal of Urology, 178*(4.1), 1440–1446.

Watkins, J. (2008). Genital herpes simplex. *Practice Nursing, 19*(6), 296–297.

Wendel, K. A., & Zenilman, J. M. (2007). Sexually transmitted diseases. In N. H. Fiebach, et al. (Eds.). *Principles of ambulatory medicine* (7th ed.). Philadelphia: Lippincott Williams & Wilkins.

Yates, M., & Vlahos, N. (2007). Endometriosis. In K. B. Fortner, et al. (Eds.). *The Johns Hopkins manual of gynecology and obstetrics.* Philadelphia: Lippincott Williams & Wilkins.

Yonkers, K. A., O'Brien, P. M., & Eriksson, E. (2008). Premenstrual syndrome. *Lancet, 371*(9619), 1200–1210.

Yigiter, M., Arda, I. S., & Hicsonmez, A. (2008). An unusual cause of paraphimosis: hemangioma of the glans penis. *Journal of Pediatric Surgery, 43*(2), e31–e33.

Zampieri, N., et al. (2007). Varicocele and adolescents: semen quality after 2 different laparoscopic procedures. *Journal of Andrology, 28*(5), 727–733.

SUGGESTED READINGS

Biro, F. M. (2007). Adolescents, sexual activity, and sexually transmitted infections. *Journal of Pediatric and Adolescent Gynecology, 20*(4), 219–220.

Daley, C. M. (2007). College students' knowledge of risk and screening recommendations for breast, cervical, and testicular cancers. *Journal of Cancer Education, 22*(2), 86–90.

Hannema, S. E., & Hughes, I. A. (2007). Regulation of Wolffian duct development. *Hormone Research, 67*(3), 142–151.

Massey, M. T., & Winterburn, S. A. (2008). Managing minor illness—vaginal discharge. *Journal of Community Nursing, 22*(1), 20–21.

Moul, J. W. (2007). Timely diagnosis of testicular cancer. *Urologic Clinics of North America, 34*(2), 109–117.

Peate, I., & Maloret, P. (2007). Testicular self-examination: the person with learning difficulties. *British Journal of Nursing, 16*(15), 931–935.

Proctor, M. L., & Murphy, P. A. (2009). Herbal and dietary therapies for primary and secondary dysmenorrhoea. *Cochrane Database of Systematic Reviews, 2009*(1), (CD002124).

Shah, A. P., et al. (2007). Recent change in the annual pattern of sexually transmitted diseases in the United States. *Chronobiology International, 24*(5), 947–960.

Varty, A. (2008). Establishing best practice for premenstrual syndrome. *Nursing Times, 104*(20), 23–24.

Vichnin, M., et al. (2007). Premenstrual syndrome (PMS) in adolescents: severity and impairment. *Journal of Pediatric and Adolescent Gynecology, 19*(6), 397–402.

Chapter 48

Nursing Care of a Family When a Child Has an Endocrine or a Metabolic Disorder

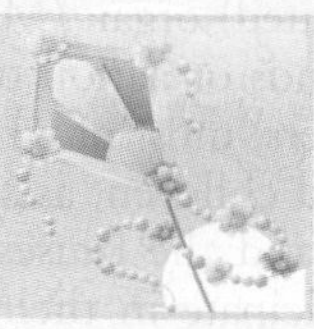

Rob Tebecco is a 16-year-old boy with type 1 diabetes whom you meet in the emergency department, where he was taken after he became comatose while ice skating. His diabetes was diagnosed when he was 7 years old. His records indicate that his disease has generally been under good control over the past years, but in the last 6 months he has "forgotten" to take his insulin at least once a week. When you ask him about this, he tells you that ice skating practice every morning and a new girlfriend have occupied his time and interrupted what used to be a strict schedule of home-cooked meals and a rigid routine.

Previous chapters described the growth and development of well children. This chapter adds information about the dramatic changes, both physical and psychosocial, that occur when children develop an endocrine or metabolic disorder. This is important information because it builds a base for care and health teaching.

Is Rob's history unusual for an adolescent? What health teaching do you think will most help him re-establish control?

KEY TERMS

- carpal spasm
- exophthalmos
- glycosuria
- hormones
- hyperglycemia
- hypoglycemia
- hypothalamus
- ketoacidosis
- latent tetany
- manifest tetany
- pedal spasm
- polydipsia
- polyuria
- sella turcica
- Somogyi phenomenon

OBJECTIVES

After mastering the contents of this chapter, you should be able to:

1. Describe the structure and function of the endocrine glands and why metabolic illnesses occur.
2. Identify National Health Goals related to childhood endocrine or metabolic disorders that nurses could help the nation achieve.
3. Analyze ways that care of a child with altered endocrine or metabolic function can be made more family centered.
4. Assess a child with a disorder of endocrine or metabolic function.
5. Formulate nursing diagnoses for a child with altered endocrine or metabolic function.
6. Develop expected outcomes for a child with endocrine or metabolic dysfunction.
7. Plan nursing care for a child with altered endocrine or metabolic function.
8. Implement nursing care such as teaching medicine administration to a child with an endocrine or metabolic disorder.
9. Evaluate expected outcomes for achievement and effectiveness of care.
10. Identify areas related to care of children with endocrine or metabolic disorders that could benefit from additional nursing research or application of evidence-based practice.
11. Synthesize knowledge of endocrine and metabolic dysfunctions and the nursing process to ensure quality maternal and child health nursing care.

The endocrine system is composed of a small group of ductless glands that work together with the neurologic system to regulate and coordinate all body systems (Fig. 48.1). The glands produce chemicals called **hormones,** which are secreted into surrounding tissue and picked up by the bloodstream, where they act individually and in concert to affect various organ systems. (The word *hormone* is from the Greek *hormaein,* which means "to set in motion.") Each gland of the endocrine system has specific functions that are necessary for regulating body processes; each hormone secreted acts on a specific target (or designated) organ (Masharani, 2009).

Dysfunction of the glands or action of the hormones results in a variety of disorders, most of which have long-term implications. Parents—and children, as soon as they are old enough—need to understand the causes and symptoms of these diseases and to participate in their long-term plan of care. National Health Goals related to endocrine and metabolic disorders in children are presented in Box 48.1.

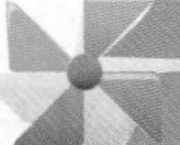

BOX 48.1 * Focus on National Health Goals

Diabetes mellitus is an endocrine disorder with serious consequences in both children and pregnant women. Several National Health Goals address reducing the incidence of this disease:

- Reduce the diabetes-related death rate from a baseline of 77 per 100,000 to no more than 46 per 100,000 people.
- Increase the proportion of persons with diabetes who receive formal diabetes education from a baseline of 45% to a target of 60% (http://www.nih.gov).

Nurses can help the nation achieve these goals by educating women about the possible effects of diabetes on pregnancy and by educating children about ways to prevent the long-term effects of the illness. Nursing research could shed additional light on these goals by asking questions such as: How should women be taught that fetal anomalies from hyperglycemia occur very early in pregnancy, so they must be certain to enter pregnancy in good glucose control? Long-term effects of diabetes are not noticeable in childhood, but how can children be educated to plan a healthy lifestyle to prevent these effects in adult life? At what age can children be expected to be responsible for glucose monitoring and insulin injection? What methods are best for encouraging children to be in charge of their own nutrition?

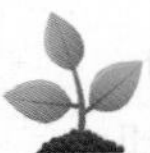

Nursing Process Overview

For Care of a Child With an Endocrine or Metabolic Disorder

Assessment

Endocrine and metabolic disorders as a group commonly cause changes in normal growth or activity patterns. This is usually detected when a child's height and weight are assessed and compared with standards for the child's age at a health visit. An acute loss in weight is often the first symptom of type 1 diabetes mellitus in children. Thyroid deficiencies or type 2 diabetes mellitus may be revealed by overweight. As more children become obese, more children develop type 2 diabetes. Pituitary difficulties may be revealed by short or unusually tall stature.

The way people view endocrine disorders can be culturally influenced. Because many of these disorders are inherited, they tend to cluster in various populations, so that either the incidence of the condition in family or friends is high, or else people know nothing about the condition. In the past, because many endocrine disorders led to changes in body appearance, particularly overgrowth or undergrowth, and because the reason for these changes was poorly understood, children with these disorders found themselves poorly accepted by peers. Being aware of the way these diseases used to be viewed aids in understanding a parent's anxiety at diagnosis of these disorders and helps with nursing care planning to include reassurance and modern concepts of therapy in education. Also, be sure to ask parents if they are using alternative therapies, because many herbs are advertised to suggest that they increase growth.

To obtain information on activity, take a day history by asking a parent or child to describe all of the child's actions on a typical day. This type of information yields clues that are helpful in distinguishing between a normally "quiet" child and one who is experiencing inactivity and chronic fatigue as a result of decreased endocrine function. For example, the quiet child lies down after school and reads; the ill child lies down and sleeps. Taking a day

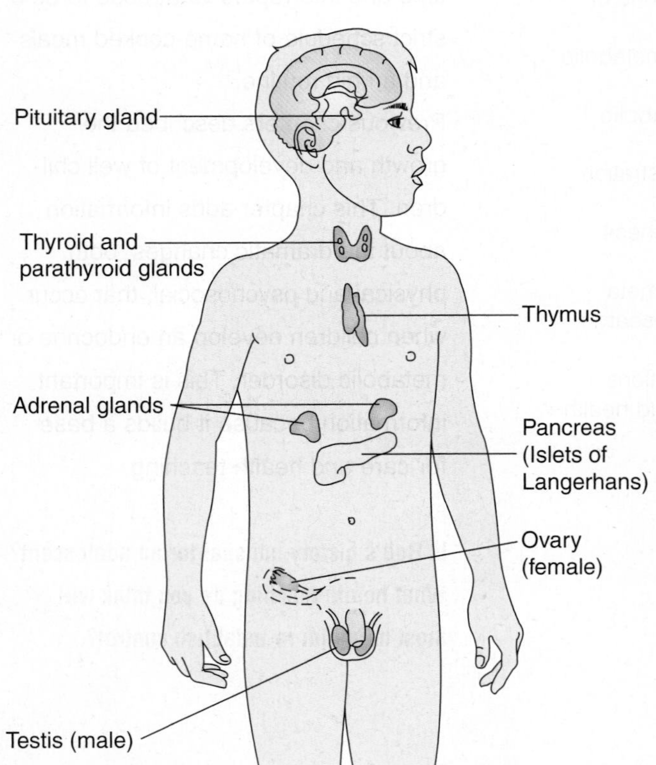

FIGURE 48.1 Location of the endocrine glands.